D0205283

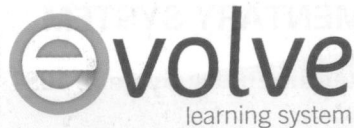
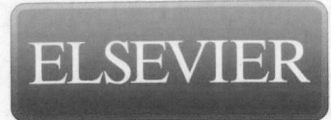
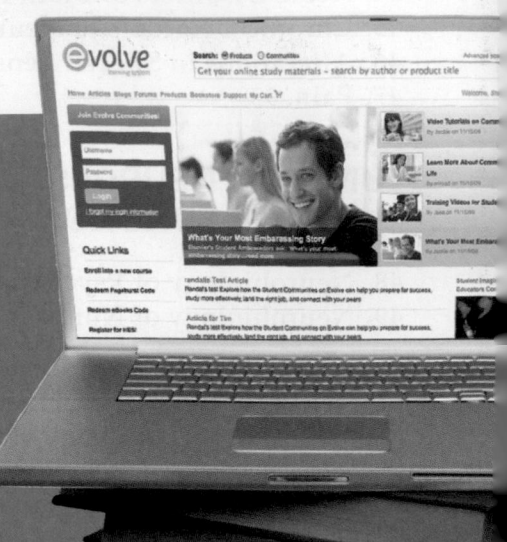

FIFTH EDITION

PATHOPHYSIOLOGY

Lee-Ellen C. Copstead, PhD, RN
Professor
Department of Nursing
College of Nursing and Health Sciences
University of Wisconsin—Eau Claire
Eau Claire, Wisconsin

Jacquelyn L. Banasik, PhD, ARNP
Associate Professor
College of Nursing
Washington State University
Spokane, Washington

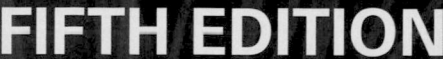

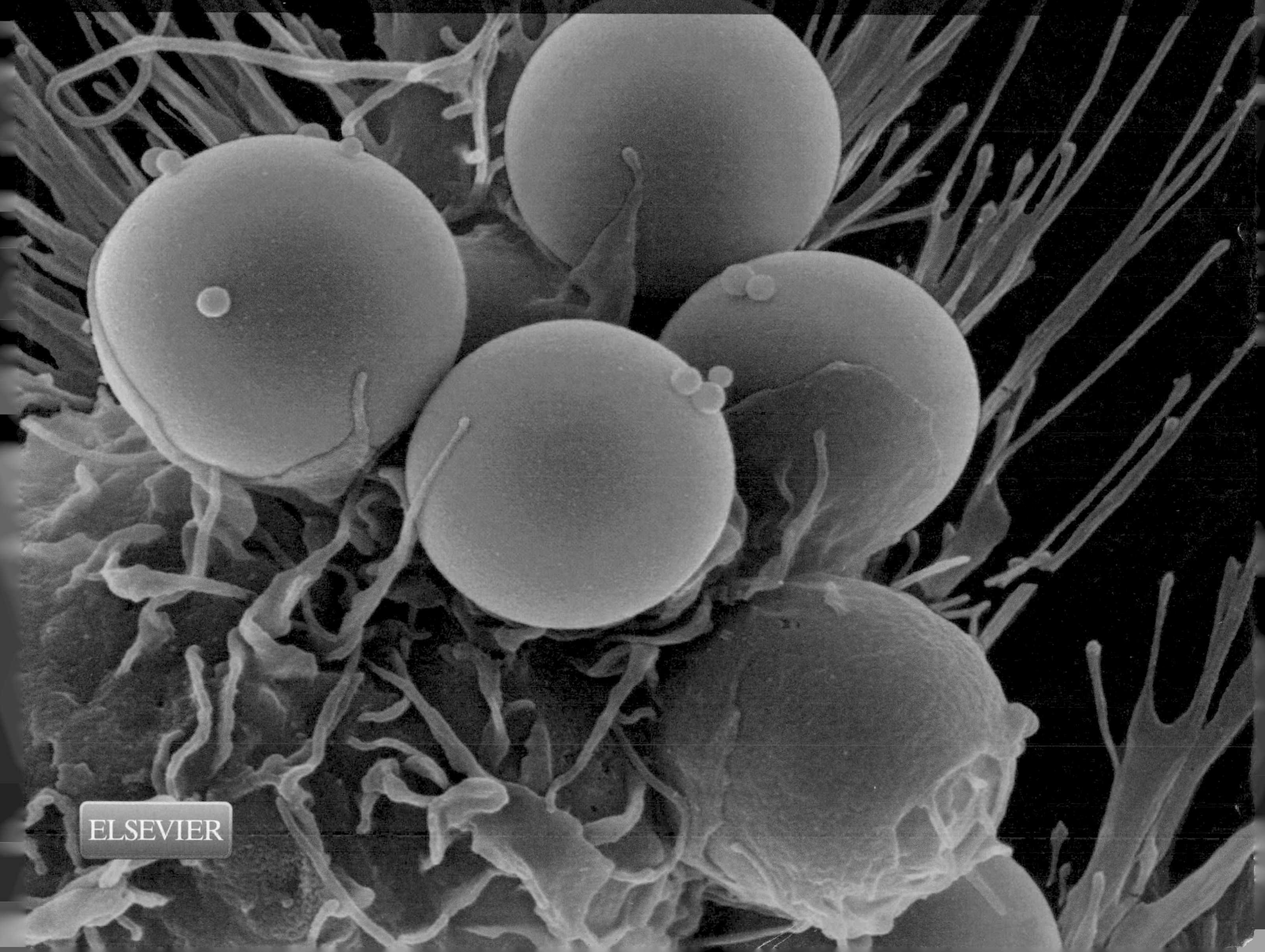

ELSEVIER

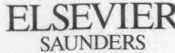
SAUNDERS

3251 Riverport Lane
St. Louis, Missouri 63043

PATHOPHYSIOLOGY, ed 5   ISBN: 978-1-4557-2650-9
Copyright © 2013 by Saunders, an imprint of Elsevier Inc.

Previous editions copyrighted 2010, 2005, 2000, 1995

Library of Congress Cataloging-in-Publication Data
Copstead, Lee Ellen.
 Pathophysiology/Lee-Ellen C. Copstead, Jacquelyn L. Banasik. -- 5th ed.
     p.; cm.
 Includes bibliographical references and index.
 ISBN 978-1-4557-2650-9 (pbk.: alk. paper)
 I. Banasik, Jacquelyn L. II. Title.
 [DNLM: 1. Disease. 2. Pathology. QZ 140]
 616.07--dc23   2012037206

Vice President and Publisher: Loren Wilson
Senior Content Strategist: Sandra Clark
Senior Content Development Specialists: Karen C. Turner and Charlene Ketchum
Senior Content Coordinator: Brooke Kannady
Publishing Service Manager: Jeffrey Patterson
Senior Project Manager: Jeanne Genz
Senior Book Designer: Amy Buxton
Multimedia Producer: Anitha Sivaraj

Printed in China

Last digit is the print number: 9 8 7 6 5 4 3 2 1

CONTRIBUTORS

Robin Y. Beeman, PhD, RN
Professor
Department of Nursing
University of Wisconsin—Eau Claire
Marshfield, Wisconsin

Cheryl L. Brandt, PhD, ACNS-BC
Professor
Department of Nursing
University of Wisconsin—Eau Claire
Eau Claire, Wisconsin

Ann Futterman Collier, PhD
Assistant Professor
Department of Psychology
Northern Arizona University
Flagstaff, Arizona

Carol L. Danning, MD
Rheumatologist
Gundersen Lutheran Health Systems
La Crosse, Wisconsin

Michael R. Diestelmeier, MD
Fellow American Academy of Dermatology
Dermatologist
Mayo Clinic Health System
Eau Claire, Wisconsin

Ruth E. Diestelmeier, RN, MSN
Clinical Instructor
Department of Nursing
University of Wisconsin—Eau Claire
Eau Claire, Wisconsin

Roberta J. Emerson, PhD, RN
Associate Professor, Retired
Washington State University
College of Nursing
Spokane, Washington

Linda Felver, PhD, RN
Associate Professor
School of Nursing
Oregon Health Sciences University
Portland, Oregon

Daniel J. Guerra, PhD, MS
Senior Scientific Consultant
Adjunct Professor, Department of Nutrition
    and Exercise Physiology
Washington State University
Spokane, Washington

Rosemary A. Jadack, PhD, RN
Professor
Department of Nursing
University of Wisconsin—Eau Claire
Eau Claire, Wisconsin

Debra A. Jansen, PhD, RN
Associate Dean, Professor
Department of Nursing
College of Nursing and Health Sciences
University of Wisconsin—Eau Claire
Eau Claire, Wisconsin

Shann Dyes Kim, PhD, RN
Regional Scientific Associate Director,
    Specialty Medicines
Novartis Pharmaceuticals
Woodinville, Washington

Marie L. Kotter, PhD
Department Chair Health Sciences
Weber State University
Ogden, Utah

Teresa G. Loftsgaarden, MSN, RN
Clinical Instructor
University of Wisconsin—Eau Claire
Eau Claire, Wisconsin

Joni D. Marsh, MN, ARNP
Family Nurse Practitioner
South Hill Family Medicine
Columbia Medical Associates
Spokane, Washington

**Benjamin J. Miller, MN, ARNP, FNP,
ACNP, PhDc**
President
Practical Healthcare Solutions, Inc.
Lolo, Montana

Carrie W. Miller, MSN, RN, CNE, IBCLC
Adjunct Faculty
Seattle University
Seattle, Washington

Nirav Y. Patel, MD, FACS
Trauma, Acute Care Surgery, Critical Care
    Surgeon
Banner Good Samaritan Medical Center
Phoenix, Arizona

Faith Young Peterson, MSN, FNP
Family Nurse Practitioner
Marsing Clinic
Terry Reilly Health Services
Marsing, Idaho

Dawn F. Rondeau, DNP, ACNP, FNP
Clinical Assistant Professor
College of Nursing
Washington State University
Vancouver, Washington
Assistant Professor
Oregon Health & Science University
Portland, Oregon

Jeffrey S. Sartin, MD
Infectious Diseases
Infectious Disease and Epidemiology
    Associates
Omaha, Nebraska

**Lorna L. Schumann, PhD, ACNP-BC,
ACNS-BC, CCRN, FAANP**
Associate Professor
College of Nursing
Washington State University
Spokane, Washington

Angela Stombaugh, PhD, FNP-BC
Assistant Professor
Department of Nursing
University of Wisconsin—Eau Claire
Eau Claire, Wisconsin

Susan G. Trevithick, RN, MS, NE-BC
Compliance Officer
VA Salt Lake City Healthcare System
Salt Lake City, Utah

Marvin J. Van Every, MD
Staff Urologist
Gundersen Clinic
La Crosse, Wisconsin

Linda D. Ward, PhD, ARNP
Assistant Professor
College of Nursing
Washington State University
Spokane, Washington

REVIEWERS

Deborah Allen, MSN, CNS, FNP-BC, AOCNP
Advanced Practice Nurse
Duke Cancer Institute
Durham, North Carolina

Nancy Burruss, PhD, RN, CNE
Associate Professor
BSN Program Director
Bellin College, School of Nursing
Green Bay, Wisconsin

Joanna Cain, BSN, BA, RN
President and Founder
Auctorial Pursuits, Inc.
Austin, Texas

Deborah Cipale, RN, MSN
Coordinator, Nursing Resource Lab
Des Moines Area Community College
Ankeny, Iowa

David Derrico, RN, MS
Assistant Clinical Professor
University of Florida College of Nursing
Gainesville, Florida

Linda Felver, PhD, RN
Associate Professor
School of Nursing
Oregon Health Sciences University
Portland, Oregon

Beth Forshee, DO, PhD
Internal Medicine Resident
Freeman Health Systems
Joplin, Missouri

Charlene Beach Gagliardi, RN, MSN
Assistant Professor
Mount St. Mary's College
Los Angeles, California

Samantha Greed, RN, BSN
Faculty Assistant
Mt. Hood Community College
Gresham, Oregon

Sandra Kaminski, MS, PA-C
Assistant Professor
School of Health & Medical Sciences
Physician Assistant Program
Seton Hall University
South Orange, New Jersey

Lori Kelly, RN, MSN, MBA
Assistant Professor of Nursing
Aquinas College
Nashville, Tennessee

Claire Leonard, BS, MS, PhD
Professor
William Paterson University
Wayne, New Jersey

Kristin Metcalf-Wilson, DNP, WHNP-BC
Instructor
University of Missouri
Sinclair School of Nursing
Columbia, Missouri

Katie Miller, BSN, MSN
Assistant Professor
College of the Albemarle
Elizabeth City, North Carolina

Rebecca Ramirez, RN, BSN, MSN
Instructor, Nursing & Medical Assisting
San Benito Consolidated Independent
   School District
San Benito, Texas

Mona Sedrak, PhD, PA-C
Associate Dean, Division of Health Sciences
Associate Professor
School of Health & Medical Sciences
Physician Assistant Program
Seton Hall University
South Orange, New Jersey

Elise Webb, RN, MSN
Coordinator/Instructor
CE Allied Health Program
Wilson Community College
Wilson, North Carolina

PREFACE

The scientific basis of pathophysiology is rapidly expanding and becoming increasingly well understood at the genetic and cellular levels. Progress in human genetics and epigenetics has transformed our understanding of physiology and disease. To be clinically relevant and useful to health care students and professionals, a text must be able to synthesize a vast amount of detailed knowledge into overarching concepts that can be applied to individual diseases. As in previous editions, the fifth edition of *Pathophysiology* gives attention to the development of practical, student-centered learning aids that support learning and mastery of content. Discussions of relevant biochemistry, genetics, and cell physiology are used to help students understand concepts at a deeper level. This fifth edition has been updated extensively with sensitivity to the unique needs of today's students to better prepare them as practitioners in an ever-changing health care environment.

ORGANIZATION

Pathophysiology is a comprehensive text and reference that uses a systems approach to content, beginning with a thorough treatment of normal physiology, followed by pathophysiology and application of concepts to specific disorders. The text is organized into 15 units, each of which includes a particular system or group of interrelated body systems and the pertinent pathophysiologic concepts and disorders.

Unit I: Pathophysiologic Processes (Chapters 1 and 2) sets the stage for understanding major elements of the pathophysiologic processes in individuals and population groups. The purpose of these chapters is to give students an appreciation for the complex nature of disease and illness, including sociocultural influences, global health considerations, and the significant contributions of stress, adaptation, and coping. The unifying concepts of pathophysiologic processes—etiology, pathogenesis, clinical manifestations, and implications for treatment of disease—are explained. A new section on telomeres and telomerase and their relationship to stress and aging is presented in Chapter 2.

Unit II: Cellular Function (Chapters 3 to 7) addresses cellular mechanisms of physiology and disease. Chapter 3 describes normal cells to give students an insight into how cells function, with an emphasis on cellular signaling and communication. Chapter 4 discusses cellular pathology and the processes of injury, apoptosis, aging, and death. Chapters 5 and 6 describe gene structure, function and regulation, development, and genetic and congenital disorders. Chapter 7 describes the cellular biology of tumor growth, focusing on the roles of proto-oncogenes and tumor suppressor genes. Revisions reflect new knowledge about apoptosis, genetics, and cancer biology.

Unit III: Defense (Chapters 8 to 12) addresses key cellular defense mechanisms and the basic processes of infectious disease, inflammation, immunity, autoimmune disease, hypersensitivity, hematologic malignancies, and HIV-AIDS. Unit III was revised to reflect new knowledge about immune mechanisms and therapy for HIV disease as well as global health considerations for HIV-AIDS.

Unit IV: Oxygen Transport, Blood Coagulation, Blood Flow, and Blood Pressure (Chapters 13 to 16) includes content pertaining to the transport of oxygen in the circulation, hemostasis, vascular regulation of flow, blood pressure regulation, and the pathologies relevant to these functions. Content on blood pressure was updated to reflect current practice recommendations.

Unit V: Cardiac Function (Chapters 17 to 20) includes concepts related to cardiac physiology and pathophysiology. Content has been updated to reflect new knowledge in the areas of apoptosis and regeneration of cardiac cells, heart failure, and shock.

Unit VI: Respiratory Function (Chapters 21 to 23) provides a thorough description of pulmonary anatomy and physiology including concepts of ventilation, perfusion, and gas exchange. Differences between obstructive and restrictive diseases are highlighted.

Unit VII: Fluid, Electrolyte, and Acid-Base Homeostasis (Chapters 24 and 25) describes concepts basic to understanding the alterations in fluid, electrolyte, and acid-base homeostasis that accompany many disease processes.

Unit VIII: Renal and Bladder Function (Chapters 26 to 29) provides a thorough description of renal anatomy and physiology, abnormalities of renal function, bladder dysfunction, and strategies for interpreting common laboratory values in the context of kidney or bladder diseases. Chapters on renal disorders, chronic kidney disease, and disorders of the urinary tract have been extensively revised.

Unit IX: Genital and Reproductive Function (Chapters 30 to 34) includes comprehensive, current information on male and female genital anatomy, embryology, and reproductive physiology as well as discussion of common disorders. Chapter 34 provides thorough coverage of common sexually transmitted infections.

Unit X: Gastrointestinal Function (Chapters 35 to 38) provides a review of normal gastrointestinal anatomy, physiology, and disorders, with separate chapters dedicated to pancreatic and biliary dysfunction and liver disease.

Unit XI: Endocrine Function, Metabolism, and Nutrition (Chapters 39 to 42) addresses alterations in endocrine control, metabolism, and nutrition. The chapter on normal endocrine physiology includes a detailed discussion of hormone synthesis, activity, and regulation. A separate chapter is dedicated to the growing problem of type 2 diabetes mellitus.

Unit XII: Neural Function (Chapters 43 to 47) includes a review of neurologic anatomy and physiology, acute and chronic neuronal disorders, disorders of special senses, and pain. Content has been updated to reflect new information on Alzheimer disease and Parkinson disease.

Unit XIII: Neuropsychological Function (Chapters 48 and 49) covers current concepts in the pathophysiology of psychobiology including anxiety, mood, thought, and personality disorders. New to the fifth edition is inclusion of global health considerations in mental health. Chapter 49 was completely rewritten to reflect current insights about disorders commonly seen in clinical practice and updated with a focused discussion of global health and pathophysiologic implications of depression.

Unit XIV: Musculoskeletal Support and Movement (Chapters 50 to 52) includes alterations in musculoskeletal support and movement, with separate chapters dedicated to normal bone and muscle anatomy and physiology, disorders of bone and muscle, and rheumatic disorders.

Unit XV: Integumentary System (Chapters 53 and 54) includes alterations affecting the largest system of the body—the integumentary system. Chapter 53 includes normal integumentary structure and function and a survey of common skin disorders. Chapter 54 covers burn injury, emphasizing the multiple stresses that are encountered in patients with these complex injuries.

FEATURES

An understanding of normal structure and function of the body is necessary for any detailed understanding of its abnormalities and pathophysiology. The first chapter in most units includes a fully illustrated *review of normal physiology*. *Global Health Considerations,* where pertinent, are highlighted in separate boxes. Changes in structure and function as a result of normal development and aging are also addressed where appropriate. Age-related concepts are highlighted in boxes titled *Geriatric Considerations* and *Pediatric Considerations*.

Each chapter opens with *Key Questions,* which are designed to develop a strong pathophysiologic knowledge base and to serve as the foundation for critical thinking. These Key Questions integrate the essential information in each chapter, emphasizing *concepts* rather than small details. *Chapter Outlines* are also included at the beginning of each chapter to help the reader locate specific content. Within every chapter, *Key Points* are identified at the end of every major discussion and are presented in short bulleted lists. These recurring summaries help readers to focus on the main points.

Nearly 900 illustrations elucidate both normal physiology and pathophysiologic changes. The entire book is in *full color,* with color used generously in the illustrations to better explain pathophysiologic concepts.

To help students master the new vocabulary of pathophysiology, key terms appear in boldface within each chapter, and these terms are defined in a comprehensive *Glossary,* which appears at the end of the text. Throughout this text, the nonpossessive forms of eponyms (e.g., Down syndrome) are used consistently when referring to the person for whom a disease is named. Clinical and laboratory values are provided in the *Appendix*.

ANCILLARIES

Student Learning Resources on Evolve

The student section of the book's website hosted on Evolve offers nearly 700 *Student Review Questions* in a variety of question formats, an *Audio Glossary, Animations* to help readers visualize pathophysiologic processes, *Case Studies with questions,* **Key Points** review, and answers to *Key Questions*. Visit the Evolve website at **http://evolve.elsevier.com/Copstead/**.

Study Guide

Pathophysiology can be a daunting subject for students because of the large volume of factual material to be learned. The student **Study Guide** is designed to help students focus on important pathophysiologic concepts. Questions to check recall of normal anatomy and physiology are included for each chapter. A number of activities that help the student focus on similarities and differences between often-confused pathologic processes are included. More than 1500 *Self-assessment test questions* with answers are included to help students check their understanding and build confidence for examinations. *Case studies,* with more than 250 questions including rationales for correct and incorrect answers, are used to help students begin to apply pathophysiologic concepts to clinical situations.

Instructor Learning Resources on Evolve

The **Instructor's Resources** on Evolve provide a number of teaching aids for instructors who require the text for their students. The materials include a *Test Bank* presented in Exam View with approximately 1200 test items, a *Teach for Nurses instructor manual* detailing the resources available to instructors for their lesson planning, a *PowerPoint lecture guide* with more than 4000 slides with integrated case studies and audience response questions to facilitate classroom presentations, and an *Image Collection* of more than 900 color images from the text.

ACKNOWLEDGMENTS

Many creative and unique efforts grace the pages of this work. It is exceedingly difficult to know how to best recognize every one. Writing this text has been possible only because of the tremendous dedication of authors, artists, reviewers, and editors. Our sincere gratitude goes to all who helped with this and previous editions. In particular, grateful appreciation is extended to all of the contributing authors—recognized experts—who gave exhaustively of their time to write chapters and create illustrations. We are also indebted to the many thoughtful experts who gave of their time to read and critique manuscripts and help ensure excellence in chapter content throughout the text.

No project of this magnitude could be accomplished without wonderfully supportive colleagues and students who provided a source of continual motivation and encouragement. We are most keenly aware of the inspiration provided by the faculty, staff, and students of Washington State University College of Nursing and the University of Wisconsin—Eau Claire College of Nursing and Health Sciences. Thank you to Assistant Professor of Nursing, Dr. Angela Stombaugh, for her contribution to the *Pediatric Considerations* boxes. Undergraduate nursing students Rachel Nerison and Anja Meerwald, and honors economics student, Laurelyn Wieseman of the University of Wisconsin—Eau Claire, deserve mention for their enthusiastic support and scholarly review of the *Global Health Considerations* boxes included in the fifth edition.

Grateful recognition is made to the staff at Elsevier. In particular, Charlene Ketchum deserves our heartfelt thanks for helping us with developmental editing through two editions of the text. As our new senior content development specialist (who picked up the reins from Charlene), Karen Turner helped with the content, illustrations, and the many details to keep our project on track; Jeanne Genz, our project manager, paid excellent attention to the copyediting, proofreading, and page layout. George Barile contributed extensively to the art program of the fifth edition. Assistant Brooke Kannady kept all of the details straight to help this edition run so smoothly. In addition, we owe grateful thanks to Nursing Editor Sandra Clark, who believed in the book and oversaw the revision of the fifth edition from beginning to end.

We would like to recognize those who provided a foundation for the revised text through their contributions to first editions: Mary Sanguinetti-Baird, Linda Belsky-Lohr, Tim Brown, Karen Carlson, Leslie Evans, Jo Annalee Irving, Debby Kaaland, Rick Madison, Maryann Pranulis, Edith Randall, Bridget Recker, Cleo Richard, Gary Smith, Pam Springer, Martha Snider, Patti Stec, Julie Symes, Lorie Wild, and Debra Winston-Heath. We also would like to thank those who contributed to the second and third editions of the book: Arnold A. Asp, Katherina P. Choka, Cynthia F. Corbett, Mark Puhlman, Barbara Bartz, Arnold Norman Cohen, Karen Groth, Christine M. Henshaw, Carolyn Hoover, Marianne Genge Jagmin, Linda Denise Oakley, Anne Roe Mealey, David Mikkelsen, Donna Bailey, Billie Marie Severtsen, and Jacqueline Siegel. Thank you also to the contributors of the fourth edition: Carolyn Spenee Cagle, Lorri Dawson, Patricia Garber, Jane Georges, Naomi Lungstrom, Sheila Smith, and Angela Starkweather.

To the late Dr. Michael J. Kirkhorn, we give acknowledgment and thanks for writing the first, second, and third edition's provocative and thoughtful essays that began each unit, and we thank Dr. Sheila Smith for her contribution to the fourth edition essays opening each of the units. We would also like to thank April Hart for her help with revising the glossary for this edition.

CONTENTS

UNIT VII FLUID, ELECTROLYTE, AND ACID-BASE HOMEOSTASIS

UNIT VIII RENAL AND BLADDER FUNCTION

UNIT X GASTROINTESTINAL FUNCTION

UNIT XI ENDOCRINE FUNCTION, METABOLISM, AND NUTRITION

UNIT XIII NEUROPSYCHOLOGICAL FUNCTION

Introduction to Pathophysiology

Lee-Ellen C. Copstead

⊖volve WEBSITE

http://evolve.elsevier.com/Copstead/
- Review Questions and Answers
- Glossary (with audio pronunciations for selected terms)
- Animations
- Case Studies
- Key Points Review

KEY QUESTIONS

- What is pathophysiology?
- How are etiology and pathogenesis used to predict clinical manifestations and response to therapy?
- How are normal and abnormal physiologic parameters defined?
- What general factors affect the expression of disease in a particular person?
- What kinds of information about disease can be gained through understanding concepts of epidemiology?

CHAPTER OUTLINE

Pathophysiology derives from the intersection of two older, related disciplines: pathology (from *pathos,* suffering) and physiology (from *physis,* nature). Pathology is the study and diagnosis of *disease* through examination of *organs, tissues, cells,* and *bodily fluids.* Physiology is the study of the mechanical, physical, and biochemical functions of living organisms. Together, as *pathophysiology,* the term refers to the study of abnormalities in physiologic functioning of living beings.

Pathophysiology seeks to reveal physiologic responses of an organism to disruptions in its internal or external environment. Because humans exhibit considerable diversity, healthy structure and function are not precisely the same in any two individuals. However, discovering the common and expected responses to abnormalities in physiologic

functioning is useful, and it allows a general prediction of clinical progression, identification of possible causes, and selection of interventions that are most likely to be helpful. Thus, pathophysiology is studied in terms of common or "classic" presentations of disorders.

Historically, descriptions of diseases were based on observations of those individuals who attracted medical attention because they exhibited abnormal signs or complained of symptoms. Over time, cases with similar presentations were noted and treatments that had been successful before were used again. In some cases, similarities among individuals pointed to possible common causes. With the advent of more sophisticated measurements of physiologic and biochemical function, such as blood pressure measurements, blood chemistry values, x-ray images, and DNA analysis, the wide variability in the expression of diseases and disorders in the population became apparent, as did the opportunity to discover diseases at earlier stages, before they were clinically obvious. Screening programs that evaluated large segments of the population revealed the complexity and diversity of disease expression, even in persons with the same genetic defect. Thus, although the study of pathophysiology is necessarily a study of the usual and expected responses of the body to a given disruption, individuals often vary significantly from a classic presentation, making the diagnostic process complex and challenging.

Advances in genomic and epigenomic characterization, innovative technologies, and revolutionary approaches to the analysis of genetic variation and function have made studies and treatments possible that were not even imaginable just a few years ago. As a result, definitions of the living world have been virtually transformed and permeate every branch of biological science. Benefits of this new biology include a deeper understanding of evolution, greater insights into immune mechanisms, and nearly every advance against cancer and acquired immunodeficiency syndrome (AIDS).

Genetic manipulation also raises sensitive and complex ethical and moral questions that did not exist half a century ago. Scientists are able to experiment with genetic manifestations and their mechanisms of action, dramatically altering medical practice, especially the management of inherited diseases. New capabilities have led to experimental treatments such as gene therapy–molecular surgery powerful enough to cure and alter the next generation. The study of pathophysiology assumes even greater significance as genetic research shows fresh insights and hopeful new treatments for human diseases.

Pathophysiology examines disturbances of normal mechanical, physical, and biochemical functions, either caused by a disease or resulting from a disease or abnormal syndrome or condition. For example, the study of a toxin released by a bacterium has evolved from the science of infectious diseases, as well as the harmful effects of that toxin on the body, one possible result being sepsis. Another example is the study of the chemical changes that take place in body tissue as the result of inflammation.

Although individual study of specific diseases undertaken in medical pathology textbooks helps students identify subtle differences between similar diseases, the study of pathophysiology is dynamic and conceptual, seeking to explain processes and relationships common to a number of pathologies. For example, the pathophysiology of inflammation, hypotension, fluid volume deficit, hypoxia, and ischemia is important to the understanding of a large number of different pathologies, but each separate process is not necessarily a specific disease.

Pathophysiology includes four interrelated topics: etiology, pathogenesis, clinical manifestations, and treatment implications—the framework used throughout this textbook. Specific diseases will be used as illustrative examples of conditions in which particular pathophysiologic processes may occur.

FRAMEWORK FOR PATHOPHYSIOLOGY

Etiology

Etiology, in its most general definition, is the study of the causes or reasons for phenomena.[1] A description of etiologic process includes the identification of those causal factors that, acting in concert, provoke a particular disease or injury. When the cause is unknown, a condition is said to be *idiopathic*. If the cause is the result of an unintended or unwanted medical treatment, the resulting condition is said to be *iatrogenic*. Most disorders are multifactorial, having several different etiologic factors that contribute to their development. For example, coronary

BOX 1-1	ETIOLOGIC CLASSIFICATION OF DISEASES

Congenital (inborn) diseases or birth defects
Degenerative diseases
Iatrogenic diseases
Idiopathic diseases
Immunologic diseases
Infectious diseases
Inherited diseases
Metabolic diseases
Neoplastic diseases
Nutritional deficiency diseases
Physical agent–induced diseases
Psychogenic diseases

heart disease is a result of the interaction of genetic predisposition, diet, exposure to cigarette smoke, elevated blood pressure, and perhaps numerous other lifestyle and hormonal factors acting in concert. None of these individual factors can be said to cause the disease. When the link between an etiologic factor and development of a disease is less than certain, but the probability is increased when the factor is present, it is termed a *risk factor*. The identification of risk factors is important for disease prevention and various levels of prevention provide focus for the epidemiology section at the end of this chapter.

Some diseases are closely linked with etiologic factors, such that they are said to be the causative agents in the disease. For example, microbial pathogens are considered to be causative agents for infectious diseases: human immunodeficiency virus causes HIV disease, influenza viruses cause the flu, and *Mycobacterium tuberculosis* causes pulmonary tuberculosis. These diseases do not occur unless the pathogen is present in the body; however, this does not mean that the infection will have the same consequences in each case, because many host factors affect the clinical course. Even when the link between disease and etiologic agent is strong, only a portion of the population exposed to the factor may develop the disease. For example, in persons who consume large quantities of alcohol and develop liver cirrhosis, it is the alcohol consumption that is considered to be the cause, yet only a portion of persons who drink heavily will develop cirrhosis.[2] Thus categorizing the probable etiologies for diseases is a long, difficult research process and, not surprisingly, the exact causes of most disorders remain incompletely understood. Several classification schemes have been proposed to categorize diseases according to etiology. Box 1-1 summarizes an example of an etiologic classification system. No classification system is truly comprehensive and some diseases fall into multiple categories. Some diseases may receive different designations in the future, as further research reveals new data.

Pathogenesis

Pathogenesis refers to the development or evolution of a disease, from the initial stimulus to the ultimate expression of the manifestations of the disease.[3] The sequence of physiologic events that occurs in response to an etiologic agent is a dynamic interplay of changes in cell, tissue, organ, and systemic function. As the ways in which intricate intercellular communication networks control physiologic function are discovered, pathogenesis is being increasingly understood on the cellular level. One of the best examples of this communication network is the immune system and its interactions with essentially every other cell in the body. A disruption in the delicate system of checks and balances between immune tolerance of normal cells and immune surveillance for abnormal cells and foreign antigens is at the root of a large number of degenerative and inflammatory diseases.

Pathologic disruptions in cellular behavior lead, in turn, to changes in organ and system function that may be detected by clinical or laboratory examination. Most pathophysiology texts take a systems approach to presenting information. This approach builds on the way in which students learn anatomy and physiology and has its roots in medical specialization. Usually the clinical examination of a patient is also conceptualized by a systems approach. Although the division into systems is useful for dividing the content into conceptual pieces, it is important to remember that the organism functions as an integrated whole and the intercellular communication networks are not confined within single systems. In summary, pathogenesis is a description of how etiologic factors are thought to alter physiologic function and lead to the development of clinical manifestations that are observed in a particular disorder or disease.

Clinical Manifestations

Manifestations of disease that are observed are termed *signs of disease.* Such objective data may be gathered by clinical examination or by biochemical analysis, diagnostic imaging, and other laboratory tests. The subjective feelings of an abnormality in the body are termed *symptoms.* By definition, symptoms are subjective and can only be reported by the affected individual to an observer. For example, the feeling of nausea is a symptom, whereas vomiting is objectively observed and is a sign. Some signs and symptoms, such as fever and headache, are nonspecific and, although they designate that something is amiss, they do not indicate a specific cause. In this case further examination and, often, laboratory tests are needed to focus on the possible causes of the signs and symptoms. Many diseases and disorders are characterized by a particular constellation of signs and symptoms, the knowledge of which is essential for accurate detection and diagnosis. When the etiology of a particular set of signs and symptoms has not yet been determined, the disorder may be termed a *syndrome.* For example, AIDS was originally detected as a set of signs and symptoms related to a deficiency of helper T cells of unknown cause, now known to be a late stage of HIV infection.[4]

The clinical manifestations of some diseases may change significantly over time, resulting in a completely different clinical presentation at different stages. Knowledge of the possible stages of a disease is helpful in making an appropriate diagnosis and anticipating the clinical course.

Stages and Clinical Course

Early in the development of a disease, the etiologic agent or agents may provoke a number of changes in biological processes that can be detected by laboratory analysis, although no recognition of these changes by the patient has occurred. The interval between exposure of a tissue to an injurious agent and the first appearance of signs and symptoms may be called a latent period or, in the case of infectious diseases, an incubation period. The prodromal period, or prodrome, refers to the appearance of the first signs and symptoms indicating the onset of a disease. Prodromal symptoms often are nonspecific, such as headache, malaise, anorexia, and nausea. During the stage of manifest illness, or the acute phase, the disease reaches its full intensity, and signs and symptoms attain their greatest severity. Sometimes during the course of a disease, the signs and symptoms may become mild or even disappear for a time. This interval may be called a silent period or latent period. For example, in the total-body irradiation syndrome, a latent period may occur between the prodrome and the stage of manifest illness. Another example is syphilis, which may have two latent periods: one occurring between the primary and secondary clinical stages and another occurring between the secondary and tertiary stages.[5]

A number of diseases have a subclinical stage, during which the patient functions normally, although the disease processes are well established. It is important to understand that the structure and function of many organs provide a large reserve or safety margin, so that functional impairment may become evident only when organ damage has become advanced. For example, chronic renal disease can completely destroy one kidney and partly destroy the other before any symptoms related to a decrease in renal function are perceived.[6]

The clinical course of a disease is often classified as acute or chronic. An acute condition has relatively severe manifestations but runs a short course measured in hours, days, or a few weeks. A chronic condition lasts for months to years. Sometimes chronic disease processes begin with an acute phase and become prolonged when the body's defenses are insufficient to overcome the causative agent or stressor. In other cases, chronic conditions develop insidiously and never have an acute phase.

Some diseases (e.g., some types of autoimmune diseases) follow a course of alternating exacerbations and remissions. An exacerbation is a relatively sudden increase in the severity of a disease or any of its signs and symptoms. A remission is an abatement or decline in severity of the signs and symptoms of a disease. If a remission is permanent (sometimes defined as longer than 5 years), the person is said to be cured.

Convalescence is the stage of recovery after a disease, injury, or surgical operation. Occasionally a disease produces a subsequent pathologic condition called a sequela (plural: sequelae). For example, the sequela of an inflammatory process might be scarring. The sequelae of acute rheumatic inflammation of the heart might be scarring and deformation of cardiac valves. In contrast, a complication of a disease is a new or separate process that may arise secondarily because of some change produced by the original problem. For example, bacterial pneumonia may be a complication of viral infection of the respiratory tract.

Treatment Implications

An understanding of the etiology, pathogenesis, and clinical consequences of a particular disorder may suggest, or "imply," that certain treatments could be helpful. For example, understanding that a person with septic shock has excessive dilation of blood vessels that contributes to hypotension implies that fluid administration would likely be helpful. In contrast, most patients with cardiogenic shock have fluid overload, and hypotension in this case is unlikely to improve with fluid administration. Care must be taken not to rely on theoretical implications when evidence-based treatment recommendations are available. When subjected to evaluation by rigorous randomized clinical trials, many treatments that seem as though they should help based on pathophysiology fail to pass the test of application.

The treatment implications discussed in pathophysiology texts usually are general statements rather than specific prescriptions. For example, the pathophysiology of heart failure is characterized by fluid overload, which implies that diuretic therapy would be useful; however, the exact selection of a drug and the dosing schedule would depend on a number of factors particular to the individual patient. Specific treatment recommendations are beyond the scope of a pathophysiology text and can be found in pharmacology and clinical practice textbooks.

KEY POINTS

- Pathophysiology includes four interrelated topics: etiology, pathogenesis, clinical manifestations, and treatment implications.
- Etiology refers to study of the proposed cause or causes of a particular disease process. Etiology is a complex notion because most diseases are multifactorial, resulting from interplay between genetic constitution and environmental influences.
- Pathogenesis refers to the proposed mechanisms whereby an etiologic stimulus leads to typically observed clinical manifestations. Pathogenesis describes the direct effects of the initiating event, as well as the usual physiologic responses and compensatory mechanisms.
- Clinical manifestations describe the signs and symptoms that typically accompany a particular pathophysiologic process. Manifestations may vary depending on the stage of the disorder, individual variation, and acuity or chronicity.
- An understanding of the etiology, pathogenesis, and clinical consequences of a particular disorder may imply that certain treatments could be helpful.

CONCEPTS OF NORMALITY IN HEALTH AND DISEASE

The ability to measure numerous structural, physiologic, biochemical, and genetic parameters in an individual allows the evaluation of information that is helpful in the diagnosis and monitoring of clinical diseases. Many of these same measures are commonly used to screen for disease or to evaluate the risks of a disease occurring in the future. To determine whether a certain finding is indicative of disease or "abnormal," it must be compared with what is "normal." The obviousness of this statement belies the difficulty in determining what is normal and the degree of deviation from normal that would be considered abnormal. Many clinical parameters are evaluated by direct observation by the examiner. Skin color and warmth, quality of pulses, briskness of pupil reactions to light, mental acuity, muscle strength, joint mobility, heart sounds, lung sounds, bowel sounds, balance, psychological affect, and level of consciousness are but a few examples of assessments that are subjectively interpreted based on the examiner's observations. Deciding whether a clinical finding is normal, a normal variation, or an abnormality indicative of a disorder is essential.

Reliability of data obtained from observation is dependent upon the examiner's skill and experience. Often the clinical examination is not sufficient to determine definitively the underlying pathophysiologic processes, and diagnostic testing is undertaken to provide more information.

Statistical Normality

Some of the variables that are measured to diagnose disease are relatively easy to declare as normal or abnormal because they occur in only two states; for example, a bone is either broken or not broken on x-ray examination. However, most diagnostic variables occur in the population according to a "bell curve" or normal distribution.[7] This means that a large enough sample taken from the population should give a good estimate of the range of values in the population. Statistics are often used to determine the standard deviation of the variable in question, and then a normal range is suggested as the mean ±2 standard deviations. This means that 95% of the values in the population are expected to fall in the normal range and 5% will be either higher or lower (Figure 1-1). The "population" chosen to serve as the normal reference population must be carefully selected to represent the individual to be tested for disease, because many variables are influenced by age and gender.

For example, bone density can be measured in the population by radiologic imaging and then a mean and standard deviation can be calculated. Women typically have lower bone density than men, and older women have lower bone density than younger women. If an elderly woman's bone density is compared to women of her own age group, it may fall within the normal range, but when compared to a group of younger women, it is more than 2 standard deviations below the mean. Which is the right comparison group to use to determine if she has osteoporosis? There is controversy on this point because, in this situation, it is difficult to determine the difference between disease and the effects of normal aging.

Often, when assessing a person's health status, a change in some value or factor is more significant than the actual value of the factor. A blood pressure of 90/70 mm Hg may not be significant if that is the usual value. However, if a person usually has a blood pressure of 120/80 mm Hg, a reading of 90/70 mm Hg could indicate a significant change. Individuals are typically evaluated more than once—generally two or three times—to establish deviation from their usual value.

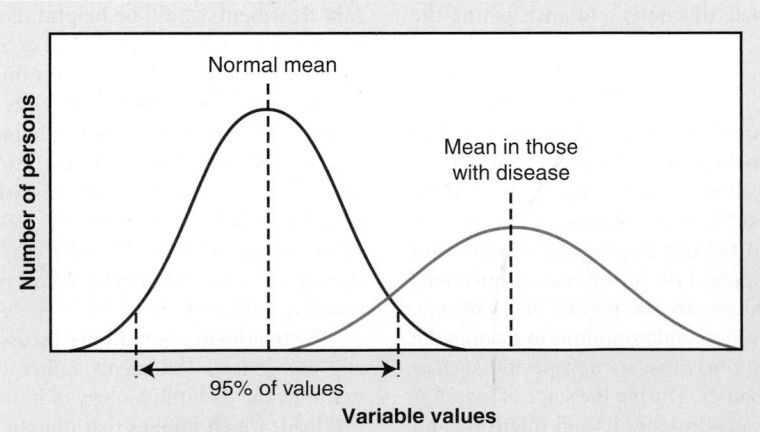

FIGURE 1-1 Representative example of a normal bell curve for a physiologic variable. Many physiologic variables are normally distributed within the population, so the mean ±2 standard deviations include 95% of the normal values in the sample. Approximately 2.5% of values will be above the normal range and 2.5% will be below it. There may be overlap between the values in a normal sample and those in the population with a disease, making interpretation difficult in some cases.

Reliability, Validity, and Predictive Value

The accurate determination of whether a specific condition is present or absent depends on the quality and adequacy of the data collected, as well as the skill of interpretation. Decisions about the data needed are based on the initial clinical presentation and a working knowledge of pathophysiology, which guide hypothesis generation about probable etiologies. During the clinical examination, data are analyzed and a number of likely explanations for the clinical presentation may emerge. These possible explanations are "probabilities" based on knowledge and past experience with similar cases. The purpose of further data collection, particularly laboratory and diagnostic testing, is to refine the initial probability estimates and identify the most likely diagnosis. The success of this approach depends on the selection of appropriate tests based on the pretest probabilities, as well as on the validity, reliability, and predictive value of the tests.

Validity, or accuracy, is the degree to which a measurement reflects the true value of the object it is intended to measure. For example, a pulse oximeter is designed to measure arterial oxygen saturation, and the closeness of the reading to a direct measurement of oxygen saturation in an arterial blood sample reflects its accuracy. Reliability, or precision, is the ability of a test to give the same result in repeated measurements. An instrument or laboratory test can be reliable, yet inaccurate. Repeated measurements with the pulse oximeter could give the same result each time, but if those values are significantly different from the "gold standard" of an arterial blood sample, the oximeter data would have poor validity.

Some measurements vary according to the reagents and laboratory methods used. For example, prothrombin time (PT) is sensitive to the reagent used. In one method of determining PT, the reagent—a substance composed of thromboplastin and calcium—is added to decalcified plasma to create a reaction resulting in clot formation. The PT is then determined by measuring the length of time it takes for clotting to occur after this reagent is added and compared to the normative average. Portions of the same blood sample sent to several different laboratories could return significantly different PT results. In fact, this is such a problem that laboratories now use a correction procedure to normalize the PT values across labs. The corrected PT value is reported as the International Normalized Ratio (INR), which has higher reliability than the PT.[8]

The predictive value of a test is the extent to which the test can differentiate between the presence or absence of a condition in an individual. The positive predictive value is an estimate of the probability that disease is present if the test is positive. The negative predictive value is an estimate of the probability that disease is absent if the test is negative. The predictive value of a test depends in part upon the sensitivity and specificity of the test and in part upon the probability of the disease being present before the test is obtained. Most tests are not perfectly specific and sensitive so the results must be interpreted probabilistically in view of the diagnostic hypotheses being tested.

Sensitivity and specificity are measures of how well a given test can discriminate between persons with and without a given condition. Sensitivity is the probability that the test will be positive when applied to a person with the condition. For example, if a kit for testing a throat swab for the presence of streptococcal infection has a sensitivity of 80%, then 20% of a group of people with streptococcal throat infection would erroneously test negative for the condition (false negative rate). Another example is the blood test for HIV antibodies, which has a sensitivity of 99% and would fail to detect the condition in only 1% of a group of individuals who had HIV antibodies in their blood. Specificity is the probability that a test will be negative when applied to a person who does not have a given condition. If the streptococcal throat swab kit has a specificity of 95%, then 5% of those tested who do not actually have the condition would erroneously test positive (false positive rate).

The importance of evaluating the accuracy and precision of data is paramount because inappropriate diagnoses and clinical management could occur if decisions are predicated on invalid or unreliable data.

The positive predictive value of a test is improved when sensitivity and specificity are high and the test is applied to individuals who have a high probability of having the condition being tested. If the likelihood of a condition in the population being tested is low (e.g., a 2% prevalence rate), then a positive result in a test with 99% specificity and 99% sensitivity would only have a 67% positive predictive value.[9] This means that testing low-likelihood or low-risk individuals would produce a high percentage of false positive results (33% in the preceding example). Therefore deciding who to test for a given condition based on the probability of the condition being present is as important as the sensitivity and specificity of the test. A good working knowledge of pathophysiology is necessary to generate the hypotheses that guide collection of appropriate data and facilitate the diagnostic process.

Individual Factors Influencing Normality

Variations in physiologic processes may be a result of factors other than disease or illness. Age, gender, genetic and ethnic background, geographic area, and time of day may influence various physiologic parameters.[10] Care must be taken to interpret "abnormal" findings with consideration of these possible confounding factors. In addition, the potential for spurious findings always exists. Thus, trends and changes in a particular individual are more reliable than single observations. Single measurements, observations, or laboratory results that seem to indicate abnormality must always be judged in the context of the entire health picture of the individual. One slightly elevated blood glucose level does not mean clinical diabetes, a single high blood pressure reading does not denote hypertension, and a temporary feeling of hopelessness does not indicate clinical depression.

Cultural Considerations

Each culture defines health and illness in a manner that reflects its experience. Cultural factors determine which signs, symptoms, or behaviors are perceived as abnormal. An infant from an impoverished culture with endemic chronic diarrhea and a degree of malnutrition would be viewed as abnormal in a progressive culture, such as a well-baby clinic in Sweden. Given cultural variations that affect definitions of normal and abnormal, the resulting pattern of behaviors or clinical manifestations affects what the culture labels as illness.[11]

Age Differences

Many biological factors vary with age, and the normal value for a person at one age may be abnormal at another. Physiologic changes, such as hair color, skin turgor (tension), and organ size, vary with age. In general, most organs shrink; exceptions are the male prostate and the heart, which enlarge with age.[12] Special sensory changes, such as severely diminished near-sight, high-tone hearing loss, and loss of taste discriminations for sweet and salty, are normal in an elderly adult and abnormal in a middle-aged adult or child. There are fewer sweat glands and less thirst perception in an elderly person than in a young adult or child. Elderly persons have diminished temperature sensations and can therefore sustain burn injuries—from a heating pad or bath water—because they do not perceive heat with the same intensity as do middle-aged adults. A resting heart rate of 120 beats per minute is normal for an infant but not for an adult.

Gender Differences

Some laboratory values, such as levels of sex and growth hormones, show gender differences. The complete blood cell count shows differences by gender in hematocrit, hemoglobin, and red blood cell (RBC) count.[13] For example, the normal range of hemoglobin concentration for adult women is lower than that for adult men—for adult women, the normal hemoglobin range is 12 to 16 g/100 ml of blood whereas for adult men the normal range is 13 to 18 g/100 ml of blood.[13] There are also gender differences in the erythrocyte sedimentation rate (ESR). Normally, in males, the ESR is less than 13 mm/hr; it is slightly higher in females.[13] There are differences by gender in creatinine values. For females, the normal serum creatinine level is 0.4 to 1.3 mg/dl; for males, the normal range is 0.6 to 1.5 mg/dl.[13] Research into gender differences also suggests that, on average, males snore more; have longer vocal cords, better daylight vision, and higher metabolic rates; and are more likely to be left-handed than females.[14] Research suggests, too, that females and males have different communication styles and respond differently to similar conditions.

Situational Differences

In some cases, a deviation from the usual value may occur as an adaptive mechanism, and whether the deviation is considered abnormal depends on the situation. For example, the RBC count increases when a person moves to a high altitude.[15] The increase is a normal adaptive response to the decreased availability of oxygen at a high altitude and is termed *acclimatization*. A similar increase in the RBC count at sea level would be abnormal.

Time Variations

Some factors vary according to the time of day; that is, they exhibit a circadian rhythm or diurnal variation. In interpreting the result of a particular test, it may be necessary to know the time at which the value was determined. For example, body temperature and plasma concentrations of certain hormones (such as growth hormone and cortisol) exhibit diurnal variation. Reflecting fluctuation in plasma levels, the peak rate in urinary excretion for a particular steroid (17-ketosteroid) occurs between 8 AM and 10 AM for persons who customarily rise early in the morning and is about two to three times greater than the lowest rate in the same people, which occurs between midnight and 2 AM, usually during sleep.[16] The urinary excretion of ions (e.g., potassium) also exhibits diurnal variation. Figure 1-2 illustrates circadian rhythms of several physiologic variables for persons living on a standard day-active schedule.

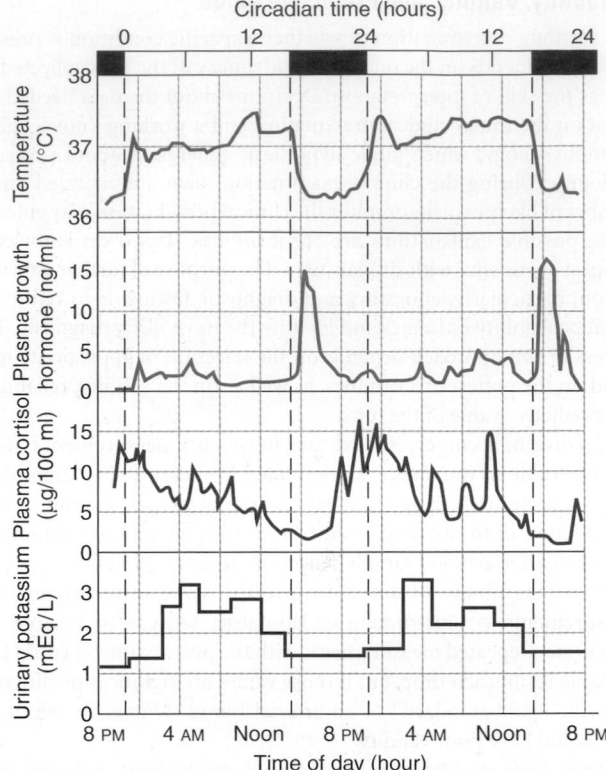

FIGURE 1-2 Circadian rhythms of several physiologic variables in a human subject depict the effect of light and dark. In an experiment with lights on (*open bars* at top) for 16 hours and off (*black bars* at top) for 8 hours, temperature readings and plasma growth hormone, plasma cortisol, and urinary potassium levels exhibit diurnal variation. (Redrawn from Vander AJ et al: *Human physiology*, ed 7, New York, 1998, McGraw-Hill.)

> **KEY POINTS**
> - Determining whether clinical findings are normal, abnormal, or normal variation is an essential but often difficult process in evaluating for the presence or absence of disease.
> - Normal ranges for laboratory tests are typically defined as the mean ±2 standard deviations; thus, 5% of the normal population may fall outside the normal range despite the absence of disease. Laboratory tests must be evaluated in concert with clinical information.
> - The predictive value of a clinical test is the extent to which it can differentiate between the presence and absence of disease in an individual. Tests with high sensitivity and specificity generally have better predictive value.
> - Variations in physiologic processes may be a result of factors other than disease or illness. Age, gender, genetic and ethnic background, geographic area, and time of day may influence various physiologic parameters.
> - Trends and changes in a particular individual are more reliable than single observations.

PATTERNS OF DISEASE IN POPULATIONS

Concepts of Epidemiology

Differences among *individuals* are, of course, very important in determining the diseases to which they are susceptible and their reactions to the diseases once contracted. But epidemiology, or the study of *patterns of disease* involving aggregates of people (Figure 1-3), provides yet another important dimension. Information may be gained by examining the occurrence, incidence, prevalence, transmission, and distribution of diseases in large groups of people or populations.

Endemic, Pandemic, and Epidemic Diseases

A disease that is native to a local region is called an *endemic disease*. If the disease is disseminated to many individuals at the same time, the situation is called an *epidemic*. *Pandemics* are epidemics that affect large geographic regions, perhaps spreading worldwide. Because of the speed and availability of human travel around the world, pandemics are more common than they once were. Almost every flu season, a new strain of influenza virus quickly spreads from one continent to another.

Aggregate Factors

Principal factors affecting patterns of disease in human populations include the following: (1) age (i.e., time in the life cycle), (2) ethnic group, (3) gender, (4) socioeconomic factors and lifestyle considerations, and (5) geographic location.

Age. In one sense, life is entirely different during the 9 months of gestation. The structures and functions of tissues are different: they are primarily dedicated to differentiation, development, and growth. Certainly the environment is different; the individual is protected from the light of day, provided with predigested food (even preoxygenated blood), suspended in a fluid buffer, and maintained at incubator temperature. This is fortunate because the developing embryo or fetus has which ethnicity is inseparably bound. For example, carcinoma of the penis is virtually unknown among Jews and Muslims who practice circumcision at an early age (avoiding the carcinogenic stimulus that arises from accumulation of smegma about the glans penis).

However, comparisons reveal significant differences in the occurrence of certain disease states in ethnic groups that seem to be more closely related to genetic predisposition than to environmental factors. For example, sickle cell anemia has a much higher rate of occurrence in African populations, whereas pernicious anemia occurs more frequently among Scandinavians and is rare among black populations worldwide.

The study of racial and ethnic group variation in disease states is the domain of medical anthropology. Volumes have been written about disease-specific differences that relate to racial or ethnic group differences. In clinical practice, recognition of diversity in disease risk by racial or ethnic group is useful in disease diagnosis, prevention, and management. Ethnic group–specific differences, where important, are presented in individual chapters.

Gender. Particular diseases of the genital system obviously show important differences between the sexes; men do not have endometriosis nor do women have hyperplasia of the prostate, and carcinoma of the breast is more common in women than in men. Pyelonephritis is more common in young women than in men of comparable age (before they develop prostatic hyperplasia) because the external urethral orifice of women is more readily contaminated, and bacteria can more easily travel up a short urethra than a long one. Less obviously related to the reproductive system, the onset of severe atherosclerosis in women is delayed nearly 20 years or more over that in men, presumably because of the protective action of estrogenic hormone.

There are also gender-specific factors that defy explanation.[17] For example, systemic lupus erythematosus is much more common in women.[18] Toxic goiter and hypothyroidism are also more common in women.[19] Rheumatoid arthritis is more common in women, but osteoarthritis affects men and women with equal frequency.[20] Thromboangitis obliterans (a chronic, recurring, inflammatory peripheral vascular disease) occurs more commonly in men.[21] Gender differences in predisposition to cancer and other diseases are presented throughout the text.

Socioeconomic factors and lifestyle considerations. The environment and the political climate of countries determine how people live and the health problems that are likely to ensue. The importance of poverty, malnutrition, overcrowding, and exposure to adverse environmental conditions, such as extremes of temperature, is obvious. Volumes have been written about the effects of socioeconomic status on disease. Sociologists study the influence of these factors. Social class influences education and occupational choices.

Disease is related to occupational exposure to such agents as coal dust, noise, or extreme stress.[22] Lifestyle considerations are closely related to socioeconomic factors. People living in the United States, for example, consume too much food, alcohol, and tobacco and do not exercise enough. Childhood obesity is a problem in the United States. Arteriosclerosis; cancer; diseases of the kidney, liver, and lungs; and accidents cause most deaths in the United States. By contrast, people living in developing nations suffer and frequently die from undernutrition and infectious diseases.

However, infectious disease is not limited to developing countries.[23] The Centers for Disease Control and Prevention (CDC) estimates that 2 million people annually acquire infections while hospitalized and 90,000 people die as a result of those infections. More than 70% of hospital-acquired infections have become resistant to at least one of the drugs commonly used to manage them, largely attributable to the overprescribing of antibiotics.[24] *Staphylococcus,* the leading cause of hospital infections, is now resistant to 95% of first-choice antibiotics and 30% of second-choice antibiotics. Poor hygiene is considered the leading

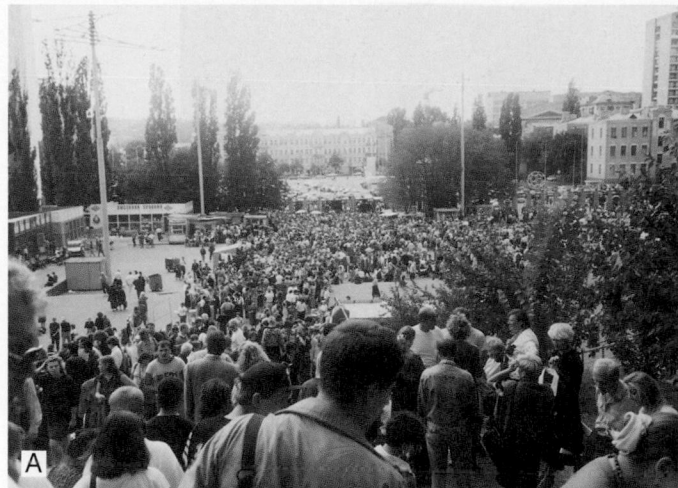

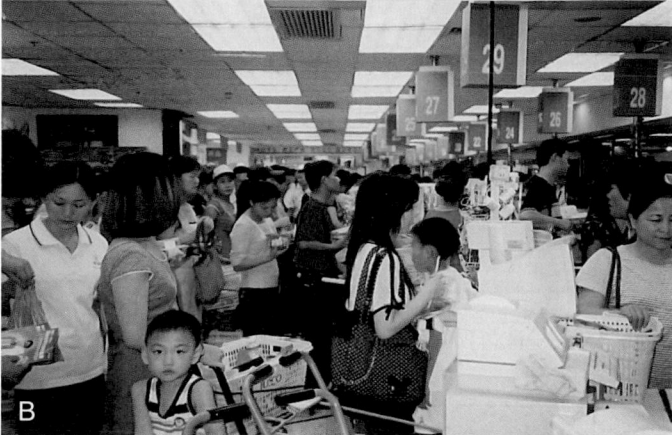

FIGURE 1-3 A, The aggregate focus in disease: influence of crowds upon disease transmission. Crowd gathered at a public market in Russia. **B,** Crowds gathered to purchase goods at a public market in Guangzhou, China. (Photographed by L-E Copstead.)

relatively few homeostatic mechanisms to protect it from environmental change. (The factors that produce disease in utero are discussed in Chapter 6.) Diseases that arise during the postuterine period of life and affect the neonate include immaturity, respiratory failure, birth injuries, congenital malformations, nutritional problems, metabolic errors, and infections. These conditions are discussed in separate chapters.

Accidents, including poisoning, take their toll in childhood. Infections in children reflect their increased susceptibility to agents of disease. Consideration of other childhood diseases is addressed in each chapter, as appropriate and given separate consideration throughout the text. The study of childhood processes and of changes that occur in this period of life is the domain of pediatrics; specific diseases that occur during maturity (ages 15 to 60) are emphasized in this text.

The changes in function that occur during the early years of life are termed *developmental processes.* Those that occur during maturity and postmaturity (age 60 and beyond) are called *aging processes.* The study of aging processes and other changes that occur during this period of life is called *gerontology.* The effects of aging on selected body systems are so important physiologically that they also receive separate consideration throughout the text. The immune, cardiac, respiratory, musculoskeletal, neurologic, special sensory, endocrine, gastrointestinal, and integumentary systems are among those affected by the process of aging.

Ethnic group. It is difficult to differentiate precisely between the effects of ethnicity on patterns of disease and the socioeconomic factors, religious practices, customs, and geographic considerations with

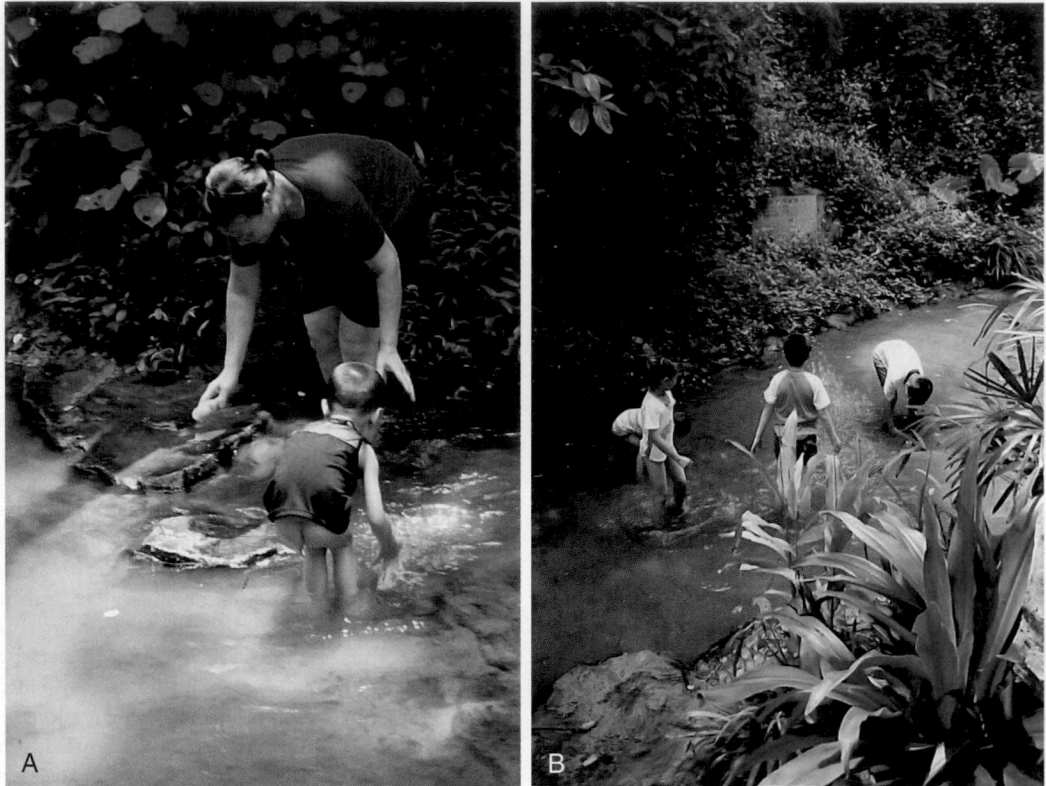

FIGURE 1-4 Risk factors for schistosomiasis include the widespread use of irrigation ditches that harbor the intermediate snail host. (Photographed in China by L-E Copstead.)

source for infections acquired during hospitalizations. Unfortunately, efforts to convince health care personnel to reduce transmission of infection through practices as simple as more frequent and thorough hand washing have met with only modest success.

The incidence of many parasitic diseases is closely tied to socioeconomic factors and lifestyle considerations. Worm infections, for example, are related to the use of human feces as fertilizer. In some areas, such as parts of Asia, Africa, and tropical America, the frequency of schistosomiasis (a parasitic infestation by blood flukes) is directly related to the widespread use of irrigation ditches that harbor the intermediate snail host.[25] There is adequate opportunity for transmission of schistosomiasis because children often play in these ditches and families wash their clothes in ditch water (Figure 1-4).

Trichinosis, a disease caused by the ingestion of *Trichinella spiralis,* occurs almost entirely from eating inadequately cooked, infected pork. People who are fond of raw meat and inadequately cooked sausage are at highest risk.

Education is often very effective in changing lifestyle patterns that contribute to disease. In Tokyo, for example, mass public education about minimizing the use of sodium—a common ingredient in most traditional Japanese cooking—has been effective in changing dietary practices.

Examples of educational efforts directed at lifestyle modification in the United States are numerous.[26-28] Antidrug, antismoking, and pro-fitness messages fill the media and are prevalent on the Internet. Choosing healthy alternatives over unhealthy ones is made easier through positive peer pressure and support groups.

Geographic location. Patterns of disease vary greatly by geographic location. Certainly there is considerable overlap with ethnicity, socioeconomic factors, and lifestyle choices, but physical environment also is an important aspect. Obviously, frostbite in Antarctica and dehydration in the Sahara are examples of disorders that are more prevalent in specific geographic settings. However, important patterns of disease

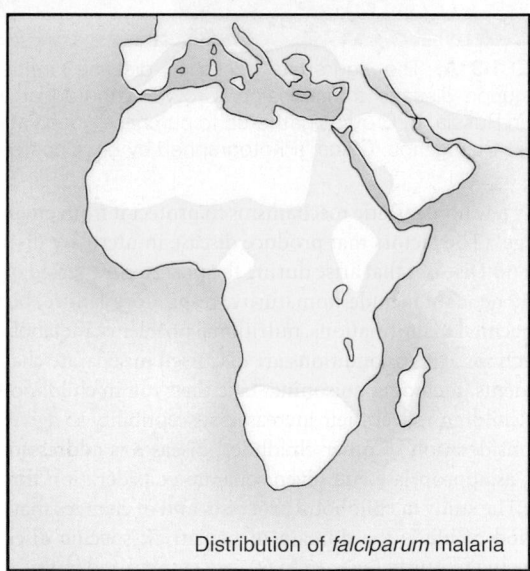

Distribution of *falciparum* malaria

FIGURE 1-5 Geographic distribution of malaria. (From Patton KT, Thibodeau GA: *Anatomy & physiology,* ed 8, St Louis, 2013, Mosby, p 113.)

occur within individual countries. For example, the incidence and type of malnutrition vary tremendously by geographic region.

Many diseases have a geographic pattern for reasons that are clear. For example, malaria, an acute and sometimes chronic infectious disease resulting from the presence of protozoan parasites within red blood cells, is transmitted to humans by the bite of an infected female *Anopheles* mosquito. The *Anopheles* mosquito can live only in certain regions of the world[29] (Figure 1-5).

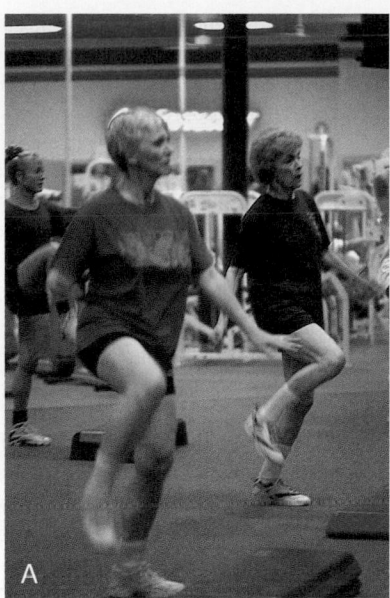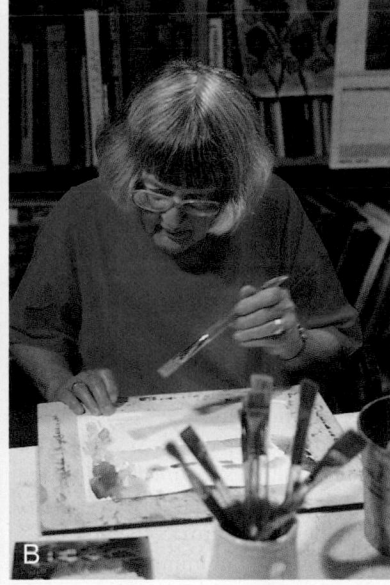

FIGURE 1-6 Healthy aging: elders exercising in an aerobics class **(A)** and painting **(B)** illustrate the concept that aging and disease are not synonymous. The artist, a healthy woman in her mid-70s, is also a breast cancer survivor. (Photographed by Therese A. Capal, Rockville, Md.)

Fungal diseases are both more common and more serious in hot, humid regions. But some infectious diseases are highly limited geographically for reasons that are not well understood. For example, bartonellosis, which is also called Carrión disease, is found only in Peru, Ecuador, Chile, and Colombia.[30] This disease resembles malaria superficially in that the minute rickettsia-like organisms invade and destroy erythrocytes. Humans are infected by the bite of the sand fly. Although conditions in other parts of the world should be favorable for this disease, it remains limited geographically.

Taking a world view, there is widespread recognition of the importance of geographic factors in influencing human disease.[31] The World Health Organization (WHO) and the National Institutes of Health (NIH) have been deeply concerned with geographic problems in disease. Consult WHO and NIH home pages on the World Wide Web for additional information. (Web locations are provided on the Evolve website.)

Levels of Prevention

The goal of health care should encompass much more than the prevention of illness. What is needed instead is some notion of positive health or physical "wholeness" that extends beyond the absence of ill health. WHO defines health as complete physical, mental, and social well-being and not merely the absence of disease or infirmity.[31] For some individuals, health implies the ability to do what they regard as worthwhile and to conduct their lives as they want. Aging and ill health are not synonymous, and many elders enjoy excellent health, even in the face of chronic disease (Figure 1-6).

Epidemiologists suggest that treatment implications fall into categories called *levels of prevention*. There are three levels of prevention: primary, secondary, and tertiary. Primary prevention is prevention of disease by altering susceptibility or reducing exposure for susceptible individuals. Secondary prevention (applicable in early disease, i.e., preclinical and clinical stages) is the early detection, screening, and management of the disease. Tertiary prevention (appropriate in the stage of advanced disease or disability) includes rehabilitative and supportive care and attempts to alleviate disability and restore effective functioning.[32]

Primary prevention. Prolongation of life has resulted largely from decreased mortality from infectious disease. Primary prevention in terms of improved nutrition, economy, housing, and sanitation for those living in developed countries is also responsible for increased longevity. Certain childhood diseases—measles, poliomyelitis, pertussis (whooping cough), and neonatal tetanus—are decreasing in prevalence, owing to a rapid increase in coverage by immunization programs. More than 120 million children younger than age 5 in India were immunized against poliomyelitis in a single day in 1996.[33] Globally, coverage of children immunized against six major childhood diseases increased from 5% in 1974 to 80% in 1995.[33] In 1985 Rotary International launched the PolioPlus program to protect children worldwide from the cruel and fatal consequences of polio. In 1988 the World Health Assembly challenged the world to eradicate polio. Since that time, Rotary International's efforts and those of partner agencies, including the WHO, the United Nations Children's Fund, the CDC, and governments around the world, have achieved a 99% reduction in the number of polio cases worldwide.[33]

The prevalence of cardiovascular diseases in developed countries (except those in Eastern Europe) is diminishing, thanks to the spread of health education and promotion. Infant and child death rates and the overall death rate are continuing to decrease globally.

High school education programs about abstinence from sex and ways to "say no" to drugs, alcohol, and tobacco are other examples of primary prevention making a difference in the lives of people. Primary prevention also includes adherence to safety precautions, such as wearing seat belts, observing the posted speed limit on highways, and taking precautions in the use of chemicals and machinery. Violent crimes involving dangerous weapons must be stopped to achieve primary prevention of the traumatic or fatal injuries they cause.

Environmental pollutants poison the body's organs. Some experts fear the emergence of an epidemic of cancer attributable to the carcinogenic chemicals afflicting the environment.[34] Public health measures to ensure clean food, air, and water prevent many diseases, including cancer. As air, water, and soil quality is improved, the risk of exposure to harmful carcinogens is minimized.

Secondary prevention. Yearly physical examinations and routine screening are examples of secondary prevention that lead to the early diagnosis of disease and, in some cases, cures. The routine use of

Papanicolaou (Pap) smears has led to a decline in the incidence of invasive cancer of the uterine cervix. Also, more women are examining their own breasts monthly for cancer; thus, earlier diagnoses are achieved.

Prenatal diagnosis of certain genetic diseases is possible. New diagnostic laboratory techniques provide definitive information for the genetic counseling of parents. This information can aid in predicting chances of involvement or noninvolvement of offspring for a given genetic disorder (e.g., Down syndrome). One technique, *amniocentesis*, consists of removing a small amount of fluid from the amniotic sac that surrounds the fetus and analyzing the cells and chemicals in the fluid. Blood samples can also be obtained from the fetus by amniocentesis; the amniotic fluid and fetal blood are then studied to determine defects in enzymes, to ascertain gender, and to measure substances associated with defects in the spinal cord and brain.

Tertiary prevention. Once a disease becomes established, treatment—within the context of traditional Western medicine—generally falls into one of the following two major categories: medical (including such measures as physical therapy, pharmacotherapy, psychotherapy, radiation therapy, chemotherapy, immunotherapy, and experimental gene therapy) and surgical. Numerous other subspecialties of medicine and surgery also have evolved to focus on a given organ or technique. In a clinical setting, a large array of professional caregivers provides rehabilitative and supportive tertiary prevention to the diseased individual. Every professional brings the perspective of his or her discipline to the caregiving situation. Each makes clinical judgments about the patient's needs and problems and decides which goals and intervention strategies are most beneficial.

KEY POINTS

- Epidemiology is the study of patterns of disease in human populations.
- Diseases may be endemic, epidemic, or pandemic depending upon location and the number of people affected.
- Aggregate factors such as age, ethnicity, gender, lifestyle, socioeconomic status, and geographic location are epidemiologic variables that influence the occurrence and transmission of disease in populations.
- Understanding the epidemiologic aspects of a disease is essential for effective prevention and treatment.

SUMMARY

Most people recognize what it is to be healthy and would define disease or illness as a change from or absence of that state. Under closer scrutiny, the concept of health is difficult to describe in simple, succinct terms. Correspondingly, the concepts of disease and illness also are complex. Environment, genetic constitution, socioeconomic status, lifestyle, and previous physical health all affect the timing and ultimate expression of disease in individuals.

Because humans exhibit considerable diversity, healthy structure and function are not precisely the same in any two individuals. By discovering common and expected patterns of responses to abnormalities, general prediction of etiology, pathogenesis, clinical manifestations, and targeted levels of prevention and intervention becomes possible.

REFERENCES

1. *Dorland's illustrated medical dictionary*, ed 32, St Louis, 2011, Elsevier.
2. Graham K et al: Alcohol-related negative consequences among drinkers around the world, *Addiction* 106(8):1391–1405, 2011.
3. MedicineNet.com. Available at http://www.medterms.com/script/main/art.asp?articlekey=6385. Accessed 12/6/2011.
4. Office of AIDS Research, National Institutes of Health. Available at http://www.oar.nih.gov/about/research/etiology/oaretio.htm. Accessed 12/6/2011.
5. Pickering LK: Syphilis. In *Red book*, Elk Grove Village, IL, 2009, American Academy of Pediatrics, pp 638–651.
6. Herzog CA et al: Cardiovascular disease in chronic kidney disease: a clinical update from kidney disease improving global outcomes (KDIGO), *Kidney Int* 9(6):572–586, 2011.
7. Clinical and Laboratory Standards Institute (CLSI): *Defining, establishing, and verifying reference intervals in the clinical laboratory: approved guideline—third edition,* Wayne, PA, 2008, Author, NCCLS document C28–A3.
8. Lindahl TL et al: INR calibration of Owren-type prothrombin time based on the relationship between PT% and INR utilizing normal plasma samples, *Thromb Haemost* 91(6):1223–1231, 2004.
9. Smith J, Winkler R, Fryback D: The first positive: computing positive predictive value at the extremes, *Ann Intern Med* 132:804–809, 2000.
10. Bocklandt S, Vilain E: Sex differences in brain and behavior: hormones versus genes, *Adv Genet* 59:245–266, 2007.
11. Gerber A, Hentzelt F, Lauterbach KW: Can evidence-based medicine implicitly rely on current concepts of disease or does it have to develop its own definition? *J Med Ethics* 33(7):394–399, 2007.
12. Linton AD, Lach HW: *Matteson & McConnell's gerontological nursing: concepts and practice*, ed 3, Philadelphia, 2006, Saunders.
13. Wu AHB: *Tietz clinical guide to laboratory tests*, ed 4, Philadelphia, 2006, Saunders.
14. Blair ML: Sex-based differences in physiology: what should we teach in the medical curriculum? *Adv Physiol Educ* 31(1):23–25, 2007.
15. Hopfl G, Ogunshola O, Gassmann M: Hypoxia and high altitude: the molecular response, *Adv Exp Med Biol* 543:89–115, 2003.
16. Buckley TM, Schatzberg AF: On the interactions of the hypothalamic-pituitary-adrenal (HPA) axis and sleep: normal HPA axis activity and circadian rhythm, exemplary sleep disorders, *J Clin Endocrinol Metab* 90(5):3106–3114, 2005.
17. Wizemann TM, Pardue M-L, editors: *Exploring the biological contributions to human health: does sex matter?* Washington, DC, April 25, 2001, Institute of Medicine Board of Health Sciences Policy.
18. Walsh SJ, Rau LM: Autoimmune diseases: a leading cause of death among young and middle-aged women in the United States, *Am J Public Health* 90(9):1463–1466, 2000.
19. Surks MI et al: Subclinical thyroid disease: scientific review and guidelines for diagnosis and management, *JAMA* 291:228–238, 2004.
20. Klippel JH: *Primer on the rheumatic diseases*, ed 13, Atlanta, 2008, Arthritis Foundation, pp 86–93, 184–190.
21. Puechal X, Fiessinger JN: Thromboangiitis obliterans or Buerger's disease: challenges for the rheumatologist, *Rheumatology (Oxford)* 46:192–199, 2007.
22. Division of Cancer Epidemiology & Genetics: *Cancer, organic solvents and other industrial chemicals,* Bethesda, MD, National Cancer Institute, U.S. National Institutes of Health. Available at http://www.cancer.gov. Accessed 12/6/2011.
23. Trends in tuberculosis incidence—United States, 2006, *JAMA* 297:1765–1767, 2007.
24. Sartin J et al: Medical management issues surrounding community-acquired pneumonia in adults, *Gundersen Lutheran Med Found J* 1(2):6–9, 2003.
25. World Health Organization: *Tropical diseases research.* Available at http://www.who.int/en/. Accessed 12/6/2011.

26. Daynard RA: Lessons from tobacco control for the obesity control movement, *J Public Health Policy* 24(3-4):274–290, 2003.

27. Wadden TA et al: Randomized trial of lifestyle modification and pharmacotherapy for obesity, *N Engl J Med* 353(20):2111–2120, 2005.

28. McCabe BW et al: Practice of health-promoting behaviors by nursing home residents, *West J Nurs Res* 27(12):1000–1016, 2005.

29. World Health Organization: *World malaria situation.* Available at http://www.who.int/en/. Accessed 12/6/2011.

30. O'Neill J: Environmental values through thick and thin, *Conserv Soc* 3:479–500, 2005.

31. World Health Organization. Available at http://www.who.int/en/. Accessed 12/6/2011.

32. Jekel JF: *Epidemiology, biostatistics, and preventive medicine*, Philadelphia, 2007, Saunders.

33. Rotary.org: *Facts about polio.*Available at http://www.rotary.org.Accessed 12/6/2011.

34. Laden F et al: Reduction in fine particulate air pollution and mortality: extended follow-up of the Harvard Six Cities study, *Am J Respir Crit Care Med* 173:667–672, 2006.

2

Homeostasis and Adaptive Responses to Stressors

Debra A. Jansen and Roberta J. Emerson

evolve WEBSITE

http://evolve.elsevier.com/Copstead/
- Review Questions and Answers
- Glossary (with audio pronunciations for selected terms)
- Animations
- Case Studies
- Key Points Review

KEY QUESTIONS

- What is the relationship between homeostasis and allostasis?
- How do the sympathetic nervous system and neuroendocrine system respond to stress?
- What are the key features of Selye's General Adaptation Syndrome?
- What factors affect the stress response?
- How does allostatic overload contribute to the development of disease?

CHAPTER OUTLINE

Survival of the human species is dependent on its ability to respond to changes in the environment. Changes in the external environment, such as moving outside from a warm house on a cold winter day, demand physiologic adjustments in the body's internal environment beyond the simple addition of layers of clothing to the outside of the body. Variations in the internal environment, such as a fever caused by infection, also necessitate physiologic responses to return the body's temperature to the normal range. The human organism maintains a variety of highly complex interactions with both internal and external environments. These interactions facilitate ongoing compensatory changes designed to support the organism physically and psychologically. This process is necessary, allowing the perpetuation of both the individual and the species. Researchers, however, have found that the body's efforts to adapt to prolonged and repeated or extraordinarily demanding environmental changes may be associated with many physical and psychological health problems. This chapter explores the historical and current perspectives of homeostasis, allostasis, and stress responses, and their relationship to illness.

HOMEOSTASIS AND ALLOSTASIS

Homeostasis

The word *homeostasis* is derived from the Greek words *homeo,* or same, and *stasis,* or stable, and means remaining stable by remaining the same.[1] Homeostasis is conceptualized as a state of being in which all systems are in balance around a particular ideal "set-point." From this perspective, bodily changes formerly seen as conflicting or detrimental are understood as adaptive or compensatory to the maintenance of homeostasis within the body as a whole. Homeostasis reflects a tendency to stabilize an organism's functional systems, despite changes both internally and externally. Deviations from homeostasis resulting from these changes require elaborate systems to support its reestablishment. A great deal of discussion exists in the literature over the past several decades criticizing the inadequacy of the definition of homeostasis to encompass the entire process of maintaining a stable state in complex organisms. But the fact remains that homeostatic concepts are an essential starting point for an exploration of stress, adaptation, and disease.

Claude Bernard, a nineteenth century French physiologist, is credited with describing the basic premise of homeostasis. He believed that the various vital physiologic mechanisms of the body had as their goal the maintenance of a uniform and constant internal environment, or *milieu intérieur*, for the body. The stability of the internal environment was deemed necessary for the survival of the person, independent or free of the external environment.[1,2] Disease occurred when the body did not respond appropriately to maintain internal stability when threatened by perceived or actual events.[1] Building on Bernard's work, Walter B. Cannon created a concept that he referred to as "homeostasis" in his 1932 book *The Wisdom of the Body*.[1-4] Homeostasis, according to Cannon, was a process in which each of the body's biochemical or physiologic variables (e.g., body temperature; oxygen, sodium, calcium, and glucose levels; and pH) was maintained within a narrow set point range. Negative feedback loops were used to sense and correct any deviations from the set point ranges for the variables, thereby supporting the survival of the individual, despite threats from the external or internal environments. These environmental threats could range from temperature extremes and water loss or gain, to "savage animals," to bacterial infection.[1,3] Box 2-1 provides examples of homeostatic systems designed to support the life of the person in the most basic sense.

Allostasis

The original concept of homeostasis, with the principle that the body attempts to achieve balance around a single optimal level or set point for a given physiologic variable, has been challenged in recent decades. The innate complexity of biological organisms requires that set points be readjusted for different circumstances (i.e., diverse situations necessitate different homeostatic set points).[5] For example, respiratory rate needs to increase when vigorously exercising or when ill with pneumonia in order to obtain more oxygen. At the same time, when responding to an internal or external environmental challenge (i.e., a stressor), *multiple* physiologic parameters may have to raise or lower their levels or actions in order to meet the demands posed by the challenge and achieve some internal stability. Desired changes in one body system, though, may be detrimental to another; these changes, however, may ultimately be needed to support the survival of the organism as a whole

at that particular point in time.[5] For instance, in shock, when the life of the organism is at risk, blood flow to essential organs (brain and heart) is maintained by reducing perfusion to the kidneys, skin, and gastrointestinal tract. Simply stated, the body is not concerned about digesting dinner or making urine when it is trying to divert resources to a struggling brain and heart.

In 1988 Sterling and Eyer introduced the concept of **allostasis** in recognition of the complexity and variable levels of activity necessary to reestablish or maintain homeostasis.[6] They described allostasis as the ability to successfully adapt to challenges. In order to survive, "an organism must *vary* all the parameters of its internal milieu and match them appropriately to environmental demands." Like homeostasis, allostasis is a derivation of the Greek words *allo,* meaning variable, and *stasis,* meaning stable. Therefore this term accentuates the role of allostatic systems in maintaining the organism's stability by being variable.[1] Allostasis is a dynamic process that supports and helps the body achieve homeostasis; homeostasis, from this perspective, is seen as a steady state. In essence, the organism's overall stability is accomplished through change.[1,7]

Allostasis involves intricate regulatory processes orchestrated by the brain.[8] Through these processes, the body's parameters are continuously reevaluated and readjusted in order to match resources to the needs dictated by the situation. These parameter readjustments (e.g., of heart rate, blood pressure, or glucose levels) entail altering multiple set points such that the person may be functioning at reduced or elevated levels or rates for numerous physiologic variables. Thus, an individual may have different set points for different circumstances (e.g., when resting versus running or when healthy versus sick). Allostasis comes into play in the complexity of social interactions, during changes in the weather, during reproduction, and even in the hibernation and migration patterns of bears and birds, as well as in critical illness.[1,6,7,9] Although the concept is occasionally challenged,[7,10] it has garnered broad support in both the physical and the behavioral sciences. It seems especially applicable to subsequent discussions of adaptation and disease.

KEY POINTS

- Contemporary concepts of homeostasis have a long history, reaching back to the ancient Greeks.
- Homeostasis is a state of equilibrium, of balance within the organism.
- Homeostatic responses refer to systems whose purpose is specifically to normalize selected physiologic variables.
- Allostasis is the overall process of adaptive change necessary to maintain survival and well-being.
- Allostasis may involve altering multiple physiologic variables in order to match the resources of the body to environmental demands. It helps the body achieve homeostasis.

STRESS AS A CONCEPT

Referring to **stress** as something of an "ambiguous" term is an understatement. Its ubiquitous use in everyday parlance is matched by its frequent presence in the health and psychology literature. Stress often is interpreted as a physical, chemical, or emotional factor that produces tension in the body or the mind ("He's experiencing a lot of stress"). But it also can mean the actual physical and mental state of tension ("I feel stressed"). Others use the term stress in relation to the response by the body to internal and external demands. Stress can be defined as a real or perceived threat to the balance of homeostasis. The neuroendocrinologist Robert Sapolsky more specifically distinguishes between the stress terminology and defines a stressor as anything that throws the body out of allostatic balance, whereas the stress response is

---

BOX 2-1   EXAMPLES OF HOMEOSTATIC SYSTEMS

Baroreceptor response to acute changes in blood pressure
Vasopressin/antidiuretic hormone release from the posterior pituitary in response to changes in serum osmolality
Hypothalamic-mediated responses to changes in body core temperature
Central chemoreceptor responses to changes in Pa_{CO_2}
Parathyroid gland response to changes in serum calcium level

the body's effort to try to restore the balance. To that end, stress is a natural outgrowth of the concept of homeostasis but is even more applicable to the dynamic concept of allostasis. Sapolsky's[5] definition also underscores an important point: The stress response by the body is meant to be helpful, at least in the short term; however, it becomes damaging when repeatedly activated or when it does not cease.

As early as the 1920s, Walter Cannon used the term stress in relation to humans and medicine. Hans Selye, however, often is erroneously credited with being the first person to borrow the term from the fields of engineering and physics and apply it to the human condition.[5] In the 1930s Selye was experimenting with assorted ovarian and placental hormonal preparations and other tissue extracts and toxic agents. He was injecting these into rats when he serendipitously uncovered a biological basis for stress.[1,5,11] Selye was expecting to find different physiologic responses in the rats, depending on which of the various substances was injected; however, to his surprise and disappointment, the same three changes occurred each time. In every animal tested, the cortex of the adrenal gland enlarged, lymphatic organs (thymus, spleen, and lymph nodes) shrank, and bleeding peptic ulcers developed in the stomach and duodenum. When Selye experimented with other noxious stimuli, such as exposing the rats to temperature extremes, surgery, or forced exercise, the same three changes occurred. Any kind of harmful physical stimuli he used produced the same observed physiologic changes. Selye termed the harmful stimuli or causative agents **stressors** and concluded that the changes observed represented a nonspecific response by the body to any noxious stimulus or demand, a general "stress" response.[11] Because so many different agents caused the same changes, Selye called this process a **general adaptation syndrome (GAS)** with three components: an *alarm reaction,* a *stage of resistance,* and a *stage of exhaustion.*[1,5,11] According to Selye, when confronted by stressors during daily life, individuals move through the first two stages repeatedly and eventually become adapted and "used to" the stressors.[11]

Selye's original conceptualization of the stress response and GAS has been criticized as being too simplistic for the complexities of humans. In particular, evidence suggests the body does not produce the same responses to all types of stressors. Depending on the type and severity of stressor, different patterns of hormone release occur, with more of some substances and less of others being produced and at different speeds and for varying lengths of time.[5,12] Moreover, Selye's early work in the 1930s concentrated on stimuli of a physical or biological nature.[11] Beginning in the 1970s, researchers began to realize that perception of these stimuli was important to individuals' responses to stress, and that responses could be physiologic, as Selye described, as well as behavioral in nature.

When stress is generated by extreme psychological or environmental demands, balance is disrupted, and allostatic reactions are initiated to restore balance.[13] The discussion that follows presents the GAS as a reflection of the responses to these diverse stimuli and incorporates much of the knowledge acquired since Selye's early pioneering work.

The General Adaptation Syndrome and Allostasis

Components of the GAS can be subdivided into three unique, largely physiologic stages (Table 2-1). Examining the stages separately is the best way to understand the entire GAS. The specific chemicals involved are among those seen today as integral to the broader view of allostatic responses to stress in the maintenance of homeostasis. All will be discussed later in the chapter.

Alarm Stage

The alarm stage has been called the **fight-or-flight response,** derived from Cannon's work, because it provides a surge of energy and physical alterations to either evade or confront danger[12] (Figure 2-1). This stage

TABLE 2-1	STAGES OF THE GENERAL ADAPTATION SYNDROME	
ALARM	**RESISTANCE**	**EXHAUSTION**
Increased secretion of glucocorticoids and responses	Eventual normalization of glucocorticoid secretion	Increased glucocorticoid secretion followed by significant reduction
Increased sympathetic nervous system activity	Eventual normalization of sympathetic nervous system activity	Diseases of adaptation
Increased secretion of epinephrine (and some norepinephrine) from adrenal medulla	Eventual normalization of epinephrine and norepinephrine secretion from adrenal medulla	Loss of resistance to stressor; possible death of organism
Fight-or-flight manifestations	Resolution of fight-or-flight manifestations	
Reduced resistance to stressors	Increased resistance (adaptation) to stressor	

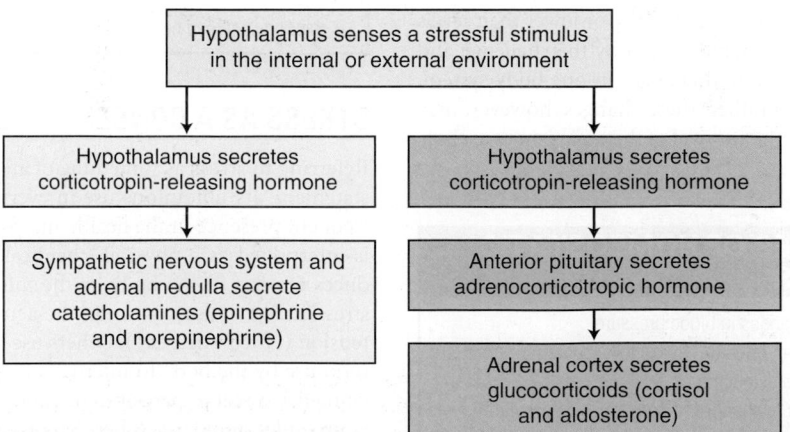

FIGURE 2-1 Steps of Selye's alarm stage of the general adaptation syndrome. (Modified from McKenry L et al: *Mosby's pharmacology in nursing,* ed 22, St Louis, 2006, Mosby.)

begins when the hypothalamus, as it monitors the internal and external environment, senses a need to activate the GAS in response to a stimulus, a stressor placing the balance of homeostasis at risk. The stressor might be physical or emotional, positive or negative—arguing with a friend, having an upper respiratory tract infection, running to catch a bus, or winning the lottery. The hypothalamus then secretes corticotropin-releasing hormone (CRH) to activate the sympathetic nervous system, which in turn also stimulates the adrenal medulla (the inner portion of the adrenal gland) to release the catecholamines—norepinephrine and epinephrine. The increased levels of catecholamines enable the body to rapidly take action to fight or flee the stressor. This series of events is part of the sympathetic-adrenal-medullary system, originally referred to as the fight-or-flight response by Walter Cannon. Additionally, the hypothalamus secretes CRH to also stimulate the anterior pituitary gland to release adrenocorticotropic hormone (ACTH). ACTH then causes the

adrenal cortex (the outer portion of the adrenal gland) to release substantial amounts of the glucocorticoids, specifically cortisol, eliciting its diverse responses, and also aldosterone. This cascade of effects is termed the **hypothalamic-pituitary-adrenal (HPA)** axis.[4] Once the pituitary gland is activated, the alarm stage progresses to the stage of resistance. This coordinated systemic response to stress is illustrated in Figure 2-2.

Allostasis is essentially the activation of these stress responses to evoke changes that return the organism to homeostasis. Mediators of allostasis include the aforementioned hormones, neurotransmitters of the HPA axis and the sympathetic-adrenal-medullary system (e.g., cortisol, epinephrine, and norepinephrine),[1,8,9] various other hormones presented later in this chapter, and also cytokines from the immune system. The alarm stage of the stress response with the release of its various hormones is meant to be helpful to the organism in overcoming the stressor, at least initially.

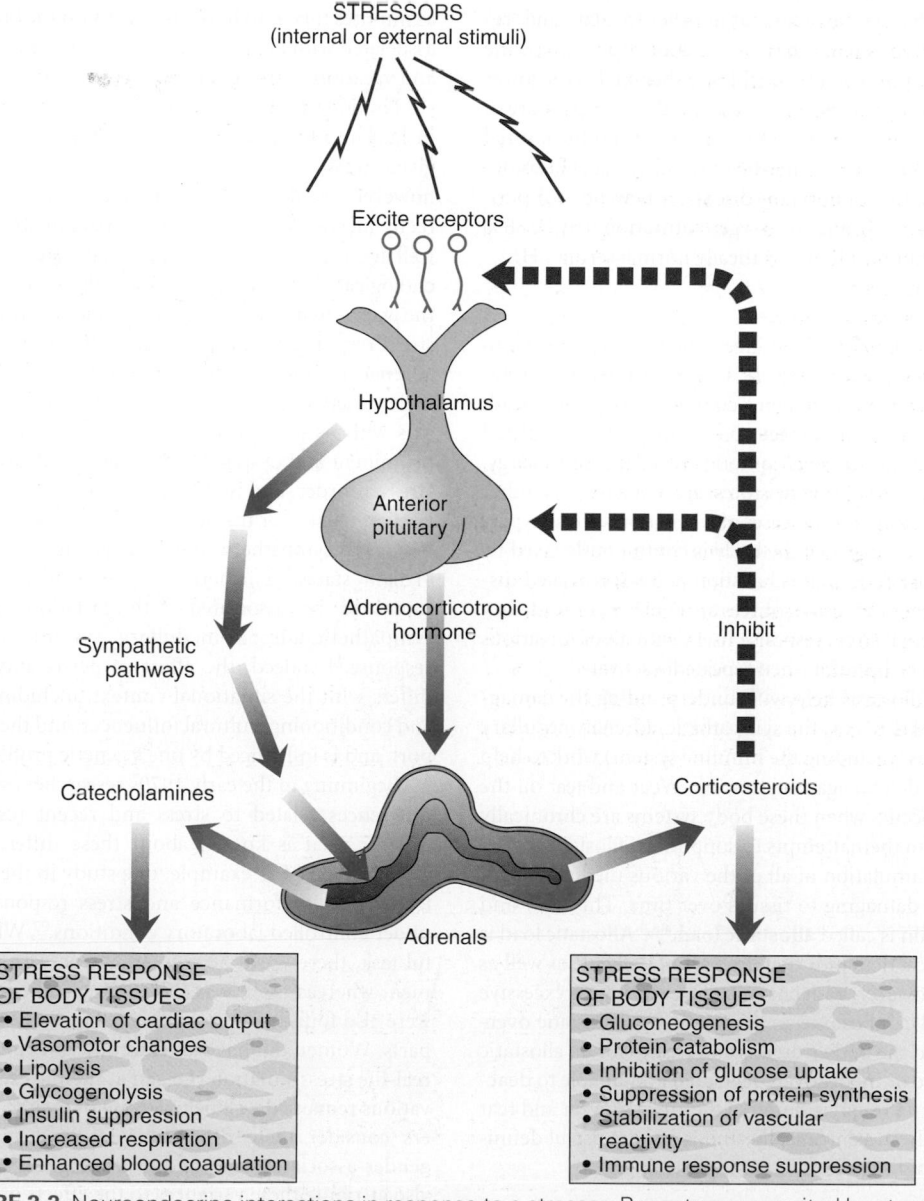

FIGURE 2-2 Neuroendocrine interactions in response to a stressor. Receptors are excited by stressful stimuli and relay the information to the hypothalamus. The hypothalamus signals the adrenal cortex (by way of the anterior pituitary) and the sympathetic pathways (by way of the autonomic nervous system). The stress response is then mediated by the catecholamines (i.e., epinephrine and norepinephrine) and by the glucocorticoids (predominantly cortisol).

Resistance or Adaptation Stage

If the alarm stage were to persist, the body would soon suffer undue wear and tear and become subject to permanent damage and even death.[11] To survive, the body must move beyond the alarm stage to a stage of resistance (also called adaptation) supportive of the allostatic return to a state of homeostasis. As the body moves into the stage of resistance, the sympathetic nervous system and adrenal medulla and cortex are functioning at full force to mobilize resources to manage the stressor. The resources include glucose, free fatty acids, and amino acids, and concentrations of all of these chemicals are elevated through the effects of cortisol and the catecholamines (i.e., epinephrine and nor-epinephrine). These resources are used for energy and as building blocks, especially the amino acids, for the later growth and repair of the organism after the stress abates. If the stressor is adequately addressed and resolved, the organism returns to its steady-state, having reattained allostatic balance.[5] This process described by Selye is clearly a part of the more recently described process of allostasis. However, with the current understanding of allostasis, it is possible that in order to adapt and re-attain homeostasis, the organism may have to function at a new baseline steady-state for different physiologic variables, either higher or lower than the previous set points. For instance, the normal partial pressure of carbon dioxide (pco_2) in the blood is 35 to 45 mm Hg and the normal oxygen saturation is greater than 94% in a healthy individual. For some-one with chronic obstructive pulmonary disease, a new normal pco_2 value might be 50 to 60 mm Hg and the oxygen saturation may be 88% to 90%, while still maintaining a homeostatically normal serum pH.

Exhaustion Stage

Exhaustion occurs when the body is no longer able to effect a return to homeostasis following prolonged exposure to noxious agents.[11] Selye postulated that when energy resources are completely depleted, death occurs because the organism is no longer able to adapt. He speculated that individuals are born with a given amount of adaptation energy. However, when these adaptive energy stores are depleted, no other resource exists to facilitate recovery. Diseases of adaptation such as hyper-tension and heart disease occur when the body is continuously taxed by stressors.[11] It is now understood that exhaustion and stress-related dis-ease do not necessarily occur because resources are depleted; instead, they can occur because the actual stress response itself, with all of its various biological mediators, can be harmful when repeatedly activated.[5]

Concepts related to allostasis help with understanding the damag-ing effects of stress. The HPA axis, the sympathetic-adrenal-medullary system, and other systems (including the immune system) work to help the person adapt to and defend against stressors. Wear and tear on the body and on the brain occurs when these body systems are chronically over- or underactivated in their attempts to support an allostatic return to homeostasis. The accumulation of all of the various mediators pro-duced by the systems is damaging to tissues over time. This wear and tear on the body and brain is called **allostatic load.**[4,8,9] Allostatic load is basically due to the typical demands that are part of daily life as well as unpredictable events. However, with chronic, unremitting, or excessive demands, allostatic load can become an overload. This allostatic over-load reflects the "cost" to the body's organs and tissues for an allostatic response that is excessive or ineffectively regulated and unable to deac-tivate.[1,7,14] It is essentially a re-envisioning of the effect of wear and tear on the body, both acutely and chronically, and is a more useful defini-tion than homeostasis in discussions of pathophysiology.

Stressors and Risk Factors

Stressors are agents or conditions that are capable of producing stress and endangering homeostasis. They initiate stress response systems in order to return to a state of allostatic balance. Every day the human organism encounters stressors. These may be external to the individual (e.g., air pollution, radiation, a motor vehicle accident) or internal (e.g., low blood glucose level or a threat to self-esteem). Common gen-eral stressors are physical (e.g., extreme hot or cold air temperature), chemical (e.g., auto exhaust), biological (e.g., bacteria and viruses), social (e.g., overcrowding and relationships), cultural (e.g., behavioral norms), or psychological (e.g., feelings of hopelessness). Stressors of an emotional or mental origin may be actually present or anticipated, or may involve the recollection of prior traumatic events. Less commonly noted but extremely powerful stressors are psychosocial experiences over which a person may have little or no personal control. Racial[15-18] and socioeconomic stressors[8,19-21] as well as childhood abuse[22] can produce many of the manifestations of stress described in this chapter.

Stressors vary in their scope, intensity, and duration. A stressor of less intensity can still have a significant impact if it persists for some time. A glass of water held at arm's length poses little stress initially, but as minutes turn into hours the stress on the body escalates. Even events associated with happiness may serve as stressors—holidays, childbirth, and vacations. Stressors of all types challenge human adaptation.

The identification of specific stressors in isolation provides little insight into today's complex global society. As noted by Sapolsky,[5] a given stressor may have its own particular pattern of hormone release; however, researchers have explored innumerable factors that can indi-rectly increase or decrease the impact of stressors. It is now generally well accepted that inherent personal characteristics as well as the psy-chological context of the situation allow for a great deal of variation in the way humans perceive and respond to stressors, and thus the type of stress response produced.[4,5] The activation of both the sympathetic-adrenal-medullary system response and the HPA axis occurs with a wide variety of physical, mental, and psychosocial stressors. The HPA axis with its glucocorticoid response, however, seems to be notably prominent and dysregulated in cases of depression and posttraumatic stress disorder, and is also active when a person's sense of self is nega-tively evaluated or the person lacks a sense of control.[5,23] On the other hand, the sympathetic system is particularly active with anxiety and vigilant states.[5] Furthermore, personality characteristics have been found to be associated with variations in cortisol release and sympathetic-adrenal-medullary system activation in the stress response.[24] Indeed, the effect of personality on the stress response differs with the situational context, including one's past experiences and conditioning, cultural influences, and the availability of social sup-port, and is influenced by one's genetic profile[4] and gender.

Beginning in the early 1970s researchers started to examine gender differences related to stress and recent research has continued to expand what is known about these differences between men and women.[14,25-29] For example, one study in the 1980s examined the dif-ferences in performance and stress responses of men and women under controlled laboratory conditions.[27] When subjected to a stress-ful task, there was a 50% to 100% increase in epinephrine release in men, whereas there was little if any increase noted in women, who were also found to perform as well or better than their male counter-parts. Women did have an elevation in epinephrine release in a more real-life stress situation (i.e., an academic examination), but these ele-vations remained well below those of men.[27] Although some research-ers consider these differences, at least in part, to be related to gender-associated roles and psychological factors,[26] other researchers also attribute these variances to the effects of the sex hormones on the stress response.[28,29]

Developmental stage of life and age also appear to relate to the way the body responds to stressors. Variations in HPA axis function are noticeable during adolescence, when sex hormone secretion is significantly elevated in both males and females.[29] A prolonged HPA activation in response to stress in childhood has been documented in both genders when compared with that of adults. This physiologic finding has been suggested to impact the vulnerability of brain development in adolescents exposed to high levels of stress during this period.[29] Adult women during the period between menarche and menopause have lower stress responses than men of the same age.[28] It has been hypothesized that this is a physiologic evolutionary effort to protect the fetus from the effects of exposure to elevated levels of cortisol, in particular. Postmenopause, the responses of both the sympathetic nervous system and the HPA axis appear to increase.[28] Clearly, stressors can affect the same person in different ways at different times over the course of a lifetime.

Risk factors alone are not inherently stressors, but rather conditions or situations that increase the likelihood of encountering or experiencing a stressor. Using a cellular phone while driving is a risk factor for having a motor vehicle accident; running in the dark is a risk factor for falling; inadequate immunization is a risk factor for certain infectious illnesses and even cancers. Risk factors include genetic predispositions and epigenetic factors, as well as early life experiences.[4,30,31] By being aware of risk factors, it is possible to decrease the probability of exposure to certain stressors and their inevitable threat to homeostasis.

KEY POINTS

- Stress is a real or perceived threat to the balance of homeostasis. The stress response is meant to restore balance.
- Selye's theory of a GAS reflects the view of a nonspecific physiologic response to stress. It incorporates three stages reflecting the changes in the body's systemic response: alarm, resistance, and exhaustion.
- Stressors are agents or conditions capable of producing stress.
- The body's response to stressors is meant to be helpful, at least initially, in terms of mobilizing resources to help manage stressors.
- Response to a stressor depends on its magnitude and the meaning that the stressor has for an individual. Stressors may be perceived as more or less stressful. Perception depends on genetic constitution, gender, past experiences and conditioning, and cultural influences. Stressors may be external or internal. They may be physical, chemical, biological, sociocultural, or psychological.
- Individuals may be more vulnerable to the effects of stressors at certain times. The developmental stage of life and the effects of other previous or concurrent stressors all contribute to the stress response.
- Risk factors are conditions or situations that increase the likelihood of encountering or experiencing a stressor.

NEUROHORMONAL MEDIATORS OF STRESS AND ADAPTATION

Numerous hormones and signaling molecules are involved in the daily maintenance of homeostasis through allostatic processes. These mediators are briefly described here, and their roles in allostasis, adaptation, and disease are discussed in later parts of this chapter. A key idea to the understanding of homeostasis is that once the challenges contributing to allostatic load have been resolved, levels of these chemicals should return to their baselines. However, in cases of allostatic overload, pathologies of a physiologic, psychological, or behavioral nature may result.

Catecholamines: Norepinephrine and Epinephrine

Cannon identified that the body's response to threats resulted in the activation of the adrenal medulla and sympathetic nervous system. He deemed this the "sympathico-adrenal system" and believed it was ultimately responsible for what he termed the *"fight-or-flight"* reaction. The purpose of the fight-or-flight reaction was the maintenance of the physical and psychological integrity of the organism.[1,3,12] The catecholamine neurotransmitters—epinephrine and norepinephrine—play integral roles in allostasis.

Release of catecholamines is initiated through the activation of the hypothalamus gland, a collection of nerve centers situated near the third ventricle close to the base of the brain (see Chapter 39). The cerebral cortex and limbic system (including the hippocampus and amygdala, important for memory and emotions) receive information regarding stressors and determine whether or not something is potentially harmful to the organism (i.e., whether it is stressful).[8] They relay the information to the hypothalamus. (It should be noted, though, that the stress response, depending on the type of stressor, may occur to some extent even in comatose and sedated individuals.[32]) In response to these stressors, the hypothalamus prompts the release of **norepinephrine** from the sympathetic branch of the autonomic nervous system and epinephrine and some norepinephrine from the adrenal medulla.[33] Norepinephrine is released by sympathetic neurons directly into the synaptic clefts near the effector organs and tissues. Preganglionic fibers from the sympathetic nervous system neurons synapse at the adrenal medulla, stimulating the release of **epinephrine** and, to a lesser extent, norepinephrine. The adrenal catecholamines are released into the bloodstream, and travel to effector organs and tissues (endocrine).[33] These circulating adrenal catecholamines have essentially the same effects as sympathetic nerve stimulation and are often seen as an extension of the sympathetic nervous system. The responses on the part of the sympathetic nervous system and the adrenal medulla may differ according to the stimulus.[12] During situations such as exposure to cold temperatures the sympathetic nervous system response with norepinephrine production dominates. Emotional distress or acute hypoglycemia, however, causes a greater response from the adrenal medulla, with increased production of epinephrine.[12]

The effects of catecholamines are profound. They affect cardiovascular function, control fluid volume by activating the renin-angiotensin-aldosterone mechanism, have a role in inflammation and immunity, and impact metabolism; and they are associated with attentiveness, arousal, and memory formation in the central nervous system.[1,30,33,34] Norepinephrine is the primary constrictor of smooth muscle in blood vessels. It therefore regulates blood flow through tissues and its distribution through the organs, as well as, importantly, maintenance of blood pressure. It also reduces gastric secretion and innervates the iris and ciliary muscles of the eyes, thereby dilating the pupils and increasing night vision and far vision.[34] Epinephrine enhances myocardial contractility and increases heart rate and venous return to the heart, thus increasing cardiac output. It additionally relaxes bronchial smooth muscle, thereby dilating the airways to enable better oxygenation. Epinephrine also has the metabolic effects of increasing glycogenolysis and the release of glucose from the liver and inhibiting insulin secretion, further elevating blood glucose levels. In the brain, the increased blood flow and availability of glucose lead to increases in mental attention and alertness. Epinephrine and norepinephrine also are able to exert immune system effects by affecting the production of cytokines by immune cells and adipose cells.[33] The effects of these catecholamines are summarized briefly in Table 2-2. For more detail, see Chapter 43.

Adrenocortical Steroids: Cortisol and Aldosterone

Among the most versatile hormones in the human body, glucocorticoids have regulatory roles in the cardiovascular system and in maintaining fluid volume, and contribute to metabolism, immunity, and inflammatory responses, brain function, and even reproduction[30]

TABLE 2-2   BRIEF SUMMARY OF EFFECTS OF CATECHOLAMINES ON TISSUES AND ORGANS OF THE BODY

TISSUE/ORGAN	CATECHOLAMINE EFFECT
Heart	Increases rate
	Increases speed of impulse conduction
	Increases contractility
Respiratory tract	Relaxes bronchial smooth muscle to dilate airway
Vascular smooth muscle	
Skin, mesenteric bed, kidneys	Constricts to reduce perfusion
Skeletal muscle, lungs, heart	Dilates to increase perfusion
Peripheral vasculature	Constricts to increase blood pressure
Gastrointestinal tract	Decreases peristalsis
	Contracts sphincters
	Decreases gastric acid secretion
Eyes	Contracts radial muscle to dilate iris and pupil
	Relaxes ciliary muscle for far vision
Liver	Glycogenolysis and gluconeogenesis for increased glucose levels and thus energy
Central nervous system	Promotes arousal, attention, and vigilance

TABLE 2-3   MAJOR EFFECTS OF GLUCOCORTICOIDS IN THE STRESS RESPONSE

Metabolism	Catabolism of muscle, fat, lymphoid tissue, skin, and bone
	Liver gluconeogenesis
	Opposes insulin in transport of glucose into cells
	Increased appetite
Fluid balance	Sodium and water retention
Inflammation and infection	Suppressed inflammatory response
	Increased neutrophil release
	Decreased new antibody release
	Decreased T lymphocyte production and function
	Decreased production of eosinophils, basophils, and monocytes
Support catecholamines	Increased epinephrine synthesis
	Enhanced vasoconstriction

(Table 2-3). Glucocorticoids are lipid-soluble hormones, allowing them to pass through cell membranes to bind with receptors in the cytosol or nucleus and initiate changes in cellular activities. Practically every body tissue has intracellular glucocorticoid receptors.[30] As opposed to the catecholamines, the onset of their effects is slower, but the duration of action is longer.[5]

The **glucocorticoids** are so named because of their significant role in glucose metabolism. The primary glucocorticoid, **cortisol,** is secreted by the adrenal cortex in response to ACTH from the anterior pituitary. Release of ACTH is itself affected by another releasing hormone, CRH, from the hypothalamus. Negative feedback loops help to maintain cortisol level within a normal range. Cortisol is able to bind

to receptors on the hypothalamus and anterior pituitary gland to suppress CRH and ACTH release when it is excessive.[23,35]

The actions of the HPA axis may synergize or antagonize the effects of the catecholamines.[30] Catecholamines facilitate the release of ACTH, therefore helping to maintain the function of the HPA axis and release of cortisol. Glucocorticoids promote adrenal medulla synthesis of epinephrine through control of the major enzyme phenylethanolamine N-methyltransferase (PNMT). Glucocorticoids also support the actions of the catecholamines in the maintenance of normal blood pressure and, therefore, cardiac output. In skeletal muscle, catecholamines antagonize the catabolic glucocorticoid effects by impeding the breakdown of somatic protein.[30] Together, the catecholamines and glucocorticoids facilitate the brain's development of memory, which is especially important when hazardous circumstances have occurred.[1,5]

The metabolic effects of cortisol are significant. Cortisol affects protein metabolism. It has an *anabolic* effect leading to increased rates of protein synthesis in the liver. However, it has a *catabolic* effect in muscle, lymphoid, and adipose tissues, and on skin and bone. This protein breakdown produces increased levels of circulating amino acids. The resulting pool of amino acids from catabolized proteins ensures their availability for the liver. Cortisol then stimulates gluconeogenesis in the liver and a sixfold to tenfold increase in the rate of amino acid conversion to ketoacids and glucose. The catabolism of adipose tissue releases free fatty acids and glycerol that also can be used for gluconeogenesis and to create ketoacids for fuel. Gluconeogenesis ensures an adequate supply of glucose for body tissues in general, but nerve cells have priority. Cortisol may act to preserve available glucose for brain nerve cell use by limiting the uptake and oxidation of glucose by other cells in the body. Cortisol also promotes appetite and food-seeking behaviors.[30]

Glucocorticoids are known for their significant role in the control of the immune response. They suppress the acute-phase response to infection and inflammation, helping to curtail the possible effects of overactivity.[30] This is accomplished by inhibiting the production of select immune cytokines (signaling molecules), by increasing the production of other cytokines, and in some cases by directly inhibiting the proliferation and activation of specific immune system cells.[30] At the same time, when the acute stress of tissue injury or infection occurs, the resulting release of glucocorticoids and catecholamines assists the movement of the necessary immune cells to the affected location.[5,30] However, with prolonged stress and chronic elevation in the levels of glucocorticoids, desensitization and down-regulation (decrease) of glucocorticoid receptors may occur on some immune cells, eventually resulting in fewer antiinflammatory effects over time.[36] In fact, continued stress can even result in proinflammatory effects. Thus the relationship of the immune system to stress is quite multifaceted and our understanding of it is evolving.

Aldosterone is the primary **mineralocorticoid** steroid hormone secreted by the adrenal cortex. Stimulation of the sympathetic nervous system activates the renin-angiotensin system, and the release of aldosterone is the final chemical outcome. The specific stressor of fluid volume depletion also activates the release of renin, similarly initiating the renin-angiotensin system. The primary effect of aldosterone, once bound to receptors in the kidneys' distal tubules and collecting ducts, is reabsorption of sodium and an increase in the excretion of potassium. Because of osmotic force, water tends to follow sodium; therefore, enhanced reabsorption of sodium leads to increased extracellular fluid volume and increased blood pressure. Endogenous glucocorticoids have a small amount of mineralocorticoid effect, but the greatest effect on circulating volume is through aldosterone. Additionally, angiotensin II, whose formation stimulates aldosterone release, is a potent vasoconstrictor. This chemical mediator provides support for the catecholamine-induced increase in blood pressure.[30]

Endorphins, Enkephalins, and Immune Cytokines

Stress naturally activates the inhibition of pain through the release of small peptides called endorphins and enkephalins.[32,37] First discovered in 1975, **endorphins** and **enkephalins** are endogenous opioids that are produced within the central nervous system and released in response to stressors, by certain foods (most notably chocolate), by laughter, and from massage or acupuncture.[38] The term *endorphin* comes from *endogenous* and *morphine*. Like the opiate drug morphine, endorphins raise the pain threshold (reduce pain) and produce sedation and euphoria. Some immune cells (T lymphocytes, granulocytes, and monocytes) also produce several types of endorphins that are released in response to stressors, CRH, antiinflammatory cytokines, and catecholamines.[37] Opioid receptors have been identified on immune cells, and when activated they modulate both immune cell proliferation and immune cell activity. In the presence of acute or chronic stress, activated immune cells (mast cells, neutrophils, macrophages, and T lymphocytes) can release proinflammatory cytokines that enhance pain.[37,39] Pain is a classic manifestation of the inflammatory response (Chapter 9). Thus the central and peripheral nervous systems and the immune system maintain an intricate "pain-related" communication that serves as part of the allostatic mechanism to return the system to homeostasis.[37]

Another example of the interaction between stress, the nervous system, and the immune system is interleukin-1, one of the cytokines secreted by macrophages and other immune cells. It is capable of impacting the production of CRH by the hypothalamus. Leukocytes are also capable of producing some of the other hormones, such as ACTH, that are involved in the signaling system.[32] Some researchers propose that stressors of relatively short duration (less than 2 hours) could augment facets of immune function, including the emigration of immune cells from the lymphoid tissues to the skin and peripheral components of the vascular system.[40] On the other hand, numerous studies over the years have shown that severe and persistent psychological stress can down-regulate, or suppress, immune functioning through innumerable and elaborate mechanisms.[5,40] Immune system suppression caused by severe or persistent stress represents a direct link between stress and illness. Expanded understanding of the interrelationships between the nervous, endocrine, and immune systems holds great promise in the identification of new therapeutic interventions.[32,40]

Sex Hormones: Estrogen, Testosterone, and Dehydroepiandrosterone

As noted previously, women during the period between menarche and menopause have a different stress response than men of the same age, and this may be attributable to influences of sex hormones on allostasis. Cortisol exerts inhibiting effects on the female reproductive system by suppressing release of gonadotropin-releasing hormone, luteinizing hormone, estradiol, and progesterone. Excessive stress appears, in general, to inhibit female reproduction.[14] However, sexual stimulation may cause the gonadal axis to be resistant to suppression by the HPA axis. Estradiol down-regulates glucocorticoid receptor binding in the brain and alters regulatory feedback control. Androgens, such as testosterone and dehydroepiandrosterone (DHEA), may also inhibit the effects of glucocorticoids.[30] Androgens oppose the catabolic effects of glucocorticoids on bone and the impact of glucocorticoids on lymphoid tissues, inflammatory cytokines, and leukocytes. DHEA interacts with numerous neurotransmitters in the brain, counteracting the depressive tendencies often noted with glucocorticoids.[30] Numerous stressful stimuli, such as illness, surgery, strenuous physical exercise, heart failure, and stressful academic programs, result in a significant reduction in circulating testosterone levels. In combination with

another hormone, vasopressin, testosterone enhances blood pressure and heart rate reactivity and augments the "fight-or-flight" response. In contrast, the hormone oxytocin (whose impact is modulated by estrogen) and the endogenous opioids are thought to produce a calming effect during times of stress, resulting in the notion that women may have a "tend and befriend" response, rather than a "fight-or-flight" response in some situations.[40-42]

Growth Hormone, Prolactin, and Oxytocin

Growth hormone (somatotropin) is released from the anterior pituitary gland and affects protein, lipid, and carbohydrate metabolism. It has anabolic effects, increasing protein synthesis and bone and muscle mass growth. It also increases fat mobilization (lipolysis) while decreasing the rate of carbohydrate utilization by peripheral tissues. Growth hormone is normally secreted in a cyclic basal pattern, primarily at night, and according to developmental stage. Growth hormone secretion is highest during adolescence and then gradually declines during middlescence. Serum levels of growth hormone also increase, at least initially, following a variety of intensely stressful physical or psychological stimuli, such as strenuous exercise or extreme fear.[43] Growth hormone appears to enhance immune function. However, continued activation of the stress response eventually results in the decreased secretion of growth hormone, accounting for stunted growth in children experiencing prolonged chronic stress.[5]

Prolactin is similar in structure to growth hormone and is also secreted from the anterior pituitary gland in response to stress,[32] sexual activity, and suckling (even in men) and breast feeding. It interferes with ovulation.[5,43] Numerous tissues have receptors for prolactin in addition to the breast, including kidney, liver, and adrenal glands. Lymphocytes also have prolactin receptors, suggesting a role for prolactin in immune regulation. A significant increase in the level of growth hormone or prolactin tends to require more intense stimuli than the stress that increases the concentrations of catecholamines and glucocorticoids.

Oxytocin is produced during childbirth, lactation, and sexual behavior (in both genders) and has been associated with promoting bonding and social attachment. Oxytocin is thought to moderate the stress response and have a calming effect, with reductions in HPA and sympathetic activation and reduced perceived anxiety. Oxytocin also may have some analgesic effects. It is synthesized by the hypothalamus and secreted by the posterior pituitary gland and other brain regions. Oxytocin is believed to have stronger effects in females in comparison to males, because of the effects of estrogen on oxytocin.[42]

Through interactions of the primary stress hormones—catecholamines and glucocorticoids—as well as numerous other mediating influences, the allostatic process needed to sustain the human organism is achieved. In some cases, these stress-related hormones have similar and synergistic effects and in others they work in opposition. This state of counterbalancing helps to facilitate allostasis, ideally returning the human organism back toward homeostasis.

KEY POINTS

- Modern views of allostatic maintenance of homeostasis in the face of stress are primarily derived from an understanding of negative feedback, as well as the roles of the sympathetic nervous system and the glucocorticoid cortisol.
- The primary role of the sympathetic nervous system is appraisal of a stressful stimulus and release of norepinephrine. Norepinephrine released from sympathetic nerve endings increases heart rate and contractility, constricts blood vessels to decrease blood flow to less essential tissues and organs and raise blood pressure, reduces gastrointestinal motility and gastric acid secretion, dilates the pupils, and inhibits insulin secretion.

- Stress simultaneously stimulates sympathetic activation of the adrenal medulla to release epinephrine. Epinephrine's actions are similar to those of norepinephrine and are particularly important for increasing cardiac performance (increased heart rate, contractility, and cardiac output), promoting the release of glucose from the liver, and enhancing bronchodilation.
- Cortisol, from the adrenal cortex, has widespread effects on numerous tissues that are both synergistic and antagonistic with catecholamines, and has an antiinflammatory role.
- Aldosterone promotes fluid volume expansion and increases blood pressure.
- Endorphins and enkephalins are released by the central nervous system (CNS) in response to painful stressors, leading to decreased perception of pain and increased sedation and euphoria. Immune cells in the periphery also contribute to pain modulation.
- Understanding the role of the immune system in response to stressors is rapidly expanding. Immune cells respond to the hormones released by the HPA axis and sympathetic nervous system. They also release cytokines that in turn affect the functioning of these stress systems.
- Sex hormones and differential release of growth hormone, prolactin, and oxytocin produce mediating effects on the stress response that may differ between genders.

ADAPTATION, COPING, AND ILLNESS

Although much has been learned about the dynamic biological systems and human/environmental interactions involved, stress is personal in that individual stress responses change with time and circumstances. Indeed, the effects of stress on each individual are impacted by genetics, socioeconomic status, environmental context, perception, developmental history, prior susceptibilities, preexisting health status, and individual coping abilities to manage stress.[1,4,8,12] Clearly, the maintenance of homeostasis requires the human organism to routinely initiate allostatic responses to the stressors of daily life, as well as the less frequent severe assaults on the integrity of the body and the mind, responsible for allostatic load. The roles of the sympathetic nervous system and the HPA axis have been defined and supportive chemical mediators described. Systemically, allostasis may be seen as beginning with some degree of the alarm stage (fight-or-flight activation), and ideally moving to an effective resolution through adaptation, ultimately culminating in a return to homeostasis. The effects of this process are seen in allostatic load and the occasional allostatic overload. The prolonged effects of allostatic overload—the long-term wear-and-tear costs of adaptation efforts—provide a conceptual foundation for examining the long-term consequences of stress to health.[14] What Selye called "diseases of adaptation" are the outcome of allostatic overload.[44]

Adaptation and Coping

Adaptation, seen from the perspective of allostasis rather than simply as Selye's stage of the GAS, broadly refers to the biopsychosocial process of changing and adjusting physiology, morphology, and behavior in response to new or altered circumstances, internal and external in origin, in one's physical and social environments.[7] The term has been intertwined with allostasis, because allostasis is a process of attaining and maintaining stability through change, and leads to a state of adaptation.[1,14] Encountering favorable or unfavorable stressors requires multiple levels of biological, personal, and social change or adaptation. **Maladaptation,** a less frequently used term, refers to ineffective, inadequate, or inappropriate change in response to new or altered circumstances. **Coping** is another term used and is most often seen as a behavioral adaptive response to a stressor. Coping mechanisms are typically culturally based, and so vary with the individual within the parameters of what is acceptable to the given culture. The coping behavior is usually dictated by the specific stressor; thus, it commonly varies with the circumstances, but individuals typically embrace a specific repertoire of coping behaviors. These behavioral adaptations allow an individual or a group to withstand successfully the stressful experience or the stress response generated by the experience. A coping strategy can be considered effective or functional if it helps resolve either the situation or the feelings. In some cases, such as exercise, the coping method can promote health.[9] A coping strategy is considered ineffective or dysfunctional if it does not achieve the desired goal. Coping that achieves unintended goals is considered dysfunctional. Being complex organisms, adaptation may result in the adoption of less than desirable coping behaviors, such as excessive eating or alcohol consumption, smoking, or other types of substance abuse.[18] Unfortunately, these dysfunctional coping behaviors can ultimately be damaging to overall health. Smoking and overeating contribute to atherosclerosis, the underlying pathophysiology of coronary artery disease and a risk factor for hypertension. Excess weight accumulated through overeating is a contributing factor for type 2 diabetes mellitus and metabolic syndrome. Although coping is customarily interpreted as behavioral adaptation only, the terms *coping* and *adapting* often are used interchangeably.

Perception and expectations of the stressor can affect its interpretation, and therefore the behavior evoked by it. Perceptions can be related to uncertainty about the meaning of the stressor. Consider the stressor of undue noise. The "bang" of a car backfiring could also be the sound of a gun being fired. Depending upon the environment and circumstances, one or the other etiology would be more expected, dictating different adaptive responses. The term *distress* describes the experience of perceiving an inability to cope with a stressor.[12] This distress further activates the HPA axis, escalating levels of circulating mediators, and may exacerbate existing allostatic load and preexisting pathophysiologic conditions.[12] For instance, the person with asthma who is experiencing an episode of acute shortness of breath is likely to become even more short of breath when discovering an inhaler is not readily available.

Adaptation to a particular stressor can occur in several ways. Loud noise is a known stressor. Yet people who live close to busy airports often reach a point at which they barely notice the noise of airplanes flying over their homes. They become *habituated* to the stressor (loud noise). One important way to habituate to a stressor is to manipulate or "train" the hypothalamus to react less forcefully to a perceived threat or stressor. Repeatedly ignoring a specific stressor prevents the inappropriate triggering of the GAS. The result is a more acceptable level of stress response. Techniques that accomplish this **desensitization** change the predominant brain waves of the individual from beta to alpha waves, which are slower and more normal. Biofeedback, visualization, and meditation are examples of therapies that use this principle. Practicing these techniques for 20 to 30 minutes daily can enhance the ability to alter how a stressor is perceived and modulate the stress response. These techniques have documented efficacy in modulating immune function.[41] Desensitization methods have been found to be beneficial for common stress-related conditions, such as migraine headache, chronic back pain, and hypertension.

Allostatic Overload and Illness

When adaptation mechanisms are inadequate or the total amount of allostatic load is excessive, overwhelming allostasis capacities, the result is allostatic overload. There are several ways in which allostatic load can accumulate in an individual: (1) repeated exposures to multiple stressors, (2) inability to habituate or adapt to the stressor, (3) unnecessarily prolonged stress response or stress

BOX 2-2 PHYSICAL AND BEHAVIORAL INDICATORS OF HIGH STRESS

Physical Indicators

Elevated blood pressure
Increased muscle tension
Elevated pulse rate
Increased respiration
Sweaty palms
Cold extremities (hands and feet)
Fatigue
Tension headache
Upset stomach: nausea, vomiting, diarrhea
Change in appetite
Change in weight
Increased blood catecholamine level
Hyperglycemia
Restlessness
Insomnia

Behavioral and Emotional Indicators

Anxiety (nonspecific fears)
Depression
Increased use of mind-altering substances (e.g., alcohol, chemical substances)
Change in eating, sleeping, or activity pattern
Mental exhaustion
Feelings of inadequacy; loss of self-esteem
Increased irritability
Loss of motivation
Decreased productivity
Inability to make good judgments
Inability to concentrate
Increased absenteeism and illness
Increased proneness to accidents

response that continues after the stressor is removed, and (4) inadequate response to the stressor that causes other stress response mediators to attempt to compensate.[8,9] Homeostasis, the steady-state that previously existed, cannot be attained. Instead, allostatic overload occurs and the resulting maladaptation can be reflected in a range of pathophysiologic states that span the traditional boundaries of health care, from psychiatric and endocrine disorders to inflammatory disease.

Hair loss, emotional tension, burnout, mouth sores, insomnia, asthma, heart palpitations, neuromuscular movement disorders (tics), tension headaches, muscle contraction backaches, digestive disorders, and irritable bladder are just a few of the common disorders that can be caused by or worsened by stress. Reproductive disorders such as menstrual irregularity in women[14] and male impotence also have been linked with the effects of allostatic overload. Box 2-2 summarizes some of the physiologic and psychological effects of excessive stress. Figure 2-3 depicts the multiple body organs and systems in which the effects of insufficient or overactive stress responses may be seen.

There is a strong physiologic basis for the role of the chemical mediators of stress in contributing to illness. Cortisol being released from the adrenal cortex supports Selye's stage of resistance or adaptation but may also be accountable for pathologic changes. The same can be said of the catecholamines and the other chemical mediators (e.g., immune cytokines).[1,45] Because these blood-borne chemicals have

such broad effects systemically, the impact of excessive or inadequate amounts is understandably wide-reaching. In some cases, the relationships have been well substantiated by research; in others, they are hypothesized based upon knowledge of the effects of these chemicals.

The relationship between excessive catecholamine levels and what have been called "stress-related" illnesses historically has often been associated with cardiovascular pathologies such as hypertension, stroke, and myocardial infarction. Abdominal fat cells are well supplied with cortisol receptors.[45] Excessive secretion of cortisol results in the collection of fat in this area. When this fat is released into the bloodstream, the resulting increase in the levels of circulating free fatty acids plays a role in cardiovascular risk.[5,45] Repeated or prolonged elevation of blood pressure, especially in combination with the metabolic effects of elevated cortisol levels, promotes the development of atherosclerosis and, ultimately, many cardiovascular pathologies.[14] Not only do catecholamines contribute to the development of atherosclerosis and hypertension, but also they increase the risk of developing cardiac dysrhythmias and sudden cardiac death, and even stress-induced cardiomyopathy.[1] They increase platelet activity, resulting in clot formation, and elevate serum lipid levels, significant factors in the pathogenesis of myocardial infarction. A growing body of evidence suggests that inflammation may mediate a link between stress and cardiovascular disease. Stress has been associated with the production of proinflammatory cytokines such as interleukin-1 (IL-1), IL-6, and tumor necrosis factor (TNF). These cytokines can trigger the production of C-reactive protein (CRP), a cytokine associated with cardiovascular disease.[39]

The field of psychoneuroimmunology has provided substantive evidence of the roles of the stress hormones in the brain. In the central nervous system, specifically the brain, the mediators of adaptation facilitate learning, memory, and neuroendocrine and autonomic regulation.[8,9,46] This heightened memory, at least in the short term, allows the individual to be more aware of the potential stressor in the future.[1,44] Chronic over- or underactivity, however, may result in atrophy and death of some nerve cells (especially in the hippocampus), impairing memory,[8,31] whereas others have been found to hypertrophy (especially in the amygdala) and undergo remodeling, resulting in an increase in fear.[1,8,44] In essence, allostatic overload results in altered and impaired cognitive function. Some evidence suggests that inflammation associated with allostatic overload may play a role in learning and memory impairment. For instance, elevated levels of interleukin-6 (IL-6), a marker of inflammation associated with stress, were inversely related to memory in a study of middle-aged adults.[8]

Stress hormones have been found to be elevated and dysregulated in major depressive illness.[31] Abnormal patterns of cortisol secretion, elevated androgen levels in women, and increased levels of growth hormone and proinflammatory cytokines have been documented in major depressive illness.[31,46] In addition, other effects of long-term cortisol dysregulation, including demineralization of bone and increased abdominal fat deposits, have been noted.[31] Researchers also have found levels of cortisol and certain cytokines from immune cells to be elevated in depressed patients with fibromyalgia[47] and multiple sclerosis.[48] Depression is common with chronic disease, and the elevated cortisol levels associated with allostatic overload may be a significant finding in association with depression and the progression of some of the diseases. Another condition, posttraumatic stress disorder (PTSD), also appears to be associated with heightened sympathetic-adrenal-medullary responses as well as alterations in the HPA axis. Evidence suggests cortisol and norepinephrine help promote long-term memory consolidation and retention of traumatic and fearful events; however, administration of

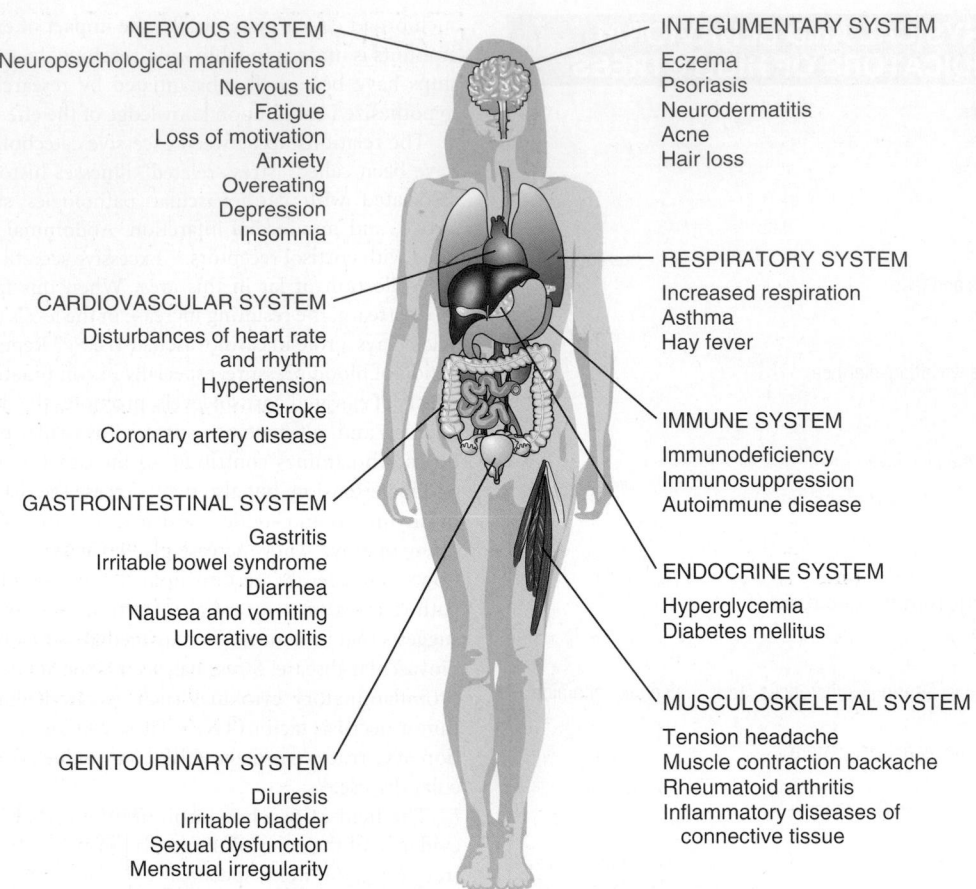

NERVOUS SYSTEM
Neuropsychological manifestations
Nervous tic
Fatigue
Loss of motivation
Anxiety
Overeating
Depression
Insomnia

CARDIOVASCULAR SYSTEM
Disturbances of heart rate
and rhythm
Hypertension
Stroke
Coronary artery disease

GASTROINTESTINAL SYSTEM
Gastritis
Irritable bowel syndrome
Diarrhea
Nausea and vomiting
Ulcerative colitis

GENITOURINARY SYSTEM
Diuresis
Irritable bladder
Sexual dysfunction
Menstrual irregularity

INTEGUMENTARY SYSTEM
Eczema
Psoriasis
Neurodermatitis
Acne
Hair loss

RESPIRATORY SYSTEM
Increased respiration
Asthma
Hay fever

IMMUNE SYSTEM
Immunodeficiency
Immunosuppression
Autoimmune disease

ENDOCRINE SYSTEM
Hyperglycemia
Diabetes mellitus

MUSCULOSKELETAL SYSTEM
Tension headache
Muscle contraction backache
Rheumatoid arthritis
Inflammatory diseases of
connective tissue

FIGURE 2-3 Effects of Allostatic Overload on Body Organs and Systems.

α- and β-blockers that interfere with the effects of norepinephrine has been shown to reduce the incidence of PTSD symptoms, although study results have been mixed.[49,50]

Allostatic mediators activate and maintain energy reserves, which is initially meant to be helpful in managing stressors. Nonetheless, obesity, diabetes, atherosclerosis, and other diseases are associated with their chronic activation.[14,45] The food-seeking behavior initiated by cortisol is beneficial in the short term, but when cortisol levels are increased by chronic stress of either a physiologic or a psychological origin, this adaptation gone awry results in obesity. Obesity is a risk factor for decreased effectiveness of glucose transport into the cells (insulin resistance), the pathophysiologic basis for type 2 diabetes.[44] Elevated cortisol levels also directly increase insulin resistance.[45] Additionally, obesity is associated with the production of proinflammatory cytokines, which also have been connected to diabetes.[45]

In acute stress, activation of the immune system allows for the coordinated defense of the body from damage.[44] At first, leukocytosis and immune function including phagocytosis and antibody production may be enhanced in order to protect the body from foreign invaders (e.g., bacteria and viruses), but then is followed quickly by immunosuppression.[1] Chronic activation of the stress mediators produces immunosuppression and increases the risk of infection[5,33,40,44] and has been implicated in the development of autoimmune diseases.[5,14] Such overactivation also prolongs existing infections and the development of secondary infections.[1] Research supports the hypothesis that physical and emotional stress and dysfunctional coping mechanisms impair both antibody and T cell–mediated responses to viruses and antiviral and antibacterial vaccines. Stressors of more than

1 month's duration have been found to be the greatest predictors of the development of colds. Cumulated evidence, in both human and animal models, supports the premise that stress-induced dysregulation of the cellular and humoral arms of the immune system increases risk of infectious disease. Stress has been found by numerous studies to accelerate the progression of human immunodeficiency virus (HIV) infection. Immune dysregulation can also include the excessive production of cytokines that have actions supporting the inflammatory response. Both physical and psychological stressors have been found to accomplish this, sensitizing the overall inflammatory response so that subsequent activations are markedly increased. This is important because many diseases are associated with inflammation: cancer, acute coronary syndrome resulting in myocardial infarction, chronic inflammatory bowel disease, and asthma, to name but a few. Wound healing also is impaired by multiple mediators of stress in excessive amounts.[5,14,39]

A new area of stress research attracting attention pertains to **telomeres** and **telomerase.** Telomeres are the tail ends of chromosomes that get shaved down with repeated cell division; and thus older cells tend to have shorter telomeres than younger ones. These cells with shortened telomeres are more susceptible to death. Telomeres are considered to be markers of "biological age" and may serve as a means of measuring a person's total accumulated exposure to stressors.[31] Chronic stress related to caregiving and lower socioeconomic status has been linked with shorter telomere length. Depression and several other diseases (e.g., cardiovascular disease) also have been associated with shortened telomeres.[31,51] This research suggests a mechanism by which stress may contribute to cell death and disease, because telomere shortening may be connected to some extent to elevated cortisol, catecholamine, and inflammatory cytokine levels produced as part of the stress response.[31] On the other hand, telomerase is an enzyme capable of lengthening telomeres and is inversely related to perceptions of stress. In one study, 30 men and women took part in a 3-month meditation retreat program aimed at reducing psychological distress. By the end of the study period, the participants had significantly higher telomerase activity levels in comparison to wait-list controls.[52] More research is needed to understand the relationships among telomeres, telomerase, stress, and stress-related diseases and coping methods, as well as aging and longevity.

KEY POINTS
- Adaptation, or allostasis, is a network of biopsychosocial processes of responding to a stressor with the goal of re-establishing homeostasis. Coping mechanisms are usually seen as behavioral adaptations to stress but are often used interchangeably with adaptation.
- The wear-and-tear effect of adaptation on the body and mind is the allostatic load. It occurs as mediators produced by the stress response systems accumulate and contribute to tissue damage over time. Allostatic load reflects the cumulative costs of adaptation.
- A number of disorders are thought to be related to excessive stress or inappropriate stress responses—allostatic overload. These are a result of the dysregulation and excessive use of the mechanisms and mediators involved in the stress response.

SUMMARY

Homeostasis is the state of balance of the body's biopsychosocial systems. Stressors evoke a stress response and initiate adaptive efforts, an allostatic process, designed to return to this steady-state. The response to stressors is affected by a wide variety of factors. Recently there has been an exponential increase in knowledge regarding the complex interactions of the HPA axis, the sympathetic nervous system, the immune system, and the chemical mediators of the stress response.

Excessive or prolonged stress and over- or underactivity of these chemical mediators produce disproportionate responses in the body, a condition of allostatic overload known as stress-induced illness. As humans strive to adapt to the constant changes of modern life, the study of stress and stress-related disease has become vital to public health and contributes to the development of increasingly sophisticated models of health and illness.

REFERENCES

1. Brame AL: Stressing the obvious? An allostatic look at critical illness, *Crit Care Med* 38:S600–S607, 2010.
2. Gross CG: Three before their time: neuroscientists whose ideas were ignored by their contemporaries, *Exp Brain Res* 192:321–334, 2009.
3. Cannon WB: *The wisdom of the body*, New York, 1932, W. W. Norton & Company.
4. Ganzel BL, Morris PA, Wethington E: Allostasis and the human brain: integrating models of stress from the social and life sciences, *Psychol Rev* 117:134–174, 2010.
5. Sapolsky RM: *Why zebras don't get ulcers*, ed 3, New York, 2004, Henry Holt.
6. Sterling P, Eyer J: Allostasis: a new paradigm to explain arousal pathology. In Fisher S, Reason J, editors: *Handbook of life stress, cognition, and health*, New York, 1988, John Wiley & Sons, pp 629–649.
7. McEwen BS, Wingfield JC: What is in a name? Integrating homeostasis, allostasis, and stress, *Horm Behav* 57:105–111, 2010.
8. McEwen BS, Gianaros PJ: Central role of the brain in stress and adaptation: links to socioeconomic status, health, and disease, *Ann NY Acad Sci* 1186:190–222, 2010.
9. McEwen BS, Gianaros PJ: Stress- and allostasis-induced brain plasticity, *Annu Rev Med* 62:431–445, 2011.
10. Romero LM, Dickens MJ, Cyr NE: The reactive scope model—a new model integrating homeostasis, allostasis, and stress, *Horm Behav* 55:375–389, 2009.
11. Selye H: *The stress of life*, New York, 1984, McGraw-Hill.
12. Goldstein DS: Adrenal responses to stress, *Cell Mol Neurobiol* 30:1433–1440, 2010.
13. Stewart JA: The detrimental effects of allostasis: allostatic load as a measure of cumulative stress, *J Physiol Anthropol* 25:133–145, 2006.
14. Groer M: Allostasis: a model for women's health. In Kendall-Tacket K, editor: *The psychoneuroimmunology of chronic disease*, Washington, DC, 2010, American Psychological Association, pp 183–218.
15. Brondolo E, ver Halen NB, Libby D, Pencille M: Racism as a psychosocial stressor. In Contrada RJ, Baum A, editors: *The handbook of stress science*, New York, 2011, Springer, pp 167–184.
16. Carter RT, Reynolds AL: Race-related stress, racial identity status attitudes, and emotional reactions of black Americans, *Cultur Divers Ethnic Minority Psychol* 17:156–162, 2011.
17. Greer TM: Coping strategies as moderators of the relationship between race- and gender-based discrimination and psychological symptoms for African American women, *J Black Psychol* 37:42–54, 2011.
18. Jackson JS, Knight KM, Rafferty JA: Race and unhealthy behaviors: chronic stress, the HPA axis, and physical and mental health disparities over the life course, *Am J Pub Health* 100:933–939, 2010.
19. Chandola T, Marmot MG: Socioeconomic status and stress. In Contrada RJ, Baum A, editors: *The handbook of stress science*, New York, 2011, Springer, pp 185–193.
20. Matthews KA, Gallo LC: Psychological perspectives on pathways linking socioeconomic status and physical health, *Annu Rev Psychol* 62:501–530, 2011.
21. Santiago CD, Wadsworth ME, Stump J: Socioeconomic status, neighborhood disadvantage, and poverty-related stress: prospective effects on psychological syndromes among diverse low-income families, *J Econ Psychol* 32:218–230, 2011.
22. Nicolson NA, Davis MC, Kruszewski D, Zautra AJ: Childhood maltreatment and diurnal cortisol patterns in women with chronic pain, *Psychosomat Med* 72:471–480, 2010.
23. Handwerger K: Differential patterns of HPA activity and reactivity in adult posttraumatic stress disorder and major depressive disorder, *Harvard Rev Psychiatry* 17:184–205, 2009.
24. Williams PG, Smith TW, Gunn HE, Uchino BN: Personality and stress: individual differences in exposure, reactivity, recovery, and restoration. In Contrada RJ, Baum A, editors: *The handbook of stress science*, New York, 2011, Springer, pp 231–245.
25. Bagley SL, Weaver TL, Buchanan TW: Sex differences in physiological and affective responses to stress in remitted depression, *Physiol Behav* 104:180–186, 2011.
26. Davis MC, Burleson MH, Kruszewski DM: Gender: its relationship to stressor exposure, cognitive appraisal/coping processes, stress responses, and health outcomes. In Contrada RJ, Baum A, editors: *The handbook of stress science*, New York, 2011, Springer, pp 247–254.
27. Frankenhaeuser M: The sympathetic-adrenal and the pituitary-adrenal response to challenge: comparison between the sexes. In Dembroski TM, Smidt TH, Blumchen G, editors: *Biobehavioral bases of coronary heart disease*, New York, 1983, Karger, pp 91–105.

28. Kajantie E, Phillips DI: The effects of sex and hormonal status on the physiological response to acute psychosocial stress, *Psychoneuroendocrinology* 31:151–178, 2006.

29. McCormick CM, Mathews IZ: HPA function in adolescence: role of sex hormones in its regulation and the enduring consequences of exposure to stressors, *Pharmacol Biochem Behav* 86:220–233, 2007.

30. McEwen BS: Interacting mediators of allostasis and allostatic load: towards an understanding of resilience in aging, *Metabolism* 52:10–16, 2003.

31. Wolkowitz OM, Epel ES, Reus VI, Mellon SH: Depression gets old fast: do stress and depression accelerate cell aging? *Depression Anxiety* 27:327–338, 2010.

32. Papathanassoglou ED, Giannakopoulou M, Mpouzika M, Bozas E, Karabinis A: Potential effects of stress in critical illness through the role of stress neuropeptides, *Nurs Crit Care* 15:204–216, 2010.

33. Dunser MW, Hasibeder WR: Sympathetic overstimulation during critical illness: adverse effects of adrenergic stress, *J Intensive Care Med* 24: 293–316, 2009.

34. Einhauser W, Koch C, Carter OL: Pupil dilation betrays the timing of decisions, *Front Hum Neurosci* 4:1–9, 2010.

35. Gillespie CF, Phifer J, Bradley B, Ressler KJ: Risk and resilience: genetic and environmental influences on development of the stress response, *Depression Anxiety* 26:984–992, 2009.

36. Stewart JS, Janicki-Deverts D, Muldoon MF, Kamarck TW: Depressive symptoms moderate the influence of hostility on serum interleukin-6 and C-reactive protein, *Psychosomat Med* 70:197–204, 2008.

37. Machelska H: Targeting of opioid-producing leukocytes for pain control, *Neuropeptides* 41:355–363, 2007.

38. Davidson MW: *The endorphin collection*, Florida State University. Available at http://micro.magnet.fsu.edu/micro/gallery/endorphin/endorphins.html.

39. Kang D, Rice M, Park N, Turner-Henson A, Downs C: Stress and inflammation: a biobehavioral approach for nursing research, *West J Nurs Res* 32:730–760, 2010.

40. Dhabhar FS: A hassle a day may keep the pathogens away: the fight-or-flight stress response and the augmentation of immune function, *Integr Comp Biol* 49:215–236, 2009.

41. Shenefelt PD: Relaxation strategies for patients during dermatologic surgery, *J Drugs Dermatol* 9:795–799, 2010.

42. Taylor SE, Master SL: Social responses to stress: the tend-and-befriend model. In Contrada RJ, Baum A, editors: *The handbook of stress science*, New York, 2011, Springer, pp 101–109.

43. Molitch ME: Anterior pituitary. In Goldman L, Schafer AI, editors: *Goldman's Cecil medicine*, ed 24, Philadelphia, 2012, Elsevier, pp 1431–1444.

44. McEwen BS: Stressed or stressed out: what is the difference? *J Psychiatry Neurosci* 30:316–318, 2005.

45. Brooks L, McCabe P, Schneiderman N: Stress and cardiometabolic syndrome. In Contrada RJ, Baum A, editors: *The handbook of stress science*, New York, 2011, Springer, pp 399–409.

46. McEwen B: Mood disorders and allostatic load, *Biol Psychiatry* 54: 200–207, 2003.

47. Van Houdenhove B, Luyten P: Stress, depression and fibromyalgia, *Acta Neurol Belg* 106:149–156, 2006.

48. Pucak ML, Carroll KA, Kerr DA, Kaplin AL: Neuropsychiatric manifestations of depression in multiple sclerosis: neuroinflammatory, neuroendocrine, and neurotrophic mechanisms in the pathogenesis of immune-mediated depression, *Dialog Clin Neurosci* 9:125–139, 2007.

49. Strawn JR, Geracioti TD: Noradrenergic dysfunction and the psychopharmacology of posttraumatic stress disorder, *Depression Anxiety* 25:260–271, 2008.

50. Shad MU, Suris AM, North CS: Novel combination strategy to optimize treatment for PTSD, *Hum Psychopharmacol* 26:4–11, 2011.

51. Epel E, Daubenmier J, Moskowitz JT, Folkman S, Blackburn E: Can meditation slow rate of cellular aging? Cognitive stress, mindfulness, and telomeres, *Ann NY Acad Sci* 1172:34–53, 2009.

52. Jacobs TL, Epel ES, Lin J, Blackburn EH, Wolkowitz OM, et al: Intensive meditation training, immune cell telomerase activity, and psychological mediators, *Psychoneuroendocrinology* 36:664–681, 2011.

Cell Structure and Function

Jacquelyn L. Banasik

⊖volve WEBSITE

KEY QUESTIONS

- What are the major cellular structures and their functions?
- How do cells acquire and use energy?
- How are substances transported across the cell membrane?
- Why is it that some cells can produce action potentials and others cannot?
- How do cells in a multicellular organism communicate with one another?
- What are the normal mechanisms of cellular growth control?

CHAPTER OUTLINE

A basic principle of biology states that the cell is the fundamental unit of life. As more diseases are understood on the cellular and molecular levels, it appears that the cell is also the fundamental unit of disease. A knowledge explosion is currently occurring in the fields of cell and molecular biology, leading to a better understanding of human physiology and the cellular aspects of disease. Detailed knowledge of cellular dysfunction has led to the development of more specific and appropriate prevention and treatment modalities for many disease processes. Thus, an understanding of cellular mechanisms is essential for health care providers and fundamental to the discussions of pathophysiologic processes presented throughout the remainder of this text.

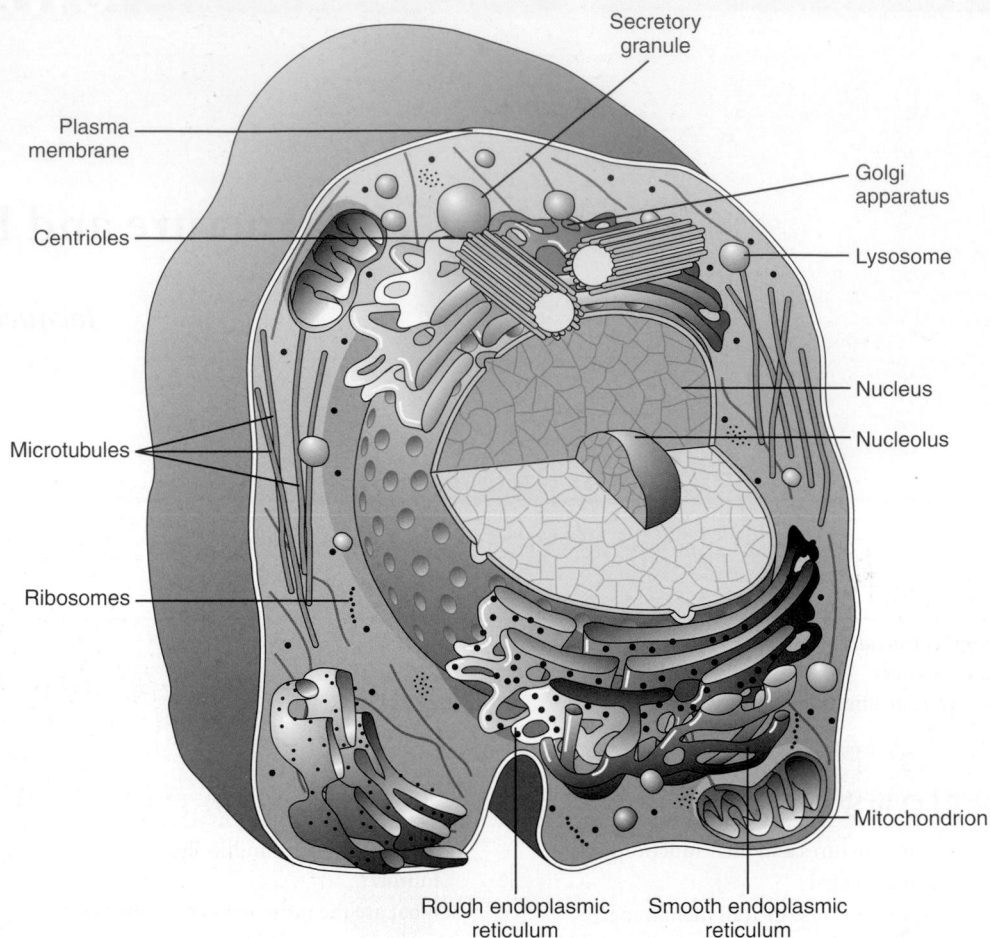

FIGURE 3-1 Structure of a typical eukaryotic cell showing intracellular organelles.

Cells are complex, membrane-bound units packed with a multitude of chemicals and macromolecules. They are able to replicate and thus form new cells and organisms. The very first cells on Earth probably arose from the spontaneous association of organic (carbon-containing) and inorganic molecules about 3.5 billion years ago.[1] Over billions of years, the self-replicating molecules now known as deoxyribonucleic acid (DNA) and ribonucleic acid (RNA) are believed to have evolved by chance association and natural selection. Development of the cell membrane created a closed compartment that provided a selective advantage for the cell and accomplished the first separation of life (inside) from nonlife (outside). In this protected environment, the early cells continued to evolve and develop. Today, a large number of different cell types exist, but many of the basic biochemical mechanisms of these cells are remarkably similar. Scientists believe that all modern cells, from bacteria to human neurons, evolved from common primordial cells.[2] It is therefore possible to unlock many of the secrets of human cellular physiology by studying easily grown and rapidly proliferating cells, such as yeasts and bacteria.

Much of our knowledge of cell physiology has derived from study of the class of cells known as prokaryotic, which includes bacteria and archaea. Prokaryotic cells are smaller and simpler than eukaryotic cells, having no defined nucleus or cytoplasmic organelles. Fungi, plants, and animals belong to the eukaryotic class of cells, which possess a membrane-bound nucleus and a host of cytoplasmic organelles (Figure 3-1). In this chapter, the essentials of eukaryotic cell structure, physiology, metabolism, and communication are reviewed.

PLASMA MEMBRANE

Membrane Structure

All cells are enclosed by a barrier composed primarily of lipid and protein called the plasma membrane (plasmalemma). This cell membrane is a highly selective filter that shields internal cell contents from the external environment. The plasma membrane performs a variety of functions, including transport of nutrients and waste products, generation of membrane potentials, and recognition, communication, and growth regulation of cells. The cell membrane is a sensor of signals and enables the cell to respond and adapt to changes in its environment.

According to the fluid mosaic model first described in the 1960s by Singer and Nicolson,[3] the plasma membrane is a dynamic assembly of lipid and protein molecules. Most of the lipids and proteins move about rapidly in the fluid structure of the membrane. As shown in Figure 3-2, the lipid molecules are arranged in a double layer, or **lipid bilayer,** which is highly impermeable to most water-soluble molecules, including ions, glucose, and proteins. A variety of proteins embedded or "dissolved" in the lipid bilayer perform most of the membrane's functions. Some membrane proteins are involved in the transport of specific molecules into and out of the cell; others function as enzymes or respond to external signals; and some serve as structural links that connect the plasma membrane to adjacent cells. The lipid structure of the plasma membrane is similar to the structure of the membrane that surrounds the cell's organelles (e.g., nucleus, mitochondria, endoplasmic reticulum, Golgi apparatus, lysosomes).

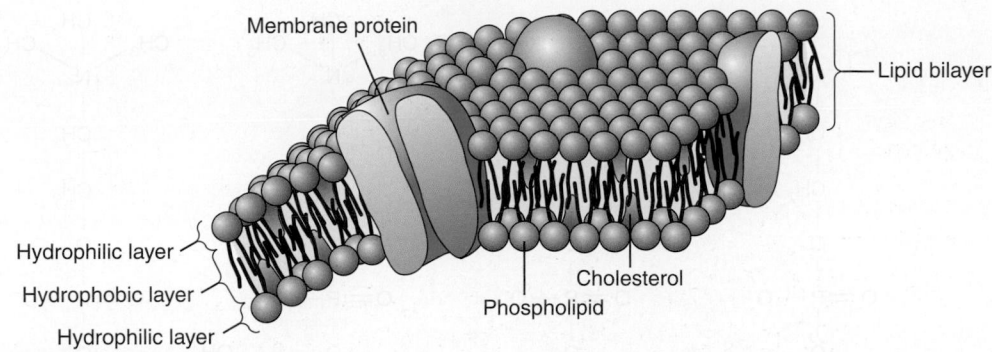

FIGURE 3-2 Section of the cell membrane showing the lipid bilayer structure and integral membrane proteins.

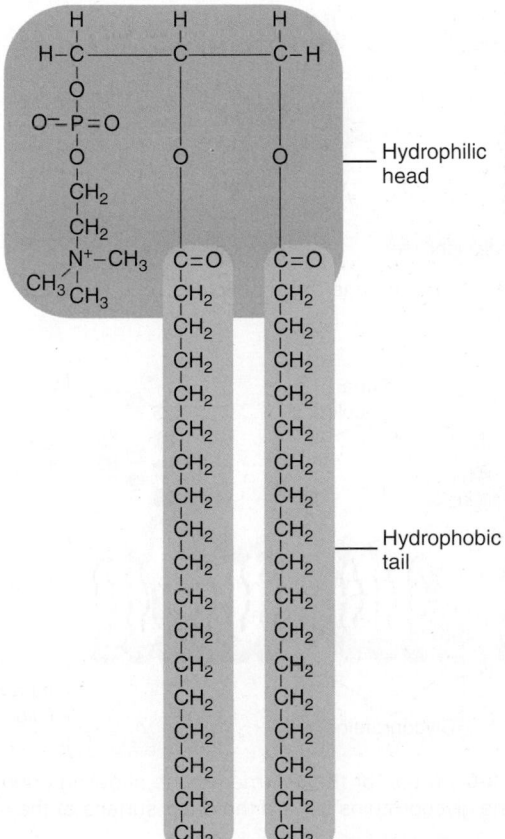

FIGURE 3-3 Schematic drawing of a typical membrane phospholipid molecule showing the amphipathic nature of the structure.

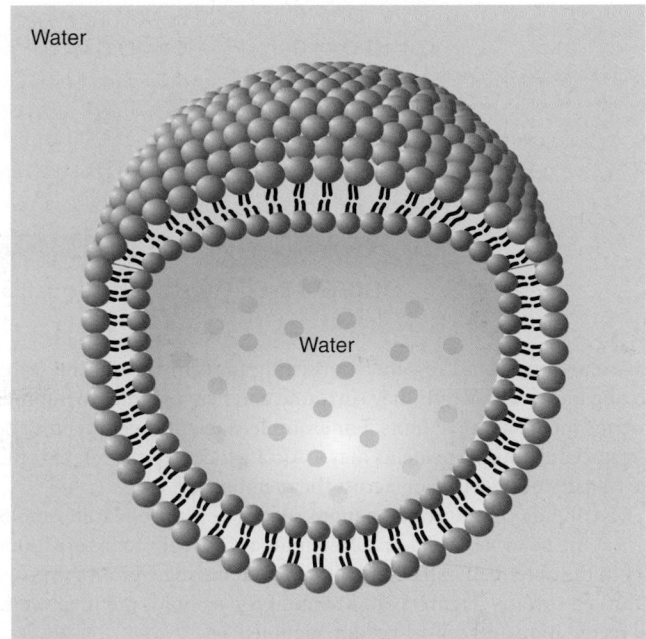

FIGURE 3-4 The amphipathic nature of membrane lipids results in bilayer structures that tend to form spheres.

Lipid Bilayer

The bilayer structure of all biological membranes is related to the special properties of lipid molecules that cause them to spontaneously assemble into bilayers. The three major types of membrane lipids are cholesterol, phospholipids, and glycolipids. All three have a molecular structure that is **amphipathic;** that is, they have a hydrophilic (water-loving) charged or polar end and a hydrophobic (water-fearing) non-polar end.[1] This amphipathic nature causes the lipids to form bilayers in aqueous solution. A typical phospholipid molecule is shown in Figure 3-3. The hydrophobic nonpolar tails tend to associate with other hydrophobic nonpolar tail groups to avoid association with polar water molecules. The hydrophilic polar head groups preferentially interact with the surrounding aqueous environment. A bilayer, with tails

sandwiched in the middle, allows both portions of the lipid molecules to be chemically "satisfied." In addition, the lipid bilayers tend to close on themselves, forming sealed, spherical compartments (Figure 3-4). If the membrane is punctured or torn, it will spontaneously reseal itself to eliminate contact of the hydrophobic tails with water.

For the most part, individual lipid and protein molecules can diffuse freely and rapidly within the plane of the bilayer. The degree of membrane fluidity depends on the lipid composition. Saturated lipids have straight tails that can pack together and tend to stiffen the membrane, whereas lipids with bent, unsaturated hydrocarbon tails tend to increase fluidity. About 50% of the lipid in eukaryotic cell membranes is cholesterol, which serves to decrease membrane permeability and prevent leakage of small water-soluble molecules. In addition to affecting fluidity by the degree of saturation of tail groups, the phospholipids that inhabit the membrane also differ in the size, shape, and charge of the polar head groups. Figure 3-5 shows the structures of the four most prevalent membrane phospholipids: phosphatidylethanolamine, phosphatidylserine, phosphatidylcholine, and sphingomyelin. Some membrane-bound proteins require specific phospholipid head groups to function properly. Some lipids—sphingolipids and cholesterol in

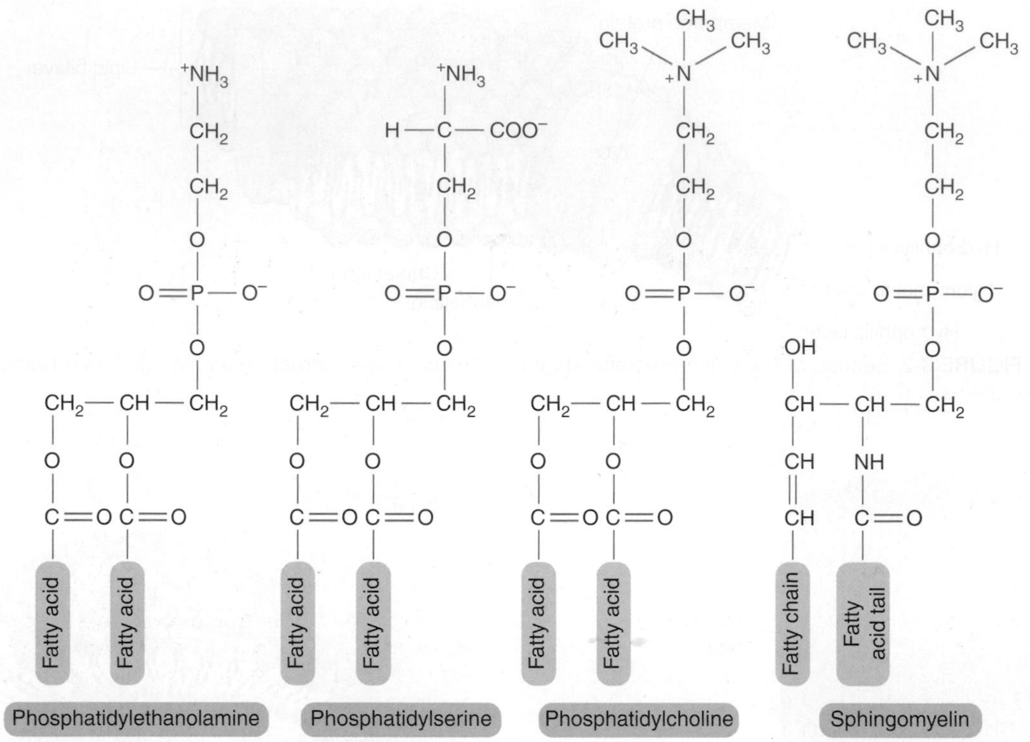

FIGURE 3-5 Chemical structures of the four most common membrane phospholipids.

Phosphatidylethanolamine Phosphatidylserine Phosphatidylcholine Sphingomyelin

particular—may bind together transiently to form rafts in the sea of moving lipids. These rafts may surround and help organize membrane proteins into functional units. For example, a membrane receptor and its intracellular target proteins may associate together in a raft to facilitate transfer of information across the membrane.[4]

Glycolipids contain one or more sugar (i.e., carbohydrate) molecules at the polar head region. Glycolipids and glycoproteins are found only in the outer half of the lipid bilayer, with the sugar groups exposed at the cell surface (Figure 3-6). Membrane glycolipids are involved in cell recognition and cell-to-cell interactions.[5]

Membrane Proteins

Approximately 50% of the mass of a typical cell membrane is composed of protein. The specific types of membrane proteins vary according to cell type and environmental conditions. Some membrane proteins, called *transmembrane proteins,* extend across the membrane bilayer and are in contact with both the extracellular and the intracellular fluids. Transmembrane proteins serve a variety of functions, including transport of charged and polar molecules into and out of cells and transduction of extracellular signals into intracellular messages. Other peripheral membrane proteins are less tightly anchored to the membrane. The common structural orientations of membrane proteins are shown in Figure 3-7. The amino acid structure of membrane proteins determines the way they are arranged in the membrane. Nonpolar amino acids tend to inhabit the hydrophobic middle of the membrane, whereas charged and polar amino acids protrude into the aqueous fluid or associate with polar lipid head groups. The three-dimensional structure of many membrane proteins is complex, with numerous twists and turns through the lipid bilayer.

The type of membrane proteins in a particular cell depends on the cell's primary functions. For example, a kidney tubule cell has a large proportion of transmembrane proteins, which are needed to perform the kidney's function of electrolyte and nutrient reabsorption. In

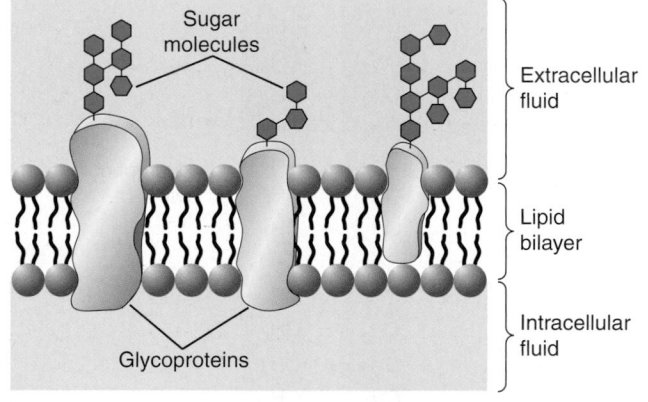

FIGURE 3-6 Portion of the cell membrane showing orientation of membrane glycoproteins toward the outer surface of the cell.

contrast, the human red blood cell (RBC) contains mainly peripheral proteins attached to the inner surface of the membrane.[6] One of these proteins, spectrin, has a long, thin, flexible rodlike shape that forms a supportive meshwork or **cytoskeleton** for the cell. It is this cytoskeleton that enables the RBC to withstand the membrane stress of being forced through small capillaries.

Although proteins and lipids are generally free to move within the plane of the cell membrane, many cells are able to confine certain proteins to specific areas. Using the example of the kidney tubule cell again, it is important for the cell to keep transport proteins on its luminal side to reabsorb filtered molecules (Figure 3-8). This segregation of particular proteins is accomplished primarily by intercellular connections called **tight junctions,** which connect neighboring cells and function like a fence to confine proteins to an area of the membrane. Membrane proteins also can be immobilized by tethering them to cytoskeleton or extracellular matrix structures.

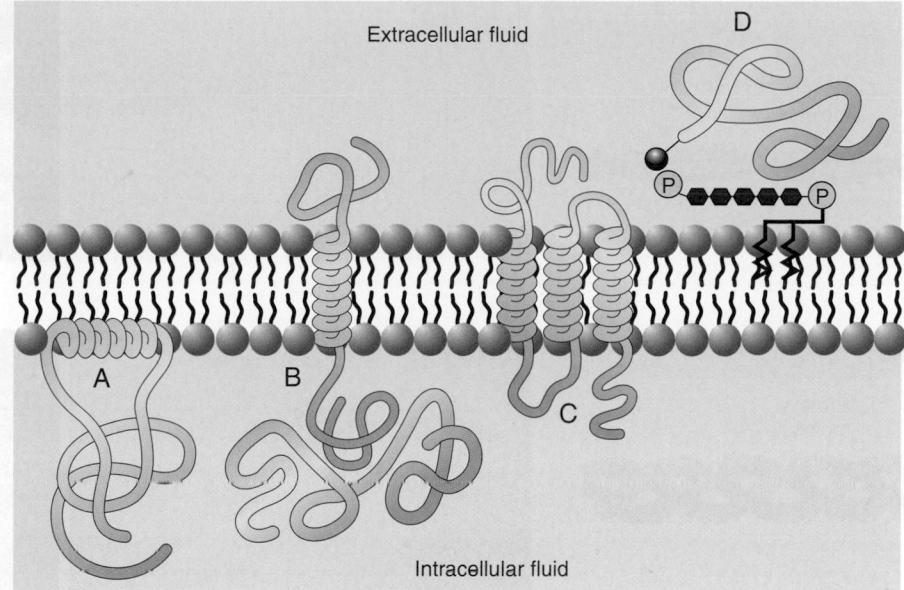

FIGURE 3-7 Structural orientation of some proteins in the cell membrane. **A,** Membrane-associated protein with noncovalent attachment to plasma lipids. **B,** Membrane protein with noncovalent attachment to another membrane protein. **C,** Transmembrane protein extending through the lipid bilayer. **D,** Covalently attached peripheral membrane protein.

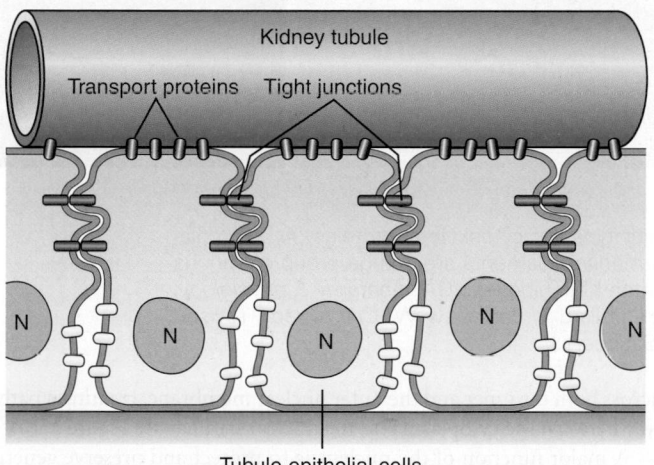

FIGURE 3-8 Transport proteins may be confined to a particular portion of the cell membrane by tight junctions. Segregation of transport proteins is important for the absorptive functions of the kidney epithelial cells. *N,* Nucleus.

KEY POINTS
- The plasma membrane is composed of a lipid bilayer that is impermeable to most water-soluble molecules, including ions, glucose, and amino acids, but permeable to lipid-soluble substances, such as oxygen and steroid hormones.
- Proteins embedded in the lipid bilayer execute most of the membrane's functions, including transport and signal transduction.

ORGANIZATION OF CELLULAR COMPARTMENTS

Cytoskeleton

Eukaryotic cells have a variety of internal compartments, or **organelles,** that are membrane bound and carry out distinct cellular functions. The cell's organelles are not free to float around haphazardly in the cytoplasmic soup; rather, they are elaborately organized by a protein network called the *cytoskeleton* (Figure 3-9).[7] The cytoskeleton maintains the cell's shape, allows cell movement, and directs the trafficking of substances within the cell. Three principal types of protein filaments make up the cytoskeleton: actin filaments, microtubules, and intermediate filaments.

All three types of filaments consist of small proteins that can assemble (polymerize) into filaments of varying length. The filament structures are dynamic and can be rapidly disassembled and reassembled according to the changing needs of the cell. Actin filaments play a pivotal role in cell movement. As one might expect, muscle cells are packed with actin filaments, which allows the cell to perform its primary function of contraction. However, nonmuscle cells also possess actin filaments that are important for complex movements of the cell membrane, such as cell crawling and phagocytosis. Such movements of the cell membrane are mediated by dense networks of actin filaments that cluster just beneath the plasma membrane and interact with specific proteins embedded in it. Actin and some of the other cytoskeletal proteins make specific contacts with and through the plasma membrane and are involved in information transfer from the extracellular environment to signaling cascades within the cell.

Organization of the cytoplasm and its organelles is achieved primarily by microtubules. In animal cells, microtubules originate at the cell center, or **centrosome,** near the nucleus and radiate out toward the cell perimeter in fine lacelike threads. Microtubules guide the orderly transport of organelles and vesicles in the cytoplasm as well as the equal distribution of chromosomes during cell division. Intermediate filaments, so named because their size is between that of microtubules and actin filaments, are strong, ropelike, fibrous proteins. A variety of intermediate filaments that differ from tissue to tissue have been identified. In addition to the three main groups of cytoskeletal filaments just described, a large number of accessory proteins are essential for cytoskeletal function. For example, the accessory protein myosin is needed to bind with actin to achieve motor functions. Different accessory proteins are present in different cell types.

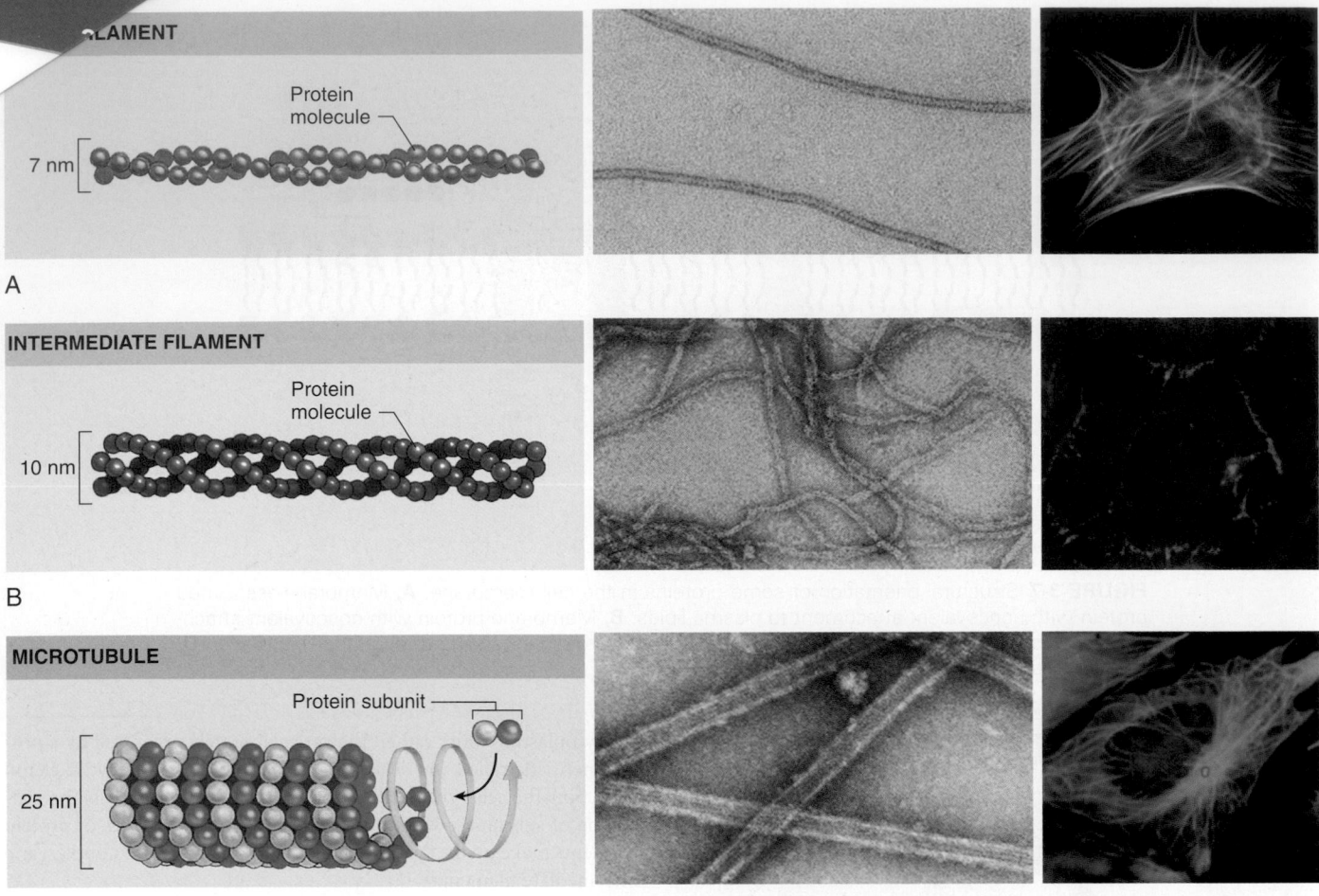

FIGURE 3-9 Schematic and micrographs of three major types of cytoskeletal proteins. **A,** Microfilaments shown are composed of actin proteins; **B,** intermediate filaments are a large group of various types of proteins; **C,** microtubules (see text). (From Patton KT, Thibodeau GA: *Anatomy & physiology,* ed 8, St. Louis, 2013, Mosby, p. 80. Micrographs from Pollard T, Earnshaw W: *Cell biology,* revised reprint, international edition, ed 1, Philadelphia, 2004, Saunders.)

Nucleus

The largest cytoplasmic organelle is the nucleus, which contains the genetic information for the cell in the form of DNA. The human genome contains approximately 23,000 genes that code for proteins, representing less than 1.3% of the total DNA structure composed of more than 6 billion base pairs.[8] The nuclear contents are enclosed and protected by the nuclear envelope, which consists of two concentric membranes. The inner membrane forms an unbroken sphere around the DNA and contains protein-binding sites that help to organize the chromosomes inside. The outer nuclear membrane is continuous with the endoplasmic reticulum (ER) (see next section) and closely resembles it in structure and function (Figure 3-10). The nucleus contains many proteins that help mediate its functions of genetic control and inheritance. These proteins, including histones, polymerases, and regulatory proteins, are manufactured in the cytosol and transported to the nucleus through holes in the membrane called *nuclear pores.* The nuclear pores are selective as to which molecules are allowed access to the nuclear compartment, and in this way they protect the genetic material from enzymes and other molecules in the cytoplasm. The nuclear pores also mediate the export of products such as RNA and ribosomes that are synthesized in the nucleus but function in the cytosol. Ribosomes are manufactured in a specialized portion of the nucleus called the *nucleolus.* Nuclear pores are complexes of proteins that span

across both the inner and the outer nuclear membrane, creating a pathway between the cytoplasm and the nuclear lamina (see Figure 3-10).

A major function of the nucleus is to protect and preserve genetic information so that it can be replicated exactly and passed on during cell division. However, the nucleus is continuously functioning even when the cell is not actively dividing. The nuclear DNA controls the production of cellular enzymes, membrane receptors, structural proteins, and other proteins that define the cell's type and behavior. (The structure and function of DNA are discussed in Chapter 5.)

During mitosis, the complex structure of the nuclear membrane and its pore-forming proteins breaks into small pieces that diffuse through the cell cytoplasm. After cell division is complete, pieces of nuclear membrane surround and gather the chromosomes and then fuse together to form a new nuclear membrane. Nuclear proteins and pore structures are then recruited back to their normal nuclear locations.[9]

Endoplasmic Reticulum

The ER is a membrane network that extends throughout the cytoplasm and is present in all eukaryotic cells (Figure 3-11). The ER is thought to have a single continuous membrane that separates the lumen of the ER from the cytosol—it could be likened to a "gastrointestinal tract" in the cell. The ER plays a central role in the synthesis of membrane components, including proteins and lipids, for the plasma membrane and

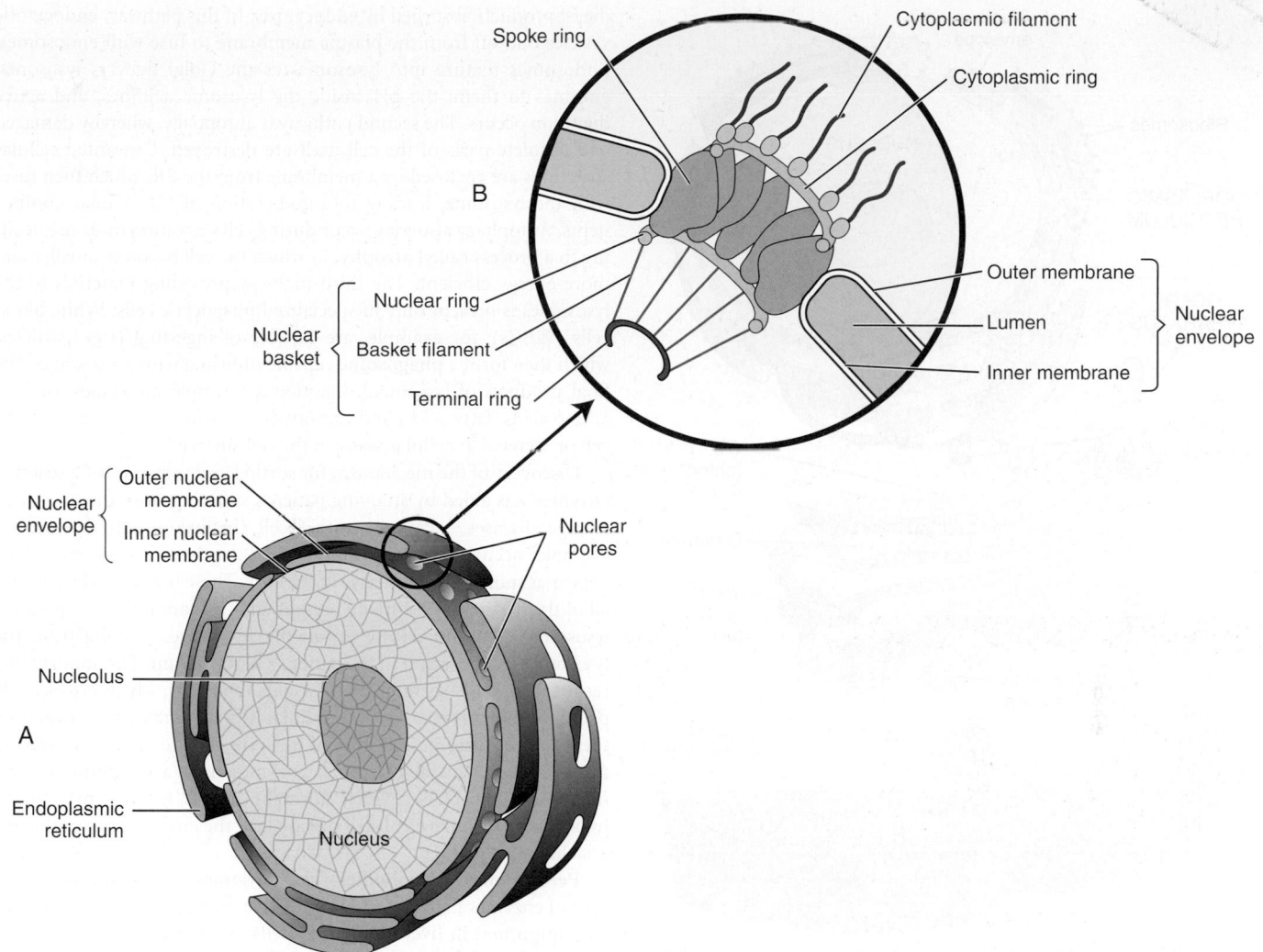

FIGURE 3-10 A, Structure of the double-membrane envelope that surrounds the cell nucleus. **B,** Detail of a nuclear pore.

cellular organelles, as well as in the synthesis of products to be secreted from the cell. The ER is divided into rough and smooth types based on its appearance under the electron microscope. The **rough ER** is coated with ribosomes along its outer surface. **Ribosomes** are complexes of protein and RNA that are formed in the nucleus and transported to the cytoplasm. Their primary function is the synthesis of proteins (see Chapter 5). Depending on the destination of the protein to be created, ribosomes may float free in the cytosol or may bind to the ER membrane. Proteins synthesized by free-floating ribosomes are released within the cytosol of the cell. Proteins to be transported into the ER have a special sequence of amino acids that directs the ribosome responsible for its synthesis to the ER membrane. Special proteins called signal recognition particles (SRPs) bind to the leading sequence of the protein and then bind to a receptor on the ER membrane. As the ribosome adds amino acids to the growing protein chain, it is pushed into the lumen of the ER through a pore in the ER membrane called a *translocon*.[10] After being processed in the ER and Golgi apparatus, the protein is eventually transported to the appropriate organelle or secreted at the cell surface. Free-floating and rough ER ribosomes are identical and interchangeable; their location depends on the amino acid structure of the protein they are producing at the time.[11]

Regions of ER that lack ribosomes are called **smooth** ER. The smooth ER is involved in lipid metabolism. Most cells have very little smooth ER, but cells specializing in the production of steroid hormones or lipoproteins may have significant amounts of smooth ER. For example, the hepatocyte (liver cell) has abundant smooth ER–containing enzymes (P450) responsible for the manufacture of lipoproteins as well as the detoxification of harmful lipid-soluble compounds, such as alcohol. The cellular smooth ER can double in surface area within a few days if large quantities of drugs or toxins enter the circulation. Cells in the adrenal cortex and gonads that produce steroid hormones also have abundant smooth ER. In addition to synthetic functions, the ER also sequesters large amounts of calcium ions by pumping them from the cytoplasm. In response to specific signals, the ER releases calcium ions as part of important second-messenger cascades. Muscle cells have extensive smooth ER (sarcoplasmic reticulum) dedicated to the sequestration of calcium. When the cell is stimulated, the sarcoplasmic reticulum releases the calcium ions needed to accomplish muscle contraction.

Golgi Apparatus

The **Golgi apparatus** or Golgi complex is composed of a stack of smooth membrane-bound compartments resembling a stack of hollow plates (see Figure 3-11). These compartments or *cisternae* are organized in a series of at least three processing compartments. The first compartment (*cis* face) lies next to the ER and receives newly

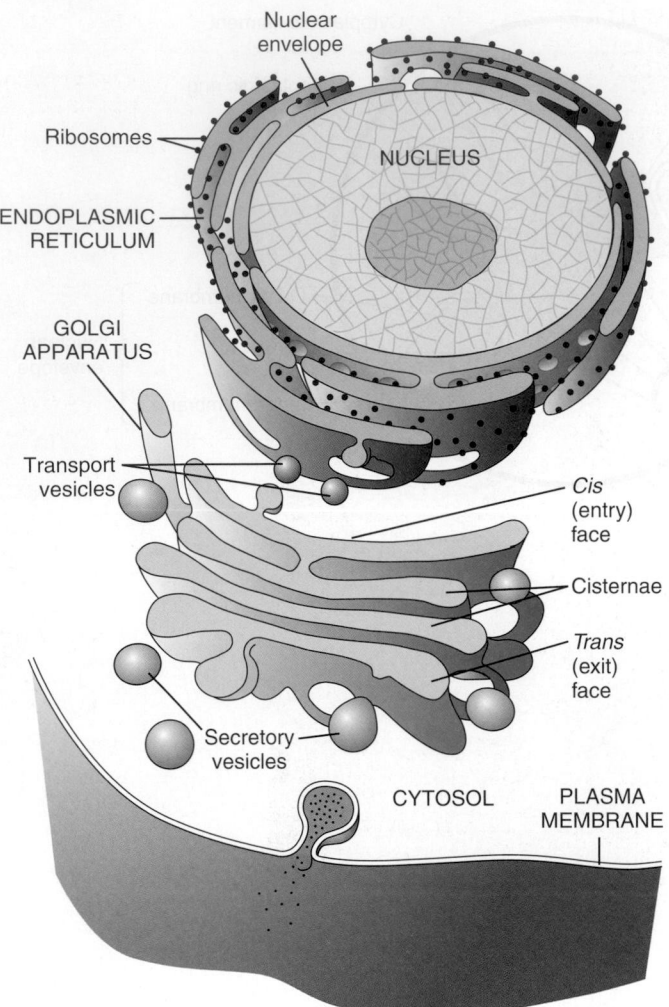

Nuclear envelope

Ribosomes

NUCLEUS

ENDOPLASMIC RETICULUM

GOLGI APPARATUS

Transport vesicles

Cis (entry) face

Cisternae

Trans (exit) face

Secretory vesicles

CYTOSOL   PLASMA MEMBRANE

FIGURE 3-11 Schematic drawing of the endoplasmic reticulum and its relationship to the Golgi apparatus and nuclear envelope.

synthesized proteins and lipids by way of ER transport vesicles. These transport vesicles are outgrowths that bud off from the ER membrane and diffuse to the Golgi, where they bind and become part of the Golgi apparatus membrane. The proteins and lipids then move through the middle compartment (medial) to the final compartment (*trans* face), where they depart for their final destination. As the lipid and protein molecules pass through the sequence of Golgi compartments, they are modified by enzymes that attach or rearrange carbohydrate molecules. After specific arrangement of these carbohydrates has occurred, the lipids and proteins are packaged into Golgi transport vesicles (secretory vesicles). The particular configuration of carbohydrate molecules on the lipid or protein is believed to serve as an "address label," directing them to the correct destination within the cell. Golgi vesicles transport their contents primarily to the plasma membrane and to lysosomes.

Lysosomes and Peroxisomes

Transport of Golgi vesicles to the membrane-bound bags of digestive enzymes known as **lysosomes** has been well described and provides a model for Golgi sorting and transport to other destinations. Lysosomes are filled with more than 40 different acid hydrolases, which are capable of digesting organic molecules, including proteins, nucleotides, fats, and carbohydrates.[12] Lysosomes obtain the materials they digest from three main pathways. The first is the pathway used to

digest products absorbed by endocytosis. In this pathway, endocytotic vesicles bud off from the plasma membrane to fuse with endosomes. Endosomes mature into lysosomes as the Golgi delivers lysosomal enzymes to them; the pH inside the lysosome acidifies, and active digestion occurs. The second pathway is autophagy, whereby damaged and obsolete parts of the cell itself are destroyed. Unwanted cellular structures are enclosed by a membrane from the ER, which then fuses with the lysosome, leading to autodigestion of the cellular components. Autophagy also may occur during cell starvation or disuse, leading to a process called **atrophy,** in which the cell becomes smaller and more energy efficient. The third pathway providing materials to the lysosomes is present only in specialized phagocytic cells. White blood cells (WBCs), for example, are capable of ingesting large particles, which then form a **phagosome** capable of fusing with a lysosome. The final products of lysosomal digestion are simple molecules, such as amino acids, fatty acids, and carbohydrates, which can be used by the cell or secreted as cellular waste at the cell surface.

Discovery of the mechanism for sorting and transport of lysosomal enzymes was aided by studying patients suffering from the lysosomal storage diseases.[13] Patients with I-cell (inclusion cell) disease, for example, accumulate large amounts of debris in lysosomes, which appear as spots or "inclusions" in the cells. These lysosomes lack nearly all of the hydrolases normally present and thus are unable to perform lysosomal digestion. However, all the hydrolases missing from the lysosomes can be found in the patient's bloodstream. The abnormality results from "mis-sorting" by the Golgi apparatus, which erroneously packages the enzymes for extracellular secretion rather than sending them to the lysosomes. Studies of this rare genetic disease resulted in the discovery that all lysosomal enzymes have a common marker, mannose-6-phosphate, which normally targets the enzymes to the lysosomes. Persons with I-cell disease lack the enzyme responsible for attaching this marker.

Peroxisomes (microbodies), like lysosomes, are membrane-bound bags of enzymes that perform degradative functions. They are particularly important in liver and kidney cells, where they detoxify various substances, such as alcohol. In contrast to lysosomes, which contain hydrolase enzymes, peroxisomes contain oxidative enzymes. These enzymes use molecular oxygen to break down organic substances by an oxidative reaction that produces hydrogen peroxide. The hydrogen peroxide is then used by another enzyme (catalase) to degrade other organic molecules, including formaldehyde and alcohol. Catalase also prevents accumulation of excess hydrogen peroxide in the cell by converting it to water and oxygen. Peroxisomes also oxidize fatty acids (β oxidation) to produce acetyl coenzyme A (acetyl CoA) that is used in cellular metabolism. Unlike lysosomes, which acquire their enzymes from Golgi vesicles, peroxisomes import enzymes directly from the cytoplasm.

Mitochondria

The **mitochondria** have been aptly called the "powerhouses of the cell" because they convert energy to forms that can be used to drive cellular reactions. A distinct feature of mitochondria is the large amount of membrane they contain. Each mitochondrion is bound by two specialized membranes. The inner membrane forms an enclosed space, called the *matrix,* which contains a concentrated mix of mitochondrial enzymes. The highly convoluted structure of the inner membrane with its numerous folds, called cristae (Figure 3-12), provides a large surface area for the important membrane-bound enzymes of the respiratory chain. These enzymes are essential to the process of oxidative phosphorylation, which generates most of the cell's **adenosine triphosphate (ATP).** The outer membrane contains numerous porin transport proteins forming large aqueous channels that make the membrane

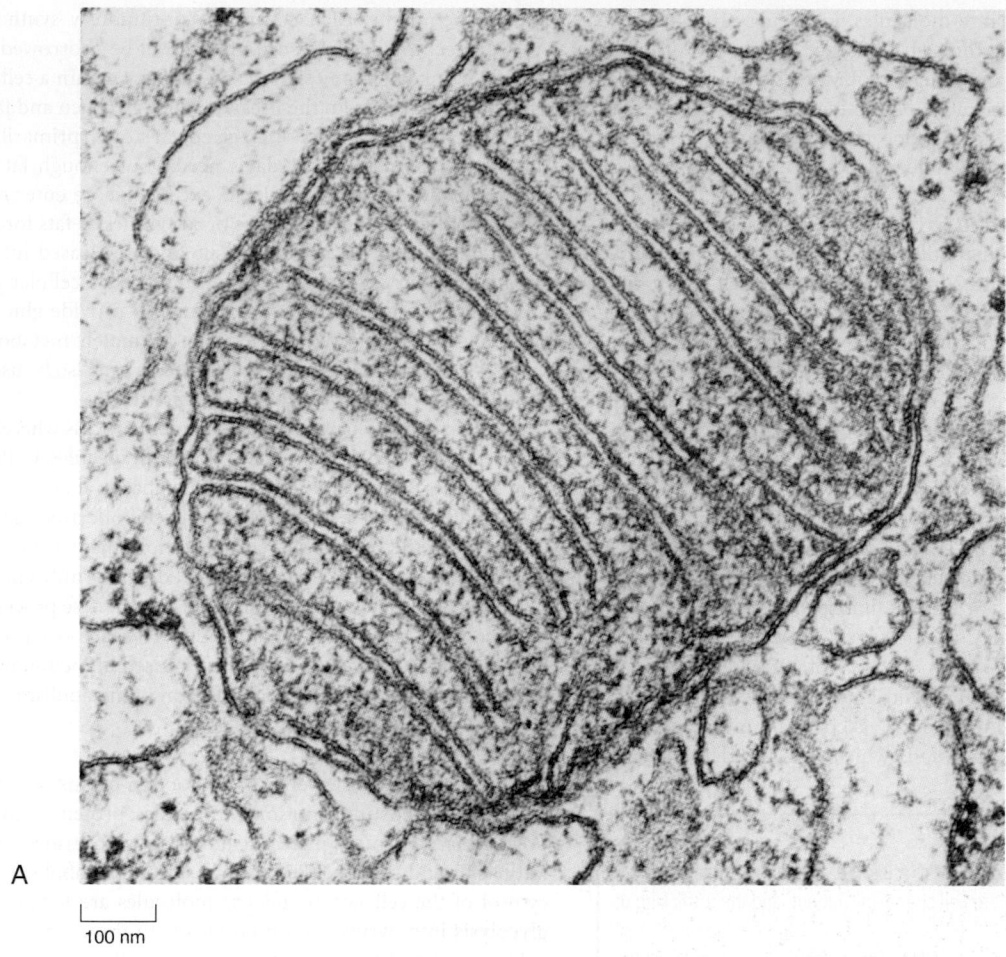

A

100 nm

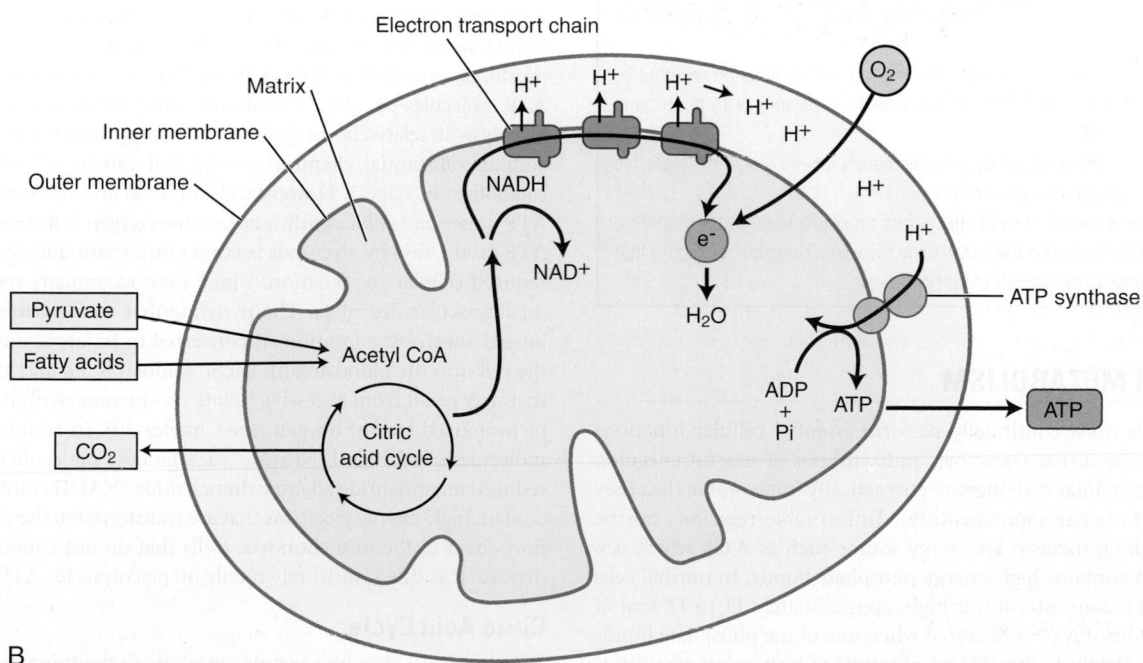

B

FIGURE 3-12 Electron micrograph **(A)** and schematic drawing **(B)** of the mitochondrial structure. The highly convoluted inner membrane provides a large surface area for membrane-bound metabolic enzymes. (**A,** From Alberts B et al, editors: *Molecular biology of the cell,* ed 5, New York, 2008, Garland Science, p 28. Micrograph courtesy Daniel S. Friend. All rights reserved. Used under license from The American Society for Cell Biology.)

porous like a sieve. Fairly large molecules, including proteins up to 5000 daltons, can pass freely through the outer membrane such that the space between the outer and inner membranes is chemically similar to the cytosol. However, the inner membrane is quite impermeable, even to small molecules and ions. Specific protein transporters are required to shuttle the necessary molecules across the inner mitochondrial membrane.

Mitochondria are believed to have originated as bacteria that were engulfed by larger cells but that still retain some of their own DNA. Mitochondrial DNA codes for 22 transfer RNA molecules, 2 ribosomal RNAs that form mitochondrial ribosomes, and 13 proteins.[14-16] During evolution the majority of mitochondrial genes were transferred to locations within the nuclear genome. Thus only a few of the mitochondrial enzymes are produced from DNA located in the mitochondria; the majority are transcribed from nuclear DNA. Nuclear genes are translated into protein in the cytoplasm and then transported to the mitochondria, whereas mitochondrial gene–derived proteins are made within the mitochondria. There are several rare disorders associated with mitochondrial gene defects (see Chapter 6). The number and location of mitochondria differ according to cell type and function. Cells with high energy needs, such as cardiac or skeletal muscle, have many mitochondria. These mitochondria may pack between adjacent muscle fibrils, such that ATP is delivered directly to the areas of unusually high energy consumption. The details of mitochondrial energy conversion are discussed in the next section. Mitochondria also have an important role in programmed cell death, called *apoptosis*, which is discussed in Chapter 4.

KEY POINTS
- The cytoskeleton is made up of actin, microtubules, and intermediate filaments. These proteins regulate cell shape, movement, and the trafficking of intracellular molecules.
- The nucleus contains the genomic DNA. These nuclear genes code for the synthesis of proteins. There are about 23,000 protein-coding genes in the human genome.
- The endoplasmic reticulum and the Golgi apparatus function together to synthesize proteins and lipids for transport to lysosomes or to the plasma membrane.
- Lysosomes and peroxisomes are membrane-bound bags of digestive enzymes that degrade intracellular debris.
- Mitochondria contain enzymes necessary for oxidative phosphorylation to produce ATP. Mitochondria have their own small number of genes that code for some of the mitochondrial proteins.

CELLULAR METABOLISM

All living cells must continually perform essential cellular functions such as movement, ion transport, and synthesis of macromolecules. Many of these cellular activities are energetically unfavorable (i.e., they are unlikely to occur spontaneously). Unfavorable reactions can be driven by linking them to an energy source such as ATP, which is a molecule that contains high-energy phosphate bonds. In normal cells where the ATP concentration is high, approximately 11 to 13 kcal of energy per mole of ATP is liberated when one of the phosphate bonds is hydrolyzed (broken with the aid of water) in a chemical reaction.[15] Enzymes throughout the cell are able to capture the energy released from ATP hydrolysis and use it to break or make other chemical bonds. In this way, ATP serves as the "energy currency" of the cell. A specific amount of ATP is "spent" to "buy" a specific amount of work. Most cells contain only a small amount of ATP, sufficient to maintain cellular activities for just a few minutes. Because ATP cannot cross the plasma membrane, each cell must continuously synthesize its own ATP to meet its energy needs; ATP cannot be "borrowed" from other cells or "banked" in any significant quantity within a cell. ATP is synthesized primarily from the breakdown of glycogen and fat.

An average adult has enough glycogen stores (primarily in liver and muscle) to supply about 1 day's needs, but enough fat to last for a month or more. After a meal, the excess glucose entering the cells is used to replenish glycogen stores or to synthesize fats for later use. Fat is stored primarily in adipose tissue and is released into the bloodstream for other cells to use when needed. When cellular glucose levels fall, glycogen and fats are broken down to provide glucose and fatty acyl molecules, respectively, which are ultimately metabolized to provide ATP. During starvation, body proteins can also be used for energy production by a process called *gluconeogenesis*.

Cellular metabolism is the biochemical process whereby foodstuffs are used to provide cellular energy and biomolecules. Cellular metabolism includes two separate and opposite phases: anabolism and catabolism. **Anabolism** refers to *energy-using* metabolic processes or pathways that result in the synthesis of complex molecules such as fats. **Catabolism** refers to the *energy-releasing* breakdown of nutrient sources such as glucose to provide ATP to the cell. Both of these processes require a long, complex series of enzymatic steps. The catabolic processes of cellular energy production are briefly discussed in the following sections. (See Chapter 42 for a detailed discussion of metabolism.)

Glycolysis

The catabolic process of energy production begins with the intestinal digestion of foodstuffs into small molecules: proteins into amino acids, polysaccharides into simple sugars (monosaccharides), and fats into fatty acids and glycerol. The second stage of catabolism occurs in the cytosol of the cell, where glucose molecules are further degraded by **glycolysis** into pyruvate (compounds with three carbon atoms). Glycolysis involves 10 enzymatic steps to break the 6-carbon glucose molecule into a pair of 3-carbon pyruvate molecules (Figure 3-13).[15] Glycolysis requires the use of two ATP molecules in the early stages but produces four ATP molecules in the later steps, for a net gain of two ATP molecules per glucose molecule. The production of ATP through glycolysis is relatively inefficient, and the pyruvate end products still contain substantial chemical energy that can be released by further catabolism in stage 3. However, glycolysis is an important provider of ATP under *anaerobic* conditions because oxygen is not required. Thus, ATP production by glycolysis becomes important during conditions of reduced cellular oxygenation, which may accompany respiratory and cardiovascular disorders. The pyruvate that accumulates during prolonged anaerobic conditions is converted to lactate and excreted from the cell into the bloodstream. Lactic acidosis is a dangerous condition that may result from excessive lactate production attributable to severe or prolonged lack of oxygen (see Chapter 20). In addition to the two molecules of ATP and pyruvate, each glucose molecule produces two reduced nicotinamide adenine dinucleotide (NADH) molecules, which contain high-energy electrons that are transferred to the electron transport chain in the mitochondria. Cells that do not contain mitochondria, such as RBCs, must rely totally on glycolysis for ATP production.

Citric Acid Cycle

For most cells, glycolysis is only a prelude to the third stage of catabolism, which takes place in the mitochondria and results in the complete oxidation of glucose to its final end products, CO_2 and H_2O. The third stage begins with the citric acid cycle (also called the Krebs cycle or the tricarboxylic acid cycle) and ends with the production of ATP by oxidative phosphorylation.[15] The purpose of the citric acid cycle is to break, by oxidation, the C-C and C-H bonds of the compounds produced in

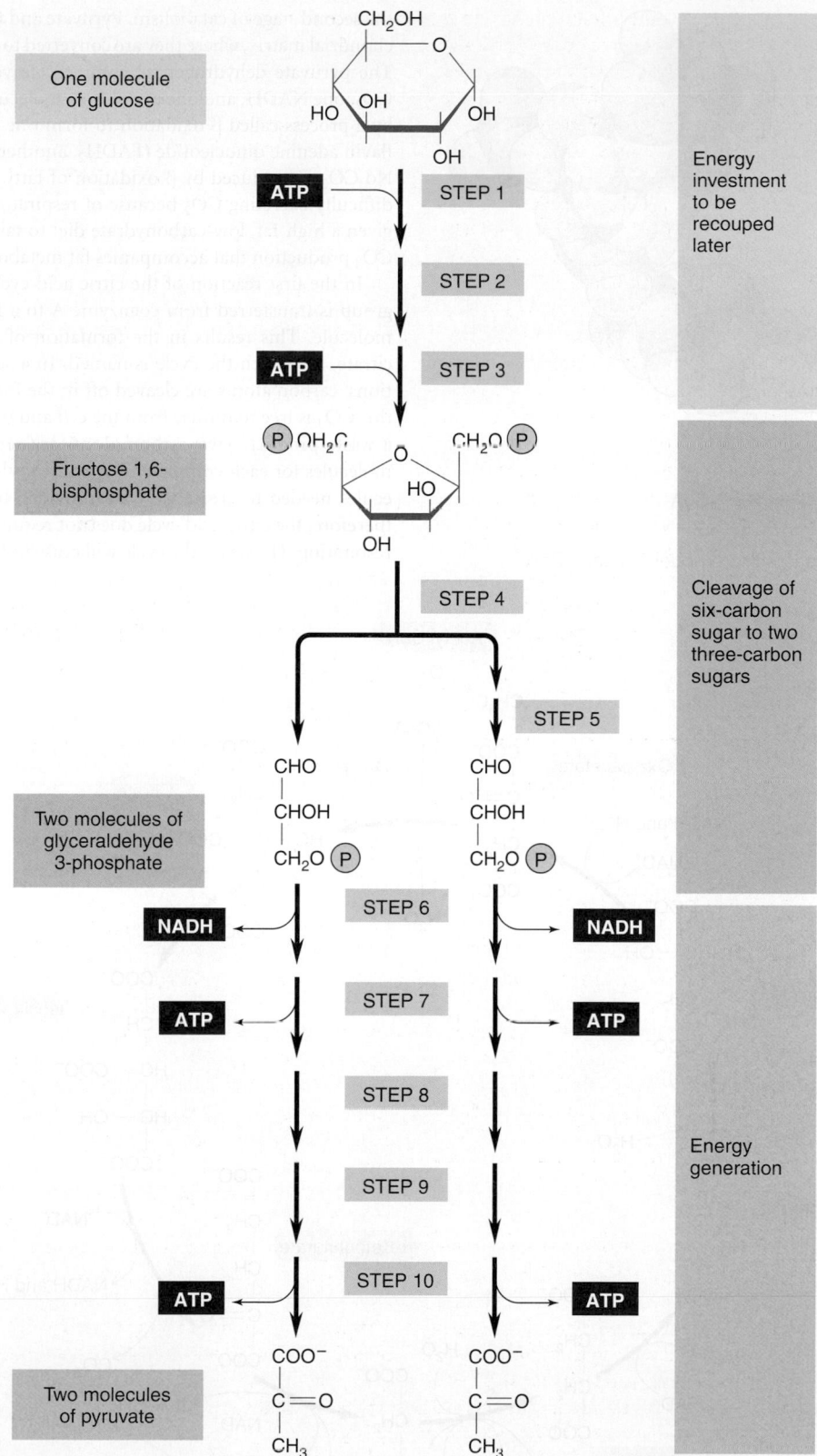

One molecule of glucose

ATP — STEP 1

Energy investment to be recouped later

STEP 2

ATP — STEP 3

Fructose 1,6-bisphosphate

STEP 4

Cleavage of six-carbon sugar to two three-carbon sugars

STEP 5

Two molecules of glyceraldehyde 3-phosphate

NADH — STEP 6 — NADH

ATP — STEP 7 — ATP

STEP 8

Energy generation

STEP 9

ATP — STEP 10 — ATP

Two molecules of pyruvate

FIGURE 3-13 Ten enzymatic steps are required in glycolysis to break glucose into two three-carbon pyruvate molecules. A net gain of two ATP molecules is achieved. (Copyright 2008 from *Molecular biology of the cell* by Alberts et al. Reproduced by permission of Garland Science/Taylor & Francis, LCC.)

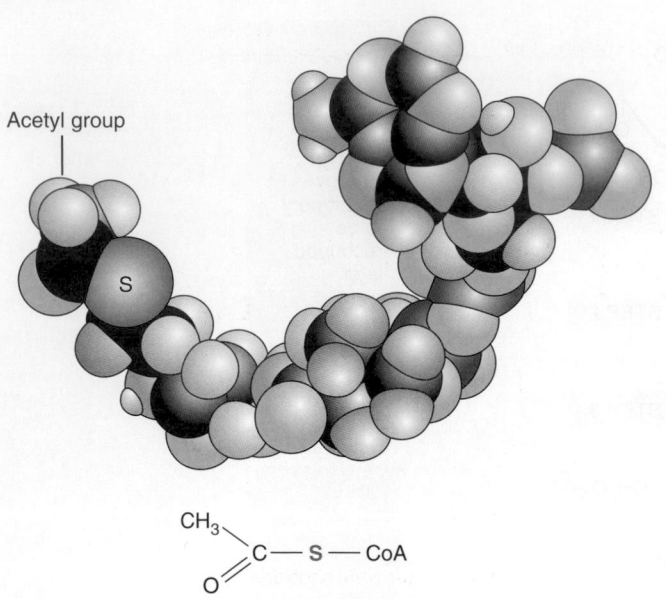

Acetyl group

$$CH_3\!-\!\underset{O}{\overset{\|}{C}}\!-\!S\!-\!CoA$$

FIGURE 3-14 Space-filling model of acetyl CoA.

the second stage of catabolism. Pyruvate and fatty acids enter the mitochondrial matrix, where they are converted to acetyl CoA (Figure 3-14). The pyruvate dehydrogenase complex cleaves pyruvate to form one CO_2, one NADH, and one acetyl CoA molecule. Fatty acids are cleaved by a process called β oxidation to form one NADH and one reduced flavin adenine dinucleotide ($FADH_2$, another type of electron carrier). No CO_2 is produced by β oxidation of fatty acids. Patients who have difficulty excreting CO_2 because of respiratory disease are sometimes given a high-fat, low-carbohydrate diet to take advantage of the lower CO_2 production that accompanies fat metabolism.

In the first reaction of the citric acid cycle, the two-carbon acetyl group is transferred from coenzyme A to a four-carbon oxaloacetate molecule. This results in the formation of the six-carbon molecule citrate, for which the cycle is named. In a series of enzymatic oxidations, carbon atoms are cleaved off in the form of CO_2 (Figure 3-15); this CO_2 is free to diffuse from the cell and be excreted by the lungs as a waste product. Two carbon atoms are removed to form two CO_2 molecules for each complete turn of the cycle. The extra oxygen molecules needed to create CO_2 are provided by the surrounding H_2O; therefore, the citric acid cycle does not require molecular oxygen from respiration. However, the cycle will cease to function in the absence of

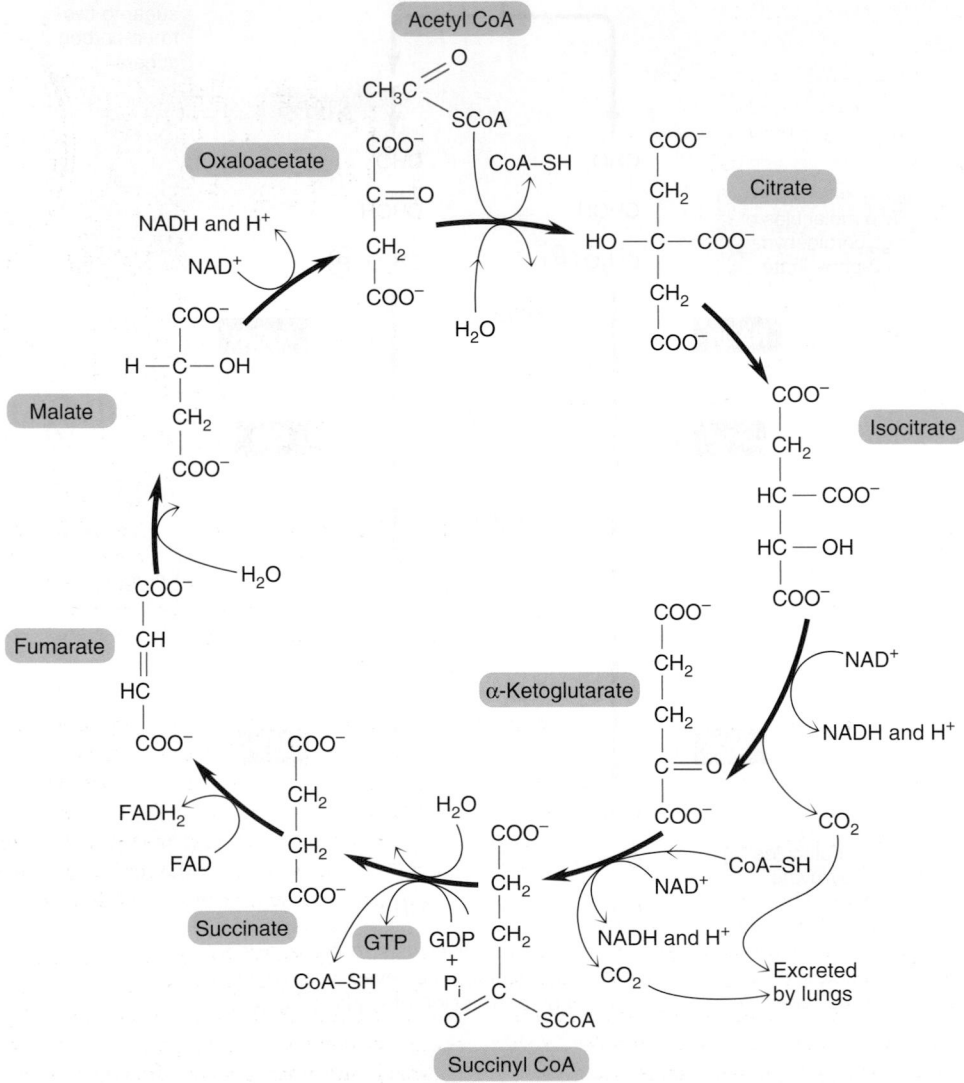

FIGURE 3-15 Chemical structures of the compounds of the citric acid cycle (Krebs cycle). In a series of enzymatic reactions, carbon atoms are cleaved to form CO_2 and high-energy hydride ions, which are carried by FAD and NAD.

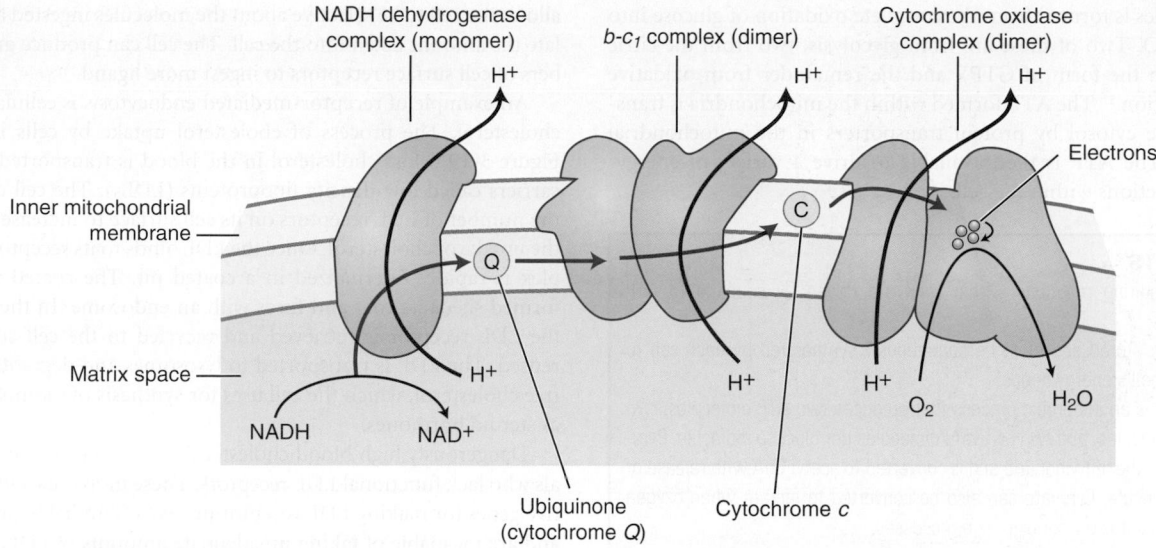

FIGURE 3-16 Representation of the electron transport chain located in the inner mitochondrial membrane. High-energy electrons are passed along the chain until they combine with oxygen to form water. The energy released at each electron transfer is used to pump H+ across the membrane.

oxygen because the carrier molecules, NADH and FADH$_2$, cannot unload their electrons onto the electron transport chain (which does require oxygen) and thus are unavailable to accept electrons from the citric acid cycle.

Although the citric acid cycle directly produces only one ATP molecule (in the form of guanosine triphosphate [GTP]) per cycle, it captures a great deal of energy in the form of activated hydride ions (H$^-$). These high-energy ions combine with larger carrier molecules, which transport them to the electron transport chain in the mitochondrial membrane. Two important carrier molecules are nicotinamide adenine dinucleotide (NAD$^+$), which becomes NADH when reduced by H$^-$, and flavin adenine dinucleotide (FAD), which becomes FADH$_2$ when reduced by H$^-$. The energy carried by these molecules is ultimately used to produce ATP through a process called *oxidative phosphorylation*. One glucose molecule provides for two turns of the cycle and produces a net of two GTP, four CO$_2$, two FADH$_2$ and six NADH.[14]

Oxidative Phosphorylation

Oxidative phosphorylation follows the processes of glycolysis and the citric acid cycle and results in the formation of ATP by the reaction adenosine diphosphate (ADP) and inorganic phosphate (P$_i$): ADP + P$_i$ → ATP. The energy to drive this unfavorable reaction is provided by the high-energy hydride ions (H$^-$) derived from the citric acid cycle. This energy is not used to form ATP directly; a series of energy transfers through reduction-oxidation (redox) reactions is required.[14,15] In eukaryotic cells, this series of energy transfers occurs along the **electron transport chain** on the inner mitochondrial membrane. The transport chain consists of three major enzyme complexes and two mobile electron carriers that shuttle electrons between the protein complexes (Figure 3-16). Respiratory chain proteins contain metal ions (iron, copper) that facilitate the transfer of electrons. The hydrogen molecules and their associated electrons are transported to the electron transport chain by the carrier molecules NADH or FADH$_2$. The path of electron flow is NADH → NADH dehydrogenase complex → ubiquinone → b-c$_1$ complex → cytochrome c → cytochrome oxidase complex. With each redox reaction the electrons pass from one complex to the next and the free energy that is released is used to pump hydrogen ions (H$^+$) out of the mitochondrial matrix. Each redox reaction provides enough energy to pump four protons (H$^+$) across the membrane.[14] At the very

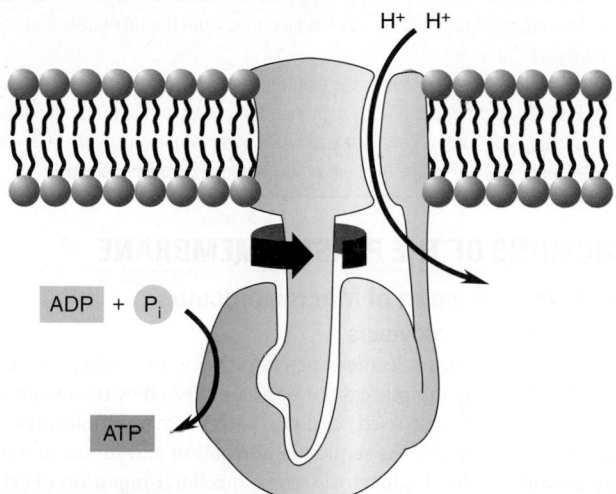

FIGURE 3-17 Inner mitochondrial ATP synthetase captures the potential energy of the H+ gradient in a manner similar to a turbine. The proton gradient drives the synthesis of ATP from adenosine diphosphate *(ADP)* and inorganic phosphate *(P$_i$)*. A 360-degree rotation of the rotor requires 12 H+ ions and produces 3 ATP molecules.

end of the transport chain, low-energy electrons are finally transferred to O$_2$ to form H$_2$O. Oxidative phosphorylation is called *aerobic* because of this oxygen-requiring step. The last enzyme in the chain, cytochrome oxidase, collects four electrons and then transfers all four at once to a molecule of O$_2$ to create two water molecules. If electrons are not transferred to oxygen in the correct ratio, then oxygen free radicals may be produced and damage the cell. Free radical generation is discussed in Chapter 4.

Thus far, little ATP synthesis has been accomplished. However, the enzymes of the transport chain have harnessed energy from the transported electrons in the form of a proton (H$^+$) gradient. Finally, the proton gradient is used to power the synthesis of ATP. A special enzyme in the inner mitochondrial membrane (ATP synthase) allows protons to flow back into the mitochondria down their electrochemical gradient. The energy of the proton flow is used to drive ATP synthesis (Figure 3-17). Under normal cellular conditions a total of about 30

ATP molecules is formed from the complete oxidation of glucose into CO_2 and H_2O. Two of these are from glycolysis, two from the citric acid cycle (in the form of GTP), and the remainder from oxidative phosphorylation.[15] The ATP formed within the mitochondria is transported to the cytosol by protein transporters in the mitochondrial membrane. The ATP is then available to drive a variety of energy-requiring reactions within the cell.

KEY POINTS
- Energy-requiring reactions within cells are driven by coupling to ATP hydrolysis.
- ATP is not stored and must be continuously synthesized by each cell to meet the cell's energy needs.
- Glycolysis is an anaerobic process that produces two ATP molecules, two NADH molecules, and two pyruvate molecules per glucose molecule. Pyruvate enters the mitochondria and is converted to acetyl CoA with release of a CO_2 molecule. Pyruvate can also be converted to lactate when oxygen supply is insufficient for oxidative processes.
- The citric acid cycle in the mitochondrial matrix oxidizes the acetyl groups supplied by acetyl CoA to form large quantities of H^- (hydride ions), which are carried to the respiratory chain by NADH and $FADH_2$.
- The respiratory chain enzymes capture the energy from electron transfer and use it to produce an H^+ (proton) gradient. Molecular oxygen is required at this stage (aerobic) to accept the electrons from the last enzyme in the transport chain.
- ATP is produced by ATP synthase, a protein in the mitochondrial membrane. ATP synthase produces ATP by capturing the energy of the proton gradient and using it to form a bond between ADP and inorganic phosphate (P_i). In total, about 30 ATP molecules are produced per glucose molecule.

FUNCTIONS OF THE PLASMA MEMBRANE

Membrane Transport of Macromolecules

Endocytosis and Exocytosis

The transport of large molecules, such as proteins and polysaccharides, across the plasma membrane cannot be accomplished by the membrane transport proteins discussed earlier. Rather, macromolecules are ingested and secreted by the sequential formation and fusion of membrane-bound vesicles. Endocytosis refers to cellular ingestion of extracellular molecules. The process of cellular secretion is called exocytosis. There are two types of endocytosis, which are differentiated by the size of the particles ingested. Pinocytosis, or "cellular drinking," is the method of ingesting fluids and small particles and is common to most cell types. Phagocytosis, or "cellular eating," involves the ingestion of large particles, such as microorganisms, and is practiced mainly by specialized phagocytic WBCs. Endocytosis begins at the cell surface by the formation of an indentation or "pit" in the plasma membrane, which is coated with special proteins, including clathrin (*coated pit*). The indentation invaginates and then pinches off a portion of the membrane to become a vesicle (Figure 3-18). Each vesicle thus formed is internalized, sheds its coat, and fuses with an endosome. The contents of these endocytic vesicles usually accumulate in lysosomes, where they are degraded.

Endocytosis of certain macromolecules is regulated by specific receptors on the cell surface. These receptors bind the molecules (ligands) to be ingested and then cluster together in coated pits. The receptor-ligand complexes are internalized by the invagination process described previously. The vesicles generally fuse with endosomes where the ligand is removed from the receptor for processing by the cell. The receptor may be degraded in the lysosome or may be recycled to the cell surface to be used again. Receptor-mediated endocytosis

allows the cell to be selective about the molecules ingested and to regulate the amount taken into the cell. The cell can produce greater numbers of cell surface receptors to ingest more ligand.

An example of receptor-mediated endocytosis is cellular uptake of cholesterol. The process of cholesterol uptake by cells is shown in Figure 3-19. Most cholesterol in the blood is transported by protein carriers called low-density lipoproteins (LDLs). The cell can regulate the number of LDL receptors on its cell surface to increase or decrease the uptake of cholesterol. Once the LDL binds to its receptor, this complex is rapidly internalized in a coated pit. The coated vesicle thus formed sheds its coat and fuses with an endosome. In the endosome, the LDL receptor is retrieved and recycled to the cell surface to be reused. The LDL is transported to lysosomes and degraded to release free cholesterol, which the cell uses for synthesis of biomolecules such as steroid hormones.

Dangerously high blood cholesterol levels occur in some individuals who lack functional LDL receptors. These individuals inherit defective genes for making LDL receptor proteins (familial hyperlipidemia) and are incapable of taking up adequate amounts of LDL. Accumulation of LDL in the blood predisposes these individuals to development of atherosclerosis and heart disease (see Chapter 18).

Exocytosis is essentially the reverse of endocytosis. Substances to be secreted from the cell are packaged in membrane-bound vesicles and travel to the inner surface of the plasma membrane. There the vesicle membrane fuses with the plasma membrane and the contents of the vesicle arrive at the cell surface. Some secreted molecules may remain embedded in the cell membrane, others may be incorporated into the extracellular matrix, and still others may enter the extracellular fluids and travel to distant sites. Many substances synthesized by the cell, including new membrane components, are constantly being packaged and secreted. This continuously operative and unregulated pathway is termed *constitutive*. In some specialized cells, selected proteins or small molecules are packaged in secretory vesicles, which remain in the cell until the cell is triggered to release them. These special secretory vesicles are typically regulated by stimulation of cell surface receptors. For example, the mast cell, a special type of WBC, releases large amounts of histamine when its cell surface receptors are activated (Chapter 9).

Membrane Transport of Small Molecules

All cells must internalize essential nutrients, excrete wastes, and regulate intracellular ion concentrations. However, the lipid bilayer is extremely impermeable to most polar and charged molecules. Transport of small water-soluble molecules is achieved by specialized transmembrane proteins called *transporter proteins*. Most membrane transporters are highly specific—a different transporter protein is required for each type of molecule to be transported. Only lipid-soluble molecules can permeate the lipid bilayer directly by simple diffusion.

Membrane transport proteins are of three basic kinds: ATP-driven pumps, carriers, and channel proteins. Channel proteins are the simplest of the three, forming a water-filled pore through the lipid bilayer. These pores are able to open and close to allow ions to pass through the membrane. The particular structure of the protein channel ensures that only ions of a certain size and charge can move through the membrane. Pumps and carrier proteins, however, bind to the solute to be transported and move it through the membrane by undergoing a structural, or conformational, change. Pumps and carriers have a transport maximum that is much lower than that of channels because they must bind to the molecules to be transported and then move them through the membrane. Pumps and carriers, which transport ions and nonelectrolyte molecules (e.g., glucose and amino acids), are also highly specific for the substances they transport.

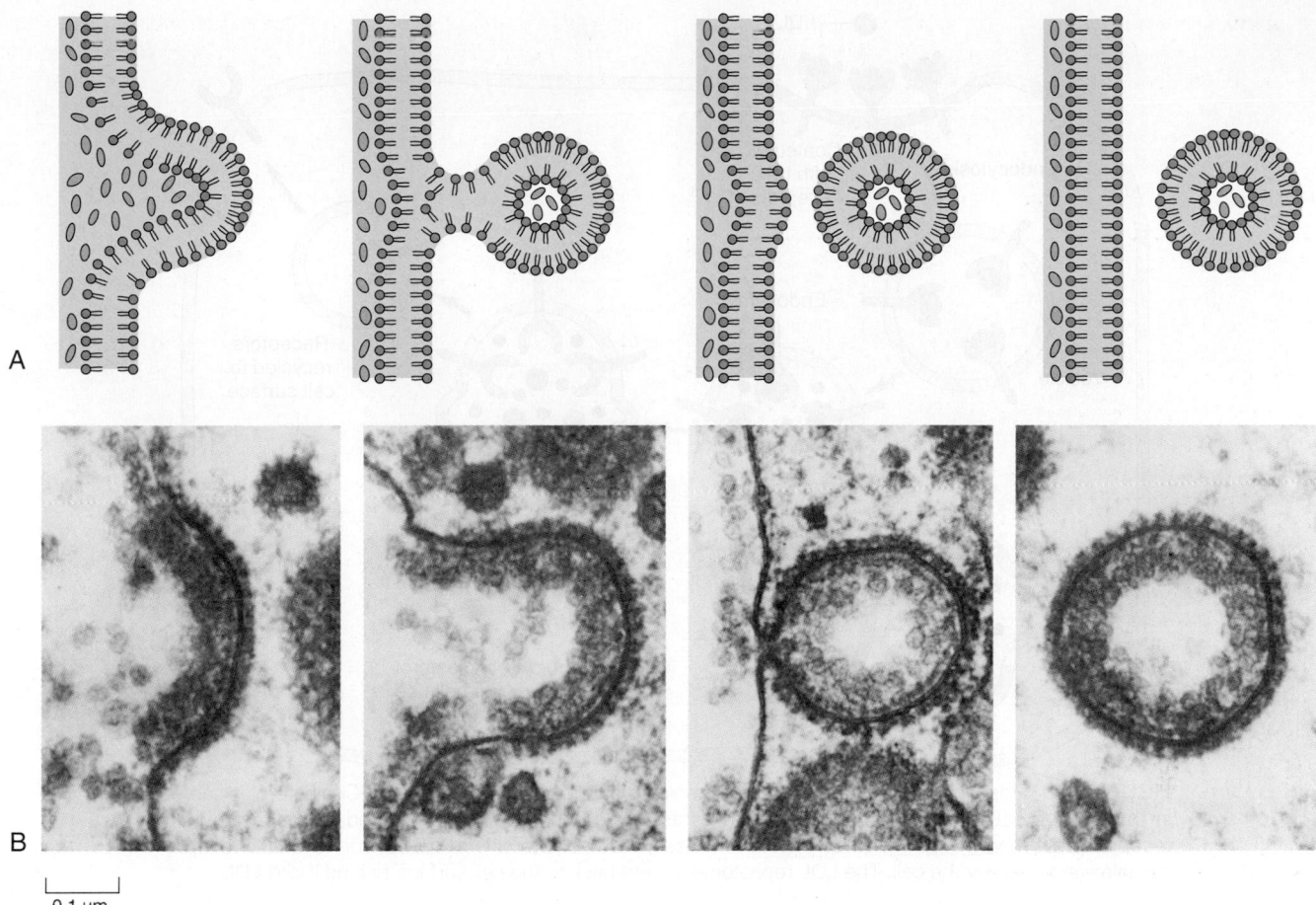

0.1 µm

FIGURE 3-18 A, Representation of the steps of endocytosis. An invagination of the membrane occurs and pinches off to form a vesicle. Exocytosis progresses in essentially the reverse sequence. **B,** Electron micrograph showing the steps of endocytosis. (**B,** From Perry M, Gilbert A: Yolk transport in the ovarian follicle of the hen *[Gallus domesticus]:* lipoprotein-like particles at the periphery of the oocyte in the rapid growth phase, *J Cell Sci* 39:257-272, 1979.)

Lipid-soluble particles can cross the lipid bilayer directly by simple diffusion through the hydrophobic lipid portion of the membrane. Polar or charged molecules must cross the membrane via protein channels or carriers. Transport through membrane proteins may be a passive or an active process. Passive transport through membrane proteins is called *facilitated diffusion.* Diffusion of ions occurs passively because of an **electrochemical gradient.** The electrochemical gradient exists because of differences in intracellular and extracellular charge and/or concentration of chemicals and is governed by laws of physics. Channel proteins only allow particles to move down their electrochemical or concentration gradients. Some carriers are passive, but others use the movement of one ion flowing down its concentration gradient (usually Na^+ moving into the cell) to move another substance uphill against its gradient.[17] This process is called *secondary active transport* because ATP is not used directly; however, ATP is necessary to run the pumps that maintain the sodium gradient. The lipid bilayer is quite impermeable to water because of its polar structure. Water moves across the plasma membrane through channels called *aquaporins.* Nearly all cells have aquaporins present in their cell membranes at all times, with the exception of a few specialized cells in the kidney tubules. Net movement of water across a membrane (osmosis) occurs in response to differences in osmotic pressure on either side of the membrane and is a passive process.

Active Transport Pumps

Active transport is the process whereby protein transport pumps move solutes across the membrane against an electrochemical or concentration gradient. Primary active transport requires metabolic energy, which is supplied by ATP hydrolysis. There are three families of ATP-driven pumps: the F-type ATPases that move H^+; the P-type adenosine triphosphatase (ATPase) that pump ions across membranes; and the ATP-binding cassette (ABC) transporters that transport a wide range of solutes. The ATP synthase located on the inner mitochondrial membrane is an example of an F-type pump; however, in that location it runs backward, allowing H^+ to run down its electrochemical gradient and using the energy to form a bond between ADP and P_i (see Figure 3-17). As a general principle, pumps, carriers, and channels can transport either direction depending on the concentration of substrate on either side of the membrane.

Sodium-potassium ion pump. The sodium-potassium (Na^+-K^+) pump is a P-type ATPase present in the plasma membranes of virtually all animal cells. It serves to maintain low sodium and high potassium concentrations in the cell. The Na^+-K^+ transporter must pump ions against a steep electrochemical gradient. Almost one third of the energy of a typical cell is consumed by the Na^+-K^+ pump. ATP hydrolysis provides the energy to drive the Na^+-K^+ transporter. The Na^+-K^+ pump behaves as an enzyme in its ability to split ATP to form ADP and P_i, leading to the protein being termed *Na^+-K^+ ATPase.*

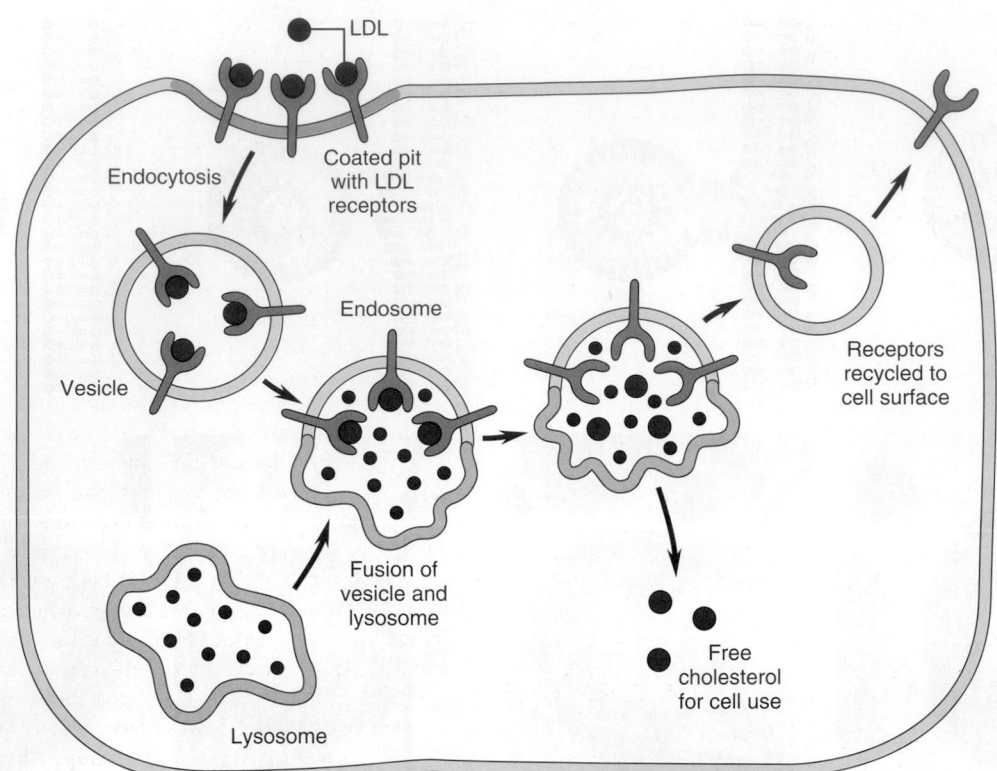

FIGURE 3-19 Steps in the process of receptor-mediated endocytosis of cholesterol. Cholesterol is carried in the blood by LDL. The uptake of LDL with its associated cholesterol is mediated by a specific LDL-receptor protein on the cell surface. Once internalized, the cholesterol is removed from the LDL-receptor complex and used by the cell. The LDL receptors are sent back to the cell surface to bind more LDL.

Transport of sodium and potassium ions through the Na^+-K^+ carrier protein is *coupled;* that is, the transfer of one ion must be accompanied by the simultaneous transport of the other ion. The transporter moves three sodium ions *out* of the cell for every two potassium ions moved *into* the cell (Figure 3-20). The Na^+-K^+ pump is important in maintaining cell volume. It controls the solute concentration inside the cell, which in turn affects the osmotic forces across the membrane. If Na^+ is allowed to accumulate within the cell, the cell will swell and could burst. The role of the Na^+-K^+ pump can be demonstrated by treating cells with digitalis, a drug that inhibits Na^+-K^+ ATPase. Cells thus treated will indeed swell and often rupture. The Na^+-K^+ pump is responsible for maintaining a steep concentration gradient for Na^+ across the plasma membrane. This gradient can be harnessed to transport small molecules across the membrane in a process called secondary active transport. Carriers that use ATP directly are engaged in primary active transport.

Membrane calcium transporters. Numerous important cellular processes, such as cell contraction and growth initiation, are dependent on the intracellular calcium ion concentration. Intracellular Ca^{2+} is normally very low and tightly regulated. Two important calcium pumps, present in the plasma membrane and in the endoplasmic reticulum (sarcoplasmic reticulum of muscle cells), function to remove Ca^{2+} from the cell cytoplasm. Similar to the Na^+-K^+ transporter, these transporters use ATP as the energy source (Figure 3-21).

If calcium ion levels in the cytoplasm become dangerously elevated, calcium pumps in the mitochondrial membrane are activated. Calcium ions are actively pumped into the mitochondria using the energy of the proton (H^+) gradient. This is the same proton gradient that the mitochondria use to synthesize ATP, and ATP production declines when the mitochondria are required to sequester Ca^{2+}. A high intracellular Ca^{2+} level is even more dangerous to the cell than a reduction in ATP production.

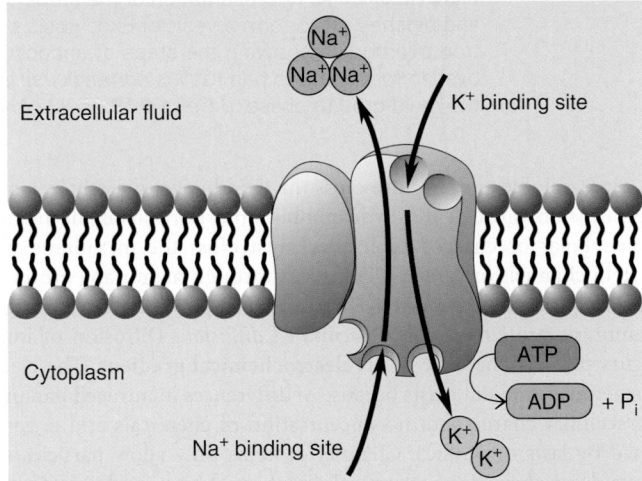

FIGURE 3-20 Schematic drawing of the sodium-potassium transport protein, which uses ATP to pump Na^+ out of the cell and K^+ into the cell against steep electrochemical gradients. This transporter is responsible for maintaining a low intracellular concentration of Na^+ and a large Na^+ gradient across the membrane. The energy of this Na^+ gradient can be harvested by other transporters to actively transport substances.

ABC transporters. Another important class of ATP-driven transporters is the ABC transporter family. These transporters all have a common ATP-binding domain, called the *ATP binding cassette* (ABC), which hydrolyzes ATP to provide energy for the transport process (Figure 3-22). This family of membrane transporters is the largest of the transporter families. A clinically important member of this family is a chloride channel in the plasma membrane of epithelial cells. A defect in this transporter is responsible for cystic fibrosis, a common genetic disorder that affects the lungs and pancreas (see Chapter 22). Bacteria use ABC transporters to pump antibiotics out of the cell, resulting in drug resistance (see Chapter 8).

Membrane Transport Carriers

Na⁺-driven carriers. In animal cells, the Na^+ gradient created by the Na^+-K^+ pump is used to power a variety of transporters by secondary active transport. An important Ca^{2+} transporter located in the plasma membrane of cardiac muscle cells uses the electrochemical gradient of Na^+ to power the transport of Ca^{2+} out of the cell (see Figure 3-21). The dependence of this calcium transporter on the sodium gradient helps

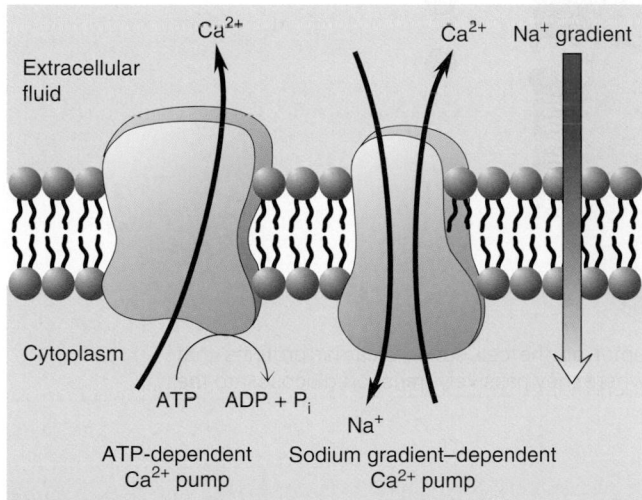

FIGURE 3-21 Two transporters of calcium ions are present in some cell membranes. One uses ATP as the energy source to pump calcium against a gradient (primary active transport). The other captures the potential energy of the sodium gradient to pump calcium out of the cell (secondary active transport).

explain the inotropic effects of the commonly prescribed drug digitalis. Digitalis is a cardiac glycoside that inhibits the Na^+-K^+ pump and allows the accumulation of intracellular Na^+. The Na^+ concentration gradient across the membrane is thus decreased, leading to less efficient calcium removal by the Na^+-dependent Ca^{2+} pump. A more forceful cardiac muscle contraction results from the increased intracellular Ca^{2+} concentration. Another example of a transporter that uses secondary active transport is the Na^+-H^+ exchange carrier, which uses the Na^+ gradient to pump out excess hydrogen ions to help maintain intracellular pH balance. The Na^+ gradient also can be used to bring substances into the cell. For example, glucose and amino acid transport into epithelial cells is coupled to Na^+ entry. As Na^+ moves through the transporter, down its electrochemical gradient, the sugar or amino acid is "dragged" along. Entry of the nutrient will not occur unless Na^+ also enters the cell. The epithelial cells that line the gut and kidney tubules have large numbers of these nutrient transporters present in the luminal (apical) surfaces of their cell membranes. In this way, large amounts of glucose and amino acids can be effectively absorbed. The reuptake of numerous types of neurotransmitters from synapses also occurs via Na^+-driven carrier proteins. The movement of Na^+ through carriers located in the presynaptic neuron drags the neurotransmitter from the synapse back into the nerve terminal, where it can be repackaged for reuse or metabolized by cellular enzymes.

Passive transport carriers. Some carriers are not linked to the Na^+ gradient and move substances across the membrane passively. The glucose transporters in many cell types belong to this class of transporters. In β cells of the pancreas, for example, the glucose transporters (Glut-1) are always present in the plasma membrane and let glucose into the cell according to its concentration in the extracellular fluid. In this way the pancreas detects blood glucose levels and releases an appropriate amount of insulin. In insulin-sensitive cells, such as muscle, liver, and adipose cells, the glucose carriers are sequestered inside the cell until insulin binds to its receptor at the cell surface. Receptor activation causes the glucose carriers (Glut-4) to move to the cell surface, where they allow passive influx of glucose (Figure 3-23).

Membrane Channel Proteins

In contrast to carrier proteins, which bind molecules and move them across the membrane by a conformational change, channel proteins

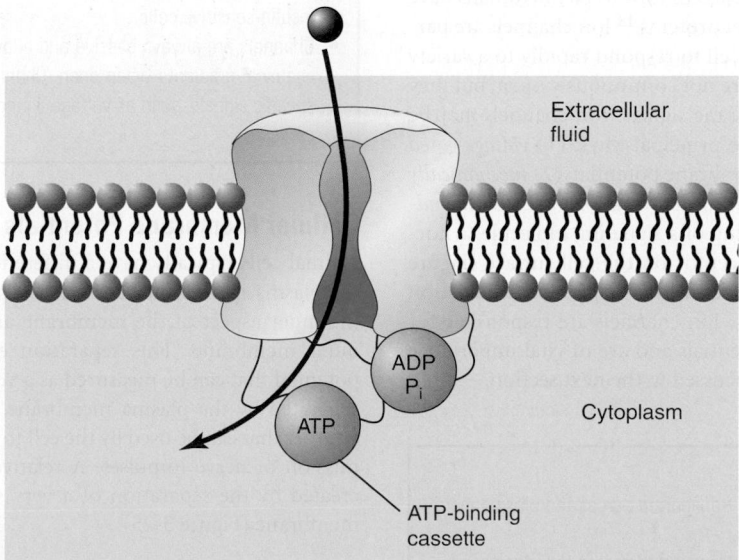

FIGURE 3-22 The ABC transporters are the largest known family of membrane transport proteins. They are characterized by an ATP-binding domain that causes a substrate pocket to be exposed first on one side of the membrane and then on the other as ATP is bound and hydrolyzed to ADP and P_i.

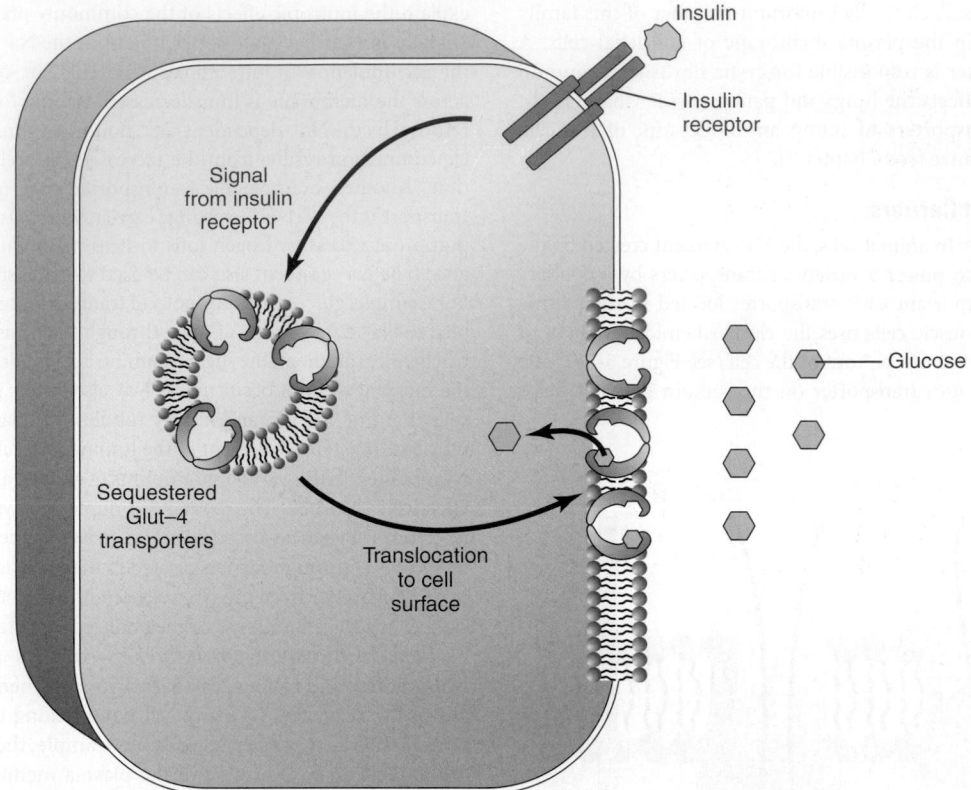

FIGURE 3-23 In response to insulin binding to its receptor on the cell surface, carrier proteins that transport glucose *(Glut-4)* are moved to the cell surface where they passively transport glucose into the cell (facilitated diffusion).

form water-filled pores in the membrane. Nearly all channel proteins are involved in transport of ions and may be referred to as ion channels. Ions can flow through the appropriate channel at very high rates (100 million ions/sec); this is much faster than carrier-mediated transport.[17] However, channels are not linked to an energy source, so ions must flow passively down an electrochemical gradient. The channel proteins in the plasma membranes of animal cells are highly selective, permitting only a particular ion or class of ions to pass. Humans have about 400 genes that encode channel proteins.[18] Ion channels are particularly important in allowing the cell to respond rapidly to a variety of external stimuli. Most channels are not continuously open, but they open and close according to membrane signals. Ion channels may be stimulated to open or close in three principal ways: (1) *voltage-gated* channels respond to a change in membrane potential; (2) *mechanically gated* channels respond to mechanical deformation; and (3) *ligand-gated* channels respond to the binding of a signaling molecule (a hormone or neurotransmitter) to a receptor on the cell surface (Figure 3-24). In addition, some channels open without apparent stimulation and are referred to as *leak* channels. Ion channels are responsible for the development of membrane potentials and are of vital importance in nerve and muscle function, as discussed in the next section.

KEY POINTS

- Large, lipid-insoluble molecules are transported across the plasma membrane by endocytosis and exocytosis.
- Small, lipid-insoluble molecules are transported across the plasma membrane by three kinds of membrane proteins: ATP-driven pumps, carriers, and channels.

- Pumps use the energy of ATP to move solutes against a gradient. Examples of ATP-driven active transport include proton pumps, Na^+-K^+ pumps, Ca^{2+} pumps, and ABC transporters.
- Carriers may be passive or use the Na^+ gradient for secondary active transport. Neurotransmitter reuptake carriers and those that transport glucose and amino acids across the gut and renal tubules are examples of Na^+-driven carriers. Passive carriers include those that allow glucose entry into insulin-sensitive cells.
- Channels are always passive and allow ions to move down their electrochemical gradients when open. Channels open and close in response to specific signals, such as voltage changes, ligand binding, and mechanical pressure.

Cellular Membrane Potentials

Animal cells typically have a difference in the electrical charge across the plasma membrane. There is a slight excess of negative ions along the inner aspect of the membrane and extra positive ions along the outer membrane. This separation of charges creates a membrane potential that can be measured as a voltage. Positive and negative ions separated by the plasma membrane have a strong attraction to one another that can be used by the cell to perform work, such as the transmission of nerve impulses. A relatively large membrane potential is created by the separation of a very small number of ions along the membrane (Figure 3-25).

Resting Membrane Potential

When there is no net ion movement across the plasma membrane, the electrical charge present inside the cell is called the *resting membrane*

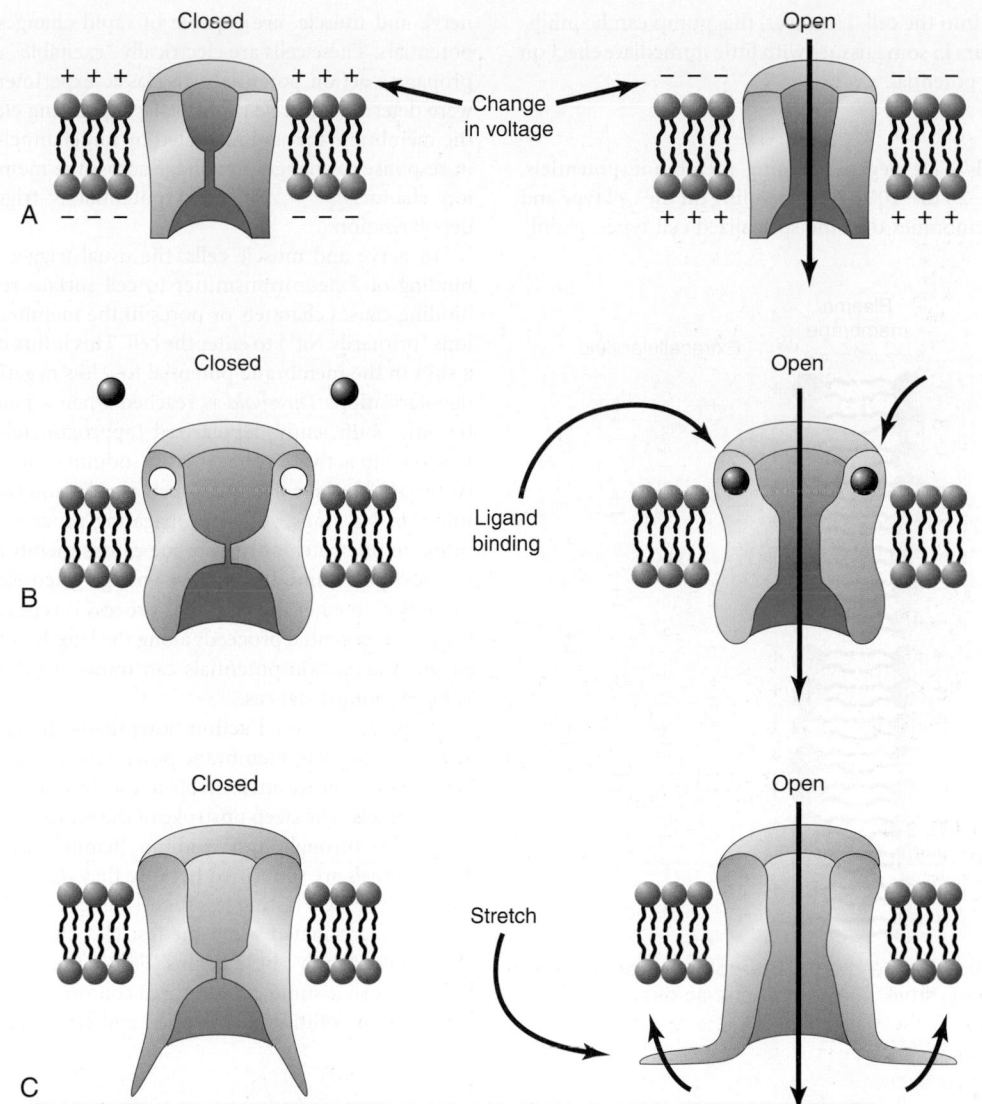

FIGURE 3-24 Gating of ion channels. **A,** Voltage-gated channel. **B,** Ligand-gated channel. **C,** Mechanically gated channel.

potential (RMP). The major determinant of the resting membrane potential is the difference in potassium ion concentration across the membrane.[17,19] The concentration of potassium inside the cell is much greater (about 30 times greater) than the extracellular potassium concentration. At rest, the membrane is permeable to K^+, but not to other positively charged cations, including Na^+ and Ca^{2+}. Potassium ions remain inside the cell because of the attraction of fixed intracellular anions (negatively charged organic molecules such as proteins and phosphates that cannot diffuse out of the cell). Because the cell membrane is impermeable to Na^+ and Ca^{2+}, only K^+ is available to balance these negative intracellular ions. Thus, two opposing forces are acting on the potassium ion. The negative cell interior attracts K^+ into the cell, whereas the huge K^+ concentration gradient favors movement of K^+ out of the cell. When the cell is at rest and not transmitting impulses these forces are balanced, and although the membrane is permeable to K^+ there is no net movement. The voltage required to exactly balance a given potassium concentration gradient can be calculated mathematically.*

The measured membrane potential is very close to that predicted mathematically and varies directly with changes in extracellular K^+ ion concentration. For example, a typical nerve cell has a normal resting potential of about -85 mV. If the extracellular K^+ level is increased, more K^+ ions will stay in the cell, owing to the reduced concentration gradient. These extra positive intracellular ions will neutralize more of the negative cellular anions, and the cell will *hypopolarize,* or become less negative. Conversely, if extracellular K^+ levels fall, more K^+ will exit the cell, owing to a greater concentration gradient. Fewer intracellular anions will be neutralized, and the cell interior will become more negative, or *hyperpolarized* (Figure 3-26). Changes in RMP can have profound effects on the ease of action potential generation in cardiac and nerve cells.

The RMP is described by the potassium equilibrium potential because the cell is relatively impermeable to other ions at rest. Under certain conditions, the membrane may become highly permeable to an ion other than potassium. The membrane potential will reflect the equilibrium potential of the most permeant ions.

Long-term maintenance of ion gradients across the cell membrane is accomplished primarily by the Na^+-K^+ pump. The Na^+-K^+ pump also contributes to the negative RMP in that it extrudes *three* Na^+ for

---

*The numeric value of the resting potential (*M*) can be calculated from the ratio of extracellular to intracellular K^+ concentration using the Nernst equation: M (in millivolts) = 61 log ($K^+_{outside} \div K^+_{inside}$).

every *two* K⁺ brought into the cell. However, this pump can be inhibited for minutes to hours in some tissues with little immediate effect on the resting membrane potential.

Action Potential

Nearly all animal cells have negative resting membrane potentials, which may vary from −20 to −200 mV, depending on the cell type and organism. The cell membranes of some specialized cell types, mainly nerve and muscle, are capable of rapid changes in their membrane potentials. These cells are electrically "excitable" and can generate and propagate action potentials. In classic experiments, action potentials were determined to be rapid, self-propagating electrical excitations of the membrane that are mediated by ion channels that open and close in response to changes in voltage across the membrane (voltage-gated ion channels).[20-24] An action potential is triggered by membrane depolarization.

In nerve and muscle cells, the usual trigger for depolarization is binding of a neurotransmitter to cell surface receptors. Transmitter binding causes channels or pores in the membrane to open, allowing ions (primarily Na⁺) to enter the cell. This influx of positive ions causes a shift in the membrane potential to a less negative value, resulting in depolarization. *Threshold* is reached when a patch of the membrane becomes sufficiently depolarized (approximately −65 mV in animal neurons) to activate voltage-gated sodium channels in the membrane. At threshold, these channels open rapidly and transiently to allow the influx of Na⁺ ions. A self-propagating process follows whereby Na⁺ influx in one patch of membrane causes membrane depolarization of the next patch and opens more voltage-gated Na⁺ channels, allowing more Na⁺ to enter the cell. This process is repeated many times while the action potential proceeds along the length of the cell (Figure 3-27). In this way, action potentials can transmit information rapidly over relatively long distances.

A typical neuronal action potential is shown in Figure 3-28. The various changes in membrane potential during the time course of the action potential are attributable to the flow of ions through membrane ion channels. The steep upstroke of the action potential corresponds to Na⁺ influx through "fast" sodium channels, as described previously. *Fast channels* are so termed because they open and close rapidly, with the entire process lasting less than 1 msec. This phase of rapid depolarization is terminated when the fast Na⁺ channels suddenly close and the repolarization phase begins. Fast Na⁺ channels are interesting in that they can assume at least three conformations (three-dimensional forms).[25] In addition to the open and closed conformations, the fast

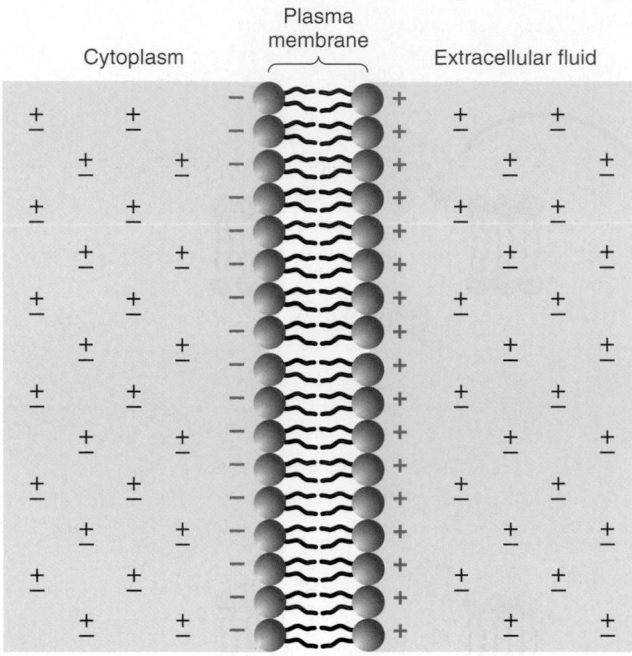

FIGURE 3-25 A relatively large membrane potential results from the separation of a very small number of ions across the plasma membrane.

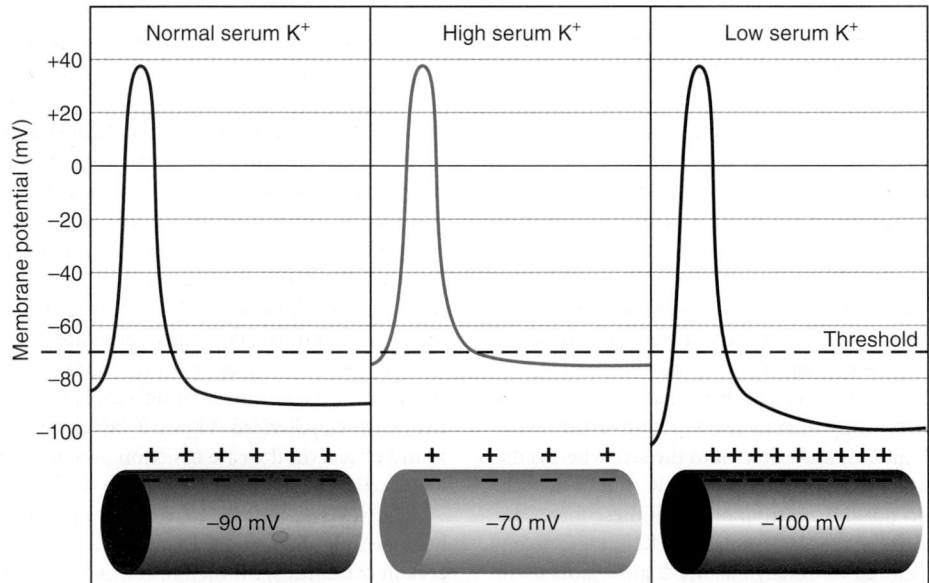

FIGURE 3-26 Effects of changes in extracellular K⁺ level on the resting membrane potential. A high level of serum K⁺ results in a hypopolarization of the membrane. A low serum K⁺ level results in membrane hyperpolarization. With high serum K⁺ levels, the resting membrane potential is closer to threshold, making it easier to achieve an action potential. A low serum K⁺ level moves the resting membrane potential away from threshold, making it more difficult to achieve an action potential.

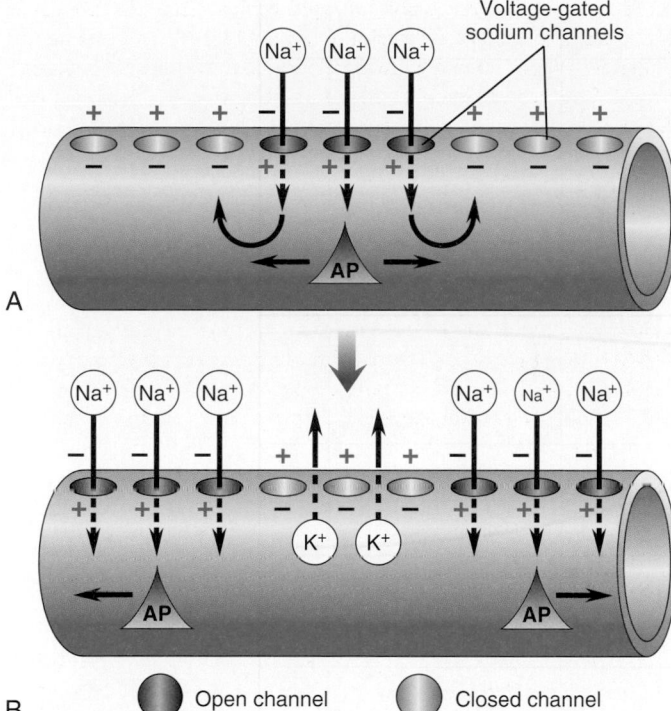

A

B   Open channel   Closed channel

FIGURE 3-27 The action potential *(AP)* in excitable cells is propagated along the membrane by the sequential opening of voltage-gated sodium channels in adjacent sections of membrane. **A,** An action potential is initiated by the opening of sodium channels in a section of membrane. **B,** The action potential is regenerated in adjacent sections of membrane as more sodium channels open. The initial segment repolarizes as sodium channels close and potassium ions move out of the cell.

Na^+ channel has a refractory form during which the channel will not reopen in response to another depolarizing stimulus (Figure 3-29). This refractory period limits the rate at which action potentials can be generated.

Two major factors contribute to cellular repolarization: sodium conductance (inflow) is stopped by closing Na^+ channels, as described previously, and K^+ conductance (outflow) through K^+ channels increases. Although cells are always permeable to K^+, during repolarization additional voltage-gated K^+ channels open allowing a higher rate of K^+ efflux. These K^+ channels respond to depolarization of the membrane in the same manner as fast Na^+ channels, but they take much longer to open and close. When K^+ channels open, K^+ flows out of the cell, owing to the concentration gradient and the loss of intracellular negativity that accompanies Na^+ influx. The outward flow of positive intracellular potassium ions helps to quickly return the membrane potential to its negative RMP value.

Action potentials in cardiac muscle cells are more complex than the neuronal ones just described. Recall that contraction depends on the presence of free intracellular calcium ions. Because Ca^{2+} carries a charge, its entry into the cell cytoplasm is reflected in the membrane potential. In skeletal muscle, most of the free cytosolic calcium ions come from intracellular stores (sarcoplasmic reticulum) that are released when the cell is depolarized. In cardiac muscle cells, Ca^{2+} entry through voltage-gated channels in the plasma membrane is also important. Calcium conductance into the cell tends to prolong the action potential, resulting in a plateau phase (Figure 3-30). This is of functional importance in cardiac tissue, because it allows time for muscular contraction before another impulse is conducted and

prevents the potentially disastrous condition of cardiac muscle tetany. (For a more thorough discussion of cardiac electrophysiology, see Chapter 17.)

KEY POINTS

- The negative value of the RMP is determined by the ratio of intracellular to extracellular K^+ ion concentration. Changes in serum K^+ concentration can have profound effects on the RMP.
- Cells with voltage-gated ion channels are excitable and can produce and conduct action potentials. An action potential results from the opening of "fast" Na^+ channels, which allows Na^+ to rush into the cell.
- Repolarization is caused by closure of Na^+ channels and efflux of K^+ from the cell. In cardiac muscle, repolarization is prolonged owing to Ca^{2+} influx through "slow" Ca^{2+} channels.

INTERCELLULAR COMMUNICATION AND GROWTH

Cell Signaling Strategies

Cells in multicellular organisms need to communicate with one another and respond to changes in the cellular environment. Coordination of growth, cell division, and the functions of various tissues and organ systems is accomplished by three principal means of communication: (1) through gap junctions that directly connect the cytoplasm of adjoining cells; (2) by direct cell-to-cell contact of plasma membranes or the extracellular molecules associated with the cell (extracellular matrix); and (3) by secretion of chemical mediators (ligands) that influence cells some distance away (Figure 3-31).[26]

Gap junctions are found in many tissues. They are connecting channels between adjacent cells that allow the passage of small molecules from one cell to the next. These junctions are formed by special transmembrane proteins called connexins that associate to form pores of about 1.5 nm in width. Small molecules, such as inorganic ions, glucose, amino acids, nucleotides, and vitamins, may pass through the pores, whereas macromolecules (e.g., proteins, polysaccharides, and nucleic acids) are too large to pass through pores. Gap junctions are particularly important in tissues in which synchronized functions are required, such as cardiac muscle contraction, vascular tone, and intestinal peristaltic movements. Gap junctions appear to be important in embryogenesis as well. Cellular differentiation may be mediated in part through chemical signaling through gap junctions. (See Chapter 5 for a discussion of the development and differentiation of tissue types.)

Direct contact of cell membrane receptors with signaling molecules present on the surface of other cells or extracellular matrix is an important means of local communication among cells in tissues. Contact-dependent signaling is particularly important for the development of the immune response. Such cell-to-cell contact during fetal development is thought to allow the cells of the immune system to discriminate between foreign and self tissues and to develop self-tolerance. If cell-to-cell contact does not occur during fetal life, the immune cells may later attack the body's own cells, leading to the development of autoimmune diseases. (See Chapter 10 for a discussion of autoimmunity.) There are four major families of cell adhesion molecules (CAMs): immunoglobulin-cell adhesion molecules (Ig-CAMs); cadherins; integrins; and selectins. These cell adhesion proteins make contacts between cells and with the extracellular matrix and provide signals that maintain cell survival and differentiated cell types (Figure 3-32).

The best understood form of cell communication is signaling through secreted molecules or *ligands*. Three strategies of intercellular chemical signaling have been described, relating to the distances over which they operate (Figure 3-33). *Synaptic* signaling is confined to the

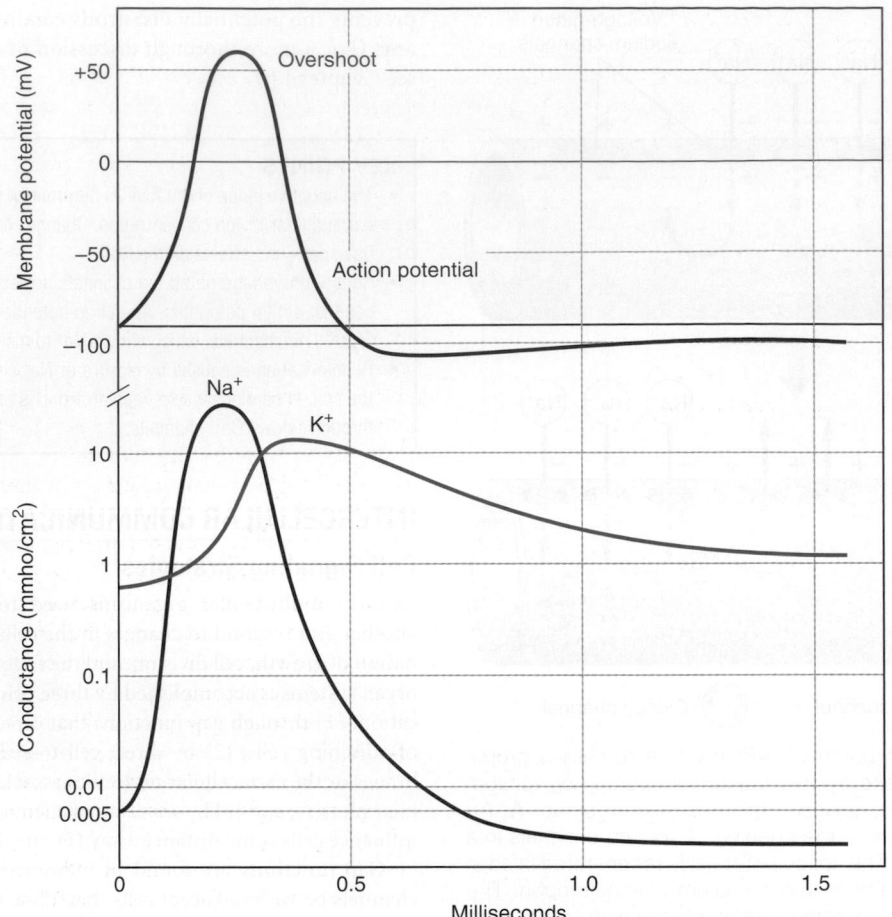

FIGURE 3-28 A typical neuronal action potential showing changes in membrane potential and the associated ion conductances. NOTE: mmho is a measure of conductance (amperes per volt), also called millisiemens (mS). The steep upstroke of the action potential is attributed to the sudden influx of Na^+ through voltage-gated "fast" sodium ion channels. Voltage-gated K^+ channels open more slowly and stay open longer to allow K^+ efflux from the cell, which aids in repolarization.

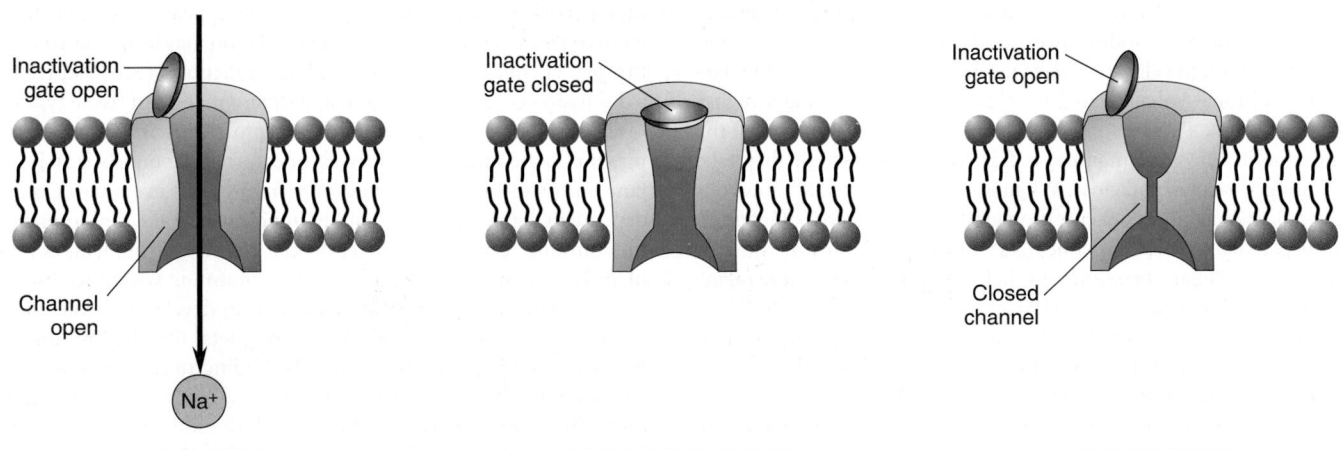

FIGURE 3-29 Three possible states of the voltage-gated sodium channel. In the open state, Na^+ is allowed to pass. In the refractory state, the channel is blocked by the inactivation gate and will not open in response to a depolarizing stimulus. In the closed state, the channel will open in response to a membrane depolarization.

cells of the nervous system and occurs at specialized junctions between the nerve cell and its target cell. The neuron secretes a chemical neurotransmitter into the space between the nerve and target cell; the neurotransmitter then diffuses across this synaptic cleft and binds receptors on the postsynaptic cell. Synaptic signaling occurs over very small distances (50 nm) and involves only one or a few postsynaptic target cells. In *paracrine* signaling, chemicals are secreted into a localized area and are rapidly destroyed, so that only cells in the immediate area are affected. Growth factors (GFs), for example, act locally to promote wound healing without affecting the growth of the entire organism. *Endocrine* signaling is accomplished by specialized endocrine cells that secrete hormones that travel via the bloodstream to target cells widely distributed throughout the body. Endocrine signaling is slow in comparison to nervous signaling, because it relies on diffusion and blood flow to target tissues.

A fourth type of signaling, *autocrine* signaling, occurs when cells are able to respond to signaling molecules that they secrete. Autocrine communication provides a feedback signal to the secreting cell and is commonly linked to pathways that regulate ligand secretion rates. Abnormal autocrine stimulation is thought to be a mechanism in some forms of cancer (see Chapter 7).

Target cells respond to ligand signaling through specific protein *receptors*. Cells can respond to a particular ligand only if they possess the appropriate receptor. For example, all cells of the body are exposed to thyroid-stimulating hormone (TSH) as it circulates in the blood, but only thyroid cells respond because they alone possess TSH receptors. However, cells that possess the same receptor may respond very differently to a particular ligand. For example, binding of acetylcholine to its receptor on a glandular cell may induce secretion, whereas binding to the same receptor on a cardiac muscle cell causes a decrease in contractile force. The cellular response to signaling molecules is regulated both by the array of receptors the cell carries and by the internal machinery to which the receptors are linked.

Cell Surface Receptor–Mediated Responses

Most hormones, local chemical mediators, and neurotransmitters are water-soluble molecules that are unable to pass through the lipid bilayer of the cell. These ligands exert their effects through binding with a receptor on the surface of the target cell, which then changes or transduces the external signal into an intracellular message. There are

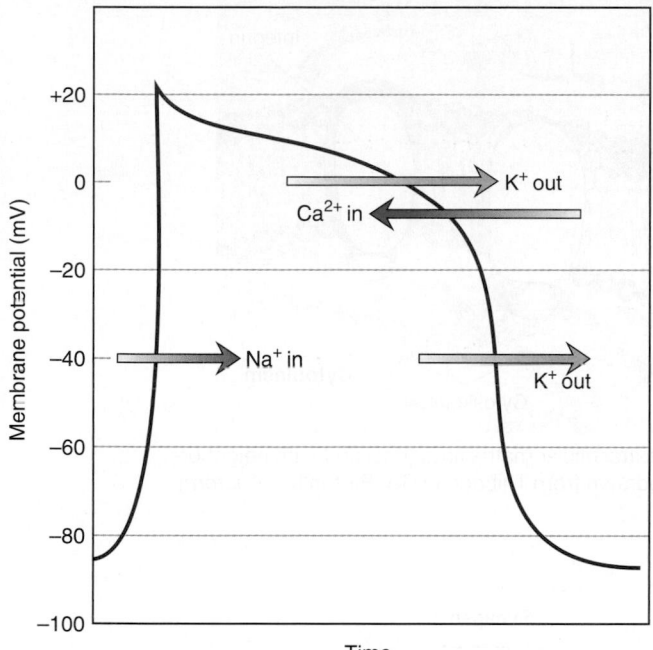

FIGURE 3-30 A typical cardiac muscle cell action potential showing the ion fluxes associated with each phase. Note that the repolarization phase is prolonged in comparison to the nerve action potential in Figure 3-28. This occurs because Ca^{2+} influx offsets the repolarizing effect of K^+ efflux and a plateau in the membrane potential is seen. When the Ca^{2+} channels close, the membrane quickly repolarizes.

REMOTE SIGNALING BY SECRETED MOLECULES

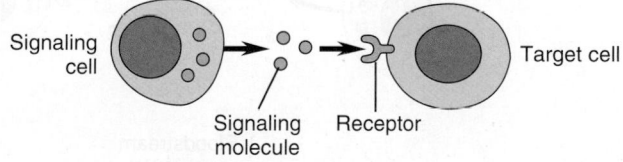

DIRECT SIGNALING BY PLASMA MEMBRANE–BOUND MOLECULES OR EXTRACELLULAR MATRIX

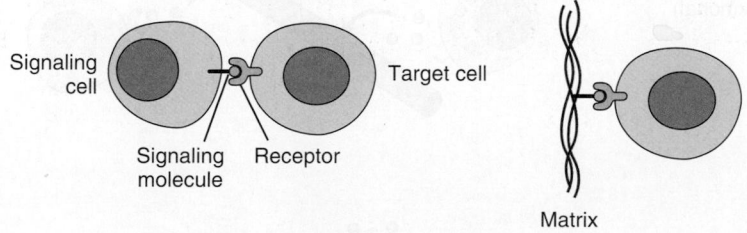

DIRECT SIGNALING VIA GAP JUNCTIONS

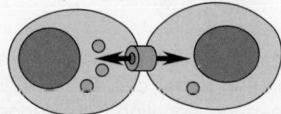

FIGURE 3-31 Methods used for intercellular communication.

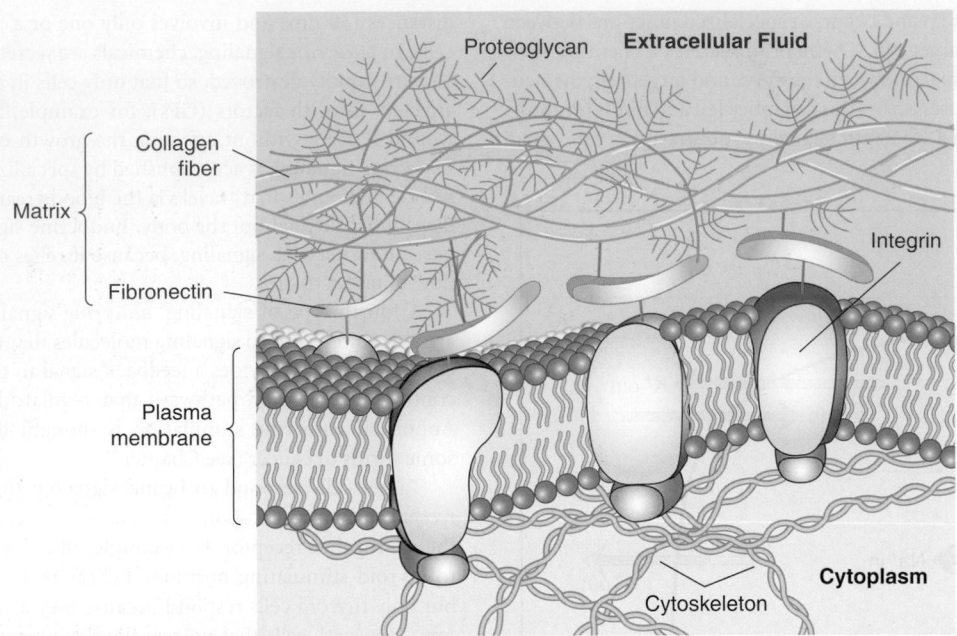

FIGURE 3-32 Cell adhesion proteins interact with the extracellular matrix (integrins) and with neighboring cells to maintain cell survival and differentiation. (Redrawn from Thibodeau GA, Patton KT: *Anatomy & physiology,* ed 6, St Louis, 2007, Mosby.)

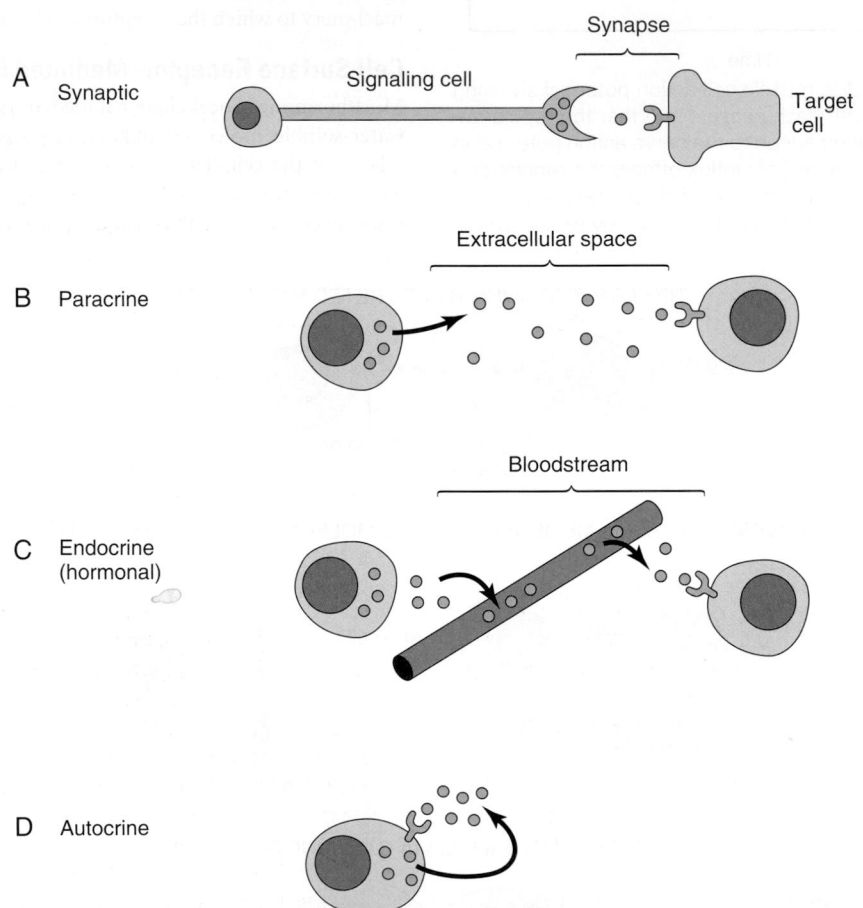

FIGURE 3-33 Signaling by secreted ligands can occur over variable distances. **A,** Synaptic signaling over a very small distance between neuron and target cell. **B,** Paracrine signaling through the extracellular fluid between cells in a tissue. **C,** Long-range signaling from endocrine cells through the bloodstream to distant targets. **D,** Localized autocrine signaling in which the secreting cell is also the target cell.

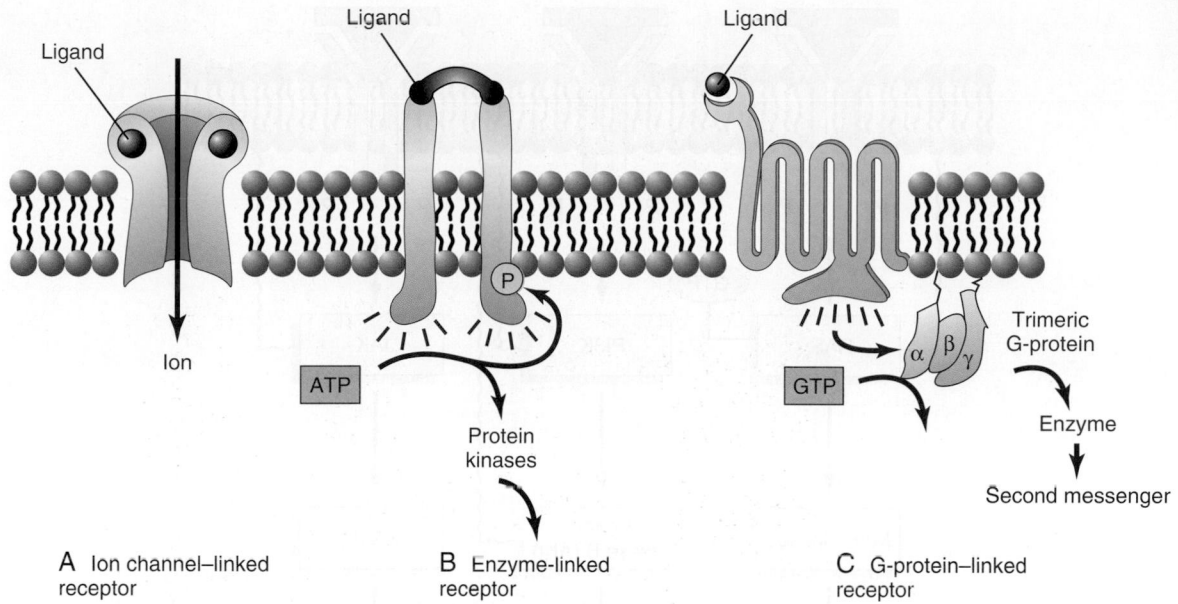

A Ion channel–linked receptor

B Enzyme-linked receptor

C G-protein–linked receptor

FIGURE 3-34 There are three major types of cell surface receptor proteins. **A,** Ion channel–linked receptors are also called ligand-gated channels. When the ligand binds, they open to allow specific ions through the membrane. **B,** Enzyme-linked receptors become activated kinases when a ligand binds to them. Kinases phosphorylate target proteins and change their activity. **C,** G-protein–linked (coupled) receptors have seven membrane-spanning segments with a ligand-binding pocket on the outside and a G-protein–activating portion on the inside. G-protein–linked receptors activate G-proteins, which in turn influence enzymes that produce second messengers.

three major classes of cell surface receptor proteins: ion channel–linked, enzyme-linked, and G-protein–coupled (Figure 3-34).[26]

Ion channel–linked receptors bind neurotransmitters, causing specific ion channels in the membrane to open or close. This type of signaling is prevalent in the nervous system, where rapid synaptic signaling between neurons is required. *Enzyme-linked* receptors catalyze enzyme reactions when they are activated by appropriate ligands. Nearly all enzyme-linked receptors function as *protein kinases;* that is, they mediate the transfer of phosphate groups from ATP (or GTP) to proteins (phosphorylate), and thus affect the activity of those proteins. The insulin receptor and most growth factor receptors are protein kinase receptors that phosphorylate and activate intracellular enzyme cascades. Enzyme-linked kinase receptors activate common kinase cascades including the PI3K-protein kinase B pathway, the RAS-MAP kinase pathway, and the JAK-STAT pathway (Figure 3-35).

A large number of signaling ligands bind to *G-protein–coupled receptors* (GPCRs). Most hormones and many drugs have their effects through G-protein–linked cascades. G-protein–coupled receptors act indirectly through a membrane-bound trimeric G-protein that binds GTP when activated by the receptor. The activated α subunit of the trimeric G-protein influences the activity of specific target enzymes. The target enzymes of G-proteins produce second messengers that trigger specific intracellular cascades and alter cell function (Figure 3-36). The α subunit of G-proteins has intrinsic enzyme activity that degrades GTP into GDP and P_i after a time. When GTP is bound, the G-protein is in the right conformation to activate its downstream targets, but when GTP is hydrolyzed to GDP and P_i, the G-protein resumes its inactive conformation and the activity of the signaling cascade is terminated.

There are three principal G-protein–coupled signaling systems that, when activated, alter the intracellular concentration of one or more second messengers (see Figure 3-36). Numerous receptors

activate trimeric G-proteins whose α subunit stimulates adenylyl cyclase to produce the second messenger cyclic adenosine monophosphate (cAMP). These G-proteins are called G_s. An increase in cAMP concentration is linked to different signaling cascades in different cell types. For example, cAMP causes glycogen breakdown in liver cells, increased force of contraction in cardiac cells, and increased secretion by glandular cells. Various cell types respond differently to the same second messenger because of differences in enzymes and other proteins in the cell.

Another important G-protein–coupled cascade is mediated by G-proteins called G_q whose α subunit stimulates the enzyme phospholipase C. Phospholipase C cleaves a membrane phospholipid (PI[4,5] P_2) to form two second messengers—inositol 1,4,5-trisphosphate (IP_3) and diacylglycerol (DAG) (see Figure 3-36). The IP_3 travels to the endoplasmic reticulum, where it stimulates the release of Ca^{2+} into the cytoplasm. The Ca^{2+} then triggers a change in cell function. DAG remains bound to the inner surface of the plasma membrane and can trigger several different intracellular cascades. Two important targets are the protein kinase C pathway and the eicosanoid pathway. Protein kinase C is a key enzyme in the growth response. The eicosanoid pathway results in the production of several arachidonic acid derivatives, including prostaglandins. These products are often secreted by the cell as signaling molecules to other nearby cells. Prostaglandins are important mediators of inflammation and platelet function.

The third trimeric G-protein type is called G_i because it is inhibitory to the production of cAMP. G-protein–coupled receptors such as the acetylcholine receptor in the heart activate G_i, whose α subunit then inhibits adenylyl cyclase (see Figure 3-36). In this case, the γβ subunit of G_i is also activated and opens membrane potassium channels in the heart, which tend to slow the heart rate.

In addition to the four second messengers already mentioned (cAMP, IP_3, DAG, and Ca^{2+}) there is a fifth called *cyclic guanosine*

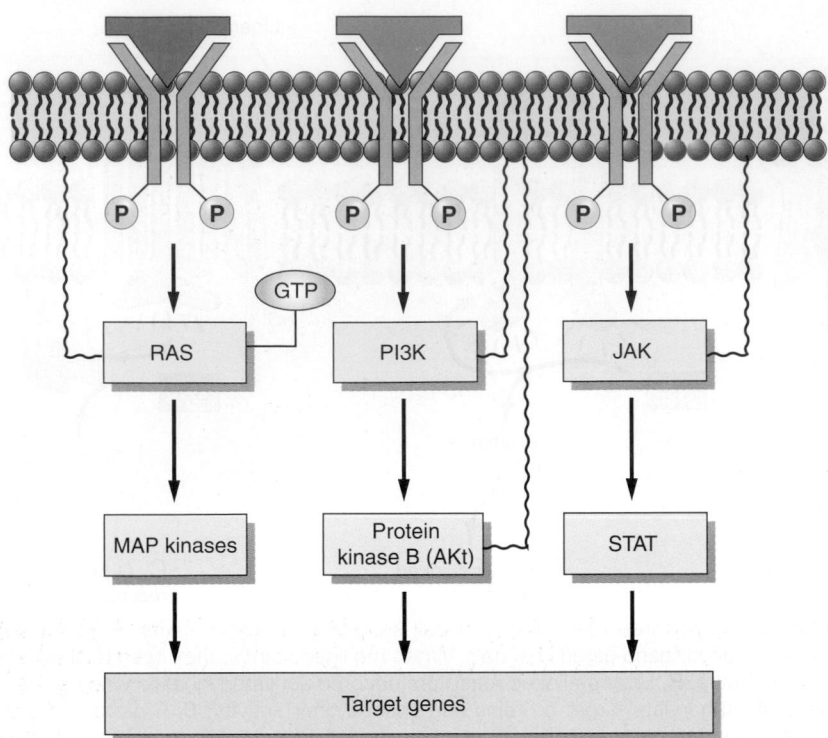

FIGURE 3-35 Many growth factor receptors activate protein kinase cascades within the cell. Three common pathways are shown. After binding of ligand, the receptor dimerizes and becomes phosphorylated. A cascade of kinase activations is initiated resulting in a change in target gene transcription. *GTP*, Guanosine triphosphate; *JAK*, janus kinase; *MAP*, mitogen-activated kinase; *PI3K*, phosphoinositide 3-kinase; *RAS*, rat sarcoma protein; *STAT*, signal transducer and activator of transcription.

monophosphate (cGMP), which is produced by the enzyme guanylyl cyclase (Figure 3-37). The primary activator of guanylyl cyclase is a small lipid-soluble gas molecule called *nitric oxide*. Nitric oxide is an important signaling molecule with widespread targets. It functions as a neurotransmitter in the brain and is an important smooth muscle relaxant in the vascular system. cGMP is also produced by a special class of enzyme-linked receptors (see Figure 3-37).

To be effective at communicating signals, all the receptor systems must be quickly turned off so that they can be responsive to the next incoming signal. A variety of strategies are used to quench the signaling cascades (Figure 3-38). For example, phosphodiesterases are enzymes that convert the cyclic nucleotides cAMP and cGMP to their inactive forms, AMP and GMP, respectively, and help to remove these second messengers soon after they are formed. Some drugs, such as caffeine and sildenafil citrate (Viagra), are phosphodiesterase inhibitors that slow the normal breakdown of cyclic nucleotides and prolong their activity. Many of the intracellular signaling cascades rely on kinases that phosphorylate their target proteins so as to change their activity. The action of kinases is countered by numerous phosphatase enzymes that quickly cleave the phosphates off the target proteins and inhibit their activity.

The cell also can regulate the activity and number of receptors on the cell surface.[26] Generally a cell decreases the number or activity of receptors when it is exposed to excessive concentrations of signaling molecules (see Figure 3-38). Receptors can be internalized in the cell where they are inactive but are available for later use, or they can be sent to lysosomes for degradation. Destruction of receptors in lysosomes is called *down-regulation*. (The production of extra receptors is called *up-regulation*.) Receptors that remain in the membrane also can be inhibited by phosphorylation, which blocks them from interacting

with their intracellular targets. Receptors that can bind ligand but do not produce a response are said to be uncoupled. The proteins that phosphorylate G-protein receptors are called G-protein–receptor kinases (GRKs). The mechanisms that "turn off" signaling cascades are vitally important to maintaining a responsive communication system.

Intracellular Receptor–Mediated Responses

A small number of hormones are lipid soluble and can pass directly through the cell membrane to interact with receptors *inside* the cell. These receptors are located in the cell cytosol (e.g., cortisol) or may be associated with the cell nucleus. Intracellular receptors are specific for a particular ligand, just as surface receptors are. Binding of the ligand causes the receptor to become activated. Because lipid-soluble ligands enter the cell directly, no second messengers are needed. An activated cytosolic steroid receptor travels to the nucleus, where it binds with specific genes and regulates their activity (Figure 3-39). Thyroid receptors are also located within the cell. Thyroid hormone enters the cell through carriers in the membrane and travels to the nucleus. The thyroid receptor is already bound to DNA in the absence of thyroid hormone. When thyroid hormone finds its nuclear receptor, the complex dissociates and removes an inhibitory influence on gene transcription. Cellular responses to these gene regulatory receptor complexes are slow in comparison to the cell surface receptor responses and generally last longer.

Regulation of Cellular Growth and Proliferation

In multicellular organisms such as humans, the growth and proliferation of cells and tissues must be strictly controlled to maintain a balance between cell birth rate and cell death rate. The system must be capable of rapidly increasing proliferation of a particular tissue to replace cells

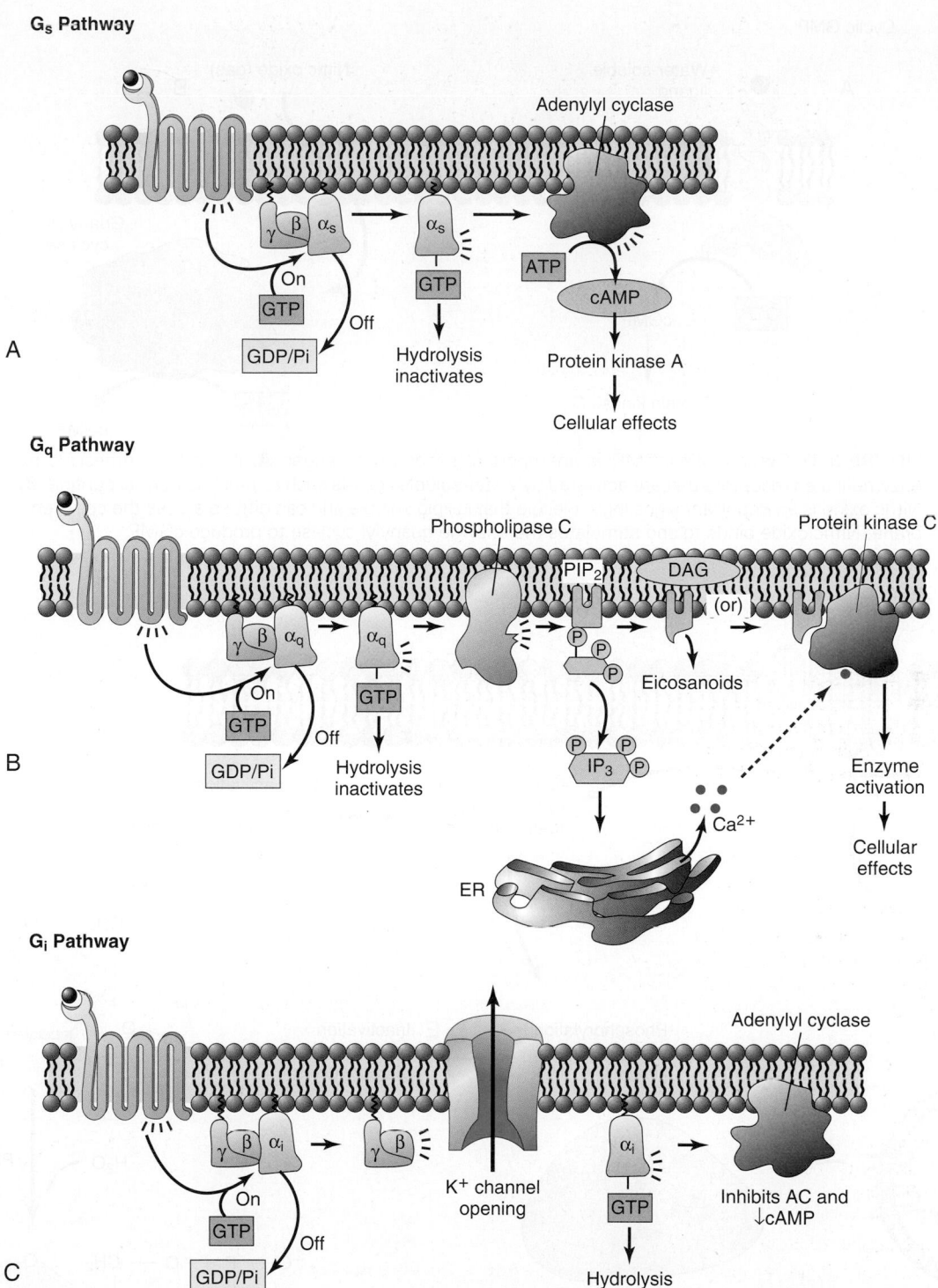

FIGURE 3-36 G-protein–coupled signaling. When the ligand binds to the receptor, an intracellular domain is changed into an active configuration that can interact with inactive trimeric G-proteins. The receptor induces the G-protein to release its bound GDP and P_i in exchange for a GTP molecule. When GTP binds to the α subunit of the G-protein, it is activated and diffuses away from the $\gamma\beta$ subunits to find its target enzyme (adenylyl cyclase *[AC]* or phospholipase C). The α GTP stimulates its target enzyme to produce a second messenger, which in turn activates a signaling cascade within the cell. After a time, the α subunit hydrolyzes its GTP to GDP and P_i and becomes inactive. The α subunit is now in the correct conformation to reassociate with the $\gamma\beta$ subunits and await another signal from the receptor. **A,** The G_s pathway increases the production of cyclic adenosine monophosphate (cAMP). **B,** The G_q pathway increases the production of inositol 1,4,5-trisphosphate *(IP3)* and diacylglycerol *(DAG)*. **C,** The G_i pathway is inhibitory to the production of cAMP. In some cases the $\gamma\beta$ subunit also has functional activity and may regulate ion channels. *ER,* Endoplasmic reticulum; *PKC,* protein kinase C.

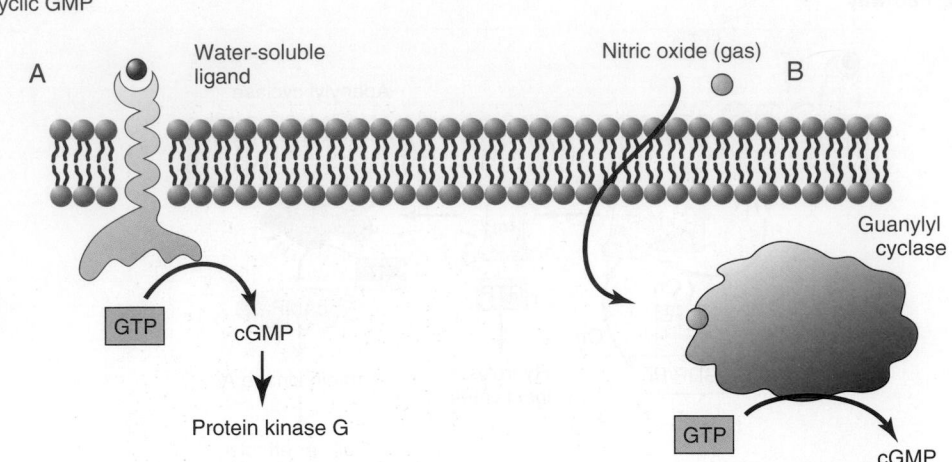

FIGURE 3-37 Cyclic GMP *(cGMP)* is an important second messenger. **A,** It can be synthesized by enzyme-linked receptors that are activated by water-soluble ligands such as atrial natriuretic peptide. **B,** Nitric oxide is an important signaling molecule that is lipid soluble and can diffuse across the cell membrane. Nitric oxide binds to and stimulates the enzyme guanylyl cyclase to produce cGMP.

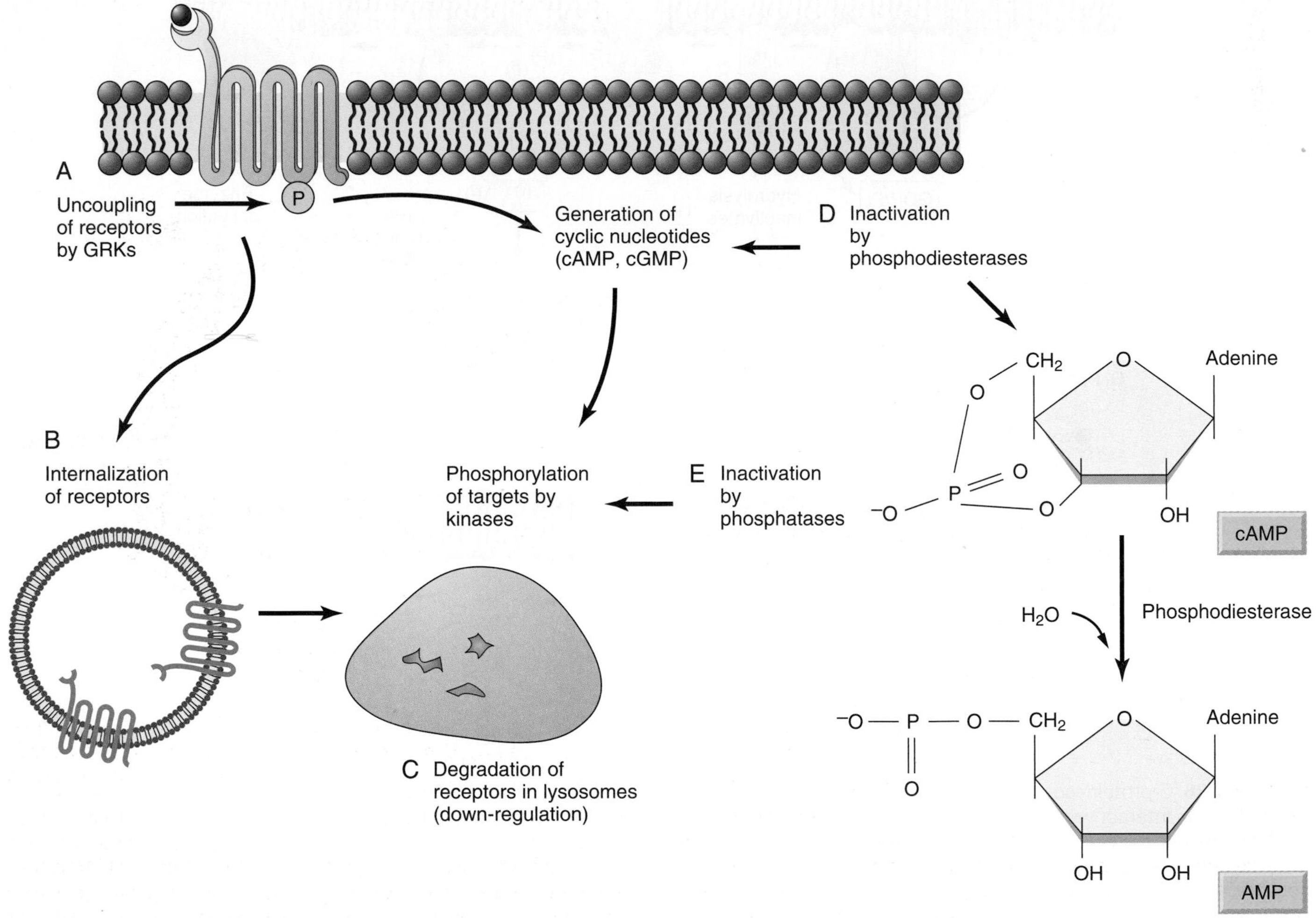

FIGURE 3-38 A variety of mechanisms exist to inhibit receptor-mediated signaling cascades. **A,** Phosphorylation of the receptor by receptor kinases such as G-protein receptor kinases *(GRKs)* uncouples the enzyme from its intracellular cascade. **B,** Receptor internalization temporarily reduces the number of receptors displayed at the cell surface. **C,** Receptor degradation results in a long-term reduction in receptors (down-regulation). **D,** The cyclic nucleotide second messengers can be degraded by phosphodiesterase enzymes to stop the intracellular cascade. **E,** Phosphatase enzymes counteract the phosphorylating activities of kinases and inhibit the intracellular cascade.

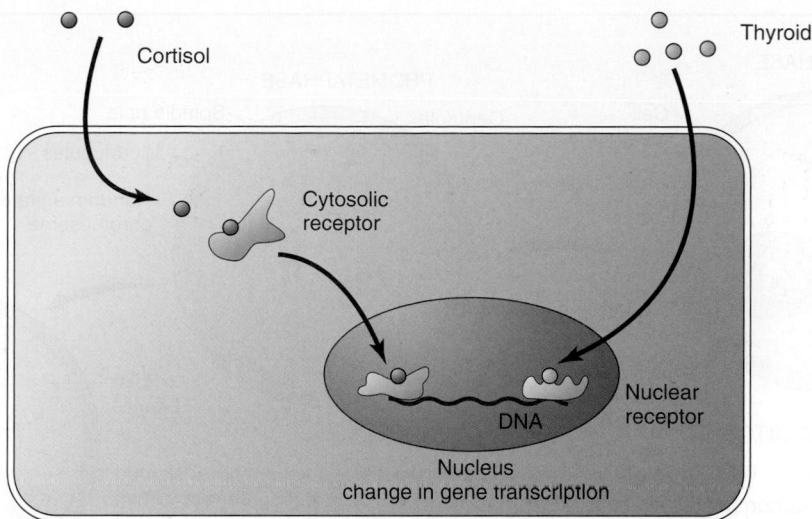

FIGURE 3-39 Lipid-soluble ligands, such as steroid hormones and gases, can diffuse across the cell membrane and interact with receptors located within the cell cytoplasm or nucleus. Thyroid hormone is not lipid soluble and enters the cell through a carrier to interact with its intracellular receptor. When the ligand binds to its intracellular receptor, it forms a functional gene regulatory protein that affects the rate of transcription of its target genes. The response of the cell to intracellular ligands is generally slow and long lasting.

lost to injury and normal wear and tear while simultaneously inhibiting unwanted growth or proliferation of other cells. Special intercellular communication systems function to regulate the replication of individual cells in the body. Two important strategies of cell cycle control have been described. First, a variety of protein mitogens and growth factors are required in specific combinations for growth and proliferation of particular cell types. Second, cells respond to spatial signals from the extracellular matrix (from integrin receptors) and neighboring cells (from cell adhesion proteins) that indicate how much room is available. When conditions favor cell proliferation, the cell proceeds through the stages of the cell cycle (Figure 3-40). Dormant cells remain in G_1 phase indefinitely. Cycling cells proceed through G_1, S phase (synthesis), G_2, M phase (mitosis), and cell division. S phase is characterized by duplication of DNA and synthesis of intracellular components in preparation for cell division. M phase, or mitosis, proceeds through six stages, beginning with prophase, in which the chromosomes condense and become visible, and ending with cytokinesis, when cell division is accomplished. The chromosomes of body cells are duplicated and distributed equally to the cell's progeny when it divides by mitosis, such that each daughter cell receives an identical full set of 46 chromosomes. The stages of mitotic cell division are explained in Figure 3-41. Mitosis is responsible for the proliferation of body cells in which little genetic variation is needed or desired. A more elaborate cell division process, meiosis, occurs in the germ cells (egg and sperm), where significant chromosomal rearrangements occur (see Chapter 6).

The **cell cycle** has been the subject of intense study in recent years because of its importance in cancer biology. Cancer cells continue to grow and divide unchecked, despite the lack of appropriate signals to stimulate them. Of particular interest are the events that prod the cell from its dormant state and cause it to begin the cycle. A simplified picture of a major component of this complex process is shown in Figure 3-42. The Rb protein (or pRb) is of central importance in preventing a cell from proceeding through the cell cycle.[27] The Rb protein functions to bind gene transcription factors called *E2F* so that they are unable to bind to DNA promoter regions and begin the processes of cell replication. The Rb protein can be induced to release the E2F transcription factors when appropriate mitogen signals arrive at the cell surface.

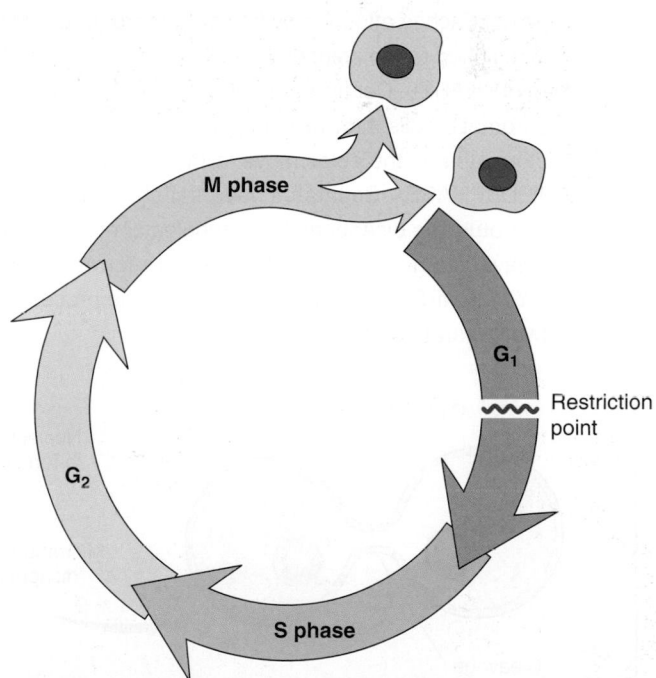

FIGURE 3-40 Events of the cell cycle. The cycle begins late in G_1 when the cell passes a restriction point. The cell then proceeds systematically through the S phase (synthesis), G_2, and M phase (mitosis).

These proliferation-promoting signals at the cell surface are transmitted to the Rb protein by way of cyclin-dependent signaling pathways within the cell. Proteins called *cyclins* accumulate in the cell and then bind to and activate cyclin-dependent kinases (cdk). The cdk then phosphorylates the Rb protein, changing its affinity for E2F so that it is released. The E2F then translocates to specific regions of DNA where it regulates more than 500 genes and promotes cell replication.[28]

To respond to a mitogen growth factor, a cell must have the corresponding receptor on its cell surface. Many cells in the body synthesize

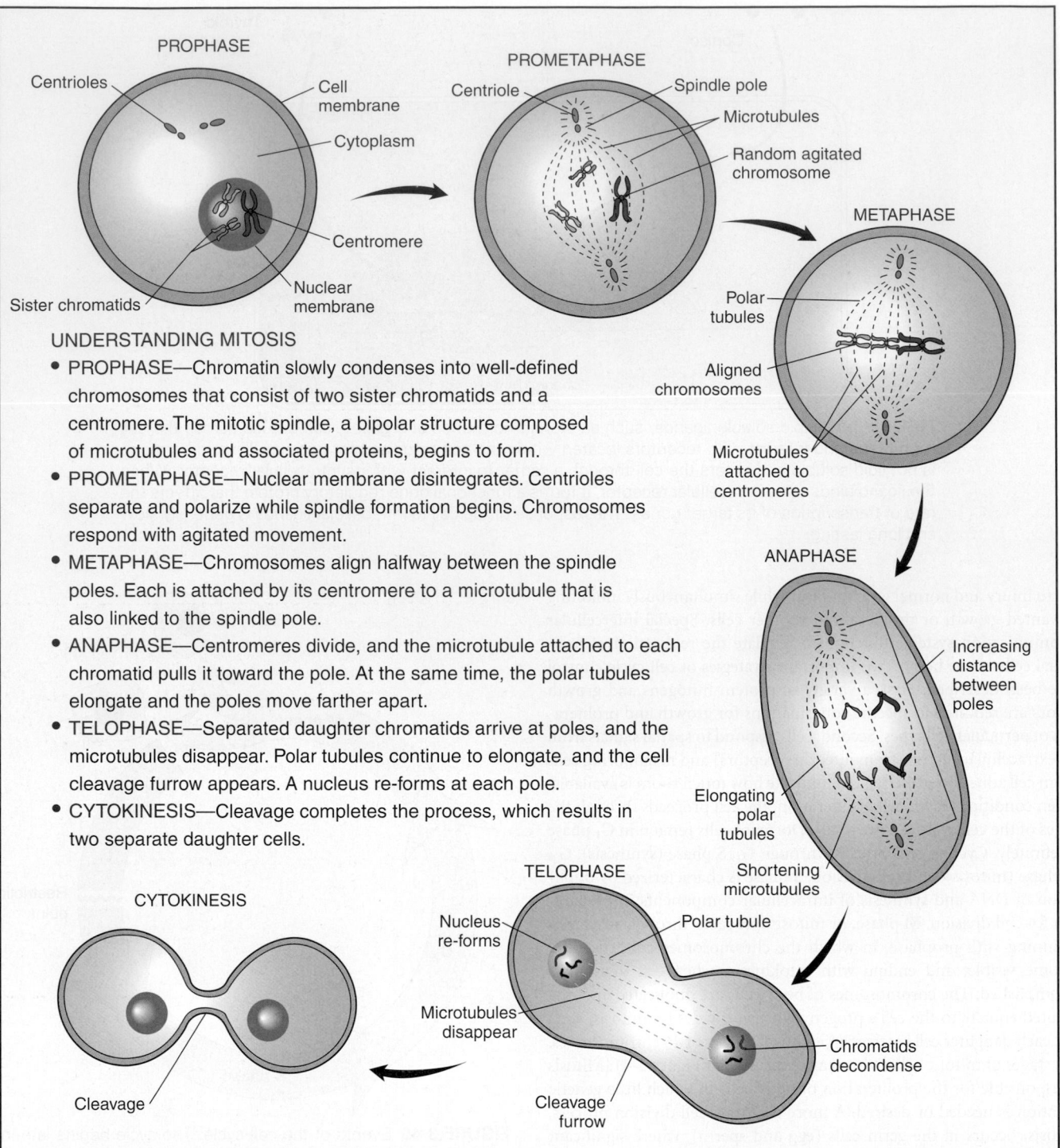

UNDERSTANDING MITOSIS

- PROPHASE—Chromatin slowly condenses into well-defined chromosomes that consist of two sister chromatids and a centromere. The mitotic spindle, a bipolar structure composed of microtubules and associated proteins, begins to form.
- PROMETAPHASE—Nuclear membrane disintegrates. Centrioles separate and polarize while spindle formation begins. Chromosomes respond with agitated movement.
- METAPHASE—Chromosomes align halfway between the spindle poles. Each is attached by its centromere to a microtubule that is also linked to the spindle pole.
- ANAPHASE—Centromeres divide, and the microtubule attached to each chromatid pulls it toward the pole. At the same time, the polar tubules elongate and the poles move farther apart.
- TELOPHASE—Separated daughter chromatids arrive at poles, and the microtubules disappear. Polar tubules continue to elongate, and the cell cleavage furrow appears. A nucleus re-forms at each pole.
- CYTOKINESIS—Cleavage completes the process, which results in two separate daughter cells.

FIGURE 3-41 Six stages of mitotic cell division. (Redrawn from Nichols FH, Zwelling E, editors: *Maternal-newborn nursing: theory and practice,* Philadelphia, 1997, Saunders, p 307.)

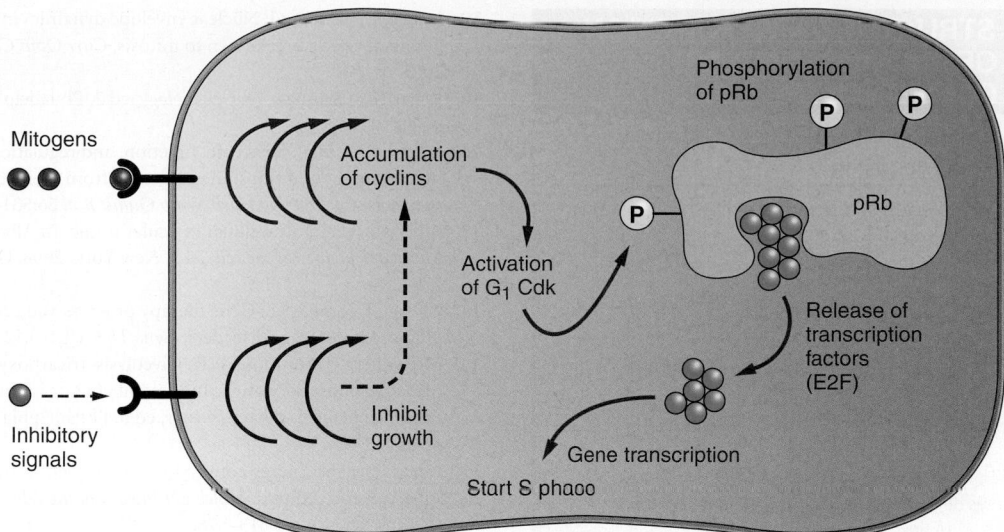

FIGURE 3-42 The mechanism of initiation of cellular replication requires appropriate stimulation by extracellular growth factors that bind their complementary receptors on the cell surface. Activation of the receptor stimulates signaling pathways within the cell that increase cyclin proteins. The cyclins bind to cyclin-dependent kinases (Cdks) to form active enzyme complexes. The active cyclin-Cdk enzymes phosphorylate Rb protein (pRb), inducing it to release E2F transcription factors that initiate replication. In the absence of appropriate growth factor signals, the Rb protein functions to inhibit unwanted cell proliferation.

and secrete mitogens, which then influence the proliferation of other cell types in a paracrine or endocrine fashion. Platelet-derived growth factor (PDGF) was one of the first mitogens to be discovered. It is secreted by platelets when they form blood clots in response to an injury. PDGF stimulates fibroblasts and smooth muscle cells in the damaged area to divide and replace cells lost to the injury. Numerous mitogens have been identified, and most cells require an appropriate combination of mitogen signals before they can enter the cell cycle. There are many signaling steps in the pathway from mitogen receptor to DNA activation. Somatic cells respond to growth factors by increasing cell size, whereas stem cell populations undergo cell division. Thus the same signaling ligands may have different effects depending on cell type and conditions. Similar signaling pathways may also trigger cell death (apoptosis) when cells have to be reduced or removed during tissue development and remodeling. The processes of abnormal cellular proliferation and cancer are further detailed in Chapter 7. The process of apoptosis is described in Chapter 4.

> **KEY POINTS**
> - Intercellular communication is accomplished by three principal means: (1) gap junctions, which directly connect the cytoplasm of adjoining cells; (2) direct cell-to-cell surface contact; and (3) secretion of chemical mediators (ligands). Most ligands are water-soluble molecules that interact with receptors on the cell surface. These receptors are of three general types: ion channel linked, enzyme linked, and G-protein coupled.
> - Binding of a ligand to a G-protein receptor controls the production of second messengers (cAMP, IP_3, DAG, Ca^{2+}) within the target cell that initiate changes in cell function.
> - Somatic cells divide by a process called *mitosis* in which daughter cells each receive an identical and complete set of 46 chromosomes.
> - Cell replication normally requires specific extracellular mitogens that activate signaling systems within the cell. Cyclin proteins and cyclin-dependent kinases alter the function of Rb protein, causing it to release transcription factors that begin the process of cell replication.

SUMMARY

Detailed knowledge of cell physiology is essential to understanding disease processes. Cells are complex, membrane-bound units that perform a variety of functions necessary to the maintenance of life. The major cell components and their functions are summarized in Table 3-1. The cell membrane is an important cellular structure that protects the cell interior and mediates information transfer to and from the extracellular environment. Proteins embedded in the membrane lipid bilayer perform most of the membrane functions, including transduction of extracellular messages, membrane transport, electrical excitation, and cell-to-cell communication.

Human cells have several important intracellular organelles. These include the cytoskeleton, which organizes the intracellular compartment; the nucleus, which holds the cell's genetic material and directs the daily activities of the cell; the endoplasmic reticulum and the Golgi apparatus, which produce, package, and transport proteins and lipids to the plasma membrane and lysosomes; the lysosomes and peroxisomes, which perform the task of intracellular digestion of organic waste; and the mitochondria, which produce cellular energy in the form of ATP. The energy released by ATP hydrolysis is used by the cell to drive the many energetically unfavorable reactions needed to maintain cellular functions. Multicellular organisms have developed complex communication systems to control cell behavior, such as growth and differentiation into specialized cell types. Disruption of these cellular processes is at the root of pathophysiologic processes and disease.

TABLE 3-1 STRUCTURE AND FUNCTION OF MAJOR CELLULAR COMPONENTS

CELLULAR STRUCTURE	FUNCTIONS
Plasma membrane	Protective barrier separates life from nonlife
	Extracellular message transduction
	Transport of materials into and out of cell
	Maintenance and transmission of membrane potentials
	Cell-to-cell recognition, interaction
Cytoskeleton	Maintenance of cell shape
	Cell movement
	Trafficking within cell
Nucleus	Protection of genetic material
	Regulation of cell type and function through control of protein synthesis
Endoplasmic reticulum	Protein and lipid synthesis
	Lipid metabolism and detoxification
Golgi apparatus	Protein and lipid modification and sorting
	Transport of proteins and lipids to appropriate destinations
Lysosomes	Hydrolytic breakdown of organic waste
Peroxisomes	Oxidative breakdown of organic waste
Mitochondria	Cellular energy production (ATP)

ATP, Adenosine triphosphate.

REFERENCES

1. Alberts B, et al: Cells and genomes. In Alberts B et al, editors: *Molecular biology of the cell*, ed 5, New York, 2008, Garland Science, pp 1–44.
2. Lahava N, Nira S, Elitzurb A: The emergence of life on Earth, *Prog Biophys Mol Biol* 75:75–120, 2001.
3. Singer SJ, Nicolson GL: The fluid mosaic model of the structure of cell membranes, *Science* 175:720–731, 1972.
4. Alberts B, et al: Membrane structure. In Alberts B et al, editors: *Molecular biology of the cell*, ed 5, New York, 2008, Garland Science, pp 617–650.
5. Moran AP, Gupta A, Joshi L: Sweet-talk: role of host glycosylation in bacterial pathogenesis of the gastrointestinal tract, *Gut* 60(10):1412–1425, 2011.
6. Meisenberg G, Simmons WH: The cytoskeleton. In Meisenberg G, Simmons WH, editors: *Principles of medical biochemistry*, ed 3, Philadelphia, 2012, Saunders, pp 198–211.
7. Alberts B, et al: The cytoskeleton. In Alberts B et al, editors: *Molecular biology of the cell*, ed 5, New York, 2008, Garland Science, pp 965–1062.
8. Meisenberg G, Simmons WH: The human genome. In Meisenberg G, Simmons WH, editors: *Principles of medical biochemistry*, ed 3, Philadelphia, 2012, Saunders, pp 93–117.
9. Lenart P, Ellenberg J: Nuclear envelope dynamics in oocytes: from germinal vesicle breakdown to mitosis, *Curr Opin Cell Biol* 15(1):88–95, 2003.
10. Pollard T, Earnshaw W: *Cell biology*, ed 2, Philadelphia, 2008, Saunders, p 348.
11. Johnson AE, et al: Structure, function, and regulation of free and membrane-bound ribosomes: the view from their substrates and products, *Cold Spring Harb Symp Quant Biol* 66:531–541, 2001.
12. Alberts B, et al: Intracellular vesicular traffic. In Alberts B et al, editors: *Molecular biology of the cell*, ed 5, New York, 2008, Garland Science, pp 779–784.
13. Cheng SH, Smith AE: Gene therapy progress and prospects: gene therapy of lysosomal storage disorders, *Gene Ther* 10(16):1275–1281, 2003.
14. Meisenberg G, Simmons WH: Glycolysis, tricarboxylic acid cycle, and oxidative phosphorylation. In Meisenberg G, Simmons WH, editors: *Principles of medical biochemistry*, ed 3, Philadelphia, 2012, Saunders, pp 347–373.
15. Alberts B, et al: Energy conversion: mitochondria and chloroplasts. In Alberts B et al, editors: *Molecular biology of the cell*, ed 5, New York, 2008, Garland Science, pp 813–878.
16. Pollard T, Earnshaw W: *Cell biology*, ed 2, Philadelphia, 2008, Saunders, p 332.
17. Alberts B, et al: Membrane transport of small molecules and the electrical properties of membranes. In Alberts B et al, editors: *Molecular biology of the cell*, ed 5, New York, 2008, Garland Science, pp 651–694.
18. Pollard T, Earnshaw W: *Cell biology*, ed 2, Philadelphia, 2008, Saunders, p 149.
19. Lamas JA, Reboreda A, Codesido V: Ionic basis of the resting membrane potential in cultured rat sympathetic neurons, *Neuroreport* 13(5):585–591, 2002.
20. Hodgkin AL: *The conduction of the nervous impulse*, Liverpool, England, 1971, Liverpool University Press.
21. Baker PF, Hodgkin AL, Shaw T: The effects of changes in internal ionic concentrations of the electrical properties of perfused giant axons, *J Physiol* 164:355–374, 1962.
22. Hodgkin AL, Huxley AF: Currents carried by sodium and potassium ions through the membrane of the giant axon of Loligo, *J Physiol* 116:449–472, 1952.
23. Hodgkin AL, Huxley AF, Katz B: Measurement of current-voltage relations in the membrane of the giant axon of Loligo, *J Physiol* 116:424–448, 1952.
24. Hodgkin AL, Katz B: The effect of sodium ions on the electrical activity of the giant axon of the squid, *J Physiol* 108:37–77, 1949.
25. Bezanilla F: Voltage sensor movements, *J Gen Physiol* 120(4):465–473, 2002.
26. Alberts B, et al: Mechanisms of cell communication. In Alberts B et al, editors: *Molecular biology of the cell*, ed 5, New York, 2008, Garland Science, pp 879–964.
27. Poznic M: Retinoblastoma protein: a central processing unit, *J Biosci* 34(2):305–312, 2009.
28. Meisenberg G, Simmons WH: Cellular growth control and cancer. In Meisenberg G, Simmons WH, editors: *Principles of medical biochemistry*, ed 3, Philadelphia, 2012, Saunders, pp 307–332.

Cell Injury, Aging, and Death

Jacquelyn L. Banasik

ⓔvolve WEBSITE

http://evolve.elsevier.com/Copstead/
- Review Questions and Answers
- Glossary (with audio pronunciations for selected terms)
- Animations
- Case Studies
- Key Points Review

KEY QUESTIONS

- What are the usual cellular responses to reversible injury?
- How are reversible and irreversible cellular injuries differentiated?
- How do necrosis and apoptosis differ?
- To what kind of injuries are cells susceptible?
- What are the usual physiologic changes of aging and how are these differentiated from disease?

CHAPTER OUTLINE

Disease and injury are increasingly being understood as cellular and genetic phenomena. Although pathophysiologic processes are often presented in terms of systemic effects and manifestations, ultimately it is the *cells* that make up the systems that are affected. Even complex multisystem disorders such as cancer ultimately are the result of alterations in cell function. As the mysterious mechanisms of diseases are understood on the cellular and molecular levels, more specific methods of diagnosis, treatment, and prevention can be developed. This chapter presents the general characteristics of cellular injury, adaptation, aging, and death that underlie the discussions of systemic pathophysiologic processes presented in later chapters of this text.

Cells are confronted by many challenges to their integrity and survival and have efficient mechanisms for coping with an altered cellular environment. Cells respond to environmental changes or injury in three general ways: (1) when the change is mild or short-lived, the cell may withstand the assault and completely return to normal. This is called a *reversible cell injury*. (2) The cell may adapt to a persistent but sublethal injury by changing its structure or function. Generally, adaptation also is reversible. (3) Cell death may occur if the injury is too severe or prolonged. Cell death is irreversible and may occur by two different processes termed *necrosis* and *apoptosis*. Necrosis is cell death caused by external injury, whereas apoptosis is triggered by intracellular signaling cascades that result in cell suicide. Necrosis is considered to be a pathologic process associated with significant tissue damage, whereas apoptosis may be a normal physiologic process in some instances and pathologic in others.

REVERSIBLE CELL INJURY

Regardless of the cause, reversible injuries and the early stages of irreversible injuries often result in cellular swelling and the accumulation of excess substances within the cell. These changes reflect the cell's inability to perform normal metabolic functions owing to insufficient cellular energy in the form of adenosine triphosphate (ATP) or dysfunction of associated metabolic enzymes. Once the acute stress or injury has been removed, by definition of a reversible injury, the cell returns to its preinjury state.

Hydropic Swelling

Cellular swelling attributable to accumulation of water, or hydropic swelling, is the first manifestation of most forms of reversible cell injury.[1] Hydropic swelling results from malfunction of the sodium-potassium (Na^+-K^+) pumps that normally maintain ionic equilibrium of the cell. Failure of the Na^+-K^+ pump results in accumulation of sodium ions within the cell, creating an osmotic gradient for water entry. Because Na^+-K^+ pump function is dependent on the presence of cellular ATP, any injury that results in insufficient energy production also will result in hydropic swelling (Figure 4-1). Hydropic swelling is characterized by a large, pale cytoplasm, dilated endoplasmic reticulum, and swollen mitochondria. With severe hydropic swelling, the endoplasmic reticulum may rupture and form large water-filled vacuoles. Generalized swelling in the cells of a particular organ will cause the organ to increase in size and weight. Organ enlargement is indicated by the suffix -*megaly* (e.g., *splenomegaly* denotes an enlarged spleen, *hepatomegaly* denotes an enlarged liver).

Intracellular Accumulations

Excess accumulations of substances in cells may result in cellular injury because the substances are toxic or provoke an immune response, or merely because they occupy space needed for cellular functions. In some cases, accumulations do not in themselves appear to be injurious but rather are indicators of cell injury. Intracellular accumulations may be categorized as (1) excessive amounts of normal intracellular substances such as fat, (2) accumulation of abnormal substances produced by the cell because of faulty metabolism or synthesis, and (3) accumulation of pigments and particles that the cell is unable to degrade (Figure 4-2).

Normal intracellular substances that tend to accumulate in injured cells include lipids, carbohydrates, glycogen, and proteins. Faulty metabolism of these substances within the cell results in excessive intracellular storage. In some cases, the enzymes required for breaking down a particular substance are absent or abnormal as a result of a genetic defect. In other cases, altered metabolism may be due to excessive intake, toxins, or other disease processes.

A common site of intracellular lipid accumulation is the liver, where many fats are normally stored, metabolized, and synthesized. Fatty liver is often associated with excessive intake of alcohol.[2] Mechanisms whereby alcohol causes fatty liver remain unclear, but it is thought to result from direct toxic effects as well as the preferential metabolism of alcohol instead of lipid (see Chapter 38 for a discussion of fatty liver). Lipids may also contribute to atherosclerotic diseases and accumulate in blood vessels, kidney, heart, and other organs. Fat-filled cells tend to compress cellular components to one side and cause the tissue to appear yellowish and greasy (Figure 4-3). In several genetic disorders, the enzymes needed to metabolize lipids are impaired; these include Tay-Sachs disease and Gaucher disease, in which lipids accumulate in neurologic tissue.

Glycosaminoglycans (mucopolysaccharides) are large carbohydrate complexes that normally compose the extracellular matrix of connective tissues. Connective tissue cells secrete most of the glycosaminoglycan into the extracellular space, but a small portion remains inside the cell and is normally degraded by lysosomal enzymes. The *mucopolysaccharidoses* are a group of genetic diseases in which the enzymatic degradation of these molecules is impaired and they collect within the cell. Mental disabilities and connective tissue disorders are common findings.

Like other disorders of accumulation, *excessive glycogen storage* can be the result of inborn errors of metabolism, but a common cause is diabetes mellitus.[1] Diabetes mellitus is associated with impaired cellular uptake of glucose, which results in high serum and urine glucose levels. Cells of the renal tubules reabsorb the excess filtered glucose and store it intracellularly as glycogen. The renal tubule cells also are a common site for abnormal accumulations of proteins. Normally, very little

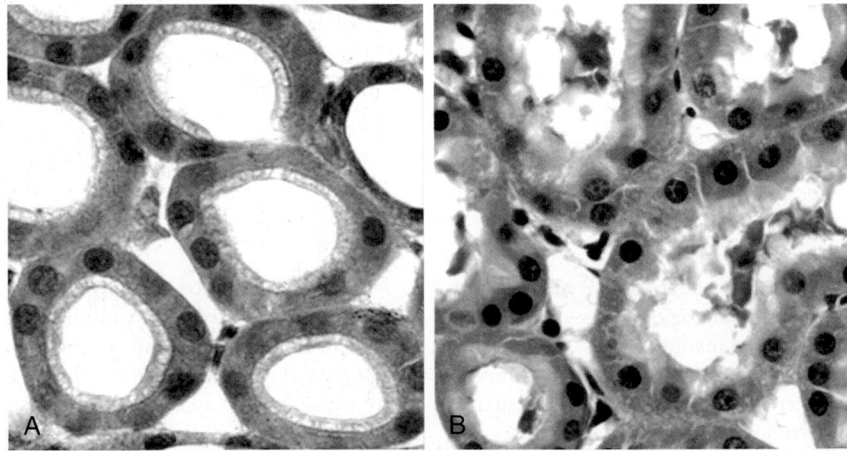

FIGURE 4-1 Cellular swelling in kidney tubule epithelial cells. **A,** Normal kidney tubule with cuboidal cells; **B,** early ischemic changes showing surface blebs and swelling of cells. (From Kumar V et al: *Robbins and Cotran pathologic basis of disease*, ed 8, Philadelphia, 2010, Saunders, p 14. Photograph courtesy Drs. Neal Pinckard and M. A. Venkatachalam, University of Texas Health Sciences Center, San Antonio, TX.)

protein escapes the bloodstream into the urine. However, with certain disorders, renal glomerular capillaries become leaky and allow proteins to pass through them. Renal tubule cells recapture some of the escaped proteins through endocytosis, resulting in abnormal accumulation.

Cellular stress may lead to accumulation and aggregation of denatured proteins. The abnormally folded intracellular proteins may cause serious cell dysfunction and death if they are allowed to persist in the cell. A family of stress proteins (also called chaperone or heat-shock proteins) is responsible for binding and refolding aberrant proteins back into their correct three-dimensional forms (Figure 4-4). If the chaperones are unsuccessful in correcting the defect, the abnormal proteins form complexes with another protein called *ubiquitin*. Ubiquitin targets the abnormal proteins to enter a proteosome complex, where they are digested into fragments that are less injurious to cells (see Figure 4-4). In some cases, the accumulated substances are not metabolized by normal intracellular enzymes. In diabetes, for instance, high serum glucose levels result in excessive glucose uptake by neuronal cells because they do not require insulin for glucose uptake.[3] (Diabetes mellitus is discussed in Chapter 41.)

Finally, a variety of pigments and inorganic particles may be present in cells. Some pigment accumulations are normal, such as the accumulation of melanin in tanned skin, whereas others signify pathophysiologic processes. Pigments may be produced by the body (endogenous) or may be introduced from outside sources (exogenous). In addition to melanin, the iron-containing substances hemosiderin and bilirubin are endogenous pigments that, when present in excessive amounts, indicate disease processes. Hemosiderin and bilirubin are derived from hemoglobin. Excessive amounts may indicate abnormal breakdown of hemoglobin-containing red blood cells (RBCs), prolonged administration of iron, and the presence of hepatobiliary disorders. Inorganic particles that may accumulate include calcium, tar, and mineral dusts such as coal, silica, iron, lead, and silver. Mineral dusts generally are inhaled and accumulate in lung tissue (Figure 4-5). Inhaled dusts cause chronic inflammatory reactions in the lung, which generally result in destruction of pulmonary alveoli and capillaries and the formation of scar tissue. Over many years, the lung may become stiff and difficult to expand because of extensive scarring (see Chapter 23).

Deposits of calcium salts occur in conditions of altered calcium intake, excretion, or metabolism. Impaired renal excretion of phosphate may result in the formation of calcium phosphate salts that are deposited in the tissues of the eye, heart, and blood vessels. Calcification of the heart valves may cause obstruction to blood flow through the heart or interfere with valve closing. Calcification of blood vessels may result in narrowing of vessels and insufficient blood flow to distal tissues. Dead

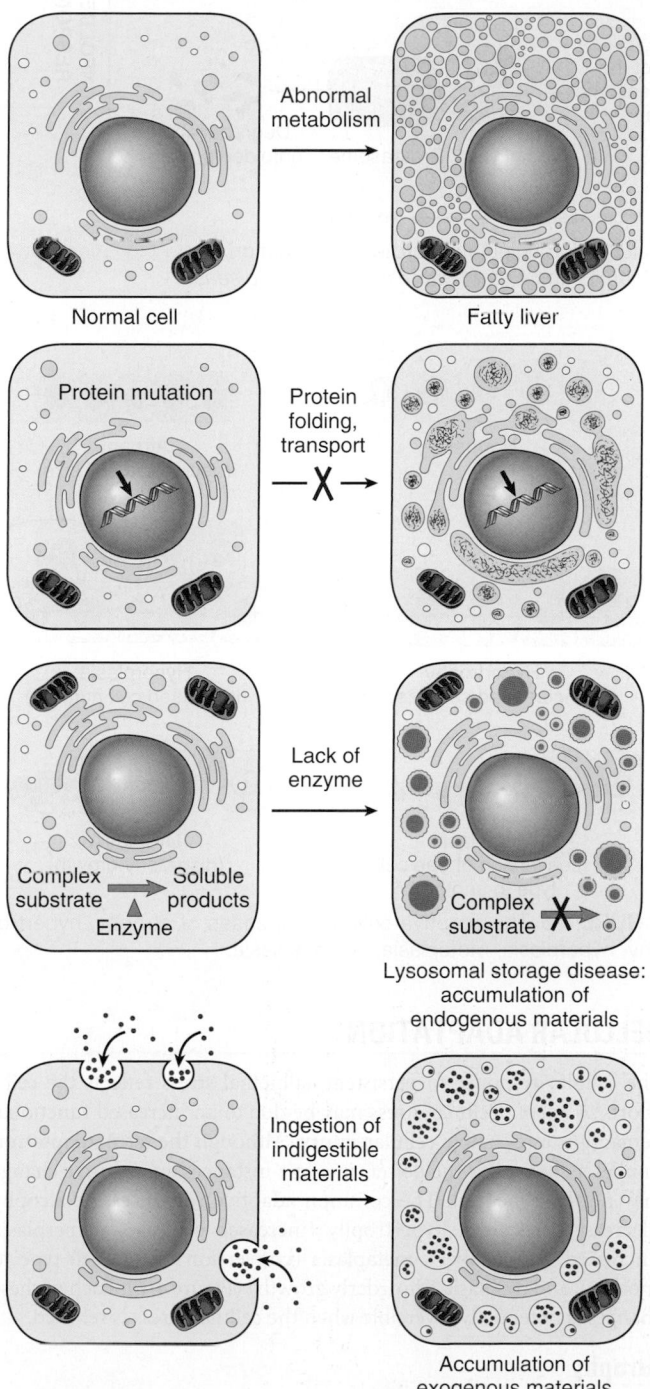

FIGURE 4-2 General mechanisms of intracellular accumulation: (1) abnormal metabolism as in fatty change in the liver, (2) mutations causing alterations in protein folding and transport so that defective proteins accumulate, (3) deficiency of critical enzyme responsible for lysosomal degradation, and (4) an inability to degrade phagocytosed particles such as coal dust. (From Kumar V et al: *Robbins and Cotran pathologic basis of disease,* ed 8, Philadelphia, 2010, Saunders, p 33.)

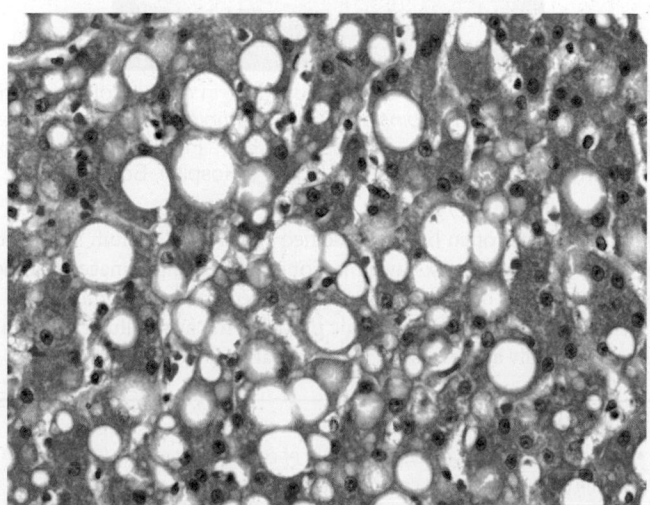

FIGURE 4-3 Fatty liver showing large intracellular vacuoles of lipid. (From Kumar V et al: *Robbins and Cotran pathologic basis of disease,* ed 8, Philadelphia, 2010, Saunders, p 34. Photograph courtesy Dr. James Crawford, Department of Pathology, University of Florida School of Medicine, Gainesville, FL.)

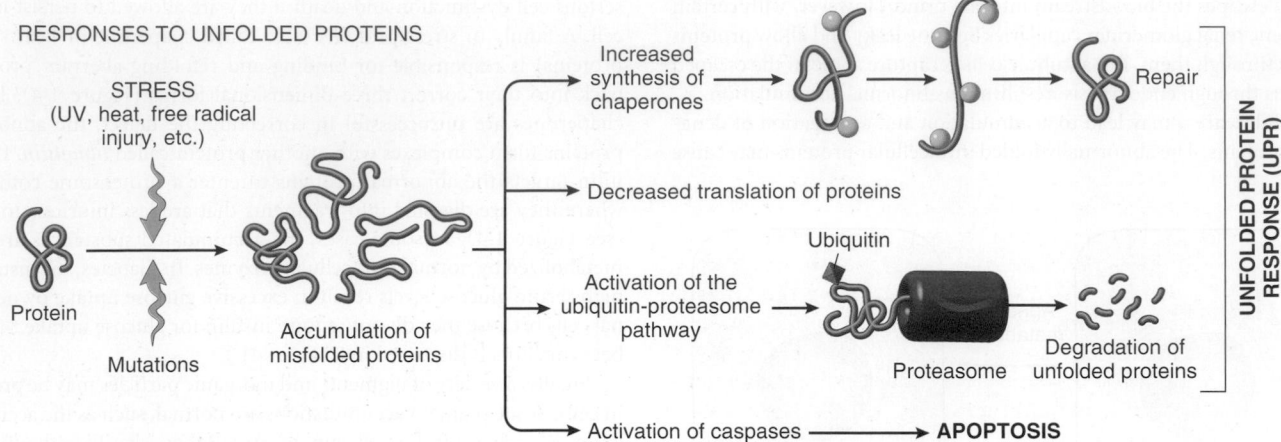

FIGURE 4-4 Roles of chaperone proteins in protein refolding and ubiquitin in protein degradation after stress-induced protein damage. (From Kumar V et al: *Robbins and Cotran pathologic basis of disease,* ed 8, Philadelphia, 2010, Saunders, p 31.)

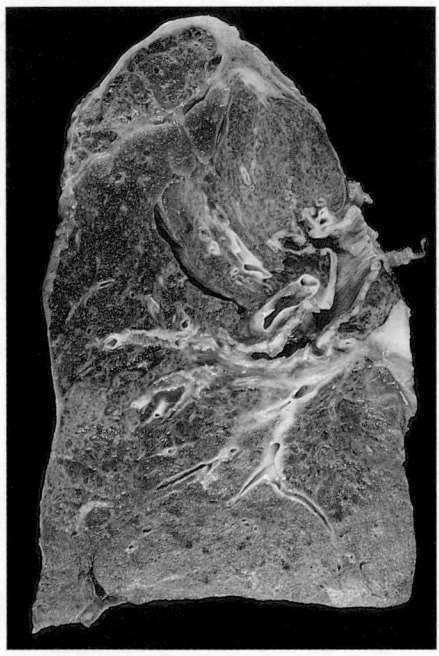

FIGURE 4-5 Accumulations of silicon dust in tissues of the lung. (From Kumar V et al: *Robbins and Cotran pathologic basis of disease,* ed 8, Philadelphia, 2010, Saunders, p 699. Photograph courtesy Dr. John Goldeski, Brigham and Women's Hospital, Boston, MA.)

and dying tissues often become calcified (filled with calcium salts) and appear as dense areas on x-ray films. For example, lung damage resulting from tuberculosis often is apparent as calcified areas, called *tubercles*.

With the exception of inorganic particles, the intracellular accumulations generally are reversible if the causative factors are removed.

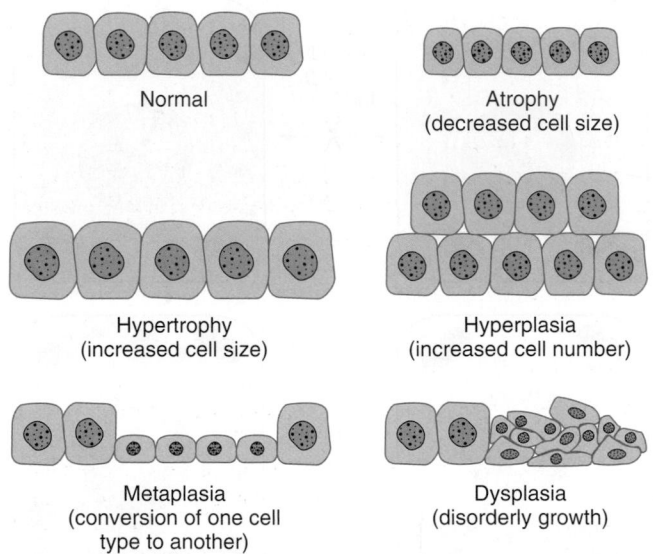

FIGURE 4-6 The adaptive cellular responses of atrophy, hypertrophy, hyperplasia, metaplasia, and dysplasia.

CELLULAR ADAPTATION

The cellular response to persistent, sublethal stress reflects the cell's efforts to adapt. Cellular stress may be due to an increased functional demand or a reversible cellular injury. Although the term **adaptation** implies a change for the better, in some instances an adaptive change may not be beneficial. The common adaptive responses are atrophy (decreased cell size), hypertrophy (increased cell size), hyperplasia (increased cell number), metaplasia (conversion of one cell type to another), and dysplasia (disorderly growth) (Figure 4-6). Each of these changes is potentially reversible when the cellular stress is relieved.

Atrophy

Atrophy occurs when cells shrink and reduce their differentiated functions in response to a variety of normal and injurious factors. The general causes of atrophy may be summarized as (1) disuse, (2) denervation, (3) ischemia, (4) nutrient starvation, (5) interruption of endocrine signals, (6) and persistent cell injury. Apparently, atrophy represents an effort by the cell to minimize its energy and nutrient consumption by decreasing the number of intracellular organelles and other structures.

> **KEY POINTS**
> - Hydropic swelling is an early indicator of cell injury. It results from Na$^+$-K$^+$ pump dysfunction at the cell membrane.
> - Intracellular accumulations of abnormal endogenous or exogenous particles indicate a disorder of cellular metabolism.
> - Damage from accumulation of abnormal intracellular protein is limited by chaperone proteins that attempt to refold the protein into its correct shape and by the ubiquitin-proteosome system that digests targeted proteins into fragments.

A common form of atrophy is the result of a reduction in functional demand, sometimes called **disuse atrophy.** For example, immobilization by bed rest or casting of an extremity results in shrinkage of skeletal muscle cells. On resumption of activity, the tissue resumes its normal size. Denervation of skeletal muscle results in a similar decrease in muscle size caused by loss of nervous stimulation. Inadequate blood supply to a tissue is known as **ischemia.** If the blood supply is totally interrupted, the cells will die, but chronic sublethal ischemia usually results in cell atrophy. The heart, brain, kidneys, and lower leg are common sites of ischemia. Atrophic changes in the lower leg attributable to ischemia include thin skin, muscle wasting, and hair loss. Atrophy also is a consequence of chronic nutrient starvation, whether the result of poor intake, absorption, or distribution to the tissues. Many glandular tissues throughout the body depend on growth-stimulating (trophic) signals to maintain size and function. For example, the adrenal cortex, thyroid, and gonads are maintained by trophic hormones from the pituitary gland and will atrophy in their absence. Atrophy that results from persistent cell injury is most commonly related to chronic inflammation and infection.

The biochemical pathways that result in cellular atrophy are imperfectly known; however, two pathways for protein degradation have been implicated. The first is the previously mentioned ubiquitin-proteosome system, which degrades targeted proteins into small fragments (see Figure 4-4). The second involves the lysosomes that may fuse with intracellular structures leading to hydrolytic degradation of the components. Certain substances apparently are resistant to degradation and remain in the lysosomal vesicles of atrophied cells. For example, lipofuscin is an age-related pigment that accumulates in residual vesicles in atrophied cells, giving them a yellow-brown appearance.

Hypertrophy

Hypertrophy is an increase in cell mass accompanied by an augmented functional capacity. Cells hypertrophy in response to increased physiologic or pathophysiologic demands. Cellular enlargement results primarily from a net increase in cellular protein content.[4] Like the other adaptive responses, hypertrophy subsides when the increased demand is removed; however, the cell may not entirely return to normal because of persistent changes in connective tissue structures. Organ enlargement may be a result of both an increase in cell size (hypertrophy) and an increase in cell number (hyperplasia). For example, an increase in skeletal muscle mass and strength in response to repeated exercise is primarily the result of hypertrophy of individual muscle cells, although some increase in cell number is also possible because muscle stem cells (satellite cells) are able to divide. Physiologic hypertrophy occurs in response to a variety of trophic hormones in sex organs—the breast and uterus, for example. Certain pathophysiologic conditions may place undue stress on some tissues, causing them to hypertrophy. Liver enlargement in response to bodily toxins and cardiac muscle enlargement in response to high blood pressure (Figure 4-7) represent hyperplastic and hypertrophic adaptations to pathologic conditions. Hypertrophic adaptation is particularly important for cells, such as differentiated muscle cells, that are unable to undergo mitotic division.

Hyperplasia

Cells that are capable of mitotic division generally increase their functional capacity by increasing the number of cells (**hyperplasia**) as well as by hypertrophy. Hyperplasia usually results from increased physiologic demands or hormonal stimulation. Persistent cell injury also may lead to hyperplasia. Examples of demand-induced hyperplasia include

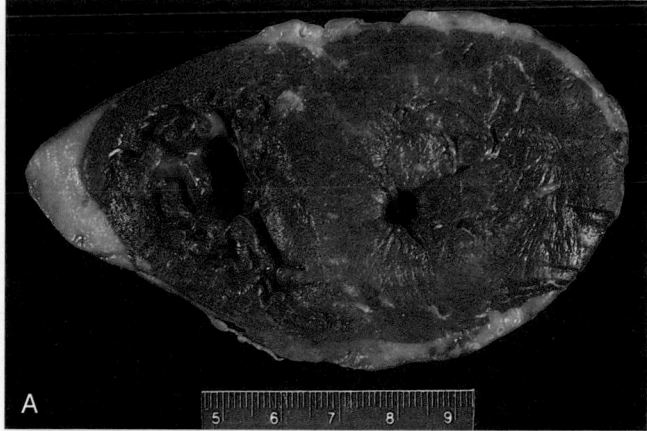
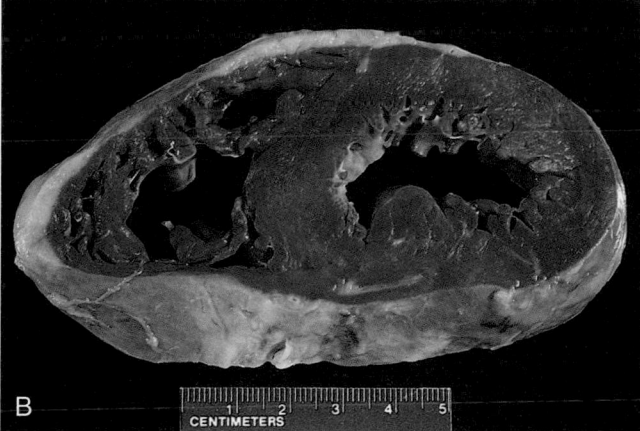

FIGURE 4-7 A, Hypertrophy of cardiac muscle in the left ventricular chamber. **B,** Compare with the thickness of the normal left ventricle. This is an example of cellular adaptation to an increased cardiac workload. (From Kumar V et al: *Robbins and Cotran pathologic basis of disease,* ed 8, Philadelphia, 2010, Saunders, p 6.)

an increase in RBC number in response to high altitude and liver enlargement in response to drug detoxification. Trophic hormones induce hyperplasia in their target tissues. Estrogen, for example, leads to an increase in the number of endometrial and uterine stromal cells. Dysregulation of hormones or growth factors can result in pathologic hyperplasia, such as that which occurs in thyroid or prostate enlargement.

Chronic irritation of epithelial cells often results in hyperplasia. Calluses and corns, for example, result from chronic frictional injury to the skin. The epithelium of the bladder commonly becomes hyperplastic in response to the chronic inflammation of cystitis.

Metaplasia

Metaplasia is the replacement of one differentiated cell type with another. This most often occurs as an adaptation to persistent injury, with the replacement cell type better able to tolerate the injurious stimulation.[1] Metaplasia is fully reversible when the injurious stimulus is removed. Metaplasia often involves the replacement of glandular epithelium with squamous epithelium. Chronic irritation of the bronchial mucosa by cigarette smoke, for example, leads to the conversion of ciliated columnar epithelium to stratified squamous epithelium. Metaplastic cells generally remain well differentiated and of the same tissue type, although cancerous transformations can occur. Some cancers of the lung, cervix, stomach, and bladder appear to derive from areas of metaplastic epithelium.

Dysplasia

Dysplasia refers to the disorganized appearance of cells because of abnormal variations in size, shape, and arrangement. Dysplasia occurs most frequently in hyperplastic squamous epithelium, but it may also be seen in the mucosa of the intestine. Dysplasia probably represents an adaptive effort gone astray. Dysplastic cells have significant potential to transform into cancerous cells and are usually regarded as *preneoplastic* lesions. (See Chapter 7 for a discussion of cancer.) Dysplasia that is severe and involves the entire thickness of the epithelium is called *carcinoma in situ*. Mild forms of dysplasia may be reversible if the inciting cause is removed.

KEY POINTS

- Adaptive cellular responses indicate cellular stress caused by altered functional demand or chronic sublethal injury.
- Hypertrophy and hyperplasia generally result from increased functional demand. Atrophy results from decreased functional demand or chronic ischemia. Metaplasia and dysplasia result from persistent injury.

IRREVERSIBLE CELL INJURY

Pathologic cellular death occurs when an injury is too severe or prolonged to allow cellular adaptation or repair. Two different processes may contribute to cell death in response to injury: necrosis and apoptosis. Necrosis usually occurs as a consequence of ischemia or toxic injury and is characterized by cell rupture, spilling of contents into the extracellular fluid, and inflammation. Apoptosis (from a Greek word meaning *falling off,* as in leaves from a tree) occurs in response to injury that does not directly kill the cell but triggers intracellular cascades that activate a cellular suicide response. Apoptotic cells generally do not rupture and are ingested by neighboring cells with minimal disruption of the tissue and without inflammation. Apoptosis is not always a pathologic process and occurs as a necessity of development and tissue remodeling.

Necrosis

Necrotic cells demonstrate typical morphologic changes, including a shrunken (pyknotic) nucleus that is subsequently degraded (karyolysis), a swollen cell volume, dispersed ribosomes, and disrupted plasma and organelle membranes (Figure 4-8). The disruption of the permeability barrier of the plasma membrane appears to be a critical event in the death of the cell.[5]

Localized injury or death of tissue is generally reflected in the entire system as the body attempts to remove dead cells and works to compensate for loss of tissue function. Several manifestations indicate that the system is responding to cellular injury and death. A general inflammatory response is often present, with general malaise, fever, increased heart rate, increased white blood cell (WBC) count, and loss of

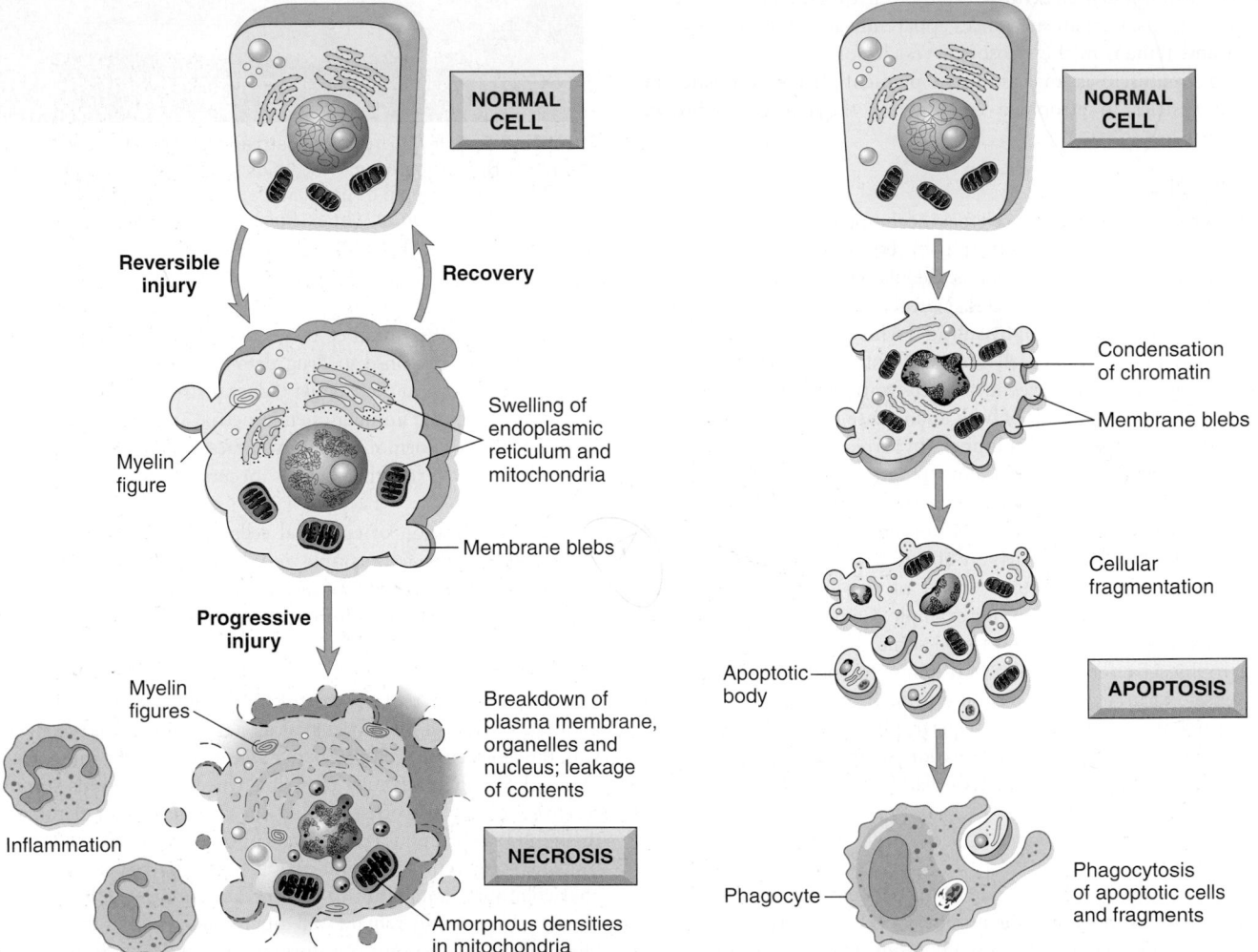

FIGURE 4-8 Comparison of cellular changes in necrosis and apoptosis. (From Kumar V et al: *Robbins and Cotran pathologic basis of disease,* ed 8, Philadelphia, 2010, Saunders, p 13.)

appetite. With the death of necrotic cells, intracellular contents are released and often find their way into the bloodstream. The presence of specific cellular enzymes in the blood is used as an indicator of the location and extent of cellular death. For example, an elevated serum amylase level indicates pancreatic damage, and an elevated creatine kinase (MB isoenzyme) or cardiac troponin level indicates myocardial damage. The location of pain caused by tissue destruction may also aid in the diagnosis of cellular death.

Four different types of tissue necrosis have been described: coagulative, liquefactive, fat, and caseous (Figure 4-9). They differ primarily in the type of tissue affected. *Coagulative* necrosis is the most common. Manifestations of coagulative necrosis are the same, regardless of the cause of cell death. In general, the steps leading to coagulative necrosis may be summarized as follows: (1) ischemic cellular injury, leading to (2) loss of the plasma membrane's ability to maintain electrochemical gradients, which results in (3) an influx of calcium ions and mitochondrial

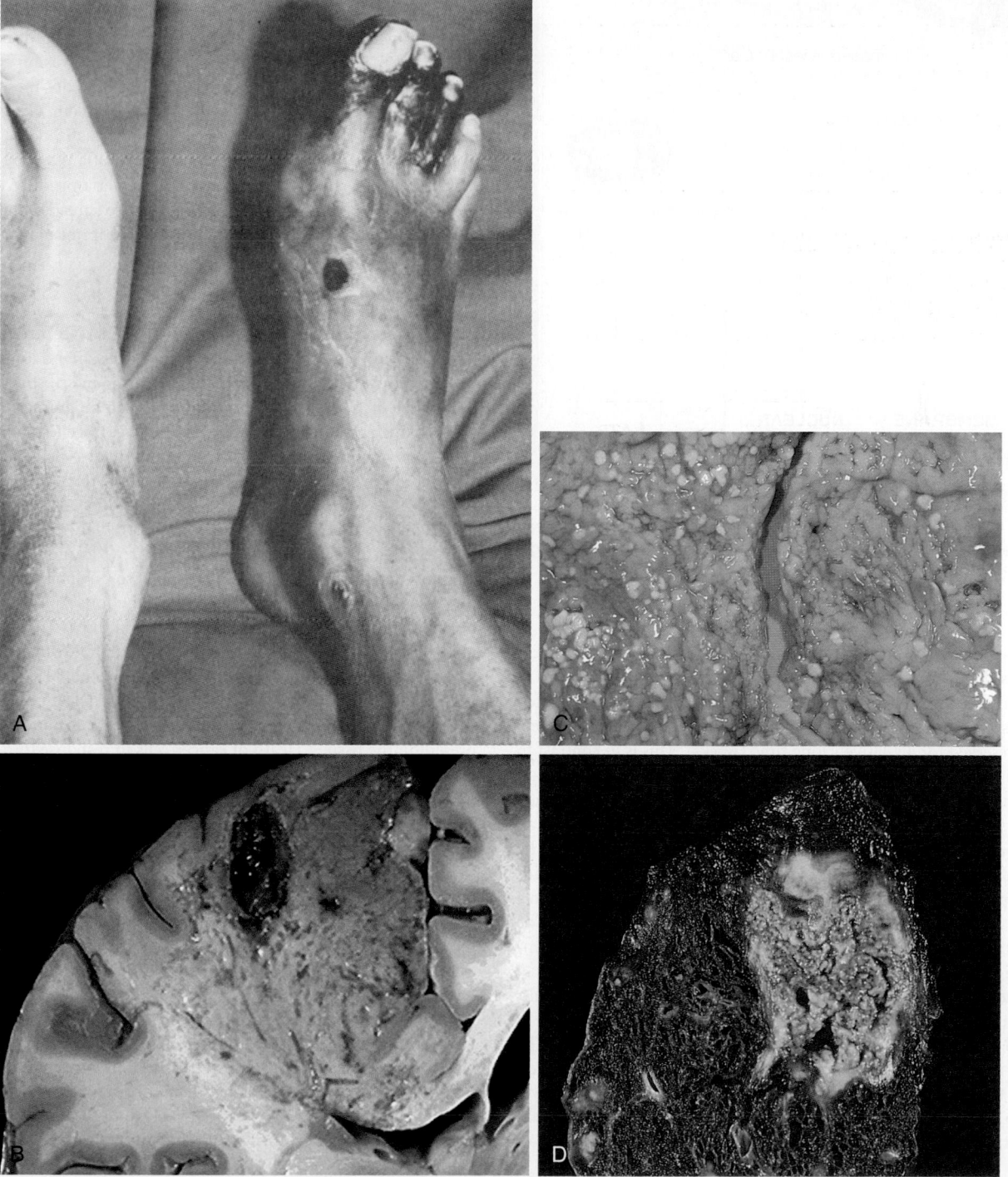

FIGURE 4-9 The four primary types of tissue necrosis. **A,** Coagulative; **B,** liquefactive; **C,** fat; **D,** caseous. (**A,** From Crowley L: *Introduction to human disease,* ed 4, Sudbury, MA, 1996, Jones and Bartlett, www.jbpub.com. Reprinted with permission. **B-D,** From Kumar V et al: *Robbins and Cotran pathologic basis of disease,* ed 8, Philadelphia, 2010, Saunders, pp 16-17.)

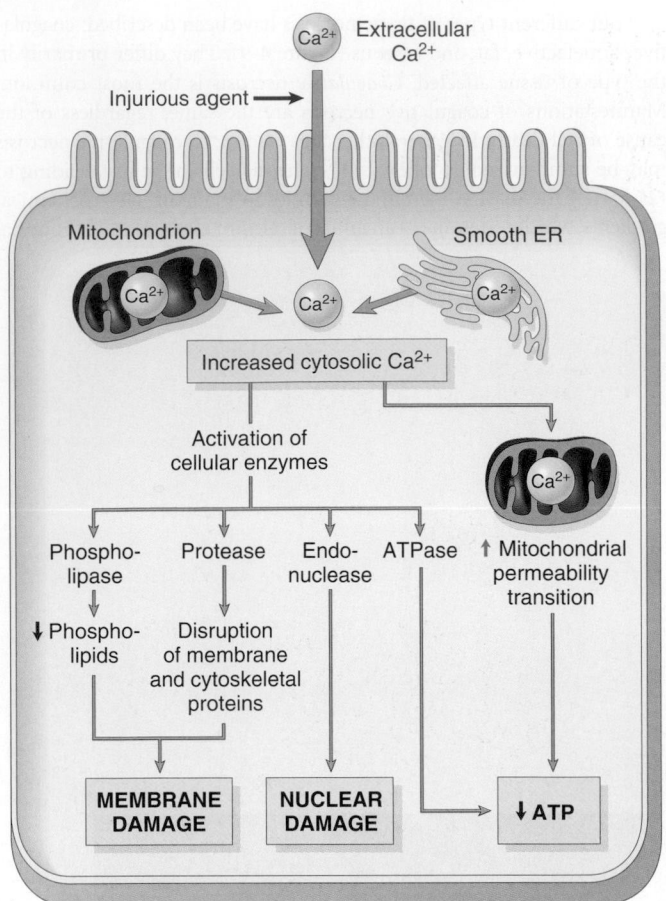

FIGURE 4-10 Cellular injury as a consequence of intracellular calcium overload. (From Kumar V et al: *Robbins and Cotran pathologic basis of disease,* ed 8, Philadelphia, 2010, Saunders, p 19.)

dysfunction, and (4) degradation of plasma membranes and nuclear structures (Figure 4-10). The area of coagulative necrosis is composed of denatured proteins and is relatively solid. The coagulated area is then slowly dissolved by proteolytic enzymes and the general tissue architecture is preserved for a relatively long time (weeks). This is in contrast to liquefactive necrosis.

When the dissolution of dead cells occurs very quickly, a liquefied area of lysosomal enzymes and dissolved tissue may result and form an abscess or cyst. This type of necrosis, called *liquefactive necrosis,* may be seen in the brain, which is rich in degradative enzymes and contains little supportive connective tissue. Liquefaction may also result from a bacterial infection that triggers a localized collection of WBCs. The phagocytic WBCs contain potent degradative enzymes that may completely digest dead cells, resulting in liquid debris.

Fat necrosis refers to death of adipose tissue and usually results from trauma or pancreatitis. The process begins with the release of activated digestive enzymes from the pancreas or injured tissue. The enzymes attack the cell membranes of fat cells, causing release of their stores of triglycerides. Pancreatic lipase can then hydrolyze the triglycerides to free fatty acids and glycerol, which precipitate as calcium soaps (saponification). Fat necrosis appears as a chalky white area of tissue.

Caseous necrosis is characteristic of lung tissue damaged by tuberculosis. The areas of dead lung tissue are white, soft, and fragile, resembling clumpy cheese. Dead cells are walled off from the rest of the lung tissue by inflammatory WBCs. In the center, the dead cells lose their

cellular structure but are not totally degraded. Necrotic debris may persist indefinitely.

Gangrene is a term used to describe cellular death involving a large area of tissue. Gangrene usually results from interruption of the major blood supply to a particular body part, such as the toes, leg, or bowel. Depending on the appearance and subsequent infection of the necrotic tissue, it is described as dry gangrene, wet gangrene, or gas gangrene. *Dry* gangrene is a form of coagulative necrosis characterized by blackened, dry, wrinkled tissue that is separated from adjacent healthy tissue by an obvious line of demarcation (see Figure 4-9, *A*). It generally occurs only on the extremities. Liquefactive necrosis may result in *wet* gangrene, which is typically found in internal organs, appears cold and black, and may be foul smelling because of the invasion of bacteria. Rapid spread of tissue damage and the release of toxins into the bloodstream make wet gangrene a life-threatening problem. *Gas* gangrene is characterized by the formation of bubbles of gas in damaged tissue. Gas gangrene is the result of infection of necrotic tissue by anaerobic bacteria of the genus *Clostridium.* These bacteria produce toxins and degradative enzymes that allow the infection to spread rapidly through the necrotic tissue. Gas gangrene may be fatal if not managed rapidly and aggressively.

Apoptosis

The number of cells in tissues is tightly regulated by controlling the rate of cell division and the rate of cell death. If cells are no longer needed, they activate a cellular death pathway resulting in cell suicide. In contrast to necrosis, which is messy and results in inflammation and collateral tissue damage, apoptosis is tidy and does not elicit inflammation. Apoptosis is not a rare event; large numbers of cells are continually undergoing programmed cell death as tissues remodel. During fetal development, for example, more than half of the nerve cells that form undergo apoptosis. It is estimated that more than 95% of the T lymphocytes that are generated in the bone marrow are induced to undergo apoptosis after reaching the thymus. These are normal physiologic processes that regulate normal system function. Apoptosis also has been implicated in pathologic cell death and disease. For example, it has been estimated that the area of tissue death following a myocardial infarction (heart attack) is about 20% necrotic and 80% apoptotic.[6] It is difficult to measure the degree of apoptotic cell death because neighboring cells rapidly ingest their apoptotic neighbors and few are ever present in the tissue.[7] Death of cancer cells in response to radiation or chemotherapy is believed to be primarily caused by apoptotic mechanisms. When the rate of apoptosis is greater than the rate of cell replacement, tissue or organ function may be impaired. Apoptosis is now recognized as a primary factor in diseases such as heart failure (Chapter 19) and dementia (Chapter 45). The mechanisms regulating apoptosis are complex, and only major concepts are included here.

There are two types of environmental or extrinsic signals that may induce apoptosis. First, apoptosis may be triggered by withdrawal of "survival" signals that normally suppress the apoptotic pathways.[7] Normal cells require a variety of signals from neighboring cells and from the extracellular matrix in order to stay alive (Figure 4-11). If these contacts or signals are removed, the cell death cascade is activated. Cancer cells are notorious for their ability to survive despite the lack of appropriate survival signals from their environment (see Chapter 7). A second mechanism of triggering apoptosis involves extracellular signals, such as the *Fas* ligand, that bind to the cell and trigger the death cascade though activation of "death receptors" (Figure 4-12).

Apoptosis can also be triggered by intrinsic pathways. Cells have ways to monitor their condition and usefulness internally. When excessive, irreparable damage occurs to the cell's DNA or other vital structures, growth and division stalls for a while to permit repair. If the

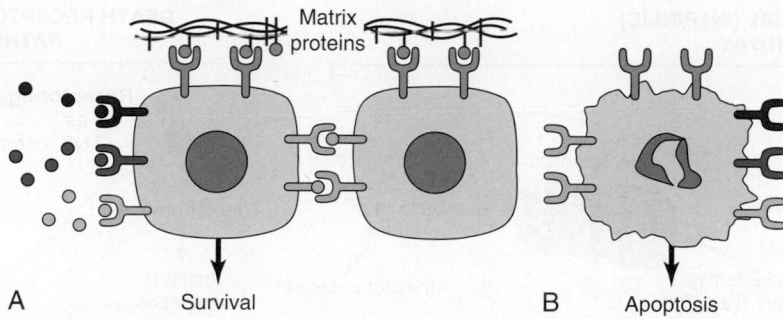

FIGURE 4-11 Each cell displays a set of receptors that enable it to respond to extracellular signals that control growth, differentiation, and survival. **A,** Extracellular signals are provided by the neighboring cells, secreted signaling molecules, and the extracellular matrix. **B,** Withdrawal of these survival signals induces the cell to initiate apoptosis.

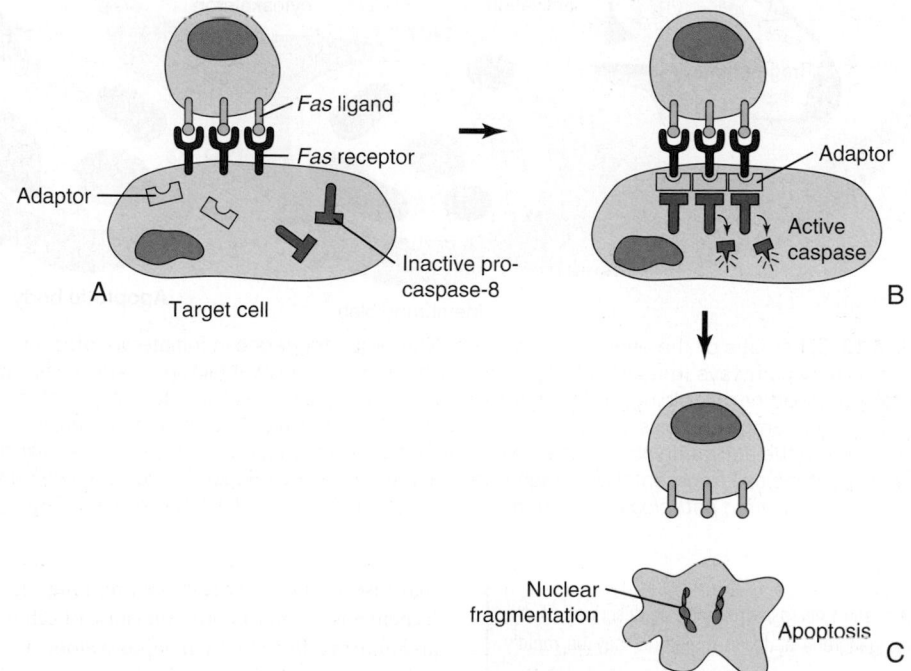

FIGURE 4-12 Induction of apoptosis by *Fas* ligand. **A,** Target cell binds to *Fas* ligand on a signaling cell. **B,** Active *Fas* receptors organize and activate caspases. **C,** The caspases degrade the nucleus and trigger cell death.

damage is too great, the cell will trigger its own death. Mitochondrial damage with leakage of cytochrome *c* into the cytoplasm is a critical activator of the intrinsic apoptotic pathway. This pathway is governed in part by a protein called p53. The amount of p53 in a cell is normally quite low but increases in response to cellular DNA damage. If high levels of p53 are sustained, apoptosis will occur.[8] Thus p53 is important in preventing the proliferation of cells with damaged DNA. A large number of cancers (50%) are associated with a mutation in the *P53* gene, which allows cancer cells to escape this monitoring system.[8]

Regardless of the initiating event, apoptosis involves numerous intracellular signals and enzymes (Figure 4-13). A family of enzymes called caspases is the main component of the proteolytic cascade that degrades key intracellular structures leading to cell death. The caspases are proenzymes that are activated in a cascade. Activation of a few *initiator* caspases at the beginning of the cascade results in a rapid domino effect of caspase activation. Some caspases cleave key proteins, such as the nuclear lamina, to destroy the nuclear envelope, whereas others activate still more enzymes that chop up the DNA. All of this

destruction is contained within an intact plasma membrane, and the cell remnants are then assimilated by its neighbors. Neighboring cells are prompted to ingest apoptotic cells because a phospholipid that is normally located only on the cytoplasmic side of a healthy cell (phosphatidylserine) flips to the outside of the lipid bilayer. This membrane lipid signals neighbors and tissue macrophages to bind and assimilate the cell components and suppresses the inflammatory response that normally accompanies phagocytosis.[7]

KEY POINTS

- Necrosis occurs when the injury is too severe or prolonged to allow adaptation and is usually a consequence of disrupted blood supply.
- Local and systemic indicators of cell death include pain, elevated serum enzyme levels, inflammation (fever, elevated WBC count, malaise), and loss of function.
- Different tissues exhibit necrosis of different types: heart (coagulative), brain (liquefactive), lung (caseous), and pancreas (fat).

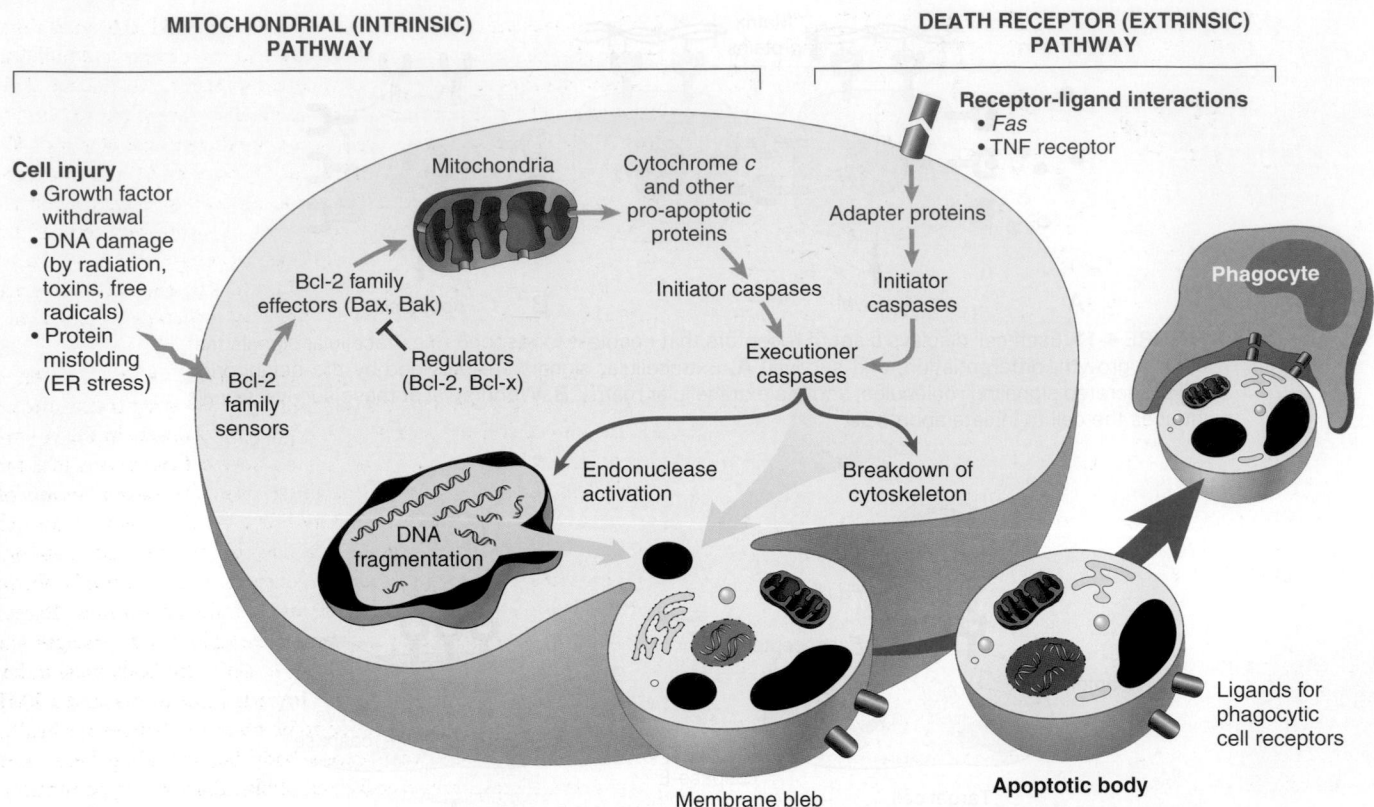

MITOCHONDRIAL (INTRINSIC) PATHWAY

DEATH RECEPTOR (EXTRINSIC) PATHWAY

FIGURE 4-13 Schematic of the events of apoptosis. Numerous triggers can initiate apoptosis through intrinsic cell injury pathways (mitochondrial), such as withdrawal of survival factors, various cell injuries, and protein overload or misfolding; or through extrinsic cell injury pathways (death receptors), such as binding to *Fas* or tumor necrosis factor receptors. A number of intracellular regulatory proteins may inhibit or promote the activation of caspases, which, when activated begin the process of cellular degradation and apoptotic cell fragmentation. Fragments are internalized by phagocytic cells. (From Kumar V et al: *Robbins and Cotran pathologic basis of disease*, ed 8, Philadelphia, 2010, Saunders, p 28.)

- Gangrene refers to a large area of necrosis that may be described as dry, wet, or gas gangrene. Gas gangrene and wet gangrene may be rapidly fatal.
- Apoptosis is cell death resulting from activation of intracellular signaling cascades that cause cell suicide. Apoptosis is tidy and not usually associated with systemic manifestations of inflammation.

ETIOLOGY OF CELLULAR INJURY

Cellular injury and death result from a variety of cellular assaults, including lack of oxygen and nutrients, infection and immune responses, chemicals, and physical and mechanical factors. The extent of cell injury and death depends in part on the duration and severity of the assault and in part on the prior condition of the cells. Well-nourished and somewhat adapted cells may withstand the injury better than cells that are poorly nourished or unadapted. Common causes of cellular injury include hypoxic injury, nutritional injury, infectious and immunologic injury, chemical injury, and physical and mechanical injury.

Ischemia and Hypoxic Injury

Living cells must receive a continuous supply of oxygen to produce ATP to power energy-requiring functions. Lack of oxygen (**hypoxia**) results in power failure within the cell. Tissue hypoxia is most often caused by *ischemia,* or the interruption of blood flow to an area, but it

may also result from heart failure, lung disease, and RBC disorders. Ischemia is the most common cause of cell injury in clinical medicine and injures cells faster than hypoxia alone. Faster injury occurs because ischemia not only disrupts the oxygen supply but also allows metabolic wastes to accumulate and deprives the cell of nutrients for glycolysis. The cellular events that follow oxygen deprivation are shown in Figure 4-14. Decreased oxygen delivery to the mitochondria causes ATP production in the cell to stall and ATP-dependent pumps, including the Na^+-K^+ and Ca^{2+} pumps, to fail. Sodium accumulation within the cell creates an osmotic gradient favoring water entry, resulting in hydropic swelling. Excess intracellular calcium collects in the mitochondria, further interfering with mitochondrial function. A small amount of ATP is produced by anaerobic glycolytic pathways, which metabolize cellular stores of glycogen. The pyruvate end products of glycolysis accumulate and are converted to lactate, causing cellular acidification. Lactate can escape into the bloodstream, resulting in **lactic acidosis,** which can be detected by laboratory tests. Cellular proteins and enzymes become progressively more dysfunctional as the pH falls. Up to a point, ischemic injury is reversible, but when the plasma, mitochondrial, and lysosomal membranes are critically damaged, cell death ensues.[1]

Cell death resulting from ischemia may be slow to develop, generally taking many minutes to hours. In fact, most cellular damage occurs after the blood supply to the tissues has been restored—a so-called *reperfusion injury.* Ischemia-reperfusion is a complex phenomenon, but three critical components have been identified: (1) calcium

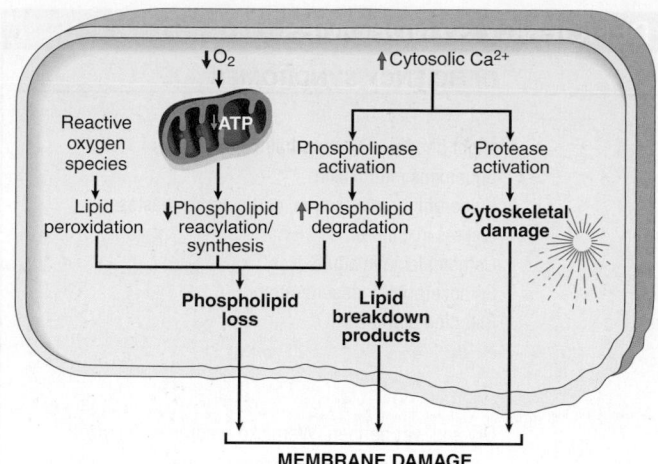

FIGURE 4-14 Mechanisms of ischemia-induced cell injury. Cellular damage often occurs through the formation of reactive oxygen radicals. (From Kumar V et al: *Robbins and Cotran pathologic basis of disease,* ed 8, Philadelphia, 2010, Saunders, p 22.)

overload, (2) formation of reactive oxygen molecules (free radicals), and (3) subsequent inflammation.

Restoration of blood flow to ischemic cells bathes them in a fluid high in calcium ions at a time when their ATP stores are depleted and they are unable to control ion flux across the cell membrane. Accumulation of calcium ions in the cytoplasm can trigger apoptosis or activate enzymes that degrade lipids in the membrane (lipid peroxidation).

The ischemic episode also primes cells for abnormal generation of reactive oxygen molecules, such as superoxide (O_2^-), peroxide (H_2O_2), and hydroxyl radicals (OH^-).[9] These reactive oxygen molecules are free radicals that have an unpaired electron in an outer orbital. They steal hydrogen atoms and form abnormal molecular bonds. Molecules that react with free radicals are in turn converted to free radicals, continuing the destructive cascade. Reactive oxygen species damage cell membranes, denature proteins, and disrupt cell chromosomes. Oxygen free radicals also have been linked to initiation of the inflammatory cascade.

Ischemia primes cells for the generation of oxygen radicals by allowing the buildup of ATP precursors, such as adenosine diphosphate (ADP) and pyruvate, during the period of hypoxia. When oxygen supply is reestablished, there is a disorganized burst of high-energy electrons that partially reduce oxygen and form oxygen radicals. The ischemia-reperfusion event frequently is followed by a generalized inflammatory state,[10] which may lead to ongoing cellular and organ damage for days and weeks following the initial event. WBCs recruited to the area release enzymes and other chemicals that further damage the cells in the area. (Mechanisms and causes of ischemic tissue injury are described further in Chapter 20.)

Nutritional Injury

Adequate amounts of fats, carbohydrates, proteins, vitamins, and minerals are essential for normal cellular function. Most of these essential nutrients must be obtained from external sources because the cell is unable to manufacture them. The cell is unable to synthesize many of the 20 amino acids needed to form the proteins of the body. Likewise, most vitamins and minerals must be obtained from exogenous sources. Cell injury results from deficiencies as well as excesses of essential nutrients.

Certain cell types are more susceptible to injury from particular nutritional imbalances. Iron deficiency, for example, primarily affects

RBCs, whereas vitamin D deficiency affects bones. All cell types must receive glucose for energy as well as fatty acid and amino acid building blocks to synthesize and repair cellular components. Nutritional deficiencies result from poor intake, altered absorption, impaired distribution by the circulatory system, or inefficient cellular uptake. Common causes of malnutrition include (1) poverty, (2) chronic alcoholism, (3) acute and chronic illness, (4) self-imposed dietary restrictions, and (5) malabsorption syndromes.[11] Vitamin deficiencies are common even in industrialized countries because of pervasive use of processed foods. Some examples of vitamin deficiency disorders are shown in Table 4-1. Deficiencies of minerals, especially iron, also are common (Table 4-2).

Nutritional excesses primarily result from excessive intake, although deficient cellular uptake by one cell type may contribute to excess nutrient delivery to other cell types. For example, in the condition of diabetes mellitus, some cell types have deficient receptors for insulin-dependent glucose uptake, which causes excessive amounts of glucose to remain in the bloodstream. As a result, cells that do not require insulin to take in glucose, such as neurons, may have abnormally high intracellular glucose levels. An excess of caloric intake above metabolic use produces overweight and obesity syndromes. Excess body fat can be estimated by measuring the ratio of body weight (in kilograms) to height (in meters squared) to derive the body mass index (BMI). A BMI greater than 27 kg/m^2 imparts a health risk and a BMI greater than 30 kg/m^2 is considered to be obesity.[12] Numerous health problems are associated with excess body fat, including heart and blood vessel disease, musculoskeletal strain, diabetes, hypertension, and gallbladder disease. Metabolism is explored in Chapter 42.

Infectious and Immunologic Injury

Bacteria and viruses are common infectious agents that may injure cells in a variety of ways. The virulence of a particular biological agent depends on its ability to gain access to the cell and its success in altering cellular functions. (See Chapter 8 for a detailed discussion of infectious processes.) Some of the injurious effects are directly due to the biological agent, but added injury may be done indirectly by triggering the body's immune response.

Most bacteria do not gain entry into the cell and so accomplish their injurious effects from the outside. (Notable exceptions include *Mycobacterium tuberculosis, Shigella, Legionella, Salmonella,* and *Chlamydia.*) Some bacteria produce and secrete powerful destructive enzymes that digest cellular membranes and connective tissues. For example, collagenase and lecithinase are produced by *Clostridium perfringens.* Other bacteria produce **exotoxins,** which interfere with specific cellular functions when released from the bacterium. *Clostridium botulinum* and *Clostridium tetani,* for example, produce life-threatening toxins that disrupt normal neuromuscular transmission. Cholera and diphtheria are well-known examples of exotoxin-related diseases. Exotoxins are primarily proteins and are generally susceptible to destruction by extremes of heat. Certain gram-negative bacteria (e.g., *Escherichia coli, Klebsiella pneumoniae*) contain another type of toxin, **endotoxin,** in their cell wall. On lysis of the bacteria, the endotoxin is released, causing fever, malaise, and even circulatory shock.[13]

The indirect cellular injury attributable to the bacteria-evoked immune response may be more damaging than the direct effects of the infectious agent. White blood cells secrete many enzymes and chemicals meant to destroy the invading organism, including histamines, kinins, complement, proteases, lymphokines, and prostaglandins. Normal body cells may be exposed to these injurious chemicals because they are too close to the site of immunologic battle. Immune cells are particularly adept at producing free radicals, which can attack host cell membranes and induce significant cell injury.

TABLE 4-1   VITAMINS: MAJOR FUNCTIONS AND DEFICIENCY SYNDROMES

VITAMIN	FUNCTIONS	DEFICIENCY SYNDROMES
Fat Soluble		
Vitamin A	A component of visual pigment	Night blindness, xerophthalmia, blindness
	Maintenance of specialized epithelia	Squamous metaplasia
	Maintenance of resistance to infection	Vulnerability to infection, particularly measles
Vitamin D	Facilitates intestinal absorption of calcium and phosphorus and mineralization of bone	Rickets in children Osteomalacia in adults
Vitamin E	Major antioxidant; scavenges free radicals	Spinocerebellar degeneration
Vitamin K	Cofactor in hepatic carboxylation of procoagulants—factors II (prothrombin), VII, IX, and X; and protein C and protein S	Bleeding diathesis
Water-Soluble		
Vitamin B_1 (thiamine)	As pyrophosphate, is coenzyme in decarboxylation reactions	Dry and wet beriberi, Wernicke syndrome, Korsakoff syndrome
Vitamin B_2 (riboflavin)	Converted to coenzymes flavin mononucleotide and flavin adenine dinucleotide, cofactors for many enzymes in intermediary metabolism	Ariboflavinosis, cheilosis, stomatitis, glossitis, dermatitis, corneal vascularization
Niacin	Incorporated into NAD and NAD phosphate; involved in a variety of redox reactions	Pellagra—"three D's": dementia, dermatitis, diarrhea
Vitamin B_6 (pyridoxine)	Derivatives serve as coenzymes in many intermediary reactions	Cheilosis, glossitis, dermatitis, peripheral neuropathy
Vitamin B_{12}	Required for normal folate metabolism and DNA synthesis Maintenance of myelinization of spinal cord tracts	Megaloblastic pernicious anemia and degeneration of posterolateral spinal cord tracts
Vitamin C	Serves in many oxidation-reduction (redox) reactions and hydroxylation of collagen	Scurvy
Folate	Essential for transfer and use of 1-carbon units in DNA synthesis	Megaloblastic anemia, neural tube defects
Pantothenic acid	Incorporated in coenzyme A	No nonexperimental syndrome recognized
Biotin	Cofactor in carboxylation reactions	No clearly defined clinical syndrome

From Kumar V et al: *Robbins and Cotran pathologic basis of disease,* ed 8, Philadelphia, 2010, Saunders, p 438.
NAD, Nicotinamide adenine dinucleotide.

TABLE 4-2   SELECTED TRACE ELEMENTS AND DEFICIENCY SYNDROMES

ELEMENT	FUNCTION	BASIS OF DEFICIENCY	CLINICAL FEATURES
Zinc	Component of enzymes, principally oxidases	Inadequate supplementation in artificial diets Interference with absorption by other dietary constituents Inborn error of metabolism	Rash around eyes, mouth, nose, and anus called acrodermatitis enteropathica Anorexia and diarrhea Growth retardation in children Depressed mental function Depressed wound healing and immune response Impaired night vision Infertility
Iron	Essential component of hemoglobin as well as a number of iron-containing metalloenzymes	Inadequate diet Chronic blood loss	Hypochromic microcytic anemia
Iodine	Component of thyroid hormone	Inadequate supply in food and water	Goiter and hypothyroidism
Copper	Component of cytochrome *c* oxidase, dopamine β-hydroxylase, tyrosine, lysyl oxidase, and unknown enzyme involved in cross-linking collagen	Inadequate supplementation in artificial diet Interference with absorption	Muscle weakness Neurologic defects Abnormal collagen cross-linking
Fluoride	Mechanism unknown	Inadequate supply in soil and water Inadequate supplementation	Dental caries
Selenium	Component of glutathione peroxidase Antioxidant with vitamin E	Inadequate amounts in soil and water	Myopathy Cardiomyopathy (Keshan disease)

From Kumar V et al: *Robbins and Cotran pathologic basis of disease,* ed 8, Philadelphia, 2010, Saunders, p 439.

Viruses are small pieces of genetic material that are able to gain entry into the cell.[14] They may be regarded as intracellular parasites that use the host cell's metabolic and synthetic machinery to survive and replicate. In some cases the virus remains in the cell for a considerable time without inflicting lethal injury. In other cases the virus causes rapid lysis and destruction of the host cell.

Virally infected cells may trigger their own destruction when they express viral proteins on the cell surface that are foreign to the host's immune system. The hepatitis B virus is an example of such an indirectly cytopathic virus that causes immune-mediated cell death. The hepatitis B virus consists of double-stranded DNA that becomes incorporated into the host cell's nucleus, where it can be transcribed by the

TABLE 4-3 HEALTH EFFECTS OF OUTDOOR AIR POLLUTANTS

POLLUTANT	POPULATIONS AT RISK	EFFECTS*
Ozone	Healthy adults and children	Decreased lung function
		Increased airway reactivity
	Athletes, outdoor workers	Lung inflammation
		Decreased exercise capacity
	Asthmatics	Increased hospitalizations
Nitrogen dioxide	Healthy adults	Increased airway reactivity
	Asthmatics	Decreased lung function
	Children	Increased respiratory tract infections
Sulfur dioxide	Healthy adults	Increased respiratory symptoms
	Patients with chronic lung disease	Increased mortality
	Asthmatics	Increased hospitalization
		Decreased lung function
Acid aerosols	Healthy adults	Altered mucociliary clearance
	Children	Increased respiratory tract infections
	Asthmatics	
		Decreased lung function
		Increased hospitalizations
Particulates	Children	Increased respiratory tract infections
	Individuals with chronic lung or heart disease	Decreased lung function
		Excess mortality
	Asthmatics	Increased attacks

From Kumar V et al: *Robbins and Cotran pathologic basis of disease,* ed 8, Philadelphia, 2010, Saunders, p 404.
*See Chapters 22 and 23 for a discussion of respiratory disorders.

TABLE 4-4 SELECTED INDOOR AIR POLLUTANTS WITH SIGNIFICANT HEALTH RISKS

POLLUTANT	SOURCE
Carbon monoxide	Fuel combustion, fire, furnace
Wood smoke	Fireplaces, woodstoves
Formaldehyde	Manufacture of construction materials
Radon	Natural ground radiation
Asbestos fibers	Old insulation, shingles
Manufactured mineral fibers	Insulation, building materials
Aerosols	Spray bottle propellants

normal DNA polymerases. The mRNA transcripts of the viral genes are transported to the cytoplasm and translated into structural proteins and enzymes, which are used to make more copies of the virus. Such virally infected cells may remain functional virus factories until they are destroyed by the host's immune system.

Chemical Injury

Toxic chemicals or poisons are plentiful in the environment (Tables 4-3 and 4-4). Some toxic chemicals cause cellular injury directly, whereas others become injurious only when metabolized into reactive chemicals by the body. Carbon tetrachloride (CCl_4) is an example of the latter.[15] Carbon tetrachloride, a formerly used dry-cleaning agent, is converted to a highly toxic **free radical,** CCl_3^-, by liver cells. The free radical is very reactive, forming abnormal chemical bonds in the cell and ultimately destroying the cellular membranes of liver cells, causing liver failure. In high doses, acetaminophen, a commonly used analgesic, may have similar toxic effects on the liver.

Many toxins are inherently reactive and do not require metabolic activation to exert their effects. Common examples are heavy metals (e.g., lead and mercury), toxic gases, corrosives, and antimetabolites. Some toxins have an affinity for a particular cell type or tissue, whereas others exert widespread systemic effects. For example, carbon monoxide binds tightly and selectively to hemoglobin, preventing the red blood cell from carrying sufficient oxygen. Lead poisoning, however, has widespread effects, including effects on nervous tissue, blood cells, and the kidney. Extremely acidic or basic chemicals are directly corrosive to cellular structures. Certain chemicals interfere with normal metabolic processes of the cell. Some of these antimetabolites have been utilized in the form of cytotoxic agents for the management of cancer.

Physical and Mechanical Injury

Injurious physical and mechanical factors include extremes of temperature, abrupt changes of atmospheric pressure, mechanical deformation, electricity, and ionizing radiation.[11]

Extremes of cold result in the hypothermic injury known as frostbite. Before actual cellular freezing, severe vasoconstriction and increased blood viscosity may result in ischemic injury. With continued exposure to cold, a rebound vasodilatory response may occur, leading to intense swelling and peripheral nerve damage. The cytoplasmic solution may freeze, resulting in the formation of intracellular ice crystals and rupture of cellular components. Frostbite generally affects the extremities, ears, and nose, and is often complicated by gangrenous necrosis.

Extremes of heat result in hyperthermic injury or burns. High temperatures cause microvascular coagulation and may accelerate metabolic processes in the cell. Burns result from direct tissue destruction by high temperatures and are classified according to the degree of tissue destruction. Burns are discussed in Chapter 54.

Abrupt changes in atmospheric pressure may result from high-altitude flying, deep-sea diving, and explosions. Pressure changes may interfere with gas exchange in the lungs, cause the formation of gas emboli in the bloodstream, collapse the thorax, and rupture internal organs. A well-known example of pressure injury is the condition of "the bends," which afflicts deep-sea divers who surface too quickly. The rapid decrease in water pressure results in the formation of bubbles of nitrogen gas in the blood, which may obstruct the circulation and cause ischemic injury.

Destruction of cells and tissues resulting from mechanical deformation ranges from mild abrasion to severe lacerating trauma. Cell death may result from direct trauma to cell membranes and resulting blood loss or from obstruction of blood flow and hypoxia. Nonpenetrating trauma generally results from physical impact with a blunt object such as a fist, a car steering wheel, or the pavement. Surgery is a common cause of tissue trauma. Other causes of penetrating trauma are bite, knife, and gun wounds. Trauma-induced inflammatory swelling may further compromise injured tissues.

Electrical injury may occur when the cells of the body act as conductors of electricity. The electrical current damages tissues in two ways: (1) by disruption of neural and cardiac impulses, and (2) by hyperthermic destruction of tissues. Resistance to the flow of electrons results in heat production, which damages the tissues. The current tends to follow the path of least resistance—through neurons and body fluids—causing violent muscle contractions, thermal injury, and coagulation in

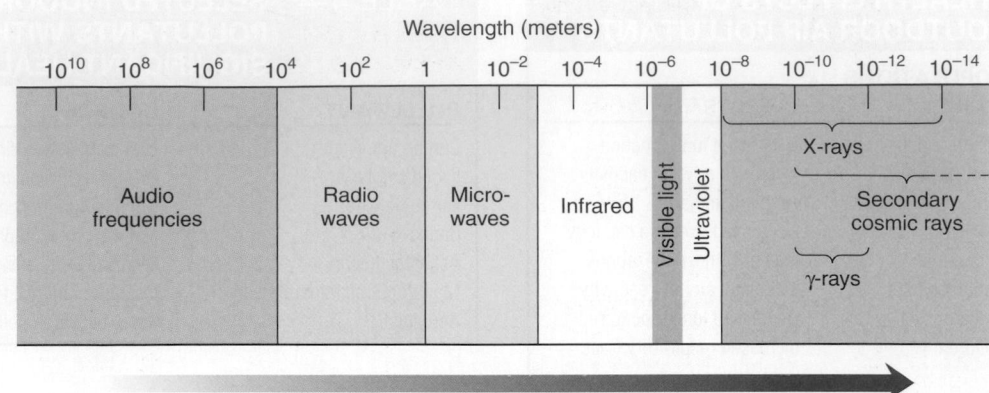

Wavelength (meters)

| 10^{10} | 10^8 | 10^6 | 10^4 | 10^2 | 1 | 10^{-2} | 10^{-4} | 10^{-6} | 10^{-8} | 10^{-10} | 10^{-12} | 10^{-14} |

Audio frequencies | Radio waves | Micro-waves | Infrared | Visible light | Ultraviolet | X-rays | Secondary cosmic rays | γ-rays

Increasing frequency and increasing energy

FIGURE 4-15 Types of electromagnetic radiation.

blood vessels. In general, greater injury is suffered with high-voltage alternating current applied to a low-resistance area (e.g., wet skin).

There are many forms of electromagnetic radiation, ranging from low-energy radio waves to high-energy γ-rays or photons (Figure 4-15). Radiation is capable of injuring cells directly by breaking chemical bonds and indirectly by generating free radicals. Cellular DNA is particularly susceptible to damage from radiation exposure.[16] A direct hit of the radiant energy on the DNA molecule may result in breakage of the chemical bonds holding the linear DNA together. This type of direct bond breakage generally results from the high-energy forms of radiation, such as x-rays and γ-rays. The molecular bonds of DNA also may be indirectly disrupted by ionizing radiation. *Ionization* refers to the ability of the radiant energy to split water molecules by knocking off orbital electrons (**radiolysis**). Radiolysis creates activated free radicals that steal electrons from other molecules and disrupt chemical bonds. Many forms of radiation are capable of ionization, but the medium-energy α and β particles that result from decay of atomic nuclei are especially destructive. Low-energy electromagnetic radiation, such as that created by microwaves, ultrasound, computers, and infrared light, cannot break chemical bonds, but it can cause rotation and vibration of atoms and molecules.[17] The rotational and vibrational energy is then converted to heat. It is probable that the resulting localized hyperthermia may result in cellular injury. Early studies reported a higher incidence of certain cancers in persons occupationally exposed to radiofrequency microwave electromagnetic radiation, but further analysis failed to confirm these findings.[11]

At the cellular level, radiation has two primary effects: (1) genetic damage and (2) acute cell destruction (Figure 4-16). The vulnerability of a tissue to radiation-induced genetic damage depends on its rate of proliferation. Genetic damage to the DNA of a long-lived, nonproliferating cell may be of little consequence, whereas tissues with rapid cellular division have less opportunity to repair damaged DNA before passing it on to the next generation of cells. (Genetic mutation is discussed in Chapter 6.) Hematopoietic, mucosal, gonadal, and fetal cells are particularly susceptible to genetic radiation damage.

Radiation-induced cell death is attributed primarily to the radiolysis of water, with resulting free radical damage to the plasma membrane. Whole-body exposure to sufficiently high levels of radiation (300 rad) results in acute radiation sickness with hematopoietic failure, destruction of the epithelial layer of the gastrointestinal tract, and neurologic dysfunction. The high levels of irradiation that cause acute radiation sickness are associated with events such as nuclear accidents and bombings. Radiation exposure from diagnostic x-rays, cosmic

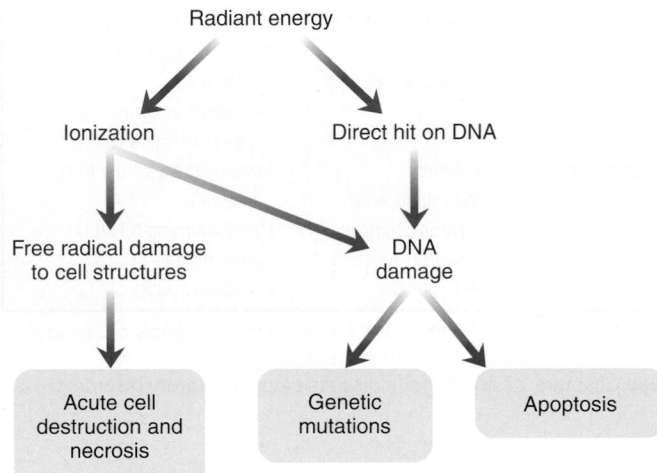

FIGURE 4-16 The mechanism of radiation-induced genetic and cell injury.

rays, and natural radiant chemicals in the earth is far below the level that would result in acute radiation sickness. The signs and symptoms of acute radiation sickness are shown in Figure 4-17. The fact that radiation induces cell death in proliferating cells is used to advantage in the management of some forms of cancer. Radiation therapy may be used when a cancerous growth is confined to a particular area. Injury associated with radiation therapy is generally localized to the irradiated area. Small arteries and arterioles in the area may be damaged, leading to blood clotting and fibrous deposits that compromise tissue perfusion. Most irradiated cells are thought to die through the process of apoptosis rather than from direct killing effects of radiation.[18] Radiation induces cell damage that triggers the apoptotic pathway in cells that cannot efficiently repair the damage. Cells most susceptible to apoptotic death are those that tend to have high rates of division.

> **KEY POINTS**
> - Hypoxia is an important cause of cell injury that usually results from poor oxygenation of the blood (hypoxemia) or inadequate delivery of blood to the cells (ischemia).
> - Reperfusion injury to cells may occur when circulation is restored, as a result of the production of partially reduced oxygen molecules that damage cell membranes and trigger immune-mediated injury.

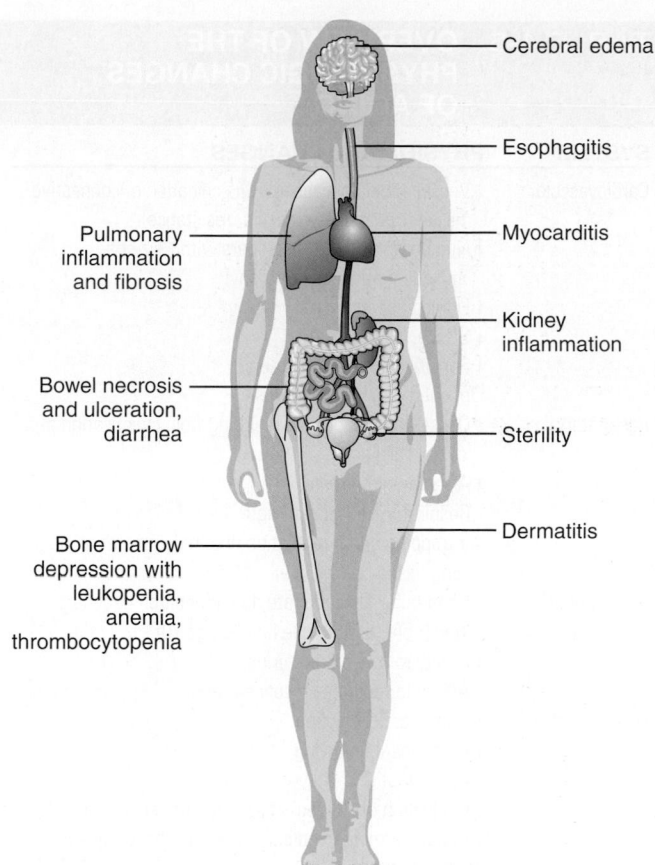

FIGURE 4-17 Signs and symptoms of acute radiation sickness.

- Nutritional injury is a common cause of dysfunction and disease. Malnutrition is rampant in many poor countries, whereas industrialized nations are facing an epidemic of obesity-related disorders, including heart disease and diabetes.
- Cellular damage attributable to infection and immunologic responses is common. Some bacteria and viruses damage cells directly, whereas others stimulate the host's immune system to destroy the host's cells.
- Chemical, physical, and mechanical factors cause cell injury in various ways. Chemicals may interfere with normal metabolic processes in the cell. Injury resulting from physical factors, such as burns and frostbite, causes direct destruction of tissues. Radiation-induced cell death is primarily a result of radiolysis of water, with resulting free radical damage to the cell membrane.

CELLULAR AGING

The inevitable process of aging and death has been the subject of interest and investigation for centuries. Despite scientific study and the search for the "fountain of youth," a satisfactory explanation for the process of cellular aging and methods for halting the aging process have not been revealed. The maximal human life span has remained constant at about 90 to 110 years, despite significant progress in the management of diseases.[19] It seems apparent that aging is distinct from disease, and that the life span is limited by the aging process itself rather than by the ravages of disease. Although the elderly are certainly more vulnerable to diseases, the aging process and disease processes are generally viewed as different phenomena. In practice, the distinction between aging and disease may be difficult to make. For example, the aging skeleton normally loses some bone mass, but too much bone

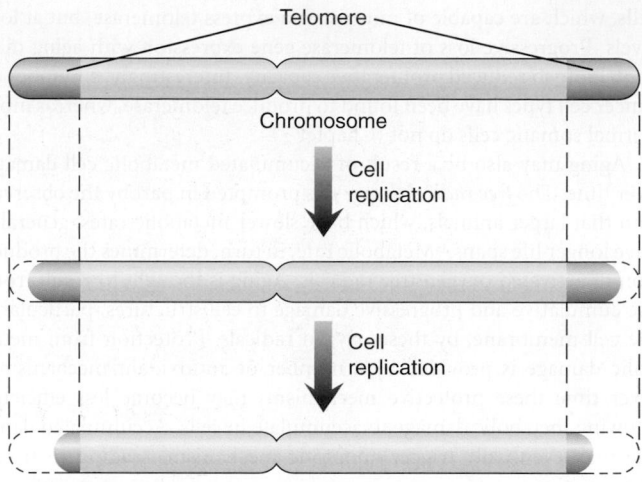

FIGURE 4-18 The end caps of the chromosomes are called *telomeres.* In most body cells, the telomeres progressively shorten with each cell replication until a critical point is reached, at which time the cell becomes dormant or dies.

loss results in osteoporosis—a disease process. Likewise, a loss of blood vessel elasticity is generally viewed as a normal aging change, but at what point does too much arterial stiffness become abnormal? This confusion results from the continued inability to identify the irreversible and universal processes of cellular aging as separate from the potentially reversible effects of disease.

Cellular Basis of Aging

Cellular aging is the cumulative result of a progressive decline in the proliferative and reparative capacity of cells coupled with exposure to environmental factors that cause accumulation of cellular and molecular damage. Several mechanisms are believed to be responsible for cellular aging. These include DNA damage, reduced proliferative capacity of stem cells, and accumulation of metabolic damage.

Damage to cellular DNA is a common phenomenon resulting from various factors, including ultraviolet radiation, oxidative stress from normal metabolism, and errors in DNA replication. A host of DNA repair mechanisms is present in normal cells to prevent accumulation of DNA damage. With aging these repair systems appear to become less able to keep pace with DNA damage, and cell replication may be inhibited or apoptosis initiated. Support for this idea comes from the premature aging syndromes that are associated with defective DNA repair mechanisms.

The *programmed senescence theory* states that aging is the result of an intrinsic genetic program. Support for the theory of a genetically programmed life span comes primarily from studies of cells in culture. In classic experiments by Hayflick, fibroblastic cells in culture were shown to undergo a finite number of cell divisions.[20] Fibroblasts taken from older individuals underwent fewer cell divisions than those from younger individuals. Given an adequate environment, the information encoded in the cellular genome is thought to dictate the number of possible cell replications, after which damaged or lost cells are no longer replaced. It has been postulated that cells undergo a finite number of replications because the chromosomes shorten slightly with each cell division until some critical point is reached (Figure 4-18), at which time the cell becomes dormant or dies. The end caps of the chromosomes, called **telomeres,** are the sections that shorten with each cell division.[21] Certain cells (germ cells, such as egg and sperm) are able to replenish their telomeres, which gives them potential immortality. The enzyme that rebuilds the telomeres has been named *telomerase.* Stem cells, which are capable of mitosis, also express telomerase, but at low levels. Progressive loss of telomerase gene expression with aging may contribute to reduced proliferative capacity. Interestingly, a number of cancer cell types have been found to produce telomerase, whereas most normal somatic cells do not (Chapter 7).

Aging may also be a result of accumulated metabolic cell damage over time. The *free radical theory* was prompted in part by the observation that larger animals, which have slower metabolic rates, generally have longer life spans.[1] Metabolic rate, in turn, determines the production of activated oxygen free radicals. Aging is thought to result from the cumulative and progressive damage to cell structures, particularly the cell membrane, by these oxygen radicals. Protection from metabolic damage is provided by a number of antioxidant mechanisms. Over time these protective mechanisms may become less efficient, allowing metabolic damage to accumulate in cells. Accumulated damage may eventually trigger apoptotic mechanisms leading to tissue degeneration.

Physiologic Changes of Aging

All the body systems show age-related changes that can be generally described as a decrease in functional reserve or inability to adapt to environmental demands. An overview of the tissue and systemic changes of aging is presented in Table 4-5. The details of age-related changes in the various body systems are described in later chapters of this book.

KEY POINTS

- Aging is theoretically distinct from disease. The maximal life span is limited by the aging process itself rather than by the ravages of disease.
- Aging is thought to be the result of accumulated DNA damage, decreased proliferative capacity of stem cells, and accumulated metabolic damage. Cells may age more quickly when DNA repair mechanisms are faulty and when metabolic damage is excessive because of reduced antioxidant activity.
- Age-related changes in body systems can generally be described as a decrease in functional reserve and a reduced ability to adapt to environmental demands.

SOMATIC DEATH

Death of the entire organism is called *somatic death*. In contrast to localized cell death, no immunologic or inflammatory response occurs in somatic death. The general features of somatic death include the absence of respiration and heartbeat. However, this definition of death is insufficient because, in some cases, breathing and cardiac activity may be restored by resuscitative efforts. Within several minutes of cardiopulmonary arrest, the characteristics of irreversible somatic death become apparent. Body temperature falls, the skin becomes pale, and blood and body fluids collect in dependent areas. Within 6 hours, the accumulation of calcium and the depletion of ATP result in perpetual actin-myosin cross-bridge formation in muscle cells. The presence of stiffened muscles throughout the body after death is called *rigor mortis.* Rigor mortis progresses to limpness or flaccidity as the tissues of the body begin to deteriorate. Tissue deterioration or putrefaction becomes apparent 24 to 48 hours after death.[22] Putrefaction is associated with the widespread release of lytic enzymes in tissues throughout the body, a process called *postmortem autolysis.*

The determination of "brain death" has become necessary because of the technological ability to keep the heart and lungs working through artificial means, even though the brain is no longer functional. Criteria

TABLE 4-5 OVERVIEW OF THE PHYSIOLOGIC CHANGES OF AGING

SYSTEM	PHYSIOLOGIC CHANGES
Cardiovascular	↓ Vessel elasticity caused by calcification of connective tissue (↑ pulmonary vascular resistance)
	↓ Number of heart muscle fibers with ↑ size of individual fibers (hypertrophy)
	↓ Filling capacity
	↓ Stroke volume
	↓ Sensitivity of baroreceptors
	Degeneration of vein valves
Respiratory	↓ Chest wall compliance resulting from calcification of costal cartilage
	↓ Alveolar ventilation
	↓ Respiratory muscle strength
	Air trapping and ↓ ventilation due to degeneration of lung tissue (↓ elasticity)
Renal/urinary	↓ Glomerular filtration rate due to nephron degeneration (↓ one third to one half by age 70)
	↓ Ability to concentrate urine
	↓ Ability to regulate H^+ concentration
Gastrointestinal	↓ Muscular contraction
	↓ Esophageal emptying
	↓ Bowel motility
	↓ Production of HCl, enzymes, and intrinsic factor
	↓ Hepatic enzyme production and metabolic capacity
	Thinning of stomach mucosa
Neurologic/sensory	Nerve cells degenerate and atrophy
	↓ Of 25-45% of neurons
	↓ Number of neurotransmitters
	↓ Rate of conduction of nerve impulses
	Loss of taste buds
	Loss of auditory hair cells and sclerosis of eardrum
Musculoskeletal	↓ Muscle mass
	↑ Bone demineralization
	↑ Joint degeneration, erosion, and calcification
Immune	↓ Inflammatory response
	↓ In T cell function owing to involution of thymus gland
Integumentary	↓ Subcutaneous fat
	↓ Elastin
	Atrophy of sweat glands
	Atrophy of epidermal arterioles causing altered temperature regulation

for determining brain death as proof of somatic death may vary by geographic area but generally include unresponsiveness, flaccidity, absence of brainstem reflexes (e.g., swallowing, gagging, pupil and eye movements), absence of respiratory effort when the subject is removed from the mechanical ventilator, absence of electrical brain waves, and lack of cerebral blood flow.

KEY POINTS

- Somatic death is characterized by the absence of respirations and heartbeat. Definitions of brain death have been established to describe death in instances in which heartbeat and respiration are maintained mechanically.
- After death, body temperature falls, blood and body fluids collect in dependent areas, and rigor mortis ensues. Within 24 to 48 hours the tissues begin to deteriorate and rigor mortis gives way to flaccidity.

SUMMARY

Cells and tissues face many challenges to survival, including injury from lack of oxygen and nutrients, infection and immune responses, chemicals, and physical and mechanical factors. Cells respond to environmental changes or injury in three general ways: (1) If the change is mild or short lived, the cell may withstand the assault and return to its preinjury status. (2) The cell may adapt to a persistent but sublethal injury by changing its structure or function. (3) Cell death by apoptosis or necrosis may occur if the injury is too severe or prolonged. Characteristics of reversible cell injury include hydropic swelling and the accumulation of abnormal substances. Cell necrosis is characterized by irreversible loss of function, release of cellular enzymes into the bloodstream, and an inflammatory response. The disruption of the permeability barrier of the plasma membrane appears to be a critical event in necrotic cellular death. Apoptosis is characterized by a tidy, noninflammatory autodigestion of the cell.

Aging is a normal physiologic process characterized by a progressive decline in functional capacity and adaptive ability. The biological basis of aging remains largely a mystery, but several theories have been proposed to explain certain aspects of the process. At present, most sources differentiate between the biological alterations of aging and the alterations consequent to disease processes. In practice, however, the distinction may be difficult to make.

REFERENCES

1. Kumar V, Abbas A, Fausto N, Aster J: Cellular responses to stress and toxic insults: adaptation, injury, and death. In Kumar V, Abbas A, Fausto N, Aster J, editors: *Robbins and Cotran pathologic basis of disease*, ed 8, Philadelphia, 2010, Saunders, pp 3–42.

2. Crawford J, Liu C: Liver and biliary tract. In Kumar V, Abbas A, Fausto N, Aster J, editors: *Robbins and Cotran pathologic basis of disease*, ed 8, Philadelphia, 2010, Saunders, pp 833–890.

3. Maitra A: The endocrine system. In Kumar V, Abbas A, Fausto N, Aster J, editors: *Robbins and Cotran pathologic basis of disease*, ed 8, Philadelphia, 2010, Saunders, pp 1097–1164.

4. Yarasheski KE: Exercise, aging, and muscle protein metabolism, *J Gerontol A Biol Sci Med Sci* 58(10):M918–M922, 2003.

5. Han SI, Kim TH, Kim YS: Role of apoptotic and necrotic cell death under physiologic conditions, *BMB Rep* 41(1):1–10, 2008.

6. Nadal-Ginard B, et al: Myocyte death, growth, and regeneration in cardiac hypertrophy and failure, *Circ Res* 92:139–150, 2003.

7. Alberts B, et al: Apoptosis. In Alberts B, et al, editors: *Molecular biology of the cell*, ed 5, New York, 2008, Garland Science, pp 1115–1129.

8. Alberts B, et al: Mechanisms of cell communication. In Alberts B, et al, editors: *Molecular biology of the cell*, ed 5, New York, 2008, Garland Science, pp 879–964.

9. Guo MF, Yu JZ, Ma CG: Mechanisms related to neuron injury and death in cerebral hypoxic ischaemia, *Folia Neuropathol* 49(2):78–87, 2011.

10. Jaeschke H: Reactive oxygen and mechanisms of inflammatory liver injury: present concepts, *J Gastroenterol Hepatol* 26(Suppl 1):173–179, 2011.

11. Kumar V, Abbas A, Fausto N, Aster J: Environmental and nutritional diseases. In Kumar V, Abbas A, Fausto N, Aster J, editors: *Robbins and Cotran pathologic basis of disease*, ed 8, Philadelphia, 2010, Saunders, pp 399–446.

12. National Institutes of Health (NIH): *Clinical guidelines on the identification, evaluation, and treatment of overweight and obesity in adults*, NIH Pub No. 98–4083, Bethesda, MD, 1998, Author.

13. Wiersinga WJ: Current insights in sepsis: from pathogenesis to new treatment targets, *Curr Opin Crit Care* 17(5):480–486, 2011.

14. McAdam A, Sharpe A: Infectious diseases. In Kumar V, Abbas A, Fausto N, Aster J, editors: *Robbins and Cotran pathologic basis of disease*, ed 8, Philadelphia, 2010, Saunders, pp 331–398.

15. Weber LW, Boll M, Stampfl A: Hepatotoxicity and mechanism of action of haloalkanes: carbon tetrachloride as a toxicological model, *Crit Rev Toxicol* 33(2):105–136, 2003.

16. Williams D: Radiation carcinogenesis: lessons from Chernobyl, *Oncogene* 27(Suppl 2):S9–S18, 2008.

17. D'Andrea JA, Ziriax JM, Adair ER: Radio frequency electromagnetic fields: mild hyperthermia and safety standards, *Prog Brain Res* 162:107–135, 2007.

18. Speirs CK, Hwang M, Kim S, Li W, Chang S, et al: Harnessing the cell death pathway for targeted cancer treatment, *Am J Cancer Res* 1(1):43–61, 2011.

19. Troen BR: The biology of aging, *Mt Sinai J Med* 70(1):3–22, 2003.

20. Hayflick L: The biology of human aging, *Adv Pathobiol* 7(2):80–99, 1980.

21. Oeseburg H, de Boer RA, van Gilst WH, van der Harst P: Telomere biology in healthy aging and disease, *Pflugers Arch* 459(2):259–268, 2010.

22. Shennan T: *Postmortems and morbid anatomy*, ed 3, Baltimore, 1935, William Wood.

Genome Structure, Regulation, and Tissue Differentiation

Jacquelyn L. Banasik

⊖volve WEBSITE

http://evolve.elsevier.com/Copstead/
- Review Questions and Answers
- Glossary (with audio pronunciations for selected terms)
- Animations
- Case Studies
- Key Points Review

KEY QUESTIONS

- How is genetic information stored in the cell and transmitted to progeny during replication?
- How does the simple 4-base structure of DNA serve as a template for synthesis of proteins that may contain 20 varieties of amino acids?
- What roles do genes play in determining cell structure and function?
- How is gene expression regulated?
- By what mechanisms can the cells of an organism, which all contain identical genes, become differentiated into divergent cell types?
- What are the general structures and functions of the four main tissue types: epithelial, connective, muscle, and nerve?

CHAPTER OUTLINE

The ability of scientists to study and manipulate genes has evolved at an incredible pace, including the complete sequencing of all 6.4 billion nucleotides in an entire human genome. A better understanding of the role that genetics plays in cellular function and disease has spurred efforts to develop therapies to correct genetic abnormalities. The science of genetics developed from the premise that invisible, information-containing elements called **genes** exist in cells and are passed on to daughter cells when a cell divides. The nature of these elements was at first difficult to imagine: what kind of molecule could direct the daily activities of the organism and be capable of nearly limitless replication? The answer to this question was discovered in the late 1940s and was almost unbelievable in its simplicity. It is now common knowledge that genetic information is stored in long chains of stable molecules called **deoxyribonucleic acid (DNA).** The human genome contains approximately 23,000 genes encoded by only four different molecules. These molecules are the deoxyribonucleotides containing the bases *adenine* (A), *cytosine* (C), *guanine* (G), and *thymine* (T). Genes are composed of varying sequences of these four bases, which are linked together by sugar-phosphate bonds. By serving as the templates for the production of body proteins, genes ultimately affect all aspects of an organism's structure and function. When the sequencing of an entire human genome was completed in 2004 it became clear that the genome

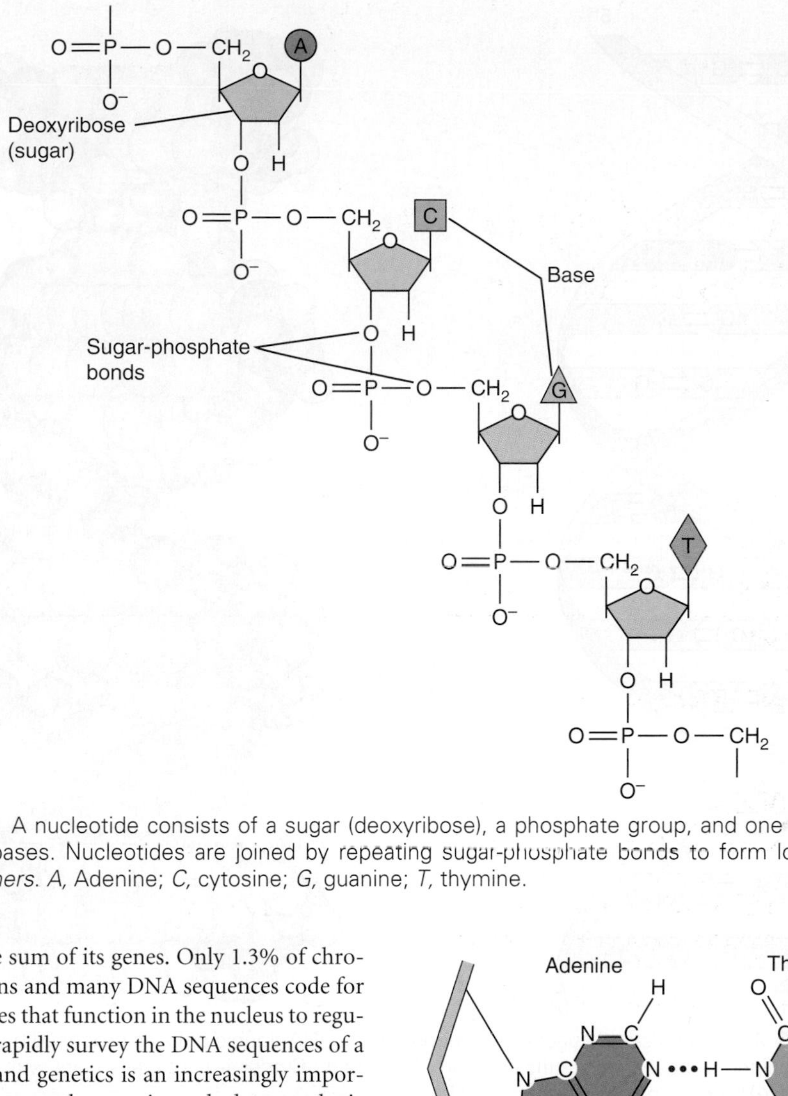

FIGURE 5-1 A nucleotide consists of a sugar (deoxyribose), a phosphate group, and one of the four nucleotide bases. Nucleotides are joined by repeating sugar-phosphate bonds to form long chains, called *polymers*. *A*, Adenine; *C*, cytosine; *G*, guanine; *T*, thymine.

is much more complex than the sum of its genes. Only 1.3% of chromosomal DNA codes for proteins and many DNA sequences code for ribonucleic acid (RNA) molecules that function in the nucleus to regulate gene function. Methods to rapidly survey the DNA sequences of a particular person are available and genetics is an increasingly important consideration in the etiology, pathogenesis, and pharmacologic treatment of a variety of diseases. However, genetic inheritance involves more than the transfer of genes from parent to offspring. For example, the nutritional exposures of grandparents may influence the metabolic physiology of grandchildren through a process known as **epigenetics.** Epigenetics is further explored in Chapter 6. Knowledge of the basic principles of genetics and gene regulation is a prerequisite to understanding not only conventional genetic diseases but also nearly every pathophysiologic process. This chapter examines the biochemistry of genes (molecular genetics), the regulation of gene expression, and the processes of tissue differentiation. Principles of genetic inheritance precede the discussion of genetic diseases in Chapter 6.

MOLECULAR GENETICS

Structure of DNA

In humans, DNA encodes genetic information in 46 long double-stranded chains of nucleotides called chromosomes.[1] The **nucleotides** consist of a 5-carbon sugar (deoxyribose), a phosphate group, and one of the four nucleotide bases (Figure 5-1). The nucleotide bases are divided into two types based on their chemical structure. The pyrimidines, cytosine and thymine, have single-ring structures. The purines, guanine and adenine, have double-ring structures (Figure 5-2). DNA polymers are formed by the chemical linkage of these nucleotides. The sugar-phosphate linkages, also called *phosphodiester bonds,* join the

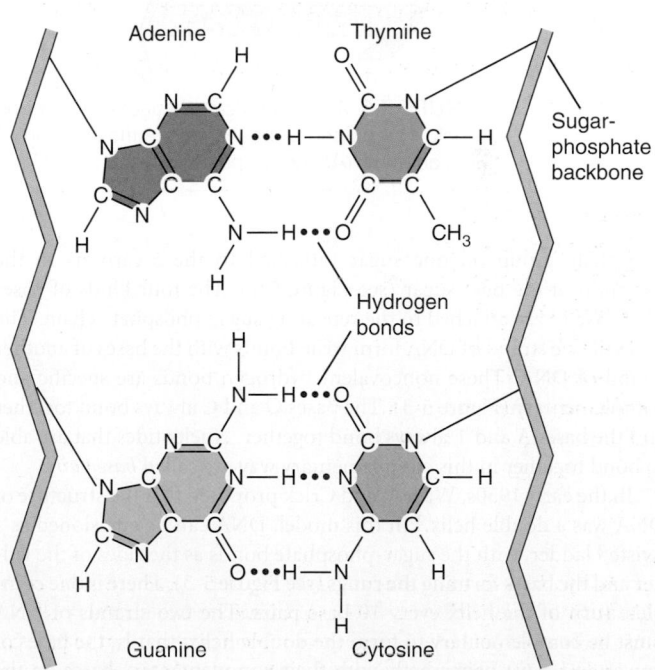

FIGURE 5-2 The two types of DNA bases are the single-ring pyrimidines and the double-ring purines. Thymine (T) and cytosine (C) are pyrimidines, and adenine (A) and guanine (G) are purines. Base pairing occurs between A and T and between C and G because of hydrogen bonds *(dots)*.

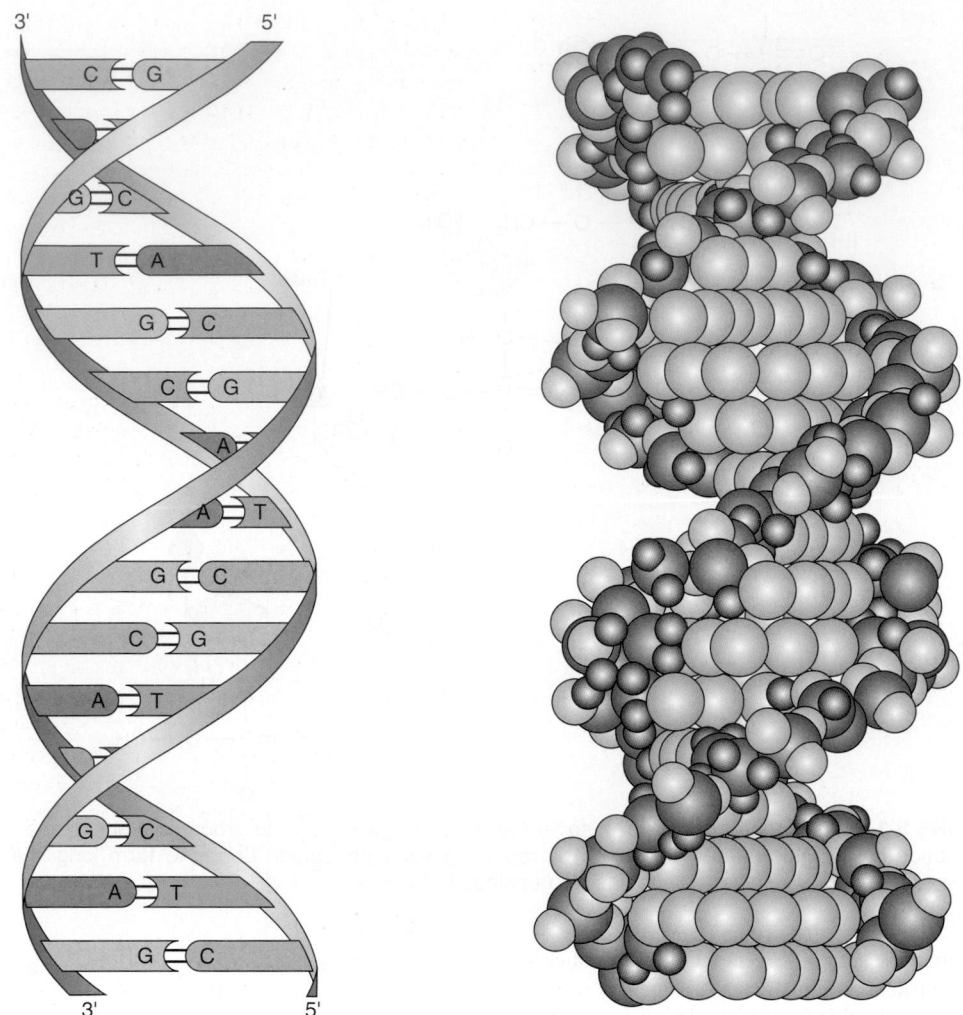

FIGURE 5-3 A schematic and space-filling model of the DNA double helix as proposed by Watson and Crick. The pairing of bases is specific and complementary: Cytosine *(C)* always pairs with guanine *(G)*, and adenine *(A)* always pairs with thymine *(T)*.

phosphate group on one sugar (attached to the 5-carbon) to the 3-carbon of the next sugar (see Figure 5-1). The four kinds of bases (A, C, G, T) are attached to the repeating sugar-phosphate chain. The bases of one strand of DNA form weak bonds with the bases of another strand of DNA. These noncovalent hydrogen bonds are specific and complementary (Figure 5-3). The bases G and C always bond together and the bases A and T always bond together. Nucleotides that are able to bond together in this complementary way are called *base pairs.*

In the early 1950s, Watson and Crick proposed that the structure of DNA was a double helix.[2] In this model, DNA can be envisioned as a twisted ladder, with the sugar-phosphate bonds as the sides of the ladder and the bases forming the rungs (see Figure 5-3). There is one complete turn of the helix every 10 base pairs. The two strands of DNA must be complementary to form the double helix; that is, the bases of one strand must pair exactly with their complementary bases on the other strand. The helix is wound around proteins called histones to form *nucleosomes* (Figure 5-4). DNA coupled to histones and other nuclear proteins is termed *chromatin.* When a cell is not dividing, the chromatin is loosely packed within the nucleus and not visible under the light microscope. During cell division, the chromatin becomes tightly condensed into the 46 chromosomes that become visible during mitosis.

The discovery of the double-helix model was profound because it immediately suggested how information transfer could be accomplished by such simple molecules. Because each DNA strand carries a nucleotide sequence that is exactly complementary to the sequence of its partner, both strands can be used as templates to create an exact copy of the original DNA double helix. When a cell divides to form two daughter cells, each daughter cell must receive a complete copy of the parent cell's DNA. The process of DNA replication requires separation of the DNA double helix by breaking the hydrogen bonds between the base pairs. Specific replication enzymes then direct the attachment of the correct (complementary) nucleotides to each of the single-stranded DNA templates. In this way, two identical copies of the original DNA double helix are formed and passed on to the two daughter cells during cell division.

DNA Replication

Although the underlying principle of gene replication is simple, the cellular machinery required to carry out the replication process is complex, involving a host of enzymes and proteins.[3] These "replication machines" can duplicate DNA at a rate of 1000 nucleotides per second and complete the duplication of the entire genome in about 8 hours.[4] The DNA double helix must first separate so that new nucleotides can

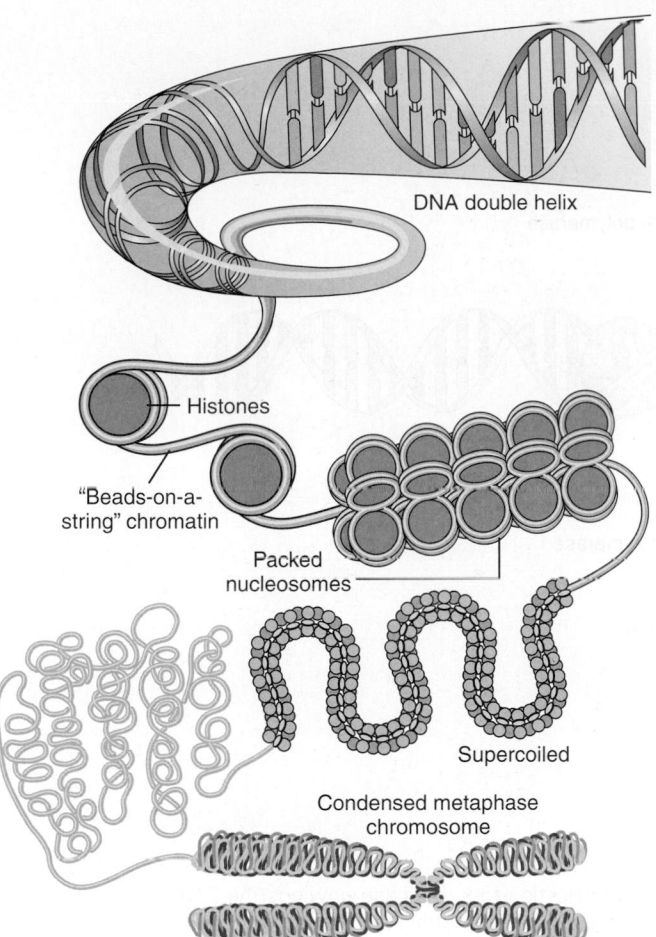

DNA double helix

Histones

"Beads-on-a-string" chromatin

Packed nucleosomes

Supercoiled

Condensed metaphase chromosome

FIGURE 5-4 DNA is packaged by wrapping around protein complexes called histones to form beadlike structures called *nucleosomes*. During cell division, the coiled DNA becomes very condensed into chromosomes that are visible under the light microscope. During interphase and when genes are being transcribed, the DNA is more loosely packaged and not visible.

be paired with the old DNA template strands. The DNA double helix is normally very stable: the base pairs are locked in place so tightly that they can withstand temperatures approaching the boiling point. In addition, DNA is wrapped around histones and bound by a host of DNA-binding proteins through which the replication machinery must navigate. DNA replication is started by special proteins (initiator proteins) that pry the DNA strands apart at specific places along the chromatin, called *replication origins*. Then special enzymes (DNA helicases) are needed to rapidly unwind and separate the DNA strands, whereas helix-destabilizing proteins (also called single-stranded DNA-binding proteins) bind to the exposed DNA strands to keep them apart until replication can be accomplished (Figure 5-5). As the DNA is unwound in the replication fork, it becomes overly twisted downstream, so another set of enzymes, topoisomerases, cuts nicks in the DNA and allows it to unwind to prevent tangling. Ligases repair the nicks.

Once a portion of the DNA double helix has been separated, an enzyme complex, DNA polymerase, binds the single strands of DNA and begins the process of forming a new complementary strand of DNA. The polymerases match the appropriate base to the template base and catalyze the formation of the sugar-phosphate bonds that form the backbone of the DNA strand. Replication proceeds along the DNA strand in one direction only: from the 3′ end toward the 5′ end.[4] The ends of the DNA strands are labeled 3′ and 5′ according to the

exposed carbon atom at that end. Because two complementary DNA strands are antiparallel, DNA replication is asymmetrical; one strand, the leading strand, is replicated as a continuous polymer, but the lagging strand must be synthesized in short sections in a "backstitching" process (see Figure 5-5). The backstitched fragments of DNA, called Okazaki fragments, are then sealed together by DNA ligase to form the unbroken DNA strand. DNA polymerase is unable to replicate DNA located at the very ends of the chromosomes (the telomeres), so another special enzyme complex, telomerase, is needed for this. The telomeres are fairly short, being composed of approximately 1000 repeats of a GGGTTA sequence. When the telomeres are replicated, one side of the double helix (3′ end) is always longer and loops around and tucks back into the strand. This prevents nuclear enzymes from mistaking the ends of the chromosomes as broken DNA ends and trying to attach them to each other. In many somatic cell types, telomerase activity is low and the cell's chromosomes become slightly shorter with each cell division. Chromosomal shortening has been proposed as a mechanism of "counting" the number of replications and may be important in cellular aging and prevention of cancer (see Chapter 7). DNA replication is said to be semiconservative because each of the two resulting DNA double helices contains one newly synthesized strand and one original (conserved) strand (Figure 5-6).

The DNA polymerase also has the ability to proofread the newly synthesized strands for errors in base pairing. If an error is detected, the enzyme will reverse, remove the incorrect nucleotide, and replace it with the correct one. The fidelity of copying during DNA replication is such that only about one error is made for every 10^9 base pair replications.[5] The self-correcting function of the DNA polymerases is extremely important because errors in replication will be transmitted to the next generation of cells.

Genetic Code

How do an organism's genes influence its structural and functional characteristics? A central theory in biology maintains that a gene directs the synthesis of a protein. It is the presence (or absence) and relative activity of various structural proteins and enzymes that produce the characteristics of the cell. This definition of genes as protein-coding elements is not entirely correct because many "genes" code for ribonucleic acid (RNA) molecules as their final functional products and some genes may code for more than one protein product through alternate splicing of the RNA messages. Protein synthesis still holds a predominant place in understanding how genes direct cell structure and function. One of the surprising outcomes of the Human Genome Project was how little of the DNA in chromosomes contains coding segments (less than 2%) and the low number of genes that exist (23,000). Before the completion of the Human Genome Project, it was estimated that the human genome contained 100,000 genes.

Proteins are composed of one or more chains of amino acids (polypeptides) that fold into complex three-dimensional structures. Cells contain 20 different types of amino acids that connect in a specific sequence to form a particular protein (Table 5-1). Each type of protein has a unique sequence of amino acids that dictates its structure and activity.

If genes are to direct the synthesis of proteins, the information contained in just four kinds of DNA nucleotide bases must code for 20 different amino acids. This so-called genetic code was deciphered in the early 1960s.[6,7] It was determined that a series of three nucleotides (triplet) was needed to code for each of the 20 amino acids. Because there are four different bases, there are 4^3, or 64, different possible triplet combinations. This is far more than needed to code for the 20 known amino acids. Three of the nucleotide triplets or **codons** do not code for amino acids and are called *stop codons* because they signal the

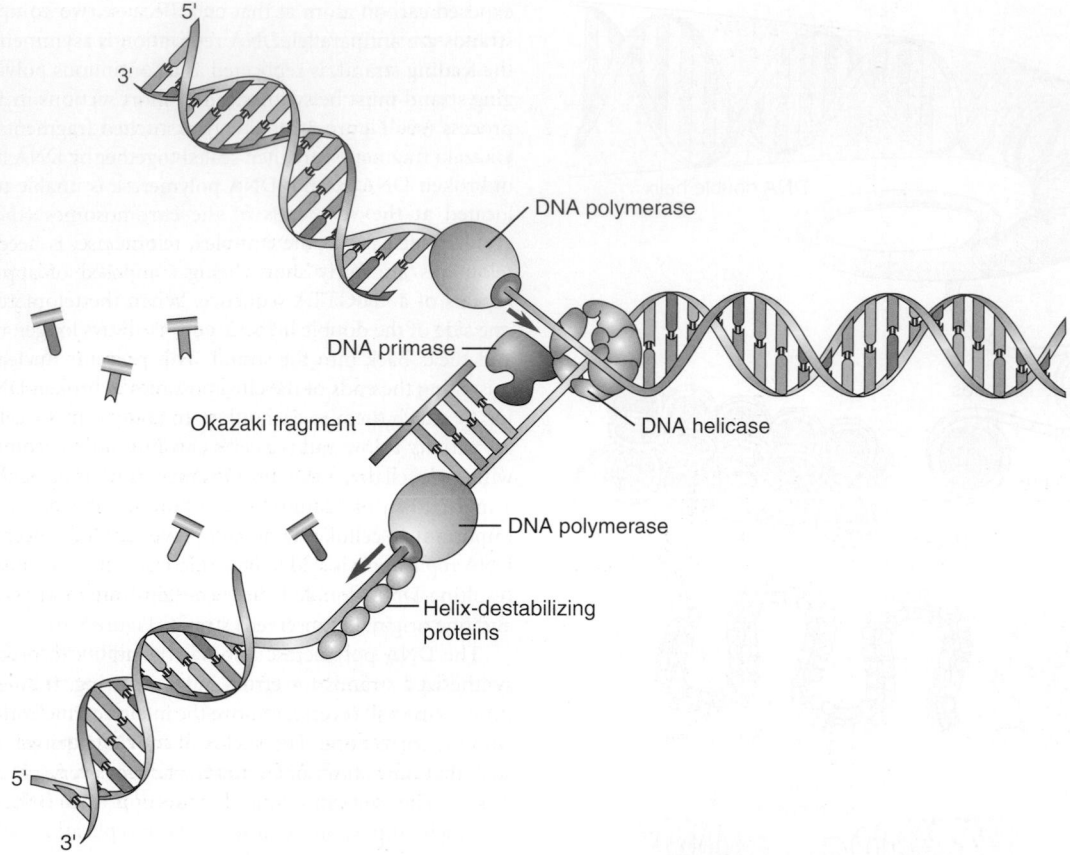

FIGURE 5-5 Summary of the major proteins of the DNA replication fork. Helicase unwinds the DNA double helix, whereas helix-destabilizing proteins keep the strands from reuniting. The leading strand (top) can be replicated in a continuous manner, whereas the lagging strand (bottom) must be synthesized in pieces. Okazaki fragments are formed in a "backstitching" direction and then sealed together with DNA ligase.

end of a protein code. The remaining 61 codons code for 1 of the 20 amino acids (see Table 5-1). Obviously, some of the amino acids are specified by more than one codon. For example, the amino acid arginine is determined by six different codons. The code has been highly conserved during evolution and is essentially the same in organisms as diverse as humans and bacteria.

Several intermediate molecules are involved in the process of DNA-directed protein synthesis, including the complex protein-synthesizing machinery of the ribosomes and several types of RNA. RNA is structurally similar to DNA, except that the sugar molecule is ribose rather than deoxyribose, and one of the four bases is different in that uracil replaces thymine. Because of the biochemical similarity of uracil and thymine, both can form base pairs with adenine. In addition, RNA can form stable single-stranded molecules, whereas DNA strands anneal together, forming a double-stranded molecule.

Several functionally different types of RNA are involved in protein synthesis and cell function. The number and variety of RNA molecules existing within the nucleus is large (Box 5-1) and the exact function of most has yet to be determined. Some perform messenger RNA (mRNA) splicing, ribosome assembly, and quality control of RNA messages before they are transferred to the cytoplasm. The roles of three types of RNA that participate in protein production are well understood. Ribosomal RNA (rRNA) is found associated with the ribosome (see Chapter 3) in the cell cytoplasm. Messenger RNA is synthesized from the DNA template in a process termed **transcription** and carries the protein code to the cytoplasm, where the proteins are manufactured. The amino acids that will be united to form proteins are carried in the cytoplasm by a

third type of RNA, transfer RNA (tRNA), which interacts with mRNA and the ribosome in a process termed **translation**.

Transcription

Transcription is the process whereby mRNA is synthesized from a single-stranded DNA template. The process is similar in some respects to DNA replication. Double-stranded DNA must be separated in the region of the gene to be copied, and specific enzyme complexes (DNA-dependent RNA polymerases) orchestrate the production of the mRNA polymer. Only one of the DNA strands contains the desired gene sequence and serves as the template for the synthesis of mRNA. This strand is called the *sense strand*. The other strand is termed the *nonsense* or *antisense strand* and is not transcribed into an RNA message.

Some genes are continuously active in certain cells, whereas others are carefully regulated in response to cellular needs and environmental signals. Special sequences of DNA near a desired gene may enhance or inhibit its rate of transcription. In general, a gene is transcribed when the RNA polymerase–enzyme complex binds to a promoter region just upstream of the gene's start point. This binding event requires the cooperative function of numerous DNA-binding proteins. Once bound at the promoter, the RNA polymerase directs the separation of the DNA double helix and catalyzes the synthesis of the RNA message by matching the appropriate RNA bases to the DNA template (Figure 5-7). The RNA message is directly complementary to the DNA sequence, except that uracil replaces thymine.

In higher organisms, the DNA template for a particular protein is littered with stretches of bases that must be removed from the original

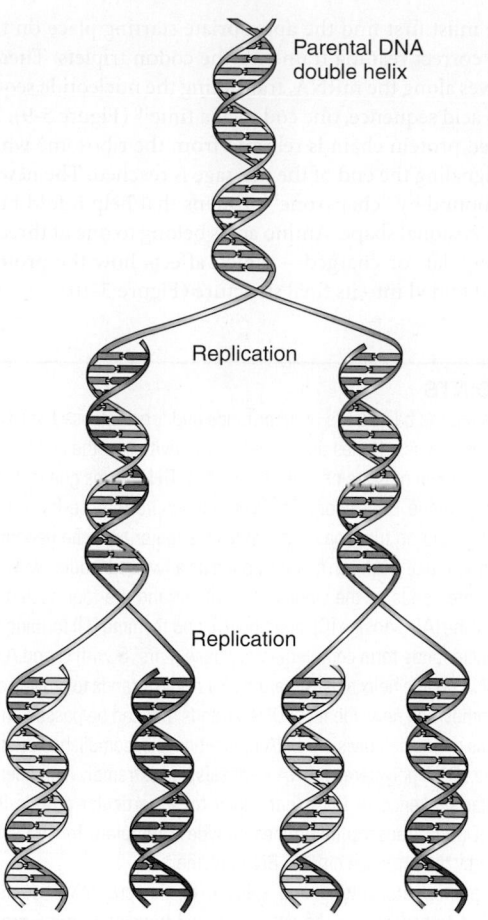

Parental DNA
double helix

Replication

Replication

FIGURE 5-6 DNA replication is semiconservative. Each of the new DNA double helices contains one newly synthesized strand and one original strand.

RNA transcript (pre-mRNA) before it can be translated into a protein. These intervening segments, called **introns,** are removed in the nucleus by a complex splicing process, resulting in an mRNA sequence that contains only the wanted segments, called **exons.** Introns range from 10 to 100,000 nucleotides in length.[8] On average, 90% of a gene is composed of introns and only 10% remains in the final mRNA transcript; thus, a single gene may contain dozens of introns that must be precisely removed. The function of introns remains largely a mystery, although they are believed to be important in the evolution of new genetic information and in gene regulation. Many of these intron sequences are conserved across species, which implies an important function. The removal of introns and splicing of the RNA transcript is mediated by a group of small RNA molecules located in specialized areas of the nucleus called the *spliceosomes.* The *snRNAs,* or small nuclear RNAs, cause the introns to loop out like a lariat, bringing the adjacent exons close together, followed by cutting and splicing. Another group of RNA-protein complex molecules called *small nuclear ribonucleoproteins* (snRNPs) attach to the pre-mRNA and prevent its escape through the nuclear envelope until all the necessary splicing has been accomplished.[9] Most pre-mRNA transcripts can be spliced in different ways to increase the number of different protein forms produced by a single gene.[8]

The processed mRNA is finally transported to the cell cytoplasm through pores in the nuclear membrane that contain complexes that inspect the mRNA for certain structural characteristics that distinguish it from RNA debris. The mRNA then directs the synthesis of a protein in cooperation with tRNA and the ribosomes. Each mRNA may serve as a template for thousands of copies of protein before it is degraded.

Translation

Translation is the process whereby messenger RNA is used to direct the synthesis of a protein. The mRNA is read in linear fashion from one end to the other, with each set of three nucleotides serving as a codon

TABLE 5-1	RNA CODONS FOR THE DIFFERENT AMINO ACIDS AND FOR START AND STOP					
AMINO ACIDS	**RNA CODONS**					
Alanine	GCU	GCC	GCA	GCG		
Arginine	CGU	CGC	CGA	CGG	AGA	AGG
Asparagine	AAU	AAC				
Aspartic acid	GAU	GAC				
Cysteine	UGU	UGC				
Glutamic acid	GAA	GAG				
Glutamine	CAA	CAG				
Glycine	GGU	GGC	GGA	GGG		
Histidine	CAU	CAC				
Isoleucine	AUU	AUC	AUA			
Leucine	CUU	CUC	CUA	CUG	UUA	UUG
Lysine	AAA	AAG				
Methionine	AUG					
Phenylalanine	UUU	UUC				
Proline	CCU	CCC	CCA	CCG		
Serine	UCU	UCC	UCA	UCG	AGC	AGU
Threonine	ACU	ACC	ACA	ACG		
Tryptophan	UGG					
Tyrosine	UAU	UAC				
Valine	GUU	GUC	GUA	GUG		
Start (CI)	AUG					
Stop (CT)	UAA	UAG	UGA			

CI, Chain initiation; *CT,* chain termination.

for a particular amino acid. The codons in the mRNA do not directly recognize the amino acids. Intermediary molecules or "translators" are required. These intermediaries are the tRNA molecules. A schematic drawing of a tRNA molecule is shown in Figure 5-8, illustrating its L-shaped, three-dimensional structure. A codon reading area (anticodon) is located at one end and an amino acid attachment at the other. A group of specialized enzymes that have a binding pocket for a particular amino acid and a reading pocket for the anticodon are needed to attach the correct amino acid to its appropriate tRNA. The anticodon is formed by a sequence of three nucleotides. Recognition between the mRNA codon and the tRNA anticodon is accomplished by the same kind of complementary base pairing as was described for DNA. The complex machinery of the ribosome is needed to align the tRNA on the mRNA and to catalyze the peptide bonds that hold the amino acids together. **Ribosomes** are large complexes of protein and RNA. Each ribosome is composed of two subunits that are first assembled in a special part of the nucleus called the *nucleolus* and then transported through the nuclear pores to the cytoplasm. The smaller subunit binds the mRNA and the tRNA, whereas the larger subunit catalyzes the formation of peptide bonds between the incoming amino acids. The

ribosome must first find the appropriate starting place on the mRNA to set the correct reading frame for the codon triplets. Then the ribosome moves along the mRNA, translating the nucleotide sequence into an amino acid sequence, one codon at a time[10] (Figure 5-9). The newly synthesized protein chain is released from the ribosome when a "stop codon" signaling the end of the message is reached. The new protein is typically bound by "chaperone" proteins that help it fold into its final three-dimensional shape. Amino acids belong to one of three groups—polar, nonpolar, or charged— which affects how the protein is processed and folded into its final structure (Figure 5-10).

BOX 5-1   TYPES OF RNA PRODUCED IN CELLS

mRNA—messenger RNA; codes for proteins

rRNA—ribosomal RNA; within ribosomes, catalyzes protein synthesis

tRNA—transfer RNA; adaptors between mRNA and amino acids in protein synthesis

snRNA—small nuclear RNA; splicing of pre-mRNA in the nucleus

snoRNA—small nucleolar RNA; processing of rRNA in the nucleolus

scaRNA—small cajal RNA; modifies snoRNA and snRNA

miRNA—micro RNA; regulates gene expression by blocking mRNA translation

siRNA—small interfering RNA; turns off gene expression through alteration in chromatin

---

KEY POINTS

- Genes are the basic units of inheritance and are composed of DNA located on chromosomes. Genes direct the daily activities of the cell by controlling the production of proteins. Less than 2% of DNA forms genes that code for proteins. Some DNA codes for RNA transcripts that perform a variety of functions, but no function is known for the majority of the genomic DNA.
- The structure of DNA can be envisioned as a twisted ladder, with the sugar-phosphate bonds as the sides of the ladder and the four nucleotide bases (adenosine [A], cytosine [C], guanine [G], and thymine [T]) forming the rungs. The nucleotides form complementary base pairs, C with G and A with T.
- The DNA double helix must separate into single strands to provide a template for synthesizing new, identical DNA strands that can be passed on to daughter cells during cell division. DNA replication is accomplished by the enzyme complex DNA polymerase. DNA synthesis has extremely high fidelity.
- A linear sequence of DNA that codes for a particular protein is called a gene. During transcription, genes provide a template for the synthesis of mRNA by the enzyme complex RNA polymerase.
- After appropriate cutting and splicing of the pre-mRNA transcript, the mRNA is transported to the cytoplasm and translated into a protein. Each nucleotide triplet (codon) in the mRNA codes for a particular amino acid. Protein synthesis is accomplished by ribosomes, which match the mRNA codon with the correct tRNA anticodon and then catalyze the peptide bond to link amino acids together into a linear protein.

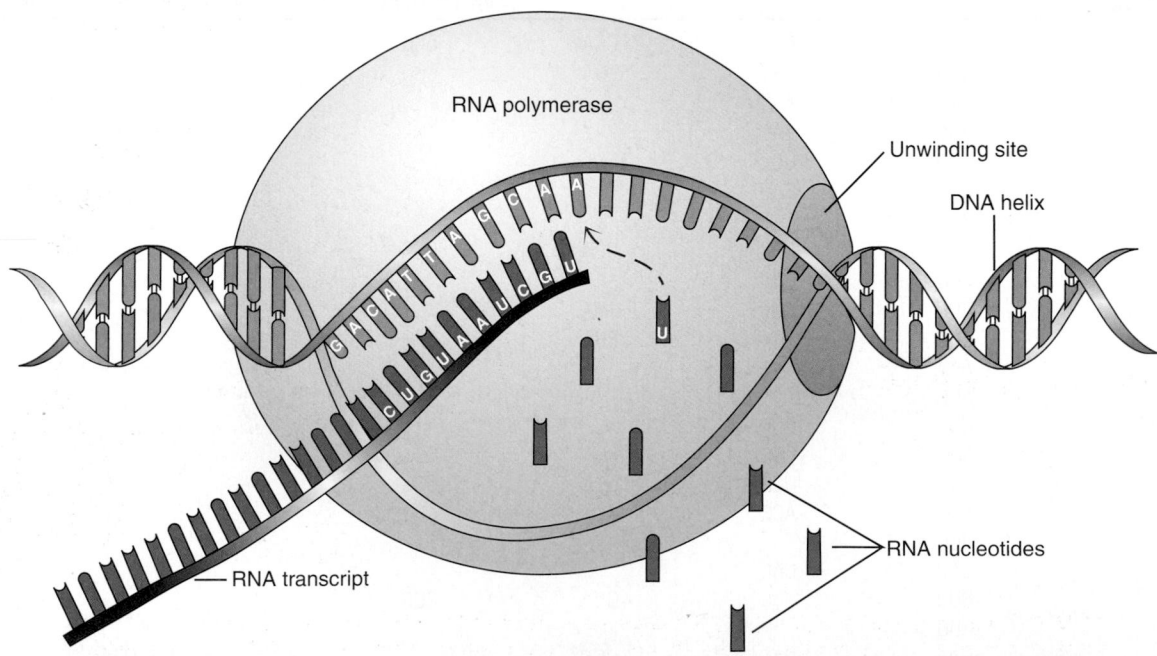

FIGURE 5-7 A moving RNA polymerase complex unwinds the DNA helix ahead of it while rewinding the DNA behind. One strand of the DNA serves as the template for the formation of mRNA.

REGULATION OF THE GENOME

The genome contains the genetic information of the cell and ultimately determines its form and function. All the various cells in a multicellular organism contain the same genes, and differences in cell type are thought to be the result of differences in DNA *expression*. To maintain the cell's phenotype, some genes must be actively transcribed, whereas others remain quiescent. In addition, the cell must be able to change the expression of certain genes to respond and adapt to changes in the cellular environment. At any one time, a cell expresses 30% to 60% of its approximately 23,000 genes.[11] There is evidence that gene expression can be regulated at each of the steps in the pathway from DNA to RNA to protein synthesis. The proteins made by a cell can be controlled in the following ways: (1) regulating the rate and timing of gene transcription; (2) controlling the way the mRNA is spliced; (3) selecting the mRNAs that are transported to the cytoplasm; (4) selecting the mRNAs that are translated by ribosomes; (5) selectively destroying certain mRNAs in the cytoplasm; or (6) selectively controlling the activity of the proteins after they have been produced.[11]

For a majority of genes, the most important regulators of expression are the transcriptional controls. Cells contain DNA-binding proteins that are able to enhance or inhibit gene expression. These gene regulatory proteins recognize and bind only particular DNA sequences and thus are specific to the genes they regulate.[12] The genome contains about 2000 different genes that code for gene regulatory proteins, each of which works in combination with others to control numerous genes. The ability to regulate gene expression allows the cell to alter its structure and function in response to signals from its environment.

Transcriptional Controls

The gene regulatory proteins described in the preceding paragraphs are thought to control gene transcription by binding near the promoter sequence of DNA, where the RNA polymerase must attach to initiate transcription of the gene.[13] Binding of the regulatory proteins may either enhance or inhibit RNA polymerase binding and subsequent transcription of the gene. This is sometimes referred to as "turning on" or "turning off" a gene. The DNA-binding proteins are able to recognize their specific binding sites because of small variations in structure of the external surface of the DNA double helix and do not require separation of the strands to bind. These regulatory DNA-binding proteins can be categorized either as positive controls that activate transcription (*activators*) or as negative controls that inhibit transcription (*repressors*).

In humans, the strategies for gene regulation are complex. Gene regulatory proteins often bind DNA segments far from the gene being regulated, and binding of several gene regulatory proteins in combination is often necessary. A critical step in initiating gene transcription in human cells is the assembly of general transcription factors at the promoter region.[14] General transcription factors are a group of DNA-binding proteins necessary for RNA polymerase activity, and initiation of transcription does not occur without them. Regulatory gene activator proteins help to collect the transcription factors at the promoter of the correct gene by first recognizing and binding to a specific DNA

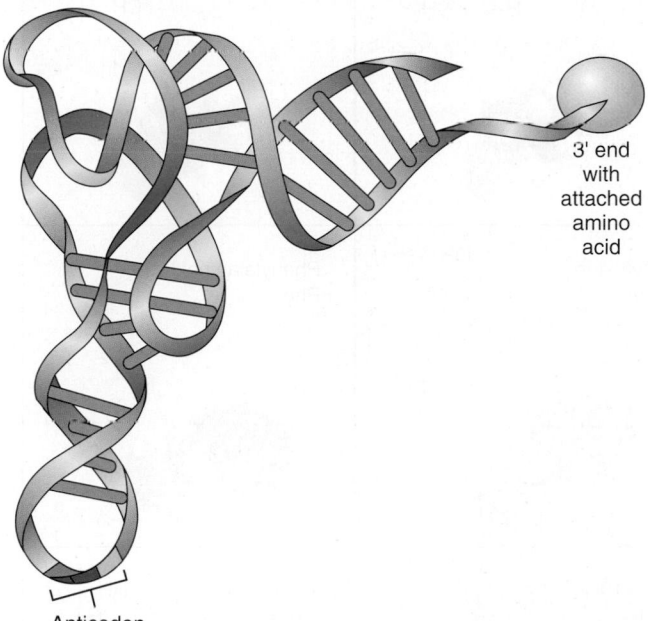

3' end with attached amino acid

Anticodon

FIGURE 5-8 Schematic drawing of a transfer RNA (tRNA) molecule. Each tRNA binds a specific amino acid, which corresponds with the three-base sequence at the anticodon end.

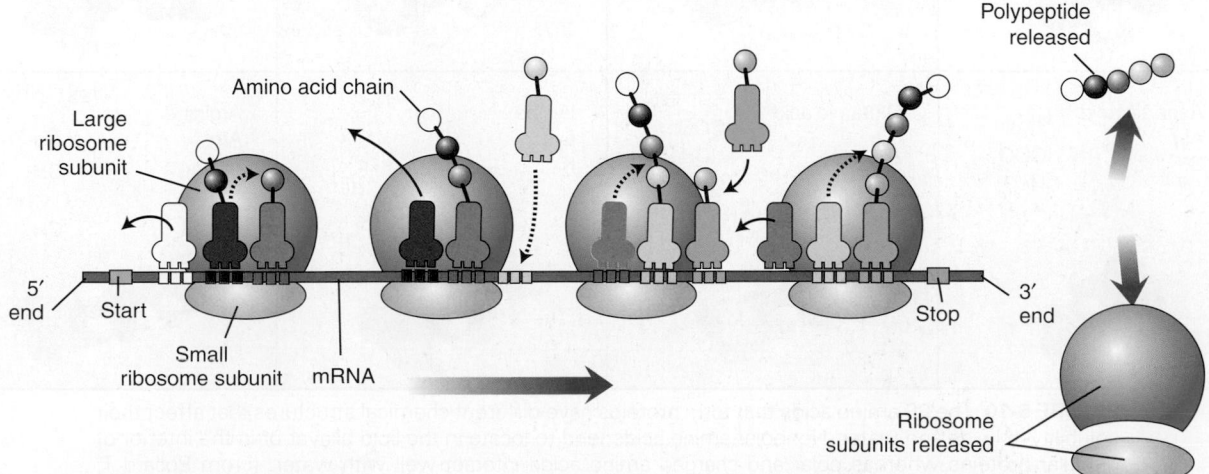

Polypeptide released

Amino acid chain

Large ribosome subunit

5' end   Start

Small ribosome subunit   mRNA

Stop   3' end

Ribosome subunits released

FIGURE 5-9 Synthesis of a protein by the ribosomes attached to a mRNA molecule. Ribosomes attach near the start codon and catalyze the formation of the peptide chain. The mRNA strand is read in groups of three nucleotides (codons) until the stop codon is reached and the peptide is released. Several ribosomes may translate a single mRNA into multiple copies of the protein.

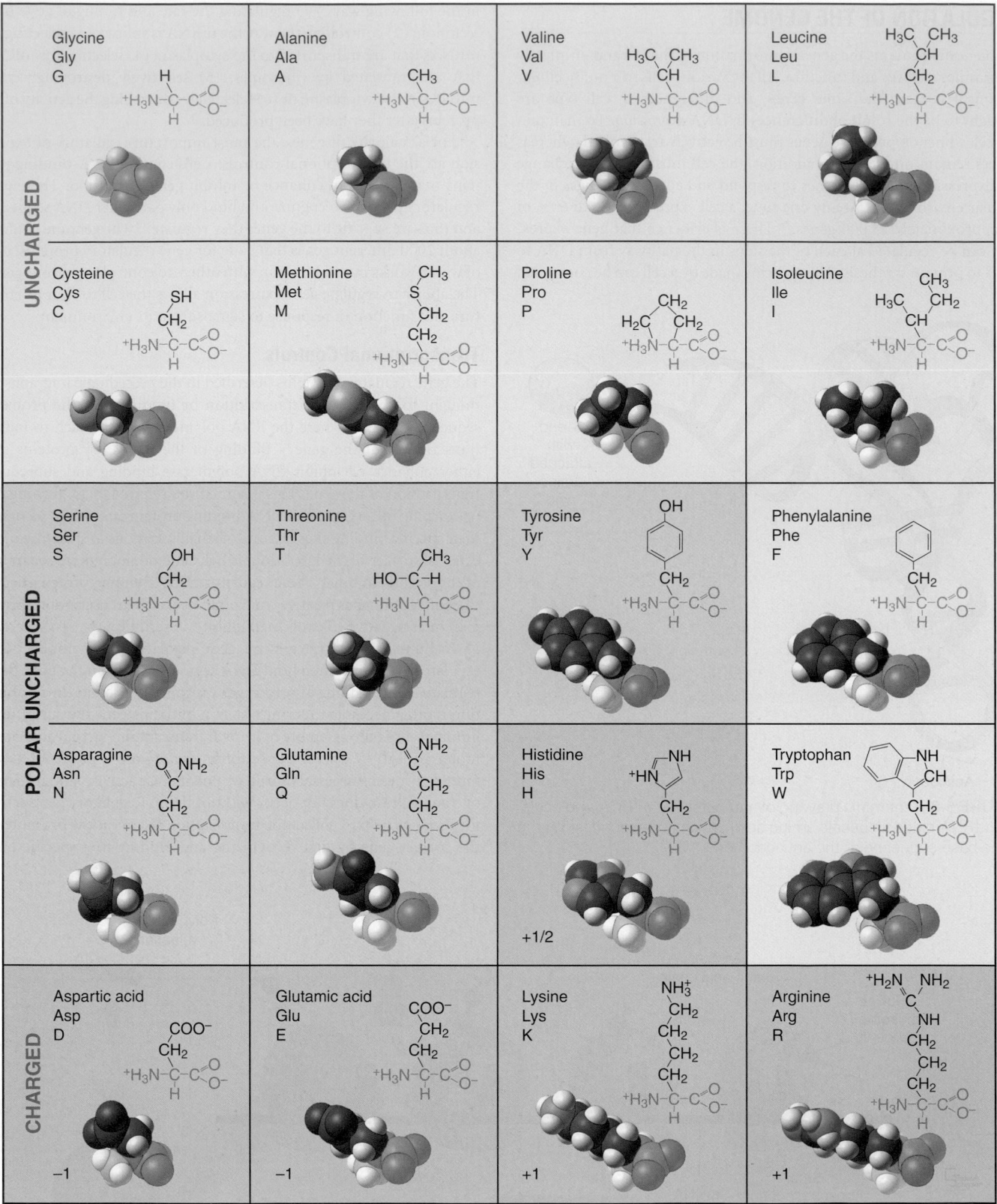

FIGURE 5-10 The 20 amino acids that form proteins have different chemical structures that affect their solubility in lipids and water. Nonpolar amino acids tend to locate in the lipid bilayer or in the interior of globular proteins whereas polar and charged amino acids interact well with water. (From Pollard T, Earnshaw W: *Cell biology*, 2007, Philadelphia, Saunders.)

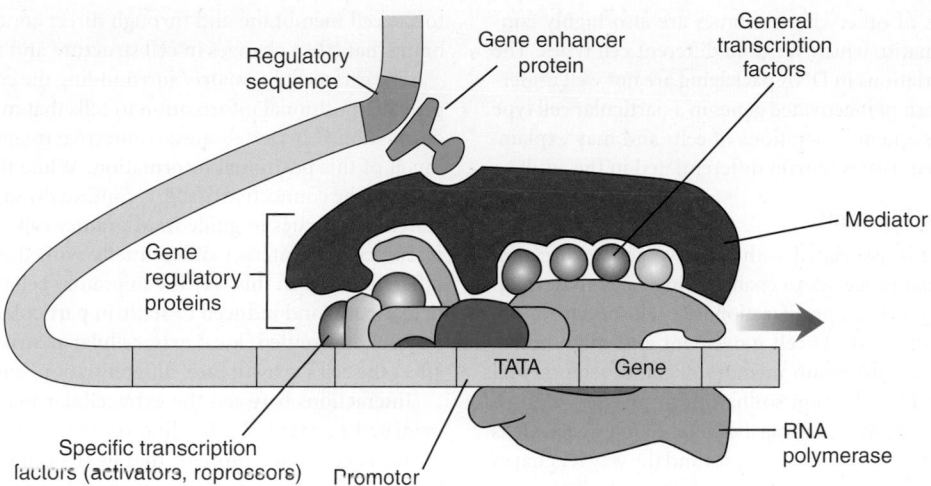

FIGURE 5-11 Gene activator proteins coordinate the assembly of general transcription factors at the promoter region of the gene to be transcribed. RNA polymerase is unable to bind and begin transcription until the requisite transcription factors are in place.

sequence and then coordinating the assembly of the transcription factors (Figure 5-11).

Inhibition of transcription is achieved by gene repressor proteins, which also recognize and bind specific DNA sequences but inhibit the assembly of transcription factors at the site. Some repressor proteins may function simply by binding to and physically blocking the promoter region, but most appear to exert their effects through more complex mechanisms, such as compacting the DNA to make it difficult to pry open, interfering with activator proteins, and binding up or inhibiting transcription factors. Inappropriate transcription of genes in a particular cell may have dire consequences for the cell or for the organism as a whole and is therefore a carefully regulated process. The presence, position, and activity of gene regulatory proteins may be regulated by various signaling cascades within the cell. Many of these signaling cascades are triggered by changes in the cell's environment, which then alter gene transcription (see Chapter 3). This process is very complex, with numerous signaling pathways often converging on a particular gene regulatory system. Even after the mRNA transcript is produced it may not be allowed to reach the ribosome for translation. Small RNA molecules called micro RNA (miRNA) and small interfering RNA (siRNA) can anneal to complementary segments of the mRNA within the nucleus. In some cases, these small RNAs regulate gene splicing, but in other cases they "silence" the gene by preventing the mRNA from being translated into a protein.

KEY POINTS

- All the cells in an individual have essentially the same DNA; however, cells differ greatly in structure and function. This occurs because genes are selectively expressed in particular cells.
- Gene expression can be regulated at any step in the pathway from DNA to RNA to protein synthesis. The most important regulators are transcriptional controls.
- A critical step for initiation of gene transcription is the assembly of general transcription factors at the promoter region of the gene.
- The actions of general transcription factors and RNA polymerase are controlled by a large number of regulatory proteins that specifically bind to DNA. The presence of certain DNA-binding proteins at specific sites can activate or repress the transcription of a particular gene in response to signals in the cell's environment.
- A number of small RNA molecules function to regulate mRNA transcription and translation.

DIFFERENTIATION OF TISSUES

Cell Diversification and Cell Memory

The cells of a multicellular organism tend to specialize to perform particular functions in coordination with other cells and tissues of the body. Cells not only must become different during development but also must remain different in the adult, after the original cues for cell diversification have disappeared. The differences among cell types are ultimately the result of the differentiating influences experienced in the embryo. Differences are maintained because the cells retain the effects of those past influences and pass the memory on to their descendants. When a skin cell divides to replace lost skin cells, the daughter cells are also skin cells; when a liver cell divides, its daughter cells are liver cells; and so on. The behavior of cells of higher organisms is governed by their genome and their present environment, as well as by their developmental history.

There is substantial evidence that the differences in tissue structure and function in a particular organism are not due to deletions or additions to the genes.[15] All the cells of an organism contain essentially the same genes. It is the expression of a relatively few tissue-specific genes that results in differences among cell types.[11] The exact mechanisms leading to the stable expression of tissue-specific genes in particular cell types are partly unknown; however, differences in DNA packaging and the combination of gene regulatory proteins passed on during cell division are thought to be important. The DNA in human cells is extensively packaged, so that 40 inches of linear DNA can be compacted to fit into the cell nucleus. However, different regions of chromosomes can be more or less condensed[1] (see Figure 5-4).

Some regions of DNA, called **heterochromatin,** are so condensed that they are not open to transcription. It is thought that the pattern of packaging as well as the DNA-binding proteins that regulate it are transmitted to progeny when a cell divides such that the pattern of gene expression is maintained as the cell's developmental memory. An example of this mechanism is the inactivation of one of the X chromosomes in females.[16] In mammals, all female cells contain two X chromosomes (XX), whereas male cells contain an X and a Y chromosome (XY). One of the X chromosomes in females is permanently inactivated early in development by condensed packaging. This apparently occurs to prevent a double dose of the X gene products. Which of the two X chromosomes is inactivated in a particular cell is a random event. However, the same X chromosome will be inactive in all of the cell's progeny. Segments of other chromosomes are also highly condensed into heterochromatin, which varies in different cell types. The processes that initiate variations in DNA packaging are not well understood; however, the pattern of inactivated genes in a particular cell type is "remembered" in subsequent generations of cells and may explain, in part, how differentiated tissues remain differentiated in the adult.

Mechanisms of Development

Embryonic development is associated with selective gene expression that controls four essential processes to enable a single cell to develop into a complex organism: (1) cell proliferation, (2) cell specialization, (3) cell-to-cell interactions, and (4) cell movement and migration.[17] Each time a cell divides it must retain memory of the developmental events that have preceded the division so that it can progress along a developmental pathway toward becoming a differentiated tissue. Cells have a genetic memory: the genes a cell expresses and the way it behaves depend on the cell's past as well as its present environment. There is no overall controlling center; each cell must make its own developmental decisions.

There are two major classes of proteins that are particularly important for multicellular development: (1) transmembrane proteins in the cell surface that participate in cell adhesion and communication; and (2) DNA-binding proteins that regulate gene transcription. Differences between cells in an embryo are a necessary prelude to development of a multicellular organism and arise in various ways. Very early in embryonic development, cells begin to divide asymmetrically so that daughter cells are not identical—those on the outside of the group of cells receive different environmental cues than those on the inside, which are surrounded by other cells. These simple differences in cell-to-cell adhesion may alter the transcription of a set of genes. The altered genetic expression will then be passed on to daughter cells in the next cell division, making them diverge further from the original cell. Subsequently, the cell will respond differently to environmental influences, which further alter the cell's structure and function. Thus cells become committed to a developmental pathway over the course of many cell divisions that transmit the history of previous exposures through sequential changes in gene expression.

Continued interactions with nearby cells, chemical gradients, and extracellular matrix components provide clues to guide the cell to its appropriate form and location in the developing organism. Chemicals that control the patterning of fields of nearby tissue are termed **morphogens.** For example, cells in the head region may specialize to secrete a "position signal" for other cells. The morphogen is progressively degraded as it diffuses through the neighboring tissue, such that it has higher concentration close to the source. A particular cell will have information regarding its proximity to the head region based on the surrounding concentration of the chemical. Morphogens are thought to be effective only over small distances. Thus the gross distinctions between head and tail, for example, must be made very early in the embryo, and morphogens can provide only a general pattern for future development. Successive levels of detail can be provided later by other positional signals.

The organization of molecules surrounding the cell surface also provides positional information. The extracellular matrix is composed of a large meshwork of molecules that is produced locally by cells in the area. Some common components include the proteins collagen and elastin, long polysaccharide chains called *glycosaminoglycans,* and a variety of peptides, growth factors, and hormones. The extracellular matrix is highly organized, with components binding to each other and to the cell membrane in specific ways. The extracellular matrix is thought to be important in cell development through its ability to screen or modulate the transport of molecules, such as growth factors,

to the cell membrane and through direct contacts with the cell membrane that effect changes in cell structure and function.[18]

The extracellular matrix surrounding the cells in different locations provides positional information to cells that must migrate to their final destination.[18] In vertebrates, connective tissue cells appear to provide much of this positional information. While the migratory cell travels through the connective tissue, it continually samples the surroundings, searching for cues to guide it. Migratory cells with specific cell surface receptors may interact differentially with the extracellular matrix in different areas. In this way the migratory cell can be guided along particular paths and induced to settle in particular areas. Once the migratory cell has settled, local extracellular matrix molecules may further affect the cell's growth rate, differentiation, and likelihood of survival.

Interactions between the extracellular matrix and nearby cells are mediated primarily by binding proteins called **integrins.**[19] Integrins are transmembrane proteins that tie the cell's cytoskeleton to particular matrix structures (see Chapter 3). They enable the cytoskeleton and extracellular matrix to communicate across the plasma membrane in specific ways. In addition to inducing cells to bind in a particular location, integrins have been shown to activate intracellular signaling pathways, which may influence cell behavior in numerous ways (e.g., cell shape, polarity, metabolism, development, and differentiation).

The steps leading to the development of differentiated tissues in a multicellular organism are such that, once differentiated, a cell type generally does not revert to earlier forms. Some cells in a tissue are terminally differentiated and have limited capacity to change form or replicate. Tissues also maintain less-differentiated stem cells that are able to proliferate depending on environmental cues. Some stem cells, located mainly in the bone marrow, are quite similar to embryonic stem cells and can be recruited into tissues where they proliferate and differentiate into tissue cells. The ability of these multipotent or pleuripotent stem cells to survive and differentiate correctly in their adopted home depends on making complex cell-to-cell and cell-to-matrix connections. In the absence of an appropriate environment, the cells will undergo apoptosis and die (see Chapter 4).

Differentiated Tissues

The more than 200 different cell types in the adult human are generally classified into 4 major tissue categories: epithelium, connective tissue, muscle, and nerve.[20] Tissue types and some of their subtypes are summarized in Table 5-2. Most of the organ systems of the body are combinations of these four tissue types mixed in a highly organized and cooperative manner.

Epithelial Tissue

Epithelial cells cover the majority of the external surfaces of the body and line the glands, blood vessels, and internal surfaces. Epithelial cells adopt a variety of shapes and functions, depending on their locations. For example, the *stratified* epithelium that composes the epidermis of the skin is several layers thick and is primarily protective in function. New epithelial skin cells are formed from stem cells in the deepest part of the epidermis, where it contacts the basal lamina. As cells mature, they move outward toward the surface until they become keratinized and finally flake away (Figure 5-12). Keratin is a tough protective protein that is present in large quantities in the outer skin layers of flattened, dead epithelial cells. The epidermis in humans is completely replaced about once per month, but turnover can occur more rapidly after injury to the skin.[20]

In addition to stratified epithelium, the epithelium may be characterized as simple or pseudostratified according to the number and arrangement of cell layers (Figure 5-13). *Simple* epithelium consists of a single layer of cells, all of which contact the basement membrane.

TABLE 5-2 MAJOR CATEGORIES AND LOCATION OF BODY TISSUES

TISSUE TYPE	LOCATIONS
Epithelial Tissue	
Simple squamous	Lining of blood vessels, pulmonary alveoli, Bowman capsule
Simple cuboidal	Thyroid, sweat, and salivary glands; kidney tubules
Simple columnar	Lining of intestine, glandular ducts
Pseudostratified (mixed cell shapes)	Male urethra, respiratory tract passages
Stratified squamous	Skin, mucous membranes
Stratified columnar	Epiglottis, anus, parts of pharynx
Stratified transitional (layers of different cell shapes)	Bladder
Connective Tissue	
Loose	Widespread locations, dermis of skin, adipose tissue, organs
Dense/supportive	Cartilage, bone, tendons, joints, fascia surrounding muscles
Hematopoietic	Bone marrow, lymph tissue, plasma
Muscle Tissue	
Skeletal	Voluntary muscles of body
Cardiac	Heart (myocardium)
Smooth	Intestine, blood vessels, bladder, uterus, airways
Myoepithelial	Mammary, sweat, and salivary glands
Nervous Tissue	
Neurons	Central and peripheral nerves
Neuroglia	Primarily central nervous system

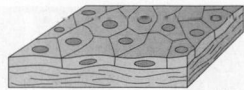
Simple squamous

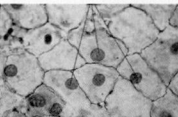
Simple squamous

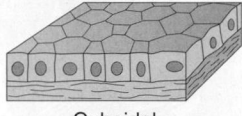
Cuboidal

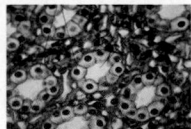
Simple cuboidal

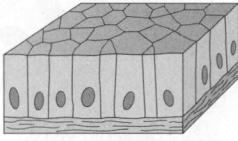
Simple columnar

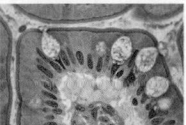
Simple columnar

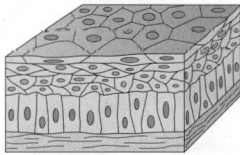
Stratified squamous

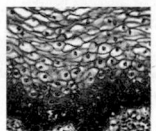
Stratified squamous

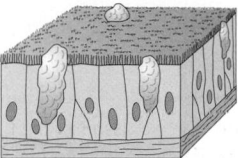
Pseudostratified ciliated columnar

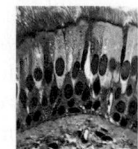
Pseudostratified

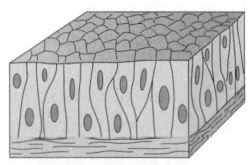
Pseudostratified columnar

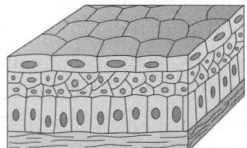
Transitional

FIGURE 5-13 Various epithelial tissue shapes and layering.

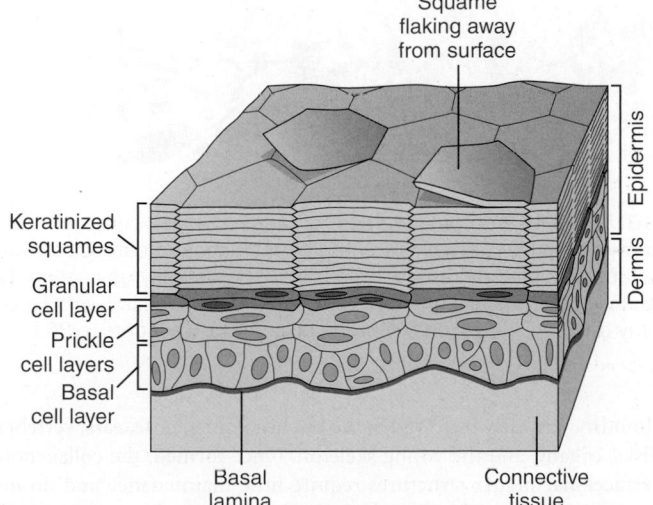

FIGURE 5-12 Organization of epidermal skin layers, showing the flattened keratinized outer layer. Epithelial cells are continually produced by stem cells at the basal lamina and then migrate to the surface.

Simple epithelium is found in the lining of blood vessels and body cavities, in many glands, and in the alveoli of the lungs. The simple epithelium that lines the blood vessels is called *endothelium*. Simple epithelium also forms the kidney tubules and lines the intestine, where absorption is its primary function. *Stratified* epithelium consists of two or more layers of epithelial cells and is found in mucous membranes, such as the mouth, and in the skin, as mentioned previously. Epithelium that appears to be more than one layer thick because of a mixture of cell shapes but is actually a single layer is called *pseudostratified* epithelium. The linings of the respiratory tract and some glands contain pseudostratified epithelium.

Epithelial cells may also be classified according to cell shape. The three basic cell shapes are squamous, cuboidal, and columnar. Squamous cells are thin in comparison to their surface area and have a flattened appearance. Cuboidal cells are approximately equal in width and height, similar to a cube. Columnar cells are a bit taller than they are wide, resembling a rectangular column. Several classifications of epithelial tissue are given in Table 5-2, using both shape and layering as criteria.

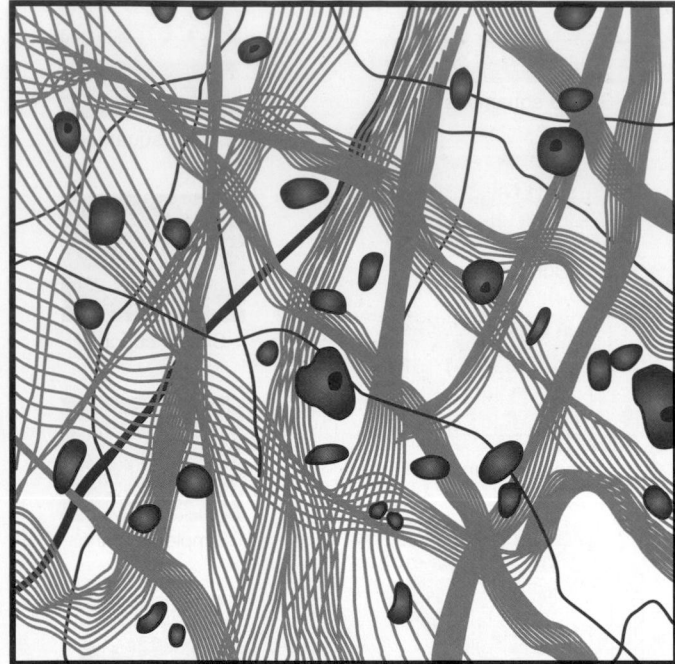

FIGURE 5-14 Schematic drawing of loose connective tissue. (From Patton KT, Thibodeau GA: *Anatomy & physiology*, ed 8, St Louis, 2013, Mosby, p 144.)

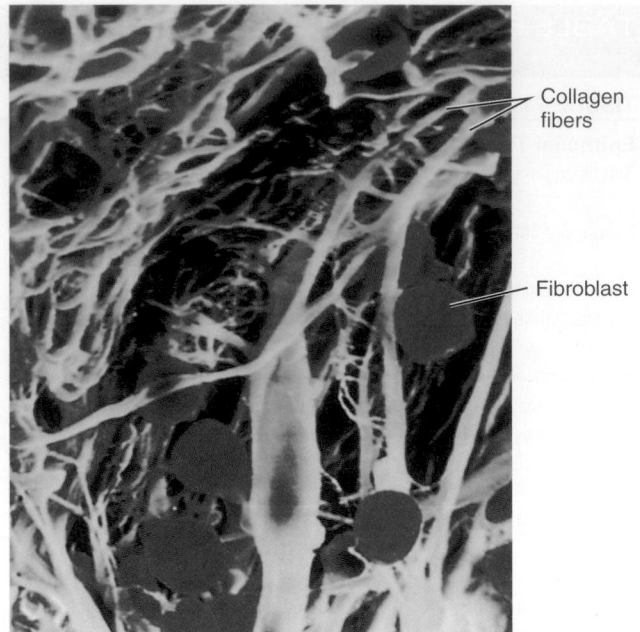

Loose connective tissue

FIGURE 5-15 Scanning electron micrograph of fibroblasts in loose connective tissue of a rat cornea. The matrix is composed primarily of collagen fibers (magnification ×440). (From Solomon EP: *Introduction to human anatomy and physiology*, ed 3, Philadelphia, 2009, Saunders, p 36.)

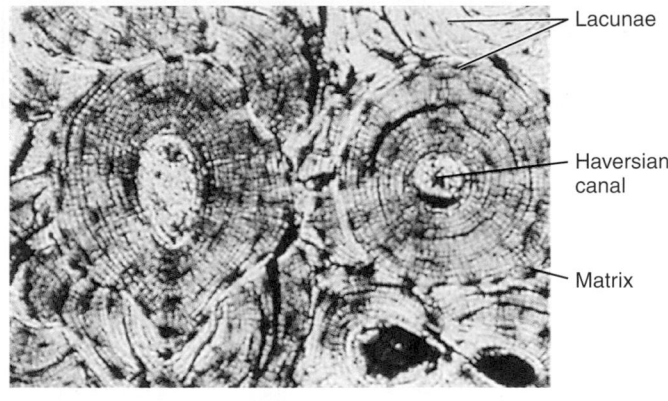

Bone

FIGURE 5-16 Photomicrograph of a section of compact bone showing circular networks formed by the action of osteoclasts and osteoblasts as they remodel the bone. The osteocytes occupy the lacunae and canals. (From Solomon EP: *Introduction to human anatomy and physiology*, ed 3, Philadelphia, 2009, Saunders, p 36.)

Connective Tissue

Connective tissue is the most abundant and diverse tissue in the body, including cell types as different as bone cells, fat cells, and blood cells.[20] Connective tissue commonly functions as a scaffold on which other cells cluster to form organs, but it does much more than hold tissues together. Connective tissue cells often form an elaborate extracellular matrix, which is thought to be important in the maintenance of cell differentiation (Figure 5-14). Connective tissue cells play an important part in the support and repair of nearly every tissue and organ in the body. Three major classifications of connective tissue are commonly identified: loose connective tissue, dense or supportive tissue, and hematopoietic tissue.

Loose connective tissue appears unstructured, with a fair amount of space between fibers of the extracellular matrix. The matrix contains a number of cell types and an elaborate meshwork of protein and other molecules (Figure 5-15). The primary protein constituents are collagen, elastin, and reticular fibers. Collagen is composed of tough, nonelastic bundles of protein fibers that are secreted by fibroblasts. It gives structural strength to skin, tendons, ligaments, and other tissues. The ability of a structure to withstand deforming and stretching forces is due, in large part, to elastin, which can return to its original length after being stretched, like a rubber band. Elastin is important to the function of structures such as the aorta, which must expand to accept the blood ejected from the heart during systole and bounce back to its original shape during diastole. Reticular fibers are short branching fibers that provide networks for the attachment of connective tissue to other cell types, such as epithelial cell attachments in glands, hematopoietic cells in bone marrow, and the parenchymal cells (functional cells) in organs. Cell types associated with loose connective tissue include the fibroblasts, mast cells, and adipocytes (fat cells).

Dense or supportive connective tissue is rich in collagen, which gives strength to structures such as cartilage, tendon, bone, and ligaments. The collagen fibers are more organized and densely packed than fibers found in loose connective tissue. Cartilage cells, or chondrocytes, may be found in the trachea, joints, nose, ears, vertebral disks, organs, and the young skeleton. Once formed, the collagenous extracellular matrix structures require little maintenance and do not receive a blood supply. Bone is a very dense form of connective tissue composed of a mixture of tough collagen fibers and solid calcium phosphate crystals in approximately equal proportions. Throughout the bone's hard extracellular matrix are channels and cavities occupied by living cells (osteocytes) (Figure 5-16). These cells incessantly model and remodel their bony environment, responding to environmental signals. These osteocytes are of two kinds: the cells that erode old bone

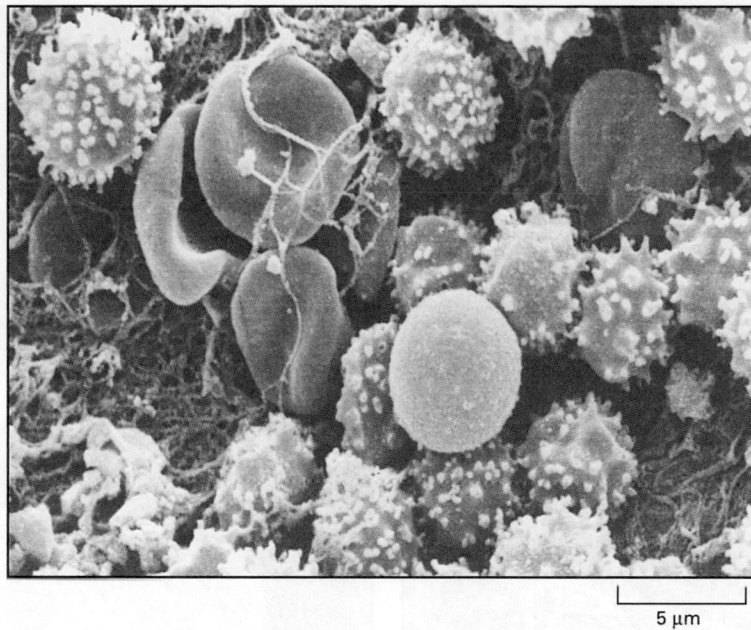

FIGURE 5-17 Scanning electron micrograph of red and white blood cells in the lumen of a blood vessel. Red blood cells are smooth and concave, whereas white blood cells are rough and rounded. (From Alberts B et al, editors: *Molecular biology of the cell,* ed 5, New York, 2008, Garland Science, p 1451. Courtesy Ray Moss.)

are called *osteoclasts,* whereas the cells that form new bone are called *osteoblasts.* Osteoblasts detect when a bone is subjected to a greater load stress and adapt by strengthening the bone mass. Conversely, when the load is removed, as during bed rest, the osteoclasts busily digest the bone, often resulting in some of the common complications of immobility. Osteoclasts, like macrophages, are derived from monocytes that are produced in the bone marrow. The monocytes travel via the bloodstream and collect at sites of bone resorption, where they fuse together to become osteoclasts.[21] Osteocyte activity is essential for bone growth and the repair of bone injuries. (See Chapter 50 for a detailed description of the musculoskeletal system.)

The blood-forming organs of the body are formed by a specialized type of connective tissue called *hematopoietic* tissue. The blood cells include the red cell, or **erythrocyte,** which is specialized for the transport of oxygen; the platelet, or **thrombocyte,** which is important in blood coagulation; and a host of white cells, or **leukocytes,** which mediate immune function. Blood-forming tissue is located in the bone marrow, spleen, and lymphatic tissue. Hematopoietic cells are necessarily nomadic, traveling to distant areas of the body and sometimes settling in a particular organ, sometimes moving continuously (Figure 5-17). Blood cells have a short life span in comparison to other cells and must continually be replenished. This is accomplished by the hematopoietic stem cells. Stem cells reside primarily in the bone marrow and are multipotent; they may differentiate into any of the blood cell types. This results in a system that can respond quickly to the changing needs of the body.

Muscle Tissue

The term *muscle* refers to tissues that are specialized for contraction. Muscle cells, or myocytes, are usually long and thin and packed with the proteins actin and myosin, which constitute the contractile apparatus. In mammals, there are four main categories of muscle cells: skeletal, cardiac, smooth, and myoepithelial (Figure 5-18).[20] Contraction in all four types depends on the presence of intracellular free calcium and

occurs because of interactions between actin and myosin filaments. Actin and myosin filaments differ among cell types with regard to amino acid sequence, arrangement within the cell, and the mechanisms that control contraction. The mechanism of muscle contraction has been called *the sliding filament hypothesis* or *cross-bridge theory.* These terms describe the interactions of the actin and myosin filaments while they form bonds and pull past each other, causing the muscle cell to shorten. Contraction is initiated by an increase in intracellular free calcium concentration and requires energy in the form of adenosine triphosphate (ATP). A detailed description of actin-myosin cross-bridging and the role of calcium, troponin, and tropomyosin can be found in Chapter 17.

Skeletal muscle is responsible for nearly all voluntary movements. Skeletal muscle cells fuse together to form long multinucleated fibers that can be huge, up to 0.5 meter (m) in length. Once fused and differentiated into mature skeletal muscle cells, they cannot enter the cell cycle and divide to produce new cells. Skeletal muscle stem cells (satellite cells) are retained in the muscle tissue and can proliferate in response to muscle damage. The actin and myosin proteins in skeletal muscle are aligned in orderly arrays, giving the tissue a striped appearance under the microscope, which in turn has led to the term *striated muscle.* Skeletal muscle contracts in response to stimulation from the motor neurons of the nervous system (see Chapter 50). As in other types of muscle, stimulation results in an increase in free calcium concentration within the cell. In skeletal muscle, the calcium originates from internal storage sites in the sarcoplasmic reticulum. Contraction is initiated when the calcium binds troponin, a regulatory protein attached to the actin filament. Because of the high energy requirements of contracting skeletal muscle, the cells are packed with energy-producing mitochondria.

Like skeletal muscle, *cardiac muscle* also has a striated appearance attributable to the systematic organization of its actin and myosin filaments. Cardiac muscle cells are linked by special structures, called *intercalated disks* and gap junctions, that cause the tissue to behave as

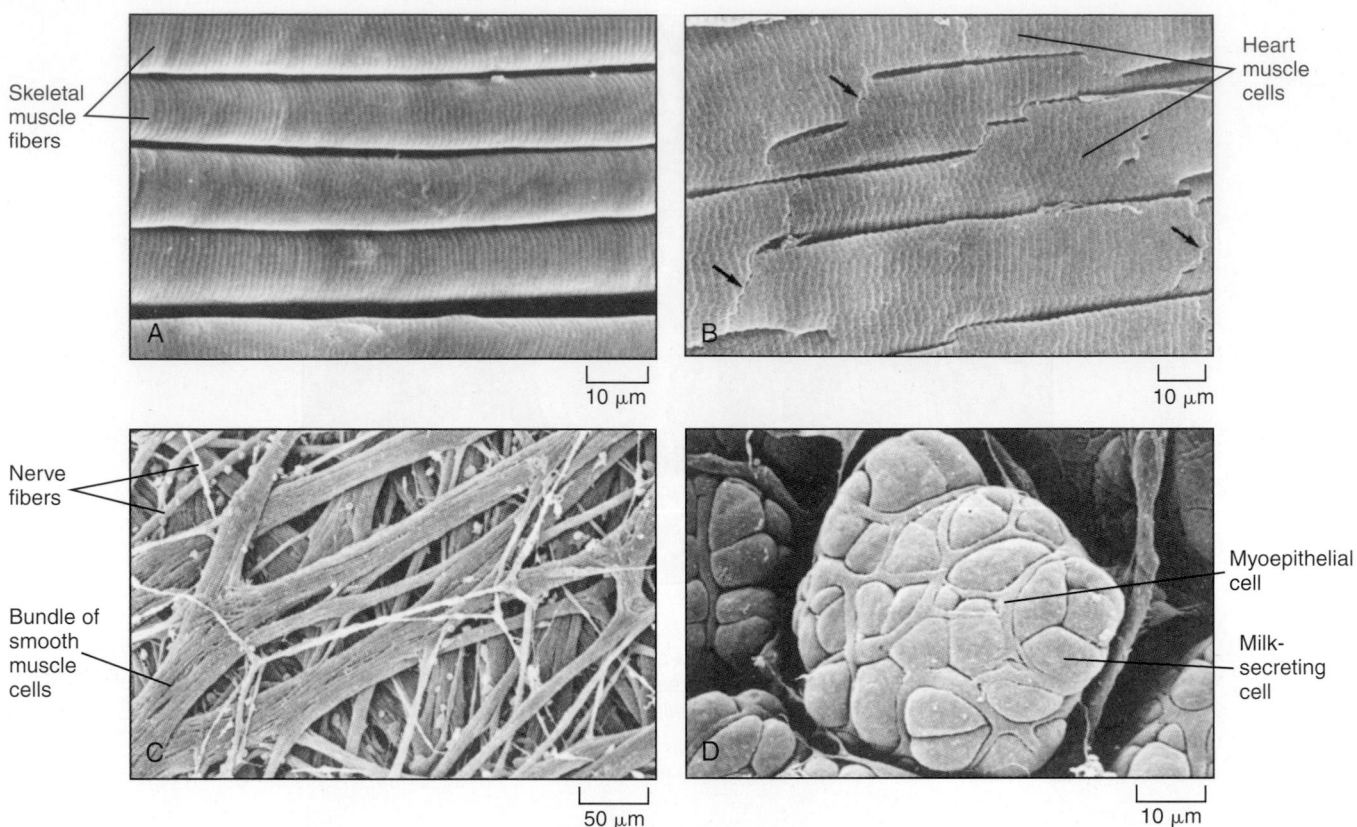

Skeletal muscle fibers

Heart muscle cells

Nerve fibers

Bundle of smooth muscle cells

Myoepithelial cell

Milk-secreting cell

10 µm

10 µm

50 µm

10 µm

FIGURE 5-18 The four classes of muscle cells. **A,** Skeletal muscle. **B,** Heart (cardiac) muscle. **C,** Smooth muscle (bladder). **D,** Myoepithelial cells in a mammary gland. (**A** and **C,** From Alberts B et al, editors: *Molecular biology of the cell,* ed 5, New York, 2008, Garland Science, p 1451. **A,** Courtesy Junzo Deskati. **B,** From Fujiwara T: Cardiac muscle. In Canal ED, editor: *Handbook of microscopic anatomy,* Berlin, 1986, Springer-Verlag. **C,** Courtesy Satoshi Nakasiro. **D,** From Nagato T et al: A scanning electron microscope study of myoepithelial cells in exocrine glands, *Cell Tissue Res* 209:1-10, 1980.)

a **syncytium:** all the cells contract synchronously. Cardiac muscle contracts in response to activation of pacemaker cells in the heart that have the special property of automaticity. *Automaticity* refers to the inherent ability of the cell to initiate an action potential without outside stimulation. The contractile mechanisms of cardiac muscle are similar to those of skeletal muscle, requiring free calcium to interact with troponin, resulting in the formation of actin-myosin crossbridges. In cardiac muscle, some of the free calcium originates from the sarcoplasmic reticulum, but diffusion into the cell through channels in the cell membrane is also necessary. These membrane calcium channels represent an important difference from skeletal muscle, because they can be manipulated by drugs (calcium channel blockers) without disrupting skeletal muscle control. (Cardiac muscle is discussed in Chapter 17.)

Smooth muscle comprises a diverse group of tissues located in organs throughout the body. Smooth muscle generally is not under voluntary control and therefore is called *involuntary muscle.* Some types of smooth muscle are able to contract intrinsically, and most are influenced by the autonomic nervous system. Smooth muscle is found in blood vessels and in the walls of hollow organs, such as those of the gastrointestinal tract, uterus, and large airways.

The structure of smooth muscle differs considerably from that of skeletal and cardiac muscle, and therefore some classification schemes consider it to be a member of the connective tissue family.[20] The actin and myosin filaments are less organized in smooth muscle, and the muscle does not have striations. Smooth muscle contraction tends to

be slower and can be maintained indefinitely. This is critical to the function of blood vessels, which must maintain a degree of contraction or vascular tone to maintain the blood pressure. Smooth muscle has no troponin and uses the protein calmodulin as the calcium-binding regulatory protein. When calmodulin binds calcium ions in the cytoplasm, it activates the enzyme myosin light chain kinase (MLCK), which phosphorylates myosin and stimulates the rate of cross-bridge formation. Actin filaments are attached to structural proteins called dense bodies that pull in the sides of the muscle cell when actin-myosin cross-bridging causes the filaments to increasingly overlap (Figure 5-19). Smooth muscle contraction is highly dependent on the diffusion of extracellular calcium into the cell through calcium channels in the plasma membrane (sarcolemma). Thus, like cardiac muscle, smooth muscle can also be affected by drugs that alter the calcium channel's ability to conduct calcium. For example, calcium channel–blocking drugs are used to cause the smooth muscle in arterial blood vessels to relax as a treatment for high blood pressure.

Myoepithelial cells represent the fourth class of muscle cells. They are located in the ducts of some glands (e.g., mammary, sweat, and salivary). Unlike all other types of muscle, myoepithelial cells lie in the epithelium and are derived from embryonic ectoderm, whereas skeletal, cardiac, and smooth muscle are derived from embryonic mesoderm. Myoepithelial cells contract in response to specific stimuli (e.g., oxytocin in the mammary gland) and serve to expel the contents from the gland.

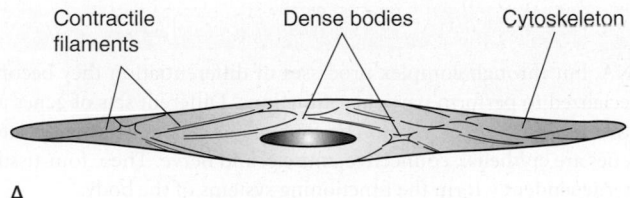

A

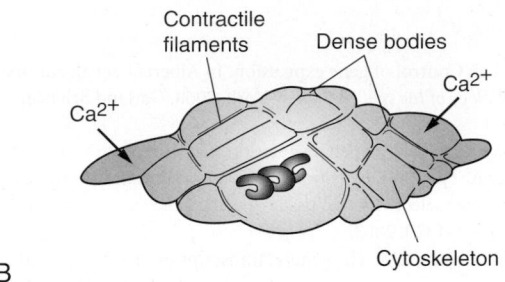

B

FIGURE 5-19 Schematic drawing of a smooth muscle cell when relaxed **(A)** and contracted **(B)**. Contraction begins with the entry of Ca^{2+} into the cell through L-type voltage-gated calcium channels. Ca^{2+} is also released from the sarcoplasmic reticulum. The calcium ions bind to cytoplasmic calmodulin to form a complex that activates myosin light chain kinase (MLCK). The kinase attaches a phosphate to the myosin head area, which stimulates its cycling activity. The myosin binds to actin filaments and tugs on them with each cross-bridge cycle. While the myosin and actin filaments pull closer together and overlap more, the muscle cell shortens. The actin filaments are attached to dense bodies that are analogous in function to the Z-disk protein in cardiac and skeletal muscle. Smooth muscle can maintain long-term actin-myosin cross-bridges that maintain a level of tone.

Nervous Tissue

Nervous tissue is widely distributed throughout the body, providing a rapid communication network between the central nervous system and various body parts. Nerve cells are specialized to generate and transmit electrical impulses very rapidly. Like muscle, nerves are excitable; they respond to stimulation by altering their electrical potentials. This excitability is caused by the presence of voltage-sensitive ion channels located in the plasma membrane of the nerve cell. Movement of ions through these channels results in the production and propagation of action potentials along the length of the neuron. Neurons communicate their action potentials to other nerve and muscle cells through synapses. At the synapse, the presynaptic neuron releases a chemical neurotransmitter into the space between itself and the next neuron (synaptic cleft), where it diffuses across and interacts with receptors on the postsynaptic neuron.

A typical neuron is composed of three parts: a cell body, an axon, and one or more dendrites (Figure 5-20). The cell body contains the nucleus and other cytoplasmic organelles. The axon is generally long (as long as 1 m) and may be encased in a myelin sheath. The axons usually conduct impulses away from the cell body, whereas the dendritic processes usually receive information and conduct impulses toward the cell body. Neurons are classified on the basis of the number of projections extending from the cell body. Neurons are terminally differentiated and incapable of replicating. However, neural stem cells are located in certain areas of the brain and may replicate to form either neurons or glial cells in response to specific signals (see Chapter 43).

In addition to neurons, nervous tissue contains a variety of supportive cells, termed **neuroglia** ("nerve glue"), that nourish, protect,

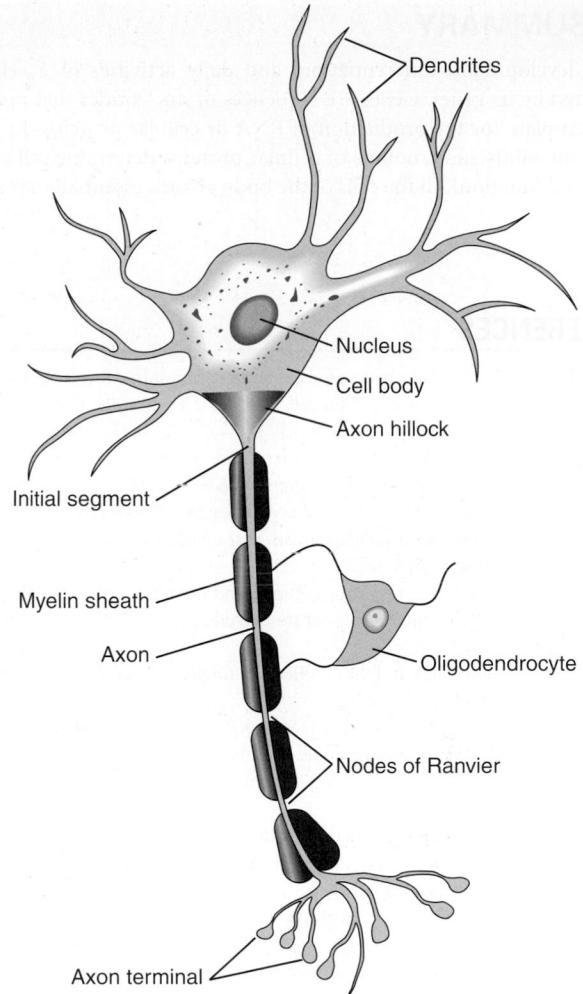

FIGURE 5-20 Diagram of a typical neuron showing the cell body, axon, and dendrites. Neurons have many shapes and sizes.

insulate, and clean up debris in the central nervous system. These include the astrocytes, oligodendroglia, ependymal cells, and microglia. (See Chapter 43 for a detailed description of nervous system anatomy and physiology.)

KEY POINTS

- The structure and function of cells are influenced by the genome and environment as well as by developmental history.
- Embryonic development is associated with selective gene expression that controls four essential processes to enable a single cell to develop into a complex organism: (1) cell proliferation; (2) cell specialization; (3) cell-to-cell interactions; and (4) cell movement and migration.
- Terminally differentiated cell types have limited capacities to divide. Some tissues, such as skin and bone marrow, maintain large numbers of stem cells, which have great capacity to proliferate. Tissues are able to recruit multipotent stem cells from the bone marrow that have the capacity to become differentiated tissue cells if given appropriate survival and developmental conditions.
- Different cell types in the adult human are classified into four major categories: epithelium (e.g., skin, glands, endothelium); connective tissue (e.g., bone, cartilage, fat, blood); muscle (e.g., skeletal, cardiac, smooth); and nervous tissue (e.g., neuronal, glial).

SUMMARY

The development, differentiation, and daily activities of a cell are directed by its genes. Genes are sequences of nucleotides that provide the template for the production of RNA or cellular proteins. In large part, the kinds and amounts of cellular proteins determine cell structure and function. All the cells of the body possess essentially the same DNA, but through complex processes of differentiation they become specialized to perform particular functions. Different sets of genes are active in different cell types. The four major classes of differentiated tissues are epithelial, connective, muscle, and nerve. These four tissues interdependently form the functioning systems of the body.

REFERENCES

1. Alberts B, et al: DNA chromosomes, and genomes. In Alberts B, et al, editors: *Molecular biology of the cell*, ed 5, New York, 2008, Garland Science, pp 195–262.
2. Watson JD, Crick FHC: Molecular structure of nucleic acids: a structure for deoxyribose nucleic acid, *Nature* 171:737–738, 1953.
3. Balakrishnan L, Bambara RA: Eukaryotic lagging strand DNA replication employs a multi-pathway mechanism that protects genome integrity, *J Biol Chem* 286(9):6865–6870, 2011.
4. Alberts B, et al, editors: DNA replication, repair and recombination. In Alberts B, et al, editors: *Molecular biology of the cell*, ed 5, New York, 2008, Garland Science, pp 263–328.
5. Kunkel TA, Bebenek K: DNA replication fidelity, *Annu Rev Biochem* 69:497–529, 2000.
6. Crick FHC: The genetic code: III, *Sci Am* 215(4):55–62, 1966.
7. Frisch L, editor: The genetic code. In *Cold Spring Harbor symposia on quantitative biology*, Cold Spring Harbor, NY, 1966, Cold Spring Harbor Laboratory.
8. Meisenberg G, Simmons WH: The human genome. In Meisenberg G, Simmons WH, editors: *Principles of medical biochemistry*, ed 3, Philadelphia, 2012, Saunders, pp 93–117.
9. Gravely BR: Sorting out the complexity of SR functions, *RNA* 6(9):1197–1211, 2000.
10. Frank J: The ribosome: a macromolecular machine par excellence, *J Chem Biol* 7:R133–R141, 2000.
11. Alberts B, et al: Control of gene expression. In Alberts B, et al, editors: *Molecular biology of the cell*, ed 5, New York, 2008, Garland Science, pp 411–499.
12. Emerson BM: Specificity of gene regulation, *Cell* 109(3):267–270, 2003.
13. Hochheimer A, Tjian R: Diversified transcription initiation complexes expand promoter selectivity and tissue-specific gene expression, *Genes Dev* 17(11):1309–1320, 2003.
14. Thomas MC, Chiang CM: The general transcription machinery and general transcription factors, *Crit Rev Biochem Mol Biol* 41:105–178, 2006.
15. Gurdon JB: The developmental capacity of nuclei taken from intestinal epithelium cells of feeding tadpoles, *J Embryol Exp Morphol* 10:622–640, 1962.
16. Bell O, Tiwari VK, Thomä NH, Schübeler D: Determinants and dynamics of genome accessibility, *Nat Rev Genet* 12(8):554–564, 2011.
17. Alberts B, et al: Development of multicellular organisms. In Alberts B, et al, editors: *Molecular biology of the cell*, ed 5, New York, 2008, Garland Science, pp 1305–1416.
18. Lock JG, Wehrle-Haller B: Cell-matrix adhesion complexes: master control machinery of cell migration, *Semin Cancer Biol* 18(1):65–67, 2008.
19. Gardiner NJ: Integrins and the extracellular matrix: key mediators of development and regeneration of the sensory nervous system, *Dev Neurobiol* 71(11):1054–1072, 2011.
20. Alberts B, et al: Specialized tissues, stem cells, and tissue renewal. In Alberts B, et al, editors: *Molecular biology of the cell*, ed 5, New York, 2008, Garland Science, pp 1417–1484.
21. Teitelbaum SL: Osteoclasts: what do they do and how do they do it? *Am J Pathol* 170(2):427–435, 2007.

Genetic and Developmental Disorders

Linda D. Ward

KEY QUESTIONS

- How are genes transmitted from parent to offspring?
- How is pedigree analysis used to determine if a trait is inherited as autosomal dominant, autosomal recessive, or X-linked?
- How might abnormal meiosis lead to alterations in chromosome number or structure?
- What are the inheritance patterns and general clinical features of some common genetic disorders?
- What is the role of the environment in the development of congenital disorders?
- What methods of genetic testing are available?

CHAPTER OUTLINE

Geneticists and parents alike have marveled at the development of a recognizable human baby, with eyes and ears, toes and fingers, from its simple beginning as a single cell containing one set of genes. Considering the enormous list of potentially disastrous genetic and environmental influences, the birth of a healthy normal child does indeed seem like a miracle. Although the risk of bearing a child with mental or physical defects is small for most parents, it is real and is often a source of worry during the prenatal period. It has been estimated that most people harbor five to eight defective genes that are recessive and therefore of little consequence until they are transmitted to offspring.[1] In addition, there are many known and unknown environmental hazards to which the parent and fetus may be exposed. Disorders that are present at birth are called *congenital*, whether the cause is genetic, environmental, or both. Some congenital disorders are associated with structural defects attributable to errors in fetal development and are called **congenital malformations.** It is estimated that about 3% of newborns have a major malformation of cosmetic or functional significance.[2,3] Malformations are frequently associated with genetic causes; however, environmental influences (teratogens) also may adversely affect the developing fetus, and in half of cases a clear explanation for a malformation cannot be found. Approximately 30% to 40% of all birth malformations are associated with genetic factors—6% are associated with chromosomal abnormalities, 8% are associated with single-gene disorders, and 20% to 30% are most likely multifactorial.[3] Some inherited genetic disorders do not become apparent until later in

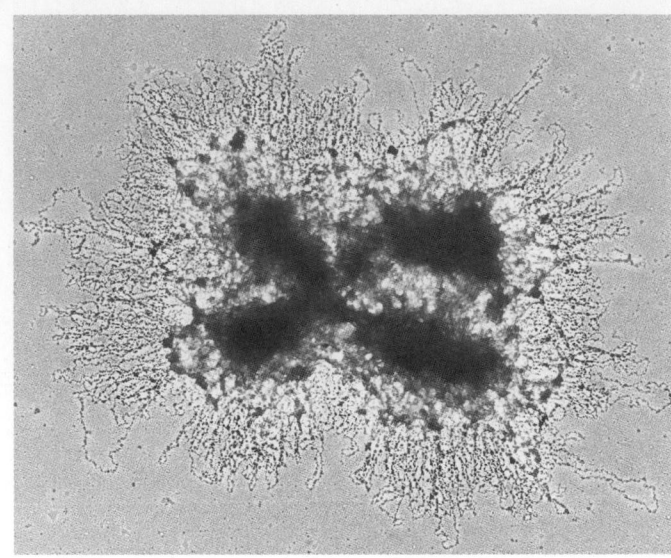

FIGURE 6-1 Scanning electron micrograph of a chromosome showing the two sister chromatids attached at the centromere. Sister chromatids separate during meiosis with one chromatid being distributed to each daughter cell. (From Pollard T et al: *Cell biology,* ed 2, Philadelphia, 2007, Saunders, p 224.)

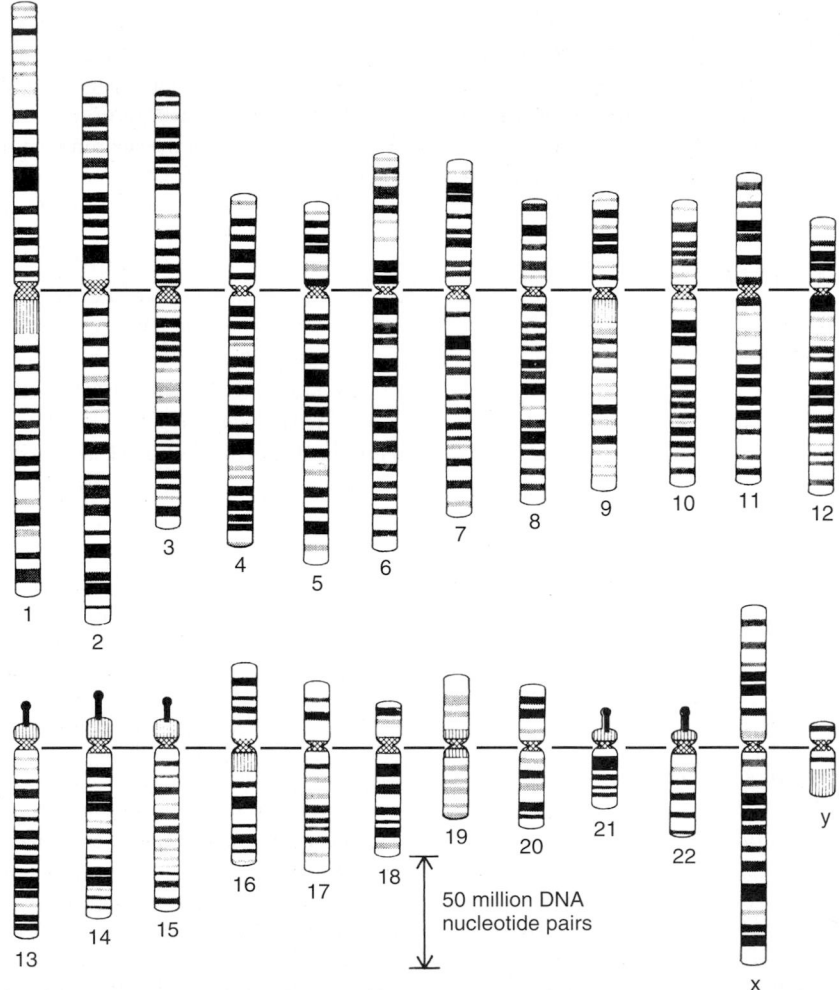

FIGURE 6-2 A standard map of the banding pattern of each of the 23 chromosomes of the human. Somatic cells contain two copies of each chromosome. The centromere region is marked by the line. (From Alberts B et al, editors: *Molecular biology of the cell,* ed 5, New York, 2008, Garland Science, p 203.)

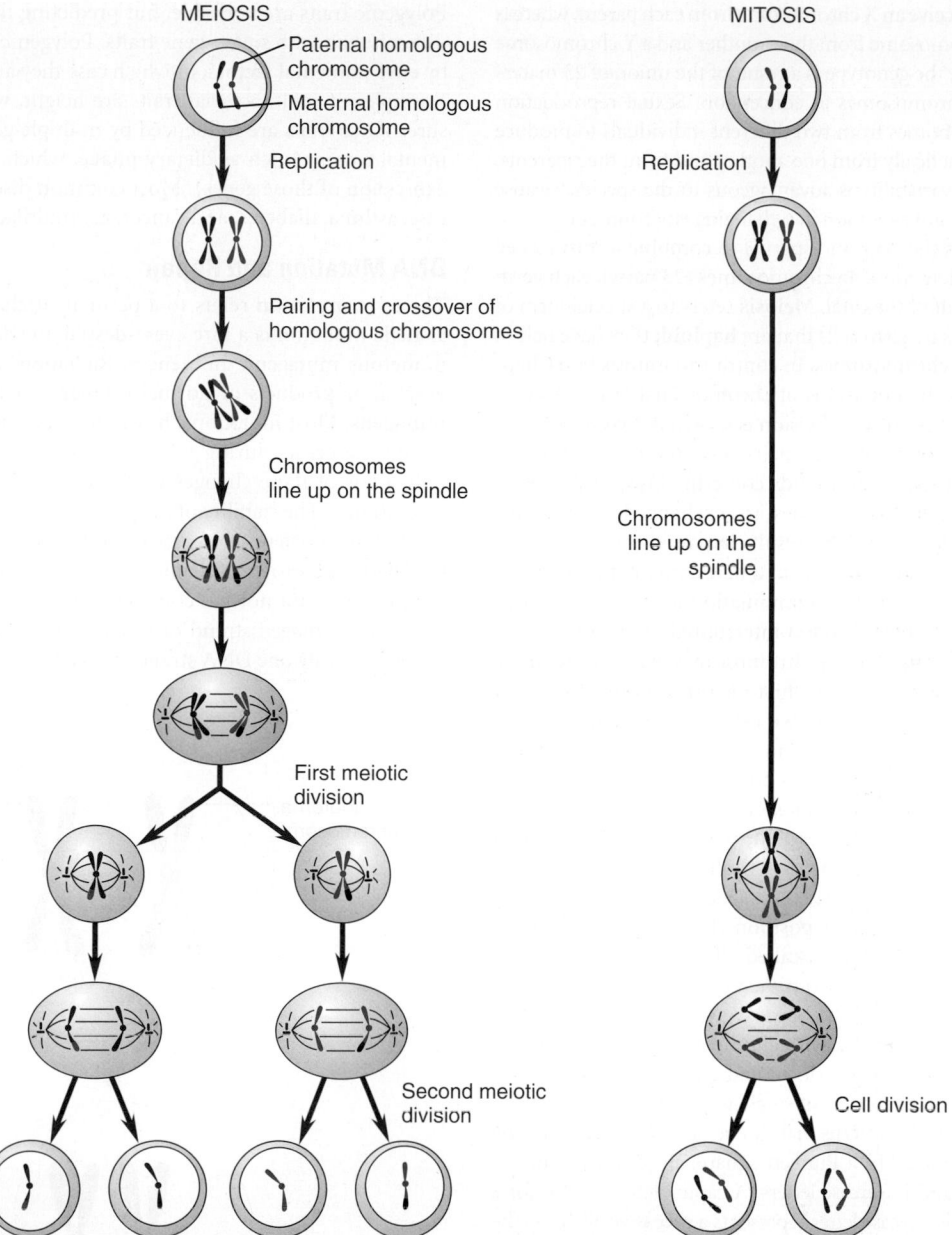

FIGURE 6-3 Comparison of meiosis and normal mitotic cell division, showing only one homologous chromosome pair. In meiosis, the homologous chromosomes form a pair and exchange sections of DNA in a process called *crossing over*. Two nuclear divisions are required in meiosis to form the haploid germ cells.

childhood or adulthood and therefore are not considered to be congenital. In this chapter, the general principles of inheritance; genetic and environmental causes of congenital disorders; and the principles of diagnosis, counseling, and gene therapy are described.

PRINCIPLES OF INHERITANCE

"Whom does the baby look like?" is frequently asked of new parents. It is common knowledge that traits tend to run in families, but Gregor Mendel, a nineteenth-century monk turned geneticist, was the first to notice that traits were transmitted in a predictable way from parent to offspring.[4] Height, weight, skin color, eye color, and hair color are some of the physical traits that characterize an individual; other inherited traits contribute to risk for disease. **Phenotype** refers to the physical and biochemical attributes of an individual that are outwardly apparent. These traits are a result of the expression of the individual's

unique genetic makeup, or **genotype.** In humans, genes are organized into 46 different chromosomes that become visible under the microscope only during cell division (see Chapter 5).

Before cell division, chromosomes look like X's of varying sizes and shapes. The X-shaped chromosome is really made up of two identical linear chromosome units, called **chromatids,** which separate during meiosis. The point at the middle of the X at which the two sister chromatids are united is the **centromere** (Figure 6-1). Human chromosomes are **diploid;** they occur as pairs. One member of the pair comes from the mother, and one member comes from the father. Under the microscope the members of a pair appear to be identical (**homologous),** although they are different in DNA sequence. Chromosomes are characterized on the basis of total size, length of the arms of the X, and characteristic banding patterns when exposed to certain stains (karyotype) (Figure 6-2).

Of the 23 pairs of chromosomes, 22 are homologous and are called **autosomes.** The remaining pair, the **sex** chromosomes, differs in males and females. Females receive an X chromosome from each parent, whereas males receive an X chromosome from their mother and a Y chromosome from their father. Thus, the genotype is a result of the union of 23 maternal and 23 paternal chromosomes at conception. Sexual reproduction allows the mixing of genomes from two different individuals to produce offspring that differ genetically from one another and from their parents. This source of genetic variability is advantageous to the species because it allows for adaptation and evolution in a changing environment.

For the 2 germ cells (i.e., egg and sperm) to combine to form a cell with the normal complement of 46 chromosomes (23 pairs), each germ cell must contribute half of the total. **Meiosis** refers to a special form of cell division that results in germ cells that are **haploid;** they have half of the normal number of chromosomes. In contrast to mitosis (see Chapter 3), meiosis involves two divisions of chromosomal DNA. A comparison of meiotic and mitotic cell division is shown in Figure 6-3.

During the first phase of meiosis, pairs of homologous chromosomes with duplicated sister chromatids come in close contact. Portions of the homologous chromosomes are exchanged in a process called *crossing over* (Figure 6-4). This results in a mixing of the maternal and paternal genes of the cell to form a new combination of genes within the chromosomes. Genetic recombination is very precise, such that genes are exchanged intact and not interrupted in the middle. On average, each homologous pair of chromosomes has one to three crossover events occurring during the first meiotic division.[5] The first cellular division of meiosis results in two cells, each with 46 chromosomes. These two cells undergo a second division in which the sister chromatids are pulled apart (similar to normal mitosis), resulting in four cells, each having only 23 chromosomes. Each of the germ cells has a different combination of genes that, when passed on through sexual reproduction, will form a new, genetically unique individual.

The genes that code for a particular gene product, such as an enzyme, are located at a particular position (locus) on the chromosome. Genes come in several forms, called alleles. A person has two alleles for each gene, one received from each parent. If both alleles are identical, the individual is said to be homozygous for that gene. If two different alleles are present, the individual is heterozygous.

Some traits involve only one gene locus and are called single-gene (or monogenic) traits. The transmission of single-gene traits from parent to offspring follows predictable patterns that can be demonstrated using the Punnett square (Figure 6-5). In a Punnett square, alleles for a gene are represented by capital and lowercase letters. A capital letter is used for a **dominant** allele, and a lowercase letter represents a **recessive** allele. As the term implies, a dominant allele will mask a recessive allele, making the associated trait apparent. A recessive trait is apparent only if *both* alleles for the trait are recessive (homozygous). Dominant genes often code for functional enzymes or structural proteins, and recessive genes code for nonfunctional ones. The Punnett square is based on the mendelian principle that all genes are inherited independently from each other in a random manner. Thus, if both parents are heterozygous for a dominant trait (Aa), the offspring will have a 25% probability of being AA, a 50% probability of being Aa, and a 25% probability of being aa. Persons having the AA and Aa genotypes will *express* the trait in a similar manner. The trait will be absent in the aa genotype. Many genetic diseases are carried on the recessive allele and are manifested only by the homozygous (aa) genotype (e.g., cystic fibrosis, phenylketonuria). Persons who are heterozygous for the disease (Aa) are said to be **carriers** because they are able to pass the defective recessive gene to their offspring even though they do not exhibit the trait.

Some alleles are not clearly dominant or recessive and result in a blending or *codominant* expression of the trait. Blood type, for example, has three distinct alleles: A, B, and O. The A and B alleles may both be expressed together, resulting in the AB blood type. Most traits result from the interaction of several gene loci and are called **polygenic**.

Polygenic traits are heritable, but predicting their occurrence is more difficult than with single-gene traits. Polygenic traits are often affected by environmental factors, in which case they are called **multifactorial.** Examples of multifactorial traits are height, weight, and blood pressure. These traits are influenced by multiple genes as well as environmental factors (such as dietary intake, which influences the ultimate expression of those genes). Most common diseases, such as heart disease, asthma, diabetes, and cancer, are multifactorial as well.

DNA Mutation and Repair

The term **mutation** refers to a permanent change in DNA structure. Genetic mutation is a rare event despite the daily exposure of cells to numerous mutagenic influences. Radiation, chemicals, viruses, and even some products of normal cellular metabolism are all potential **mutagens.** Most mutations, however, occur spontaneously as a result of copying errors during DNA replication.[3] Regardless of the cause, only a few of these changes in DNA result in permanent alterations (mutations). The stability of the genes, and thus the low mutation rate, depends on efficient DNA repair mechanisms.

There are a variety of cellular DNA repair mechanisms. Most require the presence of a normal complementary DNA template to correctly repair the damaged strand of DNA. Single-stranded breaks or loss of bases from only one DNA strand are readily repaired. Double-stranded

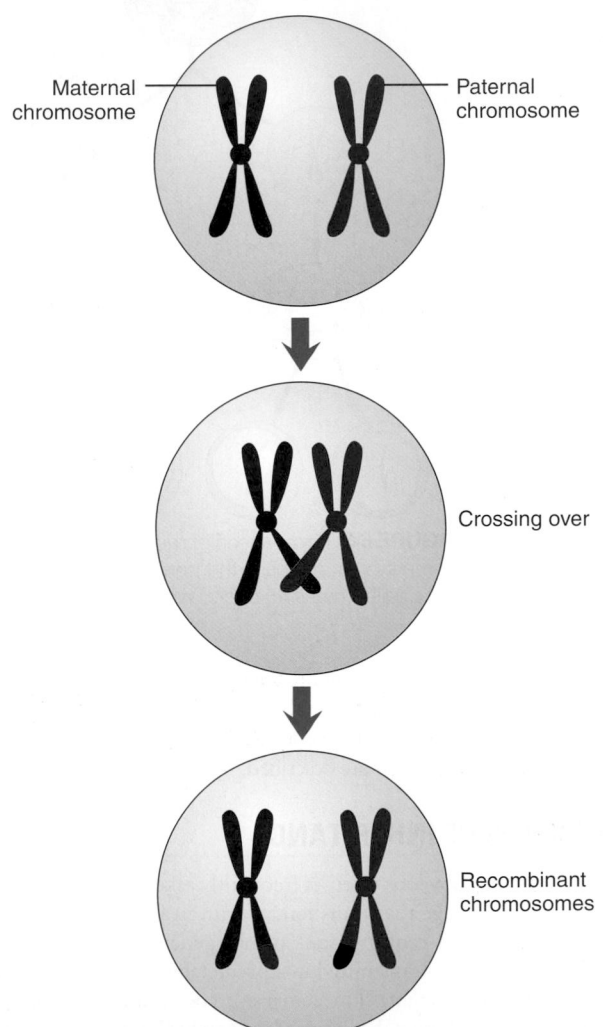

Maternal chromosome — Paternal chromosome

Crossing over

Recombinant chromosomes

FIGURE 6-4 Crossing over during meiotic prophase I results in a reassortment of genes between homologous chromosomes.

breaks, involving both strands of complementary DNA, may result in permanent loss of genetic information at the break point when the broken strands are reunited. Different types of DNA damage are detected and repaired by different enzyme systems. The steps in one type of DNA repair are shown in Figure 6-6.

Genetic mutations are generally of two types: a point mutation, which involves a single base pair substitution, or a frameshift mutation, which often changes the genetic code dramatically. A sequence of three DNA bases (codon) is required to code for each amino acid. A point mutation in the gene may cause the affected codon to signify an abnormal amino acid. The inclusion of the abnormal amino acid in the sequence of the protein may or may not be of clinical significance. Sickle cell anemia and α_1-antiprotease deficiency are examples of point mutation disorders in which a single amino acid substitution causes significant dysfunction.

A frameshift mutation is due to the addition or deletion of one or more bases, which changes the "reading frame" of the DNA sequence. The DNA sequence is normally "read" in groups of three bases, with no spaces between codons. All of the codon triplets will be changed in the DNA downstream from a frameshift mutation, resulting in a protein with a greatly altered amino acid sequence (Figure 6-7). Numerous genetic disorders are due to mutations in a gene that codes for a particular protein. These are termed *single-gene* or *mendelian* disorders. Mutations may also alter chromosome structure through loss, gain, or translocation of chromosome segments. These processes are discussed later in the chapter.

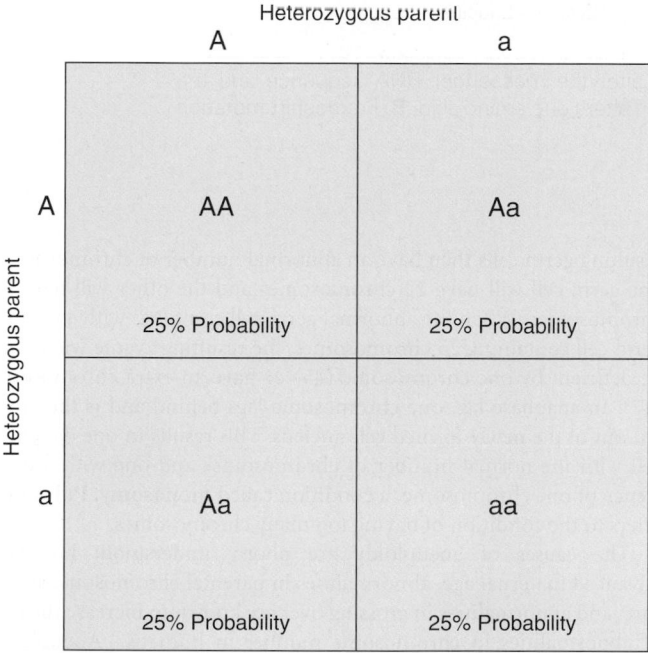

FIGURE 6-5 Punnett square shows the distribution of parental genes to their offspring. This example shows the mating of two heterozygous individuals. *A*, Dominant gene; *a*, recessive gene.

KEY POINTS

- Human DNA is organized into 46 chromosomes (23 pairs). Paired chromosomes look similar under the microscope but differ in DNA sequence. One member of each pair is inherited from the mother, and the other from the father.
- Twenty-two pairs of chromosomes are autosomes. The remaining pair, the sex chromosomes, confers maleness (XY) or femaleness (XX).
- During meiotic cell division, the chromosomes are distributed to daughter cells. Meiosis results in four daughter cells, each having half the normal number of chromosomes (23 chromosomes).
- Genes that code for a particular trait may come in several forms or alleles. Genotype refers to the particular set of alleles an individual receives. Phenotype refers to an individual's observable attributes. People with different genotypes may have similar phenotypes.
- Some traits involve only one gene locus and are called *single-gene traits*. The transmission of these traits from parent to offspring follows predictable patterns. The expression of single-gene traits is determined by whether the gene is dominant or recessive. Dominant genes usually code for functional enzymes; recessive genes do not. Most traits result from the interaction of several genes. These polygenic traits do not follow predictable patterns of inheritance.

GENETIC DISORDERS

Genetic disorders may be apparent at birth or may not be clinically evident until much later in life. The majority of genetic disorders are inherited from the affected individual's parents; however, new (de novo) mutations sometimes occur during gamete formation or arise

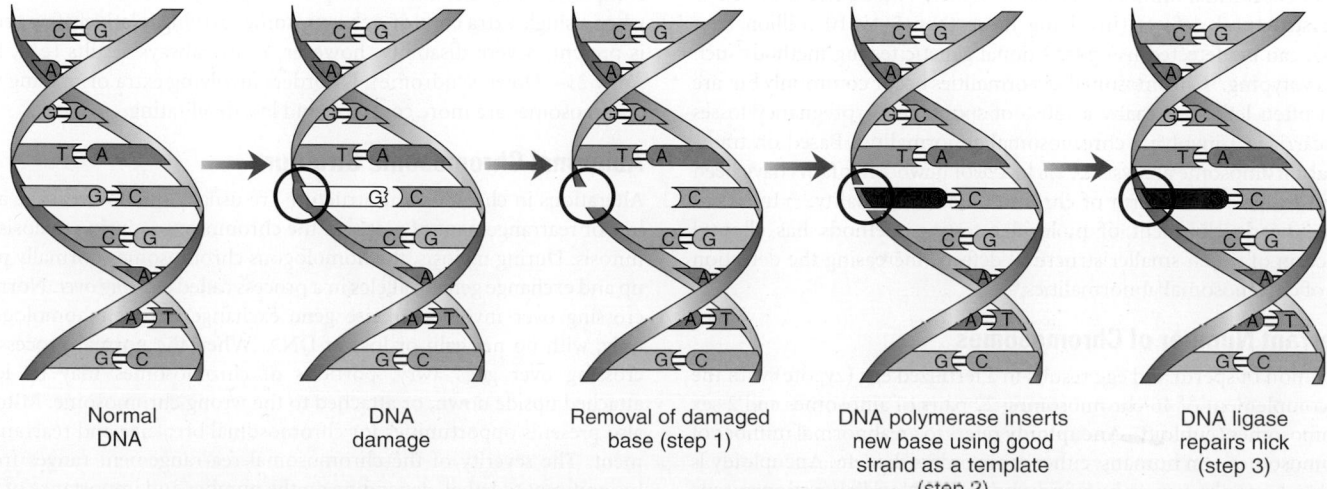

FIGURE 6-6 Steps of DNA repair. In step 1 the damaged section is removed; in steps 2 and 3 the original DNA sequence is restored.

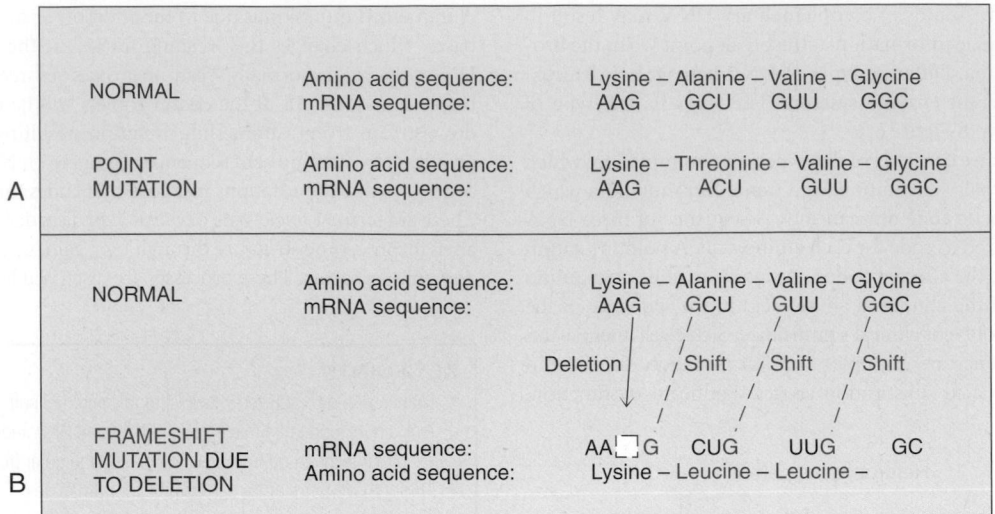

FIGURE 6-7 Schematic illustration of mutations that alter the messenger RNA sequence and the resulting protein amino acid sequence. **A,** Point mutation alters one amino acid. **B,** Frameshift mutation alters all downstream amino acids.

during fetal development. Genetic disorders encountered clinically are only a small percentage of those that occur and represent the less extreme aberrations that permit live birth.

Disorders that are genetic in origin traditionally have been divided into three groups: (1) chromosomal aberrations, (2) mendelian single-gene disorders, and (3) polygenic or multifactorial disorders. A fourth group encompasses a number of single-gene defects that do not follow classic mendelian patterns of inheritance. This group includes triplet repeat (trinucleotide) mutations, mitochondrial gene mutations, and mutations influenced by genomic imprinting. General principles of transmission and selected examples are included for each of the four groups.

CHROMOSOMAL ABNORMALITIES

Chromosomal defects are generally due to an abnormal number of chromosomes or alterations in the structure of one or more chromosomes. Errors in the separation of chromosomes during meiosis may result in abnormal numbers of chromosomes. These defects, as well as large structural defects (involving more than 5 to 10 million base pairs), can be detected using traditional genetic testing methods such as karyotyping.[6] Chromosomal abnormalities occur commonly but are most often lethal; as many as 50% of spontaneous pregnancy losses (miscarriages) involve a chromosomal abnormality.[1] Based on traditional chromosome analysis, 0.5% to 1% of newborn infants have been found to have some form of chromosomal abnormality.[1,3] In recent years, the development of molecular testing methods has allowed detection of much smaller structural defects, increasing the detection rate of chromosomal abnormalities.[6]

Aberrant Number of Chromosomes

The union of sperm and egg results in a fertilized egg (zygote) with the full complement of 46 chromosomes: 22 pairs of autosomes and 2 sex chromosomes (euploid). **Aneuploidy** refers to an abnormal number of chromosomes—in humans, either more or less than 46. Aneuploidy is most commonly caused by nondisjunction.[3] **Nondisjunction** means that paired homologous chromosomes fail to separate normally during either the first or the second meiotic division (Figure 6-8). The

resulting germ cells then have an abnormal number of chromosomes: one germ cell will have 22 chromosomes and the other will have 24 chromosomes. When the abnormal germ cell combines with a normal germ cell containing 23 chromosomes, the resulting zygote will either be deficient by one chromosome (45) or have an extra chromosome (47). In anaphase lag, one chromosome lags behind and is therefore left out of the newly formed cell nucleus. This results in one daughter cell with the normal number of chromosomes and one with a deficiency of one chromosome, a condition called **monosomy. Polysomy** refers to the condition of having too many chromosomes.

The causes of aneuploidy are poorly understood; however, advanced maternal age, abnormalities in parental chromosome structure, and abnormalities in crossing over are known to increase the risk of abnormalities in chromosome number in humans.[7] Aneuploidy occurs rather frequently during human gametogenesis; however, zygotes with abnormal chromosome numbers are usually nonviable. Approximately one third of human miscarriages involve an aneuploid fetus.[8] Although monosomy involving the autosomes is not usually compatible with life, autosomal polysomy may result in a viable fetus when a single extra copy of a chromosome carrying relatively few genes is present. Severe disability, however, nearly always results (e.g., trisomy 21—Down syndrome). Disorders involving extra or missing sex chromosomes are more common and less debilitating.

Abnormal Chromosome Structure

Alterations in chromosome structure are usually due to breakage and loss or rearrangement of pieces of the chromosomes during meiosis or mitosis. During meiosis, the homologous chromosomes normally pair up and exchange genetic alleles in a process called *crossing over.* Normal crossing over involves precise gene exchange between homologues only, with no net gain or loss of DNA. When the normal process of crossing over goes awry, portions of chromosomes may be lost, attached upside down, or attached to the wrong chromosome. Mitosis also presents opportunities for chromosomal breakage and rearrangement. The severity of the chromosomal rearrangement ranges from insignificant to lethal, depending on the number and importance of the gene loci involved. Gene locations can be described by their position on the long arm (q arm) or the short arm (p arm) of the chromatid. For

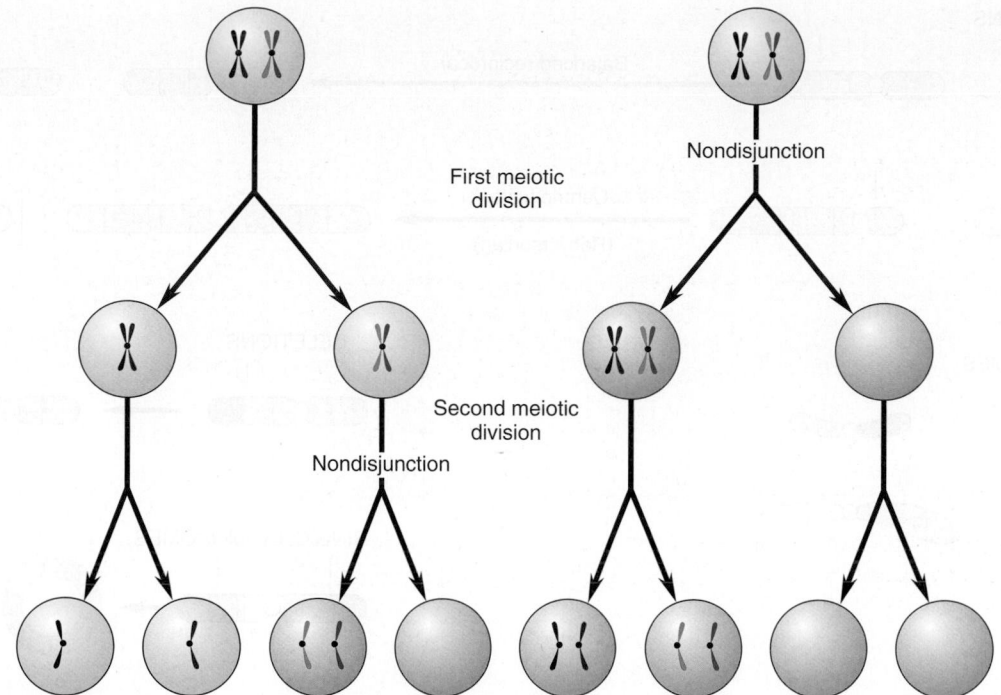

FIGURE 6-8 Mechanism of nondisjunction leading to aneuploidy. For simplicity, only one pair of chromosomes is shown.

example, the gene locus 2p13 is located on the short arm of chromosome 2 at region 1, band 3 (Figure 6-9). The common types of chromosomal rearrangements are translocations, inversions, deletions, and duplications (Figure 6-10).

Chromosomal *translocations* result from the exchange of pieces of DNA between nonhomologous chromosomes. If no genetic material is lost, as in a reciprocal translocation, the individual may have no symptoms or disorder. However, an individual with a reciprocal translocation is at increased risk of producing abnormal gametes. The exchange of a long chromatid arm for a short one results in the formation of one very large chromosome and one very small chromosome (see Figure 6-10). This is called a robertsonian translocation and is responsible for a rare hereditary form of Down syndrome, discussed later in the chapter. Isochromosomes occur when the sister chromatids separate incorrectly at the centromere such that the two identical short arms remain together, as do the two long arms.

Inversion refers to the removal and upside-down reinsertion of a section of chromosome (see Figure 6-10). Like balanced translocations, inversions involve no net loss or gain of genetic material and are often without consequence to the individual. Difficulties result, however, when homologous chromosomes attempt to pair up during meiosis. The chromosome with an inverted section may not pair up properly, resulting in duplications or loss of genes at the time of crossing over. Thus, the offspring of an individual harboring an inversion may be affected.

Loss of chromosomal material is called *deletion*. Deletions result from a break in the arm of a single chromosome, resulting in a fragment of DNA with no centromere. The piece is then lost at the next cell division. Chromosomal deletions have been associated with some forms of cancer, including retinoblastoma (see Chapter 7). Deletions at both ends of a chromatid may cause the free ends to attach to one another, forming a ring chromosome.

In contrast to a deletion, where genes are lost, *duplication* results in extra copies of a portion of DNA. The consequences of duplications are generally less severe than those from loss of genetic material.

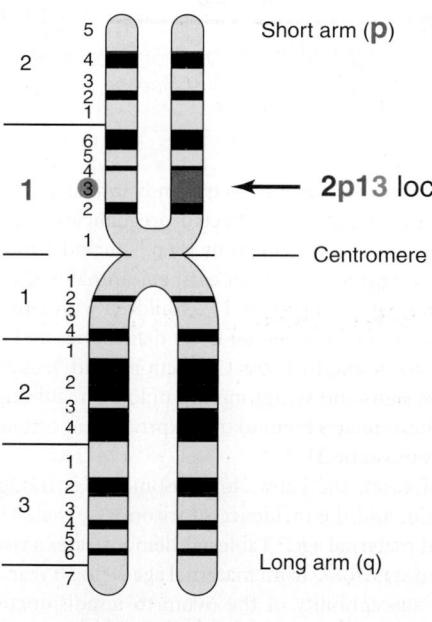

FIGURE 6-9 Metaphase chromosome showing location of centromere and long and short arms of the chromatids. Gene loci are described by the chromosome number, location on short *(p)* or long *(q)* arm, region, and band.

Examples of Autosomal Chromosome Disorders
Trisomy 21 (Down Syndrome)

Trisomy 21 is a chromosomal disorder in which individuals have an extra copy of chromosome 21. It is the most common of the chromosomal disorders and a leading cause of mental disability, occurring in about 1 in 700 live births.[3] The incidence varies among populations

TRANSLOCATIONS

Balanced reciprocal

Centric fusion
(Robertsonian)

Lost

ISOCHROMOSOMES

DELETIONS

Fragments

RING CHROMOSOMES

Fragments

INVERSIONS

Paracentric

Pericentric

DUPLICATIONS

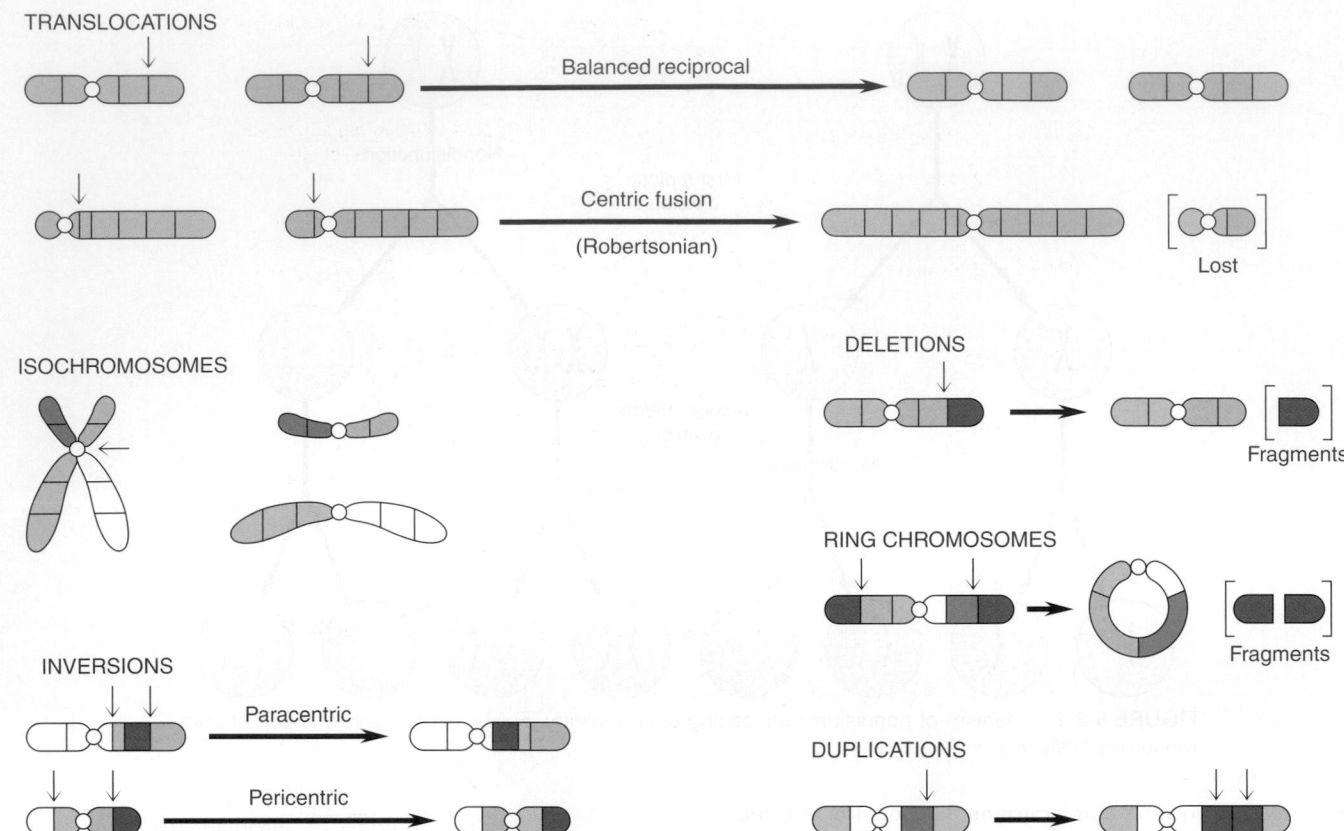

FIGURE 6-10 Types of chromosomal rearrangement. (Adapted from Kumar V et al: *Robbins and Cotran pathologic basis of disease,* ed 8, Philadelphia, 2010, Saunders, p 160.)

and over time, however, and reflects trends in maternal age, prenatal diagnosis, and termination of affected pregnancies.[9] The syndrome, first described by Langdon Down in 1866,[10] includes intellectual disability, protruding tongue, low-set ears, epicanthal folds, poor muscle tone, and short stature (Figure 6-11). Children with Down syndrome often are afflicted with congenital heart deformities and an increased susceptibility to respiratory tract infections and leukemia. Precise causes of these signs and symptoms are unknown, although the gene-dosage hypothesis relates them to overexpression of certain genes contained on chromosome 21.[11]

In 95% of cases, the extra chromosome 21 is thought to be of maternal origin, and the incidence of trisomy 21 is clearly associated with advanced maternal age.[3] Table 6-1 demonstrates a rise in the incidence of Down syndrome from maternal age 20 to 50 years. The reason for increased susceptibility of the ovum to nondisjunction with age remains unknown.

A rare form of Down syndrome (occurring in about 4% of cases) is due to a chromosomal translocation of the long arm of chromosome 21 to another chromosome. This form of Down syndrome is not associated with increased maternal age but is passed from parent to offspring. Therefore, testing for translocations in newborns with Down syndrome is recommended to determine recurrence risk for families.

Trisomy 18 (Edwards Syndrome) and Trisomy 13 (Patau Syndrome)

Trisomy of chromosomes 18 or 13 is much less common than trisomy 21 and more severe. Most affected pregnancies are lost before term, and liveborn infants usually do not survive more than a few days or

weeks.[3] It is not insignificant that the few trisomy conditions compatible with life involve chromosomes containing the smallest numbers of genes. Trisomies involving chromosomes 8, 9, and 22 also have been described but are extremely rare.

Cri du Chat Syndrome

Deletion of part of the short arm of chromosome 5 results in a syndrome characterized by severe mental retardation, round face, and congenital heart anomalies. The syndrome was so named because of the characteristic cry of the affected infant, which is caused by laryngeal malformation and resembles a cat crying. Some children afflicted with this syndrome survive to adulthood, and they generally thrive better than those with the trisomies.

Examples of Sex Chromosome Disorders
Klinefelter Syndrome

The incidence of Klinefelter syndrome is about 1 in 600 liveborn males, making it the most common sex chromosome abnormality.[12] Individuals with Klinefelter syndrome usually have an extra X chromosome (an XXY genotype). However, individuals with more than one extra X (XXXY and XXXXY) have also been described. The presence of the Y chromosome determines the sex of these individuals to be male; however, the extra X chromosomes result in abnormal sexual development and feminization. The condition is rarely diagnosed before puberty, when lack of secondary sex characteristics may become apparent. Associated symptoms reflect a lack of testosterone and include testicular atrophy and infertility, tall stature with long arms and legs, feminine hair distribution, gynecomastia (breast enlargement), high-pitched voice, and marginally impaired intelligence (Figure 6-12).[5] Testosterone

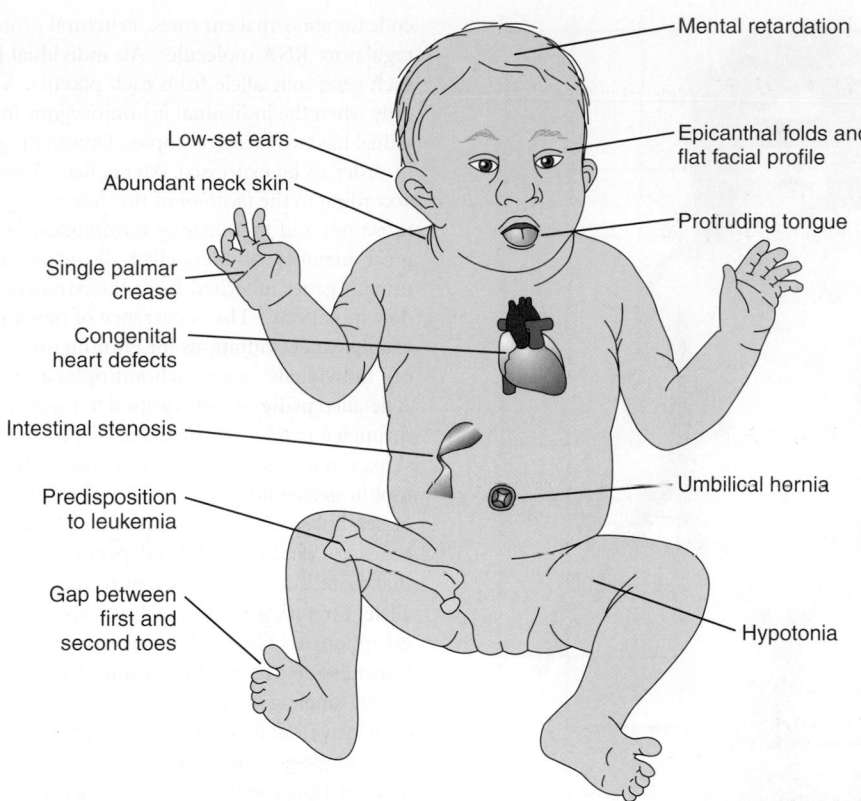

- Mental retardation
- Epicanthal folds and flat facial profile
- Protruding tongue
- Umbilical hernia
- Hypotonia
- Low-set ears
- Abundant neck skin
- Single palmar crease
- Congenital heart defects
- Intestinal stenosis
- Predisposition to leukemia
- Gap between first and second toes

FIGURE 6-11 Typical clinical manifestations of trisomy 21 (Down syndrome).

TABLE 6-1	FREQUENCY OF TRISOMY 21 (DOWN SYNDROME) IN RELATION TO MATERNAL AGE
AGE OF MOTHER AT BIRTH (YEAR)	**FREQUENCY OF TRISOMY 21 AT BIRTH**
20	1/1470
25	1/1333
30	1/935
35	1/353
37	1/200
39	1/112
41	1/68
43	1/46
45	1/36
50	1/26

Data from Morris JK et al: Comparison of models of maternal age-specific risk for Down syndrome live births, *Prenat Diagn* 23:252-258, 2003.

therapy can achieve a dramatic reduction in the feminine characteristics associated with Klinefelter syndrome.

Turner Syndrome

Also known as monosomy X, Turner syndrome is associated with the presence of only one normal X chromosome and no Y chromosome. The absence of the Y chromosome results in a female phenotype; however, the ovaries fail to develop or fail prematurely. In some cases of Turner syndrome, the second X chromosome is not entirely missing but is structurally abnormal. In the majority of cases, the missing or

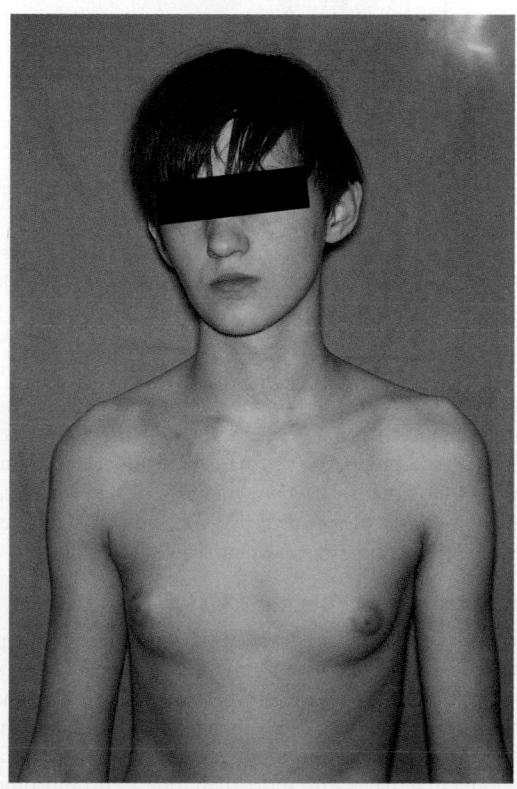

FIGURE 6-12 Typical clinical manifestations of Klinefelter syndrome. (From Moore KL, Persuad TVN: *The developing human: clinically oriented embryology,* ed 8, Philadelphia, 2007, Saunders, p 466.)

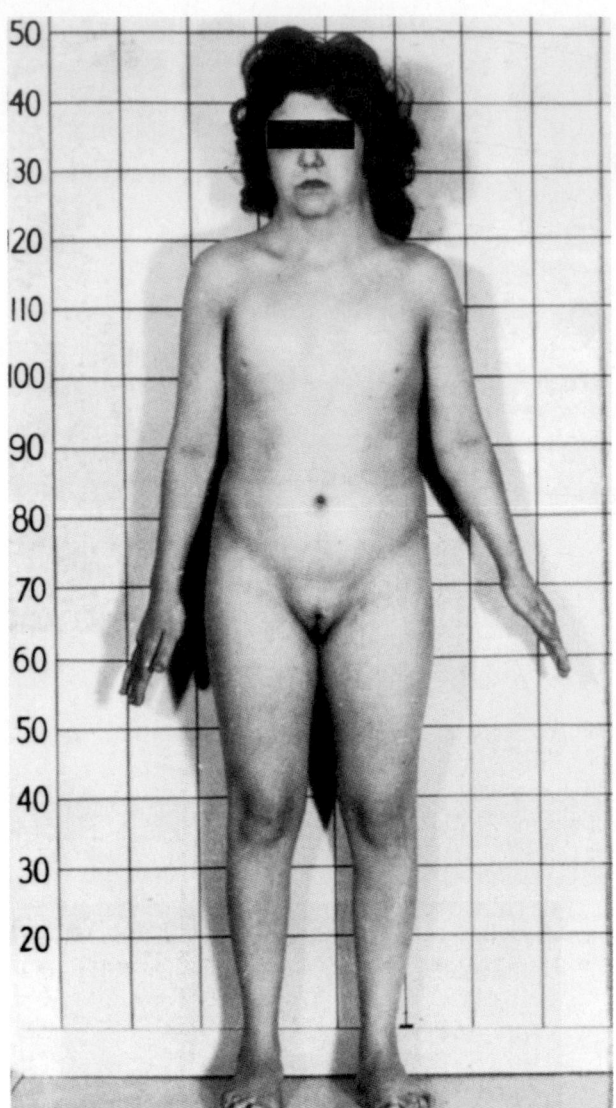

FIGURE 6-13 Typical clinical manifestations of Turner syndrome. (From Connor JM, Ferguson-Smith MA: *Essential medical genetics,* ed 5, London, 1997, Blackwell Scientific, p 123.)

damaged X chromosome is of paternal origin. Most fetuses with monosomy X are lost during pregnancy, and the incidence is about 1 in 3000 live female births.[3,5] Principal characteristics of Turner syndrome include short stature, webbing of the neck, a wide chest, lymphedema of the hands and feet at birth, congenital heart defects, and failure to develop secondary sexual characteristics[13] (Figure 6-13).

Multiple X Females and Double Y Males

A relatively common disorder of the sex chromosomes is the presence of an extra copy of the X chromosome in females (XXX) or of the Y chromosome in males (XYY). Most individuals appear normal; however, females may experience menstrual abnormalities, and males will generally be taller than average. A tendency toward mental retardation has been noted in females with more than four X chromosomes.

MENDELIAN SINGLE-GENE DISORDERS

In contrast to the chromosomal disorders described above, mendelian disorders result from mutations in single genes. The affected genes may

code for abnormal enzymes, structural proteins, regulatory proteins, or regulatory RNA molecules. An individual has two copies or alleles of each gene (one allele from each parent). A recessive gene is expressed only when the individual is homozygous for the gene; that is, the individual has two identical copies. Dominant genes require only one allele in order to be expressed. Mendelian disorders are generally classified according to the *location* of the defective gene (autosomal or sex chromosome) and the *mode of transmission* (dominant or recessive). The great majority of mendelian disorders are familial (attributable to mutant genes inherited from the parents), but 15% to 20% represent new mutations.[1] The occurrence of new mutations ranges widely. For example, new mutations for Huntington disease are rare, whereas 80% of individuals with achondroplasia represent new mutations.[1] A detailed **pedigree** may be used to trace the transmission of the disease through a family. The pedigree (Figure 6-14), showing family relationships and the members who have been affected by the disease, is a useful tool in determining the pattern of inheritance as recessive, dominant, or sex-linked. Mendelian genetics is based on the principle that single genes are randomly and independently transmitted to offspring such that there is a 50:50 chance of receiving one or the other of a parent's alleles for a particular gene. It is important to note that there are many exceptions to these rules, but they generally are useful in predicting transmission patterns for a number of single-gene disorders. More than 10,000 single-gene traits and disorders have been identified.[3] A comprehensive database of the chromosomal location and sequence of these single-gene traits and disorders, called *Online Mendelian Inheritance in Man,* can be accessed at www.ncbi.nlm.nih.gov/omim.

Autosomal Dominant Disorders

Autosomal dominant disorders are due to a mutation of a dominant gene located on one of the autosomes. Autosomal dominant disorders follow predictable patterns of inheritance (Figure 6-15), which may be summarized as follows:

- Males and females are equally affected.
- Affected individuals usually have an affected parent.
- Unaffected individuals do not transmit the disease.
- Offspring of an affected individual (with normal mate) have a 1 in 2 chance of inheriting the disease.
- The rare mating of two individuals, each carrying one copy of the defective gene (heterozygous), results in a 3 in 4 chance of producing an affected offspring.

The list of known autosomal dominant disorders is long. Many are described in later chapters as they relate to system pathophysiology. A partial list is presented in Table 6-2. In general, autosomal dominant disorders involve key structural proteins or regulatory proteins, such as membrane receptors. Marfan syndrome and Huntington disease are commonly cited examples of autosomal dominant disorders and are briefly described here.

Marfan Syndrome

Marfan syndrome is a disorder of the connective tissues of the body. Individuals with Marfan syndrome are typically tall and slender with long, thin arms and legs (Figure 6-16). Because of the long, thin fingers, this syndrome has also been called *arachnodactyly* ("spider fingers"). It is commonly suggested that President Abraham Lincoln may have had this disorder. Although skeletal and joint deformities are problematic, the cardiovascular lesions are the most life threatening. The medial layer of blood vessels, particularly the aorta, tends to be weak and susceptible to dilation and rupture. Dysfunction of the heart valves may occur from poor connective tissue support. Marfan syndrome has been traced to hundreds of different mutations in the fibrillin 1 gene on chromosome 15.[3,5] Fibrillin 1 is a glycoprotein secreted

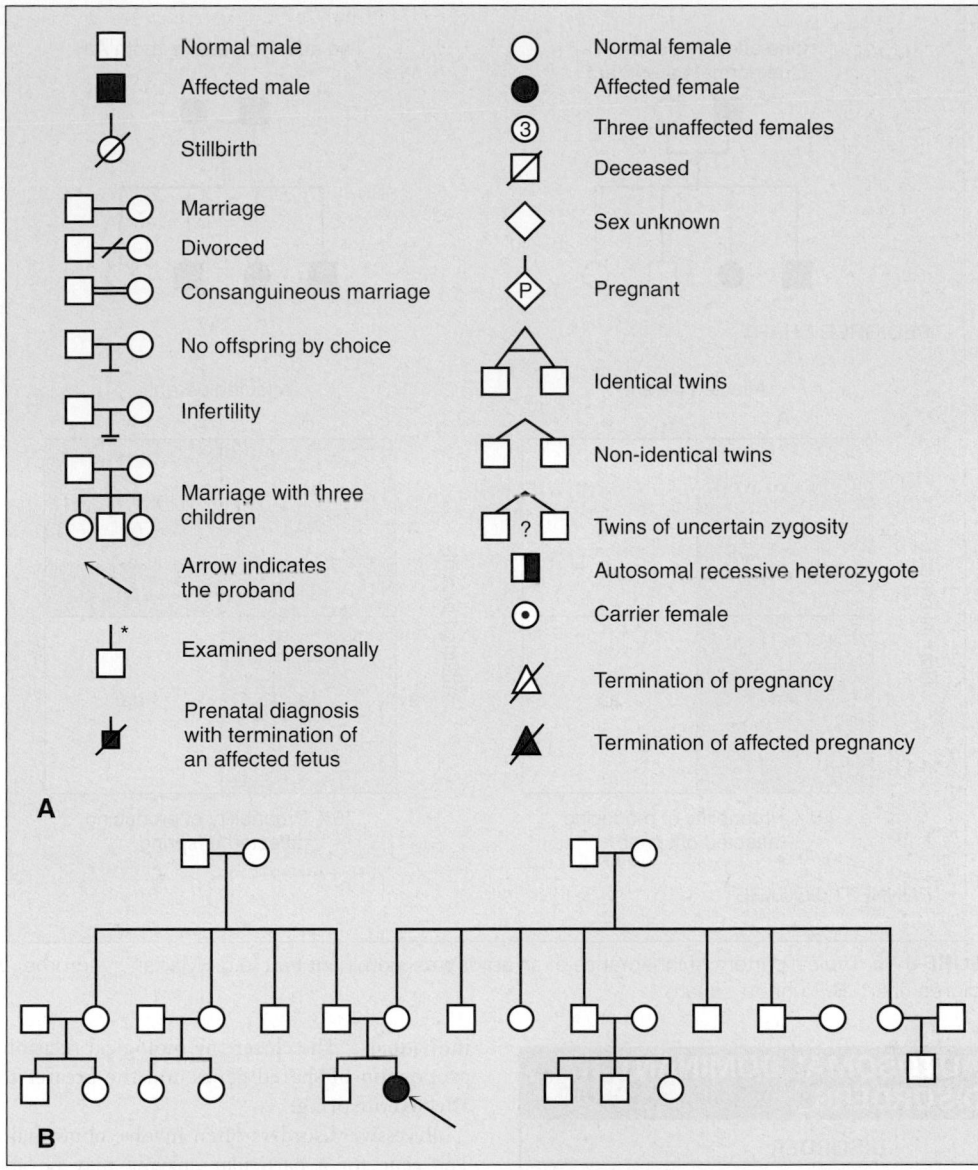

FIGURE 6-14 A, Common symbols for pedigree analysis. **B,** Typical family pedigree chart.

by fibroblasts into the extracellular matrix. It provides important scaffolding for deposition of other matrix proteins such as elastin. Marfan-type fibrillin 1 appears to be more susceptible to proteolytic degradation than normal fibrillin, leading to the weakened connective tissues typical of the disease.

Huntington Disease

Huntington disease is an autosomal dominant disease that primarily affects neurologic function. The symptoms of mental deterioration and involuntary movements of the arms and legs do not appear until approximately age 40 years. The disease was formerly called Huntington chorea (from the Greek *khoreia,* meaning "dance") because of the uncontrolled movements of the limbs. The delayed onset of symptoms means that the disease may be transmitted to offspring before the parent is aware that he or she harbors the defective gene. The prevalence rate is about 1 in 20,000 persons.[5]

The gene abnormality in Huntington disease has been localized to chromosome 4, where an abnormally large number of triplet repeats (CAG) has been noted. Triplet repeats of more than 40 are reliably associated with development of the disease, and the greater the number

of triplet repeats, the earlier the onset of symptoms.[5] The Huntington disease protein (huntingtin) has a long segment of glutamine amino acids that are coded by the CAG triplet repeat. The protein forms aggregates in brain tissue, which are thought to contribute to the pathogenesis of neurodegeneration.[5] Clinical manifestations and pathophysiology of Huntington disease are discussed in Chapter 45.

Autosomal Recessive Disorders

Autosomal recessive disorders are due to a mutation of a recessive gene located on one of the autosomes. Autosomal recessive disorders follow predictable patterns of inheritance (Figure 6-17), which may be summarized as follows:

- Males and females are equally affected.
- In most cases, the disease is not apparent in the parents or relatives of the affected individual, but both parents are carriers of the mutant recessive gene.
- Unaffected individuals may transmit the disease to offspring.
- The mating of two carriers (heterozygous) results in a 1 in 4 chance of producing an affected offspring and a 2 in 4 chance of producing an offspring who carries the disease.

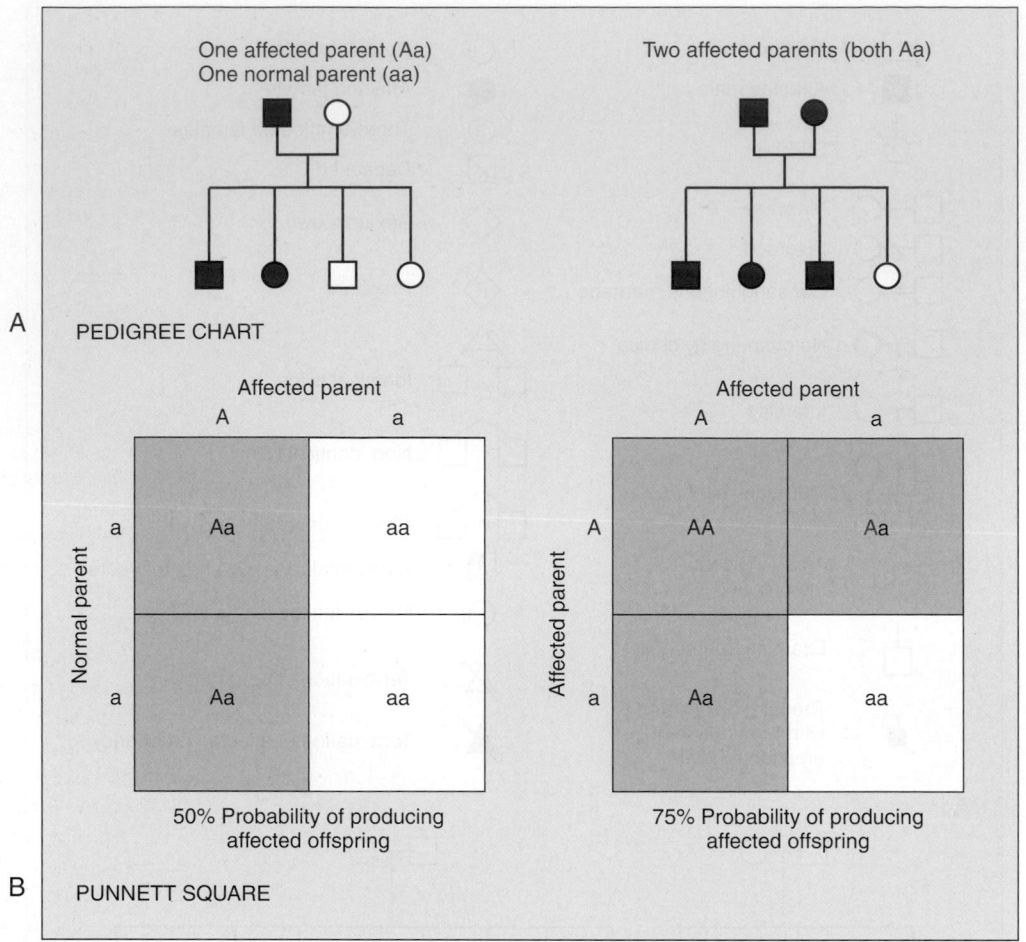

FIGURE 6-15 Typical pattern of inheritance of an autosomal dominant trait (e.g., Marfan syndrome). **A,** Pedigree chart. **B,** Punnett square.

TABLE 6-2	AUTOSOMAL DOMINANT DISORDERS
SYSTEM	**DISORDER**
Nervous	Huntington disease
	Neurofibromatosis
	Myotonic dystrophy
	Tuberous sclerosis
Urinary	Polycystic kidney disease
Gastrointestinal	Familial polyposis coli
Hematopoietic	Hereditary spherocytosis
	Von Willebrand disease
Skeletal	Marfan syndrome
	Ehlers-Danlos syndrome (some variants)
	Osteogenesis imperfecta
	Achondroplasia
Metabolic	Familial hypercholesterolemia
	Acute intermittent porphyria

From Kumar V et al: *Robbins & Cotran pathologic basis of disease,* ed 8, Philadelphia, 2010, Saunders, p 141.

It is estimated that nearly everyone carries several mutated recessive genes, and related individuals are more likely to carry the *same* recessive genes.[1] Because recessive diseases are only expressed when both alleles for a particular gene are mutant (homozygous), they are often associated with **consanguinity**—the mating of related individuals.[5] The closer the biological relationship, the greater the proportion of shared genes and the greater the risk of producing affected offspring.

Recessive disorders often involve abnormal enzymatic functions. The gene for a particular enzyme may be absent or present in a mutated, and therefore nonfunctional, form. The enzyme deficiency usually is not apparent in heterozygotes carrying one normal gene and one mutated gene because the normal gene produces enough of the necessary enzyme. In the homozygous state, neither gene for the enzyme is functional, resulting in an enzyme deficiency. A partial list of the large number of autosomal recessive disorders that have been identified is given in Table 6-3. Many of these diseases involve the inability to metabolize nutrients (inborn errors of metabolism) or to synthesize cellular components because of enzyme deficiencies. Albinism, phenylketonuria, and cystic fibrosis are described here as representative examples. Other disorders are described in the discussions of system pathophysiology in later chapters.

Albinism

Albinism refers to a lack of pigmentation of the hair, skin, and/or eyes. There are several types of albinism; all types involve disruption of melanin synthesis. Albinism is currently classified according to the affected gene. In oculocutaneous albinism, which is inherited in an autosomal recessive fashion, pigmentation of the skin, hair, and eyes is decreased.[14] Affected individuals are at risk for sunburn and skin cancer, and generally exhibit impaired vision, nystagmus (involuntary eye movements), and photosensitivity.

The cystic fibrosis gene was isolated in 1989 and mapped to chromosome 7. More than 1300 different mutations of this gene have been identified, all of which cause a defect in chloride transport across the cell membrane; however, the severity of chloride channel dysfunction varies widely with different mutations.[1] The most common mutation, accounting for about 70% of cystic fibrosis cases, is due to a deletion of three nucleotides that normally code for a phenylalanine at position 508.[3] The absence of this single amino acid apparently causes the protein to fold abnormally, preventing its release from the endoplasmic reticulum, where it is eventually degraded. A schematic of the normal chloride transporter (called *cystic fibrosis transmembrane conductance regulator* [CFTR] *protein* is shown in Figure 6-18. This transporter belongs to the family of ABC transporters that bind and hydrolyze ATP (see Chapter 3).

The discovery and characterization of the cystic fibrosis gene and CFTR protein have made it possible to envision effective gene therapy for this disorder. Clinical trials have been published, however, efficiency for delivering genes to target cells has been low.[16] Reliable genetic screening for the common forms of cystic fibrosis is readily available, making prevention and early management possible.

Sex-Linked (X-Linked) Disorders

Sex-linked disorders occur because of a mutation of the sex chromosomes. Disorders linked to the Y chromosome are extremely rare, and for that reason the terms *sex-linked* and *X-linked* are often used interchangeably. Nearly all X-linked disorders are recessive. Females express the X-linked disease only in the rare instance in which both X chromosomes carry the defective gene. Males, however, do not have the safety margin of two X chromosomes and express the disease if their one and only X chromosome is abnormal. X-linked disorders follow predictable patterns of inheritance (Figure 6-19), which are dependent on the sex of the offspring, and may be summarized as follows:

- Affected individuals are almost always male.
- Affected fathers transmit the defective gene to none of their sons but to all of their daughters.
- Unaffected males do not carry the defective gene.
- A carrier female has a 1 in 2 chance of producing an affected son and a 1 in 2 chance of producing a carrier daughter.
- Females are affected only in the rare homozygous state that may occur from the mating of an affected or carrier mother and an affected father.

Several X-linked recessive disorders have been identified, as presented in Table 6-4. A well-known example of an X-linked disease is hemophilia A.

Hemophilia A

Hemophilia A is a bleeding disorder associated with a deficiency of factor VIII, a protein necessary for blood clotting. Individuals afflicted with hemophilia A bleed easily and profusely from seemingly minor injuries (see Chapter 14). The transmission of hemophilia A in the European royal families constitutes one of the best-known pedigrees available (Figure 6-20). Queen Victoria of England was the first known carrier of the disease. A number of her male descendants were affected by it.

NONMENDELIAN SINGLE-GENE DISORDERS

Transmission of certain single-gene disorders does not follow the classic mendelian principles of random and independent assortment. Three such categories have been described: (1) disorders caused by long triplet repeat mutations, such as fragile X syndrome; (2) disorders

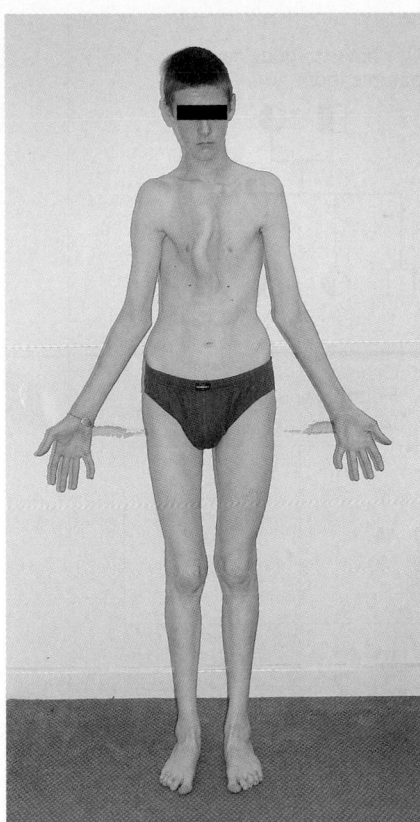

FIGURE 6-16 Clinical manifestations of Marfan syndrome. Skeletal deformities such as pectus excavatum and abnormal curvature of the thoracic spine are common findings. (From Turnpenny P: *Emory's elements of medical genetics,* ed 14, Philadelphia, 2012, Churchill Livingstone, p 301.)

Phenylketonuria

Phenylketonuria (PKU) results from an inability to metabolize the amino acid phenylalanine because of lack of the enzyme phenylalanine hydroxylase. It is one of several enzyme deficiencies that are often referred to as *inborn errors of metabolism.* The symptoms of the disorder are due to the accumulation of dietary phenylalanine in the body, which primarily affects the nervous system. Children with PKU tend to be overly irritable and tremorous and have slowly developing mental retardation. Excess phenylalanine is excreted in the urine in the form of phenylketones, hence the name phenylketonuria. Infants typically have a musty odor because of excess phenylalanine by-products in the sweat and urine. The enzyme deficiency can be detected soon after birth and managed with a low-phenylalanine diet. Because treatment must be instituted very early to prevent mental retardation, routine screening for PKU is performed at birth.

Cystic Fibrosis

Cystic fibrosis is one of the most common single-gene disorders. About 4% of Caucasian Americans harbor the defective gene, and the incidence of cystic fibrosis is approximately 1 in 3200 live births.[15] The clinical abnormalities associated with cystic fibrosis have been traced to a defect in a membrane transporter for chloride ions in epithelial cells. The alteration in chloride transport is associated with production of abnormally thick secretions in glandular tissues. The lung bronchioles and pancreatic ducts are primarily affected, often resulting in progressive destruction of these organs (see Chapter 22).

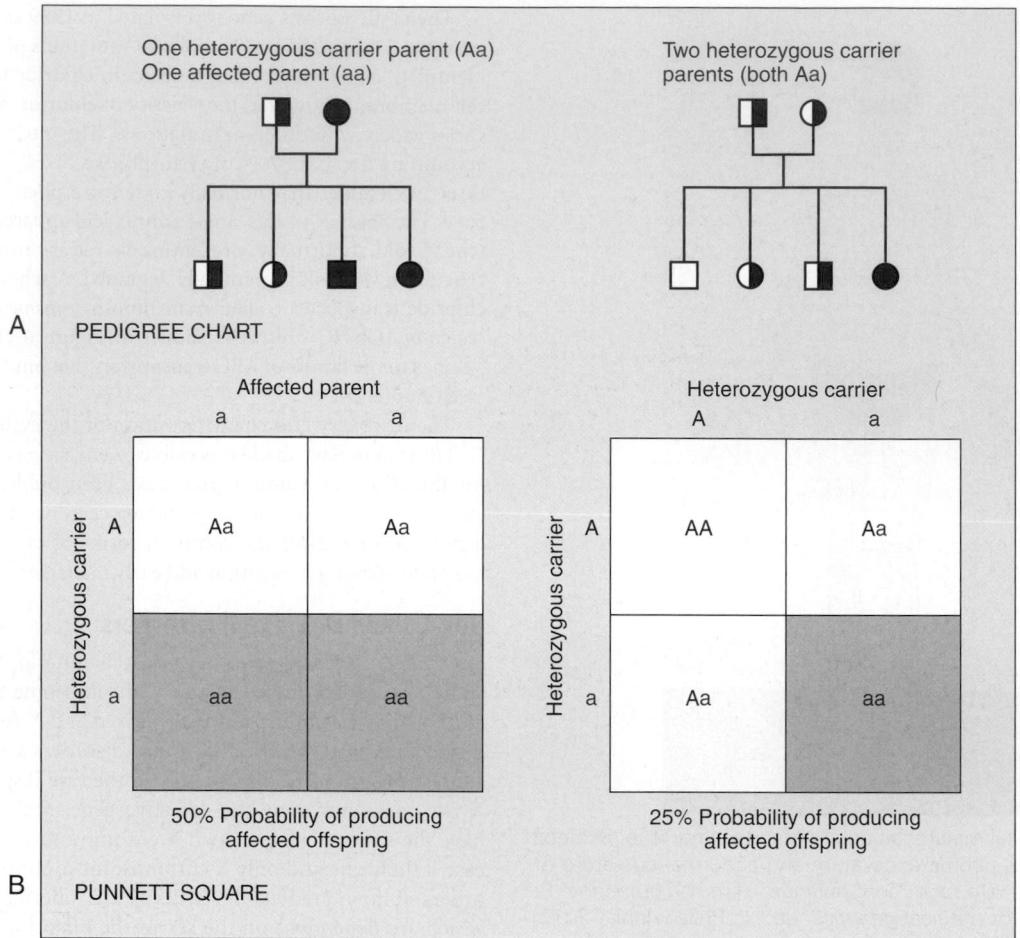

FIGURE 6-17 Typical pattern of inheritance of an autosomal recessive trait (e.g., cystic fibrosis, sickle cell anemia). **A,** Pedigree chart. **B,** Punnett square.

TABLE 6-3	AUTOSOMAL RECESSIVE DISORDERS
SYSTEM	**DISORDER**
Metabolic	Cystic fibrosis
	Phenylketonuria
	Galactosemia
	Homocystinuria
	Lysosomal storage disease
	α_1-Antitrypsin deficiency
	Wilson disease
	Hemochromatosis
	Glycogen storage diseases
Hematopoietic	Sickle cell anemia
	Thalassemias
Endocrine	Congenital adrenal hyperplasia
Skeletal	Ehlers-Danlos syndrome (some variants)
	Alkaptonuria
Nervous	Neurogenic muscular atrophies
	Friedreich ataxia
	Spinal muscular atrophy

From Kumar V et al: *Robbins & Cotran pathologic basis of disease,* ed 8, Philadelphia, 2010, Saunders, p 142.

attributable to mitochondrial DNA mutations; and (3) disorders associated with genomic imprinting.

Triplet Repeat Mutations

Fragile X syndrome is a prototypical example of disorders characterized by long repeating sequences of three nucleotides, called *triplet (or trinucleotide) repeat mutations.* Fragile X syndrome is the most common cause of familial mental retardation, exhibiting a prevalence rate of about 1 in 4000 males (1 in 8000 females).[5] A typical constriction on the long arm of the X chromosome can be detected on cytogenic studies. This narrowed area is composed of long repeating triplets of the sequence CGG. Normal individuals have an average of 29 CGG repeats at this gene locus. Persons with fragile X syndrome have significantly more: 200 to 1000 or more triplet repeats. Persons who have an intermediate number of repeats (60 to 200) are said to have a *pre*mutation and are at significant risk for producing affected offspring, although they themselves are unaffected.[1,3] The premutation is unstable and predisposed to amplification during oogenesis, but much less so during spermatogenesis.[1] As the premutation is passed on through the female lineage, the number of triplet repeats tends to increase as does the risk of mental retardation in the offspring. As might be guessed, the transmission patterns of this disorder are quite unusual. Males with fragile X syndrome tend to be more severely affected, apparently because the presence of a second X chromosome in females moderates the clinical symptoms. The protein normally produced by the fragile X gene *(FMR1)* is crucial to the development and function of cerebral neurons.[3]

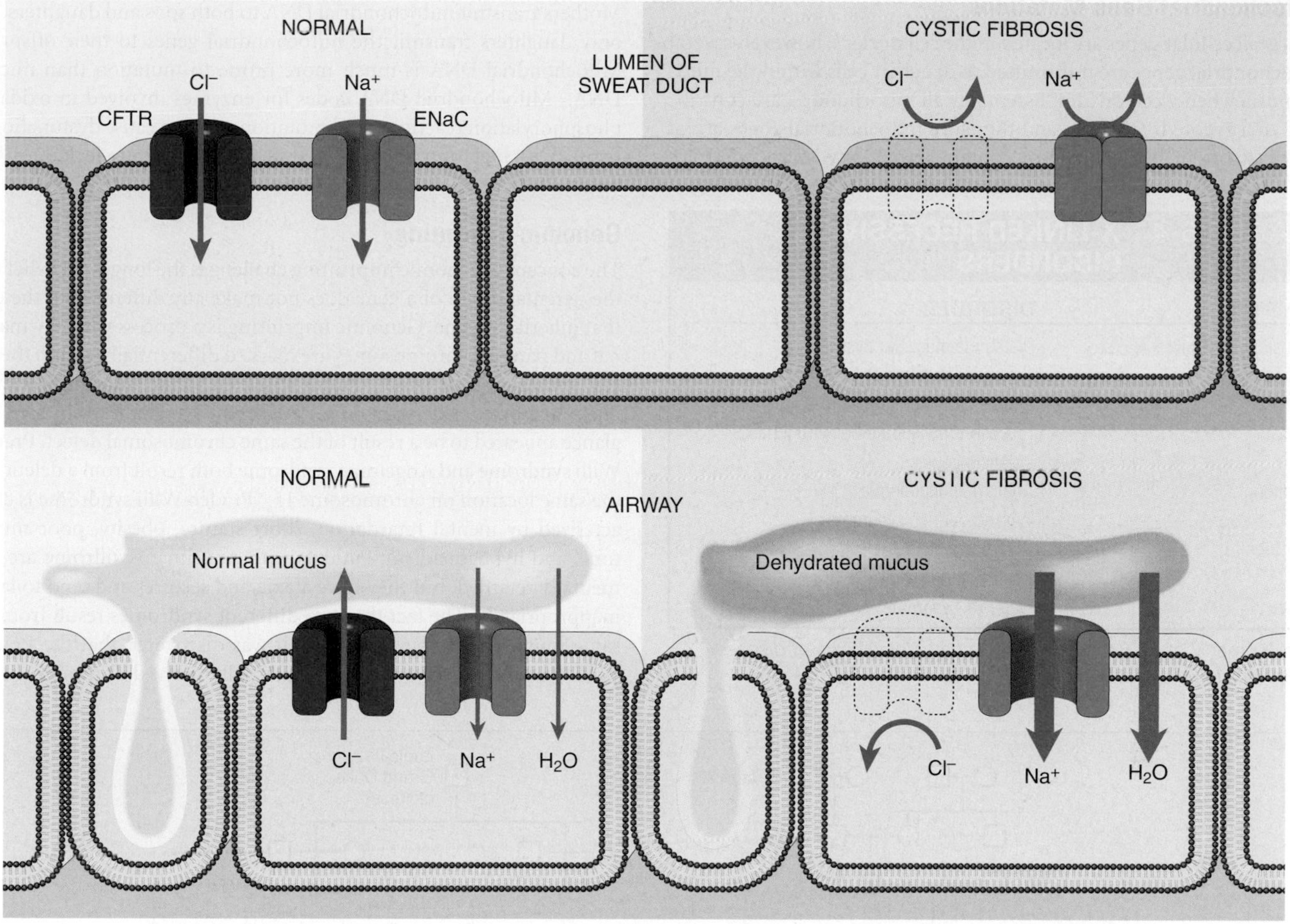

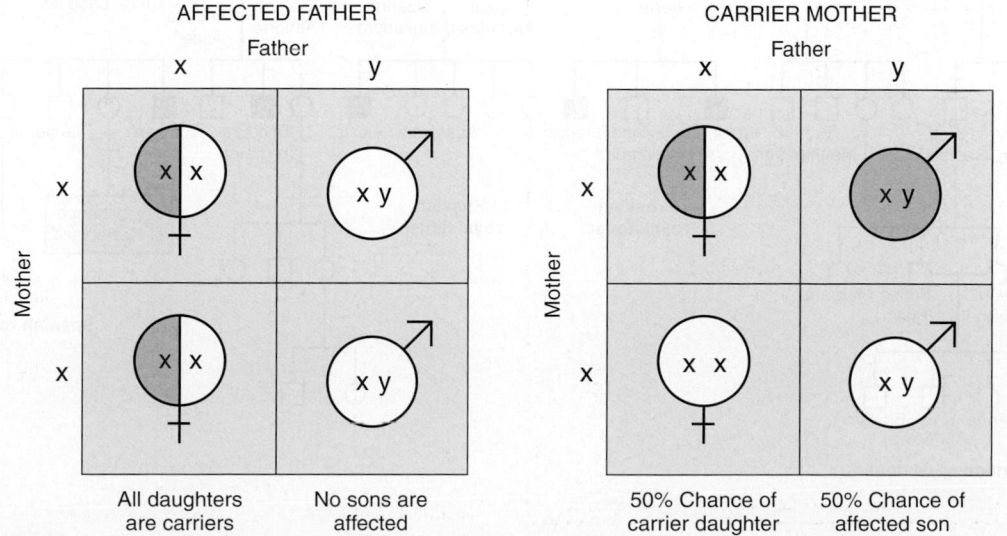

FIGURE 6-18 Schematic illustration of the cystic fibrosis transmembrane conductance regulator *(CFTR)* located in an epithelial cell. CFTR is a transmembrane protein that transports chloride from the cytoplasm into the lumen of the bronchiole. Mutations in the *CFTR* transporter gene are believed to cause the thick secretions typical of cystic fibrosis. (From Kumar V et al: *Robbins & Cotran pathologic basis of disease,* ed 8, Philadelphia, 2010, Saunders, p 467.)

FIGURE 6-19 Typical inheritance pattern for X-linked disorders. The risk of disease varies according to the gender of the offspring.

Mitochondrial Gene Mutations

Nearly all cellular genes are located in the cell nucleus; however, several mitochondrial genes are transmitted to daughter cells within the mitochondria when a cell divides. Essentially all mitochondria are contributed to a zygote by the egg, and therefore mitochondrial genes are of maternal origin because sperm contain few, if any, mitochondria.[5]

Mothers transmit mitochondrial DNA to both sons and daughters, but only daughters transmit the mitochondrial genes to their offspring. Mitochondrial DNA is much more prone to mutation than nuclear DNA.[5] Mitochondrial DNA codes for enzymes involved in oxidative phosphorylation reactions, and mutations tend to cause dysfunction in tissues with high utilization of ATP such as nerve, muscle, kidney, and liver cells.

Genomic Imprinting

The concept of genomic imprinting challenges the long-held belief that the parental origin of a gene does not make any difference to the cells that inherit the gene. Genomic imprinting is a process whereby maternal and paternal chromosomes are marked differentially within the cell (by methylation of DNA for example). Genomic imprinting can be illustrated by considering two very different syndromes, which at first glance appeared to be a result of the same chromosomal defect. Prader-Willi syndrome and Angelman syndrome both result from a deletion at the same location on chromosome 15.[5] Prader-Willi syndrome is characterized by mental retardation, short stature, obesity, poor muscle tone, and hypogonadism. Patients with Angelman syndrome are also mentally retarded, but they have ataxia and seizures and tend to laugh inappropriately. The fact that two different syndromes result from the same mutation was puzzling until it was discovered that the Prader-Willi mutation is always on the paternally derived chromosome 15,

TABLE 6-4	X-LINKED RECESSIVE DISORDERS
SYSTEM	**DISORDER**
Musculoskeletal	Duchenne muscular dystrophy
Blood	Hemophilias A and B
	Chronic granulomatous disease
	Glucose-6-phosphate dehydrogenase deficiency
Immune	Agammaglobulinemia
	Wiskott-Aldrich syndrome
Metabolic	Diabetes insipidus
	Lesch-Nyhan syndrome
Nervous	Fragile X syndrome

From Kumar V et al: *Robbins & Cotran pathologic basis of disease,* ed 8, Philadelphia, 2010, Saunders, p 142.

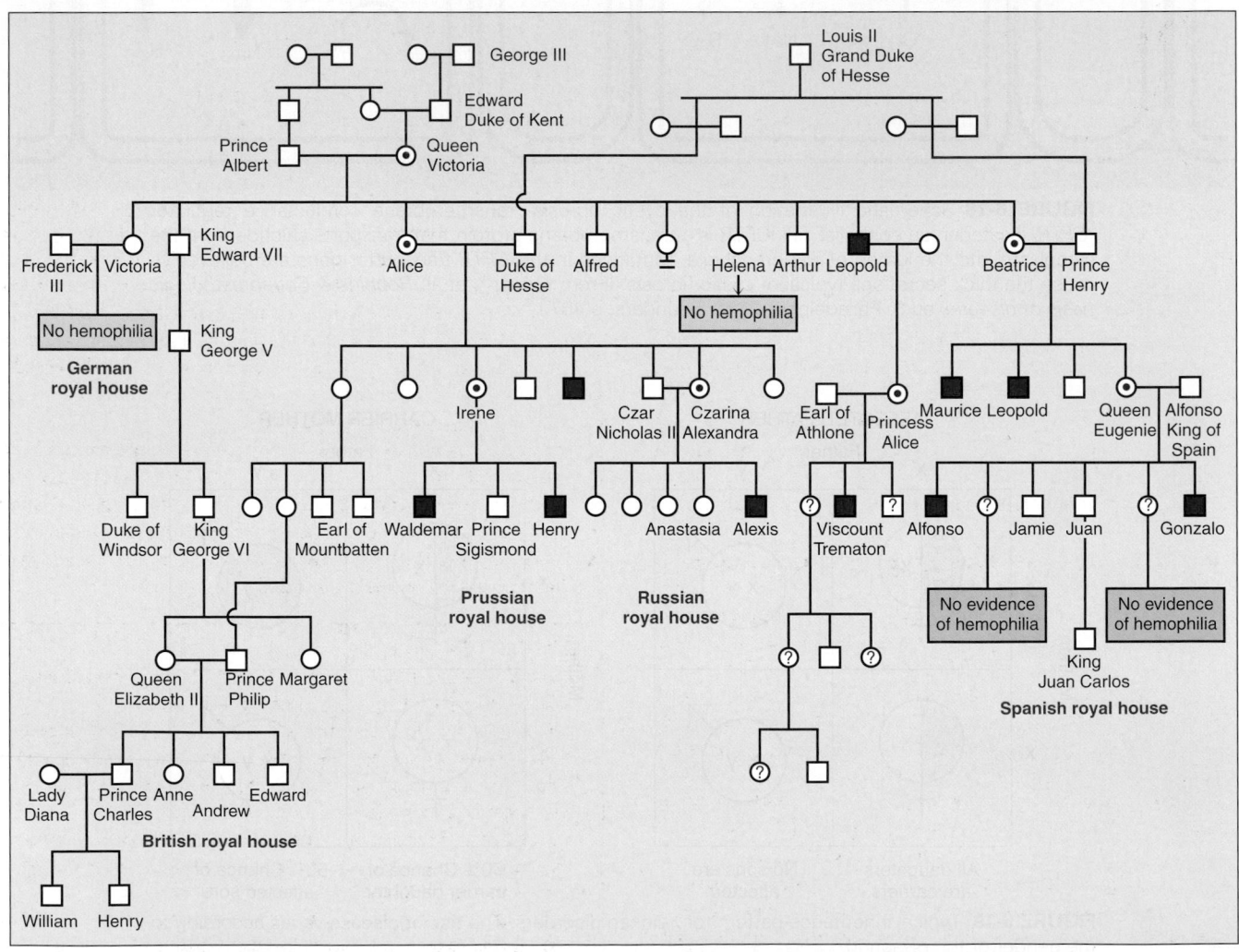

FIGURE 6-20 Pedigree chart for the transmission of the X-linked disease hemophilia A in the royal families of Europe.

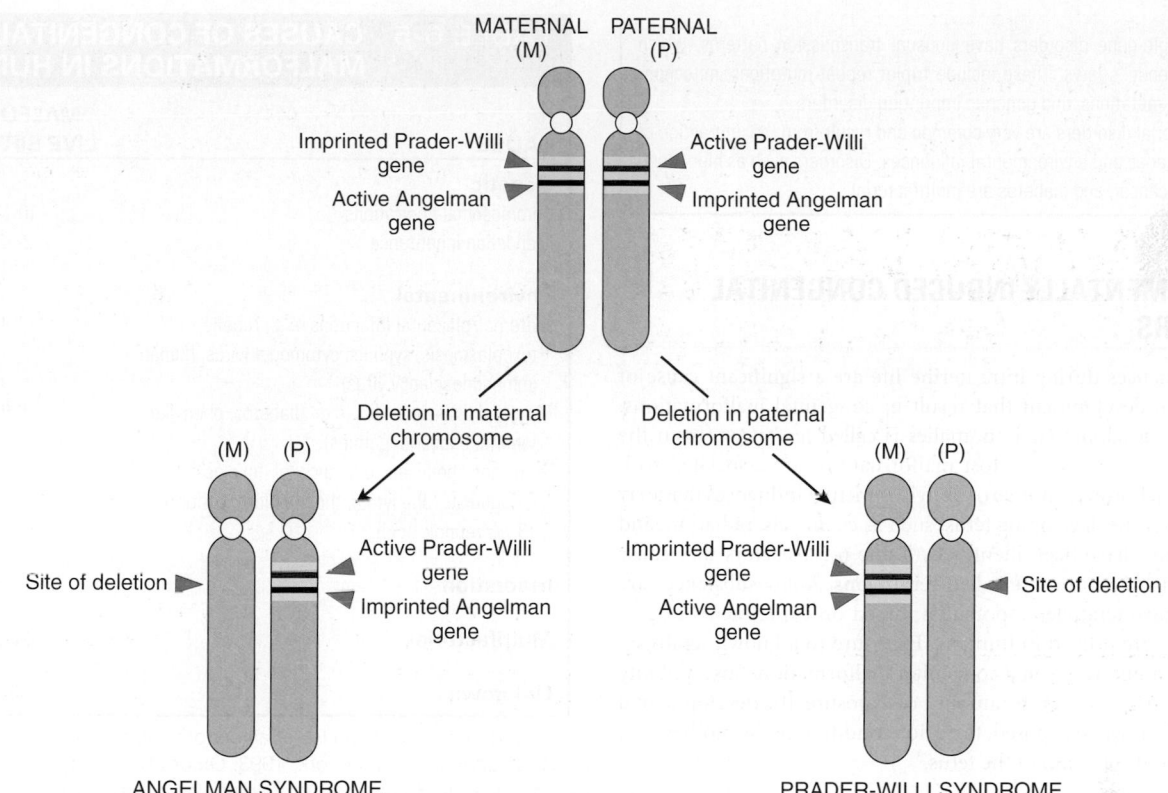

FIGURE 6-21 Angelman and Prader-Willi syndromes are examples of genetic imprinting, where the location of a mutation on the maternal or paternal homologous chromosome produces a different outcome. (From Kumar V et al: *Robbins & Cotran pathologic basis of disease,* ed 8, Philadelphia, 2010, Saunders, p 172.)

whereas the Angelman syndrome mutation is always on the maternally derived chromosome 15. Two genes are normally present in the region; the "Angelman gene" is normally active on a maternal chromosome and silent (imprinted) on the paternal chromosome, whereas the "Prader-Willi" gene is normally active on only the paternal chromosome and silent on the maternal chromosome. Thus normal cells have only one functional copy of each gene. The disorders arise when there is a deletion mutation of chromosome 15. A different syndrome arises if the area on a maternal chromosome is deleted compared to the paternal one (Figure 6 21). These findings imply that the cell is not blind to the parental origin of chromosomes and that homologous chromosomes may be marked and function differently within the cell.

POLYGENIC AND MULTIFACTORIAL DISORDERS

Most human traits develop in response to more than one gene; such traits are called *polygenic.* Environmental influence also has a role in gene expression; traits and disorders influenced by multiple genes as well as environmental factors are called *multifactorial.* Multifactorial traits do not follow clear-cut modes of inheritance but do tend to "run in families." Characteristics governed by multifactorial inheritance tend to have a range of expression in the population and demonstrate a "bell curve" distribution. They are thought to be produced by the interaction of several genes, each contributing a small additive effect and modulated by environmental influences, such as diet. Height, weight, and intelligence are multifactorial, as are most common health conditions and diseases. Most multifactorial disorders also present a range of severity, although a few disorders are either present or absent. In the latter case, it may be that a certain threshold number of defective genes must be inherited before the disease is expressed.[5]

It is extremely difficult to predict the risk of occurrence of multifactorial disorders based on family history, and empirical estimates have been derived, based on observing inheritance in the population. Recurrence risk is specific for each disorder and varies among different populations, but in general the risk is much less than that found in mendelian disorders. As an example, neural tube defects, which are multifactorial, occur in 2% to 3% of siblings of probands. Based on such a recurrence risk, parents of one affected child have a 2% to 3% chance of bearing a second affected child.[5]

In contrast to single-gene and chromosomal abnormalities, which are rare, multifactorial disorders are very common. High blood pressure, atherosclerosis, cancer, diabetes mellitus, cleft lip, and several forms of congenital heart defects are governed by multifactorial inheritance. This list is destined to grow as knowledge of the role of genetic mechanisms in cellular function and disease expands.

KEY POINTS

- Genetic disorders are of three general types: chromosomal aberrations, single-gene disorders, and polygenic/multifactorial disorders.
- Chromosome disorders result from an abnormality in number or structure. The presence of only one chromosome of a homologous pair is termed *monosomy* (e.g., Turner syndrome), and the presence of an excessive number of chromosomes is called *polysomy* (e.g., Down syndrome). Abnormal rearrangement of portions of the chromosomes (translocation, inversion, deletion, duplication) can result in loss or unusual expression of genes.
- Single-gene disorders result from mutations that alter the nucleotide sequence of one particular gene. Mendelian disorders are transmitted predictably and include autosomal dominant (e.g., Huntington disease), autosomal recessive (e.g., cystic fibrosis), and sex-linked (e.g., hemophilia) disorders.

- Some single-gene disorders have unusual transmission patterns, which violate Mendel's laws. These include triplet repeat mutations, mitochondrial DNA mutations, and genomic imprinting disorders.
- Multifactorial disorders are very common and result from the interaction of multiple genes and environmental influences. Disorders such as high blood pressure, cancer, and diabetes are multifactorial.

ENVIRONMENTALLY INDUCED CONGENITAL DISORDERS

Adverse influences during intrauterine life are a significant cause of errors in fetal development that result in congenital malformations. The study of developmental anomalies is called *teratology* (from the Greek *teras*, or "monster"). Most malformations are associated with genetic causes; however, numerous environmental influences that may adversely affect the developing fetus, such as chemicals, radiation, and viral infections, have been identified (Table 6-5). Factors that cause congenital malformation are called **teratogens.** Many substances are thought to have teratogenic potential, based on experiments in animals, but few are proved in humans. Exposure to a known teratogen may, but need not, result in a congenital malformation. Susceptibility to a teratogen depends on the amount of exposure, the developmental stage of the fetus when exposed, the prior condition of the mother, and the genetic predisposition of the fetus.[3]

Periods of Fetal Vulnerability

The timing of the exposure to a teratogen greatly influences fetal susceptibility and the resulting type of malformation. The intrauterine development of humans can be divided into two stages: (1) the embryonic period, which extends from conception to 9 weeks of development, is followed by (2) the fetal period, which continues until birth. Before the third week of gestation, exposure to a teratogen generally either damages so few cells that the embryo develops normally, or damages so many cells that the embryo cannot survive and spontaneous abortion occurs. Between the third and ninth weeks of gestation the embryo is very vulnerable to teratogenesis, with the fourth and fifth weeks being the time of peak susceptibility.[1,3] Organ development (organogenesis) occurs during this period; the process is very sensitive to injury, regardless of the cause. Each organ has a critical period during which it is most vulnerable to malformation (Figure 6-22). Unfortunately, an embryo may be exposed to teratogens during the vulnerable period because the mother does not yet realize she is pregnant. The fetal period, from 3 to 9 months, is primarily concerned with further growth and maturation of the organs, and susceptibility to errors of morphogenesis is significantly less. Fetal insults occurring after the third month are more likely to result in growth retardation or injury to normally formed organs.

Teratogenic Agents

The teratogenic potential of many agents is unknown. Several chemicals, some infections, and large doses of radiation are definitely associated with a higher risk of congenital disorders. In general, teratogens cause errors in morphogenesis by interfering with cell proliferation, migration, or differentiation. The specific mechanisms of action of most teratogens are unknown.

Chemicals and Drugs

The list of proven teratogenic chemicals and drugs includes thalidomide, alcohol, anticonvulsants, warfarin, folate antagonists, androgenic

TABLE 6-5	**CAUSES OF CONGENITAL MALFORMATIONS IN HUMANS**
CAUSE	**MALFORMED LIVE BIRTHS (%)**
Genetic	
Chromosomal aberrations	10-15
Mendelian inheritance	2-10
Environmental	
Maternal/placental infections (e.g., rubella, toxoplasmosis, syphilis, cytomegalovirus, human immunodeficiency virus)	2-3
Maternal disease states (e.g., diabetes, phenylketonuria, endocrinopathies)	6-8
Drugs and chemicals (e.g., alcohol, folic acid antagonists, phenytoin, thalidomide, warfarin, 13-*cis*-retinoic acid)	≈1
Irradiation	≈1
Multifactorial	20-25
Unknown	40-60

Adapted from Stevenson RE et al, editors: *Human malformations and related anomalies,* New York, 1993, Oxford University Press, p 115; Kumar V et al: *Robbins & Cotran pathologic basis of disease,* ed 8, Philadelphia, 2010, Saunders, p 450.

hormones, angiotensin-converting enzyme inhibitors, and organic mercury. Almost no drugs or chemicals are considered to be totally safe, and the current trend is to discourage pregnant women from using *any* drugs or chemicals. A classification system for determining relative risk of medications in pregnancy has been developed (Table 6-6). Two agents, thalidomide and alcohol, illustrate the teratogenic potential of chemicals.

In the 1960s, an increase in the incidence of congenital limb deformities was traced to maternal use of thalidomide, a tranquilizer, during early pregnancy.[3] Exposure during the vulnerable period (20 to 35 days following conception) was associated with a very high risk of fetal malformation. Typically, the arms were short and flipperlike, although deformities ranged from mild abnormalities of the digits to complete absence of the limbs. Damage to other structures, particularly the ears and heart, also occurred. Thalidomide is one of the most potent teratogens known.

The chronic ingestion of large amounts of alcohol is known to cause a group of congenital anomalies referred to as *fetal alcohol syndrome* (FAS). Fetal alcohol syndrome represents the severe end of a wide spectrum of conditions called fetal alcohol spectrum disorders (FASDs) that are associated with maternal alcohol use.[17] It is estimated that between 0.5 and 2.0 of every 1000 newborns suffer from FAS. The prevalence of FASD is estimated to be much higher, reaching 1% and much higher in populations with high alcohol use among women of childbearing age.[18] Affected infants suffer from growth retardation, developmental delay, learning and behavioral problems, malformations of the head and face, and cardiac defects, although alterations to the developing brain result in the most devastating deficits.[18,19] Multiple mechanisms for alcohol teratogenesis have been suggested.[20] Data are insufficient to determine what, if any, level of alcohol intake during pregnancy is safe. It is clear that factors other than the absolute amount of alcohol intake during pregnancy are important in determining risk of FAS. Complete abstinence from alcohol during pregnancy is recommended.

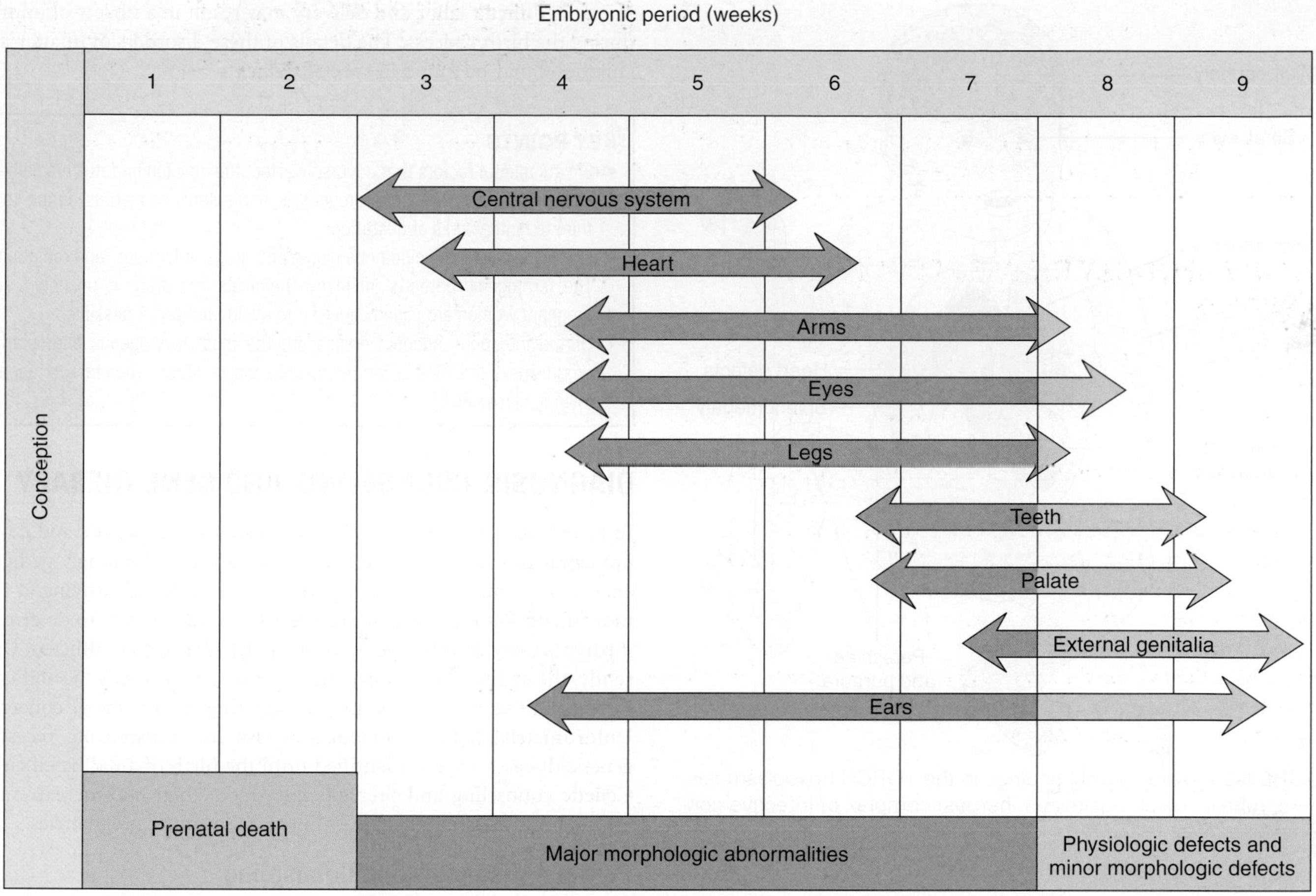

FIGURE 6-22 Vulnerable periods of fetal organ development.

TABLE 6-6 PREGNANCY CATEGORIES FOR MEDICATION ADMINISTRATION

CATEGORY	INTERPRETATION
A	Adequate and well-controlled studies in pregnant women have not shown an increased risk of fetal abnormalities to fetus in any trimester of pregnancy.
B	Animal studies have revealed no evidence of harm to fetus; however, there are no adequate and well-controlled studies in pregnant women.
	OR
	Animal studies have shown an adverse effect, but adequate and well-controlled studies in pregnant women have failed to demonstrate risk to fetus in any trimester.
C	Animal studies have shown an adverse effect, and there are no adequate and well-controlled studies in pregnant women.
	OR
	No animal studies have been conducted, and there are no adequate and well-controlled studies in pregnant women.
D	Adequate and well-controlled or observational studies in pregnant women have demonstrated risk to fetus. However, benefits of therapy may outweigh potential risk. For example, the drug may be acceptable if needed in a life-threatening situation or serious disease for which safer drugs cannot be used or are ineffective.
X	Adequate and well-controlled or observational studies in animals or pregnant women have demonstrated positive evidence of fetal abnormalities or risks. Use of the product is contraindicated in women who are or may become pregnant.

Infectious Agents

A number of perinatal infections have been implicated in the development of congenital malformations.[3] Certain viral infections appear to carry the greatest threat, although protozoa and bacteria have also been implicated. As with other teratogens, the gestational age of the fetus at the time of infection is critically important. Perhaps the best known viral teratogen is rubella. The risk period for rubella infection begins just before conception and extends to 20 weeks' gestation, after which the virus rarely crosses the placenta. Rubella-induced defects vary but typically include cataracts, deafness, and heart defects. Several other organisms cause a similar constellation of congenital defects; therefore the acronym **TORCH** was developed to alert clinicians to the potential teratogenicity of these infections. TORCH stands for **t**oxoplasmosis, **o**thers, **r**ubella, **c**ytomegalovirus, **h**erpes. The major features of the

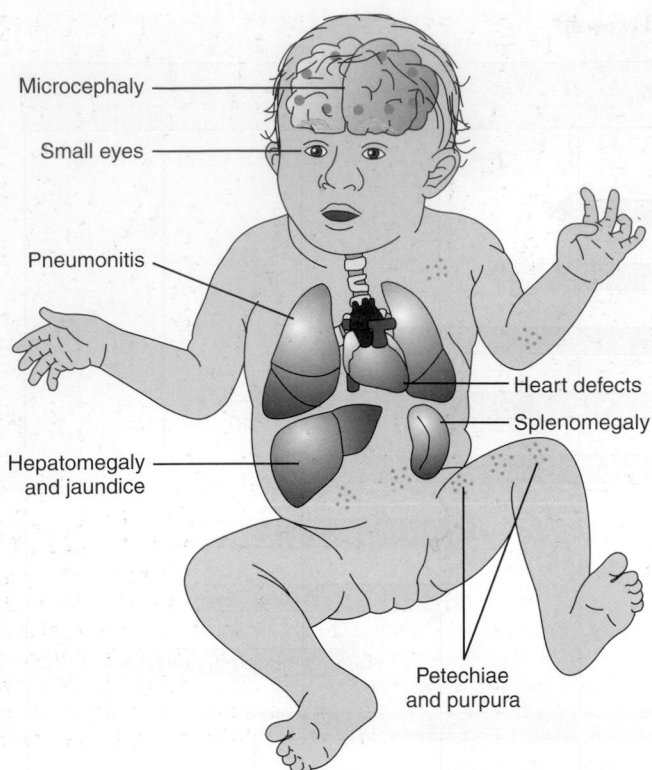

Microcephaly

Small eyes

Pneumonitis

Heart defects

Splenomegaly

Hepatomegaly and jaundice

Petechiae and purpura

FIGURE 6-23 Major clinical findings in the TORCH (toxoplasmosis, others, rubella, cytomegalovirus, herpes) complex of infective congenital disorders.

TORCH complex are shown in Figure 6-23. The category of "others" includes several less frequently seen causes: hepatitis B, coxsackievirus B, mumps, poliovirus, and others. All microorganisms of the TORCH complex are able to cross the placenta and infect the fetus.

Toxoplasmosis is a protozoal infection that can be contracted from ingestion of raw or undercooked meat and from contact with cat feces. Cytomegalovirus and herpes simplex virus are generally transmitted to the fetus by chronic carrier mothers. Cytomegalovirus and herpes simplex virus often colonize in the genital area of the mother. Infants who escape infection in utero may still acquire the virus as they pass through the birth canal (see Chapter 34).

Radiation

In addition to being mutagenic, radiation is also teratogenic. The teratogenic potential of radiation became apparent from the increased incidence of congenital malformations in children born to women who underwent irradiation of the cervix for cancer and in the children of atomic bomb victims in World War II. It is not known if lower levels of radiation, such as those used in diagnostic x-rays, are teratogenic. It is generally recommended that pregnant women avoid diagnostic x-rays or use appropriate lead shielding.

Other Disorders of Infancy

An infant may be afflicted with a variety of problems at birth that do not fall into the category of genetic or developmental malformations. These problems generally arise later in uterine life and often involve mechanical factors or problems with the health of the mother and placenta. For example, babies with low birth weight or immaturity at birth may have difficulty breathing and taking in adequate nutrition. Interruption of the placental oxygen supply because of maternal hemorrhage, sedation, or blood incompatibility may result in fetal brain

injury. A difficult labor and delivery may result in a variety of injuries during the birth process. The details of these disorders of infancy and childhood may be found in specialized texts.

> **KEY POINTS**
> - Environmental factors that adversely affect the developing fetus are called teratogens. Exposure to teratogens is particularly dangerous during the third to ninth weeks of gestation.
> - Known teratogens include chemicals and drugs, infections, and radiation. The teratogenic potential of many chemicals and drugs is unknown, so pregnant women are usually advised to avoid all drugs if possible.
> - Of the infectious agents, viruses are the most teratogenic, particularly organisms of the TORCH variety (toxoplasmosis, others, rubella, cytomegalovirus, herpesvirus).

DIAGNOSIS, COUNSELING, AND GENE THERAPY

In recent years, the ability to diagnose and manage genetic and developmental disorders has improved dramatically. Although pedigree analysis continues to be an important method for identifying at-risk individuals, for a number of disorders it is now possible to determine if parents carry defective genes or if a particular fetus is afflicted. Currently, the ability to detect genetic mutations far exceeds the ability to offer definitive genetic treatment, triggering many ethical concerns. Unfortunately, many individuals at risk for transmitting recessive genetic diseases are not identified until the birth of an afflicted child. Genetic counseling and prenatal assessment then become extremely important in assisting the family in regard to future pregnancies.

Prenatal Diagnosis and Counseling

A number of conditions are associated with a higher risk of congenital anomalies and are indications for instituting counseling and prenatal diagnostic examination. These conditions include (1) a maternal age of 35 years or greater; (2) a history of previously bearing a child with a chromosomal disorder (such as trisomy 21); (3) a known family history of X-linked disorders; (4) a family history of inborn errors of metabolism; (5) the occurrence of neural tube anomalies in a previous pregnancy; and (6) awareness that the mother is a known carrier of a recessive genetic disorder. As diagnostic methods become more cost-effective, general screening for other risk factors may be undertaken. Samples for prenatal testing of the fetus are usually obtained by amniocentesis, chorionic villus biopsy, or umbilical cord blood. Postnatal genetic analysis is usually done on peripheral blood samples of lymphocytes.

Ultrasound and amniocentesis are mainstays of prenatal diagnostic examination. **Ultrasound** is a noninvasive procedure that uses sound waves to produce a reflected image of the fetus. It is commonly used to determine gestational age, fetal position, and placental location. Ultrasound is also useful in detecting visible congenital anomalies such as spina bifida (neural tube defect); heart defects; and malformations of the face, head, body, and limbs.

Amniocentesis may be performed to determine genetic and developmental disorders not detectable by ultrasound. During amniocentesis, a needle is inserted through the abdomen or vagina and into the uterus. A sample of amniotic fluid containing skin cells shed by the fetus is removed for analysis. The amniotic fluid can be analyzed for abnormal levels of certain substances secreted by the fetus, such as α-fetoprotein, which may indicate neural tube defects. The live skin cells can be cultured and subjected to biochemical, chromosomal, and genetic analysis. Only certain genetic and developmental disorders can be reliably detected by these procedures, and they may not provide the needed information until relatively late in the pregnancy. Amniocentesis cannot generally be performed before 16 weeks' gestation. **Chorionic villus sampling (CVS)** involves the removal of a piece of tissue directly from the chorion (the outer membrane of the fetal sac). It can be performed at 8 weeks' gestation. Whether obtained via amniocentesis or CVS, fetal cells provide small amounts of DNA that can then be amplified into a larger quantity by a process called polymerase chain reaction (PCR). This DNA can then be analyzed by a variety of methods to determine the genetic sequence, the presence or absence of particular genes, or the presence of mutations. The fetal genome can be scanned for particular genes by exposing the processed DNA to microchips that are coated with thousands of genetic sequence probes in specific locations. Complementary base pairing between the probes fixed on the microchip and the DNA being tested is used to detect the presence of particular gene sequences.

Embryoscopy allows direct visualization of the embryo as early as the first trimester of pregnancy. The scope is inserted through the cervix and into the uterus. Embryoscopy can be used to identify developmental progress and to diagnose structural anomalies. An exciting application of this technique is the potential to directly manage genetic disorders with targeted gene or stem cell therapy. The early diagnosis of congenital disorders allows a greater number of treatment options. Some disorders can be managed in utero; others may require early delivery, immediate surgery, or cesarean section to minimize fetal trauma. Early warning of fetal difficulties allows parents time to prepare emotionally for the birth of the child. In some instances, termination of the pregnancy may be the treatment of choice.

Genetic Analysis and Therapy

An exciting outcome of the Human Genome Project is the potential for gene therapy—the treatment of genetic disease by replacing the defective gene with a normal, healthy gene. This idea once sounded like science fiction, but clinical trials are under way to manage a number of genetic disorders.[21] The first federally approved gene therapy procedure was performed in 1990 to treat a child who suffered from a rare condition called *severe combined immunodeficiency* (SCID) by introducing a functional gene for the enzyme adenosine deaminase. In the past, children who suffered from SCID had severely compromised immune systems and generally died from overwhelming infections unless their environment was strictly controlled. Use of gene therapy has shown some success in improving immune function and allowing these children to live in the outside world, although the safety of gene therapy is a continuing challenge.[22]

Gene therapy has the potential for alleviating human suffering by curing genetic diseases, but it is accompanied by a number of moral and ethical dilemmas. Tampering with the human gene pool could have serious implications for human evolution. There is also the potential for using the technology to create "new and improved" human beings or human clones.

Recombinant DNA Technology

Over the past 30 years, DNA has gone from being the most difficult cellular molecule to study to being the easiest. The great advances in molecular genetics during this time are due to plummeting costs of DNA sequencing and the development of recombinant DNA technologies. It is now possible to select a specific region of DNA, produce unlimited copies of it, determine its nucleotide sequence, use it to make unlimited quantities of a desired protein, or alter its DNA sequence at will (genetic engineering) and reinsert it into a living cell. These tools provide the means to decipher the nucleotide sequence of an individual human genome, to create DNA probes to explore an individual's genetic makeup for specific mutations, to mass-produce therapeutic proteins and vaccines, and to cure genetic disorders by replacing mutated genes with normally functioning ones.

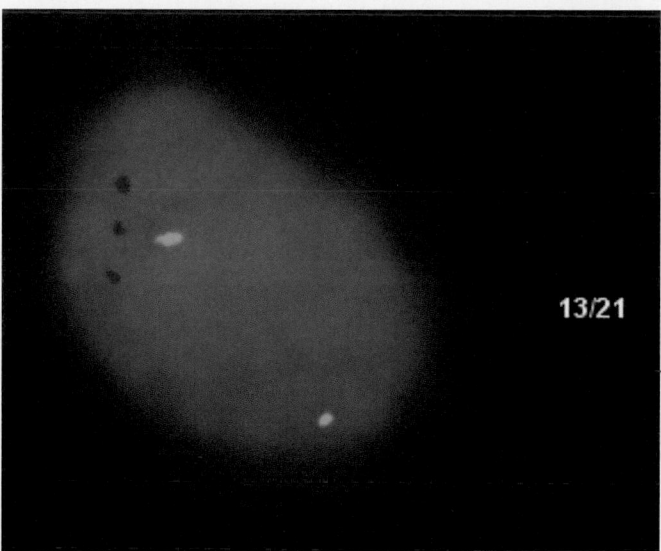

FIGURE 6-24 Fluorescence in situ hybridization assay showing an interphase nucleus. The red probe hybridized to chromosome 21 and the green probe hybridized to chromosome 13. Three copies of chromosome 21 are identified, confirming the diagnosis of trisomy 21. (From Kumar V et al: *Robbins & Cotran pathologic basis of disease,* ed 8, Philadelphia, 2010, Saunders, p 161. Photograph courtesy Dr. Stuart Schwartz, Department of Pathology, University of Chicago, Chicago, IL.)

Recombinant DNA technology comprises a number of techniques, the most important of which are briefly described here.

- The long, difficult-to-handle DNA strands are more easily studied if cut into smaller pieces. This is accomplished by using restriction enzymes that cleave DNA at specific sites. The resulting pieces can then be separated by electrophoresis according to their size. A section of DNA can be collected and efficiently sequenced by automated means.

- Nucleic acid hybridization techniques take advantage of the natural tendency for DNA and RNA to find and bind to a complementary nucleotide sequence. A labeled piece of DNA or RNA can therefore be used to search for or "probe" for its complementary sequence among the many millions of sequences in a cell or cell extract. For example, in a fluorescence in situ hybridization assay, a probe for a specific site on a chromosome is attached to a fluorescent label and incubated with a cell. The fluorescence is then examined to identify the location and number of copies of the particular chromosome sequence (Figure 6-24). Without the hybridization technique, finding a desired gene among the 3 billion base pairs in the human genome could take many years of intense effort, like finding the proverbial needle in a haystack. Hybridization is also the method behind the "gene chip assay" technology. As an outcome of the Human Genome Project, the DNA sequences for the thousands of human genes and common mutations have been identified. Specific DNA sequence probes for these genes can be synthesized and attached to a fixed position on a plate (microchip). The DNA of interest can then be exposed to the chip, and the probes will preferentially bind to DNA segments having complementary bases. The position of the probe and the degree of DNA binding can then be analyzed by computer to produce a specific genetic analysis of gene mutations.

- DNA cloning is the technique used to produce many identical copies of a DNA sequence containing a gene of interest. The availability of large quantities of a purified gene sequence makes study and gene manipulation possible. A number of different techniques can be used to clone DNA. The polymerase chain reaction (PCR) technique is very efficient if the DNA sequence is already partially known. Basically, the DNA sequence of interest is mixed with special DNA polymerases that use the DNA sequence as a template to produce double-stranded DNA. Each DNA thus produced can in turn act as a template for production of another DNA. Large quantities can be produced very rapidly by PCR. The DNA can also be cloned by inserting it into bacteria by use of a viral or plasmid vector. Bacteria that incorporate the desired gene are identified by hybridization with a labeled probe. The desired bacteria then are allowed to proliferate, making a copy of the DNA sequence along with their own genome with each cell division.

- Genetic engineering refers to a process whereby a gene of interest is altered from its original form. The altered (mutated) gene can be reintroduced into a cell to disclose its effect on cell function and thus elucidate the normal function of the original gene and its protein product. Genetic engineering has been applied to plants to increase their value as food crops. Genetically engineered cells can be turned into protein factories to produce hormones, such as insulin, in large quantity.

Gene therapy relies heavily on these techniques to facilitate identification of genetic mutations, study of gene function, and development of methods to repair or replace mutated genes. Many more applications of recombinant DNA technology will become apparent as research on the genetic basis of human function and disease proceeds.

KEY POINTS

- Risk factors that indicate the need for prenatal diagnostic examination and counseling include advanced maternal age (older than 35 years), a family history of genetic disorders, and the previous birth of a child with chromosomal or neural tube defects.
- Ultrasound, amniocentesis, and chorionic villus sampling are the mainstays of prenatal assessment for genetic disorders.
- DNA sequences that are complementary to a gene of interest can be synthesized and used to probe a genome to determine if and where the gene is present. These hybridization techniques make screening for genetic disorders relatively fast and simple.
- Gene therapy is the treatment of genetic disease by replacing defective genes with normal genes. Gene therapy is possible because of the advances attained in recombinant DNA technology over the past 30 years.

SUMMARY

Genetic and developmental disorders are responsible for a number of congenital malformations. Congenital disorders are caused by genetic and environmental factors that disrupt normal fetal development. Genetic disorders are classified as (1) chromosomal alterations, including structural and numeric abnormalities; (2) mendelian disorders, including autosomal dominant, autosomal recessive, and X-linked disorders; (3) nonmendelian single-gene disorders, including triplet repeats, mitochondrial gene defects, and genetic imprinting disorders; and (4) polygenic or multifactorial disorders. Known environmental teratogens include radiation, infectious organisms, and various chemicals and drugs. The embryo is particularly susceptible to teratogens during the period of organogenesis, which extends from the third to the ninth week of gestation. Pedigree analysis, ultrasound, amniocentesis, and chorionic villus biopsy may provide helpful information regarding genetic risk and the prenatal condition of at-risk infants. DNA sequencing of normal and mutated genes has made it possible to efficiently screen for genetic disorders and develop gene therapies for a variety of genetic diseases.

REFERENCES

1. Kumar V, Abbas A, Fausto N, Aster JC: *Pathologic basis of disease*, ed 8, Philadelphia, 2010, Saunders.
2. Bennett RL: *The practical guide to the genetic family history*, Hoboken, NJ, 2010, Wiley-Blackwell.
3. Turnpenny P, Ellard S: *Emery's elements of medical genetics*, ed 14, Philadelphia, 2012, Churchill-Livingstone.
4. Bateson W: *Mendel's principles of heredity*, London, 1902, Cambridge University Press.
5. Jorde LB, Carey JC, Bamshad MJ: *Medical genetics*, ed 4, Philadelphia, 2010, Mosby Elsevier.
6. Shaffer LG, Bejjani BA: Using microarray-based molecular cytogenetic methods to identify chromosome abnormalities, *Pediatr Ann* 38(8):440–447, 2009.
7. Hassold T, Hall H, Hunt P: The origin of human aneuploidy: where we have been, where we are going, *Hum Mol Genet* 16(2):R203–R208, 2007.
8. Compton DA: Mechanisms of aneuploidy, *Curr Opin Cell Biol* 23:109–113, 2011.
9. Neri G, Opitz JM: Down syndrome: comments and reflections on the 50th anniversary of Lejeune's discovery, *Am J Med Genet A* 149A:2647–2654, 2009.
10. Down JHL: Observations on an ethnic classification of idiots, *Clin Lect Rep London Hosp* 3:259–262, 1866.
11. Megarbane A, Ravel A, Mircher C, Sturtz F, Grattau Y, et al: The 50th anniversary of the discovery of trisomy 21: the past, present and future of research and treatment of Down syndrome, *Genet Med* 11(9):611–616, 2009.
12. Wikstrom AM, Dunkel L: Klinefelter syndrome, *Best Pract Res Clin Endocrinol Metab* 25:239–250, 2011.
13. Davenport M: Approach to the patient with Turner syndrome, *J Clin Endocrinol Metab* 25(4):1487–1495, 2010.
14. Summers CG: Albinism: classification, clinical characteristics, and recent findings, *Optom Vis Sci* 86(6):659–662, 2009.
15. Moskowitz SM, Chmiel JF, Sternen DL, Cheng E, Cutting GR: CFTR-related disorders. In Moskowitz SM, et al, editors: *GeneReviews at Gene Tests: Medical Genetic Information Resource*, 2008. Available at www.ncbi.nlm.nih.gov/books/NBK1250/. Accessed 8/12/11.
16. Davies JC, Alton EW: Gene therapy for cystic fibrosis, *Proc Am Thorac Soc* 7(6):408–414, 2010.
17. Centers for Disease Control and Prevention (CDC): *Fetal alcohol spectrum disorders*, 2010. Available at www.cdc.gov/ncbddd/fasd/facts.html. Accessed 8/15/11.
18. Riley EP, Infante A, Warren KR: Fetal alcohol spectrum disorders: an overview, *Neuropsychol Rev* 21:73–80, 2011.
19. Mattson SN, Crocker N, Nguyen TT: Fetal alcohol spectrum disorders: neuropsychological and behavioral features, *Neuropsychol Rev* 21:81–101, 2011.
20. Urban KA, Bodnar T, Butts K, Sliwowska JH, Comeau W, et al: Direct and indirect mechanisms of alcohol teratogenesis: implications for understanding alterations and brain and behavior in FASD. In Riley EP, Clarren S, Weinberg J, Jonsson E, editors: *Fetal alcohol spectrum disorder*, Weinheim, Germany, 2010, Wiley-Blackwell.
21. Kay MA: State-of-the-art gene-based therapies: the road ahead, *Nat Rev Genet* 12:316–328, 2011.
22. Fisher A, Hacein-Bey-Albina S, Cavazzana-Calvo M: Gene therapy for primary adaptive immune deficiencies, *J Allergy Clin Immunol* 127:1356–1359, 2011.

Neoplasia

Jacquelyn L. Banasik

evolve WEBSITE

KEY QUESTIONS

- How do neoplastic cells differ from normal cells?
- In what ways do benign and malignant tumors differ?
- How might overexpression of proto-oncogenes lead to abnormal cellular proliferation?
- How might underexpression of tumor suppressor genes lead to abnormal cellular proliferation?
- What properties are gained during tumor progression that contribute to malignant behavior and metastasis?
- How are tumor grading and staging used to guide the selection of cancer therapies?
- How might lifestyle and carcinogen exposure contribute to cancer risk?
- What treatment options are available for benign and malignant tumors?

CHAPTER OUTLINE

Neoplasia means "new growth." In common use, the term implies an *abnormality* of cellular growth and may be used interchangeably with the term *tumor*. It is no surprise that the discovery of a tumor in an individual can evoke feelings of disbelief, anger, and dread. Characterization of the tumor cells is of critical importance to determine whether the tumor is benign or malignant. The term *cancer* is applied only to malignant neoplasms. The diagnosis of a **benign** growth is received with great relief inasmuch as the tumor is generally easily cured. The diagnosis of a **malignant** cancer, on the other hand, may herald months of intensive and often uncomfortable treatment with uncertain outcomes. Cancer remains the second leading cause of death in the United States for both men and women.

It is increasingly clear that cancer is associated with *altered expression of cellular genes* that normally regulate cell proliferation and differentiation. A unified theory of cancer causation has emerged, and new methods for cancer therapy continue to be developed. Cancer is a complex, multifaceted disorder with each individual cancer having some unique properties. A better understanding of the molecular characteristics of individual cancers is encouraging the development of specific therapies that target each cancer's weaknesses.

BENIGN VERSUS MALIGNANT GROWTH

Characteristics of Benign and Malignant Tumors

The terms *benign* and *malignant* refer to the overall consequences of a tumor to the host. Generally, malignant tumors have the potential to kill the host if left untreated, whereas benign tumors do not. This difference is not strict because some benign tumors may be located in critical areas. For example, a benign tumor may be life threatening if it causes pressure on the brain or blocks an airway or blood vessel. Histologic examination of a tumor is the primary mode for determining its benign or malignant nature. Certain tumor characteristics have historically been shown to indicate malignant potential. Important considerations include localization of the tumor and determination of the degree of tumor cell differentiation.

Benign tumors do not invade adjacent tissue or spread to distant sites. Many benign tumors are encapsulated by connective tissue, which is an indication of strictly local growth. Any evidence that tumor cells have penetrated local tissues (invasiveness), lymphatics, or blood vessels suggests a malignant nature with potential to spread to distant sites (metastasize).

As a general rule, benign cells more closely resemble their tissue type of origin (e.g., skin, liver) than do malignant cells. The degree of tissue-specific differentiation has traditionally been used to predict malignant potential. A lack of differentiated features in a cancer cell is called **anaplasia**, and a greater degree of anaplasia is correlated with a more aggressively malignant tumor.[1] Anaplasia is indicated by variation in cell size and shape within the tumor, enlarged nuclei, abnormal mitoses, and bizarre-looking giant cells (Figure 7-1). Regardless of histologic appearance, invasion of local tissue or evidence of **metastasis** to distant sites confirms the diagnosis of malignancy.

Other differences between benign and malignant tumors have been noted (Table 7-1). Benign tumors generally grow more slowly, have little vascularity, rarely have necrotic areas, and often retain functions similar to those of the tissue of origin. Conversely, malignant tumors often grow rapidly and may initiate vessel growth in the tumor. They frequently have necrotic areas and are dysfunctional.

Tumor Terminology

General rules for the naming of tumors have been developed to indicate the tissue of origin and the benign or malignant nature of the tumor. The suffix *-oma* is used to indicate a benign tumor, whereas *carcinoma* and *sarcoma* are used to indicate malignant tumors.

TABLE 7-1	GENERAL CHARACTERISTICS OF BENIGN AND MALIGNANT TUMORS	
CHARACTERISTIC	**BENIGN**	**MALIGNANT**
Histology	Typical of tissue of origin	Anaplastic, with abnormal cell size and shape
	Few mitoses	Many mitoses
Growth rate	Slow	Rapid
Localization/metastasis	Strictly local, often encapsulated/no metastasis	Infiltrative/frequent metastases
Tumor necrosis	Rare	Common
Recurrence after treatment	Rare	Common
Prognosis	Good, unless in critical area	Poor if untreated

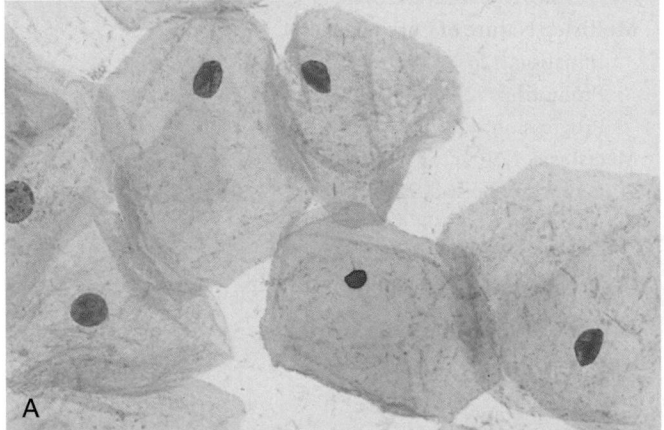 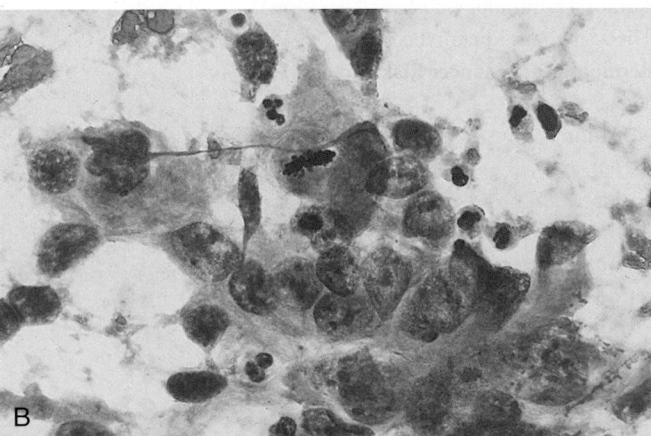

FIGURE 7-1 A, Normal Papanicolaou smear from the uterine cervix showing large, flat epithelial cells with small nuclei. **B,** Typical histologic appearance of anaplastic tumor cells showing variation in cell size and shape, with large, hyperchromic nuclei. (From Kumar V et al: *Robbins basic pathology*, ed 8, Philadelphia, 2007, Saunders, p 220. Courtesy Dr. Richard M. DeMay, Department of Pathology, University of Chicago.)

Carcinoma refers to malignant tumors of epithelial origin and sarcoma to malignant tumors of mesenchymal (nerve, bone, muscle) origin. Thus a benign tumor of glandular tissue would be called an adenoma, but a malignant tumor of the same tissue would be called an adenocarcinoma (Table 7-2). Some notable exceptions to the rules are lymphomas, hepatomas, and melanomas, which are all highly malignant despite their -*oma* suffix. Leukemia refers to a malignant growth of white blood cells. The great majority of human cancers (90%) are carcinomas from malignant transformation of epithelial cells.[2]

The Malignant Phenotype

Cells growing in normal tissue have predictable relationships with neighboring cells. In a particular tissue, the rate of cell proliferation is precisely matched to the rate of cell death. Normal cells require constant reassurance in the form of survival signals from their environment that their continued existence is desirable, and they proliferate only when space is available and appropriate mitogen-stimulating signals are present. Normal cells also respond to signals instructing them to actively destroy themselves in a process called *apoptosis* (see Chapter 4). Cancer cells, however, do not obey the rules; they have escaped the normal mechanisms of growth control. A number of antisocial properties develop in malignant cells that allow them to proliferate at the expense of other cells and tissues of the body. These abnormal behaviors can be summarized as follows:

- Cancer cells proliferate despite lack of growth-initiating signals from the environment.
- Cancer cells escape apoptotic signals and achieve a kind of immortality in that they are capable of unlimited replication.
- Cancer cells lose their differentiated features and contribute poorly or not at all to the function of their tissue.
- Cancer cells are genetically unstable and evolve by accumulating new mutations at a much faster rate than normal cells.
- Cancer cells invade their local tissue and overrun their neighbors.
- Perhaps worst of all, cancer cells gain the ability to migrate from their site of origin to colonize distant sites where they do not belong.

TABLE 7-2   NOMENCLATURE FOR NEOPLASTIC DISEASES

CELL OR TISSUE OF ORIGIN	BENIGN	MALIGNANT
Tumors of Epithelial Origin		
Squamous cells	Squamous cell papilloma	Squamous cell carcinoma
Basal cells	—	Basal cell carcinoma
Glandular or ductal epithelium	Adenoma	Adenocarcinoma
	Cystadenoma	Cystadenocarcinoma
Transitional cells	Transitional cell papilloma	Transitional cell carcinoma
Bile duct	Bile duct adenoma	Bile duct carcinoma (cholangiocarcinoma)
Liver cells	Hepatocellular adenoma	Hepatocellular carcinoma
Melanocytes	Nevus	Malignant melanoma
Renal epithelium	Renal tubular adenoma	Renal cell carcinoma
Skin adnexal glands		
Sweat glands	Sweat gland adenoma	Sweat gland carcinoma
Sebaceous glands	Sebaceous gland adenoma	Sebaceous gland carcinoma
Germ cells (testis and ovary)	—	Seminoma (dysgerminoma), embryonal carcinoma, yolk sac carcinoma
Tumors of Mesenchymal Origin		
Hematopoietic/lymphoid tissue	—	Leukemia, lymphoma, Hodgkin disease, multiple myeloma
Neural and retinal tissue		
Nerve sheath	Neurilemmoma, neurofibroma	Malignant peripheral nerve sheath tumor
Nerve cells	Ganglioneuroma	Neuroblastoma
Retinal cells (cones)	—	Retinoblastoma
Connective tissue		
Fibrous tissue	Fibromatosis (desmoid)	Fibrosarcoma
Fat	Lipoma	Liposarcoma
Bone	Osteoma	Osteogenic sarcoma
Cartilage	Chondroma	Chondrosarcoma
Muscle		
Smooth muscle	Leiomyoma	Leiomyosarcoma
Striated muscle	Rhabdomyoma	Rhabdomyosarcoma
Endothelial and related tissues		
Blood vessels	Hemangioma	Angiosarcoma
		Kaposi sarcoma
Lymph vessels	Lymphangioma	Lymphangiosarcoma
Synovium	—	Synovial sarcoma
Mesothelium	—	Malignant mesothelioma
Meninges	Meningioma	Malignant meningioma

From Murphy GP, Lawrence W, Lenhard RE, editors: *American Cancer Society textbook of clinical oncology*, Atlanta, 1995, Author, p 77. Reproduced by permission of the American Cancer Society.

Most cancers are thought to arise from stem cells that are present in tissues. Tissue stem cells are capable of unlimited proliferation, entering the cell cycle to produce two daughter cells—with one cell retaining the original stem cell properties and the other becoming a more differentiated cell, but still capable of proliferation. Normally, the partially differentiated cells can undergo only a limited number of cell divisions before they permanently leave the cell cycle and become senescent.[2] Either a stem cell or a partially differentiated cell has the potential to acquire the genetic mutations necessary to become malignant.

KEY POINTS

- Malignant tumors have the potential to kill the host, whereas benign tumors generally do not. The primary difference between malignant and benign tumors is the propensity of malignant tumors to invade adjacent tissue and spread to distant sites (metastasize).
- The suffix -*oma* is used to indicate a benign tumor (e.g., fibroma). *Carcinoma* and *sarcoma* are used to indicate malignancy (e.g., fibrosarcoma). Exceptions include melanomas, lymphomas, hepatomas, and leukemia, all of which are malignant.
- Malignant cells exhibit antisocial properties that allow them to ignore growth-controlling signals from the environment. Cancer cells proliferate excessively, become immortal, invade locally, and may travel to distant sites where they establish new colonies.

EPIDEMIOLOGY AND CANCER RISK FACTORS

Cancer accounts for approximately 25% of all deaths, which makes it the second leading cause of death in the United States. Most cancer deaths (77%) occur in persons older than 55 years. The American Cancer Society (ACS) estimates that men have almost a 1 in 2 lifetime risk of developing cancer and women have slightly higher than a 1 in 3 risk. The 5-year relative survival rate for all cancers combined is about 68%.[3] The 5-year survival rate does not distinguish between those who were cured and those who have relapsed or are still in treatment. Fortunately, the current view of cancer causation predicts that many cancers are preventable. Indeed, one third of cancer- related deaths may be attributed to lifestyle factors. Lifestyle factors of particular importance are tobacco use, nutrition, and obesity.[4] Sun exposure is a significant risk factor for skin cancer (Chapter 53), and sexual exposure to certain strains of human papillomavirus predisposes to cervical cancer (Chapter 34). The high incidence and relative ease of screening for breast, cervical, colorectal, and prostate cancers has prompted the development of guidelines for early detection of these cancers. The current recommendations for early detection of cancer in average-risk, asymptomatic persons are shown in Table 7-3. Statistics regarding some of the major forms of cancer are shown in Figure 7-2. Further discussions of particular cancers can be found in chapters relating to corresponding body systems.

Tobacco Use

The impact of tobacco use on cancer-related death can be most vividly seen by looking at cancer death rates in the United States from 1930 to 2007 (Figure 7-3). Whereas all other cancer-related death rates declined or remained relatively stable, the death rate from lung cancer increased dramatically. The increase is attributable almost entirely to smoking. Lung cancer remains the leading cause of cancer death in both men and women, accounting for 30% of all cancer deaths. Lung cancer has one of the worst survival rates of all cancers—only 15%. In addition to lung cancer, tobacco use has been linked with cancer of the pancreas, bladder, kidney, mouth, esophagus, and cervix (Figure 7-4). Smoking prevalence among adults in the United States declined from 42% in 1965 to 21% in 2004 and has remained stable at 21%, with rates being approximately 5% lower in women than in men. An estimated 45 million U.S. adults currently smoke cigarettes. Approximately 20% of high school students reported being cigarette smokers in 2009. In 2006, only 8% of college graduates were current smokers, compared to 21% in 1983.[3]

Carcinogens can be grouped into two major types: those that cause genetic damage (initiators) and those that promote growth of the tumor (promoters). Tobacco smoke contains hundreds of compounds, many of which have known genotoxicity (e.g., polycyclic aromatic hydrocarbons, nicotine derivatives) and probably serve as initiators. Tobacco smoke also contains promoters, which spur the mutant cells to proliferate. Second-hand smoke contains more than 7000 chemicals, of which 69 are known to cause cancer.[3] The American Cancer Society estimates that about 3400 nonsmoking adults die from lung cancer each year as a result of exposure to second-hand smoke.[3]

Nutrition

The scientific study of nutrition and cancer is complex, and it is not clear how single nutrients, combinations of nutrients, overnutrition and energy imbalance, or the amount and distribution of body fat affect a person's risk for specific cancers.[3] The ACS suggests a mostly plant-based diet emphasizing a variety of vegetables, fruits, and whole grains. The ACS endorses limiting the intake of red and processed meats, while controlling total caloric intake to maintain a healthy weight. Individual nutritional supplements are not recommended for cancer prevention.[3] The results of randomized clinical trials of antioxidant supplements and selenium have shown no reduction in risk for cancer, at least in generally well-nourished populations.[3]

Fat

Several epidemiologic studies performed in the 1970s and early 1980s suggested a relationship between high-fat diets and the development of breast, colon, and prostate cancer. In some studies, however, higher fat intake was found to be protective against some cancers. A pooled analysis of seven large studies found no link between fat intake and the risk of breast cancer.[5] The results of one large, randomized clinical trial investigating the effect of a low-fat diet on the occurrence of invasive breast cancer found no difference between the control and low-fat groups after 8 years of follow-up in postmenopausal women.[6] Fat or calorie intake and high production of insulin may affect breast cancer outcomes depending on tumor cell type and hormone responsiveness. Further research on the specific type of fat intake and other cofactors is needed to clarify the fat-cancer relationship. Several studies in animals have shown that regardless of fat intake, tumor growth may be inhibited by caloric restriction. Some investigators have proposed a link between high insulin production and breast cancer.

Fiber

Fiber is a general term for nondigestible dietary substances that remain in the intestinal lumen, increase fecal bulk, and improve bowel regularity. Fiber includes a diversity of compounds such as cellulose, bran, and pectin. An association between fiber intake and colorectal cancer proposed in the early 1970s was based on a study comparing the incidence of certain ailments in Americans and Africans.[7] A number of correlational and comparison studies done since that time have yielded conflicting results, and large randomized trials failed to show a benefit.[8] Part of the difficulty may be linked to the way that different studies

TABLE 7-3 SCREENING GUIDELINES FOR THE EARLY DETECTION OF CANCER IN AVERAGE-RISK ASYMPTOMATIC PEOPLE

CANCER SITE	POPULATION	TEST OR PROCEDURE	FREQUENCY
Breast	Women, age 20+	Breast self-examination	Beginning in their early 20s, women should be told about the benefits and limitations of breast self-examination (BSE). The importance of prompt reporting of any new breast symptoms to a health professional should be emphasized. Women who choose to do BSE should receive instruction and have their technique reviewed on the occasion of a periodic health examination. It is acceptable for women to choose not to do BSE or to do BSE irregularly.
		Clinical breast examination	For women in their 20s and 30s, it is recommended that clinical breast examination (CBE) be part of a periodic health examination, preferably at least every 3 years. Asymptomatic women aged 40 and over should continue to receive a clinical breast examination as part of a periodic health examination, preferably annually.
		Mammography	Begin annual mammography at age 40–50*
Colorectal[†]	Men and women, age 50+	*Tests that find polyps and cancer:* Flexible sigmoidoscopy[‡] *or*	Every 5 years starting at age 50
		Colonscopy, *or*	Every 10 years, starting at age 50
		Double-contrast barium enema (DCBD) [‡]	Every 5 years, starting at age 50
		Tests that mainly find cancer: Fecal occult blood test (FOBT) with at least 50% test sensitivity for cancer, fecal immunochemical test (FIT) with at least 50% test sensitivity for cancer,[‡,§] *or*	Annual, starting at age 50
		Stool DNA test (sDNA)[‡]	Interval uncertain, starting at age 50
Prostate	Men, age 50+	Prostate-specific antigen test (PSA) with or without digital rectal exam (DRE)	Asymptomatic men who have at least 10-year life expectancy should have an opportunity to make an informed decision with their health care provider about screening for prostate cancer after receiving information about the uncertainties, risks, and potential benefits associated with screening. Prostate cancer screening should not occur without an informed decision-making process.
Cervix	Women, age 21+	Pap test	Cervical cancer screening should begin approximately 3 years after a woman begins having vaginal intercourse, but no earlier than 21 years of age. Screening should be done every year with conventional Pap tests or every 2 years using liquid-based Pap tests. At or after age 30, women who have had three normal test results in a row may get screened every 2 to 3 years with cervical cytology (either conventional or liquid-based Pap test) alone, or every 3 years with an HPV DNA test plus cervical cytology. Women 70 years of age and older who have had three or more normal Pap tests and no abnormal Pap tests in the past 10 years and women who have had a total hysterectomy may choose to stop cervical cancer screening.
Endometrial	Women, at menopause		At the time of menopause, women at average risk should be informed about risks and symptoms of endometrial cancer and strongly encouraged to report any unexpected bleeding or spotting to their physicians.
Cancer-related checkup	Men and women age 20+		On the occasion of a periodic health examination, the cancer-related checkup should include examination for cancers of the thyroid, testicles, ovaries, lymph nodes, oral cavity, and skin, as well as health counseling about tobacco, sun exposure, diet and nutrition, risk factors, sexual practices, and environmental and occupational exposures.

American Cancer Society: *Cancer facts and figures—2012,* Atlanta, 2012, American Cancer Society; ACOG Committee on Practice Bulletins-Gynecology. *Obstet Gynecol* 114(6):1409-1429, 2009.

*Beginning at age 40, annual clinical breast examination should be performed before mammography.

[†]Individuals with a personal or family history of colorectal cancer or adenomas, inflammatory bowel disease, or high-risk genetic syndromes should continue to follow the most recent recommendations for individuals at increased or high risk.

[‡]Colonoscopy should be done if test results are positive.

[§]For FOBT or FIT used as a screening test, the take-home multiple sample method should be used. An FOBT or FIT done during a digital rectal exam in the doctor's office is not adequate for screening.

[¶]Information should be provided to men about the benefits and limitations of testing so that an informed decision can be made with the clinician's assistance.

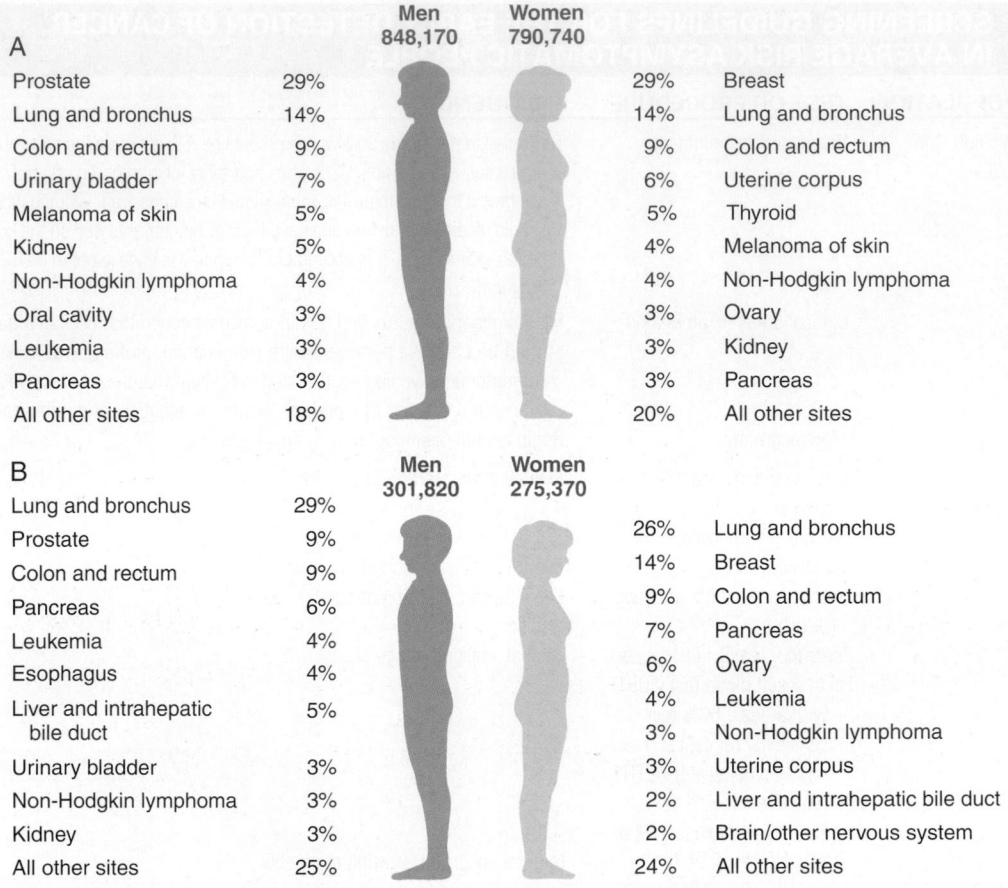

A

Prostate	29%			29%	Breast
Lung and bronchus	14%			14%	Lung and bronchus
Colon and rectum	9%			9%	Colon and rectum
Urinary bladder	7%			6%	Uterine corpus
Melanoma of skin	5%			5%	Thyroid
Kidney	5%			4%	Melanoma of skin
Non-Hodgkin lymphoma	4%			4%	Non-Hodgkin lymphoma
Oral cavity	3%			3%	Ovary
Leukemia	3%			3%	Kidney
Pancreas	3%			3%	Pancreas
All other sites	18%			20%	All other sites

Men 848,170   Women 790,740

B

Lung and bronchus	29%				
Prostate	9%			26%	Lung and bronchus
Colon and rectum	9%			14%	Breast
Pancreas	6%			9%	Colon and rectum
Leukemia	4%			7%	Pancreas
Esophagus	4%			6%	Ovary
Liver and intrahepatic bile duct	5%			4%	Leukemia
Urinary bladder	3%			3%	Non-Hodgkin lymphoma
Non-Hodgkin lymphoma	3%			3%	Uterine corpus
Kidney	3%			2%	Liver and intrahepatic bile duct
All other sites	25%			2%	Brain/other nervous system
				24%	All other sites

Men 301,820   Women 275,370

FIGURE 7-2 United States 2012 estimated new cancer cases **(A)** and estimated cancer deaths **(B)** in 10 leading sites by gender. Excludes basal and squamous cell skin cancers and in situ carcinomas except urinary bladder. (American Cancer Society: *Cancer facts and figures—2012,* Atlanta, 2012, American Cancer Society.)

define dietary fiber. Because fiber is associated with beneficial effects on digestion and elimination, fiber intake in the range of 10 to 13 g per 1000 calories consumed is generally recommended.

Alcohol

Alcohol intake has been linked to a number of cancers, including breast, esophageal, laryngeal, and liver cancer. Alcohol may exert its cancer-promoting effects through impairment of the liver's ability to metabolize harmful substances and endogenous hormones. Moderate alcohol intake has been shown to increase estrogen levels, which may account for its promoting effects on breast cancer.[9] As a carbohydrate-dense substance, alcohol may contribute to cancer risk through its effects on insulin secretion. Insulin is a general growth factor for a number of tissues. Limiting alcohol intake may provide a modest reduction in cancer risk.

Antioxidants

Until recently, the emphasis of cancer prevention has been on the identification and avoidance of cancer-causing agents. However, increasing interest has been shown in finding substances with cancer-protective properties. The fact that DNA damage is an important step in cancer initiation, coupled with the knowledge that oxygen free radicals can impart this damage, led to the idea that antioxidants may have protective effects for cancer. The specific agents tested in clinical trials included β-carotene, vitamin E, vitamin C, selenium, retinol, zinc, riboflavin, and molybdenum. None of the completed trials produced convincing evidence to justify the use of traditional antioxidant-related vitamins or minerals for cancer prevention.[10]

Vitamin A and the antioxidant trio of vitamin E, β-carotene, and vitamin C have been most widely studied. The use of antioxidants to prevent cancer sounds like a good idea; however, several large-scale studies have failed to reveal a benefit and some have found that the risk of cancer may be increased.[11,12] At present, it may be prudent to consume a diet high in natural fruit and vegetable sources of antioxidants.

> **KEY POINTS**
> - The risk of developing cancer increases with age. It is estimated that men have almost a 1 in 2 lifetime chance of developing cancer, whereas women have a little more than a 1 in 3 chance.
> - The development of many cancers is related to lifestyle, particularly tobacco use and nutrition. Smoking cessation is considered important in reducing cancer risk. Guidelines regarding nutrition are less clear. Limiting excessive calorie and alcohol intake while increasing intake of dietary fiber, fruit, and vegetables may be of benefit.

GENETIC MECHANISMS OF CANCER

Despite much progress in our understanding of how mechanisms of growth control and cellular differentiation may go awry, there is still no simple answer to the question, "What causes cancer?" It is increasingly evident, however, that cancer is primarily a disorder of gene

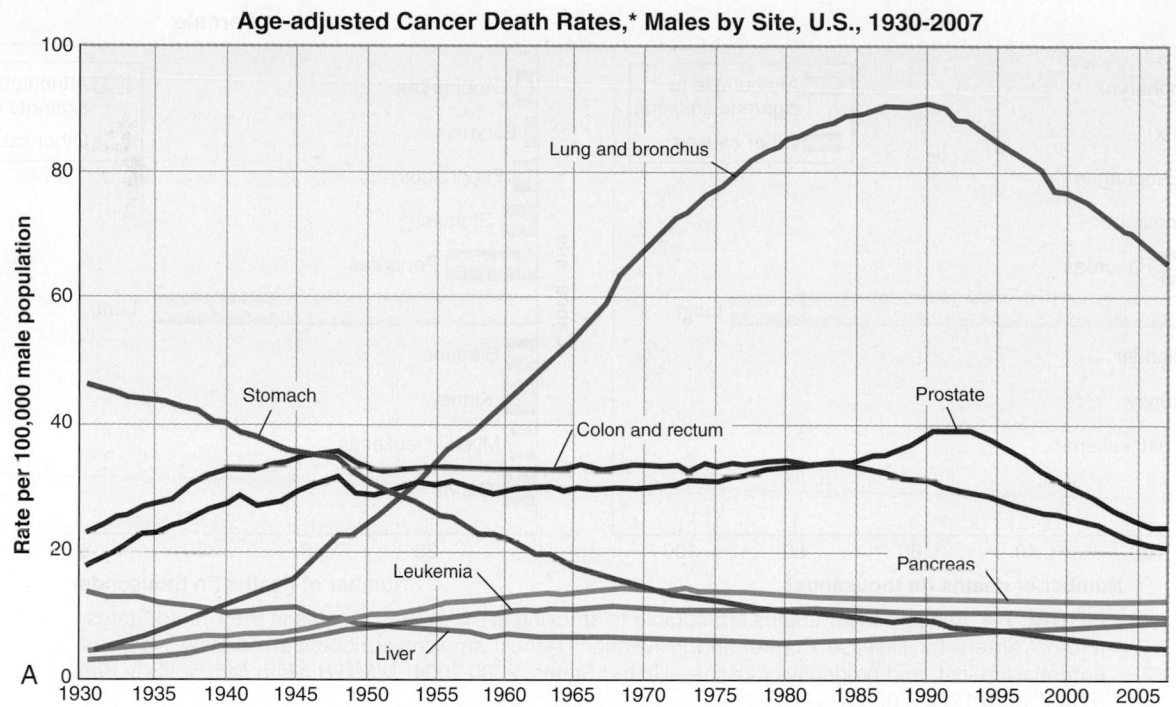

Age-adjusted Cancer Death Rates,* Males by Site, U.S., 1930-2007

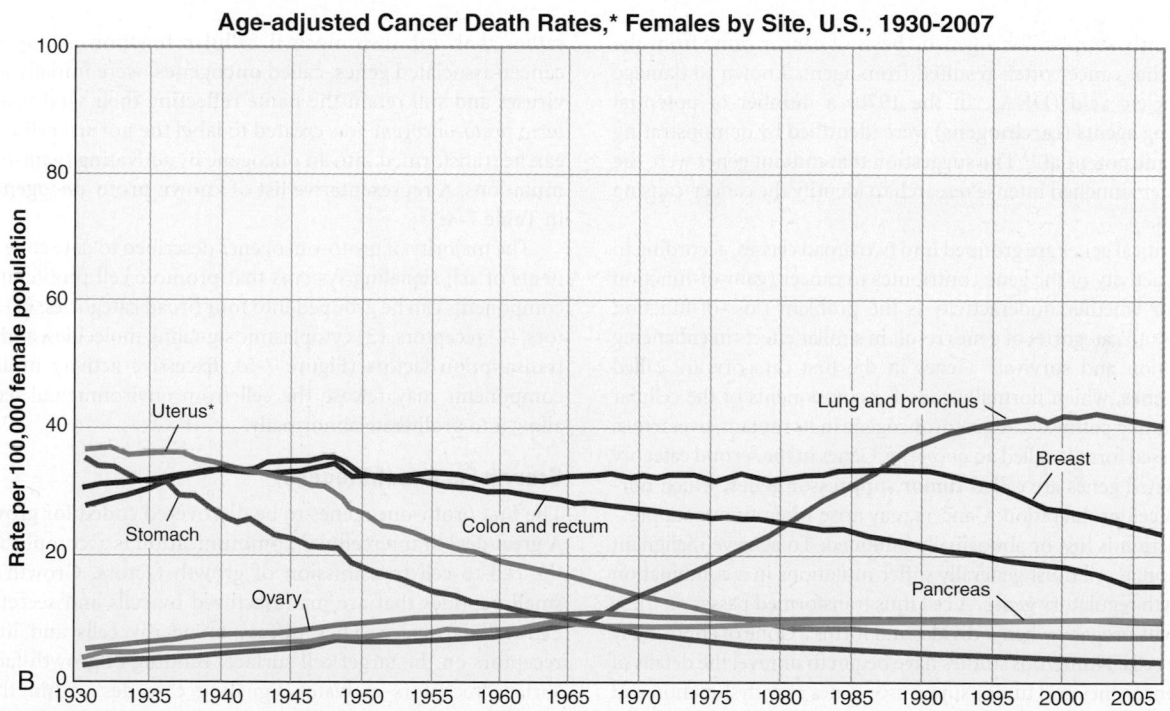

Age-adjusted Cancer Death Rates,* Females by Site, U.S., 1930-2007

*Per 100,000 age adjusted to the 2000 U.S. standard population.

Note: Due to changes in ICD coding, rumerator information has changed over time. Rates for cancer of the liver, lung and bronchus, and colon and rectum are affected by these changes.

FIGURE 7-3 United States age-adjusted cancer death rates for selected sites in men **(A)** and women **(B)** from 1930 to 2007. (American Cancer Society: *Cancer facts and figures—2012,* Atlanta, 2012, American Cancer Society.)

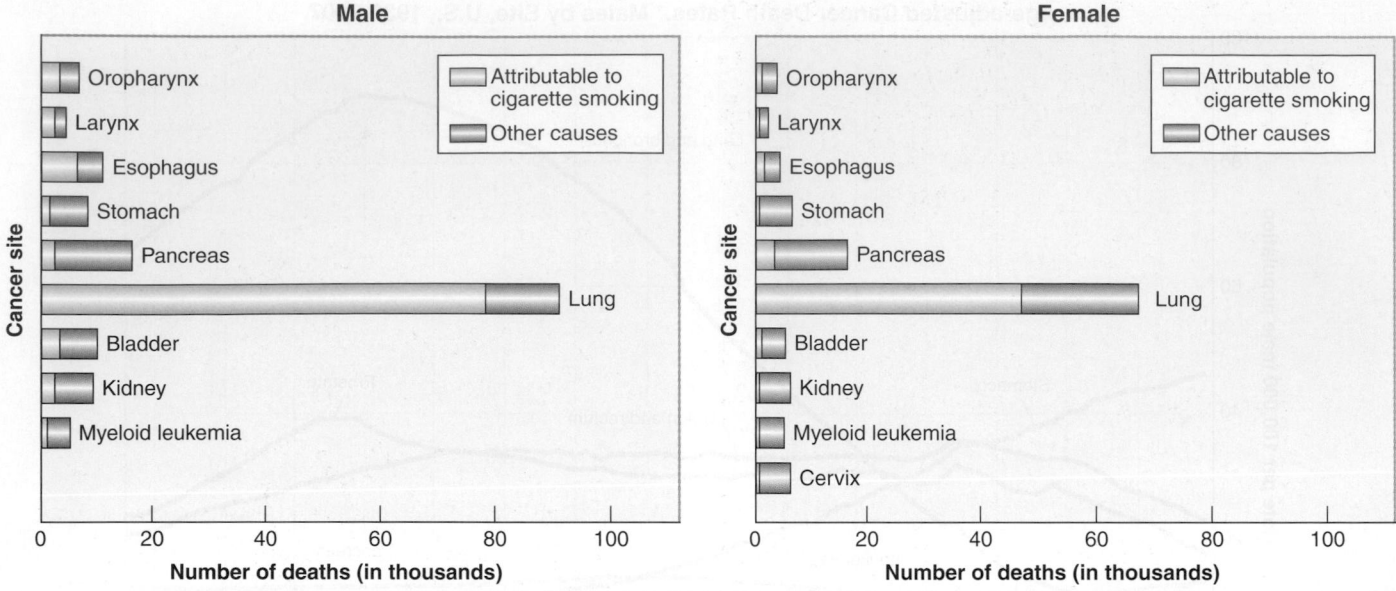

FIGURE 7-4 Annual cancer deaths attributable to smoking in males and females in the United States. (From Centers for Disease Control and Prevention: Annual smoking-attributable mortality, years of potential life lost, and productivity losses—United States, 2000-2004, *MMWR Morb Mortal Wkly Rep 57*[45]:1226-1228, 2008.)

expression. Early support for a genetic basis of cancer came from the observation that cancer often resulted from agents known to damage deoxyribonucleic acid (DNA). In the 1970s a number of potential cancer-causing agents (**carcinogens**) were identified by demonstrating their mutagenic potential.[13] The suggestion that mutant genes were the basis for cancer launched intense research to identify the cancer-causing gene or genes.

Cancer-critical genes are grouped into two broad classes, according to whether overactivity of the gene contributes to cancer (gain-of-function mutations) or whether underactivity is the problem (loss-of-function mutations). Both categories of genes result in similar effects in enhancing cell proliferation and survival.[2] Genes in the first category are called **proto-oncogenes,** which normally code for components of the cellular growth–activating pathways. A proto-oncogene in its mutant, overactive, or overexpressed form is called an *oncogene.* Genes in the second category of cancer-related genes are called **tumor suppressor genes,** which normally inhibit cell proliferation. Cancers may arise when tumor suppressor gene function is lost or abnormally inhibited. To achieve malignant transformation, a cell must generally suffer mutations in a combination of these growth regulatory genes. A cell thus transformed passes on these mutations to its progeny when it divides and forms a clone of abnormally proliferating cells. Numerous studies have begun to unravel the details of how proto-oncogenes and tumor suppressor genes may dysfunction and contribute to the malignant phenotype. In addition to the genes that regulate the cell cycle, two other categories of genes that monitor and maintain the genome contribute indirectly to the development of cancer. These are the DNA-repair genes and the genes that regulate apoptosis (see Chapter 4).

Proto-Oncogenes

Proto-oncogenes were the first of the tumor-associated genes to be discovered, and hundreds have been described to date.[2] As often happens in the study of genes, a gene associated with a disease process is identified long before its normal cellular function is elucidated. Thus genes associated with cancer are traditionally named for the cancer in which they were first discovered (in mutant form)

rather than for their normal cellular function. Many of the first cancer-associated genes, called **oncogenes,** were initially identified in viruses and still retain the name reflecting their viral discovery. The term *proto-oncogene* was created to label the normal cellular gene that can be transformed into an oncogene by activating (gain-of-function) mutations. A representative list of known proto-oncogenes is shown in Table 7-4.

The majority of proto-oncogenes described to date code for components of cell-signaling systems that promote cell proliferation.[2] These components can be grouped into four broad categories: (1) growth factors, (2) receptors, (3) cytoplasmic signaling molecules, and (4) nuclear transcription factors (Figure 7-5). Excessive activity in any of these components may release the cell from environmental feedback and allow it to proliferate abnormally.

Growth Factors (Mitogens)

The first proto-oncogenes to be discovered coded for growth factors. A great deal of intercellular communication is accomplished through the cell-to-cell transmission of growth factors. Growth factors are small peptides that are manufactured by cells and secreted into the extracellular space. They diffuse to nearby cells and interact with receptors on the target cell surface. Binding of growth factors to cell surface receptors activates signaling cascades within the cell that enhance proliferation. As a general principle, cells do not independently produce growth factors sufficient to stimulate their own proliferation. The proliferation signals must be produced by the cell's environment. The cell's environment also conveys growth-inhibiting signals. Overproduction of stimulatory growth factors by a mutant proto-oncogene can shift the balance of signals and produce excessive self-stimulated growth (**autocrine signaling**). Examples of tumor-secreted growth factors include platelet-derived growth factor (PDGF), transforming growth factor-α (TGF-α), and epidermal growth factor (EGF). Certain cancer types typically secrete particular growth factors. For example, platelet-derived growth factor is commonly oversecreted in glial cell cancers (brain tumors) and connective tissue cancers (sarcomas).

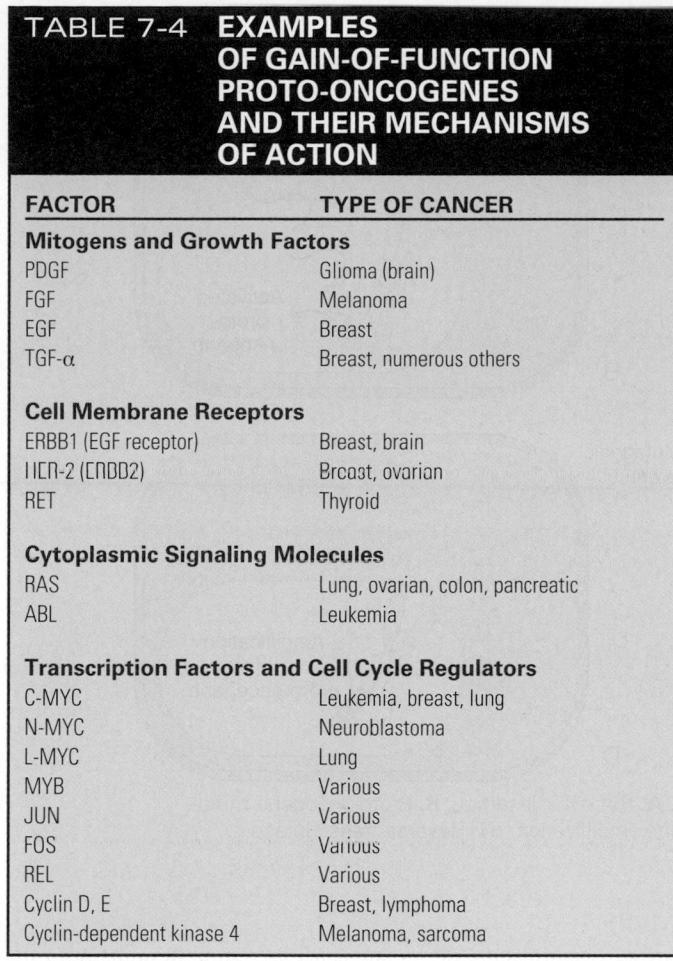

TABLE 7-4	EXAMPLES OF GAIN-OF-FUNCTION PROTO-ONCOGENES AND THEIR MECHANISMS OF ACTION
FACTOR	**TYPE OF CANCER**
Mitogens and Growth Factors	
PDGF	Glioma (brain)
FGF	Melanoma
EGF	Breast
TGF-α	Breast, numerous others
Cell Membrane Receptors	
ERBB1 (EGF receptor)	Breast, brain
HER-2 (ERBB2)	Breast, ovarian
RET	Thyroid
Cytoplasmic Signaling Molecules	
RAS	Lung, ovarian, colon, pancreatic
ABL	Leukemia
Transcription Factors and Cell Cycle Regulators	
C-MYC	Leukemia, breast, lung
N-MYC	Neuroblastoma
L-MYC	Lung
MYB	Various
JUN	Various
FOS	Various
REL	Various
Cyclin D, E	Breast, lymphoma
Cyclin-dependent kinase 4	Melanoma, sarcoma

EGF, Epidermal growth factor; *FGF,* fibroblast growth factor; *PDGF,* platelet-derived growth factor; *TGF,* transforming growth factor.

Growth Factor Receptors

Peptide growth factors (mitogens) cannot penetrate the cell membrane directly, so their presence at the cell surface must be transmitted intracellularly by cell surface receptors. Receptors are transmembrane proteins with the mitogen-binding area on the outside of the cell and an enzyme-activating area on the inside of the cell. These receptors are extremely specific; they will bind with only one particular mitogen. Binding activates a series of reactions within the cell that eventually leads to cell proliferation.

A mutational event may allow the expression of receptors that should not be present at all or allow excessive amounts of normally present receptors, or it may produce receptors with abnormally high affinity. All of these changes result in excessive responsiveness to the mitogens normally present in the cell's environment. Some mutant receptors may even be active in the absence of growth factors and spur the cell to divide despite the absence of environmental signals to do so. An important example of a receptor abnormality is the overexpression of human epidermal growth factor receptor type 2 (HER2) receptors in about 25% of breast cancers. The overactive receptors stimulate proliferation of tumor cells even when there is little or no epidermal growth factor bound to them.

Cytoplasmic Signaling Pathways

A third way in which oncogenes may facilitate proliferation is by the manufacture of excessive or abnormal components of the intracellular

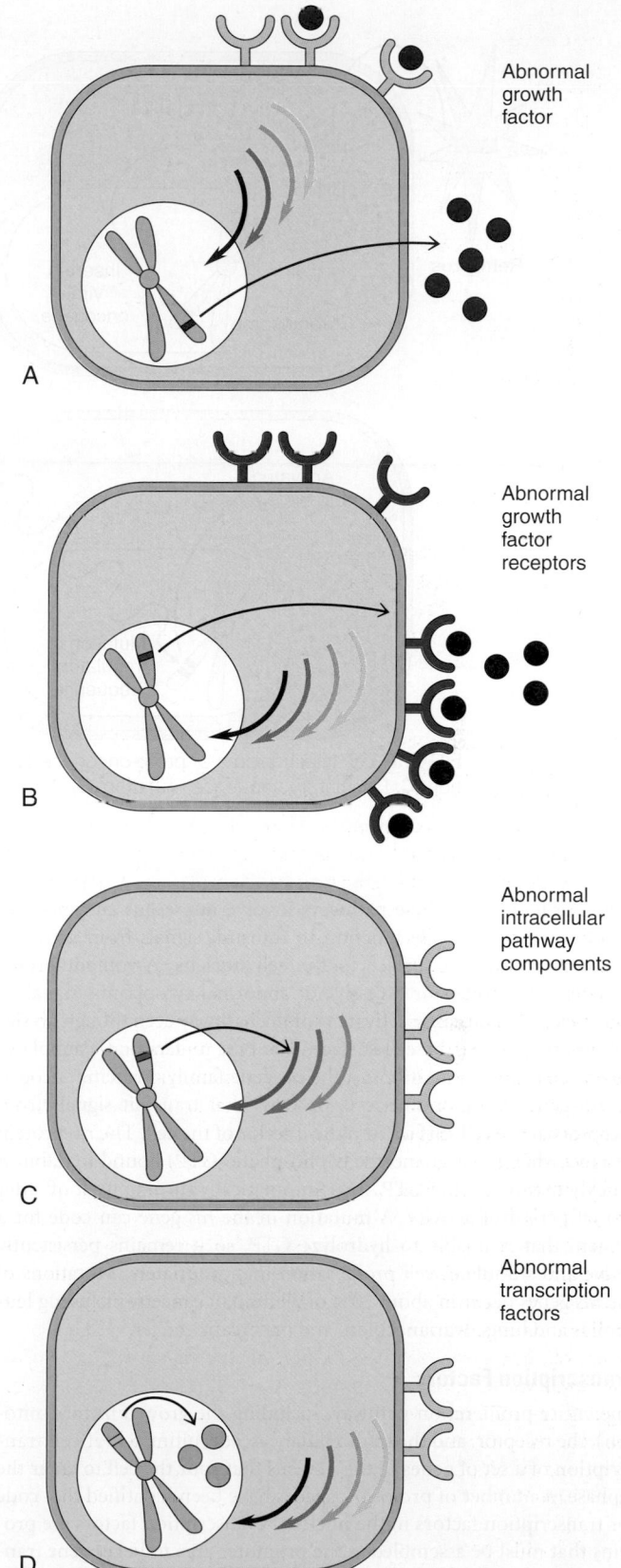

FIGURE 7-5 Possible effects of proto-oncogene activation on growth signaling pathways. **A,** Production of growth factors (mitogens). **B,** Production of growth factor receptors. **C,** Intracellular pathway disturbances. **D,** Activation of transcription factors for growth.

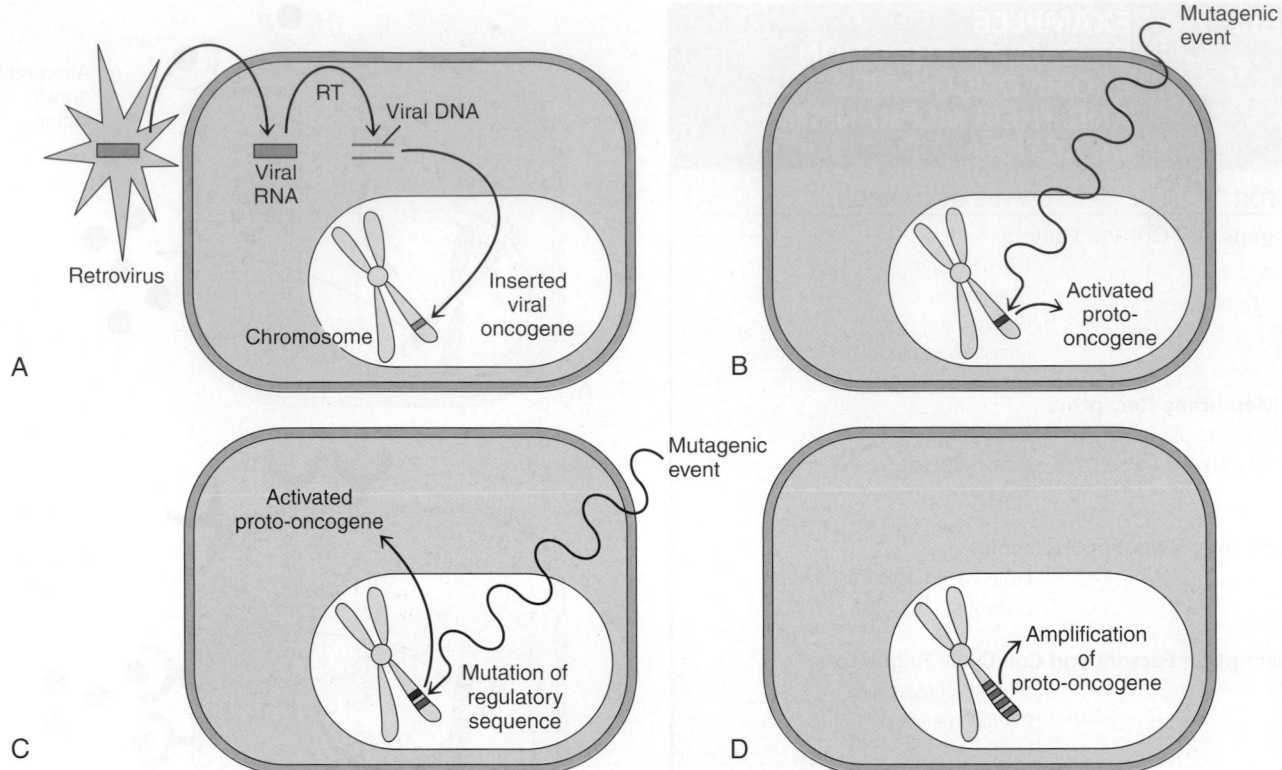

FIGURE 7-6 Mechanisms of proto-oncogene activation. **A,** Retroviral insertion. **B,** Proto-oncogene mutation. **C,** Regulatory sequence mutation. **D,** Proto-oncogene amplification. *RT,* Reverse transcriptase.

signaling pathways. These pathways involve numerous enzymes and chemicals that normally function to transmit signals from activated receptors at the cell surface to the cell nucleus. A mutant proto-oncogene that codes for excessive or abnormal cytoplasmic signaling components could cause activation of the pathway even though no signal was received at the cell surface. The best understood example of this mechanism is mutations of the *ras* gene family. Proteins encoded by *ras* genes are monomeric G-proteins that transmit signals from receptors at the cell surface into the interior of the cell. The *ras* protein is active when it has guanosine triphosphate (GTP) bound to it, but it quickly hydrolyzes the GTP, thus automatically turning itself off after a brief period of activity. A mutation in the *ras* gene can code for a protein that is unable to hydrolyze GTP, so it remains persistently active and stimulates cell proliferation inappropriately. Mutations of the *ras* genes occur in about 20% of all human cancers, including leukemias and lung, ovarian, colon, and pancreatic cancer.[1]

Transcription Factors

The entire proliferation pathway, including the growth factor (mitogen), the receptor, and the intracellular cascade, ultimately affects transcription of a set of genes in the nucleus that spur the cell to enter the S phase. A number of proto-oncogenes have been identified that code for transcription factors in the nucleus. Transcription factors are proteins that must be assembled at the promoter area to begin gene transcription (see Chapters 3 and 5). Transcription factors are normally sequestered and prevented from indiscriminate activity until appropriate signals cause their release. Mutations in transcription factor genes may cause overproduction of transcription factors or interfere with the normal mechanisms for keeping them in check. *Myc, jun,* and *fos* are examples of proto-oncogenes that code for nuclear transcription

factors. Abnormalities of the *myc* genes are found in numerous cancers, including lung and breast cancer, leukemia, and neuroblastoma.

From Proto-Oncogene to Oncogene

Proto-oncogenes become activated oncogenes when mutations alter their activity so that proliferation-promoting signals are generated inappropriately. At least four general ways in which proto-oncogenes can be activated are known (Figure 7-6): (1) Oncogenes may be introduced into the host cell by a retrovirus; (2) a proto-oncogene within the cell may suffer a mutagenic event that changes its structure and function; (3) a DNA sequence that normally regulates proto-oncogene expression may be damaged or lost and allow the proto-oncogene to become abnormally active; and (4) an error in chromosome replication may cause extra copies of the proto-oncogene to be included in the genome (amplification).

In the early 1960s it was discovered that certain viruses were associated with cancer in various animal models. Researchers speculated that a virus could introduce a mutant, cancer-causing gene (oncogene) into the host's cells. Indeed, malignant cells containing the cancer-causing viruses were shown to have incorporated a small number of viral genes into their cellular DNA.[14] The presence of these oncogenes was required to maintain the malignant state of the cell.

Only a few types of human cancers are thought to be associated with viruses. The clearest associations involve viruses called *retroviruses*. At least three retroviruses are considered to be causative factors in some human cancers: Human immunodeficiency virus is associated with Kaposi sarcoma, Epstein-Barr virus with Burkitt lymphoma, and human T lymphocyte virus type I with adult T cell leukemia-lymphoma.

Retroviruses are composed of RNA and possess a unique enzyme—reverse transcriptase—that directs the synthesis of a DNA copy of the

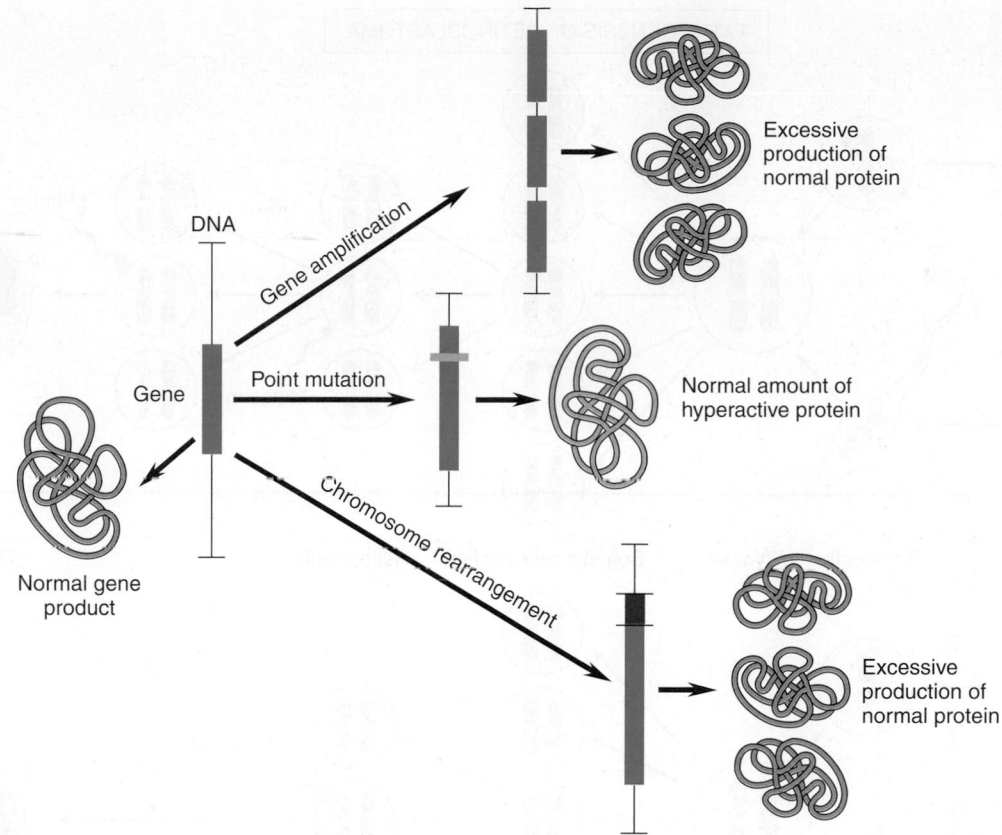

FIGURE 7-7 Overactivity of proto-oncogenes may be due to normal production of an abnormal protein (mutation in coding sequence) or excessive production of a normal protein (gene amplification or chromosome rearrangement).

viral RNA. The DNA copy can then be incorporated into the cellular DNA and become part of the host's genome. The degree of viral oncogene expression depends on where the oncogene is inserted in the host DNA. Insertion near a promoter sequence may result in continuous transcription of the oncogene. Viral oncogenes are not subject to normal DNA transcription controls and are thus not responsive to growth-suppressing signals. Where did the viral oncogenes originate? Apparently, the tendency of retroviruses to slip in and out of host genomes allows them to pick up some of the host's genes, namely, the growth-promoting proto-oncogenes.

Proto-oncogene expression is tightly regulated in a normal cell. A number of different mutations can affect proto-oncogene expression and activity. A point mutation in the coding region of the proto-oncogene can alter the structure of its protein product and make it hyperactive. An example of this mechanism is the abnormal *ras* protein described earlier. Even though the protein is synthesized in normal quantity, its activity is enhanced. Other mutations may lead to overproduction of a protein with normal structure. Gene amplification and chromosomal rearrangement during mitosis may release the proto-oncogene from its normal regulation and allow excessive transcription (Figure 7-7).

In summary, mutational events in the cell's genome may cause overexpression of normal proto-oncogene products or production of altered and hyperactive proteins. Most known oncogenes act by releasing the cell from its dependence on growth and survival signals in its environment. This effect usually is accomplished by gain-of-function abnormalities in the proliferation pathways that involve growth factors (mitogens), receptors, cytoplasmic signaling molecules, or nuclear transcription factors.

Tumor Suppressor Genes

To become malignant, cells must devise ways to evade the normal inhibitory mechanisms that keep the brakes applied to cell division. It is not enough to simply overstimulate growth-promoting signals. Critical elements of the proliferation-inhibiting pathways are defective in most cancers. The components of the inhibitory machinery are specified by the so-called *tumor suppressor genes.* Tumor suppressor genes are difficult to study because they contribute to cancer only when they are not there. The first tumor suppressor gene to be discovered was the *Rb* gene, so named because of its role in retinoblastoma, a cancer of the eye.[15] A familial form of retinoblastoma is associated with the transmission of a genetic defect; a portion of chromosome 13 is missing, which is where the *Rb* gene is normally located. An absent *Rb* gene predisposes an individual to cancer, but cancer will not develop unless the other copy of the *Rb* gene (from the other parent) is also damaged (Figure 7-8).

Since the initial discovery of the *Rb* tumor suppressor gene, researchers have compiled an impressive list of other genes that appear to function as inhibitors of cellular proliferation (Table 7-5). As with the *Rb* gene, both copies of the tumor suppressor genes usually are inactivated when cancer develops. A person who inherits a defective copy of a tumor suppressor gene from one parent has a much higher risk of cancer than a person who inherits two healthy copies. Knowledge about the sequence of many of these genes provides the opportunity to screen individuals with familial cancers to determine whether they carry a defective gene. Detection of defective tumor suppressor genes is easier than determining their normal cellular functions, but steady progress is being made.

Why do tumor suppressor genes stop functioning? As with proto-oncogene activation, genetic mutations are the usual culprits. Chromosome deletions, point mutations, or chromosome loss through

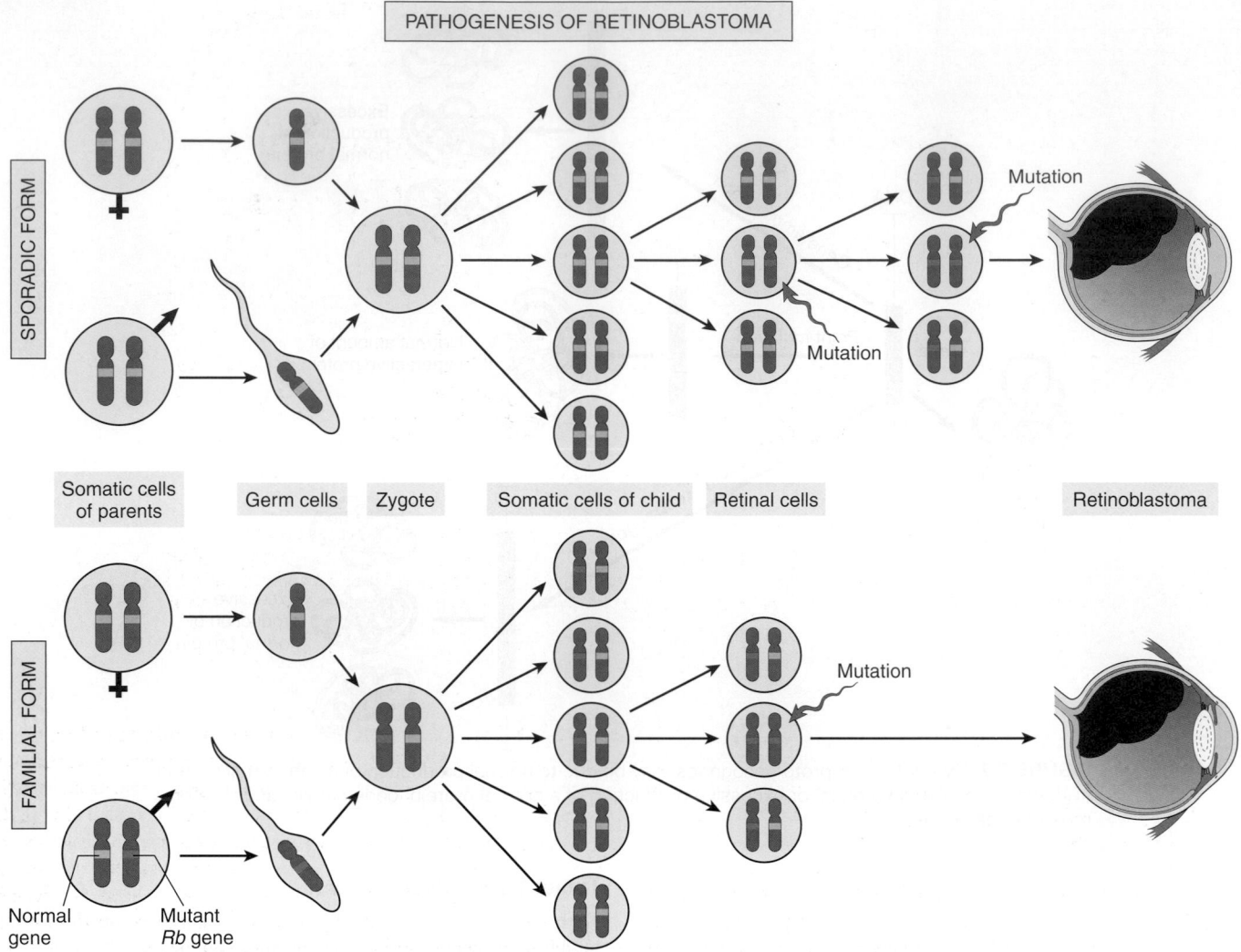

PATHOGENESIS OF RETINOBLASTOMA

SPORADIC FORM

FAMILIAL FORM

Somatic cells of parents | Germ cells | Zygote | Somatic cells of child | Retinal cells | Retinoblastoma

Mutation

Normal gene | Mutant Rb gene

FIGURE 7-8 Both DNA copies (alleles) of the *Rb* tumor suppression gene must be dysfunctional for occurrence of retinoblastoma. Inheriting a defective *Rb* gene predisposes an individual to the development of cancer because only a single mutational event is required to inactivate *pRb* function. (From Kumar V et al: *Robbins and Cotran pathologic basis of disease,* ed 8, Philadelphia, 2010, Saunders, p 288.)

TABLE 7-5 EXAMPLES OF TUMOR SUPPRESSOR GENES

GENE	CHROMOSOME LOCATION	CANCER
Rb	13q14	Retinoblastoma, sarcoma
P53	17p13	Li-Fraumeni syndrome, 50% of all tumors
DCC	18q21	Colorectal carcinoma
APC	5q21	Colorectal, stomach, pancreatic
BRCA1	17q21	Breast, ovarian
BRCA2	13q12	Breast, ovarian, prostate
WT1	11p13	Wilms tumor
WT2	11p15	Rhabdomyosarcoma
NF1	17q11	Neurofibromatosis type 1, astrocytoma
NF2	22q12	Neurofibromatosis type 2, meningioma
VHL	3p25	Renal cell carcinoma
MEN1	11q23	Multiple endocrine neoplasia
MTS1	9p21	Melanoma, leukemia, sarcomas, several carcinomas

nondisjunction may knock out tumor suppressor gene function. Tumor suppressor gene function may also be lost through an "epigenetic" process that "silences" the gene. Epigenetic influences do not change the DNA sequence (no mutation is required), but change the packaging of DNA and chemically modify it (e.g., methylation) so that the gene is inactivated. This inactivation can be passed on to daughter cells during mitosis.

The *Rb* Gene

The *Rb* gene codes for a large protein in the cell nucleus (pRb) that has been labeled the "master brake" of the cell cycle (see Chapter 3). It blocks cell division by binding transcription factors (E2F) and thereby inhibiting them from transcribing the genes that initiate the cell cycle (Figure 7-9). The Rb protein can be induced to release the transcription factors when it is sufficiently phosphorylated. Proliferation-promoting signals in the cell increase cyclin-dependent kinase (cdk) enzymes and promote pRb phosphorylation, whereas growth-inhibiting signals prevent phosphorylation. Thus an inactivating mutation of the *Rb* genes removes one of the major restraints on cell division. Defective pRb is common to a number of different cancers.

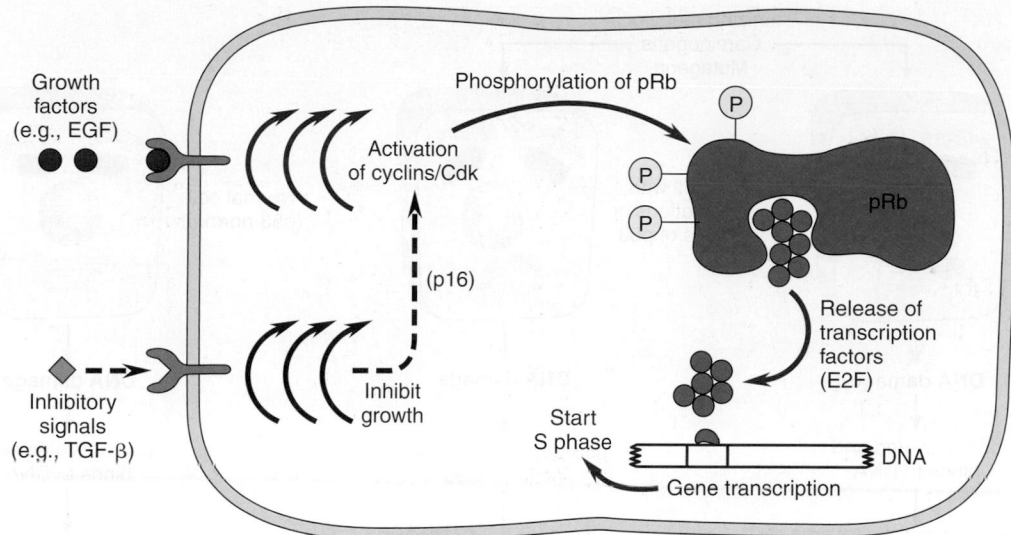

FIGURE 7-9 The Rb protein functions to bind transcription factors in the nucleus and keep them from participating in the transcription of cell cycle–related genes. pRb is induced to release its hold on the E2F transcription factors when it is sufficiently phosphorylated by cyclin-dependent kinases *(Cdk).* Cyclin-dependent kinases are activated by cyclin proteins that accumulate when growth factors bind to receptors and stimulate growth pathways. Other signals, such as transforming growth factor-β *(TGF-β),* inhibit the activity of cyclin/Cdk through activation of inhibitory proteins such as p16. A loss of pRb function removes the "major brake" on cell division. *P,* Phosphate group; *EGF,* epidermal growth factor.

The *P53* Gene

The most common tumor suppressor gene defect identified in cancer cells involves *P53,* so named because of the protein's molecular mass of 53 kilodaltons (also called TP53). More than half of all types of human tumors lack functional *P53.* The p53 protein, like pRb, inhibits cell cycling. Unlike pRb, however, normally very little p53 is found in cells, and it accumulates only after cellular, particularly DNA, damage. P53 is a transcription factor that binds to damaged DNA and regulates hundreds of genes.[1] P53 stalls cell division, presumably to allow time for DNA repair before DNA replication in the S phase (Figure 7-10). In the face of excessive damage (or other distress signals), p53 may direct the cell to initiate apoptosis. A defect in p53 function disrupts this important quality control system, allowing genetically damaged and unstable cells to survive and continue to replicate (see Figure 7-10). Genetically unstable cells have a propensity to accumulate more cancer-promoting mutations while they proliferate. The *P53* gene is important for therapeutic reasons as well. Chemotherapy- and radiation-induced cell death is mediated in large part by p53. These agents usually do not kill cancer cells directly; rather, they cause enough cellular damage in the target cell to trigger p53-mediated cell suicide. Cancer cells that lack functional p53 may therefore be resistant to some radiation and chemotherapeutic protocols.

BRCA1 and *BRCA2*

Many tumor suppressor genes have been identified through studies of inherited predisposition to certain types of cancer. The breast cancer genes *BRCA1* and *BRCA2* are important examples. Women with a family history of breast cancer and an inherited defect in the *BRCA1* gene have about a 50% risk of developing breast cancer.[16] The age of onset of inherited breast cancer is earlier than the onset of noninherited (sporadic) forms, and the prevalence of bilateral breast cancer is higher. Inherited forms of breast cancer account for only about 5% to 10% of all cases of breast cancer, but study of the genes involved is providing important insights into breast cancer biology in general.

Defects in numerous other tumor suppressor genes have been identified in certain types of cancers (see Table 7-5), including *APC* and *DCC* in colorectal cancer, *NF1* and *NF2* in neurofibromatosis, and *VHL* in renal cell cancers. The functions of tumor suppressor genes are varied, but most appear to inhibit proliferation or induce apoptosis in defective cells.

Figure 7-11 summarizes the major known cellular signaling pathways that are relevant to the development of cancer. The functions of oncogenes and tumor suppressor genes are shown to interact to determine cell proliferation, cell survival, and cell death. In general, any cellular alteration that promotes proliferation or inhibits cell death can contribute to an increased risk of tumor development.

KEY POINTS

- Cancer is thought to develop when proto-oncogenes become inappropriately activated in a cell or when tumor suppressor genes become inactivated. This change in gene function is usually due to mutations in the cell's DNA.
- Mutant proto-oncogenes disrupt the intercellular communication pathway that normally regulates cell proliferation. This disruption may occur through abnormal production of growth factors, receptors, cytoplasmic signaling molecules, or nuclear transcription factors.
- Both copies of a tumor suppressor gene usually must be inactivated to eliminate its function. Tumor suppressor genes inhibit cellular proliferation in various ways. The Rb protein serves as a "master brake" on cell proliferation by inhibiting transcription factors. *P53* inhibits cell cycling when the cell is damaged to allow time for DNA repair. *P53* is also important in initiating apoptosis of damaged or unwanted cells.

MULTISTEP NATURE OF CARCINOGENESIS

From the preceding discussion, it might seem that simply activating an oncogene in a normal cell or knocking out a tumor suppressor gene would be sufficient to transform it into a malignant cell. Such has not proved to be the case. Growth regulation of mammalian cells appears to be organized in such a manner that a single aberrant gene is unable to induce conversion to full malignancy. Different genes function in

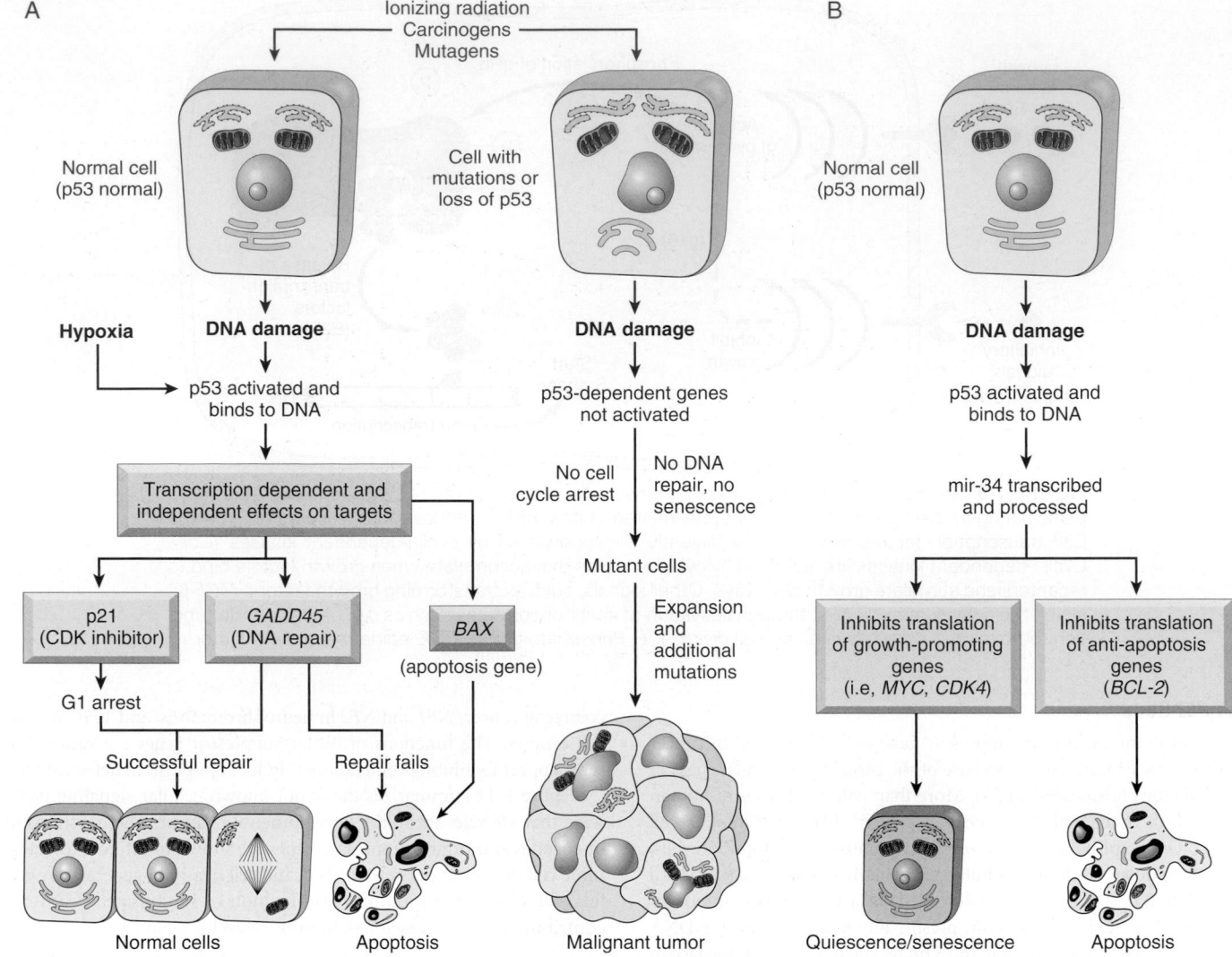

FIGURE 7-10 Role of *P53* (TP53) in maintaining the integrity of the genome. Damage to DNA in cells with functional *P53* stalls the cell cycle so that DNA can be repaired. If repair fails, then the cell undergoes apoptosis to prevent the proliferation of DNA-damaged cells. If the *P53* is not functional, genetically unstable cells may be allowed to survive and proliferate. (From Kumar V et al: *Robbins and Cotran pathologic basis of disease*, ed 8, Philadelphia, 2010, Saunders, p 291.)

distinct ways and may affect only a subset of the changes necessary to achieve full malignancy. For example, introduction of the *ras* oncogene into normal cells in culture causes them to show anchorage independence, but they are unable to form tumors when inoculated into an animal. Anchorage independence is a typical feature of most transformed cells and means that they are capable of proliferating even if they are not attached to a matrix. Normal cells will not divide and will initiate apoptosis if they do not have a space on the matrix on which to anchor themselves. Similarly, the *myc* oncogene allows cells to grow indefinitely in culture, but these immortal cells are still unable to induce tumor formation. However, when both the *ras* and the *myc* oncogenes are introduced into normal cells, they become fully malignant (Figure 7-12).[17]

These culture experiments support the clinical observation that carcinogenesis is a multistep phenomenon.[2] The steps of carcinogenesis have been labeled *initiation, promotion,* and *progression* (Figure 7-13).

Initiation

Initiating events are thought to be the genetic mutations that inappropriately activate proto-oncogenes and inactivate tumor suppressor

genes. However, the genetic mutations are not evident until the mutant cell proliferates. *Proliferation* is a requirement for cancer development, and nonproliferating cells are unlikely to cause cancer. It has been suggested that several mutations may be necessary to achieve full malignancy. The development of colorectal cancer is a well-documented example of these sequential changes (Figure 7-14). Each individual cancer is likely to have its own unique combination of mutations that eventually lead to malignant behavior.

A number of etiologic agents are considered important initiators of cancer. The term *carcinogen* is applied to agents and substances capable of inducing cancer. Some carcinogens are complete carcinogens in that they are capable of the initiation of genetic damage as well as the promotion of cellular proliferation, whereas many others are only partial carcinogens. Partial carcinogens are often promoters that stimulate growth but are incapable of causing genetic mutations sufficient to initiate cancer by themselves. Examples of known carcinogens are ultraviolet and ionizing radiation, certain viruses, asbestos, and numerous chemicals. Most known chemical carcinogens are encountered through repeated occupational exposure (Box 7-1).

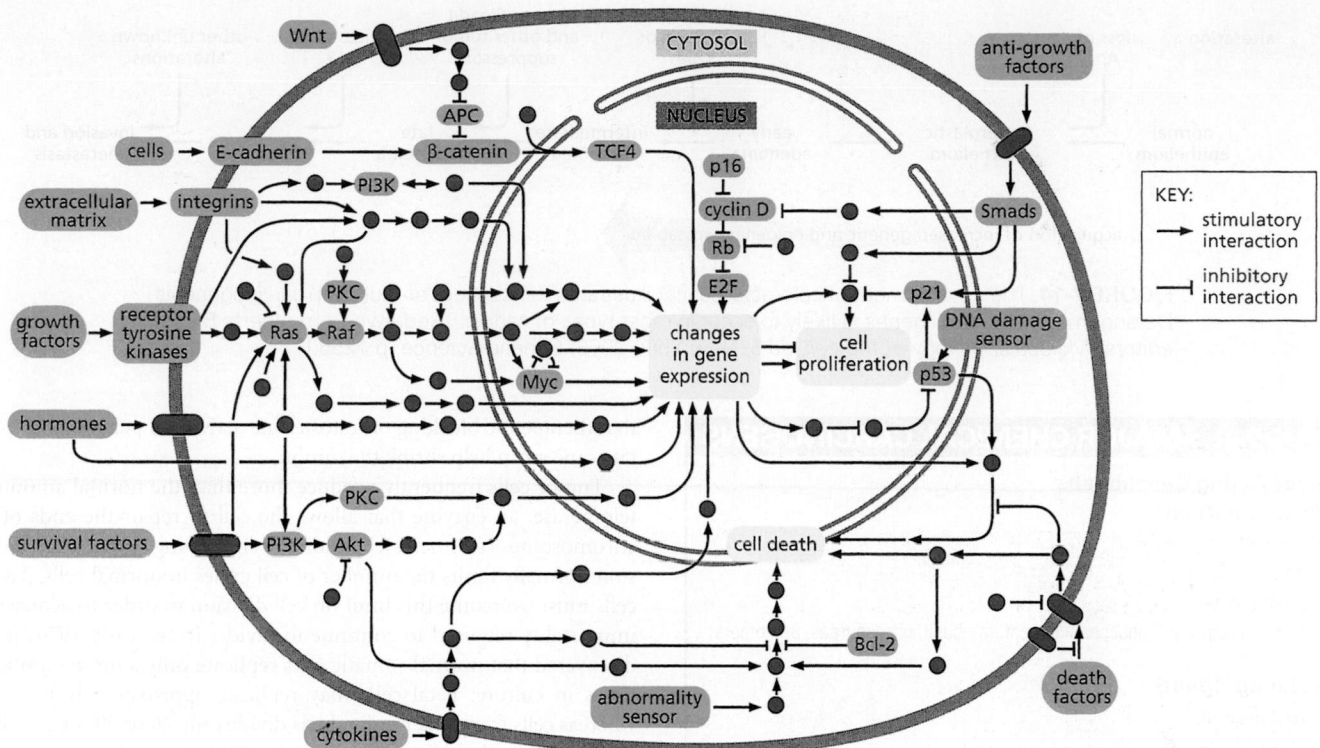

FIGURE 7-11 Diagram of the major signaling pathways relevant to human cancer. Overactivity of proto-oncogenes and underactivity of tumor suppressor genes result in enhanced cell proliferation and inhibition of appropriate cell death. More than 100 proto-oncogene products and numerous tumor suppressor gene products have been identified. (From Alberts B et al, editors: *Molecular biology of the cell,* ed 5, New York, 2008, Garland Science, p 1243.)

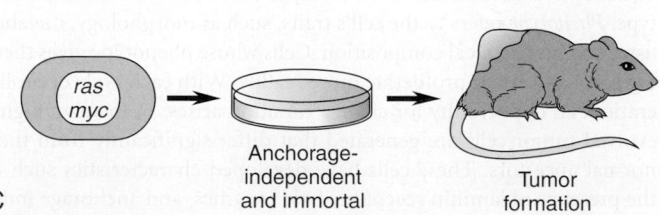

FIGURE 7-12 Synergy between oncogenes may be necessary to initiate malignant growth. **A,** The *ras* gene only. **B,** The *myc* gene only. **C,** Synergy between *ras* and *myc* genes.

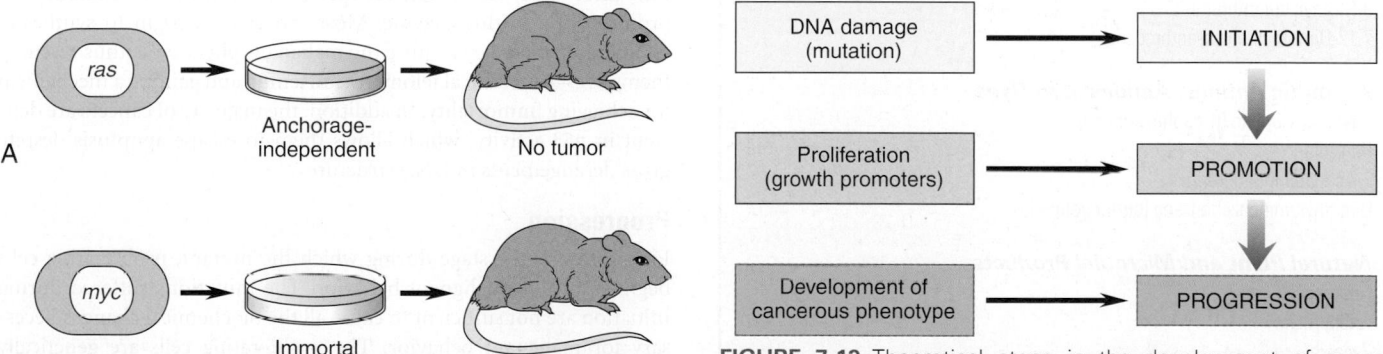

FIGURE 7-13 Theoretical steps in the development of cancer include initiation, promotion, and progression.

Promotion

Promotion is the stage during which the mutant cell proliferates. The transition from initiation to promotion may involve the activation of another oncogene or the inactivation of a tumor suppressor gene that

has kept proliferation in check. Nonmutating factors may also be important in promoting cellular proliferation. Nutritional factors and infection may provide a stimulus for cellular proliferation. As previously described, proliferation is regulated by numerous hormonal growth factors. It is not surprising, then, that hormones may act as promoters of certain types of cancer. The relationship between estrogen hormones and breast, ovarian, and uterine cancer is an important example. Epidemiologic studies indicate that the greater the number of menstrual cycles experienced, the higher the risk of these types of cancer developing. Women with early menarche, late first pregnancy, lack of breast feeding, and late menopause have a greater risk of developing breast, uterine, and ovarian cancer. This enhanced susceptibility is thought to occur in part because of the greater lifetime estrogen exposure. Estrogen is a trophic hormone for these tissues and may therefore be viewed as having promoter effects. Treatment protocols using antiestrogen agents

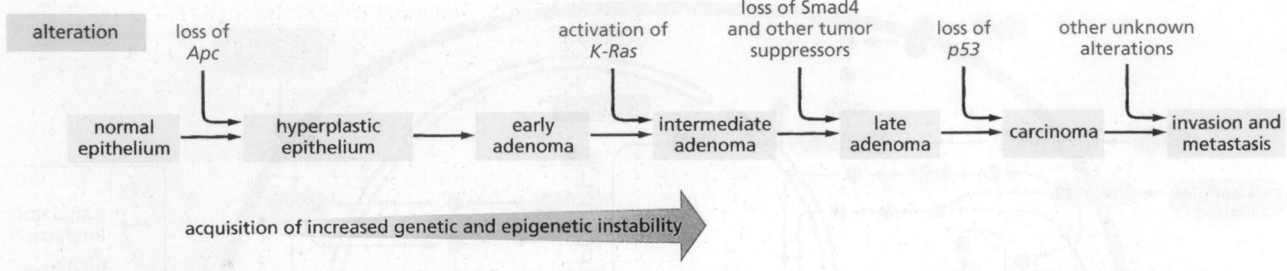

FIGURE 7-14 The development of colorectal cancer illustrates the concept of multistep carcinogenesis. Derangement of several genes is likely to occur in most types of cancer. (Redrawn from Alberts B et al, editors: *Molecular biology of the cell*, ed 5, New York, 2008, Garland Science, p 1255.)

BOX 7-1   MAJOR CHEMICAL CARCINOGENS

Direct-Acting Carcinogens
Alkylating Agents
β-Propiolactone
Dimethyl sulfate
Diepoxybutane
Anticancer drugs (cyclophosphamide, chlorambucil, nitrosoureas, and others)

Acylating Agents
1-Acetylimidazole
Dimethylcarbamoyl chloride

Procarcinogens That Require Metabolic Activation
Polycyclic and Heterocyclic Aromatic Hydrocarbons
Benz[*a*]anthracene
Benzo[*a*]pyrene
Dibenz[*a,h*]anthracene
3-Methylcholanthrene
7,12-Dimethylbenz[*a*]anthracene

Aromatic Amines, Amides, Azo Dyes
2-Naphthylamine (β-naphthylamine)
Benzidine
2-Acetylaminofluorene
Dimethylaminoazobenzene (butter yellow)

Natural Plant and Microbial Products
Aflatoxin B_1
Griseofulvin
Cycasin
Safrole
Betel nuts

Others
Nitrosamine and amides
Vinyl chloride, nickel, chromium
Insecticides, fungicides
Polychlorinated biphenyls

---

that therapeutic blocking of testosterone activity in persons with prostate cancer can help shrink the tumor.

Tumor cells frequently produce more than the normal amount of telomerase, an enzyme that allows the cell to repair the ends of the chromosomes (telomeres).[20] Telomere shortening with each cell division normally limits the number of cell cycles in normal cells. Tumor cells must overcome this limit on cell division in order to achieve the immortality required to continue to divide. In the early 1970s it was discovered that normal somatic cells replicate only a finite number of times in culture: Fetal cells may replicate approximately 80 times, whereas cells from older individuals divide only 20 or 30 times.[21] Each time a cell divides, it must replicate its DNA, but DNA polymerase is unable to copy the DNA strands all the way to the very tips of the chromosomes (called *telomeres*). The telomere thus shortens slightly with each cell division until some critical length is reached and cell division stops (see Chapter 4). Stem cells and germ cells produce an enzyme called *telomerase* that promotes synthesis of the telomere ends and permits these cell types to replicate indefinitely, but normal somatic cells produce little of this enzyme. Most cancer cells begin to synthesize telomerase while they acquire the malignant phenotype, thus rescuing themselves from critical telomere shortening and gaining a mechanism for achieving immortality. In addition, the majority of cancers are deficient in *p53* activity, which allows them to escape apoptosis despite gross derangements in DNA structure.

Progression

Progression is the stage during which the mutant, proliferating cells begin to exhibit malignant behavior. The mutations suffered during initiation are not sufficient to cause all the biochemical changes necessary for malignant behavior. The proliferating cells are genetically unstable and undergo chance mutations that give them a growth advantage. Clones of mutant cells exhibit a wide variation in phenotype. *Phenotype* refers to the cell's traits, such as morphology, metabolism, and biochemical composition. Cells whose phenotype gives them a growth advantage proliferate more readily. With each cycle of proliferation, an opportunity for chance variation arises. In the end, highly evolved tumor cells are generated that differ significantly from their normal ancestors. These cells have developed characteristics such as the presence of laminin receptors, lytic enzymes, and anchorage independence that enable them to behave malignantly.[1]

Cancer cells often have numerous abnormalities of chromosome structure, and the karyotype can be quite bizarre with bits and pieces of chromosomes attached in the wrong places and extra or missing chromosomes. An example of the chromosomes obtained from an ovarian cancer cell is shown in Figure 7-15. The color stains are specific for a particular chromosome, and each chromosome pair should be one color. Note the numerous multicolored chromosomes indicating multiple translocations of chromosome pieces.

(tamoxifen) indicate that breast cancer risk may be reduced by blocking the effects of estrogen.[18,19] However, estrogen is not considered to be carcinogenic and does not cause genetic mutations.

A similar relationship has been identified for prostate cancer and testosterone hormones. In males, testosterone is secreted primarily from the testes under the influence of pituitary gonadotropins. Testosterone is a growth factor for the prostate gland and can act as a promoter of tumor formation in this tissue. This relationship is supported by the fact

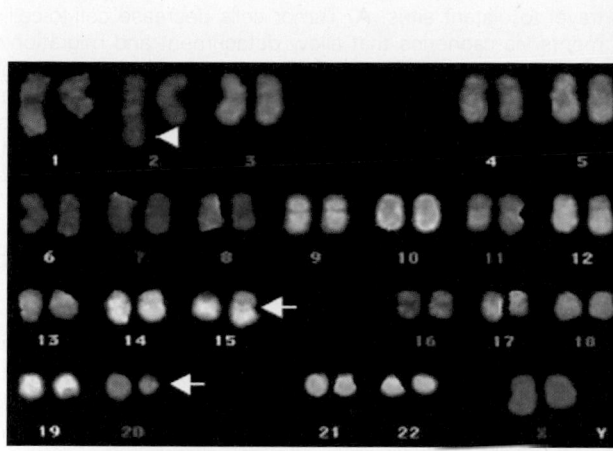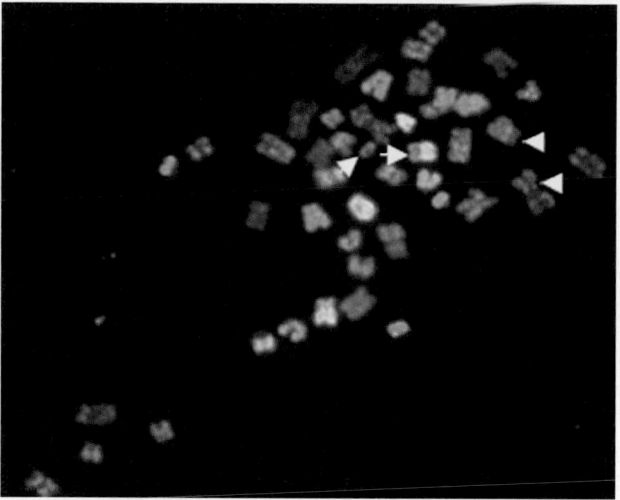

FIGURE 7-15 Fluorescent images from human ovarian cancer (CH1) cells. A representative karyotype of CH1 cell line shows the balanced *t*(15;20) chromosomes *(arrows)*. The size of one of the chromosomes 2 *(arrowhead)* is slightly bigger than normal, which contains a duplication. (From Xueying Mao et al: Subtle genomic alterations and genomic instability revealed in diploid cancer cell lines, *Cancer Lett* 267[1]:49-54, August 2008.)

The fact that conversion from a normal cell type to a malignant cell type requires multiple steps implies many opportunities to intervene in the process. Prevention of the initiating mutation may be difficult inasmuch as carcinogens are ubiquitous; however, therapies to prevent promotion and progression could render the initial mutation harmless. As the biochemical processes governing promotion and progression become clearer, strategies for blocking these stages continue to be developed.

> **KEY POINTS**
> - Full expression of cancer in a host is a multistep process. These steps have been described as initiation, promotion, and progression. The initiating event is usually from genetic mutations. Promotion refers to the stage in which the mutant cell is induced to proliferate. Progression is the stage during which the mutant, proliferating cells acquire properties that allow malignant behavior.
> - Malignant cells commonly produce telomerase, an enzyme that repairs the telomeres and may be a key for attaining immortality. The majority also have insufficient p53, which allows the tumor cells to escape apoptosis despite DNA damage.

METASTASIS

Metastasis is the process whereby cancer cells escape their tissue of origin and initiate new colonies of cancer in distant sites. For tumor cells to gain access to the blood or lymphatic circulation, they must first escape the basement membrane of the tissue of origin, move through the extracellular space, and penetrate the basement membrane of the vessel. This process is thought to involve loss of cell-to-cell adhesion and binding to matrix components such as laminin via specific laminin receptors on the tumor cell, followed by release of enzymes such as proteases and collagenases that digest the basement membrane.[22] The cancer cell then squeezes through the rift by ameboid movement. The process is repeated at the vessel basement membrane to access the blood or lymphatic vessel. When the cell reaches the tissue to be colonized, it must again traverse the basement membranes by using similar mechanisms (Figure 7-16). Once in a new tissue setting, the cancer cell colony must acquire nutrients and a blood supply and cope with an environment that may differ

considerably from its origin. In general, less differentiated cancer cells are better able to adapt to foreign tissues and survive.

Patterns of Spread

The survival of tumor cells in the circulation is not guaranteed. They may be detected by immune cells and destroyed, or they may undergo apoptosis unless they quickly find a matrix on which to adhere. Fewer than 1 in 10,000 of the cancer cells that enter the circulation survives to form a new tumor at a distant site.[22] Some tumor cell types appear to prefer specific target organs. Sometimes the pattern of metastasis is related to the circulatory flow. For example, metastatic tumors from the colon often seed the liver because they travel within the portal vein. The localization of most metastatic tumors is not so easily explained by blood flow patterns, and some tumor cells appear to "home" to specific targets. This homing tendency is poorly understood but may involve chemotactic signals from the organ to which the tumor cells respond. Cell surface receptors of the integrin and cell adhesion molecule families, which mediate cell-to-matrix and cell-to-cell adhesion, are likely to influence the choice of tissues that cancer cells invade. Dissemination via lymphatics is somewhat more predictable than distribution by blood flow. Generally, the lymph nodes that immediately drain the tissue of cancer origin are colonized first, and then the tumor cells tend to spread contiguously from node to node. Hodgkin disease, a lymphoma, is particularly noted for its orderly spread via the lymphatics.

Because tumor cells exhibit various degrees of differentiation or resemblance to the parent tissue of origin, it may be difficult to determine the metastatic cancer's tissue of origin. **Tumor markers** are substances associated with tumor cells that may be helpful in identifying their tissue type. Identification of the tissue of origin has important implications for prognosis and selection of treatment options. Tumor markers rely on the retention of at least some characteristics of the parent tissue type. Some tumor markers are released into the circulation, whereas others must be identified through biopsy of the metastatic tissue. Enzymes and other proteins that are specific to a particular cell type are commonly used as tumor markers. For example, production of thyroglobulin protein is specific for thyroid tumor cells. Melanoma cells express the antigens HMB-45 and S-100, which is helpful in identification as melanocytes. Unfortunately, most tumor markers are not very specific for cancer because the normal cells in the

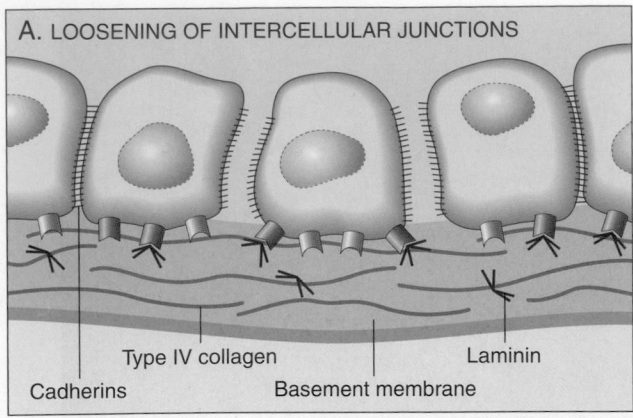

A. LOOSENING OF INTERCELLULAR JUNCTIONS

Type IV collagen
Laminin
Cadherins
Basement membrane

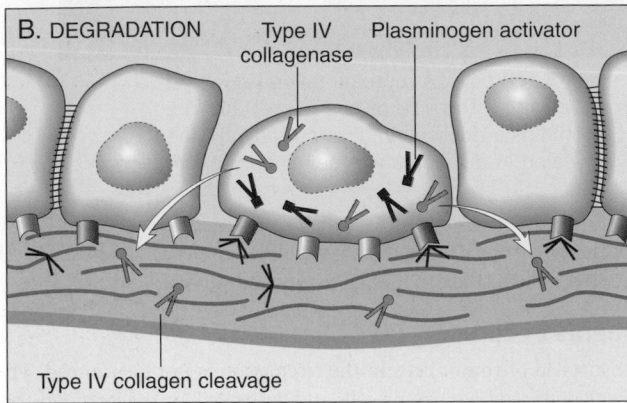

B. DEGRADATION
Type IV collagenase
Plasminogen activator

Type IV collagen cleavage

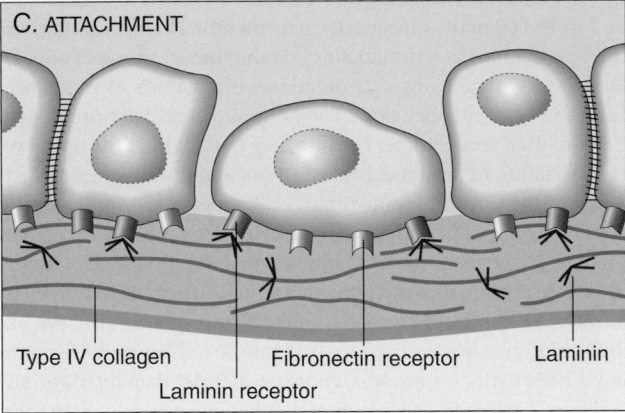

C. ATTACHMENT

Type IV collagen
Fibronectin receptor
Laminin
Laminin receptor

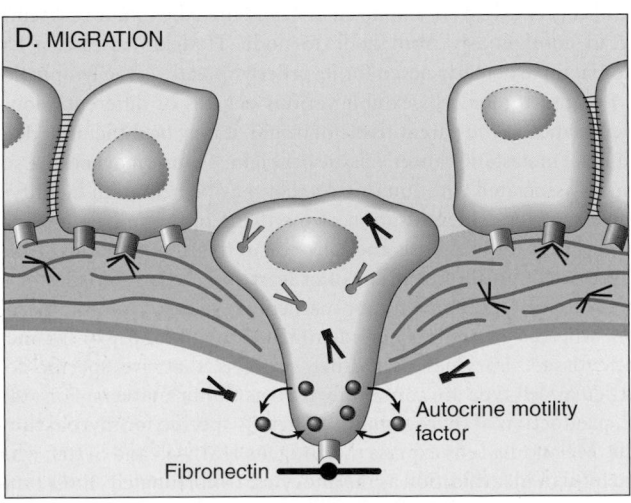

D. MIGRATION

Autocrine motility factor

Fibronectin

FIGURE 7-16 Mechanisms of tumor invasion allow tumor cells to escape the site of origin, penetrate the basement membrane, and travel to distant sites. **A,** Tumor cells decrease cell-to-cell attachments via cadherins that allow detachment and migration toward the basement membrane. **B,** Enzymes that degrade proteins are released into the area to form a rift. **C,** The tumor cell migrates away from the site of origin using laminin and fibronectin receptors to pull through the tissue. **D,** Finally the cell moves through a rift in the matrix. (From Kumar V et al: *Robbins and Cotran pathologic basis of disease,* ed 8, Philadelphia, 2010, Saunders, p 299.)

tissue of origin also produce them. Tumor markers are most useful as indicators for further diagnostic evaluation and to track the tumor activity. An increasing blood concentration of a specific tumor marker may indicate progression and proliferation of the cancer cells (increased tumor burden). See Table 7-6 for other examples of antigen, hormone, isoenzyme, and immunoglobulin markers used to identify tumor cell types.

TABLE 7-6 SELECTED TUMOR MARKERS

Hormones

Human chorionic gonadotropin	Trophoblastic tumors, nonseminomatous testicular tumors
Calcitonin	Medullary carcinoma of thyroid
Catecholamine and metabolites	Pheochromocytoma and related tumors
Ectopic hormones	Paraneoplastic syndromes

Oncofetal Antigens

α-Fetoprotein	Liver cell cancer, nonseminomatous germ cell tumors of testis
Carcinoembryonic antigen	Carcinomas of colon, pancreas, lung, stomach, and heart

Isoenzymes

Prostatic acid phosphatase	Prostate cancer
Neuron-specific enolase	Small cell cancer of lung, neuroblastoma

Specific Proteins

Immunoglobulins	Multiple myeloma and other gammopathies
Prostate-specific antigen and prostate-specific membrane antigen	Prostate cancer

Mucins and Other Glycoproteins

CA-125	Ovarian cancer
CA-19-9	Colon cancer, pancreatic cancer
CA-15-3	Breast cancer

New Molecular Markers

p53, APC, and RAS mutants in stool and serum	Colon cancer
p53 and RAS mutants in stool and serum	Pancreatic cancer
p53 and RAS mutants in sputum and serum	Lung cancer
p53 mutants in urine	Bladder cancer

Angiogenesis

Tumors cannot enlarge more than about 2 mm in diameter unless they grow blood vessels into the tumor mass to provide oxygen and nutrients. Angiogenesis is the process of forming new blood vessels. Most tumors do not induce angiogenesis until late in the stage of cancer development and so remain small and nonvascularized for years. The triggers that spur the cancer to begin angiogenesis are not completely understood. Tumor cells may begin to produce angiogenic factors such as vascular endothelial growth factor (VEGF) in response to hypoxia or other signals. VEGF stimulates proliferation of vascular endothelial cells, which then migrate to the tumor and orchestrate blood vessel development. Metastatic tumors must also initiate angiogenesis in their new locations or they will not survive. Therefore inhibition of angiogenesis is an important therapeutic goal to limit tumor growth and metastasis and continues to be an area of active research.

Grading and Staging of Tumors

Grading and staging of tumors are done to predict the clinical behavior of a malignant tumor and to guide therapy. **Grading** refers to the histologic characterization of tumor cells and is basically a determination of the degree of anaplasia. Most grading systems classify tumors into three or four classes of increasing degrees of malignancy. A greater degree of anaplasia indicates a greater malignant potential. The correlation between the grade of the tumor and its biological behavior is not perfect. Some low-grade tumors have proved to be quite malignant.

The choice of treatment modality is usually influenced more by the stage of the tumor than by its histologic grade. **Staging** describes the location and pattern of spread of a tumor within the host. Factors such as tumor size, extent of local growth, lymph node and organ involvement, and presence of distant metastases are considered. Several staging systems exist; however, the international TNM (*tumor, node, metastasis*) system is used extensively as a general framework for staging tumors.[23] Particular staging criteria vary with tumors in different organ systems. Examples of staging criteria for breast and colon cancer are shown in Tables 7-7 and 7-8.

In the past, tumor staging was based primarily on results of radiography and exploratory surgery. The availability of computed tomography (CT), magnetic resonance imaging (MRI), positron emission tomography (PET), and other highly sophisticated imaging techniques has revolutionized cancer detection. These imaging modalities allow noninvasive exploration of the tissues of the entire body. The computer-generated images can then be scrutinized for any signs of abnormality that might signal the presence of hidden tumors. CT and MRI rely primarily on detection of differences in tissue density and are therefore not totally specific for tumors. They can, however, guide the selection of sites for exploration and biopsy and potentially reduce unnecessary surgery. Positron emission tomography is a promising staging technology because it facilitates cancer detection based on molecular and biochemical processes within the tumor tissues (Figure 7-17). PET may be used in certain clinical situations in which CT has known limitations, such as differentiation of benign from malignant lymph nodes or other lesions, differentiation of residual tumor from scar tissue, or detection of unsuspected distant metastases.

Antibodies can also be used to locate cancer cells in the body. Antibodies can be raised against specific antigens present on the surface of tumor cells. The antibodies are also bound to a tracer (e.g., a radioactive isotope such as iodine-125), which can be detected by imaging. Because methods for identifying tumor antigens and raising specific antibodies have improved, this technology provides the potential for finding very small numbers of tumor cells hidden in the body.

The results of the staging procedure will determine which of the mainstays of cancer treatment—surgery, radiation therapy, or chemotherapy—may be used, singly or in combination, to destroy the cancer cells. Localized tumors may be managed with surgery and radiation therapy, whereas evidence of metastasis generally necessitates the addition of chemotherapy.

KEY POINTS

- Malignant cells produce specialized enzymes and receptors to enable them to escape their tissue of origin and metastasize.
- The spread of tumors generally occurs by way of the bloodstream or lymphatics. Tumor cells often lodge in the capillary beds of the organs that drain them, such as liver and lung. Some tumors appear to "home" to certain tissues.
- Grading and staging are done to predict tumor behavior and guide therapy. Grading is the histologic characterization of tumor cells, whereas staging describes the location and pattern of tumor spread within the host.
- The TNM staging system is used to describe the tumor size, lymph nodes affected, and degree of metastasis.

EFFECTS OF CANCER ON THE BODY

The effects of cancer on the host vary widely, depending on the location of the tumor and the extent of metastasis. Early-stage cancer may be asymptomatic. As the tumor increases in size and spreads through the body, a number of symptoms typically become apparent, including pain, cachexia, immune suppression, and infection. Once treatment has begun, patients may also suffer hair loss and sloughing of mucosal membranes. The American Cancer Society has published the seven warning signs of cancer as a way of encouraging the public to seek early evaluation of potential cancers (Box 7-2). The presentation of cancer in children differs from that in adults, and special warning signs have been identified for the pediatric population (Box 7-3).

Pain is a common and feared complication of the disease process. Pain may be due to invasion of metastatic cells into organs or bone and subsequent activation of pain and pressure receptors in these tissues. Tissue destruction and inflammation may contribute to cancer pain. Cancer treatment may contribute to overall pain because of procedures requiring biopsy and intravenous drug administration. Pain can usually be controlled through the use of analgesics. The use of patient-controlled analgesia has been effective in reducing patient fears of inadequate therapy for pain (see Chapter 47).

Cachexia refers to an overall weight loss and generalized weakness (Figure 7-18). Many factors contribute to cancer cachexia, including loss of appetite (anorexia) and increased metabolic rate. Anorexia accompanies many disease processes and may result from toxins released by the cancer cells or immune cells. Cancer patients may have aversions to specific foods and may feel full after only a few bites. Nausea and vomiting are common complications of cancer therapy and contribute to decreased nutrient intake. Despite the minimal nutrient intake, body metabolism remains high. Production of tumor necrosis factor (TNF) and other immune cytokines is thought to be important in producing the hypermetabolic state. Nutrients are mobilized from fat and protein stores in the body and consumed by the hypermetabolic cells (see Chapter 42). Some patients may require nutritional supplementation by enteral or parenteral routes.

Individuals with cancer often demonstrate deficits in immune system competence. Cancer cells secrete substances that suppress the immune system. Individuals with cancer may have reduced populations of T and B cells and may respond poorly to injected antigens. The mechanisms by which cancer cells depress immune responses are not well understood, but the prognosis for cancer recovery is poorer when the immune system is depressed. Immune cells, including cytotoxic T cells and natural killer (NK) cells, actively detect and destroy cancer cells.

TABLE 7-7 TNM STAGING CRITERIA FOR BREAST CANCER

Primary Tumor (T)

TX	Primary tumor cannot be assessed
T0	No evidence of primary tumor
Tis	Carcinoma in situ
Tis (DCIS)	Ductal carcinoma in situ
Tis (LCIS)	Lobular carcinoma in situ
Tis (Paget's)	Paget's disease of the nipple NOT associated with invasive carcinoma and/or carcinoma in situ (DCIS and/or LCIS) in the underlying breast parenchyma. Carcinomas in the breast parenchyma associated with Paget's disease are categorized based on the size and characteristics of the parenchymal disease, although the presence of Paget's should still be noted.
T1	Tumor ≤20 mm in greatest dimension
T1mi	Tumor ≤1 mm in greatest dimension
T1a	Tumor >1 mm but ≤5 mm in greatest dimension
T1b	Tumor >5 mm but ≤10 mm in greatest dimension
T1c	Tumor >10 mm but ≤20 mm in greatest dimension
T2	Tumor >20 mm but ≤50 mm in greatest dimension
T3	Tumor >50 mm in greatest dimension
T4	Tumor of any size with direct extension to chest wall and/or to skin (ulceration or skin nodules). **Note:** Invasion of dermis alone does not qualify as T4.
T4a	Extension to chest wall, not including only pectoralis muscle adherence/invasion
T4b	Ulceration and/or ipsilateral satellite nodules and/or edema (including peau d'orange) of the skin, which do not meet the criteria for inflammatory carcinoma
T4c	Both T4a and T4b
T4d	Inflammatory carcinoma

Lymph Node (N)

NX	Regional lymph nodes cannot be assessed (e.g., previously removed)
N0	No regional lymph node metastasis
N1	Metastasis to movable ipsilateral level I, II axillary lymph node(s)
N2	Metastasis in ipsilateral level I, II axillary lymph node(s) that are clinically fixed or matted; or in clinically detected ipsilateral internal mammary nodes in the *absence* of clinically evident axillary lymph node metastasis
N2a	Metastasis in ipsilateral axillary level I, II lymph nodes fixed to one another (matted) or to other structures
N2b	Metastasis only in clinically detected* ipsilateral internal mammary nodes and in the *absence* of clinically evident axillary lymph node metastasis
N3	Metastasis in ipsilateral infraclavicular (level III axillary) lymph node(s) with or without level I, II axillary lymph node involvement, or in clinically detected* ipsilateral internal mammary lymph node(s) with clinically evident level I, II axillary lymph node metastasis; or metastasis in ipsilateral supraclavicular lymph node(s) with or without axillary or internal mammary lymph node involvement
N3a	Metastasis in ipsilateral infraclavicular lymph node(s)
N3b	Metastasis in ipsilateral internal mammary lymph node(s) and axillary lymph node(s)
N3c	Metastasis in ipsilateral supraclavicular lymph node(s)

Distant Metastasis (M)

M0	No clinical or radiographic evidence of distant metastasis
cM0(i+)	No clinical or radiographic evidence of distant metastasis, but deposits of molecularly or microscopically detected tumor cells in circulating blood, bone marrow, or other nonregional nodal tissue that are no larger than 0.2 mm in a patient without symptoms or signs of metastasis
M1	Distant detectable metastasis as determined by classical clinical and radiographic means and/or histologically proven larger than 0.2 mm

Stage Grouping

Stage 0	Tis	N0	M0
Stage IA	T1	N0	M0
Stage IB	T0	N1mi	M0
	T1	N1mi	M0
Stage IIA	T0	N1	M0
	T1	N1	M0
	T2	N0	M0
Stage IIB	T2	N1	M0
	T3	N0	M0
Stage IIIA	T0	N2	M0
	T1	N2	M0
	T2	N2	M0
	T3	N1	M0
	T3	N2	M0

TABLE 7-7   TNM STAGING CRITERIA FOR BREAST CANCER—cont'd

Stage	T	N	M
Stage IIIB	T4	N0	M0
	T4	N1	M0
	T4	N2	M0
Stage IIIC	Any T	N3	M0
Stage IV	Any T	Any N	M1

From Edge SB, Byrd DR, Compton CC, Fritz AG, Greene FL et al, editors: *AJCC cancer staging handbook*, ed 7, New York, 2010, Springer-Verlag, pp 440-443.

Clinically detected is defined as detected by imaging studies (excluding lymphoscintigraphy) or by clinical examination and having characteristics highly suspicious for malignancy or a presumed pathologic macrometastasis based on fine needle aspiration biopsy with cytologic examination.

TABLE 7-8   TNM STAGING CRITERIA FOR COLON CANCER

Primary Tumor (T)

TX	Primary tumor cannot be assessed
T0	No evidence of primary tumor
Tis	Carcinoma in situ: intraepithelial or invasion of lamina propria
T1	Tumor invades submucosa
T2	Tumor invades muscularis propria
T3	Tumor invades through the muscularis propria into pericolorectal tissues
T4a	Tumor penetrates to the surface of the visceral peritoneum
T4b	Tumor directly invades or is adherent to other organs or structures

Regional Lymph Nodes (N)

NX	Regional lymph nodes cannot be assessed
N0	No regional lymph node metastasis
N1	Metastasis in 1-3 regional lymph nodes
N1a	Metastasis in one regional lymph node
N1b	Metastasis in 2-3 regional lymph nodes
N1c	Tumor deposit(s) in the subserosa, mesentery, or nonperitonealized pericolic or perirectal tissues without regional nodal metastasis
N2	Metastasis in 4 or more regional lymph nodes
N2a	Metastasis in 4-6 regional lymph nodes
N2b	Metastasis in 7 or more regional lymph nodes

Distant Metastasis (M)

M0	No distant metastasis
M1	Distant metastasis
M1a	Metastasis confined to one organ or site (e.g., liver, lung, ovary, nonregional node)
M1b	Metastasis in more than one organ/site or the peritoneum

Stage Grouping

Stage	T	N	M
Stage 0	Tis	N0	M0
Stage I	T1	N0	M0
	T2	N0	M0
Stage IIA	T3	N0	M0
Stage IIB	T4a	N0	M0
Stage IIC	T4b	N0	M0
Stage IIIA	T1-T2	N1/N1c	M0
	T1	N2a	M0
Stage IIIB	T3-T4a	N1/N1c	M0
	T2-T3	N2a	M0
	T1-T2	N2b	M0
Stage IIIC	T4a	N2a	M0
	T3-T4a	N2b	M0
	T4b	N1-N2	M0
Stage IVA	Any T	Any N	M1a
Stage IVB	Any T	Any N	M1b

From Edge SB, Byrd DR, Compton CC, Fritz AG, Greene FL et al, editors: *AJCC cancer staging handbook*, ed 7, New York, 2010, Springer-Verlag, pp 197-199.

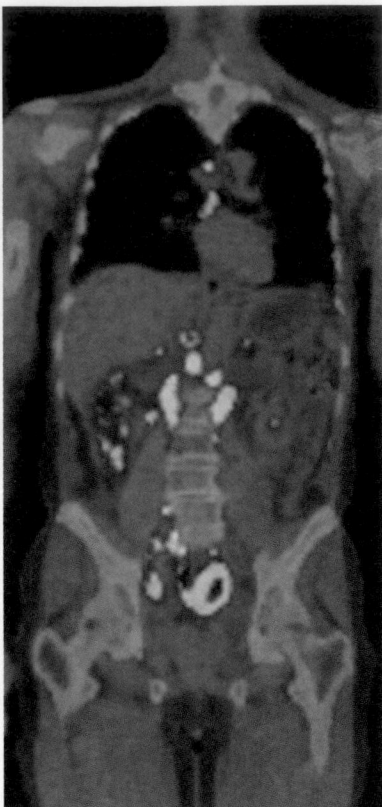

FIGURE 7-17 PET scan that detects uptake of radioactively labeled glucose is overlaid onto a CT scan background image. The yellow spots in the abdomen and mediastinum are indicative of multiple metastases of non-Hodgkin lymphoma. (From Alberts B et al, editors: *Molecular biology of the cell,* ed 5, New York, 2008, Garland Science, p 1206. Courtesy Dr. Sanjiv Sam Gambhir.)

In addition to the general immunodepressive effects of cancer, some cancer cells have developed ways to elude immune system detection.[24] For example, cancer cells can internalize their immuno-reactive cell surface antigens. Some tumors escape detection because they are coated with normal extracellular matrix molecules such as glycoproteins. The glycoproteins physically conceal the antigenic tumor markers.

Bone marrow suppression contributes to the anemia, leukopenia, and thrombocytopenia that often accompany cancer. Bone marrow suppression may be due to invasion and destruction of blood-forming cells in the bone marrow, poor nutrition, and chemotherapeutic drugs. *Anemia* refers to a deficiency in circulating red blood cells. In addition to decreased production of blood cell precursors in the bone marrow, anemia may result from chronic or acute bleeding. The signs and symptoms of anemia, such as fatigue, increased heart rate, and increased respiratory rate, are related to a decrease in oxygen-carrying capacity.

Leukopenia refers to a decrease in circulating white blood cells (leukocytes). Malignant invasion of the bone marrow is a primary cause of leukopenia, with malnutrition and chemotherapy being contributing factors. A deficiency in white blood cells reduces the patient's ability to fight infection, which is a major cause of morbidity and mortality in cancer patients. Often the offending organism is *opportunistic;* it is unable to infect an immunocompetent host and becomes virulent only when a person is immunocompromised. Infections are very difficult to manage because the host is unable to mount an effective immune response. Infections are also difficult to prevent because the majority

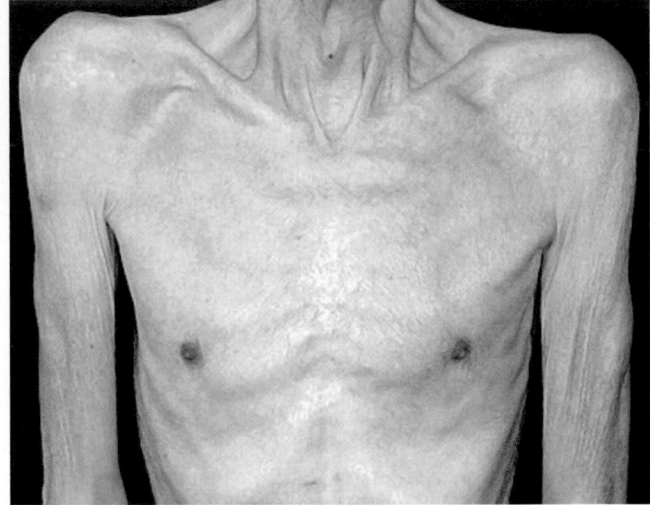

FIGURE 7-18 General emaciated appearance in cancer cachexia. (Courtesy Dr. P. Marazzi/Science Photo Library.)

of the infecting organisms are from the patient's own endogenous flora (e.g., skin, gastrointestinal tract). The development of severe leukopenia or infection during treatment may necessitate changes in the chemotherapeutic regimen to allow bone marrow recovery.

Thrombocytopenia is a deficiency in the number of circulating platelets, which are important mediators of blood clotting. Platelet deficiencies predispose to life-threatening hemorrhage. A platelet count of less than 20,000/mm^3 has been associated with spontaneous hemorrhage.

Anemia, leukopenia, and thrombocytopenia may be managed by administration of blood products containing red blood cells, white blood cells, and platelets, respectively. In fact, blood replacement therapy is used more often in cancer patients than in patients with any other medical condition. When chemotherapy is terminated, stem cells in the bone marrow generally recover and the production of blood cells resumes. In some cases, the production of red and white blood cells can be enhanced by treating the patient with specific growth factors, such as erythropoietin (Epogen) or granulocyte-stimulating factors (Neupogen).

Hair loss and the sloughing of mucosal membranes are complications of radiation therapy and chemotherapy. Treatment is designed to kill the rapidly proliferating cancer cells, but normal cells with high growth rates such as mucosal epithelia and hair follicle cells are also damaged. Damaged mucosa is a primary source of cancer pain and anorexia, and may provide a portal for the invasion of organisms from the skin or gastrointestinal tract.

Paraneoplastic syndromes are symptom complexes that cannot be explained by obvious tumor properties and occur in 10% to 15% of patients with cancer. Many of the syndromes are associated with excessive production of hormones or cytokines by the tumor. Common paraneoplastic syndromes include (1) hypercalcemia, (2) Cushing syndrome secondary to excess adrenocorticotropic hormone (ACTH) secretion, and (3) hyponatremia and water overload secondary to excess antidiuretic hormone (SIADH, syndrome of inappropriate ADH) secretion. Small cell carcinoma of the lung is commonly the culprit for excess ACTH and ADH syndromes. Hypercalcemia (elevated concentration of serum calcium) is a paraneoplastic syndrome associated with abnormal production of parathyroid hormone–related protein (PTHrP) by the tumor cells. Unexplained hypercalcemia is regarded as evidence of cancer until proven otherwise. Hypercalcemia may be a consequence of metastatic bone cancer, and in this case it would be an expected finding rather than a paraneoplastic syndrome.

If left untreated, cancer has the potential to kill the host. The cause of death is multifactorial. Infection, hemorrhage, and organ failure are the primary causes of cancer death. The failure of cancer-ridden organs such as the liver, kidney, brain, and lung results in the loss of life-sustaining functions. Treatment for cancer can also be detrimental to the host by contributing to immunosuppression and platelet deficiencies. The cumulative effects of one or more of these factors may lead to death.

KEY POINTS
- Regardless of the type of malignancy, affected individuals exhibit characteristic signs and symptoms, including pain, cachexia, bone marrow suppression, and infection.
- Bone marrow suppression is manifested as anemia, leukopenia, and thrombocytopenia.
- Immunosuppression with consequent infection is a primary cause of cancer-associated death.

CANCER THERAPY

The overall 5-year survival rate for patients with cancer is approximately 68%, with some types of cancer having much higher or lower rates.[3] Early detection of cancer, while it remains localized in the tissue of origin, is associated with the best prognosis for cure. Cure implies eradication of all cancer cells in the body and is different than the 5-year survival rate. Patients with metastatic invasion of regional lymph nodes still have a good opportunity for cure with appropriate therapy. Widespread invasion of multiple tissues and organs is associated with a poor prognosis, and therapy may be aimed at remission or palliation of symptoms rather than cure. The mainstays of cancer therapy are surgery, radiation therapy, and drug therapy. In some hormone-sensitive tumors (breast, prostate), hormonal blocking drugs may be used.

Immunotherapy and targeted molecular therapies have begun to emerge as important treatments for specific cancers. Traditional forms of treatment are not selective for cancer cells and result in unavoidable damage to normal tissue. The immune system, on the other hand, is noted for its ability to make subtle distinctions between normal and abnormal or foreign cells. Recognition of tumor cells as different from their normal counterparts is the basis of tumor immunology. Recognition depends on the expression of abnormal molecules or antigens on the cancer cell surface. Unfortunately, most tumor-associated antigens are also expressed to some degree on normal cells, which makes it difficult to develop strategies to target cancer cells selectively.

Transplantation of stem cells from the bone marrow or peripheral blood is an increasingly important aspect of cancer treatment for leukemia, lymphoma, and some solid tumors. The choice of treatment depends largely on the results of the staging procedure. A greater degree of metastasis generally requires a more aggressive therapeutic approach.

Surgery

The majority of patients with solid tumors are treated surgically, which can be curative in some localized cancers. The main benefit of surgery is removal of a tumor with minimal damage to other body cells. The surgeon generally removes a margin of normal-appearing tissue around the resected tumor to ensure complete tumor removal. Lymph nodes are subjected to biopsy and also removed if evidence of metastasis is present. Surgical resection of some tumors can be tricky if vital structures such as neurons or blood vessels are involved.

Surgery involves risks related to the effects of anesthesia, infection, and blood loss. The surgical procedure may be disfiguring or may result in loss of function. Surgical resection as the sole treatment for solid tumors is curative in a minority of patients because most patients already have undetectable metastases at the time of diagnosis.[25] Therefore, surgical resection is commonly accompanied by radiation therapy or chemotherapy. Even one remaining cancer cell could be sufficient to reinitiate tumor formation.

Radiation Therapy

Ionizing radiation is used for two principal reasons: to kill tumor cells that are not resectable because of location in a vital or inaccessible area and to kill tumor cells that may have escaped the surgeon's scalpel and remain undetected in the local area. Radiation kills cells by damaging their nuclear DNA. Cells that are rapidly cycling are more susceptible to radiation death because there is little time for DNA repair. Radiation may not kill cells directly; rather, it may initiate apoptosis. The *P53* tumor suppressor gene is an important mediator of this response. Many tumors have mutant *P53* and may be less susceptible to radiation-induced cell death.

It is difficult to kill all the cells of a large tumor by irradiation because they are heterogeneous—they are in different phases of mitosis and are cycling at different rates. A single radiation dose large enough to kill all the tumor cells would be sufficient to kill the normal cells as well. Radiation is often administered in smaller doses over several treatments and is most effective at eradicating small groups of tumor cells. It is often used in combination with surgery. Radiation is also useful for palliative reductions in tumor size. Pain from bone and brain tumors may be effectively managed with radiation therapy that shrinks the tumor. Tumors with bleeding surfaces may be coagulated with radiation to decrease blood loss.

A certain degree of destruction of normal cells in the irradiated field is expected with radiation therapy. Radiation is best used when tumor cells are regionally located. Total-body irradiation to kill tumor cells in disseminated locations is not recommended because of the likelihood of life-threatening tissue damage, although it may be used in preparation for bone marrow or peripheral stem cell transplantation.

Drug Therapy

Chemotherapy generally refers to the systemic administration of anti-cancer chemicals as treatment for cancers that are known or suspected to be disseminated in the body. Unlike surgery or radiation therapy, which is locally or regionally applied, parenterally administered chemotherapeutic drugs can find their cancer cell targets in areas throughout the entire body.

Most chemotherapeutic agents are cytotoxic because they interfere with some aspect of cell division. The more rapidly dividing cells are more susceptible to the killing effects of chemotherapeutic agents. In a large tumor mass, the rates of cell division are very diverse, with many slowly dividing cells. At any one time, only a portion of the tumor cells are in a cell cycle stage that is susceptible to chemotherapy. Several courses of chemotherapy are generally necessary to ensure that all tumor cells have been killed. It is difficult to kill slowly cycling tumor cells without also killing normal cells that are cycling at approximately the same rate. Small tumors are easier to eradicate because rates of cell division are generally faster. To prevent relapse, the "stem" cells that develop into clones of malignant cells must be destroyed. Unfortunately, stem cells may not divide as rapidly as other cells. Resection or irradiation to reduce tumor size may prompt the stem cells to divide, thus making them more susceptible to chemotherapy. Tumor cells with mutations of the *P53* gene may be resistant to chemotherapeutic agents that work by damaging DNA, so drugs that act by interfering with the cancer cell cycle in other ways may be more effective.

Chemotherapeutic agents are not selective for tumor cells, and a certain amount of normal cell death also occurs. Rapidly dividing cells, particularly those of the bone marrow, intestinal epithelia, and hair follicles, are most affected. Bone marrow depression is a most serious side effect inasmuch as it predisposes the patient to anemia, bleeding, and infection.

New approaches to cancer drug therapy have emerged that indirectly inhibit tumors rather than seeking to eradicate tumor cells directly. A promising approach is to interrupt the tumor's blood supply. To proliferate, solid tumors must be supplied by a progressively expanding network of capillaries. The development of new capillaries, called *angiogenesis,* is accomplished by migration and growth of endothelial cells. Antiangiogenic drugs block the development of new capillaries.

Immunotherapy

Harnessing the power of the immune system to fight cancer is a particularly appealing idea because of the potential for *specificity.* Current modes of immunomodulation primarily involve the use of interferons, interleukins, and monoclonal antibodies. These therapies are generally used as adjuncts to surgery, irradiation, and chemotherapy.

Interferons are glycoproteins produced by immune cells in response to viral infection. Interferons inhibit cell proliferation and are stimulatory to NK cells, T cells, and macrophages. Interferon-α has been used successfully to treat hairy cell leukemia (a rare B cell malignancy), chronic myelogenous leukemia, and multiple myeloma. Interferon therapy produces symptoms similar to those of a viral infection: fever, chills, and muscle aches.

Interleukins are peptides produced and secreted by white blood cells. They are also called lymphokines or cytokines. Interleukin-2 (IL-2) is an important cytokine secreted by activated T helper cells. It stimulates the proliferation of T cells, NK cells, and macrophages. IL-2 can be used to stimulate the growth of these immune cells in culture. Immune cells taken from a patient's blood can be grown in culture in the presence of IL-2. Then the greatly expanded number of immune cells can be given back to the patient, along with intravenous infusions of IL-2. Such treatment has been associated with regression of some tumors (melanoma, renal cell carcinoma). Because IL-2 toxicity is high

and many individuals have severe allergic reactions, the benefit of therapy must be weighed against the risks for each individual situation.

The use of monoclonal antibodies (antibodies having identical structure) in cancer therapy is currently the subject of intense investigation. Monoclonal antibodies specifically bind with target antigens and can therefore be used in several ways as treatment for cancer. Antibodies can be used to deliver a cytotoxic drug preferentially to the cancer cell and thus minimize drug interactions with normal cells. Similarly, antibodies can be used to direct other cytotoxic cells, such as NK and T cells, to tumor cells lurking in the body. Antibodies can be attached to a radioactive label and injected into a patient to screen for recurrence of tumor growth. Antibodies can also be directed against cells that support tumor growth.

Monoclonal antibodies have been developed for management of several cancers. For example, nearly 25% of breast cancers have overexpression of the HER2 receptor on the surface of malignant cells. The monoclonal antibody trastuzumab specifically binds to this HER2 protein and helps immune cells to find and kill the tumor cells. A summary of monoclonal antibody agents and their main tumor protein targets is shown in Figure 7-19.

Gene and Molecular Therapy

Because cancer is fundamentally a disorder of gene function, the use of gene therapy to alter the malignant behavior of cells may have high therapeutic potential.[26] As specific gene derangements are identified for particular tumors, gene therapy may be used to suppress overactive oncogenes or replenish missing tumor suppressor function. Current uses of gene therapy for cancer include genetic alteration of tumor cells to make them more susceptible to cytotoxic agents or immune recognition, and genetic alteration of immune cells to make them more efficient killers of tumor cells.

Tumor cells can also be made more recognizable to immune cells by insertion of genes that cause the tumor cells to express "foreign" proteins on their cell surface. This type of gene therapy has shown some benefit in melanoma and renal carcinoma. Replacement of genes for *P53* is an attractive therapy because tumor cells would be more susceptible to apoptosis. Gene replacement of other tumor suppressors such as *pRb* or *APC* in those tumors that are deficient could help inhibit tumor proliferation.

Gene therapy can be directed at cells other than tumor cells to enhance the body's cancer defenses. One such approach involves harvesting immune cells from the cancer patient, inserting IL-2 genes, and then returning the genetically enhanced immune cells to the patient. The enhanced immune cells attack the tumor cells more vigorously than normal immune cells do and have been shown to persist in the body for 6 months or longer.

At present, gene therapy is limited by difficulty in delivering the new genes to the target cells. As methods improve, gene therapy will become an increasingly important part of cancer prevention and management.

Molecular therapies that target cytoplasmic signaling pathways have also been developed. For example, in chronic myelogenous leukemia a chromosomal rearrangement results in the abnormal production of an enzyme, BCR/ABL. This enzyme stimulates cell proliferation and contributes to the overproduction of leukemic cells. An agent that specifically inhibits this enzyme (Gleevec) has dramatically improved the management of this disease. Other drugs that specifically target abnormal tumor products are under development.

Stem Cell Transplantation

Transplantation of hematologic stem cells is used to manage life-threatening disorders in which the patient's bone marrow is incapable of manufacturing white blood cells, red blood cells, or platelets. Most often, nonfunctional marrow is a consequence of the high-dose

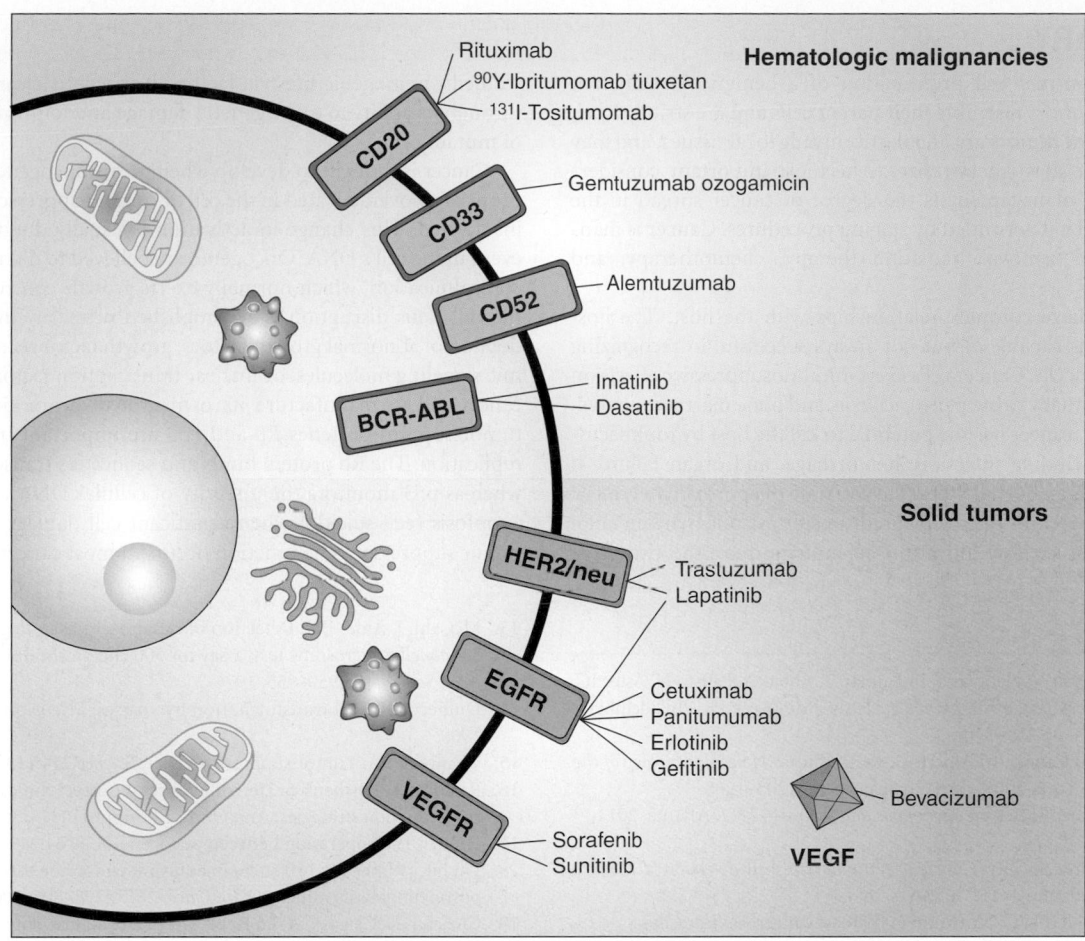

FIGURE 7-19 Cancer cells express abnormal antigens (tumor-associated antigens) on their cell surface that can activate immune cells or be used as targets for monoclonal antibodies. Numerous medications are now available that use monoclonal antibodies to target cellular proteins relevant to several different types of cancer.

chemotherapy and radiation used to manage hematologic malignancies such as leukemia and lymphoma. Stem cell transplantation also has been applied to other malignancies (e.g., breast cancer) and to nonmalignant disorders (e.g., aplastic anemia, sickle cell anemia, and thalassemia). Stem cells can be harvested from aspirates of bone marrow or from the donor's peripheral bloodstream. Bone marrow is rich in stem cells, but the peripheral blood is poor. The stem cell donor can be a tissue-matched individual (allogeneic), an identical twin (syngeneic), or the patient in question (autologous). A closer match between donor and recipient is associated with a better outcome.

Before infusion of donor stem cells, the patient's own immune cells must be suppressed to prevent transplant rejection. It is also necessary to eliminate any residual malignant cells from the body to avoid relapse of the cancer. Both of these objectives are accomplished through high-dose chemotherapy and total-body irradiation regimens, which leave the patient susceptible to severe anemia, infection, and bleeding. The therapeutic goal of stem cell transplantation is to restore immune and hematopoietic function. It may take weeks to months for the infused stem cells to reestablish themselves and begin to proliferate in their new host. During this time, the transplant recipient requires intensive monitoring and management of complications.

The success of stem cell transplantation depends on a number of factors, including the age of the patient, closeness of tissue matching, stage of cancer, and general health status of the patient before transplantation. Transplantation is an expensive undertaking but may significantly improve disease survival rates in some malignancies.[27]

KEY POINTS
- Early detection of cancer while it remains localized is associated with the best prognosis for cure. The overall 5-year survival rate for patients with cancer is about 68%.
- The mainstays of cancer therapy are surgery, radiation therapy, and chemotherapy. Surgery and radiation therapy are effective for cancers that are localized. Chemotherapy is usually the treatment of choice for cancers known or suspected to be disseminated in the body.
- Cells that divide rapidly are the most susceptible to damage from radiation therapy or chemotherapy. However, in addition to cancer cells, rapidly dividing normal cells may be killed. Cells of the bone marrow, hair follicles, and gastrointestinal mucosa are particularly susceptible.
- Immunotherapy has the potential to specifically target cancer cells. At present, interferon, IL-2, and numerous monoclonal antibodies are being used to boost the immune system's ability to locate and destroy cancer cells.
- Gene and molecular therapy may be used to alter cancer cells to suppress oncogenes, enhance tumor suppressor genes, make tumor cells more susceptible to cytotoxic agents, or interfere with the function of cancer gene products.
- Transplantation of hematopoietic stem cells is an important adjunct to cancer therapy that provides a method to restore bone marrow function after high-dose irradiation or chemotherapy.

SUMMARY

Neoplasia is abnormal cell proliferation of a benign or malignant nature. Benign tumors resemble their parent cells and are strictly local, whereas malignant tumors are anaplastic, invade local tissues, and may spread to distant sites (metastasize). The most important consideration for cancer management is the degree of cancer spread in the body, which can be determined by staging procedures. Cancer is managed by surgical removal, radiation therapy, chemotherapy, and immunotherapy.

Cancer cells have complex relationships with the host. The host immune system is capable of but not always successful in recognizing and killing cancer cells. Cancer cells exert immunosuppressive effects on the host and eventually cause pain, cachexia, and bone marrow suppression. If untreated, cancer has the potential to kill the host by multifactorial processes, including infection, hemorrhage, and organ failure. If treated, cancer has an overall 5-year survival rate of approximately 68%.

Cancer is an outcome of genetic predispositions and environmental carcinogens. Tobacco use and improper nutrition are the two most studied carcinogenic lifestyle factors. Tobacco is clearly carcinogenic through its ability to cause genetic damage and to promote the growth of mutant cells.

Cancer is thought to develop when proto-oncogenes become inappropriately overactivated in the cell or tumor suppressor genes become inactivated. This change in activation is usually due to a mutational event in the cell's DNA. Oncogenes are believed to disrupt intercellular communication, which normally exerts growth-controlling effects on the cell. This disruption is accomplished primarily through the production of abnormal growth factors, growth factor receptors, cytoplasmic signaling molecules, or nuclear transcription factors that allow the cancer cell to manufacture its own growth-promoting signals. The tumor suppressor genes *Rb* and *P53* are important inhibitors of cell replication. The Rb protein binds and sequesters transcription factors, whereas p53 monitors the integrity of cellular DNA and may initiate apoptosis (cell suicide) when significant cell damage occurs. Loss of tumor suppressor gene function occurs in most cancers.

REFERENCES

1. Stricker T, Kumar V: Neoplasia. In Kumar V, Abbas A, Fausto N, Aster JC, editors: *Robbins and Cotran pathologic basis of disease*, ed 8, Philadelphia, 2010, Saunders, pp 259–330.
2. Alberts B, et al: Cancer. In Alberts B, et al, editors: *Molecular biology of the cell*, ed 5, New York, 2008, Garland Science, pp 1205–1268.
3. American Cancer Society: *Cancer facts and figures—2011*, Atlanta, 2011, Author.
4. American Cancer Society: *Cancer prevention and early detection facts & figures 2011*, Atlanta, 2011, Author.
5. Hunter DJ, Willett WC: Nutrition and breast cancer, *Cancer Causes Control* 7(1):56–68, 1996.
6. Prentice RL, et al: Low-fat dietary pattern and risk of invasive breast cancer: the Women's Health Initiative Randomized Controlled Dietary Modification Trial, *JAMA* 295(6):629–642, 2006.
7. Burkitt DP, Walker ARP, Painter NS: Dietary fiber and disease, *JAMA* 229:1068–1074, 1974.
8. Rock CL: Primary dietary prevention: is the fiber story over? *Recent Results Cancer Res* 174:171–177, 2007.
9. McTiernan A: Behavioral risk factors in breast cancer: can risk be modified? *Oncologist* 8:326–334, 2003.
10. Goodman M, Bostick RM, Kucuk O, Jones DP: Clinical trials of antioxidants as cancer prevention agents: past, present, and future, *Free Radic Biol Med* 51(5):1068–1084, 2011.
11. Omenn GS, et al: Risk factors for lung cancer and for intervention effects in CARET, the Beta-Carotene and Retinol Efficacy Trial, *J Natl Cancer Inst* 88(21):1550–1559, 1996.
12. Albanes D, et al: Effects of Alpha-Tocopherol Beta-Carotene Cancer Prevention Study, *Am J Clin Nutr* 61:S1427–S1430, 1995.
13. McCann J, Ames BN: Detection of carcinogens as mutagens in the *Salmonella*/microsome test: assay for 300 chemicals: discussion, *Proc Natl Acad Sci USA* 73:950–955, 1976.
14. Dulbecco R: Cell transformation by viruses, *Science* 166:962–968, 1969.
15. Weinberg RA: Tumor suppressor genes, *Science* 254:1138–1146, 1991.
16. Paradiso A, Formenti S: Hereditary breast cancer: clinical features and risk reduction strategies, *Ann Oncol* 22(Suppl 1):I31–I36, 2011.
17. Hunter T: Cooperation between oncogenes, *Cell* 64:249–270, 1991.
18. Lin NU, Winer EP: Advances in adjuvant endocrine therapy for postmenopausal women, *J Clin Oncol* 26(5):798–805, 2008.
19. Cuzick J, DeCensi A, Arun B, Brown PH, et al: Preventive therapy for breast cancer: a consensus statement, *Lancet Oncol* 12(5):496–503, 2011.
20. Xu Y, He K, Goldkorn A: Telomerase targeted therapy in cancer and cancer stem cells, *Clin Adv Hematol Oncol* 9(6):442–455, 2011.
21. Hayflick L: The biology of human aging, *Adv Pathobiol* 7(2):80–99, 1980.
22. Cairns RA, Khokha R, Hill RP: Molecular mechanisms of tumor invasion and metastasis: an integrated view, *Curr Mol Med* 3(7):659–671, 2003.
23. Edge SB, Byrd DR, Compton CC, Fritz AG, Greene FL, et al, editors: *AJCC cancer staging manual*, ed 7, New York, 2010, Springer-Verlag.
24. Steidl C, Shah SP, Woolcock BW, Rui L, Kawahara M, et al: MHC class II transactivator CIITA is a recurrent gene fusion partner in lymphoid cancers, *Nature* 471(7338):377–381, 2011.
25. Coffey JC, et al: Excisional surgery for cancer cure: therapy at a cost, *Lancet Oncol* 4(12):760–768, 2003.
26. Fukazawa T, Matsuoka J, Yamatsuji T, Maeda Y, Durbin ML, et al: Adenovirus-mediated cancer gene therapy and virotherapy (Review), *Int J Mol Med* 25(1):3–10, 2010.
27. Breems DA, Löwenberg B: Acute myeloid leukemia and the position of autologous stem cell transplantation, *Semin Hematol* 44(4):259–266, 2007.

Infectious Processes

Dawn F. Rondeau

ⓔvolve WEBSITE

http://evolve.elsevier.com/Copstead/

- Review Questions and Answers
- Glossary (with audio pronunciations for selected terms)
- Animations

- Case Studies
- Key Points Review

KEY QUESTIONS

- What is the role of epidemiology in the identification, definition, and prevention of infectious diseases?
- What factors influence the transmission of infectious agents?
- How do infectious microorganisms, including bacteria, viruses, fungi, and parasites, differ in structure, life cycle, and infectious processes?

- What conditions compromise host defenses against microorganisms?
- What are opportunistic infections, and when do they develop?

CHAPTER OUTLINE

Infectious diseases can be caused by bacteria, viruses, fungi, and animal- or insect-borne parasites that enter the body by penetrating natural barriers. Viruses are the single most common cause of infectious diseases worldwide.[1] Although treatments are available for many of these diseases, development of resistant strains complicates successful treatment in some cases.

A variety of pathogens inhabit different environments such as hospitals, the food supply, water, animals, and humans. For example,

many hospitalized patients are at risk for the development of sepsis, an overwhelming infection that may lead to shock, multiple organ failure, and death. The methods for preserving the food supply have an impact on transmission of infections, as do the location, density, and sanitary practices of a population. Globalization of the world's population, with the associated rapidity and extent of air travel, has major implications for the worldwide spread of infectious agents before the infected individual becomes symptomatic or identifiable.

Infection with pathogenic microorganisms has become a tool of war and terrorism in the world. Whether it is anthrax spores sent through the mail or the threat of smallpox being introduced into an unimmunized population, methods of preventing infection have a key role in the defense of humanity.

Medications that inhibit the immune response in populations such as transplant or cancer patients, and the use of immunomodulators for treatment of diseases like rheumatoid arthritis, increase the likelihood of **opportunistic** infections. Excessive use of antibiotics in humans and domesticated animals has contributed to the emergence of treatment-resistant infections. Health care professionals have a vital role in the prevention, early detection, and management of infections.

EPIDEMIOLOGIC CONCEPTS

Epidemiology is the study of the causes, distribution, and control of disease in populations. Epidemiology evaluates where, when, and to whom a health event happens and quantifies the risk associated with a particular event.[2] The risk to a population for development of disease varies with the population. For example, in a low-income population the risks are related to poor water supply, poor sanitation, and inadequate nutrition. In affluent populations the risks of decreased physical activity, increased body fat, and poor urban air quality are more important[3] (Figure 8-1). Epidemiology is discussed in more detail in Chapter 1.

One of the first attempts to identify the cause of an infection and develop a method to prevent it was conducted by Benjamin Jesty in England in the mid-1700s. He noticed that milkmaids who developed cowpox from working with cows did not develop smallpox disease. He deduced that there was a connection between cowpox and smallpox. He exposed his wife and children to cowpox to protect them from smallpox and provided an example of the successful use of epidemiological principles and inoculation to prevent disease.[4]

Jesty also performed basic statistical analyses of the numbers of people who developed infections and the numbers who did not, using the concepts of prevalence and incidence. The prevalence of a disease is the number of people who have that disease during a year (e.g., the number of people living with human immunodeficiency virus [HIV] infection). The number of people who develop a new infection in a year is the incidence. The number of new cases within a given population is the incidence rate (e.g., 10 cases per 1000 persons).[5] A variety of other statistics can be used for surveillance, monitoring, and investigation of outbreaks.[6]

An infectious disease that has a fairly constant presence in a community and changes little from year to year, such as the sexually transmitted disease *Chlamydia*, is classified as **endemic.** A significant increase in new infections in a certain population, such as a measles outbreak at a university, is termed an epidemic. An epidemic that has spread to a large geographic area is a **pandemic.** The bubonic plague, which caused 100 million deaths worldwide in the 1300s, was a pandemic.

The study of infectious diseases requires the evaluation of many factors to determine the association of a disease with its cause. The United States Centers for Disease Control and Prevention (CDC) and the World Health Organization (WHO) have pivotal roles in identifying diseases, tracking their natural history, and defining protocols for their control and prevention. An example of how these organizations can control disease is the virtual eradication of smallpox. The World Health Organization, with the cooperation of other health organizations such as the Centers for Disease Control and Prevention, mandated immunizations for all those susceptible to the disease that were living in or traveling to areas where smallpox was prevalent. This immunization program, coupled with the lack of a viral host other than humans, led to the eradication of smallpox, except in the laboratory. Only the fear of the reintroduction of the virus into the population in a bioterrorism attack or biological warfare may mandate the continued immunization of susceptible populations such as health care workers, emergency personnel, and the military.

Transmission of Infection

The transmission of infection or disease requires an unbroken chain of events to enable one host to infect another[7] (Figure 8-2). Disease-causing organisms (**pathogens**) must live and reproduce in a reservoir. The reservoir may be a human, as in the influenza virus; an animal, as in rabies; an insect, as in West Nile virus; or soil, as in enterobiasis (pinworm infestation).

The **pathogen** must have a portal of exit and a mode of transmission from the reservoir to a susceptible host. The portal of exit

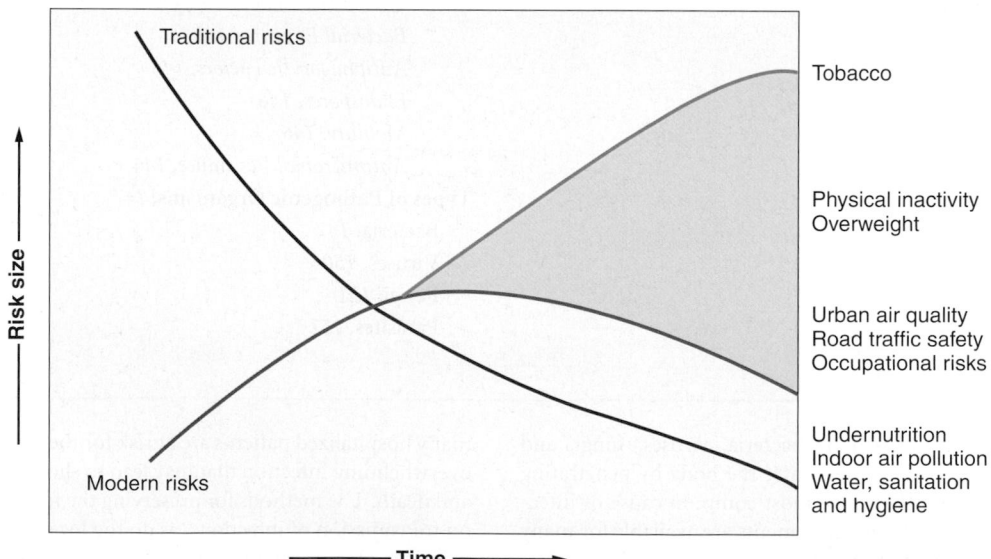

FIGURE 8-1 Traditional risks to a population compared to modern risks. (From World Health Organization: *Global health risks: mortality and burden of disease attributable to selected major risks,* 2009, available at www.who.int/healthinfo/global_burden_disease/GlobalHealthRisks_report_full.pdf.)

is usually closest to the breeding site of the organism. For example, *Neisseria gonorrhoeae,* the organism that is responsible for gonorrhea, usually resides in the urethra of an infected male and in the vaginal canal of an infected female. The microorganism is transmitted to others by sexual contact.

Control of disease acquisition depends on breaking the chain of transmission in one or more places[8] (Figure 8-3). A pathogen can be vulnerable in one or more links of the transmission chain. The goal of epidemiology is to identify these vulnerabilities and exploit them to stop disease transmission.

The ability of a pathogen to cause disease is influenced by the ability to communicate the infection, in other words the ability to spread and cause the disease. The ability to invade and multiply within the host is termed infectivity. Some pathogens have a greater ability to spread and multiply in the host, increasing their infectivity. This difference in the mechanism of action can make one pathogen much better at causing disease (pathogenicity) and some can cause very severe disease (virulence). The ability to cause disease is also influenced by the access to a host. For example, respiratory diseases caused only by exposure to droplets are much more easily transmitted than a disease that requires direct contact. Some pathogens produce toxins or endotoxins that can markedly increase the toxigenicity of the organism.[9]

Transmission of infection is defined as any mechanism by which an infectious agent is spread through the environment to another person.[7] These mechanisms can be either direct or indirect. There are three direct transmissions. The most common transmission occurs through the exchange of body fluids (droplets) from kissing or sexual intercourse. In this type of transmission droplets are spread from an infected host to the conjunctiva or mucous membranes of a second host. The second type of direct transmission occurs from the bite of an animal (e.g., rabies) or from soil (e.g., systemic mycosis) transmitting the inoculant. The third type of direct transmission occurs through the placenta when diseases such as HIV are transmitted directly to the fetus.[6]

Indirect transmissions occur as vehicle-borne, vector-borne, or airborne transfers. A vehicle-borne transfer occurs when an infectious agent is transported to the host. The vehicle could be food, water, clothing, plasma, or tissues. The agent does not require any development or multiplication and is delivered without change with the vehicle. Airborne transmission occurs with aerosols including suspensions of particles (smaller than the size of droplets), which can be carried great distances from the source for transmission. Examples are outbreaks of measles and legionnaires disease. Vector-borne transmission can occur as a mechanical or biological transfer. The mechanical transfer occurs when an insect carries an infectious agent on its feet or proboscis (Figure 8-4). In this transfer the agent does not require multiplication or development before transfer. This is in contrast to biological vector-borne transport. In this type of transmission the agent propagates and there is cyclic development before the arthropod can transmit the disease.[6]

The human body also contains a variety of microorganisms that colonize the body and are called normal flora. These flora occur naturally and have a role in defense by occupying space, competing for nutrients, stimulating cross-protective antibodies, and reducing or containing the growth of potentially disease-causing bacteria or fungi. These organisms can become pathogens and cause disease if the host defenses are altered, as in the case of patients receiving chemotherapy. For example, *Staphylococcus epidermidis* is commonly present on the skin. With an injury to the skin, or injection through the skin, this

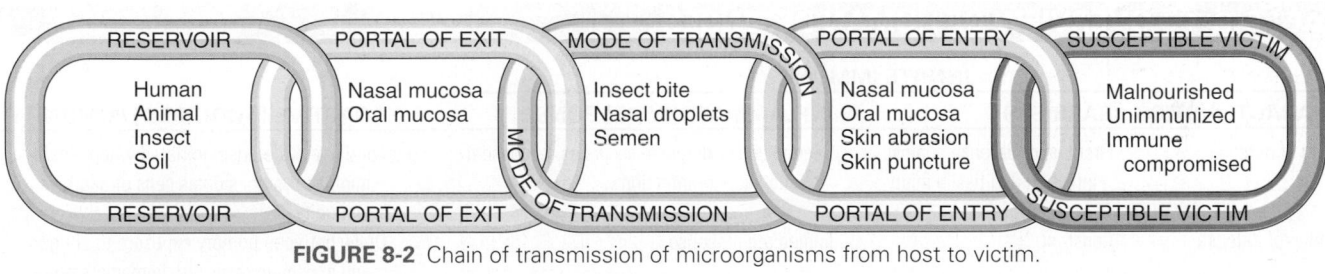

FIGURE 8-2 Chain of transmission of microorganisms from host to victim.

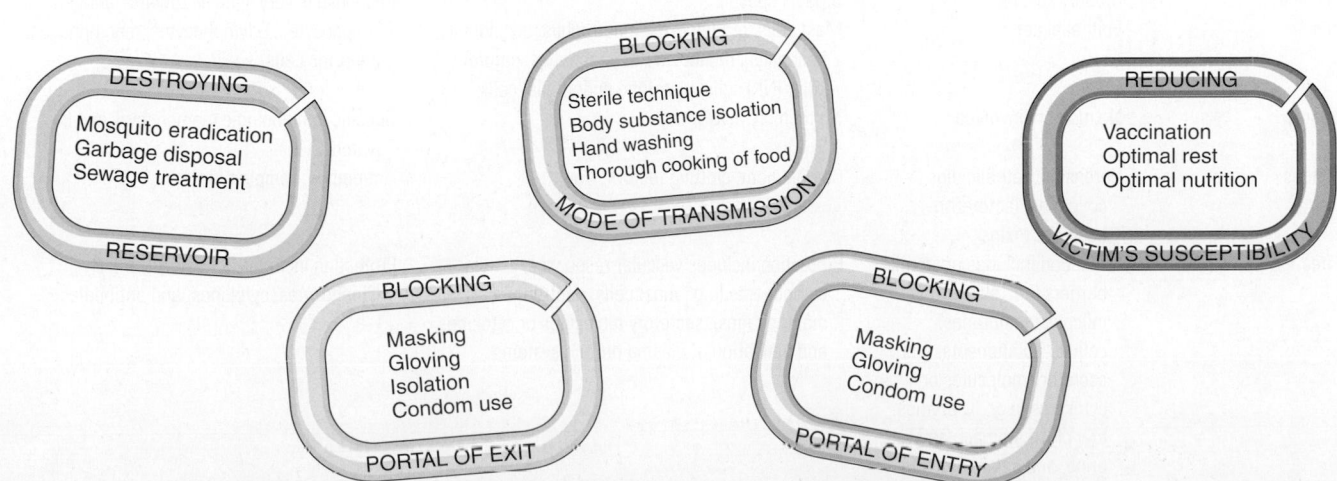

FIGURE 8-3 Breaking the chain of transmission of microorganisms from host to victim.

normal bacterial flora can be introduced to a different space in the body and then become an infectious agent.[10]

Destroying nonhuman reservoirs and vectors of the pathogen can break the chain of transmission. For example, controlling the number of mosquitoes with insecticides and other biological means is a method used to curb the spread of malaria and West Nile virus. Immunization of domesticated animals against rabies eliminates one reservoir of potential rabies transmission. Distribution of clean needles in the intravenous drug user community is aimed at removing a common transmission vector (contaminated needles) for HIV, the causative pathogen responsible for acquired immunodeficiency syndrome (AIDS).

Blocking the portal of exit can also block transmission of the pathogen. Having patients with tuberculosis wear face masks while they move through the hospital and implementing respiratory isolation techniques to stop transmission are interventions aimed at blocking the portal of exit. Standard precautions are infection-control guidelines designed to block the pathogen's portal of exit, route of transmission, and portal of entry.[2] Hand washing is one of the most effective ways to break the chain of transmission by blocking an important mode of transmission—contaminated hands. Many factors influence the risk of exposure to foreign materials and the occurrence of infection (Table 8-1).

Role of Host

The body's defense system is responsible for identifying foreign materials and neutralizing or eliminating them without injuring its own tissues.[6] Responses to a pathogen can be either innate or specific. Innate responses occur on the initial exposure to the antigen, whereas a specific response is slow to develop and more efficient on subsequent exposures. Immune responses can be modified by the characteristics of the host, including genetics, age, metabolism, anatomic, and physiologic and environmental factors[6,11] (Table 8-2). Host immune systems are discussed in greater detail in Chapter 9.

Host Characteristics
Physical and Mechanical Barriers

Intact physical barriers act as a blockade to foreign material entering the body (Figure 8-5). Epithelial cells of the skin and those that line the gastrointestinal, genitourinary, and respiratory tracts are tightly linked and provide an initial barrier to infection. Because the intestinal epithelial cell half-life is 30 hours, the constant shedding of the epidermis and mucosal membranes aids in the removal of any microorganisms that

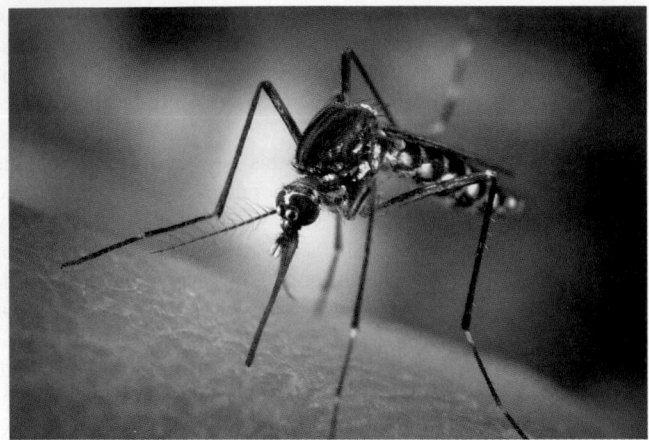

FIGURE 8-4 A female *aedes aegypti* mosquito as it breaks the surface of the host. (Courtesy James Gathany, Centers for Disease Control and Prevention, Atlanta.)

TABLE 8-1   OVERVIEW OF HUMAN DEFENSES

CHARACTERISTICS	INNATE IMMUNITY		ADAPTIVE (ACQUIRED) IMMUNITY
	BARRIERS	INFLAMMATORY RESPONSE	
Level of defense	First line of defense against infection and tissue injury	Second line of defense; occurs as response to tissue injury or infection	Third line of defense; initiated when innate immune system signals cells of adaptive immunity
Timing of defense	Constant	Immediate response	Delay between primary exposure to antigen and maximum response; immediate against secondary exposure to antigen
Specificity	Broadly specific	Broadly specific	Response is very specific toward "antigen"
Cells	Epithelial cells	Mast cells, granulocytes (neutrophils, eosinophils, basophils), monocytes/macrophages, natural killer (NK) cells, platelets, endothelial cells	T lymphocytes, B lymphocytes, macrophages, dendritic cells
Memory	No memory involved	No memory involved	Specific immunologic memory by T and B lymphocytes
Peptides	Defensins, cathelicidins, collectins, lactoferrin, bacterial toxins	Complement, clotting factors, kinins	Antibodies, complement
Protection	Protection includes anatomic barriers (i.e., skin and mucous membranes), cellular components, and secretory molecules or cytokines (e.g., lysozymes, low pH of stomach and urine, and ciliary activity)	Protection includes vascular responses, cellular components (e.g., mast cells, neutrophils, macrophages), secretory molecules or cytokines, and activation of plasma protein systems	Protection includes activated T and B lymphocytes, cytokines, and antibodies

From McCance K, Huether S: *Pathophysiology: the biologic basis for disease in adults & children,* ed 6, St Louis, 2010, Mosby.

are attached to their surfaces.[9] In addition, the high fat content of the skin inhibits the growth of bacteria and fungi. Changes in this barrier are sometimes the route for normal flora to become infectious.[12]

The mucous membrane linings of the gastrointestinal and genitourinary tracts provide a barrier separating the sterile internal body from the external environment. The lungs are protected with a layer of mucous lining. The sticky consistency of mucus traps microorganisms, and the cilia sweep the microorganisms from the body. The mucociliary system and alveolar macrophages are important for ridding the lungs of trapped microorganisms. Mechanisms such as coughing, sneezing, and urinating help to remove particles trapped on mucous membranes of the body.[9]

Biochemical barriers enhance the effectiveness of the mechanical barriers. The acidic environment of the skin, urine, and vagina inhibits bacterial growth. The secretion by the stomach of hydrochloric acid (with a pH of 1 to 2) results in the killing of microorganisms. Saliva, mucus, tears, and sweat contain antimicrobial chemicals such as lysozyme, an enzyme that destroys cell walls of gram-positive bacteria.[9] Lactoferrin is a

mucosal protein that keeps bacterial replication low by reducing the availability of free iron needed for bacterial growth. Sebaceous gland secretions act as antifungals. Immunoglobulins (immunoglobulin A [IgA], immunoglobulin G [IgG]) are present in many of the body's secretions and prevent entry of bacteria and viruses through mucous membranes.[13] (See Chapter 9 for a discussion about immunoglobulins.)

Removal or degradation of the body's mechanical and biochemical barriers creates a setting in which infection is likely. For example, burn victims who have lost portions of their skin barrier are at high risk for infection. Cellular changes induced by smoking reduce the number of cilia in the respiratory tract. The normal action of cilia in the respiratory tract in removing foreign particles is blocked by endotracheal tubes. Hospitalized patients who have incisions or intravenous and urinary catheters are at risk for infection because their skin barrier has been breached. When a urinary catheter is in place, flushing of bacteria from the urinary tract opening (meatus) is bypassed.

Risk Factors

Nutritional status. The World Health Organization (WHO) reports that inadequate nutrition is a general risk factor for disease and is a particularly important factor in tuberculosis (TB) infection.[14] Protein-energy malnutrition is associated with defects in cell-mediated immunity (specific), impaired intracellular destruction by neutrophils, reduced complement activity, and decreased levels of secretory IgA.[15] At the time of an illness, nutrition is negatively affected by decreased appetite, malabsorption, diarrhea, diversion of nutrients for immune responses, and urinary nitrogen loss, further exacerbating a malnourished state. The presence of fever increases the metabolic rate, requiring more energy and micronutrients. Malnutrition exists because of the lack of available clean and safe food. Contributing factors include decreased financial resources, inadequate housing, potentially unsafe water supplies, and the lack of or accessibility to health care.

Micronutrients are also important in immune function. Vitamin A contributes to maintenance of the epithelium and vitamin E is an antioxidant that supports the development and function of T cells.[16] Vitamin D supports innate and adaptive immunity and promotes immune protection against tuberculosis by increasing macrophage defenses.[9] Decreased availability of zinc results in a reduction in neutrophil and natural killer cell function, complement activity, and lymphocyte activity. Iron deficiency is associated with decreased cell-mediated immunity and reductions in neutrophil action. Iron deficiency is one of the most common deficiencies worldwide.[17]

Age. Age is also a variable in the ability to resist infections. Viruses such as mumps, polio, or Epstein-Barr virus (EBV) cause less severe infection in infants, whereas others such as rotaviruses result in severe illness in infants. These age-related factors may reflect the availability of immune factors or the maturity of the immune system.[12] T-cell function appears to be impaired in newborns, with the majority of the immune response provided by maternal IgG that crossed the placenta. As this immunity fades over approximately the first 6 months of life, these newborns are more at risk of serious infection. Those infants who are breast feeding will obtain secretory IgA, which does provide additional protection.[13] Immunity tends to decline in the elderly, resulting in reduced antibody responses to new antigens. The immune system may become disregulated as evidenced by the increased frequency of autoimmune diseases with age.[13]

Chronic illness and immunosuppression. Chronic illnesses such as diabetes, cancer, heart disease, and renal failure are associated with an increased risk of infection. Deaths in patients with chronic illnesses are frequently directly related to an infectious process. Diabetes alters the host's ability to resist infection. Phagocytosis is impaired with hyperglycemia, and detection of the pain of infection may be delayed because of

TABLE 8-2	HOST CHARACTERISTICS INFLUENCING INFECTION
Exposure	**Host Health**
Animals, humans, insects, parasites	Intact immune system
Environmental	Absence of chronic disease such as diabetes
Water, toxins, pollutants, radiation, sewage	Absence of genetic abnormality
Hygiene	**Nutritional Status**
Toileting, hand washing, dental care, bathing	Adequate intake of proteins, vitamins, and minerals
Social Behaviors	**Antibiotic Exposure**
Illicit drug use, alcohol, smoking	Recent use, noncompletion of course
Risk taking: sexual, sports	Development of resistance or allergy
Travel	
Exposure to vectors in undeveloped countries	

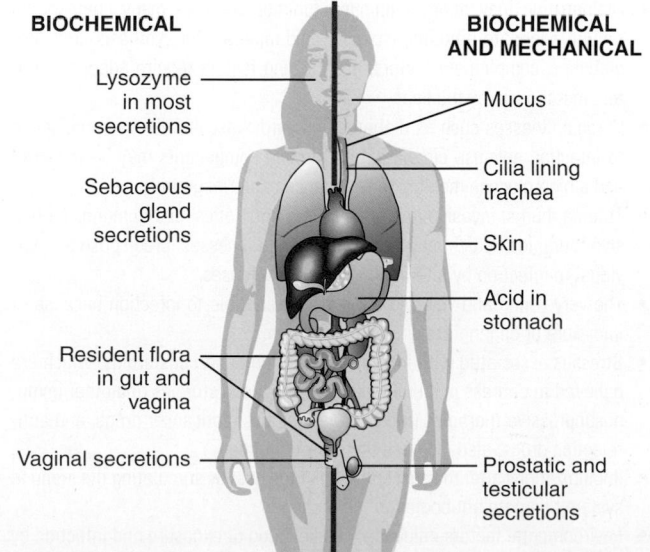

BIOCHEMICAL
- Lysozyme in most secretions
- Sebaceous gland secretions
- Resident flora in gut and vagina
- Vaginal secretions

BIOCHEMICAL AND MECHANICAL
- Mucus
- Cilia lining trachea
- Skin
- Acid in stomach
- Prostatic and testicular secretions

FIGURE 8-5 Some of the mechanical and biochemical barriers of the human body.

neuropathies. The invasiveness of the microorganisms is increased when exposed to hyperglycemic environments. This increased risk of infectious disease in a population with chronic disease is multifactorial and includes the nature of their chronic disease, medications, treatments, exposure to health care settings, and the innate genetics of the individual.

Immunocompromised patients have an increased risk of severe, rapidly progressing infections that may be unresponsive to usual treatments. Infection with pathogens that are usually not pathogenic is an indicator that a person is immunocompromised. The immunocompromised status might be a result of genetic disorders (such as hypogammaglobulinemia) or may be acquired (such as in patients who have undergone a splenectomy). The prevalence of people with transplants and medication-induced immunosuppression is increasing. Antirejection medications such as corticosteroids, cyclosporine, and tacrolimus contribute to immunosuppression in transplant patients.[18] People who take corticosteroids and immunomodulators to suppress inflammatory and autoimmune diseases are also at high risk of infection. Human immunodeficiency virus (HIV) disease is an important chronic condition that predisposes to a variety of other infections (see Chapter 12).

The physiologic response to chronic stress is thought to contribute to risk for infection. The neurohormonal alterations lead to changes in the levels of cortisol and other stress hormones that may affect immune responsiveness (see Chapter 2).

Role of Immunization

Immunization of a population is the most effective means to reduce morbidity and mortality from vaccine-preventable diseases such as hepatitis A, hepatitis B, influenza, and pneumococcal infections.[18] There are two goals of immunization. The first is to confer immunity to a host by direct exposure to the altered pathogen. The second is to decrease the number of susceptible hosts in the population, thereby limiting the possibility of transmission of the disease. By this method, known as *herd immunity,* the disease can be controlled or eliminated without immunizing everyone, as long as a high enough percentage of the population is immunized. The number of susceptible hosts in the population decreases as immunization rates increase. When a critical percentage of the susceptible population is immunized, the chain of transmission is broken and the disease outbreak averted. If the percentage of adequately immunized individuals drops, epidemics may result.

Immunization with preformed antibodies to the infectious agent provides immediate immunity. Immunizations with killed vaccines such as influenza provide immunity without the risk of infection from the agent. This type of vaccination may require several doses spaced at intervals to allow for continued development of an antibody level sufficient to prevent disease.[12] The increased prevalence of pertussis infection in recent years demonstrates the importance of continued monitoring of vaccine use. Historically, the last pertussis dose was given with the last tetanus dose of a teenaged child. Increasing occurrence rates precipitated a CDC recommendation for a booster dose for adults ages 19 to 64 years.[18] The CDC provides updates and recommendations for immunizations for adults, children, and travelers (www.cdc.gov).

Role of Environment

Multiple environmental factors affect the prevalence and transmission of various infections and infestations. For example, parasitic infections are facilitated by hot and humid climates, overcrowded living conditions, the presence of insect vectors in bed linen or clothing, improper sewage disposal or treatment (such as the use of raw human sewage as fertilizer), the lack of clean water, and the consumption of contaminated raw or undercooked meat or vegetables.

Infections may be transmitted by inhalation of polluted dust or air. For example, the fungus *Coccidioides immitis,* which causes valley fever, is pandemic in the southwestern United States. Toxoplasmosis is caused by inhalation or ingestion of dirt, sand, or litter dust contaminated with cat feces that contain the causative protozoon *Toxoplasma gondii.* The plague is still a disease of concern in many countries. It is caused by the bacterium *Yersinia pestis,* which is carried by a rodent flea.[19] There are multiple examples of foodborne illness such as *Salmonella,* with outbreaks related to improper processing, storage, or cooking of meats and raw produce.[20]

The risk factors for tuberculosis (TB) include crowded living conditions, poor nutrition, frequent contact with those who have TB, and extremes of age (i.e., infants and elderly). Those with reduced immune function attributable to HIV infection, medications, or other risks as previously listed are also at risk for TB.[21]

There are periodic outbreaks of diseases that occur related to travel, shipments of food products, and vaccination levels. Monitoring of travel from those countries with known endemic vaccine-preventable diseases is important to prevent global transmission. SARS (severe acute respiratory syndrome) was identified in 2003 in a businessman traveling from China to Vietnam. The diagnosis was made by WHO physician Dr. Carlo Urbani. This life-threatening disease required the skills of the WHO to identify it as a new and different disease. Unfortunately, Dr. Carlo Urbani died from this disease as did the original patient. This coronavirus, which is transmitted as a respiratory virus, is believed to have originated from small mammals in China and developed into a lethal disease. It is a tribute to the WHO and cooperating agencies that SARS was identified as a global health threat, and a travel advisory was issued.[22,23]

KEY POINTS

- Epidemiology is the study of health events and disease, their distribution, and associated causative factors in a defined population. Goals of epidemiology are to define a disease, identify outbreaks, assist in the development and evaluation of treatment protocols, and develop prevention strategies.
- Transmission of disease requires a chain of events that includes passing of the pathogen from the reservoir of the infection through a portal of exit to a susceptible host through a portal of entry by a circumscribed mode of transmission.
- The host has several lines of defense to prevent and fight infection. The skin and mucous membranes provide a first line of defense through mechanical and biochemical barriers. Epithelial shedding, ciliary action, acidic secretions, and enzymes help remove or destroy microorganisms before they gain access to the body.
- Malnutrition may depress immune function because many components require adequate proteins, vitamins, and minerals for synthesis. Immunoglobulins, complement factors, and clotting factors require adequate protein metabolism by the liver.
- Chronic illnesses such as diabetes and cardiovascular disease predispose to infection because circulation of immune components may be impaired and a high-glucose medium may enhance bacterial growth.
- Trauma, burns, invasive instrumentation, antibiotics, and immunosuppressive therapies, which may accompany acute illnesses, predispose an individual to infection by altering normal host defenses.
- The very young and very old are more susceptible to infection because of immature or degenerating immune function.
- Stress is associated with increased secretion of corticosteroids, which are believed to depress immune function. Exogenous steroids and other immunosuppressive therapies (radiation, antibiotics, anticancer drugs, and antirejection drugs) also increase the risk of infection.
- Immunizations alter the susceptibility of the host by stimulating the immune system to create antibodies to the pathogen.
- Environmental factors influence the likelihood of exposure and infection by microorganisms. Sanitation, air quality, living conditions, and climate are important factors.

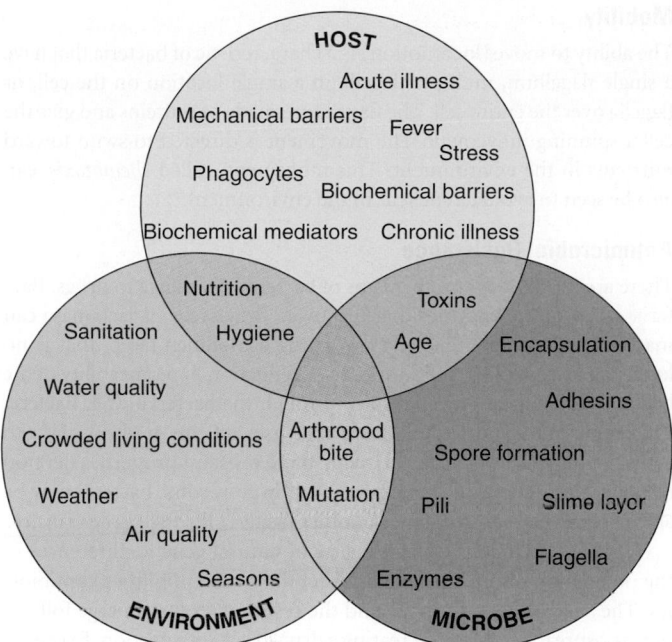

FIGURE 8-6 This depiction of the interactions of host, microbe, and environment provides a framework for understanding infectious processes.

HOST-MICROBE RELATIONSHIP

Normal Microbial Flora

The ability of the human body to resist infection requires an intact defense system. Host and environmental factors such as nutrition, age, illness, air quality, sanitation, and stress may alter the host's resistance to infection. In addition, characteristics of the pathogen such as virulence, toxins, adherence, and invasiveness may allow it to evade the human defense system and colonize.[11] This relationship between the host, the infectious agent, and the environment, as shown in Figure 8-6, is the framework for understanding infectious processes.[1]

Large numbers of microorganisms reside on the skin and in the gastrointestinal tract and vagina of the human host. These microbes can have a symbiotic relationship or just a neutral relationship to the host. Residents are those that are continually present on or in the host. Transients are acquired and may be present briefly but are removed either by host immunity or because the environment is not suited to their continued presence. Variable quantities of available nutrients, pH variability, and microbial resistance to local antibacterial substances such as bile and lysozymes influence the presence of flora (Table 8-3).

In the intestinal tract, the mouth and oral pharynx have large numbers of anaerobes, whereas the stomach, because of the presence of gastric hydrochloric acid and peptic enzymes, is inhospitable to bacteria. In the colon the quantity of bacteria is markedly increased. These primarily include anaerobes such as *Bacteroides* and *Clostridium*. The respiratory tract (beginning with the nares) contains *Staphylococcus* and *Streptococcus,* and may also potentially have pathogenic bacteria such as pneumococci, meningococci, and *Haemophilus* species. The areas below the larynx, including the trachea and bronchi, have only transient bacteria, as do the eustachian tubes. The genitourinary tract is sterile beyond the distal 1 cm of the urethra. The organisms at this site vary by age in women because of the influence of estrogenic hormones.[12]

Normal flora can cause an opportunistic infection when they reach certain areas of the body. For example, a common cause of urinary

TABLE 8-3 CLASSES OF ORGANISMS INFECTIOUS TO HUMANS

CLASS	SIZE	SITE OF REPRODUCTION	EXAMPLE
Viruses	20-300 nm	Intracellular	Poliomyelitis
Chlamydiae	200-1000 nm	Intracellular	Urethritis
Rickettsiae	300-1200 nm	Intracellular	Rocky Mountain spotted fever
Mycoplas-mas	125-350 nm	Extracellular	Atypical pneumonia
Bacteria	0.8-15 mcg	Skin	Staphylococcal wound
		Mucous membranes	
		Extracellular	infection
		Intracellular	Cholera
			Streptococcal pneumonia
			Tuberculosis
Fungi	2-200 mcg	Skin	Tinea pedis
		Mucous membranes	(athlete's foot)
		Extracellular	*Candida* (e.g.,
		Intracellular	thrush)
			Sporotrichosis
			Histoplasmosis
Protozoa	1-50 mm	Mucosal	Giardiasis
		Extracellular	Sleeping sickness
Helminths	3 mm to 10 m	Intracellular	Trichinosis
		Extracellular	Filariasis

From McCance K, Huether S: *Pathophysiology: the biologic basis for disease in adults & children,* ed 6, St Louis, 2010, Mosby.

tract infection is the migration of *Escherichia coli* from the colon into the urinary tract. If the host has reduced defenses or immune dysfunction, then normal flora can invade to become an opportunistic infection.[12]

Microorganism Characteristics

Virulence

Microorganisms possess certain characteristics that assist in their penetration and survival in the host despite the presence of an intact defense system. Virulence, toxin production, microbial adherence, and invasiveness are microorganism factors that influence the development of infection in the host.

Adherence

The ability to adhere to the contact surface is critical for the success of a microorganism. This ability is affected by the surface hydrophobicity, the net surface charge, the binding molecules on the bacteria (ligands), and the interaction with the host cell. Many bacteria, such as *E. coli,* have pili, which are hairlike structures that extend from the bacterial cell wall and help to increase attachment of the bacteria to host cells. Other bacteria, such as *Streptococcus pyogenes,* have hairlike appendages called fimbriae that extend from the cell surface and promote attachment.[24]

Invasion

Access to the host by invasion of the epithelium is important for many bacteria. These bacteria move through cellular junctions to more central tissues (e.g., *Salmonella*). Others invade certain types of cells and enter a host cell. They may stay in a vacuole (made of the host cell membrane) and may multiply in the host cell. Improvements in *in vitro* studies with tissue cultures are adding to our knowledge about these processes.[24]

Toxins and Exotoxins

Some bacteria produce a lipopolysaccharide termed a toxin. The toxins are further delineated as exotoxins (excreted by a living cell, with high concentrations in liquid) or endotoxins (an integral part of the cell wall, which is released upon cell death and sometimes during cell growth). An example is tetanus, which is caused by the toxin of *Clostridium tetani*. (Vaccines that are made to prevent these types of diseases are then called toxoids.) When the toxins are released, they have specific effects throughout the body. For example, tetanus causes release of a toxin that attaches to receptors of the motor neurons. The toxin migrates to the spinal cord and then to the brainstem with resulting paralysis. Some toxins are so powerful that very small quantities are required to produce severe effects.[24]

Bacterial Enzymes

Tissue-degrading enzymes are produced by some bacteria. These enzymes degrade certain body tissues, promoting continued disease. For example *Staphylococcus aureus* secretes coagulase, which coagulates plasma and contributes to the formation of fibrin walls around the lesions caused by these bacteria. This allows the bacteria to persist in the cellular environment. The coagulase also causes deposits of fibrin on the bacteria itself, leading to improved protection from phagocytosis.[24]

Other bacteria produce hyaluronidase, which is an enzyme that breaks down hyaluronic acid. This acid is present in connective tissue. This action helps dissemination of the bacteria through the tissues. Some bacteria are able to produce substances that are cytolysins. These cytolysins can dissolve red blood cells, tissue cells, or leukocytes. For example, group A streptococci produce streptolysin O, which lyses red blood cells.[24]

Antiphagocytic Factors

Some bacteria develop an outside coating on their surface to prevent phagocytosis. The coating can be made of host cell components or a polysaccharide capsule. In this way they are not as recognizable to leukocytes.[24] Development of a microbial slime layer also facilitates adherence and improves survival of the pathogen. A thin layer of peptidoglycan is created that can participate in the development of pili or flagella on some organisms.[24]

The identification of the production of biofilm by bacteria has changed many facets of patient treatment and prevention of disease. The biofilm is a collection of interactive bacteria that are attached to a solid surface or to each other. This collection is then encased in a polysaccharide matrix. This slimy coat on solid surfaces can involve a single species or several species. These bacteria can then be protected from the host's immune mechanisms. Measures to prevent the collection of this biofilm can reduce infection rates.[24]

Endospores

Several of the bacteria are capable of creating endospores. In responses to the depletion of nutrients such as carbon, nitrogen, or phosphorus, the cell forms an internal spore. These spores are in a resting state that is markedly resistant to heat, chemical agents, and desiccation. When the environment is more favorable spores are reactivated. Common bacteria with this ability include *Bacillus* and *Clostridium*.[24]

Mobility

The ability to move (locomotion) is a characteristic of bacteria that have a single flagellum, multiple flagella in a single location on the cell, or flagella over the entire cell. The flagella are made of proteins and give the cell a spinning movement. The movement is directed to swim toward nutrients in the environment. This movement, called *chemotaxis*, can also be seen to avoid a repellent in the environment.[24]

Antimicrobial Resistance

There are four known mechanisms of bacterial resistance to drugs. Bacteria can produce enzymes that inactivate drugs (e.g., β-lactamase can inactivate penicillins). Bacteria can create a modified target that is no longer as susceptible to the antibiotic. A reduction in permeability of the bacteria to the drug prevents entry through the bacterial wall. Bacteria can employ an export mechanism that uses an ion gradient (H^+) to actively pump out the drug.[13] Usually these resistant properties develop by chance mutations in the organisms; however, some bacteria may be able to transmit their resistance to other bacteria through gene transfer.

Resistant infections occur because of natural genetic differences in the population of organisms that affect their susceptibility to antibiotics. The susceptible strains die and the resistant strains emerge following exposure to antibiotics, creating a drug-resistant infection. Excessive use of antibiotics and subtherapeutic dosing contribute to the development of resistant infections. Relatively resistant microorganisms survive a low-dose antibiotic course to become the dominant species and may then be transmitted to other individuals.

The emergence of vancomycin-resistant *Enterococcus* (VRE) and methicillin-resistant *S. aureus* (MRSA) among others is a troubling development in infectious disease management. The emergence of MRSA was the result of a mutation of the organism and selection of resistant strains in response to antibiotics. The ability of *S. aureus* to become antibiotic resistant was first recognized following the introduction of penicillin (Table 8-4).[13] Multidrug-resistant tuberculosis has also emerged as has antiviral medication resistance, making treatment more difficult.

In summary, virulence and invasiveness factors include a variety of mechanisms that microorganisms have evolved to elude and block host defenses or assist in host invasion. These characteristics contribute to the pathogenicity of the microorganism by enabling it to penetrate natural barriers, resist death by phagocytosis, or survive antimicrobial therapy (e.g., MRSA). Examples include bacterial enzymes, encapsulation, mutation, mobility, endospore formation, and resistance to phagocytosis and antimicrobial therapy.

TABLE 8-4	HISTORICAL PROGRESSION OF *STAPHYLOCOCCUS AUREUS* RESISTANCE TO ANTIBIOTICS	
ANTIBIOTIC AND YEAR INTRODUCED	**YEAR RESISTANCE APPEARED**	
Penicillin, 1941	1940s	
Streptomycin, 1944	Mid-1940s	
Tetracycline, 1948	1950s	
Erythromycin, 1952	1950s	
Gentamicin, 1964	Mid-1970s	
Methicillin, 1959	Late 1960s	

Data from Morita MM: Methicillin-resistant *Staphylococcus aureus*: past, present and future, *Nurs Clin North Am* 28:625-637, 1993; Rosenberg J: Methicillin-resistant *Staphylococcus aureus* (MRSA) in the community: who's watching? *Lancet* 346:132-133, 1995.

KEY POINTS

- A number of microorganisms are considered resident flora because they live on or in the host without causing disease. Resident flora benefit the host by synthesizing molecules and inhibiting the growth of nonresident microorganisms. If the host's immune system is compromised, resident flora may become pathogenic and cause opportunistic infection.
- Microorganisms possess characteristics that enhance their pathogenic potential. Adherence is improved by the presence of adhesion molecules, slime layers, and pili. Escape from immune detection and destruction is enhanced by encapsulation, spore formation, mutation, use of flagella, and toxin production. Microorganisms that possess these characteristics are more virulent and thus more likely to cause disease.
- Drug resistance occurs when microorganisms undergo chance mutations that allow them to survive in the presence of an antibiotic. When the antibiotic is present, these resistant strains emerge to become the dominant species in an individual and may be transmitted to others, causing resistant infections.

TYPES OF PATHOGENIC ORGANISMS

Box 8-1 summarizes primary pathogens associated with specific infections in the human host. Photographic examples of pathogenic organisms are shown in Figure 8-7.

Bacteria

Bacteria are single-celled rigid wall organisms that have no internal organelles (Figure 8-8). Some live in the intestines of humans, and other animals, and participate in digestion. Others live in the soil and are responsible for its fertility. They degrade dead tissue into useful components for other organisms to use. Among the countless types of bacteria that exist, only a small percentage is known to be harmful to humans.[12]

"True bacteria" have a variety of shapes including cocci (spherical), bacilli (rod shaped or comma-shaped rods, e.g., *Pseudomonas aeruginosa* vibrio), or spiral (twisted rod shaped, e.g., *Spirillum*). Those classified as cocci are also seen in clusters, chains, pairs, or tetrads. The

---

BOX 8-1   EXAMPLES OF PRIMARY PATHOGENS ASSOCIATED WITH SPECIFIC INFECTIONS

Burns
Staphylococcus aureus
Streptococcus pyogenes (group A)
Pseudomonas aeruginosa
Gram-negative bacilli

Skin Infections
Staphylococcus aureus
Streptococcus pyogenes (group A)
Gram-negative bacilli
Treponema pallidum

Decubitus and Surgical Wounds
Staphylococcus aureus
Gram-negative enteric bacilli
Pseudomonas aeruginosa
Streptococcus pyogenes (group A)
Anaerobic streptococci
Clostridium spp.
Enterococcus
Bacteroides spp.

Meninges
Neisseria meningitidis
Haemophilus influenzae
Streptococcus pneumoniae
Streptococcus spp.
Escherichia coli
Gram-negative bacilli
Streptococcus pyogenes (group A)
Staphylococcus aureus
Mycobacterium tuberculosis
Listeria monocytogenes
Enterococcus (neonatal period)
Treponema pallidum
Leptospira

Brain Abscess
Streptococci (aerobic and anaerobic)
Bacteroides spp.
Staphylococcus aureus

Paranasal and Middle Ear
Streptococcus pneumoniae
Streptococcus pyogenes (group A)
Haemophilus influenzae
Gram-negative enteric bacilli
Pseudomonas aeruginosa
Anaerobic streptococci
Staphylococcus aureus

Throat
Streptococcus pyogenes (group A)
Neisseria gonorrhoeae
Bacteroides spp.
Fusobacterium
Spirochetes
Corynebacterium diphtheriae
Bordetella pertussis

Lungs
Mycoplasma pneumoniae
Streptococcus pneumoniae
Haemophilus influenzae
Staphylococcus aureus
Klebsiella
Pseudomonas aeruginosa
Gram-negative bacilli
Streptococcus pyogenes (group A)
Mycobacterium tuberculosis
Chlamydia psittaci
Legionella pneumophila
Anaerobic streptococci
Bacteroides spp.
Coxiella burnetii

Lung Abscess
Anaerobic streptococci
Bacteroides spp.
Fusobacterium
Staphylococcus aureus
Klebsiella
Gram-negative bacilli

Streptococcus pneumoniae
Enterococcus

Pleura
Staphylococcus aureus
Streptococcus pneumoniae
Haemophilus influenzae
Gram-negative bacilli
Anaerobic streptococci
Bacteroides spp.
Fusobacterium
Streptococcus pyogenes (group A)
Mycobacterium tuberculosis

Endocardium
Viridans group of streptococci
Staphylococcus aureus
Enterococcus
Other streptococci
Staphylococcus epidermidis
Gram-negative enteric bacilli
Pseudomonas aeruginosa

Peritoneum
Escherichia coli
Gram-negative bacilli
Enterococcus
Bacteroides fragilis
Anaerobic streptococci
Clostridium spp.
Streptococcus pneumoniae
Streptococcus pyogenes (group A)
Neisseria gonorrhoeae
Mycobacterium tuberculosis

Biliary Tract
Escherichia coli
Gram-negative bacilli
Enterococcus spp.
Staphylococcus aureus
Clostridium spp.
Streptococci (aerobic and anaerobic)

Continued

BOX 8-1 EXAMPLES OF PRIMARY PATHOGENS ASSOCIATED WITH SPECIFIC INFECTIONS—cont'd

Kidney and Bladder
Escherichia coli
Gram-negative bacilli
Staphylococcus aureus
Staphylococcus epidermidis
Mycobacterium tuberculosis

Urethra
Neisseria gonorrhoeae
Chlamydia trachomatis
Trichomonas vaginalis
Gram-negative enteric bacilli
Ureaplasma urealyticum

Prostate
Gram-negative enteric bacilli
Neisseria gonorrhoeae
Staphylococcus aureus

Epididymis and Testes
Gram-negative bacilli
Neisseria gonorrhoeae
Chlamydia trachomatis
Mycobacterium tuberculosis

Bone (Osteomyelitis)
Staphylococcus aureus
Salmonella
Gram-negative enteric bacilli

Streptococcus pyogenes (group A)
Mycobacterium tuberculosis
Anaerobic streptococci
Pseudomonas aeruginosa

Joints
Staphylococcus aureus
Neisseria gonorrhoeae
Streptococcus pyogenes (group A)
Gram-negative enteric bacilli
Pseudomonas aeruginosa
Streptococcus pneumoniae
Neisseria meningitidis
Haemophilus influenzae (in children)
Mycobacterium tuberculosis

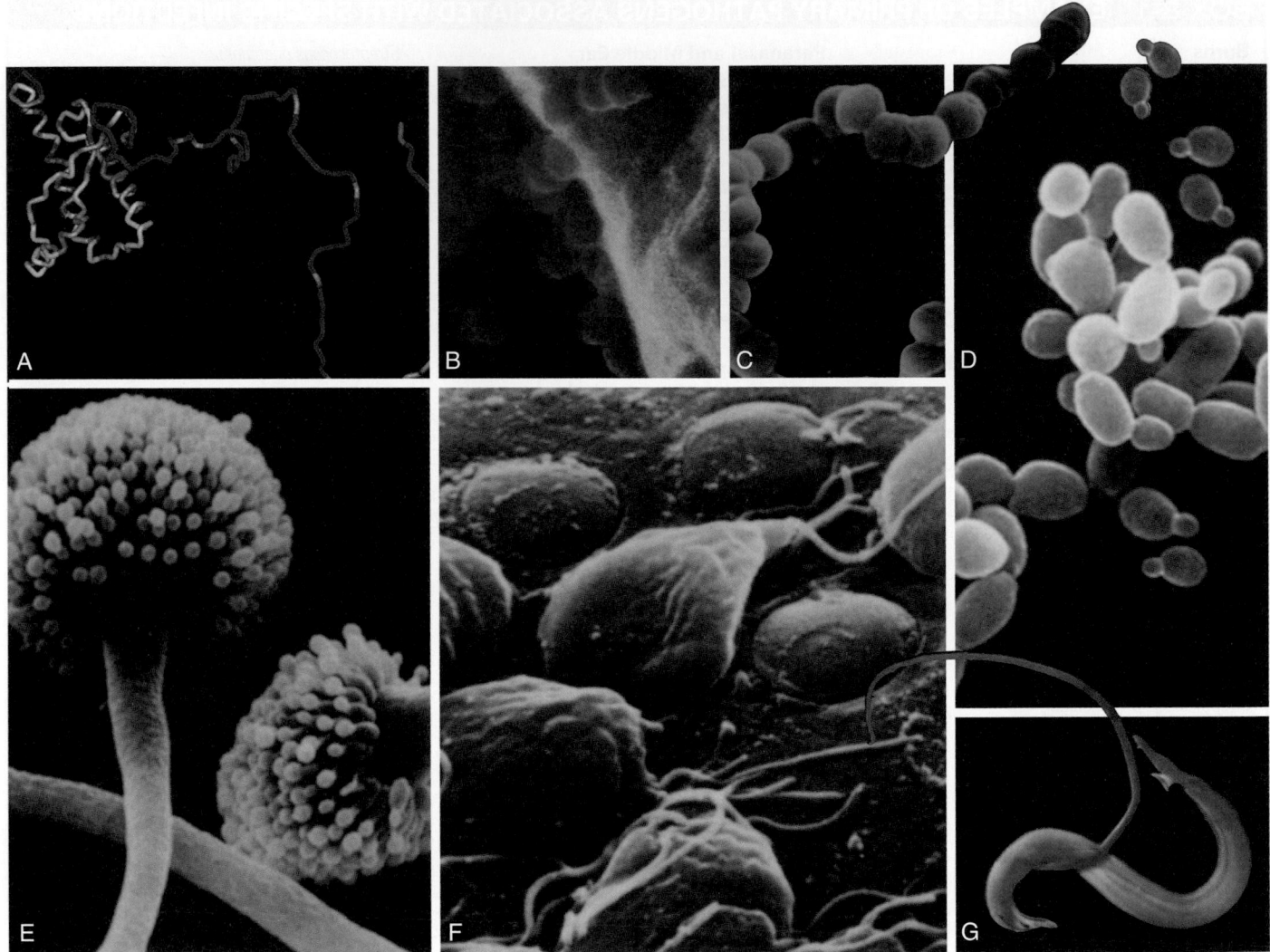

FIGURE 8-7 Examples of pathogenic organisms. **A,** Prion (infectious protein). **B,** Viruses (the human immunodeficiency virus [HIV] that causes AIDS). **C,** Bacteria (*Streptococcus* bacteria that cause strep throat and other infections). **D,** Fungi (yeast cells that commonly infect the urinary and reproductive tracts). **E,** Fungi (the mold that causes aspergillosis). **F,** Protozoa (the flagellated cells that cause traveler's diarrhea). **G,** Pathogenic animals (the parasitic worms that cause snail fever). (**A,** from Donne DG, et al: Structure of the recombinant full-length hamster prion protein PRp (29-231): the N terminus is highly flexible, *Proc Natl Acad Sci USA* 94:13452-13457, 1997. Copyright National Academy of Sciences, USA; **B,** from Lennart Nilsson; **C-G,** from Patton KT, Thibodeau GA: *Anatomy & physiology,* ed 8, St Louis, 2013, Mosby, p 26.)

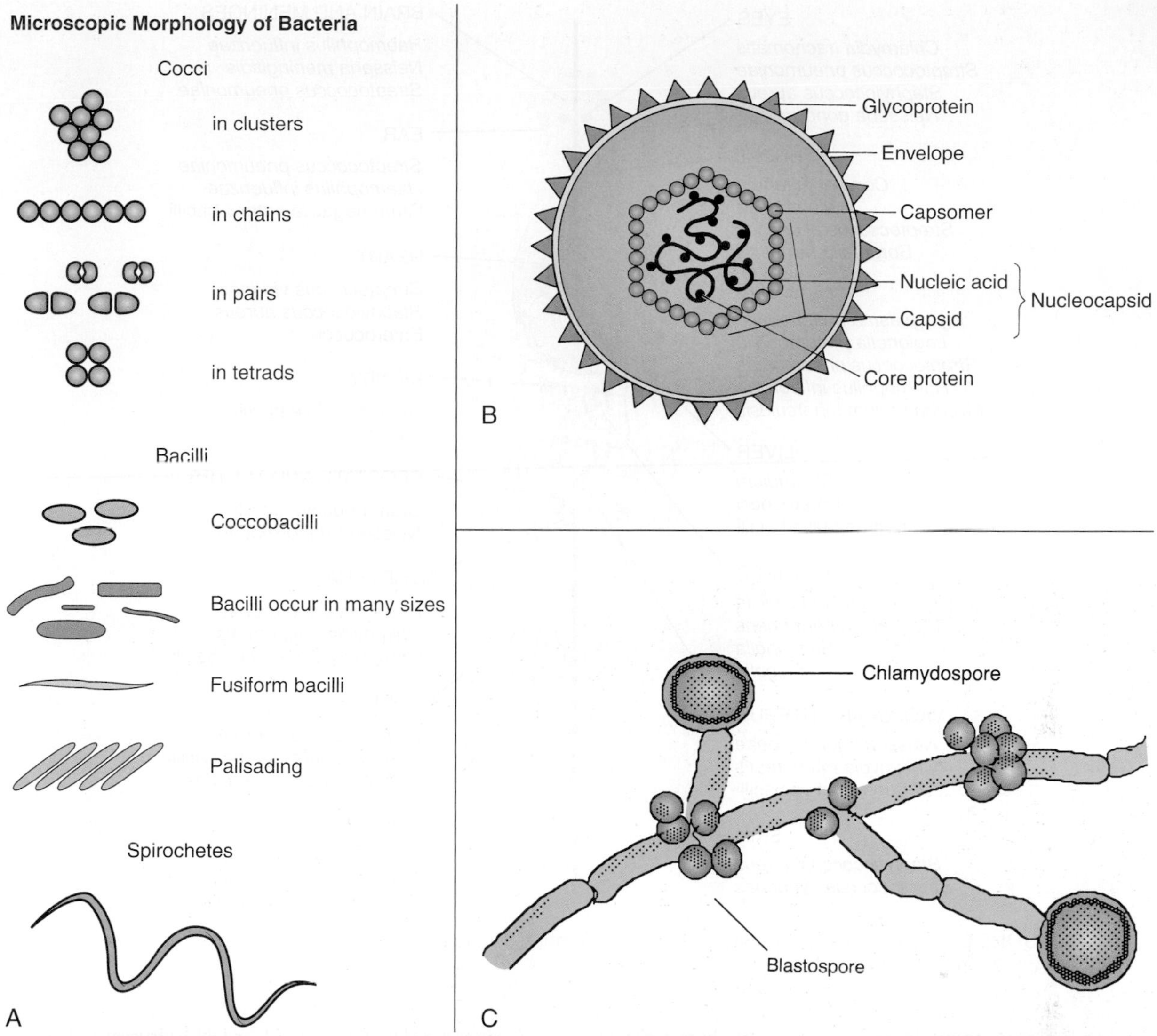

Microscopic Morphology of Bacteria

Cocci

in clusters

in chains

in pairs

in tetrads

Bacilli

Coccobacilli

Bacilli occur in many sizes

Fusiform bacilli

Palisading

Spirochetes

A

B
- Glycoprotein
- Envelope
- Capsomer
- Nucleic acid ⎫ Nucleocapsid
- Capsid ⎭
- Core protein

C
- Chlamydospore
- Blastospore

FIGURE 8-8 Types of microorganisms. **A,** Bacteria. **B,** Virus. **C,** Fungus. (**A,** from Mahon CR, et al: *Textbook of diagnostic microbiology*, ed 4, Philadelphia, 2011, Saunders; **B** and **C,** from Nisengard RJ, Newman MG: *Oral microbiology and immunology*, ed 2, Philadelphia, 1994, Saunders.)

majority of bacteria that cause disease in humans are one of these true bacteria. Filamentous bacteria may have branching structures that resemble fungi. *Mycobacterium tuberculosis* would be an example.[9]

Spirochetes (the majority of which are anaerobic) possess a motile spiral filament (e.g., *Treponema pallidum* [Figure 8-9]). Bacteria of the genus *Mycoplasma* do not have a rigid cell wall and are pleiomorphic (many formed) in shape. They are some of the smallest of the bacteria; an example is *Mycoplasma pneumoniae*, which causes an atypical pneumonia. *Rickettsia* is a genus consisting of intracellular parasites that can have a variety of shapes. This group is usually spread by vectors; an example is Rocky Mountain spotted fever caused by *Rickettsia rickettsii* transmitted by ticks. *Chlamydia* are also intracellular parasites but have a more complex life cycle, with *Chlamydia trachomatis* as an example.[9]

Bacteria are classified not only by morphology (shape) but also by the response to gram staining. Gram staining separates bacteria into gram-positive organisms, which appear dark purple under the microscope; gram-negative organisms, which appear pink; or acid-fast organisms, which resist staining but once stained resist discoloration. Further differentiation of bacteria is based on nutritional requirements (such as

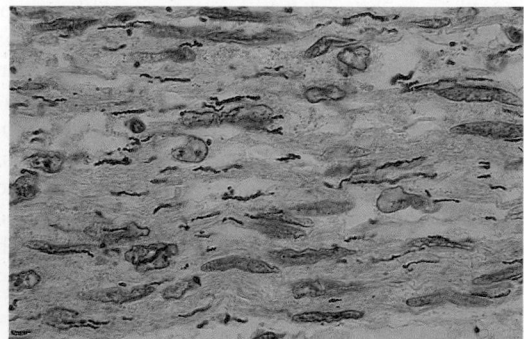

FIGURE 8-9 Spirochetes (e.g., *Treponema pallidum*): immunohistochemistry of the muscular layer in the small intestine of a newborn with congenital syphilis. Multiple spirochetes are shown in red (both cross-sections and entire treponemes can be noted [×100]). (Courtesy Jeannette Guarner, MD, and Sherif R. Zaki, MD, PhD, Centers for Disease Control and Prevention, Atlanta.)

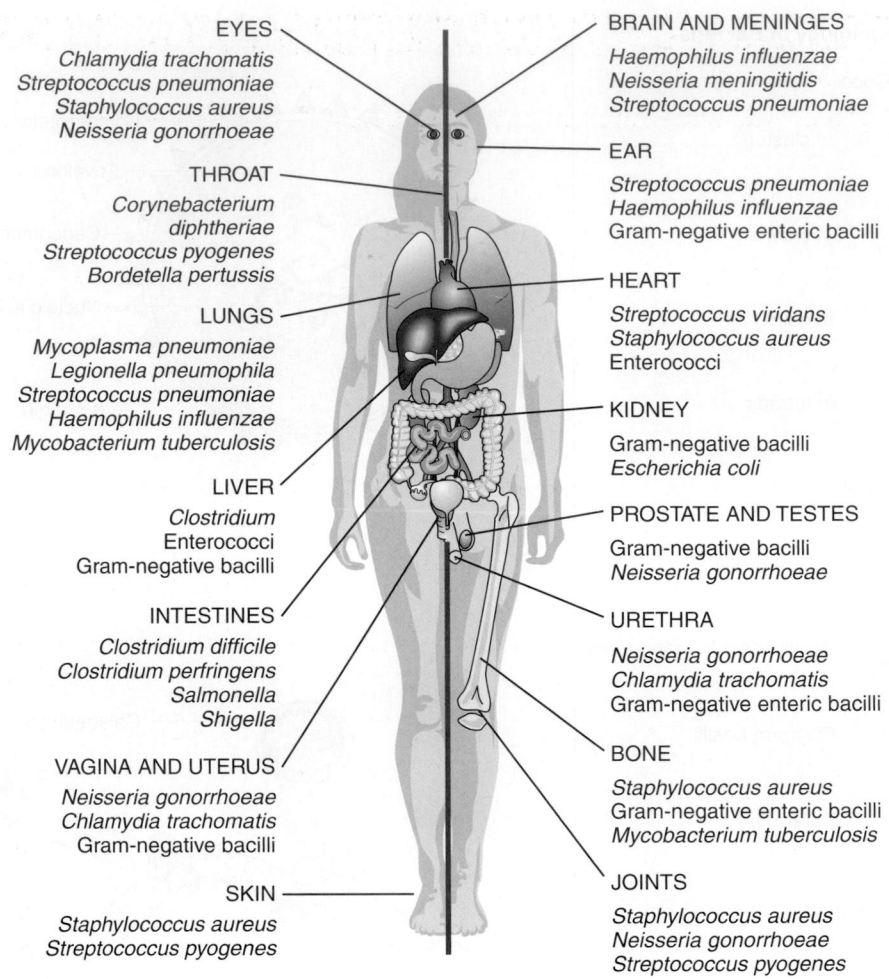

EYES

Chlamydia trachomatis
Streptococcus pneumoniae
Staphylococcus aureus
Neisseria gonorrhoeae

THROAT

Corynebacterium
diphtheriae
Streptococcus pyogenes
Bordetella pertussis

LUNGS

Mycoplasma pneumoniae
Legionella pneumophila
Streptococcus pneumoniae
Haemophilus influenzae
Mycobacterium tuberculosis

LIVER

Clostridium
Enterococci
Gram-negative bacilli

INTESTINES

Clostridium difficile
Clostridium perfringens
Salmonella
Shigella

VAGINA AND UTERUS

Neisseria gonorrhoeae
Chlamydia trachomatis
Gram-negative bacilli

SKIN

Staphylococcus aureus
Streptococcus pyogenes

BRAIN AND MENINGES

Haemophilus influenzae
Neisseria meningitidis
Streptococcus pneumoniae

EAR

Streptococcus pneumoniae
Haemophilus influenzae
Gram-negative enteric bacilli

HEART

Streptococcus viridans
Staphylococcus aureus
Enterococci

KIDNEY

Gram-negative bacilli
Escherichia coli

PROSTATE AND TESTES

Gram-negative bacilli
Neisseria gonorrhoeae

URETHRA

Neisseria gonorrhoeae
Chlamydia trachomatis
Gram-negative enteric bacilli

BONE

Staphylococcus aureus
Gram-negative enteric bacilli
Mycobacterium tuberculosis

JOINTS

Staphylococcus aureus
Neisseria gonorrhoeae
Streptococcus pyogenes

FIGURE 8-10 Examples of pathogenic bacteria classified according to the part of the human body that they commonly infect.

whether the organism is anaerobic or aerobic), on colony characteristics, and on resistance.

Figure 8-10 depicts examples of pathogenic bacteria and the areas that they commonly infect. Once they have penetrated the initial defense mechanisms, the bacteria multiply and create a colony. In an attempt to contain and eliminate the invading bacteria, an acute inflammatory reaction occurs. Phagocytic cells such as neutrophils and macrophages are recruited to the area, where they ingest and destroy the microorganisms. If these responses are insufficient to contain the infection, the bacteria move through the body in natural currents of fluids (i.e., bloodstream, lymph system, or interstitial fluids). Bacteria may move through the lymph system to the lymph nodes where they stimulate an immune response. If they are present in sufficient numbers to overwhelm the lymph nodes, circulating clumps of bacteria (emboli) can cause bacteremia and microabscesses. In severe cases, sepsis, hypotension, organ system failure, and death can occur (see Chapter 20).

Viruses

Viruses, the smallest known infective agents, range in size from 20 to 300 nm. They consist of a protein shell called the capsid and a core of genetic material made of either ribonucleic acid (RNA) or deoxyribonucleic acid (DNA). The capsid can be in many shapes including helical, icosahedral, or large pleiomorphic shapes. Some viruses also have a protective envelope surrounding the capsid. This envelope is acquired from the cell membrane of the infected host cell.

Viruses are classified as RNA or DNA viruses, and as either single-stranded (ss) or double-stranded (ds). Some RNA viruses, called retroviruses, contain the enzyme reverse transcriptase and can convert their RNA into DNA that can be incorporated into the host's DNA. The HIV virus is an example of a retrovirus (see Chapter 12). A comparison of viruses, transmission characteristics, and resulting disease processes is presented in Table 8-5.

DNA viruses (e.g., herpes simplex virus) enter the nucleus of the host cell and produce messenger RNA (mRNA) using the host cell's enzymes. Viral proteins are then formed from the messenger RNA, and the DNA of the virus is replicated by host polymerases. DNA and proteins are assembled into new viruses in the host cell. The RNA viruses replicate within the cytoplasm and most produce mRNA that is then translated into proteins and genomic RNA, from which new viruses are created.

Transmission of a virus occurs from one infected person to another or from an animal reservoir (zoonotic infection). The steps of the viral life cycle include attachment to the target cell as the initial step. The virus then penetrates the cell membrane in various ways. Once inside the host cell, the virus uses the host cell's materials to produce new viral components. The virus may be released from the host cells by budding from the cell's surface (Figure 8-11). Viruses that do not manufacture an envelope are usually released by *lysing* the host cell, thus destroying it.[25] A comparison between viruses and other microorganisms is presented in Table 8-6.

TABLE 8-5   HUMAN DISEASES CAUSED BY SPECIFIC VIRUSES

BALTIMORE CLASSIFICATION	FAMILY	VIRUS	ENVELOPE	MAIN ROUTE OF TRANSMISSION	DISEASE
dsDNA	Adenoviruses	Adenovirus	No	Droplet contact	Acute febrile pharyngitis
	Herpesviruses	Herpes simplex type 1 (HSV-1)	Yes	Direct contact with saliva or lesions	Lesions in mouth, pharynx, conjunctivitis
		Herpes simplex type 2 (HSV-2)	Yes	Sexually, contact with lesions during birth	Sores on labia, meningitis in children
		Herpes simplex type 8 (HSV-8)	Yes	Sexually?, body fluids	Kaposi sarcoma
		Epstein-Barr virus (EBV)	Yes	Saliva	Mononucleosis, Burkitt lymphoma
		Cytomegalovirus (CMV)	Yes	Body fluids, mother's milk, transplacental	Mononucleosis, congenital infection
		Varicella-zoster virus (VZV)	Yes	Droplet contact	Chickenpox, shingles
ssDNA	Papovaviruses	Papillomavirus	No	Direct contact	Warts, cervical carcinoma
dsRNA	Reoviruses	Rotavirus	No	Fecal-oral	Severe diarrhea
ssRNA+	Picornaviruses	Coxsackievirus	No	Fecal-oral, droplet contact	Nonspecific febrile illness, conjunctivitis, meningitis
		Hepatitis A virus	No	Fecal-oral	Acute hepatitis
		Poliovirus	No	Fecal-oral	Poliomyelitis
		Rhinovirus	No	Droplet contact	Common cold
	Flaviviruses	Hepatitis C virus	Yes	Blood, sexually	Acute or chronic hepatitis, hepatocellular carcinoma
		Yellow fever virus	Yes	Mosquito vector	Yellow fever
		Dengue virus	Yes	Mosquito vector	Dengue fever
		West Nile virus	Yes	Mosquito vector	Meningitis, encephalitis
	Togaviruses	Rubella virus	Yes	Droplet contact, transplacental	Acute or congenital rubella
	Coronaviruses	SARS	Yes	Droplets in aerosol or direct contact	Severe respiratory disease
	Caliciviruses	Norovirus	No	Fecal-oral	Gastroenteritis
ssRNA−	Orthomyxoviruses	Influenzavirus	Yes	Droplet contact	Influenza
	Paramyxoviruses	Measles virus	Yes	Droplet contact	Measles
		Mumps virus	Yes	Droplet contact	Mumps
		Parainfluenza	Yes	Droplet contact	Croup, pneumonia, common cold
		Respiratory syncytial virus (RSV)	Yes	Droplet contact, hand-to-mouth	Pneumonia, influenza-like syndrome
	Rhabdoviruses	Rabies virus	Yes	Animal bite, droplet contact	Rabies
	Bunyaviruses	Hantavirus	Yes	Aerosolized animal fecal material	Viral hemorrhagic fever
	Filoviruses	Ebola virus	Yes	Direct contact with body fluids	Viral hemorrhagic fever
		Marburg	Yes	Direct contact with body fluids	Viral hemorrhagic fever
	Arenavirus	Lassa virus	Yes	Aerosolized animal fecal material	Viral hemorrhagic fever
ssRNA+ with RT	Retroviruses	HIV	Yes	Sexually, blood products	AIDS
dsDNA with RT	Hepadna viruses	Hepatitis B virus	Yes	All body fluids	Acute or chronic hepatitis, hepatocellular carcinoma

From McCance K, Huether S: *Pathophysiology: the biologic basis for disease in adults & children*, ed 6, St Louis, 2010, Mosby.
AIDS, Acquired immunodeficiency syndrome; *DNA,* deoxyribonucleic acid; *ds,* double-stranded; *HIV,* human immunodeficiency virus; *RNA,* ribonucleic acid; *RT,* reverse transcriptase; *SARS,* severe acute respiratory syndrome; *ss* single-stranded.

Fungi

Fungi are eukaryotic microorganisms with the ability to form complex structures with thick rigid cell walls. They can grow as a mold with branched filaments or as a meshwork-type structure. Yeasts are a type of fungi with ovoid or spherical shapes. In contrast to bacteria, which have no organelles, the cytosol of fungi does contain organelles. Infections caused by fungi are called mycotic infections, or **mycoses.** Fungi cause infection first by colonizing the area. The fungus adheres to and proliferates on the site of infection. The next phase requires invasion of the epithelium. Anything that breaks the integrity of the skin (e.g., maceration) facilitates the invasion. Polymorphonuclear leukocytes attempt to phagocytize and digest the

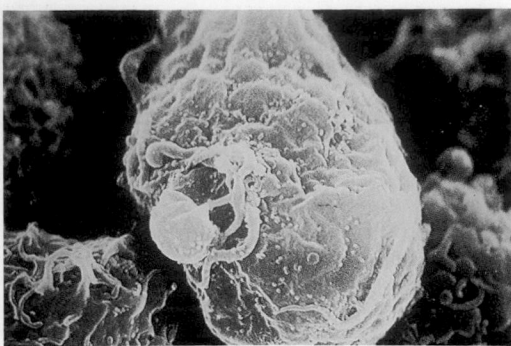

FIGURE 8-11 Scanning electron micrograph of HIV-1–infected T4 lymphocyte. Large numbers of HIV virions are budding from the plasma membrane of the lymphocytes. (Courtesy Centers for Disease Control and Prevention, Atlanta.)

invading fungi. Neutrophils, monocytes, and eosinophils can destroy fungi in the body.

Certain fungi live in the body as normal flora (e.g., *Candida*). When the body's defense mechanisms are compromised, they can overgrow and cause local or systemic infections. Patients who have been given antibiotics lose some of their normal flora along with the targeted pathogen. The fungi that are not affected by the antibiotic overgrow to fill that niche. Some patients suffering from AIDS, leukemia, alcoholism, drug abuse, and malnutrition or those being treated with immunosuppressive agents lack a well-functioning immune system that prevents fungi from overgrowing, and are therefore more susceptible to fungal infections (opportunistic fungi). When the environment contains more nutrients on which the fungi can grow, such as the hyperglycemic bloodstream of a diabetic patient or the vaginal tract of a female taking antibiotics, fungi can overgrow and cause infections. *Pneumocystis carinii* was reclassified as a fungus in 2006, and renamed to *Pneumocystis jiroveci*. This opportunistic infection is commonly associated with HIV disease.[9]

Superficial mycoses, such as those caused by dermatophytes (e.g., tinea pedis), occur only on superficial, dead, keratinized tissue like hair, epidermis, and nails. Cutaneous fungi do not invade the tissues but do result in an inflammatory response, as in *tinea pedis (athlete's foot)*. Subcutaneous mycoses occur when fungi are introduced into subcutaneous tissues and can be seen in ulcers or abscesses on the skin. Systemic infections are invasive to lungs and other organs (e.g., *Cryptococcus neoformans*). Systemic treatment is used more commonly for the immunocompromised patient or for the patient with disseminated disease because skin infection is usually self-limited. Topical antifungal drugs may be used to treat these superficial infections. Table 8-7 summarizes some examples of fungal infections.

Systemic mycoses may occur in both healthy and immunocompromised hosts. Because the fungi causing systemic infections are usually found in soil, these infections tend to be endemic to certain regions where the fungus is found. Infection is caused by inhalation of dust containing the fungus. Because of the endemic nature of these fungi, large segments of the population in the area may have been exposed and infected without any symptoms. If symptoms develop, they are usually self-limiting and mild. However, for those with compromised immune systems, the disease becomes severe and disseminated. Examples of systemic mycoses are histoplasmosis, blastomycosis, and coccidiomycosis.[12] *Histoplasma capsulatum* is a fungus that commonly occurs in soil in the central and eastern United States. *Histoplasma* also occurs in soil rich with chicken feces or bat guano. Humans and animals exposed to dust storms in endemic areas or contaminated with these feces are most likely to be infected. They may also have positive histoplasmin skin tests and may show calcified sites of infection in their lungs.[12]

Parasites

Parasites establish themselves with another organism and benefit from the other organism. They range in size from a small unicellular protozoan to large worms. Parasites are representative of four families of the animal kingdom: protozoa, or single-celled animals (Figure 8-12); nemathelminths, or roundworms; platyhelminths, or flatworms; and arthropoda, or invertebrate animals with jointed appendages. These parasites live on or in the human body during some part of their life cycle. Parasites and protozoa are rarely transmitted by human contact; usually they are disseminated through a vector where the parasite or protozoan spends part of its life cycle. For example, malaria (*Plasmodium* sp.) is transmitted by mosquitoes. Many of the protozoal infections are transmitted through contaminated water or food and require ingestion (e.g., *Giardia lamblia*). Some parasites have specific surface glycoproteins that influence their ability to enter macrophages.

Host resistance depends on macrophages, neutrophils, eosinophils, and platelets, which kill both protozoa and worms. T cells are required to develop immunity against these organisms. The symptoms of parasitic infection depend on the area in which the infestation develops. Protozoan infestation (amebiasis) of the gastrointestinal tract produces cramping, abdominal pain, and bloody diarrhea. Infestation of the blood produces fever, chills, rigor, and later anemia, all of which are associated with malaria (*Plasmodium* infection). Acute pruritus and rash occur after infection of the skin with *Sarcoptes scabiei* (scabies).[9]

Identification of the infectious agent is usually accomplished either by visualization of the adult parasite, by direct observation of the area (inspection of the skin or hair), or by microscopic examination of blood, feces, or tissue samples. Table 8-8 summarizes various parasitic infections of humans, including the common name, location, symptoms, and mode of transmission.

TABLE 8-6	COMPARISON OF VIRUSES AND OTHER MICROORGANISMS			
ORGANISM	GROWS IN NONLIVING MEDIA	CONTAINS BOTH DNA AND RNA	CONTAINS RIBOSOMES	SENSITIVE TO ANTIBIOTICS
Bacteria	Yes	Yes	Yes	Yes
Mycoplasmas	Yes	Yes	Yes	Yes
Rickettsiae	No	Yes	Yes	Yes
Chlamydiae	No	Yes	Yes	Yes
Viruses	No	No	No	No

TABLE 8-7 FUNGAL INFECTIONS

INFECTION	DISTRIBUTION	MODE OF TRANSMISSION	VECTOR	SYMPTOMS	PRIMARY SITE(S)	SECONDARY SITE(S)
Cryptococcosis	Everywhere	Inhalation	Pigeon feces	Fever, cough, weight loss, pleuritic pain, CNS disturbances	Pulmonary system	Meninges, skin, bone
Candidiasis	Normal flora	Ever present	N/A	Mucocutaneous pain and pruritus at site of infection	Fungemia, endocarditis	Kidneys, eyes, heart
Phycomycosis (mucormycosis)	Everywhere	Inhalation, ingestion, wound contamination	Decayed matter, soil	Rhinocerebral mucormycosis: destruction of CN II, IV, V, VI; erosion of carotid artery; meningitis; brain abscess. Pulmonary mucormycosis: dyspnea, chest pain, hemoptysis	Nose, brain, lung	Rare
Histoplasmosis	River valleys (e.g., California), southwestern USA (Arizona, Nevada)	Inhalation	Bird and bat feces	Flulike: cough, fever, myalgias, weight loss, anemia, leukopenia, thrombocytopenia, painful oropharyngeal ulcers	Pulmonary system	Bone marrow
Coccidioidomycosis (San Joaquin Valley fever)	Semiarid USA (e.g., California), southwestern USA (Arizona, Nevada)	Inhalation	Dust, dirt	Cough, fever, pleuritic chest pain, weight loss, dyspnea, chest pain, CNS disturbances	Pulmonary system	Skin, bone, joints, meninges
Blastomycosis	Southeastern USA, south central USA, midwestern USA, Great Lakes region	Inhalation	Unknown	Flulike: pleuritic chest pain, arthralgias, erythema nodosum, weight loss, fever, cough, chest pain	Pulmonary system	Skin, bone, joints, male GU tract
Aspergillosis	Everywhere	Inhalation	Decaying vegetation	Dyspnea, chest pain, hemoptysis, wheezing	Pulmonary system	Brain, kidney, liver

CN, Cranial nerve; *CNS,* central nervous system; *GU,* genitourinary; *N/A,* not applicable.

KEY POINTS

- Microorganisms responsible for infections in humans include bacteria, viruses, fungi, and parasites.
- Bacteria are characterized according to shape (cocci, rods, spirals), reaction to stains (gram negative, gram positive, acid fast), and oxygen requirements (aerobic, anaerobic).
- Viruses are small pieces of genetic material (DNA, RNA) with associated proteins and lipids. The smallest infective agents known, viruses are intracellular pathogens that use the host's energy sources and enzymes to replicate. Viral replication may or may not destroy the host cell. DNA viruses may be incorporated directly into the host genome. RNA viruses serve as templates for the production of viral RNA and proteins.
- Retroviruses are RNA viruses that contain a special enzyme called *reverse transcriptase* that mediates the synthesis of a DNA copy of the RNA virus. The DNA can then be incorporated into the host genome and passed on to daughter cells when the cell divides.
- Fungal infections can be superficial (e.g., ringworm, athlete's foot), subcutaneous (e.g., sporotrichosis), or systemic (e.g., histoplasmosis). Systemic fungal infections tend to be more serious and usually do not occur unless the host's immune system is compromised.
- Parasites include protozoa, helminthes (roundworms, flatworms), and arthropods. Manifestations of parasitic infections vary depending on the organism and site of infection. Common sites of parasitic infestation are the skin and gastrointestinal tract.

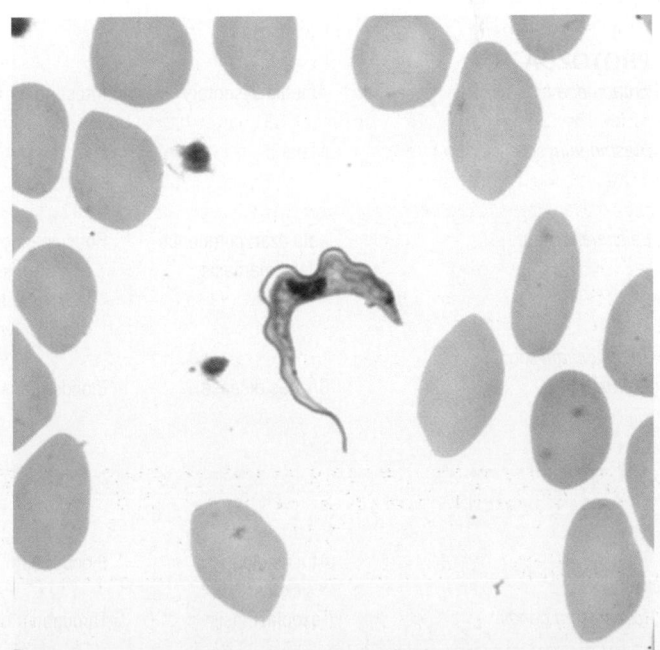

FIGURE 8-12 *Trypanosoma brucei* parasite in a blood smear. Giemsa-stained light photomicrograph. (Courtesy Blaine Mathison, Centers for Disease Control and Prevention, Atlanta.)

TABLE 8-8 PARASITIC INFECTIONS

PARASITIC AGENT	COMMON NAME OF DISEASE	LOCATION OF INFECTION	SYMPTOMS	MODE OF TRANSMISSION
HELMINTHS (WORMS)				
Nematodes (Roundworms)				
Ancylostoma duodenale	Hookworm	Blood vessels of gut	Anemia	Skin penetration
Ascaris lumbricoides	Giant roundworm	Small intestine, lungs	Pneumonitis (rare), intestinal obstruction (rare)	Oral (fecal contamination), autoinfection
Enterobius vermicularis	Pinworm	Cecum	Anal pruritus	Oral
Onchocerca volvulus	River blindness	Skin, eye	Blindness	Insect inoculation
Strongyloides stercoralis	Strongyloidiasis	Small intestine, lungs	Eosinophilia, urticaria, rash, abdominal pain, pneumonitis	Skin penetration, autoinfection
Trichinella spiralis	Trichinosis	Muscles	Muscular pain, eosinophilia, fever, periorbital edema	Oral (infected meat)
Trichuris trichiura	Whipworm	Intestine	Rectal prolapse	Oral (fecal contamination)
Wuchereria bancrofti	Filariasis	Lymphatics	Elephantiasis	Insect (mosquito)
Trematodes (Flukes)				
Clonorchis sinensis	Liver fluke	Liver	Biliary obstruction (rare)	Oral (raw fish)
Fasciola hepatica	Liver fluke	Liver	Fever, right upper quadrant abdominal pain, eosinophilia	Oral
Fasciolopsis buski	Intestinal fluke	Liver	Abdominal pain, diarrhea	Oral
Paragonimus westermani	Lung fluke	Lung, intestine	Eosinophilia, cough, chest pain, bronchitis	Oral (poorly cooked freshwater crab or crayfish)
Schistosoma haematobium	Blood fluke	Urinary tract	Acute: rash, fever, cough, chest pain, chills	Skin inoculation
Schistosoma japonicum	Blood fluke	Mesenteric blood vessels	Hepatomegaly, splenomegaly	Skin inoculation
Schistosoma mansoni	Blood fluke	Mesenteric blood vessels	Lymphadenopathy, eosinophilia	Skin inoculation
Cestodes (Tapeworms)				
Diphyllobothrium latum	Fish tapeworm	Intestine	Megaloblastic anemia	Oral (poorly cooked fish)
Taenia saginata	Beef tapeworm	Intestine	Mild abdominal pain	Oral (poorly cooked beef)
Taenia solium	Pork tapeworm	Intestine	Mild abdominal pain	Oral (poorly cooked pork)
Echinococcus granulosus	Hydatid cyst	Lung, liver	Cholestasis, liver congestion and atrophy, biliary obstruction	Oral (inoculation with sheep, cattle, or dog feces)
PROTOZOA				
Entamoeba histolytica	Amebic dysentery	Intestine	Bloody, mucoid diarrhea; colicky abdominal pain	Contaminated water, raw vegetables
Plasmodium spp.	Malaria	Liver, erythrocytes	High fever, chills, rigor, anemia, headache, malaise, chest pain, abdominal pain	Female *Anopheles* mosquito
Leishmania spp.	Kala azar; cutaneous leishmaniasis	Reticuloendothelial cells of body disseminates to spleen, liver, bone marrow, lymph glands	Chronic: abdominal discomfort, ascites, fever, weakness, pallor, weight loss, cough Acute: sudden fever, chills	All transmission accomplished through bite of sandflies after biting specific infected mammals
Trypanosoma spp.				
T. cruzi	Chagas disease	Bloodstream	Local inflammation, lymphadenopathy, muscular necrosis including myocardium (heart failure), esophagus, and colon (dilation); fever, malaise, anorexia, edema of face	Insects—hematophagous *Triatoma* (blood drinking)
T. brucei	African sleeping sickness	Bloodstream	Fever, malaise, headache, rash, CNS disturbances	*Glossina* flies (tsetse flies)
Toxoplasma gondii	Toxoplasmosis	Throughout body	Acute: usually asymptomatic Immunosuppressed: encephalitis, myocarditis, pneumonitis	Eating raw or undercooked meat, poultry, or dairy foods; oral inoculation with cat feces

TABLE 8-8 PARASITIC INFECTIONS—cont'd

PARASITIC AGENT	COMMON NAME OF DISEASE	LOCATION OF INFECTION	SYMPTOMS	MODE OF TRANSMISSION
Giardia lamblia	Epidemic diarrhea	Intestine	Newborn: impaired vision, neurologic disorders Acute: self-limited diarrhea; occasionally malabsorption with weight loss	Fecal contamination of water; person to person
Trichomonas vaginalis	Trichomoniasis (vaginitis)	Vagina	Irritation, discharge	Sexually transmitted
ECTOPARASITES **Pediculus humanus**				
Var. corporis	Body louse	All hair-covered parts of body	Pruritus Nits at base of hair shaft	Person to person, by fomites
Var. capitis	Head louse	Head area		
Pediculus pubis	Pubic louse	Pubic area		
Sarcoptes scabiei (var. hominis)	Scabies	Skin	Pruritus, worse at night; linear burrows in folds of fingers, elbows, knees, axillae, pelvic girdle	Person to person
Maggots (larvae of dipterous flies)	Myiasis	Necrotic tissue	Depends on location of infestation	Dipterous flies
Chiggers (mites)		Skin	Intense pruritus, hemorrhagic papules	Inhabit dogs, rabbits, cats, rats; foul cheese, flour, house dust
Ticks		Skin	Can transmit tick paralysis, Lyme disease	Reside in wooded and grassy areas

SUMMARY

The process of transmission of infection can be thought of as a chain with links that flow from the host or reservoir of the microorganism to the next susceptible victim. The goal of infection control is to block transmission of the microorganism to susceptible victims by severing the chain at one or more links.

Four basic types of microorganisms exist: bacteria, or single-celled organisms with cellular organelles that allow them to live independently in the environment; viruses, or tiny genetic parasites that require the host cell to replicate and spread; fungi that may cause superficial or sytemic mycotic infections; and parasites, which include protozoa, roundworms, flatworms, and arthropods. These organisms can be helpful or harmful to the host. When harmful, a microorganism is considered pathogenic. The study of pathogenic organisms and the way that they spread is called *epidemiology*.

The host-microbe relationship is determined by the characteristics of both the microorganism and the host. Microorganism factors that affect the relationship include the requirement for the microbe to kill the host cell in order to propagate, the reaction of the host to the invading microorganism and its endotoxins, and the ability of the microorganism to live independently from the host in the environment. Multiple host factors such as the integrity of barriers to transmission, nutritional status, age, and drug regimen all have an impact on this relationship.

Health care professionals have a key role in the prevention, surveillance, and early detection of infectious processes in hospital and community settings. The identification of high-risk individuals who are more susceptible to infection will assist in earlier detection of the manifestations of infection. Management of infections requires optimizing the client's host defense system and is supplemented by targeted pharmacologic and nutritional interventions.

REFERENCES

1. Mandell GL, Bennett JE, Dolin R: *Principles and practice of infectious diseases*, ed 6, Philadelphia, 2004, Churchill Livingstone.
2. Porta M: *Dictionary of epidemiology*, ed 5, New York, 2009, Oxford University Press.
3. WHO: *Global health risks: mortality and burden of disease attributable as elected major risks.* Available at www.who.int/healthinfo/global_burden_disease/GlobalHealthRisks_report_full.pdf/.
4. Merrill RM: *Introduction to epidemiology*, ed 5, Sudbury, MA, 2010, Jones and Bartlett.
5. Andresen E, Bouldin ED: *2010 Public health foundations concepts and practices*, San Francisco, 2010, Jossey-Bass.
6. Mandell GL, Bennett JE, Dolin R: *Mandell, Douglas and Bennett's principles and practice of infectious diseases*, ed 7, Philadelphia, 2009, Churchill Livingstone.
7. Heymann DL, Nunn M: *Control of communicable diseases manual*, ed 19, Washington, DC, 2008, American Public Health Association.
8. Garner JS: *Guideline for isolation precautions: preventing transmission of infectious agents in healthcare settings.* Available at www.cdc.gov/ncidod/dhaqp/guidelines/isolation2007.pdf.
9. McCance KL, Huether SE, Brasher VL, Rote NS: *Pathophysiology: the biologic basis for disease in adults & children*, ed 6, St Louis, MO, 2010, Mosby.
10. Deipirio JR, Talbert RL, Yee GC, Matzke GR, Wells BG, et al: *Pharmacotherapy: a pathophysiologic approach*, ed 8, New York, 2011, McGraw-Hill.
11. Kindt TJ, Osborne BA, Goldsby RA: *Kuby immunology*, ed 6, New York, 2006, WH Freeman.
12. Ryan K, Ray CG, Ahmad N, Drew WL, Plorde J: *Sherris medical microbiology*, ed 5, New York, 2010, McGraw-Hill.
13. Levinson W: *Review of medical microbiology and immunology*, ed 11, New York, 2010, McGraw-Hill.
14. *Nutrition and TB* from WHO, 2010. Available at www.who.int/nutrition/topics/meeting_nutrition_and_tb/en/index.html. Accessed 9/1/11.
15. Schiable UE, Kaufmann SHE: Malnutrition and infection: complex mechanisms and global impacts, *PLoS Med* 4(5):115, 2007.
16. Goldstein EJC: The interaction between nutrition and infection, *Clin Infect Dis* 46:1582–1588, 2008.
17. Halter J, Ouslander J, Tinetti M, Sudenski S, High K, et al: *Hazzard's geriatric medicine and gerontology*, ed 6, New York, 2009, McGraw-Hill.
18. McPhee SJ, Papadakis M, Rabow MW: *2011 Current medical diagnosis and treatment*, New York, 2011, McGraw-Hill.
19. *The plague.* Available at www.cdc.gov/ncidod/dvbid/plague/index.htm.
20. *Salmonella.* Available at www.cdc.gov/salmonella/.
21. *Pulmonary tuberculosis.* Available at www.ncbi.nlm.nih.gov/pubmedhealth/PMH0001141/.
22. *Travel guidelines.* Available at wwwnc.cdc.gov/travel/.
23. *Severe acute respiratory syndrome (SARS).* Available at www.ncbi.nlm.nih.gov/pubmedhealth/PMH0004460/.
24. Brooks G, Carroll KC, Butel J, Morse S, et al: *Jawetz, Melnick & Adleberg's medical microbiology*, ed 25, New York, 2010, McGraw-Hill.
25. Delves PJ, Martin SJ, Burton DR, Toitt IM: *Roitt's essential immunology*, ed 11, Boston, 2006, Blackwell Publishing.

Inflammation and Immunity

Jacquelyn L. Banasik

⊖volve WEBSITE

KEY QUESTIONS

- What are the major organs and cellular components of the body's defense against foreign antigens?
- How do immune cells communicate through cell-to-cell interactions and through secreted cytokines?
- How do innate and adaptive immune mechanisms differ?
- How do macrophages, granulocytes, and lymphocytes work together to locate, recognize, and eliminate pathogens?
- What is the role of MHC class I and II proteins in cell-mediated immunity?
- Why is an immune response usually more effective on subsequent exposure to an antigen than after the first exposure?
- How do noncellular immune system components, including antibodies, complement, and clotting factors, aid the immune response?

CHAPTER OUTLINE

The immune system is a complex network of cells and tissues that work together to protect the body against foreign invaders. The wide variety of potential pathogens requires a defense system that is diversified and adaptable. Several types of white blood cells (WBCs) are of primary importance in localizing, recognizing, and eliminating foreign substances. These immune cells are strategically situated in diverse locations so that pathogens may be detected quickly. The dispersed nature of these defensive cells necessitates a complex system of intercellular communication to effectively mobilize reinforcements to areas of need. A tremendous amount of information has accumulated about how immune cells communicate and the processes that enable them to migrate to particular locations. The impact of this research goes far beyond the traditional immune disorders such as immunodeficiency diseases and hypersensitivity reactions. The immune system has been implicated in the pathogenesis of disorders as diverse as atherosclerosis, myocardial infarction, shock, diabetes, and stroke. Therefore, an understanding of immune function is fundamental to the study of a wide variety of diseases. This chapter describes the organs and cells that constitute the immune system, the mechanisms of action of innate and adaptive defenses, and the communication processes whereby immune cells achieve a coordinated response. Underreactions and overreactions of the immune system, immune system malignancies, and human immunodeficiency virus disease are described in Chapters 10, 11, and 12, respectively.

COMPONENTS OF THE IMMUNE SYSTEM

The structures of the immune system include (1) skin and mucous membranes; (2) the mononuclear phagocyte system; (3) the lymphoid system, including spleen, thymus gland, and lymph nodes; and (4) bone marrow. All these structures are inhabited by different types of WBCs (leukocytes) that mediate **inflammation** and **immunity.** Leukocytes are responsible for locating and eliminating pathogens and foreign molecules. They are aided in their task of bodily defense by a number of chemical mediators, including **complement, kinins,** clotting factors, **cytokines, and chemokines.**

Components of the immune system are often categorized into specific or innate defenses according to the mechanisms whereby antigens are recognized. Innate defenses require no previous exposure to mount an effective response against an **antigen,** and a wide variety of different antigens are recognized. Natural killer (NK) cells and phagocytic cells such as **neutrophils** and **macrophages** are mediators of innate defenses. In contrast, specific defenses respond more effectively on second exposure to an antigen (adaptive) and are highly selective in the ability to recognize antigens. B lymphocytes (B cells) and T lymphocytes (T cells) are the agents of specific immunity.

Although separating immune components into specific and innate systems is helpful for studying inflammation and immunity, it is an artificial division because they function in a highly integrated manner.

The approach used in this chapter is to first describe the major components of the immune system, discuss innate and specific adaptive defenses separately, and then summarize the integrated function of the entire system and its regulation.

EPITHELIAL BARRIERS

The skin and mucous membranes are sometimes called the "first line of defense" because they are frequently the initial sites of microbial invasion. Intact epithelia in skin and mucous membranes provide mechanical and chemical barriers that prevent microorganisms from gaining access to the body's tissues. The skin epithelium produces antimicrobial peptides called *defensins* that can kill a wide variety of bacteria and fungi. The intestinal epithelium produces another form of bactericidal peptide called *cryptocidins* that prevent bacteria from colonizing the intestinal wall.[1] Resident microorganisms may aid in providing this line of defense by making conditions inhospitable for pathogens (see Chapter 8). Disruption of the normal epithelial barriers increases the likelihood that pathogens will successfully establish an infection. Physical trauma (e.g., burns, lacerations, erosions) and biochemical alterations (e.g., pH changes, increased glucose concentration, decreased enzyme production) predispose to infection. Pathogens that breach the skin or mucous membranes are generally first detected by cells of the mononuclear phagocyte system. These cells are thought to originate from monocytes produced in the bone marrow. Specialized antibody-secreting cells also locate to the mucous membranes where they produce antibodies of the immunoglobulin A (IgA) class. IgA antibodies bind antigens on the mucosal surface and prevent them from entering more deeply into the tissues.

MONONUCLEAR PHAGOCYTE SYSTEM

The mononuclear phagocyte system (previously called the reticuloendothelial system) is composed of dendritic cells, monocytes, and macrophages that are widely distributed throughout the body. Monocytes from the circulating blood migrate to organs and tissues to become macrophages. Macrophages are found throughout the body and are assigned various names according to the tissues in which they are located, such as alveolar macrophages in the lungs, microglial cells in the brain, Kupffer cells in the liver, and histiocytes in connective tissue (Figure 9-1). Dendritic cells are a monocyte-derived cell type that specializes in capturing and presenting antigens to T cells. Dendritic cells are strategically located in subcutaneous and submucosal tissues.

Macrophages and dendritic cells are often the first immune system cells to encounter a pathogen or foreign antigen after it has entered the body, and they are instrumental in communicating news of the invasion to other immune cells. This communication is accomplished through secretion of chemical signaling molecules called *cytokines* and

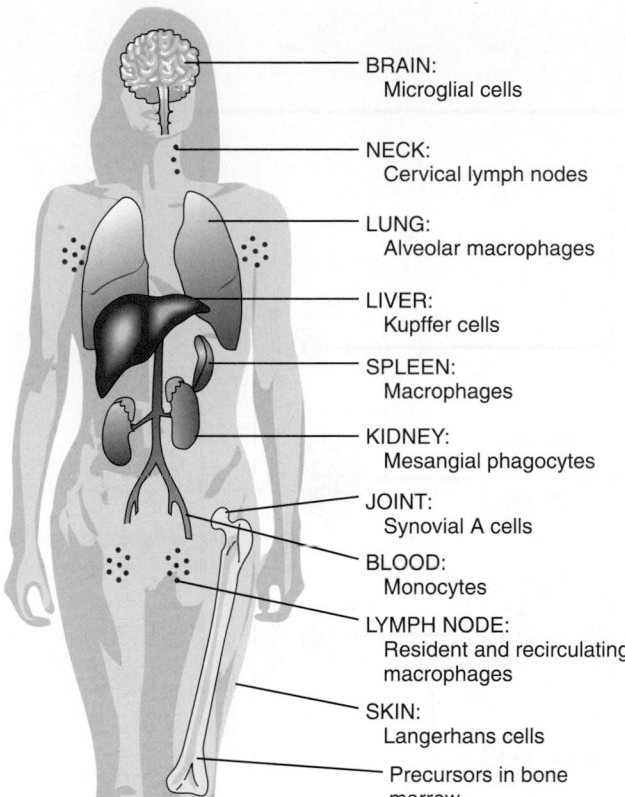

BRAIN:
Microglial cells

NECK:
Cervical lymph nodes

LUNG:
Alveolar macrophages

LIVER:
Kupffer cells

SPLEEN:
Macrophages

KIDNEY:
Mesangial phagocytes

JOINT:
Synovial A cells

BLOOD:
Monocytes

LYMPH NODE:
Resident and recirculating
macrophages

SKIN:
Langerhans cells

Precursors in bone
marrow

FIGURE 9-1 Cells of the mononuclear phagocyte system. (Redrawn from Schindler LW: *Understanding the immune system,* NIH Pub No. 92-529, Bethesda, MD, 1991, U.S. Department of Health and Human Services, p 9.)

by presentation of captured antigen to the specific, adaptive immune cells. Dendritic cells specialize in antigen presentation and are able to migrate quickly to lymphoid tissues when they have captured antigens. Macrophages have many other roles in the immune response in addition to their sentry function. Macrophages are powerful phagocytes, each capable of ingesting numerous microbes. Macrophages are called on to clean up the area in which dead neutrophils and inflammatory debris have accumulated after an inflammatory reaction, and they have a role in wound healing.

LYMPHOID SYSTEM

The primary lymphoid organs are the bone marrow and thymus gland, which are the structures where lymphocytes develop. All types of lymphocytes are produced from stem cells in the bone marrow (Figure 9-2). T lymphocytes then migrate to the thymus for development, whereas B lymphocytes and NK cells stay in the marrow to develop. NK cells are a population of lymphocytes that lack both T-cell and B-cell markers. NK cells are produced and released from the bone marrow and function in innate immune responses. NK cells are found mainly in the circulation and spleen. Once mature, T and B lymphocytes migrate to the secondary lymphoid organs where they await activation by antigens. Secondary lymphoid organs include the tonsils, spleen, lymph nodes, and Peyer patches (Figure 9-3).

Primary Lymphoid Organs

Bone marrow is contained in all the bones of the body. The primary function of bone marrow is **hematopoiesis,** or the formation of blood cells. There are two kinds of bone marrow: red and yellow. Hematopoiesis is

carried out by red (functioning) marrow. By adulthood, red marrow is confined to the pelvis, sternum, ribs, cranium, ends of the long bones, and vertebral spine. Yellow or fatty bone marrow is found in the remaining bones. It normally does not contribute to hematopoiesis in the adult, but can be recruited to become red marrow again under conditions of increased need for hematopoiesis.[2]

B lymphocytes (B cells) are produced and develop in the bone marrow. B cells migrate from the outer edges toward the center of the bone marrow as they develop. Pre-B cells are subjected to a highly selective quality control process, and less than 25% of the developing B cells are allowed to survive. During migration through the bone marrow, immature B cells are exposed to self antigens. B cells that do not bind to any antigens continue to develop into mature B cells. If immature B cells encounter antigens to which they bind while still in the bone marrow, a series of events is triggered to induce self-tolerance. The immature B cell is stimulated to reactivate the genetic recombination machinery in an attempt to produce a new B-cell receptor (BCR) that does not bind to self antigens. If this receptor editing attempt fails to alter binding sufficiently, the immature B cell will undergo apoptosis in the bone marrow.[3] Mature B cells that leave the bone marrow to colonize secondary lymphoid organs are called *naive* B cells because they have not yet encountered antigen.

T lymphocytes (T cells) develop in the thymus, which is located in the anterior mediastinum overlying the heart. Pre-T cells initially enter the outer aspect (cortex) of the thymus lobules, and many die while they migrate to the center (medulla) of the thymus. The selection process for T cells is even more rigorous than that for B cells; only about 5% of the cells entering the thymus survive to reenter the circulation and colonize secondary lymphoid organs. The thymus is relatively large at birth and steadily atrophies after puberty.[4] The thymus produces interleukin-7 (IL-7), a cytokine that promotes T cell proliferation.

Secondary Lymphoid Organs

Once mature, lymphocytes leave their primary lymphoid organs and travel through the blood to localize in peripheral, or secondary, lymphoid tissues, including lymph nodes, spleen, tonsils, and Peyer patches in the intestine. These naive T cells and B cells express specific receptor proteins on their cell surfaces that allow them to migrate or "home" to specific locations in lymph tissue. Most mature T lymphocytes are in constant circulation through lymphatic tissues and the bloodstream. It has been estimated that a lymphocyte makes a circuit from the blood to tissues to lymphatics and back to the bloodstream once or twice per day.[3] Antigens can be carried to the naive cells in the lymph nodes by the specialized antigen-presenting dendritic cells. When exposed to an appropriate antigen, T cells and B cells migrate toward each other within the lymph nodes and begin to proliferate. Activated T cells may then migrate to lymph vessels and travel to the bloodstream, where they are dispersed throughout the system. The majority of B cells stay in the lymph node, where they mature into antibody-secreting plasma cells. Lymphocyte recirculation and homing is regulated by binding interactions between various types of cell adhesion molecules (CAMs) including selectins, integrins, and addressins.[3]

Tonsils

Tonsils are aggregates of lymphoid tissue located in the mouth and pharynx. The tonsils are strategically located at the entrance to the digestive and respiratory tracts, where they are likely to encounter microorganisms. Unlike lymph nodes, tonsils have no afferent (incoming) lymphatic vessels. They do have efferent lymphatic drainage so that activated lymphocytes from the tonsils can migrate to other lymphoid organs. Tonsils normally make an important contribution to

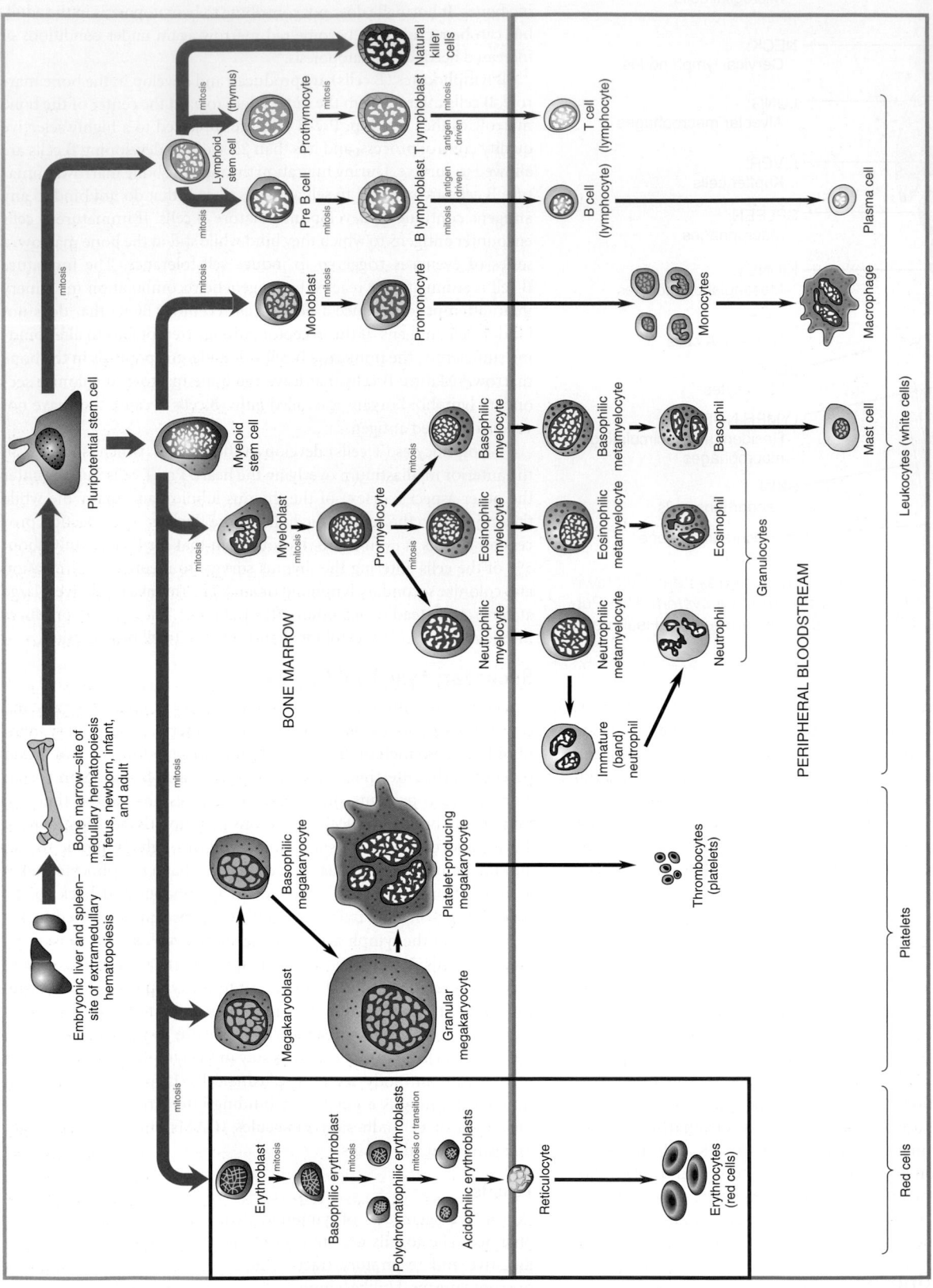

FIGURE 9-2 Maturation of human blood cells showing pathways of cell differentiation from the pluripotent stem cell to mature granulocytes, monocytes, lymphocytes, thrombocytes, and erythrocytes. Production begins in embryo blood islands in the yolk sac. As the embryo matures, production shifts to the liver, spleen, and bone marrow. In an adult, nearly all hematopoiesis occurs in the bone marrow. The two major differentiation pathways are the myeloid pathway and the lymphoid pathway. The lymphoid pathway produces lymphocytes, whereas the myeloid pathway produces granulocytes, monocytes, platelets, and red blood cells.

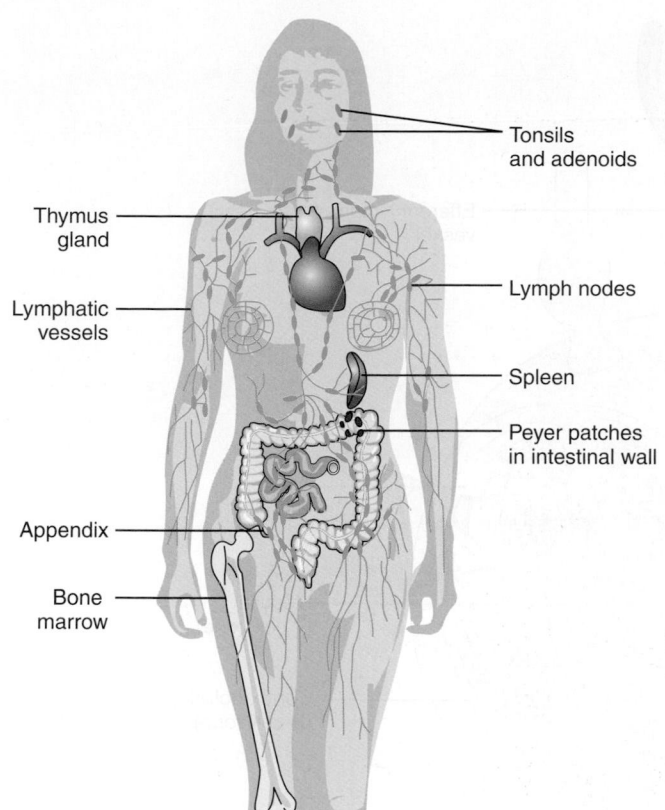

FIGURE 9-3 Principal organs of the lymphoid system.

Tonsils and adenoids

Thymus gland

Lymphatic vessels

Lymph nodes

Spleen

Peyer patches in intestinal wall

Appendix

Bone marrow

immune function; however, they may occasionally become chronically infected, and surgical removal (tonsillectomy) is then helpful.

Spleen

The spleen is located under the diaphragm on the left side of the body. It measures about 12 cm in length, which makes it the largest of the lymphoid organs. The spleen provides an important filtering function for blood. The tissue structure of the spleen is similar to that of lymph nodes. It is surrounded by a capsule of connective tissue and filled with a meshwork of red pulp and localized masses of lymphocytes called *white pulp*. Within the red pulp are many blood-filled sinuses lined with macrophages. Macrophages filter out foreign substances and old red blood cells. Lymphocytes located in the white pulp are in a strategic position to come in contact with blood-borne antigens. Lymphocytes thus activated in the spleen can migrate to other lymphoid organs via efferent lymphatics. Like the tonsils, the spleen does not have afferent lymphatic vessels.

Lymph Nodes and Lymphatics

The lymphatic vessels begin with small, closed-ended lymphatic capillaries in direct contact with the interstitial fluid surrounding cells and tissues. Lymphatics pick up fluid and proteins that escape the bloodstream and return them to the circulation by way of the right lymphatic and thoracic ducts. Along the way from lymphatic capillaries to the thoracic ducts, lymph flows through specialized structures called *lymph nodes*. Lymph nodes are found primarily in the neck, axilla, thorax, abdomen, and groin. They often become tender and palpable when responding to foreign invaders. Projections of connective tissue called *trabeculae* divide the interior of the lymph node into compartments (Figure 9-4). Lymph nodes contain large numbers of B and T lymphocytes and macrophages. B cells are the predominant cell type in

the cortical follicles, whereas T cells predominate in the area just under the cortex called the *paracortex*. The central region, or medulla, is populated by macrophages, B cells, and plasma cells (antibody-secreting B cells). Lymph fluid flows through the nodes in a way that allows these immune cells to filter, detect, and react to foreign material.

Peyer Patches

Aggregates of lymphoid tissue can be found scattered throughout the body, particularly in the gastrointestinal, respiratory, and urogenital tracts. These structures are analogous to lymph nodes, but they are not encapsulated and contain primarily B cells. Because of their location, these structures have been termed *mucosa-associated lymphoid tissue* (MALT) or *gut-associated lymphoid tissue* (GALT). These structures, also called *Peyer patches*, are of particular importance in producing antibodies to microorganisms that tend to invade mucosal tissue.

LEUKOCYTES

Leukocytes, or WBCs, are the primary effector cells of the immune system. Each of the different types of leukocytes found in blood has a special job to perform. All leukocytes, as well as red blood cells and platelets, are formed from stem cells in the bone marrow. Stem cells can produce daughter cells that differentiate along several different pathways to become mature cell types (see Figure 9-2). The first major differentiation step produces either a lymphoid stem cell or a myeloid stem cell. Lymphoid stem cells further differentiate to form B and T lymphocytes and NK cells. Myeloid stem cells can produce a variety of cell types, including red blood cells, platelets, monocytes, dendritic cells, and **granulocytes.** Monocytes that migrate from the blood into tissues are called *macrophages*. Granulocytes are further divided into neutrophils, eosinophils, and basophils. Basophils are precursors of the mast cells located in tissues.

Development of these cell types is influenced by hormonal signaling molecules called *cytokines*. Cytokines are produced locally in the bone marrow and by various other cells. Certain cytokines stimulate stem cell growth, proliferation, and differentiation into particular cell types. The WBC count and differential are commonly measured laboratory tests used to evaluate white blood cell production. A normal WBC count and differential are shown in Table 9-1. The general features of each of the WBC types are summarized in the following sections.

Neutrophils

Neutrophils are circulating granulocytes that are also known as *polymorphonuclear leukocytes* (polys or PMNs). They account for 60% to 80% of the total WBC count. Neutrophils normally have two to five nuclear lobes and coarse, clumped chromatin. Neutrophils arise from bone marrow stem cells and undergo several stages of maturation. As illustrated in Figure 9-2, these stages, from least to most mature, are myeloblast, promyelocyte, metamyelocyte, band cell, and mature segmented neutrophil.

Neutrophils stored in the bone marrow outnumber, by about 10-fold, the quantity of circulating neutrophils. An adult produces more than 1×10^{11} neutrophils each day.[1] These stored neutrophils are released into the circulation, where they have a half-life of 4 to 10 hours. Neutrophils that are not recruited into tissues within about 6 hours undergo programmed cell death (apoptosis). Neutrophils are early responders to an acute bacterial infection and arrive in large numbers very quickly. They are phagocytes that engulf and degrade microorganisms. Circulating neutrophils have receptors on their cell surfaces that enable them to bind to endothelial cells in areas of inflammation. These receptors, called *L-selectins*, allow neutrophils to adhere and roll along

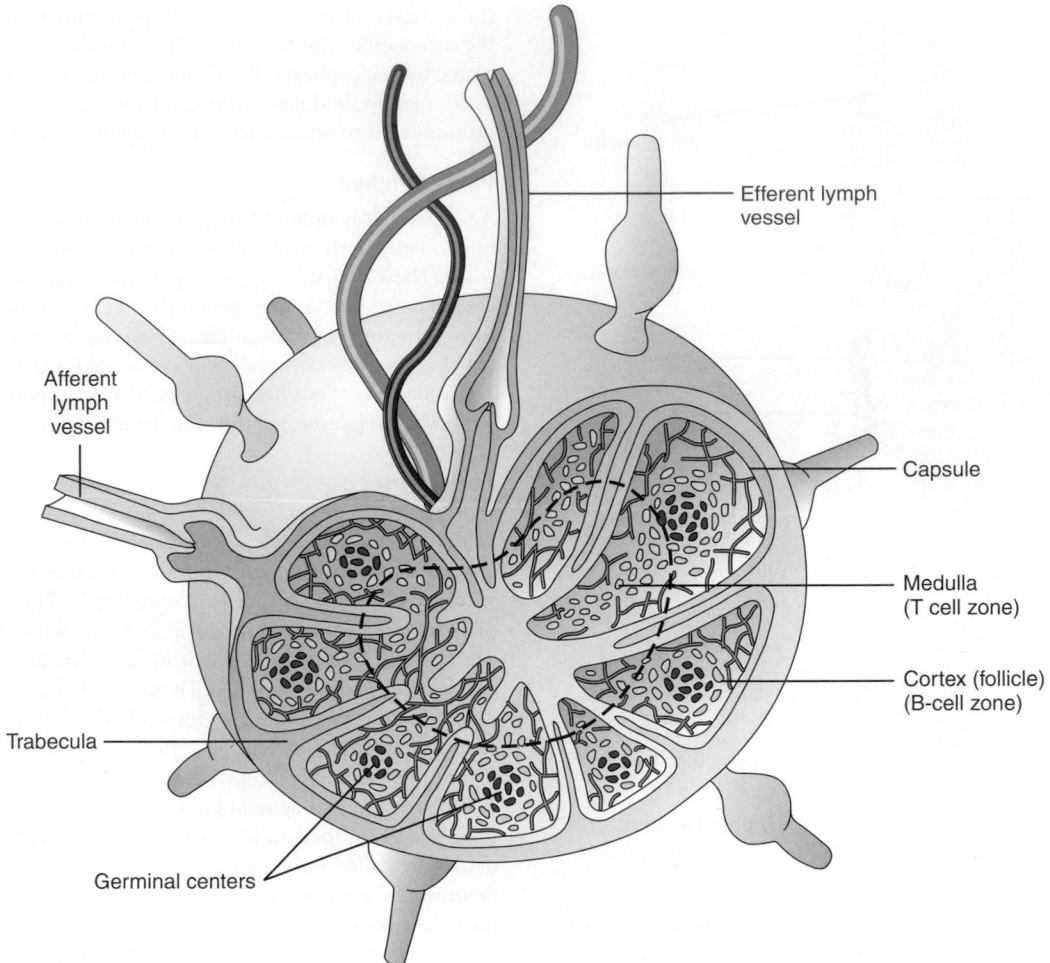

FIGURE 9-4 Schematic drawing of a typical lymph node showing afferent and efferent lymph vessels, as well as B-cell and T-cell zones.

TABLE 9-1	LEUKOCYTE PROPORTIONS AND FUNCTIONS	
TYPE	**PERCENTAGE***	**ROLE IN INFLAMMATION**
Neutrophils	60-80	First to appear after injury, phagocytosis
Lymphocytes	20-30	Immune response
Monocytes (macrophages)	3-8	Phagocytosis
Eosinophils	1-6	Allergic reactions, parasite infection
Basophils	0-2	Contain histamine, mediate type I allergic reactions, initiate inflammation

*Total white cell count, 3500 to 10,000/μL.

the capillary surface.[5] Other interactions between neutrophil integrin receptors and extracellular matrix then facilitate movement of neutrophils through the capillary wall and into the tissue. Neutrophils are attracted to areas of inflammation and bacterial products by **chemotactic** factors such as complement fragments and cytokines. This process is discussed in more depth in the section titled Inflammation.

Initially during an acute infection, **neutrophilia,** or an increase in the number of circulating neutrophils, occurs as the bone marrow releases stored neutrophils. As neutrophils are consumed and demand exceeds production, an increase in the number of immature (band) neutrophils occurs. Bands are identified by their lack of nuclear segmentation. This increase in band cells is referred to as a "shift to the left of normal" (Figure 9-5). Traditionally, the band count has been used to differentiate bacterial from viral infections, and a greater shift to the left is viewed as a more severe infection. The utility of using the band count for these purposes has been called into question because the specificity is poor.[6]

Neutrophils produce potent chemical mediators that enable them to destroy microorganisms. Numerous toxins released by neutrophils have been identified, including oxidizing free radicals, defensins, and proteolytic enzymes, such as elastase.[7] Because of the ability to generate free radicals and release enzymes, neutrophils can cause extensive damage to normal tissue during their inflammatory response.

Eosinophils

Eosinophils are circulating granulocytes that have two nuclear lobes and stain brilliant red-orange with eosin. They constitute 1% to 6% of the total WBC count. Eosinophils mature in the bone marrow (3 to 6 days) and circulate in the blood for about 30 minutes. They have a half-life of 12 days in tissue. Eosinophils arise from myeloid stem cells and undergo a maturation process similar to that of neutrophils.

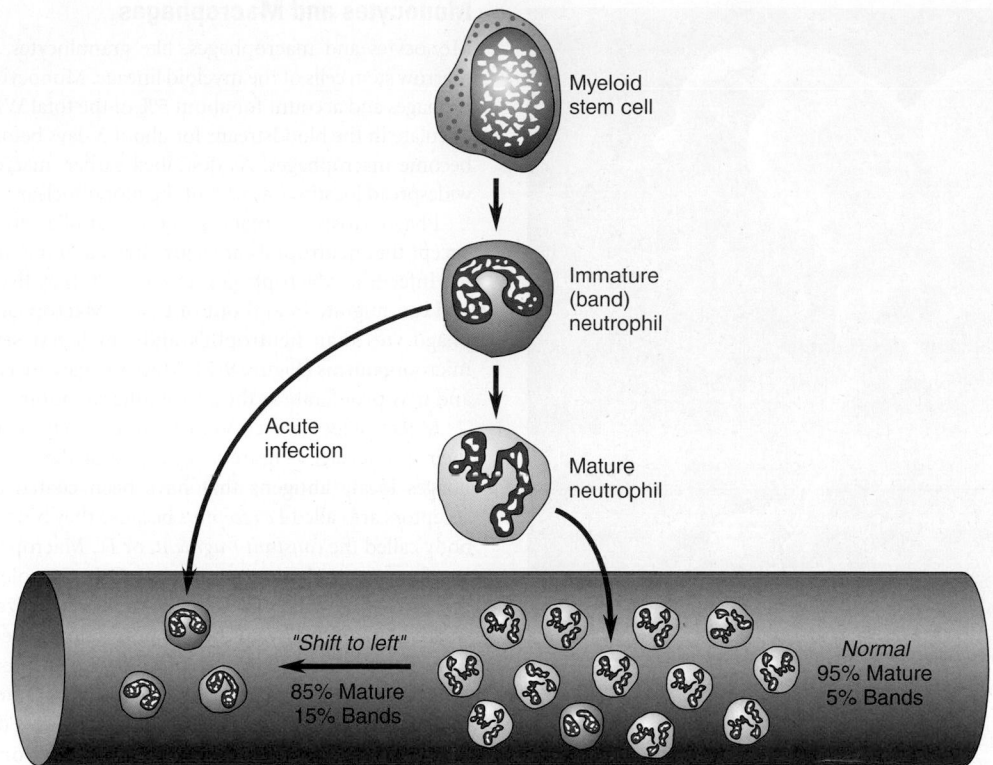

Myeloid
stem cell

Immature
(band)
neutrophil

Mature
neutrophil

Acute
infection

"Shift to left"

85% Mature
15% Bands

Normal
95% Mature
5% Bands

FIGURE 9-5 Inflammatory cytokines stimulate the release of more immature neutrophils, called *bands,* from the bone marrow. An increased ratio of bands to mature neutrophils is termed a "shift to the left." This clinical term evolved from the practice of listing bands to the left of mature cells on the laboratory report sheet. A shift to the left is commonly seen with acute bacterial infections.

Eosinophils are particularly associated with an increase in number during allergic reactions and infection by intestinal parasites. The role of eosinophils in allergic reactions is less well characterized than that of mast cells. Eosinophils are recruited into areas of inflammation by the chemokine eotaxin, which is produced by epithelial cells.[3] Eosinophils release inflammatory chemicals, such as lysosomal enzymes, peroxidase, major basic protein, and cationic protein. The primary function of eosinophils is to kill parasitic helminths (worms). Helminths are too large to be phagocytosed by neutrophils or macrophages, and their exterior is resistant to attack by complement or mast cell products. Eosinophils produce specialized molecules such as major basic protein and eosinophil cationic protein, which may be more effective against helminths.[1] Eosinophils recognize helminths that have been opsonized (coated) with IgE antibody. They bind to the IgE and then release their stored chemicals onto the surface of the opsonized helminth. Parasitic infections are a significant problem in much of the world, with one third of the population being affected.

Basophils and Mast Cells

Basophils are granulocytes characterized by granules that stain blue with basophilic dyes. Basophils account for 0% to 2% of the total leukocyte count. Basophils are structurally similar to mast cells. Mature basophils circulate in the vascular system, whereas mast cells are found in connective tissue, especially around blood vessels and under mucosal surfaces. When stimulated by cytokines, mature basophils can migrate to connective tissue, but once in the tissue, basophils (then called mast cells) do not reenter the circulation.

The average basophil life span is measured in days, whereas mast cells can live for weeks to months. Mast cells and basophils have IgE receptors that allow them to bind and display IgE antibodies on their cell surfaces. When an appropriate stimulus occurs, such as antigen binding to the IgE antibodies, mast cells and basophils release granules (**degranulate**) containing proinflammatory chemicals.

Mast cell and basophil granules contain histamine, platelet-activating factor, and other vasoactive amines that are important mediators of immediate hypersensitivity responses (Figure 9-6). Degranulation of mast cells and basophils begins the inflammatory response that is characteristically associated with allergic reactions. Mast cells and basophils are also involved in wound healing and chronic inflammatory conditions (see Chapter 10).

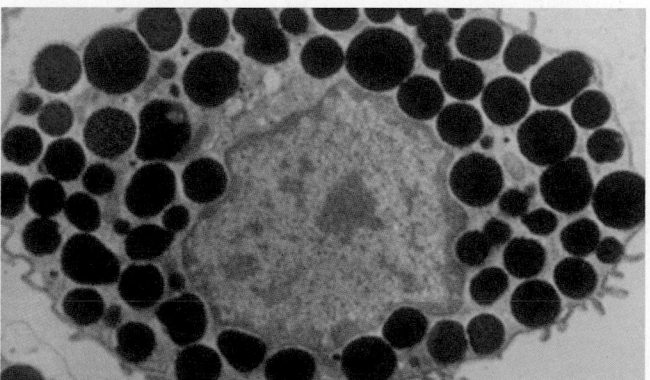

FIGURE 9-6 Micrograph of a mast cell showing a large yellow nucleus and numerous packets containing histamine, which are colored red. (Roitt IM, Brostoff Male, DK: *Immunology,* ed 3, St Louis, 1993, Mosby.)

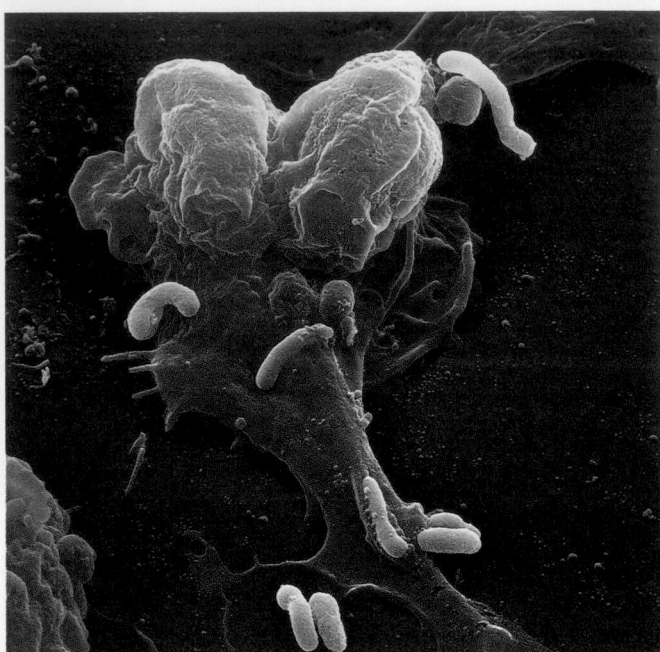

FIGURE 9-7 Scanning electron micrograph of a macrophage *(red)* attaching to and phagocytizing bacteria *(yellow)*. (From Nairn R, Helbert M: *Immunology for medical students,* ed 2, St Louis, 2007, Mosby, p 3. With permission from Juergen Berger, Max-Planck Institute, and the Science Photo Library.)

Monocytes and Macrophages

Monocytes and macrophages, like granulocytes, originate from bone marrow stem cells of the myeloid lineage. Monocytes are immature macrophages and account for about 5% of the total WBC count. Monocytes circulate in the bloodstream for about 3 days before they enter tissue to become macrophages. As described earlier, macrophages are found in widespread locations as part of the mononuclear phagocyte system.

Phagocytosis by macrophages is similar to that by neutrophils except that neutrophils are short-lived and die in the process of fighting infection. Macrophages, in contrast, may live for months to years and can migrate in and out of tissue. Macrophages are more efficient phagocytes than neutrophils and can ingest several times as many microorganisms (Figure 9-7). Macrophages are capable of cell division and may proliferate at the site of inflammation.

Macrophages are covered with a variety of receptor proteins on their cell surface (Figure 9-8). Some of these receptors help macrophages locate antigens that have been coated by antibodies. These receptors are called *Fc receptors* because they bind to the part of an antibody called the *constant fragment,* or *Fc.* Macrophages also have receptors for the complement component C3b. Complement, like antibodies, can coat an antigen and make it more recognizable to macrophages. Coating of antigen by antibodies or by complement is called **opsonization.** Macrophages have receptors that help them recognize bacteria directly. These innate pattern-recognition receptors bind to particular molecules prevalent in the bacterial cell wall. For example, mannose receptors and numerous Toll-like receptors on macrophages allow them to recognize common microbial structures (see Figure 9-8).

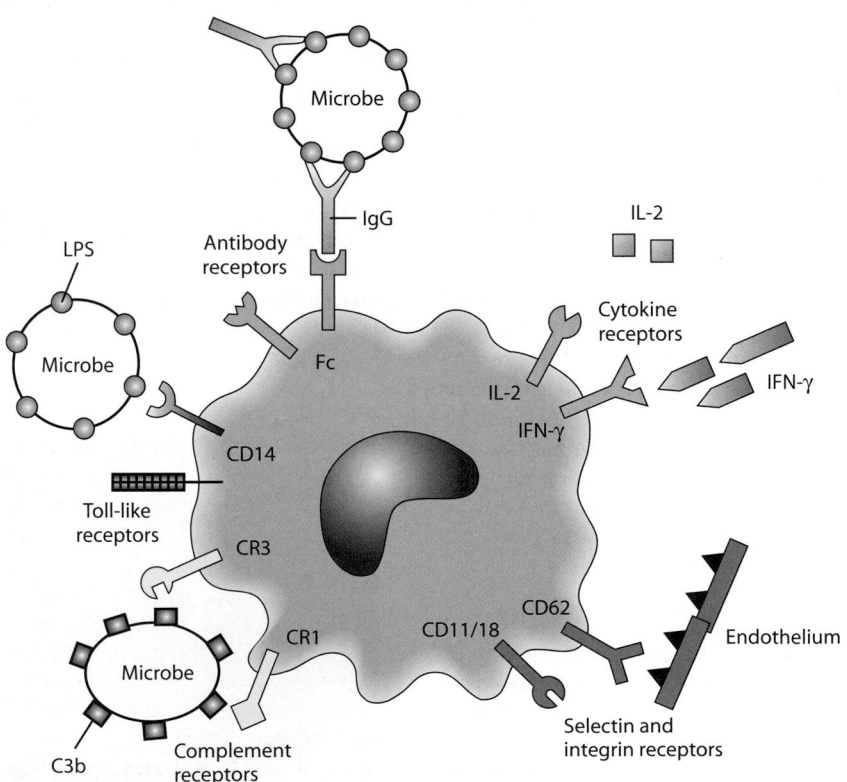

FIGURE 9-8 Macrophage surface receptors. Macrophages display receptors for a number of extracellular molecules that enhance their function such as cytokines, complement, selectins, integrins, and antibody *(Fc).* Toll-like receptors recognize patterns of microbial components and trigger intracellular signaling cascades in the macrophage. *IFN-γ,* Interferon-γ; *IL,* interleukin; *LPS,* lipopolysaccharide.

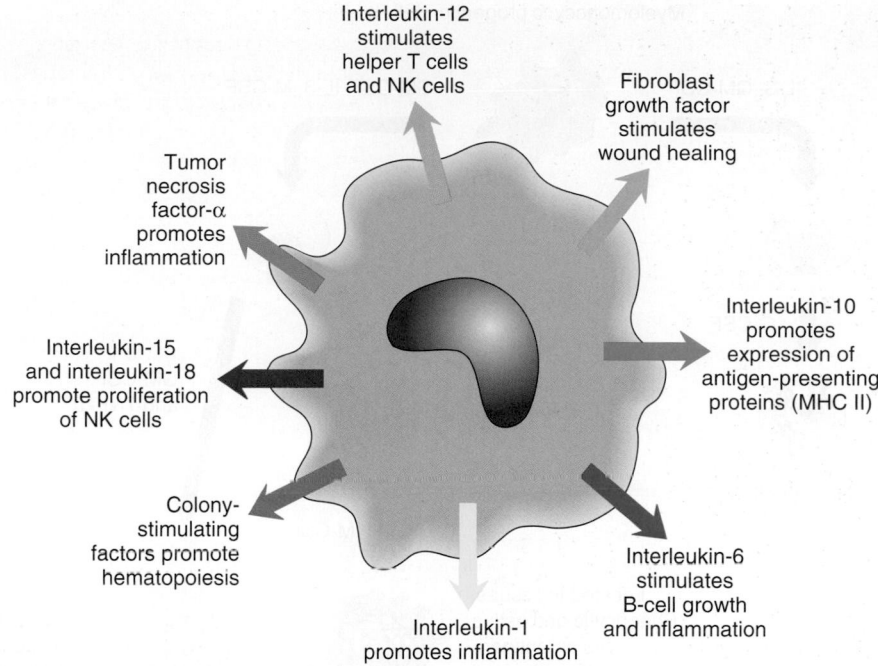

FIGURE 9-9 Macrophages are of central importance in initiating inflammation and recruitment of other leukocytes to areas of need. Macrophages secrete a variety of cytokines that induce inflammation and chemotaxis. Some macrophage cytokines stimulate the growth and differentiation of other white blood cell types.

Other receptors, called *selectins* and *integrins,* help macrophages adhere to capillary walls, and enter and move through tissue. Integrin receptors bind to proteins in the extracellular matrix and help macrophages target or "home" to certain areas.

In addition to their phagocytic function, macrophages have important secretory function. Some of the substances secreted by macrophages are cytokines, which help to coordinate the activities of other immune cells (Figure 9-9). Macrophage cytokines include IL-1, IL-6, IL-12, and tumor necrosis factor-α (TNF-α). These cytokines promote inflammation, as well as the activity of other WBCs, including neutrophils and lymphocytes (see the section titled Cytokines and Chemokines).

Macrophages secrete a number of proteins that are important in wound healing. Some of these proteins are enzymes that degrade tissue (e.g., collagenase, elastase, plasminogen activator), whereas others stimulate the growth of new granulation tissue (e.g., fibroblast growth factor, angiogenic factors).

A third function of macrophages, in addition to phagocytosis and secretion, is antigen presentation. For T cells to recognize antigens, these antigens must first be processed and presented on the surface of an antigen-presenting cell such as dendritic cells, macrophages, or B cells. Macrophages accomplish this task by first engulfing the antigen, then processing it into smaller pieces, and finally combining the antigen fragments with special membrane proteins. The antigen complexes are then displayed on the macrophage cell surface, where T lymphocytes (T helper cells) can recognize and become activated by them. Antigen presentation is explored in more detail in the section titled Specific Adaptive Immunity.

Dendritic Cells

Dendritic cells are derived in the bone marrow from the same progenitor cells that produce monocytes and macrophages (Figure 9-10) and are structurally and functionally similar to macrophages (Figure 9-11). Dendritic cells derive their name from an unusual shape that has extensive projections from the surface. Dendritic cells are located throughout the body as part of the mononuclear phagocyte system. They function primarily as antigen-presenting cells, capturing antigen in tissues and then migrating to lymphoid areas to present antigen to T cells. Some types of dendritic cells produce chemical messengers called *type I interferon* (IFN-α and IFN-β) in response to viral infections. Type I interferons suppress the viral replication machinery in nearby cells and help stop the local spread of the virus.

Lymphocytes

The three major types of lymphocytes are NK cells, T cells, and B cells. NK cells function in innate immunity, whereas B and T lymphocytes are the cells responsible for specific, adaptive immunity. B and T cells have the capacity to proliferate into "memory cells," which provide long-lasting immunity against specific antigens. NK, T, and B cells are derived from a common lymphoid stem cell in the bone marrow that is stimulated to proliferate by bone marrow–derived cytokines including IL-7. T cells then migrate to the thymus, where they mature. B cells remain in the bone marrow during their maturation phase. NK cells are released into the circulation. Together NK, B, and T lymphocytes compose approximately 20% of the total WBC count. Mature NK cells circulate and populate the spleen, whereas T and B cells migrate to secondary lymphoid organs.

Structurally, lymphocytes are small, round cells with a large, round nucleus. Despite their relatively uniform appearance, lymphocytes can be sorted into a number of subpopulations based on characteristic surface proteins called *cluster of differentiation (CD) markers*. More than 350 different CD markers have been identified thus far, with different immune cell types displaying different combinations on their cell surfaces. Lymphocytes have many complex and differentiated functions, and only the major lymphocyte subtypes are discussed in this chapter.

Natural Killer Cells

NK cells have no B- or T-cell markers and are not dependent on the thymus for development. NK cells are considered to be innate immune

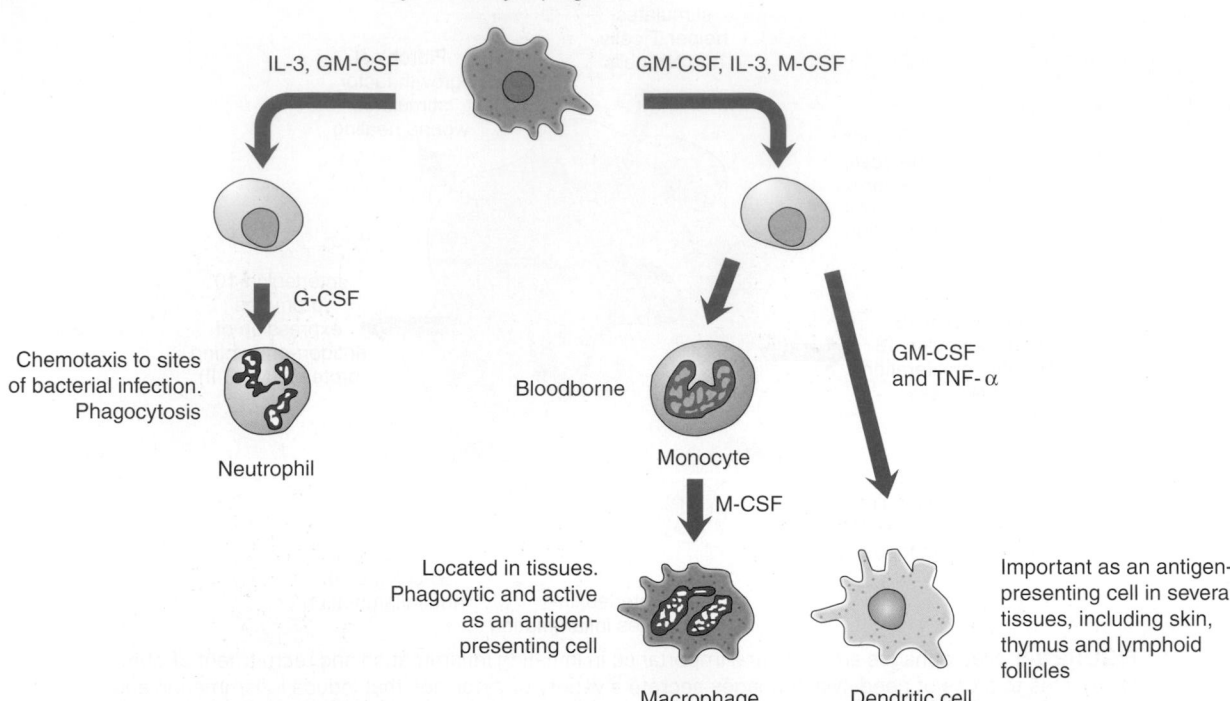

Myelomonocytic progenitor cell

IL-3, GM-CSF   GM-CSF, IL-3, M-CSF

G-CSF

Chemotaxis to sites
of bacterial infection.
Phagocytosis

Neutrophil

Bloodborne

Monocyte

M-CSF

GM-CSF
and TNF-α

Located in tissues.
Phagocytic and active
as an antigen-
presenting cell

Important as an antigen-
presenting cell in several
tissues, including skin,
thymus and lymphoid
follicles

Macrophage   Dendritic cell

FIGURE 9-10 Development of dendritic cells from a myelomonocytic progenitor cell and precursor cells in common with monocytes and macrophages. (Redrawn from Nairn R, Helbert M: *Immunology for medical students,* ed 2, St Louis, 2007, Mosby, p 81.)

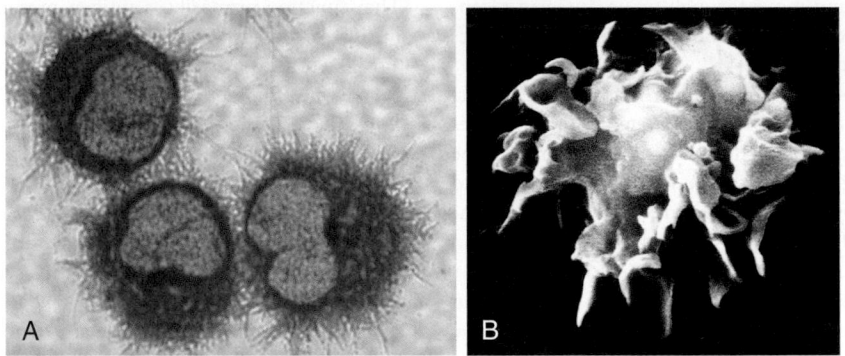

FIGURE 9-11 Dendritic cell morphology. **A,** Light micrograph of resting dendritic cells from the bone marrow. **B,** Scanning electron micrograph of a mature dendritic cell showing extensive projections of the cell membrane. (From Abbas AK, et al: *Cellular and molecular immunology,* ed 7, Philadelphia, 2012, Saunders, p 115. Courtesy of Dr. Y-J Liu, MD, Anderson Cancer Center, Houston, TX.)

cells because they can effectively kill tumor cells and virally infected cells without previous exposure. NK cells kill their target cells by a mechanism similar to that used by cytotoxic T cells. Unlike T and B cells, NK cells can respond to a variety of antigens and are therefore not specific for a particular antigen. Like neutrophils and macrophages, NK cells recognize antibody-coated target cells with their Fc receptors. This process is called *antibody-dependent cell-mediated cytotoxicity* (ADCC). NK cells also target virally infected cells and tumor cells. They are thought to be able to recognize virally infected cells through innate pattern-recognition receptors; however, only those cells that lack certain normal self proteins on their cell surface (major histocompatibility complex I, or MHC I, proteins) are targeted for killing.[3] Cells that display normal MHC I on their cell surfaces are protected from NK cell cytotoxicity, but will be susceptible to killing by cytotoxic T cells that recognize viral antigen displayed on the MHC I proteins.

T Lymphocytes

Two major classes of T lymphocytes can be differentiated by the presence or absence of CD4 and CD8 surface proteins (Figure 9-12). T cells that possess CD4 proteins (CD4+) are called T helper cells. T helper cells interact with antigens presented on the surface of specialized antigen-presenting cells such as dendritic cells, macrophages, and B cells. T helper cells can be further divided into subclasses called T_H1, T_H2, and T_H17 based on the types of cytokines that they secrete (Figure 9-13). The T_H1 subset of T helper cells develops in response to IL-12 from macrophages and, when activated, secretes cytokines that activate other T cells (IL-2) and macrophages (interferon-γ [IFN-γ]). T_H2 cells develop in response to IL-4 from activated T helper cells and secrete cytokines that stimulate B-cell proliferation and antibody production (e.g., IL-4, IL-5, IL-10, IL-13).[8] The T_H17 subclass, as its name implies, secretes IL-17, which is a proinflammatory cytokine.

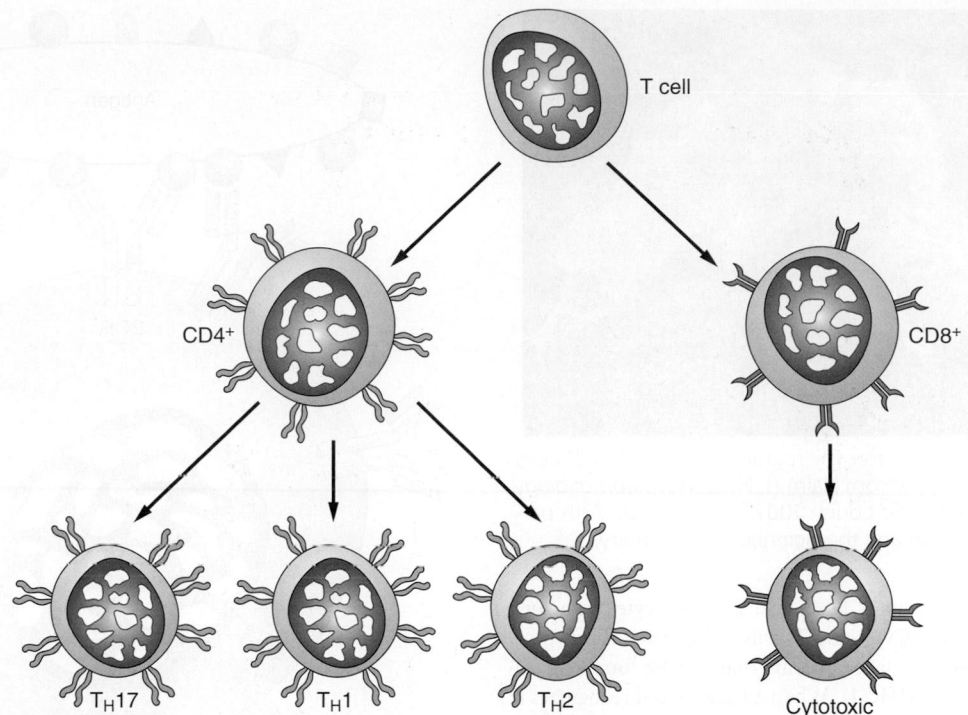

FIGURE 9-12 Two major classes of T lymphocytes can be differentiated by CD markers on the cell surface. T helper cells have CD4 markers, whereas cytotoxic T cells have CD8 markers. CD4 cells can be further differentiated into T_H1, T_H2 and T_H17, which secrete different cytokines. CD8 cells are cytotoxic T cells.

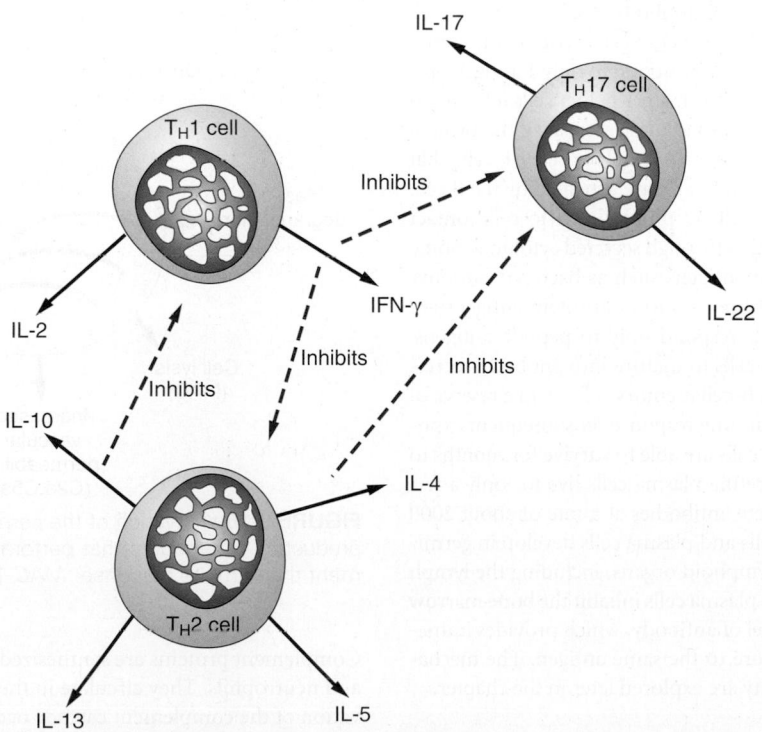

FIGURE 9-13 Three types of T helper cells, T_H1, T_H2, and T_H17 secrete different cytokines. T_H1 cells secrete interleukin-2 and interferon-γ, which stimulate T cells and macrophages. T_H2 cells secrete a number of cytokines that affect B cells. T_H17 cells secrete a proinflammatory cytokine, IL-17. T_H1, T_H2, and T_H17 cells inhibit the release of cytokines from one another and thus help regulate the immune response. *IFN-γ*, Interferon-γ; *IL*, interleukin.

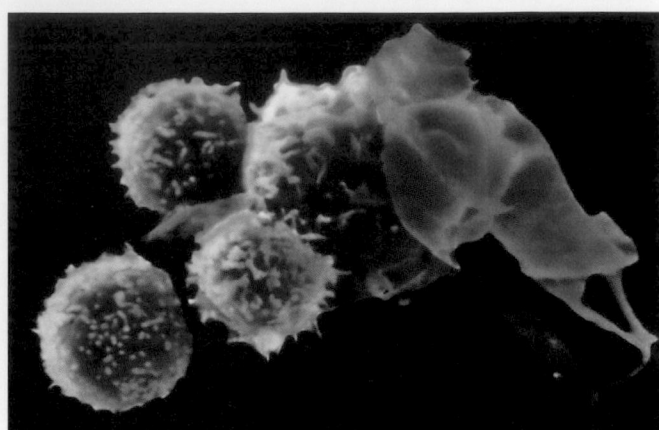

FIGURE 9-14 Scanning electron micrograph of activated T cells *(blue)* and a tumor cell *(red)*. (From Nairn R, Helbert M: *Immunology for medical students,* ed 2, St Louis, 2007, Mosby, p 3. With permission from BSIP Lecaque and the Science Photo Library.)

The presence of CD8 protein (CD8$^+$) on a T lymphocyte characterizes it as a cytotoxic T cell. Cytotoxic T cells recognize antigen presented in association with surface proteins that can be found on all nucleated cells of the body (MHC I). When a CD8$^+$ T cell recognizes a foreign antigen on a cell, the antigen-presenting cell is killed, thus the name *cytotoxic T cell.* CD8$^+$ cells are particularly effective at destroying virally infected cells, foreign cells, and mutant cells (Figure 9-14). Proliferation of activated cytotoxic T cells is enhanced by T helper cell cytokines, particularly IL-2.

B Lymphocytes

B cells are distinguished from other lymphocytes by their ability to produce antibodies and by the presence of antibody-like receptors (B-cell receptors [BCRs]) on their cell surfaces. Each B cell carries many copies (100,000) of identical BCRs and is able to respond to only 1 antigen **epitope**[9] (Figure 9-15). B cells require "help" from T helper cells to respond efficiently to protein antigens. B cells bind and internalize the protein antigen, and then process and present it to T helper cells. T cells that recognize the presented peptides bind to and are activated by the B cell. T-cell help is provided to the B cell by physical cell-to-cell contact through coreceptor binding, as well as through secreted cytokines. Some B cells can respond to nonprotein antigens such as bacterial carbohydrate and lipid molecules. B-cell responses to nonprotein antigens are T-cell independent because T cells respond only to peptide antigens. Exposure to antigens stimulates B cells to mature into antibody-secreting plasma cells and memory cells. B-cell memory cells form a reserve of cells that can quickly mount an immune response on subsequent exposure to the same antigen. Memory cells are able to survive for months to years, whereas most antibody-secreting plasma cells live for only a few days. Plasma cells are able to secrete antibodies at a rate of about 2000 per second per cell.[9] Memory B cells and plasma cells develop in germinal centers located in secondary lymphoid organs, including the lymph nodes and spleen. A few long-lived plasma cells inhabit the bone marrow and continue to produce a low level of antibody, which provides immediate protection on second exposure to the same antigen. The mechanisms of specific adaptive immunity are explored later in the chapter.

CHEMICAL MEDIATORS OF IMMUNE FUNCTION

Complement

The complement system consists of about 20 plasma proteins that interact to enhance inflammation, chemotaxis, and lysis of target cells.

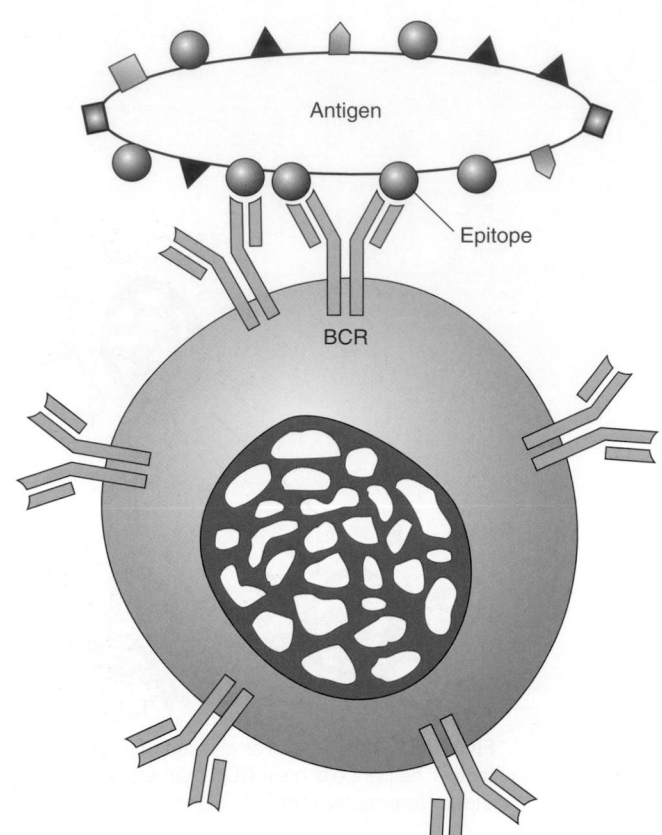

FIGURE 9-15 Typical B cell showing a number of identical B-cell receptors *(BCRs)* on the cell surface. Each BCR is capable of binding to two identical antigen epitopes.

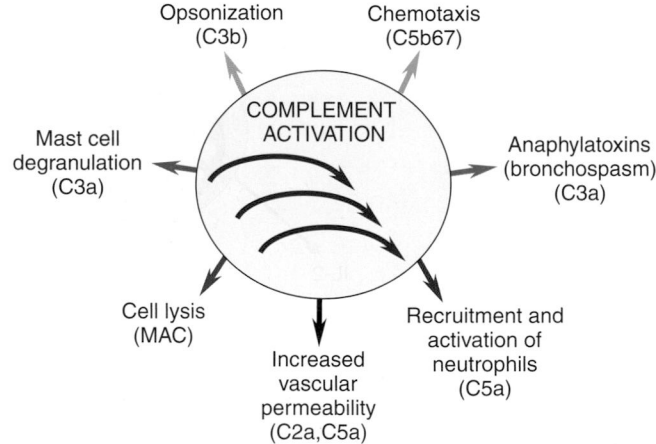

FIGURE 9-16 Activation of the complement cascade results in the production of products that perform a variety of functions to augment the immune response. *MAC,* Membrane attack complex.

Complement proteins are synthesized in the liver and by macrophages and neutrophils. They circulate in the blood in an inactive form. Activation of the complement cascade occurs via three different pathways: classical, alternative, and lectin. In all three pathways, the inactive complement proteins are converted to their active form in a sequence of reactions. Major actions of complement proteins include cell lysis, facilitation of phagocytosis by opsonization, inflammation, and chemotaxis (Figure 9-16).

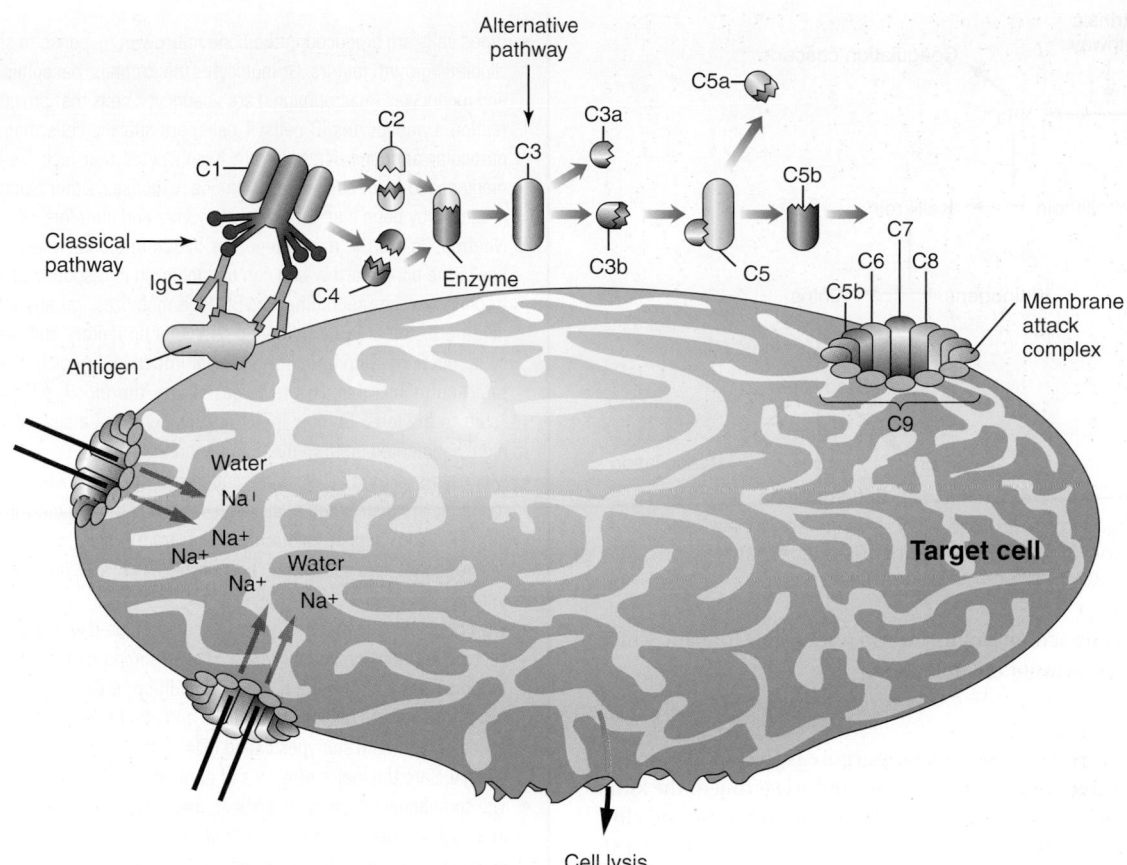

FIGURE 9-17 Complement cascade. The cascade is activated by the first complement molecule, C1, which binds an antigen-antibody complex. This event begins a domino effect, with each of the remaining complement proteins performing its part in the attack sequence. The end result is a hole in the membrane of the offending cell and destruction of the cell. Activation of the complement cascade results in the formation of membrane attack complexes that insert in the cell membrane. These pore-like structures allow sodium and water influx, which causes the cell to swell and rupture. (Redrawn from Schindler LW: *Understanding the immune system*, NIH Pub. No. 92-529, Bethesda, MD, 1991, U.S. Department of Health and Human Services, p 11.)

The classical pathway is usually triggered by IgG or IgM antibody-antigen complexes. The alternative pathway can be initiated on first exposure to an antigen. Lipopolysaccharide, in bacterial cell walls, and bacterial endotoxin are effective triggers of the alternative pathway. In the classical pathway, an antibody hooked onto an antigen combines with C1, the first of the complement proteins. This step sets in motion a domino effect called the *complement cascade* (Figure 9-17). The alternative pathway begins with the activation of C3. The alternative pathway can be activated on first exposure and is part of the innate immune response.[10] The lectin pathway also can be triggered on first exposure. Lectin is a circulating biomolecule that binds mannose on bacterial cell walls and triggers complement activation at C2 and C4. C3 spontaneously degrades into active C3b fragments in plasma. If microbial cell surfaces are present, the C3b fragment can bind directly to the microbe. Two other complement proteins, factors B and D, combine with C3b to initiate the alternative pathway. C3 is the most important and plentiful of the complement proteins. C3 divides into two fragments called C3a and C3b. C3a is a proinflammatory protein that causes histamine release from mast cells, contraction of smooth muscle, and increased endothelial cell permeability. C3b initiates the next step in the cascade by cleaving C5 into its active fragments C5a and C5b. Complement protein fragment C5a is both a powerful inflammatory chemical and a potent chemotactic agent. C5a chemotaxis stimulates neutrophils and monocytes to migrate to the inflamed tissue. C5a also activates

neutrophils by triggering their oxidative activity and increasing their glucose uptake.

The C5b fragment combines with C6, C7, C8, and multiple units of C9 to form a large porelike structure (C5b6789) called the *membrane attack complex*. The membrane attack complex has a direct cytotoxic effect by attacking cell membranes and disrupting the lipid bilayer. This action allows free movement of sodium and water into the target cell, which causes it to rupture (see Figure 9-17). The complement system is a potent inflammatory and cytotoxic system that is carefully regulated by eight known inhibitory factors.[3] Normal host cells produce membrane and inhibitory plasma proteins that prevent complement binding to their surface (e.g., C1 inhibitor, protein S).

Kinins

Bradykinin and kallidin are two of the many kinins present in the body. Kinins are small polypeptides that cause powerful vasodilation. They are especially active in the inflammatory process. The kinin system is linked to the clotting system via the Hageman factor (XII) and is activated with the activation of clotting.[1] The first step in this process is the conversion of factor XII to factor XIIa (Figure 9-18). Factor XIIa converts a substance known as prekallikrein to kallikrein. Kallikrein converts precursor substances known as kininogens to kinins. The most prevalent is kallidin, which is then converted to bradykinin. Activated kinins cause increased vascular permeability, vasodilation, and

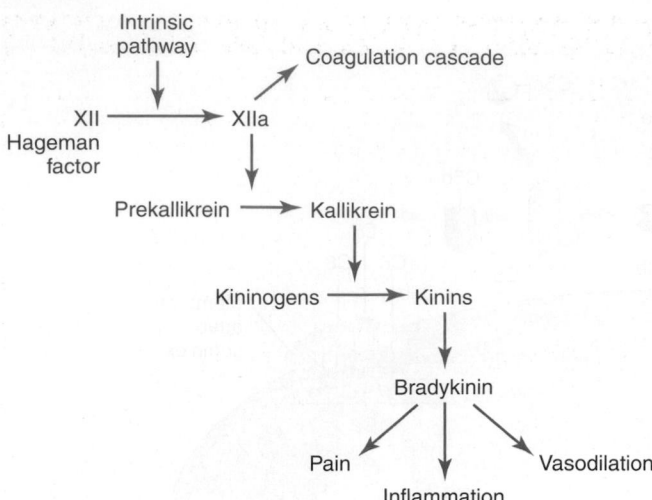

FIGURE 9-18 Common linkage of the kinin and coagulation systems through the activation of factor XII (Hageman factor). *XIIa,* Activated factor XII.

smooth muscle contraction. Kinins are also responsible for pain, which is one of the classic signs of inflammation.

Clotting Factors

The blood coagulation cascade's major purpose is to stop bleeding. It is also intimately involved in inflammation and triggering of the kinin system. The key linkage between the inflammatory response and clotting system is activated factor XII (Hageman factor) (see Figure 9-18). (The blood coagulation cascade is discussed in detail in Chapter 14.) Activation of the coagulation cascade results in the formation of insoluble fibrin strands, which provide an effective barrier to the spread of infection. Clot formation also activates the fibrinolytic cascade, which splits fibrin proteins. Some of the fibrin degradation products are chemotactic signals for neutrophils.

Cytokines and Chemokines

Cytokines are polypeptide signaling molecules that affect the function of other cells by stimulating surface receptors. Cytokines function in a complex intercellular communication network. WBC cytokines have previously had many names, including monokines, lymphokines, and interleukins, depending on their cell of origin. The number of known cytokines is large and growing; they can be grouped according to their source and function (Table 9-2).

Macrophages and T helper cells are the main sources of immune system cytokines. These cytokines generally function as chemotactic factors (chemokines), antiviral factors, mediators of inflammation, hematopoietic factors, or activation signals for specific types of WBCs. The major cytokines produced by macrophages are shown in Figure 9-9. T helper cells of the T_H1 subclass produce two main cytokines, IL-2 and IFN-γ, whereas T_H2 cells secrete a number of cytokines important to B-cell function (see Figure 9-13). Cytokines function to enhance and coordinate both innate and specific immune defenses. They are discussed in more detail in the sections that follow.

KEY POINTS

- The primary lymphoid organs are the thymus and bone marrow. T cells develop in the thymus, whereas B cells develop in the bone marrow. Mature lymphocytes then migrate to secondary lymphoid structures, including the spleen and lymph nodes.

- Blood cells are produced in the bone marrow in response to specific hematopoietic growth factors. Granulocytes (neutrophils, basophils, eosinophils) and monocytes (macrophages) are phagocytic cells that provide innate protection. Lymphocytes (B cells, T cells) are specific cells that react only to particular antigens. NK cells are lymphocytes that lack T cell and B-cell markers and function in innate immune responses. Other blood components produced by bone marrow are erythrocytes and platelets.
- Neutrophils are the most numerous WBCs in blood. A large storage pool lies in the bone marrow and can be mobilized in response to antigen. Neutrophils are the predominant WBC type mobilized in early infection. They migrate to the area by following chemotactic factors and perform phagocytic functions. During acute bacterial infection, larger numbers of immature neutrophils (bands) are released into the blood, which is termed a "shift to the left." Chronic infections may produce a shift to the right with more segmented neutrophils than normal.
- Monocytes located in tissue are called *macrophages*. Monocytes and macrophages are distributed in strategic locations throughout the body, including the skin, lungs, gastrointestinal tract, liver, spleen, and lymph. Macrophages are powerful phagocytes and are predominant in late inflammation.
- T lymphocytes, the major effectors of cell-mediated immunity, interact with specific antigens on cell surfaces. They are important in immunity against foreign, infected, or mutant cells. In addition, they secrete cytokines that boost the immune response of B cells and other cell types. T cells are composed of two main subtypes called CD4 (helper) and CD8 (cytotoxic). B lymphocytes are the major effectors of antibody-mediated immunity.
- The complement system consists of about 20 plasma proteins that interact in a cascade fashion to produce important mediators of inflammation and immunity. The cascade can be activated by microbial antigens (alternative pathway) or by antigen-antibody complexes (classical pathway).
- Cytokines are peptide factors released by immune cells. They have many functions, including as inflammatory mediators, chemotaxins, intercellular communication signals, growth factors, and growth inhibitors. Macrophages and lymphocytes are important sources of immune cytokines.

INNATE DEFENSES AND INFLAMMATION

Inflammation occurs when cells are injured, regardless of the cause of the injury. It is a protective mechanism that also begins the healing process. The inflammatory response has three purposes: (1) to neutralize and destroy invading and harmful agents, (2) to limit the spread of harmful agents to other tissue, and (3) to prepare any damaged tissue for repair. Inflammatory reactions increase capillary permeability such that phagocytic cells, complement, and antibodies can leave the bloodstream and enter tissues where they are needed.

Five cardinal signs of inflammation have been described: (1) redness (rubor), (2) swelling (tumor), (3) heat (calor), (4) pain (dolor), and (5) loss of function (functio laesa). The suffix *-itis* is commonly used to describe conditions associated with inflammation. For example, appendicitis, tendonitis, and nephritis refer to inflammation of the appendix, tendon, and kidney, respectively.

Inflammation can be caused by many conditions. Any injury to tissue will evoke an inflammatory response. Injury can arise from sources outside the body (exogenous) or from sources inside the body (endogenous). Surgery, trauma, burns, and skin injury from chemicals are all examples of exogenous injuries. Endogenous injuries may result from tissue ischemia such as myocardial infarction or pulmonary embolism.

Inflammation and infection are commonly confused because they often coexist. Under normal conditions, infection is always accompanied by inflammation; however, not all inflammation involves an

TABLE 9-2 SELECTED IMMUNE CYTOKINES AND THEIR FUNCTIONS

CYTOKINE	ORIGIN	FUNCTION
IFN-α	Macrophages and induced by RNA or DNA viruses and by single- or double-stranded polyribonucleotides	Inhibits virus replication, toxic to cancer cells, stimulates leukocytes, facilitates NK cell activity, produces fever, increases B- and T-cell activity
IFN-β	Fibroblasts and induced by RNA or DNA viruses and by single- or double-stranded polyribonucleotides	Inhibits virus replication, toxic to cancer cells, facilitates NK cell activity, produces fever
IFN-γ	T cells (T$_H$1 and CD8$^+$) and NK cells	Inhibits virus replication, promotes antigen expression, activates macrophages, inhibits cell growth, induces myeloid cell lines, promotes B cell switch to IgG
IL-1	Mononuclear phagocyte	Stimulates T cells and macrophages, induces acute phase reaction of inflammation, produces fever; similar to TNF and endogenous pyrogen
IL-2	T helper cells (T$_H$1)	Promotes growth of T cells, enhances function of NK cells, assists T-cell maturation in thymus and B-cell proliferation
IL-3	T cells, endothelial cells, fibroblasts, other cells	Induces proliferation and differentiation of other lymphocytes, pluripotent stem cells, mast cells, and granulocytes
IL-4	T helper cells (T$_H$2)	Promotes T-cell/B-cell interactions, promotes synthesis of IgE by B-cell and T$_H$2 cell growth, promotes mast cell and hematopoietic cell growth
IL-5	T helper cells (T$_H$2)	Promotes growth and differentiation of B cells to secrete IgA, induces differentiation of eosinophils
IL-6	Mononuclear phagocytes, T helper cells (T$_H$2), tumors, and nonlymphoid cells (e.g., endothelium)	Promotes immunoglobulin secretion by B cells, induces fever, promotes release of inflammation factors from liver cells, promotes differentiation of hematopoietic stem cells and nerve cells
IL-7	Stromal cells in bone marrow	Stimulates immature lymphocytes to divide to produce B and T cells
IL-8	Macrophages	Enhances inflammation and chemotaxis (CXCL chemokine)
IL-9	T$_H$2 cells	Enhances growth of T helper cells
IL-10	T cells and macrophages	Inhibits activation of macrophages and dendritic cells, inhibits IL-12 production
IL-11	Stromal cells in bone marrow	Stimulates platelet production
IL-12	Macrophages, dendritic cells	Enhances T$_H$1 cell activities and release of IFN-γ by T cells and NK cells
IL-13	T$_H$2 cells	Stimulates B-cell growth and IgF production, suppresses macrophages
IL-14	T cells	Induces B-cell proliferation
IL-15	Macrophages (esp. viral infection)	Similar actions to IL-2, enhances proliferation of T cells (CD8) and NK cells
IL-16	CD8$^+$ T cells	CD4$^+$ cell chemotaxis, suppresses viral replication of HIV
IL-17	CD4$^+$ T cells	Stimulates production of colony-stimulating factors and chemokines
IL-18	Macrophages in response to microbes	Increases NK cell proliferation and secretion of IFN-γ by T$_H$1
IL-19	Macrophages	Stimulates macrophage IL-1 secretion
IL-20	Monocytes	Stimulates hematopoietic stem cells
IL-21	T$_H$2 and T$_H$17 cells	Activates B cells, stimulates production of NK cells
IL-22	T$_H$17 cells	Epithelial cells, increased barrier function, defensin production
IL-23	Macrophages and dendritic cells	Similar to IL-12, stimulates cell-mediated immunity
IL-24	Monocytes, T cells	Monocyte inflammatory cytokine production
IL-25	T$_H$2 cells	Stimulates production of cytokines by T$_H$2 cells
IL-26	T cells, monocytes	Uncertain
IL-27	Macrophages and dendritic cells	Inhibits T$_H$1 cells
TNF-α	Macrophages	Induces leukocytosis, fever, weight loss, inflammation, necrosis of some tumors; stimulates lymphokine synthesis; activates macrophages; toxic to viruses and tumor cells
TNF-β	T cells	Inhibits B-cell and T-cell proliferation
G-CSF, M-CSF, GM-CSF	Macrophages, T cells, fibroblasts	Stimulates granulocyte and monocyte production in bone marrow
TGF-β	T cells, macrophages	Inhibits T cells, B cells, and macrophages
Chemokines		
CXCL 1-16	Macrophages and various cells in tissues	Recruitment of neutrophils, macrophages, lymphocytes
CCL 1-28	Macrophages and various cells in tissues	Recruitment of neutrophils, macrophages, lymphocytes

GM-CSF, Granulocyte-macrophage colony-stimulating factor; *HIV*, human immunodeficiency virus; *IFN*, interferon; *IL*, interleukin; *NK*, natural killer; *TNF*, tumor necrosis factor; *TGF*, transforming growth factor.

infectious agent. For example, inflammation can occur with sprain injuries to joints, myocardial infarction, sterile surgical incisions, thrombophlebitis, and blister formation as a result of either temperature extremes or mechanical trauma.

Inflammation may be categorized as either acute or chronic. Acute inflammation is short in duration, lasting less than 2 weeks, and involves a discrete set of events. Chronic inflammation tends to be more diffuse, extends over a longer period, and may result in the formation of scar tissue and deformity.

INFLAMMATION

The inflammatory response is remarkably the same, regardless of the cause. Events in the inflammatory process include (1) increased vascular permeability, (2) recruitment and emigration of leukocytes, and

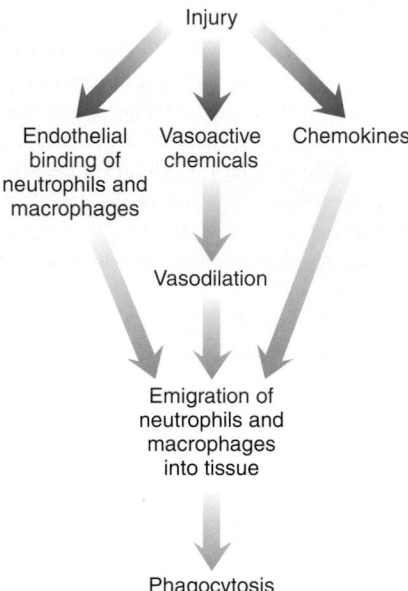

FIGURE 9-19 Tissue injury stimulates the release of a number of chemical mediators that promote vasodilation, chemotaxis, and binding of neutrophils and macrophages to area capillaries. These events facilitate the emigration of neutrophils and macrophages into the tissue, where they begin phagocytosis.

(3) phagocytosis of antigens and debris. The inflammatory response is outlined in Figure 9-19.

Increased Vascular Permeability

Immediately after injury, the precapillary arterioles around the injured area contract briefly, which causes a short period of vasoconstriction. The amount of vasoconstriction depends on the degree of vascular injury and is usually of little significance.[11] Vasoconstriction is followed by a prolonged period of vasodilation caused by release of chemical mediators from injured tissues.

Vasoactive chemicals released during the inflammatory process include histamine, prostaglandins, and leukotrienes (Table 9-3). Mast cells are an important source of these inflammatory chemicals. Mast cells in the area of injury degranulate and release packets of histamine and other inflammatory chemicals. One of the early actions of these mediators is to vasodilate and cause endothelial cells to begin contraction and rounding up, thus increasing capillary permeability. The greater volume of blood increases the amount of pressure within the blood vessels (hydrostatic pressure). The increased pressure along with increased permeability pushes fluid out of the blood vessels and into the surrounding tissue, contributing to local swelling. Because of the dilated blood vessels and open capillaries, more blood is carried to the injured area and contributes to the redness, pain, heat, and swelling of inflammation (Figure 9-20).

Histamine is an early mediator of this inflammatory response. It is such a potent vasodilator that it can cause significant reductions in blood pressure when released in excessive amounts. Histamine also causes bronchial constriction and mucus production. Histamine receptor blocking agents are widely used in allergic reactions, such as skin reactions and hay fever, to suppress these inflammatory actions of histamine.

Prostaglandins and leukotrienes are phospholipid compounds formed from arachidonic acid. The prostaglandins involved in inflammation contribute to vasodilation and increased permeability (Figure 9-21). Prostaglandin D_2 also acts as a chemotactic factor and stimulates neutrophil emigration. Prostaglandins cause pain by enhancing the sensitivity of pain receptors.[11] They arise from the cyclooxygenase pathway and can be inhibited by drugs that block enzymes in this pathway, such as aspirin.

Five types of leukotrienes are generated from the lipoxygenase pathway: A_4, B_4, C_4, D_4, and E_4. Leukotriene B_4 is a potent chemotactic agent that causes aggregation of leukocytes; leukotrienes C_4, D_4, and E_4

TABLE 9-3 MEDIATORS OF ACUTE INFLAMMATION

| MEDIATOR | VASODILATION | INCREASED PERMEABILITY | | CHEMOTAXIS | OPSONIN | PAIN |
		IMMEDIATE	SUSTAINED			
Histamine	+	+++	−	−	−	−
Serotonin (5-HT)	+	+	−	−	−	−
Bradykinin	+	+	−	−	−	++
Complement 3a	−	+	−	−	−	−
Complement 3b	−	−	−	−	+++	−
Complement 5a	−	+	−	+++	−	−
Prostaglandin (E_2)	+++	+	+?	−	−	−
Leukotrienes (B_4, D_4)	−	+++	+?	+++	−	−
Lysosomal proteases	−	−	++*	−	−	−
Oxygen free radicals	−	−	++*	−	−	−

Data from Roitt I et al: *Immunology,* ed 6, St Louis, 2001, Mosby.
*Proteases and oxygen-based free radicals derived from neutrophils are believed to mediate a sustained increase in permeability by means of their damage to endothelial cells.

are inflammatory and cause smooth muscle contraction, bronchospasm, and increased vascular permeability.[11] Leukotriene receptor blocking agents can be used to inhibit the inflammatory actions of these chemicals.

During the early phase of tissue inflammation, platelets move into the site and adhere to exposed vascular collagen. The platelets release fibronectin to form a meshwork trap and stimulate the intrinsic

clotting cascade to help reduce bleeding. Platelets release a number of peptide growth factors, including platelet-derived growth factor and insulin-like growth factor.[12] Platelet-derived growth factor stimulates fibroblast cell proliferation, and insulin-like growth factor type 1 is a potent vascular endothelial cell chemotactic factor. Triggering of the blood coagulation cascade also occurs and leads to the formation of a fibrin clot. Usually, early clot formation occurs within several minutes. Fibrin is also deposited in the lymph system, where it causes lymphatic blockage. Lymphatic blockage "walls off" the area of inflammation from the surrounding tissue and delays the spread of toxins.

The vascular changes that occur soon after injury are beneficial to the injured tissue because irritating or toxic agents are diluted by the fluid that leaks out of the blood vessels into surrounding tissue. In addition, when the fluid leaves the blood vessels, the remaining blood becomes viscous (thick) and circulation is slowed, facilitating neutrophil emigration.

Emigration of Leukocytes

As blood flows through areas of inflammation, neutrophils move to the sides of the blood vessels and roll along the endothelium of the vessel wall. This process is referred to as *margination* or *pavementing*. Normally, neutrophils slide past the capillary endothelial cells and do not stick. Injured tissue triggers the expression of adhesion molecules on the surface of endothelial cells, and the adhesion molecules bind to receptors on neutrophils (Figure 9-22). These receptors, called *selectin and chemokine receptors,* help neutrophils stick and roll along the

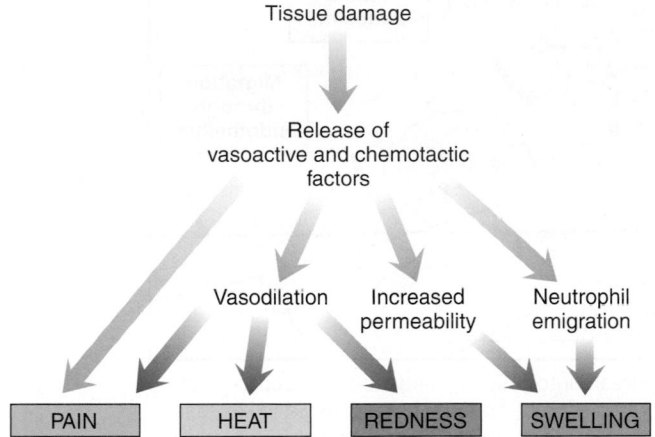

FIGURE 9-20 Cardinal signs of acute inflammation result mainly from vasodilation and increased vascular permeability.

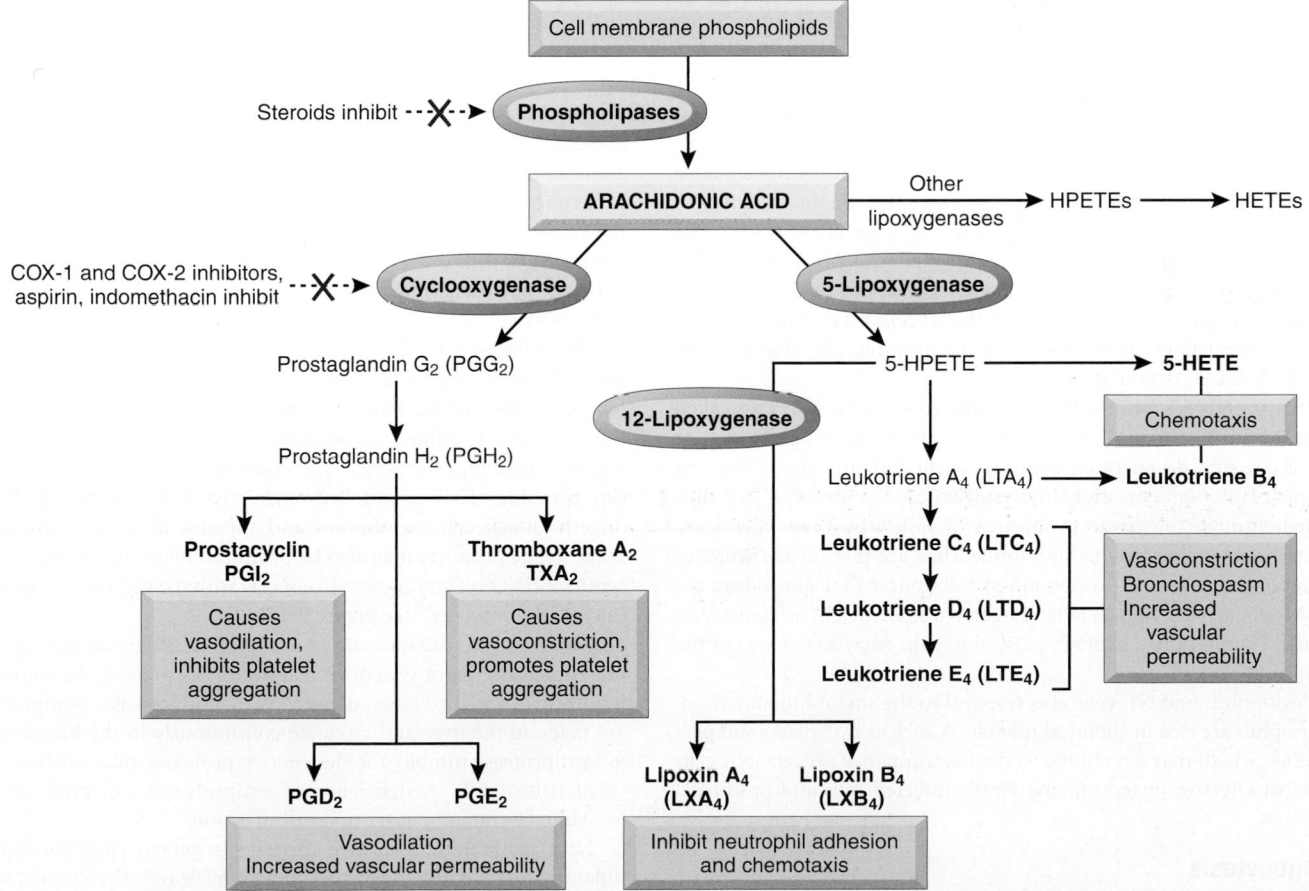

FIGURE 9-21 Generation of prostaglandins, thromboxane, and leukotrienes from arachidonic acid, and roles in inflammation. *HETEs,* Hydroeicosatetraenoic acids; *HPETEs,* hydroperoxyeicosatetraenoic acids. (From Kumar V et al: *Robbins and Cotran pathologic basis of disease,* ed 8, Philadelphia, 2010, Saunders, p 58.)

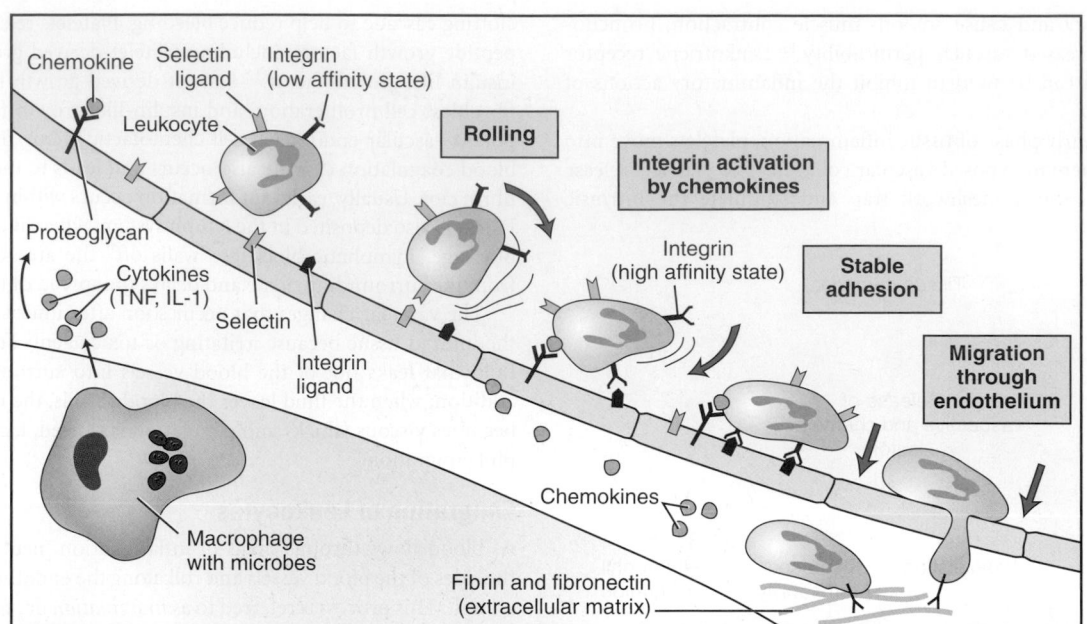

FIGURE 9-22 Emigration of neutrophils from the bloodstream into tissue is mediated by receptor interactions with the capillary endothelium. With inflammation and injury, endothelial cells begin to express binding molecules on their cell surfaces (selectins). Leukocytes also have selectins, which can bind to endothelial adhesion proteins. The selectin interactions cause the leukocytes to stick and roll. Chemokines on the surface of endothelial cells interact with neutrophils (and macrophages) to increase the binding affinity of integrin receptors on leukocytes. Firm attachment and diapedesis through the capillary wall is facilitated by integrins, which allow the neutrophils to bind to endothelial cells and extracellular matrix and then pull themselves into the tissue. *IL,* Interleukin; *TNF,* tumor necrosis factor.

capillary endothelial surface.[5] Binding to and subsequent movement through the capillary wall are accomplished by another group of receptors called *integrins.* Chemokines present on the endothelium enhance the binding affinity of integrins so the neutrophil can attach firmly to the vessel wall. The process of passing through the blood vessel walls and migrating to the inflamed tissue is referred to as *emigration* or *diapedesis.* Diapedesis begins within a few minutes to hours of injury. Even though the spaces between endothelial cells lining the vessels are much smaller than the neutrophils, neutrophils are able to slide through a small portion at a time.

Neutrophils are attracted to the inflamed tissue by a process called **chemotaxis.** Biochemical mediators that attract neutrophils include bacterial toxins, degenerative products of the inflamed tissue, the C5a complement fragment, and other substances. Neutrophils are thus guided through the tissue to an area of injury by these chemicals. Because neutrophils are highly mobile, they are first on the scene to begin phagocytosis and production of collagenase to degrade dead tissue. Monocytes are slightly slower to arrive at an area of inflammation but use a similar process of emigration to gain entry to the area of tissue injury.

Eosinophils and NK cells also respond to the site of inflammation. Eosinophils are rich in chemical mediators such as hydrolases and peroxidases, which may contribute to the inflammatory process. NK cells are most effective in recognizing virally infected cells and opsonized microbes.

Phagocytosis

Once neutrophils and monocytes (macrophages) enter the tissue, they begin the process of phagocytosis (Figure 9-23). These cells produce a wide variety of enzymes that digest protein structures. Some of these enzymes include lysozyme, neutral proteases, collagenase, elastase, and

acid hydrolases. Neutrophils and macrophages specialize in collagen and extracellular matrix degradation. Peptide bonds are cleaved in the extracellular matrix by collagenase, elastase, proteinase, and gelatinase. If the microbe is small enough to be internalized, it will be captured by the phagocyte and endocytosed into a phagosome. The phagosome then merges with a lysosome containing degradative enzymes. Large antigens may trigger the neutrophil to release its degradative enzymes extracellularly, causing damage to local tissues.

Oxidizing agents, the most destructive of the inflammatory cell products, are formed as a result of the phagocyte oxidase enzyme system on the membrane of the lysosome. Neutrophils are capable of synthesizing and assailing microorganisms with these oxidizing agents, which include the following oxygen radicals: superoxide (O_2^-), hydrogen peroxide (H_2O_2), and hydroxyl ions (OH^-). Oxidizing agents directly attack cell membranes and thereby increase permeability. Nitric oxide products may also be produced by inducible nitric oxide synthase (iNOS) and function in concert with oxygen radicals to attack microbial molecules[1] (see Figure 9-23).

Because acute inflammation can cause severe tissue damage, it is not surprising that a system of inactivators is present. An important inhibitor of inflammatory damage is α_1-antiprotease. Antiproteases are made in the liver and circulate continuously in the bloodstream. α_1-Antiprotease inhibits the destructive proteases released from activated neutrophils. A deficiency of antiproteases can predispose an individual to inflammatory tissue destruction.

Neutrophils have a limited capacity to phagocytose foreign and inflammatory debris. Once the neutrophil leaves the circulation to fight an infection, it is unable to return and will die at the site. When phagocytosis is incomplete, a collection of dead neutrophils, bacteria, and cellular debris, called *pus,* may form at the site. Macrophages are left with the job of removing spent neutrophils and preparing the site

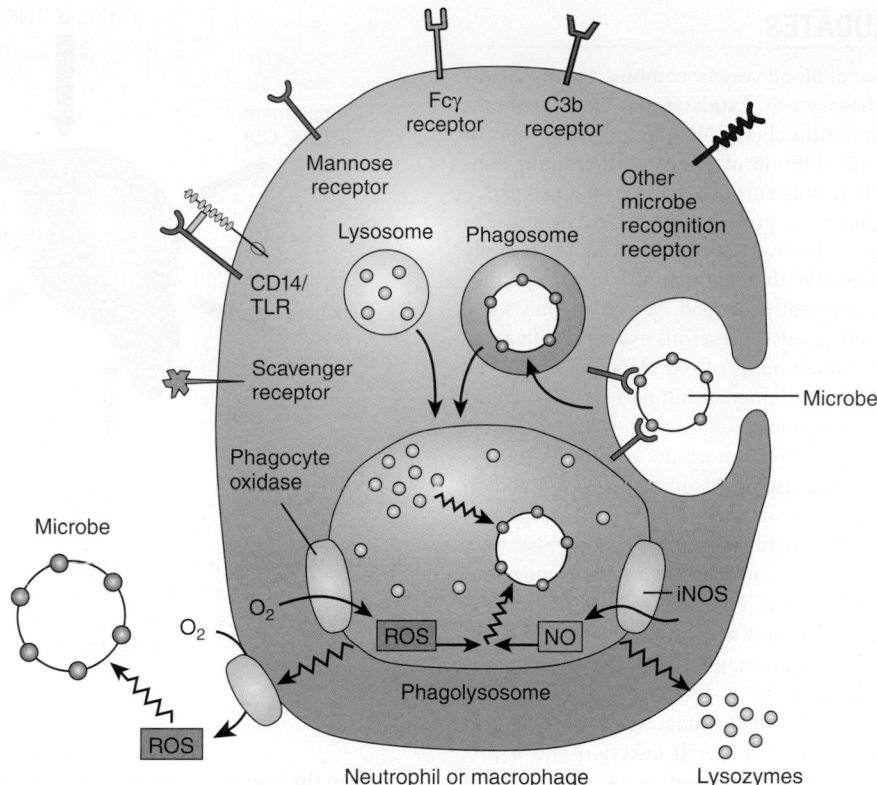

FIGURE 9-23 Neutrophils and macrophages have a number of different receptors on their surface that enable them to bind to components of microbes or to opsonins like IgG and complement. Bound microbes are internalized into phagosomes that fuse with lysosomes containing numerous enzymes. Some of these enzymes degrade proteins (proteolytic), and others such as oxidase and inducible nitric oxide synthase *(iNOS)* produce free radicals that attack molecular bonds. When phagocytes are strongly stimulated or microbes are too large to internalize, the lysosomal enzymes may be activated or released at the cell surface, causing tissue damage and inflammation. *ROS,* Reactive oxygen species.

for healing. A predominance of monocytes and macrophages in an inflamed area signals the beginning of chronic inflammation.

Chronic Inflammation

Macrophages are essential for wound healing because of their phagocytic and debridement functions. Macrophages produce proteases that help in removing foreign protein from the wound. Macrophages also release tissue thromboplastin to facilitate hemostasis and stimulate fibroblast activity. Macrophages secrete other peptide growth factors such as angiogenic factor, which encourages the growth of new blood vessels. Macrophages also phagocytose spent neutrophils and their degradation products so they do not interfere with healing. Prolonged inflammation may impair healing and result in an accumulation of macrophages, fibroblasts, and collagen, called a *granuloma*. Granulomas are usually evident on examination of tissue biopsy as clusters of macrophages surrounding particulate matter or resistant microbes such as *Mycobacterium tuberculosis*. Fibrosis and scarring are evident because normal parenchyma is replaced with fibrous tissue.

HEALING

Healing of tissues following inflammation can occur in different ways over time. Usually the reconstructive phase begins 3 to 4 days after injury and persists for 2 weeks. The major cells involved in this phase include fibroblasts, endothelial cells, and myofibroblasts.

Fibroblasts are found all over the body and are thought to originate in mesenchymal primitive tissue. They synthesize connective tissue and are able to migrate. Fibroblasts are stimulated to make collagen, proteoglycans, and fibronectin by a variety of growth factors.[12] Macrophages secrete lactate and release growth factors that stimulate fibroblasts. Fibroblasts respond to contact and density inhibition and thereby facilitate orderly cellular growth. Myofibroblasts develop at the wound edge and induce wound contraction.

Endothelial cells grow into the connective tissue gel stimulated by angiogenic substances. They usually develop capillary beds from existing vessels. The new capillaries can transport nutrients for tissue repair and wound healing. However, because the new capillaries are leaky, they contribute to continuing edema.

Regeneration of damaged tissue into the preexisting tissue type requires survival of the basement membrane and tissue stem cells. Some cell types regenerate constantly; among these types are the epithelial cells of the skin and mucous membranes, bone marrow cells, and lymphoid cells. Cells of the liver, pancreas, endocrine glands, and renal tubules are also able to regenerate when necessary. However, some cell types, such as neurons and muscle cells, regenerate poorly. The maturation phase of wound healing occurs several weeks after the injury and may last for 2 years or more. It is characterized by wound remodeling by fibroblasts, macrophages, neutrophils, and eosinophils. Wound remodeling is the process of collagen deposition and lysis with debridement of the wound edges. During this phase the wound changes color from bright red to pink to whitish. As long as a wound is pink, the maturation phase is not completed.

INFLAMMATORY EXUDATES

Exudate is fluid that leaks out of blood vessels, combined with neutrophils and the debris from phagocytosis. Exudates may vary in composition, but all types have similar functions, including (1) transport of leukocytes and antibodies, (2) dilution of toxins and irritating substances, and (3) transport of the nutrients necessary for tissue repair.

Serous exudate is watery, has a low protein content, and is similar to the fluid that collects under a blister. This type of exudate generally accompanies mild inflammation. With mild inflammation, the permeability of the blood vessels is not greatly changed. As a result, only some protein molecules escape from vessels, and serous exudate, with a low protein content, develops. Small amounts of red blood cells may leak into the serous fluid with capillary injury, resulting in a pink-tinged drainage called *serosanguineous* drainage.

With greater injury, more inflammation occurs and the blood vessels become more permeable. Because of this increased permeability, more protein can pass through the vessel walls. Fibrinogen, a large protein molecule, can pass through a highly permeable blood vessel wall. *Fibrinous exudate* is sticky and thick and may have to be removed to allow healing; otherwise, scar tissue and adhesions may develop. However, in some instances fibrinous exudate may be beneficial. In the case of acute appendicitis, fibrinous exudate may actually wall off and localize the infection and prevent its spread.

Purulent exudate is called pus. Purulent exudate generally occurs in severe inflammation accompanied by bacterial infection and is primarily composed of neutrophils, protein, and tissue debris. Large pockets of purulent exudate, called abscesses, must generally be removed or drained for healing to take place.

Hemorrhagic exudate has a large component of red blood cells. This type of exudate is usually present with the most severe inflammation. Hemorrhagic exudate occurs with severe leakage from blood vessels or after necrosis or breakdown of blood vessels.

SYSTEMIC MANIFESTATIONS OF INFLAMMATION

Inflammation is associated with both localized and systemic signs and symptoms. The localized symptoms, described previously, occur with both acute and chronic inflammation. Depending on the magnitude of injury and the resistance of the individual, localized inflammation can lead to systemic involvement. Systemic responses include fever, neutrophilia (increased blood neutrophil count), lethargy, and muscle catabolism. Three macrophage-derived cytokines—IL-1, IL-6, and TNF-α—are responsible for most of the systemic effects of inflammation.[11]

TNF-α and IL-1 act on the brain to raise body temperature, induce sleep, and suppress appetite. By raising the set point for body temperature, these cytokines induce conservation of heat through vasoconstriction, as well as increased heat production through shivering. An increase in body temperature is assumed to improve the immune response; however, the mechanism is unclear. IL-1 is responsible for stimulating the release of neutrophils from bone marrow storage sites, thus producing neutrophilia. All three cytokines act on skeletal muscle to enhance protein catabolism, which provides an available pool of amino acids for efficient antibody production by plasma cells.

The liver is an important target for IL-1, IL-6, and TNF-α. These cytokines induce the liver to release a number of proteins collectively called *acute phase proteins*, which include complement components, clotting factors, and protease inhibitors (Figure 9-24). Two of the most important acute phase proteins are C-reactive protein (CRP) and serum amyloid A. CRP binds to phospholipids on bacterial cell membranes and acts as an opsonin to facilitate phagocytosis.[3]

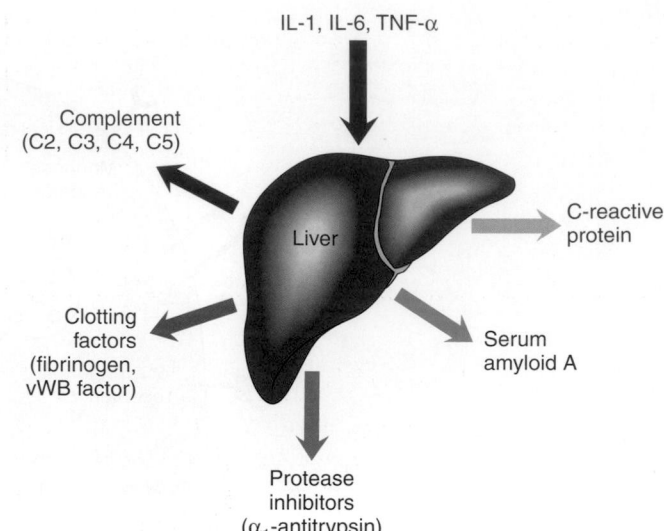

FIGURE 9-24 The liver is a target for three important cytokines: interleukin-1 *(IL-1)*, interleukin-6 *(IL-6)*, and tumor necrosis factor-α *(TNF-α)*. In response to these cytokines, the liver releases a number of proteins, collectively called *acute phase proteins*. *vWB, von Willebrand factor.*

When the liver releases acute phase proteins, the level of fibrinogen in the serum is increased. Fibrinogen coats the surface of red blood cells and reduces their charge so that they aggregate more readily. A blood test called the *erythrocyte sedimentation rate* (ESR, "sed rate") provides a simple measure of the level of inflammation in an individual. Thus an elevated ESR indicates the presence of inflammation in the body. The greater the inflammation, the faster the red blood cells precipitate to the bottom of a test tube and the higher the ESR. The ESR is a nonspecific but clinically useful indicator of inflammation. Serum CRP activity is also used as a nonspecific indicator of inflammation in a manner similar to the ESR.

KEY POINTS

- Previous exposure to foreign antigens is not required for the activation of innate immune defenses. Inflammation is an important aspect of innate immunity that involves localization of harmful agents and the movement of phagocytic cells to the area. Classic manifestations of inflammation are redness, swelling, heat, pain, and loss of function.
- Inflammatory chemicals such as histamine, prostaglandins, and leukotrienes are released from injured tissues, mast cells, macrophages, and neutrophils. These chemicals increase vascular permeability, vasodilate, and attract immune cells to the area (chemotaxis).
- Phagocytes migrate to the inflamed area, collect at the side of the vessel, and squeeze through into the tissue. Emigration of neutrophils and macrophages is facilitated by chemokines, selectins, and integrins present on the surface of endothelial cells and leukocytes. Neutrophils arrive in large numbers in acute bacterial infection and begin active phagocytosis. Neutrophils and macrophages produce proteolytic enzymes and oxidizing agents to destroy and digest antigens. With chronic inflammation, macrophages and lymphocytes predominate.
- Healing is mediated by growth factors released from platelets and immune cells that stimulate fibroblasts to divide and manufacture extracellular matrix proteins. Endothelial cells respond to angiogenic growth factors by forming capillary networks.

- Inflammatory exudate functions to transport immune cells, antibodies, and nutrients to the tissue and dilute the offending substances. Serous exudate is watery and low in protein; fibrinous exudate is thick, sticky, and high in protein; purulent exudate contains infective organisms, leukocytes, and cellular debris; and hemorrhagic exudate contains red blood cells.
- Systemic manifestations of inflammation include fever, neutrophilia, lethargy, muscle catabolism, increased acute phase proteins (CRP), and increased ESR. These responses are attributable to the IL-1, IL-6, and TNF-α released from macrophages and inflamed tissues.

SPECIFIC ADAPTIVE IMMUNITY

The specific immune system uses remarkably effective and adaptive defense mechanisms capable of recognizing foreign invaders, destroying them, and retaining a memory of the encounter such that an even more effective defense (adaptive) will be achieved after subsequent exposure. As previously described, B and T lymphocytes are the cellular mediators of specific adaptive immunity. B cells are said to provide "humoral" immunity because the antibodies they produce are found in body fluids, or "humors." T cells provide "cell-mediated" immunity because they recognize antigen presented on the surface of cells. To achieve immunity against specific antigens, B and T lymphocytes must be capable of recognizing an enormous range of foreign antigen yet not be reactive to self tissues.

Differentiation between self and nonself requires a complex lymphocyte development process in which self-reactive lymphocytes are destroyed and potentially useful lymphocytes are preserved. The MHC proteins have a primary role in enabling lymphocytes to react to foreign antigen while remaining tolerant to self antigen. Self-tolerance is not always effectively maintained, and impairment in self-tolerance can result in the development of autoimmune disorders (see Chapter 10).

MAJOR HISTOCOMPATIBILITY COMPLEX

A cluster of genes on chromosome 6 is known as the **major histocompatibility complex (MHC)**. In humans, the MHC is also known as the **human leukocyte antigen (HLA)** complex. The proteins made by these genes are displayed on the surface of body cells and mark them as "self." The MHC contains three classes of genes: I, II, and III (Figure 9-25). Class I and II genes code for proteins that display or "present" antigens on the surface of cells. Antigen presentation is a vital first step in the initiation of an immune response. T lymphocytes cannot recognize foreign antigens unless they are displayed on MHC proteins on the surface of a cell. Class III genes code for a variety of proteins, many of which are of importance to inflammatory reactions, including several complement proteins.

A great deal of **polymorphism** is found in the MHC class I and II genes, which means that it is very unlikely that one individual will have exactly the same MHC genotype as another individual. For example, three gene loci for MHC class I proteins (A, B, C) are located on each chromosome 6, and an individual inherits one chromosome from each parent for a total of six MHC class I genes. Each of these genes has many different forms (alleles) such that each of the six is likely to be different (Figure 9-26). Related individuals will generally be more similar but not identical (unless identical twins). The "matching" of MHC gene expression is an important consideration for tissue and organ transplantation. The closer the match is, the less likely that the host will reject the transplant. An individual also receives six MHC class II genes that are expressed on specialized antigen-presenting cells, such as dendritic cells, macrophages, and B cells. Because of the potential for

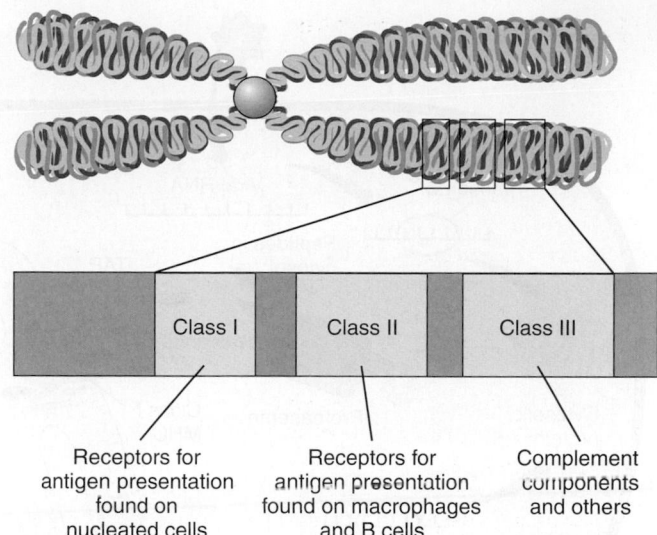

FIGURE 9-25 Major histocompatibility complex genes are categorized into three main groups known as class I, II, and III. Class I and II genes code for antigen-presenting proteins, whereas class III genes code for a heterogeneous group of proteins, many of which serve immune functions.

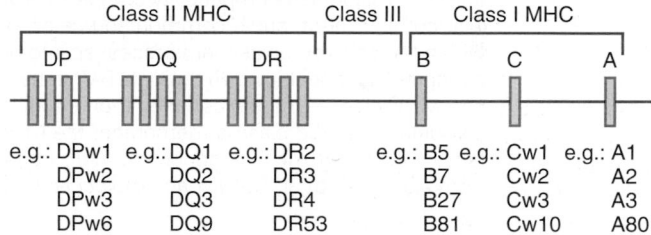

FIGURE 9-26 Each individual receives six class I major histocompatibility complex (*MHC*) genes including pairs of *A*, *B*, and *C* genes. One member of the pair is inherited from each parent. MHC class I genes are expressed in all nucleated cells of the body. Each individual also receives six class II MHC genes, three from each parent. However, class II proteins are composed of 2 polypeptide chains such that an individual may have 10 to 20 different MHC class II protein molecules. Class II MHC proteins are expressed on the surface of specialized antigen-presenting cells like macrophages, dendritic cells, and B cells. The structure of an individual's MHC proteins is assessed to determine the "tissue type" when matching for tissue transplantation procedures.

mixing and matching of class II MHC gene products, an individual may express 10 to 20 different MHC class II proteins.[1] The MHC class I and II proteins on the surface of cells display both self and foreign antigens for inspection by T cells. Cells displaying foreign antigens stimulate an immune response, whereas those displaying self antigens do not. Genetic diversity in MHC gene expression is believed to be important to the preservation of a species because new pathogens are likely to encounter at least some individuals with MHC genotypes that can recognize and eliminate these pathogens.

ANTIGEN PRESENTATION BY MHC

Nucleated cells in the body are capable of expressing MHC class I proteins on their cell surfaces, whereas only certain specialized cells, primarily dendritic cells, macrophages, and B cells, are able to express MHC class II proteins. Cytotoxic T cells are able to recognize antigen

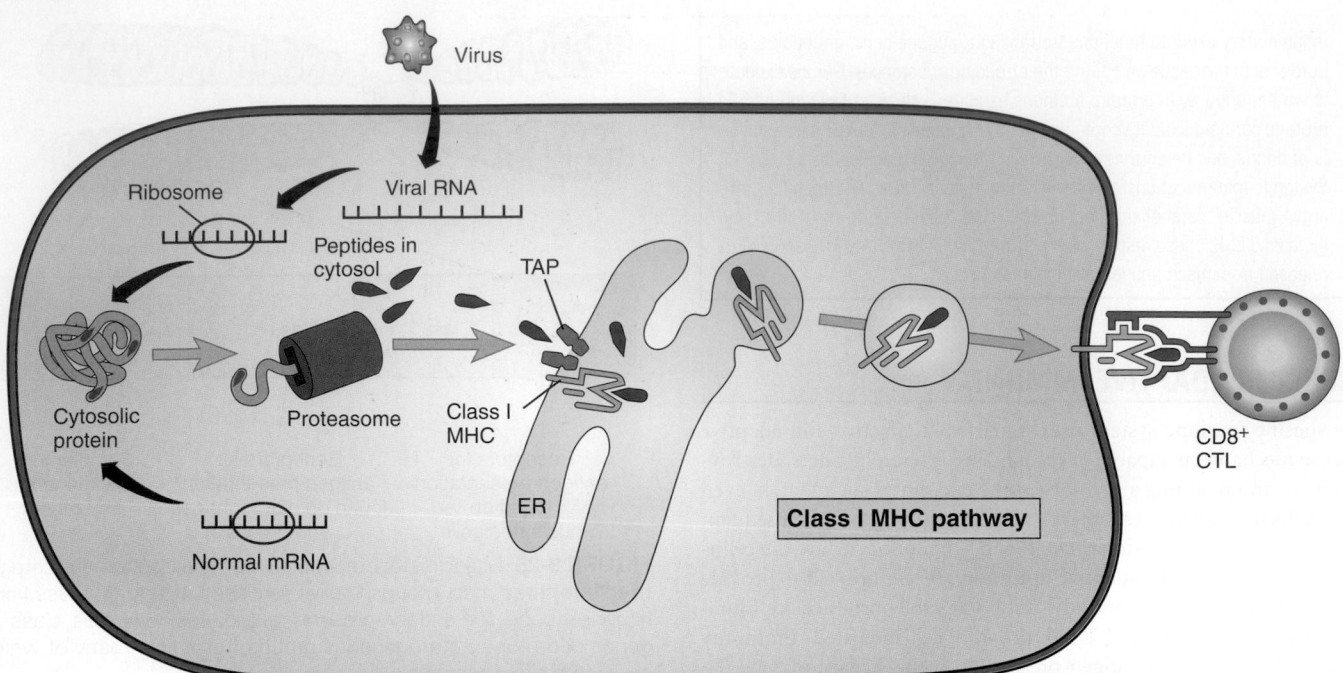

FIGURE 9-27 Nearly all nucleated cells of the body are able to process and display antigen in association with major histocompatibility complex *(MHC)* class I protein. The antigens come from the intracellular compartment, and a common source of foreign antigen is viral infection. The viral proteins made within the cell's cytoplasm are processed into peptide fragments in the proteasome and then enter the endoplasmic reticulum *(ER)* through TAP transporters. There they combine with MHC class I proteins. The MHC class I–antigen complex then shuttles to the cell surface within a vesicle. When the vesicle combines with the plasma membrane, the MHC class I–antigen complex is displayed on the cell surface. *CTL,* Cytotoxic T lymphocyte; *TAP,* transporter associated with antigen processing. (Redrawn from Abbas AK et al: *Cellular and molecular immunology,* ed 7, Philadelphia, 2012, Saunders, p 131.)

bound to MHC class I proteins, whereas T helper cells recognize antigen bound to MHC class II proteins. T cells are screened during development in the thymus so that they recognize and are tolerant to self MHC proteins and do not react to self peptides displayed by self MHC proteins. This concept is explored further in the section Mechanisms of Cell-Mediated Immunity. The sources of antigen, mechanism of antigen processing, and T-cell response to antigen are quite different for MHC I and MHC II reactions.

MHC Class I Presentation

Nucleated cells continuously produce MHC class I proteins on the rough endoplasmic reticulum (ER), where they are combined with various peptide fragments that are present in the cytoplasm. These peptides result from degradation of normal intracellular proteins. The MHC I–peptide complexes are cycled to the cell surface for inspection by T cells. Normal MHCs displaying normal cellular proteins are ignored by T cells. If abnormal proteins are produced in the cell, then the MHC I–peptide complex will be recognized as foreign and an immune response will occur. The peptide antigens presented on MHC I are of intracellular origin. Because viruses are able to gain access to cells directly, viral protein is a common source of foreign MHC class I antigens. Abnormal intracellular proteins produced by mutant cells may also be presented on MHC I, thus targeting them for immune destruction. Before intracellular proteins can be presented at the cell surface, they must be processed and transported to the ER, where they are combined with newly synthesized MHC class I protein (Figure 9-27). Peptide fragments are generated in the cytoplasmic proteasomes and escorted through the ER by special transporters called *transporters associated with antigen processing* (TAPs). The TAPs are located near

the MHC I complexes on the ER membrane and target the peptides to the MHC I–binding cleft. The MHC I–binding cleft can accommodate peptide fragments of 8 to 11 amino acids[1] (Figure 9-28). The MHC I–antigen complexes then travel to the cell membrane, where they are displayed. Recognition of foreign antigen in association with the MHC I protein on the cell surface targets the presenting cell for destruction by cytotoxic T cells. When the cytotoxic T cell binds to the MHC I–antigen complex, it is stimulated to release enzymes and pore-forming proteins (perforins) that lyse the target cell. Cytotoxic T cells can only recognize an antigen if it is physically bound to an MHC class I molecule. Cytotoxic T cells are thus said to be MHC class I restricted.

MHC Class II Presentation

MHC class II proteins are used to present antigens obtained from extracellular sources. Extracellular antigens must first be engulfed by the antigen-presenting cell. Cells of the monocyte-macrophage lineage, dendritic cells, and B cells are responsible for presenting antigen by MHC II. Macrophages and dendritic cells obtain foreign antigens by phagocytosis and are thus able to process and present a large number of different antigens. They are said to be "nonspecific" for this reason. B cells, on the other hand, are very particular about the antigens that they engulf. The antigen must specifically bind to the BCR to be ingested by a B cell. Each B cell has only one type of BCR and therefore processes and presents only one specific antigen. The specificity of the BCR corresponds to the antibody that the activated B cell will produce. The process of B-cell activation is explored in the section titled Mechanisms of Humoral Immunity.

After the antigen-presenting cell has ingested an antigen, it is degraded into fragments within the cellular phagosomes (endocytic vesicle). MHC

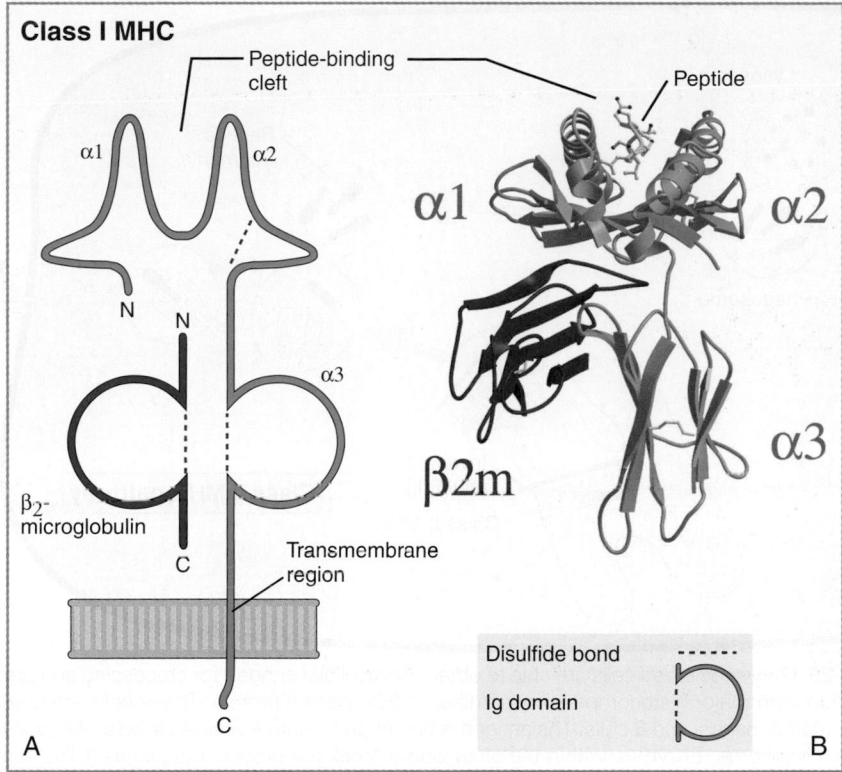

FIGURE 9-28 Schematic **(A)** and ribbon **(B)** diagrams of the class I major histocompatibility complex molecule. Note that the peptide-binding cleft is formed from one polypeptide chain that restricts the size of peptide in the pocket to 8 to 11 amino acids. (From Abbas AK et al: *Cellular and molecular immunology,* ed 7, Philadelphia, 2012, Saunders, p 123.)

II proteins are synthesized on the rough ER and pick up an antigen from the phagosome on their way to the plasma membrane (Figure 9-29). The class II MHC molecule is formed by two protein chains, and the binding cleft is more flexible than that of MHC I proteins (Figure 9-30). Peptides displayed by MHC class II proteins range in size from 10 to 30 amino acids.[1] The MHC II–antigen complexes are then displayed at the cell surface where T helper cells can detect them. T helper cells can only recognize a foreign antigen if it is physically bound to an MHC II protein. T helper cells are thus said to be MHC II restricted. Naive T cells located in lymph nodes are usually presented with antigen by dendritic cells. Dendritic cells populate the body surfaces and mucous membranes. When they engulf antigen, they break their tissue attachments and migrate to lymph nodes where they interact with T helper cells.

MECHANISMS OF CELL-MEDIATED IMMUNITY

T cells are able to recognize foreign antigen displayed on the surface of antigen-presenting cells through specialized receptors called *T cell receptors* (TCRs). Each T cell has tens of thousands of identical TCRs on its cell surface.[9] Each T cell is thus able to recognize and respond to only a single antigenic epitope. This property is what makes T cells specific. The binding specificity of the TCR is randomly determined by recombination and rearrangement within the genes that code for the TCR-binding domain. Billions of different TCR amino acid sequences are possible, thus providing a tremendous diversity of potential antigen-binding specificities. This diversity increases the likelihood that one or more T cells will have the right TCRs to allow recognition of any of the various pathogens that may gain access to the body. The drawback to this random approach is that many TCRs will be useless or may bind self antigens. A rigorous selection process occurs in the thymus such

that self-reactive T cells are eliminated. This selection process requires at least two steps. In the first, T cells must demonstrate an ability to recognize self MHC proteins displayed on the surface of specialized thymic cells. Portions of the TCR must make appropriate contact with the MHC protein, or the T cell will not be able to respond to antigens presented on the cell surface.[13] The expression of either CD4 or CD8 on the T cell helps determine which class of MHC the T cell must fit. T cells that do not have functional TCRs undergo apoptosis in the thymus. The second requirement is that the TCR does not bind tightly to MHC proteins that are displaying normal self-derived peptides. Tight binding to self peptides also triggers the cell to initiate apoptosis. T cells that pass these tests migrate to secondary lymphoid tissues to await foreign antigens. Exposure of a T cell to its corresponding antigen results in expansion of the T cell into a clone of cells that all recognize the same antigen. This process ensures that useful T cells are maintained in the body as memory cells, whereas T cells that do not encounter antigen will not proliferate. Members of the T-cell clone migrate to lymphoid organs throughout the body, where they can respond rapidly should the same antigen reenter the system. The life span of mature T cells is long, but the numbers of memory cells in a clone will decline over time. However, intermittent exposure to the antigen is likely to occur and will stimulate proliferation and maintain immunity.

The two major types of T cells, T helper cells and cytotoxic T cells, react very differently to activation of their TCRs by antigen and are therefore described separately in the following sections.

T Helper Cells (CD4+)

T helper cells recognize antigen in association with MHC class II molecules. The CD4 protein is needed to enable T helper cells to bind the MHC II protein, whereas the TCR recognizes the specific antigen being

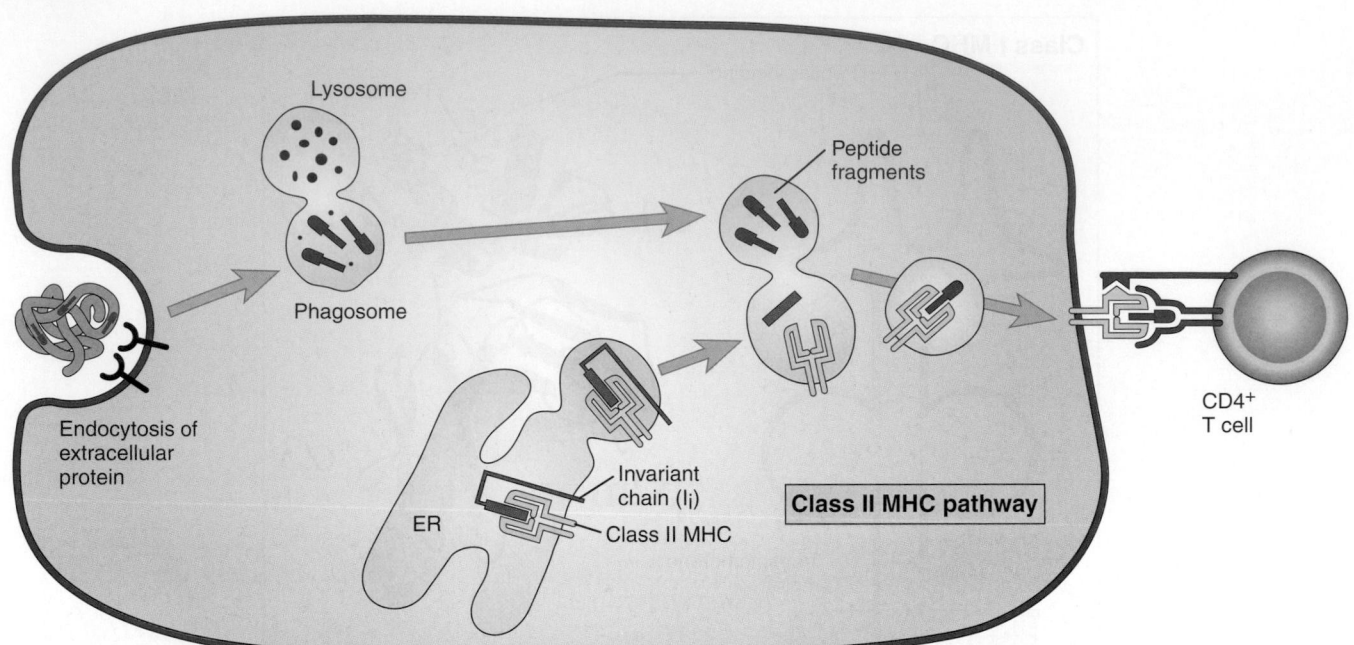

FIGURE 9-29 Only specialized cells are able to obtain extracellular antigen for processing and presentation in association with major histocompatibility complex *(MHC)* class II protein. These cells are primarily dendritic cells, macrophages, and B cells. The antigen is first engulfed into a vesicle called a *phagosome,* which fuses with a lysosome. Enzymes within the phagosome break the protein into pieces. MHC II molecules are synthesized on the endoplasmic reticulum *(ER)* and then transported to the phagosome in a vesicle. The binding cleft of the MHC II protein is complexed with a blocking protein to prevent it from retrieving peptide before it reaches the phagosome. The phagosome and vesicle fuse, and the MHC II loses its blocking protein and picks up an antigen peptide. The complex then migrates to the cell surface and combines with the cell membrane. The MHC II–antigen complex is then displayed on the cell surface. (Redrawn from Abbas AK et al: *Cellular and molecular immunology,* ed 7, Philadelphia, 2012, Saunders, p 130.)

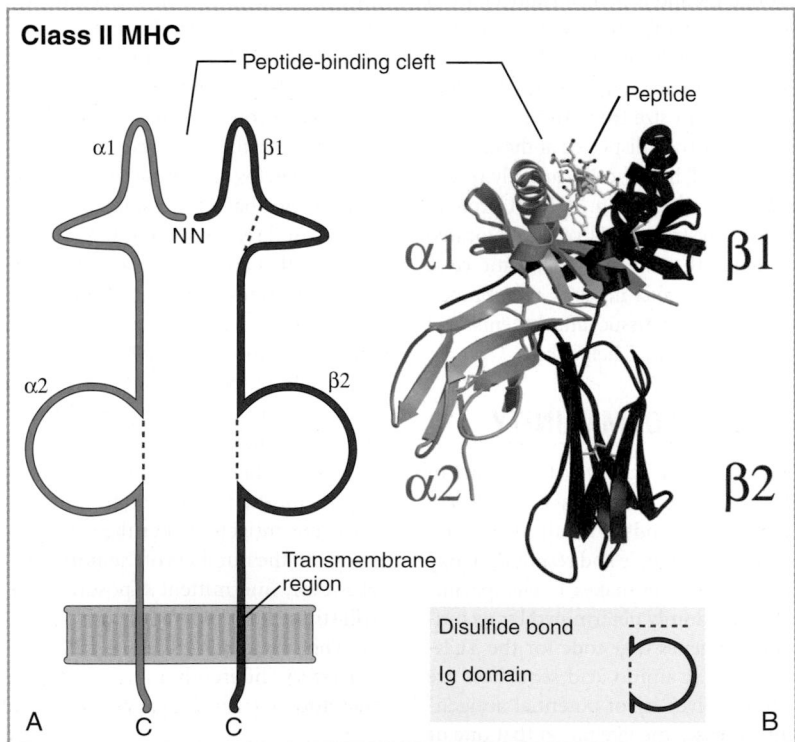

FIGURE 9-30 Schematic **(A)** and ribbon **(B)** diagrams of the class II major histocompatibility complex *(MHC)* molecule. Note that the peptide-binding cleft is formed from 2 separate polypeptide chains, which allows the size of peptide in the pocket to be 10 to 30 amino acids. (From Abbas AK et al: *Cellular and molecular immunology,* ed 7, Philadelphia, 2012, Saunders, p 125.)

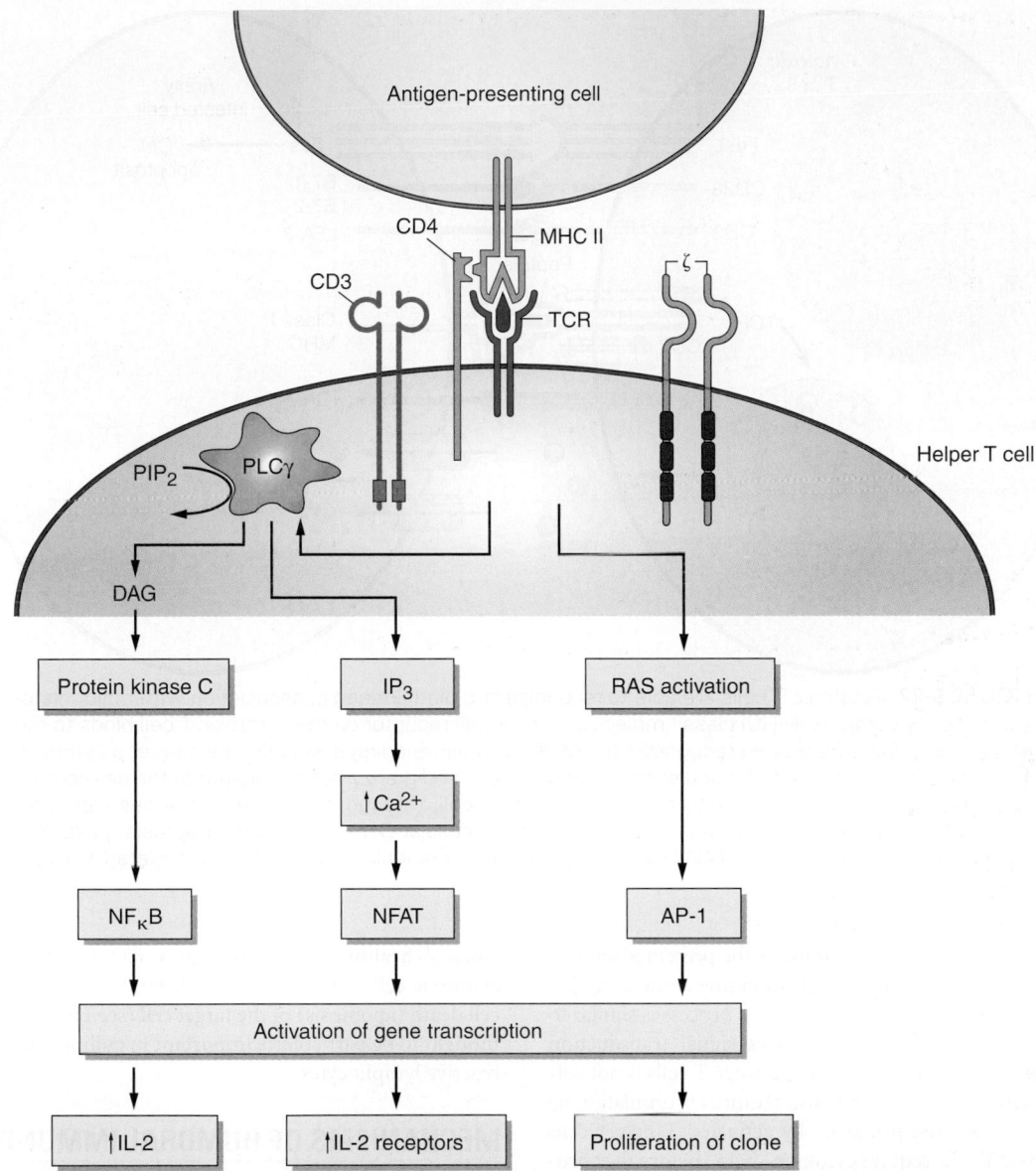

FIGURE 9-31 T helper cells can recognize and bind antigen in association with major histocompatibility complex *(MHC)* class II molecules. The T cell receptor *(TCR)* on the T helper cell binds to the antigen, and the CD4 protein recognizes the MHC class II protein. Binding is very specific because the TCR must match the antigen fragment precisely. Once binding is achieved, CD3 and ζ proteins associated with the TCR are activated to initiate intracellular enzyme cascades. Major signaling pathways in activated T cells are shown. These ultimately result in activity of transcription factors and changes in gene activity. *AP-1,* Activation protein-1; *DAG,* diacylglycerol; *IP₃,* inositol 1,4,5-trisphosphate; *NFAT,* nuclear factor of activated T cells; *NF$_\kappa$B,* nuclear factor kappa B; *PIP₂,* phosphatidylinositol 4,5-bisphosphate; *PLCγ,* phospholipase C-γ.

presented (Figure 9-31). Binding of the TCR to its corresponding antigen generates a signaling cascade in the cytoplasm of the T helper cell. The TCR is linked to this signaling cascade through another protein called *CD3.* Stimulation of CD3 results in the activation of enzymes (kinases) in the cytoplasm that mediate the production of two second messengers: inositol trisphosphate (IP_3) and diacylglycerol (DAG) (see Chapter 3). Inositol trisphosphate initiates a rise in the concentration of intracellular calcium ions, which also act as second messengers to change cell behavior. Other protein kinases turn on the genes for cytokines (e.g., IL-2, IFN-γ, and others), IL-2 receptors, and other cell surface proteins. As previously mentioned, the subtypes of T helper cells (i.e., T_H1, T_H2, and T_H17) secrete somewhat different amounts and

types of cytokines. These cytokines provide the "help" that T helper cells give to other cells of the immune system. For example, IL-2 activates helper and cytotoxic T cells, NK cells, and macrophages; and IFN-γ is a potent activator of macrophages. IL-2 and IFN-γ are the main cytokines secreted by T_H1 cells. The cytokines secreted by T_H2 cells have stimulatory effects on B cells (e.g., IL-4, IL-5, IL-6, IL-13). In addition, when a B cell is serving as the antigen-presenting cell, T helper cells provide specific B cell help through direct cell-to-cell contact by receptor proteins.

Cytotoxic T Cells (CD8⁺)

Cytotoxic T cells recognize antigen displayed in association with MHC class I protein. The CD8 protein is needed to facilitate binding to the

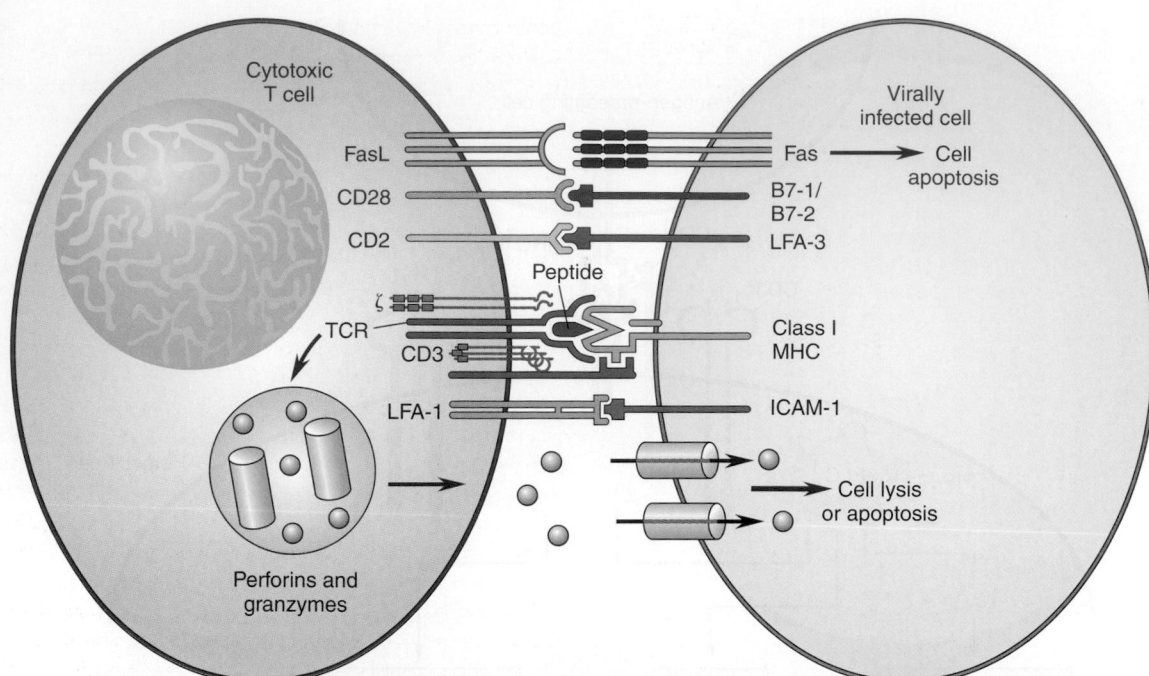

FIGURE 9-32 Cytotoxic T cells are able to recognize and bind antigen in association with major histocompatibility complex (MHC) class I molecules. The T cell receptor on the cytotoxic T cell binds to the antigen, and the CD8 protein recognizes the MHC I protein. Binding is specific. Binding of a cytotoxic T cell to its target stimulates granules containing perforin and granzymes to migrate to the cell contact site. Perforins then assemble into pores on the target cell, through which the granzymes can enter the target cell cytoplasm. The granzymes interrupt the cellular DNA and trigger apoptosis. *FasL,* Fas ligand (CD95L); *ICAM,* intercellular adhesion molecule; *LFA,* leukocyte function–associated antigen; *TCR,* T cell receptor.

MHC I, whereas the TCR specifically recognizes the presented antigen (Figure 9-32). Binding of the TCR to its corresponding antigen triggers a number of responses in the cytotoxic T cell. This process is similar to that described for T helper cells and involves signal transduction through CD3 proteins. Antigen binding by cytotoxic T cells is not sufficient to activate them. Cytotoxic T cells also require costimulation by IL-2 cytokines. IL-2 is secreted primarily by activated T helper cells (T_H1). Thus, cytotoxic T cells require cytokine "help" before they proliferate effectively. Cytokines are generally not enough to induce significant proliferation of target cells unless other coactivators are also presented by target cells (see Figure 9-32). Once activated, cytotoxic T cells proliferate into memory cells as well as effector cells. Effector cells accomplish their cytotoxic functions in two ways: through perforins and through CD95.

Perforins are proteins manufactured in the cytotoxic T cell and stored in granules (vesicles) within the cytoplasm. A number of proteolytic enzymes (granzymes) are located in the granules along with the perforins. Binding to the target cell causes the granules to migrate to the contact site, where they are released onto the target cell membrane. The perforins assemble into pores, which then allow the granzymes to move into the target cell. Granzymes degrade DNA and trigger target cell death (apoptosis).

Perforins function in a similar manner to the complement membrane attack complex previously described. It is not entirely clear how the cytotoxic T cell manages to escape injury in this process. Presumably, the perforins and granzymes are focused on the target cell in some controlled manner.

The CD95 protein on cytotoxic T cells is called the *CD95 ligand* (CD95L) or the *Fas ligand (FasL)*.[14] It can bind specifically to complementary CD95 proteins (Fas) found on the surface of target cells.

Normal, healthy cells do not express CD95 and are not recognized by cytotoxic cells. Binding of the CD95L to CD95 triggers programmed cell death (apoptosis) of the target cell (see Figure 9-32). This system is thought to be particularly important in culling senescent cells and self-reactive lymphocytes.

MECHANISMS OF HUMORAL IMMUNITY

B cells are responsible for antibody-mediated (humoral) immunity. B cells have two major subpopulations: memory cells and plasma cells. Memory B cells contain antigen receptors and function in a manner similar to memory T cells. In other words, memory of exposure to an antigen is stored in a clone of memory B cells. When exposed to the same type of antigen in the future, these memory B cells are able to respond rapidly with appropriate antibodies.

Some B cells differentiate into short-lived antibody-producing factories called *plasma cells*. All of the plasma cells in a clone secrete antibodies with identical antigen-binding specificity (monoclonal antibody). The secreted antibodies circulate in the blood and body fluids and bind specifically to the antigen that triggered their production. Once antigen is cleared, the population of plasma cells declines and the antibody concentration (titer) falls. However, some long-lived plasma cells migrate to the bone marrow where they continue to secrete a level of antibody sufficient to provide immediate protection upon the next exposure to the same antigen.[1]

Antigen Recognition by B Cells

During their development in the bone marrow, B cells begin to express BCRs on their cell surfaces. The structure of the antigen-binding area on the BCR is randomly determined in a manner similar to that

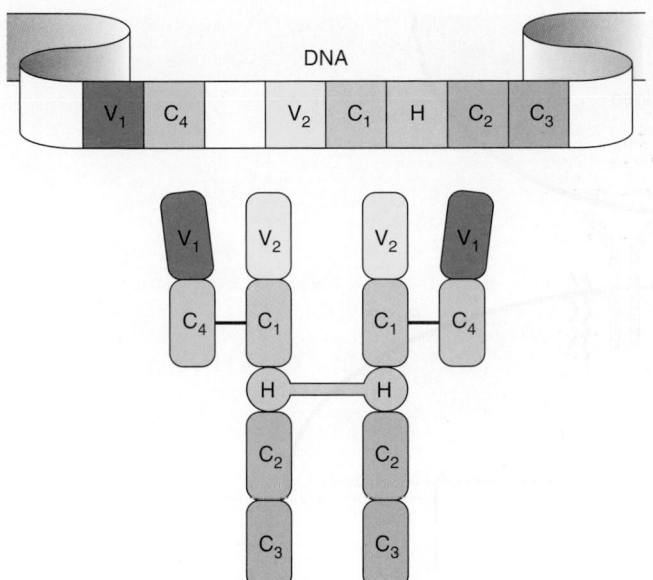

FIGURE 9-33 Two major classes of genes are responsible for coding for the variable *(V)* and constant *(C)* regions of an antibody. Variable genes code for the antibody region that binds to antigen. Constant genes form the stem of the antibody and are the same for any antibody of a given class.

described for TCRs. Each BCR is coded for by two distinct types of genes: one for the variable region, which makes up the antigen-binding site, and one for the constant region, which is essentially the same for all antibodies of a given class (Figure 9-33). The structure of the BCR bound to the B-cell surface is similar to the structure of IgM. Rearrangement, recombination, and selective splicing of variable region genes allow for great diversity of BCR binding specificities. The potential number of different BCR structures is enormous. Some of these combinations are unsuitable for BCR assembly, and it has been estimated that a typical human B-cell population can recognize approximately 10^{11} different antigenic epitopes.[3] As is the case with T cells, useful B cells—ones activated by antigen—will be preserved in the body, whereas B cells that encounter no antigen will not proliferate. Binding of an antigen to the B cell results in the cross-linking of two surface BCR proteins and initiates an intracellular cascade. These cascades activate transcription factors within the B cell (NFκB, NFAT, AP-1) that regulate genes involved in proliferation and differentiation of the B cell (Figure 9-34).

The growth and activity of B cells that recognize protein antigens are regulated by helper T cells. Binding of antigen to the B cell's BCR is a necessary but insufficient stimulus to produce an effective B-cell clone in most cases. To be effectively activated, the B cell must engulf some of the antigen, process it, and present it to T helper cells. This activity will initiate cell-to-cell contact between the B cell and its complementary T-cell helper. A number of receptor interactions bind the T cells and B cells together, in addition to the main MHC II–TCR interaction, and include CD80-CD28 and CD154-CD40 (Figure 9-35). These cell-to-cell binding interactions stimulate intracellular signaling pathways in the B cell (and T helper cell) that promote clonal expansion and differentiation. B cells also require certain cytokines to proliferate and begin antibody synthesis. B cells are quite dependent on T cell help during the initial exposure to antigen (primary response), but less so on subsequent exposures. Some types of B cells have BCRs that bind nonprotein antigens, such as bacterial carbohydrates and lipids. Because T cells only recognize peptides, these types of B-cell responses are T-cell independent. Other costimulatory signals, such as the

complement fragment C3d on the antigen, may provide the necessary costimulation to achieve a B-cell response and antibody production. It is doubtful that memory cells are formed in this process[1] (Figure 9-36).

Antibody Structure

Each antibody (immunoglobulin) molecule contains two identical light polypeptide chains joined by disulfide bonds to two identical heavy polypeptide chains. The geometry of the relationship between the heavy (H) and light (L) chains forms a Y-like structure. The H chains form the stem of the Y, and the L chains are on the outside of the arms of the Y. The antigen-binding end of the antibody is often called *Fab* (antigen-binding fragment), whereas the stem is called *Fc* (constant fragment). It is the structure of the constant fragment that determines the antibody class.

Antibodies are differentiated into five classes: IgG, IgM, IgA, IgD, and IgE. The structure and properties of the immunoglobulin classes are listed in Table 9-4. IgG and IgE circulate as single molecules or monomers; IgA is a dimer (two antibodies joined together); and IgM consists of five antibody molecules joined together to form a pentamer. IgD is found mainly on the B-cell plasma membrane and does not circulate in significant quantity. IgD is thought to participate in signal transduction across the B-cell membrane along with the BCR. Different antibody classes serve different immune functions in the body.

IgG, the most common type of immunoglobulin, accounts for 75% to 80% of all immunoglobulins. It is found in nearly equal proportions in the intravascular and interstitial compartments and has a long half-life of about 3 weeks.[15] IgG is the smallest of the immunoglobulins and can more easily escape the bloodstream to enter the interstitial fluid surrounding tissues.

IgM accounts for about 10% of circulating immunoglobulins and is predominantly found in the intravascular pool.[15] Its large pentamer structure prevents it from migrating through the capillary wall. IgM has a half-life of 10 days. It is the first immunoglobulin to be produced on exposure to antigens or after immunization and is the major antibody found on B-cell surfaces. IgM is the antibody class that works best to activate complement, which is important for cytotoxic functions in the immune system. Only one molecule of IgM is needed to activate complement, whereas two molecules of IgG are needed to activate complement.

IgA is produced by plasma cells located in the tissue under the skin and mucous membranes. IgA is primarily found in saliva, tears, tracheobronchial secretions, colostrum, breast milk, and gastrointestinal and genitourinary secretions. Transport of IgA into secretions is facilitated by binding to a secretory component produced by epithelial cells. This complex is called *secretory IgA* (Figure 9-37). The half-life of IgA is about 6 days.[15]

IgD is found in trace amounts in the serum (1%) and is located primarily on the membranes of B cells along with IgM. IgD has a half-life of 3 days.[15] IgD functions as a cellular antigen receptor acting to stimulate the B cell to multiply, differentiate, and secrete other specific immunoglobulins.

IgE is found bound by its Fc tail to receptors on the surface of basophils and mast cells (Figure 9-38). Only trace amounts of IgE are identified in the serum. IgE has a half-life of 2 days.[13] It has a role in immunity against helminthic parasites (worms) and is responsible for initiating inflammatory and allergic reactions (e.g., asthma, hay fever). IgE functions as a signaling molecule and causes mast cell degranulation when antigen is detected at the mast cell surface (see Chapter 10).

Class Switching and Affinity Maturation

During the course of an antibody response, the class of antibody manufactured by a particular B cell usually changes. The antigen-binding

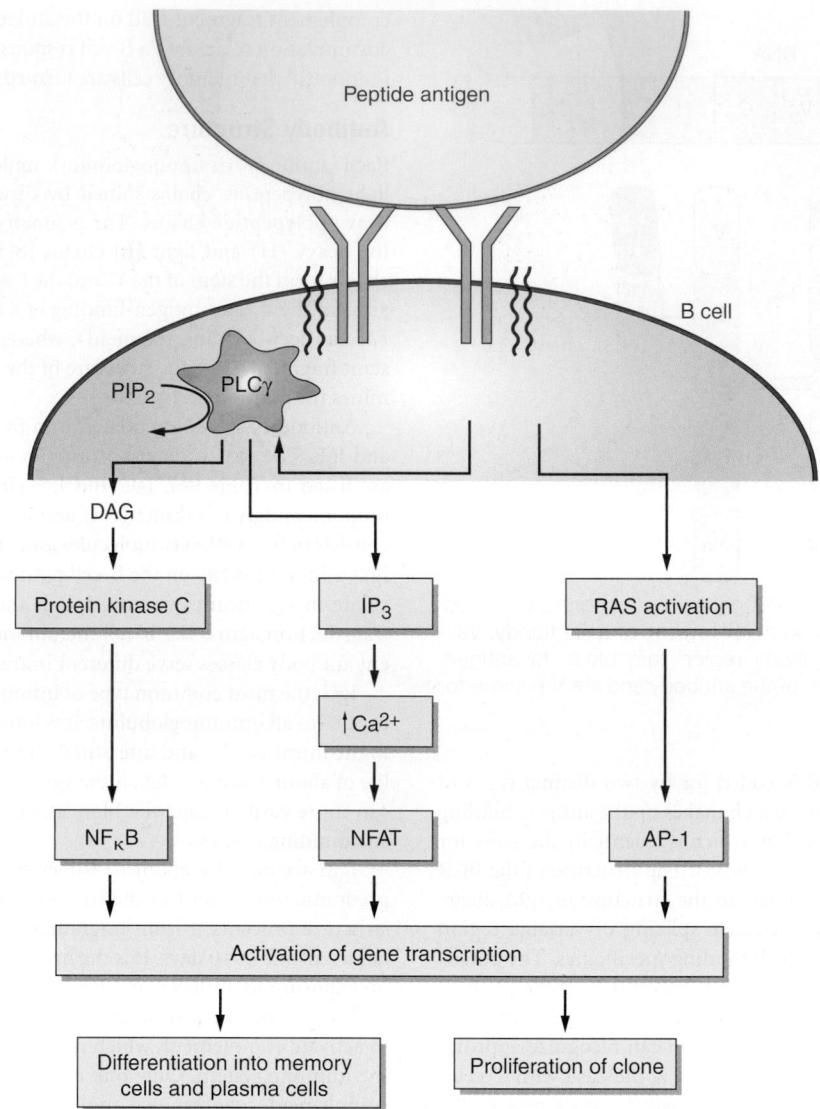

FIGURE 9-34 Major signaling pathways in B cells. Cross-linking of two surface B-cell receptors initiates intracellular pathways that subsequently activate several transcription factors leading to altered gene activity. *AP-1*, Activation protein-1; *DAG*, diacylglycerol; *IP₃*, inositol 1,4,5-trisphosphate; *NFAT*, nuclear factor of activated T cells; *NF_κB*, nuclear factor kappa B; *PIP₂*, phosphatidylinositol 4,5-bisphosphate; *PLCγ*, phospholipase C-γ.

site does not change significantly and remains specific for the particular antigen that initiated the response. To switch class, the B cell selects different constant region genes to splice to the antigen-binding fragment. Thus, most B cells begin by using genes that code for IgM and IgD. Then the B cell switches to produce IgG, IgE, or IgA.[16] The triggers that determine the class of antibody a particular B cell will produce are not completely understood. Some cytokines have a role in class switching. For example, IFN-γ promotes IgG production, IL-4 promotes IgE production, and transforming growth factor-β (TGF-β) promotes IgA production[16] (Figure 9-39).

Knowledge about the normal progression of class switching may be helpful in determining whether an infectious process is acute or chronic. For example, a person newly infected with hepatitis B virus would be expected to have primarily IgM antihepatitis B antibodies, whereas in chronic or previous infection, B cells would switch class to produce mainly IgG. The relative concentrations of antihepatitis B IgM and IgG can help identify the time of onset of the infection.

Over the course of a B cell antibody response, the affinity with which the antibodies bind to antigen often increases. This is thought to occur because of a process called *affinity maturation* during which B cells undergo a hypermutation response producing random changes in the antigen-binding pocket of the BCR.[17] Those that bind antigen most avidly are stimulated to proliferate to a greater extent. Thus, the antibodies formed later in an immune response are more efficient in binding antigen at lower and lower concentrations. Affinity maturation occurs in specialized germinal centers in the lymph nodes.

Antibody Functions

Antibodies function in a number of ways to enhance the localization and removal of antigens from the body. These functions can generally be summarized as precipitation, agglutination, neutralization, opsonization, and complement activation. Precipitation and agglutination occur because each arm of the immunoglobulin Y structure can bind an antigenic epitope. This structure allows the antibodies and antigens to bind together into large insoluble complexes that precipitate out of

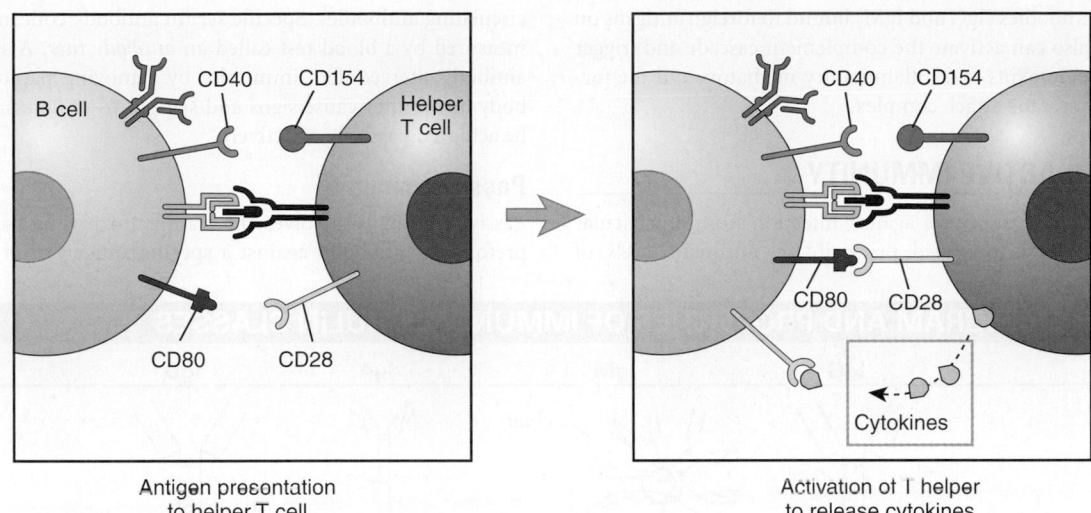

FIGURE 9-35 Activation of a B cell requires T helper cell "help." This help is given through a number of cell-to-cell interactions via receptors, as well as through the secretion of cytokines that stimulate B-cell growth and differentiation.

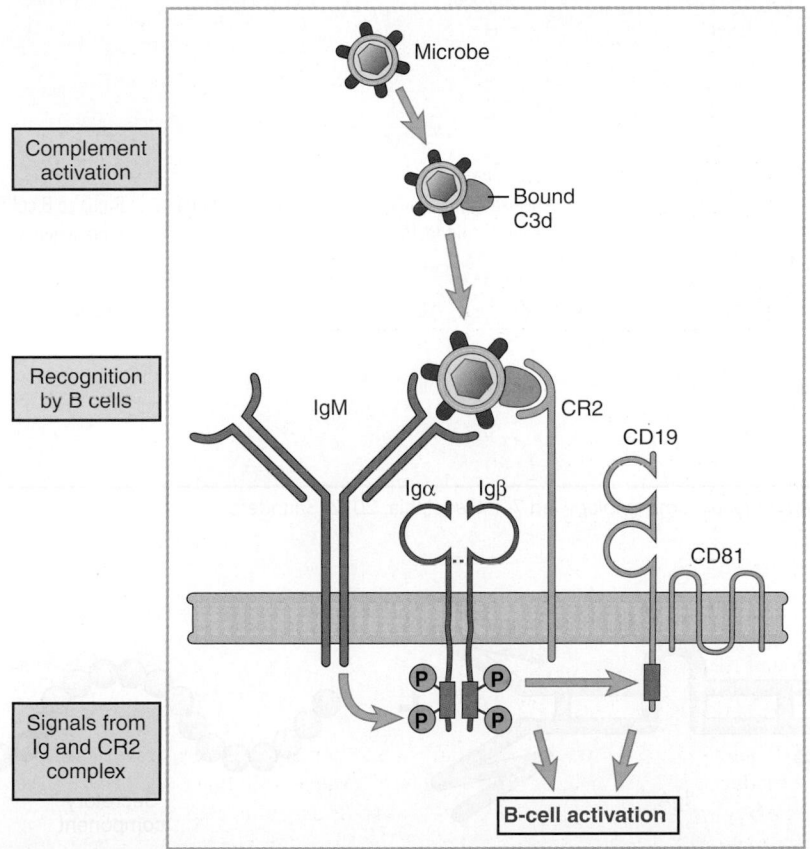

FIGURE 9-36 In response to nonprotein antigens (T-cell independent), B cells can be activated by complement opsonins on the microbial antigen. The complement-receptor *(CR)* interaction provides a costimulatory signal to the B-cell receptor–antigen signal. (Redrawn from Abbas AK et al: *Cellular and molecular immunology,* ed 7, Philadelphia, 2012, Saunders, p 161.)

body fluids (Figure 9-40). Agglutination refers to the same process as applied to cellular antigens rather than soluble antigens. It is efficient for phagocytic cells to find the large complexes and clear them from the system.

Antibodies can function as antitoxins by neutralizing bacterial toxin. This role is accomplished by binding the toxins before they can interact with cells or by covering the active portions of the toxin and inactivating it. Some antibodies are effective opsonins. They coat the foreign antigen and thereby make it more recognizable to phagocytic cells. Macrophages, neutrophils, eosinophils, and NK cells have receptors for the Fc ends of the antibodies, which help them bind to opsonized antigens. Antibodies thus make the innate phagocytic processes more efficient. Antibodies (IgG and IgM) bound to foreign antigens on cell membranes also can activate the complement cascade and trigger the release of chemotaxins and inflammatory mediators and the formation of the membrane attack complex.

PASSIVE AND ACTIVE IMMUNITY

Immunity is a state of resistance against infection from a particular pathogen. Immunity is provided primarily by adequate levels of

circulating antibodies. Specific serum antibody concentrations can be measured by a blood test called an *antibody titer*. A sufficiently high antibody titer confers immunity by removing pathogens from the body before they cause signs and symptoms of illness. Immunity can be achieved passively or actively.

Passive Immunity

Passive immunity involves the transfer of plasma (sera) containing preformed antibodies against a specific antigen from a protected or

---

TABLE 9-4   DIAGRAM AND PROPERTIES OF IMMUNOGLOBULIN CLASSES

Property	IgG	IgM	IgA	IgD	IgE
Half-life (days)	23-25	5	6	3	2.5
Percent total immunoglobulin	80	6	13	0-1	0.002
Molecular weight (daltons)	146,000	900,000	160,000	184,000	200,000
Complement fixation	++	+++	–	–	–
Placental transfer	+++	–	–	–	–
Receptor for macrophage	+++	–	–	–	–
Reaction with staph protein A	+++	–	–	–	–
Passive cutaneous anaphylaxis	+++	–	–	–	+
Transported across epithelium	–	Occasionally	+	–	–
Prominent antibody activity	Anti-Rh against infections	ABO isoaggulutinins, rheumatoid factor	Against infections	Binds to B cells in presence of IgM	Mast cell sensitization, cytophilic antibody skin sensitizing antibody
Cell-Binding Functions					
Mononuclear cells	+	–	–	–	?/+
Neutrophils	+	–	+	–	–
Mast cells/basophils	–	–	–	–	+++
T cells/B cells	+	+	+	+	+
Platelets	+	+	–	–	?

Data from Abbas AK: *Cellular and molecular immunology,* ed 7, Philadelphia, 2012, Saunders.

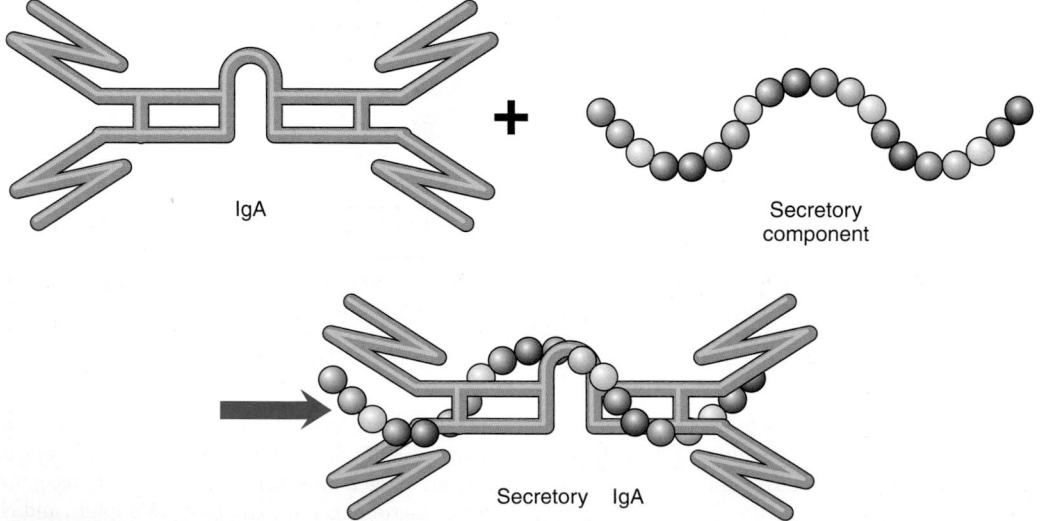

FIGURE 9-37 IgA is often combined with a protein called *secretory component,* which helps bind two IgA molecules together at their Fc ends.

immunized person to an unprotected or nonimmunized person. As a treatment, this is indicated in the following situations: (1) when B cell immunodeficiency exists; (2) when highly susceptible persons are exposed to a disease without adequate time for active immunization; and (3) when antibody injection may alleviate or suppress the effects of an antigenic toxin.

Passive transfer of antibodies can occur in a variety of ways. In the fetus, certain maternal IgG antibodies can cross the placental barrier. Most of the time these antibodies are beneficial and assist the newborn in resisting pathogens. However, in some cases these antibodies can be damaging to the fetus, as occurs in hemolytic disease of the newborn. In this disorder, maternal antibodies bind to and lyse fetal red blood cells (see Chapters 10 and 13).

Antibody, complement, and macrophage function is deficient at birth. Newborns who are breast fed may have improved immune function. Newborns receive IgA antibodies through breast milk. The infant's immature gastrointestinal tract and low proteolytic enzyme activity do not destroy all protein, which allows some of the IgA antibodies to be

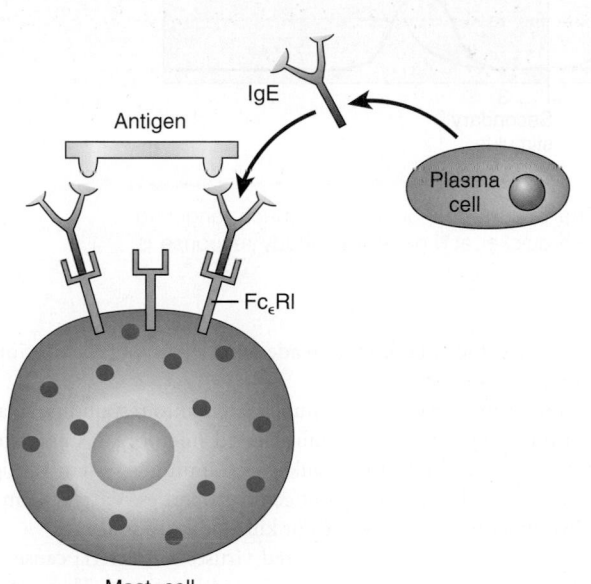

FIGURE 9-38 Mast cells bind IgE antibody with their Fc receptors ($Fc_\epsilon RI$) and display the IgE on the cell surface, where they are available to bind antigens.

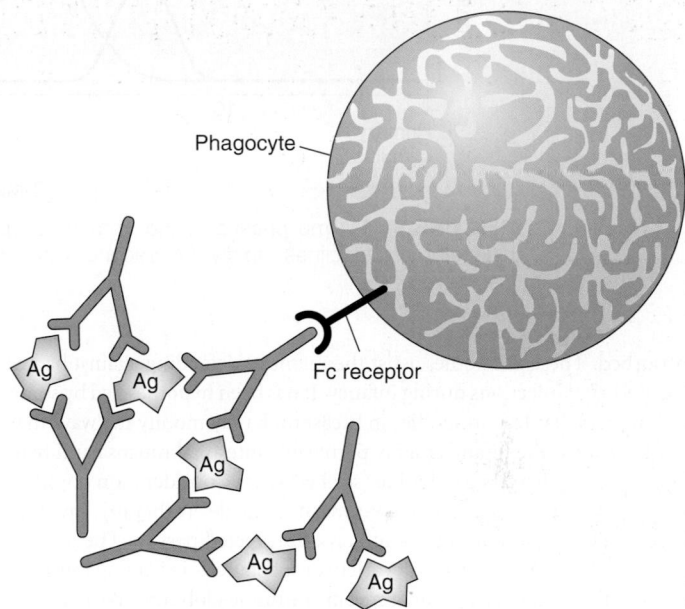

FIGURE 9-40 Large antigen *(Ag)*-antibody complexes tend to precipitate out of solution, which makes it easier for phagocytic cells to find and eliminate the antigens.

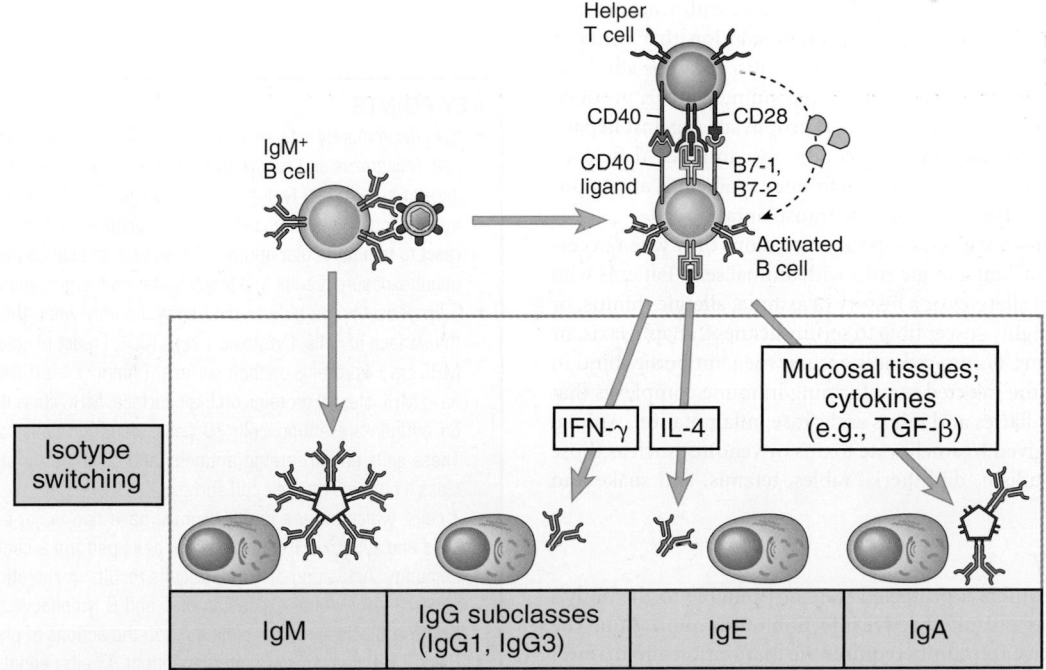

FIGURE 9-39 Activated B cells undergo class switching from IgM to IgG, IgE, or IgA. Class switching is influenced by the presence of specific cytokines. *IFN*, Interferon; *IL*, interleukin; *TGF*, transforming growth factor. (Redrawn from Abbas AK et al: *Cellular and molecular immunology*, ed 7, Philadelphia, 2012, Saunders, p 257.)

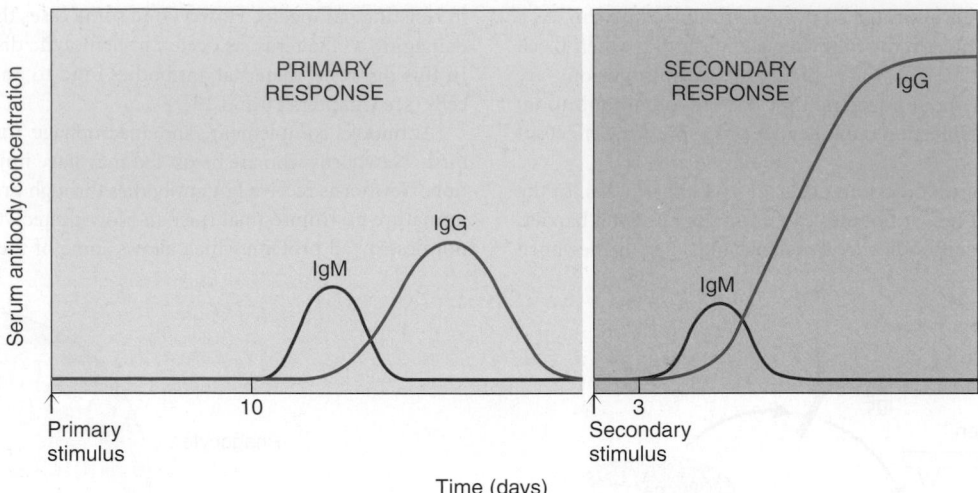

FIGURE 9-41 Time phases in the immune response. The primary response takes much longer to develop and declines rapidly. On second exposure, a much quicker and greater antibody response is achieved.

absorbed. These antibodies assist the infant in defending against bacterial and viral infections during infancy. It has been hypothesized by some researchers that IgA antibodies in breast milk may modify the ways that proteins cross the infant's highly permeable intestinal mucosa and help prevent food allergies in later life (see Pediatrics Consideration box).[18]

Another method of passive immunity, called serotherapy, involves direct injection of antibodies into an unprotected person. The unprotected individual can receive a variety of substances, including immune globulin (human) such as IgG; specific immune globulins like hepatitis B immune globulin (human) or rabies immune globulin (human); plasma containing all human antibodies; or animal antibodies such as diphtheria antitoxin, tetanus antitoxin, botulism antitoxin, and antirabies serum.

Human immune globulin contains mostly IgG with traces of IgA and IgM. It is a sterile, concentrated protein solution that contains antibodies from the pooled plasma of many adults. It can be administered intramuscularly or intravenously, depending on the product. Human immune globulins may be used as prophylaxis against hepatitis B and as therapy for the following conditions: antibody deficiency disorders, pediatric acquired immunodeficiency syndrome, and hypogammaglobulinemia after bone marrow transplantation.

Animal antibodies are given in specific situations only when necessary because of significant allergic risks with animal sera. Patients who have specific animal allergies or a history of asthma, allergic rhinitis, or other allergies are highly susceptible to serum sickness, anaphylaxis, or acute febrile reactions. Serum sickness occurs when antibodies bind to foreign proteins in the injected sera, forming immune complexes that precipitate into capillaries and joints and cause inflammation. Animal antibodies may be given to ameliorate toxins or venoms, such as those associated with botulism, diphtheria, rabies, tetanus, and snake and spider bites.

Active Immunity

Active immunity confers a protected state attributable to the body's immune response as a result of active infection or immunization. The development of active immunity requires the maturation and maintenance of memory B cells. On second exposure to antigen, the antibody response is much greater and more rapid (Figure 9-41). Exposure to antigen can be achieved through active infection or through immunization. The immune system must be exposed to the antigen at a sufficient dose for an adequate length of time to stimulate an immune response.

Immunization tricks the immune system into responding to a perceived infection. Vaccines contain altered microorganisms or toxins that retain their ability to stimulate the immune system (antigenic properties) but do not have pathogenic properties. Vaccines can contain live and attenuated (altered) or killed infectious agents.

Vaccines that contain live, altered viruses or bacteria cause active infection but little injury to the vaccinated individual. These vaccines mimic a natural immune response, activating B and T cells, and provide good humoral and cellular immunity with longer lasting memory and often lifetime immunity. Examples of vaccines registered in the United States are listed in Box 9-1.

KEY POINTS

- Specific immunity refers to functions of B and T lymphocytes. Each lymphocyte recognizes and reacts to only one particular antigen. On initial exposure to an antigen, lymphocytes undergo clonal expansion; consequently, many lymphocytes are distributed throughout the body to recognize and react to that particular antigen. These cells are called *memory cells*. Subsequent exposure results in a much faster and larger lymphocyte response.

- T lymphocytes are able to bind antigens only when they are displayed on the surface of cells. Cytotoxic T cells (CD8+) react to cells that have foreign MHC class I proteins on their surface. T helper cells (CD4+) bind to cells that have MHC class II proteins on their surface. MHC class II proteins are found on antigen-presenting cells (B cells, dendritic cells, and macrophages). These cells engulf foreign antigens and combine the antigens with MHC class II proteins on their cell surface.

- T cells, which mature in the thymus, have two major subgroups: T helper cells and cytotoxic T cells. T helper cells perform a central role in specific immunity. Activation of T helper cells results in secretion of the cytokines necessary for clonal expansion of T and B lymphocytes. Cytotoxic T cells locate and lyse abnormal cells through the actions of perforins.

- B and T cell functions are interdependent. T cells cannot respond to soluble antigens. B cells can process free antigen and present it to T cells. On first exposure, B cells are minimally activated by antigen unless they are stimulated by cytokines and coreceptors from T cells.

Changes in the Immune System in Infants

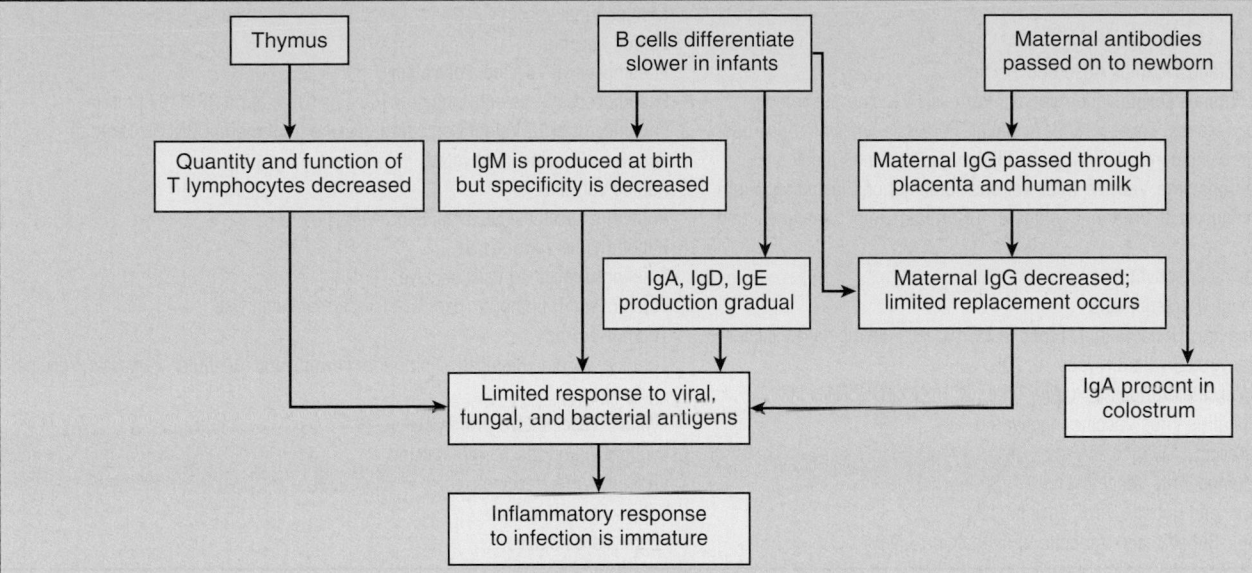

The immune system is immature in an infant. Infants generally do not produce immunoglobulin (Ig) until the beginning of the second month of life and then production is slow (Hockenberry and Wilson, 2011). IgM is produced at birth but specificity is decreased, limiting the infant's ability to fight some antigens. IgM reaches adult levels by 9 to 12 months. IgA, IgD, and IgE begin gradual production in the second month of life and reach adult levels around early childhood.

Infants rely on maternal antibodies for production until their own immune system can mature. Maternal IgG is passed through the placenta and breast milk and for the first 3 months provides protection to the infant from antigens to which the mother has been exposed. IgG levels decline after 4 months and remain low until 6 months of age. Forty percent of infants achieve adult levels of

IgG by 1 year of age with the remaining reaching adult IgG levels by 4 years of age. IgA is present in the colostrum and believed to protect the infant's gastrointestinal tract until more IgA can be produced.

The thymus is large in infants and decreases in size over childhood. By the end of adolescence, the thymus shrivels and its function declines. The infant's immune response is immature resulting in a limited response to viral, fungal, and bacterial antigens in the infant.

Reference

Hockenberry MJ, Wilson D: *Wong's nursing care of infants and children*, ed 8, St Louis, 2011, Mosby.

- B lymphocytes mature in bone marrow and lymph tissue. B cells have receptors on their surfaces that can bind antigens. Each B cell binds only one particular antigen. With appropriate T helper cell "help," antigen binding causes the B cell to divide (clonal expansion). Some of the daughter cells become plasma cells, which actively produce and secrete antibodies. Other daughter cells (memory cells) resemble the original cell and are distributed in lymph throughout the body. On subsequent exposure to the antigen, antibody production is rapid.
- Antibodies are proteins that specifically bind a particular antigen. Antibodies have several functions, including precipitation, agglutination, neutralization, opsonization, and complement activation.
- The five major antibody classes are IgG, IgM, IgA, IgD, and IgE. Antibody class is determined by the structure of the Fc portion. IgG is the most prevalent antibody class (75%). IgM is the first kind to be produced on antigen exposure. IgA is found primarily in body secretions. IgD is present on the B-cell membrane and functions in signal transduction. IgE binds to basophil and mast cell membranes and mediates inflammation and allergy.
- Administration of preformed antibodies confers passive immunity. Passive immunity provides immediate but temporary protection. Active immunity occurs when individuals are exposed to antigen that stimulates their own lymphocytes to produce memory cells. Active immunity confers long-term protection but may take several weeks to develop.

INTEGRATED FUNCTION AND REGULATION OF THE IMMUNE SYSTEM

The innate and adaptive cells of the immune system work interdependently to protect the host from foreign antigens. Efficient interdependent function depends on a complex communication network that allows coordination of various immune components. One of the reasons that the immune system uses such a complex communication system is to ensure that normal healthy tissue is not injured. The destructive powers of the immune system must be tightly regulated to avoid undue tissue damage. These regulatory controls can be affected by aging and disease. The effects of aging on immune function are described in Geriatric Considerations: Changes in the Immune System. In the following sections, major events in the immune response to a new antigen are summarized and mechanisms of immune regulation are described.

INTEGRATED RESPONSE TO NEW ANTIGEN

A new antigen entering the body through the skin or mucous membranes will generally encounter tissue macrophages and dendritic cells stationed in strategic locations in the body as part of the mononuclear phagocyte system. Macrophages initiate activity of both innate and

BOX 9-1 SELECTED VACCINES AVAILABLE FOR IMMUNIZATION IN THE UNITED STATES

Adenovirus Type 4 and Type 7 Vaccine, Live, Oral

Anthrax Vaccine Adsorbed

BCG Vaccine

Diphtheria and Tetanus Toxoids Adsorbed

Diphtheria and Tetanus Toxoids and Acellular Pertussis Vaccine Adsorbed

Diphtheria and Tetanus Toxoids and Acellular Pertussis Vaccine Adsorbed, Hepatitis B (recombinant) and Inactivated Poliovirus Vaccine Combined

Haemophilus b Conjugate Vaccine (plus various combinations including: Diphtheria, Meningococcal Protein Conjugate, Tetanus Toxoid Conjugate, and Hepatitis B)

Hepatitis A Vaccine, Inactivated

Hepatitis B Vaccine (Recombinant)

Human Papillomavirus Quadrivalent (Types 6, 11, 16, 18) Recombinant Vaccine

Human Papillomavirus Bivalent (Types 16, 18)

Influenza Virus Vaccine (Various including Types A, H1N1, B, H5N1)

Japanese Encephalitis Virus Vaccine Inactivated

Measles Virus Vaccine, Live

Measles and Mumps Virus Vaccine, Live

Measles, Mumps, and Rubella Virus Vaccine, Live

Measles, Mumps, Rubella, and Varicella Virus Vaccine, Live

Meningococcal Polysaccharide Vaccine, Groups A, C, Y, and W-135 Combined

Mumps Virus Vaccine Live

Plague Vaccine

Pneumococcal Vaccine, Polyvalent

Pneumococcal 7-Valent Conjugate Vaccine (Diphtheria CRM197 Protein)

Pneumococcal 13-Valent Conjugate Vaccine (Diphtheria CRM197 Protein)

Poliovirus Vaccine Inactivated

Rabies Vaccine

Rotavirus Vaccine, Live, Oral, Pentavalent

Rubella Virus Vaccine Live

Smallpox (Vaccinia) Vaccine, Live

Tetanus and Diphtheria Toxoids Adsorbed for Adult Use

Tetanus Toxoid

Tetanus Toxoid, Reduced Diphtheria Toxoid, and Acellular Pertussis Vaccine Adsorbed

Typhoid Vaccine Live Oral Ty21a

Typhoid Vi Polysaccharide Vaccine

Varicella Virus Vaccine Live

Yellow Fever Vaccine

Zoster Vaccine, Live

Data from www.fda.gov/BiologicsBloodVaccines/Vaccines/ApprovedProducts/ucm093833.htm.

GERIATRIC CONSIDERATIONS

Changes in the Immune System

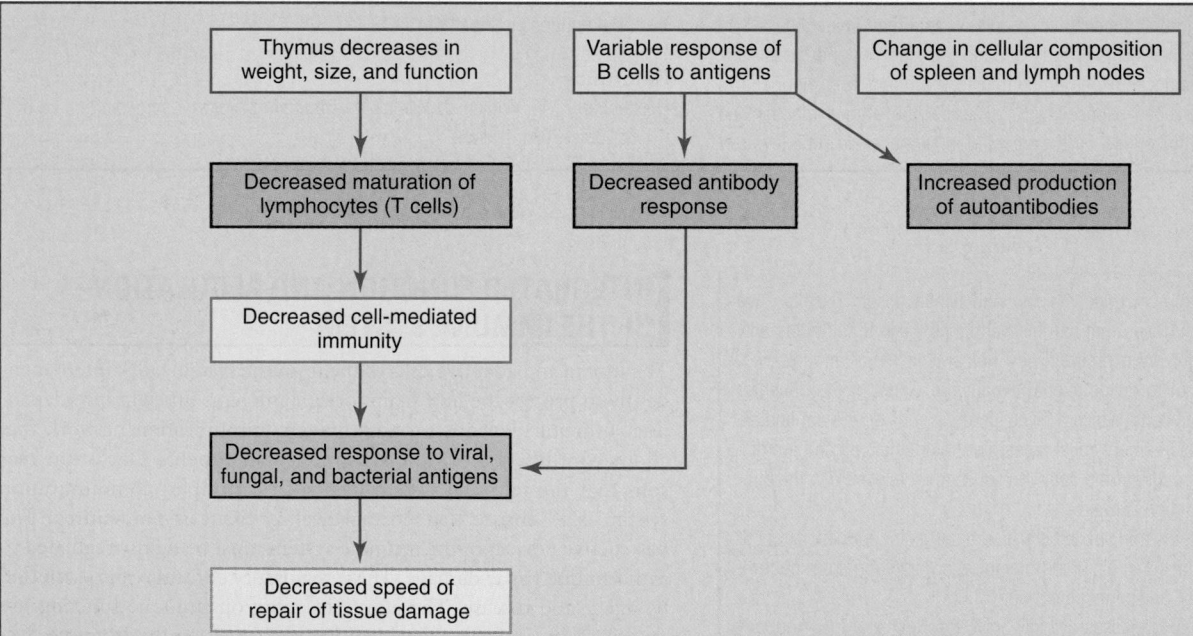

In the elderly, immune system function is altered with a decreased ability to respond to antigenic stimulation. The elderly are able to respond to infections with previously produced "remembered" antibodies. However, they are less able to respond to new antigens. As a result of these changes, there is decreased speed of repair of tissue damage and increased vulnerability to disease. The cells of the immune system in elderly persons are not able to proliferate or reproduce as effectively as those in younger persons. Although the total number of T cells remains the same, T-cell function is decreased. T cells are less able to proliferate and have decreased cytotoxicity. Antibody production also decreases, especially antibodies such as IgG. There is also a rise in autoantibody production, which may influence the increase in autoimmune disease in the elderly. Thymus size decreases after puberty, causing a decline in thymic hormone production, decreased T-cell differentiation, and reduced T cell–related B-cell differentiation. Usually thymic hormone secretions stop after age 60 years. However, the role of thymus involution in elderly immune system changes is currently uncertain.

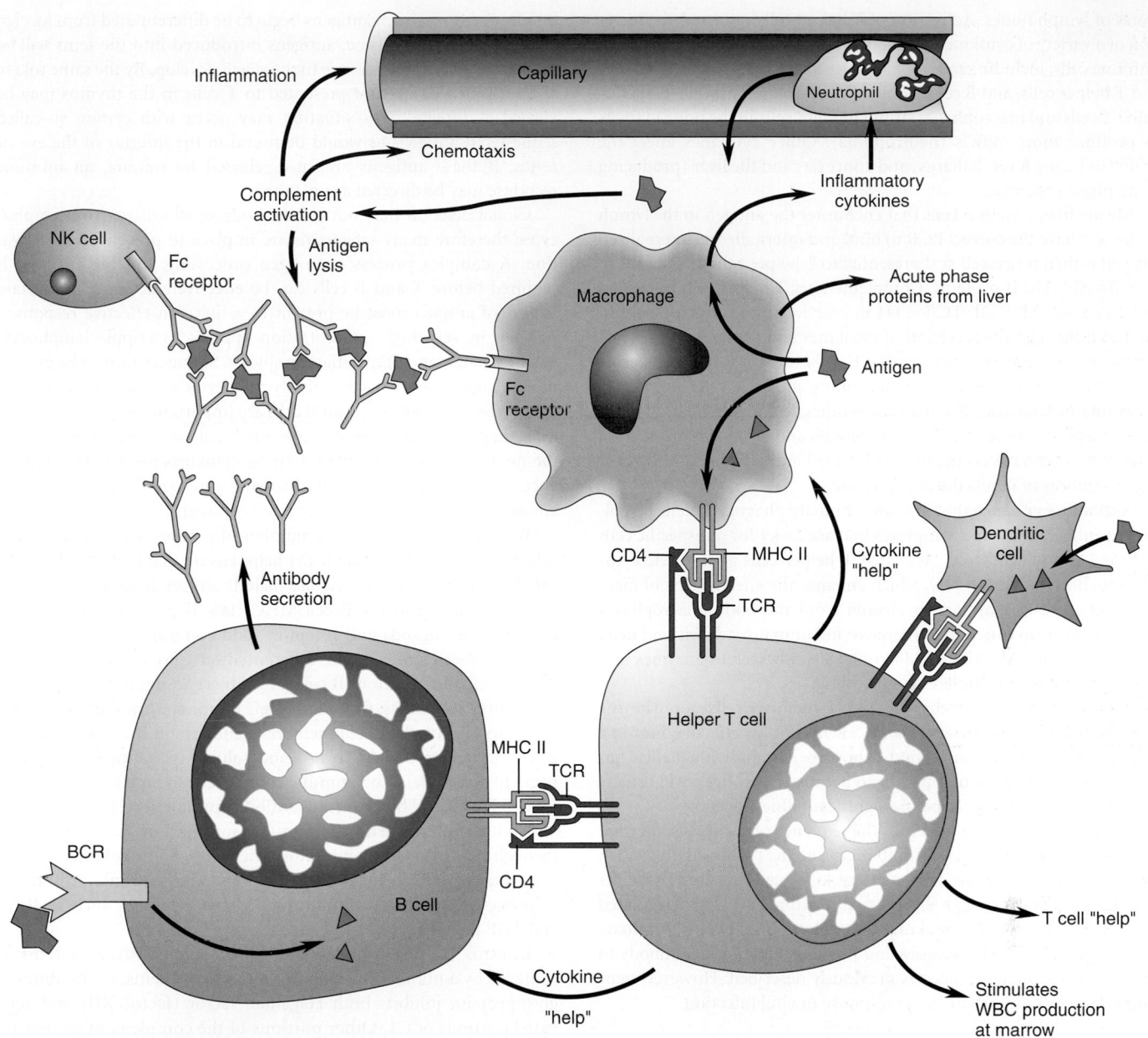

FIGURE 9-42 Diagram showing the integrated function of a number of immune components. Note that the macrophage is at the center of many immune functions, including chemotaxis and inflammation, presentation of antigen to T cells, and phagocytosis of antibody-antigen complexes. *BCR*, B-cell receptor; *MHC*, major histocompatibility complex; *NK*, natural killer; *TCR*, T cell receptor; *WBC*, white blood cell.

specific immune components (Figure 9-42). First, activated macrophages release cytokines that initiate inflammation and chemotaxis. Some of these cytokines (TNF-α, IL-1) induce capillary endothelial cells to express selectins and integrin ligands that help circulating leukocytes adhere to the capillary wall (margination) and then move into the tissue locations of antigens (emigration). Neutrophils, macrophages, and NK cells are attracted to the infected area by chemotactic factors, some of which are released by macrophages, whereas others are products of the complement cascade and tissue injury. The complement cascade is activated by the alternative pathway on primary exposure to an antigen. Complement fragments C3a and C5a are potent inflammatory agents. Complement activation also results in the formation of membrane attack complexes that directly lyse cellular antigens.

Tissue injury associated with the infectious process also activates both the coagulation cascade, which forms a fibrin meshwork to help entrap and localize the agent, and the kinin system, which promotes vasodilation to increase blood flow to the area. A number of other vasodilatory chemicals may be released from mast cells in the area when they degranulate. These inflammatory chemicals lead to the classic manifestations of inflammation: warmth, swelling, redness, pain, and loss of function. Neutrophils, macrophages, and NK cells that emigrate to the tissue find their targets through innate receptors on their cell surfaces. Thus, they are as effective on first exposure to an antigen as they are on subsequent exposures. These receptors bind to complement opsonins and molecules expressed on microbes such as lipopolysaccharide and mannose. NK cells release cytotoxins onto their targets; macrophages and neutrophils phagocytose and digest their targets.

Dendritic cells and macrophages ingest protein antigens to process and present them to T helper cells in association with MHC class II proteins. Dendritic cells move from the tissue and travel to the T-cell zones of lymph nodes. Activation of T helper cells results in the secretion of a variety of cytokines that boost the growth and activity of many immune cells, including macrophages, neutrophils, NK cells, cytotoxic and T helper cells, and B cells. Some of the cytokines produced by activated T cells and macrophages stimulate stem cells in the bone marrow to produce more WBCs (neutrophilia). Other cytokines affect the brain (inducing fever, lethargy, and anorexia) and the liver (producing acute phase proteins).

Meanwhile, certain B cells that encounter the antigen in the lymph nodes will have the correct BCR to bind and internalize it. Internalized antigen is then processed and presented to T helper cells in association with B-cell MHC II proteins. Complementary T helper cells then bind the B cell (via MHC II–TCR–CD4 interactions) and provide help to the B cell through the secretion of cytokines and through coreceptor-mediated second-messenger signals. B cells thus activated proliferate into a clone of cells, with some becoming memory cells and others becoming plasma cells. Plasma cells synthesize and secrete antibodies that specifically bind the antigen. Significant antibody production takes 10 to 14 days to occur, and the infected individual may have signs and symptoms of illness during this time.

Antibodies enhance the function of innate phagocytic cells by collecting antigen into large complexes that are easier for nonspecific cells to locate and phagocytose. Activated T helper cells also secrete cytokines such as IL-2 and IFN-γ, which enhance the effectiveness of macrophages. After the antigen is cleared from the body, macrophages perform clean-up functions to remove inflammatory debris and dead neutrophils from the tissue. Macrophages also secrete enzymes and growth factors that stimulate tissue healing.

After the primary infection, B and T memory cells populate the body in much larger numbers and can mount an effective immune response very quickly on second exposure. The individual then has immunity for the particular pathogen because the antigen will usually be cleared from the system before significant illness occurs.

If the infectious agent is a virus, the sequence of events is somewhat different. Virally infected cells initiate cytotoxic T cell activity, which serves to kill the infected cells. Natural killer cells are important for detecting and destroying virally infected cells that have down-regulated their MHC I proteins, making themselves invisible to cytotoxic T cells.[19] Helper T cell responses and B-cell production of antibody to the virus occur by the processes previously described. However, neutrophils are less important in the response to viral infection.

REGULATION OF IMMUNE FUNCTION

The mechanisms that promote inflammation and enhance immune function are much better understood than those that negatively regulate these processes. However, the mechanisms for inactivating an immune response and keeping inflammation in check are just as important. The destructive powers of the immune system can cause severe tissue damage unless carefully controlled.

Inhibition of immune responses occurs in a number of different ways. The process of inducing tolerance to self antigens is of primary importance. Because both T and B lymphocytes produce antigen-binding receptors by a random process, generation of self-reactive lymphocytes cannot be prevented. As previously mentioned, B and T cells are subjected to a rigorous selection process as they mature in the bone marrow and thymus, respectively. Several theories have been proposed to explain how self-reactive cells are detected and eliminated. The clonal deletion theory suggests that cells in the thymus process and present self antigens to developing T cells. Those lymphocytes that avidly bind self antigens are triggered to initiate programmed cell death (apoptosis).[20] There appears to be a critical time in fetal development when self antigens begin to be differentiated from foreign antigens. Before that time, antigens introduced into the fetus will be viewed as "self" and tolerance to them will develop. By the same token, self antigens that are not presented to T cells in the thymus may be viewed as foreign. This situation may occur with certain so-called sequestered antigens as would be found in the interior of the eye or testes. If these antigens are later released by trauma, an immune response may be directed against them.

Clonal deletion may not rid the body of all self-reactive lymphocytes; therefore many safeguards are in place to prevent their activation. A complex process of antigen processing and presentation is required before T and B cells can be effectively activated. A certain "dose" of antigen must be present to achieve an effective response.[1] Antigen in very high concentration appears to cripple lymphocyte responsiveness and may initiate apoptosis. Self antigens may be present in such high quantity that reactive lymphocytes are killed. Because dendritic cells, macrophages, and B cells are important antigen-presenting cells, they can exert some influence on T cell activation by controlling the dose of antigen presented. Certain cytokines are known to influence the production of MHC proteins and can therefore alter the amount of antigen to which T cells are exposed.

B-cell activation requires a number of costimulatory signals from different sources. This complexity helps ensure that B cells will be activated appropriately. These signals include antigen binding to the BCR, T helper binding to the B cell MHC class II protein, expression of costimulatory ligands and receptors, and secretion of cytokines that promote B-cell growth and differentiation into memory cells and plasma cells. In addition, B cells are subject to negative feedback by circulating antibodies. Circulating IgG antibodies can bind to special receptors (Fc) on the B-cell membrane and inhibit B-cell activity.[21] As B cells switch from IgM to IgG and soluble IgG-antigen complexes begin to accumulate, the immune complexes can bind to the Fc receptors on B cells and block further antibody production (Figure 9-43).

Another mechanism of immune suppression is accomplished through cells that secrete inhibitory chemicals. Some subtypes of CD4 T cells may perform regulatory functions. They can inhibit immune responses by secreting immunosuppressive cytokines such as IL-10 and TGF-β.

Control of the complement, kinin, and clotting systems is achieved by a number of inhibitory binding proteins. C1 inhibitor, a glycoprotein, inhibits both Hageman factor (factor XII) and activated portions of C1. Other portions of the complement system are regulated by other binding proteins (e.g., factor I, factor H, and S protein). S protein is of particular importance. It prevents the complement membrane attack complex from attaching to and lysing cell membranes.

The production of oxygen free radicals by neutrophils can be inhibited through a number of antioxidant enzymes, including superoxide dismutase, glutathione peroxidase, and catalase. Vitamin E and β-carotene are fat-soluble vitamins that react with oxygen free radicals and prevent membrane damage. Uric acid and vitamin C neutralize oxidizing agents in the cytoplasm.[22] Neutrophils also release proteolytic enzymes that injure tissues. Protease inhibitors synthesized by the liver, such as α_1-antitrypsin, help reduce excessive protein destruction.

The neuroendocrine system also has a role in immune regulation. Immune cells have receptors for glucocorticoid hormones and a number of neuropeptides, including enkephalins, endorphins, adrenocorticotropic hormone, oxytocin, somatostatin, and substance P.[23,24] It is a well-known phenomenon that stress and depression can lead to reduced immune function. Some of these hormones are believed to be responsible for this effect. The immune system also affects the nervous

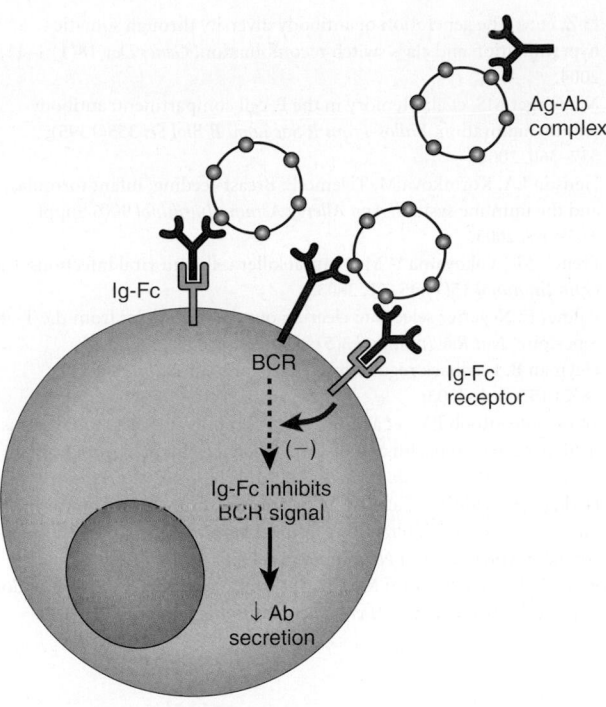

FIGURE 9-43 IgG antibody can bind to antigen to form antigen-antibody *(Ag-Ab)* complexes that attach to special Fc receptors on the surface of B cells. Binding of the antigen-antibody complexes in this manner inhibits B-cell production of antibody. This process is called *negative-feedback regulation. BCR,* B-cell receptor.

system through secreted cytokines such as IL-1 and TNF-α, which induce sleep and malaise.

One of the most important mechanisms of terminating an immune reaction is the elimination of the inciting antigen. As the antigen is cleared, levels of many of the cytokines and costimulators are reduced so that "survival signals" are no longer given to lymphocyte populations and they undergo apoptosis.

Despite these complex and effective regulatory mechanisms, immune and inflammatory disorders are extremely common. Chapter 10 describes the pathophysiology of the common overreactions and underreactions of the immune system.

KEY POINTS

- Specific and innate immune cells work together to protect the body from foreign antigens. Macrophages and dendritic cells play a central role because they are commonly the first immune cells to encounter the antigen. Macrophages secrete cytokines that stimulate WBC production and help WBCs locate the area. Tissue reactions activate the clotting cascade and kinin system, which help to localize the antigen and promote movement of fluid and immune cells into the tissue.
- Macrophages and dendritic cells are antigen-presenting cells that engulf and display antigen on their cell surface in association with MHC class II proteins. T helper cells are specifically activated by these antigen-presenting cells. T helper cells secrete cytokines that promote the production of WBCs in the marrow, initiate proliferation of mature B and T cells, and stimulate the phagocytic potential of macrophages and neutrophils.
- B-cell proliferation and antibody secretion usually require T cell help. B cells internalize and present antigen to T cells, which then stimulate B-cell proliferation. B cells secrete antibodies that help phagocytic cells localize and destroy antigens.
- The immune response to primary exposure is slow and often insufficient to prevent illness. Memory cells that develop during primary exposure can mount a more effective response on subsequent exposure and usually prevent manifestations of illness.
- T and B lymphocytes must be tolerant to self. T lymphocytes capable of reacting with self tissue are thought to be destroyed or permanently inactivated during development in the thymus. One theory suggests that lymphocytes must come in contact with all self antigens during development, and those that do not specifically bind self antigens are allowed to survive.
- B cells are subject to careful regulation by T helper cells and by negative feedback from high concentrations of circulating antigen-antibody complexes.
- Mechanisms to inhibit and control the immune response include activation of regulatory T-cell cytokines, complement inhibitors, circulating antiproteases, and antioxidants as well as degradation of inflammatory mediators.

SUMMARY

Cells and tissues throughout the body participate in defense against foreign antigens. Some components of the immune system are able to react to a large number of foreign invaders upon first exposure. These innate components are essential for protecting the body while the specific immune defenses are being activated. Innate defenses include physical and biochemical barriers of the skin and mucous membranes, cells of the mononuclear phagocyte system, neutrophils, NK cells, and a large number of chemical mediators such as complement, clotting factors, kinin, and cytokines. Immunity to specific antigens is provided by B and T lymphocytes. T helper cells are important regulators of the immune system because they secrete cytokines that enhance T cell, B cell, and macrophage function.

The forces of inflammation and immunity must be carefully controlled to prevent excessive tissue damage. Extensive measures are used to rid the body of self-reactive lymphocytes and to control reactions once a foreign antigen has been cleared. A well-functioning immune system not only successfully protects against foreign invaders and learns from the process so that it is even more effective on subsequent exposure, but also leaves healthy normal tissue unharmed.

REFERENCES

1. Abbas AK, Lichtman AH, Pillai S: *Cellular and molecular immunology,* ed 7, Philadelphia, 2012, Saunders.
2. Patton KT, Thibodeau GA: *Anatomy & physiology,* ed 7, St Louis, 2010, Mosby.
3. Nairn R, Helbert M: *Immunology for medical students,* ed 2, St Louis, 2007, Mosby.
4. Lydyard PM, Grossi CE: Cells, tissues and organs of the immune system. In Male D, Brostoff J, Roth D, Roitt I, editors: *Immunology,* ed 7, St Louis, 2006, Mosby, pp 15–45.
5. McIntyre TM, et al: Cell-cell interactions: leukocyte-endothelial interactions, *Curr Opin Hematol* 10(2):150–158, 2003.
6. Cornbleet PJ: Clinical utility of the band count, *Clin Lab Med* 22(1): 101–136, 2002.

7. Aldridge AJ: Role of the neutrophil in septic shock and the adult respiratory distress syndrome, *Eur J Surg* 168(4):204–214, 2002.

8. Agnello D, et al: Cytokines and transcription factors that regulate T helper cell differentiation: new players and new insights, *J Clin Immunol* 23(3):147–161, 2003.

9. Hall JE: Resistance of the body to infection: II. Immunity and allergy. In *Guyton and Hall textbook of medical physiology*, ed 12, Philadelphia, 2011, Saunders.

10. Blatteis CM, et al: Signaling the brain in systemic inflammation: the role of complement, *Front Biosci* 9:915–931, 2004.

11. Kumar V, Abbas A, Fausto N, Aster J: Acute and chronic inflammation. In Kumar V, Abbas A, Fausto N, Aster J, editors: *Robbins and Cotran pathologic basis of disease*, ed 8, Philadelphia, 2010, Saunders, pp 43–78.

12. Kumar V, Abbas A, Fausto N, Aster J: Tissue renewal, repair and regeneration. In Kumar V, Abbas A, Fausto N, Aster J, editors: *Robbins and Cotran pathologic basis of disease*, ed 8, Philadelphia, 2010, Saunders, pp 79–110.

13. Faro J, et al: The impact of thymic antigen diversity on the size of the selected T cell repertoire, *J Immunol* 172(4):2247–2255, 2004.

14. Kojima Y, et al: Localization of Fas ligand in cytoplasmic granules of CD8+ cytotoxic T lymphocytes and natural killer cells: participation of Fas ligand in granule exocytosis model of cytotoxicity, *Biochem Biophys Res Commun* 296(2):328–336, 2002.

15. Jefferis R: Antibodies. In Male D, Brostoff J, Roth D, Roitt I, editors: *Immunology*, ed 7, St Louis, 2006, Mosby, pp 59–86.

16. Li Z, et al: The generation of antibody diversity through somatic hypermutation and class switch recombination, *Genes Dev* 18(1):1–11, 2004.

17. Neuberger MS, et al: Memory in the B-cell compartment: antibody affinity maturation, *Philos Trans R Soc Lond B Biol Sci* 355(1395): 357–360, 2000.

18. Hanson LA, Korotkova M, Telemo E: Breast-feeding, infant formulas, and the immune system, *Ann Allergy Asthma Immunol* 90(6 Suppl 3):59–63, 2003.

19. French AR, Yokoyama WM: Natural killer cells and viral infections, *Curr Opin Immunol* 15(1):45–51, 2003.

20. Palmer E: Negative selection: clearing out the bad apples from the T-cell repertoire, *Nat Rev Immunol* 3(5):383–391, 2003.

21. Heyman B: Feedback regulation by IgG antibodies, *Immunol Lett* 88(2):157–161, 2003.

22. Winklhofer-Roob BM, et al: Effects of vitamin E and carotenoid status on oxidative stress in health and disease. Evidence obtained from human intervention studies, *Mol Aspects Med* 24(6):391–402, 2003.

23. Haddad JJ, Saade NE, Safieh-Garabedian B: Cytokines and neuro-immune-endocrine interactions: a role for the hypothalamic-pituitary-adrenal revolving axis, *J Neuroimmunol* 133(1-2):1–19, 2002.

24. Pert CB, Dreher HE, Ruff MR: The psychosomatic network: foundations of mind-body medicine, *Altern Ther Health Med* 4(4):30–41, 1998.

Alterations in Immune Function

Faith Young Peterson

evolve WEBSITE

http://evolve.elsevier.com/Copstead/

- Review Questions and Answers
- Glossary (with audio pronunciations for selected terms)
- Animations

- Case Studies
- Key Points Review

KEY QUESTIONS

- What are the potential mechanisms whereby erroneous reaction of the immune system with self tissue leads to autoimmune diseases?
- How do type I, II, III, and IV hypersensitivity reactions differ according to the immune cell types involved and the mechanism of tissue injury?
- What are the common features of autoimmune disorders and certain types of hypersensitivity disorders?

- How are hypersensitivity disorders detected, prevented, and treated?
- How do the etiologic processes of primary and secondary immune deficiency disorders differ?
- What are the clinical features of the common immunodeficiency disorders?

CHAPTER OUTLINE

The purposes of the immune system are to defend the body against invasion or infection by foreign substances called **antigens,** and to patrol for and destroy cells that are abnormal or damaged. Normally, the immune system works efficiently to accomplish these purposes, but in some situations inappropriate immune responses lead to disease.

These disorders can be divided into two general categories: (1) excessive immune responses and (2) deficient immune responses. The category of excessive immune responses includes disorders in which the immune system is overfunctioning or hyperfunctioning. Examples are autoimmunity and hypersensitivity disorders.

The category of deficient immune responses includes disorders in which the immune response is ineffective because of disease-causing genotypes or secondary/acquired dysfunction. Examples of deficient immune responses are severe combined immunodeficiency (SCID) syndrome, DiGeorge syndrome, and selective immunoglobulin A (IgA) deficiency. Human immunodeficiency virus/acquired immunodeficiency syndrome (HIV/AIDS) is a primary acquired immunodeficiency disorder that is discussed in Chapter 12. The secondary immunodeficiencies associated with white blood cell malignancies are included in Chapter 11.

EXCESSIVE IMMUNE RESPONSES

Excessive immune response disorders result from a functional increase in the activity of the immune system involving multiple, interacting immune cells. Autoimmunity and hypersensitivity are types of excessive immune response disorders. They are often related, and both may be present in patients with excessive immune responses. It may be helpful to think of autoimmunity as a way of describing the *etiologic process,* or cause, of abnormal excessive immune responses toward self tissues. Hypersensitivity disorders describe *mechanisms* of injury, or how the injury occurs, which may or may not involve autoimmunity. Autoimmunity is a general term that is used when the immune system attacks its own tissues. Most autoimmune reactions toward self tissues are mediated through type II (cytotoxic) and III (immune-complex) hypersensitivity mechanisms. For this reason, many autoimmune diseases also are considered hypersensitivity reactions. For example, myasthenia gravis is both an autoimmune disease and a type II hypersensitivity reaction. Immune complex glomerulonephritis is both an autoimmune disease and a type III hypersensitivity reaction. When hypersensitivity reactions occur in response to foreign antigens, such as bee venom, they are not autoimmune.

The causes of immune system overreactions are poorly understood. Interplay between genetic factors, including major histocompatibility complex (MHC) genes, and environmental factors is thought to be important in the development of autoimmune disorders. Most hypersensitivity disorders have familial tendencies also, but the specific genes and environmental agents remain to be discovered. Some evidence suggests that excessive immune responses may be the result of glucocorticoid resistance in target tissues. For example, the number of glucocorticoid receptors in circulating leukocytes is decreased 50% in patients with rheumatoid arthritis. This decrease in receptors would prevent adequate suppression of leukocyte activity and could further enhance inflammation.

AUTOIMMUNITY

Autoimmunity occurs when the immune system recognizes a person's own cells ("self") as foreign and mounts an immune response that injures self tissues. It is a failure of self tolerance. Identification and tolerance of self antigens occur during embryonic development. The adaptive immune response is the responsibility of antigen-specific

T cells and B cells that learn to identify "self" in the thymus and bone marrow.[1] The thymus gland is principally responsible for eliminating self-reactive cells.[1] During this time, aggressive or intolerant self-reactive (autoreactive) lymphocytes are eliminated or suppressed (see Chapter 9). However, a small number of T cells escape thymic control, and move into the peripheral circulation. The immune system has other peripheral "checkpoints" to detect, limit, and control these "self" or "auto" reactive T cells.[1] Autoimmune diseases result when self tolerance is lost and reactions between self antigens and the immune system occur causing dysregulation of proinflammatory and antiinflammatory mediators, cytokines, $CD4^+$ and $CD8^+$ T cells, B cells, and ubiquitin-editing enzyme A20 in dendritic cells.

Several theories have been proposed to explain how various immune system components and environmental triggers might interact to produce autoimmunity. However, no single theory can fully explain the loss of self tolerance that occurs in autoimmune diseases. A number of genetic and environmental factors interacting together contribute to the development of autoimmunity. The triggers for autoimmunity are not known exactly because autoimmune diseases are mediated by a variety of mechanisms, biochemical and cellular events, and responses to those events.

The theory of antigenic mimicry emphasizes the similarities between certain molecular segments of foreign antigens called *epitopes* and the person's own cells. For example, all cells, whether self or foreign, are composed of proteins, carbohydrates, nucleic acids, and lipids. Certain viruses and bacteria evolve to look like "self" and use "molecular mimicry" to slip past the immune system defenses. Self cells with the same or similar molecular segments as these foreign epitopes can "fit" lymphocyte receptors. Therefore, these self antigens or autoantigens can be attacked as foreign under certain circumstances when the normal cell has been altered, such as by a viral infection that stimulates the immune response.[2] The persistent presence of these autoantigens then acts as a constant source of stimulation to the immune system.[2] A recent study of the molecular mimicry theory established an epidemiologic association between *Campylobacter jejuni* enteritis and the subsequent development of Guillain-Barré syndrome.[2] This theory is also suggested as a cause of rheumatic heart disease attributable to cross-reactions between streptococcal antigens and human proteins.[3] In both cases, autoantigens have been identified following exposure to bacterial or viral infection.

Another theory proposes that release of sequestered antigens triggers the autoimmune response. This theory suggests that certain self antigens are isolated from the immune system within an organ during the neonatal period. They are not in contact with antigen-processing cells during the embryonic period when self tolerance usually occurs. These hidden self antigens or sequestered proteins that are normally sheltered from immune recognition occur in sites such as the cornea of the eye, the testicles, or other areas not drained by lymphatics. If and when these sites are damaged later in life, the hidden or sequestered proteins are exposed to the immune system, which does not recognize them as self. Therefore, the damaged cells are attacked.

A number of T cell theories of autoimmunity have been proposed, including thymus gland defects, decreased suppressor T cell function, and altered T helper cells. The theories attributing autoimmunity to thymus gland defects state that maturation and differentiation of T cells are affected either by decreased hormone secretion or by failure of the thymus to expose T cells to all self products. The thymus gland is responsible for exposing developing T cells to self products produced in the thymus or carried to the thymus gland. If some self products are not exposed to the developing T cells, the product will not be recognized as self and will subsequently be attacked. However, recent evidence demonstrates that not all T cells mature in the thymus. Thus not all T cells may experience or "learn" to recognize "self."[4] This lack of exposure to self products is thought to be a major factor in the development of generalized autoimmune diseases such as systemic lupus erythematosus (SLE). Thymus dysfunction in "programming" self-tolerance to pancreatic insulin-secreting islet β cells along with increased effector T cells and decreased regulatory T cells is thought to be the cause of autoimmune type 1 diabetes mellitus.[5]

The theory attributing autoimmunity to decreased or lost regulatory/suppressor T cell (Treg) activity states that decreased numbers of Treg cells fail to repress immunoglobulin activity. It is unclear in this theory if Treg cells are lost or if they are "reprogrammed" when exposed to inflammation.[6] Some data suggest that Treg cells lose their forkhead box p3(FOXP3) protein and are transformed into effector T cells.[6] It is also unclear if this disruption in the number of, or activity of, T cells may also be the result of genetic mutations. For example, a mutation of the transcription factor (FOXP3) causes impaired development and function of CD4$^+$ T cells, which can lead to autoimmune inflammation. T helper cells 22 (Th22 cells) are a newly identified subset of T cells that are important mediators of chronic inflammation and autoimmunity by inducing the production of inflammatory cytokines (ll17a, ll17f, ll22, ll26) by CCR6$^+$ cells.[7]

A number of B cell theories of autoimmunity also have been proposed. The theory attributing autoimmunity to escape of B cell tolerance proposes that certain B cells lose their responsiveness to suppressor T-cell messages. The B cell activation theories, which are well supported clinically and experimentally, suggest that extrinsic factors or intrinsic, genetic B cell defects cause autoantibody production and an increase in the number and activity of B cells. A number of extrinsic factors, including viruses, bacteria, antibiotics, proteolytic enzymes, and lipopolysaccharides, have been found to be B-cell activating factors that could trigger autoantibody production.

Research has linked mast cells to autoimmunity as well as hypersensitivity. Mast cells reside in most mucous membranes waiting for foreign proteins or bacteria to invade. Their cell membranes are studded with bacteria-sensing proteins, called Toll-like receptors, which cause release of up to 10,000 different chemicals in response to activation. Mast cells release the cytokine interleukin-1 (IL-1), attracting and enlisting inflammation-inducing cells to joints and leaking fluid into joints in the autoimmune disease of rheumatoid arthritis. They are also thought to be involved in development of irritable bowel syndrome and other functional gastrointestinal disorders.

Genetic Factors

Genetic predisposition seems to be an important factor in the development of autoimmune disorders. Gender, which is genetically determined, also influences the expression of autoimmune disorders. The exact mechanisms of gender and genetic influence on autoimmune expression have not been established, but the relationship is significant. Females are at significantly higher risk for developing autoimmunity compared to males. Different cytokine profiles can be associated with autoimmunity. Those with genetically low levels of tumor necrosis factor-α (TNF-α) and high levels of IL-10 may be more tolerant than those with normal levels.

The role of genetics is also supported by the observation that certain human major histocompatibility complex (MHC) genes located on chromosome 6p21 (also called human leukocyte antigen [HLA] genes) are frequently associated with certain autoimmune disorders (Table 10-1). The MHC gene region demonstrates a high level of polymorphism. One of the strongest correlations of MHC molecules with autoimmune disease is the linkage between the HLA-B27 phenotype and ankylosing spondylitis. In this case, 95% of all people with ankylosing spondylitis have a positive B27 phenotype. However, not everyone with a positive B27 phenotype develops ankylosing spondylitis, both because of differences in the way antigen is presented to the immune system and because of environmental factors. Other diseases are associated with different MHC phenotypes, but the correlation between risk for disease and presence of the disease marker is much lower. For example, Addison disease is associated with the HLA-DR3 phenotype, but it has only a 6% risk correlation. Juvenile rheumatoid arthritis is strongly associated with HLA-DR5.

There may also be disease-causing genotypes or genetic factors affecting expression of immune factors. For example, the lymphoid protein tyrosine phosphatase nonreceptor type 22 gene is associated with type 1 diabetes and other autoimmune disease. Tumor necrosis factor-α (TNF-α) is involved in acute and chronic inflammation, autoimmunity, and malignancies. Of special interest is the *FOXP3* gene, which is expressed by CD4$^+$ regulatory T cells. *FOXP3* deficiency is associated with both primary immune deficiency disorders and autoimmune disorders owing to its effect on regulatory T-cell immune function.

Environmental Triggers

Chronic or multiple viral or bacterial infections may trigger the development of autoimmune disease in susceptible persons. Viruses can activate B cells, decrease the function of T cells, contribute to the development of antigenic mimicry, or insert viral components on cell surfaces and trigger immune reactions. For example, Epstein-Barr virus, cytomegalovirus, and bacteria such as *Campylobacter jejuni* and *Helicobacter pylori* have been frequently cited as potential triggers of autoimmune disease.

Environmental stress and occupational stress can affect the immune system because of their relationship to the neuroendocrine system,

TABLE 10-1	MAJOR HISTOCOMPATIBILITY GENES AND AUTOIMMUNE DISEASE			
DISEASE	**HLA (MHC) ANTIGEN**	**FREQUENCY IN PATIENTS (%)**	**FREQUENCY IN CONTROLS (%)**	**RELATIVE RISK**
Ankylosing spondylitis				
Caucasians	B27	89	43	69
Japanese	B27	85	<1	207
Rheumatoid arthritis	DR4	68	25	3.8
Graves disease	Dw3	56	25	3.7
Type 1 diabetes mellitus	DR3/DR4 heterozygous			33
Systemic lupus erythematosus	DR4	73	33	5
Narcolepsy	DR2	100	34	358

Data from Tierney LM, McPhee SJ, Papadakis MA, editors: *Current medical diagnosis and treatment*, ed 46, New York, 2007, Lange/McGraw-Hill.

leading to inflammation or lymphokine release that activates T cells. Neuroendocrine and immune system interaction during life stress, such as shift work or workplace stress, promotes the synthesis and overproduction of proinflammatory cytokines. In genetically susceptible persons, this increase in systemic and local proinflammatory cytokines may affect the system's balance enough to trigger autoimmune disease. There are also other linkages between the neuroendocrine and immune systems.

Although the etiology of autoimmunity continues to be investigated, the mechanisms whereby autoantibodies injure tissues are better understood. The autoantibodies produced by autoimmune disorders affect tissue by the mechanisms described for type II and type III hypersensitivity reactions found later in this chapter.

Pharmacotherapies

Immunosuppressive therapy is a common treatment for autoimmune disease. Because autoimmunity is expressed in different ways, the immunosuppressive treatment for each type of autoimmune disease is individualized, depending on disease expression. Immunosuppressive therapy, including corticosteroids and certain cytotoxic chemotherapeutic agents, has become an increasingly important treatment choice. These drugs are essential for inhibiting excessive or aberrant immune responses. The ideal immunosuppressive medication would be an agent that inhibits only the abnormal immune response without limiting the positive and protective functions of the immune system or causing any organ toxicity. Unfortunately, no immunosuppressive medication with these specific properties yet exists.

Immunosuppressive agents include corticosteroids, tumor necrosis factor inhibitors, immunomodulators, and cytotoxins. Corticosteroids decrease the number of lymphocytes and decrease antibody formation, as well as alter the functional activities of lymphocytes. They also have many other activities as a result of their glucocorticoid function. Corticosteroids tend to be used in the treatment of many autoimmune diseases and are the oldest of the immunosuppressive drugs. The adverse effects that occur during corticosteroid use often limit their extended use over time. The common side effects include hypercorticism with changes in fat distribution and buffalo hump formation, suppression of the HPA axis (hypothalamic-pituitary-adrenal axis), congestive heart failure, hypertension, emotional changes, thinning of skin, petechiae, diabetes mellitus, menstrual irregularities, electrolyte imbalances, liver and pancreatic dysfunction, exophthalmos, glaucoma, loss of muscle mass, and muscle weakness. Because corticosteroids affect the HPA system, gradual withdrawal by tapering the dose over time is necessary when discontinuing long-term therapy.

Cytotoxins, such as methotrexate, are used to manage autoimmune disorders because of their ability to kill actively proliferating lymphocytes after they are transformed from their resting G_0 state. The key to the use of cytotoxins is to effectively apply their killing activity without damaging the rest of the body. Cyclosporine (Sandimmune) is a more selective immunosuppressant that reversibly suppresses T-helper cells in the G_0 or G_1 phase of the cell cycle without killing them. As a result, it inhibits the development of killer or cytotoxic T cells without decreasing the numbers of cells. It also impairs the ability of T cells to respond effectively to foreign antigens. It is used to suppress reactions during tissue or organ transplantation. Frequent side effects include edema, hypertension, headache, hirsutism, elevated triglyceride levels, gastrointestinal effects, nephropathy, infection, emotional changes, gynecomastia, leukopenia, anemia, and hepatotoxicity.

Tumor necrosis factor (TNF) inhibitors or immunomodulators, such as etanercept (Enbrel) or infliximab (Remicade), are used as disease modifiers that bind to and block the activity of TNF-α and TNF-β. They may also modulate TNF-mediated responses, such as leukocyte migration and expression of adhesion molecules. The most common side effects of TNF inhibitors include headache, gastrointestinal changes, injection site skin reactions, respiratory tract infections, edema, dizziness, dyspepsia, and weakness.

Therapeutic plasmapheresis is another type of therapy occasionally used in the management of autoimmune diseases. Plasmapheresis is analogous to dialysis and involves the selective filtering or removal of plasma or a plasma cell type as well as protein-bound toxic substances. The patient's whole blood is filtered, blood cells and platelets are returned, and the plasma component containing the autoantibodies is removed and replaced with 5% albumin or another colloid solution. According to the American Society for Apheresis, this type of therapy has been effective in the management of diseases such as myasthenia gravis, thrombocytopenia purpura, multiple sclerosis, and Rh-negative hemolytic disease of the newborn. Plasmapheresis is generally well tolerated; however, there are both major and minor risks involved in the process. Some of the risks include insertion of large intravenous (IV) catheters to perform the procedure, decrease in serum ionized calcium concentration, shifts of fluid levels, and risks of infection and bleeding from loss of coagulation factors.

KEY POINTS

- Autoimmune disorders occur when the immune system erroneously reacts with "self" tissues. These disorders are thought to be polygenic and multifactorial; however, the exact etiologic process is unknown.
- The antigenic mimicry theory involves the alteration of viruses or bacteria to look like "self" and the precipitation of immune reactions.
- The theory involving release of sequestered antigens suggests that self antigens that do not come in direct contact with lymphocytes during fetal development may cause autoimmune reactions if they are subsequently released from sequestration.
- Abnormal production of subclasses of T lymphocytes, particularly suppressor T cells, has been proposed as a reason for the development of autoimmunity, as well as the development of abnormal B cells that do not respond to suppressor T cell signals.
- Genetic factors such as female gender and MHC genes are associated with certain autoimmune disorders.
- Autoantibodies injure body tissues through the mechanisms described for type II and type III hypersensitivity reactions.

HYPERSENSITIVITY

Hypersensitivity is a normal immune response that is inappropriately triggered or excessive or produces undesirable effects on the body. The basic mechanism that triggers hypersensitivity is a specific antigen-antibody reaction or a specific antigen-lymphocyte interaction. Four classes or types of hypersensitivity are differentiated. Each type is characterized by a specific cellular or antibody response. Hypersensitivity types I, II, and III are mediated by antibodies produced by B lymphocytes. Type IV hypersensitivity is mediated by T cells. Hypersensitivity reactions are specific to a particular antigen and usually do not occur on first exposure to the antigen. Although the diseases or syndromes associated with each type differ in their clinical signs and symptoms, the underlying pathophysiologic process is similar within each type. In Table 10-2 the four major types of hypersensitivity are contrasted. The complex interactions between immune system inflammatory mediators, cytokines, T cells, B cells, and mast cells characterize hypersensitivity reactions.

TABLE 10-2   THE FOUR TYPES OF HYPERSENSITIVITY

CHARACTERISTIC	TYPE I: ATOPIC, ANAPHYLACTIC	TYPE II: CYTOTOXIC, CYTOLYTIC	TYPE III: IMMUNE COMPLEX (ARTHUS REACTION)	TYPE IV: DELAYED HYPERSENSITIVITY
Mediated by:	IgE	IgM or IgG	IgG	T_{DTH} lymphocytes
Complement activation	No	Yes	Yes	No
Immune response	Ag plus IgE, leading to mast cell degranulation	Surface Ag and Ab, leading to killer cell cytotoxic action or complement-mediated lysis	Ag-Ab complex in tissues; complement activated and PMNs attracted	Ag-sensitized T cells release lymphokines, leading to inflammatory reactions, and attract macrophages, which release mediator
Peak action	15-30 min	15-30 min	6 hr	24-48 hr
Serum transferability	Yes	Yes	Yes	No
Cell transferability	No	No	No	Yes (T cells)
Genetic mechanisms	Familial High IgE lovol HLA-linked *Ir* genes General hyperresponsiveness	HLA linked in some cases	Familial (autoimmune) HLA specificities	Unknown
Causes of reaction	T cell deficiency Abnormal mediator feedback Environmental factors and Ag	Exposure to Ag or foreign tissue, cells, or graft	Persistent infection— microbe Ag Extrinsic environmental Ag Autoimmunity—self Ag	Intradermal Ag Epidermal Ag Dermal Ag
Manifestation (examples)	Asthma, rhinitis, atopic eczema, bee sting reaction	ABO transfusions, hemolytic disease of newborn, myasthenia gravis	Glomerulonephritis, SLE, farmer's lung arthritis, vasculitis	Guillain-Barré disease, tuberculin test, contact dermatitis, multiple sclerosis

Ab, Antibody; *Ag,* antigen; *DTH,* delayed-type hypersensitivity; *Ig,* immunoglobulin; *HLA,* human leukocyte antigen; *PMN,* polymorphonuclear leukocyte; *SLE,* systemic lupus erythematosus.

Type I Hypersensitivity

Etiology. Genetic mechanisms influence type I hypersensitivity with strong genetic or hereditary linkage regarding the IgE response to antigens (allergens). This genetic component involves both the ability to respond to an allergen and the general ability to produce an IgE antibody response. For example, children born to two allergic parents have a 50% chance of being allergic. Children born to one nonallergic and one allergic parent have a 30% chance of being allergic. It has been identified that total IgE concentration is higher in patients with atopic rhinitis or asthma compared to nonatopic patients.[8]

Pathogenesis. Type I hypersensitivity is also known as immediate hypersensitivity, because the reaction is immediate. It is a sensitization reaction characterized by signs and symptoms of an allergic reaction that usually occurs 15 to 30 minutes after exposure to an antigen (allergen).

At the cellular level, immunoglobulin E (IgE) is the principal antibody mediating this reaction. IgE is produced by specialized plasma B cells and circulates in very small amounts in the blood. When an individual is exposed to an allergen, selected plasma B cells produce allergen-specific IgE. It usually takes repeated exposures to the allergen to cause significant levels of IgE to be present in the blood. Environmental pollutants may play a role by increasing mucosal permeability and enhancing antigen (allergen) entry into the body. This increased entry would subsequently increase IgE responsiveness.

Mast cells and basophils are the principal effector cells, although there are many other cells with histamine and other inflammatory mediators that can be involved in the reaction. These may include neutrophils, eosinophils, lymphocytes, macrophages, epithelial cells, and endothelial cells. Mast cells are found throughout the body in all loose connective tissue. They are covered with IgE receptors—up to 500,000 on their cell surfaces—and they are filled with vesicles or granules containing potent vasoactive, proinflammatory chemical mediators (especially histamine) that produce inflammation when they are released. The IgE receptors on mast cells bind the Fc portion of an IgE antibody. The IgE antigen-binding sites are then displayed on the mast cell surface, where they can bind to antigens that pass by the mast cell (Figure 10-1). This process makes the mast cells responsive to particular antigens.

The initial incident during a type I hypersensitivity response is the cross-linking of two IgE receptors to one antigen on the mast cell located at the site of the allergen's entry into the body (see Figure 10-1). Cross-linking of IgE and the antigen causes an increase in intracellular calcium (Ca^{2+}) concentration that results in immediate, massive, local mast cell degranulation of preformed and newly formed proinflammatory mediators. The release of mediators causes an inflammatory response.

Mast cells, basophils, and other effector cells release many chemicals. Some of the mediators are preformed and stored in vesicles, such as histamine, heparin, proteolytic enzymes, and chemotactic factors. Other mediators are formed during the degranulation process. Examples of newly formed mediators include superoxide, prostaglandins, thromboxanes, leukotrienes, bradykinin, and interleukins (see Chapter 9).

One of the most important mediators of type I hypersensitivity is histamine. Histamine binds to H_1 (histamine 1), H_2, H_3, and H_4 receptors, which are located on many types of cells. Mast cells have receptors for H_1, H_2, and H_3, with H_1 receptors being the most active. Basophils express predominantly H_2 receptors, whereas neutrophils and eosinophils have both H_1 and H_2 receptors. Recent evidence shows that H_1 and H_2 receptors are present on monocytes and macrophages, with an increase in H_1 receptors when monocytes differentiate into macrophages. Histamine binding to H_1 receptors triggers increased vascular

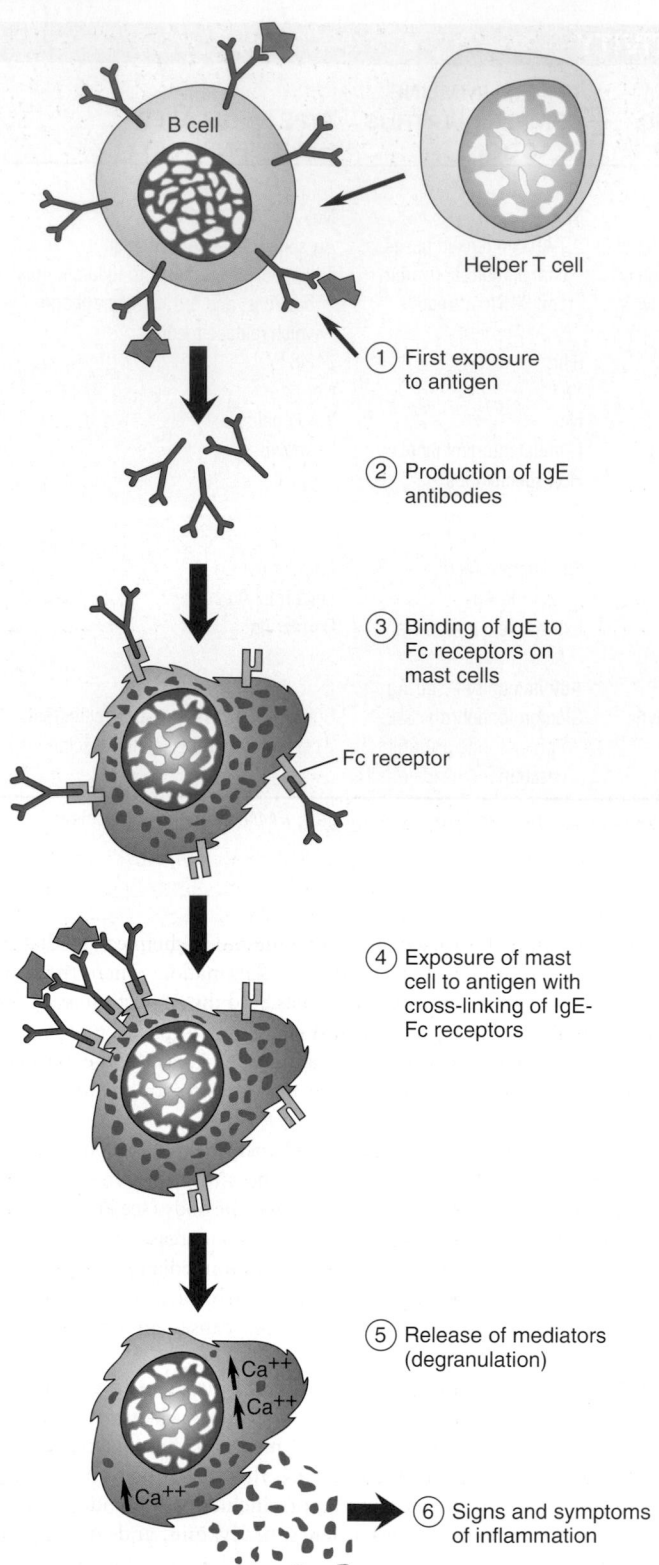

① First exposure to antigen

② Production of IgE antibodies

③ Binding of IgE to Fc receptors on mast cells

— Fc receptor

④ Exposure of mast cell to antigen with cross-linking of IgE-Fc receptors

⑤ Release of mediators (degranulation)

⑥ Signs and symptoms of inflammation

FIGURE 10-1 Type I hypersensitivity reaction.

concentrations has an inhibitory effect on inflammatory cells, decreasing degranulation and decreasing neutrophil chemotaxis. The H_3 receptors are located in the brain, in the spinal cord, and on sensory neurons such as postganglionic cholinergic nerves in lung bronchi. The H_4 receptors are found on immune system cells such as dendritic cells, eosinophils, T cells, monocytes, macrophages, and natural killer cells as well as in hematopoietic cells such as the spleen, thymus, bone marrow, and blood leukocytes. H_4 receptors are highly attracted to histamine and are also involved in chemotaxis and inflammatory responses.

The proteolytic enzymes kininogenase and tryptase activate the kinin pathway and C3 activates the complement cascade via the alternative pathway. Heparin decreases clot formation. The chemotactic factors recruit or activate other inflammatory and immune cells. Leukotrienes cause smooth muscle contraction and increase vascular permeability.

Clinical manifestations. Manifestations of an immediate hypersensitivity reaction vary in severity and intensity. For many people, type I hypersensitivity reactions are annoying, such as hives (urticaria), seasonal allergic rhinitis, eczema, or mild bronchoconstriction. In other people, the symptoms are more problematic, including tightening of the throat, localized edema, wheezing, and tachycardia, such as is associated with localized angioedema reactions or severe airway reactions. In a very small number of highly allergic people, the type I hypersensitivity reaction can be expressed as a life-threatening allergic reaction known as anaphylaxis such as that associated with bee stings and seafood or peanut allergic reactions. Common allergenic medications, insects, and foods that can trigger type I hypersensitivity reactions are listed in Box 10-1.

permeability, vasodilation (flushing), urticaria formation (hives), smooth muscle constriction (bronchoconstriction), increased mucus secretion and pruritus (increased itching), and increased gut permeability. The activation of H_2 receptors has opposing effects to H_1 receptors in some tissues and causes smooth muscle relaxation in the lower airways, augments gastric acid secretion from parietal cells, and in high

Treatment. Treatment for type I hypersensitivity primarily involves pharmacologic management with antihistamines, β-adrenergics, corticosteroids, anticholinergics, and anti–immunoglobulin E therapy (IgE blocker therapy). Antihistamines such as diphenhydramine (Benadryl) are used to block the effect of histamine. This action decreases vascular permeability and bronchoconstriction. β-Adrenergic sympathomimetics are used to decrease bronchoconstriction and bronchospasm. **Epinephrine** is an adrenergic agent (α, β$_1$, and β$_2$) given subcutaneously or intravenously during acute allergic reactions, especially after food or bee sting reactions. Most patients with severe allergies to food or insect bites are given prescriptions for epinephrine in the form of EpiPen with an autoinjector. Corticosteroids are used to decrease the inflammatory response. Anticholinergics are used to block the parasympathetic system and thus allow greater sympathetic activity. This action indirectly causes bronchodilation. Anti–immunoglobulin E therapy (omalizumab) may be used for persons with severe persistent asthma. Omalizumab (Xolair) is a subcutaneously injected, monoclonal anti-IgE antibody that binds to the IgE molecule, thus inhibiting the binding of IgE to mast cells and basophils and promoting downregulation of IgE receptors. It is used to improve asthma control in patients with moderate to severe persistent asthma not controlled with inhaled corticosteroids. It is used in children 12 years or older and in adults.

Prevention. Some protective, proactive actions taken during pregnancy are thought to decrease the likelihood that type I hypersensitivity will develop in children from families with a history of allergies. These actions include avoiding foods to which the mother is allergic, limiting excesses of one type of food during the last trimester of pregnancy, avoiding whole eggs during the last month before delivery and while breast feeding, and limiting cow's milk to two glasses per day. Other actions that may be helpful during the child's infancy include avoiding exposure to environmental pollution, breast feeding for a minimum of 6 months, supplementing the child's diet with non–cow's milk products such as soy milk, giving solid foods only after the infant is 6 months old, keeping the infant's room as free of dust and molds as possible, and keeping pets (dogs, cats, birds) out of the home.

Pharmacotherapeutic prevention. Another avenue for prevention of type I hypersensitivity reactions involves the use of desensitization therapy (immunotherapy). Desensitization, or immunotherapy, is more successful in patients with hay fever than in those with other types of allergies. It involves both environmental control of external allergens and titrated pharmacologic exposure to allergens. Environmental control involves a systematic plan to decrease exposure to house dust, molds, and animal dander. Pets are kept out of the house. The person must avoid food allergens, wool carpets, goose down or feather pillows, dried plants, and exposure to other animal and vegetable products. The person is urged to use air conditioning and electronic air filters.

Pharmacologic desensitization involves injecting a person with sufficient antigen (allergen) on a regular basis over a course of months or years, followed by periodic maintenance or booster therapy. Gradually the dose is increased until the person can tolerate the allergen without a type I hypersensitivity reaction. The goal of this therapy is a change in immunoglobulins so that there is an increase in IgG- and IgA-blocking antibodies, no increase in IgE during allergy season, decreased basophil reactivity, and decreased lymphocyte reactivity to allergens.

Type II Hypersensitivity

Etiology and pathogenesis. Type II hypersensitivity, also known as tissue-specific, cytotoxic, or cytolytic hypersensitivity, is characterized by antibodies that attack antigens on the surface of specific cells or tissues. Often the reaction is immediate (15 to 30 minutes after

TABLE 10-3	DISEASE AND AUTOANTIBODIES ASSOCIATED WITH TYPE II HYPERSENSITIVITY
DISEASE	**ANTIGEN/AUTOANTIBODY**
Type 1 diabetes	Islet cells
Insulin-resistant diabetic states	Insulin receptor
Myasthenia gravis	Acetylcholine receptor
Addison disease	Adrenal epithelial cells
Autoimmune hemolytic anemia	Red blood cell membrane
Immune thrombocytopenic purpura	Platelet membrane
Autoimmune neutropenia	Neutrophil antigens
Pernicious anemia	Intrinsic factor, gastric parietal cells
Lymphocytic thyroiditis	Thyroglobulin
Graves disease	Receptor for thyroid-stimulating hormone
Pemphigus vulgaris	Desmosomes
Hyperacute graft rejection	Donor antigens

exposure to the antigen). However, it can occur over time, such as in thyroiditis or myasthenia gravis. The mechanisms that encompass type II tissue-specific hypersensitivity all occur after the binding of antibody to tissue-specific antigens. The reaction is mediated by the complement system and a variety of effector cells, including tissue macrophages, platelets, natural killer cells, neutrophils, and eosinophils. IgG and IgM are the principal antibodies. Examples of this type of hypersensitivity reaction include ABO transfusion reactions, hemolytic disease of the newborn, myasthenia gravis, thyroiditis, hyperacute graft rejection, and autoimmune hemolytic anemia (Table 10-3). Transfusion reactions, hemolytic disease of the newborn, and graft rejection are examples of **isoimmunity (alloimmunity)**, a condition in which the immune system reacts against antigens on tissues from other members of the same species.

The initial mechanism during a type II hypersensitivity response is exposure to antigen on the surface of foreign cells. The Fab portion of IgG or IgM antibodies binds to antigens on the target foreign cell to form an antigen-antibody complex (Figure 10-2). (Refer also to Chapter 9 for a discussion of IgG and IgM antibodies.) The Fc region of the IgG or IgM antibodies protrudes away from the cell membrane surface. The Fc region then acts as a bridge between the antigen and complement or the effector cells. This antigen-antibody binding with Fc bridging is the key and leads to lysis of the cell by one of several mechanisms. One mechanism is complement-mediated lysis. Complement-mediated lysis occurs through the classical pathway for activation of complement. The classical pathway of complement generates the activated complement component C3b via splitting of C4 and C2 by C1 (Chapter 9). The activated complement component C3b is bound to the target cell by the Fc region of IgG or IgM. C3b increases opsonization, which in turn increases the capacity of the system to allow lysis by other effector cells or by complement itself. Lysis of the foreign cell by complement occurs via the C5-C9 membrane attack complex (MAC), which disrupts the plasma membrane of the cell.

Transfusion Reaction

An example of this type of mechanism is an acute hemolytic blood transfusion reaction. It occurs when a person receives blood from someone with a different blood group type (Table 10-4). In this case, the recipient of the blood transfusion has antibodies to the donor's

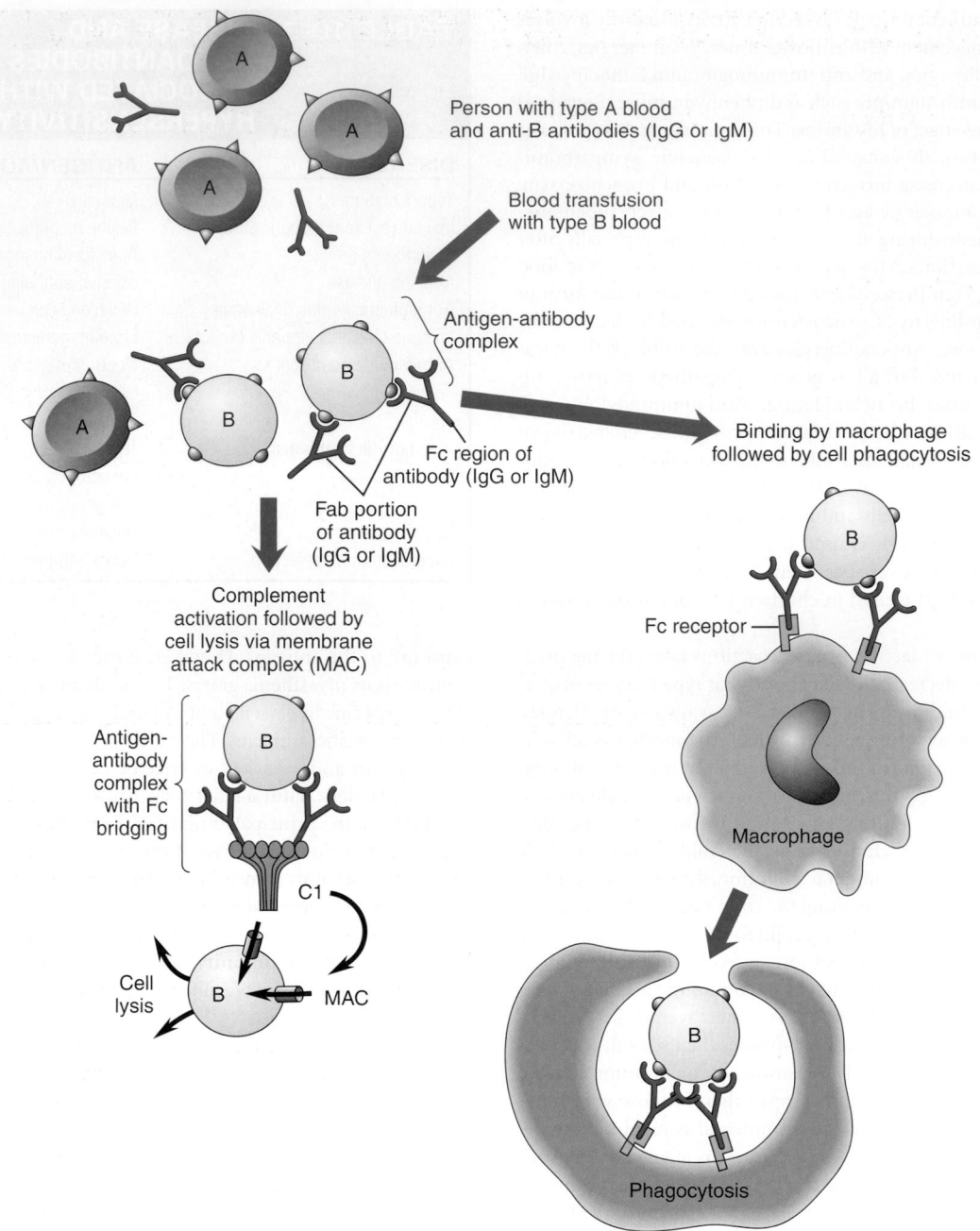

FIGURE 10-2 Type II hypersensitivity reactions.

red blood cell (RBC) antigens. For example, if a person with type A blood having type A antigens and anti-B antibodies incorrectly receives type B blood with B antigens and anti-A antibodies, the anti-B antibodies will attach to the surface of the infused type B red blood cells and the anti-A antibodies in the infusion will attach to the surface of the circulating type A red blood cells. This event will stimulate the destruction of large numbers of red blood cells. The resulting signs and symptoms of this major blood group reaction include fever, chills, flushing, tachycardia, hypotension, low back pain, pleuritic chest pain, nausea, vomiting, restlessness, anxiety, oliguria, and headache. The reaction may progress to anaphylaxis, shock, and death.

Transfusion reactions are not always immediate. They may be delayed from a few days to 2 weeks especially in persons requiring periodic transfusions such as in sickle cell anemia or thalassemia.[9] In many cases, antibodies occur as a result of blood component exposure from multiple transfusions. Delayed reactions can also occur as a result of transplantation. In delayed transfusion reactions, often the mechanism of action is related to differences in erythrocyte (RBC) antigens between blood donors rather than differences in the major ABO blood groups.[9] There are many hundreds of RBC antigens that have been identified; fortunately, most of them are rare. In the case of sickle cell anemia, RBC antigens between blood donors of European descent and patients of Afro-Caribbean descent can result in the development of alloantibodies when exposed.[9] The resulting type II hypersensitivity reaction causes the destruction of both the donor's and the recipient's RBCs along with the symptoms of acute hemolysis and severe vaso-occlusive crisis.

TABLE 10-4 · MAJOR BLOOD GROUPS

PHENOTYPE	GENE LOCI	FREQUENCY (%)	ANTIGENS	ANTIBODIES IN SERUM
		BLOOD GROUP		
A	1	42	A	Anti-B
B	1	8	B	Anti-A
AB	1	3	A and B	None
O	1	47	H	Anti-A, anti-B
Other Major Blood Group Systems				
Rhesus (Rh)		Three closely linked loci: Major antigen = RhD	C, D, E, c, d, e	
		Rh+	85	Cde, CDE
		Rh–	15	Cde, CdE
Kell	1		K or k	
		K	9	K
		K	91	k
MN	1		M or N	
		MM	28	MM
		MN	50	MN
		NN	22	NN
Duffy	1		Fy^a, Fy^b, Fy	
		Fy^aFy^b	46	Fy^a, Fy^b
		Fy^a	20	Fy^a
		Fy^b	34	Fy^b
		Fy	0.1	Fy

Hemolytic Disease of the Newborn

A second mechanism for antigen-antibody binding in type II hypersensitivity reactions is direct destruction by Fc-bearing effector cells, such as macrophages. The macrophage can link to exposed Fc antibody regions. Once this bridging occurs, the foreign cell is phagocytized and destroyed by lysosomes within the effector cell. This can be mediated with or without complement involvement. An example of this type of mechanism is hemolytic disease of the newborn (erythroblastosis fetalis).

This condition occurs during pregnancy when an Rh-negative mother is sensitized to the Rh-positive red cell group antigens of her fetus because of exposure during her current or a previous pregnancy. The mother's IgG Rh-positive antibodies cross the placental barrier and attack the red blood cells of the fetus. The mother's exposure occurs when mixing of fetal and maternal blood takes place. This can occur during an episode of antepartal bleeding or trauma to the placenta, during birth, or during miscarriage of an Rh-positive child. Of these situations, the most likely time for mixing of fetal and maternal blood is at the time of delivery. After this exposure, Rh-positive antibodies gradually develop in the mother and can affect her subsequent children. It takes as little as 1 cm^3 of fetal blood exposure for antibodies to Rh-positive red blood cells to develop in the mother. Usually, the first Rh-positive child is not affected unless placental tearing or leakage into the mother's circulation occurs during pregnancy.

Antibody screens are routinely performed during pregnancy to determine a mother's Rh status including indirect Coombs test and identification of specific antibodies. If the mother is Rh-negative, RhoGAM is administered at 28 weeks, after any prenatal bleeding, and at delivery for prevention of Rh-positive antibodies. RhoGAM contains antibodies against Rh antigens on fetal blood cells and is given to the mother to destroy fetal cells that may be present in her circulation before her immune system becomes activated and begins to produce anti-Rh antibodies. RhoGAM is not effective if the mother already has a positive antibody titer for fetal Rh antigens.

If the mother is Rh-negative, already has fetal Rh antibodies (i.e., is sensitized), and is carrying an Rh-positive fetus, she will not exhibit any significant physiologic effects except some discomfort from potential polyhydramnios. The mother may experience psychological distress. Most of the symptoms of Rh sensitization occur in the fetus, including signs of anemia, hypoxia, decreased fetal activity, ascites, congestive heart failure, and an elevated baseline heart rate of 180 beats/minute or greater with late decelerations. As a result, there is frequent fetal surveillance by 26 weeks' gestation including assessment of fetal heart rate, biweekly performance of nonstress tests, execution of serial amniocenteses to measure levels of bilirubin, and/or direct evaluation of fetal hemoglobin and hematocrit levels by means of percutaneous umbilical blood sampling. If fetal anemia becomes severe any time after 18 weeks' gestation, an intrauterine blood transfusion may be necessary to try to prolong the time the fetus is able to stay in utero. After 34 weeks, the fetus is often taken by cesarean section.

Myasthenia Gravis

A third mechanism for antigen-antibody binding is seen in myasthenia gravis, an autoimmune disease of the neuromuscular junction. In this case, antibodies form primarily to the acetylcholine receptor (AChR), and less frequently to muscle-specific kinase (MuSK) or low-density lipoprotein receptor–related protein 4 (Lrp4) on muscle membrane surfaces, primarily the motor end-plate[10] (Figure 10-3). With antigen-antibody formation at the receptor site, complement is activated and disrupts the muscle cell membrane. Effector cells are not thought to be involved in this type II hypersensitivity reaction. The thymus gland is believed to be the site of anti–acetylcholine receptor antibody development.[11] It also sustains the autoimmune, hypersensitivity reaction.[11] The loss of acetylcholine stimulation at the motor end-plate causes the extreme muscular weakness associated with myasthenia gravis. The major symptoms of myasthenia gravis include ptosis, diplopia, and muscle weakness after exercise that resolves with rest.

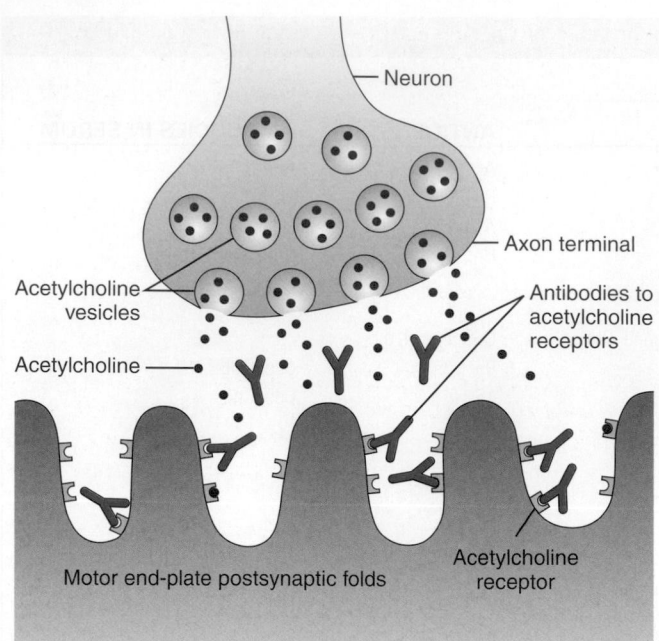

FIGURE 10-3 Type II hypersensitivity reaction in a person with myasthenia gravis. Having limited receptors available for acetylcholine impairs neuromuscular transmission.

Graves Disease and Thyroiditis

A fourth mechanism for antigen-antibody binding in type II hypersensitivity reactions is also mediated by effector cells. The effector cells in this case do not directly engulf and destroy the complex because the tissue is too large for this process. Therefore, the effector cells, such as neutrophils, bind to the target cells and block the receptors from normal functioning, causing injury to or malfunction of the involved tissue. Lymphocytic thyroiditis and Graves disease (toxic diffuse goiter) are examples of this type of disorder. In Graves disease, the autoantibody attacks the thyroid-stimulating hormone (TSH) receptor and causes the cells to malfunction, producing excess thyroxine (T_4) and triiodothyronine (T_3) by stimulation of the cells. This causes the symptoms of hyperthyroidism including tachycardia, fatigue, weight loss, tremor, heat intolerance, diarrhea, and emotional/mental changes.

Hyperacute Graft Rejection

Another type II hypersensitivity mechanism for antigen-antibody binding that involves both effector cells and complement is the hyperacute graft rejection that affects transplanted tissues. It occurs when the transplanted donor tissue has an antigen to which the recipient has preformed antibodies. For example, when tissue from a blood type A or B donor is transplanted into a blood type O recipient, the recipient has anti-A and anti-B antibodies. These antibodies will immediately attack the foreign transplanted tissue.

Onset begins immediately after revascularization of the transplanted tissue. At this time, the blood supply from the patient is established in the newly transplanted organ. The patient's antibodies attack the foreign protein antigens and form an antigen-antibody complex. Effector cell infiltration and complement-mediated lysis of donor tissues, inflammation, vascular thrombosis, and hemorrhage occur. The reaction happens so quickly that within 48 hours after transplantation the graft tissue is no longer functioning.

To prevent hyperacute graft rejection, tissue and blood typing of donors and recipients of transplanted tissue is extensive. Lists of potential recipients are matched to donors through organ donation laboratories both regionally and nationally. Only rarely has hyperacute graft rejection occurred because of an error in tissue or blood typing.

Type III Hypersensitivity

Etiology. Type III hypersensitivity results from failure of the immune and phagocytic systems to effectively remove antigen-antibody immune complexes and is not tissue specific. It is also known as an immune complex reaction. Type III hypersensitivity is characterized by antigen-antibody complex deposition into tissues, with consequent activation of complement and a subsequent self-sustaining inflammatory reaction. It is not an immediate reaction; it occurs over a period of several hours or longer (i.e., glomerulonephritis) and is often ongoing.

Three possible scenarios can precipitate type III hypersensitivity. First, a recent history of infection or persistent low-grade infection by a microbial or viral agent can stimulate a weak antibody response. The continuing nature of persistent infection or untreated/undertreated infection provides a source of circulating antigen. The antigen and antibody response leads to chronic immune complex production. These immune complexes are not successfully removed from the blood and are deposited in many sites, including blood vessels, glomeruli, and joints. Second, an extrinsic environmental antigen from molds, plants, or animals can be inhaled into the lung, where it is exposed to antibody in the body fluid. This inhalation of antigen causes antigen-antibody complex formation in alveoli with immune complex deposition in the alveolar walls. Third, an autoimmune process can develop in which autoantibodies attack self antigens. In this case, the body forms both parts of the immune complex. Autoantibodies to either circulating or tissue-fixed self antigens may be produced. Because the self antigens persist over time, chronic immune complex production and deposition in tissues take place.

The mechanism of injury in type III hypersensitivity reactions is from activation of complement and other proinflammatory mediators in response to the antigen-antibody complex deposition. The antibody-antigen complex deposition does not cause the injury. The tissue injury is caused by an inflammatory reaction to the antibody-antigen complex. Therefore, it is not a tissue-specific reaction. The onset of this reaction occurs up to 6 or more hours after exposure to the antigen. IgG and IgM are the principal antibodies. The principal effector cells are neutrophils and mast cells. The principal mediator of the reaction is complement. Examples of type III hypersensitivity reaction include systemic lupus erythematosus, immune complex glomerulonephritis, serum sickness, and drug-induced vasculitis. Diseases associated with type III hypersensitivity are listed in Table 10-5.

Pathogenesis. Type III hypersensitivity reactions tend to be ongoing with variations in symptoms based on the fluctuation of antibody to antigen ratios, the amount of complement available to mediate the inflammation, and the dynamic nature of the antibody-antigen reaction. It is sometimes difficult to differentiate between type II and type III hypersensitivity reactions. The key differences between a type II and a type III reaction are the location of antigen and the mechanism of injury. As previously described, type II reactions occur in response to tissue-specific antigen located on cell surfaces and involve direct cell death or malfunction from the antigen-antibody reaction. Type III hypersensitivity reactions involve antigens forming antigen-antibody complexes that precipitate out of the blood or body fluid and are deposited into tissues.

Type III hypersensitivity reactions involve a sequential process that begins with interaction between a circulating soluble antigen and soluble antibody or between an insoluble antigen and a soluble antibody. Depending on the concentration of antigen and antibody, multiple cross-linking of antigen and antibody occurs and immune complexes are formed. Most immune complexes are removed effectively before they can cause injury. In type III hypersensitivity, the immune complexes are not removed, which causes an inflammatory process and thus leads to tissue injury.

When both antigen and antibody are small or intermediate in size and soluble, the immune complex precipitates out of the body fluid and is deposited into tissues. When only the antibody is soluble, the antibody reacts with fixed antigen in the tissues. Then the antibody within the complex links with the complement system by its Fc receptors (Figure 10-4).

Activation of the classic complement cascade causes release of C3a and C5a, as well as the membrane attack complex. C3a stimulates the release of histamine from mast cells, indirectly increasing vascular permeability and vasodilation. Bronchial smooth muscle contraction

occurs, resulting in bronchial constriction, wheezing, and coughing. C3a also causes the endothelial cells to become more round, thereby increasing vascular permeability. The increased vascular permeability leads to edema formation, which provides more space for the movement of cellular inflammatory components. It also dilutes and limits the duration of action of mediators. C5a is an even more powerful component than C3a. It causes a powerful release of proinflammatory mediators with actions that are identical with those of C3a. It is also a powerful chemotactic agent for neutrophils and causes a respiratory burst within neutrophils in which oxygen consumption is increased to 50 times normal along with increased glucose uptake and procoagulant activity.

As a result of the activation of complement, neutrophils, macrophages, and mast cells are attracted to the area and are activated. These cells begin lysis and destruction of tissue via the release of cytokines and the inflammatory response. The inflammation causes tissue destruction, scarring, and further reaction of the immune system against the damaged tissue (see Figure 10-4). The persistence of the inflammation is due to the ongoing release of autoantigen particles in the damaged tissue that stimulate autoreactive B cells, leading to the formation and deposition of more immune complexes.[12]

Tissue deposition. Antigen-antibody complex deposition in tissues is affected by a number of factors including size and clearance rate.[12] Smaller immune complexes are able to circulate for longer periods, which may increase the immune response. However, small complexes also can be removed more easily because they can pass through the glomerular basement membrane. The very large complexes can be phagocytized more easily because they are easily marked or fixed by complement and bound to red blood cells. The large complexes can then be transported to the liver, where they are phagocytized by the reticuloendothelial system—particularly the Kupffer cells in the liver—and easily removed from the system. However, large complexes can become stuck in the kidney where they are unable to cross the glomerular basement membrane.

Increased vascular permeability as a result of histamine or other vasoactive mediator release is also hypothesized to be an important factor in tissue deposition. Researchers have found that small immune complexes can be deposited in tissues treated with vasoactive mediators. Sites of increased turbulence and blood pressure tend to have increased immune complex deposition. These sites include the glomerular capillaries, joint linings, ciliary body, pulmonary alveolar membranes, and vascular endothelial linings, especially around curves or bifurcations.

Intermediate-sized immune complexes tend to be deposited because they do not fix complement well, do not bind with red blood cells well

TABLE 10-5	DISEASES ASSOCIATED WITH TYPE III HYPERSENSITIVITY
DISEASE	**ANTIGEN**
Immune complex glomerulonephritis	GBM, exogenous antigens, drugs
SLE	Double-stranded DNA, DNA-histone complex, Sm, RNP, Ro:SSA, La:SSB, centromere
SLE-associated glomerulonephritis	Double-stranded DNA, DNA-histone complex, Sm, RNP, Ro:SSA, La:SSB
Acute allergic alveolitis	Various puffball spores from moldy dwellings
Farmer's lung disease	Thermophilic *Actinomycetes* from contaminated hay or grains
Chemical worker's lung	Isocyanates
Still disease— postinfectious arthritis	RANA, or none identified
Rheumatoid arthritis	RANA
Serum sickness	Lymphocytes or thymocytes from heterologous serum
Henoch-Schönlein purpura	Upper respiratory tract viruses, drugs (antibiotics and thiazides), foods (milk, fish, eggs, rice, nuts, beans), and immunizations
Drug-induced vasculitis	Drugs (antibiotics and thiazides)
Polyarteritis nodosa	Antineutrophil cytoplasmic
Wegener granulomatosus	Antineutrophil cytoplasmic
Goodpasture syndrome	GBM

GBM, Glomerular basement membrane; *La,* Lane; *RANA,* rheumatoid arthritis nuclear antigen; *RNP,* ribonucleoprotein; *Ro,* Robert; *SLE,* systemic lupus erythematosus; *Sm,* Smith; *SS,* single stranded.

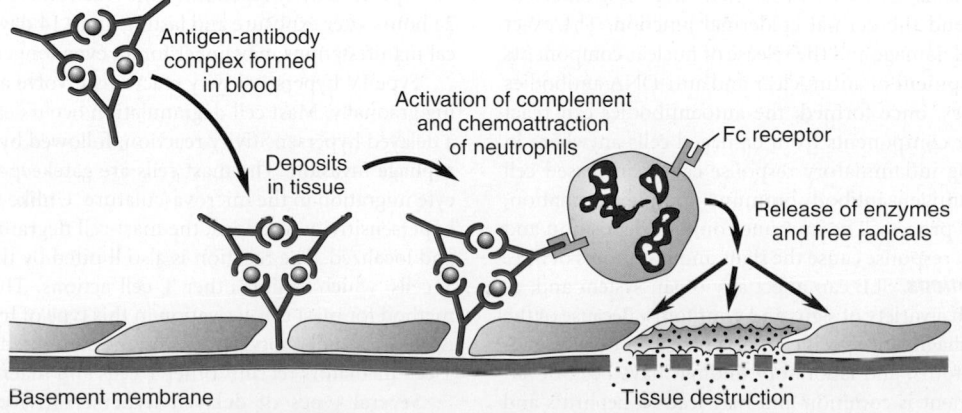

FIGURE 10-4 Type III hypersensitivity reaction.

after fixation, and are not readily removed by the mononuclear phagocyte system. Large numbers of any size immune complex can be deposited if they are so numerous that the phagocytic cells are overwhelmed. Deposition of immune complexes also depends on their immunoglobulin class and the affinity between the antigen and antibody. Finally, deposition may be affected by the type of antigen or by the relationship between the immune complex and sites with increased collagen. Because DNA and collagen have strong affinity, an increased quantity of DNA–anti-DNA immune complexes may be deposited in collagen membranes, such as in the kidney. The electrical charge of the immune complex may affect where it is deposited. For example, a positively charged immune complex may be attracted by a negatively charged basement membrane.

Immune Complex Glomerulonephritis

Etiology. Immune complex glomerulonephritis (an inflammatory renal disorder) is an example of a type III hypersensitivity reaction typically occurring 10 to 14 days after infection with a *Streptococcus* or *Staphylococcal* bacterial strain. It involves the interaction of soluble exogenous antigen with soluble antibody and is the cause of most glomerulonephritis cases. The circulating immune complex is then deposited in the glomerular capillary wall and mesangium.

Clinical manifestations and treatment. This deposition causes damage to the glomerular basement membrane with resultant proteinuria, hematuria, hypertension, oliguria, and red cell casts in the urine (see Chapter 27). In some types of glomerulonephritis, the patient may have nephrotic syndrome and acute renal failure that may progress to chronic renal failure.

Treatment of glomerulonephritis involves the use of corticosteroids and other medications to decrease inflammation. Antihistamines and antiserotonins have been tried in attempts to decrease vasoactive mediators and vascular permeability. Anticoagulants and antiplatelet medications such as aspirin, as well as plasmapheresis, are currently being studied. In plasmapheresis, plasma is removed from the blood and fresh frozen plasma or albumin is used to replace the withdrawn plasma.

Systemic Lupus Erythematosus

Etiology. Systemic lupus erythematosus (SLE) is another example of a type III hypersensitivity reaction caused by autoantibody production. SLE tends to occur more frequently in women than in men (ratio of 7:1) and with an incidence of 20 cases per 100,000 persons. It is primarily characterized by the development of antibodies against nuclear antigens such as DNA, deoxyribonucleohistone, and RNA. Production of autoantibodies to red blood cells, neutrophils, platelets, lymphocytes, and other organs or tissues may also occur.

In SLE, antinuclear antibodies (ANAs) and anti-DNA autoantibodies attach to components of the nucleus to form immune complexes that are deposited on collagen-rich tissues, including the glomerular basement membrane and the dermal-epidermal junction. The exact mechanism causing cell damage and the release of nuclear components and subsequent development of antinuclear and anti-DNA antibodies is not known. However, once formed, the autoantibodies can react with DNA and nuclear components from damaged cells anywhere in the body. The resulting inflammatory response causes increased cell damage and further antigen-antibody immune complex formation, thus leading to a cyclic process. The immune complex deposition and resulting inflammatory response cause the signs and symptoms of SLE.

Clinical manifestations. SLE can affect any organ system and, as such, it can present with a variety of signs and symptoms. Because of the variable presentation, diagnostic specific criteria based on the presence of specific signs, symptoms, and laboratory findings have been developed. Kidney involvement is common and may lead to nephritis and glomerulonephritis. Skin symptoms are wide ranging and include malar

"butterfly" rash, erythematous rash on exposed skin, purpura, alopecia, mucosal ulcerations, subcutaneous nodules, and splinter hemorrhages. The malar butterfly rash occurs across the nose onto the cheeks in approximately 26% of patients with acute SLE. The butterfly rash can be flat or raised and always spares the nasolabial folds. The rash that occurs on sun-exposed skin can be superficial to indurated and is nonpruritic. It can occur on the face, chest, shoulders, extensor surfaces of the arms, and backs of the hands. The color ranges from red to reddish purple. Most patients have symptoms of arthritis or polyarthralgia. Other symptoms include pleurisy, pericarditis, restrictive pulmonary disease, retinal changes, thrombocytopenia, anemia, and gastrointestinal ulceration. Central nervous system involvement includes neuritis, seizures, depression, or psychosis. A positive ANA test is usually present with positive anti-DNA (antibody to native DNA) and anti-Sm (antibody to Smith nuclear antigen) (see Chapter 52 for more information).

Treatment. Treatment of SLE depends upon the organ system affected and includes administration of nonsteroidal antiinflammatory agents such as aspirin, systemic corticosteroids, and antimalarials such as hydroxychloroquine (Plaquenil). Antimalarials are a cornerstone of treatment for SLE because of their effectiveness. The major side effect of antimalarials is ocular toxicity, which can be prevented by limiting therapy to 10 years or less, not exceeding 6.5 mg/kg/day dosages, and undergoing yearly ophthalmic evaluations. Other side effects include myopathy, pigmentation changes, gastrointestinal effects, liver enzyme changes, dizziness, and emotional changes. Corticosteroids decrease inflammation and provide immunosuppression, which can decrease symptoms and add to the patient's quality of life. If the patient does not respond to corticosteroids, immunosuppressives or cytotoxic agents can be used. Antibiotics are commonly prescribed because of frequent infections secondary to immune system compromise. There are new biological therapies being developed to target cytokines, and decrease immune system activation. Sunscreens with maximum sun protection factor (SPF) values are necessary to prevent photosensitivity reactions. Patients are also encouraged to avoid direct sunlight from 10 AM until at least 3 PM.

Type IV Hypersensitivity

Type IV hypersensitivity is also known as delayed hypersensitivity. Delayed hypersensitivity is characterized by tissue damage resulting from a delayed cellular reaction to an antigen. Unlike other hypersensitivity reactions, primary antibody involvement is absent. The principal mediators are lymphocytes, including T helper cells (Th) that mediate the reaction by releasing lymphokines (cytokines) and/or antigen-sensitized cytotoxic T cells (Tc) that can directly kill cells. The principal effector cells are lymphocytes and macrophages, with mast cells involved in the early phases. Neutrophils are not involved in type IV hypersensitivity reactions. This reaction is slow in onset, beginning 24 hours after exposure and lasting up to 14 days after exposure. Clinical manifestations may linger for an even longer period.

Type IV hypersensitivity reactions involve a series of events evolving gradually. Mast cell degranulation occurs early in the evolution of a delayed hypersensitivity reaction, followed by lymphocyte and macrophage invasion. The mast cells are gatekeepers that regulate leukocyte migration in the microvasculature. Unlike that occurring in type I hypersensitivity reactions, the mast cell degranulation is more limited and localized. The reaction is also limited by the action of suppressor T cells, which inhibit other T-cell actions. The justification and the method for mast cell activation in this type of hypersensitivity reaction is not well understood. However, the combined action of mast cell and T cell mediators recruits other T cells and macrophages to the site.

Several types of delayed hypersensitivity reactions are recognized, including cutaneous basophil hypersensitivity (Jones-Mote sensitivity), contact hypersensitivity, tuberculin-type hypersensitivity, and granulomatous hypersensitivity.

Cutaneous Basophil Hypersensitivity

Cutaneous basophil is the most rapid type of delayed hypersensitivity reaction. It is a lymphocyte-mediated basophil reaction. Soluble antigen that has been injected intradermally or antigens introduced into the dermis trigger T-cell activation and subsequent release of cytokines and activation of basophils, which infiltrate the area. The reaction peaks with skin swelling in 24 hours and can last 7 to 10 days. An example of this type of hypersensitivity is skin graft reactions and rejection.

Contact Hypersensitivity

Contact hypersensitivity is the most familiar type IV hypersensitivity. It is an immune or inflammatory response to a wide variety of plant oils, chemicals, ointments, clothing, cosmetics, dyes, and adhesives.

Contact hypersensitivity is an epidermal phenomenon. As a delayed reaction, it peaks in 48 to 72 hours. The reaction is slow because the skin-penetrating antigen is very small and in an incomplete form. This incomplete, lipid-soluble antigen is called a **hapten.** The hapten must first penetrate the epidermis, where it links with a normal body protein, called a *carrier*. Only after the hapten combines with the carrier is it a complete antigen—often called a hapten conjugate.

The complete antigen is processed by dermal dendritic cells located in the suprabasal epidermis. The dermal dendritic cells move to the local lymph channel, where they migrate to the regional lymph node. Within the lymph node, the dermal dendritic cells display the now processed complete antigen to CD4$^+$ T cells in the paracortex. Then the antigen-sensitized CD4$^+$ T cells release lymphokines, which initiate an inflammatory response and attract other effector cells. The primary lymphokines include IL-2, IL-3, interferon, TNF, and macrophage-stimulating factors (Figure 10-5).

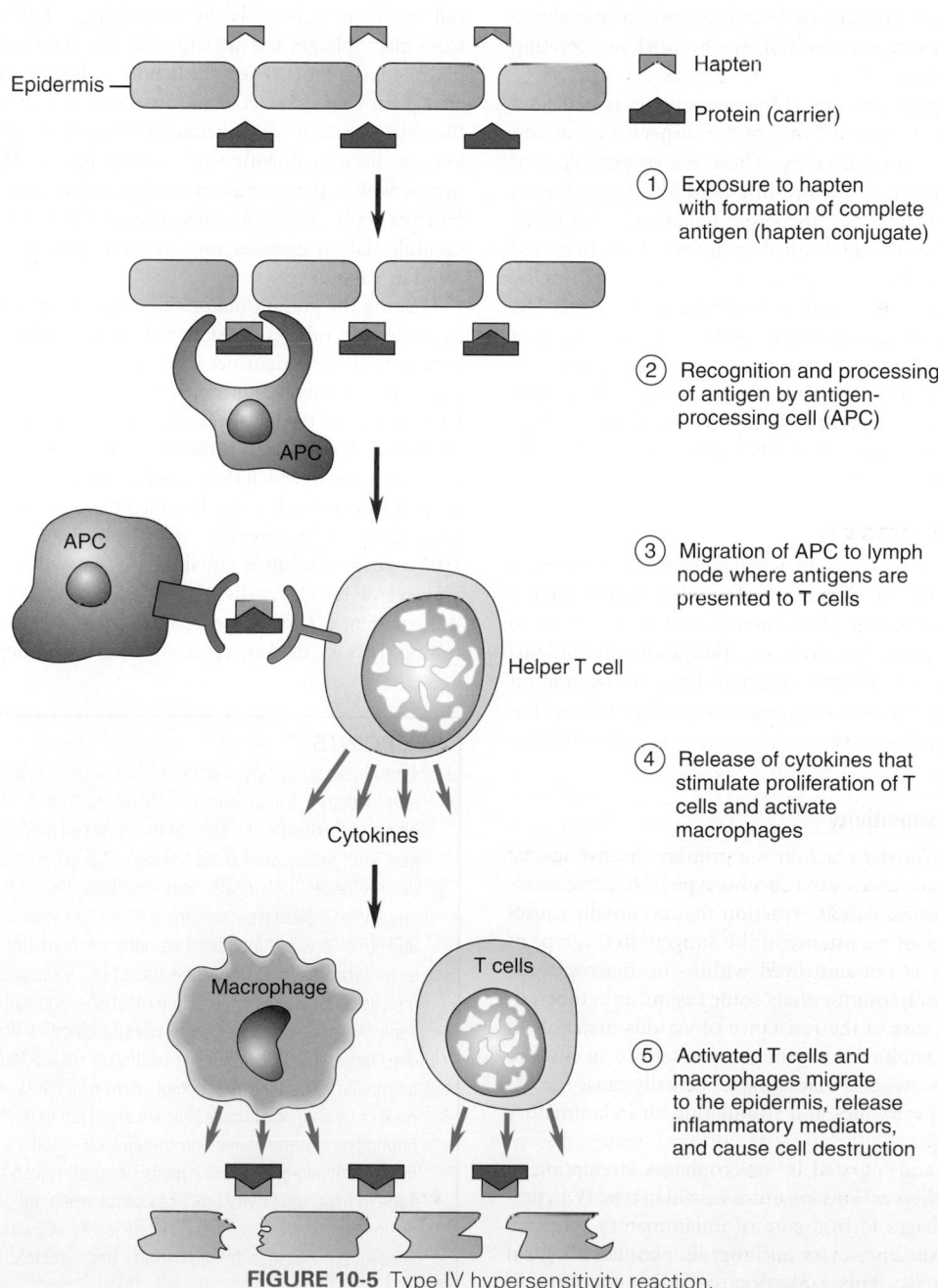

FIGURE 10-5 Type IV hypersensitivity reaction.

Lymphokines (cytokines) and prostaglandins are important in contact hypersensitivity. The presentation of antigen to T cells causes the lymphokine cascade of vasoactive and cytoactive substances. These substances cause inflammation as well as activation of other cells. After about 72 hours, the reaction begins to decrease because of degradation of the antigen and production of prostaglandin E, which inhibits IL-1 and IL-2 production.

After primary exposure or immunization, a cellular reaction takes place at each subsequent exposure site. Cross-reactivity with related substances also occurs in contact hypersensitivity. For example, a person with contact dermatitis to nickel will react when exposed to a variety of nickel alloys, including the metal in earrings, zippers, snaps, and belt buckles. Skin symptoms resulting from contact dermatitis include redness (erythema), edema, pruritus, and blisters. People with sensitivities may also experience respiratory symptoms if exposed to aerosolized hapten. This situation could occur when a person is downwind from burning poison ivy or burning tires. Delayed hypersensitivity reaction (type IV) caused by exposure to the compounds in latex gloves is an occupational risk in surgeons and nurses who work in operating rooms.

Patch testing for diagnosis of contact hypersensitivity is indicated when symptoms persist despite avoidance of the suspected agent and with appropriate use of topical therapy. There are several types of patch tests including open and closed testing used by dermatologists and allergists. In open patch testing, the suspected allergen is applied twice daily to the upper arm and left uncovered for 2 days. In closed patch tests, the suspected allergen is applied to the skin away from the original site of eruption and is covered with an adhesive bandage. The bandage is then removed in 2 days. The results are graded according to response. A 1+ positive patch test response involves erythema of the entire area of exposure. Patchy pustular responses are not positive and are irritant reactions. A 2+ patch test response involves erythema and vesicles. A 3+ patch test response involves erythema, vesicles, and bullae.

Tuberculin-Type Hypersensitivity

Tuberculin-type hypersensitivity occurs when someone who has been previously infected by tuberculosis is exposed to tuberculin antigen in a tuberculin test. It is a dermal phenomenon that peaks in 48 to 72 hours. The person experiences erythema, induration, and inflammation at the site of the intradermal injection. Because the amount injected is so small, the reaction disappears when the antigen has degraded. However, people with severe reactions may experience tissue necrosis at the site.

Granulomatous Hypersensitivity

Granulomatous hypersensitivity reaction is a primary defense against intracellular infections and represents a chronic type IV hypersensitivity reaction. It is a protective defense reaction that eventually causes tissue destruction because of persistence of the antigen. In this type of hypersensitivity, antigen is not destroyed within the macrophages, either because of failure of lysosome-phagosome fusion, as in tuberculosis and leprosy, or because of the resistance of various materials to internal lysozymes, as in retained suture material or talc. In an effort to protect the host, lymphocytes and macrophages actually cause the tissue damage by releasing cytokines and stimulating an inflammatory response.

Antigen is engulfed and ingested by macrophages attempting to destroy the antigen, but these actions are unsuccessful in type IV hypersensitivity. The macrophages form a core of inflammatory cells that include lymphocytes, tissue histiocytes, eosinophils, plasma cells, giant cells, and epithelioid cells. This collection of inflammatory cells develops into a ball-like mass called a granuloma. The predominant cell in the granuloma is the macrophage. Epithelioid cells originate from macrophages and are large, flat cells with a large amount of endoplasmic reticulum. When epithelioid cells fuse, they form multinucleated giant cells. This core is surrounded by lymphocytes. Gradually, fibroblastic activity and increased collagen synthesis cause the granuloma to become fibrotic with scar formation. Often, central necrosis occurs within the granuloma and is called *caseous* or *cheesy necrosis*. Patients with granulomatous diseases have a variety of symptoms. Granulomatous diseases and the pathogens associated with them are listed in Table 10-6.

Testing for granulomatous diseases also involves skin testing. For example, the tuberculin skin test (i.e., Mantoux or purified protein derivative [PPD]) identifies infection but is not diagnostic of active disease. The test involves *intradermal* injection of 0.1 ml of PPD into the volar surface of the left forearm. There should be a clear bleb at the site of the test. The skin test is then read in 48 to 72 hours. A negative PPD skin test is one in which there is either no reaction or only redness at the site. A positive result is one in which there is equal to or greater than 10 to 15 mm of induration (or tissue firmness) at the site. In patients with HIV a positive result is equal to or greater than 5 mm of induration. However, if the HIV patient's CD4+ cell count is low (<200 cells/μL), or if the patient is febrile or elderly, there may be no reaction to any skin testing. This is called anergy and causes a false negative in many cases.

TABLE 10-6	GRANULOMATOUS DISEASE ASSOCIATED WITH TYPE IV HYPERSENSITIVITY
DISEASE	**BACTERIUM**
Tuberculosis	*Mycobacterium tuberculosis*
Leprosy	*Mycobacterium leprae*
Histoplasmosis	*Histoplasma capsulatum*
Coccidioidomycosis	*Coccidioides immitis*
Brucellosis	*Brucella abortus*
	Brucella suis (less common)
	Brucella melitensis (less common)
Tularemia	*Francisella (Pasteurella) tularensis*

KEY POINTS

- Type I hypersensitivity is an immediate allergic or anaphylactic type of reaction mediated primarily by sensitized mast cells. The reaction is initiated when IgE antibodies located on the mast cell membrane are bound by antigen, with subsequent cross-linking of IgE receptors. Mast cell degranulation releases chemicals that mediate the signs and symptoms of anaphylaxis. Released histamine, kinin, prostaglandins, interleukins, and leukotrienes cause increased vascular permeability, vasodilation, hypotension, urticaria, and bronchoconstriction. Examples of type I reactions include drug reactions, bee sting reactions, and asthma.
- Type II hypersensitivity occurs when antibodies are formed against antigens on cell surfaces, usually resulting in lysis of target cells. Cell lysis may be mediated by activated complement fragments (membrane attack complex) or by phagocytic cells that are attracted to target cells by the attached antibodies. Examples include transfusion reactions, erythroblastosis fetalis, myasthenia gravis, and hyperacute graft rejection.
- Type III hypersensitivity reactions occur when antigen-antibody complexes are deposited in tissues and result in the activation of complement and subsequent tissue inflammation and destruction. Antigen-antibody

complexes activate the complement cascade and subsequently attract phagocytic cells to the tissue. History of persistent low-grade infections, inhalation of antigens into alveoli, and autoimmune production of antibodies may result in chronic production of antigen-antibody complexes. Examples include glomerulonephritis and SLE.

- Type IV hypersensitivity reactions are T-cell mediated and do not require antibody production, in contrast to type I, II, and III reactions. Sensitized T cells react with altered or foreign cells and initiate inflammation. Contact dermatitis, tuberculin reactions, transplant rejection, and graft-versus-host disease are examples.

DEFICIENT IMMUNE RESPONSES

Deficient immune responses result from a functional decrease in one or more components of the immune system. These disorders can affect lymphocytes, antibodies, phagocytes, and complement proteins. Two types of immune deficiency are differentiated: primary and secondary. Primary disorders are immune deficiencies not attributable to other causes; these may be congenital or acquired. Examples of primary immunodeficiency disorders include severe combined immunodeficiency (SCID) syndrome, DiGeorge syndrome, selective IgA deficiency, and AIDS. Persons with a primary immunodeficiency can be predisposed to multiple deficiencies, as in agammaglobulinemia or SCID, or can have a single phenotype deficiency predisposing to a specific infection, such as disorders of the IL-12–interferon-γ (IFN-γ) circuit, which predispose to infections caused by mycobacteria.[14] Secondary immunodeficiency disorders are a consequence of non–immune system disorders or treatments that secondarily affect

immune function. Examples of secondary disorders include those associated with hyperlipidemia or malnutrition, medical treatments such as cancer chemotherapy, or biopsychosocial stress such as postsurgical immune system problems.

PRIMARY IMMUNODEFICIENCY DISORDERS

Primary immunodeficiency disorders (PIDs) include congenital phenotypes that result from abnormal development or maturation of immune cells, as well as acquired primary disorders of immune cells such as HIV/AIDS. AIDS is described in Chapter 12 and only the congenital forms of primary immunodeficiency are included here. The classic view of primary congenital immunodeficiency disorders is that they are rare genetic disorders that are often sex linked. The most common primary disorders are listed in Table 10-7. However, there are strong genetic epidemiologic data suggesting that most people have some inborn errors of immunity that may vary in clinical significance and severity. This novel observation is changing how we view immunodeficiency (Table 10 8).[13] The first clinical indicators of immunodeficiency disorders are the signs and symptoms of infection, and the disorders are often first suspected when an individual has severe recurrent, unusual, or unmanageable infections.

B-Cell and T-Cell Combined Disorders
Severe Combined Immunodeficiency Disorders

Etiology and pathogenesis. (SCIDs) are inherited primary immunodeficiency disorders and are characterized by the absence or dysfunction of T cells affecting both cellular and humoral adaptive immunity.[14] Depending on the genetic defect, B cells may be present (T B+) or absent (T-B−), and there is wide phenotypic and immunologic variability.[14] As

TABLE 10-7 PRIMARY CONGENITAL IMMUNODEFICIENCY DISORDERS

DISORDER	FUNCTIONAL DEFICIENCY	ERROR
Bruton X-linked agammaglobulinemia	B cells; antibody	*BTK gene mutant*
Common variable (acquired) hypogammaglobulinemia	B cells; antibody	Unknown: possible *CARMA1* variant and *BOB1* variant
Selective IgA deficiency	B cells; IgA antibody	Unknown: possible alterations in transmembrane activator, calcium modulator, and cycophilin ligand interactor gene
Secretory component deficiency—chronic mucocutaneous candidiasis	B cells; secretory IgA antibody	Autosomal recessive deficiency in IL-17RA; autosomal dominant deficiency of IL-17F
Selective IgM deficiency	IgM antibody	Unknown
Selective deficiency of IgG subclasses	IgG antibody subclass	Unknown
Transient hypogammaglobulinemia of infancy	Low antibodies	Unknown
X-Linked lymphoproliferative disease or Duncan X-linked lymphoproliferative disease	Anti–Epstein-Barr virus–linked antigen antibody	Mutations in *SH2D1A* and *XIAP (BIRC4)*
DiGeorge syndrome (congenital thymic hypoplasia or aplasia)	Primarily T cells	Chromosome 22q11.2 Deletion syndrome
Autosomal recessive SCID	T cells, antibody	Defects of JAK3
X-Linked recessive, T-B+ SCID	T cells, antibody	Defects of *IL2RG* gene
T-B− SCID (reticular dysgenesis)	T cells, antibody, granulocytes	Mutations of *RAG1* or *RAG2*
MHC class II expression deficiency (rare lymphocyte syndrome)	T cells, antibody	Impaired gene regulation and lack of HLA class II gene expression Probable: class II transactivator and regulatory factor X5
Wiskott-Aldrich syndrome (immunodeficiency with eczema and thrombocytopenia)	Antibody, T cells	Defect of short arm of X chromosome at Xp11.3 mutation of *WASP* gene
Chédiak-Higashi syndrome	Natural killer cells, phagocytic cells, granulocytes, platelets	Autosomal recessive disorder; *CHS1/L4ST* gene on chromosome 1
Chronic granulomatous disease of childhood	Phagocytic cells (neutrophils)	Mutations in genes *CYBA, NCF-1, NCF-2, CYBB*

BTK, Bruton tyrosine kinase; *JAK,* Janus kinase; *MHC,* major histocompatibility complex; *SCID,* severe combined immunodeficiency; *WASP,* WAS protein.

TABLE 10-8   PARADIGM SHIFT IN PRIMARY IMMUNODEFICIENCIES

PRIMARY IMMUNODEFICIENCIES	CONVENTIONAL VIEW	CONTEMPORARY VIEW
Patient and Population Levels		
Frequency	Rare	Common
Occurrence	Familial	Sporadic
Age at onset	Childhood	Adulthood
Prognosis	Spontaneously worsening	Spontaneously improving
Phenotype Level		
Disease-defining clinical phenotypes	Opportunistic infections	Other infections and phenotypes
Number of phenotypes per patient	High	Low (even single)
Number of episodes per patient	High	Low (even single)
Disease-causing cellular phenotypes	Hematopoietic	Nonhematopoietic
Genotype Level		
Disease-causing genes per patient	One (monogenic, mendelian)	A few (oligogenic, major genes)
Mode of mendelian inheritance	Autosomal and X-linked recessive	Autosomal dominant
Clinical penetrance	Complete	Incomplete
Mutations	Inherited from parental genome	Germ line de novo or somatic

From Casanova JL, Abel L: Primary immunodeficiencies: a field in its infancy, *Science* 317(5838):618, 2007.

such, these disorders vary in their severity and clinical features. T-B+ SCID is caused by mutations in cytokine-mediated signaling. The majority of these patients have X-linked SCID caused by mutations in the *IL2RG* gene that is responsible for encoding common γ chain, which is needed by several cytokine receptors.[14] Other T-B+ SCID patients have mutations in one of the four *CD3* genes.[14] T-B− SCID patients have a defect caused by mutations of recombination activating genes 1 or 2 (*RAG1* or *RAG2*), both of which are involved in the process of antigen receptor gene assembly. The three major types of SCIDs are classical SCID, atypical SCID, and Omenn syndrome.

The most severe form of T-B− SCID, called classical SCID or *reticular dysgenesis,* is characterized by failure of all white blood cell development. Infants with reticular dysgenesis have failure of both lymphocyte and granulocyte development. Although the fetus grows normally, the infant is severely affected with absent lymphoid tissue, absent T lymphocytes, and absent immunoglobulins. The T-B+ SCID X-linked recessive type is the most common type (50% of cases), affecting boys more often than girls. These infants lack circulating T cells and usually have a normal to increased number of B cells that do not function normally. The enzymes or other essential components necessary for immune cell functioning are deficient, particularly enzymes linked with purine nucleoside phosphorylase or adenosine deaminase metabolism. As a result, the infant accumulates toxic metabolites of purine or adenosine that affect lymphocytes. Antibody titers are decreased because of lack of antibody formation after immunization. T cells are low in number (less than 1000/µL) or absent. Some infants have increased numbers of B cells, but they are unable to function normally because of poor antibody production with decreased synthesis of IgG, IgM, and IgA. Generally, most patients have small, hypoplastic thymus glands indicative of poor or absent T cell development. Because complete failure of lymphoid and myeloid stem cells during fetal development is not generally compatible with life, many infants die in utero or shortly after birth.

Clinical manifestations and treatment. Infants with these syndromes are usually ill within 3 months of age and often have thrush, severe *Candida* diaper dermatitis, or infections causing otitis, pneumonia, and diarrhea. They are prone to sepsis, opportunistic infections with such pathogens as *Candida albicans* or *Pneumocystis jiroveci (carinii),* infections with such viruses as cytomegalovirus (CMV) or herpesvirus, and common childhood diseases such as varicella and measles.

Because of their severity, infections in infants with SCID are medical emergencies. T-B− SCID patients have an overall worse outcome than T-B+ SCID patients.[14]

Infants suspected of having SCID should be placed in protective isolation and all staff involved in the infants' care should be vigilant about following proper hand washing procedures and avoiding exposure to infections. Breast feeding is encouraged if the mother is CMV negative and without active infection. Curative therapy involves hematopoietic stem cell transplantation with either umbilical cord blood or bone marrow preferably from HLA-haploidentical siblings.[14] Other therapies include chemotherapy conditioning regimens, long-term immunoglobulin therapy, enzyme replacement therapy, and gene therapy.[14]

Wiskott-Aldrich Syndrome

Etiology and pathogenesis. Wiskott-Aldrich syndrome is an X-linked immunodeficiency disorder that affects both T cells and B cells. The gene deficiency is caused by a mutation of the WAS protein *(WASP)* gene and has been mapped to the short arm of the X chromosome at Xpll.23. The *WASP* gene is involved in cytoplasmic signaling and in reorganization of the actin cytoskeleton. In this syndrome, IgM concentration is decreased. Other antibody concentrations are variable, with IgE and IgA levels usually elevated and IgG level normal to low. This antibody variability is the result of increased antibody catabolism. Platelet deficiency is also associated with Wiskott-Aldrich syndrome. T cells are present but function deficiently. Affected infants have particular difficulty mounting immune responses to protein and polysaccharide antigens, including bacterial cell walls (e.g., *Pseudomonas aeruginosa, Staphylococcus pneumoniae*).

Clinical manifestations and treatment. Wiskott-Aldrich syndrome is clinically characterized by the presence of eczema, thrombocytopenic purpura, and infection. Affected children are prone to pneumococcal infections, including pneumonia, meningitis, otitis media, and sepsis. They are also subject to renal disease, malignancies, and systemic autoimmunity.[15] The average age of these infants at death is 3.5 years without treatment.

Infants with Wiskott-Aldrich syndrome are treated with antibody replacement therapy, and antibiotic therapy. Bone marrow transplantation, stem cell transplantation, and gene therapy are options used to manage this disorder in affected children.

T-Cell Disorders

DiGeorge Syndrome or 22q11.2 Deletion Syndrome

Etiology and pathogenesis. 22q11.2 Deletion syndrome, previously known as DiGeorge syndrome, or thymic hypoplasia, is a developmental T-cell disorder associated with total or partial loss of thymus gland function. The development of this syndrome is caused by a chromosomal 22q11.2 deletion (del 22q11). It is the most common microdeletion syndrome with an estimated prevalence of 1 in 4000 live births.[16] Male and female children are equally affected.[16] There may also be associated genetic modifiers that vary in clinical presentation. In this disorder, the aplastic or hypoplastic thymus is unable to assist in the maturation of T cells. Therefore, T cells are deficient. B cells are normal.

Clinical manifestations and treatment. Because 22q11.2 deletion syndrome is a congenital disorder of fetal organ development, it is often associated with other congenital problems, such as developmental delay, cardiac and great vessel anomalies, hypoparathyroidism with hypocalcemia, hypothyroidism, esophageal atresia or reflux, urogenital anomalies, and unusual facial features, including mandibular hypoplasia, short forehead, and protuberant or low-set ears.[15] With partial loss of thymus function, the individual may not have trouble with infections. However, recurrent infections occur in up to 40% of patients and up to 1% of patients have severe immunodeficiency that resembles SCID with total loss of thymus function.[16] This increases the risk of fetal loss or infant death. For these children, thymic transplantation has been helpful in reestablishing T-cell populations. Specific treatments and therapies are needed for the management of these patients.

Chronic Mucocutaneous Candidiasis

Etiology and pathogenesis. Chronic mucocutaneous candidiasis is a T-cell disorder caused by one of two genetic etiologies. The first is an autosomal recessive deficiency in a specific cytokine receptor: interleukin-17 receptor A (IL-17RA), which causes complete lack of cellular responsiveness to the inflammatory cytokines IL-17A and IL-17F.[17] The second etiology is an autosomal dominant deficiency of the cytokine IL-17F, which is partial and allows some cytokine activity.[17] As a result of these deficiencies, chronic mucocutaneous candidiasis is characterized by a selective deficiency of cell-mediated immunity against *Candida albicans* and, to a lesser extent, *Staphylococcus aureus*. In this case, T cells do not produce the correct cytokines needed for the cell-mediated immunity to *C. albicans*. This causes persistent or recurrent severe skin, nail, and mucous membrane infections with *C. albicans*. B-cell and T-cell functions are usually normal, except for the inability of the T cells to respond to *Candida* infections. Occasionally IgA or other antibody levels may be affected.

Clinical manifestations and treatment. The goal of treatment is to reduce the severity of skin and mucous membrane infection and to decrease the disfigurement from infection and scarring. Treatment involves antifungal therapy. This disorder is also associated with an autoimmune disorder called *autoimmune polyendocrinopathy-candidiasis-ectodermal dystrophy* (APECED).[18] The most common components of APECED are chronic mucocutaneous candidiasis, hypoparathyroidism, and Addison disease (see Chapter 40).

B-Cell Disorders

IgA Deficiency

Etiology and pathogenesis. The most common B-cell primary immunodeficiency disorder is selective IgA deficiency. This disorder affects 1 in 2000 persons.[19] It is a B-cell disorder characterized by failure of IgA-bearing lymphocytes to become plasma cells, with resulting lack of secretory IgA in the serum. Genetically, it can be an autosomal recessive or autosomal dominant disease. The B-cell level is normal but there is a lack of B-cell response to interleukins (IL-4, IL-6, IL-7, or IL-10).[19]

Clinical manifestations and treatment. People with this disorder are prone to respiratory, gastrointestinal, and genitourinary tract infections. They tend to have many autoantibodies (including anti-IgA antibodies), with a high incidence of vascular, endocrine, and collagen autoimmune diseases.[20] They often react to cow's milk, and inflammatory bowel conditions such as celiac disease can develop. Because they have severe allergic reactions to blood or blood products containing IgA, exogenous IgA replacement is contraindicated. Treatment includes prevention of infection and management of infection with appropriate antibiotics.

Bruton X-Linked Agammaglobulinemia

Etiology and pathogenesis. Bruton X-linked agammaglobulinemia (XLA), or congenital hypogammaglobulinemia, is a B-cell genetic disorder caused by a lack of normal B-cell development in the bone marrow. The disorder is linked to a mutation of the gene *btk* (Bruton tyrosine kinase) located on the long arm of the X chromosome at position Xq21.3 to Xq22. In 1952 it was the first genetic immunodeficiency disorder identified. This mutation occurs in a cytoplasmic signal-transducing molecule encoded by the *btk* gene, which results in B-cell deficiency. The B-cell deficiency causes decreased serum concentrations of IgG and no detectable IgA or IgM. The number of CD4[+] memory T cells is decreased.[21] The decreased number of CD4[+] T cells is believed to be due to the lack of B cells and supports the importance of B-cell and T-cell immune system interaction.[21] The thymus functions normally. Plasmocytes are absent and reticuloendothelial tissue and lymphoid organs (e.g., tonsils, spleen, Peyer patches, lymph nodes) are poorly developed.[19] The disease is characterized by recurrent bacterial infection and profound hypogammaglobulinemia resulting from decreased numbers of circulating B cells. Male infants are affected, but this disorder is typically diagnosed after the infant reaches 9 to 12 months of age because of passive maternal IgG protection. The frequency of the disease is 1:250,000 males.[19] Females are carriers.

Clinical manifestations and treatment. Frequent infections, most often attributable to *Haemophilus influenzae* and *Streptococcus pneumoniae*, occur in patients, causing pneumonia, otitis media, meningitis, sinusitis, and septicemia. The recurrent infections can lead to tissue destruction and injury.

Treatment of this disorder includes implementation of antibiotic therapy and prophylactic antibiotics as well as monthly administration of immunoglobulin infusions. However, passive immunotherapy is not always effective. Many children die before the age of 6. If the child survives to adulthood, life expectancy is decreased. Chronic lung disease and large joint arthritis are common in adults with XLA. Currently, curative hematopoietic stem cell–based gene therapy is advocated to correct B cell and myeloid deficiencies.[22] Children who have been diagnosed with XLA should not be immunized with live virus vaccine.[19]

Transient Hypogammaglobulinemia

Transient hypogammaglobulinemia of infancy is a self-limiting condition in which the infant is slow to acquire normal immunoglobulin levels. The infant experiences a lengthened period of low IgG, IgM, and IgA levels after birth. Normal IgG production begins only after 2 months of life and increases slowly as maternal immunoglobins are metabolized.[19] Affected infants can demonstrate normal immunoglobulin levels and immune system function by approximately age 3. During the period of low antibody levels, they are more susceptible to infections, particularly respiratory tract infections.

Common Variable Immunodeficiency

Common variable immunodeficiency (CVI) is a B-cell disorder characterized by low titers of immunoglobulins, particularly IgG and IgA, with 50% of affected individuals also experiencing low titers of IgM.[19] The primary defect is the inability of B cells to differentiate into plasma cells. The exact genetic defect is unknown but there are mutations in genes that encode the production of antibody subclasses and interleukins.[19] This disease is usually not recognized until the second or third decade of life with an incidence of 1:10,000-50,000.[19] Males and females are equally affected.

Clinical manifestations and treatment. CVI is characterized by chronic infections, particularly respiratory tract disorders including sinusitis, otitis, laryngitis, and pneumonia. The most frequent pathogens involved are encapsulated bacteria such as *S. pneumoniae* and *H. influenzae*. Infections of the gastrointestinal tract also occur from *Giardia* and *Salmonella*. There is an increased incidence of gastric adenocarcinoma, lymphoma, and lymphoproliferative disease as well as autoimmune diseases including autoimmune thrombocytopenia purpura, arthritis, and thyroiditis. Treatment involves intravenous or subcutaneous administration of immunoglobulin every 2 to 4 weeks, use of corticosteroids, and prompt treatment with antibiotics as needed.

SECONDARY IMMUNODEFICIENCY DISORDERS

A number of physical, psychosocial, nutritional, environmental, and pharmacologic factors can singly or in combination lead to the development of secondary immunodeficiency disorders. Many of these linkages are discussed in Chapter 8.

The direct and indirect linkages between the brain and the endocrine and immune systems are well known. As a result, excessive or defective neuroendocrine responses can lead to disease. For example, an excessive neuroendocrine response to stress with increased secretion of corticosteroids boosts a person's susceptibility to infectious agents and tumors but enhances resistance to autoimmune disease. On the other hand, a defective neuroendocrine response to stress with low corticosteroid levels enhances autoimmune disease and inhibits infections and tumors. Individuals experiencing physical and psychosocial stress, decreased social support, depression, and bereavement show decreased immune system functioning.

Morbidity and surgery also affect the function of the immune system. After surgery, T-cell and B-cell numbers decrease. This temporary deficiency can last up to 1 month and is most likely a result of the stress of surgery. Some types of surgery, such as splenic surgery, actually reduce the effectiveness of the immune system. Removal of the spleen reduces serum IgM and the antibody response to encapsulated bacteria (e.g., *S. pneumoniae, H. influenzae, S. aureus*). Disease states such as diabetes mellitus, drug- or alcohol-induced cirrhosis, severe burns, severe trauma, sickle cell anemia, malignancies, and severe infections are associated with secondary immune deficiencies. For example, when blood glucose level rises in patients with diabetes mellitus, white blood cell response to infection declines.

Pregnancy requires immune adaptation in order to be successful. Pregnancy's pro-inflammatory state requires careful control of the immune response and failure to adapt can lead to spontaneous abortion or preeclampsia.[23] During pregnancy, many factors are released from the placenta that influence the immune system, B-cell and T-cell function, and cytokine balance.[22] For example, syncytiotrophoblast microvesicles (STBMs) are shed from the placenta into the maternal circulation. These microvesicles bind to monocytes and B cells and induce cytokine release. Both proinflammatory and antiinflammatory cytokines are released, which prevents excessive inflammation.[23]

A number of pharmaceuticals affect the functioning of the immune system. Cytotoxins and other cancer pharmacotherapeutic drugs cause a state of generalized immunosuppression. For example, methotrexate is a phase-specific cytotoxin in which cells are killed only if they are in the S, or DNA-synthetic, phase. Cyclophosphamide is toxic to cells in any mitotic phase, although it is better at killing active cells. Anesthetics (e.g., halothane, cyclopropane, nitrous oxide, ether), alcohol, antibiotics, antithyroids, anticonvulsants, antihistamines, and steroids decrease cellular or humoral immunity by various methods. For example, chronic nitrous oxide toxicity leads to cell-mediated immune deficits. Therapeutic radiation (x-rays) also affects the immune system by destroying rapidly proliferating cells. When T-cell and B-cell clones are needed, irradiation eliminates these cells, thus blunting or reducing the effectiveness of the body's response.

A number of studies have linked immune system competency and nutritional status. Malnutritional states can lead to protein depletion, as well as carbohydrate, lipid, vitamin, and mineral deficiencies. Protein and calorie depletion causes T-cell reductions and dysfunction. Antibodies are composed of proteins, levels of which are also low in a state of depletion. Low levels of zinc, an enzyme cofactor needed for lymphocyte function, as well as low levels of folic acid and vitamins B_6, A, D, and E can result in T-cell and B-cell dysfunction. Overnutrition, especially hyperlipidemia, can lead to lymphocyte and granulocyte dysfunction. Nutritional balance is best for the development of all stem cells, the recognition and processing of antigens, and the attainment of optimal immune cell function.

In the elderly, immune system function is altered. The response to antigenic stimulation is variable. The elderly are less able to respond to "new" antigenic stimuli. The cells of the immune system in the elderly are not able to proliferate or reproduce as effectively as in younger persons. Although the total number of T cells remains the same, T-cell function is decreased. T cells are less capable of proliferating and have decreased cytotoxicity. Antibody production also decreases. A rise also is seen in autoantibody production, which may influence the increase in autoimmune disease in the elderly.

KEY POINTS

- Primary deficiencies in immune function may be from congenital, genetic, or acquired defects that directly affect immune cell function.
- Secondary deficiencies are conditions that impair immune function as a result of other nonimmune system disorders, such as poor nutrition, pregnancy, stress, or drugs, that secondarily suppress immune function.
- Primary genetic immunodeficiency disorders are fairly common, with most causing moderate immune impairment that may not be diagnosed. Severe congenital immunodeficiency disorders are less common, but clinically significant. Impairment in T cells and B cells results in SCID. Functional B and T lymphocytes are lacking, and infants with SCID easily succumb to sepsis and opportunistic infections. Other types of primary immunodeficiency disorders affect a particular cell type: DiGeorge syndrome (now called 22q11.2 deletion syndrome) occurs with T-cell agenesis related to a lack of thymus function; chronic mucocutaneous candidiasis is caused by abnormal T cells that cannot respond to *Candida;* and selective IgA deficiency is caused by B-cell abnormality.
- Problems in neuroendocrine and immune system interactions are a cause of secondary immunodeficiencies. Excessive neuroendocrine response to stress with increased corticosteroid production increases susceptibility to infection.
- Medications such as cytotoxins and other cancer pharmacotherapeutic drugs cause generalized secondary immunosuppression. However, other medications, such as anesthetics, alcohol, antibiotics, and steroids, also affect the immune response and can lead to secondary immunosuppression.
- Malnutrition, a major cause of immune system dysfunction, leads to lymphocyte dysfunction and altered stem cell development.

SUMMARY

Human beings live in internal and external environments teeming with antigens capable of producing immunologic responses. Contact with an antigen or antigens usually leads to induction of a normal protective immune response. However, some individuals experience disease caused by either excessive or deficient immune responses.

Both excessive and deficient immune reactions are damaging to tissue. The tissues that are affected depend on the type of antigen, the type of antigen exposure, and the degree of immune responsiveness. In children with immune system dysfunction caused by genetic or embryonic defects, the lack or dysfunction of T cells, B cells, and antibodies can lead to lethal or recurrent infections that severely limit the child's ability to interact with the environment. As a result of their immune disorder, some of these children may never reach maturity. In the elderly, malnutrition, medications, and decreased immune system function as a result of aging, surgery, stress, decreased social support, depression, and bereavement lead to increased infections and autoimmune disease. Autoimmune disease is a type of excessive immune reaction in which the immune system reacts against the body's own cells.

Excessive immune reactions are common and involve a complex interplay between antigen and components of the immune system. Hypersensitivity disorders are differentiated by the cell type involved and the time course of the reaction. For example, type I hypersensitivity is a rapid response caused by a host of lethal chemicals generated by but involving only one antibody, IgE, and one effector cell, the mast cell. It is an antigen-antibody reaction causing the release of potent chemicals that can lead to extreme, even life-threatening reactions in susceptible individuals. Type II hypersensitivity is also immediate but is tissue specific involving IgG and IgM antibodies, a host of effector cells, and the complement system. It is a linkage between antigen on target cells and the Fab portion of IgG or IgM antibodies. Examples include blood transfusion reactions, hemolytic anemia, and myasthenia gravis.

Type III hypersensitivity reactions, which involve IgG as the major antibody and neutrophils and mast cells as the effector cells, take several hours to develop. These reactions involve the deposition of antigen antibody immune complexes into tissue and activation of the complement system. This reaction is a deposition problem that depends on the solubility of the antigen-antibody complex and the vascular system. The tissues that have the antigen-antibody complex deposited into them become inflamed. SLE is the major example of type III hypersensitivity. Type IV hypersensitivity takes days to develop and involves cytotoxic T cells but no antibodies. Examples include poison ivy, contact dermatitis, and organ transplant rejection.

REFERENCES

1. Hoyne GF: Mechanisms that regulate peripheral immune responses to control organ-specific autoimmunity, *Clin Dev Immunol,* 294968, 2011, April 28, 2011.
2. Shahrizaila N, Yuki N: Guillain-Barré syndrome animal model: the first proof of molecular mimicry in human autoimmune disorder, *J Biomed Biotechnol* 2011:829129, 2011.
3. Guilherme L, et al: Rheumatic heart disease: mediation by complex immune events, *Adv Clin Chem* 53:31–50, 2011.
4. Fink PJ, Hendricks DW: Post-thymic maturation: young T cells assert their individuality, *Nat Rev Immunol* 11(8):544–549, 2011.
5. Greenen V, et al: Thymic self-antigens for the design of a negative/tolerogenic self-vaccination against type 1 diabetes, *Curr Opin Pharmacol* 10(4):461–472, 2010.
6. Bailey-Bucktrout SL, Bluestone JA: Regulatory T cells: stability revisited, *Trends Immunol* 32(7):301–306, 2011.
7. Wan Q, et al: Cytokine signals through PI-3 kinase pathway modulate TH17 cytokine production by CCR6+ human memory T cells, *J Exp Med* 208(9):1875–1887, 2011.
8. Ciebiada M, et al: SICAM-1 and TNF-α in asthma and rhinitis: relationship with the presence of atopy, *J Asthma* 48(7):660–666, 2011.
9. de Montalembert M, et al: Delayed hemolytic transfusion reaction in children with sickle cell disease, *Haematologica* 96(6):801–807, 2011.
10. Higuchi O, et al: Autoantibodies to low-density lipoprotein receptor-related protein 4 in myasthenia gravis, *Ann Neurol* 69(2):18–22, 2011.
11. Cavalcante P, et al: The thymus in myasthenia gravis: site of "innate autoimmunity"? *Muscle Nerve* 44(4):467–484, 2011.
12. Arazi A, Neumann AU: Modeling immune complex-mediated autoimmune inflammation, *J Theor Biol* 267(3):426–436, 2010.
13. Casanova JL, Abel L: Primary immunodeficiencies: a field in its infancy, *Science* 317(5838):617–619, 2007.
14. van der Burg M, Gennergy AR: The expanding clinical and immunological spectrum of severe combined immunodeficiency, *Eur J Pediatr* 170(5):561–571, 2011.
15. Becker-Herman S, et al: WASp-deficient B cells play a critical, cell-intrinsic role in triggering autoimmunity, *J Exp Med* 208(10): 2033–2042, 2011.
16. Bassett AS, et al: Practical guidelines for managing patients with 22q11.2 Deletion Syndrome, *J Pediatr* 159(2):332–339, 2011.
17. Puel A, et al: Chronic mucocutaneous candidiasis in humans with inborn errors of interleukin-17 immunity, *Science* 332(6025):65–68, 2011.
18. Akirav EM, et al: The role of AIRE in human autoimmune disease, *Nat Rev Endocrinol* 7(1):25–33, 2011.
19. Moise A, et al: Primary immunodeficiencies of the B lymphocyte, *J Med Life* 3(1):60–63, 2010.
20. Jorgensen GH, et al: Association of immunoglobulin A deficiency and elevated thyrotropin-receptor autoantibodies in two Nordic countries, *Hum Immunol* 72(2):166–172, 2011.
21. Martini H, et al: Importance of B cell co-stimulation in CD4(+) T cell differentiation: X-linked agammaglobulinaemia, a human model, *Clin Exp Immunol* 164(3):381–387, 2011.
22. Hendriks RW, et al: Biology and novel treatment options for XLA, the most common monogenetic immunodeficiency in man, *Expert Opin Ther Targets* 15(8):1003–1021, 2011.
23. Southcombe J, et al: The immunomodulatory role of syncytiotrophoblast microvesicles, *PLoS One* 6(5):320245, May 2011.

11

Malignant Disorders of White Blood Cells

Marie L. Kotter and Jacquelyn L. Banasik

evolve WEBSITE

http://evolve.elsevier.com/Copstead/

- Review Questions and Answers
- Glossary (with audio pronunciations for selected terms)
- Animations
- Case Studies
- Key Points Review

KEY QUESTIONS

- How do the various types of leukemia, lymphoma, and plasma cell myelomas differ based on the type of malignant transformation?
- How do the clinical presentations, prognosis, and management of types of acute and chronic leukemia differ?
- Why are malignant disorders of white blood cells commonly associated with bone marrow depression?
- How is Hodgkin disease clinically and histologically differentiated from other types of lymphoma?
- What is the purpose and process of staging procedures for lymphomas?
- What clinical and laboratory findings would suggest a diagnosis of plasma cell myeloma?

CHAPTER OUTLINE

Leukemia, lymphoma, and plasma cell myeloma (multiple myeloma) are common neoplastic disorders of the bone marrow and lymphoid tissues. Depending on the location and specific types of white blood cells involved, these malignancies can be further divided into a number of specific subtypes. Leukemias can be conceptualized as circulating tumors that are disseminated from the beginning of the disease process and primarily involve the blood and bone marrow. Lymphoma tends to localize in lymph tissues but is often disseminated to other sites at the time of diagnosis. Plasma cell myeloma is a malignant transformation of B cell plasma cells and has a predilection to form localized tumors in bony structures.

Malignancies of the blood-forming tissues and lymphatic structures often present with nonspecific symptoms. Malaise, weakness, unexplained fever, night sweats, and recurrent infections should raise suspicion of malignancy. Enlarged, nontender lymph nodes (lymphadenopathy) are a common finding in lymphoma and some leukemias. Often, white blood cell malignancies are found by chance during routine assessment of the complete blood cell count (CBC). A very high total white blood cell count or the presence of abnormal cell types should precipitate an assessment for hematologic cell malignancy. In general, earlier detection of malignancy is associated with a better prognosis for cure.

BOX 11-1 WHO CLASSIFICATION (2008) OF MYELOID NEOPLASMS

Myeloproliferative Diseases (MPD)
Chronic myelogenous leukemia, Philadelphia chromosome (Ph1) (t[;22][qq34;q11], bcr/abl)+
Chronic neutrophilic leukemia
Chronic eosinophilic leukemia/hypereosinophilic syndrome
Primary myelofibrosis
Polycythemia vera
Essential thrombocythemia
Myeloproliferative neoplasms, unclassifiable
Mastocytosis

Myelodysplastic/Myeloproliferative Diseases
Chronic myelomonocytic leukemia (CMML)
Atypical chronic myelogenous leukemia (aCML)
Juvenile myelomonocytic leukemia (JMML)
Myelodysplastic/myeloproliferative neoplasms, unclassifiable

Myelodysplastic Syndromes
Refractory cytopenia with unilineage dysplasia
Refractory neutropenia
Refractory thrombocytopenia
Refractory anemia (RA)
  With ringed sideroblasts
  Without ringed sideroblasts
Refractory cytopenia (myelodysplastic syndrome) with multilineage dysplasia (RCMD)
Refractory anemia (myelodysplastic syndrome) with excess blasts (RAEB)
Myelodysplastic syndromes associated with isolated del(5q)
Myelodysplastic syndrome, unclassifiable

Acute Myeloid Leukemias (AML)
Acute myeloid leukemias with recurrent cytogenetic translocations
  AML with t(8;21)(q22;q22), AML1(CBF_)/ETO
    Acute promyelocytic leukemia (AML with t(15;17)(q22;q11-12) and variants, PML/RAR_)
    AML with abnormal bone marrow eosinophils (inv(16)(p13q22) or t(16;16)(p13;q11), CBF_/MYHIIX)
    AML with 11q23 (MLL) abnormalities
Acute myeloid leukemia with multilineage dysplasia
  With prior myelodysplastic syndrome
  Without prior myelodysplastic syndrome
Acute megakaryoblastic leukemia with t(1;22)(p13;q13), RBM 15-MKL1
Acute myeloid leukemia and myelodysplastic syndrome, therapy related
Other types

Acute Myeloid Leukemia (AML) Not Otherwise Categorized
AML minimally differentiated
AML without maturation
AML with maturation
Acute myelomonocytic leukemia
Acute monocytic leukemia
Acute erythroid leukemia
Acute megakaryocytic leukemia
Acute basophilic leukemia
Acute panmyelosis with myelofibrosis
AML associated with Down syndrome

Acute Biphenotypic Leukemias

From Hoffbrand AV, Moss PAH: World Health Organization classification of tumours of the haematopoietic and lymphoid tissues, *Essential haematology*, ed 6, Oxford, England, 2011, Blackwell, p 427.

CLASSIFICATION OF HEMATOLOGIC NEOPLASMS

Various classification schemes have been used to group hematologic neoplasms, with clinicians favoring schemes that use clinical findings and pathologists preferring morphologic criteria. With the advent of technologies to identify specific genetic alterations and molecular characteristics of neoplastic cells, the traditional classification systems have become less useful. However, many clinicians and organizations, such as the American Cancer Society, continue to use traditional groupings to collect statistics and to provide information to the public. The approach used in this chapter incorporates the most recent World Health Organization (WHO) classifications for hematologic neoplasms and also includes common clinical terminology. A major force behind the adoption of the WHO classification is the recognition that lymphoid leukemias and lymphomas are not separate disorders but represent different stages of the same biological disease. Thus, the major categories of the WHO system are based on the cell type of the neoplasm, rather than its location in the body.[1] Neoplasms involving cells of the myeloid lineage (Box 11-1) are separated from those of the lymphoid lineage (Box 11-2). The myeloid lineage includes red blood cells, platelets, monocytes, and granulocytes; the lymphoid lineage includes B cells, T cells, and natural killer (NK) cells (Figure 11-1). There are four major categories of myeloid neoplasms: myeloproliferative diseases; myelodysplastic/proliferative diseases; myelodysplastic syndromes; and acute myeloid leukemia (AML). There are three major categories of lymphoid neoplasms: B-cell neoplasm; T-cell and NK-cell neoplasm; and Hodgkin disease. The term non-Hodgkin lymphoma is still in clinical usage and refers to lymphomas of B-cell, T-cell, and NK-cell origin. Non-Hodgkin lymphoma includes such a large and diverse group of malignancies that it has little relevance to prognosis or treatment. The WHO classification does not use this term. Other classification systems in current use include the FAB (French-American-British) system for subtypes of myeloid leukemia (Table 11-1). There are many etiologic, pathogenic, and treatment similarities among the hematologic malignancies, and these are addressed in a general way first, followed by sections concentrating on specific diseases.

ETIOLOGY OF MYELOID AND LYMPHOID NEOPLASMS

As in other malignant processes, the exact cause of hematologic neoplasms is unknown. The basic mechanism of malignant transformation involves mutation of cells, which disrupts growth control and differentiation pathways. These processes are thought to be similar to those described for solid tumors (see Chapter 7).

Viruses have long been suspected as mutagenic agents in some neoplasms, particularly retroviruses and herpesviruses. Close associations have been found between a small number of viruses and particular malignancies. For example, human T-cell leukemia virus (HTLV-1) is linked to the development of adult T cell lymphoma/leukemia and human immunodeficiency virus (HIV) is linked to B-cell lymphomas. Epstein-Barr virus (EBV) has been implicated in both Hodgkin disease and Burkitt lymphoma.[2] Effective immune surveillance is thought to

BOX 11-2 WHO CLASSIFICATION OF LYMPHOID NEOPLASMS

Precursor Lymphoid Neoplasms
Precursor B lymphoblastic leukemia/lymphomas (precursor B-cell ALL)
  Precursor T lymphoblastic leukemia/lymphoma

Mature (Peripheral) B-Cell Neoplasms*
B cell chronic lymphocytic leukemia/small lymphocytic lymphoma
B cell prolymphocytic leukemia
Lymphoplasmacytic lymphoma
Splenic marginal zone B-cell lymphoma (6 villous lymphocytes)
Hairy cell leukemia variant
Plasma cell myeloma/plasmacytoma
Waldenström macroglobulinemia
Heavy-chain diseases
Extranodal marginal zone B-cell lymphoma of MALT type
Nodal marginal zone B-cell lymphoma (6 monocytoid B cells)
Follicular lymphoma
Mantle cell lymphoma
Epstein-Barr virus positive DLBCL of the elderly
Large B-cell lymphoma arising in HHV8-associated multicentric
  Castleman disease
Primary mediastinal (thymic) large B-cell lymphoma
Primary effusion lymphoma
Burkitt lymphoma/Burkitt cell leukemia

Mature T-Cell and NK-Cell Neoplasms
Mature (peripheral) T-cell neoplasms
  T-cell prolymphocytic leukemia
  T-cell granular lymphocytic leukemia
Aggressive NK-cell leukemia
Adult T-cell lymphoma/leukemia (HTLV1+)
Extranodal NK/T-cell lymphoma, nasal type
Enteropathy-type T-cell lymphoma
Hepatosplenic γδ T-cell lymphoma
Subcutaneous panniculitis-like T-cell lymphoma
Mycosis fungoides
Sézary syndrome
Primary cutaneous anaplastic large cell lymphoma
Peripheral T-cell lymphoma, not otherwise characterized
Angioimmunoblastic T-cell lymphoma
Anaplastic large cell lymphomas (ALK positive or ALK negative)

Hodgkin Lymphoma (Hodgkin Disease)
Nodular lymphocyte predominance Hodgkin lymphoma
Classical Hodgkin lymphoma
  Nodular sclerosis Hodgkin lymphoma (Grades 1 and 2)
  Lymphocyte-rich classical Hodgkin lymphoma
  Mixed cellularity Hodgkin lymphoma
  Lymphocyte depletion Hodgkin lymphoma

From Hoffbrand AV, Moss PAH: World Health Organization classification of tumours of the haematopoietic and lymphoid tissues, *Essential haematology,* ed 6, Oxford, England, 2011, Blackwell, pp 428-429.
*B- and T/NK-cell neoplasms are grouped according to major clinical presentations (predominantly disseminated/leukemic, primary extranodal, predominantly nodal).

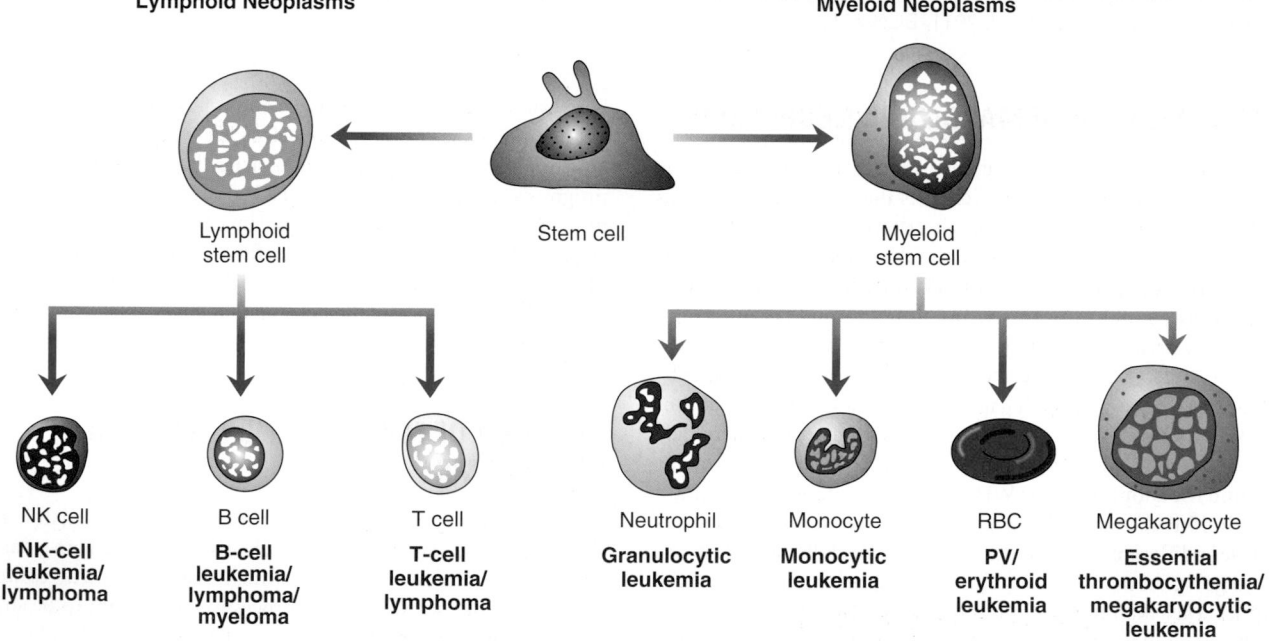

FIGURE 11-1 Division of hematologic neoplasms into myeloid and lymphoid lineages. *PV,* Polycythemia vera.

keep proliferation in check and prevent progression in immunocompetent individuals.

Radiation exposure is an important etiologic factor for leukemia and lymphoma. Because of the relatively high turnover of hematologic cells, they are more susceptible to radiation-induced damage than most other cell types. An acute whole-body dose of radiation like that which occurs with nuclear explosions is known to increase the risk of leukemia. In Japanese survivors of the atomic bomb, the estimated lifetime risk of leukemia is 0.85%, sixfold higher than the norm.[3] There are substantial uncertainties about the risk of low-level, long-term

TABLE 11-1 FAB CLASSIFICATION OF ACUTE MYELOBLASTIC (MYELOCYTIC) LEUKEMIAS

CLASS	MORPHOLOGY	COMMENTS
M0: Minimally differentiated AML	Blasts lack definitive cytologic and cytochemical markers of myeloblasts but express myeloid lineage antigens	2% to 3% of AML
M1: AML without differentiation	Very immature myeloblasts predominate; few granules or Auer rods	20% of AML; Ph chromosome present in 10% to 15% of cases, worsens prognosis
M2: AML with differentiation	Myeloblasts and promyelocytes predominate; Auer rods commonly present	30% of AML; presence of t(8;21) translocation associated with good prognosis
M3: Acute promyelocytic leukemia	Hypergranular promyelocytes, often with many Auer rods per cell; may have reniform or bilobed nuclei	5% to 10% of AML; disseminated intravascular coagulation common; presence of t(15;17) translocation is characteristic; responds to retinoic acid therapy
M4: Acute myelomonocytic leukemia	Myelocytic and monocytic differentiation evident; myeloid elements resemble M2; peripheral monocytosis	20% to 30% of AML; presence of inv16 or del16q associated with better prognosis
M5: Acute monocytic leukemia	Monoblasts (peroxidase negative, esterase positive) and promonocytes predominate	10% of AML; usually in children and young adults; gum infiltration common; associated with abnormalities of chromosome 11q23
M6: Acute erythroleukemia	Bizarre, multinucleated, megaloblastoid erythroblasts predominate; myeloblasts also present	5% of AML; high blood counts and organ infiltration are rare; affected persons are of advanced age
M7: Acute megakaryocytic leukemia	Blasts of megakaryocytic lineage predominate; react with antiplatelet antibodies; myelofibrosis or increased bone marrow reticulin	

From Kumar V, Cotran RS, Robbins SL, editors: *Basic pathology,* ed 7, Philadelphia, 2003, Saunders, p 437.
AML, Acute myeloblastic (myelocytic) leukemia; *FAB,* French-American-British; *Ph,* Philadelphia.

exposure to radiation. The average annual exposure from usual sources including cosmic rays and medical procedures is very low and estimated to account for less than 5% of leukemia cases.

Despite intensive scrutiny only a small number of chemicals have been shown unequivocally to increase the risk of hematologic malignancies. Benzene has been implicated in numerous studies as has cigarette smoking. Other suggested carcinogens have failed to be confirmed, including exposure to hair dye, alcohol, and marijuana.[4] On the other hand, a study from the Children's Cancer Group found a link between high maternal intake of products high in bioflavonoids (beans, fresh vegetables, and fruit) and an increased incidence of infant leukemia.[5] These bioflavonoids were enzyme inhibitors (topoisomerase II inhibitors) that caused DNA cleavage and chromosome translocations. Many of the antineoplastic drugs used to treat cancers, especially the alkylating agents, are significant factors in the development of posttreatment hematologic neoplasia. Any drugs that suppress the bone marrow or immune function are also believed to predispose to the emergence of malignancies.

A number of disease conditions have been linked to the development of leukemia, although the mechanisms are unclear. A reduction or alteration in normal hematopoiesis, as occurs in such disorders as Fanconi anemia and aplastic anemia (see Chapter 13), is associated with a higher incidence of leukemia. A higher risk also has been noted in some genetic diseases, including Down syndrome and Klinefelter syndrome (see Chapter 6).

GENERAL PRINCIPLES OF MANAGEMENT

Diagnosis of Hematologic Neoplasms

Manifestations of hematologic neoplasms vary somewhat, depending upon the cell type involved. Common manifestations are shown in Box 11-3. Clinical symptoms are related to bone marrow suppression and organ dysfunction secondary to leukemic infiltration. Bone marrow suppression results in varying degrees of **leukopenia, anemia, and thrombocytopenia.** These three deficiencies cause the most common clinical manifestations and may prompt the patient to seek care.

BOX 11-3 COMMON MANIFESTATIONS OF HEMATOLOGIC MALIGNANCIES

History
Fever
Weight loss
Night sweats
Itching (pruritus)
Fatigue
Bone pain (sternum, tibia, femur, back)
Abdominal fullness
Bleeding episodes (epistaxis, menorrhagia)
Bruising, petechiae
Frequent infections
Headache, nausea, vomiting

Physical
Enlarged spleen
Enlarged liver
Enlarged lymph nodes
Hyperplasia of gums

Laboratory
Anemia or polycythemia
Thrombocytopenia or thrombocythemia
Leukopenia or leukocytosis
Blasts on peripheral blood smear
Elevated uric acid level
Elevated alkaline phosphatase level
Hypercalcemia

Anemia, with a hematocrit level of 25% to 30% or a hemoglobin level of 8 to 10 g/dl, may manifest with pallor, fatigue, malaise, shortness of breath, and decreased activity tolerance. The severity of symptoms is determined by the rate of red blood cell decrease as well as the absolute deficiency. Chronically low hemoglobin and hematocrit values may be better tolerated than a drastic drop in these measurements. Depending on symptoms, transfusion may be indicated when the hematocrit level falls below 30%.

Thrombocytopenia, with a platelet count less than 20,000 cells/μL, can manifest as petechiae, easy bruising, bleeding gums, occult hematuria, or retinal hemorrhages. Spontaneous intracranial bleeding can occur and may be fatal. In general, the risk of bleeding increases proportionately to the fall in platelet count. Platelet transfusion may be given when the risk of bleeding is high.

Insufficient numbers of functional leukocytes leaves the patient at high risk for development of infection and the complete blood count is routinely monitored. **Neutropenia** is an absolute neutrophil count less than 500 cells/μL, and an affected patient requires protective isolation (neutropenic precautions) to prevent infection. Infections may be caused by bacterial, viral, fungal, or protozoal organisms. Often, the microorganisms are of the opportunistic variety. That is, they are part of the patient's own flora, which normally do not cause disease unless the host's immune system becomes incompetent. It is very difficult to protect patients from their own flora, and infection is the most common cause of death in the immunocompromised leukemic patient. The presence of infection is suspected if fever develops. Infections are managed aggressively with antibiotic agents to prevent development of life-threatening sepsis.

Infiltrative manifestations include lymphadenopathy, joint swelling and pain, weight loss, anorexia, hepatomegaly, and splenomegaly. Sternal tenderness is frequently present in chronic myeloid leukemia (CML). Gingival hyperplasia occurs in acute myeloid leukemia (AML). Meningeal involvement is frequently encountered in children with acute lymphoid leukemia (ALL). Central nervous system (CNS) infiltration can occur with any type of leukemia and may be difficult to manage because of the poor ability of chemotherapeutic agents to cross the blood-brain barrier. CNS involvement can present with increased intracranial pressure, seizures, or changes in mental ability. Increased intracranial pressure should be suspected in the leukemia patient who complains of nausea, vomiting, headache, and visual changes.

A key aspect of diagnosis is the evaluation of a peripheral blood sample. Blood cell number and morphologic evaluation are indicative; however, definitive diagnosis is usually made after bone marrow aspiration or lymph node biopsy. Malignant cells can be subtyped according to genetic and molecular characteristics to better determine prognosis and choice of treatment.[6]

Principles of Treatment

To make informed treatment decisions, patients and their families need information about the nature and prognosis of their disease as well as about the risks and benefits of various treatment options. Many treatment protocols are experimental, and the outcomes may be uncertain. Sometimes the side effects of treatment as well as its limited efficacy will weigh in favor of palliative care. Treatment decisions are complex and stressful for all concerned. A great deal of support must be available during the diagnostic, treatment, and monitoring phases.

The management of hematologic malignancies relies primarily on the use of combination chemotherapy to eradicate malignant cells and stem cell transplant to rescue and restore bone marrow function. In some cases radiation and tissue-specific drug therapy may be indicated. Unfortunately, the treatment regimen usually causes many serious side effects that must be monitored and treated.

The goal of chemotherapy is to induce long-term remission, that is, the absence of any detectable neoplastic cells in the body. A complete remission (CR) is defined as a return to normal hematopoiesis with normal red blood cell, neutrophil, and platelet counts and no detectable neoplastic cells. For leukemia, the bone marrow must have less than 5% blasts, which are the most immature bone marrow cells, and be maintained for at least 4 weeks.[7] CR is not synonymous with cure. Therefore, most treatment protocols include several cycles of chemotherapy to eradicate the undetected cells. The choice of antineoplastic agents varies with the type of neoplasia and the stage of clinical disease. Most chemotherapeutic agents work by disrupting some aspect of DNA synthesis or cell replication and induce **apoptosis** (cell suicide; see Chapter 4). In general, rapidly dividing cells are more susceptible to apoptosis because they have less time for repair. Neoplasms with genetic defects that impair apoptotic pathways may be more difficult to eradicate and require more intense therapy. Unfortunately, these high doses are toxic to normal stem cells as well and can produce fatal bone marrow failure. Therefore, to effect a cure, high-dose chemotherapy is often followed by bone marrow "rescue" with transplantation of functional stem cells.

Chemotherapy usually includes two or three treatment phases: (1) remission induction phase, (2) postremission or consolidation phase, and (3) remission maintenance phase. The aim of treatment during the remission induction phase is to eliminate all detectable neoplastic cells and achieve a CR. Postremission consolidation therapy begins after CR is attained in an attempt to eliminate the population of undetected cells that may have escaped initial induction phase treatment. Maintenance phase treatment is used in the management of some neoplasms to prolong the remission interval. Intermittent chemotherapy may be continued for 2 to 3 years after initial induction of remission. Drugs that target the neoplastic cells specifically, such as monoclonal antibodies or molecular therapies, are generally less toxic than other agents and may be used for long-term maintenance in patients with residual disease.

In children and adults, the CNS can act as a sanctuary for neoplastic cells in diseases such as acute lymphoblastic and acute myeloblastic leukemias. This makes conventional routes of chemotherapy unsuccessful, because they do not permit drugs to cross the blood-brain barrier efficiently. Chemotherapeutic agents administered into the cerebrospinal fluid (CSF) via lumbar puncture (intrathecal route) can effectively eliminate leukemic cells in the CNS. This therapy carries significant risk for temporary or permanent neurologic damage. A number of different chemotherapeutic agents can be administered safely by the intrathecal route, including methotrexate.[8]

Prevention and Management of Complications

Maintenance of adequate nutrition in patients with hematologic malignancy is a major challenge. Anorexia, weight loss, nausea, vomiting, and **stomatitis** are common findings, especially during the treatment phase. Children and adolescents receiving chemotherapy may experience significant growth delay, and measures to maintain protein and caloric intake are necessary. Newer antiemetic agents have been helpful in reducing nausea, vomiting, and anorexia associated with chemotherapy and should be considered in patients experiencing these symptoms.

Infection is the most troublesome of complications for the patient who is immunosuppressed by either disease or treatments. Constant vigilance in prevention, early detection, and rapid management of infections can profoundly affect the outcome of chemotherapy. The length of time that a patient remains neutropenic can be shortened with the use of growth factors to stimulate bone marrow production of granulocytes.

Bone marrow transplantation (BMT) has been an important part of the management of certain leukemias for many years. The intense chemotherapy used to induce remission can lead to bone marrow failure. Stem cells can be reintroduced into the host's bone marrow by bone marrow transplantation. The transplanted cells are given intravenously; they find their way to the host's bone marrow, where they establish residence and begin to produce functional white blood cells, red blood cells, and platelets. A close match between donor and host is necessary for a successful transplantation. Otherwise, the transplanted cells can mount an immune attack on the host's tissues—a life-threatening problem called *graft-versus-host disease* (see Chapter 10). In past years, bone transplantation was obtained by aspiration from the marrow of a suitable donor and this is still appropriate in some cases. *Peripheral stem cell transplantation* allows stem cells to be harvested from the circulating bloodstream. This procedure can be used to collect stem cells from the patient's own blood to be stored and then reinfused after chemotherapy and irradiation. This type of transplant is called *autologous,* whereas a transplant from a closely matched relative is called *allogeneic* (Figure 11-2). Use of autologous transplants eliminates the problem of graft-versus-host disease and reduces transplant-related mortality, but the potential for disease recurrence is higher than with allogeneic transplants.

It has been noted that in AML and CML, transplantation with allogeneic cells is much more successful in curing leukemia than is autologous transplantation. Transplanted cells in the allograft are thought to detect and kill leukemic cells in a process termed *graft versus leukemia.* Autologous transplants are appropriate in some cases, especially when a matched donor is not available, because they may extend life even though cure is unlikely. Autologous transplants are well tolerated and cause fewer complications than allografts. Methods to purify a patient's collected peripheral blood by selectively removing neoplastic cells are available to reduce the risk of reintroducing malignant cells during autologous transplantation. Increased availability of stem cell transplants allows patients to undergo more intensive chemotherapy, aimed at cure rather than palliation, based on the knowledge that bone marrow rescue is possible.

Anemia is a common complication of leukemia and chemotherapy. Red blood cell production by the bone marrow is suppressed, but the size and shape of red blood cells present in the blood are normal. This is called *normocytic,* normochromic anemia. Administration of erythropoietin growth factors can enhance red blood cell production and moderate anemic episodes. However, patients frequently require red blood cell transfusion therapy to maintain adequate red blood cell counts. Patients with frequent or significant bleeding episodes are also

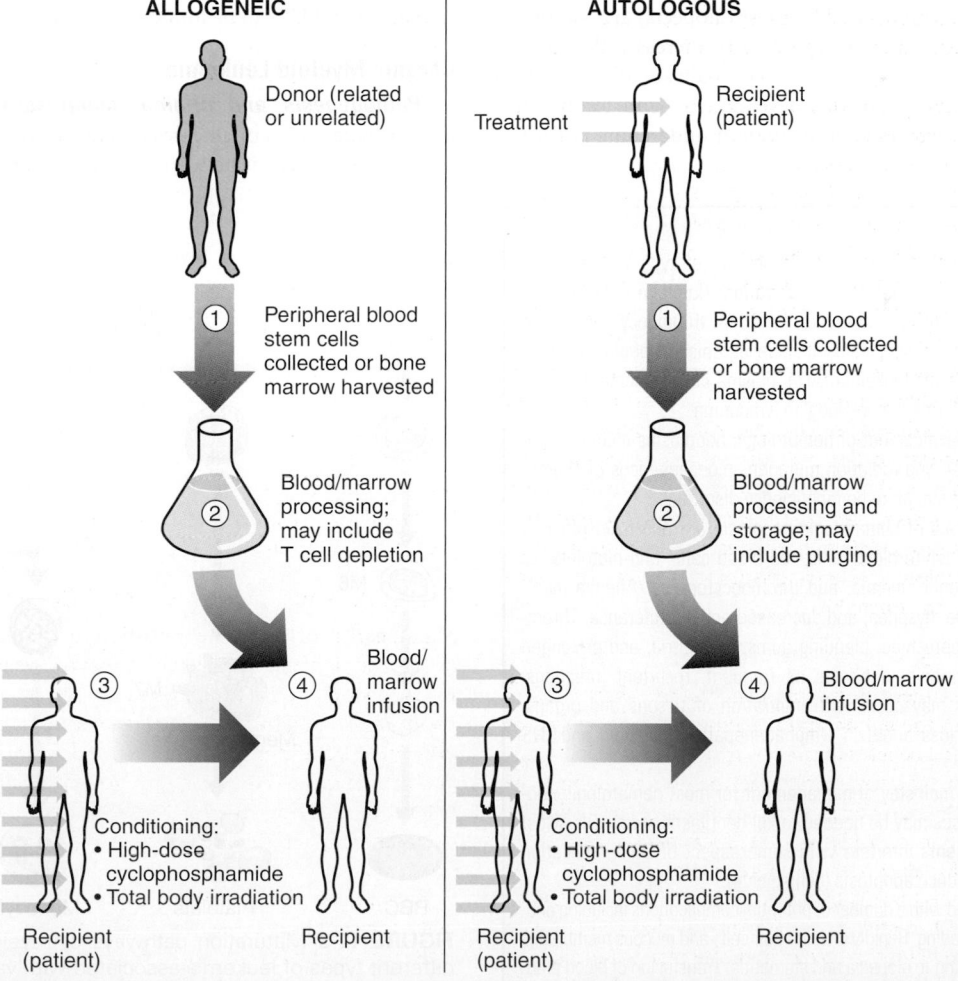

FIGURE 11-2 Procedures for allogeneic and autologous stem cell transplantation. For nonmyeloblative (reduced intensity) allogeneic stem cell transplantation, lower doses of chemotherapy with or without radiotherapy are used. (From Rodak B et al: *Hematology: clinical principles and application,* ed 4, Philadelphia, 2012, Saunders.)

predisposed to severe anemia, and efforts to prevent bleeding will help to minimize anemia.

Platelet deficiency (thrombocytopenia) with resultant hemorrhage can be a life-threatening complication of leukemia and chemotherapy. In patients at high risk of bleeding, fresh frozen plasma or pooled platelets may be given to inhibit bleeding. Patients must be protected from trauma and may be placed on activity restrictions.

Pain is a common complication of the diagnostic and treatment protocols used in the cancer patient as well as of the disease process itself. Pain most commonly involves the bones and joints, and is due to pressure caused by infiltration and accumulation of neoplastic cells in the bone marrow. *Hemarthrosis* (bleeding into joints) can cause acute episodes of joint pain. Chemotherapy may help reduce bone pain, as the number of neoplastic cells is reduced drastically. Patients are subjected to numerous painful procedures during diagnosis, treatment, and monitoring. Frequent collection of blood and bone marrow samples, placement of intravenous access lines for drug administration, and manifestation of unpleasant drug side effects all contribute to the pain experience. Nausea and mouth pain (stomatitis) are frequent complaints during chemotherapy. Pain management with a variety of strategies, including narcotic and nonnarcotic drugs, distraction, and biofeedback, is generally helpful. (See Chapter 47 for a discussion of pain and pain management.)

Epithelial cells, with normally high rates of turnover, are particularly susceptible to damage by radiation and chemotherapy. Sloughing of skin and mucous membranes and hair loss (alopecia) are common. Loss of skin and mucous membrane integrity increases the risk of infection and can contribute significantly to the pain and discomfort of treatment. Abnormalities in growth, development, and fertility are complications of particular concern in children undergoing radiation and chemotherapy.

MYELOID NEOPLASMS

Myeloid neoplasms result from transformation and proliferation of a precursor stem cell in the bone marrow (Figure 11-3). The progeny of the aberrant stem cell clone accumulate in the bone marrow and are released into the circulation. In many cases, the abnormal stem cell is multipotent and causes the overproduction of more than one cell type, resulting in myeloproliferative disease. The cells produced in myeloproliferative diseases are usually functional and have a normal morphologic appearance. The common myeloproliferative diseases are chronic myeloid leukemia (CML), polycythemia vera (PV), and essential thrombocythemia (ET), referring respectively to an excess of granulocytes, red blood cells, and platelets. These insidious and indolent disorders have few clinical symptoms and are commonly discovered on routine CBC analysis. Common features of CML, PV, and ET include involvement of a multipotent hematopoietic progenitor cell; hypercellularity of marrow; overproduction of one or more functional blood cells; chromosomal abnormalities involving chromosomes 1, 8, 9, 13, and 20; and eventual spontaneous conversion to AML or development of marrow fibrosis.[9]

In contrast to the myeloproliferative diseases, the myelodysplastic syndromes and AML are characterized by neoplastic cells that are morphologically and functionally abnormal. The prognosis for myelodysplastic syndromes and AML is poor, and intensive treatment is necessary to extend life. AML and CML are described next. A discussion of PV and ET can be found in Chapters 13 and 14, respectively.

Chronic Myeloid Leukemia

Pathogenesis and clinical manifestations. CML represents approximately 15% of all cases of leukemia in the United States. The average age of onset is between 40 and 50 years, and CML occurs only

---

KEY POINTS

- Classification of the types of leukemia is based on cell type involved (lymphoid or myeloid) and degree of cell maturation. Common myeloid neoplasms include CML, polycythemia vera, essential thrombocythemia, and AML. Common lymphoid neoplasms include chronic lymphoid leukemia (CLL), acute lymphoblastic leukemia (ALL), plasma cell myeloma, Hodgkin disease, and various forms of non-Hodgkin lymphoma.
- Risk factors for the development of hematologic neoplasms include exposure to chemical, viral, and radiation mutagens; consequences of chemotherapy drugs; and effects of immunodeficiency disorders.
- Common manifestations of hematologic neoplasia are due to insufficient production of normal white blood cells, red blood cells, and platelets, as evidenced by leukopenia, anemia, and thrombocytopenia. Anemia manifests as pallor, fatigue, dyspnea, and decreased activity tolerance. Thrombocytopenia causes petechiae, bleeding gums, hematuria, and prolonged bleeding time. Leukopenia manifests as frequent, recurrent infections. Other manifestations may occur with infiltration of tissues and organs. These include weight loss, anorexia, lymphadenopathy, bone pain, and CNS dysfunction.
- Chemotherapy is the mainstay of management for most hematologic neoplasms. Several courses may be needed to kill neoplastic stem cells. Most chemotherapeutic agents interfere with some aspect of DNA replication and cell division to induce apoptosis (cell suicide).
- Treatment is associated with a number of potential complications including anemia, infection, and bleeding. Rapidly dividing hair cells and mucous membranes are also affected, leading to alopecia and stomatitis. Transfusion of blood products or stimulation of endogenous production with colony-stimulating factors and erythropoietin may be necessary. Bone marrow transplantation may be undertaken in some cases to restore stem cell function.

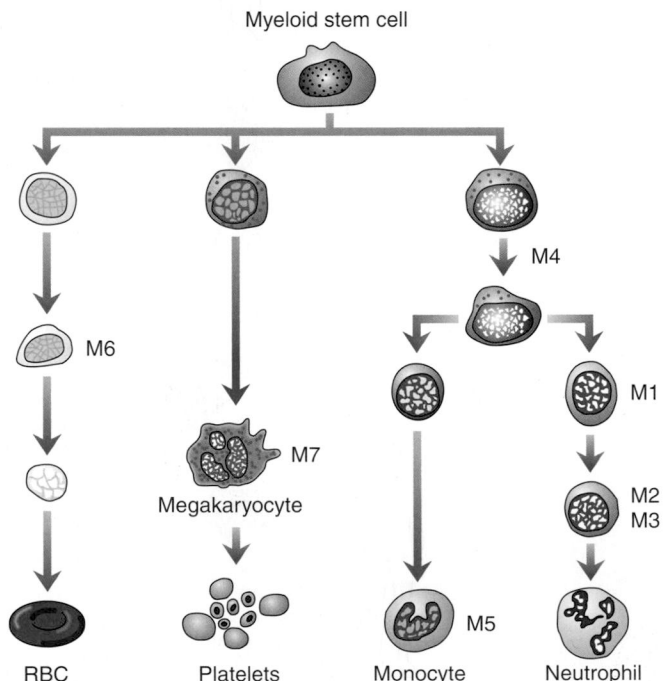

FIGURE 11-3 Maturation pathways of myeloid cells showing the different types of leukemia associated with various stages of development. M1, M2, and M3 types result in granulocytic leukemia; M4 has characteristics of monocytic and granulocytic leukemia; M5 is monocytic; M6 is associated with erythroid leukemia; and M7 is associated with megakaryocytic leukemia. *RBC,* Red blood cell.

occasionally in childhood and adolescence.[10] The majority of CML cases are characterized by malignant granulocytes that carry a unique chromosomal abnormality, the Philadelphia chromosome (Ph+). The Philadelphia chromosome is formed because of a balanced translocation between chromosomes 9 and 22 (Figure 11-4). The translocation causes two genes to be juxtaposed, resulting in a new fusion gene called *bcr-abl*. This mutation is thought to be critical in the development of CML. Molecular studies have revealed that the protein product of the fusion gene is a functional enzyme that spurs cell proliferation and reduces apoptotic cell death. CML is unusual among human cancers because a single oncogene *(bcr/abl)* is capable of conferring a malignant state.[11] Numerous mutations are necessary for development of most other cancers (see Chapter 7). The cells in CML are more mature than those found in AML, as noted by the greater degree of nuclear segmentation (Figure 11-5).

The usual clinical presentation of CML includes a high granulocyte count on the CBC and splenomegaly. Symptoms, when present, may include fatigue, weight loss, diaphoresis, bleeding, and abdominal discomfort from the enlarged spleen.

Prognosis and treatment. CML does not respond well to chemotherapy. Although most patients will achieve a temporary remission, the overall survival time is poor. In untreated patients the median survival is about 2 years.[12] After discovery of the fusion protein *(bcr/abl)*, drugs targeted to inhibit its action were developed (e.g., imatinib). The goal of anti-*bcr/abl* therapy is to reduce the number of leukemic cells with the *bcr/abl* phenotype to undetectable levels. It is not known whether imatinib can cure CML or what duration of treatment is necessary to permanently suppress the leukemic cell population. Some patients with CML have developed drug resistance against imatinib, and research is ongoing. The only known curative treatment is **allogeneic** bone marrow transplantation from a suitable donor. It is believed that the donor cells detect and kill the host's leukemic cells. Even with a human leukocyte antigen (HLA)–identical sibling donor, the probability of transplant-related mortality is about 25% and the likelihood of long-term disease-free survival is 50% to 60%.[11,12] Transplant-related mortality is about 50% if the HLA-matched donor is unrelated.[11] Bone marrow transplantation with cells harvested from the patient's own blood (autografting) during the early stages of CML may also be done, but it is less effective in curing the disease. For those not able to undergo stem cell transplantation, standard chemotherapy during the chronic phase may be instituted. Chemotherapy may include hydroxyurea, interferon-α (IFN-α), cytosine arabinoside (cytarabine, Ara-C), and

imatinib. Once CML has progressed to the blast phase, essentially becoming AML, the prognosis is very poor regardless of treatment, with an expected median survival of 3 to 4 months.

Acute Myeloid Leukemia

Pathogenesis and clinical manifestations. AML is primarily a disease of adults, comprising 80% of cases of acute leukemia in this population while accounting for only 20% of the cases of acute leukemia of childhood.[10] The median age at presentation is 64 years. Like CML, AML is a malignant disorder associated with transformation of a myeloid stem cell. The bone marrow aspirate must have more than 20% blasts to be classified as AML.[13] AML can present in a variety of ways because of the potential for myeloid stem cells to produce different cell types. Thus, AML has a number of subtypes. These are identified by the stage at which cell development stops (see Figure 11-3). The French, American, British (FAB) system for classifying AML as M0 through M7 is in common use (see Table 11-1). Acute granulocytic leukemia is the most common type of disorder, and the term is often used interchangeably with AML. Myeloblastic cells have a large, nonsegmented nucleus and fine chromatin (Figure 11-6). AML is also subtyped according to genetic abnormalities. Worse outcomes are noted with loss of *TP53* or *RB* tumor suppressor gene function. The World Health Organization (WHO) classification of AML recognizes four common types of genetic abnormalities (and one other) (see Box 11-1). Most are chromosomal translocations or inversions. If cytogenetic class is not apparent, then AML is classified by morphologic characteristics, including myeloid cell of origin and degree of differentiation or maturation. Correct classification increases the accuracy of prognosis and may influence the choice of treatment.

AML presents in a manner very similar to that of ALL, and the two are difficult to distinguish by clinical findings alone. Acute leukemia causes bone pain, anemia, thrombocytopenia, and increased susceptibility to infection. The skin, the genitourinary and gastrointestinal systems, and the respiratory tract are common infection sites. The onset of symptoms is abrupt, with most patients seeking care within a few weeks of disease onset. The prognosis is much worse for AML than for ALL, with fewer than 50% of children and only about 30% of adults achieving long-term survival.[6,14] An exception is the promyelocytic

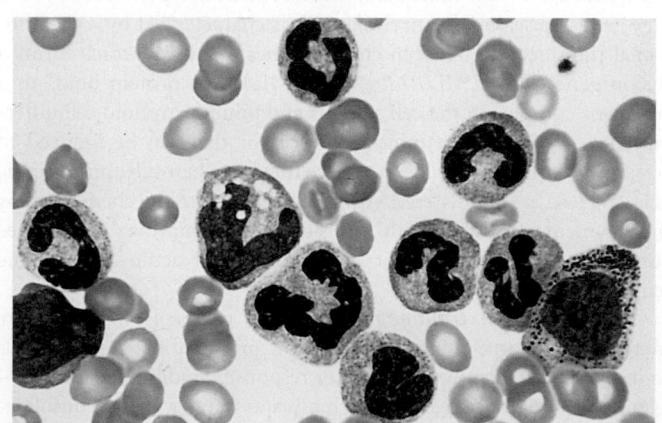

FIGURE 11-5 Peripheral blood smear from a patient with chronic myeloid leukemia (CML). Note that a greater degree of neutrophil segmentation is found in CML than in acute myelogenous leukemia (see Figure 11-6), reflecting a more advanced stage of development. (From Kumar V et al, editors: *Robbins basic pathology,* ed 8, Philadelphia, 2007, Saunders, p 464. Photograph courtesy Dr. Robert W. McKenna, Department of Pathology, University of Texas Southwestern Medical School, Dallas, TX.)

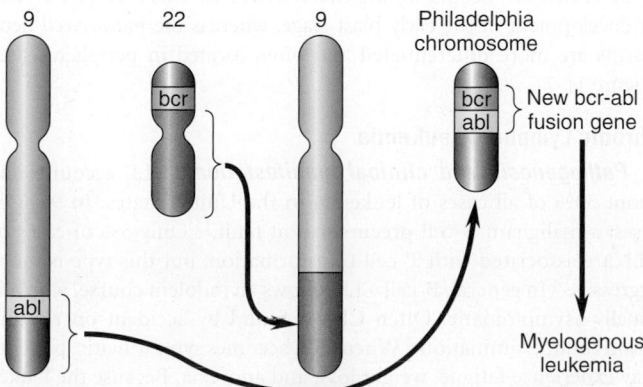

FIGURE 11-4 Balanced translocation between chromosomes 9 and 22 results in the formation of a Philadelphia chromosome. The translocation causes two genes, *abl* and *bcr,* to become juxtaposed, resulting in a fusion gene. This fusion gene, *bcr-abl,* is thought to be essential for the development of chronic myeloid leukemia.

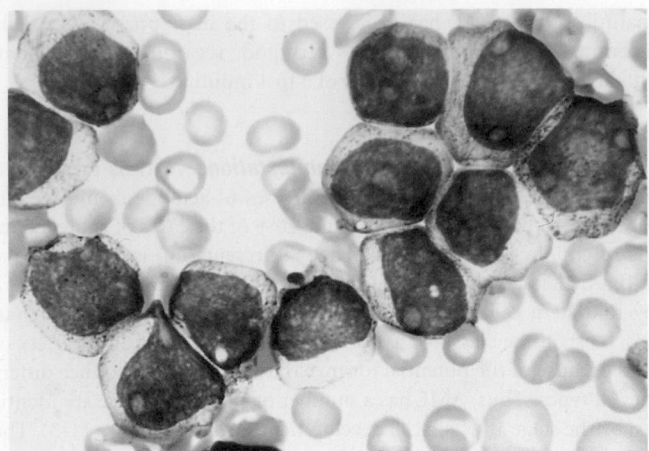

FIGURE 11-6 Peripheral blood smear showing typical cells of acute myelogenous leukemia. (From Kumar V et al, editors: *Robbins basic pathology*, ed 8, Philadelphia, 2007, Saunders, p 448.)

TABLE 11-2	COMPARISON OF ACUTE AND CHRONIC LEUKEMIAS	
	ACUTE	**CHRONIC**
Age	All ages	Adult
Clinical onset	Sudden	Insidious
Course of untreated disease	Weeks to months	Months to years
Predominant cell	Blasts, some mature forms	Mature forms
Anemia	Mild to severe	Mild
Thrombocytopenia	Mild to severe	Mild
WBC count	Variable	Increased

Adopted from McKenzie S: *Clinical laboratory hematology*, Upper Saddle River, NJ, 2004, Pearson, p 482.

subtype of AML. Although it accounts for only 10% to 15% of AML cases, acute promyelocytic leukemia (APL) deserves special consideration because it is the most curable of all AML subtypes, with a 70% to 80% 5-year disease-free survival.[6] APL is characterized by a chromosomal translocation between chromosomes 8 and 21, which forms a fusion gene called *PML/RARα*. The PML/RARα protein binds to a repressor complex in the cell nucleus and inhibits myeloid cell differentiation. RARα is a retinoic acid receptor that can be induced to release its inhibitory hold on differentiation when *all-trans*-retinoic acid (ATRA) is administered. Addition of ATRA to the chemotherapy management of patients with APL significantly improves disease-free survival[6] (see Table 11-2 for a comparison of acute and chronic leukemias).

Prognosis and treatment. Treatment protocols for AML are increasingly incorporating the cytogenetic profile of the leukemic cells to individualize therapy and monitor response. Traditionally the management of AML has two phases: remission induction and consolidation/postremission. A CR is attempted in the remission induction phase, with an attempt to eliminate any undetected residual leukemic cells during the consolidation/postremission phase. Patients with AML who are able to complete only one or two cycles of their chemotherapy because of toxicity almost invariably have recurrence of leukemia even when CR was achieved. To induce remission, most protocols use two cycles of a combination of agents (e.g., idarubicin + Ara-C + etoposide, called the ICE protocol; or daunorubicin + Ara-C + 6-thioguanine,

called the DAT protocol). Postremission therapy commonly includes high-dose Ara-C in younger patients whereas the elderly require lower dose regimens. Drug treatment is constantly being evaluated and altered to obtain better outcomes. At present patients younger than 60 years have a 4-year survival of 30% to 40%, whereas elderly patients have a 2-year survival of 20%.[6] With the advent of allogeneic stem cell transplantation, the chances for cure may improve; however, procedure-related mortality is 10% to 25%. New therapies using monoclonal antibodies to detect and destroy leukemic cells have been used and show promise for improving outcomes in AML.

> **KEY POINTS**
> - CML is a myeloproliferative disorder that affects adults primarily, has an insidious onset, and responds poorly to chemotherapy. CML is characterized by the presence of a gene translocation (Philadelphia chromosome) that produces a fusion gene called *bcr-abl*. The product of this gene is thought to be responsible for producing the malignancy. This molecular abnormality is the target of new drug therapies to eliminate neoplastic cells. The prognosis of CML remains relatively poor but may be improved with allogeneic bone marrow transplantation in which transplanted cells destroy leukemic cells.
> - AML affects adults primarily, has an acute onset, responds fairly well to treatment, and has a prognosis somewhat worse than that of ALL. AML is usually a malignancy of granulocytes, although other myeloid cell types may be affected. Several gene abnormalities have been identified in AML that may indicate better or worse prognosis. The median survival of patients younger than 60 years is 30% to 40% at 4 years.

LYMPHOID NEOPLASMS

The lymphoid neoplasms include malignant transformations of B cells, T cells, and NK cells. When present in blood and bone marrow, lymphoid neoplasms are called *leukemias*, and when they are localized in lymphoid tissues they are called *lymphomas*. The location of lymphoid neoplasms is a consequence of the stage of the disease. The WHO classification uses cell type rather than stage to classify the lymphoid neoplasms, resulting in some difficulty with the traditional conceptualization of leukemias and lymphomas. The factors that determine whether a particular neoplastic cell will present as leukemia or as lymphoma are not presently known. Subcategories of the B-cell and T-cell/NK-groups are based on the maturity of the neoplastic cells (see Box 11-2). The *precursor cell* neoplasms are characterized by cells that have arrested development in the early blast stage, whereas the *mature cell* neoplasms are more differentiated and often located in peripheral sites (Figure 11-7).

Chronic Lymphoid Leukemia

Pathogenesis and clinical manifestations. CLL accounts for about 30% of all cases of leukemia in the United States. In 95% of cases, a malignant B-cell precursor is at fault.[15] Only 5% of cases of CLL are associated with T-cell transformation, but this type is more aggressive.[4] In general, B-cell CLL follows an indolent course, which is usually asymptomatic. Often CLL is found by accident on routine blood count examinations. When CLL becomes symptomatic, patients may experience fatigue, weight loss, and anorexia. Because the leukemic B cells do not produce antibodies normally, an increased susceptibility to certain types of infection may occur. Malignant lymphocytes invade lymphoid tissues and bone marrow, disrupting function. Lymphoid invasion often presents as enlarged, painless lymph nodes (lymphadenopathy) or enlarged spleen (splenomegaly). Bone marrow

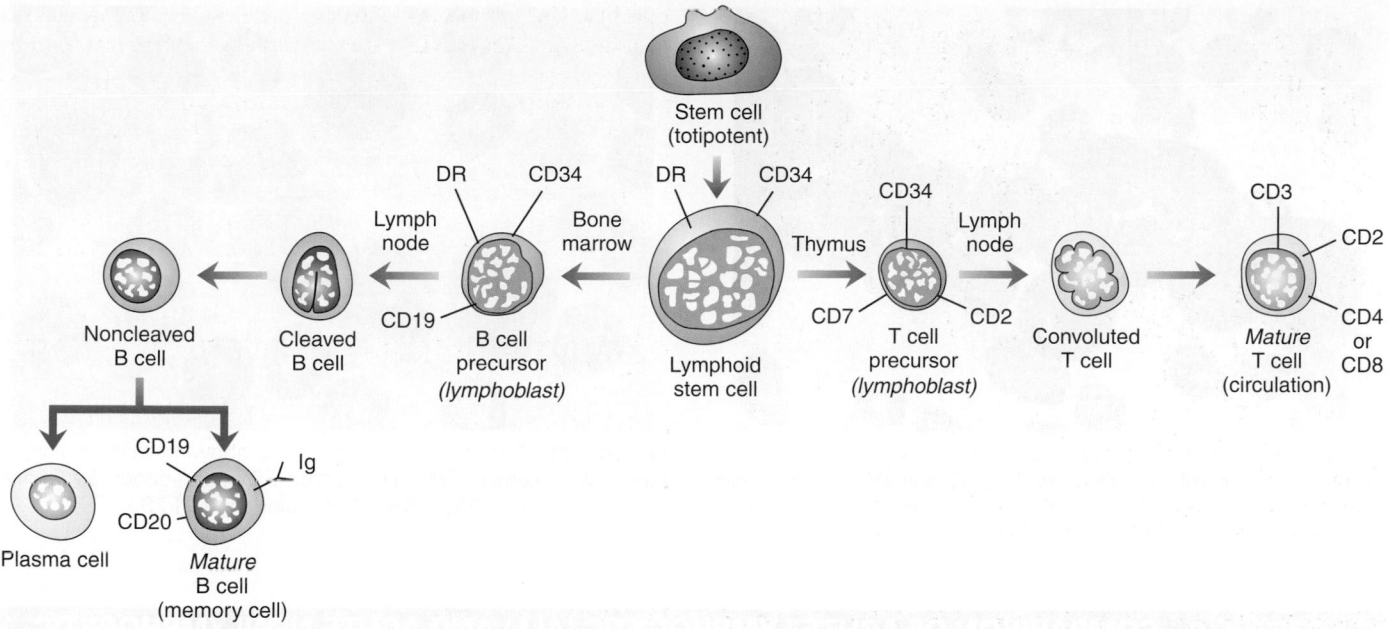

FIGURE 11-7 Maturation pathways of T and B lymphocytes showing the stages at which lymphocyte development is typically arrested in leukemia. Different markers are present on the surface of B cells and T cells at progressive stages of development, which are helpful in identifying the neoplastic cell type and maturity.

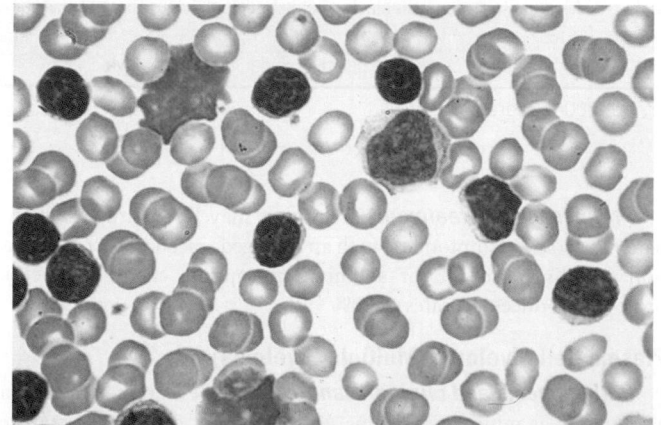

FIGURE 11-8 Bone marrow aspirate showing small lymphocytes with condensed nuclear chromatin typical of chronic lymphocytic leukemia, B-cell type. (From Henderson ES et al, editors: *Leukemia,* ed 7, Philadelphia, 2003, Saunders, color plate 11-28.)

infiltration reduces the production of other cells, including red blood cells and platelets. A typical slide of a bone marrow aspirate from a patient with CLL is shown in Figure 11-8. Note the preponderance of lymphoid cells. CLL cells are characterized by defective apoptosis and therefore have extended life spans. They are derived from mature peripheral B cells (see Table 11-3 for a comparison of acute and chronic leukemias).

Prognosis and treatment. Certain genetic mutations confer better or worse prognosis. A mutation in the variable region of the immunoglobulin gene (IgV) is associated with a median survival of 24 years or more; those without this mutation have a median survival of less than 8 years.[15] CLL cell types demonstrating short telomere lengths and TP53 dysfunction have poor outcomes. Since the average age of patients with CLL is about 65 to 70 years, those with indolent disease may not be treated; they are more likely to die of another disorder

rather than CLL. Patients with cell types likely to progress rapidly may receive chemotherapy to induce remission. Those without complete response may consider stem cell transplantation to prolong the duration of remission.

Acute Lymphoblastic Leukemia/Lymphoma

Pathogenesis and clinical manifestations. ALL is a malignant disorder of the lymphoid cell lineage. The great majority of cases are the result of malignant transformation of B cells (80%), with the remainder involving T cells.[16] The abnormal cells resemble immature lymphocytes, called *lymphoblasts* (Figure 11-9). Most lymphoblastic neoplasms present as leukemias, but lymphoblastic lymphomas are thought to be the same disease at a different stage. B cell leukemias are categorized into cytogenetic groups based on common chromosomal translocations. One of these transformations results in the *bcr/abl* fusion gene discussed previously in the context of CML. Three other types of translocations also form fusion genes that produce abnormal signaling components. These gene derangements have different prognoses and may respond differently to alternative treatment protocols.

Lymphoblasts do not mature and accumulate in large numbers in the blood and bone marrow. At least 20% of the bone marrow cells must be leukemic lymphoblasts to meet the diagnostic criteria for ALL.[16] The space occupied by the accumulation of leukemic cells in the bone marrow prohibits the production of normal red blood cells, platelets, and leukocytes. Circulating blasts are poorly functioning cells and do not provide effective immunocompetence (see Table 11-3 for a comparison of acute lymphocytic leukemia [ALL] and acute nonlymphocytic leukemia [ANLL]).

ALL is primarily a disorder of children. It is the most common malignancy and the second leading cause of death in this population.[17,18] The peak incidence occurs between the ages of 3 and 7 years. A second peak occurs in middle age. The onset of symptoms is abrupt, with complaints of bone pain, bruising, fever, and infection being common. Children may refuse to walk and their parents may report

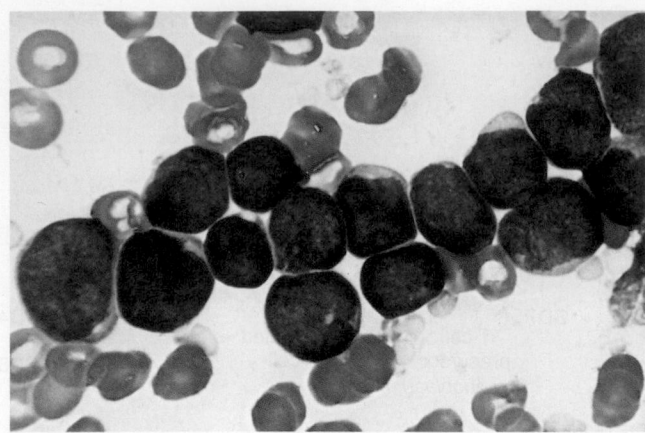

FIGURE 11-9 Peripheral blood smear showing typical cells of acute lymphocytic leukemia. (From Kumar V et al, editors: *Robbins basic pathology*, ed 8, Philadelphia, 2007, Saunders, p 448.)

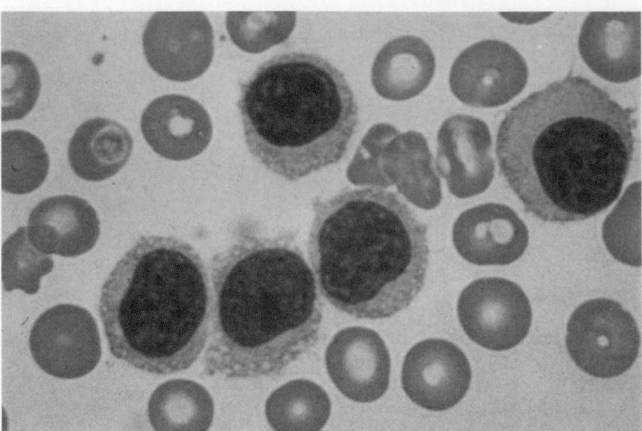

FIGURE 11-10 Peripheral blood smear showing cells typical of hairy cell leukemia. (From Henderson ES et al, editors: *Leukemia*, ed 7, Philadelphia, 2003, Saunders, color plate 11-29.)

TABLE 11-3 COMPARISON OF ACUTE LYMPHOCYTIC (ALL) AND ACUTE NONLYMPHOCYTIC LEUKEMIA (ANLL)

	ALL	ANLL
Age	Common in children	Common in adults
Hematology results	Anemia, neutropenia, thrombocytopenia	Anemia, neutropenia, thrombocytopenia
Cell morphology	Small to medium lymphoblasts, fine chromatin, indistinct nucleoli	Medium to large myeloblasts, distinct nucleoli, clear chromatin, Auer rods
Cytochemistry	PAS positive, peroxidase negative, Sudan black B negative	PAS negative, peroxidase positive, Sudan black B positive

Adopted from McKenzie S: *Clinical laboratory hematology*, Upper Saddle River, NJ, 2004, Pearson, p 487.
PAS, Periodic acid–Schiff reaction.

loss of appetite, fatigue, and abdominal pain. The spleen, liver, and lymph nodes may be enlarged from leukemic infiltration. A small number of children (3%) may present with CNS signs from leukemic infiltration of brain tissues.[19]

Prognosis and treatment. ALL is highly curable in the pediatric population, but less so in adults. The 5-year survival rate is 85% in children and 30% to 50% in adults.[19] Certain forms of ALL are more responsive to therapy. For example, children with pre-B cell type have a 90% cure rate, whereas those with mature B-cell or immature T-cell leukemia have a poorer prognosis.

Chemotherapy is used for remission induction. Postremission chemotherapy with or without stem cell transplantation is indicated for most patients.[20] In general, adults with ALL require more intense therapy than children to achieve complete remission (CR). Monoclonal antibodies may be used in patients whose tumors express specific antigens.

Hairy Cell Leukemia

Pathogenesis and clinical manifestations. Hairy cell leukemia is a rare, chronic type of leukemia. The disease represents about 2% of adult leukemias, but it is of interest because of its highly treatable nature. The median age at presentation is about 55 years and there is a 5-to-1 predominance of males.[21] Hairy cell leukemia has a B-cell phenotype and is characterized by the presence of peculiar cells with hairlike projections on their surface (Figure 11-10). At diagnosis, patients have hairy cells in the peripheral blood as well as reduced numbers of granulocytes, platelets, and red blood cells. Splenomegaly is a common finding, being present in 90% of patients.

Prognosis and treatment. Treatment may be instituted when a patient becomes symptomatic with an enlarged spleen, recurrent infection, bleeding disorder, or anemia. Appropriate chemotherapeutic protocol produces CR rates of 80%.[22]

Plasma Cell Myeloma (Multiple Myeloma)

Pathogenesis and clinical manifestations. Plasma cell myeloma, also known as multiple myeloma, is a malignant disorder of mature, antibody-secreting B lymphocytes, called *plasma cells.* Malignant plasma cells have a predilection to invade bone and form multiple tumor sites. Other tissues may be targeted also, including lymph nodes, liver, spleen, and kidneys. Plasma cell myeloma occurs exclusively in the adult population, usually affecting individuals older than 40 years, with a median age at presentation of 65 years.[23] Men are affected more often than women.

As with other forms of neoplasia, the exact etiologic process of plasma cell myeloma is unknown, but abnormalities in chromosome structure and number are commonly found.[23] The malignant plasma cells all belong to a single clone, and the excessive antibodies they produce are identical monoclonal antibodies. These accumulate in the bloodstream and can be detected by serum protein electrophoresis. Normally, serum antibodies are of many forms (polyclonal) and show a varied distribution of size on the electrophoresis test. In plasma cell myeloma, there is a large amount of one type of antibody, which forms a characteristic spike (Figure 11-11). Excessive production of light-chain antibody fragments by malignant plasma cells results in their accumulation in blood and urine. When found in urine, these light-chain fragments are called **Bence Jones protein.** In addition to helping

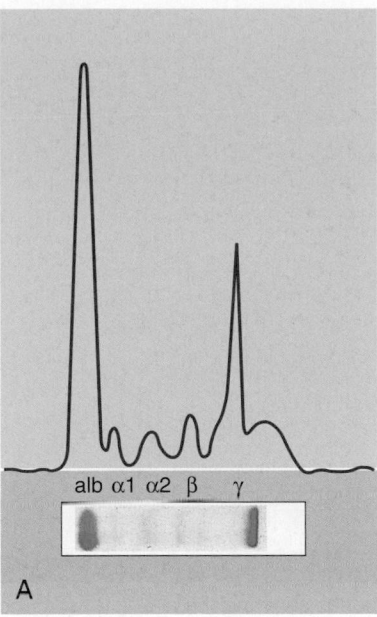
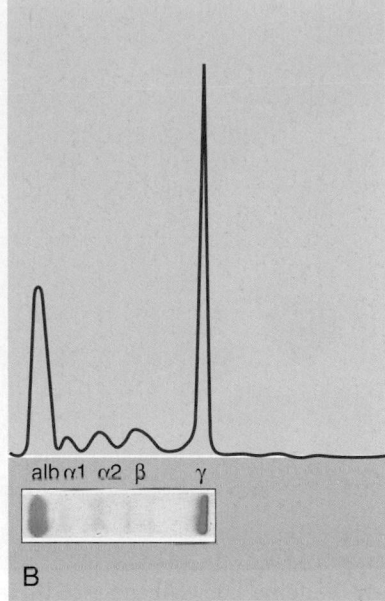

FIGURE 11-11 Serum protein electrophoresis comparing abnormal myeloma protein in the γ region typical of benign monoclonal gammopathy **(A)** with the large quantity of monoclonal antibody (spike) γ typical of plasma cell myeloma **(B)**. (From Skarin AT: *Atlas of diagnostic oncology*, London, 2003, Gower Medical, pp 536-537.)

to confirm the diagnosis, Bence Jones protein is important to the pathogenesis of plasma cell myeloma because it can accumulate in the kidneys and cause kidney damage. Malignant plasma cells tend to accumulate in bone where they enhance osteoclastic activity and produce bone lesions.[23] Pathologic fractures, especially compression fractures of the vertebral column, are common. Bone destruction releases calcium into the bloodstream, with resultant hypercalcemia.

Most of the clinical manifestations of multiple myeloma are due to bone and renal damage. The diagnosis of plasma cell myeloma is suspected based on the monoclonal antibody peak, the presence of Bence Jones protein, hypercalcemia, and evidence of bone lesions. The diagnosis is confirmed by bone marrow biopsy. Normally, the plasma cell component of the marrow comprises about 5%. In multiple myeloma, plasma cells may occupy 30% to 95% of the bone marrow (Figure 11-12). A minimum of at least 10% to 15% bone marrow plasma cells is necessary for the diagnosis of plasma cell myeloma.[23] The likelihood of bone marrow dysfunction increases as the plasma cell component increases. Normal production of erythrocytes, platelets, and leukocytes can be impaired to varying degrees.

The onset of plasma cell myeloma is generally slow and insidious. A premalignant stage of plasma cell myeloma is apparent in some individuals who have excess production of monoclonal antibodies but no evidence of bone lesions or Bence Jones protein in the urine. This stage is called monoclonal gammopathy of undetermined significance (MGUS). Approximately 25% of patients with MGUS progress to malignant disease.[17] Affected individuals remain asymptomatic until the disease is fairly advanced. The asymptomatic stage often lasts for many years after malignant transformation. During this time the only complaint may be frequent infections. Diagnosis during the asymptomatic phase is usually made because protein in the urine or high serum calcium levels are found on routine examination. Bone pain is usually the first symptom. Sometimes the evaluation of a fracture or back pain leads to the identification of myeloma. Anemia, recurrent infections, and bleeding tendencies are suggestive of bone marrow depression.

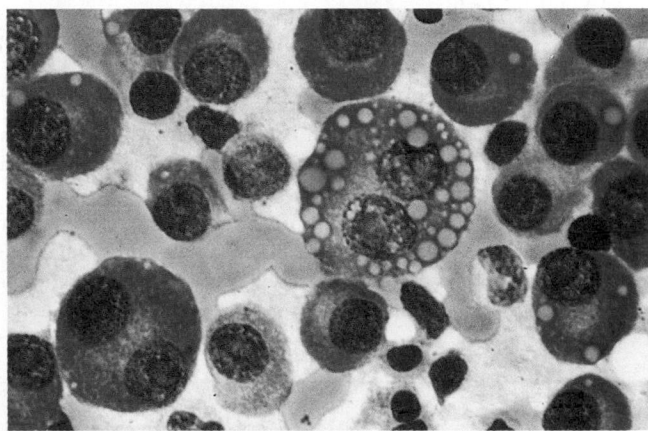

FIGURE 11-12 Bone marrow aspirate from a patient with multiple myeloma showing a large number of abnormal plasma cells with multiple nuclei and cytoplasmic droplets. (From Kumar V et al, editors: *Robbins basic pathology*, ed 8, Philadelphia, 2007, Saunders, p 455.)

Renal insufficiency is a complication experienced by approximately 50% of patients with plasma cell myeloma.[23] Impairment of renal function is due to a combination of factors, including hyperproteinemia, high levels of Bence Jones protein, hypercalcemia, and hyperuricemia. Renal function may continue to decline over time, culminating in end-stage renal disease (chronic renal failure).

Bone involvement is a consistent feature of plasma cell myeloma. Radiologic studies of ribs, spine, skull, and pelvis show a characteristic "honeycomb" appearance, attributable to lucid areas of demineralized bone (Figure 11-13). Minimal trauma is likely to result in fractures. Sometimes fractures occur with no known trauma; these are called *pathologic* fractures.

Prognosis and treatment. Antineoplastic agents may be used to induce and maintain a remission in plasma cell proliferation. The best

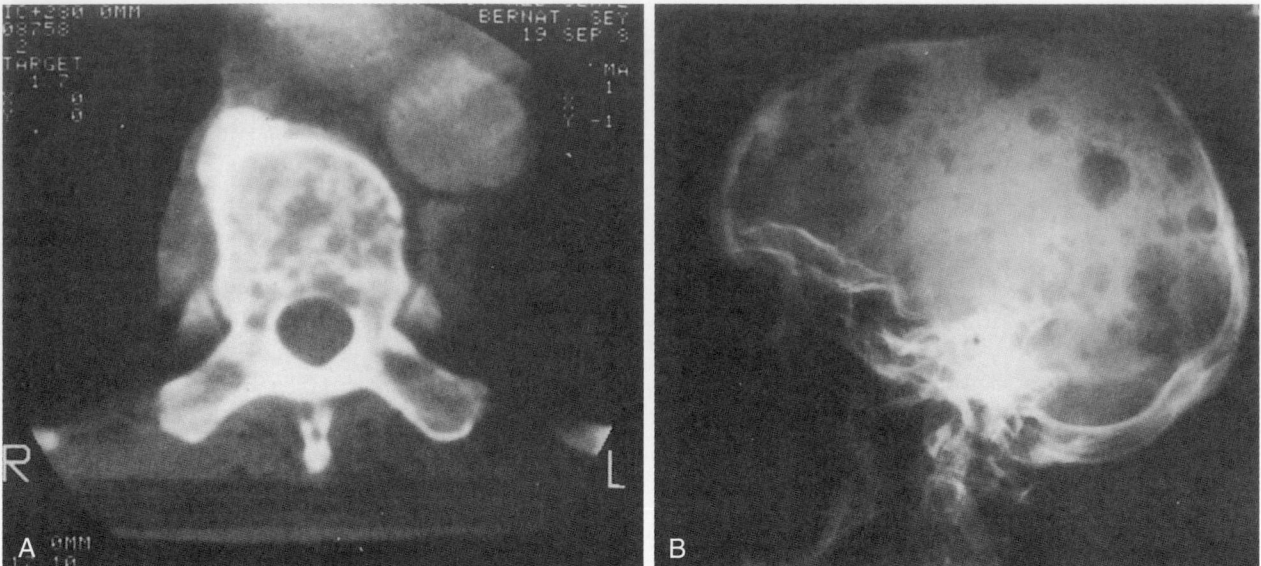

FIGURE 11-13 Vertebral body **(A)** and skull **(B)** radiographs showing the characteristic "honeycomb" appearance of demineralized bone associated with multiple myeloma. (Courtesy Marvin J. Stone, MD, Sammons Cancer Center, Baylor University Medical Center, Dallas, TX.)

chemotherapy regimen has not yet been determined. The remission induction rate with these agents is about 60%, with a median survival of about 3 years after initiation of therapy.[23] High-dose chemotherapy followed by allogeneic bone marrow transplantation is becoming more common and offers a better CR rate. However, the death rate associated with transplantation is high (approximately 40% to 50%).[17] Autologous stem cell transplantation is considered to be the optimal initial therapy for most patients. Pharmacologic management of renal dysfunction is often necessary.

Chronic bone pain is a common problem in the myeloma patient that may require use of multiple remedies. Narcotic and nonnarcotic pain relievers are often necessary. Localized application of radiation to bone lesions may reduce bone pain in some cases.

KEY POINTS

- CLL is a neoplastic transformation of a mature, peripheral B cell that affects adults primarily and has an insidious onset. CLL is usually asymptomatic. Disease in certain genotypes is associated with long survival times and does not require therapy; in other cases, disease is progressive and may be managed with stem cell transplantation or administration of monoclonal antibodies.
- ALL affects children primarily, has an acute onset, responds well to therapy, and has a good prognosis. ALL is associated with transformation of precursor "blasts" in the bone marrow. ALL often manifests with bone pain, infections, and a tendency to bleeding. A significant number of children with ALL have CNS involvement and intrathecal chemotherapy is necessary.
- Plasma cell myeloma is due to malignant transformation of antibody-secreting B lymphocytes. It primarily affects older adults. The onset of symptoms is insidious, with most patients experiencing a 4- to 10-year period of clinical latency. Some patients have a preneoplastic phase called monoclonal gammopathy of undetermined significance. When present, symptoms include bone pain, pathologic fractures, anemia, thrombocytopenia, leukopenia, and renal insufficiency. Malignant plasma cells all secrete the same monoclonal antibody, and detection of this antibody in the blood or urine (Bence Jones protein) aids in diagnosis.

Hodgkin Disease

Hodgkin disease represents about 30% of all cases of malignant lymphoma, accounting for approximately 7000 new cases annually in the United States.[10] It occurs across the age continuum, with half of cases occurring in persons between the ages of 20 and 40 years. The overall incidence of Hodgkin disease is higher in males, who have a worse prognosis. The overall 5-year survival rate for treated Hodgkin disease, including all stages, is about 85%.[10]

Pathogenesis and clinical manifestations. Hodgkin disease is a malignant disorder of the lymph nodes characterized by the presence of **Reed-Sternberg** cells on histologic examination. Reed-Sternberg cells originate from B cells in the germinal centers of lymph nodes.[24] Reed-Sternberg cells are malignant, but they tend to grow and spread in a very predictable manner. This predictability differentiates Hodgkin disease from other types of lymphoma. Hodgkin disease usually metastasizes along contiguous lymphatic pathways (Figure 11-14). Epstein-Barr virus is frequently found in the genome of transformed Reed-Sternberg cells and is thought to be important in the pathogenesis of Hodgkin disease. The malignant cells are clonal, originating from a single mutant precursor cell, and usually present in a single node or localized chain of nodes. In addition to malignant Reed-Sternberg cells, inflammatory cells accumulate within the node (Figure 11-15) such that Reed-Sternberg cells constitute only a small minority (2%) of the cells in the lymph node tumor.[24]

There are two types of Hodgkin disease: (1) the rare lymphocyte predominance type, which accounts for 5% of cases, and (2) the classical type (cHD) representing the other 95%. The classical type can be divided further into four subtypes according to the relative number of reactive cells in the tumor. The histologic pattern does not seem to predict the prognosis. The stage of Hodgkin disease is more relevant.[24]

Clinical manifestations of Hodgkin disease are dependent on the site of origin as well as on the stage of dissemination. Lymphomas often are asymptomatic in the early stages. The usual clinical presentation includes painless lymphadenopathy that may be accompanied by fever, night sweats, pruritus, weight loss, and malaise. Usually enlargement occurs in lymph nodes above the diaphragm, the cervical nodes being the most common site (Figure 11-16). Other supradiaphragmatic nodes are the supraclavicular, axillary, and mediastinal nodes. Less commonly,

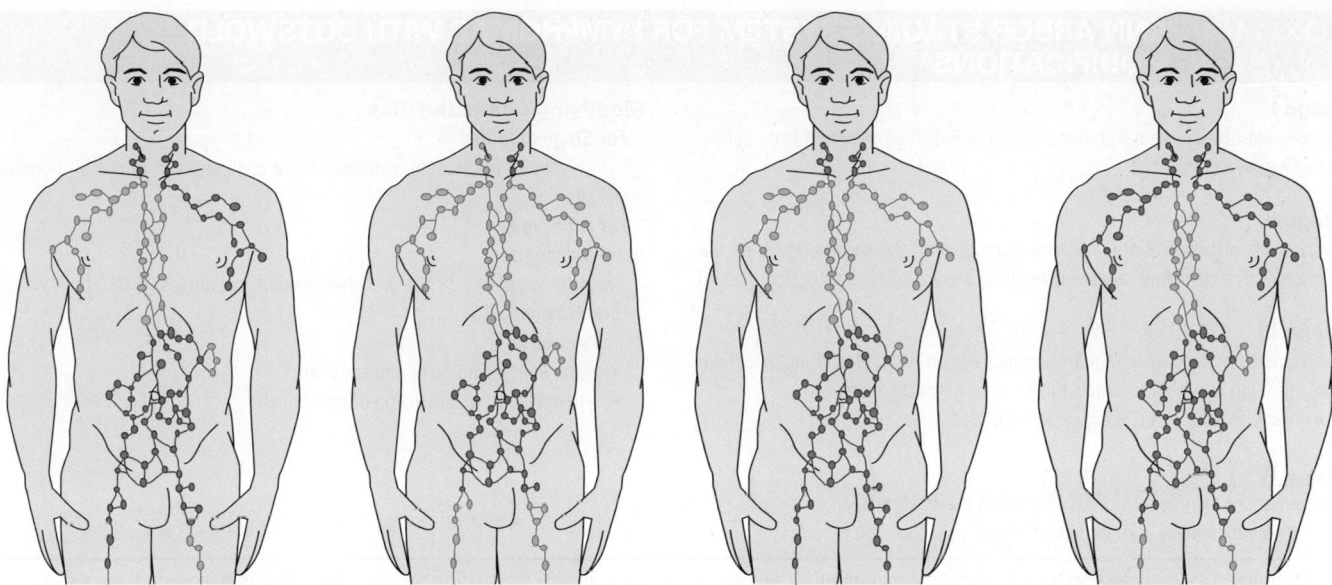

FIGURE 11-14 Schematic drawing showing the orderly, contiguous, and predictable spread of Hodgkin disease. (Redrawn and modified from Rosenberg SA: Hodgkin disease: no stage beyond cure, *Hosp Pract* 21[8]:97, 1986. After original illustrations by Bunji Tagawa.)

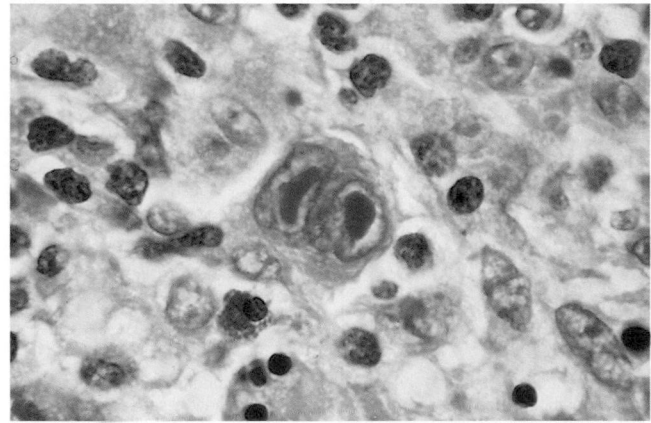

FIGURE 11-15 Histologic sample showing the typical binucleate Reed-Sternberg cells found in Hodgkin disease. An eosinophil can be seen below the Reed-Sternberg cell. (From Kumar V et al, editors: *Robbins basic pathology,* ed 8, Philadelphia, 2007, Saunders, p 457. Courtesy Dr. Robert W. McKenna, Department of Pathology, University of Texas Southwestern Medical School, Dallas, TX.)

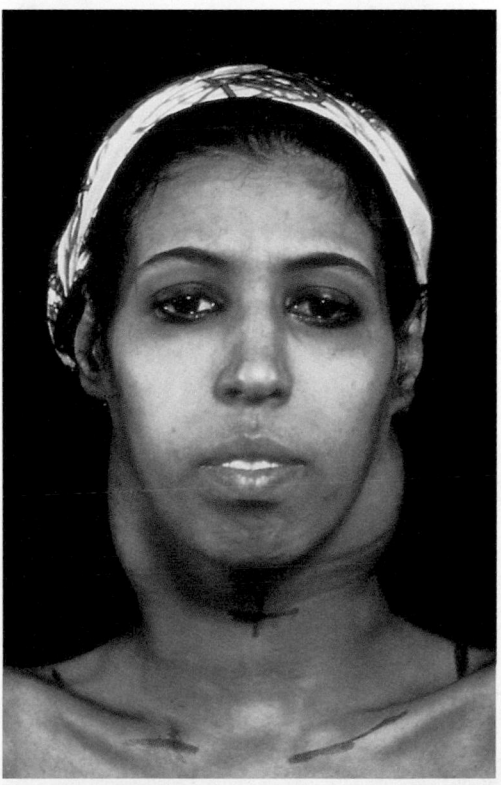

FIGURE 11-16 Hodgkin disease (stage IIA). Marked enlargement of cervical lymph nodes is present in this patient. It is usually painless and may be confined to only one area or may affect two or more areas. (From Skarin AT: *Atlas of diagnostic oncology,* London, 2003, Gower Medical, p 482.)

nodes below the diaphragm are the primary site. The inguinal nodes are the most common subdiaphragmatic site. As the disease spreads from the site of origin, other lymph nodes and lymphatic tissues may become involved, including the spleen and bone marrow. Staging procedures are performed to determine the extent of metastasis at the time of diagnosis. Staging dictates the treatment modality best suited to provide the patient with the greatest chance for long-term survival.

Prognosis and treatment. The staging protocol commonly used today was first adopted in 1971 at the Ann Arbor symposium and modified later in 1989 at the Cotswold meeting (Box 11-4).[25,26] The same procedure is also used for staging non-Hodgkin lymphomas. This protocol uses the presence or absence of certain clinical symptoms as well as the locations of affected nodes to determine the clinical stage of disease. The four stages are shown in Figure 11-17. The letter A denotes the absence of clinical symptoms, whereas the letter B is used when symptoms are present at the time of staging. These symptoms

include loss of more than 10% of body weight, unexplained fevers, and night sweats. The clinical stage (CS) is based on history, physical examination, and noninvasive procedures such as computed tomography (CT) scanning. The pathologic stage (PS) is determined by the results of invasive procedures such as laparotomy and tissue biopsy. The stage

BOX 11-4 ANN ARBOR STAGING SYSTEM FOR LYMPHOMAS WITH COTSWOLD MODIFICATIONS*

Stage I

Involvement of a single lymph node region or lymphoid structure (e.g., spleen, thymus, Waldeyer ring)

Stage II

Involvement of two or more lymph node regions on the same side of the diaphragm. The number of anatomic regions is indicated by a subscript (e.g., II_3).

Stage III

Involvement of lymph node regions or structures on both sides of the diaphragm
- III_1: with or without splenic, hilar, celiac, or portal nodes
- III_2: with para-aortic, iliac, mesenteric nodes

Stage IV

Involvement of extranodal site(s) beyond that designated "E"
The site is indicated by a letter code followed by a plus sign (+)

Modifying Characteristics
For Stages I to III
E: Involvement of a single, extranodal site contiguous or proximal to known nodal site
For All Stages
A: No symptoms
B: Fever (temperature >38° C), drenching sweats, weight loss (>10% body weight over 6 months)
X: Bulky disease
- >One third widening of mediastinum
- >10 cm maximal dimension of nodal mass

*Clinical stage (CS) is based on history, physical examination, laboratory studies, and CT scans. Pathologic stage (PS) is based on tissue sampling obtained through invasive procedures such as laparotomy and biopsy.

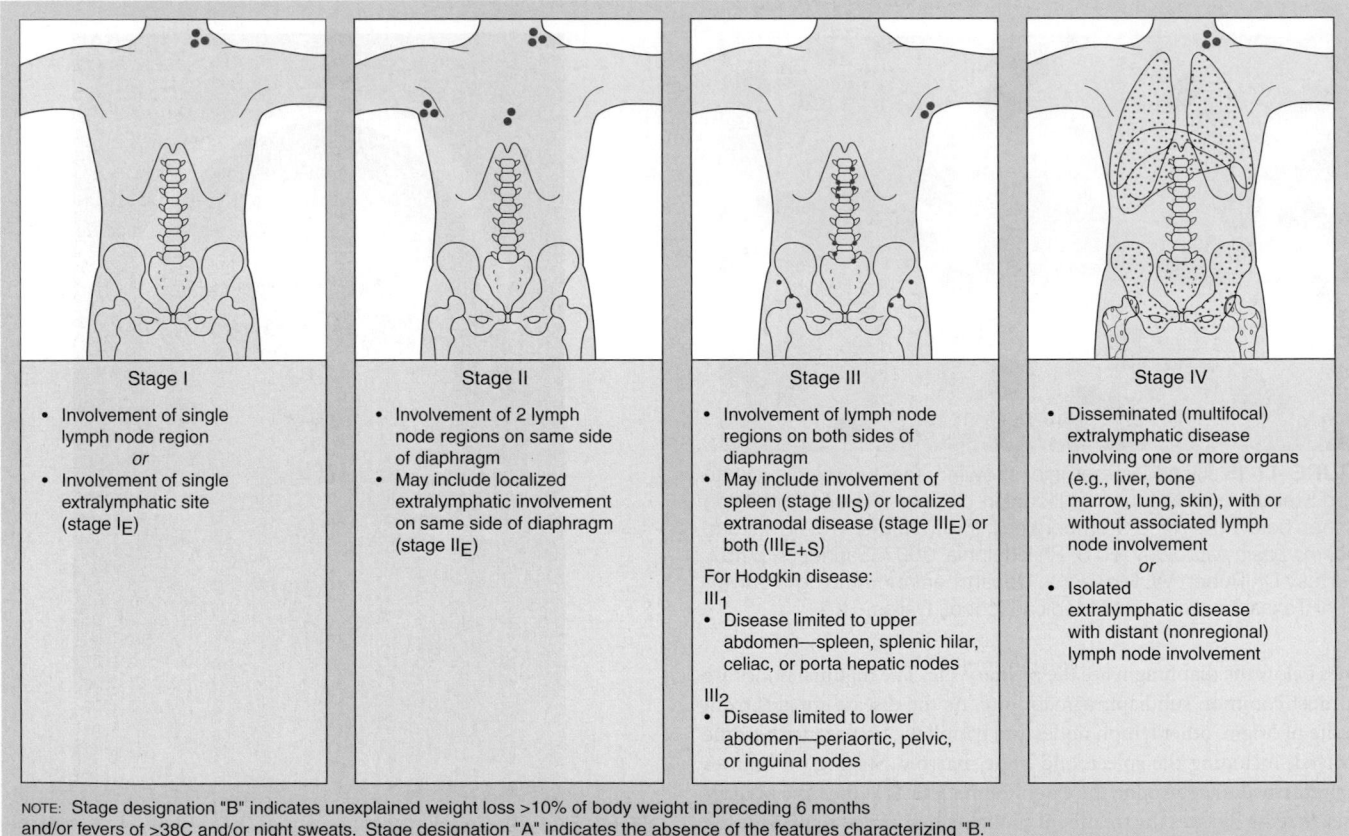

Stage I	Stage II	Stage III	Stage IV
• Involvement of single lymph node region *or* • Involvement of single extralymphatic site (stage I_E)	• Involvement of 2 lymph node regions on same side of diaphragm • May include localized extralymphatic involvement on same side of diaphragm (stage II_E)	• Involvement of lymph node regions on both sides of diaphragm • May include involvement of spleen (stage III_S) or localized extranodal disease (stage III_E) or both (III_{E+S}) For Hodgkin disease: III_1 • Disease limited to upper abdomen—spleen, splenic hilar, celiac, or porta hepatic nodes III_2 • Disease limited to lower abdomen—periaortic, pelvic, or inguinal nodes	• Disseminated (multifocal) extralymphatic disease involving one or more organs (e.g., liver, bone marrow, lung, skin), with or without associated lymph node involvement *or* • Isolated extralymphatic disease with distant (nonregional) lymph node involvement

NOTE: Stage designation "B" indicates unexplained weight loss >10% of body weight in preceding 6 months and/or fevers of >38C and/or night sweats. Stage designation "A" indicates the absence of the features characterizing "B."

FIGURE 11-17 Depiction of the locations of malignant cells in the various stages of lymphoma using the Ann Arbor staging system. (From Skarin AT: *Atlas of diagnostic oncology,* London, 2003, Gower Medical, p 479.)

dictates the treatment modalities used. In general, localized tumors are more amenable to application of radiation therapy, whereas disseminated disease responds better to systemic chemotherapeutic agents. Since Hodgkin disease often is detected while localized, radiation therapy is commonly used, with good results (Figure 11-18).

Patients with nonbulky, stage IA or IIA disease may be candidates for radiation as sole therapy. However, a relatively high rate of relapse has been noted, and combined chemotherapy with limited field radiation is often used.[27] Patients with bulky disease, "B" symptoms, or stage III and IV disease require chemotherapy with or without

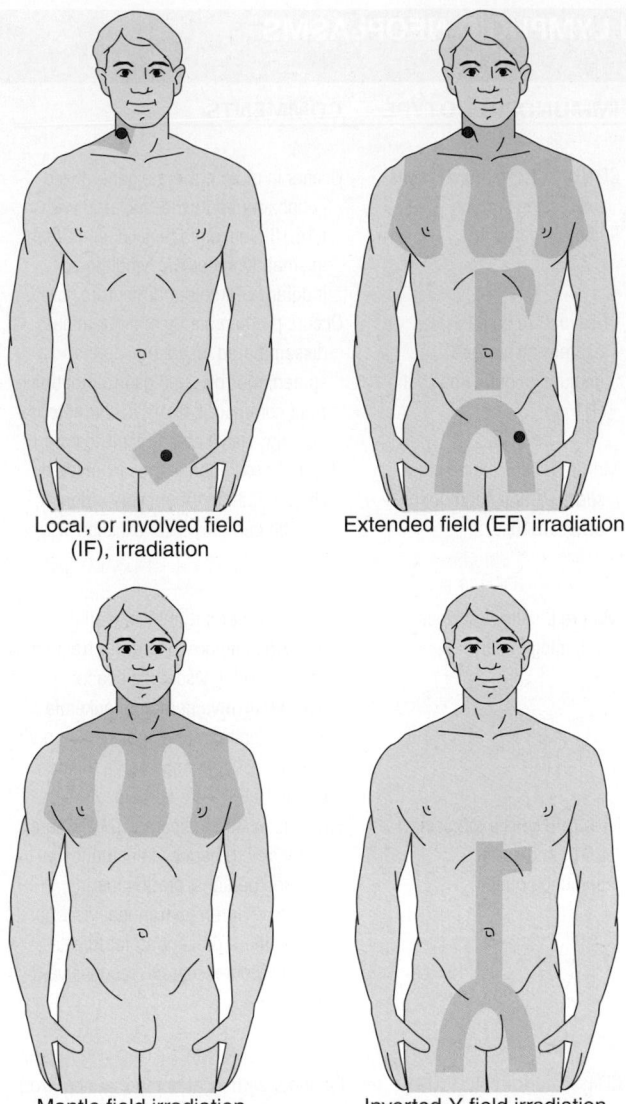

Local, or involved field (IF), irradiation

Extended field (EF) irradiation

Mantle field irradiation

Inverted-Y field irradiation

FIGURE 11-18 Typical radiation fields for lymphoma. Different fields of radiation may be used depending on the location of disease.

radiation. In early stage disease appropriate treatment produces a 90% 10-year disease-free survival. More aggressive chemotherapy is indicated for patients with advanced Hodgkin disease.

B-Cell, T-Cell, and NK-Cell Lymphoma (Non-Hodgkin)

The malignancies included in the classification of non-Hodgkin lymphoma are those that do not have the characteristic Reed-Sternberg cells found in Hodgkin disease. The majority of cases of non-Hodgkin lymphoma arise from lymph nodes, but they can originate in any lymphoid tissue. With the exception of a few subtypes, most cases of non-Hodgkin lymphoma occur in older adults (95%), and males are at a slightly higher risk than females. The incidence of non-Hodgkin lymphoma is on the rise, particularly in areas with large AIDS populations. More than 50,000 new cases of non-Hodgkin lymphoma are diagnosed annually in the United States.[9] The lifetime risk of developing this disease is about 1 in 50.

Most cases of non-Hodgkin lymphoma arise from B cells, T cells, or NK cells. Some of the more common types of non-Hodgkin lymphoma are summarized in Table 11-4. The prognosis and recommended treatment protocols vary according to type. A general schema for grouping non-Hodgkin lymphoma according to indolent or aggressive types is

in common usage.[28] Generally, indolent disease is associated with longer survival times whereas aggressive lymphomas tend to be disseminated at presentation and carry a generally poorer prognosis. As a group, the non-Hodgkin types of lymphoma are more likely to spread early and unpredictably in comparison with Hodgkin disease.

Pathogenesis and clinical manifestations. The etiologic process of non-Hodgkin lymphoma is thought to be similar to that of other malignant transformations. The tumor cells are all derived from a single mutant precursor cell and are clonal. Viruses are suspected in the development of some types of lymphoma. In particular, Burkitt lymphoma is strongly associated with the presence of Epstein-Barr virus.[2] Adult T-cell lymphomas are associated with infection by human T cell leukemia virus, type 1 (HTLV-1).[2] The overall 5-year survival rate for all types of non-Hodgkin lymphomas combined is about 50%.[10]

Most patients with non-Hodgkin lymphoma present with advanced disease (stage III or IV). Clinical manifestations may include painless lymphadenopathy, fever, night sweats, weight loss, malaise, and pruritus (similar to Hodgkin disease). A comparison of the features of Hodgkin disease and non-Hodgkin lymphoma is shown in Table 11-5. Extranodal involvement occurs early in the course of non-Hodgkin lymphoma, and patients may present with infiltrative disease of the skin, gastrointestinal tract, bone, or bone marrow. Complications occur more frequently than in Hodgkin disease. Two of the most serious oncology emergencies are obstruction of the superior vena cava and spinal cord compression. Infection, bone metastasis, and joint effusions are also common. Staging of non-Hodgkin lymphoma is done in the same way as for Hodgkin disease, and the classification system is not different. Earlier clinical stages are associated with the best prognosis for survival.

Prognosis and treatment. The effectiveness of therapy for non-Hodgkin lymphoma is variable. Favorable outcomes are likely in stage I and II disease. However, non-Hodgkin lymphoma is likely to present as stage III or IV disease, which has a poor prognosis. Therapeutic management is determined by the clinical stage, histologic type, patient age, and bone marrow integrity at the time of diagnosis.[29] Radiation, chemotherapy, and tissue-specific therapies such as monoclonal antibodies and bone marrow transplants may all be applicable.

KEY POINTS

- Hodgkin disease is characterized by malignant transformation of B cells in lymph nodes, called *Reed-Sternberg cells*. The spread of malignant cells occurs along predictable, contiguous pathways. Most commonly, a single cervical lymph node is involved initially, with slow progression to nearby nodes.
- Non-Hodgkin lymphoma constitutes a diverse group of malignant diseases of lymphoid tissue. The characteristic Reed-Sternberg cell of Hodgkin disease is not present. Non-Hodgkin lymphoma is unpredictable in its spread and is often disseminated at diagnosis.
- Manifestations of Hodgkin disease and non-Hodgkin lymphoma are similar. These include painless lymph node enlargement, fever, night sweats, and weight loss. Early stage disease is often asymptomatic.
- Staging is done to determine the degree of dissemination of disease. When affected lymph nodes are localized to one area (stage I) or one side of the diaphragm (stage II), the prognosis for cure is very good. Dissemination to lymph nodes above and below the diaphragm (stage III) or to extralymphatic organs or tissues (stage IV) carries a poorer prognosis.
- Radiation of the involved field is commonly used for malignant lymphoma in early stages. More disseminated disease may be treated with chemotherapeutic protocols. Non-Hodgkin lymphoma is routinely treated with chemotherapy because the disease is often well advanced at the time of diagnosis. Treatment may lead to bone marrow suppression and may predispose the patient to anemia, thrombocytopenia, and leukopenia.

TABLE 11-4 SUMMARY OF THE MORE COMMON LYMPHOID NEOPLASMS (NON-HODGKIN TYPE)

ENTITY	FREQUENCY	SALIENT MORPHOLOGY	IMMUNOPHENOTYPE	COMMENTS
B-Cell Lymphoma				
Follicular lymphoma	40% of adult lymphomas	Germinal center cells arranged in a follicular pattern	$CD10^+$, $BCL2^+$ mature B cells expressing surface immunoglobulin	Occurs in older patients; generalized lymphadenopathy; associated with t(14;18); leukemia less common than in small lymphocytic lymphoma; indolent course but difficult to cure
Mantle cell lymphoma	3% to 4% of adult lymphomas	Diffuse or vaguely nodular pattern with small cleaved cells	$CD5^+$ mature B cells expressing surface immunoglobulin and cyclin D1	Occurs predominantly in older males; disseminated disease in nodes, spleen, marrow, and gastrointestinal tract common; t(11;14) is characteristic; aggressive and difficult to cure
Extranodal marginal zone lymphoma (MALT lymphoma)	About 5% of adult lymphomas; more common in parts of Europe (Italy)	Variable; small round to irregular lymphocytes predominate; 40% show plasmacytic differentiation; B cells invade epithelium in small nests (lymphoepithelial lesions)	Mature B cells expressing surface immunoglobulin $CD5^-$, $CD10^-$	Occurs at extranodal sites involved by chronic inflammation; very indolent; may be cured by local excision
Diffuse large B-cell lymphoma	40% to 50% of adult lymphomas	Various cell types; predominantly large germinal center–like cells; others with immunoblastic morphology	Mature B cells, ± surface immunoglobulin	Occurs in older patients as well as pediatric age group; greater frequency of extranodal, visceral disease; marrow involvement and leukemia very uncommon at diagnosis and poor prognostic sign; aggressive tumors, but up to 50% are curable
Burkitt lymphoma	<1% of lymphomas in United States	Cells intermediate in size between small lymphocytes and immunoblasts; prominent nucleoli; high mitotic rate; starry sky appearance caused by high rate of apoptosis	Mature B cells expressing CD10 and surface immunoglobulin	Endemic in Africa; sporadic elsewhere; increased frequency in immunosuppressed persons; predominantly affects children; extranodal visceral involvement presenting features; rapidly progressive but responsive to therapy
T-Cell Lymphoma				
Mycosis fungoides/Sézary syndrome	Most common type of cutaneous lymphoma	Variable; in most cases, small cells with markedly convoluted nuclei predominate; cells often infiltrate epidermis (Pautrier abscess)	$CD4^+$ mature T cells ($CD3^+$)	Presents with local or more generalized skin involvement; very indolent course; Sézary syndrome associated with diffuse erythroderma and peripheral blood involvement
Peripheral T-cell lymphoma, not otherwise specified	Most common type of T-cell lymphoma in adults	Variable; usually a spectrum of small to large tumor cells with irregular nuclei	Mature T-cell phenotype ($CD3^+$)	Not clearly a specific entity; often presents as disseminated disease; generally poor prognosis

Modified from Kumar V et al, editors: *Robbins basic pathology,* ed 8, Philadelphia, 2007, Saunders, p 448-449.
MALT, Mucosa-associated lymphoid tissue.

TABLE 11-5 CLINICAL DIFFERENCES IN HODGKIN DISEASE AND NON-HODGKIN LYMPHOMA

CHARACTERISTIC	HODGKIN DISEASE	NON-HODGKIN LYMPHOMA
Pattern of spread	Contiguous spread	Noncontiguous spread
Extranodal disease	Uncommon	More common involvement of gastrointestinal tract, testes, bone marrow
Site of disease	Mediastinal involvement common	Mediastinal involvement less common
	Bone marrow involvement uncommon	Bone marrow involvement common
	Liver involvement uncommon	Liver involvement common
Extent of disease	Often localized	Rarely localized
B symptoms	Common	Uncommon

SUMMARY

Malignant disorders of white blood cells are classified according to cell type and fall into two major categories: myeloid neoplasms and lymphoid neoplasms. Myeloid neoplasms commonly present as leukemia and usually involve transformation of granulocytes. Lymphoid neoplasms may present as leukemia, lymphoma, or plasma cell myeloma. Leukemia is a malignant neoplasm of immature stem cells that is characterized by diffuse replacement of the bone marrow by neoplastic blasts. In most cases the leukemic cells overflow into the bloodstream, where they may be seen in large numbers. These cells may also infiltrate the liver, spleen, lymph nodes, and other tissues throughout the body. Lymphoma is characterized by malignancy of cells found in lymphoid tissues and usually arises in the lymph nodes. Hodgkin disease is a special category of malignant lymphoma that is characterized by the presence of Reed-Sternberg cells. Hodgkin disease is more predictable in its spread than the non-Hodgkin types of lymphoma, and it is generally curable in the early stages. Non-Hodgkin lymphoma types comprise a large number of different disorders that involve malignant transformation of B cells, T cells, or NK cells. As with Hodgkin disease, earlier stages are more easily cured. However, the non-Hodgkin lymphomas tend to be unpredictable in their dissemination, and the prognosis is less certain. Plasma cell myeloma is a malignant transformation of mature, antibody-secreting B cells. Malignant plasma cells are monoclonal and all produce identical antibodies, which accumulate in the blood. These cells have a predilection to settle in skeletal structures, where they cause bone demineralization and destruction. Hypercalcemia, bone fractures (pathologic fractures), and renal damage are common complications of plasma cell myeloma. Treatment for the various types of hematologic neoplasms continues to evolve, and excellent disease-free survival is commonly achieved when the disease is diagnosed in the early stages.

REFERENCES

1. Jaffe ES, Harris NL, Stein H, Vardiman JW, editors: *Pathology and genetics of tumours of haematopoietic and lymphoid tissues*, Lyon, France, 2001, IARC Press.
2. Schulz TF, Neil JC: Viruses and leukemia. In Henderson ES, Lister TA, Greaves MF, editors: *Leukemia*, ed 7, Philadelphia, 2002, Saunders, pp 200–225.
3. Boice JD Jr: Radiation-induced leukemia. In Henderson ES, Lister TA, Greaves MF, editors: *Leukemia*, ed 7, Philadelphia, 2002, Saunders, pp 152–169.
4. Pedersen-Bjergaard J: Chemicals and leukemia. In Henderson ES, Lister TA, Greaves MF, editors: *Leukemia*, ed 7, Philadelphia, 2002, Saunders, pp 171–199.
5. Ross JA, Potter JD, Reaman GH, Pendergrass TW, Robison LL: Maternal exposure to potential inhibitors of DNA topoisomerase II and infant leukemia (United States): a report from the Children's Cancer Group, *Cancer Causes Control* 7(6):581–590, 1996.
6. McKenzie SB: *Clinical laboratory hematology*, Upper Saddle River, NJ, 2004, Pearson Education.
7. Lowenberg B, Griffin JD, Tallman MS: Acute myeloid leukemia and acute promyelocytic leukemia, *Hematology* 82–101, 2003. doi: 10.1182/asheducation-2003.1.82.
8. Gaynon PS, Siegel SE: Childhood acute lymphoblastic leukemia. In Henderson ES, Lister TA, Greaves MF, editors: *Leukemia*, ed 7, Philadelphia, 2002, Saunders, pp 601–620.
9. Spivak JL, et al: Chronic myeloproliferative disorders, *Hematology* 200–224, 2003. doi: 10.1182/asheducation-2003.1.200.
10. American Cancer Society: *Cancer facts and figures, 2003*, Atlanta, 2003, Author.
11. Melo JV, Hughes TP, Apperley JF: Chronic myeloid leukemia, *Hematology* 132–152, 2003. doi: 10.1182/asheducation-2003.1.132.
12. Barnett MJ, Eaves CJ: Chronic myeloid leukemia. In Henderson ES, Lister TA, Greaves MF, editors: *Leukemia*, ed 7, Philadelphia, 2002, Saunders, pp 583–600.
13. Hoffbrand AV, Moss PAH: The World Health Organization (WHO) classification of the tumors of haematopoietic and lymphoid tissues. In *Essential haematology*, ed 6, Oxford, England, 2011, Blackwell.
14. Robatiner A, Lister TA: Acute myelogenous leukemia. In Henderson ES, Lister TA, Greaves MF, editors: *Leukemia*, ed 7, Philadelphia, 2002, Saunders, pp 485–517.
15. Keating MJ: Chronic lymphocytic leukemia. In Henderson ES, Lister TA, Greaves MF, editors: *Leukemia*, ed 7, Philadelphia, 2002, Saunders, pp 656–691.
16. Keating MJ, et al: Biology and treatment of chronic lymphocytic leukemia, *Hematology* 153–175, 2003. doi: 10.1182/ashwducation-2003.1.153.
17. Aster JC: The hematopoietic and lymphoid systems. In Kumar V, Abbas AK, Fausto N, Mitchell R, editors: *Robbins basic pathology*, ed 8, Philadelphia, 2007, Saunders, pp 421–478.
18. McKenzie SB: *Clinical laboratory hematology*, Upper Saddle River, NJ, 2004, Pearson Education.
19. Gaynon PS, Siegel SE: Childhood acute lymphoblastic leukemia. In Henderson ES, Lister TA, Greaves MF, editors: *Leukemia*, ed 7, Philadelphia, 2002, Saunders, pp 601–620.
20. Joel SP, Robatiner A: Pharmacology of antileukemic drugs. In Henderson ES, Lister TA, Greaves MF, editors: *Leukemia*, ed 7, Philadelphia, 2002, Saunders, pp 394–440.
21. Hoffman M, Rai K: Hairy cell leukemia. In Henderson ES, Lister TA, Greaves MF, editors: *Leukemia*, ed 7, Philadelphia, 2002, Saunders, pp 693–703.
22. Linker CA: Blood. In Tierney LM, McPhee SJ, Papadakis MA, editors: *Current medical diagnosis and treatment*, ed 46, New York, 2007, McGraw-Hill, pp 493–547.
23. Barille-Nion S, et al: Advances in biology and therapy of multiple myeloma, *Hematology* 248–278, 2003. doi: 10.1182/asheducation-2003.1.248.
24. Diehl V, Stein H, Hummel M, Zollinger R, Connors JM: Hodgkin's lymphoma: biology and treatment strategies for primary, refractory and relapsed disease, *Hematology* 225–247, 2003. doi: 10.1182/asheducation-2003.1.225.
25. Carbone PP, Kaplan HS, Musshoff K, Smithers DW, Tubiana M: Report of the Committee on Hodgkin's Disease Staging Classification, *Cancer Res* 31:1860–1861, 1971.
26. Lister TA, et al: Report of a committee convened to discuss the evaluation and staging of patients with Hodgkin's disease: Cotswolds Meeting, *J Clin Oncol* 7(11):1630–1636, 1989.
27. National Cancer Institute: *Adult Hodgkin lymphoma (PDQ)*. Available at www.cancer.gov/cancertopics/pdq/treatment/adulthodgkins/HealthProfessional. Accessed 7/8/10.
28. National Cancer Institute: *Non-Hodgkin lymphoma (PDQ): National Cancer Institute*. Available at www.cancer.gov/cancertopics/pdq/treatment/adult-nonhodgkins/HealthProfessional. Accessed 7/28/11.
29. Vose JM, Chiu BCH, Cheson BD, Dancey J, Wright J: Update on epidemiology and therapeutics for non-Hodgkin's lymphoma, *Hematology* 241–262, 2002. doi: 10.1182/asheducation-2002.1.241.

HIV Disease and AIDS

Faith Young Peterson

evolve WEBSITE

http://evolve.elsevier.com/Copstead/

- Review Questions and Answers
- Glossary (with audio pronunciations for selected terms)
- Disease Profiles
- Animations

- Case Studies
- WebLinks
- Key Points Review

KEY QUESTIONS

- What are the common modes of HIV transmission and how can infection be prevented?
- What is the scope of the HIV/AIDS epidemic in the United States and the world?
- How does infection with HIV lead to progressive immunodeficiency and AIDS?
- How has knowledge of the HIV life cycle led to the development of multidrug treatment strategies?

- How are CD4+ cell counts and various clinical findings used to classify the stages of HIV disease and AIDS?
- What are the common systemic manifestations of AIDS and associated opportunistic infections?
- What are the current treatment recommendations for HIV disease and AIDS?

CHAPTER OUTLINE

This chapter focuses on HIV disease and AIDS—from epidemiology to pathogenesis and management. Human immunodeficiency virus (HIV), an infectious organism, is the prototypical public health infectious disease of the late twentieth century. Originally thought to be a rapid killer, it does not act like other infectious organisms that overwhelm the immune system. HIV infection triggers chronic widespread and diverse organ involvement with varying signs and symptoms. It encompasses all of the armamentarium of a viral infection that has completed the evolutionary progression from animal to human. HIV has done more than just confuse and captivate scientists and health professionals; it also has mobilized risk groups and placed medicine and society at a crossroads of opinion. In this epidemic, the lines between privacy and public health and between morality and compassion have been debated. HIV disease is complex, but in its complexity it has opened the door to better understanding of the immune system.

Human immunodeficiency virus (HIV) infection and **acquired immunodeficiency syndrome (AIDS)** are acquired immunodeficiency disorders resulting in defective immune functioning. The hallmark of HIV infection is defective cell-mediated immunity, especially the decrease in CD4[+] or T helper/inducer lymphocytes. CD4[+] T cells are necessary for appropriate immune responsiveness because they are the cells that mediate between the antigen-presenting cells and other immune cells, such as B cells and other T cells. CD4[+] lymphocytes are characterized by the presence of the CD4 receptor.

EPIDEMIOLOGY

HIV infection is a primary immunodeficiency disease caused by the retroviruses HIV type 1 and HIV type 2. Despite research and public health surveillance and prevention activities, the virus has continued mutating and spreading globally. HIV infects people worldwide. However, HIV infection is increasingly becoming a disease of poor, uneducated, or undereducated people of color. Since its identification in the early 1980s, the HIV global epidemic continues with an estimated 33.3 million people living with HIV worldwide as of 2010 and a total of 1.8 million AIDS deaths worldwide in 2009.[1] Selected aspects of the global impact of HIV and AIDS are illustrated in Table 12-1.

The total adult prevalence is now 0.8% of the adult population of the world.[1] Of the 33.3 million people infected with HIV, women comprise 15.9 million and children <15 years old comprise 2.5 million.[1] According to the World Health Organization (WHO), the number of new HIV infections globally declined 19% over the past decade, attributable to expanded and improved HIV programs.[1] However, HIV infection rates continue to increase in sub-Saharan Africa as well as in eastern Europe and central Asia. In third world countries, those infected with HIV have more limited access to testing and medication for treatment, as well as limited information for prevention because of the effects of gender inequity and harmful social norms that drive transmission.[1] For example, only 37% of those infected in sub-Saharan Africa receive antiretroviral therapy compared to 50% in Latin America and the Caribbean.[1]

In the United States, more than 1 million people have been diagnosed with HIV/AIDS since the beginning of the epidemic.[2] It is estimated by the Centers for Disease Control and Prevention (CDC) that there are 663,084 persons living with HIV/AIDS in the United States, with 56,000 new HIV infections diagnosed yearly.[2] In the United States and other industrialized countries where access to medication, care, and prevention is greater, the number of patients diagnosed with and dying from AIDS is stable or declining (Figure 12-1). The proportion of people living 3 or more years after an AIDS diagnosis in the United States has increased. However, the CDC estimates that up to 25% of the people who are infected with HIV in the United States may be unaware that they are infected.

Current statistics show that of the people diagnosed with HIV/AIDS in the United States, racial and ethnic minorities, women of color, and men who have sex with men (MSM) are disproportionately affected.[2] Overall, there has been a decrease in the rates of new diagnoses between 1998 and 2007 by 20.7%—from 18.4 to 14.6 new cases per 100,000 population.[3] Among racial and ethnic groups, most of the new cases are in black non-Hispanics, followed by Hispanics.[3-5] Males had a higher rate of diagnoses (21.9 per 100,000 in 2007) than females (7.6 per 100,000 population).[3] According to the CDC, 75% of new HIV infections occur in men and of those 50% occur in men who have sex with men (MSM).[4] The highest rates of new diagnoses of HIV are in black men and women, with a lifetime risk of 1 in 16 for black males and 1 in 30 for black females compared to 1 in 104 for white males and 1 in 588 for white females.[5] The rate of diagnoses also varied by state, with the District of Columbia having 154.6 new cases per 100,000 population, which is the highest rate in the country.[3] It is thought that noninjection drugs (such as crack cocaine or methamphetamine) may also contribute to the spread of HIV/AIDS because of sex trading for drugs, shelter, or money. Ninety percent of children younger than age 13 are infected perinatally.[6] Ten to eleven percent of HIV cases are in people older than age 50 often as a result of a decreased perception of risk. As a result, older adults are often diagnosed later with a death rate that is higher than in other age groups.

History

In 1981 the first descriptions of immunodeficiency disease in previously healthy persons appeared in the medical literature. At that time, previously healthy young homosexual men in increasing numbers contracted unusual diseases for their age group, such as *Pneumocystis jiroveci (carinii)* pneumonia (PCP) and Kaposi sarcoma, that researchers identified as HIV. The first evidence of alternative forms of transmission of the virus by blood and blood products appeared in 1982. All these early patients were shown to have a type of HIV virus called HIV-1. It was at this time that the term *acquired immunodeficiency syndrome (AIDS)* was first used. However, the specific retrovirus causing HIV infection and AIDS was not isolated until the early to mid-1980s. The timeline of HIV history is found in Table 12-2.

Types of HIV

HIV is a type of retrovirus from the subfamily Lentivirinae, with *Lentivirus* being its only genus. This subfamily is so named from the Latin word *lentus,* meaning "slow," because infection develops gradually. HIV-2, a related but distinct retrovirus, was later identified in 1986 and is most closely related to simian immunodeficiency virus. HIV-2 is differentiated from HIV-1 by a longer clinical latency period from the onset of infection to the development of symptoms. It is also characterized by having lower plasma HIV-2 viral loads and lower mortality rates and by generally being a milder form of the disease.[6] HIV-2 infection can progress to AIDS, even though it appears to be less virulent than HIV-1. It is also possible to be coinfected with both HIV-1 and HIV-2.[6]

Both HIV-1 and HIV-2 are found worldwide. They are similar in structure and function but are differentiated from each other by their envelope glycoproteins, point of origin, and latency periods. The point of origin for HIV-1 is Central Africa and for HIV-2 it is West Africa. HIV-1 is the causative organism of most cases found in Central Africa, the United States, Europe, and Australia. HIV-2 is found primarily in West Africa or in countries with strong socioeconomic ties to West Africa (e.g., France, Spain, Portugal, and former Portuguese colonies).[6]

Many subspecies or strains of HIV also exist because of the rapid rate of HIV virion mutation. The subspecies may exist in different hosts, as well as within an individual host. Currently, at least 10 subtypes of HIV-1 have been identified: group N (YBF30), group O, and

TABLE 12-1 GLOBAL HEALTH CONSIDERATIONS FOR HIV/AIDS

COUNTRY/ REGION	PREVALENCE OF DISEASE	CULTURAL FACTORS	MOST COMMON MEANS OF TRANSMISSION	TREATMENT	ECONOMIC/SOCIAL IMPACT
Sub-Saharan Africa*	22.5 million people affected. This region carries 70% of the world's HIV/AIDS burden Adult prevalence % = 5.0% Adult and child deaths due to AIDS = 1.3 million	Gender inequalities: Males dominate sexual decision making and women are disproportionately infected	Heterosexual sex and mother-to-child transmission	Treatment available, but not affordable for most people Treatment coverage: 37% (3,911,000)	Life expectancy has decreased dramatically and population is beginning to bottleneck Reversing the progress in poverty reduction Stigma associated with disease causes people to lose property
East Asia/ China†	770,000 people affected Adult prevalence % = 0.1% Adult and child deaths due to AIDS = 36,000	Growing male demographic has led to a growing sex industry	Intravenous drug use, prostitution, and transmission through migrant workers	Medical coverage in rural areas is poor, so a large proportion of the population must pay out of pocket. Treatment coverage: 31%	Cost of therapy generally exceeds annual income Stigma is so great that many people do not disclose their HIV status to their families and thus do not seek treatment
North America	1.5 million people affected Adult prevalence % = 0.5%	Continued stigma	Men having sex with men (MSM), intravenous drug use, heterosexual transmission and prostitution	Treatment available to most people	Cost of therapy is high but programs are available for assistance
Western and Central Europe	820,000 people affected Adult prevalence % = 0.2% Adult and child deaths due to AIDS = 76,000	Continued stigma	MSM, intravenous drug use, heterosexual transmission and prostitution	Treatment available to most people	
South and Southeast Asia	4.1 million people affected Adult prevalence % = 0.3% Adult and child deaths due to AIDS =260,000	Stigma Drug use and prostitution high in some areas such as Thailand	MSM, intravenous drug use, prostitution	Cambodia and Thailand have 50-80% antiretroviral coverage	
Central and South America	1.4 million people affected Adult prevalence % = 0.5% Adult and child deaths due to AIDS = 58,000	Men who have sex with men are highly stigmatized, so prevention efforts overlook this group. Drug use is commonplace	MSM, intravenous drug use, and prostitution	50-80% of infected people are receiving antiretroviral therapy. The government provides therapy for free.	Government has had a strong and positive response to the epidemic: Its efforts have reduced stigma, improved social reintegration, and reduced HIV prevalence among high risk populations.

*USAID (2010). HIV/AIDS health profile. *USAID From the American People.* Retrieved from http://www.usaid.gov/our_work/global_health/aids/Countries/lac/brazil.pdf. WHO HIV/AIDS Statistics.
†Self service a la mode. *Business China, 36*(13), 5-6, 2010.

group M with 8 subtypes (A, B, C, D, E, F, G, H). Research is currently focusing on the identification of HIV subtypes and strains in different populations and geographic areas. For example, in the United States, Europe, and Australia, most infected persons have HIV-1, subtype B, whereas in India, HIV-2 is found near Goa, and HIV-1 strains A, B, and C are also present.[6]

Transmission

HIV-1 and HIV-2 are relatively weak viruses outside of the body. HIV viruses can infect people through three major types of transmission: sexual transmission via semen or vaginal and cervical secretions through homosexual, bisexual, or heterosexual intercourse; parenteral transmission via blood, blood products, or blood-contaminated needles or syringes; and perinatal transmission in utero, during delivery, or in breast milk. Of these forms of transmission, sexual transmission through unprotected vaginal or anal intercourse is the most common mode of infection globally. In very low titers, HIV is known to be present but has not been shown to be transmitted via urine, saliva, tears, cerebrospinal fluid, amniotic fluid, and feces. HIV is not known to be transmitted via aerosol routes. In the United States, those at greatest risk of HIV infection include (1) men having sex with men (MSM); (2) intravenous drug users (IVDs) who share needles or syringes; (3) sexual partners of those in high-risk groups, particularly heterosexual women; and (4) infants born to infected mothers. Heterosexual intercourse with infected partners, contact with contaminated blood, and prenatal or perinatal exposure of the infant prenatally are the major routes of transmission of HIV in Africa, South and Southeast Asia, and developing countries.[1] In these countries, an equal proportion of males and females are infected.

Common modes of transmission include needle/syringe sharing between intravenous drug users, unprotected sex with infected partners, recipients of HIV-contaminated blood or blood products or infected semen during artificial insemination, unanticipated needle or scalpel

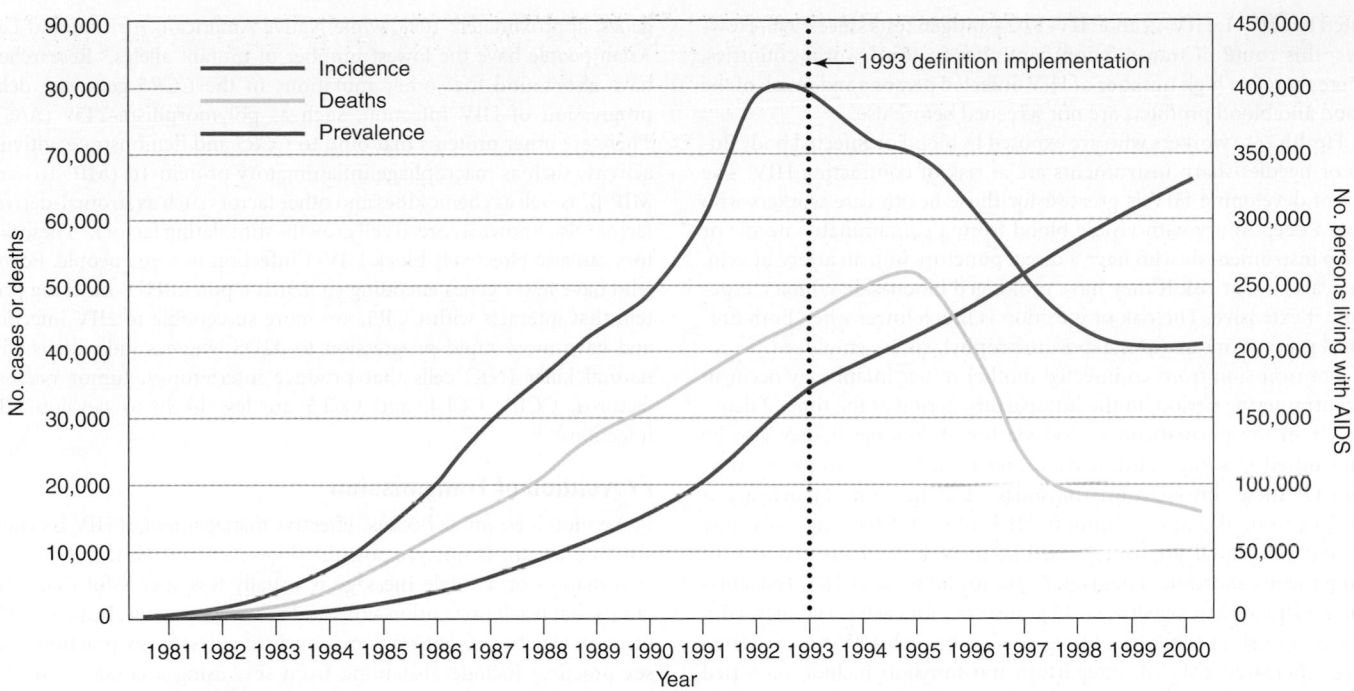

FIGURE 12-1 Estimated AIDS incidence and deaths among persons with AIDS, by year of diagnosis or death and year-end prevalence, United States, 1981 to 2000. Data were adjusted for delays in reporting of cases and deaths. (From Update: AIDS—United States, 2000, *MMWR Morb Mortal Wkly Rep* 51[27]:592-595, 2002.)

TABLE 12-2 HIV HISTORY TIMELINE

1900	Retroviruses identified as cause of cancer in chickens
1930s	HIV-1 precursor virus crossed species from chimpanzees to humans during hunting from contact with infected chimpanzee blood
1950s	Positive tests on serum from man in Leopoldville (now Kinshasa) Congo
1960s	Virus reaches Haiti
1968	First case in U.S. in sexually active 15-year-old African-American male in St. Louis
1980	First retrovirus identified in humans affecting T cells (human T cell lymphocytic virus, HTLV-1)
1981	Syndrome of HIV first reported in healthy young homosexual men in LA and New York
1982	Identification of HIV transmission by blood/blood products with first use of term AIDS
	Syndrome also identified in women, infants, Haitians, and persons who had received blood or blood products
1983	CDC publishes first Blood and Body Fluid Precautions
	First WHO meeting on AIDS
1985	First HIV-1 antibody testing (ELISA and Western Blot)
	First international conference on AIDS
1987	HIV-2 identified in visitor to U.S. from West Africa
	First anti-HIV drug approved
	CDC revises guidelines with identification of mucocutaneous exposure – "Universal Blood and Body Fluid Precautions"
1988	World Health Organization (WHO) declares December 1 as World AIDS Day
1994	CDC announces that AIDS is leading cause of death among Americans 25 to 44 years old
1996	Combination antiretroviral therapy (HAART) is introduced
1999	Researchers discover origins of HIV-1 from chimpanzee species (see 1930s)
2006	WHO declares March 8 as National Women's & Girls HIV/AIDS Awareness Day
	SMART trial found that episodic antiretroviral therapy more than doubles risk of AIDS or death in people with HIV infection

injury during care or surgical treatment of infected patients, and neonatal transmission from an infected mother to her infant. In both men and women, concomitant sexually transmitted diseases or genital lesions increase the risk of HIV infection. In women, high-risk heterosexual contact is influenced by lack of HIV knowledge, low socioeconomic status, low perception of risk, concomitant drug or alcohol use, relationship dynamics such as fear of abuse or loss of relationship, and the increased biological vulnerability of HIV contraction during vaginal

intercourse, especially in the presence of other sexually transmitted diseases or vaginal inflammation. In both men and women, the use of non-injection drugs (such as crack cocaine) contributes to HIV transmission by decreasing inhibition, allowing the person to engage in risky sexual behaviors or to trade sexual relations for drugs, money, or shelter.

Blood bank screening and testing procedures have nearly eliminated the transmission of HIV-contaminated blood in the United States. In the United States, all blood and blood products have been tested by HIV-1, HIV-2, and HIV-1 p24 antigen tests since 1996. However, this route of transmission continues in third world countries, where there is a high number of HIV-infected persons and much of the blood and blood products are not screened before use.

Health care workers who are exposed to blood or infected body fluids or needles/sharp instruments are at risk of contracting HIV. The risk of developing HIV is greatest for those health care workers who have a deep injury with visible blood from a contaminated needle or sharp instrument or who have a direct puncture into an artery or vein. They also are at risk if they have prolonged blood-skin contact, especially if extensive. The risk of infection is much lower when both universal precautions and postexposure prophylaxis are employed.

Transmission from an infected mother to her infant may occur in the intrauterine period, in the intrapartum period at the time of delivery, or in the postpartum period via breast feeding; it may also be transmitted in some cultures from saliva attributable to premastication. Of these, intrapartum transmission at the time of delivery is thought to be the most common. HIV infection does not cause any specific congenital abnormalities, but there is an increased risk of spontaneous abortion. The overall risk to the fetus of HIV transmission is estimated to be between 15% and 40% for each pregnancy, with increasing risk in subsequent pregnancies for each HIV-positive fetus born. Increased risks of antepartum transmission include increased maternal viral load or high viremia during early infection, advanced maternal clinical disease as evidenced by low CD4+ counts, and breaks in the placental barrier. Increased risks of intrapartum transmission include high maternal viral load at the time of delivery, prolonged ruptured membranes (more than 4 hours), infant exposure to blood/secretions, abruptio placentae, infant prematurity, and the presence of coinfections. The rate of HIV perinatal transmission is reduced with the use of antiretroviral therapy during pregnancy and during the first months of the infant's life.

Routine social contact with people who are HIV positive does not increase one's risk of HIV infection. The following examples are safe practices and will not cause exposure to HIV infection: using public restrooms, swimming in public swimming pools, touching or hugging someone who is HIV positive, and eating with community utensils or in restaurants. Insects such as mosquitoes cannot transmit the HIV virus to humans.

Exposure to HIV does not mean that one will contract HIV or AIDS, and it does not mean rapid progression. The interacting forces between viral and host factors influence whether a person will contract HIV infection, particularly the amount and virulence of the virus and the host's response by T cell–mediated cytotoxicity or by cytokines. For example, a woman's plasma viral load may predict the amount of her genital HIV viral shedding, which may influence the exposure to HIV virion by her sexual partner.[7] In studies of patients with hemophilia who received tainted blood products, 10% to 25% of the individuals evaded infection. Because of genetic differences that either increase or decrease susceptibility to the infection, the risk of acquiring HIV and the response to infection also vary within populations.[8] Despite infection for more than 10 years, some infected individuals remain symptom free; and some individuals, despite high-risk exposure, do not exhibit any signs of infection or immunodeficiency.[8]

Researchers have identified an HIV resistance mutation of the *CCR5* gene, called *CCR5-delta 32*, which is associated with natural resistance to HIV infection in certain people.[8] When inherited from both parents, the mutant *CCR5-delta 32* gene appears to protect individuals from infection even after multiple exposures. When only one gene is inherited, the progression to AIDS tends to be slower.[8] The *CCR5* gene is not equally distributed among people. Persons of Caucasian-American and Caucasian-European descent have the highest number of mutant allele

genes, approximately 10%, while Native American, African, and East Asian people have the lowest number of mutant alleles.[8] Researchers have also found that other mutations in the *CCR5* gene can delay progression of HIV infection, such as polymorphism-2459 (A/G).[8] There are other proteins that bind to *CCR5* and demonstrate antiviral activity, such as macrophage inflammatory protein-1α (MIP-1α) and MIP-β, as well as chemokines and other factors such as stromal-derived factor (also known as pre-B cell growth–stimulating factor).[9] These factors can also effectively block HIV-1 infection in some people. People who have fewer genes encoding CCL3L1, a potent HIV-blocking protein that interacts with CCR5, are more susceptible to HIV infection and have more rapid progression to AIDS whereas individuals with natural killer (NK) cells that produce interferon-γ, tumor necrosis factor-α, CCL3, CCL4, and CCL5 are less likely to develop HIV infection.[8-10]

Prevention of Transmission

Prevention is essential, because effective management of HIV is expensive and a cure is not yet possible. However, one-time exposure to information or a single message is usually less successful than programs that teach prevention skills and reinforce positive behavior. The primary way to prevent transmission is to use safe sex practices. Safe sex practices include abstaining from sex, using a condom (barrier protection) during sexual intercourse, avoiding multiple sexual partners, and knowing the HIV status of all sexual partners. It is important that education regarding safe sex practices be tailored to appropriate age groups, ethnicity, culture, and sexual preference. Patient visits to health care providers are an excellent opportunity to encourage individual HIV protection.

Spermicides such as nonoxynol 9 or C31G do not inactivate HIV or other sexually transmitted microorganisms. No studies suggest any benefit from using progestins such as levonorgestrel (Norplant) or medroxyprogesterone (Depo-Provera), the diaphragm, or oral contraceptives to prevent HIV transmission. The early use of antepartum and intrapartum antiretroviral therapy and avoidance of breast feeding can prevent maternal-child HIV infection.

HIV infection in drug users can be prevented with the use of sterile needles via improved access to clean needles and avoidance of dirty or shared needles. Such intervention includes needle/syringe exchange programs for IVDs and cleaning of dirty needles with bleach before use. When using bleach, the user must rinse out all blood first; then fill the needle and syringe with full-strength bleach at least three times for 30 to 60 seconds.

Medical and health care personnel are at risk through occupational exposure to blood and body fluids. Self-protection through the use of standard precautions can decrease risk by reducing exposure. Health care providers should carefully wash their hands before and immediately after patient contact even when using gloves. It is essential to wear disposable gloves for any actual or potential contact with blood or body secretions, when handling items contaminated with blood or body fluids, when performing finger sticks or heel sticks, or when the health care provider has scratches or cuts on the hand.

Gowns or plastic aprons, masks, goggles, or face shields should be worn to protect the face and clothing when there is risk of splashes and airborne droplets of blood or body fluids. Protective gear should be changed between patients. Careful prevention of parenteral exposure when using needles or other equipment should be emphasized. Needles and sharp implements should be disposed in rigid, puncture-proof containers. Such implements should not be bent, broken, or recapped before disposal. In combative patients who must have blood drawn or injections given, careful use of humane and limited restraint devices may be necessary to prevent injury to the involved health care workers. Resuscitation bags and masks should be readily available to minimize the need for mouth-to-mouth procedures.

Unfortunately, accidents necessitating the development of postexposure prevention protocols do occur. If a health care worker sustains an injury with significant exposure to HIV-infected blood or body fluids such as a needle stick, a workplace postexposure prevention protocol should be followed immediately. According to the U.S. Public Health Service and National Institutes of Health (NIH), the selection of a drug regimen for HIV postexposure prophylaxis must balance the risk for infection against potential toxicities and side effects of the medication(s). As such, consultation with an infectious disease provider is recommended. Treatment usually depends on knowledge of the viral status and/or viral load of the exposure source; this information will help determine the appropriate antiretroviral therapy regimen that should be implemented. Often postexposure protocols involve the administration of two or three medications. The length of administration of the agents depends on multiple factors and may be 4 weeks or longer. This same protocol has been advocated for use as post-sexual exposure prophylaxis.

KEY POINTS

- HIV disease is a primary immunodeficiency disorder caused by viral infection of CD4+ cells. It is a major health concern because it causes chronic, severe, long-term disease in industrialized countries with access to medication, care, and prevention. In third world countries where therapy is unavailable, the prognosis for HIV is very poor and death is more likely.
- HIV types 1 and 2 are retroviruses that primarily infect CD4+ lymphocytes and macrophages. HIV-1 is the primary causative virus infecting persons in Central Africa, the United States, Europe, and Australia.
- HIV is acquired primarily through sexual transmission via semen and vaginal and cervical secretions; through parenteral transmission via blood, blood products, and contaminated needles/syringes; and through perinatal transmission from an infected mother to her infant antepartum, intrapartum, and postpartum via breast milk.
- HIV is known to be present in but is not believed to be transmitted via urine, saliva, tears, cerebrospinal fluid, amniotic fluid, feces, or aerosols.
- Those at greatest risk of HIV infection include homosexual and bisexual men, IVDs who share needles or syringes, sexual partners of those in high-risk groups, and infants born to infected mothers.
- The use of safe sex practices (such as condoms) and safe parenteral practices (such as sterile needles/syringes) decreases the risk of infection.
- Exposure to blood and body fluids of infected individuals through skin, mucous membranes, and accidental needle sticks is the primary risk factor for health care workers. The universal use of standard precautions decreases the risk of infection.
- After significant accidental exposure to HIV-infected blood or body fluids, it is recommended that health care workers receive postexposure antiretroviral medication as soon as possible after exposure and as needed for 4 weeks following the incident.

ETIOLOGY

HIV Structure

HIV is an RNA retrovirus that causes a defect in cell-mediated immunity that may progress to AIDS. The viral RNA must be converted to DNA before the viral genes can be expressed to make copies of the RNA virus. Like other retroviruses, HIV differs from DNA viruses in that the RNA genome cannot replicate without undergoing conversion into DNA.

HIV consists of a core or nucleocapsid containing two strands or chains of RNA, protein, and enzymes surrounded and protected by a spherical lipid bilayer viral envelope that is 0.0001 mm in diameter. Between the envelope and core is a protein layer called p17. The nucleocapsid or core is composed of a protein called p24. Within the nucleocapsid, the two strands of RNA compose the HIV genome (Figure 12-2). The HIV genome consists of at least nine genes. The *gag* gene encodes the core antigen proteins. The *pol* gene encodes reverse transcriptase proteins. The *env* gene encodes the viral envelope protein glycoprotein gp160, which is split into two fragments, gp120 and gp41, by cellular protease.

Several other genes have been identified, including *tat, rev, nef, vif, vpr,* and *vpu*. These genes are primarily regulatory genes. The *tat* gene encodes proteins that regulate HIV replication and can accelerate HIV viral protein production. It is controlled by *tat*-binding protein. The *rev* gene encodes proteins that regulate viral messenger RNA expression. Rev proteins inhibit regulatory proteins, allowing the transport of HIV RNA from the nucleus. Rev proteins also enhance viral structural gene production. The *vif* (virion infectivity factor) gene appears to increase the ability of the virus to infect other cells. It suppresses the human protein (CEM 15) that inhibits HIV-1.

The HIV genome contains all the information regulating the virus's structural format and growth during its life cycle. The enzymes within the core also are very important because they facilitate the conversion of RNA to DNA. This conversion is the means of information transfer. The enzymes include reverse transcriptase, integrase, and protease. Reverse transcriptase is composed of two associated enzymes called polymerase and ribonuclease. It is the unique enzyme in HIV that allows the virus to copy RNA into DNA. Protease is a complex enzyme that works as a "molecular scissors." It splits the other viral components by a process known as autocatalysis. Immature, noninfectious virions containing inactive gag/pol, a long precursor protein, are released in the plasma, where they are cleaved by protease into smaller active units. Protease also clips p55, the core gag viral protein precursor, into smaller molecules and is needed to facilitate final mature viral assembly for HIV to be infectious.[11] In other words, HIV infection does not occur unless *protease* activates the virions.

The viral envelope consists of a membrane derived from the host cell. Viral glycoprotein studs protruding from the cell membrane make it look like a studded ball (Figure 12-3). Gp120 and gp41 are the two HIV envelope proteins that cover the viral particle surface. Gp120 is

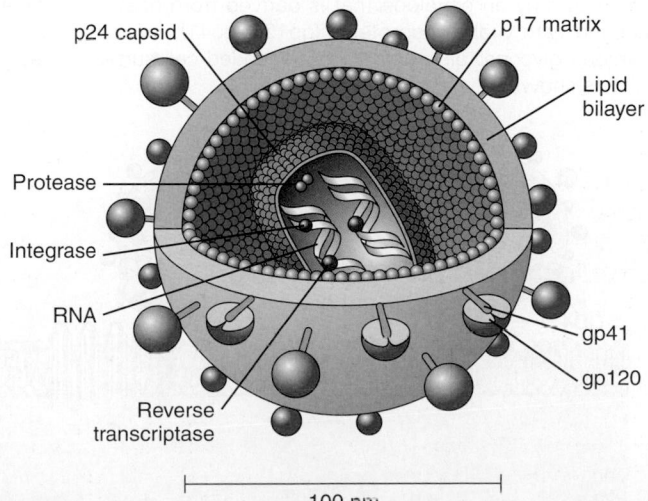

FIGURE 12-2 HIV particle showing the p24 capsid protein surrounding the two strands of viral RNA.

the most external and distal part of each "stud," whereas gp41 is the bridge that holds it onto the virion surface. The surface envelope also contains other cell surface proteins derived from the host cell containing adhesion molecules. Although the viral particle (virion) is nearly spherical, great diversity is found in size and shape, such as comet-shaped virions and virions with tails.

HIV Binding and Infection

Once inside the body, HIV particles are attracted to cells with receptors on their surface called CD4. The HIV envelope protein gp120 specifically binds to the CD4 receptor. The specific CD4+ cells that are attracted to the virus change over time. The CD4 receptor is found on many types of cells, including T cells, microglial cells, monocyte-macrophages, follicular dendritic cells, immortalized B cells, retinal cells, Langerhans cells in the skin, bone marrow stem cells, cervical cells, bone marrow–derived circulating dendritic cells, and enterochromaffin cells in the colon, duodenum, and rectum. Of these cells, the CD4+ T helper/inducer cells and macrophages are most often implicated and involved in the process of infection. Figure 12-4 illustrates a group of HIV-infected CD4+ cells imaged by scanning electron micrography. Initially the virus is attracted to macrophages and the virus is called "M tropic." Later the virus either becomes dual tropic and affects both macrophages and T cells, or becomes "T tropic" and affects primarily T cells. During heterosexual transmission of HIV, the virus is attracted to Langerhans cells in the mucosal membranes mediated through the CD4/CCR5 pathway.[12] Later the virus becomes attracted to other cells in the body, primarily T cells, and is "T tropic."

Usually T cells are infected before the onset of symptoms. CD4+ T cells are composed of two subsets: T helper-1 (T_H1) and T helper-2 (T_H2). The T_H1 subset produces interferon-γ and interleukin-2 (IL-2). The T_H2 subset produces IL-4, IL-6, and IL-10. Of these two subsets, the one that is markedly decreased in advanced disease is T_H1.

However, CD4 alone is not sufficient for fusion of the virion and host cell. A number of important coreceptors on the target cells called chemokines are necessary for the virus to gain entry into cells.[13] These important chemokine coreceptors must be present for the virion to fuse with the host cell. The chemokine called CCR5 must be present for the HIV particles to bind to the CD4+ cells in early infection during the M-tropic phase, and another chemokine receptor named CXCR4 must be present in later infection during the T-tropic phase.[13] Since 1996 when the coreceptors were first discovered, a number of other coreceptors have been identified, including APJ, CCR2b, CCR3, CCR8, CCR9, CX3CR1, CXCR4, GPR1, GPR15, STRL33, US28, and V28. The function of most of these coreceptors is unknown. It is hypothesized that some of the coreceptors may be needed for various strains of HIV, for HIV infection in infants and children, or for infection of the brain and nervous system.

The gp120 portion of the virion envelope must combine with the first receptor, CD4, and then change shape by refolding. In the second shape, it combines with the second receptor, either CCR5 or CXCR4, to fuse with the cell. Once the HIV particle is bound to both the CD4 receptor and the chemokine receptor on the host cell, gp41 implants itself in the cell membrane (Figure 12-5). This sequence of events causes the viral particle and the cell to fuse. The core of the virus is then injected into the cytoplasm of the host cell and infection is produced. The gp120 portion of the virion envelope is "hyper-variable in

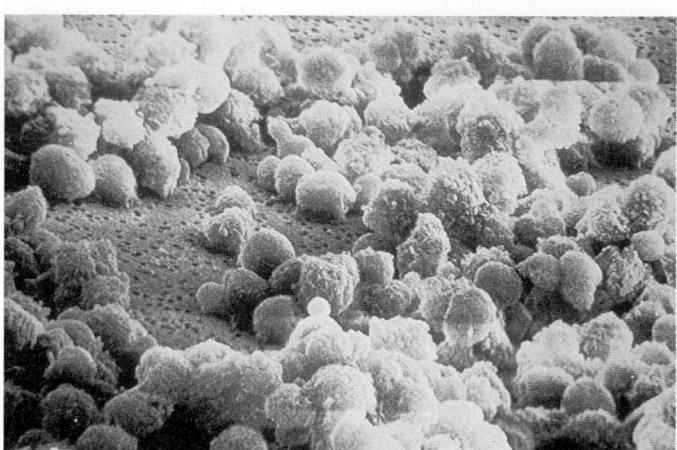

FIGURE 12-4 Scanning electron micrograph (low magnification) of a population of HIV-infected lymphocytes. (Courtesy Centers for Disease Control and Prevention, Atlanta.)

FIGURE 12-3 Schematic view of a retrovirus particle. The core is surrounded by an envelope that is derived from host membranes enriched with viral glycoproteins (gp120, gp41). Interaction of the envelope glycoproteins with a host-encoded cell surface receptor (CD4) is shown.

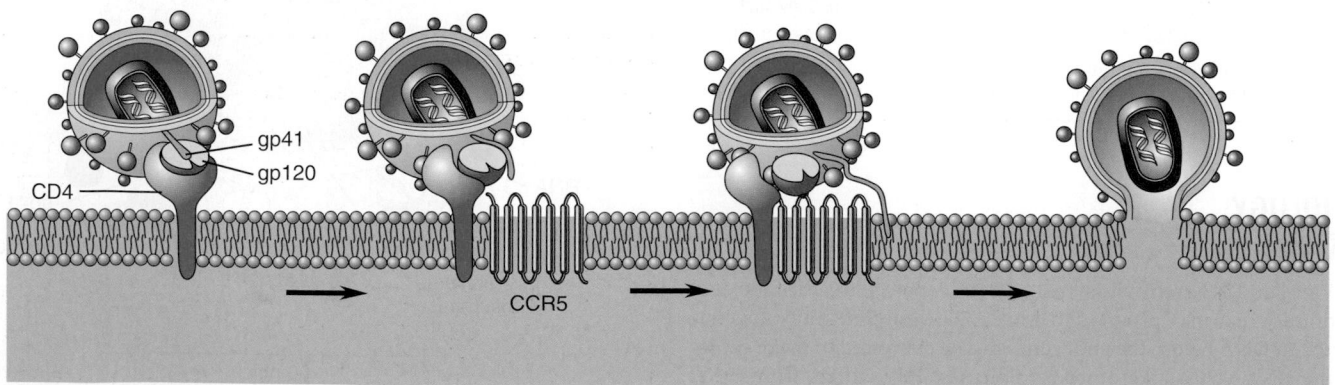

FIGURE 12-5 Early HIV infection, M tropic. In HIV infection, the virus must bind both a CD4 receptor and a coreceptor to fuse with the host cell. In the M-tropic phase, the key coreceptor is CCR5.

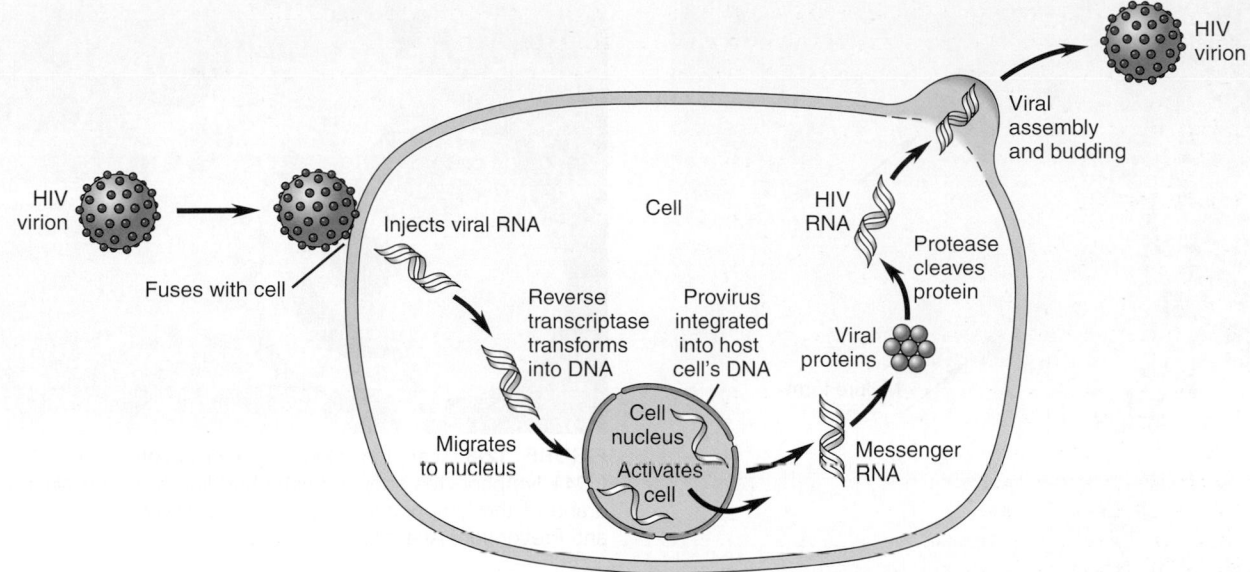

FIGURE 12-6 HIV life cycle. A schematic representation from the time of initial HIV fusion with a host cell, to integration into the host cell's DNA, and ending with the replication of a new virion.

sequence," which allows for the flexibility of the protein loops that permits the virion to escape neutralizing antibodies.[13]

Once in the cytoplasm, a single-stranded DNA copy is made by reverse transcriptase from the viral RNA. Using the single-stranded DNA as a template, DNA polymerase copies it to make a second DNA strand and destroys the original RNA strands. The accuracy of DNA transcription is poor, with mutations occurring frequently. This tendency to mutate makes HIV highly resistant to antiviral medications.

Once formed, the new viral DNA, called viral provirus or preintegration complexes (PICs), migrates to the cell nucleus and is actively transported in the nuclear compartment.[14] Inside the nucleus, integrase splices the viral DNA, or **provirus,** into the host cell's DNA. Once in the host cell's DNA, the viral DNA is replicated together with the host cell's DNA during every cell division. Now the viral DNA is permanently part of the host cell's DNA (Figure 12-6).

The process of building new virus particles begins within the host cell's DNA. Segments at the end of the viral genome instruct the host cell to make RNA copies of the viral DNA. Some of the genes direct the host cell to manufacture viral envelope proteins (gene name: *env*) and enzymes (gene name: *pol*), whereas other RNA strands become future genetic material (gene name: *gag*). The HIV DNA then hijacks cellular protein pathways to produce the proteins needed for replication of HIV.[14] In the nucleus of the cell, there is an interaction between the host cellular kinases and the HIV DNA that affects the HIV replication cycle.[14-15] Sometimes the host cell produces kinases or factors that aid viral integration and sometimes there are kinases or factors that inhibit viral integration by recognizing and neutralizing infecting retroviral DNA.[15] New studies are also demonstrating that not all proviral DNA is integrated into the cell's DNA and yet the proviral DNA can still synthesize viral gene products and replicate within the cell assisted by the expression of *tat* and *nef*.[15]

To cause further infection, the viral RNA must be produced, leave the nucleus, and migrate to the cell surface. Rev proteins along with a human protein called CRM1 aid in the process of transporting the viral RNA proteins from the cell nucleus. A human RNA helicase enzyme, DDX3, helps to straighten HIV's twisted strand of RNA before threading it through a small pore in the nucleus. The assembly of new virus particles, called **virions,** occurs at the cell membrane. Three proteins are produced and migrate to the cell periphery, attach to the cell membrane,

and cause the viral material to bud out from the membrane. The protein-cutting enzyme protease separates the envelope proteins from enzymes and RNA genetic material and binds the viral core (Figure 12-7). Therefore, the completed virion has a host cell membrane from which the envelope proteins gp120 and gp41 protrude like spikes.

When CD4+ cells decline, the diversity of CD4+ cells is affected. With antiretroviral therapy, the naive T cells that can respond to new infections persist in low numbers despite an increase in memory T cells. Therefore, persons with HIV who are receiving antiretroviral therapy can respond to old but not new infections. This phase is indicative of deterioration in immune system function despite any temporary increase in CD4+ cell counts and decreased viral load from antiretroviral therapy.

Exposure to HIV-1 in epithelial cells (genital and gastrointestinal) and subsequent transmission and infection following exposure are incompletely understood. These processes involve multiple and complex interactions between HIV, cytokines, and CD4 cells. With HIV exposure, proinflammatory cytokines are produced by epithelial cells. Among the proinflammatory cytokines, tumor necrosis factor-α (TNF-α) is produced, which impairs the tight epithelial junctional barrier and allows migration of HIV and bacteria to move or translocate across the epithelium.[15] Infection in the presence of inflammation is also influenced by the presence of CD4+ macrophages or Langerhans cells that lie directly under the epithelial cells. Macrophages may also release tumor necrosis factor or other cytokines stimulating other antigen-presenting cells, or T cells.[16]

KEY POINTS

- HIV is an RNA virus known as a retrovirus. It must undergo reverse transcription within infected cells to form viral DNA.
- HIV consists of a nucleocapsid containing two strands of RNA, protein, and enzymes surrounded by a spherical lipid bilayer viral envelope. At least nine genes comprise the HIV genome.
- The HIV genome contains all the information regulating the virus's structural format and growth, including the conversion of RNA to DNA.
- The enzymes needed to convert HIV RNA to DNA include reverse transcriptase, integrase, and protease.
- HIV gains access to CD4+ cells by attaching to the CD4 receptor on the cell surface. Viral envelope protein gp120 and coreceptor chemokines such as CCR5 or CXCR4 mediate attachment.

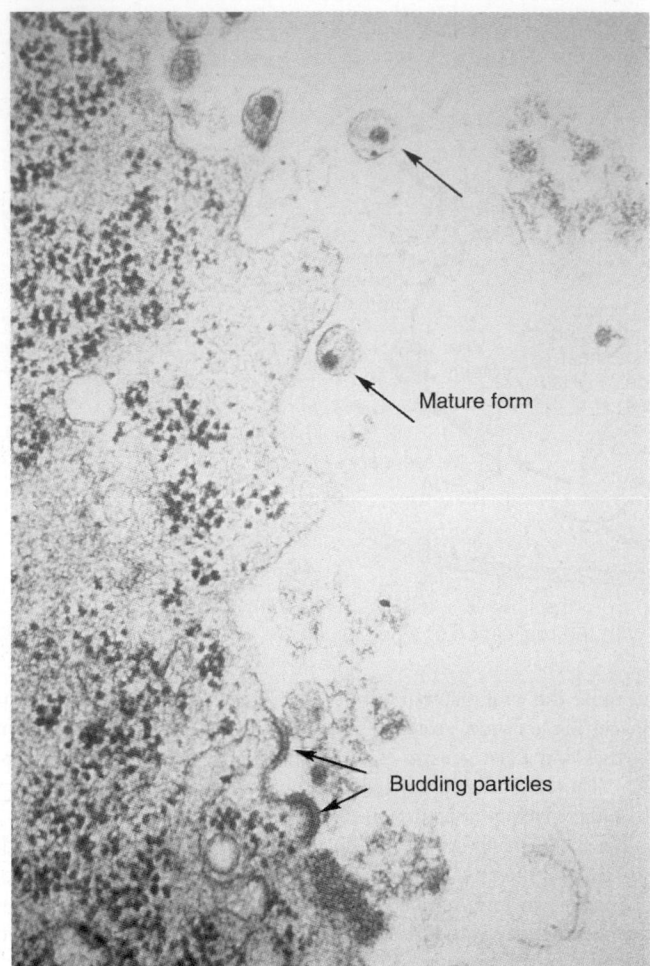

FIGURE 12-7 HIV-1/lymphadenopathy virus found in a hemophiliac patient with AIDS. Virus particles range in size from 90 to 120 nm. Viral budding and the production of new virions are facilitated by protease. (Courtesy Centers for Disease Control and Prevention, Atlanta.)

PATHOGENESIS

Effect of HIV on Immune Cells at the Cellular Level

The hallmark of HIV infection is the decrease in the number of CD4+ T helper/inducer lymphocytes. T helper/inducer cells are necessary for appropriate immune responsiveness because they are the cells that mediate between the antigen-presenting cells, other immune cells such as B cells, and other T cells. During acute and chronic untreated HIV infection, the immune system is in a hyperactive state with high T-cell death, nonspecific T cell activation, polyclonal activation of B cells, and elevated levels of proinflammatory cytokines.[17]

Macrophages have CD4 receptors and act as both targets and reservoirs for HIV. As the infection progresses, they become more functionally impaired with defective phagocytosis and chemotaxis, abnormal antigen presentation, and abnormal cytokine production. They also contribute to the T-cell decline by increasing CD4+ cell death.

Humoral immune system dysfunction is also present, although the effect of HIV on antibody-producing B cells is more poorly understood. There are changes in B cell structure and function. B cell numbers usually remain normal but they are progressively dysfunctional with overproduction of nonessential antibodies, as well as failure to respond appropriately to normal immune system signals.[18]

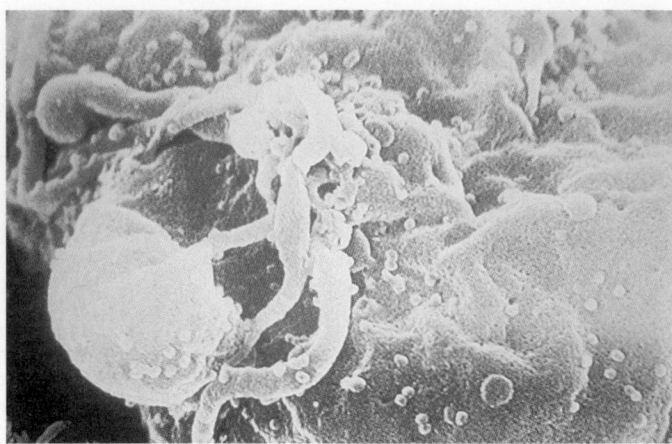

FIGURE 12-8 Scanning electron micrograph of HIV-1–infected CD4+ lymphocytes showing virus budding from the plasma membrane of the lymphocytes. (Courtesy Centers for Disease Control and Prevention, Atlanta.)

Immunoglobulin G1 (IgG1) and IgG3 levels are usually elevated, causing hypergammaglobulinemia. IgM levels are elevated in early infection, whereas IgA levels are elevated in late infection. Despite these elevations, the responsiveness to bacterial cell wall (polysaccharide) antigens that require CD4+ cell activation of B cells is decreased. Immune complexes are increased, and B-cell differentiation and response to antigens are decreased. Autoantibodies, especially against erythrocytes, platelets, lymphocytes, neutrophils, nuclear proteins, myelin, and spermatozoa, occur either in association with disease processes (e.g., HIV-associated thrombocytopenia) or spontaneously. HIV antibodies are produced, but they are ineffective against the disease. Also B cells have an increased risk of cell death through apoptosis.[16]

The envelope glycoproteins (gp120 and gp41) on the surface of HIV virions are the reason for successful HIV infection. The immunogenic portions of the viral envelope glycoproteins are well disguised and variable—most likely because of the large amount of carbohydrate on the surface of gp120.[13] Within the human body, high-carbohydrate substances look like "self" to the immune system. Therefore, the virus "hides" under the cover of the glycosylation. Another factor that allows HIV envelope proteins to escape the early antibodies is the way that gp120 and gp41 are bound together. Although the interface between gp120 and gp41 is an area that is highly immunogenic, the gp120 and gp41 molecules are noncovalently bonded together. Early antibodies cannot bind the assembled, functional envelope glycoprotein complex. Later, neutralizing antibodies are effective against the complex, but by that time the infection is well established.

Viral Production and Cell Death

A key element in the success of HIV infection is that HIV replicates prolifically from the onset of infection. It generates so many virions that it overwhelms the body's defenses. Because HIV is primarily a mucosal disease, the gastrointestinal (GI) tract is the major site of HIV replication.[17] Within the first 3 to 6 weeks and continuing throughout the infection, HIV replication is high in the lamina propria CD4 T cells of the GI tract.[17] HIV infection is characterized by a high level of virion turnover (HIV replication) and a high level of CD4+ cell turnover (host cell death). HIV-infected CD4+ cells undergo viral budding to generate and produce new virions (Figure 12-8). At least 10 billion HIV particles are produced and destroyed each day, with a plasma virus half-life of 6 hours and an acutely infected T-cell half-life of 1.1 days. Total T-cell numbers in acute HIV infection decline sharply, but with continuing infection blood T-cell numbers rebound slightly as a result of antiviral immune responses whereas GI T cell numbers remain low. In children infected with HIV, the virus is more aggressive and leads more rapidly to immune system dysfunction.

The production of new virus is variable between individuals and dependent on the host's cellular activity, as well as the interaction between HIV regulatory genes *(tat, nef, rev, vif)*. In some cells, such as T cells, HIV can lie dormant until activated. In other cells, such as macrophages and monocytes, RNA copies of HIV are consistently being made and released, initially without destruction of the host cell. Other host cellular factors that influence viral production of HIV include inhibition by other proteins or low concentrations of initiation factors.

There are other proteins in the body that can repress or inhibit HIV-1 if present in the cell. One of these is the delta 32 mutation in the *CCR5* gene, which involves the chemokine coreceptor needed for HIV to infect cells.[18] Other inflammatory proteins from macrophages decrease the probability of becoming infected with HIV-1 and promote recovery of the CD4 cells after starting therapy, including macrophage inflammatory protein-1α (MIP-1α/CCL3) and macrophage inflammatory protein-1β (MIP-1β/CCL4).[18] HLA-B57 and HLA-B27, part of the major histocompatibility complex alleles, have been found to target several gag epitopes inducing cytolytic destruction of infected cells.[18] Natural killer (NK) cells and macrophages secrete soluble factors that can inhibit HIV infection including TNF-α, interferon, and chemokines CCL3, CCL4, and CCL5. The chemokines tend to compete with the virus for cell adhesion because of their attraction to CCR5.[18] Interferon type 1 also inhibits HIV cell adhesion and induces apoptosis of HIV-1–infected CD4 T cells.[18] These factors have been associated with lower viral loads and improved survival.

Long-term survivors with HIV often have a lower viral load and strong CD8[+] killer T-cell activity. The CD8[+] killer T-cell activity suppresses viral replication and thus slows progression of the disease, especially in the early stages of the disease. It is also thought that a strong immunologic defense preserves the manufacture of CD4[+] T cells that especially recognize and react to HIV. If this ability is lost, these cells may not regenerate, even with treatment. The presence of a weaker strain of HIV, particularly during the M-tropic phase, may also lead to longer survival.

Once viral production starts or restarts in activated cells, death of the infected cells may occur by a variety of mechanisms. Cells may die from the accumulation of intracellular viral DNA or from the loss of normal cellular protein synthesis because of the infection. Some cell death may occur due to the action of natural killer T cells. Most methods of host cell death involve the envelope protein gp120 or immune processes. Cross-linking of CD4 and gp120 can trigger automatic preprogrammed T-cell death **(apoptosis)**. *Apoptosis is the major mechanism of CD4 T cell depletion.*[19] CD4 and gp120 cross-linking can also cause the cell to stop dividing and decreases the cell's ability to fight new infections—a condition called **anergy.** Profuse viral production with multiple CD4 receptors in close proximity can rip holes in the cell membrane and cause host cell death (Figure 12-9). Multiple virion buds with gp120 on their surfaces attach to the surrounding host cell membrane CD4 receptors. This attachment causes tearing of the host cell membrane with subsequent cellular edema and death.[17] Viral proteins, such as *nef, vpr,* or *tat,* also contribute to the causes of cell death in HIV. Microvesicles containing *nef* protein released into the blood can cause *nef*-induced apoptosis associated with death receptors on a cell surface or by triggering the intrinsic pathway.[17] *Tat* protein can disrupt mitochondrial function, and trigger extrinsic and intrinsic

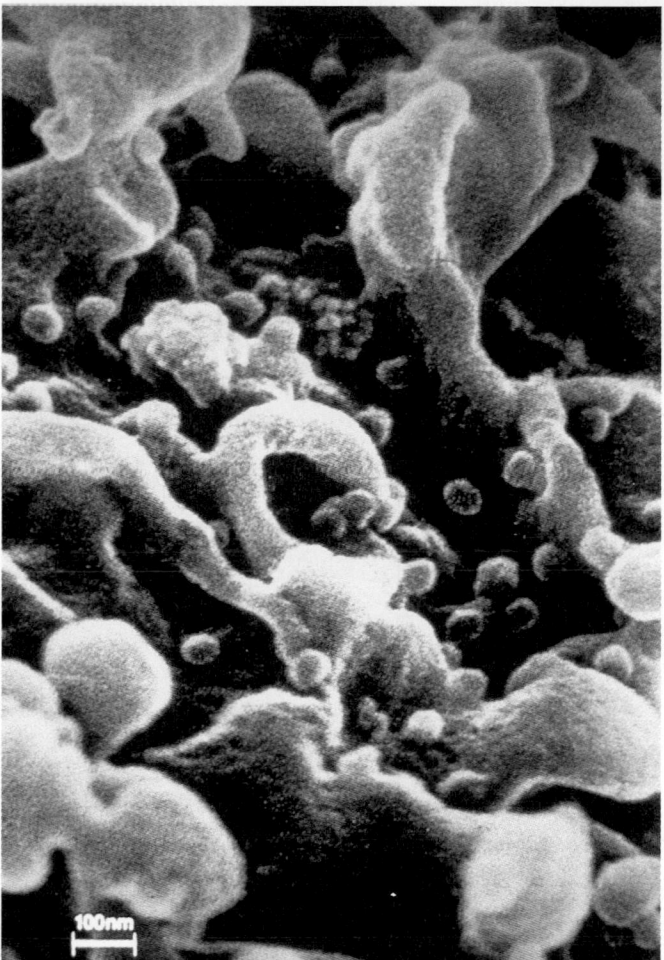

FIGURE 12-9 High magnification of a CD4+ lymphocyte infected with HIV-1. Note the large number of budding HIV virions, which can lead to host cell death by membrane tearing or syncytium formation. (Courtesy Centers for Disease Control and Prevention, Atlanta.)

apoptosis pathways.[17] *Vpr* either directly or indirectly causes induction of apoptosis because it causes cell cycle arrest and/or the intrinsic pathway.[17]

Another process of cell death occurs when multiple uninfected cells become fused together with infected cells by the virus. This mass of cells, called a **syncytium,** can lead to a large number of cell deaths from a single event. During the T-tropic phase, there is a greater tendency to produce syncytia, causing even faster depletion of T cells. Myeloid-derived dendritic cells (MDDCs) aid in the formation of syncytia when they patrol the body, engulfing the virus and presenting the virus to T cells. During this presentation, virus, receptors, and coreceptors are in close proximity, facilitating infection as well as the development of a syncytium.

Cell death can occur when the immune system makes antibodies to the viral envelope protein. When gp120 is shed, it can bind to uninfected CD4 receptors. The immune system then attacks the uninfected but antibody-coated cells via the complement system (antibody-dependent cellular cytotoxicity) or killer T cells. Cell death can also be secondary to a type III hypersensitivity reaction. As discussed earlier, gp120 and gp41 hide from the immune system because of the large amount of carbohydrate on the surface of gp120 and gp 41. The binding and glycosylation of gp120 and gp41 cause them to have characteristics

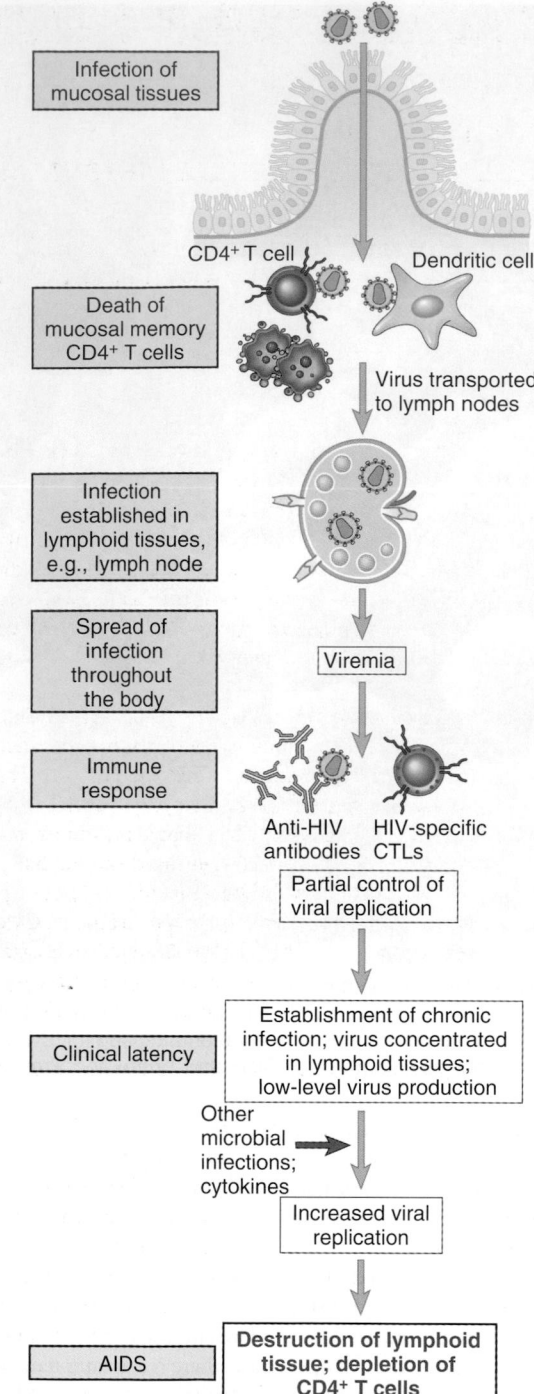

Infection of mucosal tissues

CD4⁺ T cell

Dendritic cell

Death of mucosal memory CD4⁺ T cells

Virus transported to lymph nodes

Infection established in lymphoid tissues, e.g., lymph node

Spread of infection throughout the body

Viremia

Immune response

Anti-HIV antibodies

HIV-specific CTLs

Partial control of viral replication

Clinical latency

Establishment of chronic infection; virus concentrated in lymphoid tissues; low-level virus production

Other microbial infections; cytokines

Increased viral replication

AIDS

Destruction of lymphoid tissue; depletion of CD4⁺ T cells

FIGURE 12-10 Progression of HIV infection. The clinical stages of HIV disease correlate with a progressive spread of HIV from the initial site of infection to lymphoid tissues throughout the body. The immune response of the host temporarily controls acute infection but does not prevent the establishment of chronic infection of cells in the lymphoid tissues. Cytokine stimuli induced by other microbes serve to enhance HIV production and progression to AIDS. *CTLs,* Cytotoxic T lymphocytes. (From Abbas AK et al: *Cellular and molecular immunology,* ed 6, Philadelphia, 2007, Saunders, p 481.)

similar to those of major histocompatibility class (MHC) antigens. In this case, immune system cells may fail to recognize the difference between gp120 and "self MHC markers" causing them to attack normal cells as "nonself." This phenomenon causes immune cells to attack and destroy large numbers of T cells. Cells also may be affected by T cell–mediated cytotoxicity or by cytokines and inflammation resulting from infection.

Progression of HIV Infection from Seroconversion to AIDS

HIV disease infection progresses over time to AIDS with many manifestations. AIDS is a syndrome, not a disease, which means that the virus can express itself in many ways. No one symptom typifies either HIV infection or AIDS. However, groups of signs and symptoms are useful in staging progress of the infection. HIV is characterized by two major phases: acute and chronic.

Once the HIV virion enters the body, it rapidly replicates (Figure 12-10). HIV is present in the blood and cerebrospinal fluid but is not detected by usual laboratory tests because no antibodies have formed yet. Usually no symptoms are present. It is a time of rapid virus replication with widespread attack of CD4+ T cells in mucosal membranes, especially in the gastrointestinal (GI) system. The person is infectious but does not know it.

Seroconversion occurs when sufficient antibodies are detected in the blood, usually between 3 weeks and 6 months after exposure (range: 3 weeks to 14 months). At the time of seroconversion, the person experiences signs and symptoms of acute retroviral syndrome or primary HIV infection. Up to 80% of people newly infected with HIV have flulike symptoms that can mimic other viral illnesses. At this time, the symptoms of primary HIV infection include flulike or mononucleosis-like symptoms, such as fever, chills, headaches, nausea, vomiting, fatigue, weakness, arthralgias, sore throat, stiff neck, photophobia, irritability, and rash. The rash is not the same in everyone and may be maculopapular, vesicular, or urticarial. Encephalopathy may even develop. The CD4⁺ T-cell count is greater than 400 cells/μL. The number of white blood cells, including lymphocytes, is decreased except for an increased number of CD8⁺ T cells. The number of platelets is also decreased. The person has an elevated erythrocyte sedimentation rate. During this period, the HIV count in the blood and genital fluids is high and the individual is very infectious. Then, after 1 to 4 weeks, the symptoms disappear. However, HIV is still present and the person continues to be infectious throughout the rest of the course of the infection.

After this period of seroconversion, the patient experiences the clinical latency period, which may last for longer than 10 years (range: 3 to 12 years). During this period, seeded HIV replicates in the lymph nodes and gradually destroys lymph tissue over time. Antiviral immune activity is ongoing. Production of virus is maintained or stabilized at a set level. The person feels well but may experience chronic lymphadenopathy (enlargement of lymph nodes for more than 3 months) or mild general symptoms, including lack of energy, weight loss, frequent fevers, and sweats. The CD4⁺ T-cell count is greater than 400 cells/μL. Stabilization of the serum level of virus at a certain point is attributable to the antiviral response, the number of CD4⁺ cells, and the virulence of the HIV strain. During this period of asymptomatic or mild infection, large numbers of virions are produced, destroying the body's immune system. Up to 2 million viral particles can be produced daily. The lymphadenopathy is caused by a vigorous immune response against HIV infection. The key point is that although the infection is clinically asymptomatic or mildly symptomatic, the virus is active, not latent.

Immediately after the latency period of infection, a period of rapid virus production occurs for up to 18 months. It is hypothesized that the

TABLE 12-3   CDC HIV/AIDS CLASSIFICATION MATRIX

| | CLINICAL CATEGORIES | | |
CD4+ T CELL CATEGORIES	A ASYMPTOMATIC ACUTE HIV	B SYMPTOMATIC, NOT A OR C	C AIDS INDICATOR
≥500/μL	A1	B1	C1
200-499/μL	A2	B2	C2
<200/μL AIDS indicator T-cell count	A3	B3	C3

From Centers for Disease Control and Prevention: 1993 Revised Classification System for HIV Infection and Expanded Surveillance Case Definition for AIDS Among Adolescents and Adults, *MMWR Morb Mortal Wkly Rep* 41(RR-17):1-6, 1993.

destroyed lymph nodes are no longer capable of removing or holding virus, thus allowing viral escape into the bloodstream (viremia). During this time, a persistent and continuous drop in the CD4+ T cell count to less than 400/μL is taking place. The antiviral innate immune activity is less effective as the viral load (level of virus in the blood) increases. Also during this time, HIV can persist for years in pools of resting, memory CD4+ T cells. This pool of CD4+ T cells carries only provirus DNA and lacks HIV surface antigens, so they are not detected or destroyed by the immune system.

As the viral loads increase and the immune system declines, the patient enters the stage of symptomatic, chronic HIV infection. At this time, the patient progresses from partially responding to skin testing (partial anergy) to complete anergy with no response to skin testing. Severe viral or fungal infections of the skin and mucous membranes develop. Oral and genital herpes simplex infections, including shingles or candidiasis (yeast) infections, usually develop, as well as oral hairy leukoplakia. The patient also may have persistent skin rashes or flaky skin, short-term memory loss, or pelvic inflammatory disease that does not respond to treatment. Children tend to have growth delays and frequent illnesses. The person may develop cytomegalovirus (CMV) infection, Epstein-Barr virus infection, or both, as well as other opportunistic infections.

An HIV-infected person is not diagnosed with AIDS until the CD4+ T-cell count is less than 200/μL. At that time, the person typically has one or more opportunistic infections, including *Pneumocystis carinii* pneumonia (PCP), *Toxoplasma gondii*–associated neural toxoplasmosis, cryptosporidiosis (gastroenteritis), and *Mycobacterium tuberculosis*. The person usually has one or more tumors or cancers, including Kaposi sarcoma (a connective tissue skin cancer), lymphomas, or cancer of the rectum or tongue. General symptoms of opportunistic infections include coughing or shortness of breath; difficult or painful swallowing (dysphagia); cognitive symptoms such as confusion, forgetfulness, or lack of coordination; seizures; fever; vision loss; severe headaches; and gastrointestinal symptoms such as abdominal cramps, nausea and vomiting, severe and persistent diarrhea, and weight loss, causing extreme fatigue.

Disease progression in infants and children is determined by the timing of the child's infection, the viral load, the child's immune response, and the viral virulence. In general, children with HIV progress more rapidly than adults. Most children fall into two distinct groups: rapid disease progression or slower disease progression. In those with rapidly progressing disease, symptoms develop within the first 6 months of life, sustained decreases in CD4+ T-cell counts are noted, and AIDS develops within the first 2 years of life. Early aggressive treatment in perinatally infected infants may slow disease progression and prolong immune function. Children with AIDS generally manifest the same opportunistic infections as adults and also may have severe forms of common childhood diseases, such as conjunctivitis, otitis media, and tonsillitis.

CDC HIV Classification System

The CDC HIV classification system is a simple matrix classification system for adults and children and is the preferred method of staging. In this system, CD4+ T-cell counts are linked with clinical symptomatology. The CDC has defined three CD4+ T-cell categories and three clinical categories that are mutually exclusive. The CD4+ T-cell categories define three T-cell ranges. In category 1, the CD4+ T-cell count is greater than or equal to 500/μL; in category 2, the CD4+ T-cell counts range from 200 to 499/μL; and in category 3, the CD4+ T-cell count is less than 200/μL.[20]

In adults, the clinical categories are labeled A through C. Category A includes a variety of clinical conditions, such as asymptomatic, persistent generalized lymphadenopathy and a history of or current acute HIV infection with accompanying illness. Category B includes conditions that are secondary to impaired cell-mediated immunity, such as candidiasis (oral or vaginal), fever, persistent diarrhea, oral hairy leukoplakia, shingles, idiopathic thrombocytopenic purpura, pelvic inflammatory disease, listeriosis, and peripheral neuropathy. Category C includes conditions that are listed in the AIDS surveillance case definition. An individual in category C will remain in this category. The CDC classification matrix is shown in Table 12-3. An HIV-positive person with a CD4+ count less than 200/μL or a category C AIDS indicator condition is diagnosed with AIDS. A list of AIDS indicator conditions is shown in Box 12-1.

In children, category N is an asymptomatic phase with no signs or symptoms of disease. Category A is a mildly symptomatic phase with two or more of the following conditions: lymphadenopathy, hepatomegaly, splenomegaly, dermatitis, parotitis, or recurrent/persistent upper respiratory tract infection, sinusitis, or otitis media. Category B is a moderately symptomatic phase in which the child exhibits some opportunistic infections as a result of impaired cell-mediated immunity or impaired bone marrow function. These conditions include anemia, thrombocytopenia, bacterial meningitis, pneumonia or sepsis, candidiasis, thrush, CMV, diarrhea, hepatitis, herpes simplex infection, herpes zoster infection, leiomyosarcoma, nephropathy, persistent fever, toxoplasmosis, and varicella. The category C phase is severely symptomatic with AIDS. The revised pediatric HIV classification system based on age-specific CD4+ T-cell counts and percentage is shown in Table 12-4.

DIAGNOSTIC TESTING

To diagnose HIV infection, laboratory tests such as the enzyme-linked immunosorbent assay (ELISA) and the Western blot are used to detect the presence of HIV antibodies. The ELISA test result is positive for HIV antibodies if the blood or oral mucosal transudate of an infected person reacts with the surface antigen of a killed HIV virus. The ELISA test uses purified viral proteins placed on plastic beads or in multiwell trays. When

BOX 12-1 CONDITIONS INDICATIVE OF AIDS IN HIV-INFECTED PERSONS

- Candidiasis of bronchi, trachea, or lungs
- Candidiasis, esophageal
- Cervical cancer, invasive*
- Coccidioidomycosis, disseminated or extrapulmonary
- Cryptococcosis, extrapulmonary
- Cryptosporidiosis, chronic intestinal (greater than 1 month's duration)
- Cytomegalovirus disease (other than liver, spleen, or nodes)
- Cytomegalovirus retinitis (with loss of vision)
- Encephalopathy, HIV-related
- Herpes simplex: chronic ulcer(s) (greater than 1 month's duration); or bronchitis, pneumonitis, or esophagitis
- Histoplasmosis, disseminated or extrapulmonary
- Isosporiasis, chronic intestinal (greater than 1 month's duration)
- Kaposi sarcoma
- Lymphoma, Burkitt (or equivalent term)
- Lymphoma, immunoblastic (or equivalent term)
- Lymphoma, primary, of brain
- *Mycobacterium avium complex* or *M. kansasii,* disseminated or extrapulmonary
- *Mycobacterium tuberculosis,* any site (pulmonary* or extrapulmonary)
- *Mycobacterium,* other species or unidentified species, disseminated or extrapulmonary
- *Pneumocystis carinii* pneumonia
- Pneumonia, recurrent*
- Progressive multifocal leukoencephalopathy
- Salmonella septicemia, recurrent
- Toxoplasmosis of brain
- Wasting syndrome attributable to HIV

From Appendix B of the 1993 Revised Classification System for HIV Infection and Expanded Surveillance Case Definition for AIDS Among Adolescents and Adults, *MMWR* 41(RR-17).
*Added in the 1993 expansion of the AIDS surveillance case definition.

TABLE 12-4 REVISED PEDIATRIC HIV CLASSIFICATION MATRIX*

IMMUNE CATEGORIES	CD4+ T-CELL COUNTS		
	<12 MO	**1-5 YR**	**6-12 YR**
Category 1: No suppression	>1500/µL >25%	>1000/µL >25%	>500/µL >25%
Category 2: Moderate suppression	750-1499/µL 15-24%	500-999/ml 15-24%	200-499/µL 15-24%
Category 3: Severe suppression	<750/µL <15%	<500/µL <15%	<200/µL <15%

From Foundation for Care Management, Dunn JM, editor: Special considerations in treating HIV positive children, *HIV Hotline* 7(5):7-12, 1997.
*Based on age-specific CD4+ count per microliter and percentage.

the test serum or oral mucosal transudate from a patient is contacted by the purified viral proteins, an antigen-antibody reaction occurs. Antihuman antibody added to the reaction can be detected colorimetrically and indicates whether any antigen-antibody compounds have formed. This test is highly sensitive (more than 99%) and specific (more than 99%) in high-risk populations. For the test to be specific, however, it must be performed with both HIV-1 and HIV-2 viral antigens.

When the ELISA test result is positive, a second test, the Western blot, is used to confirm the presence of HIV antibodies. The Western blot test uses an expensive process called *electrophoresis,* so usually it is used only as a confirmatory test. This test identifies specific antibodies against the HIV protein antigens. The specificity of this test in combination with the ELISA is greater than 99.9%. The problem with this additional testing is that the patient must wait up to 1 to 2 weeks for confirmation.

A rapid, fingerstick-based HIV assay is being used as well: OraQuick Rapid HIV-1. Antibody test results can be obtained in about 20 minutes. However, positive results must be confirmed by a Western blot. It is also important to remember that false-negative tests can occur during the initial period of HIV infection before seroconversion.

Testing neonates for HIV is difficult because of maternal transmission of IgG antibodies against HIV. These passive maternal antibodies cross the placenta and can last as long as 15 months. Therefore, the best method to determine whether a neonate has HIV is to culture the virus from blood and peripheral tissue.

MONITORING THE PROGRESSION OF HIV

After initial diagnosis of HIV, other laboratory tests need to be performed to stage the disease and assist in the selection and monitoring of appropriate drug treatments. One of the most important of these tests is the CD4+ T-cell count, which monitors HIV disease status.[6] The CD4+ count is a specific indicator of disease progression of HIV to AIDS. As the CD4+ T-cell count declines, the risk of progression to AIDS and development of opportunistic infections and malignancies increases. Highly virulent communicable diseases can still occur when the CD4+ count is high. However, when the CD4+ T-cell count drops below 200 cells/µL, the number and severity of low-virulence diseases and opportunistic infections increase. It is at this level that many patients begin taking prophylactic medications to prevent opportunistic and other infections. Also used is the CD4+ lymphocyte percentage, which is more stable and has less variation over time. When the CD4+ lymphocyte percentage is less than 20%, the risk of developing AIDS is higher.

Another useful test is the plasma HIV RNA or viral load. This test indicates the amount of viral replication, and helps predict disease progression. The level of HIV RNA in plasma is the strongest predictor of outcome over time. When the plasma HIV RNA content is low, the risk of disease progression declines. The plasma viral load helps the clinician to assess the effectiveness of various therapies and is the basis for initiating more aggressive therapies to decrease the viral load. Usually, HIV RNA levels should drop after the onset of therapy and by 6 months should be undetectable in the plasma. The viral load assay counts copies of HIV RNA in 1 ml of plasma and is either a reverse transcriptase polymerase chain reaction (RT-PCR) or a branched DNA (bDNA) assay. Because each virion contains two strands of RNA, the actual virion level is half the HIV RNA counted. Tests are currently sensitive to 50 copies per milliliter.

Genotypic resistance testing is now part of routine management of HIV infection and is usually part of the initial evaluation of HIV.[6] Genotypic testing identifies viral mutations, whereas phenotypic testing identifies the concentration of antiretroviral drug needed to inhibit viral replication in culture medium. Ideally this testing can help to determine the best drugs to be given to the patient. Genotypic resistance tests specifically examine protease and reverse transcriptase and are now used even when the viral loads are less than 1000 copies/ml.[21] These tests are expensive, which can limit their use in some populations.

Another common test is an anergy test or a delayed hypersensitivity (type IV) test for such organisms as *M. tuberculosis* or mumps or measles virus. In early HIV infection, these skin test results are normal. However, in advanced cases, the patient will have no response to testing because of the loss of macrophage and CD4+ T-cell functioning.

BOX 12-2 TESTS USED TO EVALUATE PROGRESSION OF HIV INFECTION

Complete Blood Cell Count with Differential
At entry into care and every 3-6 months
White blood cell count normal to decreased
Lymphopenia (<30% of normal number of WBCs)
Thrombocytopenia (decreased platelet count)

CD4+ Count
At entry into care and every 3-6 months
Reduced CD4+/CD8+ T cell ratio
CD4+ (helper) lymphocytes decreased
CD8+ lymphocytes increased

Resistance Testing
At entry into care, and before initiation of or any modification in HAART
Determines viral resistance to HAART

Quantitative Immunoglobulin
As needed depending on immune function
IgG increased
IgA frequently increased

Chemistry Panel
At entry into care and every 6-12 months
Lactate dehydrogenase increased (all fractions)
Serum albumin decreased
Total protein increased
Cholesterol decreased
AST and ALT elevated
Total bilirubin elevated
Serum glucose elevated

Lipid Panel
At entry into care and, if abnormal, every 6-12 months
Total cholesterol increased
Triglycerides increased
LDL cholesterol increased

Anergy Panel
As needed
Nonreactive (anergic) or poorly reactive to infectious agents or environmental materials (e.g., pokeweed, phytohemagglutinin mitogens and antigens, mumps, *Candida*)

Urinalysis
At entry into care and as needed
To detect urinary tract infections or hematuria

Hepatitis B Serology
At entry into care and as needed
To detect the presence of hepatitis B

Blood Cultures
As needed
To detect septicemia

Chest Radiograph
At entry into care and as needed
To detect *Pneumocystis jiroveci (carinii)* infection or tuberculosis

HLA-B5701 Testing
If considering use of abacavir

Tropism Testing
If considering use of CCR5 antagonist

Pregnancy Testing
If female at entry into care and as needed
To detect early pregnancy

ALT, Alanine aminotransferase; *AST,* aspartate aminotransferase; *HAART,* highly active antiretroviral therapy.
Data from DHHS Panel on Antiretroviral Guidelines for Adults and Adolescents: *Adult and adolescent treatment guidelines,* Office of AIDS Research Advisory Council, Department of Health and Human Services, p 6, October 14, 2011.

Two other tests may be used: β_2-microglobulin and p24 antigen. β_2-Microglobulin is a cell surface protein that indicates macrophage stimulation. Levels greater than 3.5 mg/L are associated with rapid progression of the disease. P24 antigen is indicative of active HIV replication and confirms the diagnosis of HIV infection. It is positive before seroconversion and may be used before confirmation of the disease by ELISA. It is also elevated in later stages of the disease, a period when antibody testing may be unreliable.

Other laboratory and diagnostic tests can assist in the identification, monitoring, and treatment of persons infected with HIV, including a complete blood cell count (CBC), a chemistry panel or screen, and chest radiographs. These tests are routinely used to detect infections and changes in a patient's physiologic status (Box 12-2). The CBC detects the development of anemia (as a result of infection, chronic illness, or secondary to therapy) and neutropenia and thrombocytopenia, which may occur in advanced stages of the disease. In addition to the aforementioned tests, it is important to measure serologic values for hepatitis A, B, and C viruses as well as to obtain screening tests for sexually transmitted infections in light of the risk of coinfection.[6]

KEY POINTS
- HIV virions are attracted to cells with CD4 receptors such as T cells, microglial cells, monocyte-macrophages, follicular dendritic cells, immortalized B cells, retinal cells, Langerhans cells in the skin, bone marrow stem cells, cervical cells, bone marrow–derived circulating dendritic cells, and enterochromaffin cells in the colon, duodenum, and rectum.
- The hallmark of AIDS is a decrease in the number of CD4+ cells, including T helper lymphocytes and macrophages, especially in mucosal membranes. B cell responsiveness is decreased because of dependence on T helper cell cytokines.
- The key element in HIV infection is the high level of virion production and the high level of CD4+ cell death.
- CD4+ cell death occurs via several mechanisms. Cross-linking of CD4 receptors by viruses may result in T-cell death, apoptosis, or anergy. Virions may cause the linkage of infected and uninfected cells, followed by cell fusion and death. B cells may form antibodies against infected T cells. Viral budding may cause excessive loss of cell membranes.

- Laboratory testing for HIV is accomplished by using either the ELISA or the Western blot test. Usually the ELISA test is performed first. If it is positive, the Western blot test is performed to confirm the presence of specific antibodies against HIV protein antigens.
- HIV is an infectious disease that progresses to AIDS and is characterized by different clinical manifestations at each stage. Individuals move through the stages at different rates.
- Flulike symptoms and the formation of anti-HIV antibodies (seroconversion) characterize the early stage of viral seeding. Next, symptoms of early immune dysfunction are present, including lymphadenopathy, fever, and night sweats. A surge in viral production and a drop in the CD4$^+$ lymphocyte count follow this stage.
- In the later stages, CD4$^+$ counts continue to fall and the person is subject to a number of opportunistic infections and tumor formation. An HIV-positive individual is diagnosed with AIDS when the CD4$^+$ T-cell count is less than 200/μL or when a category C AIDS indicator condition is present.
- Children often have rapidly progressive disease, with onset of AIDS between ages 4 and 8 years.

BOX 12-3   COMMON AGENTS OF INFECTION IN PATIENTS WITH AIDS

Viruses
Herpes simplex 1 and 2
Herpes zoster
JC virus
Epstein-Barr virus
Human papillomavirus
Varicella
Adenovirus

Bacteria
Campylobacter spp.
Shigella spp.
Neisseria spp.
Salmonella spp.
Chlamydia spp.
Staphylococcus spp.
Haemophilus influenzae spp.
Legionella spp.

Treponema spp.
Mycobacterium spp.

Fungi
Candida albicans
Cryptococcus neoformans
Histoplasma capsulatum
Coccidioides immitis
Nocardia

Protozoa
Pneumocystis jiroveci (carinii)
Toxoplasma gondii
Isospora belli
Cryptosporidium
Giardia lamblia
Entamoeba histolytica

Data from Stites DP, Terr AI: *Basic and clinical immunology*, ed 7, Los Altos, CA, 1991, Appleton & Lange; Ungvarski PJ, Schmidt J: AIDS patients under attack, *RN* 55(11):35-44, 1992; Anastasi JK, Rivera JL: Identify the skin manifestations of H.I.V., *Nursing* 92(11):58-61, 1992.

CLINICAL MANIFESTATIONS

HIV affects all body systems, particularly the integumentary, pulmonary, gastrointestinal (GI), neurologic, and ocular systems. GI manifestations develop in nearly all persons with HIV because of the major effect of HIV infection on the GI system. Pulmonary and cutaneous symptoms develop in approximately 50% to 75% of all persons with HIV, and neurologic symptoms develop in 50% to 60%. Box 12-3 outlines the common agents of infection in patients with AIDS.

Systemic Manifestations

As implied in the classification systems presented earlier, the course of HIV infection parallels the functioning of the immune system. As immune function declines, the number of opportunistic infections and malignancies increases and the normal functioning of organ systems declines.

One of the most significant systemic symptoms is malnutrition or wasting syndrome. In Africa, HIV is known as "slim disease" because of the wasting. Malnutrition is defined as unintended, involuntary loss of greater than 10% body weight. The systemic symptoms attributable to HIV infection malnutrition include major muscle wasting, weight loss, and loss of vitamins, minerals, and other nutrients. HIV malnutrition is the result of a combination of factors, including an elevated metabolic rate with increased resting energy expenditure (REE), chronic inflammation, malabsorption, anorexia, decreased intake of food, and the effect of multiple opportunistic insults.[22,23] There is a 10% to 30% increase in resting metabolic rate attributable to secondary infections or elevated plasma viral load.[23] In addition, levels of tumor necrosis factor, interleukin-1, interleukin-6, and other proinflammatory cytokines are elevated in HIV infection, causing anorexia as well as increased metabolism of fat.[23] Malabsorption is affected by the loss of GI-associated lymphoid tissue (especially during the initial phase of HIV infection) impairing the integrity of the epithelial mucosal barrier and predisposing to secondary infections of the GI tract.[23] Low basal metabolic index (BMI), failure to regain weight after weight loss, and continued weight loss after the start of medication hasten disease progression and are risk factors for increased mortality.[22,23] In children, growth failure is indicative of poor outcomes and mortality.[23] Malnutrition is a leading cause of death among AIDS patients worldwide. Prevention is key—involving assessment of nutritional parameters as well as nutritional education/counseling and exercise. A patient's body mass index, weight, waist-to-hip ratio, mid-arm circumference, calorie and protein intake, and prealbumin, serum albumin, and triglyceride levels are frequently measured.

To prevent or delay the wasting process, some medications have been used, including anabolic steroids, growth hormone treatments, cytokine inhibitors, and appetite stimulants.[23] Ketotifen is a tumor necrosis factor inhibitor and antihistamine that is used because its side effects are appetite stimulation and weight gain. Thalidomide, which is also a tumor necrosis factor inhibitor, appears to be effective against wasting syndrome and increases fat-free mass. Oxandrolone is an anabolic steroid designed specifically to promote weight gain, particularly lean body mass. Megestrol acetate (Megace), a progestational agent, and dronabinol, an antiemetic, are often used to decrease nausea and increase appetite. Use of human growth hormone (somatropin, Serostim) may also be given to increase lean body mass.

Vitamins A, C, D, and E; the B vitamins; zinc; selenium; sulfur-containing amino acids; and other antioxidants are also prescribed. The use of these nutrients can prevent the up-regulation of inflammatory cytokines and thereby decrease inflammation. High-protein, high-calorie meals and snacks are recommended, along with nutritional supplements to meet the required amounts of energy, protein, and micronutrients needed as a result of increased metabolic rates (REE). High-fat foods should be avoided because they increase diarrhea, as can lactose-containing foods. Nutritional supplements (Ensure, Nitrofuel, Sustacal Plus, Advera, Lipisorb), which provide both protein and calories, are full of nutrients and can be formulated either with or without lactose and with or without medium-chain triglyceride oil (a more easily digested fat). Implementation of total parenteral nutrition (TPN), including gastrostomy or jejunostomy tube feedings, is reserved for those with severe malnutrition and GI manifestations.[27]

Gastrointestinal Manifestations

GI manifestations are nearly universal in persons with HIV. In fact, the GI tract is the major target organ in HIV infection. HIV may be a significant direct pathogen in the GI tract. The major HIV GI complication is chronic diarrhea, which increases with decreasing CD4$^+$ counts.[24] The diarrhea, often watery or bloody, causes malabsorption and consequently severe weight loss. This complication of HIV-related malnutrition causes muscle loss leading to increased morbidity and risk of death. Antiemetics and antidiarrheals are often useful in controlling symptoms.

Whenever chronic diarrhea or other GI symptoms develop in a patient with HIV, it is important to determine the cause. GI symptoms can be the result of multiple opportunistic infectious agents and are rarely the result of tumors occurring in the GI tract. Some of the most significant infectious agents are viruses such as CMV and herpes simplex; fungi such as *Candida;* bacteria such as *Salmonella, Shigella, Clostridium difficile, Chlamydia trachomatis,* and *Campylobacter;* and parasites such as *Giardia, Isospora, Entamoeba histolytica,* and *Cryptosporidium.* GI symptoms include chronic diarrhea, oral candidiasis, anorexia, nausea, vomiting, mucous membrane ulcers, retrosternal pain on swallowing, abdominal pain, and low levels of serum vitamin B_{12}. Ulcerations occur as a primary manifestation or secondary to the inflammation. Treatment involves the use of disease-appropriate antimicrobials, depending on the offending organism.

A common cause of diarrhea is the protozoa *Cryptosporidium,* which infects the intestinal epithelial lining. This organism is transmitted via water, food, animals, and other humans. The onset is generally acute and associated with explosive diarrhea within 4 to 14 days after infection. In nonimmunocompromised persons, the symptoms last up to 2 weeks, but in immunocompromised persons, the diarrhea and symptoms can persist indefinitely. Cryptosporidiosis causes nausea, vomiting, severe watery nonbloody diarrhea (more than 15 to 20 L), abdominal pain, cramping, electrolyte disturbances, and dehydration.

Diagnosis is made by stool examination for ova and parasites and by bacterial culture and sensitivity. Antibiotic treatment is not always effective, but antimicrobials such as the macrolides have been used. In the acute phase, some patients must be given intravenous hydration for support. Thereafter, increased oral intake along with low-residue, high-protein, high-calorie diets and loperamide (Imodium) 2 mg tablets, up to 16 to 18 tablets or 36 mg per day, are used to help control the diarrhea.

Prevention of *Cryptosporidium* infection is most important. Preventive activities include routine testing of well water, using water filters at home, avoiding ice or unfiltered tap water both at home and in restaurants, and avoiding fresh fruits or vegetables rinsed with unfiltered water. Fruits and vegetables can be washed in bottled water, filtered water, or water with 20 drops of 2% iodine per gallon.

Oropharyngeal and esophageal *Candida albicans* infections occur in most patients with HIV during the course of their disease. Most often, oral *candidiasis* is pseudomembranous in type, with white plaques that bleed when removed and leave an erythematous surface. *Candida* oropharyngeal lesions produce pain and discomfort during eating, loss of taste, and **xerostomia (dry mouth).** *Candida* esophageal lesions cause pain with swallowing, dysphagia, and a feeling of "throat swelling." These lesions lead to worsening wasting syndrome. Management of oropharyngeal *candidiasis* includes the use of topical antifungal agents (such as clotrimazole or nystatin) in a suspension or lozenges, whereas management of esophageal *candidiasis* includes antifungal agents by oral or intravenous routes of administration. Side effects include an unpleasant taste and GI side effects, with inconvenient dosing regimens (up to six times per day).

Pulmonary Manifestations

Pulmonary manifestations are a major source of morbidity and mortality in AIDS patients. Pulmonary diseases include opportunistic pneumonias, such as those associated with *P. jiroveci (carinii),* CMV, *M. tuberculosis, Histoplasma,* or *Staphylococcus,* as well as parenchymal lung diseases including Kaposi sarcoma, lymphoma, nonspecific pneumonitis, and adult respiratory distress syndrome. Infection with *M. tuberculosis* occurs in 4% of patients with HIV and is particularly problematic in third world countries where the tuberculosis comorbidity

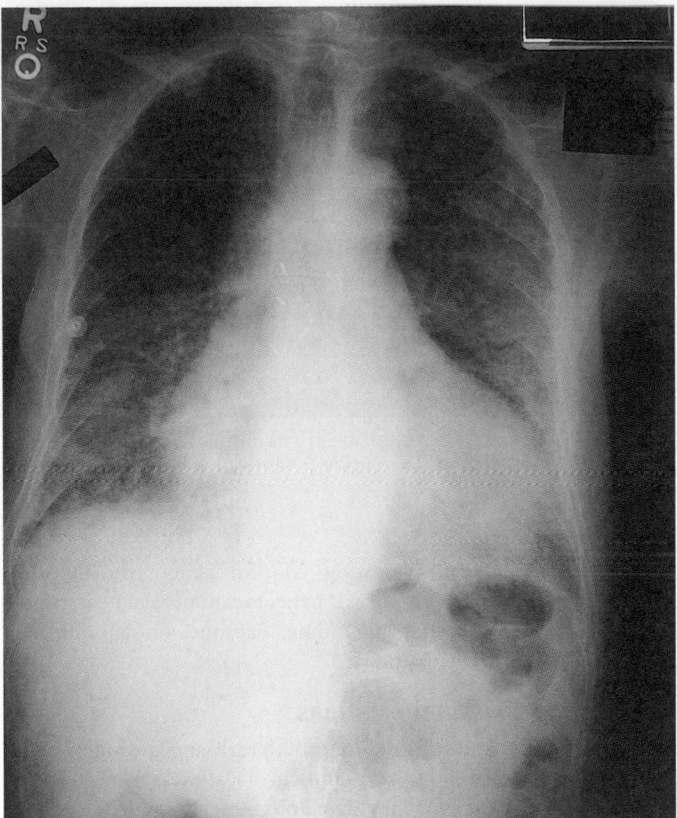

FIGURE 12-11 *Pneumocystis jiroveci (carinii).* A chest radiograph shows bilateral lower lobe interstitial infiltrates. (Courtesy Dr. Paula Karvalho, Veterans Administration Medical Center, Boise, Idaho.)

rates are up to 50%. Patients with HIV have an increased risk of being infected with a multidrug-resistant type of tuberculosis organism.

PCP is a common initial opportunistic infection in HIV and is an AIDS-defining diagnosis in the United States and Europe. However, the incidence of *P. carinii* has decreased with the use of prophylaxis. *P. carinii* is a fungus (renamed *P. jiroveci*). This organism prefers alveolar environments and infects most people during early childhood. Children usually have *Pneumocystis* antibodies by 2 to 3 years of age, but the organism does not cause disease in immunocompetent persons. With immunodeficiency and CD4+ T-cell counts below 200/µL, *Pneumocystis* becomes activated and causes PCP. The nonspecific symptoms of PCP include flu-like fever, fatigue, and weight loss. The major pulmonary feature of PCP is severe hypoxemia with a PaO_2 less than 60 mm Hg. The most severe pulmonary symptoms are similar to those of adult respiratory distress syndrome (Figure 12-11). These symptoms include decreased phospholipid (surfactant) production, early dry cough, dyspnea, tachypnea, chest discomfort, and marked pallor and cyanosis.

Diagnosis of PCP is by chest radiography, and organisms are identified in sputum with Wright-Giemsa stain. *Pneumocystis* cannot be cultured.[25] Sputum is induced by using 3% saline via nebulizer, and patients must avoid brushing their teeth, using mouthwash, or eating for 8 hours before expectoration of a sputum sample. Other tests that can be performed include bronchoalveolar lavage or biopsy and gallium scanning. Treatment usually includes the use of intravenous or oral trimethoprim-sulfamethoxazole (Bactrim, Septra) and parenteral and aerosolized pentamidine (NebuPent, Pentam 300).

To prevent PCP infections by prophylaxis, patients with CD4+ counts of less than 200 cells/µL are given trimethoprim-sulfamethoxazole tablets either daily or three times per week to prevent the recurrence of infection. This is a very effective suppressive therapy that prevents life-threatening

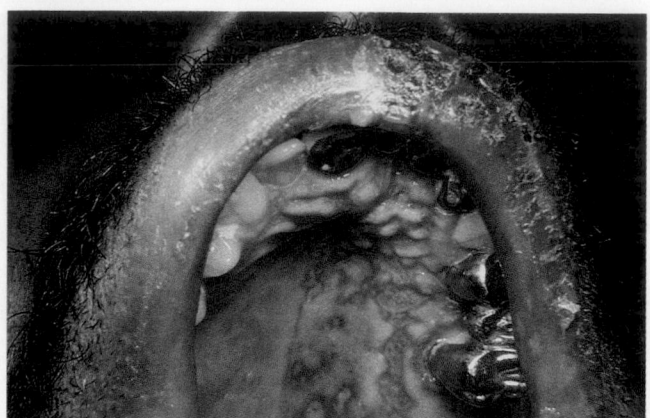

FIGURE 12-12 Herpes zoster in an HIV-infected individual. (From Callen JP: *Color atlas of dermatology,* Philadelphia, 1993, Saunders, p 382.)

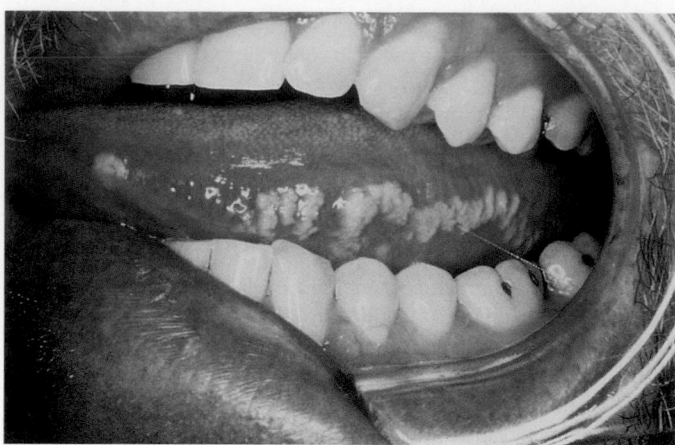

FIGURE 12-13 Oral hairy leukoplakia, a manifestation of Epstein-Barr virus infection in HIV-infected individuals. (From Callen JP: *Color atlas of dermatology,* Philadelphia, 1993, Saunders, p 377.)

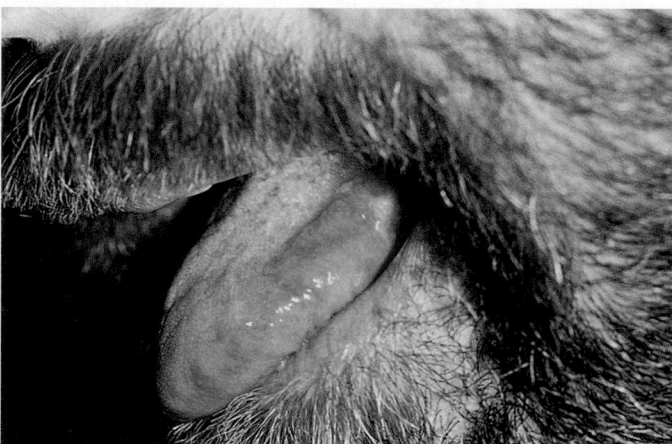

FIGURE 12-14 *Candida albicans* in an HIV-infected person. (From Callen JP: *Color atlas of dermatology,* Philadelphia, 1993, Saunders, p 386.)

PCP. However, there is growing concern about trimethoprim-sulfamethoxazole drug resistance. If patients cannot tolerate it, substitutes include aerosolized pentamidine, dapsone, or dapsone with pyrimethamine and leucovorin.

Mucocutaneous Manifestations

Mucocutaneous manifestations occur both early and late in the course of HIV infection. The early viral exanthem of HIV infection, associated with seroconversion, is an erythematous, fine maculopapular rash found on the face, trunk, and arms. It is a self-limited manifestation that occurs in 40% to 60% of all HIV-infected persons. It is generally seen within 2 to 6 weeks of exposure and lasts up to 1 to 2 weeks. It is associated with mild pruritus, fever, malaise, night sweats, fatigue, pharyngitis, weight loss, diarrhea, headache, and lymphadenopathy.

Other mucocutaneous manifestations may be allergic, infectious, or neoplastic in origin. Cutaneous symptoms depend on the cause and location. Allergic causes may be the result of drug reactions or the development of seborrheic dermatitis, psoriasis, or skin-colored papular eruptions.

Viral causes include herpes simplex virus, varicella-zoster virus, Epstein-Barr virus, and human papillomavirus (Figure 12-12). The development of genital warts (condylomata acuminata) from human papillomavirus is an early symptom of HIV disease in women. For mucocutaneous viral infections, acyclovir (Zovirax) or vidarabine is the recommended antiviral agent.

Oral hairy leukoplakia is an example of an oral mucous membrane infection first described in 1984. It occurs only in immunosuppressed individuals and is associated with Epstein-Barr virus. It occurs in up to 50% of patients with untreated HIV, especially when the CD4+ count declines. Oral hairy leukoplakia is characterized by white to gray thickened, raised lesions with vertical folds, corrugations, or "hairs" that form on the tongue and buccal mucosa. Usually they form on the sides of the tongue (Figure 12-13). These lesions cannot be removed with a tongue blade, which differentiates this infection from oral candidiasis or thrush. They are not usually painful. There is no specific treatment for oral hairy leukoplakia. It will often resolve with treatment of the HIV infection with improvement in the CD4+ cell count.[26]

In HIV-infected persons, herpes simplex viruses 1 and 2 cause the formation of large groups of painful vesicles on an erythematous base. The HSV-1/-2 vesicles then rupture, crust, and become large, ulcerative, and occasionally necrotic. They are chronic and painfully persistent, and usually occur on the genitalia, digits, and perianal or perioral areas. Herpes simplex virus may produce protein that enhances the replication of HIV.

Bacterial infectious causes of mucocutaneous manifestations include *Mycobacterium avium* or *Staphylococcus aureus. Staphylococcus* is a common bacterial skin infection in patients with HIV associated with folliculitis, furuncles (boils), or bullous impetigo. Occasionally sepsis may occur. Treatment includes application of topical antibiotics, use of an antibacterial soap, and administration of systemic antibiotics, either oral or intravenous, as needed. Abscesses usually are surgically opened and drained.

Fungal skin infectious agents include *Candida, Cryptococcus,* or *Histoplasma* (Figure 12-14). Vaginal candidiasis is the most common early skin symptom in HIV-positive women. Other infectious agents include parasites such as the mites that cause scabies. Treatment is with topical, oral, or intravenous antifungal or antiparasitic agents, depending on the severity of the infection.

Neoplasms can also occur, including Kaposi sarcoma, squamous cell carcinoma, basal cell carcinoma, or cutaneous lymphomas. Kaposi sarcoma is an AIDS-related malignancy that affects the skin and mucous membranes, lymphatics, and other internal organs. It is one of the few neoplasms indicative of immune system dysfunction. Since 1981, Kaposi sarcoma is the most common tumor found in HIV-infected homosexual men. It rarely occurs in other high-risk groups or in women in the United States. The skin lesions of Kaposi sarcoma are individual tumors that begin as flat or macular subcutaneous patches.

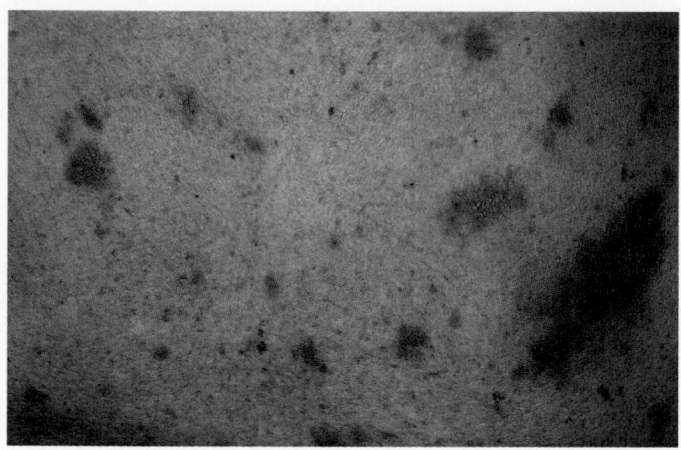

FIGURE 12-15 HIV-associated Kaposi sarcoma in the macular stage. (From Callen JP: *Color atlas of dermatology*, Philadelphia, 1993, Saunders, p 55.)

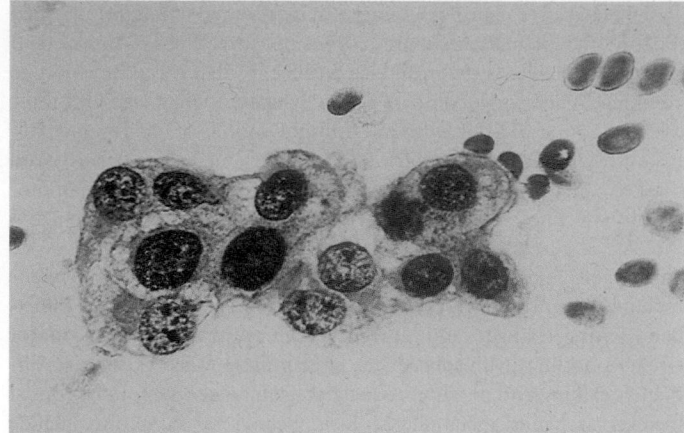

FIGURE 12-17 Cervical dysplasia. Women with AIDS require more frequent monitoring because cervical dysplasia commonly occurs and progresses rapidly.

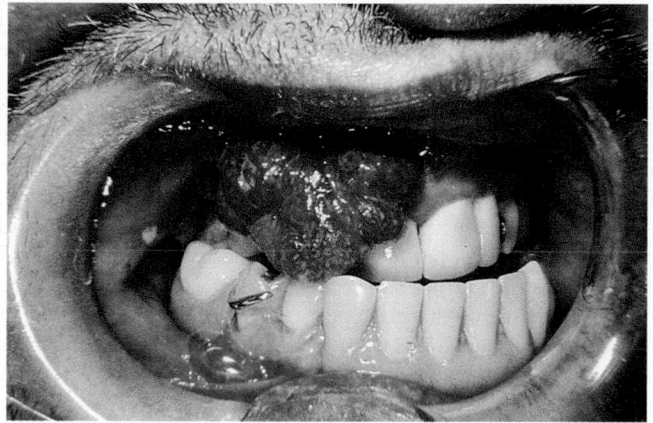

FIGURE 12-16 HIV-associated Kaposi sarcoma in the nodular stage. (From Callen JP: *Color atlas of dermatology*, Philadelphia, 1993, Saunders, p 379.)

The patches initially range from light pink to deep purple and are painless, nonblanching, and nonpruritic (Figure 12-15). The lesions evolve from patches into thickened plaques or large nodules that may change to brown over time, especially in darkly pigmented persons. They may occur anywhere on the body, and usually begin on the head—face, eyelids, conjunctivae, pinnae, scalp, or buccal membranes (Figure 12-16). Lesions range in size from a few millimeters to coalesced patches covering large areas of the body. The lesions are highly vascular but do not bleed excessively. The lesions also may occur internally in either the lungs or the intestines in approximately 40% of patients.

Kaposi sarcoma is managed with radiation therapy and medications, including chemotherapy. Surgery is rarely indicated except to remove large, uncomfortable lesions. Radiation therapy is used primarily for oral or cutaneous lesions. Mitotic inhibitors (e.g., vinblastine, vincristine) or immunomodulators (e.g., interferon-α) have been useful chemotherapeutic agents in the management of Kaposi sarcoma. Smaller lesions may be managed with intralesional injections of a mitotic inhibitor. Those with the best prognosis tend to have limited disease, no other opportunistic infections, and no weight loss, fevers, or night sweats.

Gynecologic Manifestations

The primary genital barrier to HIV virus is the genital epithelial cell (GEC). When pro-inflammatory cytokines are produced in response to HIV virus, the usually tight epithelial junction barrier becomes impaired allowing HIV virus to move across the epithelium.[16] The gynecologic manifestations of HIV disease are marked by persistent monilial vaginitis secondary to *C. albicans,* cervical dysplasia, and neoplasia, as well as pelvic inflammatory disease. Cervical dysplasia affects 40% of HIV-infected women (Figure 12-17). Cervical dysplasia has no symptoms, but the cell changes can lead to neoplasia (cancer). Therefore, either Papanicolaou smears or colposcopic examinations should be performed every 6 months to detect cervical cancer early in HIV-positive women. Cervical cancer is particularly aggressive in women with HIV. Pelvic inflammatory disease (PID) is common in HIV-positive women. PID is caused by a variety of organisms, including *C. trachomatis,* and is managed with antibiotics.

Neurologic Manifestations

Neurologic manifestations are often the reason that people with HIV seek treatment. HIV invades the neurologic system early in the course of its infection, infecting glial cells, endothelial cells, and brain macrophages—particularly microglial cells, which are the main cellular targets of HIV in the brain. Microglial HIV infection results in elevated levels of the enzyme *glutaminase,* which produces increased extracellular glutamate concentrations leading to increased neurotoxicity.[27] Central and peripheral nervous system manifestations are caused by HIV infection directly, as a result of infectious agents causing meningitis, or secondary to neoplasms causing space-occupying lesions. Opportunistic infectious agents affecting the neurologic system include *Toxoplasma* and *Cryptococcus.* A variety of peripheral neuropathies can result from HIV infection directly, although some may be caused by herpes zoster infection.

HIV encephalopathy (AIDS dementia complex, subacute, or AIDS encephalopathy) is the most common neurologic manifestation. HIV encephalopathy is caused directly or indirectly by HIV infection or viral products, by cytokine-related cellular damage, and by the competition or interference between gp120 and neuroleukin, a nerve growth factor. This disorder can affect both adults and children. It occurs when other opportunistic infections begin to appear later in the disease process. HIV encephalopathy is a syndrome characterized by progressive cognitive impairment or subcortical dementia. In other words, the patient is alert but demented and confused. Computed tomography shows diffuse atrophy in the cerebral cortex, widened sulci, ventricular enlargement, and shrinking of the basal ganglia. Cerebrospinal fluid analysis shows elevated protein and abnormal IgG levels.

The cognitive neurologic symptoms associated with HIV encephalopathy include inattentiveness, confusion, forgetfulness, loss of concentration, slower verbal response, headache, apathy, and inability to complete or perform complex tasks. Symptoms may wax and wane over the course of a day, with intermittent periods of lucidity and confusion. Symptoms can progress to global dementia associated with marked memory impairment and disorientation. Before motor strength declines, the patient may forget time, place, person, and activities, leading to safety issues such as wandering, leaving appliances on, and forgetting to take medications. The associated focal motor deficits include slower motor responses, clumsiness, weakness, loss of balance, handwriting changes, and slurred speech. With progression, motor strength declines with subsequent large muscle weakness causing difficulty walking and moving. Associated generalized symptoms consist of fever and mild metabolic acidosis. Behavioral symptoms include personality changes, social withdrawal, depression, poor hygiene and grooming, lack of insight, apathy, agitation, and, less commonly, anxiety and hyperactivity. In children, head circumference does not increase with age. As the disorder progresses, the neurologic symptoms become more severe. Ataxia, hypertonia, tremors, and incontinence appear. The person may be alert but cognitively impaired, mute, and paraplegic. Hemianopia (partial blindness), myoclonus, and seizures also may develop. The person may become comatose and lethargic with other systemic dysfunctions. Management of HIV encephalopathy includes treatment with antiretroviral agents and neuroleptics (to control agitation) as well as coordination of home and environmental safety plans and patient/family support.

Ocular Manifestations

Ocular manifestations of HIV infection may be of infectious or noninfectious origin. Noninfectious causes of ocular problems include HIV retinopathy and malignancy. Infectious causes include bacteria such as *Treponema pallidum* (syphilis) and *Staphylococcus;* fungi including *Candida, Cryptococcus,* and *Histoplasma;* protozoa such as *Pneumocystis* and *Toxoplasma;* and viruses such as herpes simplex and CMV.

The most severe type of ocular infection is CMV retinitis. After an insidious onset, ocular CMV causes perivascular hemorrhages, fluffy exudates, and vasculitis in the retina, leading to destruction and necrosis of the retina with resulting blindness. Treatment of CMV retinitis involves the use of anti-CMV agents (e.g., ganciclovir) intravenously and the use of oral anti-CMV agents for prophylaxis. An intraocular sustained-release anti-CMV implant is also available for the management of acute and chronic CMV retinitis.

HIV-associated retinopathy causes the development of cotton-wool spots and microvascular retinal changes. Cotton-wool spots are small, indistinct white spots with associated hemorrhage. These changes are not as severe as CMV retinitis and may remit spontaneously.

Cardiovascular Manifestations

Cardiovascular disease is the second most frequent cause of death after cancer in persons with HIV.[28] Increased cardiovascular risk is an important treatment consideration in an aging HIV-positive population with either untreated or treated HIV infection. The 2006 Strategies for Management of Antiretroviral Therapy (SMART) study found that cardiovascular events, hypertriglyceridemia, and lipidemia were the result of HIV infection and not just caused by medications for HIV. This study determined that cardiovascular and renal diseases were higher in those not treated effectively with antiretroviral medications. Therefore, lipid abnormalities and cardiovascular disease are due either to HIV immunosuppression and HIV viremia or to highly active antiretroviral therapy (HAART), or both. Hypertriglyceridemia and lipogenesis are the result of inflammatory responses to HIV infection secondary to elevated serum interferon-α (IFN-α) level as well as decreased triglyceride clearance from the blood in HIV infection.[29] Antiretroviral therapies also cause dyslipidemias primarily because of the effects on hepatocytes.[29]

The treatment of HIV-associated dyslipidemia includes education/counseling on heart-healthy diet, exercise, and smoking cessation; management of hypertension and diabetes if present; treatment of dyslipidemia with medications as needed; and use of antiplatelet agents.[29] The treatment of dyslipidemia includes the use of fish oils, fibrates, statins, niacin, and ezetimibe.[29] Of the statins, atorvastatin and pravastatin (Pravachol) are less likely to cause adverse interactions with HAART medications. Fibrates, such as gemfibrozil, are generally well tolerated and do not interact adversely with most HAART medications. Ezetimibe, in combination with Pravachol, appears to benefit most patients. However, ezetimibe, which blocks cholesterol absorption in the intestine, does not appear to lower lipid levels alone. [29]

Manifestations in Other Systems

Renal impairment can also occur with HIV infection. HIV can affect the kidneys and cause AIDS-associated nephropathy (AIDS-related glomerulopathy or HIV-associated nephropathy [HIVAN]), drug-induced ischemia, and renal failure. Hematologically, individuals with HIV have anemia, thrombocytopenia, and granulocytopenia. Liver dysfunction is also a problem in persons with HIV because there is an increased risk of concomitant hepatitis C or B (HCV/HBV) infection. This comorbidity of HIV/HCV or HIV/HBV causes increased mortality from end-stage liver disease. Also compounding liver dysfunction in patients with HIV is the effect of multiple medications on the liver itself.

HIV-related endocrine dysfunction is usually associated with inflammation; changes in hormone secretion secondary to the stress response; destruction of endocrine tissue from infection, cancer, or inflammation; use of pharmacologic agents; or the effect of severe illness on hormonal function and metabolic homeostasis.[30] Insulin resistance is a major metabolic complication of antiretroviral therapy. Insulin resistance can be either direct (from insulin signal interference at the cellular level) or indirect (from antiretroviral therapy and lipid dysfunction).[31] It leads to abnormal glucose metabolism and the development of diabetes mellitus. The adrenal gland is another organ affected by HIV infection because of increased adrenal secretion of cortisol with stress. Injury to the adrenal gland rarely leads to frank cortisol deficiencies. Levels of thyroid hormones (e.g., triiodothyronine [T_3], thyroxine [T_4], and thyroid-stimulating hormone [TSH]) may be elevated or decreased. Hypogonadism can be primary in HIV infection or secondary to antiretroviral therapy.

Adipose tissue endocrine function is also affected by HIV infection and antiretroviral therapy. This dysfunction may cause the development of HIV-1 HAART-associated lipodystrophy syndrome (HALS) in some persons. It is characterized by subcutaneous adipose tissue atrophy, dorsocervical fat ("buffalo hump") accumulation, and visceral adipose tissue hypertrophy.[32] The cause of this dysfunction is multifactorial due to the effects on systemic metabolism, as well as enhanced production of proinflammatory cytokines and excessive free fatty acid release.[32] Not all people treated with antiretroviral therapy develop lipodystrophy. It is suspected that there may be a genetic component or predisposition to development.[33] At this time, the treatment and causes of adipose tissue dysfunction are still being researched.

Rheumatologic manifestations of HIV infection are varied, encompassing osteoporosis, osteopenia, and musculoskeletal infections (infectious arthritis and osteomyelitis). Musculoskeletal infections are caused by a decrease in the number of T cells. The most common infectious organisms include *S. aureus, Streptococcus pneumoniae, C. albicans, Mycobacterium kansasii,* and *Mycobacterium avium-intracellulare.* Other manifestations are caused by immune-mediated arthritis (such as Reiter disease, psoriatic arthritis, and undifferentiated spondyloarthropathy syndromes) or occur as a direct result of the immune response to HIV (including polymyositis, vasculitis, and immune complex diseases related to the production of autoantibodies). The increasing incidence of osteopenia, osteoporosis, and osteonecrosis in the HIV population is significant and may be due either to HIV infection or to antiretroviral therapy. Treatment includes using bisphosphonate medications and selective estrogen receptor modulators as well as risk factor modification.

Manifestations in Children

Children with HIV become symptomatic much faster than adults—usually within their first year of life. Because of the invasion of virus, children's growth and development are markedly affected, including physical growth retardation with failure to thrive, impaired intellectual development, and impaired motor functioning with decreased coordination. The infant develops normally until the virus begins its nervous system invasion. After that time, neurologic impairment is characterized by development of weakness, loss of previously accomplished developmental milestones, hypotonia, or hypertonia. Extensive candidiasis without any relationship to antibiotic therapy may be an early symptom. Respiratory problems, including the development of PCP, are common.

More serious bacterial and viral infections also develop in children who undergo repeated bouts of communicable diseases such as chickenpox or measles. As a result, it is recommended that children obtain vaccinations. In a recent meta-analysis of the safety of measles vaccination, the vaccination using live virus appears to be safe in HIV-infected children as early as 6 months of age.[34]

Because lactose intolerance is common in HIV-infected children, soy formulas are often used. Dairy products may be introduced into the diet gradually, as tolerated. Children need particular attention to their diet; increased intake of calories and protein, as well as nutrient-rich snacks such as raisins and peanuts for growth and development, is advisable.

KEY POINTS

- All body systems are affected by HIV.
- Early HIV infection is characterized by fever, chills, headaches, nausea, vomiting, diarrhea, fatigue, weakness, arthralgia, sore throat, stiff neck, photophobia, irritability, and rash.
- The most significant systemic symptom is malnutrition or wasting, which is due to a combination of factors, including an elevated metabolic rate, chronic inflammation, malabsorption, anorexia, and the effect of multiple opportunistic insults.
- GI symptoms occur frequently in patients with HIV. Symptoms include diarrhea caused by *Cryptosporidium* or other agents, ulceration, and candidiasis, as well as multiple opportunistic infections.
- Pulmonary symptoms include opportunistic pneumonias (particularly PCP), tuberculosis, and adult respiratory distress syndrome.
- Mucocutaneous symptoms occur both early and late in the course of HIV infection. One of the first symptoms is the viral exanthem that occurs during the primary infection. Other manifestations may be allergic; infectious, such as candidiasis or herpes, human papillomavirus, and Epstein-Barr virus infections; or neoplastic, such as Kaposi sarcoma.
- Neurologic manifestations include peripheral neuropathy, encephalopathy with dementia, headache, apathy, and focal deficits.
- Gynecologic manifestations include persistent monilial vaginitis, cervical dysplasia, and pelvic inflammatory disease.
- Ocular manifestations include HIV-associated retinopathy, CMV retinitis, malignancy, and a variety of infectious causes.
- Children with HIV have growth and development problems, including impaired physical growth, intellectual development, and motor functioning.

TREATMENT

Antiretroviral Therapy Recommendations

The goal of medication and therapeutic management of HIV/AIDS is to delay disease progression, restore or preserve immunologic function, suppress plasma HIV viral load, minimize clinical manifestations, reduce morbidity, prolong survival, and prevent HIV transmission.[6] Drug management of HIV infection has evolved from monotherapy, or therapy with one agent, to the use of multiple medications, called antiretroviral therapy (ART) or highly active antiretroviral therapy (HAART). This polydrug therapy approach involves the administration of multiple antiretroviral agents. It provides better viral suppression, thereby decreasing viral load, increasing CD4+ counts, and decreasing resistance for a longer period. The objective of HAART is to provide the greatest viral suppression for the longest time to prevent viral mutations. This approach makes good sense. If one drug blocks 90% of viral replication, the others may eliminate the rest of the resistant virions. However, even with HAART, complete viral eradication is not possible with current treatment strategies. It has also been found that continuous HIV therapy is more beneficial than treatment interruption with prolonged drug treatment holidays.

Antiretroviral therapy in HIV infection is more successful in some patients than others, depending on both internal and external factors. Some important factors include prescribing the appropriate polydrug therapy and ensuring maximal convenience of therapy, aiding patient adherence to the treatment regimen. Other factors include early identification of HIV infection with low baseline viremia and higher baseline CD4+ count, usually >200 cells/mm³.[6] However, there are also unknown factors involving the response of individual patients to the therapy, including the rate of reduction of viremia in response to treatment.[6] People who present for treatment later in HIV infection with higher viremia and lower CD4+ counts tend to have increased morbidity, increased progression, and decreased immune system responses, as well as poor adherence to therapy.

HIV drug treatment failures are the result of HIV resistance, which is a widespread problem and concern. Failure of HIV drug treatment is usually caused by poor adherence to HAART, poor toleration of the drugs, prior exposure to single or multiple antiretroviral drug therapy, or counteracting interactions among the drugs used. It is easy to see why persons taking the multidrug regimen may fail to comply with nutritional and drug therapy because of the sheer volume of drugs to be taken in a day. A person infected with HIV may take up to 13 to 30 pills per day; he or she must also remember which medications should be taken with food or on an empty stomach and which medications cannot be taken together simultaneously. In addition, some persons with HIV/AIDS may be demented because of the disease or may be homeless or addicted to intravenous drugs, any of which limits the person's ability to adhere to the strict treatment regimens. Finally, some of the treatments for opportunistic infection or cancer involve many other drugs: intravenous, oral, and intracavital. Multidrug therapy retails at approximately $900 to $1400 per month. Patient compliance with complicated drug therapy that has many side effects and high cost is often variable. Virus resistance increases with treatment protocol noncompliance. Therefore, the key appears to be encouraging patient compliance by tailoring medication regimens that improve tolerability and convenience.

Current recommendations for antiretroviral therapy for HIV per U.S. Department of Health and Human Services (USDHHS) guidelines (October 14, 2011) include initiation of therapy for all persons

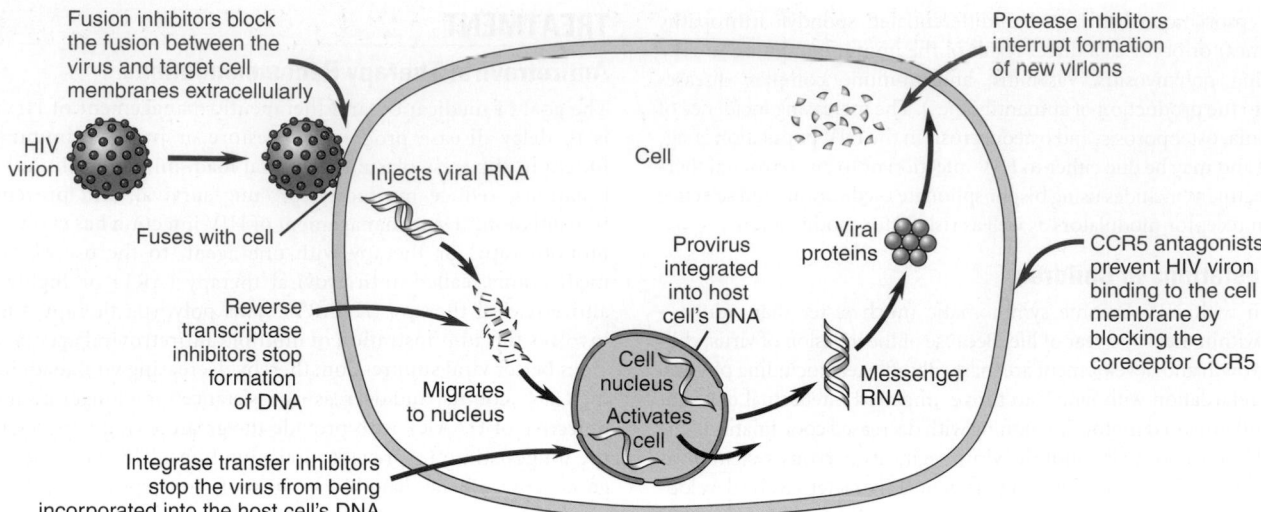

FIGURE 12-18 Antiretroviral therapy. The stages in the life cycle of HIV in which antiretroviral therapy is effective are shown.

with AIDS-defining illness or severe symptoms at any CD4+ count or viral load, for all asymptomatic HIV-infected persons with a CD4+ cell count <350 cells/mm³, and for all persons with HIV-associated nephropathy or hepatitis B virus (HBV) coinfection.[11] Antiretroviral therapy is recommended but not mandated for patients with CD4+ cell counts between 350 and 500 cells/mm³. In asymptomatic HIV-infected persons who have a CD4+ cell count greater than 500/μL some clinicians may delay treatment until after patient consultation. The USDHHS panel was evenly divided, with 50% favoring early treatment and the other 50% viewing treatment as optional. Early antiretroviral treatment seems to be better tolerated by patients and helps to prolong life, but it is imperative that patients starting antiretroviral therapy be committed to life-long treatment and adherence to therapy with knowledge of the risks and benefits of therapy.

Some of the current medications available to adults with HIV have not been recommended for children younger than 13 years. In the past, treatment for infants and children was often delayed weeks or months; this is because virion levels are usually not detectable for up to 2 weeks after birth. Some clinicians recommend intensive therapy for all infants born to HIV-positive women even though the infant may not have infection. This controversial method is not universal but does take into consideration the rapid progression of infection in infants.

The major classes of antiretroviral medications are nucleoside reverse transcriptase inhibitors (NRTIs) (nucleoside analogues), nonnucleoside reverse transcriptase inhibitors (NNRTIs) (nonnucleoside analogues), protease inhibitors (PIs), fusion inhibitors, integrase strand transfer inhibitors (INSTIs), and CCR5 antagonists. The current optimal combination of medications is multidrug therapy with two nucleoside analogues (NRTIs) and one active drug from one of the following classes: protease inhibitors (PIs) boosted with ritonavir (RTV), a nonnucleoside reverse transcriptase inhibitor (NNRTI, which is called protease-sparing regimen), an integrase strand transfer inhibitor (INSTI), or a CCR5 antagonist. Viral resistance to treatment is reduced by the complete suppression of the virus with multiple drugs (Figure 12-18). In general, there are now a variety of antiretroviral medication choices available to meet patient needs, tolerance, and cost concerns (Table 12-5).

Nucleoside Reverse Transcriptase Inhibitors

NRTIs resemble the natural substances used by the virus to build HIV DNA. NRTIs prevent HIV replication by preventing HIV DNA synthesis and have been found to slow progression of the disease. Nucleoside analogues include zidovudine, didanosine, zalcitabine, stavudine, lamivudine, and abacavir. All must be converted to an active state intracellularly.

Nonnucleoside Reverse Transcriptase Inhibitors

NNRTIs also inhibit reverse transcriptase, but by a different mechanism. Drugs in this class include efavirenz (Sustiva), nevirapine (Viramune), and delavirdine (Rescriptor). These medications need not be converted intracellularly to be activated. The greatest benefit is that they are potent antiretrovirals. The biggest problem is that they affect the cytochrome P-450 system, which increases drug interactions and must be given cautiously. They can only be administered in combination with other antiretrovirals.

Protease Inhibitors

PIs attack at another phase in the viral life cycle. These medications inhibit the enzyme protease, whose action is to clip the viral protein precursors to the appropriate size. These precursors are essential for HIV maturation, infection, and replication. Protease inhibitor therapy is extremely expensive, with a retail price of approximately $6000 to $8000 per year. Protease inhibitors are never used as single agents because of the potential for a patient to develop resistance. PIs have poor central nervous system (CNS) penetration.

Fusion Inhibitors

Fusion inhibitors (e.g., enfuvirtide [Fuzeon, ENF]) work extracellularly by blocking fusion between viral and target cell membranes. They are always used with other treatment regimens to decrease viral load, never as monotherapy. They increase the effects of protease inhibitors. They are given only by subcutaneous injection. The pediatric dosage is weight-based and given twice daily. The adult dose is usually 90 mg twice daily.

CCR5 Antagonists

CCR5 antagonists are best suited for earlier infection when the CCR5 tropic virus (M-tropic phase) predominates (see Figure 12-5).

TABLE 12-5 ANTIRETROVIRAL THERAPY

CLASS	GENERIC NAME (TRADE NAME)	USE IN PREGNANCY OR CHILDREN	SIDE EFFECTS	MONITORING
Nucleoside reverse transcriptase inhibitors	Zidovudine (AZT, Retrovir) Lamivudine (3TC, Epivir) Didanosine (ddl, Videx)	Pregnancy Class B or C: approved and used in pregnancy as early as 10 weeks' gestation Can be given to infants and children	Pancreatitis, bone marrow toxicity, anemia/ neutropenia, peripheral neuropathy, dyslipidemia, insulin resistance, hepatic toxicity, headache, nausea, vomiting, diarrhea, insomnia, malaise, myalgia, hypersensitivity, lactic acidosis, osteopenia, confusion	Liver function studies, CBC, metabolic panel studies (chem 14)
Nonnucleoside reverse transcriptase inhibitors	Efavirenz (Sustiva) Nevirapine (Viramune) Delavirdine (Rescriptor)	Pregnancy Class D: not approved d/t teratogenic and CNS defects Avoid during lactation Approved in children over 3 yr	CNS effects, dizziness, drowsiness, concentration problems, insomnia, vivid dreams, depression, headache, maculo-papular rash, nausea, vomiting, diarrhea, myalgia, hyperlipidemia, hyperglycemia, liver enzyme elevations, Stevens-Johnson syndrome, hepatitis	Liver function studies, CBC, chem 14, lipid function; take between 6 and 9 PM to sleep through side effects
Protease inhibitors	Ritonavir (Norvir) Atazanavir (Reyataz) Nelfinavir (Viracept)	Pregnancy Class B or C: approved in pregnancy and in children Avoid during lactation	Hyperlipidemia, lipid abnormalities, lipodystrophy, elevated LFTs/uric acid, dizziness, anxiety, bleeding, pancreatitis, MI, stroke, weakness, asthenia, headache, nausea, diarrhea, vomiting, anorexia, abdominal pain, taste perversion, paresthesias	Liver function studies, CBC, chem 14, lipid function, uric acid levels; must take with food
Fusion inhibitor	Enfuvirtide (ENF, Fuzeon)	Pregnancy Class B: approved Approved in children older than 6 yr	Fatigue, insomnia, diarrhea, nausea, abdominal pain, anorexia, elevated CPK, myalgia, cough, bacterial pneumonia, flulike syndrome, thrombocytopenia, hyperlipid-emia, elevated LFTs	Liver function studies, chem 14, lipid function
CCR5 antagonist	Maraviroc (Selzentry)	Pregnancy Class B: approved Approved in adolescents 16 yr and older	Hepatotoxicity, hypersensitivity reactions, fever, cough, vascular hypertensive disorder, dizziness, insomnia, pruritus, lipodystrophy, elevated LFTs, peripheral neuropathy, myalgia	Liver function studies, CBC, chem 14, lipid function
Integrase transfer inhibitor	Raltegravir (Isentress)	Pregnancy Class C: not approved Approved in adolescents 16 yr and older	Myopathy, rhabdomyolysis, hyperlipidemia, hypertension, fatigue, dizziness, elevated glucose/lipase/LFTs/creatinine, anemia, thrombocytopenia	Liver function studies, CBC, chem 14, lipid function, uric acid levels

CBC, Complete blood cell count; *CNS,* central nervous system; *CPK,* creatine phosphokinase; *d/t,* due to; *LFTs,* liver function tests; *MI,* myocardial infarction; *yr,* year.

This medication acts to prevent infection by blocking the coreceptor CCR5 and preventing HIV binding to the cell membrane. Tropism testing is necessary before treatment with this medication. It is always given with other antiretroviral medications.

Integrase Strand Transfer Inhibitors

INSTIs are the newest class of antiretroviral medications. These medications target and inhibit *integrase* encoded by the viral *pol* gene. The first INSTI approved by the U.S. Food and Drug Administration (FDA) was raltegravir (Isentress).

Other Treatments and Vaccines

Antibiotics, antivirals, antifungals, antiparasitics, and antimycobacterial medications are administered as needed to treat the many opportunistic infections that are secondary to HIV infection. Human granulocyte colony–stimulating factor (filgrastim [Neupogen]) may be used to improve nonspecific immunity by increasing the number of neutrophils in persons with neutropenia. This agent is particularly helpful in decreasing medication-induced neutropenia. It is given daily in a subcutaneous dose calculated according to the patient's weight (usually 5 μg/kg). However, it is of questionable value because it may act as a growth factor for cancers. Epoetin alfa (erythropoietin) is used to manage medication-induced anemia. The starting dosage is 8000 units subcutaneously per week and may be increased to 48,000 units/ week until the hematocrit is 35% to 40%. An associated side effect is hypertension. Intravenous immunoglobulin can sometimes be used in HIV-infected children with T-cell counts greater than 200/μL. It helps to decrease the incidence of serious bacterial, minor bacterial, viral, and opportunistic infections. Interferon alfa-2b (Intron A) is used to treat AIDS-related Kaposi sarcoma in adults. The usual dosage is 30 million units/m² three times per week. Other studies are being conducted in an effort to find ways to rebuild the immune system. Researchers want to make sure that the T cells cloned after initiation of antiretroviral therapy will respond to both new and old infections.

Prevention of HIV infection by vaccine-conferred active immunity is the ultimate goal of current research. This task is extremely difficult because of HIV strain variability and HIV mutation frequency. To date, none of the vaccine trials have been successful and several have been stopped in phase II. In September 2007, Merck stopped the AIDS vaccine trial (STEP study) that focused on killer T cells, because 24 of 741 patients became infected with HIV as a result of the vaccine. Ongoing research is being carried out in an effort to quantify the effectiveness of other vaccines in stimulating both cellular and humoral responses to HIV. The most recent trial (RV144 Thai) in September 2009 focused on neutralizing antibodies.[35] This regimen provided some modest protection to HIV-1 infection but neutralizing antibodies were not induced.[35] At this time, there is no effective or efficacious vaccine available for prevention of HIV.

KEY POINTS

- Management of HIV and AIDS includes the use of antiretroviral medications, including NRTIs, NNRTIs, PIs, fusion inhibitors, INSTIs, and CCR5 antagonists.
- The current optimal combination of medications is multidrug therapy with two nucleoside analogues (NRTIs) and one active drug from one of the following classes: protease inhibitors (PIs) boosted with ritonavir (RTV), a non-nucleoside reverse transcriptase inhibitor (NNRTI), an integrase strand transfer inhibitor (INSTI), or a CCR5 antagonist.
- Efforts to stimulate immune function with peptide growth factors and the development of vaccines are under investigation.
- Aggressive treatment of opportunistic infections with appropriate antibiotics and antivirals is a large part of the treatment regimen.

SUMMARY

HIV is an RNA virus that primarily infects and destroys the immune system. In so doing, it destroys one of the basic foundations of human regulation and protection. HIV decreases the body's ability to fight organisms, opens the door to opportunistic infections, and allows neoplasms to emerge. HIV can infect anyone of any age. The ultimate intracellular pathogen, it slowly destroys the host while manufacturing billions of copies of itself. Study of this virus has improved our understanding of the immune system as well as of cellular function.

REFERENCES

1. UNAIDS: *Global health sector strategy on HIV/AIDS 2011-2015*, Geneva, 2011, WHO.
2. National Institutes of Health: *HIV infection and AIDS factsheet*, Bethesda, MD, June 2007, U.S. Department of Health and Human Services.
3. National Center for Health Statistics, CDC and Health Resources and Services Administration: *Final review Healthy People 2010*, Bethesda, MD, October 2011, U.S. Department of Health and Human Services.
4. National Center for Health Statistics, CDC and Health Resources and Services Administration: *Healthy People 2020 guidelines*, Bethesda, MD, October 2011, U.S. Department of Health and Human Services.
5. Sutton M, et al: A review of the Centers for Disease Control and Prevention's response to the HIV/AIDS crisis among blacks in the United States, 1981-2009, *Am J Pub Health* 99(suppl 2):S351–S359, 2009.
6. DHHS Panel on Antiretroviral Guidelines for Adults and Adolescents: *Adult and adolescent treatment guidelines*, October 14, 2011, Office of AIDS Research Advisory Council, Department of Health and Human Services. pp 1–130.
7. Jaspan HB, et al: Immune activation in the female genital tract during HIV infection predicts mucosal CD4 depletion and HIV shedding, *J Infect Dis* 204(10):1550–1556, November 2011.
8. Taborda-Vanegas N, et al: Genetic and immunological factors involved in natural resistance to HIV-1 infection, *Open Virol J* 5:35–43, May 11, 2011.
9. Adachi T, et al: Identification of a unique CXCR4 epitope whose ligation inhibits infection by both CXCR4 and CCR5 tropic human immunodeficiency type-1 viruses, *Retrovirology* 8(1):84, October 22, 2011.
10. Pitha PM: Innate antiviral response: role in HIV-1 infection, *Viruses* 3(7):1179–1203, July 2011.
11. Sakuragi J: What's going on post-budding? *Uirusu* 61(1):91–98, June 2011.
12. Kawamura T: Langerhans cell and HIV, *Nihon Rinsho Meneski Gakkai Kaishi* 34(2):70–75, 2011.
13. Cicala C, et al: HIV-1 envelope, integrins and co-receptor use in mucosal transmission of HIV, *J Trans Med* 9(suppl 1):S2, January 27, 2011.
14. Francis AC, et al: Role of phosphorylation in the nuclear biology of HIV-1, *Curr Med Chem* 18(19):2904–2912, 2011.
15. Sloan RD, Wainberg MA: The role of unintegrated DNA in HIV infection, *Retrovirology* 8:52, 2011.
16. Kaushic C: HIV-1 infection in the female reproductive tract: role of interactions between HIV-1 and genital epithelial cells, *Am J Reprod Immunol* 65(3):253–260, March 2011.
17. Fevrier M, et al: CD4+ T cell depletion in human immunodeficiency virus (HIV) infection: role of apoptosis, *Viruses* 3(5):586–612, May 12, 2011.
18. Shen X, Tomaras GD: Alterations of the B-cell response by HIV-1 replication, *Curr HIV/AIDS Rep* 8(1):23–30, March 2011.
19. Taborda-Vanegas N, et al: Genetic and immunological factors involved in natural resistance to HIV-1 infection, *Open Virol J* 5:35–43, May 11, 2011.
20. Centers for Disease Control and Prevention: 1993 Revised Classification System for HIV Infection and Expanded Surveillance Case Definition for AIDS Among Adolescents and Adults, *MMWR Morb Mortal Wkly Rep* 41(RR-17):1–6, 1992.
21. Dunn DT, et al: Genotypic resistance testing in routine clinical care, *Curr Opin HIV AIDS* 6(4):251–257, July 2011.
22. Sztam KA, et al: Macronutrient supplementation and food prices in HIV treatment, *J Nutr* 140(1):S213–S223, January 2010.
23. Koethe JR, Heimburger DC: Nutritional aspects of HIV-associated wasting in sub-Saharan Africa, *Am J Clin Nutr* 91(4):S1138–S1142, April 2010.
24. Beatty GW: Diarrhea in patients infected with HIV presenting to the emergency department, *Emerg Med Clin North Am* 28(2):299–310, May 2010.
25. Huang L, et al: HIV-associated *Pneumocystis* pneumonia, *Proc Am Thorac Soc* 8(3):294–300, June 2011.
26. Kreuter A, Wieland U: Oral hairy leukoplakia: a clinical indicator of immunosuppression, *CMAJ* 183(8):932, May 17, 2011.
27. Huang Y, et al: Glutaminase dysregulation in HIV-1-infected human microglia mediates neurotoxicity: relevant to HIV-1-associated neurocognitive disorders, *J Neurosci* 31(42):15195–15204, October 19, 2011.
28. Giannarelli C, et al: Cardiovascular implications of HIV-induced dyslipidemia, *Atherosclerosis*, June 13, 2011 (Epub ahead of print).
29. Feeney ER, Mallon PW: HIV and HAART-associated dyslipidemia, *Cardiovasc Med J* 5:49–63, 2011.
30. Brown TT: The effects of HIV-1 infection on endocrine organs, *Best Pract Res Clin Endocrinol Metab* 25(3):403–413, June 2011.
31. Feeney ER, Mallon PW: Insulin resistance in treated HIV infection, *Best Pract Res Clin Endocrinol Metab* 25(3):443–458, June 2011.
32. Giralt M, et al: Adipose tissue biology and HIV-infection, *Best Pract Res Clin Endocrinol Metab* 25(3):487–499, June 2011.
33. Vidal R, et al: Pharmacogenetics of the lipodystrophy syndrome associated with HIV infection and combination antiretroviral therapy, *Expert Opin Drug Metab Toxicol* 7(11):1365–1382, November 7, 2011.
34. Scott P, et al: Measles vaccination in HIV-infected children: systematic review and meta-analysis of safety and immunogenicity, *J Infect Dis* 204(suppl 1):S164–S178, July 2011.
35. Munier CM, et al: HIV vaccines: progress to date, *Drugs* 71(4):387–414, March 5, 2011.

Alterations in Oxygen Transport

Marie L. Kotter and Susan G. Trevithick

KEY QUESTIONS

- What factors are necessary for normal red blood cell production?
- How are oxygen and carbon dioxide transported in the circulation?
- How are laboratory tests used to detect anemia and polycythemia?
- What are the general effects of anemia on body systems?

- How are history, clinical manifestations, and laboratory studies used to differentiate the various forms of anemia?
- How are history, clinical manifestations, and laboratory studies used to differentiate the various forms of polycythemia?
- What are the appropriate treatment measures for each of the common types of anemia and polycythemia?

CHAPTER OUTLINE

Blood is a critical body fluid composed of formed elements and cells suspended in plasma that circulates through the cardiovascular system. As the primary transport system of the body, blood is involved in the physiologic and pathologic activities of all organs. The **red blood cell (RBC),** or **erythrocyte,** is essential to oxygen transport within the circulatory system. Red blood cells contain large numbers of hemoglobin molecules, which are designed to move oxygen efficiently from the lungs to other body tissues. Hemoglobin also aids in acid-base balance.

In addition, RBCs carry carbon dioxide wastes away from the cells and back to the lungs for expiration.

COMPOSITION OF BLOOD

The total blood volume averages 75.5 ml/kg in men and 66.5 ml/kg in women, which is 5 to 6 L or 7% to 8% of body weight. The blood cells comprise approximately 45% and the blood plasma 55% of the blood

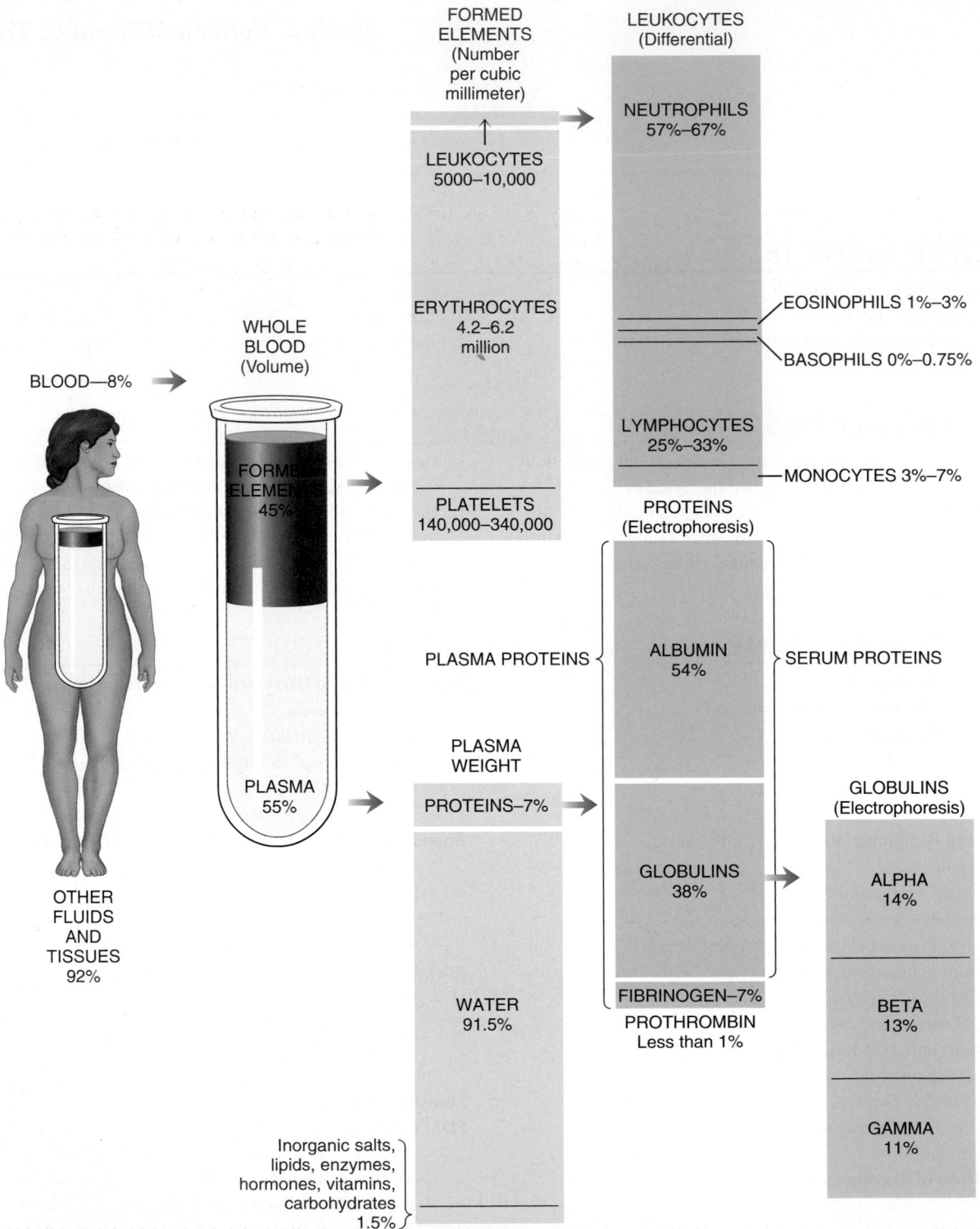

FIGURE 13-1 Composition of blood in the normal adult.

volume. Blood **plasma** is composed of about 92% water and 7% plasma proteins (Figure 13-1). The arterial pH of normal blood is 7.35 to 7.45.

Organic and Inorganic Components

The plasma proteins are formed mainly in the liver. They are unable to leave the vascular space under normal circumstances and assist in regulating blood volume and the body's fluid balance. Plasma proteins contribute to colloid osmotic pressure, which is important in maintaining blood pressure. There are three general types of plasma proteins. The first is serum albumin, which is an essential factor in maintaining blood volume and pressure. The second is serum globulin, which is composed of three general fractions: the α fraction is associated with the transport of bilirubin, lipids, and steroids; the β fraction is associated with the transport of iron and copper in plasma; and the γ fraction contains the antibody molecules. Fibrinogen is the third major type of plasma protein. It is the inactive precursor of fibrin, which forms the framework of blood clots. Regulatory proteins, such as hormones and enzymes, are also present in the plasma. Diffusible nonorganic substances, such as sodium chloride, calcium, potassium, iodine, and iron, are used by body cells and constitute 0.9% of plasma. Diffusible organic constituents, such as urea, uric acid, xanthine, creatine, creatinine, and ammonia, are products of tissue metabolism that are transported from the tissues to the kidneys and skin for excretion. Also included in this category are nutritive organic materials, such as amino acids, glucose, fats, and cholesterol, which are foodstuffs in solution absorbed from the gastrointestinal (GI) tract. They are transported to other body tissues for utilization and storage (Table 13-1).[1]

Cellular Components

The amounts of the different cellular components in the blood vary with age. Table 13-2 gives normal values from birth to 21 years.[2]

TABLE 13-1 ORGANIC AND INORGANIC COMPONENTS OF BLOOD

CONSTITUENT	AMOUNT/CONCENTRATION	MAJOR FUNCTIONS
Water	92% of plasma weight	Medium for carrying all other constituents
Electrolytes	Total <1% of plasma weight	Keep H_2O in extracellular compartment; act as buffers; function in membrane excitability
Na^+	136-145 mEq/L (142 mM)	
K^+	3.5-5 mEq/L (4 mM)	
Ca^{2+}	4.5-5.5 mEq/L (2.5 mM)	
Mg^{2+}	1.5-2.5 mEq/L (1.5 mM)	
Cl^-	100-106 mEq/L (103 mM)	
HCO_3^-	27 mEq/L (27 mM)	
Phosphate (mostly HPO_4^{2-})	3-4.5 mEq/L (1 mM)	
SO_4^{2-}	0.5-1.5 mEq/L (0.5 mM)	
Proteins	6-8 g/dl (2.5 mM)	
Albumin	3.5-5.5 g/dl	Provides colloid osmotic pressure of plasma; acts as buffers; bind other plasma constituents (e.g., lipids, hormones, vitamins, metals)
Globulins	1.5-0.3 g/dl	Enzymes; enzyme precursors; antibodies (immune globulins); hormones
Fibrinogen	0.2-0.4 g/dl	Clotting factor
Gases, arterial plasma		
CO_2 content	22-30 mmol/L of plasma	By-product of metabolism; most CO_2 content is from HCO_3^- and acts as buffer
O_2	PaO_2, 80 mm Hg or greater (arterial); $P\bar{v}O_2$, 30-40 mm Hg (venous)	Oxygenation
N_2	0.9 ml/dl	By-product of protein catabolism
Nutrients		Provide nutrition and substances for tissue repair
Glucose and other carbohydrates	70-105 mg/dl (5.6 mM)	
Total amino acids	40 mg/dl (2 mM)	
Total lipids	450 mg/dl (7.5 mM)	
Cholesterol	150-250 mg/dl (4-7 mM)	
Individual vitamins	0.0001-2.5 mg/dl	
Individual trace elements	0.001-0.3 mg/dl	
Waste products		
Urea (BUN)	10-20 mg/dl (5.7 mM)	End product of protein catabolism
Creatinine	0.7-1.5 mg/dl (0.09 mM)	End product of energy metabolism
Uric acid	2.5-8 mg/dl (0.3 mM)	End product of protein metabolism
Bilirubin	0.3-1.1 mg/dl	End product of red blood cell destruction
Direct conjugated	0.1-0.5 mg/dl	
Indirect unconjugated	0.1-0.7 mg/dl	
Individual hormones	0.000001-0.05 mg/dl	Functions specific to target tissue

Adapted with permission from Vander AJ et al: *Human physiology: the mechanisms of body function*, ed 7, New York, 1998, McGraw-Hill.

TABLE 13-2 AGE-RELATED CHANGES IN HEMATOLOGIC VALUES

AGE	HEMOGLOBIN (g)	HEMATOCRIT (%)	RBC COUNT (millions/mm³)	PLATELETS (thousands/ mm³)	RETICULOCYTES (%)
Birth	17.6	55	5.5	350.0	5.0
24 hr	18.0	56	5.3	400.0	5.2
1 wk	17.0	54	5.0	300.0	1.0
2 mo	12.4	30	4.3	260.0	0.5
6 mo	11.5	34	4.6	250.0	0.8
2 yr	12.9	40	4.8	250.0	1.0
6 yr	14.1	42	4.8	250.0	1.0
14 yr	15.0	M: 45; F: 42	5.1	250.0	1.0
21 yr	15.0	M: 45; F: 42	5.1	250.0	1.0

Data from Platt W: *Color atlas and textbook of hematology,* ed 2, Philadelphia, 1979, Lippincott, p 4. Reproduced by permission of William R. Platt, MD.

TABLE 13-3 CHARACTERISTICS OF BLOOD CELLS

CELL	STRUCTURAL CHARACTERISTICS	NORMAL AMOUNTS IN CIRCULATING BLOOD*	FUNCTION	LIFE SPAN
Erythrocyte (red blood cell)	Nonnucleated biconcave disk containing hemoglobin	Males: $4.7\text{-}6.1 \times 10^{12}$/L Females: $4.2\text{-}5.4 \times 10^{12}$/L	Gas transport to and from tissue cells and lungs	80-120 days
Leukocyte (white blood cell)	Nucleated cell	$4.8\text{-}10.8 \times 10^9$/L	Body defense mechanisms	See below
Lymphocyte	Mononuclear immunocyte	$1.2\text{-}3.4 \times 10^9$/L; 20-44% leukocyte differential	Humoral and cell-mediated immunity	Days or years, depending on type
Neutrophil	Segmented polymorphonuclear granulocyte with neutrophilic granules	$1.4\text{-}6.5 \times 10^9$/L; 50-70% leukocyte differential	Phagocytosis, particularly during early phase of inflammation	5 days
Eosinophil	Segmented polymorphonuclear granulocyte with eosinophilic granules	$0\text{-}0.7 \times 10^9$/L; 0-4% leukocyte differential	Phagocytosis, antibody-mediated defense against parasites; participates in mucosal immune response	Unknown
Basophil	Segmented polymorphonuclear granulocyte with basophilic granules	$0\text{-}0.2 \times 10^9$/L; 0-2% leukocyte differential	Transport and release of heparin and histamine; involved in immune and inflammatory responses	Unknown
Monocyte-macrophage	Large mononuclear phagocyte	$0.11\text{-}0.59 \times 10^9$/L; 2%-9% leukocyte differential	Phagocytosis; process and present antigens	Months to years

WBC COUNT (cells/mm³)	PMN COUNT, ADULT	BAND FORMS (%)	EOSINOPHILS (%)	BASOPHILS (%)	LYMPHOCYTES (%)	MONOCYTES (%)
9000-30,000 (avg., 18,000)	9400 (52%)	9.1	2.2	0.6	31	5.8
9400-34,000 (avg., 19,045)	9800 (52%)	9.2	2.4	0.5	31	5.8
5000-21,000 (avg., 12,279)	4700 (39%)	6.8	4.1	0.4	41	9.1
5500-18,000 (avg., 11,000)	3300 (30%)	4.4	2.7	0.5	57	5.9
6000-17,500 (avg., 11,900)	3300 (28%)	3.8	2.5	0.4	61	4.8
6000-17,000 (avg., 10,680)	3200 (30%)	3.0	2.6	0.5	59	5.0
5000-14,500 (avg., 8500)	4000 (48%)	3.0	2.7	0.6	42	4.7
4500-13,000 (avg., 7900)	4200 (53%)	3.0	2.5	0.5	37	4.7
4500-11,000 (avg., 7400)	4200 (56%)	3.0	2.7	0.5	34	4.0

TABLE 13-3	CHARACTERISTICS OF BLOOD CELLS—cont'd			
CELL	**STRUCTURAL CHARACTERISTICS**	**NORMAL AMOUNTS IN CIRCULATING BLOOD***	**FUNCTION**	**LIFE SPAN**
Platelet	Discoid cytoplasmic fragment derived from megakaryocytes	130-400 × 10⁹/L	Hemostasis following vascular injury; forms hemostatic plug, provides cofactors, maintains vascular endothelium	9.5 days

Illustrations from Patton KT, Thibodeau GA: *Anatomy & physiology*, ed 8, St Louis, 2013, Mosby, p. 606.
*Given in SI units.

Erythrocytes

Of the cellular elements of blood (Table 13-3), **RBCs,** or **erythrocytes,** are the most numerous, with normal concentrations ranging from 4.2 to 6.2 million cells/mm³. RBCs are responsible for transporting oxygen to the tissues, and participate in both removing carbon dioxide from the tissues and buffering blood pH. They have no cytoplasmic organelles, nucleus, mitochondria, or ribosomes. Therefore, RBCs cannot synthesize protein or carry out oxidative reactions. Instead the erythrocyte's cytoplasm consists of a solution containing proteins, hemoglobin, and electrolytes that regulates diffusion through the cellular membrane. RBCs live for 80 to 120 days in the circulation; then they die and are replaced. Hemoglobin is the main functional constituent of the red cell. It is a protein that enables the blood to transport 100 times more oxygen than could be transported in plasma alone. An enzyme inside RBCs, carbonic anhydrase, is responsible for the buffering mechanism of red cells.[3]

The erythrocyte's size and shape also contribute to its function as a gas carrier (Figure 13-2). It is a small, biconcave disk (about 7.2 μm in diameter) that must circulate through splenic sinusoids and capillaries, which are only 2 μm in diameter. This remarkable feat is accomplished through a property called *reversible deformability,* which allows the RBC to assume a torpedo-like conformation and then return to a biconcave disk shape.[3]

Leukocytes

White blood cells (WBCs), or **leukocytes,** protect the body by phagocytosis of microorganisms and other debris and participate in immune antibody formation. Leukocytes act primarily in the tissues but are also transported in the circulatory and lymphatic systems. The average adult has approximately 5000 to 10,000 leukocytes per cubic millimeter of blood. Monocytes and granulocytes are WBCs that share a common lineage with RBCs and platelets. Because of the interrelationship of RBCs, WBCs, and

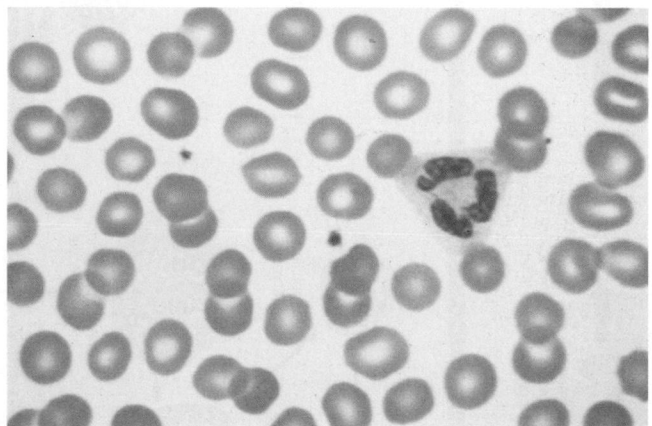

FIGURE 13-2 Mature erythrocytes. A mature neutrophil is also shown. (Courtesy Beth Payne, Sacred Heart Medical Center, Spokane, WA.)

platelets, which are all derived from the myeloid stem cell (Figure 13-3), abnormalities in these cells are seen in some red cell diseases.[4] Leukocyte structure and function are discussed in detail in Chapter 9.

Platelets

Platelets are essential in the formation of blood clots and in the control of bleeding. They are not cells but are circulating cytoplasmic fragments of megakaryocytes and are incapable of mitotic division. They contain cytoplasmic granules that release biochemical mediators involved in the hemostatic process. Normally, 150,000 to 400,000 platelets/mm³ circulate freely in the blood. An additional one third of the body's platelets are in a reserve pool in the spleen. The average life span of platelets in the peripheral blood is approximately 4 to 5 days.[5]

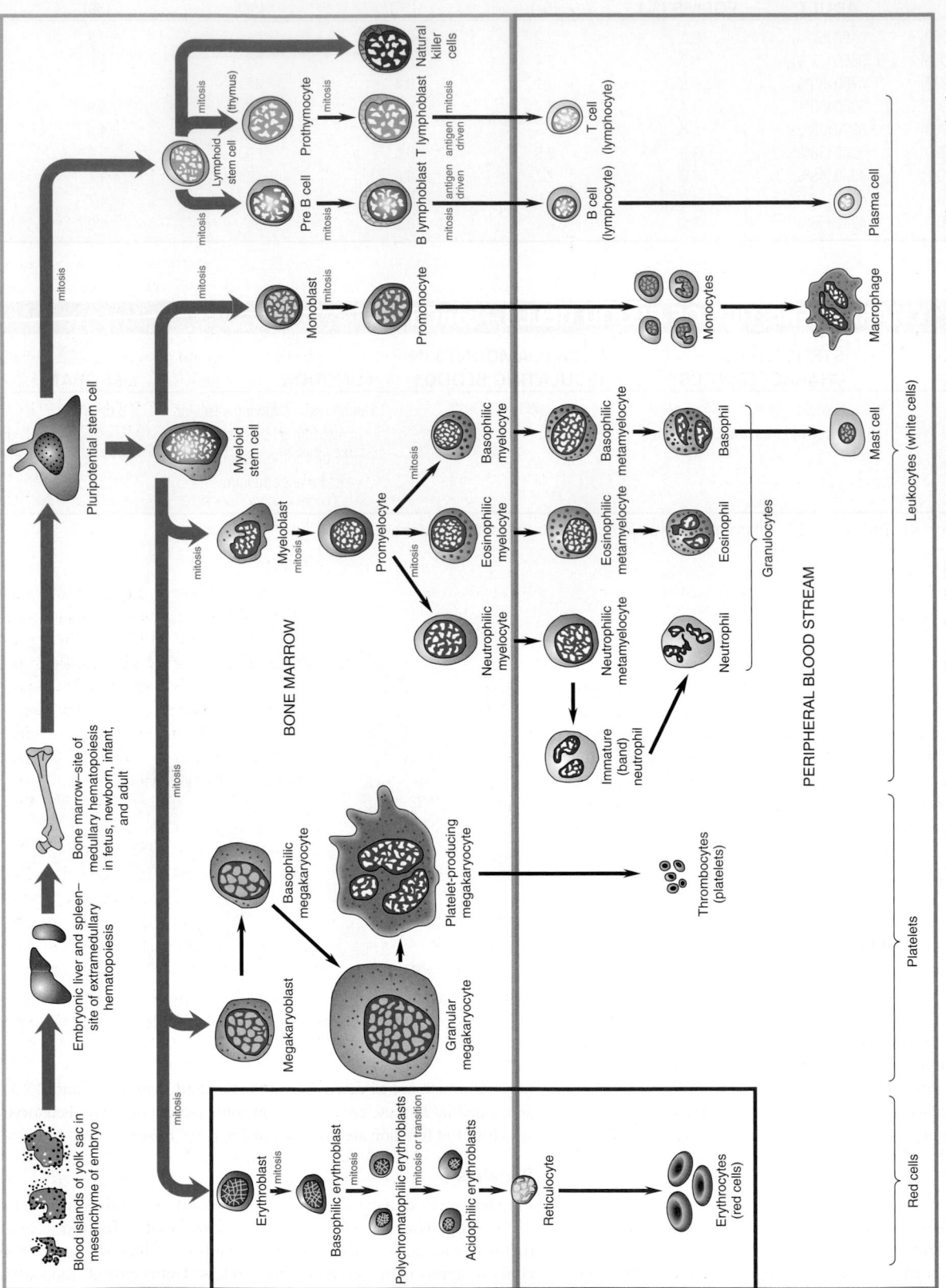

FIGURE 13-3 Maturation of human blood cells. Probable pathways of blood cell differentiation from the pluripotential stem cell to mature leukocytes, erythrocytes, and platelets. Production of cells begins in embryo blood islands of the yolk sac. As the embryo matures, production shifts to the liver and spleen (extramedullary hematopoiesis) and progresses to bone marrow (medullary hematopoiesis). In an adult, all production is in the bone marrow. Current thinking is that all cell production begins with a pluripotential stem cell, which differentiates into either a myeloid stem cell or a lymphoid stem cell, which then differentiates into a specific blast cell. For example, red cell differentiation begins with the proerythroblast, which matures into a basophilic erythroblast, to a polychromatophilic erythroblast, and to an acidophilic erythroblast, all of which are found in the bone marrow. Red cell differentiation concludes with production of reticulocytes and mature red cells (erythrocytes), which normally are found only in the peripheral blood.

STRUCTURE AND FUNCTION OF RED BLOOD CELLS

The cellular components of blood originate in the yolk sac mesenchyme, move to the liver and spleen during fetal life, and finally are limited to the marrow of the body skeleton (Figure 13-4). Bone marrow provides a special environment for hematopoietic cell proliferation and maturation. Developing cells are held in a fine reticular meshwork, which provides free access to plasma nutrients but retains developing cells until their maturity allows penetration of the endothelial barrier. In times of need, immature cells (reticulocytes and nucleated red blood cells, or NRBCs) are released early into the circulation; their presence in increased numbers is a sign that the hematopoietic system is stressed or is experiencing disease.[2]

Hematopoiesis

Hematopoiesis is the developmental process leading from pluripotential stem cells to mature, differentiated red cells, neutrophils, eosinophils, basophils, monocytes, and platelets. **Lymphopoiesis** describes this process for lymphocytes. Both hematopoietic and lymphopoietic stem cells probably derive from a single totipotent stem cell pool in fetal development, but it is uncertain if this is the functioning stem cell after birth (Figure 13-5). Research suggests that a pluripotential stem cell that is stimulated by erythropoietin and other poietins to cause further differentiation into separate cell lines may be the primary stem cell in adults.[6]

Hematopoiesis is a two-stage process that involves mitotic division (proliferation) and maturation (differentiation). Each type of blood cell has stem cells that undergo mitosis when stimulated by a specific biochemical signal, indicating that the number of circulating cells has decreased. Medullary or bone marrow hematopoiesis continues throughout life and can be accelerated by several mechanisms, including (1) an increase in differentiation of daughter cells, (2) an increase in number of stem cells, and (3) conversion of yellow (fatty) bone marrow (which does not produce cells) to red marrow (which does produce cells). Marrow conversion is stimulated by erythropoietin, which is the hormone from the kidney that stimulates erythrocyte production. In adults, extramedullary hematopoiesis, or production of blood cells in tissue other than bone, is usually due to disease.[7]

Erythrocyte development is shown in detail in Figure 13-3. During this process, the cell changes from a large nucleated cell, rich in ribosomes, to a reticulocyte, which is a small disk that has lost its nucleus. The reticulocyte (Figure 13-6) leaves the marrow, enters the bloodstream, and matures into an erythrocyte in 24 to 48 hours. During this period, mitochondria and ribosomes disappear; the cell can no longer synthesize hemoglobin, and it relies on glycolysis for adenosine triphosphate (ATP) production. The normal reticulocyte count is 1% of the total RBC count.

This makes it a useful test to determine effective erythropoietic activity[7] because erythropoietin stimulates uncommitted stem cells to differentiate into proerythroblasts.

Hemoglobin Synthesis

The immature red cell can be viewed as a factory for hemoglobin synthesis. In a mature red cell, **hemoglobin,** the oxygen-carrying protein, composes about 90% of the cell's dry weight in the form of approximately 300 hemoglobin molecules.[3] Hemoglobin that is carrying oxygen is called oxyhemoglobin. Hemoglobin is composed of two pairs of polypeptide chains—the globins. Each globin has an attached heme molecule that is composed of iron plus a protoporphyrin molecule (Figure 13-7).[8]

After dietary iron is absorbed in the duodenum and proximal jejunum, it is transported through the plasma by the protein transferrin to transferrin iron receptors on the RBC membrane. The transferrin-receptor complex is engulfed by the cell into an invagination of the cell surface. The invagination becomes sealed off and forms an intracytoplasmic vacuole. Iron is then released and either stored as ferritin or used to synthesize heme (Figure 13-8).[2] About 67% of total body iron is bound to heme in erythrocytes and muscle cells, and 30% is stored bound to ferritin or hemosiderin-containing macrophages and hepatic parenchymal cells. The remaining 3% is lost daily in urine, sweat, bile, and epithelial cells that are shed in the intestines. The mitochondria are responsible for the synthesis of protoporphyrin. The final heme molecule consists of four porphyrin moieties assembled in a ring structure around a central iron molecule.[2]

Hemoglobin Synthesis in Infants

When an infant is born many mechanisms occur to decrease the infant's hemoglobin level. At birth, erythropoietin, a hormone that stimulates red blood cell production, disappears from blood plasma; there is an increase in arterial oxygen saturation and the infant is born with immature bone marrow. These mechanisms cause a slow rate of red blood cell production at birth. In addition, infants primarily have fetal hemoglobin, accounting for about 70% of their total hemoglobin. Although fetal hemoglobin is a more efficient oxygen carrier, it has a shorter life span than adult hemoglobin. This causes red blood cells to be turned over every 70 to 90 days, instead of 120 days for adult red blood cells. Fetal hemoglobin may suppress production of erythropoietin.

Hemoglobin levels gradually decrease in the infant over the first 2 to 3 months because of the rapid destruction of fetal hemoglobin, decreased red blood cell production and depressed erythropoietin production. Additionally, the infant experiences rapid growth during this time, which creates quick expansion of blood volume that further dilutes the supply of hemoglobin. Maternal iron stores are rapidly depleting at this time and the baby's iron stores will gradually diminish by 6 months.

As fetal hemoglobin is metabolized, the iron is released and stored. The body has enough iron to synthesize hemoglobin, but there is no stimulation to create hemoglobin at this time. Hemoglobin levels will continue to decrease until the oxygen needs of the tissues in the body are depleted enough to stimulate erythropoietin production. Release of erythropoietin causes erythropoiesis to resume. Adult hemoglobin is made at this time with the iron stored in the body. Hemoglobin levels will steadily increase in the infant starting about 6 months of age as fetal hemoglobin is replaced by adult hemoglobin.[9]

Globin is assembled from two pairs of polypeptide chains produced on specific ribosomes. The protein chain produced in fetal life is altered after birth by sequential gene suppression and activation. At birth, red cells contain mainly fetal hemoglobin (hemoglobin F), which is composed of two α chains and two γ chains. Hemoglobin F is a more efficient gas carrier under decreased oxygen tension than hemoglobin A and releases CO_2 more readily. Within 120 days, fetal hemoglobin disappears

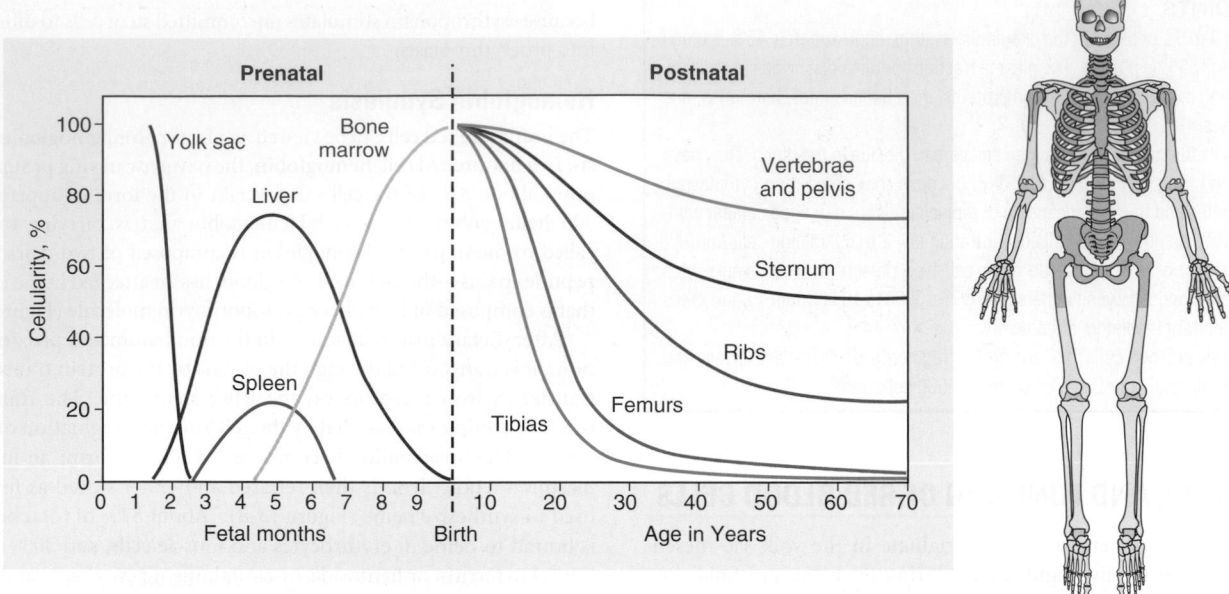

FIGURE 13-4 Location of active marrow growth in the fetus and adult. During fetal development, hematopoiesis is first established in the yolk sac mesenchyme, later moves to the liver and spleen, and finally is limited to the bony skeleton. From infancy to adulthood, there is progressive restriction of productive marrow to the axial skeleton and proximal ends of the long bones, which appear as shaded areas on the drawing of the skeleton.

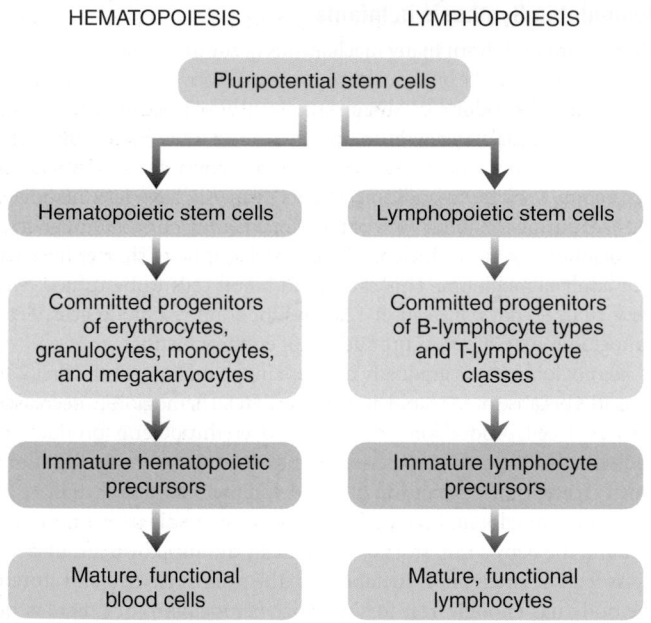

FIGURE 13-5 Stem cells and normal hematopoiesis.

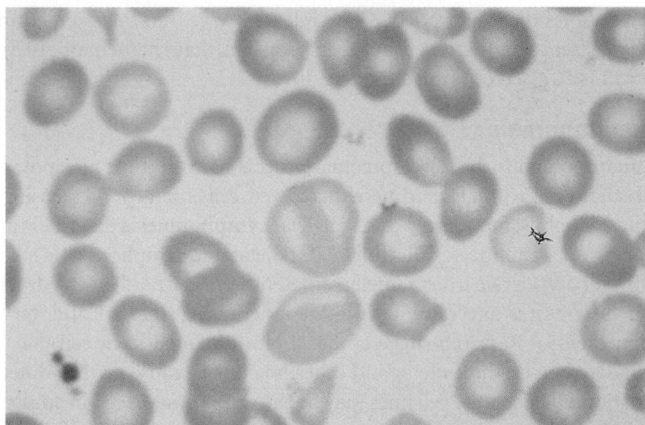

FIGURE 13-6 Reticulocytes seen on peripheral blood smear. The two reticulocytes in the center still contain remnants of intracellular organelles. (Courtesy Beth Payne, Sacred Heart Medical Center, Spokane, WA.)

and is replaced by adult hemoglobin (hemoglobin A) (Figure 13-9). This switch is the result of globin genes and is not well understood. Hemoglobin A is composed of two α chains and two β chains and constitutes 97% of the hemoglobin found in adults. Hemoglobin A_2 comprises 2% to 3% of hemoglobin found in adults and is composed of $\alpha_2\delta_2$.[8,9]

Several hundred hemoglobinopathies have been described that have changes in the two α chains and two β chains. Most are characterized by the substitution of only one amino acid and are classified by the polypeptide chain in which the substitution occurs.[8]

Nutritional Requirements for Erythropoiesis

In addition to iron, which is required for hemoglobin synthesis, the normal development of erythrocytes requires adequate supplies of protein, vitamins, and minerals. Erythropoiesis cannot proceed in the absence of vitamins, especially B_{12}, folate, B_6, riboflavin, pantothenic acid, niacin, ascorbic acid, and vitamin E. Folates and vitamin B_{12} (cobalamin) are absorbed from food by the ileal mucosa. Folate deficiencies or vitamin B_{12} deficiencies lead to impaired DNA synthesis in erythroid cells because the vitamins are coenzymes in a large number of key reactions in cellular metabolism. Absorption of vitamin B_{12} requires intrinsic factor in the gastric juice. Intrinsic factor is secreted by the stomach parietal cells and binds to vitamin B_{12}. The complex then moves down the gastrointestinal tract to the ileum, where it attaches to specific receptor sites on the ileum mucosal cell. It is absorbed into the cell, released, and transported in the blood to the tissues and liver.[10,11]

Energy and Maintenance of Erythrocytes

For the RBC to perform efficiently and survive in the circulation for the full 120-day life span, it must have a source of energy. Without an energy source, ion pumps fail and the RBC becomes sodium logged

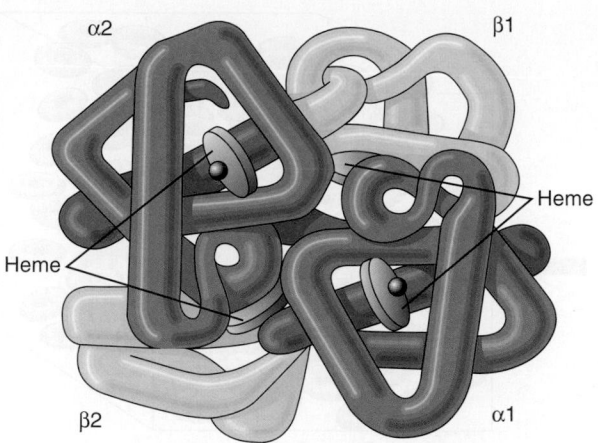

FIGURE 13-7 Molecular structure of hemoglobin. The molecule is a spherical tetramer weighing approximately 64,500 daltons. It contains two α- and two β-polypeptide chains and four heme groups.

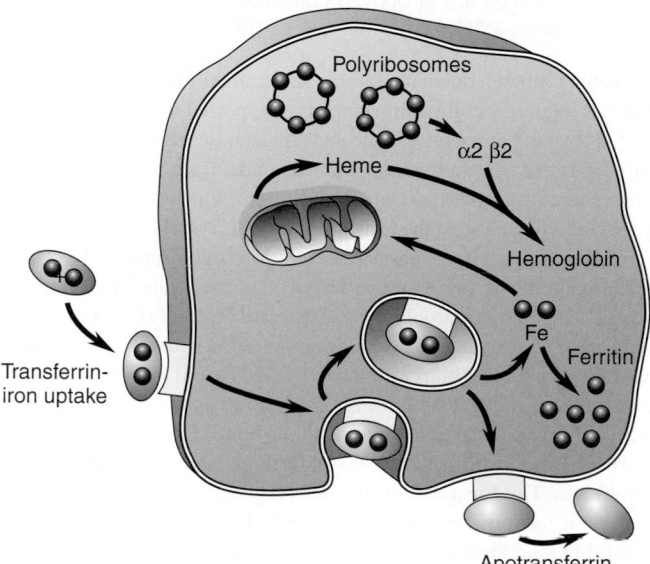

FIGURE 13-8 Intracellular pathways for iron uptake and incorporation into hemoglobin in erythroblasts in the bone marrow. The iron-transferrin complex is picked up by a membrane-associated receptor and brought into the cell by invagination and formation of an intracytoplasmic vacuole. The iron is then released and stored as intracytoplasmic ferritin or used to synthesize heme, the precursor of hemoglobin. The transferrin-receptor complex is returned to the cell membrane, where the apotransferrin is expelled back into the circulation. (Redrawn from Hillman RS, Finch CA, editors: *Red cell manual*, ed 6, Philadelphia, 1992, FA Davis, p 8.)

and potassium depleted. The shape changes from a biconcave disk to a sphere, and it is quickly removed from the circulation by the filtering action of the spleen and the mononuclear phagocyte system. The metabolism of the RBC is limited because of the absence of a nucleus, mitochondria, and other subcellular organelles. Although the binding, transport, and release of O_2 and CO_2 is a passive process that does not require energy, other energy-dependent metabolic processes occur that are essential to RBC viability. The chief metabolic pathway, accounting for about 90% of the glucose used, is the anaerobic or Embden-Meyerhof pathway. The Embden-Meyerhof pathway provides ATP for regulation of intracellular Na^+, K^+, Ca^{2+}, and Mg^{2+} concentrations via cation pumps. About 10% of the glucose undergoes aerobic glycolysis in the hexose monophosphate shunt. The hexose monophosphate shunt provides nicotinamide adenine dinucleotide

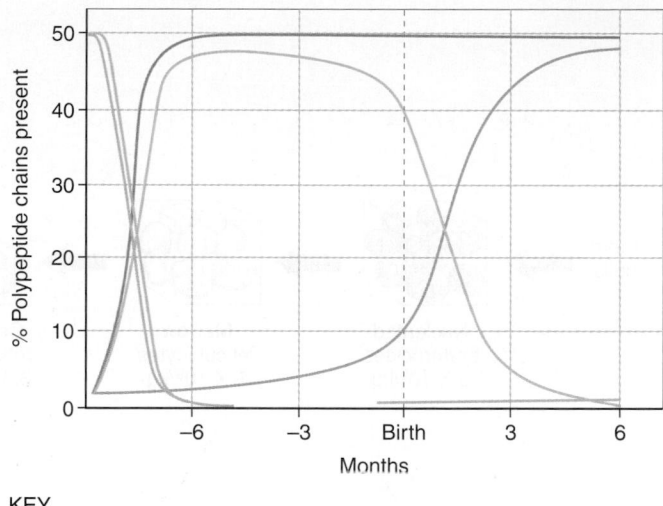

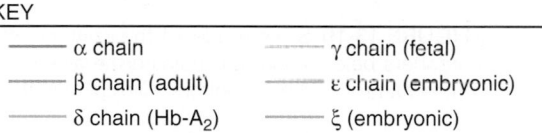

— α chain
— β chain (adult)
— δ chain (Hb-A₂)
— γ chain (fetal)
— ε chain (embryonic)
— ξ (embryonic)

FIGURE 13-9 Changes in hemoglobin with development. Sequential suppression and activation of individual globin genes in the immediate postnatal period result in a switch from fetal hemoglobin (hemoglobin F: two α chains and two γ chains) to adult hemoglobin (hemoglobin A: two α chains and two β chains). A small amount of hemoglobin A_2 (two α chains and two δ chains) is also present in the adult. (From Young NS et al, editors: *Clinical hematology*, Philadelphia, 2006, Mosby, p 24.)

phosphate (NADPH) and glutathione (GSH) to reduce cellular oxidants. This protects the cell from permanent oxidant injury. The methemoglobin reductase pathway protects hemoglobin from oxidation via NADH and methemoglobin reductase. Last, the Rapoport-Luebering pathway forms 2,3-diphosphoglycerate (2,3-DPG), which facilitates oxygen release to the tissues. These pathways contribute energy for maintaining (1) high intracellular K^+, low intracellular Na^+, and very low intracellular Ca^{2+} levels (cation pumps); (2) reduced hemoglobin concentration; (3) high levels of reduced GSH; and (4) membrane integrity and deformability.[2] Deficiencies of enzymes that regulate these pathways can be due to natural causes, such as the normal aging process, or to an inherited deficiency of an enzyme.[3,12]

Red cell membrane structures are matrices formed from a double layer of phospholipids. In the red cell membrane, the globular proteins floating on the "sea of lipids" form a protein network on the cytoplasmic surface of the membrane. Half of the mass of the membrane is lipid, which is partially responsible for many of its physical characteristics. Both passive cation permeability and mechanical flexibility can be significantly influenced by changing the lipid composition of the membrane. Maintenance and renewal of membrane lipids in well-developed RBCs is important, and problems in these pathways result in premature cell death.[13]

Red Cell Production

When blood is described as a single body system, it is called the **erythron** (Figure 13-10). The erythron includes the blood cells and their bone marrow precursors. The size of the erythron increases or decreases based on the erythropoietic process and the pathologic changes in red cells seen in anemia.[14] **Erythropoiesis** is controlled by a system sensitive to alterations in the concentration of hemoglobin in the blood. A decrease in hemoglobin level decreases the tissue oxygen tension in the kidney. In response to this hypoxia, the kidney secretes a hormone, **erythropoietin,** that stimulates primitive stem cells in the bone marrow to differentiate into proerythroblasts or pronormoblasts, thereby increasing the

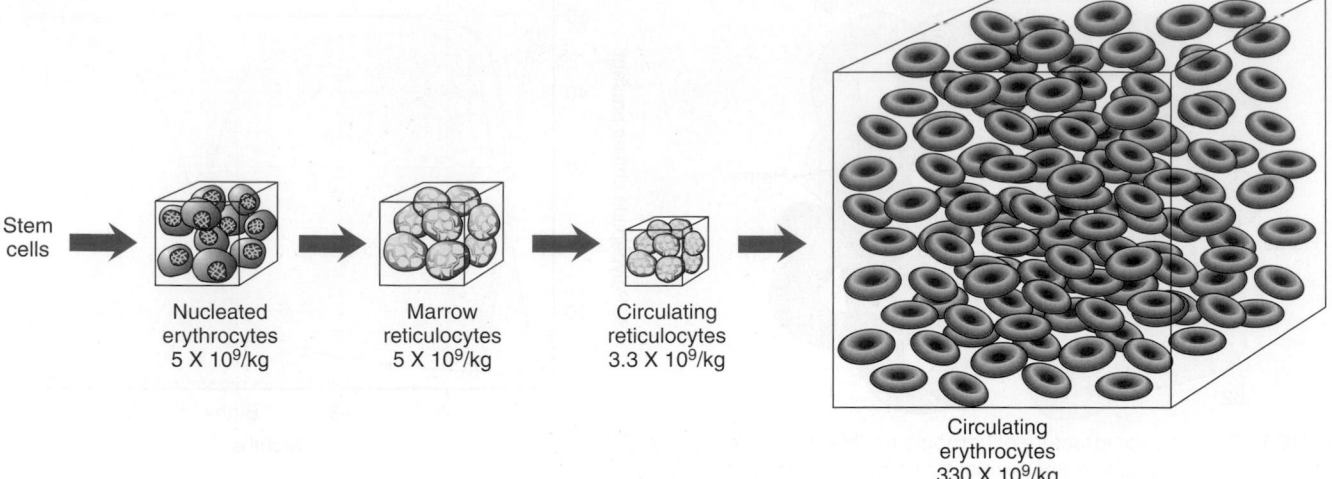

Stem cells → Nucleated erythrocytes 5 X 10^9/kg → Marrow reticulocytes 5 X 10^9/kg → Circulating reticulocytes 3.3 X 10^9/kg → Circulating erythrocytes 330 X 10^9/kg

FIGURE 13-10 Scale model of the erythron, showing the relative proportions of each component. The numbers below each box indicate the average number of cells per kilogram of body weight. (Redrawn from Wintrobe M et al, editors: *Clinical hematology*, ed 8, Philadelphia, 1981, Lea & Febiger, p 109.)

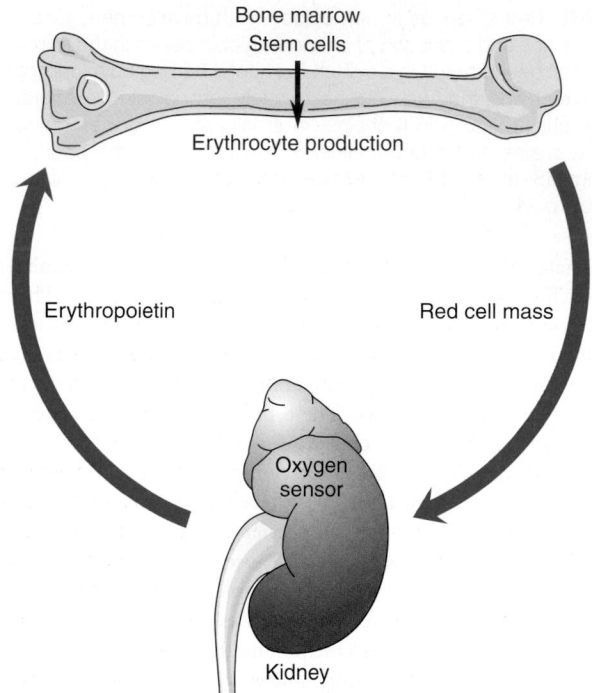

Bone marrow
Stem cells
Erythrocyte production
Erythropoietin
Red cell mass
Oxygen sensor
Kidney

FIGURE 13-11 Feedback circuit illustrating the role of erythropoietin in the regulation of red cell mass.

erythron (Figure 13-11).[3,15] Hypoxia from a low hemoglobin level and other causes, such as high altitudes, can also initiate this response.

Red Cell Destruction

While the red cell ages, the various enzyme activities decrease, amounts of membrane lipids decrease, levels of hemoglobin A_2 and methemoglobin increase, and changes in cell size occur. **Methemoglobin** is formed when the iron of the hemoglobin molecule is oxidized to the ferric state (Fe^{3+}). The cell loses its ability to deform and becomes increasingly fragile. These aging red cells are then removed by the mononuclear phagocytic system. The red cells are digested by proteolytic and lipolytic enzymes in phagolysosomes of macrophages. Almost 80% to 90% of this process occurs in macrophages of the spleen and liver. Only 10% to 20% of normal destruction occurs intravascularly.[3,16]

Globin is broken down into amino acids, and the iron is recycled. Porphyrin is reduced to **bilirubin,** which is transported to the liver and conjugated by the enzyme glucuronyl transferase. Finally, conjugated bilirubin is excreted in the bile as glucuronide. Bacteria in the intestine convert conjugated bilirubin into urobilinogen, which is excreted primarily in the stool but also in the urine (Figure 13-12). Any condition causing increased red cell destruction increases the load of bilirubin to be cleared, which leads to increased serum levels of unconjugated bilirubin and increased excretion of urobilinogen. Increased levels of circulating bilirubin give the skin a yellowish tone, which is called *jaundice*. In newborns, the albumin levels for bilirubin transport are low and the amount of liver glucuronidase available for bilirubin conjugation is low, which may cause an accumulation of toxic unconjugated bilirubin. Unconjugated bilirubin is toxic because in this form it is lipid soluble and can easily cross cell membranes. This form of bilirubin has a high affinity for basal ganglia of the central nervous system. The conjugated form of bilirubin is water soluble but lipid insoluble so it cannot cross cell membranes.[3,16]

KEY POINTS

- Red cell development from pluripotential stem cells in the bone marrow is stimulated by a hormone growth factor called *erythropoietin.* Erythropoietin is secreted into the bloodstream by kidney cells in response to low oxygen tension in the blood.
- During development, red cells lose their nuclei and other cytoplasmic organelles. A reticulocyte is an immature red cell that still retains some cellular organelles. An increased blood reticulocyte count is a useful indicator of increased red cell production.
- Hemoglobin is the major component of red cells. It is composed of two pairs of polypeptide chains, each of which has a heme molecule attached. Oxygen can bind reversibly to an iron molecule at the center of each heme. When fully saturated, a hemoglobin molecule carries four oxygen molecules, and is referred to as *oxyhemoglobin.*
- Red cell production requires adequate amounts of several nutrients, particularly iron, vitamin B_{12}, and folate. Lack of intrinsic factor inhibits absorption of B_{12} from the small intestine and is a risk factor for anemia.
- Red cells rely on glycolysis for energy production because they do not contain mitochondria. As energy production declines because of red cell aging and loss of essential glycolytic enzymes, the cell swells, is trapped in the spleen, and is removed from the circulation. Red cell degradation releases bilirubin, a toxic substance that is conjugated in the liver and excreted in urine and bile.

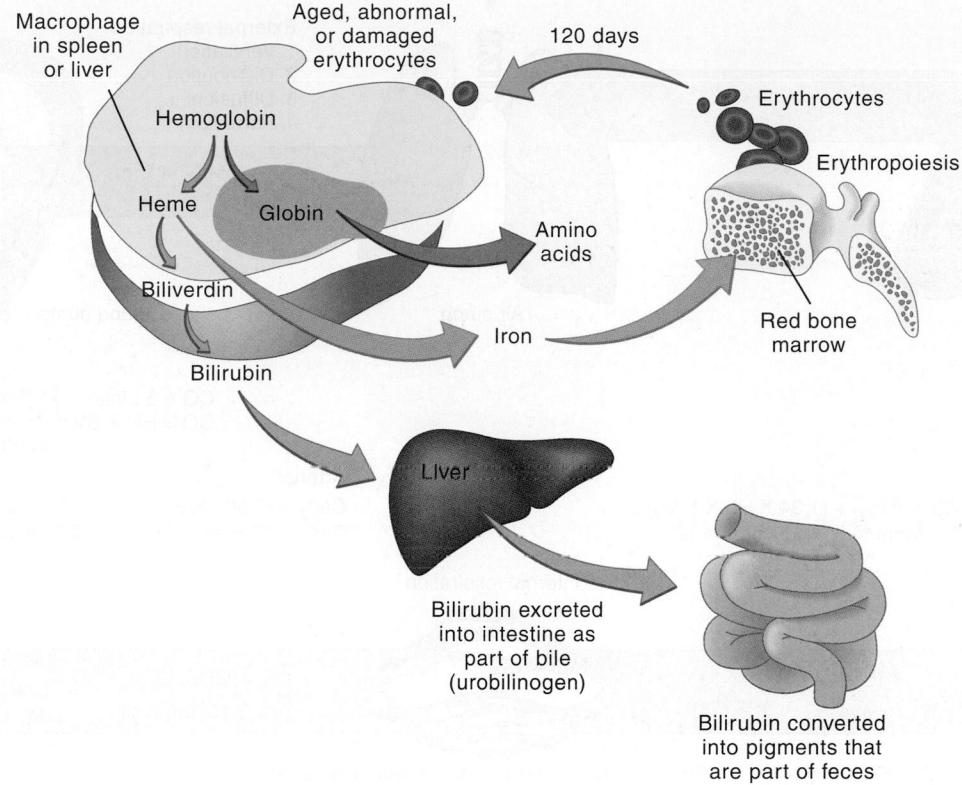

FIGURE 13-12 Most hemoglobin degradation occurs in the macrophages of the spleen. The globin and iron portions are conserved and reused. Heme is reduced to bilirubin, eventually degraded to urobilinogen, and excreted in the feces. Thus, indirect indicators of erythrocyte or erythrocyte destruction include the blood bilirubin level and urobilinogen concentration in the feces. (From Thibodeau GA, Patton KT: *Anatomy & physiology*, ed 6, St Louis, 2007, Mosby, p 654.)

GAS TRANSPORT AND ACID-BASE BALANCE

RBCs have many important functions in the body related to gas transport and acid-base balance.[3,16,17] RBCs contain hemoglobin, which is responsible for oxygen transport to the body tissues.[3,16] Oxygen combines with the heme portion of hemoglobin to form oxyhemoglobin in a loose and reversible bond in the pulmonary capillary attributable to a high partial pressure of oxygen (PO_2) and is carried to the tissues with a low PO_2, where it is released.[17] Large quantities of carbonic anhydrase in RBCs catalyze the reaction between CO_2 produced by cellular metabolism in the tissues and water to form carbonic acid, which dissociates into hydrogen and bicarbonate ions for elimination by the lungs and kidneys. Approximately 90% of the CO_2 in the arterial blood and 60% of the CO_2 in the venous blood are transported as bicarbonate. Finally, the hemoglobin protein directly binds with the remaining CO_2 to form carbaminohemoglobin for CO_2 transport. Carbamino compounds are acid-base buffers responsible for as much as 50% of the whole blood–buffering power.[3,16]

Oxygen Transport

Transport of oxygen to the body tissues and removal of carbon dioxide is a complex process involving interdependent function of the lungs, heart, and blood (Figure 13-13). Approximately 97% of oxygen in the blood is transported on red cells loosely and reversibly combined with hemoglobin (oxyhemoglobin), and 3% is dissolved in plasma. Each hemoglobin molecule can bind four atoms of oxygen. Despite a combining potential of 1.39 ml of oxygen per gram of hemoglobin in pure hemoglobin, a maximum of about 1.34 ml of oxygen per gram of hemoglobin is available, owing to a reduction of about 4% by impurities such as methemoglobin. The blood of an average person contains approximately 15 g of hemoglobin per 100 ml of blood. Therefore, in the average person, the hemoglobin in 100 ml of blood can combine with approximately 20 ml of oxygen if the hemoglobin is 100% saturated. This value is expressed as 20 vol%.[17,18]

The partial pressure of oxygen (PO_2) reflects the pressure or tension that oxygen exerts when it is dissolved in blood. Partial pressure is measured in millimeters of mercury (mm Hg). In the pulmonary capillaries, where PO_2 is high, oxygen binds efficiently with hemoglobin, but in the tissue capillaries, where PO_2 is low, oxygen is released from hemoglobin. The partial pressure affects the tendency of oxygen to bind with hemoglobin.[19] The partial pressure of oxygen in arterial blood (PaO_2) is usually 80 to 100 mm Hg, whereas the partial pressure of oxygen in venous blood ($P\bar{v}O_2$) is usually 35 to 40 mm Hg. The amount of hemoglobin bound to oxygen relative to the total amount of hemoglobin is expressed as the oxygen saturation, in a percentage.[19,20] Saturation of arterial blood with oxygen ($S\bar{a}O_2$) is normally 95% to 100%, whereas that of venous blood ($S\bar{v}O_2$) is 60% to 80%.[17-20]

The oxygen-hemoglobin dissociation curve (Figure 13-14) describes the relationship between PO_2 and SO_2. The upper part of the curve represents oxygen uptake in the lungs and demonstrates that significant changes in PO_2 result in only small changes in SO_2 to help ensure adequate oxygen delivery to the tissues.[18,19] On the steep lower portion of the curve, reflecting the venous blood, small changes in venous PO_2 result in large changes in $S\bar{v}O_2$.[19] Therefore, the tissues are protected with an available oxygen reserve as large quantities of oxygen are released from the blood for relatively small decreases in PO_2. Normally, tissue PO_2 does not rise above 40 mm Hg to enhance diffusion of oxygen from the blood to the tissues. The strength of the bond between hemoglobin and oxygen is called the *oxygen-hemoglobin affinity*. For

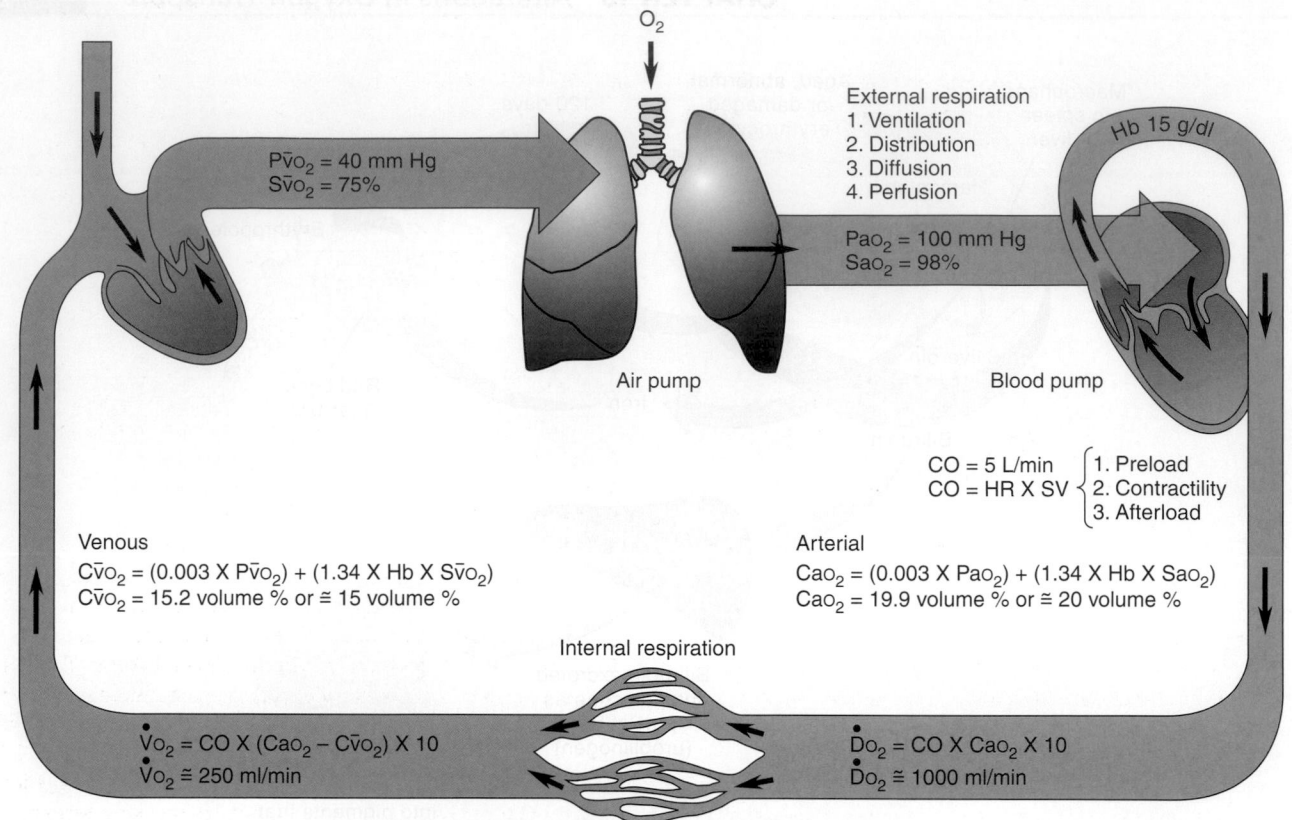

FIGURE 13-13 Oxygen transport. Diffusion of oxygen into the pulmonary capillaries occurs when alveolar PO_2 exceeds capillary PO_2. Maintenance of this gradient is dependent on adequate alveolar ventilation and perfusion. Delivery of oxygenated blood to the tissues $(\dot{D}O_2)$ is determined by the content of oxygen in the blood (CaO_2) and the cardiac output (CO). The difference between arterial and venous oxygen is a reflection of oxygen consumption by tissues $(\dot{V}O_2)$. *Hb*, Hemoglobin; *HR*, heart rate; *SV*, stroke volume.

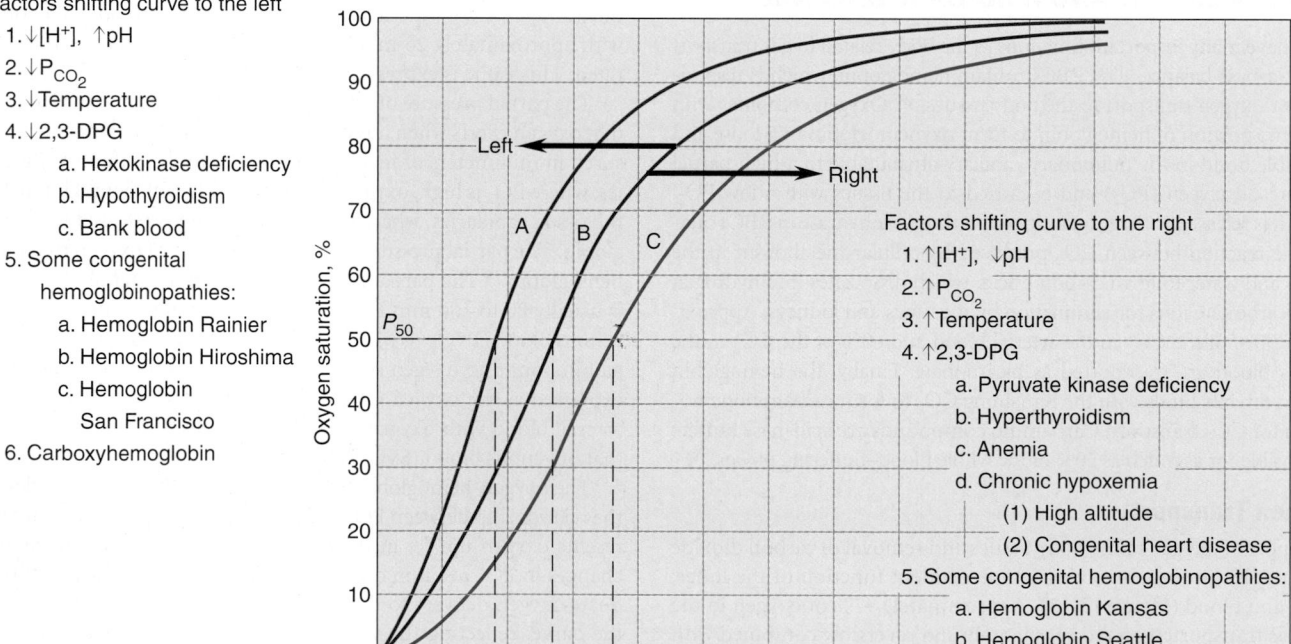

FIGURE 13-14 Oxygen-hemoglobin dissociation curve: factors affecting hemoglobin's affinity for oxygen. Curve *B* is the standard oxyhemoglobin dissociation curve. Factors that shift the curve to the left are represented in curve *A;* factors that shift the curve to the right are represented in curve *C. 2,3-DPG,* 2,3-Diphosphoglycerate. (Redrawn from Gottlieb JE: Breathing and gas exchange. In Kinney MR et al, editors: *AACN's clinical reference for critical care nursing,* ed 3, New York, 1993, McGraw-Hill, p 672.)

any given PO_2, hemoglobin saturation will be higher when affinity is increased and saturation will be lower when affinity is decreased. Changes in hemoglobin affinity are represented by shifts in the oxyhemoglobin dissociation curve (see Figure 13-14). Shifts in the oxyhemoglobin curve affect the ability of hemoglobin to bind O_2 in the lungs and release it in the tissues. The ability of hemoglobin to release oxygen to the tissues is commonly assessed at point P_{50} on the oxygen-hemoglobin dissociation curve. The P_{50} is the PO_2 at which 50% of the hemoglobin is saturated. A decrease in oxygen affinity (shift to the right on the oxyhemoglobin dissociation curve) or an increase in oxygen affinity (shift to the left) can be caused by the conditions listed in Figure 13-14.[18]

A shift of the oxyhemoglobin dissociation curve attributable to changes in the blood levels of PCO_2 and the H^+ concentration is important to enhance oxygen uptake by the blood in the lungs and the release of oxygen from the hemoglobin to the body tissues. This is called the *Bohr effect*.[17]

A shift of the oxyhemoglobin dissociation curve to the right enhances oxygen release to the cell. The shift provides the increase in oxygen delivery that is needed during exercise and other types of stress, as well as in chronic disease states. A shift of the oxyhemoglobin dissociation curve to the left is seen with a decrease in H^+ ion concentration, with a decrease in PCO_2, with an increase in pH, with a decrease in temperature, with a decrease in 2,3-DPG concentration, in some congenital hemoglobinopathies, and with increased carboxyhemoglobin concentration.

Another important factor affecting O_2 delivery to tissues is the arterial oxygen content (CaO_2).[17,18,20] Arterial blood oxygen content (CaO_2) and venous blood oxygen content (CvO_2) can be calculated by adding the amount of oxygen combined with hemoglobin, and the amount of oxygen dissolved in plasma (Table 13-4).

Oxygen delivery, or ($\dot{D}O_2$), is the amount of oxygen (in milliliters) delivered per minute to the tissues.[18] It is calculated by multiplying the arterial oxygen content (CaO_2) by the cardiac output (CO). Cardiac output is usually between 4 and 8 L/min. Therefore, oxygen delivery is approximately 1000 ml/min.

Oxygen consumption ($\dot{V}O_2$) is the amount of oxygen consumed by the tissues and is measured in milliliters of oxygen per minute. Once the oxygen reaches the tissues, oxygen consumption is controlled by the rate of energy expenditure within the cells or the rate at which adenosine diphosphate (ADP) is formed from ATP to provide energy. The increasing concentration of ADP enhances the metabolic utilization of oxygen.[17] Oxygen consumption can be determined by subtracting the oxygen remaining in the venous blood (CvO_2) from the oxygen delivered to the tissues by the arteries (CaO_2), and is known as the *Fick equation*.[20]

Gas values (pressure and content) relative to the oxygenation of blood are summarized in Table 13-4.

Carbon Dioxide Transport

RBCs are also important in the transport of carbon dioxide in the blood. Carbon dioxide, a by-product of cellular metabolism, is transported in three forms in the blood: (1) as dissolved gas, (2) as bicarbonate ion (HCO_3^-), and (3) in association with hemoglobin (Figure 13-15).[17] The partial pressure of carbon dioxide (PCO_2) reflects the pressure or tension that carbon dioxide exerts when it is dissolved in the blood. Partial pressure is measured in millimeters of mercury (mm Hg). In the pulmonary capillaries, carbon dioxide easily dissociates from hemoglobin and then diffuses across the alveolar membrane into the alveolar sacs. In the body tissues, the carbon dioxide inside the cells diffuses into the blood and attaches to the hemoglobin as oxygen is released to the tissues. The partial pressure of carbon dioxide in the arterial blood ($PaCO_2$) is usually 40 mm Hg and in the venous blood ($PvCO_2$) it is usually 45 mm Hg.[17] These differences are much smaller than those of oxygen, but carbon dioxide diffuses much more readily. Dissolved carbon dioxide combines slowly with water in the plasma to form carbonic

acid (H_2CO_3), but in the red cell the presence of carbonic anhydrase acting as a catalyst significantly accelerates this reaction.[17,20] Carbonic acid rapidly dissociates into hydrogen ions (H^+) and bicarbonate ions (HCO_3^-).[17,20] As the concentration of HCO_3^- in the red cell increases, it diffuses into the plasma, whereas the H^+ remains. This increase in intracellular cation concentration causes the anion chloride to diffuse from the plasma into the red cell to maintain electrical neutrality. This is referred to as the **chloride shift**.[18]

Hemoglobin provides an excellent acid-base buffer by reacting with the free hydrogen ions and directly with carbon dioxide to form carbaminohemoglobin ($HbCO_2$), which is easily dissociated in the lungs to yield free carbon dioxide for exhalation.[17] Unloading of oxygen in the tissue facilitates the loading of carbon dioxide and is referred to as the *Haldane effect*.[17,18]

Alterations in Oxygen Transport

There must be sufficient circulating hemoglobin mass to meet the metabolic needs of the body. A feedback mechanism ensures that when the amount of oxygen reaching the tissues decreases, a compensatory increase occurs in the production of red cells.[3] The feedback mechanism regulating RBC production is under the control of erythropoietin. As stem cells differentiate into the erythroid committed line, the most primitive stem cell is referred to as the erythroid burst-forming unit (BFU-E), which is controlled by growth factors derived from T lymphocytes and macrophages and, to a lesser degree, by erythropoietin.[2,4] The BFU-E further differentiates into erythroid colony-forming units (CFU-E) more responsive to erythropoietin, and subsequently into normoblasts and mature RBCs.[2-4] The majority of erythropoietin is actively secreted by the kidney. Another 10% of erythropoietin is formed elsewhere in the body.[2-4]

KEY POINTS

- Nearly all (97%) of the oxygen transported in blood is bound to hemoglobin within the red cells. Only 3% is dissolved in plasma. It is this 3% that is measured as PaO_2. At a normal PaO_2, hemoglobin is 95% to 100% saturated with oxygen. About 25% of the bound oxygen is unloaded to the tissues, resulting in a venous hemoglobin saturation of about 75%.
- The oxyhemoglobin dissociation curve describes the relationship between the partial pressure of oxygen and hemoglobin saturation. In the lung, where PO_2 is high (100 mm Hg), oxygen is loaded onto hemoglobin. In the tissues, where PO_2 is low (40 mm Hg), oxygen is unloaded from hemoglobin to tissues.
- The affinity of hemoglobin for oxygen is affected by temperature, acid-base status, 2,3-DPG levels, and carbon dioxide concentration. Affinity decreases at the tissue level because of increased levels of acid, 2,3-DPG, and carbon dioxide. This shift to the right of the oxyhemoglobin dissociation curve enhances unloading of oxygen to the tissue. A shift to the left occurs in the lungs, where blood is more alkalotic and carbon dioxide levels are lower. The increased affinity of hemoglobin for oxygen at the lung facilitates oxygen binding.
- The oxygen content of arterial blood is calculated by adding the amount bound to hemoglobin (Hb) plus the amount dissolved in plasma: $CaO_2 = (Hb \times 1.34 \times SaO_2) + (PaO_2 \times 0.003)$. Oxygen delivery to the body tissues is calculated by multiplying CaO_2 by cardiac output (CO): $\dot{D}O_2 = CaO_2 \times CO \times 10$.
- The consumption of oxygen by tissues can be estimated using the Fick equation: $\dot{V}O_2 = CO \times (CaO_2 - C\overline{V}O_2) \times 10$. Oxygen consumption increases with increased tissue metabolism.
- Hemoglobin is an important factor in carbon dioxide transport in the blood. In the tissues, hemoglobin binds carbon dioxide to form carbaminohemoglobin, which then releases carbon dioxide in the lungs. RBCs contain the enzyme carbonic anhydrase, which greatly increases conversion of carbon dioxide and water into HCO_3^- and H^+ at the tissue level. In the lungs, the reaction proceeds in reverse, producing carbon dioxide, which is eliminated by the lungs.

TABLE 13-4 GAS VALUES SIGNIFICANT TO THE OXYGENATION OF BLOOD

GAS VALUES	DESCRIPTION	MEASUREMENT/ REFLECTION	CALCULATION/FORMULA	NORMAL VALUE/ FORMULA
CaO_2	Arterial blood oxygen content is amount of oxygen carried in arterial blood	Measured in milliliters of oxygen per deciliter of blood (ml/dl), or vol%	Sum of oxyhemoglobin (15 Hb g/100 ml × 1.34 ml O_2/g Hb × 97.5% arterial saturation = 19.6 vol%) + amount of oxygen dissolved in plasma (PaO_2 = 100 mm Hg × 0.003 vol%/mm Hg = 0.3 vol%)	~20 vol% Formula: 19.6 vol% oxyhemoglobin + 0.3 vol% dissolved in plasma = 19.9 vol%
$C\bar{v}O_2$	Venous blood oxygen content is amount of oxygen carried in venous blood	Measured in milliliters of oxygen per deciliter of blood (ml/dl), or vol%	Sum of oxyhemoglobin (15 Hb/100 ml × 1.34 ml O_2/g Hb × 75% venous saturation = 15.0 vol%) + amount of oxygen dissolved in plasma ($C\bar{v}O_2$ = 40 mm Hg × 0.003 vol%/mm Hg = 0.12 vol%)	~15 vol% Formula: 15 vol% oxyhemoglobin + 0.12 vol% dissolved in plasma = approximately 15 vol%
$\dot{D}O_2$	Oxygen delivery or transport is amount of oxygen delivered to tissues	Measured in milliliters of oxygen per minute (ml/min)	*Normal arterial:* $\dot{D}O_2$ = cardiac output (L / min) × CaO_2 × 10 *Normal venous:* $\dot{D}O_2$ = cardiac output (L / min) × $C\bar{v}O_2$ × 10	*Normal arterial:* ~1000 ml of O_2/min *Normal venous:* ~750 ml of O_2/min
PaO_2	Partial pressure of oxygen in arterial blood	Measured in millimeters of mercury (mm Hg) Reflects tension or pressure that is exerted by oxygen when it is dissolved in plasma		Normal PaO_2 is 80-100 mm Hg
$PaCO_2$	Partial pressure of carbon dioxide in arterial blood	Measured in millimeters of mercury (mm Hg) Reflects tension or pressure that is exerted by carbon dioxide when it is dissolved in plasma		Normal $PaCO_2$ is 35-45 mm Hg
$P\bar{v}O_2$	Partial pressure of oxygen in venous blood	Measured in millimeters of mercury (mm Hg) Reflects tension or pressure that is exerted by oxygen when it is dissolved in plasma		Normal $P\bar{v}O_2$ is 35-40 mm Hg
$P\bar{v}CO_2$	Partial pressure of carbon dioxide in venous blood	Measured in millimeters of mercury (mm Hg) Reflects tension or pressure that is exerted by carbon dioxide when it is dissolved in plasma		Normal $P\bar{v}CO_2$ is 41-51 mm Hg
SaO_2	Amount of hemoglobin bound to oxygen relative to total amount of hemoglobin, both reduced and bound, in arterial blood	Expressed as percentage		Normal SaO_2 is 95-100%
$S\bar{v}O_2$	Amount of hemoglobin bound to oxygen relative to total amount of hemoglobin, both reduced and bound, in venous blood	Expressed as percentage		Normal $S\bar{v}O_2$ is 60-80%
$\dot{V}O_2$	Oxygen consumption is amount of oxygen consumed by tissues	Measured in milliliters of oxygen per minute (ml/min) Oxygen consumption is derived from difference between arterial oxygen transport and venous oxygen transport	$\dot{V}O_2$ = cardiac output × (CaO_2 − $C\bar{v}O_2$) × 10	Normal $\dot{V}O_2$ is 200-250 ml of O_2/min

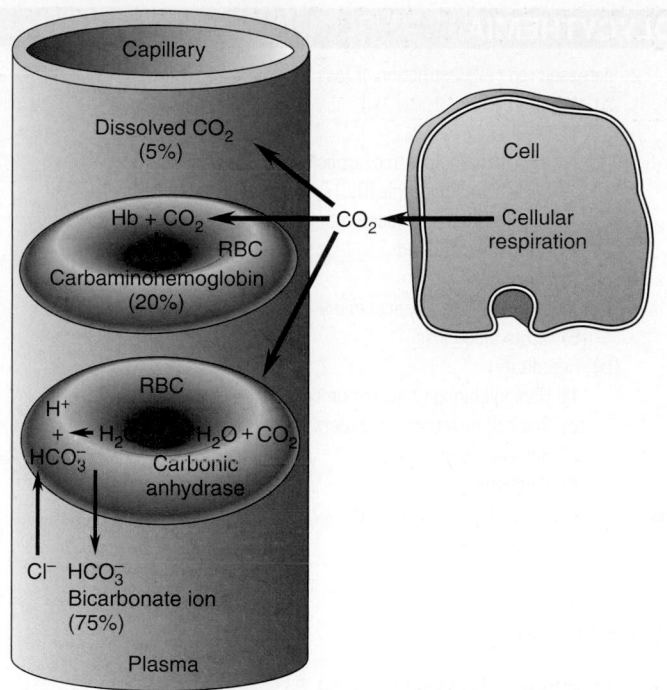

FIGURE 13-15 Carbon dioxide is transported in three forms in the blood. Transportation of CO_2 (1) as dissolved gas, (2) as bicarbonate ion (HCO_3^-), and (3) in association with hemoglobin (Hb).

Factors that decrease hemoglobin mass (such as anemia) or decrease arterial saturation (such as hypoxia from either cardiac or pulmonary conditions) impair oxygen delivery to the body tissues. This stimulates an increased release of erythropoietin and the production of RBCs.[3] Figure 13-16 illustrates the compensatory regulation of erythropoiesis that is seen in hypoxia, anemia, and polycythemia.

ANEMIA

Erythrocyte disorders are divided into two groups: (1) **anemia,** defined as a deficit of red cells, and (2) **polycythemia,** defined as an excess of red cells (Box 13-1).[21,22] An anemic patient has tissue hypoxia attributable to the low oxygen-carrying capacity of the blood. In contrast, a patient with polycythemia has increased blood viscosity and volume attributable to the increase in the number of RBCs.[22] (Polycythemia is discussed in greater detail later in this chapter.) Table 13-5 presents the laboratory findings for erythrocyte disorders in terms of relative anemia, absolute anemia caused by decreased RBC production, and absolute anemia caused by increased RBC destruction.

Relative anemia is characterized by normal total red cell mass with disturbances in the regulation of plasma volume. For example, in pregnant women the average plasma volume is 43% greater than in nonpregnant women, which causes a "dilutional anemia."[21]

Absolute anemia includes those types of anemia with an actual decrease in numbers of red cells. This can be caused by decreased production of red cells or increased destruction of red cells.[21]

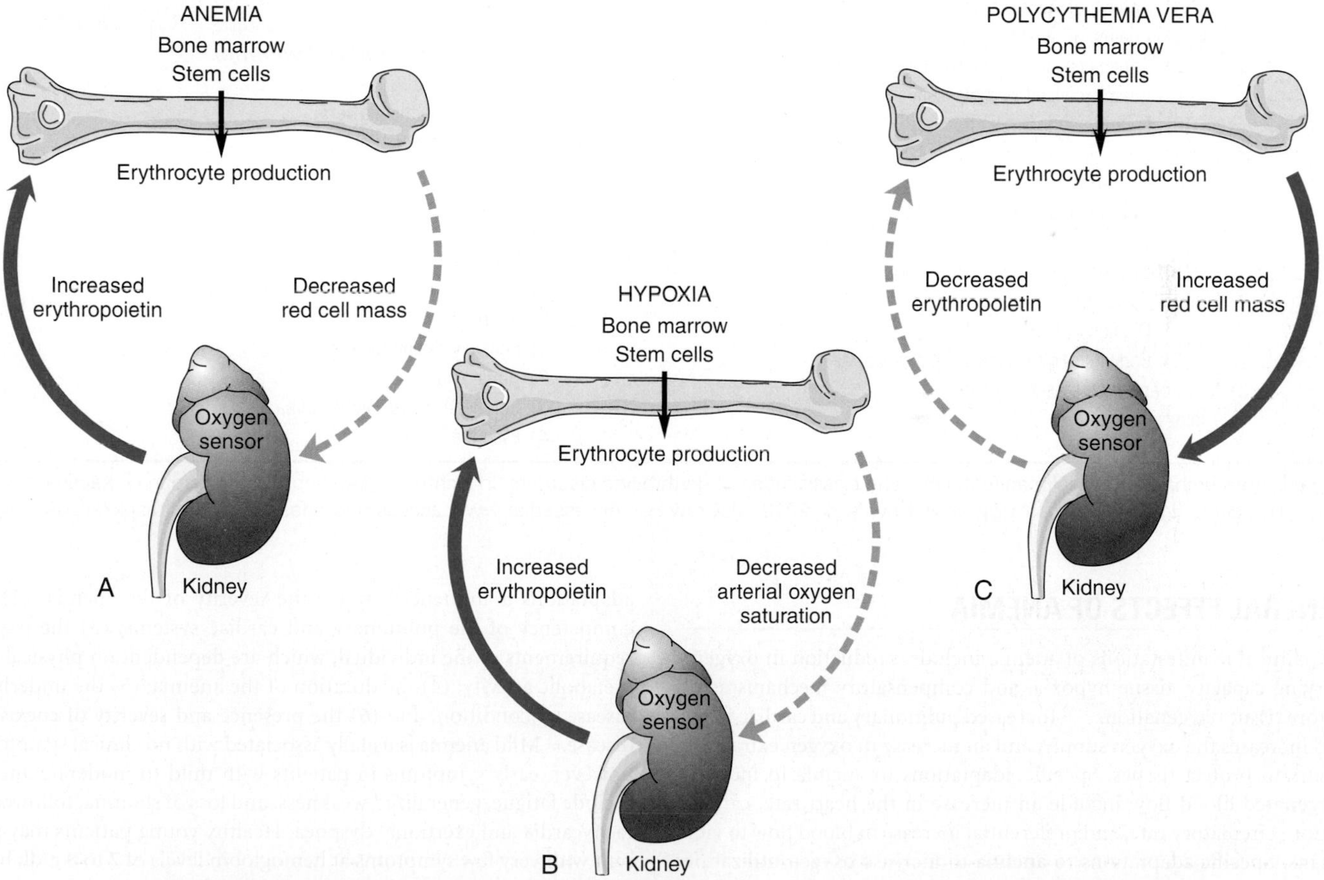

FIGURE 13-16 Alterations in the erythropoietin feedback circuit. Any factor decreasing oxygen delivery to the oxygen sensor cells results in increased secretion of erythropoietin and a compensatory increase in erythrocyte production as illustrated in **(A)** for anemia, with a decrease in erythrocyte mass; and in **(B)** for hypoxia, with a decrease in arterial oxygen saturation. An increase in erythrocyte mass, as occurs with polycythemia vera **(C),** decreases erythropoietin production.

BOX 13-1   CLASSIFICATION OF ANEMIA AND POLYCYTHEMIA

I. Anemia

A. Absolute

1. Decreased red cell production
   (a) Acquired
       1) Pluripotent stem cell failure
          a) Aplastic anemia
             {1} Radiation induced
             {2} Drugs and chemicals
             {3} Viruses
             {4} Idiopathic
          b) Anemia of leukemia and myelodysplastic syndrome
          c) Anemia associated with marrow infiltration
          d) Anemia associated with chemotherapy
       2) Erythroid progenitor cell failure
          a) Pure red cell aplasia
          b) Endocrine disorders
          c) Acquired sideroblastic anemia
       3) Functional impairment of erythroid progenitors
             {1} Megaloblastic anemias
          a) B_{12} deficiency
          b) Folate deficiency
          c) Acute megaloblastic anemia due to nitrous oxide
          d) Drug-induced megaloblastic anemia
             {2} Iron deficiency anemia
             {3} Anemia from other nutritional deficiencies
             {4} Anemia of chronic disease
             {5} Anemia of renal failure
             {6} Anemia caused by chemical agents
             {7} Anemia caused by thalassemias
             {8} Erythropoietin antibodies
   (b) Hereditary
       1) Pluripotent stem cell failure
             {1} Fanconi anemia
             {2} Shwachman syndrome
             {3} Dyskeratosis congenita
       2) Erythroid progenitor cell failure
             {1} Diamond-Blackfan syndrome
             {2} Congenital dyserythropoietic syndrome
       3) Hereditary sideroblastic anemia
       4) Thalassemias

2. Increased red cell destruction or loss
   (a) Acquired
       1) Mechanical
          a) Macroangiopathic (artificial heart valves)
          b) Microangiopathic (DIC)
          c) Parasites and microorganisms
       2) Antibody mediated
       3) Hypersplenism
       4) Chemical and physical injury
       5) Acute blood loss
   (b) Hereditary
       1) Hemoglobinopathies (sickle cell)
       2) Red cell membrane disorders
       3) Red cell enzyme defects
       4) Porphyrias

B. Relative (increased plasma volume)
   1. Macroglobulinemia
   2. Pregnancy
   3. Athletes
   4. Postflight astronauts

II. Polycythemia (Erythrocytosis)

A. Relative (decreased plasma volume)

1. Dehydration
2. Diuretics
3. Stress or smoker's erythrocytosis

B. Absolute (increased red cell volume)

1. Primary polycythemia
   (a) Acquired (polycythemia vera)
   (b) Hereditary congenital polycythemia
2. Secondary polycythemia
   (a) Appropriate
       1) Altitude
       2) Cardiopulmonary disorders
       3) Increased hemoglobin affinity for oxygen
   (b) Inappropriate
       1) Renal cysts and tumors
       2) Hepatoma
       3) Cerebellar hemangioblastoma
       4) Essential

Adapted from Prchal JT: Clinical manifestations and classification of erythrocyte disorders. In Lichtman MA, Kipps TJ, Seligsohn U, Kaushansky K, Prchal JT, editors: *Williams hematology,* ed 8, New York, 2010, McGraw-Hill. Accessed at www.accessmedicine.com/content.aspx?aID=6108487.

GENERAL EFFECTS OF ANEMIA

The clinical manifestations of anemia include a reduction in oxygen-carrying capacity, tissue hypoxia, and compensatory mechanisms to restore tissue oxygenation.[21,22] Increased pulmonary and cardiac function increases the oxygen supply, and an increase in oxygen extraction occurs to protect tissues. Specific adaptations to anemia to increase oxygenated blood flow include an increase in the heart rate, cardiac output, circulatory rate, and preferential increase in blood flow to vital organs. Specific adaptations to anemia to increase oxygen utilization by tissues include an increase in 2,3-DPG concentration in erythrocytes and a decreased oxygen affinity of hemoglobin in tissues. Selective tissue perfusion provides shunting to vital organs in short-term compensation, and increased erythropoietic activity is stimulated to provide long-term compensation.[6] The extent of the physiologic adaptations is influenced by (1) the severity of the anemia; (2) the competency of the pulmonary and cardiac systems; (3) the oxygen requirements of the individual, which are dependent on physical and metabolic activity; (4) the duration of the anemia; (5) the underlying disease or condition; and (6) the presence and severity of coexisting disease.[21] Mild anemia is usually associated with no clinical symptoms; however, early symptoms in patients with mild to moderate anemia include fatigue, generalized weakness, and loss of stamina, followed by tachycardia and exertional dyspnea. Healthy young patients may present with very few symptoms at hemoglobin levels of 7 to 8 g/dl; however, elderly patients and patients with cardiovascular or pulmonary disease may have symptoms with even modest degrees of anemia and hemoglobin levels of 9 to 11 g/dl. Specific symptoms related to moderate to severe anemia are orthostatic and nonorthostatic hypotension, vasoconstriction, pallor, tachypnea, dyspnea, tachycardia, transient

TABLE 13-5 **LABORATORY FINDINGS FOR ERYTHROCYTE DISORDERS**

DISEASE	HCT	HB	MCV	MCH	MCHC	RETIC	RBC	WBC	PLT	BLOOD SMEAR	OTHER LABORATORY TESTS	OTHER DIAGNOSTIC CHARACTERISTICS
Relative anemia	Low	Low	Normal	Low	Low	Normal	Low	Low	Low	Normal	Plasma volume increased, causing relative decrease in number of cells	Increased volume can be caused by pregnancy, splenomegaly, IV infusions

Absolute Anemia Caused by Decreased Production

DISEASE	HCT	HB	MCV	MCH	MCHC	RETIC	RBC	WBC	PLT	BLOOD SMEAR	OTHER LABORATORY TESTS	OTHER DIAGNOSTIC CHARACTERISTICS
Aplastic anemia	Low	Low	Normal	Low	Low	Low	Low	Low	Low	Normocytic, hypochromic RBCs; lack of neutrophils; increased lymphocytes	HbF may be increased; erythropoietin increased; bone marrow aplastic	Specific cause should be identified and removed from environment
Chronic renal failure	Low	Low	Normal	Normal	Normal	Low	Low	Normal	Normal	Normocytic, normochromic RBCs; RBCs often have spicules	Erythropoietin decreased; bone marrow production suppressed	Kidney tests abnormal
Pernicious anemia	Low	Low	High	High	Normal	Low	Low	Low	Low	Oval macrocytes; hypersegmented segs	Decreased B_{12} level; positive Schilling test	Neurologic symptoms; increased bilirubin
Folate deficiency	Low	Low	High	High	Normal	Low	Low	Low	Low	Oval macrocytes; hypersegmented segs	Decreased folic acid level; negative Schilling test	No neurologic symptoms
Iron deficiency	Low	Low	Low	Low	Low	Normal or high	Low	Normal	Normal	Microcytic, hypochromic RBCs	Serum iron decreased; iron-binding	Bone marrow iron decreased
Thalassemia	Low	Low	Low	Low	Low	High	Low	Normal	Normal	Microcytic, hypochromic RBCs	Decreased osmotic fragility; hemoglobin electrophoresis diagnostic; serum iron, TIBC, and ferritin normal	Hereditary disease

Absolute Anemia Caused by Increased Destruction
Intrinsic Abnormality

DISEASE	HCT	HB	MCV	MCH	MCHC	RETIC	RBC	WBC	PLT	BLOOD SMEAR	OTHER LABORATORY TESTS	OTHER DIAGNOSTIC CHARACTERISTICS
Sickle cell	Low	Low	Normal	Normal	Normal	High	Low	Normal	Normal	Normocytic, normochromic RBC target cells; sickle cells; NRBCs	HbS present on electrophoresis	Hereditary disease
Hereditary spherocytosis	Low	Low	Normal	Normal	Normal to high	High	Low	Normal	Normal	Spherocytes present	Bilirubin elevated; haptoglobins reduced; abnormal RBC fragility	Hereditary disease

Continued

TABLE 13-5 LABORATORY FINDINGS FOR ERYTHROCYTE DISORDERS—cont'd

DISEASE	HCT	HB	MCV	MCH	MCHC	RETIC	RBC	WBC	PLT	BLOOD SMEAR	OTHER LABORATORY TESTS	OTHER DIAGNOSTIC CHARACTERISTICS
G6PD deficiency	Low	Low	Normal	Normal	Normal	High	Low	High	Normal	Heinz body smear positive	Tests only abnormal in hemolytic episodes	Hereditary disease
Extrinsic Abnormality												
HDNB	Low	Low	Normal	Normal	Normal	High	Low	High	Normal	Spherocytes, NRBCs	Bilirubin elevated; Coombs test positive; urinary urobilinogen increased	Jaundice; edema; hepatosplenomegaly
Antibody-mediated drug reactions	Low	Low	Normal	Normal	Normal	High	Low	Normal	Normal	Polychromatic RBCs due to increased reticulocytes	Bilirubin elevated; Coombs test positive; urinary urobilinogen increased	Jaundice
Acute blood loss	Normal to low	Normal to low	Normal	Normal	Normal	High	Normal to low	Normal to low	Normal to low	Appears normal until reticulocytes increase	Values depend on severity of hemorrhage and when blood is drawn	
Polycythemias												
Relative polycythemia	High	High	Normal	Normal	Normal	Normal	High	High	High	Normal	Plasma volume decreased, causing relative increase in number of blood cells	Decrease in volume
Absolute polycythemia vera	High	High	Normal	Normal	Normal	High	High	High	High	Teardrops, macrocytes, and NRBCs may be present; shift to left on differential	O₂ saturation normal; bone marrow hypercellular; all three cell lines increased	
Secondary polycythemia	High	High	Normal	Normal	Normal	High	High	Normal	Normal	Normal	Hypoxemia may be evident; serum erythropoietin elevated	Lung disease may be present

G6PD, Glucose-6-phosphate dehydrogenase; *Hb,* hemoglobin; *Hct,* hematocrit; *HDNB,* hemolytic disease of the newborn; *MCH,* mean corpuscular hemoglobin; *MCHC,* mean corpuscular hemoglobin concentration; *MCV,* mean corpuscular volume; *NRBC,* nucleated red blood cell; *PLT,* platelet; *RBC,* red blood cell; *RETIC,* reticulocytosis; *Segs,* segmented neutrophils; *TIBC,* total iron binding capacity; *WBC,* white blood cell.

murmurs, angina pectoris, heart failure, intermittent claudication, night cramps in muscles, headache, lightheadedness, tinnitus, roaring in the ears, and faintness.[6]

ANEMIA RELATED TO DECREASED RED CELL PRODUCTION

Aplastic Anemia

Etiology and pathogenesis. Aplastic anemia is a stem cell disorder that is characterized by a reduction of hematopoietic tissue in the bone marrow, fatty marrow replacement, and pancytopenia. The decrease in functional bone marrow mass is usually caused by toxic, radiant, or immunologic injury to the bone marrow stem cells, which causes a decrease in the levels of red cells, white cells, and platelets, or **pancytopenia.**[23]

Aplastic anemia can be classified as acquired or familial. Acquired aplastic anemia can be caused by chemical and physical agents, such as those listed in Table 13-6. Other causes include certain viral infections (e.g., hepatitis, Epstein-Barr virus, human immunodeficiency virus [HIV], dengue), some mycobacterial infections, diffuse eosinophilic

fasciitis, pregnancy, Simmonds disease, and sclerosis of the thyroid. Familial aplastic anemia is associated with Fanconi constitutional pancytopenia, pancreatic deficiency in children, and putative hereditary defect in cellular uptake of folate.[24]

Laboratory features. Pancytopenia is characterized by low red cell, white cell, and platelet counts. The magnitude of the **granulocytopenia** is very important for the immediate prognosis. An absolute granulocyte count of less than 200/mm^3 results in immediate susceptibility to infectious complications. Coagulation tests are generally normal except for the bleeding time, which reflects the low platelet count.[24] The ultimate diagnosis of aplastic anemia rests on the interpretation of an adequate bone marrow biopsy specimen, although important clues to the cause of pancytopenia can be obtained from the history, physical examination, and laboratory data. Pancytopenia that is not primarily hematologic in origin but secondary to other disease processes is usually an obvious diagnosis.[25]

Clinical manifestations. Aplastic anemia is a disease of the young with most patients presenting between 15 and 25 years of age. Another age group likely to present with aplastic anemia are those ≥60 years old. The most common form of aplastic anemia is iatrogenic—resulting from

TABLE 13-6 DRUGS ASSOCIATED WITH APLASTIC ANEMIA*

CATEGORY	HIGH RISK	MODERATE RISK	LOW RISK
Analgesic			Phenacetin, aspirin, salicylamide
Antidysrhythmic			Quinidine, tocainide
Antiarthritic		Gold salts	Colchicine
Anticonvulsant		Carbamazepine, hydantoin, felbamate	Ethosuximide, phenacemide, primidone, trimethadione, sodium valproate
Antihistamine			Chlorpheniramine, pyrilamine, tripelennamine
Antihypertensive			Captopril, methyldopa
Anti-inflammatory		Penicillamine, phenylbutazone, oxyphenbutazone	Diclofenac, ibuprofen, indomethacin, naproxen, sulindac
Antimicrobial			
Antibacterial		Chloramphenicol	Dapsone, methicillin, penicillin, streptomycin, β-lactam antibiotics
Antifungal			Amphotericin, flucytosine
Antiprotozoal		Quinacrine	Chloroquine, mepacrine, pyrimethamine
Antineoplastic			
Alkylating agents	Busulfan, cyclophosphamide, melphalan, nitrogen mustard		
Antimetabolites	Fluorouracil, mercaptopurine, methotrexate		
Cytotoxic antibiotics	Daunorubicin, doxorubicin, mitoxantrone		
Antiplatelet			Ticlopidine
Antithyroid			Carbimazole, methimazole, methylthiouracil, potassium perchlorate, propylthiouracil, sodium thiocyanate
Sedative and tranquilizer			Chlordiazepoxide, chlorpromazine (and other phenothiazines), lithium, meprobamate, methyprylon
Sulfonamides and derivatives			
Antibacterial			Numerous sulfonamides
Diuretic		Acetazolamide	Chlorothiazide, furosemide
Hypoglycemic			Chlorpropamide, tolbutamide
Miscellaneous			Allopurinol, interferon, pentoxifylline

From Segel GB: Aplastic anemia. In Lichtman MA et al, editors: *Williams hematology,* ed 7, New York, 2006, McGraw-Hill, p 421. This list was compiled from the AMA Registry, Publications of the International Agranulocytosis and Aplastic Anemia Study, other reviews and studies, previous compilations of offending agents, and selected reports.
*Drugs that invariably cause marrow aplasia with high doses are termed high risk; drugs with 30 or more reported cases are listed as moderate risk; others are less often associated with aplastic anemia (low risk).

a transient marrow failure following treatment with cytotoxic chemo-therapeutic drugs or irradiation. Certain chemical or physical agents directly injure proliferating and quiescent hematopoietic cells.[25] The onset is usually insidious, and patients often present only after the late manifestations of pancytopenia are evident. The symptoms attributable to the gradual decrease in the number of RBCs include weakness, fatigue, lethargy, pallor, dyspnea, palpitations, onset of transient murmurs, and tachycardia of anemia. Fever, chills, and bacterial infections (particularly in the mouth or perirectal area) are seen secondary to neutropenia. Petechiae, bruising, nosebleeds, retinal hemorrhage, and increased menstrual flow are manifestations of thrombocytopenia.[23]

Treatment. Treatment for aplastic anemia is multifaceted and dependent on the etiology and severity of the disease. Treatment includes (1) identification and avoidance of further toxin exposure; (2) human leukocyte antigen (HLA) and ABO typing of family members to identify serologically defined loci and potential bone marrow transplant donors; (3) maintenance of minimally essential levels of hemoglobin and platelets; (4) prevention and management of infection; (5) determination of efficacy of bone marrow transplantation; and (6) implementation of other forms of therapy, such as immunosuppressive therapy or stimulation of hematopoiesis and bone marrow regeneration in patients not suited for transplantation.[23-26] In patients with severe disease, the major curative approach is allogeneic bone marrow transplantation; however, only one third of all patients have compatible donors.[23-26] Preparative regimens using cyclophosphamide and antithymocyte globulin followed by post-transplant immunosuppression with cyclosporine and methyltrexate as prophylaxis against graft-versus-host disease (GVHD) have resulted in a 90% disease-free survival rate at 2 years for patients with bone marrow transplants derived from an HLA-matched sibling donor.[27]

Course and prognosis. Bone marrow transplantation is highly successful and curative for 80% to 85% of untransfused patients and 55% to 60% of patients with multiple previous transfusions.[27] Approximately 20% to 30% of transplantation survivors with multiple previous transfusions experience severe GVHD, which can be significantly improved by immunosuppressive therapy in 50% to 70% of patients.[22] The risk of graft failure in patients who have not been transfused is less than 5%. Prognosis is related to the absolute neutrophil count and the platelet count. Children respond better than adults with both bone marrow transplantation and immunosuppression therapy, especially in patients with mild to moderate disease. Aplastic anemia is usually fatal unless managed with bone marrow transplantation.[23-27]

Anemia of Chronic Renal Failure

Etiology and pathogenesis. The anemia of chronic renal failure occurs primarily from failure of the renal endocrine function, which causes impaired erythropoietin production and bone marrow compensation, and secondarily from failure of the renal excretory function, leading to hemolysis, bone marrow cell depression, and blood loss.[28]

Laboratory features. This anemia is characterized by a decreased red cell count and low hemoglobin and hematocrit values. Some red cells appear grossly deformed with a few large spicules (Figure 13-17). The total leukocyte differential cell count, leukocyte counts, and platelet count are usually normal. The red cell indices—mean corpuscular volume (MCV), mean corpuscular hemoglobin (MCH), and mean corpuscular hemoglobin concentration (MCHC)—are also normal.[28,29]

Clinical manifestations. Any of the clinical manifestations described earlier (see General Effects of Anemia) may be evident in chronic renal failure. The hematocrit falls in proportion to the degree of renal insufficiency, and uremia occurs as the glomerular filtration rate drops below 40 ml/min. Signs and symptoms of anemia usually manifest when the hematocrit decreases to ≤20%.[29]

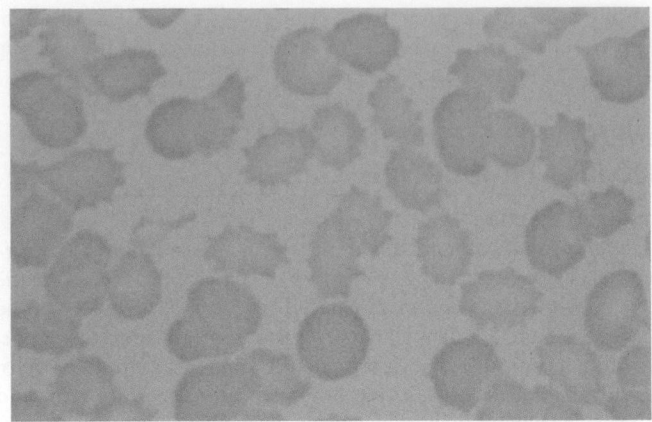

FIGURE 13-17 Burr cells found in acute kidney disease. (Courtesy Beth Payne, Sacred Heart Medical Center, Spokane, WA.)

Treatment. Therapy consists of dialysis when the glomerular filtration rate is less than 15 ml/min, and erythropoietin is administered to achieve the target hematocrit concentration of 33% to 36% and hemoglobin level of 11 to 12 g/dl. However, excessive correction of the hemoglobin level to greater than 12 g/dl may be associated with an increased incidence of cardiovascular and thromboembolic events. Therefore, the use of erythropoiesis-stimulating agents to increase hemoglobin values to greater than 12 g/dl is not routinely recommended.[30] The hematocrit and hemoglobin values are monitored at least every 2 weeks to ensure adequate oxygen-carrying capacity and minimize an increased respiratory rate and heart rate. When the target hematocrit is achieved, adult patients can be maintained by administering 50 to 100 units per kilogram per week in divided doses. Pediatric patients younger than 5 years usually require higher initial and maintenance doses.[28-33] Patients with chronic renal failure are also prone to nutritional anemias (lack of iron, folate, and B_{12}) because of dietary restrictions and anorexia. Patient replacement of iron, folate, and B_{12} to adequate levels should be considered a treatment goal. Some patients may fail to respond or may be resistant to the effects of erythropoietin. The most common cause for a failure in response is iron deficiency anemia.[30]

Course and prognosis. More than 95% of patients respond to erythropoietin therapy. Patients who do not respond or first respond when larger doses are given should be evaluated for an adequate iron supply, infection, or excessive splenic hemolysis.[28-33]

Anemia Related to Vitamin B_{12} (Cobalamin) or Folate Deficiency

Etiology and pathogenesis. The anemia resulting from a deficiency of either vitamin B_{12} (cobalamin) or folate is caused by a disruption in DNA synthesis of the blast cells in the bone marrow. This disruption produces very large abnormal bone marrow cells called **megaloblasts.** In the peripheral blood, the red cells are larger than normal (**macrocytic**), the granulocytes are hypersegmented, and the numbers of red cells, white cells, and platelets are decreased.[34,35] All of these signs can be seen on the peripheral blood smear.

The classic anemia in this classification is pernicious anemia. The fundamental defect causing pernicious anemia is the lack of intrinsic factor. Without it, vitamin B_{12} cannot be absorbed, thus leading to vitamin B_{12} deficiency. This deficiency results in disordered nucleic acid metabolism, which causes **megaloblastic dysplasia,** a condition involving abnormal production and maturation of red cell, white cell, and platelet systems. There is strong evidence that pernicious anemia develops as a result of genetically determined autoimmune disease, which is manifested by serum and gastric juice antibodies against intrinsic factor and parietal cells.[34] The biochemical basis of the neurologic lesions in pernicious anemia is not known. There can be peripheral nerve degeneration, degeneration of the posterior columns of the spinal cord, or both. There is some evidence of abnormal fatty acid metabolism in the peripheral nerves and degeneration of the white matter in the spinal cord in animals.[34,35]

Folate deficiencies resemble vitamin B_{12} deficiencies except for the neurologic disease, which is more characteristic of vitamin B_{12} deficiency. Folate deficiencies are usually the result of dietary deficiencies, alcoholism and cirrhosis, pregnancy, or infancy.

Laboratory features. The peripheral blood shows low RBC counts of 500,000 to 750,000 cells/mm³, low WBC counts of 4000 to 5000 cells/mm³, and low platelet counts of 50,000 cells/mm³. These counts are usually not as low as those seen in aplastic anemia. The bone marrow shows megaloblastic dysplasia, which results in a peripheral blood picture of macrocytosis and hypersegmented neutrophils. The red cell indices reveal normal MCH and MCHC and increased MCV. The Schilling test, which measures excretion of radioactive vitamin B_{12}, indicates low levels, and the serum level of vitamin B_{12} is low. Gastric analysis indicates a lack of free hydrochloric acid in the gastric juice (achlorhydria).[34,35]

Clinical manifestations. The clinical features of vitamin B_{12} deficiency include paranoid ideation, dementia, cognitive dysfunction, delusions, and hallucinations, often referred to as "megaloblastic madness."[34] The neurologic abnormalities include symmetric paresthesias of the feet and hands with vibratory sense and proprioception disturbances. The paresthesias progress to spastic ataxia as a result of degenerative changes of the dorsal and lateral columns of the spinal cord. Cerebral signs include irritability, somnolence, memory impairment, and perversion of taste, smell, and vision.[34,35] Manifestations of pure folate deficiency include a blunted affect in general demeanor with evidence of depression, sleep deprivation, and irritability. History of circumstances likely to result in folic acid deficiency includes poor or fad diet, frank malabsorption, or alcoholism. In folate deficiency, cerebral symptoms, such as irritability, memory loss, and personality changes, are seen.[34,35] Clinical manifestations that are seen in both vitamin B_{12} and folate deficiencies include pedal edema, nocturia, tachypnea, dyspnea, and tachycardia associated with heart congestion; glossitis, weight loss, malabsorption, and episodic or chronic diarrhea with steatorrhea are gastrointestinal manifestations. Musculoskeletal symptoms of arthralgia and frank arthritis are seen in autoimmune diseases; nocturnal pain and upper and/or lower extremity cramps often indicate spinothalamic tract involvement. Dermatologic symptoms include blotchy brown skin pigmentation, especially in nail beds and skin creases. When this is associated with vitiligo, autoimmune processes should be suspected.[34,35]

Recent research has reported an association between low folate levels and the risk of neural tube defects and abnormalities of the heart, urinary tract, and limbs in neonates. These data support the routine supplementation before pregnancy of all women who might become pregnant with 1.0 mg/day of folic acid.[34,35] This is the largest dose that will not mask vitamin B_{12} deficiency.

Treatment. Routine treatment with full doses of parenteral vitamin B_{12} (1 mg/day) and oral folate (1 to 5 mg/day) before the cause of the deficiency is identified should only be used in critically ill patients. In managing the anemia related to vitamin B_{12} or folate deficiency, it is important to (1) recognize that megaloblastic anemia is present; (2) ascertain if vitamin B_{12}, folate, or a combined deficiency is the cause; and (3) diagnose the underlying disease and mechanism responsible for the deficiency. In vitamin B_{12} and folic acid deficiency anemia, replacement therapy for vitamin B_{12} is oral cobalamin and folic acid. Transfusion therapy may be indicated in elderly or critically ill patients. Hypokalemia should be managed with potassium supplements to prevent sudden death, reportedly associated with a sharp drop in serum potassium level seen in vitamin B_{12} therapy.[34,35]

Course and prognosis. The majority of patients respond well to replacement therapy; however, continued assessment and monitoring of these patients is essential to prevent hematologic or neurologic relapse secondary to inadequate therapy.[34,35] In patients with neurologic signs and symptoms, the reversibility of the neurologic damage is slow, with a maximal response requiring up to 6 months. Further substantial increases in recovery are unlikely after 12 months. In 90% of patients with subacute combined degeneration, major improvement is seen.[34] The degree of functional recovery is inversely related to the extent of the disease and duration of the signs and symptoms. Patients with signs and symptoms of less than 3 months' duration may have complete reversal.[34,35]

Iron Deficiency Anemia

Etiology and pathogenesis. Iron deficiency, the most common nutritional deficiency in the world, is the most common cause of anemia. Iron deficiency results in the unavailability of iron for hemoglobin synthesis. This may be due to low intake, diminished absorption (such as from chronic disease), physiologic increase in requirements (such as during pregnancy), excessive iron loss (such as from acute or chronic hemorrhage), or chronic renal failure, hemodialysis, and idiopathic iron loss. The most common cause in men is occult gastrointestinal bleeding and in women is menorrhagia. Iron is one of the most carefully conserved body substances, and under normal conditions very little is lost except as a result of bleeding. Normal dietary requirements, if 10% is absorbed, are as follows: adult men, 12 mg/day; adult women ages 14 to 30 years, 15 mg/day; and adult women ages 60 years or more, 10 mg/day. Pregnant women require up to 30 mg/day, and children require 10 mg/day. A normal diet supplies the adult with about 10 to 15 mg/day.[36-40]

Laboratory features. In latent iron deficiency there may be no anemia; however, after patients receive iron, they respond with a significant increase in blood hemoglobin level. In a typical case caused by chronic bleeding, the reduction in hemoglobin concentration is proportionately greater than the reduction in the red cell count. The red cells are smaller and paler than normal RBCs because of the decreased amount of hemoglobin and are described as **hypochromic, microcytic red cells.** Therefore, the red cell indices MCV, MCH, and MCHC are decreased. The white cell counts are usually normal. The platelet count varies, depending on the cause of the deficiency. In severely anemic children and infants, thrombocytopenia may be present. In patients who are bleeding, thrombocytosis may be present. The serum ferritin level is decreased to less than 10 ng/ml, the serum iron level is decreased, total iron binding capacity (TIBC) is increased, and tissue iron stores are decreased.[36-40]

Clinical manifestations. Patients with iron deficiency may present with (a) no signs or symptoms, only seeking medical attention because of abnormalities noted on laboratory tests; (b) features of the underlying disorder responsible for the development of iron deficiency; or (c) manifestations common to all anemias, such as pallor, weakness, fatigue, dyspnea, palpitations, new and transient heart murmurs, irritability, headaches, or lightheadedness. Patients may also present with (d) one or more of the few signs and symptoms considered highly specific for iron deficiency, including pagophagia or pica (craving for nonfood substances such as dirt, clay, ice, laundry starch, cardboard, or hair), koilonychias (spoon-shaped nails), and blue sclerae. In addition, a high prevalence of iron deficiency with or without anemia has been reported among patients with restless legs syndrome (Ekbom syndrome), especially in the elderly.[39] In severe cases, gastrointestinal symptoms are seen, such as glossitis, dysphagia, erosions at the corners of the mouth, esophageal webbing, and atrophic gastritis, as well as changes in the fingernails, conjunctival pallor, and splenomegaly.[36-40]

Treatment. To maintain a normal iron balance in the body, men need to absorb 1.0 to 1.5 mg/day and women need to absorb 2 to 3 mg/day because of iron losses with menstruation. The goal of therapy for iron deficiency anemia is to supply sufficient iron to repair the hemoglobin deficit and to replenish iron stores. Oral iron is the treatment of choice for almost all patients because of its effectiveness, safety, and economy and should always be given preference over parenteral iron for initial treatment.[39] Iron deficiency anemia is managed with oral administration of ferrous sulfate taken separately from meals in three or four divided doses and supplying a daily total of 150 to 200 mg of elemental iron in adults or 3 mg of iron per kilogram of body weight in children until hematologic normality is reached.[39] Infants may be given 50 to 100 mg daily in divided doses. Thereafter it is important to continue the treatment for 4 to 6 months to build iron stores. Urgent treatment may be accomplished with the administration to intravenous ferric gluconate following a test dose to determine possible hypersensitivity. Patients undergoing dialysis should have a serum ferritin level greater than 100 μg/L to optimize their response to erythropoietin administration. Although iron therapy remediates the iron deficiency anemia, the underlying cause must be determined and corrected.[36-40]

Course and prognosis. The symptoms may be alleviated in the first few days of treatment. The reticulocyte count is an index of erythropoiesis. The reticulocyte count increases as the RBC production increases and usually reaches maximal levels in 7 to 12 days, and the hemoglobin level is usually normal by 2 months after initiation of therapy.[36-40] Failure to obtain a complete and characteristic response to iron therapy should cause the clinician to review the findings and reevaluate the patient. One possible problem is an incorrect diagnosis, when the anemia of chronic disease is mistaken for the anemia of iron deficiency.[39] The prognosis is excellent if the underlying cause is benign; however, even in patients with incurable disease states, management of iron deficiency anemia with iron therapy can increase the comfort level.[36-40]

ANEMIA RELATED TO INHERITED DISORDERS OF THE RED CELL

Thalassemia

Anemia can also be caused by increased RBC destruction, or **hemolysis.** Hemolytic anemias are characterized by decreased red cell survival rates. The thalassemias are examples of a type of anemia caused by decreased red cell survival rates. The red cells produced are abnormal and prone to destruction. This destruction is based on an intrinsic defect in the red cells.[41-44]

Etiology and pathogenesis. The thalassemias are a group of diseases associated with the presence of mutant genes that suppress the rate of synthesis of globin chains. Thalassemias are classified according to the polypeptide chain or chains with deficient synthesis, such as α-thalassemia or β-thalassemia.[41-44] There are two main classes of thalassemia, α and β, in which the α- and β-globin genes are involved, and rarer forms caused by abnormalities of other globin genes. These conditions all have in common an imbalanced rate of production of the globin chains of adult hemoglobin—excess α chains in β-thalassemia and excess β chains in α-thalassemia. Several hundred different mutations at the α- and β-globin loci have been defined as the cause of the reduced or absent output of α or β chains. The high frequency and genetic diversity of the thalassemias are related to past or present heterozygote resistance to malaria.[41] A deficiency in one or more polypeptide chains causes decreased hemoglobin synthesis and an imbalance between α-chain and non–α-chain production. Because of the lack of hemoglobin, the anemia is severe, and the peripheral cells are microcytic and hypochromic. The disruption of the globin balance causes the normal chains to accumulate and precipitate within the cytoplasm. This damages the cell membranes, which leads to premature cell destruction. The most clinically severe form of the thalassemias is *thalassemia major,* which occurs in homozygous patients. *Thalassemia minor* is the term used to describe the heterozygous carrier state. For example, in homozygous β-thalassemia, the deficiency of β-chain synthesis results in the accumulation of α chains, which aggregate to form insoluble inclusions in bone marrow erythroid precursors (Figure 13-18). These inclusions cause early destruction of 70% to 85% of marrow erythroblasts. In response to this massive destruction, erythroid cell proliferation in homozygous β-thalassemia is significant.[41-44]

Patients who are significantly anemic have an increased intestinal iron absorption that is related to the degree of expansion of the RBC precursor population. This can be decreased with blood transfusions. The iron accumulates in the Kupffer cells of the liver, the macrophages in the spleen, and the parenchymal cells of the liver.[41]

Laboratory features. Laboratory values vary, depending on the severity of the imbalance, which is determined by the genetic pattern. Because of the decrease in hemoglobin level, the red cells are hypochromic and microcytic, and red cell indices—MCV, MCH, and MCHC—are decreased. Many target cells are present. In homozygous or major syndromes, the hemoglobin concentration is often less than 7 g/dl, and there are nucleated red cells in the peripheral blood. The leukocyte number is usually increased but the platelet number is normal. The bone marrow is hypercellular, with profound erythroblastic hyperplasia. There is evidence of hemolysis with increased unconjugated bilirubin levels and increased excretion of urobilin and urobilinogen. Hemoglobin electrophoresis is performed to determine the type of abnormal hemoglobin. An increased level of fetal hemoglobin ranging from 10%

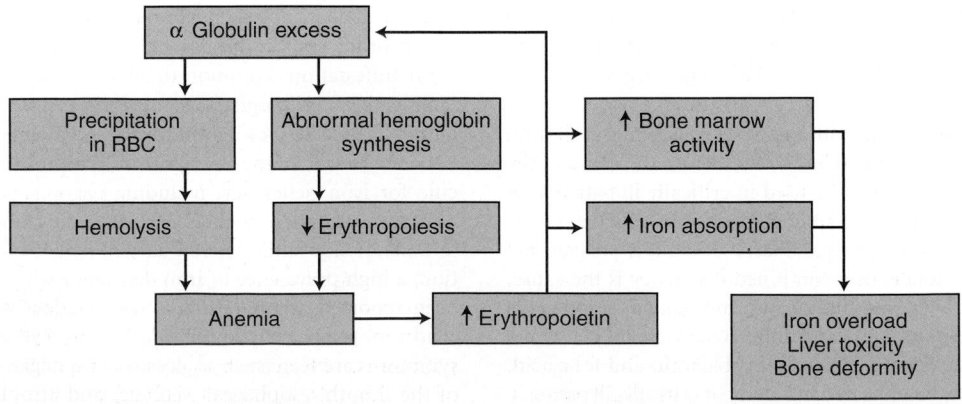

FIGURE 13-18 Pathophysiology of β-thalassemia.

to 90% is characteristic of homozygous α-thalassemia. No hemoglobin α is produced. Excess γ chains form γ4 homotetramers or Bart's hemoglobin. Excess β chains form β4 homotetramers or hemoglobin H.[41-44]

Clinical manifestations. Patients may have any of the clinical manifestations described earlier (see General Effects of Anemia). The clinical findings are the result of deficient α-globin production in α-thalassemia or α-globin chain excess and persistent hemoglobin F production in β-thalassemia.[41-44]

α-Thalassemia is found primarily in Asian individuals; however, it has also been documented in increasing numbers in individuals of Mediterranean or African descent. Usually patients with α-thalassemia minor are silent carriers or present with mild to moderate anemia. They are recognized during familial studies following the identification of a family member with Bart's hemoglobin hydrops fetalis or hemoglobin H disease (α-thalassemia major). Infants with Bart's hemoglobin hydrops fetalis are pale and edematous and have hepatomegaly, splenomegaly, and ascites. Individuals with hemoglobin H disease have typical facies and bone changes seen in β-thalassemia, splenomegaly, and hepatomegaly.[41-43]

β-Thalassemia occurs mainly in individuals of Mediterranean descent and presents as thalassemia major, intermedia, or minor. It is also seen in the Middle East, parts of India and Pakistan, and throughout Southeast Asia. Untreated patients with thalassemia major have skull bone deformities from intramedullary and extramedullary bone marrow expansion, mongoloid facies, bowing and **rarefaction** of long bones, extension of bone marrow into paraspinal or intraabdominal tumors, **icterus,** hepatomegaly, splenomegaly, and cardiac failure or endocrinopathies, such as diabetes mellitus and hypogonadism from excessive intestinal iron absorption. Patients with thalassemia intermedia show fewer effects of iron overload, growth retardation, marrow expansion, and splenomegaly; however, deforming bone and joint disease, chronic leg ulceration, and infection are common in this form of thalassemia. Thalassemia minor is usually relatively asymptomatic.[41-44]

Treatment. Because the carrier states for the thalassemias can be identified and affected fetuses can be diagnosed by DNA analysis after the ninth to tenth week of gestation, these conditions are widely amenable to prenatal diagnosis. Currently, bone marrow transplantation is the only way in which they can be cured. Symptomatic management is based on regular blood transfusions, iron chelation therapy, and the judicious use of splenectomy.[41] Children with thalassemia are treated with blood transfusion therapy to maintain a hemoglobin level of 11 to 13 g/dl to ensure normal growth and development and to avoid skeletal deformities. Patients should be tested for the presence of hepatitis B antibodies and immunized if they test negative. Splenectomy is recommended in children 6 to 7 years of age or in adolescents when their transfusion requirements exceed 1.5 times normal (>200 ml/kg/yr). Before splenectomy, children should be immunized with polyvalent pneumococcal vaccine, *Haemophilus influenzae,* and *Neisseria meningitidis.* Iron supplements are avoided, and chelation therapy is started when the serum ferritin levels reach 1000 μg/dl. Vitamin C is required for management of iron overload. Bone marrow transplantation has been used with success in severe β-thalassemia. The best candidates are younger children, because older children have high rejection and mortality rates.[41-44] Two experimental approaches are currently being pursued in the search for more effective therapy of the thalassemias: (1) reactivation or augmentation of fetal hemoglobin production and (2) somatic gene therapy.[41]

Course and prognosis. Infants with Bart's hemoglobin hydrops fetalis inherit an α-thalassemia gene from both parents who only have the α-thalassemia trait. These infants are usually stillborn or die within hours to days of birth. Some patients with hemoglobin H disease live a full life. Patients with β-thalassemia intermedia can expect to live until middle age; however, iron loading and crippling bone disease occur in the third and fourth decades. Children with adequate treatment with

iron chelation before bone marrow transplantation have disease-free survival rates up to 95%, whereas older patients and those exhibiting more than one risk factor have a rejection-free survival rate of less than 75%. Treatments under investigation include manipulation of globin gene expression with drugs such as 5-azacytidine, hydroxyurea, erythropoietin, or butyrate analogues and gene therapy directed at replacing or compensating for the defective β-globin alleles. Because this is a genetically transmitted disease, it is important for patients and parents to receive appropriate genetic counseling.[41-44]

Sickle Cell Anemia

Etiology and pathogenesis. Sickle cell anemia is a genetically determined defect of hemoglobin synthesis. Sickle cell disease is a disorder in which patients inherit specific mutated variants of the β-globin gene that lead to hemoglobin polymerization. The sickle mutation of the β-globin gene results in the production of an abnormal hemoglobin called sickle hemoglobin S (HbS). In hemoglobin S, valine is substituted for glutamic acid in the sixth position of the β chain, rather than the normal configuration. This apparently minor change in the molecular structure causes profound changes in hemoglobin stability and solubility. Under decreased oxygen tension, hemoglobin S undergoes polymerization, which causes the red cell to assume a sickled shape (Figure 13-19). Patients who are homozygous produce only hemoglobin S. No hemoglobin A is synthesized because all the β chains are S chains, which

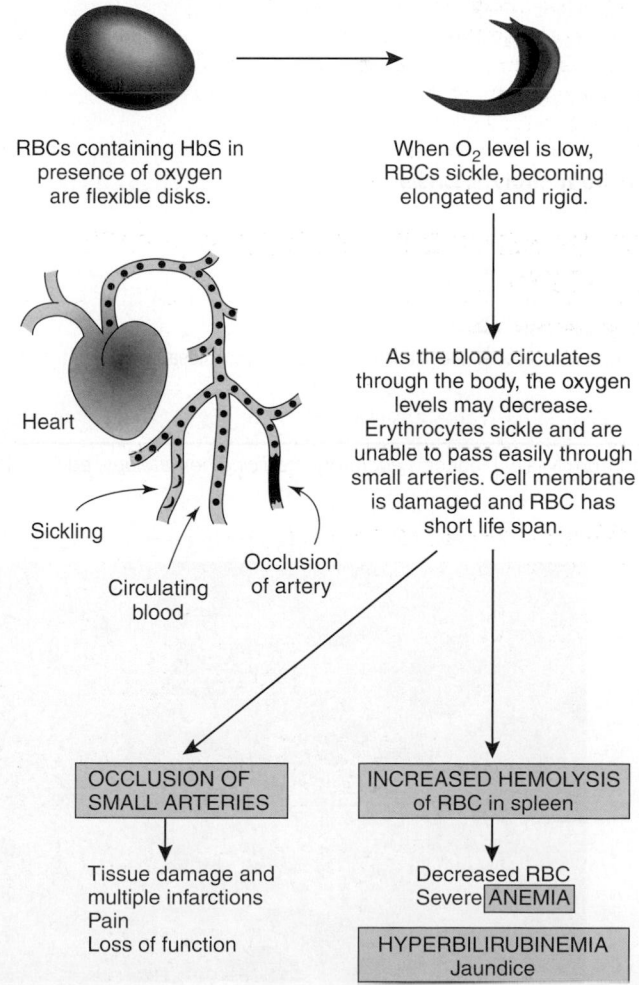

RBCs containing HbS in presence of oxygen are flexible disks.

When O_2 level is low, RBCs sickle, becoming elongated and rigid.

Heart

Sickling

Circulating blood

Occlusion of artery

As the blood circulates through the body, the oxygen levels may decrease. Erythrocytes sickle and are unable to pass easily through small arteries. Cell membrane is damaged and RBC has short life span.

OCCLUSION OF SMALL ARTERIES

INCREASED HEMOLYSIS of RBC in spleen

Tissue damage and multiple infarctions
Pain
Loss of function

Decreased RBC
Severe ANEMIA

HYPERBILIRUBINEMIA Jaundice

FIGURE 13-19 Sickle cell anemia: effects of sickling. *HbS,* Hemoglobin S; *RBC,* red blood cell. (From Gould BE: *Pathophysiology for the health professions,* ed 2, Philadelphia, 2002, Saunders, p 247.)

combine with normal α chains to form hemoglobin S. In heterozygous patients with sickle cell trait, both normal and S chains are formed. Because fewer abnormal chains are produced than normal ones, the amount of hemoglobin A usually exceeds that of hemoglobin S. The sickle mutation has undergone positive selection during human evolution because individuals with one copy of the sickle gene and one normal β-globin gene (sickle cell trait) have a survival advantage in malaria-endemic regions. The preferential sickling of cells with malarial parasites reduces the number of parasites and allows children with sickle cell trait who are infected with these parasites to reach reproductive age. This has provided a selective advantage to the hemoglobin S trait, thereby preventing S from being genetically eliminated.[45-48]

The pathogenetic signs and symptoms of sickle cell disease all relate to the red cell sickling. Sickled red cells have a decreased survival time, which causes anemia, and sickled cells cause vascular occlusion, which results in capillary stasis, venous thrombosis, and arterial emboli. The most dangerous feature of sickle cell anemia is the occurrence of acute episodes of "crisis," which can be hemolytic or vascular (Box 13-2).[45-48]

Laboratory features. The laboratory features in sickle cell anemia are distinctive. The anemia is usually severe, with red cells of different shapes and sizes. Target red cells are present, and occasionally sickled cells can be seen on smears (Figure 13-20). Red cell breakdown products are increased, which increases serum bilirubin, urobilinogen, and urobilin levels. Acute hemolytic crisis is characterized by hemoglobinuria, leukocytosis, and normoblastosis; diffuse intravascular coagulation may develop.[45-48]

Clinical manifestations. Chronic hemolytic anemia, recurrent painful episodes, and acute and chronic organ dysfunction particularly of the spleen, bones, brain, kidneys, lungs, skin, and heart are the cardinal features of sickle cell anemia. Sickle cell anemia and sickle cell trait are found almost entirely in the black race.[45-48] Hemolysis of the sickle cells occurs in the spleen or vascular space, and vaso-occlusive

---

BOX 13-2 COMPLICATIONS OF SICKLE CELL ANEMIA

Decreased RBC Survival
Anemia
Reticulocytosis
Hyperbilirubinemia
Increased pigment excretion
Cholelithiasis
Hyperplastic bone marrow
Osteoporosis
Osteosclerosis
Siderosis

Acute Hemolytic Crisis
Leukocytosis
Reticulocytosis
Hyperbilirubinemia
Hemoglobinuria
Normoblastosis
Diffuse intravascular coagulation (consumption coagulopathy)

Vascular Occlusion (Capillary Stasis, Venous Thrombosis, Arterial Emboli)
Splenomegaly
Splenic infarction
Splenic atrophy
Hepatomegaly
Cirrhosis
Hematuria
Sickle cell dactylitis
Aseptic necrosis of bones
Infarction of bone marrow
Infarction of various organs (brain)
Priapism
Skin ulcers
Pulmonary embolism

Painful Crisis (Occlusive Vascular Crisis)
Fever
Pain
Sudden death

Data from Miale J, editor: *Laboratory medicine hematology,* ed 6, St Louis, 1982, Mosby, p 637.

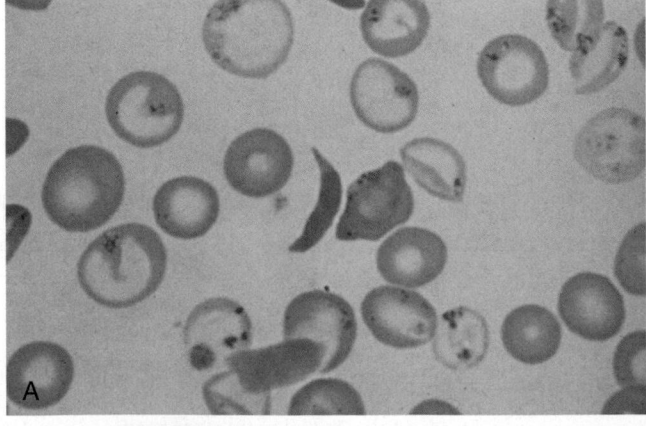 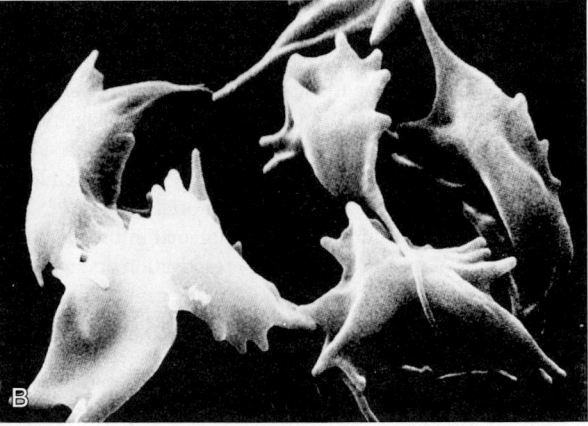

FIGURE 13-20 A, Blood smear showing sickle cells in sickle cell anemia. B, Scanning electron micrograph of deoxygenated sickled red cells. **(A,** Courtesy Beth Payne, Sacred Heart Medical Center, Spokane, WA. **B,** From Young NS et al, editors: *Clinical hematology,* Philadelphia, 2006, Mosby, p 39.)

events occur in the small capillaries and venules caused by sickle cells.[45] The red cell life span is already shortened by the sickling and may precipitate a hemolytic crisis with jaundice. Sudden massive pooling of red cells, particularly in the spleen, can create a sequestration crisis, which is thought to result in the deaths that occur in the first years of life.[45-48] Infarctive crises or painful episodes are a result of obstruction of blood vessels, tissue hypoxia, and tissue death, and may occur throughout the body. Vaso-occlusive events are described in Table 13-7. Children with sickle cell anemia are shorter and experience delayed puberty, but they attain normal height with late adolescent growth. Bony abnormalities, "hand-foot" syndrome with periostitis of the metacarpal and metatarsal bones, splenomegaly, inability to concentrate urine, priapism with subsequent impotence, underdeveloped genitalia and hypogonadism, hepatomegaly, jaundice, gallstones, tachycardia, acute chest syndrome (fever, chest pain, increasing WBC count, and pulmonary infiltrates), retinal vessel obstruction, cerebrovascular accidents, leg ulcers, and infections are all seen in sickle cell disease patients. Pregnant women may exhibit signs of pyelonephritis, pulmonary infarction, pneumonia, antepartum hemorrhage, premature fetal delivery, and fetal death.[45-48]

Treatment. Stem cell transplantation is curative and the treatment of choice. Currently there are no safe, effective antisickling agents, and treatment is primarily supportive. To avoid precipitation of a vaso-occlusive crisis, it is important to prevent dehydration, infection, fever, acidosis, hypoxemia, and cold exposure.[45-48] Because salicylates impose an acid load, acetaminophen is the preferred antipyretic.[46] Vaccination for pneumococcal pneumonia should be done before 2 years of age in patients with sickle cell anemia and booster vaccinations given 3 to 5 years later. Penicillin prophylaxis is important to prevent streptococcal pneumonia and pneumococcal septicemia. Other vaccinations include *Haemophilus influenzae* type B and hepatitis B. Transfusions are used to restore normal hematocrit levels, and splenectomy is performed in children with sequestration syndrome. Treatment with oral hydroxyurea reduces leukocyte, polymorphonuclear (PMN), reticulocyte, and sickle cell counts while increasing the hemoglobin and hematocrit levels and resulting in fewer acute painful episodes. Appropriate treatment of pain is important. During pregnancy, folic acid should be given to prevent neural tube defects. If iron deficiency is present, iron supplements should also be administered. Transfusion should be used only when clinical and hematologic indicators are present.[45-48]

Course and prognosis. Successful bone marrow stem cell transplantation cures sickle cell anemia. Bone marrow transplantation from a sibling-matched donor has a 94% survival rate and an 84% event-free survival rate. Sickle cell anemia is a serious disorder, and without stem cell transplantation many patients die in childhood, especially in sequestration crisis. In young children with sickle cell anemia, there is a 30% incidence of splenic sequestration crisis with a 15% death rate. Functional hyposplenia predisposes individuals to infections, such as pneumonia and chronic pyelonephritis with renal failure. Heart failure, bone marrow and fat emboli, shock, and organ failure are common causes of death. In developed countries, patients who have not undergone stem cell transplantation may survive into the third and fourth decades, whereas survival past childhood in underdeveloped countries is unusual.[45-48] The survival rates have increased dramatically because of stem cell transplantation, newborn screening, early diagnosis, preventive measures to avoid sequestration crisis, and patient education.[45-48]

Hereditary Spherocytosis

Etiology and pathogenesis. In hereditary spherocytosis, the red cells have defective red cell membrane skeletons, altered membrane properties, and altered cell metabolism. This causes them to have a decreased survival time in patients with an intact spleen. The disease is inherited as an autosomal dominant trait and is characterized by red cells that are fragile microspherocytes. In addition, there is increased destruction of **spherocytes** (abnormal spherical erythrocytes) in the spleen. Patients have anemia, intermittent jaundice, splenomegaly, and uniform responsiveness to splenectomy. The principal cellular defect is a loss of membrane surface area attributable to defects of several membrane proteins, including ankyrin, band 3, α-spectrin, and β-spectrin.[49-52]

Laboratory features. The concentration of hemoglobin within the red cells is increased. Reticulocytosis is present, and microspherocytes are seen on the blood smear. Osmotic fragility is increased, and serum unconjugated bilirubin level is increased. Following splenectomy, the hemoglobin level is in the high-normal range.[49-52]

Clinical manifestations. Hereditary spherocytosis is the most common hereditary hemolytic anemia and is most common in people with a northern European background. The major clinical manifestations are anemia, jaundice, splenomegaly, bile pigment gallstones, and

TABLE 13-7	VASO-OCCLUSIVE CONSEQUENCES OF SICKLE CELL DISEASE	
EVENT	**INCIDENCE**	**FEATURES**
Acute		
Painful episodes	>50% of patients with HbSS and HbS β-thalassemia	Mild to severe pain; one or several areas
Chest syndrome	10-20% of adults	Difficult to distinguish from pneumonia; may involve entire lung
Priapism	10-40% of males	Can have a more chronic form; causes impotence
Cerebrovascular accidents	1-10% of children	Usually subarachnoid bleeding in adults
Hepatopathy	<2% of adults	Bilirubin may reach >80 mg/dl
Chronic		
Aseptic bone necrosis	10-25% of adults	Hips and shoulders, common in HbSC
Proliferative retinopathy	50% of adults with HbSC; <5% HbSS 10%	Can lead to retinal detachment
Leg ulcers		Can be severe and disabling
Functional asplenia and autosplenectomy	Starts in infancy; >90% of adults with HbSS	Predispose to sepsis
Nephropathy	Renal failure in older patients	Nephritic syndrome, renal failure

Adapted from Sternberg MH: Hemoglobinopathies and thalassemias. In Stein JH et al, editors: *Internal medicine,* ed 5, St Louis, 1998, Mosby, p 658. *HbS,* Hemoglobin S (sickle hemoglobin); *HbSC,* hemoglobin SC disease; *HbSS,* hemoglobin SS (sickle cell anemia).

chronic leg ulcers. The anemia is usually mild because of compensation by the erythropoietic bone marrow cells. Aplastic crisis precipitated by an infection may be seen with associated fever, abdominal discomfort, nausea, vomiting, rapidly increasing weakness, pallor, tachycardia, low blood pressure, and shock.[49-52]

Treatment. Treatment usually consists of splenectomy in children with severe cases (hemoglobin concentration <8 g/dl and reticulocyte count >10%) and children with moderate disease reflected (hemoglobin concentration 8 to 11 g/dl and reticulocyte count of 8% to 10%) when the anemia compromises physical activity. All children undergoing splenectomy should be immunized with polyvalent pneumococcal vaccine, *Haemophilus influenzae*, and *Neisseria meningitidis*. Oral penicillin should be given for several years after splenectomy to prevent pneumococcal sepsis. Folic acid therapy to prevent folate deficiency is necessary as well. Transfusion is usually indicated only in aplastic crisis.[49-52]

Course and prognosis. Most patients have no or mild anemia, fluctuating degrees of jaundice, and episodes of aplastic or hemolytic anemia. Splenectomy is usually curative; however, the subsequent risk of acquiring a serious infection is significant.[49-52]

Glucose-6-Phosphate Dehydrogenase Deficiency

Etiology and pathogenesis. An example of an RBC intracellular defect caused by an enzyme deficiency is glucose-6-phosphate dehydrogenase (G6PD) deficiency. The energy required for RBC membrane function and cellular integrity is derived from the anaerobic metabolism of glucose. Traditionally, hemolytic anemias caused by enzyme deficiencies have been called nonspherocytic to distinguish them from classic hereditary spherocytosis. When black soldiers receiving the antimalarial drug primaquine began suffering hemolytic episodes, a type of hemolytic anemia caused by a deficiency of G6PD (an enzyme in the red cell glycolytic pathway) was discovered. When G6PD-deficient RBCs are challenged by one of several drugs, glutathione is depleted and glucose utilization is inhibited. These events cause RBC membrane damage, which results in removal of the damaged cells by mononuclear phagocytes. Except in rare instances, G6PD-deficient persons do not have hemolytic anemia unless challenged by drugs.[53-58] G6PD deficiency is the most common metabolic disease of the RBC, affecting hundreds of millions of people worldwide. This gene is found in 11% of African-American males and in Sephardic Jews. Because the responsible gene is an X-linked recessive gene, close relatives of affected individuals should be screened. Because G6PD deficiency is found in areas where malaria was once endemic, G6PD deficiency is thought to have conferred selective advantage against *Plasmodium falciparum* malaria infection.[58]

Laboratory features. Usually this anemia is first recognized during or after an infectious illness or following exposure to a suspect drug or chemical. The hematologic tests reflect the severity of the hemolytic episode. The diagnosis of G6PD deficiency is based on the generation of NADPH from NADP as detected either by quantitative spectrophotometric analysis or by a rapid fluorescent screening test.[53-58]

Clinical manifestations. Most individuals have no clinical manifestations of this disease. When such manifestations occur, hemolytic anemia is triggered by drug administration, infection, diabetic acidosis, the newborn period, and, in one subset, exposure to fava beans.[53-58]

Treatment. Treatment is usually preventive and consists of avoidance of drugs that trigger hemolytic episodes and aggressive infection management. Some patients may require transfusion therapy or exchange transfusion in the case of life-threatening hemolysis.[53-58]

Course and prognosis. The prognosis is generally good since the episodes of hemolytic crisis are usually self-limiting, except in fava bean–susceptible individuals, in whom shock may develop in a short time.[55]

ANEMIA RELATED TO EXTRINSIC RED CELL DESTRUCTION OR LOSS

The final category of types of absolute anemia includes those caused by extrinsic abnormalities. The most important of these category types is immune hemolytic anemia caused by antibodies to red cells. Immune hemolytic anemias are further subdivided into those caused by isoantibodies, which may be the result of accidental immunization of individuals (e.g., hemolytic disease of the newborn), and those caused by autoantibodies (in individuals whose bodies create antibodies against their own red cells).[59-64]

Hemolytic Disease of the Newborn

Etiology and pathogenesis. When fetal red cells cross the placenta, they may stimulate the production of maternal antibodies against antigens on the fetal red cell not inherited from the mother. These maternal antibodies cross into the fetal circulation and cause destruction of fetal cells. In severe cases, hydrops fetalis may result. Fetal-maternal ABO incompatibility is the most common cause of hemolytic disease of the newborn (HDNB), but Rh incompatibility is clinically more important because of the severity of the hemolytic disease in the fetus. With the introduction of Rh treatment, the total incidence of HDNB in Rh-negative women has been greatly reduced.[60,63]

Laboratory features. Anemia, **reticulocytosis** (an increased number of circulating reticulocytes), and nucleated red cells are seen in the peripheral blood of the infant. There is a rough correlation between the hemoglobin levels and the severity of the disease. Untreated infants may experience a rapid drop in hemoglobin levels after birth. Leukocytosis is present, but platelet counts are usually normal. Infants with severe disease may have thrombocytopenia. Serum bilirubin, a hemolytic breakdown product, is readily transferred across the placenta. At birth, the infant's total bilirubin level reflects both the severity of the hemolytic process and the ability of the infant's liver enzyme system to conjugate and excrete bilirubin. Cord blood red cells show a characteristic positive direct antiglobulin test (**Coombs test),** reflecting the maternal antibodies attached to the infant's red cells.[60,63]

During pregnancy, laboratory tests of amniotic fluid for bilirubin and antibodies and tests of the mother's peripheral blood for maternal sensitization are useful in predicting whether infants will be affected by HDNB.[60,63]

Clinical manifestations. The clinical manifestations of HDNB are hemolytic anemia, extramedullary erythropoiesis, and hyperbilirubinemia. Jaundice, petechial hemorrhages, hepatomegaly, splenomegaly, heart failure (with pulmonary edema, pleural effusions, ascites, and edema), kernicterus (a condition in the newborn marked by severe neural symptoms, associated with high levels of bilirubin in the blood), and diffuse intravascular coagulation are seen in these infants. Many infants die in utero.[60,63]

Treatment. A standard dose of anti-Rh immunoglobulin (RhoGAM) is given to the mother before or after delivery. This immunoglobulin destroys the infant's RBCs before they can sensitize the mother. This dose protects the mother against 30 ml of Rh-positive blood. Amniocentesis and fetal blood sampling are used to evaluate the severity of the disease. In severe cases, in utero transfusion and early delivery have been performed on fetuses with severe **erythroblastosis.** Exchange transfusion lowers the serum bilirubin level and the antibody content of the neonatal blood and removes cells susceptible to hemolysis. Phototherapy and phenobarbital are used to lower the bilirubin level.[60,63]

Course and prognosis. The consequences of HDNB range from death, to possible retardation, to a barely perceptible hemolytic process. Severe anemia correlates with equally severe hyperbilirubinemia and

TABLE 13-8	MECHANISMS OF DRUG-INDUCED HEMOLYSIS OR POSITIVE DIRECT ANTIGLOBULIN TEST			
	DRUG ABSORPTION	**NEOANTIGEN**	**AUTOIMMUNE**	**NONIMMUNE ABSORPTION**
Prototype drug	Penicillin	Quinidine/stibophen	α-Methyldopa	First-generation cephalosporins
Role of drug	Cell-bound hapten	Antibody binds drug + RBC	Induces drug-independent RBC antibody	Modifies RBC membrane; absorbs proteins nonantibody-specifically
Typical DAT	IgG	C3	IgG	Nonimmunoglobulin
Antibody reactions	Reacts only with drug-coated cells	Reacts only with drug present	Drug independent; panagglutinin	No antibody present
Typical clinical presentation	Subacute onset; mild to severe hemolysis	Acute onset; severe hemolysis	Insidious onset; chronic mild hemolysis	No hemolysis

From Greer JP et al, editors: *Wintrobe's clinical hematology*, ed 11, Philadelphia, 2004, Lippincott Williams & Wilkins, p 1176.
C3, Complement third component; *DAT*, direct antiglobulin test; *IgG*, immunoglobulin G; *RBC*, red blood cell.

high risk of central nervous system complications.[60,63] Many infants appear normal at birth, only to develop jaundice within 2 to 3 hours. Petechial hemorrhages develop soon after birth, and kernicterus is usually seen late in the second day of significant jaundice. Successful Rho-GAM administration prevention programs have reduced the perinatal death rate to about 1% to 2%.[60,63]

Antibody-Mediated Drug Reactions

Etiology and pathogenesis. Drug-induced immune hemolytic anemia is an example of a disease in which exposure to a drug causes destruction and lysis of the sensitized person's own red cells. Drugs can lead to red cell hemolysis by four different immune mechanisms (Table 13-8).[53,59,61,62,64]

Hapten mechanisms. In the hapten mechanism, which is seen with penicillin, cephalosporins, and tetracycline, the drug combines with a component of the RBC membrane. An antibody is developed against the drug. When the drug is given again, it coats the red cells, and the antibody attaches to the drug–red cell complex. The antigen-antibody complex then causes hemolysis.[53,59,61,62,64]

Neoantigen formation. The old terminology for neoantigen formation is *immune complex formation*. In this situation, the drug combines with the RBC membrane and the antibody reacts with the new antigenic sites created by the combination of the drug and membrane. The RBC is hemolyzed. The immune complex can also bind to platelet and leukocyte membranes, causing anemia, leukopenia, and thrombocytopenia. Quinidine, hydrochlorothiazide; sulfonamides, isoniazid, tetracycline, and cephalosporin are common drugs that cause this type of reaction.[53,59,61,62,64]

Membrane modification. In membrane modification, seen in cephalosporin sensitivity, the drug alters the RBC membrane protein. Plasma proteins attach to the altered RBC protein and cause a positive serologic test but no cell hemolysis.[61]

Autoantibody induction. This mechanism was first studied in cases of hemolytic anemia with patients who were taking the antihypertensive agent methyldopa (Aldomet). The drug appears to induce antibody formation to red cell membrane Rh antigens. About 29% of the patients receiving this drug develop a positive antiglobulin test response.[53,59,61,62,64]

Laboratory features. The laboratory features for all mechanisms show increased red cell turnover and anemia if hemolysis exceeds the rate of RBC production. Serologic tests, such as the direct antiglobulin test, will be positive. In hapten antibody–mediated drug reactions and

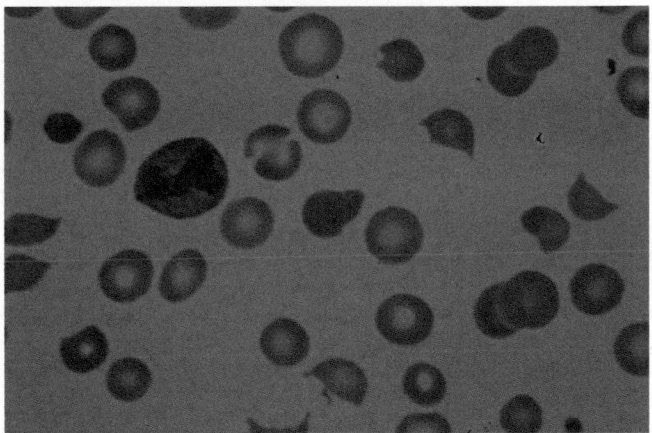

FIGURE 13-21 Schistocytes are fragments of red blood cells produced by hemolytic pathologies. (Courtesy Beth Payne, Sacred Heart Medical Center, Spokane, WA.)

in immune complex formation, the antiglobulin reaction is positive for immunoglobulins. In autoantibody induction, the antiglobulin reaction is positive for complement. Fragmented RBCs may be seen on the peripheral blood smear. These fragments are called *schistocytes* (Figure 13-21). Leukopenia and thrombocytopenia are sometimes seen with drug-induced platelet or leukocyte destruction.[53,59,61,62,64]

Clinical manifestations. Types of immune drug-induced hemolytic anemia vary in symptoms and severity, depending on the mechanism involved. Hapten (e.g., penicillin) and autoimmune (e.g., methyldopa) drug-induced hemolytic anemias have an insidious onset of symptoms over a period of weeks. The neoantigen formation (e.g., quinine or quinidine) may present with sudden, severe hemolysis with hemoglobinuria and result in acute renal failure. Other clinical manifestations include acute respiratory distress syndrome and respiratory arrest.[53,59,61,62,64]

Treatment. Recognition and discontinuation of the responsible drug are usually the only treatment necessary. Steroid therapy and transfusions may be required in cases of severe hemolysis.[53,59,61,62,64]

Course and prognosis. Immune hemolytic anemia attributable to drugs is usually mild and the prognosis is good; however, with severe hemolysis, death can occur.[53,59,61,62,64] Laboratory findings for erythrocyte disorders are summarized in Table 13-5.

Acute Blood Loss

Etiology and pathogenesis. Acute blood loss anemia may present after trauma or secondary to a disease process. Acute blood loss anemia rapidly decreases the overall blood volume and impairs oxygen delivery.[65,66]

Laboratory features. A decrease occurs in both hematocrit level and hemoglobin concentration attributable to blood loss. The hematocrit level is less than 40% in men and less than 37% in women. The hemoglobin concentration is less than 14 g/dl in men and less than 12 g/dl in women.[65] Anemia may not be apparent in the early stages because the cells and plasma are diminishing simultaneously. As replacement fluids move into the intravascular space, the anemia becomes apparent in later laboratory tests. The cells have normal MCV, MCH, and MCHC values.

Clinical manifestations. In a normal 70-kg person with a 5000-ml total blood volume, 10% loss of blood (500 ml) rarely causes any clinical signs except occasional vasovagal syncope. A 20% loss (1000 ml) usually causes no clinical symptoms at rest, but tachycardia is seen with exercise, and a slight postural drop in blood pressure occurs.[65,66] A person with a 30% loss (1500 ml) usually presents with flat neck veins when supine, postural hypotension, and exercise tachycardia. A 40% loss (2000 ml) causes the central venous pressure, cardiac output, and arterial blood pressure to fall below normal while the patient is supine and at rest, with associated air hunger, tachycardia, and cold, clammy skin. A 50% loss of total blood volume (2500 ml) often causes shock and death.[65,66]

Treatment. Blood volume replacement therapy with crystalloid solutions, colloid solutions (plasma protein, albumin, or dextran), and fresh whole blood is essential in the early management of acute hemorrhage to restore blood volume and to prevent shock. Complete reliance on fresh whole blood for managing acute blood loss is contraindicated and should be reserved for patients with a low red cell mass, in whom tissue hypoxia is a threat. Replacement of red cell mass by increased red cell production is a gradual process, which occurs over 2 to 5 days as the marrow stem cells proliferate and mature. Maximal red cell production is seen by the tenth day after hemorrhage.[65,66]

Course and prognosis. With adequate replacement therapy, the prognosis is excellent; however, the underlying cause must be identified and managed.

Other Extrinsic Abnormalities

Other *mechanisms,* such as mechanical heart valves or cardiopulmonary bypass machines, may cause physical damage to the red cells, resulting in hemolysis. Drugs and chemicals, physical agents (e.g., burns), or infectious diseases (e.g., malaria) may result in anemia. Venom from bee and wasp stings, spider and scorpion bites, and snake bites has been associated with hemolytic anemia. Finally, hypersplenism and splenomegaly can cause anemia, leukopenia, or **thrombocytopenia** severe enough to require splenectomy.[67]

KEY POINTS

- The general effects of anemia are due to tissue hypoxia and efforts to compensate for low oxygen-carrying capacity. Vasoconstriction, pallor, tachypnea, dyspnea, tachycardia, ischemic pain, lethargy, and lightheadedness may be present. In addition, signs and symptoms relating to the specific cause of the anemia may be present. These accompanying manifestations are helpful in determining the cause of the anemia.
- Anemia may be due to abnormally low production of red cells and/or excessive loss or destruction. Decreased production of red cells may be due to stem cell failure (aplastic anemia), lack of erythropoietin (renal disease), or nutritional deficiencies of iron, vitamin B_{12}, or folate. Excessive red cell loss may be due to hemolysis (e.g., ABO and Rh incompatibility, drugs) or bleeding (e.g., surgery, trauma). Inherited disorders of red cells often impair production and increase destruction of red cells.

- Determination of the cause of anemia is based on the history, differential signs and symptoms, and results of laboratory studies. The important differentiating features of the major types of anemia are as follows:
  - *Aplastic anemia:* History of toxic or radiation injury to bone marrow. Accompanying leukopenia and thrombocytopenia. Red cells are normocytic and normochromic.
  - *Chronic renal failure:* History of renal disease. Decreased erythropoietin level and erythropoietin responsiveness. Red cells are normocytic and normochromic.
  - *Vitamin B_{12} and folate deficiency:* History of poor nutrient intake or gastrointestinal disease. Accompanying neurologic dysfunction. Red cells are megaloblastic (macrocytic).
  - *Iron deficiency:* History of poor nutrient intake or chronic blood loss. Decreased serum ferritin and iron levels. Red cells are microcytic and hypochromic.
  - *Hemolytic:* History of ABO or Rh incompatibility or drug exposure. Increased bilirubin level, jaundice, positive direct antiglobulin test. Red cells are normocytic and normochromic.
  - *Acute blood loss:* History of trauma, surgery, or known bleeding. Accompanying manifestations of volume depletion. Red cells are normal. Anemia may not be apparent until fluid loss is replaced.
- Inherited disorders of the red cell (thalassemia, sickle cell anemia, spherocytosis, G6PD deficiency) predispose red cells to early destruction because of abnormalities in hemoglobin structure, cell shape, membrane structure, or energy production. Manifestations of hemolysis (e.g., bilirubin, jaundice) are often present.
- The general management of anemia is aimed at removing the cause, if possible; restoring oxygen-carrying capacity with blood transfusion when necessary; and preventing the complications of ischemia (e.g., with rest, oxygen therapy) and hemolysis (e.g., increased fluid intake, management of high bilirubin levels).

TRANSFUSION THERAPY

Medical indications for transfusion therapy are restoration or maintenance of oxygen-carrying capacity, blood volume, hemostasis, and leukocyte function. Red cell transfusions are administered to improve tissue oxygenation in the context of anemia or acute blood loss. Adaptive responses to a declining hemoglobin concentration include increased cardiac output, augmented oxygen extraction, blood flow redistribution to the heart and brain, a right shift in the oxyhemoglobin dissociation curve, and increased red cell production by the marrow. These compensatory mechanisms help to ensure continued oxygen delivery.[17-20] A summary of blood components, indications, actions, contraindications, precautions, and hazards is presented in Table 13-9.[66,68] Before transfusion therapy can occur, various donor tests are performed on the blood unit sample. These include ABO and Rh(D); syphilis; HIV antigen and antibodies; hepatitis B and C antigens; and human T-cell lymphotropic virus. Blood centers, which are producing plasma for fractionation, also test for alanine aminotransferase.[68] Specific pretransfusion testing using blood samples from the recipient and the donor unit must be done to ensure that the blood component will not harm the recipient and that the blood component will have an acceptable survival time when transfused. ABO and Rh typing and RBC antibody detection tests are performed, and then a cross-match between the donor unit and the recipient is performed.[68] Types of transfusion reactions, signs and symptoms, usual causes, treatment, and precautions are summarized in Table 13-10. Two serious complications of transfusion therapy include transfusion-related acute lung injury (TRALI) and transfusion-related circulatory overload (TACO). TRALI is a syndrome of acute hypoxia as a result of noncardiogenic pulmonary edema that follows transfusion. All blood components have been implicated in TRALI, but plasma-containing products are more prevalent. Supportive care is the mainstay of therapy in TRALI with (1) oxygen supplementation, (2) aggressive respiratory support, and (3) intravenous administration of fluids as well as vasopressors, which are essential for blood pressure support. Corticosteroids can be beneficial and diuretics should be avoided in TRALI. TACO is defined as an expansion in the intravascular volume when the infused blood components and/or other fluids exceed the cardiovascular ability to handle the additional workload, and results in congestive heart failure. Diuretics are given in TACO along with the supportive care noted previously.[66,68]

POLYCYTHEMIA

In polycythemia, red cells are present in excess, increasing blood viscosity, which in turn causes clinical manifestations such as hypertension. The three types of polycythemia are classified according to cause. *Polycythemia vera* is associated with neoplastic transformation of bone marrow stem cells. *Secondary polycythemia* is due to chronic hypoxemia, with a resultant increase in erythropoietin production. *Relative polycythemia* is due to dehydration, which causes a spurious increase in the RBC count.[69,73]

Polycythemia Vera

Etiology and pathogenesis. Polycythemia vera or primary polycythemia is a type of chronic **panmyelosis** (see Chapter 11) and is part of the spectrum of myeloproliferative disorders. Polycythemia vera arises from the transformation of a single stem cell into a cell with a selective growth advantage that gradually becomes the predominant source of marrow precursors. There is an overproduction of normal red cells, white cells, and platelets. As with many malignancies, the cause is unknown. Possible mechanisms for the proliferation include (1) unregulated neoplastic proliferation of stem cells, (2) presence of abnormal myeloproliferative factor acting on normal stem cells, and (3) increase of stem cell sensitivity to erythropoietin and other hematopoietins.[69,73] Some researchers have postulated that it is damage to the undifferentiated stem cell by a virus, radiation, drugs, or other agents that causes mutation and subsequent neoplastic transformation.[69,73]

Laboratory features. The diagnosis depends primarily on results of laboratory studies, which show an absolute increase in red cell mass and leukocytosis and thrombocytosis. The bone marrow shows **hyperplasia** of red cells, white cells, and platelets and extension of active hematopoietic marrow into bones of the extremities. Uric acid concentration is increased because of excessive cell proliferation, which results in the destruction of an increased number of cells. Arterial oxygen saturation is normal, which differentiates polycythemia vera from the more common secondary (hypoxemic) polycythemia. Additional findings include elevated serum vitamin B_{12} and elevated leukocyte alkaline phosphatase levels (Figure 13-22).[69,73]

Clinical manifestations. Symptoms include headache, backache, weakness, fatigue on exertion, pruritus, dizziness, sweating, visual disturbances, weight loss, paresthesias, dyspnea, joint complaints, and epigastric distress and pressure.[69,73] Common clinical manifestations include hypertension, thrombosis, and mucosal hemorrhage attributable to engorgement of retinal and sublingual veins, but each phase of the disease presents somewhat differently. Most of the clinical symptoms of polycythemia vera are related to the increased red cell mass, which gives rise to an increased blood viscosity. The liver and spleen become congested, which increases the risk of clots, acidosis, and organ infarction. The onset is insidious, with variable manifestations in virtually any organ system. Clinical symptoms appear between 60 and 80 years of age, and they appear more often in men and Caucasians. The disorder is rarely seen in children. In the preerythrocytic or developmental phase, hepatosplenomegaly, night sweats, and postbathing pruritus are common. Other patients experience mild thrombohemorrhagic symptoms or **erythromelalgia** (painful erythematous palms and soles from an increased number of circulating platelets).[69,73]

The evolution of polycythemia vera is shown in Figure 13-23. The phases include an asymptomatic phase, a plethoric or erythrocytic phase, an inactive phase, and a spent phase when anemia develops. The final evolutionary phase of polycythemia vera is that of acute myeloid leukemia.[69,73]

In the erythrocytic phase, occlusive vascular lesions, such as transient ischemic attacks, cerebrovascular accidents (strokes), myocardial ischemia or infarctions, portal venous obstruction, or superficial venous thrombosis, occur and may be the first indication of the presence of the disease. The hyperviscosity produces symptoms of reduced cerebral blood flow, such as headaches, dizziness, and visual disturbances. Walking may induce leg pain and spasm, called *intermittent claudication.*[69,73]

Mucosal hemorrhagic manifestations include epistaxis, ecchymosis, and gastrointestinal and genitourinary bleeding. Progressive splenomegaly, intermittent claudication, peptic ulcer, hyperuricemia, and gout are often seen. The most striking feature is a ruddy or florid face, telangiectasis (chronic dilation of capillaries and small arterial branches, producing small, reddish tumors of the skin) of the cheeks and nose, and purplish cyanosis of the lips and ears. Hypertension is seen in about half of patients. Distention of the retinal veins with a dark purple coloration is another important clinical finding. As the disease develops into the spent or postpolycythemia myeloid metaplasia phase, many patients complain only of **asthenia;** however, progressive hepatosplenomegaly, severe anemia, hemorrhage (particularly cutaneous), weight loss, and wasting often occur. The final phase is the development of acute myeloid leukemia.[69,73]

Treatment. There is no cure. Treatment is directed at reducing the increased blood volume, blood viscosity, red cell mass, and platelet counts by use of phlebotomy and myelosuppressive therapy with radioactive phosphorus and chemotherapeutic agents. Phlebotomy of 450 to 500 ml every 2 to 4 days until a normal hematocrit level is reached alleviates many symptoms for most patients. Phlebotomy of only 200 to 300 ml should be considered for elderly patients or those with cardiovascular disease. In the past, a hematocrit of 50% was used as the upper limit of hematocrit tolerated before phlebotomy was used. Studies have found that increased vascular complications, decreased cerebral blood flow, and decreased mental alertness occurred when hematocrit levels exceeded 45%. Hematocrit levels should be maintained at 42% for females and 45% for males. Phlebotomy is effective in controlling red cell mass, but myelosuppressive therapy is needed when the platelet count increases to more than 800,000-1,000,000/μL to control hepatosplenomegaly and thrombocytosis. The agent of choice for myelosuppressive therapy is hydroxyurea, but radioactive phosphorus is also used. Hyperuricemia is treated with allopurinol (100 to 300 mg/day), pegylated interferon (90 to 180 μg/week), or interferon-α (3 × 106 units three times a week; alter dose depending on response and toxicity). Pegylated interferon, which can be administered once weekly, should be considered. As the disease progresses, thrombosis or hemorrhage, systemic symptoms, severe pruritus refractory to histamine antagonists, and painful splenomegaly occur and a splenectomy is indicated.[69,73]

Course and prognosis. Unmanaged polycythemia vera has a poor prognosis, with a survival of less than 2 years. The prognosis depends on the nature and severity of the complications, the duration of the

Text continued on p. 288

TABLE 13-9 SUMMARY OF BLOOD COMPONENTS

COMPONENT*	MAJOR INDICATIONS	ACTION	NOT INDICATED FOR THESE CONDITIONS	SPECIAL PRECAUTIONS	HAZARDS	RATE OF INFUSION
Whole blood	Symptomatic anemia with large volume deficit	Increases oxygen-carrying capacity Increases blood volume	Condition responsive to specific component Treatment of coagulopathy	Must be ABO identical; labile coagulation factors deteriorate within 24 hr after collection	Infectious diseases Hemolytic, septic/toxic, allergic, febrile reactions TACO TRALI TA-GVHD	For massive loss, as fast as patient can tolerate
Whole blood irradiated	See *Whole blood* Increased risk for TA-GVHD	See *Whole blood* Donor lymphocytes are inactivated, reducing risk of TA-GVHD	See *Whole blood*	See *Whole blood*	See *Whole blood*	See *Whole blood*
RBCs; RBCs (adenine-saline added)†	Symptomatic anemia	Increases oxygen-carrying capacity	Pharmacologically treatable anemia Coagulation deficiency Volume expansion	Must be ABO-compatible	Infectious diseases Hemolytic, septic/toxic, allergic, febrile reactions TACO TRALI TA-GVHD	As patient can tolerate, but <4 hr
RBCs, deglycerolized	See *RBCs* IgA deficiency with anaphylactoid reactions	See *RBCs* Deglycerolization removes plasma proteins Risk of allergic and febrile reactions reduced	See *RBCs*	See *RBCs*	See RBCs Hemolysis due to incomplete deglycerolization can occur	See *RBCs*
RBCs, irradiated	See *RBCs* Increased risk for TA-GVHD	See *RBCs* Donor lymphocytes are inactivated, reducing risk of TA-GVHD	See *RBCs*	See *RBCs*	See *RBCs*	See *RBCs*
RBCs, leukocytes reduced; apheresis red blood cells, leukocytes reduced	Symptomatic anemia Reduces risk of febrile reactions	Increases oxygen-carrying capacity Reduces risk of febrile reactions from leukocyte antibodies, HLA alloimmunization, and CMV infection	Pharmacologically treatable anemia; coagulation deficiency Leukocyte reduction should not be used to prevent TA-GVHD	Must be ABO-compatible Hypotensive reaction may occur if bedside leukocyte reduction filter is used	Infectious diseases Hemolytic, septic/toxic, allergic reactions (unless plasma also removed [e.g., by washing]) TACO TRALI TA-GVHD	As patient can tolerate, but <4 hr
RBCs washed	See *RBCs* IgA deficiency with anaphylactoid reactions Recurrent severe allergic reactions to unwashed red cell products	See *RBCs* Washing reduces plasma proteins Risk of allergic reactions may be reduced	See *RBCs*	See *RBCs*	See *RBCs*	See *RBCs*
Fresh-frozen plasma (FFP)	Clinically significant deficit of labile and stable plasma protein coagulation factors and TTP	Source of labile and nonlabile plasma proteins, including all coagulation factors	Volume expansion Coagulopathy can be more effectively treated with specific therapy	Must be ABO-compatible	Infectious diseases Hemolytic, septic/toxic, allergic, febrile reactions TACO TRALI TA-GVHD	<4 hr

Liquid plasma, plasma, and thawed plasma	Bleeding patients with deficit of stable coagulation factors	Source of plasma proteins and nonlabile factors	Deficit of labile coagulation factors or volume replacement	Must be ABO-compatible	Infectious diseases Allergic reactions TACO TRALI	<4 hr
Plasma, cryoprecipitate reduced	TTP	See *FFP* Deficient in fibrinogen; factors I, VIII, vWF, and XIII Deficient in high molecular weight vWF multimers as compared to FFP	Volume expansion Deficiency of coagulation factors known to be depleted in this product, fibrinogen, and factors I, VIII, vWF, and XIII	Must be ABO-compatible	See *FFP*	<4 hr
Cryoprecipitated AHF; pooled cryoprecipitated AHF	Provides fibrinogen, vWF, factor XIII, and factor VIII	Provides fibrinogen, vWF, factor XIII[‡]	Deficit of any plasma protein other than those enriched in cryoprecipitated AHF	Frequent repeat doses may be necessary	Infectious diseases Allergic reactions	<4 hr
Platelets; platelets pooled	Bleeding from thrombocytopenia or platelet function abnormality Prevention of bleeding from marrow hypoplasia	Improves hemostasis	Plasma coagulation deficits Some conditions with rapid platelet destruction (e.g., ITP, TTP) unless life-threatening hemorrhage	Must be ABO-compatible with plasma Should not use some filters (check manufacturer's instructions)	Infectious diseases Hemolytic, septic/toxic, allergic, febrile reactions TACO TRALI TA-GVHD	<4 hr
Platelets, apheresis[‡]	See *Platelets*	See *Platelets* May be HLA or other antigen selected	See *Platelets*	See *Platelets*	See *Platelets*	See *Platelets*
Platelets, irradiated; platelets, pooled irradiated; platelets, apheresis irradiated	See *Platelets* Increased risk of TA-GVHD	See *Platelets* Donor lymphocytes are inactivated, reducing risk of TA-GVHD	See *Platelets*	See *Platelets*	See *Platelets*	See *Platelets*
Platelets, leukocytes reduced; pooled platelets, leukocytes reduced; apheresis platelets, leukocytes reduced	See *Platelets* Reduction of febrile reactions; reduction of HLA alloimmunization	See *Platelets* Reduction of leukocytes reduces risk of febrile reactions, HLA alloimmunization, and CMV infection	See *Platelets* Leukocyte reduction; should not be used to prevent TA-GVHD	See *Platelets*	See *Platelets*	See *Platelets*
Granulocytes, apheresis	See *Platelets* Neutropenia with infection, unresponsive to appropriate antibiotics	Provides granulocytes with or without platelets	Infection responsive to antibiotics, eventual marrow recovery not expected	Must be ABO-compatible Should not use some filters (check manufacturer's instructions); do not use depth-type microaggregate filters	Infectious diseases Hemolytic, allergic, febrile reactions TACO TRALI TA-GVHD	One unit over 2-4-hr period Observe closely for reactions
Granulocytes, pheresis irradiated; granulocytes, platelets irradiated	See *Granulocytes*; see *Platelets*	Provides granulocytes with or without platelets	See *Granulocytes*; see *Platelets*	See *Granulocytes*; see *Platelets*	See *Granulocytes*; see *Platelets*	See *Granulocytes*; see *Platelets*

*For all cellular components there is a risk that the recipient may become alloimmunized.

[†]RBCs and platelets may be processed in a manner that yields leukocyte-reduced components for which the main indications are prevention of febrile, nonhemolytic transfusion reactions and prevention of leukocyte alloimmunization. Risks are the same as those for standard components, except for reduced risk of febrile reactions.

[‡]When virus-inactivated concentrates are not available.

AHF, Antihemophilic factor; *CMV*, cytomegalovirus; *FFP*, fresh-frozen plasma; *HLA*, human leukocyte antigen; *ITP*, idiopathic thrombocytopenic purpura; *TACO*, transfusion-associated circulatory overload; *TA-GVHD*, transfusion-associated graft-versus-host disease; *TRALI*, transfusion-related acute lung injury; *TTP*, thrombotic thrombocytopenic purpura; *vWF*, von Willebrand factor.

TABLE 13-10 TRANSFUSION REACTIONS

TYPE	SIGNS AND SYMPTOMS	USUAL CAUSE	TREATMENT	PRECAUTIONS
Acute intravascular hemolytic (immune)	Hemoglobinemia and hemoglobinuria, fever, chills, anxiety, shock, disseminated intravascular coagulation (DIC), dyspnea, chest pain, flank pain, nausea/vomiting, headache, pain at needle site and along venous tract	Incompatibility because of clerical errors; involves ABO (primarily) or other erythrocyte antigen-antibody incompatibility	Stop transfusion; hydrate; support blood pressure and respiration; induce diuresis; treat shock and DIC	Positively identify donor and recipient blood types and groups before transfusion is begun; verify with one other nurse or physician. Transfuse blood slowly for first 15-20 min and/or initial one-fifth volume of blood; remain with patient. In event of signs or symptoms, stop transfusion immediately, maintain patent IV line, and notify physician. Save donor blood to re–cross-match with patient's blood. Monitor blood pressure for shock. Insert urinary catheter and monitor hourly outputs. Send sample of patient's blood and urine to laboratory to determine presence of hemoglobin (indicates intravascular hemolysis). Observe for signs of hemorrhage resulting from DIC. Support medical therapies to reverse shock.
Delayed extravascular hemolytic (immune)	Fever, malaise, indirect hyperbilirubinemia, increased urine urobilinogen, falling hematocrit and hemoglobin	Occurs in previously RBC-alloimmunized patients in whom antigen on transfused red cells provokes anamnestic production of antibody; destruction of RBCs; usually involves non-ABO antigen-antibody incompatibility occurring 2-14 days post-transfusion	Monitor hematocrit, renal function, coagulation profile; no acute treatment generally required	Observe for post-transfusion anemia and decreasing benefit from successive transfusion.
Graft versus host disease (GVHD) or TA-GHVD		Viable T lymphocytes react against tissue antigens in recipient Immunocompromised recipients most at risk		Use γ-irradiated components to prevent TA-GVHD.
Febrile	Fever, chills, rarely hypotension	Antibodies to leukocytes or plasma proteins	Stop transfusion; give antipyretics, acetaminophen (or aspirin if patient not thrombocytopenic)	Use of leukocyte-poor RBCs is less likely to cause reaction.
Allergic	Urticaria (hives), flushing, wheezing, laryngeal edema, rarely hypotension or anaphylaxis	Antibodies to plasma proteins	Stop transfusion; give antihistamine; if severe, give epinephrine and/or steroids	Administer pretransfusion antihistamine; use washed RBC components.
Hypervolemic or TACO	Dyspnea, rales, hypertension, pulmonary edema, cardiac dysrhythmias, precordial pain, cyanosis, dry cough, distended neck veins	Transfusion-associated circulatory overload from too rapid or excessive blood transfusion	Induce diuresis; phlebotomy; support cardiorespiratory system as needed	Transfuse blood slowly. Prevent overload by using packed RBCs or administering divided amounts of blood. Use infusion pump to regulate and maintain flow rate. If signs of overload, stop transfusion immediately. Place patient in semi-Fowler position to increase venous resistance.

TRALI	Acute onset of hypoxemia within 6 hr of a blood or blood component transfusion; dyspnea, pulmonary edema, normal cardiac pressures	Anti-HLA or antileukocyte antibodies	Support blood pressure and aggressive respiratory support that may require intubation and mechanical ventilation	Use washed RBCs; avoid unnecessary transfusion.
Hypothermia	Chills, low temperature, irregular heart rate, possible cardiac arrest	Rapid infusion of cold blood products	Monitor temperature; if markedly subnormal, stop transfusion	Allow blood to warm at room temperature (<1 hr). Use an electric warming coil to rapidly warm blood.
Electrolyte disturbances, hyperkalemia	Nausea, diarrhea, muscular weakness, flaccid paralysis, paresthesia of extremities, bradycardia, apprehension, cardiac arrest	Massive transfusions or in patients with renal problems	Kayexalate enemas if potassium >5.0 mEq/L	Use washed RBCs or fresh blood if patient at risk.
Citrate intoxication (hypocalcemia)	Tingling in fingers, tetany, muscular cramps, carpopedal spasm, hyperactive reflexes, convulsions	Massive transfusion of blood	Stop transfusion; administer IV calcium if severe	Infuse blood slowly (citrate reaction less likely to occur). If signs of tetany occur, clamp tubing immediately, maintain patent intravenous line, and notify physician.
Air emboli	Sudden difficulty in breathing, sharp pain in chest, apprehension, respiratory or cardiac arrest	Air emboli from blood administered under pressure	Stop transfusion; turn patient on left side; aspirate right atrial/ ventricular air emboli	When infusing blood under pressure before container is empty: if air is observed in tubing, clamp tubing immediately below air bubble, clear tubing of air by aspirating air with syringe or disconnecting tubing and allowing blood to flow until air has escaped.
Bacterial sepsis	Shock, chills, high fever	Bacterial contamination of blood component or endotoxin reaction seen more commonly with platelet components stored at room temperature	Stop transfusion; support blood pressure; give antibiotics	Use care in blood collection and storage.
Delayed reactions, transmission of infection	Signs of infection after transfusion (e.g., jaundice from hepatitis; bacterial or toxin contamination— high fever, severe headache or substernal pain, hypotension, intense flushing, vomiting/diarrhea)	Hepatitis, AIDS, malaria, syphilis, bacteria, viruses, other	Stop transfusion; do culture and sensitivity tests; treat specific infection	Blood is tested for HBsAg (hepatitis B), syphilis, and, in most centers, HIV (AIDS); positive units are destroyed. Individuals at risk for carrying certain viruses are deferred from donation. Observe for signs of infection.

Adapted with permission from Wong L, editor: *Nursing care of infants and children,* ed 8, St Louis, 2007, Mosby, pp 1513-1514; and American Association of Blood Banks, American Red Cross, America's Blood Centers and the Armed Services Blood Program: *Circular of information for the use of human blood and blood components,* Washington, DC, December 2009, American Red Cross.

Diagnostic Algorithm for Polycythemia Based on Serum Epo Level

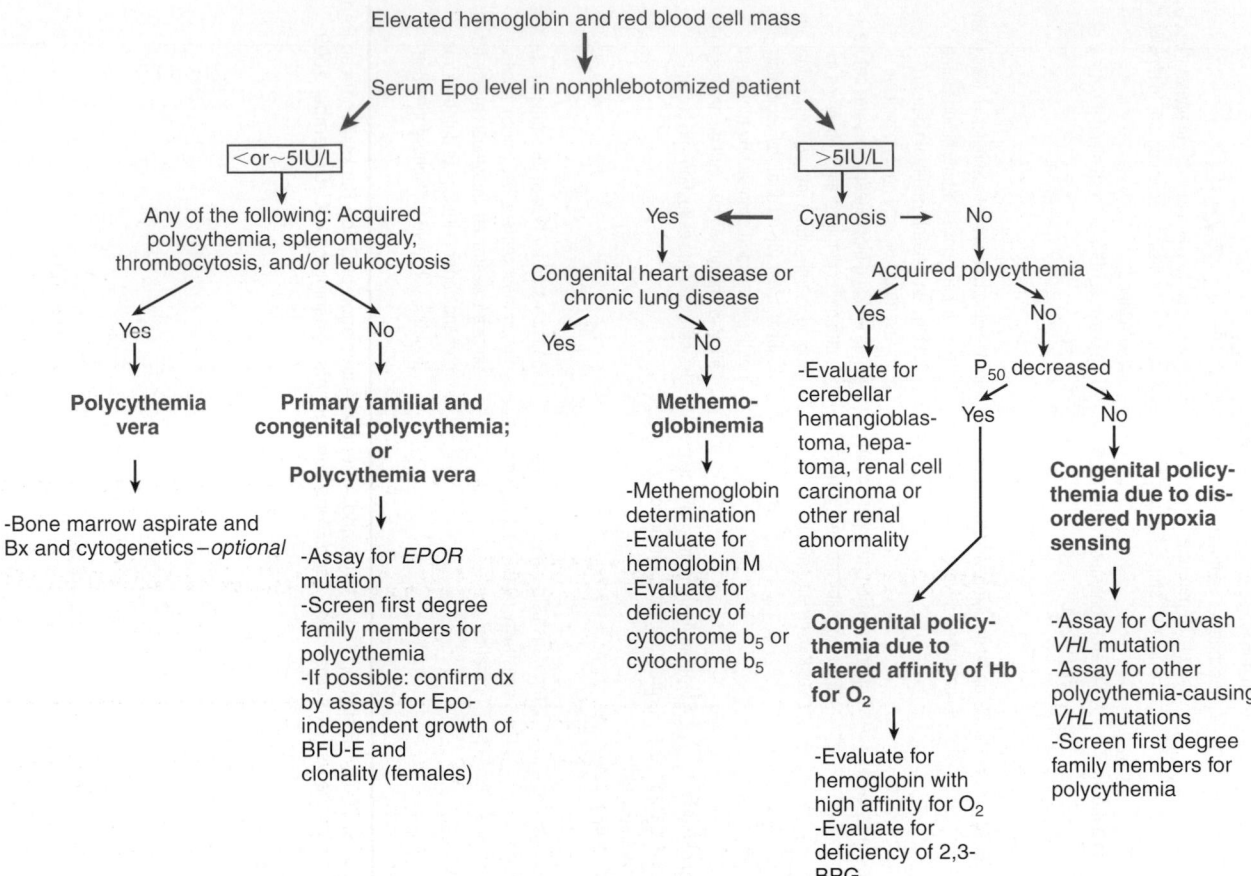

FIGURE 13-22 Algorithm showing differentiating features of different forms of polycythemia. *BFU-E,* Burst-forming unit-erythroid; *2,3-BPG,* 2,3-bisphosphoglycerate; *Epo,* erythropoietin; *EPOR,* erythropoietin receptor gene; *VHL,* von Hippel-Landau gene. (From Lichtman MA et al, editors: *Williams hematology,* ed 7, New York, 2006, McGraw-Hill, p 791.)

erythrocytotic phase, and the duration of the acute myeloid leukemia phase. Treatment in the erythrocytotic phase is essential, or the patient is at extremely high risk for thromboses. The development of thrombosis, hemorrhage, and myeloproliferative syndromes is common. Treated patients have a median survival of 10 to 15 years, with the most common causes of death being thrombosis, hemorrhage, leukemia, and other myeloproliferative conditions.[69-73]

Secondary Polycythemia

Etiology and pathogenesis. Secondary polycythemia is absolute erythrocytosis caused by increased stimulation of RBC production, usually in response to tissue hypoxia caused by, for example, high altitude or lung disease. There are other less common types of secondary polycythemia that are caused by renal or other organ tumors, which cause an increase in erythropoietin production.[69-70,74]

Because this type of polycythemia demonstrates an increase in red cell mass with no involvement of other marrow elements, it is most commonly seen in association with a known hypoxic stimulus, increased erythropoietin concentration, or excess levels of adrenocortical steroids or androgens.[69-70,74]

Laboratory features. The laboratory findings confirm increased red cell production with no increase in white cells or platelets. Erythropoietin levels are increased.[69-70,74]

Clinical manifestations. The symptoms are those of the underlying disease state, such as cardiovascular disease with right-to-left shunt, chronic lung disease or alveolar hypoventilation, low barometric pressure and/or high altitude, or abnormal hemoglobin concentration.[69-70,74]

Treatment. Because this condition is a physiologic compensation, the clinical treatment is directed at identifying and managing the underlying cause. Phlebotomy has been used to reduce cardiovascular work and appears to be helpful in both cardiovascular and chronic obstructive pulmonary disease. Oxygen administration is helpful in chronic lung diseases.[69-70,74]

Course and prognosis. The course and prognosis are influenced by the underlying disease process.

Relative Polycythemia

Etiology and pathogenesis. **Relative** (spurious) **polycythemia** is characterized by an increased hematocrit level in the presence of normal or decreased total RBC mass. Two types of patients manifest this characteristic. In the first group, the laboratory finding is secondary to an obvious disturbance in fluid balance such as is seen in severe dehydration or endocrinologic disorders. Patients in the other group, often described as having stress polycythemia, present with hypertension, increased hematocrit levels, and no increase in total RBC mass or obvious fluid loss. Research is continuing on the etiologic process and pathogenesis.[69,74,75]

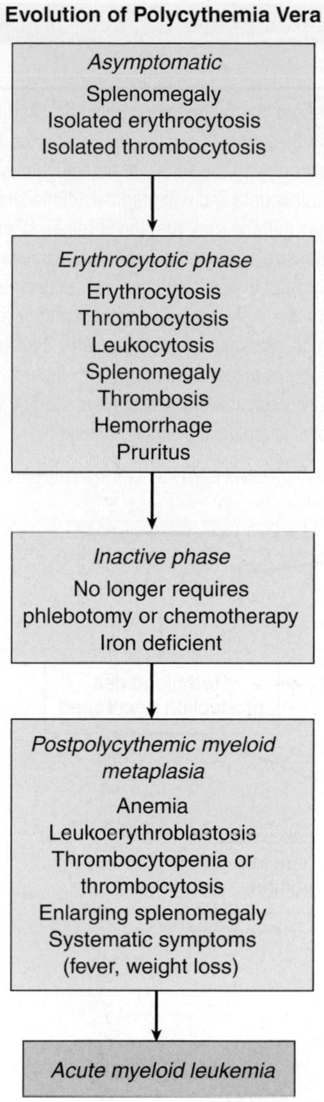

Evolution of Polycythemia Vera

Asymptomatic
Splenomegaly
Isolated erythrocytosis
Isolated thrombocytosis

↓

Erythrocytotic phase
Erythrocytosis
Thrombocytosis
Leukocytosis
Splenomegaly
Thrombosis
Hemorrhage
Pruritus

↓

Inactive phase
No longer requires
phlebotomy or chemotherapy
Iron deficient

↓

Postpolycythemic myeloid metaplasia
Anemia
Leukoerythroblastosis
Thrombocytopenia or
thrombocytosis
Enlarging splenomegaly
Systematic symptoms
(fever, weight loss)

↓

Acute myeloid leukemia

FIGURE 13-23 Clinical evolution of polycythemia vera. (From Hoffman R et al, editors: *Hematology: basic principles and practice,* ed 4, New York, 2005, Churchill Livingstone, p 1216.)

Laboratory features. All hematologic tests are normal except for elevated hematocrit and hemoglobin levels and RBC count. The size and color of the red cell are normal. Increased levels of cholesterol and uric acid are common.[70,74,75]

Clinical manifestations. The manifestations are contingent on the underlying cause. In dehydration, the patient will have flat neck veins, decreased skin turgor, thirst, tachycardia, and, in severe cases, low cardiac output and blood pressure. If the underlying condition is stress related, the symptoms are those of a catecholamine stress response. Patients are usually Caucasian middle-aged men. In patients with spurious polycythemia caused by smoking, the problem is usually chronic, and the symptoms attributable to the hyperviscosity described for polycythemia vera are often found.[70,74,75]

Treatment. Because this is a spurious form of polycythemia, it is important to recognize and manage the underlying cause. Fluid administration and management will resolve dehydration; however, spurious polycythemia is likely to be associated with a long-term condition that will require concurrent medical management. When the condition is a result of stress, identification of the stressors and stress management are indicated, with long-term follow-up. In spurious polycythemia attributable to smoking, the patient must stop smoking in order for the condition to resolve.[70,74,75]

Course and prognosis. The long-term prognosis is excellent if the underlying condition is identified and resolved, but patients with chronic anxiety or an inability to quit smoking may experience the same complications related to erythrocytosis as are seen in polycythemia vera.[70,74,75]

KEY POINTS

- Three types of polycythemia have been identified, according to cause. Polycythemia vera is associated with neoplastic transformation of bone marrow stem cells. Secondary polycythemia is due to chronic hypoxemia, with a resultant increase in erythropoietin production. Relative polycythemia is due to dehydration, which causes a spurious increase in RBC count.
- Differential diagnosis of the type of polycythemia is based on the history and accompanying manifestations:
  - *Polycythemia vera:* Absence of hypoxemia and dehydration, accompanied by leukocytosis and thrombocytosis.
  - *Secondary polycythemia:* History of lung disease or living at high altitude. Hypoxemia evident on blood gas evaluation. Erythropoietin level is elevated.
  - *Relative polycythemia:* History of fluid loss or poor intake. Accompanying manifestations of dehydration.
- Treatment of polycythemia is aimed at removing the cause, if possible. Phlebotomy and bone marrow–suppressing agents may be used for polycythemia vera. Major complications of polycythemia are increased blood viscosity and the risk of thrombi.

PEDIATRIC CONSIDERATIONS

Hemoglobin Synthesis in Infants

When an infant is born many mechanisms occur to decrease the infant's hemoglobin level. At birth, erythropoietin, a hormone that stimulates red blood cell production, disappears from blood plasma; there is an increase in arterial oxygen saturation and the infant is born with immature bone marrow. These mechanisms cause a slow rate of red blood cell production at birth. In addition, infants primarily have fetal hemoglobin, accounting for about 70% of their total hemoglobin. Although fetal hemoglobin is a more efficient oxygen carrier, it has a shorter life span than adult hemoglobin. This causes red blood cells to be turned over every 70 to 90 days, instead of 120 days for adult red blood cells. Also, fetal hemoglobin is thought to suppress production of erythropoietin.

Hemoglobin levels gradually decrease in the infant over the first 2 to 3 months because of the rapid destruction of fetal hemoglobin, decreased red blood cell production, and depressed erythropoietin production. Additionally, the infant experiences rapid growth during this time, which creates quick expansion of blood volume that further dilutes the supply of hemoglobin. Maternal iron stores are rapidly depleting at this time and will gradually diminish by 6 months.

As fetal hemoglobin is metabolized, the iron is released and stored. The body has enough iron to synthesize hemoglobin, but it is not stimulated to create hemoglobin at this time. Hemoglobin levels will continue to decrease until the oxygen needs of the tissues in the body are sufficiently depleted enough to stimulate erythropoietin production. Release of erythropoietin causes erythropoiesis to resume. Adult hemoglobin is made at this time with the iron stored in the body. Hemoglobin level will increase steadily in the infant starting around 6 months of age and fetal hemoglobin is replaced by adult hemoglobin.

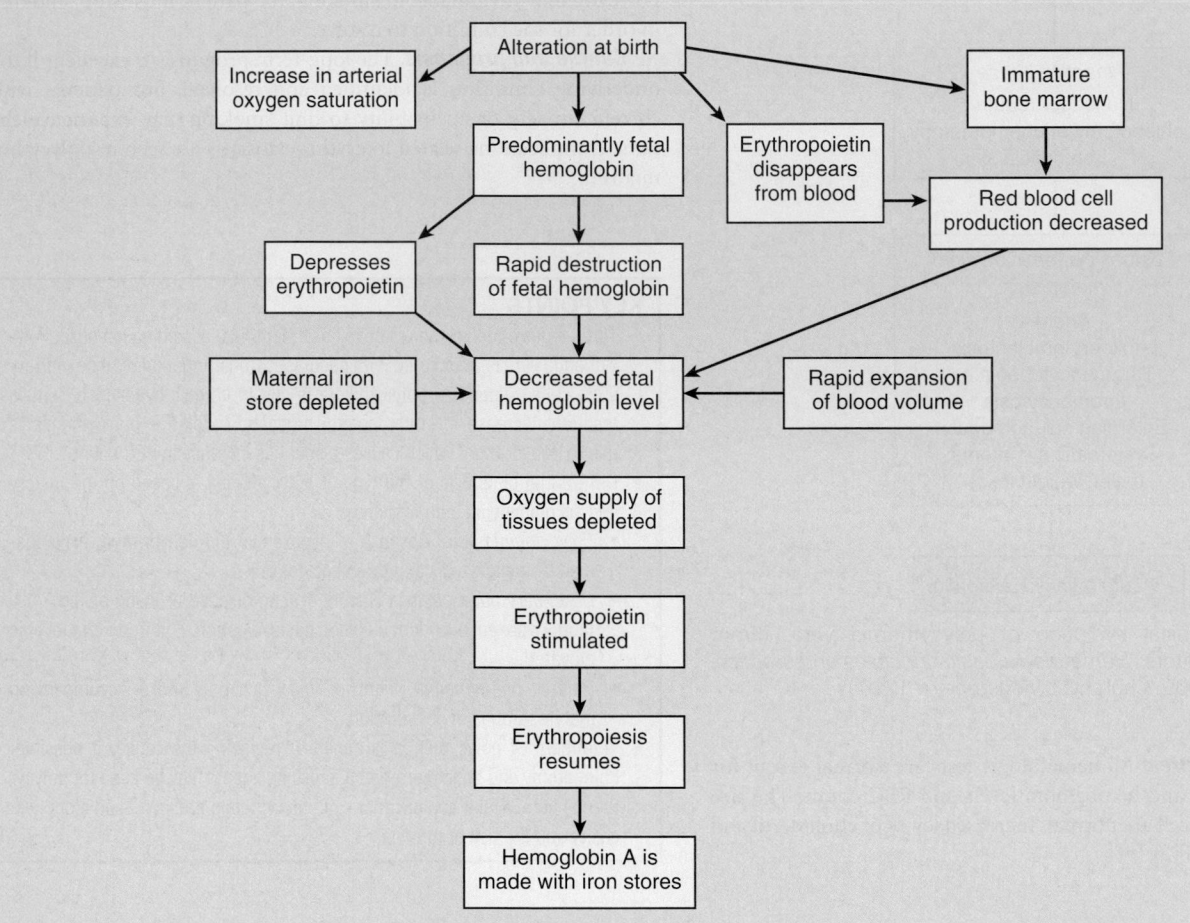

SUMMARY

The purpose of the erythron is to ensure adequate oxygen delivery with respect to oxygen demand. This is enhanced by the unique ability of hemoglobin in RBCs to carry and release oxygen at a suitable tension to support energy-generating systems in the body tissues. Anemia, a deficit in RBCs, poses a serious threat to oxygen transport and to the ability of the body to receive adequate oxygenation. Intense research in RBC physiology and pathophysiology continually yields new information for a better understanding of erythrocyte disorders, improved treatment modalities, and improved prognoses.

REFERENCES

1. Platt W: Introduction to hematology. In Platt W, editor: *Color atlas and textbook of hematology*, Philadelphia, 1979, Lippincott, pp 1–6.

2. Hillman RS, Finch CA: General characteristics of the erythron. In Hillman RS, Finch CA, editors: *Red cell manual*, ed 7, Philadelphia, 1996, FA Davis, p 8.

3. Prchal JT: Production of erythrocytes. In Lichtman MA, Kipps TJ, Seligsohn U, Kaushansky K, Prchal JT, editors: *Williams hematology*, ed 8, New York, 2010, McGraw-Hill. Accessed at www.accessmedicine.com/content.aspx?aID=6129311, August 2011.

4. Ryan DH: Examination of blood cells. In Lichtman MA, Kipps TJ, Seligsohn U, Kaushansky K, Prchal JT, editors: *Williams hematology*, ed 8, New York, 2010, McGraw-Hill. Accessed at www.accessmedicine.com/content.aspx?aID=6106433, August 2011.

5. Monroe DM, Hoffman M, Roberts HR: Molecular biology and biochemistry of the coagulation factors and pathways of hemostasis. In Lichtman MA, Kipps TJ, Seligsohn U, Kaushansky K, Prchal JT, editors. *Williams hematology*, ed 8, New York, 2010, McGraw-Hill. Accessed at www.accessmedicine.com/content.aspx?aID=6233396, August 2011.

6. Kaushansky K: Hematopoietic stem cells, progenitors, and cytokines. In Lichtman MA, Kipps TJ, Seligsohn U, Kaushansky K, Prchal JT, editors: *Williams hematology*, ed 8, New York, 2010, McGraw-Hill. Accessed at www.accessmedicine.com/content.aspx?aID=6105821, August 2011.

7. Diggs L, Sturm D, Bell A: *The morphology of human blood cells*, Abbott Park, IL, 1985, Abbott Laboratories, 1–86.

8. Nagel RL: Disorders of hemoglobin function and stability. In Handin RL, Lux SE, Stossel TP, editors: *Blood: principles and practice of hematology*, ed 2, Philadelphia, 2003, Lippincott, pp 1597–1654.

9. Telen MJ, Kaufman RE: The mature erythrocyte. In Greer JP, et al, editors: *Wintrobe's clinical hematology*, ed 12, Philadelphia, 2009, Lippincott Williams & Wilkins, pp 126–155.

10. McKenzie SB: Megaloblastic and nonmegaloblastic macrocytic anemias. In *Textbook of hematology*, ed 2, Baltimore, 1996, Williams & Wilkins, pp 177–199.

11. Carmel R, Rosenblatt DS: Disorders of cobalamin and folate metabolism. In Handin RL, Lux SE, Stossel TP, editors: *Blood: principles and practice of hematology*, ed 2, Philadelphia, 2003, Lippincott, pp 1361–1398.

12. Beutler E: Composition of the erythrocyte. In Lichtman MA, Kipps TJ, Seligsohn U, Kaushansky K, Prchal JT, editors: *Williams hematology*, ed 8, New York, 2010, McGraw-Hill. Accessed at www.accessmedicine.com/content.aspx?aID=6107043, August 2011.

13. Bull BS, Herrmann PC: Morphology of the erythron. In Lichtman MA, Kipps TJ, Seligsohn U, Kaushansky K, Prchal JT, editors: *Williams hematology*, ed 8, New York, 2010, McGraw-Hill. Accessed at www.accessmedicine.com/content.aspx?aID=6119772, August 2011.

14. Dessypris EN, Sawyer ST: Erythropoiesis. In Greer JP, et al, editors: *Wintrobe's clinical hematology*, ed 12, Philadelphia, 2009, Lippincott Williams & Wilkins, pp 106–125.

15. Papayannopoulou T, Migliaccio AR, Abkowitz JL, D'Andrea A, et al: Biology of erythropoiesis erythroid differentiation, and maturation. In Hoffman RL, et al, editors: *Hematology: basic principles and practice*, ed 5, New York, 2008, Churchill Livingstone. Accessed at www.mdconsult.com, August 2011.

16. Hall JE: Red blood cells, anemia, polycythemia. In Hall JE, editor: *Guyton and Hall textbook of medical physiology*, ed 12, Philadelphia, 2011, Saunders, pp 413–422.

17. Hall JE: Transport of oxygen and carbon dioxide in blood and tissue fluids. In Hall JE, editor: *Guyton and Hall textbook of medical physiology*, ed 12, Philadelphia, 2011, Saunders, pp 495–504.

18. Ellstrom K: The pulmonary system. In Alspach JG, editor: *Core curriculum for critical care nursing*, ed 6, St Louis, 2006, Saunders, pp 45–183.

19. American Edwards Laboratories: *Continuous SvO2 monitoring: theory and applications*, Irvine, CA, n.d., The Laboratories.

20. Ahrens TS, Powers KC: Pulmonary clinical physiology. In Kinney MR, Packa DR, Dunbar SB, editors: *AACN's clinical reference for critical care nursing*, ed 4, St Louis, 1998, Mosby, pp 491–516.

21. Prchal JT: Clinical manifestations and classification of erythrocyte disorders. In Lichtman MA, Kipps TJ, Seligsohn U, Kaushansky K, Prchal JT, editors: *Williams hematology*, ed 8, New York, 2010, McGraw-Hill. Accessed at www.accessmedicine.com/content.aspx?aID=6108487, August 2011.

22. Linker CA, Damon LE: Blood disorders. In McPhee SJ, Papadakis MA, editors: *Current medical diagnosis & treatment 2011*, New York, 2011, McGraw-Hill. Accessed at www.accessmedicine.com/content.aspx?aID=5476, August 2011.

23. Segel GB, Lichtman MA: Aplastic anemia: acquired and inherited. In Lichtman MA, Kipps TJ, Seligsohn U, Kaushansky K, Prchal JT, editors: *Williams hematology*, ed 8, New York, 2010, McGraw-Hill. Accessed at www.accessmedicine.com/content.aspx?aID=6107317, August 2011.

24. Guinan EC, Shimamura A: Acquired aplastic anemia. In Greer JP, et al, editors: *Wintrobe's clinical hematology*, ed 12, Philadelphia, 2009, Lippincott Williams & Wilkins, pp 1185–1195.

25. Young NS, Maciejewski JP: Aplastic anemia. In Hoffman RL, et al, editors: *Hematology: basic principles and practice*, ed 5, New York, 2008, Churchill Livingstone. Accessed at www.mdconsult.com, August 2011.

26. Bagby GC: Aplastic anemia and related bone marrow failure states. In Goldman L, Schaefer AI, editors: *Goldman's Cecil medicine*, ed 24, Philadelphia, 2011, Saunders. Accessed at www.mdconsult.com, August 2011.

27. Lowsky R, Negrin RS: Principles of hematopoietic cell transplantation. In Lichtman MA, Kipps TJ, Seligsohn U, Kaushansky K, Prchal JT, editors: *Williams hematology*, ed 8, New York, 2010, McGraw-Hill. Accessed at www.accessmedicine.com/content.aspx?aID=6128003, August 2011.

28. Caro J, Outschoorn UM: Anemia of chronic renal disease. In Lichtman MA, Kipps TJ, Seligsohn U, Kaushansky K, Prchal JT, editors: *Williams hematology*, ed 8, New York, 2010, McGraw-Hill. Accessed at www.accessmedicine.com/content.aspx?aID=6108595, August 2011.

29. Fauci AS, Braunwald E, Kasper DL, Hauser SL, Longo DL, et al: Chronic kidney disease. In Fauci AS, Braunwald E, Kasper DL, Hauser SL, Longo DL, et al, editors: *Harrison's principles of internal medicine*, ed 17, New York, 2008, McGraw-Hill. Accessed at www.accessmedicine.com/content.aspx?aID=2880823, August 2011.

30. Marks PW, Rosovsky R: Hematologic manifestations of systemic disease: liver and renal disease. In Hoffman R, et al, editors: *Hematology: basic principles and practice*, ed 5, New York, 2008, Churchill Livingstone. Accessed at www.mdconsult.com, August 2011.

31. Tolkoff-Rubin N: Treatment of irreversible renal failure. In Goldman L, Schaefer AI, editors: *Goldman's Cecil medicine*, ed 24, Philadelphia, 2011, Saunders. Accessed at www.mdconsult.com, August 2011.

32. Means RT: Anemias secondary to chronic disease and systemic disorders. In Greer JP, et al, editors: *Wintrobe's clinical hematology*, ed 12, Philadelphia, 2009, Lippincott Williams & Wilkins, pp 1221–1238.

33. Mitch WE: Chronic kidney disease. In Goldman L, Schaefer AI, editors: *Goldman's Cecil medicine*, ed 24, Philadelphia, 2011, Saunders. Accessed at www.mdconsult.com, August 2011.

34. Antony AC: Megaloblastic anemias. In Hoffman R, et al, editors: *Hematology: basic principles and practice*, ed 5, New York, 2008, Churchill Livingstone. Accessed at www.mdconsult.com, August 2011.

35. Green R: Folate, cobalamin, and megaloblastic anemias. In Lichtman MA, Kipps TJ, Seligsohn U, Kaushansky K, Prchal JT, editors: *Williams hematology*, ed 8, New York, 2010, McGraw-Hill. Accessed at www.accessmedicine.com/content.aspx?aID=6129579, August 2011.

36. Andrews NC: Iron deficiency and related disorders. In Greer JP, et al, editors: *Wintrobe's clinical hematology*, ed 12, Philadelphia, 2009, Lippincott Williams & Wilkins, pp 810–834.

37. Fauci AS, et al: Iron deficiency and other hypoproliferative anemias. In Fauci AS, et al: *Harrison's principles of internal medicine*, ed 17. http://www.accessmedicine.com/content.aspx?aID=2872958, August 2011.

38. Beutler E: Disorders of iron metabolism. In Lichtman MA, Kipps TJ, Seligsohn U, Kaushansky K, Prchals, JT: *Williams hematology*, 8e. http://www.accessmedicine.com/content.aspx?aID=6110247, August 2011.

39. Brittenham GM: Disorders of iron metabolism: iron deficiency and overload. In Hoffman R, et al, editors: *Hematology: basic principles and practice*, ed 5, New York, 2008, Churchill Livingstone. Accessed at www.mdconsult.com, August 2011.

40. Ginder GD: Microcytic and hypochromic anemias. In Goldman L, Schaefer AI, editors: *Goldman's Cecil medicine*, ed 24, Philadelphia, 2011, Saunders. Accessed at www.mdconsult.com, August 2011.

41. Weatherall DJ: The thalassemias: disorders of globin synthesis. In Lichtman MA, Kipps TJ, Seligsohn U, Kaushansky K, Prchal JT, editors: *Williams hematology*, ed 8, New York, 2010, McGraw-Hill. Accessed at www.accessmedicine.com/content.aspx?aID=6123722, August 2011.

42. Borgna-Pignatti C, Galanello R: The thalassemias and related disorders: quantitative disorders of hemoglobin synthesis. In Greer JP, et al, editors: *Wintrobe's clinical hematology*, ed 12, Philadelphia, 2009, Lippincott Williams & Wilkins, pp 1083–1131.

43. Cappellini MD: Thalassemias. In Goldman L, Schaefer AI, editors: *Goldman's Cecil medicine*, ed 24, Philadelphia, 2011, Saunders. Accessed at www.mdconsult.com, August 2011.

44. Fauci AS, Braunwald E, Kasper DL, Hauser SL, Longo DL, Jameson JL, Loscalzo J: Disorders of hemoglobin. In Fauci AS, Brunwald E, Kasper DL, Hauser SL, Longo DL, Jameson JL, Loscalzo J: *Harrison's principles of internal medicine*, ed 17, New York, 2008, McGraw-Hill.

45. Natarajan Kavita, Townes Tim M, Abdullah Kutlar: Disorders of hemoglobin structure: Sickle cell anemia and related abnormalities. In Lichtman MA, Kipps TJ, Seligsohn U, Kaushansky K, Prchals JT: *Williams hematology*, 8e. http://www.accessmedicine.com/content.aspx?aID=6130552, August 2011.

46. Steinberg MH: Hemoglobins with altered oxygen affinity, unstable hemoglobins, M-hemoglobins, and dyshemoglobinemias. In Greer JP, et al, editors: *Wintrobe's clinical hematology*, ed 12, Philadelphia, 2009, Lippincott Williams & Wilkins, pp 1132–1142.

47. Sauntharajah Y, Vichinsky EP: Sickle cell disease—clinical features and management. In Hoffman R, et al, editors: *Hematology: basic principles and practice*, ed 5, New York, 2008, Churchill Livingstone. Accessed at www.mdconsult.com, August 2011.

48. Steinberg MH: Sickle cell disease and other hemoglobinopathies. In Goldman L, Schaefer AI, editors: *Goldman's Cecil medicine*, ed 24, Philadelphia, 2011, Saunders. Accessed at www.mdconsult.com, August 2011.

49. Gallagher Patrick G: The red blood cell membrane and its disorders: Hereditary spherocytosis, elliptocytosis and related diseases. In Lichtman MA, Kipps TJ, Seligsohn U, Kaushansky K, Prchal JT: *Williams hematology*, 8e. http://www.accessmedicine.com/content.aspx?aID+6244171. Accessed August 2011.

50. Golan DE: Hemolytic anemias: red cell membrane and metabolic defects. In Goldman L, Schaefer AI, editors: *Goldman's Cecil medicine*, ed 24, Philadelphia, 2011, Saunders. Accessed at www.mdconsult.com, August 2011.

51. Gallagher PG, Glader BE: Hereditary spherocytosis, elliptocytosis, disorders associated with abnormalities of erythrocyte membrane. In Greer JP, et al, editors: *Wintrobe's clinical hematology*, ed 12, Philadelphia, 2009, Lippincott Williams & Wilkins, pp 911–932.

52. Gallagher PG, Jarolim P: Red blood cell membrane disorders. In Hoffman R, et al, editors: *Hematology: basic principles and practice*, ed 5, New York, 2008, Churchill Livingstone. Accessed at www.mdconsult.com, August 2011.

53. Fauci AS, Braunwald E, Kasper DL, Hauser SL, Longo DL, et al: Hemolytic anemias and anemia due to acute blood loss. In Fauci AS, Braunwald E, Kasper DL, Hauser SL, Longo DL, et al, editors: *Harrison's principles of internal medicine*, ed 17, New York, 2008, McGraw-Hill. Accessed at www.accessmedicine.com/content.aspx?aID=2889894, August 2011.

54. Vulliamy TJ, Luzzatto L: Glucose-6-phosphate dehydrogenase deficiency and related disorders. In Handin RL, Lux SE, Stossel TP, editors: *Blood: principles and practice of hematology*, ed 2, Philadelphia, 2003, Lippincott, pp 1921–1950.

55. van Solinge WW, van Wijk R: Disorders of red cells resulting from enzyme abnormalities. In Lichtman MA, Kipps TJ, Seligsohn U, Kaushansky K, Prchal JT, editors: *Williams hematology*, ed 8, New York, 2010, McGraw-Hill. Accessed at www.accessmedicine.com/content.aspx?aID=6120127, August 2011.

56. Gregg XT, Prchal JT: Red cell enzymopathies. In Hoffman R, et al, editors: *Hematology: basic principles and practice*, ed 5, New York, 2008, Churchill Livingstone. Accessed at www.mdconsult.com, August 2011.

57. Gallagher PG: Hemolytic anemias: red cell membrane and metabolic defects. In Goldman L, Schaefer AI, editors: *Goldman's Cecil medicine*, ed 24, Philadelphia, 2011, Saunders. Accessed at www.mdconsult.com, August 2011.

58. Glader BE: Hereditary hemolytic anemia due to red blood cell enzyme disorders. In Greer JP, et al, editors: *Wintrobe's clinical hematology*, ed 12, Philadelphia, 2009, Lippincott Williams & Wilkins, pp 933–955.

59. Friedberg RC, Johari VP: Autoimmune hemolytic anemias. In Greer JP, et al, editors: *Wintrobe's clinical hematology*, ed 12, Philadelphia, 2009, Lippincott Williams & Wilkins, pp 956–977.

60. Ramasethu J, Luban NL: Alloimmune hemolytic disease of the fetus and newborn. In Lichtman MA, Kipps TJ, Seligsohn U, Kaushansky K, Prchal JT, editors: *Williams hematology*, ed 8, New York, 2010, McGraw-Hill. Accessed at www.accessmedicine.com/content.aspx?aID=6131386, August 2011.

61. Packman CH: Hemolytic anemia resulting from immune injury. In Lichtman MA, Kipps TJ, Seligsohn U, Kaushansky K, Prchal JT, editors: *Williams hematology*, ed 8, New York, 2010, McGraw-Hill. Accessed at www.accessmedicine.com/content.aspx?aID=6116067, August 2011.

62. Hansen CN, Rosenberg AF: Drug-induced hematologic disorders. In DiPiro JT, Talbert RL, Yee GC, Matzke GR, Wells BG, et al, editors: *Pharmacotherapy: a pathophysiologic approach*, ed 8, New York, 2011, McGraw-Hill. Accessed at www.accesspharmacy.com/content.aspx?aID=8000685, August 2011.

63. Eder AF, Manno CS: Alloimmune hemolytic disease of the fetus and newborn. In Greer JP, et al, editors: *Wintrobe's clinical hematology*, ed 12, Philadelphia, 2009, Lippincott Williams & Wilkins, pp 978–997.

64. Powers A, Siberstein LE: Autoimmune hemolytic anemia. In Hoffman R, et al, editors: *Hematology: basic principles and practice*, ed 5, New York, 2008, Churchill Livingstone. Accessed at www.mdconsult.com, August 2011.

65. Seligsohn U, Kaushansky K: Classification, clinical manifestation and evaluation of disorders of hemostasis. In Lichtman MA, Kipps TJ, Seligsohn U, Kaushansky K, Prchal JT, editors: *Williams hematology*, ed 8, New York, 2010, McGraw-Hill. Accessed at www.accessmedicine.com/content.aspx?aID=6123085, August 2011.

66. Galel S, Nguyen DD, Magali JF, Goodnough LT, Viele MK: Transfusion medicine. In Greer JP, et al, editors: *Wintrobe's clinical hematology*, ed 12, Philadelphia, 2009, Lippincott Williams & Wilkins, pp 672–721.

67. Bull BS, Herrmann PC: Hemolytic anemia resulting from chemical and physical agents. In Lichtman MA, Kipps TJ, Seligsohn U, Kaushansky K, Prchal JT, editors: *Williams hematology*, ed 8, New York, 2010, McGraw-Hill. Accessed at www.accessmedicine.com/content.aspx?aID=6111475, August 2011.

68. American Association of Blood Banks, American Red Cross, America's Blood Centers and the Armed Services Blood Program: *Circular of information for the use of human blood and blood components*, Washington, DC, December 2009, American Red Cross.

69. Prchal JT: Primary and secondary polycythemias (erythrocytosis). In Lichtman MA, Kipps TJ, Seligsohn U, Kaushansky K, Prchal JT, editors: *Williams hematology*, ed 8, New York, 2010, McGraw-Hill. Accessed at www.accessmedicine.com/content.aspx?aID=6131859, August 2011.

70. Means RT: Erythrocytosis. In Greer JP, et al, editors: *Wintrobe's clinical hematology*, ed 12, Philadelphia, 2009, Lippincott Williams & Wilkins, pp 1261–1272.

71. Hoffman R, Xu M, Finazzi G, Barbui T: Polycythemias. In Hoffman R, et al, editors: *Hematology: basic principles and practice*, ed 5, New York, 2008, Churchill Livingstone. Accessed at www.mdconsult.com, August 2011.

72. Gilliland DG, Dunbar CL: Myelodysplastic syndromes. In Handin RL, Lux SE, Stossel TP, editors: *Blood: principles and practice of hematology*, ed 2, Philadelphia, 2003, Lippincott, pp 335–377.

73. Fauci AS, Braunwald E, Kasper DL, Hauser SL, Longo DL, et al: Polycythemia vera and other myeloproliferative diseases. In Fauci AS, Braunwald E, Kasper DL, Hauser SL, Longo DL, et al, editors: *Harrison's principles of internal medicine*, ed 17, New York, 2008, McGraw-Hill. Accessed at www.accessmedicine.com/content.aspx?aID=2865885, August 2011.

74. Means RT: Polycythemia vera. In Greer JP, et al, editors: *Wintrobe's clinical hematology*, ed 12, Philadelphia, 2009, Lippincott Williams & Wilkins, pp 2031–2044.

75. McCullough J: Blood procurement and screening. In Lichtman MA, Kipps TJ, Seligsohn U, Kaushansky K, Prchal JT, editors: *Williams hematology*, ed 8, New York, 2010, McGraw-Hill. Accessed at www.accessmedicine.com/content.aspx?aID=6132879, August 2011.

Alterations in Hemostasis and Blood Coagulation

Robin Beeman and Roberta J. Emerson

evolve WEBSITE

http://evolve.elsevier.com/Copstead/
- Review Questions and Answers
- Glossary (with audio pronunciations for selected terms)
- Animations
- Case Studies
- Key Points Review

KEY QUESTIONS

- How do platelets and factors of the clotting cascade contribute to hemostasis?
- What findings from the patient history, physical examination, or laboratory studies would indicate a potential bleeding disorder?
- How are laboratory tests used to differentiate the various coagulation disorders?
- What vascular alterations result in abnormalities of hemostasis?
- What are the common causes of platelet deficiencies, excesses, and dysfunction?
- What are the common causes of inherited and acquired disorders of coagulation?

CHAPTER OUTLINE

The term **hemostasis** means arrest of bleeding or prevention of blood loss after a blood vessel is injured. Hemostasis is accomplished via a complex interaction involving the vessel wall, circulating platelets, and plasma coagulation proteins. If hemostasis is inadequate, bleeding results; if hemostasis is excessive, inappropriate clotting or thrombosis results.

This chapter reviews the process of hemostasis and describes how that process is evaluated by means of clinical assessment and laboratory tests. The focus of this chapter is disorders of hemostasis and coagulation that result in bleeding. Disorders that result in thrombosis are discussed in Chapter 15.

THE PROCESS OF HEMOSTASIS

Stages of Hemostasis

Primary hemostasis, the initial response to vascular injury, involves the interaction between platelets and the endothelium of the injured blood vessel. The immediate response of the vessel to trauma is vasoconstriction to reduce blood loss. Although nervous reflex may play a part, this vasoconstriction results primarily from local myogenic spasm that may last from minutes to hours. The more trauma to the vessel, the greater the degree of vascular spasm.[1]

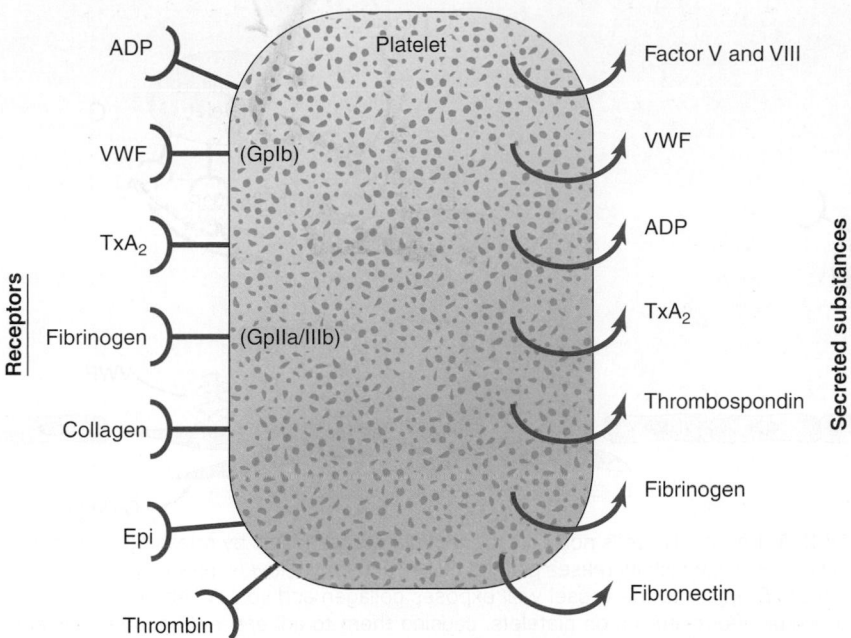

FIGURE 14-1 Platelets are complex cell fragments containing numerous chemical mediators that are released when platelets are activated. Platelets display a variety of cell surface receptors that mediate both adhesion to exposed subendothelium and aggregation with other platelets. *ADP*, Adenosine diphosphate; *Epi*, epinephrine; *TxA$_2$*, thromboxane A$_2$; *vWF*, von Willebrand factor.

The second component of primary hemostasis is formation of a platelet plug. Platelets not only adhere to endothelial collagen exposed by injury but also aggregate (clump together) at the site of vessel injury. The formation of this platelet plug is usually completed within 3 to 7 minutes.

Secondary hemostasis involves the formation of a fibrin clot, or **coagulation,** at the site of injury to maintain the hemostasis already initiated. Clotting factors are activated via the **intrinsic pathway** or **extrinsic pathway,** and participate in a series of events that catalyze or facilitate the conversion of fibrinogen to fibrin.[1] This process takes an average of 3 to 10 minutes.

Clot retraction, the final stage of clot formation, occurs when the components of the fibrin clot—the platelet plug, fibrin strands, and trapped red blood cells—are compressed or contracted to form a firm clot. This stage takes approximately 1 hour.

Platelets

Platelets have an integral role in hemostasis; thus, it is important to review their nature and function (Figure 14-1). A normal platelet count is between 150,000 and 400,000 platelets/mm^3 of blood. Platelets, also known as *thrombocytes,* are the smallest of the formed elements in the blood. They are produced in the bone marrow from megakaryocytes, which are derived from the pluripotent stem cell. Most of the platelets are found in the circulation and about 25% are sequestered in the liver and spleen.[3] Factors such as the stress response, epinephrine, and exercise may stimulate platelet production. The average life span of a platelet is 7 to 12 days. On completion of its life span, a platelet is eliminated from the circulation by the tissue macrophage system.[1-3]

Platelets play a complex role in the process of hemostasis. Initially, platelets adhere to subendothelial collagen exposed by trauma (Figure 14-2). After adhesion, the platelets become activated and initiate degranulation, the release of α granules and dense bodies. α granules release platelet thrombospondin, fibrinogen, fibronectin, von Willebrand factor (VWF), and coagulation factors V and VIII. The dense

granules release adenosine diphosphate (ADP), adenosine triphosphate (ATP), and serotonin. The presence of ADP and collagen encourages arachidonic acid formation, which leads to formation of thromboxane A$_2$ (TxA$_2$, a potent platelet aggregation agonist). Aspirin and other cyclooxygenase enzyme inhibitors can be used to block this cascade. Thromboxane A$_2$ stimulates the glycoprotein IIb/IIIa (GpIIb/IIIa) receptors on platelets to be expressed and further promotes platelet adhesion. The glycoprotein IIb/IIIa blockers (e.g., eptifibatide) are useful antiplatelet agents.[2-5]

In addition to the major role platelets play in primary hemostasis, they are also involved in secondary hemostasis and clot retraction. Platelets catalyze interactions between activated coagulation factors, accelerating the conversion of prothrombin to thrombin. Platelets also have a role in clot retraction.

Blood Coagulation Factors

With the exception of tissue factor (factor III; tissue thromboplastin) and calcium, blood coagulation factors are plasma proteins that circulate in the bloodstream in an inactive state. These factors are listed in Table 14-1 according to the internationally standardized nomenclature. The factors are numbered in the order of their discovery, not the order in which they participate in the clotting cascade. Factors with both active and inactive forms are differentiated with the letter "a" after the Roman numeral to designate the active form.

The liver is responsible for the synthesis of coagulation factors, with the exception of part of factor VIII. Factors II, VII, IX, and X; protein C; and protein S are dependent on vitamin K for synthesis and normal activity. Some of the coagulation proteins also can be synthesized by other cells, such as megakaryocytes and endothelial cells.[4,5] Antithrombin III (ATIII) and protein C are protein complexes that promote anticoagulation. Antithrombin is a potent anticoagulant that binds to and inactivates free thrombin, preventing its binding and cleaving of fibrinogen. Protein C, a plasma protein that inactivates factors V and VIII, prevents clot formation. Protein S assists protein C in binding to phospholipase and stimulates release of tissue plasminogen activator,

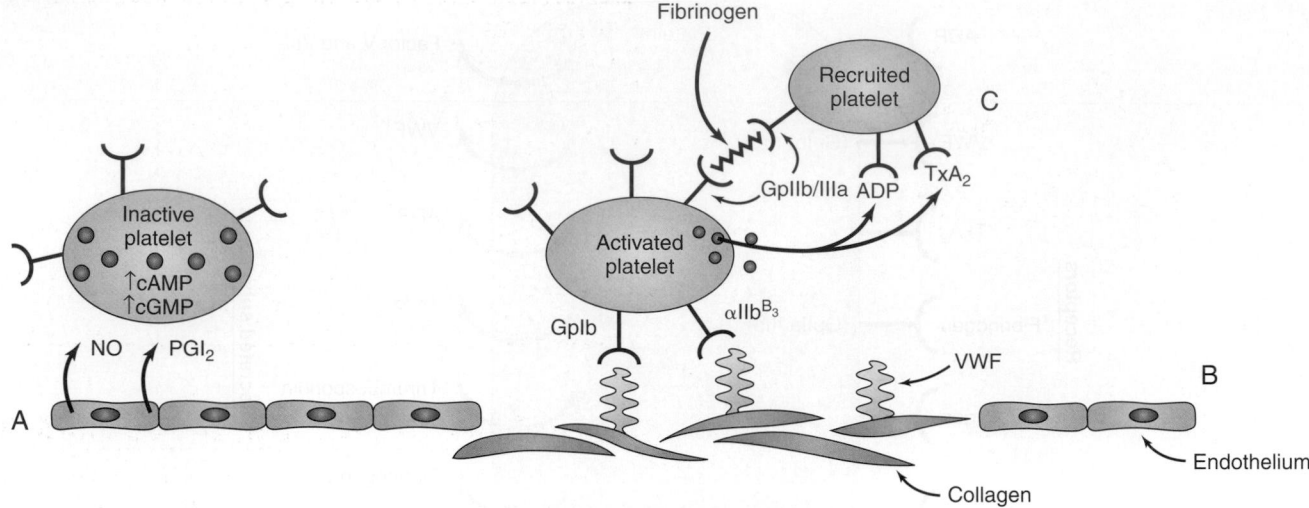

FIGURE 14-2 A, Endothelial cells normally prevent platelet adhesion by releasing nitric oxide (NO) and prostaglandin I₂ (PGI₂), which increases platelet cGMP and cAMP levels, reducing the likelihood of their being activated. **B,** Injury to the vessel wall exposes collagen and von Willebrand factor (vWF), which are bound by specific receptors on platelets, causing them to adhere and become activated. **C,** Activated platelets release numerous chemical mediators that bind to and stimulate other nearby platelets. Groups of platelets aggregate together by binding to fibrinogen molecules through their GpIIb/IIIa receptors. *ADP,* Adenosine diphosphate; *TxA₂,* thromboxane A₂.

TABLE 14-1	THE CLOTTING FACTORS
FACTOR	**ACTION**
I: Fibrinogen	Factor I is converted to fibrin by the enzyme thrombin. Individual fibrin molecules form fibrin threads, which are the scaffold for clot formation and wound healing.
II: Prothrombin	Factor II is the inactive precursor of thrombin. Prothrombin is activated to thrombin by coagulation factor X (Stuart-Prower factor). After it is activated, thrombin converts fibrinogen (coagulation factor I) into fibrin and activates factors V and VIII. Synthesis is vitamin K–dependent.
III: Tissue thromboplastin	Factor III interacts with factor VII to initiate the extrinsic clotting cascade.
IV: Calcium	Calcium (Ca^{2+}), a divalent cation, is a cofactor for most of the enzyme-activated processes required in blood coagulation. Calcium also enhances platelet aggregation and makes red blood cells clump together.
V: Proaccelerin	Factor V is a cofactor for activated factor X, which is essential for converting prothrombin to thrombin.
VI: Discovered to be an artifact	No factor VI is involved in blood coagulation.
VII: Proconvertin	Factor VII activates factors IX and X, which are essential in converting prothrombin to thrombin. Synthesis is vitamin K–dependent.
VIII: Antihemophilic factor	Factor VIII together with activated factor IX enzymatically activates factor X. In addition, factor VIII combines with another protein (von Willebrand factor) to help platelets adhere to capillary walls in areas of tissue injury.
IX: Plasma thromboplastin component (Christmas factor)	Factor IX, when activated, activates factor X to convert prothrombin to thrombin. This factor is essential in the common pathway between the intrinsic and extrinsic clotting cascades. A lack of factor IX is the basis for hemophilia B. Synthesis is vitamin K–dependent.
X: Stuart-Prower factor	Factor X, when activated, converts prothrombin into thrombin. Synthesis is vitamin K–dependent.
XI: Plasma thromboplastin antecedent	Factor XI, when activated, assists in the activation of factor IX. However, a similar factor must exist in tissues. People who are deficient in factor XI have mild bleeding problems after surgery but do not bleed excessively as a result of trauma.
XII: Hageman factor	Factor XII is critically important in the intrinsic pathway for the activation of factor XI.
XIII: Fibrin-stabilizing factor	Factor XIII assists in forming cross-links among the fibrin threads to form a strong fibrin clot.

From Ignatavicius DD, Workman ML: *Medical surgical nursing: patient-centered collaborative care,* ed 7, Philadelphia, 2013, Saunders, p 860.

initiating fibrinolysis.[4,5] Low-molecular-weight heparins and heparin work by enhancing the activity of antithrombin III (Figure 14-3).

Fibrin Clot

In normal hemostasis, the fibrin clot is produced through activation of the intrinsic or extrinsic pathway and, in turn, the common final pathway. Effective hemostasis is the result of interactions between all of these pathways and is commonly referred to as the *coagulation cascade.*

Figure 14-4 illustrates the coagulation cascade. The intrinsic pathway of coagulation begins when blood comes into contact with altered vascular endothelium or another negatively charged surface, such as

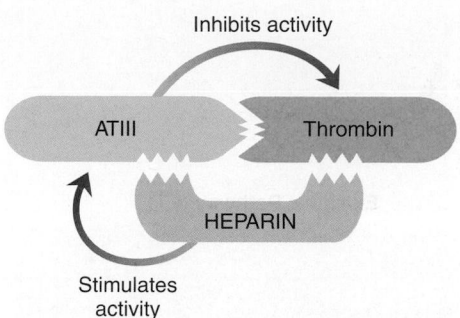

FIGURE 14-3 Antithrombin III (ATIII) can bind and neutralize the activity of thrombin. Heparin is a catalyst that increases the activity of ATIII, making it more effective. Thrombin is a potent inducer of clot formation; thus, ATIII and heparin have significant anticoagulant properties.

glass. This contact phase of coagulation involves four factors: (1) factor XII, (2) high-molecular-weight kininogen (HMWK), (3) prekallikrein, and (4) factor XI. Factor XII is activated to factor XIIa, which in turn activates XI to XIa and prekallikrein to its active form, kallikrein (KAL). Kallikrein liberates bradykinin from HMWK. The release of bradykinin produces an initial vasodilation followed by release of angiotensin II and vasoconstriction. The major role of factor XIa is activation of factor IX to factor IXa in the presence of calcium. Factor IXa then activates factor X to factor Xa in the presence of factor VIII, calcium, and phospholipid. This activation usually takes place on the membrane of stimulated platelets. The common final pathway is initiated by factor Xa.

The extrinsic pathway of coagulation begins when the vascular wall is traumatized, as in a crush injury. Tissue factor (factor III) from injured tissue activates factor VII. Factor VIIa activates factor X to Xa, which in turn initiates the common final pathway. Factor VIIa also activates factor IX in the intrinsic system.

The common final pathway of coagulation is initiated by factor X, which is activated by both the intrinsic and extrinsic pathways. Factor Xa, in the presence of factor V, calcium, and phospholipid, converts prothrombin (factor II) to thrombin. This conversion is facilitated by the presence of activated platelets. Thrombin then cleaves fibrinogen to form an insoluble fibrin clot. Thrombin also activates factor XIII, which promotes fibrin stabilization. The clot is further stabilized by clot retraction. Thrombin also helps to perpetuate the clotting cascade by continuing to activate factors V and VIII.

Fibrinolysis

At the same time the fibrin clot is forming, the process of **fibrinolysis** or clot dissolution is initiated (Figure 14-5). Factor XII, HMWK, kallikrein, and thrombin are involved in the release of plasminogen activators. The plasminogen activators cleave plasminogen, a plasma protein that has been incorporated into the fibrin clot, to its active form, plasmin. Plasmin digests fibrinogen and fibrin and inactivates blood coagulation factors V and VIII. Fibrin split products, or fibrin degradation products, result from the dissolution of the fibrin clot.

The control of fibrinolysis is complex. The Kupffer cells of the liver and macrophages located in the spleen and bone marrow clear the circulation of activated clotting factors and fibrin degradation products. Antiplasmins that inhibit plasmin exist to prevent inappropriate fibrinolysis. All these factors and mechanisms are present to create a balance between clot production and clot dissolution.

KEY POINTS
- Hemostasis involves several critical steps. These include vasospasm, formation of a platelet plug, and activation of the clotting cascade to form a fibrin clot.
- Factors released from platelets contribute to hemostasis by enhancing vasoconstriction, platelet aggregation, and vessel repair.
- Fibrin clot formation can be initiated by the intrinsic or extrinsic pathway. Each pathway requires the sequential activation of specific clotting factors, ultimately resulting in enzymatic cleavage of fibrinogen to form an insoluble fibrin clot.
- Initiation of fibrinolysis occurs simultaneously with clot formation to prevent excessive clotting and vessel occlusion.

EVALUATION OF HEMOSTASIS AND COAGULATION

Data obtained from clinical assessment and laboratory tests facilitate the identification and evaluation of a hemostatic abnormality. Evaluation of a patient for a bleeding tendency is indicated in the following circumstances: when there is a personal or family history of bleeding; during active bleeding that is unresponsive to standard interventions; as part of screening before surgery; and for ongoing evaluation of anticoagulation therapy. A bleeding tendency may be inherited or acquired, and may result from defects in blood vessels, platelets, or coagulation factors. The purpose of the evaluation process is to determine if a problem exists and to ascertain the underlying cause so that appropriate management can be initiated.

Clinical Assessment

Both the family history and the personal history are important in the evaluation of a bleeding problem (Table 14-2). A family history of bleeding in males is often linked to one of the types of hemophilia, which accounts for the majority of serious inherited coagulation problems.[4,5] The location, severity, duration, and setting in which bleeding occurs are also important clues to the type of defect that is present. Bleeding associated with vascular or platelet defects usually occurs immediately after trauma (e.g., dental extraction), involves skin or mucous membranes, and is brief. Delayed bleeding or bleeding into muscles or joints is more typical of a coagulation defect.[5-8]

Systemic diseases, such as renal failure, liver disease, systemic lupus erythematosus, and malignancies, may be associated with a bleeding problem. Medication history, including use of over-the-counter medications, is another important aspect in the evaluation of a hemostatic defect. A common cause of acquired bleeding problems is drug ingestion. Specific drugs that alter hemostasis include aspirin and aspirin-containing preparations, nonsteroidal antiinflammatory agents, some antibiotics, anticoagulants, alcohol, and chemotherapeutic and thrombolytic agents.

Many of the physical findings of bleeding are manifested in the skin and mucous membranes. The individual may appear pale or jaundiced. Pallor is associated with a marked decrease in hemoglobin level; jaundice is associated with liver or gallbladder disease, possible coagulation disorders, and excessive red blood cell destruction.

Petechiae are flat, pinpoint, nonblanching red or purple spots caused by capillary hemorrhages in the skin and mucous membranes (Figure 14-6). Petechiae are commonly seen with vascular and platelet disorders. They are usually present on dependent areas of the body, such as the legs, or on areas constricted by tight clothing. Not all petechiae indicate a bleeding problem. Petechiae found on other body areas not constricted by tight clothing, such as the abdomen or thorax, may be associated with infectious disease or other pathophysiologic sources. Petechiae may be seen in the newborn as a result of the trauma of delivery, not as a result of a bleeding problem.

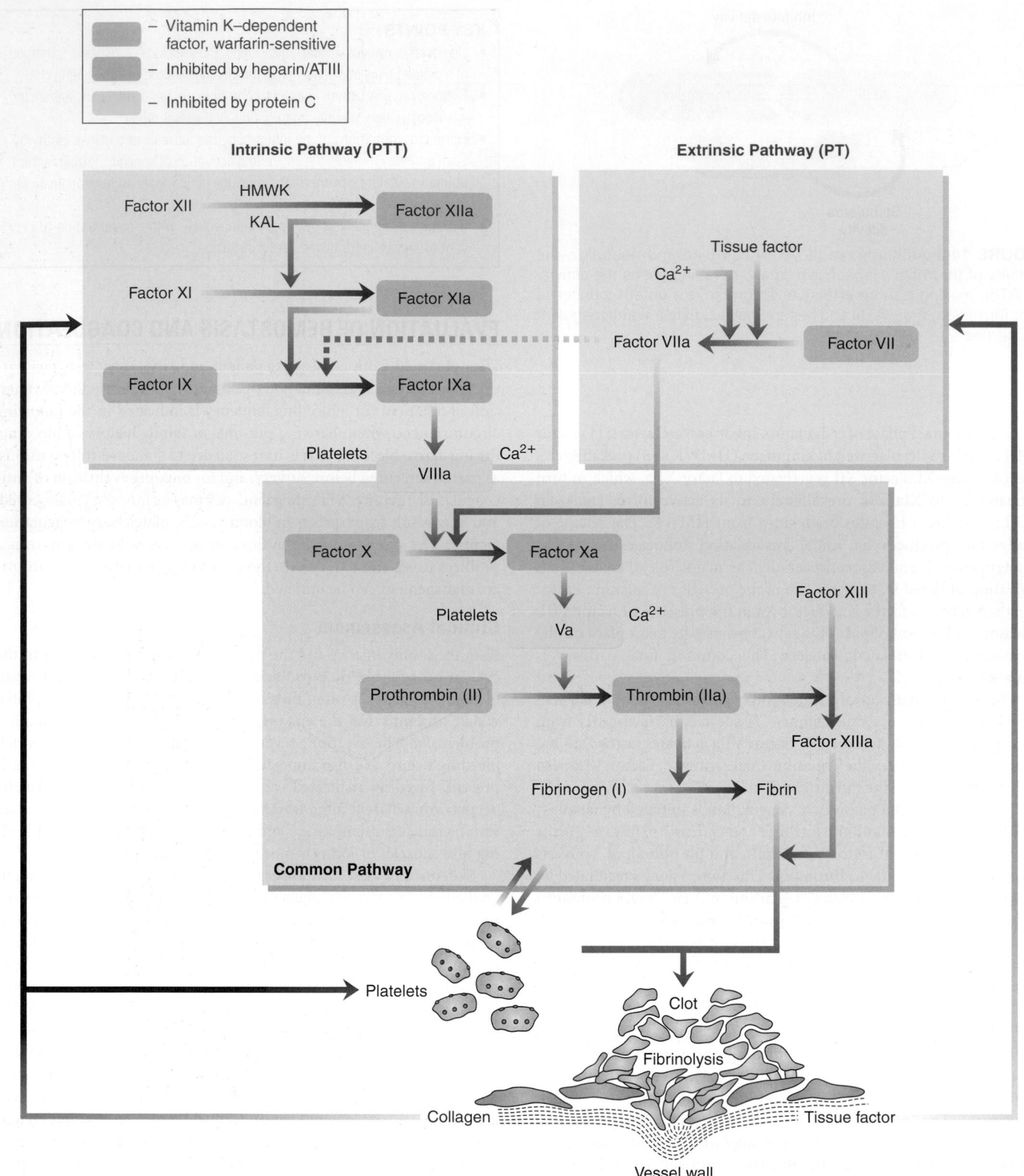

FIGURE 14-4 Coagulation cascade. *PT,* Prothrombin time; *PTT,* partial thromboplastin time.

When petechiae occur in groups or patches, the term **purpura** is used (Figure 14-7). Purpuric lesions are often pruritic (itchy). Fever and malaise may be present, as may effusions into joints or viscera, manifested by joint or abdominal pain.

Ecchymosis occurs when blood escapes into the tissues, producing a bruise (Figure 14-8). If the area is raised, it is called a **hematoma.**

Hemarthrosis, manifested by swelling and pain, is bleeding into a joint. Large ecchymoses, hematomas, and hemarthroses are seen in coagulation disorders.

Telangiectasia is a lesion created by dilation of capillaries and small arteries, typically on the lips, tongue, tips of the fingers and toes, and sometimes in visceral vessels (Figure 14-9). These thin, dilated, tortuous

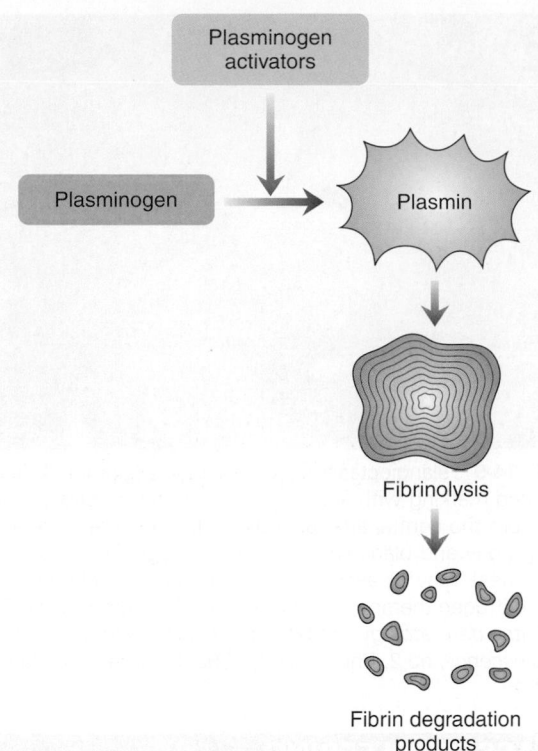

FIGURE 14-5 Fibrinolysis. Plasmin, activated from plasminogen, enzymatically cleaves fibrin proteins in the clot. This results in fibrin split products, which can be measured.

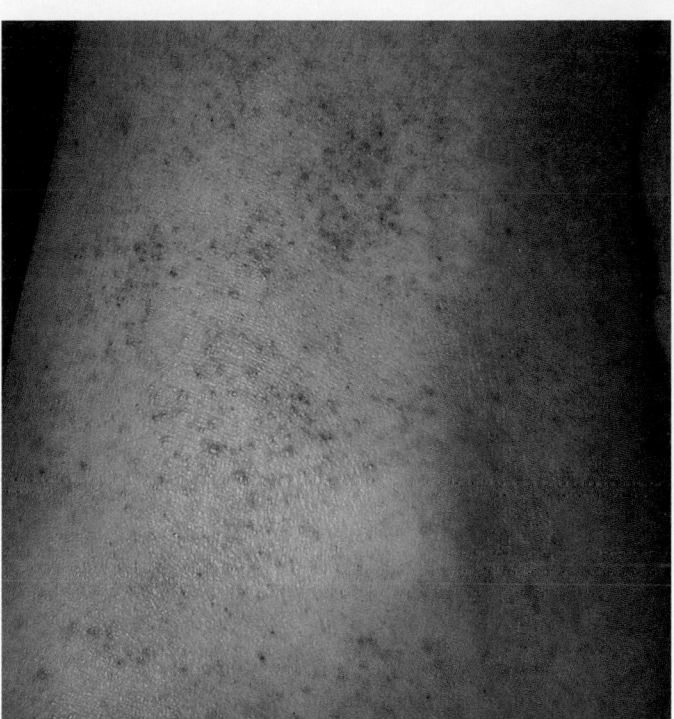

FIGURE 14-6 Petechiae. (From Dockery GL: *Cutaneous disorders of the lower extremity*, Philadelphia, 1997, Saunders.)

TABLE 14-2	CLUES FROM PATIENT HISTORY REGARDING BLEEDING DISORDERS
CLUE FROM PATIENT HISTORY	**POSSIBLE CAUSE**
Family history of bleeding in both males and females	von Willebrand disease
Family history of bleeding in males	Hemophilia A or B
Newly acquired bruising	Drugs (especially aspirin and NSAIDs, anticoagulant therapy), thrombocytopenia
Excessive bleeding/bruising during/after surgery	Mild-severe deficiency of coagulation factors, von Willebrand disease; thrombocytopenia, drug ingestion
Bleeding following initial hemostasis	Factor XIII deficiency

NSAIDs, Nonsteroidal antiinflammatory drugs.

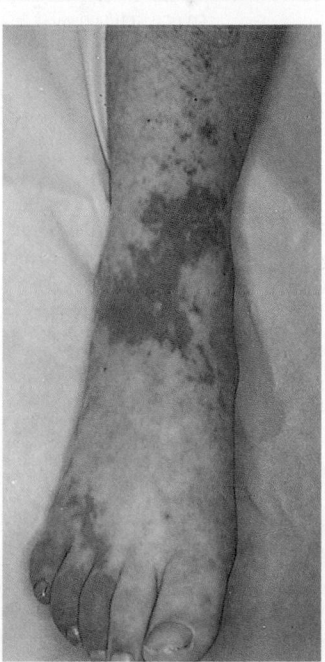

FIGURE 14-7 Purpura. (From Hurwitz S: *Clinical pediatric dermatology: a textbook of skin disorders of childhood and adolescence,* ed 2, Philadelphia, 1993, Saunders, p 269.)

vessels are red to violet in color, blanch with pressure, and tend to bleed with minimal trauma. Spider telangiectasia branch into the subcutaneous and dermal layers of the skin and are often associated with liver disease.

Other significant findings indicative of a bleeding disorder include blood (bright red, rusty, or black) in drainage or excreta, such as feces (**hematochezia** or **melena**), urine (**hematuria**), vomitus (**hematemesis**), nasal drainage (**epistaxis**), gastric drainage, or sputum (**hemoptysis**). Excessive menstrual bleeding may occur (**menorrhagia**). Acute abdominal or flank pain may indicate internal bleeding. Hypovolemia from bleeding may produce a shock state and present as hypotension, tachycardia, pallor, altered mentation, and decreased urine output. The two sites at which bleeding is most life threatening are the oropharynx

(resulting in airway compromise) and within the brain tissue. One of the leading causes of death in patients experiencing severe disorders of coagulation is intracerebral hemorrhage.[5]

Laboratory Tests

Many laboratory tests are available to aid in the diagnosis of hemostasis problems (Table 14-3). Basic screening includes a complete blood

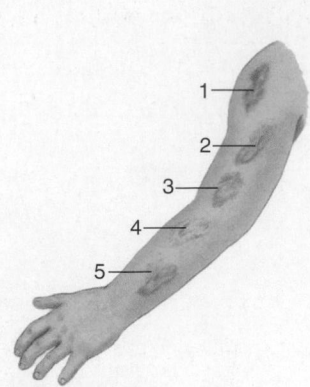

FIGURE 14-8 Ecchymosis. A large patch of capillary bleeding into tissues. Color in a light-skinned person is first red-blue or purple *(1)* immediately after or within 24 hours of trauma and generally progresses to blue to purple *(2)*, blue-green *(3)*, yellow *(4)*, and brown to disappearing *(5)*. (From Jarvis C: *Physical examination and health assessment,* ed 6, Philadelphia, 2012, Saunders.)

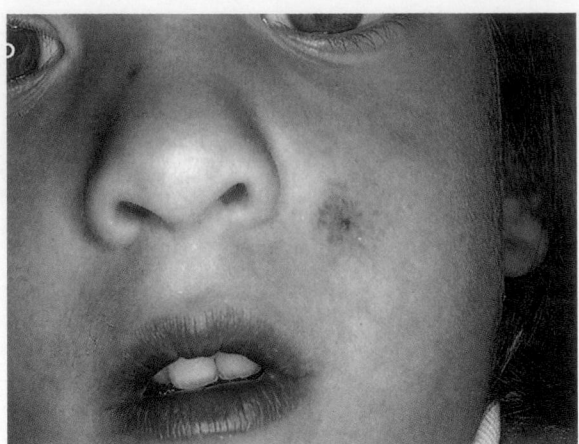

FIGURE 14-9 Telangiectasia (spider or star angioma). A fiery red, star-shaped marking with a solid circular center. Capillary radiations extend from the central arterial body. With pressure, note a central pulsating body and blanching of extended legs. Develops on face, neck, or chest; may be associated with pregnancy, chronic liver disease, or estrogen therapy, or may be normal. (From Hurwitz S: *Clinical pediatric dermatology: a textbook of skin disorders in childhood and adolescence,* ed 2, Philadelphia, 1993, Saunders, p 266.)

TABLE 14-3 SELECT LABORATORY TESTS USED TO ASSESS BLEEDING

TEST	NORMAL VALUE*	PURPOSE OR SIGNIFICANCE
Platelet count	150,000-400,000/mm³	Determines number of platelets; decreased in ITP, anemias, DIC, infection, chemotherapy; increased in leukemia, cancer, splenectomy
Bleeding time	3-10 min	Assesses platelet and vascular response; increased in thrombocytopenia, vascular defects, severe liver disease, DIC, von Willebrand disease, aspirin ingestion
Prothrombin time	10-14 sec; 100%	Evaluates extrinsic pathway of coagulation; increased in vitamin K deficiency, hemorrhagic disease of the newborn, liver disease, DIC, anticoagulant therapy. Evaluates all coagulation factors except VIII and XII.
International normalized ratio	1.5 (low-level anticoagulation for atrial fibrillation) 2.0-3.0 (medium-level anticoagulation for DVT, pulmonary embolism, MI, stroke prophylaxis) 2.5-3.5 (high-level anticoagulation for mechanical heart valve)	Evaluates extrinsic pathway of coagulation (as prothrombin time); provides uniformity worldwide, independent of reagents
Activated partial thromboplastin time	33-45 sec	Evaluates intrinsic pathway of coagulation; increased in hemophilia, vitamin K deficiency, liver disease, DIC, circulating anticoagulants, heparin therapy
Thrombin time	15 sec, or control + 5 sec	Measures conversion of fibrinogen to fibrin; increased in DIC, liver disease, low fibrinogen <100 mg/dl, multiple myeloma
Fibrinogen	200-400 mg/dl	Measures fibrinogen level; decreased in liver disease, DIC
Fibrin split products or fibrin degradation products†	<3 µg/ml	Measures by-products from breakdown of fibrin clot; increased in DIC, hypoxia, leukemia, thromboembolic disorders
Clot retraction†	1hr: evidence of shrinking and increased firmness 24hr: 50% of volume is clot, 50% is serum	Approximate measure of platelet function; decreased in thrombocytopenia, von Willebrand disease
Platelet aggregation†	Visible aggregates form in <5 min	Measures rate and percentage of aggregation; decreased in mononucleosis, ITP, von Willebrand disease, leukemia, aspirin ingestion, thrombasthenia, Bernard-Soulier syndrome
Tourniquet test (Rumpel-Leede test, capillary fragility test)†	No petechiae or occasional petechiae	Evaluates vascular fragility and platelet function; positive test in thrombocytopenia, vascular purpuras, thrombasthenia
Euglobulin lysis time†	No lysis of fibrin clot at 37° C for 3 hr; clot is observed for 24 hr	Assesses fibrinolysis; increased lysis in DIC, incompatible blood transfusion, cirrhosis, cancer, obstetric complications
Plasma D-dimer assay	<200 ng/ml	Assesses fibrinolysis; increased in DVT, pulmonary embolism (highly nonspecific), DIC (high negative predictive value)

*Value may vary, depending on source.
†Tests not included in a routine coagulation screen.
DIC, Disseminated intravascular coagulation; *DVT,* deep vein thrombosis; *ITP,* immune thrombocytopenic purpura; *MI,* myocardial infarction.

TABLE 14-4 ALTERATIONS IN LABORATORY VALUES SEEN WITH MAJOR DISORDERS OF HEMOSTASIS

	LABORATORY ALTERATIONS							
DISORDER	PLATELET COUNT	BLEEDING TIME	PT/INR	aPTT	TT	FSP	FVIII	FIX
Idiopathic thrombocytopenic purpura	↓	Prolonged	N	N	N	N	N	N
Hemophilia A	N	N/Prolonged	N	↑	↑	↓	↓	N
Hemophilia B	N	N/Prolonged	N	↑	↑	N	N	↓
von Willebrand disease	N	Prolonged	N	↑	↑	N	↓	N
Vitamin K deficiency	N	Prolonged	↑	N/↑	↑	N	N	N/↓
Disseminated intravascular coagulation	↓	Prolonged	↑	↑	↑	↑	↓	↓
ASA/NSAIDs	N	Prolonged	N	N	N	N	N	N
Heparin	N/↓	Prolonged	N	↑	↑	N	N	N
Coumadin	N	Prolonged	↑	N/↑	↓	N	N	N
Vascular purpura	N	N/Prolonged	N	N	N	N	N	N
Liver disease	N/↓	Prolonged	↑	N/↑	N	N	N	N/↓

aPTT, Activated partial thromboplastin time; *ASA*, acetylsalicylic acid; *FIX*, factor IX; *FSP*, fibrin split products; *FVIII*, factor VIII; *INR*, International normal ratio; *N*, normal; *NSAIDs*, nonsteroidal antiinflammatory drugs; *PT*, prothrombin time; *TT*, thrombin time.

cell count (CBC), including a platelet count and peripheral blood smear, bleeding time, prothrombin time (PT) or international normalized ratio (INR), activated partial thromboplastin time (aPTT), and thrombin time. These screening tests evaluate both primary and secondary hemostasis. The CBC determines if anemia is present, the platelet count determines the number of platelets, and the peripheral smear indicates the number and gross morphologic characteristics of platelets. The bleeding time evaluates vascular status and platelet function. The PT and INR assess the extrinsic pathway of coagulation, and the aPTT assesses the intrinsic pathway. Reporting prothrombin activity as a percentage of PT in seconds can pose difficulty in the adjustment of anticoagulation therapy because the PT varies with each laboratory and the reagent used at that lab. Laboratories have tried to compensate for this variation by using the ratio of the patient's value to the laboratory's control value, which again varied with the reagent. The INR is a standardized PT value used worldwide that controls for this reagent variability. Thrombin time measures the time needed to convert fibrinogen to fibrin; this reflects the quantity and quality of fibrinogen as well as the influence of any inhibitors. The D-dimer assay reflects fibrinolysis.

Further laboratory investigation is necessary if abnormalities are identified on the screening tests or if, despite normal screening test results, a bleeding problem obviously exists. Specific tests are available to assess abnormal platelet function, the presence of circulating anticoagulants or fibrin split products, and the levels of individual coagulation factors. Table 14-4 reflects the alterations in laboratory values seen with the major disorders of hemostasis.

KEY POINTS
- Bleeding tendencies may be inherited or acquired. Abnormal bleeding, liver disease, and anticoagulant drug use may be important risk factors. Physical findings of petechiae, purpura, ecchymoses, telangiectasia, and occult or frank bleeding are indicative.
- Usual laboratory tests include platelet count, bleeding time, PT/INR (extrinsic pathway), and activated partial thromboplastin time (intrinsic pathway).

VASCULAR AND PLATELET DISORDERS

Vascular Disorders

Vascular disorders of hemostasis and coagulation are those in which the primary cause of bleeding is a problem with the vascular component of primary hemostasis. The vascular defect may be acquired (e.g., related to ingestion of a specific drug) or inherited.

Vascular Purpura

Etiology. Vascular purpura is a disorder in which purpura—patches of petechiae, or pinpoint hemorrhages, on the skin—are present. The primary cause of the purpura, or more extensive bleeding in some cases, is an abnormality of the vessels or the tissues that support them (see Figure 14-7).

Allergic purpura (anaphylactoid purpura, Henoch-Schönlein purpura) is most often seen in children between the ages of 4 and 7.[9-11] Drug-induced purpura may result from many drugs, including atropine, chloral hydrate, and other sedatives; sulfa drugs; procaine penicillin; and warfarin (Coumadin). Purpuric lesions and perhaps severe hemorrhage are components of Ehlers-Danlos syndrome and osteogenesis imperfecta, both of which are inherited disorders of connective tissue.[12,13] Acquired disorders of connective tissue such as scurvy (vitamin C deficiency), senile purpura (seen in the elderly), and corticosteroid purpura (associated with chronic steroid drug therapy) may also result in purpuric lesions.

Pathogenesis. The allergic purpuras are thought to result from an autoimmune process that produces inflammation or vasculitis of small vessels. As a result, perivascular infiltration and serosanguineous effusion occur into surrounding tissues to produce the characteristic purpuric lesion. The pathophysiologic process of drug-induced purpura is not well understood. An autoimmune process has been proposed.

Structural abnormalities of vessels and perivascular supportive tissue provide the mechanism for bleeding in many of the vascular purpuras. These abnormalities may be inherited or acquired. In Ehlers-Danlos syndrome and osteogenesis imperfecta, the vascular abnormality is thought to result from decreased amounts or poor quality of collagen and elastin; both are necessary for perivascular support.

Vitamin C deficiency, which causes scurvy, results in defective collagen synthesis. The lack of proper collagen support for the vessels leads to bleeding. In the elderly (senile purpura), loss of subcutaneous fat and changes in connective tissue allow for more mobility of the skin. Shearing force then causes rupture of small vessels. Steroids induce catabolism of proteins in supportive tissues, decreasing the mechanical strength of the microvasculature.

Clinical manifestations. The purpuric lesions characteristically appear and fade or disappear in groups. The lesions are not elevated and do not blanch with pressure.

With allergic purpura, the lesions tend to be palpable and are found on the proximal extremities, especially on the legs and buttocks; they may be accompanied by fever, pruritus, arthralgia, and paresthesia. Bleeding from the lesions themselves and generalized bleeding are uncommon. Usually, allergic purpura is self-limited, and the prognosis is good.

Generalized purpura is characteristic of drug-induced vascular purpura. The lesions quickly subside when the drug is discontinued. Other bleeding manifestations are uncommon.

The purpuric lesions associated with inherited connective tissue disorders, such as Ehlers-Danlos syndrome, often are accompanied by large ecchymoses and hematomas. Although not common, bleeding into the brain tissue may result in cerebrovascular accident (stroke).[12,13]

The purpuric lesions seen with scurvy typically occur around hair follicles and on the medial surfaces of the thighs and buttocks. Ecchymoses and large hematomas may also occur.

Senile purpura and corticosteroid purpura generally occur on the dorsum of the hands and forearms and are aggravated by trauma. Other bleeding is uncommon.

Diagnosis and treatment. The diagnosis of vascular purpura is one of exclusion after platelet disorders and coagulation disorders have been ruled out. An abnormal tourniquet test (positive Rumpel-Leede test) in the setting of a normal or increased bleeding time, normal platelet count, and normal coagulation study results suggest a problem with the vascular component of hemostasis. The tourniquet test is an assessment for abnormal capillary fragility. To perform the test, a blood pressure cuff is applied and inflated to a point between the systolic and diastolic blood pressures for 5 minutes. The test is positive if there are more than 20 petechiae per square inch.

Treatment for vascular purpura includes removal or avoidance of the causative agent if one is identified (e.g., penicillin) and interventions to relieve symptoms such as pruritus. If more extensive bleeding accompanies the purpura, identification of the cause and interventions to control the bleeding are necessary.

Hereditary Hemorrhagic Telangiectasia

Etiology. A telangiectasia is a dilated or tortuous small blood vessel, found in the skin or mucous membranes, that has a tendency to bleed spontaneously or following minor trauma (see Figure 14-9). Hereditary hemorrhagic telangiectasia (Osler-Weber-Rendu disease) is transmitted as an autosomal dominant trait; the vascular abnormalities can be seen in children but become more prominent after puberty, peaking between the fourth and fifth decades. As the telangiectases—the skin spots resulting from the vascular lesion—become more prominent, the frequency and severity of the bleeding increase.[14]

Pathogenesis. The telangiectases result from an abnormality in vascular development. The vessel wall is composed of a single layer of endothelium; thus, support and contractile properties are deficient, leading to spontaneous bleeding or bleeding as a result of minor trauma.[14] Any mucosal surface (e.g., respiratory, gastrointestinal, and genitourinary tracts) may be involved. Arteriovenous malformations in the lung, liver, and brain are the most serious complications.[14,15]

Clinical manifestations. Bright red or purple lesions, ranging from pinpoint to 3 mm in diameter, can be found on the nasal mucous membranes, lips, palate, tongue, face, trunk, palms of the hands, and the soles of the feet. A hallmark symptom is recurrent nosebleeds (epistaxis), with increasing frequency as the patient ages. The severity of the disorder is linked to age of onset.[14,15] Typically the lesions are flat and blanch with pressure. The most common clinical problem is mucous membrane bleeding, especially epistaxis. However, bleeding may occur from telangiectases in any area. Frequent bleeding episodes may result in anemia.[14,15]

Diagnosis and treatment. The diagnosis is confirmed by the presence of multiple telangiectases, repeated episodes of bleeding, or a family history of bleeding in both genders. If telangiectases are not easily visible, the diagnosis is more difficult to make.

Treatment is primarily supportive and includes humidification of the nasal cavity, use of topical hemostatic agents or cauterization if the bleeding site is accessible, tamponade of the nasal cavity, use of iron replacement therapy, laser treatment for cutaneous lesions, embolization, and administration of estrogen or estrogen with progesterone for epistaxis. Tranexamic acid is used for controlling severe hemorrhage.[14,15] Blood transfusions or surgical intervention for uncontrolled bleeding may be considered in selected cases.[14,15]

Platelet Disorders

Platelet disorders of hemostasis and coagulation are those in which the primary cause of bleeding is an abnormality in the quantity or the quality of platelets.

Thrombocytopenia

Etiology. **Thrombocytopenia** is a common cause of generalized bleeding. Some of the many causes of thrombocytopenia are listed in Box 14-1.

Immune thrombocytopenia (ITP), previously called idiopathic thrombocytopenic purpura, is an acquired immune-mediated disorder. Formerly classified as either "acute" or "chronic," ITP is now

---

BOX 14-1 SOME CAUSES OF THROMBOCYTOPENIA

Decreased Platelet Production
Folate/B_{12} deficiency
Radiation therapy
Chemotherapy
Drugs (e.g., alcohol, thiazides, phenytoin)
Aplastic anemia
Cancer in bone marrow

Decreased Platelet Survival
Drugs (e.g., thiazides, digoxin, heparin, furosemide, certain antibiotics)
Mechanical prosthetic heart valves
Viral and bacterial infections
Circulating immune complexes
Increased destruction in the spleen
Disseminated intravascular coagulation

Splenic Sequestration (Pooling)
Splenomegaly
Hypothermia

Platelet Dilution
Massive transfusions with blood stored for more than 24 hours

classified according to the duration of the disease: "newly diagnosed," "persistent" (lasting 3 to 12 months), or "chronic" (lasting 12 months or longer). ITP occurs at any age and in both genders until mid-life, when it is more common in women 30 to 60 years of age.[16-18] ITP in children may follow a viral illness or have no evidence of previous illness, and typically spontaneously resolves in 6 months.[17,18] ITP in adults has a more insidious onset and tends to be more chronic.[16,18] A pregnant woman with ITP can deliver a thrombocytopenic infant because the antiplatelet antibody crosses the placenta. Adult ITP may precede or occur in association with diseases of altered immunity, such as systemic lupus erythematosus (see Chapter 10), lymphoproliferative disease (see Chapter 11), or acquired immunodeficiency syndrome (AIDS) (see Chapter 12).

Pathogenesis. Four general mechanisms are responsible for thrombocytopenia: decreased platelet production, decreased platelet survival, splenic sequestration (pooling), and intravascular dilution of circulating platelets (see Box 14-1). Regardless of the mechanism responsible, there are fewer platelets available, and inadequate hemostasis is the potential result.

Platelets are produced by bone marrow megakaryocytes. Production declines when the number of megakaryocytes is reduced or when the process of platelet production (thrombocytopoiesis) is ineffective. Although numerous causes of decreased platelet production are listed in Box 14-1, drugs are often responsible. Bone marrow suppression from chemotherapy, recent immunizations, and alcohol ingestion are common causes of platelet level reduction.[16,18]

The average life span of a platelet is 7 to 9 days. Decreased platelet survival may be the result of an antibody-mediated immune mechanism that destroys platelets (e.g., ITP, a possible adverse effect of heparin) or the result of increased consumption of platelets, as seen in DIC. Direct trauma to platelets from vascular or valvular prostheses also may be responsible for decreased platelet survival.

Normally, about 25% of the total number of platelets can be found in the spleen and the remaining 75% are circulating. When the spleen is enlarged (splenomegaly), as much as 90% of the platelets may be pooled or sequestered in the spleen; thus, the circulating number of platelets is markedly decreased.[3,5] If the spleen cannot be palpated on physical examination, platelet sequestration can be ruled out as the primary mechanism of the thrombocytopenia.

The final mechanism responsible for thrombocytopenia is dilution of circulating platelets by administration of massive transfusions. Platelets degenerate in stored blood after 24 hours; thus, when a large amount of blood deficient in platelets is transfused, thrombocytopenia results.

Clinical manifestations. Clinical manifestations of thrombocytopenia are generally absent[3,5] until the platelet count drops below 100,000/mm³. Petechiae and purpura are prominent with platelet counts below 50,000/mm³. Spontaneous mucosal, deep tissue, and intracranial bleeding[3,5] may be seen with platelet counts less than 20,000/mm³, though recent evidence suggests serious bleeding[17,18] is more likely to occur at platelet counts less than 10,000/mm³.

New research is exploring fatigue as a common symptom among patients with ITP.[19]

Diagnosis. Thrombocytopenia is diagnosed by the presence of a low platelet count on peripheral blood laboratory examination. The bleeding time is prolonged and clot retraction is poor or absent. PT/INR, partial thromboplastin time, and other coagulation studies are normal. The CBC will indicate if the thrombocytopenia is isolated or if an associated problem, such as anemia or leukopenia, is present. Gross morphologic analysis of platelets, evaluated from the peripheral blood smear, and bone marrow examination provide additional information regarding the mechanism for the thrombocytopenia. Because many

drugs are associated with thrombocytopenia, careful review of all medications the patient is taking is also necessary in the search for the cause of the thrombocytopenia.

Treatment. The treatment for thrombocytopenia is based on the identified cause or mechanism and may include any of the following: discontinuation of any suspected drug; avoidance of aspirin and pharmacodynamically similar drugs that alter normal platelet function; and administration of corticosteroids, immunosuppressants, intravenous immunoglobulin (IVIg), rituximab, and thrombin receptor agonists such as romiplostim and eltrombopag to increase platelet production.[18] Splenectomy may be helpful in some cases because it results in removal of a major site of platelet destruction and eliminates a source for production of antiplatelet antibodies.

Thrombocytosis

Etiology. Thrombocytosis is generally defined as a platelet count greater than 400,000/mm³. Transitory thrombocytosis is seen following stress or physical exercise. Secondary or reactive thrombocytosis occurs as a response to hemorrhage, inflammatory diseases, malignancy, infection, hemolysis, or splenectomy. Primary thrombocytosis is seen with polycythemia vera and chronic granulocytic leukemia.[3,5]

Pathogenesis. In all types of thrombocytosis, the number of platelets is increased, but the mechanism of the increase varies. Transitory thrombocytosis results from release of preformed platelets, not increased production. As the name implies, the elevation in platelet count is transient. Secondary thrombocytosis results from an actual increase in platelet production via an unknown mechanism. With primary thrombocytosis, there is abnormal proliferation of megakaryocytes in the bone marrow, resulting in as much as a 15-fold increase in platelet production.

Clinical manifestations. In general, transitory thrombocytosis and secondary thrombocytosis do not result in hemorrhage or thrombotic complications. Hemorrhage into the skin and mucous membranes and gastrointestinal bleeding may be seen with primary thrombocytosis. The pathogenesis of excessive bleeding in the presence of excessive levels of platelets is not well understood. Thrombosis resulting in peripheral vascular ischemia or pulmonary embolism may further complicate the clinical picture. Thromboembolic events are the most common cause of death. However, the course of thrombocytosis is benign in most patients.

Diagnosis and treatment. The diagnosis is made on the basis of a high platelet count. Bleeding time may be normal or prolonged, and platelet aggregation is normal or impaired. The history and clinical presentation, as well as additional laboratory tests such as bone marrow examination, aid in determining the type of thrombocytosis.

No treatment is necessary with transitory and secondary thrombocytosis. To manage primary thrombocytosis, the use of cytotoxic agents or interferon may be used.[4] Antiplatelet therapy (e.g., aspirin or dipyridamole) also may be used. In the presence of acute bleeding or thrombosis, plasma exchange may be used to temporarily control the platelet count.

Qualitative Platelet Disorders

Etiology. Although the number of platelets may be normal, the ability of the platelets to function in the hemostatic process may be abnormal; thus, a qualitative platelet disorder is present. Inherited defects in platelet function, such as Bernard-Soulier syndrome (giant platelet syndrome), von Willebrand disease, and thrombasthenia (Glanzmann disease), are rare. In contrast, acquired disorders of platelet function are common; they are often associated with drugs, especially aspirin; with renal failure; or with a coexisting hematologic disease, such as leukemia.

Pathogenesis. Whether the qualitative platelet disorder is inherited or acquired, at least one aspect of platelet function (adhesion, aggregation, or release reaction) is abnormal and a bleeding tendency results. In both Bernard-Soulier syndrome and von Willebrand disease, platelet adhesion is abnormal. Platelet aggregation is the problem in thrombasthenia, owing to the absence of the fibrinogen receptor necessary for normal platelet aggregation. Aspirin and other nonsteroidal antiinflammatory agents inhibit production of thromboxane A_2 and thus impair both platelet aggregation and the platelet release reaction.

Clinical manifestations. The clinical presentation of a qualitative platelet disorder is some form of bleeding tendency, such as petechiae or purpura on skin and mucous membranes, epistaxis, gastrointestinal bleeding, or menorrhagia. Acquired platelet function defects also may result in excessive bleeding during and following surgical procedures.

Diagnosis and treatment. With qualitative platelet defects, the bleeding time is prolonged but the platelet count and other routine coagulation screening test results are normal. Although a bleeding time greater than 10 minutes is associated with a slight increase in bleeding tendency, the risk is not significantly increased until the bleeding time exceeds 15 or 20 minutes.[5,7]

Special laboratory tests that more specifically evaluate platelet function, such as platelet aggregation studies, are necessary to determine the exact cause of bleeding.[7] Coexisting hematologic defects may make diagnosis of a platelet defect difficult.

If the platelet disorder is drug induced, the offending drug is discontinued. Transfusion with normal platelets is the usual intervention if treatment is necessary because of bleeding. Administration of desmopressin or cryoprecipitate is the treatment of choice when von Willebrand disease is the underlying cause of bleeding, as well as for patients with aspirin overdose and cirrhosis.[5,7] von Willebrand disease is described in greater detail in the following section.

KEY POINTS

- Disorders of the vasculature that result in altered hemostasis include inflammation (allergic purpura), structural abnormalities (collagen diseases), and weakened vessel walls (telangiectasia).
- An insufficient quantity of platelets (fewer than 50,000/mm^3) results from decreased production, sequestration, increased destruction, or dilution. Important causes of thrombocytopenia include autoimmune destruction (ITP), DIC, and mechanical destruction (artificial valves).
- Excessive quantity of platelets (more than 400,000/mm^3) results from excessive production (proliferation of bone marrow cells). Thrombocythemia may result in excessive coagulation with thrombosis or excessive bleeding.
- A normal platelet count does not ensure adequate platelet function. Platelet adhesion, aggregation, and degranulation may be abnormal, resulting in a prolonged bleeding time. The usual cause is drug related (e.g., aspirin); rarely, the platelet defect is inherited (e.g., von Willebrand disease).

COAGULATION DISORDERS

Coagulation disorders or **coagulopathies** are defects of the normal clotting mechanism. They may cause bleeding as a result of problems with the formation, stabilization, or lysis of the fibrin clot. Alternatively, the coagulation disorder may be attributable to inappropriate activation of the coagulation cascade, producing excessive clot formation.

Hemophilia

Etiology. Hemophilia is rare in the general population, but it is the most common severe inherited coagulation disorder. Excessive bleeding following circumcision or the formation of a hematoma after vitamin K injection leads to the diagnosis in the neonate. Some children will not develop bleeding problems until they begin crawling or walking.

Hemophilia A, the classic form of the disease, accounts for approximately 85% of cases of clinical hemophilia. Hemophilia A is caused by factor VIII deficiency.[1,20-22] The majority of patients inherit this X-linked recessive disorder; hemophilia is transmitted by an asymptomatic carrier female to an affected son. Approximately 20% of patients with hemophilia A have a negative family history because of a spontaneous mutation of the hemophilic gene.

Less common than hemophilia A is hemophilia B, also known as Christmas disease. Factor IX is deficient in this form of hemophilia.[20,21]

Hemophilia is often classified according to the extent to which the specific coagulation factor (factor VIII or IX) is deficient. Patients with severe hemophilia have less than 1% normal coagulation factor activity; patients with moderate hemophilia, 1% to 5% normal coagulation factor activity; and patients with mild hemophilia, 5% to 40% normal coagulation factor activity.[20,22]

Of critical concern in the hemophilic patient is intracranial hemorrhage and other serious bleeding episodes. Because of advances in treatment, however, a normal life span is possible for many.

Pathogenesis. Hemophilia A results from factor deficiency or the abnormal function of factor VIII. Hemophilia B results from factor deficiency or the abnormal function of factor IX. A deficiency or malfunction in either factor interferes with the normal sequence of events in the intrinsic pathway of coagulation and, in turn, the eventual production of a fibrin clot. Inability to form a fibrin clot results in bleeding.

Clinical manifestations. Once clinical evidence of bleeding is present, hemophilia A and hemophilia B are indistinguishable. Patients with mild hemophilia may not experience symptoms until stressed by surgery or trauma. Prolonged bleeding from relatively minor trauma and occasional spontaneous bleeding episodes are characteristic of moderate hemophilia. With severe hemophilia, frequent episodes of spontaneous bleeding are likely.

Any of the following clinical manifestations may occur: easy bruising, prolonged bleeding from the nasal or oral mucosa, deep tissue hematomas, hemarthrosis, bleeding into muscles in the extremities, spontaneous hematuria, gastrointestinal bleeding, and intracranial bleeding. The hallmark of hemophilia is hemarthrosis. Knees, ankles, and elbows are the most often affected. Repeated episodes of hemarthrosis may result in joint deformity.[4,20-22]

Major long-term complications of hemophilia include progressive joint deformity as a result of repeated hemarthroses, hepatitis B or C, cirrhosis, and HIV infection related to repeated transfusions or administration of virus-contaminated factor concentrates.

Diagnosis and treatment. Hemophilia is considered as the cause of bleeding when the family history is positive for bleeding in males, there is a history of joint bleeding and hematomas, and joint deformity is present on physical examination. Laboratory tests consistent with hemophilia include a normal or slightly prolonged bleeding time, a normal PT/INR, and a prolonged aPTT. Factor assay verifies a deficiency in factor VIII or IX. Early in pregnancy, chorionic villus biopsy or amniocentesis may be done to identify factor deficiency, making prenatal diagnosis of hemophilia possible.[5]

The patient and family must learn about hemophilia, including recognition and appropriate response to bleeding episodes, lifestyle changes that will be necessary, and the genetic nature of disease transmission. Prevention of injury and avoidance of aspirin and aspirin-like drugs, which alter platelet function, are important parts of treatment. Joint bleeding is managed by immobilization of the limb and application of ice.

With dental procedures requiring administration of a local anesthetic, prophylactic administration of factor VIII should be considered in the patient with hemophilia A. Bleeding episodes from hemophilia A are managed primarily by the administration of cryoprecipitate or other preparations of factor VIII concentrate. Recombinant DNA–derived factor concentrates contain no viruses and are now available. In addition, desmopressin and antifibrinolytics (e.g., tranexamic acid and aminocaproic acid) are possibilities to treat mild bleeding episodes.[20,22] The goal of therapy is to obtain a factor VIII level of at least 40% to 60% for joint and most muscle bleeding, and 80% to 100% for iliopsoas muscle, throat or neck, central nervous system (CNS), or gastrointestinal bleeding.[20] Up to 20% of patients with severe hemophilia develop factor VIII inhibitor, an antibody that rapidly inactivates transfused factor VIII.[20,22] Plasmapheresis and immunosuppressive therapy are sometimes necessary to maintain adequate factor VIII levels in these patients.

Mild to moderate bleeding resulting from hemophilia B is managed with the administration of fresh or fresh frozen plasma or cryoprecipitate. Use of Konyne 80 or Proplex T, both of which are concentrates containing factors II, VII, IX, and X, is another therapeutic option. These concentrates are now treated in a variety of fashions (heat, pasteurization, solvent detergents, immunoaffinity purification) to prevent transmission of viruses. Their use was previously associated with the transmission of human immunodeficiency virus (HIV) and hepatitis viruses.[20,22] Mononine is a newer, highly purified factor IX concentrate that appears to be safe in terms of both adverse effects and viral transmission.[20]

von Willebrand Disease

Etiology. von Willebrand disease is inherited as an autosomal dominant disorder of factor VIII carrier protein and platelet dysfunction. In rare cases, von Willebrand disease is an autosomal recessive disorder.[7,23,24] Several less common subtypes of the disease have been identified, but all have some defect in von Willebrand factor, a plasma protein. von Willebrand disease occurs in both females and males. Bleeding manifestations of the disease tend to become more severe with age.

Pathogenesis. von Willebrand factor and factor VIII normally circulate in plasma as a complex. von Willebrand factor is necessary for stabilization of factor VIII in the circulation and for normal adherence of platelets to damaged vascular endothelium.[7,23,24] In von Willebrand disease, the level of von Willebrand factor is decreased or absent. Serum levels of factor VIII range from mildly to severely reduced. Absence of platelet adhesion at the site of vascular injury and deficient factor VIII activity in the intrinsic coagulation pathway contribute to the bleeding seen in von Willebrand disease.

Clinical manifestations. Epistaxis, mucosal bleeding, ecchymoses, gastrointestinal bleeding, and menorrhagia are common clinical manifestations of von Willebrand disease. Once hemostasis is achieved, it can usually be maintained. Hemarthrosis is rare. Although not common, von Willebrand disease should be considered as a possible cause of excessive surgical bleeding. Bleeding manifestations may decrease during pregnancy because levels of von Willebrand factor and factor VIII rise during this time.[23]

Diagnosis and treatment. The history and clinical presentation initially suggest the possibility of von Willebrand disease as the cause of bleeding. Laboratory tests consistent with the disease include a prolonged bleeding time, prolonged aPTT, normal platelet count, and normal PT/INR. More specialized testing will verify that the level of plasma von Willebrand factor is decreased and that factor VIII activity is reduced.

Mild forms of classic von Willebrand disease can be managed with desmopressin, which causes release of von Willebrand factor and factor VIII from vascular endothelial cells.[7,23] Excessive menstrual bleeding can be treated with hormonal suppression therapy. Severe bleeding is addressed by using cryoprecipitate that contains both factor VIII and von Willebrand factor. Humate-P, a recombinant replacement therapy, is now available. Aspirin and aspirin-containing drugs, which inhibit normal platelet function in hemostasis, should be avoided in patients with von Willebrand disease.[7,22,24]

Complications of therapy for severe von Willebrand disease include hepatitis and AIDS, related to transfusions with blood products. Antibodies that inhibit the activity of von Willebrand factor may develop, but this is rare.

Vitamin K Deficiency Bleeding in Infancy

Etiology. As the name implies, this coagulation disorder is seen in the newborn, typically 48 to 72 hours after birth, through 6 months of age.[25,26] Hemorrhagic disease of the newborn is more common in breast-fed babies (who do not receive vitamin K supplement) than in formula-fed babies. It is rare in Western countries because of routine administration of vitamin K to newborns.

Pathogenesis. This bleeding disorder results from a deficiency of the vitamin K–dependent coagulation factors II, VII, IX, and X. The levels of these factors are approximately 50% of normal in umbilical cord blood and they decline rapidly after birth, reaching their lowest levels at 48 to 72 hours. In a small number of infants, the decline is so significant that severe bleeding occurs. After 72 hours, the levels of these coagulation factors gradually increase over the course of several weeks. This increase is primarily caused by absorption of vitamin K from the diet. The vitamin K content of human milk is very low compared with standard infant formulas; therefore, breast-fed babies need vitamin K supplementation.[25,26]

Hepatic immaturity may also contribute to hemorrhagic disease of the newborn. The liver may be unable to initially produce adequate levels of the vitamin K–dependent coagulation factors.[27]

Clinical manifestations. Evidence of bleeding, such as melena (tarry, black feces composed of partially digested blood), bleeding from the umbilicus, and hematuria, appears on the second or third day of life. Life-threatening complications include intracranial hemorrhage and hypovolemic shock.

Diagnosis and treatment. The diagnosis is primarily based on the clinical presentation, particularly the timing of the onset of bleeding. The PT/INR is prolonged; levels of vitamin K–dependent clotting factors are decreased.

Prophylactic administration of vitamin K to the newborn prevents the severe decline of the vitamin K–dependent coagulation factors and largely eliminates this coagulation disorder.

If evidence of hemorrhage is present, vitamin K should be administered. For severe hemorrhage, fresh plasma will replenish the deficient coagulation factors and stop the bleeding. Fresh whole blood will correct severe anemia and shock.

Premature infants may experience bleeding attributable to platelet abnormalities and a deficiency in several coagulation factors. Because of hepatic immaturity, vitamin K is ineffective therapy in these infants. Fresh plasma is the treatment of choice for the premature infant with bleeding complications.

Acquired Vitamin K Deficiency

Etiology. Acquired vitamin K deficiency may result in bleeding as a result of a coagulation defect. Vitamin K, a fat-soluble vitamin, is obtained by the ingestion of specific foods (e.g., liver, cheese, butter, egg yolks, and green, leafy vegetables) and by a synthetic process occurring in the intestinal flora. Vitamin K is then absorbed by the intestine and stored in the liver. Normal absorption is dependent on bile acids and adequate mucosal function in the intestine. Vitamin K is necessary for normal synthesis and function of coagulation proteins (factors II, VII, IX, and X) as well as coagulation inhibitors (proteins C and S).

Vitamin K deficiency, with its associated risk for bleeding, may occur with the following: malnutrition, malabsorption (including biliary disease), chronic hepatic disease, antibiotic therapy, and oral anticoagulation therapy.

Pathogenesis. One of the many functions of the liver is the synthesis and transport of bile, which is necessary for fat digestion and normal absorption in the small intestine. Vitamin K is a fat-soluble vitamin; if fat malabsorption occurs because of a lack of bile, vitamin K is not absorbed, resulting in a vitamin K deficiency. In the newborn, especially the premature infant, vitamin K deficiency may be related to liver immaturity and the lack of vitamin K synthesis by the intestine until the gut is colonized with the flora that produce vitamin K. Coumadin-type drugs are vitamin K antagonists that inhibit the normal activity of vitamin K in the synthesis of clotting factors. The net effect is decreased clotting factor activity.

Although vitamin K is deficient, the liver continues to synthesize the vitamin K–dependent coagulation factors. However, the coagulation activity of these factors is impaired, resulting in bleeding.

Clinical manifestations. Evidence of bleeding may present in a variety of ways, including mucosal and gastrointestinal bleeding, ecchymoses, menorrhagia, and hematuria. Surgical bleeding may be a significant problem in the patient with a vitamin K deficiency.

Diagnosis and treatment. Vitamin K deficiency should be considered as the cause for bleeding when the PT/INR is increased but other coagulation studies are normal. Of the vitamin K–dependent clotting factors, factor VII (extrinsic pathway) has the shortest half-life; thus, the PT/INR is prolonged first. Ultimately, the aPTT also will be prolonged as clotting factors in the intrinsic pathway become deficient.

Parenteral administration of vitamin K rapidly restores levels in the liver.[25,26] Fresh frozen plasma, with an immediate supply of clotting factors, is the treatment of choice for severe hemorrhage. Correction or removal of the cause of vitamin K deficiency also is an important part of therapy.

Disseminated Intravascular Coagulation (DIC)

Etiology. DIC is an acquired hemorrhagic syndrome in which both clotting and bleeding occur simultaneously (Figure 14-10). This syndrome is also known as "disseminated intravascular coagulopathy" or "disseminated intravascular consumption" in some references. Widespread clotting in small vessels leads to consumption of the clotting factors and platelets, which in turn leads to bleeding. DIC is either chronic or acute. The chronic form is seen mainly in the cancer patient with malignancy and presents in a less severe form with bleeding tendencies that are mild to moderate and thrombotic episodes.[27,28] The liver and bone marrow have sufficient time to replenish consumed factors and platelets, which leads to a more pronounced thrombotic problem.[8] Acute DIC occurs secondary to a variety of factors, including malignancy, sepsis, snake bite, abruptio placentae, trauma and crushing injuries, transfusions of incompatible blood, burns, shock, and severe liver disease.[5,27,28] DIC is estimated to occur in 1 of every 900 to 2400 adult admissions in large, urban hospitals. Death rates are reported to range from 50% to 80%.

Pathogenesis. DIC represents a paradox of both thrombosis and hemorrhage. Accelerated intravascular clotting in small vessels is initiated by contact of the blood with damaged vascular endothelium (sepsis, burns), release of procoagulant substances into the blood (snake venom, malignancy), generation of procoagulants in the blood

(incompatible blood transfusion), or stagnant blood flow (shock). Coagulation factors, especially prothrombin, platelets, factor V, and factor VIII, are rapidly consumed. At the same time, the fibrinolytic system is activated to break down the clots. The fibrin degradation products or fibrin split products that result act as circulating anticoagulants. The combination of coagulation, anticoagulation, and fibrinolysis ultimately leads to hemorrhage.[27,28]

Clinical manifestations. Although both bleeding and clotting are part of the syndrome, initially bleeding is more apparent clinically. Petechiae and ecchymoses on skin and mucous membranes, as well as bleeding from orifices and any site of injury, such as venipuncture and injection sites, may be present. Acrocyanosis (cold, mottled fingers and toes) may be apparent attributable to thrombi formation in the microvasculature of the extremities. Thrombi in the pulmonary microcirculation (small vessels) may result in dyspnea, hemoptysis, and crackles or rales, as blood fills alveoli. Patients with DIC are also predisposed to acute renal failure because of the presence of microthrombi in the renal microvasculature.

Diagnosis and treatment. The diagnosis of DIC is based on a high index of suspicion drawn from the history and presenting signs and symptoms. The typical clinical picture described previously, plus the presence of a predisposing cause, should make DIC a consideration in the differential diagnosis. Abnormal coagulation studies that help confirm the diagnosis include increased values for bleeding time, PT/INR, aPTT, fibrin split products, and thrombin time as well as decreased measurements for the fibrinogen level and platelet count. D-Dimer (a fibrin degradation product) is one of the most useful tests to measure fibrinolysis; this in conjunction with an elevated antithrombin complex is indicative of DIC.[7,27,28]

The cornerstone of treatment for DIC is removal or correction of the underlying cause and support of major organ systems. Replacement of depleted clotting factors with fresh frozen plasma, packed red blood cells, platelets, or cryoprecipitate may be necessary. Antifibrinolytics (aminocaproic acid) may be used if there is life-threatening hemorrhage.[25] Some studies have had promising results in decreasing

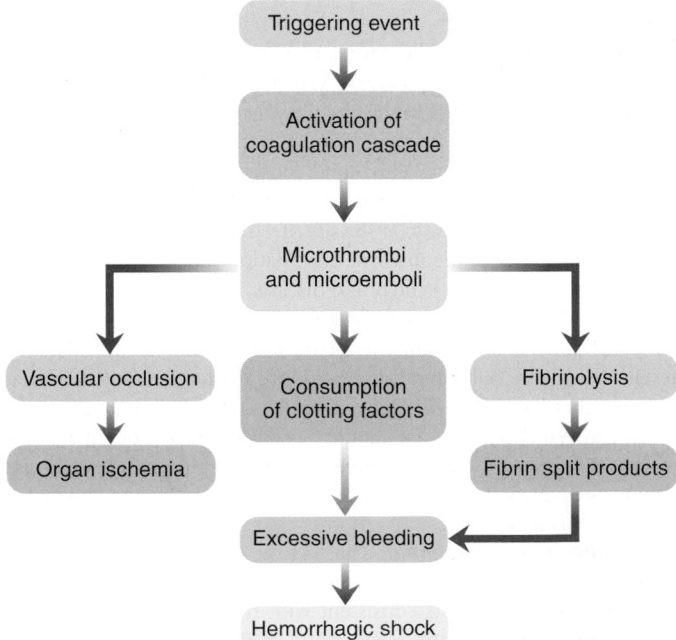

FIGURE 14-10 Pathophysiology of disseminated intravascular coagulation. Clotting and bleeding occur simultaneously, resulting in organ ischemia and hemorrhagic shock.

mortality with administration of antithrombin concentrate or activated protein C. Improved mortality was seen in the groups with higher severity ratings.[28] Although controversial, heparin may be used to minimize further consumption of clotting factors. The purpose of heparin therapy is to stop thrombin formation, thus preventing microemboli. Low-dose subcutaneous heparin appears to be as effective as high-dose heparin with fewer complications. Heparin has been found useful in chronic DIC.[28]

Hepatic Disease

Etiology. A common complication of many hepatic disorders is abnormal hemostasis. With the exception of part of the antihemophilic factor, all plasma protein clotting factors and fibrinolytic factors and their inhibitors are synthesized totally or predominantly by the liver.[3,5,25] If liver function is altered by disease, bleeding is one manifestation.

Pathogenesis. Several factors may contribute to the abnormal hemostasis seen in liver disease. Liver disease alters the synthesis and transport of bile, which is necessary for normal fat digestion and absorption. Impaired absorption and metabolism of vitamin K, which is fat soluble, results in decreased hepatic synthesis of coagulation factors II, VII, IX, and X. Altered liver function also results in decreased synthesis of fibrinogen and factors V and XI.[28] A deficiency in any of the coagulation factors can interrupt the normal process of fibrin clot formation. In addition to synthesis of coagulation factors, the liver also has a role in removing activated coagulation and fibrinolytic proteins from the circulation. Failure to filter these proteins adequately may result in an imbalance between clot formation and clot dissolution (fibrinolysis), manifesting clinically as DIC.[25,28] Liver disease also may alter normal production of inhibitors of coagulation (antithrombin III, proteins C and S), which contributes to the hypercoagulable component of DIC.[27]

Another factor contributing to the bleeding associated with liver disease is thrombocytopenia. A low platelet count is common in liver disease. The exact mechanism is unknown but may relate to the splenomegaly associated with portal hypertension.[27] Sequestration of platelets in the enlarged spleen depletes the number of platelets circulating and available for normal hemostasis. The portal hypertension that develops as blood flow through the liver is retarded adds to the bleeding problem. While pressure in collateral circulatory beds increases, bleeding is manifested as esophageal varices and hemorrhoids (see Chapter 38).

Clinical manifestations. Patients with chronic, rather than acute, liver disease are more likely to have clinical evidence of a bleeding problem. Typical clinical features may include any of the following: petechiae, ecchymoses, spider telangiectasia, bleeding from venipuncture sites or esophageal varices, and gastrointestinal bleeding. DIC may complicate the clinical presentation. Bleeding may not be a problem until the patient has surgery or a biopsy.

Diagnosis and treatment. The patient with liver disease and associated bleeding will commonly have a decreased platelet count, normal or decreased fibrinogen levels, and prolonged PT/INR and aPTT values. More specific coagulation studies may be indicated in some situations.

Treatment may be instituted prophylactically before surgery or biopsy, or it may be mandated by a bleeding episode. The degree of abnormality on coagulation tests or the severity of the bleeding will influence the aggressiveness of therapy. Because of the high likelihood of vitamin K deficiency, administration of vitamin K may be the initial intervention. Platelet infusions are appropriate if significant thrombocytopenia is present. Fresh frozen plasma is the primary replacement product used to supply coagulation factors. Administration of large quantities of plasma carries the risk of precipitating hepatic encephalopathy and fluid overload. Transfusions of whole blood or, more commonly, packed red blood cells may be necessary to manage anemia from bleeding of significant proportions.

KEY POINTS
- Coagulation disorders result from defects in the clotting cascade or fibrinolytic process. These disorders may be inherited or acquired.
- Hemophilia is an inherited bleeding disorder that results from deficient clotting factor production. The most common types are hemophilia A (factor VIII) and hemophilia B (factor IX).
- von Willebrand disease is an inherited bleeding disorder caused by abnormal factor VIII carrier protein production. The disease results in a deficiency of factor VIII in the circulation and decreased platelet function.
- Vitamin K deficiency is associated with several coagulation disorders, including hemorrhagic disease of the newborn and bleeding related to malnutrition and liver disease. Vitamin K is a necessary cofactor for liver production of factors II, VII, IX, and X.
- DIC is an acquired bleeding syndrome associated with a number of etiologic factors, including trauma, malignancy, burns, shock, and abruptio placentae. DIC is characterized by widespread clot formation in small vessels. Clotting factors and platelets are consumed, leaving the patient with deficient resources for appropriate clot formation. The platelet count and fibrinogen levels are typically decreased, and values for PT, aPTT, thrombin time, bleeding time, and fibrin split products are elevated.

SUMMARY

The presence of unexpected overt or covert bleeding may signal an acquired or inherited problem with hemostasis. A review of normal hemostasis, as well as information on selected disorders of hemostasis and coagulation, has been presented in this chapter. With a sound knowledge base, the health care professional is in a position to play a key role in the recognition, diagnosis, and management of a bleeding problem.

REFERENCES

1. Hall JE: *Guyton and Hall textbook of medical physiology*, ed 12, Philadelphia, 2011, Saunders.
2. Quinn M: Platelet physiology. In Quinn M, et al: *Platelet function*, New York, 2010, Humana Press.
3. Pagana KD, Pagana TJ: *Mosby's manual of diagnostic and laboratory tests*, ed 4, St Louis, 2011, Mosby.
4. McCance K, Huether S, Brashers V, Rote N: *Pathophysiology the biologic basis for disease in adults & children*, ed 6, St Louis, 2010, Mosby Elsevier.
5. Fauci A: *Harrison's principles of internal medicine*, ed 17, New York, 2008, McGraw-Hill.
6. Israels SJ, Kahr WH, Blanchette VS, Luban NL, Rivard GE, et al: Platelet disorders in children: a diagnostic approach, *Pediatr Blood Cancer* 56(6):975–983, 2011.
7. Bolton-Maggs P, et al: A review of inherited platelet disorders with guidelines for their management, on behalf of the UKHCDO, *Br J Haemotol* 135:603–633, 2006.
8. George J: Platelets, *Lancet* 355:1531–1539, 2000.
9. Gallo RL: Vascular purpuras. In Kaushansky K, et al, editors: *Williams hematology*, ed 8, New York, 2010, McGraw-Hill.
10. Roberts P, et al: Henoch-Schönlein purpura: a review article, *South Med J* 100(8):821–824, 2007.
11. Dillon M: Henoch-Schönlein purpura: recent advances, *Clin Exp Rheumatol* 25:566-558, 2007.
12. Germain D: Ehlers-Danlos syndrome type IV, *Orphanet J Rare Dis* 2:32–40, 2007.
13. Shimaoka Y, Kosho T, et al: Clinical and genetic features of 20 Japanese patients with vascular-type Ehlers-Danlos syndrome, *Br J Dermatol* 163(4):704–710, 2010.
14. McDonald J, Bayrack-Toydemir P, Pyeritz R: Hereditary hemorrhagic telangiectasia: an overview of diagnosis, management and pathogenesis, *Genet Med* 13(7):607–616, 2011.
15. Faughnan M, et al: International guidelines for the diagnosis and management of hereditary haemorrhagic telangiectasia, *J Med Genet* 48:73–87, 2011.
16. Stasi R, Newland A: ITP: a historical perspective, *Br J Haemotol* 153(4):437–450, 2011.
17. Segal G, Feig S: Controversies in the diagnosis and management of childhood acute immune thrombocytopenic purpura, *Pediatr Blood Cancer* 53:318–324, 2009.
18. Provan D, et al: International consensus report on the investigation and management of primary immune thrombocytopenia, *Blood* 115:168–186, 2010. doi:10.1182.
19. Newton J, et al: Fatigue in adult patients with primary immune thrombocytopenia, *Eur J Haemotol* 86:420–429, 2011.
20. Stachnik J: Hemophilia: etiology, complications, and current management, *Formulary* 45:218–227, 2010.
21. Kasper C, Lin C: Prevalence of sporadic and familial haemophilia, *Haemophilia* 13:90–92, 2007.
22. World Federation of Hemophilia: *Guidelines for the management of hemophilia*, 2005. Available at, www.wfh.org/2/docs/Publications/Diagnosis_and_Treatment/Guidelines_Mng_Hemophilia.pdf. Accessed July 31, 2011.
23. Pacheco L, et al: von Willebrand disease and pregnancy: a practical approach for the diagnosis and treatment, *Am J Obstet Gynecol* 203(3):194–200, 2010.
24. Lima H: The diagnosis and management of von Willebrand disease, *Infusion* 16(6):1–11, 2010.
25. Van Winckel M, et al: Vitamin K an update for the paediatrician, *Eur J Pediatr* 168(2):127–134, 2009.
26. Lippi G, Franchini M: Vitamin K in neonates: facts and myths, *Blood Transfus* 9:4–9, 2011.
27. Hoffman R, et al: *Hematology basic principles and practices*, ed 5, Philadelphia, 2009, Churchill Livingstone Elsevier.
28. Levi M: Disseminated intravascular coagulation, *Crit Care Med* 35(9):2191–2195, 2007.

Alterations in Blood Flow

Teresa Grigsby Loftsgaarden

⊝volve WEBSITE

http://evolve.elsevier.com/Copstead/
- Review Questions and Answers
- Glossary (with audio pronunciations for selected terms)
- Animations
- Case Studies
- Key Points Review

KEY QUESTIONS

- How do the structures of arteries, veins, capillaries, and lymphatics differ, and how do these differences reflect the functions of each?
- What is the relationship among vessel resistance, blood pressure, and blood flow?
- How is vascular resistance regulated centrally by the autonomic nervous system and locally by tissues?
- What are the determinants of transcapillary exchange of fluids, electrolytes, and nutrients?
- How do arterial and venous obstructions develop?
- What are the clinical consequences of acute and chronic arterial obstruction?
- What are the clinical consequences of superficial and deep venous obstructions?

CHAPTER OUTLINE

The primary functions of the circulatory system are the transportation of oxygen and nutrients and the removal of metabolic waste products within the body. To perform these functions, a complex circuitry of vessels traverses the body (Figure 15-1), powered by the pumping action of the heart. Propulsion of blood through the lungs is provided by the right ventricle, whereas systemic blood flow is driven by the left ventricle.

Nutrients are absorbed into the blood as it moves through the gastrointestinal tract via the splanchnic circulation. Oxygen uptake and the release of carbon dioxide occur in the specialized vascular bed of the pulmonary circulation. The liver, with its extensive blood supply, has a major role in metabolism and generation of metabolic waste products. These, and other metabolic by-products, are carried by the

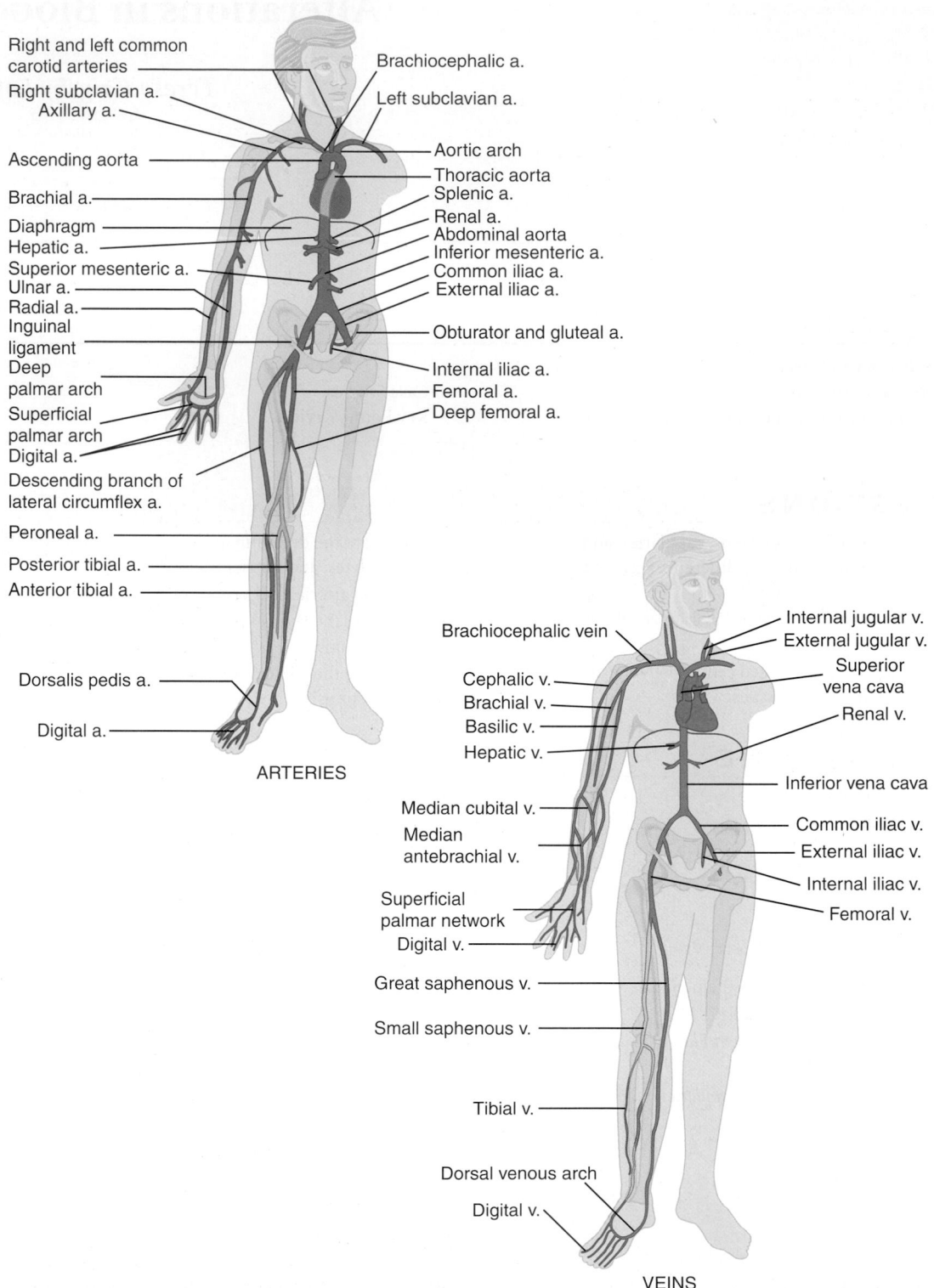

FIGURE 15-1 The primary systemic arterial and venous circulatory networks. *a.,* Artery; *v.,* vein. (From Black JM, Hawks J: *Medical-surgical nursing: clinical management for positive outcomes,* ed 8, Philadelphia, 2008, Saunders, p 1273.)

blood to the kidneys for elimination. Inadequate circulation in the lungs, liver, or kidneys may interfere with the removal of metabolic wastes from the body. Effective transportation of oxygen and nutrients and removal of waste materials depend on proper functioning of the circulatory system.

Aging produces significant changes in the circulatory system, altering the ability of the system to carry out its functions and increasing susceptibility to certain disease processes. The effects of the aging process on the circulatory system are summarized in Geriatric Considerations: Changes in the Circulatory System.

ORGANIZATION OF THE CIRCULATORY AND LYMPHATIC SYSTEMS

After passing through the pulmonary circulatory system and leaving the left ventricle, blood flows through a graduated series of tubes to tissues of the body before returning to the right side of the heart. The powerful left ventricle propels the blood to the aorta, arteries, arterioles, and, finally, to the capillary beds. Here the proximity of capillary endothelium to the other cells of the body facilitates movement of nutrients and oxygen into the cells and removal of cellular metabolic wastes. Capillary blood is then collected by venules, which flow into

veins, returning blood to the venae cavae and the right side of the heart (Figure 15-2). The complete process, moving approximately 5 L of blood through the entire circuit, takes only about 1 minute.

The lymphatic circulation is a specialized system of channels and tissues (nodes). It is not arranged in a circuit, as is the vascular system. Instead, the lymphatic vessels begin blindly, deep in the connective tissue. One of the functions of the lymphatic system is to reabsorb fluid that leaks out of the vascular network into the interstitium and return it to the general circulation. During the process of cellular exchange within the capillary bed, some fluid moves into the interstitium and fails to return to the vascular bed. This lost fluid can amount to as much as 2 to 4 L/day. At this circulatory level, lymphatic vessels lie in close proximity to the capillary vasculature. The fluid, now called *lymph*, is absorbed by the lymphatic vessels and returned to the venous circulation by way of the thoracic duct and the right lymphatic duct (Figure 15-3). Lymphatic drainage of the breast is illustrated in Figure 15-4.

Vessel Structure

To perform their specialized functions, the blood and lymphatic vessels are different in their structure. Knowledge of the morphology of these vessels is essential for an understanding of the alterations in function produced by disease.

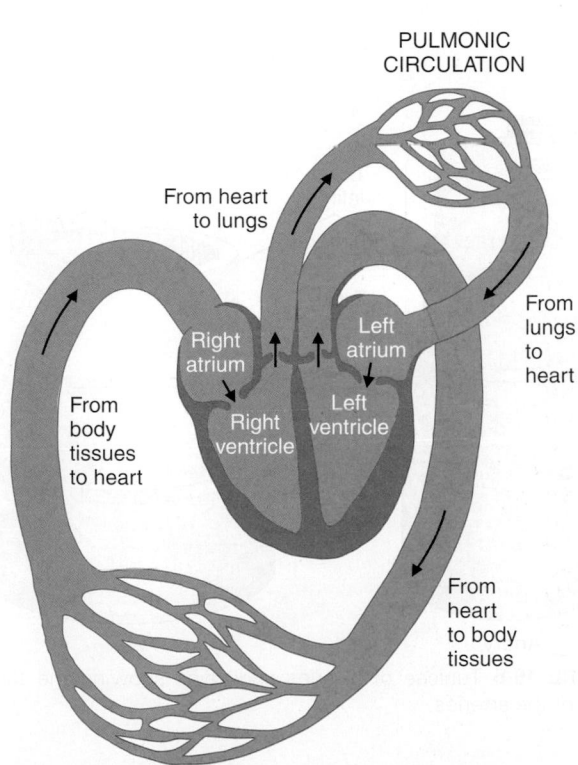

FIGURE 15-2 The circulatory system. Beginning from the body tissues, blood returns to the right side of the heart, through the right atria to the right ventricle, which propels it into the lungs. In the lungs, the metabolic waste carbon dioxide is removed and oxygen is replenished. Oxygenated blood leaves the pulmonic circulation and returns to the heart via the left atrium and then to the left ventricle. From the left side of the heart, the oxygenated blood enters the systemic circulation, where oxygen is delivered to the tissues in exchange for metabolic wastes. (From Black JM, Hawks J. *Medical-surgical nursing: clinical management for positive outcomes*, ed 8, Philadelphia, 2008, Saunders, p 1344.)

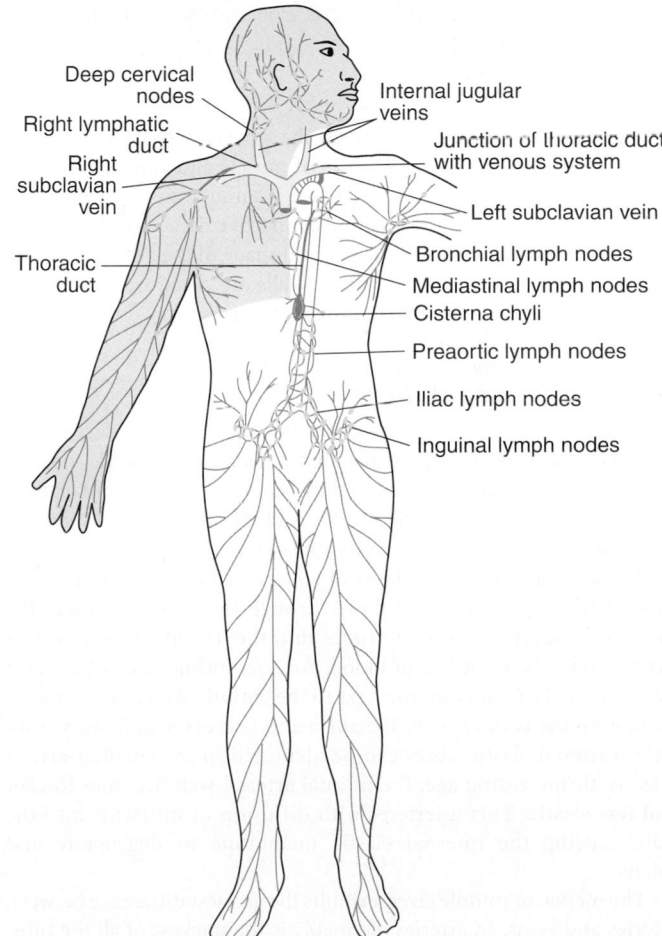

FIGURE 15-3 Anatomy of the lymphatic system. Lymphatic capillaries collect the excess fluid from the vascular capillaries, returning it to the venous circulation at the junction of the internal jugular and subclavian veins. (From Monahan FD et al: Phipps' medical-surgical nursing: health and illness perspectives, ed 8, Philadelphia, 2007, Mosby, p 936.)

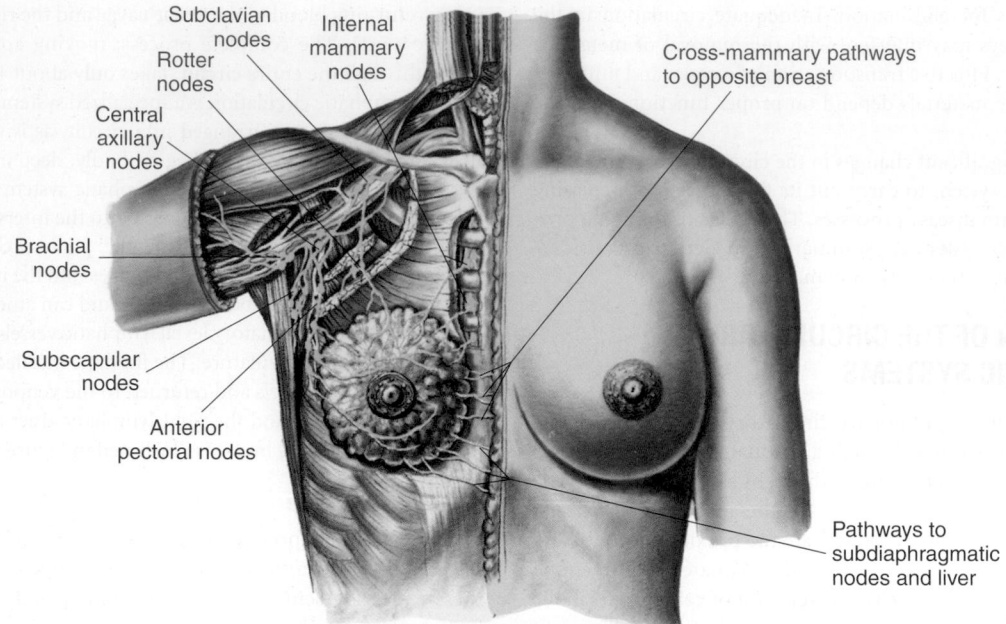

FIGURE 15-4 Lymphatic drainage of the breast to the axillary and subclavian nodes, then to the jugular and subclavian veins. (From Monahan FD et al: *Phipps' medical-surgical nursing: health and illness perspectives,* ed 8, Philadelphia, 2007, Mosby, p 1661.)

The primary differences between the smaller arterial and venous vessels are in terms of the quantities of muscle and connective tissue present. In arterioles, the principal tissue is smooth muscle, whereas in venules, smooth muscle is scarce and connective tissue dominates. The composition of the walls and the size and shape of the vessels also vary in larger arteries and veins. Capillary walls are composed of a single layer of endothelial cells. These simple structures carry out extraordinarily complex functions.

Anatomy of Arteries and Veins

The walls of both arteries and veins are composed of three microscopically distinct layers, or tunicae: the intima, the media, and the adventitia. The histologic constituents of these tunicae are similar in arteries and veins (Figure 15-5). Generally, the walls of veins are not as thick as the walls of arteries, but the lumina are larger.

The intima consists of a layer of endothelial cells that is in direct contact with the blood as it flows through the vessel. Periodically, the intimal layer of veins protrudes into the lumen, creating valves that prevent the backflow of blood. Arterial intima is characterized by an inner elastic membrane next to the endothelial cells. This elastic membrane is thickest in the aorta and decreases in density until only scattered elastic fibers can be identified in the smallest arterioles. With increasing age, the intimal arterial wall becomes thicker and less elastic. This interferes with diffusion of nutrients into the wall, causing the internal elastic membrane to degenerate and calcify.

The media, or middle layer, exhibits the greatest difference between arteries and veins. In arteries the media is the thickest of all the tunicae. Large arteries have smooth muscle fibers arranged in a circular pattern and interspersed with elastic fibers. Progressing from arteries to ever-smaller arterioles, the smooth muscle remains but the elastic tissue disappears. This thick, smooth muscle layer is responsible for the firmness and limited distensibility of arterial vessels. With advancing age, changes in the intima result in decreased nutrition reaching

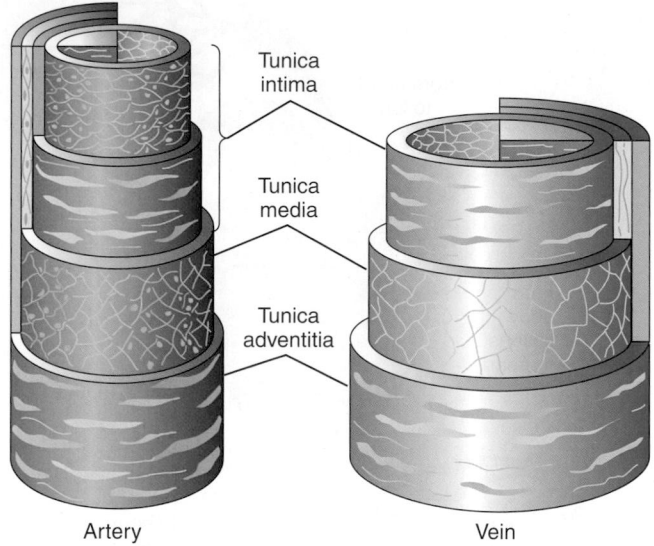

FIGURE 15-5 Tunicae of arteries and veins showing the thicker walls of the arteries.

the media, causing degeneration of the smooth muscle tissue. In veins, the media also has smooth muscle, usually arranged in a circular pattern with some longitudinal strands. The quantity of smooth muscle decreases as the veins become larger. Venous media also contains collagenous connective tissue, but elastic tissue is rare except in the largest veins.

In veins, the adventitia is the thickest of the tunicae. It is composed of collagenous connective tissue and longitudinal smooth muscle. In larger arteries there is a discernible external elastic membrane in the adventitia. This membrane disappears as the arteries decrease in diameter. Arterial adventitia consists predominantly of collagenous

GERIATRIC CONSIDERATIONS
Changes in the Circulatory System

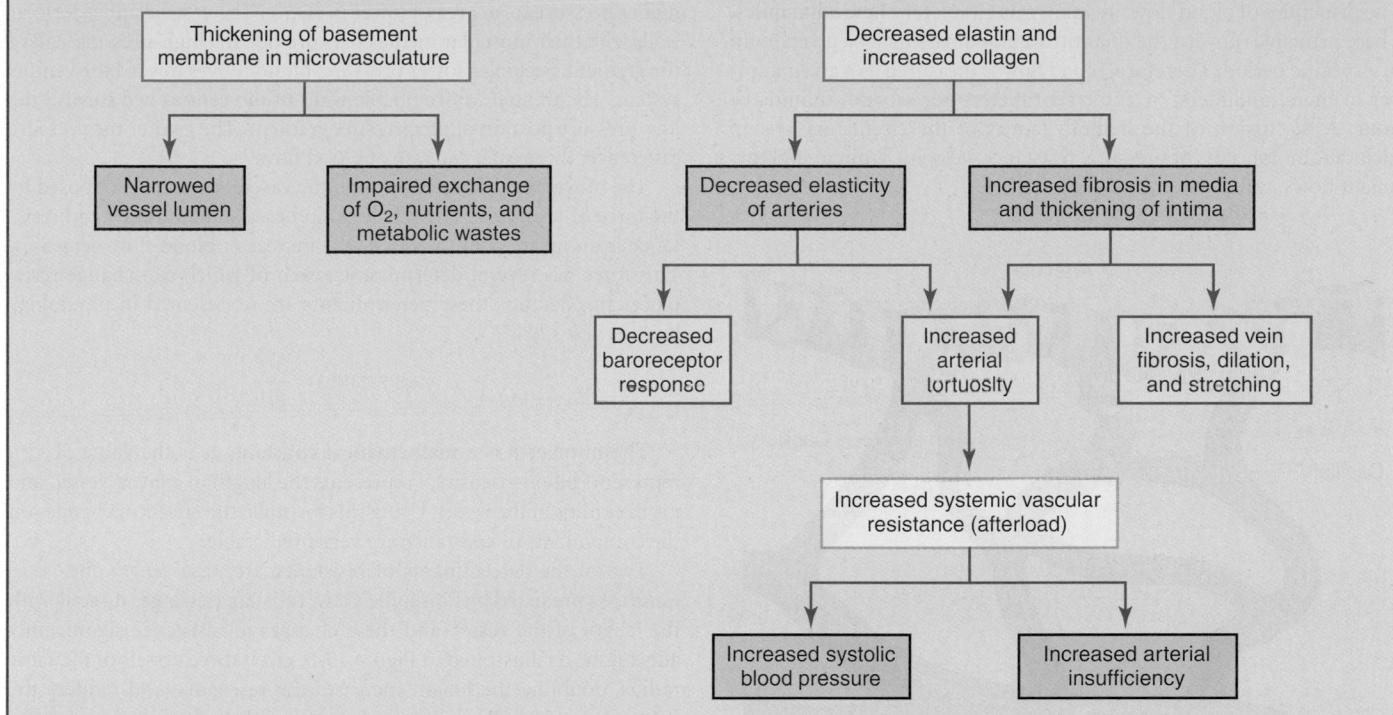

In the aging individual, changes occur throughout the vascular bed. The microvascular bed demonstrates thickening of the basement membrane. This change narrows the vessel lumen and impairs the free exchange of oxygen, nutrients, and metabolic wastes at the cellular level.

In both arteries and veins, the vascular changes occur first in the proximal portions. The intima becomes fibrotic and the endothelial cell variation increases. In the media, the amount of elastin and smooth muscle is reduced, whereas the amount of fibrotic and collagen tissue increases. With collagen cross-linking, the vessel walls lose elastic flexibility and recoil, becoming more stiff and less

compliant. They become inflexible tubes with an increase in systemic vascular resistance (SVR). The increased SVR causes a reduction in tissue and organ blood flow and decreased perfusion.

Baroreceptor function is reduced because of decreased sensitivity of the receptors and diminished responsiveness of the vessels attributable to their rigidity. These factors decrease the body's ability to respond to hypotensive and hypertensive stimuli. The decreased compliance of the systemic vascular system increases afterload, forcing the left ventricle of the heart to work harder to meet the metabolic demands of the body.

connective tissue. Some larger vessels also contain isolated, longitudinally arranged fibers of smooth muscle.

Anatomy of Capillaries

Capillaries are composed of a single thickness of endothelial cells attached to a protein network called the basement membrane. Moving from the end of an arteriole to the beginning of a venule, capillaries narrow to a diameter barely sufficient for a single red blood cell (RBC) to pass through the aperture. In some tissues, one or two smooth muscle cells form a precapillary sphincter that controls flow through the vessel (Figure 15-6).

There are spaces between the endothelial cells that vary in size among organ systems. These spaces, or pores, permit certain constituents to pass in and out of the capillaries. For example, capillary beds in the brain have little or no spaces and permit the passage of only certain molecules. The space between endothelial cells of the brain is so small that it is referred to as the *blood-brain barrier*. In parts of the kidneys, however, capillaries are more porous, allowing much larger molecules to move between the circulation and the filtrate (urine). The size of these spaces determines the *capillary permeability* of a specific capillary bed.

Lymphatic Structure

Lymphatic vessels are thin walled and most resemble veins in their appearance. Like their counterparts in the circulatory system, they range in size from lymphatic capillaries to vessels of increasing diameter. Like veins, lymphatics have intermittent valves composed of folds of their inner layer that extend into the lumen (Figure 15-7). The walls of lymphatic capillaries contain contractile fibers that are stimulated when stretched, causing the vessels to contract and propel lymph along the vessel.

KEY POINTS

- Arteries and veins have three distinct layers. The intima, the innermost layer, is composed of a single layer of endothelial cells. The media, or middle layer, is composed of smooth muscle and elastin. Media is thicker in arteries than in veins. The adventitia, the outermost layer, is composed of supporting connective tissue.
- Capillaries have only a single layer of endothelial cells attached to a basement membrane. The permeability of capillaries is determined by the tightness of the endothelial cell connection.
- Lymphatic vessels resemble veins, having thin walls and valves.

PRINCIPLES OF FLOW

Hemodynamics of the Circulatory System

The principles of blood flow are known as circulatory **hemodynamics.** These principles govern the quantity of blood passing by a given point in a specific period. Therefore, blood flow is measured as a given number of liters, milliliters, or cubic centimeters per second, minute, or hour. A discussion of the hemodynamics of the circulatory system includes the concepts of pressure, resistance, velocity, laminar and turbulent flows, wall tension, and compliance.

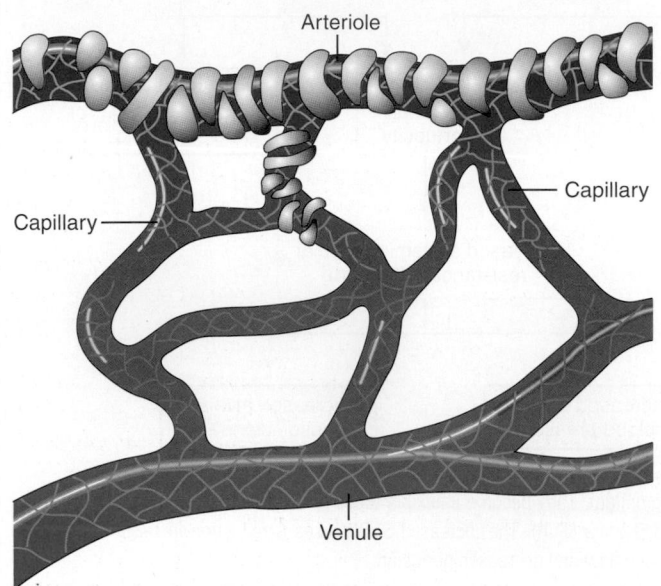

FIGURE 15-6 Capillary network.

Blood Flow, Pressure, and Resistance

Blood flow is accomplished by movement along a pressure gradient within the vascular bed. This means that blood moves from an area of higher pressure to an area of lower pressure. The arterial and arteriolar walls with their muscular media coats provide the high-pressure end of the gradient. Seeking a lower pressure, blood moves toward the venous system. The thinner, more pliable walls of the venous bed furnish the low-pressure portion of the pressure gradient. The greater the pressure difference, the greater the rate of blood flow.

The movement of blood through the vascular system is opposed by the force of *resistance.* The relationship between blood flow and resistance is an inverse one: as resistance increases, blood flow decreases. This force has several determinants, each of which can change resistance considerably; these determinants are represented in physiology by *Poiseuille's law:*

$$\text{Resistance} = \frac{8nl}{\pi r^4}$$

The number 8 is a mathematical constant, as is the value of π; n represents blood viscosity, l represents the length of a given vessel, and r is the radius of the vessel. Using this formula, the effects of changes on the components of resistance are very predictable.

Two of the determinants of resistance are *vessel length* and *vessel radius.* As predicted by Poiseuille's law, resistance changes directly with the length of the vessel, and these changes in resistance significantly affect flow. As illustrated in Figure 15-8, given three vessels of the same radius, doubling the length increases the resistance and reduces the flow (Q) by 50%. Reducing the vessel length by half decreases resistance and increases the flow by 100%. These changes in flow occur when the pressure gradient remains constant and are caused solely by variations in vessel length. Resistance decreases as the radius of a vessel increases and resistance is inversely related to the fourth power of the radius of a vessel, or r^4. Therefore, increasing a vessel's radius markedly

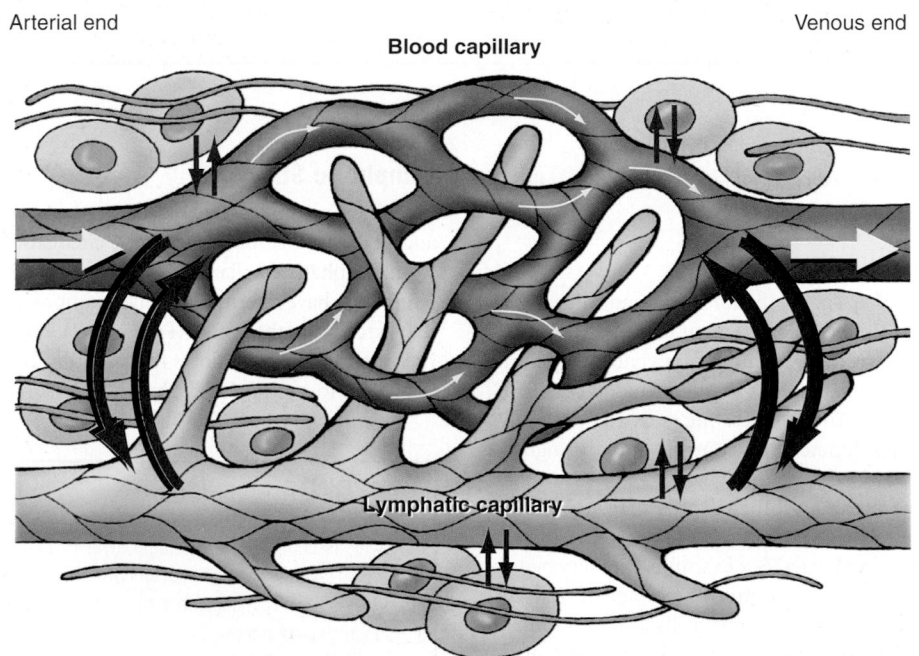

FIGURE 15-7 Lymphatic network. The lymphatic system is integrally related to the systemic vascular system. Excess fluid and plasma diffuse between the capillaries, interstitial spaces, and lymphatic vessels. Because lymphatic capillaries have larger spaces between endothelial cells, they can remove excess interstitial fluid or plasma that venous capillaries cannot reabsorb.

reduces resistance and produces an exponential increase in blood flow. Figure 15-9 demonstrates the effect of doubling the radius of a vessel on the flow of blood if all other factors related to flow are held constant. The resulting flow of blood is 16 times greater in the greater diameter vessel.

Although there is variability in the length of vessels throughout the circulatory system, vessels are incapable of altering their own length. They do, however, possess a considerable ability to change their diameters, and many disease processes (e.g., arteriosclerosis) and drug therapies (e.g., vasopressors) are associated with changes in the size of the vessel lumen. Even minor changes will produce major alterations in resistance and, hence, blood flow. This makes changes in diameter the most important determinant of resistance.

The third determinant of resistance is the *viscosity* of the blood itself, represented in Poiseuille's law as *n*. Viscosity is defined as the thickness of a fluid. When the blood is more viscous, the friction between the cells and the liquid increases, and an increase in resistance to flow is produced. Blood is composed of a suspension of cellular material and plasma. Approximately 99% of the cellular constituents of the blood are RBCs. The ratio of RBCs to plasma is presented in the laboratory value *hematocrit*. Increasing the number of RBCs or decreasing the plasma component results in more viscous blood (increased hematocrit value), more resistance, and a slowing of blood flow. This is what occurs in dehydration, when the plasma component is relatively decreased, or in polycythemia, when the number of RBCs increases.

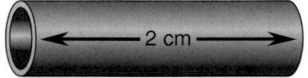

Q = 10 ml/sec

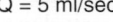

Q = 5 ml/sec

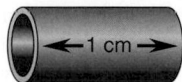

Q = 20 ml/sec

FIGURE 15-8 Relationship of vessel length to blood flow *(Q)* with a constant pressure gradient.

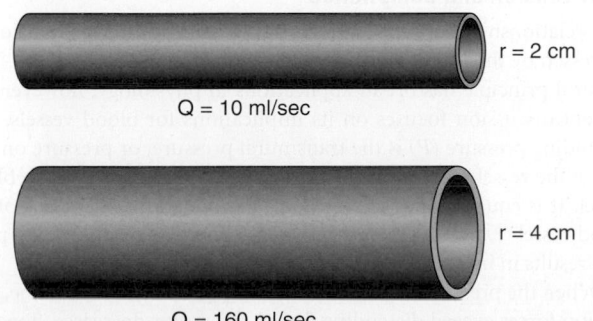

r = 2 cm

Q = 10 ml/sec

r = 4 cm

Q = 160 ml/sec

FIGURE 15-9 Relationship of vessel radius *(r)* to blood flow *(Q)* with a constant pressure gradient.

The relationship between the variables of driving pressure and resistance and their effect on blood flow is expressed by *Ohm's law,* as follows:

$$Q = P/R$$

Here, Q is the blood flow, P is the pressure difference between two points, and R is resistance. Altering any one of the determinants of resistance (vessel length, vessel radius, or blood viscosity) produces a change in flow. According to Ohm's law, a change in the pressure difference within the circulatory system also results in a change in the flow of blood. The arterioles are the major site of resistance in the vascular system and require a greater pressure to maintain blood flow. As the resistance decreases across the systemic vasculature, less pressure is necessary to maintain blood flow (Figure 15-10). *Total peripheral resistance* refers to the resistance throughout the entire vascular system. It can be calculated on the basis of the pressure difference between the arteries and the veins. Clinically, systemic vascular resistance (SVR) is used to specifically denote resistance peripheral to the heart and lungs. Because the primary determinant of SVR is the resistance vessels (arterioles), diseases or drug therapies that affect these vessels have the most profound impact on the SVR. Any condition that produces an increase in SVR, such as hypertension, requires more work for the heart to overcome the elevated resistance and eject its volume of blood (see Chapter 16). This increased workload means that the heart needs more oxygen and nutrients. When SVR is pathologically decreased, the blood is distributed over a larger area and blood flow slows dramatically. Individual organs, such as the kidney and brain, may not obtain sufficient blood flow to meet metabolic needs. This is what occurs in distributive shock states (see Chapter 20).

Velocity and Laminar and Turbulent Flow

As previously discussed, blood flow is defined as the volume of blood that passes by a given point in a given unit of time. *Velocity* is a measure

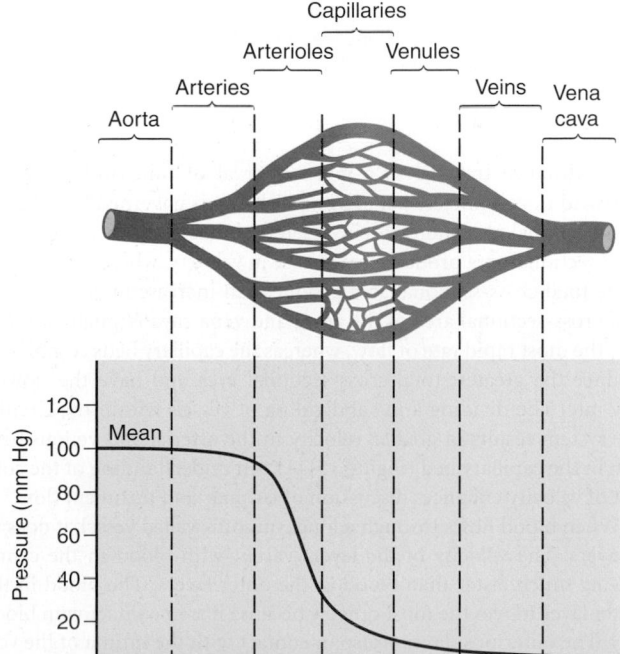

FIGURE 15-10 Mean pressure changes within the systemic vasculature. A significant decrease in pressure occurs as blood flows through the arterioles into the capillaries. The figure illustrates the role of the arterioles in the determination of vascular resistance. Because of the large number of capillaries, total resistance is not increased with the decreased radius of the capillaries.

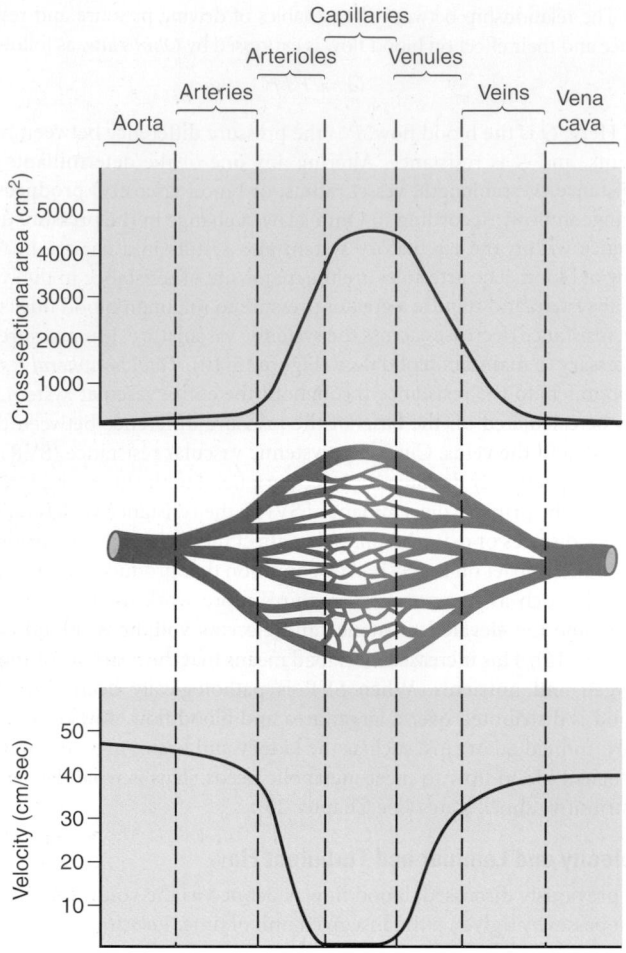

FIGURE 15-11 Effect of increasing cross-sectional area on the velocity of blood flow. Increased cross-sectional area in the capillary bed results in a significant decrease in velocity when compared to the arterial and venous networks.

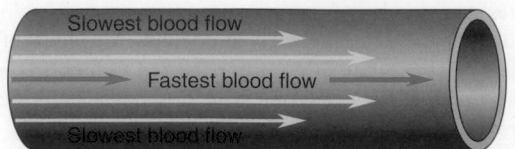

FIGURE 15-12 Parabolic profile of laminar blood flow.

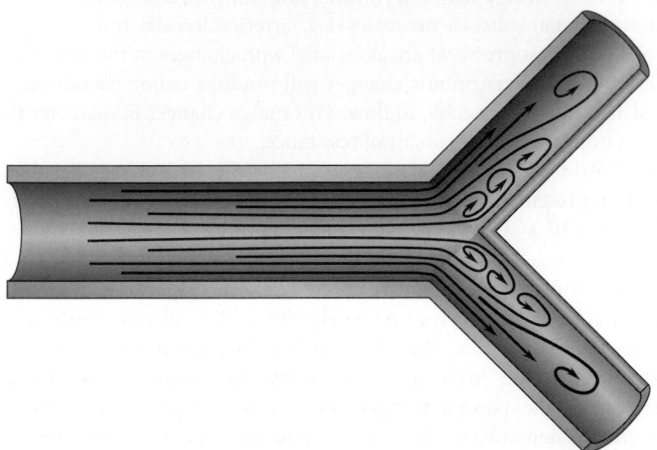

FIGURE 15-13 Turbulent flow generated at a blood vessel bifurcation.

of the distance traveled in a given interval of time and is usually expressed in centimeters per second. Velocity is governed by the total cross-sectional area and varies inversely with it. An increase in the total cross-sectional area produces a decrease in velocity, whereas a decrease in the total cross-sectional area produces an increase in velocity. The total cross-sectional area of the aorta and vena cava is small and they have the most rapid rate of flow, whereas the capillary beds combine to produce the greatest total cross-sectional area and have the slowest flow rate. The dividing and subdividing of vessels within the circulatory system results in greater velocity in the arterial and venous beds than in the capillary bed (Figure 15-11). An understanding of the concept of velocity enhances discussion of laminar and turbulent flow.

When blood flows through a long, smooth-walled vessel, it does so in layers. The velocity of the layers varies, with blood in the center moving much faster than blood in the outer layers. The blood in the center layer moves the most quickly because it is in contact with blood only. The outermost layer is also in contact with the intima of the vessel wall, which exerts friction against the cellular components of the blood. Many blood cells stick to the intima; this layer may flow only minimally. Layers of blood between this outer layer and the central core of blood slide over one another with increasing velocity. This is referred to as the *parabolic profile of laminar flow* and is illustrated in Figure 15-12.

The streamlined nature of laminar flow is disrupted by normal anatomy and by pathologic processes creating turbulent flow. Turbulent flow is an interruption in the forward current of blood flow by crosswise flow (Figure 15-13). The propensity for turbulent flow increases with increasing velocity and increased vessel radius, so that some turbulence can be predicted at the aortic root and in the branches of major arteries. The same process can be seen in a river, where boulders interrupting the flow produce whirlpools and the characteristic roar of rapids. In the human body, turbulent flow through blood vessels can be auscultated as a **bruit.** Sometimes it can be palpated as well, and then it is called a **thrill.** This turbulence may be the result of a normal increase in velocity or be attributable to blood moving through vessels that branch at a sharp angle. Pathologically, turbulence results if blood flows around an obstruction in the vessel or over a roughened intimal surface. Regardless of cause, turbulent flow alters the parabolic profile seen with laminar flow, slowing velocity around the source of the turbulence. This slowing can cause cellular components of the blood to adhere to one another, to the turbulent focus itself, and to the intimal wall, promoting the formation of a blood clot (**thrombus**).

Wall Tension and Compliance

The relationship between distending pressure and wall tension is expressed by the *law of Laplace* and is illustrated in Figure 15-14. This physical principle has broad applications in physiology; however, the present discussion focuses on its implications for blood vessels. The distending pressure *(P)* is the transmural pressure, or pressure on one side of the vessel wall minus the pressure on the other side of the blood vessel. It is equal to the wall tension *(T)* divided by the radius of the blood vessel *(r).* In summary, an increase in radius or distending pressure results in increased wall tension.

When the pressure of the blood in the vessel begins to decline, wall tension forces exceed distending forces, the radius decreases, flow rate declines, and resistance increases. The distending pressure may fall to a point at which it is no longer possible to hold the blood vessel open. If

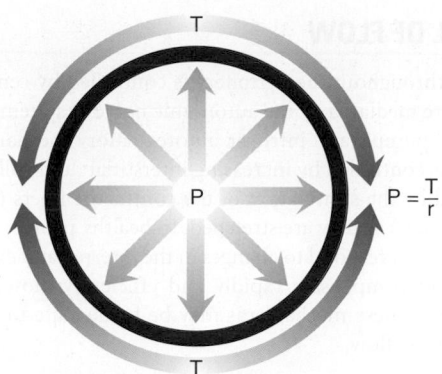

FIGURE 15-14 Law of Laplace as applied to a blood vessel. Distending pressure *(P)* is the difference between the pressures on either side of the vessel and is equal to the wall tension *(T)* divided by the radius of the blood vessel *(r)*.

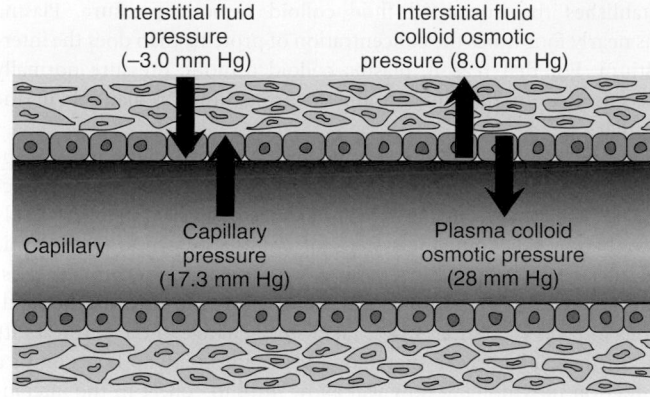

FIGURE 15-15 Components of the capillary pressure gradient. Filtration reflects the difference between the combined forces that push fluid out of the capillary (capillary pressure and interstitial fluid colloid osmotic pressure) and those that attempt to hold fluid in the capillary (plasma colloid osmotic pressure and interstitial fluid pressure).

the pressure reaches 20 mm Hg, a point called the *critical* closing pressure, blood flow ceases entirely.

The smaller the radius of the blood vessel, as in a capillary when compared to an artery or a vein, the less tension is needed in the wall to equalize the distending pressure. Wall tensions decrease rapidly from 170,000 dynes/cm in the aorta to 16 dynes/cm in the capillaries, rising to 21,000 dynes/cm in the vena cava.

Wall tension is a product of the elasticity of the vessel and is a force that opposes the distending pressure. The manner in which wall tension in a given vessel responds to changes in distending pressures is based on its compliance. Compliance reflects the distensibility of a blood vessel—its ability to accept an increased volume of blood. The large quantity of muscle tissue in much of the arterial system limits its distensibility. Veins, however, are highly distensible and compliant, capable of holding a large quantity of blood at a low pressure. Because of this quality, veins are referred to as *capacitance vessels*. When the body is at rest, 75% of the total blood volume is found in the systemic venous system.

Dynamics in the Microcirculation: Capillaries and Lymphatics

The smallest vessels of the vascular system and the lymphatic vessels are commonly referred to as the *microcirculation*. The primary function of the capillary bed is essentially the essence of the entire circulatory system: the exchange of gases and nutrients. Blood flow in the capillary bed is largely laminar, with minimal turbulence at bifurcations. Within each organ or tissue in the body, capillary blood flow is related to the driving force, which is the difference between arterial and venous pressures, and inversely related to resistance.

The exchange of materials across the capillary endothelium through the interstitial space, to or from the cells, occurs on an ongoing basis. Substances pass between tissue interstitial fluid and capillary blood by moving along a concentration gradient (diffusion), whereas fluid moves according to a pressure gradient (filtration). As fluid moves through the interstitial space, most of it returns to the capillary bed. Normally, approximately 10% of the fluid remains in the interstitium and is absorbed by the adjacent lymphatic system to be returned to the general circulation. Alteration in the pressure gradient responsible for filtration can allow an excessive amount of fluid to escape into the interstitial space. Increased fluid accumulation in the interstitial space also can occur when the lymphatic flow is impaired or when capillaries become more permeable and "leak" fluid. These are the pathophysiologic mechanisms that result in **edema.**

The pressure gradient between the capillary and the interstitium is produced and maintained in accord with the balance of four distinct forces or pressures: (1) capillary hydrostatic pressure (P_{cap}), (2) interstitial fluid colloid osmotic pressure (π_{tissue}), (3) plasma colloid osmotic pressure (π_{cap}), and (4) interstitial fluid pressure (P_{tissue}) (Figure 15-15). This delicate balance of forces is summarized by *Starling's hypothesis,* which states that the net filtration is equal to the combined forces fostering filtration minus the combined forces opposing filtration. Using the normal values shown in Figure 15-15, each component of the formula and the resulting net filtration pressure are shown below:

$$\text{Pressures favoring filtration} = P_{cap} + \pi_{tissue}$$

$$(+17.3 \text{ mm Hg}) + (+8.0 \text{ mm Hg}) = 25.3 \text{ mm Hg}$$

$$\text{Pressures opposing filtration} = P_{tissue} + \pi_{cap}$$

$$(-3.0 \text{ mm Hg}) + (28 \text{ mm Hg}) = 25.0 \text{ mm Hg}$$

$$\text{Net filtration pressure} = (P_{cap} + \pi_{tissue}) - (P_{tissue} + \pi_{cap})$$

$$(+25.3 \text{ mm Hg}) - (+25.0 \text{ mm Hg}) = +0.3 \text{ mm Hg}$$

Clinically, capillary fluid pressure and plasma colloid osmotic pressure are the most important concepts to a discussion of pathophysiology. Capillary fluid pressure is the blood pressure in the capillary. It is the force pushing fluid from the capillary into the interstitium and is often called the *hydrostatic pressure*. The strength of this force depends on the blood pressure and the resistance within the arterial and venous systems. Pathologic conditions resulting in an increase in either the blood pressure or the resistance to flow can alter this force, increasing it and propelling more fluid into the interstitial space, resulting in the formation of edema.

Plasma proteins are responsible for the plasma colloid osmotic pressure, the primary force resulting in fluid remaining in the capillary. Most plasma proteins normally remain in the capillaries because they are such large molecules that they cannot move through the capillary spaces. The vast majority of plasma protein, by weight, is albumin. Although globulins and fibrinogen have greater molecular weight, albumin is present in plasma in greater quantity. The number of dissolved molecules in the plasma determines the *plasma colloid osmotic pressure.* The number of dissolved molecules in the interstitial space establishes the interstitial fluid colloid osmotic pressure. Plasma has nearly four times the concentration of proteins than does the interstitium. For that reason, plasma colloid osmotic pressure normally exceeds that in the interstitium, favoring fluids remaining in the capillaries.

As previously illustrated, the net filtration pressure in a typical capillary is 0.3 mm Hg. This pressure difference is responsible for producing the fluid excess in the interstitial space, which is then normally absorbed by the lymphatic system for eventual return to the systemic vascular circulation. If the pressures are altered, an even greater pressure gradient may be produced and more fluid moves from the capillaries into the interstitial space. Likewise, a change in the permeability (K) of the capillary wall that allows plasma proteins to leak out, or a reduction in lymphatic flow will allow fluid to collect in the interstitium. In each case, the result is edema, which can occur with many pathologic conditions. When the pathology is an impairment of lymphatic flow allowing fluid to collect in the interstitium, it is more specifically termed **lymphedema.**

Once absorbed into the lymphatic system, interstitial fluid is referred to as *lymph.* It is similar in composition to interstitial fluid but has a lower concentration of protein. Molecules of fat and bacteria are also found in lymph. Lymph circulates throughout the body at a rate of approximately 3 L/day. Lymphatic flow can be increased in several ways: by increasing the capillary pressure, decreasing the plasma colloid osmotic pressure, increasing the interstitial fluid colloid osmotic pressure, or increasing the permeability of the capillaries. The interstitial fluid hydrostatic pressure increases (becomes less negative) when any of these factors changes, producing an increase in lymphatic flow.[1]

KEY POINTS

- Physical laws govern the flow of blood through the circulatory system. Predictions regarding blood flow, blood pressure, and resistance to flow can be made using these laws. The important relationships may be summarized as follows:
  - Flow = pressure/resistance
  - Blood pressure = flow (cardiac output) × resistance
  - Resistance = pressure/flow
- The main factors affecting resistance to flow are the radius and length of the vessels, and blood viscosity and turbulence. Usually, the radius of the vessel is the most important determinant of resistance. It affects resistance inversely and to the fourth power. A small decrease in radius results in a large increase in resistance.
- The velocity of blood flow varies inversely with the total cross-sectional area of the vascular bed. The capillaries have the greatest total cross-sectional area and, therefore, the slowest flow.
- Laplace's law describes the relationships among wall tension, distending pressure, and vessel radius (P = T/r; T = Pr). An increase in radius or distending pressure results in increased wall tension. At critical closing pressure, wall tension overwhelms distending pressure and blood flow ceases.
- The transcapillary exchange of fluid and nutrients is accomplished by the processes of diffusion and filtration. Diffusion refers to movement of solute and is determined by capillary permeability and the size of the concentration gradient. Filtration refers to movement of fluid and is affected in the following ways:
  - Increased capillary fluid pressure and interstitial fluid colloid osmotic pressure enhance filtration.
  - Increased interstitial fluid pressure and plasma colloid osmotic pressure oppose filtration.
  - Increased permeability (K) enhances filtration.

CONTROL OF FLOW

Blood flow throughout the periphery is controlled by central mechanisms that are mediated by the autonomic nervous system, the venous and thoracic pumps, and intrinsic autoregulatory mechanisms. Lymphatic flow is controlled by increasing interstitial fluid colloid osmotic pressure and by the stimulation of the contractile fibers (often called *lymphatic pumps*) as they are stretched. In healthy people, these mechanisms of control respond to changes in the internal and external environments and compensate rapidly and efficiently; however, during states of illness these mechanisms may be inadequate to compensate for alterations in flow.

Control of Blood Flow
Extrinsic Mechanisms

The autonomic nervous system provides the primary extrinsic control of blood flow through the sympathetic nervous system (SNS). Although parasympathetic nervous system (PSNS) innervation is important to the regulation of the heart, it is not important to the regulation of peripheral resistance. Within the medulla, groups of neurons form the *vasomotor center.* This area plays a major role in the maintenance of blood pressure (see Chapter 16). The vasomotor center responds to direct stimulation and to afferent stimuli of both an excitatory and an inhibitory nature. A basal rate of discharge from the vasomotor center results in a continuous minimal level of contraction of vascular smooth muscle, referred to as *vasomotor tone.*

All blood vessels except the small venules and capillaries contain smooth muscle that is innervated by adrenergic fibers from the SNS. Because arteries have the most smooth muscle, they are most affected by SNS stimulation. Veins, by contrast, have little neural innervation, and venoconstriction has a minor role in controlling blood flow except in the skin and the splanchnic circulatory bed of the gut. In general, the release of norepinephrine, the SNS postganglionic neurotransmitter, results in arterial vasoconstriction via the α_1 receptors located on the vascular smooth muscle walls. Likewise, drugs that mimic the α_1-receptor response (α_1 agonists) produce vasoconstriction, increasing vasomotor tone and diastolic blood pressure. Administration of an α_1 antagonist results in the blockade of these receptors and results in vasodilation of the arterial bed, reducing blood pressure.

Although the β_2-adrenergic receptors located on blood vessels in skeletal muscle produce vasodilation when stimulated, they are only minimally affected by endogenous norepinephrine from the SNS. Epinephrine, the endogenous catecholamine released by the adrenal medulla, or its exogenous pharmacologic equivalent (adrenalin), stimulates these receptors, producing vasodilation. Therefore, their major role is not so much to maintain vasomotor tone but to increase nutrient and oxygen supplies to skeletal muscles during periods of increased demand.

Blood flow through the venous system into the right side of the heart is maintained by the pressure gradient from the veins and by the venous and thoracic pumps. Blood is propelled through the circuit, pushed by the force of left ventricular contraction, and moves forward toward the low-pressure side of the pump on the right side of the heart. In the peripheral veins, what is known as the *venous pump* is activated by skeletal muscle activity. Folds in the intimal wall of the veins create valves. Contraction of the skeletal muscles bordering the veins compresses them, forcing the valves open and propelling venous blood back toward the heart. Instigation of the venous pump significantly facilitates venous return. Patients who are immobilized by bed rest lose this valuable mechanism, which results in a decrease in cardiac preload to the right heart and increased work of the heart to maintain the cardiac output. The *thoracic pump* acts to increase venous return to the heart as intrathoracic pressure changes with breathing. Inspiration increases negative intrathoracic pressure, resulting in more venous return (see Chapter 17).

Intrinsic Mechanisms

Autoregulation refers to the ability of blood vessels within organs to maintain a relatively constant blood flow, regardless of changes in arterial pressure. This flow is *relatively* constant because it does have limits; there is a range within which it is maintained, and the range varies slightly from organ to organ. Several processes contribute to the autoregulation of perfusion to meet the needs of individual organs within the body.

It is known that as vascular smooth muscle is stretched, it contracts. Therefore, as arterial pressure rises and arterial walls stretch, contraction is stimulated, producing vasoconstriction. Resistance to flow is also increased with stretch by early closing of precapillary sphincters. This process certainly may contribute to autoregulation, but it is not the primary mechanism.

Over the past several decades, a great deal has been learned about the endothelium of blood vessels. The previous perceptions of the endothelium as an inactive structure, whose function was no more than acting as a barrier between the blood and the more functional layers of the vessel wall, have been proven incorrect.[2] We now understand that the endothelium is a major participant in vascular tone and growth of vascular smooth muscle.[2] The endothelium tissue plays an active role in the immune and inflammatory processes (see Chapter 9), platelet activity in normal coagulation and thrombus formation (see Chapter 14), and arteriosclerosis,[2-4] discussed later in this chapter. In a discussion of autoregulation, the key is the endothelial role in modulating vascular smooth muscle to produce vasoconstriction or vasodilation. The endothelium is capable of sensing alterations of a chemical or physical nature within the vessel and responding to these stimuli directly or through the release of signals that initiate change.[3] Almost all of the vasodilation occurs because of the effect of nitric oxide (NO). NO is a gas present in most body tissues and is produced by the cells of the vascular endothelium. As a gas, it diffuses from the endothelium to the smooth muscle cells, binding to intracellular receptors to impact cytoplasmic Ca^{++} concentration and produce vasodilation.[3-5] Deficits of nitric oxide, or a decreased responsiveness, have been the focus of considerable recent research into the pathogenesis of hypertension (Chapter 16) and heart disease (Chapter 18).[2-7] Other relaxing factors produced by the endothelium include prostacyclin, and endothelium-derived hyperpolarizing factor.[6] Angiotensin II, endothelin, oxygen-derived free radicals, prostacyclin H_2, and thromboxane A_2 are among the constricting factors. The role of angiotensin II (AII) as a constricting factor has been the focus of considerable recent research.[7] Because drugs that block the effects of AII are available and in widespread use, the ability of these drugs to improve peripheral vascular blood flow has been an important finding.[7] In addition to substances produced by the endothelium itself, metabolic by-products (metabolites) or substrates have been found to exert a direct effect, altering blood flow to the area.[1] Metabolites might include carbon dioxide or lactic acid. Histamine and prostaglandins are examples of metabolic substrates. Other substances, such as acetylcholine, bradykinin, histamine, and substance P, exert their effect by increasing the formation of nitric oxide or are themselves generated by nitric oxide.[7] These various chemicals create a balance of forces in health. They may also be affected by aging, disease, or pharmacologic interventions.

A local increase in blood flow is referred to as **hyperemia.** The increase in local blood flow in response to increased metabolic demand is called *active* or *functional* hyperemia. *Reactive* hyperemia occurs when a temporary reduction in blood flow is reversed. The body responds by briefly increasing circulation to the area, resulting in the characteristic flushing seen, for instance, when a tourniquet is removed. The *tissue pressure hypothesis* of autoregulation postulates that an acute increase in the pressure within the arterial system causes an increase in interstitial volume and pressure. This increased tissue pressure, external to the vasculature, results in compression of small vessels, which increases resistance and reduces flow.

Control of Lymphatic Flow

The movement of lymph is expedited by lymphatic pumps. This is a general concept that encompasses the pumping action of the lymphatics themselves and the pumping effect on the lymphatic vessels produced by activity external to them. Like veins, lymphatic vessels have valves on their intimal surface that allow forward movement of fluid to join the venous return to the systemic circulation. Compression of lymphatic channels by adjacent skeletal muscles, the smooth muscle of organs, and the pulsatile movement of arteries force lymph forward. Intrathoracic pressure changes related to breathing increase lymphatic return as well as venous return. Lymphatic flow is therefore enhanced by increased physical activity, increased blood pressure, or increased respiratory rate. Lymphatic contractions are thought to be the primary factor in lymphatic flow. Lymph is propelled forward when lymphatic capillaries contract in response to being stretched. The rate of contractions increases as the volume of lymph increases.

KEY POINTS

- The blood flow through a particular vascular bed is regulated centrally by the autonomic nervous system and locally by the organ or tissue.
- In most vascular beds, the SNS causes constriction, which increases resistance and reduces flow. Smooth muscle cells in these vascular beds have α_1 receptors that bind the SNS neurotransmitter norepinephrine, causing contraction. There is no significant parasympathetic innervation of systemic vessels.
- Autoregulation refers to a tissue's ability to regulate its own flow. Autoregulation allows a tissue to maintain optimal flow despite changes in blood pressure or metabolic demands. In instances of high blood pressure or decreased metabolic demand, the arterioles and precapillary sphincters that control flow to the tissue constrict, reducing flow. In instances of low blood pressure or high demand, vessels dilate, increasing flow.
- Lymphatic vessels maintain flow by contracting when stretched with lymph. Intraluminal valves prevent backflow. External compression by contracting muscles enhances lymph flow.

GENERAL MECHANISMS THAT CAUSE ALTERED FLOW

A reduction in flow through the systemic vasculature results in the impaired ability to transport gases and nutrients to and from body tissues. Cells of the body vary in their oxygen demands. *Hypoxia,* an insufficient supply of oxygen, can occur for many reasons, such as a decrease in hemoglobin formation (see Chapter 13) or diminished oxygen transport in the lungs (see Chapter 21). When hypoxia is a result of a decrease in flow through the arterial system, it is called *ischemia.* Impairment in flow through the venous system interferes with the removal of metabolic waste products and causes fluid pressure to accumulate in the system, a condition known as *venous engorgement* or *venous obstruction.* When the lymphatic circulation is altered, the resulting fluid and pressure changes may be visible locally or systemically.

Blood Vessels: Obstructions

Pathologic processes affecting blood flow may involve impedance of the arterial or venous system. Some obstructions to flow are specific to either the arterial or the venous portion of the system, but most can occur in some form in both. Obstructions to flow that may interfere with arterial or venous flow are presented in detail in the following discussion. Those that are specifically related to one or the other are detailed more fully later in the chapter.

Thrombus

A thrombus is a stationary blood clot formed within a vessel or a chamber of the heart. Thrombosis is initiated by a change in the blood vessel resulting in localized stasis of flow. Inflammation of blood vessels may be the stimulus for thrombosis in either arteries or veins.

Etiology. Thrombosis refers to the pathologic formation of clots at these sites, to differentiate it from the clotting process that takes place as a homeostatic mechanism. Thrombi (blood clots) are composed of aggregated platelets, clotting factors, and fibrin that adhere to vessel walls.[1,8] Thrombi may form in the chambers of the heart in association with certain abnormal heart rhythms (see Chapter 19), following a myocardial infarction, or as a result of damage to heart valves or replacement of heart valves with artificial ones (see Chapter 18). More commonly, thrombi develop in either the arterial or the venous peripheral circulatory systems. Activation of the coagulation cascade within the vessel produces a hypercoagulable state resulting in thrombosis (see Chapter 14, Figure 14-4). Certain drugs, such as oral contraceptives, increase the tendency to form thrombi as well. Thrombosis is also more likely to occur when blood flow slows dramatically or becomes more turbulent, or if there is damage to intimal walls, creating a roughened surface.

Pathogenesis

Arterial. The significance of thrombosis rests in the ability of a clot within a blood vessel to reduce flow and increase turbulence, which enhances thrombus enlargement and the formation of more thrombi. The results of reduced blood flow vary depending on whether the arterial or venous system is involved. If the thrombus forms in the arterial system, decreased distal flow can result in **ischemia.** This is significant in several pathologic conditions, such as acute arterial occlusion (discussed in this chapter). Other examples of arterial thrombosis are explored elsewhere in this text (e.g., myocardial infarction, Chapter 18; stroke, Chapter 44).

Venous. In the venous system, thrombosis alters venous return, impairing removal of metabolic wastes and producing swelling (edema). When inflammation occurs in a vein (**phlebitis**) and is accompanied by the formation of a thrombus, it is called **thrombophlebitis.** The most common cause of thrombophlebitis is the inflammation produced by the presence of a needle or catheter used for intravenous therapy. Thrombosis may also be initiated by a generalized reduction in flow and the accompanying release of vasoactive substances that occur in shock states (see Chapter 20). Systemic derangement in coagulation takes place in disseminated intravascular coagulation, resulting in thrombosis in the microcirculation throughout the body (see Chapter 14). Risk factors associated with both arterial and venous thrombosis are listed in Box 15-1.

Clinical manifestations and treatment. Arterial thrombosis is usually manifested by intermittent claudication (pain with activity) in the affected limb that improves with rest. The limb might also be cool to touch and cyanotic. A late sign is a painful arterial ulcer found usually around one toe.[8]

Symptoms for venous thrombosis may be absent or may be life threatening secondary to pulmonary embolism. Other signs include calf or groin tenderness and swelling of the affected limb with associated

---

BOX 15-1 RISK FACTORS COMMONLY ASSOCIATED WITH THROMBOSIS

General (Arterial and Venous)
Hypercoagulable conditions
- Polycythemia
- Dehydration
- Platelet aggregation

Pump failure
- Heart failure
- Shock

Dysrhythmias
Aging

Trauma, including surgery
Drugs
- Anesthetic agents
- Oral contraceptives
- Tobacco

Arterial
Arteriosclerosis/atherosclerosis

Venous
Immobilization/sedentary lifestyle

---

increased skin temperature. Pain in the calf with dorsiflexion of the foot (Homan sign) appears in 10% of those with thrombophlebitis.

Interventions in the management of thrombus formation may be medical or surgical. Ideally, thrombosis is prevented in high-risk individuals through pharmacologic and other medical interventions. The prophylactic (preventive) interventions may include oral or parenteral anticoagulant therapy, or drugs to block platelet activation and/or aggregation.[9] Risk factors must be addressed. Once a thrombus has formed, anticoagulant therapy at a therapeutic level is initiated to prevent the enlargement of the thrombus and formation of further thrombi. However, these drugs are not effective in dissolving an existing clot. These clots must be removed by the body's own fibrinolytic process, surgically removed, or dissolved by intravenous thrombolytic agents. Anticoagulant therapy is currently used for patients with thrombi in coronary and pulmonary arteries, peripheral arteries in the legs, and cerebral arteries. Their use must be closely supervised; patients receiving thrombolytic therapy are usually in critical care settings.[9] Additional medical prophylactic interventions may include the use of antiembolic stockings or sequential compression devices for immobilized patients, and initiation of ambulation as soon as possible. Surgical interventions, such as removal of the thrombus, may be an option.

Because thrombi partially or completely occlude flow through the involved vessel, they can produce ischemia distal to that point in an artery or congestion proximally in a vein. A thrombus that only partially occludes a vessel continues to be affected by the force of blood flow. Eventually, it may break free from the vessel wall and become an embolus.

Embolus

An embolus is a collection of material that forms a clot within the bloodstream. This traveling clot is propelled forward in the circulatory system by blood flow to a distant point, where it lodges to produce a new site of obstruction.

Etiology and pathogenesis. An embolus is most often a blood clot, a **thromboembolus,** having begun as a thrombus that was subsequently dislodged from the vessel intima or from the valvular leaflets in the heart, or having formed within a chamber of the heart. Thromboemboli from the left side of the heart exit the aorta and most commonly lodge in a cerebral artery, resulting in a *stroke* (see Chapter 44). But most thromboemboli originate in the deep veins of the pelvis and lower extremities. They traverse the venous circulation and return to the right side of the heart, eventually lodging in the arterial side of the pulmonary vasculature and resulting in a pulmonary embolism (see

Chapter 21). A thromboembolus from the right side of the heart will also result in a pulmonary embolism. Thromboemboli from the venous circulation are the most common cause of pulmonary emboli, but the cause may be nonthrombotic, as is the case for tumor, fat, air, amniotic fluid, or bacterial emboli; these are less frequent and are further examined later in this discussion.

Clinical manifestations. An embolism exiting the left ventricle may lodge in the cerebral vasculature, leading to an ischemic stroke. Manifestations differ depending on the area of the brain affected. Symptoms include loss of cognitive function, motor changes, and different levels of sensory loss (see Chapter 44). More often, an embolism leaving the right ventricle lodges in the pulmonary vasculature. This pulmonary embolism may be asymptomatic or present with various signs and symptoms, many of which are vague and nonspecific.[10] Most common is the sudden onset of shortness of breath (dyspnea), increased respiratory rate, and chest pain. It may be a cause of sudden death.[10]

Treatment. Embolectomy, the surgical removal of an embolus, is usually confined to thromboemboli. The use of this surgical technique is contingent on the location of the embolus. In patients who experience repeated emboli, usually originating from the peripheral venous system, a filter (e.g., Greenfield filter) may be surgically implanted in the inferior vena cava.[10] As the blood passes through the filter, emboli are trapped and cannot progress into the pulmonary circulation. The body's own thrombolytic enzyme, plasmin, then destroys the trapped emboli.

Emboli produced by other causes. Various other materials, some totally foreign to the bloodstream, can also form emboli if present in sufficient quantity. Fat emboli are aggregates of fat molecules released into the blood after trauma or surgery involving bone. Most frequently the long bones of the legs are the source of these emboli. Increased pressure generated within the traumatized bone by the inflammatory response forces molecules of fat from the interior of the bone into the bloodstream. Malignant neoplasms can metastasize by various means, one of which is via the blood as tumor emboli. Collections of bacteria and infectious exudate may break free from a source within the circulation, such as the leaflets of the valves of the heart in bacterial endocarditis. Once in the bloodstream, the bacterial emboli continue to travel, eventually occluding circulation and becoming a new site of infection. Air from the external environment is a foreign material when found in the bloodstream as air emboli. Bubbles of air, having most likely entered the blood through an intravenous catheter, come to rest in small blood vessels and obstruct perfusion. It is difficult to identify the specific volume of air that can sufficiently obstruct flow to result in deleterious effects in humans. In animal studies, the quantity of air needed to produce death varies, partially affected by the speed with which it is injected. Under some circumstances, a 5-ml injection of air will result in death of animal models. At other times, a 100-ml bolus of air will not produce adverse effects.[11]

Increased pressure in the abdomen generated during labor and delivery may force amniotic fluid into the bloodstream as emboli. Here the emboli cause a different set of problems. Amniotic fluid cannot perform the functions of the blood in carrying gases and nutrients, but as a fluid, it does not produce obstruction to flow. Instead, the proteins and cells in amniotic fluid act as antigens, initiating an immune response.

Vasospasm

Vasospasm is a sudden constriction of arterial smooth muscle that results in an obstruction to flow. In some cases, vasospasm is sufficient to produce hypoxia distally, as in variant (Prinzmetal) angina (see Chapter 18) or vasospasm of cerebral vessels following a hemorrhagic stroke (see Chapter 44). Frequently, the cause of vasospasm is unknown. Certain individuals may be unusually sensitive to hormonal changes or food additives, which may result in vasospasm of cerebral arteries. The vasodilation following cerebral vasospasm is thought to contribute to migraine headaches. Vasospasm may also be mediated by environmental factors, such as exposure to cold or emotional stress, producing a localized response.

Inflammation

Vasculitis is inflammation of the intima of an artery. Inflammation of the lining of a vein is called **phlebitis.** If superficial, these inflammations may be visible as reddened, tender streaks on the skin. Of more significance is their potential to serve as foci for the thrombotic process.

Arteritis *(angiitis)* is a specific term that identifies an inflammatory process of autoimmune origin in arteries. The initiating stimulus is frequently an infectious process that is viral or bacterial (especially streptococcal), or an adverse response to drugs such as sulfonamides or phenothiazines.

Mechanical Compression

A variety of forces external to the vascular system may result in partial or complete obstruction of blood flow. Trauma may produce direct pressure on a blood vessel, resulting in occlusion. This same effect may result from constriction from casts or tight dressings. Swelling secondary to bleeding or edema within a fascial compartment created by fascial tissue surrounding groups of muscle, or external compression of the compartment by a tight cast, eventually compromises the circulation distally, producing *compartment syndrome* (see Chapter 51). Prolonged occlusion produces neurovascular alterations that can be assessed before the ischemia is irreversible. These alterations are identical to those of acute arterial occlusion, discussed later in this chapter. In an untreated patient, compartment syndrome can result in prolonged hypoxia, ischemia, and necrosis of tissues.

Blood Vessels: Structural Alterations

An assortment of conditions affecting blood vessel structure will produce alterations in blood flow. The structure of arteries or veins may be changed secondary to congenital anomalies or pathologic processes triggered later in life.

Types of Structural Alterations

Valvular incompetence. The intimal folds of veins that form the valves can be damaged, interfering with the effective flow of blood through a portion of the venous system (**valvular incompetence).** The subsequent pathologic processes may affect superficial veins (**varicose veins**) or deep veins (**chronic venous insufficiency),** resulting in severe tissue hypoxia and venous stasis ulcers.

Arteriosclerosis/atherosclerosis. **Arteriosclerosis** is a complex condition that produces structural changes in arteries. **Atherosclerosis,** a specific type of arteriosclerosis, produces an increase in the number of smooth muscle cells and a collection of lipids within the intima of medium- and large-size arteries. This process eventually narrows the lumina and decreases their ability to dilate. Atherosclerotic changes are responsible for or contribute to many diseases throughout the body such as hypertension, renal failure, coronary artery disease (CAD), and cerebrovascular disease.

Aneurysms. An **aneurysm** is a localized dilation of an arterial wall. Aneurysms vary in the severity of their consequences, depending on their size, type, and location. All aneurysms produce an alteration in flow attributable to the changes in vessel diameter. More significant, however, is the fact that the aneurysm represents a weakened area in the artery that may eventually rupture.

Arteriovenous fistulas. An **arteriovenous fistula (AVF)** is an abnormal communication between arteries and veins. It is usually congenital in origin but may result from traumatic injury. Symptoms depend on the size and location of the fistula. Because AVFs provide a shortcut between the two vascular systems, they can result in alterations in oxygenation to the involved tissues and systemic hemodynamic changes. One of the most common and serious types of AVFs is an **arteriovenous malformation (AVM).** An AVM is a tangled knot of arteries and veins found most commonly within the brain vasculature. AVMs may be the underlying cause of such conditions as headaches, hemorrhagic stroke, dementia, or seizures (see Chapters 44 and 45).

Lymphatic Vessels

The lymphatic collection system may be overwhelmed when changes in capillary or interstitial oncotic pressures increase filtration into tissues. The result is **edema,** the collection of an excessive amount of fluid in the interstitial spaces. A wide variety of conditions can result in edema.

When lymphatic flow is altered because of impairment in the circulation of lymph itself, the condition is called **lymphedema.** The result is also an excessive quantity of fluid in the interstitium, but the underlying cause is an obstruction to flow.

KEY POINTS

- Altered blood flow results from obstructive processes. Obstruction results in reduced flow beyond the obstruction (downstream) and increased pressure before the obstruction (upstream).
- In the arterial system, obstruction manifests primarily as distal ischemia. In the venous system, obstruction manifests as edema.
- The causes of vessel obstruction include thrombi, emboli, vasospasm, external compression (e.g., compartment syndrome), and structural alterations (e.g., atherosclerotic plaques, aneurysms).
- Alterations in pressures within the circulatory system or interstitium produce edema, whereas an impairment of the lymphatic system results in lymphedema.

ALTERATIONS IN ARTERIAL FLOW

Alterations in arterial flow result from obstruction (arteriosclerosis/atherosclerosis, inflammation, vasospasm, thrombi, emboli, and acute occlusion) or mechanical alterations (AVFs and aneurysms).

Arteriosclerosis/Atherosclerosis

Etiology and pathogenesis. **Arteriosclerosis** is a generic term meaning "hardening of the arteries" and broadly includes three pathologic processes: Mönckeberg sclerosis (medial calcific sclerosis), arteriolar sclerosis, and atherosclerosis. Mönckeberg sclerosis is a noninflammatory, degenerative disorder in which the media of small- and medium-size arteries becomes calcified.[12] The disease is a risk factor for cardiovascular disease, but the pathology is independent of atherosclerosis. The intimal layer is not a part of the pathogenesis; although the vessel becomes increasingly thickened and rigid, it remains patent because of the changes in the medial layer.[12] Arteriolar sclerosis is characterized by thickening and luminal narrowing of the small arteries that occurs in association with hypertension. However, because hypertension is primarily associated with atherosclerotic changes, this particular pathology is rarely addressed. Atherosclerosis, the most common arteriosclerotic process, affects intermediate-size and large arteries. Smooth muscle cells and lipids collect along the intimal surface, producing a narrowing of the luminal diameter and a reduction in flow (Figure 15-16).

Atherosclerosis is the dominant type of arteriosclerosis. The word is derived from two Greek words: *athero* (gruel or paste) and *sclerosis* (hardness).[13] It is the pathologic origin for the vast majority of arterial disease that is ultimately the leading cause of death in the United States and western Europe, and is increasing in developing countries.[14] Atherosclerosis tends to develop in large- and medium-size arteries, most frequently the coronary, cerebral, carotid, and femoral arteries and the aorta. Most of the mortality associated with atherosclerosis is the result of occlusion of coronary arteries (CAD), producing myocardial ischemia and infarction.[15] The remainder of atherosclerosis-related deaths is secondary to thrombotic or hemorrhagic processes, primarily in the brain (stroke) and extremities, although other organ systems including the kidneys, liver, and gastrointestinal tract are also affected. When atherosclerosis involves the peripheral vascular system, it is most often the lower extremities, and the disease process may be called

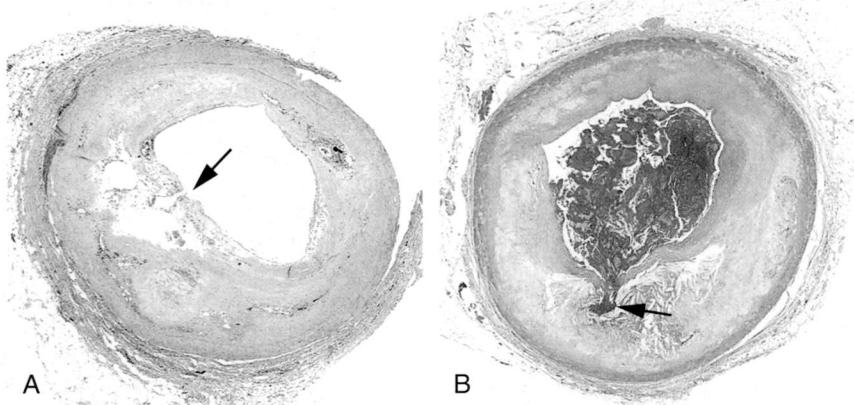

FIGURE 15-16 Atherosclerotic plaque rupture. **A,** Plaque rupture without superimposed thrombus, in a patient who died suddenly. **B,** Acute coronary thrombosis superimposed on an atherosclerotic plaque with focal disruption of the fibrous cap, triggering a fatal myocardial infarction. In both panels **A** and **B,** an *arrow* points to the site of plaque rupture. (**A,** From Kumar V et al: *Robbins basic pathology,* ed 8, Philadelphia, 2007, Saunders, p 351. **B,** Reproduced from Schoen FJ: *Interventional and surgical cardiovascular pathology: clinical correlations and basic principles,* Philadelphia, 1989, Saunders, p 61.)

atherosclerosis obliterans.[8,16,17] Box 15-2 lists the manifestations of this arterial peripheral vascular disease. With arterial occlusion, patients may complain of pain with activity (*intermittent claudication*; Figure 15-17) and also have pain at rest with advanced disease. Peripheral pulses are diminished. Ulceration may occur (Figure 15-18).[8,16-18] Research results from the classic Framingham Study identified the development of lower extremity arterial disease in 5% of the subjects over the course of the 24-year data collection interval.[18]

> ## BOX 15-2 CLINICAL MANIFESTATIONS OF ARTERIAL PERIPHERAL VASCULAR DISEASE
>
> **Skin Assessment**
> - Cool or cold to touch
> - Decreased or absent hair growth
> - Dry, thin, glossy appearance
> - Thickened nails
> - Pallor when elevated, rubor when dependent
> - Diminished or absent pulses
>
> **Pain Assessment**
> - Sharp and stabbing
> - Intensified with activity
> - Relieved by rest or dependency
>
> **Ulcer Assessment**
> - Severely painful
> - Pale, gray base
> - Well-defined edges
> - Located on heels, lateral malleolus, between distal portions of phalanges, pretibial area

Because of the breadth of diseases known to be associated with atherosclerosis, a great deal of research has been accomplished and an understanding of many of the significant aspects of its pathogenesis has evolved. These are summarized in Figure 15-19. The process is initiated by damage to the endothelial surface of the arterial intima, initiating an inflammatory response and an increase in the vessel wall permeability.[19] Many of the risk factors for atherosclerosis discussed later may be initiators of this vessel injury. The increased permeability of the vessel wall allows low-density serum lipoproteins to breach the intimal layer. Leukocytes also are drawn to the site, and along with the endothelial cells, they oxidize the lipids, producing further damage to the vessel wall. Simultaneously, platelets aggregate at the site of injury. They are activated, releasing platelet-derived growth factor (PDGF), which stimulates growth of smooth muscle cells. Media smooth muscle cells, normally confined to the other tunicae, are drawn to the intima where they proliferate. The result is an atherosclerotic *plaque,* primarily composed of smooth muscle cells, lipoproteins, and inflammatory debris. While the plaques slowly enlarge, the orifice of the artery is decreased and perfusion is diminished. In coronary artery disease, the plaque may also acutely rupture, initiating thrombus formation and acute loss of perfusion (see Chapter 18).

Risk factors. Risk factors for the development of atherosclerosis are categorized as modifiable or nonmodifiable, according to the degree to which they can be altered (Box 15-3). Historically, health care has focused on preventing atherosclerosis by the manipulation of predisposing modifiable factors. It often is difficult to isolate the effect of a single risk factor because they usually occur in combination.

The most frequently cited prospective research into atherosclerotic risk factors began in 1948 in Framingham, Massachusetts.[18] Initially, 5209 men and women between the ages of 30 and 59 volunteered to be subjects in the study, the purpose of which was to identify factors associated with the development of atherosclerosis over time. The Framingham Study remains ongoing, with researchers now studying the children and grandchildren of the original participants. Much of the available information regarding atherosclerotic risk factors has its origins in the results of this research.

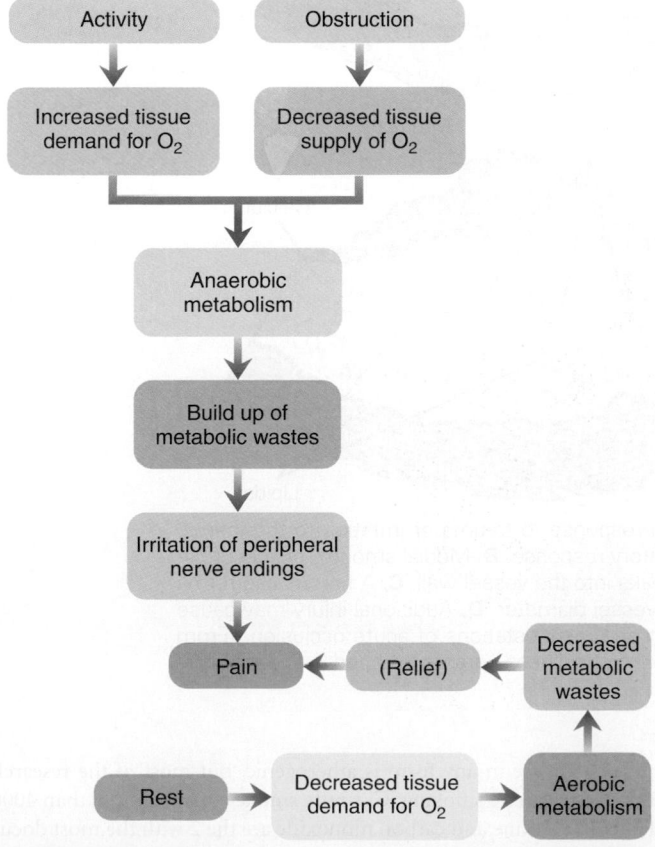

FIGURE 15-17 Pathophysiologic process of intermittent claudication and its relief.

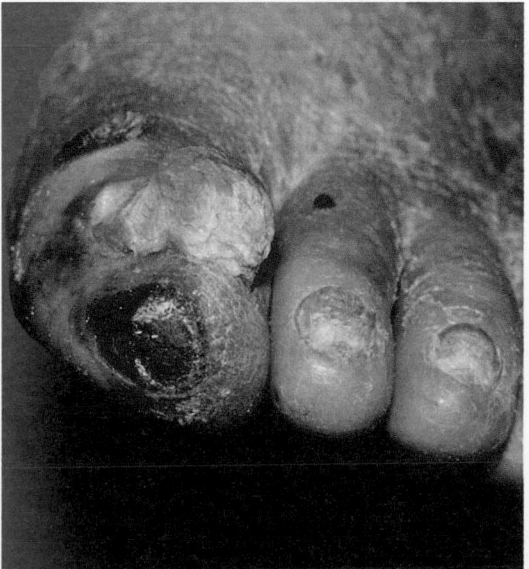

FIGURE 15-18 Arterial ulcer. (From Zipes DP et al: *Braunwald's heart disease: a textbook of cardiovascular medicine,* ed 7, Philadelphia, 2005, Saunders, p 1444.)

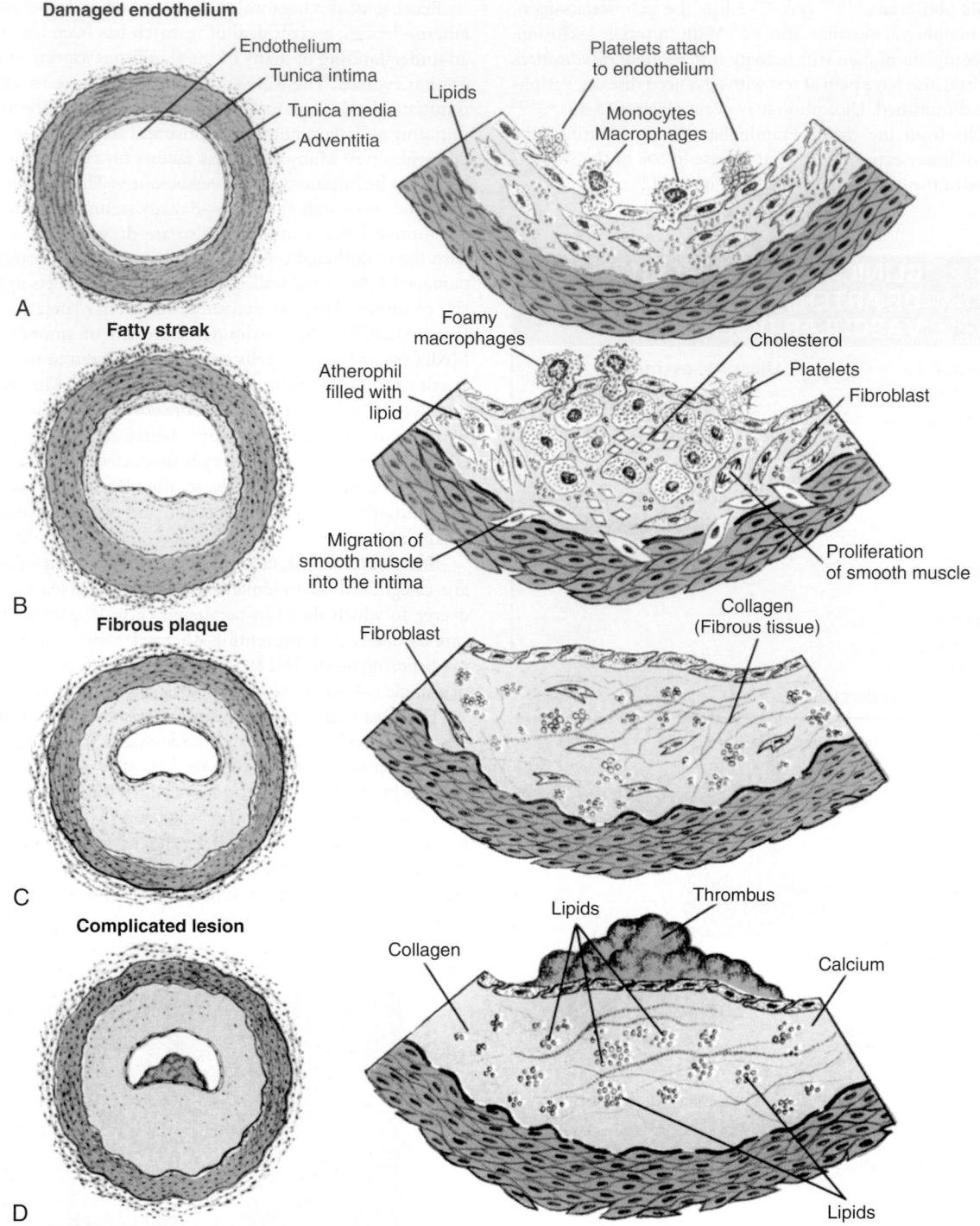

FIGURE 15-19 Pathogenesis of atherosclerosis. **A,** In response to trauma or irritation to the intima, injury stimulates platelet aggregation and the inflammatory response. **B,** Medial smooth muscle proliferates and migrates into the intima; LDL cholesterol leaks into the vessel wall. **C,** A fibrous cap forms over the plaque; the lesion slowly grows to decrease vessel diameter. **D,** Additional injury may cause rupture of the plaque, resulting in thrombus formation and manifestations of acute occlusion. (From Monahan FD et al: Phipps' medical-surgical nursing: health and illness perspectives, ed 8, Philadelphia, 2007, Mosby, p 750.)

Modifiable risk factors. Fortunately, there are far more modifiable risk factors than nonmodifiable ones and the changes individuals make have documented effects in risk reduction for cardiovascular disease. Unfortunately, lifestyle changes are often difficult to make and to maintain.

Tobacco use in any form is atherogenic, but most of the research addresses cigarette smoking. Cigarette smoke contains more than 4000 elements; nicotine and carbon monoxide are the 2 with the most documented damage to blood vessels.[20] Exposure to both active and passive smoke has been found to cause injury, although the precise mechanisms

BOX 15-3   RISK FACTORS ASSOCIATED WITH ATHEROSCLEROSIS

Modifiable Risk Factors
- Smoking
- Elevated blood pressure
- Glucose intolerance
- Elevated cholesterol and low-density lipoproteins
- Decreased physical activity
- Obesity
- Weight fluctuations
- Ineffective stress management

Nonmodifiable Risk Factors
- Age
- Gender
- Ethnicity
- Heredity

have not yet been elucidated. What is known is that cigarette smoking produces injury to the endothelium, generates superoxide anions, decreases both the production and the bioavailability of nitric oxide, and increases the production and release of endothelin. The result is dysfunction of the endothelium, increased tendency to form thromboses, and accelerated atherosclerosis.[20,21] Nicotine also elevates levels of low-density lipoprotein (LDL) cholesterol and triglycerides, and decreases levels of high-density lipoproteins (HDLs). It produces vasospasm and increased platelet aggregation, which can decrease myocardial oxygen supply. Endogenous catecholamines are released with smoking, increasing blood pressure and heart rate, which produce an increase in myocardial oxygen demand. Specifically, smoking increases the risk of coronary heart disease to two to four times normal. Even smoking only a few cigarettes per day is correlated with an increased risk.[22] This risk is even greater if the individual has hypertension, hypercholesterolemia, glucose intolerance, or diabetes because these conditions have a synergistic effect with smoking. Death rates after a myocardial infarction are higher among smokers. Cessation of smoking results in a 50% risk reduction from coronary heart disease within the first year, and a risk equal to that in nonsmokers after 10 years.

Hypertension is both a risk factor for the development of atherosclerosis and an outcome of it.[23] Increases in both systolic and diastolic blood pressure are associated with an increased incidence of atherosclerosis. Diastolic blood pressure elevations are probably more significant because they represent the status of the cardiovascular system when it is at rest. Control of hypertension reduces the injury it produces to the vessel walls and, at a minimum, decreases the rate of atherosclerotic formations. Hypertension is often found in the presence of other risk factors.[23] (See Chapter 16 for a discussion of hypertension.)

Cholesterol, the lipoproteins, and triglycerides are important in the discussion of atherosclerosis. Cholesterol is a necessary component of cellular membranes and is used in the manufacture of steroids within the body.[1] Approximately 40% to 50% of the body's cholesterol is absorbed; the remainder is synthesized by the liver utilizing dietary saturated fats.[24] Cholesterol, like other fats in the bloodstream, is highly insoluble and is transported to and from the body's cells within lipoprotein shells.[24] Although there are several forms of lipoproteins, low-density lipoprotein (LDL) and high-density lipoprotein (HDL) are most important in the discussion of atherosclerosis. Receptors on the surface of the LDL molecule bind with receptors on cell membranes, allowing the molecule to be absorbed into the cell. These receptors abound in the muscle cells of arteries. The protein coat is dissolved and the cholesterol is then used to meet the body's cellular needs. The excess cholesterol that is not removed is stored and acts as a cellular irritant, participating in endothelial injury and plaque formation. Since the early 1990s, evidence of the cardiovascular benefit of controlling serum lipid levels has been mounting.[25] The precise mechanism is

unclear, but the correlation between high serum levels of LDL and cholesterol is clearly significant in the development of atherosclerosis.[24-27] HDL seems to serve as a protective mechanism in the formation of atherosclerosis.[25,26] It is postulated that HDL can remove cholesterol from formations in the arterial walls and transport it back to the liver.[1] Consequently, serum lipid profiles are closely supervised. An acceptable total cholesterol level for an adult who has no coronary disease is less than 200 mg/dl.[27] Levels of LDL-C (low-density lipoprotein cholesterol) are felt to be detrimental if greater than 160 mg/dl. In those with known coronary disease, an LDL-C value of less than 100 mg/dl is thought to be beneficial. Protective levels of HDL are those greater than 45 mg/dl for men and greater than 55 mg/dl for women. A major intervention related to atherosclerosis is encouraging the consumption of a low-fat diet, with those fats being primarily polyunsaturated (from vegetable sources as opposed to animal). Additionally, exercise and weight control are effective in improving lipid profiles. Pharmacologic management of elevated levels of serum lipids is encouraged as a prophylactic intervention.[27]

Glucose intolerance/metabolic syndrome and diabetes mellitus have been found to be associated with elevations in LDL levels and reduced levels of HDL, hypertension, and atherosclerosis.[25,28,29] Glucose intolerance is often a precursor of diabetes mellitus, a disease in which an absolute lack of or a significantly decreased response to insulin produces a derangement in metabolism (see Chapter 41). Atherosclerosis is highly correlated with glucose intolerance, probably because of the alterations in carbohydrate and fat metabolism and the direct damage to vessel basement membrane with elevated blood glucose levels. The incidence of atherosclerotic diseases is much higher among those with diabetes mellitus than in the general population. It does not appear to be related to the degree of hyperglycemia, yet glycemic control has been found to decrease the incidence of acute myocardial infarction.[23,27,28]

Obesity, defined as a body weight 30% or greater than ideal, is thought to be a contributing risk factor for atherosclerosis in that it may accelerate the process. Abdominally distributed obesity is a greater risk than an increase in BMI (body mass index).[22] A desirable waist circumference for men is less than 40 inches, and less than 35 inches for women. Weight gain is associated with increasing serum cholesterol and LDL levels, increasing systolic blood pressure, glucose intolerance, and a sedentary lifestyle.[22]

Physical activity has been found to increase HDL levels, collateral circulation, and vessel size, and to decrease total cholesterol levels, glucose intolerance, body weight, and blood pressure.[22] Clearly, all these findings can retard the development and mitigate the severity of atherosclerosis. Research likewise substantiates physical inactivity as a risk factor for cardiovascular disease.

Stress and mental health have historically received considerable attention as risk factors for atherosclerosis, and this continues to be the case.[22] It is extremely difficult to isolate these factors and examine them quantitatively and qualitatively. Stress results in the release of endogenous catecholamines that contribute to the increased work of the cardiovascular system. Subjectively, the rushed, stressed person is less inclined to exercise and eat wisely and more inclined to smoke and be hypertensive. Recently, depression has been identified as a cardiovascular risk factor.[22] Both stress and depression also may contribute to a delay in seeking treatment.

The importance of managing modifiable risk factors in the reduction of cardiovascular risk cannot be overstated. Recent research continues to substantiate the interrelationship of these risk factors.[29] When dietary fat intake is reduced, concomitant reductions in total serum cholesterol, LDL levels and body weight are predicted. These factors all interact with exercise to predict a decrease in the perception of stress. Stress management is related both to decreased measurements for body weight, total cholesterol and triglycerides, and hemoglobin A_{1C} (an indicator of diabetic glycemic control) and to increased measurements of HDL. Clearly, not only is the reduction of a single risk factor meaningful, but also there is an interactive, additive effect among risk factors.[29]

Nonmodifiable risk factors. Certain risk factors are not modifiable and cannot be manipulated for prevention or to decrease the severity of atherosclerosis and cardiovascular disease. Age, gender, ethnicity, and genetics are interrelated, and their impact as risk factors can be modulated by lifestyle changes.

With aging, changes occur in the arterial walls (see Geriatric Considerations) that predispose to the development of atherosclerosis. Men have a higher incidence of atherosclerosis earlier in life than women, but following menopause, the incidence and prevalence of cardiovascular disease equalize.[15,22] Postmenopausal status is often seen as an independent risk factor for cardiovascular disease, generating increased attention in research regarding the potential cardioprotective role of estrogen.[22,30] At this time, studies indicate postmenopausal women taking either estrogen alone or in combination with progesterone have an increased risk of thrombotic events (myocardial infarction, deep vein thrombosis, ischemic stroke) and of breast cancer. Consequently, such interventions are not recommended for cardiovascular risk reduction.[30]

A strong family history of CAD is an important predictor of its occurrence and subsequent prognosis.[22] The specific mechanism is uncertain, but most likely it is a combination of genetic and environmental factors. Certain of the modifiable risk factors are also known to have a genetic component.

Studies of ethnicity as a nonmodifiable risk factor associated with atherosclerosis have predominantly focused on the increased incidence of CAD and hypertension among black Americans compared with white Americans.[15] Degree of risk differs between Caucasians, African-Americans, Hispanics, and Asians.[31] Prevalence of smoking, diabetes, and hypertension is greater for African-Americans and Hispanics, whereas Caucasians are more likely to have abnormal serum lipid levels. After correction for age, gender, risk factors, and pharmacologic treatment of hyperlipidemia, one study reported the least amount of coronary artery calcification to be among Asian men and women.[31] Historically, American Indians have had very low rates of cardiovascular disease.[32] However, it is now the leading cause of death in this population, with the majority of cardiovascular disease cases in those with diabetes, which has a very high incidence in this population.[32] These disparities highlight the overlap of genetic and environmental factors and illustrate how ethnicity, as an isolated independent variable, is very difficult to evaluate.

Clinical manifestations and diagnosis. Disease manifestations vary with the tissues involved and the severity of altered flow. Atherosclerosis is an underlying pathologic condition for much of the hypertension, renal disease, cardiac disease, peripheral arterial disease, and stroke seen in health care practice.

Approaches to diagnosis and treatment of decreased organ or tissue function vary. Patient history and physical assessment provide significant information. Noninvasive tests such as Doppler flow studies may identify areas of occlusion or diminished flow.[28,33] *Plethysmography* may be used to measure changes in the relative size of extremities associated with blood flow. Ankle pressures are obtained with a blood pressure cuff and Doppler ultrasonography and compared with brachial blood pressures in the ankle-brachial (A/B) index. A normal A/B index is greater than or equal to 1.0; an index less than 1.0 is indicative of diminished arterial flow in the lower extremities. Exercise or stress testing may be performed to evaluate the pain of arterial occlusive disease

(intermittent claudication). Angiography—the radiologic study of blood flow—is the most frequently used diagnostic examination.[28,33] (See Chapter 18 for a discussion of coronary artery disease, Chapter 16 for a discussion of hypertension, Chapter 28 for a discussion of renal failure, and Chapter 44 for a discussion of stroke.)

Treatment. Identification of and interventions directed toward modifiable risk factors are the major thrusts of treatment, regardless of the organs or tissues affected. Nonpharmacologic interventions, such as reduction of body weight, cessation of smoking, implementation of an exercise program, and consumption of a low-fat diet, are the first-line actions.[22,28] Drug therapy to decrease hypercholesterolemia is considered when the nonpharmacologic approaches are found to be ineffective or inadequate, or the presence of additional risk factors indicates that the patient would benefit from such interventions.[22,25,27,28]

A wide variety of additional interventions may be undertaken, depending upon the specific disorder and organ involved. Balloon angioplasty, the surgical radiologic fragmentation of atherosclerotic plaques by inflation of a specially equipped catheter, is commonly performed on both coronary and peripheral arteries.[28] Laser angioplasty is being combined with balloon angioplasty to create an opening in significantly obstructed peripheral vessels before the balloon is inflated. Balloon angioplasty with stent placement is being used. Currently, when balloon angioplasty of the coronary arteries is unacceptable or fails to result in satisfactory improvement, coronary artery bypass graft (CABG) surgery is performed. Peripheral arterial bypass grafts are common interventions for the lower extremities and are named for their sites of origin and termination (e.g., aortofemoral, femoropopliteal).

Thromboangiitis Obliterans (Buerger Disease)

Thromboangiitis obliterans (Buerger disease) is a rare inflammatory condition affecting both small- and medium-size arteries and veins of the upper and lower extremities, producing varying degrees of obstruction.[34,35] Although both arteries and veins are involved, the signs and symptoms relate to obstruction of arterial flow (see Box 15-2).[34,35] The rarity of this disease impacts the availability of research funding; therefore, progress in understanding the pathogenesis is limited.[34] What is known is that this vasculitis is strongly associated with smoking, and that smoking cessation is essential to effective treatment.[34,35] Additionally, pharmacologic interventions currently use prostaglandins. New approaches to angiogenesis have resulted in the development of significant collateral circulation and marked clinical improvement. If patients do not abstain from smoking, the disease is progressive and amputation may be necessary.[34,35]

Raynaud Syndrome

An extreme vasoconstriction producing cessation of flow to the fingers and toes produces the characteristic signs and symptoms of Raynaud syndrome.[36,37] Sometimes earlobes or the tip of the nose are also affected.[37] Attacks are recurrent, usually beginning in adolescence.[36] They are most often initiated by cold or emotional distress.[36,37] The phenomenon is classically characterized by a series of color changes in the involved area, starting with white, corresponding to the vasoconstriction.[37] The affected area then becomes cyanotic, with the desaturation of blood remaining in the area. Finally, the tissue flushes red (reactive hyperemia) with the resumption of perfusion. The attack also commonly affects local nerve function, causing pain and/or numbness.[37]

Raynaud syndrome is more prevalent among women, presenting between puberty and menopause, and there appears to be a genetic predisposition.[36,37] Women have an increase in sympathetic tone of the vessels of the skin, causing young women to have basal cutaneous flows that are half those of young men.[37] Knowledge regarding the complex regulation of local perfusion has expanded over the years since the condition was identified by Maurice Raynaud in 1862.[36,37] The pathogenesis is an interplay of intrinsic structural factors (e.g., inflammatory activation and damage), extrinsic neuroregulation, locally produced mediators, and soluble mediators (including estrogen).[36,37]

Various treatment modalities have been used with differing degrees of success.[36,37] Because the precise cause of Raynaud syndrome is unknown, interventions have been directed to enhancing the circulation. Biofeedback and relaxation techniques may be beneficial. The most widely used drugs are calcium channel blockers, which produce vasodilation by interfering with calcium influx into vascular smooth muscle cells. Sympatholytic drugs have been studied and found to be more effective than placebos. Prostaglandin therapy has proved helpful. Persons with the syndrome are urged to protect themselves from cold temperatures, vibration, and nicotine, and to use stress reduction interventions.[36,37]

Aneurysms

As described previously, aneurysms are localized arterial dilations. The arterial wall deteriorates until it is weakened sufficiently to bulge outward. The underlying cause may be atherosclerotic changes in the vessel, a congenital weakness, or a weakening induced by infection, inflammation, or traumatic injury.[38,39] Aneurysms are most frequently found in the cerebral circulation (circle of Willis or posterior circulation) and in the thoracic and abdominal aorta.[38] Estimates are that between 10 and 15 million individuals are treated for cerebral aneurysms annually, with rupture occurring in 30,000. Mortality and morbidity associated with ruptured cerebral aneurysms are high, so early diagnosis and treatment are most desirable.[38]

Classifications. Aneurysms are classified as true or false, depending on the layers of the arterial wall involved (Figure 15-20). In *true aneurysms,* all three tunicae are involved (intima, media, and adventitia), whereas in *false aneurysms,* at least one tunica is left unaffected. In a false aneurysm, the muscle tissue and fascia often confine the leaking blood, which enhances thrombus formation. False aneurysms are most often caused by trauma rather than vessel disease. True aneurysms are further divided by their shape and their size. In *saccular aneurysms,* the weakening is confined to one side of the vessel, producing a lateral ballooning. *Fusiform aneurysms* represent weakening on both sides of the vessel wall—a central ballooning. A *berry aneurysm* is the most common cerebral aneurysm; it is shaped like a berry, with a neck or stem.[38]

All aneurysms can affect blood flow. Cerebral aneurysms are addressed in detail in Chapter 44. Of significant clinical concern is the *dissecting aortic aneurysm* (see Figure 15-20). Here the tear in the arterial wall creates a channel for blood flow. The tear may be between the intima and media or between the media and adventitia. As more blood escapes into the space, the layers are separated from one another in both directions from the leak, and as the vessel becomes progressively weaker, it may rupture. Rupture can be explained by the law of Laplace—as the radius of the vessel increases, the tension in the wall increases. Rupture of a major vessel such as the aorta carries a high mortality.[39]

Clinical manifestations and diagnosis. Signs and symptoms of a leaking or ruptured cerebral aneurysm are associated with increasing intracranial pressure and hemorrhagic stroke. Dissecting aortic aneurysms often present as sudden, severe, tearing pain that radiates into the back or abdomen. The patient may show signs and symptoms of shock. Renal blood flow or perfusion of the spinal nerves may be compromised, if the descending abdominal aorta is affected. Renal failure or paraplegia may result. If the ascending aorta is affected, arterial blood flow to the head and upper extremities may be affected.

Diagnostic tests are somewhat dependent upon location.[33] Computed tomography (CT) and transesophageal echocardiography (TEE)

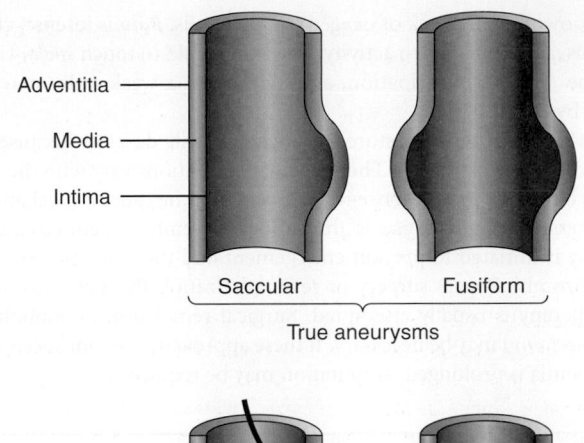
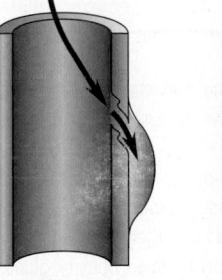
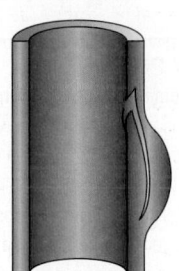

FIGURE 15-20 Classification of aneurysms. All three tunicae are involved in true aneurysms (fusiform and saccular). In false aneurysms, blood escapes between tunica layers and they separate. The muscle and fascia confine the leak; a thrombus forms and seals the leak. In a dissecting aneurysm, a tear in the intima creates a channel into which blood leaks, creating a hematoma. Continued expansion of the hematoma further separates the intima from the other layers, weakening the vessel.

are the most common diagnostic modalities for aortic aneurysms. TEE has proven to be reliable and is immediately available in an emergency setting. For cerebral aneurysms, CT, magnetic resonance imaging (MRI), and cerebral angiography are used.[33,38]

Treatment. Dissecting aortic aneurysms are emergency situations and may be managed medically, surgically, or both. Medical intervention is directed at lowering the blood pressure to decrease the speed and severity of the dissection. Vasodilators are often administered parenterally. Surgical intervention involves resection (removal) of the aneurysm and insertion of a prosthetic graft. This procedure may require an open approach, but as with many surgeries, it may be done with a series of smaller incisions in an endovascular approach.[39] If the aneurysm is extremely large, it may be inoperable.

A variety of interventions are used for cerebral aneurysms; these are briefly addressed in Chapter 44.

Acute Arterial Occlusion

Acute arterial occlusion is an emergency, because it may result in such profound ischemia that the involved limb becomes gangrenous and sepsis may result. Acute arterial occlusion may be caused by a thrombus or embolus lodging in a major artery, or by external mechanical compression producing compartment syndrome. The result is an effective absence of arterial circulation to the extremity. Although it is usually attributable to a thrombus or an embolus, it may occur with vasospastic disease or trauma, as a complication of vascular surgery, or from swelling within a cast or tight dressing.[40]

The classic signs and symptoms of acute arterial occlusion are known as the *six Ps. Pallor* occurs in the involved extremity. The patient may complain of *paresthesia,* and some degree of *paralysis* may be noted, owing to the lack of oxygen to nerve cells. *Pain* is intense, continuous, and unrelated to activity. The skin is cold to touch *(polar)* and may be *pulseless* by palpation, although often a weak pulse may be noted by Doppler.

Perfusion must be restored or necrosis will develop because of ischemia to the extremity. The specific interventions vary with the etiology. Dressings may be loosened or casts cut if the cause is mechanical compression. If the cause is thrombotic or embolic, anticoagulant therapy is initiated to prevent enlargement and the formation of further thrombi. Bypass surgery or revascularization through thrombolytic therapy is usually attempted. Surgical removal of an embolism *(embolectomy)* may be necessary. If these approaches are not successful or ischemia is prolonged, amputation may be required.

KEY POINTS

- Common causes of arterial obstruction are atherosclerosis, inflammation, vasospasm, and aneurysms. Emboli are the usual cause of acute arterial occlusion.
- Atherosclerosis is the most common cause of chronic progressive arterial obstruction. Several risk factors for the development of atherosclerosis have been proposed, among them smoking, hyperlipidemia, male gender, advancing age, sedentary lifestyle, obesity, glucose intolerance, and a family history of cardiovascular disease.
- Acute arterial obstruction is accompanied by the classic manifestations known as the six Ps: pallor, paresthesia, paralysis, pain, pulselessness, and polar (cold to touch).

ALTERATIONS IN VENOUS FLOW

Pathologic venous conditions are the result of obstruction to flow (deep vein thrombosis) or structural alterations (valvular incompetence) and are primarily seen in the lower extremities.

Valvular Incompetence

Etiology and pathogenesis. The intimal surface of veins periodically folds into valves to facilitate efficient flow (Figure 15-21). When the valves are open, blood is propelled forward by the pressure changes exerted by the skeletal muscles and the intraabdominal and intrathoracic pumps. When this pressure decreases, backward flow of blood is prevented by proper closure of the valves (valvular competency). Valvular

incompetence results in *venous insufficiency.* When the superficial veins are involved, the disorder is called **varicose veins. Chronic venous insufficiency** occurs when the deep veins are affected.

The cause of valvular incompetence is the overstretching of the valves as a result of excessive venous pressures. Veins are designed as low-pressure systems. After the blood leaves the high-pressure arterial bed, it passes into the fine capillary network, which slows flow and reduces the pressure. Blood flow through the veins is essentially accomplished by forces outside the veins—the skeletal muscle, intraabdominal and intrathoracic pumps. The highly distensible vein walls are capable of expanding to create a reservoir of blood. When the pressure against which the pumps must push is elevated for a prolonged period, the veins stretch and the valve cusps can no longer meet. Backflow results in further engorgement of the involved veins. The process is most frequently seen in people whose occupations require them to stand for long periods. The effect of gravity on venous flow accentuates the problem. Obesity and pregnancy also elevate venous pressure and may contribute to varicosity formation. As much as 10% of the European and North American population have valvular incompetence.[41]

Clinical manifestations and treatment. Symptoms may include a feeling of heaviness or tension and pruritus. Thrombi can promote valve obstruction and further thrombus formation. In prolonged insufficiency, edema and stasis dermatitis (discoloration along the lower calf to ankle) may develop. Long-term insufficiency can lead to ulcer formation.[41,42]

Prevention interventions include stopping smoking and beginning a walking program. Regular exercise has been shown to decrease future cardiovascular events.[28] Drugs that interfere with platelet aggregation may be initiated, or revascularization procedures may be attempted.[9,28]

Varicose Veins

Etiology and pathogenesis. Varicosities are superficial, darkened, raised, and tortuous veins (Figure 15-22). The greater saphenous vein is primarily affected, although varicosities may also develop in the

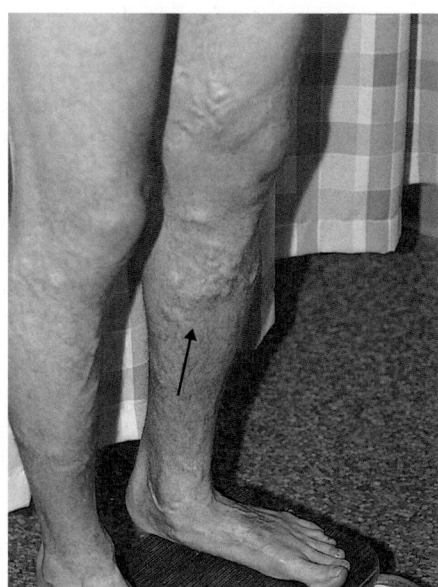

FIGURE 15-22 Varicose veins. Varicosities are best observed when the patient is standing because standing increases the pressure and causes the tortuous veins to become more visible. (From Black JM, Hawks J: *Medical-surgical nursing: clinical management for positive outcomes,* ed 8, Philadelphia, 2008, Saunders, p 1336.)

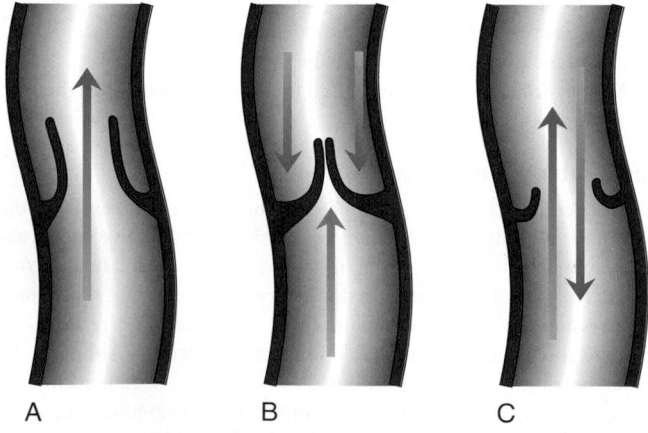

A   B   C

FIGURE 15-21 The venous valves. **A,** Open valves permit forward blood flow. **B,** Closed valves prevent backflow of blood. **C,** Incompetent valves, unable to close fully, allow blood to flow backward, producing venous insufficiency.

lesser saphenous veins. Impaired venous return results in increased capillary pressure, and the involved limb may become edematous.

Clinical manifestations and treatment. Patients may complain of an aching, heavy discomfort, but they are primarily disturbed by the appearance of the varicosities. Venous ulcers may develop.[41,42]

Many of the diagnostic tests used for the arterial system are used for the identification of venous disease. The patient history and physical assessment provide important baseline information. Doppler ultrasound and impedance plethysmography are among the most frequently used assessment tools.[33]

Conservative medical interventions are designed to reduce venous pressure and enhance the venous pump, especially the skeletal muscle pump. Patients are encouraged to elevate their legs whenever possible and to avoid standing for long periods. Elastic stockings can facilitate venous return by enhancing the skeletal muscle pump. When sitting, patients are urged to not cross their knees or ankles. Exercise, particularly walking or swimming, is suggested. If appropriate, weight reduction is recommended.

More aggressive interventions may be initiated in severe cases, as illustrated in Figure 15-22. *Sclerotherapy* involves the injection of a chemical that initiates an inflammatory process and subsequent compression dressings force the lumen to collapse.[28] The intima adheres to itself and heals, and the vein is obliterated. Collateral venous circulation meets the need for venous return from the extremity. Surgical interventions include *vein stripping* and *vein ligation*. These are commonly performed as outpatient procedures and are often combined with sclerotherapy. Both of these treatment modalities depend on the presence of adequate deep venous structures to provide alternate routes for venous drainage.[28]

Chronic Venous Insufficiency

Etiology and pathogenesis. **Chronic venous insufficiency** results when valvular incompetence involves the deep veins (superficial femoral, anterior and posterior tibial, peroneal) of the legs.[42] Communicating or perforating veins provide direct access between the superficial and deep veins.[1,42] Because the pressure in the superficial veins remains elevated for a prolonged period, the deep veins are eventually affected.[42] Individuals with chronic venous insufficiency often also have heart disease and a history of extremity trauma and phlebitis. Previous deep vein thrombosis is a risk factor.[42]

Clinical manifestations and treatment. Venous stasis ulcers also develop as superficial veins rupture with the increased pressures associated with activity.[41,42] The skin pigmentation becomes brown as small veins rupture, leaking red blood cells, which are eventually broken down. Defining characteristics of chronic venous insufficiency are listed in Box 15-4.

Chronic venous insufficiency is primarily diagnosed clinically, but if necessary, ultrasound is considered the best method of evaluation.[42] Many of the diagnostic techniques described for varicose veins may prove helpful, including Doppler ultrasound and impedance plethysmography.[42] Treatment of venous ulcers is challenging and incorporates the use of compression as its foundation.[41,42] Venous ulcers are prone to secondary infection, usually by *Staphylococcus aureus*, *Pseudomonas aeruginosa*, or β-hemolytic streptococci, requiring systemic antibiotic therapy.[41] Other interventions previously described for superficial varicosities also are used for chronic venous insufficiency.

Deep Vein Thrombosis

Etiology and pathogenesis. The pathophysiologic process of thrombus formation has been previously described. Acute venous obstruction is most frequently secondary to a thrombus in a deep vein of the lower extremities. Upper extremities are less frequently affected by deep vein thrombosis.

Clinical manifestations and treatment. Deep vein thrombosis of the legs may be asymptomatic. Signs and symptoms, if present, typically include edema, manifestations of local inflammation, and possible dilated superficial veins secondary to the increased venous pressure.[28] Pain may be present owing to pressure on adjacent nerves and the inflammatory process.

Deep vein thrombosis is treated aggressively; deep vein thrombosis of the lower extremities and pelvic veins is the most frequent source of pulmonary emboli. Patients are often hospitalized so that intravenous anticoagulation therapy may be initiated; otherwise, they are treated on an outpatient basis with oral anticoagulants.[9,28] Patients who have previously developed deep vein thromboses are at risk for further hypercoagulation and may undergo long-term prophylactic anticoagulation with antiplatelet therapy and parenteral anticoagulants with subsequent hospitalization for any reason.[9,28]

KEY POINTS

- Common causes of venous obstruction are incompetent valves (as may occur with obesity, pregnancy, right heart failure, or prolonged standing), producing varicose veins and chronic venous insufficiency, and obstruction by deep vein thrombosis.
- Edema, venous stasis ulcers, and pain usually accompany chronic venous obstruction.
- Deep vein thrombosis is potentially life threatening because of the likelihood of embolization to the pulmonary circulation. It is treated aggressively with the administration of anticoagulants.

ALTERATIONS IN LYMPHATIC FLOW

Lymphedema

Etiology and pathogenesis. Lymphedema occurs when the normal flow of lymph is obstructed or altered in some fashion (Figure 15-23).[43] This results in the collection of lymphatic fluid in the interstitium, initiating an inflammatory response, hypertrophy of subcutaneous adipose tissue, and fibrotic changes.[43] Primary lymphedema

---

BOX 15-4 DEFINING CHARACTERISTICS OF CHRONIC VENOUS INSUFFICIENCY

Skin Assessment
- Warm, tough, and thickened to touch
- Pigmented areas, reddish brown
- Edema, especially at end of day
- Visible healed ulcers
- Evidence of varicose veins may be present

Pain Assessment
- Aching, cramping
- Sometimes decreases with ambulation
- Relieved by elevation

Ulcer Assessment
- Moderately painful
- Pink-red base
- Irregular, uneven edges
- Located on medial malleolus

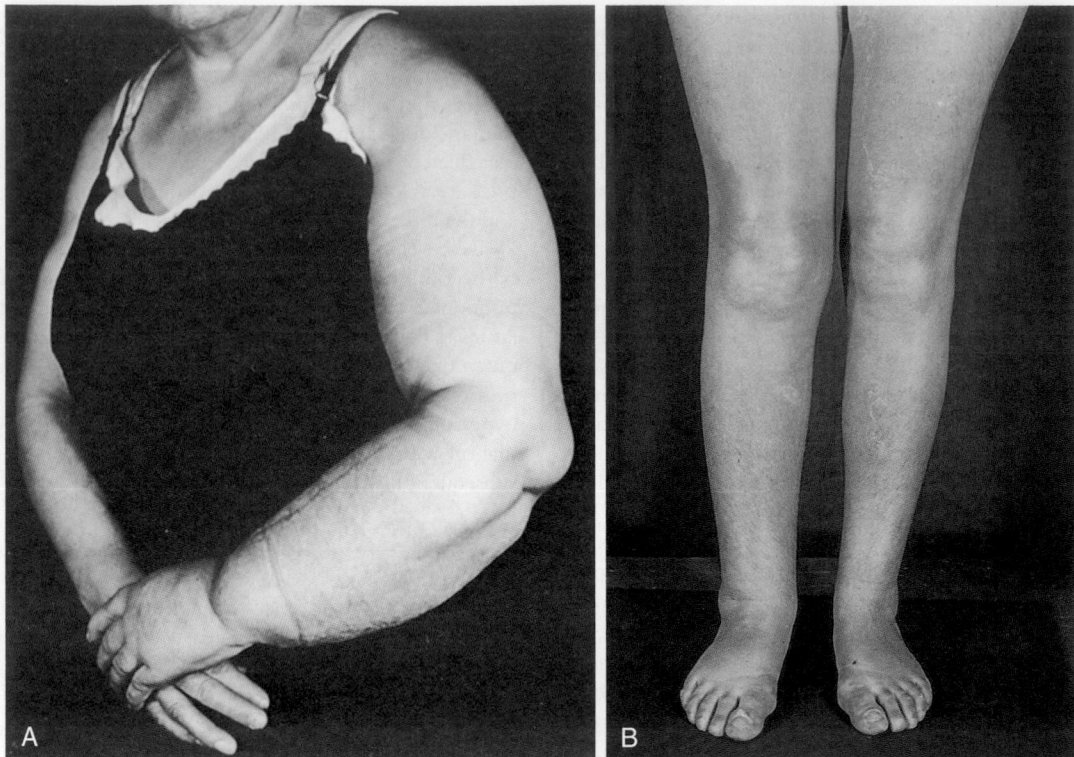

FIGURE 15-23 Types of lymphedema. **A,** Lymphedema of an arm secondary to surgical alterations in the lymphatic system associated with mastectomy. **B,** Lymphedema of a leg. (From Black JM, Hawks J: *Medical-surgical nursing: clinical management for positive outcomes,* ed 8, Philadelphia, 2008, Saunders, p 1339.)

is related to a congenital anomaly or dysfunction of the lymphatic system. Secondary lymphedema develops in association with a disease process or is iatrogenic (a consequence of medical intervention) in origin. Throughout the world, secondary lymphedema is most commonly caused by an infection by filarial worms that migrate to the nodes of the lymphatic system, producing an obstruction of flow. Infection by this nematode *(Wuchereria bancrofti)* affects more than 90 million people worldwide. In the United States, secondary lymphedema is most frequently caused by the surgical removal of lymph nodes, as with breast cancer, or by the destruction of the lymphatics from radiation therapy in the management of various malignancies.[43] This has been reported to develop in 24% to 49% of women after mastectomy and in 4% to 28% of women after lumpectomy.[43]

    Clinical manifestations, diagnosis, and treatment. Most often, lymphedema affects the extremities, but it may be found in the region of the head and neck, trunk, or genitalia.[43] Initially it presents as a soft, pitting edema but as it progresses the inflammatory response is activated and lipogenesis, fat deposition, and fibrotic changes occur.[43] Without early diagnosis and treatment, lymphedema may progress from an acute problem to a chronic one, where congestion produces thick and roughened skin *(brawny edema)* and a large deformed limb.

    Diagnosis is primarily one of exclusion, with other causes of localized edema being ruled out.[43] A complete history and physical examination will allow the elimination of cardiac, renal, and peripheral vascular etiologies. The primary diagnostic test uses the injection of radioisotopes (lymphoscintigram) to assess the overall function of the lymphatic system. Ultrasound, duplex ultrasound, CT, and MRI are additional options and produce unique results.[43]

    There is no cure for lymphedema; interventions are both medical and surgical.[43] Medical treatment includes use of external pneumatic compression devices, elastic stockings, and exercise. Decongestive lymphatic therapy (DLT) or complete decongestive physiotherapy (CDP) combines skin care, massage, compression dressings, and exercise. For many individuals, this therapy results in a 40% to 60% reduction in edema. At this time, no medication has been approved for lymphedema therapy by the Food and Drug Administration (FDA); although diuretics have been used with minimal effect, they are not recommended. Surgical interventions are limited to very select patients, as they may actually be harmful. Resections (debulking) remove subcutaneous tissue and bypass procedures use lymphatic-venous anastomosis.[43] A new approach involves the use of liposuction for the removal of subcutaneous fatty tissue.[43]

KEY POINTS
- Obstruction of lymph flow is most commonly the result of surgical removal of, or radiation damage to, lymphatic vessels during treatment of cancer.
- Manifestations of lymphatic obstruction include regional edema and thickened subcutaneous tissue.

SUMMARY

The circulatory system is organized to facilitate its dual functions of oxygen and nutrient transport and metabolic waste product removal. The arrangement and unique structure of the circulatory vessels permit these functions to be accomplished.

An understanding of the principles and control of flow aids in the comprehension of the pathologic conditions that result in alterations in flow. Principles of flow, or the hemodynamics of the circulation, include concepts and physical laws relating to relationships of flow, pressure and resistance, velocity, laminar and turbulent flow, and wall tension and compliance. Control of blood flow occurs through both extrinsic and intrinsic mechanisms. Lymphatic flow is controlled through the lymphatic pump system, governed by skeletal muscle, and the smooth muscle of organs and arteries.

Pathophysiologic changes that result in alterations in blood flow can be classified as being caused by either obstruction (thrombosis, emboli, vasospasm, inflammation, mechanical compression) or structural alterations (valvular incompetence, arteriosclerosis/atherosclerosis, aneurysms, AVFs). Conditions that produce alterations in arterial or venous flow are the result of one of these primary processes. Pathology of the lymphatic system is essentially the result of disruption of the normal pressure relationships or an obstruction within the circulatory system; proper functioning of the lymphatic system depends on the appropriate functioning of the vascular system.

REFERENCES

1. Guyton AC, Hall JE: *Textbook of medical physiology*, ed 12, Philadelphia, 2011, Saunders.
2. Mensah GA: Healthy endothelium: the scientific basis for cardiovascular health promotion and chronic disease prevention, *Vasc Pharmacol* 46:310–314, 2007.
3. Victor VM, et al: Regulation of oxygen distribution in tissues by endothelial nitric oxide, *Circ Res* 104:1178–1183, 2009.
4. Rajendran S, Chirkov YY: Platelet hyperaggregability: impaired responsiveness to nitric oxide ("platlet NO resistance") as a therapeutic target, *Cardiovasc Drugs Ther 22(3):EPub*, 2008, .
5. Nohria A, et al: Rho kinase inhibition improves endothelial function in human subjects with coronary artery disease, *Circ Res* 291:1426–1432, 2006.
6. Warnholtz A, et al: AT 1-receptor blockade with irbesartan improves peripheral but not coronary endothelial dysfunction in patients with stable coronary artery disease, *Atherosclerosis* 194:439–445, 2007.
7. Oka RK: Peripheral arterial disease in older adults: management of cardiovascular disease risk factors, *J Cardiovasc Nurs* 21:S15–S20, 2006.
8. McKenry L, Tessier E, Hogan MA: *Mosby's pharmacology in nursing*, ed 22, Philadelphia, 2006, Mosby.
9. Cloutier LM: Diagnosis of pulmonary embolism, *Clin J Oncol Nurs* 11:343–348, 2007.
10. Ganong WF: *Review of medical physiology*, ed 23, New York, 2009, McGraw-Hill.
11. Couri CBE, et al: Mönckeberg's sclerosis—is the artery the only target of calcification? *BMC Cardiovasc Disord* 5:34, 2005. Available at www.biomedcentral.com/1471-2261/5/342005. Accessed 8/11/11.
12. American Heart Association: *Atherosclerosis*. Available at www.heart.org/HEARTORG/Conditions/Cholesterol/WhyCholesterolMatters/Atherosclerosis_UCM_305564_Article.jsp.Accessed 8/11/11.
13. Bukhman G, Kidder A: Cardiovascular health and global equity, *Am J Pub Health* 98:44–54, 2008.
14. Roger VL, et al: Heart disease and stroke statistics 2011 update: a report from the American Heart Association, *Circulation* 123(4):e18, e209, 2011 Feb1. Accessed 8/11/11.
15. DiSabatino A, Vassey J: Innovations in PAD therapy: make sure you're up to date on peripheral arterial disease, *Nursing* 38:10–13, 2008.
16. Coughlin PA, et al: Risk factor awareness in patients with peripheral arterial disease, *J Cardiovasc Surg* 48:735–740, 2007.
17. Dawber TR: *The Framingham Study: the epidemiology of atherosclerotic disease*, Cambridge, MA, 1980, Harvard University Press.
18. Libby P: Inflammatory mechanisms: the molecular basis of inflammation and disease, *Nutr Rev* 65:S140–S146, 2007.
19. Mazzone P, et al: Pathophysiological impact of cigarette smoke exposure on the cerebrovascular system with a focus on the blood-brain barrier: expanding the awareness of smoking toxicity in an underappreciated area, *Int J Environ Res Public Health* 7:4111–4126, 2010.
20. Mercado C, Jaimes EA: Cigarette smoking as a risk factor for atherosclerosis and renal disease: novel pathogenic insights, *Curr Hyperten Rep* 9:66–72, 2007.
21. Cheek D, Sherrod M, Tester J: Women and heart disease: what's new? *Nursing* 38:36–42, 2008.
22. Chobanian AV: Seventh Report of the Joint National Committee on Prevention, Detection, Evaluation, and Treatment of High Blood Pressure: the JNC 7 complete report, *Hypertension* 42:1206–1252, 2003.
23. Pottie A: Measuring cholesterol levels, *Nurs Stand* 21:42–47, 2007.
24. Keevil JG, et al: Implications of cardiac risk and low-density lipoprotein cholesterol distributions in the United States for the diagnosis and treatment of dyslipidemia: data from National Health and Nutrition Examination Survey 1999-2002, *Circulation* 115:1363–1370, 2007. Epub.
25. Evered A: Understanding cholesterol and its role in heart disease, *Nurs Times* 103:28–29, 2007.
26. Stone NJ, Bilek S, Rosenbaum S: Recent National Cholesterol Education Program Adult Treatment Panel III Update: Adjustments and options, *Am J Cardiol* 96(suppl):53E–59E, 2005.
27. Monahan FD, et al: *Phipps' medical-surgical nursing: health and illness perspectives*, ed 8, Philadelphia, 2007, Mosby.
28. Daubenmier JJ, et al: The contribution of changes in diet, exercise, and stress management to changes in coronary risk in women and men in the multisite lifestyle intervention program, *Ann Behav Med* 33:57–68, 2007.
29. Rossouw J, et al: Postmenopausal hormone therapy and risk of cardiovascular disease by age and years since menopause, *JAMA* 297:1465–1477, 2007.
30. Budoff MJ, et al: Ethnic differences of the presence and severity of coronary atherosclerosis, *Atherosclerosis* 187:343–350, 2006.
31. Carson AP, et al: Ethnic differences in hypertension incidence among middle aged and older adults: the multi ethnic study of atherosclerosis, *Hypertension* 57:1101–1107, 2011.
32. Pagana KD, Pagana TJ: *Mosby's manual of diagnostic and laboratory tests*, ed 3, St Louis, 2008, Mosby.
33. Piazza G, Creager MA: Thromboangiitis obliterans, *Circulation* 121(16):1851–1861, 2010.
34. Puéchal X, Fiessinger JN: Thromboangiitis obliterans or Buerger's disease: challenges for the rheumatologist, *Rheumatology (Oxford)* 46:192–199, 2007.
35. Baumhakel M, Böhm M: Recent achievements in the management of Raynaud's phenomenon, *Vasc Health Risk Manag* 6:207–210, 2010.
36. Cooke JP, Marshall JM: Mechanisms of Raynaud's disease, *Vasc Med* 10:293–307, 2005.
37. Wright I: Cerebral aneurysm—treatment and perioperative nursing care, *AORN J* 85:1172–1186, 2007.
38. Donato G, et al: Abdominal aortic aneurysm repair in octogenarians: mith (sic) or reality? *J Cardiovasc Surg* 48:697–703, 2007.
39. Klonaris C, et al: Changing patterns in the etiology of acute lower limb ischemia, *Int Angiol* 26:49–52, 2007.
40. Grey JE, Enoch S, Harding KG: Venous and arterial leg ulcers, *BMJ* 332:347–350, 2006.
41. Etufugh CN, Phillips TJ: Venous ulcers, *Clin Dermatol* 25:121–130, 2007.
42. Warren AG, et al: Lymphedema: a comprehensive review, *Ann Plast Surg* 59:464–472, 2007.
43. Gary DE: Lymphedema diagnosis and management, *J Am Acad Nurse Pract* 19:72–78, 2007.

Alterations in Blood Pressure

Robin Beeman

evolve WEBSITE

http://evolve.elsevier.com/Copstead/
- Review Questions and Answers
- Glossary (with audio pronunciations for selected terms)
- Animations
- Case Studies
- Key Points Review

KEY QUESTIONS

- How do changes in cardiac output and systemic vascular resistance affect blood pressure?
- How is blood pressure regulated on a short- and long-term basis?
- What are the risk factors for the development of primary hypertension?
- How is secondary hypertension defined, and what are the common etiologies?
- How is hypertension detected, classified, and managed?

- What are the end-organ consequences of inadequately controlled hypertension?
- What are the differences between hypertensive emergency and hypertensive urgency and how are they managed?
- What are the risk factors for orthostatic hypotension, and how is the condition managed?

CHAPTER OUTLINE

Meeting the needs of the body's tissues for oxygen and nutrients requires both adequate blood flow at the tissue level and sufficient perfusion pressure systemically to force that blood forward. The systemic arterial blood pressure provides that momentum, and the tissues depend on its preservation to ensure their metabolic needs are met. This maintenance requires a complex regulatory system. The body's organs can be damaged if the perfusion pressure is insufficient or if it is excessive.

ARTERIAL BLOOD PRESSURE

As described in Chapter 15, oxygenated blood is propelled from the left side of the heart into the arterial circulatory system, and following a pressure gradient, travels to the capillary beds of the body's tissues (Figure 16-1). There, oxygen and nutrients are exchanged for metabolic wastes, and the blood then returns to the right side of the heart via the venous circulatory system, where it passes through the lungs to

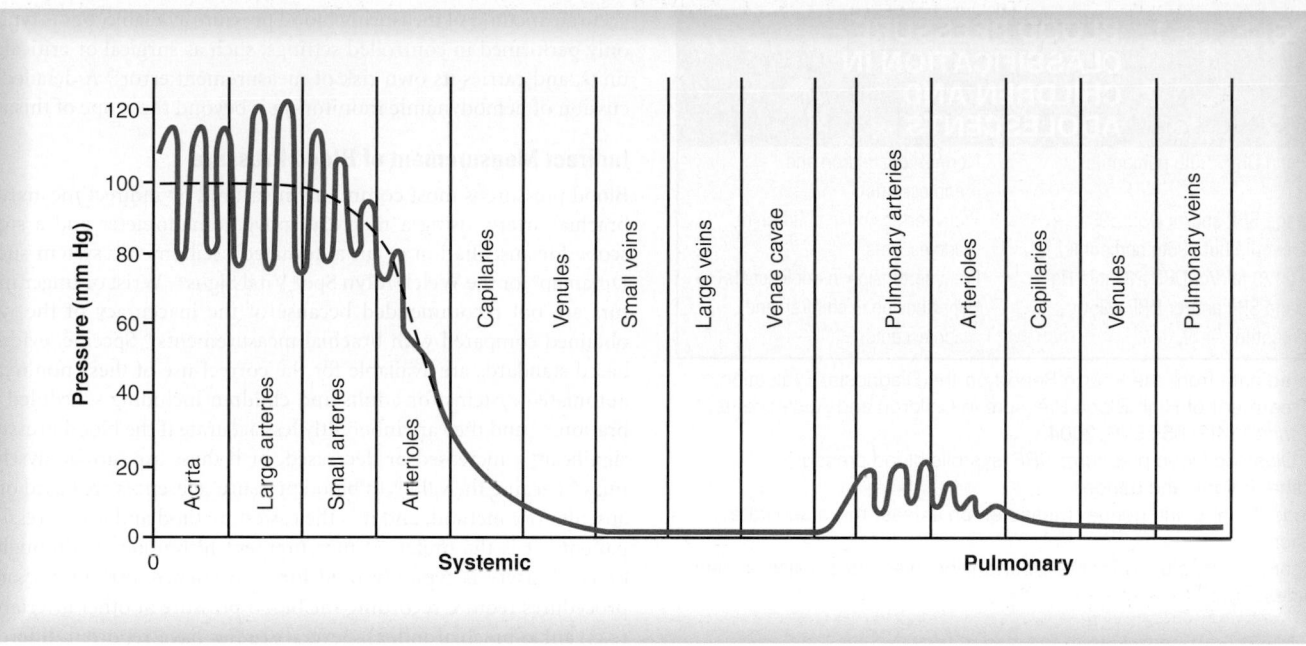

FIGURE 16-1 Normal pressures throughout the vascular system in the supine position. (From Hall JE: *Guyton and Hall Textbook of medical physiology,* ed 12, Philadelphia, 2011, Saunders.)

repeat the process. It is the pressure difference between the left and right sides of the heart that produces the gradient allowing this systemic movement of blood. The arterial blood pressure is produced by the force of left ventricular contraction overcoming the resistance of the aorta to open the aortic valve, and is the pressure maintained in the arterial system throughout the cardiac cycle.

Determinants of Systemic Blood Pressure

The systemic arterial blood pressure is the physiologic result of the cardiac output and the resistance to the ejection of blood from the heart.[1] Cardiac output (CO) is the product of two variables: stroke volume (SV) and heart rate (HR) (CO = SV × HR). SV is the specific volume of blood leaving the heart with each contraction, which itself is determined by the volume of blood in the heart before systole (end-diastolic volume) and the contractility of the myocardium.[1] The end-diastolic volume is determined by the amount of blood returned to the heart between contractions, and is typically called the heart's *preload.* Stroke volume multiplied by the number of contractions of the heart per minute (heart rate) determines the amount of blood leaving the heart—the cardiac output, measured in liters per minute. The resistance to ejection into the arterial circulation is known as the *systemic vascular resistance* (SVR) and is determined by the radius of arteries and the degree of vessel compliance. SVR is synonymous with cardiac *afterload,* and can be altered by constricting or relaxing (dilating) arterial smooth muscle. It can be calculated by using a derivation of Poiseuille's law (see Chapter 15). This physical law states that in a tube with laminar flow, resistance is primarily determined by three factors: the radius of the tube, the length of the tube, and the viscosity of the fluid. Applied to SVR, because the viscosity of the blood and the total length of the arterial system are normally relatively constant, the radius of the arterioles becomes the major determinant of resistance. Therefore, the formula for blood pressure is: BP = CO × SVR. Alteration in any one of these variables will result in a change in blood pressure. This basic concept is important to normal physiologic function, disorders of blood pressure, and the therapeutic interventions undertaken to treat them. The pulmonary vascular bed contributes minimally to total systemic

resistance and is seen as a separate resistance system, called pulmonary vascular resistance (PVR). It has its own pathology discussed in Chapter 21.

Measurement of Blood Pressure
Components of Blood Pressure Measurement

Arterial blood pressure is measured from its highest point during cardiac systole to its lowest during diastole. These are referred to as *systolic pressure* and *diastolic pressure,* respectively, and are measured in millimeters of mercury (mm Hg). During ventricular contraction, the pressure in the aorta rises to an average peak value of approximately 110 mm Hg in the adult[1] (see Figure 16-1). Whatever this peak pressure may be, it is referred to as the systolic blood pressure. The smooth muscle of the aorta passively recoils from this point, ejecting blood forward into the peripheral arteries at that given pressure. Stroke volume is the primary factor impacting systolic pressure; an increase or decrease in SV produces a corresponding change in systolic blood pressure. During ventricular diastole, the pressure in the arterial system falls to an average minimum value of 70 mm Hg in the adult. The value of this minimum pressure is called the *diastolic blood pressure.* SVR is the major determinant of diastolic blood pressure; an increase or decrease in diastolic pressure is the result of a corresponding increase or decrease in arterial resistance (SVR). The difference between systolic and diastolic blood pressure is termed the *pulse pressure.*[1] Therefore, the pulse pressure for a systolic pressure of 110 mm Hg and a diastolic pressure of 70 mm Hg would be 40 mm Hg.

Systolic and diastolic values are normed by age. Standards for the identification of normal blood pressure and levels of abnormal elevation have been established. The most precise standards for children are those based on height, age, and gender[2,3] (Table 16-1). Standards for blood pressure have likewise been determined for the adult[4] (Table 16-2).

Mean arterial pressure (MAP) is the calculated average pressure within the circulatory system throughout the cardiac cycle. Because more time is spent in diastole than in systole, MAP is not the arithmetic average of diastolic and systolic pressure but rather reflects the relative

TABLE 16-1 BLOOD PRESSURE CLASSIFICATION IN CHILDREN AND ADOLESCENTS

SBP and DBP <90th percentile*	Normal for children and adolescents
Average SBP and/or DBP ≥90th percentile but <95th percentile†	Prehypertension in children or adolescents
SBP ≥120 and/or DBP ≥80 mm Hg	Prehypertension in adolescents‡
Average SBP and/or DBP ≥95th percentile†	Hypertension in children and adolescents

Selected data from the Fourth Report on the Diagnosis, Evaluation, and Treatment of High Blood Pressure in Children and Adolescents, *Pediatrics* 114(2):555-576, 2004.
DBP, Diastolic blood pressure; *SBP*, systolic blood pressure.
*For age, height, and gender.
†For age, height, and gender measured on at least three separate occasions.
‡The same criteria used for prehypertension in adults are also applied to adolescents.

TABLE 16-2 BLOOD PRESSURE CLASSIFICATION IN ADULTS

CATEGORY	SBP (mm Hg)*	DBP (mm Hg)*
Normal	<120	<80
Prehypertension	120-139	80-89
Stage 1 hypertension	140-159	90-99
Stage 2 hypertension	≥160	≥100

From Chobanian AV: Seventh Report of the Joint National Committee on Prevention, Detection, Evaluation, and Treatment of High Blood Pressure: The JNC 7 Complete Report, *Hypertension* 42:1206-1252, 2003.
DBP, Diastolic blood pressure; *SBP*, systolic blood pressure.
*Classification determined by the higher value.

time spent in each portion of the cardiac cycle.[5] The calculation may be performed by computer during direct arterial blood pressure measurement, as described below, but is most conveniently determined by a simple formula using the values of blood pressure obtained indirectly. Several formulas are available, and they may use systolic, diastolic, or pulse pressures; the most common formula uses the systolic and diastolic pressures as follows:

$$\frac{(2 \times \text{diastolic pressure}) + \text{systolic pressure}}{3}$$

For a person with a systolic pressure of 110 mm Hg and a diastolic pressure of 70 mm Hg, the MAP would be:

$$(2 \times 70) + 110 = 250/3 \text{ or approximately 83 mm Hg}$$

MAP is used clinically as part of cardiovascular assessment and in the incremental adjustment (titration) of parenterally administered vasoactive drugs.

Direct Measurement of Blood Pressure

Direct measurement of blood pressure is one aspect of hemodynamic monitoring and requires an intraarterial catheter and specialized equipment to transduce the arterial fluid pulsations into electrical signals. The catheter most often is placed in the radial artery. These signals are then displayed on a computer screen as waveforms, and the systolic, diastolic, and MAPs are digitally represented. This is the most accurate method of measuring blood pressure available, but is typically only performed in controlled settings, such as surgical or critical care units, and carries its own risk of measurement error.[5] A detailed discussion of hemodynamic monitoring is beyond the scope of this text.

Indirect Measurement of Blood Pressure

Blood pressure is most commonly measured by indirect means at the brachial artery, using a mercury sphygmomanometer and a stethoscope for auscultation or an automated oscillometric system such as Dinamap® or the Welch Allyn Spot Vital Signs®. Wrist or finger monitors are not recommended because of the inaccuracy of the values obtained compared with brachial measurements.[6] Specific, evidence-based standards are available for the correct use of these noninvasive automated systems for adults and children including scheduled calibration,[6-8] and they are inherently less accurate if the blood pressure is significantly increased or decreased, or if there are cardiac dysrhythmias.[8] Because the values in blood pressure references are based on the auscultatory method, and it is the easiest method and least stressful to patients, it is the preferred measurement technique.[7,9] Although the brachial artery is typically used for convenience, certain assessment procedures require recording the blood pressure at other arterial sites (e.g., ankle-brachial index). Several studies have reported differences between the right and left arm pressures, but no pattern of differences is evident.[6] Other studies report that in the absence of disease, systolic pressures do not differ significantly at a clinical or statistical level between the right and left arms.[10] In practice, it is recommended that blood pressures be initially taken in both arms and the arm with the highest value be recorded.[6] In situations such as a shock state, when systolic and diastolic pressures cannot be auscultated, the systolic pressure alone may be obtained by palpation or by amplification of the pulse using ultrasound technology (Doppler pressure).

Auscultated and oscillometric blood pressure measurements are burdened with the potential of measurement error, in both reliability and validity (Table 16-3). This dictates the need for careful technique, and in most cases enhances the value of trend data as opposed to individual readings. The individual patient's heart rate, degree of arterial compliance, and dynamics of blood flow may vary over time. Inappropriate blood pressure cuff size, arm position, and both the visual and auditory acuity of the clinician may impact the accuracy of individual readings.[9] An additional source of error has been named the "white coat effect" for the elevation of blood pressure when taken in a clinic or office environment.[3,11] First described in 1897 by Scipione Riva-Rocci, who was the first to document assessing the systolic pressure by palpating the brachial artery,[12] these situational elevations in blood pressure are of concern because treatment may be initiated based on inaccurate data.[11] This condition is most common in older individuals of either gender, but may occur at any age.[6] Pickering and colleagues report that in approximately 15% to 20% of patients with stage I hypertension, elevated blood pressure may only be persistent under these circumstances. Significant pressure differences have been found using the automatic noninvasive technology between the supine, 45-degree elevation of the head of the bed, and sitting position in the same patient,[13] and between multiple body positions using the auscultatory method.[6,14] Normal values are based on the subject being seated, with the back supported and the arm at heart level. Specific recommendations regarding all aspects of indirect measurement are provided by the American Heart Association,[6] and sources of error within pediatric populations also have been documented.[15]

The recommended approach for obtaining an auscultated blood pressure is a two-step approach, beginning with inflating the cuff to the point at which the pressure obliterates the palpated radial pulse (systolic pressure). The pressure is completely released and after 15 to

TABLE 16-3   INTRINSIC AND EXTRINSIC FACTORS THAT INFLUENCE INDIRECT BLOOD PRESSURE ACCURACY

FACTOR	EFFECT ON BLOOD PRESSURE MEASUREMENT
Intrinsic Factors	
Heart rate	Elevated or decreased
Arterial compliance	Elevated or decreased
Alterations in flow dynamics	Elevated or decreased
Respiratory rate	Normal increase on inspiration
Extrinsic Factors	
Cuff	
Too small	Falsely elevated
Too large	Falsely decreased
Supine position	≈5 mm Hg lower DBP
Seated, back not supported	≈6 mm Hg increased DBP
Crossed legs	Increased SBP 2-8 mm Hg
Seated, arm position	
Above heart	Falsely decreased
Below heart	Falsely elevated
Inadequately supported	Falsely elevated
Excessive stethoscope pressure	Diastolic pressure falsely decreased
<1 min between measurements	Falsely elevated
Deflation rate >3 mm Hg/sec	Falsely decreased SBP and increased DBP
Exercise, eating, smoking, intake of caffeine ≤30 minutes before measurement	Falsely elevated
Talking during measurement	Falsely elevated
"White coat effect"/anxiety	Falsely elevated
Decrease in recorder auditory or visual acuity	Falsely elevated or decreased
Recorder bias	Falsely elevated or decreased

TABLE 16-4   KOROTKOFF SOUNDS

PHASE	DESCRIPTION
I	Initiation of clear tapping sounds—systolic blood pressure
II	Murmuring or swishing sounds
III	Increase in intensity and crispness of sounds
IV	Muffling of sounds
V	Disappearance of sounds—diastolic blood pressure

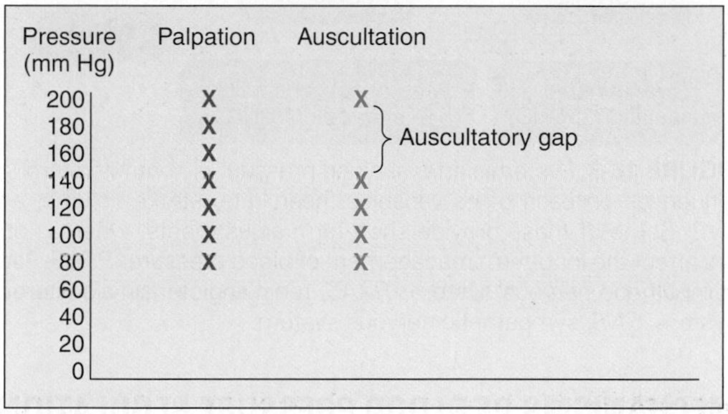

FIGURE 16-2 Auscultatory gap. Palpating the blood pressure (BP) before auscultation allows assessment of the true systolic BP. Palpated BP equals 200/P. The same result can often be obtained by elevating the arm overhead for 30 seconds before inflating the cuff. Auscultated BP when the cuff is inflated to only 180 mm Hg results in a falsely low value of 140/80 mm Hg.

intraarterial pressure fluctuations associated with hypertension (Figure 16-2) and can often be eliminated by elevating the arm above the level of the head for 30 seconds before cuff inflation. This approach is postulated to enhance the audibility of Korotkoff sounds by increasing arterial flow following the increase in venous return.[6]

Increasingly, self-monitoring of blood pressure is being performed at home. Potential sources of error as well as optimal schemes of measuring and recording have been identified.[16-18] It has been found that the values documented in this setting are more accurate, if correctly obtained, because of the elimination of the white coat effect.[3,11,18]

30 seconds the cuff is reinflated to 30 mm Hg above that point, and then gradually deflated while the clinician listens through the stethoscope with the diaphragm placed over the brachial artery and monitors the position of the mercury in the sphygmomanometer. The return of blood flow through the artery is signaled by the sounds produced by the turbulent flow through the partially occluded artery and named after the Russian physician who first described them in 1905 (*Korotkoff sounds*).[12] This sound is recorded as the systolic pressure. As the pressure continues to be released, sounds change in intensity until the point at which the Korotkoff sounds disappear, which is noted as the diastolic pressure (Table 16-4). Nurse researchers in Britain found statistically significantly lower diastolic values using this approach compared with a one-step approach.[9] In this approach, the systolic pressure was estimated by palpating the brachial artery during cuff inflation, and inflation continued 30 mm Hg beyond that point before proceeding with deflation. It was postulated that the first inflation and occlusion produced a reactive vasodilation that could be responsible for this difference.[9] Regardless, the auscultation of Korotkoff sounds results in systolic values that are lower than those obtained by direct, intraarterial blood pressure measurement.[6] Older patients often have a period during measurement when the Korotkoff sounds disappear, returning 20 to 40 mm Hg later. This *auscultatory gap* may be attributed to

KEY POINTS

- Systemic arterial blood pressure varies with the cardiac cycle. The highest pressure (systolic) corresponds to ejection of blood from the left ventricle into the aorta. The lowest point in pressure (diastolic) occurs at the end of diastole, just before the next ventricular contraction.
- Blood pressure is the product of the CO (HR × SV) and SVR. Changes in any of these variables will change blood pressure. The arterioles create most of the resistance in the vascular system; changes in the diameter of these vessels profoundly affect SVR and therefore blood pressure.
- The difference between the systolic and diastolic pressures is called the *pulse pressure*. The average pressure within the systemic arterial system is the MAP, mathematically derived from the two pressure values.
- Blood pressure can be directly measured by placement of a catheter within an artery and utilization of specific computer software. More routinely it is measured by auscultation. Systolic pressure is recorded as the onset of the Korotkoff sounds, and their disappearance is recorded as the diastolic pressure.
- Erroneous blood pressure values may be obtained because of a missed auscultatory gap, hydrostatic pressure changes associated with arm position, inappropriate cuff size, observer error, and other factors.

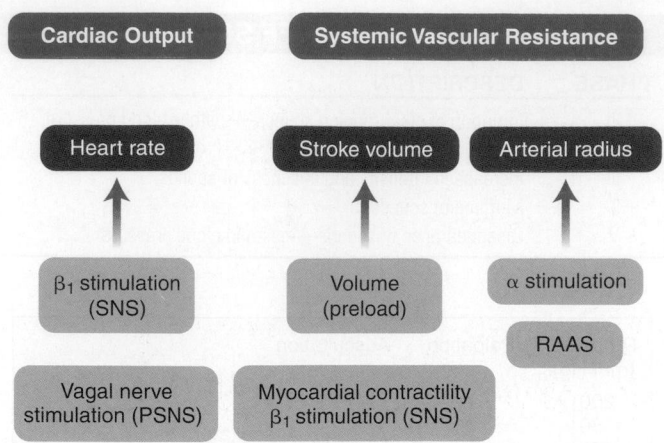

FIGURE 16-3 Systemic arterial blood pressure is controlled through influences on each of its variables: heart rate, stroke volume, and SVR. Some of these provide short-term adjustments, whereas others affect the long-term management of blood pressure. *PSNS,* Parasympathetic nervous system; *RAAS,* renin-angiotensin-aldosterone system; *SNS,* sympathetic nervous system.

MECHANISMS OF BLOOD PRESSURE REGULATION

Arterial blood pressure is physiologically controlled on both a short-term and a long-term basis. Regulation of blood pressure is achieved through changes in factors that impact the primary determinants of blood pressure: heart rate, stroke volume, and SVR (Figure 16-3). These variables are affected by a complex interplay between neural, humoral, and renal factors to maintain stability in the face of ever-changing internal and external environmental demands. An understanding of these mechanisms is essential to exploring pathophysiologic alterations. Blood pressure normally fluctuates over the course of 24 hours owing to physiologic changes associated with circadian rhythm.

Short-term Regulation of Systemic Blood Pressure

Changes in blood pressure must occur quickly to accommodate behavioral changes (e.g., position changes, exercise), emotional changes (e.g., fear, anxiety), and physiologic changes (e.g., fever, volume depletion). Changes in physical activity require the most frequent alterations, and rapid adjustments are initiated in seconds so that the arterial blood pressure may be increased to twice the normal value within 5 to 10 seconds.[1] This short-term regulation is mediated by the sympathetic branch of the autonomic nervous system (the sympathetic nervous system, SNS). Activation of the SNS influences both heart rate and SVR. The force of contraction is primarily a factor of the circulating volume (preload) and affects long-term regulation of arterial blood pressure.

Modifications in systemic blood pressure are made by activation of the SNS directly or indirectly through stimulation of the baroreceptor reflex. (Autoregulatory changes in pressure at a local level, at the tissues of body organs, are discussed in more detail in Chapter 15.) These SNS activities related to the distribution and pressure of blood are directed through the vasomotor center in the medulla of the brainstem while the lower centers of the brain monitor the body's internal and external environments.[1] The vasomotor center is directly activated by such stimuli as fever or external stressors to evoke increased activity and elevate systemic arterial blood pressure.

The autonomic nervous system maintains a basal level of arteriolar smooth muscle tone through the SNS, and provides heart rate control through a balance of SNS and parasympathetic nervous system (PSNS) activity. Stimulation of the SNS results in the increased release of the

neurotransmitters epinephrine and norepinephrine. At the smooth muscle of the arterial system, these neurotransmitters bind to α_1 receptors to initiate vasoconstriction and an increase in SVR. Stimulation of the PSNS has almost no effect on most systemic vessels, other than venodilation in localized areas such as the face, producing a blush.[1] Receptors within the brain (α_2) provide negative feedback regulation, decreasing the central release of epinephrine and norepinephrine in response to stimulation. In the heart, the binding of these neurotransmitters to β_1 receptors results in an increase in the rate of firing at the sinoatrial (SA) node, increasing the heart rate in response to increased demands. The PSNS is responsible for maintaining a slower heart rate during periods of rest.[1]

Indirectly, the vasomotor center is stimulated by a decreased rate of discharge by *baroreceptors*. Pressure-sensitive receptors (baroreceptors) are found in the vessel walls of nearly all large arteries in the thorax and neck, but are particularly plentiful in the sinuses of the carotid arteries and in the arch of the aorta.[1] Signals from the aorta travel through cranial nerve X and those from the carotids are transmitted through cranial nerve IX; both terminate in the vasomotor center of the medulla. These specialized receptors are sensitive to changes in MAP. They transmit impulses continuously, altering their rate of discharge in response to changes in MAP. Their response to these changes is very brisk, especially when pressure changes occur rapidly, which makes them the perfect mechanism to respond to variations in body position and minimize the gravity-induced decreases in pressure in the upper body.[1] A decrease in sensed pressure induces a decrease in action potential formation by the baroreceptors. This causes the vasomotor center to increase SNS outflow to the heart and arterial bed and to decrease PSNS stimulation to the heart. The net result is an increase in both heart rate and SVR, producing an increase in blood pressure. An increase in sensed pressure results in an increased rate of firing by the baroreceptors and a negative feedback response, lowering systemic arterial pressure. The responsiveness of the baroreflex declines with age; age-related stiffening of the arterial walls has been implicated along with contributions from pathologic conditions such as hypertension and diabetes mellitus, which are more common in the older population.[1,19] The results of animal studies indicate that the overall effect of the baroreflex is a reduction of the minute-to-minute fluctuations in arterial blood pressure by 33% of what it would be without this mechanism.[1] There is abundant evidence that within 1 to 2 days of exposure to chronic elevations of blood pressure, baroreceptors reset to the new level and the rate of discharge begins to decrease and then slowly returns to the norm despite an elevated baseline pressure.[11,19] This finding suggests that the baroreflex may contribute to long-term blood pressure regulation through the SNS stimulation of the kidneys[1] discussed in the next section.

Receptors in the carotid and aortic arterials respond to chemical signals of hypoxia (H^+ and CO_2 level elevations) that occur when arterial pressure declines. These chemoreceptors stimulate the medullary vasomotor center to increase SNS activity. However, this mechanism responds significantly only when systolic pressures decrease below 80 mm Hg, so blood pressure can be prevented from falling even lower.[20]

Long-term Regulation of Systemic Blood Pressure

The regulation of arterial blood pressure on a long-term basis, week after week and month after month, is accomplished through the interplay of neural, hormonal and renal interaction[21,22] and is intimately connected with the body's fluid volume homeostasis.[1] The balance of the intake of water and sodium with their excretion by the kidney remains the central feature of long-term blood pressure maintenance. Historically, the role of the renin-angiotensin-aldosterone system

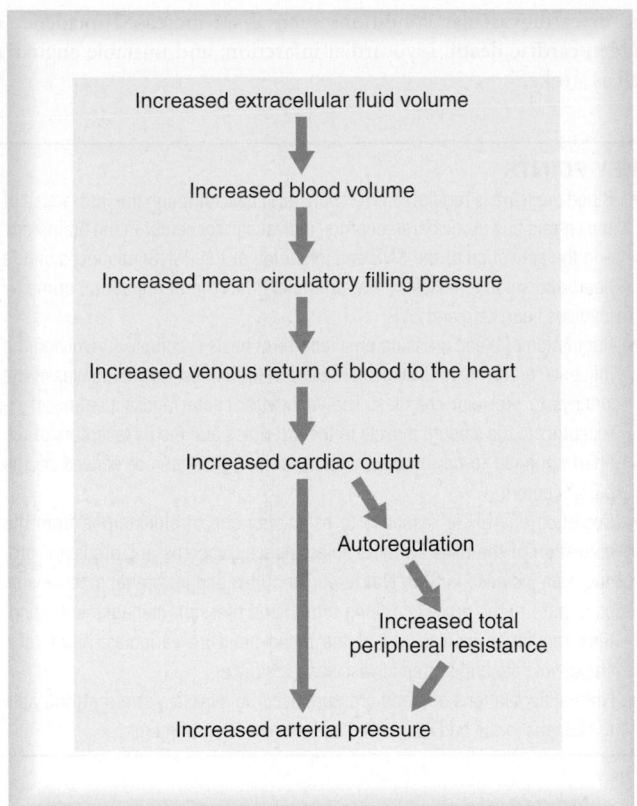

FIGURE 16-4 Mechanism by which an increase in extracellular fluid volume results in an increase in systemic arterial pressure. (From Hall JE: *Guyton and Hall Textbook of medical physiology,* ed 12, Philadelphia, 2011, Saunders.)

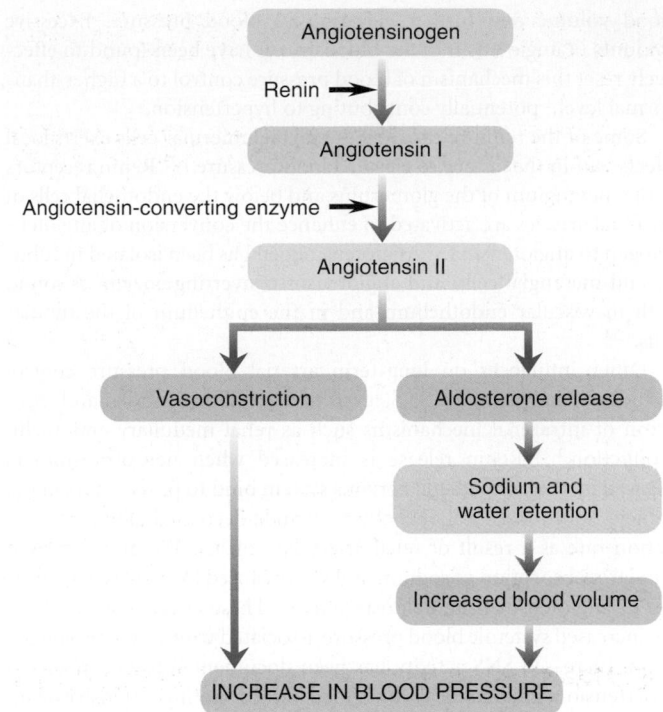

FIGURE 16-5 The renin-angiotensin-aldosterone system (RAAS) and its systemic effects.

(RAAS) has been seen as the primary contributor to this process, and although it continues to be a major determinant, mechanisms involving the baroreflex and the vasomotor center in the brainstem as well as localized renal systems are receiving increased attention in research.[1,21,22]

An increase in extracellular fluid (ECF) volume, because of increased intake or decreased excretion, results in an increase in cardiac output; when combined with the volume-induced increase in systemic vascular resistance, this results in an elevation in the arterial blood pressure (Figure 16-4). Body tissues initiate their local autoregulation mechanisms, constricting arterioles to protect against high-flow damage, which further contributes to the overall arterial resistance in the body. Unless fluid intake or renal functions are abnormal, this increase in systemic vascular resistance will not result in a prolonged elevation in arterial pressure.[1] The kidneys will respond quickly, increasing excretion of sodium and water and normalizing pressure within a matter of hours. This physiologic regulatory response may be disrupted if the renal vasculature is constricted, as occurs in hypertension.[1]

Because sodium is not as rapidly eliminated by the kidney as water, elevations in sodium intake are more likely to elevate arterial pressure.[1] Excess sodium also adds to the body's fluid volume by several mechanisms. Sodium increases the osmolality of the ECF and activates the central thirst center, causing an increase in water intake. The increased serum osmolality will be sensed by the hypothalamus and posterior pituitary, causing the release of antidiuretic hormone (ADH) into the bloodstream. Once ADH arrives in the renal vasculature, it binds to receptors in the collecting ducts, resulting in the enhanced reabsorption of water in order to decrease osmolality (Chapter 26).

The physiologic mechanisms of the RAAS are tightly controlled and interdependent (Figure 16-5). Prorenin, the inactive form of renin, is synthesized and stored by specialized smooth muscle cells located in the afferent arterioles of the kidney situated immediately proximal to the glomeruli.[1] Known as the *juxtaglomerular cells,* these cells are stimulated by a decrease in arterial pressure to enzymatically cleave the precursor, and release the activated renin enzyme into the vascular bed of the kidney. Most of the renin travels into the general circulation where it acts on a circulating plasma protein called *angiotensinogen,* resulting in the release of angiotensin I, a peptide possessing minimal vasoconstrictive capacity.[1] Angiotensin I continues to be created by renin for about 30 to 60 minutes, until renin is removed from the body. While the blood carrying angiotensin I circulates through the pulmonary vessels, an enzyme produced by the vascular endothelium (angiotensin-converting enzyme [ACE]) comes in contact with angiotensin I, and two amino acids are fragmented from angiotensin I to produce angiotensin II.[1] Inactivated in minutes by angiotensinases, continued production of angiotensin II maintains the profound effects it initiates. Angiotensin II is an extremely potent vasoconstrictor, primarily of the arterial bed but also slightly affecting the venous system. The SVR is therefore increased, raising blood pressure. The vasoconstrictive response to angiotensin II requires about 20 minutes to reach maximal capacity, but is capable of elevating arterial pressure to 50% of normal after severe hemorrhage.[1] The enhanced venous return attributable to the elevated SVR improves cardiac function by increasing myocardial fiber stretch, producing increased contractility and therefore stroke volume. Angiotensin II also is an intermediary for an additional means of raising blood pressure—increasing circulating volume to significantly increase venous return to the heart and therefore stroke volume. Angiotensin II in the general circulation reaches the cortex of the adrenal glands, stimulating the release of the hormone aldosterone. Aldosterone circulates to the kidneys where it binds to receptors in the renal tubules, causing the kidneys to reabsorb more sodium. Water follows the sodium back into the bloodstream. The result is an increase in blood volume and further elevation in blood pressure. Excessive amounts of angiotensin in the bloodstream have been found to effectively reset this mechanism of blood pressure control to a higher-than-normal level,[1] potentially contributing to hypertension.

Some of the renin released by the juxtaglomerular cells exerts local effects within the kidney to elevate blood pressure.[1,23] Renin receptors in the mesangium of the glomerulus and below the endothelial cells of the renal arteries are activated to enhance the conversion of angiotensinogen to angiotensin I.[23] Angiotensinogen has been isolated in tubular and mesangial cells, and angiotensin-converting enzyme is found both in vascular endothelium and in the epithelium of the tubular cells.[1,23]

Other influences on long-term arterial blood pressure control include the activity of the SNS, levels of natriuretic peptides, and regulation of intrarenal mechanisms such as renal medullary endothelin production.[1,23] Renin release is increased when neurotransmitters released by the sympathetic nervous system bind to β_1 receptors in the kidney. Additional local SNS effects include decreased glomerular filtration rate as a result of renal arteriolar constriction and increased tubular reabsorption of sodium and water caused by increased quantities of angiotensin II and aldosterone.[1,23] These effects contribute to the increased systemic blood pressure associated with severe prolonged stress. Increased SNS activity has been documented to be present in hypertension, and its role is confirmed because antihypertensive drugs that affect autonomic control of heart rate and systemic vascular resistance are so clearly effective in treatment.[1] A number of natriuretic hormones play a role in arterial pressure through their effects on ECF volume regulation; most important of these is atrial natriuretic peptide (ANP).[1] Increased volume in the atria of the heart triggers stretch receptors and stimulates the release of ANP into the bloodstream by cardiac muscle fibers. ANP causes the kidneys to increase water and sodium excretion by increasing glomerular filtration rate (GFR) and decreasing sodium reabsorption so both sodium and water remain in the filtrate.[1] This diuretic effect reduces circulating volume and therefore blood pressure. Endothelin-1 (ET-1) is a peptide produced in the renal medulla.[22] ET-1 binds to receptors within the kidney, initiating an autocrine-induced vasodilatory response affecting renal perfusion, water and electrolyte movement, and release of renin. This makes ET-1 an important participant in normal systemic blood pressure control, and levels have been found to be decreased in hypertension.[22] Most likely, long-term blood pressure control is a reflection of the unified contributions of all the factors discussed here, and more are yet to be identified.

Normal Fluctuations in Systemic Blood Pressure

Many homeostatic mechanisms of the body undergo daily variations in their function governed by an area of the brain called the *suprachiasmatic nuclei*—the body's internal clock. Brain wave activity, cell regeneration, cortisol release, body temperature, heart rate, and blood pressure are only a few of the more than 100 circadian rhythms.[24] In the case of blood pressure, it is known that it rises before awakening (morning surge), is highest in the middle of the morning, then begins to fall, and reaches its lowest level at night (nocturnal dip).[25] In their recent review of the available research, Peixoto and White[25] found these basic fluctuations to be primarily determined by internal neural and hormonal regulation, as well as by external environmental factors such as sodium intake and physical activity. Additional factors known to impact the normal rhythmic changes in blood pressure include lifestyle influences such as alcohol consumption and cigarette smoking, as well as cognitive activity and emotional state. Elevated blood pressure levels at specific points within the circadian rhythm have been documented to be associated with the development of diabetic nephropathy

and of cardiovascular conditions such as an increased incidence of sudden cardiac death, myocardial infarction, and unstable angina, as well as stroke.[25]

KEY POINTS

- Blood pressure is regulated on a short-term basis through the interaction of the carotid and aortic baroreceptors, the vasomotor center in the brainstem, and the activation of the SNS and inhibition of the PSNS influences on the heart and smooth muscle in the arterioles. Short-term regulation primarily involves heart rate and SVR.
- Regulation of blood pressure on a long-term basis is complex, involving the influence of the nervous system, release of hormones, and responses of the kidneys to pressure changes. The vasomotor center and activation of α_1 receptors in the smooth muscle of the arterioles and the β_1 receptors of the heart continue to be involved when pressure changes are sensed by the baroreceptors.
- Secretion of ADH in response to osmolality and of aldosterone from the activation of the RAAS affects fluid balance, whereas angiotensin II produces an increase in SVR. Natriuretic peptides and intrarenal mechanisms contribute to the process of long-term blood pressure management. Long-term regulation involves all of the blood pressure variables: heart rate, stroke volume, and systemic vascular resistance.
- Normal fluctuations of blood pressure occur in a cyclic pattern attributable to changes in the body's internal and external environments.

HYPERTENSION

The current and projected global prevalence of hypertension is stunning. Hypertension is the most common primary diagnosis in the United States.[4] About 30% of adults in the United States have high blood pressure. The prevalence of high blood pressure remains higher among non-Hispanic black adults compared with non-Hispanic white and Mexican-American adults.[26] In 2000, more than 25% of the entire world population was hypertensive.[26] Using the 2000 estimate of 972 million adults with hypertension, projections are for this number to increase by 60%—to 29% of the 2025 world population, that is, 1.56 billion individuals! Changes in the standard of living of those in developing countries mirror the trends in economically developed ones: increasing obesity and sedentary lifestyles.[26] Increased consumption of alcohol, cigarette smoking, and diets deficient in fruits and vegetables will contribute further to the problem of escalating hypertension worldwide.[27] Hypertension will soon affect more than 50% of the adult population in the majority of the world. India and Asia have the lowest current and projected prevalence, whereas the former Socialist Republics, sub-Saharan Africa, the Caribbean, and Latin America have the highest rates.[26] Given that the risks to health begin with blood pressure elevations of 115/75 mm Hg, the future impact of hypertension is profound.[26] Hypertension increases morbidity and mortality associated with heart disease, kidney disease, peripheral vascular disease, and stroke.[27] It is responsible for a worldwide annual death rate of 7 million,[27] and it will be the most common risk factor worldwide by 2020.[27] An understanding of the types and causes of hypertension and the interventions associated with its treatment is essential to having an impact on the current and future effects of this disease.

Definition and Classification

The standard for the definition and classification of hypertension in adults continues to be drawn from the *Seventh Report of the Joint National Committee on Prevention, Detection, Evaluation, and Treatment of High Blood Pressure*, published in 2003.[4] For those individuals age 18 years and older, normal blood pressure is defined as <120 mm Hg systolic and <80 mm Hg diastolic; stage 1 hypertension begins at a systolic pressure of 140 mm Hg or a diastolic pressure of 90 mm Hg (see Table 16-2). The range of pressures between normal blood pressure and stage 1 hypertension has been identified as *prehypertension* as part of efforts to initiate interventions early enough to prevent or at least slow the progression of the disease process. These values differ from those established by the World Health Organization, International Society of Hypertension, and European Society of Hypertension/European Society of Cardiology[6] in that those used in the United States are more conservative, identifying both normal and elevated levels at lower values. Standards for children and adolescents also have been established (see Table 16-1). Differing etiologies and risk factors have led to the differentiation of two major types of hypertension: primary and secondary.

Primary Hypertension

Primary hypertension, also called *essential hypertension,* does not have a clearly identifiable known etiology and is therefore an idiopathic disorder. This differentiates primary from secondary hypertension, in which blood pressure elevation occurs secondarily to another, identifiable cause. Primary hypertension is by far the most common form of the disease, representing somewhere between 90% and 95% of the known cases.[1] Early diagnosis and intervention for adults with hypertension has been a major focus of health care for many decades; the more recent escalating incidence in children has generated alarm. Primary hypertension is increasing in prevalence among children and adolescents and is associated with positive family history of hypertension, obesity, and lifestyle factors. The prevalence of HTN in children and adolescents is determined to be 3.5%.[28,29] Primary hypertension is rare before children reach the age of 10 years. At this point, most of the hypertension diagnosed in preadolescents has a secondary etiology; by adolescence, 85% to 95% of the cases are primary hypertension.[31-33]

Subtypes

Primary hypertension has one of several presentations: isolated systolic hypertension (ISH) in which the systolic BP is ≥140 mm Hg and the diastolic pressure remains <90 mm Hg; isolated diastolic hypertension (IDH) in which the diastolic pressure is ≥90 mm Hg with a systolic pressure of <140 mm Hg; and the combination of systolic and diastolic hypertension (SDH) occurring when both systolic and diastolic pressures exceed prehypertension values. The differing subtypes are more prevalent in specific populations, and researchers increasingly focus on subtypes in long-term outcome predictions and interventions.[6,33-34] The evidence overwhelmingly supports SBP as the major risk for subsequent cardiovascular disease.[4]

Risk Factors

In Western populations, there is a 90% lifetime risk for the development of hypertension.[26] Many of the risk factors for hypertension have been known for decades and because so many are modifiable by lifestyle changes, targeted interventions are urged to address them. Other factors remain nonmodifiable, yet predictive of the development of hypertension. Ample data indicate that primary hypertension arises as a consequence of the interplay of several genes and environmental factors.[35] Hypertension risk factors are listed in Table 16-5.

Increasing age is a nonmodifiable risk and an independent risk factor for hypertension beginning at mid-adulthood.[35] Normal aging produces a rising systolic pressure over the course of a lifetime, whereas diastolic pressure increases for approximately 50 years, levels off during the sixth decade, and remains stable or declines thereafter.[4,34] ISH is the dominant subtype of hypertension in those older than age 55.[34] Changes normally associated with aging are profiled in Geriatric

TABLE 16-5	RISK FACTORS FOR THE DEVELOPMENT OF PRIMARY HYPERTENSION
NONMODIFIABLE RISK FACTORS	**MODIFIABLE RISK FACTORS**
Increasing age	Obesity
Family history	Sedentary lifestyle
	Metabolic syndrome
	Dietary factors
	• Increased fat intake
	• Increased sodium intake
	• Inadequate potassium intake
	• Inadequate calcium intake
	Tobacco use
	Laboratory data
	• Elevated blood glucose
	• Elevated total cholesterol
	• Elevated triglycerides
	• Decreased high-density lipids (HDL)
	• Elevated low-density lipids (LDL)

Considerations: Changes in the Circulatory System in Chapter 15. The level of the systolic pressure, MAP, and the difference between systolic and diastolic pressures (pulse pressure), among other factors, are used to guide pharmacologic interventions.[6] Given this normal age-related development of hypertension, most early and subsequent data related to the increased risk of mortality and morbidity are based on this population, and systolic pressure elevation clearly affects risk more than diastolic, as noted in the earliest and most famous cardiovascular research in the Framingham Study.[4]

Age is not a risk factor for hypertension in childhood or adolescence. Hypertension does occur in these age groups, however, and the distribution of subtypes and the proposed bases and prognosis are worth noting. Determination of hypertension is based on the normal expectations for the child's age, gender, and height (see Table 16-1). Although isolated diastolic hypertension (IDH) is more common among younger adults, ISH can occur.[6,36] ISH in adolescents and young adults (<45 years of age) has been attributed to the increased elasticity of their arteries in the face of rapid growth; this produces an increase in brachial systolic pressure, although aortic pressure is unchanged.[6] Others have found an increase in stroke volume with or without aortic stiffening to be the basis of ISH in this age group.[37,38] IDH often seems to develop in prehypertensive young adults,[33] and the prognosis remains open to debate.[6,33,39,40] One study found that IDH does not appear to predict the development of ISH but is a strong predictor of the later development of SDH.[33] The report of a review of the literature indicated that below the age of 50, diastolic pressure was a greater predictor of coronary artery disease (CAD), whereas CAD risk in those age 60 and older was greater with elevated systolic pressure.[40] In children, hypertension is a risk both for adult hypertension and for subsequent development of adult cardiovascular disease.[31,36]

Another significant nonmodifiable risk factor is ethnicity, which combines race with genetics. Adult African Americans have the highest risk, but there is controversy about this finding for the pediatric population.[36] A concrete reason for this finding in adults continues to elude researchers, although increased salt sensitivity seems most likely.[37] The number of individual genes and their signaling pathways and organizational arrangements that affect the control of blood pressure are vast[39] and beyond the scope of this book. Despite the identification of the

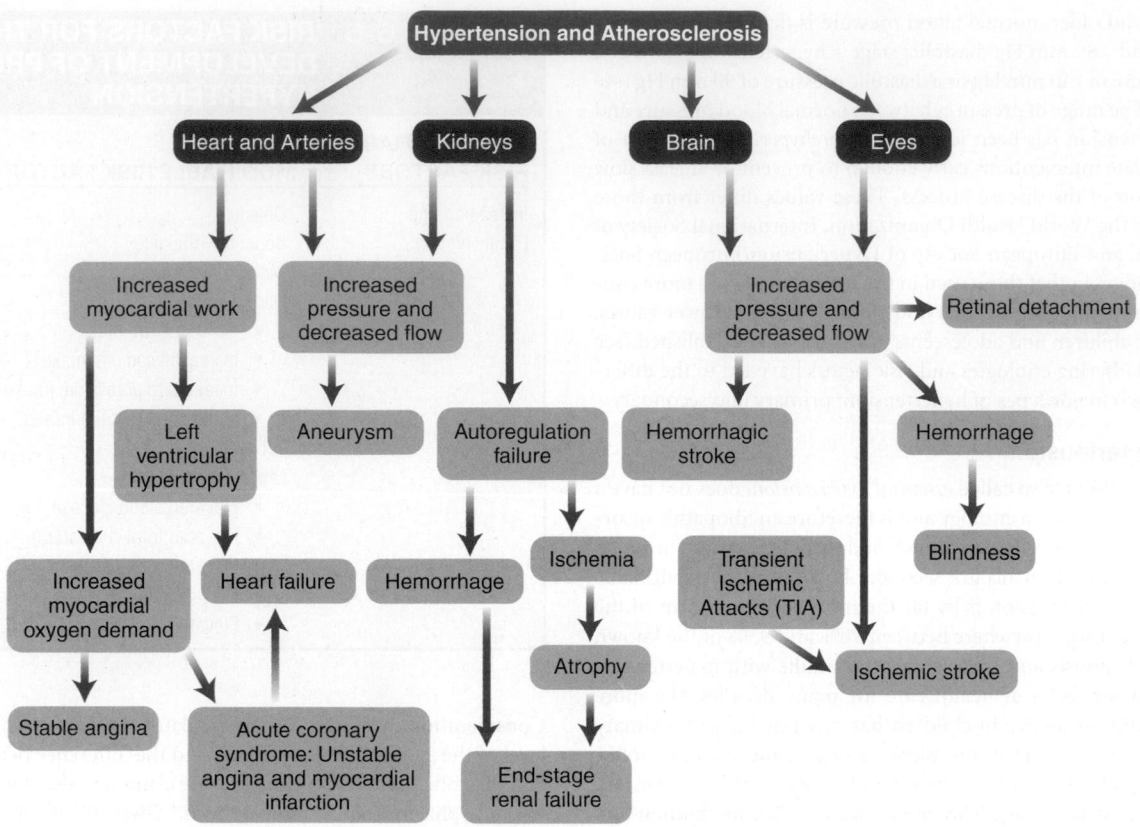

FIGURE 16-6 Effects of chronic hypertension and atherosclerosis on target end-organs.

genetic role in hypertension, specifying the mechanisms themselves is a challenge.[39] Genetics may be responsible for low renin levels and salt sensitivity, heightened responses to angiotensin II, altered amounts or responses to local tissue factors such as endothelin and nitric oxide, and any number of mechanisms accounting for primary hypertension that have been proposed.[22,37] At the same time, none of the currently identified genetic disorders has been demonstrated to be accountable for a noteworthy quantity of hypertension in the general population, either as individual genes or as several genes working in concert.[4] A family history of hypertension is a risk factor in both adults and children.[32]

Modifiable risk factors are often called *lifestyle factors* in acknowledgment of the role of individual choice in both their development and their control. Both weight gain and obesity are significant risk factors for all subtypes of primary hypertension at all ages.[32,33,41] Obesity has reached epidemic proportions and represents between 65% and 75% of the overall risk for the development of hypertension.[1,41] Diet and activity levels contribute to the development and continuation of obesity in all age groups. Diets high in fat and sodium and low in potassium and in fruits have been found to increase the risk of developing hypertension.[1,31,36,37] Obesity not only increases the risk of hypertension but also is a risk factor for hyperlipidemia, salt sensitivity, and insulin resistance.[31] Known as *metabolic syndrome* and characterized by elevated circulating insulin and lipid levels, hypertension, and obesity, this condition was previously only identified as a risk factor for hypertension in adults but is now becoming more common in children. It has been estimated that the prevalence of metabolic syndrome is 7% in adolescents at risk for becoming overweight, 29% in overweight adolescents, and 50% in severely obese adolescents.[42] Elevated blood glucose levels, diabetes mellitus, and elevated total cholesterol level, as well as smoking and excessive alcohol intake, are all implicated as risk factors for hypertension.[4,27,31,40]

Recently, the apparent increased incidence of childhood and adolescent hypertension has spawned research into predictors of the development of hypertension from the maternally-provided intrauterine environment through the childhood and adolescent period. Maternal smoking, pregnancy-induced hypertension, and maternal dietary habits have been shown to influence the later development of hypertension.[41-42,44] Low birth weight,[31] followed later by rapid growth in both height and weight, seems to be more common in the history findings of patients with hypertension.[43] Lower socioeconomic level of the mother[43] and inadequate dietary calcium intake during pregnancy appear to increase the risk for later development of hypertension,[46] whereas breast feeding seems to act as a protective factor against hypertension.[42,43]

Outcomes

End-organ damage. The great concern for the prevention, early identification, and treatment of hypertension is because of the harm it may cause in body tissues and organs and the resulting significant morbidity and mortality (Figure 16-6). This end-organ damage is a function of both the stage of hypertension and its duration.[4] Unfortunately, early hypertension causes no overt clinical manifestations, and individuals may have considerable end-organ damage before the diagnosis is made. This has earned hypertension the moniker of the "silent killer" and explains the rationale for screening programs to encourage early diagnosis. Hypertension is an important independent risk factor for the development of renal failure, stroke, and CAD.[4,40] CAD and hypertension heighten the risk of angina, myocardial infarction, and heart failure. As the systolic and diastolic pressures rise from normal levels, mortality from ischemic heart disease and stroke also increases linearly and progressively.[4]

Cardiovascular disease is the most commonly recognized outcome of hypertension. For those older than age 50 years, SBP ≥140 mm Hg presents a far greater risk for the development of cardiovascular disease than does an elevated diastolic blood pressure. Risk for the initial occurrence of cardiovascular disease begins with a blood pressure of 115/75 mm Hg, and with each incremental increase of 20/10 mm Hg, the risk doubles.[44-46]

Hypertension itself is directly harmful to the arterial system, but it also acts in concert with the other risk factors associated with the development and acceleration of atherosclerosis.[31,35,40] Atherosclerosis is the underlying pathophysiologic basis of coronary artery disease (see Chapter 15). Evidence of atherosclerosis has been found in adolescents and very young children.[31] The increased tension that high blood pressure generates on the walls of arteries precipitates an increase in the accumulation of collagen as well as reduction, fragmentation, and breakage of elastin fibers.[40] An ongoing low level of inflammation occurs in arteries exposed to hypertension, and combined with the dyslipidemia commonly seen, the development of atherosclerotic plaques is escalated.[40] CAD predisposes to stable angina and the acute coronary syndrome of unstable angina and myocardial infarction (see Chapter 18).

Hypertension reflects an elevation in SVR; rising afterload increases myocardial oxygen demand and overall cardiac workload. In an effort to compensate for this increased effort, the left ventricle hypertrophies.[40] The development of left ventricular hypertrophy also has been noted in children and adolescents.[4] The CAD typically found in association with hypertension limits the supply of oxygen to the heart, and this combination of increased demand and decreased supply predisposes the heart to ischemia.[40] Ischemia may result in stable or unstable angina, or myocardial infarction. Myocardial infarction and left ventricular hypertrophy increase the risk for the development of heart failure (see Chapter 19). Patients may seek health care intervention because of these conditions so that the presence of hypertension is discovered only secondarily.

The atherosclerotic process described previously with coronary artery disease (Chapter 15) is likely to be the basis for the damage to the microcirculation of the kidneys that develops with chronic hypertension.[40] Within a proscribed MAP, healthy kidneys are able to autoregulate blood flow delivered to the glomerulus, but with prolonged or severe hypertension this regulatory ability is lost and glomerular damage ensues.[1,35] Damage to the glomerulus allows large molecules not normally filtered out of the bloodstream to appear in the urine. The presence of microalbuminuria (proteinuria) is reflective of increased glomerular permeability and an early indicator of hypertensive renal injury. At this point, the patient is usually asymptomatic, but if interventions for blood pressure control are not initiated, renal impairment progresses, culminating in end-stage renal disease (ESRD), which requires long-term renal dialysis or transplantation.[47]

Identifiable damage to the kidneys is often preceded by changes in the microcirculation of the retina of the eye.[35] Atherosclerosis also contributes to the retinal injury produced by hypertension. The result may be retinal detachment or hemorrhage, which can cause blindness.

Hypertension and the accelerated development of atherosclerosis affect arteries of all sizes throughout the body. Decreased flow or rupture of weakened blood vessels within the brain results in strokes. Ischemic strokes are associated with atherosclerosis, whereas hypertension is the major risk factor for hemorrhagic strokes. This type of stroke results in high morbidity and mortality. Hypertension is also the primary risk factor for the development and rupture of aortic aneurysms. The peripheral arteries of the lower extremities are common targets of atherosclerosis, and the resulting peripheral vascular arterial disease is the source of significant impairment of independence and mobility and potential amputation in the elderly.[35]

Treatment Interventions

Effective treatment of hypertension results in decreased morbidity and mortality associated with cardiovascular, cerebrovascular, and renal disease.[4,35,47] However, the goal of normal systolic and diastolic pressures is not attained for many patients with hypertension. The problem appears to be even greater in Europe, where only 5% to 12% achieve control compared with 27% in the United States.[48] Cumulative data from clinical drug trials indicate the risk of stroke can be reduced 35% to 40% by decreasing blood pressure, myocardial infarction 20% to 25%, and heart failure by more than 50%.[4] Approaches to treatment are affected by several factors including the patient's age, stage of hypertension, identified risk factors, concomitant disorders, ethnicity, and medication history. Interventions fall into two categories: lifestyle alterations and pharmacologic interventions. The overall approach to treatment is detailed in Figure 16-7. Although an in-depth discussion of treatments is beyond the scope of this book, they are summarized in the following text.

Lifestyle alterations assume special importance because addressing modifiable risk factors has a documented effect in preventing hypertension from developing, as well as treating it in adults[4] and children.[2] Primary prevention of hypertension could have a profound influence on the morbidity and mortality associated with end-organ damage throughout the world and includes lifestyle changes and effective screening procedures to facilitate early diagnosis. These lifestyle changes are listed in Table 16-6. Weight loss is clearly an important intervention, with profound evidence that it reduces cardiovascular mortality.[41] The efficacy of exercise in blood pressure control is also well substantiated by research.[49] Brisk exercise of at least 30 minutes most days of the week plus the acceptance of the Dietary Approaches to Stop Hypertension (DASH) diet address a number of hypertensive risk factors.[4] Because they have been found to augment drug efficacy, these lifestyle adjustments also are included for those who require medication interventions for primary hypertension[4]; however, it is unlikely that lifestyle interventions alone will be sufficient for those with stage 1 hypertension.[26]

Drug therapy for hypertension addresses one or more of the variables responsible for blood pressure: heart rate, SVR, and stroke volume, which is primarily a function of the volume of blood returned to the heart during diastole. This is reflected in how the classifications of oral medications used in the treatment of hypertension are listed in Box 16-1. Figure 16-8 identifies comorbid conditions that require the use of specific medications.[4] Combination drugs, taking advantage of the effects of more than one classification without increasing the total number of medications a patient is taking, are becoming increasingly popular.[35] Because there is considerable variation in individual response to antihypertensive drug therapy, long-term monitoring is essential and alterations in treatment may be necessary.[35,50]

Secondary Hypertension

When hypertension is found to have a specific identifiable cause, it is termed *secondary hypertension*. The cause may be a specific pathology or condition that results in hypertension, or the development of high blood pressure may be the result of the ingestion of certain drugs, foods, or chemicals. Conditions associated with secondary hypertension are listed in Box 16-2. Some common substances that increase blood pressure are shown in Box 16-3.

In infants and preschool children, hypertension is usually of a secondary etiology and primary hypertension is rare.[31,36] In a study of 220 hypertensive children, 85% of the cases were found to be of a secondary etiology.[36] The four variables independently associated with primary hypertension were absence of signs and symptoms, normal serum creatinine level, family history of hypertension, and elevated body weight.[36] In the diagnostic assessment of adults, secondary

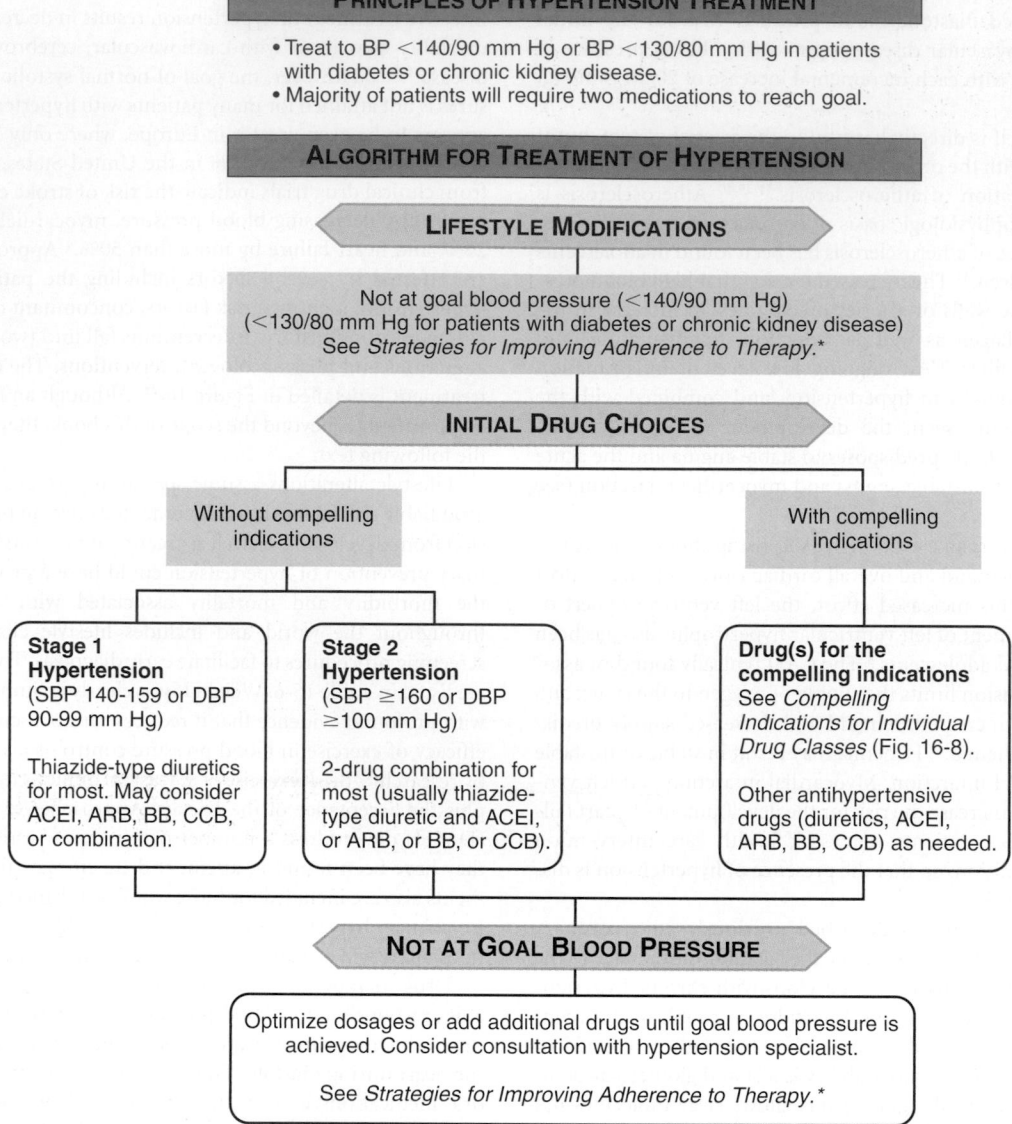

FIGURE 16-7 Treatment recommendations for primary hypertension. (From U.S. Department of Health and Human Services [National Institutes of Health, National Heart, Lung, and Blood Institute]: *The Seventh Report of the Joint National Committee on Prevention, Detection, Evaluation, and Treatment of High Blood Pressure [JNC7]*, NIH Pub No. 03-5231, May 2003.) *ACEI,* Angiotensin-converting enzyme inhibitor; *ARB,* angiotensin receptor blocker; *BB,* β-blocker; *BP,* blood pressure; *CCB,* calcium channel blocker; *DBP,* diastolic blood pressure; *SBP,* systolic blood pressure.

etiologies should be ruled out, but from the age of 18 years, primary hypertension is far more common. Interventions for secondary hypertension are directed at removing the cause, if possible. Drug therapy may be indicated, using the same agents previously discussed in the treatment of primary hypertension. As with primary hypertension, both the severity of the elevation as well as its duration must be considered because they heighten the risks for end-organ damage. The most common etiologies of secondary hypertension are discussed next.

Renal disease may be the result of a disease process either involving the parenchyma of the kidney or involving its vascular system. Hypertension is a risk factor for the development of renal failure, but it can

also develop secondary to renal pathologies. In adults with renal disease, hypertension is common and develops early, primarily as a result of heightened SNS activity.[21] In children one of the most common causes of hypertension is renal disorders; however, by the age of 12 to 18, the major cause becomes idiopathic primary hypertension.[31] As renal disease progresses, the kidneys' ability to excrete sodium effectively is lost and the renin-angiotensin-aldosterone system as well as the SNS are inappropriately activated. Renal artery stenosis should be considered in the diagnostic evaluation of new-onset hypertension in patients younger than 30 or older than 55 years, and an abdominal bruit is often found on auscultation.[4]

TABLE 16-6 LIFESTYLE MODIFICATIONS TO PREVENT AND TREAT PRIMARY HYPERTENSION IN ADULTS*

MODIFICATION	RECOMMENDATION	RANGE OF SBP REDUCTION[†]
Weight reduction	Attain and maintain BMI of 18.5-24.9 kg/m²	5-20 mm Hg/10 kg
DASH diet	High in fruits and vegetables and low-fat dairy products with decreased total and saturated fat	8-14 mm Hg
Decreased sodium intake	No more than 100 mmol/day (2.4 gm sodium or 6 gm sodium chloride)	2-8 mm Hg
Exercise plan	Regular aerobic activity for at least 30 min/day most days of week	4-9 mm Hg
Moderate intake of alcohol	≤2 drinks/day for men ≤1 drink/day for women	2-4 mm Hg

Modified from Chobanian AV: Seventh Report of the Joint National Committee on Prevention, Detection, Evaluation, and Treatment of High Blood Pressure: The JNC 7 Complete Report, *Hypertension* 42:1206-1252, 2003, p 1217.
BMI, Body mass index; *DASH,* Dietary Approaches to Stop Hypertension.
*Smoking cessation increases the overall reduction in cardiovascular risk.
[†]Results vary based on individual response, amount, and time of modification accomplished.

Another common cause of hypertension in children younger than age 6, along with renal disease, is coarctation of the aorta.[31] Without treatment, median life expectancy is only 31 years, with death from hypertension-related systemic effects.[48-51] It is for this reason that palpation of peripheral pulses and measurement of blood pressure in both arms are recommended both in routine pediatric physical examinations and in physical examinations in those whom hypertension is present.[2,52] Early diagnosis facilitates early surgical intervention, reducing both premature mortality and end-organ damage.[52] Hypertension persists after surgical repair in 20% to 30% of patients, but the pathophysiologic basis of this finding has yet to be determined.[51,53] Unfortunately, this means that these individuals remain at risk for the long-term effects and increased mortality associated with hypertension.

Hypertension arises in 5% to 12% of all pregnancies, depending upon the source,[6] and is the most frequent medical diagnosis for this condition.[6] Hypertension during this time is of foremost concern because of increased risk of maternal, fetal, and neonatal morbidity and mortality.[4] Preterm labor, abruptio placentae, disseminated intravascular coagulation, hemorrhagic stroke, liver failure, and acute renal failure are all potential outcomes of hypertension during pregnancy.[54] When hypertension is diagnosed during pregnancy, it is classified into one of four categories: chronic hypertension (preexisting), preeclampsia, chronic hypertension with superimposed preeclampsia, or gestational hypertension.[4,54] Pharmacologic interventions are used cautiously, and lifestyle interventions such as limiting salt intake and avoiding the use of alcohol or tobacco may be sufficient.[4,54]

Obstructive sleep apnea (OSA) is closely associated with obesity; it is found in 2% to 4% of adults, and hypertension is present in 45% to

BOX 16-1 DRUG CLASSIFICATIONS USED TO TREAT HYPERTENSION AND THE VARIABLES THEY AFFECT

Reduce Stroke Volume
Thiazide diuretics
Loop diuretics
Potassium-sparing diuretics
Aldosterone receptor blockers
Angiotensin (ACE) inhibitors
Angiotensin II receptor blockers
Venodilators

Reduce Systemic Vascular Resistance
Combination α₁- and β-blockers
Angiotensin-converting enzyme (ACE) inhibitors
Angiotensin II receptor blockers
Calcium channel blockers
α₁-Blockers
Central α₂ agonists
Direct-acting vasodilators (arterial)

Decrease Heart Rate
β-Blockers
Combination α₁- and β-blockers

Compelling Indication	Diuretic	BB	ACEI	ARB	CCB	Aldo ANT
Heart failure	●	●	●	●		●
Post–myocardial infarction		●	●			●
High coronary disease risk	●	●	●		●	
Diabetes	●	●	●	●	●	
Chronic kidney disease			●	●		
Recurrent stroke prevention	●		●			

FIGURE 16-8 Compelling indications for the use of individual drug classes in the treatment of hypertension. (From U.S. Department of Health and Human Services [National Institutes of Health, National Heart, Lung, and Blood Institute]: *The Seventh Report of the Joint National Committee on Prevention, Detection, Evaluation, and Treatment of High Blood Pressure [JNC7],* NIH Pub. No. 03-5231, May 2003.) *ACEI,* Angiotensin-converting enzyme inhibitor; *Aldo ANT,* aldosterone antagonist; *ARB,* angiotensin receptor blocker; *BB,* β-blocker; *CCB,* calcium channel blocker.

60% of those diagnosed with OSA.[4,55] Historically, there has been debate as to whether OSA itself was an etiologic factor in hypertension, or whether obesity simply increased the risk of both. Researchers now take the position that the potential causality between hypertension and OSA entails both an independent role of OSA in chronic blood pressure elevation as well as the obesity-hypertension linkage.[4] Certain molecular mechanisms including increased vasomotor activity mediated by angiotensin II, endothelin, and nitric oxide may occur in both.[56,57] Obstructive sleep apnea increases the risk of obesity in patients who were not originally overweight.[4] The severity of OSA has a direct relationship to the level of blood pressure elevation[4] and when untreated mortality and morbidity resulting from cardiovascular pathologies is increased.[55] A milder form of OSA is found in children, and evidence is increasing that it too is associated with discernible cardiovascular abnormalities including hypertension, decreased arterial distensibility, and left ventricular hypertrophy.[58,59]

BOX 16-2 COMMON PATHOLOGIC CAUSES OF SECONDARY HYPERTENSION IN CHILDREN AND ADULTS

Renal (Parenchymal or Vascular)
Renal artery stenosis
Renal failure* (end-stage renal failure attributable to any etiology; acute renal failure)
Polycystic kidney disease
Glomerulonephritis*
Hypertensive nephrosclerosis

Cardiovascular
Coarctation of the aorta*

Tumors
Pheochromocytoma*
Neuroblastoma*
Wilms tumor*
Adrenal adenocarcinoma*

Endocrine
Hyperthyroidism*
Cushing disease*
Congenital adrenal hyperplasia*
Primary hyperaldosteronism*

Neurologic
Guillain-Barré syndrome*
Increased intracranial pressure*

Other
Systemic arteritis (e.g., Henoch-Schönlein purpura)
Sleep apnea*

*Also seen in children

BOX 16-3 SUBSTANCES KNOWN TO CAUSE HYPERTENSION

Over-the-Counter Drugs, Prescription Drugs, and Illicit Drugs
Sympathomimetic agents (e.g., decongestants, amphetamines)
Glucocorticoids
Cocaine
Calcineurin inhibitors (e.g., cyclosporine, tacrolimus)
Oral contraceptives, especially if high in estrogen
Nonsteroidal antiinflammatory drugs
Erythropoietin
Antidepressants
Phenylpropanolamine analogues (e.g., ma huang, "herbal ecstasy")
Nicotine (and withdrawal)
Anabolic steroids
Narcotic withdrawal
Ergotamine
St. John's wort

Foods
Foods containing tryptophan or tyramine
- Chicken liver
- Pickled herring
- Yeast extract
- Lima beans
- Aged cheeses
- Beer and wine

Caffeine
Sodium chloride
Alcohol
Licorice

Chemical Elements
Lead
Mercury
Lithium salts
Thallium and other heavy metals

Pheochromocytoma is a catecholamine-secreting tumor of the adrenal medulla that generates hypertension on either a short-term or a long-term basis.[60] The condition is rare, although well-recognized; it can result in angina, myocardial infarction, acute heart failure, dilated cardiomyopathy, cerebral ischemia or hemorrhagic stroke, and cardiac dysrhythmias.[61] Treatment involves control of blood pressure pharmacologically, and then surgical removal of the tumor.

Hypertension is a predictable finding in primary hyperaldosteronism. Most frequently it is caused by a hypersecreting benign adenoma of the adrenal cortex or either unilateral or bilateral idiopathic adrenal hyperplasia.[62] Although evidence exists that aldosterone is produced by other body tissues, hormone from the adrenal gland represents by far the majority of circulating aldosterone.[63] The ratio of aldosterone to renin may be genetically influenced, but this has not been consistently documented.[64] For decades, hyperaldosteronism was thought to be a rare cause of hypertension; it is now known to be the most common form of secondary hypertension,[62] responsible for at least 12% of all cases, and it is believed that this number would be higher with improved screening.[65] Screening for hyperaldosteronism is recommended for hypertensive patients with decreased potassium levels or those found to be refractive to three or more antihypertensive agents.[65] Diagnosis requires measurement of serum aldosterone and renin levels.[62] Surgical removal of the involved adrenal gland results in a cure for 30% to 60% of cases and improved blood pressure levels in the remainder. Removal of one or both adrenal glands in bilateral disease rarely appears curative, so bilateral disease is treated medically with agents that block aldosterone's binding sites in the kidney.[62]

Hypertensive Emergencies and Urgency

Acute rises in blood pressure are identified by several names, complicating discussion of the condition. *Hypertensive crisis* was the term introduced to replace the initial term *malignant hypertension*, which originated as early as 1914.[66] Sixty-five million Americans have been diagnosed with hypertension, and about 1% of these will experience a hypertensive crisis during their lifetime.[66] At least 500,000 Americans are evaluated for hypertensive crises annually.[66] Most cases seem to be caused by secondary hypertension or poorly or uncontrolled primary hypertension.[66] Some other notable etiologies for hypertensive crisis include autonomic dysfunction, as is seen in Guillain-Barré syndrome, and autonomic dysreflexia, which can manifest in patients with high spinal cord injuries as well as in patients discontinuing certain drugs, such as β-blockers.[66,67] When *hypertensive crisis* is used today, two subgroups are differentiated: *hypertensive emergency* and *hypertensive urgency*. In both cases, the DBP is usually >120 mm Hg.[66] Hypertensive emergencies are situations characterized by a sudden increase in either or both systolic and diastolic pressures accompanied by evidence of acute end-organ damage.[66-68] These same references use the term *hypertensive urgency* to describe similar blood pressure elevations, but without the end-organ damage. The differentiation is necessary because it is the presence of end-organ damage and not the level of the blood pressure that usually determines the treatment.[66,68-69]

Hypertensive emergencies can occur in the previously undiagnosed patient or the patient with chronic hypertension; these emergencies are twice as common in males as in females,[70] and elderly African Americans have the highest incidence.[69] Hypertensive emergencies can occur at any age and are estimated to be responsible for more than 25% of emergency department visits.[71] Of all the end-organ damage with which hypertensive emergencies are associated, abnormalities of the central nervous system are the most frequent. These include ischemic stroke, encephalopathy, and subarachnoid or intracerebral hemorrhages. Acute heart failure, including acute pulmonary edema, myocardial infarction, and aortic dissection are the common cardiovascular complications, and retinopathy is a frequent finding.[66] From a pathophysiologic standpoint, hypertensive emergencies are the result of multiple factors including an abrupt release of catecholamines, mechanical stress producing endothelial damage, inappropriate activation of the renin-angiotensin-aldosterone system, and oxidative stress.[66] These changes overwhelm the normal autoregulatory mechanisms and result in a sudden and significant increase in systemic vascular resistance, initiating an inflammatory response.[66] Because of the evidence of end-organ damage, recommendations are for the rapid but controlled reduction of blood pressure using primarily parenteral antihypertensive agents closely monitored in a critical care setting.[66-68,72] The standard goal is to decrease the DBP to 100 to 110 mm Hg or about a 25% decrease in the MAP.[66,67]

Hypertensive urgency is actually more common than hypertensive emergency.[66] The approach to treatment of hypertensive urgency, when end-organ damage is not evident, is quite different. Once measurement error is eliminated, other sources of rapid-onset reactive hypertension should be ruled out. These may include anxiety, pain, abrupt withdrawal of alcohol or antihypertensive medications, postoperative hypertension especially following cardiac and vascular surgery, and full bladder.[66-68] In some of these cases, interventions other than antihypertensive drugs are indicated. In patients with hypertensive urgency, rapidly decreasing blood pressure has been associated with a substantial mortality.[66] Blood pressure in these patients is usually brought under control over 24 to 48 hours through the use of oral medications,[66,67] although there are indications for more aggressive intervention with parenteral agents.[67,72]

KEY POINTS

- Primary hypertension has no identifiable etiology, but risk factors include age; dietary factors including excess sodium and obesity; ethnicity and family history; sedentary lifestyle; and tobacco use.
- In adults, a normal blood pressure is <120 mm Hg systolic and <80 mm Hg diastolic pressure. Stage 1 hypertension begins with a systolic pressure of 140 mm Hg or a diastolic pressure of 90 mm Hg. Between these values, the individual is said to have prehypertension, and interventions related to lifestyle changes should be initiated for primary hypertension.
- Treatment of primary hypertension includes lifestyle modifications and drug therapy. Lifestyle changes address the modifiable risk factors. Drug therapy targets one or more of the variables of blood pressure: heart rate, stroke volume, and SVR.
- In secondary hypertension, the elevated blood pressure is the result of identifiable pathologic conditions, or certain drugs or foods. It is less common in adults, but is the major cause of hypertension in children. The underlying cause must be treated; drug interventions may also be necessary.
- Hypertension is usually asymptomatic until there is significant damage to vulnerable organs or tissues. This process is augmented by atherosclerosis in the coronary, renal, and cerebral arteries. Ultimately, hypertension increases the risk of stroke, angina, myocardial infarction, heart failure, renal failure, and blindness caused by retinopathy.
- Extreme and rapidly developing hypertension is divided into two groups: emergency, where there is evidence of end-organ damage; and urgency, where there is not. Urgencies are treated more slowly and with oral medications; emergencies require hospitalization and more rapid acting interventions.

LOW BLOOD PRESSURE

The mechanism for short-term maintenance of blood pressure described previously is designed to respond rapidly to changes in both internal and external environments. Over the course of the day, this system of increased autonomic activity usually accommodates changes in activity, especially changes in position. Recall that when moving from a supine position to sitting or standing, gravity pulls blood away from the upper body and stimulates the baroreceptors in the carotid arteries and aortic arch; 500 to 1000 ml of a person's circulating blood volume pools in the venous system of the lower extremities.[73] Messages transmitted from these receptors to the vasomotor center of the brain result in SNS activation, increasing both heart rate and arterial smooth muscle tone. The effect of these SNS-mediated responses to position change is the rapid increase in blood pressure and improved perfusion to the upper body, especially the brain. When this mechanism fails to produce this response in a timely fashion, the drop in blood pressure with position change is called *orthostatic hypotension*, and may have serious consequences.

Orthostatic hypotension (OH) (postural) is a widespread but often unrecognized disorder with potentially serious consequences. It has been reported to occur in 6% to 30% of healthy elderly persons with normal blood pressures.[74-77] When perfusion is not rapidly returned to the brain, dizziness, blurred vision, fainting (syncope), and injury from falls are familiar outcomes.[74-76] But OH can have even more serious consequences. It has been demonstrated to be associated with cardiovascular disease, and research results indicate it may predict stroke, cognitive impairment, and death.[75,79]

The standard definition of orthostatic hypotension is a decrease in systolic blood pressure of ≥20 mm Hg or a decrease in systolic pressure that is ≥10 mm Hg within 3 minutes of moving to an upright position.[74-76] Other references state that an excessive increase in heart rate, by 20 to 30 beats/minute, is also diagnostic.[75] Some researchers have found that the response can be delayed well beyond that timeframe in the elderly, perhaps up to 10 minutes or more.[76]

An ineffective response to position change may be associated with problems within the nervous system resulting from a number of pathologies, a vasovagal reaction, depletion in circulating volume, or cardiac dysrhythmias.[75] It can also occur as an adverse effect of drug therapy, most frequently antihypertensive, tricyclic antidepressant, and pain medications.[73,77] The elderly are at special risk of OH when they are taking these medications. They also commonly have an inadequate fluid intake, age-related decreases in autonomic nervous system function, and disorders such as Parkinson disease and diabetes with which postural hypotension is associated.[75] Orthostatic hypotension also is more common in the presence of arterial stiffness, which may be caused by an alteration in baroreceptor sensitivity.[19] Alcohol ingestion and exposure to heat will also cause vasodilation and may precipitate orthostatic hypotension.[73]

A normal response to the SNS activation by the baroreceptors depends on effective functioning of all components of the system. Damage to the vasomotor center or neurons within the central or peripheral nervous system may be responsible for a lack of sufficient response. This may be caused by disease or blunted responses associated with normal aging, prolonged bed rest, or medications. The prevalence of OH in Parkinson disease has been reported to be 37% to 58%.[75] Direct damage to nerve fibers by elevated blood glucose levels in diabetes or an autoimmune injury as in multiple sclerosis can blunt the response, as well as impaired transmission resulting from spinal cord injury. Altered sensitivity of the baroreceptors has been well documented.[77] The vasovagal response is a paradoxical increase in parasympathetic activity and a decrease in sympathetic activity resulting in bradycardia and vasodilation rather than an increase in heart rate and vasoconstriction. This contradictory response can be triggered by other stimuli such as stress, painful or unpleasant events, and activities such as coughing that increase intraabdominal or intrathoracic pressures. Dysrhythmias that impair cardiac output or an inadequate volume in the vascular space to respond to vasoconstriction signals will both also produce OH. Volume depletion as occurs in hemorrhage, burns, or severe diarrhea may reach a point where normal compensatory responses to position changes are inadequate; this happens after about a 30% volume loss.[1] The development of postural changes in vital signs is a useful clinical indicator of inadequate circulating volume.

Because orthostatic hypotension is often caused by physiologic conditions that are not amenable to modification, patients must be taught how to make changes to avoid initiating the response or reducing its impact. In addition to changing positions slowly to reduce the initial drop in blood pressure, patients are encouraged to avoid hot environments (baths or saunas), because of their vasodilating effects, and large or carbohydrate-heavy meals, because postprandial hypotension can result from the increased blood volume drawn to the splanchnic bed. When symptoms begin, before fainting, actions can be taken to prevent the progression of OH. Squatting, bending forward to lower the head, or crossing the legs while tightening calf, thigh, and buttocks muscles may counter the effects. Elastic compression stockings and abdominal binders have documented value, as does elevating the head of the bed. Unless contraindicated, liberal intake of both salt and fluids is encouraged.[78-79] Medication history should be carefully reviewed; a thorough history and physical examination, chemistry panel and blood count, and 12-lead electrocardiogram (ECG) should be carried out. Elderly patients may find use of a cane with a folded tripod seat or a walker equipped with a seat helpful to reduced OH-related falls.

> **KEY POINTS**
> - Orthostatic hypotension is an extreme response to the change from supine to upright position, where the activation of the short-term control mechanisms is slow or inadequate in its response. Heart rate and diastolic and systolic blood pressures are more affected by gravitational effects of position change than is normally expected.
> - Orthostatic hypotension results in dizziness, blurred vision, confusion, and possible syncope, which may cause injuries secondary to falls. OH is associated with cardiovascular disease and is a risk factor for stroke, cognitive impairment, and death.
> - Orthostatic hypotension may be the result of a number of pathologies involving the baroreceptor response, damage to the vasomotor center or the peripheral nervous system, a vasovagal reaction, or cardiac dysrhythmias, or it may be an adverse drug effect. Most often it occurs because of insufficient circulating volume.
> - Nonpharmaceutical interventions may be used if the cause cannot be ameliorated.

SUMMARY

Adequate perfusion of body organs and tissues depends on the maintenance of arterial blood pressure. This is accomplished through the highly orchestrated interaction of multiple systems on both a short-term and a long-term basis.

Blood pressure may be elevated secondary to other pathologic conditions, or to food or drug ingestion. Secondary hypertension is treated by managing the causative factors, although medication also may be necessary. More commonly the etiology is not discernible, although risk factors are identified, and primary hypertension is diagnosed.

Primary hypertension affects millions of Americans and is a public health concern worldwide. Once identified, lifestyle modifications and pharmaceutical interventions are initiated to avoid the significant pathologic outcomes to body organs.

When the mechanism for short-term blood pressure regulation fails to adequately respond to position changes, the resulting orthostatic hypotension can cause syncope and potential injury. If the cause cannot be identified and treated, accommodations can be used to decrease its occurrence and minimize risks.

REFERENCES

1. Hall JE: *Guyton and Hall textbook of medical physiology*, ed 12, Philadelphia, 2011, Saunders.
2. National High Blood Pressure Education Program Working Group on High Blood Pressure in Children and Adolescents: The fourth report on the diagnosis, evaluation, and treatment of high blood pressure in children and adolescents, *Pediatrics* 114(Suppl 4th report):555–576, 2004.
3. Urbina E, et al: Ambulatory blood pressure monitoring in children and adolescents: recommendations for standard assessment: a scientific statement from the American Heart Association Atherosclerosis, Hypertension and Obesity Youth Committee of the Council on Cardiac Disease in the Young and the Council for High Blood Pressure Research, *Hypertension* 52:433–451, 2008.
4. U.S. Department of Health and Human Services, National Institutes of Health, National Heart, Lung, and Blood Institute: *The Seventh Report of the Joint National Committee on Prevention, Detection, Evaluation, and Treatment of High Blood Pressure*, 2004, NIH Pub No. 04–5230. Available at www.nhlbi.nih.gov/guidelines/hypertension/jnc7full.pdf.
5. Headley JM: Arterial pressure-based technologies: a new trend in cardiac output monitoring, *Crit Care Nurs Clin North Am* 18(2):179–187, 2006.
6. Pickering TG, et al: Recommendations for blood pressure measurement in humans and experimental animals, I: Blood pressure measurement in humans: a statement for professionals from the Subcommittee of Professional and Public Education of the American Heart Association Council on High Blood Pressure Research, *Hypertension* 45:142–161, 2005.
7. Schell KA: Evidence-based practice: noninvasive blood pressure measurement in children, *Pediatr Nurs* 32(3):263–267, 2006.
8. American Association of Critical-Care Nurses: Practice alert: noninvasive blood pressure monitoring, *AACN News* 23(6):4–5, 2006.
9. Jones S, Simpson H, Ahmed H: A comparison of two methods of blood pressure measurement, *Br J Nurs* 15(17):948–951, 2006.
10. Eguchi K, et al: Consistency of blood pressure differences between the left and right arms, *Arch Intern Med* 167:388–393, 2007.
11. Parati G, Mancia G: Assessing the white-coat effect: which blood pressure measurement should be considered? *J Hypertens* 24:29–31, 2006.
12. O'Rourke MF, Seward JB: Central arterial pressure and arterial pressure pulse: new views entering the second century after Korotkov, *Mayo Clin Proc* 81(8):1057–1068, 2006.

13. Cicolini G, Gagliardi G, Ballone E: Effects of Fowlers body position on blood pressure measurement, *J Clin Nurs* 19(23-24):3581–3583, 2010.
14. Eşer I, et al: Issues in clinical nursing: the effect of different body positions on blood pressure, *J Clin Nurs* 16:137–140, 2006.
15. Podoll A, et al: Inaccuracy in pediatric outpatient blood pressure measurement, *Pediatrics* 119(3):e538–e543, 2007. Available at www.pediatrics.org/cgi/content/full/119/3/e538. Accessed 8/30/07.
16. Godwin M, et al: A primary care pragmatic cluster randomized trial of the use of home blood pressure monitoring on blood pressure levels in hypertensive patients with above target blood pressure, *Fam Pract* 27:135–142, 2010.
17. Shaw J, et al: Are stroke patients' reports of home blood pressure readings reliable? Cross sectional study, *Fam Pract* 28:118–122, 2011.
18. Argarwal R, et al: Role of home blood pressure monitoring in overcoming therapeutic inertia and improving hypertension control: a systematic review and meta-analysis, *Hypertension* 57(1):29–38, 2011.
19. Mattace-Raso F, et al: Arterial stiffness, cardiovagal baroreflex sensitivity in older adults: the Rotterdam study, *J Hypertens* 25(7):1421–1426, 2007.
20. Grassi G, et al: Baroreflex function in hypertension: consequences of antihypertensive therapy, *Prog Cardiovasc Dis* 48(6):407–415, 2006.
21. Charkoudian N, Rabbitts J: Sympathetic neural mechanisms in human cardiovascular health and disease, *Mayo Clin Proc* 84(9):822–830, 2009.
22. Kohan DE: Endothelin, hypertension and chronic kidney disease: new insights, *Curr Opin Nephrol Hypertens* 19:134–139, 2010.
23. Siragy HM: Angiotensin II compartmentalization within the kidney: effects of salt diet and blood pressure alterations, *Curr Opin Nephrol Hypertens* 15:50–53, 2006.
24. Public Library of Science (June 18): Circadian rhythms dominate all life functions, *Science Daily*, 2007 Available at, www.sciencedaily.com/releases/2007/06/070615075550.htm. Accessed 8/25/07.
25. Peixoto AJ, White WB: Circadian blood pressure: clinical implications based on the pathophysiology of its variability, *Kidney Int* 71(9):855–860, 2007.
26. Williams B: The year in hypertension, *J Am Coll Cardiol* 48(8):1698–1711, 2006.
27. Reid CM, Thrift AG: Hypertension 2020: confronting tomorrow's problem today, *Clin Exp Pharmacol Physiol* 32:374–376, 2005.
28. Yoon S, Ostchega Y, Louis T: *Recent trends in the prevalence of high blood pressure and its treatment and control, 1999-2008*, NCHS Data Brief No. 48, Hyattsville, MD, 2010, National Center for Health Statistics.
29. Chioler A, et al: Has high blood pressure increased in children in response to the obesity epidemic? *Pediatrics* 119:544–553, 2007.
30. Yoon EY, et al: Medical management of children with primary hypertension by pediatric subspecialists, *Pediatr Nephrol* 24:147–153, 2009.
31. McCrindle BW: Assessment and management of hypertension in children and adolescents, *Nature Rev Cardiol* 7:155–163, 2010.
32. Falkner B: Hypertension in children and adolescents: epidemiology and natural history, *Pediatr Nephrol* 25:1219–1224, 2010.
33. Franklin SS, et al: Predictors of new-onset diastolic and systolic hypertension: The Framingham Heart Study, *Circulation* 111(9):1121–1127, 2005.
34. Bouvet CB, et al: Arterial stiffness as a therapeutic target for isolated systolic hypertension: focus on vascular calcifications and fibrosis, *Curr Hypertens Rev* 6(1):20–31, 2010.
35. Aronow W, et al: ACCF/AHA 2011 expert consensus document on hypertension in the elderly: a report of the American College of Cardiology foundation task force on clinical expert consensus documents, *Circulation* 123:2434–2506, 2011.
36. Gomez R, et al: Primary versus secondary hypertension in children followed up at an outpatient tertiary unit, *Pediatr Nephrol* 26:441–447, 2011.
37. Narchi H: Assessment and management of hypertension in children and adolescents: part B—investigation and management, *J Med Sci* 4(1):14–24, 2011.
38. McEniery CM, et al: Increased stroke volume and aortic stiffness contribute to isolated systolic hypertension in young adults, *Hypertension* 46:221–226, 2005.
39. Ingelfinger JR: The molecular basis of pediatric hypertension, *Pediatr Clin North Am* 53:1011–1028, 2006.
40. Rosendorff C, et al: Treatment of hypertension in the prevention and management of ischemic heart disease, *Circulation* 115:2761–2788, 2007.
41. Mathew B: Obesity-hypertension: emerging concepts in pathophysiology and treatment, *Am J Med Sci* 334(1):23–30, 2007.
42. Spiotta RT, Luma GB: Evaluating obesity and cardiovascular risk factors in children and adolescents, *Am Fam Physician* 78(9):1052–1058, 2008.
43. Lawlor DA, Smith GD: Early life determinants of adult blood pressure, *Curr Opin Nephrol Hypertens* 14:259–264, 2005.
44. Adrogué H, Madias NE: Sodium and potassium in the pathogenesis of hypertension, *N Engl J Med* 356(19):1966–1978, 2007.
45. Vehaskari VM: Developmental origins of adult hypertension: new insights into the role of the kidney, *Pediatr Nephrol* 22:490–495, 2007.
46. Bergel E, Barros A: Effect of maternal calcium intake during pregnancy on children's blood pressure: a systematic review of the literature, *BMC Pediatr* 7(Article 15), 2007. Available at www.biomedcentral.com/1471-2431/7/15. Accessed 8/30/07.
47. Tanemoto M: Regulatory mechanism of "K^+ recycling" for Na^+ reabsorption in renal tubules, *Clin Exp Nephrol* 11:1–6, 2007.
48. Kennedy S: Clinical update: essential hypertension—recent changes in management, *Community Pract* 79(1):23–24, 2006.
49. Fagard RH, Cornelissen VA: Effect of exercise on blood pressure control in hypertensive patients, *Eur J Cardiovasc Prev Rehabil* 14:12–17, 2007.
50. Materson BJ: Variability in response to antihypertensive drugs, *Am J Med* 120(4A):S10–S20, 2007.
51. Polson JW, et al: Evidence for cardiovascular autonomic dysfunction in neonates with coarctation of the aorta, *Circulation* 113:2844–2850, 2006.
52. Cay S, Metin F, Korkmaz S: A common cause of secondary hypertension: coarctation of the aorta, *Heart* 92:734, 2006.
53. De Caro E, et al: Aortic arch geometry and exercise-induced hypertension in aortic coarctation, *Am J Cardiol* 99:1284–1287, 2007.
54. Frishman WH, et al: Pathophysiology and medical management of systemic hypertension in pregnancy, *Cardiol Rev* 13(6):274–284, 2005.
55. Yu S, et al: Effect of revised UPPP surgery on ambulatory blood pressure in sleep apnea patients with hypertension and oropharyngeal obstruction, *Clin Exp Hypertens* 32:49–53, 2010.
56. Smith ML, Pacchia CF: Sleep apnoea and hypertension: role of chemoreflexes in humans, *Exp Physiol* 92(1):45–50, 2007.
57. Weiss JW, Liu Y, Huang J: Physiological basis for a causal relationship of obstructive sleep apnoea to hypertension, *Exp Physiol* 92:21–28, 2007.
58. Driscoll DM, et al: Acute cardiovascular changes with obstructive events in children with sleep disorder breathing, *SLEEP* 32(10):1265–1271, 2009.
59. Chan DK, Chow AS, Kwok K: Childhood sleep-disordered breathing and its implications for cardiac and vascular diseases, *J Paediatr Child Health* 41:640–646, 2005.
60. Fernandes GH, et al: Delayed diagnosis of pheochromocytoma associated with chronic kidney disease, *Indian J Nephrol* 20(3):166–167, 2010.
61. Lin PC, et al: Pheochromocytoma underlying hypertension, stroke, and dilated cardiomyopathy, *Tex Heart Inst J* 34:244–246, 2007.
62. Young WF: Primary aldosteronism: renaissance of a syndrome, *Clin Endocrinol* 66:607–618, 2007.
63. Sowers JR, Whaley-Connell A, Epstein M, et al: Narrative review: the emerging clinical implications of the role of aldosterone in the metabolic syndrome and resistant hypertension, *Ann Intern Med* 150:776–783, 2009.
64. Newton-Cheh C, et al: Clinical and genetic correlates of aldosterone-to-renin ratio and relations to blood pressure in a community sample, *Hypertension* 49:846–856, 2007.
65. Doi S, et al: Optimal use and interpretation of the aldosterone renin ratio to detect aldosterone excess in hypertension, *J Hum Hypertens* 20(7):482–489, 2006.
66. Rodriguez MA, Kumar SK, DeCaro M: Hypertensive crisis, *Cardiol Rev* 18:102–107, 2010.
67. Shanahan A, Linas S, Anderson M: How should hypertensive emergencies be managed? *Hospitalist*, August 2010.
68. Angelats E, Bauer E: Hypertension, hypertensive crisis, and hypertensive emergency: approaches to emergency department care, *Emergencias* 22:209–219, 2010.

69. Marik PE, Varon J: Hypertensive crises: challenges and management, *Chest* 131:1949–1962, 2007.

70. Schulenburg M: Management of hypertensive emergencies: implications for the critical care nurse, *Crit Care Nurs Q* 30(2):86–93, 2007.

71. Feldstein C: Management of hypertensive crises, *Am J Ther* 14:135–139, 2007.

72. Chandar J, Zilleruelo G: Hypertensive crisis in children, *Pediatr Nephrol*, 2011. doi:10.1007/s00467-011-1964-0.

73. Thomson P, Wright J, Chakravarthi R: Non-pharmacological treatments for orthostatic hypotension, *Age Ageing* 40:292–293, 2011.

74. Zesiewicz TA, et al: Practice parameter: treatment of nonmotor symptoms of Parkinson disease, *Am Acad Neurol* 74:924–931, 2010.

75. Sathyapalan T, Atkin SL: Postural hypotension, *Br Med J* 342:1–3, 2011.

76. Task Force for the Diagnosis and Management of Syncope of the European Society of Cardiology: Guidelines for the diagnosis and management of syncope (version 2009), *Eur Heart J* 30(21):2631–2671, 2009.

77. Baliga R, Prabhu G: Orthostatic hypotension in healthy elderly: is it a myth? *North Am J Med Sci* 2(9):416–418, 2010.

78. Meuleman J: Diagnosis and treatment of chronic orthostatic hypotension, *Clin Geriatr* 19(4):29–32, 2011.

79. Cooke J, et al: The changing face of orthostatic and neurocardiogenic syncope with age, *QJM Int J Med* 104(8):689–695, 2011.

Cardiac Function

Jacquelyn L. Banasik

evolve WEBSITE

http://evolve.elsevier.com/Copstead/

- Review Questions and Answers
- Glossary (with audio pronunciations for selected terms)
- Animations
- Case Studies
- Key Points Review

KEY QUESTIONS

- How are events of the cardiac cycle reflected in pressure and volume changes within the cardiac chambers?
- What factors affect the blood supply to myocardial tissue?
- How does sarcomere cross-bridge formation lead to muscle cell contraction?
- What is the process of excitation-contraction coupling in heart muscle cells?
- How are action potentials generated and conducted in myocardial and pacemaker cells?

- How does the electrocardiogram relate to impulse conduction through the heart?
- How do heart rate, preload, afterload, and contractility affect cardiac output and cardiac workload?
- What diagnostic tests are used to evaluate cardiac structure and function?

CHAPTER OUTLINE

CHAPTER OUTLINE—cont'd

The primary function of the heart is to produce the driving force that propels blood through the vessels of the circulatory system. Along with the lungs, the heart works to distribute oxygenated blood and nutrients to tissues and organs of the body. Complex regulatory mechanisms function to match the cardiac output with the metabolic needs of the tissues. Cardiac dysfunction can lead to abnormal function or death of cells in tissues throughout the body. Cardiovascular disease is the leading cause of mortality in the United States, and a significant proportion of the population suffers from physical limitations associated with impaired cardiac function. Familiarity with cardiac anatomy and physiology is requisite to understanding cardiac diseases and therapy.

CARDIOVASCULAR ANATOMY

Heart

The heart is located in the **mediastinum,** suspended between the lungs, behind the sternum, and in front of the vertebral column, thoracic aorta, and esophagus (Figure 17-1).[1] When viewed from the front, the heart appears to be rotated to the left, so that the right atrium and right ventricle are most anterior. The base of the heart protrudes somewhat into the right side of the chest and is relatively fixed in place by its attachments to the great vessels. The apex of the heart lies primarily in the left side of the chest and is directed forward toward the anterior chest wall. With each heartbeat, a characteristic thrust, or point of maximal impulse (PMI), is generated and can be palpated where the apex strikes against the chest. The PMI is normally located on the left side of the chest where the fifth intercostal space and midclavicular line intersect. Variations in heart size and position within the chest may be related to age, body size, shape, weight, or pathologic conditions of the heart and other nearby structures.

Functionally important cardiac tissues include connective tissues, which form the fibrous skeleton and valves; cardiac muscle, which produces the contractile force; and epithelial tissue, which lines the cardiac chambers and covers the outer surfaces of the heart. The fibrous skeleton includes an extensive network of matrix that supports cardiac cells and four rings that provide a firm scaffold for attachment of the cardiac valves. Four cardiac valves control the direction of blood flow through the heart (Figure 17-2). The **mitral valve** (bicuspid) directs blood flow from the left atrium to the left ventricle, whereas the **tricuspid valve** directs blood from the right atrium to the right ventricle. The edges of these atrioventricular (AV) valves are attached to rings formed by the fibrous skeleton. Valve leaflets are tethered to papillary muscles of the ventricular chambers by connective tissues called **chordae tendineae. Papillary muscles** attach to ventricular walls and help prevent the valve leaflets from bending backward into the atria during ventricular contraction (Figure 17-3). The AV valves open passively during diastole when the pressure of blood in the atria exceeds that in the ventricles. Ventricular contraction reverses the pressure gradient and causes AV valves to snap shut, preventing blood from flowing backward into the atria.

Two semilunar valves are located in the ventricular outflow tracts. The **pulmonic valve** lies between the right ventricle and pulmonary artery, and the **aortic valve** lies between the left ventricle and aorta. Compared to the AV valves, the semilunar valves are thicker and are not supported by fibrous cords. They open and close passively according to pressure gradients, just as the AV valves do. When intraventricular pressures exceed pulmonary and aortic pressures, the semilunar valves remain open and then close when ventricular pressures fall below aortic and pulmonary artery pressures.

The cardiac muscle layer (**myocardium**) produces the contractile force that pushes blood through the circulatory system. Heart muscle

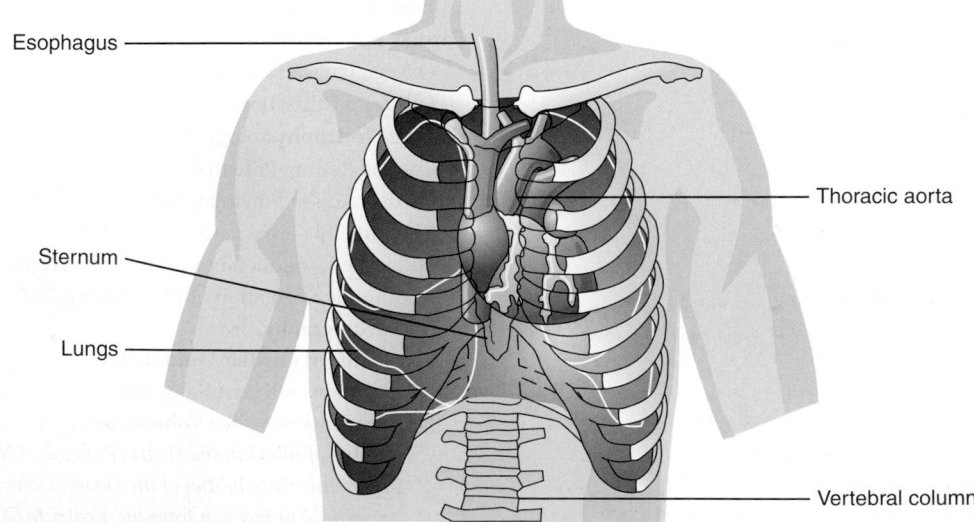

FIGURE 17-1 Position of the heart in the mediastinum. The base of the heart protrudes into the right side of the chest, whereas the apex lies in the lower left side of the chest.

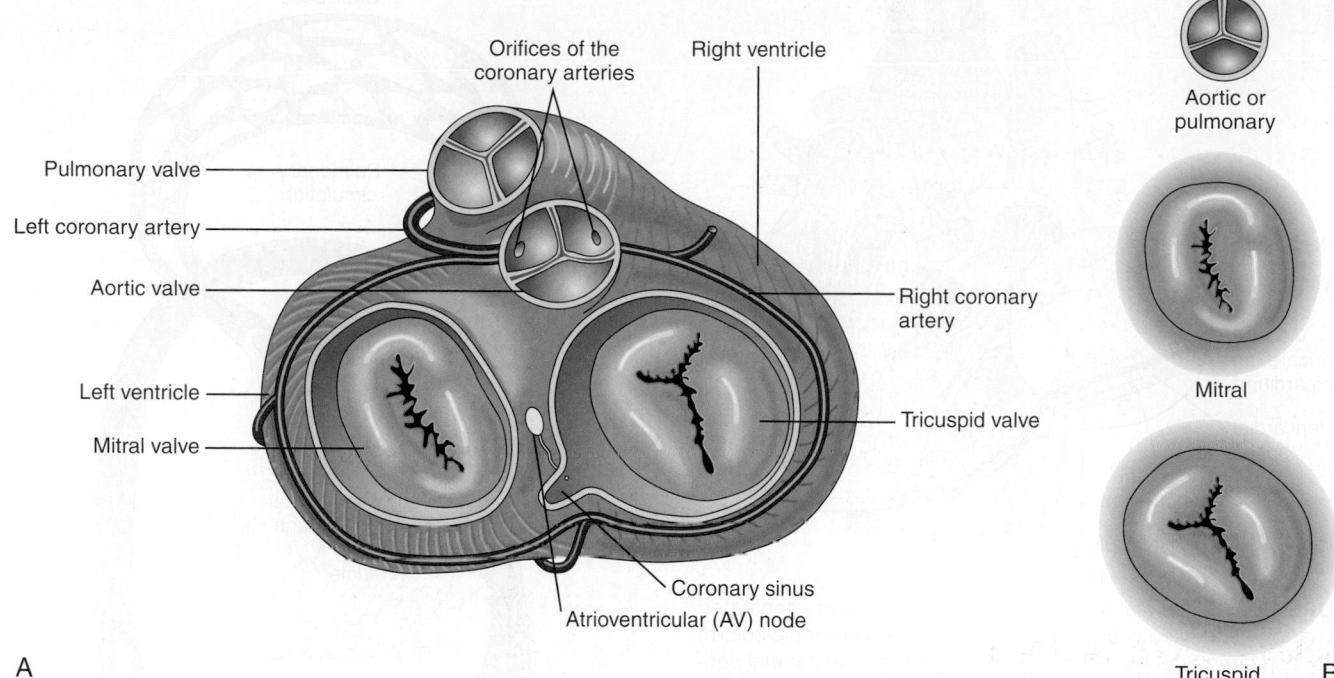

FIGURE 17-2 A, Position of the heart valves as viewed from above. **B,** Configuration of the heart valves showing the two cusps of the mitral valve and the three cusps of the tricuspid valve. The pulmonary and aortic valves have three leaflets.

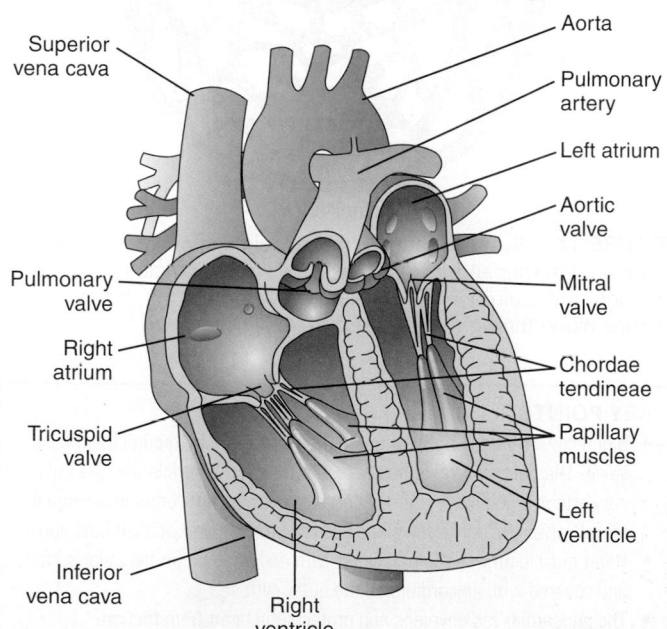

FIGURE 17-3 Chordae tendineae and papillary muscles attach the mitral and tricuspid valve leaflets to the ventricular myocardium.

TABLE 17-1	NORMAL PRESSURES IN THE HEART	
LOCATION	**PRESSURE (mm Hg)***
Right atrium	0-8
Right ventricle	15-28/0-8
Pulmonary artery	15-28/4-12
Left atrium	4-12
Left ventricle	100-120/4-12
Aorta	100-120/60-80

*Right and left atrial pressures listed as means; other pressures written as systolic/diastolic.

is organized into four separate chambers of varying muscular wall thickness, reflecting the degree of pressure each chamber must generate to pump blood. Atria serve primarily as conduits and have a thinner layer of muscle than the ventricles. The left ventricular muscle is two to three times thicker than that of the right ventricle because higher pressures are required to eject blood into the systemic circulation than into the pulmonic system. Normal chamber pressures are

shown in Table 17-1. Alterations in chamber pressures may reflect pathologic cardiovascular changes such as valvular disorders, blood volume abnormalities, and heart failure (see Chapters 18 and 19).

Cardiac chambers and valves are lined by a layer of squamous epithelial cells called the **endocardium.** The endocardial layer provides a smooth surface that prevents clotting and minimizes trauma to red blood cells. The endocardium is continuous with the endothelium of the vascular system. Outer surfaces of the heart are also covered by a layer of epithelial cells called the **epicardium,** which is part of a protective covering called the pericardium. The **pericardium** is composed of two layers that envelop the heart like a sac (Figure 17-4). The inner layer (visceral pericardium or epicardium) is attached directly to the heart's outer surface, whereas an outer layer (parietal pericardium) forms a sac around the heart. The parietal pericardium is composed of an epithelial layer and a tough fibrous layer.

Visceral and parietal pericardial layers are separated by a thin, fluid-filled space (pericardial space) that usually contains 10 to 30 ml of serous fluid. This fluid lubricates pericardial surfaces and reduces friction while

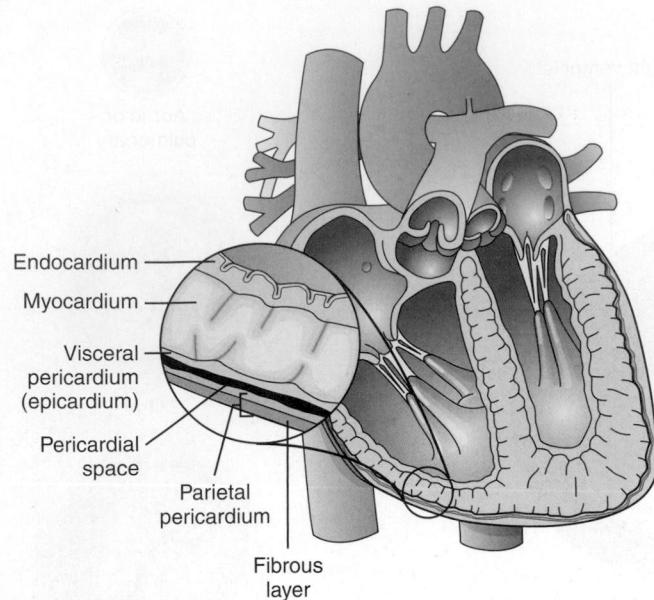

FIGURE 17-4 Pericardial sac is composed of two layers separated by a narrow fluid-filled space. The visceral pericardium (epicardium) is attached directly to the heart's surface, whereas the parietal pericardium forms the outer layer of the sac.

the layers slide against one another during cardiac contraction. Accumulations of fluid in the pericardial space or inflammation of the pericardial sac can restrict cardiac filling and impair cardiac output.

Circulatory System

The circulatory systems of the lungs and body can be viewed as two separate but interdependent systems (Figure 17-5). The left-sided heart chambers produce the force to propel blood through the vessels of the systemic (body) circulation. The left atrium receives oxygenated blood from the lungs by way of the pulmonary veins and delivers it to the left ventricle. This oxygenated blood is pumped by the left ventricle into the aorta, which supplies the arteries of the systemic circulation. Venous blood is collected from capillary networks of the body and returned to the right atrium by way of the vena cavae. Blood from the head returns to the right atrium through the superior vena cava; blood from the body returns via the inferior vena cava. There are no valves between the vena cavae and the right atrium, and the atrial pressure waves that are generated during the cardiac cycle cause characteristic visible pulsations in the jugular veins. An increased right atrial pressure may be observed as distention within the jugular veins.

The right side of the heart receives deoxygenated blood from the systemic circulation and pumps it through the lungs by way of the pulmonary artery. The pulmonary artery divides into left and right branches, which subdivide to supply blood to pulmonary capillary beds. Exchange of respiratory gases occurs at the pulmonary capillaries so that blood delivered to the left atrium by the pulmonary veins is well oxygenated.

Blood flow through the left and right heart chambers is connected in series such that the output of one becomes the input of the other. Thus, the functions of the right and left sides of the heart are interdependent. Failure of one side of the heart to pump efficiently soon leads to dysfunction of the other side.

Characteristic changes in the anatomy and physiologic functioning of the heart and circulatory systems occur with aging (see Geriatric Considerations: Changes in the Heart). In general, these changes result in a decreased cardiac reserve and a greater predisposition to cardiac muscle ischemia.

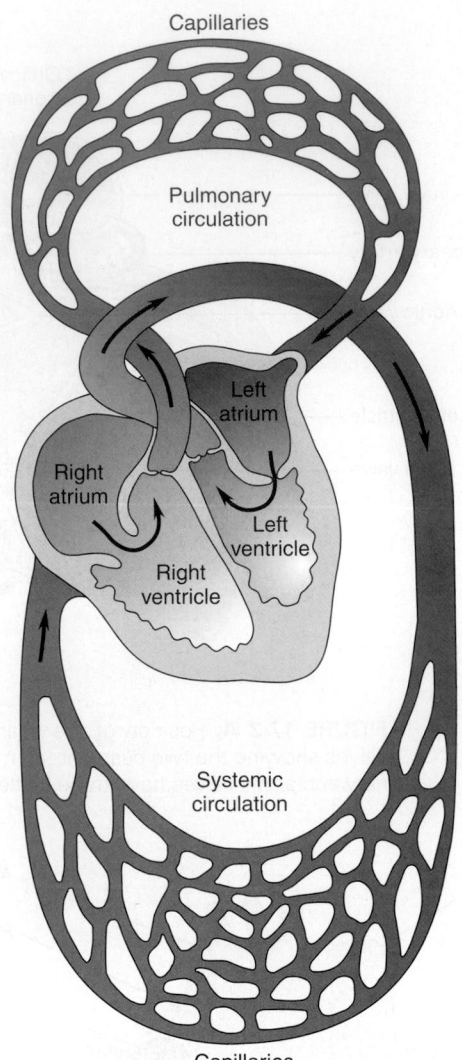

FIGURE 17-5 Systemic and pulmonary circulations viewed as separate but interdependent systems. The right ventricle pumps blood through the pulmonary vasculature, whereas the left ventricle pumps blood through the systemic circulation.

KEY POINTS
- Blood flows from the right atrium to the right ventricle through the tricuspid valve. The pulmonic valve lies between the right ventricle and the pulmonary artery. Blood flows from the left atrium to the left ventricle through the mitral valve. The aortic valve lies between the left ventricle and the aorta.
- Heart muscle (myocardium) is lined with endothelium on the inner surface and covered with epicardium on the outer surface.
- The pericardial sac envelops and protects the heart from friction.
- The right-sided heart chambers pump deoxygenated (venous) blood through the lungs. The left-sided heart chambers pump oxygenated blood through the systemic circulation.

CARDIAC CYCLE

Each heartbeat is composed of a period of ventricular contraction (**systole**) followed by a period of relaxation (**diastole**). The interval from one heartbeat to the next is called a **cardiac cycle** and includes ventricular, atrial, and aortic (or pulmonic) events. Each of these events is associated with characteristic pressure changes within the cardiac chambers.[2]

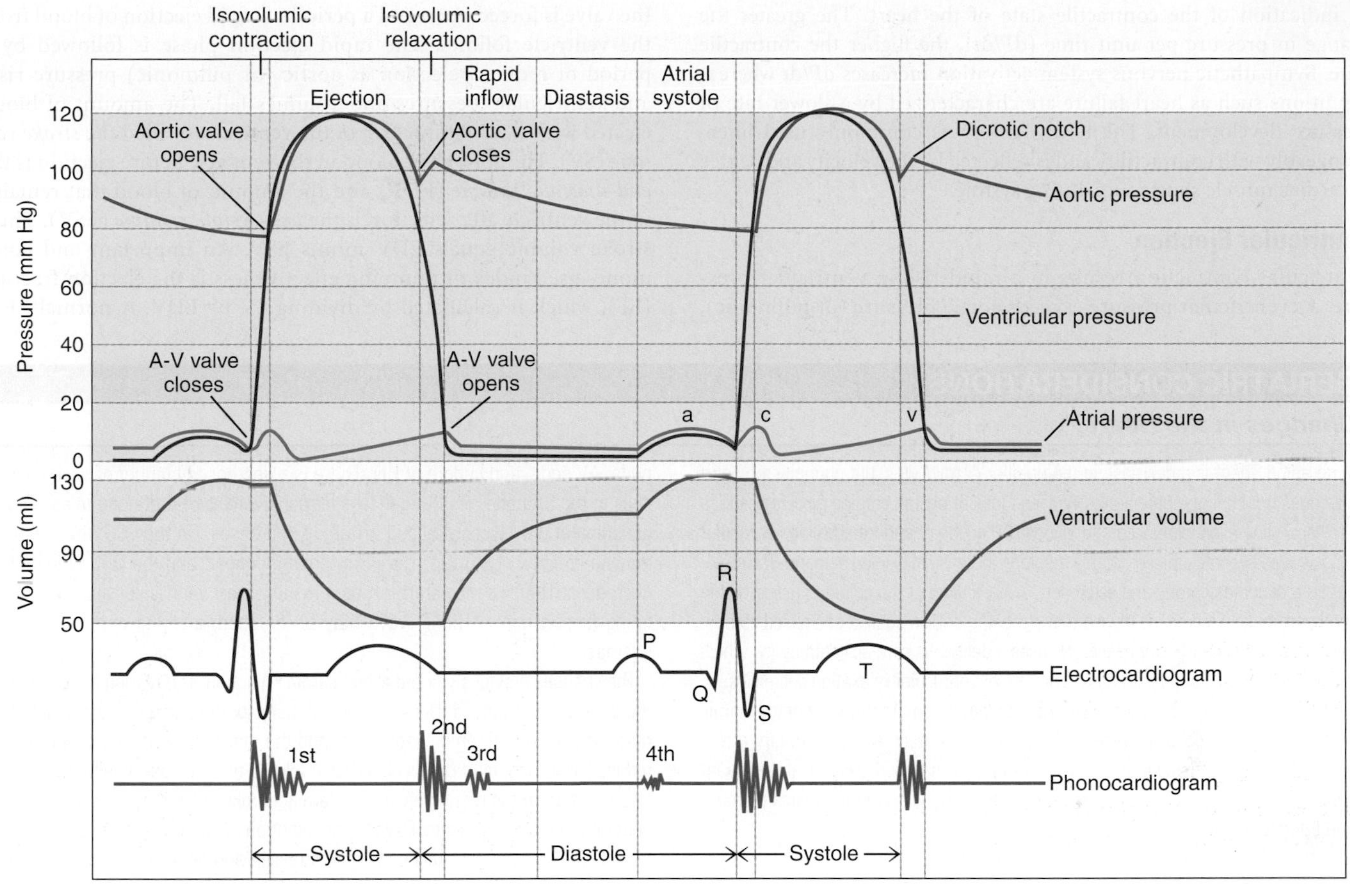

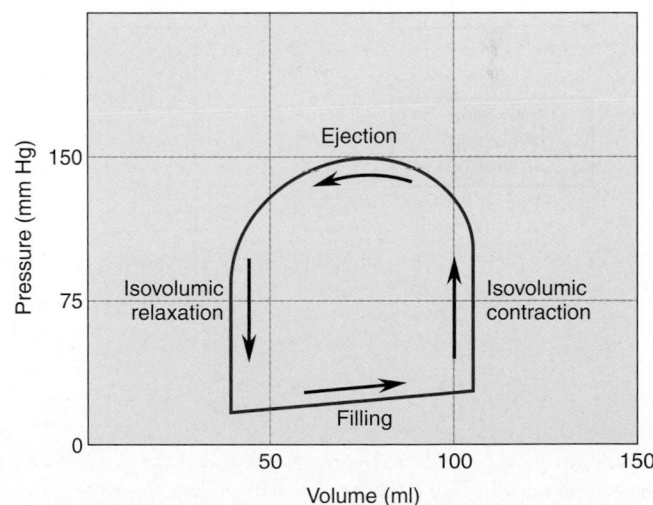

FIGURE 17-6 Events of the cardiac cycle showing relationships among left atrial and ventricular pressures, ventricular volume, and aortic pressure. An identical set of events occurs on the right side of the heart, although pressures are lower.

Pressure changes result in valvular opening and closing and unidirectional movement of blood through the heart. The various events of the cardiac cycle are illustrated as a function of time in Figure 17-6. Another method of graphing ventricular function is the pressure-volume loop (Figure 17-7). Pressure-volume loops are useful for assessing the relationships between pressure and volume at various points in the cardiac cycle to evaluate left ventricular function. Abnormalities in these waveforms may occur with diseases of the cardiac valves, changes in blood volume, or changes in pumping capacity of the heart (see Chapter 18). These waveforms are commonly monitored with specialized cardiac catheters in patients with cardiac or hemodynamic disorders.

The cardiac cycle can be described sequentially, beginning with ventricular filling. During diastole the ventricles are relaxed and blood flows in from the atria through open AV valves. Initially, ventricular filling occurs passively because of a pressure gradient between the atria and ventricles. Toward the end of ventricular diastole, the atria contract, squeezing more blood through the AV valves into the ventricles. The "atrial kick" provided by atrial contraction is particularly important during fast heart rates, when the time for ventricular filling is shortened; the atrial contraction helps to load the ventricle quickly to prevent a reduction in stroke volume. Ventricular events include isovolumic contraction, ejection, and isovolumic relaxation. Each of these cycle events is further described in the following sections.

Isovolumic Contraction

Immediately following atrial systole the ventricles begin to contract, causing intraventricular pressure to rise and the AV valves to close. AV

FIGURE 17-7 Pressure-volume loop showing changes in left ventricular volume and pressure during the cardiac cycle.

valve closure produces a sound that can be heard at the chest wall and is termed S_1. Ventricular pressure rises rapidly during isovolumic contraction because all four cardiac valves are closed, and the volume of blood within the ventricular chamber is forcefully compressed by the powerful ventricular myocardium (see Figure 17-6, *red tracing*). Volume remains constant during this phase. The rate of rise in pressure is an indication of the contractile state of the heart. The greater the change in pressure per unit time (d*P*/d*t*), the higher the contractile state. Sympathetic nervous system activation increases d*P*/d*t* whereas conditions such as heart failure are characterized by a slower rate of pressure development. The term *inotropy* is commonly used interchangeably with contractility and is reflected by the velocity and degree of cardiac muscle shortening during systole.

Ventricular Ejection

Ventricular contraction results in a rapid rise in ventricular pressure. As ventricular pressure exceeds aortic pressure (or pulmonic), the valve is forced open and a period of rapid ejection of blood from the ventricle follows. The rapid ejection phase is followed by a period of reduced ejection as aortic (or pulmonic) pressure rises and ventricular pressures and volumes fall. The amount of blood ejected with each contraction of the ventricle is called the *stroke volume* (SV). The volume of blood in the ventricle before ejection is the *end-diastolic volume* (EDV) and the amount of blood that remains in the ventricle after ejection is the *end-systolic volume* (ESV). Thus, stroke volume equals EDV minus ESV. An important and commonly used index of pumping effectiveness is the ejection fraction (EF), which is calculated by dividing SV by EDV. A normal EF is

GERIATRIC CONSIDERATIONS

Changes in the Heart

With aging, there is a decrease in the number of myocytes, but normally the heart size does not change appreciably. With the loss of overall cardiac muscle tissue, a corresponding expansion occurs in myocardial collagen and fat. The left ventricular muscle wall becomes thicker, with a resulting increase in oxygen demand. The endocardium becomes fibrotic and sclerosed. Cross-linking of the collagen tissue within the heart muscle increases myocardial stiffening, which causes decreased compliance. The decrease in compliance produces a decline in cardiac contractility, which reduces the heart's pumping ability. The rate of ventricular relaxation decreases.

Fibrotic changes in cardiac valves result from a combination of hemodynamic stress and generalized thickening. There is also a decrease in coronary artery blood flow to the myocardium, which affects myocardial oxygen and nutrient supply. The myocardial cells increase in size, with increased lipofuscin pigment and lipid deposition.

Within the specialized electrical conduction tissue, there is loss of myocytes and fibrosis of conduction pathways, especially in the sinoatrial (SA)

node, AV node, and bundle of His. There is a decreased number of pacemaker cells in the SA node, resulting in less responsiveness of that node to adrenergic stimulation. Myocardial cell irritability increases. On the ECG, the P wave may be notched or slurred. The PR interval is longer, and the QRS amplitude decreases. The axis may shift left as a result of left ventricular muscle thickening (hypertrophy). The T wave may be notched, and the amplitude may decrease.

The changes previously noted affect cardiac function. The resting heart rate in the elderly is unchanged. During stress or exercise, the aging heart is unable to respond quickly with an elevated rate, and the maximal heart rate elevation is reduced. Once the heart rate is elevated, it takes a much longer time for the heart rate to return to the resting level. The cardiac stroke volume and cardiac output generally decrease with age. Oxygen consumption in the myocardium is reduced, resulting in less efficient function when stressed and an overall decreased cardiac reserve.

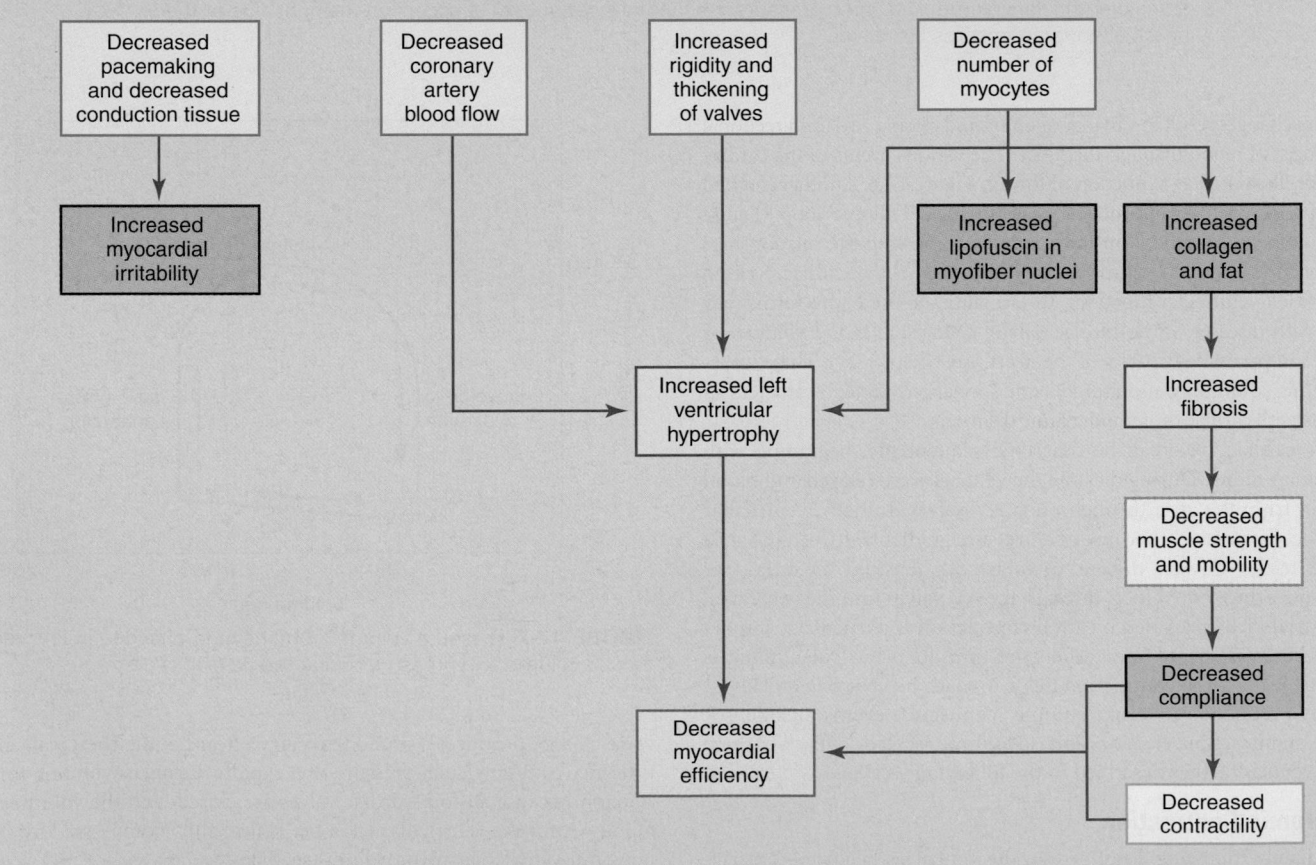

60% to 80%; patients with systolic heart failure often have an EF of less than 40%.

Isovolumic

The isovolu~~me~~ [stopped here] ~~sure in respo~~ AV valves o~~pen~~ ume remain~~s~~ valves rema~~ins~~ second heart sound, S_2. Opening of the AV valves signals the beginning of rapid ventricular filling and the start of another cardiac cycle. The rate of ventricular relaxation is indicated by the drop in ventricular pressure per unit time and is called the $-dP/dt$. The rate and degree of ventricular relaxation is called *lusitropy* and is an energy-requiring process that reflects the efficiency of calcium removal from the cytoplasm. Rapid relaxation is necessary to allow the ventricle to fill quickly and at a low pressure before the next systole. Impaired relaxation (lusitropic dysfunction) is a common finding in patients with heart failure and contributes to the symptoms of congestion (see Chapter 19). Because relaxation of the ventricle is an energy-requiring process, it may become impaired when blood flow and oxygen delivery to the heart are inadequate.

Atrial Events

Atrial pressure waves have three characteristic curves: *a*, *c*, and *v* (see Figure 17-6, *green tracing*). The *a* wave corresponds to atrial contraction, which immediately precedes AV valve closure. The *c* wave occurs early in ventricular systole and is thought to represent bulging of AV valves into the atrial chambers. The *v* waves have a gradual incline, which represents filling of the atrium as blood returns from the circulation. The *v* wave drops rapidly as atrial pressure is relieved by AV valve opening. A large *v* wave is often associated with inadequate closure of the AV valve, resulting in regurgitation of ventricular blood back into the atrium during ventricular systole. The mean right atrial pressure, also called the *central venous pressure* (CVP), is commonly measured as an indicator of the blood volume in the heart, which is dependent in part on the amount of blood being returned from the systemic circulation.

Aortic and Pulmonary Artery Events

Aortic and pulmonary artery pressures rise and fall in relation to the cardiac cycle. Arterial pressures fall to their lowest value just before semilunar valve opening. This lowest pressure is called *diastolic blood pressure*. Arterial pressure reaches its maximum during ventricular ejection and is called *systolic blood pressure*. A characteristic notch (*dicrotic notch*) in the arterial pressure curve may be seen as the semilunar valves close (see Figure 17-6, *blue tracing*).

The difference in aortic pressure between systole and diastole is partly dependent on the aorta's elastic characteristics. During systole, the aorta stretches to accommodate blood ejected by the ventricle. The stretched aorta has "stored" or potential energy that is released during diastole to maintain driving pressure and to keep blood flowing continuously through the circulation. Aortic stiffening, as occurs with aging or arteriosclerosis, may result in higher systolic and lower diastolic blood pressures attributable to loss of aortic elastic properties.[3] When aortic or pulmonic pressures are chronically elevated, the ventricles must generate more pressure to open the semilunar valves and eject the stroke volume. Over time this extra effort required to increase the pressure can damage the heart muscle and lead to hypertrophy or failure.

CORONARY CIRCULATION

Anatomy of the Coronary Vessels

The blood supply to heart muscle is provided by the coronary arteries (Figure 17-8). Right and left coronary artery openings are located in the sinuses of Valsalva, in the aortic root, just beyond the aortic valve.[2] The right coronary artery originates near the aortic valve's anterior cusp and passes diagonally toward the right ventricle in the AV groove. In approximately 50% of the population, the right coronary artery gives rise to a posterior descending vessel that supplies blood to the heart's posterior aspect. In 20% of the population, the left coronary artery is dominant in supplying blood to the ventricles, and in 30% of the population the right and left coronary arteries deliver about the same amount of blood and neither is dominant.[3] The *left main coronary artery* arises near the aortic posterior cusp and travels a short distance anteriorly before dividing into the *left anterior descending* and *circumflex* branches. The anterior descending branch supplies septal, anterior, and apical areas of the left ventricle, whereas the circumflex artery supplies the lateral and posterior left ventricle. The three major coronary arteries give rise to a number of smaller branches that penetrate the myocardium and branch into small arterioles and capillaries. Regular exercise and stable atherosclerotic plaques in the coronary arteries are thought to stimulate the development of more extensive collateral circulation in the heart. Collateral vessels may help limit infarct size in patients suffering acute coronary occlusions (see Chapter 18). Areas supplied by divisions of the coronary arteries are listed in Table 17-2. Most of the heart's capillary beds drain into the coronary veins, which then empty into the right atrium through the coronary sinus (Figure 17-9).

Regulation of Coronary Blood Flow

Blood flow through coronary vessels is determined by the same physical principles that govern flow through other vessels of the body, namely, driving pressure and vascular resistance to flow.[3] According to Ohm's law, an increase in driving pressure (P) increases blood flow (Q), whereas an increase in resistance (R) reduces blood flow: $Q = P/R$ (see Chapter 15). Driving pressure through the coronary arteries is determined by aortic blood pressure and right atrial pressure. This relationship can be expressed in the following equation:

$$\text{Coronary driving pressure } (P) = \text{ABP} - \text{RAP}$$

where ABP is aortic blood pressure and RAP is right atrial pressure. Thus, an increase in aortic pressure enhances coronary blood flow, whereas an increase in right atrial pressure opposes coronary flow.

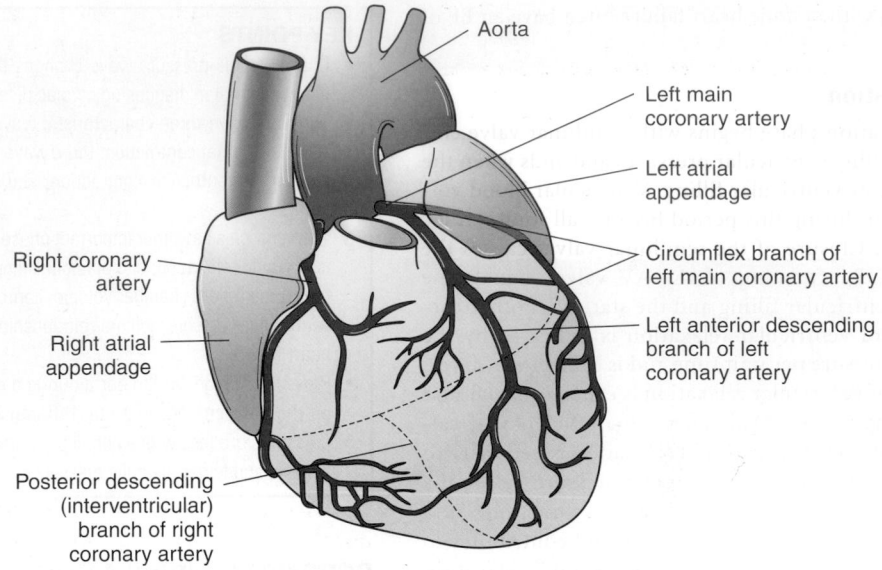

A

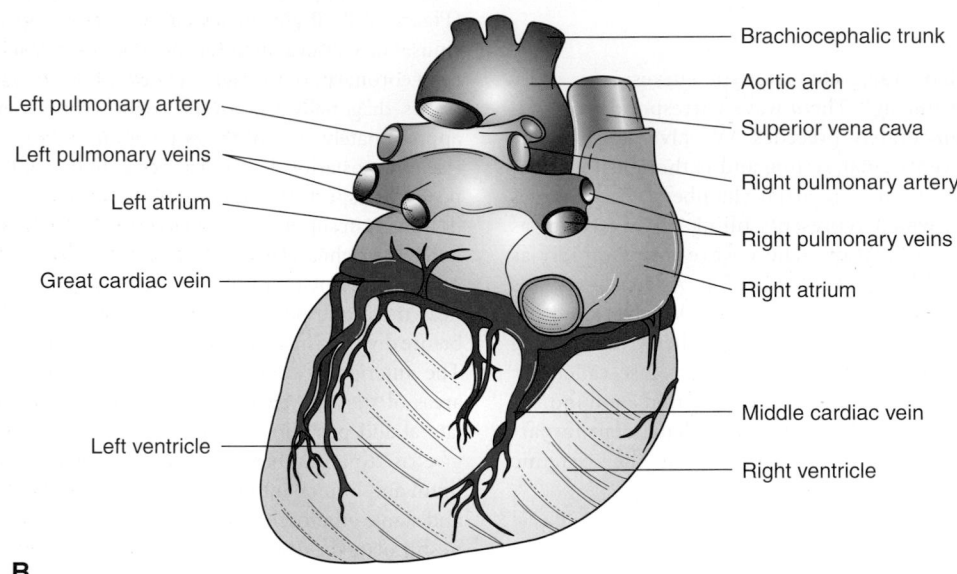

B

FIGURE 17-8 Coronary arteries supplying the heart. The right coronary artery supplies the right atrium, ventricle, and posterior aspect of the left ventricle in most individuals. The left coronary artery divides into the left anterior descending and circumflex arteries, which perfuse the left ventricle. **A,** Anterior view. **B,** Posterior view.

Coronary vascular resistance *(R)* has two major determinants: (1) coronary artery diameter and (2) the varying degrees of external compression attributable to myocardial contraction and relaxation. Coronary artery diameter is continuously adjusted to maintain blood flow at a level adequate for myocardial demands. **Autoregulation** is the term used to describe the intrinsic ability of the arteries to adjust blood flow according to tissue needs. Vessel dilation *(vasodilation)* occurs in response to increased tissue metabolism or reduced driving pressure, whereas decreased metabolic activity or increased driving pressure results in a decreased vessel diameter *(vasoconstriction)*.

The mechanism of autoregulation can be explained by the metabolic hypothesis, which proposes that increased metabolism, reduced oxygen concentration, or decreased blood flow results in a buildup of vasodilatory chemicals in the vessel. Smooth muscle encircling the vessel relaxes in response to the presence of the chemicals, increasing vessel diameter. Several vasodilating substances have been proposed, including potassium ions, hydrogen ions, carbon dioxide, nitric oxide, prostaglandins, and adenosine. The endothelial cells that line vessels are known to secrete a variety of relaxing and constricting factors, which may contribute to autoregulation.[4] Vasodilatory substances are washed away as blood flow increases in response to increased vessel diameter. A declining level of vasodilatory chemicals results in vasoconstriction. Thus, vessel diameter is continuously adjusted according to concentrations of vasodilatory chemicals, which are directly related to the tissue's metabolic activity.

TABLE 17-2 AREAS SUPPLIED BY THE CORONARY ARTERIES

ARTERY	AREA SUPPLIED
Right coronary	Right atrium (55% of persons)
	Right ventricle
	Intraventricular septum
	Sinus node (55% of persons)
	Atrioventricular node
	Bundle of His
Left anterior descending	Right atrium (45% of persons)
	Right ventricle (minor)
	Left ventricle (anterior, apex)
	Anterior papillary muscles
	Right and left bundle branches
	Intraventricular septum
Left circumflex	Left atrium
	Left ventricle (posterior, anterior)
	Sinus node (45% of persons)

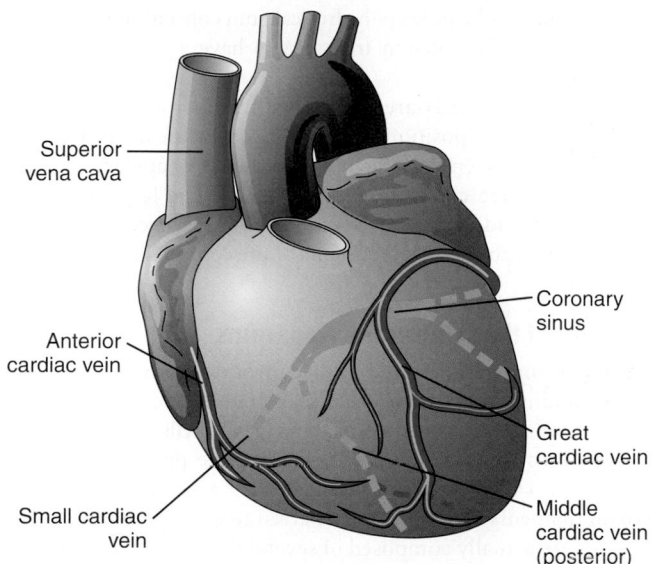

FIGURE 17-9 Venous drainage of the heart. Coronary veins drain blood from the myocardial capillary bed and deliver it into the right atrium.

One mechanism for autoregulation of coronary blood flow involves an ATP-sensitive potassium channel in vascular smooth muscle.[5] When ATP levels rise in response to increased coronary flow, the channel closes, making it easier to depolarize the cell and contract vascular smooth muscle. Contraction of vascular smooth muscle reduces the diameter of the coronary arteries and reduces blood flow. The opposite also occurs: a reduction in ATP level, due to low flow or increased metabolism, opens the K^+ channels. Potassium then leaks out of the vascular smooth muscle and short-circuits the depolarizing influences. This inhibits vascular contraction, leading to vasodilation and increased coronary blood flow. Adenosine also contributes to regulation of the ATP-sensitive K^+ channels, causing vasodilation when adenosine levels are elevated.

Nitric oxide (NO) produced by endothelial cells lining the coronary arteries is an important regulator of coronary blood flow. NO is a diffusible gas produced by the enzyme inducible nitric oxide synthase in response to numerous stimuli including hypoxemia and platelet factors. NO is a potent vasodilator, and inhibition of its production is associated with reduced coronary blood flow. Many known risk factors for coronary heart disease have been shown to impair nitric oxide–dependent vasodilation of coronary arteries.[5]

Vessel diameter also is regulated by the autonomic nervous system. The coronary arteries are primarily innervated by sympathetic nerves, but they also receive a small amount of parasympathetic innervation. The sympathetic neurotransmitter norepinephrine (NE) binds to both α_1 and β_2 receptors in coronary arteries; α_1 stimulation results in vasoconstriction, whereas β_2 stimulation dilates. Under normal conditions the vasodilator response predominates, but in pathologic states, excessive α_1-mediated constriction can occur. The increased metabolic activity associated with sympathetic nervous system stimulation generally causes autoregulatory vasodilation and overrides the direct effect of norepinephrine on the vessels. Parasympathetic activity contributes to vasodilation by promoting the production of nitric oxide by coronary endothelial cells.

In addition to vessel diameter, coronary resistance is affected by myocardial contraction. During systole, cardiac muscle compression creates a marked rise in coronary resistance that reduces coronary blood flow (perfusion). Blood flow to the left ventricle is greatly decreased during systole because of the pressures generated by the thick muscular layer. Blood vessels that penetrate the myocardium to supply the innermost endocardial areas are more compressed during contraction than are outer epicardial vessels. Even though coronary artery driving pressure is greatest during ventricular systole, little blood flow reaches the left ventricle because of the high external pressure applied to the coronary vessels as the myocardium contracts. Therefore, most myocardial blood flow occurs during the diastolic interval between ventricular contractions. The time the heart spends in diastole is directly related to heart rate. Faster heart rates reduce diastolic time and decrease coronary artery blood flow.

Cardiac muscle needs a continuous supply of oxygen and nutrients to perform its pumping functions. A disruption in cardiac blood flow (*ischemia*) generally results in some degree of pump failure and damage to cardiac tissues. Myocardial ischemia may be caused by conditions that reduce coronary blood flow or increase myocardial demands for oxygen. These include (1) reduced driving pressure (e.g., low aortic blood pressure or high right atrial pressure), (2) reduced vessel diameter (e.g., myocardial hypertrophy, arteriosclerosis, thrombosis, vasoconstricting chemicals), (3) reduced perfusion time (e.g., high heart rates, some dysrhythmias), and (4) increased metabolic demands (e.g., fever, sepsis, anemia).

KEY POINTS

- The right and left coronary arteries originate from the aortic root, within the sinuses of Valsalva. In most people the right coronary artery perfuses the right ventricle, AV node, sinoatrial (SA) node, and right atrium.
- The left coronary artery divides into the left circumflex artery and left anterior descending artery, which perfuse the left atrium and ventricle.
- Coronary blood flow is regulated centrally by the autonomic nervous system and locally by autoregulation. The amount of coronary flow depends on driving pressure and coronary resistance. Coronary resistance is dependent on vessel diameter.
- Adenosine and nitric oxide are two important vasodilating chemicals that are produced in response to inadequate oxygen delivery to the heart and help to increase blood flow to meet metabolic demands.
- Although driving pressure is highest during systole, there is little coronary flow to the left ventricle because of vessel compression by the contracting myocardium. Most coronary blood flow to endocardial areas of the ventricles occurs during diastole.

CARDIAC MYOCYTES

Cardiac muscle cells are divided into two general types: working cells, which have primarily mechanical pumping functions, and electrical cells, which primarily transmit electrical impulses. Both types are *excitable*: they are able to produce and transmit action potentials. Working myocardial cells are packed with contractile filaments and compose the bulk of the atrial and ventricular muscle. Electrical cells function to initiate and coordinate contraction of the working cells. Differentiated cardiac myocytes are unable to enter the cell cycle to proliferate; however, they can increase in size and synthesize more contractile proteins (hypertrophy). New myocardial cells can be formed from stem cells that have the potential to divide. Stem cells may be recruited from the circulation and stimulated to divide and mature into myocytes within the myocardium. Conditions that increase myocardial cell death are thought to stimulate recruitment of stem cells into the myocardium. A high turnover rate of cardiac myocytes occurs, and increases with age, suggesting that the entire population of cells within the heart is completely replaced 11 to 15 times over a lifetime.[6] When the rate of myocardial cell loss exceeds replacement by stem cells, the condition of heart failure may ensue (see Chapter 19).

Myocyte Structure

Typical myocardial cells (myocytes) are illustrated in Figure 17-10. Cardiac myocytes are described as muscle "fibers" because of their long, narrow shape. The plasma membrane (sarcolemma) of one cardiac cell is joined end-to-end with its neighbors by intercalated disks, which contain gap junctions that allow the rapid passage of electrical impulses from one cell to the next. The intercalated disks permit the many separate cells of the myocardium to function together in a coordinated

manner. This arrangement is called a *functional syncytium*. The sarcolemma also forms membrane-lined channels that penetrate the cell and become the transverse tubules (T tubules) (Figure 17-11). The T tubules permit extracellular fluid and ions to diffuse near intracellular structures. Movement of ions across the sarcolemma is an essential part of cellular excitation and the subsequent contraction of intracellular elements. Cellular contractile elements are simultaneously activated because signals at the cell surface are rapidly transmitted internally by the T tubules.[7]

The sarcoplasmic reticulum (SR) is an extensive labyrinth of hollow membrane that stores significant amounts of intracellular calcium. It contains Ca^{2+}-sensitive channels that open briefly during depolarization and allow calcium ions to flow into the cytoplasm. An action potential traveling along the T tubule opens voltage-sensitive calcium ion channels (L type) in the plasma membrane. The Ca^{2+} ions that enter the cell through these channels interact with receptors on the SR membrane called *ryanodine receptors* (see Figure 17-11, *B*). Activation of these receptors opens calcium gates on the SR, and Ca^{2+} rushes into the cytoplasm to initiate contraction. The SR also contains powerful sarcoplasmic endoplasmic reticulum calcium ATPase (SERCA) pumps that recover calcium ions from the cytoplasm and return them to the SR. Inside the SR, calcium is bound to specialized proteins including calsequestrin. This helps keep the free calcium concentration in the SR lower such that the calcium transporters have a lower gradient to pump against.

Cardiac muscle cells are packed with numerous mitochondria that are strategically positioned along the contractile fibers of the cell. The heart is also endowed with an extensive capillary network, approximately one capillary per muscle cell. The large number of mitochondria and abundant oxygen supply are necessary to keep pace with the high ATP requirements of the contractile elements and ion pumps.

Structure of the Contractile Apparatus

Microscopic inspection of the cardiac myocyte reveals a typical pattern of banding called *striation*.[8] This striated appearance is due to an organized structure of the proteins (myofibrils) of the contractile apparatus (Figure 17-12). The contractile proteins, actin and myosin, are called *filaments* because they are long and narrow. **Myosin** filaments are larger and referred to as *thick filaments. Thin filaments* are actually composed of several different types of protein bundled together. **Actin** is the primary constituent of thin filaments, with smaller amounts of the proteins **tropomyosin** and **troponin** bound to it.

The thick and thin filaments are specifically arranged in contractile units called *sarcomeres* (Figure 17-13). Sarcomeres are defined by dark bands called *Z disks* (also called Z lines), which lie perpendicular to actin and myosin filaments. A sarcomere extends from one Z disk to the next. Thin actin filaments are attached to Z disks and extend from them. The I bands (isotropic) are light in color and correspond to the position of thin actin filaments extending in both directions from the Z disk. Thick myosin filaments lie parallel to and between the thin filaments. They are held in place by a very large and elastic protein called *titin* that extends from the Z disk to the center of the sarcomere. Each myosin filament is surrounded by six thin filaments (see Figure 17-13). An efficient, synchronized contraction is enhanced by this precise arrangement of contractile elements.

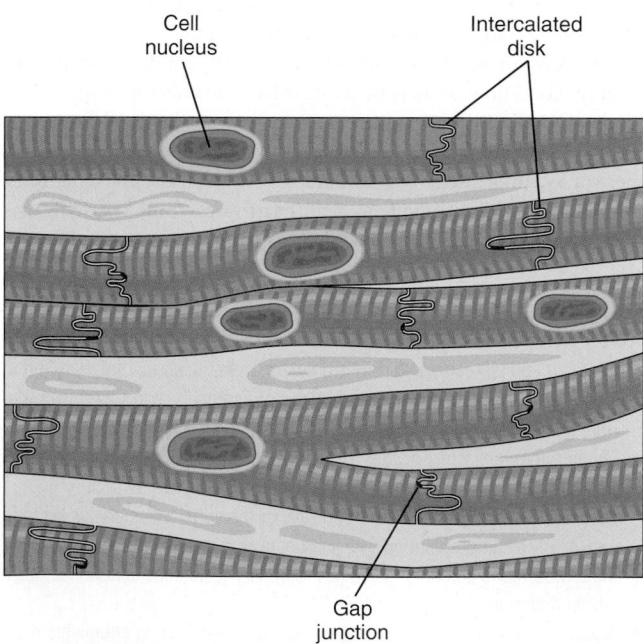

Cell nucleus

Intercalated disk

Gap junction

FIGURE 17-10 Myocardial cells, showing long narrow shape and interconnecting junctions, forming a functional syncytium. The end of one muscle cell is fused to the next by intercalated disks. Within these connections are specialized proteins that form a fluid-filled pore (gap junction) between the fused cells. Ions can travel through the gap junctions to transport changes in membrane potential from one cell to the next.

Characteristics of Contractile Filaments

Myosin molecules are composed of six polypeptide chains: two heavy (H) chains and four light (L) chains. These light and heavy

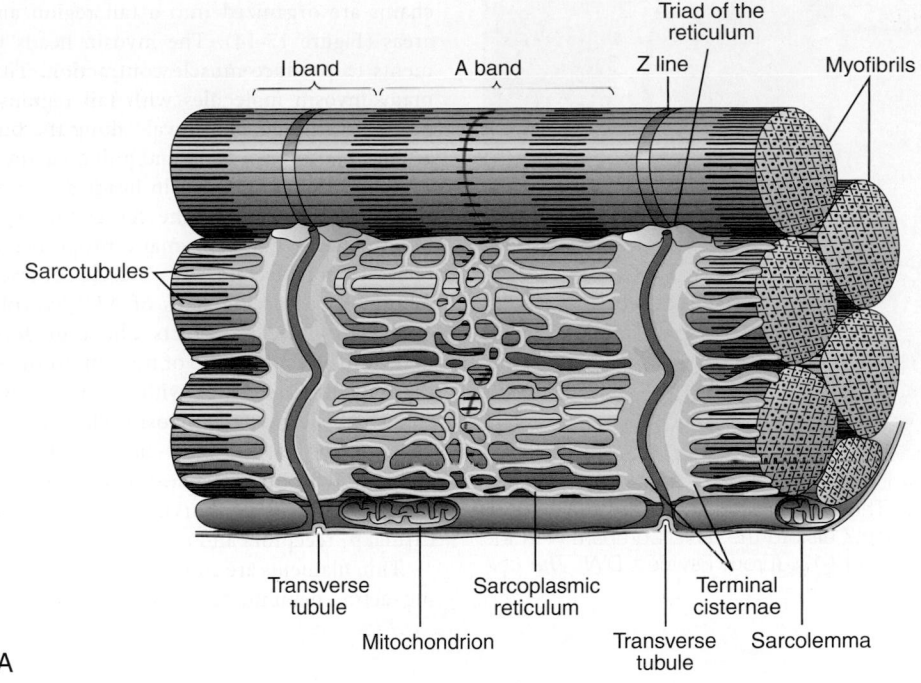

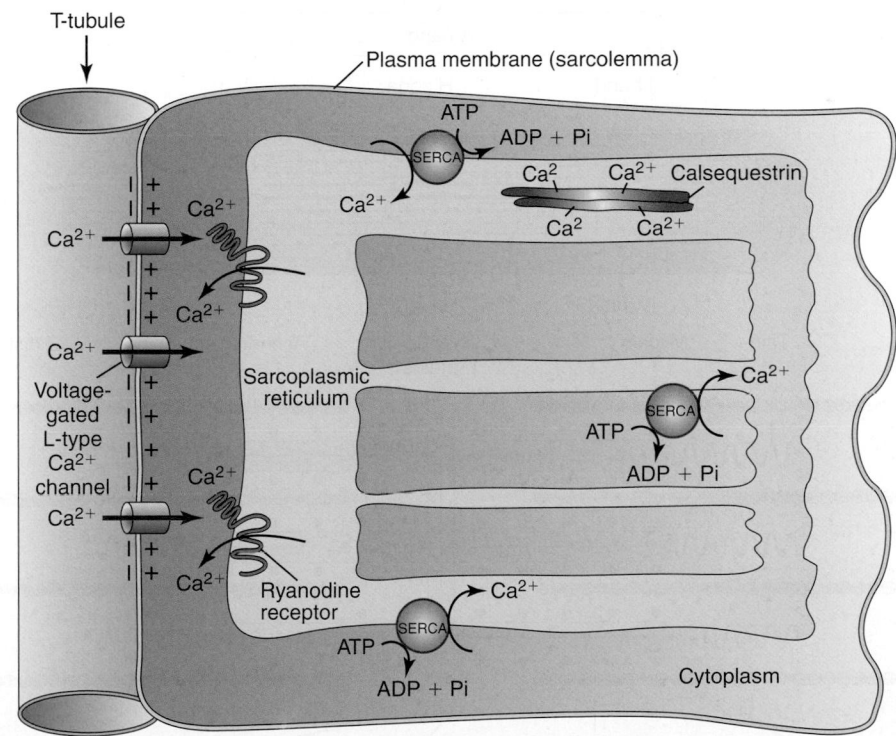

FIGURE 17-11 A, Schematic diagram of a portion of a cardiac myocyte showing the transverse tubules (T tubules), which extend at right angles from the plasma membrane (sarcolemma) into the cell interior. The T tubules are extensions of the plasma membrane that bring the extracellular fluid into juxtaposition with the terminal ends of the sarcoplasmic reticulum (SR). The T tubule with the SR on either side of it is called the *triad of the reticulum*. **B,** Calcium ions that enter the cytoplasm through voltage-gated L-type channels on the T-tubule membrane interact with the ryanodine receptors on the sarcoplasmic reticulum. The activated ryanodine receptors allow calcium ions to flow into the cell cytoplasm where they initiate contraction. As soon as they are released, calcium ions are rapidly captured by the sarcoplasmic endoplasmic reticulum calcium ATPase *(SERCA)* pumps on the SR membrane.

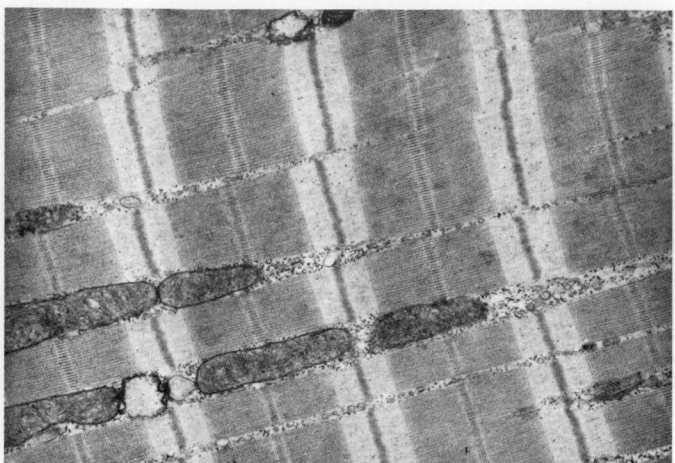

FIGURE 17-12 Electron micrograph of muscle fibrils showing characteristic banding pattern. The dark vertical lines are the Z disks. A sarcomere extends from one Z disk to the next. Compare with the schematic drawing in Figure 17-13. (From Fawcett DW: *The cell*, Philadelphia, 1981, Saunders.)

chains are organized into a tail region and two globular "head" areas (Figure 17-14). The myosin heads interact with actin filaments to produce muscle contraction. Thick filaments consist of many myosin molecules with tail regions bundled together and heads protruding at intervals along the bundle. The head regions are flexible and can bend and pull on actin filaments to accomplish muscle contraction. Myosin heads are oriented in opposite directions on either side of the center tail region (see Figure 17-14). Myosin heads have enzymatic properties and can cleave ATP to release energy necessary for muscle contraction. Different forms of myosin have varying rates of ATP hydrolysis, which affects how quickly the muscle contracts. The serum level of thyroid hormone is known to affect the type of myosin produced in heart cells. Hyperthyroidism is associated with a fast-cycling type and hypothyroidism with a slow type of myosin. The rate of myosin cycling can also be regulated at the light chain of the myosin protein. Cellular enzymes that attach a phosphate to the light chain accelerate the rate of cycling. Phosphorylation is increased by activation of myocardial β_1 receptors and enhances contractility.[8]

Thin filaments are composed of several different proteins, including actin, nebulin, tropomyosin, and troponin. Actin filaments

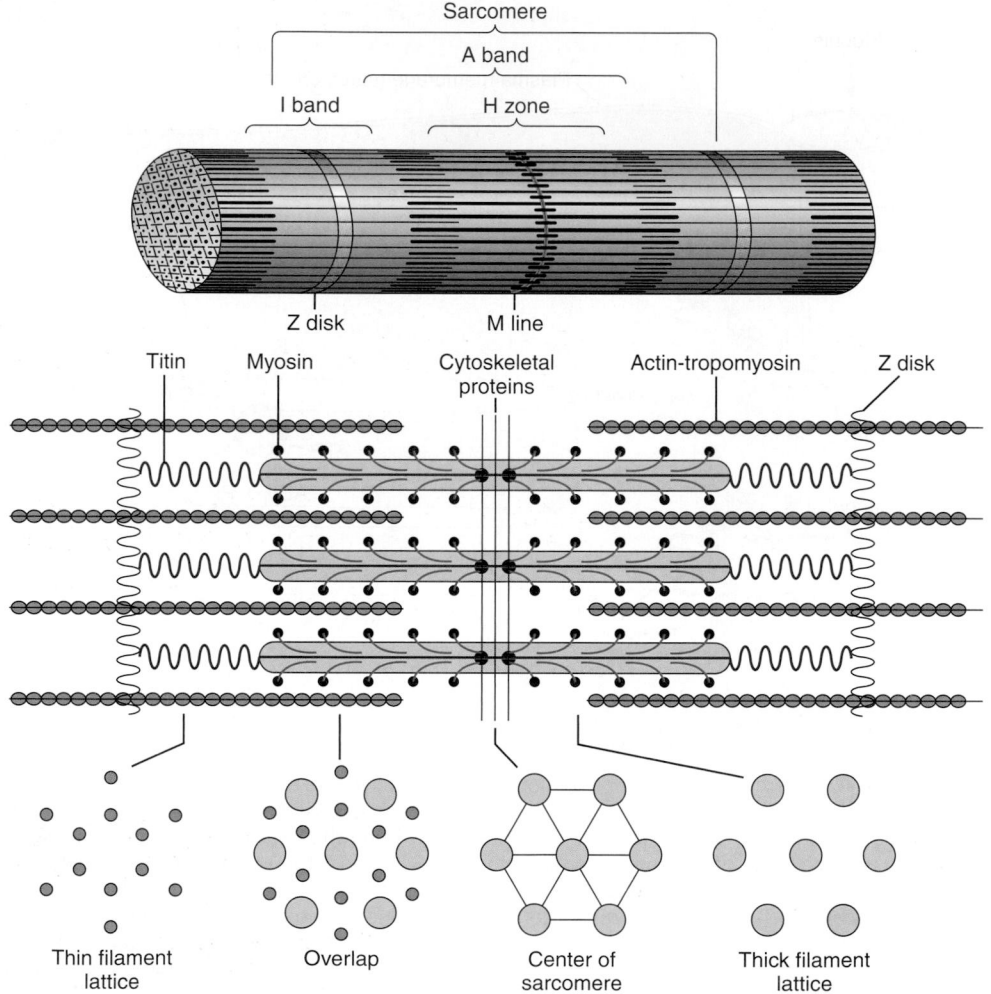

FIGURE 17-13 Thick and thin filaments are organized into contractile units called *sarcomeres*. A sarcomere extends from one Z disk to the next and represents the fundamental unit of muscle contraction. See text for description of bands, zones, and lines. Overlap of thick and thin filaments in each area is shown in cross-section at the bottom. Each thick filament interacts with six thin filaments that surround it.

are actually polymers of many globular actin proteins that are attached end-to-end, like two strings of beads, and then twisted together to form a helix (Figure 17-15). Each of the actin beads has a site that can bind with myosin heads. Nebulin is a long protein that extends the entire length of the thin filament and is thought to regulate the length of the actin polymer such that all of the thin filaments are the same size. Tropomyosins are long, slender proteins that bind to a string of six or seven actin beads.[9] When myocardial muscle is relaxed, tropomyosin molecules inhibit the myosin-binding sites on the actin beads. A third protein complex, troponin, is attached to the thin filament and regulates the availability of

binding sites on the actin filament by controlling the position of tropomyosin. Each troponin is composed of three subunits, called troponins T, I, and C. Troponin T binds to tropomyosin, troponin I participates in the inhibitory actions of tropomyosin, and troponin C binds up to four molecules of Ca^{2+}. As described in the following section, tropomyosin and troponin are important regulatory proteins that control the activities of actin and myosin filaments. The specific isoforms (amino acid sequences) of troponins T and I present in heart tissue differ from those in other types of cells, and their presence in the serum can be used to detect myocardial infarction (see Chapter 18).

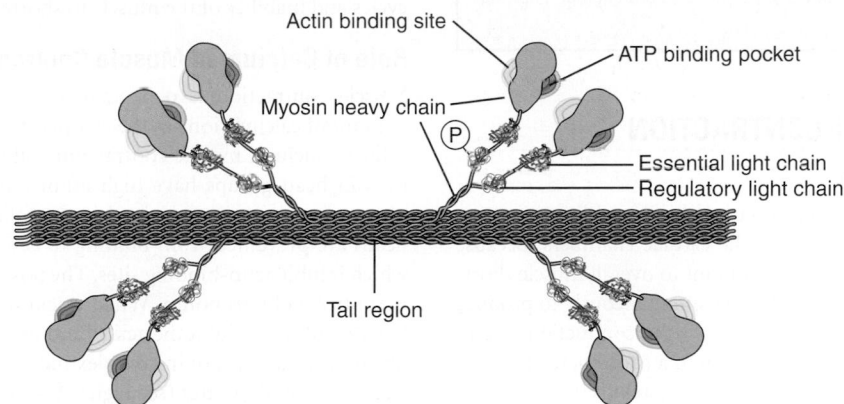

FIGURE 17-14 Thick filament of the sarcomere is composed of myosin proteins. Myosin head groups are oriented in opposite directions on either side of the center tail region. Phosphorylation *(P)* of the regulatory light chain increases myosin activity and rate of cross-bridge cycling.

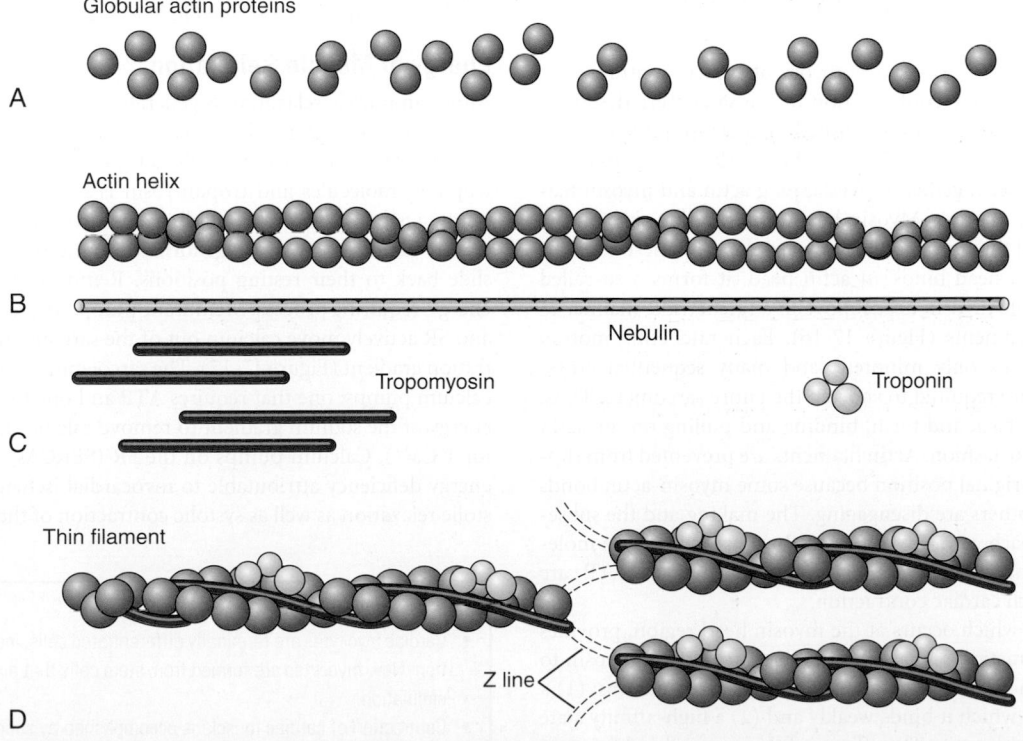

FIGURE 17-15 Schematic drawing of the proteins that comprise the thin filament. **A,** Globular actin proteins combine to form long double-helix filaments. **B,** Nebulin (nebulette) is a long cytoskeletal protein that extends the length of the thin filament and is thought to regulate filament length. **C** and **D,** The proteins troponin and tropomyosin combine with the actin helix to form the thin filament.

MOLECULAR BASIS OF CONTRACTION

Overview of Contraction

The heart's pumping action is accomplished by the additive contractions of the many myocytes that form the cardiac chambers. Because each myocyte contributes only a small amount to overall muscle shortening, all cells of the chamber must shorten simultaneously to produce a forceful contraction. The specialized cells of the conduction system function to stimulate myocardial contraction in a coordinated way. An action potential traveling down the conduction system is the usual trigger for contraction. Cardiac myocyte depolarization causes ion channels in the plasma membrane and T tubules to open, permitting sodium and calcium entry and release of calcium from the SR. The presence of free calcium in the sarcoplasm (muscle cytoplasm) results in contraction. These events describe the process of *excitation-contraction coupling*.

Sliding Filament/Cross-Bridge Theory of Muscle Contraction

The sliding filament, or cross-bridge, theory of muscle contraction is suggested by the anatomic configuration of the sarcomere described earlier. Muscle shortening is accomplished by increasing the amount of overlap of actin and myosin filaments. The Z disks at the ends of the sarcomere move closer together as overlapping actin and myosin filaments pull past one another. Myosin heads grip binding sites on the actin beads and pull the thin filaments toward the sarcomere's center. Each time a myosin head binds an actin bead, it forms a so-called **cross-bridge.** Flexible myosin heads move in a ratchet-like manner to tug on the actin filaments (Figure 17-16). Each ratcheting motion moves actin filaments only minutely, and many sequential cross-bridge formations are required to shorten the entire sarcomere. Thus, myosin heads bend back and forth, binding and pulling on the actin filaments in a steplike fashion. Actin filaments are prevented from slipping back to their original position because some myosin-actin bonds are forming while others are disengaging. The making and the subsequent breaking of each actin-myosin cross-bridge requires one molecule of ATP. Consequently, tremendous quantities of ATP are hydrolyzed with each cardiac contraction.

ATP hydrolysis, which occurs at the myosin head region, provides the energy for contraction and also affects the capability of myosin to bind actin.[7] Myosin has two functional states or conformations: (1) a low-affinity state in which it binds weakly and (2) a high-affinity state in which it avidly binds actin. The affinity of the myosin head for actin depends on whether ATP is bound (low affinity) or ADP and inorganic phosphate (P_i) are bound (high affinity). A proposed sequence of cross-bridge cycling is as follows (see Figure 17-16):

1. Free myosin heads bind ATP and hydrolyze it to ADP and P_i, which remain on the myosin. Myosin heads now have a high affinity for actin and are in a high-energy conformation.
2. If binding sites on actin are accessible, myosin binds to the actin.
3. Binding results in release of ADP and P_i and a ratchet movement of the myosin as it assumes its low-energy conformation, which shortens the sarcomere (power stroke).
4. With loss of ADP and P_i, myosin can bind another molecule of ATP. The myosin heads with ATP bound now have a low affinity for actin and are released from the binding site. ATP is again hydrolyzed to ADP and P_i, and another cross-bridge cycle is initiated.

Continued cross-bridge cycling is dependent on the availability of ATP and calcium ions. A lack of ATP results in fewer cross-bridge cycles and inability of the muscle to shorten normally.

Role of Calcium in Muscle Contraction

Muscle contraction is dependent on the presence of an adequate amount of calcium ions in the cytoplasm. In the absence of free intracellular calcium, muscle contraction will not take place, even though myosin head groups have high affinity for actin-binding sites. This phenomenon can be explained in the following way. At rest, myosin heads are prevented from binding to actin by tropomyosin proteins, which inhibit actin-binding sites. The position of tropomyosin protein is controlled by troponin. When calcium is absent, troponin induces tropomyosin to inhibit the actin-binding sites. When calcium binds to troponin C, the troponin complex induces tropomyosin to move and expose the binding sites (see Figure 17-16, *A* and *B*). Cross-bridge formation immediately ensues because myosin heads have high affinity for these sites in the relaxed state. The concentration of free calcium ions in the myocardial cell determines how many actin sites are exposed and for how long, and therefore, determines the number of cross-bridges and extent of contraction. The release of Ca^{2+} into the cytoplasm is regulated by numerous neurotransmitters and hormones that affect contractility as described in later sections of this chapter.

Energy of Muscle Relaxation

Although muscle relaxation is generally viewed as a passive phenomenon, it actually requires significant energy to pump calcium ions out of the cytoplasm. As calcium levels fall, calcium diffuses away from the troponin molecules and tropomyosin is induced to cover the actin-binding sites. With actin-binding sites covered, myosin heads are unable to initiate cross-bridge formation, and thick and thin filaments slide back to their resting positions. Removal of calcium ions is an energy-requiring process. Membrane pumps located in the sarcolemma and SR actively move calcium out of the sarcoplasm against a concentration gradient (Figure 17-17). The sarcolemma contains two different calcium pumps: one that requires ATP and one that uses the potential energy of the sodium gradient to remove calcium from the cell (3 Na^+ for 1 Ca^{2+}). Calcium pumps on the SR (SERCAs) require ATP. Thus energy deficiency attributable to myocardial ischemia can impair diastolic relaxation as well as systolic contraction of the heart muscle.

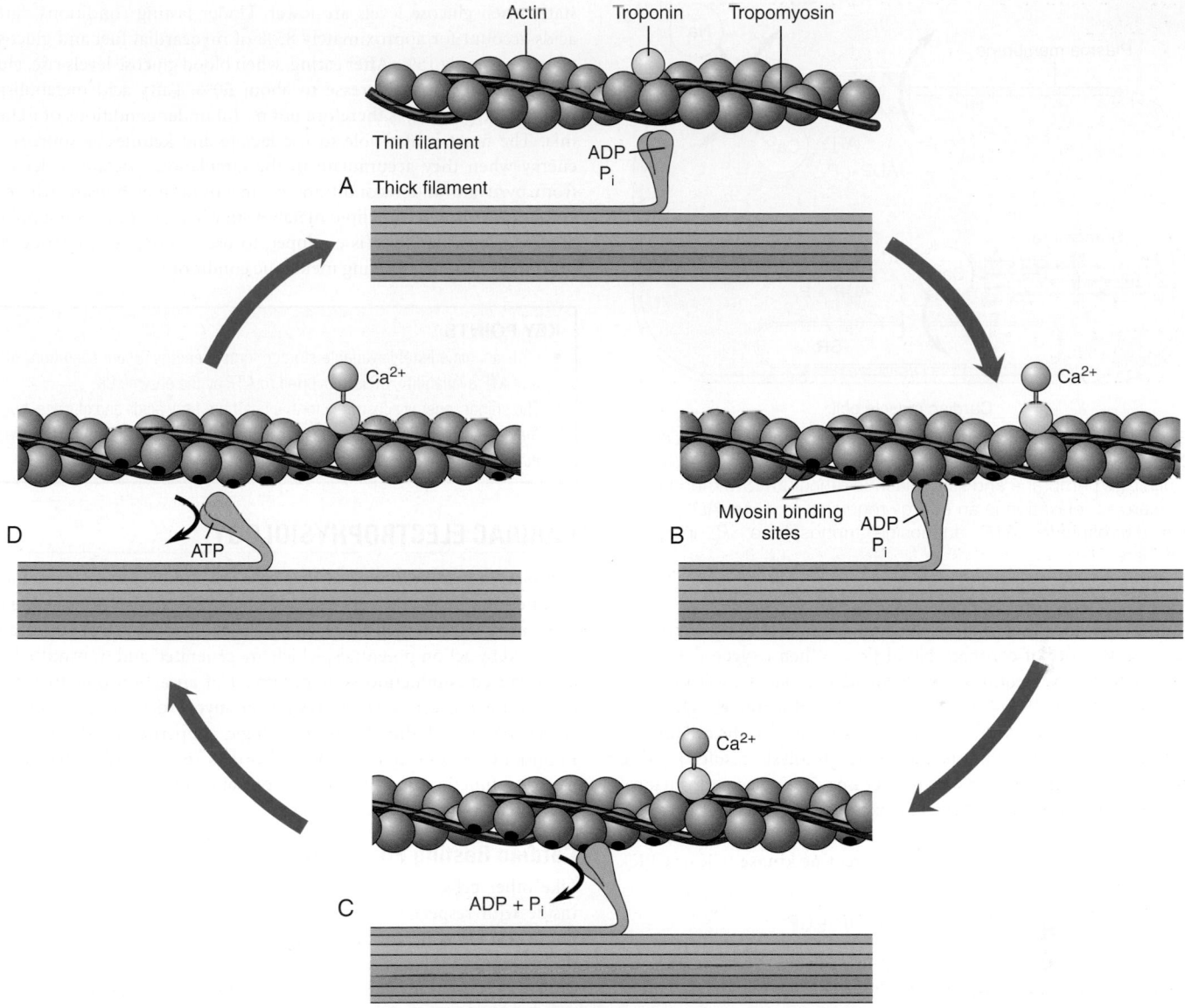

FIGURE 17-16 Cross-bridge cycle of muscle contraction. **A,** The myosin head has hydrolyzed its bound adenosine triphosphate *(ATP)* to adenosine diphosphate *(ADP)* and inorganic phosphate *(P$_i$)*, which remain on the myosin. In this state the myosin has high affinity for actin but cannot bind because the actin-binding sites are not accessible. **B,** When calcium ions enter the cell and bind to troponin, the tropomyosin-blocking protein moves to allow myosin to bind actin, forming a cross-bridge. **C,** The act of binding changes the shape of myosin so that ADP and P$_i$ are released. The "power stroke" is accomplished by movement of the myosin neck region. **D,** When a new molecule of ATP binds to the myosin, it changes to a low-affinity state and releases from the actin. ATP is again hydrolyzed to ADP and P$_i$ to restart the cycle. Each cross-bridge cycle uses one ATP molecule.

- ATP hydrolysis provides the energy for cross-bridging and also affects the affinity of myosin for actin. Myosin has high affinity for actin when ADP and P$_i$ are bound, and low affinity when ATP is bound. Myosin cycles between high- and low-affinity states, making and breaking cross-bridges with the actin filament.
- The presence of intracellular free calcium ion (Ca^{2+}) is necessary for muscle contraction to occur. When Ca^{2+} is absent, actin-binding sites are inhibited and inaccessible for cross-bridging. Binding of Ca^{2+} to troponin induces the movement of tropomyosin to expose actin-binding sites and allow cross-bridge formation.
- Muscle relaxation (lusitropy) is due to removal of Ca^{2+} from the cytoplasm. This is an energy-requiring process.

CARDIAC ENERGY METABOLISM

The heart, like other tissues in the body, utilizes energy from ATP hydrolysis to drive its energy-requiring functions. Synthesis of ATP in cardiac muscle cells is accomplished by the same glycolytic and oxidative reactions described in detail in Chapter 3.

Oxygen Utilization

Because the heart is continuously active, its energy requirements are considerable. Very little ATP is stored in myocardial cells, so that a continuous supply of oxygen and nutrients is necessary to support ongoing ATP synthesis. Even under normal resting conditions, the heart extracts a large portion of oxygen from the blood perfusing it.

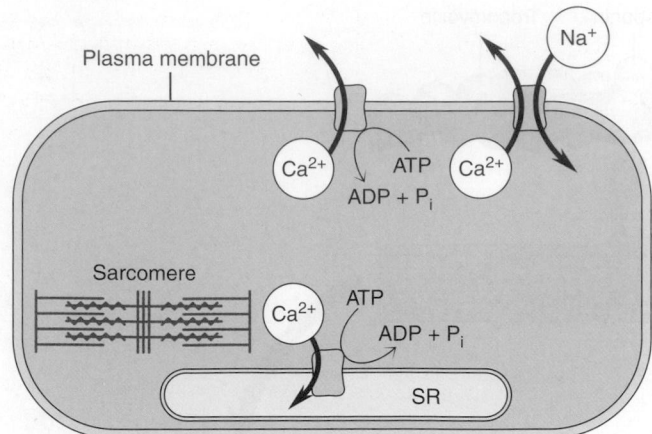

Cardiac muscle cell

FIGURE 17-17 Calcium ions *(Ca²⁺)* are removed from the cardiac muscle cell cytoplasm by energy-dependent protein transporters in the plasma membrane and sarcoplasmic reticulum *(SR)* membrane. Thus cardiac relaxation is an energy-requiring process. *ADP,* Adenosine diphosphate; *ATP,* adenosine triphosphate; *Pᵢ,* inorganic phosphate.

Conditions of increased oxygen demand, therefore, must be met by increasing the rate of coronary blood flow. When oxygen delivery is insufficient to meet requirements for oxidative phosphorylation, the cell must rely on ATP produced by glycolysis. Unfortunately, glycolysis results in production of only enough ATP to maintain the cell for seconds to minutes. In addition, anaerobic glycolysis results in local buildup of lactic acid, which may further impair cardiac performance.

Under conditions of relative ATP excess, myocardial cells are able to transfer energy to a storage form called *creatine phosphate* (CP). This transfer is accomplished by the enzyme **creatine kinase** (CK or CPK), in the following reaction:

$$ATP + creatine \leftrightarrow ADP + CP$$

Although amounts of cellular CP are limited, they provide an immediate source of energy when cellular ATP levels drop acutely. Under conditions of ischemia, the enzymatic reaction would proceed in reverse, utilizing CP and adenosine diphosphate (ADP) to produce ATP, for immediate use by the cell. This phosphate transfer reaction is important during fluctuations in ATP supply because it does not require the presence of oxygen.

The enzyme CK is also useful in the diagnosis of myocardial cell damage. Myocardial cells that lose membrane integrity (necrosis) leak their enzymes into extracellular fluid and eventually into the bloodstream. Elevated levels of blood CK are indicative of the degree of acute myocardial cell death. Different types of tissue contain different forms of CK (isoenzymes). The MB form of CK is found in cardiac muscle, and elevated serum levels of this enzyme are indicative of myocardial infarction.[9] Other intracellular proteins, including troponin and myoglobin, are released during myocardial cell death and also can be used as markers of myocardial infarction (see Chapter 18).

Substrate Utilization

The primary foodstuffs that provide fuel for energy-producing enzymatic processes in cardiac muscle are glucose and fatty acids.[7] Amino acids are less important metabolic substrates for cardiac muscle except during states of starvation. The amount of fatty acids and glucose utilized by heart muscle cells depends on their relative concentrations in the blood. Fatty acids are the preferred fuel, particularly in a fasting state, when glucose levels are lower. Under fasting conditions, fatty acids account for approximately 85% of myocardial fuel and glucose contributes only 15%. After eating, when blood glucose levels rise, glucose utilization may increase to about 50%. Fatty acid metabolism requires oxygen and is therefore not useful under conditions of ischemia. The heart is also able to use lactate and ketones as sources of energy when they accumulate in the circulation. Lactate is derived from pyruvate under conditions of anaerobic metabolism, whereas ketones are formed from lipid metabolism when carbohydrate supplies are low. Thus, the heart is equipped to use a variety of substrates to produce ATP under varying metabolic conditions.

KEY POINTS

- CP is an immediately available storage form of energy. Under conditions of low ATP availability, CP is converted to ATP by the enzyme CK.
- The primary energy substrates for the heart are fatty acids and glucose, but the heart can utilize a variety of sources to produce energy depending on the nutrients available in the circulation.

CARDIAC ELECTROPHYSIOLOGY

The plasma membranes of cardiac cells are endowed with special ion channels that make the cells excitable. Excitable tissues are capable of generating and conducting action potentials. The heart is rhythmically activated by action potentials, which are generated and transmitted by a specialized conduction system. Spread of an action potential over cardiac muscle cell surfaces results in myocardial contraction. An understanding of the electrophysiologic properties of the heart is important because many cardiac disorders result in disturbances in electrical function that produce abnormal conduction pathways, dysrhythmias, and conduction blocks.

Cardiac Resting Potential

Like other cells, resting cardiac cells are negatively charged on the inside with respect to the outside (see Chapter 3). A difference in potassium ion concentration across the cell membrane is the primary determinant of the resting membrane potential. Atrial and ventricular muscle cells generally have a resting membrane potential of −85 to −95 mV. Pacemaker cells in the SA node are less polarized, having a resting membrane potential of about −60 mV. An increase in the concentration of extracellular potassium ion tends to hypopolarize the cell (make it less negative), and a lower-than-normal extracellular potassium concentration tends to hyperpolarize the cell (make it more negative). The degree of polarization is an important determinant of the ease with which an action potential can be initiated. Abnormalities in serum potassium level are a common source of cardiac dysrhythmias.

Cardiac Action Potential

Depolarization of cardiac cells to a threshold point results in activation of voltage-sensitive ion channels in the membrane. A myocardial action potential (Figure 17-18) results from movement of ions through these open voltage-gated channels. The action potential in atrial and ventricular cells has five characteristic phases.[10] Atrial action potentials are shorter in duration because they have a reduced phase 2 compared with ventricular cells.

Phase 0. Phase 0 begins when the membrane potential approaches threshold and voltage-gated "fast" sodium channels open momentarily. As a result of a steep electrochemical gradient for sodium entry, rapid influx of sodium ions occurs. Sodium entry depolarizes the cell by neutralizing the difference in charge (polarity) across the membrane. A steep depolarizing deflection (upstroke) is recorded. Class I

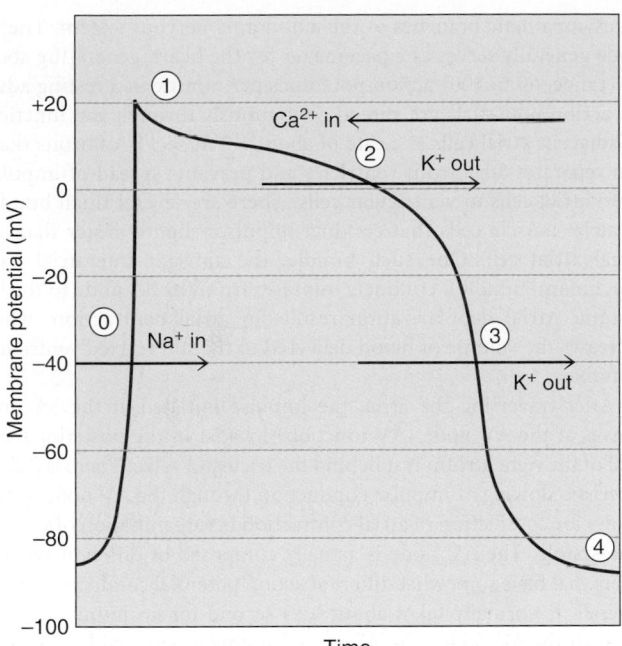

FIGURE 17-18 Ventricular myocardial action potential has five characteristic phases, representing changes in ion movement through the plasma membrane. *Phase 0:* Rapid upstroke attributable to sodium influx. *Phase 1:* Slight repolarization attributable to closure of sodium channels and initiation of potassium efflux. *Phase 2:* Plateau attributable to offsetting influx of calcium and efflux of potassium. *Phase 3:* Rapid repolarization attributable to closure of calcium channels and increased potassium efflux. *Phase 4:* Resting membrane potential reestablished attributable to closure of all voltage-sensitive channels.

antidysrhythmic agents such as quinidine and lidocaine block voltage-gated sodium channels and interfere with phase 0 depolarization (see Chapter 19).[11]

Phase 1. Phase 1 is identified as a small repolarizing deflection that corresponds to closure of the fast sodium channels and transient efflux of potassium from the cell through K+ channels. The interior of the cell is now more positively charged than at rest, which induces potassium ions to leave the cell.

Phase 2. Phase 2 is also called the *plateau phase* because little change in membrane potential occurs during this time, even though ions continue to move across the membrane. Phase 2 is primarily associated with an influx of calcium ions, which is offset by an efflux of potassium ions. The ability of K+ to leave the cell down its electrochemical gradient is inhibited during the plateau phase by a relative inhibition of a subset of potassium channels. This is sometimes called potassium *rectification.* Chloride also may leave the cell during this phase. The voltage-gated calcium channels open and close slowly in comparison to fast sodium channels and are thus referred to as slow channels or L-type channels (long-lasting).

The calcium that enters the cell during phase 2 is linked to muscle contraction as previously described. The L-type calcium channels can be modified by agonists that prolong the open phase, such as catecholamines, and by antagonists that shorten the open phase, such as acetylcholine. Calcium channel–blocking agents (class IV antidysrhythmic agents) are used commonly in patients with cardiovascular diseases to inhibit calcium influx.[11] β-Blockers (class II antidysrhythmics) also reduce calcium ion influx during phase 2 by indirectly inhibiting calcium channels.

Phase 3. Phase 3 is characterized by a rapid return to the resting membrane potential. This is accomplished by closure of the slow

calcium channels and continued and even more rapid efflux of potassium ions from the cell through a variety of potassium channels. Sodium channels remain absolutely refractory during phases 1, 2, and early 3. The latter part of phase 3 represents a *relative refractory period,* when sodium channels may be induced to open, but a larger than normal depolarizing stimulus is required. If an abnormally early (premature) depolarization occurs during the relative refractory period, it will be conducted more slowly than usual because few fast Na+ channels are ready to be activated. Slow conduction through the myocardium predisposes to cardiac dysrhythmias, such as ventricular fibrillation (see Chapter 19). Class III antidysrhythmic agents, such as amiodarone, increase the refractory period by inhibiting opening of potassium channels during phase 3.[11]

Phase 4. Phase 4 of the ventricular myocyte action potential corresponds to the period of time between action potentials when no changes in membrane voltage are evident and the resting membrane potential is present. The resting membrane potential in ventricular myocardial cells is flat, and they do not spontaneously depolarize. In contrast, cells in the pacemaker and conduction system automatically depolarize and have a sloping phase 4. The Na+-K+ pump and Ca2+ pump work continuously throughout all phases to reestablish the internal and external concentrations of sodium, potassium, and calcium ions.

Rhythmicity of Myocardial Cells

Rhythmicity and automaticity refer to regular, spontaneous generation of action potentials. Rhythmic pacemaker cells have a recognizable action potential that is characterized by a sloping phase 4 (Figure 17-19), in contrast to the flat phase 4 of ventricular muscle cells. A requirement for rhythmicity is that the cell membrane has channels that automatically open during phase 4. These channels begin to open as the membrane potential becomes more negative during the repolarization phase.[10] Progressive channel opening makes the pacemaker cells leaky to Na+, Ca2+, and K+. Gradually the flow of positive ions into a cell offsets the repolarizing currents and depolarizes the membrane, resulting in generation of an action potential. One contributor to the automatic depolarization during phase 4 is the I_f channel. The I_f channels originally were named for a "funny" current and later discovered to be sodium channels that are activated by membrane repolarization. Channels that allow calcium and potassium leakage are also operative during phase 4 in pacemaker cells. Late in phase 4, an increase in calcium ion influx occurs through voltage-gated calcium channels called *T type,* for "transient." These channels open and close more quickly than the L-type calcium channels that open during the action potential. Spontaneous release of Ca2+ from the sarcoplasmic reticulum also contributes to depolarization by activating the 3Na+/Ca2+ exchanger and promoting Na+ influx.[10] Many of these channels can be regulated by various means, including autonomic neurotransmitters, in order to change heart rate. An action potential is initiated when phase 4 depolarization reaches the threshold for opening of voltage-gated, L-type, slow calcium channels. Repolarization is achieved in large part by an exodus of potassium ions from the cell.

The rate of rhythmic discharge is determined by the relative influx of Na+ and Ca2+ versus the efflux of K+. In a normal heart, a cell with the fastest rate of spontaneous depolarization becomes the pacemaker for the rest of the heart. Cells in the SA node, located in the right atrium, generally function as the heart's pacemaker because they have the fastest rate of spontaneous depolarization. However, other cells in the conduction system are also capable of spontaneous depolarization and may initiate an action potential in certain circumstances.

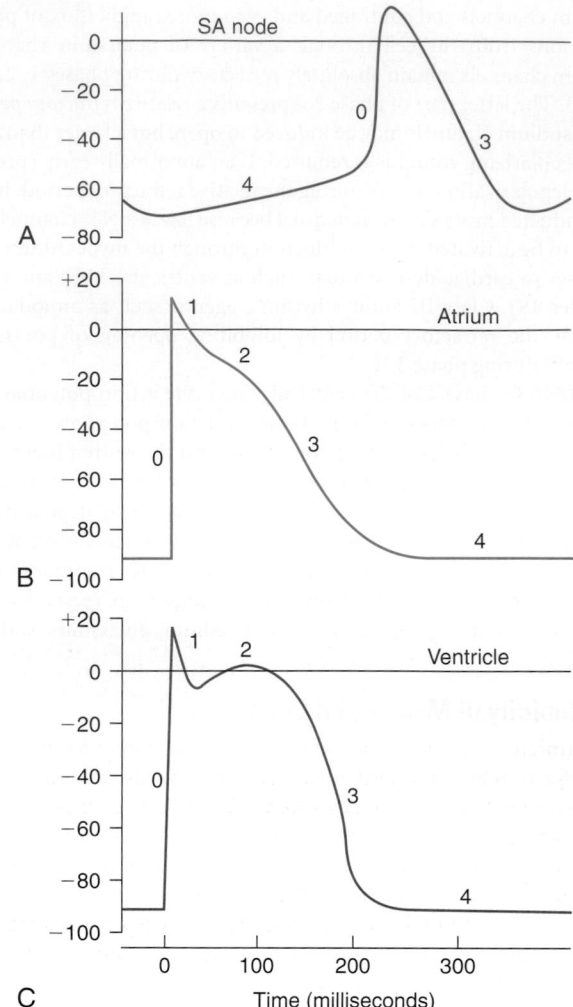

FIGURE 17-19 Rhythmic cells **(A)** have a sloping phase 4, in contrast to the flat phase 4 of the atrial **(B)** and ventricular **(C)** muscle cells. Spontaneous depolarization during phase 4 allows pacemaker cells to develop action potentials automatically. *SA,* Sinoatrial. (Adapted from Hoffman BF, Cranefield PF: *Electrophysiology of the heart,* New York, 1960, McGraw-Hill.)

The steepness of the slope of phase 4 depolarization determines the rate of action potential generation and therefore heart rate. Several factors determine the steepness of the slope, including membrane permeability to sodium, calcium, and potassium. For example, an increase in potassium ions leaving the cell would slow depolarization and result in a slower rate. Rhythmicity may be influenced by the autonomic nervous system, drugs, and electrolyte balance. These conditions are discussed in the following sections.

Specialized Conduction System of the Heart

Some myocardial cells are specialized to conduct action potentials throughout the heart in an organized and rapid manner. These cells constitute the conduction system of the heart, as shown in Figure 17-20. Normal excitation of the heart follows a pathway beginning with the SA node, atrial internodal pathways, AV node, bundle of His, ventricular bundle branches, and, finally, Purkinje fibers.

The SA node is located in the right atrium near the superior vena cava inlet. It receives innervation from sympathetic and parasympathetic branches of the autonomic nervous system. The SA node generally serves as a pacemaker for the heart, generating about 70 (range, 60 to 100) action potentials per minute in a resting adult. SA action potentials are spread contiguously through gap junctions to adjacent atrial cells at a rate of about 1.0 m/sec.[10] A fibrous skeleton separates atria from ventricles and prevents spread of impulses from atrial cells to ventricular cells. There are several small bundles of atrial muscle cells that conduct impulses slightly faster than the usual atrial cell. One such bundle, the anterior interatrial band (Bachmann bundle), conducts impulses from the SA node to the left atrium. Atrial depolarization results in atrial contraction, which increases the volume of blood delivered to the still relaxed ventricular chambers.

After traversing the atria, the impulse initiated at the SA node arrives at the AV node (AV junction) located in the posterior septal wall of the right atrium just behind the tricuspid valve. There is a characteristic slowing of impulse conduction through the AV node, which allows for completion of atrial contraction before initiation of ventricular systole. The AV node is actually composed of different types of fibers that have somewhat different action potential conduction times. Overall, it normally takes about 0.13 second for an impulse to pass through the AV node. The AV node is richly innervated by the autonomic nervous system. The AV node spontaneously depolarizes at a rate of 40 to 60 times per minute and usually becomes the heart's pacemaker if the SA node fails.

Purkinje cells (fibers), which lead from the AV node to ventricular myocardium, are vastly different from AV nodal cells. They are large and well structured to conduct impulses very rapidly. After penetrating the AV fibrous barrier, the bundle of Purkinje fibers travels 5 to 15 mm down the intraventricular septum toward the apex. The main bundle then divides into left and right bundle branches, which travel down the left and right sides of the intraventricular septum. Successive branches of Purkinje fibers penetrate the ventricular muscle mass from the endocardial side. Intraventricular septal areas are depolarized first, followed by apical muscle and finally the lateral walls (Figure 17-21). Early septal depolarization allows the septum to contract first and provide a stable wall against which the left and right ventricles can contract.[10] The total time elapsed between main bundle branch and terminal Purkinje fiber depolarization is only 0.03 second. Therefore, the entire ventricular endocardium is activated almost simultaneously. Purkinje fibers are capable of spontaneous depolarization at a rate of 15 to 40 times per minute and may become pacemakers for the heart if impulses from the SA and AV nodes are interrupted.

Action potentials are rapidly transmitted from the terminal Purkinje fibers to cardiac muscle fibers and then spread contiguously from cell to cell through gap junctions in the ventricular muscle. Approximately 0.03 second is required for the impulse to be transmitted through the ventricular myocardium.[10] Impulses normally travel from the terminations of Purkinje fibers at endocardial surfaces toward the epicardial surfaces. Depolarization of the right ventricle is accomplished slightly sooner than the left because of differences in muscle mass. Depolarization of the ventricular myocardium is followed by contraction and ejection of blood from the ventricles.

The capability of faster pacemakers to suppress the automatic discharge of slower pacemakers is called *overdrive suppression.* A slower pacemaker may be revealed if the normal pacemaker is suddenly interrupted. Sometimes it takes time for the slower pacemaker to "kick in" and begin pacing at its intrinsic rate. A previously rapid rate of depolarization apparently enhances the activity of membrane Na^+-K^+ pumps, resulting in a period of hyperpolarization (more negative

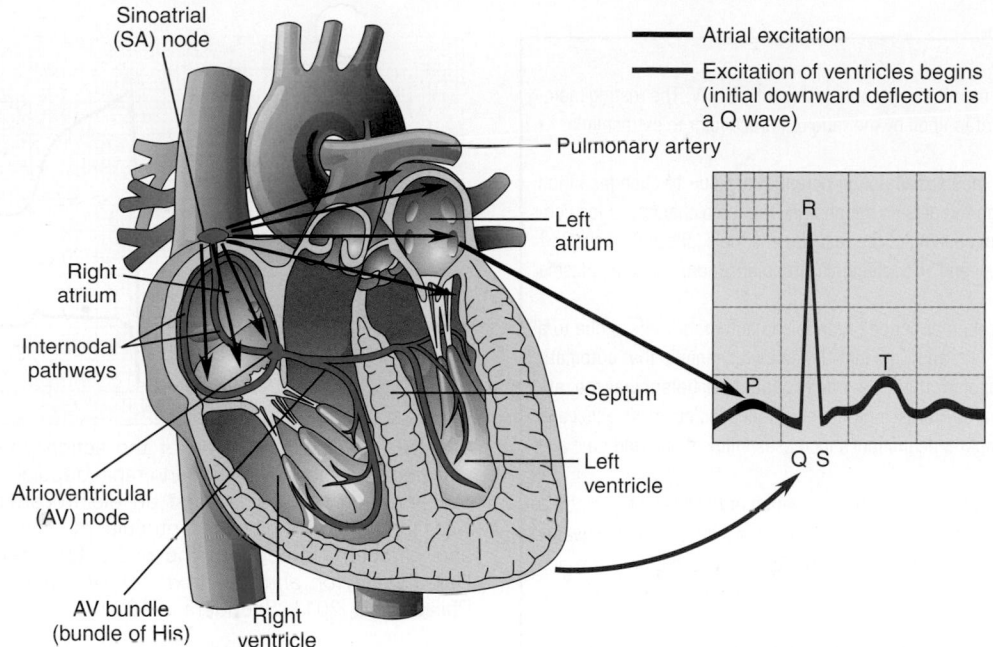

FIGURE 17-20 Schematic drawing of the conduction system of the heart. An impulse normally is generated in the sinus node and travels through the atria to the AV node, down the bundle of His and Purkinje fibers, and to the ventricular myocardium. Recording of the depolarizing and repolarizing currents in the heart with electrodes on the surface of the body produces characteristic waveforms.

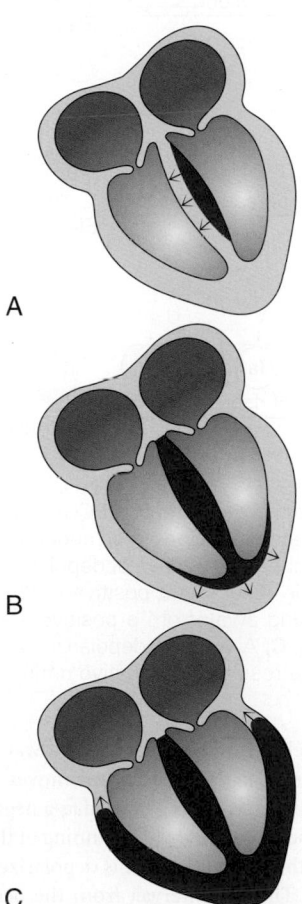

FIGURE 17-21 Sequence of ventricular depolarization showing septal depolarization in a left-to-right direction **(A)**, followed by apical depolarization in an endocardial to epicardial direction **(B)**, and, finally, depolarization of the lateral walls **(C)**. Repolarization proceeds in the opposite direction.

resting potential) when the faster pacemaker suddenly stops. Thus, it takes slightly longer to reach threshold and initiate the first action potential.

Autonomic Regulation of Rhythmicity

Both sympathetic and parasympathetic nerves supply the heart. Sympathetic innervation is widespread to all areas, including the ventricular myocardium. Parasympathetic innervation, by way of the vagus nerves, is localized primarily in SA and AV nodal areas. The right vagus nerve supplies the SA node, whereas the left vagus nerve supplies the AV node.[12] The autonomic nervous system exerts control over heart rate and velocity of impulse conduction. In general, sympathetic activation increases heart rate (*chronotropic effect*) and increases speed of conduction (*dromotropic effect*) as well as inducing heart muscle to contract more forcefully (*inotropic effect*) and relax more quickly (*lusitropic effect*). These effects are achieved by release of NE from sympathetic nerve endings. Binding of NE to β receptors on heart muscle cell membranes increases production of cAMP, which regulates several membrane channels and pumps and increases depolarizing ion currents.

Parasympathetic stimulation primarily results in a reduction in heart rate and speed of action potential conduction. Acetylcholine is the neurotransmitter released by parasympathetic nerve endings. Acetylcholine binding to muscarinic receptors on heart cells inhibits cAMP production and increases membrane permeability to potassium ions, allowing them to leak from the cell. The resulting hyperpolarization makes it more difficult to reach threshold and initiate an action potential. The resting heart is normally under a predominant parasympathetic influence, which results in an SA discharge rate of about 70 beats/min. If parasympathetic activity is blocked, the spontaneous discharge rate of SA nodal cells increases to about 100 beats/min. An increase in vagal activity can reduce heart rate significantly. Breath holding, bearing down during defecation, and pressing on the carotid arteries may increase vagal tone and reduce heart rate. This is sometimes called a *vasovagal response* and may lead to dizziness and fainting.

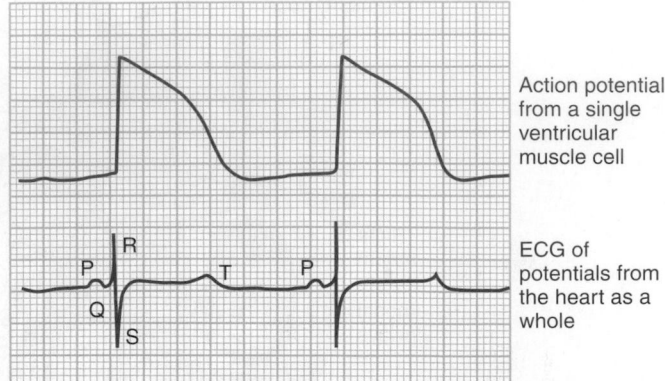

FIGURE 17-22 Comparison of the action potential from a single ventricular muscle cell, showing rapid depolarization and prolonged repolarization phases, against an electrocardiogram of potentials from the heart as a whole. Ventricular myocytes remain depolarized and refractory throughout the entire QT interval. (Redrawn from Hall JE: *Guyton and Hall textbook of medical physiology*, ed 12, Philadelphia, 2011, Saunders, p 122.)

ELECTROCARDIOGRAPHY

As action potentials spread from cell to cell throughout the myocardium, an electrical current is transmitted to the body surface and can be detected by electrodes placed on the skin.[13,14] A recording of these electrical currents is called an *electrocardiogram* (ECG). The ECG is a useful indicator of abnormalities of the heart's conduction system. Irregularities in initiation of impulses, conduction rates, and conduction pathways can be identified. The ECG has a different appearance than the cardiac action potential described previously because it registers depolarizing and repolarizing currents in the whole heart rather than the activity of individual myocytes (Figure 17-22).

Electrical currents traveling through the heart have both direction and magnitude and are often described as *vectors*. At any instant, electrical currents are moving in various directions through different regions of the heart. Waveforms recorded at the ECG electrodes are algebraic sums of all of these vectors. Patterns of electrical activity shown on the ECG vary according to the placement of electrodes on the body. In general, a wave of depolarization moving toward a positive recording electrode will register as an upward deflection on the ECG. A wave of repolarization moving away from a positive electrode also will register as an upward deflection on the ECG. A downward deflection results from a wave of depolarization moving away from a positive electrode (Figure 17-23). Placement of a recording electrode on the lower-left extremity (lead II) results in the typical ECG pattern shown in Figure 17-24. A description of the usual electrode placements is included in the section Tests of Cardiac Function at the end of this chapter.

Each deflection on the ECG has a normal characteristic shape and time interval (see Figure 17-24). The three major wave complexes are the *P wave*, which corresponds to atrial depolarization, the *QRS complex*, which represents ventricular depolarization, and the *T wave*, which reflects ventricular repolarization. The PR interval, between the beginning of the P wave and the beginning of the QRS complex, includes atrial, AV node, and His Purkinje fiber depolarization. The normal sequence of ventricular depolarization begins with the septum, followed by the apex, and, finally, the base of the ventricular walls. Septal depolarization begins on the left septal surface and then travels toward the right, resulting in a small negative deflection, the *Q wave* in lead II (Figure 17-25). A large upright *R wave* corresponds to a wave of

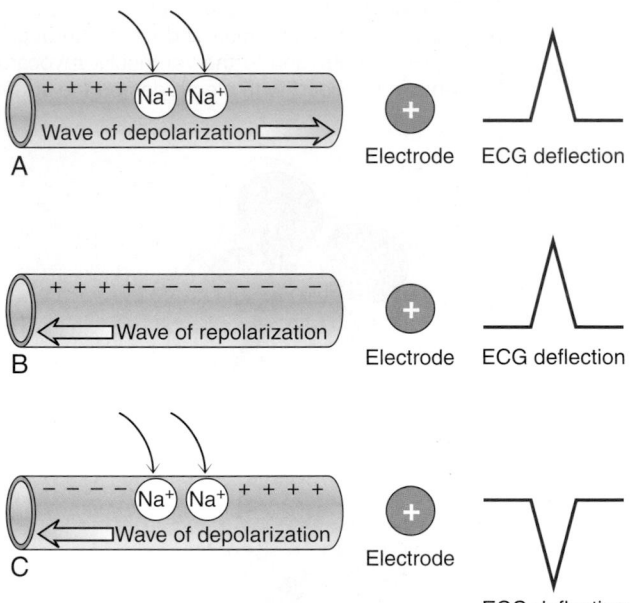

FIGURE 17-23 Electrocardiographic *(ECG)* waveforms may be positive (upward) or negative (downward), depending on the location of electrodes on the chest. **A,** A wave of depolarization moving toward a positive electrode results in a positive deflection. **B,** A wave of repolarization moving away from a positive electrode results in a positive deflection. **C,** A wave of depolarization moving away from a positive electrode results in a negative deflection.

depolarization traveling down the ventricles toward the apex. Depolarization of the ventricular base, because it moves in a direction away from the lower limb electrode, is recorded as a negative *S wave*. The ST interval, between the S wave and the beginning of the T wave, is isoelectric (flat), because the entire ventricle is depolarized and no detectable current is flowing. The QT interval, from the beginning of the QRS complex to the end of the T wave, is commonly measured as an indicator of ventricular systole. The T wave is normally upright in lead II, representing a wave of repolarization moving away from a positive electrode. In some patients, particularly those with slow heart rates, the T wave is followed by a small positive deflection, called a *U wave*. Prominent U waves also are a sign of a low potassium level. Abnormalities in

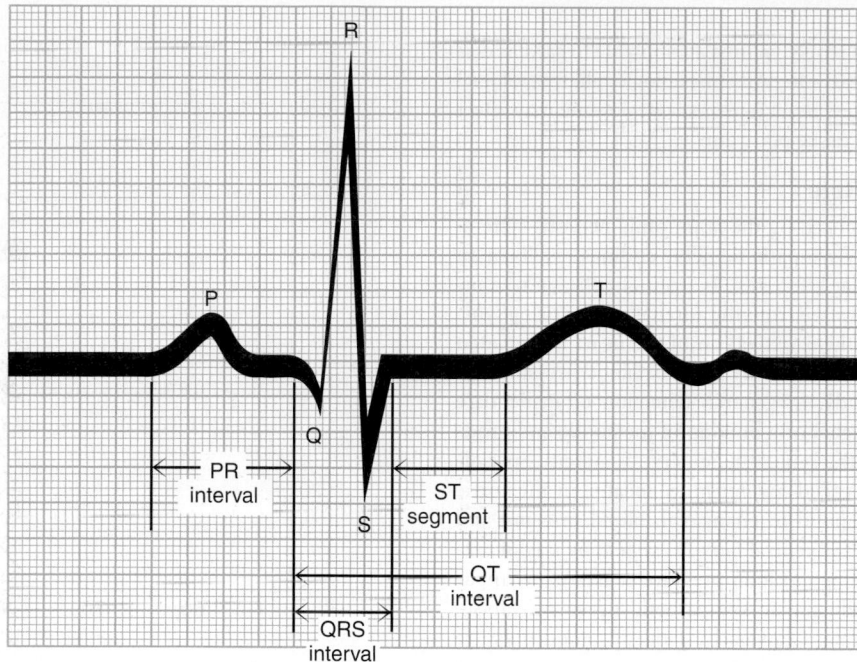

FIGURE 17-24 Usual electrocardiographic pattern recorded from lead II, showing characteristic waves and intervals.

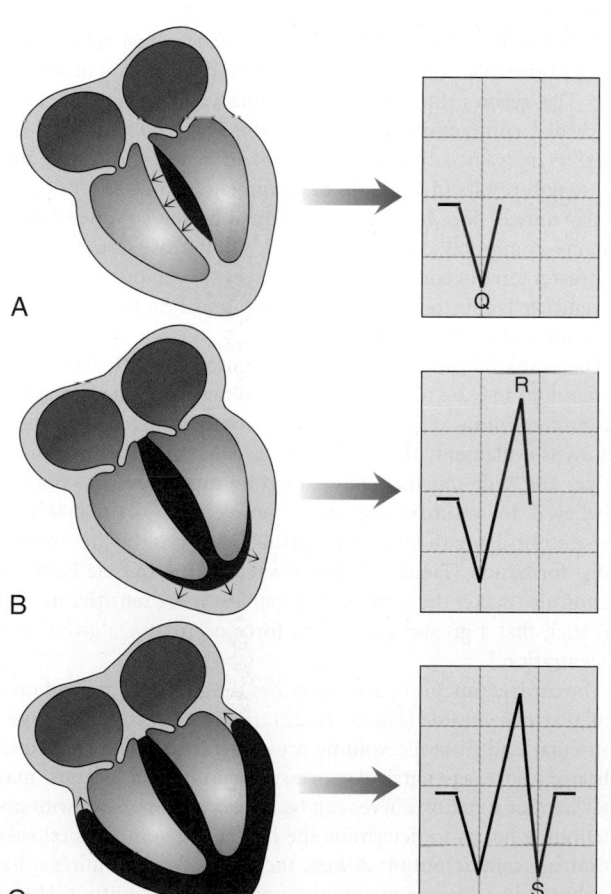

FIGURE 17-25 QRS complex results from the sequence of ventricular depolarization. **A,** In lead II, septal depolarization is in a direction away from the positive electrode, resulting in a negative Q wave. **B,** Depolarization of the apex of the heart is in a direction toward the positive electrode, resulting in a large positive R wave. **C,** Depolarization of the lateral walls and base of the ventricles is in a direction away from the positive electrode, resulting in a negative S wave.

any time intervals may indicate abnormal conduction pathways and enhanced or slowed conduction times. Rhythm disturbances are discussed in detail in Chapter 19.

> **KEY POINTS**
> - The ECG represents an algebraic sum of all depolarizing and repolarizing currents occurring in the heart. ECGs are useful for detecting conduction and rhythm disturbances.
> - The major deflections of the ECG are:
>   P wave: atrial depolarization
>   PR interval: atrial, AV node, and Purkinje depolarization
>   Q wave: septal depolarization
>   R wave: apical depolarization
>   S wave: depolarization of lateral walls (base)
>   T wave: ventricular repolarization

DETERMINANTS OF CARDIAC OUTPUT

Cardiac output is a measure of the amount of blood pumped out of the heart each minute. Because the heart's primary function is to pump enough blood to circulate oxygen and nutrients to tissues, the cardiac output is an extremely important indicator of cardiovascular health. Normal resting cardiac output is approximately 5 to 6 L/min, but it varies with body size and age. Cardiac output is often indexed to body surface area in an attempt to adjust for these differences (cardiac index = cardiac output/body surface area). A normal cardiac index ranges from 2.8 to 3.3 $L/min/m^2$. Regardless of the actual number of liters of blood pumped per minute, the adequacy of tissue perfusion is ultimately important.

Cardiac output is a product of heart rate and stroke volume (CO = HR × SV). **Stroke volume** refers to the amount of blood ejected from the ventricle with each contraction. An increase in heart rate (to a point) and/or an increase in stroke volume will result in a greater cardiac output. Conversely, a low heart rate and/or a decreased stroke volume will cause cardiac output to fall. To a certain extent, a change in one factor can be compensated for by a change in the other, thus maintaining cardiac output at a constant level. For example, it is common for an individual with limited stroke volume attributable to cardiac disease to have a high resting heart rate. Any physiologic, pharmacologic, or pathologic process that alters heart rate or stroke volume may affect cardiac output and therefore tissue perfusion.

Determinants of Heart Rate

Heart rate is primarily influenced by the autonomic nervous system. Release of norepinephrine by sympathetic nerve endings results in an increased heart rate. A similar effect results from circulating norepinephrine and epinephrine released from the adrenal gland during sympathetic stimulation. Sympathetic activation of the heart is regulated by several reflex pathways that constantly monitor blood pressure and metabolic activity in the body. In general, detection of inadequate blood pressure, a lack of oxygen, or a buildup of metabolic end products results in activation of the sympathetic nervous system. Specialized sensory nerve endings, called *baroreceptors*, located in the aortic arch and carotid arteries respond to changes in blood pressure and transmit this information to the central nervous system by way of cranial nerves IX and X. A decline in blood pressure causes parasympathetic system inhibition and cardiac sympathetic nerve activation, resulting in a rise in heart rate. Conversely, a rise in blood pressure causes the heart rate to fall because of parasympathetic activation and sympathetic inhibition. Under normal resting conditions, the heart rate is under parasympathetic influence, with a usual rate of approximately 70 beats/min.

In addition to baroreceptors, other sensory fibers that detect pressure are located in the cardiac chambers. These sensory receptors respond to changes in intrachamber pressure, which reflect the volume of blood in the chamber. Atrial or ventricular overdistention suppresses parasympathetic influence and increases heart rate (Bainbridge reflex).[12] Heart rate may also be influenced by higher central nervous system (CNS) activities that do not involve reflex pathways. Anxiety, fear, stress, excitement, trauma, and fever may activate the sympathetic system, for example. A variety of drugs can mimic or block the effects of both sympathetic and parasympathetic systems and therefore influence heart rate (see Chapter 18).

In general, an increase in heart rate results in an increase in cardiac output; however, at very high heart rates, cardiac output may actually fall. At high heart rates (e.g., more than 200 beats/min in the young, even lower in the adult), the time for diastolic ventricular filling can be significantly reduced, resulting in a low stroke volume. The benefit of increased heart rate is therefore undermined by impaired pumping efficiency.

Determinants of Stroke Volume

Three major factors influence stroke volume: (1) the volume of blood in the heart (**preload**), (2) the contractile capabilities of heart muscle (**contractility**), and (3) the impedance opposing ejection of blood from the ventricle (**afterload**). Each of these factors is in turn influenced by many other physiologic, pharmacologic, and sometimes pathologic variables.

Volume of Blood in the Heart (Preload)

The heart can only pump as much blood as is delivered to it by the circulatory system. Blood returning to the heart from the circulation is often called venous return. Normally, venous return is equal to cardiac output because the circulatory system is just that—a circuit. However, there may be inequalities over several heartbeats when changes in blood volume or blood distribution occur. The heart is well suited to adjust to these beat-to-beat changes in venous return such that the healthy heart pumps essentially whatever amount is delivered to it.

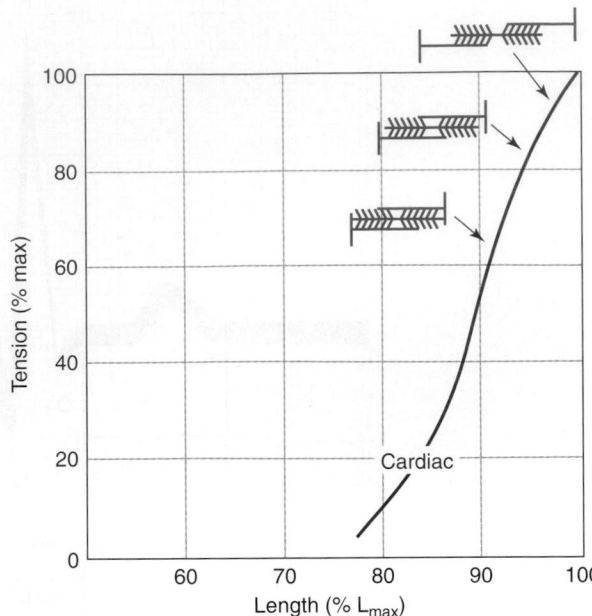

FIGURE 17-26 Force of muscle contraction depends in part on its resting length before activation. At optimal lengths, the greatest tension is developed, and cross-bridge formation is enhanced.

The amount of blood present in the ventricles just before contraction (end-diastolic volume) is an important determinant of stroke volume. The relationship between diastolic volume and the force of myocardial contraction is known as the **Frank-Starling law of the heart**.[2,15] In essence, this law states that an increase in resting muscle fiber length results in a greater development of muscle tension. Ventricular muscle fiber length is determined by the volume of blood it contains, commonly called the *preload*. An increase in preload results in a greater force of contraction and a larger stroke volume. In this way, the ventricle is able to adjust its stroke volume, beat by beat, according to the amount of blood to be pumped.

The Frank-Starling law of the heart (also called the *length-tension relationship*) may be understood by recalling the molecular structure of contractile units of heart muscle. For contraction to occur, the actin and myosin filaments that make up the sarcomere must form crossbridges and slide together. Stretching the muscle before contraction is believed to optimize the space between the actin and myosin filaments, bringing them closer together, and resulting in more crossbridge formation (Figure 17-26). Stretching the muscle before contraction also makes the contractile apparatus more sensitive to calcium ions such that a greater contractile force occurs for a given calcium concentration.[2]

The cardiac function curve describes the effects of preload on ventricular stroke volume (Figure 17-27). In practice, stroke volume and ventricular end-diastolic volume are difficult to measure, and other indicators, such as ventricular pressure and cardiac output, may be used. Cardiac function curves can be measured in persons with poorly functioning hearts to determine the best filling volume (preload) for optimizing cardiac output. Often, the failing heart requires a higher than normal preload to maintain a normal cardiac output. However, there are limits to the improvement in stroke volume with increased diastolic filling, and beyond that point the curve will flatten. On the flat part of the curve, an increase in preload increases the workload of the heart, but does not provide an improvement in output. The workload imposed on the heart chambers by preload is sometimes called the *volume work of the heart*. An increase in preload increases the volume

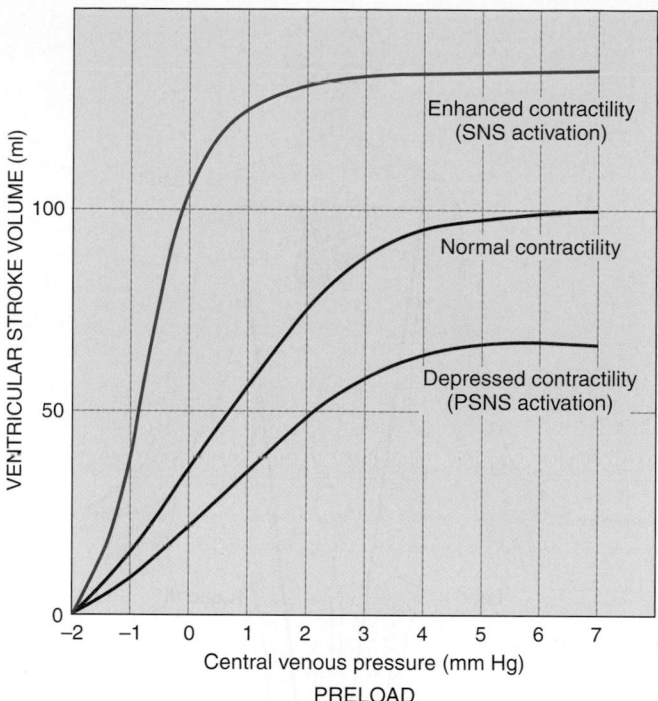

FIGURE 17-27 Cardiac function curves showing the dependence of ventricular stroke volume on preload. Different hearts have different cardiac function curves and may respond differently to the same degree of preload. *PSNS*, Parasympathetic nervous system; *SNS*, sympathetic nervous system.

work of the heart, which must be met by increased oxygen uptake to maintain adequate ATP production.

Contractile Capabilities of the Heart (Contractility)

Heart muscle contractility depends on several factors, including (1) the amount of contractile proteins in the muscle cells, (2) the availability of ATP, and (3) the availability of free calcium ions in the cytoplasm. Contractility is, by definition, independent of fiber end-diastolic length and is therefore not affected by preload. Given an adequate ATP supply, the contractile state of the normal myocardium is primarily determined by factors that increase the availability of free calcium ions within the myocardial cell. In general, an increased intracellular free calcium level can be accomplished by enhanced release from internal stores, enhanced entry from extracellular fluid, and reduced rates of extrusion across the plasma membrane.

A variety of agents that increase contractility, called *positive inotropes*, are associated with increased intracellular calcium levels in the heart. These include the sympathetic neurotransmitters norepinephrine and epinephrine, thyroid hormone, caffeine, digitalis, and many others. Agents that depress contractility, called *negative inotropes*, achieve their effects by reducing intracellular calcium levels. These agents include L-type calcium channel blockers, parasympathomimetics, and sympathetic blocking drugs. The baroreceptor reflex, described previously in relation to heart rate, is also an important regulator of stroke volume through its effects on contractility. Positive inotropic agents increase ATP utilization by the myocardium, whereas negative inotropes decrease myocardial workload and reduce ATP requirements.

Cardiac disease may adversely affect contractility because of an inadequate oxygen supply or because of loss of myocardial pumping cells. These disorders are discussed in Chapter 18.

Impedance to Ejection from the Ventricle (Afterload)

The third major determinant of stroke volume is afterload, which refers to the impedance or resistance that must be overcome to eject blood from the chamber. Left ventricular afterload is determined primarily by aortic blood pressure. Because high blood pressure increases left ventricular afterload, vasodilating agents that reduce blood pressure can significantly decrease afterload. Normally the aortic valve offers little impedance to flow; however, aortic valve narrowing may significantly increase afterload. An increase in afterload will result in a decrease in stroke volume unless contractility or preload (or both) is adjusted to compensate. Conversely, a decrease in afterload will allow a larger than normal volume of blood to be ejected from the heart, requiring less myocardial work. The work done by the heart to overcome afterload is often called the *pressure work of the heart*. An increase in afterload increases pressure work and requires greater tension development within the walls of the chamber (wall stress). Increased wall stress not only increases myocardial workload and oxygen consumption but also, if prolonged, may trigger structural changes leading to hypertrophy of myocytes.

The ventricles normally eject about 60% to 70% of their end-diastolic volume during contraction; the remaining 30% to 40% remains in the ventricle. **Ejection fraction** is influenced by afterload as well as preload and contractile state. A reduced ejection fraction is a common finding in persons suffering from myocardial infarction. Ejection fractions less than 40% indicate significant myocardial impairment and may be associated with systolic heart failure (see Chapter 19).

Cardiac Workload

The oxygen requirements of the heart are related to the amount of energy (ATP) exerted to perform its pumping function. The four determinants of cardiac output described in the previous section—heart rate, preload, contractility, and afterload—are also the major determinants of cardiac energy requirements. An increase in any of these four factors will increase ATP requirements and therefore cardiac cell oxygen requirements. High afterload is most detrimental, because it greatly increases cardiac work without producing a higher cardiac output. When oxygen supply to the heart is impaired, as in coronary atherosclerosis, it may be beneficial to reduce myocardial oxygen demand by reducing cardiac workload. This may be accomplished by reductions in heart rate, preload, afterload, and contractility.

KEY POINTS

- Cardiac output is the product of the heart rate times the stroke volume (CO = HR × SV). An increase in heart rate or stroke volume will increase cardiac output. An increase in heart rate can compensate for a decrease in stroke volume.
- Heart rate is controlled primarily by the autonomic nervous system. Factors that increase heart rate include low blood pressure (baroreceptors), acidemia (chemoreceptors), atrial and ventricular overdistention (Bainbridge reflex), and emotions. Activation of the vagus nerve will decrease heart rate.
- Stroke volume is influenced by preload. According to the Frank-Starling law, increased preload stretches the sarcomere, resulting in more forceful contraction.
- Increased contractility increases stroke volume by causing a greater percentage of the ventricular volume to be ejected. Any factor that enhances the availability of cytoplasmic free Ca^{2+} will increase contractility.
- Increased afterload will decrease stroke volume. Afterload is determined primarily by the resistance of the arterial system. Vasoconstriction and high aortic pressure increase afterload.
- Any factor that increases heart rate, preload, contractility, or afterload will increase the workload of the heart.

ENDOCRINE FUNCTION OF THE HEART

In addition to its pumping function, the heart also has an endocrine function: secretion of natriuretic peptides.[16] Atrial natriuretic peptide (ANP) is synthesized by myocytes in the atria and released in response to atrial stretch. Increased atrial stretch occurs when blood volume becomes excessive. The ventricles produce a related peptide called B-type natriuretic peptide (BNP) when they are chronically overdistended. An elevated BNP value is a marker for congestive heart failure.[16] ANP and BNP cause enhanced excretion of sodium and water by the kidney. In general, the effects of the natriuretic peptides are antagonistic to those of the renin-angiotensin-aldosterone system (see Chapter 26).

TESTS OF CARDIAC FUNCTION

In addition to patient history, laboratory results, and physical assessment, a number of diagnostic tests may be employed to evaluate cardiac function.[17] The ECG is routinely obtained and provides information about the heart's conduction patterns. Echocardiography and nuclear cardiography are tests that use various modes to image the heart. A more direct assessment of cardiac function can be obtained by cardiac catheterization. In addition, a number of methods have been developed to quantify myocardial blood flow. Each of these studies is briefly described in this section.

Electrocardiography

The ECG graphically indicates electrical currents generated by cardiac cells. The current is registered by skin electrodes placed in particular positions on the body.[14] The standard ECG has 12 different leads that are obtained through 10 skin electrodes: 3 standard bipolar limb leads, 3 augmented unipolar limb leads, and 6 unipolar chest leads. Bipolar leads represent a difference in electrical potential between two electrodes, one positive and one negative. Augmented unipolar limb leads represent a difference in potential between one electrode and the average of the other two limb electrodes. Unipolar chest leads represent a difference in potential between the chest electrode and a location at the center of the heart. Each lead provides a different ECG because of its particular "view" of current flow through the heart.

The three standard bipolar limb leads are lead I, lead II, and lead III (Figure 17-28): lead I measures the current between the right arm and left arm, lead II measures the current between the right arm and left leg, and lead III measures the current between the left arm and left leg. A normal ECG from leads I, II, and III is illustrated in Figure 17-29.

Electrode placement for the augmented unipolar limb leads is illustrated in Figure 17-30. Unipolar limb lead electrodes provide the positive pole: lead aV_R is recorded from the right arm, lead aV_L is recorded from the left arm, and lead aV_F is recorded from the left leg. In these leads, *a* stands for augmented; *V* stands for voltage; and *R, L,* and *F* indicate the location of the unipolar lead (*right* arm, *left* arm, and *foot* [left]). A normal ECG from these leads is illustrated in Figure 17-31.

Precordial unipolar chest leads are recorded from electrodes placed in six positions over the heart on the anterior chest (Figure 17-32). Chest leads are designated as V_1, V_2, V_3, V_4, V_5, and V_6. The normal ECG from the chest leads is shown in Figure 17-33. The chest leads provide a horizontal view of the heart, whereas the limb leads provide a view of the frontal plane.

Twelve-lead ECGs are usually recorded for a short period of time when the patient is resting. Sequential ECGs are useful for

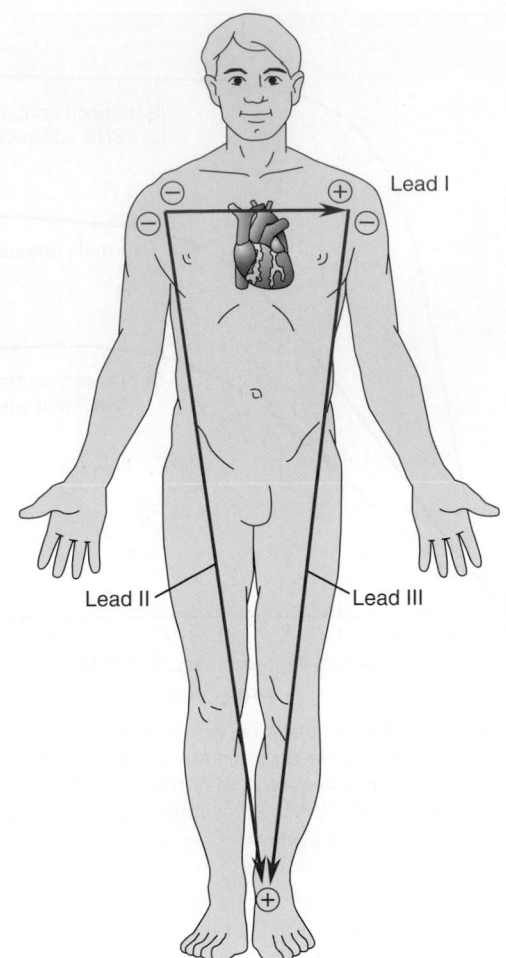

FIGURE 17-28 Positions of standard bipolar limb leads I, II, and III. The positive (+) lead is the recording lead.

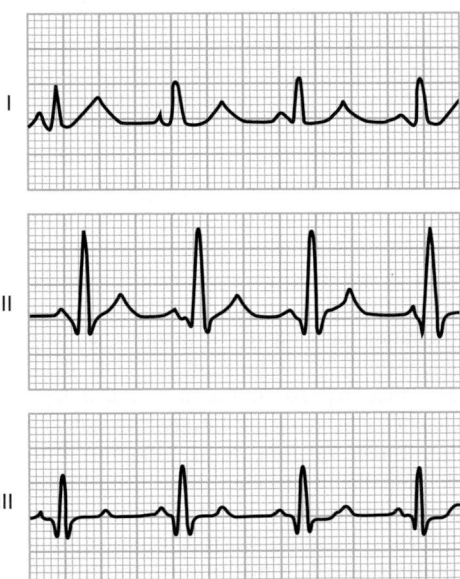

FIGURE 17-29 Normal electrocardiogram recorded from the three standard bipolar limb leads. The R wave is normally upright in leads I, II, and III. (Redrawn from Hall JE: *Guyton and Hall textbook of medical physiology*, ed 12, Philadelphia, 2011, Saunders, p 126.)

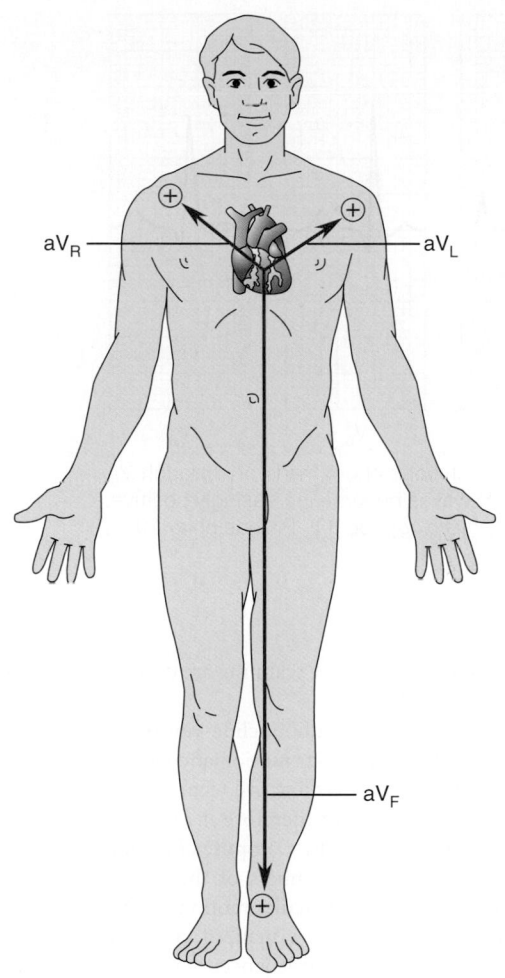

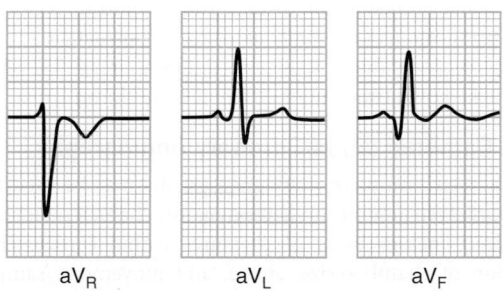

FIGURE 17-30 Unipolar augmented leads aV_R, aV_L, and aV_F.

FIGURE 17-31 Normal electrocardiogram recorded from the three unipolar augmented leads. The aV_R lead is characterized by a large S wave and an inverted T wave. The aV_L and aV_F leads have an upright R wave and T wave.

determining changes over time. In some cases it is necessary to monitor the ECG recording for an extended period to capture rhythm problems that occur infrequently or with particular activities. This is accomplished by continuous ambulatory monitoring (e.g., Holter monitoring) over a 24- to 48-hour period. An ECG can also be recorded during exercise to monitor the effects of exercise stress on cardiovascular function. An exercise test (stress test) is usually performed while the subject progressively increases his or her effort on a treadmill or stationary bicycle. The exercise ECG is particularly useful for assessing the adequacy of coronary circulation when the

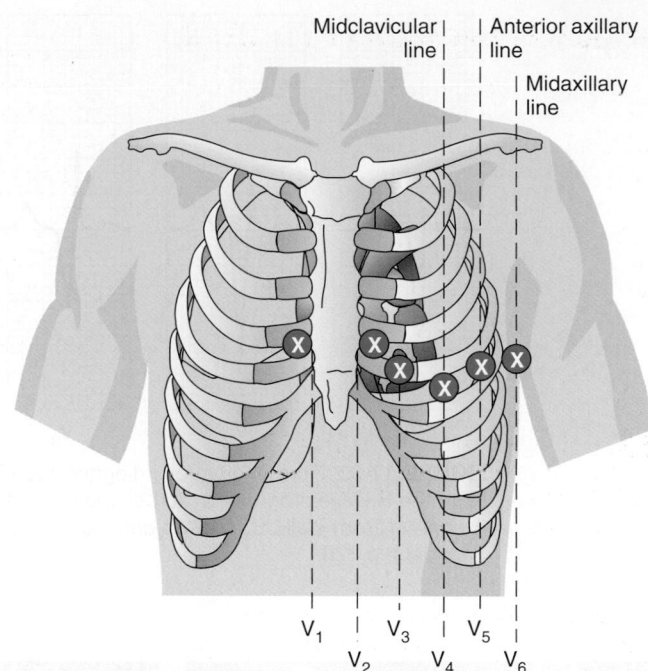

FIGURE 17-32 Unipolar chest (precordial) leads V_1 through V_6.

myocardial workload is increased. Impaired myocardial oxygen delivery may be evident on the ECG as ST segment elevation or depression and abnormal T waves.

Magnetic Resonance Imaging and Computed Tomography

Magnetic resonance imaging (MRI) and computed tomography (CT) are useful for imaging cardiac structures.[1] Myocardial thickening, pericardial sac disease, valvular structures, and congenital malformations may be visualized by MRI. Contrast-enhanced imaging identifies acute and chronic myocardial infarcts with high specificity and sensitivity. MRI and CT are used to detect coronary plaque burden and assess vulnerable plaque morphology in the arterial walls. Excessive plaque burden and unstable plaques are correlated with a greater degree of coronary atherosclerosis and may be used to predict coronary artery disease risk or progression.

Echocardiography

Echocardiography uses reflected sound waves (ultrasound) to provide an image of cardiac structure and motion within the chest. The cardiac echo is obtained by placing a blunt probe on the chest surface that transmits and receives high-frequency sound waves. Sound waves traveling through chest and heart structures are reflected back to the receiving probe. The time between sound wave emission and detection of reflected waves is used to calculate distances between the probe and reflecting tissue. The sound waves are not heard or felt by the subject and have no known detrimental effects on tissues. The probe is moved across the chest to assess cardiac structures of interest, and recordings are videotaped for later viewing.

Echocardiograms are particularly useful for diagnosis of heart enlargement, valvular disorders, collections of fluid in the pericardial space, cardiac tumors, and abnormalities in left ventricular motion. Estimations of ejection fraction and assessments of ventricular systolic and diastolic function can be made noninvasively by echocardiogram. An echocardiogram is shown in Figure 17-34.

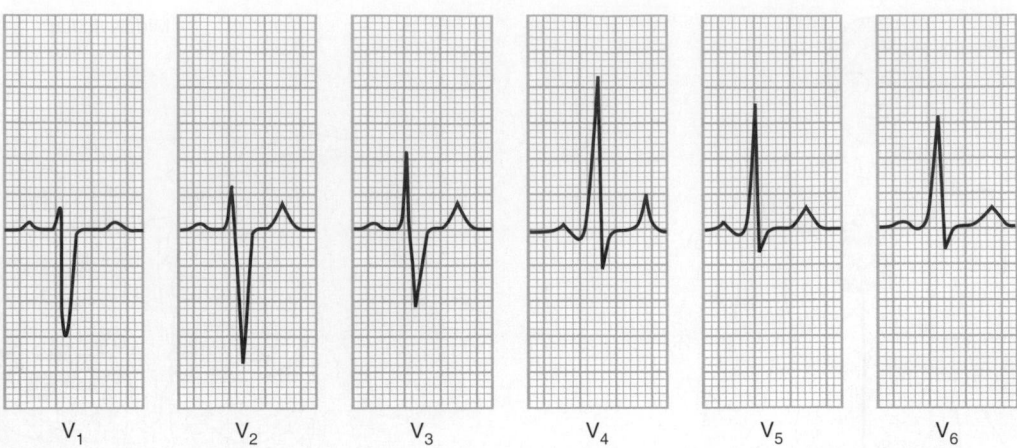

V_1 V_2 V_3 V_4 V_5 V_6

FIGURE 17-33 Normal electrocardiogram recorded from the six unipolar chest leads, V_1 through V_6. Note the R wave progression across the precordial leads as the R waves become increasingly positive. (Redrawn from Hall JE: *Guyton and Hall textbook of medical physiology*, ed 11, Philadelphia, 2011, Saunders, p 126.)

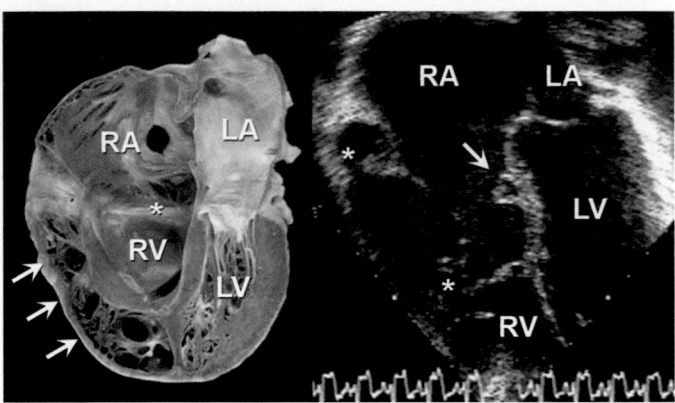

FIGURE 17-34 Pathology specimen *(left)* and echocardiography image *(right)* of heart with enlarged right atrium and right ventricle. *LA*, Left atrium; *LV*, left ventricle; *RA*, right atrium; *RV*, right ventricle. (From Connolly H, Oh J: Echocardiography. In Bonow R et al, editors: *Braunwald's heart disease: a textbook of cardiovascular medicine*, ed 9, vol 1, Philadelphia, 2012, Saunders, p 264.)

Nuclear Cardiography

Radioactive substances injected into the bloodstream can be used to trace the patterns of blood flow in the heart. Radiation exposure is minimal, because very small amounts of radioactive substances are used. Radioactive tracers can be linked to substances that accumulate in normal myocardial cells while the tracer is delivered by coronary blood flow. Areas with impaired perfusion will absorb less radioactivity and appear as "cold spots" on the scan. Scanning usually is done using single-photon emission computed tomography (SPECT), which images numerous slices through the heart, or by planar imaging, which gives an overall picture in one plane only.

Thallium-201 (^{201}Tl) and technetium-99 labeled compounds (^{99m}Tc sestamibi) are used to assess the adequacy of blood flow to cardiac tissues. After injection of the radioactive compound, the heart is scanned to visualize the amount of radioactivity absorbed by cardiac tissues. Healthy cardiac tissues that receive adequate blood supply actively accumulate these isotopes. Areas of inadequate blood flow or infarcted tissue do not accumulate isotopes and appear as cold spots on

the scan. Resting and exercise scanning are done to assess for exercise-induced perfusion defects.

Gated pool scanning (radionuclide ventriculogram) is used primarily to assess left ventricular motion and ejection fraction. Before it is injected intravenously, radioactive technetium is attached to albumin or red blood cells, and therefore it remains in the bloodstream and is not absorbed by cells. Computer imaging is used to analyze blood flow through the chambers of the heart over many cardiac cycles. The dynamics of ventricular motion, such as hypercontractility or hypocontractility, may be visualized. Separate radionuclide ventriculogram evaluation has largely been replaced by SPECT scanning that allows simultaneous evaluation of perfusion and left ventricular function.

Positron emission tomography (PET) scans may also be used to evaluate cardiac perfusion and metabolism. Radiotracers can be incorporated into substances normally used in cellular metabolic processes, such as glucose. Metabolic activity in different areas of the heart can then be tracked over time under different conditions.

Cardiac Catheterization/Coronary Angiography

Cardiac catheterization/coronary angiography may be used to determine important structural and hemodynamic characteristics because it affords direct measurement of pressures within cardiac chambers; visualization of chamber size, shape, and movement; sampling for blood oxygen content in various heart regions; measurement of cardiac output and ejection fraction; and visualization and management of coronary artery obstructions.[18]

Cardiac catheterization angiography is associated with several serious risks, including bleeding, dysrhythmias, heart perforation, and coronary ischemia. The advent of noninvasive high-resolution MRI, echocardiograms, and SPECT scanning has replaced the need for cardiac catheterization in many instances; however, the value of information supplied is generally believed to outweigh the risks in certain cases. Catheterization is frequently used for interventions to rapidly improve coronary blood supply and to evaluate suspected or confirmed coronary artery disease, valvular dysfunction, congenital defects, left ventricular dysfunction, and coronary bypass graft patency.

Assessment of the left side of the heart, including the coronary arteries, is achieved by passing a catheter through a femoral or

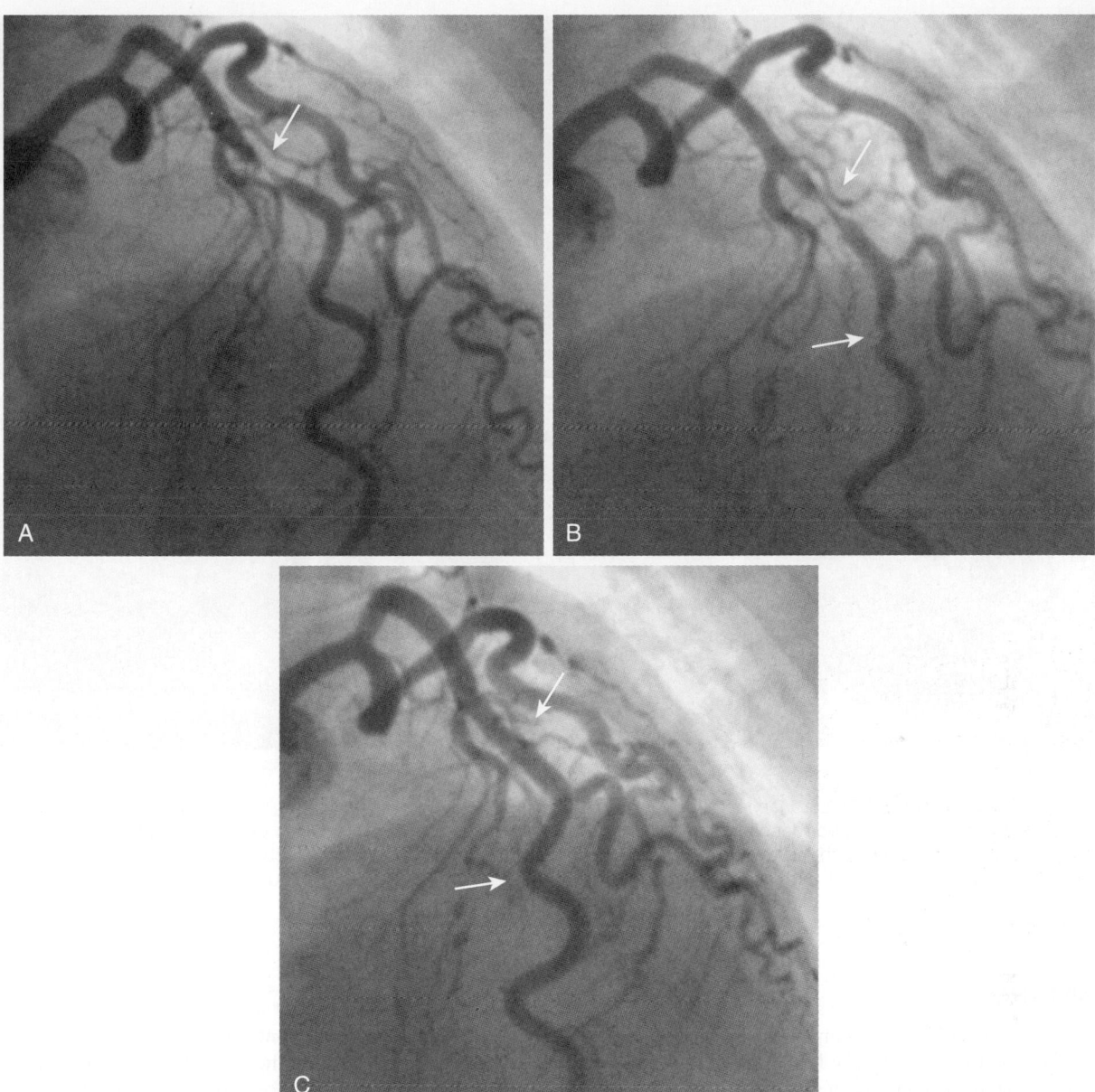

FIGURE 17-35 Coronary artery angiography. The *arrows* show an area of obstruction of the coronary artery. (From Popma J: Coronary arteriography. In Bonow R et al, editors: *Braunwald's heart disease: a textbook of cardiovascular medicine,* ed 9, vol 1, Philadelphia, 2012, Saunders, p 428.)

brachial artery into the aorta. The catheter is then manipulated into the left ventricle or left atrium to assess chamber pressures, and a ventriculogram is obtained. Contrast dye injected into the ventricular chamber is monitored fluoroscopically to assess ventricular function. The catheter is usually pulled back into the aorta and then advanced into one or more of the coronary arteries. The patency of the coronary arteries can be visualized by injecting contrast dye into them and monitoring by fluoroscopy (Figure 17-35). When contrast dye is in the coronary artery, a period of cardiac ischemia is produced during which the patient may experience angina, dysrhythmias, and coronary spasms. Coronary catheterization may also be done to insert a probe for obtaining intracoronary ultrasounds. Ultrasounds are useful for assessing plaque morphologic characteristics (Figure 17-36).

Right-sided heart catheterization is done to evaluate right-sided heart structures. The catheter is introduced into a vein, usually femoral,

then threaded through the inferior vena cava and into the heart. Pressures and blood samples are obtained as the catheter is advanced into the right atrium, ventricle, and pulmonary artery. Right heart catheterization is useful in assessing tricuspid and pulmonary valve disorders, pulmonary hypertension, septal defects, and right ventricular function.

Coronary angiography is commonly followed by interventions to treat detected abnormalities. The coronary catheter can be used to direct thrombolytic agents to the site of coronary thrombosis and rapidly restore blood flow to ischemic areas. Laser therapy, coronary balloon angioplasty, and stent placement can also be performed during coronary angiography. These methods clear the coronary obstruction through thermal and mechanical means. The success of these approaches to management of coronary obstruction depends largely on how soon after an ischemic event they are performed (Chapter 18).

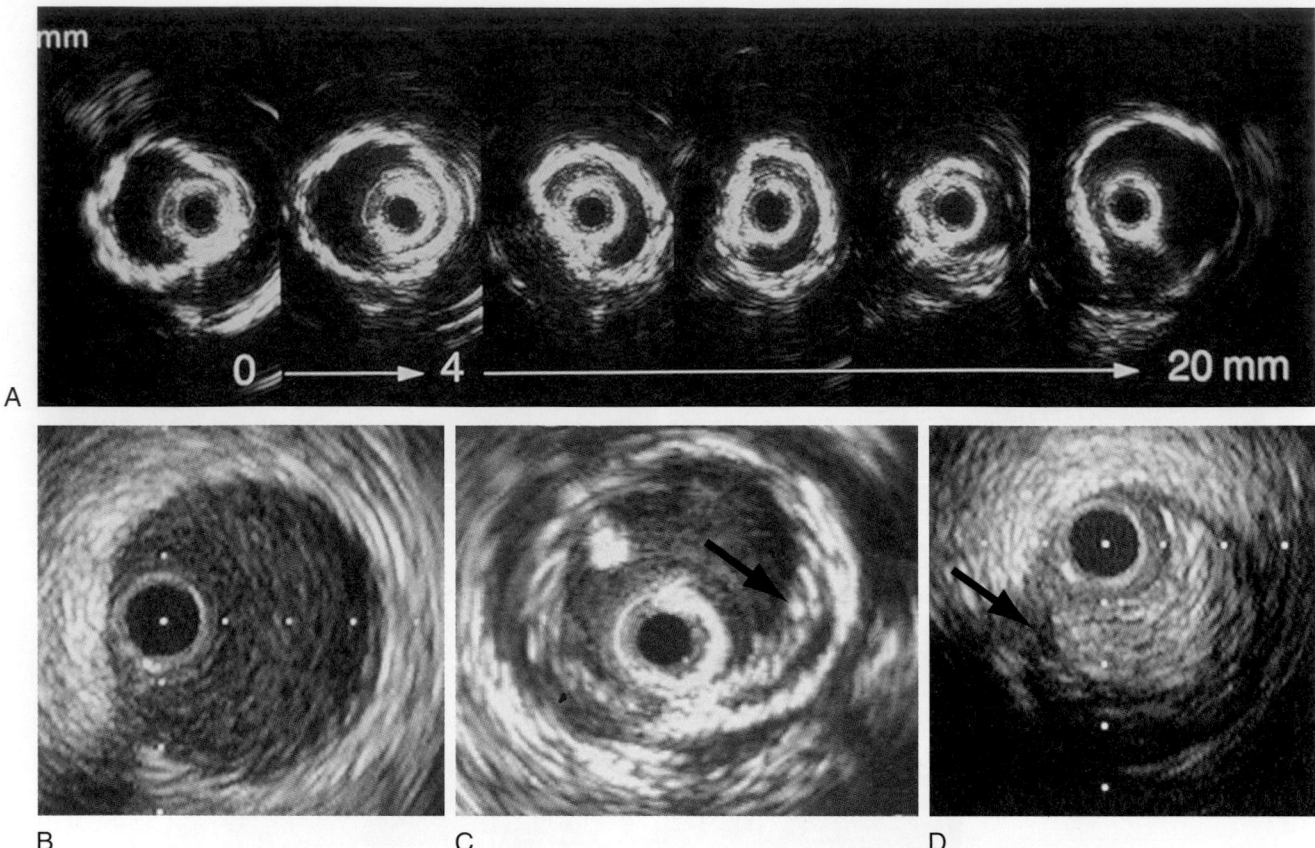

FIGURE 17-36 Intracoronary ultrasonographic examples of plaque morphology. **A,** Concentric calcification of the left anterior descending artery. **B,** A normal vessel wall. **C,** Fibrous cap on coronary plaque. **D,** A soft plaque with rupture of the fibrous cap. (From Braunwald E, Zipes D, Libby P, editors: *Braunwald's heart disease: a textbook of cardiovascular medicine,* ed 6, Philadelphia, 2001, Saunders, p 416.)

SUMMARY

The heart's primary function is to pump sufficient blood to deliver oxygen and nutrients to the body. The heart may be viewed as two separate pumps: a right-sided pump that perfuses the lungs and a left-sided pump that perfuses the systemic circulation. The left ventricle must generate higher pressures and therefore has a thicker myocardial mass and higher energy requirements. Because little ATP storage in cardiac cells is possible, the coronary arteries must deliver a steady supply of oxygen and nutrients. Cardiac contraction can be described by the sliding filament/cross-bridge theory and occurs only in the presence of ATP and free calcium ions. Factors that enhance intracellular calcium ion concentration will result in generation of a greater contractile force.

A coordinated cardiac contraction is possible because the heart's conduction system activates the chambers in a sequential manner. The sinoatrial node is the usual pacemaker because it has the highest intrinsic rate of diastolic depolarization. The diastolic depolarization rate is strongly influenced by the autonomic nervous system. The ECG shows the electrical activity of the heart and is a useful indicator of cardiac conduction abnormalities.

The ultimate indicator of cardiac function is the cardiac output, which is the product of heart rate and stroke volume. The autonomic nervous system is the main regulator of heart rate, whereas stroke volume is influenced by preload, afterload, and contractility. These factors are also the primary determinants of myocardial work and energy expenditure.

REFERENCES

1. Strandring S: *Gray's anatomy,* ed 40, London, 2009, Churchill Livingstone.
2. Opie LH, Hasenfuss G: Mechanisms of cardiac contraction and relaxation. In Bonow R, Mann D, Zipes D, et al: *Braunwald's heart disease: a textbook of cardiovascular medicine,* ed 9, Philadelphia, 2012, Saunders, pp 459–486.
3. Koeppen B, Stanton B: Properties of the vasculature. In Koeppen B, Stanton B, editors: *Berne & Levy physiology,* ed 6, St Louis, 2010, Mosby, pp 330–369.
4. Barrett K, Ganong WF: *Review of medical physiology,* New York, 2010, McGraw-Hill.
5. Canty JM: Coronary blood flow and myocardial ischemia. In Bonow R, Mann D, Zipes D, et al, editors: *Braunwald's heart disease: a textbook of cardiovascular medicine,* ed 9, Philadelphia, 2012, Saunders, pp 1049–1075.
6. Hosoda T, Rota M, Kajstura J, et al: Role of stem cells in cardiovascular biology, *J Thromb Haemostasis* 9(suppl 1):151–161, 2011.
7. Koeppen B, Stanton B: Cardiac muscle. In Koeppen B, Stanton B, editors: *Berne & Levy physiology,* ed 6, St Louis, 2010, Mosby, pp 256–267.
8. Pollard TD, Earnshaw WC: Muscles. In Pollard TD, Earnshaw WC, editors: *Cell biology,* Philadelphia, 2008, Saunders, pp 705–725.

9. Panteghini M, et al: Use of biochemical biomarkers in acute coronary syndromes. IFCC Scientific Division, Committee on Standardization of Markers of Cardiac Damage, International Federation of Clinical Chemistry, *Clin Chem Lab Med* 37:683–693, 1999.

10. Koeppen B, Stanton B: Elements of cardiac function. In Koeppen B, Stanton B, editors: *Berne & Levy physiology*, ed 6, St Louis, 2010, Mosby, pp 292–329.

11. Sanoski CA, Bauman JL: Arrhythmias. In Dipiro JT, et al, editors: *Pharmacotherapy: a pathophysiologic approach*, ed 8, New York, 2011, McGraw-Hill, pp 273–310.

12. Koeppen B, Stanton B: Regulation of the heart and vasculature. In Kopppen B, Stanton B, editors: *Berne & Levy physiology*, ed 6, St Louis, 2010, Mosby, pp 370–392.

13. Conover MB: *Understanding electrocardiography*, ed 8, St Louis, 2003, Mosby.

14. Mirvis DM, Goldberger AL: Electrocardiography. In Bonow R, Mann D, Zipes D, et al, editors: *Braunwald's heart disease: a textbook of cardiovascular medicine*, ed 9, Philadelphia, 2012, Saunders, pp 126–165.

15. Starling EH: *The Linacre lecture on the law of the heart*, London, 1918, Longmans Green.

16. Clerico A, Giannoni A, Vittorini S, Passino C: Thirty years of the heart as an endocrine organ: physiological role and clinical utility of cardiac natriuretic hormones, *Am J Physiol Heart Circ Physiol* 301(1):H12–H20, 2011.

17. Fang JC, O'Gara PT: The history and physical examination: an evidence-based approach. In Bonow R, Mann D, Zipes D, et al, editors: *Braunwald's heart disease: a textbook of cardiovascular medicine*, ed 9, Philadelphia, 2012, Saunders, pp 107–125.

18. Popma J: Coronary arteriography. In Bonow R, Mann D, Zipes D, et al, editors: *Braunwald's heart disease: a textbook of cardiovascular medicine*, ed 9, vol 1, Philadelphia, 2012, Saunders, pp 406–440.

CHAPTER
18

Alterations in Cardiac Function

Shann D. Kim and Jacquelyn L. Banasik

evolve WEBSITE

http://evolve.elsevier.com/Copstead/
- Review Questions and Answers
- Glossary (with audio pronunciations for selected terms)
- Animations
- Case Studies
- Key Points Review

KEY QUESTIONS

- What is the role of injury, inflammation, and lipid oxidation in coronary plaque initiation and progression?
- What factors alter the balance between myocardial oxygen supply and demand?
- How do the clinical features of the coronary heart disease syndromes differ?
- How do valvular disorders alter cardiac pressure dynamics and workload?
- What are the similarities and differences among the cardiomyopathies and myocarditis?
- How do pericarditis and pericardial effusions differ in regard to cause and significance?
- What factors determine whether a congenital heart defect will produce cyanosis?

CHAPTER OUTLINE

The incidence of cardiovascular disease (CVD) increased rapidly in the United States during the last century, but the death rates from CVD declined between 1998 and 2008 by 30.6%.[1] Mortality data from 2007 showed that CVD accounted for 32.8% of all deaths. Approximately half of these deaths are due to coronary heart disease (CHD), whereas stroke, high blood pressure, heart failure, and others claim the remainder. Since the late 1960s, however, a decline in cardiac mortality has been achieved in the United States because of improvements in treatment and prevention. More than 16 million people living today have a history of angina pectoris or myocardial infarction (MI).[1] Men and women are equally represented, although women tend to be older when their heart disease becomes apparent. In 2008, the direct and indirect economic cost of cardiovascular diseases, including stroke, was estimated at $297.7 billion annually.[1] CHD is the most important cardiovascular disorder in terms of numbers affected and economic impact.

CORONARY HEART DISEASE

CHD is also called ischemic heart disease (IHD) and coronary artery disease (CAD) in some sources. These terms are related because CHD is characterized by insufficient delivery of oxygenated blood to the myocardium (ischemia) because of atherosclerotic coronary arteries (CAD). The American Heart Association compiles statistics under the heading of CHD, which includes the diagnoses of angina pectoris and myocardial infarction. CHD caused about one in six deaths in the United States in 2008.[1] Other sequelae of CHD include dysrhythmias, sudden cardiac death, and heart failure. When metabolic demand for oxygen exceeds supply, the myocardium becomes ischemic, which leads to a dysfunction in cardiac pumping and predisposes to abnormal heart rhythms. If the ischemic episode is severe or prolonged, irreversible damage to myocardial cells may result in MI.

Etiology of Coronary Heart Disease

Atherosclerosis of coronary arteries is the source of nearly all CHD. Atherosclerosis causes progressive narrowing of the arterial lumen and predisposes to a number of processes that can precipitate myocardial ischemia, including thrombus formation, coronary vasospasm, and endothelial cell dysfunction. Uncommon causes of cardiac ischemia include abnormalities of blood oxygen content (e.g., respiratory failure) and poor perfusion pressure through the coronary arteries (e.g., hypotension, hypovolemia). Occasionally, patients experience the signs and symptoms of cardiac ischemia but show no evidence of significant coronary artery atherosclerosis when evaluated by angiography. These patients are thought to have abnormalities of the microcirculation. Abnormal vascular regulation by endothelial cells in small vessels of the heart has been suggested as a probable mechanism. Endothelial cells secrete variable quantities of vascular relaxing and contracting factors and play a key role in controlling myocardial blood flow. Abnormalities of the microcirculation are more difficult to detect than coronary artery plaque, which is evident on coronary angiography. As evaluation methods improve, disorders of the microcirculation are likely to be more frequently recognized as factors contributing to CHD.

Mechanisms of Coronary Atherosclerosis

Knowledge about mechanisms of plaque formation in the coronary arteries has rapidly accumulated in recent years. Epidemiologic studies reported in the 1960s suggested associations among certain traits and habits and the development of CHD. More recent studies have confirmed and expanded on these *risk factors*, which include several major risks (e.g., age, family history, abnormal lipid levels, cigarette smoking, hypertension, diabetes, and obesity) and numerous probable risks (Box 18-1).[2] Although males and females succumb to heart disease in equal numbers, male gender is a risk factor for earlier development of heart disease, on average about 10 years earlier. The risk factors for CHD are the same as those for atherosclerosis in other arteries and are discussed in Chapter 15.

The observation that atherosclerotic plaque is composed primarily of lipid prompted the idea that abnormal lipid metabolism was a probable culprit in the development of CHD, and a great deal of attention has

---

BOX 18-1   RISK FACTORS FOR CORONARY HEART DISEASE

Nonmodifiable Risks

Age: ≥45 years for men; ≥55 years for women
Gender: male
Family history of premature coronary heart disease
- Myocardial infarction or sudden cardiac death in male first-degree relative at age less than 55 years or female first-degree relative at age less than 65 years

Lipid Risk Factors

Total cholesterol >200 mg/dl
LDL cholesterol >130 mg/dl
Triglycerides >150 mg/dl
HDL cholesterol <40 mg/dl

Nonlipid Risk Factors

Hypertension >140/90 mm Hg
Cigarette smoking
Thrombogenic state
Diabetes
Obesity
Physical inactivity
Poor diet (atherogenic)

Probable Risk Factors (Emerging)

Lipoprotein(a)
Small LDL particles (pattern B)
HDL subtypes
Apolipoprotein B
Homocysteine
Fibrinogen
High-sensitivity C-reactive protein
Impaired fasting glucose (100-125 mg/dl)

Data from *NCEP III Guidelines*, 2002, NIH Pub. No. 02-5215.
HDL, High-density lipoprotein; *LDL,* low-density lipoprotein.

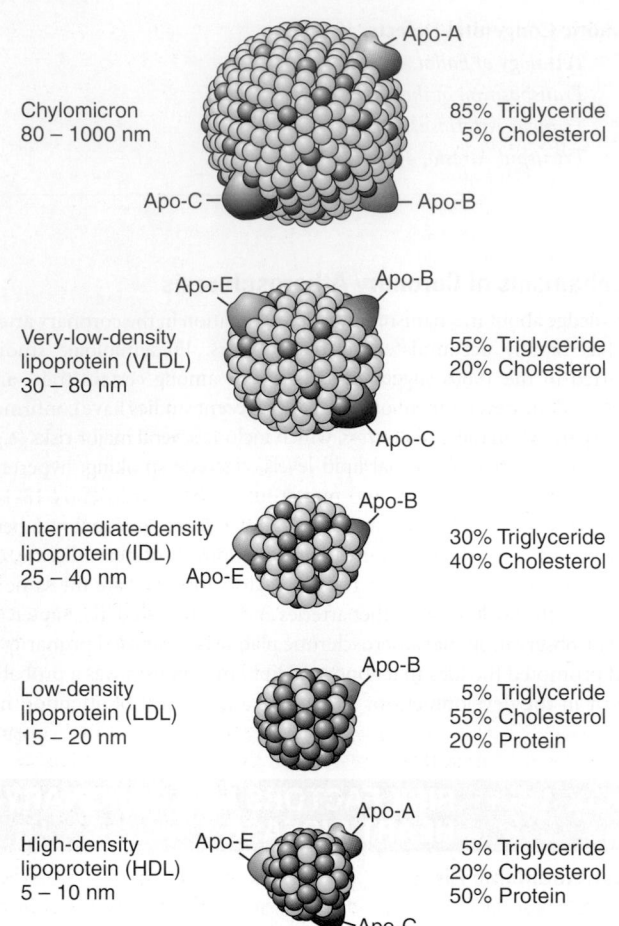

FIGURE 18-1 Serum lipoprotein fractions showing lipid composition and apoprotein components. Binding of lipoproteins to receptors is mediated through apoproteins.

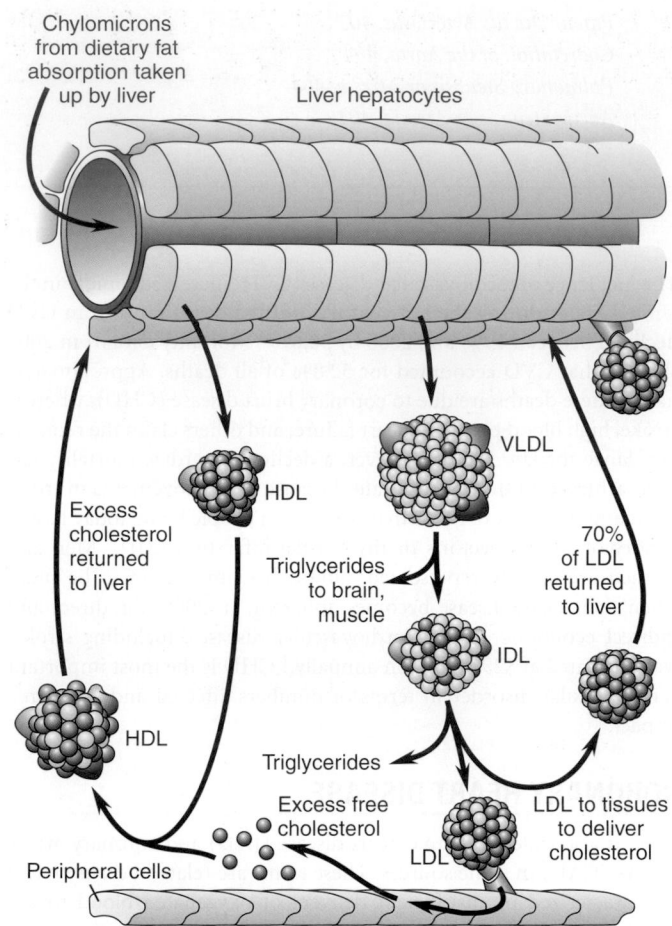

FIGURE 18-2 Schematic of lipoprotein metabolism in the body. Chylomicrons from dietary fat absorption are taken up by the liver and resynthesized into high-density lipoprotein *(HDL)* and very-low-density lipoprotein *(VLDL)*. HDL circulates to the peripheral tissues and takes up excess cholesterol for transport back to the liver. Triglycerides are removed for tissue use from VLDL, which becomes intermediate-density lipoprotein *(IDL)*. More triglyceride removal leads to the formation of low-density lipoprotein *(LDL)*. LDL is absorbed by peripheral tissues to obtain cholesterol. About 70% of the circulating LDL returns to the liver.

been focused on therapies to reduce levels of serum cholesterol in individuals with dyslipidemia. Lipids are transported through the bloodstream in combination with specific proteins (**apoproteins**). Certain lipid-protein molecules (**lipoproteins**) are associated with a greater risk of atherosclerosis. The five major kinds of lipoproteins are shown in Figure 18-1. High levels of low-density lipoproteins (LDLs), which are high in cholesterol, have been associated with the highest risk. Very-low-density lipoproteins, which have large amounts of triglycerides, also appear to increase the risk. High-density lipoproteins, on the other hand, have been correlated with a decreased risk of atherosclerosis.[2]

High-density lipoproteins are thought to transport cholesterol from the peripheral tissues back to the liver, thus removing atheromatous plaque. The role of low-density and, indirectly, very-low-density lipoproteins is to transport cholesterol to the peripheral tissues (Figure 18-2). Cholesterol uptake by peripheral cells is mediated by LDL receptors on cell surfaces that bind and promote endocytosis of cholesterol. The liver normally binds and internalizes about 75% of the circulating LDL cholesterol.

Extreme cases of hyperlipidemia occur in individuals who have genetic derangements in lipid metabolism. These disorders run in families, and some are associated with the development of severe coronary atherosclerosis at a young age unless aggressively managed. The most common form of genetic hyperlipidemia (familial hypercholesterolemia) is associated with a defect in the LDL receptor on liver cells.[3] Inability of the liver to efficiently remove cholesterol from the bloodstream results in hyperlipidemia. Genetic disorders of lipid metabolism

are described in Table 18-1. Even when lipid metabolism is normal, a high-fat diet can overwhelm the liver's ability to clear LDL cholesterol from the circulation and results in hyperlipidemia. Dietary fat restriction may be beneficial in reducing cholesterol level in this case.

Atherosclerotic plaque formation is initiated by injury to the coronary artery endothelium. The specific cause of endothelial dysfunction in the early stage of atherosclerosis is uncertain; however, several potential mechanisms have been described. These include chronic hemodynamic wall stress, which may explain the typical localization of plaques at arterial branch points and the role of hypertension as a risk factor; toxins from cigarette smoke; circulating inflammatory cytokines; and hyperlipidemia. Once the injury occurs, the endothelium may become more permeable and recruit leukocytes (Figure 18-3). LDLs leak through the endothelium and into the vessel wall (insudation) where they are oxidized by endothelial cells and macrophages.[4] Oxidized lipids are damaging to the endothelial and smooth muscle cells, and stimulate the recruitment of macrophages into the vessel wall, where they engulf the lipids. Lipid-filled macrophages are called *foam cells*. The macrophages and foam cells release inflammatory mediators and growth factors that attract more leukocytes and

TABLE 18-1 · GENETIC LIPOPROTEIN DISORDERS

DISORDER	GENE
LDL Particles	
Familial hypercholesterolemia	*LDL-R*
Familial defective ApoB-100	*ApoB*
Autosomal dominant hypercholesterolemia	*PCSK9*
Autosomal recessive hypercholesterolemia	*ARH*
Abetalipoproteinemia	*MTP*
Hypobetalipoproteinemia	*ApoB*
Familial sitosterolemia	*ABCG5/ABCG8*
Familial LP(a) hyperlipoproteinemia	*Apo(a)*
Remnant Lipoproteins	
Dysbetalipoproteinemia type III	*ApoE*
Hepatic lipase deficiency	*HL*
Triglyceride-Rich Lipoproteins	
Lipoprotein lipase deficiency	*LPL*
ApoC-II deficiency	*ApoC-II*
Apo-AV	*ApoA-V*
Familial hypertriglyceridemia	Polygenic
Familial combined hyperlipidemia	Polygenic
HDL Particles	
Apo-A1 deficiency	*Apo-A1*
Tangier disease, familial HDL deficiency	*ABCA1*
Familial LCAT deficiency syndromes	*LCAT*
CETP deficiency	*CETP*
Niemann-Pick disease types A and B	*SMPD1*
Niemann-Pick disease type C	*NPC1*

Adapted from Genest J, Libby P: Lipoprotein disorders and cardiovascular disease. In Bonow R, Mann D, Zipes D et al, editors: *Braunwald's heart disease: a textbook of cardiovascular medicine*, ed 9, Philadelphia, 2012, Saunders, p 983.
CETP, Cholesteryl ester transfer protein; *HDL,* high-density lipoprotein; *LCAT,* lecithin cholesterol acyltransferase; *LDL,* low-density lipoprotein; *Lp(a),* lipoprotein a.

stimulate smooth muscle proliferation. Excess lipid and debris begins to accumulate within the vessel wall and to coalesce into a pool called the *lipid core* (Figure 18-4). Atherosclerotic plaques with large lipid cores are fragile and prone to rupture. Rupture of a plaque exposes subendothelial proteins and initiates platelet aggregation and thrombus formation. Thrombi may be asymptomatic if they are small and do not occlude the artery. Components of the thrombus may be incorporated into the plaque, causing it to enlarge. Older plaques have significant collagen and fibrin, which form a cap and tend to make the plaque more stable. Numerous therapies aimed at stabilizing vulnerable plaques and preventing thrombus formation have been studied in clinical trials. Lipid-lowering therapy is a mainstay of treatment and prevention for atherosclerosis. Targets for serum LDL cholesterol levels have been developed by the National Cholesterol Education Program (NCEP) Adult Treatment Panel (NCEP III) based on the presence of known CHD or risk factors (Table 18-2).[5] An update to the NCEP III is expected in 2012. In addition to risk factor modification, therapies to reduce plaque inflammation, inhibit lipid oxidation, and prevent thrombosis are in common use (Table 18-3). A major aim of therapy is to stabilize the plaques, making them less prone to rupture.

Atherosclerotic lesions generally increase in size over many years and progressively occlude the lumen of vessels. A significant reduction in blood flow can result when plaque occupies 75% or more of the arterial lumen. Clinically significant atherosclerotic plaque may be located anywhere within the three major coronary arteries or major secondary branches. All three coronary arteries are often simultaneously affected, although some individuals have only one or two diseased vessels. Surprisingly, the extent and severity of atherosclerotic lesions are not good predictors of the severity of ischemia.

Atherosclerotic coronary lesions have been characterized and attempts made to correlate the anatomic descriptions with plaque development and behavior. Typically atherosclerotic lesions begin as fatty streaks and progress to small regions of medial wall thickening with scattered macrophages at a young age. These lesions are considered to be precursor lesions and are not symptomatic.[6] As the plaques acquire more free lipid within the arterial wall, they are more vulnerable to rupture, thrombus formation, and progressive plaque growth. These are considered to be advanced lesions and carry a significant risk of producing disruptions in coronary blood flow. Critical narrowing of the coronary lumen over time or sudden rupture of a plaque followed by thrombus formation causes the clinical syndromes of CHD, including angina, infarction, ischemic cardiomyopathy, and sudden cardiac arrest.

Stable plaques usually are asymptomatic or may be associated with exercise-induced angina pain (stable angina pectoris). However, plaques are vulnerable to rupture or erosion, which can initiate thrombus formation and acute coronary occlusion. A variety of factors have been identified as markers of increased plaque vulnerability. These factors include (1) active inflammation within the plaque; (2) a large lipid core with a thin cap; (3) endothelial denudation (erosion) with superficial platelet adherence; (4) fissured or ruptured cap; and (5) severe stenosis predisposing to high shear stress.[7] Acute coronary syndrome (ACS), or unstable angina or MI, as well as sudden cardiac arrest, is nearly always associated with acute disruption of a vulnerable plaque. Because the types of plaques that are most vulnerable often do not significantly obstruct the lumen before they rupture, ACS frequently occurs in individuals whose disease had been asymptomatic. Patients with a high risk for or known presence of vulnerable plaques benefit from therapies such as lipid-lowering agents (to stabilize plaques) and antiplatelet agents (to prevent thrombosis).[8]

Pathophysiology of Ischemia

Ischemia of cardiac cells occurs when the oxygen supply is insufficient to meet metabolic demands. Myocardial cells are unable to store much energy in the form of adenosine triphosphate (ATP) and must therefore continuously receive a supply of oxygen for aerobic synthesis of ATP. ATP is essential for powering myocardial contraction as well as for cell maintenance. Because the heart is unable to slow its activity when ATP supplies dwindle, a steady flow of oxygen is essential.

Factors that decrease myocardial oxygen supply or increase myocardial oxygen demand can upset the balance and result in cellular ischemia. Thus, the critical factors in meeting cellular demands for oxygen are (1) the rate of coronary perfusion and (2) the myocardial workload. Coronary perfusion can be impaired in several ways, including (1) large, stable atherosclerotic plaque, (2) acute platelet aggregation and thrombosis, (3) vasospasm, (4) failure of autoregulation by the microcirculation, and (5) poor perfusion pressure.

Myocardial workload depends on heart rate, preload, afterload, and contractility (see Chapter 17). An increase in any of these variables increases myocardial oxygen requirements and may precipitate ischemia. However, even conditions resulting in very high myocardial oxygen consumption will seldom lead to ischemia unless some underlying impairment in coronary perfusion is present.

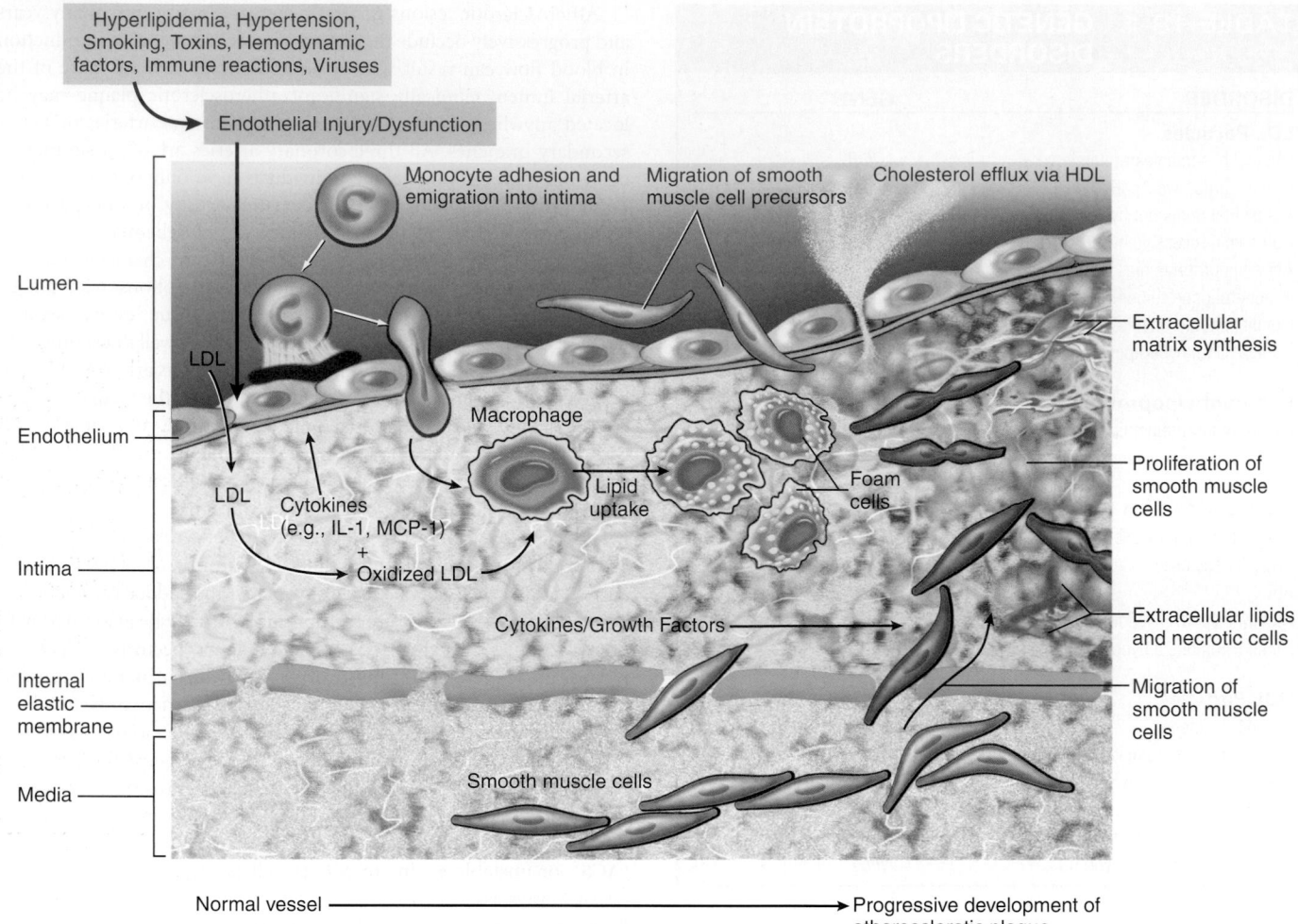

Hyperlipidemia, Hypertension, Smoking, Toxins, Hemodynamic factors, Immune reactions, Viruses

Endothelial Injury/Dysfunction

Monocyte adhesion and emigration into intima

Migration of smooth muscle cell precursors

Cholesterol efflux via HDL

Lumen

LDL

Endothelium

LDL

Macrophage

Lipid uptake

Foam cells

Cytokines (e.g., IL-1, MCP-1) + Oxidized LDL

Intima

Cytokines/Growth Factors

Internal elastic membrane

Media

Smooth muscle cells

Extracellular matrix synthesis

Proliferation of smooth muscle cells

Extracellular lipids and necrotic cells

Migration of smooth muscle cells

Normal vessel ⟶ Progressive development of atherosclerotic plaque

FIGURE 18-3 Sequence of events in the arteriolar wall associated with development of atherosclerosis. Note that smooth muscle cells migrate from the intima through the internal elastic membrane and into the intimal layer where they proliferate in response to growth factors. Macrophages in the intima release signals that alter the endothelial cell layer and induce expression of cell adhesion molecules that recruit monocytes into the tissue. (From Kumar V et al, editors: *Robbins and Cotran pathologic basis of disease*, ed 8, Philadelphia, 2010, Saunders, p 501.)

One or more of the aforementioned mechanisms are operative in producing clinically significant myocardial ischemia resulting in the acute or chronic coronary syndromes. Advanced fibrous plaque is thought to produce intermittent ischemia when 75% or more of the arterial lumen is occluded.[9] Because fibrous plaque progresses slowly over many years, the heart can develop alternative pathways for myocardial blood flow. This collateral circulation can preserve blood flow despite almost total occlusion of the coronary artery. Thus, stable fibrous plaque may produce no symptoms of ischemia unless the demand of the heart for oxygen is suddenly elevated, as occurs in exercise or stress. When the onset of ischemia is predictable with certain activities and subsides with rest, the patient is said to have a chronic coronary syndrome, called *classic* or *stable angina pectoris*.

ACS occurs when sudden obstruction of coronary blood flow results in acute myocardial ischemia. Acute obstruction is usually associated with the formation of a clot in the coronary artery at the site of a vulnerable plaque. Rupture of the plaque exposes a rough area composed of collagen and other molecules that are thrombogenic. A high fibrinogen level, as occurs in smokers, and enhanced platelet adhesiveness, as occurs in hyperlipidemia, may enhance the risk of thrombus

formation. Clot formation begins with adherence of platelets to the ruptured plaque. The platelets that initially attach release chemicals that attract more platelets, which aggregate and form a plug. The coagulation cascade may also be initiated and result in the formation of a platelet-fibrin clot that may occlude the vessel or break loose and travel farther along the vessel. Chemicals released by activated platelets include several vasoactive products (e.g., serotonin, thromboxane) that may contribute to spasm of the coronary vessel, further reducing blood flow.

Thrombosis occurs suddenly and may partially or completely obstruct the artery and cause acute ischemia. The ACS may present as unstable angina, MI, or sudden cardiac arrest. Appreciation of the role thrombus formation plays in coronary obstruction has resulted in the prophylactic use of antithrombotics, such as aspirin. Research indicates that the long-term use of small doses of aspirin reduces mortality from ischemic heart disease.[10]

Vasospasm usually occurs in areas of atherosclerotic plaque, but is also proposed as a mechanism of ischemia in patients who have anginal signs and symptoms but no significant amount of fibrous plaque in the coronary arteries. *Variant*, or *Prinzmetal*, angina is the term applied

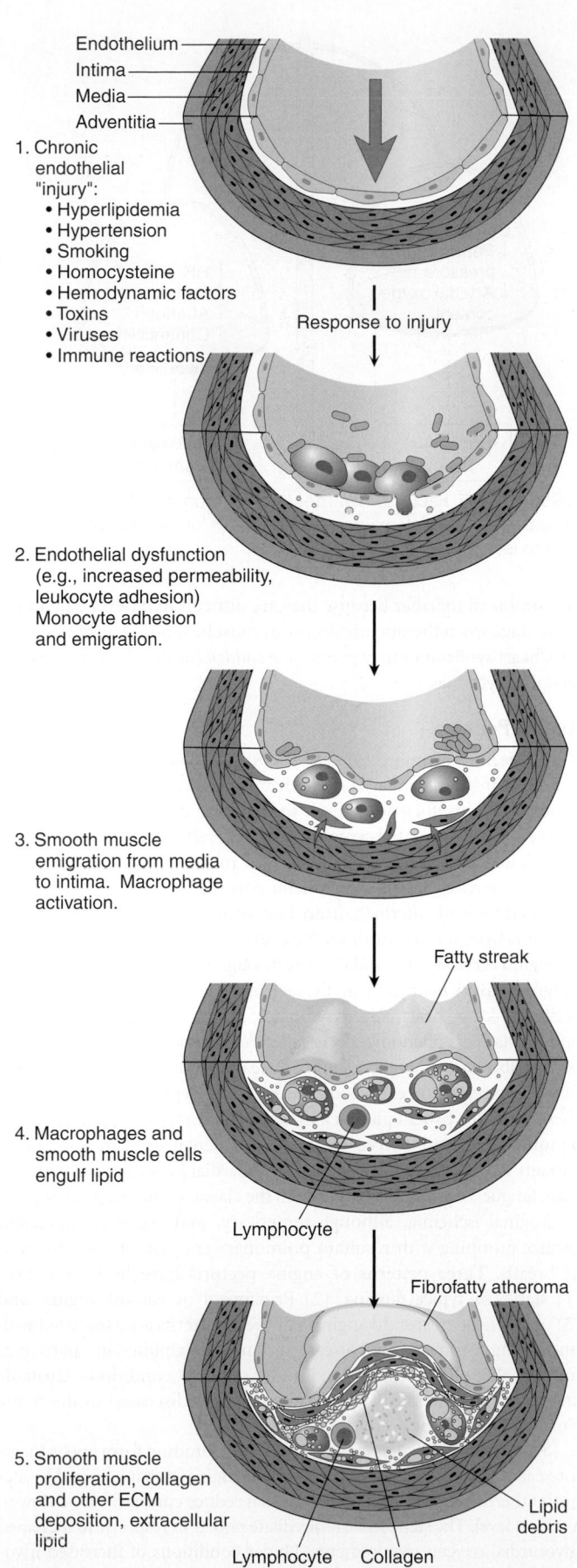

Endothelium
Intima
Media
Adventitia

1. Chronic endothelial "injury":
   • Hyperlipidemia
   • Hypertension
   • Smoking
   • Homocysteine
   • Hemodynamic factors
   • Toxins
   • Viruses
   • Immune reactions

Response to injury

2. Endothelial dysfunction (e.g., increased permeability, leukocyte adhesion) Monocyte adhesion and emigration.

3. Smooth muscle emigration from media to intima. Macrophage activation.

Fatty streak

4. Macrophages and smooth muscle cells engulf lipid

Lymphocyte

Fibrofatty atheroma

5. Smooth muscle proliferation, collagen and other ECM deposition, extracellular lipid

Lymphocyte   Collagen   Lipid debris

FIGURE 18-4 Pathogenesis of atherosclerosis. *1,* Chronic endothelial injury leads to *2. 2,* Endothelial dysfunction, permeability, and inflammation. *3,* Activated monocytes infiltrate the arterial wall and smooth muscle proliferates. *4,* Macrophages engulf lipid to become foam cells. *5,* A lipid core forms in the arterial wall and a fibrous cap evolves. (From Kumar V et al, editors: *Robbins and Cotran pathologic basis of disease,* ed 8, Philadelphia, 2010, Saunders, p 499.)

TABLE 18-2	**RECOMMENDED SERUM LOW-DENSITY LIPOPROTEIN TARGETS TO REDUCE THE RISK OF CORONARY HEART DISEASE**	
PATIENT RISK CATEGORY	**LDL-C CUT POINT FOR INITIATING DRUG THERAPY (mg/dl)**	**LDL-C GOAL (mg/dl)**
High risk: CHD present or CHD risk equivalent (≥2 risks plus 10-year risk >20%)	>100	<100 (optional <70)
Moderately high risk: ≥2 risks and 10-year risk 10-20%	≥130	<130
Moderate risk: ≥2 risks and 10-year risk <10%	≥160	<130
Lower risk: ≤1 risk	≥190	<160

From National Cholesterol Education Program: Third Report of the Expert Panel on Detection, Evaluation, and Treatment of High Blood Cholesterol in Adults (Adult Treatment Panel III), *Circulation* 110.227-239, 2004. *CHD,* Coronary heart disease; *LDL-C,* low-density lipoprotein cholesterol.

TABLE 18-3	**ACTIONS OF THERAPIES TO REDUCE CORONARY HEART DISEASE**	
THERAPY	**MAJOR ACTIONS**	**OTHER ACTIONS**
Angiotensin inhibitors (ACEI, ARB)	Improve endothelial function	Antioxidant (LDL), antiinflammatory
Statins	Decrease LDL-C, increase HDL-C	Improve endothelial function, antiinflammatory, antioxidant (LDL)
Fish oil (omega-3)	Decreases LDL-C, increases HDL-C	Inhibits thrombosis
Fibrates	Improve endothelial function	Increase HDL
Aspirin	Inhibits thrombosis, antiinflammatory	
Exercise	Increases HDL	Improves endothelial function

ACEI, Angiotensin-converting enzyme inhibitor; *ARB,* angiotensin II receptor blocker; *HDL-C,* high-density lipoprotein cholesterol; *LDL-C,* low-density lipoprotein cholesterol.

to vasospasm-initiated anginal symptoms. The etiology of spasm in vessels having no significant atherosclerotic plaques is unclear, but usually responds promptly to vasodilating agents. Intense vasospasm can occur in response to certain drugs, such as cocaine.

As previously mentioned, endothelial cells are important regulators of vascular tone. They secrete variable amounts of constricting and relaxing factors to control tissue perfusion. This autoregulation of blood flow allows the microvasculature to dilate when the need for oxygen in a particular area is increased. Failure of endothelial cells to appropriately regulate flow is a potential mechanism of myocardial ischemia.[11] Endothelial cells can be damaged by circulating toxins from cigarette smoke, immune cells, and infectious agents. Inflammatory disorders that may alter endothelial cell function include lupus erythematosus, Kawasaki syndrome, and polyarteritis nodosa. The importance of inflammatory processes in the pathogenesis of CHD has been recognized, resulting in efforts to find markers (e.g., serum high-sensitivity C-reactive protein) and methods to reduce inflammation in those at risk.

Even if the coronary arteries and microcirculation are functioning properly, coronary perfusion may still be inadequate if perfusion pressure is low. Recall from Chapter 17 that coronary blood flow occurs primarily during diastole and depends on the driving pressure in the aorta. A fall in aortic blood pressure can significantly reduce coronary perfusion, particularly in vessels with high resistance to flow. Conditions such as shock, hemorrhage, and anesthesia may be associated with a decline in blood pressure, which decreases driving pressure and coronary perfusion and results in myocardial ischemia. However, the most common cause of cardiac ischemia is atherosclerotic coronary arteries.

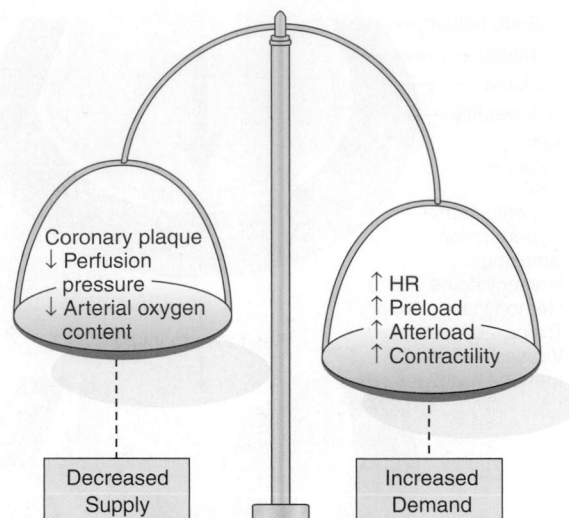

FIGURE 18-5 Factors that decrease coronary blood supply or increase myocardial oxygen demand can upset the balance and lead to ischemia and anginal pain.

are combined together because they are difficult to differentiate in the acute stage when therapeutic decisions must be made. Any of the coronary heart syndromes may precipitate *sudden cardiac death* and associated dysrhythmias.

Angina Pectoris

Angina pectoris literally means *chest pain* and is associated with intermittent myocardial ischemia. The length and the severity of the myocardial ischemia are insufficient to result in the acute death of cells. Bouts of chest pain and associated symptoms are generally recurrent and may be precipitated by conditions that increase myocardial oxygen demand, such as exercise, stress, sympathetic nervous system activation, and increased preload, afterload, heart rate, or muscle mass. Ischemic pain receptors from the myocardium travel to the central nervous system with the eighth cervical nerve and the first through fourth thoracic dorsal root ganglia. Sensory neurons from the jaw, neck, and arm also travel in these nerve trunks, so heart pain may be perceived as emanating from these body parts. This phenomenon is called *referred pain.* Anginal pain may be described as burning, crushing, squeezing, or choking. Pain is sometimes represented by expressions such as "an elephant is sitting on my chest" or by the patient placing a tight fist on the chest. Anginal pain may be mistakenly attributed to indigestion or dental pain. In some cases, patients have atypical symptoms of myocardial ischemia, such as back pain, fatigue, or weakness, rather than the classic symptom of chest pain.

Anginal ischemia, although temporary, may result in inefficient cardiac pumping with resultant pulmonary congestion and shortness of breath. Three patterns of angina pectoris have been described: (1) stable or typical angina, (2) Prinzmetal or variant angina, and (3) unstable or crescendo angina. All these patterns are associated with underlying coronary vessel disease and may be exhibited in a particular individual at different times and under different conditions. Unstable angina may progress to acute ischemia and is discussed in the Acute Coronary Syndrome section along with MI.

Stable angina. *Stable angina* is the most common form and is therefore called *classic* or *typical angina.* Stable angina is characterized by stenotic atherosclerotic coronary vessels that reduce coronary blood flow to a critical level. The stenosed arteries dilate poorly in response to increased myocardial oxygen requirements. Under conditions of increased myocardial workload, such as during physical exertion or emotional strain, coronary perfusion is inadequate and ischemia results (Figure 18-5). The

---

KEY POINTS

- Cardiac ischemia occurs when the heart's demand for oxygenated blood exceeds its supply. In most cases, ischemia is a result of impaired blood flow through the coronary arteries.
- CHD is associated with coronary atherosclerosis. Risk factors for CHD are the same as those for atherosclerosis of other arteries and include advancing age, male gender, family history, hyperlipidemia, diabetes, smoking, hypertension, and obesity. Endothelial injury and inflammation and lipid accumulation in the intima are thought to be the primary initiators of coronary atherosclerosis.
- Early atherosclerotic lesions are asymptomatic precursor lesions in which lipids begin to accumulate in the arterial wall. Advanced lesions may cause symptoms because of progressive arterial occlusion or acute plaque disruption and thrombus formation.
- Vulnerable plaques may rupture or become eroded, which stimulates clot formation on the plaque. Plaques with a large lipid core, thin cap, or high shear stress are vulnerable plaques.
- Chronic occlusion of a coronary vessel is associated with the clinical syndrome of stable angina. Acute occlusion is associated with plaque disruption and thrombus formation and results in ACS (unstable angina or MI).
- Myocardial ischemia may uncommonly be caused by coronary vasospasm, hypoxemia, or low perfusion pressure from volume depletion or shock.

Clinical Features and Management of Coronary Syndromes

Five syndromes can be differentiated according to the severity and onset of cardiac symptoms. Stable *angina pectoris* and *ischemic cardiomyopathy* are chronic syndromes that usually progress slowly and are a consequence of chronic obstruction from stable atherosclerotic plaques. ACS has an abrupt onset and life-threatening consequences and is associated with acute changes in plaque morphology and thrombosis. ACS includes *unstable angina* and *MI.* Unstable angina and MI

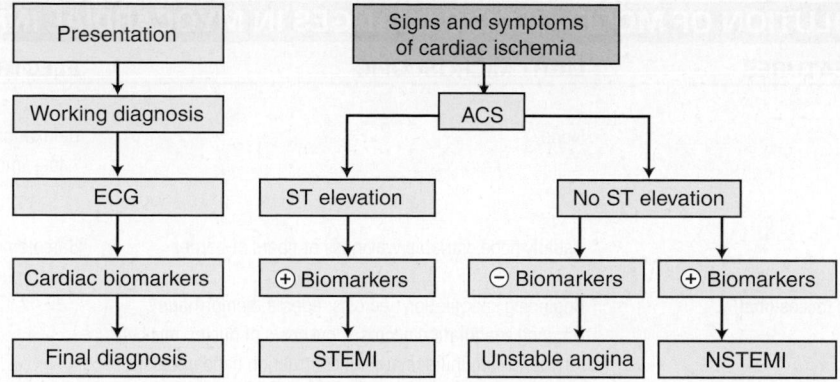

FIGURE 18-6 The etiologies of acute coronary syndrome (ACS) are difficult to differentiate by presenting symptoms because all involve some degree of myocardial ischemia. The electrocardiogram (ECG) is used to distinguish those patients with ST elevation from those with no ST elevation. Serum levels of cardiac biomarkers are then used to make a final diagnosis. Most patients with ACS characterized by ST elevation are diagnosed with MI (STEMI), and a proportion of patients with no ST elevation also will have elevated serum markers and are diagnosed with MI (NSTEMI). Patients who do not exhibit serum enzyme elevations are usually diagnosed with unstable angina.

onset of anginal pain is generally predictable and elicited by similar stimuli each time. Stable angina is generally relieved by rest and nitroglycerin, a drug that causes coronary and peripheral vasodilation, reduces preload, and, consequently, reduces myocardial workload.

Prinzmetal variant angina. Prinzmetal variant angina is characterized by unpredictable attacks of anginal pain. Although most individuals with Prinzmetal angina have significant coronary atherosclerosis, the onset of ischemic symptoms is unrelated to physical or emotional exertion, heart rate, or other obvious causes of increased myocardial oxygen demand. Vasospasm has been identified as the probable mechanism leading to variant angina, although the cause of the vasospasm is unknown. Proposed mechanisms include atherosclerosis-induced hypercontractility, abnormal secretion of vasospastic chemicals by local mast cells, and abnormal calcium flux across vascular smooth muscle. Variant angina responds well to treatment with calcium channel–blocking drugs, which inhibit vascular smooth muscle contraction.

Patients with angina are at risk for developing ACS and need aggressive treatment for risk factor reduction and therapies to reduce the risk of plaque rupture, thrombosis, and dysrhythmia.

Acute Coronary Syndrome

Unstable angina and MI are difficult to distinguish on the basis of clinical manifestations and are lumped together as ACS. Both are characterized by chest pain that may be more severe and lasts longer than the patient's typical angina and may occur in individuals whose disease was previously asymptomatic. In both cases, plaque rupture with subsequent acute thrombus development is thought to occur. In unstable angina, the occlusion is partial or the clot is dissolved before the death of myocardial tissue. In MI, the occlusion is complete and the thrombus persists long enough for development of irreversible damage to myocardial cells resulting in necrosis. In the past, differentiation of unstable angina and MI was based on laboratory evaluation of serum biomarker levels (e.g., MB band of creatine kinase [CK-MB], troponins I and T). If cardiac biomarkers were elevated, which is indicative of necrosis, a diagnosis of MI was made; if not, a diagnosis of unstable angina was appropriate. In a time when monitoring and management of complications were the mainstay of treatment, this approach worked well. With the advent of reperfusion therapy, which is effective only if administered early in the course of infarction, the distinction between unstable angina and MI has become less clinically relevant. Because unstable angina and MI present a similar clinical picture in

the acute phase, they have been combined in treatment protocols for ACS (Figure 18-6).[12] Patients with chest pain and evidence of acute ischemia on the electrocardiogram (ECG) (ST-segment elevation [STEMI]) are candidates for acute reperfusion therapy. Patients presenting with symptoms of unstable angina and no ST elevation on the ECG may not benefit from reperfusion strategies, and antiplatelet drugs are a cornerstone of therapy.[13] Differentiation between unstable angina and NSTEMI (non ST elevation MI) is made after obtaining cardiac necrosis markers; those patients with elevations are diagnosed with NSTEMI and those without elevations are diagnosed with unstable angina.

Etiology and pathogenesis. MI results when prolonged or total disruption of blood flow to the myocardium causes cellular death by necrosis or apoptosis. Acute MI is an important form of CHD resulting in more than 150,000 deaths annually in the United States.[1] It is estimated that an American male has a greater than 1 in 5 chance of sustaining an MI or fatal ischemic event before the age of 65. An MI may occur at any age, but the frequency rises with advancing age. Females younger than 45 years have a sixfold lesser risk of MI than men of the same age. After menopause, the rate of MI in women approaches that of their male counterparts and becomes essentially equal by age 80.[9]

As previously described, the initiating event in most MIs is believed to be development of a thrombus on top of an ulcerated or cracked atherosclerotic plaque. The initiating event is a sudden change in structure of the plaque. Platelets passing by the surface of the ruptured plaque adhere to it, initiate formation of a platelet plug, and activate the clotting cascade. The resultant thrombus grows until it occludes the vessel and triggers the transmural MI.

The thrombus theory of acute MI was controversial for many years because only 50% of persons dying of MI had a demonstrable thrombus at autopsy. Then DeWood and coworkers[14] demonstrated that about 90% of persons with acute MI had an intracoronary thrombus within 4 hours of the onset of symptoms, but only 60% had thrombi 12 to 24 hours later. This observation suggested that the thrombus was quickly dissolved by natural mechanisms after the occlusive event. Further support for the thrombus theory comes from the effectiveness of reperfusion therapies that successfully restore flow through obstructed coronary vessels and significantly reduce mortality.[15]

The cellular consequences of an acute interruption in blood flow to the myocardium do not occur instantaneously or uniformly. Acute occlusion causes a range of cellular events, depending on the availability

TABLE 18-4 EVOLUTION OF MORPHOLOGIC CHANGES IN MYOCARDIAL INFARCTION

TIME	GROSS FEATURES	LIGHT MICROSCOPIC	ELECTRON MICROSCOPIC
Reversible Injury			
0-½ hr	None	None	Relaxation of myofibrils; glycogen loss; mitochondrial swelling
Irreversible Injury			
½-4 hr	None	Usually none; variable waviness of fibers at border	Sarcolemmal disruption; mitochondrial amorphous densities
4-12 hr	Dark mottling (occasional)	Beginning coagulation necrosis; edema; hemorrhage	
12-24 hr	Dark mottling	Ongoing coagulation necrosis; pyknosis of nuclei; myocyte hypereosinophilia; marginal contraction band necrosis; beginning neutrophilic infiltrate	
1-3 days	Mottling with yellow-tan infarct center	Coagulation necrosis, with loss of nuclei and striations; interstitial infiltrate of neutrophils	
3-7 days	Hyperemic border; central yellow-tan softening	Beginning disintegration of dead myofibers, with dying neutrophils; early phagocytosis of dead cells by macrophages at infarct border	
7-10 days	Maximally yellow-tan and soft, with depressed red-tan margins	Well-developed phagocytosis of dead cells; early formation of fibrovascular granulation tissue at margins	
10-14 days	Red-gray depressed infarct borders	Well-established granulation tissue with new blood vessels and collagen deposition	
2-8 weeks	Gray-white scar, progressive from border toward core of infarct	Increased collagen deposition, with decreased cellularity	
>2 mo	Scarring complete	Dense collagenous scar	

From Kumar V et al: *Robbins and Cotran pathologic basis of disease,* ed 9, Philadelphia, 2010, Saunders, p 550.

and adequacy of collateral blood flow, the relative workload, and the length of time that flow is interrupted. A typical myocardial infarct has several zones composed of cells in various stages of ischemia and death.

Experiments in animal models indicate that complete occlusion of a coronary vessel results in a predictable pattern of cellular dysfunction and death.[9] Depletion of ATP in acutely ischemic cells begins immediately, followed within 1 to 2 minutes by an impaired ability to contract. Within 10 minutes, cellular concentrations of ATP fall to half of normal, and irreversible cell injury occurs after 30 to 40 minutes of complete occlusion (Table 18-4). Ischemic necrosis begins in the subendocardial zone and spreads across the ventricular wall toward epicardial surfaces. Epicardial areas are spared for longer periods because they have the greatest collateral network of arterial vessels. The ultimate size of the infarcted tissue depends on the extent, duration, and severity of ischemia. Areas of necrosis may be intermixed with or surrounded by zones of reversibly injured cells that are marginally perfused by collaterals. Injured cells die both from necrosis and from apoptosis.[3] Restoring perfusion to potentially salvageable cells is an important focus of treatment. (See Chapter 4 for a discussion of necrosis and apoptosis.)

Nearly all infarcts are located in the left ventricular walls. Isolated right ventricular infarction occurs in only 1% to 3% of MIs. Occlusion of the left anterior descending artery causes 40% to 50% of acute MIs, the right coronary artery contributes another 30% to 40%, and the left circumflex contributes 15% to 20%.[9] The locations of the resulting infarcts are shown in Table 18-5. It is common for individuals with coronary heart disease to suffer from more than one MI during their lifetime.

The area of necrosis resulting from MI undergoes a series of morphologic changes as the infarct ages.[9] These morphologic changes generally cannot be detected on gross examination until 6 to 12 hours after infarct. After 18 to 24 hours, the area of infarction becomes paler than surrounding tissues. Thereafter, the area of infarction becomes obvious because it turns yellowish and soft with a rim of red vascular connective tissue (Figure 18-7). At 1 to 2 weeks, the necrotic tissue is progressively

TABLE 18-5 LOCATION OF MYOCARDIAL INFARCTION ACCORDING TO CORONARY ARTERY AFFECTED

ARTERIAL OBSTRUCTION	LOCATION OF INFARCT
Left anterior descending (40-50% of infarcts)	Anterior wall of LV near apex Anterior two thirds of interventricular septum
Right coronary (30-40% of infarcts)	Posterior wall of LV Posterior one third of interventricular septum
Left circumflex (15-20% of infarcts)	Lateral wall of LV

Data from Kumar V et al: *Robbins and Cotran pathologic basis of disease,* ed 8, Philadelphia, 2010, Saunders, p 551.
LV, Left ventricle.

degraded and cleared from the site. Infarcted myocardium is particularly weakened and susceptible to rupture at this time. By 6 weeks, the necrotic tissue has been replaced by tough fibrous scar tissue.

Diagnosis of MI. The diagnosis of MI is based on three primary indicators: signs and symptoms, electrocardiographic changes, and elevations in the levels of specific marker proteins in the blood. Other diagnostic examinations such as cardiac catheterization, echocardiography, and radionuclide scintigraphy may also be performed to provide additional information (see Chapter 17).

Severe crushing, excruciating chest pain that may radiate to the arm, shoulder, jaw, or back is the harbinger of MI. Pain is commonly accompanied by nausea, vomiting, diaphoresis (sweating), and shortness of breath. In contrast to anginal pain, infarction pain generally lasts more than 15 minutes and is not relieved by rest or nitroglycerin.

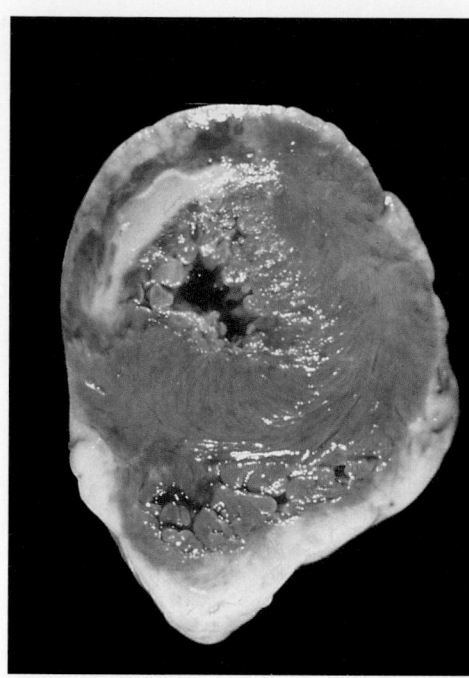

FIGURE 18-7 This photograph of a 5- to 7-day-old posterolateral infarction clearly shows a large, pale yellow lesion surrounded by a dark red zone of inflammation. (From Kumar V et al, editors: *Robbins basic pathology*, ed 7, Philadelphia, 2003, Saunders, p 369.)

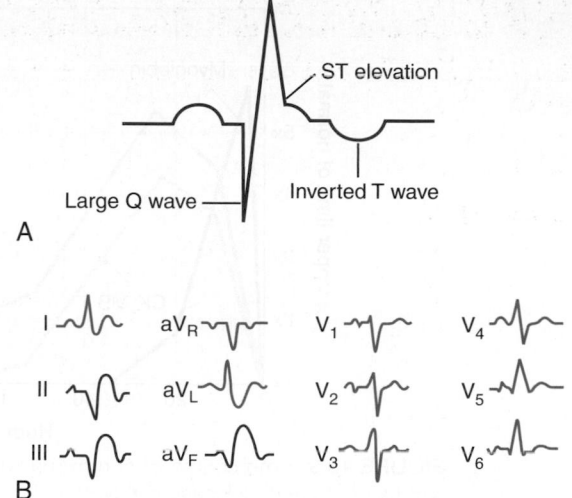

FIGURE 18-8 A, Typical ECG infarction pattern showing abnormally large Q wave, ST elevation, and inverted T wave. **B,** Typical ECG in acute inferior myocardial infarction. Note the Q waves and ST-segment elevation in leads II, III, and aV$_F$.

In some instances, however, the MI is entirely asymptomatic and may elude detection. Asymptomatic MI has been called *silent MI* and may be detected only serendipitously at a later date. Pain may be difficult to assess in individuals with atypical presentations or a tendency to ignore or deny their symptoms. Thus, although pain is an important indicator of acute ischemia, other clinical information is often needed to correctly distinguish between angina, infarction, and noncardiac sources of pain. Women, the elderly, and patients with diabetic neuropathies more commonly complain of atypical symptoms, including fatigue, nausea, back pain, and abdominal discomfort. Atypical complaints in patients with CHD risk factors should prompt a high suspicion of MI.

Electrocardiographic changes. Myocardial ischemia and infarction often result in characteristic changes on ECG waveforms. Injury and ischemia are indicated on the ECG by ST-segment changes. ST-segment elevation is thought to represent acute cellular injury and ischemia. The presence of ST-segment elevation on the ECG indicates that the ischemic injury is ongoing and that efforts to improve perfusion or reduce oxygen demand may be effective in preserving myocardial muscle mass. Until measurements of specific serum markers of infarction are obtained, these patients are regarded as having unstable angina/STEMI in treatment protocols for ACS. Infarcted muscle that is necrotic and no longer electrically active is indicated by the appearance of abnormally deep (>0.1 mV) or wide (>0.03 seconds) Q waves and inverted T waves (Figure 18-8). These changes are very specific for MI and, when present, are diagnostic. Q waves are usually persistent findings, whereas ST-segment and T wave changes may resolve over time. Q waves take time to develop and may not be present in the acute phase of an MI.

Dysrhythmias and the characteristic ST-segment changes that accompany MI are attributed to injured and ischemic cells that have not yet become necrotic. Reversibly injured cells have limited ATP supplies to power membrane pumps and are predisposed to leakage of ions across their cell membranes. Abnormal ion flux may result in continuous current flow even when the heart is at rest. This current leak may be seen on the ECG as ST-segment elevation.

The 12-lead ECG is used to localize the injured region of the left ventricle. Various leads of the 12-lead ECG "view" different regions of the heart. Abnormalities such as Q waves and ST-segment elevation in a particular lead or leads indicate that the damage is localized to the part of the left ventricle "seen" by that lead. MIs may thus be described as anterior, lateral, posterior, septal, inferior, or a combination of these sites. (The 12-lead ECG is described in Chapter 17.)

In some cases, patients presenting with ACS do not have ST elevation on the ECG. They may have ST depression or T wave changes. Some of these patients will develop elevated serum markers indicating MI. These patients have NSTEMI. The infarct size is generally smaller, and the outcomes are better than those in patients with STEMI.[13]

Serum markers. The appearance of certain proteins in the blood after myocardial cell death is a very sensitive and reliable indicator of MI. Myocardial cell death leads to elevated serum levels of myoglobin, troponin, lactate dehydrogenase, and creatine kinase.[9] Cardiac cells contain particular forms of these proteins called *isoforms*. An increase in the concentration of these proteins suggests leakage from fatally damaged cells that have lost plasma membrane integrity. Cardiac biomarkers have a slightly different amino acid sequence than other cell types. In particular, myocytes contain the isoforms CK-MB, troponin I, and troponin T. An elevated level of serum CK-MB is a highly specific indicator of MI and considered to be diagnostic. However, the level of CK-MB remains elevated for only 48 to 72 hours after MI. Two proteins that comprise part of the cardiac cell contractile apparatus, troponins I and T, have become the markers of choice for detecting MI. Cardiac troponin levels become elevated in serum at about the same time as the CK-MB level, but they remain elevated for a longer period. Cardiac troponins I and T are highly sensitive and specific for cardiac cell death but less helpful in detecting new infarction (reinfarction) because levels remain elevated for a prolonged period (Figure 18-9). Cardiac myoglobin levels are elevated in serum very quickly after MI and may be helpful in early detection; however, cardiac myoglobin is less specific than the other markers. All serum markers are useful diagnostically only during the acute period of MI. Patients with ACS who do not develop elevations of these serum markers are diagnosed with unstable angina.

Clinical course. In addition to chest pain, electrocardiographic abnormalities, and serum protein marker elevations, a person experiencing an MI may exhibit signs of cardiac inflammation, including

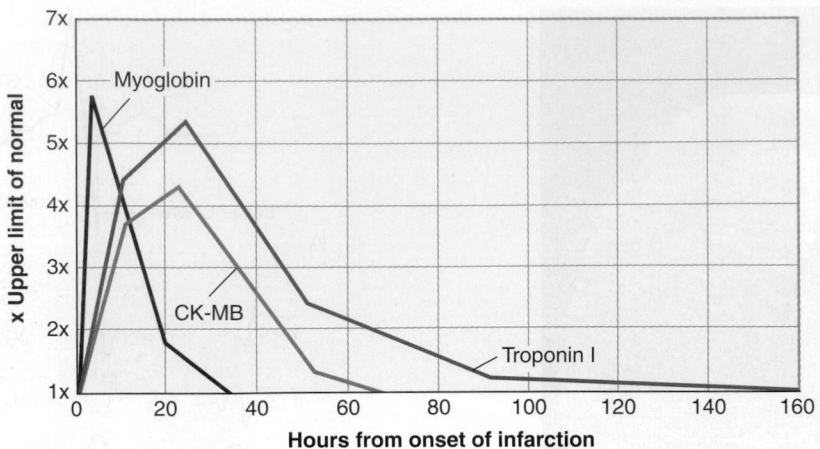

FIGURE 18-9 Time course of serum marker protein elevations after acute myocardial infarction. The MB band of creatine kinase (CK-MB) and troponin I are the most specific of the protein markers. Myoglobin is an early marker but is not very specific.

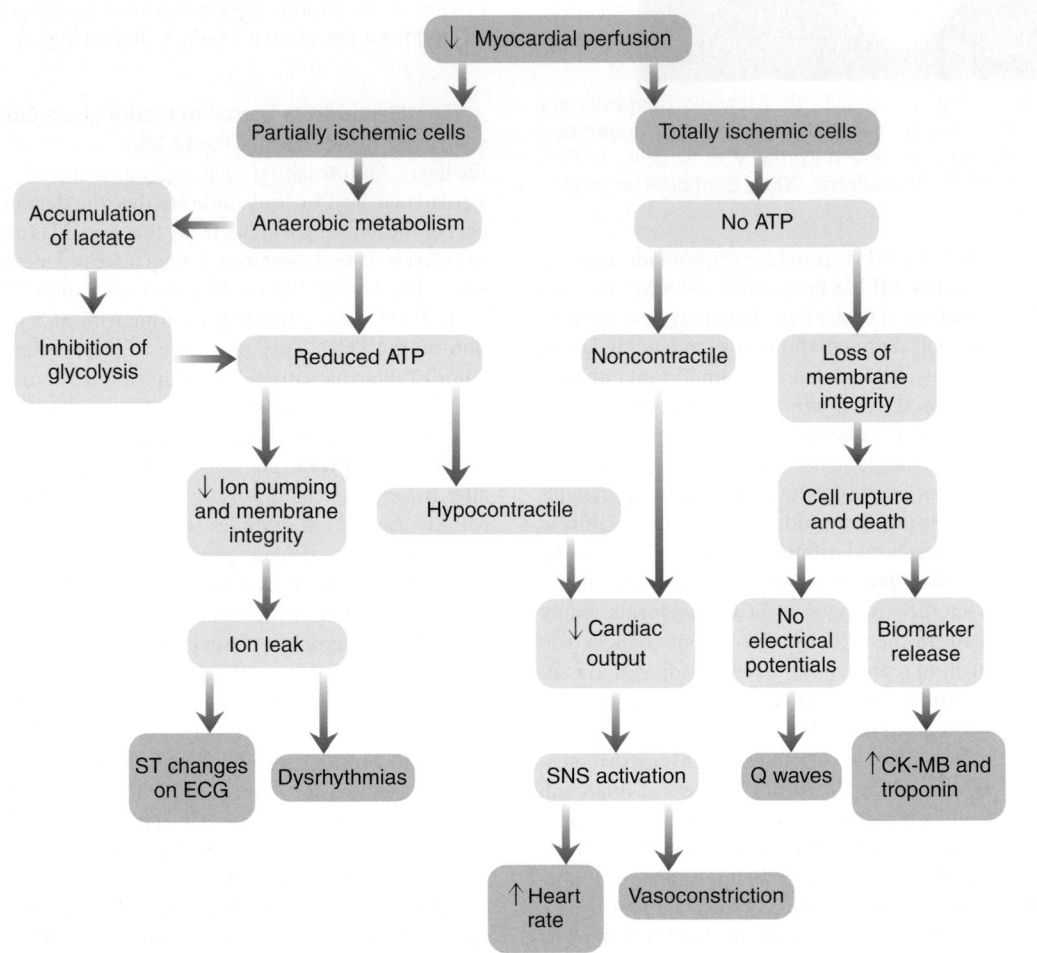

FIGURE 18-10 Summary of events after myocardial infarction. ATP, Adenosine triphosphate; CK-MB, MB band of creatine kinase; *ECG*, electrocardiography; *SNS*, sympathetic nervous system.

fever, leukocytosis, and an elevated sedimentation rate. Symptoms of circulatory inadequacy, including fatigue, restlessness, anxiety, and weakness, may be present.

The events associated with MI are summarized in Figure 18-10. Note that totally ischemic cells, which die and become electrically silent, are the source of the clinical findings of Q waves and also release the indicative serum marker proteins (CK-MB, troponins). Partially ischemic cells are potentially salvageable but are unable to maintain normal ion flux across the cell membrane. Abnormal ion flux is responsible for the ST-segment changes in acute ischemia and also predisposes to a variety of cardiac dysrhythmias, including ventricular ectopy and conduction blocks (see Chapter 19).

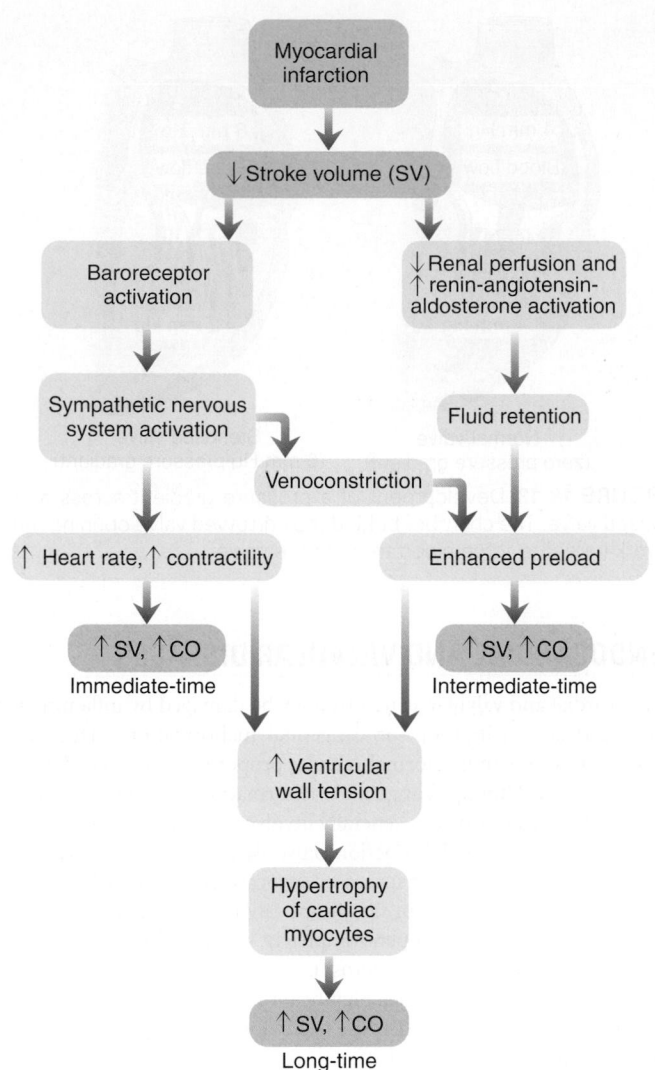

FIGURE 18-11 Compensatory responses to increase stroke volume *(SV)* and maintain cardiac output *(CO)* after myocardial infarction.

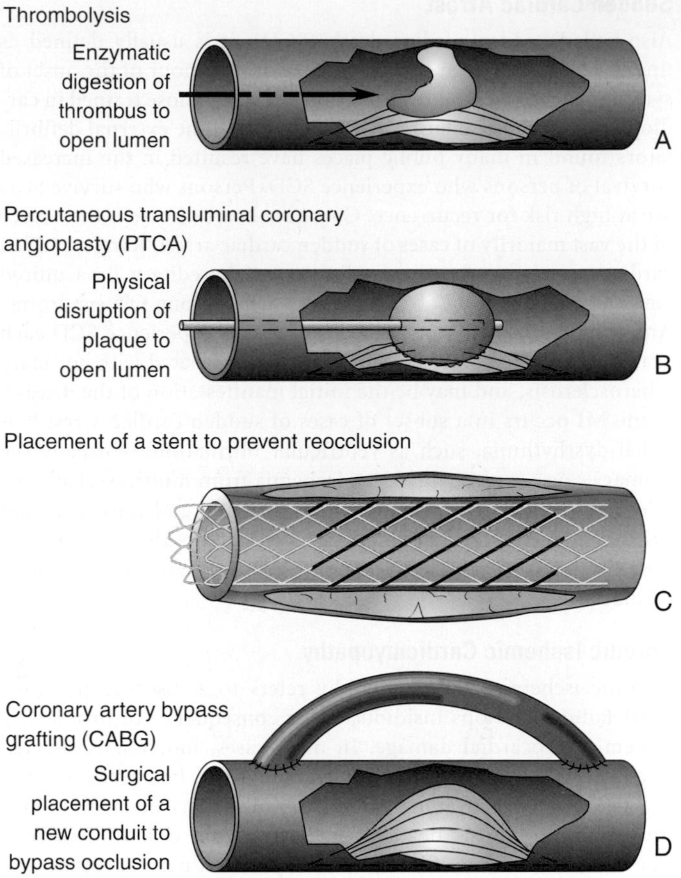

Thrombolysis

Enzymatic digestion of thrombus to open lumen

A

Percutaneous transluminal coronary angioplasty (PTCA)

Physical disruption of plaque to open lumen

B

Placement of a stent to prevent reocclusion

C

Coronary artery bypass grafting (CABG)

Surgical placement of a new conduit to bypass occlusion

D

FIGURE 18-12 Management of blocked coronary arteries includes **(A)** thrombolysis with drugs such as streptokinase and tissue plasminogen activator; **(B)** plaque disruption with percutaneous transluminal coronary angioplasty, followed by anticoagulation or stent placement; **(C)** placement of a stent to prevent reocclusion; and **(D)** coronary artery bypass grafting—surgical placement of a new conduit to bypass the occluded area of the artery.

Neither partially ischemic nor totally ischemic cells are able to contract effectively, and poor stroke volume leads to a drop in cardiac output. Decreased stroke volume triggers a number of compensatory actions designed to improve cardiac output. In particular, activation of the sympathetic nervous system increases the heart rate, contractility, blood pressure, and fluid retention by the kidney. Unfortunately, these compensatory efforts impose a greater workload on the heart and may contribute to further ischemic damage. Compensatory mechanisms are shown in Figure 18-11 and include sympathetic nervous system activation, enhanced preload, and hypertrophy of cardiac myocytes.

Prognosis and treatment. An overall prognosis for acute MI is difficult to determine because many variables affect the outcome, including the extent and location of the infarct, previous cardiovascular health, age, and the presence of other disease processes. Of particular importance is how quickly treatment is sought. Most deaths from MI occur before the victim reaches the hospital. The in-hospital mortality rate of MI is about 10%.[9] In approximately 25% of cases, an MI is not accompanied by any complications (uncomplicated MI) and the patient recovers rapidly. However, the remaining 75% of MIs are followed by one or more complications.[9] Potential complications include cardiac dysrhythmias, heart failure, cardiogenic shock, ventricular rupture, pericarditis, and thromboembolism.

Treatment for MI is directed at decreasing myocardial oxygen demand and increasing myocardial oxygen supply while monitoring and managing complications as they arise. Measures to reduce myocardial workload frequently include preload and afterload reduction, heart rate control, pain relief, and activity restriction. Sympathetic antagonists, nitrates, and morphine sulfate are the mainstays of drug therapy. Measures to increase oxygen delivery to ischemic areas include oxygen administration, antiplatelet therapy with aspirin and other antiplatelet agents, thrombolytic (fibrinolytic) drugs, anticoagulants, angioplasty, stent placement, and coronary artery bypass grafting (CABG) (Figure 18-12). Therapies aimed at opening the blocked coronary artery are called reperfusion therapies.

Early detection and management of dysrhythmias and conduction disorders are an important part of the immediate care of a patient with MI. Many dysrhythmias are life threatening and, at the very least, lead to decreased cardiac output or increased myocardial workload. Continuous electrocardiographic monitoring is generally the standard of care because of the high incidence of electrical disturbances after MI. Common dysrhythmias and conduction disorders are described in Chapter 19.

Sudden Cardiac Arrest

Also called sudden cardiac death (SCD), it is usually defined as unexpected death from cardiac causes within 1 hour of the onset of symptoms.[16] Successful resuscitation efforts by those trained in cardiopulmonary resuscitation (CPR) and use of the external defibrillators found in many public places have resulted in the increased survival of persons who experience SCD. Persons who survive SCD are at high risk for recurrence. Coronary heart disease is the source of the vast majority of cases of sudden cardiac arrest. Rarely, sudden cardiac arrest may be a complication of hereditary or acquired structural or electrical abnormalities, such as long QT syndrome. An estimated 300,000 to 400,000 individuals experience SCD each year in the United States.[1] Most cases are associated with coronary atherosclerosis, and may be the initial manifestation of the disease. Acute MI occurs in a subset of cases of sudden cardiac arrest.[16] A lethal dysrhythmia, such as ventricular fibrillation, is usually the primary cause (see Chapter 19). Ischemia from multivessel atherosclerosis, diffuse myocardial atrophy, scarring and fibrosis of old MI tissue, and electrolyte imbalances are factors that may predispose the heart to the electrical abnormalities that lead to sudden cardiac arrest.

Chronic Ischemic Cardiomyopathy

Chronic ischemic cardiomyopathy refers to a disorder in which heart failure develops insidiously as a consequence of progressive ischemic myocardial damage. In most cases, individuals affected have a history of angina or MI, often many years before the onset of heart failure. Heart failure appears to be a consequence of slow, progressive apoptotic death of myocytes from chronic ischemia. The disease is usually found in elderly individuals. Atrophic and dead cells are scattered throughout the myocardium rather than being localized, as occurs with MI. The prognosis for patients with chronic ischemic cardiomyopathy is quite poor, with death from heart failure the common outcome. Heart failure is further discussed in Chapter 19.

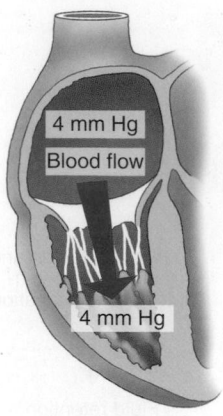
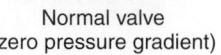
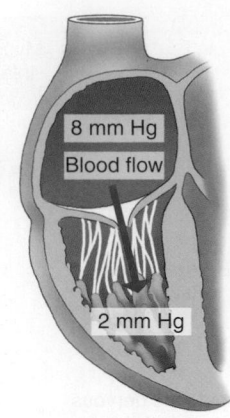

Normal valve   Stenosed valve
(zero pressure gradient)   (6 mm Hg pressure gradient)

FIGURE 18-13 Development of a pressure gradient across a stenosed valve. The chamber behind the narrowed valve opening must work harder to force blood through the valve.

ENDOCARDIAL AND VALVULAR DISEASES

Endocardial and valvular structures may be damaged by inflammation and scarring, calcification, or congenital malformations. These processes interfere with the normal valvular property of unimpeded, unidirectional flow. Although congenital malformations may affect any valve, acquired valvular disorders generally involve the mitral or aortic valves. Abnormalities in valvular function cause altered hemodynamics in the heart and generally result in increased myocardial workload. Ultimately, heart failure may result from significant valvular dysfunction.

Normally, heart valves open completely, so blood flows through with little or no pressure difference across the valve. Failure of a valve to open completely is termed **stenosis.** Significant hemodynamic consequences generally begin to occur when the valve opening is reduced to half its normal diameter. The severity of stenosis can be estimated by the degree of pressure gradient across the valve (Figure 18-13). Stenosis results in extra pressure work for the heart because blood must be forced through the high resistance of a narrow valve opening. Stenosis generally progresses slowly over years to decades, which allows time for affected heart chambers to compensate through myocardial cell hypertrophy.

Regurgitation (insufficiency) refers to the inability of a valve to close completely, thereby allowing blood to flow backward across the valve when no flow should be occurring. Regurgitation may develop suddenly from valvular infection or rupture of a supporting papillary muscle. Sudden regurgitation is poorly tolerated inasmuch as little compensation is possible. Regurgitation results in extra volume work for the heart because more blood must be pumped to maintain adequate forward flow.

Diseased valves may exhibit elements of both stenosis and regurgitation, although one problem usually predominates. Postinflammatory scarring from rheumatic heart disease and valvular calcification with aging are the primary causes of stenosis (Figure 18-14). A wide variety of diseases of the endocardium may lead to valvular regurgitation, including rheumatic heart disease and infective endocarditis, which are discussed later in this chapter. Damaged valves are susceptible to infection, and antibiotic prophylaxis may be indicated for dental, surgical, and diagnostic procedures. The major causes of acquired mitral and aortic valvular diseases are listed in Table 18-6. Valvular disorders are often associated with abnormal turbulence of blood flow that produces heart sounds called *murmurs.* Careful assessment of the location and character of a murmur can help identify the underlying

---

KEY POINTS

- The clinical syndromes of CHD include angina pectoris, ACS (unstable angina, NSTEMI, STEMI), chronic ischemic cardiomyopathy, and sudden cardiac arrest. These conditions are associated with advanced coronary atherosclerosis.
- Angina is characterized by intermittent bouts of chest pain triggered by exertion and generally relieved by rest. No permanent myocardial damage occurs.
- Prolonged or severe ischemia results in MI that is characterized by severe, unrelieved chest pain, nausea and vomiting, diaphoresis, shortness of breath, and inflammation (e.g., fever, increased white blood cell count, increased sedimentation rate).
- Serum protein marker elevations and electrocardiographic changes are diagnostic of MI. The most specific and sensitive serum markers are increased levels of CK-MB and troponins I and T. ECG changes include ST-segment elevation, large Q waves, and inverted T waves.
- A drop in cardiac output as a result of MI triggers a number of compensatory responses, including sympathetic activation. The sympathetic nervous system increases the heart rate, contractility, and blood pressure, all of which increase myocardial workload.
- Treatment of acute ischemia usually includes efforts to decrease myocardial oxygen demand (e.g., sympathetic antagonists, rest, heart rate control, pain relief, afterload reduction) and increase oxygen delivery (e.g., thrombolysis, angioplasty, coronary artery bypass grafting).

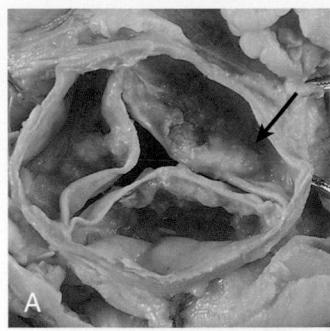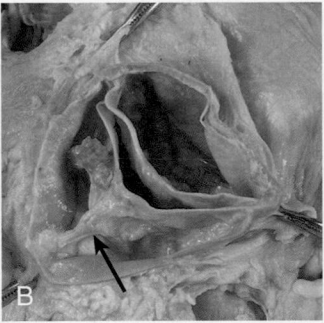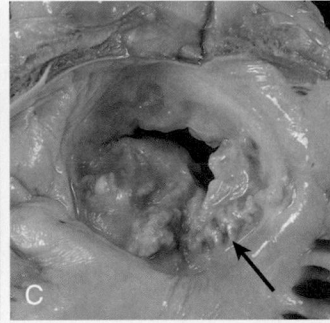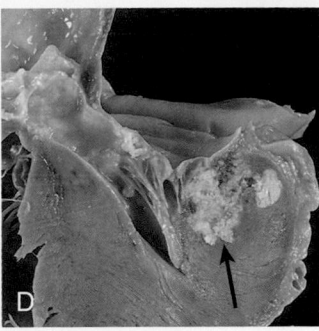

FIGURE 18-14 Valvular degeneration and calcification. **A,** Calcific aortic stenosis of previously normal (three-cusp) valve. **B,** Calcific aortic stenosis of congenital bicuspid valve. **C,** Mitral valve calcification. **D,** Cut section of valve from **C.** (From Kumar V et al, editors: *Robbins and Cotran pathologic basis of disease,* ed 8, Philadelphia, 2010, Saunders, p 562.)

TABLE 18-6   MAJOR ETIOLOGIES OF ACQUIRED HEART VALVE DISEASE

MITRAL VALVE DISEASE	AORTIC VALVE DISEASE
Mitral Stenosis	**Aortic Stenosis**
Postinflammatory scarring (rheumatic heart disease)	Postinflammatory scarring (rheumatic heart disease)
	Senile calcific aortic stenosis
	Calcification of a congenitally deformed valve
Mitral Regurgitation	**Aortic Regurgitation**
Abnormalities of leaflets and commissures:	Postinflammatory scarring (rheumatic heart disease)
Postinflammatory scarring	Infective endocarditis
Infective endocarditis	Marfan syndrome
Mitral valve prolapse	Aortic disease:
Drugs (e.g., Fen-Phen)	Degenerative aortic dilation
Abnormalities of the tensor apparatus:	Syphilitic aortitis
Rupture of papillary muscle	Ankylosing spondylitis
Papillary muscle dysfunction (fibrosis)	Rheumatoid arthritis
Rupture of chordae tendineae	Marfan syndrome
Abnormalities of left ventricular cavity and/or annulus:	
LV enlargement (myocarditis, dilated cardiomyopathy)	
Calcification of mitral ring	

Modified from Schoen FJ: Surgical pathology of removed natural and prosthetic heart valves, *Hum Pathol* 18(6):558-567, 1987; and from Kumar V et al: *Robbins and Cotran pathologic basis of disease,* ed 8, Philadelphia, 2010, Saunders, p 561.
LV, Left ventricle.

TABLE 18-7   DEFINING CHARACTERISTICS OF MURMURS

VALVE DISORDER	QUALITY	LOCATION, RADIATION
Mitral stenosis	Low-pitched rumble, diastolic	At apex
Mitral regurgitation	Loud, pansystolic, high pitched, blowing	Loudest at apex, transmitted to left axilla
Aortic stenosis	Harsh, midsystolic, crescendo-decrescendo	Right second intercostal space, transmitted to neck
Aortic regurgitation	Faint, blowing, diastolic	Left sternal border, aortic area, apex

valvular abnormality. Defining characteristics of common valve disorders are described in Table 18-7.

Disorders of the Mitral Valve

Three important disorders of the mitral valve are stenosis, regurgitation, and mitral valve prolapse.

Mitral Stenosis

In *mitral stenosis* the flow of blood from the left atrium into the left ventricle is impaired. Mitral stenosis is therefore characterized by an abnormal left atrial–left ventricular pressure gradient during ventricular diastole (Figure 18-15). Normally the pressures in the atrium and ventricle are nearly equal during ventricular diastole when the mitral valve is open. Figure 18-15 shows that with mitral valve stenosis, atrial pressure remains higher than ventricular pressure throughout diastole. As the stenosis worsens, the pressure gradient often increases. In normal adults the area of the mitral valve orifice is 4 to 6 cm^2, and symptoms of stenosis do not appear until the orifice is narrowed to 2 cm^2. When the mitral valve orifice narrows to 1 cm^2, a critical stenosis is present and a pressure gradient of 20 mm Hg or more usually develops across the valve.[17] Increased pressure work of the left atrium leads to atrial chamber enlargement and hypertrophy. Progressive narrowing of the mitral valve may lead to markedly elevated left atrial pressures and subsequent increased pulmonary vascular pressure. If uncorrected, mitral stenosis may result in chronic pulmonary hypertension, right ventricular hypertrophy, and right-sided heart failure.

The signs and symptoms of mitral stenosis are due to congestion of blood volume and increased pressure in the left atrium and pulmonary circulation, as well as decreased stroke volume of the left ventricle because of deficient filling. Symptoms are exacerbated by conditions that further decrease left ventricular filling such as an increased heart rate. Atrial dysrhythmias such as atrial fibrillation are common because of excessive atrial volume. Atrial enlargement and fibrillation also predispose to the development of atrial clots, which may dislodge and result in systemic embolization and stroke. Signs and symptoms of mitral stenosis secondary to pulmonary congestion may include orthopnea, cough, dyspnea on exertion, paroxysmal nocturnal dyspnea, abnormal

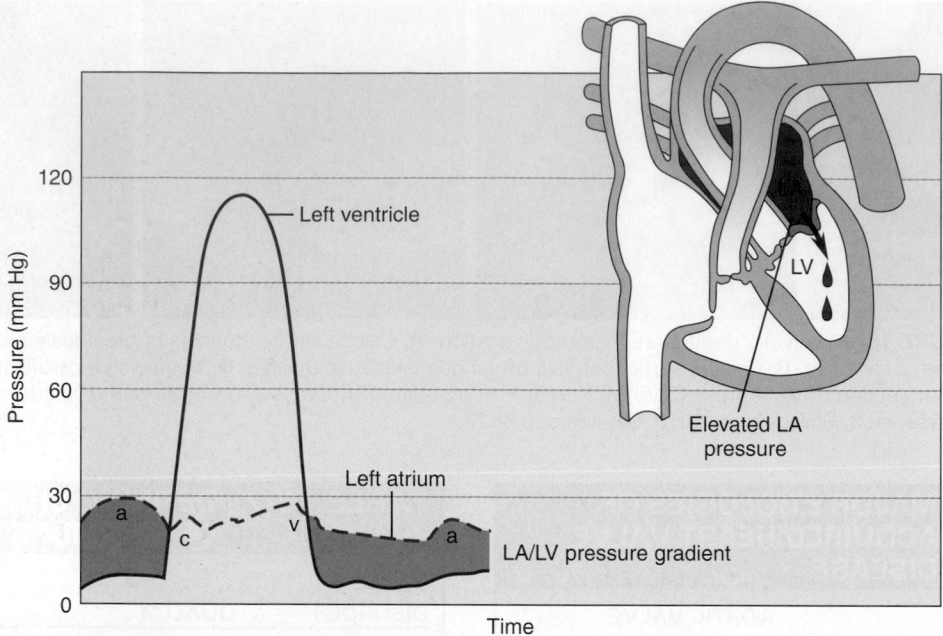

FIGURE 18-15 Mitral stenosis is characterized by an abnormal left atrial *(LA)*–to–left ventricular *(LV)* pressure gradient during ventricular diastole *(shaded area)*.

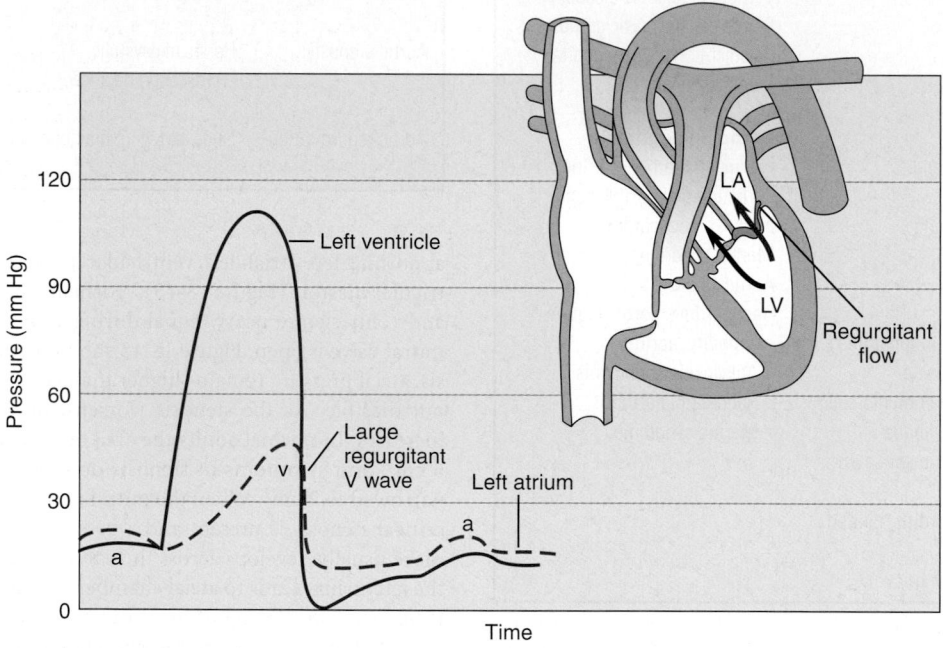

FIGURE 18-16 Mitral regurgitation causes characteristic giant V waves on the left atrial *(LA)* pressure monitor. *LV,* left ventricular.

breath sounds, and poor arterial oxygenation. Reduced left ventricular stroke volume may be apparent as fatigue, poor activity tolerance, and weakness. Exertional dyspnea is the most common complaint. Blood rushing through the narrowed mitral valve during ventricular diastole can sometimes be heard as a low-pitched, rumbling diastolic murmur at the heart's apex. In many cases, an opening snap may also be heard.

Mitral Regurgitation

Mitral regurgitation is characterized by backflow of blood from the left ventricle to the left atrium during ventricular systole. Elevation of left atrial volume and pressure by regurgitant flow leads to characteristic

giant V waves on the atrial pressure monitor (Figure 18-16). The severity of mitral insufficiency is related to the amount of left ventricular stroke volume that is regurgitant and depends, in part, on the aortic resistance to flow (afterload). A high afterload increases the amount of regurgitant flow. The left ventricle must pump a greater volume to compensate for the regurgitant flow and maintain an effective stroke volume. Both the left atrium and the left ventricle generally dilate and hypertrophy to compensate for the extra volume that they are required to pump. In most patients with mitral regurgitation, compensation is maintained for many years before symptoms occur.[17] If severe and uncorrected, mitral regurgitation may eventually lead to left-sided heart failure. The signs and symptoms of mitral regurgitation are similar to those described for mitral stenosis and result from pulmonary congestion and poor cardiac output. Chronic weakness and fatigue are common complaints. The murmur of mitral regurgitation usually occurs throughout ventricular systole (pansystolic), radiates toward the left axilla, and has a high-pitched blowing character. The arterial pulse may be helpful in distinguishing the systolic murmur of mitral regurgitation from that of aortic stenosis. The upstroke of the pulse is sharp and full in mitral regurgitation, whereas it is weaker and delayed in aortic stenosis.

Mitral Valve Prolapse

Approximately 2% to 3% of the population have mitral valves that balloon into the left atrium during ventricular systole.[17] This condition is called *mitral valve prolapse* (Figure 18-17). Women are affected twice as often as men. In a great majority of cases, the disorder is asymptomatic and diagnosed only incidentally on routine physical examination. In some cases, the prolapse is sufficient to cause a degree of mitral regurgitation. The cause of this valvular abnormality is uncertain, although it is commonly associated with other connective tissue disorders such as Marfan syndrome or scoliosis.

The finding of 2 mm or more displacement of the mitral valve leaflets above the annulus on echocardiogram is an important diagnostic criterion.[17] Mitral valve prolapse may be detected by a midsystolic click or systolic murmur. Individuals whose disease is symptomatic may experience palpitations, rhythm abnormalities, dizziness, fatigue, dyspnea, chest pain, or psychiatric manifestations such as depression and anxiety. The large majority of affected persons have no untoward effects and most are unaware of their condition. Complications of mitral valve prolapse are relatively rare and include infective endocarditis, sudden cardiac arrest, cerebral embolic events, and progression to mitral regurgitation.

Disorders of the Aortic Valve

The primary disorders of the aortic valve are stenosis and regurgitation.

Aortic Stenosis

With the decline in incidence of rheumatic fever, the predominant cause of aortic stenosis is age-related calcification. The hallmark of this disorder is the formation of calcium deposits on the aortic cusps (see Figure 18-14). Calcification is particularly common in patients with a congenital bicuspid aortic valve. Aortic calcifications accumulate over several decades and generally become clinically apparent in individuals 70 to 90 years old. Rheumatic heart disease, on the other hand, occurs primarily in children and young adults and now accounts for only a small percentage of cases of acquired aortic stenosis in the United States.

Aortic stenosis results in obstruction to aortic outflow from the left ventricle into the aorta during systole. This condition is characterized by a left ventricular–aortic pressure gradient during ventricular ejection (Figure 18-18). The left ventricle produces high systolic pressure to overcome resistance of the stenotic aortic valve. The slow development of aortic stenosis allows the heart to maintain stroke volume by compensatory left ventricular hypertrophy. The combination of high left ventricular pressure and hypertrophy predisposes the heart to ischemia and attacks of anginal pain. Continued high left ventricular afterload from a stenotic aortic valve may lead to left-sided heart failure.

Critical obstruction is characterized by a mean systolic pressure gradient exceeding 40 mm Hg and an effective aortic valve orifice less than 25% of normal (<1.0 cm^2 in an average-sized adult).[17] The symptoms of aortic stenosis are due to diminished cardiac output, with pulmonary complications occurring later as the left ventricle fails. Syncope, fatigue, low systolic blood pressure, and faint pulses are common signs and symptoms. Angina occurs frequently in patients with

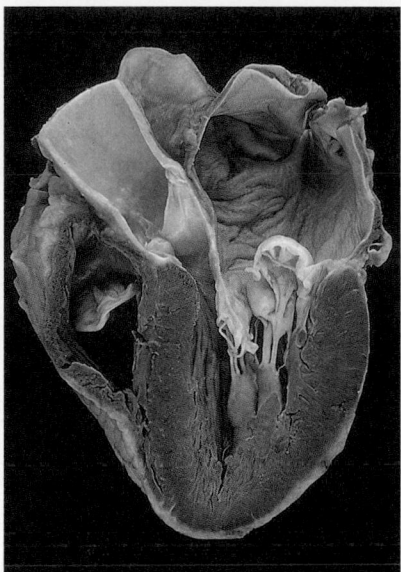

FIGURE 18-17 Appearance of mitral valve prolapse. Note how the valve balloons up into the left atrium. (From Kumar V et al, editors: *Robbins and Cotran pathologic basis of disease*, ed 8, Philadelphia, 2010, Saunders, p 564. Courtesy William D. Edwards, MD, Mayo Clinic, Rochester, MN.)

critical aortic stenosis and is often initiated by exertion and relieved by rest. Angina is thought to occur because of thickening of the ventricular wall with reduced perfusion and high intraventricular wall tension. Syncope and "graying out" spells may occur when cerebral perfusion is inadequate. The onset of atrial fibrillation or heart block may precipitate worsening of symptoms. A characteristic murmur occurs during ventricular systole and varies in intensity, progressively getting louder and then diminishing (crescendo-decrescendo). The murmur of aortic stenosis generally radiates to the neck. The heart rate is usually slow to allow for a necessarily long ejection phase, and a prominent S_4 is usually present. Surgical correction is indicated for symptomatic aortic stenosis because medical therapy is not effective.

Aortic Regurgitation

Aortic regurgitation results from an incompetent aortic valve that allows blood to leak back from the aorta into the left ventricle during diastole. Causes of aortic regurgitation are similar to those of mitral regurgitation (see Table 18-6). Valvular incompetence may be secondary to an abnormal aortic valve or to aortic root dilation with widening of the aorta such that the valve leaflets no longer appose. Aortic root dilation is a more common cause of aortic regurgitation than primary valvular disease.[17] The aorta may dilate because of degenerative changes with aging or as a consequence of connective tissue disease. The left ventricle becomes volume overloaded because it contains its usual preload, received from the atrium, plus regurgitant blood from the aorta. The left ventricle compensates for this extra volume work with hypertrophy and dilation. A larger than normal stroke volume is thus achieved and produces a high systolic blood pressure. Diastolic blood pressure is generally lower than normal because of rapid runoff of blood into the ventricle. The large stroke volume and rapid decline in diastolic blood pressure result in a bounding peripheral pulsation, and the head may bob with each systole (Figure 18-19).

Aortic insufficiency is characterized by a high-pitched blowing murmur during ventricular diastole. Patients may complain of palpitations and a throbbing or pounding heart because of the large ventricular stroke volume. The major complication of aortic regurgitation is left-sided

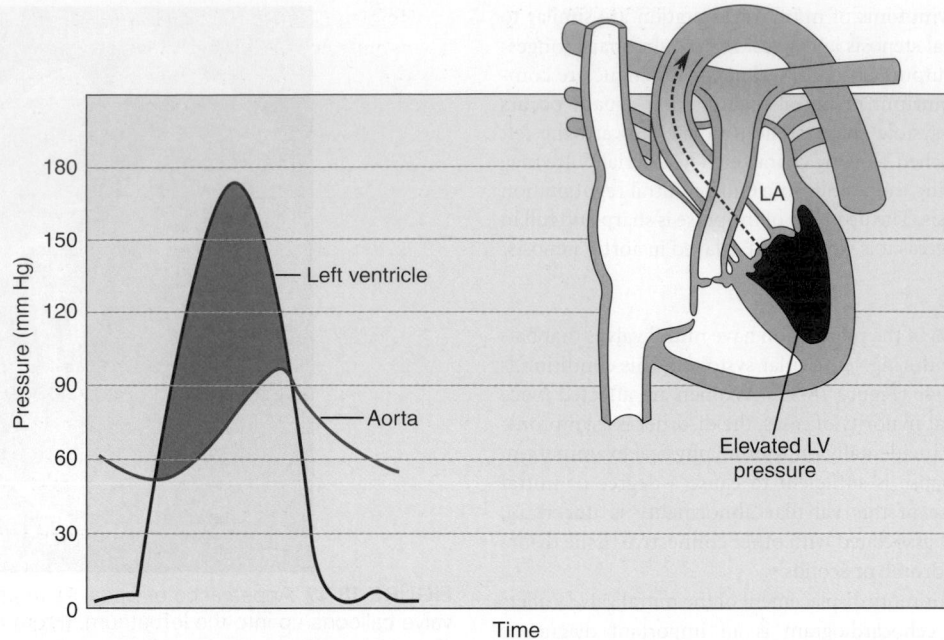

FIGURE 18-18 Aortic stenosis is characterized by an abnormal left ventricular *(LV)*–to–aortic pressure gradient *(shaded area)*. *LA,* Left atrium.

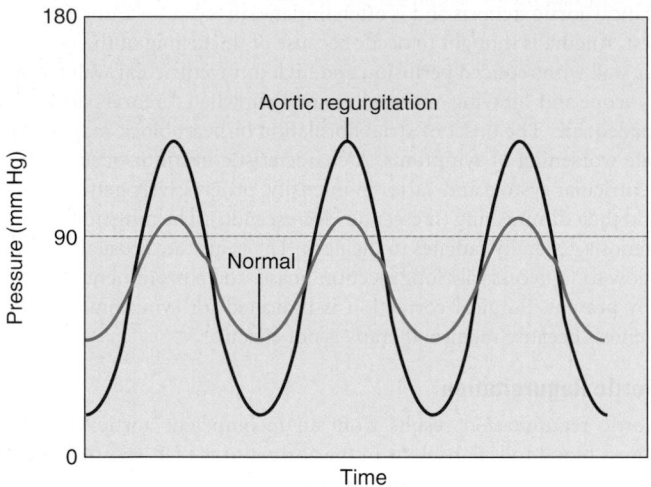

FIGURE 18-19 Typical arterial pressure fluctuation in aortic regurgitation showing a high systolic pressure and a low diastolic pressure.

heart failure as a result of the high ventricular workload. However, chronic aortic regurgitation is well tolerated for years, and asymptomatic individuals can delay valve replacement surgery. Acute aortic regurgitation is poorly tolerated and necessitates immediate correction.

Diseases of the Endocardium
Rheumatic Heart Disease

Rheumatic heart disease is an uncommon but serious consequence of rheumatic fever. The incidence of rheumatic fever has steadily declined in the United States, but the disease still affects an estimated 15 million people worldwide.[18] Rheumatic fever is an acute inflammatory disease that follows infection with group A β-hemolytic streptococci.

Damage is due to an immune attack on the individual's own tissues. For incompletely understood reasons, antibodies against the streptococcal antigens are also directed against self tissues, possibly because of an immune hypersensitivity reaction resulting from cross-reactivity between streptococcal antigens and certain tissue molecules. Epitopes on the bacterial surface are similar to proteins on cardiac myosin, valve, skin, joint, and brain tissue. Most individuals with group A β-hemolytic streptococcal infection do not develop rheumatic fever, and a number of genetic factors are associated with development of the disease.[9]

The acute infection occurs primarily in children and is accompanied by fever and a sore throat. In only 3% of children with pharyngeal streptococcal infection does rheumatic fever eventually develop.[9] Prompt initiation of antibiotic therapy is often effective in primary prevention of rheumatic fever. Rheumatic fever diffusely affects connective tissue in joints, the heart, and the skin. The central nervous system and kidney are also frequently involved. Inflammation of the heart usually includes all layers and results in carditis. Endocardial inflammation results in valvular swelling, erosions, and clumping of platelets and fibrin on valve leaflets. Scarring and shortening of valvular structures become progressively more severe. The myocardium and pericardium may show signs of rheumatic inflammation; however, if there is no associated valvular inflammation the diagnosis is unlikely to be rheumatic fever. Other hallmarks of rheumatic fever include joint inflammation, involuntary movements (Sydenham chorea), and a distinctive truncal rash. An elevated antibody titer against streptococcal products (antistreptolysin O, anti-DNase B) may help confirm the diagnosis. Unfortunately, individuals who experience rheumatic fever have a high chance of recurrence if they have another pharyngeal streptococcal infection.[19] Prophylactic antibiotic therapy is recommended for individuals who develop rheumatic fever.

Infective Endocarditis

Infective endocarditis is caused by invasion and colonization of endocardial structures by microorganisms with resulting inflammation. A variety of organisms are known to have an affinity for the endocardium and for the cardiac valves in particular. Valvular lesions include growths of microorganisms enmeshed in fibrin deposits. These growths are called *vegetations*. They may become quite large, interfering with valvular function and predisposing to embolus formation. The most common bacterial culprits are several strains of *Streptococcus* and *Staphylococcus aureus*. A requisite

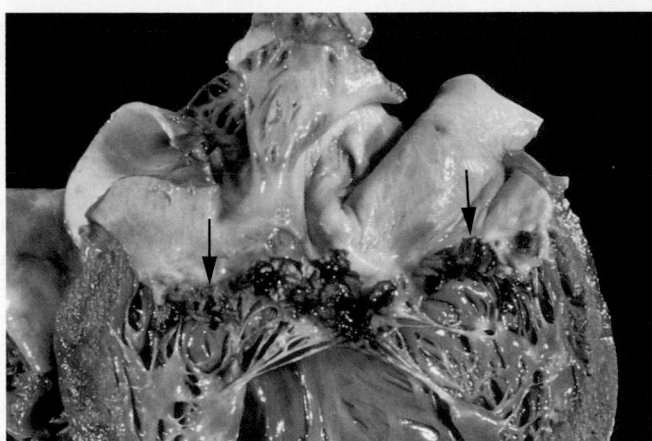

FIGURE 18-20 Mitral valve endocarditis from subacute bacterial infection with *Streptococcus viridans*. The left ventricle contains numerous abscesses formed by seeding from vegetations traveling in the coronary arteries. (From Kumar V et al, editors: *Robbins and Cotran pathologic basis of disease,* ed 8, Philadelphia, 2010, Saunders, p 568.)

for infective endocarditis is invasion of the bloodstream by infective organisms. The portal of entry may be obvious, as with an overt infection, intravenous drug abuse, or invasive surgical or dental procedures. Sometimes the source may be less obvious, such as the gastrointestinal tract or the oral cavity. Once the organism enters the circulation, several factors influence its ability to attack endocardial structures and cause disease.

Acute infective endocarditis may theoretically develop in any individual if host resistance is low, if the organism is highly virulent, and if the bacterial invasion is sufficiently large. Acute infective endocarditis usually affects individuals with previously normal valves and leads to death in a large percentage of patients. The overall mortality rate for infective endocarditis is between 13% and 20%.[20] However, mortality rates vary with the type of infective organism, with *Pseudomonas aeruginosa* endocarditis having greater than 50% mortality. Intravenous drug abusers are particularly susceptible to acute infective endocarditis. *Subacute* infective endocarditis has a more insidious onset and generally affects individuals with some preexisting propensity for valvular colonization. The offending organisms are less virulent. Rheumatic heart disease, congenital heart abnormalities, mitral valve prolapse, calcified valves, and prosthetic valves are important predisposing factors. Immunosuppression and repeated exposure through intravenous drug abuse are other predisposing influences. *S. aureus, Staphylococcus epidermidis,* and *Candida,* which colonize the skin, are common offenders in intravenous drug users. The valves on the right side of the heart commonly are infected in this population.

Organisms associated with subacute infective endocarditis usually are not virulent enough to attack normal healthy endocardium but are able to gain a foothold in hearts with some underlying predisposition. Preexisting cardiac disease may allow the formation of platelet-fibrin deposits on the valves because of abnormal or stagnant blood flow patterns. These deposits become the site of organism attachment. Antibodies against the invader may further assist attachment by causing clustering of organisms.

The diagnostic findings in both acute and subacute infective endocarditis are much the same. Large, bulky, bacteria-laden vegetations hang from the heart valves and adjacent endocardial surfaces (Figure 18-20). In addition to the risk of embolization, vegetations may cause erosion or perforation of the underlying valve leaflet. In acute forms, adjacent myocardium may be eroded and abscessed. With time, valvular vegetations become fibrotic and calcified.

Unfortunately, the clinical features of subacute infective endocarditis are quite nonspecific, with low-grade fever the most consistent sign. Nonspecific fatigue, weight loss, and flulike symptoms may be the only clues. Positive blood cultures may help confirm the diagnosis. In contrast, acute infective endocarditis has a more obvious onset with fever, chills, malaise, and, frequently, a heart murmur. Complications such as valvular insufficiency, myocardial abscess, embolization, and renal disease generally occur early in the course of the disease. The interval between initiation of bacteremia and the onset of symptoms is less than 2 weeks in the majority of cases.[20] Management of the acute and subacute types centers on antibiotic therapy, with surgical replacement of valves when indicated. Prevention through prophylactic antibiotic therapy in individuals at risk is an important consideration.

The endocardium is prey to many other disorders, such as systemic lupus erythematosus (an immunologic disease), calcium deposition secondary to renal disease, and nonbacterial thrombotic endocarditis secondary to hypercoagulable states associated with cancer.

> **KEY POINTS**
> - Valvular disorders are of two primary types. Failure of stenotic valves to open properly causes an abnormal pressure gradient across the valve and increases the pressure work of the heart. Regurgitant valves allow blood to flow backward across the valve and result in extra volume work for the heart.
> - Mitral stenosis is characterized by a large left atrial–to–left ventricular pressure gradient during ventricular diastole. Mitral stenosis leads to left atrial and pulmonary congestion.
> - Mitral regurgitation is characterized by large V waves in the left atrial pressure tracing and a loud systolic murmur that radiates to the left axilla. Mitral regurgitation increases the work of the left atrium and ventricle and can lead to left-sided heart failure.
> - Aortic stenosis results in obstruction to the outflow of blood from the left ventricle. It is characterized by a large left ventricular–to–aortic pressure gradient and a crescendo-decrescendo murmur during systole that radiates to the neck. The extra pressure work can lead to left ventricular hypertrophy and failure.
> - Aortic regurgitation is characterized by a high systolic and low diastolic blood pressure and a bounding pulse. The murmur of aortic regurgitation occurs during diastole. Left ventricular failure may result because of the high-volume work.
> - Rheumatic heart disease results from immune-mediated damage to the endocardium after group A β-hemolytic streptococcal infection.
> - Acute and subacute infective endocarditis results in the growth of bacteria-laden vegetations on heart valves. In addition to valvular erosion and scarring, embolization may occur.

MYOCARDIAL DISEASES

In addition to the diseases already discussed, which secondarily affect the myocardium as a consequence of inadequate blood supply or endocardial infection, two additional categories of diseases of heart muscle are *myocarditis* and *cardiomyopathy*. Myocarditis is an inflammatory disorder of the heart muscle characterized by necrosis and degeneration of heart muscle cells. Cardiomyopathy includes several disorders of the heart muscle that may be genetic or acquired but are noninflammatory. The division of these categories is somewhat arbitrary; however, the clinical course of myocarditis is generally acute and stormy, with recovery or death from cardiac failure occurring weeks to months after the onset of symptoms. In contrast, the cardiomyopathies generally evolve more insidiously over years, with few symptoms until the heart slips into failure.

Myocarditis

Myocarditis is characterized by inflammation, leukocyte infiltration, and necrosis of cardiac muscle cells. Causes of myocarditis are many and include microbial agents, several forms of immune-mediated disease, and several physical agents. The more common causes of myocarditis are listed in Box 18-2. The true incidence of myocarditis is unknown because the diagnosis relies largely on circumstantial evidence.

Most cases of myocarditis in the Northern hemisphere are associated with viral infections.[21] Cardiac involvement generally appears days or weeks after a viral infection elsewhere in the body. Documenting a viral cause is often impossible, but a rising antibody titer supports the diagnosis. The mechanism of viral myocarditis is incompletely understood. Direct viral cytotoxicity may occur to some extent, and the virus may evoke an immune response directed against the heart. Most investigators currently believe the second mechanism to be most important. In some countries, nonviral organisms are more commonly associated with myocarditis. For example, the protozoan *Trypanosoma cruzi*, which is endemic in areas of Central and South America, infects about 18 million persons worldwide.[21] A myocarditis called *Chagas disease* eventually develops in a large number of infected individuals and is an important cause of cardiovascular death in endemic countries.

In some cases of myocarditis, the immune system reaction against the myocardium appears to be the primary cause. Antibodies or activated lymphocytes are formed against heart tissue. Several drugs, including penicillin, tend to evoke a hyperactive immune response in some individuals and may cause an allergic-type reaction that affects the myocardium. Myocarditis accompanies some autoimmune disorders, such as systemic lupus erythematosus (SLE) and polymyositis. Toxins

and chemical causes of myocarditis include cocaine, chemotherapeutic agents, snake bite and insect venoms, lead, and numerous others. Regardless of the specific cause, inflammation of cardiac muscle is characteristic.

Acute myocarditis is commonly characterized by left ventricular dysfunction or general dilation of all four heart chambers. The ventricular myocardium is "flabby" with patchy or diffuse necrotic lesions. The heart muscle appears inflamed and edematous with white blood cell infiltrates. Endocardial structures are usually normal. The clinical course of acute myocarditis varies in severity from asymptomatic to rapidly evolving heart failure. Generalized symptoms related to the inflammatory process may be present, as well as electrocardiographic changes caused by myocardial cell death. Common presenting symptoms include fatigue, dyspnea on exertion, and dysrhythmia with associated palpitations. Many persons recover completely, whereas others have progressive disease that is manifested years later as dilated cardiomyopathy. Thus myocarditis and the cardiomyopathic forms of myocardial disease overlap and are difficult to separate. Therapy is supportive and usually includes therapy for heart failure (see Chapter 19). Immunosuppressive therapy may be considered for myocarditis associated with autoimmune disease or hypersensitivity reactions.

Cardiomyopathy

Cardiomyopathies can be classified by cause or by functional impairments. Those with known causes have been classified as specific cardiomyopathy by the World Health Organization (Table 18-8).[22] Those cardiomyopathies with uncertain cause are classified based on their predominant pathophysiologic features. The major functional classes are the dilated, hypertrophic, and restrictive forms (Figure 18-21). The terms *primary cardiomyopathy* for dysfunction of unknown cause and *secondary cardiomyopathy* for myocardial dysfunction of known cause are also in clinical use. Definitions of primary cardiomyopathy usually exclude hypertensive, ischemic, congenital, valvular, pericardial, and inflammatory myocardial disorders; however, classification of cardiomyopathy continues to evolve as more is understood about the genetic contributions to the condition.

Dilated Cardiomyopathy

Dilated or congestive cardiomyopathy (DCM) is characterized by cardiac failure associated with dilation of one or both ventricular chambers. Numerous factors are suspected in the initiation of dilated cardiomyopathy, including alcohol toxicity, genetic abnormality, pregnancy, and postviral myocarditis. Alcohol and its metabolites are toxic to heart muscle cells and are associated with thiamine and other nutritional deficiencies. Peripartum cardiomyopathy is the term applied to cases of dilated cardiomyopathy discovered just before or just after delivery. The etiology is unclear; however, inflammatory factors are implicated and a high incidence of lymphocytic activation has been reported. A risk of recurrence in subsequent pregnancies has been noted.

In some cases, dilated cardiomyopathy runs in families and has a presumed genetic basis. At least 20% of patients with DCM have a first-degree relative with signs of DCM.[23] Inherited genetic defects in the protein structure of the myocardial cytoskeleton appear to be contributory in most genetic forms of DCM.

Postviral myocarditis is an attractive pathogenic mechanism for dilated cardiomyopathy, as previously discussed. Myocardial biopsy specimens often reveal signs of inflammatory injury; however, progression from acute myocarditis to dilated cardiomyopathy is difficult to document. A variety of other causes have been proposed as well. In fact, dilated cardiomyopathy is a bit of a catch-all term invoked to cover cases of dilated congestive failure having no well-defined origin.

Histologic examination of hearts with dilated cardiomyopathy reveals nonspecific changes in the majority of cases.[23] Hypertrophied

---

BOX 18-2   ETIOLOGIC AGENTS OF MYOCARDITIS

Viral (Most Common)
Adenovirus
Coxsackie virus/Enterovirus
Cytomegalovirus
Parvovirus B19
Hepatitis C virus
Influenza virus
Human immunodeficiency virus
Herpes virus
Epstein-Barr virus
Mixed infections

Bacterial
Myobacterial species
Chlamydia pneumoniae
Streptococcal species
Mycoplasma pneumoniae
Treponema pallidum

Fungal
Aspergillus
Candida
Coccidioides
Cryptococcus
Histoplasma

Protozoal
Trypanosoma cruzi

Parasitic
Schistosomiasis
Larva migrans

Toxins
Anthracyclines
Cocaine

Hypersensitivity
Clozapine
Sulfonamides
Cephalosporins
Penicillins
Tricyclic antidepressants

Autoimmune Activation
Smallpox vaccination
Giant cell myocarditis
Churg-Strauss syndrome
Sjögren syndrome
Inflammatory bowel disease
Celiac disease
Sarcoidosis
Systemic lupus erythematosus
Takayasu arteritis
Wegener granulomatosis

From Liu P, Schultheiss HP: Myocarditis. In Bonow R, Mann D, Zipes D et al, editors: *Braunwald's heart disease: a textbook of cardiovascular medicine*, ed 9, Philadelphia, 2012, Saunders, p 1597.

TABLE 18-8 CLASSIFICATION OF THE CARDIOMYOPATHIES

DISORDER	DESCRIPTION
Dilated cardiomyopathy	Dilatation and impaired contraction of left or both ventricles. Caused by familial/genetic, viral and/or immune, alcoholic/toxic, or unknown factors, or is associated with recognized cardiovascular disease.
Hypertrophic cardiomyopathy	Left and/or right ventricular hypertrophy, often asymmetric, which usually involves interventricular septum. Mutations in sarcoplasmic proteins cause disease in many patients.
Restrictive cardiomyopathy	Restricted filling and reduced diastolic size of either or both ventricles with normal or near-normal systolic function. Is idiopathic or associated with other disease (e.g., amyloidosis, endomyocardial disease).
Dysrhythmogenic right ventricular	Progressive fibrofatty replacement of right, and to some degree left, ventricular cardiomyopathy myocardium. Familial disease is common.
Unclassified cardiomyopathy	Diseases that do not fit readily into any category. Examples include systolic dysfunction with minimal dilatation, mitochondrial disease, and fibroelastosis.
Specific Cardiomyopathies	
Ischemic cardiomyopathy	Presents as dilated cardiomyopathy with depressed ventricular function not explained by extent of coronary artery obstructions or ischemic damage.
Valvular cardiomyopathy	Presents as ventricular dysfunction that is out of proportion to abnormal loading conditions produced by valvular stenosis and/or regurgitation.
Hypertensive cardiomyopathy	Presents with left ventricular hypertrophy with features of cardiac failure attributable to systolic or diastolic dysfunction.
Inflammatory cardiomyopathy	Cardiac dysfunction as a consequence of myocarditis.
Metabolic cardiomyopathy	Includes a wide variety of causes, including endocrine abnormalities, glycogen storage disease, deficiencies (such as hypokalemia), and nutritional disorders.
General systemic disease	Includes connective tissue disorders and infiltrative diseases such as sarcoidosis and leukemia.
Muscular dystrophies	Includes Duchenne, Becker-type, and myotonic dystrophies.
Neuromuscular disorders	Includes Friedreich ataxia, Noonan syndrome, and lentiginosis.
Sensitivity and toxic reactions	Includes reactions to alcohol, catecholamines, anthracyclines, irradiation, and others.
Peripartal cardiomyopathy	First becomes manifest in peripartum period, but it is likely a heterogeneous group.

Derived from *Circulation* 112:1825-1852, 2005. ACC/AHA 2005 Guideline Update for the Diagnosis and Management of Chronic Heart Failure in the Adult. Reprinted with permission. Table: Stages in the Development of HF/recommended therapy by stage. Copyright © 2007 American Heart Association.

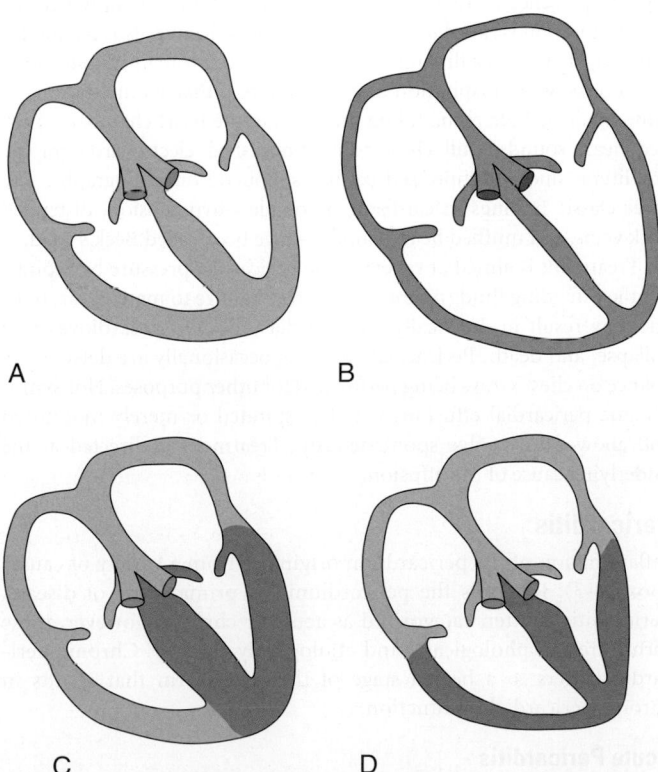

FIGURE 18-21 The three types of cardiomyopathy. **A,** Normal heart. **B,** Dilated cardiomyopathy demonstrating enlargement of all four chambers. **C,** Hypertrophic cardiomyopathy showing a thickened left ventricle. **D,** Restrictive cardiomyopathy characterized by a small left ventricular volume.

or atrophied myocytes may be apparent, along with mild fibrosis. The clinical picture is one of slowly progressing biventricular heart failure with low ejection fraction (EF). Annual mortality rates vary widely from 10% to 50% depending on the etiology of DCM.

Hypertrophic Cardiomyopathy

In contrast to dilated cardiomyopathy, hypertrophic cardiomyopathy (HCM) is characterized by a thickened, hyperkinetic ventricular muscle mass. The hypertrophy is often not uniform throughout the heart, and in about 25% of patients the septum is most affected and causes a dynamic aortic outflow obstruction. The left ventricle is usually more involved than the right.

Substantial evidence suggests that this form of cardiomyopathy is transmitted genetically in an autosomal dominant pattern.[9] Abnormalities of cardiac sarcomere proteins have been identified in several familial forms of the disease. Abnormalities in genes coding for myosin heavy chain, myosin-binding protein C, and troponin T account for 70% to 80% of HCM cases.[9] The remaining third of cases are thought to have mutations in other cytoskeletal proteins. Although the genetic basis of hypertrophic cardiomyopathy is well established, the events leading from cytoskeletal protein mutations to clinical disease are poorly understood.

There is wide variation in the expression of HCM. It may be asymptomatic or may be associated with symptoms of ventricular outflow obstruction or impaired diastolic filling. Outflow obstruction is particularly problematic when the myocardial hypertrophy is localized in the subaortic septal region. Strenuous activity may precipitate profound outflow obstruction, negligible stroke volume, and sudden death. Other factors contributing to reduced stroke volume are the smaller intraventricular chamber size and a noncompliant ventricle characteristic of diastolic dysfunction with preserved EF. The most common symptoms of HCM are dyspnea and angina. Microscopically, the hypertrophied muscle cells appear disorganized and haphazardly oriented into whorls rather than the usual linear arrangement.

The clinical course of HCM is variable, with most patients experiencing little change in cardiac function over many years. Surgery to thin the septal thickening (myectomy) is rarely performed any longer because this technique has been superseded by drug therapy. In general, drugs that increase myocardial contractility or heart rate are avoided because they further impair diastolic filling and worsen aortic outflow obstruction. β-Adrenergic antagonists and calcium channel–blocking drugs may be used to dampen the hypercontractility. Normal life expectancy is possible. Myocardial ischemia is common, and the risk of sudden cardiac arrest is significant. Patients who die suddenly from HCM usually have fatal dysrhythmias that may occur when sedentary but are frequently associated with vigorous physical exertion.[23]

Restrictive Cardiomyopathy

Restrictive cardiomyopathy (RCM) is the rarest form and is characterized by a stiff, fibrotic ventricle with impaired diastolic filling. In about 50% of cases, RCM can be attributed to specific clinical disorders, the most common being amyloidosis—abnormal deposition of amyloid protein in tissues. The mechanisms proposed for development of other cases include sarcoidosis, genetic inheritance (e.g., hemochromatosis), scleroderma, radiation injury, and exposure to agents that promote fibrosis (e.g., serotonin).[23] Regardless of the specific cause, the myocardium becomes fibrosed, rigid, and noncompliant. The major difficulty is restricted diastolic filling with resultant low stroke volume and heart failure. Exercise intolerance, dyspnea, and weakness may be present. RCM is difficult to manage effectively because no specific therapy is available for most types.

Specific Cardiomyopathy

Cardiomyopathies of presumed known origin constitute the category of specific cardiomyopathy (see Table 18-8). The specific cardiomyopathies present functionally as dilated, hypertrophic, or restrictive disorders, and the symptoms are consistent with the functional categories previously described.

KEY POINTS

- Myocarditis is an inflammatory disorder characterized by scattered necrotic and dead heart muscle cells. Most cases are associated with viral infection. The major complication of myocarditis is left ventricular dysfunction and dilation of the heart chambers, with reduced contractility.
- Cardiomyopathies encompass a number of disorders of heart muscle that may be genetic or acquired. In many cases the exact cause is unknown.
- Dilated cardiomyopathy is characterized by enlargement of both ventricular chambers, reduced contractility, and low EF.
- Hypertrophic cardiomyopathy primarily affects the left ventricle and ventricular septum. Genetic mutations in sarcomere proteins are suspected in most cases. Conditions that increase contractility of the heart (exercise, drugs) can result in obstruction of ventricular outflow and reduced cardiac output. EF is preserved, and diastolic dysfunction is predominant. Patients with HCM have a significant risk of sudden cardiac arrest.
- Restrictive cardiomyopathy is characterized by a stiff, fibrotic left ventricle that resists diastolic filling. Decreased cardiac output and left-sided heart failure can result.

PERICARDIAL DISEASES

Pericardial disorders are rarely isolated processes of primary cause; rather, they are sequelae of other disorders such as systemic infection, trauma, metabolic derangement, or neoplasia. Despite the diversity of causative factors, pericardial involvement may be asymptomatic, manifested as an accumulation of fluid in the pericardial sac, or as painful inflammation of pericardial structures.

Pericardial Effusion

An accumulation of noninflammatory fluid in the pericardial sac is called *pericardial effusion*. Normally, the pericardial space contains only 30 to 50 ml of thin, clear fluid. Under pathologic conditions, as much as 500 ml may accumulate. The compositions of the usual types of effusions are as follows:

Serous—a transudate secondary to heart failure or hypoproteinemia
Serosanguineous—a mixture of serous fluid and blood that may follow blunt chest trauma, heart surgery, or cardiopulmonary resuscitation
Chylous—a collection of lymph from obstruction of lymphatic drainage
Blood—hemopericardium usually resulting from penetrating trauma to the heart

Cardiac Tamponade

The accumulation of pericardial fluid is generally without clinical significance except as an indicator of underlying disease processes. However, if the fluid accumulation is large or occurs suddenly, the life-threatening condition of cardiac tamponade may ensue. *Tamponade* refers to external compression of the heart chambers such that filling is impaired.

Signs and symptoms of cardiac tamponade include reduced stroke volume and compensatory increases in heart rate. Systemic venous congestion occurs because blood is prevented from entering the compressed heart by way of the superior and inferior venae cavae. Venous congestion may be apparent as distended neck veins. Changes in intrathoracic pressure during respiration may have exaggerated effects on cardiac filling. The presence of waxing and waning of blood pressure in synchrony with respiration is called *pulsus paradoxus*. Significant pulsus paradoxus is usually defined as a difference of 10 mm Hg or more in systolic blood pressure between inspiration and expiration. Other manifestations of tamponade include rising filling pressures in the heart chambers, muffled heart sounds, dull chest pain, diminished electrocardiographic amplitude, and a compressed cardiac silhouette on radiographs. The three classic findings in cardiac tamponade—hypotension, distended neck veins, and muffled heart sounds—have been called Beck's triad.

Treatment is aimed at relieving the pericardial pressure by aspirating the offending fluid (*pericardiocentesis*). Failure to manage tamponade may result in drastically reduced diastolic filling, cardiovascular collapse, and death. Pericardial effusions occasionally are detected by chance on chest x-rays being performed for other purposes. Nonsymptomatic pericardial effusions may be aspirated or merely monitored and allowed to resolve spontaneously. Treatment is directed at the underlying cause of the effusion.

Pericarditis

Inflammation of the pericardium originates from a variety of causes (Box 18-3). Rarely is the pericardium the primary site of disease. Pericarditis is often categorized as acute or chronic; however, these forms are morphologically and etiologically similar.[9] Chronic pericarditis refers to a healed stage of the acute form that results in chronic pericardial dysfunction.

Acute Pericarditis

It is estimated that 80% of cases of acute pericarditis are idiopathic, and most of these are presumed to be viral.[24] Uncomplicated acute pericarditis typically resolves spontaneously within 2 weeks and nonsteroidal antiinflammatory agents (NSAIDs) may be the only therapy

BOX 18-3   CATEGORIES OF PERICARDIAL DISEASE AND SELECTED SPECIFIC CAUSES

Idiopathic*

Infectious

Viral* (echovirus, coxsackievirus, adenovirus, cytomegalovirus, hepatitis B, infectious mononucleosis, HIV/AIDS)

Bacterial* (*Pneumococcus, Staphylococcus, Streptococcus, Mycoplasma,* Lyme disease, *Haemophilus influenzae, Neisseria meningitidis,* and others)

Mycobacteria* (*Mycobacterium tuberculosis, Mycobacterium avium-intracellulare*)

Fungal (histoplasmosis, coccidioidomycosis)

Protozoal

Immune-Inflammatory

Connective tissue disease* (systemic lupus erythematosus, rheumatoid arthritis, scleroderma, mixed)

Arteritis (polyarteritis nodosa, temporal arteritis)

Inflammatory bowel disease

Early post-myocardial infarction

Late post-myocardial infarction (Dressler syndrome),* late postcardiotomy/thoracotomy*

Late post-trauma*

Drug induced* (procainamide, hydralazine, isoniazid, cyclosporine, others)

Neoplastic Disease

Primary: mesothelioma, fibrosarcoma, lipoma, others

Secondary*: breast and lung carcinoma, lymphomas, Kaposi sarcoma

Radiation Induced*

Early Post–Cardiac Surgery and Post–Orthotopic Heart Transplantation

Hemopericardium

Trauma

Post–myocardial infarction free wall rupture

Device and procedure related: percutaneous coronary procedures, implantable defibrillators, pacemakers, post–dysrhythmia ablation, post–atrial septal defect closure, post–valve repair or replacement

Dissecting aortic aneurysm

Trauma

Blunt and penetrating,* post-cardiopulmonary resuscitation*

Congenital

Cysts, congenital absence

Miscellaneous

Cholesterol ("gold paint" pericarditis)

Chronic renal failure, dialysis related

Chylopericardium

Hypothyroidism and hyperthyroidism

Amyloidosis

Aortic dissection

From LeWinter M, Tischler MD: Pericardial diseases. In Bonow R, Mann D, Zipes D et al, editors: *Braunwald's heart disease: a textbook of cardiovascular medicine,* ed 9, Philadelphia, 2012, Saunders, p 1653.
*Etiologies that can present as acute pericarditis.
HIV/AIDS, Human immunodeficiency virus/acquired immunodeficiency syndrome.

used. A small number of cases may be complicated by significant pericardial effusion or by persistent or recurrent inflammation, and may require hospitalization for more thorough diagnostic investigation to determine the specific etiology and more intensive therapy.

The symptoms of acute pericarditis are associated with the systemic effects of inflammation and pericardial damage and include fever, leukocytosis, malaise, and tachycardia. Acute pericarditis almost always presents with chest pain and may be confused with anginal pain. Adhesion and friction between the visceral and parietal pericardial layers cause pain that may radiate to the back and be associated with esophageal discomfort and dysphagia (difficulty swallowing). Rubbing of the pericardial layers may be heard as a friction rub. The rub can be transient and intermittent and may sound squeaky or like scratchy sandpaper. Epicardial injury from pericarditis may be apparent on the ECG as ST-segment elevation. Treatment is generally symptom oriented and includes medications to relieve pain and minimize inflammation.

In the past, MI was a common cause of pericarditis, but the incidence of both acute post-MI pericarditis and the delayed pericarditis of Dressler syndrome has decreased with the advent of early reperfusion therapy for MI.[24] Acute post-MI pericarditis occurs within a few days of an MI in which the infarction involves the epicardial surfaces of the heart (transmural MI). The inflammation of the necrotic heart muscle extends to adjacent pericardial structures, causing them to become inflamed as well. The degree of pericardial involvement reflects the size of the MI. In contrast, late pericarditis, occurring 1 week to a few months after the MI (Dressler syndrome), is believed to be an autoimmune reaction caused by exposure of the immune system to damaged myocardial tissue. The presence of antimyocardial antibodies has been demonstrated, and the pericardial inflammation is diffuse and not localized to the area of myocardial injury.

Chronic Pericarditis

Healing of an acute form of pericardial inflammation may result in chronic (healed) pericardial dysfunction of two principal kinds: adhesive mediastinopericarditis and constrictive pericarditis. Adhesive mediastinopericarditis is usually a consequence of suppurative or caseous pericarditis or a complication of previous cardiac surgery. It may also follow significant irradiation of the chest. The pericardial sac is destroyed and the external aspect of the heart adheres to surrounding mediastinal structures. The workload of the heart increases significantly because contraction is opposed by the attached surrounding structures.

Constrictive pericarditis may be a result of previous suppurative or caseous pericarditis, commonly secondary to tuberculosis. However, in many cases the cause of pericardial dysfunction is unknown. The pericardial sac becomes dense, nonelastic, fibrous, and scarred. It encases the heart like a stiff cage and impairs diastolic filling. The constrictive process generally occurs slowly and may be quite advanced by the time symptoms occur.

Symptoms may include exercise intolerance, weakness, fatigue, and systemic venous congestion. Treatment is aimed at relieving the constriction by removal of pericardium (pericardectomy) and administration of inotropic agents to improve cardiac contractility.

CONGENITAL HEART DISEASES

Congenital heart disease is an abnormality of the heart that is present from birth. A wide variety of defects have been described, and only the pathophysiology of the most common defects will be included. A brief description of fetal cardiac development is a necessary prelude to a discussion of congenital heart diseases.

Embryologic Development

Development of the heart involves a complex orchestration of formation and resorption of structures. Abnormalities in the development of four important heart structures are at the root of most of the common heart defects: (1) development of the atrial septum, (2) development of the ventricular septum, (3) division of the main outflow tract (truncus arteriosus) into the pulmonary and aortic arteries, and (4) development of the valves. Each of these processes is briefly reviewed.

The primitive heart begins as an enlarged tube much like a blood vessel. The tube has three layers. The inner luminal layer is thin and composed of endothelial cells. This layer will eventually line the inner chambers of the heart and valves. The outermost layer is also thin and is called the *myoepicardial mantle.* The outer mantle will form the epicardial and muscular structures of the heart. In between these two thin layers of cells is a thick layer of gelatinous substance called *cardiac jelly.* Cardiac jelly is the precursor to endocardial cushion tissue, which is important in the formation of membranes in the heart, including the septa that separate the four chambers of the heart.

By day 23, the heart tube begins to beat. The tube folds on itself to form an asymmetric loop structure (Figure 18-22). One bulge of the loop forms a primitive single atrium, another forms the future left ventricle, and a third forms the future right ventricle and common ventricular outflow tract (truncus arteriosus). The common atrium is divided into right and left atria by growth of the interatrial septum. Atrial septation occurs in several steps. First, the *septum primum* is formed passively in the superior surface by an indentation caused by the overlying truncus arteriosus (Figure 18-23). Next, the superior and inferior endocardial cushions grow and extend toward each other. These flaps of tissue overlap but do not fuse so that blood can pass through from the right atrium to the left atrium. A reverse in the direction of flow, as occurs at birth, normally would push the flap shut and close the hole (see Pediatrics Considerations box). This flaplike opening, called the *ostium secundum,* remains open throughout fetal life and is later called the *foramen ovale.*

Septal formation between the ventricles follows a similar pattern. The lower portion of the interventricular septum is formed by circular growth and fusing of the muscular ventricular walls. Then the muscular septum proliferates upward toward the atria. The inferior endocardial

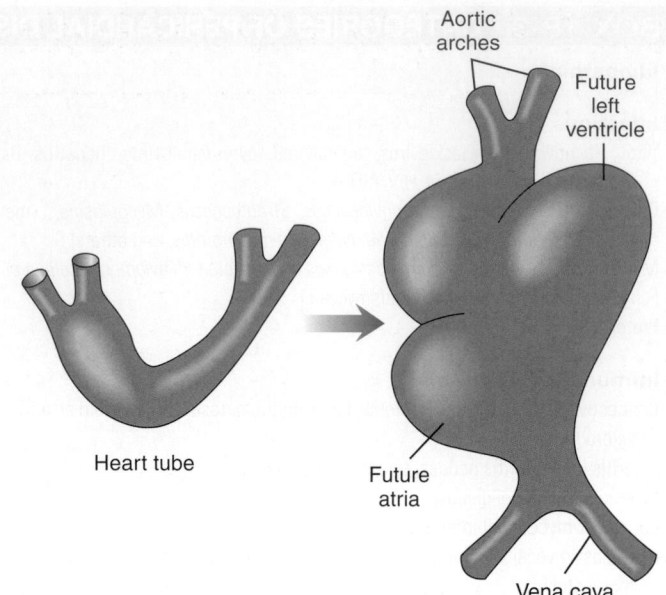

FIGURE 18-22 Asymmetric loop structure in early embryonic development of the heart.

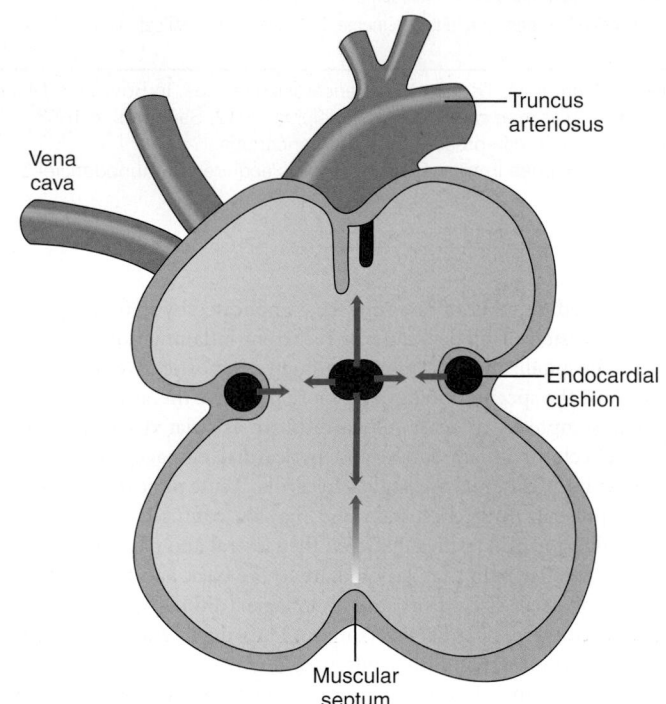

FIGURE 18-23 Formation of the intracardiac septa.

cushion tissue also grows downward to meet the uplifting muscular septum (see Figure 18-23).

At about the same time that the atrial and ventricular septal structures are being elaborated, the common ventricular outflow tract, the truncus arteriosus, is divided into the pulmonary and aortic channels. This process is accomplished by growth and eventual fusion of mounds of endocardial cushions located in the wall of the truncus arteriosus. The truncal endocardial cushions go on to form the semilunar valves as well (Figure 18-24).

PEDIATRIC CONSIDERATIONS
Changes in Newborn Heart

When a newborn takes his or her first breath, several changes occur. The alveoli of the lungs expand with the inspired oxygen dilating the pulmonary vessels, which decreases pulmonary vascular resistance. Pulmonary blood flow increases because of this dilation. The increased pulmonary blood flow is from the right side of the heart. Because of this increased flow, the pressures in the right atrium, right ventricle, and pulmonary arteries are decreased. Simultaneously, the umbilical cord is clamped, which increases systemic vascular resistance and increases blood volume. The pressure in the left side of the heart increases as more blood returns to the left atrium from the pulmonary veins related to the clamping. Since the pressure gradient has shifted with higher pressure in the left side of the heart, the circulation of blood through the fetal shunts is reversed.

Foramen ovale closure occurs because of the decreased blood flow from the placenta related to cord clamping. The blood flow from the placenta holds the foramen ovale open before birth. The change in the pressure gradient closes the foramen ovale at or soon after birth. When this closure occurs blood from the right ventricle flows entirely into the pulmonary circulation.

Increased oxygen concentration of the blood is the critical factor in closure of the ductus arteriosus. Bradykinin is signaled to be released by high oxygen concentration in blood from the initial aeration of the lungs. Bradykinin has contractile effects on smooth muscle and forces the ductus arteriosus walls to constrict. The secretion of endogenous prostaglandin E and prostacyclin, which maintain the patency of the ductus arteriosus during gestation, is decreased after birth, which further diminishes the opening of the ductus arteriosus. In addition, decreased pulmonary vascular resistance decreases the blood flow from the ductus arteriosus. Functional closure of the ductus arteriosus occurs 4 days after birth, but may be delayed in preterm or ill infants.

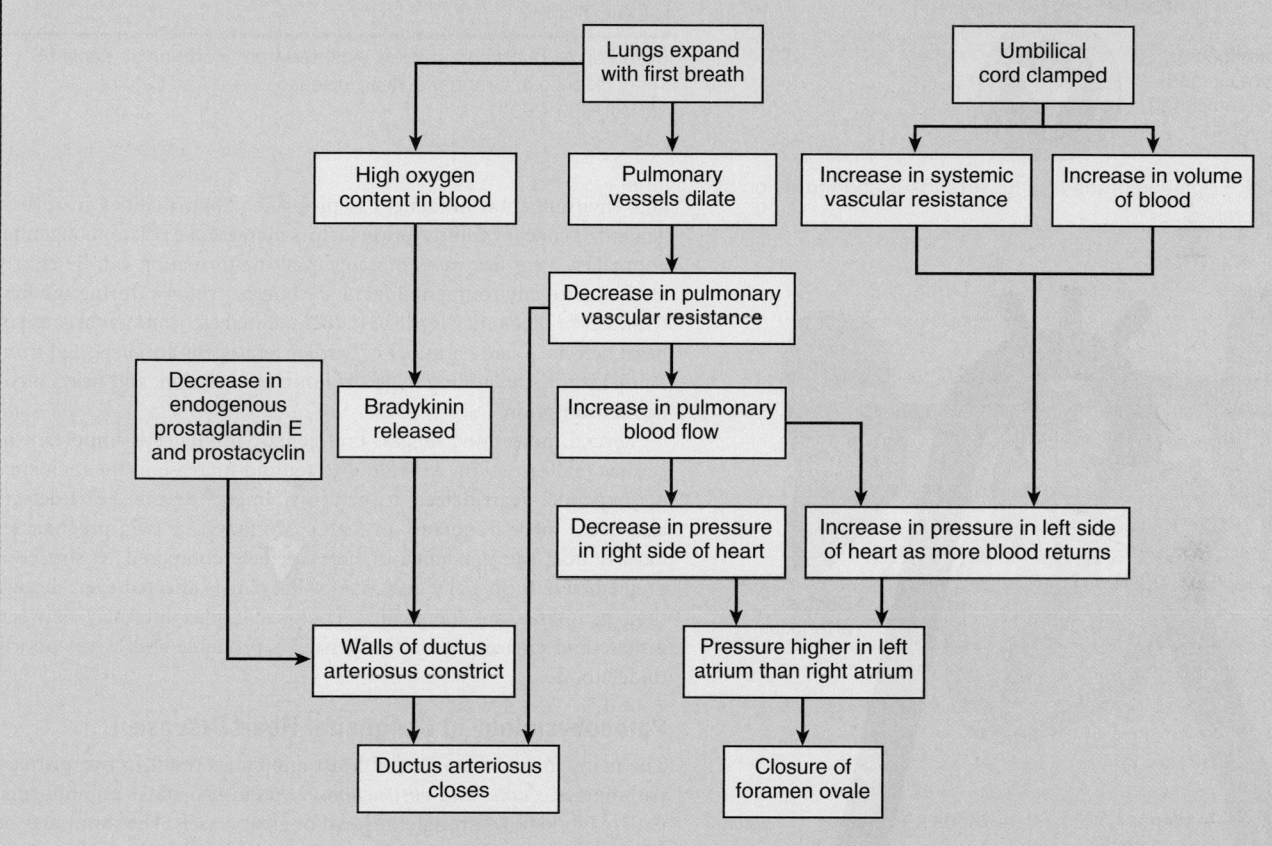

The atrioventricular septum and valves are similarly formed by growth and fusion of the right and left lateral cushions. Superior and inferior cushions also contribute to formation of the septum between the atria and ventricles. Leaflets of the valves are initially formed by lumps of cushion material, which are replaced by muscle tissue from the ventricular wall. The muscle tissue also forms the chordae tendineae and papillary muscle structures. Eventually, the muscle cells of the leaflets and chordae tendineae are replaced by tough, fibrous connective tissue.

When the embryonic heart is fully developed, two important passageways still permit blood flow to bypass the lungs (Figure 18-25).

The foramen ovale lies between the left and right atria and allows blood to bypass the right ventricle. Blood flows right to left through the atrial opening because the pressure in the left atrium is low. High resistance of the deflated lungs also causes right ventricular pressure to be high, which impedes right ventricular filling. The other important structure is the ductus arteriosus, a channel that connects the pulmonary artery and the aorta. Blood flows from the pulmonary artery into the aorta during fetal life because of high vascular resistance in the collapsed lungs. Both these communications generally close after birth when the lungs inflate and the resistance on the right side of the heart falls. Clamping the umbilical cord also serves to increase systemic vascular

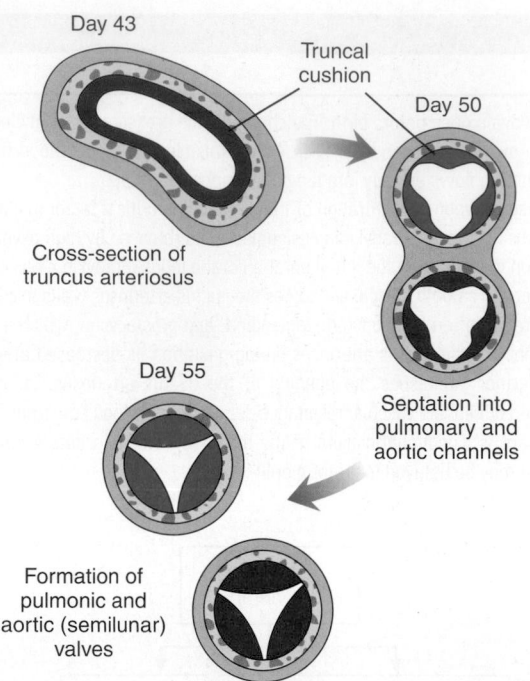

FIGURE 18-24 Septation of the truncus arteriosus and formation of the semilunar valves.

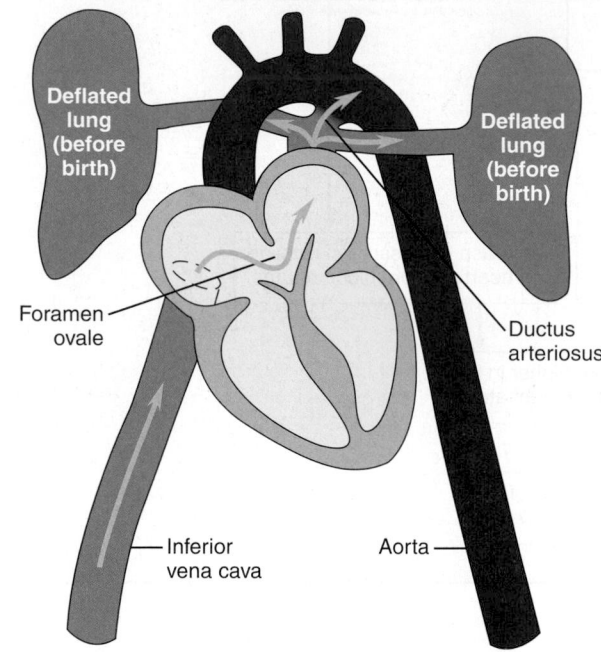

FIGURE 18-25 Fully developed embryonic heart showing the foramen ovale and ductus arteriosus. These structures allow blood to bypass the pulmonary circulation during fetal life.

resistance, which further augments the reverse in pressure gradient, with left heart pressures now exceeding those on the right.

Etiology and Incidence of Congenital Heart Disease

Congenital heart disease is the most common heart disorder in children, with an overall incidence of about 1.0% of all live births.[9] The most common heart defects are listed in Table 18-9, with approximate frequencies of occurrence. In the majority of cases, the cause of the heart defect is unknown. Multifactorial inheritance with both genetic

TABLE 18-9	RELATIVE FREQUENCY OF OCCURRENCE OF CARDIAC MALFORMATIONS AT BIRTH
DISEASE	**PERCENTAGE**
Ventricular septal defect	42
Atrial septal defect	10
Pulmonic stenosis	8
Patent ductus arteriosus	7
Tetralogy of Fallot	5
Coarctation of the aorta	5
Atrioventricular septal defect	4
Aortic stenosis	4
Complete transposition of the great arteries	4
Persistent truncus arteriosus	1
Anomalous pulmonary venous connection	1
Tricuspid atresia	1

Based on 44 published studies. Adapted from Hoffman JI, Kaplan S: The incidence of congenital heart disease, *J Am Coll Cardiol* 39(12):1890, 2002.

and environmental influences is probable. Abnormalities in several genes that code for transcription factors increase the risk for congenital anomalies. Very few cases of congenital malformation can be clearly attributed to environmental factors. Maternal rubella during the first trimester of pregnancy is the best documented environmental cause of heart defects. A large number of cardiac teratogens are suspected from animal studies, including hypoxia, ionizing radiation, and heavy alcohol consumption.

Several indications suggest that genetic influence is important in cardiac malformation. A twofold to tenfold increase in the incidence of congenital heart defects is seen in siblings.[25] Several heart defects also occur more frequently in males. Monozygotic twin pregnancies have double the incidence of heart defects compared to singleton pregnancies, but usually only one of the pair is affected even though their genotypes are identical.[25] Thus a complex interplay between genetic and environmental influences is probable and as yet poorly understood.

Pathophysiology of Congenital Heart Disease

The many forms of congenital heart anomalies result in two primary pathologies: *shunts* and *obstructions*.[26] A shunt denotes an abnormal path of blood flow through the heart or great vessels. The shunt may be further characterized as *right-to-left* or *left-to-right* to indicate the direction of abnormal blood flow. Right-to-left shunts allow unoxygenated blood from the right side of the heart to enter the left side and systemic circulation without first passing through the lungs. Infants with right-to-left shunting of blood generally have some degree of cyanosis because of the decreased oxygen content of the arterial blood (cyanotic defect). Conversely, a left-to-right shunt occurs when oxygenated blood from the left side of the heart or aorta flows back into the right side to be recirculated through the lungs. The blood reaching the systemic circulation is oxygenated and the infant is not cyanotic (acyanotic defect). However, the right side of the heart has an increased workload because of the extra shunt blood. In time, the overload of the right side of the heart can result in right ventricular hypertrophy and high right-sided heart pressures. A left-to-right shunt may then progress to a more dangerous right-to-left shunt when right heart pressures exceed left heart pressures. Congenital disorders causing abnormal blood flow through the heart include atrial septal defect, ventricular septal defect, patent ductus arteriosus, tetralogy of Fallot, transposition of the great arteries, truncus arteriosus, and tricuspid atresia.

Some heart anomalies produce obstructions to blood flow because of abnormal narrowings. Stenosis or atresia (failure to develop) of valves and coarctation of the aorta are the most common obstructive defects. Obstructions do not result in cyanosis but generally increase the workload of the affected chamber. Heart failure is a potential consequence of congenital heart defects and presents differently in infants and children than in adults (Box 18-4).

In addition to being classified according to pathologic features as obstructions or shunts, heart defects are also classified according to the clinical manifestation of cyanosis. Acyanotic disorders include the obstructive disorders and left-to-right shunts. The cyanotic category includes abnormalities causing right-to-left shunts. Specific heart defects are described further and follow this categorization.

Acyanotic Congenital Defects
Atrial Septal Defect
During the third to fifth week of fetal development, the left and right atria are separated by flaps of tissue that become the atrial septum. The foramen ovale remains patent during intrauterine life such that blood may pass from the right to the left atrium and bypass the uninflated and nonfunctional lungs. The foramen ovale normally remains open in utero because pressure on the right side of the heart is higher than that on the left. With birth, however, the pressure gradient reverses as the lungs inflate and greatly reduce pulmonary vascular resistance. The higher left-sided pressure forces the flap shut, and fusion of the foramen ovale membrane normally occurs. The majority of atrial septal defects occur at the location of the foramen ovale. The abnormal septal opening may be of variable size. Small defects (1 cm) are well tolerated. Even larger atrial septal defects may be asymptomatic for many years as long as the shunt flow is left to right and therefore acyanotic (Figure 18-26).

The long-term increase in pulmonary blood flow may eventually lead to pulmonary hypertension, right ventricular hypertrophy, and a reversal of the shunt to a right-to-left pattern. Cyanosis, respiratory difficulty, and right-sided heart failure may ensue. Large or symptomatic atrial septal defects are commonly repaired surgically early in life, before pulmonary complications occur.

Ventricular Septal Defect
A ventricular septal defect is the most common congenital cardiac anomaly.[9] It is frequently associated with other cardiac defects such as tetralogy of Fallot, transposition of the great arteries, and atrial septal defects. The ventricular septum develops between the fifth and sixth weeks of fetal life as the membrane derived from the endocardial cushion fuses with the muscular septum.

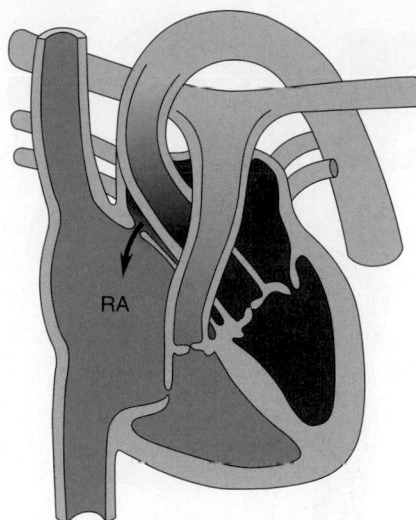

FIGURE 18-26 Atrial septal defect. Blood flow through the defect is usually left to right and produces an acyanotic shunt.

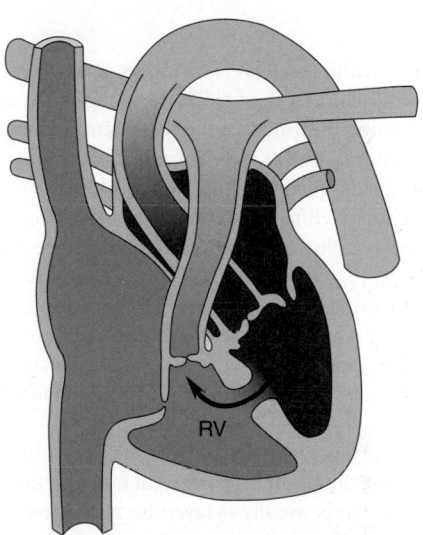

FIGURE 18-27 Ventricular septal defect. Blood flow through the defect is usually left to right and produces an acyanotic shunt.

The majority of ventricular septal defects are located in the membranous septum, very close to the bundle of His. As with atrial septal defects, the functional significance depends largely on the size of the defect. The shunt is initially left to right because left-sided heart pressures are higher (Figure 18-27). With the increase in pulmonary blood flow, pulmonary hypertension and right ventricular hypertrophy may result and cause a reversal of the shunt.

Large ventricular septal defects may be apparent at birth because of rapidly developing right-sided heart failure and a loud systolic murmur. Large, symptomatic defects in infants or moderate defects in older children are repaired surgically to avoid progression to pulmonary vascular disease. Small ventricular septal defects in infants are generally not immediately repaired because of the tendency of such defects to close spontaneously.

Patent Ductus Arteriosus
The ductus arteriosus is a normal channel between the pulmonary artery and the aorta that remains open during intrauterine life (Figure 18-28). Within 1 to 2 days after birth, the ductus arteriosus closes

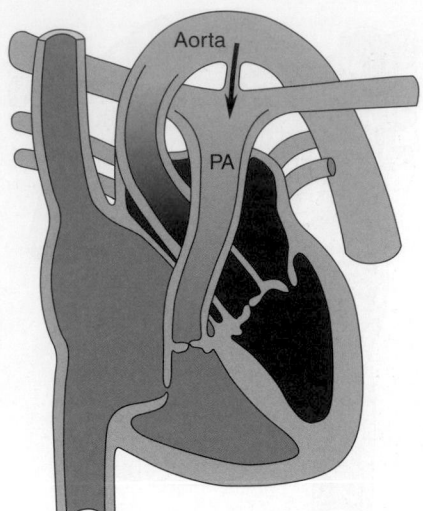

FIGURE 18-28 Patent ductus arteriosus. Blood flow through the ductus is usually from the aorta to the pulmonary artery and produces an acyanotic shunt.

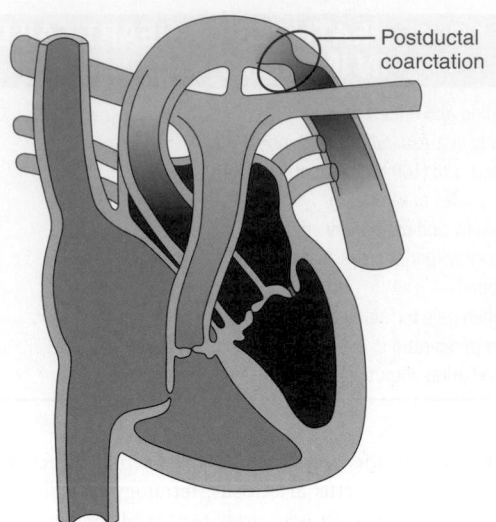

FIGURE 18-29 Coarctation of the aorta. The arterial narrowing can produce a weaker pulse in the lower extremities.

functionally, and within a few weeks it closes permanently. The ductus arteriosus allows blood to flow from the pulmonary artery into the aorta, thus bypassing the lungs. Low oxygen tension and local production of prostaglandins appear to be important in maintaining patency of the channel during fetal life. After birth, flow through the ductus arteriosus switches to left to right because of the higher pressure in the aorta. This change in flow direction brings oxygenated blood through the ductus arteriosus and stimulates it to close. A reduction in prostaglandin E production after birth appears to contribute to constriction and closure. In many cases the reason for abnormal continued patency of the ductus arteriosus after birth is not well understood. Conditions that cause low blood oxygen tension may contribute to continued patency.

Most often a patent ductus arteriosus has no clinical significance early in life because the shunt is left to right and no cyanosis is evident. Surgical management is usually delayed because these defects tend to close spontaneously. Prostaglandin inhibitors may be given to induce closure of the defect. Continued patency of the ductus arteriosus is usually obvious because of a harsh, grinding systolic murmur and often a systolic thrill (vibration). Surgical closure of the patent ductus arteriosus is done as soon as it becomes evident that spontaneous closure is unlikely. As with other left-to-right shunt disorders, uncorrected patent ductus arteriosus results in pulmonary hypertension complicated by respiratory and right-sided heart failure. Eventual reversal of the shunt to a right-to-left pattern results in cyanosis. Because the ductus is usually located distal to the origin of the subclavian artery, the lower extremities may show cyanosis whereas the upper extremities remain pink.

Coarctation of the Aorta

Coarctation refers to a narrowing or stricture that may impede blood flow. Coarctation of the aorta is a common heart defect that affects males three to four times more frequently than females. Narrowing of the aorta may occur anywhere along its length; however, in most cases the coarctation is located just before or just after the ductus arteriosus (Figure 18-29). Preductal coarctation (proximal to the ductus arteriosus) is usually more severe and often associated with other anomalies. In some instances, the aortic stricture is so severe that blood flow to the lower part of the body must be maintained solely by flow through

the ductus arteriosus. This situation results in a very high workload for the right side of the heart and may lead to heart failure in the early neonatal period. Blood supply to the arms and head is unaffected because these arteries arise proximal to the stricture. Postductal coarctation is generally less severe and may remain unrecognized until adulthood.

The upper extremities typically have an elevated blood pressure, whereas the lower extremities have weak pulses and low blood pressure. An important part of assessment of the newborn is comparison of pulses in the upper and lower extremities to assess for symmetry. All types of coarctation are usually accompanied by systolic murmurs and ventricular hypertrophy. The stricture can be repaired surgically by resection of the narrowed region. If left untreated, significant coarctation may lead to congestive heart failure, intracranial hemorrhage, or aortic rupture.

Pulmonary Stenosis or Atresia

Isolated pulmonary stenosis and atresia are included in the category of acyanotic defects because they do not themselves result in cyanosis. However, they often occur in conjunction with other anomalies that allow survival into the neonatal period. The other defects may allow shunting of blood and result in cyanosis. In pulmonary atresia, no communication is found between the right ventricle and the lungs, so that blood must enter the lungs by first traveling through a septal opening and then through a patent ductus arteriosus. The right ventricle is typically underdeveloped (hypoplasia), and the atrial septal defect is large. Pulmonary stenosis can be mild to severe, depending on the extent of narrowing of the pulmonic valve. Pulmonary stenosis is usually due to abnormal fusion of the valvular cusps. Right ventricular hypertrophy occurs secondary to the high ventricular afterload caused by the narrowed outflow opening. Isolated pulmonary stenosis is easily corrected by surgery; however, the prognosis depends in large part on the health of the right ventricle.

Aortic Stenosis or Atresia

Congenital aortic atresia is rare and not compatible with survival. Depending on its severity, aortic stenosis is correctable and associated with a good prognosis. Aortic stenosis may involve the valvular cusps or the subvalvular fibrous ring just below the cusps. The narrowed aortic outflow tract results in a high left ventricular afterload, which causes

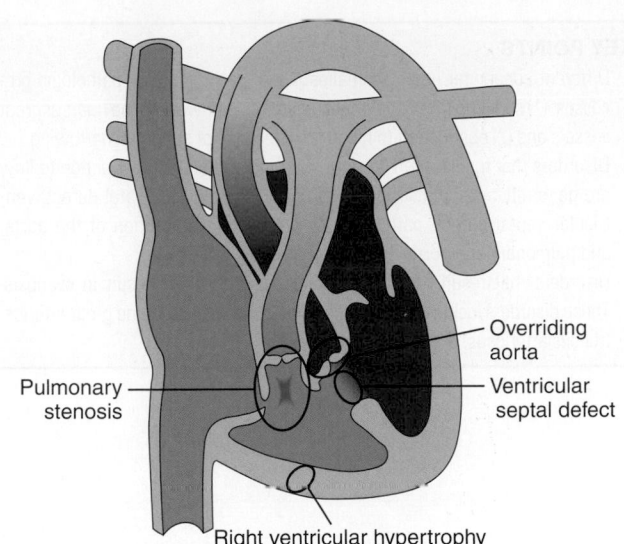

FIGURE 18-30 Tetralogy of Fallot showing the four characteristic abnormalities: pulmonary stenosis, ventricular septal defect, overriding aorta, and right ventricular hypertrophy. Tetralogy of Fallot is a cyanotic defect.

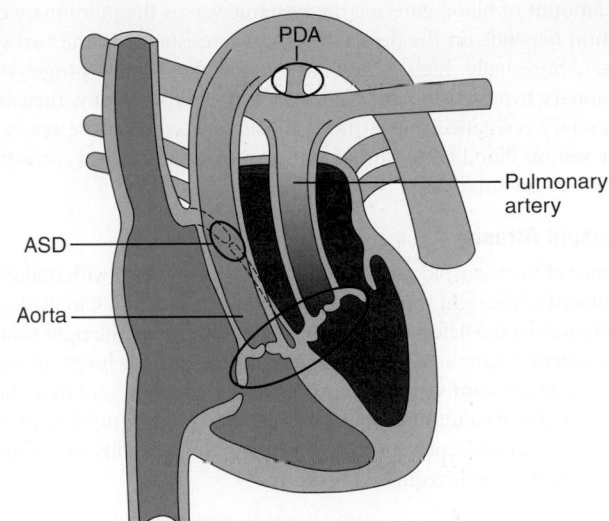

FIGURE 18-31 Transposition of the great arteries. Two separate circulations are formed, which is incompatible with life unless mixing of blood occurs through other defects. *ASD*, Atrial septal defect; *PDA*, patent ductus arteriosus.

the left ventricle to enlarge. A prominent systolic murmur is usually apparent. Surgical replacement is the definitive treatment if the stenosis is severe, progresses, or becomes symptomatic.

Cyanotic Congenital Defects
Tetralogy of Fallot

The four defining features of tetralogy of Fallot are: (1) a ventricular septal defect; (2) an aorta positioned above the ventricular septal opening (overriding aorta); (3) pulmonary stenosis that obstructs right ventricular outflow; and (4) right ventricular hypertrophy (Figure 18-30).

The severity of the symptoms is related primarily to the degree of pulmonary stenosis. The heart is generally enlarged because of the extensive right ventricular hypertrophy. Even if the condition is untreated, individuals with tetralogy of Fallot may live into adulthood. The defect often results in cyanosis because the overriding aorta receives unoxygenated blood from the right side of the heart as well as oxygenated blood from the left side. The degree of cyanosis depends on the amount of blood received from the right side, which in turn depends on the degree of pulmonic obstruction. Surgical correction of the defects is usually recommended because prolonged noncorrective management carries the risk of infective endocarditis and secondary polycythemia.

Transposition of the Great Arteries

In the most common form of transposition of the great arteries, the aorta arises from the right ventricle and the pulmonary artery arises from the left ventricle (Figure 18-31). This anomaly results in the formation of two separate, noncommunicating circulations. The right side of the heart receives blood from the systemic circulation and recirculates it through the body by way of the aorta. Blood reaching the body has not passed through the lungs and is therefore not oxygenated. The left side of the heart receives oxygenated blood from the lungs and then recirculates it through the lungs by way of the pulmonary artery. Unless some mixing of these separate circulations takes place through other heart defects, such as septal defects, transposition is not compatible with life.

Nearly all infants who survive the neonatal period have an interatrial opening, and most also have a patent ductus arteriosus. A good

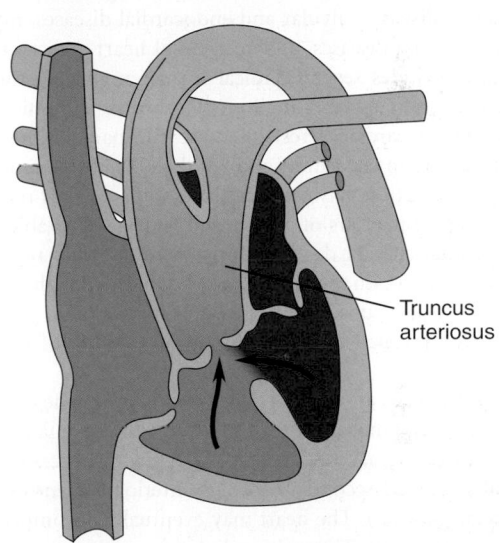

FIGURE 18-32 Truncus arteriosus is a cyanotic defect. Failure of septation results in a common outflow tract from the ventricles. A ventricular septal defect is also present.

deal of mixing must be maintained after birth for the infant to survive. Surgery may be directed at improving the mixing of systemic and pulmonary blood by enlarging or creating openings in the heart. Corrective surgery in which the aorta and pulmonary arteries are excised from the heart and sutured to the opposite ventricular outflow tract is the treatment of choice. The coronary arteries must also be reimplanted into the new left ventricular outflow tract in this procedure.

Truncus Arteriosus

Truncus arteriosus is a congenital malformation in which failure of the pulmonary artery and aorta to separate results in formation of one large vessel that receives blood from both the right and left ventricles (Figure 18-32). A large ventricular septal defect and a single valvular structure are present and lead to the single large artery. Mixing of blood from the right and left sides of the heart results in systemic cyanosis.

The amount of blood entering the systemic versus the pulmonary circulation depends on the degree of vascular resistance in the two systems. Abnormally high pulmonary blood flow may progress to pulmonary hypertension and right ventricular hypertrophy. Increased pulmonary resistance causes the cyanosis to become more severe as more venous blood enters the systemic circulation. Surgical correction is required for survival.

Tricuspid Atresia

Absence of the tricuspid valve is almost always associated with underdevelopment of the right ventricle and an atrial septal defect. Circulation is maintained by the defect, which allows blood to bypass the right ventricle. A patent ductus arteriosus is required to perfuse the lungs. In some cases, a concomitant ventricular septal defect is present and may allow some blood to pass into the right ventricle and enter the pulmonary circulation. Cyanosis is present from birth, and the mortality rate is high. Surgical correction is required for survival.

> **KEY POINTS**
> - Different congenital heart anomalies result in two primary pathologic processes: (1) shunting of blood through abnormal pathways in the heart or great vessels and (2) obstruction to blood flow because of abnormal narrowing.
> - Disorders that result in left-to-right shunting of blood or obstruction to flow are generally acyanotic. These disorders include atrial septal defect, ventricular septal defect, patent ductus arteriosus, coarctation of the aorta, and pulmonary and aortic stenosis or atresia.
> - Disorders that result in right-to-left shunting of blood result in cyanosis. These disorders include tetralogy of Fallot, transposition of the great arteries, truncus arteriosus, and tricuspid atresia.

■ SUMMARY

A variety of disease processes may interfere with the heart's ability to provide the body with oxygenated blood. Among these processes are coronary heart disease, valvular and endocardial diseases, myocardial diseases, pericardial diseases, and congenital heart defects. Coronary heart disease includes several clinical forms: angina pectoris, acute coronary syndrome (unstable angina, MI), chronic ischemic heart disease, and sudden cardiac arrest. Stenotic coronary lesions obstruct blood flow to the myocardium and result in these ischemic clinical syndromes. Distinction between unstable angina and MI relies on the presence of serum markers of myocardial damage. Unstable angina is ischemia without cellular death and therefore does not result in biomarker elevation. MI, on the other hand, is associated with the death of myocardial cells and subsequent release of intracellular components. MI may be complicated by dysrhythmias and failure of the heart to pump efficiently.

Valvular disorders are of two types: those that impede flow because of stenosis and those that allow regurgitation because of failure to close completely. The general consequence of valvular disorders is increased myocardial workload secondary to high afterload (stenosis) or high preload (regurgitation). The heart may eventually decompensate and proceed to heart failure. The endocardial diseases rheumatic heart disease and infective endocarditis also primarily affect the heart valves and create stenosis and regurgitation.

Disorders of the myocardium include myocarditis, which is an inflammatory process, and cardiomyopathy, which is a noninflammatory process, usually of unknown cause. Most cases of myocarditis are viral; however, it is the immune system's response to the virus that appears to cause myocardial damage. Myocarditis results in a dilated, flabby heart with decreased pumping efficiency. The cardiomyopathies are a diverse group of disorders that may be classified as primary (having unknown cause) and specific (caused by a known disease process). Cardiomyopathies include a dilated form, a hypertrophic form, and a restrictive form. The primary problem in the dilated form is poor contractility of all heart chambers. The hypertrophic form may cause left ventricular outflow obstruction that interferes with cardiac output and increases left ventricular strain. Dysfunction in the restrictive form is caused by poor diastolic filling as a result of a stiff, fibrosed ventricular chamber.

Pericardial disorders include accumulations of fluid in the pericardial sac and acute and chronic forms of pericarditis. Pericardial fluid may be serous, serosanguineous, chylous, or frank blood. Pericardial accumulations are usually of little consequence except as indicators of underlying pathophysiologic processes. However, if the accumulation is large or rapid, it may compress the heart and interfere with diastolic filling—a process called *cardiac tamponade*. Pericarditis refers to inflammation of the pericardium. It is usually secondary to other disease processes. Pericardial inflammation generally causes pain and may be associated with a friction rub. Chronic pericarditis can cause erosion of the pericardial sac such that the epicardial layer of the heart may become fused to other mediastinal structures. Alternatively, chronic pericarditis may cause the pericardial sac to become fibrotic and noncompliant such that it restricts expansion of the heart during diastolic filling.

A number of heart disorders may be present at birth and can be categorized as obstructions or shunts and as cyanotic or acyanotic. In general, disorders that allow unoxygenated blood from the right heart to enter the systemic circulation (right-to-left shunt) cause cyanosis. Examples of cyanotic defects include tetralogy of Fallot, transposition of the great arteries, truncus arteriosus, and tricuspid atresia. Examples of acyanotic defects are coarctation of the aorta, atrial and ventricular septal defects, and patent ductus arteriosus.

All heart diseases discussed in this chapter may be complicated by heart failure. Heart failure occurs when the pumping efficiency of the heart is decreased such that cardiac output is subnormal. It is often accompanied by congestion of the lungs or the systemic venous system. Heart failure is discussed in Chapter 19.

REFERENCES

1. American Heart Association: *Heart disease and stroke statistics—2012 update*, Dallas, 2012, The Association.
2. National Cholesterol Education Program (NCEP): *Third Report of the Expert Panel on Detection, Evaluation, and Treatment of High Blood Cholesterol in Adults (Adult Treatment Panel III)*, Bethesda, MD, 2002, National Heart, Lung, and Blood Institute, National Institutes of Health.
3. Canty JM: Coronary blood flow and myocardial ischemia. In Bonow R, Mann D, Zipes D, et al, editors: *Braunwald's heart disease: a textbook of cardiovascular medicine*, ed 9, Philadelphia, 2012, Elsevier, pp 1049–1075.
4. Mitchell RN, Schoen FJ: Blood vessels. In Kumar V, Abbas A, Fausto N, Aster J, editors: *Robbins and Cotran pathologic basis of disease*, ed 8, Philadelphia, 2010, Saunders, pp 487–528.
5. Grundy SM et al, National Heart, Lung, and Blood Institute, American College of Cardiology Foundation, American Heart Association: Implications of recent clinical trials for the National Cholesterol Education Program Adult Treatment Panel III guidelines, *Circulation* 110(2):227–239, 2004.
6. Stary HC, et al: A definition of initial, fatty streak, and intermediate lesions of atherosclerosis. A report from the Committee on Vascular Lesions of the Council on Arteriosclerosis, American Heart Association, *Circulation* 89(5):2462–2478, 1994.
7. Antman EM: ST-Segment elevation myocardial infarction: pathology, pathophysiology and clinical features. In Bonow R, Mann D, Zipes D, et al, editors: *Braunwald's heart disease: a textbook of cardiovascular medicine*, ed 9, Philadelphia, 2012, Saunders, pp 1087–1110.
8. Finn AV, Nakano M, Narula J, et al: Concept of vulnerable/unstable plaque, *Arterioscler Thromb Vasc Biol* 30:1282–1292, 2010.
9. Schoen FJ, Mitchell R: The heart. In Kumar V, Abbas A, Fausto N, Aster J, editors: *Robbins and Cotran pathologic basis of disease*, ed 8, Philadelphia, 2010, Saunders, pp 529–588.
10. Wolff T, Miller T, Ko S: Aspirin for the primary prevention of cardiovascular events: an update of the evidence for the US Preventative Services Task Force, *Ann Intern Med* 150(6):405–410, 2009.
11. Hadi HA, Carr CS, Al Suwaidi J: Endothelial dysfunction: cardiovascular risk factors, therapy, and outcome, *Vasc Health Risk Manag* 1(3):183–198, 2005.
12. Jois P: NSTEMI and STEMI: therapeutic updates 2011, *Emerg Med Rep* 32(1), 2011.
13. Wright RS, et al: 2011 ACC/AHA focused update of the guidelines for the management of patients with unstable angina/non–ST-elevation myocardial infarction (Updating the 2007 guideline): a report of the American College of Cardiology Foundation/American Heart Association Task Force on Practice Guidelines (Writing Committee to Revise the 2002 Guidelines for the Management of Patients With Unstable Angina/Non–ST-Elevation Myocardial Infarction): developed in collaboration with the American College of Emergency Physicians, American College of Physicians, Society for Cardiovascular Angiography and Interventions, and Society of Thoracic Surgeons, *J Am Coll Cardiol* 57(19):1920–1959, 2011.
14. DeWood MA, et al: Prevalence of total coronary occlusion during the early hours of transmural myocardial infarction, *N Engl J Med* 303(16):897–902, 1980.
15. Kushner FG, et al: 2009 Focused updates: ACC/AHA guidelines for the management of patients with ST-elevation myocardial infarction (Updating the 2004 Guideline and 2007 Focused Update) and ACC/AHA/SCAI Guidelines on percutaneous coronary intervention (Updating the 2005 Guideline and 2007 Focused Update): a report of the American College of Cardiology Foundation, *J Am Coll Cardiol* 54(23):2205–2241, 2009.
16. Kong MH, Fonorow GC, Peterson ED, et al: Systematic review of the incidence of sudden cardiac death in the United States, *J Am Coll Cardiol* 57:794–901, 2011.
17. Otto CM, Bonow RO: Valvular heart disease. In Bonow R, Mann D, Zipes D, et al: *Braunwald's heart disease: a textbook of cardiovascular medicine*, ed 9, Philadelphia, 2012, Saunders, pp 1468–1539.
18. Marijon E, Ou P, Celermajer DS, et al: Prevalence of rheumatic heart disease detected by echocardiographic screening, *N Engl J Med* 357:470, 2007.
19. Raju BS, Turi ZG: Rheumatic fever. In Bonow R, Mann D, Zipes D, et al, editors: *Braunwald's heart disease: a textbook of cardiovascular medicine*, ed 9, Philadelphia, 2012, Saunders, pp 1868–1875.
20. Karchmer AW: Infective endocarditis. In Bonow R, Mann D, Zipes D, et al, editors: *Braunwald's heart disease: a textbook of cardiovascular medicine*, ed 9, Philadelphia, 2012, Saunders, pp 1540–1560.
21. Liu P, Schultheiss HP: Myocarditis. In Bonow R, Mann D, Zipes D, et al, editors: *Braunwald's heart disease: a textbook of cardiovascular medicine*, ed 9, Philadelphia, 2012, Saunders, pp 1595–1610.
22. Richardson P, et al: Report of the 1995 World Health Organization/International Society and Federation of Cardiology Task Force on the Definition and Classification of Cardiomyopathies, *Circulation* 93(5):841–842, 1996.
23. Hare J: The dilated, restrictive, and infiltrative cardiomyopathies. In Bonow R, Mann D, Zipes D, et al, editors: *Braunwald's heart disease: a textbook of cardiovascular medicine*, ed 9, Philadelphia, 2012, Saunders, pp 1561–1581.
24. LeWinter M, Tischler M: Pericardial diseases. In Bonow R, Mann D, Zipes D, et al, editors: *Braunwald's heart disease: a textbook of cardiovascular medicine*, ed 9, Philadelphia, 2012, Saunders, pp 1651–1671.
25. Newman TB: Etiology of ventricular septal defects: an epidemiologic approach, *Pediatrics* 76(5):741–749, 1985.
26. Webb GD, Smallhorn JF, Therrien J, Redington A: Congenital heart disease. In Bonow R, Mann D, Zipes D, et al, editors: *Braunwald's heart disease: a textbook of cardiovascular medicine*, ed 9, Philadelphia, 2012, Saunders, pp 1411–1467.

Heart Failure and Dysrhythmias: Common Sequelae of Cardiac Diseases

Shann D. Kim and Jacquelyn L. Banasik

evolve WEBSITE

http://evolve.elsevier.com/Copstead/

- Review Questions and Answers
- Glossary (with audio pronunciations for selected terms)
- Animations
- Case Studies
- Key Points Review

KEY QUESTIONS

- What are the common predisposing factors for development of heart failure?
- How does heart failure with primarily systolic dysfunction differ from heart failure with primarily diastolic dysfunction?
- How do the compensatory responses triggered in heart failure work to restore cardiac output?
- What are the clinical manifestations of heart failure?
- How are preload, afterload, and contractility managed therapeutically in the patient with heart failure?
- What are the characteristic electrocardiographic features of the common cardiac dysrhythmias?
- What is the clinical significance and usual treatment of each of the common cardiac dysrhythmias?

CHAPTER OUTLINE

Heart failure (HF) and cardiac dysrhythmias (arrhythmias) may occur in association with cardiac diseases from a number of different causes. *Heart failure* refers to the inability of the heart to maintain sufficient cardiac output to optimally meet metabolic demands of tissues and organs, and is the end stage of most cardiac diseases. Heart failure involves multiple organ systems and is a progressive syndrome. If the contracting ability of the heart is impaired, then blood flow to the systemic circulation will be reduced, and congestion of blood can occur in the pulmonary venous circulation. In patients with HF, these symptoms of fluid overload are described as *congestive heart failure* (CHF), a term used as a diagnosis in some cases. The term CHF may also be used to differentiate chronic heart failure from acute heart failure. This chapter includes the chronic forms of heart failure; acute heart failure is discussed in Chapter 20 because it commonly results in cardiogenic shock. Disturbances in electrical activity of the heart may signify underlying pathophysiologic processes and may also lead to insufficient cardiac output. Neither heart failure nor dysrhythmia is a primary cardiac disease; therefore, underlying pathophysiologic processes must be investigated.

Heart failure is the fastest-growing cardiac disorder; it affects about 5.7 million Americans. More than 550,000 new cases are diagnosed in the United States each year, with an incidence of 10 per 1000 population after age 65.[1] Heart failure is the most common reason for hospitalization in patients older than 65 years.[2] The increasing incidence and hospitalization rates of HF reflect aging of the U.S. population, as well as better treatment and an improved survival rate after myocardial infarction (MI).[1,3]

HEART FAILURE

Pathogenesis and Diagnosis

A large number of cardiac disorders, including most of those discussed in Chapter 18, can lead to the development of heart failure. Coronary artery disease (CAD) is responsible for 60% to 75% of HF cases, and hypertension (HTN) contributes to nearly 75% of HF cases. CAD contributes to HF progression through mechanisms that include endothelial dysfunction, ischemia, and infarction. CAD and HTN interact to increase the risk of HF.[1] In recent years, the impact of obesity and type 2 diabetes mellitus (T2DM) has become important. T2DM is known to accelerate atherosclerosis, and is frequently associated with HTN. Less common causes of HF include dilated cardiomyopathy, congenital heart defects, valvular disorders, respiratory diseases, anemia, and hyperthyroidism. The diagnosis of heart failure is based on the presence of a constellation of signs and symptoms that are characteristic of the syndrome. However, different sets of criteria are in use, including the Framingham Criteria and Minnesota Heart Failure Criteria.[4] Commonly used criteria for identifying heart failure include the presence of dyspnea, pulmonary rales, cardiomegaly, pulmonary edema, S_3 heart sound, and tachycardia (greater than 120 beats/min), although many other criteria may be applied. No single diagnostic test is available for HF. The diagnosis should be based on a thorough medical history and physical examination.[1]

CHF is generally classified as systolic or diastolic heart failure.[5,6,7] Regardless of specific cause, the pathophysiologic state of heart failure results from the impaired ability of myocardial fibers to contract (systolic failure), relax (diastolic failure), or both.[7] Until the late 1980s, systolic dysfunction was thought to be the primary problem in all forms of HF. However, epidemiologic studies have shown that about half of patients with chronic HF have preserved systolic function, but impaired diastolic function.[8,9] The severity and differentiation of heart failure patients with systolic failure or preserved systolic function is based primarily on the left ventricular ejection fraction (EF). Ejection

fraction is calculated by dividing stroke volume by end-diastolic volume. A normal EF is 60% to 80%. Patients with systolic failure have characteristically low ejection fractions (<40%). Patients with EF greater than 50% do not have significant systolic dysfunction and are categorized as HF with normal EF (HFnlEF). The majority of patients diagnosed with heart failure who have an EF greater than 50% have diastolic dysfunction.[8,9] Many patients with low EF also have impaired diastolic function. In general, patients with low EF but no congestive symptoms have a survival rate about the same as those with preserved EF who have congestive symptoms. The highest mortality occurs in patients with both low EF and congestive symptoms.

The overall mortality for heart failure is high with about 50% (42% to 65% in various studies) of patients dying within 5 years of diagnosis.[2,5,6] Survival rates vary significantly between genders, with men having a 35% survival rate at 5 years and women having a 53% survival rate. The median survival time after diagnosis is 1.7 years in men and 3.2 years in women.[6]

Systolic Dysfunction

Patients with systolic dysfunction have reduced myocardial contractility evidenced by a low EF and a reduced dP/dt during ventricular systole. The dP/dt is a measure of **inotropy**—how quickly the ventricle can develop a forceful contraction. The nature of the impaired contractility is only partially understood; however, myocyte loss, mechanical derangements of myocardial cells, and dysregulation of neurohormones are believed to be critical elements.[10]

Impaired contractility attributable to myocardial infarction (MI) is a common cause of heart failure.[11] MI, with cell death and loss of contractile elements, reduces the heart's contractile force. The degree of pump failure is related to the amount of heart muscle lost. In patients with heart failure, myocardial cells are also subject to high rates of apoptosis or programmed cell death. Apoptosis can be triggered by excessive stimulation by certain neurohormones and by ischemia. Over time, the loss of myocardial cells contributes to reduced contractility. In severe systolic HF, the EF may fall below 15% or 20%. In general, the prognosis worsens as EF decreases. Symptomatic patients with systolic heart failure often have impaired diastolic function, which is associated with a higher mortality rate.[7]

Inadequate supplies of oxygen to the contracting cells may impair contractility because each myosin cross-bridge cycle requires a molecule of adenosine triphosphate (ATP). When ATP production is low, fewer cross-bridge cycles are completed with each contraction, which results in a reduced EF.

β_1-Receptor down-regulation is thought to be an important mechanism of impaired systolic function. Chronic overexcitation of cardiac β_1 receptors by sympathetic neurotransmitters (e.g., norepinephrine) leads to a reduction in the number of β_1 receptors, and results in a myocardium that is less responsive to sympathetic stimulation and adrenergic drug therapy. β_1-Receptor blocking agents have been shown to improve EF and also to reduce mortality, which lend support to the view that chronic excessive sympathetic nervous system (SNS) activation is detrimental to cardiac function.[12-14]

Diastolic Dysfunction

Coronary artery disease and hypertension are the two main causes of diastolic dysfunction, just as they are the primary causes of systolic failure. Why the same disease processes result in different cardiac dynamics in different individuals is not known. Some patients have isolated systolic failure, whereas others have isolated diastolic failure. Some patients exhibit both abnormal systolic and diastolic function. HF with normal EF is more common in women, the elderly, and those with no history of MI.[7] Diastolic failure is a disorder of myocardial relaxation.

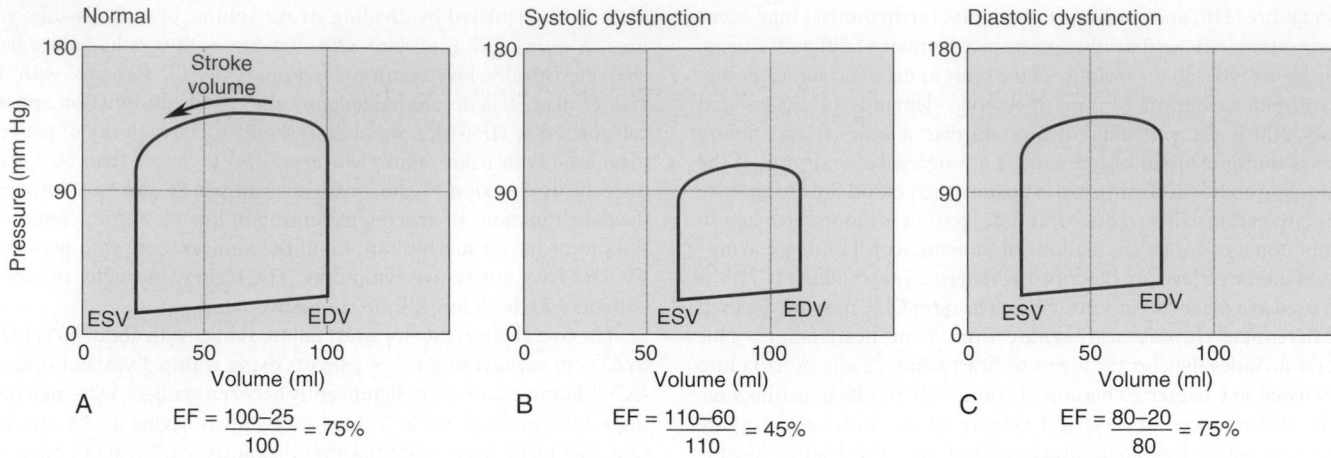

FIGURE 19-1 Comparison of the left ventricular pressure-volume loop in normal heart **(A)**, systolic dysfunction **(B)**, and diastolic dysfunction **(C)**. Note that end-diastolic *pressure* is higher than normal in both systolic and diastolic failure, but end-diastolic *volume* is lower in diastolic dysfunction. *EDV*, End-diastolic volume; *EF*, ejection fraction; *ESV*, end-systolic volume.

In this condition, the left ventricle is excessively noncompliant and does not fill effectively. Two separate functional processes occur during the diastolic relaxation phase: The first is an energy-requiring process (**lusitropy**) that removes free calcium ions from the cytoplasm by pumping them back into the sarcoplasmic reticulum and across the cell membrane into the extracellular fluid. Removal of calcium ions inhibits cross-bridge formation and allows the thick and thin filaments of the sarcomere to passively slide apart. Ischemia, with subsequent ATP deficiency, interferes with the efficiency of calcium ion removal and can impair the active phase of diastolic relaxation.

The second process is passive stretch of the ventricular myocardium to accommodate filling. Passive compliance of the ventricle can be decreased by deposition of fibrin and collagen during scar formation or by hypertrophic thickening of the ventricular wall. Both active and passive processes may be impaired together and are difficult to distinguish clinically.

The hallmark of HF with normal EF is that the patient exhibits clinical manifestations of HF, including low cardiac output, pulmonary congestion, and edema formation, but has a normal EF (usually defined as greater than 50%), indicating absence of significant systolic impairment.[8,9] Because prognosis and treatment recommendations may differ, an echocardiogram to measure EF is recommended in all patients with HF to determine the presence of isolated diastolic dysfunction from systolic failure.[11,13] A comparison of the left ventricular pressure-volume loop in systolic and diastolic dysfunction is shown in Figure 19-1. Systolic failure is characterized by higher than normal diastolic volume and low EF, whereas the pressure-volume loop in diastolic failure indicates poor compliance with a lower diastolic volume at a higher than normal pressure.

KEY POINTS
- HF is the end stage of most cardiac disorders. HF occurs when the heart is unable to provide sufficient cardiac output to meet normal metabolic functions of the body.
- The most common cause of HF is myocardial ischemia from coronary artery disease, followed by hypertension and dilated cardiomyopathy.
- Impaired contractility resulting in systolic failure is frequently associated with HF. The biochemical basis of impaired contractility involves loss of cardiac muscle cells, β_1-receptor down-regulation, and reduced ATP production.

- In about half of HF patients, systolic function is preserved and diastolic dysfunction predominates. HF with normal EF is particularly likely to develop in the elderly, in women, and in those without a history of MI.
- Left ventricular pressure-volume loops characterize the differences in systolic and diastolic dysfunction. High diastolic volume and reduced EF indicate systolic failure, whereas diastolic failure is characterized by higher diastolic pressure and low volume.

Compensatory Mechanisms and Remodeling

When the heart fails to provide adequate cardiac output to meet tissue demands, a number of compensatory mechanisms are triggered. In the short term, these mechanisms are helpful in restoring cardiac output toward normal levels, but in the long term, they are detrimental to cardiac structure and function. Much of the current management of HF is aimed at attenuating the harmful consequences of these compensatory responses.[7] Three main compensatory mechanisms are activated in heart failure: SNS activation, increased preload, and myocardial hypertrophy (Figure 19-2).

Sympathetic Nervous System Activation

Sympathetic activation of the heart is primarily a result of baroreceptor reflex stimulation. The baroreceptors (pressoreceptors), located in the aorta and carotid arteries, detect a fall in pressure because of diminished stroke volume and transmit this information to the central nervous system (CNS). The CNS increases activity in the sympathetic nerves to the heart, resulting in increased heart rate and contractility. However, because of impaired contractile ability, the failing heart may have reduced responsiveness to sympathetic activation. Sympathetic activation also causes venoconstriction, which redistributes blood and increases cardiac preload. Sympathetic constriction of arterioles helps to maintain blood pressure when cardiac output is reduced. Specialized cells in the kidney called *juxtaglomerular cells* also receive SNS stimulation when cardiac output falls. The juxtaglomerular cells release renin and initiate the renin-angiotensin-aldosterone cascade, leading to salt and water retention by the kidney. Sympathetic activation is an early and immediate compensatory response to insufficient cardiac output.

Sympathetic activation is a very effective means for increasing cardiac output in an acute process, such as volume depletion. However, in heart failure, sympathetic activation becomes a chronic process that is ultimately deleterious. A major problem with excessive sympathetic

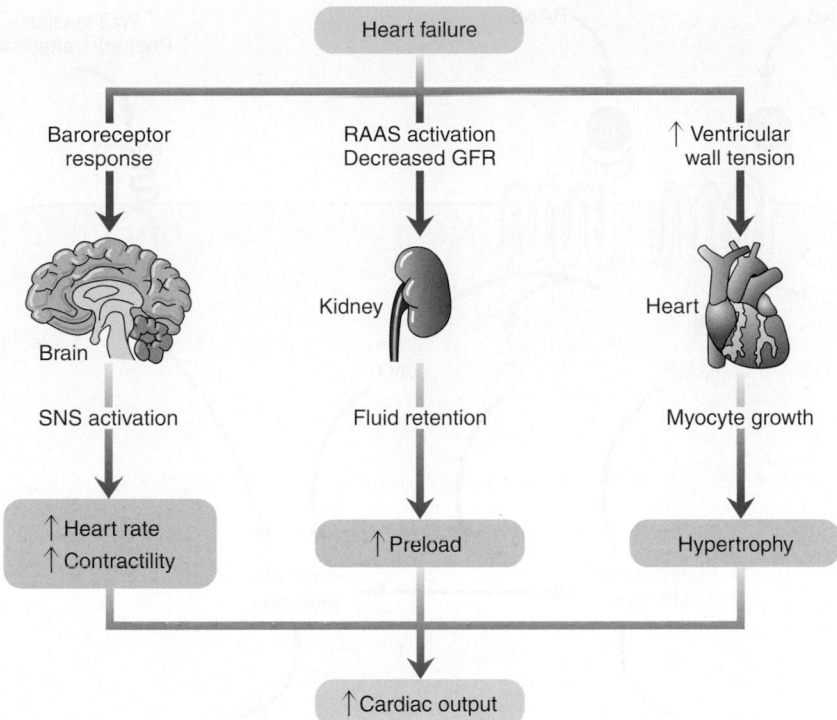

FIGURE 19-2 Major compensatory mechanisms in heart failure that act to restore cardiac output. *GFR,* Glomerular filtration rate; *RAAS,* renin-angiotensin-aldosterone system; *SNS,* sympathetic nervous system.

activation is that afterload on the left ventricle can be increased significantly. A high afterload increases cardiac workload and may decrease stroke volume. Therefore, treatment of high blood pressure is important to improve cardiac function in patients with HF.[8]

Drugs that block β_1 receptors have been advocated in the management of HF to inhibit the cardiac effects of sympathetic activation. Many clinicians had been reluctant to use β-blockers in patients with HF because these drugs are negative inotropes and have the potential to reduce cardiac output. In HF, where cardiac output is already low, the use of a negative inotrope would seem to be contraindicated. However, several randomized clinical trials have reported an improved mortality rate in patients receiving certain β_1-blockers, and they are now recommended as standard therapy in most HF guidelines.[6,13] Long-term SNS stimulation of the heart may contribute to heart failure progression and remodeling of the cardiac tissue. Remodeling is a process of myocyte loss, hypertrophy of remaining cells, and interstitial fibrosis (Figure 19-3). The remodeled tissue is less functional and may predispose to worsening failure and cardiac dysrhythmias.

Increased Preload

Increased **preload** in the cardiac chambers is initially a consequence of reduced EF with a resultant increase in residual end-systolic volume. Subsequently, decreased cardiac output to the kidney reduces glomerular filtration, resulting in fluid conservation. In addition, the renin-angiotensin-aldosterone system (RAAS) is activated because of reduced blood flow to the kidney and SNS activation of the juxtaglomerular cells. Angiotensin II (AII) and aldosterone enhance sodium and water reabsorption by the kidney, contributing to an elevated blood volume. Increased preload is a compensatory mechanism that enhances the ability of the myocardium to contract forcefully. An enlarged chamber volume causes the myocardial fibers to lengthen during diastole, which results in greater fiber shortening during contraction (Frank-Starling mechanism).[12] The diastolic length of the

muscle fibers is thought to determine the number of effective cross-bridge cycles that can be accomplished during systole.[10] Thus, up to a point, an increase in the volume or preload of the heart will result in a greater force of contraction (Figure 19-4). The cardiac function curve flattens out at a certain point, and minimal benefit is obtained despite increasing preload. Patients with systolic failure have a cardiac function curve that is flat and shifted to the right of normal. Thus, they require a higher preload to achieve a given stroke volume. However, patients with HF often retain so much volume that their hearts are functioning on the flat part of the curve. These patients benefit from preload reduction, which will decrease systemic and pulmonary congestive symptoms and cardiac workload with little or no reduction in cardiac output. Diuretics are commonly used to achieve moderate preload reduction.

Myocardial Hypertrophy and Remodeling

Hypertrophy of cardiac muscle cells is the third mechanism of compensation and generally takes much longer to occur than preload enhancement or sympathetic activation. Hypertrophy appears to result, in part, from a chronic elevation of myocardial wall tension.[10] Wall tension may be high as a result of increased diastolic blood volume (high preload) or as a consequence of high systolic pressures generated in the chamber (to overcome high afterload). The relationship between myocardial wall tension and intrachamber pressure and diameter is described by the law of Laplace: tension = (transmural pressure × radius)/wall thickness. When the ventricular chamber enlarges and pressures increase, more tension is created in the ventricular muscle wall (Figure 19-5). The development of high systolic pressures in the ventricle may be necessary to overcome a high afterload, such as occurs with arterial hypertension and aortic valve stenosis. The hypertrophy of contractile elements in the myocardium increases the heart's pumping force and helps to reduce the wall tension of the heart toward normal levels. In general, an increase in chamber diameter because of excessive preload is thought to contribute

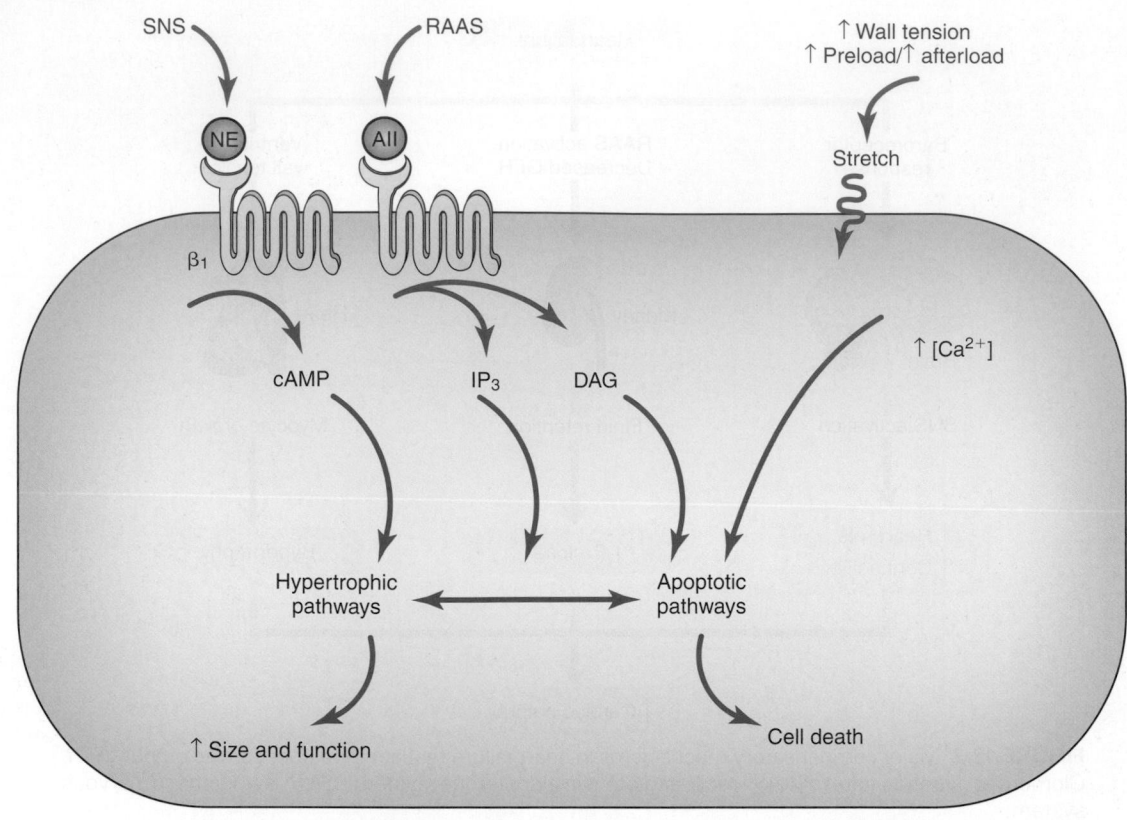

FIGURE 19-3 Mechanisms of ventricular remodeling in heart failure. Activation of β_1 receptors and *AII* receptors along with stretch of the cell membrane trigger signaling cascades. Under some conditions these triggers lead to effective hypertrophy and an increase in size and function, and in others they trigger apoptotic cell death. *AII,* Angiotensin II; *cAMP,* cyclic adenosine monophosphate; *DAG,* diacylglycerol; *IP₃,* 1,4,5-inositol trisphosphate; *NE,* norepinephrine; *RAAS,* renin-angiotensin-aldosterone system; *SNS,* sympathetic nervous system.

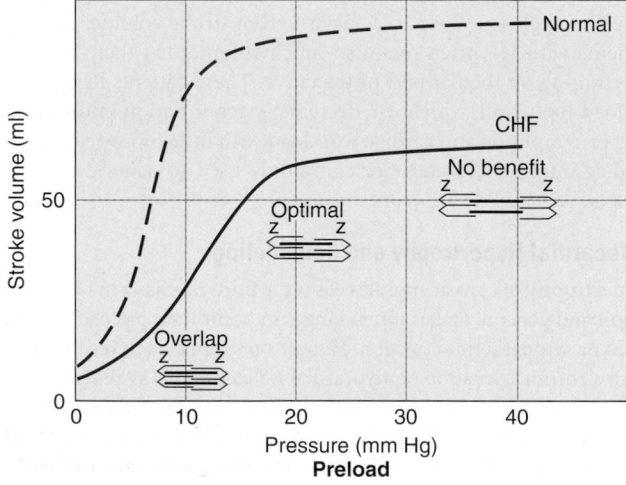

FIGURE 19-4 Effect of increased preload on sarcomere length and stroke volume. Systolic failure results in a shift of the curve to the right and a dampening of maximal stroke volume. A greater preload is required to achieve a given stroke volume compared with the normal ventricle. *CHF,* Congestive heart failure.

to eccentric hypertrophy in which the muscle fibers elongate.[7,10] High afterload results in concentric hypertrophy in which the muscle fibers grow in diameter and thicken the ventricular wall (Figure 19-6).

Neurohormones, which include norepinephrine (NE) and angiotensin (Ang II), also have hypertrophic effects on the heart. Circulating

Ang II levels are higher than normal in HF because of poor kidney perfusion, which triggers production of Ang II through the RAAS. In heart failure, Ang II is also produced locally in the heart. Ang II binds to the angiotensin type 1 (AT1) receptor on cardiac myocytes to activate genes in various growth pathways. Initially, hypertrophy may help the heart compensate for acute loss of myocardial tissue from MI or help maintain cardiac function during chronic hypertension. But over time, the signals that promote hypertrophy are thought to trigger a type of ventricular remodeling that contributes to progression of heart failure. Pathologic remodeling includes loss of myocardial cells through apoptosis and production of fibrous changes in the heart that stiffen the ventricles and contribute to diastolic failure (Figure 19-7). In addition to NE and Ang II, a number of immune cytokines have been implicated in cardiac remodeling.[7,11,12]

Evidence for a role of Ang II in remodeling comes from drug studies in which Ang II production is inhibited or the actions of Ang II are blocked at the AT1 receptor. An important enzyme in the pathway of Ang II production is angiotensin-converting enzyme (ACE). Drugs called ACE inhibitors (ACEIs) have been developed to inhibit the activity of this enzyme and prevent formation of Ang II. Another drug class, angiotensin type 1 receptor blockers (ARBs), binds to this Ang II receptor and blocks the intracellular actions of Ang II. ARBs were developed as a more selective means of RAAS inhibition, and to improve the safety and tolerability profile of ACE inhibitors. Both ACE inhibitors and ARBs have been shown to significantly reduce HF mortality, and both drug classes are used as standard therapy in HF.[1,4,6] In general, ARBs are prescribed if a patient is intolerant of ACE inhibitors.

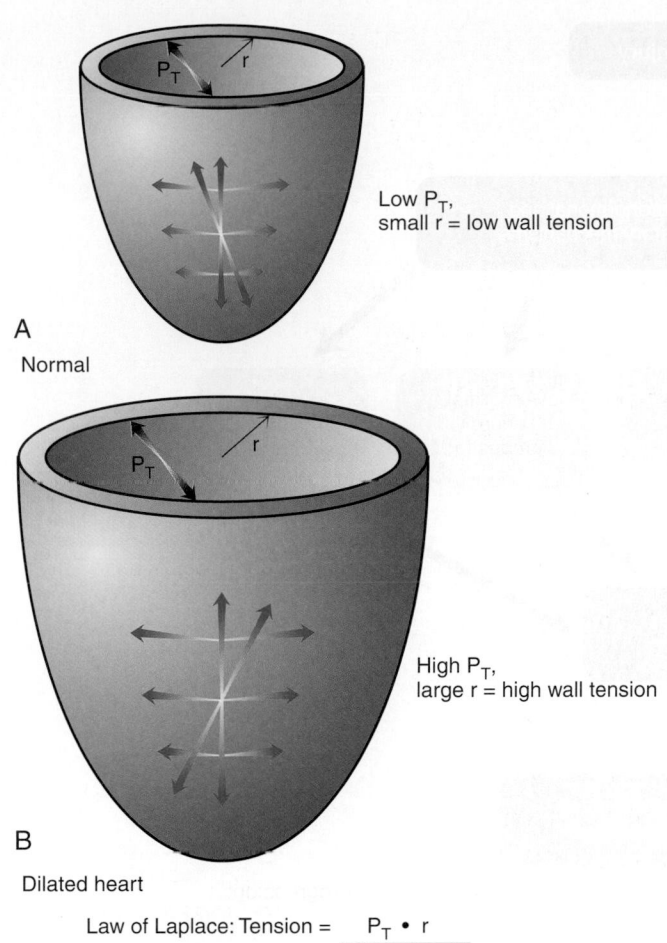

FIGURE 19-5 Mechanism of myocardial hypertrophy attributable to increased ventricular wall tension. According to the law of Laplace, an increase in chamber radius or pressure will increase wall tension. The hypertrophic response increases wall thickness and helps to relieve wall tension. **A,** Heart with normal radius *(r)* and intraventricular pressure. **B,** Heart with enlarged chamber and high intraventricular pressure. P_T, Transmural pressure.

$$\text{Law of Laplace: Tension} = \frac{P_T \bullet r}{\text{wall thickness}}$$

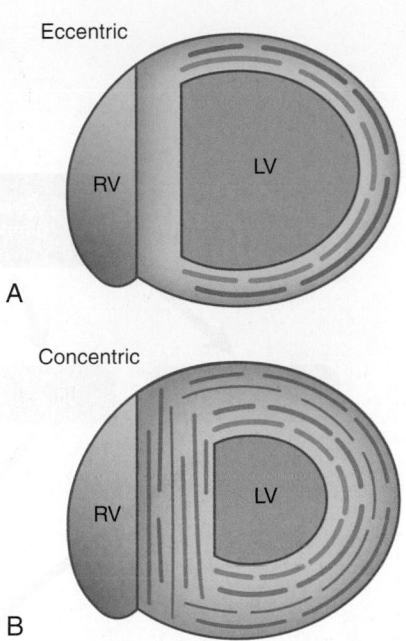

FIGURE 19-6 Forms of ventricular hypertrophy. **A,** Eccentric, in which muscle fibers grow in length and the chamber diameter increases. **B,** Concentric, in which muscle fibers grow in diameter and the ventricular wall becomes thicker. *LV,* Left ventricle; *RV,* right ventricle.

In summary, enhanced preload and cardiac hypertrophy may allow a heart to compensate for reduced ventricular function for an extended period. Unfortunately, these compensatory mechanisms, which serve to restore cardiac output to the tissues, also result in an increase in myocardial work and oxygen requirements and appear to cause pathologic remodeling. Progression and decompensation may occur when the primary disease plus the superimposed burdens of compensation overwhelm the heart's ability to generate adequate contractile force. The focus of therapy for HF is to maintain a state of compensation by minimizing cardiac work while optimizing cardiac output and preventing or delaying ventricular remodeling.

> **KEY POINTS**
> - Compensatory mechanisms are activated in heart failure in an attempt to improve cardiac output. Unfortunately, these responses also increase myocardial workload and may perpetuate the heart failure. Treatment for HF is aimed at attenuating the harmful effects of the compensatory responses.
> - Sympathetic activation is an early response to reduced cardiac output. Sympathetic nervous system activation increases heart rate, contractility, arterial vasoconstriction, and renin release. The failing heart generally has reduced responsiveness to SNS neurotransmitters because of β_1-receptor down-regulation.

> - Decreased cardiac output reduces kidney perfusion and leads to activation of the renin-angiotensin-aldosterone system and volume retention. Extra blood volume increases cardiac preload. Higher preload results in more forceful ejection of blood from the heart (Frank-Starling law) and improves cardiac output.
> - Cardiac hypertrophy is stimulated by elevated myocardial wall tension and the growth-promoting actions of neurohormones, such as NE and Ang II. Hypertrophy adds contractile filaments and improves contractile force.
> - The mechanisms that enable the heart to compensate for reduced stroke volume are detrimental in the long term. Excessive neurohormones, volume overload, and high wall tension contribute to abnormal ventricular remodeling. Gradually, the ventricle loses myocytes and accumulates fibrotic tissue. The remaining myocytes are usually hypertrophied and less efficient. These processes lead to progression of HF over time.

Clinical Manifestations

The clinical presentation of HF differs depending on which ventricle (left, right, or both) is failing to pump blood adequately. Left ventricular failure is the most common presentation of HF. Because of circulatory dynamics, left ventricular failure often leads to right ventricular failure—a condition termed *biventricular failure.* The etiologic process, clinical manifestations, and management of isolated right ventricular failure differ substantially from those for left ventricular and biventricular failure. Recall that the right side of the heart receives blood from the systemic venous circulation and pumps blood into the pulmonary system, whereas the left side of the heart receives blood from the pulmonary circulation and delivers it to the systemic arterial system (Figure 19-8). Insufficient cardiac pumping is manifested by poor cardiac output, called *forward failure,* and by congestion of blood behind the pumping chamber, called *backward failure.* The clinical manifestations of left and right ventricular failure differ as a result of the anatomic location of the "backward" or congestive processes, but the forward effects of low cardiac output are the same.

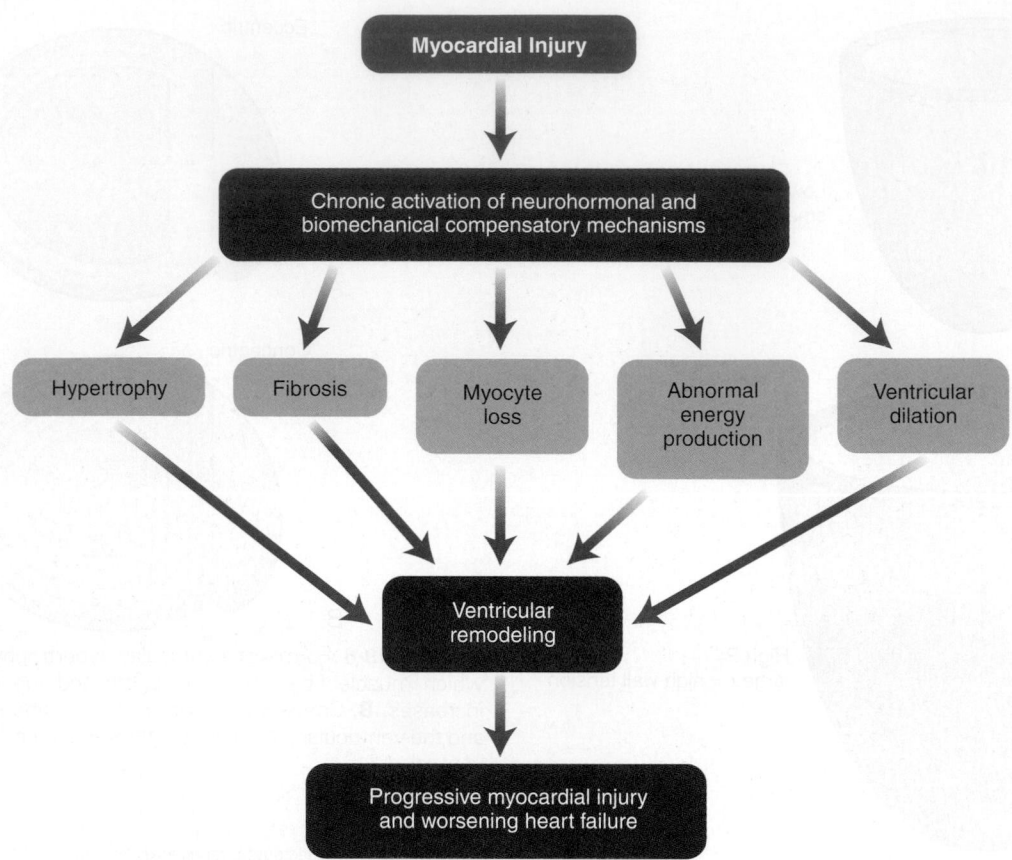

FIGURE 19-7 Mechanisms of cardiac remodeling that contribute to heart failure progression.

The *forward* effects of HF are due to insufficient cardiac output with diminished delivery of oxygen and nutrients to peripheral tissues and organs. Inadequate perfusion of the brain may lead to restlessness, mental fatigue, confusion, anxiety, and impaired memory. Generalized fatigue, activity intolerance, and lethargy may be present.

Reduced perfusion of the kidney results in a decline in urine output (oliguria) with subsequent fluid retention. Activation of the RAAS contributes to conservation of sodium and water by the kidney, and may also cause blood vessel constriction. Constriction of blood vessels serves to maintain blood pressure and redistribute reduced cardiac output to vital organs. However, this vasoconstriction also increases afterload, so the damaged left ventricle must generate more force to pump the same volume of blood. Depending on how much the afterload increases, the damaged left ventricle may not be able to pump sufficient quantities of blood into the circulation. If renal blood flow becomes severely limited, the patient with left ventricular failure may develop kidney failure. Forward failure also results in activation of the SNS because of the baroreceptor reflex. Sympathetic activation contributes to blood vessel constriction and helps maintain blood pressure in the face of reduced cardiac output; however, as with Ang II, SNS activation increases left ventricular afterload. SNS activation results in a compensatory increase in heart rate that may augment cardiac output to some extent, but also raises myocardial ATP consumption.

Left-Sided Heart Failure

Left-sided heart failure is most often associated with left ventricular infarction and systemic hypertension.[7,8] The *backward effects* of left-sided heart failure may produce dramatic clinical symptoms attributable to pulmonary dysfunction (Figure 19-9). Ineffective pumping of the left ventricle results in an accumulation of blood within the pulmonary circulation. As hydrostatic pressure builds within the pulmonary veins and capillaries, fluid is forced from the capillaries into interstitial and alveolar spaces, causing edema. Pulmonary congestion and edema are associated with a number of clinical findings (Figure 19-10). **Dyspnea,** or breathlessness, occurs early in the progression of left-sided heart failure and may be considered the cardinal symptom. Difficulty breathing may be exacerbated by activity (dyspnea on exertion), lying down (**orthopnea** and **paroxysmal nocturnal dyspnea),** and blood volume expansion from excessive salt or fluid intake. Orthopnea and paroxysmal nocturnal dyspnea are due in part to a redistribution of blood volume from the periphery to the heart when the individual lies down. The failing left ventricle is unable to effectively pump extra volume, and pulmonary congestion is worsened. The severity of orthopnea may be quantified by the degree of head elevation (e.g., number of pillows) used to relieve dyspnea. Paroxysmal nocturnal dyspnea refers to intermittent attacks of severe dyspnea during the night and is a most distressing form of orthopnea. The individual experiences a feeling of suffocation and panic at not being able to overcome the dyspnea. Sitting or standing helps to relieve the dyspnea because blood pools in the extremities, reducing pulmonary hydrostatic pressure and congestion.

Clinical signs of pulmonary congestion include cough, respiratory crackles (rales), hypoxemia, and high left atrial pressure (LAP). Cough results from bronchial irritation associated with congestion. In severe cases, sputum may be blood tinged, from breakage of fragile capillaries, and frothy, from fluid buildup in the alveoli. The severity of pulmonary edema can be estimated from the location of crackles within the lung fields. Crackles are abnormal sounds caused by the movement of air through partially fluid-filled alveoli. Edema fluid collects in dependent lung fields because of gravity and progressively moves up the lung as

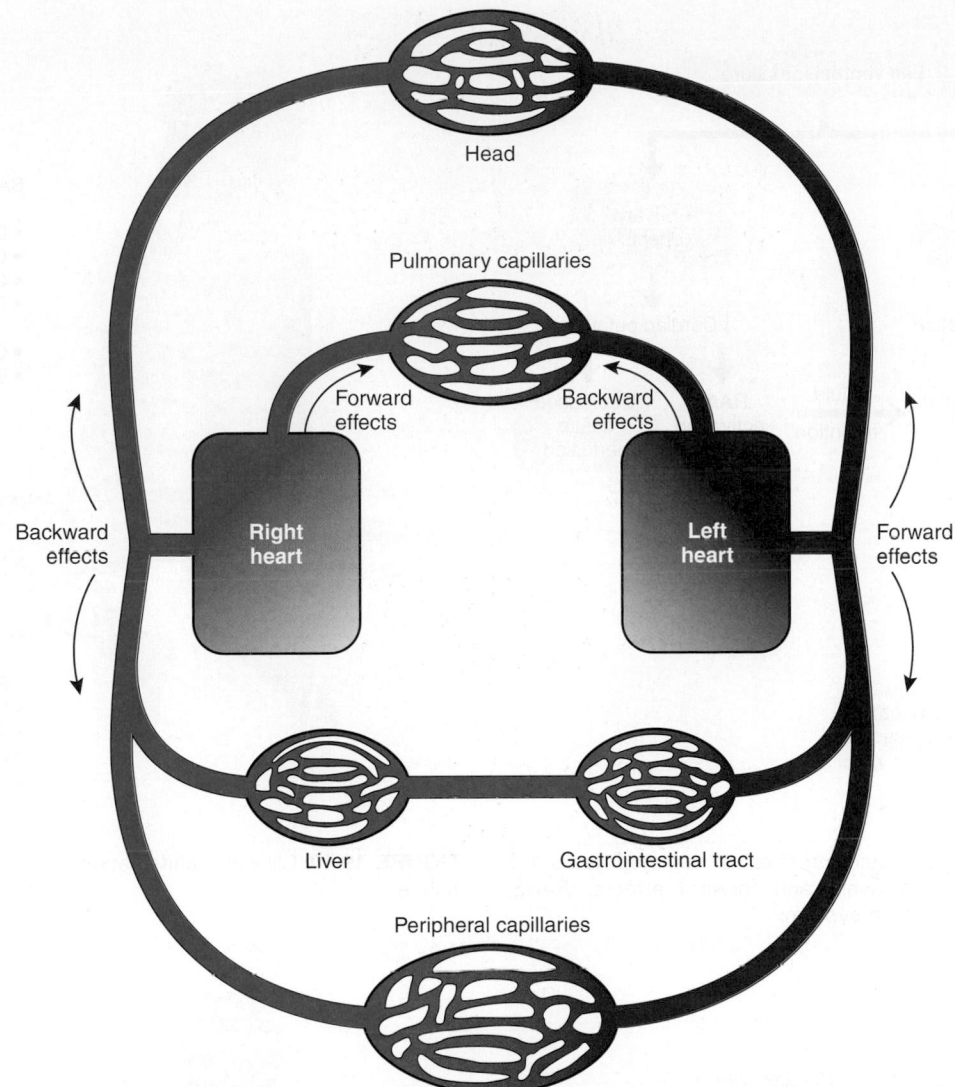

FIGURE 19-8 Systemic and pulmonary circulations viewed as separate but interdependent systems.

more edema fluid accumulates. For example, in mild pulmonary edema, crackles might be heard with a stethoscope only at the base of the upright lung, but with increasing severity they become apparent in the lower third to half of the lung. Fluid in the alveoli and interstitial spaces also interferes with alveolar-capillary gas exchange and results in some degree of hypoxemia. Hypoxemia may be detected by arterial blood gas analysis or pulse oximetry and may be apparent clinically as cyanosis. **Cyanosis** refers to a blue coloration of the skin typically seen around the mouth (circumoral cyanosis) and results from the presence of significant amounts of desaturated hemoglobin in the blood. Cyanosis is a late sign, and is clinically evident only when a large amount (about 5 g/dl) of hemoglobin is deoxygenated (less than or equal to 75% saturated).

Elevated LAP is a common finding in left-sided heart failure because of excessive blood volume and the compensatory responses of atrial dilation and hypertrophy. Atrial pressure can be estimated by inserting a balloon-tipped catheter (Swan-Ganz) into the pulmonary artery. If LAP acutely increases to 25 mm Hg (normal is 4 to 12 mm Hg), increased capillary filtration leads to pulmonary edema. Patients with chronic elevations in LAP associated with chronic HF are more resistant to developing acute pulmonary edema, and may not experience symptoms until pressures approach 40 mm Hg.[7] On x-ray, findings of fluid overload include an enlarged heart and engorged pulmonary capillaries and lymphatic vessels.

Acute cardiogenic pulmonary edema is a life-threatening condition associated with left ventricular failure that severely impairs gas exchange, producing dramatic signs and symptoms. The patient exhibits severe dyspnea and anxiety, and a bolt-upright posture is usually assumed in order to maximize respiratory effort. Bubbly crackles may be heard all the way up the lung from the bases to the apices, and pink frothy sputum may be expectorated or well up from the trachea into the nose and mouth. Anxiety and hypoxemia contribute to tachycardia, which may worsen the pumping efficiency of the failing heart. Cyanosis and symptoms of tissue hypoxia are usually apparent. The immediate treatment is aimed at reducing the fluid volume in the lungs and supporting oxygenation.

Right-Sided Heart Failure

Because the right and left ventricles function in series, left ventricular failure eventually increases the workload on the right ventricle. Consequently, the right ventricle may fail. The etiology of right ventricular failure must include all the causes of left ventricular failure. Isolated right ventricular failure is rare and is usually a consequence of right ventricular infarction or pulmonary disease. Only 3% of MIs occur in the right ventricle; however, right ventricular infarctions are often poorly tolerated and difficult to manage.[7] Pulmonary disorders that result in increased pulmonary vascular resistance impose a high

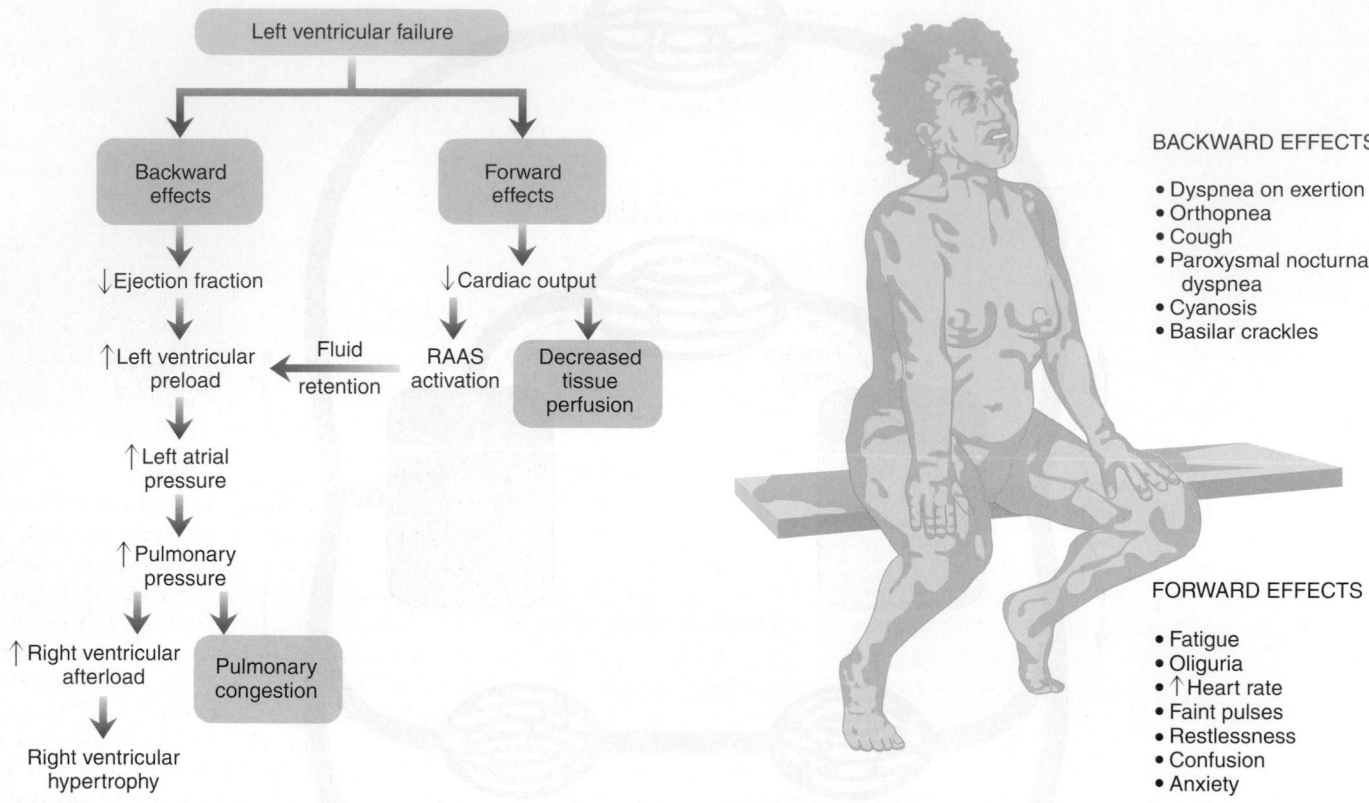

FIGURE 19-9 Pathophysiologic process of isolated left-sided heart failure, showing backward and forward effects. *RAAS,* Renin-angiotensin-aldosterone system.

BACKWARD EFFECTS

- Dyspnea on exertion
- Orthopnea
- Cough
- Paroxysmal nocturnal dyspnea
- Cyanosis
- Basilar crackles

FORWARD EFFECTS

- Fatigue
- Oliguria
- ↑ Heart rate
- Faint pulses
- Restlessness
- Confusion
- Anxiety

FIGURE 19-10 Clinical manifestations of isolated left-sided heart failure.

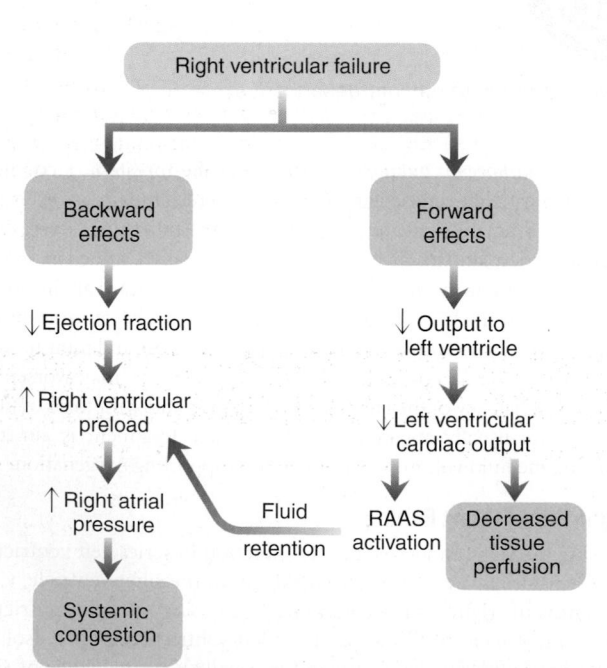

FIGURE 19-11 Pathophysiologic process of isolated right-sided heart failure, showing backward and forward effects. *RAAS,* Renin-angiotensin-aldosterone system.

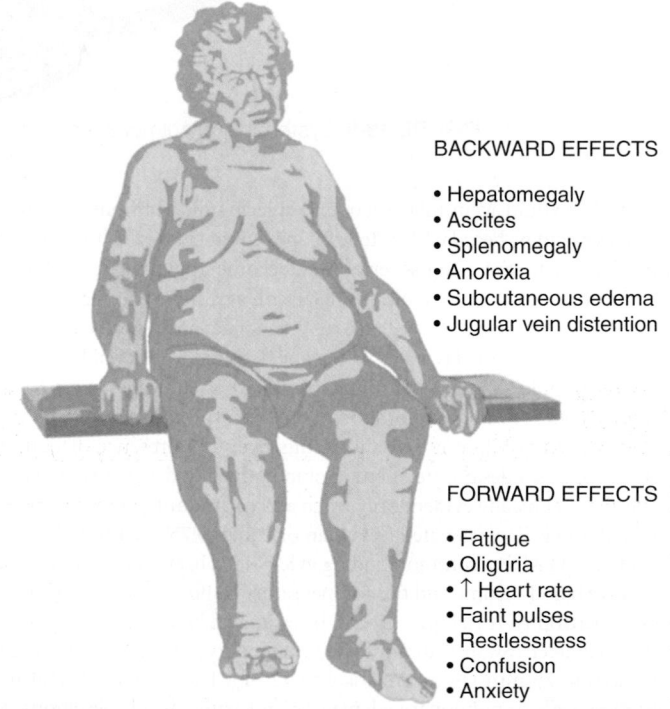

BACKWARD EFFECTS

- Hepatomegaly
- Ascites
- Splenomegaly
- Anorexia
- Subcutaneous edema
- Jugular vein distention

FORWARD EFFECTS

- Fatigue
- Oliguria
- ↑ Heart rate
- Faint pulses
- Restlessness
- Confusion
- Anxiety

FIGURE 19-12 Clinical manifestations of isolated right-sided heart failure.

afterload on the right ventricle. The resultant right ventricular hypertrophy, called **cor pulmonale,** may progress to right ventricular failure as the lung disease worsens.

Any lung disorder that decreases the total cross-sectional area of the lung vasculature can increase pulmonary vascular resistance and produce right ventricular strain. Hypoxemia, for example, causes the pulmonary arterioles to constrict, which increases pulmonary resistance. Constriction or blockage of the vascular bed, such as occurs with pulmonary hypertension or pulmonary embolus, similarly reduces the cross-sectional area of the pulmonary vasculature and leads to increased pulmonary resistance. If the increase in pulmonary resistance and right ventricular workload occurs gradually, the right ventricle can compensate by increasing preload and hypertrophy. However, the thin musculature of the right ventricle has limited ability to adjust to acute changes in workload, as would occur with a right ventricular infarction or large pulmonary embolus.

As with left-sided heart failure, congestion of blood occurs behind the failing right ventricle because of inefficiency of the pump. The *backward effects* of right-sided heart failure are due to congestion in the systemic venous system (Figure 19-11). Systemic venous congestion results in impaired function of the liver, portal system, spleen, kidneys, peripheral subcutaneous tissues, and brain (Figure 19-12).

The liver is usually somewhat increased in size and weight, but individual hepatocytes may show signs of atrophy and necrosis attributable to chronic passive congestion.[7] Impedance to blood flow through the liver may cause hydrostatic pressure to build in the portal system, leading to edema formation in the peritoneal cavity (ascites). Increased pressure in the portal system is reflected back to the spleen and gastrointestinal tract. The spleen is generally enlarged (congestive splenomegaly), and gastrointestinal symptoms such as anorexia and abdominal discomfort may be present.

Increased systemic venous pressure causes congestion of the kidneys, which contributes to the decreased glomerular filtration and fluid retention. Fluid retention may be perpetuated by the congested liver, which is unable to metabolize plasma aldosterone normally.[7] Excess fluid volume and venous congestion caused by right-sided heart failure result in subcutaneous edema. Edema is usually particularly apparent in the lower extremities or sacral area if the patient is supine.

Drainage of venous blood from the head and neck by way of the superior vena cava is also impeded by right-sided heart failure. The jugular veins may be abnormally distended, and mental functioning may be impaired. The hepatojugular reflux test can be done to assess the severity of right-sided heart failure. The liver is manually compressed, causing a sudden increase in venous blood returning to the right heart, while jugular neck veins are observed for sudden distention. In the absence of right-sided heart failure, the sudden increase in venous return would enter the heart unimpeded and no neck vein distention would be apparent.

Biventricular Heart Failure

In many cases, heart failure is not isolated to one side of the heart. Biventricular failure is most often a result of primary left ventricular failure that has progressed to right-sided heart failure. With biventricular failure, cardiac output is reduced and pulmonary congestion exists as a result of left-sided heart failure, as well as systemic venous congestion attributable to right-sided heart failure.

Class and Stage of Heart Failure

A variety of clinical criteria have been used to aid in the diagnosis of HF, but to date, no diagnostic test has been universally accepted. A commonly suggested tool for detecting heart failure in previously undiagnosed individuals is called FACES of heart failure: *f*atigue, *a*ctivity limitation, *c*ongestion, *e*dema, *s*hortness of breath. These are classic findings in HF and, if present, indicate a need for further diagnostic assessment. Traditionally, a patient with suspected HF would be diagnosed by x-ray and echocardiography. Echocardiography is the gold standard for evaluation of HF, and is able to measure chamber size, volume, and dynamics during diastole and systole, as well as determine ejection fraction. A blood test for B-type natriuretic peptide (BNP) may also be used to help identify patients with HF. BNP is synthesized by left ventricular myocytes under conditions of increased left ventricular wall stress. A significant correlation between the amount of plasma BNP or the BNP precursor, N-terminal pro-BNP (NT-proBNP), and the severity of HF has been documented.[15]

The severity of symptoms can be used to assign a heart failure class (New York Heart Association classes [NYHA] I to IV).[15] Another classification scheme has been proposed by the American Heart Association (AHA) to allow inclusion of patients at high risk for heart failure but whose disease is not yet symptomatic. By including this pre–heart failure group, efforts aimed at prevention may be instituted in more patients. Class and stage are used to determine prognosis, therapy, and monitoring in HF. These two classification schemes are compared in Table 19-1.

TABLE 19-1	COMPARISON OF ACC/AHA STAGES OF HEART FAILURE AND NEW YORK HEART ASSOCIATION CLASSES		
ACC/AHA STAGE	**DESCRIPTION**	**CLINICAL CLUES**	**NYHA CLASS**
A	Patients at high risk of developing HF	Coronary artery disease, hypertension, diabetes, dyslipidemia, family history of cardiomyopathy	Not applicable
B	Patients who have structural heart disease but have never manifested signs or symptoms of HF	Left ventricular hypertrophy (by ECG or echo), valvular disease, past myocardial infarction	I
C	Patients who have current or previous symptoms of HF	Dyspnea, fatigue, exercise intolerance, prior HF hospitalization	II-III
D	Patients with advanced structural heart disease and marked symptoms of HF at rest	End-stage, awaiting transplant, receiving palliative care	IV

Adapted from Hunt SA et al: American College of Cardiology; American Heart Association: 2009 focused update incorporated into the ACC/AHA 2005 guidelines for the diagnosis and management of heart failure in adults: summary article, *J Am Coll Cardiol* 53(15):e3-e62, 2009.
HF, Heart failure.

Treatment

Therapy for HF is aimed at improving cardiac output while minimizing congestive symptoms and cardiac workload. These objectives are obtained by manipulating preload, afterload, and contractility. When possible, specific treatment is undertaken to correct the underlying cause of the heart failure.

Despite the large number of pharmacologic agents being used in the management of HF, only a few have been associated with significant improvement in mortality risk, particularly ACE inhibitors, ARBs, aldosterone antagonists, and certain β_1-blockers (Table 19-2).[16] A classification system has been developed by the AHA and American College of Cardiology (ACC), and suggests therapy goals and treatments for the four stages of heart failure (Figure 19-13).

A better understanding of the underlying molecular mechanisms of HF is needed to improve pharmacologic management. Little research has been conducted to determine the best treatment for patients with primarily diastolic failure, and treatment recommendations are similar.[3] Many patients with HF have signs and symptoms of elevated preload attributable to an expanded intravascular volume and a reduced EF. According to the Frank-Starling law, an elevated preload is desirable to enhance systolic shortening and improve cardiac output. Unfortunately, high preload exacerbates congestive symptoms and adds to the workload of an already damaged heart. Thus, the aim of therapy is to optimize preload, so that congestive symptoms are minimized, but cardiac output is not compromised. The right ventricle is particularly sensitive to reductions in preload, and care must be taken to avoid a significant drop in right ventricular output when intravascular volume is decreased. Drugs, such as diuretics, may be administered to reduce intravascular volume. Diuretics promote the excretion of fluid by increasing renal blood flow, blocking sodium and chloride reabsorption, or both. Patients may also be instructed to modify salt and fluid intake.

With the exception of digitalis, positive inotropic agents are avoided in chronic heart failure because they are associated with higher mortality. However, when improving cardiac output is necessary to avoid shock, positive inotropic agents may be used. Positive inotropes work by increasing the availability of intracellular calcium ions during systole. Drugs that mimic SNS effects, such as norepinephrine, isoproterenol, dobutamine, and dopamine, may be used to improve cardiac output, but have a potential for dramatically increasing myocardial oxygen consumption.

Digitalis or a related cardiac glycoside may be used for symptom management of heart failure. Cardiac glycosides directly inhibit the sodium-potassium pump present in the cell membrane of all cells. This results in an increase in intracellular sodium accumulation and a decrease in the gradient for sodium entry into the cell. A diminished sodium gradient slows the sodium-dependent calcium pump that normally removes intracellular calcium. This allows more calcium to remain in the cell, thus strengthening myocardial contraction. Digitalis also slows the heart rate through parasympathetic system activation and promotes sodium and water excretion through improved cardiac output to the kidney. Depletion of serum potassium (hypokalemia) may potentiate digitalis toxicity. Unlike the other positive inotropic agents, digitalis does not appear to increase mortality.[17] Digitalis also does not improve mortality and is not recommended as routine therapy.[1,6,13,17]

Patients with enlarged hearts and conduction delays may benefit from pacemakers, which help to synchronize ventricular contraction. A wide QRS complex is the usual indication for resynchronization therapy in the HF patient. Pacing electrodes are placed in the atrium and both ventricles to allow coordinated depolarization of the heart muscle. Many patients experience significant improvement in congestive symptoms and activity tolerance with resynchronization.

TABLE 19-2 **INHIBITORS OF THE RENIN-ANGIOTENSIN-ALDOSTERONE SYSTEM AND β-BLOCKERS COMMONLY USED FOR THE TREATMENT OF PATIENTS WITH HEART FAILURE WITH LOW EJECTION FRACTION**

DRUG	INITIAL DAILY DOSE(S)	TARGET DAILY DOSE
ACE Inhibitors		
Captopril	6.25 mg 3 times	50 mg 3 times
Enalapril	2.5 mg twice	10 mg twice
Fosinopril	5-10 mg once	80 mg once
Lisinopril	2.5-5 mg once	20 mg once
Quinapril	5 mg twice	80 mg once
Ramipril	1.25-2.5 mg once	10 mg once
Trandolapril	1 mg once	4 mg once
Angiotensin Receptor Blockers		
Candesartan	4-8 mg once	32 mg once
Losartan	12.5-25 mg once	150 mg once
Valsartan	40 mg twice	160 mg twice
Aldosterone Antagonists		
Spironolactone	12.5-25 mg once	25 mg once
Eplerenone	25 mg once	50 mg once
β-Blockers		
Bisoprolol	1.25 mg once	10 mg once
Carvedilol	3.125 mg twice	25 mg twice
Carvedilol CR	10 mg once	80 mg once
Metoprolol succinate (CR/XL)	12.5-25 mg once	200 mg once

From Lindenfield J, Albert NM, Boehmer JP et al: Executive summary: HFSA 2010 comprehensive heart failure practice guidelines, *J Card Fail* 16:475-539, 2010.

ACE, Angiotensin-converting enzyme; *CR,* controlled-release; *kg,* kilogram(s); *mg,* milligram(s); *XL,* extended-release.

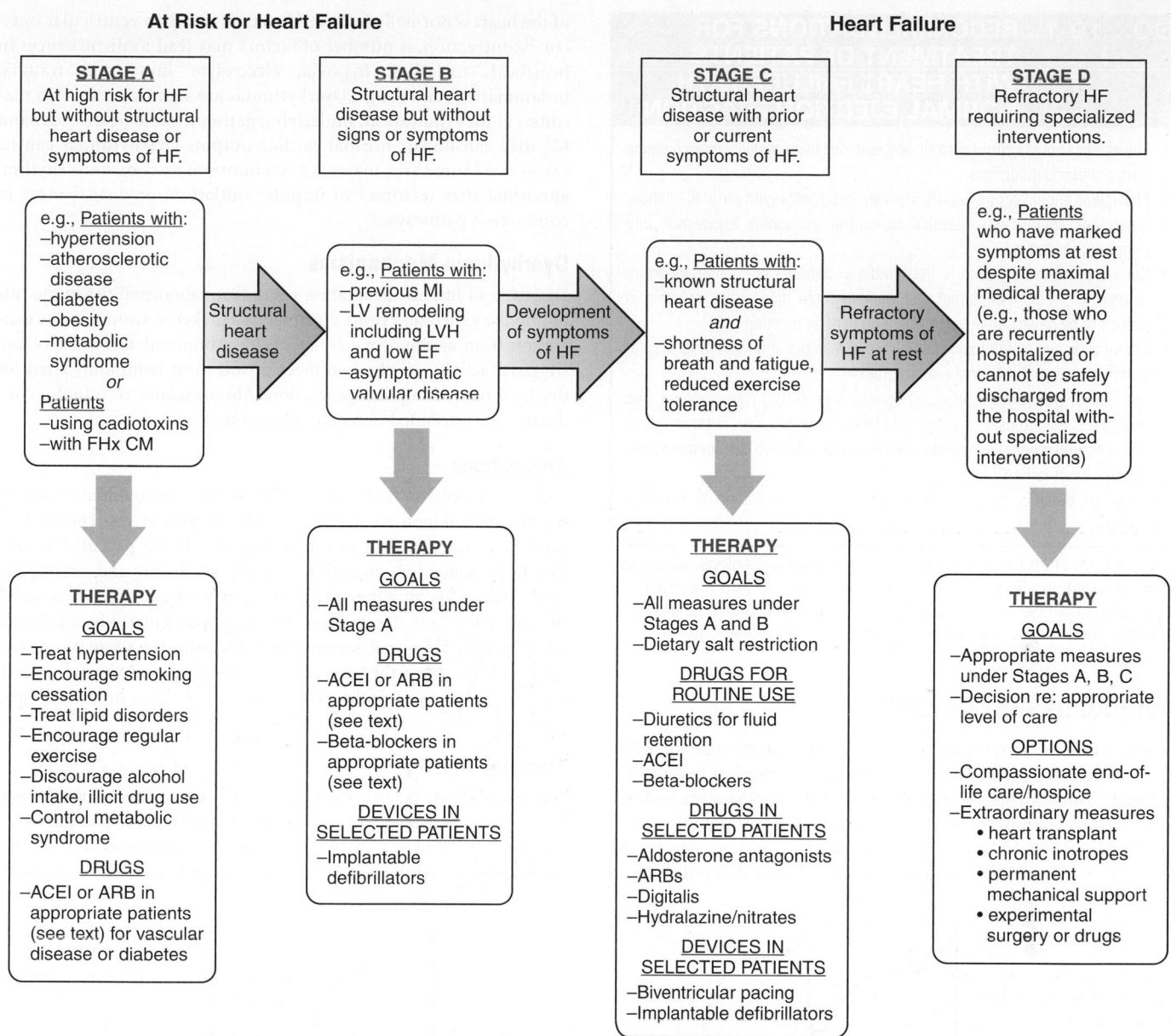

FIGURE 19-13 Stages of heart failure and recommended therapy according to stage. *ACEI,* Angiotensin-converting enzyme inhibitor; *ARB,* angiotensin receptor blocker; *FHx CM,* family history of cardiomyopathy. (From Hunt SA et al: American College of Cardiology; American Heart Association: 2009 focused update incorporated into the ACC/AHA 2005 guidelines for the diagnosis and management of heart failure in adults: summary article, *J Am Coll Cardiol* 53[15]:e3-e62, 2009.)

Little research has been conducted to determine the best treatment for patients with HF and normal EF who have primarily diastolic failure. The effectiveness of renin-angiotensin-aldosterone system blocking agents, β_1-blockers, and digitalis in this population is not well established. Treatment goals are aimed at controlling etiologic factors, such as hypertension and rhythm abnormalities, as well as managing symptoms (Box 19-1).

KEY POINTS
- The primary aims of treatment are to improve cardiac output, minimize congestive symptoms, and prevent progression.
- ACE inhibitors, ARBs, and some β_1-blocking agents have been shown to improve mortality risk in patients with HF characterized by low EF.

- Diuretics alleviate congestive symptoms and reduce cardiac workload by reducing preload.
- Myocardial contractility may be improved acutely by positive inotropic drugs, such as β agonists; however, long-term use is associated with higher mortality. An exception is digitalis, which has positive inotropic effects, does not appear to alter mortality, and may improve symptoms in some patients.
- Resynchronization of ventricular depolarization with pacemakers may improve contraction in patients with wide QRS complexes.
- Few studies are available to guide therapy in patients with HF characterized by normal EF. Efforts to improve etiologic factors, such as atherosclerosis, hypertension, type 2 diabetes, and atrial dysrhythmias, are recommended.

Adapted from Hunt SA et al: American College of Cardiology; American Heart Association: 2009 focused update incorporated into the ACC/AHA 2005 guidelines for the diagnosis and management of heart failure in adults: summary article, *J Am Coll Cardiol* 53(15):e3-e62, 2009.

CARDIAC DYSRHYTHMIAS

Dysrhythmia or arrhythmia refers to a cardiac rhythm abnormality affecting impulse generation or conduction. A normal heartbeat is initiated at an appropriate rate in the sinoatrial (SA) node and follows a consistent pathway of depolarization through the atria, atrioventricular (AV) node, His-Purkinje system, and, finally, the ventricular myocardium (see Chapter 17). Electrical depolarization of the heart is normally followed by atrial and then ventricular muscular contraction. A number of factors may lead to disturbances in heartbeat, including hypoxia, electrolyte imbalance, trauma, inflammation, and drugs. Dysrhythmias are significant for two reasons: (1) they indicate an underlying pathophysiologic disorder and (2) they can impair normal cardiac output. Dysrhythmias can be categorized into three major types: abnormal rates of sinus rhythm, abnormal sites (ectopic) of impulse initiation, or disturbances in conduction pathways.

Dysrhythmia Mechanisms

Disorders of impulse generation result from abnormalities in the *rate* of impulse generation from a normal pacemaker or from impulse generation from an abnormal *(ectopic)* site. Abnormal automaticity and triggered activity are the two mechanisms most commonly cited for dysrhythmias of impulse generation. Abnormalities of impulse conduction are attributed to reentry phenomena.

Automaticity

Failure to repolarize to normal resting membrane potential or plasma membrane leakiness to sodium or calcium ions at rest (phase 4) is thought to cause a shift in the resting membrane potential toward threshold, generating an action potential. Ischemia and subsequent ATP deficiency reduce the cell's ability to control electrolyte flux across the cell membrane. Electrolyte imbalance, particularly hypokalemia, contributes to abnormal automaticity. Alterations in spontaneous calcium ion flux from the sarcoplasmic reticulum and the subsequent triggering of calcium influx across the plasma membrane may also contribute to abnormal automaticity (see Chapter 17).

Triggered Activity

Triggered activity occurs when an impulse is generated during or just after repolarization because of a depolarizing oscillation of the membrane potential (Figure 19-14). Early afterdepolarizations occur during the relative refractory period of phase 3 in patients with abnormally

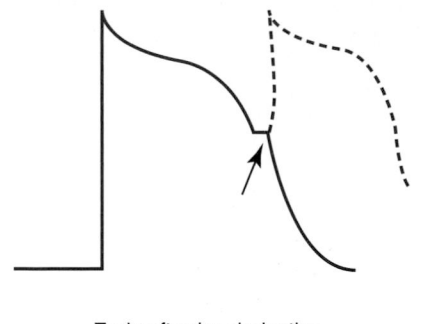
Early afterdepolarization

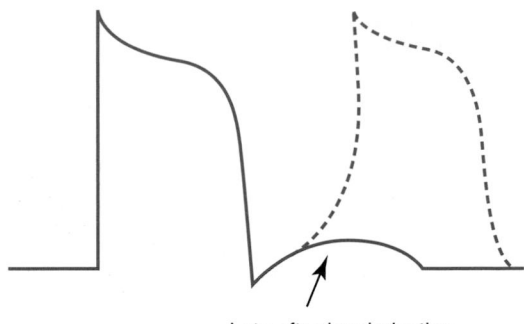
Late afterdepolarization

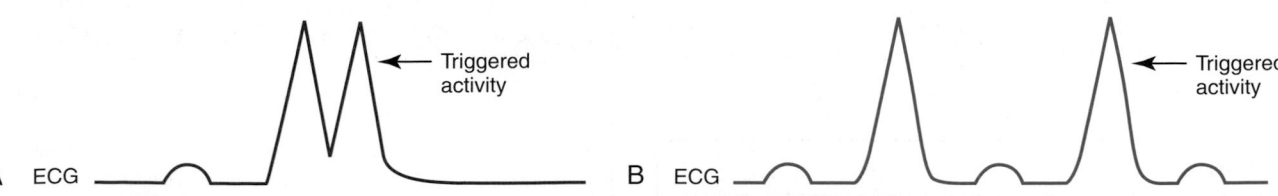

A ECG — Triggered activity

B ECG — Triggered activity

FIGURE 19-14 Mechanisms of triggered activity. **A,** Early afterdepolarization in ventricular cell showing triggered action potential during the repolarization phase. The electrocardiogram *(ECG)* shows an R wave occurring on top of the T wave (R-on-T phenomenon). **B,** Late or delayed afterdepolarization occurs after the repolarization phase has been completed and results in an early beat after the T wave. If the late afterdepolarization does not reach threshold, no triggered beat will occur.

long repolarization times (prolonged QT syndrome). The prolonged action potential is thought to allow some of the voltage-gated calcium channels to reopen during phase 3 and trigger another impulse[18] (see Figure 19-14, *A*). Delayed or late afterdepolarizations occur after the repolarization phase is complete and are seen as oscillating depolarizing waves on the ECG (see Figure 19-14, *B*). If the delayed afterdepolarization reaches threshold, it will trigger an action potential. Digitalis toxicity and excessive catecholamine stimulation may contribute to this mechanism. Delayed afterdepolarizations are thought to occur because calcium ions are spontaneously released from the sarcoplasmic reticulum after repolarization. An increase in intracellular free Ca^{2+} concentration during phase 4 can trigger Ca^{2+} influx across the plasma membrane and release more Ca^{2+} from the sarcoplasmic reticulum, resulting in an action potential.[18] A number of genetic abnormalities in intracellular calcium handling have been associated with triggered activity mechanisms.

Reentry

Reentry is thought to be the culprit in most tachydysrhythmias, including atrial and ventricular tachycardia, flutter, and fibrillation. Reentry is a complex process in which a cardiac impulse continues to depolarize in a part of the heart after the main impulse has finished its path and the majority of the fibers have repolarized. If the errant impulse proceeds slowly enough, it may eventually meet with nonrefractory cells and initiate an extra, ectopic cardiac depolarization. Reentry processes are produced when electrical conduction in a portion of the heart is abnormally slowed (functional) or has an unusually long pathway (anatomic). A number of theories have been proposed to describe the generation and conduction of reentry depolarizations including specific subsets of cells that continue to produce waves of activation or more general involvement of the myocardial tissue in propagating waves of conduction. The rate of conduction is controlled in part by the density and structure of gap junctions that connect the cardiac cells together. Recall that a wave of depolarization moves from cell to cell through these gap junctions; however, different regions of the heart may have different gap junction properties that predispose to different conduction rates. Mutations in the genes that code for gap junction proteins (connexins) may increase the predisposition to dysrhythmias.[19] Reentry depolarizations may

occur as complex spiral waves in which the activating wavefront follows or "chases" its repolarizing tail (Figure 19-15). If the wavefront encounters only refractory tissue, the reentrant process suddenly terminates.[19] Myocardial ischemia and electrolyte abnormalities predispose to reentry mechanisms.

Dysrhythmia Analysis

ECG recording paper is specifically designed to allow easy measurement of waveform amplitude and duration (Figure 19-16). Each small box on the ECG paper represents an amplitude of 0.1 mV and a duration of 0.04 second (paper speed at 25 mm/sec).[20] Larger boxes are also marked on the paper and correspond to 0.5 mV in amplitude (five small boxes) and 0.2 second in duration (five small boxes). These markings allow measurement of waveform amplitude, duration, and heart rate. Rhythm strips presented in this chapter are from a single lead only (usually lead II), but it should be emphasized that thorough ECG interpretation often requires several leads to provide different views of electrical conduction through the heart. (Lead placement is discussed in Chapter 17.)

Normal Sinus Rhythm

Before one proceeds to the interpretation of dysrhythmias, the features of normal sinus rhythm must be understood. Normal sinus rhythm is generally defined as an impulse rate between 60 and 100 per minute that begins in the sinus node and follows the normal conduction pathway. Characteristics of normal sinus rhythm are listed in Table 19-3. The rhythm shown in Figure 19-17 is regular; there is a P wave for every QRS complex; the PR, QRS, and QT intervals are of normal duration; and there are no "funny-looking" beats.

There are several methods for determining heart rate using the rhythm strip. The easiest but least accurate method is to count the number of QRS complexes within 6 seconds and multiply by 10. Electrocardiogram (ECG) paper has 3 second marks along the top that can be used to determine a 6-second interval. A more accurate method for determining heart rate is to count the number of small boxes between complexes. The number of boxes is divided by 1500 to determine heart rate because there are 1500 small boxes per minute (1500 × 0.04 second = 60 seconds). Neither of these methods is accurate with irregular rhythms,

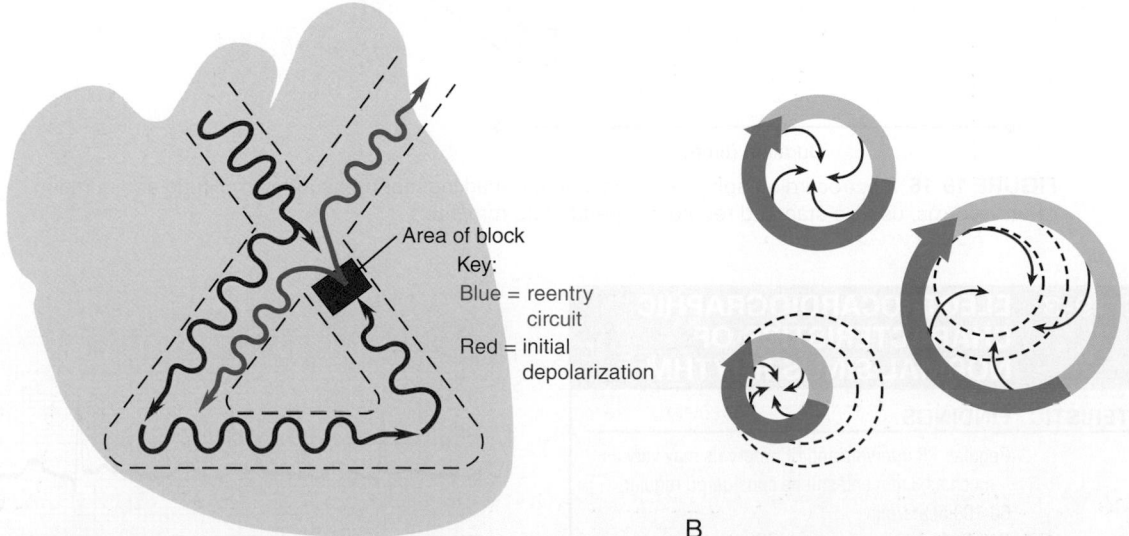

A   B

FIGURE 19-15 Mechanism of reentry. **A,** A wave of depolarization that travels slowly or by an abnormal pathway may encounter myocardium that has had time to recover and can restimulate it. **B,** This may result in an extra beat, or the depolarization may continuously "chase its tail" in a circuit, causing defibrillation. The circuit can be relatively fixed or can wander into various "wavelets."

so heart rate must be calculated for a longer interval, usually 1 minute. With this understanding of rate calculation and methods to measure the duration and amplitude of waveforms, one can analyze dysrhythmias.

KEY POINTS

- Dysrhythmias are initiated by three types of depolarizing mechanisms: abnormal automaticity, triggered activity from afterdepolarizations, and reentrant circuits.
- Measurement of ECG waveform amplitude, duration, and frequency is necessary to analyze cardiac rhythms. ECG paper is marked in small boxes representing 0.1 mV of amplitude and 0.04 second of duration.
- Normal sinus rhythm is characterized by regular PP and RR intervals, a rate of 60 to 100 beats/min, and normal PR (0.12 to 0.20 second) and QRS (0.04 to 0.10 second) intervals.

Abnormal Rates of Sinus Rhythm
Sinus Tachycardia

Sinus tachycardia is an abnormally fast heart rate of greater than 100 beats/min (Figure 19-18). A number of factors, including sympathetic activation, decreased parasympathetic activity, fever, hyperthyroidism, pain, increased metabolism, low blood pressure, and hypoxia, can lead to sinus tachycardia, making it a very common dysrhythmia. Sinus tachycardia often is a compensatory response to increased demand for cardiac output or reduced stroke volume. Treatment is aimed at correcting the underlying cause. In some instances, however, the rate can become so high that ventricular filling is impaired and cardiac output is compromised. The heart rate at which this occurs will vary depending on age and cardiac function. Sympatholytic agents or calcium channel–blocking agents may then be indicated.

Sinus Bradycardia

Traditionally a heart rate of less than 60 beats/min is called *bradycardia;* however, lower rates are commonly encountered in physically trained individuals. Sinus bradycardia results from slowed impulse generation by the sinus node in response to increased parasympathetic activity, sleep, drugs, increased stroke volume, or acute hypertension (baroreceptor reflex). Important features of sinus bradycardia are shown in Figure 19-19. Sinus bradycardia may be a normal finding in well-conditioned individuals who have large resting stroke volumes. Abnormal parasympathetic activation can result from pain (vasovagal response), carotid sinus massage, endotracheal suctioning, and the Valsalva maneuver (bearing down). Slow heart rates may be well tolerated by some individuals and not require treatment. If the slow heart rate precipitates low cardiac output, it is usually treated with sympathomimetic or parasympatholytic drugs.

Sinus Arrhythmia

A degree of variability in the heart rate, or sinus arrhythmia, is a normal finding associated with fluctuations in autonomic influences and respiratory dynamics. Sinus arrhythmia can be particularly pronounced in children. Sinus arrhythmia must be differentiated from a sinus node irregularity called *sick sinus syndrome,* in which alternating periods of sinus bradycardia and tachycardia occur (Figure 19-20). Sick sinus syndrome may necessitate implantation of a permanent pacemaker. Sinus arrhythmia is a normal finding and thus requires no treatment.

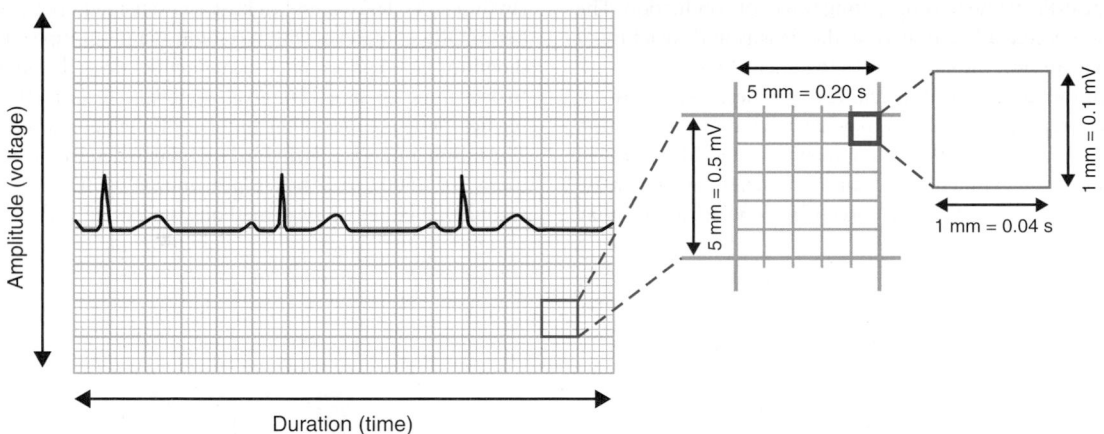

FIGURE 19-16 Electrocardiographic strip showing the markings for measuring amplitude and duration of waveforms, using a standard recording speed of 25 mm/sec.

TABLE 19-3	ELECTROCARDIOGRAPHIC CHARACTERISTICS OF NORMAL SINUS RHYTHM
CHARACTERISTIC	**FINDINGS**
Rhythm	Regular, PP intervals and RR intervals may vary as much as 3 mm and still be considered regular
Rate	60-100 beats/min
P waves	One P wave preceding each QRS
PR interval	0.12-0.20 sec, constant
QRS duration	0.04-0.10 sec, constant
QT interval	0.40 sec (varies with rate)

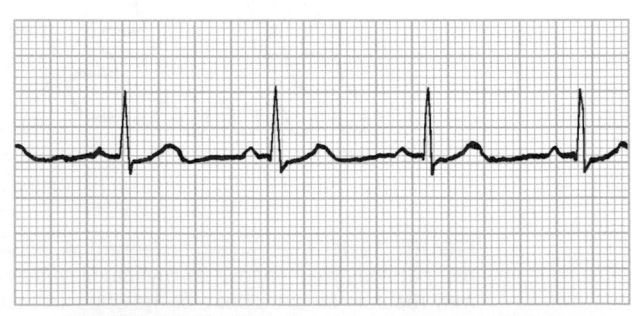

FIGURE 19-17 Normal sinus rhythm (rate, 64/min).

Sinus Arrest

The absence of impulse initiation in the heart results in electrical *asystole*. It is characterized by a flat ECG lacking recognizable waveforms (Figure 19-21). Electrical asystole results in mechanical asystole and zero cardiac output. An escape rhythm from a slower pacemaker will generally begin to fire after several seconds of sinus arrest. Sinus arrest may result from MI, electrical shock, electrolyte disturbances, acidosis, and extreme parasympathetic activity. Prolonged complete electrical asystole is unlikely, and fine ventricular fibrillation may be the underlying rhythm. Sinus arrest may be treatable with a cardiac pacemaker.

> ### KEY POINTS
> - Sinus tachycardia (more than 100 beats/min) usually occurs from sympathetic activation of the heart. SNS activation may be compensatory (e.g., occurring in the setting of low blood pressure, low cardiac output, or hypoxemia) or may be due to pain and anxiety.
> - Sinus bradycardia (less than 60 beats/min) usually occurs in response to parasympathetic activity. Bradycardia is treated if the slow heart rate precipitates inadequate cardiac output.
> - Sinus arrhythmia is usually normal and more pronounced in young persons than in older adults.
> - Sinus arrest may lead to prolonged intervals of electrical asystole and zero stroke volume until another pacemaker begins to fire. An artificial pacemaker may be required.

Abnormal Site of Impulse Initiation

Initiation of a cardiac impulse at a site other than the SA node occurs primarily for two reasons. First, SA node failure may allow a slower pacemaker to take over. Takeover by a slower pacemaker is called an *escape rhythm*. Second, enhanced excitability, triggered activity, or reentrant circuits may cause a premature depolarization and override the SA node.

Escape Rhythms

Escape beats can originate in the AV nodal region or in the ventricular Purkinje fibers. A junctional escape rhythm originates in the AV node, has a rate of 40 to 60 per minute, and has a normal QRS configuration (Figure 19-22). A ventricular escape rhythm originates in the Purkinje fibers, has a rate of 15 to 40 per minute, and is characterized by an abnormally wide QRS complex on the ECG (Figure 19-23). An important clue to identifying escape rhythms is the absence of normal P waves and PR intervals. After the impulse is generated in the Purkinje or nodal cell, it can be conducted backward to the atria (retrograde P wave). Thus, a P wave, if present, may be inverted and located before,

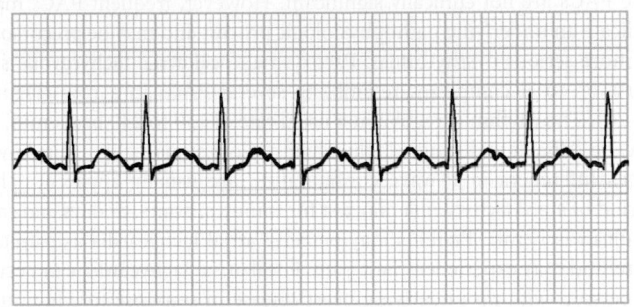

FIGURE 19-18 Sinus tachycardia (rate, 150/min).

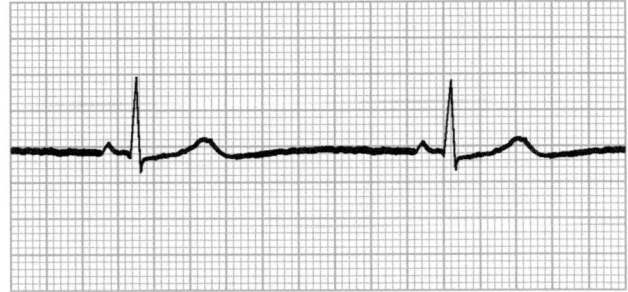

FIGURE 19-19 Sinus bradycardia (rate, 35/min).

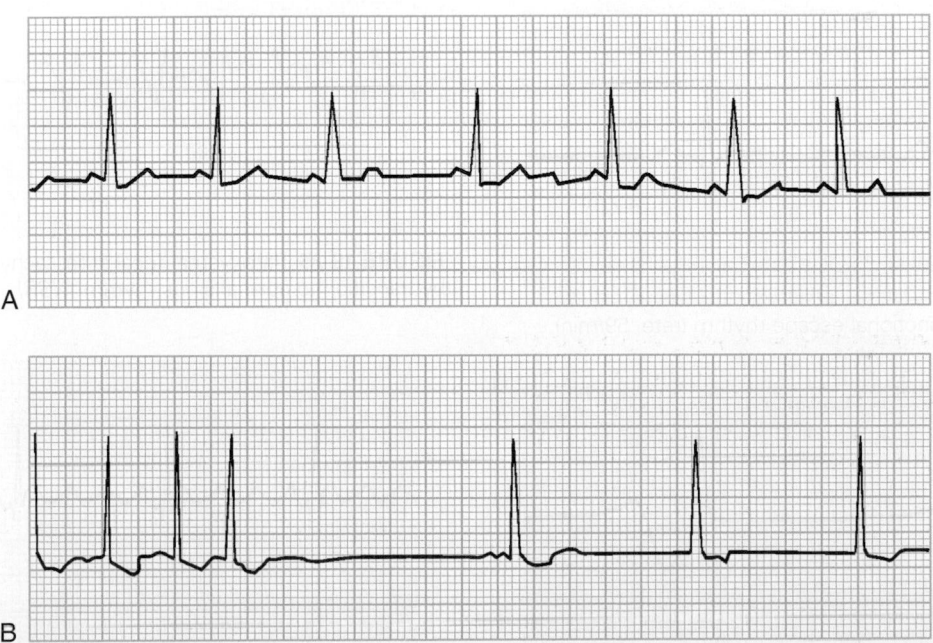

FIGURE 19-20 A, Sinus arrhythmia is a normal finding that may be particularly pronounced in children. **B,** Sick sinus syndrome. The strip shows alternating periods of tachycardia and bradycardia.

during, or after the QRS complex. Escape rhythms are usually poorly tolerated because they are slow and associated with decreased cardiac output. Failure of the sinus node can be managed with a pacemaker.

Atrial Dysrhythmias

Premature atrial complexes and tachycardia. Premature atrial complexes (PACs) originate in the atria but not at the SA node. The PAC occurs earlier than normal, is preceded by a P wave, and has a normal QRS configuration (Figure 19-24). P waves preceding the PAC usually have a different shape (morphology) than the sinus beats. Sometimes the PAC is not conducted through the AV node to the ventricle and is not followed by a QRS complex (nonconducted P wave). Isolated or rare PACs are not clinically significant. However, frequent PACs may indicate an underlying pathophysiologic process and may be precursors to more serious dysrhythmias. Paroxysmal focal atrial tachycardia is a burst of atrial complexes resembling several PACs in a row (Figure 19-25). The rhythm is regular at a usual rate of 130 to 240 beats/min. It may be difficult to distinguish this rhythm from sinus tachycardia; however, differences in P-wave configuration are usually apparent. The period of atrial tachycardia may last for minutes, hours, or days and can result in ischemia. Patients may perceive atrial tachycardia as palpitations and may experience chest pain. Focal atrial tachycardia can occur in persons with no underlying heart disease in response to emotional stress or drugs. An episode may start as a PAC that has an abnormally

slow conduction time through the atria and AV node. This is thought to allow the wave of depolarization to reexcite previously depolarized cells, resulting in reentry and perpetuation of the abnormal rhythm.

Atrial flutter and fibrillation. **Atrial flutter** is typically manifested by a rapid atrial rate of 240 to 350 beats/min and a characteristic sawtooth pattern of atrial depolarizations (Figure 19-26). There is overlap in the mechanism of atrial tachycardia and atrial flutter, and several types of flutter have been described. These are commonly categorized according to atrial rate; type I (typical) has rates of 240 to 350 beats per minute, and type II has rates in excess of 350 beats per minute. The QRS configuration is normal; however, some of the atrial depolarizations do not conduct through the AV node, resulting in a slower ventricular rate. The ventricular rate may be irregular if there is a variable block or may be regular if there is a uniform block, such as 2:1 or 3:1. Reentry is the probable mechanism for typical atrial flutter. Persons exhibiting atrial flutter usually have underlying heart disease, fluid overload, or atrial ischemia.

Atrial fibrillation is a completely disorganized and irregular atrial rhythm accompanied by an irregular ventricular rhythm of variable rate (Figure 19-27). The atrial impulses appear as small, squiggly waves of

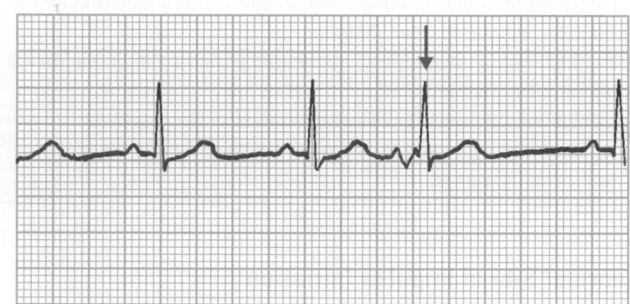

FIGURE 19-24 Premature atrial complex *(arrow)*. Note early P wave and different P wave morphology.

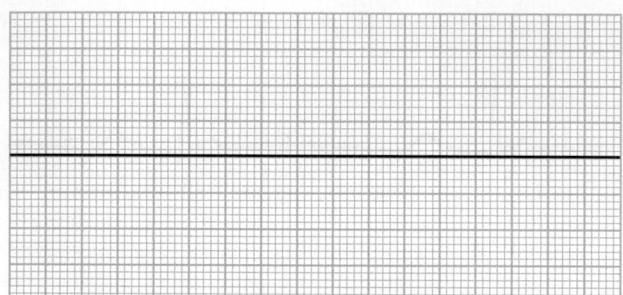

FIGURE 19-21 Electrical asystole.

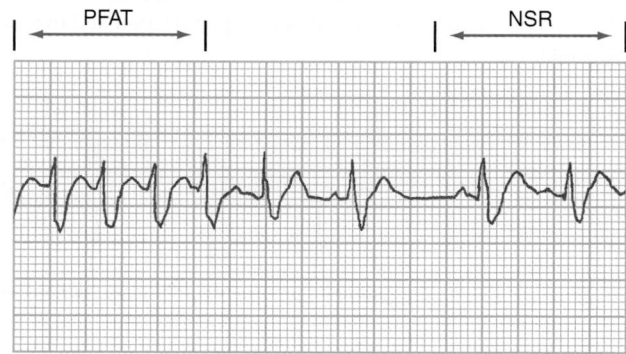

FIGURE 19-25 Paroxysmal focal atrial tachycardia *(PFAT)* followed by transition to normal sinus rhythm *(NSR)*.

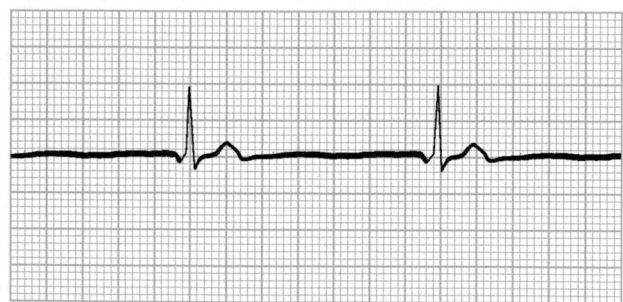

FIGURE 19-22 Junctional escape rhythm (rate, 59/min).

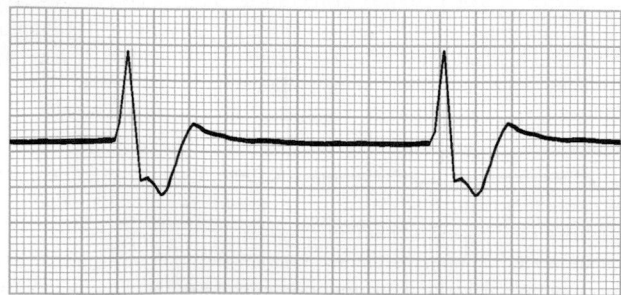

FIGURE 19-23 Ventricular escape rhythm (rate, 33/min).

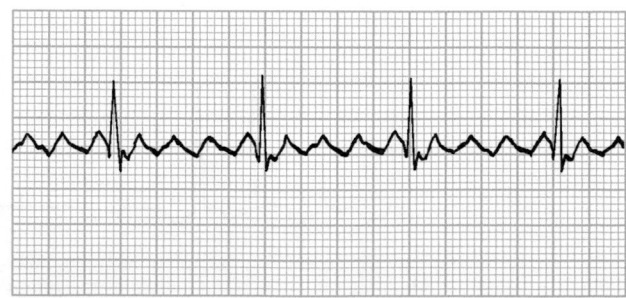

FIGURE 19-26 Atrial flutter with four atrial depolarizations to one ventricular depolarization.

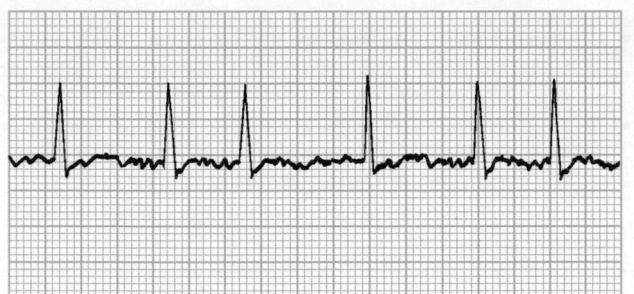

FIGURE 19-27 Atrial fibrillation showing an irregularly irregular ventricular response.

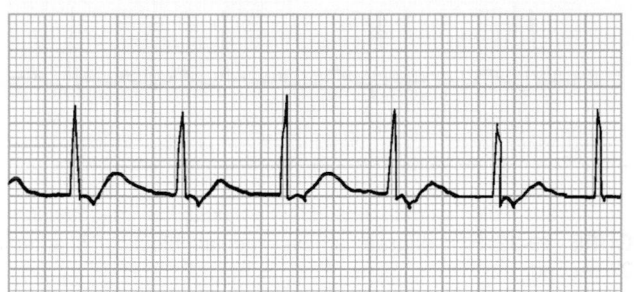

FIGURE 19-28 Junctional tachycardia (rate, 108/min). Note that P waves follow the QRS waves because of retrograde depolarization spreading from the atrioventricular node to the atria. This rhythm may also be called supraventricular tachycardia.

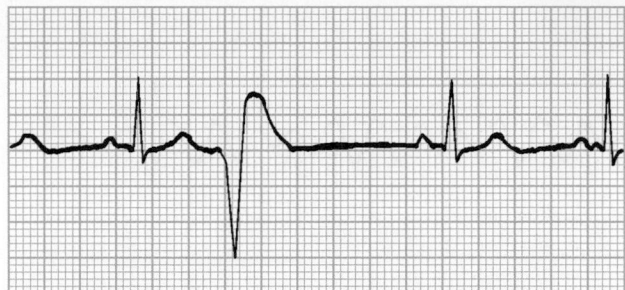

FIGURE 19-29 Premature ventricular complex.

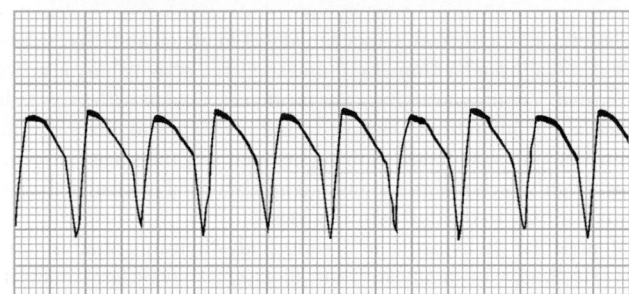

FIGURE 19-30 Ventricular tachycardia (rate, 178/min).

various sizes and shapes. Atrial fibrillation is sustained by multiple reentrant "wavelets" that continually change in size and direction. The majority of atrial depolarizations are blocked at the AV node, with few reaching the ventricles and initiating ventricular contraction. Atrial fibrillation causes the atria to quiver rather than to contract forcefully. This allows blood to become stagnant in the atria and may lead to formation of thrombi. Atrial fibrillation may occur intermittently or be sustained in the long term. Patients with chronic atrial fibrillation often are treated with anticoagulant medications to prevent atrial clot formation. Atrial fibrillation is a significant risk factor for cerebrovascular stroke. Patients with heart failure may experience more symptoms when they are in atrial fibrillation because the usual "atrial kick" that normally adds 15% to 20% more blood to the ventricle before systole is lost and therefore cardiac output may be reduced. Cardioversion with an electrical shock to the chest is commonly used to manage atrial fibrillation. Numerous antidysrhythmic agents can be used to convert atrial fibrillation to sinus rhythm or control the ventricular response rate, including calcium channel blockers, β-blockers, digitalis, and amiodarone.

Junctional Dysrhythmias

Premature junctional complexes can be initiated in two junctional zones: in the area just proximal to the AV node, where atrial fibers enter; or in the area just distal to the AV node, where nodal fibers enter the bundle of His. The impulse spreads upward into the atrium, causing a P wave, and downward into the ventricle, causing a normally configured QRS complex. The P wave may precede, follow, or be buried in the QRS complex. Premature junctional beats have the same clinical significance as PACs and are generally well tolerated.

Junctional tachycardia is a rapid junctional discharge in the range of 70 to 140 beats/min (Figure 19-28). The rhythm resembles a series of junctional premature beats, with P waves preceding, following, or buried in the QRS complexes. Differentiation of the electrocardiographic pattern produced by junctional tachycardia from that

produced by atrial tachycardia is often difficult, and the term *supraventricular tachycardia* may be used for both.

Ventricular Dysrhythmias

Premature ventricular complexes. Premature ventricular complexes (PVCs) arise from the ventricular myocardium. The impulse depolarizes the ventricles but does not activate the atria or depolarize the sinus node. Thus, the normal rhythm of sinus discharge is not disturbed. The normal sinus impulse is generally buried in the bizarre-looking QRS complex from the premature ventricular beat. The sinus impulse does not result in a QRS complex because the ventricles are refractory from the premature depolarization. The next sinus beat occurs just when it would have occurred normally if there had been no premature beat. Thus, the interval between the sinus beat preceding the premature beat and the sinus beat following the premature beat is twice the regular interval (Figure 19-29). This is known as a *compensatory pause* and helps confirm the diagnosis of PVCs. The QRS of the premature complex is prolonged (more than 0.10 second) and bizarre in appearance. The T wave is usually in a direction opposite to the main QRS deflection. Premature ventricular beats are commonly associated with coronary artery disease, drug overdose, and electrolyte disturbances—particularly hypokalemia and hypomagnesemia. The clinical significance depends in part on the frequency of the premature beats. The PVCs may occur at regular intervals, such as bigeminy (every other beat) or trigeminy (every third beat). With high frequency, cardiac output may be compromised. Frequent PVCs may be managed with antidysrhythmic drugs, such as amiodarone. However, prophylactic use of antidysrhythmic drugs in patients with asymptomatic disease is not recommended. In some groups (e.g., after MI), certain antidysrhythmics have been linked to higher mortality.[19]

Ventricular tachycardia. Ventricular tachycardia consists of 3 or more consecutive ventricular complexes at a rate greater than 100 beats/min (Figure 19-30). The rhythm is fairly regular, and the complexes generally have the same configuration (monomorphic). With rapid rates, it may be difficult to distinguish the QRS complexes from the ST segments and T waves, and the ECG depicts a series of large, wide, undulating waves. The sinus node usually continues to discharge independently of the ventricular rhythm, and P waves, if seen, are not associated with the QRS complexes.

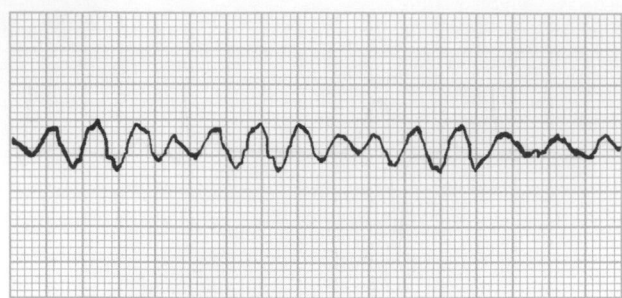

FIGURE 19-31 Ventricular fibrillation.

Reentry is the probable mechanism of ventricular tachycardia in most cases, although automaticity and triggered activity have also been implicated. Ventricular tachycardia is often associated with myocardial ischemia and infarction. Damage to the myocardium alters conduction times and conduction pathways, which sets the stage for reentry loops. High catecholamine levels and an abnormal electrolyte balance may contribute to the dysrhythmogenesis.

Ventricular tachycardia is a serious dysrhythmia that is nearly always indicative of significant heart disease. It may be fatal unless it is successfully and rapidly managed. Ventricular tachycardia may compromise cardiac output, resulting in loss of consciousness. Treatment consists of administration of antidysrhythmic drugs and, if necessary, cardiopulmonary resuscitation and electrical cardioversion.

Ventricular fibrillation. Ventricular fibrillation is a rapid, uncoordinated cardiac rhythm that results in ventricular quivering and lack of effective contraction. The rhythm is generally easily identified, particularly when assessment of the patient indicates absence of pulse and loss of consciousness. The ECG is rapid and erratic, with no identifiable QRS complexes (Figure 19-31). Ventricular fibrillation results in death if not reversed within minutes.

The same conditions that result in ventricular tachycardia may cause ventricular fibrillation. A critically timed premature beat or accelerating ventricular tachycardia may be the precursor to ventricular fibrillation. The ventricular depolarization is thought to be fractionated into a number of localized reentrant currents within the myocardial mass. The uncoordinated depolarizations are sustained because of variability in conduction velocities and refractory periods.

Ventricular fibrillation must be rapidly identified and managed with cardiopulmonary resuscitation and defibrillation with electrical current. Defibrillation differs from cardioversion in that the administration of current is not synchronized with the R wave and the amount of energy delivered is greater (200 to 350 J). The earlier the defibrillation is performed, the better is the chance for successful resuscitation. In some instances, the ventricular fibrillation pattern is very fine and is similar to the tracing seen in atrial arrest. Defibrillation is still indicated. Defibrillation and cardiopulmonary resuscitation are usually followed by administration of antidysrhythmic drugs.

KEY POINTS

- Failure of the SA node to generate impulses may result in a junctional or ventricular escape rhythm. These rhythms are slow and may be poorly tolerated. Absence of P waves is important in determination of escape rhythms.
- In most cases, premature beats and ectopic rhythms are attributed to reentry mechanisms. Reentry circuits may be established when portions of the heart have abnormal conduction rates or pathways. Enhanced automaticity and triggered activity are alternative mechanisms for generation of ectopic complexes.

- Atrial dysrhythmias include premature atrial complexes, tachycardia, flutter, and fibrillation. Atrial dysrhythmias are usually well tolerated unless the ventricular response rate is significantly altered.
- Junctional tachycardias are difficult to distinguish from atrial tachycardias and they are often regarded together as supraventricular tachycardias.
- Frequent PVCs, ventricular tachycardia, and ventricular fibrillation are associated with a significant fall in cardiac output and must be rapidly diagnosed and managed.

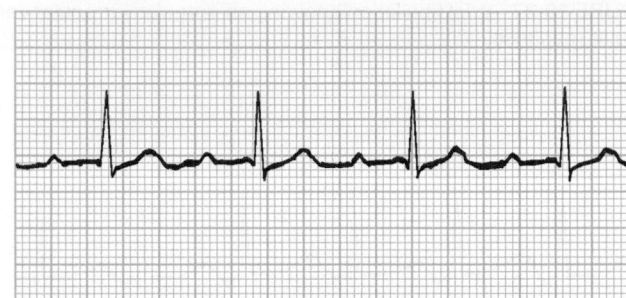

FIGURE 19-32 First-degree atrioventricular block. PR interval, 0.32 second.

Conduction Pathway Disturbances

Disorders of cardiac impulse conduction include delays, blocks, and abnormal pathways. Cardiac ischemia and infarction commonly are associated with conduction blocks and delays, whereas abnormal pathways are usually congenital.

Disturbances of Atrioventricular Conduction

A disturbance in conduction between the sinus impulse and its associated ventricular response has been called *atrioventricular block.* The conduction may be abnormally slowed or completely blocked. The AV block results from a functional or pathologic defect in the AV node, bundle of His, or bundle branches. Three categories of AV block have traditionally been described: first-degree block, second-degree block (which includes types I and II), and third-degree (complete) block. These AV conduction disorders are associated with different pathologic processes and clinical implications.

First-degree block is generally identified by a prolonged PR interval (more than 0.20 second) on the ECG (Figure 19-32). The rhythm remains regular, and each P wave is associated with a QRS complex. First-degree block is a common finding and may occur in the absence of organic heart disease. Drugs and organic heart disorders, such as myocardial ischemia and congenital heart defects, may cause first-degree block. First-degree block is generally monitored but is not actively managed except to alleviate the underlying cause if possible.

Second-degree block is diagnosed when some of the atrial impulses are not conducted to the ventricles. Two types of second-degree block are identified by the pattern of nonconducted impulses. Type I (Mobitz type I, Wenckebach) is associated with progressively lengthening PR intervals until one P wave is not conducted (dropped beat). The pattern repeats, causing the QRS complexes to occur in groups. The PP intervals are constant, whereas the RR intervals vary (Figure 19-33). Type I second-degree block is usually due to reversible ischemia of the AV node, often associated with acute MI. The ischemic node is slow to recover after each depolarization, resulting in a longer and longer nodal delay until one impulse is not conducted. This gives the AV node time to recover, and the next atrial impulse is conducted more quickly, with a nearly normal PR interval, beginning the cycle again. Treatment

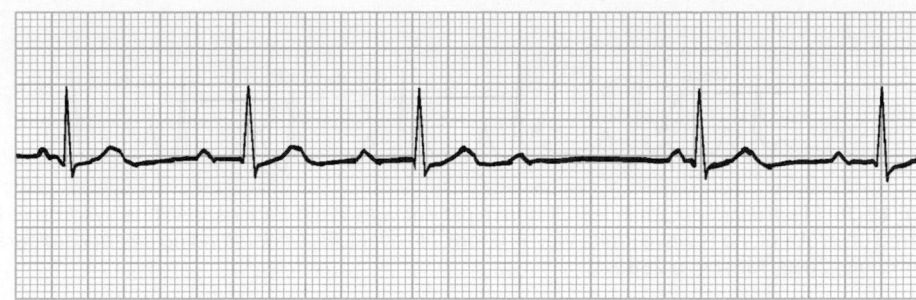

FIGURE 19-33 Second-degree atrioventricular block, type I (Wenckebach, Mobitz type I). Note the progressive lengthening of the PR interval until one P wave is not conducted (dropped).

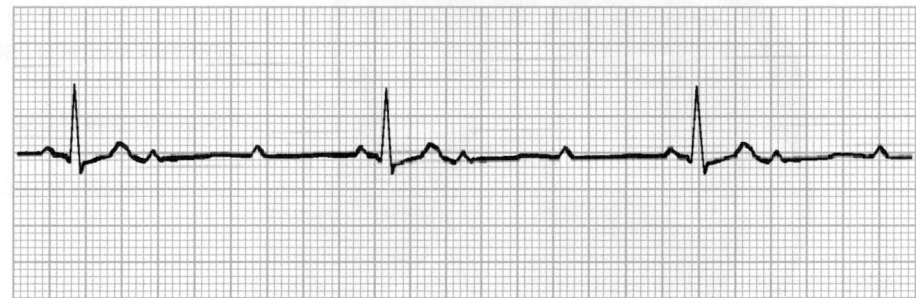

FIGURE 19-34 Second-degree atrioventricular (AV) block, type II (Mobitz type II). Every third P wave is followed by a QRS complex. The other P waves are not conducted through the AV node. The PR interval on conducted impulses is constant.

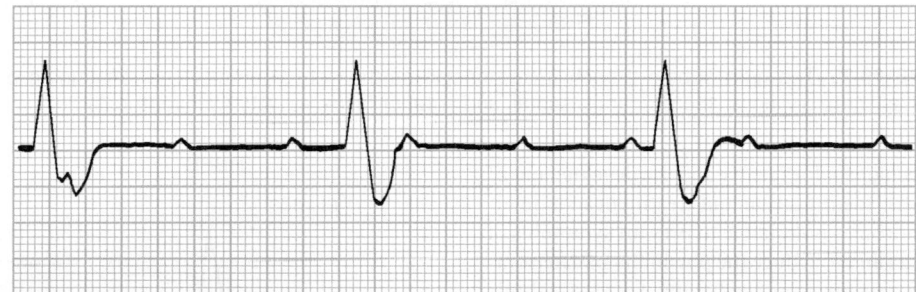

FIGURE 19-35 Complete third-degree atrioventricular block. Note that there is no relationship between P waves and QRS complexes because the atria and ventricles are depolarizing independently.

is rarely required. If the block progresses to a type II block, a pacemaker may be required.

Type II second-degree block is identified by the presence of nonconducted P waves (dropped beats) with a consistent PR interval (Figure 19-34). The QRS complex is usually, but not always, wide (0.12 second or greater). Type II block is generally associated with pathologic lesion of the bundle of His, the right bundle branch, or both. It is the bundle branch block that causes the QRS complexes to be abnormally wide. Type II second-degree block is less common than type I but is more serious. It is usually associated with anterior septal MI or fibrosis of the conduction system. Type II block may progress to complete heart block with slow ventricular escape rhythm and poor cardiac output. Type II block may also result in severe bradycardia because of the number of dropped beats. Symptomatic type II block may require implantation of a pacemaker.

Third-degree block may occur as a result of a pathologic lesion of the AV node, bundle of His, or bundle branches. No impulses are conducted from the atria to the ventricles, and a junctional or ventricular escape rhythm is evident. The ECG shows regularly occurring P waves

that are totally independent of the ventricular rhythm (Figure 19-35). If the QRS complex is narrow, the block is most likely in the AV node, proximal to the bundle of His. A prolonged QRS interval (more than 0.12 second) indicates pathology distal to the bundle of His, within the bundle branches. The severity of symptoms is determined primarily by the heart rate, with slower rhythms being more serious. A pacemaker is generally required.

Abnormal Conduction Pathways

Some individuals have congenital abnormalities of the cardiac conduction system called *accessory pathways*. These extra conduction tracts provide alternative pathways for depolarization of the heart, resulting in abnormally early ventricular depolarizations following atrial depolarizations. The best known of these preexcitation syndromes is Wolff-Parkinson-White syndrome. This syndrome is caused by accessory pathways that originate in the atria, bypass the AV node, and enter a site in the ventricular myocardium. This results in more rapid activation of the ventricle, a short PR interval, initial slurring of the QRS (δ wave), and a wide QRS complex (Figure 19-36). The accessory

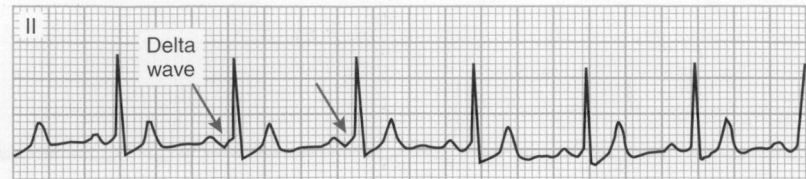

FIGURE 19-36 Electrocardiogram in lead II from a patient with Wolff-Parkinson-White syndrome. Note the slurred upstroke of the R wave (delta wave). (From Conover MB: *Understanding electrocardiography,* ed 8, St Louis, 2003, Mosby, p 288.)

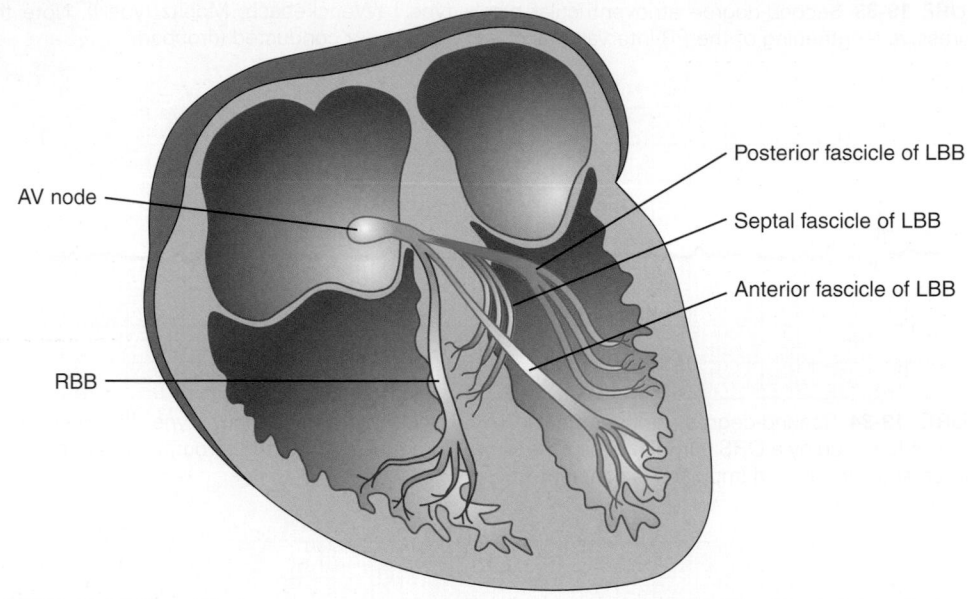

FIGURE 19-37 The right bundle branch *(RBB)* innervates the right ventricle. The left bundle branch *(LBB)* has three divisions: the posterior, septal, and anterior fascicles. *AV,* Atrioventricular.

pathway may provide a mechanism for reentry and the development of supraventricular tachycardia. Identification and treatment of individuals with preexcitation syndromes is desirable to prevent symptoms of supraventricular tachycardia and to reduce the possibility of deterioration of the rhythm to atrial or ventricular fibrillation. Antidysrhythmic agents and measures to interrupt the pathway, such as vagal stimulation or ablation, may be used.

Intraventricular Conduction Defects

Abnormal conduction of impulses through the intraventricular bundle branches is called *bundle branch block.* The two primary bundles are the right bundle branch, which supplies the right ventricle, and the left bundle branch, which supplies the left ventricle. The left bundle branch is further divided into three fascicles: anterior, posterior, and septal (Figure 19-37). These supply the anterior, posterior, and septal portions of the left ventricle, respectively. Slowed or obstructed conduction occurring in one or more of these bundles results in abnormal ventricular depolarization and wide, bizarre-appearing QRS complexes. Bundle branch blocks are best detected with ECG leads V_1 and V_6.

Right bundle branch block may be present in almost any form of heart disease. It is occasionally found in individuals having no clinical evidence of heart disease. Right bundle branch block can progress to complete heart block in some cases. The electrocardiographic pattern is indicative of blocked conduction to the right ventricle such that the left ventricle depolarizes first, then spreads to the right ventricle. Right bundle branch block is classically associated with a late R wave in lead V_1 and an S wave in V_6. These changes are compared with the normal V_1 and V_6 in Figure 19-38.

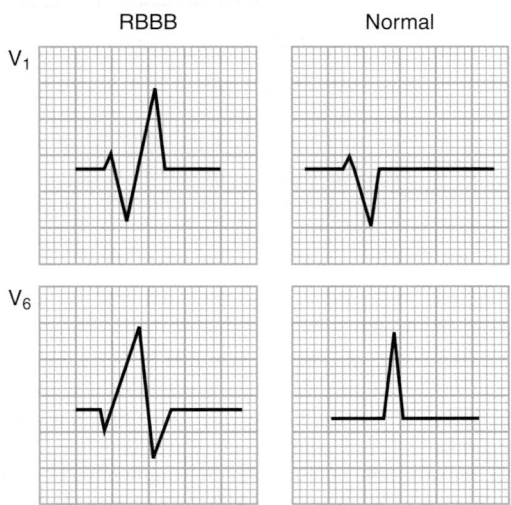

FIGURE 19-38 Right bundle branch block pattern. Note late R wave in V_1 and abnormal S wave in V_6.

Left bundle branch block causes a delay in left ventricular depolarization. The right ventricle is activated first through the right bundle branch, followed by right-to-left activation of the septum and, finally, left ventricular activation. The QRS complex is abnormally wide (more than 0.12 second) but has a nearly normal deflection pattern in V_1 and V_6. In V_1, the small R wave normally associated with septal depolarization is absent, and V_6 consists of a wide R wave (Figure 19-39).

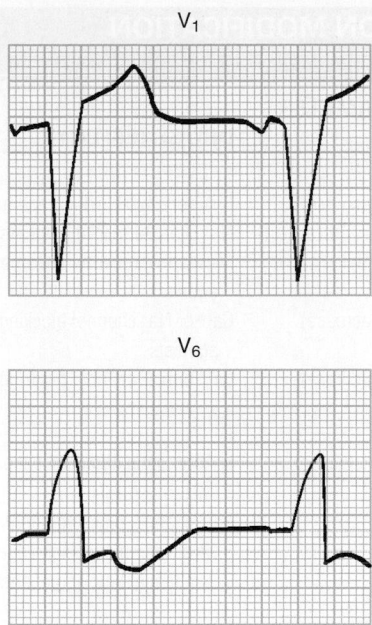

FIGURE 19-39 Left bundle branch block pattern. Note wide S wave in V_1 and wide R wave in V_6.

KEY POINTS

- Disturbances of AV conduction are generally referred to as AV blocks. First-degree block is characterized by a prolonged PR interval and usually requires no treatment.
- Two types of second-degree block have been identified. Type I (Wenckebach) is characterized by progressive prolongation of the PR interval until one P wave is not conducted. Type I block is associated with AV nodal ischemia. Type II second-degree block is identified by a rhythm showing a consistent PR interval with some nonconducted P waves. This block is more serious because it has a tendency to progress to complete AV (third-degree) block.
- Third-degree or complete heart block is diagnosed when there is no apparent association between atrial and ventricular conduction. This rhythm is serious, because it is typically associated with slow ventricular rhythm and poor cardiac output.
- Accessory conduction pathways are suspected in persons exhibiting preexcitation syndromes such as Wolff-Parkinson-White syndrome. Severe tachycardias and other reentrant rhythms may occur.
- Disturbances of intraventricular conduction (bundle branch blocks) are characterized by wide, bizarre-looking QRS complexes. Any of the three ventricular fascicles may be affected (right bundle, left anterior fascicle, or left posterior fascicle).

Left anterior fascicular block is also called *anterior hemiblock*. Impaired conduction in the anterior fascicle causes the posterior aspect of the left ventricle to be activated first, followed by spread through the left ventricular myocardium in an upward and leftward direction. The electrocardiographic pattern shows small initial R waves followed by large S waves in leads II and III. The duration of the QRS complex is within normal limits.

Left posterior fascicular block (hemiblock) is due to a block in the posterior fascicle of the left bundle, which causes the anterior left ventricle to be activated first, followed by spread in a downward and rightward direction. The electrocardiographic findings include Q wave in leads II, III, and aV_F and R wave in leads I and aV_L. These electrocardiographic findings may mimic ventricular hypertrophy or inferolateral MI, making recognition difficult.

Slowed or obstructed conduction may occur simultaneously in more than one bundle or fascicle, leading to the terms *bifascicular block* and *trifascicular block*. For example, a right bundle branch block occurring in conjunction with a left posterior hemiblock is called a *bilateral* or *bifascicular block*. Trifascicular block refers to a bifascicular bundle block (most commonly right bundle branch block with left anterior hemiblock) in addition to a first-degree block (prolonged PR interval). The prolonged PR interval is usually due to incomplete block in the left posterior fascicle. Complete trifascicular block would make it impossible for a supraventricular depolarization to activate the ventricles and would be a third-degree or complete heart block.

Treatment

Dysrhythmias are generally treated if they produce significant symptoms or are expected to progress to a more serious level. A number of antidysrhythmic drugs have proved effective in managing many dysrhythmias; however, most have also been shown to cause dysrhythmias (prodysrhythmic).[19] These drugs alter the properties of ion movement across cardiac membranes and affect automaticity as well as the rate and duration of depolarization and repolarization. The major electrophysiologic classes of antidysrhythmic (antiarrhythmic) compounds are summarized in Table 19-4. Treatment may also include measures to improve cardiac output, including pacemakers and drugs to improve contractility and blood pressure. Dysrhythmias causing severely reduced cardiac output, such as severe bradycardia, asystole, ventricular tachycardia, and ventricular fibrillation, require cardiopulmonary resuscitation until an effective cardiac rhythm is established.

Ablation procedures may be effective in eliminating a focus of dysrhythmia generation if one can be identified. An electrophysiologic study is done to evoke and analyze the dysrhythmia, followed by interruption (ablation) of the area generating it. Ablation is accomplished with high-frequency radio waves (radioablation) or by surgical excision. The electrophysiologic study requires insertion of electrodes directly into the heart by way of a venous or arterial catheter. The electrodes are used to record activity in specific locations and to deliver electric shocks to initiate or terminate an abnormal rhythm.[21] This test is useful in assessing responses to drug therapy and in identifying risk for sudden cardiac arrest. Those at high risk may benefit from insertion of implantable defibrillators that detect lethal rhythms and apply an electric shock to convert the rhythm.

TABLE 19-4 CLASSIFICATION OF DRUG ACTIONS BASED ON MODIFICATION OF VULNERABLE PARAMETER

MECHANISM	DYSRHYTHMIA	VULNERABLE PARAMETER (EFFECT)	DRUGS (EFFECT)
Automaticity			
Enhanced normal	Inappropriate sinus tachycardia	Phase 4 depolarization (decrease)	β-Adrenergic blocking agents
	Some idiopathic ventricular tachycardias		Na^+ channel blocking agents
Abnormal	Atrial tachycardia	Maximum diastolic potential (hyperpolarization)	Muscarinic receptor subtype 2 (M_2) agonists
		Phase 4 depolarization (decrease)	Ca^{2+} or Na^+ channel blocking agents; M_2 agonists
	Accelerated idioventricular rhythms	Phase 4 depolarization (decrease)	Ca^{2+} or Na^+ channel blocking agents
Triggered Activity			
Early afterdepolarization (EAD)	Torsades de pointes	Action potential duration (shorten)	β-Adrenergic agonists, vagolytic agents (increase rate)
		EAD (suppress)	Ca^{2+} channel blocking agents; Mg^{2+}; β-adrenergic blocking agents
Delayed afterdepolarization (DAD)	Digitalis-induced dysrhythmias	Calcium overload (unload)	Ca^{2+} channel blocking agents
		DAD (suppress)	Na^+ channel blocking agents
	Right ventricular outflow tract ventricular tachycardia	Calcium overload (unload)	β-Adrenergic blocking agents
		DAD (suppress)	Ca^{2+} channel blocking agents; adenosine
Na^+ Channel–Dependent Reentry			
Long excitable gap	Typical atrial flutter	Conduction and excitability (depress)	Types IA, IC Na^+ channel blocking agents
	Circus movement tachycardia in Wolff-Parkinson-White syndrome (WPW)	Conduction and excitability (depress)	Types IA, IC Na^+ channel blocking agents
	Sustained uniform ventricular tachycardia	Conduction and excitability (depress)	Na^+ channel blocking agents
Short excitable gap	Atypical atrial flutter	Refractory period (prolong)	K^+ channel blocking agents
	Atrial fibrillation	Refractory period (prolong)	K^+ channel blocking agents
	Circus movement tachycardia in WPW	Refractory period (prolong)	Amiodarone, sotalol
	Polymorphic and uniform ventricular tachycardia	Refractory period (prolong)	Type IA Na^+ channel blocking agents
	Bundle branch reentry	Refractory period (prolong)	Type IA Na^+ channel blocking agents; amiodarone
	Ventricular fibrillation	Refractory period (prolong)	K^+ channel blocking agents
Ca^{2+} Channel–Dependent Reentry			
	Atrioventricular nodal reentrant tachycardia	Conduction and excitability (depress)	Ca^{2+} channel blocking agents
	Circus movement tachycardia in WPW	Conduction and excitability (depress)	Ca^{2+} channel blocking agents
	Verapamil-sensitive ventricular tachycardia	Conduction and excitability (depress)	Ca^{2+} channel blocking agents

From the Task Force for the Working Group on Arrhythmias of the European Society of Cardiology: The Sicilian gambit: a new approach to the classification of antiarrhythmic drugs based on their actions on arrhythmogenic mechanisms, *Circulation* 84:1831, 1991. Copyright © 1991, American Heart Association.

SUMMARY

Heart failure may result from a number of cardiac and noncardiac disorders that diminish myocardial contractility or impose an excessive workload on the heart. Heart failure is a clinical diagnosis based on characteristic signs and symptoms. Decreased cardiac output to the tissues results in decreased renal blood flow, fluid retention, activity intolerance, and mental fatigue. Backward effects are due to congestion of blood behind the ineffectively pumping ventricle. With left-sided heart failure, the congestion is located in the lungs and produces a number of signs and symptoms, including dyspnea, orthopnea, hypoxemia, crackles, and frank pulmonary edema. Isolated right-sided heart failure causes congestion in the systemic venous system leading to congestion and dysfunction of the liver, spleen, and kidney, as well as peripheral subcutaneous edema and distended neck veins. In the early stages HF may be asymptomatic, and attention to risk factors and early structural abnormalities of the heart may allow early intervention. Two types of HF have been described based on EF. Those with low ejection fraction are commonly described as having systolic failure. Those with normal EF, usually defined as greater than 50%, usually have diastolic failure. Many patients with low EF have both systolic and diastolic dysfunction.

Three major compensatory mechanisms operate to maintain cardiac output in the failing heart: (1) sympathetic activation, (2) increased preload, and (3) cardiac muscle cell hypertrophy. Unfortunately, these mechanisms also increase myocardial workload and oxygen requirements and may trigger neurohormonal dysregulation and ventricular remodeling associated with HF progression and decompensation. Progression of HF is related to myocardial remodeling characterized by myocyte loss and myocardial fibrosis. Therapies that slow the remodeling process may slow the progression of heart failure. The primary aims of therapy are to improve cardiac output, minimize congestive symptoms and cardiac workload, and slow the detrimental remodeling process.

Dysrhythmia refers to an abnormality of electrical impulse generation or conduction. Dysrhythmias may occur in association with a number of cardiac and noncardiac disorders. Disturbances in electrical activity of the heart can indicate underlying pathophysiologic processes but are not themselves primary medical diseases. Dysrhythmias are significant because they can signal underlying pathophysiologic disorders and can disrupt normal cardiac output. Dysrhythmias can be categorized into three major types: (1) abnormal rates of sinus rhythm, (2) abnormal sites of impulse initiation, and (3) disturbances in conduction pathways. Treatment for dysrhythmias centers on maintaining adequate cardiac output, providing antidysrhythmic drugs as needed, and diagnosing and managing the underlying pathologic process.

REFERENCES

1. Lindenfield J, Albert NM, Boehmer JP, et al: Executive summary: HFSA 2010 comprehensive heart failure practice guidelines, *J Card Fail* 16:475–539, 2010.
2. American Heart Association: *Heart disease and stroke statistics—2011 update*, Dallas, 2011, The Association.
3. Fang J, Mensah G, Croft JB, Keenan NL: Heart failure-related hospitalization in the US. 1979-2004, *J Am Coll Cardiol* 52:428–434, 2008.
4. Kim J, Jacobs DR Jr, Luepker RV, et al: Prognostic value of a novel classification scheme for heart failure: the Minnesota Heart Failure Criteria, *Am J Epidemiol* 164(2):184–193, 2006.
5. Loehr LR, Rosamond WD, Chang PP, et al: Heart failure incidence and survival (from the Atherosclerosis Risk in Communities Study), *Am J Cardiol* 101(7):1016–1022, 2008.
6. Swedberg K, Cleland J, Dargie H, et al: Guidelines for the diagnosis and treatment of chronic heart failure: executive summary (update 2005): The Task Force for the Diagnosis and Treatment of Chronic Heart Failure of the European Society of Cardiology, *Eur Heart J* 26:1115, 2005.
7. Mann DL: Pathophysiology of heart failure. In Bonow R, Mann D, Zipes D, et al, editors: *Braunwald's heart disease: a textbook of cardiovascular medicine*, ed 9, Philadelphia, 2012, Elsevier, pp 487–503.
8. Bursi F, Weston SA, Redfield MM, et al: Systolic and diastolic heart failure: differences and similarities, *JAMA* 296(18):2209–2216, 2007.
9. Redfield MM: Heart failure with normal ejection fraction. In Bonow R, Mann D, Zipes D, et al, editors: *Braunwald's heart disease: a textbook of cardiovascular medicine*, ed 9, Philadelphia, 2012, Elsevier, pp 586–599.
10. Opie LH, Hasenfuss G: Mechanisms of cardiac contraction and relaxation. In Bonow R, Mann D, Zipes D, et al, editors: *Braunwald's heart disease: a textbook of cardiovascular medicine*, ed 9, Philadelphia, 2012, Elsevier, pp 459–483.
11. Mann DL: Management of heart failure with reduced ejection fraction. In Bonow R, Mann D, Zipes D, et al, editors: *Braunwald's heart disease: a textbook of cardiovascular medicine*, ed 9, Philadelphia, 2012, Elsevier, pp 459–483.
12. Parker RB, Cavallari LH: Systolic heart failure. In Dipiro JT, et al, editors: *Pharmacotherapy: a pathophysiologic approach*, ed 8, New York, 2011, McGraw-Hill, pp 137–172.
13. Hunt SA et al, American College of Cardiology; American Heart Association: 2009 focused update incorporated into the ACC/AHA 2005 guidelines for the diagnosis and management of heart failure in adults: summary article, *J Am Coll Cardiol* 53(15):e3–e62, 2009.
14. Fowler MB, Lottes SR, Nelson JJ, et al: β-Blocker dosing in community-based treatment of heart failure, *Am Heart J* 153(6):1029–1036, 2007.
15. Kim HN, Januzzi JL: Biomarkers and prognosis. In Bonow R, Mann D, Zipes D, et al, editors: *Braunwald's heart disease: a textbook of cardiovascular medicine*, ed 9, Philadelphia, 2012, Elsevier, pp 544–547.
16. Krum H, Teerlink JR: Medical therapy for congestive heart failure, *Lancet* 378(9792):713–721, 2011.
17. The Digitalis Investigation Group: The effect of digoxin on mortality and morbidity in patients with heart failure. *N Engl J Med* 336(8):525–533, 1997.
18. Sanoski CA, Bauman JL: The arrhythmias. In Dipiro JT, et al, editors: *Pharmacotherapy: a pathophysiologic approach*, ed 8, New York, 2011, McGraw-Hill, pp 273–310.
19. Rubart M, Zipes DP: Genesis of cardiac arrhythmias: electrophysiological considerations. In Bonow R, Mann D, Zipes D, et al: *Braunwald's heart disease: a textbook of cardiovascular medicine*, ed 9, Philadelphia, 2012, Elsevier, pp 653–686.
20. Conover MB: *Understanding electrocardiography*, ed 8, St Louis, 2003, Mosby.
21. Miller JM, Zipes DP: Therapy for cardiac arrhythmias. In Bonow R, Mann D, Zipes D, et al, editors: *Braunwald's heart disease: a textbook of cardiovascular medicine*, ed 9, Philadelphia, 2012, Elsevier, pp 710–744.

Shock

Shann D. Kim

evolve WEBSITE

KEY QUESTIONS

- What are the common causes of cardiogenic, hypovolemic, obstructive, and distributive shock?
- What are the common cellular and tissue responses to shock of any cause?
- How does the body try to compensate for insufficient cardiac output during shock states?
- How do clinical and hemodynamic findings differ among types of shock?
- What is the role of the immune system in septic shock and the progressive stage of other types of shock?
- How is shock managed?
- Why does shock have high mortality?

CHAPTER OUTLINE

Shock is a life-threatening condition characterized by insufficient delivery of oxygenated blood to the microcirculation, resulting in tissue hypoxia and cellular dysfunction. In 1895, John Collins Warren described shock as a momentary pause in the act of death.[1] In spite of advances in the understanding and management of shock, it still has a high rate of mortality. This chapter presents an overview of circulatory shock, including the major causes, cellular and systemic pathogenesis, clinical manifestations, and general therapeutic management.

PATHOGENESIS OF SHOCK

Shock is characterized by an imbalance between oxygen supply and oxygen requirements at the cellular level.[2] When the cell does not have adequate amounts of oxygen and nutrients, it is unable to meet its metabolic demands. Cellular hypoxia results in impaired cellular function and may progress to irreversible organ damage and death. The causes of circulatory shock classically are divided into four general types: cardiogenic, obstructive, hypovolemic, and distributive.[3]

BOX 20-1 ETIOLOGY OF CIRCULATORY SHOCK

Cardiogenic Shock
Myocardial infarction
Cardiomyopathy
Valvular heart disease
Ventricular rupture
Congenital heart defects
Papillary muscle rupture

Obstructive Shock
Pulmonary embolism
Cardiac tamponade
Tension pneumothorax
Dissecting aortic aneurysm

Hypovolemic Shock
Acute hemorrhage
Dehydration from vomiting, diarrhea
Overuse of diuretics
Burns
Pancreatitis

Distributive Shock
Anaphylaxis
Neurotrauma
Spinal cord trauma
Spinal anesthesia
Sepsis

TABLE 20-1 COMPARISON OF CLINICAL FINDINGS IN DIFFERENT TYPES OF SHOCK

PARAMETER	CARDIOGENIC	HYPOVOLEMIC	SEPTIC
Hypotension	Yes	Yes	Yes
Systemic vascular resistance	High	High	Low
Cardiac output	Low	Low	High
Cardiac preload	High	Low	Low
Venous oxygen saturation	Low	Low	High
Urine output	Low	Low	Low
Skin temperature	Cool	Cool	Warm

Each of these types is associated with a number of primary causes (Box 20-1). Cardiogenic shock results from heart disorders that cause inadequate cardiac output despite sufficient vascular volume. Obstructive shock develops when circulatory blockage disrupts cardiac output, such as a large pulmonary embolus or cardiac tamponade. Because the causes of obstructive shock are associated with failure of the heart to pump sufficiently, some sources include obstructive shock within the category of cardiogenic shock. Hypovolemic shock is associated with loss of blood volume as a result of hemorrhage or excessive loss of extracellular fluids, such as through vomiting, diarrhea, or excessive diuresis. Distributive shock is characterized by a greatly expanded vascular space because of inappropriate vasodilation. Vasodilation leads to hypotension and altered perfusion of tissues. Anaphylactic, neurogenic, and septic are forms of distributive shock. Each type of shock has certain unique features (Table 20-1), but all are associated with impaired tissue oxygenation that can progress to refractory shock and organ failure.

Impaired Tissue Oxygenation

The common denominator of all forms of shock is impaired oxygen utilization by cells, which disrupts function and, if ongoing or severe, may lead to cell death, organ dysfunction, and stimulation of inflammatory reactions. Recent discoveries about the contribution of inflammatory reactions in the pathogenesis of shock have provided new insight into this complicated syndrome.

The reason for impaired oxygen utilization by cells differs with the various types of shock, but the outcomes are similar. A continuous supply of oxygen is needed by cells to allow sufficient production of energy in the form of adenosine triphosphate (ATP). Inadequate oxygen availability at the cellular level quickly impairs aerobic metabolism of glucose, fatty acids, and amino acids and causes the cells to rely on the relatively inefficient processes of glycolysis to produce cellular ATP. (A review of ATP synthesis can be found in Chapter 3.) Glycolysis is the enzymatic process of converting glucose to pyruvate, with the net production of two ATP molecules per glucose molecule. If oxygen were available, pyruvate would normally enter the mitochondria and proceed through the citric acid cycle. In the absence of cellular oxygen, the citric acid cycle is inhibited and pyruvate accumulates in the cytoplasm. Pyruvate accumulation would quickly inhibit further glycolysis and shut down ATP production entirely if not for the conversion of pyruvate to *lactate*. Lactate diffuses from the cell and into the extracellular fluid, and accumulation of lactate in the bloodstream (more than 5 to 6 mmol/L) is considered a sign of significant tissue hypoxia.[4,5]

An inadequate supply of cellular ATP inhibits energy-requiring cellular functions, including maintenance of ion concentrations across the plasma membrane. Because of their steep electrochemical gradients, extracellular sodium and calcium ions tend to leak into the cell. ATP-dependent pumps in the cell membrane are needed to continuously pump these ions back out. Failure of ion pumps leads to sodium and water accumulation in the cell (hydropic swelling) and an excess of intracellular free calcium. Intracellular calcium ions trigger a cascade of cellular events that further impair energy production and plasma membrane integrity. Cell death from oxygen deprivation takes from minutes to several hours, depending on the rate of cellular metabolic activity. However, even a short period of oxygen deprivation often sets in motion a complex cascade of events that lead to further cell damage (Figure 20-1). Two important aspects of this cascade are (1) formation of oxygen free radicals, and (2) induction of inflammatory cytokines.

Ischemic cells may produce oxygen free radicals when oxygen supplies are restored. This process has been called *reperfusion injury*. Reactive oxygen molecules include superoxide (O_2^-), peroxide (H_2O_2), hydroxyl radicals (OH^-), and singlet oxygen (O). These molecules are unstable and will attack membrane structures, denature proteins, and damage DNA. Another source of oxygen free radicals is immune cells, particularly neutrophils, which are recruited to the area of tissue injury. Thus, cellular injury may continue and progress long after the initial hypoxic insult has been resolved.

The role that immune cytokines play in shock has been studied extensively in septic shock. The roles of these cytokines are thought to be similar in the late stages of other types of shock as well. Macrophages and tissue cells are stimulated to release inflammatory cytokines in response to hypoxic tissue injury and, in the case of septic shock, in response to endotoxin or other microorganism antigens.[6] The levels of tumor necrosis factor-α (TNF-α) and interleukin-1 (IL-1) cytokines in particular have been shown to increase in the bloodstream

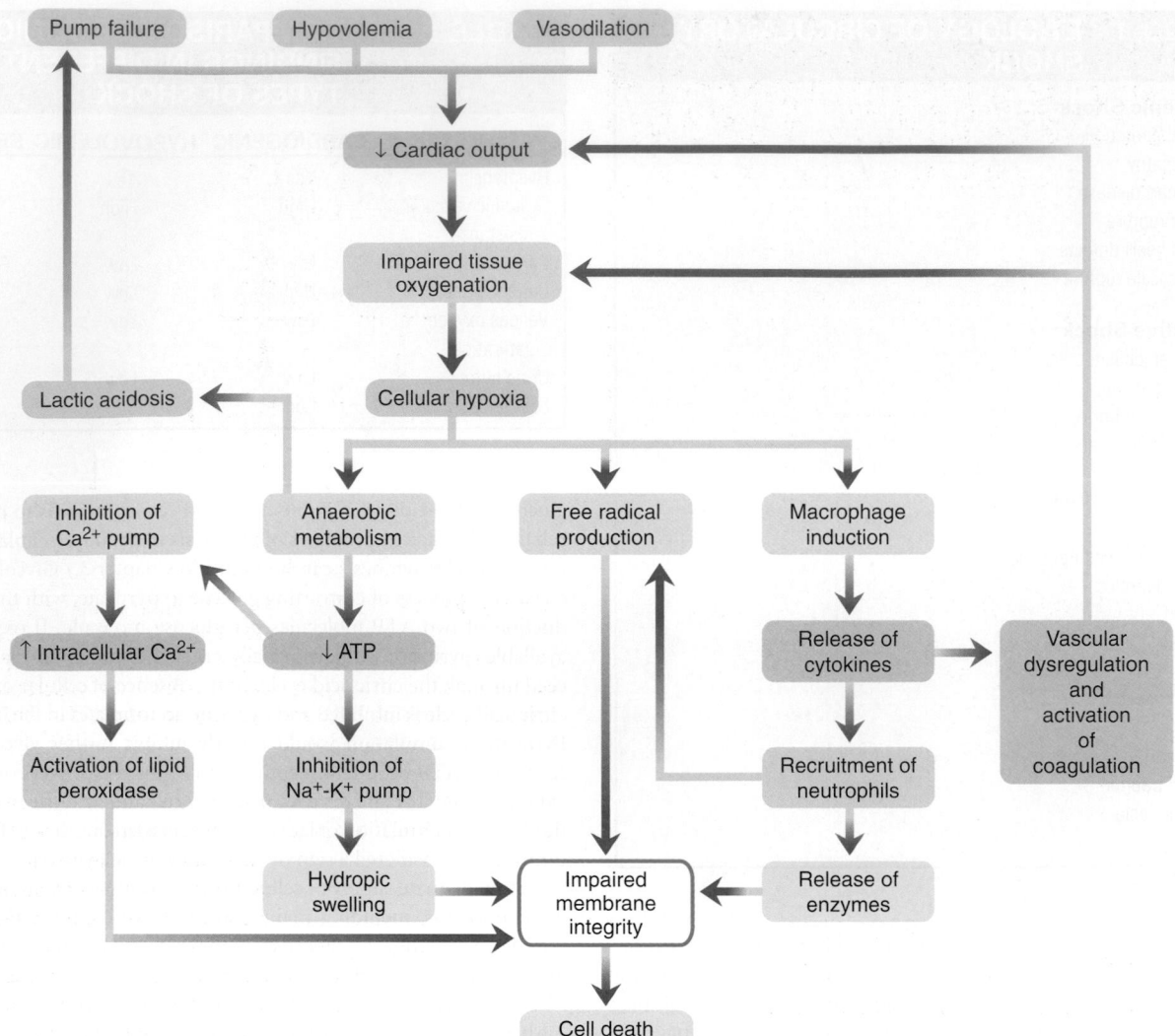

FIGURE 20-1 Shock is a complex process involving cellular hypoxia, free radical formation, and systemic inflammation. All forms of shock are associated with impaired tissue oxygenation, which triggers a cascade of events leading to tissue injury and death. *ATP,* Adenosine triphosphate.

of patients with septic shock, and these cytokines are thought to be important mediators of vascular failure and progressive organ damage.[6] Numerous other immune cytokines and neurohormonal mediators have been implicated in the pathogenesis of shock (Table 20-2). These mediators represent potential therapeutic targets for a disorder that is notoriously difficult to manage effectively.

A hallmark of shock is failure of the microcirculation to appropriately autoregulate blood flow. Normal tissues are able to match blood flow with metabolic needs across a wide range of blood pressures. This property ensures that blood flow is evenly distributed to tissues according to metabolic needs. In shock, autoregulation fails, leading to an abnormal distribution of blood flow.[7] Some capillary beds receive inadequate flow and become progressively more hypoxic, whereas other vascular routes are excessively dilated and receive too much flow. Advances in technology have allowed direct visualization of capillary flow through tissue beds and confirmed the presence of perfusion abnormalities in the microcirculation. These abnormalities differ depending on the primary cause of shock.[7] In cases of reduced cardiac output resulting from hypovolemic or cardiogenic shock, there is a homogeneous reduction in blood flow through a given tissue's arterioles, capillaries, and venules that is directly related to the severity of cardiac output reduction. In

distributive shock states, such as septic shock, the degree of microcirculatory flow is heterogeneous within a tissue, with some capillaries being closed and others open. Often there is high flow rate through some of the venules and the degree of microcirculatory dysfunction is poorly correlated with systemic hemodynamics. Overall, this imbalance leads to a so-called *oxygen debt* in the tissues. It has been suggested that the overall oxygen debt can be estimated clinically by the serum lactate level and degree of metabolic acidosis, both of which imply a switch to anaerobic metabolism by oxygen-deprived tissues.[5]

In septic shock, immune cytokines are believed to be at the root of the microcirculatory maldistribution problem. TNF-α, IL-1, and other inflammatory mediators induce vascular cells to produce excessive amounts of the vasodilator nitric oxide.[6] Nitric oxide in normal quantity is thought to be protective for tissues during shock, whereas excessive production is detrimental. Nitric oxide is produced in endothelial cells and vascular smooth muscle by two enzymes: nitric oxide synthase (NOS) and inducible nitric oxide synthase (iNOS). TNF-α and IL-1 increase the activity of iNOS and thereby cause excessive production of nitric oxide (Figure 20-2). Efforts to minimize the microcirculatory oxygen debt in early shock and to quickly restore adequate microcirculatory blood flow distribution, as evidenced by normalized

TABLE 20-2	IMMUNE CYTOKINES AND NEUROHORMONES ASSOCIATED WITH CIRCULATORY SHOCK
MEDIATOR	**ASSOCIATED DYSFUNCTION**
IL-1α	Inflammation, vasodilation, vascular leakiness
IL-1β	Inflammation, vasodilation, vascular leakiness
IL-6	Fever, increased acute phase protein
TNF-α	Inflammation, neutrophil activation
IL-10	Antiinflammatory, may suppress shock
TGF-β	Fibrosis, pulmonary edema
PAF	Platelet activation, chemotaxis
PAI-1	Increased clotting, thrombosis
Substance P	Proinflammatory
Chemokines	Neutrophil recruitment and binding to vessel endothelium
Nitric oxide	Vasodilator
C5a	Chemotactic
Protein C	Inhibits thrombus formation
Vasopressin	Improves vascular tone and responsiveness to NE/E
Cortisol	Antiinflammatory, improves vascular response to NE/E
Endothelin	Vasoconstriction
Adrenomedullin	Vasodilation
Norepinephrine	Vasoconstriction
Epinephrine	Inotropic, bronchodilation
Leukotrienes	Inflammation, bronchospasm
Histamine	Increased vascular permeability, edema
Heparin	Inhibits action of histamine
Angiotensin II	Vasoconstriction
Heat-shock proteins	Protect protein structure and function, inhibit apoptosis

E, Epinephrine; *IL,* interleukin; *NE,* norepinephrine; *PAF,* platelet-activating factor; *PAI,* plasminogen activator inhibitor; *TGF,* transforming growth factor; *TNF,* tumor necrosis factor.

serum lactate concentration and acid-base balance, are an important focus of therapy for all types of shock.

Compensatory Mechanisms and Stages of Shock

A number of compensatory responses are set in motion to restore tissue perfusion and oxygenation in the early stage of shock. Historically, these responses to shock have been divided into three clinical stages: compensated shock, progressive shock, and refractory shock. Although these stages may be useful for determining prognosis and the likelihood of the patient's recovering, shock is viewed as a continuum in which compensatory mechanisms become progressively less effective as function of the microcirculation becomes increasingly impaired.

Insufficient cardiac output and decreased effective tissue perfusion are early defects in all types of shock. Insufficient cardiac output may be a consequence of an ineffective cardiac pump (cardiogenic, obstructive) or insufficient blood volume to fill the vascular space (hypovolemic, distributive). A number of compensatory mechanisms are triggered in response to inadequate cardiac output in an attempt to restore adequate perfusion pressure (Figure 20-3). Baroreceptors located in the aorta and carotid arteries quickly sense the decrease in pressure and transmit signals to the vasomotor center in the brainstem medulla. Stimulation of the sympathetic nervous system (SNS) results in increased cardiac output and vascular resistance. Because blood pressure is determined by the

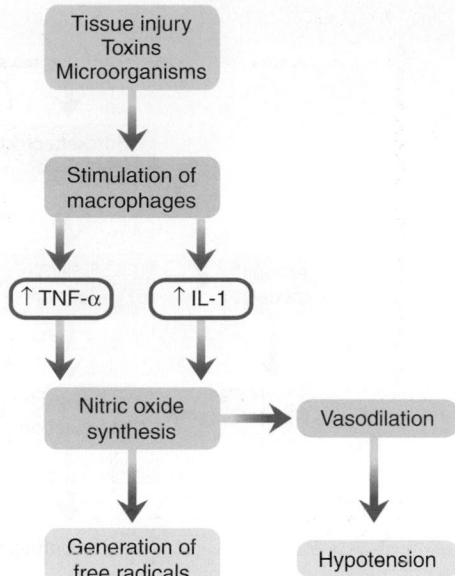

FIGURE 20-2 Excess production of nitric oxide is an important mechanism of vascular failure in shock. The tumor necrosis factor-α and interleukin-1 cytokines are promoters of inducible nitric oxide synthase. These cytokines are released from macrophages that have been activated by tissue injury or toxins. *IL-1,* Interleukin-1; *TNF-α,* tumor necrosis factor-α.

product of cardiac output and vascular resistance, an increase in one or both of these factors will help restore blood pressure. The SNS increases cardiac output through several mechanisms. The adrenal medulla is stimulated to release increased amounts of the catecholamines epinephrine and norepinephrine (NE), which circulate to the heart and stimulate β_1 receptors. The β_1 receptors respond by increasing the heart rate and force of contraction in an attempt to increase cardiac output. The SNS also enhances venous return to the heart by constricting systemic arterioles and venules. Arterial vasoconstriction reduces flow through the capillary bed, which causes hydrostatic pressure in the capillaries to fall. Fluid reabsorption from interstitial spaces helps increase blood volume and improve preload. Blood vessels in the skin, kidneys, and gastrointestinal tract constrict and shunt blood to the heart and brain.

The SNS stimulates cells in the kidney to release renin, which triggers the renin-angiotensin-aldosterone system (RAAS). Renin is also secreted from the kidneys in response to decreased blood flow and pressure in the afferent arterioles. Renin triggers the formation of angiotensin II, which is a potent vasoconstrictor and also stimulates kidney nephrons to conserve sodium and water. Conservation of volume by the kidney is further enhanced by aldosterone, which is secreted from the adrenal cortex in response to angiotensin II (Ang II). Reabsorption of fluid from the kidney helps increase blood volume and enhances venous return to the heart. Another hormone, antidiuretic hormone (vasopressin), is secreted from the posterior pituitary in response to reduced blood volume. Antidiuretic hormone stimulates the kidney tubules to reabsorb water and improves the vascular response to catecholamines. In shock, urine output may fall to zero as the kidneys attempt to conserve fluid to maintain blood volume and cardiac output. Unfortunately, the kidney tubules often sustain damage because of the low-flow state, which may result in the complication of acute renal failure.

These compensatory mechanisms work well in the early stage of hypovolemic shock and may maintain blood pressure within the normal range until the volume of blood loss becomes too great (Figure 20-4). In other forms of shock, compensatory mechanisms are less effective in restoring cardiac output. In cardiogenic shock, the compensatory responses may

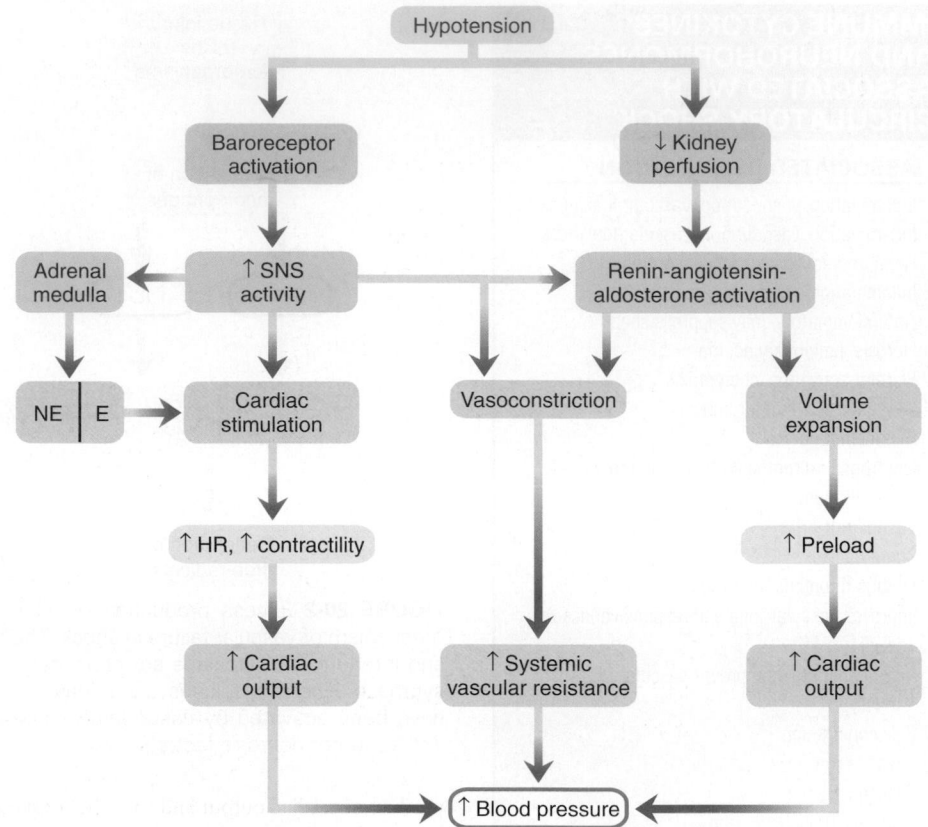

FIGURE 20-3 Compensatory mechanisms are triggered in shock to help maintain arterial blood pressure despite a fall in cardiac output. *E,* Epinephrine; *HR,* heart rate; *NE,* norepinephrine; *SNS,* sympathetic nervous system.

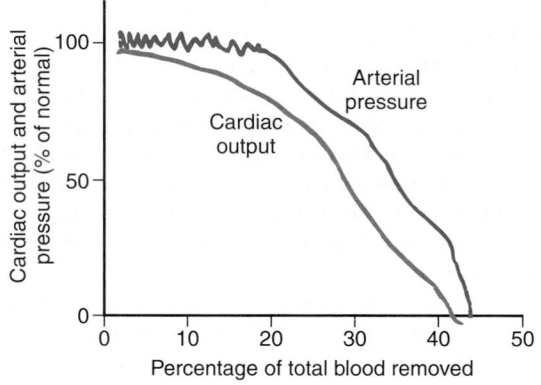

FIGURE 20-4 In early stages of hypovolemia, blood pressure is stable even though cardiac output is falling. When volume losses equal about 25% of the total blood volume, blood pressure falls precipitously. (Redrawn from Hall JE: *Guyton and Hall textbook of medical physiology,* ed 12, Philadelphia, 2011, Saunders, p 274.)

worsen the already high preload and impose a greater workload on the failing heart. In distributive shock, the vasculature is not responsive to SNS signals to constrict. Blood pools in the peripheral tissues, which makes it difficult for the heart to maintain cardiac output despite sympathetic stimulation to increase the heart rate and contractility.

The early, compensated stage of shock may be difficult to detect clinically (Figure 20-5). A high index of suspicion is needed in patients with heart failure, trauma, blood loss, and severe infection. In addition, the following clinical findings may be present:
- A narrow pulse pressure with or without hypotension
- Tachycardia greater than 100 beats/min
- Fast and deep respirations
- Decreased urinary output
- Increased urine specific gravity
- Cool, clammy skin
- Altered mentation
- Dilated pupils

At some point, which is highly variable and differs among individuals depending on age, comorbidities, and specific etiology, the compensatory mechanisms can no longer sustain adequate perfusion to tissues and cells begin to suffer significant hypoxic injury. This condition is sometimes called the *progressive stage of shock.* Active therapeutic intervention is required at this stage or the patient will probably not survive. As previously described, reduced delivery of oxygen to tissues results in hypoxic injury, free radical damage, and stimulation of the inflammatory response. Lactic acidosis may occur during the progressive stage of shock. In addition to being a marker of anaerobic metabolism, lactate can alter the acid-base balance of the blood and create metabolic acidosis. Metabolic acidosis places a greater burden on the respiratory and renal systems and may contribute to further dysfunction. Metabolic acidosis can affect electrolyte balance and contribute to cardiac dysrhythmias and conduction disturbances. In addition, myocardial depressant factors are released that impair myocardial contractility.[8] These factors contribute to reduced cardiac output and a progressive cycle of worsening tissue hypoxia.

As shock continues to progress, the vascular system begins to fail. Arterioles become unresponsive to catecholamines and previously constricted vascular beds begin to dilate. Widespread dilation and low cardiac output combine to produce severe hypotension. The low blood pressure is not sufficient for organ perfusion. At this stage the effects of shock produce more shock processes. Tissue

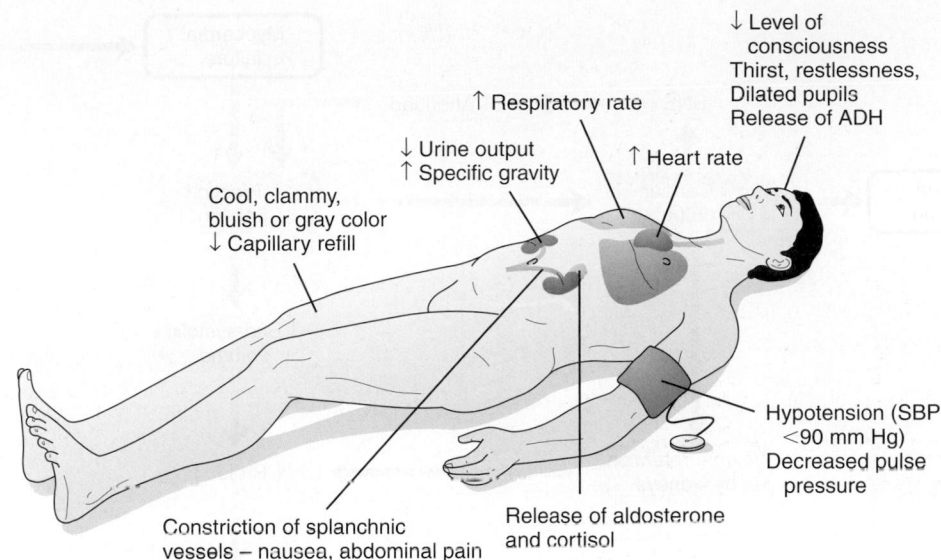

FIGURE 20-5 Classical manifestations of shock. *ADH,* Antidiuretic hormone; *SBP,* systolic blood pressure.

damage often activates the clotting cascade, which contributes to sluggish blood flow, vascular thrombosis, and more severe tissue ischemia. Release of inflammatory mediators, along with vascular occlusion, may precipitate organ failure. The kidney, liver, and lung are particularly susceptible. At some point, the stage of refractory shock occurs and the patient becomes unresponsive to therapeutic interventions.

The progressive stage of shock is characterized by the following clinical manifestations:
- Low blood pressure, usually lower than 90 mm Hg
- Narrow pulse pressure
- Tachycardia
- Acute renal failure (e.g., oliguria, increased levels of blood urea nitrogen and serum creatinine)
- Decreased level of consciousness
- Increased respiratory rates
- Metabolic and respiratory acidosis with hypoxemia

KEY POINTS
- Shock represents a diverse group of life-threatening circulatory conditions. The common factor among all types of shock is hypoperfusion and impaired cellular oxygen utilization. Inadequate cellular oxygenation may result from decreased cardiac output, maldistribution of blood flow, or reduced blood oxygen content.
- During the compensatory stage of shock, homeostatic mechanisms are sufficient to maintain adequate tissue perfusion despite a reduction in cardiac output. Manifestations of SNS activation are an elevated heart rate, increased myocardial stimulation, bronchodilation, vasoconstriction, cool clammy skin, dilated pupils, and decreased urine output. Blood pressure is maintained even though cardiac output has fallen.
- During the progressive stage of shock, compensatory mechanisms begin to fail and hypotension and progressive tissue hypoxia result. Shift of cells to anaerobic metabolism results in lactate production and metabolic acidosis. A lack of cellular ATP production leads to cellular swelling, dysfunction, and death. Generation of oxygen free radicals, release of inflammatory cytokines, and activation of the clotting cascade lead to further cellular and organ dysfunction.

TYPES OF SHOCK

In addition to the general pathophysiology of shock just described, each type of shock has special features that affect prevention, diagnosis, and treatment. These features are briefly reviewed here, and the reader is referred to the specific chapters that describe the primary disorders that predispose to shock, including cardiogenic (Chapters 18 and 19), hypovolemic (Chapter 24), anaphylactic (Chapter 10), neurogenic (Chapter 44), and septic (Chapter 8).

Cardiogenic Shock

Etiology and pathogenesis. Cardiogenic shock occurs primarily as a result of severe dysfunction of the left, right, or both ventricles that results in inadequate cardiac pumping. The most common cause of cardiogenic shock is myocardial infarction resulting in a significant dysfunction or loss (greater than 40%) of left ventricular myocardium.[9] Other causes of cardiogenic shock include right ventricular myocardial infarction, end-stage cardiomyopathy, papillary muscle dysfunction, free wall rupture, and congenital heart defects.

The low cardiac output state is associated with a high left ventricular diastolic filling pressure (preload), a finding that differentiates cardiogenic from hypovolemic forms of shock (Figure 20-6). High left ventricular preload leads to movement of fluid from the pulmonary vascular beds into the pulmonary interstitial space, which initially results in interstitial pulmonary edema and later in alveolar pulmonary edema.

The SNS is stimulated as a compensatory mechanism to increase cardiac output. The result is an increase in heart rate and systemic vascular resistance. High systemic vascular resistance increases the workload on the heart. Activation of the RAAS results in further increases in resistance and preload. The net effect of the activation of compensatory mechanisms is to increase myocardial workload and oxygen demand. Consequently, the compensatory responses can precipitate further cardiac damage and cause a progressive decline in cardiac output.

Clinical manifestations. Sympathetic nervous stimulation increases the heart rate and vascular resistance, which maintain blood pressure even though cardiac output has decreased. As compensatory mechanisms fail, systolic blood pressure falls and diastolic pressure increases

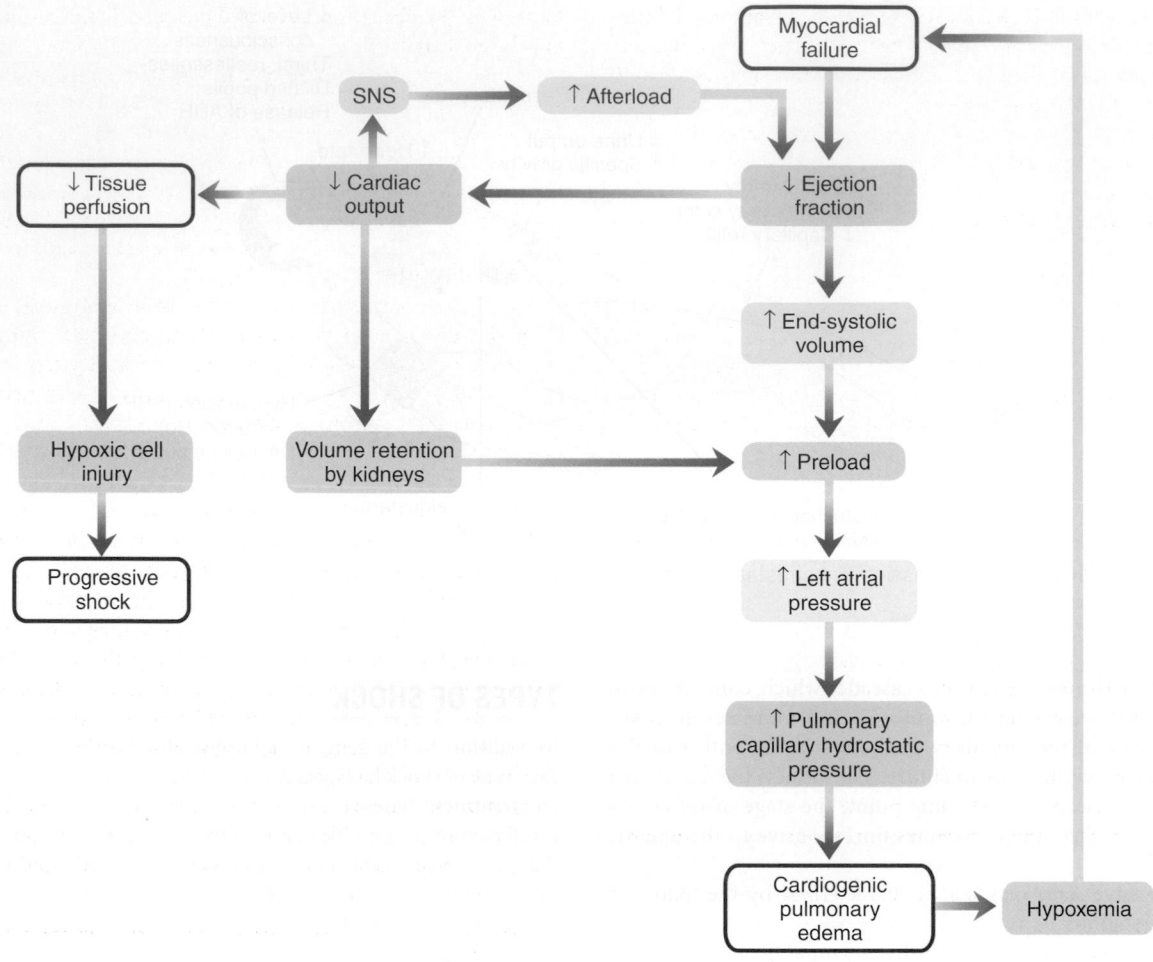

FIGURE 20-6 Cardiogenic shock results in decreased tissue perfusion and cardiogenic pulmonary edema because of reduced myocardial function, usually associated with left ventricular failure. *SNS,* Sympathetic nervous system.

(as a result of the sympathetic stimulation), thus narrowing the pulse pressure. Heart rates exceed 100 beats/min. Peripheral vasoconstriction occurs and produces cool, clammy skin. Auscultation of the lungs reveals coarse crackles resulting from pulmonary edema. An S_3 summation gallop may be audible over the left apex as a result of increased preload in the left ventricle.

Frequent assessments of cardiac output and cardiac index are helpful in the clinical treatment of a patient in cardiogenic shock. A pulmonary artery catheter may be inserted to measure cardiac index and left heart filling pressures (e.g., pulmonary capillary occlusion pressure). Pulmonary artery pressures are increased, with the pulmonary capillary occlusion pressure typically being greater than 15 mm Hg (normal, less than 12 mm Hg).[9] When pulmonary capillary occlusion pressure acutely increases, pulmonary congestion may develop because fluid shifts from the capillary into the interstitial and alveolar spaces. Patients with chronic congestive heart failure may not develop pulmonary edema until pulmonary occlusion pressures exceed 20 to 40 mm Hg. Arterial blood gas values initially demonstrate a respiratory alkalosis secondary to hyperventilation. As pulmonary edema progresses, respiratory acidosis with hypoxemia may occur. Hypoxemia further impairs myocardial function.

Determination of mixed venous oxygen levels in blood samples obtained from the pulmonary artery catheter is helpful in assessing the adequacy of cardiac output. Decreased tissue oxygen delivery because of low cardiac output increases the degree of oxygen extraction. Mixed

venous blood samples show decreased venous oxygen saturation (SvO_2) with a decreased cardiac output. An increase in mixed venous oxygenation would be expected with improved cardiac output.

Treatment. Cardiogenic shock is difficult to manage because the underlying myocardial damage is often not reversible. Prevention of cardiogenic shock through measures to limit infarct size during acute myocardial ischemia is desirable. Early efforts to restore coronary perfusion are associated with a decrease in the incidence of cardiogenic shock after myocardial infarction.[9,10] (A discussion of reperfusion therapy can be found in Chapter 18.)

The goal of treatment for cardiogenic shock is to decrease myocardial oxygen demands, increase myocardial oxygen delivery, and increase cardiac output. It is difficult to achieve these goals because interventions to increase cardiac output tend to increase myocardial oxygen demands.

Pharmacotherapy. Positive inotropic drugs are frequently used in the management of cardiogenic shock to increase contractility. Positive inotropes include β-adrenergic agonists such as NE, dobutamine, and dopamine and phosphodiesterase inhibitors that prevent the degradation of cyclic adenosine monophosphate (cAMP). These drugs have the ability to increase contractility, increase cardiac output, and increase tissue perfusion; however, these drugs increase myocardial oxygen demand. NE is the natural neurotransmitter of the sympathetic nerves and mimics SNS activation by increasing heart rate, contractility, and vascular resistance. Dobutamine increases contractility by stimulating β receptors. However, unlike NE or dopamine, dobutamine has minimal α-receptor activity. The major effect of dobutamine is on contractility rather than heart rate. Dobutamine may contribute to a decrease in vascular resistance and must be used with caution in hypotensive patients.[11] Vasodilators may be used to decrease the workload of the heart by decreasing left ventricular afterload. Examples of commonly used vasodilators include nitroprusside and nitroglycerin.

Mechanical assist devices. Cardiogenic shock is sometimes managed by mechanical assist devices. For temporary management, **intraaortic** balloon counterpulsation may be indicated.[12] A catheter with a balloon at the distal segment is inserted through the femoral artery and positioned in the aorta just distal to the left subclavian artery. The balloon is connected to a console that triggers the balloon to inflate in diastole and deflate in systole. The effect of balloon inflation during diastole is to increase perfusion pressure of the coronary arteries. Sudden deflation of the balloon just before ventricular systole creates a vacuum effect in the aorta that reduces left ventricular afterload. A reduction in afterload decreases left ventricular workload and increases stroke volume. Balloon counterpulsation restricts mobility and is associated with a number of vascular complications. Long-term management of patients with low cardiac output can be achieved with mechanical pumps that take over the function of the ventricle or ventricles (ventricular assist devices). Ventricular assist devices (VADs) are commonly used in patients waiting for a heart transplant. In some cases, the temporary decrease in cardiac workload afforded by the VAD is associated with significant improvement in cardiac structure and function, and the device can be removed.

KEY POINTS

- Cardiogenic shock is usually a result of severe ventricular dysfunction associated with myocardial infarction. Other causes include cardiomyopathy, ventricular rupture, and congenital heart defects.
- Diagnostic features of cardiogenic shock include decreased cardiac output as a result of left ventricular dysfunction, along with elevated left ventricular end-diastolic pressure, S_3 heart sounds, and pulmonary edema. Sympathetic activation leads to an increased heart rate, vasoconstriction, and a narrow pulse pressure.
- Low cardiac output leads to reduced oxygen delivery to tissues. Tissues extract a greater percentage of oxygen from the delivered blood, which leads to reduced Svo_2.
- Therapy is aimed at improving cardiac output and myocardial oxygen delivery while reducing cardiac workload. Pharmacologic treatment often includes the use of inotropic agents, afterload-reducing agents (e.g., vasodilators), and preload-reducing agents, such as venodilators and diuretics. Intraaortic balloon counterpulsation may be used to reduce afterload and improve coronary artery perfusion. Ventricular assist devices may be used for longer-term circulatory support, whereas heart transplantation provides definitive treatment.

Obstructive Shock

Etiology. Obstructive shock develops when the heart is prevented from pumping because of a mechanical obstruction to blood flow. Impaired ventricular filling leads to reduced cardiac output and signs and symptoms similar to cardiogenic shock, and is considered by many to be a form of cardiogenic shock. Causes of mechanical obstruction include pulmonary embolism, cardiac tamponade, and tension pneumothorax. Prompt relief of the obstruction is necessary to restore cardiac output and prevent cardiovascular collapse.

Clinical manifestations. Obstructive shock is usually characterized by manifestations of right-sided heart failure. Depending on the location of the obstruction, elevated pressures in the cardiac chambers may be evident.

Pulmonary embolism results in elevated right-sided heart pressures, but left-sided pressures remain normal to low. Pulmonary emboli are usually generated in the veins of the lower extremities in patients with immobility, trauma, or hypercoagulable states. Pulmonary embolism is manifested as sudden, severe dyspnea and deteriorating arterial blood gas values. A perfusion scan of the lung may demonstrate an area of reduced blood flow. Pulmonary emboli are not generally detectable by chest radiographs.

Cardiac tamponade, which results from an accumulation of fluid in the pericardial sac, causes elevation of pressures on both the right side and the left side of the heart. Despite the elevated pressure, preload in the heart chambers is low, as is stroke volume. The elevated pressure is due to external compression of the heart chambers. Risks for the development of cardiac tamponade include pericarditis, blunt trauma to the chest, and cardiac surgical procedures. In pericarditis, a pericardial friction rub can sometimes be heard and may help with the diagnosis.

Tension pneumothorax results in shifting and compression of mediastinal structures, including the heart, which compromises left ventricular filling. Accumulation of air in the pleural space may occur because of trauma or spontaneous rupture of lung parenchyma. A tension pneumothorax develops when the air in the pleural space begins to exert a positive pressure on lung and mediastinal structures. A deviated trachea and decreased or absent breath sounds may occur. Arterial blood gas values can deteriorate rapidly. Tension pneumothorax is detectable by chest radiography.

Treatment. Management of obstructive shock is aimed at identifying and removing the offending obstruction. Compensatory mechanisms are generally ineffective in obstructive shock, and the patient's condition may deteriorate rapidly.

KEY POINTS

- Obstructive shock results from mechanical obstructions that prevent effective cardiac filling and stroke volume.
- Pulmonary embolism, cardiac tamponade, and tension pneumothorax are common causes of obstructive shock.
- Prompt management of the underlying obstruction is necessary to prevent cardiovascular collapse.

Hypovolemic Shock

Etiology and classification. Hypovolemic shock results when circulating blood volume is inadequate to perfuse tissues.[13] The pathogenesis of early stage hypovolemic shock is straightforward: decreased intravascular volume leads to a decrease in venous return, which causes a decrease in cardiac output (Figure 20-7). The decrease in cardiac output results in decreased tissue perfusion and decreased oxygen delivery.

Circulatory volume deficits may be the result of internal or external losses. Internal losses can result from internal hemorrhage, fracture of long bones, or leakage of fluid into the interstitial spaces. External losses can result from external hemorrhage, burns, severe vomiting and diarrhea, or diuresis. External hemorrhage is the most common cause of hypovolemic shock.

The American College of Surgeons stratifies hemorrhagic shock into four classes according to the degree of blood volume lost (Table 20-3).[3] These values are based on a 70-kg adult and are guidelines that may not apply to all patients with hemorrhage, depending on etiology, rate of blood loss, and comorbidities.

The initial stage hemorrhage (Class I) occurs with blood loss up to 750 ml or 15% of total blood volume. Compensatory mechanisms maintain cardiac output, and the patient's vital signs remain within the normal range. Class II compensated hemorrhage is categorized as blood loss between 750 and 1500 ml (15% to 30% of total blood volume). The patient becomes anxious and restless. Blood pressure remains normal when the patient is supine but decreases upon standing (orthostatic hypotension). The heart rate is between 100 and 120 beats/min. The respiratory rate is normal to mildly increased. Urine output is between 20 and 30 ml/hr. The capillary refill time may be prolonged. (The capillary blanch test is performed by depressing a patient's fingernail and observing how long after release the skin color takes to return to normal. Normal capillary refill times are less than 2 seconds.)

Class III hemorrhage (progressive stage) is blood loss between 30% and 40% of total blood volume (1500 to 2000 ml). The patient is anxious and confused. Blood pressure is decreased with a narrow pulse pressure. The heart rate is greater than 120 beats/min. Respiratory rates are between 30 and 40 respirations/min. Urine output is 5 to 20 ml/hr. The capillary refill test is prolonged.

Severe Class IV hemorrhage (refractory stage) occurs when more than 40% of total blood volume is lost (2000 ml or more). The patient

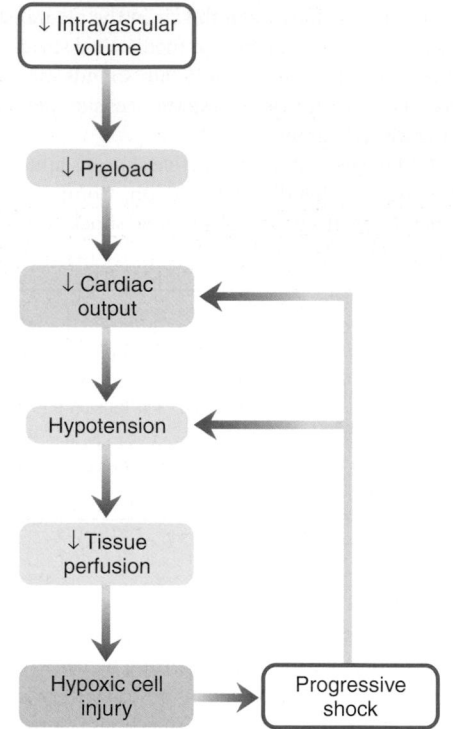

FIGURE 20-7 Pathogenesis of Hypovolemic Shock.

is lethargic and has severe hypotension with a narrow pulse pressure. The heart rate usually exceeds 140 beats/min, and the respiratory rate is markedly increased. Urine output is negligible. The capillary refill test is prolonged.

The clinical features of other forms of hypovolemic shock are similar to those of hemorrhagic shock, although the volume loss has usually occurred more gradually.

Clinical manifestations. The cardiac output and cardiac index are found to be decreased. Pulmonary artery pressures and pulmonary capillary wedge pressures are decreased because of the decreased preload. The finding of a low preload distinguishes hypovolemic shock from cardiogenic shock. In cardiogenic shock, preload is high and cardiac output is low. In hypovolemic shock, preload and cardiac output are both low.

Systemic vascular resistance is increased as a result of sympathetic activation. This increase is a compensatory mechanism in hypovolemia to maintain perfusion pressure. SvO_2 may be decreased because of decreased oxygen delivery and increased oxygen extraction.

Treatment. The first intervention for hemorrhagic shock is to control the source of blood loss. Second, volume losses are replaced with appropriate fluids to normalize blood pressure, cardiac output, and perfusion of the microvasculature. In severe, uncontrolled hemorrhage, efforts to increase blood pressure should be postponed until the hemorrhage is under control.[13] Otherwise, the increased blood pressure may worsen the hemorrhage. In all types of hypovolemic shock, fluid replacement is the primary therapy. The three main types of fluid therapy agents are colloids, crystalloids, and blood products. There continues to be controversy about which type of fluid is the most appropriate for resuscitation of hypovolemic shock.

Colloids are solutions that increase the serum colloid osmotic pressure within the vascular compartment. Increased colloid pressure pulls fluid from the interstitium into the vascular space. Examples of colloid solutions are normal human serum albumin, dextran, and hetastarch. Colloids generally are not recommended for hypovolemic shock unless the patient has significant interstitial edema.

Crystalloids are solutions that contain electrolytes. Isotonic solutions such as lactated Ringer solution or normal saline solution are commonly used crystalloid solutions. Isotonic fluids are preferred over hypotonic solutions because isotonic solutions remain in the extracellular space and are more effective in increasing blood volume. Isotonic crystalloid fluids are preferred for volume resuscitation in hypovolemic shock that is not associated with severe anemia.[14]

When significant anemia accompanies hypovolemia, *blood products* may be the treatment of choice. In hemorrhagic shock, whole blood or packed red blood cells (RBCs) with saline may be given to replace blood volume loss. Significant anemia may contribute to tissue hypoxia simply because of reduced oxygen-carrying capacity; however, recent research suggests that RBCs may also regulate capillary blood flow by

TABLE 20-3	**CLASSIFICATION OF HEMORRHAGIC SHOCK**			
	CLASS I (INITIAL STAGE)	**CLASS II (COMPENSATED STAGE)**	**CLASS III (PROGRESSIVE STAGE)**	**CLASS IV (REFRACTORY STAGE)**
Blood loss (ml)	≤750 (15%)	750-1500 (15-30%)	1500-2000 (30-40%)	>2000 (>40%)
Clinical features	Minimal tachycardia	Tachycardia	Tachycardia	Marked tachycardia
	Normal or increased pulse pressure	Tachypnea	Tachypnea	Decreased systolic blood pressure
		Decreased pulse pressure	Decreased systolic blood pressure	Narrowed pulse pressure
		Cool, clammy skin	Oliguria	Markedly decreased urinary output
		Delayed capillary refill	Changes in mental status such as confusion and agitation	Loss of consciousness
		Slight anxiety		Cold, pale skin

releasing vasodilating substances, including ATP, into the microcirculation under conditions of hypoxia. Significant reduction in RBC flow through capillaries has been suggested as a mechanism for further impairing microcirculatory function.[2]

In general, pharmacologic agents are not indicated for hypovolemia. Restoration of blood volume is essential. However, in some cases of shock, blood pressure remains low despite large amounts of fluid replacement, so vasoconstrictor agents must be used to support blood pressure.

KEY POINTS

- Hypovolemic shock results from inadequate circulating blood volume precipitated by hemorrhage, burns, dehydration, or leakage of fluid into interstitial spaces.
- The classic features of hypovolemic shock are the result of low cardiac output and low intracardiac pressures. Manifestations are due primarily to SNS activation: elevated heart rate, vasoconstriction, and increased myocardial contractility.
- The severity of symptoms of hemorrhagic shock correlates with the amount of blood loss; however, there is significant variation in the clinical presentation of hypovolemic and hemorrhagic shock and careful assessment is required to diagnose it in the early stages.
- Therapy for hypovolemic shock is aimed at fluid replacement and control of the source of volume loss. Colloids, isotonic crystalloids, and blood products may be used as replacement fluids.

Distributive Shock

Distributive shock is characterized by an abnormally expanded vascular space caused by excessive vasodilation. Vasodilation results in peripheral pooling of blood in the venous capacitance vessels and creates a relative hypovolemia. Preload and stroke volume are insufficient to maintain perfusion of the brain and tissues. Anaphylactic, neurogenic, and septic are the types of distributive shock. All are characterized by vasodilation and profound hypotension, but the cause and pathogenesis of each type differ significantly.

Anaphylactic Shock

Etiology and pathogenesis. Type I anaphylactic reactions involve an antigen/immunoglobulin E (IgE) antibody reaction on the surface of mast cells and basophils. IgE antibodies attach to receptor sites on these cells, where they await activation by specific antigens. Exposure to that antigen causes receptors on mast cells and basophils to crosslink and become activated. A host of vasoactive chemicals are released, including histamines, leukotrienes, bradykinins, and prostaglandins.[15] These substances result in bronchoconstriction, peripheral vasodilation, and increased capillary permeability. (A detailed discussion of type I anaphylaxis can be found in Chapter 10.) In some cases, mast cell degranulation is triggered by a mechanism that does not involve IgE. These reactions may be called *anaphylactoid* (Box 20-2).

Most type I anaphylactic reactions are mild and do not result in shock. Even in more severe anaphylaxis, prompt treatment can prevent the shock syndrome.[16] Shock occurs when peripheral dilation is massive, and a type of hypovolemic shock is precipitated. In this case, blood volume may be normal but the sudden enlargement of the vascular space causes blood to pool in the periphery. In some cases, there is also significant leakage of fluid from the bloodstream into the interstitial spaces.[15] Both of these conditions cause cardiac preload to drop, followed by a decrease in cardiac output.

Clinical manifestations. The onset of symptoms is usually within 2 to 30 minutes of exposure to the antigen; however, symptoms may not develop for several hours.[15] The clinical presentation can vary widely in severity depending on the stimulus and rapidity of therapy. Initially the patient appears very anxious, with an increased heart rate and respiratory rate. Hypotension, urticaria (hives), pruritus (itching), and angioedema then develop. Often the patient has a sense of impending doom. Bronchoconstriction causes wheezing and cyanosis, and laryngeal edema results in hoarseness and stridor.

Prevention and treatment. Prevention of anaphylactic shock is achieved by avoidance of precipitating allergens. Anaphylactic shock is most frequently associated with antibiotic therapy, in particular β-lactams.[15] Other common causes include other types of drugs, peanuts and tree nuts, insect stings, and snake bites (see Box 20-2). More than one third of cases are of unknown cause. Anaphylaxis is not a reportable disease, and the incidence is unknown; however, the estimated risk of occurrence is 1% to 3% per person in the United States.[15]

Initial therapy for anaphylactic shock is directed to removing the inciting antigen if possible. Airway management and circulatory support are critical. Tracheal intubation and assisted ventilation may be needed. Bronchodilators can be used to manage bronchospasm. Epinephrine is helpful in stabilizing mast cells to prevent further release of inflammatory mediators and increasing blood pressure.[15] Intravenous fluid therapy is used to increase intravascular volume and fill the enlarged vascular space. Increased preload will enhance cardiac output. A vasopressor may be given in an attempt to constrict the arterioles and raise blood pressure. Steroids may be given for their antiinflammatory effects, but their onset of action tends to be slow. Antihistamines may be administered to block histamine receptors, although their effectiveness is reduced once

---

BOX 20-2   COMMON TRIGGERS OF ANAPHYLAXIS

Anaphylactic (IgE-Dependent)

Foods
- Peanuts
- Tree nuts
- Crustaceans (crab, shrimp)

Medications
- β-Lactam antibiotics
- Other antibiotics
- Aspirin and other nonsteroidal antiinflammatory drugs

Venoms
- Bee sting
- Snake bite

Animal proteins
- Cat
- Dog
- Horse

Anaphylactoid (IgE-Independent)

Radiocontrast media

Opioids

Muscle relaxants

Temperature
- Cold
- Heat

Transfusion reactions
- IgG
- IgM

Unidentified Triggers

Idiopathic

symptoms are present and the inflammatory mediators have been released.[15] New therapeutics are being developed to target endotoxin and proinflammatory cytokines.[16] Response to therapy for anaphylactic shock is usually rapid with a good outcome if instituted early; however, approximately 1% of anaphylactic episodes are fatal, and the majority of these are associated with antibiotics and nut allergies.[15]

Neurogenic Shock

Neurogenic shock is often transitory. It may result from depression of the vasomotor center in the medulla or from interruption of sympathetic nerve fibers in the spinal cord. Causes of neurogenic shock include brain trauma that results in depression of the vasomotor center, spinal cord injury, high spinal anesthesia, and drug overdose.

Interruption of the neural pathway for the baroreceptor reflex results in loss of sympathetic tone in the vasculature. Profound peripheral vasodilation of both arterioles and veins occurs and leads to peripheral pooling of blood and hypotension. Decreased venous return to the heart results in decreased cardiac output and hypotension. Body position greatly influences the development of neurogenic shock. When the body is horizontal, venous return may be adequate and cardiac output and blood pressure are sufficient. However, when an upright position is assumed, peripheral pooling from gravitational effects causes a severe drop in cardiac output and blood pressure. Syncope and fainting will follow unless measures are taken to redistribute the blood. Elevation of the legs, slow position changes, and the use of pressure stockings on the legs may help prevent peripheral pooling. Vasoconstricting drugs and fluid expansion may sometimes be used to increase blood pressure if mechanical measures are ineffective. The outcome of neurogenic shock depends in large part on the severity of neurologic injury. Shock resulting from head trauma has a poor prognosis, whereas acute neurogenic shock associated with spinal cord injuries may resolve as spinal cord reflexes return in the weeks following the injury.

Septic Shock

Septic shock is a common cause of death in intensive care units in the United States, and the incidence continues to increase. Large numbers of immunocompromised individuals in the population and extensive use of invasive technology contribute to the high rates of septic shock. The mortality associated with septic shock averages between 30% and 50% in various clinical trial registries.[17,18] High mortality is in part because of the underlying diseases that often accompany sepsis, such as trauma, peritonitis, cancer, and immunodeficiency diseases.

Etiology. Sepsis results from the presence of microorganisms in the bloodstream (bacteremia). However, most cases of bacteremia do not result in shock. Normally, the body's defense systems effectively destroy the bacteria and prevent widespread dissemination of the infection. Immunocompromised individuals are prone to disseminated infections called *bacteremia* (the term *septicemia* is still in clinical use, but is discouraged because of imprecise meaning). When the body's response to infection or other insults results in systemic signs and symptoms of widespread inflammation, the term *systemic inflammatory response syndrome* (SIRS) is applied. Septic shock is a severe systemic inflammatory reaction to infection that results in abnormal vasodilation, hypotension, and tissue hypoxia attributable to the maldistribution of blood flow. Confusion about the meaning of the terms bacteremia, sepsis, septic shock, and SIRS prompted the planning of a consensus conference to provide definitions for clinical and research purposes (Table 20-4).[19]

Patients at high risk for septic shock include the very young and the elderly. Patients in these age groups are less likely to be able to destroy invading microorganisms. Patients who are debilitated, malnourished, or immunocompromised by acquired immunodeficiency syndrome or chemotherapy or have chronic health problems are also at increased risk. Medical interventions that predispose a patient to septic shock include the use of invasive lines, catheters, and procedures; surgery; and immunosuppressive therapy.

Pathogenesis. Septic shock commonly is associated with gram-negative infections. Gram-negative bacteria include *Escherichia coli, Klebsiella pneumoniae, Enterobacter aerogenes, Serratia marcescens, Pseudomonas aeruginosa,* and *Proteus* species.[20] Gram-positive organisms (*Staphylococcus aureus, Staphylococcus epidermidis, Streptococcus pneumoniae*) and fungi (*Candida* species) are also important causes of septic shock. A frequent portal of entry is the genitourinary tract. Other entry sites include the gastrointestinal tract, the respiratory tract, and the skin.

TABLE 20-4 DEFINITIONS RELATED TO SEPSIS

CONDITION	DEFINITION
Bacteremia (fungemia)	Presence of viable bacteria (fungi) in bloodstream
Infection	Inflammatory response to invasion of normally sterile host tissue by microorganisms
Systemic inflammatory response syndrome (SIRS)	Systemic inflammatory response to a variety of clinical insults that can be infectious or noninfectious; response is manifested by two or more of the following conditions: T >38° C (100.4° F) or <36° C (96.8° F); HR >90 beats/min; RR >20 breaths/min or $Paco_2$ <32 torr; WBC >12,000 cells/mm^3, <4000 cells/mm^3, or >10% immature (band) forms; positive fluid balance (>20 ml/kg over 24 hr); hyperglycemia; plasma C-reactive protein/procalcitonin >2 SD above normal value; arterial hypotension; cardiac index >3.5 L/min; arterial hypoxemia; acute oliguria; creatinine increase >0.5 mg/dl; coagulation abnormalities; ileus; platelets <100,000/μL; bilirubin >4 mg/dl; hyperlactatemia; decreased capillary refill
Sepsis	SIRS secondary to infection
Severe sepsis	Sepsis associated with one or more organ dysfunctions, hypoperfusion, or hypotension; hypoperfusion and perfusion abnormalities may include, but are not limited to, lactic acidosis, oliguria, or acute alteration in mental status
Septic shock	Sepsis with persistent hypotension despite fluid resuscitation, along with presence of perfusion abnormalities; patients taking inotropic or vasopressor agents may not be hypotensive at the time perfusion abnormalities are measured
Refractory septic shock	Persistent septic shock requiring dopamine >15 mcg/kg/min to maintain mean arterial blood pressure
Multiple organ dysfunction syndrome (MODS)	Presence of altered organ function requiring intervention to maintain homeostasis

HR, Heart rate; *Paco$_2$,* arterial carbon dioxide tension; *RR,* respiratory rate; *SD,* standard deviation; *T,* temperature; *torr,* mm Hg; *WBC,* white blood cell count.
Adapted from Dipiro JT et al, editors: *Pharmacotherapy: a pathophysiologic approach,* ed 8, New York, 2011, McGraw-Hill, p 2042.

Gram-negative bacteria have within their cell walls a lipopolysaccharide or **endotoxin.** The cell wall is composed of an O antigen side chain, an R core, and an inner lipid A, the toxic component of the endotoxin.[20] Endotoxins are released into the blood during bacterial cell lysis and initiate a chain of pathophysiologic events. Macrophages are stimulated by endotoxin to release inflammatory cytokines, including TNF-α and IL-1.[6] As previously described, TNF-α and IL-1 are thought to be major factors in the pathogenesis of septic shock because they stimulate release of more immune cytokines and the overproduction of nitric oxide.

Macrophage cytokines activate neutrophils and platelets, which release many toxic mediators such as platelet-activating factor, oxygen free radicals, and proteolytic enzymes.[6] Activation of the arachidonic acid cascade in neutrophils and platelets results in prostaglandin, leukotriene, thromboxane, and prostacyclin release, all of which have profound effects on vascular smooth muscle. Increased levels of thromboxanes A_2 and B_2 produce pulmonary vasoconstriction, mediate bronchoconstriction, and act as potent platelet aggregators. Prostacyclin is a potent vasodilator and may contribute to the development of hypotension.

A number of other inflammatory cascades are activated in septic shock. The complement system is activated with release of C5a and C3a, and can produce microemboli and endothelial cell destruction. Histamine, a potent vasodilator, is released by mast cells. Histamine also increases capillary permeability, which enhances edema formation. The coagulation system is activated and may enhance the development of thrombi. The kinin system is activated and bradykinin is released, which results in vasodilation and increased capillary permeability. All these immune responses are normal reactions to microbial invasion and are necessary for eradicating infections. In overabundance, however, these mechanisms constitute a systemic inflammatory response that can result in shock. The major components of the complex pathophysiologic processes of septic shock are illustrated in Figure 20-8.

Septic shock is associated with profound peripheral vasodilation. Systemic vascular resistance is decreased, and despite the increased cardiac output, blood pressure falls. The veins also dilate, and intravascular pooling occurs in the venous capacitance system. Because of maldistribution of blood flow, some portions of the

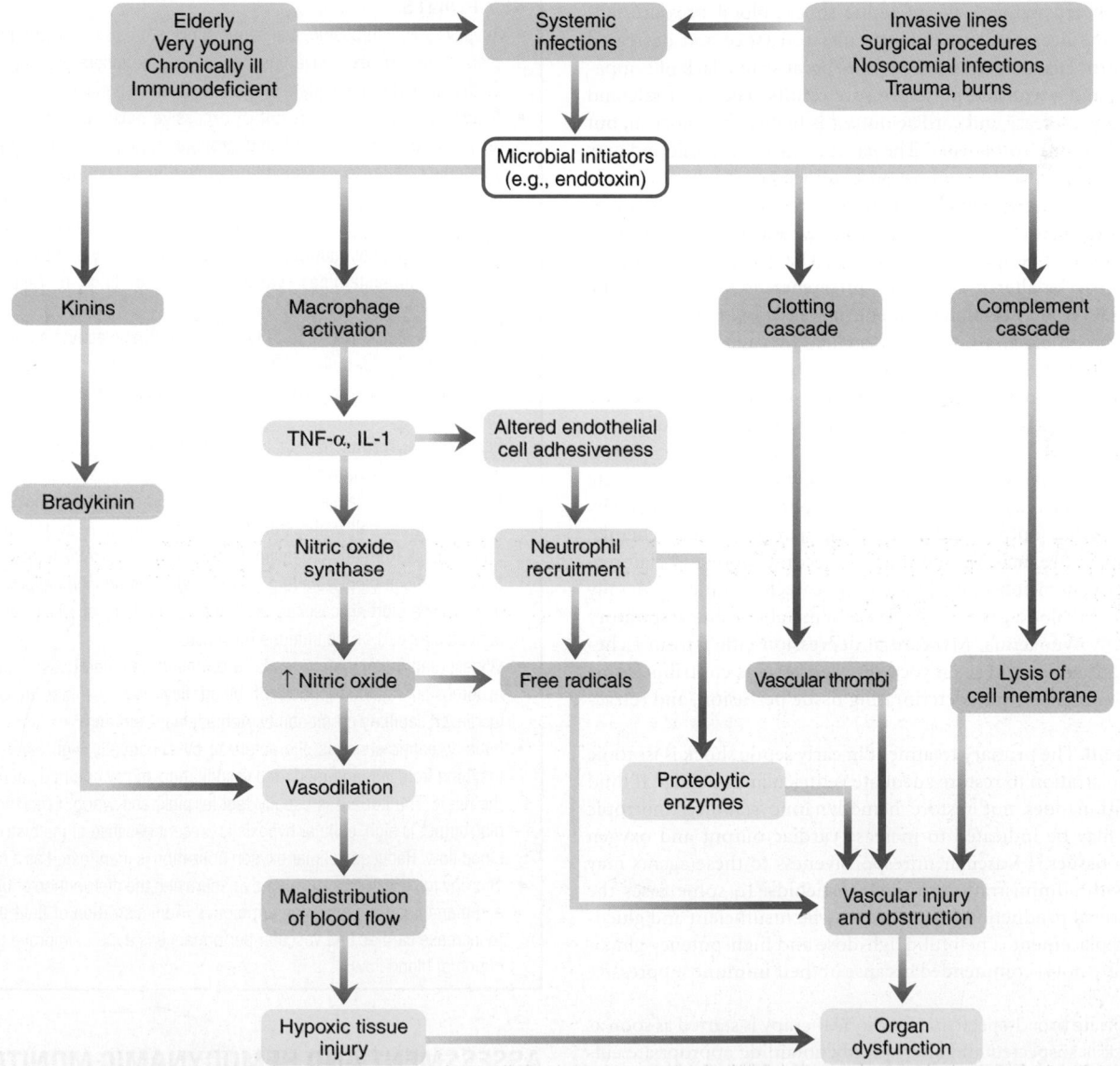

FIGURE 20-8 Pathophysiologic process of septic shock. Septic shock is characterized by immune-mediated mechanisms of cellular injury and organ dysfunction. *IL-1,* Interleukin-1; *TNF-α,* tumor necrosis factor-α.

tissue are underperfused and some are overperfused. Excessive flow to areas of lower metabolic demand limits oxygen extraction, which contributes to a common finding of lower overall oxygen consumption. In the initial stage of septic shock, a relative hypovolemia is present because of the increased size of the vascular compartment. Fluid administration to increase preload to a central venous pressure between 8 and 12 mm Hg is advocated at this stage, even though cardiac output may already be quite high.[21] Cardiac output between 8 and 12 L/min is common in early septic shock. Even this level of cardiac output may be inadequate to perfuse the expanded vascular bed.

The generalized inflammatory response triggered in septic shock affects capillary permeability. Increased capillary permeability results in fluid movement out of the vascular beds into the interstitial space. Generalized soft-tissue edema occurs and can interfere with tissue oxygenation and organ function.

Clinical manifestations. In contrast to other forms of shock, the clinical manifestation of early septic shock is a hyperdynamic state characterized by high cardiac output and warm extremities (see Table 20-1).

In the hyperdynamic stage of septic shock, blood pressure falls because of the decreased systemic vascular resistance and decreased venous return. Diastolic pressure declines because of a lack of sympathetic tone, and a widened pulse pressure results. The heart rate and stroke volume increase and cardiac output is higher than normal, but the patient remains hypotensive. The patient is usually febrile and may have associated chills. In contrast to cardiogenic and hypovolemic shock in which the peripheral circulation is reduced and extremities are cool and constricted, the skin is pink and warm to the touch in sepsis as a result of peripheral vasodilation. The patient's level of consciousness may be altered as a result of cerebral ischemia. In septic shock, Svo_2 levels may be higher than normal because of the maldistribution of blood flow. Abnormal vasodilation causes greater flow through areas with low metabolic activity. Oxygen consumption by tissues is decreased because metabolically active tissues do not receive enough flow. Lactic acidosis may be present because of tissue hypoxemia.

In the progressive stage of septic shock, some patients deteriorate to a hypodynamic phase. The hypodynamic phase is characterized by decreased cardiac output and the development of organ ischemia. The pulse pressure narrows and the skin becomes cool and clammy. Profound hypotension unresponsive to catecholamines generally occurs. Arterial blood gas analysis reveals a metabolic and respiratory acidosis with hypoxemia. Myocardial depression either from ischemia or from toxins acting as myocardial depressants contributes to a decreasing cardiac output, deteriorating tissue perfusion, and refractory shock.

Treatment. The primary treatment in early septic shock is isotonic fluid administration to restore adequate ventricular preload.[21] If fluid administration does not restore hemodynamic stability, inotropic treatment may be indicated to increase cardiac output and oxygen delivery to tissues.[21] Vascular unresponsiveness to these agents may improve with administration of glucocorticoids. In some cases the normal adrenal production of cortisol may be insufficient and glucocorticoid replacement is helpful. High-dose and high-potency glucocorticoids are not recommended because of their immunosuppressive activity.[21]

Appropriate broad-spectrum antibiotic therapy is started as soon as septic shock is suspected and after quickly obtaining appropriate cultures. Positive blood cultures can be used to narrow the antibiotic regimen to cover the specific microbes; however, blood cultures are negative in about 50% of cases despite the probable presence of systemic microorganisms.[21] Eradication of the inciting organism reduces the stimulus perpetuating SIRS. Shock itself may propagate sepsis by impairing circulation to the intestinal wall and allowing resident microorganisms to traverse from the colon to the bloodstream. Antibiotic selection for septic shock must be modified as new infective organisms are detected.

Because the inflammatory response is believed to be a critical aspect of septic shock, numerous agents designed to inhibit various components of SIRS have been investigated. Unfortunately, nearly all of these agents have failed to provide significant benefit. Some subgroups of septic patients may be helped by these agents, but overall the trials have been disappointing. Activated protein C is currently recommended for those with severe sepsis and a high-risk score for mortality.[21] Protein C has both antiinflammatory and antithrombotic actions, which may be helpful in sepsis, but the complication of bleeding is common. Therapy for septic shock is complicated and requires intensive monitoring and treatment of complications. These aspects are discussed in the next sections of this chapter.

KEY POINTS

- Anaphylactic, neurogenic, and septic shock are types of distributive shock characterized by excessive vasodilation and peripheral pooling of blood. Cardiac output is inadequate because of reduced preload.
- Anaphylactic shock is a result of excessive mast cell degranulation in response to antigen. Mast cell degranulation usually is mediated by IgE antibodies. Release of vasodilatory mediators such as histamine into the circulation by mast cells results in severe hypotension. Urticaria, bronchoconstriction, stridor, wheezing, and itching are usually present. Treatment includes maintenance of airway patency and the use of epinephrine, antihistamines, vasopressors, and fluids to restore blood pressure.
- Neurogenic shock results from loss of sympathetic activation of arteriolar smooth muscle. Medullary depression from brain injury, drug overdose, or lesions of sympathetic nerve fibers, such as spinal cord injury, are the usual causes.
- Septic shock results from a severe systemic inflammatory response to infection. Gram-negative bacteria, gram-positive bacteria, and fungal infections are common causes of septic shock. In gram-negative shock, endotoxins in bacterial cell walls stimulate massive immune system activation. Septic shock from any organism is characterized by release of large numbers of immune mediators (e.g., cytokines) resulting in widespread inflammation. The clotting cascade, complement system, and kinin system are activated as part of the immune response.
- Widespread inflammation leads to profound peripheral vasodilation with hypotension, maldistribution of blood flow with cellular hypoxia, and increased capillary permeability with edema formation.
- Initially, septic shock is characterized by abnormally high cardiac output resulting from immune-mediated vasodilation and sympathetic activation of the heart. The patient is usually febrile, pink, and warm. Even though cardiac output is high, cellular hypoxia is present because of maldistribution of blood flow. Reduced cellular oxygen utilization is manifested as a high Svo_2.
- Therapy for septic shock is aimed at improving the distribution of blood flow and managing infection with antibiotics. Administration of fluid and drugs to increase cardiac and vascular performance is done to improve the distribution of blood flow.

ASSESSMENT AND HEMODYNAMIC MONITORING

Astute assessment and appropriate hemodynamic monitoring are essential for the prevention, detection, and management of shock.

Although new methods of direct visualization of capillary flow are in development, it is not clinically feasible to directly measure the adequacy of cellular oxygenation in all of the body tissues. A number of indirect measures and clinical signs and symptoms are used to help indicate when tissue hypoxia is probably occurring. These same parameters are used to tailor therapy and assess outcomes of that therapy.

Most hospitalized patients experiencing shock will have monitoring devices in place to facilitate assessment of cardiac output, blood pressure, preload, vascular resistance, arterial oxygen content, and venous oxygen content. In addition, frequent measurement of serum lactate concentration, acid-base status, and urine output can be used to indirectly assess the severity of tissue hypoperfusion and hypoxemia.

An understanding of hemodynamic principles and monitoring techniques is helpful to the discussion of shock states. A more thorough discussion can be found in Chapters 15 and 17, and only the main points are reviewed here. The most important factors determining adequate tissue oxygenation are cardiac output, arterial oxygen content, and distribution of blood flow.

Cardiac Output

When the cardiac index falls below 2.2 L/min/m^2, the potential for inadequate tissue perfusion is high.[9] The cardiac index is the cardiac output divided by the body surface area. Cardiac output is the product of heart rate and stroke volume. Stroke volume is the amount of blood ejected by the ventricle with each heartbeat. Stroke volume is influenced by three major factors: preload, contractility, and afterload. *Preload* is the amount of blood in the ventricle at the end of diastole. In patients with low preload, a significant improvement in cardiac output often can be achieved by administering blood or intravenous fluids.

Afterload is the aortic impedance that the left ventricle must overcome to eject blood during systole. The major factors determining aortic impedance are the patency of the aortic valve and the resistance in the systemic vascular system. As resistance to left ventricular ejection increases, stroke volume decreases. Conversely, as resistance falls, stroke volume increases. In patients with high afterload, vasodilating agents may be useful in reducing the workload on the left ventricle. Care must be taken not to lower arterial blood pressure excessively, which would reduce perfusion.

Contractility is the inherent state of activation of cardiac muscle fibers. Contractility depends on the amount of free calcium ions available in the cardiac muscle cells after each electrical impulse. Contractility is influenced by sympathetic and parasympathetic nervous system neurotransmitters and other hormones and drugs. Contractility also depends on the amount of muscle mass and is influenced by myocardial ischemia and necrosis, and myocardial depressant factors that may be released by tissues in shock. Contractility can be increased by measures that increase myocardial perfusion and oxygenation, as well as by use of positive inotropic agents.

Most of the therapeutic interventions aimed at increasing cardiac output also increase myocardial workload and myocardial oxygen consumption. Especially in cardiogenic shock, these parameters must be carefully monitored and manipulated to avoid further cardiac compromise.

Arterial Oxygen Content

Oxygen delivery ($\dot{D}o_2$) can be determined by multiplying cardiac output and arterial oxygen content (Cao_2). Cao_2 is the sum of dissolved oxygen and oxygen bound to hemoglobin. Adequate gas exchange in the pulmonary capillaries is necessary to fully saturate hemoglobin with oxygen. Impaired ventilation may result in reduced Cao_2 and impair $\dot{D}o_2$. Mechanical ventilation and supplemental oxygen administration may be used to improve arterial oxygen saturation. For patients with low levels of hemoglobin, blood transfusion may significantly improve $\dot{D}o_2$.

A concept closely related to $\dot{D}o_2$ is **oxygen consumption** ($\dot{V}o_2$). Whereas $\dot{D}o_2$ is a measure of the oxygen delivered to the tissues each minute, $\dot{V}o_2$ is the amount of oxygen actually used by the tissues per minute. In a normal physiologic state, only about 25% of the oxygen delivered is taken up by tissues, which leaves about 75% of the oxygen to return to the heart in venous blood. When $\dot{D}o_2$ falls because of low cardiac output, tissues extract a greater percentage of the oxygen delivered such that the amount returning in venous blood is lower. When distribution of blood flow and tissue extraction of oxygen are impaired, as in septic shock, oxygen consumption falls and the amount of oxygen returning in venous blood will be higher than it should be. The amount of oxygen returning to the heart in venous blood can be measured by a special catheter in the pulmonary artery that detects venous oxygen saturation (Svo_2). Outcomes of therapy to improve $\dot{D}o_2$ can be assessed by monitoring Svo_2. In cardiogenic shock, for example, one would expect to see Svo_2 increase from a low value back toward 75% as cardiac output improves. In septic shock, one would expect to see Svo_2 decrease from a high value back toward 75% as distribution of blood flow to metabolically active tissues improves.

Hemodynamic Monitoring

Sophisticated monitoring equipment is available to assess the hemodynamic status of patients in shock. A flow-directed, pulmonary artery catheter can be inserted through the jugular or subclavian vein to allow measurement of intracardiac pressures, cardiac output, and Svo_2 (Figure 20-9). A catheter lumen in the right atrium allows measurement of right atrial pressure. Right atrial pressure is used to indicate right ventricular end-diastolic volume or preload. The primary value of monitoring right atrial pressure is in the management of blood volume. A low right atrial pressure is associated with a low preload and may indicate a need for extracellular volume replacement to enhance cardiac output. Conversely, a high right atrial pressure may indicate a need for extracellular volume reduction to decrease cardiac workload and congestive symptoms.

Another catheter lumen located in the pulmonary artery allows measurement of pulmonary artery pressure. Measurement of pulmonary artery pressure is helpful in assessing pulmonary complications of shock. An increase in pulmonary artery pressure may occur in progressive shock as the lungs react to inflammatory mediators and become edematous. In the absence of lung disease, pulmonary artery diastolic pressure reflects left atrial pressure. Assessment of left atrial pressure is important because it indicates left ventricular preload—an important determinant of cardiac output. A more accurate assessment of left atrial pressure can be obtained by using a small balloon at the tip of the catheter to obtain a pulmonary capillary occlusion pressure. When the balloon is inflated, the catheter tip floats into a small pulmonary artery and wedges itself there. The balloon blocks the arterial pressure events behind it and allows measurement of pressure in the capillary. Pulmonary capillary occlusion pressure is a direct reflection of left atrial pressure. Low left atrial pressure indicates reduced left ventricular preload and may signify the need for extracellular volume replacement.

> **KEY POINTS**
> - Hemodynamic monitoring during shock states is helpful for assessing cardiac output, volume status, oxygen delivery, and oxygen consumption. The pressures usually monitored include right atrial pressure, pulmonary artery pressure, and left atrial pressure.
> - Hemodynamic monitoring is used to guide management of cardiac preload, afterload, and contractility to optimize cardiac output, while minimizing cardiac workload.

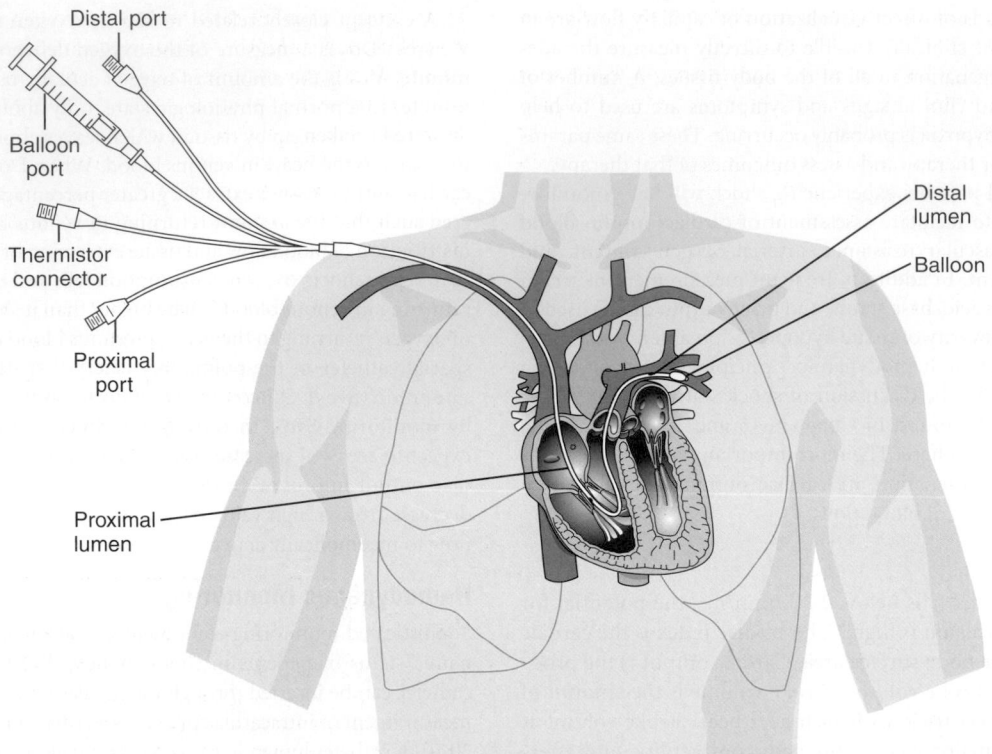

FIGURE 20-9 Properly positioned pulmonary artery catheter showing the proximal port in the right atrium and the distal port in the pulmonary artery. Cardiac output determinations can be made by injecting hypothermic solution into the proximal port and measuring the degree of warm-up near the distal port. A balloon at the end of the catheter can be intermittently inflated to measure pulmonary capillary occlusion pressure. When the balloon is inflated, it will float into a small artery and wedge there. Then the distal port measures the pressure in the capillary, which is a direct reflection of left atrial pressure.

- Normally, about 25% of the oxygen in arterial blood is extracted by the tissues, so the mixed venous oxygen saturation (Svo_2) is approximately 75%. Low cardiac output may result in greater oxygen extraction and lower Svo_2; maldistribution of flow, as occurs in septic shock, may result in less oxygen extraction and higher Svo_2.

COMPLICATIONS OF SHOCK

The pathologic process of the shock state and the effects on other organs may precipitate life-threatening complications. In severe shock of any cause, particularly in septic shock, a generalized inflammatory reaction may occur and is thought to contribute to the organ damage associated with shock states. Complications associated with shock include acute respiratory distress syndrome (ARDS), disseminated intravascular coagulation (DIC), acute renal failure, and multiple organ dysfunction syndrome (MODS). Damage to organ systems may be ongoing even after the initial precipitating event has been addressed. Inflammatory cytokines are thought to mediate this organ damage by altering metabolism, recruiting neutrophils, initiating the coagulation cascade, and altering capillary permeability. The complexities of this syndrome are being slowly unraveled as the mechanisms of immune signaling are better understood.

ACUTE RESPIRATORY DISTRESS SYNDROME

ARDS, a form of respiratory failure, is most commonly associated with septic shock. ARDS is characterized by the development of refractory hypoxemia, decreased pulmonary compliance, and radiologic evidence of pulmonary edema associated with normal cardiac preload (noncardiogenic pulmonary edema). The mortality in patients with shock that is complicated by ARDS ranges from 34% to 64%.[22] The primary cause of death in ARDS patients is multiple organ failure, not severe hypoxemia.

The lungs are a common target of immune-mediated damage in all types of shock. Tissue ischemia, even in areas distant from the lungs, leads to neutrophil migration to pulmonary capillaries.[4] Neutrophils release destructive proteolytic enzymes, produce oxygen free radicals, and secrete inflammatory chemicals that make pulmonary capillaries leaky. A protein-rich inflammatory exudate leaks into the interstitial spaces and alveoli of the lung, where it interferes with pulmonary gas exchange. Inflammation may also damage type II pneumocytes, which normally produce surfactant. Surfactant deficiency alters alveolar surface tension and causes smaller alveoli to collapse. The effort to breathe is very great in patients with ARDS because of pulmonary edema and alveolar collapse (atelectasis). Further discussion of ARDS and its clinical manifestations can be found in Chapter 23.

DISSEMINATED INTRAVASCULAR COAGULATION

DIC is a serious complication of septic shock characterized by abnormal clot formation in the microvasculature throughout the body. DIC is thought to result from immune activation of the clotting cascade. Obstruction of blood flow by small clots in the microcirculation leads to ischemic tissue damage. In addition, widespread clot formation consumes platelets and clotting factors, which leaves the patient at risk for serious bleeding. Laboratory assessment of the platelet count and clotting function is helpful in detecting and monitoring DIC. The platelet count and fibrinogen levels are typically low, whereas levels of fibrin degradation products (e.g., D-dimer) are elevated. Measures of the intrinsic and extrinsic clotting cascades demonstrate an elevated partial thromboplastin time and prothrombin time.

The clinical features of DIC are variable, depending on the location and severity of vascular thrombi. Vascular obstruction may be manifested as acute ischemia of the fingers and toes, with pain, pallor, and poor capillary refill. Obstruction of the kidney, liver, spleen, and lung by clots may result in signs and symptoms of organ failure. Patients may demonstrate various degrees of bleeding. Intravenous lines and catheters may begin to ooze around insertion sites. Previously stable incision lines may begin to bleed, and hematuria and hemoptysis may be present. Spontaneous intracranial hemorrhage is a particularly disastrous complication of DIC. Further discussion of DIC can be found in Chapter 14.

ACUTE RENAL FAILURE

In shock, the kidneys undergo prolonged periods of hypoperfusion. Vasoconstriction of the afferent arterioles causes decreased glomerular blood flow, decreased glomerular hydrostatic pressure, and decreased glomerular filtration rates. Hypoxic cellular damage occurs after 15 to 20 minutes of acute ischemia and results in necrosis of tubular epithelial cells. Acute tubular necrosis (ATN) is associated with decreased urinary excretion of waste products such as creatinine and urea. Rapidly increasing blood urea nitrogen and serum creatinine concentrations are indicative of ATN.

Urine output quickly falls toward zero, and the kidneys do not respond to fluids or diuretics. Renal tubular epithelial cell casts in the urine indicate sloughing of tubular cells. ATN is potentially reversible, although renal function must generally be supported for a time with dialysis. Recovery of tubular function begins 1 to 2 weeks after the initial injury and may take up to 1 year to be completed. Further discussion of ATN can be found in Chapter 28.

MULTIPLE ORGAN DYSFUNCTION SYNDROME

When organ dysfunction develops in two or more systems, the term *MODS* may be applied. When the patient sustains multiple organ injury from a primary insult such as trauma, the term *primary MODS* is used. *Secondary MODS* is associated with SIRS and usually develops days to weeks after the primary insult. Sepsis and septic shock are the most common causes of secondary MODS. Mortality from MODS differs depending on the number of organs affected; involvement of two organ systems carries a 54% mortality, and involvement of five organs carries a 100% mortality.[21] In MODS, the body is unable to maintain homeostasis, and intensive intervention is necessary to maintain life.

As with other manifestations of septic shock, MODS is thought to be initiated by immune mechanisms that are overactive and destructive. Immune cytokines affect endothelium throughout the body and cause recruitment of neutrophils and activation of inflammation in vascular beds. Ongoing inflammation leads to tissue destruction and organ dysfunction. Inflammatory cytokines and stress hormones stimulate an increased body metabolism, which places a greater demand on already dysfunctional organs.

> **KEY POINTS**
> - Shock states result in reduced or inadequate cellular oxygen consumption and may affect all organs and systems in the body. Complications of shock can be viewed as inflammatory in nature. Inflammation is triggered by hypoxic injury to cells, by antigen, or by endotoxin. Excessive or inappropriate immune system responses lead to leaking capillaries, damage from proteolytic enzymes, and systemic activation of the clotting, complement, and kinin systems.
> - Respiratory failure and kidney failure are commonly associated with shock. Inappropriate activation of the clotting cascade may result in DIC. MODS may occur with widespread cellular hypoxia and necrosis.

SUMMARY

Shock is a life-threatening syndrome associated with high mortality. Early identification of patients at risk and initiation of therapeutic measures may decrease the development of shock syndrome. Four major categories of circulatory shock have been described: cardiogenic, obstructive, hypovolemic, and distributive. Although each type of shock has specific characteristics, all are associated with a deficiency of cellular oxygen consumption. Tissue ischemia leads to hypoxic cellular dysfunction and death, generation of oxygen free radicals, and stimulation of a systemic inflammatory response. In late-stage shock and in septic shock, ongoing systemic inflammation leads to progressive organ dysfunction and can precipitate a number of shock complications, including ARDS, DIC, ATN, and MODS. Ongoing research into effective ways to improve microcirculatory function and intervene in the inflammatory cascade is needed to improve outcomes.

REFERENCES

1. Warren JC: *Surgical pathology and therapeutics*, Philadelphia, 1895, Saunders.
2. Ellis CG, Jagger J, Sharpe M: The microcirculation as a functional system, *Crit Care* 9(Suppl 4):S3–S8, 2005.
3. American College of Surgeons: *Advanced trauma life support course for physicians*, Chicago, 2008, Author.
4. Devlin JW, Matzke GR: Acid-base disorders. In Dipiro JT, et al, editors: *Pharmacotherapy: a pathophysiologic approach*, ed 8, New York, 2011, McGraw-Hill, pp 923–942.
5. Rixen D, Siegel JH: Bench-to-bedside review: oxygen debt and its metabolic correlates as quantifiers of the severity of hemorrhagic and post-traumatic shock, *Crit Care* 9(5):441–453, 2005.
6. Andrades ME, Movina A, Spasic S, Spasojevic I: Bench-to-bedside review: sepsis—from the redox point of view, *Crit Care* 15(5):230, 2011.
7. Elbers PW, Ince C: Bench-to-bedside review: mechanisms of critical illness—classifying microcirculatory flow abnormalities in distributive shock, *Crit Care* 10(4):221–228, 2006.
8. Deleston D, Opal SM: Future perspectives on regulating pro- and anti-inflammatory responses in sepsis, *Contrib Microbiol* 17:137–156, 2011.
9. Topalian S, Ginsberg F, Parrillo JE: Cardiogenic shock, *Crit Care Med* 36(Suppl 1):S66–S74, 2008.
10. Hochman JS, et al: Early revascularization in acute myocardial infarction complicated by cardiogenic shock. SHOCK Investigators. Should we emergently revascularize occluded coronaries for cardiogenic shock? *N Engl J Med* 341(9):625–634, 1999.
11. MacLaren R, Rudis MI, Dasta JF: Use of vasopressors and inotropes in the pharmacotherapy of shock. In Dipiro JT, et al, editors: *Pharmacotherapy: a pathophysiologic approach*, ed 8, New York, 2011, McGraw-Hill, pp 399–420.

12. Trost JC, Hillis LD: Intra-aortic balloon counterpulsation, *Am J Cardiol* 97:1391–1398, 2006.

13. Shoemaker WC, et al: Resuscitation from severe hemorrhage, *Crit Care Med* 24(Suppl):S12–S23, 1996.

14. Erstad BL: Hypovolemic shock. In Dipiro JT, et al, editors: *Pharmacotherapy: a pathophysiologic approach*, ed 8, New York, 2011, McGraw-Hill, pp 421–436.

15. Simons FE: Anaphylaxis, *J Allergy Clin Immunol* 125:S161, 2010.

16. Levy MM, Dellinger RP, Townsend SR, et al: The Surviving Sepsis Campaign: results of an international guideline-based performance improvement program targeting sever sepsis, *Intensive Care Med* 36:222–231, 2010.

17. Dellinger RP: Cardiovascular management of septic shock, *Crit Care Med* 31(3):946–955, 2003.

18. Dhainaut JF: International integrated database for the evaluation of severe sepsis (INDEPTH): clinical evaluation committee report on the safety of drotrecogin alfa (activated) therapy, *Curr Med Res Opin* 24(4):1187–1197, 2008.

19. Levy MM, et al: 2001 SCCM/ESICM/ACCP/ATS/SIS International Sepsis Definitions Conference, *Crit Care Med* 31(4):1250–1256, 2003.

20. Kang-Birken SL, Killgore-Smith K: Severe sepsis and septic shock. In Dipiro JT, et al, editors: *Pharmacotherapy: a pathophysiologic approach*, ed 8, New York, 2011, McGraw-Hill, pp 2041–2054.

21. Dellinger RP, et al: Surviving sepsis campaign: international guidelines for management of severe sepsis and septic shock: 2008, *Crit Care Med* 36(1):296–327, 2008.

22. Del Sorbo L, Slutsky AS: Acute respiratory distress syndrome and multiple organ failure, *Curr Opin Crit Care* 17(1):1–6, 2011.

Respiratory Function and Alterations in Gas Exchange

Lorna L. Schumann

⊖volve WEBSITE

KEY QUESTIONS

- How do the structures involved in gas exchange in the lungs differ from conducting structures?
- What factors determine the work of breathing?
- How are alveolar ventilation and oxygenation estimated and assessed?
- What factors affect the distribution of ventilation and perfusion in the lungs?
- How are oxygen and carbon dioxide transported in the circulation?
- What pathophysiologic factors might alter ventilation-perfusion matching in the lungs?
- What are the risk factors and complications of pulmonary venous thromboembolism and hypertension?
- What are the various types of pulmonary malignancies?

CHAPTER OUTLINE

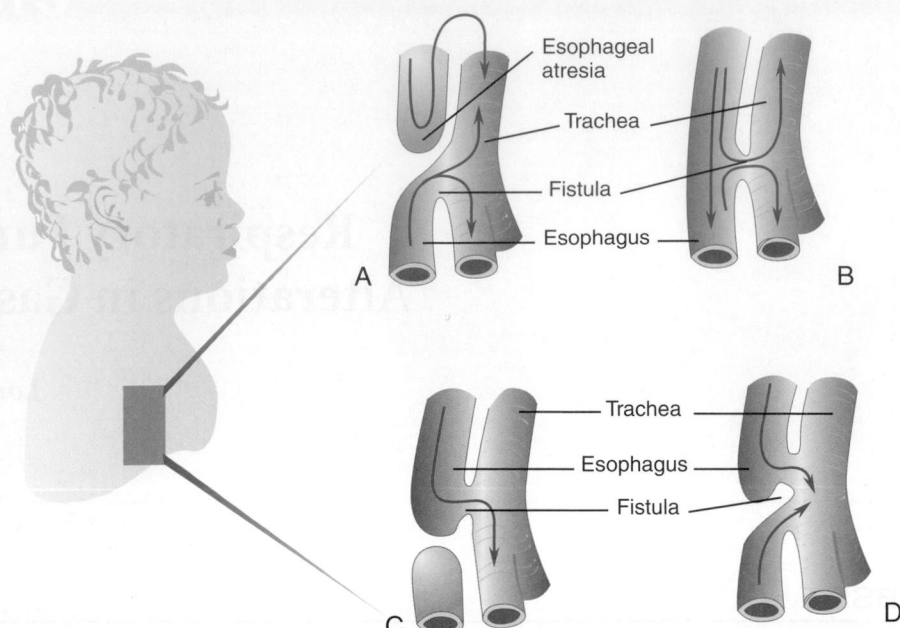

FIGURE 21-1 Four primary types of tracheoesophageal fistulas. **A,** The most common type, with complete atresia (blind pouch) of the esophagus. **B,** A common opening between the trachea and esophagus. **C,** An opening from an esophageal pouch into the trachea. **D,** A double opening from two unconnected ends of the esophagus. *Arrows* indicate flow of fluid from the esophagus to the trachea.

The primary function of the lungs is gas exchange. Oxygen is transported to the body tissues, and carbon dioxide, a waste product, is transported out of the body. The exchange of these gases takes place at the alveolar-capillary membrane. For effective gas exchange to occur, the processes of ventilation, perfusion, and diffusion must occur simultaneously at the alveolar-capillary interface. Problems with any of these three processes can result in hypoxemia (low arterial oxygen concentration) or hypercarbia (high arterial carbon dioxide concentration). An understanding of the anatomy and physiology of pulmonary gas exchange is necessary for learning about the pathophysiologic processes that follow.

FUNCTIONAL ANATOMY

Development of the Pulmonary System

Initially, the laryngotracheal diverticulum includes the esophagus and the trachea as a single tube. Then longitudinal ridges begin to develop along the tube and form a septum (wall), which separates the esophagus from the trachea. Failure of this septum to develop leads to a tracheoesophageal fistula (abnormal opening), leaving a communication between the esophagus and the trachea. This abnormality occurs about once in every 2500 births. Approximately 90% of the cases of esophageal atresia (blind pouch) are of the type seen in Figure 21-1, *A*. Parts *B* through *D* show variations of tracheoesophageal fistulas.[1]

As the laryngotracheal tube continues to elongate, the lung bud divides into two bronchial buds, which become the bronchi and the right and left lungs. The right bronchus becomes larger than the left. The right mainstem bronchus is normally more vertical than the left because it is the main continuation of the laryngotracheal tube and branches off the trachea at a 20-degree angle. The left bronchus branches off the trachea at an angle of 40 to 60 degrees. This normal anatomic development increases the chances that an inhaled foreign body will lodge in the right mainstem bronchus rather than the left.

Fetal lung development can be divided into the following four periods:

1. During the pseudoglandular period (5 to 17 weeks) the bronchial divisions are differentiated, and the major elements of lung tissue are present except for those involved in gas exchange: the respiratory bronchioles and alveoli.
2. During the canalicular period (16 to 25 weeks) the bronchi and bronchioles enlarge and vascularization of lung tissue takes place. At the end of this period, respiration is possible because of the development of respiratory bronchioles and primitive alveoli. Alveoli are grapelike sacs in which gas exchange occurs. Type II pneumocytes (epithelial cells that are on the internal surface of alveoli) begin to secrete surfactant at the end of this period. Surfactant is a phospholipid essential for maintaining alveolar patency.
3. During the terminal sac period (24 weeks to birth), terminal air sacs become thinner, preparing the lung tissue for gas exchange. Proliferation of pulmonary capillaries is also prominent during this period. Infants born prematurely in the early weeks of this period (25 to 28 weeks) are susceptible to the development of respiratory distress syndrome (RDS) because of the immaturity of the pulmonary structures.
4. The alveolar period (late fetal life to 8 years) is the final period of lung development when alveolar ducts form from terminal sacs and alveoli mature by increasing in size and number. Approximately one eighth to one sixth of the adult number of alveoli are present at birth.[1] During this growth period, there is a lack of structural collateral pathways necessary for maintaining open airways. This may make the individual more susceptible to atelectasis (incomplete expansion) and obstruction. Lung damage during this period may cause permanent defects in lung development.[1]

Upper Airway Structures

The respiratory system can be divided into two major anatomic areas: the upper airway and the lower airway. The upper airway consists of

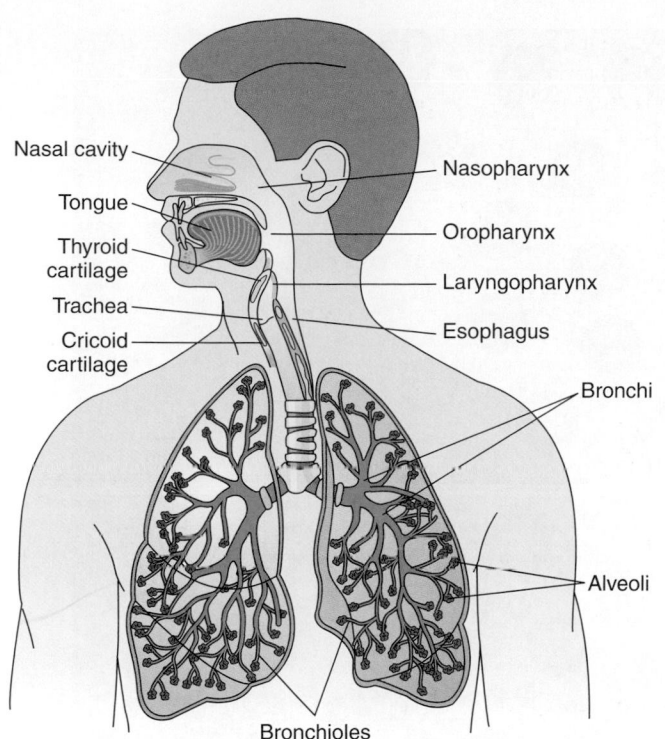

FIGURE 21-2 Sagittal view diagram of the nasopharyngeal cavity (nasal cavity, nasopharynx, oropharynx, and laryngopharynx) and the respiratory passages beginning at the trachea and ending at the alveoli.

the nasopharyngeal cavity (nasopharynx, oropharynx, laryngopharynx) (Figure 21-2). The lower airway contains the larynx, trachea, bronchi, bronchopulmonary segments, terminal bronchioles, and the acinus (the alveolar region supplied by one terminal bronchiole, which includes numerous alveoli) (see Figure 21-2).

The nasal cavity conducts gases to and from the lungs, and filters, warms, and humidifies the air. It is a rigid box composed of two-thirds cartilage and one-third bone, which prevents collapse during movement of air. The convoluted turbinates (cone-shaped bones) of the nasal cavity are highly vascular, and their blood flow forms an efficient heat exchanger. Evaporation of water from the turbinate surface and from the mucus secreted by mucosal glands raises the water vapor of the inspired air to normal saturation. Therefore, air is warmed to body temperature and humidified.

Air is filtered by the large hairs (vibrissae) of the nasal cavity and cilia that line the nasal cavity. The cilia sweep foreign particles trapped by mucus into the nasopharynx, where they are swallowed or expectorated. An electron micrograph of the tracheobronchial lining is shown in Figure 21-3. Pseudostratified ciliated columnar epithelium lines the trachea and bronchi. Goblet cells and mucus-producing glands are contained in this area and are responsible for synthesizing approximately 100 ml/day in the adult, more with disease. The composition of mucus is 95% water with the remaining 5% consisting of mucopolysaccharides, mucoproteins, and lipids. Maintenance of water content and fluid balance is important to the mobilization of secretions. A child has more mucus-producing glands and therefore produces more mucus than an adult. Consequently, in an ill child the overproduction of mucus in combination with small airway size may precipitate tracheobronchial obstruction.[2,3]

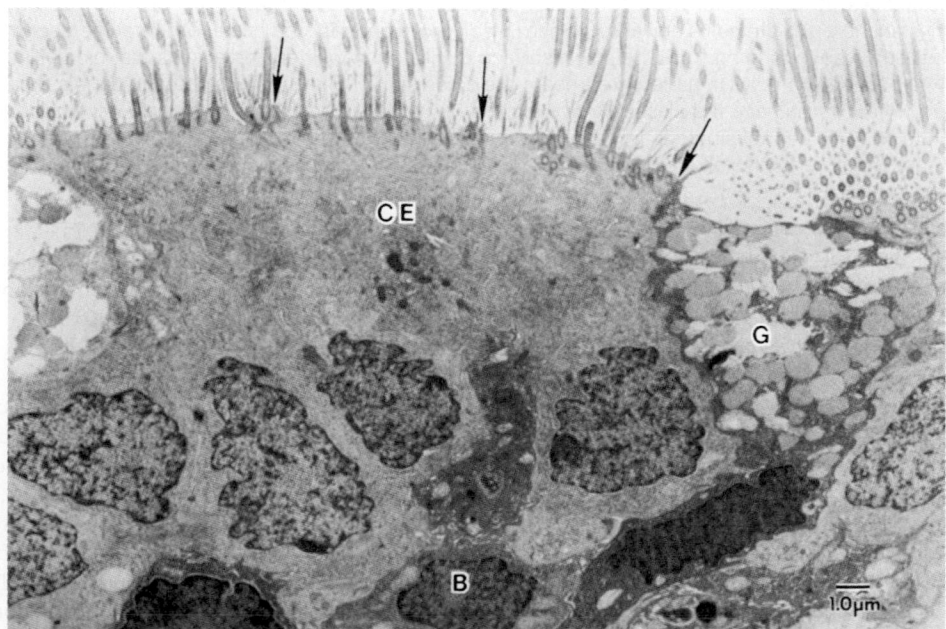

FIGURE 21-3 Cells composing the bronchial epithelium are ciliated epithelial cells *(CE)*, goblet cells *(G)*, and basal cells *(B)*. Goblet cells have abundant mucus granules in the cytoplasm, and their apical surface is devoid of cilia. Basal cells, as their name indicates, are located along the abluminal portion of the lining epithelium, adjacent to the basal lamina. The arrows at the apical surface of the airway cells indicate the location of junctional complexes between contiguous epithelial cells. (Human lung surgical specimen, transmission electron microscopy.) (From Murray JF, Nadel JA: *Textbook of respiratory medicine,* ed 4, Philadelphia, 2005, Elsevier.)

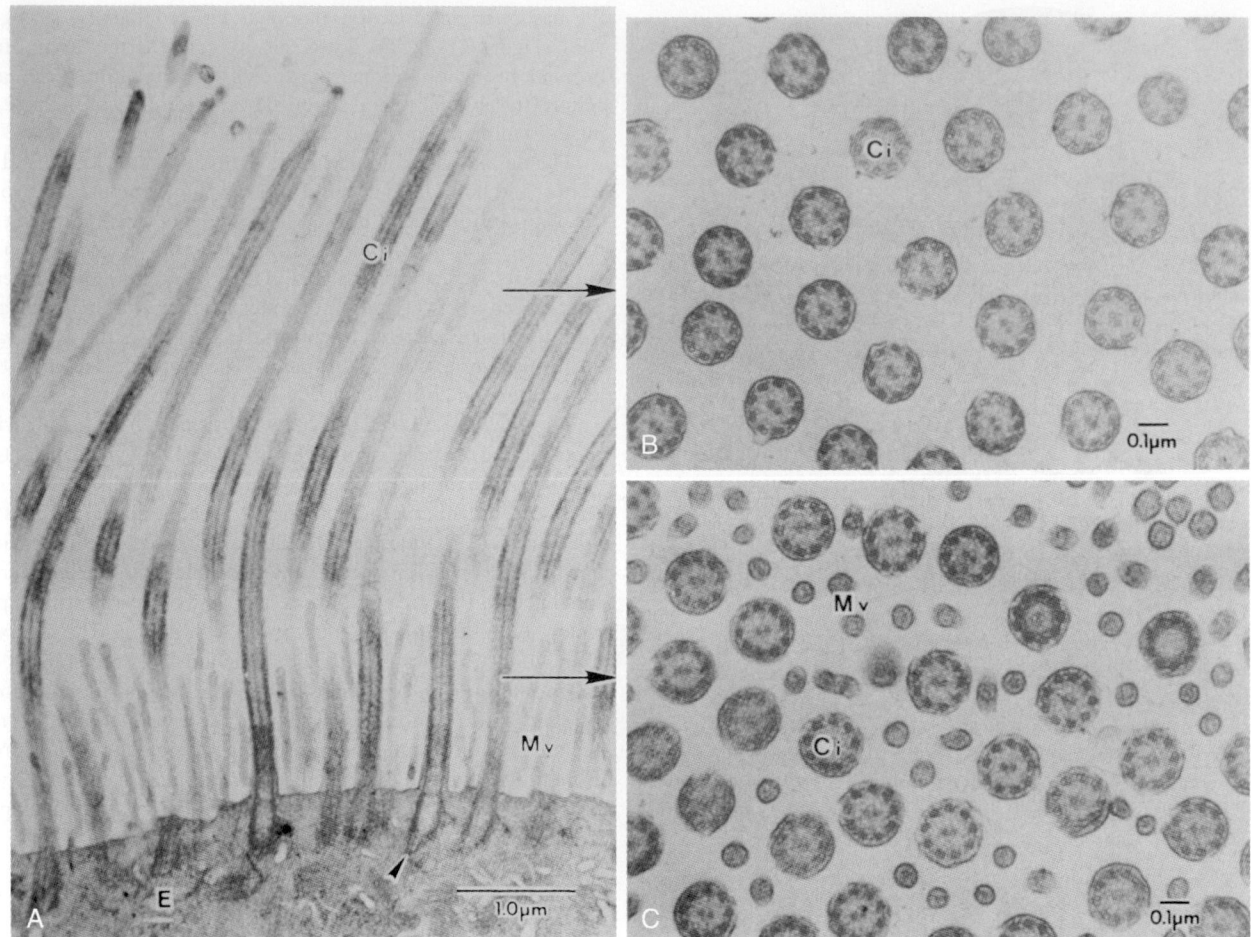

FIGURE 21-4 A, Electron micrograph shows the ultrastructural characteristics of cilia *(Ci)* on airway epithelial cells *(E)*. Each cilium has a long slender shaft that ends with a conical tip. The base of the cilium is anchored in the cell's apical cytoplasm by a curved and tapered basal foot (modified centriole; *arrowhead*). Also extending from the apical surface of ciliated airway epithelial cells are microvilli *(Mv)*. The two horizontal arrows in panel **A** represent the cross-sectional planes illustrated in panels **B** and **C**. **B** and **C,** Airway cilia have the classic microtubular arrangement of motile cilia, namely, nine peripheral doublets and two central singlets. Microvilli are randomly distributed among the cilia. (Human lung surgical specimen, transmission electron microscopy.) (From Murray JF, Nadel JA: *Textbook of respiratory medicine*, ed 4, Philadelphia, 2005, Elsevier.)

Cilia (Figure 21-4) beat in a sweeping motion like oars rowing a boat at approximately 1000 to 1500 strokes per minute.[2,3] Mucociliary transport (movement of mucus upward) is a primary defense mechanism of the tracheobronchial tree. Inhaled particles, bacteria, and macrophages are removed from the respiratory tract by ciliary clearance and the cough reflex. Ciliary function is impaired by smoking, alcohol ingestion, hypothermia, hyperthermia, cold air, low humidity, starvation, anesthetics, corticosteroids, noxious gases, the common cold, and increased mucus production.[2,3]

The four paranasal sinuses are air-containing spaces adjacent to the nasal passages that provide speech resonance and increase the surface area for heat and water vapor exchange. The sinuses are swept clean by mucociliary action when the communicating passages that connect them with the nasal passages remain open.

The eustachian tube between the middle ear and the posterior nasopharynx maintains the air in the middle ear at atmospheric pressure. To prevent secretions or food from entering the middle ear during swallowing, the pharyngeal muscles close the eustachian tube briefly. The nasal end of the eustachian tube is surrounded by flexible cartilage arranged in a spiral configuration. The muscles surrounding the eustachian cartilage close the opening by pulling the cartilage tighter. Because the tube is shorter in children, the potential for otitis media (infection of the middle ear) is increased.[2,3]

Lower Airway Structures

After air passes through the nasal cavity or oral cavity into the pharynx, it moves into the larynx and finally into the tracheobronchial tree. The acinus (Figure 21-5) is located at the end of the tracheobronchial tree and is composed of bronchioles, alveolar ducts, and alveoli.

The larynx is the transition area between the upper and lower airways. Anatomically it is considered part of the lower airway, but functionally it is similar to the upper airway. The larynx contains the epiglottis, vocal cords, and cartilages. The anatomic arrangement of the larynx functions to prevent aspiration during swallowing and to assist in phonation and coughing. Each vocal cord is attached anteriorly to the thyroid cartilage and posteriorly to the arytenoid cartilage. Vibration of the cords leads to phonation. Food is prevented from entering the trachea during swallowing by closure of the epiglottis. If food or fluid should bypass the epiglottis and enter the tracheobronchial tree, the cough reflex is initiated. The majority of cough receptors lie at the

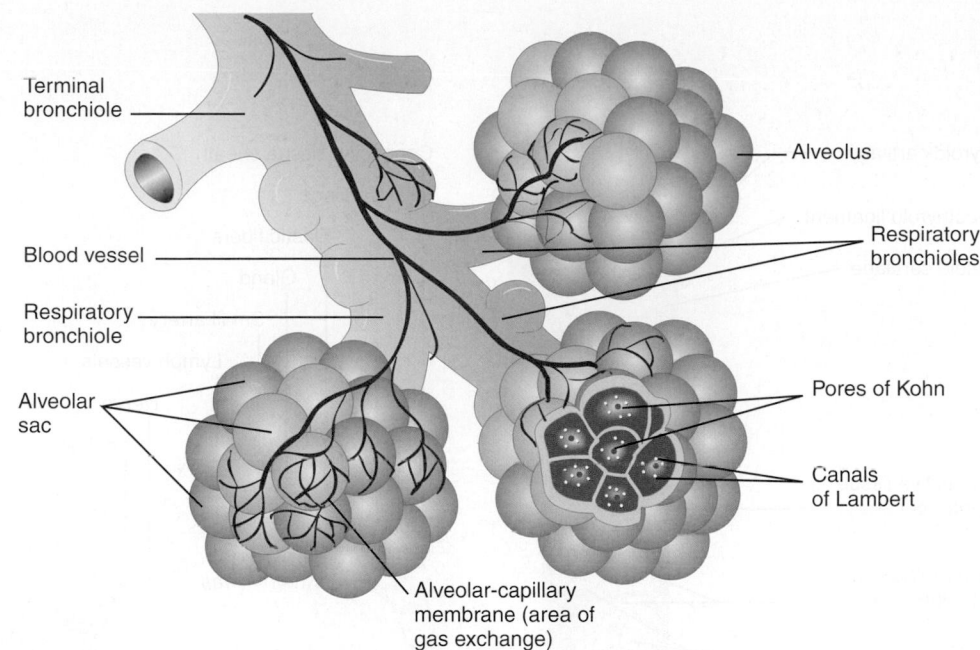

FIGURE 21-5 A portion of the lower respiratory tract, including a terminal bronchiole, respiratory bronchioles, and alveoli, where interchange of O_2 and CO_2 occurs between the thin walls of the alveoli and the capillary membrane.

carina. A cough reflex is produced when the epiglottis and vocal cords close tightly against air entrapped in the lungs. Occasionally, individuals cough hard enough to break a rib. When the expiratory muscles contract forcefully against the closed epiglottis and vocal cords, a pressure of approximately 100 mm Hg is created. When the cords and epiglottis suddenly open, the high-pressure buildup is allowed to escape. This reflex rapidly removes foreign matter from the tracheobronchial tree.[2,3]

The major cartilages of the larynx are the thyroid, cricoid, and arytenoid. The thyroid cartilage is a large shield-shaped cartilage often referred to as the *Adam's apple.* Immediately below the thyroid cartilage is the site for emergency opening (cricothyroidotomy) of the tracheal passageway. The cricoid cartilage lies below the thyroid cartilage and is the narrowest point in the airway of a child. It is the only complete tracheal ring, and because of its narrowness in the small child's airway, an endotracheal tube cuff is not necessary for required intubation of the airway.

The trachea, bronchi, and bronchioles make up the conducting airways that allow passage of gases to and from the gas exchange units (alveoli). These conducting airways comprise a proportionately larger amount of the total airway system in the infant and child than in the adult. The trachea (Figure 21-6) contains incomplete cartilaginous rings; it is approximately 11 to 13 cm long and lies between the cricoid cartilage and the carina (ridge located at the lower end of the trachea). Individual variations in tracheal shape include U, circular, D, C, triangular, and elliptical (Figure 21-7). Of 111 adult tracheas studied, the incidence of shapes in order of frequency was 48.6% C, 27% U, 12.6% D, 8.2% elliptical, 1.8% circular, and 1.8% triangular.[4] These tracheal variations may affect ventilation of patients who have endotracheal tubes in their airways and require mechanical ventilation.

The trachea divides into two mainstem (primary) bronchi, which contain cartilage and smooth muscle. Viewing the body anteriorly, the carina is located at the angle of Louis, between the sternum and manubrium at the second intercostal space.

The small size of the conducting airway in the infant and child makes even a small decrease in the size of the lumen from an obstruction

critical to airway conduction.[5] Primary bronchi further divide into five (secondary) lobar branches, three to the right lung and two to the left lung. Each lobar branch enters a lobe of the lung and further divides into bronchopulmonary segments (10 segments in the right lung, 9 segments in the left lung) (Figure 21-8).[2,3] Each bronchopulmonary segment is composed of 50 or more terminal bronchioles (conducting airways), which branch into respiratory bronchioles, where gas exchange begins.

Terminal bronchioles, which include the conducting airways, further subdivide into two or more respiratory bronchioles in which gas exchange begins. The respiratory bronchioles divide into two or more alveolar ducts, which in turn supply several alveoli.

Nervous system control of the bronchi and bronchioles is mediated by the autonomic nervous system. Stimulation of the parasympathetic nervous system via the vagus nerve leads to constriction (by means of acetylcholine receptors) of bronchial smooth muscle. Stimulation of the sympathetic nervous system leads to relaxation of bronchial smooth muscle. Sympathetic stimulation is mediated by β_2-adrenergic receptors, which are under the control of circulating catecholamines.[5] (See the discussion in the Neurologic Control of Ventilation section later in this chapter for additional information.)

The lung is fully developed by the eighth year of life.[1,2] The large alveolar surface area in conjunction with pulmonary surfactant, a phospholipid produced by type II alveolar cells, lowers surface tension and facilitates gas exchange. Two other types of cells are found: type I alveolar cells (type I pneumocytes), which are the epithelial structural cells of the alveoli, and alveolar macrophages, which act as a defense mechanism by phagocytizing particles in the alveoli. Alveolar macrophages can be damaged by cigarette smoking and by inhalation of silica (SiO_2).

Adult lungs contain approximately 300 million alveoli, and the newborn lung contains one eighth to one sixth the adult number.[1-3] An elderly person may also have a reduction in the number of alveoli as part of the normal aging process, but many elderly people retain the same number of alveoli they had as a younger adult.

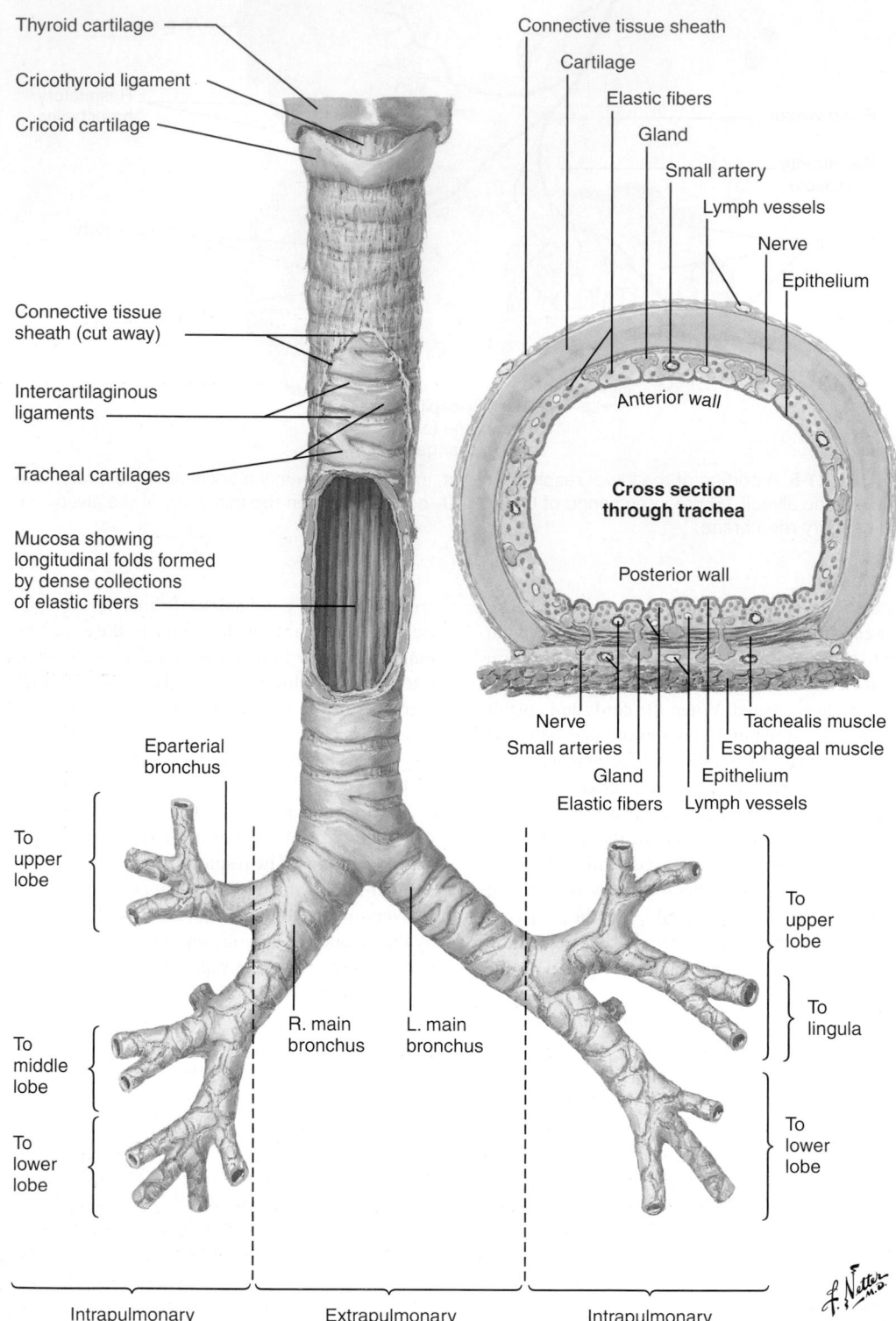

Thyroid cartilage

Cricothyroid ligament

Cricoid cartilage

Connective tissue sheath (cut away)

Intercartilaginous ligaments

Tracheal cartilages

Mucosa showing longitudinal folds formed by dense collections of elastic fibers

Connective tissue sheath

Cartilage

Elastic fibers

Gland

Small artery

Lymph vessels

Nerve

Epithelium

Anterior wall

Cross section through trachea

Posterior wall

Nerve

Small arteries

Gland

Elastic fibers

Tachealis muscle

Esophageal muscle

Epithelium

Lymph vessels

Eparterial bronchus

To upper lobe

To middle lobe

To lower lobe

R. main bronchus

L. main bronchus

To upper lobe

To lingula

To lower lobe

Intrapulmonary

Extrapulmonary

Intrapulmonary

FIGURE 21-6 Anterior diagram of the trachea and major bronchi. *L*, Left; *R*, right. (Netter illustration from www.netterimages.com. Copyright © Elsevier Inc. All rights reserved.)

Gas exchange occurs in the alveolar units (see Figure 21-5) where oxygen (O_2) and carbon dioxide (CO_2) transfer across the alveolar-capillary membrane. The partial pressures of gases in the alveoli are termed P_{AO_2} for oxygen and P_{ACO_2} for carbon dioxide. The partial pressures of gases in the blood are termed P_{AO_2} for oxygen and P_{ACO_2} for carbon dioxide. Collateral alveolar ventilation can also occur through holes in the alveolar walls, called the pores of Kohn or canals of Lambert. A small child has less collateral ventilation, because of fewer pores of Kohn.[6] The alveolar membrane is thicker in the neonate and reaches the adult thinness of 0.5 mm by the age of 8 years. This thinner membrane may allow increased transfer of O_2. The healthy older adult has very thin-walled, enlarged air sacs and fewer capillaries than a younger adult.[2,7] Respiratory system changes associated with normal aging are described in Geriatric Considerations: Changes in the Respiratory System.

Pulmonary Circulation

Blood supply to the lungs comes from two sources: the bronchial artery system, which supplies a small amount of oxygenated blood to the pleura and lung tissues, and the pulmonary artery system, which provides a vast capillary network for O_2 and CO_2 exchange. The capillary networks of the neonate, young child, and elderly person are less than those in the average healthy adult. Oxygen-depleted (unoxygenated) blood leaves the right ventricle by way of the pulmonary artery trunk, which branches into the right and left pulmonary arteries. The pulmonary arteries further divide into smaller arteries and arterioles that feed into the capillary network where gas exchange occurs from the alveolar-capillary membrane. Pulmonary artery blood is unoxygenated, and blood in the pulmonary veins is oxygenated. The opposite is true in the rest of the body, where the arterial blood is oxygenated and the venous blood is unoxygenated.

GERIATRIC CONSIDERATIONS

Changes in the Respiratory System

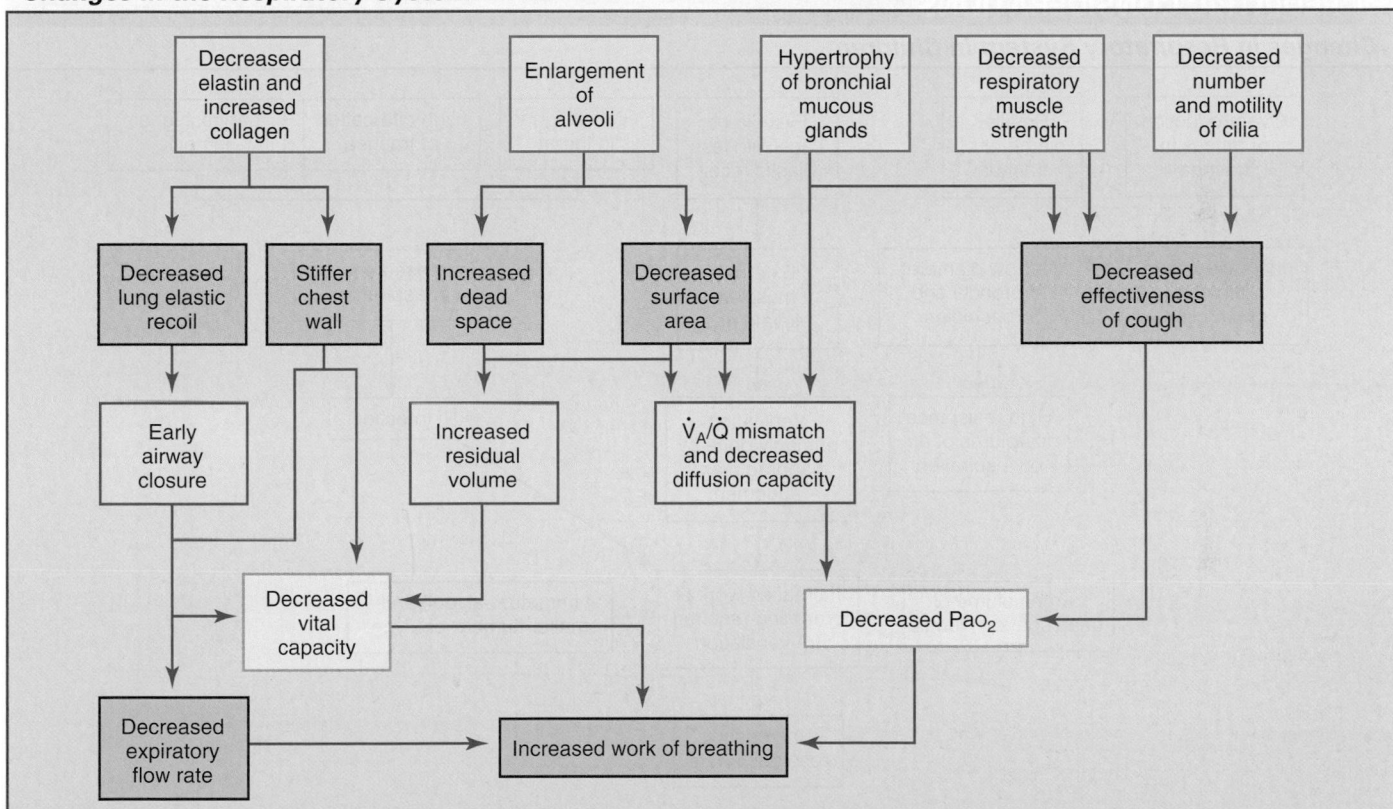

With aging, the result of all pulmonary changes is an increase in the work of breathing. The lungs show a reduction in the amount of elastin and an increase in collagen concentration, leading to decreased elastic recoil and increased compliance. These changes lead to increased residual volume and early airway closure. The chest wall becomes stiffer or more rigid as a result of rib and cartilaginous calcification. The strength of the diaphragm, intercostal muscles, and accessory muscles declines. The stiff chest wall and diminished respiratory muscle strength cause other functional changes, including an increase in dead space and decreased expiratory flow rates and vital capacity.

There is a reduction in the number and motility of cilia, resulting in a decrease in respiratory clearance. There is an increase in and hypertrophy of bronchial mucous glands. The decreased respiratory muscle strength, increased mucus production, increased chest wall stiffness, and loss of cilia together reduce cough effectiveness.

Within the lungs, there is enlargement of alveoli and respiratory bronchioles with subsequent decreased surface area. The arterial blood flow through the pulmonary vessels decreases proportionally to changes in cardiac output. The loss of elastic recoil causes the enlarged respiratory bronchioles to collapse or close before the alveoli empty. Alveolar enlargement, along with reduced pulmonary artery blood flow and early airway closure, lowers diffusion capacity and the amount of gas exchange. It also increases air trapping and residual volume.

Because of chest wall stiffness and lung rigidity, apical ventilation increases in the elderly, whereas basilar ventilation decreases. Ventilation-perfusion mismatch occurs as a result of increasing apical ventilation with poor apical capillary blood flow. The result of these changes leads to reduced arterial oxygen pressure (P_{AO_2}). Because of increased ventilation-perfusion mismatch, the P_{AO_2} may decrease when the elderly individual reclines.

The capillary network is a low-pressure system that can expand two to three times the normal size before a significant increase in pulmonary capillary pressures is detectable. The normal pulmonary arterial pressure in a healthy adult is about 22/8 to 25/8 mm Hg. The mean pulmonary arterial pressure is approximately 15 mm Hg. This compares with the high pressure of the systemic circulation, which is normally considered to be 120/80 mm Hg, with a mean arterial pressure of 96 mm Hg.

Under normal resting conditions, some pulmonary capillaries are closed and not perfused (filled with blood). The pulmonary circulation has two mechanisms for lowering pulmonary vascular resistance, when vascular pressures are increased because of increased blood flow (Figure 21-9).[2,3,5] The first mechanism is recruitment, which allows opening of previously closed capillary vessels. The second mechanism is distention, which allows for widening of capillary vessels.

Another factor influencing pulmonary circulation is the fluid balance of the lung tissues. Fluid balance is regulated by the hydrostatic pressure, colloid osmotic pressure, and capillary permeability. When capillary hydrostatic pressure exceeds colloid osmotic pressure, fluid moves from the capillary to the interstitium. If the fluid shift is not controlled, the fluid volume will continue to increase until fluid is moved into the alveoli. Alveolar edema is more serious than interstitial edema (fluid in the interstitial space), because of its negative effects on gas exchange. Pulmonary interstitial and alveolar edema is common in disease processes such as congestive heart failure and infectious diseases of the lung. Other disease processes that also increase capillary permeability are acute respiratory distress syndrome (ARDS) and infant respiratory distress syndrome. (See Chapter 23 for further discussion.)

Age-Related Variations

Structural and physiologic variations occur at each end of the age continuum. A summary of anatomic and physiologic respiratory variations by age group is presented in Table 21-1.[8] Pediatric considerations are shown in the box below.

PEDIATRIC CONSIDERATIONS

Changes in Respiratory System in Children

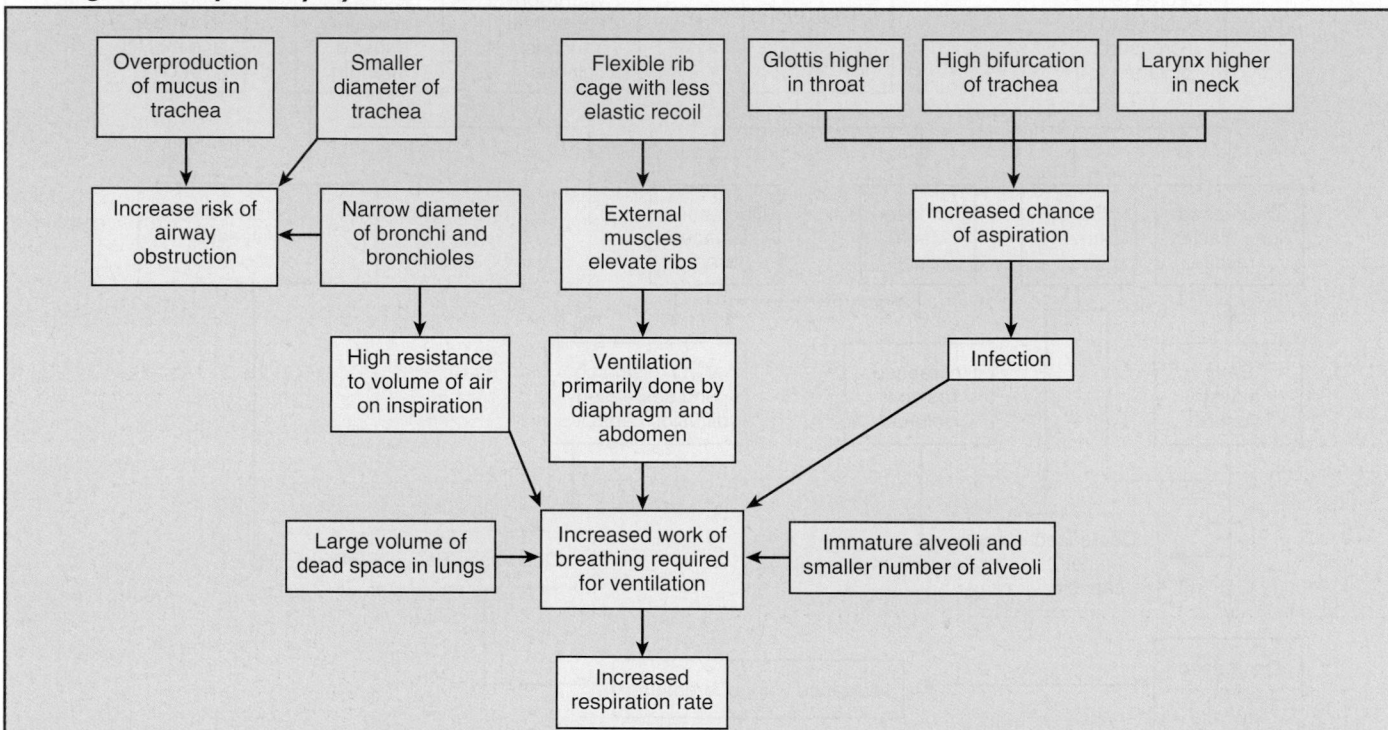

The respiratory system in children is very different than that of the adult, which makes the child susceptible to airway obstruction, aspiration, and infection. The trachea in the infant has more mucus-producing glands, which can create an overproduction of mucus in the infant. The trachea lumen, bronchi, and bronchioles are also smaller with a more narrow diameter. The excess mucus and more narrow respiratory structures increase the risk of airway obstruction in the child. The positioning of respiratory structures in the infant increases the chance of aspiration. The glottis is higher in the throat of an infant compared to a 5-year-old child (MacGregor, 2008). The trachea bifurcates at the third thoracic vertebra compared to the sixth in adults (MacGregor, 2008) and the larynx is located higher in the neck of the infant. Aspiration can lead to infection in the child and increase the work of breathing.

The infant has to work harder for ventilation of the lungs because of several factors. The more narrow diameter of bronchi and bronchioles creates a higher resistance to volume of air on inspiration. The large volume of dead space in the lungs requires the infant to breathe faster to meet oxygen demands. Compared to an adult, the alveoli are smaller and immature, which decreases the area for gas exchange to occur in the lungs. The number of alveoli and the size increase as the child ages. The flexible ribcage is unable to support the lungs adequately because it has less elastic recoil. The intercostal muscles of the ribcage also work inefficiently. The external intercostal muscles elevate the ribs for inspiration, whereas the internal intercostal muscles cannot lift the chest wall and do not help with inspiration. The infant depends on the diaphragm and abdomen for ventilation to compensate for the lack of intercostal muscle strength. All of these factors increase the work of breathing required for ventilation and the infant compensates by increasing his or her respiratory rate. By age 8 years the lungs are fully developed and the child's respiratory system begins to resemble the adult's respiratory system (MacGregor, 2008).

From MacGregor J: *Introduction to the anatomy and physiology of children: a guide for students of nursing, child care and health,* ed 2, New York, 2008, Routledge.

KEY POINTS

- Respiratory system development begins at about day 26 of gestation. Abnormal development of the septum during this time can lead to tracheo-esophageal fistula. At 25 weeks' gestation, the fetal lungs have developed sufficiently to allow respiration, although alveolar development and surfactant production are just beginning.
- The upper airway includes the nasopharynx, oropharynx, and laryngopharynx. The primary functions of the upper airway are to warm, filter, and humidify inspired air.
- The lower airway includes structures below the larynx—the trachea, bronchi, bronchioles, and alveoli. The larynx functions to prevent aspiration during swallowing and is the location of the vocal cords.
- The trachea, bronchi, and bronchioles serve as conducting passageways for air. They do not engage in gas exchange. Sympathetic influence on these airways causes relaxation (by means of β_2-adrenergic receptors), and parasympathetic influence causes constriction (by means of acetylcholine receptors).
- Exchange of respiratory gases occurs in the alveoli. The epithelial cells that comprise the alveoli are called *type I cells* (type I pneumocytes). Type II pneumocytes produce surfactant in the alveoli. The grapelike structure of the alveoli provides a huge surface area for gas exchange.
- The upper and lower airways are lined with cilia, which move rhythmically to transport mucus and trapped debris out of the respiratory tree. Ciliary function is impaired by a number of factors, including smoking, alcohol consumption, low humidity, and anesthesia.
- The lungs are perfused by two sources: bronchial arteries bring a small amount of oxygenated blood to nourish lung tissues; pulmonary arteries transport the entire cardiac output of the right ventricle to the alveoli for gas exchange.
- The lung has a large reserve capacity for gas exchange. At rest, some of the pulmonary capillaries are not perfused. During periods of high lung blood flow (such as high cardiac output during exercise), previously unperfused capillaries are recruited, and already perfused capillaries become distended.
- Filtration of fluid through pulmonary capillaries is influenced by hydrostatic pressure and colloid osmotic pressure in the same way as other capillaries. Excessive filtration can lead to pulmonary edema, which interferes with normal gas exchange.

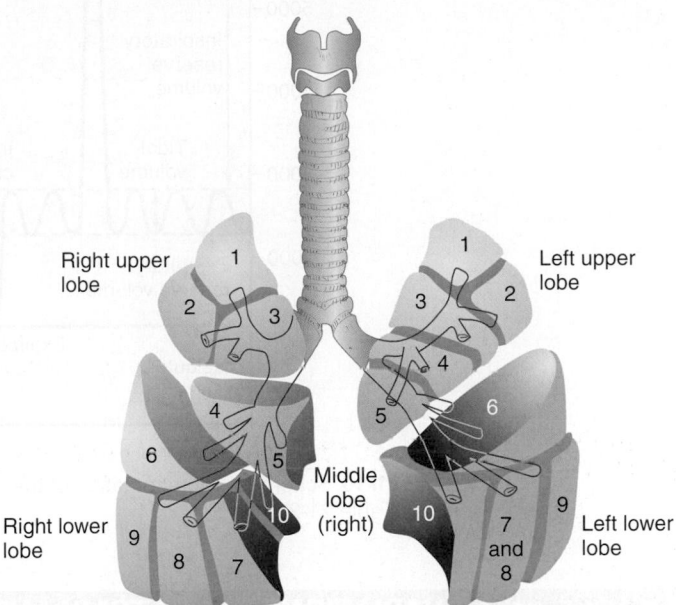

FIGURE 21-8 Bronchopulmonary segments of the human lung. Right and left upper lobes: *1,* apical segment; *2,* posterior segment; *3,* anterior segment. Left upper lobe: *4,* superior segment; *5,* inferior segment. Middle lobe (right): *4,* lateral segment; *5,* medial segment. Right and left lower lobes: *6,* superior (apical) segment; *7,* medial basal segment; *8,* anterior basal segment (on left, *7* and *8* combine to form the anteromedial basal segment); *9,* lateral basal segment. (*10,* posterior basal segment visible in medial view; not shown here.)

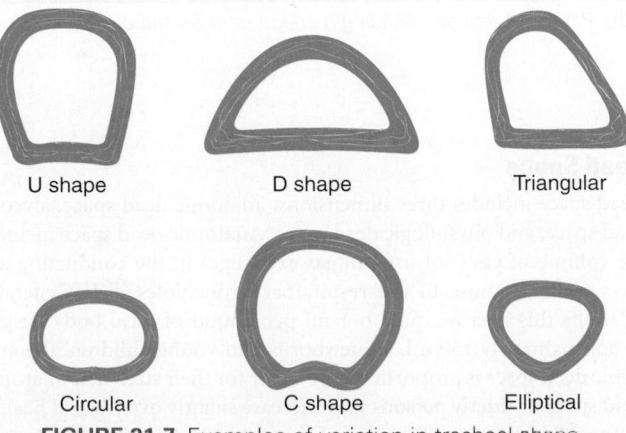

FIGURE 21-7 Examples of variation in tracheal shape.

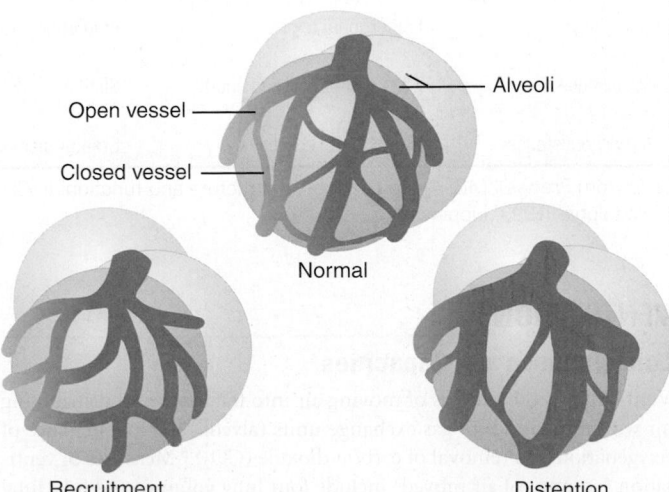

FIGURE 21-9 Two mechanisms for lowering pulmonary vascular resistance in capillary vessels. Recruitment allows for opening of previously closed capillaries. Distention allows for widening of capillary vessels.

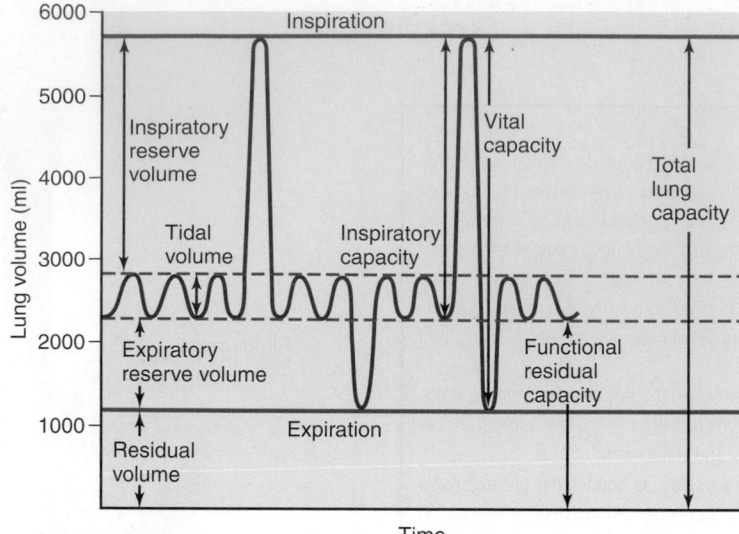

FIGURE 21-10 Schematic representation of the various lung volumes and capacities for a healthy adult (see also Table 21-2).

TABLE 21-1	**VARIATIONS IN ANATOMY AND PHYSIOLOGY OF THE RESPIRATORY SYSTEM BY AGE GROUP**			
	YOUNG NEWBORNS	**CHILDREN**	**ADULTS**	**ELDERLY (OVER 60 YEARS OLD)**
Pao_2 (mm Hg)	60-70	90-100	90-100	70-80
$Paco_2$ (mm Hg)	45-50	35-45	35-45	35-45
pH	7.3-7.4 (depends on Apgar score)	7.35-7.45	7.35-7.45	7.30-7.45
Bicarbonate (mEq/L)	20-26	22-28	24-30	24-30
Anatomic dead space	Proportional to size	Proportional to size	≈150 ml	≈150-200 ml
Number of alveoli	12.5-16.5% of adult number	Adult number by 8 years old	300,000/lung	≤300,000/lung
Thickness of alveolar membrane	Thicker than adult	Adult by 8 years old	<0.5 μm	Thinner than adult
Number of capillaries	Less than adult	Adult by 8 years old	Adult	Less than adult
Vital capacity	Proportionately less than adult	Proportional to size	4.7 L	Less than adult
Tidal volume	Proportional to size	Proportional to size	500 ml	Less than adult (30% less by age 80 years)
Compliance	More compliant than adult	Similar to adult	Static compliance (90-100 ml/cm H_2O)	Less compliant
Airway resistance	Greater than adult	Greater than adult	1.0-1.5 cm H_2O/L/sec	Adult level or less

Data from Fretwell ME: Aging changes in structure and function. In Carnevali DL, Patrick M, editors: *Nursing management for the elderly*, ed 3, Philadelphia, 1993, Lippincott.

VENTILATION

Lung Volumes and Capacities

Ventilation is the process of moving air into the lungs and distributing air within the lungs to gas exchange units (alveoli) for maintenance of oxygenation and removal of carbon dioxide (CO_2).[5] Measures of ventilation (amount of air moved) include four lung volumes and four lung capacities. Figure 21-10 schematically presents the various lung volumes and capacities; Table 21-2 defines each term and provides further details.

Lung volumes and capacities vary according to the individual's body size, age (decreased in the neonate, young child, and the elderly),[7-9] and body position (supine versus upright). Testing of pulmonary function to measure these volumes and capacities is covered under the Diagnostic Tests section in Chapter 22. Other measures important to ventilation are dead space, minute ventilation, and alveolar ventilation.

Dead Space

Dead space includes three dimensions: anatomic dead space, alveolar dead space, and physiologic dead space. Anatomic dead space includes the volume of gas (not used in gas exchange) in the conducting airways from the nose to the respiratory bronchioles.[5,10,11] Generally, in adults this area is equal to 1 ml per pound of *ideal* body weight, or approximately 150 ml. In newborns and young children, the anatomic dead space is proportionally larger for their size.[6] The anatomic dead space of elderly persons may increase slightly over that of healthy young adults because of the loss of alveolar sacs. Alveolar dead space is composed of ventilated, but unperfused areas of the lung, and is often referred to as *wasted ventilation*.[5] Physiologic dead space (functional dead space) is the sum of the anatomic dead space and alveolar dead space.[7,11] Approximately one third of each breath occupies dead space.

TABLE 21-2 LUNG VOLUMES AND CAPACITIES

TERM	DEFINITION (TYPICAL VOLUME)
Lung Volumes	
Tidal volume	A normal breath (≈500 ml) or amount of gas entering or leaving lung during normal breathing
Inspiratory reserve volume	Amount of gas a person is able to inspire above a normal breath (e.g., maximal deep breath, ≈3 L)
Expiratory reserve volume	Amount of gas expired beyond tidal volume (≈1.2 L)
Residual volume	Volume of gas left in lungs at end of a maximal expiration (≈1.2 L)
Lung Capacities	
Vital capacity	Total volume of gas that can be exhaled during maximal expiration (≈4.8 L)
Inspiratory capacity	Amount of gas that can be inspired from a resting expiration (≈3.5 L)
Functional residual capacity	Amount of gas left in lungs at end of a normal expiration (≈2.4 L)
Total lung capacity	Amount of gas contained in lungs at maximal inspiration (≈6.0 L)

Minute Ventilation

Minute ventilation is the product of tidal volume (milliliters of air inhaled with each breath) times respiratory rate per minute. For example, a person with a tidal volume of 500 ml who is breathing at a rate of 15 breaths/minute has a minute ventilation of 7500 ml (see Table 21-2 for typical volumes).

Alveolar Ventilation/Oxygenation

By comparison, alveolar ventilation ($\dot{V}_A$) equals the difference between tidal volume (V_T) and anatomic dead space volume (V_D) multiplied by the respiratory rate (RR) per minute.[10]

$$\text{Alveolar ventilation } (\dot{V}_A) = (V_T - V_D) \times RR$$

Because alveolar ventilation is affected by both the anatomic dead space and the respiratory rate, slow deep breathing yields greater alveolar ventilation than rapid shallow respiration. The patient breathing 25 times/minute at a V_T of 200 ml would have alveolar ventilation as follows:

$$(200 \text{ ml} - 150 \text{ ml [anatomic dead space]}) \times 25 \text{ breaths / minute} = 1250 \text{ ml}$$

A patient breathing 10 times/minute at a V_T of 600 ml would have an alveolar ventilation of

$$(600 \text{ ml} - 150 \text{ ml}) \times 10 = 4500 \text{ ml}$$

The partial pressure of oxygen in the alveoli (P_{AO_2}) is the driving force to move O_2 into the blood and is estimated with the following equation:

$$P_{AO_2} = F_{IO_2}(P_B - 47) - (P_{aCO_2} \div 0.8)$$

where F_{IO_2} is the fraction of inspired oxygen, P_B is the barometric pressure, 47 is the constant for water vapor pressure (mm Hg), 0.8 is the respiratory quotient, and P_{aCO_2} is the laboratory measurement of arterial CO_2 pressure (mm Hg).

The value for P_{AO_2} is normally very close to that for P_{aO_2}. The difference between alveolar and arterial oxygen tensions is called the Alveolar-arterial Difference in oxygen ($A - aDo_2$). A large $A - aDo_2$ value indicates poor matching of alveolar ventilation with alveolar blood flow ($\dot{V}_A/Q$ matching)

For example, the calculation of $A - aDo_2$ for a person at sea level ($P_B = 760$ mm Hg) breathing room air ($F_{IO_2} = 0.21$) with $P_{aO_2} = 75$ mm Hg and $P_{aCO_2} = 40$ mm Hg is

$$P_{AO_2} = 0.21(760 - 47) - (40/0.8) = 150 - 50 = 100$$

Therefore, using the arterial blood gas value obtained for the P_{aO_2} and the calculated P_{AO_2} of 100, a difference of 25 mm Hg is determined:

$$A - aDo_2 = 100 - 75 = 25 \text{ mm Hg}$$

This large of a difference indicates a significant problem with gas exchange.

In critical care settings, it is useful to calculate the $A - aDo_2$ value to monitor the efficacy of oxygen exchange across the lung. The normal $A - aDo_2$ gradient in a normal, healthy young adult is less than 10 mm Hg at room air, but it increases with age and increasing F_{IO_2}. A rising $A - aDo_2$ value indicates worsening lung function, even though hypoxemia (P_{aO_2} lower than 80 mm Hg at sea level) may not necessarily be present.

Hypoxemia that is primarily caused by hypoventilation suggests that the lung is normal, and treatment that increases ventilation will remedy the problem. This type of hypoxemia is characterized by a normal $A - aDo_2$ value.

A simple method of calculating expected P_{AO_2} is the "law of 5's." By multiplying the F_{IO_2} (%) by 5, the care provider has an estimate of what the oxygen level should be under normal, healthy conditions (e.g., $5 \times 21\%$ room air = 105).

Mechanics of Breathing

The mechanics of breathing include the concepts of airway resistance, lung compliance, and opposing lung forces (elastic recoil versus chest wall expansion) of the lung. These factors affect the overall performance of gas exchange and the work of breathing.

The lungs have a natural recoil tendency, whereas the chest wall favors the expanded state. During inspiration, the chest wall muscles (external intercostals) contract, elevating the ribs as the diaphragm moves downward. These two actions create a negative intrapleural pressure that causes the lung to expand. During expiration, the lung deflates passively because of the elastic recoil (elastic fibers in the lung tissue) and relaxation of the diaphragm. During heavy breathing, as seen with exercise, the elastic forces are not strong enough to cause the necessary rapid expiration, so abdominal muscles contract, pushing the abdominal contents upward, compressing the lungs.[3] Figure 21-11 shows the interaction of lung forces during inspiration and expiration. In the normal, healthy resting individual, expiration is accomplished almost entirely by relaxation of the diaphragm.[5] At the end of a normal expiration, the alveoli still contain some air volume, known as the *functional residual capacity*. If the alveoli were allowed to empty completely, the high surface tension in the alveoli would make it more difficult to reinflate them and add significantly to the work of breathing. In the absence of surfactant, which reduces alveolar surface tension, the alveoli tend to collapse—a condition called *atelectasis*. Excessive surface tension can increase the work of breathing so much that mechanical ventilation may be required. This is often the case in ARDS and in infant respiratory distress syndrome (see Chapter 23).

Airway Resistance

Airway resistance is determined by the relationship between driving pressure and flow. It is influenced by airway radius and the pattern of gas flow. Resistance increases as the radius of the airway tube decreases. Resistance is calculated by the following formula:

$$\text{Resistance} = \text{driving pressure} \div \text{rate of airflow}$$

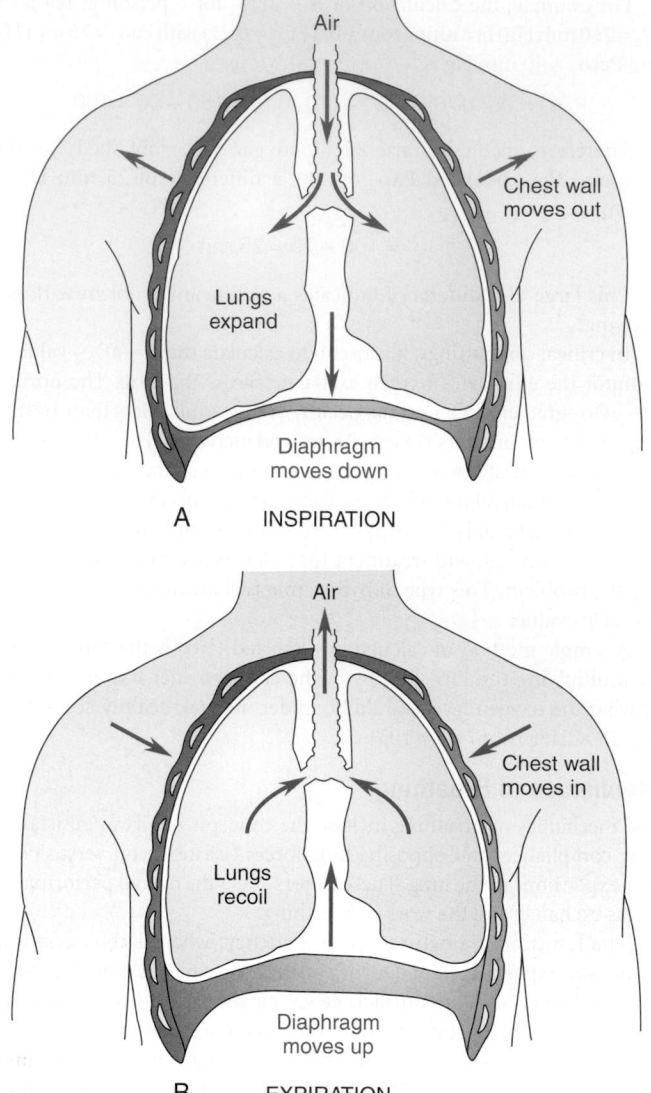

A INSPIRATION

B EXPIRATION

FIGURE 21-11 Lung forces during inspiration and expiration. **A,** During inspiration, the respiratory muscles contract, the chest wall expands, and air flows into the lungs. **B,** During expiration, the respiratory muscles relax, the lungs recoil, and air flows passively out of the lungs.

The radius of the airway decreases from the trachea to the terminal bronchioles. As mucus builds up in the airway, the passage is narrowed, and resistance to airflow increases. Other factors affecting airway resistance include stress, pulmonary conditioning, and age.

The trachea and bronchi contain cartilage and small amounts of muscle. The cartilage assists in maintaining airway passage stability, thus preventing airway collapse. The bronchioles and terminal bronchioles do not contain cartilage, but have increased amounts of smooth muscle that are innervated by the autonomic nervous system. Stimulation of cholinergic fibers leads to bronchoconstriction. Stimulation of the β_2-adrenergic receptors leads to bronchodilation. The bronchial muscles function to maintain an even distribution of ventilation. A circadian rhythm is associated with bronchial tone, with maximal bronchodilation occurring at about 6 pm and maximal bronchoconstriction occurring at 6 AM.[2]

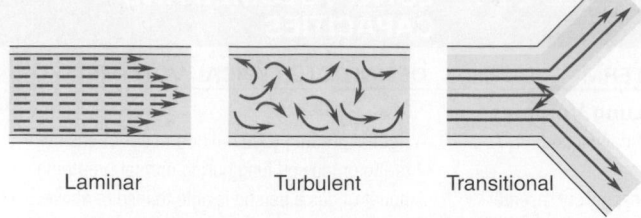

Laminar   Turbulent   Transitional

FIGURE 21-12 Patterns of gas flow.

Airway resistance is also affected by the pattern of gas flow (Figure 21-12). Air movement from the nasal cavity through the large bronchi occurs by turbulent flow, which creates friction and increases resistance. Bronchospasm in the smaller airways and high gas flow also create turbulent flow. Laminar flow occurs in the small airways of the lung and creates minimal resistance to airflow. Transitional flow (mixed pattern of flow) occurs in the larger airways, especially at bifurcations. The highest airway resistance is at the nose, because of turbulent flow with high velocities of airflow. Airway resistance is even higher in the newborn than the adult and continues to be greater than that of the adult up to the age of 5 years. Resistance changes very little in the elderly lung.[6,12,13]

Lung Compliance

Lung compliance is another factor that influences the work of breathing. Compliance represents lung expandability and the ease of lung inflation. It is best illustrated by the effort required to blow up a new balloon as compared to blowing up a balloon that has been inflated many times before. It is a measure of the relationship between pressure and volume. It is represented by the formula:

$$\text{Compliance} = \text{change in volume} \div \text{change in pressure}$$

Two factors associated with compliance are chest wall expandability and lung expandability. Lung compliance can be measured in the static (motionless) or dynamic state. Effective static compliance is determined by dividing the pressure required to deliver a volume of gas by the tidal volume as delivered by a ventilator. A more accurate measurement of compliance requires the insertion of an esophageal balloon. Normal static compliance in a healthy young adult would be 90 to 100 ml/cm H_2O.

Compliance provides an estimate of airway resistance and elasticity. Lung compliance is increased in neonates and children younger than 3.5 years because of their chest wall flexibility.[6] Lung compliance may decrease in the elderly because of increasing chest wall rigidity from calcification of costal cartilages, reduced mobility of ribs, and partial contraction of inspiratory muscles.[11,12] Changes in the thoracic vertebrae and intervertebral disks also lead to decreased expansion of the chest wall in the elderly.[7,8,12] Disease processes that make the lung stiffer and decrease respiratory function include pneumonia, pulmonary edema, atelectasis, ARDS, and pulmonary fibrosis. Other factors that decrease compliance by decreasing chest wall distensibility are obesity, abdominal distention, pregnancy, kyphoscoliosis, and abdominal surgery (attributable to decreased respiratory effort from surgical pain). Lung compliance may be increased by loss of the lung's elastic fibers that occurs with age and obstructive lung diseases.[11,12] An abnormally high lung compliance, with loss of elastic recoil increases the work of breathing by requiring greater effort to expel air from the lungs during exhalation (see Chapter 22).

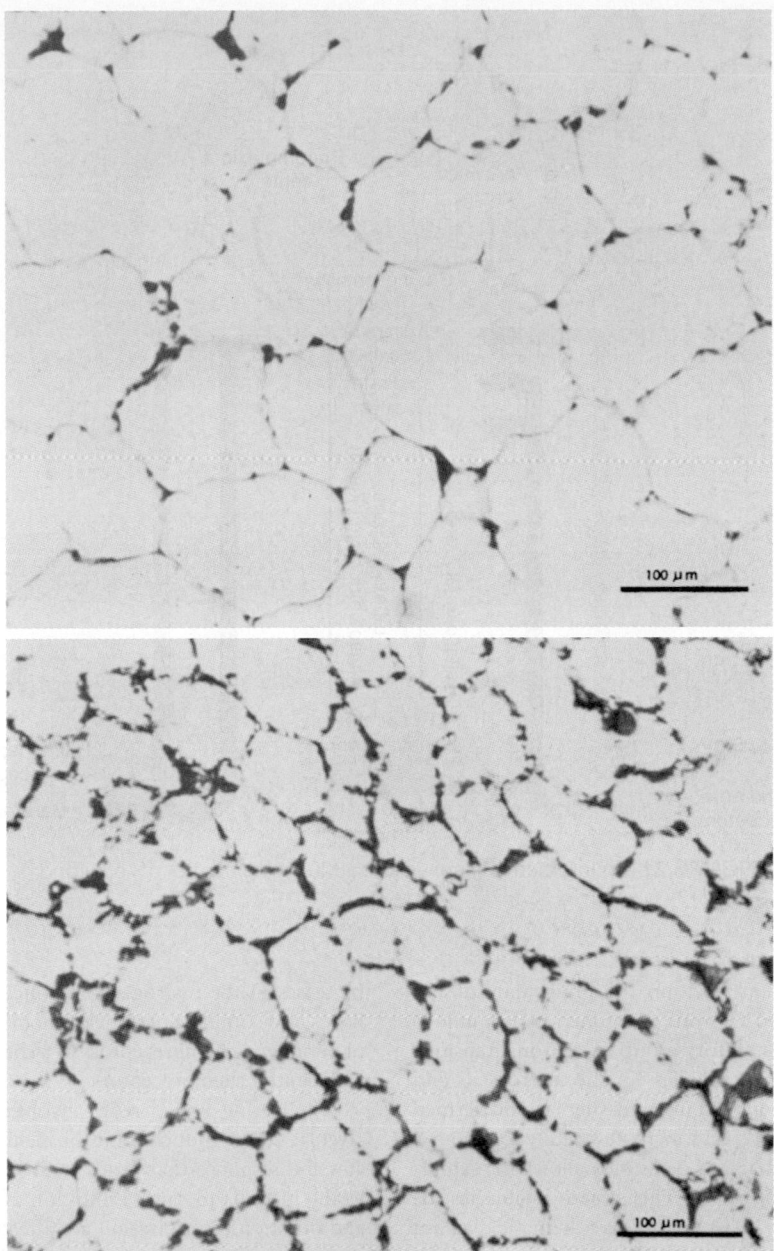

FIGURE 21-13 Sections of lung from the apex *(upper panel)* and 20 cm below the apex *(lower panel)* obtained from a greyhound dog lung (specimens frozen in a vertical position). The upper panel illustrates alveoli in the apex *(zone 1)* of the lung in the upright position: the air sacs are large, and blood flow is diminished. The lower panel represents the base of the lung zone with optimal ventilation and perfusion (×188). (From Murray JF: *The normal lung,* ed 2, Philadelphia, Saunders, p. 110. Courtesy Jon B. Glazier, MD.)

Distribution of Ventilation

Distribution of ventilation is affected by body position. In the upright individual, the alveoli at the apices (top) of the lung are much larger than those at the base. Figure 21-13 shows the variation in structural size of alveoli at the apex compared with that at the base. In the healthy upright individual, ventilation is greatest near the bottom of the lung and decreases toward the apices.[5] These regional differences are less in a supine person. The greater lung expansion at the bases results from a greater compliance of the alveoli at the bases and the downward displacement of the diaphragm, which expands the lower lobes more than the upper lobes. When an individual is in the supine lateral position, ventilation is best in the dependent part of the lung fields, but the difference is not as great as that seen in the upright lung.

Neurologic Control of Ventilation

Respiration is influenced by a number of factors. These include neural control centers, chemoreceptors, lung receptors, proprioceptors, and pressure receptors. The factors that regulate respiration are reviewed in this section.

Neural control of the respiratory system is located in the medulla oblongata and the pons, which is commonly referred to as the *respiratory center.* Efferent nerve impulses travel from the brainstem by way of the phrenic nerve to the diaphragm to stimulate muscular contractions for inspiration.

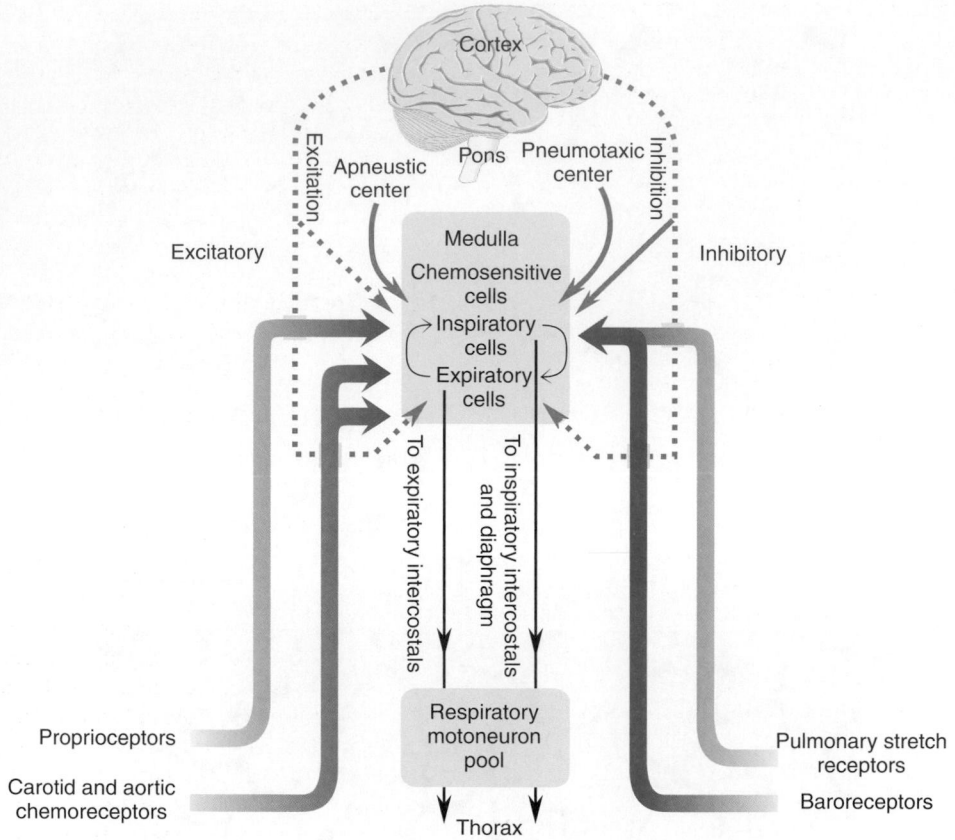

FIGURE 21-14 Interactive mechanisms influencing control of respiration.

The medullary respiratory center within the brainstem consists of two groups of widely dispersed neurons that function as a unit to regulate breathing. The dorsal respiratory group of neurons transmits impulses that stimulate inspiratory muscles (in the intercostals and diaphragm). The impulses are generated in increasing fashion, termed a *ramp signal*. Impulses begin slowly and increase steadily for about 2 seconds. Abrupt cessation of signals for 3 seconds allows for expiration, and then the cycle begins again.[2,3,5] This system establishes the basic respiratory rhythm. Figure 21-14 provides a schematic diagram of these interactive mechanisms on respiratory control.

The pneumotaxic center of the upper pons (see Figure 21-14) appears to influence the rate of respiration and ends inspiration by inhibition of the inspiratory ramp. In addition, input from the spinal cord, cortex, and midbrain contributes to the normal smooth pattern of respiration. The apneustic center of the lower pons (demonstrated to exist in dogs) influences the pattern of respiration and may function to provide an extra driving force for the inspiratory neurons, thus prolonging inspiration.

Sensory inputs to the respiratory control center include central chemoreceptors, peripheral chemoreceptors, Hering-Breuer stretch receptors, proprioceptors, baroreceptors, and environmental sensations.

The central chemoreceptors within the medullary center respond to changes in CO_2 level and pH. A stimulus to breathe occurs when a small increase in arterial carbon dioxide tension ($Paco_2$) leads to stimulation of respiration. Alveolar ventilation can increase 10-fold with an acute rise in $Paco_2$.

The peripheral chemoreceptors located in the aortic arch and carotid bodies respond primarily to decreases in arterial O_2 concentration.

Increases in the hydrogen ion concentration (decreased pH) or the $Paco_2$ also stimulate peripheral chemoreceptors, however the response of peripheral chemoreceptors to a change in $Paco_2$ is minor compared with central chemoreceptors.

The Hering-Breuer reflex involves stretch receptors located in the alveolar septa, bronchi, and bronchioles. Inflation of the lung initiates the response that sends neuronal impulses up the vagus nerve to the medulla to cause inhibition of inspiration. Therefore, the rate and duration of inspiration are affected. This reflex is primarily seen in neonates (less so in adults) and at high tidal volumes (greater than 1500 ml) and prevents overinflation of the lung.[2,3,5]

Proprioceptors located in the muscles and tendons of movable joints respond to body movement (exercise). Body movement, such as with exercise, leads to stimulation of respiration (rate and depth) to maintain oxygen levels.[3]

Baroreceptors located in the aortic arch and carotid arteries respond to changes in blood pressure. The aortic arch transmits impulses through the vagus nerve, and the carotid bodies transmit impulses through the glossopharyngeal nerve. An increase in arterial blood pressure leads to inhibition of respiration. A decrease in mean arterial blood pressure below 80 mm Hg leads to stimulation of respiration.

Environmental factors also influence respiration. Individuals demonstrate changes in respiration related to such factors as a cold shower, a pin prick, stress, or airway irritation from air pollution and smoking. Infection and fever also increase the respiratory rate. During normal breathing, energy expenditure is only 3% to 5% of total energy expenditure. During exercise and in patients with high airway resistance energy, expenditure can increase to 50%.

PULMONARY BLOOD FLOW

Pulmonary Vasculature

Perfusion (blood flow) is the second process of respiration, the first being alveolar ventilation. The pulmonary circulation is a low-pressure system (25/8 mm Hg). The volume of blood in the lungs is about 450 ml or 9% of the total amount of blood in the body. This volume can vary from one half normal to twice normal.[3] Unoxygenated blood from the right ventricle is pumped into the main pulmonary artery and then into its branches, which divide into capillary beds throughout lung tissue. The capillary beds surround the alveoli and allow for diffusion of O_2 and CO_2.

Distribution of Blood Flow

Distribution of blood flow (perfusion) is uneven and is affected by body position and exercise. When a person is upright, blood flow is decreased in the upper regions of the lungs (apices), when compared to the lower regions (bases). When a person assumes the supine position, blood flow to the posterior dependent portion of the lung is higher than to the anterior lung, although the redistribution of blood flow is less dramatic than that seen in the upright lung.

The effect of gravity on the lung has led to the concept of lung zones.[5] Figure 21-15 depicts three lung zones. Zone 1 reflects blood flow in the apices of the lung. Blood flow is minimal at the apices because the enlarged alveolar sacs create an alveolar pressure that is higher than capillary pressure, leading to pulmonary capillary collapse. Zone 2, the middle region of the lung, has a pulmonary arterial pressure greater than the pressure inside the alveoli during ventricular systole, but this may fall below alveolar pressure during diastole. Thus, zone 2 is characterized by intermittent perfusion.

Zone 3 is continuously perfused throughout the entire cardiac cycle. Pulmonary arterial pressure is greater than pulmonary venous pressure, which in turn is greater than alveolar pressure. In this zone, capillary vessels are distended and vascular resistance is low.[5,6]

Normally, 1% to 2% of the cardiac output bypasses (right-to-left shunt) alveolar ventilation, creating a decrease in arterial oxygen pressure by 3 to 5 mm Hg.[3,10] In bronchial anastomotic diseases, the amount of shunting may rise to 10% to 20%.[10]

Ventilation-Perfusion Ratios

The discussion about distribution of ventilation and perfusion indicates that the best overall ventilation and perfusion occurs in the dependent lung fields. A factor important to the concepts of ventilation and perfusion is the matching of an adequate volume of air in the alveoli to adequate pulmonary blood flow. In the ideal state, 4 L/min of alveolar ventilation is matched to 5 L/min of capillary blood flow in the lungs, creating a normal alveolar ventilation-to-perfusion ratio ($\dot{V}_A/\dot{Q}$) of 0.8 (Box 21-1). Two major factors that affect this normal $\dot{V}_A/\dot{Q}$ ratio are right-to-left shunt and regional ventilation and perfusion changes. Other factors influencing the ratio are position changes, exercise, bed rest, and lung disease.

To review, in a normal person in the upright position, ventilation and perfusion are lower in the upper lung (apex) than the lower lung (base). In the apex, alveoli are large and receive limited blood flow, whereas in the base, alveoli are smaller and allow for greater expansion of capillaries and thus more blood flow. In the apex, $\dot{V}_A/\dot{Q}$ is as much as 2.5 times the ideal value, causing a moderate degree of physiologic dead space. In the base, $\dot{V}_A/\dot{Q}$ is as low as 0.6 times the ideal value, representing lower volumes of air where the blood flow exceeds ventilation. During exercise, blood flow to the upper lung region increases dramatically, thus decreasing physiologic dead space. With bed rest, the dependent area of the lungs becomes the back region in the supine position, so that blood flow is increased to that region and alveoli are smaller.

The three types of ventilation-perfusion imbalances are: (1) high $\dot{V}_A/\dot{Q}$, (2) low $\dot{V}_A/\dot{Q}$, and (3) true shunt. High $\dot{V}_A/\dot{Q}$ is conceptually related to physiologic dead space and zone 1, in which the alveolar unit is ventilated but not perfused. High $\dot{V}_A/\dot{Q}$ units have a low Pco_2 and normal Pao_2 and can be viewed as a respiratory reserve, which can be used if perfusion is restored.

Low $\dot{V}_A/\dot{Q}$ is conceptually related to lower Pao_2 (hypoxemia). Low $\dot{V}_A/\dot{Q}$ occurs regionally in areas where the airways are partially obstructed and airflow rates are low. Although an increase in total ventilation results in a decrease in alveolar CO_2 concentration, the increment in Pao_2 and O_2 content in end-capillary blood is minimal.[5,13,14] Low $\dot{V}_A/\dot{Q}$ is responsive to treatment with oxygen, because the airways are only partially obstructed, so it is possible for oxygen to enter the alveoli by diffusion.

True shunt, which is a right-to-left shunting of unoxygenated blood through the pulmonary circulation, contributes to lowering of Pao_2. Normally, in a healthy person, there is a small physiologic shunt of less than 5% of cardiac output because of bronchial, thebesian and other veins that bypass the alveoli. In patients with acute respiratory failure

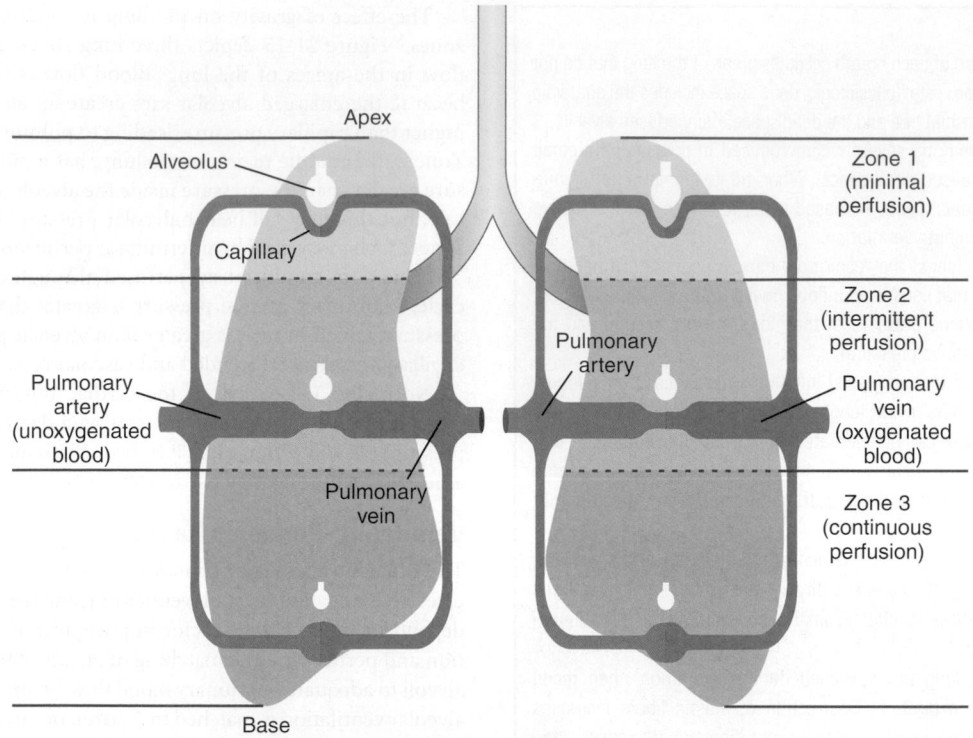

FIGURE 21-15 Schematic representation of the three lung zones in which different hemodynamic conditions govern blood flow (see text for discussion).

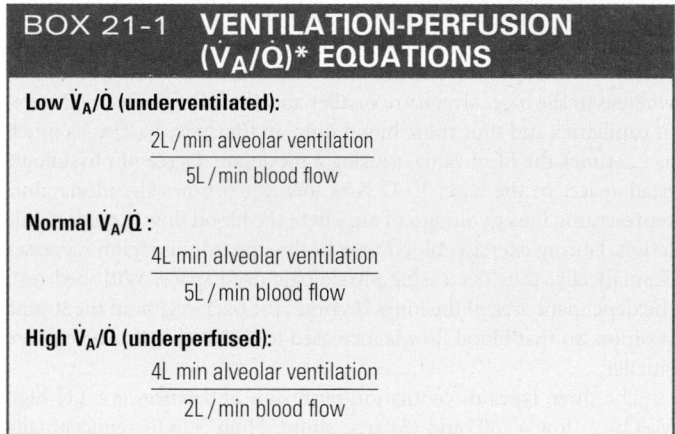

BOX 21-1 VENTILATION-PERFUSION ($\dot{V}_A/\dot{Q}$)* EQUATIONS

Low $\dot{V}_A/\dot{Q}$ (underventilated):

$$\frac{2L/min\ alveolar\ ventilation}{5L/min\ blood\ flow}$$

Normal $\dot{V}_A/\dot{Q}$:

$$\frac{4L\ min\ alveolar\ ventilation}{5L/min\ blood\ flow}$$

High $\dot{V}_A/\dot{Q}$ (underperfused):

$$\frac{4L\ min\ alveolar\ ventilation}{2L/min\ blood\ flow}$$

*$\dot{V}_A/\dot{Q}$, where $\dot{V}_A$ = alveolar ventilation and $\dot{Q}$ = blood flow.

(ARF), physiologic shunt may rise to more than 50%.[14] Although pulmonary shunt is similar to low $\dot{V}_A/\dot{Q}$ in affecting low arterial oxygen levels, true shunt is not responsive to oxygen therapy because the alveoli are collapsed or consolidated and oxygen cannot gain entry into them. See the Acute Respiratory Failure section for details.

Hypoxic Vasoconstriction

Alveolar hypoxia leads to a normal compensatory hypoxic vasoconstriction of the pulmonary vessels passing through poorly ventilated portions of the lungs. Blood is diverted from areas of low alveolar oxygen concentration to areas of higher oxygen concentration as a means of compensatory adaptation. By diverting blood flow to areas of higher oxygen concentration, the negative effects on gas exchange

are reduced. Low alveolar oxygen concentration leads to contraction of smooth muscle in the walls of the small pulmonary arterioles.[5]

> **KEY POINTS**
> - Distribution of blood flow is affected by gravity such that perfusion is greatest in dependent lung fields.
> - Zones of the lung describe regional differences in perfusion. Zone 1 has no perfusion and is equivalent to dead space; zone 2 is intermittently perfused; zone 3 is continuously perfused throughout the cardiac cycle.
> - Optimal alveolar-capillary gas exchange depends on matching of ventilation and perfusion at the alveolus. Abnormalities in $\dot{V}_A/\dot{Q}$ matching can result in inadequate oxygenation of the blood and insufficient CO_2 removal. Three types of regional $\dot{V}_A/\dot{Q}$ imbalance have been described: high $\dot{V}_A/\dot{Q}$ (dead space), low $\dot{V}_A/\dot{Q}$ (poor ventilation), and intrapulmonary true shunt (no ventilation).
> - Vessels in lung areas that are poorly ventilated, and therefore hypoxic, will constrict to minimize imbalances by diverting blood to better ventilated areas. This is termed *hypoxic vasoconstriction*.

DIFFUSION AND TRANSPORT OF RESPIRATORY GASES

Barriers to Diffusion

Diffusion is the passive movement of gas from a high-concentration area to a low-concentration area. Diffusion occurs because of the random, kinetic motion of molecules through the respiratory membranes and fluids.[3] The alveolar-capillary membrane, also known as the respiratory membrane, through which O_2 and CO_2 must diffuse consists of six barriers (Figure 21-16). The membrane averages

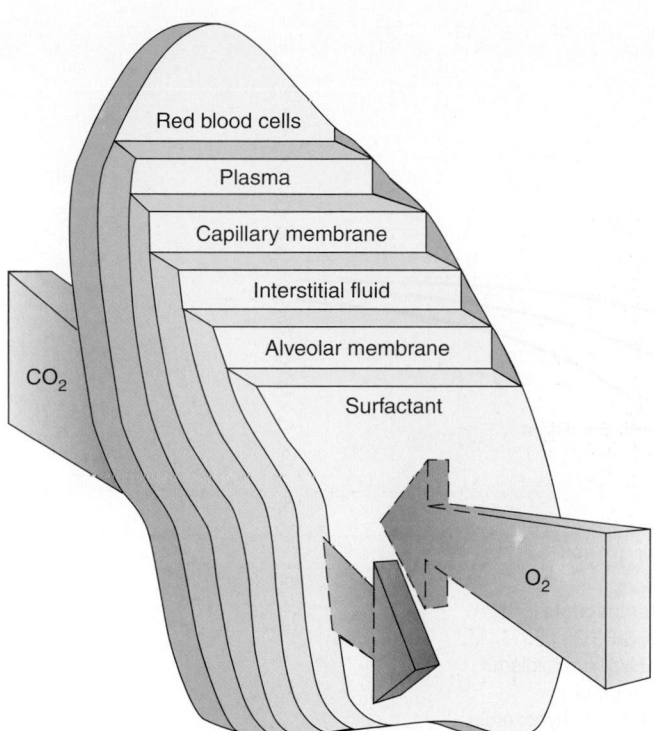

FIGURE 21-16 Schematic representing the six barriers through which O_2 and CO_2 must diffuse for gas exchange to occur.

about 0.6 micrometer in thickness.[3] For O_2 to reach the hemoglobin molecule, it must pass through surfactant, the alveolar membrane, interstitial fluid, the capillary membrane, plasma, and the red blood cell (RBC) membrane. The rate of diffusion of a gas is proportional to the tissue area and the difference in gas partial pressure between the two sides of alveoli, and inversely proportional to the tissue thickness through which the gas must move. Oxygen diffuses into the blood from the alveoli, and CO_2 diffuses out of the blood into the alveoli. Under normal conditions, O_2 and CO_2 move across the alveolar-capillary membrane in only 0.25 second. The RBC spends about 0.75 second within the pulmonary capillary system surrounding the alveoli, thus allowing an extra 0.50 second of exchange time. Even with mild disease processes, O_2 and CO_2 have adequate time for transfer. Oxygen concentration in the alveoli, as well as its partial pressure, is controlled by (1) the rate of absorption in the blood and (2) the rate of entry of new oxygen into the lungs by the ventilation process.[3]

Under abnormal conditions, such as thickening of the alveolar-capillary membrane (pneumonia, pulmonary edema, and interstitial lung disease) and decreased available surface area (emphysema), the diffusion capacity of the lung tissue is impaired. Diffusion capacity may be further impaired by increased physical activity, because of the decreased time spent by the RBCs in the pulmonary capillary system. Thickening of the alveolar-capillary membrane also occurs with aging. However, barriers to diffusion are rarely a primary cause of abnormal Pao_2 or $Paco_2$; abnormal diffusion of gases is usually secondary to $\dot{V}_A/\dot{Q}$ mismatch.

CO_2 is more diffusible than O_2, because of its greater solubility.[5] Factors that determine the ability and the speed of a gas to diffuse include the available surface area of alveoli and capillaries, the integrity of the capillary and alveolar membranes, the availability of hemoglobin to transport oxygen, the solubility of the gas, the diffusion coefficient of the gas, and the differences in partial pressure of the gases on each side of the alveolar membrane. For example, because CO_2 is 24 times more soluble than O_2, it diffuses 20 times more rapidly and requires a lower partial pressure for exchange.

The decreased diffusing capacity seen in the aged person is further compromised by a decrease in the number of pulmonary capillaries and decreased lung volume and capacities. The end result is a decreased Pao_2 and increased $\dot{V}_A/\dot{Q}$ mismatch. The Pao_2 value drops about 3 to 5 mm Hg for each decade after age 30 years.[5] Therefore, an 80-year-old individual could be expected to have a Pao_2 of 75 mm Hg. Diffusion is also decreased in the newborn because of the thickness of the alveolar membrane.[6] In a healthy adult, the Pao_2 value would be 90 to 100 mm Hg (see Table 21-1 for variations in respiratory anatomy and physiology by age grouping).

Oxygen Transport

Oxygen is transported to the tissues by two mechanisms: (1) dissolved in plasma and (2) bound to the hemoglobin molecule. Only about 0.3 ml of O_2 per 100 ml is carried dissolved in the plasma.[5] The remaining O_2 is transported on the hemoglobin molecule. A high concentration (partial pressure) of O_2 in the pulmonary capillaries causes O_2 to bind to the hemoglobin molecule. Heme is an iron-porphyrin compound that joins with the four polypeptide chains of the protein globin. Oxygen binds to iron in each of the four heme sites to form oxyhemoglobin. At the tissue level where the partial pressure of O_2 is low, O_2 is released from the hemoglobin molecule. Depending on tissue needs, 25% of the oxygen is normally unloaded at the tissues in a resting individual, which results in venous blood being 75% saturated with oxygen.

When hemoglobin is fully bound to O_2 it is nearly 100% saturated and yields a Pao_2 of 95 to 100 mm Hg. Increasing alveolar O_2 concentration above this level will have no further effect on increasing the amount of O_2 carried on the hemoglobin molecule (Figure 21-17). Oxygen binds when there is a high affinity of hemoglobin for oxygen (at the lungs) and releases when the affinity is decreased at the tissue level to maintain adequate metabolic processes. When Pao_2 is less than 60 mm Hg, saturation of hemoglobin with oxygen (Sao_2) falls steeply (see Figure 21-17). The oxyhemoglobin dissociation curve diagram shows the effects of increases and decreases in O_2 affinity at any Pao_2 level. Decreased O_2 affinity, also termed a *shift to the right*, aids in the release of O_2 from the hemoglobin molecule, thus facilitating movement of O_2 from the blood to the tissues. Factors that shift the curve to the right include acidosis, hyperthermia, increased $Paco_2$ value, and increased 2,3-bisphosphoglycerate (2,3-BPG) concentration, which is an end product of RBC metabolism. The availability of O_2 is also decreased by reduced cardiac output and anemia.[3]

Increased O_2 affinity, termed a *shift to the left*, represents a tighter binding of O_2 to the hemoglobin molecule that helps loading of oxygen in the lungs, however it may impair delivery to the tissues. Although an increased affinity for O_2 reflects a higher percentage of saturated hemoglobin, its ineffective release in the tissues may be profound. Factors that affect hemoglobin affinity and shift the curve to the left (increased affinity) include alkalosis, hypothermia, decreased $Paco_2$ value, and decreased 2,3-BPG concentration.

Cao_2 is the sum of dissolved oxygen in the plasma plus the oxygen carried on the hemoglobin (Hb) molecule. (See Chapter 13 for a more detailed discussion of oxygen carriage and transport.) Normal arterial blood oxygen content (Cao_2) is 20 ml of O_2 per 100 ml of blood (vol%) and can be calculated by the following formula:

$$Cao_2 \ (vol\%) = [Hb(g/dl) \times 1.34(ml \ of \ O_2/g \ of \ Hb) \times Sao_2] + (Pao_2 \times 0.003)$$

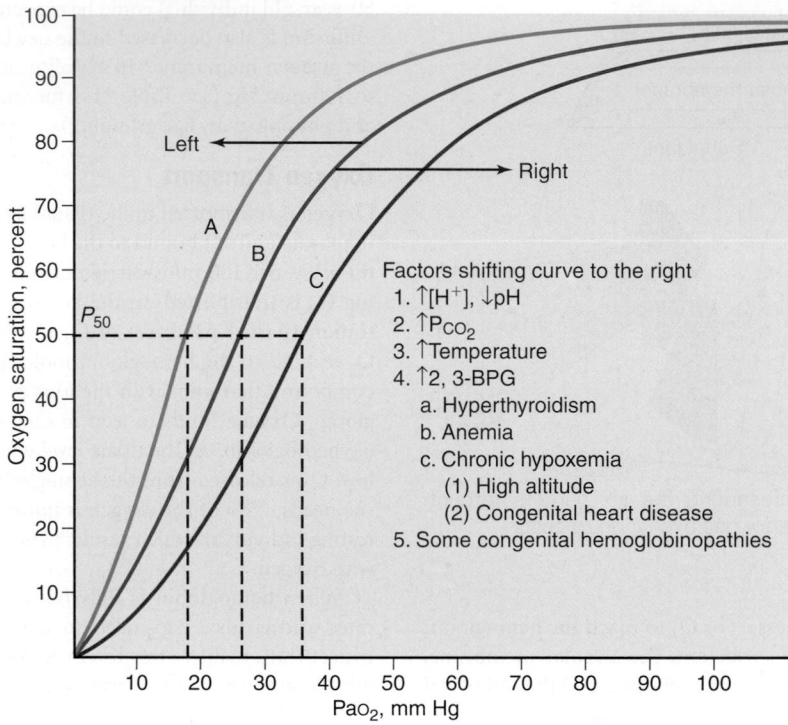

Factors shifting curve to the left
1. ↓[H⁺], ↑pH
2. ↓Pco₂
3. ↓Temperature
4. ↓2, 3-BPG
   a. Hypothyroidism
   b. Bank blood
5. Some congenital hemoglobinopathies
6. Carboxyhemoglobin

Factors shifting curve to the right
1. ↑[H⁺], ↓pH
2. ↑Pco₂
3. ↑Temperature
4. ↑2, 3-BPG
   a. Hyperthyroidism
   b. Anemia
   c. Chronic hypoxemia
      (1) High altitude
      (2) Congenital heart disease
5. Some congenital hemoglobinopathies

FIGURE 21-17 Oxyhemoglobin dissociation curve showing factors affecting hemoglobin's affinity for oxygen. Curve *B* is the standard curve under normal conditions. Curve *A* shows a shift to the left, which represents an increased affinity of hemoglobin for oxygen. Curve *C* demonstrates a shift to the right, which represents a decreased affinity. (From Gottlieb JE: Breathing and gas exchange. In Kinney MR, Packa DR, Dunbar SB, editors: *AACN's clinical reference for critical care nursing*, ed 4, New York, 1998, McGraw-Hill, p 672.)

Carbon Dioxide Transport

Carbon dioxide, a byproduct of cellular metabolism, is transported in the blood in three ways: dissolved in plasma (5% to 10% of the total CO_2 transport); as bicarbonate (60% to 70%); and as carbamino compounds on the hemoglobin molecule (20% to 30%). The greatest bulk of CO_2 transport is in the bicarbonate form. In the presence of the RBC enzyme carbonic anhydrase, CO_2 combines with water to form carbonic acid, which in turn almost instantaneously breaks down into bicarbonate ions and hydrogen ions. The released hydrogen ions attach to the hemoglobin molecule, while the bicarbonate ion diffuses into the plasma. Chloride ions in the surrounding plasma shift into the RBC (chloride shift). This chemical process is reversed when the venous blood reaches the lungs, so that CO_2 can diffuse across the alveolar membrane to be exhaled.

KEY POINTS
- Oxygen and CO_2 diffuse quickly across alveolar-capillary membranes. Complete equilibration of gases occurs in the first third of the capillary under normal conditions. Diffusion may be incomplete when the alveolar-capillary membrane is abnormally thickened or capillary blood flow is extremely rapid.
- Carbon dioxide is more soluble and diffuses more quickly than O_2. Disorders of diffusion often affect O_2 transfer earlier and more significantly than CO_2 transfer.

- Oxygen is carried in the blood in two forms: dissolved in solution ($Pao_2 \times 0.003$) and bound to hemoglobin ($Hb \times Sao_2 \times 1.34$). Significantly more O_2 is bound than dissolved. Low hemoglobin level and low hemoglobin saturation profoundly affect the O_2 content in the blood.
- The oxyhemoglobin saturation curve describes the relationship between Pao_2 and hemoglobin saturation. At a Pao_2 of 90 to 100 mm Hg, hemoglobin is fully saturated. An increase in Pao_2 above this level does not significantly improve O_2 content.
- The affinity of hemoglobin for O_2 is affected by temperature, acid-base status, 2,3-BPG levels, and CO_2 concentration. Affinity decreases at the tissue level because of increased concentrations of H^+ ions, 2,3-BPG, and CO_2. This "shift to the right" enhances the unloading of O_2 at the tissue. A "shift to the left" occurs at the lung, where the blood is more alkalotic and CO_2 levels are lower. Increased affinity of hemoglobin in the lung enhances oxygen binding.
- Carbon dioxide is transported in the blood in three major forms: dissolved, as carbaminohemoglobin, and as bicarbonate ion. The most important of these is bicarbonate ion, which is formed from the combination of CO_2 and H_2O, producing carbonic acid (H_2CO_3). Carbonic acid dissociates into HCO_3^- and H^+. At the lung, the reaction proceeds in the reverse direction to form CO_2, which diffuses into the alveoli.

ALTERATIONS IN PULMONARY FUNCTION

Partial pressures of arterial O_2 in the newborn (60 to 70 mm Hg) and elderly (70 to 80 mm Hg) are less than those in the adult. The lower O_2 pressure is well tolerated in the newborn, because of the presence of fetal hemoglobin, which has decreased binding of 2,3-BPG, thus facilitating oxygen transfer by shifting the oxygen dissociation curve to the left. The newborn also has a higher hemoglobin concentration (20 to 21 g/dl) for the first few weeks after birth. Therefore, oxygenation is not normally a problem. The lower Pao_2 of the newborn is also associated with an increased $Paco_2$. Other blood gas values (see Table 21-1) show little difference from those of adults unless an oxygenation problem is present, such as infant respiratory distress syndrome or congenital heart disease.

Hypoventilation and Hyperventilation

Hypoventilation occurs when delivery of air to the alveoli is insufficient to meet the need to provide oxygen and remove carbon dioxide. It is influenced by decreased rate and depth of respiration. Hypoventilation results in increased $Paco_2$ (>45 mm Hg) and resultant hypoxemia due to increased alveolar carbon dioxide, which displaces oxygen.[12] Causes may be drugs, such as morphine or barbiturates (which depress the central respiratory drive), or disorders such as obesity (pickwickian syndrome), myasthenia gravis, obstructive sleep apnea, chest wall damage, or paralysis of respiratory muscles (especially the diaphragm).[5] Pain related to surgery of the thorax or abdomen often results in hypoventilation secondary to decreased inspiration.

Hyperventilation is an increase in the amount of air entering the alveoli, leading to hypocapnia ($Paco_2$ <35 mm Hg).[5,13] A physiologic cause of hyperventilation is hypoxic stimulation of peripheral chemoreceptors. Pain, fever, and anxiety are common causes of hyperventilation. Less common causes include obstructive and restrictive lung diseases, sepsis, and brainstem injury (central neurogenic hyperventilation). Hyperventilation is a normal physiologic response to high altitude as a compensatory mechanism to decrease $Paco_2$. Low $Paco_2$ leads to a greater ability to bind oxygen to hemoglobin (shift to the left) despite low oxygen pressure in the inspired air at high altitude.

Ineffective gas exchange from ventilatory failure occurs when an adequate volume of gas is maldistributed, minute ventilation is decreased, and/or alveolar hypoventilation occurs. Maldistribution of gas occurs in patients with emphysema, in which gas exchange occurs only in some alveolar units.[5] In the healthy lung, some maldistribution of gas occurs because of gravitational forces on the lung, as previously discussed. In addition to the gravitational forces, airway resistance affects distribution of gases. In obstructive pulmonary diseases, increased airway resistance develops in localized regions because of (1) obstruction of airways from increased sputum production, (2) mucosal hypertrophy and edema, (3) loss of structural integrity of the airway, and (4) narrowing of the airway from bronchial smooth muscle contraction, when there is hyperactivity of the airways.[5] During expiration, air leaves the areas of least resistance first, thus creating areas of maldistribution of gas.

Hypoxemia and Hypoxia

Two terms frequently used in discussing decreased Pao_2 are *hypoxemia* and *hypoxia*. Hypoxemia refers to deficient levels of blood oxygen as measured by low arterial O_2 concentration and low hemoglobin saturation as measured by arterial blood gases or pulse oximetry (O_2 saturation). Hypoxia refers to a decrease in tissue oxygenation. Tissue hypoxia is difficult to measure, but may be assumed when either blood flow or Pao_2 is abnormally low. A decrease in blood flow leads to a decrease in oxygen delivery.

Resultant types of hypoxia can be classified into four categories: hypoxic hypoxia, anemic hypoxia, circulatory hypoxia, and histotoxic hypoxia. Hypoxic hypoxia occurs when the Pao_2 is decreased despite normal O_2-carrying capacity.[6] Causes include high altitude, hypoventilation, and airway obstruction. Oxygen therapy usually provides adequate treatment.

Anemic hypoxia results from a decrease in O_2-carrying capacity. Any disorder resulting in low hemoglobin concentration can cause anemic hypoxia.

Circulatory hypoxia results from a low cardiac output state in which the O_2-carrying capacity is normal, but blood flow is reduced. Examples of circulatory hypoxia include shock, cardiac arrest, severe blood loss, thyrotoxicosis, and congestive heart failure.

The final classification is histotoxic hypoxia, which occurs when interference of a toxic substance leads to the inability of tissues to utilize available oxygen. Cyanide poisoning is an example of histotoxic hypoxia.

Ineffective gas exchange occurs when ventilation and perfusion are mismatched, when diffusion abnormalities exist, and when right-to-left shunt exists. During periods of normal perfusion not all capillaries are open; however, the capillary system has the ability to recruit (open up) more capillaries and to distend (expand) capillaries already in use (see Figure 21-9) to increase alveolar blood flow when it is needed as a compensatory mechanism. In addition, 1% to 3% of the total blood flow in the lung is not oxygenated because the thebesian, pleural, and bronchial veins drain unoxygenated blood into the left side of the heart and into the pulmonary veins.

Areas of low ventilation-perfusion (see Box 21-1) may have normal perfusion, but receive inadequate alveolar ventilation (Figure 21-18, *A*). These areas are similar to shunting of unoxygenated pulmonary arterial blood through totally unventilated units except that they are responsive to oxygen therapy. Areas of high ventilation-perfusion (see Figure 21-18, *B*) may have adequate ventilation (high oxygen level in the alveoli), but have areas of decreased perfusion. This effect is similar to having increased dead space, clinically represented by areas of ventilation without blood flow. Although it is difficult clinically to differentiate diffusion defects from shunt effect, abnormalities occur in patients who have thickening of the alveolar-capillary membrane. Examples of diseases with thickened membranes include Goodpasture syndrome, systemic lupus erythematosus, sarcoidosis, diffuse interstitial fibrosis, and alveolar cell carcinoma.[3]

Ineffective gas exchange is also seen in patients with true pulmonary shunt (see Figure 21-18, *C*). A shunt effect results from blood flowing from the right side to the left side of the heart without passing through ventilated areas of the lung. Anatomic shunts may occur in patients with ventricular septal defects, atrial septal defects, and patent ductus arteriosus. Localized pneumonia and adult respiratory distress syndrome (ARDS) result in intrapulmonary shunts because of $\dot{V}_A/\dot{Q}$ mismatch, in which alveoli are perfused but not ventilated.

Acute Respiratory Failure (ARF)

Acute respiratory failure (ARF) is defined as a state of disturbed gas exchange resulting in abnormal arterial blood gas values: a Pao_2 value less than 60 mm Hg (hypoxemia), and a $Paco_2$ value greater than 50 mm Hg (hypercapnia) with a pH less than 7.30 when the patient is breathing room air.[1,13-15] Patients with respiratory failure can be divided into three categories: (1) those with failure of respiration or oxygenation leading to hypoxemia and normal or low carbon dioxide levels; (2) those with failure of ventilation leading to hypercapnia; and (3) those with a combination of respiratory and ventilatory failure.

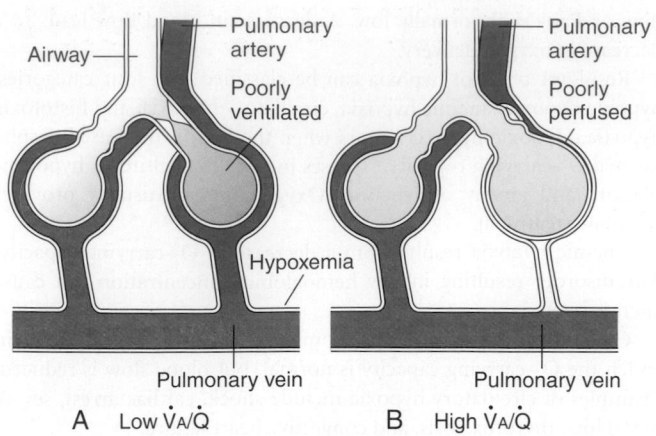

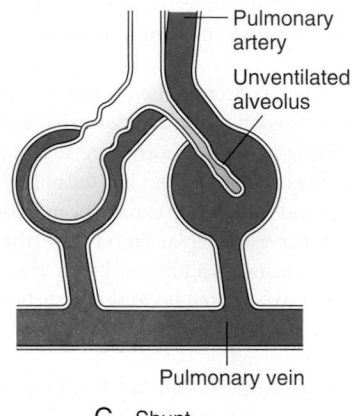

FIGURE 21-18 Ventilation-perfusion abnormalities. **A,** Low $\dot{V}_A/\dot{Q}$ areas that are well perfused but underventilated. **B,** High $\dot{V}_A/\dot{Q}$ areas that are well ventilated but underperfused. **C,** Shunt areas that have no ventilation but are perfused (blood flow passes unventilated alveoli).

Etiology. The precise pathophysiologic mechanism of ARF depends on the cause or causes of the disease process. A number of conditions may cause respiratory failure (Box 21-2), including disorders of the neuromuscular chest apparatus (poliomyelitis, Guillain-Barré syndrome, quadriplegia, hemiplegia), disorders affecting the chest skeletal system (kyphoscoliosis), and chest trauma (rib and sternal fractures). Shock (e.g., septic, hypovolemic), pulmonary emboli (PE), and pulmonary edema may also lead to respiratory failure. Extreme obesity may lead to alveolar hypoventilation, resulting in respiratory failure. The most common lung diseases causing ARF are advanced emphysema, pneumonia, asthma, and ARDS.

In general, the development of hypoxemia is related to poorly matched ventilation and perfusion. The development of hypercapnia is related to inadequate alveolar ventilation in relation to production of carbon dioxide.

Clinical manifestations. Clinical features of ARF vary with the cause. General features of hypoxia and hypercapnia include headache, dyspnea, confusion, decreased level of consciousness, restlessness, agitation, dizziness, tremors, and initial hypertension, followed by hypotension and tachycardia.[13] Early signs include rapid, shallow breathing with increased inspiratory muscle movement. Late findings include cyanosis, nasal flaring, and sternal and intercostal retractions.[1,5,7,12] The increased work of breathing may lead to cool, clammy skin, dysrhythmias, and decreased capillary refill time.

Diagnosis. Diagnostic tests include measurement of arterial blood gases and chest radiography. A Pao_2 of less than 60 mm Hg and a $Paco_2$ of greater than 50 mm Hg on room air are common findings.[12,13] Chest radiographic findings depend on the disease process. Other supporting tests include an electrolyte panel with evidence of electrolyte imbalance such as low potassium and low sodium concentrations, and a complete blood cell count with evidence of increased numbers of white blood cells associated with infection or decreased levels of red blood cells and hemoglobin attributable to anemia.

Treatment. Maintaining ventilatory support by maintaining airway patency and ensuring adequate alveolar ventilation is the primary goal of therapy. Mechanical ventilation may be the initial treatment, followed by management of the underlying cause. If a neuromuscular problem or skeletal weakness is present, assisted ventilation with a positive-pressure volume ventilator is indicated to maintain airway patency and ensure adequate alveolar ventilation.

The primary goal of therapy is to provide adequate oxygenation at the cellular level by maintaining a Pao_2 greater than 60 mm Hg (oxygen saturation, 90%). Specific interventions depend on the cause. If acute respiratory failure is caused by chronic obstructive pulmonary disease, then vigorous management of bronchospasm and possible infection is required using a combination of methylxanthines, β_2 agonists, corticosteroids (controversial), and antibiotics. Heart failure or hypotension may require drug therapy. Diuretics may be given for volume reduction depending on the fluid volume status of the patient. Hypotension should be managed promptly with volume replacement and/or vasopressors. The use of corticosteroids in high doses for the first 24 to 48 hours of the disease process is controversial, because no conclusive evidence of efficacy is available.[12-14]

General supportive care consists of providing adequate nutrition to maintain fluid and electrolyte balance, offering pain management and emotional support, and preventing complications of gastrointestinal stress and bed rest. Developing a method of communication with ventilated patients is also very important. High-calorie, high-protein, low-carbohydrate nutritional support is recommended. A diet high in carbohydrates should be avoided because of its tendency to increase carbon dioxide production.[13] (See Chapter 23 for specific treatments for ARDS and infant respiratory distress syndrome.)

KEY POINTS

- Ventilatory failure occurs when alveolar ventilation is insufficient to accomplish adequate gas exchange. Ventilatory failure may result from decreased respiratory rate, decreased tidal volume, or increased dead space. Arterial blood gas analyses demonstrate hypercarbia and hypoxemia.

- A general deficiency of O_2 in the blood (hypoxemia) results from poor diffusion at the alveoli (hypoxic hypoxia) or anemia (anemic hypoxia). Tissue hypoxia may be due to general hypoxemia or poor perfusion (circulatory hypoxia) or result from poor uptake of O_2 by the tissue (histotoxic hypoxia).

- Oxygenation failure occurs when diffusion of gases across the alveolar-capillary interface is impaired. Oxygenation failure may be due to mismatching, right-to-left shunt, or excessive barriers to diffusion. Arterial blood gas values demonstrate hypoxemia but not necessarily hypercarbia.

- Acute respiratory failure is generally diagnosed from arterial blood gas disturbances. The usual defining values are a Pao_2 less than 60 mm Hg and a $Paco_2$ greater than 50 mm Hg when the subject is breathing room air.

- Conditions that predispose an individual to hypoventilation, ventilation-perfusion mismatch, or right-to-left shunt may lead to respiratory failure

BOX 21-2 CAUSES OF ACUTE RESPIRATORY FAILURE

Central Nervous System
Drug overdose (sedative, hypnotic, opioid, anesthetic)
Cerebral vascular accident (stroke)
Hypothyroidism
Central nervous system infections
Brain trauma
Brain tumor

Neuromuscular Diseases and Related Disorders
Guillain-Barré syndrome
Myasthenia gravis
Multiple sclerosis
Muscular dystrophy
Myxedema
Poliomyelitis
Polymyositis
Drug or toxin induced
- Botulism
- Aminoglycosides
- Organophosphates
- Neuromuscular blocking agents
Tetanus
Amyotrophic lateral sclerosis
Quadriplegia
Hemiplegia

Chest Wall and Diaphragm
Trauma (thoracic/abdominal)
Kyphoscoliosis

Upper abdominal or thoracic surgery
Pleural effusion
Hemothorax/pneumothorax/chylothorax
Massive ascites

Airways
Laryngospasm
Foreign body aspiration
Asthma
Acute exacerbation of chronic bronchitis or emphysema

Pulmonary Parenchymal Diseases
Lung contusion
Aspiration
Pneumonia
Interstitial lung diseases
Emphysema
Pulmonary fibrosis
Acute respiratory distress syndrome
Infant respiratory distress syndrome
Pulmonary emboli (blood, fat, air, amniotic fluid)
Cardiac and noncardiac pulmonary edema
Shock
Increased CO_2 production
- Fever
- Infection
- Hyperthyroidism
- Drugs

- (e.g., drugs, neuromuscular weakness, chest wall deformities or trauma, and parenchymal lung diseases).
- Manifestations of respiratory failure are due to tissue hypoxia and compensatory responses and include confusion, tremors, hypotension, depressed consciousness, tachypnea, and tachycardia.
- The goal of therapy is to reduce tissue hypoxia by maintaining Pao_2 above 60 mm Hg. Depending on the underlying disease process, this may require mechanical ventilation, supplemental oxygen administration, nutritional supplementation, and utilization of bronchodilators and antibiotics.

ALTERATIONS IN PULMONARY VASCULATURE

Pulmonary Hypertension

Etiology. Normally the pulmonary circulation is a high-flow, low-pressure system. Pulmonary hypertension is defined as a sustained increase in pulmonary artery pressure above 25 mm Hg systolic resting and above 30 mm Hg systolic with exercise. In some cases of pulmonary hypertension, systolic pressures may be as high as 60 to 110 mm Hg. Two broad types of pulmonary hypertension exist: primary (idiopathic) and secondary. Primary pulmonary hypertension (PPH) is relatively rare (1300 per 1 million people), rapidly progressive, and more common in women than men (1.7:1 ratio). PPH usually presents in the third to fourth decade of life.[16] The cause is unknown, but can be associated with portal hypertension of cirrhosis, use of appetite-suppressant drugs, and human immunodeficiency virus infection. Most cases are sporadic and may be familial[14] (6% to 12% of cases); however, mutations in the genes that code for members of the tumor growth factor-β family of receptors

on chromosome 2q33 have been found in some cases.[16] The long-term prognosis is poor, and medical management is usually ineffective.

Secondary pulmonary hypertension results from a known disease process or pathophysiologic condition. Increased pulmonary blood flow, increased resistance to blood flow, and increased left atrial pressure are the three major mechanisms resulting in pulmonary hypertension. Of these, increased resistance to blood flow is the most common cause and is attributable to hypoxic vasoconstriction as seen in chronic bronchitis and advanced emphysema.[15,16] Box 21-3 lists the major causes of secondary pulmonary hypertension.

Pathogenesis. Chronic exposure to the mechanisms listed in Box 21-3 (except PPH) results in morphologic changes within the arterial lumen. Initially, the walls of the small pulmonary vessels thicken because of an increase in the muscle. This initial response is thought to occur as a result of local tissue hypoxia, acidosis, or both.

As the underlying pathologic process intensifies, the internal layer of the pulmonary artery wall becomes fibrotic, with further muscle thickening. In addition, muscle development occurs in vessels that are normally nonmuscular. Pulmonary atherosclerosis is present in major pulmonary vessels as well.

Sustained pulmonary hypertension (mean pulmonary arterial pressure of 27 to 60 mm Hg) results in the formation of plexiform (network of blood vessels) lesions. These nodular lesions are composed of irregular, interconnecting blood channels that further impede an already compromised pulmonary vasculature. Tissue necrosis and hemorrhage often result.

Clinical manifestations. The clinical manifestations of pulmonary hypertension vary according to the severity and duration of the underlying pathologic process. Because of the normal distensibility of

BOX 21-3 MECHANISMS OF SECONDARY PULMONARY HYPERTENSION

Increased Pulmonary Vascular Resistance

Vasoconstrictive
- Alveolar hypoxia attributable to bronchitis or emphysema
- Acidosis
- High altitude
- Thromboembolic causes from obstruction or release of histamine, serotonin, or catecholamines
- Hypoxia attributable to neuromuscular disease, obesity, obstructive sleep apnea, or kyphoscoliosis

Obstructive
- Embolism (blood clots, fat emboli, amniotic emboli, tumor cells, or foreign body)

Obliterative (loss of capillary bed)
- Emphysema
- Lung resection
- Pulmonary fibrosis
- Collagen vascular disease
- Vasculitis

Increased Left Atrial Pressure

Mitral stenosis, mitral regurgitation
Left ventricular failure
Constrictive pericarditis

Increased Pulmonary Blood Flow/Viscosity

Atrial septal defects
Ventricular septal defects
Polycythemia
Sickle cell disease
Patent ductus arteriosus
Congenital heart disease

Other

Portal hypertension/liver cirrhosis
Appetite-suppressant drugs
HIV
Schistosomiasis
Sarcoidosis

nerve by an engorged pulmonary artery (Ortner syndrome) may occur.

Diagnosis. Pulmonary artery catheters are used to obtain accurate pulmonary arterial pressure measurements in patients at rest and during exercise. Unfortunately, even if mild pulmonary hypertension is present, pulmonary arterial pressure values are usually normal at rest. Pulmonary arterial pressures measured in the exercising subject would be the optimal diagnostic tool. However, the feasibility of exercising a patient with invasive central line monitoring is problematic. The pulmonary artery catheter could become wedged and necrosis could occur, or the catheter could slip back into the ventricle and irritate the myocardium, causing ventricular dysrhythmias. Stress testing without exercise may be done in the cardiac catheterization laboratory by using medications to increase cardiac output.

A chest radiograph, although usually normal in cases of mild pulmonary hypertension, is one of the earliest diagnostic tools to suggest the presence of moderate to severe hypertension. Enlargement of the pulmonary arteries and right ventricle, as well as abnormal vessel contours, is indicative of hypertensive disease. The 12-lead electrocardiogram (ECG) shows evidence of right ventricular hypertrophy. The two-dimensional echocardiogram (a noninvasive technique) can also provide evidence of pulmonary hypertension. Echocardiography may reveal mitral stenosis, left atrial myxoma, and right heart enlargement. Further diagnostic tests should be done to exclude causes of secondary pulmonary hypertension.

Treatment. The major treatment for pulmonary hypertension is early identification and control of the underlying disease process. In the case of left-to-right shunts, surgical closure of an atrial septal defect or patent ductus arteriosus may be indicated. Because the most common cause of pulmonary hypertension is related to increased pulmonary vascular resistance, treatment is often directed at reversing vasoconstriction by administering supplemental oxygen and avoiding vigorous exercise and pregnancy. Depending on the stage of hypertension, vasodilators and diuretics are commonly used in an attempt to control the symptoms. These medical regimens have produced inconsistent results.[15,16]

Advanced stages of primary pulmonary hypertension are irreversible. The only feasible intervention is lung or heart-lung transplantation. Continuous long-term infusion of prostacyclin (epoprostenol, treprostinil) is being used for its potent vasodilatory effect on the pulmonary vessels. It improves exercise capacity, quality of life, and long-term survival.[16]

Pulmonary Venous Thromboembolism

Etiology. A pulmonary embolus (PE) is undissolved detached material that occludes blood vessels of the pulmonary vasculature. As a result, circulation distal to the obstructed area is impaired. Approximately 650,000 patients are affected annually, with an estimated mortality of 50,000 annually. Of those who experience fatal PE, 8% to 10% die within 1 hour of the onset of initial symptoms.[18-20]

More than 90% of pulmonary thromboemboli originate in the deep veins of the lower extremities.[17,18] Other sources of PE include fat, air, and amniotic fluid. The types of emboli and their causes are summarized in Table 21-3.

Virchow, a pathologist of the 1800s, discovered three physiologic factors that predispose patients to thrombus formation, increasing the risk of PE. The three factors, commonly referred to as *Virchow's triad*, are venous stasis (sluggish blood flow), hypercoagulability, and damage to the venous wall (intimal injury). Several predisposing factors enhance the probability of thrombus development and the subsequent risk for PE. Using Virchow's triad, predisposing factors have been categorized under each of the three components (Box 21-4). The most common

pulmonary capillaries and the ability of the lung to recruit additional reserve capillary beds with increased pressure or flow, the condition often remains asymptomatic until significant damage to pulmonary vasculature has occurred. Exercise intolerance (because of progressive loss of pulmonary capillary distention and recruitment capabilities) is often one of the earliest clinical symptoms. Patients may also experience syncope, increasing dyspnea, chest pain on exertion, fatigue, hemoptysis, and pulmonary edema. Eventually, cor pulmonale (right-sided heart enlargement secondary to primary lung disease) and right ventricular failure will develop if persistent, severe pulmonary hypertension continues, because of persistent backpressure to the right-sided heart chambers. (See the discussion of cor pulmonale and heart failure in Chapter 19.) Common signs and symptoms of pulmonary hypertension are dyspnea (60% of cases),[16] syncope, chest pain, jugular venous distention, a systolic ejection click, narrowing or a splitting of S_2 an S_4, and accentuation of the pulmonary component of the second heart sound (P_2).[11,14,16,17] In advanced cases, tricuspid and pulmonary valve insufficiency are present.[14,16] Development of a hoarse voice attributable to compression of the recurrent laryngeal

TABLE 21-3 EMBOLISM TYPES AND CAUSES

EMBOLISM TYPE	CAUSE
Thrombotic	Blood clots develop in venous system, predominantly in thighs and legs
Fat	Globules of fat secondary to fractures of pelvis or long bones
Amniotic fluid	Collections of fluid, hair, or other debris related to complicated labor, especially in older, multiparous women
Air	Venous access through IV catheters
Tumor	Fragments from malignant tissue
Foreign material	Foreign bodies (bullets, sutures, catheter tips, orally prepared medications injected IV)
Septic	Infected tissue or related substances (fungal/bacterial)
Parasitic	Parasites present in lung vasculature

BOX 21-4 FACTORS PREDISPOSING TO PULMONARY EMBOLISM OF VIRCHOW'S TRIAD

Venous Stasis

Extended bed rest (delayed venous removal of activated clotting factors)
Postoperative state
Immobility (activated clotting factors)
Vascular disorders (thrombophlebitis of lower extremities and pelvic area)
Congestive heart failure (venous backflow/stasis)
Cardiac dysrhythmias (atrial fibrillation)
Dehydration
Prolonged air travel
Obesity

Hypercoagulability

Oral contraceptives (estrogen therapy), hormone replacement therapy
Pregnancy, early puerperium
Polycythemia (chronic high altitude; chronic pulmonary disease with decreased Pao_2 and increased $Paco_2$)
Malignant pathologic processes, visceral cancer
Cigarette smoking
Inherited resistance to activated protein C
Deficiency of protein S
Deficiency of antithrombin III
Prothrombin gene mutation
Presence of antiphospholipid antibodies (lupus), anticoagulant and anticardiolipin antibodies

Damage to Vessel Wall (Intimal Injury)

Blunt trauma
Penetrating wounds
Bone fractures with soft-tissue injury
Surgical procedures (hip, pelvic, abdominal, cardiovascular)
Obstetric manipulations during labor and delivery
Burns
Central venous catheter

risk factors for venous thromboembolus formation are immobility, trauma, pregnancy, cancer, heart failure, and estrogen use.[19,20]

Pathogenesis. Thrombi are dislodged from their point of origin by multiple mechanisms, including direct trauma, exercise and muscle action, and changes in blood flow. Regardless of whether the emboli are blood clots or an alternative type of material (see Table 21-3), once they are released into the venous system, the undissolved material travels to the pulmonary vasculature.[13] The lower lobes are frequently involved because of high blood flow.[14] The impact of pulmonary emboli on the cardiopulmonary circulation depends on the size and cross-sectional area of circulatory impairment. If the embolus occludes less than 25% of the pulmonary vessels in a healthy individual, no physiologic changes may be seen. When the occlusive area approaches 25% to 30%, pulmonary arterial pressures may begin to rise, with potential right-sided heart failure.[16,17] In the patient without any underlying pulmonary pathology, 50% of the cross-sectional pulmonary circulation must be impaired before dangerously high pulmonary arterial pressures are generated. Because of the large pulmonary capillary reserve, significant damage is necessary before pulmonary decompensation occurs.[14]

Pulmonary arterial pressures increase because of vasoconstriction from actual mechanical obstruction of blood vessels and the release of serotonin and neural sympathetic stimulation in a combined neurohormonal response. Right-sided heart failure occurs because of the high resistance generated by the pulmonary vasculature. Eventually, hypotension occurs as a result of diminished cardiac output.[16]

Actual pulmonary infarction (death of lung parenchyma) occurs only in about 10% to 15% of cases of PE.[16] Pulmonary necrosis is rare, because three sources are available for oxygen supply: the pulmonary arterial circulation, the bronchial arterial circulation, and the airways. Significant underlying pulmonary or cardiac impairment (chronic obstructive pulmonary disease, mitral stenosis) increases the risk for occurrence of pulmonary infarctions.[14,16]

Clinical manifestations. Presenting symptoms depend on the size of the embolus, as well as on any underlying cardiopulmonary pathologic conditions. Initial symptoms may include restlessness, apprehension, and anxiety. The most common symptom is dyspnea (75% to 85% of patients).[14,18] In addition, tachycardia (23%) and tachypnea (30%) are often present. Sudden dyspnea and severe chest pain are usually associated with medium-sized to massive pulmonary emboli. Chest pain may be nonpleuritic or pleuritic (infarction).[18] Pain on inspiration is seen in 65% to 75% of patients.[15] Hemoptysis may or may not occur. As the clinical picture worsens, patients experience heart failure, shock, and respiratory arrest.

Diagnosis. Because PE is often misdiagnosed, the clinician should have a high index of suspicion when clinical manifestations, combined with factors predisposing to pulmonary embolism (see Box 21-4), are noted.[19,20] Although no simple noninvasive test has both high specificity and high sensitivity, the $\dot{V}_A/\dot{Q}$ lung scan is one of the tests performed to determine the presence of a PE. The scan determines if a mismatch exists between ventilation and perfusion. Adequate ventilation with impaired perfusion (blood flow) to the pulmonary vasculature (mismatch) is indicative of PE, if the scan is performed within 8 hours of symptom onset. Helical angiography is replacing lung scans as the initial diagnostic test for pulmonary thromboembolism. This noninvasive test requires administration of radiocontrast dye.[13,18]

Other screening tools, such as arterial blood gas analyses, ECGs, chest radiographs, and cardiac enzyme determinations, are valuable for ruling out related pathologic processes. Arterial blood gases generally reveal decreased Pao_2 and $Paco_2$ and increased pH. A chest radiograph may be normal or show an elevated diaphragm, pleural effusion, infiltrates, or atelectasis. An ECG is abnormal in 70% to 85% of cases with acute PE.[14,18] Common electrocardiographic findings are sinus tachycardia, nonspecific T wave and ST-segment changes, and T-wave inversion.[18] The probability of a PE can be estimated by the use of Wells rules (Box 21-5).

The conclusive diagnostic test for PE is pulmonary arteriography, but is rarely done. This invasive procedure involves the injection of radiopaque material into the pulmonary artery. If an intraluminal filling deficit can be identified, the test is considered diagnostic for PE. A duplex ultrasonography of the lower extremities to determine the site of deep vein thrombosis should also be performed.

Treatment. The primary intervention for PE is prevention. Patients who are at risk for developing one of the factors of Virchow's triad must be treated prophylactically. In the case of prolonged bed rest, active range-of-motion exercises as well as prophylactic low-dose subcutaneous sodium heparin or low-molecular-weight heparins may be used. Intraoperative and postoperative graded compression stockings and intermittent pneumatic leg compression are beneficial in reducing the risk of PE.[13]

Patients with suspected or confirmed PE are given supplemental oxygen or ventilator support with immediate activity limitations to decrease oxygen demand. A continuous heparin IV drip is used as a mainstay of therapy.[13] Although heparin does not dissolve the clot, formation of new clots is prevented. Heparin may also stimulate the intrinsic fibrinolytic system, enhancing the degradation of the PE. Thrombolytic therapy may be used to dissolve the emboli. However, thrombolytics create an increased risk of bleeding, and unless the patient has a massive embolism and is hemodynamically unstable, they are not used.[17]

If patients are thought to be releasing multiple emboli despite adequate heparin therapy, an umbrella filter (Mobin-Uddin) or a "bird's nest" filter may be placed in the inferior vena cava to trap emboli as they migrate toward the pulmonary vasculature.[13,19] Inferior vena cava filters reliably prevent recurrent PE with a recurrence rate of about 1% at 12 days.[19] An embolectomy may be performed on an emergency basis if the hemodynamic consequences of the emboli are life threatening and the patient has refractory hypotension.

KEY POINTS

- Pulmonary hypertension usually results from conditions that increase the resistance of the pulmonary vasculature. Disorders that reduce the total cross-sectional area of the lung increase resistance and promote pulmonary hypertension. Destruction of capillaries (emphysema), blockage of vessels (emboli), and vasoconstriction (hypoxemia) are common examples.
- Pulmonary hypertension may occur when left atrial pressure is elevated. Pulmonary arterial pressure must increase to maintain the driving pressure necessary to propel blood through the pulmonary circulation. The excessive pulmonary blood flow that accompanies left-to-right shunting of blood through heart defects may also lead to pulmonary hypertension.
- Cor pulmonale (right ventricular hypertrophy) and right-sided heart failure may develop with sustained high pulmonary vascular resistance. Few symptoms of pulmonary hypertension are manifested until the right side of the heart is affected.

- Treatment centers on efforts to ameliorate the underlying cause if possible (e.g., closure of heart defects, administration of oxygen to reduce hypoxic vasoconstriction). Vasodilators and diuretics may be used to reduce pulmonary arterial pressure and decrease strain on the right side of the heart.
- Pulmonary emboli result in obstruction of blood flow through part of the pulmonary system. When emboli are large or multiple, a significant increase in pulmonary pressure may result, causing right ventricular failure.
- Emboli may be composed of fat, air, amniotic fluid, or thrombi (blood clots). Thrombi are the most common cause. Thrombi generally form in the leg under conditions of venous stasis, enhanced coagulation, or vascular trauma.
- Pulmonary embolism is suspected with sudden dyspnea and chest pain. Symptoms of right-sided heart failure may be present when emboli are large. A ventilation-perfusion scan may be done to confirm the diagnosis.
- Prophylactic anticoagulation in persons at risk for thrombus formation is important to prevent PE. Postoperative pneumatic leg compression also reduces the risk of thrombus formation. Bed rest, oxygen administration, and thrombolytic and anticoagulation therapy are the mainstays of therapy for acute PE. Ventilator support and measures to improve the functioning of the right side of the heart may be necessary in severe cases.

PULMONARY MALIGNANCIES

Etiology. The incidence of lung cancer in the United States has been increasing in recent years, with greater than 200,000 new cases per year.[21,22] The four major types of lung cancer are large cell carcinoma, small cell carcinoma, squamous cell carcinoma, and adenocarcinoma. Another type of lung cancer is bronchoalveolar, which comprises 5% of lung cancers. Lung cancer is responsible for more than 32% of cancer deaths in men and greater than 25% of cancer deaths in women.[13,21] Among women there has been a 600% increase in the incidence of lung cancer over the last 80 years. Tobacco smoking is the major cause (85%) of lung cancer, with approximately 160,000 deaths reported per year. About 3800 deaths per year are reported in nonsmokers who receive secondary smoke from the environment.[21-24] The remaining percentage of lung cancer is not attributable to smoking. Individuals at highest risk for developing lung cancer are those who started smoking before the age of 25 years, have smoked one or more packs of cigarettes a day for 20 years, work under conditions of asbestos exposure, and are older than 50 years.[21-24] (See Chapter 7 for further discussion of cancer.)

Pathogenesis. Squamous cell epidermoid carcinoma (20% to 30% of cases) usually originates (in two thirds of cases) in the central bronchi near the hilus as an intraluminal growth.[13,21,22] Cytologic examination of sputum reveals the squamous cell carcinoma, leading to earlier detection of this cancer than with other lung neoplasms. The tumor normally doubles its volume in 100 days and, as it advances, metastasizes to regional lymph nodes in the area.[13]

Adenocarcinomas (35% to 40% of cases) usually appear in the periphery of the lung and are not as amenable to early detection as squamous cell carcinoma. Adenocarcinomas are characterized by acinar bronchoalveolar and papillary tumors. Doubling time is about 180 days, with metastasis occurring to distant organs, which may be due to aerosol transmission in the case of bronchoalveolar (2% of cases) carcinoma.[13,21,22]

Large cell carcinomas (10% to 15% of cases) develop in the lung periphery and are similar to adenocarcinoma. The tumor cells are large and are arranged in nests or clusters. The tumor doubles in size about every 100 days and metastasizes to distant organs.[13,21,22]

Small cell (oat cell) carcinoma (15% to 20% of cases) tends to originate extrinsically in the central bronchus region, thus compressing and narrowing the bronchi. The narrowing may lead to signs and symptoms of obstruction of a central airway, leading to wheezing. This type of tumor is associated with a lesion on chromosome 3, and grows rapidly, doubling in about 33 days.[13] Widespread metastasis is common with small cell carcinomas and they are the most resistant to therapy.

Bronchoalveolar (5%) carcinoma tends to originate in the periphery and metastasize through the lymphatics. There is no correlation with cigarette smoking.

Clinical manifestations. Clinical features vary according to the type and the location of the tumor, and whether it has metastasized. Approximately 10% to 25% of cases are asymptomatic.[13] Signs and symptoms can be classified as intrathoracic or extrathoracic.

Extrathoracic manifestations are weight loss, fatigue, anorexia, anemia, and clubbing. Facial and upper extremity edema is noted in cases of tumor compression of the superior vena cava. Superior vena cava syndrome is most commonly caused by bronchogenic carcinoma.[21]

Intrathoracic manifestations include dyspnea, cough, chest pain, hemoptysis, and increased sputum production (with bronchoalveolar carcinoma). Hoarseness may be evident and is caused by pressure of the tumor on the recurrent laryngeal nerve. Phrenic nerve involvement (1% of lung cancer patients) leads to paralysis of the hemidiaphragm on the affected side and the potential for development of atelectasis and pneumonia. Clinical findings of endobronchial obstruction include atelectasis, postobstructive pneumonia, pleural effusion (12% to 33%), and Horner syndrome (miosis, ipsilateral ptosis, and dyshidrosis).[13] Abdominal breathing measures are taught to the patient who does not recover diaphragmatic function from damage to the phrenic nerve.[13] Extension of the cancer cells to the pleural cavity may cause pleural effusion.

Diagnosis. Pulmonary function tests may show increased volumes in moderately advanced cases of bronchial carcinoma.[14] Because the tumor blocks the airway, an obstructive pattern of pulmonary disease may lead to increased or decreased functional residual capacity attributable to the effect of the mass lesion.

The definitive diagnosis of cancer requires positive cytologic or histologic findings. Bronchoscopy washings are a common method of diagnosing lung cancer in patients whose lesions are centrally located. Pleural fluid samples show positive findings in 50% to 65% of patients with malignant pleural effusion.[13] Histologic examination of tissue after biopsy of the pleura, lung tissue, or mediastinal lymph nodes may also be helpful in diagnosing lung cancer. (See Chapter 7 for discussion of tumor classification.)

Chest radiographs show abnormal findings in nearly all patients with lung cancer. Common findings are hilar (squamous cell) and/or peripheral (adenocarcinoma) masses, atelectasis, mediastinal widening, infiltrates, pleural effusions, and cavitation (squamous cell epidermoid carcinoma). Chest studies are helpful in evaluating tumor size and nodal involvement. Computed tomography (CT) scans of the chest are used for staging and for follow-up study after treatment. Positron emission tomography (PET) scanning with ^{18}F-labeled fluorodeoxyglucose, a metabolic marker of malignant tissue, is superior to CT scan in detecting mediastinal and distant metastases in non–small cell lung cancer.[21]

KEY POINTS
- Cigarette smoking is the major cause of lung cancer. Lung cancer is usually disseminated at the time of diagnosis and is associated with a high mortality.
- Lung cancers can develop in the bronchial tree (small cell, squamous cell) or in the parenchyma (large cell, adenocarcinoma).
- Lung cancer may be advanced before symptoms become troublesome. Manifestations include cough, hemoptysis, hoarseness, chest pain, and pleural effusion. The diagnosis is based on examination of cells from bronchial secretions or tissue biopsy. Pulmonary masses may be detected by plain radiography or computed tomography of the chest.
- As with other cancers, treatment includes surgical removal of resectable tumors followed by radiation therapy and/or chemotherapy.

Treatment. Primary treatment options for pulmonary neoplasms are surgery, chemotherapy, radiation therapy, laser therapy, and tissue-specific therapies for airway lesions. Patients are also strongly encouraged to stop smoking.[21,23]

The treatment of choice for non–small cell carcinoma is surgery. For nonoperable neoplasms, radiation therapy is the secondary choice. Radiotherapy improves survival in patients with nonresectable non–small cell carcinoma.[13,21] Combination chemotherapy is the therapy of choice in patients with extensive small cell carcinoma.[13,21] Combined chemotherapy and chest radiation therapy has proved effective as a cure for patients in whom disease was detected early. Radiation therapy is also used for palliation of symptoms. (See Chapter 7 for other treatment options.)

SUMMARY

The primary function of the respiratory system is oxygenation of the tissues. This function is accomplished by the movement of O_2 from the atmosphere through the airways to alveolar sacs. The inhaled air is warmed, humidified, and filtered in the upper airway on its way to the alveoli. Once in the alveoli, diffusion of O_2 and CO_2, a gaseous waste product, occurs and O_2 is transported by means of hemoglobin molecules to the tissues. The respiratory system has numerous control mechanisms that influence its function. For example, the respiratory control centers may be inhibited when a person has a brain injury, thus producing inadequate respiration. Failure of oxygenation is seen in acute respiratory failure. Acute respiratory failure, defined as a Pao_2 less than 60 mm Hg and a $Paco_2$

greater than 50 mm Hg at room air, occurs in individuals who have developed ventilation-perfusion mismatching, right-to-left shunt, or hypoventilation. Diseases affecting the pulmonary vasculature include pulmonary hypertension and pulmonary embolism. Pulmonary hypertension is associated with disease processes (e.g., emphysema, PE, hypoxemia) that increase pulmonary vascular resistance. Pulmonary emboli result in obstruction to blood flow in the pulmonary vasculature. The health or disease of a patient's cardiovascular, renal, and hematologic systems also affects the functioning of the respiratory system. Health care professionals have a key role in the prevention and management of respiratory disease and in patient and family education.

REFERENCES

1. Moore KL, Persaud TVN: *The developing human: clinically oriented embryology*, ed 9, Philadelphia, 2008, Saunders.
2. Barrett KE: *Ganong's review of medical physiology*, ed 23, Los Altos, CA, 2010, Lange.
3. Hall JE: *Guyton and Hall Textbook of medical physiology*, ed 12, Philadelphia, 2011, Saunders.
4. Mackenzie CF: Compromises in the choice of orotracheal or nasotracheal intubation and tracheostomy, *Heart Lung* 12:485–492, 1983.
5. West JB: *Respiratory physiology: the essentials*, ed 8, Philadelphia, 2008, Lippincott Williams & Wilkins.
6. Kliegman RM, Behrman RE, Jenson HB, et al, editors: *Nelson textbook of pediatrics*, ed 18, Philadelphia, 2011, Saunders.
7. Kumar V, Abbas AK, Aster J, editors: *Robbins & Cotran pathologic basis of disease*, ed 8, Philadelphia, 2010, Saunders.
8. Fretwell ME: Aging changes in structure and function. In Carnevali DL, Patrick M, editors: *Nursing management for the elderly*, ed 3, Philadelphia, 1993, Lippincott.
9. Allen SC: The respiratory system. In Fillit HM, Rockwood K, Woodhouse K, editors: *Brocklehurst's textbook of geriatric medicine and gerontology*, ed 7, New York, 2010, Churchill Livingstone.
10. Clouter MM, Throll RS: The respiratory system. In *Berne & Levy physiology*, ed 7, St Louis, 2009, Mosby.
11. Rossi A, et al: Aging and the respiratory system, *Aging* 8(3):143–161, 1996.
12. Foster C, Mistry N, Peddi P, Sharma S, editors: *The Washington manual of medical therapeutics*, ed 33, Philadelphia, 2010, Lippincott Williams & Wilkins.
13. Chestnutt MS, Prendergast TJ: Pulmonary disorders. In McPhee SJ, Papadakis MA, Rabow MW, editors: *Current medical diagnosis and treatment*, ed 46, New York, 2011, Lange/McGraw-Hill, pp 239–317.
14. West JB: *Pulmonary pathophysiology: the essentials*, ed 7, Philadelphia, 2008, Lippincott Williams & Wilkins.
15. West JB: *Pulmonary physiology and pathophysiology: an integrated case-based approach*, ed 2, Philadelphia, 2007, Lippincott Williams & Wilkins.
16. Martin DW, Choudhary G: Pulmonary hypertension. In Ferri FF, editor: *Ferri's clinical advisor: instant diagnosis and treatment*, St Louis, 2012, Mosby, pp 854–856.
17. Whelan CA: Pulmonary hypertension. In Buttaro TM, Trybulski J, Polgar-Bailey P, et al, editors: *Primary care: a collaborative practice*, ed 3, St Louis, 2008, Mosby, pp 477–480.
18. Troncales FD, Ferri FF, Choudhary G: Pulmonary embolism. In Ferri FF, editor: *Ferri's clinical advisor: instant diagnosis and treatment*, St Louis, 2012, Mosby, pp 283–285.
19. Kearon C: Venous thromboembolism. In Bope ET, Kellerman RD, Rakel RE, editors: *Conn's current therapy 2011*, Philadelphia, 2011, Saunders, pp 280–287.
20. Smiley CM, Polgar-Bailey P: Chest pain (non-cardiac). In Buttaro TM, Trybulski J, Polgar-Bailey P, et al, editors: *Primary care: a collaborative practice*, ed 3, St Louis, 2008, Mosby, pp 425–427.
21. Ferri FF: Lung neoplasm. In Ferri FF, editor: *Ferri's clinical advisor: instant diagnosis and treatment*, St Louis, 2012, Mosby, pp 514–516.
22. Theodore PR, Jablons D: Thoracic wall, pleura, mediastinum, and diaphragm. In Doherty GM, editor: *Current surgical diagnosis and treatment*, ed 13, New York, 2010, Lange/McGraw-Hill, pp 305–358.
23. Winland-Brown JE, Porter BO, Thomas DJ: Respiratory problems. In Dunphy LM, Winland-Brown JE, Porter BO, et al, editors: *Primary care: the art and science of advanced practice nursing*, ed 3, Philadelphia, 2011, FA Davis, pp 304–393.
24. Kretzke RA, Patel MA: Primary lung cancer. In Bope ET, Kellerman RD, Rakel RE, editors: *Conn's current therapy 2011*, Philadelphia, 2011, Saunders, pp 250–254.

Obstructive Pulmonary Disorders

Lorna L. Schumann

evolve WEBSITE

http://evolve.elsevier.com/Copstead/
- Case Studies
- Disease Profiles

- WebLinks
- Key Points Review
- Online Course (Module 12)

KEY QUESTIONS

- What are the clinical manifestations and common causes of acute airway obstruction?
- What is the role of inflammation in the development of asthma?
- How does the underlying genetic defect in cystic fibrosis lead to pulmonary and exocrine gland dysfunction?
- How does smoking cause both the alveolar destruction of emphysema and the bronchial damage of chronic bronchitis?

- What is the rationale for using drugs such as β_2 agonists, acetylcholine antagonists, leukotriene inhibitors, corticosteroids, and mast cell stabilizers to manage obstructive pulmonary disorders?
- What pulmonary function test abnormalities are characteristic of obstructive pulmonary disorders?

CHAPTER OUTLINE

Obstructive lung diseases are manifested by increased resistance to airflow. Obstructive diseases of the lung can be classified into those involving (1) obstruction from conditions in the wall of the lumen (e.g., asthma, bronchitis), (2) obstruction resulting from increasing pressure around the outside of the airway lumen (e.g., emphysema secondary to loss of lung tissue and elasticity, enlarged lymph node, or tumor), and (3) obstruction of the airway lumen (e.g., presence of a foreign body, excessive secretions, aspiration of fluids).[1,2]

These classifications are mainly terms of convenience, because many respiratory disease processes involve several areas of the pulmonary system. Involvement of the airways produces narrowing of the passages so that airflow obstruction occurs. The major obstructive airway diseases are asthma, bronchitis, and emphysema.

OBSTRUCTION FROM CONDITIONS IN THE WALL OF THE LUMEN

Asthma

Etiology. Asthma is a lung disease characterized by (a) airway obstruction that is reversible (but not completely in some patients); (b) airway inflammation; and (c) increased airway reactivity to a variety of stimuli.[2,3] In terms of symptoms, asthma is defined by paroxysms of diffuse wheezing, dyspnea, and cough, resulting from spasmodic contractions of the bronchi. Airway inflammation leads to epithelial denudation, collagen deposition beneath the basement membrane, mast cell activation, mucosal edema, increased viscid secretions, and smooth muscle contraction. With proper treatment, most patients with asthma can control the disease and prevent development of emphysema or bronchitis. Asthma occurs in about 5% to 12% of the U.S. population and is common among children and adults.[2-6] Asthma is the most common chronic disease of childhood.[6,7] High-risk populations include African Americans, inner-city dwellers, and premature or low-birth-weight children.[5,7] The pathophysiology of both intrinsic (non-allergic, sometimes referred to as *adult onset*) and extrinsic (allergic, sometimes referred to as *pediatric onset*) asthma is thought to involve inflammation of the airways. Most cases of asthma can be triggered both by allergens and by stimuli, such as exercise and exposure to cold air. The terms *intrinsic* and *extrinsic* are still used, but many prefer the terms *non-allergic* and *allergic*. The clinical features of all forms are similar.

Asthma is associated with the release of inflammatory chemicals from mast cells in the airways. The mechanisms stimulating mast cell release are allergic, immunoglobulin E (IgE)-mediated triggers for extrinsic/allergic asthma (Figure 22-1). Intrinsic/non-allergic asthma occurs in patients who have no history of allergy.[8] Allergic asthma (extrinsic) comprises approximately one third to one half of all cases.[8,9] Asthma is often associated with a history of hay fever or eczema (atopy), a positive family history of the disease, and positive skin test reactions to allergens (dust mites, cat/dog dander, industrial chemicals).[8,10] Pharmacologic therapy, allergen-specific immunotherapy, and environmental control are usually beneficial.[6,9] Refer to Chapter 10 for details about IgE-mediated mechanisms and hyposensitization methods.

Intrinsic/non-allergic asthma frequently develops in middle age and has a less favorable prognosis. Respiratory tract infections or psychological factors appear to be contributory, whereas antigen-antibody reactions appear to have less of a role in the disease process, although IgE levels may be elevated.[8-10] Attacks are often severe, and patients have a variable response to medical therapy.[10] Allergen-specific immunotherapy and environmental control measures are *not* usually helpful. Airways are hyperreactive, and patients may present with extreme dyspnea, orthopnea, and agitation.

Exercise-induced asthma is common, especially in children and adolescents.[8,9] Bronchospasm often occurs within 3 minutes after the end of exercise and usually resolves in 60 minutes.[9,10] Heat loss, water loss, and increased osmolarity of the lower respiratory mucosa are believed to stimulate mediator release from basophils and tissue mast cells. This mediator release produces airway smooth muscle contraction. Running, jogging, and playing tennis are the most common instigators of exercise-induced asthma. Bicycling and swimming are much less likely to induce symptoms.

Occupational asthma may be accompanied by positive skin test reactions to protein allergens in the work environment. Occupational exposures to allergens, such as fumes from plastic, formaldehyde, isocyanates, some metals, textiles, engine exhaust, sulfur dioxide, fluoride, and western red cedar dust, *do not* provoke skin reactions.[10,11] To prove hypersensitivity, it may be necessary to conduct challenge tests in the patient by inhalation of the suspected dust or fumes in a controlled environment. The individual affected by occupational asthma tends to have progressively more severe attacks with subsequent exposures. Symptoms may clear over a weekend or vacation and recur when the individual returns to the work environment.[10] This repeated history often is sufficient to establish the diagnosis. Hyposensitization in most cases of occupational asthma is ineffective because of lack of an IgE antibody reaction and because the chemicals that cause symptoms usually are toxic when injected.[10,11]

Drug-induced asthma can produce symptoms ranging from mild rhinorrhea to respiratory arrest requiring mechanical ventilation. In patients with nasal polyps, sinusitis, and asthma, ingestion of aspirin may induce severe or occasionally fatal asthmatic attacks. Sometimes anaphylactoid reactions cause a decrease in blood pressure, itching (pruritus), rhinorrhea, or a rash after aspirin ingestion. Aspirin intolerance with asthma usually occurs in adults. Attacks may occur within minutes of ingestion or may be delayed up to 12 hours. Nonsteroidal antiinflammatory drugs such as indomethacin (Indocin), ibuprofen (Motrin, Advil), and related drugs may also induce asthma in the aspirin-intolerant patient. Aspirin reactions are not immunologically mediated. Therefore, skin testing is not useful for diagnosing aspirin intolerance. Because aspirin and nonsteroidal antiinflammatory drugs inhibit the conversion of arachidonic acid to prostaglandins, it is possible that aspirin shunts arachidonic acid breakdown products to the leukotriene system. Leukotrienes, released from mast cells, are slow-reacting substances of anaphylaxis with powerful bronchoconstriction activity (see Figure 22-1). Avoidance is the most practical approach to this problem because testing can be dangerous.

Asthma can occur from ingestion of food additives. Tartrazine (yellow dye no. 5), which is used to color pharmaceuticals, hair products, and food products, may also produce severe asthma in susceptible persons. A complete list of drugs containing tartrazine can be obtained from the Food and Drug Administration.

Monosodium glutamate (MSG), used as a flavor enhancer in foods, can produce faintness, nausea, sweating, a fall in blood pressure, and, occasionally, asthma. Sodium or potassium metabisulfite, used to preserve fruits, vegetables, and meats, can cause anaphylactoid reactions. A challenge with the chemical may be necessary to establish a diagnosis, as metabisulfites are widespread in our society.

Hops in beer have also been implicated in causing severe bronchospasm. Skin reactivity does not occur, and the mechanism of the problem is not IgE mediated. The diagnosis involves a history of exposure followed by symptoms.

Pathogenesis. The immunohistopathologic features of asthma include denudation of airway epithelium, collagen deposition beneath the basement membrane, edema, mast cell activation, and inflammatory cell infiltration by neutrophils, eosinophils, and lymphocytes.[1,3] Inflammation of the airway contributes to acute bronchospasm (bronchoconstriction), mucosal edema, mucous plug formation, and airway

A   **SENSITIZATION TO ALLERGEN**

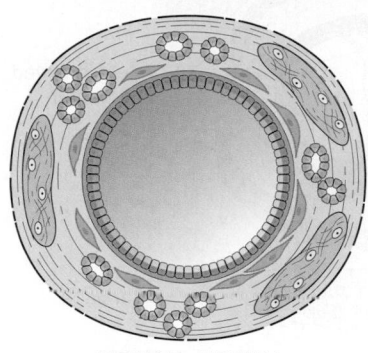

NORMAL AIRWAY

B   **ALLERGEN-TRIGGERED ASTHMA**

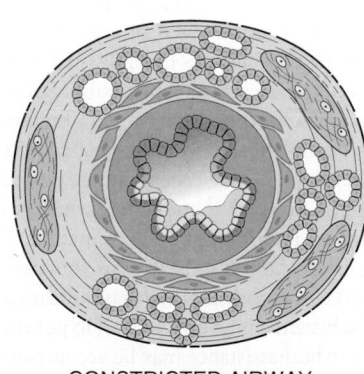

CONSTRICTED AIRWAY IN ASTHMA

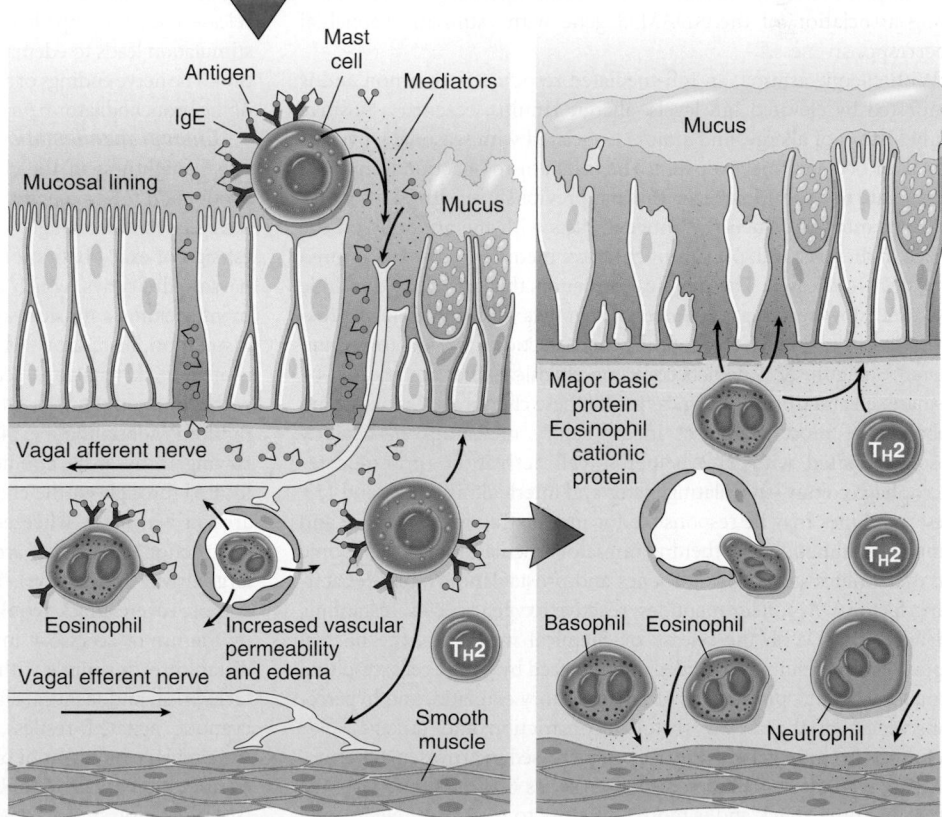

B   **IMMEDIATE PHASE (MINUTES)**

C   **LATE PHASE (HOURS)**

FIGURE 22-1 A, Sensitization to allergen. Inhaled allergens elicit a T$_H$2-dominated response favoring IgE production and eosinophil recruitment. **B,** Allergen-triggered asthma (immediate phase). On reexposure to antigen, the immediate reaction is triggered by cross-linking of IgE bound to receptors on mast cells in the airways. These cells release preformed mediators that inflame epithelial cells. Antigen then enters the mucosa to activate mucosal mast cells and eosinophils, which in turn release additional inflammatory mediators. **C,** Late phase. The arrival of recruited leukocytes signals the initiation of the late phase of asthma and more mediator release, which cause damage to epithelium. (From Kumar V et al, editors: *Robbins basic pathology,* ed 9, Philadelphia, 2013, Saunders.)

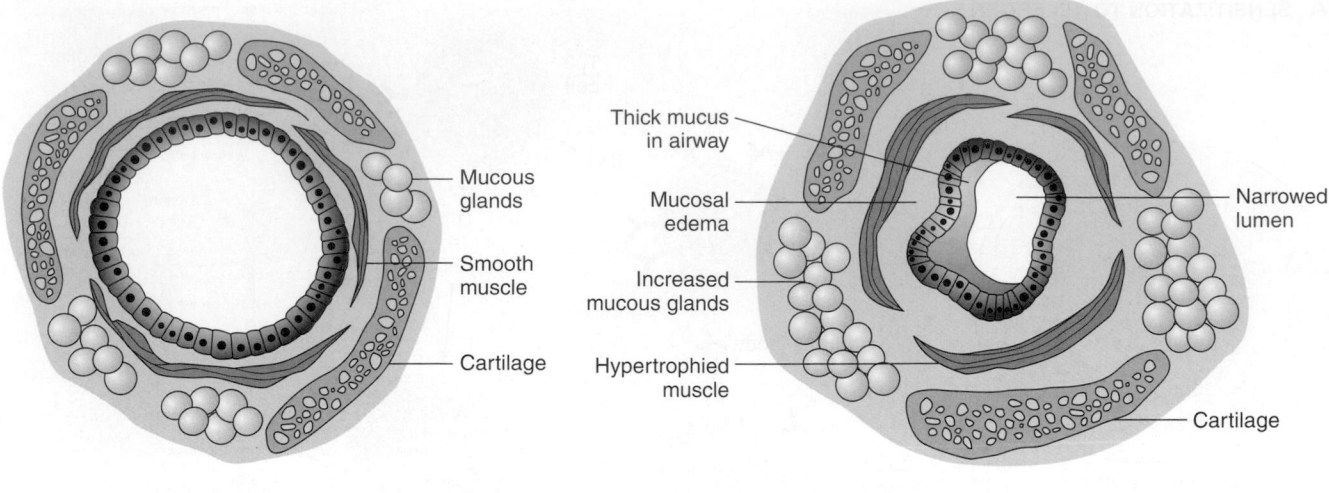

NORMAL   ASTHMA

FIGURE 22-2 Common bronchial wall remodeling changes in asthma are hypertrophied smooth muscle, edema, mucous gland hypertrophy, and mucus in the lumen.

wall remodeling (Figure 22-2). Genetic predisposition (chromosomes 5, 11, 14) for atopy and structural predisposition (smaller airways) are the strongest predisposing factors for developing asthma.[3,5] There is a strong association of the *ADAM33* gene with asthmatic bronchial hyperresponsiveness.[8]

With allergic asthma, an IgE-mediated response is common and is manifested by elevated IgE levels, allergic rhinitis, eczema, a positive family history of allergy, and attacks associated with seasonal, environmental, or occupational exposure. The mechanism of action is initiated by exposure to a specific antigen that has previously sensitized mast cells in airway mucosa. When the antigen reacts with the antibody on the surface of the mast cell, packets of chemical mediator substances stored in the cell are released. The chemical mediators that are released include histamine, slow-reacting substances of anaphylaxis (leukotrienes), prostaglandins, bradykinins, eosinophilic chemotactic factor, serotonin, and others.[1-3,7] Figure 22-1 depicts common chemicals that are released by the mast cell and the physiologic effect of these chemicals. Cytokines are probably the most important inflammatory mediators, particularly those associated with T_H2 helper T cell activation (granulocyte-macrophage colony–stimulating factor and interleukins 3, 4, 5, and 13). These cytokines may be responsible for modulating inflammatory and immune cell function.[1,2] Other inflammatory mediators are arachidonic acid metabolites such as leukotrienes and prostaglandins, platelet activating factor (PAF), neuropeptides, reactive oxygen species, histamine, and adenosine. With the release of chemical mediators, the normal respiratory epithelium is denuded and replaced by goblet cells, resulting in mucosal edema, production of inflammatory exudates, and hyperresponsiveness of the airway (bronchoconstriction and leakage).[2,12,13] Alterations in epithelial integrity lead to increased microvascular permeability. A secondary mediator response occurs 6 to 12 hours after the primary asthma attack and is more refractory to treatment. Neutrophil chemotactic factor may be the cause of this secondary response.[10]

Histologic changes in the epithelial basement membrane occur over time. The basement membrane is a complex structure that separates endothelial cells from underlying stroma. The membrane provides tensile strength and physical support to surrounding structures.[8] It also functions as a filter and as a site for cell attachment. In a classic study by Hogg in 1982, the width of the basement membrane was shown to thicken in asthmatic patients over time.[12] The width seen in asthmatic patients is 17.5 μm, whereas that seen in healthy subjects is 7 μm. Airway remodeling

has been detected pathologically. Declines in pulmonary function over time can progress to chronic obstructive pulmonary disease (COPD).[10] Figure 22-1 depicts the pathogenesis of asthma in relation to mast cell release and parasympathetic stimulation by way of the vagus nerve. Vagal stimulation leads to edema, mucus hypersecretion, and bronchoconstriction. The nerve endings of asthmatic patients have been found to be devoid of the bronchodilator neuropeptide vasoactive intestinal peptide.[10]

Clinical manifestations. Common symptoms are wheezing, feelings of tightness of the chest, dyspnea, cough, and increased sputum production.[10] Some patients have only a chronic dry cough, and others have a productive cough.[9] Especially in children, cough is often the earliest sign of exacerbation of asthma. Wheezing is caused by vibration in narrowed airways, which act like the vibrating reed of a wind instrument, yielding a musical sound.[14] Because airways naturally widen with inspiration, inspiratory wheezes reflect increased constriction. Sputum is often thick, tenacious, scant, and viscid (sticky). Physical findings vary with the severity of the attack. A mild attack may be associated with a random monophonic expiratory wheezing associated with airway narrowing, tachycardia, and tachypnea. Random monophonic wheezes are located throughout the chest and are intermittent on examination. The area in which the wheezes are heard best is indicative of the area of obstruction (e.g., if they are heard best at the mouth, this is indicative of large airway obstruction).[14,15] Tachycardia is an early sign of hypoxemia. A more severe attack requiring medical assistance may be accompanied by the use of accessory muscles of respiration, intercostal retractions, distant breath sounds with inspiratory wheezing, orthopnea, agitation, tachypnea, and tachycardia. In the severe state, the patient may appear cyanotic, agitated, restless, and confused. The intensity of wheezing is *not* a reliable indicator of blockage of airflow. The measurement of peak expiratory flow rate (PEFR) is the best indicator of reduction in airflow (see discussion under Diagnosis). PEFRs are affected by weight, height, age, gender, ethnicity, posture, effort, smoking, and circadian rhythm. A PEFR of less than 80 L/min indicates severe obstruction.[9,16] When obstruction is the tightest, the patient cannot move enough air with enough velocity to make wheezing sounds. Isolated inspiratory wheezing may be an indicator of large airway obstruction caused by mucus or laryngeal obstruction.[4] A patient with severe respiratory distress, prolonged expiration (indicating that the person is having difficulty moving air out of the lungs), neck and intercostal retractions, and minimal air sounds is critically ill and requires emergency intervention.

Components of Severity		Classification of Asthma Severity ≥12 years of age			
			Persistent		
		Intermittent	Mild	Moderate	Severe
Impairment Normal FEV$_1$/FVC: 8–19 yr 85% 20–39 yr 80% 40–59 yr 75% 60–80 yr 70%	Symptoms	≤2 days/week	>2 days/week but not daily	Daily	Throughout the day
	Nighttime awakenings	≤2x/month	3–4x/month	>1x/week but not nightly	Often 7x/week
	Short-acting beta$_2$-agonist use for symptoms control (not prevention of EIB)	≤2 days/week	>2 days/week but not daily, and not more than 1x on any day	Daily	Several times per day
	Interference with normal activity	None	Minor limitation	Some limitation	Extremely limited
	Lung function	• Normal FEV$_1$ between exacerbations • FEV$_1$ >80% predicted • FEV$_1$/FVC normal	• FEV$_1$ >80% predicted • FEV$_1$/FVC normal	• FEV$_1$ >60% but <80% predicted • FEV$_1$/FVC reduced 5%	• FEV$_1$ <60% predicted • FEV$_1$/FVC reduced >5%
Risk	Exacerbations requiring oral systemic corticosteroids	0–1 year (see note)	≥2/year (see note) →————————————→		
		←————— Consider severity and interval since last exacerbation. —————→ Frequency and severity may fluctuate over time for patients in any severity category. Relative annual risk of exacerbations may be related to FEV$_1$.			
Recommended Step for Initiating Treatment (See Figure 22-5 for treatment steps.)		Step 1	Step 2	Step 3 and consider short course of oral systemic corticosteroids	Step 4 or 5
		In 2–6 weeks, evaluate level of asthma control that is achieved and adjust therapy accordingly.			

Key: *FEV$_1$*, forced expiratory volume in 1 second; *FVC*, forced vital capacity; *ICU*, intensive care unit

Notes:

■ The stepwise approach is meant to assist, not replace, the clinical decision making required to meet individual patient needs.

■ Level of severity is determined by assessment of both impairment and risk. Assess impairment domain by patient's/caregiver's recall of previous 2-4 weeks and spirometry. Assign severity to the most severe category in which any feature occurs.

■ At present, there are inadequate data to correspond frequencies of exacerbations with different levels of asthma severity. In general, more frequent and intense exacerbations (e.g., requiring urgent, unscheduled care, hospitalization, or ICU admission) indicate greater underlying disease severity. For treatment purposes, patients who had ≥2 exacerbations requiring oral systematic corticosteroids in the past year may be considered the same as patients who have persistent asthma.

FIGURE 22-3 Classifying asthma severity and initiating treatment in youths ≥12 years of age and adults who are not currently taking long-term control medicines. (From National Institute of Health's National Heart, Lung, and Blood Institute: 2007 National Asthma Education and Prevention Program: *Expert Panel Report 3: guidelines for the diagnosis and management of asthma*, p 344, Figure 4-6.)

Diagnosis. The diagnosis of asthma is based on history, physical findings, sputum examination, pulmonary function tests, blood gas analysis, and chest radiography. Radiographic findings may be normal or may show evidence of hyperinflation with flattening of the diaphragm in progressive disease.[8] Abnormal physical findings include cough, wheezing, a hyperinflated chest, and decreased breath sounds. Asthmatic sputum samples reveal Charcot-Leyden crystals (formed from crystallized enzymes from eosinophilic membranes), eosinophils, and Curschmann spirals (mucous casts of bronchioles).

Forced expiratory volumes decrease during asthma attacks. PEFR is measured to determine the index of airway function. The PEFR is the maximal flow of expired air attained during a forced vital capacity (FVC) procedure.[15] The evaluation of asthma should include the measurement of forced expiratory volume over 1 second (FEV$_1$), FVC, and the FEV$_1$/FVC ratio before and after administration of a short-acting

bronchodilator.[8] Airflow obstruction is indicated by a FEV$_1$/FVC ratio of less than 75%.[9] Classification of asthma severity and control (Figures 22-3 and 22-4) is based on presenting symptoms, frequency of nighttime symptoms, and lung function.[2] Figure 22-5 shows stepped therapy for asthma based on classification.

Arterial blood gas values may be normal during a mild attack, but as the bronchospasm increases in intensity, respiratory alkalosis and hypoxemia become prominent findings. Elevation of arterial partial pressure of carbon dioxide (Paco$_2$) is a poor prognostic sign, indicating that the patient's ability to continue breathing at a rapid rate has diminished and that exhaustion is imminent.

Respiratory failure may be manifested by severe respiratory distress in a patient who shows no radiographic evidence of pneumothorax. As the patient improves, the wheezing becomes louder. When wheezing is no longer heard after an asthma attack, pulmonary function tests may

Components of Control		Classification of Asthma Control (≥12 years of age)		
		Well Controlled	**Not Well Controlled**	**Very Poorly Controlled**
Impairment	Symptoms	≤2 days/week	>2 days/week	Throughout the day
	Nighttime awakenings	≤2x/month	1–3x/week	≥4x/week
	Interference with normal activity	None	Some limitation	Extremely limited
	Short-acting beta₂-agonist use for symptom control (not prevention of EIB)	≤2 days/week	>2 days/week	Several times per day
	FEV_1 or peak flow	>80% predicted/ personal best	60–80% predicted/ personal best	<60% predicted/ personal best
	Validated questionnaires ATAQ ACQ ACT	0 ≤0.75* ≥20	1–2 ≥1.5 16–19	3–4 N/A ≤15
Risk	Exacerbations requiring oral systemic corticosteroids	0–1 year	≥2/year (see note)	
		Consider severity and interval since last exacerbation		
	Progressive loss of lung function	Evaluation requires long-term followup care		
	Treatment-related adverse effects	Medication side effects can vary in intensity from none to very troublesome and worrisome. The level of intensity does not correlate to specific levels of control but should be considered in the overall assessment of risk.		
Recommended Action for Treatment (See Figure 22-5 for treatment steps.)		• Maintain current step. • Regular followups every 1–6 months to maintain control. • Consider step down if well controlled for at least 3 months	• Step up 1 step and • Reevaluate in 2–6 weeks. • For side effects, consider alternative treatment options.	• Consider short course of oral systemic corticosteroids, • Step up 1–2 steps, and • Reevaluate in 2 weeks. • For side effects, consider alternative treatment options.

*ACQ values of 0.76–1.4 are indeterminate regarding well-controlled asthma.
Key: *EIB*, exercise-induced bronchospasm; *ICU*, intensive care unit

Notes:

■ The stepwise approach is meant to assist, not replace, the clinical decision making required to meet individual patient needs.

■ The level of control is based on the most severe impairment or risk category. Assess impairment domain by patient's recall of previous 2-4 weeks and by spirometry/peak flow measures. Symptom assessment for longer periods should reflect a global assessment, such as inquiring whether the patient's asthma is better or worse since the last visit.

■ At present, there are inadequate data to correspond frequencies of exacerbations with different levels of asthma control. In general, more frequent and intense exacerbations (e.g., requiring urgent, unscheduled care, hospitalization, or ICU admission) indicate poorer disease control. For treatment purposes, patients who had ≥2 exacerbations requiring oral systemic corticosteroids in the past year may be considered the same as patients who have not-well-controlled asthma, even in the absence of impairment levels consistent with not-well-controlled asthma.

■ Check NIH website for information on ATAQ, ACQ and ACT questionnaires.

■ Before step up in therapy:
— Review adherence to medication, inhaler technique, environmental control, and comorbid conditions.
— If an alternative treatment option was used in a step, discontinue and use the preferred treatment for that step.

FIGURE 22-4 Assessing asthma control and adjusting therapy in youths ≥12 years of age and adults. (From National Institute of Health's National Heart, Lung, and Blood Institute: 2007 National Asthma Education and Prevention Program: *Expert Panel Report 3: guidelines for the diagnosis and management of asthma*, p 345, Figure 4-7.)

continue to show obstructive changes for several weeks. Some patients have a slight monophonic wheeze continuously between asthma bouts and still are comfortable and functional.[14]

Determination of allergens is done by skin testing or inhalation of suspected allergens. Skin testing is usually more helpful in young patients who have extrinsic asthma. Bronchial provocation testing with histamine or methacholine[9] may be useful in confirming the diagnosis of asthma in certain cases (see the Diagnostic Tests section later in the chapter).

A complete blood cell count can show an elevated number of white blood cells (WBCs) with an increased number of eosinophils. Eosinophils are prominent in the cellular infiltrate of the bronchioles, the sputum, and the peripheral blood. A decline in the total eosinophil count is a valuable measure of effectiveness of corticosteroid treatment. With effective treatment, the total eosinophil count is depressed below 10/μL.[1,9]

Treatment. Patients should be taught to avoid the objects in the environment that trigger asthma attacks. Environmental control

Intermittent Asthma	**Persistent Asthma: Daily Medication** Consult with asthma specialist if step 4 care or higher is required. Consider consultation at step 3.

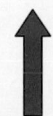

Step 1

Preferred:

SABA PRN

Step 2

Preferred:

Low-dose ICS

Alternative:

Cromolyn, LTRA, Nedocromil, or Theophylline

Step 3

Preferred:

Low-dose ICS + LABA **OR** Medium-dose ICS

Alternative:

Low-dose ICS + either LTRA, Theophylline, or Zileuton

Step 4

Preferred:

Medium-dose ICS + LABA

Alternative:

Medium-dose ICS + either LTRA, Theophylline, or Zileuton

Step 5

Preferred:

High-dose ICS + LABA

AND

Consider Omalizumab for patients who have allergies

Step 6

Preferred:

High-dose ICS + LABA + oral corticosteroid

AND

Consider Omalizumab for patients who have allergies

Step up if needed

(first, check adherence, environmental control, and comorbid conditions)

Assess control

Step down if possible

(and asthma is well controlled at least 3 months)

Each step:	Patient education, environmental control, and management of comorbidities.
Steps 2–4:	Consider subcutaneous allergen immunotherapy for patients who have allergic asthma (see notes).

Quick-Relief Medication for All Patients

- SABA as needed for symptoms. Intensity of treatment depends on severity of symptoms: up to 3 treatments at 20-minute intervals as needed. Short course of oral systemic corticosteroids may be needed.
- Use of SABA >2 days a week for symptom relief (not prevention of EIB) generally indicates inadequate control and the need to step up treatment.

Key: **Alphabetical order is used when more than one treatment option is listed within either preferred or alternative therapy.** *EIB*, exercise-induced bronchospasm; *ICS*, inhaled corticosteroid; *LABA*, long-acting inhaled beta$_2$-agonist, *LTRA*, leukotriene receptor antagonist; *PNR*, as needed; *SABA*, inhaled short-acting beta$_2$-agonist.

Notes:

- The stepwise approach is meant to assist, not replace, the clinical decisionmaking required to meet individual patient needs.
- If alternative treatment is used and response is inadequate, discontinue it and use the preferred treatment before stepping up.
- Zileuton is a less desirable alternative due to limited studies as adjunctive therapy and the need to monitor liver function. Theophylline requires monitoring of serum concentration levels.
- In step 6, before oral systemic corticosteroids are introduced, a trial of high-dose ICS + LABA + either LTRA, theophylline, or zileuton may be considered, although this approach has not been studied in clinical trials.
- Steps 1, 2, and 3 preferred therapies are based on Evidence A; step 3 alternative therapy is based on Evidence A for LTRA, Evidence B for theophylline, and Evidence D for zileuton. Step 4 preferred therapy is based on Evidence B, and alternative therapy is based on Evidence B for LTRA and theophylline and Evidence D for zileuton. Step 5 preferred therapy is based on Evidence B. Step 6 preferred therapy is based on (EPR—2 1997) and Evidence B for omalizumab.
- Immunotherapy for steps 2-4 is based on Evidence B for house-dust mites, animal danders, and pollens; evidence is weak or lacking for molds and cockroaches. Evidence is strongest for immunotherapy with single allergens. The role of allergy in asthma is greater in children than in adults.
- Clinicians who administer immunotherapy or omalizumab should be prepared and equipped to identify and treat anaphylaxis that may occur.

FIGURE 22-5 Stepwise approach for managing asthma in youths ≥12 years of age and adults. (From National Institute of Health's National Heart, Lung, and Blood Institute: 2007 National Asthma Education and Prevention Program: *Expert Panel Report 3: guidelines for the diagnosis and management of asthma*, p 343, Figure 4-5.)

includes control of dust; removal of allergens such as feathers, molds, and animal dander; and, in some cases, removal of rugs and carpets. Other environmental control factors that help some patients include the use of air purifiers and air conditioners. The patient should also be taught preventive therapy in regard to smoking cessation and

avoidance of passive smoke, aerosols, and odors. Patients should seek early treatment for respiratory tract infections.[17]

Pharmacologic therapy for all three major obstructive disorders is similar and focuses on decreasing inflammation and bronchoconstriction, including β$_2$ agonists, corticosteroids, leukotriene modifiers, and

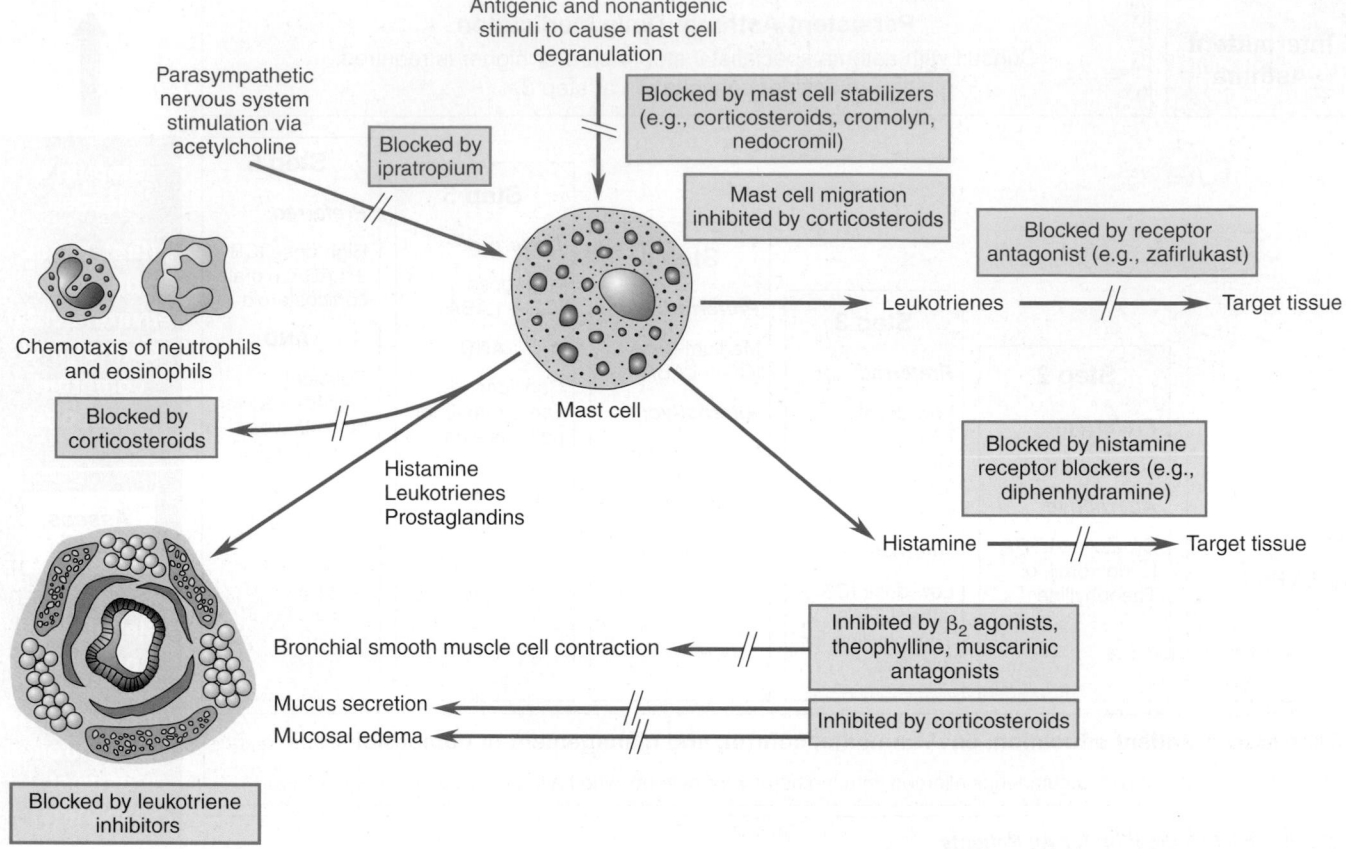

FIGURE 22-6 Pathophysiologic basis of asthma and site of action of drugs used in management.

mast cell inhibitors (Figure 22-6). Other therapies used in patients with more severe asthma include home oxygen therapy and home administration of small-volume nebulizer treatments via intermittent positive-pressure ventilation. At home, peak flow monitoring is helpful to parents or patients in determining a treatment plan and when to seek medical assistance. Peak flow meters are also helpful in monitoring progress of the patient with around-the-clock therapy.[10]

Allergen-specific immunotherapy (hyposensitization) may be used as an adjunct to other therapies. The allergen is first identified by testing with purified allergens using the scratch, prick, or intradermal method. Desensitization therapy has been shown in controlled studies to reduce the frequency and severity of asthmatic episodes when a single offending allergen can be identified.[10]

Status asthmaticus (severe attack unresponsive to routine therapy) requires more rapid and intense therapy, which may include epinephrine, subcutaneous terbutaline, and/or aminophylline. Once airflow has improved, aerosol bronchodilating inhalers may be used. Intravenous corticosteroids are the mainstay of therapy. Oxygen therapy with or without mechanical ventilation may be necessary in severe cases.

The more patients understand about their asthma, the better they are at self-managing their symptoms. Educational materials are available from the American Lung Association, the Asthma and Allergy Foundation of America, and the National Institute of Allergy and Infectious Diseases.

> **KEY POINTS**
> - An asthma episode may range in severity from mild to life threatening, depending on the degree of airway obstruction. With intense narrowing of the bronchi, severe hypoxemia may result.

> - Several types of asthma have been identified. Non-allergic (intrinsic) asthma is precipitated by exercise, stress, and exposure to pulmonary irritants, but no specific allergen can be identified. Drugs such as aspirin and exposure to occupational allergens have also been identified as etiologic agents.
> - Allergic (extrinsic) asthma is mediated by IgE, which is produced in response to specific antigens. The IgE binds to mast cells and causes them to release inflammatory chemicals in response to antigen. Skin testing may be helpful in identifying suspected allergens.
> - Prevention of asthma attacks is an important part of therapy. Avoidance of precipitating factors and use of prophylactic drug therapy are recommended. Bronchodilators, corticosteroids, and oxygen therapy are mainstays of treatment for an acute attack.

Acute Bronchitis

Etiology. Acute inflammation of the trachea and bronchi is produced most commonly (80% of the 12 million cases per year in the United States) by a variety of viruses such as influenza virus A or B, parainfluenza virus, respiratory syncytial virus, coronavirus, rhinovirus, Coxsackie virus, and adenovirus. Nonviral causes include *Streptococcus pneumoniae, Haemophilus influenzae,* mycoplasma, moraxella, and *Chlamydia pneumoniae.*[7,8] Numerous other pathogens as well as heat, smoke inhalation, inhalation of irritant chemicals (e.g., sulfur dioxide or chlorine, bromine, or fluorine gases), and allergic reactions have also been identified.[18] Highest incidences are noted in smokers, young children, and the elderly, with a prevalence in the winter months.[8,19] The swelling of bronchial mucosa in children associated with obstruction, respiratory distress, and wheezing is known as *asthmatic bronchitis.* Acute bronchitis differs from bronchiolitis in the size

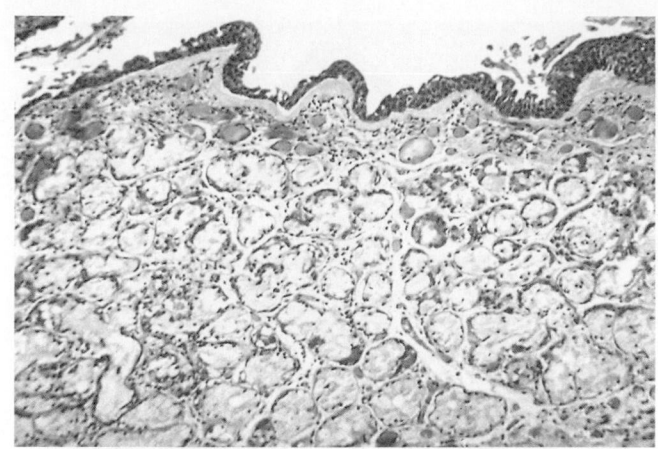

FIGURE 22-7 Histologic features of chronic bronchitis. (Lumen of bronchus is above.) Note slight desquamation of mucosal epithelial cells and marked thickening (approximately twice the normal thickness) of mucous gland layer. Vascular congestion is evident. (From Kumar V et al: *Robbins basic pathology,* ed 9, Philadelphia, 2013, Saunders.)

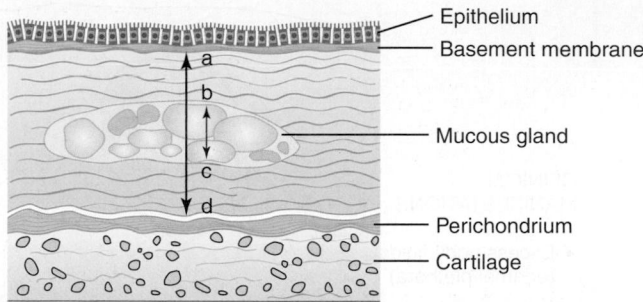

FIGURE 22-8 Structure of a normal bronchial wall. In chronic bronchitis, the thickness of the mucous glands increases and can be expressed as the Reid index, given by the following formula: (b − c)/(a − d). The ratio is normally less than 0.4. A ratio of 0.7 indicates severe bronchitis.

of the airways affected (i.e., trachea and bronchi as opposed to the small bronchioli).[20]

Pathogenesis. The airways become inflamed and narrowed from capillary dilation, swelling from exudation of fluid, infiltration with inflammatory cells, increased mucus production, loss of ciliary function, and loss of portions of the ciliated epithelium. Many viruses and mycoplasmal bacteria inhibit macrophages and lymphocytes, temporarily promoting secondary bacterial invasion. Microorganisms may also induce long-lasting hyperirritability of the respiratory tract with associated episodes of bronchospasm.

Clinical manifestations. The presentation of acute bronchitis is usually mild and self-limited, requiring only supportive treatment. Cough may be productive or nonproductive. Associated symptoms include low-grade fever, substernal chest discomfort, sore throat, postnasal drip, and fatigue. In children, the smaller airways are easily obstructed by inflammation, so that severe obstruction may occur.[8] The smallness of airways in proportion to body size is due to a smaller lumen in relation to the vessel wall. Associated inflammation of the larynx and trachea produces croup (see Croup Syndrome section in this chapter for further details).

Diagnosis. Diagnosis of acute bronchitis is usually based on the clinical presentation, with recent onset of cough being the distinctive hallmark. Neither the appearance of purulent sputum nor the determination of an increased WBC count is a reliable diagnostic indicator. A chest radiograph is required to distinguish acute bronchitis (normal radiograph) from pneumonia (pulmonary infiltrates on radiograph).

Treatment. Acute bronchitis is predominantly caused by viruses (rhinovirus, coronavirus, adenovirus, influenza virus). Viral infections do not respond to antimicrobial therapy, and symptoms resolve spontaneously in most normal, otherwise healthy individuals. Acute bronchitis caused by bacterial organisms responds well to antibiotic therapy. Codeine-containing medications are helpful in relieving the cough associated with bronchitis that interferes with sleep. Nonpharmacologic recommendations are to increase fluid intake, avoid smoke, and use a vaporizer in the bedroom.

The dangers of acute bronchitis include the potential for bacterial invasion, which can worsen symptoms in patients with chronic obstructive pulmonary disease (COPD) and precipitate serious infections in elderly patients or those with debilitating disease.

Chronic Bronchitis

Etiology. The next two sections of this chapter present chronic bronchitis and emphysema. Characteristic pathologic and clinical findings are described for each of these classifications. Clinically, pure forms of emphysema and chronic bronchitis are rare, and most patients present a combination of both of these obstructive processes. Patients with emphysema and chronic bronchitis constitute most cases of COPD.

The major causes of chronic bronchitis are cigarette smoking (90% of cases),[12] repeated airway infections, genetic predisposition, and inhalation of physical or chemical irritants.[8,9,21,22]

Chronic bronchitis (also referred to as type B COPD or the "blue bloater"[8,9,21]) is diagnosed *symptomatically* by hypersecretion of bronchial mucus and a chronic or recurrent productive cough of more than 3 months' duration and occurring each year for 2 or more successive years in patients in whom other causes have been excluded.[9] For patients with chronic bronchitis and emphysema, airway obstruction is persistent and irreversible. The National Center for Health Statistics reports a 3:1 ratio of annual cases of chronic bronchitis to emphysema.[23]

Pathogenesis. Pathologic changes in the airway include chronic inflammation and swelling of the bronchial mucosa resulting in scarring, increased fibrosis of the mucous membrane, hyperplasia of bronchial mucous glands and goblet cells, hypertrophy of bronchial glands and goblet cells, and increased bronchial wall thickness, which potentiates obstruction to airflow. Inflammation appears to predominantly be the result of neutrophil activity.[21] Interleukin-8 levels are elevated, indicating sustained attraction of neutrophils to the site of inflammation. CD8 T-lymphocyte levels are also elevated. During acute exacerbations, bronchial biopsy specimens have a 30-fold increase in the number of eosinophils.[21] Figures 22-7 and 22-8 show the histologic changes seen in chronic bronchitis. Hypertrophy of mucosal glands and goblet cells leads to increased mucus production; the mucus then combines with purulent exudate to form bronchial plugs. Chronic bronchitis patients often display bacterial colonization with *H. influenzae* and *S. pneumoniae.*[21] The mucociliary clearance action is impaired or lost, and some areas of ciliated columnar epithelium are replaced by squamous cells.[21] Ciliary dysfunction occurs because of a decreased number of cilia and decreased action of available cilia.

Often the inflammatory and fibrotic changes extend into the surrounding alveoli. The narrowed airways and the mucous plugs prevent proper oxygenation and potentiate airway obstruction. High airflow resistance increases the work of breathing, leading to increased oxygen demands. In areas of greater obstruction to airflow, alveoli empty and fill more slowly, leading to ventilation-perfusion ($\dot{V}_A/\dot{Q}$) mismatch, thus

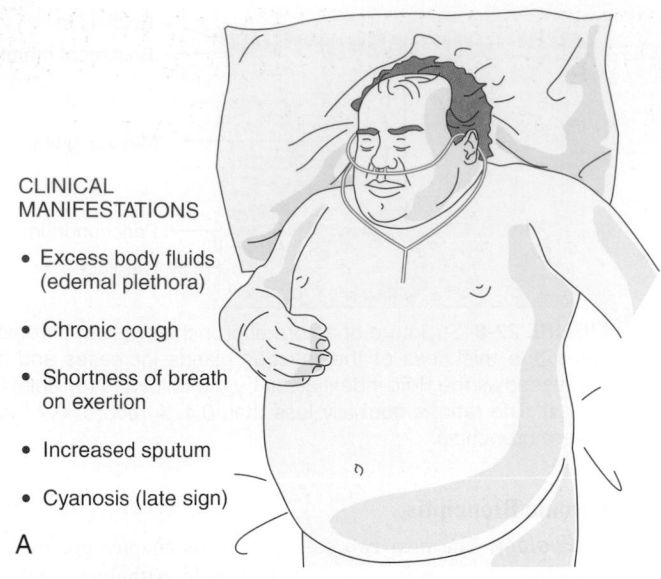

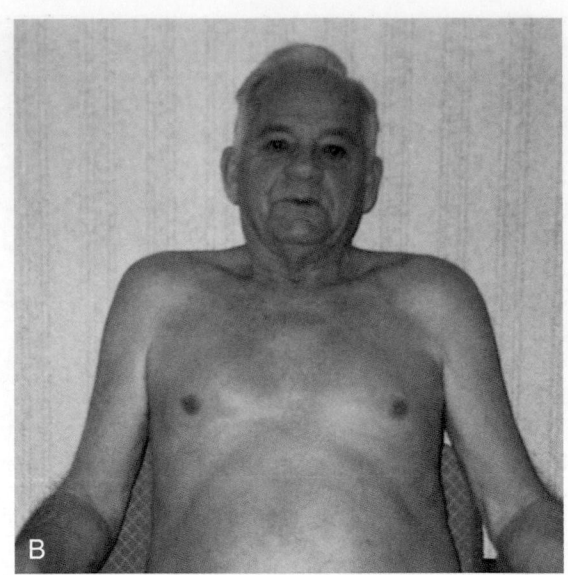

CLINICAL MANIFESTATIONS

- Excess body fluids (edemal plethora)
- Chronic cough
- Shortness of breath on exertion
- Increased sputum
- Cyanosis (late sign)

A

B

FIGURE 22-9 A, A "blue bloater" with edema from right-sided heart failure. **B,** A patient with chronic obstructive bronchitis. Note the stocky build and the presence of pursed-lip breathing and barrel chest. The slight gynecomastia is a side effect of corticosteroid therapy. The patient's shoulders are raised because of shortness of breath and increased work of breathing. (**B,** From Black JM, Hawks SJ: *Medical-surgical nursing: clinical management for positive outcomes,* ed 8, Philadelphia, 2008, Saunders, p 1581.)

lowering arterial oxygenation. The chronic bronchitis patient may appear as the "blue bloater" (Figure 22-9), characterizing the pathophysiologic process of oxygen desaturation (cyanosis) and edema associated with right-sided heart failure in advanced disease or exacerbations.

The involvement of small pulmonary arteries related to inflammation in the bronchial walls and the compensatory vasoconstriction of pulmonary blood vessels from hypoxia produce pulmonary hypertension. In addition, widespread bronchial narrowing and mucous plugging produce ventilation-perfusion mismatch with hypoxemia and hypercarbia from impeded ventilation. The combination of hypoxia and hypercarbia increases pulmonary artery resistance and pulmonary hypertension.[21] While the process of pulmonary hypertension continues, right ventricular end-diastolic pressures increase, leading to right ventricular dilation (cor pulmonale) and right-sided heart failure. An enlarged right heart results in increased venous pressure, liver engorgement, and dependent edema. Manifestations of heart failure may occur during exacerbations of bronchitis and subside with appropriate treatment.[9,21]

Destruction of bronchial walls results in dilation of airway sacs. This is termed *bronchiectasis*. Causes of bronchial wall destruction include infection from severe streptococcal or staphylococcal pneumonia, repeated bouts of acute bronchitis, infection with the mold *Aspergillus fumigatus,* presence of mucous plugs or foreign bodies, or deficiencies in immunologic response. (Refer to the Bronchiectasis section later in this chapter for a more detailed description of this disease process.) The dilated sacs contain pools of infected secretion that do not clear themselves and serve as sources of further infection that can spread to adjacent lung fields by the lymphatics or venous drainage to other areas of the body, commonly the brain. If bronchiectatic lesions are localized, surgical resection of the affected portions of lung may be helpful.

Clinical manifestations. The typical patient is an overweight man or woman (1:2 male to female ratio) in his or her thirties or forties[9,21,22,24] (or older) who presents with shortness of breath on exertion, excessive amounts of sputum, chronic cough, evidence of excess body fluids (edema, hypervolemia), and a history of smoking. In addition, the patient often complains of chills, malaise, muscle aches, fatigue, loss of libido, and insomnia.

Sputum production may be variable and worsens with respiratory tract infection. Cough and sputum production are most severe in the mornings. Gradually, patients develop progressive shortness of breath on exertion. Most patients do not seek help until dyspnea becomes troublesome. By the time dyspnea on exertion is present, the disease is well advanced.[21,22]

In the end-stage disease process, the patient presents with signs of right-sided heart failure (distended neck veins, right ventricular heave, right ventricular gallop, and peripheral edema).[21] Hypoxia leads to pulmonary hypertension. Cyanosis is a late sign.

Diagnosis. Measures used to confirm the diagnosis include chest radiography, which may show increased bronchial vascular markings, congested lung fields, an enlarged horizontal cardiac silhouette, and evidence of previous pulmonary infection. Pulmonary function tests show normal total lung capacity (TLC), increased residual volume (RV), and decreased FEV_1. Early pulmonary function testing before the onset of symptoms shows increased closing volume and a decrease in the maximal midexpiratory flow rate.[21] Arterial blood gas (ABG) evaluation may show elevated $PaCO_2$ and decreased PaO_2 (often below 65 mm Hg); abnormal ABGs develop early in the disease process. The electrocardiogram may reveal atrial dysrhythmias and evidence of right ventricular hypertrophy. Secondary polycythemia (increased numbers of red blood cells) related to continuous or nocturnal hypoxemia is common.[9,21] Hypoxemia leads to a compensatory production of red blood cells in an attempt to carry more oxygen to the body tissues.

Depending on the severity of the disease, the physical examination may reveal scattered crackles, rhonchi, and wheezes; use of accessory muscles to breathe; jugular vein distention; clubbing; and pedal and ankle edema. Table 22-1 lists the distinguishing features of both emphysema and chronic bronchitis.

Treatment. Because bronchitis and emphysema are most frequently seen in combination, the therapies are similar. The overall goals are to (1) block the progression of the disease, (2) return the patient to optimal respiratory function, and (3) return the patient to usual activities of daily living.

TABLE 22-1	COMMON DISTINGUISHING FEATURES OF EMPHYSEMA AND CHRONIC BRONCHITIS*	
PATIENT DATA	**EMPHYSEMA (COPD TYPE A)**	**BRONCHITIS (COPD TYPE B)**
History		
Lifestyle	Smoker	Smoker
Weight	Weight loss	Overweight
Onset of symptoms	Usually after age 50 years	Usually after age 40 years
Sputum	Mild, mucoid	Excessive, purulent
Cough	Minimal or absent	Chronic; more severe in mornings
Dyspnea	Progressive exertional dyspnea	Mild to moderate, but may gradually progress to severe exertional dyspnea
Patient complaints	Dyspnea on exertion, fatigue, insomnia	Chronic cough with mucopurulent sputum, chills, malaise, muscle aches, fatigue, insomnia, loss of libido
Physical Signs		
Edema	Absent	Present
Central cyanosis	Absent	Present in advanced disease
Use of accessory muscles to breathe	Present	Absent until end stage
Body build	Thin, wasted	Stocky, overweight
Anteroposterior chest diameter	"Barrel chest," 1:1 ratio anteroposterior chest diameter	Normal
Auscultation of chest	Decreased breath sounds, decreased heart sounds, prolonged expiration	Wheezes, crackles, rhonchi, depending on severity of disease
Percussion	Hyperresonance	Normal
Jugular vein distention	Absent	Present
Other	Pursed-lip breathing	Evidence of right-sided heart failure (cor pulmonale)
General Diagnostic Tests		
Chest radiography	Narrowed mediastinum; normal or small vertical heart; hyperinflation; low, flat diaphragm; presence of blebs or bullae	Congested lung fields, increased bronchial vascular markings, enlarged horizontal heart
Arterial blood gas analysis	Decreased Pao_2 (60-80 mm Hg); increased $Paco_2$ with advancing disease	Decreased Pao_2 (<65 mm Hg); increased $Paco_2$
Electrocardiography	Normal or tall symmetric P waves; tachycardia, if hypoxic	Right axis deviation, right ventricular hypertrophy, atrial dysrhythmias
Hematocrit	Normal	Polycythemia
Pulmonary Function Tests		
Functional residual capacity	Increased	Normal or slight increase
Residual volume	Increased	Increased
Total lung capacity	Increased	Normal
Forced expiratory volume	Decreased	Decreased
Vital capacity	Decreased	Normal or slight decrease
Static lung compliance	Increased	Normal

*Clinically, features of bronchitis and emphysema are not clear-cut because most patients with COPD have a combined disease process.
COPD, Chronic obstructive pulmonary disease.

Pharmacologic treatment involves the use of inhaled short-acting β_2 agonists and inhaled anticholinergic bronchodilators, cough suppressants, and antimicrobial agents for infections. Inhaled or oral corticosteroids may also be used in the treatment of some patients for acute exacerbations. Theophylline products are used less frequently because of their narrow therapeutic range and toxicity. However, many patients derive significant benefits from theophylline.[21,22]

Low-dose oxygen therapy is recommended for patients with Pao_2 levels less than 55 mm Hg.[21,22] Mechanical ventilation may become necessary to get the patient over a crisis period of acute exacerbation. Although traditionally the mechanism of carbon dioxide retention with oxygen therapy was thought to be related to a diminished ventilatory drive, current research suggests that oxygen therapy may instead cause increased $\dot{V}_A/\dot{Q}$ imbalance, precipitating a rise in carbon dioxide concentration. It is important to remember that not all patients with a history of COPD are carbon dioxide retainers and most can use oxygen safely. Home oxygen therapy has been demonstrated to retard the development of pulmonary hypertension and cor pulmonale in chronic bronchitis.[9,21] Portable oxygen saturation monitors for evaluating the effectiveness of oxygen administration at home may also be used.

Smoking cessation is essential to decreasing the progression of the disease. A reduction in exposure to inhaled pulmonary irritants is also advised.[22] Supportive therapies include adequate rest, proper hydration (8 to 12 glasses of water per day unless the patient has congestive heart failure), and physical reconditioning programs using a treadmill or stationary bicycle. Alternating rest and exercise improves results on pulmonary function tests. Walking has proved to be the best form of exercise for increasing duration and intensity of activity. All COPD patients also benefit from yearly influenza vaccine and pneumococcal vaccine.

KEY POINTS

- Acute bronchitis results from temporary inflammation of the tracheobronchial tree. Inflammation may be due to viral, bacterial, fungal, or chemical causes. Symptoms are caused by narrowing of inflamed airways and increased mucus production. Dyspnea on exertion and cough are common.
- Chronic bronchitis is an inflammatory disorder of the airways that most commonly results from long-term cigarette smoking. It is defined as a productive cough lasting more than 3 months per year for 2 or more consecutive years. Resultant airway damage is not reversible.
- Chronic bronchitis is associated with persistent narrowing of the airways attributable to chronic inflammation, scarring, and excessive mucus production. Airway obstruction leads to poor ventilation of alveoli and impaired exchange of oxygen

and carbon dioxide. Blood gases are characterized by low Pa_{O_2} and high Pa_{CO_2} values. Persistent hypoxemia causes a compensatory increase in red blood cell production (polycythemia). Cyanosis may be evident.

- Alveolar hypoxia leads to generalized pulmonary vasoconstriction, pulmonary hypertension, and right ventricular hypertrophy (cor pulmonale) in the person with chronic bronchitis. Right-sided heart failure may occur because of the high pulmonary resistance.
- The management of chronic bronchitis centers on removing the etiologic factors (e.g., cigarette smoke), providing bronchodilator therapy, removing secretions, preventing respiratory muscle fatigue, and providing low-dose supplemental oxygen. High-dose oxygen must be used cautiously because it may increase $\dot{V}_A/\dot{Q}$ imbalance and Pa_{CO_2} levels in some patients.

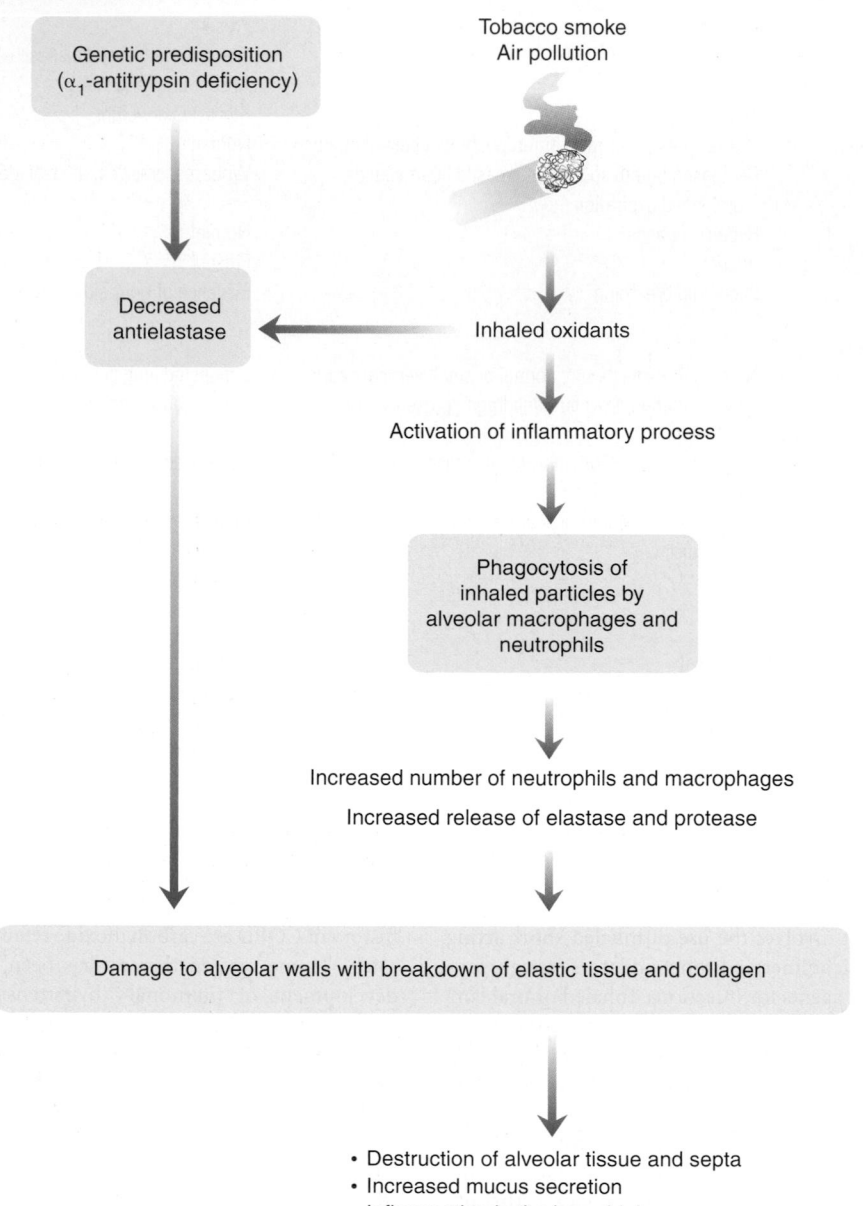

FIGURE 22-10 Pathogenesis of smoke-induced emphysema.

OBSTRUCTION RELATED TO LOSS OF LUNG PARENCHYMA

Emphysema

Etiology. Emphysema (also referred to as type A COPD or the "pink puffer") is defined *pathologically* by destructive changes of the alveolar walls and abnormal enlargement of the distal air sacs.[8,9,21,22] Emphysema is frequently associated with chronic bronchitis. According to the National Center for Health Statistics (2005 data), of the 12.7 million Americans with COPD, 8.9 million primarily have chronic bronchitis and 3.8 million primarily have emphysema.[24] The etiologies of emphysema include smoking, air pollution, certain occupations (e.g., welding, mining, and working with or near asbestos), and α_1-antitrypsin deficiency (1%). Emphysema tends to develop over a long period and thus is seen more frequently in persons older than 50. Cigarette smoking in excess of 70 pack-years is highly predictive of COPD.[21] The normal aging process, starting at about age 30, reflects changes similar to those seen in emphysema, including a loss of alveoli, an increase in the size of alveolar ducts, a loss of gas-exchanging surface area (4% per decade), and a decrease in bronchiolar musculature.[21]

When emphysema occurs in young to middle-aged adults or before the age of 50 in a smoker, it may be associated with a deficiency of α_1-antitrypsin activity in the lung. α_1-Antitrypsin deficiency is a hereditary disorder characterized by low serum levels (25 to 50 mg/dl) of α_1-antitrypsin.[21,22] α_1-Antitrypsin is a protective enzyme that inhibits proteolytic breakdown of alveolar tissue. The protease enzymes (neutrophil-derived elastase) that break down lung protein are released from neutrophils that migrate to the lung during inflammation, causing alveolar wall destruction.[21]

Emphysema may follow bacterial lung infections, which involve secretion of proteases that destroy the elastin proteins responsible for the normal elasticity of the lung tissue. Bacterial infections block mechanisms that normally inhibit the release of proteolytic enzymes from degenerating neutrophilic granulocytes.

Pathogenesis. The pathologic changes leading to alveolar destruction are associated with the release of proteolytic enzymes from inflammatory cells such as neutrophils and macrophages. Smoking is commonly associated with emphysema. Smoking causes alveolar damage in two ways: (1) it leads to inflammation in the lung tissue (parenchyma), thus initiating a chain of events leading to the release of proteolytic enzymes that directly damage alveolar tissue; and (2) it inactivates α_1-antitrypsin, which normally acts to protect the lung parenchyma.[21,22] Figure 22-10 illustrates the pathogenesis of emphysema.

With the loss of alveolar walls, there is also a marked reduction in the pulmonary capillary bed, which is essential for exchange of oxygen and carbon dioxide between the alveolar air and capillary blood. There is also a loss of elastic tissue in the lung, which leads to a decrease in the size of the smaller bronchioles. The loss of lung tissue leads to a loss of *radial traction*, which normally holds the airway open, and to increasing pressure around the outside of the airway lumen, which in turn increases airway resistance and decreases airflow. Figure 22-11 shows the effect of decreased radial traction on the size of small bronchioles. Air then becomes trapped in distal alveoli, leading to distended air sacs, which adds to the collapsing pressure on more proximal bronchi and increases airway obstruction. Loss of alveolar walls and air trapping leads to the formation of bullae (large, thin-walled cysts in the lung) that further rob the lung of its gas transport function. The histologic appearance of the lung and lung tissue from typical emphysematous patients is shown in Figures 22-12 and 22-13.

Three major classifications of emphysema exist: (1) centriacinar (also called *centrilobular*), which is associated with both smoking and chronic bronchitis and destroys the respiratory bronchioles; (2) panacinar (also called *panlobular*), which destroys the alveoli; and (3) paraseptal, which affects the peripheral lobules. Some of the classifications of emphysema and the topographic distribution of emphysema in lung tissue are shown in Figure 22-14.

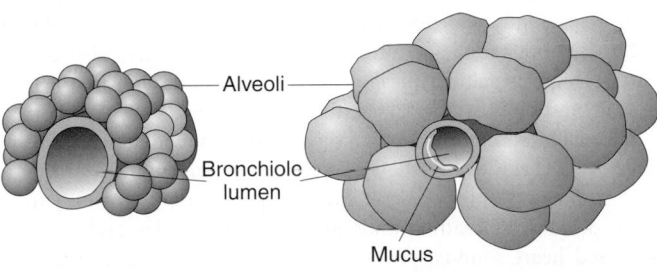

A NORMAL   B EMPHYSEMA

FIGURE 22-11 Loss of radial traction in emphysema leads to airway collapse. **A,** Terminal bronchiole in cross-section. **B,** Terminal bronchiole with narrowed lumen resulting from loss of surrounding alveoli, leading to decreased radial traction and airway collapse.

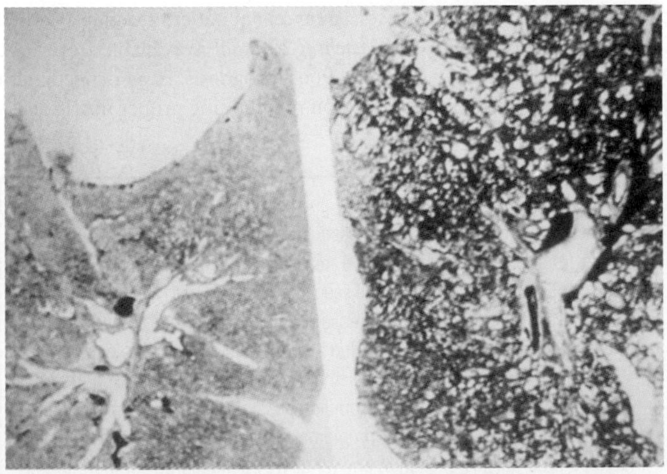

FIGURE 22-12 Gross appearance of emphysematous lung. *Left,* Normal lung tissue from a nonsmoker. *Right,* Lung tissue from a smoker who has developed emphysema.

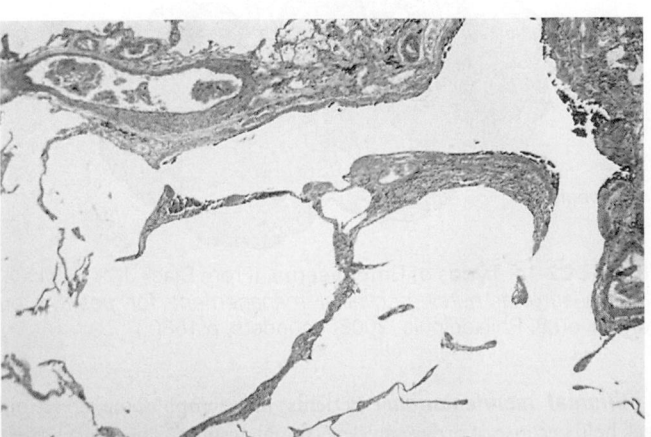

FIGURE 22-13 Pulmonary emphysema. There is a marked enlargement of air spaces with thinning and destruction of alveolar septa. (From Kumar V et al: *Robbins basic pathology*, ed 9, Philadelphia, 2013, Saunders.)

NORMAL LUNGS

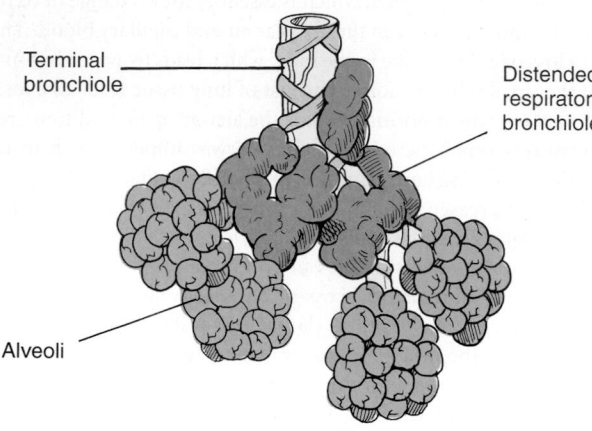

Terminal bronchiole

Respiratory bronchiole

Alveoli

CENTRIACINAR EMPHYSEMA

Terminal bronchiole

Distended respiratory bronchiole

Alveoli

PANACINAR EMPHYSEMA

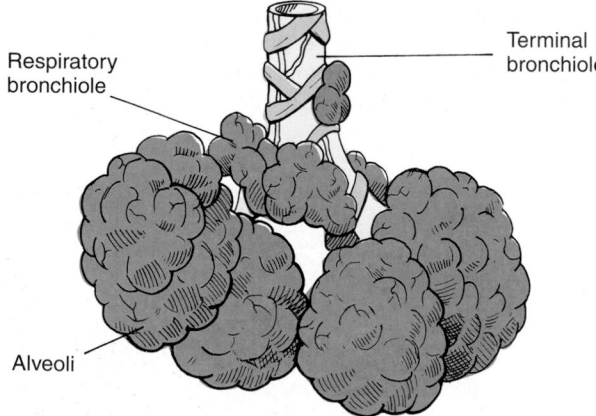

Respiratory bronchiole

Terminal bronchiole

Alveoli

FIGURE 22-14 Types of Emphysema. (From Black JM, Hawks SJ: *Medical-surgical nursing: clinical management for positive outcomes,* ed 8, Philadelphia, 2008, Saunders, p 1580.)

Clinical manifestations. Patients with emphysema commonly seek help because of progressive exertional dyspnea. The typical patient with advanced disease is a thin man or woman around 55 years of age who has complained of increasing shortness of breath for the past 3 to 4 years. As with chronic bronchitis, the incidence of emphysema is increasing in women who smoke. Patients become thin due to

increased respiratory effort and resulting caloric expenditure with decreased ability to consume adequate calories. The difficulty in breathing is evidenced by the use of accessory muscles to breathe, progressive dyspnea, and the use of pursed-lip breathing in an effort to exhale more air over a longer period of time before the small airways collapse. Cough may be minimal or absent. Digital clubbing is common. The appearance of overinflation (barrel chest) is from an increase in lung volume, which can be confirmed by pulmonary function testing. With the loss of alveolar walls and the formation of bullae, the patient is at risk for developing a pneumothorax and may present with chest pain on the affected side and dyspnea. Decreased arterial oxygen saturation remains minor until late in the course of the disease. Late in the disease process, the major symptom is dyspnea on exertion. These patients may be referred to as "pink puffers" (Figure 22-15), a term related to the physiologic matching of ventilation and perfusion that allows near normal gas exchange. Ventilation-perfusion matching and a sustained high respiratory effort produce a relatively normal arterial oxygen level until late stages of the disease.[1,2,9,21,22]

Diagnosis. The diagnosis of emphysema is based on the patient's history and physical findings, pulmonary function tests, chest radiographs, arterial blood gases, and electrocardiogram. Changes seen on pulmonary function tests include an increased functional residual capacity, increased RV, increased TLC, decreased FEV_1, and decreased FVC.[9,21] Chest radiographs show hyperinflation; a low, flat diaphragm; the presence of blebs or bullae; a narrow mediastinum; and a normal or small "vertical" heart (see Table 22-1). Electrocardiographic findings may be normal or show tall P waves. Sinus tachycardia may be the first sign of decreased oxygenation. Supraventricular dysrhythmias (atrial tachycardia, atrial flutter, and atrial fibrillation) and ventricular irregularities may also occur.[9] Arterial blood gas values typically reveal a mild decrease in Pao_2 (65 to 75 mm Hg) and a low or normal $Paco_2$ until late stages.[25]

Physical examination shows a thin, wasted individual who is using accessory muscles to breathe and sits slightly hunched forward in an effort to breathe better. Auscultation and percussion of the lung fields reveal decreased breath sounds and lack of crackles and rhonchi, decreased heart sounds, prolonged expiration, decreased diaphragmatic excursion, and hyperresonance of the chest. Pursed-lip breathing, chronic morning cough because of mucus buildup at night, and an increased anteroposterior chest diameter (barrel chest) are also common findings. Weight loss occurs because of anorexia and lack of energy to eat. Bronchoconstriction leads to wheezing.

Treatment. Refer to the Treatment section under Chronic Bronchitis earlier in this chapter for detailed treatment modalities common to both chronic obstructive lung diseases. An excellent patient teaching manual called *Better Breathing: A Self-Teaching Manual* is available from PAL Medical, Inc., Maitland, Florida. Poor prognosis is associated with weight loss, so treatment is focused on maintaining proper nutrition.

KEY POINTS

- Emphysema is a form of chronic obstructive pulmonary disease (COPD) that results from destruction of alveoli and small airways. Emphysema occurs primarily in cigarette smokers and is often seen in association with chronic bronchitis.
- Alveolar destruction is due to release of inflammatory proteolytic enzymes that degrade lung proteins. Smoking also inhibits a protective enzyme, α_1-antitrypsin, that normally inhibits the proteolytic enzymes. Genetic deficiency of α_1-antitrypsin is an uncommon possible cause of emphysema.
- Emphysema causes two major problems with respiration: (1) a decrease in surface area for gas exchange and (2) airway collapse attributable to loss of radial traction. Airway collapse is greater on expiration, resulting in air trapping and hyperinflation.

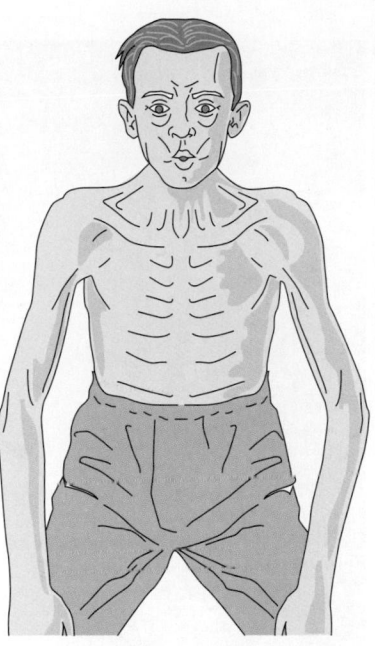

CLINICAL
MANIFESTATIONS

- Use of accessory muscles to breathe

- Pursed-lip breathing

- Minimal or absent cough

- Leaning forward to breathe

- Barrel chest

- Digital clubbing

- Dyspnea on exertion (late sign)

A

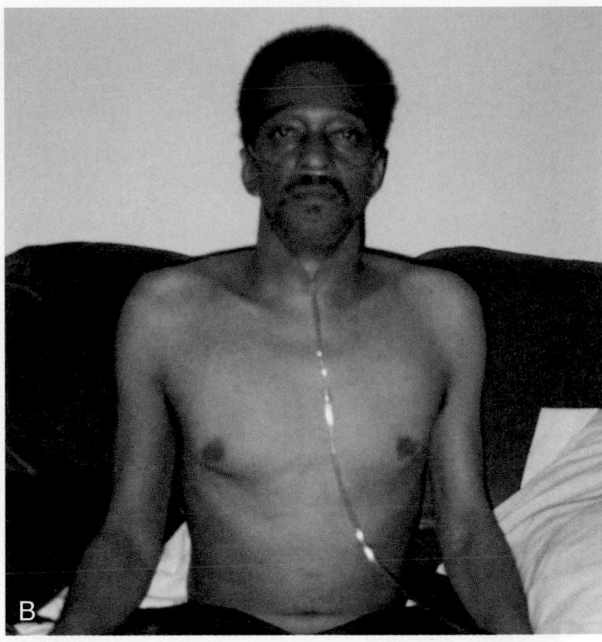

B

FIGURE 22-15 A, The "pink puffer." Note the use of accessory muscles and pursed-lip breathing in an effort to get more air out of the lungs. **B,** A patient with emphysema. Note the thin appearance and the presence of continuous oxygen therapy. The use of accessory muscles of respiration (neck and shoulder muscles) reflects the patient's shortness of breath and increased work of breathing necessary to increase minute ventilation and to maintain adequate arterial blood gas values. (**B,** From Black JM, Hawks SJ: *Medical-surgical nursing: clinical management for positive outcomes,* ed 8, Philadelphia, 2008, Saunders, p 1581.)

- Emphysema is characterized by dyspnea, weight loss, use of accessory muscles to breathe, a low, flat diaphragm, and a barrel chest. Cyanosis is not present until late stages of the disease. By sustaining high ventilatory effort, a patient can have blood oxygen levels that are generally maintained near normal. Carbon dioxide levels may be normal or low as a result of hyperventilation until late in the disease.

- Therapy for emphysema is similar to that for chronic bronchitis. Cessation of smoking is necessary to prevent progression of the disease. Present damage is irreversible. Oxygen therapy improves activity tolerance and quality of life.

OBSTRUCTION OF THE AIRWAY LUMEN

Bronchiectasis

Etiology. Bronchiectasis means dilation of bronchi. It is either acquired or congenital, and is classified as both an obstructive and a suppurative (pus-forming) disorder. Acquired bronchiectasis is now rare in the United States because of rapid diagnosis and management of bronchopulmonary infections. Fifty percent of the cases of bronchiectasis are associated with cystic fibrosis.[26] Children are at higher risk for development of bronchiectasis because of anatomic factors such as small, soft, elastic bronchi. Bronchi in children are easily damaged by overinflation and distention from inflammation and infection.

Bronchiectasis can be classified according to bronchial shape: saccular (with cavity-like dilatations) or cylindrical, and with widening of the bronchial walls. A fusiform shape is a combination of saccular and cylindrical changes. These anatomic changes are shown in Figure 22-16. Little clinical or pathophysiologic difference in the three types has been demonstrated.

Pathogenesis. Bronchiectasis is characterized by recurrent infection and inflammation of bronchial walls, which leads to persistent

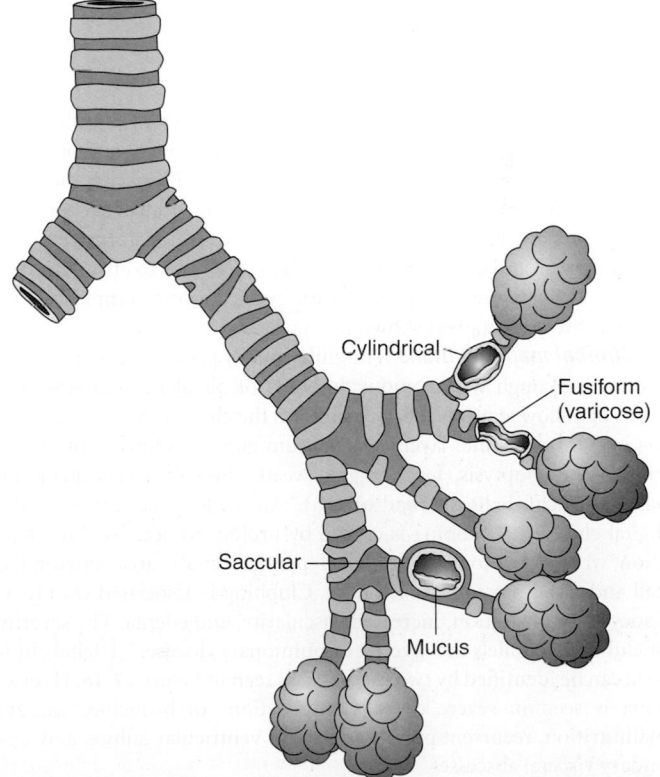

FIGURE 22-16 Bronchial dilatations attributable to bronchiectasis. The saccular form occurs in the segmental bronchi, which are severely dilated and end blindly. The varicose form resembles varicose veins with irregular dilatations and constriction. The cylindrical form shows uniform slight dilatation.

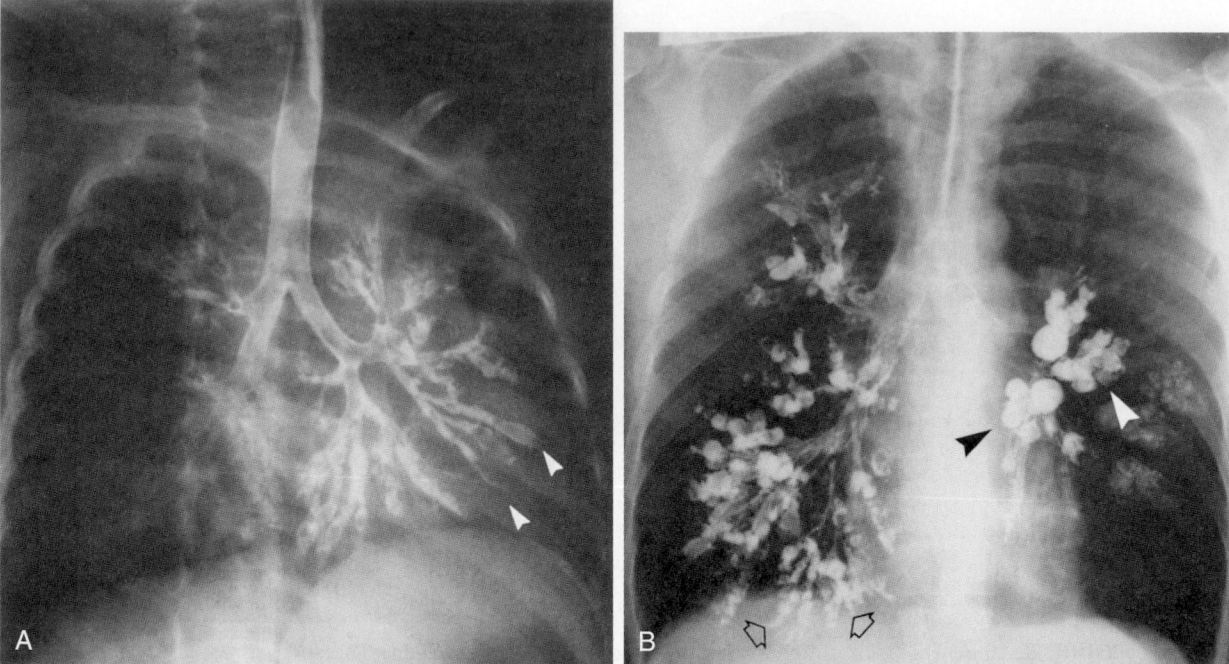

FIGURE 22-17 Bronchographic features of varicose and cystic bronchiectasis. **A,** A left tracheobronchogram in a shallow posterior oblique projection reveals mild dilatation and slightly irregular bronchi that terminate after four to six generations of branchings from the trachea in a squared or bulbous appearance *(arrowheads)*. The findings are those of varicose bronchiectasis. **B,** A bilateral tracheobronchogram in the anteroposterior projection demonstrates a multitude of contrast material–filled cystic spaces resembling a cluster of grapes *(arrowheads)*, a characteristic feature of cystic bronchiectasis. Note that the cystic spaces appear after only two to three bronchial generations. Less severe bronchiectasis of the varicose type is present in the right lower lobe *(open arrows)*. (From Fraser RG et al: *Diagnosis of diseases of the chest,* ed 3, vol 3, Philadelphia, 1990, Saunders, p 2199.)

dilatation of the medium-sized bronchi and bronchioles. Inflammation results in destruction of the walls of central bronchi and obliteration of peripheral bronchi and bronchioles.[23] *H. influenzae* is the most common cause of bacterial infections.[23,26] The destructive process leads to loss of ciliated columnar epithelium, with transformation to a squamous cell and pus formation, which in turn leads to obstruction of airflow. Lung tissue of a patient with cystic fibrosis complicated by varicose bronchiectasis is shown in Figure 22-17.

Clinical manifestations. The child usually presents with a chronic productive cough with copious amounts of purulent, foul-smelling, green or yellow sputum. The sputum has the characteristic of separating into three distinct layers in a sputum cup.[23,26] Other clinical features are hemoptysis, fever, night sweats, moist crackles including bases, rhonchi, halitosis (bad breath), skin pallor, and, infrequently, digital clubbing. Clubbing is caused by prolonged decreased oxygenation, which leads to fibrous tissue hyperplasia in the area between the nail and distal portion of each digit. Clubbing is associated with lymphocytic extravasation, increased vascularity, and edema. The severity of clubbing parallels the severity of pulmonary disease.[20] Digital clubbing can be identified by two methods, as seen in Figure 22-18. Hypoxemia is seen in severe cases. Complications of bronchiectasis are malnutrition, recurrent pneumonia, right ventricular failure, and secondary visceral abscesses.[9]

Diagnosis. Generally, the diagnosis of bronchiectasis is based on a history of chronic productive cough. The patient complains about producing copious amounts of foul-smelling, purulent sputum. Radiographic abnormalities may reveal small cysts, thickening of bronchial walls, and increased bronchial markings (areas of intensity showing bronchi, which are usually not distinct). Pulmonary function tests show decreased airflow and vital capacity in advanced cases. Arterial blood gas analyses reveal decreased PaO_2 and increased $PaCO_2$ values from obstruction to airflow. High-resolution computed tomography is the test of choice for diagnosing bronchiectasis.[9]

Treatment. Antibiotic therapy accompanied by inhalation of bronchodilators followed by vigorous chest percussion and postural drainage is the mainstay of treatment. Proper hydration and nutrition are important in promoting liquefaction of secretions and preventing increased susceptibility to infection resulting from malnutrition. Maintaining adequate nutrition is problematic because of fatigue and the energy required for eating. (Refer to the Cystic Fibrosis section later in the chapter for further discussion on treatment.) In severe cases, when other measures fail, bronchoscopy with bronchial lavage may be necessary to remove thick, purulent secretions. In the child with severe saccular bronchiectasis, removal of the affected area of the lung may be necessary. Patient education materials can be obtained from the Cystic Fibrosis Foundation.[27] Childhood immunizations have led to a decreased incidence of bronchiectasis attributable to pertussis.[28]

Bronchiolitis

Etiology. Bronchiolitis is characterized by widespread inflammation of bronchioles attributable to infectious agents such as respiratory syncytial virus (RSV) (50% of cases),[28] influenza virus (type A, B, or C), or bacteria (*H. influenzae,* pneumococci, or hemolytic streptococci), and occasionally is produced by allergic reactions. RSV infection is a common cause of hospitalization in infants.[23] Other organisms that may cause bronchiolitis include mycoplasma, chlamydia, ureaplasma,

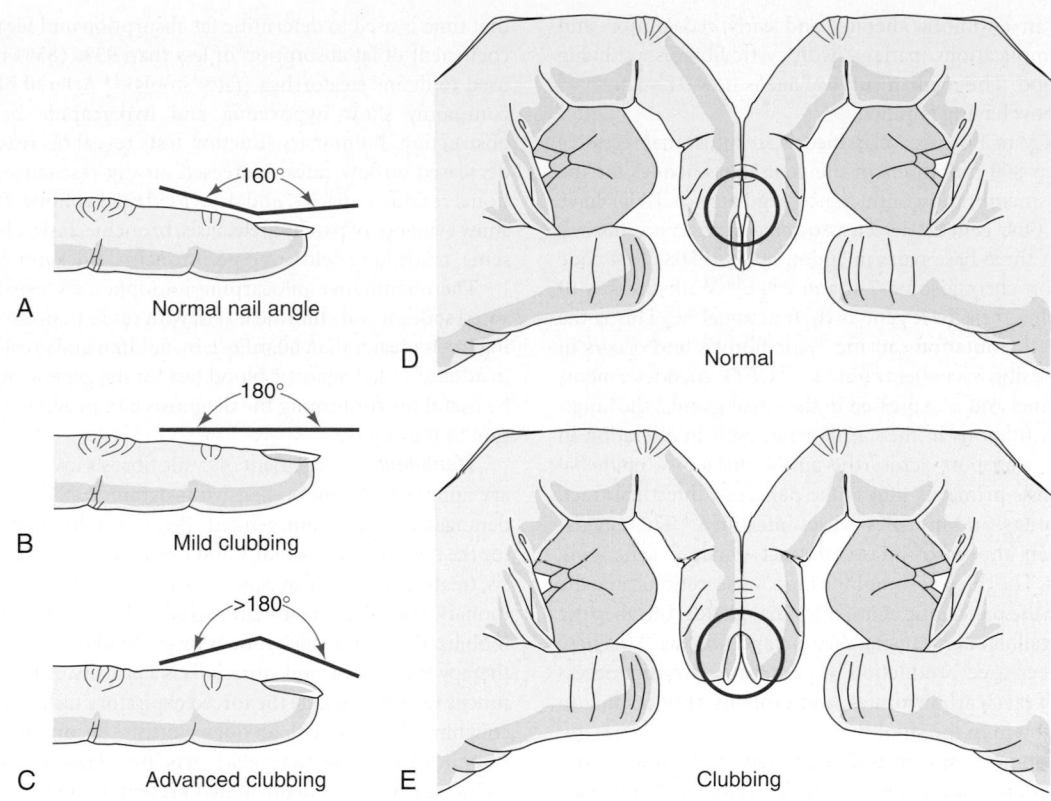

FIGURE 22-18 Clubbing. **A,** Normal fingernail angle is 160 degrees. **B,** Early mild clubbing appears as a flattened angle between nail and skin (180 degrees). **C,** Advanced clubbing shows a rounded (clubbed) fingertip and nail. To assess clubbing by Schamroth's diagnostic method (**D** and **E**), place the nails of the second digits together. Obliteration of the normal diamond-shaped space between the nails is an abnormal finding, signifying clubbing.

and *Pneumocystis (carinii) jiroveci*.[29] RSV occurs in yearly epidemics in winter to spring, usually in children younger than 2 years.[30] The average incubation period is 5 days, with inoculation occurring through the nose and eyes.[9,29] In adults, bronchiolitis is commonly associated with smoking, toxic fumes, and immunosuppression.[9]

Pathogenesis. Once initiated by the causal agent, proliferation and necrosis of bronchiolar epithelium occur, producing obstruction and increased mucus production.[9] Production of thick, tenacious mucus leads to airway obstruction, atelectasis, and hyperinflation. Three possible mechanisms of airway obstruction may follow the inflammatory process. They include (1) development of inflammatory exudate, which may displace surfactant, leading to airway obstruction; (2) release of chemical mediators, which may produce bronchiolar constriction; and (3) development of inflammation, which may induce fibrosis and narrowing of the airway.[1,23] Goblet cell metaplasia and increased bronchial muscle mass may also occur, resulting in further airway narrowing.

Clinical manifestations. The severity and course of the disease are variable, ranging from mild to fatal. Common clinical features include wheezing attributable to bronchospasm, crackles, decreased breath sounds, retractions, increased sputum, dyspnea, tachypnea (rapid, shallow respirations), and low-grade fever. Otitis media is a common complication often associated with *S. pneumoniae*.[29]

Diagnosis. Patients commonly have an elevated WBC count. The chest radiograph may show enlarged air sacs, interstitial infiltrates, atelectasis, or severe hyperinflation. Pulmonary function tests reveal severe obstruction to airflow. Rapid diagnosis of RSV may be made by identifying the viral antigen from nasal washings or nasal swab culture of secretions, using an enzyme-linked immunosorbent assay or immunofluorescent assay.

Treatment. Adequate oxygenation is maintained by providing humidified oxygen, monitoring blood gases or oxygen saturation, and administering oral, inhaled, or intravenous bronchodilator agents and, in selected cases, corticosteroids.[23] General information about pharmacologic agents commonly used in the management of various respiratory disorders is listed in other texts. Use of these agents depends on the severity of the diagnosis and prescriber preference.

Other therapies include sedation for anxiety, hydration, and the administration of appropriate antivirals and antibiotics. Patients are encouraged to stop smoking and to avoid passive smoke exposure. The use of eye-nose goggles by health care workers is recommended to control the spread of RSV. The virus is spread through the air or by contact with secretions from the eye, nose, or mouth, and transmission may not be prevented by the use of masks and gowns.

Cystic Fibrosis

Etiology. Cystic fibrosis (mucoviscidosis) is an autosomal recessive disorder of the exocrine glands. It is the most common genetic lung disease in the United States, with an incidence of 1 in 2000 to 3300 Caucasian births.[9,23,26,31] One in 25 Caucasians are heterozygous carriers of the cystic fibrosis gene.[9] The incidence in African Americans is rare (1 in 17,000 live births), and in Native Americans the incidence is 1 in 80,000 births.[31,32] It is almost never seen in the Asian population.[16,32] About 35% of the 30,000 cases of cystic fibrosis in the United States involve individuals older than 18 years.[9,16] Cystic fibrosis can be classified either as an airflow obstructive disorder or as a suppurative (pus-forming) disorder. Hypersecretion of abnormal, thick mucus that obstructs exocrine glands and ducts is a characteristic finding in the disease.[8]

With advances in antibiotic therapy and early recognition and management of complications, patients with cystic fibrosis are living longer into adulthood. The median survival age is now 31 years.[9,23,26] Some patients are now having families.

Pathogenesis. Cystic fibrosis is classified as an autosomal recessive disorder. More than 800 mutations in the gene that encodes for the cystic fibrosis transmembrane conductance regulator (CFTR) have been described.[9,23] One genetic defect associated with cystic fibrosis involves deletion of three base pairs in codon 508 (AF508) that code for phenylalanine on chromosome 7 (band q31).[16] With the loss of these three base pairs, the *CFTR* gene is dysfunctional.[9,23] This is the most common genetic mutation causing cystic fibrosis and occurs in 60% to 75% of cystic fibrosis patients tested.[9,23] *CFTR* encodes a membrane chloride channel and is expressed in the sweat glands, the lungs, and the pancreas. Mutations in the *CFTR* gene result in alteration in chloride and water transport across the apical surface of epithelial cells.[9,23] Cystic fibrosis primarily affects the pancreas, intestinal tract, sweat glands, and lungs, and in males causes infertility.[28] The mucus-producing glands in the gastrointestinal tract enlarge, generating excessive secretions. The thick eosinophilic mucous secretions plug the glands and ducts of the pancreatic acini, intestinal glands, intrahepatic bile ducts, and the gallbladder, causing dilation and fibrosis.[31,32] These changes result in decreased production of pancreatic enzymes necessary for digestion of fats, carbohydrates, and proteins, thus leading to increased fat and protein in the stool.[31,32]

The bronchopulmonary system is also affected by the thick, tenacious mucus that results from failure of chloride channels to function in the apical membranes of mucosal cells. Decreased flow of ions and water results in viscid mucus.[9,32] High concentrations of DNA in airway secretions (attributable to inflammation and lysis of neutrophils) increase sputum viscosity.[9,31,32] The thick mucus causes airway obstruction, atelectasis, and hyperinflation and also decreases ciliary action, thus contributing to mucus stasis, which provides a medium for pulmonary infection. Sweat glands, salivary glands, and lacrimal glands are also affected, leading to high concentrations of sodium and chloride in these secretions.[9,31,32]

Clinical manifestations. Typical findings include a history of cough in a young adult or child; thick, tenacious sputum; recurrent pulmonary infections (commonly *Pseudomonas aeruginosa*); and recurrent episodes of bronchitis. These processes ultimately progress to pneumonia and bronchiectasis, right-sided heart failure (cor pulmonale), and exercise intolerance.

Physical examination may reveal digital clubbing (late sign), dyspnea, tachypnea, sternal retractions, unequal breath sounds, moist basilar crackles and rhonchi, and a barrel chest that is hyperresonant to percussion.[9] Other findings that may be present are pancreatic insufficiency (85% to 90%), cirrhosis of the liver (15% to 20%), diabetes mellitus (8% to 15%), gallstones (30% to 35%), nasal polyps (15%), and failure of development of the vas deferens in males.[9,16,23,31-33] Infants frequently present with a history of multiple respiratory tract infections, meconium ileus (stool retained in intestine), failure to thrive, jaundice, salt depletion, and edema.[9,16,23]

Nutritional assessment reveals depleted fat stores, steatorrhea (fatty stools), anorexia, decreased growth rate in children (weight, height, head circumference), and decreased midarm indices.[16,23]

Diagnosis. The diagnosis of cystic fibrosis is based on clinical and laboratory findings. Diagnostic studies that are routinely performed include arterial blood gas measurements, pulmonary function tests, sputum culture and sensitivity with Gram stain, and chest radiography. Specific diagnostic tests for cystic fibrosis include stool examination for fat, pilocarpine iontophoresis (sweat test), and genetic testing. A 72-hour stool collection combined with the dietary history during that time is used to determine fat absorption and fecal fat excretion. A coefficient of fat absorption of less than 95% (85% in infants) can be used to define steatorrhea (fatty stools).[34] Arterial blood gas analyses commonly show hypoxemia and hypercapnia because of airway obstruction. Pulmonary function tests reveal decreased vital capacity, decreased airflow rates, increased airway resistance, increased functional residual capacity, and decreased tidal volume. Chest radiographs show evidence of patchy atelectasis, bronchiectasis, obstructive emphysema, cystic lung fields, and peribronchial thickening.[1,16,23,31-33]

The quantitative pilocarpine iontophoresis sweat test reveals elevated sodium and chloride levels, with more than 98% of patients having levels greater than 60 mEq/L in children and greater than 80 mEq/L in adults.[8,33] A diagnostic blood test for the genetic marker AF508 may be useful for confirming the diagnosis and providing genetic information to the family.[8]

Treatment. Management of cystic fibrosis involves an interdisciplinary approach. A comprehensive program that focuses on multiorgan derangements is recommended. Because pulmonary disease accounts for the majority of morbidity and mortality associated with cystic fibrosis, treatment is aimed at aggressive pharmacologic management of pulmonary infection. Treatment includes the use of bronchodilators, and mobilization of the thick mucus by postural drainage and chest physiotherapy (percussion and vibration) is a priority. Alternative methods for mucus removal include the forced expiratory technique, which involves coughing (huffing) with an open glottis.[33] Recombinant human deoxyribonuclease I (dornase alfa) acts by digesting extracellular DNA (released from lysed neutrophils) present in the viscid sputum of cystic fibrosis patients to decrease the viscoelasticity of sputum, thus improving pulmonary function and decreasing the risk of infection.[8,9,33,35]

High-dose antibiotic therapy is used for acute exacerbations of respiratory tract infections to decrease bacterial growth in the lungs. An annual influenza vaccine is recommended because of the increased risk of complications associated with infection.[9,31]

Nutritional therapy includes unrestricted fat consumption (approximately 30% of caloric intake), ingestion of a high-protein diet, and use of vitamin supplements (especially the fat-soluble vitamins A, D, E, and K). Other pharmacologic therapy related to nutrition is aimed at replacement of pancreatic enzymes (pancreatin or pancrelipase). Maintenance of weight in children with cystic fibrosis often requires an intake of 150% of the normal calories recommended for healthy children.[31] In some cases, enteral feedings or intravenous nutrition may be necessary on a short-term basis. Salt supplementation may be necessary in hot weather.

Heart-lung or lung transplantation is currently the only definitive treatment.[9] More than 200 cystic fibrosis patients worldwide have undergone transplantation, with a 3-year survival of 55%.[9] Patients receiving transplants showed marked improvement in mobility, energy, and quality of life.

Identification of the disease-related gene, the cystic fibrosis transmembrane conductance regulator gene *(CFTR),* has advanced prospects for corrective gene therapy. One limiting factor is that the therapeutic gene has a short-term expression.

Acute Tracheobronchial Obstruction

Etiology. Acute tracheobronchial obstruction requires immediate treatment. Causes frequently include aspiration of a foreign body (e.g., a piece of meat, peanut, coin), malpositioned endotracheal tube, laryngospasm, epiglottitis, trauma, swelling from smoke inhalation, postsurgical blood clot, and compression of the bronchus or trachea by tumors or enlarged lymph nodes. With inhaled foreign bodies, the right side of the lung is affected more often than the left because of the angle of the anatomic extension of the right main bronchus from the trachea.

Pathogenesis. Obstruction by one of the etiologic agents listed earlier can be partial or complete. The health care worker must be prepared to assess the situation rapidly and act immediately to clear the airway.

Clinical manifestations. With complete obstruction, no air movement will be heard on auscultation, but the patient may still be making inspiratory chest movements. Other clinical features of complete obstruction include inability to talk, tachycardia, cyanosis, and rapid progression to unconsciousness unless the problem is quickly reversed.

With partial obstruction of the airway, the patient usually presents with stridor, sternal and intercostal retractions, wheezing, nasal flaring, tachypnea, dyspnea, tachycardia, and use of accessory muscles to breathe. Cyanosis is a late sign that usually indicates exhaustion or complete obstruction.

Diagnosis. The diagnosis of airway obstruction is based on clinical features and arterial blood gas analyses. Arterial blood gas values frequently show hypoxemia and hypercarbia. Chest radiographs may reveal the location of the obstruction.

Treatment. Treatment involves opening the obstructed airway as quickly as possible. Blows to the patient's back or use of abdominal thrusts (previously called the Heimlich maneuver) may be necessary for the foreign body to be expelled. Aspirated contents occluding the airway are suctioned to relieve obstruction. If these methods are unsuccessful, an emergency tracheostomy should be performed in the case of a suspected upper airway obstruction in the subglottic region or above.

Epiglottitis

Etiology. Epiglottitis is a rapidly progressive cellulitis of the epiglottis and adjacent soft tissues. Acute epiglottitis is suspected when odynophagia (pain with swallowing) seems out of proportion to pharyngeal findings. Inability to swallow saliva with evidence of drooling is common. Epiglottitis is classified as a subtype of croup. The causative organism is primarily *H. influenzae* type B (Hib). It is most often seen in children 2 to 4 years old. Pneumococci, streptococci, and staphylococci are also causal agents.[23,36] The role of viruses in epiglottitis is unclear.[36]

Pathogenesis. The infecting agent localizes in the supraglottic area in the epiglottis and pharyngeal structures, causing rapid and potentially fatal inflammation with swelling and airway obstruction.

Clinical manifestations. The patient frequently presents with acute respiratory difficulty that has progressed rapidly over several hours. Common signs and symptoms include drooling, dysphagia, rapid onset of fever, dysphonia, inspiratory stridor, and inspiratory retractions. The child often sits in a "sniffing dog" position, which provides the best airway patency. The oropharynx is edematous and cherry red.[28,36]

Diagnosis. Definitive diagnosis is obtained by direct or fiberoptic visualization of the epiglottis. Lateral neck radiographs assist in making a definitive diagnosis and reveal a classic "thumbprint sign" (swollen epiglottis that looks like a thumbprint). A complete blood count may reveal leukocytosis with a shift to the left.[36]

Treatment. This condition is a true medical emergency and may necessitate intubation. Antibiotic therapy should be started immediately. Preventive treatment with the Hib vaccine has been the key to decreasing the incidence of this disease.

Croup Syndrome

Etiology. Croup syndrome describes a number of acute viral and inflammatory diseases of the larynx. Croup diseases include laryngotracheobronchitis (viral croup) and bacterial tracheitis. Viral croup affects the larynx, trachea, and bronchi. It is often caused by parainfluenza virus type 1. Other potential infecting organisms include parainfluenza types 2 and 3, RSV, influenza virus, adenovirus, and *Mycoplasma pneumoniae.*[23] Croup usually occurs in the fall and early winter, affecting children ages 6 months to 3 years.[35]

Pathogenesis. The infectious agent causes inflammation along the entire airway, leading to edema formation in the subglottic area.[1,2]

Clinical manifestations. The child presents with a history of upper respiratory tract infection or cold that has developed into a barking cough with stridor. Fever is low grade or absent. In severe cases the child may present with stridor at rest, retractions, and cyanosis.

Diagnosis. Diagnosis is based on clinical manifestations and lateral neck films to rule out epiglottitis. Direct laryngoscopy is also used to confirm the presence of epiglottitis because the clinical presentation is similar to that of croup. Lateral neck radiographs show subglottic narrowing and a normal epiglottis. The classic steeple sign associated with viral croup shows narrowing below the vocal cords.[23,37]

Treatment. Supportive treatment is used for viral croup. Mist therapy, oral hydration, and avoidance of stimulation are used in outpatient therapy. Hospitalized children are managed with oxygen therapy and pulse oximetry. Nebulized epinephrine is effective in relieving airway obstruction. Endotracheal intubation may be required for children with respiratory failure.

KEY POINTS

- Obstructive disorders are associated with increased resistance to airflow, particularly during exhalation.
- Bronchiectasis is associated with recurrent inflammation of the bronchial walls, chronic cough, and aneurysm-like dilatations of the bronchioles. These bronchiolar dilatations serve as pockets of infection, producing purulent, foul-smelling sputum. Treatment centers on use of antibiotic therapy and removal of secretions.
- Bronchiolitis refers to widespread bronchiolar inflammation, often associated with smoking and a number of infectious agents. Inflammation results in mucosal swelling, excessive mucus production, and bronchial muscle constriction—all of which narrow the airway lumen and may lead to wheezing and dyspnea. Treatment centers on administration of bronchodilating agents and management of the underlying cause.
- Cystic fibrosis is an autosomal recessive disorder of exocrine glands and mucus cells. Secretions are excessively thick because of insufficient chloride and water transport. Thick secretions cause airway obstruction, atelectasis, and air trapping. Associated symptoms resulting from dysfunction of the exocrine pancreas are apparent. Treatment centers on removal of secretions and provision of antibiotic therapy for complicating respiratory tract infections.
- Obstruction of the trachea or large bronchi may occur acutely, requiring immediate treatment. Usual causes include foreign body aspiration, trauma, and inflammation. With complete obstruction, no movement of air occurs, even though inspiratory efforts may be observed. Partial airway obstruction is associated with wheezing, retractions, and stridor. Treatment centers on removing the obstruction, if possible, or creating a patent airway by a tracheostomy.
- Epiglottitis is a medical emergency. *Haemophilus influenzae* type B, the primary organism associated with epiglottitis, invades the supraglottic structures (epiglottis and arytenoids), causing inflammation and edema, leading to obstruction. Key points in the clinical diagnosis are rapid onset of fever, pain and difficulty swallowing, and drooling. Lateral neck x-ray films reveal a classic thumbprint sign, which is indicative of epiglottal

swelling. Airway maintenance via endotracheal intubation or tracheostomy and antibiotic therapy are the primary treatments. The Hib vaccine has greatly decreased the number of cases seen in the pediatric population.
- Croup is usually from a viral infection of the subglottic area. Children ages 6 months to 3 years present with cough and stridor following an upper respiratory tract infection. Humidification, oxygenation, and inhaled epinephrine are the primary treatment modalities.

DIAGNOSTIC TESTS

Pulmonary Function Testing

The primary criterion in diagnosing obstructive disease is the demonstration of obstruction to airflow in the lungs. Table 22-2 lists common ventilatory parameters referred to in spirometry.

Spirometry is performed by asking the patient to inhale deeply and then to exhale as quickly as possible until maximal air is exhaled. The total volume of air exhaled is known as the *forced vital capacity (FVC)*. To determine flow, the time required for exhaling the air is also measured. The volume exhaled in the first second is a reliable and reproducible index of obstructive airway disease. This value is the *forced expiratory volume in 1 second* (FEV_1). Figure 22-19 presents spirogram examples of normal, restrictive, and obstructive graphs for FEV_1 and FVC. For all spirometric studies, normal values are based on large population studies of healthy volunteers and are adjusted for height, weight, age, and gender. Results are compared to predicted values and reported as percent of predicted.

A simple formula has been developed to define and quantify airflow obstruction. If the FEV_1/FVC ratio is 75% or greater, no significant obstruction of airflow is present. If the value obtained is between 60% and 70%, then mild obstruction of airflow is present. Moderate obstruction is defined as a value of 50% to 60%; and severe obstruction is present when the FEV_1/FVC ratio is less than 50%. Therefore, using a spirometer and measuring both volume and time, the diagnosis of chronic obstructive pulmonary disease can be made and the severity quantified.

From the spirometric ventilatory measurements (see Table 22-2), other determinations of airflow can be made from the middle to later parts of a FVC maneuver. These measures are helpful in determining the presence of small airways disease. Some investigators believe that small airways disease may be a precursor to the development of chronic bronchitis and emphysema.[1,21]

Frequently, an inhaled bronchodilator, such as albuterol or metaproterenol, may be given, with testing repeated in 15 to 20 minutes. If the FEV_1 improves by 15% or more, the patient is considered to have a

TABLE 22-2 COMMON VENTILATORY PARAMETERS MEASURED BY SPIROMETRY

PARAMETER*	DEFINITION
Tidal volume	Volume of air inspired and expired with a normal breath (400-500 ml or 5 ml/kg of body weight)
Residual volume	Volume of gas left in lung after maximal expiration; stabilizes alveoli
Vital capacity or forced vital capacity (FVC)	Maximal air that can be expired after a maximal inspiratory effort; includes inspiratory reserve volume, tidal volume, and expiratory reserve volume
Functional residual capacity	Volume of air left in lungs after a normal expiration; includes expiratory reserve volume and residual volume
Forced expiratory flow rate (FEF_{25}, FEF_{50}, FEF_{75})	Volume of air forcibly exhaled per unit time (liters per second or liters per minute) at 25%, 50%, and 75% of FVC
Peak expiratory flow rate	Highest rate of flow sustained for 10 msec or more at which air can be expelled from lungs

*See Figures 21-10 and 22-19 for normal values.

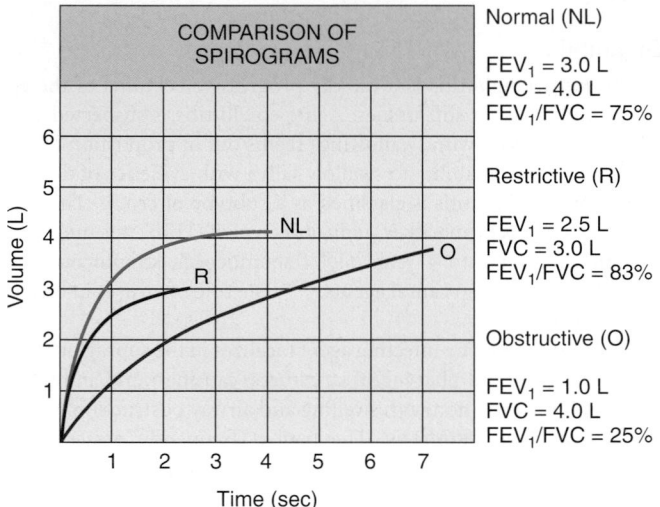

FIGURE 22-19 Comparison of spirograms for normal lungs, restrictive lung disease, and obstructive lung disease. *FEV_1*, Forced expiratory volume in 1 second; *FVC*, forced vital capacity.

TABLE 22-3 NORMAL ARTERIAL BLOOD GAS VALUES

PARAMETER	ADULT*	PREGNANCY	NEWBORN	COPD (LATE FINDINGS)
Pao_2 (mm Hg)	80-100	75-100	60-70	Decreased
$Paco_2$ (mm Hg)	34-45	30-37	35-45	Increased
pH	7.35-7.45	7.35-7.45	7.30-7.40	Decreased
HCO_3^- (mEq/L)	24-30	20-26	20-26	Increased
Base excess (mEq/L)	±2	—	—	—
O_2 saturation (%)	96-100	95-100	90-100	Decreased

*For elderly patients, Pao_2 can be estimated by the following formulas[24]: 104 − (patient's age × 0.42) for patients lying supine; and 104 − (patient's age × 0.27) for patients sitting.
COPD, Chronic obstructive pulmonary disease.

positive bronchodilator response, indicative of partially reversible bronchospasm of the smooth muscles of the airways. This is most often the case with asthma or asthmatic bronchitis.

A second pulmonary function test known as the *diffusion capacity* measures the ability of the alveolar gases to diffuse into the capillary blood. The technical details of this test are beyond the scope of this book, but it is a valuable test for determining either thickening (fibrosis) of the alveolocapillary membrane or destruction (emphysema) of the membrane.

By breathing mixtures of an inert gas, such as helium, the TLC can be determined. This volume is composed of the FVC and the RV. The RV is the volume of air that remains in the lung after a person has forcefully exhaled all of the air from the lungs (see Figure 21-10). RV/TLC is normally 30% to 35%. In some patients with airflow obstruction, air tends to get trapped in the lungs, thereby increasing the RV and resulting in overinflation of lung tissue.

Arterial blood gases are also useful as a pulmonary function measurement. Using these values, a careful assessment of both the oxygenation and the acid-base status can be determined. The normal pH is 7.40, the normal $Paco_2$ is 40 mm Hg, and the normal Pao_2, at sea level, is 80 to 100 mm Hg. In COPD, especially in the severe stage, Pao_2 falls and $Paco_2$ rises. Table 22-3 lists normal arterial blood gas values for various groups. A thorough discussion of arterial blood gas analysis can be found in Chapter 25.

Bronchial Provocation Tests

The controlled induction of bronchospasm by inhalation of various agents is occasionally used to identify patients with hyperreactive airways and to prove whether certain inhaled substances can produce bronchospasm. Usually a series of inhalations is administered, followed by a series of ventilation measurements. Generally the test is stopped when the FEV_1 falls at least 20% more than the control measurement. This should only be done where emergency support services are available. Bronchoprovocation is contraindicated if the patient is already exhibiting symptoms or requires continual asthma medication. Allergens can be administered as solutions, dusts, or fumes. The amount administered should be no more than the patient would normally encounter in the environment. If symptoms occur, they can be readily reversed by two to four inhalations of albuterol or metaproterenol.

General hyperreactivity of the bronchi can be detected by having the patient inhale histamine phosphate solutions or methacholine (related to acetylcholine) or nebulized distilled water. A decline of more than 20% in the FEV_1 is indicative of hyperreactivity.

KEY POINTS
- Obstructive disorders are associated with characteristic abnormalities on pulmonary function testing. These include the following:
- Decreased FEV_1
- Low FEV_1/FVC ratio (<70%)
- Improvement in FEV_1 after use of a bronchodilator (asthma)
- Increased residual volume
- Increased functional residual capacity

■ SUMMARY

Health care professionals have a key role in the management of respiratory disorders in the hospital and in the community. Obstructive pulmonary diseases presented in this chapter include airway obstruction, obstruction from conditions affecting the tracheobronchial walls, and loss of lung parenchyma (emphysema). Obstructive pulmonary disorders are characterized by increased resistance to airflow. With bronchiectasis, obstruction is due to inflammation, infection, and dilatation of the bronchioles. Similarly, bronchiolitis is associated with inflammation; however, in this situation, inflammation leads to mucosal edema and excessive mucus production. Airway obstruction from cystic fibrosis is related to production of excessive, thick secretions. Obstruction of the airway in croup is the result of edema and increased secretions caused by viral infection. Similarly, epiglottitis is an infectious process requiring emergency treatment. The primary organism causing epiglottitis is *H. influenzae*. The incidence of epiglottitis has been greatly reduced with the advent of the Hib vaccine.

An inflammatory process is also seen in asthma and bronchitis. The inflammation is associated with increased mucus production and edema of the tracheal bronchial mucosa in asthma and bronchitis. Bronchospasm of the tracheobronchial tree attributable to exposure to allergens, pulmonary irritants, stress, and exercise may result in hypoxemia. Obstruction to airflow in emphysema is due to loss of alveoli and small airways. The most common cause is cigarette smoking.

REFERENCES

1. West JB: *Pulmonary pathophysiology: the essentials*, ed 7, Philadelphia, 2008, Lippincott Williams & Wilkins.
2. West JB: *Pulmonary physiology and pathophysiology: an integrated case-based approach*, ed 2, Philadelphia, 2007, Lippincott Williams & Wilkins.
3. National Asthma Education and Prevention Program Expert Panel: *Report II guidelines for diagnosis and management of asthma*, Washington, DC, 2006, U.S. Department of Health and Human Services. Update.
4. Vura-Weis DE: Allergies and asthma. In Sloane PD, Slatt LM, et al, editors: *Essentials of family medicine*, ed 5, Philadelphia, 2011, Lippincott Williams & Wilkins, pp 745–768.
5. Brooks AM: Asthma. In Garfunkel LC, Kaczorowski J, Christy C, editors: *Mosby's pediatric clinical advisor: instant diagnosis and treatment*, St Louis, 2002, Mosby, pp 171–173.
6. Kolski GB: Asthma in children. In Rakel RE, Bope ET, editors: *Conn's current therapy, 2008*, Philadelphia, 2008, Saunders, pp 759–765.
7. Lester MR: Asthma in children. In Rakel RE, Bope ET, editors: *Conn's current therapy, 2008*, Philadelphia, 2008, Saunders.
8. Ferri FF: Asthma. In Ferri FF, editor: *Ferri's clinical advisor: instant diagnosis and treatment*, St Louis, 2007, Mosby, pp 89–91.
9. Chesnutt MS, Prendergast TJ: Lung. In Tierney LM, McPhee SJ, Papadakis MA, editors: *Current medical diagnosis and treatment*, ed 46, New York, 2007, Lange/McGraw-Hill, pp 222–315.
10. Goroll AH, Mulley AG: Management of asthma. In Goroll AH, Mulley AG, editors: *Primary care medicine: office evaluation and management of the adult patient*, ed 5, Philadelphia, 2006, Lippincott Williams & Wilkins, pp 357–370.
11. Binstadt BA, Schneider L: Allergic disorders and immunodeficiency. In Graef JW, editor: *Manual of pediatric therapeutics*, ed 7, Philadelphia, 2007, Lippincott-Raven, pp 500–516.

12. Hogg JC: The pathophysiology of asthma, *Chest* 82:s8–s11, 1982.

13. Guyton AC, Hall JE: *Textbook of medical physiology*, ed 11, Philadelphia, 2005, Saunders.

14. Prendergast TJ, et al: Pulmonary disease. In McPhee S, Lingappa VA, Ganong WF, et al, editors: *Pathophysiology of disease: an introduction to clinical medicine*, ed 5, New York, 2005, McGraw-Hill.

15. Williams PV: Management of asthma, *Clin Symp* 49(3):2–32, 1997.

16. Jaskiewicz J: Cystic fibrosis. In Garfunkel LC, Kaczorowski J, Christy C, editors: *Mosby's pediatric clinical advisor: instant diagnosis and treatment*, St Louis, 2002, Mosby, pp 263–264.

17. Boguniewicz M, Leung DYM: Allergic disorders. In Hay WW, et al, editors: *Current pediatric diagnosis and treatment*, ed 18, New York, 2007, Lange/McGraw-Hill, pp 1049–1077.

18. Mainous AG, Hueston WJ: Acute respiratory infections. In Sloane PD, et al, editors: *Essentials of family medicine*, ed 5, Philadelphia, 2011, Lippincott Williams & Wilkins, pp 769–785.

19. Kormis WA: Approach to the patient with acute bronchitis or pneumonia in the ambulatory setting. In Goroll AH, Mulley AG, editors: *Primary care medicine: office evaluation and management of the adult patient*, ed 5, Philadelphia, 2006, Lippincott Williams & Wilkins, pp 388–397.

20. Weiss EF: Clubbing. In Greene HL, et al, editors: *Clinical medicine*, ed 2, St Louis, 1996, Mosby, pp 563–566.

21. Goroll AJ, Mulley AG: Management of chronic obstructive pulmonary disease. In Goroll AH, Mulley AG, editors: *Primary care medicine: office evaluation and management of the adult patient*, ed 5, Philadelphia, 2006, Lippincott Williams & Wilkins, pp 345–356.

22. Garcia JA, Jenkinson SG: Management of chronic obstructive pulmonary disease. In Rakel RE, Bope ET, editors: *Conn's current therapy, 2008*, Philadelphia, 2008, Saunders, pp 225–230.

23. Kerby GS, et al: Respiratory tract and mediastinum. In Hay WW, et al, editors: *Current pediatric diagnosis and treatment*, ed 18, New York, 2007, Lange/McGraw-Hill, pp 493–541.

24. National Center for Health Statistics: *Chronic obstructive pulmonary disease (COPD)*. Available at www.cdc.gov/nchs/fastats/copd.htm. Accessed February 2007.

25. Johnston CB, et al: Geriatric medicine. In Tierney LM, McPhee SJ, Papadakis MA, editors: *Current medical diagnosis and treatment*, ed 46, New York, 2007, Lange/McGraw-Hill, pp 51–67.

26. Ferri FF: Bronchiectasis. In Ferri FF, editor: *Ferri's clinical advisor: instant diagnosis and treatment*, St Louis, 2007, Mosby, p 138.

27. Cystic Fibrosis Foundation, 6931 Arlington Rd, Suite 2000, Bethesda, MD 20814; 800-344-4823. Available at www.cff.org.

28. Behrman RE, Kliegman RM, Jenson HB: *Pocket companion to accompany Nelson textbook of pediatrics*, ed 16, Philadelphia, 2001, Saunders, pp 505–506.

29. Shandera WX, Koo H: Infectious diseases: viral and rickettsial. In Tierney LM, McPhee SJ, Papadakis MA, editors: *Current medical diagnosis and treatment*, ed 46, New York, 2007, Lange/McGraw-Hill, pp 1378–1430.

30. Chen S: Respiratory syncytial virus/bronchiolitis. In Garfunkel LC, Kaczorowski J, Christy C, editors: *Mosby's pediatric clinical advisor: instant diagnosis and treatment*, St Louis, 2002, Mosby, pp 635–636.

31. Froh DK: Cystic fibrosis. In Rakel RE, Bope ET, editors: *Conn's current therapy, 2008*, Philadelphia, 2008, Saunders, pp 230–233.

32. Fishman DS, Bousuares A: Management of nutritional gastrointestinal and hepatic disorders. In Graef JW, editor: *Manual of pediatric therapeutics*, ed 7, Philadelphia, 2007, Lippincott-Raven, p 359.

33. Yusen RD, et al: Pulmonary diseases. In Ahya SN, Flood K, Paranjothi S, editors: *Washington manual of medical therapeutics*, ed 32, Philadelphia, 2007, Lippincott Williams & Wilkins, pp 245–289.

34. Bluth MG, Hardin RE, Tenner S, et al: Laboratory diagnosis of gastrointestinal and pancreatic disorders. In McPherson RA, Pincus MR, editors: *Henry's clinical diagnosis and management by laboratory methods*, ed 21, Philadelphia, 2006, Saunders, p 291.

35. Yusen RD, Lefrak SS: Pulmonary II: diseases. In Lin TL, Rypkema SW, editors: *The Washington manual of ambulatory therapeutics*, ed 31, Philadelphia, 2002, Lippincott Williams & Wilkins, pp 202–226.

36. Opal SM, Lieber JJ: Epiglottitis. In Ferri FF, editor: *Ferri's clinical advisor: instant diagnosis and treatment*, St Louis, 2007, Mosby, pp 309–310.

37. Jackson MA, Vahle H: Croup. In Garfunkel LC, Kaczorowski J, Christy C, editors: *Mosby's pediatric clinical advisor: instant diagnosis and treatment*, St Louis, 2002, Mosby, pp 259–260.

Restrictive Pulmonary Disorders

Lorna L. Schumann

evolve WEBSITE

http://evolve.elsevier.com/Copstead/
- Review Questions and Answers
- Glossary (with audio pronunciations for selected terms)

- Animations
- Case Studies
- Key Points Review

KEY QUESTIONS

- How do fibrotic lung disorders develop?
- How is the pathogenesis of acute (adult) respiratory distress syndrome similar to that of infant respiratory distress syndrome?
- How do abnormal accumulations in the pleural space affect lung function?

- What neuromuscular disorders are associated with reduced lung compliance?
- What is the pathogenesis of tuberculosis?
- What pulmonary function test abnormalities are characteristic of restrictive pulmonary disorders?

CHAPTER OUTLINE

Restrictive pulmonary diseases result from decreased expansion of the lungs attributable to alterations in the lung parenchyma, pleura, chest wall, or neuromuscular function. These disorders may be classified as pulmonary or extrapulmonary and represent acute or chronic patterns of lung dysfunction, rather than a single clinical disease. Table 23-1 lists the various disease processes that can be classified as restrictive. These diseases are characterized by a decrease in total lung capacity (TLC), vital capacity (VC), functional residual capacity (FRC), and residual volume (RV). The greater the decrease in lung volume, the greater the severity of the disease.[1] Blood gas analysis often shows decreased arterial partial pressure of oxygen (Pao_2) and normal or decreased arterial partial pressure of carbon dioxide ($Paco_2$), resulting in increased pH (respiratory alkalosis). This chapter presents information related to restrictive pulmonary diseases, including lung parenchyma disorders, pleural space disorders, neuromuscular and chest wall disorders, pneumonia, and tuberculosis. Specific lung parenchyma disorders, including interstitial fibrosis, sarcoidosis, hypersensitivity pneumonitis, and pneumoconiosis, as well as atelectatic disorders, including acute (adult) respiratory distress syndrome (ARDS) and infant respiratory distress syndrome (IRDS), are presented. Pleural space disorders, divided into pneumothorax and pleural effusions, are discussed. The section on neuromuscular and chest wall disorders is divided into neuromuscular weakness, chest wall deformities, and obesity. The final section presents etiologic factors, pathogenesis, clinical manifestations, diagnosis, and management of pneumonia, tuberculosis, and severe acute respiratory syndrome (SARS). Table 23-2 describes variations in respiratory parameters that affect restrictive lung disease in infant and elderly populations.

TABLE 23-1　RESTRICTIVE PULMONARY DISORDERS

DISORDER TYPE	REPRESENTATIVE EXAMPLES
Diseases of the Lung Parenchyma	
Neoplastic disease	—
Pneumonia	Pneumonia (viral, bacterial, fungal), hypersensitivity pneumonitis
Granulomatous disease	Sarcoidosis, tuberculosis, coccidioidomycosis, blastomycosis
Pneumoconioses	Occupational lung disease
Acute interstitial pneumonitis	—
Collagen disease	Rheumatoid arthritis, scleroderma, systemic lupus erythematosus
Atelectasis	—
Pulmonary resection	—
Vascular Diseases	Pulmonary edema, pulmonary embolism
Acute respiratory distress syndrome	—
Diseases of Extrapulmonary Restriction	
Chest wall disease	Kyphoscoliosis, ankylosing spondylitis, obesity
Neuromuscular disease	Quadriplegia, hemiplegia, Guillain-Barré syndrome, myasthenia gravis, amyotrophic lateral sclerosis, muscular dystrophy
Pleural diseases	Pleural effusion, hemothorax, pneumothorax, chylothorax
Other	Abdominal distention, surgery, pregnancy

LUNG PARENCHYMA DISORDERS

FIBROTIC INTERSTITIAL LUNG DISEASES

The term *interstitial lung disease* describes a group of more than 180 disorders characterized by acute, subacute, or chronic infiltration of alveolar walls by cells, fluid, and connective tissue.[1-4] If left untreated, the inflammatory process may progress to irreversible fibrosis.[4] The incidence of interstitial lung disease is 20 cases per 100,000 persons in the general population and 175 per 100,000 in people more than 75 years of age.[3]

Diffuse Interstitial Lung Disease

Etiology. Diffuse interstitial lung disease (*diffuse interstitial pulmonary fibrosis*) is the name typically used for restrictive diseases characterized by thickening of the alveolar interstitium.[2] Synonyms frequently presented in the literature include *interstitial pneumonia, diffuse parenchymal lung disease, Hamman-Rich syndrome, intrinsic fibrosing alveolitis, cryptogenic fibrosing alveolitis,* and *idiopathic pulmonary fibrosis.*

Pathogenesis. Pathogenesis of the disease is not well understood, but is possibly related to an immune reaction that usually begins with injury to the alveolar epithelial or capillary endothelial cells.[1,2] Pathophysiologic changes may include interstitial and alveolar wall thickening and increased collagen bundles in the interstitium (Figure 23-1). Lung tissue becomes infiltrated by lymphocytes, macrophages, and plasma cells. Persistent alveolitis may lead to obliteration of alveolar capillaries, reorganization of the lung parenchyma, and irreversible fibrosis.[2] These changes in turn lead to the formation of large air-filled sacs (cysts) accompanied by dilated terminal and respiratory bronchioles. The immune response noted in interstitial lung disease is characterized by three pathologic patterns in the alveoli: inflammation, fibrosis, and destruction.

The inflammatory pattern occurs early and is potentially reversible.[4,5] The triggering event (occupational exposure, tobacco abuse, drug ingestion, connective tissue disease) causes an inflammatory response leading to increased numbers of inflammatory cells (neutrophils, lymphocytes, macrophages).[1,2,4] An associated injury to the alveolar capillary basement membrane from the triggering event leads to increased membrane permeability and movement of fluid and debris into the alveoli. The initial injury, in association with the inflammatory pattern, leads to fibroblastic proliferation and deposition of large amounts of collagen. The fibrotic pattern is manifested by increases in the number of mesenchymal cells and fibroblasts in the interstitium, and alveolar walls become thickened with increased amounts of fibrous tissue.[5,6] Physiologic restriction leads to reduced compliance and increased elastic recoil. The lung destruction pattern is manifested by loss of alveolar walls. Radiographically, this appears as a "honeycomb lung" and indicates end-stage disease.[2] Ground-glass appearance on chest radiograph is often an early finding.[3] The fibrotic and honeycomb patterns respond poorly to treatment.[5]

Clinical manifestations. The most common patient complaint is progressive dyspnea with nonproductive cough.[3,5] Clinical features also include rapid, shallow breathing; dyspnea; clubbing of the nail beds (40% to 80% cases)[4]; bibasilar end-expiratory[3,4] crackles (Velcro rales); and marked dyspnea with exercise. Cyanosis is a late finding. Anorexia and weight loss are noted on physical exam. While the disease progresses, patients exhibit an inability to increase cardiac output with exercise as evidenced by low maximal heart rate and high peripheral vascular resistance. Arterial oxygen desaturation occurs with exercise.[4]

Diagnosis. Chest radiographs show a honeycomb appearance and a coarse reticular pattern indicating late stage of disease.[2,3,5,6] Ground-glass haziness is indicative of the presence of infiltrates. High-resolution computed tomography (HRCT) and bronchoalveolar lavage are the primary diagnostic tests used to evaluate interstitial lung disease.[6] Open lung biopsy or transbronchial biopsy and gallium-67 scanning may be used for diagnostic evaluation.[3] Results of pulmonary function tests are usually consistent with restrictive lung disease (decreased vital capacity, reduced total lung capacity, and decreased diffusing capacity).[3]

Treatment. The patient should be encouraged to avoid tobacco use and environmental exposure to the offending agent.[2-4] Primary therapy consists of administration of antiinflammatory and immunosuppressive agents. Immunosuppressive agents have been useful in reducing the dosage of corticosteroids required. Oxygen therapy is needed in patients with hypoxemia. Lung transplantation has been successful in selected patients.[3,5-9]

Sarcoidosis

Etiology. Sarcoidosis is categorized as an acute or chronic systemic disease of unknown cause, although an immunologic basis appears likely.[1,9] A common feature of sarcoidosis is the presence of CD4+ T cells.[9] Activation of the alveolar macrophage from an unknown antigen trigger is a possible cause.[1] The acute process occurs more commonly in women in the second or third decades of life.[1,2] The chronic form is seen more commonly in the third to fourth decades of life, with the highest incidence seen in North American blacks (35.5/100,000) and northern European whites (11.9/100,000).[2] Having a first-degree relative with sarcoidosis increases the risk for disease fivefold.[9]

Pathogenesis. The disease is characterized by the development of multiple, uniform, noncaseating epithelioid granulomas that affect multiple organ systems, most commonly lymph nodes and lung tissue. Noncaseating granulomas are fibrotic and surrounded by large histiocytes.[1,2,9] Sarcoid granulomas may also develop in the bronchial airways. Abnormal T cell function is noted with this disease.[9] Other systems/organs frequently involved are the skin, eyes, spleen, liver, kidney, and bone marrow.[1,9]

Clinical manifestations. Sarcoidosis is characterized by malaise, fatigue, weight loss, fever, chest discomfort, dyspnea of insidious onset, and a dry, nonproductive cough.[2,9] Other features include erythema nodosum (lesions marked by the formation of painful nodes on the lower extremities); macules, papules, hyperpigmentation, and subcutaneous nodules; hepatosplenomegaly; and lymphadenopathy. Patients with acute disease usually present with enlarged lymph nodes and arthritis, although some patients experience no symptoms.[9] Skin lesions and lacrimal and parotid gland involvement are also noted in the acute process.[1] Iritis, uveitis (65% of patients), blurred vision, conjunctivitis, and ocular discomfort may develop.[9]

Diagnosis. Common laboratory findings in patients with sarcoidosis include leukopenia, anemia, increased eosinophil count, elevated sedimentation rate, and increased calcium levels (seen in 11% of patients).[2,9] Serum levels of liver enzymes may also be elevated. Approximately 70% of patients exhibit anergy (decreased sensitivity to specific antigens such as *Trichophyton, Candida,* mumps virus, and tuberculin).[2] Patients with active disease also demonstrate elevated levels of angiotensin-converting enzyme (40% to 80% of cases).[2] Chest radiographs can be used to differentiate stages of the disease process: stage 0, normal; stage I, hilar adenopathy alone; stage II, hilar adenopathy and bilateral pulmonary infiltrates; and stage III, pulmonary infiltrates without adenopathy. Stage IV is characterized by advanced fibrosis with evidence of honeycombing, hilar retraction, bullae, cysts, and emphysema.[7] Gallium-67

TABLE 23-2 AGE-RELATED FEATURES CONTRIBUTING TO RESTRICTIVE LUNG DISEASE

ANATOMIC SITE	IMPACT ON RESTRICTIVE DISEASE
Infant	
Sternum and ribs are cartilaginous with soft chest wall	Diminishes effect of restrictive disease in infants
Ribs are horizontally oriented so that ribs move in and out easily	Diminishes effect of restrictive disease in infants
Accessory muscles of respiration are poorly developed	Majority of respiratory movement relies on diaphragm; restrictive diseases that compromise diaphragmatic excursion affect respiratory status; e.g., thoracic or abdominal surgery, paralysis, and abdominal masses all affect diaphragmatic excursion
Diaphragm rests horizontally and draws lower ribs inward in supine position so that diaphragmatic excursion is decreased	Leads to compromised effort of breathing
Cartilage of infant larynx is soft, so airway is compressed when neck is flexed or hyperextended	Increases airway resistance
During first month of life, neonate is obligate nose breather	Nasal obstruction may lead to respiratory distress from decreased airflow
Small diameter of airway leads to increased resistance to airflow	Mucus or edema in the airway may lead to significant increase in resistance and decrease in airway diameter
Fewer alveoli than in adults, leading to decreased radial traction applied to airways	Increased tendency of airways to collapse
Pores of Kohn and channels of Lambert are underdeveloped, leading to fewer collateral ventilation pathways	May lead to respiratory compromise, reducing ventilatory support with restrictive diseases
Elderly	
Decreased ciliary activity	Increased incidence of infection; decreased mucus clearance in all types of respiratory disorders
Decreased chest wall compliance and decreased lung elasticity in some areas of lung	Leads to a reduction in lung volume; leads to decreased expansion of lungs and to decreased matching of ventilation and perfusion
Decreased stress tolerance	Increased incidence of disease and trauma with age
Decreased muscle tone	Decreased physical conditioning
Impaired immunity as evidenced by decreased T cell function; increased autoantibodies	Decreased resistance to infection
Decreased oxygen uptake	Decreased oxygen level in blood
Decreased vital capacity	Decreased alveolar expansion
Decreased cough reflex	Impaired ability to clear secretions and inhaled particulate matter

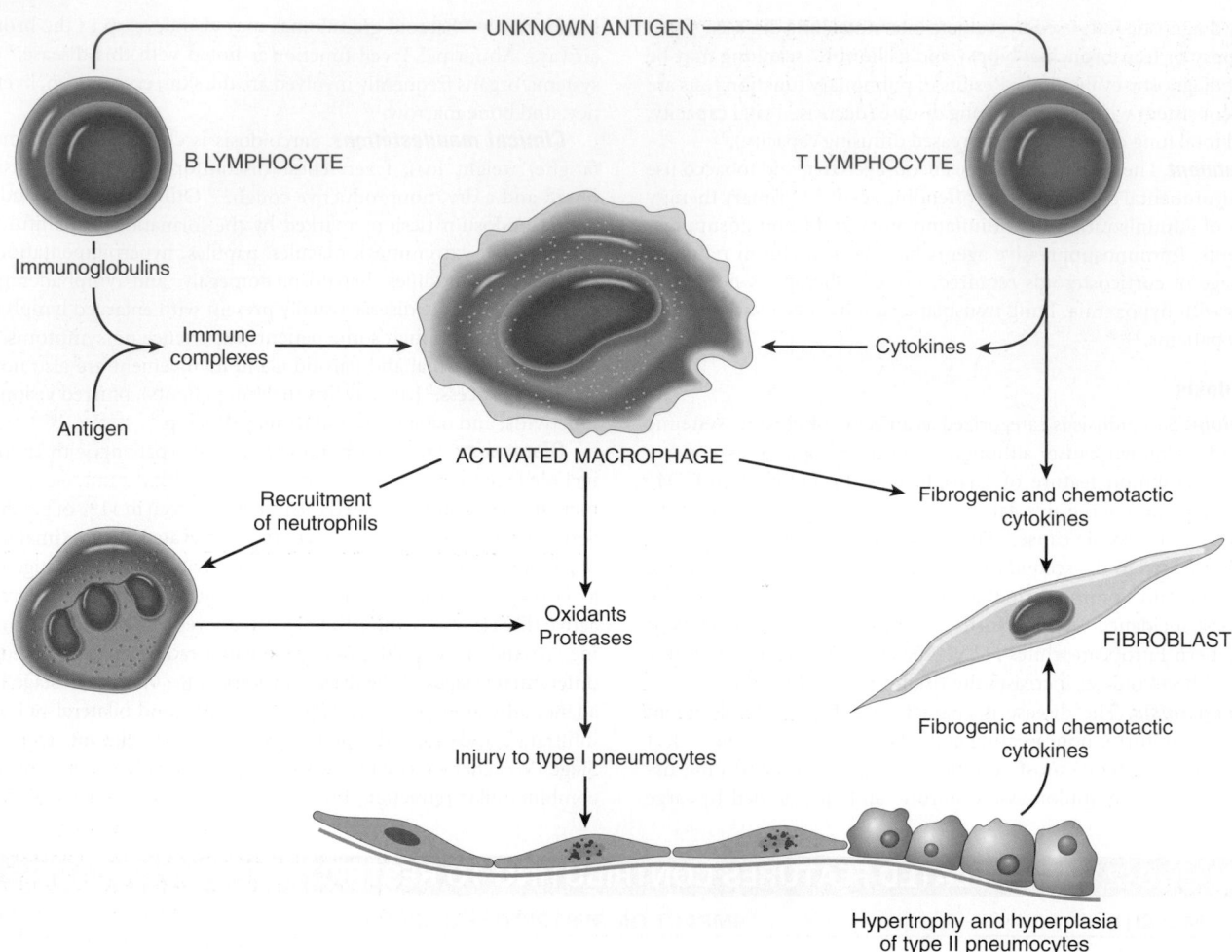

FIGURE 23-1 Possible schema of the pathogenesis of idiopathic pulmonary fibrosis. (From Kumar V et al, editors: *Robbin's basic pathology,* ed 8, Philadelphia, 2007, Saunders, p 483.)

scans will localize areas of granulomatous infiltrates. Pleural effusion is noted in 10% of cases of sarcoidosis.[1,2,9] Pulmonary function test results may be normal or show evidence of restrictive disease and/or obstructive disease.[9] Transbronchial lung biopsy demonstrates noncaseating granulomas, thus providing a definitive diagnosis (75% to 90% cases). Bronchoalveolar lavage may be used to monitor cell content in patients with sarcoidosis.[1,9] The lavage fluid is characterized by increased lymphocytes and a high CD4/CD8 cell ratio.[2]

Treatment. Administration of corticosteroids and management of symptoms is the mainstay of treatment for patients whose disease process does not resolve spontaneously and in whom progressive lung disease or evidence of extrapulmonary sarcoidosis develops. For patients with progressive disease that does not respond to corticosteroids, immunosuppressive agents may be used.[9] Hydroxychloroquine is effective for treatment of disfiguring skin lesions, hypercalcemia, and neurologic involvement.[9] The prognosis is best for stage I disease. Death attributable to pulmonary insufficiency occurs in about 5% to 7% of patients.[2,9]

Hypersensitivity Pneumonitis

Etiology. Hypersensitivity pneumonitis, also called *extrinsic allergic alveolitis,* is classified as a restrictive and occupational disease. Numerous (greater than 300) inhaled organic agents are responsible for the inflammatory process.[10] Table 23-3 lists various allergens related to the disease. Unlike other pulmonary diseases, hypersensitivity pneumonitis has a predominance in nonsmokers (80% to 95% of cases).[10]

Pathogenesis. The causative agent is suggested by the patient's history and confirmed by demonstration of precipitating antibodies in the serum directed to the causative antigen. The causative antigen combines with the serum antibody in the alveolar walls, leading to a type III hypersensitivity reaction. Type III hypersensitivity diseases are caused by the formation of antigen-antibody complexes[1,10] (see Chapter 10). These antigen-antibody complexes then elicit the granulomatous inflammation that leads to lung tissue injury, as evidenced by thickening of alveolar walls; formation of exudate in the bronchiolar lumen; and infiltration by lymphocytes, plasma cells, and eosinophils.[1,10,11] Fibrotic lung changes occur in advanced cases. Many individuals develop precipitating antibodies (precipitin) from organic dust exposure, but only a few develop pneumonitis.[11] Genetic predisposition may be involved in an exaggerated response to the offending agent. Experiments in animals show that a delayed hypersensitivity (type IV) reaction to the antigen is also required before pneumonitis can occur.[11]

Clinical manifestations. In the acute stage of the disease, symptoms start 4 to 6 hours after exposure and resolve in 18 to 24 hours.[10] General symptoms may include chills, sweating, shivering, myalgias, nausea, lethargy, headache, and malaise.[1,11,12] The patient may have a fever. Respiratory symptoms may include dyspnea at rest, dry cough, tachypnea, and chest discomfort. Physical findings may include cyanosis (a late sign) and crackles (rales) in the lung bases.[1,3]

In the chronic form, progressive diffuse pulmonary fibrosis develops in the upper lobes—the hallmark of the disease.[1] In the intermediate

TABLE 23-3 CAUSES OF HYPERSENSITIVITY PNEUMONITIS

DISEASE	ANTIGEN	ALLERGEN SOURCE
Farmer's lung	*Thermophila, Actinomyces*	Moldy hay, silage
Bird fancier's lung	Parakeet, pigeon, chicken	Bird excreta, feathers, and animal protein
Bagassosis	Thermophilic bacteria	Moldy sugarcane pulp
Mushroom, cork, maple bark, or malt hypersensitivity; cheese maker's lung, redwood lung	Various fungi	Handling moldy products
Grain handler's lung	Wheat weevil	Insect-infected grain
Pituitary extract hypersensitivity	Heterologous pituitary and serum proteins	—
Fish-meat worker's lung	Protein, fungi	Animal food
Humidifier lung (fever)	Thermophilic bacteria, amoebae, and fungi	Humidifiers and evaporative air coolers

form, the disease may manifest with acute febrile episodes and progressive pulmonary fibrosis with cough, dyspnea, fatigue, and, eventually, cor pulmonale (right-sided heart enlargement attributable to lung disorders).[10]

Diagnosis. During the acute/subacute phase, transient bilateral pulmonary infiltrates or increased bronchial markings with alveolar nodular infiltrates may be found on chest radiographs. In the chronic phase, diffuse reticulonodular infiltrates and fibrosis are present.[11] Skin testing with the causative antigen may produce a red, indurated, hemorrhagic reaction 4 to 12 hours after injection that lasts several days.[1] This reaction suggests precipitin-mediated sensitivity. Skin testing for most precipitating antigens is impractical because most produce irritating reactions before the precipitin reaction occurs, and many individuals without the disease have precipitating antibodies. Common laboratory findings include an increased white blood cell count and a decreased Pao_2. Elevations in erythrocyte sedimentation rate and the level of C-reactive protein are often present. Hypoxemia worsens with exercise. Pulmonary function tests show decreased lung volumes, diffusing capacity, and static compliance.[1,10]

Treatment. The goal of therapy is to identify the offending agent and prevent further exposure. This may require a change in environment or occupation. Oral corticosteroids may be used to decrease the inflammatory process.[10,12]

KEY POINTS
- Diffuse interstitial pulmonary fibrosis is a restrictive disorder characterized by thickening of the alveolar interstitium. The disorder is an immune-mediated disorder that follows an initial lung injury.
- Lung tissues are characteristically infiltrated by immune cells (macrophages and lymphocytes). Excess fibrin deposition results in stiff, noncompliant lungs. Vital capacity, tidal volume, FRC, and diffusion capacity are generally reduced. Respiratory rate increases to compensate for the small tidal volume.
- Treatment centers on administration of drugs to depress immune system activity, such as corticosteroids.

- Sarcoidosis is a restrictive disorder associated with abnormal protein deposits (granulomas) in the lung. Granulomas are fibrotic and are associated with immune cells (histiocytes). The cause is unknown.
- Symptoms include progressive dyspnea, fever, enlarged lymph nodes, and generalized symptoms of inflammation. Pulmonary lymph nodes may be primarily affected, with progression to parenchymal involvement. Pulmonary function test results are consistent with a restrictive disorder, demonstrating reduced lung volumes and increased respiratory rate.
- Treatment centers on alleviation of the symptoms. Corticosteroids may be used to reduce inflammation.
- Hypersensitivity pneumonitis includes a group of inflammatory lung disorders associated with inhalation of organic particles. Antibodies are produced in response to the inhaled particles; then antigen-antibody complexes deposit in the lung, initiating inflammation and granuloma production.
- Hypersensitivity pneumonitis is characterized by general symptoms of inflammation (e.g., fever, chills, malaise), dyspnea, dry cough, and tachypnea. Chronic exposure leads to progressive fibrosis and pulmonary dysfunction characteristic of restrictive parenchymal disease.

Occupational Lung Diseases

Etiology. Occupational lung diseases result from the inhalation of toxic gases or foreign particles. Traditionally, occupational lung diseases included pathologic conditions that were associated with the effects of exposure to inhaled dusts. However, a holistic approach to these diseases requires consideration of atmospheric pollutants as well as natural genetic resistance and compliance with health maintenance behaviors. The distinction between occupational and environmental respiratory diseases is becoming increasingly difficult. The integration of multiple environmental areas (home, work, and leisure) further compounds the complexity of defining occupational respiratory diseases. Although atmospheric pollutants (toxic gases) are not discussed in detail here, their impact on occupational respiratory diseases must not be minimized. The sources, potential clinical manifestations, and potential pathologic processes associated with common atmospheric pollutants are presented in Table 23-4.

Pneumoconiosis is defined as parenchymal lung disease caused by the inhalation of inorganic dust particles. The greater the exposure to the dust, the worse the pathologic consequences. Anthracosis (coal miner's lung or black lung), silicosis (silica inhalation), asbestosis (asbestos inhalation), and acute beryllium disease are common examples of occupational lung diseases. However, exposure to several other dusts may also impair respiratory function. Included in this list are antimony ore, barium, iron, tin, fuller's earth (clay), kaolin (china clay), and talc. Hairdressers exposed to bleach and hair spray are at risk for developing obstructive lung disease. Asthma caused by occupational exposures is seen in 16.3% of all adult-onset asthma.[13] Many workers are exposed to "pathogenic dust" through the processing, packaging, or manufacturing of a specific product.[10,14] Predisposing factors such as history of preexisting lung disease, exposure to atmospheric pollutants, duration of dust exposure, amount of dust concentration, and size of dust particles affect the onset and severity of the respiratory impairment.

Pathogenesis. The respiratory tract is protected by two interrelated systems: the mucociliary system and alveolar macrophages. The inhalation of inorganic particles has little effect on the mucociliary system. However, atmospheric pollutants (sulfur oxides, nitrogen oxides, and tobacco smoke) interfere with and can paralyze ciliary action.[1] As a result, the clearance effect is impaired, and inorganic particles cannot be removed. Alveolar macrophages attempt to engulf and remove inorganic dust by one of the following methods: (1) migrating to small airways to use the mucociliary escalator; (2) engulfing dust and exiting through the lymph and/or blood system; (3) passing through bronchial walls, depositing dust particles in extraalveolar tissue; or (4) destroying the particle (silica).[1,14]

Macrophage impairment is the primary mechanism through which inorganic particles initiate lung diseases. In an attempt to maintain a sterile alveolar environment, macrophages secrete lysozymes to control foreign particle activity. These enzymes, released in response to the particulate stimuli, eventually damage the alveolar walls, which may cause deposition of fibrous materials. Although the type of inorganic particle inhaled individualizes the pathophysiologic response, the general response is similar in the context of occupational lung diseases. Silica is one of the most toxic particles to alveolar macrophages. Dense deposits of collagen material are formed around the silica particles, resulting in marked fibrotic tissue deposition and restrictive lung disease. Coal dust and asbestos initiate a similar, although less severe, response. The pathologic processes and clinical features for each of the major occupational lung diseases are summarized in Table 23-5.

Clinical manifestations. Pneumoconioses (anthracosis, asbestosis, silicosis) generally produce no symptoms in the early stages. Physical evidence of the disease occurs when the pulmonary circulation is impaired because of increased pulmonary vascular resistance or development of a pulmonary infection. Workers may remain symptom free for up to 10 to 20 years with chronic exposure.[1,2,14] Once again, symptom manifestation is dependent on the predisposing factors. As pneumoconioses progress, patients present with a progressive, productive cough and dyspnea, especially with exercise. In addition, patients may complain of progressive weakness and fatigue. Clubbing of fingers may also be present. Late clinical features include chronic hypoxemia, cor pulmonale, and respiratory failure.

Diagnosis. The reliability of pulmonary changes noted on chest radiographs varies with the severity of the disease. When the patient is symptom free, no changes may be noted. However, as the pneumoconioses progress, micronodular mottling and haziness become apparent.[1] In addition, nodules, fibroses, and calcifications resulting from dust particle deposition are noted. Pneumoconioses usually produce one of three radiographic findings: nodular, reticular, or linear. However, because of the insidious progression of occupational lung diseases, radiographs negative for lung disease do not exclude the presence of the disease process. Changes in pulmonary function tests demonstrate predominantly restrictive impairment (see Figure 22-19) with a component of obstructive functional impairment, depending on the severity and type of dust inhalation.[1]

Finally, hypoxemia is evident from arterial blood gas measurements in the late disease stages. Falling Pao_2 levels are accompanied by decreased $Paco_2$ levels as the body initially compensates for the hypoxemia with an increased respiratory drive. However, as the disease progresses, both hypoxemia and hypercapnia are evident.

Treatment. Preventive measures are the key to limiting the onset and severity of occupational lung diseases. Adherence to federal standards for exposure to dust and particulate matter, as well as continuing education of workers and employers, could dramatically impact the incidence of respiratory diseases. The use of respirators and water sprays for miners to decrease airborne particles in mines are two prevention techniques. Early evaluation of a work environment predisposed to occupational lung diseases is where "treatment" must begin.[14] Two primary goals in the management of active occupational lung diseases are to prevent further parenchymal damage and to relieve

TABLE 23-4 COMMON ATMOSPHERIC POLLUTANTS CONTRIBUTING TO LUNG DISEASE

POLLUTANT	SOURCE	CLINICAL MANIFESTATIONS	POTENTIAL DISEASE PROCESSES
Carbon monoxide	Automobile exhaust (incomplete fossil fuel combustion)	Lethargy, impairs mental skills, cherry-red mucous membranes, headache	Hypoxemia, respiratory failure
Sulfur oxides	Factories (corrosive, poisonous by-products of combustion of sulfur-containing fuels)	Inflamed mucous membranes, eyes, upper respiratory tract, bronchial mucosa; cough	Pulmonary edema, bronchitis
Photochemical oxidants (ozone, hydrocarbons, or nitrogen oxides)	By-product of exposure of hydrocarbons and/or nitrogen oxides (from fossil fuel combustion with high temperatures) to sunlight	Inflammation of eyes, upper respiratory tract; cough	Tracheitis, bronchitis, pulmonary edema
Cigarette smoke	Cigarettes (carbon monoxide, nicotine, "tars")	Impaired exercise tolerance, decreased mental activity, tachycardia, hypertension, sweating	Bronchial carcinoma, chronic bronchitis, emphysema, coronary heart disease
Particulate matter	Factories/power stations; small particles, visible smoke and soot	Cough; dyspnea; itchy, watery eyes; irritated mucous membranes	Bronchitis, tracheitis, asthma

TABLE 23-5 MAJOR OCCUPATIONAL LUNG PNEUMOCONIOSES

PNEUMOCONIOSES	PATHOLOGIC FINDINGS	CLINICAL FEATURES
Anthracosis (coal miner's lung)	*Early:* Collection of coal particles with small amount of dilation of airway *Late:* Progressive, massive fibrosis, with condensed areas of black fibrous tissue	*Early:* Minimal to no symptoms; may be seen with dyspnea with cough but often due to unrelated bronchitis or emphysema *Late:* Worsening dyspnea on exertion, productive cough, respiratory failure
Silicosis	Dense collagen deposits in respiratory bronchioles and alveoli and along lymphatics	*Early:* No symptoms noted *Late:* Productive cough, dyspnea, especially with exercise; increased risk for tuberculosis
Asbestosis	Fibrous deposits secondary to long, thin fibers, allowing deep lung penetration	Progressive dyspnea on exertion, weakness, clubbing of fingers; pleural thickening with plaque development

signs and symptoms, when possible. Ideally, if the problematic dust can be identified, the individual should be removed from the environment. However, if a job change is unrealistic, every possible measure must be implemented to prevent further inhalation of dust particles. Included in this treatment is the evaluation of current health maintenance behaviors. Treatment consists of corticosteroids, inhaled bronchodilators, oxygen therapy, and respiratory treatments (intermittent positive-pressure ventilation, postural drainage, and deep breathing exercises). The effectiveness and utilization of these therapies depend on the patient's condition and the stage of disease. Rarely are those pathologic conditions reversed with medical treatment. The primary goal is to halt symptom progression.

KEY POINTS

- Occupational lung diseases result from chronic inhalation of gases and inert particles. Commonly identified particles include coal, silica, and asbestos. Smoking and environmental pollutants may be contributing factors because they depress the ciliary function necessary to remove inhaled particles.
- The presence of inert particles in the alveoli initiates macrophage activity and inflammation. Inert particles cannot be digested by phagocytes, so they are walled off by deposition of fibrous proteins.
- Manifestations of pneumoconioses are related to the restrictive nature of the pulmonary dysfunction. Progressive dyspnea, decreased vital capacity and FRC, and increased respiratory rate are common. Blood gas analyses show progressive hypoxemia; carbon dioxide levels may remain normal or low until late in the disease.
- Treatment includes prevention of further exposure and administration of corticosteroids, bronchodilators, and oxygen therapy.

ATELECTATIC DISORDERS

Acute (Adult) Respiratory Distress Syndrome

Etiology. Acute (adult) respiratory distress syndrome is characterized by damage to the alveolar-capillary membrane. In the United States there are more than 150,000 cases per year. Mortality statistics range from 30% to 63%.[1,2,15,16] Clinically, ARDS is associated with a decline in the Pao_2 that is refractory (does not respond) to supplemental oxygen therapy. Damage to the alveolar-capillary membrane causes widespread protein-rich alveolar infiltrates (visible on chest radiographs) and severe dyspnea. Patients who recover from the acute injury can expect to return to relatively normal lung function.[1,15] Follow-up studies (9 months to 4 years) in ARDS survivors show a mild restrictive pulmonary function accompanied by cough, dyspnea, and excess sputum production.[2,4] Some individuals continue to have abnormalities in diffusing capacity, oxygenation, and lung mechanics.[2,4] ARDS is associated with severe trauma, sepsis (greater than 40% of cases), aspiration of gastric acid (greater than 30% of cases), fat emboli syndrome, and shock from any cause (Box 23-1). The precise mechanism of lung injury is not known, but the common denominator appears to be increased permeability of the pulmonary vasculature and flooding of the alveoli with proteinaceous fluid, leading to the development of protein-rich pulmonary edema (noncardiogenic pulmonary edema). The acute lung injury triggers the immune system to activate the complement system and to initiate neutrophil sequestration in the lung (Figure 23-2).

Pathogenesis. The pathogenetic sequence of events in ARDS is shown in Figure 23-2. The initial injury to the alveolar-capillary membrane may be caused by direct damage, as seen in aspiration of acidic gastric contents, or by indirect damage, as occurs in shock from any cause. Therapeutic interventions (high oxygen and overhydration) may act to compound the effects of the initial lung injury. The resulting injury leads to an increase in alveolar-capillary permeability, which results in interstitial and alveolar edema. The four characteristic pathophysiologic abnormalities of ARDS involve: (1) injury to the alveoli from a wide variety of disorders, (2) changes in alveolar diameter, (3) injury to the pulmonary circulation, and (4) disruptions in oxygen transport and utilization.[15,16] Common findings in this type of injury include (1) severe hypoxemia caused by intrapulmonary shunting of blood; (2) a decrease in lung compliance; (3) a decrease in FRC; (4) diffuse, fluffy alveolar infiltrates on the chest radiograph; and (5) noncardiogenic pulmonary edema.[1,9,15,16]

BOX 23-1 MAJOR DISORDERS ASSOCIATED WITH ARDS

Shock (any process leading to a low blood flow state)
- Infectious causes
- Sepsis syndrome (primarily from gram-negative bacteria) with or without sustained hypotension (>40% cases)
- Pneumonia (viral, bacterial, fungal, mycobacterial)
- Miliary tuberculosis
- Bronchiolitis obliterans—organizing pneumonia

Trauma: pulmonary contusion

Embolism
- Fat emboli
- Air emboli
- Thrombus formation
- Amniotic fluid embolism

Head injury (increased intracranial pressure)

Aspiration (>30% of cases)
- Gastric contents
- Drowning (fresh/salt water)

Drug overdose
- Heroin
- Methadone
- Propoxyphene
- Barbiturates, salicylates, thiazides, colchicine

Inhaled toxins
- Smoke inhalation
- High concentrations of oxygen (iatrogenic)
- Corrosive chemicals (ammonia, sulfur dioxide, chlorine, nitrogen dioxide)
- Free-base cocaine smoking

Radiation

Hematologic disorders
- Disseminated intravascular coagulation
- Massive blood transfusion
- Post-cardiopulmonary bypass
- Thrombotic thrombocytopenic purpura

Metabolic disorders
- Pancreatitis
- Uremia
- Paraquat ingestion

Burns

Cancer

Anaphylaxis

Eclampsia

Radiation pneumonitis

High-altitude exposure

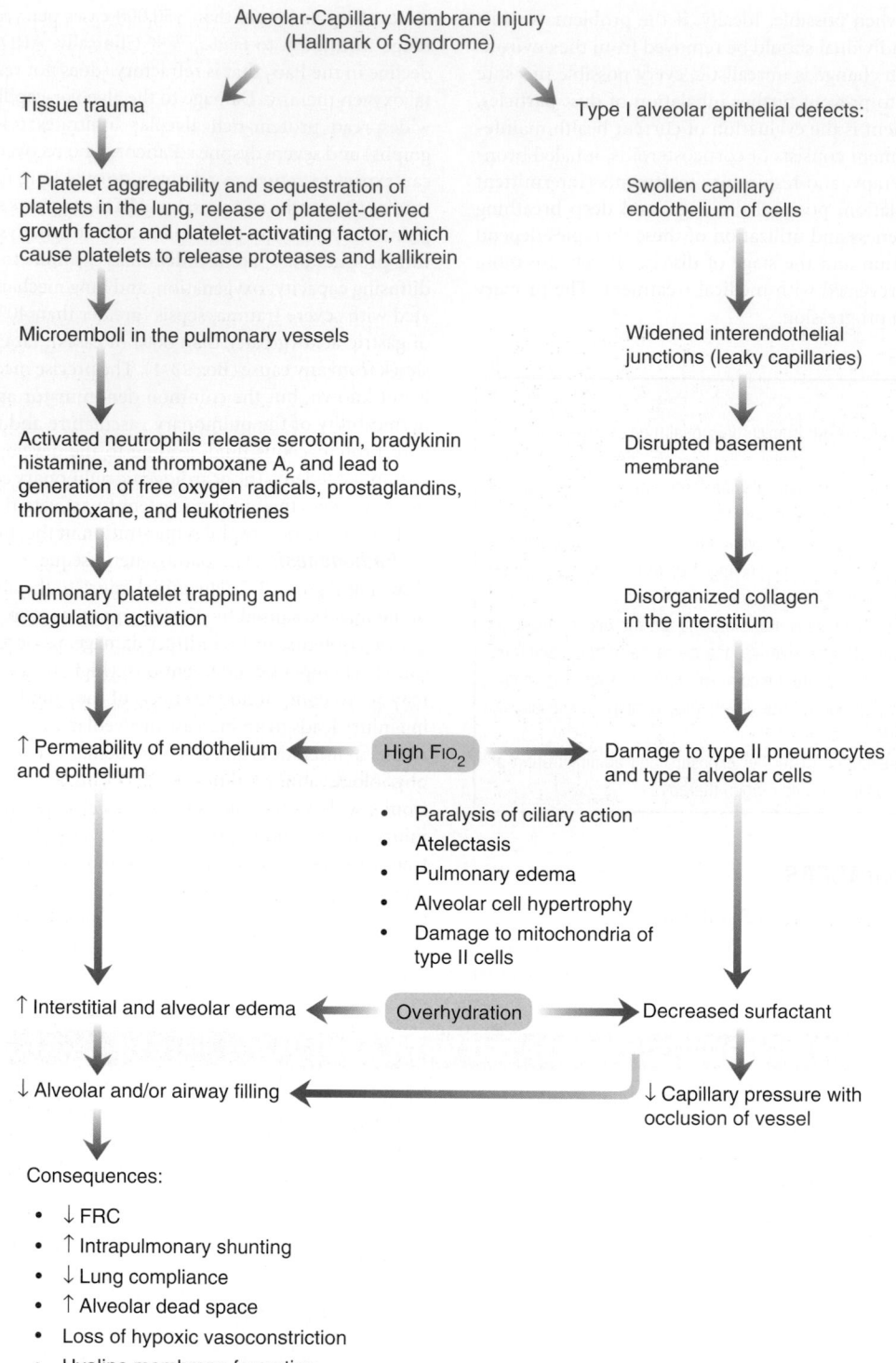

FIGURE 23-2 Pathogenesis of acute respiratory distress syndrome. *FRC,* Functional residual capacity.

The mechanism by which the FRC is decreased appears to be the result of stiff, noncompliant lungs associated with the presence of alveolar edema and exudate, which exaggerate surface tension forces.[1,2,15,16] Early alveolar closure and continued closure lead to atelectasis and loss of lung volume.[1] The decrease in lung compliance, often severe in ARDS, is reflected in the high ventilatory pressures required to deliver an adequate volume of gas. It is thought that this decrease in lung compliance is due to loss or inactivation of surfactant with subsequent increased

recoil pressure of the lungs.[1,2,15,16] In addition, proteinaceous fluid fills the alveoli and impairs ventilation. Figure 23-3 shows alveolar damage attributable to ARDS. Alveoli contain dense proteinaceous debris, desquamated cells, and hyaline membranes. The decrease in Pao_2 is a result of perfusion of large numbers of alveoli that are poorly ventilated (areas of low ventilation-perfusion ratio) or not ventilated (areas of shunt).

Clinical manifestations. The clinical features of ARDS usually include a history of a precipitating event that has led to a low blood volume state ("shock" state) 1 or 2 days before the onset of respiratory failure. The patient may complain of sudden marked respiratory distress.[1,2] Early signs and symptoms include a slight increase in pulse rate, dyspnea, and a low Pao_2. The initial presenting sign may be shallow, rapid breathing. With progression of the disease, the patient demonstrates tachycardia, tachypnea, hypotension, marked restlessness, decreased mental status, and production of frothy secretions. On auscultation of lung fields, crackles and rhonchi are heard. The patient may be using accessory muscles to breathe and demonstrating intercostal and sternal retractions. A late sign is cyanosis.

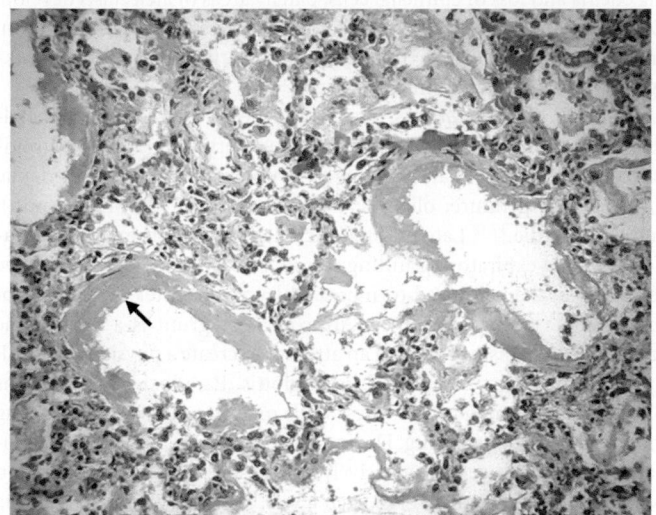

FIGURE 23-3 Diffuse alveolar damage (acute respiratory distress syndrome), shown in photomicrograph. Some of the alveoli are collapsed; others are distended. Many contain dense proteinaceous debris, desquamated cells, and hyaline membranes *(arrow).* (From Kumar V et al, editors: *Robbin's basic pathology,* ed 8, Philadelphia, 2007, Saunders, p 483.)

Diagnosis. The hallmark of ARDS is hypoxemia that is refractory to increasing levels of supplemental oxygen. Uncorrected hypoxemia is associated with hypotension, decreased urine output, respiratory and metabolic acidosis, and eventual cardiopulmonary arrest. Arterial blood gas determinations reveal hypoxia, acidosis, and hypercapnia.[16] The chest radiograph may initially be normal but progresses to a bilateral diffuse "whiteout" (Figure 23-4) indicative of diffuse alveolar infiltrates. The infiltrates characteristically spare the costophrenic angles.[2] Blood and urine cultures will help determine if infection is the etiology. Pulmonary function tests show a marked decreased in FRC, decreased lung volumes, decreased lung compliance, and a ventilation-perfusion $(\dot{V}_A/\dot{Q})$ mismatch with a large right-to-left shunt.[1] Histologic changes found on open lung biopsy reveal atelectasis, hyaline membranes, cellular debris, and interstitial and alveolar edema[1,15,16] (see Figure 23-3).

Treatment. The management of ARDS entails identifying the underlying cause, addressing the cause (e.g., sepsis), maintaining fluid and electrolyte balance, and providing adequate oxygenation with the use of a volume ventilator utilizing pressure support and positive end-expiratory pressure (PEEP). Patients may require fraction of inspired oxygen (Fio_2) levels of 1.0. The goal is to keep the Pao_2 value above 60 mm Hg. Because of increased permeability of the alveolar-capillary membrane, excessive fluid administration can produce or intensify pulmonary edema. High-frequency jet ventilation (HFJV), inverse ratio ventilation (IRV), and inhaled nitric oxide administration have also been used to treat ARDS.[4,16] ARDS can be prevented experimentally by blocking systemic inflammatory cells. Numerous agents have been investigated.[16]

Infant Respiratory Distress Syndrome

Etiology. Infant respiratory distress syndrome, also known as *hyaline membrane disease,* has features similar to those of ARDS. It is a syndrome of premature neonates, characterized by hemorrhagic pulmonary edema, patchy atelectasis, and hyaline (glassy) membranes.[1] Hypoxemia that is refractory to increasing levels of oxygen supplementation is the hallmark of the syndrome. The incidence is 60% in infants

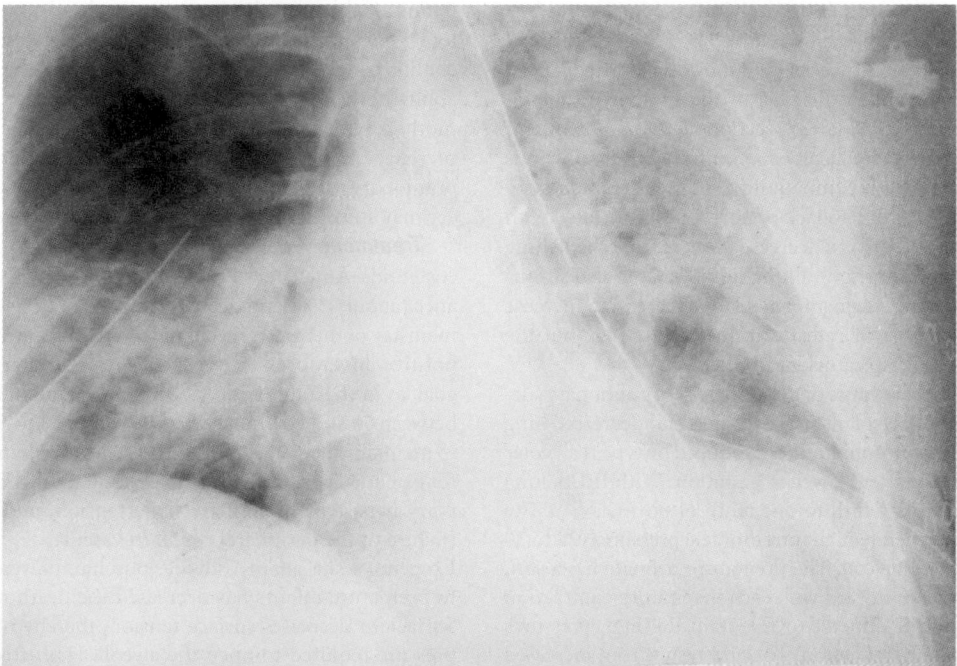

FIGURE 23-4 Chest radiograph of a 28-year-old man who was involved in an automobile accident. The patient presented with multiple bilateral rib fractures and bilateral pneumothorax. Within 24 hours, severe acute respiratory distress syndrome developed (note diffuse "whiteout").

Alteration of surface tension forces, normally maintained by surfactant, causes further leakage of proteinaceous fluid into the alveoli. This fluid contains fibrin and cellular debris, which causes hyaline membrane formation. Surfactant normally decreases surface tension in the alveolus during expiration, allowing the alveolus to remain partially open, thus maintaining FRC.[18] A secondary cause of IRDS is immaturity of the capillary blood supply, which leads to $\dot{V}_A/\dot{Q}$ mismatch, thus adding to the problems of hypoxemia and metabolic acidosis. In addition, a right-to-left shunt from an open foramen ovale or patent ductus arteriosus may increase the hypoxemia.[2] Histologically, there is progressive damage to the basement membrane and respiratory epithelial cells. With increasing edema and loss of epithelial cells, patchy areas of atelectasis develop. Cellular damage from the disease process, excess fluid administration, and high values of Fio_2 lead to increased capillary permeability and leakage of high-protein fluid into the alveoli.

Clinical manifestations. The typical neonate presents with shallow respirations; intercostal, subcostal, or sternal retractions; diminished breath sounds; flaring of nares; hypotension; peripheral edema; low body temperature; oliguria; tachypnea (60 to 120 breaths/min); and bradycardia.[17,18] Late findings include frothy sputum, central cyanosis, and an expiratory grunting sound. Nasal flaring is a physiologic response mechanism used to increase airway diameter in an attempt to overcome airway resistance. An expiratory grunt is a physiologic response mechanism reflecting an attempt to create a physiologic PEEP by exhaling against a partially closed glottis. Paradoxical respirations ("see-saw" movement of the chest wall) may also be noted, indicating increased work of breathing. During the first 48 to 72 hours of life, neonates with IRDS need progressively higher levels of Fio_2 to maintain adequate (60 to 80 mm Hg) oxygen levels.[17,18,20] As work of breathing increases and oxygen levels decrease, metabolic acidosis occurs.[21]

Diagnosis. Initial arterial blood gas determinations reveal hypoxemia and metabolic acidosis attributable to lactic acid formation by hypoxic tissues. As the disease progresses, hypercapnia and respiratory acidosis develop. Chest radiographs progress from normal, shortly after birth, to a diffuse whiteout or ground-glass appearance indicative of diffuse bilateral atelectasis and alveolar edema. Generalized hypoinflation of the lungs is also seen on chest x-ray. Measurement of the lecithin/sphingomyelin (L/S) ratio and the desaturated phosphatidylcholine concentration in amniotic fluid may be done to determine the ability of the fetus to secrete surfactant. If the L/S ratio is ≥2:1 (3:1 in mothers with diabetes), the incidence of RDS is less than 5%.[22] The presence of phosphatidylglycerol in the amniotic fluid is indicative of pulmonary maturity.[22] Administration of glucocorticoids before delivery may stimulate lung maturation and improve the L/S ratio.

Treatment. Prevention of IRDS is aimed at the use of prenatal corticosteroids. Antenatal steroids significantly increase respiratory compliance (about 23%) and decrease the risk of development of IRDS.[23] The mainstay of therapy is mechanical ventilation with PEEP or continuous positive-airway pressure. Prevention is a primary goal. The therapeutic goal, as in the adult with ARDS, is to maintain adequate oxygen levels between 50 and 90 mm Hg.[1,2,20] The lowest Fio_2 settings should be used to maintain adequate arterial oxygen levels. High Fio_2 (100%) delivered for extended periods of time may result in further alveolar damage, primary persistent pulmonary hypertension, and retrolental fibroplasia (failure of the peripheral retina to vascularize, leading to blindness).[20] Exogenous surfactant (bovine, porcine, or synthetic) administration to premature infants has decreased the death rate in IRDS by 50%.[17] Surfactant decreases surface tension, thereby reducing the amount of pressure required to open the alveoli. High-frequency ventilation has proved to be effective in infants with severe IRDS by providing more uniform lung inflation, improving lung mechanics, and enhancing gas exchange. Infants receiving high-frequency ventilation require lower

born at less than 30 weeks' gestation who are not treated with corticosteroids and decreases to 35% for infants receiving antenatal steroids.[17] The incidence in infants older than 34 weeks is 5%.[17,18] High-risk factors include birth earlier than 25 weeks' gestation, birth at advanced gestational age, poorly controlled diabetes in the mother, deliveries after antepartum hemorrhage, cesarean section without antecedent labor, or the presence of perinatal asphyxia, multiple births, previous infant with RDS, and Rh factor incompatibility.[17] The increased risk of respiratory morbidity may be due to lack of hormones associated with labor. During normal labor there is a decrease in secretion of fetal lung liquid and an increase in absorption of lung liquid. Labor also stimulates the release of surfactant. During normal labor there is an increase in catecholamine release. Loss of catecholamine release may put the neonate at increased risk of respiratory morbidity.[19]

Pathogenesis. The primary cause of IRDS is a lack of pulmonary surfactant, leading to increased alveolar surface tension and decreased lung compliance.[17] Surfactant, a phospholipid, is produced by type II alveolar cells in increasing quantities after 32 weeks' gestation. With IRDS, lung compliance is decreased to one fifth to one tenth of normal.[1,17,18] The neonate with IRDS must generate high intrathoracic pressures (25 to 30 mm Hg) to maintain patent alveoli. The premature neonate has a soft, compliant chest that is drawn inward with each inspiratory contraction of the diaphragm, making it difficult to maintain the high pressures needed to ensure adequate oxygenation. The end result from increased work of breathing and decreased ventilation is progressive atelectasis, increased pulmonary vascular resistance, profound hypoxemia, and acidosis.[1] Surfactant also functions to maintain pulmonary fluid balance.

mcan airway pressures and have better gas exchange than those ventilated conventionally.[21] General supportive therapy of adequate intravenous nutrition, fluid and electrolyte balance, minimal handling, and a neutral thermal environment should be maintained. Broad-spectrum antibiotics are prescribed for infections after cultures have been done or prophylactically until blood cultures prove negative.[20]

KEY POINTS

- The symptoms of IRDS are similar to those of ARDS. IRDS occurs most commonly in premature infants born before adequate development of their surfactant-producing pneumocytes (25 weeks' gestation). The maturity of surfactant-producing cells can be estimated from the L/S ratio in amniotic fluid. An L/S ratio of less than 2:1 is associated with a higher risk of IRDS.
- Lack of surfactant causes atelectasis and increased work of breathing as a result of high alveolar surface tension. Leakage of inflammatory exudate into the alveoli results in formation of hyaline membranes
- Symptoms of IRDS include nasal flaring, expiratory grunt, thoracic retractions, and rapid, shallow respirations. Chest radiographs demonstrate a "whiteout." As in ARDS, blood gas values are poor, indicating severe hypoxemia and acidosis.
- Therapy for IRDS includes supportive measures, such as mechanical ventilation with PEEP or continuous positive airway pressure, and use of supplemental oxygen as well as specific measures to increase alveolar surfactant levels.

PLEURAL SPACE DISORDERS

Pneumothorax

Etiology. Spontaneous pneumothorax (SP) is characterized by the accumulation of air in the pleural space. A primary pneumothorax is classified as spontaneous, occurring mainly in tall, thin men between ages 20 and 40 years without underlying disease factors.[1,2,24] Cigarette smoking increases the risk of spontaneous pneumothorax.[24] A secondary pneumothorax occurs as a result of complications from preexisting pulmonary disease (such as asthma, emphysema, cystic fibrosis, infectious disease [pneumonia or tuberculosis], or interstitial lung disease). In the United States, there are approximately 20,000 new cases annually. SP is 6 times more common in men than women.[24] A specific category of secondary pneumothorax associated with menstruation is called *catamenial pneumothorax* (pathogenesis unknown). A catamenial pneumothorax occurs primarily in the right hemothorax, and is associated with endometriosis.[25] A third classification (tension pneumothorax) is traumatic in origin, resulting from penetrating or nonpenetrating injury. A tension pneumothorax is a medical emergency. Other examples of traumatic pneumothorax have iatrogenic causes, such as placement of central lines, thoracentesis (6%),[26] percutaneous lung biopsy, and mechanical ventilation.[2]

Pathogenesis. Primary spontaneous pneumothorax (Figure 23-5) results from rupture of small subpleural blebs in the apices.[1] When

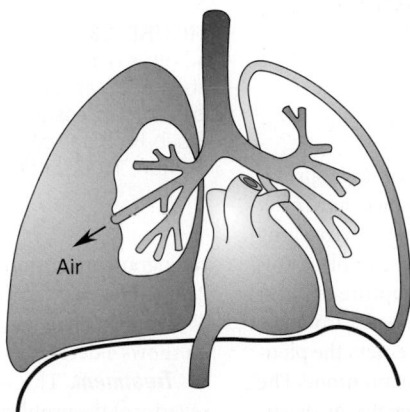

SPONTANEOUS PNEUMOTHORAX

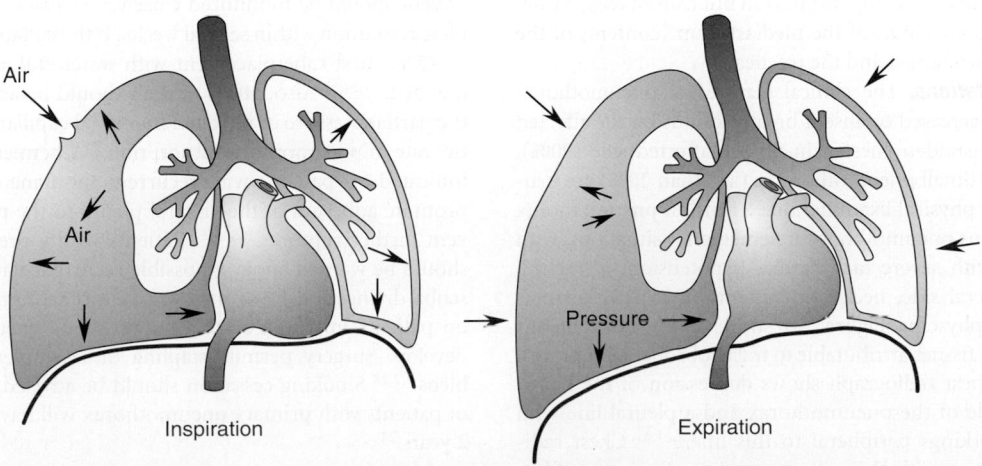

Inspiration   Expiration

TENSION PNEUMOTHORAX

FIGURE 23-5 *Top,* Spontaneous pneumothorax. *Bottom,* Tension pneumothorax: air builds up under pressure, leading to collapse of the ipsilateral lung and shift of the mediastinum to the contralateral side.

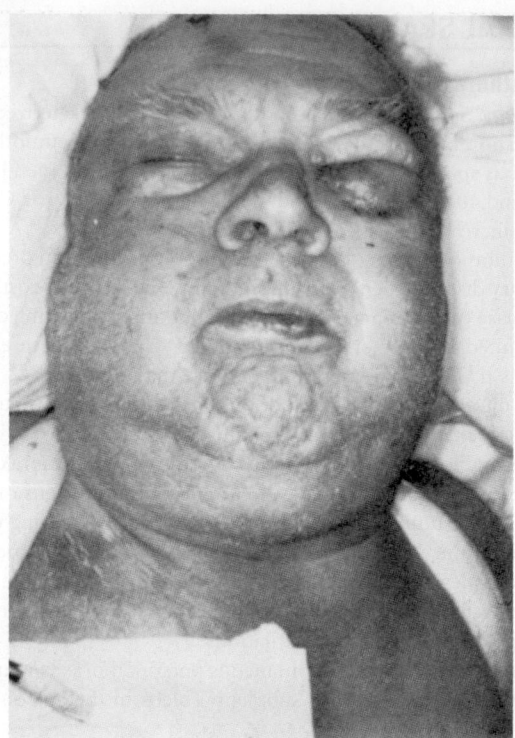

FIGURE 23-6 Subcutaneous emphysema (air in the tissues) from tracheobronchial disruption and injuries of the esophagus. (From Kirsh MM, Sloan H: *Blunt chest trauma: general principles and management,* Boston, 1977, Little, Brown, p 109.)

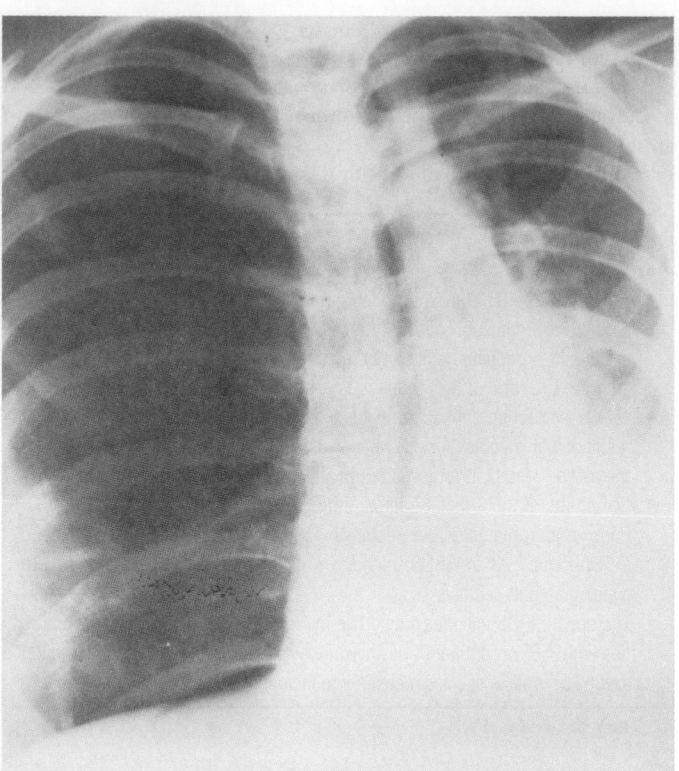

FIGURE 23-7 Upright posteroanterior chest radiograph showing a right-sided tension pneumothorax. Note marked deviation of trachea and cardiac silhouette into the left side of the chest. There is also depression of the right hemidiaphragm. (From Kirsh MM, Sloan H: *Blunt chest trauma: general principles and management,* Boston, 1977, Little, Brown, p 62.)

air enters the pleural space, the lung collapses and the rib cage springs out.[1] The subpleural blebs are believed to occur in the apices as a result of negative mechanical pressures in the upper third of the upright lung field. Secondary pneumothorax occurs as a result of complications from an underlying lung problem and may be due to rupture of a cyst or bleb.[1,2] Tension pneumothorax (see Figure 23-5) results from the buildup of air under pressure in the pleural space. Air enters the pleural space during inspiration but cannot escape during expiration.[1] The lung on the ipsilateral (same) side collapses and forces the mediastinum toward the contralateral (opposite) side, thus decreasing venous return and cardiac output (see Figure 23-5). With an open, "sucking" chest wall wound, air enters during inspiration but cannot escape during expiration, leading to a shift of the mediastinum (contents of the septum between the two lungs) and the trachea.

Clinical manifestations. The clinical features of pneumothorax include tachycardia, decreased or absent breath sounds on the affected side, hyperresonance, sudden chest pain on the affected side (90%), and dyspnea (80%).[24] Small pneumothoraces (less than 20%) are usually not detectable on physical examination.[25] Tension pneumothorax and a large spontaneous pneumothorax are emergency situations, with patients presenting with severe tachycardia, hypotension, a tracheal shift to the contralateral side, neck vein distention, hyperresonance, and subcutaneous emphysema. Figure 23-6 shows severe subcutaneous emphysema (air in the tissues attributable to tracheobronchial rupture).

Diagnosis. The chest radiograph shows depression of the hemidiaphragm on the side of the pneumothorax and a pleural line with absence of vessel markings peripheral to this line.[2,24,25] Chest radiography should be done with the patient standing. Expiratory films show a better demarcation of the pleural line than inspiratory films. The diagnosis may be based on clinical features without radiographic confirmation. However, a chest radiograph is usually obtained. A chest

radiograph in tension pneumothorax shows a mediastinal shift (Figure 23-7). The electrocardiogram may show axis deviations, nonspecific ST-segment changes, and T-wave inversion.[27] Arterial blood gas analysis shows a decreased Pao_2 and acute respiratory alkalosis.

Treatment. The management of pneumothorax depends on the severity of the problem and the cause of the air leak. If the lung collapse is less than 15% to 25%, the patient may or may not be hospitalized. Typically, the patient is treated symptomatically.[2,25] A nonhospitalized patient should be monitored closely.[27,28] The expectation is for complete resolution within several weeks. If the collapse is greater than 15% to 25%, chest tube placement with water seal and suction is recommended.[1,2,24,28] Also, 100% oxygen should be administered to reduce the partial pressure of nitrogen in pleural capillaries, thus quadrupling the rate of pneumothorax absorption.[24] Chemical pleurodesis may be indicated for patients with recurrent spontaneous pneumothorax to promote adhesion of the visceral pleura to the parietal pleura to prevent further ruptures.[1,2,26,27] Patients with a previous pneumothorax should be warned about a possible recurrence at high altitudes, from scuba diving, and from smoking. A thoracotomy may be performed on patients in whom further spontaneous pneumothorax and blebs develop. Surgery permits stapling or laser pleurodesis of ruptured blebs.[1,2,28] Smoking cessation should be advised. Approximately 25% of patients with primary pneumothorax will have a recurrence within 2 years.[24]

Pleural Effusion

Etiology. Pleural effusion is not a disease, but a pathologic collection of fluid or pus in the pleural cavity as a result of another disease process. Normally, 5 to 15 ml of serous fluid is contained in the pleural space.[2] There is a constant movement of pleural fluid from parietal pleural capillaries to the pleural space, which is then reabsorbed into the parietal pleural lymphatics. The pleural membrane is a porous mesenchymal serous membrane that allows for movement of interstitial fluid. The fluid has a mucoid characteristic allowing for easy movement of the lungs.[29] The five major types of pleural effusion are: (1) transudates, (2) exudates, (3) empyema attributable to infection in the pleural space, (4) hemothorax or hemorrhagic pleural effusions, and (5) chylothorax or lymphatic pleural effusions.[2] Transudates have low concentrations of both protein (ratio of pleural fluid protein to serum protein is less than 0.5) and lactate dehydrogenase (LDH; pleural fluid LDH/serum LDH ratio less than 0.6), and have a specific gravity below 1.016.[30,31] Transudates are frequently associated with severe heart failure or other edematous states, such as cirrhosis with ascites, nephrotic syndrome, and myxedema.[2] Exudates have high concentrations of both protein (>0.5 mg/dl) and LDH (pleural fluid LDH/serum LDH ratio >0.6).[28,30-32] Common causes of exudates are malignancies, infections (especially pneumonia), pulmonary embolism, sarcoidosis, post–myocardial infarction syndrome, and pancreatic disease. Empyema is a high-protein exudative effusion resulting from infection in the pleural space. Hemothorax (the presence of blood in the pleural space) is often the result of chest trauma. Hemorrhagic pleural effusion contains a mixture of blood and pleural fluid. If the hematocrit of the fluid is greater than 50% of the hematocrit of peripheral blood, the fluid collection is called a *hemothorax*.[1,2] Chylothorax or chylous pleural effusion is an exudative process that develops from trauma as a result of leakage of chyle (lymph fluid) from the thoracic duct or from rheumatoid pleural effusion or tuberculous pleuritis.[1,2]

Pathogenesis. Pathophysiologic changes associated with the various types of effusions relate to changes in pleural capillary hydrostatic pressure, colloid oncotic pressure, or intrapleural pressure. Transudates can be caused by increased hydrostatic or decreased oncotic pressure. Exudates are associated with increased production of fluid as a result of increased permeability of the pleural membrane (inflammation) or impaired lymphatic drainage.[2,30,31] The imbalance in these pressures is associated with fluid formation exceeding fluid removal.

Clinical manifestations. Clinical features vary depending on the cause and size of the effusion. Small effusions may be asymptomatic (which is common) in patients with less than 300 ml of fluid in the pleural cavity.[28,30] General features include dyspnea, pleuritic pain that is sharp and worsens with inspiration, dry cough, decreased chest wall movement, absence of breath sounds, dullness to percussion, and decreased tactile fremitus over the affected area.[28,32] The most useful physical findings are dullness to percussion and tactile fremitus.[33] A massive pleural effusion may lead to a contralateral tracheal shift.[28]

Diagnosis. Thoracentesis should be done to analyze the fluid and to reduce the amount of fluid in the pleural cavity. Evaluation of the pleural fluid is done to determine its characteristics, which acts as an additional indicator of its origin. Pleural fluid should be analyzed for chemistry (pH, LDH, and glucose) and presence of pathogenic bacteria. Chest radiography should be done to detect pleural-based densities, infiltrates, signs of congestive heart failure (CHF), hilar adenopathy, and loculation of fluid. Computed tomography and ultrasonographic tests assist in the diagnosis of complicated effusions and distinguish a mass from a large effusion.[28,30-32] Ultrasonography is also useful for thoracentesis guidance.

Treatment. Treatment is directed at the underlying cause of the effusion and relief of symptoms. Closed chest tube drainage in adults or thoracentesis is indicated if the effusion is large. Closed chest drainage in pediatric cases is controversial.[25] A thoracotomy to control bleeding may be required in patients with excessive bleeding (greater than 200 ml/hr).[34]

> **KEY POINTS**
> - The pleural space is usually a potential space, containing only a small amount of fluid for lubrication. Accumulations of air (pneumothorax), pus (empyema), blood (hemothorax), lymph (chylothorax), or transudate in the pleural space can restrict lung expansion.
> - Tension pneumothorax occurs when pleural air progressively accumulates and develops a positive pressure in the pleura. The ipsilateral (same side) lung collapses, and mediastinal structures (trachea, heart) are shifted to the opposite side. Breath sounds are diminished or absent on the affected side.
> - Tension pneumothorax and a large, simple (spontaneous) pneumothorax are medical emergencies requiring treatment to remove pleural air and reexpand the lung. This usually requires insertion of a chest tube. Chemical pleurodesis may be done in persons prone to spontaneous pneumothorax.
> - A number of disease processes may result in accumulation of fluid in the pleural space. Analysis of the type of fluid (e.g., transudates, exudates, blood, pus) indicates the underlying disease process. General manifestations include dyspnea, cough, pleuritic pain, and diminished breath sounds and dullness to percussion over the effusion.

NEUROMUSCULAR, CHEST WALL, AND OBESITY DISORDERS

NEUROMUSCULAR DISORDERS

Diseases affecting the muscles of respiration or their nerve supply can lead to dyspnea and respiratory failure. Table 23-6 summarizes the features of these disorders.

Poliomyelitis

Poliomyelitis is a viral disease in which the poliovirus attacks motor nerve cells of the spinal cord and brainstem. The incidence of poliomyelitis in the United States is approximately eight cases per year. All of these cases have been related to the oral polio vaccine (OPV).[35] The diaphragm and intercostal muscles can be affected, resulting in weakness or paralysis and respiratory failure. At least 95% of infections are asymptomatic.[35] Patients with minor symptoms present with fever, headache, vomiting, diarrhea, constipation, and sore throat.[36] Respiratory muscle function generally recovers, although occasionally patients have chronic respiratory insufficiency from previous disease. As the result of mass vaccination of the population, new cases are quite rare and usually occur in unvaccinated immigrants.[35]

Amyotrophic Lateral Sclerosis

Amyotrophic lateral sclerosis (ALS) is a degenerative disease of the nervous system that involves both upper and lower motor neurons. ALS occurs in males more than females (2:1) and has a prevalence of 0.5 to 2 cases in 100,000 persons. Onset is often between the ages of 50 and 70 years of age. Only 5% of ALS cases are familial.[37] Commonly, muscles innervated by both spinal nerves and cranial nerves are affected. Clinically, progressive muscle weakness and wasting develop, eventually leading to profound weakness of respiratory muscles and death. Although the course of the disease is variable from patient to patient, the natural history is one of irreversibility and progressive deterioration[2,37] (see Chapter 45).

Muscular Dystrophies

Duchenne muscular dystrophy is a hereditary disease, passed from mothers to sons (X-linked recessive) and occurs in 1 per 3500 male births. The disease is characterized by progressive muscular weakness, initially in the lower extremities, and wasting. In later years (twenties

TABLE 23-6 NEUROMUSCULAR DISORDERS AFFECTING THE RESPIRATORY SYSTEM

DISEASE	ETIOLOGY	PATHOPHYSIOLOGY	CLINICAL FEATURES
Poliomyelitis (myelitis is inflammation of spinal cord)	Develops from an enteral virus acquired by ingestion or respiratory droplet	After a 1- to 3-week period, virus invades intestinal blood supply; once in circulation, virus invades all areas of body; invasion of central nervous system leads to neural damage and initiation of an inflammatory reaction	General symptoms are tremors, muscle weakness; bulbar poliomyelitis affects respiratory muscle nerves, leading to respiratory paralysis; patients usually exhibit shoulder girdle paralysis first, followed by intercostal and diaphragm muscle paralysis; paralysis may be rapid or slowly progressive; also seen are diplopia, facial weakness, dysphagia, difficulty chewing, nasal voice, and loss of gag reflex
Amyotrophic lateral sclerosis	Cause unknown; current theories include autoimmune disease and a slow virus	Affects anterior horn cells of both upper and lower motor neurons	Progressive weakness affecting distal more than proximal muscles; atrophy, fasciculations, and spasticity are noted; involvement of respiratory muscles leads to respiratory dysfunction requiring mechanical ventilation
Muscular dystrophies (most common is Duchenne type)	Hereditary disease (X-linked recessive) passed from mothers to sons	Progressive muscular weakness noted initially in lower extremity muscles; in later years (twenties and thirties) respiratory muscles become involved; patients are at risk for respiratory tract infections	Progressive muscular weakness and wasting; skeletal deformities are also common; involvement of respiratory muscles (diaphragm, intercostals, and accessory muscles) leads to hypoxia and hypercapnia
Guillain-Barré syndrome (acute idiopathic polyneuropathy)	Exact cause unknown, but thought to be an autoimmune disease triggered by a viral infection	Disease usually follows an infection or vaccination; peripheral nerves are affected, leading to neural inflammation, demyelination, and axon destruction	Progressive weakness and loss of motor function beginning in feet and legs and ascending upward; sensory loss may also be noted but is not as dramatic as motor loss; loss of respiratory muscle control leads to respiratory failure, which frequently requires mechanical ventilation; autonomic nervous system symptoms may also be noted (tachycardia, dysrhythmias, hypotension or hypertension, loss of ability to sweat)
Myasthenia gravis	Considered an autoimmune disease with both humoral (B cell) and cell-mediated (T cell) components	Autoantibodies and T cells bind to and damage acetylcholine receptors, leading to decreased functioning of receptors	Common symptoms are diplopia, ptosis, difficulty swallowing, increased weakness with activity, nasal voice, slurred speech, and weakness of proximal extremities; as disease progresses, respiratory muscles become involved, leading to respiratory failure; pneumonia may result from respiratory failure and immobility

to thirties), respiratory muscles become involved, leading to hypoxia, hypercapnia, and frequent respiratory tract infections (see Chapter 51).[2]

Guillain-Barré Syndrome

Guillain-Barré syndrome, also called *acute polyneuritis*, is a disorder that is presumed to have an immunologic basis. Infection involving *Campylobacter jejuni* often precedes the diagnosis. Guillain-Barré syndrome is characterized by demyelination of peripheral nerves. Frequently, patients have a history of recent viral or bacterial illness (66% of cases) followed by development of ascending paralysis.[38] Clinically, weakness and paralysis begin symmetrically in the lower extremities and progress or ascend proximally to the upper extremities and trunk. In severe cases, respiratory muscle weakness accompanies limb and trunk symptoms. Generally, the natural history of the disease leads to recovery, with minor residual motor deficits occurring in 15% to 20% of patients. Mortality is about 5% to 10% worldwide (see Chapter 45).[38]

Myasthenia Gravis

Patients with myasthenia gravis experience weakness and fatigue of voluntary muscles, most frequently those innervated by cranial nerves, but peripheral and respiratory muscles can also be affected. The hallmark of the disorder is weakness made worse by exercise and improved by rest. The incidence in the United States is 2 to 5 cases per year per 1 million persons. Females are more affected than males (3:2). The primary abnormality is found at the neuromuscular junction, where transmission of impulses from nerve to muscle is impaired by a

decreased number of receptors on the muscle. Although myasthenia gravis is a chronic illness, the manifestations can often be managed by appropriate therapy, and individual episodes of respiratory failure are potentially reversible.[2] Respiratory failure in this disorder can be due to increasing severity of illness or overmedication (see Chapter 51).

CHEST WALL DEFORMITIES

Kyphoscoliosis

Etiology. Kyphoscoliosis may develop from an unknown cause (idiopathic) or may be related to congenital (Pott disease) or neuromuscular disease (muscular dystrophy, Marfan syndrome, neurofibromatosis, Friedreich ataxia, or poliomyelitis).[39] Most idiopathic cases of scoliosis are found in adolescents (11 years or older). The female to male ratio is 7:1.[40]

Pathogenesis. Commonly, a bony deformity of the chest wall occurs as a result of kyphosis (hunchback appearance; posterior curvature deformity) and scoliosis (lateral curvature deformity) (Figure 23-8). The higher the deformity in the vertebral column, the greater the compromise of respiratory status. Lung volumes are compressed, leading to atelectasis, $\dot{V}_A/\dot{Q}$ mismatch, and hypoxemia.[2]

Clinical manifestations. Common clinical features include dyspnea on exertion; rapid, shallow breathing; and chest wall deformity as evidenced by ribs protruding backward, flaring on the convex side, and being crowded on the concave side. Hypoxemia develops later, and eventually carbon dioxide retention occurs.[1]

Diagnosis. Diagnostic findings include hypercapnia, hypoxemia (due to $\dot{V}_A/\dot{Q}$ mismatch), and decreased lung volumes and lung capacities as

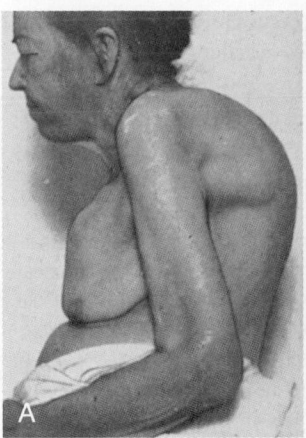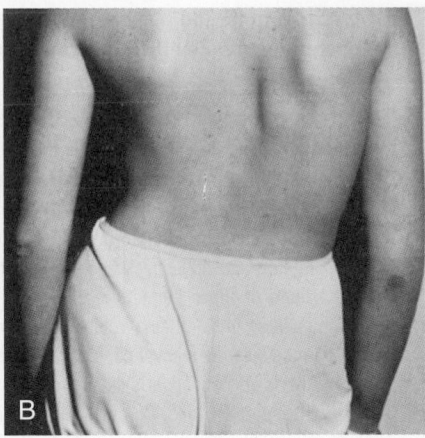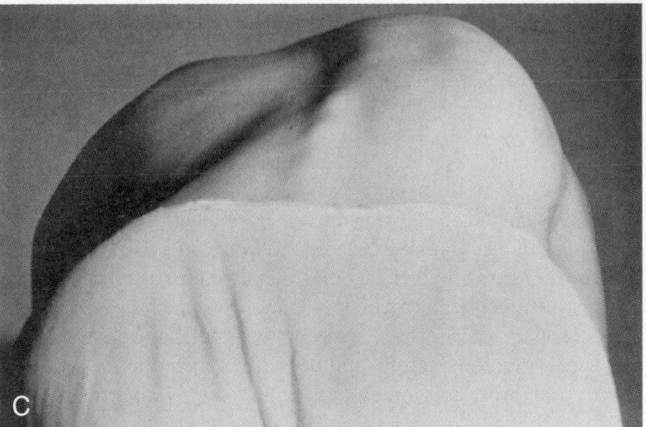

FIGURE 23-8 Kyphosis **(A)** and scoliosis **(B** and **C)** are structural deformities that can interfere with ventilation. (From Delp MH, Manning RT, editors: *Major's physical diagnosis,* ed 9, Philadelphia, 1981, Saunders.)

evidenced by decreased values on pulmonary function tests. Also noted are increased pulmonary arterial pressures because of the associated pulmonary hypoxemia. Radiographs show accentuated bony curves.[1,39,40] Screening for scoliosis and kyphoscoliosis in school-aged children has proved to be an excellent method of early diagnosis of these conditions.

Treatment. Treatment depends on the severity of the deformity and the age of the patient. Kyphosis in elderly persons, especially women, is commonly because of osteoporosis. Curvatures of less than 20 degrees should be monitored on a regular basis.[40] A postural exercise program for mild scoliosis and external braces for moderate scoliosis are recommended. For more advanced cases with curvatures greater than 40 degrees, electrical stimulation of the paraspinal muscles, spinal fusion, and spinal instrumentation (Harrington rod) placement for surgical stabilization are recommended treatments. Curvatures of greater than 60 degrees correlate with poor pulmonary function in later life.[40]

Ankylosing Spondylitis

Etiology. Ankylosing spondylitis occurs in both genders (male/female ratio of 3:1) and is commonly seen in the second or third decade of life.[1,41] It is characterized by chronic inflammation at the site of ligamentous insertion into the spine or sacroiliac joints. The precise cause is unknown. Ninety percent of patients with the disease have a positive HLA-B27 antigen (Chapter 10).[41] The respiratory system is affected by limited chest expansion and by the formation of pulmonary fibrosis in the upper lobes, which later develops into bronchiectasis and cavitation.[41] Transient acute arthritis of the peripheral joints occurs in about 50% of cases.[41]

Pathogenesis. Ankylosing spondylitis is a progressive inflammatory disease leading to immobility of the vertebral joints and fixation of the ribs.[1] The inflammatory process affects the articular processes, costovertebral joints, and sacroiliac joints by inducing a fibrotic response leading to joint calcification, ligament ossification, and skeletal immobility.

Clinical manifestations. Initial symptoms include low to middle back pain and stiffness that is more severe after prolonged rest. With exercise, the pain and stiffness decrease. As the disease process advances, rib cage movement is greatly reduced, leading to restrictive lung dysfunction.

Chest wall muscular atrophy is common and leads to further restriction of rib cage expansion. Breathing is largely accomplished by excursion of the diaphragm as the rib cage becomes immobilized. Associated problems seen with the disease include arthritis, uveitis, spondylitic heart disease, pulmonary fibrosis, and polyarteritis.[41]

Diagnosis. Pulmonary function tests show decreased vital capacity, decreased total lung capacity, and decreased compliance of the respiratory system, mainly the chest wall. Radiographs show destruction of cartilage, erosion of bone, calcification, and bony bridging of joint margins. The earliest radiologic changes are usually seen in the sacroiliac joints.[41] Laboratory findings, although not diagnostic of the disease, include an elevated sedimentation rate in 85% of cases as well as a decreased red blood cell count and an increased white blood cell count. HLA-B27 antigen is seen in 90% of cases.[41] However, 8% to 10% of the normal population have a positive HLA-B27.[41]

Treatment. General therapy includes development of an exercise program that includes breathing exercises and mobility exercises. Pharmacologic management with nonsteroidal antiinflammatory agents provides symptomatic relief of pain and stiffness and promotes function.

Flail Chest

Etiology. Flail chest results from multiple rib fractures as a result of trauma to the chest wall. The ribs are fractured at two distant sites, resulting in an unstable, free-floating chest wall segment that moves paradoxically inward on inspiration and outward on expiration. Bilateral costochondral separation and sternal fractures can also cause a flail segment.[42] Flail chest frequently occurs from the impact of the driver's chest with the steering wheel during an automobile accident.

Pathogenesis. Chest wall instability attributable to fracture at two distant sites on the same rib leads to an impairment of negative intrapleural pressure generation, causing decreased lung expansion on inspiration. The trauma commonly results in lung parenchymal injury, which may lead to pulmonary contusion, decreased lung compliance, and respiratory failure.[42] Interstitial and alveolar hemorrhage leads to abnormalities.

Clinical manifestations. Patients present after a trauma with paradoxical motion of the chest wall, either unilateral or bilateral. The injury to the chest wall is identified by careful inspection and palpation. Common features are marked shortness of breath, pain on inspiration, hypotension, cyanosis, and hypoxemia. The arterial Po_2 value is often low before clinical symptoms appear.[42] Pneumothorax, hemothorax, and subcutaneous emphysema are common (see Figure 23-5).

Diagnosis and treatment. Serial blood gas results help determine the treatment regimen. Flail chest, with large flail segments, resulting in acute respiratory failure is managed with mechanical ventilation.[35] Mechanical ventilation is achieved by positive pressure, which causes the entire chest, including the flail section, to move as a unit rather than paradoxically. Pain management may be accomplished by continuous epidural anesthesia.[42]

Disorders of Obesity

Etiology. *Obesity* is defined as excessive body fat, with a body mass index (BMI) greater than 30 kg/m^2 based on body weight and height. Overweight is defined as a BMI of 25 to 29.9 kg/m^2.[43] Obesity results from excessive caloric intake and/or reduced caloric expenditure. The National Health and Nutrition Exam survey reported that 59.4% of men and 49.9% of women are overweight. The findings for obesity were 19.9% of men and 25.1% of women.[44,45] A higher prevalence of obesity was found in blacks than in whites and in persons with lower incomes than in those with higher incomes.[43-45] Obese patients are at risk for a variety of disorders, the most common of which are diabetes mellitus, coronary artery disease, degenerative joint disease, gallstones, certain cancers (colon, rectum, and prostate in men; uterus, biliary tract, breast, and ovary in women), and pulmonary impairment. Persons with a BMI of ≥30 kg/m^2 have an all-cause increase in mortality of 50% to 100% compared to persons with a BMI between 20 and 25 kg/m^2.[43]

Pathogenesis. Endocrine causes of obesity are rare.[10] Hypothyroidism, the use of corticosteroids, and hypothalamic lesions all can lead to weight gain; however, the major cause of obesity is excess caloric intake in relation to caloric expenditure. Several hormones act on brain receptors to regulate appetite and metabolism. Leptin binds to brain receptors, causing the release of neuropeptides that promote satiety and increase metabolic rate. Ghrelin stimulates appetite. Genetic diseases such as familial partial lipodystrophy, Prader-Willi syndrome, Laurence-Moon syndrome, Bardet-Biedl syndrome, and Cohen syndrome are associated with obesity.[43-46] Obesity may be associated with hypoventilation. The mechanisms of obesity hypoventilation are reduced ventilatory drive and increased work of breathing. Some patients are thought to have an abnormality in the central nervous system.[1] In addition, the increased abdominal size can force the abdominal contents upward into the chest cavity, thus decreasing lung expansion and diaphragmatic shortening. Obesity hypoventilation is also called pickwickian syndrome, named after the obese boy in *Pickwick Papers* written by Charles Dickens. Pickwickian syndrome is associated with hypoventilation and airway obstruction.[1] An additional factor that contributes to the overall clinical picture in many obese patients is upper airway obstruction during sleep, the obstructive form of sleep apnea syndrome. Soft-tissue deposits in the neck and tissues surrounding the upper airway predispose the person to episodes of complete upper airway obstruction during sleep. In a large percentage of cases, the daytime somnolence that occurs in patients who have the obesity hypoventilation syndrome is related to obstructive sleep apnea.[44]

Clinical manifestations. Obesity hypoventilation is characterized by decreased alveolar ventilation, somnolence, severe hypoxemia, polycythemia, and cor pulmonale. Patients complain of daytime somnolence, impotence, shortness of breath, headache, and enuresis.

Diagnosis. The diagnosis of obesity is self-evident on examination. Tests for hypothyroidism, Cushing syndrome, insulinoma, diabetes, and hyperlipidemia may be done to identify comorbid factors.[43] For persons with hypoventilation, arterial blood gas analyses may reveal hypoxemia and hypercapnia. Chest wall compliance, vital capacity, total lung capacity, and expiratory reserve volume are all decreased. Patients may also have an increased red blood cell count and show signs and symptoms of cor pulmonale and pulmonary hypertension.

Treatment. Primary treatment for obesity consists of a weight loss program that includes the family members. Caloric intake that promotes an energy deficit of 500 to 1000 kcal/day is recommended. Aerobic exercise preserves lean body mass and increases energy expenditure.[43,44] Oxygen delivery through a nasal cannula or mechanical ventilation may be necessary for patients with morbid obesity. Surgical intervention with gastric stapling or gastric bypass to decrease the gastric volume and size has proved successful in some patients.[1] These operations are intended to permanently curtail food intake.

KEY POINTS

- Neuromuscular diseases affect the muscles of respiration, leading to muscular weakness, increased risk of pulmonary infections, and respiratory failure.
- Kyphoscoliosis is a deformity of the bony structure of the chest wall characterized by hunchback and lateral curvature of the spine. The abnormal shape of the chest interferes with the normal mechanics of breathing, resulting in small lung volumes, compression atelectasis, and hypoxemia. Compensatory tachypnea is usually present.
- Ankylosing spondylitis is a progressive inflammatory disease affecting vertebrae and ribs. Chronic inflammation leads to chest wall fibrosis and immobility. Chest wall muscle atrophy and rib cage stiffening result in pulmonary dysfunction characteristic of restrictive disorders.
- Obesity may interfere with the normal mechanics of breathing because of excessive chest weight and abdominal impingement on the chest cavity. Pickwickian syndrome is a disorder of obesity associated with hypoventilation and upper airway obstruction during sleep.

INFECTION OR INFLAMMATION OF THE LUNG

Pneumonia

Etiology. The term *pneumonia* (from the Greek *pneuma,* which means "breath") refers to an inflammatory reaction in the alveoli and interstitium of the lung, usually caused by an infectious agent. Pneumonia can result from three different sources: (1) aspiration of oropharyngeal secretions composed of normal bacterial flora and/or gastric contents (25% to 35% of all pneumonias); (2) inhalation of contaminants (virus, *Mycoplasma*); or (3) contamination from the systemic circulation.[2,47-49]

There are several ways to classify pneumonia. Pneumonias are typically classified as community acquired or hospital acquired. The incidence of community-acquired pneumonia is 1 in 100 persons. Approximately 15% to 20% of persons presenting with pneumonia require hospitilization.[50] Pneumonia is further classified as bacterial, atypical, and viral. The bacterial pneumonias may be grouped as either gram-positive or gram-negative, based on the staining characteristics of the organism. *Staphylococcus* and *Streptococcus* (including pneumococci) are the predominant gram-positive organisms. Gram-negative bacteria that may cause pneumonia include *Haemophilus influenzae, Klebsiella* species, *Pseudomonas aeruginosa, Serratia marcescens, Escherichia coli,* and *Proteus* species.

Patients at risk of pneumonia include the elderly; those with a diminished gag reflex; seriously ill, hospitalized patients; hypoxic patients; and immunocompromised patients.[50] Anaerobic bacteria may present clinically as a lung abscess, necrotizing pneumonia, or empyema. These diseases are usually caused by aspiration of normal oral bacteria (such as *Bacteroides* and *Fusobacterium*) into the lung.[2] Mycoplasmal pneumonia is more commonly seen in the summer and fall in young adults. About half of the cases of pneumonia in persons between 5 and 20 years of age can be classified as mycoplasmal pneumonia. Other causes of pneumonia occur less frequently in the general population. Legionnaires disease, for example, is a severe systemic illness characterized by fever, diarrhea, abdominal pain, liver and kidney failure, and pulmonary infiltrates. The causative organism for legionnaires disease lives in water and is transmitted by means of potable water, condensers, and cooling towers.[2] The current treatment of choice is administration of a macrolide antibiotic. Patients whose immune systems have been compromised by disease or by drug therapy may be susceptible to the development of opportunistic pneumonia.[50] For example, *Pneumocystis (carinii) jiroveci* pneumonia, an opportunistic fungal infection, is commonly found in patients with cancer or with human immunodeficiency virus (HIV). (See Chapter 12 for further discussion of acquired immunodeficiency syndrome [AIDS].)

Aspergillus, an opportunistic fungus that is widespread in nature, may cause progressive pneumonia. *Aspergillus* is released from the walls of old buildings under reconstruction. Attention should be given when old hospitals are renovated and when susceptible patients are located in a reconstruction area.[49] To assist the reader in differentiating among the various types of pneumonia, Table 23-7 presents the etiologic factors, common clinical features with age-related characteristics, radiologic findings, and antibiotic therapies for 11 forms of the disease.[2] There are many other types of pneumonia that are not listed.

Pathogenesis. Normally, pulmonary defense mechanisms (immune responses, cough reflex, sneezing, mucociliary clearance) protect individuals from pneumonia. Community-acquired pneumonia occurs when defense mechanisms are compromised.[2,46] A highly virulent organism may also overwhelm a person's defense mechanisms. Community-acquired pneumonias are commonly bacterial in origin.[46] After microbial agents enter the lung, they multiply and trigger pulmonary inflammation. Alveolar air spaces fill with an exudative fluid, and inflammatory cells invade the alveolar septa. Acute bacterial pneumonia may be associated with significant $\dot{V}_A/\dot{Q}$ mismatching and hypoxemia because inflammatory exudate collects in the alveolar spaces. Alveolar exudate tends to consolidate and becomes difficult to expectorate. Viral pneumonia does not produce exudative fluids.[2] Figure 23-9 shows the histologic progression of acute bacterial pneumonia. Patients with chronic illnesses and those who are immobile or immunosuppressed or have a decreased level of consciousness are at

TABLE 23-7 DIFFERENTIATING FEATURES OF TYPES OF PNEUMONIA

ETIOLOGIC ORGANISM	COMMON CLINICAL FEATURES	CHEST RADIOGRAPH	ANTIBIOTIC TREATMENT
Staphylococcus aureus; gram-positive cocci in clumps	Follows upper respiratory tract infection; fever, chills, pleuritic chest pain, cough, yellow purulent sputum; seen in patients in chronic care facilities	Consolidation, may have cavitation	Methicillin-susceptible strains: nafcillin or oxacillin with or without rifampin; methicillin-resistant strains: vancomycin with or without rifampin; alternative choice: cephalosporins, clindamycin, vancomycin
Streptococcus pneumoniae (pneumococcus); gram-positive diplococci	More common in alcoholics; also seen with chronic cardiopulmonary disease; fever, chills, pleuritic chest pain, cough, rust-colored sputum	Patchy infiltrates	Procaine penicillin G or aqueous penicillin G, amoxicillin; alternative choice: macrolides, cephalosporins, doxycycline, quinolones; prophylactic vaccine available
Haemophilus influenzae; pleomorphic gram-negative coccobacilli	Upper respiratory tract symptoms, fever, vomiting, irritability, cough, purulent sputum, dyspnea; affects children and older adults; affects people with chronic cardiorespiratory problems	Consolidation	Cefotaxime, ceftriaxone, doxycycline, azithromycin, TMP-SMX; alternative choice: quinolones or clarithromycin
Klebsiella pneumoniae; gram-negative encapsulated rods	Seen frequently in middle-aged men and associated with alcoholism and diabetes mellitus; rust-colored sputum	Consolidation	Aminoglycoside plus third-generation cephalosporin; alternative: aztreonam, imipenem, quinolone
Pseudomonas aeruginosa; gram-negative rods	Chronic obstructive pulmonary disease, cystic fibrosis, and mechanical ventilation; fever, chills, and copious greenish, foul-smelling sputum	Infiltrates, small pleural effusion	Aminoglycoside plus ticarcillin/clavulanate or piperacillin/tazobactam or aztreonam or imipenem
Escherichia coli; gram-negative rods	Complication of gastrointestinal surgery	Infiltrates, may have pleural effusion	Aminoglycoside plus third-generation cephalosporin; alternative: aztreonam, imipenem, quinolone
Virus	Fever, malaise, headache, nonproductive cough	Patchy infiltrates	Amantadine, rimantadine
Legionella species; no bacteria	Acute onset with fever, diarrhea, myalgia, and abdominal pain	Consolidation	Macrolides with or without rifampin; alternative: TMP-SMX, quinolone
Mycoplasma pneumoniae (atypical pneumonia); monocytes and neutrophils; no bacteria	Ages 5-25 years; most common in young adults; associated with otitis media and myringitis; sore throat, headache, myalgia, dry cough, fatigue, low-grade fever	Infiltrates	Erythromycin, doxycycline; alternative: quinolone or other macrolide
Pneumocystis (carinii) jiroveci (fungus)	Immunosuppressed patients (infants, children, and adults); 60% of patients have AIDS	Diffuse infiltrates, or chest x-ray may appear normal	TMP-SMX or pentamidine; isethionate plus prednisone; alternative: dapsone plus TMP-SMX, clindamycin plus primaquine
Anaerobic pneumonia (aspiration pneumonia); mixed flora	Predisposition to aspiration, fever, weight loss, malaise; risk increases with decreased level of consciousness, artificial airway, and sedation; seen in individuals with poor dental hygiene	Infiltrates in dependent lung fields	Penicillin G; alternative choices: clindamycin, metronidazole, cefoxitin

AIDS, Acquired immunodeficiency syndrome; *TMP-SMX,* trimethoprim-sulfamethoxazole.

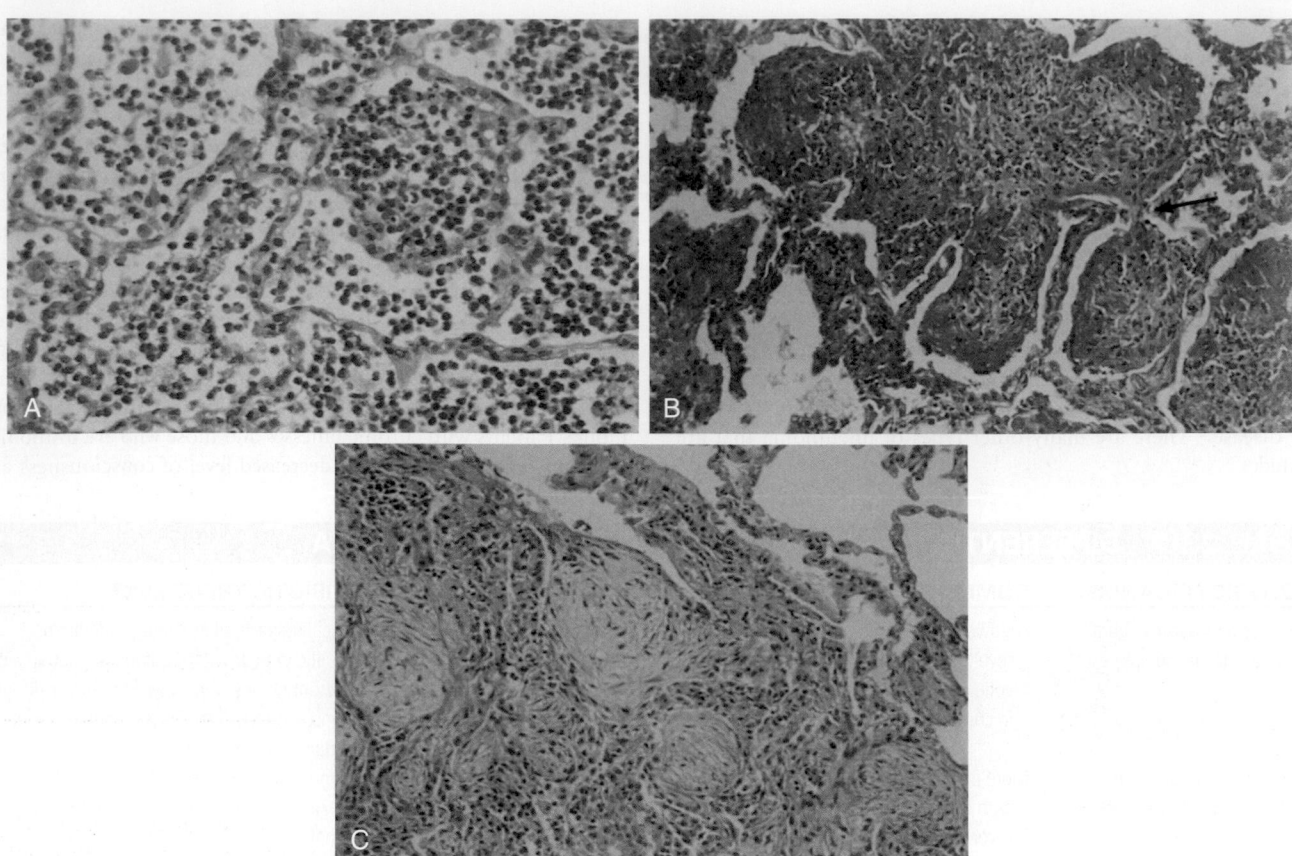

FIGURE 23-9 A, Acute bacterial pneumonia. The congested septal capillaries and extensive neutrophil exudation into the alveoli correspond to early red hepatization. Fibrin nets have not yet formed. **B,** Early organization of intraalveolar exudate, seen in areas to be streaming through pores of Kohn. **C,** Advanced organizing pneumonia corresponding to gray hepatization and featuring transformation of exudates to fibromyxoid masses richly infiltrated by macrophages and fibroblasts. (From Kumar V et al, editors: *Robbin's basic pathology,* ed 9, Philadelphia, 2013, Saunders.)

highest risk for developing pneumonia.[26] Disruption of the body's normal defense mechanisms leads to increased risk of pneumonia. Other patients at risk are those who have undergone thoracic or abdominal surgery or have received a general anesthetic.

Clinical manifestations. Clinically, the pathogenic cause, severity of the disease, and age of the patient may cause variations in the presentation of pneumonia. Some patients present with fever only.[30] Crackles (rales) and bronchial breath sounds may be heard over the affected lung tissue. Patients may present with chills, cough, purulent sputum, and an abnormal chest radiograph. Patients with viral pneumonia may present with an upper respiratory prodrome (fever, coryza, cough, hoarseness) accompanied by wheezing and/or rales.[26] Typical features of *Chlamydia* pneumonia are cough, tachypnea, rales, wheezes, and absence of fever. *Mycoplasma* pneumonia is a common cause of pneumonia in older children and adults.[26] Signs and symptoms include fever, cough, headache, and malaise.

Diagnosis. The chest radiograph demonstrates parenchymal infiltrates (white shadows) in the involved area, indicative of inflammatory alveolar processes.[2,26,47] In a patient with symptoms and clinical findings of pneumonia, a Gram stain of expectorated sputum from deep in the lungs may be obtained to distinguish bacterial from viral pneumonia and gram-negative from gram-positive organisms. If the patient had been previously healthy, the cause of the majority of these infections would be either viral, mycoplasmal, or the gram-positive pneumococcal bacterium. However, if the patient had been hospitalized or has other illnesses such as emphysema, diabetes, or alcoholism, then gram-negative organisms should be suspected.

"CURB-65" may be used to determine whether the patient should be hospitalized. "CURB-65" includes (1) *c*onfusion, (2) B*U*N >19.6 mg/dl, (3) *r*espiratory rate >30 breaths/min, (4) systolic *b*lood pressure (BP) <90 mm Hg and diastolic BP ≤60 mm Hg, and (5) age ≥65 years. Blood cultures are positive in approximately 20% of hospitalized patients.[49] Because 24 to 48 hours may be required for culture of the etiologic agent, antibiotic therapy should be started empirically.[2] Once culture and sensitivity results are obtained, antibiotic therapy may be changed. Diagnosis is based on the chest radiograph, white blood cell count (greater than 15,000/μL for acute bacterial pneumonia[26]), and sputum culture, coupled with clinical features of fever with recurrent chills, cough, dyspnea, and rales.

Treatment. Once the organism has been cultured, specific antibiotic selection is based on sensitivity of the organism to different antibiotics. Empirical treatment, before culture results for community-acquired pneumonia, consists of levofloxacin or a macrolide antibiotic. Table 23-7 presents treatment options.[49] The chest x-ray should be repeated 6 to 8 weeks after the infection has been treated.[50]

Severe Acute Respiratory Syndrome

Severe acute respiratory syndrome (SARS) was first reported in February 2003 as a severe form of pneumonia occurring in Asia. In that year, the disease spread to more than two dozen countries in North America, South America, Europe, and Asia before the global outbreak was contained.[51,52] According to the World Health Organization, a total of 8089 people became sick with SARS worldwide and 774 died. Extensive efforts at identification and containment prevented further spread of the disease, and the epidemic abated in mid-2003. Only eight confirmed SARS cases occurred in the United States during the epidemic.[51,52] Active global surveillance for SARS in human beings had detected no further confirmed person-to-person transmission of the disease between July 2003 and August 2004. However, two cases of SARS occurred in persons working in laboratories in southern China.

Etiology. SARS is caused by a coronavirus called SARS-associated coronavirus (SARS-CoV).[51,52] The primary mode of transmission appears to be through close person-to-person contact, most likely through respiratory droplets that are produced when a person coughs or sneezes. The virus also can spread through contact with contaminated objects or surfaces followed by touching the mouth, nose, or eyes.

Pathogenesis. The SARS virus epidemic was associated with milder disease in infants and children, and most of those with severe respiratory forms of the disease were adults. The median incubation period is about 4 to 6 days, and most patients become ill within 10 days after exposure.[50,51] Early clinical features of SARS are similar to those of other viral illnesses and include systemic signs and symptoms of an inflammatory response including fever, headache, and muscle aches. Respiratory complaints are also nonspecific and include nonproductive cough and shortness of breath. Nearly all patients develop radiographic evidence of pneumonia by days 7 to 10 of the illness, and the majority also develop lymphopenia (reduced number of lymphocytes in the blood).[51,52] The pneumonia can be severe with significant hypoxemia and an overall mortality of about 10%. In persons older than 60 years, the mortality may be close to 50%.[51,52]

Clinical manifestations. Most patients present with fever (temperature >100.4° F), myalgias, headache, nonproductive cough, and dyspnea, often without symptoms of an upper respiratory tract infection (no nasal drainage). Evidence of pneumonia on chest x-ray is usually apparent within 1 week of symptom onset. Lymphopenia may be evident on the complete blood count differential. There are no specific clinical manifestations for SARS, and it is unlikely as a cause of pneumonia unless there is a known history of exposure or travel to high-risk areas (mainland China, Hong Kong, or Taiwan). In the severe form of the disease, arterial blood gases reflect poor ventilation (low Pao_2 and increased $Paco_2$ measurements).

Diagnosis. No specific laboratory or clinical clues differentiate SARS-associated pneumonia from other forms of pneumonia at presentation of the patient. Early recognition and containment rely on a high index of suspicion based on clinical and epidemiologic factors. The vast majority of SARS cases during the epidemic had a clear history of exposure to a SARS patient or to a setting in which SARS-CoV transmission was known to have occurred. Patients presenting with manifestations of viral pneumonia severe enough to require hospitalization and a history of possible exposure should be tested for SARS. If known cases of SARS are occurring in the world, a lower threshold for testing may be instituted. Although not diagnostic, the following laboratory abnormalities have been seen in some patients with SARS: lymphopenia with a normal or low white blood cell count, elevated levels of liver enzymes, elevated creatine kinase concentration, elevated lactate dehydrogenase concentration, and prolonged activated partial thromboplastin time. Definitive diagnosis requires laboratory confirmation of SARS-CoV.[50,51] Respiratory specimens (e.g., from the nasopharynx, oropharynx, and sputum), blood, and stool can be tested for the presence of SARS virus.

Treatment. Currently, there are no definitive treatment recommendations for SARS. Patients with symptoms of pneumonia requiring hospitalization need supportive care, which may include administration of supplemental oxygen and mechanical ventilation. Evaluation for and treatment of other possible sources of pneumonia that may be responsive to antimicrobial therapy are recommended. Isolation precautions should be instituted in cases suspicious for SARS and discontinued only after consultation with local public health authorities.

KEY POINTS

- Pneumonia is an inflammation of the lung that is usually associated with an infectious agent. The most common types of pneumonia are bacterial, mycoplasmal, and viral. A productive cough is the primary differentiating feature between bacterial pneumonia and viral pneumonia, in which coughing is nonproductive.
- Acute bacterial pneumonia may be associated with significant $\dot{V}_A/\dot{Q}$ mismatching and poor blood gas values because inflammatory exudate collects in the alveolar spaces. Alveolar exudate tends to consolidate and becomes difficult to expectorate. Viral pneumonia does not produce exudative fluids.
- Manifestations of bacterial pneumonia may include fever, chills, cough with purulent sputum, crackles, and areas of consolidation on chest radiograph. Dyspnea may be significant.
- The treatment of bacterial pneumonia centers on antibiotic therapy to eliminate the organism and supportive therapy to enhance ventilation and oxygenation. Most cases of viral pneumonia (influenza) are managed symptomatically, because no effective antibiotic therapy is available.
- Fungal and protozoal pneumonias are uncommon and tend to occur in immunocompromised individuals.
- SARS is an acute respiratory tract infection caused by a coronavirus. The pneumonia is severe and has a mortality of 10%.

Pulmonary Tuberculosis

Etiology. Worldwide, 3 million people die of tuberculosis each year. There are an estimated 10 million people in the United States infected with tuberculosis.[2,53] More than 90% of cases involve reactivation of prior infection; the remainder are new infections. The majority of new cases occur in malnourished individuals, those living in overcrowded conditions, immunosuppressed individuals, incarcerated persons, immigrants (36% of new cases in the United States),[53] and elderly persons. Two thirds of all new cases are found in racial and ethnic minorities.[53] During the past 40 years, there has been a shift in the care of such patients from specialized tuberculosis hospitals to outpatient therapy. Hospitalization of such patients may be necessary with implementation of isolation precautions for a period of 2 to 4 weeks (longer for multidrug-resistant tuberculosis [MDR-TB]). In some countries, specialized tuberculosis hospitals have reopened owing to increasing resistance of the organism to treatment and an increasing number of cases. India and China account for nearly 50% of MDR-TB cases worldwide.[53] Tuberculosis cases should be reported to local and state health departments.

Tuberculosis is caused by the bacterium *Mycobacterium tuberculosis*, an acid-fast aerobic bacillus. Any organ system can be affected by the disease, but the most common sites are the lungs and the lymph nodes. Tuberculosis is subdivided into two major classifications: primary (usually clinically and radiographically silent[2]) and reactivating. Primary disease (initial infection) may lie dormant for many years or decades.[2] When the person's immune system becomes impaired, reactivation may occur. HIV, corticosteroid use, silicosis, and diabetes mellitus have been found to be associated with reactivation.[2] Reactivation may occur many years after the primary infection. Distant organ systems may be involved as a result of hematogenous spread during the primary or reactivation phase of infection. In addition, there may be disseminated disease, known as miliary tuberculosis, again resulting from hematogenous dissemination of the organisms. Strains of *M. tuberculosis* are becoming resistant to one or more first-line antituberculosis drugs.[45] MDR-TB accounts for 15% of the tuberculosis cases in the United States. Mortality rates range from 70% to 90% in hospitals or correctional facilities in Florida and New York, with a median survival of 4 to 16 weeks.[2] Entry into the body

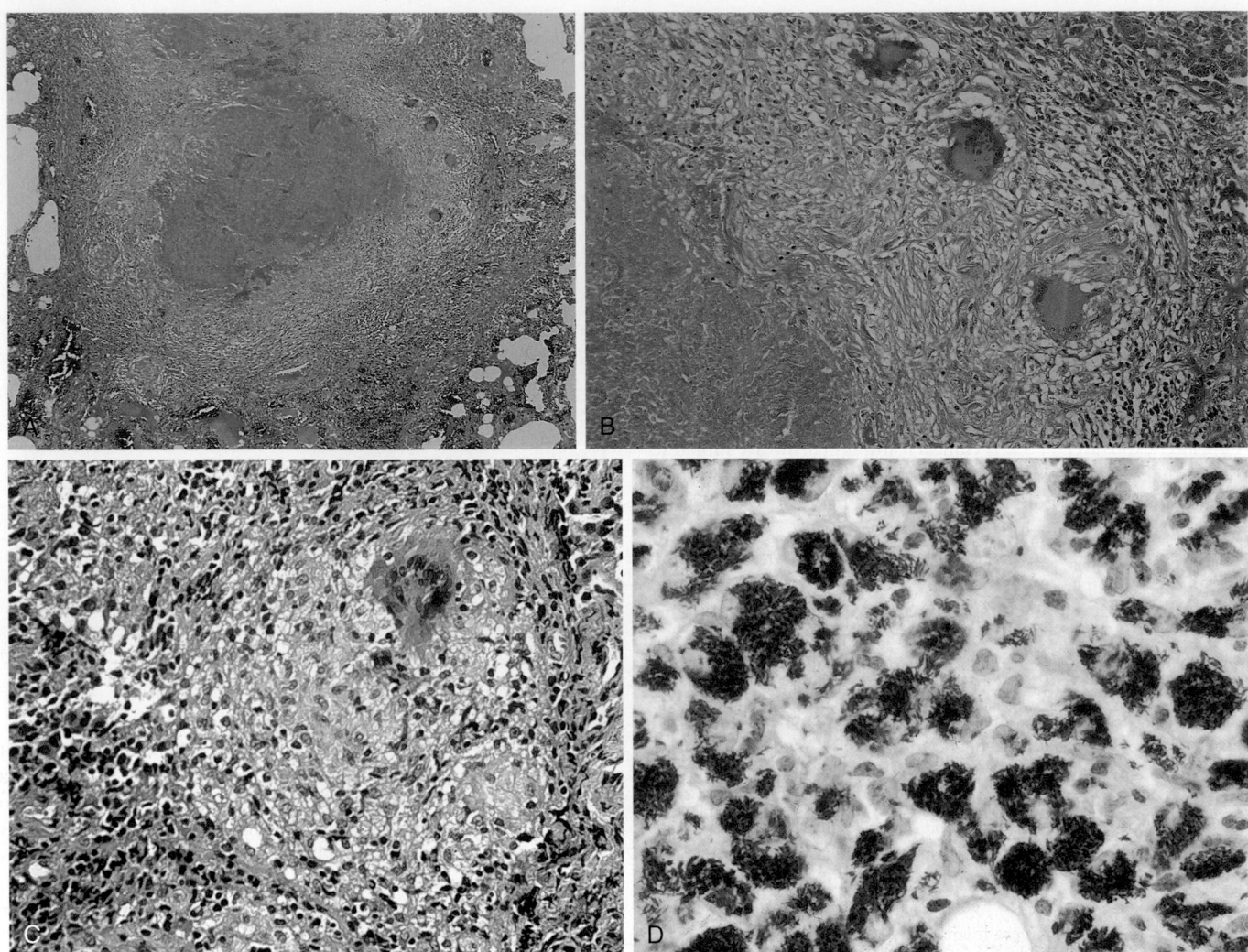

FIGURE 23-10 Morphologic spectrum of tuberculosis. A characteristic tubercle at low magnification **(A)** and in detail **(B)** illustrates central granular caseation surrounded by epithelioid and multinucleated giant cells. This is the usual response seen in patients who have developed cell-mediated immunity to the organism. Occasionally, even in immunocompetent individuals, tubercular granulomas may not show central caseation **(C)**. Therefore, irrespective of the presence or absence of caseous necrosis, special stains for acid-fast organisms need to be performed when granulomas are present in histologic sections. In immunosuppressed individuals, tuberculosis may not elicit a granulomatous response ("nonreactive tuberculosis"); instead, sheets of foamy histiocytes are seen, packed with mycobacteria that are demonstrable with acid-fast stains **(D)**. (From Kumar V et al, editors: *Robbin's basic pathology,* ed 8, Philadelphia, 2007, Saunders, p 519. **D,** Courtesy Dr. Dominick Cavuoti, Department of Pathology, University of Texas Southwestern Medical School, Dallas.)

is by inhalation of small (2 to 10 μm) droplets containing the bacteria. Infected droplets are expelled when an infected person coughs, sneezes, or talks.

Pathogenesis. After entrance of *Mycobacterium* into the lung tissue of the susceptible person, alveolar macrophages ingest and process the microorganisms. The organisms either are destroyed or persist and multiply. Once the infection becomes established, lymphatic and hematogenous dissemination occurs. T cells and macrophages surround the organisms in granulomas that limit multiplication and spread.[53] Dormant organisms persist for years. Reactivation may occur if the patient's immune system becomes impaired.[2,53] *Mycobacterium tuberculosis* is a slow-growing aerobic, non–spore-forming, nonmobile bacillus. It has a lipid-rich cell wall that lacks pigment and produces niacin growth in liquid media (BACTEC), requiring 9 to 16 days for culture results.[53] The pathologic manifestation of

pulmonary tuberculosis is the Ghon tubercle or complex, which has parenchymal and lymph components. The parenchymal component is composed of a well-circumscribed necrotic nodule that later becomes fibrotic and calcified. The lymph component is found in the lymph nodes. Primary pulmonary tuberculosis is shown in Figure 23-10.

Clinical manifestations. Clinical features of reactivated disease include a history of contact with an infected person, low-grade fever, cough, night sweats, fatigue, weight loss, malaise, and anorexia. Chronic cough is the most common symptom.[2,54] As the disease progresses, the patient develops a productive cough with purulent sputum. Physical examination of the lung fields reveals apical crackles (rales) (*M. tuberculosis* organisms prefer lung apices because of the higher concentration of oxygen in the apices) or bronchial breath sounds over the region of lung consolidation. The patient appears malnourished and chronically ill.[2] Common sites of extrapulmonary tuberculosis are

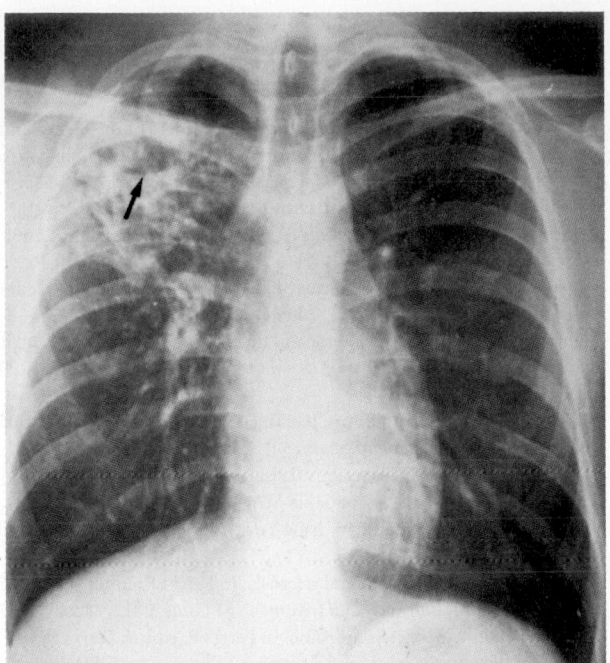

FIGURE 23-11 Cavitary pulmonary tuberculosis in a 23-year-old man. (From Kersten LD: *Comprehensive respiratory nursing*, Philadelphia, 1989, Saunders, p 146.)

the peritoneum, gastrointestinal tract, liver, spleen, bone, joints, lymph nodes, central nervous system, and genitourinary system.[54] (Refer to Chapter 12 for a discussion of tuberculosis in HIV-infected patients.) Results of pulmonary function tests are characteristic of restrictive diseases, with decreased lung volumes and decreased compliance.

Diagnosis. Definitive diagnosis is made by results of sputum culture or by identification of the organism by DNA or RNA amplification techniques.[54] Three consecutive morning sputum specimens are obtained to identify the slow-growing acid-fast bacillus. Expectoration of sputum in the early morning is ideal because the sputum is more concentrated and more plentiful. Cultures require 1 to 3 weeks for determination.[54] Gastric washings or bronchial washings may also be used for diagnostic culturing. Chest radiographs usually show nodules with infiltrates in the lung apex and posterior segments of the upper lobes. Elderly patients may present with lower lobe infiltrates with or without pleural effusion. Figure 23-11 shows the radiographic appearance of cavitary tuberculosis in a 23-year-old man. A miliary pattern (diffuse, small nodular densities) is seen with dissemination of the organism in miliary tuberculosis.[2] Another diagnostic test is the tuberculin

(Mantoux test) skin test (5 tuberculin units/0.1 ml of purified protein derivative [PPD] injected intradermally). This test does not distinguish between current disease and past infection. If the induration in a person with HIV infection is 5 mm or greater, if the patient has close contact with individuals with tuberculosis, and if the patient has a chest radiograph consistent with tuberculosis, the likelihood of active disease is high.[1] An induration of 10 mm or greater is the reaction size for other high-risk individuals, such as intravenous drug abusers, individuals who are debilitated, children younger than 4 years or with immunosuppression, and individuals living in countries with a high incidence of the disease (Asia, Africa, Latin America). An induration of 15 mm or greater is considered positive for tuberculosis in all other persons.[2,54]

False-positive PPD results may occur in persons with other mycobacterial infections or if they have received bacille Calmette-Guérin (BCG), a live attenuated strain of *Mycobacterium bovis* that provides active immunity against tuberculosis. False-negative results may also occur in patients who are malnourished, elderly, or immunocompromised.[2] Immunocompromised patients may not be able to mount a response (wheal) to injection of the organism.

Treatment. Primary therapy for active tuberculosis consists of (1) administering multiple drugs to which the organism is susceptible; (2) adding at least two new agents to the drug regimen, when treatment failure is suspected; (3) providing the safest, most effective therapy for the shortest period of time; and (4) ensuring adherence to therapy by utilizing directly observed therapy.[2] Nonadherence to therapy because of adverse drug reactions is a major cause of treatment failure. HIV-negative individuals without MDR-TB are typically treated for 6 to 9 months.

> **KEY POINTS**
> - Tuberculosis is caused by inhalation or ingestion of the bacterium *Mycobacterium tuberculosis*. The organism spreads through the lymph and blood. Bacteria are ingested by macrophages and walled off by inflammatory proteins (granulomas). The organisms may not be killed and can persist in a dormant state for years. These walled-off areas of inflammatory cells and bacteria become fibrotic and calcified, forming Ghon tubercles—the hallmark of tuberculosis.
> - Symptoms are somewhat nonspecific: low-grade fever, cough, night sweats, fatigue, and weight loss. With progression of the disease, the cough is productive of purulent sputum.
> - The diagnosis is based on a positive purified protein derivative skin test for tuberculosis, positive sputum cultures, and characteristic nodules on chest radiographs.
> - Antibiotics are used for managing tuberculosis. Drug therapy continues for 9 to 12 months for active disease and may be used for shorter periods in persons exposed to tuberculosis but having no active disease.

SUMMARY

Restrictive pulmonary disorders are those in which lung expansion is restricted. Restrictions are commonly caused by diseases that affect the lung parenchyma (e.g., diffuse interstitial pulmonary fibrosis), chest wall disorders, neuromuscular disorders, pleural space disorders, pneumonia, and tuberculosis. These diseases are characterized by a reduced vital capacity and a small residual lung volume. They differ from obstructive diseases, covered in Chapter 22, in that airway resistance is not increased.

REFERENCES

1. West JB: *Pulmonary pathophysiology: the essentials*, ed 7, Philadelphia, 2007, Lippincott Williams & Wilkins.
2. Chesnutt MS, Prendergart TJ: Pulmonary disorders. In McPhee SI, Papadakis MA, editors: *Current medical diagnosis and treatment*, ed 46, New York, 2007, Lange/McGraw-Hill, pp 285–286.
3. Shih G, Gleit C: Interstitial lung disease. In Ferri FF, editor: *Ferri's clinical advisor: instant diagnosis and treatment*, St Louis, 2012, Mosby, p 555.
4. Yusen RD, Mayse ML, Chakinala M, et al: Pulmonary diseases. In Cooper DH, et al, editors: *The Washington manual of medical therapeutics*, ed 32, Philadelphia, 2007, Lippincott Williams & Wilkins, pp 245–289.

5. Goroll AH, Mulley AG: Management of sarcoidosis: evaluation of interstitial lung disease. In Goroll AH, Mulley AG, editors: *Primary care medicine: office evaluation and management of the adult patient*, ed 5, Philadelphia, 2006, Lippincott Williams & Wilkins, pp 384–387.

6. King TE, Schwartz MJ: Approach to diagnosis and management of the idiopathic interstitial pneumonias. In Mason RJ, Broaddus VC, Murray JF, et al, editors: *Murray and Nadel's textbook of respiratory medicine*, ed 4, Philadelphia, 2005, Saunders, pp 1571–1608.

7. Ferreria A, Garvey C, Conners GL, et al: Pulmonary rehabilitation in interstitial lung disease, *Chest* 135(2):442–477, 2009.

8. Costabel U: Ask the expert—diffuse interstitial lung disease, *Breathe* 4(2):165–172, 2007.

9. Ferri FF: Sarcoidosis. In Ferri FF, editor: *Ferri's clinical advisor: instant diagnosis and treatment*, St Louis, 2011, Mosby, pp 907–908.

10. Zacharisen MC: Hypersensitivity pneumonitis. In Rakel RE, Bope ET, editors: *Conn's current therapy*, Philadelphia, 2008, Elsevier, pp 276–278.

11. Thurlbeck WM, Miller RR: The respiratory system. In Rubin E, Farber JL, editors: *Essential pathology*, ed 3, Philadelphia, 2001, Lippincott Williams & Wilkins, pp 542–627.

12. O'Conner CJ, Kramer K: Hypersensitivity pneumonitis. In Ferri FF, editor: *Ferri's clinical advisor: instant diagnosis and treatment*, St Louis, 2011, Mosby, pp 513–514.

13. Toren K, Blanc PD: Asthma caused by occupational exposures is common—a systematic analysis of estimates of the population—attributable fraction, *BMC Pulm Med* 9:7, 2009.

14. Oliver LC, Stoeckle JD: Evaluation and prevention of occupational and environmental respiratory disease. In Goroll AH, Mulley AG, editors: *Primary care medicine: office evaluation and management of the adult patient*, ed 5, Philadelphia, 2006, Lippincott Williams & Wilkins, pp 309–314.

15. West JB: *Pulmonary physiology and pathophysiology: an integrated, case-based approach*, ed 2, Philadelphia, 2007, Lippincott Williams & Wilkins.

16. Ferri FF: Acute respiratory distress syndrome. In Ferri FF, editor: *Ferri's clinical advisor: instant diagnosis and treatment*, St Louis, 2011, Mosby, pp 35–36.

17. Irvine LA: Neonatology. In Gunn VL, Nochyba C, editors: *The Harriet Lane handbook*, ed 17, Philadelphia, 2005, Mosby.

18. Carpenter TC, Dobyns EL, Grayck EN, et al: Critical care. In Hay WW, et al, editors: *Current pediatrics: diagnosis and treatment*, ed 18, New York, 2007, Lange/McGraw-Hill, pp 368–372.

19. Hansen AK, Wisborg K, Uldberg N, Henriksen TB: Risk of respiratory morbidity in term infants delivered by elective caesarean section: cohort study, *BMJ, 2007*. Online First, 1–7.

20. *Neonatal handbook: respiratory distress syndrome*. Available at www.netsvic.org.au/nets/handbook/index.cfm. Accessed February 2012.

21. Pramanik A: *Respiratory distress syndrome*. Available at http://emedicine.medscape.com/article/976034-overview. Accessed February 2012.

22. Pagana KD, Pagana TJ: *Mosby's diagnostic and laboratory test reference*, ed 8, St Louis, 2007, Elsevier.

23. McEvoy C, Schilling D, Peters D, Tillotson C, Spitale P, et al: Respiratory compliance in preterm infants after single rescue of antenatal steroids: a randomized controlled trial, *Am J Obstet Gynecol* 202(6), 544.e1-9, 2010.

24. Regnante R, Korr K: Pneumothorax, spontaneous. In Ferri FF, editor: *Ferri's clinical advisor: instant diagnosis and treatment*, St Louis, 2007, Mosby, pp 702–703.

25. Gordon CE, Feller-Kopman D, Balk EM, Smetana GW: Pneumothorax following thoracentesis, *Arch Intern Med* 170(4):332–339, 2010.

26. Thilo EN, Rosenberg AA: The newborn infant. In Hay WW, et al, editors: *Current pediatrics: diagnosis and treatment*, ed 18, New York, 2007, Lange/McGraw-Hill, pp 1–64.

27. Kerby GS, Accurso FJ, Deterding RR, et al: Respiratory tract and mediastinum. In Hay WW, et al, editors: *Current pediatrics: diagnosis and treatment*, ed 18, New York, 2007, Lange/McGraw-Hill, pp 493–541.

28. Theodore PR, Jablons D: Thoracic wall, pleura, mediastinum and lung. In Doherty GM, editor: *Current surgical diagnosis and treatment*, ed 12, New York, 2005, Lange/McGraw-Hill, pp 325–389.

29. Guyton AC, Hall JE: *Textbook of medical physiology*, ed 11, Philadelphia, 2006, Elsevier.

30. Goroll AH, Mulley AG: Evaluation of pleural effusions. In Goroll AH, Mulley AG, editors: *Primary care medicine: office evaluation and management of the adult patient*, ed 5, Philadelphia, 2006, Lippincott Williams & Wilkins, pp 329–334.

31. Kerby GS, Accurso FJ, Deterding RR, et al: Disorders of the pleura and pleural cavity. In Hay WW, et al, editors: *Current pediatrics: diagnosis and treatment*, ed 18, New York, 2007, Lange/McGraw-Hill, pp 534–535.

32. Cassivi SD, McKellar SH: Pleural effusion and empyema thoracic. In Rakel RE, Bope ET, editors: *Conn's current therapy*, Philadelphia, 2008, Elsevier, pp 248–250.

33. Wong CL, Holroyd-Loduc J, Straus SE: Does this patient have a pleural effusion? *JAMA* 301(3):309–317, 2009.

34. Light RW: Disorders of the pleura and mediastinum. In Fauci AS, et al, editors: *Harrison's principles of internal medicine*, ed 17, New York, 2008, McGraw-Hill, pp 1658–1661.

35. Mikolich DJ, Fort GG: Poliomyelitis. In Ferri FF, editor: *Ferri's clinical advisor: instant diagnosis and treatment*, St Louis, 2012, Mosby, p 802.

36. Shandera WX, Koo H: Infectious diseases: viral and rickettsial. In Tierney LM, McPhee SI, Papadakis MA, editors: *Current medical diagnosis and treatment*, ed 46, New York, 2007, Lange/McGraw-Hill, pp 1378–1430.

37. Harrison T: Amyotrophic lateral sclerosis. In Ferri FF, editor: *Ferri's clinical advisor: instant diagnosis and treatment*, St Louis, 2012, Mosby, p 57.

38. Ubogu EE: Guillain-Barré syndrome. In Ferri FF, editor: *Ferri's clinical advisor: instant diagnosis and treatment*, St Louis, 2007, Mosby, pp 367–368.

39. Eilert RE: Orthopedics. In Hay WW, et al, editors: *Current pediatrics: diagnosis and treatment*, ed 18, New York, 2007, Lange/McGraw-Hill, pp 787–805.

40. Mercier LR: Scoliosis. In Ferri FF, editor: *Ferri's clinical advisor: instant diagnosis and treatment*, St Louis, 2007, Mosby, p 808.

41. Hellmann DB, Stone JH: Arthritis and musculoskeletal disorders. In Tierney LM, McPhee SI, Papadakis MA, editors: *Current medical diagnosis and treatment*, New York, 2007, Lange/McGraw-Hill, pp 807–825.

42. Hemmila MR, Wahl WL: Management of the injured patient. In Doherty GM, editor: *Current surgical diagnosis and treatment*, ed 12, New York, 2006, Lange/McGraw-Hill, pp 207–244.

43. Iannuccilli J: Obesity. In Ferri FF, editor: *Ferri's clinical advisor: instant diagnosis and treatment*, St Louis, 2007, Mosby, pp 615–617.

44. Baron RB: Nutrition. In Tierney LM, McPhee SI, Papadakis MA, editors: *Current medical diagnosis and treatment*, ed 46, New York, 2007, Lange/McGraw-Hill, pp 1279–1310.

45. The National Health and Nutrition Examination Survey (NHANES): *Analytic and reporting guidelines*. Available at www.cdc.gov/nchs/data/nhanes_20_04/nhanes_analytic_guidelines_dec_2005.pdf.

46. Fitzgerald PA: Endocrinology. In Tierney LM, McPhee SI, Papadakis MA, editors: *Current medical diagnosis and treatment*, ed 46, New York, 2007, Lange/McGraw-Hill, pp 1123–1218.

47. Manden LA, Wanderink R, et al: Pneumonia. In Fauci AS, editor: *Harrison's principles of internal medicine*, ed 17, New York, 2008, McGraw-Hill, pp 1619–1629.

48. Hatipoglu U, Rubinstein I: Bacterial pneumonia. In Rakel RE, Bope ET, editors: *Conn's current therapy*, Philadelphia, 2008, Elsevier, pp 253–260.

49. Kerby GS, Accurso FJ, Deterding RR, et al: Acquired disorders involving the alveoli. In Hay WW, et al, editors: *Current pediatrics: diagnosis and treatment*, ed 18, New York, 2007, Lange/McGraw-Hill, pp 517–521.

50. Ferri FF: Bacterial pneumonia. In Ferri FF, editor: *Ferri's clinical advisor: instant diagnosis and treatment*, St Louis, 2012, Mosby, pp 792–793.

51. Centers for Disease Control and Prevention: *Severe acute respiratory syndrome*. Available at www.cdc.gov/ncidod/sars/2007.

52. Ferri FF: Severe acute respiratory syndrome. In Ferri FF, editor: *Ferri's clinical advisor: instant diagnosis and treatment*, St Louis, 2007, Mosby, pp 818–819.

53. Opal SM, Alonso GO: Tuberculosis, pulmonary. In Ferri FF, editor: *Ferri's clinical advisor: instant diagnosis and treatment*, St Louis, 2007, Mosby, pp 923–926.

54. Sharma SK, Mohan A: Tuberculosis and other mycobacterial diseases. In Rakel RE, Bope ET, editors: *Conn's current therapy*, Philadelphia, 2008, Elsevier, pp 278–287.

Fluid and Electrolyte Homeostasis and Imbalances

Linda Felver

⊖volve WEBSITE

http://evolve.elsevier.com/Copstead/

- Review Questions and Answers
- Glossary (with audio pronunciations for selected terms)
- Animations

- Case Studies
- Key Points Review

KEY QUESTIONS

- What physiologic and pathophysiologic conditions predispose an individual to disturbances in fluid intake?
- How do the compositions of plasma and interstitial fluids differ? How are they similar?
- What regulates water and electrolyte movement between plasma and interstitial fluids? Across cell membranes?
- What are the usual and pathologic routes of fluid exit from the body?
- Under what conditions are extracellular volume deficit and excess likely to occur, and what are the characteristic clinical findings?

- Under what conditions are hyponatremia (water excess) and hypernatremia (water deficit) likely to occur, and what are the characteristic clinical findings?
- What capillary-level mechanisms cause edema?
- What physiologic and pathophysiologic conditions can lead to alterations in electrolyte intake, absorption, distribution, or excretion? How do these differ between specific electrolytes?
- What are the characteristic clinical findings of plasma excesses and deficits of potassium, calcium, magnesium, and phosphate ions?

CHAPTER OUTLINE

The fluid of the body flows in arteries, veins, and lymph vessels; it is secreted into specialized compartments as diverse as joints, cerebral ventricles, and the intestinal lumen; it both surrounds and permeates the cells. Body fluid serves as a lubricant and as a solvent for the chemical reactions that we call *metabolism;* it transports oxygen, nutrients, chemical messengers, and waste products to their destinations; it plays an important role in the regulation of body temperature. Because the fluid within the body is so widespread and serves so many functions, it is not surprising that abnormalities in the volume, concentration, or electrolyte composition of body fluid cause clinical problems.

Disorders of fluid or electrolyte homeostasis occur as a result of many different pathophysiologic conditions. In severe cases, these disorders cause death. Although these disorders develop from many specific causes in different patient populations, these specific causes fall into general categories that arise from the principles of normal fluid and electrolyte homeostasis. This chapter first presents the principles of normal fluid homeostasis and then, building on that foundation, continues with a discussion of fluid imbalances. Similarly, it explains the principles of electrolyte homeostasis before presenting plasma electrolyte imbalances.

BODY FLUID HOMEOSTASIS

The term **body fluid,** as used in this chapter, pertains to water within the body and the particles dissolved in it. The body fluid is contained in two major compartments: **extracellular** (outside the cells) and **intracellular** (inside the cells). In all age groups except infants, approximately two thirds of body fluid is intracellular.[1] The other one third of body fluid is extracellular. Infants have more extracellular fluid than intracellular fluid; this proportion reverses within a few months as the infant grows. The extracellular fluid lies between the cells (**interstitial** compartment), in the blood vessels (**vascular** compartment), in dense connective tissue and bone, and in several minor compartments that are collectively termed the **transcellular** fluids (e.g., synovial, cerebrospinal, and gastrointestinal fluids). The major body fluid compartments are depicted in Figure 24-1.

The fluids in the various body compartments have different compositions, although their total particle concentration is equal. The intracellular fluid is relatively rich in potassium and magnesium ions,

inorganic and organic phosphates, and proteins. It is relatively low in sodium and chloride ions. In contrast, the extracellular fluid in the vascular and interstitial compartments is relatively rich in sodium, chloride, and bicarbonate ions and relatively low in potassium, magnesium, and phosphate ions. The vascular portion of the extracellular fluid contains many proteins, whereas the interstitial and transcellular portions of the extracellular fluid contain very few proteins. Most transcellular fluids are secreted by epithelial cells; their composition varies according to their function.

Total body water is the total amount of water in all fluid compartments. The percentage of body weight that is water varies according to a person's age and proportion of body fat (Figure 24-2). A full-term newborn infant is about 75% water by weight. (Preterm infants have an even higher percentage of water.) This percentage decreases with age. In a standard adult man, body water is about 60% of body weight. The percentage is less (about 50%) in women because they have a greater proportion of body fat than men of the same weight. In obese adults, with a much larger proportion of body fat, less of the body weight is water. With normal aging there is a relative increase in body fat, so that in older men, 50% of the body weight is typically composed of water; in older women, it is even less.

One liter of water weighs 1 kg (2.2 lb). Thus, a lean, middle-aged, healthy adult man who weighs 70 kg (154 lb) has approximately 42 L of body water. Of this amount, approximately 25 L is intracellular water. The approximately 17 L of extracellular water is distributed as 3 L of plasma water, 8 L of interstitial and lymph water, 5 L of water trapped in dense connective tissue and bone, and 1 L of transcellular water.

Fluid homeostasis is a dynamic process. This process may be viewed as the net result of four subprocesses: *fluid intake, fluid absorption, fluid distribution,* and *fluid excretion.* In some individuals who have pathophysiologic conditions, loss of fluid through abnormal routes also occurs. The interplay of these subprocesses is fluid homeostasis (Figure 24-3).

Fluid Intake and Absorption

Fluid intake is entry of fluid into the body by any route. People normally ingest fluids orally, both by drinking and by eating (water contained in food). They also synthesize a small amount of water through cellular metabolism of the foods they eat. Fluid intake by drinking is

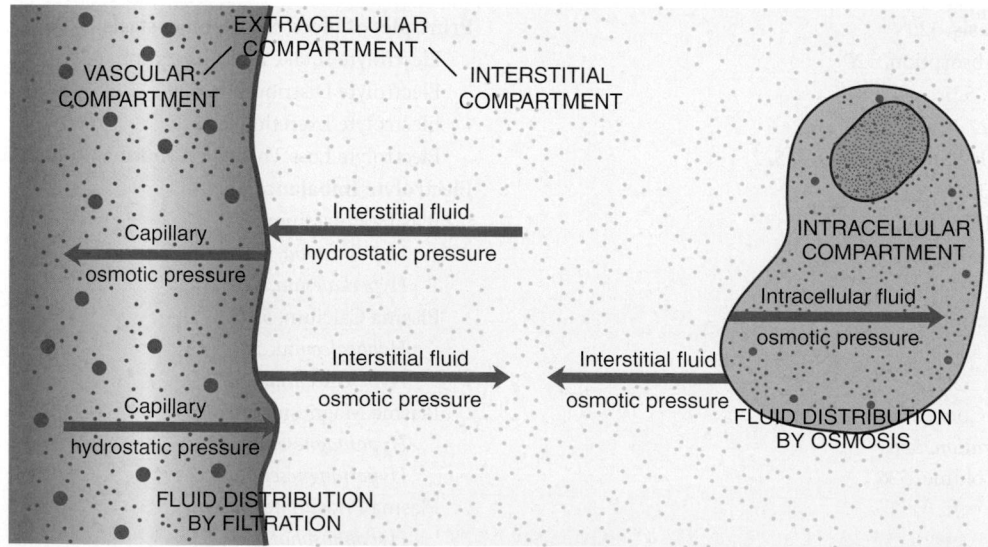

FIGURE 24-1 Factors that influence body fluid distribution. Fluid distribution between the vascular and interstitial compartments is the net result of filtration across permeable capillaries. The distribution of fluid between the interstitial and intracellular compartments occurs by osmosis rather than by filtration.

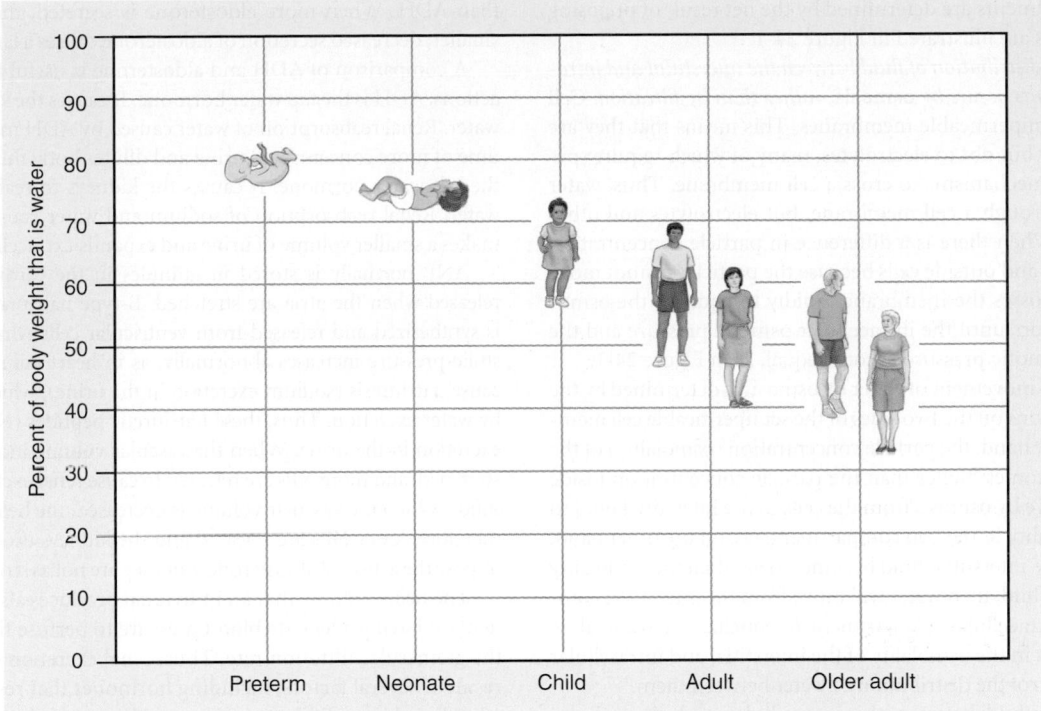

FIGURE 24-2 Percentage of total body water by age. The percentage of body weight that is water is high in infancy and decreases with increasing age.

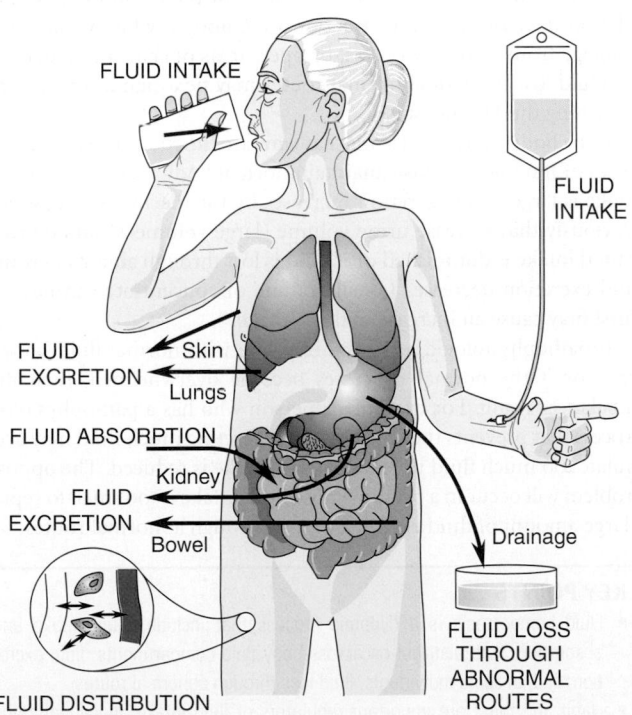

FIGURE 24-3 Fluid homeostasis. Fluid homeostasis is the interplay of fluid intake and absorption, fluid distribution, fluid excretion, and fluid loss through abnormal routes.

influenced by habit, social factors, and thirst. Physiologic triggers of thirst include increased **osmolality** (concentratedness) of extracellular fluid (osmoreceptor-mediated thirst); decreased circulating blood volume (baroreceptor-mediated and angiotensin II–mediated thirst); and dryness of the mucous membranes of the mouth and possibly other

visceral signals.[2] In older adults, cerebral osmoreceptor-mediated thirst diminishes; thus, older adults who do not have a habit of drinking fluids throughout the day may not have sufficient fluid intake to meet their needs.[3]

Additional routes of fluid intake that may occur in patients who have various pathophysiologic conditions include intravenous intake; intake tubes into the gastrointestinal tract, other body cavities, subcutaneous tissue, or bone marrow; rectal intake (such as tap water enema); and, occasionally, intake through the lungs (such as near-drowning). Health care professionals often control fluid intake by many of these routes.

Unless fluid intake occurs intravenously, the fluid must be absorbed before it reaches the vascular compartment. Fluid absorption from the gastrointestinal tract partially depends on osmotic forces generated by absorption of electrolytes and other particles.

Fluid Distribution

Much of the fluid that reaches the vascular compartment then distributes into other fluid compartments. *Fluid distribution between the vascular and interstitial compartments is the net result of* **filtration** *across permeable capillaries.* At the capillary level, two forces tend to move fluid from the capillaries into the interstitial compartment: capillary hydrostatic pressure (the outward push of vascular fluid against the capillary walls) and interstitial fluid osmotic pressure (the inward-pulling force of particles in the interstitial fluid). Concurrently, two forces tend to move fluid from the interstitial compartment into the capillaries: capillary osmotic pressure (the inward-pulling force of particles in vascular fluid) and interstitial fluid hydrostatic pressure (the outward push of interstitial fluid against the outside of the capillary walls).[1]

The distribution of fluid between the vascular and interstitial compartments is analogous to two groups of people pushing on opposite sides of a swinging door—the strongest "push" will determine in which direction the door will swing. Thus, at any one point along a capillary, the direction and amount of fluid flow between the vascular and interstitial compartments are determined by the net result of opposing forces. These forces are illustrated in Figure 24-1.

In contrast, *the distribution of fluid between the interstitial and intracellular compartments occurs by* **osmosis,** *rather than by filtration.* Cell membranes are semipermeable membranes. This means that they are permeable to water but not to electrolytes, many of which require specialized transport mechanisms to cross a cell membrane. Thus, water can move freely through a cell membrane, but electrolytes and other particles cannot. When there is a difference in particle concentration (osmolality) inside and outside cells because the particles cannot move freely, the *water* crosses the membrane rapidly to equalize the osmolality. Osmosis occurs until the intracellular osmotic pressure and the interstitial fluid osmotic pressure become equal, as in Figure 24-1.

The direction of movement of water by osmosis is determined by the particle concentrations on the two sides of the semipermeable cell membrane. If, on the one hand, the particle concentration (osmolality) of the interstitial fluid becomes higher than the particle concentration inside cells, water will move by osmosis from the cells to the interstitial fluid to equalize the osmolality in the two compartments. If, on the other hand, the osmolality of the interstitial fluid becomes lower than the osmolality of the intracellular fluid, then water will move from the interstitial compartment to the intracellular compartment to equalize the osmolality. In this way, changes in the osmolality of the interstitial and intracellular compartments control the distribution of water between them.[1]

Distribution of fluid between the intracellular and transcellular compartments is controlled by processes within the epithelial cells that secrete these fluids.

Fluid Excretion

The fourth component of fluid homeostasis is fluid excretion. Fluid excretion normally occurs through the urinary tract, bowels, lungs, and skin. Fluid is excreted through the skin as visible sweat (which may or may not occur) and as insensible perspiration (which always occurs). Another obligatory route of excretion of water is through the lungs as a person exhales. Fecal excretion of fluid occurs with normal bowel function and increases dramatically in a person who has diarrhea. In most circumstances, the largest volume of fluid is excreted in the urine.

The amount of fluid excreted in the urine is controlled primarily by the hormones antidiuretic hormone (ADH), aldosterone, and natriuretic peptides (e.g., A-type natriuretic peptide [ANP]), and to a lesser degree by minor hormones such as renal prostaglandins and by the renal sympathetic nerves. ADH is synthesized by cells in the supraoptic and paraventricular nuclei of the hypothalamus. The axons of these cells extend down the median eminence of the pituitary stalk. The release of ADH thus occurs from the posterior pituitary gland. Factors that increase release of ADH into the blood include increased osmolality (concentratedness) of the extracellular fluid, decreased circulating fluid volume, pain, nausea, and physiologic and psychological stressors. The hormone circulates to the distal tubules and collecting ducts in the kidneys where, consistent with its name, ADH causes reabsorption of water that dilutes the blood and other body fluids. Reabsorption of water decreases the urine volume and makes the urine concentrated, thus decreasing fluid excretion. Factors that decrease ADH release (such as decreased osmolality of the extracellular fluid and ethanol intake) allow a large, dilute urine volume.

Aldosterone is another hormone that influences urine volume. Aldosterone is synthesized and secreted by cells in the adrenal cortex. The major stimuli for its release are angiotensin II (from the renin-angiotensin system, which is activated by decreased circulating blood volume) and an increased concentration of potassium ions in the plasma.[4] Aldosterone causes the renal tubules to reabsorb sodium and water (saline), which expands the extracellular fluid volume. This renal action decreases fluid excretion, although by a different mechanism

than ADH. When more aldosterone is secreted, the urine volume is smaller; decreased secretion of aldosterone causes a larger urine volume.

A comparison of ADH and aldosterone is useful to remember their actions. ADH is the tap water hormone. It causes the kidneys to reabsorb water. Renal reabsorption of water caused by ADH makes a smaller volume of more concentrated urine and dilutes body fluids. Aldosterone is the salt water hormone. It causes the kidneys to reabsorb sodium and water. Renal reabsorption of sodium and water caused by aldosterone makes a smaller volume of urine and expands extracellular fluid volume.

ANP normally is stored in granules in the cardiac atrial cells and released when the atria are stretched. B-type natriuretic peptide (BNP) is synthesized and released from ventricular cells when ventricular diastolic pressure increases abnormally, as in heart failure. ANP and BNP cause natriuresis (sodium excretion in the urine), which is accompanied by water excretion. Thus, these natriuretic peptides (NPs) promote fluid excretion in the urine. When the vascular volume increases, the heart is stretched, and more NPs are released to cause renal excretion of the excess fluid.[5] When the vascular volume is decreased, the heart is less stretched; therefore, fewer NPs are released and the kidneys excrete less fluid. NPs oppose the action of aldosterone, but they are not as strong as aldosterone.

The urine volume that an individual produces also is highly dependent on having adequate blood pressure to perfuse the kidneys and on the glomerular filtration rate. Thus, renal excretion of fluid is the end result of several factors, including hormones that respond to different stimuli and have different actions on the renal tubules.

Fluid Loss Through Abnormal Routes

People who have pathophysiologic conditions often experience loss of fluid through abnormal routes. Examples of these routes are emesis; tubes in the gastrointestinal tract or other body cavities; hemorrhage; drainage from fistulas, wounds, or open areas of skin; and paracentesis. Fluid lost through abnormal routes may be a significant factor in disturbing fluid homeostasis.

If the body's physiologic mechanisms are functioning well, the processes of fluid homeostasis maintain normal body fluid status. If fluid intake is large, fluid excretion increases by the mechanisms described previously that increase urine volume (large volume of dilute urine). If fluid intake is diminished or if fluid is lost through abnormal routes, fluid excretion decreases (small volume of concentrated urine), and thirst may cause an increase in fluid intake.

If pathophysiologic processes interfere with normal fluid homeostasis or if the normal processes become overwhelmed, then fluid imbalances result. For example, a person who has a pathophysiologic process that prevents the kidneys from excreting much fluid may accumulate too much fluid unless the fluid intake is reduced. The opposite problem will occur in a person whose fluid intake is too small to replace a large amount of fluid excreted or lost through abnormal routes.

KEY POINTS

- Fluid homeostasis is a dynamic process that includes fluid intake and absorption, fluid distribution across body fluid compartments, fluid excretion, and, in some individuals, fluid loss through abnormal routes.
- Habit and thirst are important regulators of fluid intake. Individuals who are unable to control their own fluid intake (such as those receiving fluids intravenously and immobile or unconscious patients) are at high risk for fluid imbalance.
- Fluid (water and small particles) moves back and forth between the vascular and interstitial areas by filtration at the capillaries. Capillary hydrostatic pressure is the primary force promoting fluid movement from the capillaries to the interstitial fluid. Plasma colloid osmotic pressure is the primary force that causes interstitial fluid to move back into the capillaries.

- Water moves in and out of cells by osmosis. Electrolytes do not move freely across cell membranes but are transported by membrane channels and carriers.
- Fluid excretion may be visible (urine, feces, sweat) or invisible (respiration and insensible perspiration). Fluid loss may occur through abnormal routes such as emesis and wound drainage. To maintain fluid balance, fluid intake must counterbalance fluid excretion and loss through abnormal routes.
- Healthy kidneys adjust fluid excretion in response to blood pressure and several hormones. Aldosterone induces the kidneys to conserve saline (salt and water), which expands the extracellular fluid volume; natriuretic peptides (ANP and BNP) promote saline excretion. ADH causes the kidneys to retain water, thus concentrating the urine and diluting the body fluids. Urine volume and concentration are important indicators of body fluid balance.

FLUID IMBALANCES

If fluid homeostasis is disturbed by pathophysiologic processes or other factors (such as medications), fluid imbalances may occur. Fluid imbalances fall into two major categories: imbalances of extracellular fluid volume (**saline imbalances**) and imbalances of body fluid concentration (**water imbalances**).

Extracellular Fluid Volume

In some circumstances, individuals have too much or too little extracellular fluid. These disorders are called **extracellular fluid volume (ECV) imbalances** because they involve a change in the *amount* (volume) of the extracellular fluid. These disorders also are termed *saline imbalances* because they are disorders of **isotonic** salt water. (Isotonic saline is salt water in the same concentration as the normal plasma concentration.) In an ECV imbalance, the *concentration* of the extracellular fluid may be normal; there is simply too much or too little of it. Some individuals have an ECV imbalance and an imbalance of body fluid concentration at the same time. In this case, both the volume and serum sodium concentration of the extracellular fluid are abnormal. This section discusses only the isotonic volume imbalances; the concentration imbalances are discussed separately because they may occur separately.

Volume Deficit

ECV deficit is caused by removal of a sodium-containing fluid from the body. It is a decrease in saline (isotonic salt water) in the same concentration as the normal extracellular fluid, which is why the condition sometimes is termed **saline deficit**. In an uncomplicated ECV deficit, the serum sodium concentration is normal. The *concentration* of the extracellular fluid is normal; the *amount* of the extracellular fluid is abnormally decreased (Figure 24-4).

Etiology. Specific causes of ECV deficit are listed in Box 24-1. All causes of ECV deficit involve removal of a sodium-containing fluid from the extracellular compartment. The sodium-containing fluid usually is removed from the body; however, it may be sequestered in a "third space" in the body that is outside the extracellular compartment. For example, ascites (fluid in the peritoneal cavity) that develops rapidly may deplete the ECV. Another example is fluid that accumulates rapidly in the bowel during an acute intestinal obstruction. Although the fluid in these examples remains in the body, it no longer is part of the extracellular fluid, and signs and symptoms of ECV deficit occur.

Clinical manifestations. Signs and symptoms of ECV deficit are the result of decreased fluid volume in the vascular and interstitial areas. These clinical manifestations include sudden weight loss, postural blood pressure decrease with concurrent increased heart rate, flat neck veins (or veins collapsing with inspiration) when a patient is supine, prolonged small-vein filling time, prolonged capillary refill time, lightheadedness, dizziness, syncope, and oliguria. If the kidneys are responding

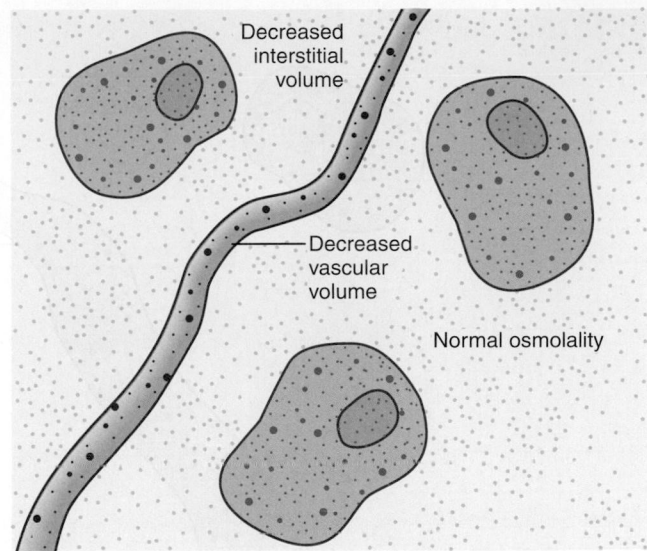

FIGURE 24-4 Extracellular fluid volume deficit. Decreased volume of extracellular fluid in vascular and interstitial compartments is characteristic of extracellular fluid volume deficit.

BOX 24-1	CAUSES OF EXTRACELLULAR FLUID VOLUME DEFICIT

Gastrointestinal Excretion or Loss of Sodium-Containing Fluid
Emesis
Diarrhea (includes laxative abuse)
Gastric suction or intestinal decompression
Fistula drainage

Renal Excretion of Sodium-Containing Fluid
Adrenal insufficiency
Salt-wasting renal disorders
Extensive diuretic use
Bed rest

Other Loss of a Sodium-Containing Fluid
Hemorrhage
Massive diaphoresis
Third-space fluid accumulation
Paracentesis and similar procedures
Burns

normally, the small volume of urine will be concentrated (and thus quite yellow). An ECV deficit that develops slowly also may be manifested by decreased skin turgor (skin tenting when it is pinched up over the sternum), dryness of oral mucous membranes between cheek and gum, hard stools, soft sunken eyeballs, longitudinal furrows in the tongue, and absence of tears and sweat. An infant who develops ECV deficit has a sunken fontanel; neck veins are not reliably assessed in infants.

Sudden weight loss is a sensitive measure of ECV deficit. One liter of saline weighs 1 kg; therefore, a person who loses 1 kg in 24 hours has excreted 1 L of fluid or lost it through an abnormal route. It is not possible to lose a kilogram of fat overnight; a sudden weight loss of this magnitude results only from fluid loss, if the body weight is measured accurately. An ECV deficit may occur without a weight loss if fluid is sequestered in a third space somewhere in the body, as with ascites or intestinal obstruction.

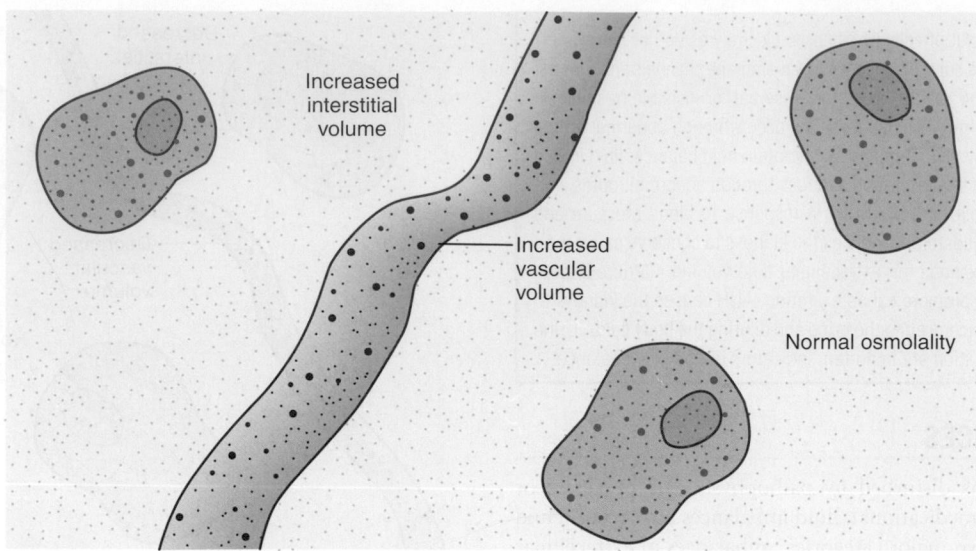

FIGURE 24-5 Extracellular fluid volume excess. Increased volume of extracellular fluid in vascular and interstitial compartments is characteristic of extracellular fluid volume excess.

BOX 24-2   CAUSES OF EXTRACELLULAR FLUID VOLUME EXCESS

Excessive Intravenous Infusion of Sodium-Containing Isotonic Solutions
Normal saline (0.9% sodium chloride)
Ringer injection
Lactated Ringer injection

Renal Retention of Sodium and Water
Primary hyperaldosteronism
Chronic heart failure
Cirrhosis
Acute glomerulonephritis
Chronic end-stage renal disease
Cushing disease
Corticosteroid therapy

A postural blood pressure decrease with concurrent increased heart rate that is measured when a previously supine person stands, or sits with legs dependent, is a good indicator of fluid volume depletion in the vascular compartment. Severe ECV deficit may lead to hypovolemic shock, which can be fatal if not treated effectively with fluid replacement.

Volume Excess

ECV excess is essentially the opposite of an ECV deficit. It is the condition in which the amount of extracellular fluid is abnormally increased. Both the vascular and the interstitial areas have too much isotonic fluid (Figure 24-5). In an uncomplicated ECV excess, the *concentration* of the extracellular fluid is normal, but an excessive *amount* of that fluid is present.

Etiology. ECV excess is caused by addition or retention of saline (salt water in the same concentration as normal plasma). For this reason, it sometimes is termed **saline excess.** As mentioned previously, the hormone aldosterone causes the kidneys to retain saline. ECV excess, therefore, may be caused by conditions that involve excessive aldosterone secretion. For example, increased aldosterone secretion is a compensatory mechanism that commonly accompanies chronic heart failure and eventually leads to ECV excess.[6] Additional causes of ECV excess are presented in Box 24-2.

Clinical manifestations. Signs and symptoms of ECV excess are sudden weight gain, edema, and manifestations of circulatory overload: bounding pulse, neck vein distention in a person in the upright position, crackles in the dependent portions of the lungs, dyspnea, orthopnea, and even the frothy sputum of pulmonary edema. An infant who develops ECV excess has a bulging fontanel; assessment of neck veins is not effective in infants.

Sudden weight gain is a sensitive measure of ECV excess. It is impossible to gain a kilogram of fat overnight; such a sudden weight gain is an accumulation of saline. People who eat salty food in a restaurant weigh more the next day because the water they drank combined with the salt in the food to make isotonic saline. The isotonic saline expands the extracellular fluid, causing a mild saline excess until it is excreted by the kidneys. This is the reason that low-sodium diets are prescribed for people who have pathophysiologic processes that cause saline excess (e.g., compensated heart failure).

Body Fluid Concentration

In contrast to the ECV disorders just discussed, imbalances of body fluid concentration are disorders of the *concentration* rather than of the *amount* of extracellular fluid. Body fluid concentration disorders also are called **water imbalances.** The serum sodium concentration reflects the osmolality (concentratedness) of the blood. Imbalances of body fluid concentration are recognized by abnormal serum sodium concentration. The normal serum sodium concentration is 135 to 145 mEq/L (may vary slightly with different laboratories). Many individuals develop imbalances of both ECV and serum sodium concentration at the same time. Isolated imbalances of serum sodium concentration may also occur. This section discusses the concentration imbalances separately.

Hyponatremia

Natrium is the Latin word for sodium. A serum sodium concentration below the lower limit of normal indicates hyponatremia. When hyponatremia is present, the extracellular fluid contains relatively too much water for the amount of sodium ions present; it is more dilute than normal.

Etiology. Hyponatremia is caused by factors that produce a relative excess of water in proportion to salt in the extracellular fluid. Because the serum sodium concentration reflects the osmolality of the blood, the reduced serum sodium concentration of hyponatremia

BOX 24-3 CAUSES OF HYPONATREMIA

Gain of Relatively More Water Than Salt

Excessive antidiuretic hormone

Excessive intravenous infusion of 5% dextrose in water (D_5W)

Hypotonic irrigating solutions

Tap water enemas

Psychogenic polydipsia (compulsive water drinking)

Forced excessive water ingestion (child abuse or club initiation)

Excessive beer ingestion (beer potomania)

Near-drowning in fresh water

Selective serotonin reuptake inhibitors (SSRIs)

Loss of Relatively More Salt Than Water

Diuretics, especially thiazides

Salt-wasting renal disease

Replacement of water but not salt lost through emesis, diarrhea, gastric suction, diaphoresis, or burns

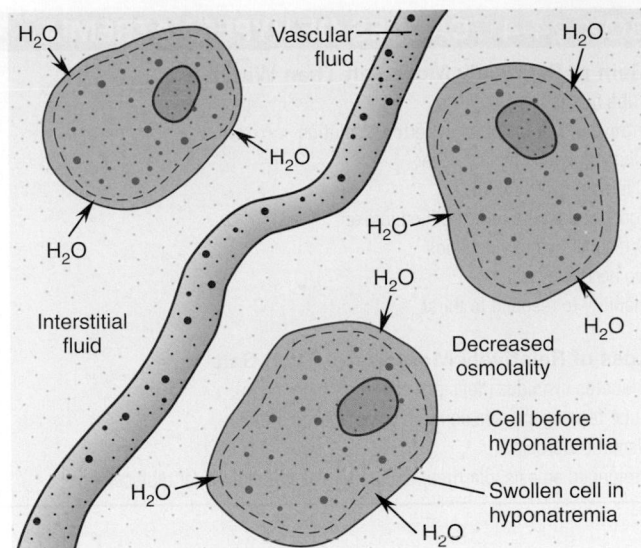

FIGURE 24-6 Cell swelling in hyponatremia. Decreased osmolality (concentration) of extracellular fluid in hyponatremia causes water to move into cells by osmosis.

indicates that the extracellular fluid has a reduced osmolality; it is too dilute. Hyponatremia also is called *hypotonic syndrome, hypoosmolality,* and *water intoxication.* All of these terms reflect the abnormally dilute concentration of the extracellular fluid that results when the normal proportion of salt to water in the extracellular fluid is disrupted by gaining more water than salt or losing relatively more salt than water.

A *gain of relatively more water than salt* will cause hyponatremia. As mentioned previously, the hormone ADH causes the kidneys to retain water (not sodium and water) in the body. This hormone is part of the system that normally regulates the osmolality of extracellular fluid. However, circumstances that cause prolonged or excessive release of ADH cause the kidneys to retain too much water, which effectively dilutes the blood; hyponatremia is the result. ADH secretion is excessive in the syndrome of inappropriate secretion of ADH (SIADH). ADH also may be produced **ectopically.** For example, small cell (oat cell) carcinoma is a type of lung tumor that frequently synthesizes and releases ADH. This ectopic production of ADH from a tumor is not subject to the feedback inhibition of normal ADH release, so inappropriate amounts of ADH are released. With continually high levels of ADH being produced by the tumor, the kidneys retain excessive amounts of water—a gain of water relative to salt. Pain, nausea, and other physical and psychological stressors also increase ADH release, which can be significant in hospitalized patients, especially in the postoperative period. Recent research links the proinflammatory cytokine interleukin-6 (IL-6) to increased ADH release during inflammatory conditions.[7] Although it is difficult to drink enough water to cause hyponatremia, water intake that exceeds renal excretory capacity is seen in some situations. For example, the hyponatremia of beer potomania arises when people habitually drink 14 or more cans of beer daily with very little food intake.[8] Factors that cause hyponatremia by gain of water relative to salt are presented in Box 24-3.

Hyponatremia also may be caused by a *loss of relatively more salt than water.* If salt is removed from the body while water remains, then the extracellular fluid once again will become too dilute; hyponatremia results. Factors that cause hyponatremia by loss of salt relative to water also are presented in Box 24-3. Although Box 24-3 separates causes of hyponatremia into two categories, some types of hyponatremia are due to simultaneous gain of water and loss of salt. For example, hyponatremia in marathon runners occurs from loss of salt through heavy sweating and gain of water from excessive water intake plus inappropriate renal water reabsorption caused by increased ADH secretion.[9]

Clinical manifestations. Clinical manifestations of hyponatremia are nonspecific manifestations of central nervous system dysfunction.[10] They vary from malaise, anorexia, nausea, vomiting, and headache to confusion, lethargy, seizures, and coma. Profound hyponatremia causes fatal cerebral herniation. The signs and symptoms are caused by swelling of neurons and glial cells as a result of the decreased osmolality of extracellular fluid. When the extracellular fluid becomes too dilute, the intracellular fluid initially is more concentrated. Therefore, water moves into cells by osmosis (Figure 24-6). The severity of the signs and symptoms depends on how rapidly hyponatremia develops as well as on the absolute value of the serum sodium concentration. A rapid decrease in osmolality produces more severe manifestations than a slow decline, other factors being equal.

Hypernatremia

Hypernatremia is a serum sodium concentration above the upper limit of normal (145 mEq/L). When hypernatremia is present, the extracellular fluid contains relatively too little water for the amount of sodium ions present; it is too concentrated. Hypernatremia also is called *water deficit, hypertonic syndrome,* and *hyperosmolality.* These terms all reflect the relative deficit of water to salt in the extracellular fluid that occurs in hypernatremia.

Etiology. Hypernatremia is caused by a *gain of relatively more salt than water* or by a *loss of relatively more water than salt.* Both of these processes cause the body fluids to become too concentrated. Patients who receive concentrated tube feedings without enough water, especially older adults, are at high risk for hypernatremia because they gain relatively more solute than water, which causes an obligatory loss of relatively more water than salt in the urine. Hypernatremia can be prevented in these individuals by administering water between feedings. Other specific factors that cause hypernatremia are presented in Box 24-4 under the two major categories.

Clinical manifestations. Signs and symptoms of hypernatremia are similar to those of hyponatremia in that they are nonspecific manifestations of central nervous system dysfunction.[10] In hypernatremia, the increased osmolality of the extracellular fluid causes neurons and glial cells to shrivel because water moves from the cells to the interstitial fluid by osmosis (Figure 24-7). The dysfunction ranges from confusion and lethargy to seizures and coma. Thirst and oliguria (except for hypernatremia of renal origin) are common. Severe hypernatremia may cause death.

BOX 24-4   CAUSES OF HYPERNATREMIA

Gain of Relatively More Salt Than Water
Tube feeding
Intravenous infusion of hypertonic solution
Near-drowning in salt water
Overuse of salt tablets
Food intake with reduced fluid intake
Difficulty swallowing fluids
No access to water
Inability to respond to thirst

Loss of Relatively More Water Than Salt
Diabetes insipidus (deficient antidiuretic hormone)
Tube feeding (causes obligate water loss in urine)
Osmotic diuresis
Prolonged emesis, diarrhea, or diaphoresis without water replacement

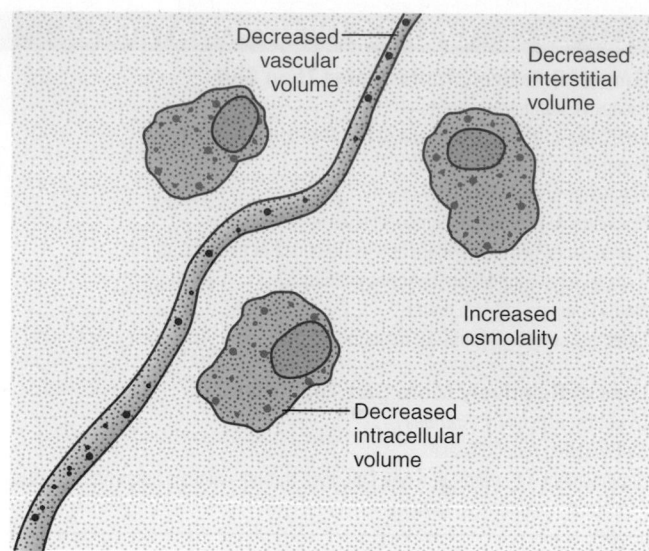

FIGURE 24-8 Clinical dehydration. Decreased volume of extracellular fluid in vascular and interstitial compartments plus cell shriveling from increased osmolality of extracellular fluid are combined in clinical dehydration.

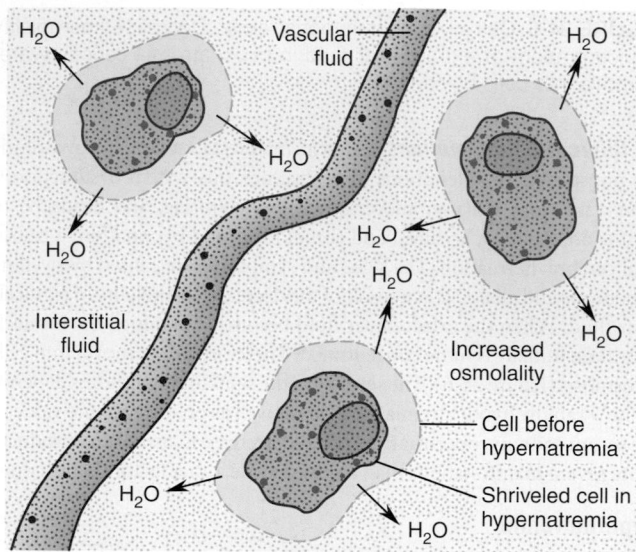

FIGURE 24-7 Cell shriveling in hypernatremia. Increased osmolality (concentration) of extracellular fluid in hypernatremia causes water to move from cells by osmosis.

BOX 24-5   SIGNS AND SYMPTOMS OF CLINICAL DEHYDRATION

Sudden weight loss
Postural blood pressure decrease with concurrent increased heart rate
Lightheadedness, dizziness, or syncope upon standing
Flat neck veins when supine or neck veins that collapse during inspiration (older children and adults)
Sunken fontanel (infants)
Rapid, thready pulse
Prolonged small-vein filling time
Prolonged capillary refill time
Oliguria
Decreased skin turgor
Dryness of oral mucous membranes
Absence of sweat and tears
Hard stools
Soft, sunken eyeballs
Longitudinal furrows in the tongue
Thirst
Increased serum sodium concentration
Confusion, lethargy
Coma
Hypovolemic shock

Both Volume and Concentration
Clinical Dehydration

Clinical dehydration is a combination of two fluid disorders: ECV deficit and hypernatremia. A person who has clinical dehydration has too small a volume of fluid in the extracellular compartment (vascular and interstitial), and the body fluids are too concentrated (Figure 24-8).

Etiology. Clinical dehydration occurs commonly in individuals who have vomiting and diarrhea and do not know how (or are unable) to replace the salt and the water that is exiting the body. Fluid excreted in diarrhea and lost by vomiting, plus the normal daily respiratory, skin, and urine excretion, is the equivalent of hypotonic sodium-containing fluid (isotonic saline with extra water added). Removal of the saline portion of this fluid from the body causes ECV deficit, and removal of the extra water from the body causes hypernatremia. The combination of these two imbalances is clinical dehydration.

Clinical manifestations. Signs and symptoms of clinical dehydration are the combination of the signs and symptoms of the two separate disorders. Therefore, a person who is clinically dehydrated will have clinical manifestations as listed in Box 24-5. Infants and older adults are at highest risk for clinical dehydration, although it can occur at any age.

Interstitial Fluid Volume
Edema

Edema is an excess of fluid in the interstitial compartment. It may be a manifestation of ECV excess or it may arise from other mechanisms. Forces that determine the distribution of fluid between the vascular and interstitial compartments are described previously in this chapter (see the Fluid Distribution section). An increase in the forces that tend to move fluid from the capillaries into the interstitial compartment or a decrease in forces that tend to move fluid from the interstitial compartment into the capillaries will cause edema by altering normal fluid distribution between the vascular and interstitial compartments.

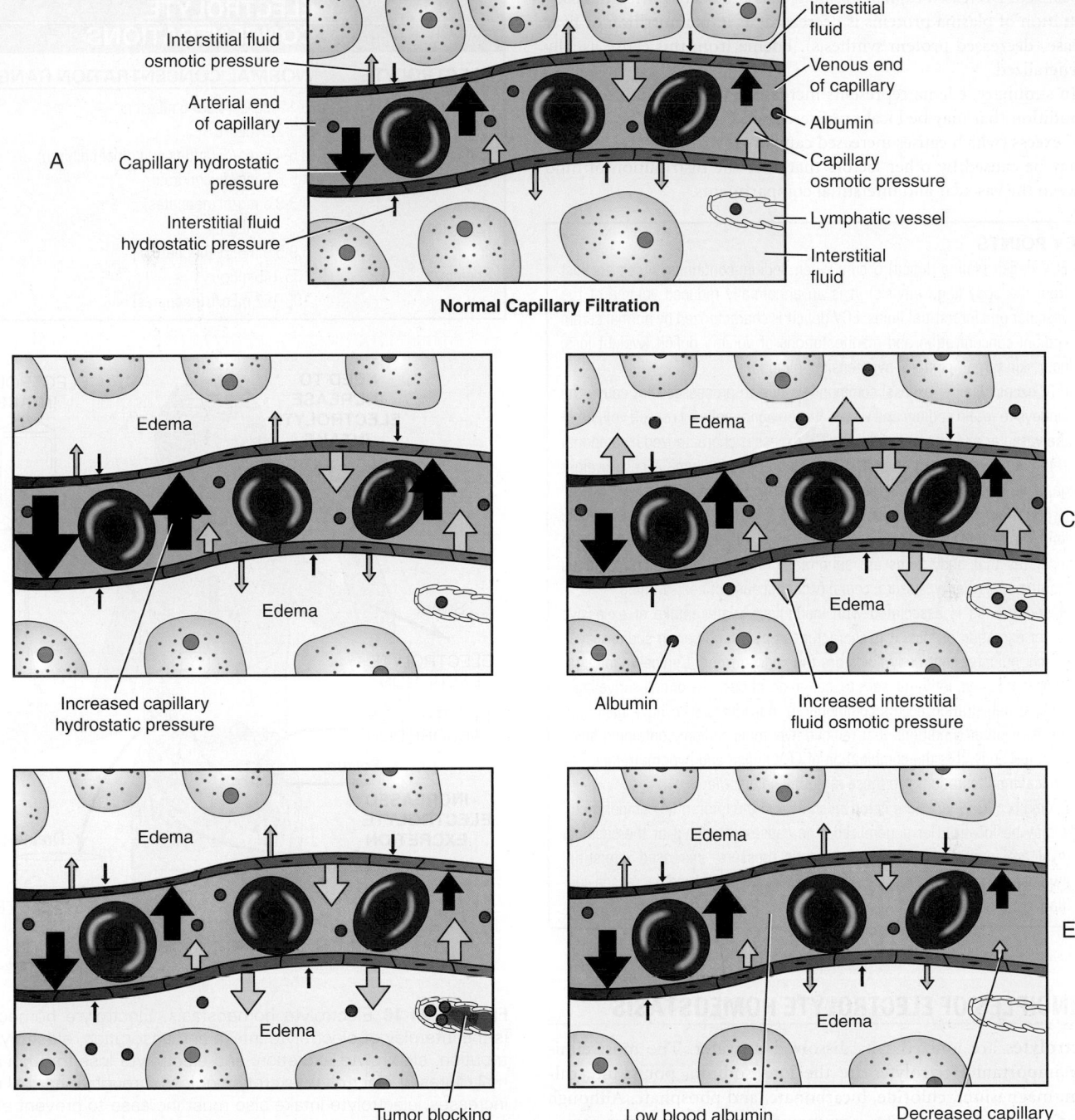

FIGURE 24-9 Causes of edema. **A,** Normal capillary filtration without edema. **B,** Edema caused by increased capillary hydrostatic pressure. **C,** Edema caused by increased interstitial fluid osmotic pressure from increased capillary permeability. **D,** Edema caused by blocked lymphatic drainage. **E,** Edema caused by decreased capillary osmotic pressure from hypoalbuminemia.

Thus, edema may arise from increased capillary hydrostatic pressure, increased interstitial fluid osmotic pressure, blockage of lymphatic drainage, or decreased capillary osmotic pressure (Figure 24-9). Edema may be localized or generalized (existing in many areas of the body simultaneously).

Increased capillary hydrostatic pressure is caused by increased ECV, by the increased local capillary flow that accompanies inflammation, and by venous congestion. *Increased interstitial fluid osmotic pressure*

occurs when inflammation increases vascular permeability and proteins leak into the interstitial fluid. Lymphatic drainage normally removes minute amounts of protein that enter the interstitial fluid. *Blockage of lymphatic drainage* (e.g., by a tumor, parasites, fibrosis from radiation therapy, or surgical removal of lymph nodes) also causes edema when the interstitial accumulation of protein increases interstitial fluid osmotic pressure.[11] This type of edema is called lymphedema and may be persistent.[12] Edema caused by increased interstitial fluid osmotic pressure or blockage of lymphatic drainage frequently is localized. *Decreased capillary osmotic pressure* occurs when the concentration of plasma proteins is decreased, as in malnutrition or liver disease (decreased protein synthesis). Edema from this cause usually is generalized.

In summary, edema represents increased interstitial fluid volume, a condition that may be local or generalized. Edema may be a sign of ECV excess (which causes increased capillary hydrostatic pressure), or it may be caused by other factors that alter the distribution of fluid between the vascular and interstitial compartments.

KEY POINTS

- ECV deficit (saline deficit) occurs when sodium-containing fluids are lost from the body (e.g., emesis). It is an abnormally reduced volume of the vascular and interstitial fluids. ECV deficit is characterized by normal serum sodium concentration and manifestations of volume deficit (weight loss, poor skin turgor, postural hypotension, oliguria).
- ECV excess (saline excess) commonly is due to processes that cause the kidneys to retain sodium and water. It is an abnormally increased volume of the vascular and interstitial fluids. ECV excess is characterized by a normal serum sodium concentration and manifestations of volume excess (weight gain, peripheral edema, distended neck veins, dyspnea).
- Hyponatremia is associated with excessive ADH secretion or hypotonic fluid intake. It is characterized by a low serum sodium concentration, which indicates that body fluids are abnormally dilute. Clinical manifestations (confusion, lethargy, seizure, coma) occur because of cell swelling.
- Hypernatremia is associated with inadequate water intake or excessive water excretion or loss. It is characterized by a high serum sodium level, which indicates that body fluids are too concentrated. Clinical manifestations (confusion, lethargy, seizure, coma) occur because of cell shriveling.
- Clinical dehydration occurs commonly in individuals who have gastroenteritis or other conditions that remove hypotonic sodium-containing fluids from the body. It is the combination of ECV deficit and hypernatremia. The clinical manifestations are those of both fluid disorders.
- Edema occurs when there is too much fluid in the interstitial compartment. It may be localized or generalized. The causes of edema at the capillary level are increased capillary hydrostatic pressure, increased interstitial fluid osmotic pressure, blockage of lymphatic drainage, and decreased capillary osmotic pressure.

PRINCIPLES OF ELECTROLYTE HOMEOSTASIS

Electrolytes are ionized salts dissolved in water. The most clinically important electrolytes are the ions sodium, potassium, calcium, magnesium, chloride, bicarbonate, and phosphate. Although sodium ions are electrolytes, serum sodium imbalances are osmolality (concentration) imbalances, as explained previously in this chapter. This section discusses homeostasis and imbalances of potassium, calcium, magnesium, and phosphate ions. Bicarbonate is discussed in Chapter 25 because it is important in acid-base balance and imbalances.

The concentration of an electrolyte in the plasma is different from its concentration inside cells. For normal body function, the electrolyte concentration must be normal in both areas. In clinical situations, the plasma (or serum) concentration of an electrolyte is measured. Normal serum electrolyte concentrations are listed in Table 24-1. The concentration of an electrolyte in the plasma is the net result of four processes: *electrolyte intake, electrolyte absorption, electrolyte distribution,* and *electrolyte excretion.* These processes work together in a dynamic fashion to maintain electrolyte concentrations within their

TABLE 24-1	NORMAL SERUM ELECTROLYTE CONCENTRATIONS	
ELECTROLYTE	**NORMAL CONCENTRATION RANGE**
Calcium (total)	9-11 mg/dl (4.5-5.5 mEq/L)
Magnesium	1.5-2.5 mEq/L
Phosphate	2.5-4.5 mg/dl (adults and older children)
	4.5-6.5 mg/dl (children)
	4.3-9.3 mg/dl (neonates)
Potassium	3.5-5.0 mEq/L
	3.9-5.9 mEq/L (neonates)
Sodium	135-145 mEq/L
	135-162 mEq/L (neonates)

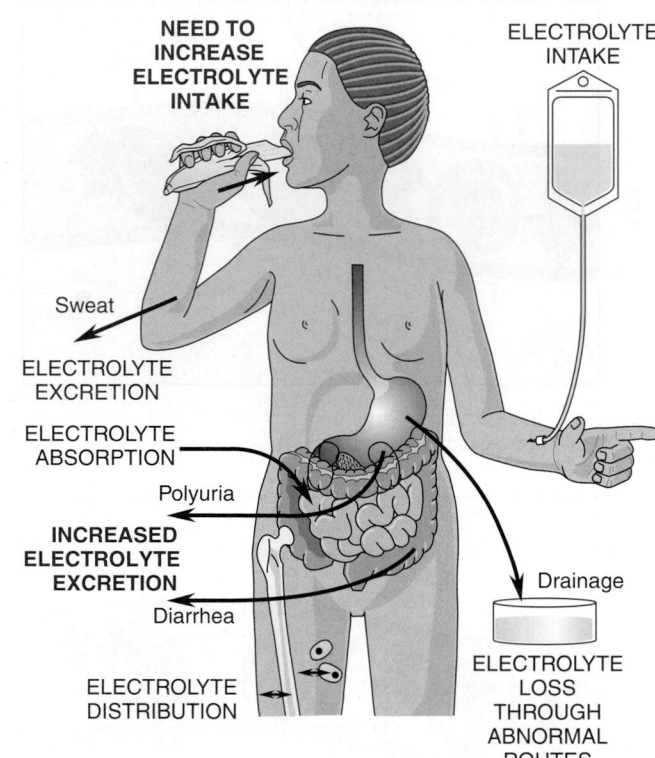

FIGURE 24-10 Electrolyte homeostasis. Electrolyte homeostasis is the interplay of electrolyte intake and absorption, electrolyte distribution, electrolyte excretion, and electrolyte loss through abnormal routes. If electrolyte excretion or loss through abnormal routes increases, electrolyte intake also must increase to prevent electrolyte imbalance.

normal limits (Figure 24-10). Thus, if intake of a specific electrolyte increases, excretion of that electrolyte also may increase and normalize the plasma levels. Similarly, if electrolyte intake decreases dramatically, electrolytes may be redistributed into the plasma to maintain the normal plasma concentration.

Electrolyte Intake and Absorption

Electrolyte intake normally occurs orally, through food and drink. It is important to remember that oral medications (e.g., magnesium antacids) also may be an important source of electrolyte intake. Intravenous fluids and nutritional solutions are common sources of parenteral intake of electrolytes. Blood transfusions may provide significant amounts of electrolytes. Less common, but important if it occurs, is intramuscular injection of the electrolyte magnesium.

Some patients have electrolyte intake through tubes into body cavities. The most obvious examples are nasogastric and gastrointestinal feeding tubes, but more unusual situations may cause significant electrolyte intake in specific individuals (e.g., irrigation of the renal pelvis with magnesium-rich solutions). Rarely, electrolyte intake may occur through such unusual routes as the lungs (e.g., near-drowning in salt water, which is rich in magnesium) or the skin (e.g., through application of ointments to large areas of broken or burned skin). Electrolyte intake is controlled by the individual and by health care providers.

If electrolyte intake occurs orally, the electrolyte must be absorbed before it is physiologically useful. Absorption of some electrolytes, such as potassium ions, depends on concentration gradients. Absorption of other electrolytes, such as calcium, depends on the availability of binding proteins, which is influenced by the activity of vitamin D.[1] The contents of the gastrointestinal tract may influence electrolyte absorption. Many agents bind electrolytes and prevent them from being absorbed. For example, undigested fat in the intestines binds calcium and magnesium ions contained in food and prevents them from being absorbed. The pH of intestinal contents also influences the absorption of certain electrolytes, especially calcium ions. Medications often alter electrolyte absorption. Surgical removal of portions of the gastrointestinal tract can decrease electrolyte absorption.

Electrolyte Distribution

Every fluid compartment contains electrolytes. However, the electrolyte composition differs in these various compartments. The concentrations of potassium, magnesium, and phosphate ions are higher inside cells than in the fluid outside the cells. Although calcium ion concentration is higher inside cells, much of the intracellular calcium is bound to other molecules; the concentration of physiologically active ionized calcium ions is higher in the extracellular fluid. The bones serve as an important reservoir of calcium, magnesium, and phosphate ions. The cells and the bones are often called the *electrolyte pools.*

Distribution of electrolytes between the extracellular fluid and the electrolyte pools is influenced primarily by hormones such as epinephrine (potassium ions), insulin (potassium and phosphate ions), and parathyroid hormone (calcium ions). Certain medications also influence electrolyte distribution. Significant movement of electrolytes between the cells and the extracellular fluid may occur within minutes.[1] In the absence of changes in electrolyte intake and excretion, a shift of electrolytes from the extracellular fluid into the electrolyte pools will decrease the plasma electrolyte concentration. Conversely, a shift of electrolyte from an electrolyte pool into the extracellular fluid will increase the plasma electrolyte concentration.

Electrolyte Excretion

Electrolyte excretion occurs through urine, feces, and sweat. Urinary excretion of some electrolytes is influenced by hormones (e.g., aldosterone increases potassium ion excretion), although factors such as the flow rate of renal tubular fluid are also influential. Many different medications alter the rate of urinary excretion of electrolytes.[13] For example, commonly used drugs that increase urinary excretion of potassium include corticosteroids, such as prednisone, and potassium-wasting diuretics, such as furosemide and hydrochlorothiazide. Drugs that increase urinary magnesium excretion include diuretics and aminoglycoside antibiotics, such as gentamicin. Conversely, thiazide diuretics, such as hydrochlorothiazide, decrease urinary excretion of calcium.

Fecal excretion of electrolytes is influenced by the type of feces produced. Diarrhea increases the excretion of potassium and magnesium

ions in particular. The composition of the feces also influences the amount of electrolyte excretion. Undigested fat in the intestines binds calcium and magnesium ions that are secreted into the gastrointestinal tract and prevents them from being reabsorbed. Thus, these electrolytes are excreted in the feces.

Electrolyte Loss Through Abnormal Routes

When electrolytes exit the body through routes other than the normal urine, feces, and sweat, this may be termed *electrolyte loss through abnormal routes.* This factor alters electrolyte homeostasis in patients who have diverse pathophysiologic conditions. Examples of electrolyte loss through abnormal routes are emesis, nasogastric suction, paracentesis, hemodialysis, wound drainage, and fistula drainage. Loss of electrolytes through abnormal routes may be uncontrollable or may result from therapeutic procedures.

Electrolyte homeostasis is a dynamic interplay between the processes of electrolyte intake, electrolyte absorption, electrolyte distribution, and electrolyte excretion. In some people, electrolyte loss through abnormal routes becomes an important factor that requires adjustment of electrolyte intake and/or electrolyte excretion to prevent development of electrolyte imbalances. Individuals who have acute or chronic illnesses have many factors that tend to cause electrolyte imbalances by disrupting or interfering with electrolyte intake, absorption, distribution, or excretion. As a result, they may develop single or multiple electrolyte imbalances.

> **KEY POINTS**
> - The electrolyte composition of the body is maintained by a careful balance of electrolyte intake, absorption, distribution, and excretion. Electrolyte imbalances result from disruption of one or more of these processes or from electrolyte loss through abnormal routes.
> - The plasma concentration of an electrolyte may not reflect the intracellular concentration. Cells contain higher concentrations of potassium, calcium, magnesium, and phosphate ions, whereas the extracellular fluid contains higher concentrations of sodium, chloride, and bicarbonate ions.

ELECTROLYTE IMBALANCES

Electrolyte imbalances are widespread in many pathophysiologic conditions. An electrolyte imbalance may be a total body imbalance or it may be an imbalance in the distribution of electrolytes within compartments, with the total body amount remaining normal. Based on the principles of electrolyte homeostasis explained in the previous section of this chapter, an excess of electrolytes in the extracellular fluid may be caused by increased electrolyte intake or absorption, shift of electrolytes from an electrolyte pool into the extracellular fluid, and decreased electrolyte excretion, either singly or in combination. Conversely, a deficit of electrolytes in the extracellular fluid may be caused by decreased electrolyte intake or absorption, shift of electrolytes from the extracellular fluid to an electrolyte pool, increased electrolyte excretion, loss of electrolytes through abnormal routes, or some combination of these factors.

Plasma Potassium

The normal concentration of potassium ions in serum is 3.5 to 5.0 mEq/L (may vary slightly with different laboratories), except in neonates, in whom it may be higher. Most of the potassium ions in the body are inside cells; the standard serum potassium measurement gives only the concentration of the small portion of potassium ions in the extracellular fluid. Because a number of factors cause potassium ions to move into or out of body cells, concentration of potassium in the plasma and total body potassium content are not necessarily correlated. Whether or not they are accompanied by total body potassium imbalances, plasma potassium imbalances may cause clinically significant signs and symptoms.

Hypokalemia

Hypokalemia denotes a decreased potassium ion concentration in the extracellular fluid. A decrease in the plasma potassium concentration does not necessarily denote a decrease in total body potassium. Thus, hypokalemia may coexist with a total body potassium deficit, a total body potassium excess, or a normal total body potassium ion concentration.

Etiology. Hypokalemia is caused by factors that decrease potassium intake, shift potassium from the extracellular fluid into the cells, increase potassium excretion through the normal routes, and cause potassium loss from the body by some abnormal route. Potassium-wasting diuretics and corticosteroids such as prednisone are well-known causes of hypokalemia from increased renal potassium excretion. The hormone aldosterone increases potassium excretion in urine; hypokalemia is associated with pathophysiologic conditions such as compensated heart failure and cirrhosis that are accompanied by increased aldosterone levels. Black licorice contains a substance that increases renal potassium excretion. Many traditional Chinese medicines and other herbal preparations contain black licorice, and excessive ingestion of these agents or black licorice candy leads to hypokalemia.[14] In many cases, several factors lead to hypokalemia. For example, some people follow a fad diet (decreased potassium intake) and abuse diuretics (increased potassium excretion) in an attempt to lose weight. Specific causes of hypokalemia are listed in Box 24-6.

Clinical manifestations. The resting membrane potential of muscle cells is determined by the ratio of intracellular to extracellular potassium ion concentration. For this reason, potassium imbalances cause altered function of muscles (skeletal, smooth, and cardiac). In hypokalemia, both smooth and skeletal muscle cells are hyperpolarized (more electrical charge than usual across the cell membrane). Therefore, these muscles are less reactive to stimuli. The resulting clinical manifestations include abdominal distention, diminished bowel sounds, paralytic ileus, postural hypotension, skeletal muscle weakness, and flaccid paralysis. The skeletal muscle weakness of hypokalemia is bilateral weakness that typically begins in the lower extremities and ascends. It may involve the respiratory muscles, causing respiratory paralysis more commonly than does hyperkalemia.

Many types of cardiac dysrhythmias arise from hypokalemia. Cardiac muscle cells usually become hyperpolarized with hypokalemia. However, with very low plasma potassium concentrations, hypopolarization of cardiac muscle occurs, most likely because of decreased potassium conductance. Hypokalemia also increases the rate of diastolic depolarization, which may give rise to ectopic beats, decreases conduction velocity in the atrioventricular node, prolongs cardiac action potentials by decreasing the rate of repolarization, shortens the absolute refractory period, and prolongs the relative refractory period.[15] Cardiac dysrhythmias in severe hypokalemia may cause sudden cardiac death.[16]

Hypokalemia also may cause polyuria by interfering with the action of ADH at the renal tubules. The plasma potassium concentration at which the various clinical manifestations of hypokalemia appear depends on individual responsiveness and the presence of other concurrent electrolyte and acid-base disorders. Chronic hypokalemia can cause rhabdomyolysis (skeletal muscle breakdown), selective myocardial cell necrosis, and nephropathy.[17]

BOX 24-6 CAUSES OF HYPOKALEMIA

Decreased Potassium Intake
Anorexia
NPO (nothing by mouth) orders and intravenous solutions without potassium
Fasting
Unbalanced diet

Shift of Potassium from Extracellular Fluid to Cells
Alkalosis
Excess insulin (e.g., during total parenteral nutrition)
Excess β-adrenergic stimulation
Hypokalemic familial periodic paralysis

Increased Potassium Excretion Through Normal Routes
Renal Route
Potassium-wasting diuretics
Corticosteroid therapy
Cushing disease
Hyperaldosteronism
Excessive ingestion of black licorice (glycyrrhizin)
Hypomagnesemia
Parenteral ticarcillin or similar agents
Amphotericin B, cisplatin, cyclosporine, and many other drugs

Fecal Route
Diarrhea (includes laxative abuse)

Skin Route
Excessive diaphoresis

Loss of Potassium Through Abnormal Routes
Emesis
Gastric suction
Fistula drainage

Hyperkalemia

If the serum potassium concentration rises above 5.0 mEq/L (the upper limit of normal), hyperkalemia is present. Hyperkalemia denotes an elevation of potassium ion concentration in the extracellular fluid. As mentioned previously, most of the potassium ions in the body are inside cells, and many factors cause potassium ions to move into or out of the cells. Thus, total body potassium content may be increased, normal, or decreased in hyperkalemia, depending on its cause.

Etiology. Hyperkalemia is caused by factors that increase potassium intake, shift potassium from the cells into the extracellular fluid, and decrease potassium excretion. For example, massive blood transfusion can cause hyperkalemia by increased potassium intake because the transfused fluid surrounding the red blood cells (RBCs) is high in potassium that was released from the RBCs during storage.[18] Large numbers of potassium ions shifting from cells into the extracellular fluid after a crushing injury or massive cell death from cytotoxic chemotherapy will cause hyperkalemia.[19] People who take two or more drugs that can increase plasma potassium concentration need monitoring for hyperkalemia.[20] Several factors together can cause hyperkalemia, such as when an individual who develops decreased potassium excretion because of oliguric chronic kidney disease continues to have a normal dietary potassium intake.[21] Specific causes of hyperkalemia are summarized by category in Box 24-7.

Clinical manifestations. As might be expected from the role of potassium ions in establishment of the resting membrane potential of muscle cells, hyperkalemia causes muscle dysfunction. As hyperkalemia develops, smooth muscle and skeletal muscle cells become hypopolarized.

BOX 24-7   CAUSES OF HYPERKALEMIA

Increased Potassium Intake
Excessive or too-rapid intravenous potassium infusion
Insufficiently mixed intravenous potassium infusion
Large transfusion of stored blood
Massive doses of potassium penicillin G

Shift of Potassium from Cells to Extracellular Fluid
Acidosis caused by nonorganic acids
Insufficient insulin
Crushing injury
Cytotoxic drugs (tumor lysis syndrome)
Hyperkalemic periodic paralysis
β-Adrenergic blockade and prolonged strenuous exercise

Decreased Potassium Excretion
Oliguria (such as in hypovolemia, acute kidney injury, or chronic end-stage renal disease)
Potassium-sparing diuretics
Adrenal insufficiency
Renin-deficient states
Drugs that reduce aldosterone effects (direct renin inhibitors, angiotensin-converting enzyme [ACE] inhibitors, angiotensin II receptor antagonists, and selective aldosterone blockers)
Nephrotoxic drugs

BOX 24-8   CAUSES OF HYPOCALCEMIA

Decreased Calcium Intake or Absorption
Diet with insufficient calcium and vitamin D
Chronic kidney disease (deficient activated vitamin D)
Excessive dietary phytates or oxalates
Steatorrhea
Pancreatitis
Chronic diarrhea (includes laxative abuse)
Malabsorption syndromes

Decreased Physiologic Availability of Calcium
Hypoparathyroidism
Excessive phosphate intake
Tumor lysis syndrome (high phosphate)
Hypomagnesemia
Alkalosis
Large transfusion of citrated blood or fresh frozen plasma
Rapid infusion of plasma expanders that bind calcium
Elevated plasma free fatty acids
Chronic kidney disease

Increased Calcium Excretion Through Normal Routes
Steatorrhea
Pancreatitis

The main clinical manifestation at this stage is mild intestinal cramping and diarrhea, which occurs only in some individuals. As hyperkalemia worsens, skeletal muscle cells become hypopolarized to the extent that their resting membrane potentials lie above their threshold potential; once they have discharged, they are unable to contract again. This situation causes the typical skeletal muscle weakness and flaccid paralysis of hyperkalemia. The skeletal muscle weakness is an ascending weakness that appears first in the lower extremities.[22] Both hypokalemia and hyperkalemia cause skeletal muscle weakness and/or paralysis, but the underlying alterations in the resting membrane potentials are different.

Cardiac muscle undergoes the same changes in resting membrane potential as skeletal muscle in hyperkalemia. In addition, hyperkalemia decreases the duration and rate of rise of cardiac action potentials and decreases conduction velocity in the heart. These pathophysiologic mechanisms underlie the cardiac dysrhythmias of hyperkalemia.[15] Severe hyperkalemia causes cardiac arrest.[23]

The plasma potassium concentration at which each of these clinical manifestations occurs varies, depending on the rapidity of rise of the potassium concentration, the causes of the hyperkalemia, and other concurrent electrolyte or acid-base imbalances. Patients who have chronic end-stage renal disease often undergo potassium adaptation and have relatively mild symptoms at high plasma potassium concentrations that would be disabling in other persons. The mechanisms of potassium adaptation include increased aldosterone levels that increase potassium excretion by the colon and shift potassium ions from extracellular fluid into cells, helping to normalize resting membrane potentials.

Plasma Calcium

Calcium in the plasma is present in three forms: some calcium ions are bound to plasma proteins (such as albumin); some are bound to small organic ions (such as citrate); and the rest are unbound. Only the free ionized calcium is physiologically active. Two laboratory measurements are available for calcium: total serum calcium and ionized calcium. The *total serum calcium* measurement includes all of the calcium (bound plus unbound). The normal range of total serum calcium concentration in adults is 9 to 11 mg/dl or 4.5 to 5.5 mEq/L (may vary slightly with different laboratories). Unless a calcium value specifies ionized calcium, it is total calcium. The *ionized calcium* measurement includes only the unbound ionized form. The normal range of ionized calcium in adults is 4.0 to 5.0 mg/dl, about half of the total calcium (varies with different laboratories). Clinically significant calcium imbalances are caused by alterations in the plasma concentration of unbound ionized calcium.

Hypocalcemia

Hypocalcemia occurs if the serum calcium concentration drops below the lower limit of normal. If the fraction of unbound ionized calcium in the blood is decreased by more calcium binding to plasma proteins or other organic ions such as citrate, the total serum calcium concentration (the usual laboratory measurement) may be normal, but *ionized* hypocalcemia is present and may cause signs and symptoms. Ionized hypocalcemia is common with massive transfusion of blood or fresh frozen plasma because citrate is part of the anticoagulant used to preserve both of these solutions.[24]

Etiology. Hypocalcemia is caused by factors that decrease calcium intake or absorption, decrease the physiologic availability of calcium, and increase calcium excretion. For example, hypocalcemia in pancreatitis arises from impaired fat digestion caused by lack of pancreatic lipase in the intestines. Both dietary calcium and calcium ions secreted into the intestine from the extracellular fluid bind to undigested fat in the intestine and are excreted in the feces. Thus, both decreased calcium absorption and increased calcium excretion play a part in hypocalcemia associated with pancreatitis. In addition, calcium ions can bind to necrotic tissue in the pancreas, decreasing their physiologic availability. Ionized hypocalcemia is common in intensive care unit patients, again due to multiple factors.[25] Parathyroid hormone increases plasma calcium concentration; people who have hypoparathyroidism thus develop hypocalcemia. Box 24-8 lists specific causes of hypocalcemia organized according to the general etiologic factors.

Clinical manifestations. Calcium ions play an important role in determining the speed of ion fluxes through nerve and muscle cell membranes. Thus, calcium imbalances alter normal neuromuscular excitability. Clinical manifestations of hypocalcemia are those of increased neuromuscular excitability: positive Trousseau sign, positive Chvostek sign, paresthesias, muscle twitching and cramping, hyperactive reflexes, carpal spasm, pedal spasm, tetany, laryngospasm, seizures, and cardiac dysrhythmias.[26] The increased neuromuscular excitability of hypocalcemia is caused by a decrease in the threshold potential of excitable cells, so that action potentials are generated more easily. Cardiac effects of hypocalcemia arise from the prolonged plateau phase of the cardiac action potential, impaired atrioventricular and intraventricular conduction, and impaired myocardial contractility, which can cause heart failure.[15,27]

Positive Trousseau sign is occurrence of a carpal spasm after occlusion of arterial blood flow to the hand for approximately 3 minutes. Positive Chvostek sign is spasm of muscles in the cheek and corner of the mouth produced by tapping the facial nerve in front of the ear. Positive Trousseau and Chvostek signs are general indicators of increased neuromuscular excitability from any cause, so they must be interpreted in the context of other clinical manifestations and specific risk factors for hypocalcemia. Chvostek sign may be positive in neonates without electrolyte imbalances.

Hypercalcemia

Hypercalcemia occurs when the serum calcium concentration rises above the upper limit of normal (11 mg/dl or 5.5 mEq/L). It indicates an elevation of the calcium concentration of the extracellular fluid.

Etiology. Hypercalcemia is caused by factors that increase calcium intake or absorption, cause a shift of calcium from bone to extracellular fluid, and decrease calcium excretion. Because parathyroid hormone shifts calcium out of bone, hyperparathyroidism causes hypercalcemia. Many malignant tumors produce chemicals that circulate in the blood and shift calcium from bones into extracellular fluid.[28] These bone-resorbing factors include parathyroid hormone–related peptide and prostaglandins. In addition, circulating factors in malignancy may decrease renal excretion of calcium ions, which also contributes to hypercalcemia. Specific causes of hypercalcemia are listed by category in Box 24-9.

Clinical manifestations. Hypercalcemia causes decreased neuromuscular excitability. Clinical manifestations of hypercalcemia include anorexia, nausea, emesis, constipation, fatigue, polyuria, muscle

---

BOX 24-9   CAUSES OF HYPERCALCEMIA

Increased Calcium Intake or Absorption
Milk-alkali syndrome
Vitamin D overdose (includes shark cartilage supplements)

Shift of Calcium from Bone to Extracellular Fluid
Hyperparathyroidism
Immobilization
Paget disease
Bone tumors
Multiple myeloma
Leukemia
Nonosseous malignancies that produce bone-resorbing factors

Decreased Calcium Excretion
Thiazide diuretics
Familial hypocalciuric hypercalcemia

---

weakness, diminished reflexes, headache, confusion, lethargy, personality change, and cardiac dysrhythmias. The decreased neuromuscular excitability is caused by elevation of the threshold potential of excitable cells. Cardiac effects of hypercalcemia include shortened plateau phase of the action potential, increased rate of diastolic depolarization of sinus node cells, and delayed atrioventricular conduction.[15] Renal calculi may occur as a result of the high calcium concentration of the urine. Hypercalcemia caused by bone resorption may lead to pathologic fractures.

Plasma Magnesium

The normal serum magnesium concentration is 1.5 to 2.5 mEq/L (may vary slightly with different laboratories). Similarly to calcium, magnesium ions also are present in the blood as bound (physiologically inactive) and unbound ionized (physiologically active) forms. Measurement of ionized magnesium levels is available in some research settings. Plasma magnesium concentration imbalances may occur concurrent with or in the absence of total body magnesium content imbalances.

Hypomagnesemia

If the serum magnesium concentration decreases below the lower limit of normal (1.5 mEq/L), hypomagnesemia is present. Hypomagnesemia indicates a decreased magnesium concentration of the extracellular fluid and does not necessarily indicate a total body magnesium deficit (although the two may occur concurrently).

Etiology. Causes of hypomagnesemia are decreased magnesium intake or absorption, decreased physiologic availability of magnesium, increased magnesium excretion, and loss of magnesium by an abnormal route. Chronic alcoholism is a major risk factor for hypomagnesemia because it is associated with decreased magnesium intake, decreased physiologic availability of magnesium, increased urinary and fecal magnesium excretion, and magnesium loss through emesis.[29] Hypomagnesemia often causes hypokalemia by increasing urinary excretion of potassium. In such cases, correction of hypomagnesemia is necessary before the hypokalemia can be corrected. Specific causes of hypomagnesemia are listed in Box 24-10.

Clinical manifestations. Magnesium ions in the extracellular fluid normally depress the release of acetylcholine at neuromuscular junctions. If too few magnesium ions are present, excessive amounts of acetylcholine are released (Figure 24-11). Therefore, the clinical manifestations of hypomagnesemia are those of increased neuromuscular excitability. Such manifestations may include insomnia, hyperactive reflexes, muscle cramps, muscle twitching, grimacing, positive Chvostek sign, positive Trousseau sign, nystagmus, dysphagia, ataxia, tetany, and seizures. Cardiac dysrhythmias also occur.

Hypomagnesemia causes decreased activity of the enzyme that drives the Na^+-K^+ pump in cell membranes, so that intracellular potassium concentration decreases in the myocardium. Increased spontaneous firing in the sinus node, shortening of the absolute refractory period, and lengthening of the relative refractory period contribute to cardiac dysrhythmias in hypomagnesemia.[15]

Hypermagnesemia

If the serum magnesium concentration rises above the upper limit of normal (2.5 mEq/L), hypermagnesemia is present. Hypermagnesemia indicates an excess of magnesium in the extracellular fluid.

Etiology. The major causes of hypermagnesemia are increased magnesium intake and decreased magnesium excretion. Shift of magnesium from bones to extracellular fluid is seen transiently in some stages of hyperparathyroidism. More commonly, hypermagnesemia from excessive intake of magnesium in laxatives and antacids occurs in people of any age who have unrecognized renal impairment or receive high doses.[30] Older adults are at high risk from these magnesium-containing medications. Individuals who have oliguria, as in chronic end-stage renal disease, are another high-risk group for development of hypermagnesemia. Specific causes of hypermagnesemia are summarized in Box 24-11.

BOX 24-10 CAUSES OF HYPOMAGNESEMIA

Decreased Magnesium Intake or Absorption
Chronic alcoholism
Malnutrition
Prolonged intravenous therapy without magnesium supplementation
Ileal resection
Chronic diarrhea (includes laxative abuse)
Malabsorption syndromes
Steatorrhea
Pancreatitis

Decreased Physiologic Availability of Magnesium
Elevated plasma free fatty acids

Increased Magnesium Excretion Through Normal Routes
Renal Route
Diabetic ketoacidosis
Chronic alcoholism
Hyperaldosteronism
Diuretic therapy
Aminoglycoside (e.g., gentamicin) toxicity
Amphotericin B, cisplatin, and many other drugs

Fecal Route
Steatorrhea
Pancreatitis

Magnesium Loss Through Abnormal Routes
Emesis
Gastric suction
Fistula drainage

Clinical manifestations. Too many magnesium ions in the extracellular fluid depress neuromuscular function by decreasing the release of acetylcholine at neuromuscular junctions (see Figure 24-11). Thus manifestations of hypermagnesemia include decreased deep tendon reflexes, lethargy, hypotension, flushing, diaphoresis, drowsiness, flaccid paralysis, respiratory depression, bradycardia, cardiac dysrhythmias, and even cardiac arrest. Mechanisms that cause the cardiac effects of hypermagnesemia include decreased cardiac conduction and depression of membrane excitability.[15]

Plasma Phosphate

The normal range of phosphate concentration in adult plasma is 2.5 to 4.5 mg/dl (may vary slightly with different laboratories). Symptomatic phosphate imbalances are less common than other electrolyte imbalances, but, like other electrolyte imbalances, they may be fatal if untreated.

Hypophosphatemia

Hypophosphatemia is present when the phosphate concentration in the plasma decreases below the lower limit of normal (2.5 mg/dl). However, the clinical manifestations of hypophosphatemia are often not observed unless the plasma phosphate concentration is less than 1.0 mg/dl. Persons whose plasma phosphate concentration is less than 1.0 mg/dl are said to have *severe symptomatic hypophosphatemia.*

Etiology. Hypophosphatemia is caused by factors that decrease phosphate intake, shift phosphate from extracellular fluid to cells,

---

BOX 24-11 CAUSES OF HYPERMAGNESEMIA

Increased Magnesium Intake or Absorption
Ingestion or aspiration of seawater
Excessive ingestion of magnesium-containing medications (e.g., laxatives, antacids)
Excessive intravenous infusion of magnesium

Decreased Magnesium Excretion
Oliguric renal disease
Adrenal insufficiency

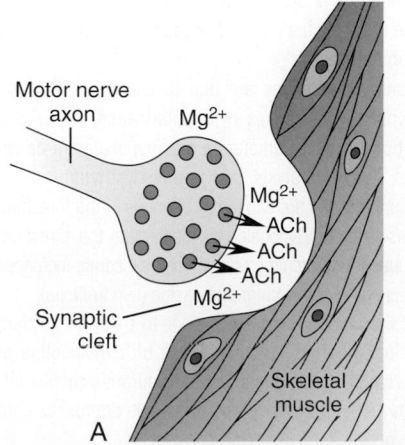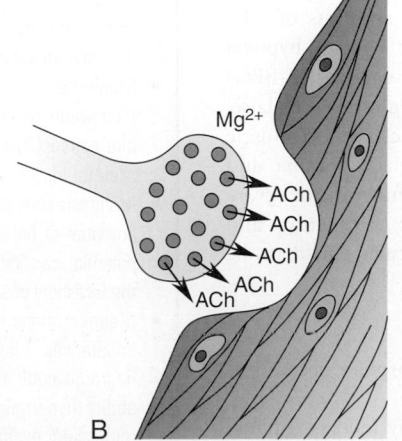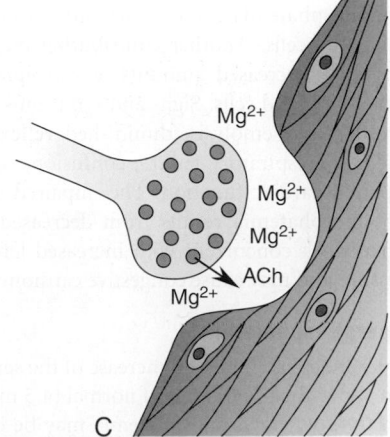

FIGURE 24-11 Acetylcholine (ACh) release at neuromuscular junctions is altered in magnesium imbalances. **A,** Normal magnesium concentration suppresses the release of acetylcholine at neuromuscular junctions to normal levels. **B,** In hypomagnesemia, more acetylcholine is released at neuromuscular junctions, causing increased neuromuscular excitability. **C,** In hypermagnesemia, less acetylcholine is released at neuromuscular junctions, causing decreased neuromuscular excitability.

BOX 24-12 CAUSES OF HYPOPHOSPHATEMIA

Decreased Phosphate Intake or Absorption
Chronic alcoholism
Chronic diarrhea
Malabsorption syndromes
Excessive or long-term use of antacids that bind phosphate

Shift of Phosphate from Extracellular Fluid to Cells
Refeeding after starvation (includes anorexia nervosa)
Total parenteral nutrition
Hyperventilation (respiratory alkalosis)
Insulin
Epinephrine
Intravenous glucose, fructose, bicarbonate, or lactate

Increased Phosphate Excretion Through the Normal Renal Route
Alcohol withdrawal
Diuretic phase after extensive burns
Diabetic ketoacidosis
Diuretic therapy

Phosphate Loss Through Abnormal Routes
Emesis
Hemodialysis

BOX 24-13 CAUSES OF HYPERPHOSPHATEMIA

Increased Phosphate Intake or Absorption
Overzealous phosphate therapy
Excessive use of phosphate-containing enemas or laxatives

Shift of Phosphate from Cells to Extracellular Fluid
Tumor lysis syndrome
Crushing injury
Rhabdomyolysis

Decreased Phosphate Excretion
End-stage renal disease
Oliguric acute kidney injury
Adrenal insufficiency

increase phosphate excretion, and cause loss of phosphate through abnormal routes. Frequently, many factors combine to produce severe symptomatic hypophosphatemia. Any factor that causes a rapid increase in cellular metabolism will cause phosphate to shift from extracellular fluid into cells. Patients who are severely malnourished (such as cancer patients with advanced disease) are at high risk for severe symptomatic hypophosphatemia after nutritional replacement is started because of their increased cellular metabolism and previously depleted phosphate stores.[31] Specific factors that cause hypophosphatemia are summarized in Box 24-12.

Clinical manifestations. Phosphate is an important component of adenosine triphosphate (ATP), the major source of energy for many cellular processes. The signs and symptoms of severe symptomatic hypophosphatemia are due, in part, to decreased amounts of ATP within the cells. Another contributing mechanism is tissue hypoxia caused by decreased amounts of 2,3-biphosphoglycerate (2,3-BPG) in the red blood cells. Signs and symptoms include anorexia, malaise, paresthesias, hemolysis, diminished reflexes, muscle aches, muscle weakness, respiratory failure, confusion, stupor, seizures, coma, and impaired cardiac function. The impaired cardiac function of severe hypophosphatemia results from decreased cardiac contractility and stroke work concurrent with increased left ventricular end-diastolic pressure and may cause congestive cardiomyopathy.[15]

Hyperphosphatemia

Hyperphosphatemia is an increase of the serum phosphate concentration above the upper limit of normal (4.5 mg/dl).

Etiology. Hyperphosphatemia may be caused by increased phosphate intake, shift of phosphate from cells or bones to extracellular fluid, and decreased phosphate excretion. Examples of specific causes in these categories are listed in Box 24-13. Hyperphosphatemia is common in people who have oliguric renal disease, either acute or chronic. In chronic kidney disease, renal phosphate excretion is severely decreased but intestinal absorption of dietary phosphate continues. In addition, elevated parathyroid hormone in chronic kidney disease shifts phosphate from bones into extracellular fluid.[32]

Clinical manifestations. Clinical manifestations of hyperphosphatemia depend on the effect of the elevated phosphate ion concentration on calcium ions. Typically, hyperphosphatemia causes hypocalcemia. The signs and symptoms are thus the manifestations of increased neuromuscular excitability that were presented in the discussion of hypocalcemia. However, in some patients, especially those who have chronic kidney disease, hyperphosphatemia causes deposition of calcium phosphate salts in the soft tissues of the body. These patients develop signs and symptoms such as aching and stiffness of joints, itching (pruritus), and conjunctivitis, depending on the areas in which these salts precipitate.

KEY POINTS

- Plasma electrolyte deficits are caused by factors that decrease electrolyte intake or absorption, shift electrolytes from the extracellular fluid to an electrolyte pool, increase electrolyte excretion, and cause loss of electrolytes through abnormal routes.
- Plasma electrolyte excesses are caused by factors that increase electrolyte intake or absorption, shift electrolytes from an electrolyte pool to the extracellular fluid, and decrease electrolyte excretion.
- Abnormalities in plasma electrolyte concentrations may profoundly affect cellular function. Excitable cells, such as nerve and muscle, are particularly sensitive to electrolyte imbalances.
- Manifestations of potassium imbalances are due to changes in resting membrane potentials. Hypokalemia causes hyperpolarization; hyperkalemia causes hypopolarization. Both hyperkalemia and hypokalemia cause skeletal muscle weakness, flaccid paralysis, and cardiac dysrhythmias.
- Manifestations of calcium imbalances are caused by changes in the threshold potential of nerve and muscle cells. Hypocalcemia decreases the threshold potential, causing hyperexcitability (twitching, tetany); hypercalcemia increases the threshold potential, causing neuromuscular depression (hyporeflexia).
- Manifestations of magnesium imbalances are similar to those of calcium imbalances. Magnesium ions normally inhibit release of acetylcholine at neuromuscular junctions. Hypomagnesemia increases neuromuscular excitability (hyperreflexia and twitching), and hypermagnesemia depresses neuromuscular excitability (hyporeflexia and flaccid paralysis).
- Severe symptomatic hypophosphatemia is characterized by manifestations of generalized cellular ATP deficiency. Hyperphosphatemia may cause hypocalcemia, with resulting increased neuromuscular excitability, or it may be associated with precipitation of calcium phosphate into soft tissues of the body.

SUMMARY

This chapter presents the principles of fluid and electrolyte homeostasis and imbalances. The boxes below summarize pediatric and geriatric considerations, respectively. Fluid and electrolyte homeostasis involves the continuous interplay of intake, absorption, distribution, and excretion of fluid and electrolytes. Loss of fluid and electrolytes through abnormal routes may also occur. When the normal mechanisms are impaired or overwhelmed, fluid and electrolyte imbalances occur. Fluid imbalances may involve the volume or the concentration of body fluid. Plasma electrolyte imbalances may be deficits or excesses and may not reflect total body electrolyte deficits or excesses. Signs and symptoms of fluid and electrolyte imbalances are summarized in Table 24-2. The pathophysiology of specific fluid and electrolyte imbalances can be derived from a working knowledge of normal fluid and electrolyte homeostasis.

PEDIATRIC CONSIDERATIONS

Fluid and Electrolyte Homeostasis and Imbalances

- Infants have more extracellular fluid than intracellular fluid; this proportion reverses by a few months of age.
- About 75% of the body weight of a term infant is water; this percentage is even higher in preterm infants. The percentage of body weight that is water decreases as the child ages.
- In the first few days after birth, an infant loses fluid equal to 5% to 10% of its body weight; this is a normal process during adjustment to extrauterine life.
- Neonates have a high metabolic rate and thus a high turnover rate of water.
- Infants have increased insensible water excretion caused by proportionately large body surface area, proportionately large respiratory mucosa surface area, vasomotor immaturity, and increased skin permeability. Preterm infants have even greater insensible water excretion through the skin because of flaccid extended posture (and thus greater exposed body surface area) and greater vasomotor immaturity.
- Use of phototherapy and radiant heat warmers increases insensible water excretion.
- Glomerular filtration rate is lower in infants than in adults.
- The kidneys of infants have limited ability to concentrate urine or to dilute it; thus, infants are unable to excrete a large load of water effectively or to conserve fluid when needed.

- Infants communicate thirst by crying, which may not be understood by their caregivers.
- Assessment of extracellular volume imbalances in infants should focus on the tension of the fontanel rather than the degree of filling of neck veins.
- Infants whose caregivers use powdered formula are at high risk for hypernatremia if the formula is reconstituted with extra powder to "strengthen" the baby.
- Laboratory normal ranges of electrolytes generally are wider for infants than older children and adults.
- Neonatal hypocalcemia may occur in infants who needed resuscitation at birth or have high-risk conditions.
- Preterm infants may have reduced body calcium stores because fetal calcium stores are built during the last trimester of pregnancy; these infants have increased incidence of neonatal hypocalcemia.
- Assessment of increased neuromuscular excitability (hypocalcemia and hypomagnesemia) in infants should not include Chvostek sign; this sign is often positive in normal neonates. Increased neuromuscular excitability in infants includes jitteriness, hyperactive reflexes, and a high-pitched cry.
- Neonates whose mothers were given magnesium sulfate for eclampsia in the 24 hours before birth may be born with hypermagnesemia. Hypermagnesemic infants lie in a flaccid, extended posture.

GERIATRIC CONSIDERATIONS

Fluid and Electrolyte Homeostasis and Imbalances

- Older adults have less body water than middle-aged adults because body composition changes with increasing age (decreased muscle mass, increased fat in internal organs). About 50% of the body weight of a lean older man is water and about 45% of the body weight of a lean older woman is water; the percentage is lower in obese older adults.
- Glomerular filtration rate is lower in older adults than in middle-aged adults.
- The kidneys of older adults are less able to concentrate urine and thus less able to conserve fluid when needed. This decreased ability to concentrate urine is also responsible for nocturia, since a larger than normal volume of urine is produced at night.
- Older adults have a reduced thirst response when the osmolality of body fluids increases; thus, they may not be aware that they are becoming dehydrated.

- Older adults are a high-risk group for clinical dehydration.
- Decreased skin turgor is not reliable as a sign of extracellular fluid volume depletion in older adults, because of age-related changes in collagen and elastin. Decreased skin turgor (skin tenting when pinched) may occur in older adults who have normal fluid volume.
- Older adults who receive tube feedings are at higher risk for hypernatremia than middle-aged adults.
- Older adults probably absorb more magnesium from antacids and cathartics than do middle-aged adults. With age-related changes in renal excretion, older adults who use oral magnesium laxatives or antacids regularly are at high risk for hypermagnesemia.

TABLE 24-2   SUMMARY OF SIGNS AND SYMPTOMS OF FLUID AND ELECTROLYTE IMBALANCES

IMBALANCE	HEART	BLOOD VESSELS	INTERSTITIAL AREA	CNS	LUNGS
↓ Extracellular volume	Tachycardia	Postural blood pressure decrease with concurrent heart rate increase, flat neck veins, ↑ small-vein filling time, thready pulse	↓ Skin turgor; soft, sunken eyeballs; longitudinal furrows in tongue	Lightheadedness, syncope	
↑ Extracellular volume		Distended neck veins, bounding pulse	Edema		Crackles, dyspnea, orthopnea, frothy sputum
↓ Na+				Confusion, lethargy, coma, seizures	
↑ Na+				Confusion, lethargy, coma, seizures	
↓ K+	Dysrhythmias	Postural hypotension			
↑ K+	Dysrhythmias, cardiac arrest				
↓ Ca++	Dysrhythmias, impaired myocardial contractility			Seizures	
↑ Ca++	Dysrhythmias			Confusion, lethargy, personality change	
↓ Mg++	Dysrhythmias			Insomnia, seizures	
↑ Mg++	Bradycardia, dysrhythmias, cardiac arrest	Hypotension, flushing		Drowsiness, lethargy	Respiratory depression
↓ Pi	Impaired cardiac function, decreased cardiac output			Confusion, stupor, coma, seizures	Respiratory failure
↑ Pi (may cause ↓ Ca++)					

CNS, Central nervous system; *ECV,* extracellular fluid volume; *Pi,* inorganic phosphate.

SKELETAL MUSCLE	NEUROMUSCULAR EXCITABILITY	GASTROINTESTINAL TRACT	KIDNEYS	OTHER
		Dry oral mucous membranes, hard stools	Oliguria	Sudden weight loss, sunken fontanel (infants), no tears or sweat, thirst with severe ↓ ECV
		Hepatomegaly		Sudden weight gain, bulging fontanel (infants)
		Anorexia, nausea, emesis		Malaise, headache
			Oliguria	Thirst
Ascending weakness, flaccid paralysis		Abdominal distention, bloating, ↓ bowel sounds, constipation, paralytic ileus	Polyuria	
Ascending weakness, flaccid paralysis		Mild cramping, diarrhea		
Twitching, cramping, carpal spasm, pedal spasm	Increased excitability, Trousseau sign, Chvostek sign, paresthesias, hyperactive reflexes, tetany			Laryngospasm
Weakness	Decreased excitability, depressed reflexes	Anorexia, nausea, emesis, constipation	Polyuria	Fatigue, headache
Twitching, cramping, grimacing, tremors	Increased excitability, Trousseau sign, Chvostek sign, hyperactive reflexes, tetany	Dysphagia		Nystagmus, ataxia
Flaccid paralysis	Depressed reflexes			Diaphoresis
Aching, weakness	Paresthesias, depressed reflexes	Anorexia		Malaise, hemolysis
			If Ca++ remains high, damage from deposition of crystals	If Ca++ remains high, pruritus, conjunctivitis, arthritis

REFERENCES

1. Hall JE: *Guyton and Hall textbook of medical physiology*, ed 12, Philadelphia, 2011, Saunders Elsevier.

2. Thornton SN: Thirst and hydration: physiology and consequences of dysfunction, *Physiol Behav* 100:15–21, 2010.

3. Waldreus N, Sjostrand F, Hahn RG: Thirst in the elderly with and without heart failure, *Arch Gerontol Geriatr* 53:174–178, 2011.

4. Thomas W, Harvey BJ: Mechanisms underlying rapid aldosterone effects in the kidney, *Ann Rev Physiol* 73:335–357, 2011.

5. Potter LR: Natriuretic peptide metabolism, clearance and degradation, *FEBS J* 278:1808–1817, 2011.

6. Longo D, Fauchi A, Kasper D, et al, editors: *Harrison's principles of internal medicine*, ed 18, New York, 2012, McGraw-Hill.

7. Swart RM, Hoorn EJ, Betjes MG, et al: Hyponatremia and inflammation: the emerging role of interleukin-6 in osmoregulation, *Nephron Physiol* 118(2):45–51, 2011.

8. Sanghvi S, Kellerman P, Nanovic L: Beer potomania: an unusual cause of hyponatremia at high risk of complications from rapid correction, *Am J Kidney Dis* 50:673–680, 2007.

9. Kipps C, Sharma S, Pedoe DT: The incidence of exercise-associated hyponatraemia in the London marathon, *Brit J Sports Med* 45:14–19, 2011.

10. Yee AH, Rabinstein AA: Neurologic presentations of acid-base imbalance, electrolyte abnormalities, and endocrine emergencies, *Neurol Clin* 28:1–16, 2010.

11. Tassenoy A, De Mey J, De Ridder F, et al: Postmastectomy lymphoedema: different patterns of fluid distribution visualised by ultrasound imaging compared with magnetic resonance imaging, *Physiother* 97:234–243, 2011.

12. Schulte-Merker S, Sabine A, Petrova TV: Lymphatic vascular morphogenesis in development, physiology, and disease, *J Cell Biol* 193:607–618, 2011.

13. Katzung T, Masters S, Trevor A: *Basic and clinical pharmacology*, ed 12, New York, 2012, Lange Medical Books/McGraw-Hill.

14. Pant P, Nadimpalli L, Singh M, et al: A case of severe hypokalemic paralysis and hypertension: licorice-induced hypokalemic paralysis, *Am J Kidney Dis* 55(6):A35–A37, 2010.

15. Felver L: Fluid and electrolyte and acid-base balance and imbalance. In Woods SL, et al, editors: *Cardiac nursing*, ed 6, Philadelphia, 2010, Lippincott, Williams & Wilkins, pp 153–176.

16. Yorgun H, Aksoy H, Sendur MA, et al: Brugada syndrome with aborted sudden cardiac death related to liquorice-induced hypokalemia, *Med Princ Pract* 19:485–489, 2010.

17. Kasap B, Soylu A, Cetin BS, et al: Acute kidney injury following hypokalemic rhabdomyolysis: complication of chronic heavy cola consumption in an adolescent boy, *Eur J Pediatr* 169:107–111, 2010.

18. Vraets A, Lin Y, Callum JL: Transfusion-associated hyperkalemia, *Transfus Med Rev* 25:184–196, 2011.

19. Howard SC, Jones DP, Pui CH: The tumor lysis syndrome, *New Engl J Med* 364:1844–1854, 2011.

20. Uijtendaal EV, Zwart-van Rijkom JE, van Solinge WW, et al: Frequency of laboratory measurement and hyperkalaemia in hospitalised patients using serum potassium concentration increasing drugs, *Eur J Clin Pharmacol* 67:933–940, 2011.

21. Allsopp K: Caring for patients with kidney failure, *Emerg Nurse* 18(10):12–15, 2011.

22. Hamilton D, Cicovic S, Rassie M: Hyperkalaemic paralysis, *New Z Med J* 124(1333):55–57, 2011.

23. El-Sherif N, Turitto G: Electrolyte disorders and arrhythmogenesis, *Cardiol J* 18:233–245, 2011.

24. Ho KM, Leonard AD: Concentration-dependent effect of hypocalcaemia on mortality of patients with critical bleeding requiring massive transfusion: a cohort study, *Anaesth Intensive Care* 39:46–54, 2011.

25. Buckley MS, Leblanc JM, Cawley MJ: Electrolyte disturbances associated with commonly prescribed medications in the intensive care unit, *Crit Care Med* 38(6 suppl):S253–S264, 2010.

26. Rehman HU, Wunder S: Trousseau sign in hypocalcemia, *CMAJ* 183:E498, 2011.

27. Solzbach U, Kitterer HR, Haas H: Reversible congestive heart failure in severe hypocalcemia, *Herz* 35:507–510, 2010.

28. Lameire N, Van Biesen W, Vanholder R: Electrolyte disturbances and acute kidney injury in patients with cancer, *Semin Nephrol* 30:534–547, 2010.

29. Yanagawa Y, Suzuki C, Imamura T: Recovery of paralysis in association with an improvement of hypomagnesemia due to alcoholism, *Am J Emerg Med* 29:242.e1-242.e2, 2011.

30. Nordt SP, Chen J, Clark RF: Severe hypermagnesemia after enteral administration of Epsom salts, *Am J Health Sys Pharm* 68:1384–1385, 2011.

31. Zeki S, Culkin A, Gabe SM, et al: Refeeding hypophosphataemia is more common in enteral than parenteral feeding in adult in patients, *Clin Nutr* 30:365–368, 2011.

32. Molony DA, Stephens BW: Derangements in phosphate metabolism in chronic kidney diseases/endstage renal disease: therapeutic considerations, *Adv Chronic Kidney Dis* 18:120–131, 2011.

Acid-Base Homeostasis and Imbalances

Linda Felver

evolve WEBSITE

http://evolve.elsevier.com/Copstead/

- Review Questions and Answers
- Glossary (with audio pronunciations for selected terms)
- Animations
- Case Studies
- Key Points Review

KEY QUESTIONS

- What are the chemistry and functional importance of the bicarbonate buffer system?
- What is the role of the respiratory system in regulating carbonic acid (carbon dioxide)?
- What is the role of the kidneys in regulating bicarbonate ion and acids other than carbonic acid?
- How do the lungs compensate for acid-base imbalances caused by altered levels of metabolic acids?
- How do the kidneys compensate for acid-base imbalances caused by altered levels of carbonic acid?
- How are arterial blood gas values used to categorize an acid-base disorder as acidosis or alkalosis, respiratory or metabolic, compensated or uncompensated?
- What pathophysiologic conditions predispose an individual to each of the four primary acid-base imbalances?

CHAPTER OUTLINE

When the pH of body fluids becomes abnormal, cellular function is impaired. The pH of a fluid reflects its degree of acidity or alkalinity. Technically, pH is the negative logarithm of the hydrogen ion (H^+) concentration. The normal hydrogen ion concentration of the blood is about 40 nmol/L (40×10^{-9} mol/L)—a very small number.[1] The pH (negative logarithm) of this number is 7.40, which is easier to use in clinical settings. An alteration in pH is a change in the hydrogen ion concentration. A high pH indicates few hydrogen ions, meaning that the solution is alkaline (basic). A low pH indicates a large amount of hydrogen ions, meaning that the solution is acidic.

An acid releases hydrogen ions. The more hydrogen ions present, the more acidic the solution. The normal pH of adult blood ranges from 7.35 to 7.45 (may vary slightly with different laboratories). The range is somewhat wider in infants and children. Table 25-1 lists normal laboratory values for pH and other acid-base parameters. If the blood and other body fluids become too acidic (reflected by pH decreased below the lower limit of the normal range), dysfunction occurs; if the pH of the blood falls below 6.9, death is likely to occur. Similarly, if the body fluids become too alkaline, as reflected by pH increased above the upper limit of the normal range, dysfunction also occurs. If the pH of the blood rises above 7.8, death is likely.

Normal cellular metabolism continually releases acids (carbonic and metabolic) that must be excreted from the body to prevent body

TABLE 25-1	NORMAL LABORATORY VALUES FOR ACID-BASE PARAMETERS	
CHARACTERISTIC	**NORMAL RANGE**
$Paco_2$ (arterial blood)	36-44 mm Hg (adults)
	30-34 mm Hg (infants)
HCO_3^- (serum)	22-26 mEq/L (adults)
	19-23 mEq/L (infants)
pH (arterial blood)	7.35-7.45 (adults)
	7.11-7.36 (neonates)
	7.36-7.41 (infants)

fluids from becoming too acidic. This chapter discusses the normal mechanisms of acid-base homeostasis and the acid-base imbalances that arise when these homeostatic mechanisms become dysfunctional or overwhelmed.

ACID-BASE HOMEOSTASIS

Three major mechanisms regulate the acid-base status of the body: buffers, the respiratory system, and the renal system. Laboratory measurements such as arterial blood gas values are useful indicators of the acid-base status of extracellular fluids. The partial pressure of carbon dioxide in arterial blood ($Paco_2$) is an indicator of the respiratory component of acid-base balance. The plasma bicarbonate ion (HCO_3^-) concentration is an indicator of the renal (metabolic) component of acid-base balance.[1] The pH of the blood indicates the net result of normal acid-base regulation, any acid-base imbalance, and the body's compensatory responses. It is important to remember that the pH measured clinically is that of the blood and may not reflect the pH inside cells or in cerebrospinal fluid.

Buffers

Buffers are chemicals that help control the pH of body fluids. Each buffer system consists of a weak acid, which releases hydrogen ions when the fluid is too alkaline, and a base, which takes up hydrogen ions when the fluid is too acidic. In this way, potential changes in pH are adjusted immediately by the action of buffers. All body fluids contain buffers. Chief among them are bicarbonate buffers (in the extracellular fluid), phosphate buffers (in intracellular fluid and urine), hemoglobin buffers (inside erythrocytes), and protein buffers (in intracellular fluid and the blood). These buffers are the first line of defense against pH imbalances.

The bicarbonate buffer system is the most important buffer in the extracellular fluid. Bicarbonate ion (HCO_3^-) is the base portion and carbonic acid (H_2CO_3) is the weak acid portion. These two components of the bicarbonate buffer system are in chemical equilibrium in the extracellular fluid.[2] If too much acid (e.g., lactic acid) is present, the bicarbonate ions take up hydrogen ions (H^+) released by the acid and become carbonic acid. Through the action of the enzyme carbonic anhydrase, the carbonic acid then is excreted through the respiratory system in the form of carbon dioxide and water. Thus the excess acid is neutralized when bicarbonate ions are used in the buffering process.

$$HCO_3^- + H^+ \rightleftharpoons H_2CO_3 \xrightarrow{\text{carbonic anhydrase}} CO_2 + H_2O$$

Conversely, if too little acid is present in the extracellular fluid, the carbonic acid portion of the bicarbonate buffer system releases

hydrogen ions. This action helps to keep the pH from becoming too high or at least minimizes the increase.

$$H_2CO_3 \rightleftharpoons HCO_3^- + H^+$$

The pH of any fluid is determined by the relative amounts of acids and bases contained in it. For the pH of the blood to be within the normal range, the ratio of bicarbonate ions to carbonic acid must be 20:1, which means that 20 bicarbonate ions must be present for every carbonic acid molecule. This relationship is explained formally by the Henderson-Hasselbalch equation, which is a mathematical description of the pH of a buffered solution, here written specifically for the bicarbonate buffer system.

$$pH = pK_a + \log \frac{[HCO_3^-]}{[H_2CO_3]}$$

Square brackets, used throughout this chapter, are a standard notation for concentration. pKa is the dissociation constant for any particular acid; it equals 6.1 for carbonic acid.[2] If the normal 20:1 ratio of bicarbonate ions to carbonic acid is present, the pH will be 7.4.

$$pH = 6.1 + \log 20$$

$$pH = 6.1 + 1.3$$

$$pH = 7.4$$

The 20:1 ratio of bicarbonate ions to carbonic acid necessary for a normal pH is an important concept in understanding the compensatory mechanisms for acid-base imbalances that are discussed later in this chapter.

Respiratory Contribution

The respiratory system is the second defense against acid-base disorders. Body cells continuously produce carbon dioxide (CO_2). Together, CO_2 and water (H_2O) make carbonic acid (H_2CO_3). The lungs excrete carbon dioxide and water from the body. Therefore, during the process of exhalation the lungs effectively excrete carbonic acid. The respiratory system adjusts the amount of carbonic acid that remains in the body by altering rate and depth of respiration.

The rate and depth of respiration are influenced strongly by chemoreceptors that sense the $Paco_2$, Pao_2, and pH of the blood. If too much carbonic acid begins to accumulate in the blood of a healthy person, the rate and depth of respiration increase and excess carbonic acid is removed. This response corrects the imbalance and restores blood chemistry to normal. If, on the other hand, too little carbonic acid is present in the blood, the rate and depth of respiration decrease to retain carbonic acid until it once more is present in normal amounts. Again, the imbalance is corrected and the blood chemistry returns to normal. Thus the body's correction of a carbonic acid excess or deficit is dependent on normal function of all components of the respiratory system, including the chemoreceptors, respiratory neurons in the brainstem, motor nerves to respiratory muscles, diaphragm and other respiratory muscles, chest wall, and, of course, the airways, lungs, and pulmonary circulation. In older adults, the chemoreceptor response to increased $Paco_2$ may occur more slowly.

The $Paco_2$ indicates how effectively the respiratory system is excreting carbonic acid. If the $Paco_2$ is elevated above the upper limit of the normal range, carbonic acid has accumulated in the blood. In other words, the respiratory rate and depth have been insufficient or lung disease has prevented sufficient carbonic acid (carbon dioxide and water) excretion.[3] Similarly, if the $Paco_2$ is decreased below the

| TABLE 25-2 | **RESPIRATORY RESPONSES TO CHANGES IN CARBONIC AND METABOLIC ACIDS** | |

STIMULUS	RESPIRATORY RESPONSE	RESULT
Increased Pa_{CO_2}, decreased pH	Hyperventilation	Correction of imbalance
Decreased Pa_{CO_2}, increased pH	Hypoventilation	Correction of imbalance
Decreased pH from excess of metabolic acids	Hyperventilation	Compensation for imbalance
Increased pH from deficit of metabolic acids	Hypoventilation	Compensation for imbalance

lower limit of the normal range, the lungs have excreted more carbonic acid than usual. In other words, the respiratory rate and depth have been excessive.[4]

Carbonic acid is known as a volatile acid because it can be excreted as gases (CO_2 and H_2O). It is the only volatile acid in the body. Other acids that accumulate in the body, such as lactic acid and acetoacetic acid, are nonvolatile. They are organic acids that have no gaseous form. The lungs can excrete only carbonic acid; they cannot excrete nonvolatile acids that may accumulate in the body. If a nonvolatile acid (such as lactic acid) accumulates in the blood, the rate and depth of respiration will increase because the excess hydrogen ions stimulate the chemoreceptors. This hyperventilation does not excrete lactic acid (which would correct the problem), but it does remove carbonic acid from the blood. Removing carbonic acid from the blood when another acid is present in excess helps keep the pH from dropping too low. However, this response makes other values abnormal. The respiratory response to an imbalance of any acid except carbonic acid is called *compensation*. A compensatory response does not correct a pH disorder but it does compensate for it by adjusting the pH back toward normal, even though other blood chemistry values are made abnormal in the process.

The compensatory response to a deficit of any acid except carbonic acid is hypoventilation.[1,5] By decreasing rate and depth of respiration, the body retains carbonic acid. This carbonic acid accumulation helps keep blood pH from rising to a fatal level when another acid is deficient in the body. Respiratory compensation for an imbalance of metabolic acid begins in minutes but requires at least several hours for full effectiveness. Respiratory responses to changes in carbonic and metabolic acids are summarized in Table 25-2.

Renal Contribution

The third defense against acid-base disorders is the kidneys. The kidneys can excrete any acid from the body except carbonic acid (which is excreted by the lungs). These acids that are not carbonic acid are called metabolic acids because cells continuously produce them during normal metabolism. The kidneys normally excrete metabolic acids. If a metabolic acid begins to accumulate in the blood, the kidneys increase their acid excretion mechanisms to correct the problem. If a metabolic acid is deficient in the blood, the kidneys slow their acid excretion mechanisms to allow acid to accumulate to normal levels. The body's ability to correct an excess or deficit of a metabolic acid depends on normal function of the renal system. Infants excrete more bicarbonate in their urine than do older children or adults; their kidneys are less effective in excreting acid. The renal response to a large acid load also is less efficient in older adults.

The kidneys have several mechanisms that accomplish acid excretion.[2] Understanding these mechanisms requires a knowledge of basic renal physiology. Briefly, at the glomerulus, fluid filtered from the blood enters the glomerular (Bowman) capsule, which is the beginning of the nephron. The cells that line the lumen of the renal tubule modify the fluid inside the nephron (renal tubular fluid). Renal tubular fluid that passes through the entire nephron becomes the urine. Renal tubular epithelial cells have different membrane structures on opposite sides of the cells. The luminal membrane (next to the renal tubular fluid) contains different transporter proteins than the basolateral membrane (next to the interstitial fluid). This structure allows these cells to secrete certain substances into the renal tubular fluid and move other substances into the interstitial fluid.

In the proximal tubules, renal tubular epithelial cells excrete metabolic acid by secreting both the anion portion of the metabolic acid (e.g., lactate) and the hydrogen ions into the tubule lumen. For every hydrogen ion (H^+) that is secreted into the renal tubular fluid, one bicarbonate ion (HCO_3^-) is moved into the interstitial fluid.[6] The fluid filtered from the blood at the glomerulus contains many bicarbonate ions and most or all of that bicarbonate is reabsorbed (returned to the blood) during secretion of hydrogen ions. Renal tubular cells are able to secrete additional hydrogen ions into the tubular fluid to excrete large amounts of hydrogen ions from metabolic acid.

Once the H^+ are in the renal tubular fluid, most of them combine with other chemicals: bicarbonate ions, which were filtered at the glomerulus, as described previously; urine buffers, such as phosphate, which were filtered at the glomerulus; or ammonia (NH_3), which is produced by renal tubular cells. Net H^+ excretion occurs after HCO_3^- has been reabsorbed in the amount that was filtered at the glomerulus. Thus net H^+ excretion is accomplished in the form of buffered H^+ (called *titratable acidity*) and H^+ attached to ammonia (ammonium ions, NH_4^+). Figure 25-1 illustrates these processes. Some of these processes operate also in the thick ascending limb of the loop of Henle and the distal nephron, where the intracellular chemistry differs slightly but the overall processes are the same.

When the kidneys need to excrete more hydrogen ions, renal tubular cells increase their production of ammonia (NH_3). Ammonia, a gas, moves easily into the renal tubular fluid where it combines with hydrogen ions to become ammonium ions (NH_4^+). Ammonium ions are not lipid soluble, so they do not cross easily from the renal tubular fluid back to the blood. Only free hydrogen ions contribute to the acidity of the urine, not those that are part of ammonium ions. Consequently, increased production of ammonia is an effective way of excreting more hydrogen ions in the renal tubular fluid without making the urine too acidic.

The concentration of HCO_3^- in plasma reflects the effectiveness of renal regulation of metabolic acids. If metabolic acids are accumulating in the blood, they will be buffered by HCO_3^- and the HCO_3^- concentration will drop below normal. Thus, a decreased concentration of HCO_3^- in plasma indicates a relative excess of metabolic acids. An increased HCO_3^- concentration in the plasma indicates a relative deficit of metabolic acids (in other words, a relative excess of base).

Although the kidneys are unable to excrete carbonic acid, they can compensate for carbonic acid imbalances by adjusting the excretion of metabolic acids.[7] For example, if carbonic acid accumulates in the blood, the kidneys can increase the excretion of metabolic acids. This compensatory action helps keep the pH of the blood from becoming too abnormal. Similarly, if a deficit of carbonic acid in the blood is prolonged, the kidneys will decrease the excretion of metabolic acids. As these metabolic acids accumulate in the blood, they will compensate for the lack of carbonic acid and return the pH of the blood toward normal. The body's compensatory response to an imbalance of one

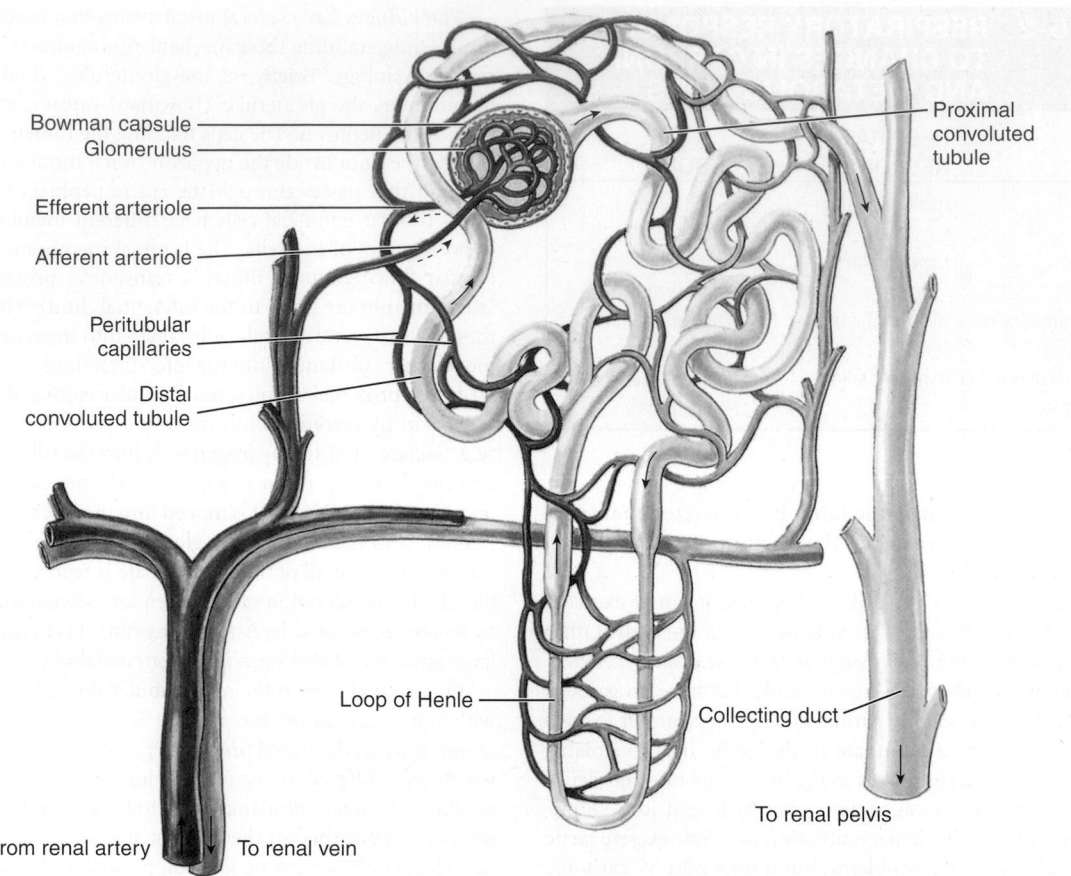

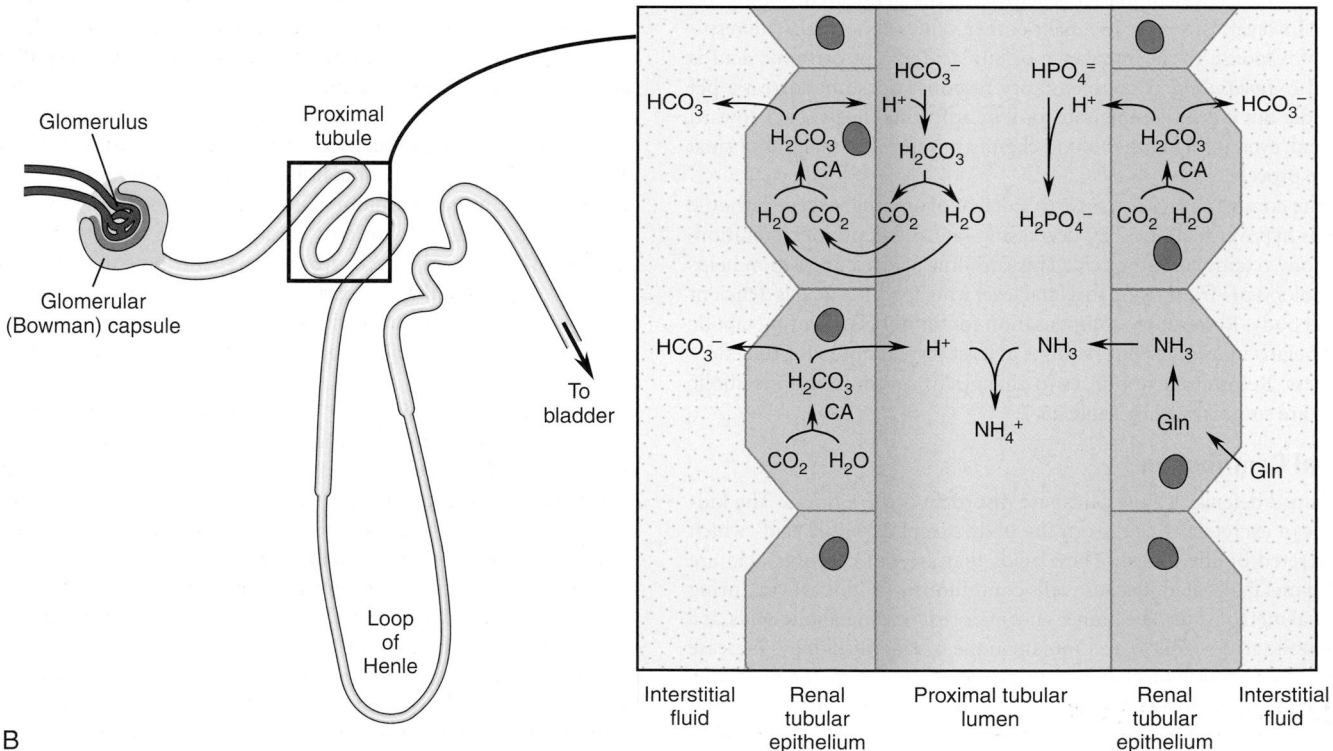

FIGURE 25-1 A, Diagram of a nephron. **B,** Renal proximal tubule mechanisms for excretion of metabolic acid. Hydrogen ions secreted into the renal tubular lumen combine with filtered bicarbonate (which then is reabsorbed), buffers (phosphate buffer illustrated here), or ammonia (forming ammonium ions). *CA,* Carbonic anhydrase, an enzyme; *Gln,* glutamine, an amino acid. **(A,** From Solomon EP: *Introduction to human anatomy and physiology,* ed 3, St Louis, 2009, Mosby, p 266.)

TABLE 25-3 RENAL RESPONSES TO CHANGES IN METABOLIC AND CARBONIC ACIDS

STIMULUS	RENAL RESPONSE	RESULT
Decreased pH from excess of metabolic acids	Secrete more H^+ into renal tubules Make more ammonia	Correction of imbalance
Increased pH from deficit of metabolic acids	Secrete fewer H^+ into renal tubules Excrete HCO_3^- Make less ammonia	Correction of imbalance
Decreased pH from excess of carbonic acid	Secrete more H^+ into renal tubules Make more ammonia	Compensation for imbalance
Increased pH from deficit of carbonic acid	Secrete fewer H^+ into renal tubules Excrete HCO_3^- Make less ammonia	Compensation for imbalance

kind of acid thus returns the pH of the blood toward normal by creating an imbalance of another kind of acid. The renal compensatory response to an imbalance of carbonic acid requires several days to be fully operative. Renal responses to changes in metabolic and carbonic acids are summarized in Table 25-3.

KEY POINTS

- Normal cellular metabolism produces both carbon dioxide and metabolic acids. Carbon dioxide (CO_2) combines with water (H_2O) to form carbonic acid (H_2CO_3). Both carbonic and metabolic acids must be excreted to maintain acid-base homeostasis.
- Buffers are chemicals (a weak acid plus its base) that prevent large changes in pH by releasing or taking up hydrogen ions (H^+). The bicarbonate buffer system is the most important buffer in the extracellular fluid. The normal ratio of bicarbonate to carbonic acid is 20:1. Any deviation from this ratio alters the pH of the blood.
- The lungs excrete carbon dioxide. Rate and depth of respiration normally are adjusted by chemoreceptors in response to acid-base and oxygen status. Increased ventilation (hyperventilation) decreases the amount of carbon dioxide in blood and thus reduces the amount of carbonic acid. Decreased ventilation (hypoventilation) allows carbon dioxide to accumulate and thus increases the amount of carbonic acid in the blood.
- The kidneys excrete metabolic acids. They can secrete H^+ into the renal tubular fluid and retain HCO_3^- in the body or may allow some HCO_3^- to be excreted, depending on homeostatic demands. Most H^+ in the urine is buffered (titratable acidity) or in the form of ammonium ions. The concentration of HCO_3^- in plasma reflects the relative amount of metabolic acid in the blood.
- The lungs compensate for acid-base imbalances resulting from altered levels of metabolic acids; the kidneys compensate for acid-base imbalances resulting from altered levels of carbonic acid. With compensation, the pH returns toward normal but $Paco_2$ and HCO_3^- levels are abnormal.

ACID-BASE IMBALANCES

The four primary acid-base disorders are metabolic acidosis, respiratory acidosis, metabolic alkalosis, and respiratory alkalosis. *Acidosis* is the presence of a condition that tends to decrease the pH of the blood below normal (make the blood relatively more acidic). If blood pH actually is decreased, *acidemia* also is present. *Alkalosis* is the presence

BOX 25-1 COMMON CAUSES OF METABOLIC ACIDOSIS

Increase in Metabolic Acid
Ketoacidosis (diabetes mellitus, starvation, alcoholism)
Severe hyperthyroidism
Burns
Circulatory shock
Tissue anoxia (lactic acidosis)
Oliguric acute kidney injury or end-stage chronic kidney disease
Excessive intake of acids or acid precursors (e.g., salicylates, methanol, ethylene glycol)

Decrease in Base (Bicarbonate)
Severe or prolonged diarrhea
Gastrointestinal fistula that drains intestinal or pancreatic secretions
Intestinal decompression
Renal tubular acidosis

of any factor that tends to increase the pH of the blood above normal (make the blood relatively more alkaline). The term *alkalemia* denotes an increased blood pH. The pathophysiology of the four primary acid-base disorders can be reasoned logically from the principles of acid-base homeostasis.

Metabolic Acidosis

Etiology. Metabolic acidosis is a condition that tends to cause a relative excess of any acid except carbonic acid.[8] Metabolic acidosis may be caused by an increase in acid (not carbonic), by a decrease in base, or by a combination of the two. These mechanisms decrease the normal 20:1 ratio of HCO_3^- to H_2CO_3.

An increase of any acid except carbonic acid will decrease the normal ratio of bicarbonate to carbonic acid because the bicarbonate ions are used up in buffering the excess acid. For example, when caloric intake is insufficient, as with prolonged fasting, the body begins to use its fat stores for energy. If too little glucose is ingested, the fat is metabolized incompletely and ketoacids accumulate in the blood. This condition is termed *starvation ketoacidosis.*[9]

Bicarbonate ions are a type of base. Any condition that causes excessive removal of bicarbonate ions from the body may cause metabolic acidosis. For example, the intestinal fluid is rich in bicarbonate ions, which originate from pancreatic secretions. Diarrhea causes removal of this base from the body and thus contributes to the development of metabolic acidosis.[10]

Other causes of metabolic acidosis are listed in Box 25-1 under the two general mechanisms discussed: increase in metabolic acid (any acid except carbonic acid) and decrease in base (bicarbonate). Either mechanism tends to make the blood overly acidic. The pathophysiology of diarrhea and other disorders that may cause metabolic acidosis is discussed in other chapters of this text.

Clinical manifestations. Signs and symptoms of metabolic acidosis include headache, abdominal pain, and central nervous system depression (confusion, lethargy, stupor, coma).[11]

Central nervous system depression that occurs in patients with metabolic acidosis is due primarily to the decreased pH of the cerebrospinal and interstitial fluid in the brain. When the pH of the interstitial fluid falls, intracellular pH decreases, the protein structure and enzyme activity in cells are altered, and cellular dysfunction results. Other factors specific to the cause of the acidosis also may induce central nervous system depression, such as hyperosmolality with diabetic ketoacidosis. Severe metabolic acidosis predisposes to tachycardia, ventricular dysrhythmias (from myocardial intracellular acidity), and decreased cardiac contractility, which may be fatal.[8] Death from brainstem dysfunction usually occurs when the pH falls below 6.9.

Arterial blood gases in metabolic acidosis show a bicarbonate concentration below normal. If metabolic acidosis is uncompensated, the pH also is below normal because the usual 20:1 ratio is decreased.

Uncompensated metabolic acidosis:

$$\frac{\text{Decreased [HCO}_3^-]}{\text{Unchanged [H}_2\text{CO}_3]} = \text{pH low}$$

Compensatory response. The respiratory compensation for metabolic acidosis is hyperventilation. The low blood pH stimulates the peripheral chemoreceptors, which then stimulate ventilatory neurons in the brainstem.[2] The end result is increased rate and depth of respiration. As the rate and depth of respiration increase, more carbonic acid (carbon dioxide and water) is excreted. Although hyperventilation does not remove metabolic acid from the body, it does change the ratio of bicarbonate ions to carbonic acid in a favorable direction. Because the bicarbonate ion concentration already is decreased by the

metabolic acidosis, the compensatory decrease in carbonic acid brings the ratio (and thus the pH) back toward normal.

The arterial blood gases of a person who has compensated metabolic acidosis show decreased bicarbonate concentration (the primary imbalance), decreased Paco2 (compensation), and decreased or even normal pH, depending on the degree of compensation. A flowchart for interpreting laboratory measures specific to acid-base imbalances is presented in Figure 25-2. Sample laboratory values for people with metabolic acidosis are presented in Table 25-4.

Compensated metabolic acidosis:

$$\frac{\text{Decreased [HCO}_3^-] \; (\text{primary})}{\text{Decreased [H}_2\text{CO}_3] \; (\text{compensatory})} = \begin{array}{l}\text{pH somewhat low} \\ (\text{partially compensated}) \\ \textit{or} \text{ pH in the normal range} \\ (\text{fully compensated})\end{array}$$

Respiratory Acidosis

Etiology. Respiratory acidosis is a condition that tends to cause an excess of carbonic acid.[8] This condition is aptly named because

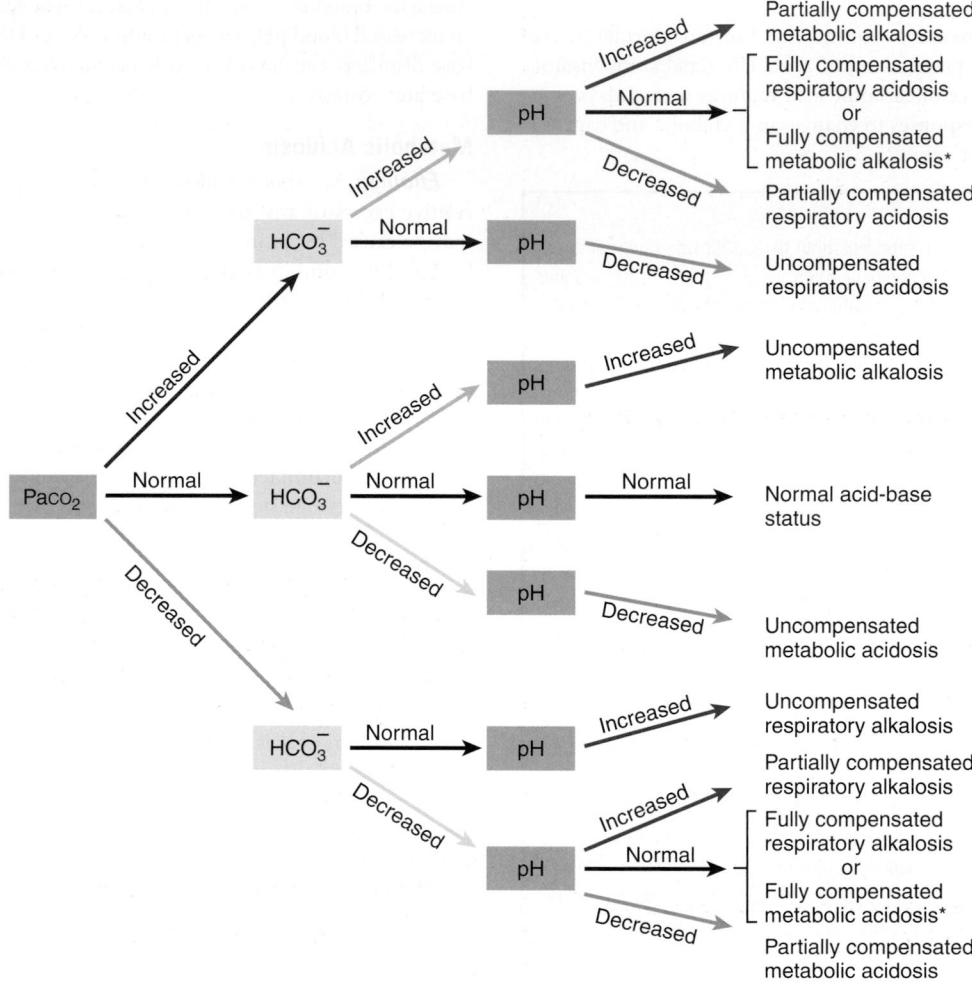

*To differentiate between possible fully compensated imbalances with the pH in the normal range, look at the previous laboratory values for the patient. If no previous values are available, choose the acidosis if the pH is below 7.40 and the alkalosis if the pH is above 7.40.

FIGURE 25-2 Flowchart for interpretation of laboratory measurements specific for acid-base imbalances. Use this flowchart to determine the primary acid-base imbalance from a set of laboratory values. Begin on the left with Paco2 and follow the arrows. This flowchart does not include mixed acid-base imbalances.

carbonic acid is excreted by the lungs in the form of carbon dioxide and water during exhalation.

Respiratory acidosis is caused by factors that impair the respiratory excretion of carbonic acid. Such factors include impaired gas exchange, inadequate neuromuscular function, and impairment of respiratory control in the brainstem. Box 25-2 provides examples of factors that may cause respiratory acidosis. These factors all decrease the normal 20:1 ratio of bicarbonate ion to carbonic acid (and thus decrease the pH of the blood) by increasing the carbonic acid portion of the ratio. Chronic respiratory acidosis often develops in people

who have type B chronic obstructive pulmonary disease (COPD). If an acute respiratory infection also develops, the acidosis may worsen.[3] Such a condition is termed *acute-on-chronic respiratory acidosis*. The pathophysiology of COPD and other disorders that may cause respiratory acidosis is discussed in other chapters of this text.

Clinical manifestations. Signs and symptoms of respiratory acidosis are headache, tachycardia, cardiac dysrhythmias, and neurologic abnormalities such as blurred vision, tremors, vertigo, disorientation, lethargy, or somnolence.

Headache occurs because of dilation of blood vessels in the brain. This cerebral vasodilation increases cerebrospinal fluid pressure; papilledema may result. Neurologic manifestations usually are more prominent in patients with respiratory acidosis than in those with metabolic acidosis because carbonic acid (in the form of carbon dioxide and water) crosses the blood-brain barrier relatively easily.[11] The neurologic manifestations are due to the decreased pH of the cerebrospinal fluid and interstitial fluid in the brain. This decreased interstitial fluid pH causes decreased intracellular pH, with resulting cellular dysfunction. Cardiac dysrhythmias in patients with respiratory acidosis occur because of decreased pH inside myocardial cells.[8] Severe respiratory acidosis causes peripheral vasodilation and hypotension may result, especially if cardiac dysrhythmias also are present.

Arterial blood gases in patients with respiratory acidosis show $Paco_2$ above normal. If respiratory acidosis is uncompensated, the pH is below normal because the usual 20:1 ratio is decreased.[1]

Uncompensated respiratory acidosis:

$$\frac{\text{Unchanged [HCO}_3^-]}{\text{Increased [H}_2\text{CO}_3]} = \text{pH low}$$

Compensatory response. The compensatory response to respiratory acidosis is increased renal excretion of metabolic acid. This mechanism requires several days to be effective. Although the kidneys cannot excrete carbonic acid, their ability to excrete more metabolic acid changes the ratio of bicarbonate ions to carbonic acid in a favorable direction so that the pH moves toward normal. As the kidneys excrete more metabolic acid, the bicarbonate concentration increases because fewer bicarbonate ions are used for buffering. Because carbonic acid concentration already is increased, the compensatory

TABLE 25-4	SAMPLE LABORATORY VALUES FOR PEOPLE WITH ACID-BASE IMBALANCES
LABORATORY VALUE FOR IMBALANCE	**EXPLANATION**
Partially Compensated Metabolic Acidosis (Diabetic Ketoacidosis)	
$Paco_2$ 30 mm Hg	Decreased because of compensatory hyperventilation
HCO_3^- 12 mEq/L	Decreased because of buffering of ketoacids
pH 7.22	Decreased because of excess metabolic acids; would be even lower without respiratory compensation
Uncompensated Respiratory Acidosis (Acute Asthma Episode)	
$Paco_2$ 55 mm Hg	Increased because of impaired gas exchange
HCO_3^- 24 mEq/L	Normal; renal compensation has not yet occurred in this acute condition
pH 7.26	Decreased because of excess carbonic acid
Fully Compensated Respiratory Acidosis (Type B COPD)	
$Paco_2$ 60 mm Hg	Increased because of impaired gas exchange
HCO_3^- 36 mEq/L	Increased because of renal compensation in this chronic condition
pH 7.35	Normal because of renal compensation, but below 7.4
Uncompensated Metabolic Alkalosis (Repeated Emesis and ECV Depletion)	
$Paco_2$ 42 mm Hg	Normal, but increasing because of compensatory hypoventilation
HCO_3^- 36 mEq/L	Increased because of loss of H^+ from emesis and renal retention of HCO_3^- from ECV depletion
pH 7.52	Increased because of metabolic acid deficit
Uncompensated Respiratory Alkalosis (Hypoxemia from Pulmonary Embolism)	
$Paco_2$ 28 mm Hg	Decreased because of hyperventilation caused by chemoreceptor response to decreased Pao_2
HCO_3^- 24 mEq/L	Normal; renal compensation has not yet occurred in this acute condition
pH 7.52	Increased because of carbonic acid deficit

ECV, Extracellular fluid volume.

BOX 25-2	COMMON CAUSES OF RESPIRATORY ACIDOSIS (HYPOVENTILATION)

Impaired Gas Exchange
Type B chronic obstructive pulmonary disease (COPD)
End-stage type A COPD
Bacterial pneumonia
Severe asthma episode
Pulmonary edema
Acute (adult) respiratory distress syndrome

Impaired Neuromuscular Function
Guillain-Barré syndrome
Chest injury or surgery (pain limits ventilation)
Hypokalemic respiratory muscle weakness
Severe kyphoscoliosis
Respiratory muscle fatigue

Impaired Respiratory Control (Brainstem)
Respiratory depressant drugs (opioids, barbiturates)

BOX 25-3 COMMON CAUSES OF METABOLIC ALKALOSIS

Increase in Base (Bicarbonate)

Excessive intake of bicarbonate or bicarbonate precursors (acetate, citrate, lactate)

Massive transfusion with citrated blood

Mild or moderate extracellular fluid volume deficit

Decrease in Metabolic Acid

Emesis

Gastric suction

Mild or moderate extracellular fluid volume deficit

Hyperaldosteronism

Hypokalemia

---

increase in bicarbonate concentration tends to normalize the ratio of HCO_3^- to H_2CO_3. The arterial blood gases of a person who has compensated respiratory acidosis show increased $Paco_2$ (the primary imbalance), increased bicarbonate concentration (compensation), and decreased or even normal pH, depending on the degree of compensation. Table 25-4 presents sample laboratory values for people with respiratory acidosis.

Compensated respiratory acidosis:

$$\frac{\text{Increased }[HCO_3^-]\text{ (compensatory)}}{\text{Increased }[H_2CO_3]\text{ (primary)}} = \begin{array}{l} \text{pH somewhat low} \\ \text{(partially compensated)} \\ or\text{ pH in the normal range} \\ \text{(fully compensated)} \end{array}$$

Metabolic Alkalosis

Etiology. Metabolic alkalosis is a condition that tends to cause a relative deficit of any acid except carbonic acid.[8] Metabolic alkalosis may be caused by an increase in base (bicarbonate), by a decrease in acid, or by a combination of the two. Bicarbonate may be ingested in antacids such as baking soda and over-the-counter bicarbonate products (e.g., effervescent antacids). With overuse of these agents, enough bicarbonate is absorbed from the gastrointestinal tract to increase the blood bicarbonate concentration, thus increasing the pH.[12]

In addition to a gain in bicarbonate, metabolic alkalosis also may be caused by a decrease in acid. The stomach is a major reservoir of acid. Emesis and gastric suction remove acid from the body and create a relative excess of base; this situation is, by definition, metabolic alkalosis.[13] Increased renal excretion of acid with retention of bicarbonate occurs in extracellular fluid volume deficit. Metabolic alkalosis caused by mild or moderate extracellular fluid volume deficit often is called *contraction alkalosis* and is common during diuretic therapy.[14] (Severe extracellular fluid volume deficit is associated with tissue anoxia, circulatory shock, and metabolic acidosis.) Hypokalemia causes metabolic alkalosis by shifting hydrogen ions into cells and increasing renal excretion of acid.[15]

Causes of metabolic alkalosis are summarized in Box 25-3. The pathophysiology of the disorders that may cause metabolic alkalosis is discussed in other chapters of this text.

Clinical manifestations. Signs and symptoms in patients who have metabolic alkalosis may arise from the extracellular fluid volume depletion that caused the alkalosis. Thus postural hypotension may be present. Hypokalemia frequently coexists with metabolic alkalosis.[15] As described previously, hypokalemia may cause metabolic alkalosis. In addition, metabolic alkalosis that arises from another cause frequently

induces hypokalemia by shifting potassium ions into cells. Regardless of whether the hypokalemia preceded or followed the metabolic alkalosis, the bilateral muscle weakness of hypokalemia frequently is evident in individuals who have metabolic alkalosis.

In people who experience signs and symptoms from the metabolic alkalosis itself, the initial manifestations are those of increased neuromuscular excitability. Fingers and toes may tingle; signs of tetany may progress to seizures.[11] Increased interstitial pH causes increased excitability of nerve cell membranes. In addition, alkalosis causes more ionized calcium to bind to albumin, thus causing an ionized hypocalcemia that contributes to increased neuromuscular excitability. People who develop metabolic alkalosis may become quite belligerent. With severe metabolic alkalosis, initial excitation may change to central nervous system depression. Confusion, lethargy, and coma may ensue from dysfunction of brain cells. Death usually occurs when the pH is around 7.8.[16] The plasma bicarbonate concentration is elevated in people who have metabolic alkalosis.

Uncompensated metabolic alkalosis:

$$\frac{\text{Increased }[HCO_3^-]}{\text{Unchanged }[H_2CO_3]} = \text{pH high}$$

Compensatory response. The compensatory response to metabolic alkalosis is hypoventilation.[5] This shallow breathing retains carbonic acid within the body, thus increasing the lower portion of the bicarbonate ion to carbonic acid ratio. Because the upper portion of the ratio has been increased by the elevated bicarbonate concentration of metabolic alkalosis, the respiratory compensation tends to move the pH toward normal. However, respiratory compensation for metabolic alkalosis usually is incomplete. The need for oxygen drives ventilation, even though the increased pH tends to depress it. Thus the arterial blood gases of a person who has compensated metabolic alkalosis usually show increased bicarbonate concentration (the primary imbalance), increased $Paco_2$ (compensation), and increased pH. Table 25-4 presents sample laboratory values for people with metabolic alkalosis.

Compensated metabolic alkalosis:

$$\frac{\text{Increased }[HCO_3^-]\text{ (primary)}}{\text{Increased }[H_2CO_3]\text{ (compensatory)}} = \begin{array}{l}\text{pH somewhat high} \\ \text{(partially compensated)}\end{array}$$

Respiratory Alkalosis

Etiology. Respiratory alkalosis is a condition that tends to cause a carbonic acid deficit.[8] With a deficit of carbonic acid, the blood is relatively too alkaline.

Respiratory alkalosis is caused by hyperventilation.[4] Carbonic acid is excreted during exhalation; when respirations are excessively rapid and deep (hyperventilation), too much carbonic acid is excreted. The resulting deficit of carbonic acid is respiratory alkalosis. For example, in gram-negative sepsis, respiratory neurons in the brainstem often are stimulated abnormally, causing hyperventilation. Hypoxemia, acute pain, and psychological distress are important clinical causes of hyperventilation that leads to respiratory alkalosis. Other causes of hyperventilation (and thus of respiratory alkalosis) are listed in Box 25-4.

Clinical manifestations. Clinical manifestations of respiratory alkalosis arise from increased neuromuscular excitability. Paresthesias (numbness and tingling) often occur in the fingers and around the mouth; carpal and pedal spasms may occur. Increased extracellular pH has a direct effect of increasing membrane excitability in both central and peripheral neurons. In addition, increased pH of

---

BOX 25-4 COMMON CAUSES OF RESPIRATORY ALKALOSIS (HYPERVENTILATION)

Hypoxemia
Acute pain
Anxiety, psychological distress
Prolonged sobbing
Alcohol withdrawal
Stimulation of the brainstem (salicylate overdose, meningitis, head injury, gram-negative sepsis)

---

the cerebrospinal fluid and cerebral interstitial fluid alters brain cell function, causing excitation and/or confusion in some people.[11] Respiratory alkalosis causes cerebral vasoconstriction, which reduces blood flow in the brain.[17] The alkalosis also decreases the availability of ionized calcium, which contributes to increased neuromuscular excitability.

The increased excretion of carbonic acid in people with respiratory alkalosis causes the Pa_{CO_2} to be abnormally low. If the imbalance is uncompensated, the pH is abnormally high.

Uncompensated respiratory alkalosis:

$$\frac{\text{Unchanged } [HCO_3^-]}{\text{Decreased } [H_2CO_3]} = \text{pH high}$$

Compensatory response. The compensatory response to respiratory alkalosis is decreased renal excretion of metabolic acid.[7] As metabolic acids accumulate in the blood, the bicarbonate ion concentration decreases because bicarbonate ions are used for buffering. Because the carbonic acid concentration already is decreased, renal compensation for respiratory alkalosis tends to return the ratio of bicarbonate ions to carbonic acid, and thus the pH, toward normal. Renal compensatory mechanisms take several days to be fully effective. Many of the causes of respiratory alkalosis, such as acute hypoxemia, pain, and psychological distress, are short-lived; for that reason, they may not be compensated renally. Arterial blood gases of a person who has compensated respiratory alkalosis show decreased Pa_{CO_2} (the primary imbalance), decreased bicarbonate concentration (compensation), and increased or (rarely) normal pH, depending on the degree of compensation. Table 25-4 presents sample laboratory values for people with respiratory alkalosis.

Compensated respiratory alkalosis:

$$\frac{\text{Decreased } [HCO_3^-]\ \text{(compensatory)}}{\text{Decreased } [H_2CO_3]\ \text{(primary)}} = \begin{array}{l}\text{pH somewhat high}\\\text{(partially compensated)}\\\textit{or}\ \text{pH in the normal range}\\\text{(fully compensated)}\end{array}$$

Mixed Acid-Base Imbalances

In most people, only one of the four primary imbalances discussed in this chapter arises at a time. If the imbalance persists, a compensatory imbalance arises as well. This situation was discussed previously in this chapter. Occasionally, however, two primary imbalances arise in the same person. This latter situation is termed a *mixed acid-base imbalance.*[18] For example, a patient who has bacterial pneumonia may develop respiratory acidosis. If severe *Clostridium difficile*–associated diarrhea develops during antibiotic therapy for the pneumonia, a concurrent metabolic acidosis may arise. In this mixed imbalance, the pH is likely to be very low because the two types of primary acidosis impair the effectiveness of the usual compensatory mechanisms. Specifically, the usual compensatory mechanism for metabolic acidosis is hyperventilation, which causes increased excretion of carbonic acid from the body. With bacterial pneumonia, however, the effectiveness of alveolar ventilation already is impaired and carbonic acid is being retained in the blood. Analogously, patients who have both types of primary alkalosis often have a very high pH because their usual compensatory mechanisms are impeded by the concurrent acid-base disorders.

Mixed acid-base disorders may also occur with a nearly normal pH if a primary acidosis and a primary alkalosis are involved. An example of this type of mixed disorder is a head-injured patient whose treatment includes hyperventilation by mechanical ventilation to reduce intracranial pressure (respiratory alkalosis) but who at the same time has a metabolic acidosis from oliguric acute kidney injury. In this situation, the Pa_{CO_2} is decreased (respiratory alkalosis), the plasma bicarbonate concentration is decreased (metabolic acidosis), and the pH depends on the relative severity of the two imbalances.

KEY POINTS

- Acidosis is a condition that tends to cause a relative excess of acid. Alkalosis is a condition that tends to cause a relative excess of base (bicarbonate).
- Metabolic acidosis is characterized by pH below 7.40 and abnormally low HCO_3^- concentration. It is caused by processes that lead to metabolic acid accumulation (e.g., lactic acidosis) or loss of HCO_3^- (e.g., diarrhea). Compensatory hyperventilation decreases the Pa_{CO_2}.
- Metabolic alkalosis is characterized by pH above 7.40 and abnormally high HCO_3^- concentration. It is caused by processes that lead to metabolic acid loss (e.g., vomiting) or gain of HCO_3^- (e.g., bicarbonate antacids). Compensatory hypoventilation increases the Pa_{CO_2}.
- Respiratory acidosis is characterized by pH below 7.40 and abnormally high Pa_{CO_2}. It is caused by processes that lead to hypoventilation by impairing gas exchange (e.g., lung diseases), neuromuscular function of the chest (e.g., hypokalemic muscle paralysis), or respiratory control mechanisms in the brainstem (e.g., opioid overdose). Compensatory excretion of H^+ and retention of HCO_3^- by the kidneys increase the HCO_3^- concentration.
- Respiratory alkalosis is characterized by pH above 7.40 and abnormally low Pa_{CO_2}. It is caused by processes that lead to hyperventilation (e.g., hypoxemia, pain, anxiety). Compensatory retention of H^+ and excretion of HCO_3^- by the kidneys decrease the HCO_3^- concentration.
- Mixed acid-base disorders occur when two primary acid-base disorders are present independently. They may arise from simultaneous dysfunction of the respiratory system and kidneys. Depending on the combination of disorders, the pH may be nearly normal or grossly abnormal.

SUMMARY

Acid-base homeostasis involves the interplay of buffers, the respiratory system, and renal mechanisms. Metabolic acids are produced continually by cellular metabolism. These metabolic acids enter the blood, where they are buffered, and eventually are excreted by the kidneys. In healthy people, the kidneys adjust the rate of excretion of metabolic acids to meet the demands of the acid load being produced. The concentration of bicarbonate ions in the blood indicates the effectiveness of renal excretion of metabolic acids. Cellular metabolism also produces carbonic acid (carbon dioxide and water) that is excreted by the lungs. In healthy people, changes in the respiratory rate and depth adjust the rate of excretion of carbonic acid appropriately. The $Paco_2$ indicates the effectiveness of respiratory excretion of carbonic acid.

If one of the two acid excretion mechanisms becomes dysfunctional or overwhelmed, the other mechanism can produce a compensatory response that will help normalize the pH of the extracellular fluid, even though it will not correct the acid-base imbalance. Thus the kidneys adjust their excretion of metabolic acids when respiratory excretion of carbonic acid is altered abnormally. Similarly, the respiratory system adjusts the rate of excretion of carbonic acid if renal excretion of metabolic acids is impaired or overwhelmed. The pH of the blood at any time is the net result of the operation of these regulatory and compensatory mechanisms.

Primary acid-base imbalances arise when the normal regulatory mechanisms for acid-base homeostasis become impaired or are overwhelmed by a large acid or alkaline load. Pediatric and geriatric considerations are summarized in the boxes below. Primary metabolic acidosis arises when the kidneys are unable to excrete enough metabolic acid, or bicarbonate is lost from the body. The compensatory response to metabolic acidosis is hyperventilation. Primary respiratory acidosis arises when the lungs are unable to excrete enough carbonic acid. The compensatory response to respiratory acidosis is increased renal excretion of metabolic acid.

Primary metabolic alkalosis arises when the kidneys excrete too much metabolic acid or there is a gain of bicarbonate. The compensatory response to metabolic alkalosis is hypoventilation. Primary respiratory alkalosis arises when the lungs excrete too much carbonic acid. The compensatory response to sustained respiratory alkalosis is decreased renal excretion of metabolic acid. The $Paco_2$ reflects the respiratory component of an acid-base imbalance; the plasma bicarbonate concentration reflects the metabolic (renal) component of an acid-base imbalance.

A mixed acid-base imbalance occurs when two primary imbalances exist at the same time. The two primary imbalances may drive the pH to an extremely abnormal value or may nearly cancel each other's effect on the pH, although the $Paco_2$ and plasma bicarbonate concentration may still be very abnormal.

PEDIATRIC CONSIDERATIONS

Acid-Base Imbalance

- Neonates often have mild metabolic acidosis. Infants younger than 1 month have a reduced ability to excrete a large acid load; their kidneys are less able to reabsorb bicarbonate, they produce less ammonia, and urinary buffers are limited in quantity. These factors increase the risk of metabolic acidosis from acid accumulation.
- Adolescents with eating disorders may develop metabolic alkalosis from repeated emesis and hypokalemia or metabolic acidosis from starvation and laxative-induced chronic diarrhea.

GERIATRIC CONSIDERATIONS

Acid-Base Imbalance

- The chemoreceptor response to increased $Paco_2$ (hyperventilation) is delayed in older adults, which may delay their ability to correct respiratory acidosis.
- Older adults are at increased risk of respiratory depression (and thus respiratory acidosis) from barbiturates because of increased drug half-life.
- Older adults' kidneys are less able to excrete a large acid load, which increases the risk for metabolic acidosis from acid accumulation.
- Diarrhea from chronic laxative overuse may contribute to metabolic acidosis.

REFERENCES

1. Rose BD, Post TW: *Clinical physiology of acid-base and electrolyte disorders,* ed 6, New York, 2013, McGraw-Hill.
2. Hall JE: *Guyton and Hall textbook of medical physiology,* ed 12, Philadelphia, 2011, Saunders Elsevier.
3. Nava S, Grassi M, Fanfulla F, et al: Non-invasive ventilation in elderly patients with acute hypercapnic respiratory failure: a randomised controlled trial, *Age Ageing* 40:444–450, 2011.
4. Schuchmann S, Hauck S, Henning S, et al: Respiratory alkalosis in children with febrile seizures, *Epilepsia* 52:1949–1955, 2011.
5. Pappano D: Alkalosis-induced respiratory depression from infantile hypertrophic pyloric stenosis, *Pediatr Emerg Care* 27:124, 2011.
6. Boron WF: Acid-base transport by the renal proximal tubule, *J Am Soc Nephrol* 17:2368–2382, 2006.
7. Madias NE: Renal acidification responses to respiratory acid-base disorders, *J Nephrol* 23(suppl 16):S85–S91, 2010.
8. Felver L: Fluid and electrolyte and acid-base balance and imbalance. In Woods SL, et al, editors: *Cardiac nursing,* ed 6, Philadelphia, 2010, Lippincott, Williams & Wilkins, pp 153–176.
9. Patel A, Felstead D, Doraiswami M, et al: Acute starvation in pregnancy: a cause of severe metabolic acidosis, *Int J Obstet Anesth* 20:253–256, 2011.
10. Han JJ, Yim HE, Lee JH, et al: Albumin versus normal saline for dehydrated term infants with metabolic acidosis due to acute diarrhea, *J Perinatol* 29:444–447, 2009.
11. Yee AH, Rabinstein AA: Neurologic presentations of acid-base imbalance, electrolyte abnormalities, and endocrine emergencies, *Neurol Clin* 28:1–16, 2010.
12. Ajbani K, Chansky ME, Baumann BM: Homespun remedy, homespun toxicity: baking soda ingestion for dyspepsia, *J Emerg Med* 40(4):e71–e74, 2011.
13. Huber L, Gennari FJ: Severe metabolic alkalosis in a hemodialysis patient, *Am J Kidney Dis* 58:144–149, 2011.
14. Sarafidis PA, Georgianos PI, Lasaridis AN: Diuretics in clinical practice. Part II: electrolyte and acid-base disorders complicating diuretic therapy, *Expert Opinion Drug Safety* 9:259–273, 2010.
15. Gennari FJ: Pathophysiology of metabolic alkalosis: a new classification based on the centrality of stimulated collecting duct ion transport, *Am J Kidney Dis* 58:626–636, 2011.
16. Tugrul S, Telci L, Yildirim A, et al: Case report of severe metabolic alkalosis: life-compatible new level, *J Trauma-Injury Inf Crit Care* 68(3):E61–E63, 2010.
17. Carrera E, Kim DJ, Castellani G, et al: Effect of hyper- and hypocapnia on cerebral arterial compliance in normal subjects, *J Neuroimaging* 21:121–125, 2011.
18. Halperin ML, Goldstein MB, Kamel KS: *Fluid, electrolyte and acid-base physiology: a problem-based approach,* ed 4, St Louis, 2010, Saunders Elsevier.

Renal Function

Jacquelyn L. Banasik

evolve WEBSITE

http://evolve.elsevier.com/Copstead/
- Review Questions and Answers
- Glossary (with audio pronunciations for selected terms)
- Animations
- Case Studies
- Key Points Review

KEY QUESTIONS

- How does the structure of the glomerulus determine the composition of the tubular filtrate?
- What factors determine glomerular filtration rate?
- How do individual nephrons regulate their glomerular filtration rates?
- How are solutes and water transported across the renal tubular epithelium?
- What is the role of the kidney in fluid, electrolyte, and acid-base balance?
- How does renal function change across the life span?
- How are laboratory and diagnostic tests used to evaluate renal function and disease?

CHAPTER OUTLINE

The kidneys are responsible for maintaining fluid and electrolyte homeostasis and ridding the body of water-soluble wastes. To accomplish these functions, the kidneys filter more than 7 L of fluid per hour, then reabsorb about 99%, producing a small amount of urine containing a high concentration of wastes.[1] The kidneys can alter the amount and composition of urine to keep blood volume and electrolyte composition within normal limits. In addition, the kidneys perform two important endocrine functions: production of erythropoietin, which is a regulator of red blood cell quantity, and activation of vitamin D, which is a cofactor for intestinal calcium absorption.

Most individuals have two kidneys, each containing approximately one million **nephrons,** which provide a large renal reserve. The nephron is the functional unit of the kidney, performing all filtration, reabsorption, and secretory functions. Removal of 50% of a person's nephrons, as occurs with kidney donation, results in no significant impairment of renal function, although renal reserve is reduced.[2,3] Serious renal impairment generally does not occur until between 75% and 90% of the total nephrons have been damaged. Thus, clinical findings may not be evident until late in the course of chronic kidney disease. A number of laboratory and diagnostic tests are used to assess renal structure and function and to identify disease processes. These are briefly described at the end of this chapter. Kidney diseases, renal failure, and abnormalities of the bladder are discussed in Chapters 27, 28, and 29, respectively. A discussion of fluid and electrolyte imbalances and acid-base disturbances can be found in Chapters 24 and 25, respectively. The essentials of kidney structure and nephron function are presented in this chapter.

RENAL ANATOMY

The urinary system consists of the kidneys, ureters, urinary bladder, and urethra (Figure 26-1). The kidneys are located in the **retroperitoneal** space in the posterior abdomen. One kidney is on each side of the vertebral column between the level of the twelfth thoracic and third lumbar vertebrae. The costovertebral angle (CVA), the point at which the bottom of the rib cage meets the spine, is commonly used as an external landmark for finding kidney position during physical examination.[4] The right kidney is located beneath the liver and is placed slightly lower than the left kidney.

The kidneys are protected and surrounded by strong back and flank muscles, fascia, and fat. The kidneys are somewhat mobile and can be injured by high-impact activities, such as bouncing along on horseback or on a mountain bike, or by direct trauma, as might occur from falls or blunt trauma. Kidney hemorrhage results in bleeding into the retroperitoneal space but not into the peritoneal cavity.

The kidneys drain urine into the ureters by gravity flow and the ureters provide peristaltic action to move urine along to the bladder where it is stored. The two principal parts of the bladder are the body and the neck. The body stores urine and is made up of smooth muscle known as detrusor muscle. Detrusor muscle extends in all directions throughout the bladder and contracts as a unit in response to initiation of action potentials. The urinary bladder collects 300 to 500 ml before stretch receptors signal a need for bladder emptying. Urine is drained from the bladder by the urethra when the internal and external sphincters are relaxed. Innervation and control of bladder function are discussed in detail in Chapter 29.

An adult kidney weighs approximately 115 to 170 g; is 11 cm long, 6 cm wide, and 3 cm thick; and is shaped like a red kidney bean, with the concave portion, termed the **hilum,** facing the vertebral column.[5] A thin, fibrous capsule covers each kidney and encloses blood vessels, lymphatic vessels, and nerve fibers, including pain receptors. Lymphatic vessels, blood vessels, and nerves enter and exit the kidney through the hilum.

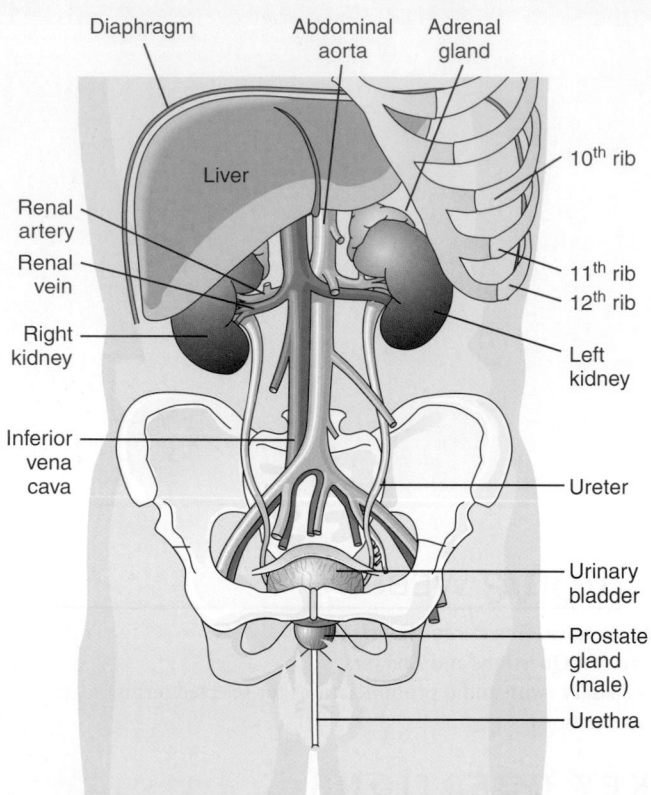

FIGURE 26-1 Structure of the urinary tract. The kidneys are located in the retroperitoneal space in the posterior abdominal cavity, in contact with the diaphragm and covered on the upper portions by ribs.

Renal Parenchyma

On cross-section, the kidney is seen to contain three principal areas: the pelvis, the medulla, and the cortex (Figure 26-2). The renal pelvis is a large collecting area for the urine that drains from the many collecting ducts of the nephrons. The minor (smaller) calices collect urine as it drains from the papilla of the renal pyramids. The normal kidney has 8 to 18 minor calices and 2 to 3 major calices.[1] The major calices are large collecting spaces located between the minor calices and the upper part of the ureter.

The medulla contains 8 to 18 renal pyramids, the bases of which are adjacent to the outer cortex, whereas the apices open into the minor calices. The pyramids consist of collecting tubules, collecting ducts, long loops of Henle, and vasa recta. The papillae are the openings at the tips of the renal pyramids through which urine exits the collecting ducts.

The renal cortex, which is the outer rim of the kidney, is about 1 cm thick. The cortex contains all of the glomeruli as well as 85% of the nephron tubules. Fifteen percent of nephrons send their loops of Henle deep into the medulla and are called **juxtamedullary nephrons.** Columns of cortical tissue are found between the medullary pyramids and provide the passageway for the interlobar arteries.

Renal Lymphatics and Innervation

There are two lymphatic systems in the kidney. One system is composed of vessels that are located both in the renal capsule and immediately under the capsule in the outer cortex. The other lymphatic system is composed of vessels that accompany and wrap around the arterial blood vessels. All the lymphatic vessels, as well as blood vessels and

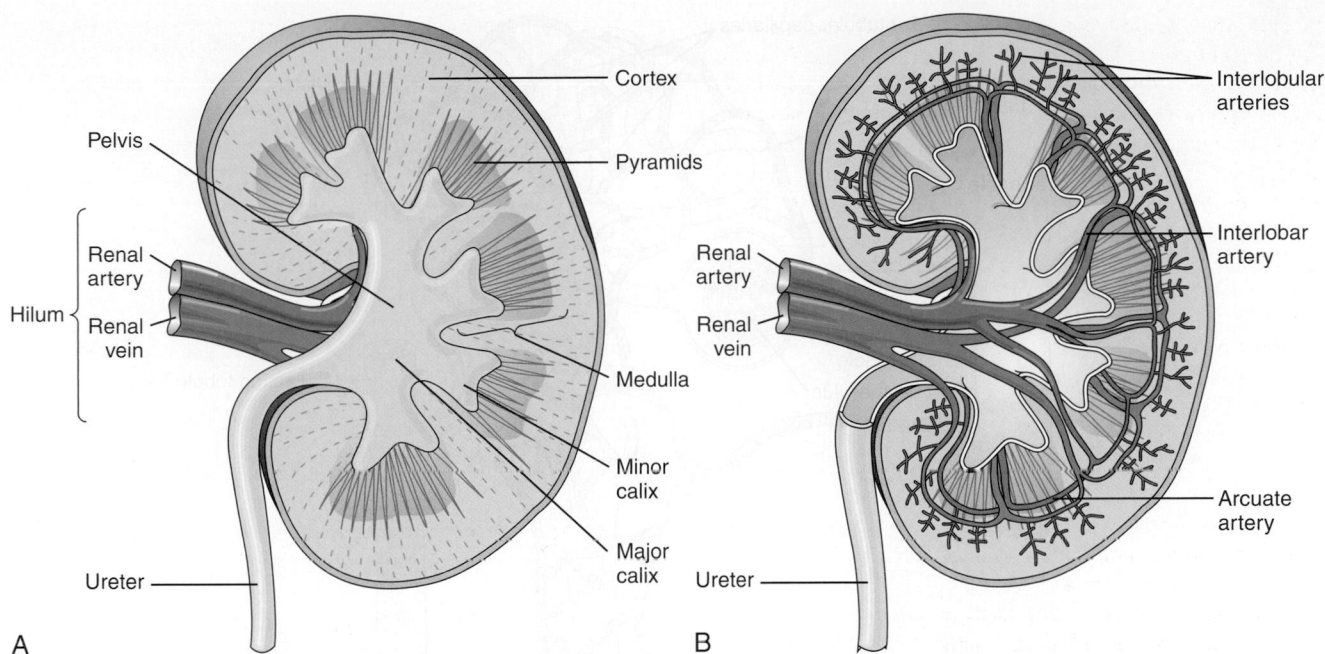

FIGURE 26-2 A, Cross-section of the kidney showing the renal pelvis, medullary pyramids, and cortex. Normal kidneys have 8 to 18 renal pyramids and a corresponding number of minor calices. The major calices drain urine into the ureter. Blood vessels, lymphatic vessels, and nerves enter and exit through the hilum. **B,** The arterial blood supply to the kidney is derived from the renal arteries, which branch from the abdominal aorta and enter the kidney through the hilus. The renal artery branches to form several interlobar arteries, which travel toward the cortex in the renal columns. The interlobar arteries branch to form the arcuate arteries, which divide further to form the interlobular arteries. Interlobular arteries branch multiple times to provide the afferent arterioles for each of the kidney's million nephrons.

nerves, exit the kidney through the hilum, and lymph drains into the paraaortic lymph nodes.

The kidneys are innervated by the sympathetic division of the autonomic nervous system. The lesser splanchnic nerves come from the renal plexuses, which are located next to the renal arteries. These nerve fibers travel with the renal arterial blood vessels and terminate in smooth muscle of the afferent and efferent arterioles, proximal and distal tubules, and the renin-secreting juxtaglomerular cells.[1,5] Stimulation of the sympathetic nervous system results in renal vasoconstriction and renin release. The renal capsule and all structures between the renal pelvis and urinary meatus are innervated with pain receptors (see Chapter 27).

Renal Blood Supply

Approximately 25% of the cardiac output is delivered to the kidneys, the majority of which circulates through the cortex, while only 1% to 2% perfuses the medulla.[5] Total renal blood flow in both kidneys is approximately 1250 ml/min. Blood flows to the kidneys from the abdominal aorta through the renal arteries, which then divide into several interlobar arteries.[5] The interlobar arteries travel in the renal columns adjacent to the pyramids (see Figure 26-2). When the interlobar arteries reach the border of the medulla and the cortex, they branch into the arcuate arteries. The arcuate arteries then travel along the cortical medullary border parallel to the renal capsule. The arcuate arteries branch further to form small interlobular arteries, which penetrate the cortex and branch extensively to form the afferent arterioles. The afferent arterioles divide to form glomerular capillaries, which coalesce to form the efferent arterioles (Figure 26-3). The efferent arterioles branch again to form a second capillary bed. The peritubular capillaries wrap around the proximal and distal convoluted tubules (Figure 26-4). Some capillaries, called *vasa recta*, dip down into the medulla to surround the loops of Henle and collecting ducts. The

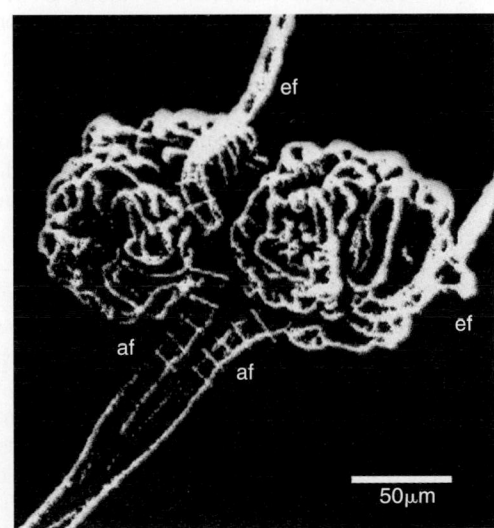

FIGURE 26-3 Scanning electron micrograph showing branching of an interlobular artery into two afferent arterioles *(af)*, with associated glomerular tufts and efferent arterioles *(ef)*. (From Kimura K et al: Effects of atrial natriuretic peptide on renal arterioles: morphometric analysis using microvascular casts, *Am J Physiol* 259:F936, 1990. Used with permission.)

vasa recta have a specialized loop structure that enables them to pick up interstitial fluid without excessive removal of interstitial solutes. Solutes and water move into and out of the vasa recta passively such that the descending limb gains solute as it dips into the highly concentrated medulla, but then most of the solute is lost as the ascending loop makes its way back up to the cortex.

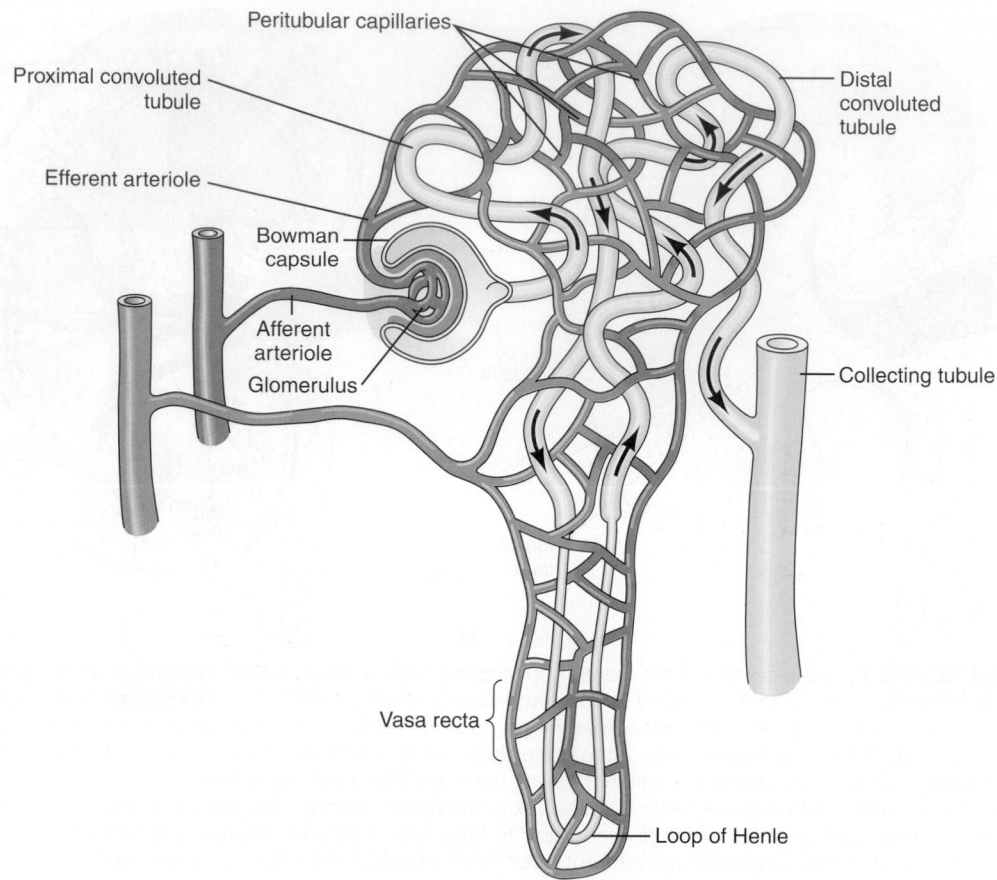

Peritubular capillaries

Proximal convoluted tubule

Efferent arteriole

Bowman capsule

Afferent arteriole

Glomerulus

Distal convoluted tubule

Collecting tubule

Vasa recta

Loop of Henle

FIGURE 26-4 The nephron tubule is covered by peritubular capillaries and vasa recta, which pick up the fluid and solutes that have been reabsorbed by the tubular epithelium and return them to the general circulation.

The capillaries of the peritubular system and the vasa recta join together and drain into interlobular venules. The veins that drain blood from the kidney run parallel to the arteries and are similarly named (Figure 26-5).

KEY POINTS

- The kidneys are located in the retroperitoneal space, just under the diaphragm. The right kidney is slightly lower than the left. The costovertebral angle is an external landmark useful for locating the kidneys.
- The kidney can be divided into three principal anatomic sections: the pelvis, the medulla, and the cortex. The pelvis is composed of urinary collecting structures, called *calices*. The medulla is the middle portion and contains the renal pyramids. The cortex is the outer portion and contains glomeruli and nephron tubules.
- The kidneys are supplied with lymphatics to drain excess interstitial fluid and proteins and with sympathetic neurons to regulate blood supply and renin release.
- Blood is supplied to the kidneys by the renal artery, which divides several times to form the interlobar, arcuate, and interlobular arteries. The interlobular arteries branch multiple times to form afferent arterioles for each of the millions of kidney glomeruli.
- Each nephron has its own afferent arteriole, capillary network or tuft, and efferent arteriole. Efferent arterioles continue on to form peritubular capillaries, or vasa recta, which wrap around nephron structures and eventually drain into the renal veins. The loop structure of the vasa recta enables them to pick up interstitial fluid without removing excessive solute.

OVERVIEW OF NEPHRON STRUCTURE AND FUNCTION

Most of the physiologic functioning of the kidney can be understood by examining the function of an individual nephron. Thus, the nephron is said to be the functional unit of the kidney. Nephrons are organized in parallel such that each must accomplish all the necessary processing before releasing urine into the collecting ducts. Complex autoregulatory mechanisms ensure that the workload is evenly distributed among the kidneys' many nephrons.

As the unit of kidney function, a nephron must accomplish three major functions: (1) filtration of water-soluble substances from the blood; (2) reabsorption of filtered nutrients, water, and electrolytes; and (3) secretion of wastes or excess substances into the filtrate. Different segments of the nephron are specialized to accomplish each of these processes. Each nephron is composed of a glomerulus, which includes the capillary tuft and Bowman capsule, and a tubule, which includes the proximal convoluted tubule, loop of Henle, distal convoluted tubule, and collecting tubule (Figure 26-6). The nephron tubule is composed of a single layer of epithelial cells with an apical side facing the lumen and a basolateral side facing the interstitial space and capillaries (Figure 26-7). The epithelial cells in each segment of the tubule are specialized for certain functions (Table 26-1). Nearly all cells in the nephron have a single cilium that protrudes from the apical surface into the lumen of the tubule. These cilia are mechanoreceptors and chemoreceptors that sense flow rate and composition of the tubular filtrate. Stimulation of the cilium triggers signaling cascades within

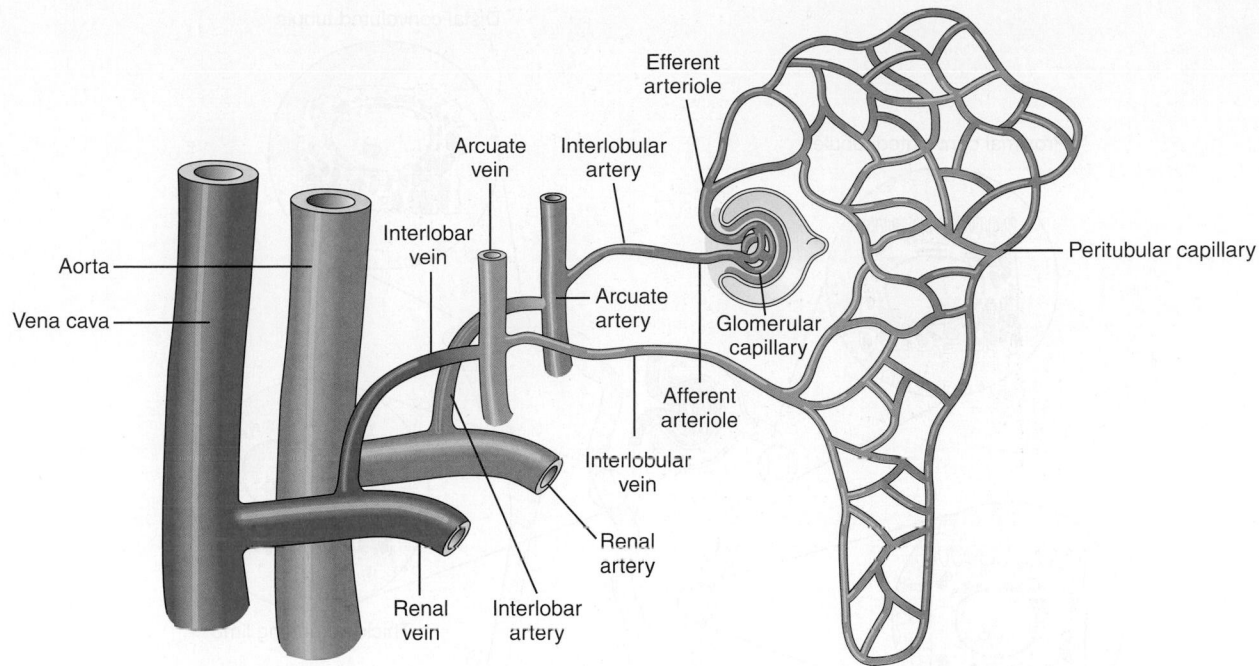

FIGURE 26-5 The venous vessels of the kidney parallel the arterial vessels and are similarly named.

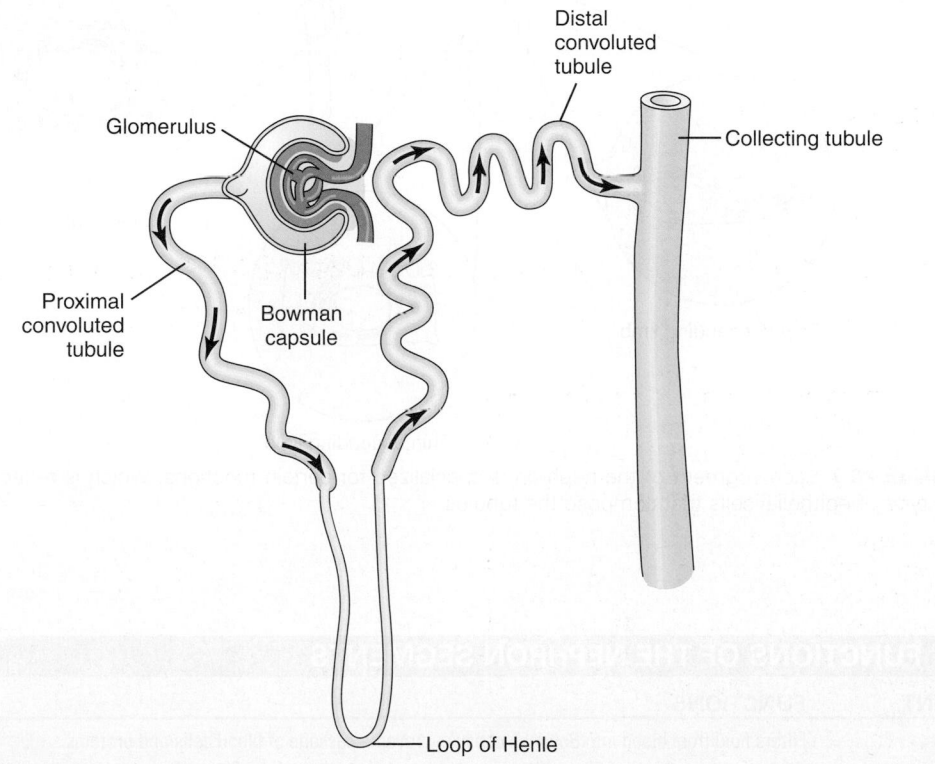

FIGURE 26-6 The nephron is composed of a glomerulus, proximal convoluted tubule, loop of Henle, distal convoluted tubule, and collecting tubule. Filtration occurs at the glomerulus, and the remaining tubule segments perform reabsorption and secretion functions.

the tubule cells that regulate cell proliferation, differentiation, and apoptosis. Abnormalities in cilia signaling function have been found in patients with polycystic kidney disease, associated with mutations in genes *(polycystin, PKD1, PKD2)* that code for cilia membrane proteins (see Chapter 27).

Glomerulus

The glomerulus is the site of fluid filtration from the blood to the nephron tubule. It is formed by a capillary tuft, which lies between the afferent and efferent arterioles, and by the surrounding epithelial cells of Bowman capsule. The outer layer of the glomerular capsule

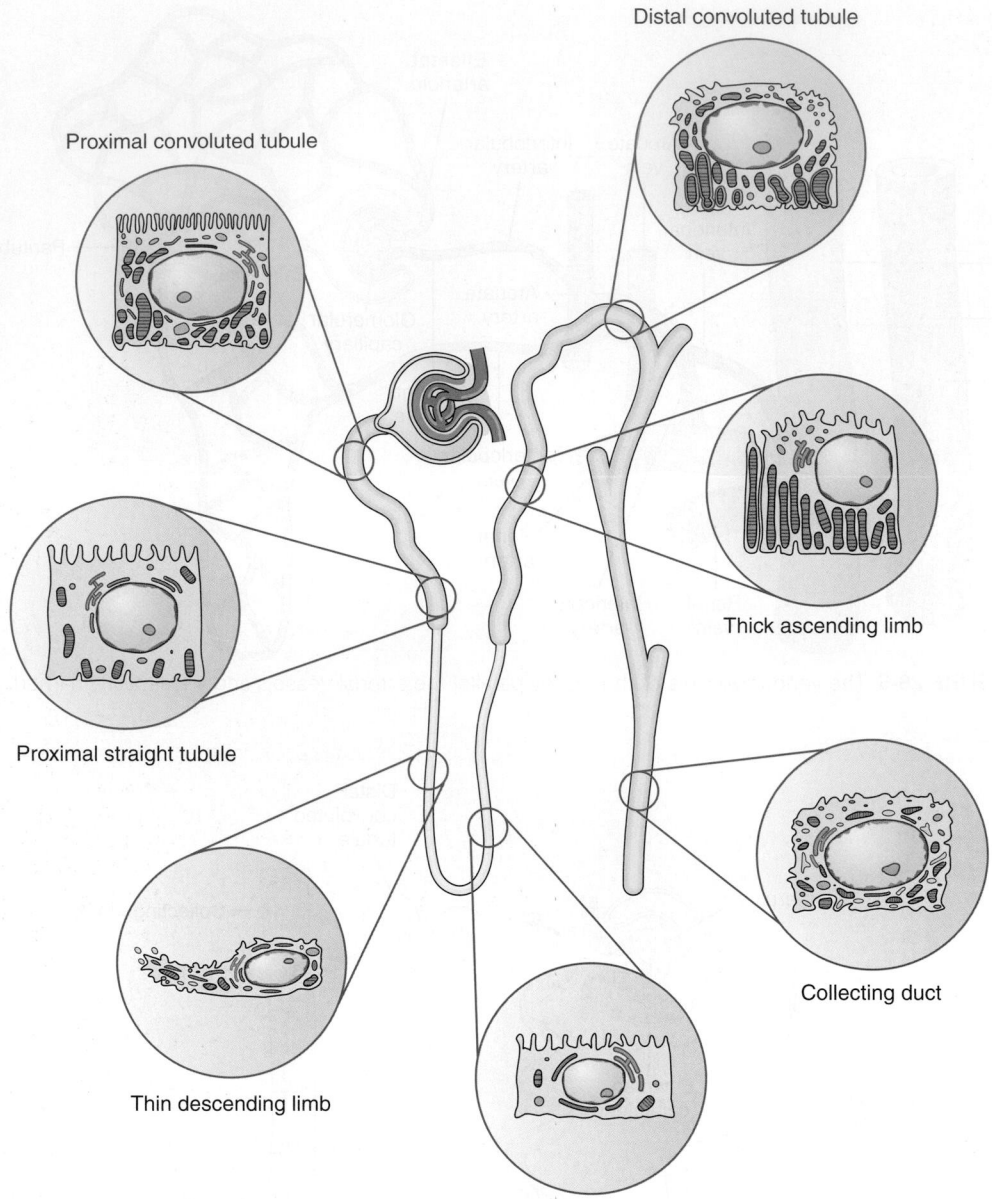

FIGURE 26-7 Each segment of the nephron is specialized for certain functions, which is reflected in the type of epithelial cells that compose the tubules.

TABLE 26-1 FUNCTIONS OF THE NEPHRON SEGMENTS	
NEPHRON SEGMENT	**FUNCTIONS**
Glomerulus	Filters fluid from blood into Bowman capsule; prevents passage of blood cells and proteins
Proximal convoluted tubule	Transports two thirds of filtered water and electrolytes and all of the filtered bicarbonate, glucose, amino acids, and vitamins from filtrate to interstitium
Descending loop of Henle	Transports water; delivers a concentrated filtrate to ascending loop of Henle
Ascending loop of Henle	Actively transports Na^+, K^+, Cl^- to produce a hypoosmotic filtrate and a high interstitial osmolality
Distal convoluted tubule	Transports Na^+, Cl^-, water, and urea; responsive to aldosterone; site of macula densa regulation of GFR; secretes H^+ and K^+
Collecting tubule	Passively transports water under influence of ADH; secretes H^+ and K^+

ADH, Antidiuretic hormone; *GFR,* glomerular filtration rate.

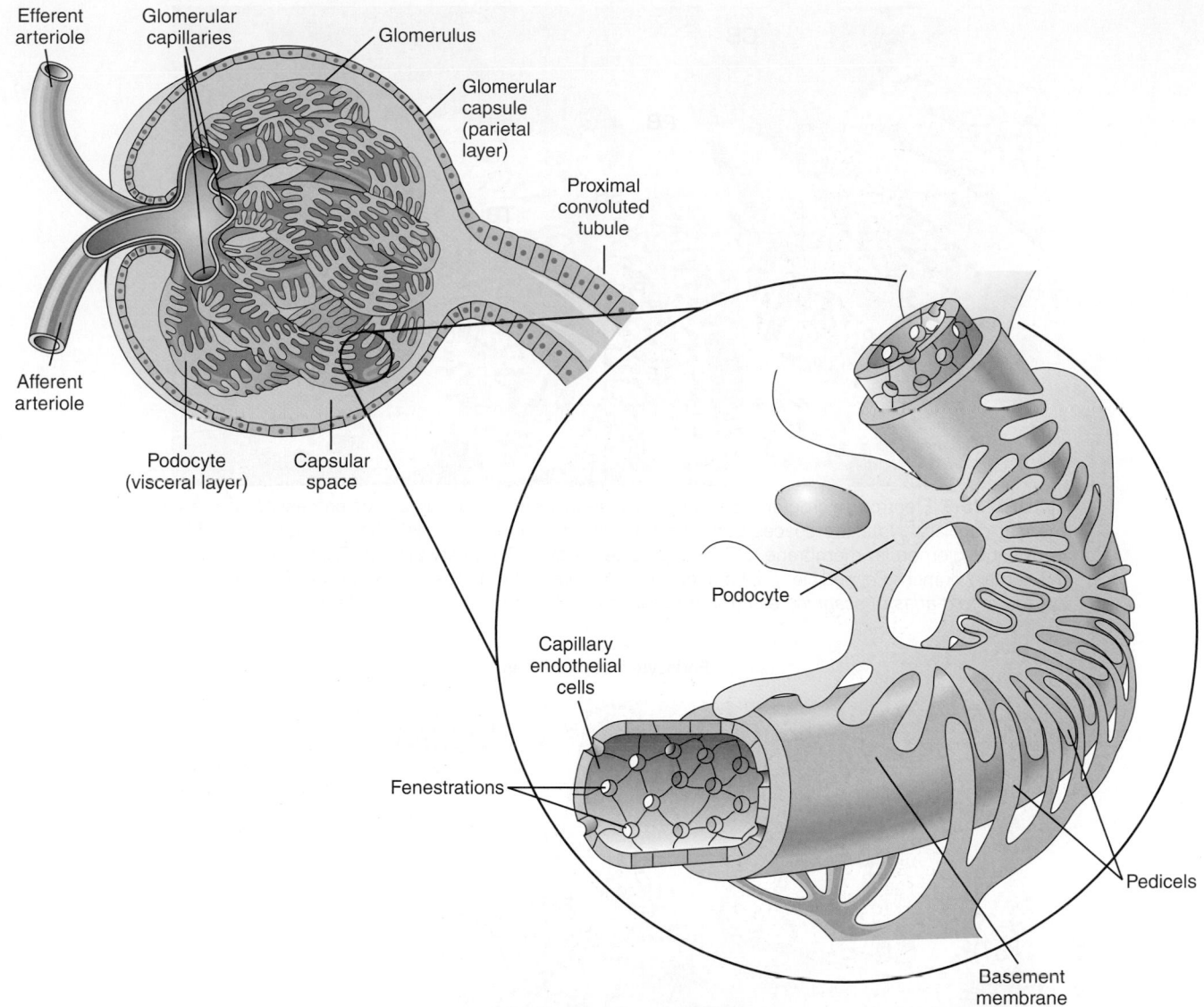

Efferent
arteriole

Glomerular
capillaries

Glomerulus

Glomerular
capsule
(parietal
layer)

Proximal
convoluted
tubule

Afferent
arteriole

Podocyte
(visceral layer)

Capsular
space

Podocyte

Capillary
endothelial
cells

Fenestrations

Pedicels

Basement
membrane

FIGURE 26-8 Structure of the glomerulus, including the afferent and efferent arterioles, capillary tuft, and surrounding epithelial membrane of Bowman capsule. The enlargement shows the glomerular membrane to be composed of the endothelial cells of the capillary, the podocytes of Bowman capsule, and the basement membrane between them.

is called the *parietal layer* and consists of a single thickness of epithelial cells resting on a layer of basement membrane (Figure 26-8). The inner (visceral) layer of the capsule is composed of specialized epithelial cells called *podocytes*. Podocytes have foot processes (pedicels) that surround the glomerular capillary walls (Figure 26-9). Between the podocyte and the capillary endothelium is a layer of extracellular matrix called the *basement membrane* (see Figure 26-8).

Spaces between the endothelial cells are called *fenestra,* and spaces between the podocyte foot processes are called *slit pores.* These intercellular spaces provide the surface area for glomerular filtration and make the glomeruli considerably more permeable than other capillaries in the body (Figure 26-10). The basement membrane is an important selectivity barrier of the glomerulus, preventing plasma proteins, erythrocytes, leukocytes, and platelets from passing through. Cells are too large to pass through pores, and plasma proteins are negatively charged and repelled to some extent by the basement membrane. Slit pores have a thin diaphragm of extracellular proteins

that restricts the filtration of plasma proteins that make it through the basement membrane.[5] *Nephrin*, podocin, NEPH1, CD2AP, and others are important proteins in the slit pores as demonstrated by the proteinuria (protein in urine) that occurs when they are genetically mutated (Figure 26-11).[5] Proteins and blood cells are not usually present in the urine. If the glomerulus is injured, blood cells and proteins may filter through and be found in urine. Proteinuria is an important sign of basement membrane dysfunction. Except for the lack of proteins and cells, the glomerular filtrate is very similar in composition to plasma.

Another important component of the glomerulus is the mesangium, which includes mesangial cells and mesangial matrix. Mesangial cells have a number of functions including provision of structural support for glomerular capillaries, secretion of matrix proteins, phagocytosis, and regulation of the **glomerular filtration rate (GFR).** By contracting and relaxing, mesangial cells can alter the available surface area for filtration and affect GFR. The GFR averages about 125 ml/min.

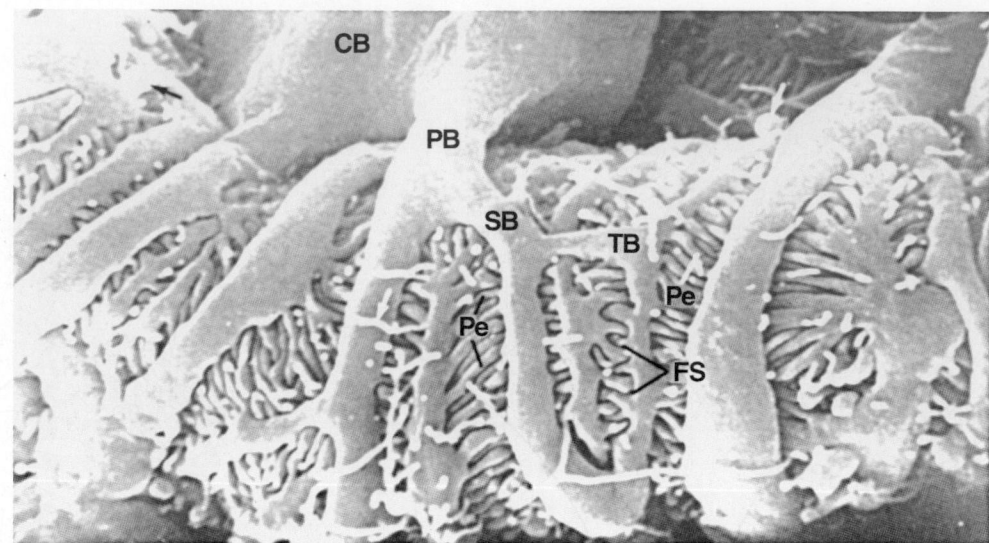

FIGURE 26-9 Electron micrograph showing a close-up view of podocyte foot processes of the glomerular capillary. Note the spaces between the podocyte foot processes that contribute to a highly permeable glomerular membrane. *CB*, Podocyte cell body; *PB*, primary branch; *SB*, secondary branch; *TB*, tertiary branch; *Pe*, pedicle; *FS*, filtration slits (slit pores). (From Kessel RG, Kardon RH: *Tissues and organs: a text-atlas of scanning electron microscopy*, San Francisco, 1979, WH Freeman.)

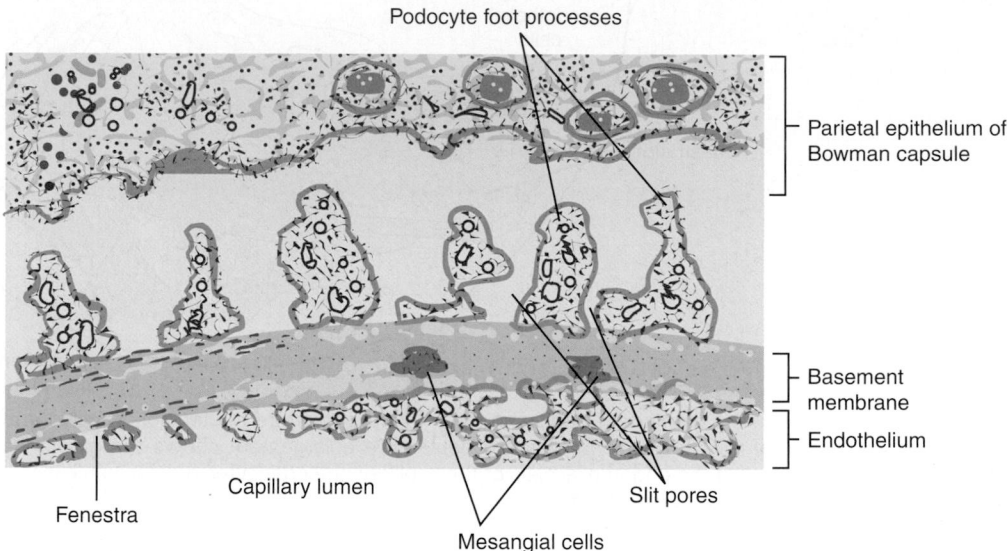

FIGURE 26-10 Section of the glomerular membrane showing the large spaces between the endothelial cells and podocyte foot processes. Filtration occurs through the fenestra and slit pores. The basement membrane provides the principal selectivity barrier of the glomerulus.

Proximal Convoluted Tubule

The Bowman capsule drains the glomerular filtrate directly into the proximal tubule segment, where two thirds of the water and electrolytes are rapidly transported from the filtrate to the interstitium for reabsorption by peritubular capillaries[6] (Figure 26-12). Nutrients, vitamins, and small proteins normally are reabsorbed completely in the early proximal tubule. The early proximal tubule is the site of most bicarbonate ion reabsorption, whereas chloride ion is reabsorbed in the late proximal tubule. The proximal tubule consists of cuboidal epithelium that is convoluted to provide a greater surface area for reabsorption. The epithelial cells in this segment have microvilli that form a brush border next to the filtrate and substantially increase the apical surface area. Proximal tubule cells have high adenosine triphosphate

(ATP) requirements because most reabsorption utilizes active transport mechanisms that are dependent on Na^+-K^+ ion pumps in the basolateral membrane. Details of some of these transport mechanisms are discussed in subsequent sections. Water is reabsorbed passively through paracellular transport between the tubular cells and through water channels in the tubule cell membranes made of proteins called *aquaporin 1*. Reabsorption of solutes creates the osmotic force for passive water reabsorption.

Loop of Henle

The loop of Henle is divided into the descending and ascending limbs, which differ significantly in structure and function. The descending limb receives filtrate from the proximal convoluted tubule and delivers it to the ascending limb. The thin descending limb is permeable to

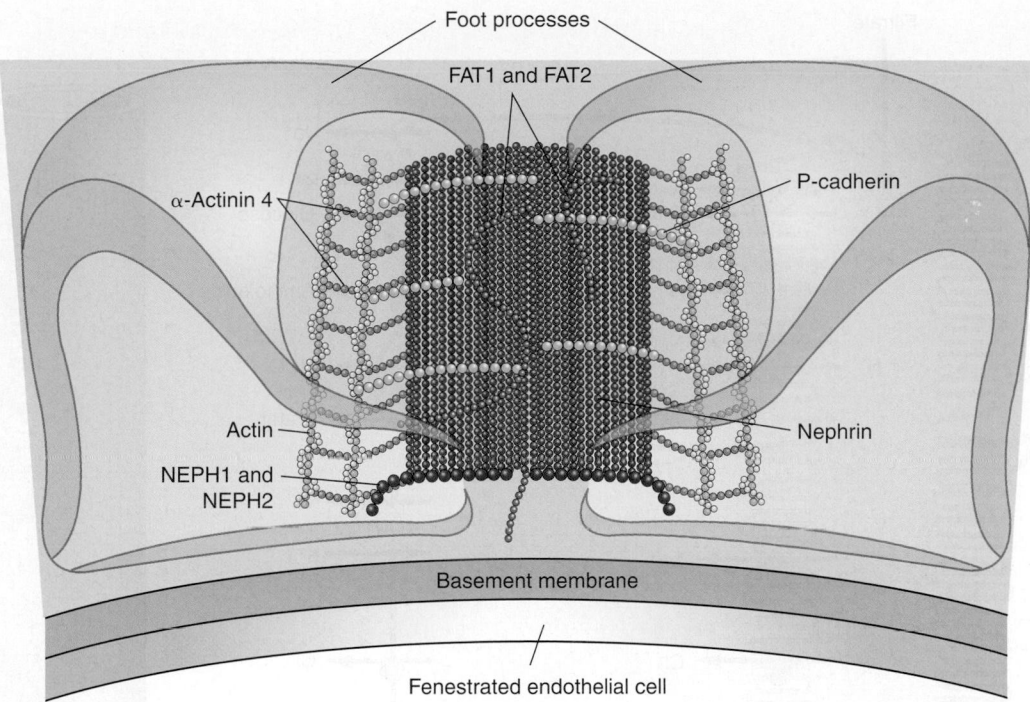

FIGURE 26-11 Diagram of the major proteins that constitute the matrix in the slit pore between renal podocyte foot processes.

water, but the thin and thick ascending part of the loop is not.[6] The thick ascending segment contains powerful membrane pumps that cotransport ions (Na⁺, K⁺, 2Cl⁻) from the filtrate and deposit them in the interstitial fluid surrounding the loops of Henle and collecting ducts (Figure 26-13). About 15% of nephrons have extra-long loops of Henle that dip down into the medulla (juxtamedullary nephrons). These nephrons are vital for creating concentrated urine.

The loop formation of the loop of Henle creates a countercurrent mechanism, which allows the ascending loop of Henle to create a high interstitial gradient in the medulla of the kidney (Figure 26-14). Because the ascending loop is impermeable to water, water cannot follow the Na⁺, K⁺, and Cl⁻ ions that are pumped into the interstitium. The descending loop is permeable to water, and water will be drawn out by the extra ions that were pumped into the interstitium by the ascending limb. Thus, the filtrate that reaches the ascending limb will be more concentrated than the original filtrate. Delivery of a more concentrated filtrate to the ascending limb allows the Na⁺-K⁺-2Cl⁻ cotransporter to pump out a greater number of ions and reach an even higher interstitial gradient (Figure 26-15). This countercurrent mechanism creates a maximal osmolarity of about 600 mOsm/L at the tip of the loop of Henle as compared with the usual extracellular osmolarity of 280 to 300 mOsm/L at the cortex. Another 600 mOsm/L is contributed by the accumulation of urea particles in the interstitium.[6] Urea moves passively from the filtrate into the interstitium down its concentration gradient. Urea becomes concentrated in the tubule filtrate when electrolytes and water are removed in the proximal tubule and loop of Henle. An overall interstitial osmolarity is generated that begins in the cortex at about 300 mOsm/L and increases progressively to about 1200 mOsm/L at a point deep in the medulla. This high interstitial osmolarity provides a gradient for water reabsorption from the collecting ducts as they pass through the medulla on their way to the renal pelvis. The maximal interstitial gradient attained is dependent on the length of the loops of Henle. In some animals that survive in dry climates, such as the desert mouse, very long loops of Henle create a much higher interstitial osmolarity, which allows formation of extremely concentrated

urine. Fluid that is reabsorbed from collecting tubules into the medullary interstitium is picked up by the specialized capillary network called the vasa recta and returned to the venous circulation. Like other capillaries, the vasa recta passively exchange ions according to concentration gradients and passively reabsorb fluid by filtration forces. The loop structure of the vasa recta allows the capillary to passively leak accumulated solute back into the interstitium as the capillary makes its way back to the cortex from the medulla. This process minimizes the washout of the interstitial osmolality and has been called the *countercurrent exchange mechanism.*

Distal Convoluted Tubule

The filtrate that reaches the distal tubule is normally hypoosmotic (100 mOsm/L) in comparison with plasma (280 mOsm/L) because electrolytes have been removed by the pumps in the ascending loop of Henle.[7] At this point in the nephron, only 10% of the original glomerular filtrate volume remains, and further reabsorption in the distal tubule is largely under hormonal control. Aldosterone and angiotensin II (AII) stimulate the tubule cells to reabsorb sodium and water, whereas atrial natriuretic peptide (ANP) and urodilatin inhibit reabsorption.

Collecting Duct

The distal tubules of several nephrons empty into a single collecting tubule, which then merges into progressively larger and fewer collecting ducts that run parallel to the loops of Henle. Eventually the collecting ducts form the medullary pyramids, which empty into the minor calices through the papilla. The collecting ducts travel through the high interstitial gradient of the medulla on their way to the renal pelvis. The collecting ducts have two cell types called *principle cells (P cells)* and *intercalated cells (I cells)*. The majority of cells are the P type that responds to antidiuretic hormone. In the presence of antidiuretic hormone (ADH), more than 99% of the original filtrate is reabsorbed by the time it reaches the renal pelvis, creating 30 to 60 ml of concentrated urine per hour. The I cells participate in acid-base balance by regulating the secretion of acid.

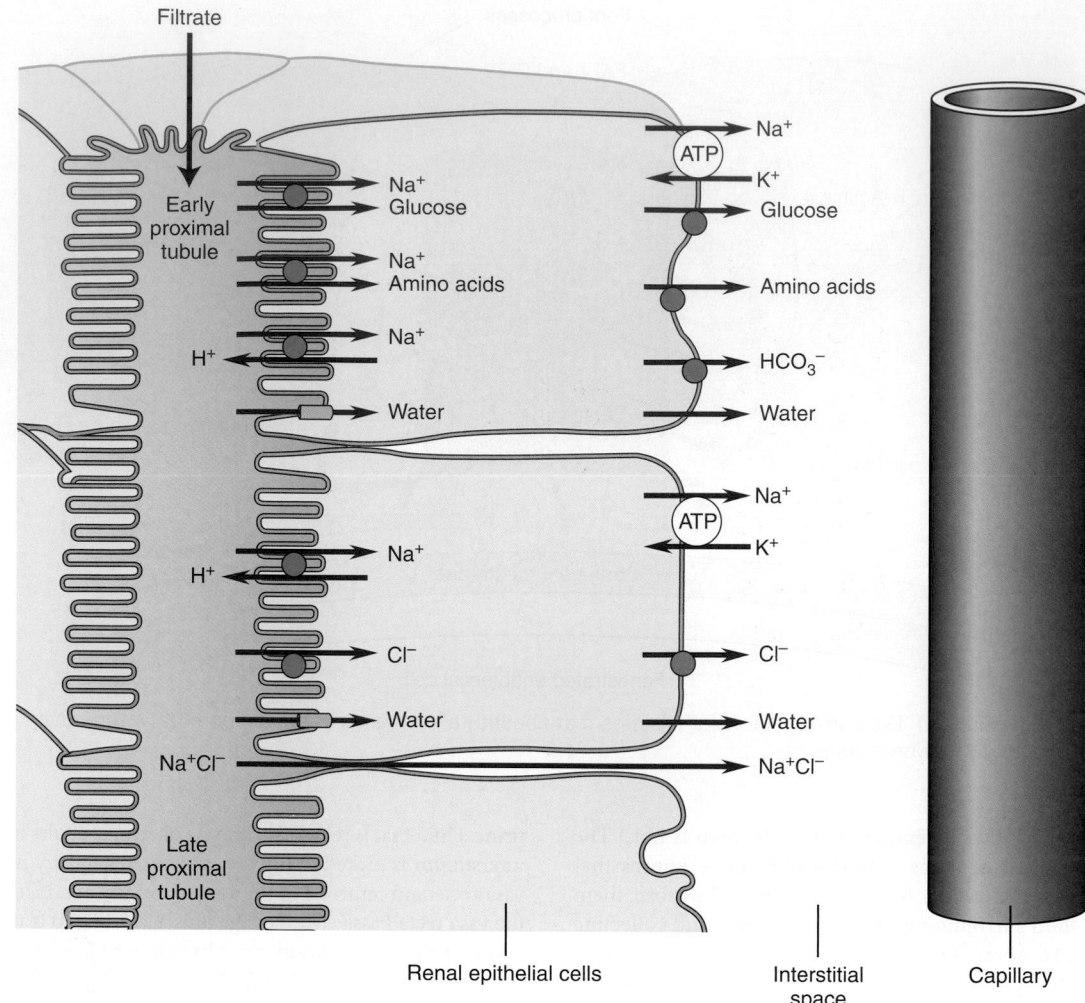

FIGURE 26-12 The proximal convoluted tubule has numerous membrane transporters that function to reabsorb filtered glucose, amino acids, water, and electrolytes. The early proximal tubule reabsorbs nearly all of the filtered bicarbonate ions, whereas the late proximal tubule reabsorbs chloride ions.

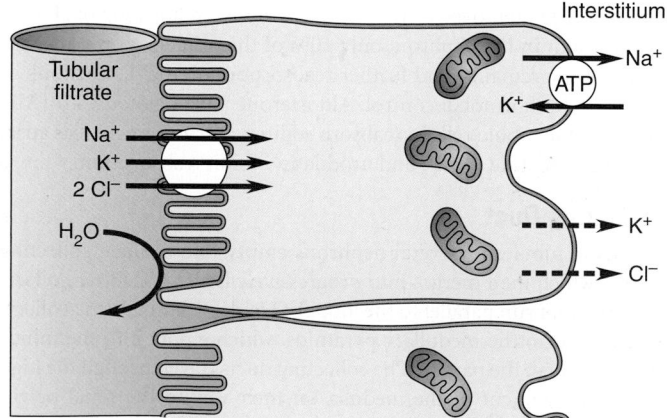

FIGURE 26-13 The epithelial cells of the thick ascending loop of Henle possess powerful ion pumps that cotransport Na^+, K^+, and $2Cl^-$ ions from the filtrate into the cell. The Na^+ is then pumped out of the basolateral membrane and into the interstitium. The loop of Henle ion cotransporter is responsible for creating a highly concentrated medullary interstitium.

REGULATION OF GLOMERULAR FILTRATION

The GFR is determined by the filtration pressure in the glomeruli and by the permeable surface area of the glomerular membrane (K_f). Filtration pressure varies considerably from the afferent end of the glomerulus to the efferent end and is difficult to measure directly. The average net filtration pressure for the capillary as a whole is about 10 mm Hg, and the permeability constant K_f is about 12.5 ml/min per mm Hg. GFR is the product of filtration pressure and K_f (10 mm Hg × 12.5 ml/min per mm Hg = 125 ml/min).[1,5] The GFR is determined by the physical principles of filtration across a capillary membrane (Figure 26-16). These values are not easily measured in patients, so a global assessment of GFR is used clinically to assess renal function (see Tests of Renal Structure and Function); however, understanding the principles that underlie the global clinical measurement is essential to anticipation and prevention of impaired GFR.

Physics of Filtration

Filtration rate is affected by factors that alter hydrostatic and oncotic pressure on either side of the glomerular membrane, as shown by the following filtration equation:

$$GFR = K_f[(P_{GC} + \pi_{BC}) - (P_{BC} + \pi_{GC})]$$

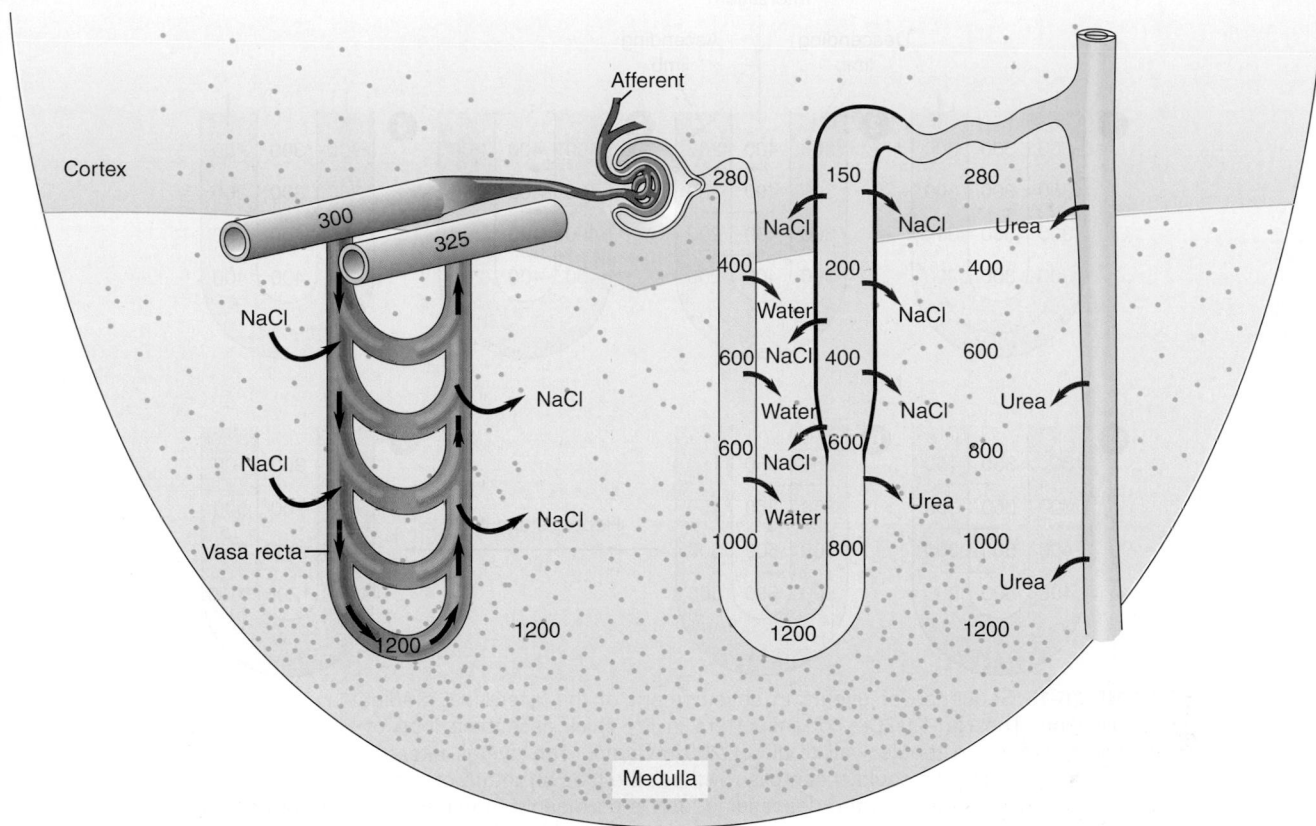

FIGURE 26-14 Mechanism of countercurrent multiplication. Ion pumps in the ascending loop of Henle create an interstitial gradient in the medulla of the kidney. The separation of solute from water in the ascending loop of Henle also produces a dilute tubular fluid allowing the excretion of excess water by making a dilute urine in the absence of antidiuretic hormone (ADH). NaCl accumulation in the interstitium contributes about half of the total osmolality. Urea particles in the interstitium contribute the other half of the particles that produce the normal interstitial gradient in the medulla. As water is removed from the collecting duct (in the presence of ADH), urea becomes more concentrated and moves passively down its gradient into the interstitium. The specialized loop structure of the vasa recta allows it to pick up interstitial water from the medulla without significant solute removal. Although solutes are acquired in the descending segment of the vasa recta, they passively diffuse back out as the ascending segment reaches the cortex. This process is called *countercurrent exchange*.

where P_{GC} is glomerular capillary hydrostatic pressure (mm Hg); π_{BC} is oncotic pressure in the Bowman capsule (mm Hg); P_{BC} is Bowman capsule hydrostatic pressure (mm Hg); and π_{GC} is oncotic pressure in the glomerular capillary (mm Hg). The following is an illustrative example resulting in a normal GFR of 125 ml/min:

$$GFR = 12.5[(60 + 0) - (18 + 32)]$$

$$GFR = 125\,ml/min$$

The main driving force for filtration is hydrostatic pressure in the glomerular capillaries. The glomerular capillary hydrostatic pressure exerts a force against the glomerular capillary walls. As blood circulates through the capillaries, the hydrostatic pressure pushes blood against the walls, and fluid is filtered out. The hydrostatic pressure remains fairly constant along the length of the capillary and exerts an average force of approximately 60 mm Hg.[1]

The glomerular capillary oncotic (colloid osmotic) pressure exists because proteins are present in the blood. Plasma proteins are negatively charged and attract positive ions, which subsequently attract water. Because ions and water are attracted to the proteins and are not pushed against the capillary wall, the glomerular capillary colloidal osmotic pressure opposes filtration by holding water and ions in the capillaries. The glomerular oncotic pressure is lower at the afferent end and becomes progressively higher along the length of the capillary (see Figure 26-16).

The hydrostatic pressure in Bowman capsule is determined by the volume of filtrate present in the capsule. This pressure exerts a force against the walls of Bowman capsule and the glomerular capillaries and opposes filtration. The normal Bowman capsule hydrostatic pressure is about 18 mm Hg. Normally plasma proteins do not filter into Bowman capsule. If they did filter, then they would create Bowman capsule oncotic pressure. This pressure would enhance glomerular filtration because proteins attract cations and water. In a healthy kidney, this pressure is negligible.

In summary, the net filtration pressure across the glomerular membrane is approximately 18 mm Hg. The filtration pressure is higher at the afferent arteriole side of the capillary and diminishes as the blood reaches the efferent end. This occurs because the capillary oncotic pressure is lower at the afferent end. As blood passes through the capillaries, continued filtration leaves a greater concentration of proteins in the capillaries, which raises the oncotic pressure. As blood reaches the efferent arterioles, filtration may cease.

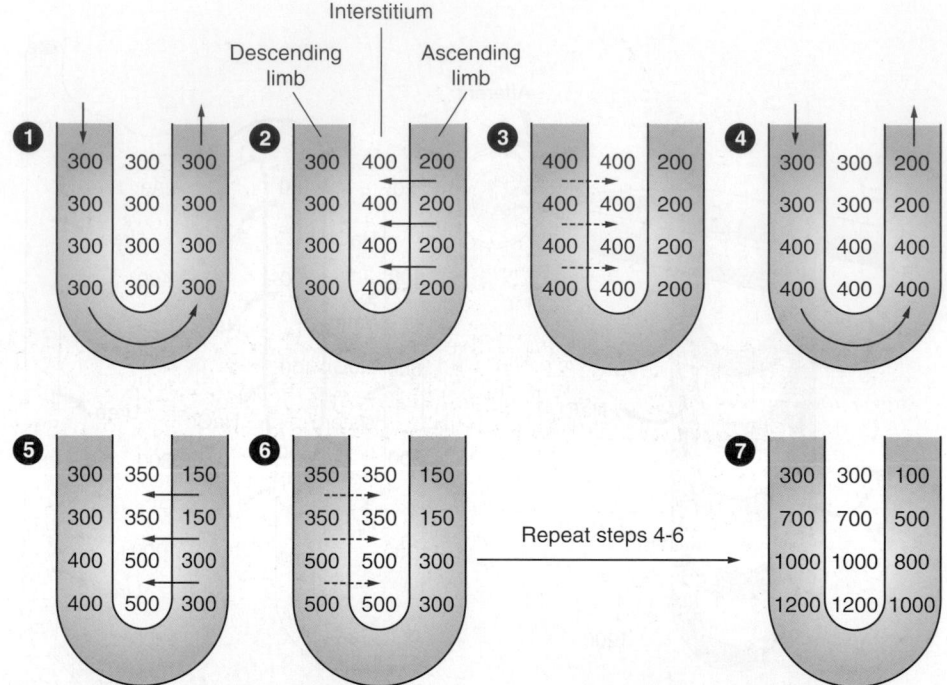

FIGURE 26-15 Sequence of events in development of the interstitial gradient by countercurrent multiplication. The Na^+-K^+-$2Cl^-$ cotransporters in the thick ascending loop of Henle can produce a gradient across the tubule wall of about 200 mOsm/L. The overall interstitial solute gradient is higher than these pumps could accomplish without the loop structure of the tubule. Countercurrent multiplication occurs because the descending loop is permeable to water and equilibrates with the rising interstitial solute concentration. Thus the filtrate reaching the ascending loop is increasingly concentrated with each step *(1-7)*, allowing the ascending loop to further increase the osmolality of the interstitial fluid.

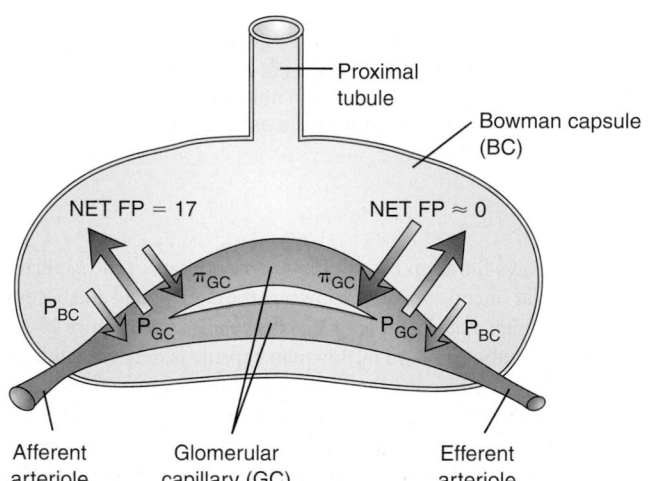

FIGURE 26-16 Net filtration is higher at the afferent end of the glomerular capillary because the hydrostatic blood pressure in the capillary exceeds the pressure in Bowman capsule and the oncotic pressure in the capillary. Toward the efferent end of the capillary, the filtration pressure is low because the oncotic pressure of the blood is high and offsets the hydrostatic blood pressure. Capillary oncotic pressure gets progressively higher along the capillary because fluid is filtering out of the blood into Bowman capsule and leaving the proteins behind so they become more concentrated and exert a greater oncotic pressure. *FP*, Filtration pressure; π, oncotic pressure; *P*, hydrostatic pressure.

Factors Affecting Filtration Pressure

One of the most important physiologic regulators of GFR is blood volume.[1] When blood volume increases because of fluid intake, the blood pressure rises slightly and causes glomerular hydrostatic pressure to increase. GFR increases, and the extra fluid is pushed into the filtrate to be excreted from the body. The opposite also occurs: when blood volume is decreased, capillary hydrostatic pressure falls, resulting in a lower GFR, and fluid is conserved. The glomerular capillary is protected from large swings in blood pressure by autoregulation. Autoregulation adjusts the arteriolar resistance to maintain a relatively steady rate of blood flow despite changes in perfusion pressure. Autoregulation is effective when arterial blood pressure varies between 75 and 160 mm Hg.[1] Autoregulation of renal blood flow is achieved in part by a stretch response in the vascular smooth muscle of the afferent arterioles. When blood pressure increases, the vascular smooth muscle cells reflexively constrict to keep blood flow at about the same rate. This mechanism is called *myogenic autoregulation.*

Other factors can affect GFR by altering the pressure within Bowman capsule or affecting plasma oncotic pressure. Obstruction in the tubules or collecting ducts can significantly elevate the pressure in Bowman capsule. According to the filtration equation, GFR would fall because filtration pressure would be reduced. Because plasma oncotic pressure is determined primarily by the concentration of plasma proteins, a low serum albumin concentration would increase GFR.

Although K_f is called a constant, it is subject to change for physiologic and pathologic reasons. Specialized mesangial cells located in the glomerulus are thought to be important regulators of K_f. These

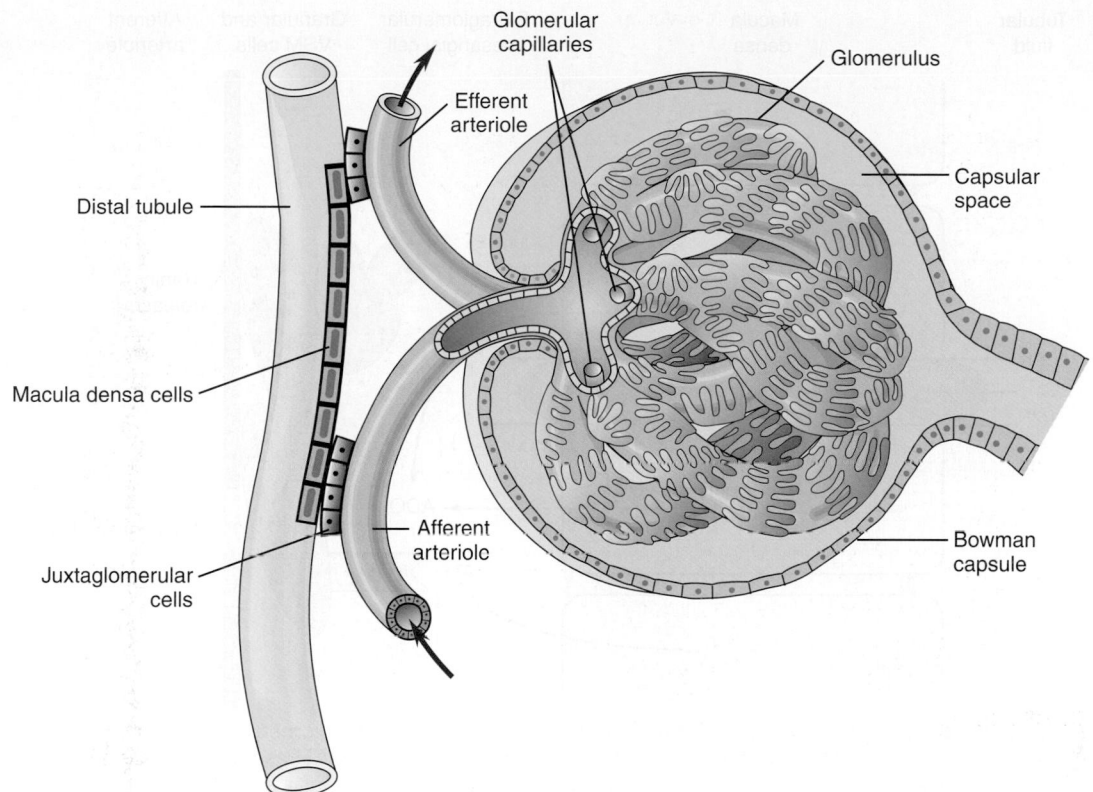

FIGURE 26-17 The juxtaglomerular apparatus is composed of the macula densa cells of the distal tubule, the afferent and efferent arterioles, and the renin-secreting juxtaglomerular cells. Macula densa cells sample the distal filtrate for NaCl content and send signals to the glomerulus to adjust glomerular filtration rate.

cells contract and relax in response to various stimuli and alter the surface area for filtration.[8] Contraction squeezes the capillary cells together and reduces GFR, whereas relaxation allows the permeable surface area to expand. Disease processes that damage the glomerular membrane also can affect permeability. Sclerotic processes reduce K_f, whereas some inflammatory injuries may increase it.

Tubuloglomerular Feedback

Each nephron is able to regulate its own individual GFR through a process termed *tubuloglomerular feedback*. A specialized group of cells forms the regulatory structure, called the **juxtaglomerular apparatus.** The juxtaglomerular apparatus is composed of the glomerulus, the macula densa, and specialized juxtaglomerular cells, which are located around the glomerular arterioles (Figure 26-17). The macula densa cells are located near the end of the thick ascending loop of Henle, which loops up to come in contact with the glomerulus and juxtaglomerular cells.

Macula densa cells sense changes in the amount of NaCl delivered to the tubule. When glomerular filtration is increased, a higher load of NaCl is delivered to the distal tubule. The mechanism whereby macula densa cells sense GFR is not completely understood, but NaCl delivery to the macula densa cells is a critical part of the process. Macula densa cells possess the same Na-Cl-K transporters as other cells in the thick ascending limb and when NaCl delivery is high, more is transported into the cells through this transporter (Figure 26-18). The macula densa cells increase the activity of the Na-K pump in the basal membrane, which stimulates production of adenosine and ATP. Adenosine stimulates contraction of afferent arterioles and relaxation of efferent arterioles, thus decreasing filtration at the glomerulus.[5]

Tubuloglomerular feedback helps to distribute GFR evenly among the kidneys' 2 million nephrons.

The juxtaglomerular cells that surround the afferent arteriole are also thought to be mediators of tubuloglomerular feedback. The juxtaglomerular cells produce and release **renin,** an enzyme that converts angiotensinogen to angiotensin I (AI). Angiotensin I is then converted to angiotensin II (AII) by endothelial cells in the glomerular capillary, which possesses angiotensin-converting enzyme (ACE) activity. AII is a potent vasoconstrictor that constricts both afferent and efferent arterioles.[9] The signals that pass from the macula densa to the glomerulus to regulate tubuloglomerular feedback are not completely known; however, in addition to roles for adenosine and ATP, release of prostaglandins and nitric oxide has been demonstrated.[10] Some prostaglandins have vasodilating activities, whereas others are vasoconstrictors.

The importance of prostaglandins and AII in regulating GFR is supported by the observation that drugs that inhibit their activity interfere with tubuloglomerular feedback in some persons. For example, ACE inhibitors block AII production and may interfere with constriction of the efferent arteriole. This can be particularly detrimental to renal function in patients who require high filtration pressures, such as those with polycystic kidney disease or collecting system obstructions. Drugs that inhibit cyclooxygenase, such as aspirin and nonsteroidal antiinflammatory drugs, interfere with prostaglandin production and may precipitate excessive renovascular constriction in some patients.[11]

Effects of Glucose and Amino Acids

The amount of glucose and amino acids filtered into the tubular fluid may alter GFR through the tubuloglomerular feedback mechanism.

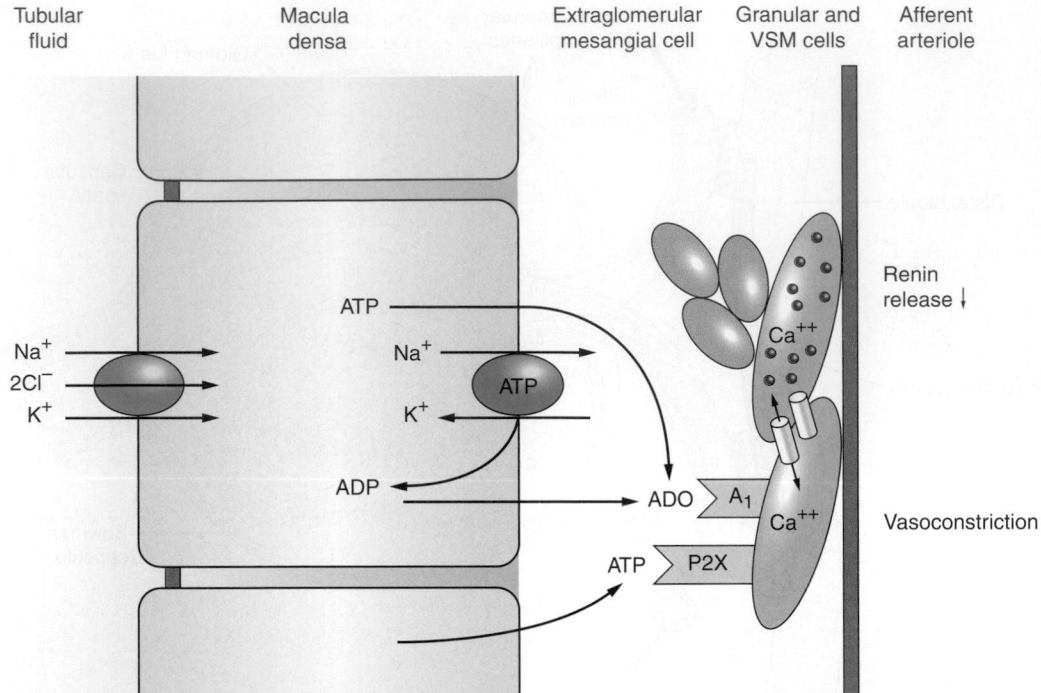

FIGURE 26-18 Mechanism of NaCl sensing by macula densa cells in tubuloglomerular feedback. Entry of ions through the apical Na-K-Cl transporter stimulates activity of the Na-K-ATPase pump on the basal side and stimulates production of ATP and adenosine. Receptors on vascular smooth muscle cells (VSM) of the afferent arterioles bind to ATP and adenosine and cause vasoconstriction. Renin release from the juxtaglomerular cells is also inhibited, thus reducing the amount of angiotensin II that reaches the efferent arteriole. The efferent arteriole becomes less constricted. Afferent constriction and efferent dilation reduce the filtration pressure in the glomerulus, reduce filtration, and reduce the delivery of NaCl to the macula densa. *ADO*, Adenosine; *A1*, adenosine-1 receptor; *P2X*, purineoreceptor (ATP receptor).

Both glucose and amino acids are filtered freely through the glomerular membrane and then are reabsorbed by active transport processes in the proximal tubule. Reabsorption occurs through transporters that use sodium ion entry into the cell to actively cotransport glucose and amino acids. The greater the load of tubular glucose and amino acids, the greater the amount of sodium reabsorbed by the proximal tubule. Fewer sodium ions are transported to the macula densa cells in the distal tubule, and the macula densa perceives this as a need to increase GFR.[5] In addition, chronically high serum glucose concentrations, as occurs in poorly controlled diabetes mellitus, may induce excessive nitric oxide production, producing hyperfiltration, excessive GFR, and damage to the glomerulus.

Role of Mesangial Cells

Mesangial cells are located around the glomerular capillaries and are thought to regulate the surface area available for glomerular filtration.[9] Contraction of the mesangial cells reduces surface area, and relaxation increases it. Mesangial cells are responsive to glomerular stretch and are stimulated to contract when more blood enters the glomerulus. This response provides a negative feedback that decreases surface area when filtration pressure is increased. In addition, mesangial cells respond to a number of chemical mediators, including AII and endothelin (peptides that favor mesangial contraction) and ANP and nitric oxide (substances that favor relaxation). Mesangial cells thus may regulate GFR by altering the filtration constant K_f.

TRANSPORT ACROSS RENAL TUBULES

Reabsorption and secretion of substances across the nephron tubule are accomplished by two routes: the *transcellular* and the *paracellular* routes. Transcellular transport uses specific transporter proteins in the membranes of the tubular epithelial cells to move substances between

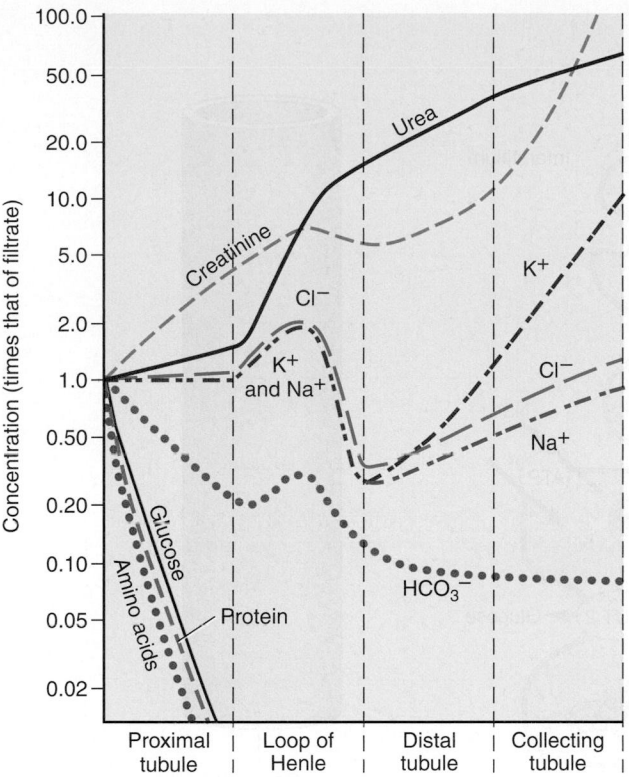

FIGURE 26-19 Summary of nutrient and electrolyte composition of the filtrate in each segment of the nephron. Two thirds of the filtrate is reabsorbed in the proximal tubule. (Adapted from Hall JE, editor: *Guyton and Hall textbook of medical physiology,* ed 12, Philadelphia, 2011, Saunders, p 334.)

the tubular filtrate and the interstitial fluid. Most of these transport processes are dependent on Na^+ reabsorption and made possible by the Na^+-K^+ pump in the basolateral membrane. Paracellular transport refers to movement of substances through the tight junctions that hold the tubular epithelial cells together. Substances using the paracellular route therefore do not traverse the cell membrane and instead move passively through the spaces between cells. *Reabsorption* is the process of transporting a substance from the filtrate into the renal capillaries and requires several transport steps. First, the substance is moved from the filtrate into the tubular cell through transporters on the apical surface of the cell; then it passes through another transporter on the basolateral side of the tubular cell and into the interstitium. From the interstitium, it moves passively by diffusion or filtration into the capillary. In general, the reabsorption of cations, especially sodium, provides an electrical gradient to pull anions across the tubule and into the interstitium. Reabsorption of ions and solutes creates an osmotic force to pull water passively across the renal epithelium. A summary of transport in the various tubule segments is shown in Figure 26-19. The details of glucose, bicarbonate, H^+, and K^+ transport are described as important representative examples.

Reabsorption of Glucose

Glucose is filtered freely across the glomerular membrane such that the tubular load (in milligrams per minute) is determined by the product of serum glucose concentration (in milligrams per milliliter) and GFR (in milliliters per minute). Normally, all of the filtered glucose is reabsorbed in the proximal tubule by a sodium-dependent cotransporter called SGLT 2 (Figure 26-20). The transport proteins have a maximal rate of transport that can be exceeded if the tubular load of glucose is too

great. The transport maximum for normal kidneys is about 375 mg/min.[6] A tubular load of glucose in excess of this amount results in glycosuria. In fact, some spillage of glucose begins at a much lower tubular load because of the uneven distribution of GFR to individual nephrons or differences in the number of transporters in different nephrons. Some nephrons with higher GFR or fewer transporters may exceed their transport maxima, whereas other nephrons are working below capacity. The point at which glucose begins to spill into the urine is called the *renal threshold.* In normal kidneys with a GFR of 125 ml/min, the renal threshold will be reached when serum glucose concentration approaches 180 mg/dl, but significant glycosuria will not occur until the transport maximum is reached at a serum glucose level of about 300 mg/dl. Persons with low GFR associated with renal disease may not experience spillage of glucose until the serum glucose level is much higher, and glycosuria is not a reliable indicator of serum glucose level in these individuals. For example, a patient with a GFR of 50 ml/min and a serum glucose concentration of 300 mg/dl will have a tubular glucose load of only 150 mg/min, which is well below the normal renal threshold. No glycosuria would occur despite the high serum glucose level.

Regulation of Acid-Base Balance

The kidney tubules have an important role in maintaining the pH of the blood. In addition to excreting excess H^+, the kidneys also regulate the concentration of bicarbonate (HCO_3^-) in the blood. The pH of the blood normally ranges between 7.35 and 7.45 and is determined by the ratio of acid (H_2CO_3) to base (HCO_3^-). The lungs and kidneys work together to maintain this balance. Metabolic processes create an excess of acid, which is excreted by the lungs in the form of CO_2 and by the kidneys in the form of H^+. In addition, HCO_3^- is filtered freely through the glomerulus and must be efficiently reabsorbed to maintain acid-base balance. Most HCO_3^- is reabsorbed in the proximal tubule; however, the distal segment also participates in regulating HCO_3^- and H^+ transport.

Reabsorption of HCO_3^- is complex because it is not directly transported across the apical membrane; rather, it is combined with H^+ in the tubule to form H_2CO_3, which dissociates into CO_2 and water (Figure 26-21). The H^+ for this reaction is secreted into the filtrate in exchange for Na^+. Carbonic anhydrase present in the brush border of the proximal tubule cell catalyzes the reaction. Carbon dioxide is lipid soluble and diffuses passively into the tubular cell. Once inside, intracellular carbonic anhydrase catalyzes the reverse reaction to once again form HCO_3^- and H^+. The HCO_3^- is transported out through the basolateral membrane, whereas the H^+ is recycled to the tubular fluid to bind with another HCO_3^-. The energy to power this reabsorptive process is provided by the Na^+-K^+ pump, which keeps intracellular Na^+ concentration low so that the sodium gradient can continue to move H^+ into the tubule lumen through the Na^+-H^+ exchanger.

Normally, all of the filtered HCO_3^- is reabsorbed by this mechanism to help maintain acid-base balance.[12] Excess H^+ ions that find no HCO_3^- in the filtrate with which to bind are excreted in the urine, and urine is normally acidic. The number of H^+ ions that can be excreted in urine is limited to a pH of about 4.0. However, urine buffers, including HPO_4^{2-} and NH_3, are secreted into the filtrate and bind with excess H^+, greatly increasing the ability of the kidney to excrete an acid load (see Figure 26-21). Ammonia (NH_3) is produced by the renal epithelium via metabolism of amino acids. Ammonia binds to H^+ to form ammonium ion (NH_4^+), whereas HPO_4^{2-} binds to H^+ to form $H_2PO_4^-$. The amino acid glutamine can also be metabolized to generate new HCO_3^- with the concurrent production of NH_4^+ that must be excreted in the urine.

Renal Compensation Process

In some cases, the kidneys are called on to compensate for an abnormality in lung function. The lungs normally regulate the amount of carbon

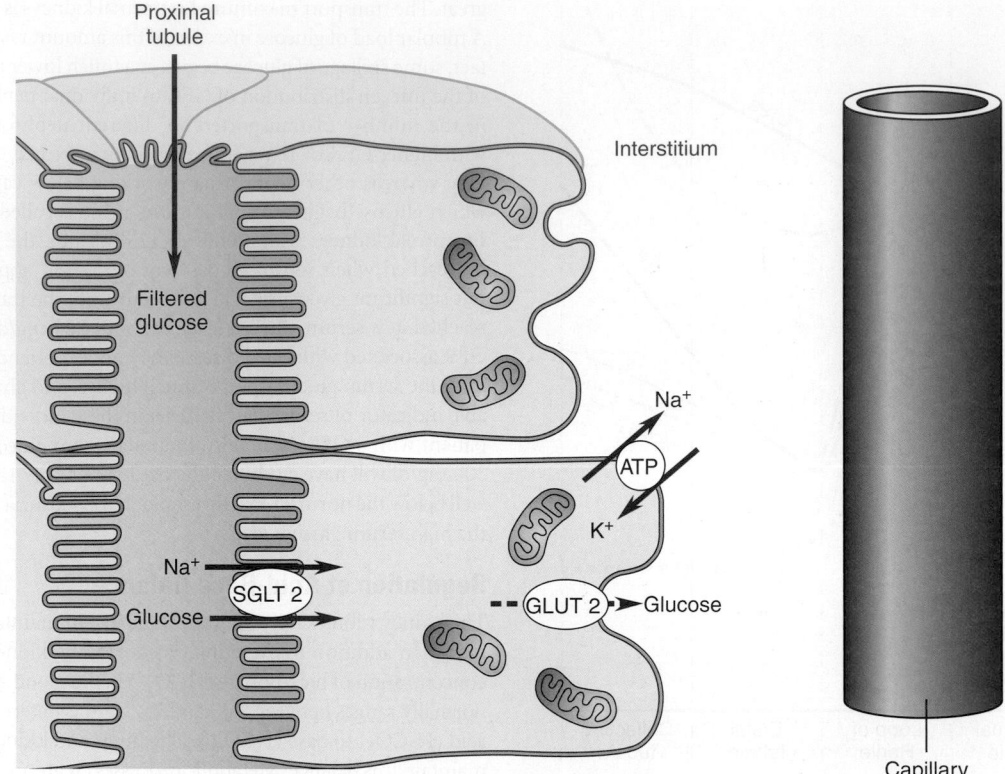

FIGURE 26-20 The glucose transporter in the proximal tubule *(SGLT 2)* is dependent on sodium reabsorption from the filtrate. The Na⁺-K⁺ pump in the basolateral membrane keeps the intracellular sodium level low and maintains a gradient for sodium and glucose reabsorption. Glucose diffuses out of the tubule cell and back into the interstitial fluid through passive carrier proteins *(GLUT 2)*. *ATP,* Adenosine triphosphate.

dioxide in the blood ($Paco_2$). When $Paco_2$ is high, more carbonic acid is formed, and the blood pH becomes acidic. The kidneys compensate by excreting more H^+ and by creating new HCO_3^- to enhance the buffering capacity of the blood. These HCO_3^- ions are additional to those already being reabsorbed from the filtrate and are, thus, new. First, excess circulating CO_2 from respiratory acidosis diffuses into the renal cell and is converted to HCO_3^- and H^+ by the enzyme carbonic anhydrase. The new HCO_3^- is sent back to the bloodstream, and the new H^+ is secreted into the urine filtrate, where it binds with a renal buffer and is excreted. As mentioned previously, new HCO_3^- also can be formed by the metabolism of glutamine, and the new HCO_3^- is sent back to the bloodstream (see Figure 26-21). Gradually, the creation of new HCO_3^- in this way increases the serum HCO_3^- concentration and restores the pH toward normal. This process may take hours to days.

The kidneys are also able to compensate for respiratory alkalosis by excreting some of the filtered HCO_3^-. Alkalosis reduces the number of H^+ ions available for transport into the filtrate. Some of the filtered HCO_3^- escapes the proximal tubule without being converted to CO_2 and is excreted in the urine.

Secretion of Potassium

There is normally a net excess of potassium from dietary sources that must be excreted by the kidneys. The primary transporter responsible for this process is the Na⁺-K⁺ pump in the basolateral cell membrane. The Na⁺-K⁺ pump moves K^+ into the tubular cell and increases the gradient for diffusion of K^+ through the apical membrane and into the filtrate (Figure 26-22). Principle cells in the distal tubule and collecting duct are the site of potassium excretion. The activity of Na⁺-K⁺ pumps

in these segments is sensitive to aldosterone, a steroid hormone secreted by the adrenal cortex. Aldosterone increases reabsorption of Na^+ and water and excretion of K^+. Potassium excretion also is affected by the activity of the K⁺-H⁺ exchanger and by the plasma K^+ concentration.

KEY POINTS

- Reabsorption across the tubular epithelium occurs by transcellular and paracellular routes. The transcellular route utilizes transporters in the apical and basolateral membranes of tubular cells to move substances from the filtrate, through the cell, to the interstitium. The paracellular route allows passive transport of substances between the tubular cells. Renal capillaries passing through the interstitium passively take up substances through filtration and diffusion and return them to the venous circulation.

- Reabsorption of glucose is accomplished by proximal tubule cell sodium-dependent transporters. These transporters have transport maxima that can be overwhelmed by excessive tubular loads of glucose, in which case glycosuria results.

- The kidneys participate in acid-base regulation through secretion of excess H^+ and reabsorption and creation of HCO_3^-. Urine buffers HPO_4^{2-} and NH_3 bind excess H^+ and increase the ability of the kidney to excrete an acid load.

- HCO_3^- is not directly reabsorbed across the renal epithelium; it is first converted to CO_2 by the enzyme carbonic anhydrase. The H^+ ions needed for this reaction are provided by Na⁺-H⁺ pumps on the apical cell membrane.

- Secretion of potassium ions is promoted by activity of the Na⁺-K⁺ pump on the basolateral cell membrane. In the distal tubule, these pumps are regulated by aldosterone, which increases potassium excretion.

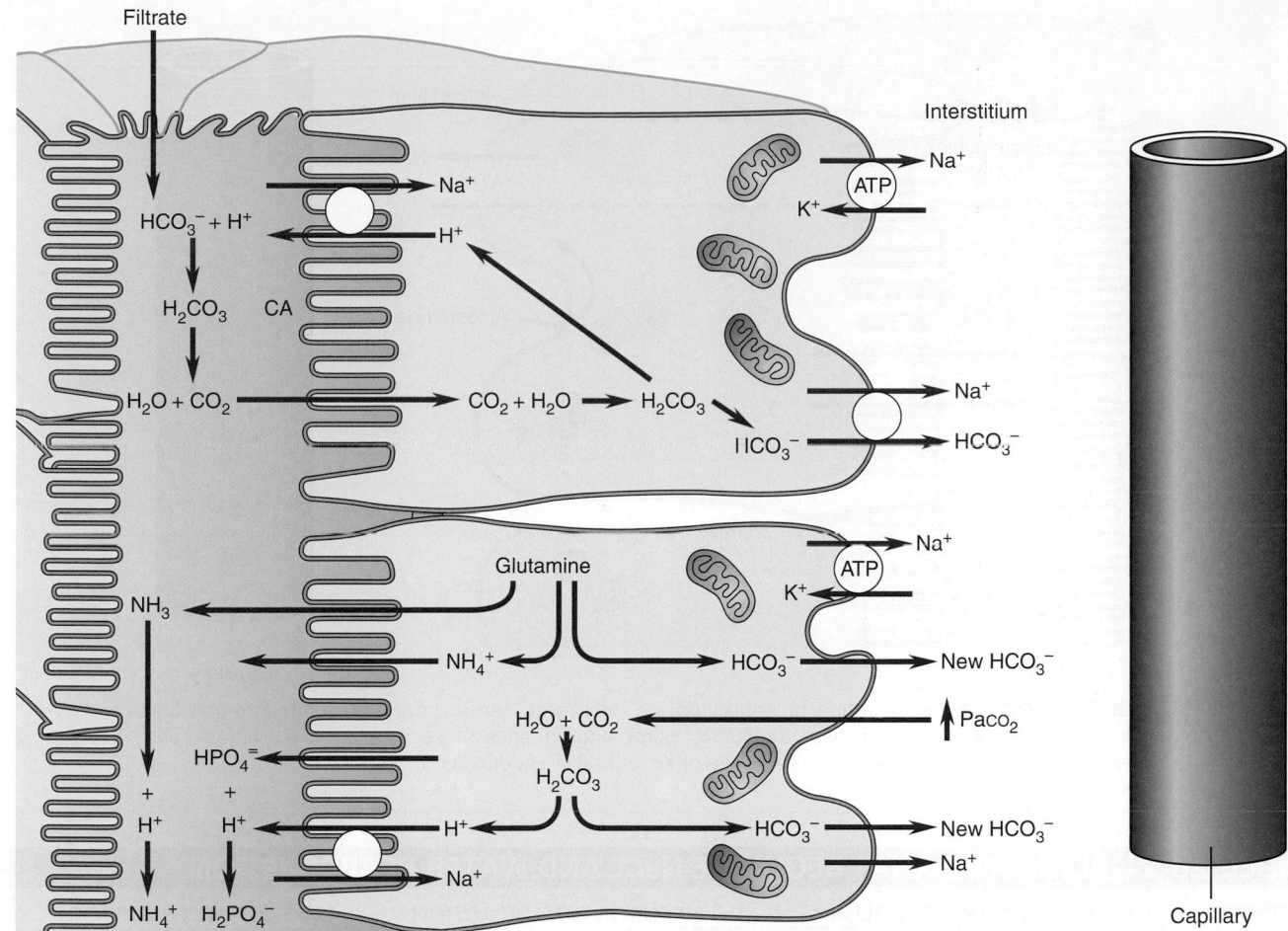

FIGURE 26-21 Bicarbonate ion reabsorption across the renal tubule. Filtered HCO_3^- is combined with secreted H^+ to form carbonic acid, which dissociates into water and carbon dioxide. Carbon dioxide is lipid soluble and diffuses into the cells, where the reverse reaction converts it back to HCO_3^- and H^+. The bicarbonate ion moves out of the basolateral membrane and returns to the bloodstream, whereas the H^+ is returned to the lumen to bind with another HCO_3^- ion. Excess H^+ ions are excreted in the urine in combination with phosphate and ammonia buffers. The kidney is able to create new bicarbonate as needed to maintain pH balance. *ATP*, Adenosine triphosphate; *CA*, carbonic anhydrase.

REGULATION OF BLOOD VOLUME AND OSMOLALITY

The kidneys play a vital role in maintaining normal blood volume and osmolality. As previously discussed, changes in blood volume alter the pressure in the glomerulus and affect GFR. An increase in blood volume results in a pressure diuresis, whereas a fall in blood volume reduces urine output. The kidney tubules are responsive to a number of hormonal signals that fine-tune tubular reabsorption (Table 26-2). These hormones include ADH, aldosterone, AII, ANP, urodilatin, uroguanylin, and guanylin. Antidiuretic hormone is the principal regulator of osmolality, and the others regulate extracellular volume by increasing or decreasing NaCl and water reabsorption.

Antidiuretic Hormone

ADH (also called vasopressin) is secreted from the posterior pituitary when osmoreceptors located in the hypothalamus detect a high osmolality of the extracellular fluid. Principle cells in the collecting tubules respond to ADH by translocating water pores called *aquaporin 2* to the apical membrane (Figure 26-23). These pores make the

tubule permeable to water and allow water to be reabsorbed from the urinary filtrate. The high interstitial gradient of the medulla provides the osmotic force for water reabsorption. Recall that this gradient was formed by the action of powerful ion pumps in the thick ascending limb of the loop of Henle.

As water is reabsorbed into the medullary interstitium, it creates a high tissue pressure that pushes fluid into the vasa recta. The vasa recta return the reabsorbed water to the general circulation. The reabsorbed water dilutes the blood and reduces osmolality. Osmoreceptors in the brain detect the reduced osmolality and inhibit further production of ADH. When blood osmolality is too low, ADH secretion is completely inhibited, and the collecting tubules become impermeable to water. Water is not reabsorbed from the filtrate, and a large quantity of dilute urine is produced. Loss of water in excess of solute returns the blood osmolality toward normal.

An insufficiency of ADH secondary to pituitary damage results in the condition of *diabetes insipidus* in which large volumes of dilute urine are excreted, leading to severe fluid imbalances. A similar problem occurs when the collecting tubules are unresponsive to ADH. This condition is called *nephrogenic diabetes insipidus* and usually

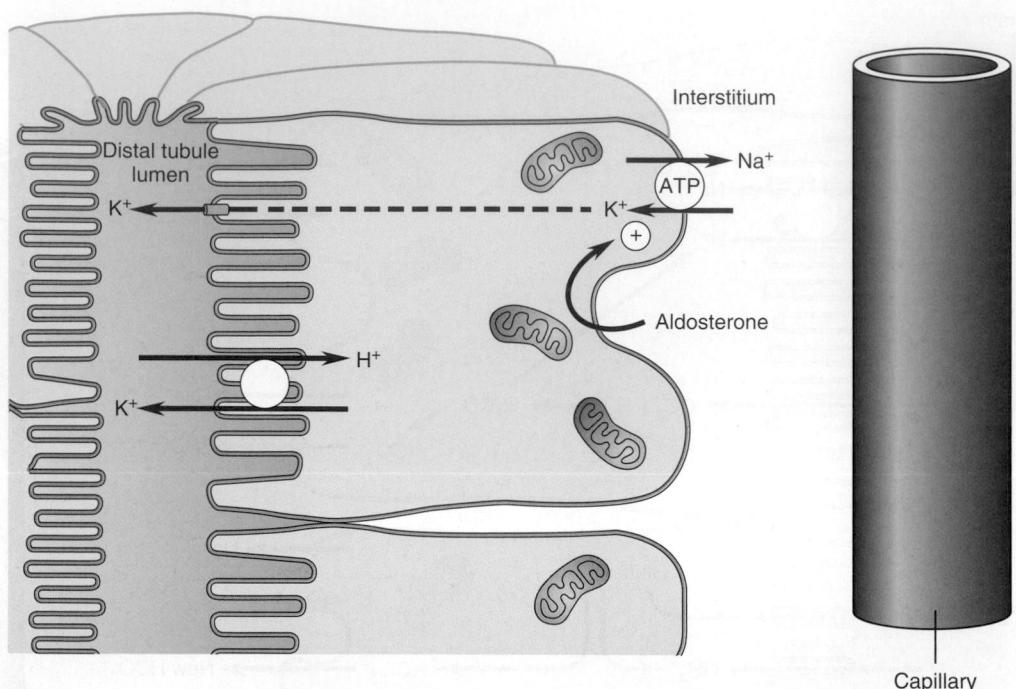

FIGURE 26-22 Tubular secretion of potassium ion. Increased serum potassium concentration and aldosterone increase the activity of the Na+-K+ pump and enhance K+ secretion into the filtrate. The H+-K+ exchanger also regulates the secretion of K+ ions. *ATP,* Adenosine triphosphate.

TABLE 26-2	HORMONES THAT REGULATE NaCL AND WATER REABSORPTION		
HORMONE	**MAJOR STIMULUS**	**NEPHRON SITE OF ACTION**	**EFFECTS ON TRANSPORT**
Angiotensin II	↑ Renin	PT, TAL, DT/CD	↑ NaCl and H_2O reabsorption
Aldosterone	↑ Angiotensin II, ↑ [K+]p	TAL, DT/CD	↑ NaCl and H_2O reabsorption*
ANP, BNP, urodilatin	↑ ECFV	CD	↓ H_2O and NaCl reabsorption
Uroguanylin, guanylin	Oral ingestion of NaCl	PT, CD	↓ H_2O and NaCl reabsorption
Sympathetic nerves	↓ ECFV	PT, TAL, DT/CD	↑ NaCl and H_2O reabsorption*
Dopamine	↑ ECFV	PT	↓ H_2O and NaCl reabsorption
ADH	↑ P_{osm}, ↓ ECFV	DT/CD	↑ H_2O reabsorption*

Data from Koeppen B, Stanton B: *Berne & Levy physiology,* ed 6, Philadelphia, 2010, Mosby, p. 610.
ADH, Antidiuretic hormone; *ANP,* atrial natriuretic peptide; *BNP,* B-type natriuretic peptide; *BP,* blood pressure; *CD,* collecting duct; *DT,* distal tubule; *ECFV,* extracellular fluid volume; *[K+]p,* plasma K+ concentration; *P_{osm},* plasma osmolality; *PT,* proximal tubule; *TAL,* thick ascending limb.
*The effect on H_2O reabsorption does not include the thick ascending limb or the early portion of the distal tube.

results from genetic defects in either the ADH receptor (V_2) or the aquaporin 2 genes.[5]

Aldosterone, Angiotensin II, Natriuretic Peptides, Urodilatin, Uroguanylin, and Guanylin

Aldosterone, AII, ANP, urodilatin, uroguanylin, and guanylin alter blood volume without affecting its concentration. Aldosterone and AII increase reabsorption of Na+, which provides a gradient for water reabsorption. Because salt and water are reabsorbed together, the osmolality of the reabsorbed fluid is isosmotic with plasma.

AII and aldosterone are produced when the juxtaglomerular cells in the kidney are stimulated to release renin. Renin is released in response to (1) decreased blood flow to the kidney, (2) reduced serum sodium levels, and (3) activation of sympathetic nerves to the juxtaglomerular cells.[5] Renin begins a cascade of reactions that result in the production of AII and aldosterone. When AII and aldosterone restore blood volume and blood pressure to normal, the stimuli for renin release are removed and the concentrations of AII and aldosterone fall.

ANP is released from atrial cells in the heart when the chamber is overstretched by excessive blood volume. ANP inhibits all of the actions of AII and results in loss of sodium and water in the urine. Thus, ANP reduces extracellular volume, but the fluid losses are isosmotic with plasma, and blood osmolality remains unchanged. Urodilatin is a peptide that is secreted by distal and collecting tubule cells in response to increased circulating volume.[6] It is very similar in structure and function to ANP and inhibits Na+ and water reabsorption by the collecting duct.

Uroguanylin and guanylin are peptide hormones produced by neuroendocrine cells in the intestine in response to NaCl ingestion. The targets for these hormones are guanylyl cyclase receptors located on cells in the proximal tubule and collecting duct. Binding to these receptors generates cGMP, which inhibits Na+, Cl−, and water reabsorption and produces an effect similar to that of natriuretic peptides and urodilatin.

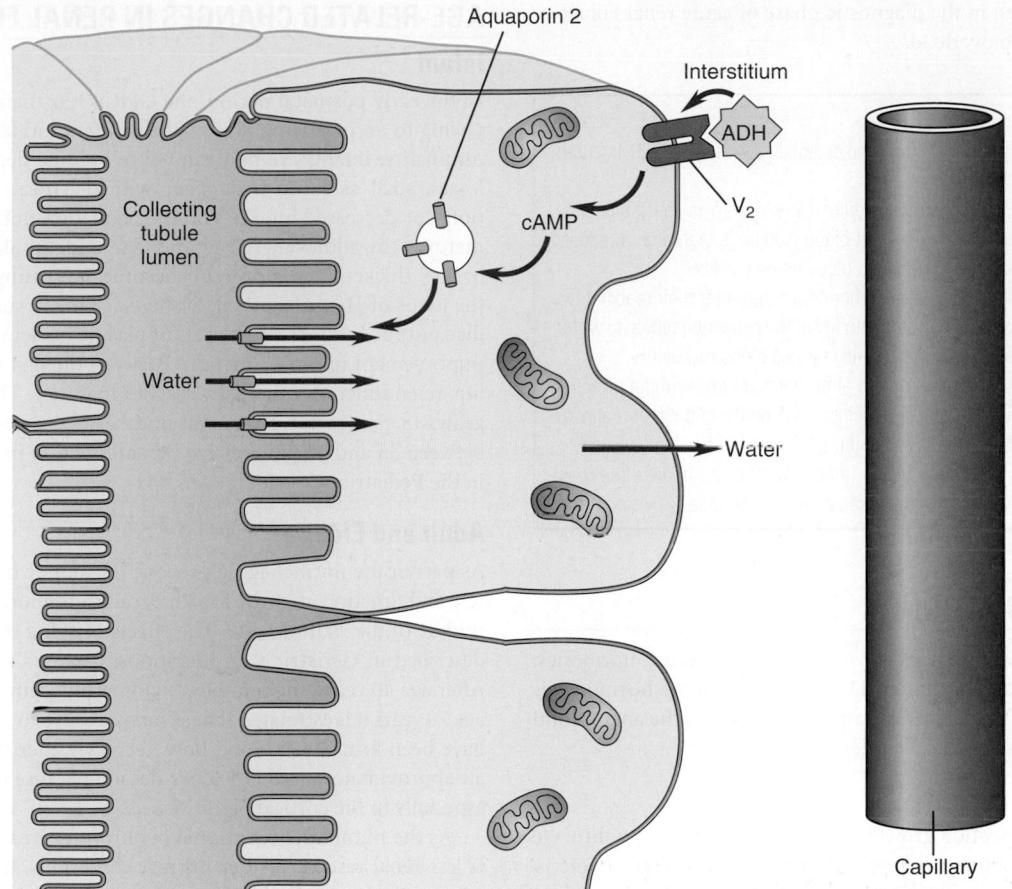

FIGURE 26-23 Antidiuretic hormone *(ADH)* action on the collecting tubule epithelium. ADH binds to receptors on the basolateral cell membrane, resulting in translocation of water pores (aquaporin 2) to the apical surface. Increased water permeability results in reabsorption of water from the filtrate and into the interstitium. *cAMP,* Cyclic adenosine monophosphate; *V_2,* vasopressin-2 receptor.

Diuretic Agents

The ability of the kidneys to reabsorb fluid can be inhibited by drugs that block sodium and water reabsorption. These agents are called *diuretics* and include osmotic diuretics, ACE inhibitors, loop diuretics, thiazide-like diuretics, and inhibitors of aldosterone activity (Table 26-3).[13] Diuretics work by altering osmotic gradients in the kidney tubules so that reabsorption of water is inhibited. Recall that water always moves passively according to an osmotic gradient. When the solute content of the filtrate is elevated, reabsorption of water is inhibited, resulting in a larger output of urine.

Osmotic diuretics (e.g., mannitol) are filtered through the glomerulus and are not reabsorbed by the tubules. The osmolality of the filtrate is increased by the presence of the solute, and more water remains in the tubule and is excreted in the urine. ACE inhibitors (e.g., captopril) inhibit the formation of AII and aldosterone, which normally stimulate the kidney tubules to reabsorb Na^+. In the absence of these hormones, more Na^+ stays in the urinary filtrate, resulting in less reabsorption of water.

Loop diuretics (e.g., furosemide) block the Na^+-K^+-$2Cl^-$ pumps in the ascending loop of Henle. The ions that would normally have been pumped into the interstitium stay in the filtrate and hold water with them. In addition, the maintenance of the high interstitial gradient in the medulla may be impaired. Washout of the gradient reduces the force for water reabsorption from the collecting ducts.

Thiazide-like diuretics (e.g., hydrochlorothiazide) block Na^+ reabsorption in the distal tubule. Sodium ions remain in the filtrate and oppose the action of the interstitial osmotic gradient.

All of these agents also increase the excretion of K^+ and are called *potassium-wasting diuretics.* Patients receiving chronic diuretic therapy with these agents usually require potassium replacement therapy.

In contrast, the aldosterone-blocking agents (e.g., spironolactone) are potassium sparing. Recall that aldosterone increases activity of the Na^+-K^+ pumps on the basolateral membrane of the distal tubule cells. These pumps promote Na^+ and water reabsorption and potassium secretion. Blockage of aldosterone reduces the activity of these pumps and results in less sodium and water reabsorption as well as less potassium excretion. Significant elevations in serum K^+ concentration can occur with these agents.

Diuretics are used primarily in the management of high blood pressure (see Chapter 16) and congestive heart failure (see Chapter 19), but

TABLE 26-3	COMMONLY USED DIURETICS
DIURETIC	**ACTION**
Osmotic diuretics	Increase solute load in tubule
ACE inhibitors	Block production of AII and aldosterone
Loop diuretics	Block Na^+-K^+-$2Cl^-$ transporter in ascending loop of Henle
Thiazide-like diuretics	Block Na^+ reabsorption in distal tubule
Aldosterone inhibitors	Block action of aldosterone on distal tubule Na^+-K^+ transporters

they also may be used in the diagnostic phase of acute renal failure or to manage potassium overload.

> **KEY POINTS**
> - The kidneys regulate blood volume and osmolality by altering GFR and reabsorption from the urinary filtrate.
> - Changes in blood volume alter the filtration pressure in the glomerulus, resulting in a pressure diuresis when blood volume is high and in reduced filtration and fluid conservation when blood volume is low.
> - The kidney tubules are responsive to hormones that alter their reabsorptive properties. ADH increases the permeability of the collecting tubule to water, resulting in increased reabsorption and reduced blood osmolality.
> - Aldosterone, AII, ANP, and urodilatin alter blood volume without affecting blood osmolality. Aldosterone and AII increase sodium and water reabsorption, whereas ANP and urodilatin inhibit their reabsorption.
> - Diuretics alter the osmolality of the urinary filtrate and oppose the reabsorption of water, resulting in an increase in urine volume.

ENDOCRINE FUNCTIONS

The kidney is the source of two important endocrine hormones: erythropoietin and active vitamin D. Secretion of these hormones is impaired in chronic kidney disease and contributes to the anemia and osteodystrophy found in this disorder (see Chapter 28).

Erythropoietin

Erythropoietin is a peptide growth factor that stimulates erythrocyte development in the bone marrow. The regulation of erythropoietin secretion is not completely understood; however, hypoxemia and decreased circulating red cell mass are known to increase its release (see Chapter 13). Erythropoietin is commercially available in a recombinant form that can be given parenterally. The anemia of chronic kidney disease usually responds well to erythropoietin replacement therapy.

Vitamin D

Synthesis of active vitamin D is an interdependent function of the skin, liver, and kidney. The precursors to active vitamin D can be formed in the skin in response to the ultraviolet rays in sunlight, or they can be ingested in fortified food products. These precursors (cholecalciferol) then must undergo a series of two hydroxylations to become active. The first occurs in the liver, resulting in the formation of 25-hydroxycholecalciferol. The kidney performs the second hydroxylation to form 1,25-dihydroxycholecalciferol, which is the active form of vitamin D. Vitamin D is a necessary cofactor for calcium absorption from the intestine. It may also facilitate calcium reabsorption in the kidney tubules.

In chronic kidney disease, the production of active vitamin D is impaired, resulting in poor calcium absorption from the intestine and low serum calcium levels. A low serum calcium level is the stimulus for parathyroid hormone release, resulting in removal of calcium and phosphate from the bones. Eventually excessive parathyroid hormone activity leads to the condition of osteodystrophy and predisposes to skeletal fractures (see Chapter 28).

> **KEY POINTS**
> - The kidney secretes two important endocrine hormones: erythropoietin, a growth factor for red blood cells, and active vitamin D, a necessary cofactor for calcium absorption from the intestine.
> - In chronic kidney disease, impaired production of these hormones results in anemia and osteodystrophy.

AGE-RELATED CHANGES IN RENAL FUNCTION

Infant

In the early postnatal period, the GFR is less than half the adult rate. Owing to an immature ability of the infant kidneys to regulate urine osmolality, infants are predisposed to volume depletion during fluid losses, such as those that occur with diarrhea, fever, fluid restrictions, or decreased intake. Volume regulation improves as the kidney matures. In addition, the glomerular and tubular basement membranes thicken, the glomeruli become increasingly permeable, and the loops of Henle lengthen. Systemic changes, such as increased cardiac output and increased levels of plasma proteins, also influence the improvement in renal function. Between the first and second years of life, renal function essentially reaches maturity. Thereafter the kidney grows in proportion to overall body growth, reaching maximal size between 35 and 40 years of age. Renal function in infants is described in the Pediatrics Considerations box.

Adult and Elderly

As part of the normal aging process, the kidney begins to diminish in size and function after the fourth decade and more significantly by the middle of the sixth decade. The effects of aging on renal function are described in Geriatric Considerations: Changes in the Renal System. After age 40 years, the number of glomeruli begins to decrease, and by age 70 years it is estimated that as many as 30% to 50% of the glomeruli have been lost. Renal blood flow decreases after the fourth decade at an approximate rate of 10% per decade because of vascular changes, especially in the cortical blood vessels.

As the number of functional nephrons decreases with aging, there is less renal reserve. Under normal conditions, the kidney functions adequately; however, elderly people are much more susceptible to fluid and electrolyte imbalances and renal damage. The elderly are also very susceptible to kidney damage from drugs and medications, including contrast media. Consequently, it is essential that renal function be evaluated before, during, and after they receive these agents or substances.

> **KEY POINTS**
> - Renal function is impaired at both ends of the life span. Infants have reduced ability to make concentrated urine because of kidney immaturity. Aged individuals have reduced numbers of functioning nephrons, reduced renal blood flow and GFR, and decreased ability to conserve salt and water.
> - The very young and very old are at increased risk for fluid and electrolyte imbalances and drug toxicity.

TESTS OF RENAL STRUCTURE AND FUNCTION

Urinalysis, serum **creatinine level,** blood urea nitrogen (BUN) levels, and tests of GFR are most helpful in evaluating kidney function, whereas other diagnostic tests are best for evaluating kidney structure.

Urine and Blood Studies

Routine assessment of urine is commonly performed to screen for a variety of kidney and metabolic disorders. Serum creatinine and BUN levels are used to monitor the progression of renal disease or to screen for occult renal insufficiency.

Urinalysis

Most often urinalysis is done on a single voided sample; however, longer collections may be done for quantitative analysis. Urinalysis assesses urine color, clarity, odor, specific gravity, pH, and concentrations of glucose, ketones, protein, and sediment (including cells,

PEDIATRIC CONSIDERATIONS

Changes in the Kidneys in Infants

At birth, the loss of placental blood flow and the rapid increase in renal blood flow lead to high vascular resistance in the kidneys. The immature kidneys respond by temporarily reducing renal blood flow and filtration to compensate. The filtration capacity of the glomeruli is reduced. The kidneys cannot adequately concentrate urine to conserve body water. This makes the child susceptible to water loss. In the first 24 hours of life, the newborn will have decreased urine output. Ninety-five percent of infants will pass urine in the first 24 hours of life, although the amount is small (about 20 ml) (Hockenberry & Wilson, 2011). As the infant increases the number and volume of feedings in the first few weeks of life, the capillary resistance is reduced and filtration is increased by the glomeruli.

The kidneys have small immature nephrons. The nephrons are lined with cuboid epithelium, which limits the function of the nephrons. The cuboid epithelium is not replaced by pavement epithelium and fully functioning until after the first year of life (MacGregor, 2008). The immaturity of the nephrons also makes the distal convoluted tubules resistant to aldosterone. The immature nephrons also have short loops of Henle, where water and sodium levels are normally adjusted. The short loops of Henle and the resistance to aldosterone make it difficult for an infant to excrete excess sodium. The presence of excess sodium increases the interstitial osmolality, which will decrease the glomerular filtration rate in the infant. The decreased glomerular filtration rate contributes to the reduced production of urine that is seen with the infant. As the child grows and the kidney matures, the glomerular filtration rate will increase. The glomerular filtration rate triples by 9 months of age and reaches 30% of adult values by 2 years of age (MacGregor, 2008).

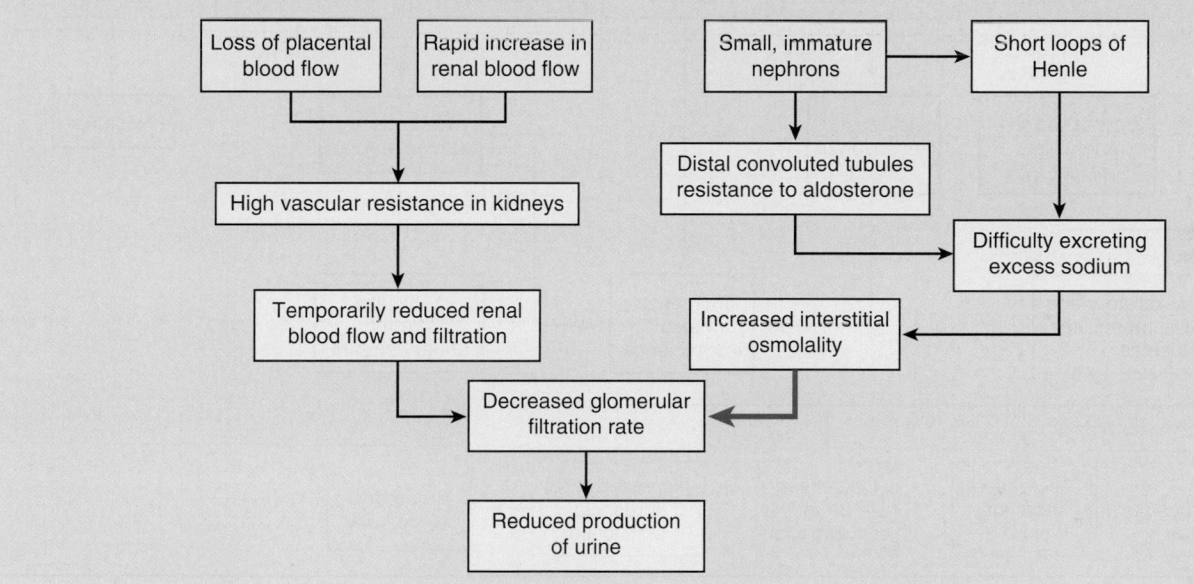

Hockenberry MJ, Wilson D: *Wong's nursing care of infants and children,* ed 9, St Louis, 2011, Mosby. MacGregor J: *Introduction to the anatomy and physiology of children: a guide for students of nursing, child care and health,* ed 2, New York, 2008, Routledge.

crystals, **casts,** and bacteria or other organisms). The first urine voided in the morning is the most concentrated, due to overnight fasting, and therefore is the best specimen to use for a routine or baseline urinalysis, especially to assess pH, osmolality, and sediment (Table 26-4).

A 24-hour urine collection measures the total quantity of a substance or substances excreted in a day. This is helpful for evaluating substances that are excreted in varying concentrations throughout the day, such as hormones, creatinine, protein, urea, and glucose.

Urine microscopy and culture and sensitivity tests assess the urine for the presence of microorganisms and accompanying cells and to determine the medications or drugs to which the organisms are most sensitive. For these tests, a few milliliters of urine is collected by the clean-catch method and placed into a sterile container.

Urine is approximately 95% water and contains varying amounts of water-soluble waste products. Freshly voided urine has a slight odor attributable to the breakdown of urea to ammonia. If urine stands for a period of time or has a large bacteria population, it will have a strong ammonia smell. The ingestion and excretion of certain foods, such as asparagus, or of certain medications, such as vitamins, may cause urine to have a different odor.

The pale yellow to amber color of urine is due to the presence of urochrome pigments. Urine color can change because of the presence of cells or because of an increased urine concentration. The presence of red blood cells (RBCs), or hematuria, can cause urine color to range from brown to bright red. White blood cells (WBCs) can make urine look cloudy. Concentrated urine is usually dark yellow to orange. Certain foods and drugs can change urine color. For instance, if beets have been eaten, the urine may be burgundy, and if the individual has taken phenazopyridine (Pyridium), the urine may be orange.

Normally, urine is clear and slightly acidic, although the pH range is 4.5 to 8.0. Urine allowed to stand undisturbed will become cloudy and alkaline because of the breakdown of urea to ammonia, which increases the pH. Cloudiness can result from the presence of cells, bacteria, crystals, casts, or fat substances.

Urine specific gravity and urine osmolality are measures of the concentration of solute in the urine. Urine specific gravity varies with the amount of solids in the urine, such as cells, casts, and microorganisms, but urine osmolality is not affected by these substances. Thus, urine osmolality is a more accurate measure of the kidneys' ability to concentrate and dilute the urine. The range for specific gravity is 1.003 to 1.030, with the higher number indicating a more concentrated urine. Usually urine osmolality and specific gravity vary throughout the day and from day to day. Results that remain fixed over consecutive voidings and days could be an indicator of renal disease.

GERIATRIC CONSIDERATIONS

Changes in the Renal System

In the aging individual, there is a 30% to 50% decrease in the number, size, weight, and function of the nephrons, with an accompanying reduction in the size and weight of the kidney. There is increasing interstitial fibrosis of the renal afferent arterioles. Loss of nephrons and diminished renal blood flow contribute to a decrease in the glomerular filtration rate (GFR).

There is also a decrease in the length and the excretory and reabsorptive capabilities of the tubules. The tubule changes affect the countercurrent mechanism, leading to significant changes in urine concentration, excretion, and absorption. Specifically, the changes include reduced urine concentration,

decreased sodium retention, diminished drug and metabolite excretion, decreased hydrogen ion (H^+) secretion, and increased renal threshold for glucose. With aging, the kidney does not respond quickly to correct pH or sodium imbalances.

With aging, urinary muscles weaken, and sphincter tone and bladder capacity decrease. This increased muscular weakness can lead to a rise in the residual volume in the bladder and difficulty in starting the urinary stream. The length of the urethra decreases. There is also less bladder innervation and a reduced sensation of filling. A loss of the diurnal excretory pattern induces nocturia.

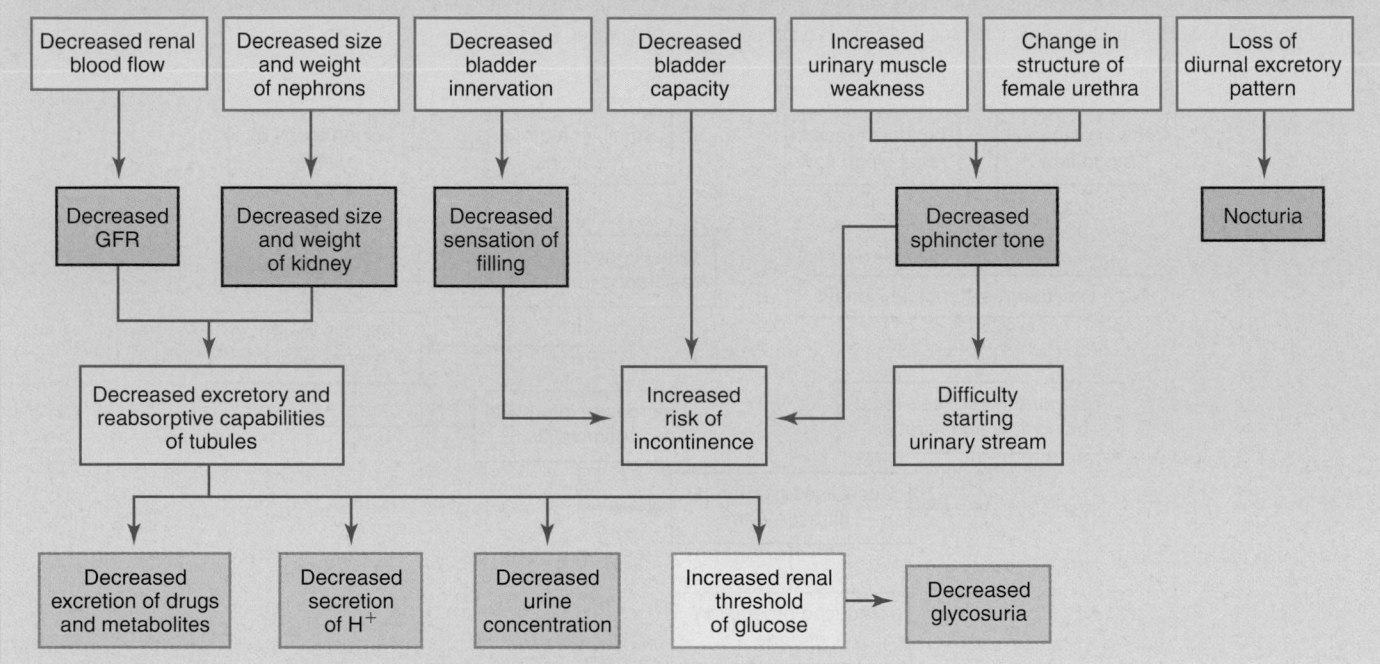

TABLE 26-4	NORMAL COMPOSITION OF URINE
CHARACTERISTICS	**NORMAL VALUE**
Color	Light yellow to amber
pH	Acidic
Specific gravity	1.003-1.030
Red blood cells	<5/HPF
White blood cells	<5/HPF
Protein	Negative
Glucose	Negative
Ketones	Negative
Nitrites	Negative
Casts	None
Crystals	None

HPF, High-powered field.

Normal urine contains little or no protein. A small amount of protein in the urine is insignificant, but excretion of more than 150 mg per 24 hours should be investigated, because it could indicate glomerular capillary disease. Proteinuria can cause urine to be foamy.

Glycosuria, or glucose in the urine, is abnormal and usually indicates hyperglycemia (elevated blood glucose level), which can occur with diabetes mellitus or following an excessive ingestion of sugar. Rarely does glycosuria indicate renal disease.

A few epithelial cells, erythrocytes, leukocytes, and bacteria are normally found in urine. Fewer than 5 RBCs or WBCs per high-powered field is considered to be within normal limits. An excess of any of these cells may indicate a pathologic process; however, collection technique and presence of menstrual blood may be confounding factors.

Crystals and stones are not usually found in the urine. Either can originate anywhere along the urinary tract. If found in the urine, their composition should be identified and the urinary tract assessed for more crystals and stones (see Chapter 27).

When urinary casts are present, they provide important clues for differentiating renal diseases. Casts are formed in the nephron tubule and are composed of a protein meshwork with entrapped cells or cell fragments. Cells in the thick ascending loop of Henle produce and secrete small amounts of a glycoprotein, called *Tamm-Horsfall* protein (also called *uromodulin*), into the tubular lumen. This protein forms the meshwork that entraps cells in the tubule to form casts and is found in normal urine. Normal protein casts that do not have cells in them are called agranular casts. There are many types of abnormal casts, each associated with certain renal pathologic conditions. For example, WBC casts are associated with renal infections (pyelonephritis); RBC casts indicate inflammation of the glomerulus (glomerulonephritis); and epithelial cell casts indicate sloughing of tubular cells (acute tubular necrosis).

Serum Creatinine and Blood Urea Nitrogen

Creatinine is an end product of muscle metabolism that is excreted exclusively by the kidney. The serum creatinine level averages approximately 0.7 to 1.5 mg/dl and is relatively constant throughout the day and from day to day. Creatinine levels are slightly higher in men than in women because of men's larger muscle mass.

Serum creatinine level is a fairly reliable indicator of renal function because it is affected by only two factors: (1) the rate of creatinine produced from muscle, which is relatively constant in the absence of muscle breakdown; and (2) the rate of creatinine excreted by the kidney, which is determined primarily by the GFR. Therefore, the GFR is reflected in the serum creatinine level. For instance, when the GFR decreases by half, the concentration of creatinine in the serum doubles. A rise in serum creatinine level indicates a decrease in renal function.

Urea is an end product of protein metabolism. It is excreted primarily by the kidney and measured in the blood as **blood urea nitrogen (BUN)**. The BUN averages approximately 10 to 20 mg/dl and rises with a decrease in renal function, a decrease in fluid volume, and an increase in catabolism and dietary protein intake. When a change in renal function occurs, the BUN measurement tends to change more rapidly than the creatinine level; however, the BUN value is less specific. Often BUN and creatinine are measured together, and the ratio is determined. Acute changes in GFR are reflected in a higher BUN-to-creatinine ratio, usually greater than 20:1.

Measures of Glomerular Filtration Rate

GFR is an important parameter in the assessment of renal function. GFR is commonly measured by evaluating the clearance of a filterable substance from the plasma. Creatinine clearance is frequently used to assess GFR, but it is not completely accurate because some secretion and reabsorption occurs in the nephron tubules. At low GFR, creatinine clearance is quite unreliable. The accuracy of creatinine clearance tests can be improved by administration of cimetidine, a drug that blocks the tubular secretion of creatinine.[14]

A more accurate measurement of GFR is obtained by using inulin, an inert substance that is filtered freely at the glomerulus and is completely unaffected by tubular secretion and reabsorption. The use of inulin is more expensive and cumbersome than creatinine clearance because it must be injected. The formula for measuring clearance is the same regardless of the marker substance used. Creatinine clearance is used in the following example, but the corresponding values for inulin can be substituted in the equation.

Creatinine clearance estimates the GFR by measuring the amount of blood that is cleared of creatinine each minute. Usually a 24-hour urine specimen and a blood specimen at the midpoint of the urine collection are used to determine creatinine clearance; however, shorter intervals can be used. The measured values are calculated in the following formula:

$$\text{Clearance} = \frac{\text{Urine volume (ml/min)} \times \text{urinary creatinine (mg/dl)}}{\text{Plasma creatinine (mg/dl)}}$$

An estimate of GFR called the *Modification of Diet in Renal Disease study equation* (MDRD) can be made using only patient demographics and serum creatinine value (S_{cr}).[15] This estimate is based on an average body surface area for an adult of 1.73 m². It does not require urine collection, making it simple compared to other measures of clearance:

$$\text{GFR (ml/min/1.73 m}^2) = 186 \times (S_{cr})^{-1.154} \times (\text{Age})^{-0.203}$$
$$\times (0.742 \text{ if female}) \times (1.210 \text{ if African American})$$

Diagnostic Tests

Although studies of urine and blood are good indicators of renal function, they often are not adequate to determine the underlying pathologic process. Diagnostic tests are helpful in assessing structural abnormalities, such as tumors or obstructions, congenital anomalies, perfusion defects, and histologic abnormalities. Sometimes a combination of diagnostic tests is necessary.

Kidney, Ureter, and Bladder Roentgenography

A kidney, ureter, and bladder (KUB) roentgenography is a plain radiograph (x-ray) taken of the abdomen to visualize the kidneys, ureters, and bladder. A KUB study shows the position, shape, size, and number of macroscopic or gross renal, ureteral, and bladder structures and surrounding bones. In addition, foreign bodies, radiopaque objects, stones, and neoplasms can be seen on KUB. The KUB may serve as a screening examination to inform further diagnostic testing.

Intravenous Urography/Pyelography

During intravenous urography, also called intravenous pyelography (IVP), an iodine-containing radiopaque dye is injected into a vein; it circulates through the kidney and is excreted in the urine. A rapid series of radiographs is made as the dye is being excreted. This test shows the size, shape, and location of urinary tract structures and can be used to evaluate renal excretory function. The dye is **nephrotoxic,** meaning poisonous to the kidney, and allergenic to some people. A state of hydration helps the dye to pass through the kidney and prevents renal damage. Because fecal matter and gas in the intestinal tract will interfere with visualization of the kidneys and ureters on the radiographs, a laxative or enema may be indicated before IVP.

Radionuclide Studies

Renograms and renal scans are diagnostic studies that use radioactive isotopes to assess kidney structure and function. In general, the renogram is more useful for assessing function, whereas the renal scan is better at detecting structural anomalies. During a renogram procedure, a small amount of filterable radioactive material is administered intravenously. It circulates through the kidney and is excreted in the urine. While the radionuclide circulates through the renal vessels and nephrons, a radiation detection probe counts the activity of the radioactive substance and simultaneously creates a graphic record of the activity. This test assesses renal function by measuring renal blood flow, glomerular filtration, and tubular secretion.

The renal scan uses a radionuclide that tends to accumulate in areas that are well perfused by blood. The renal scan images depict the concentration of the radionuclide in the kidney and provide anatomic and some physiologic information. In the presence of tumors or nonfunctioning areas, the radioactive material will not be detected by the scan.

A more dynamic assessment of renal physiology can be obtained using positron emission tomography (PET) or single-photon emission computed tomography (SPECT). These modalities use scintigraphic imaging to view the kidney and can pick up subtle, dynamic changes. Regional differences in GFR, for example, can be detected by PET scan.

Ultrasonography

Ultrasonography is a noninvasive, painless procedure that uses high-frequency sound waves to image renal structures. The sound waves are at a frequency above the limit of human hearing. Ultrasound is used because its short wavelength produces a more detailed picture or image than other types of sound waves. A probe with a transducer inside is held against the back and emits ultrasound waves that travel through tissue to the kidney and reflect off the kidney, back to the probe. Ultrasonography demonstrates gross renal anatomy, true kidney depth, structural abnormalities, and perirenal masses, and it can be used to distinguish between a fluid-filled cyst and a solid tumor.

Computed Tomography

Computed tomography (CT) combines roentgenography with computer technology and is a noninvasive, painless procedure. Instead of using broad x-ray beams, CT uses thin x-ray beams, each about 10 degrees apart. The information obtained during scanning is transmitted to a computer, which constructs a tomograph and calculates its density. Because the kidneys are located deep within the abdominal cavity, they opacify better after an IV injection of a contrast agent. CT shows more detail than ultrasonography. CT can demonstrate perirenal and renal masses, renal vascular disorders, and filling defects of the collecting system.

Magnetic Resonance Imaging

Magnetic resonance imaging (MRI) is a painless, noninvasive procedure that does not use x-rays or radioactive markers. The imager applies a strong magnetic field that causes protons to align themselves with the magnetic field. Pulses of radio waves are emitted that cause the magnetic fields to rotate or resonate. The rotating fields induce electrical signals that the computer analyzes and uses to create images or pictures on a screen. The renal images are available in all planes and show more detail than the images achievable with CT. Newer methods of MRI have been developed to obtain dynamic images using the movement of contrast dye through the kidney. Sequential fast-pulse imaging (functional MRI) allows assessment of obstructions, vascular disorders, and renal insufficiency.

Renal Biopsy

The purpose of a kidney biopsy is to obtain renal tissue that may be studied to determine the nature and extent of renal disease for diagnosis, management, and prognosis. The renal tissue is studied histologically by light and electron microscopy and immunofluorescence. Some indications for a kidney biopsy are persistent proteinuria, hematuria originating from the kidney, unexplained acute renal failure, glomerular disease, renal mass, rejection of a transplanted kidney, and renal involvement in systemic disease.

KEY POINTS

- Urinalysis provides important information about kidney function. Normal urine is clear, pale yellow to amber, and slightly acidic, and it may contain a few cells. Urine osmolality and specific gravity normally vary over the course of the day, depending on fluid intake. Urine is abnormal if it is cloudy or malodorous or contains protein, RBCs, crystals, stones, or casts. A fixed osmolality or specific gravity may indicate renal impairment.
- Serum creatinine and BUN measurements are useful indicators of renal function. Serum creatinine level is a more reliable indicator of renal function than BUN measurement. In conditions of reduced GFR, serum creatinine and BUN levels increase.
- GFR can be estimated by measuring the clearance of a filterable substance from the urine. Creatinine clearance is frequently used for this purpose, but it is not completely accurate because of some tubular processing. Inulin clearance provides a more accurate measurement of GFR. The MDRD is a simple calculated method of estimating GFR using serum creatinine values.
- Diagnostic studies used to evaluate kidney structure and function include plain radiography, pyelography, radionuclide studies, ultrasound, CT, and MRI. Renal biopsy may be performed to obtain tissue for histologic examination.

■ SUMMARY

The kidneys have a vital role in excreting water-soluble waste products and maintaining fluid, electrolyte, and acid-base homeostasis. To perform these functions, the kidneys must have a sufficient GFR. Most waste products are removed by filtration rather than by secretion; thus, a reduced GFR results in accumulation of wastes in the blood. The kidney has a large renal reserve and accomplishes its functions well until more than 75% of the nephron mass is dysfunctional.

The nephron is the structural and functional unit of the kidney. It performs three essential functions: filtration, secretion, and reabsorption. Filtration occurs at the glomerulus at a rate of about 125 ml/min. The composition of filtrate is similar to that of blood except that proteins and blood cells are absent. Normally 99% of the filtrate

is reabsorbed along the nephron tubules, resulting in the elimination of 30 to 60 ml/hr of concentrated urine. Each nephron regulates its own GFR through tubuloglomerular feedback to prevent overloading its reabsorptive capacities.

The kidneys are responsive to a number of endocrine hormones that regulate blood osmolality and volume, including ADH, aldosterone, AII, ANP, urodilatin, uroguanylin, and guanylin. In addition, the kidneys produce two important endocrine hormones: erythropoietin and vitamin D. Urinalysis, serum creatinine and BUN levels, and tests of GFR are important indicators of renal function. Structural abnormalities can be assessed by a variety of imaging techniques.

REFERENCES

1. Hall JE: Urine formation by the kidneys: I. Glomerular filtration, renal blood flow, and their control. In Hall JE, editor: *Guyton and Hall textbook of medical physiology*, ed 12, Philadelphia, 2011, Saunders, pp 303–322.
2. Ramcharan T, Matas AJ: Long-term (20-37 years) follow-up of living kidney donors, *Am J Transplant* 2(10):959–964, 2002.
3. Fehrman-Ekholm I, Kvarnström N, Söfteland JM, Lennerling A, Rizell M, et al: Post-nephrectomy development of renal function in living kidney donors: a cross-sectional retrospective study, *Nephrol Dial Transplant* 26(7):2377–2381, 2011.
4. Jarvis C: *Physical examination and health assessment*, ed 6, Philadelphia, 2012, Saunders.
5. Stanton BA, Koeppen BM: Elements of renal function. In Koeppen BM, Stanton BA, editors: *Berne & Levy physiology*, ed 6, Philadelphia, 2010, Mosby, pp 557–577.
6. Hall JE: Urine formation by the kidneys: II. Tubular reabsorption and secretion. In Hall JE, editor: *Guyton and Hall textbook of medical physiology*, ed 12, Philadelphia, 2011, Saunders, pp 323–343.
7. Hall JE: Urine concentration and dilution: regulation of extracellular fluid osmolarity and sodium concentration. In Hall JE, editor: *Guyton and Hall textbook of medical physiology*, ed 12, Philadelphia, 2011, Saunders, pp 345–360.
8. Stockand JD, Sansom SC: Glomerular mesangial cells: electrophysiology and regulation of contraction, *Physiol Rev* 78:723–744, 1998.
9. Castrop H: Mediators of tubuloglomerular feedback regulation of glomerular filtration: ATP and adenosine, *Acta Physiol (Oxford)* 189(1):3–14, 2007.

10. Schnermann J, Levine DZ: Paracrine factors in tubuloglomerular feedback: adenosine, ATP, and nitric oxide, *Annu Rev Physiol* 65:501–529, 2003.

11. Harris RC: COX-2 and the kidney, *J Cardiovasc Pharmacol* 47(suppl 1):S37–S42, 2006.

12. Hall JE: Acid-base regulation. In Hall JE, editor: *Guyton and Hall textbook of medical physiology*, ed 12, Philadelphia, 2011, Saunders, pp 379–396.

13. Saseen JJ, Maclaughlin EJ: Hypertension. In Dipiro JT, et al, editors: *Pharmacotherapy: a pathophysiologic approach*, ed 8, New York, 2011, McGraw-Hill, pp 101–136.

14. Kabat-Koperska J, Safranow K, Gołembiewska E, et al: Creatinine clearance after cimetidine administration: is it useful in the monitoring of the function of transplanted kidney? *Ren Fail* 29(6):667–672, 2007.

15. Levey AS, Bosch JP, Lewis JB, et al: A more accurate method to estimate glomerular filtration rate from serum creatinine: a new prediction equation. Modification of Diet in Renal Disease Study Group, *Ann Intern Med* 130(6):461–470, 1999.

Intrarenal Disorders

Robin Beeman and Roberta J. Emerson

evolve WEBSITE

http://evolve.elsevier.com/Copstead/
- Review Questions and Answers
- Glossary (with audio pronunciations for selected terms)
- Animations
- Case Studies
- Key Points Review

KEY QUESTIONS

- How are the locations of renal pain, findings on urinalysis, and results of other diagnostic tests used to differentiate the causes of kidney disease?
- How are renal tumors differentiated, detected, and managed?
- How do autosomal dominant and autosomal recessive forms of polycystic kidney disease differ?
- What risk factors and clinical findings are associated with pyelonephritis?
- What physiologic and pathophysiologic disorders predispose to the formation of renal calculi of differing compositions?
- How are the various forms of glomerulonephritis differentiated?
- What laboratory and clinical findings suggest a diagnosis of nephrotic syndrome?

CHAPTER OUTLINE

Functional kidneys are necessary for the removal of waste products from the blood and the maintenance of fluid, electrolyte, and acid-base balance despite wide variations in intake and losses. Systemic disorders that alter the delivery of blood flow to the kidney may adversely affect the kidney's ability to perform its filtering and homeostatic functions. In addition, many disorders occur primarily within the kidney and have the potential to result in chronic kidney disease or end-stage renal disease (ESRD). In general, these disorders can be categorized as (1) congenital, (2) neoplastic, (3) infectious, (4) obstructive, and (5) glomerular.

COMMON MANIFESTATIONS OF KIDNEY DISEASE

Pain

Thorough pain assessment is an essential component of the history and physical examination of any patient. The results can be useful in localizing the etiology of the pain, but assessment is also challenging because pain perceived as coming from the abdomen can originate from many varied organs and tissues within the abdomen or extraabdominally (see Chapter 47). Pain associated with the urinary tract may originate from the lower urinary tract (ureters, bladder, or urethra) or the kidney itself. Renal or kidney pain is also referred to as nephralgia (-*algia* is from the Greek *algos,* meaning pain). Extensive damage to a kidney can occur without nephralgia because most of the kidney lacks pain receptors. However, the renal capsule is innervated by nociceptors, and when a disease process causes it to be distended, inflamed, or punctured, a dull to sharp pain is felt. Distention or inflammation produces a dull, constant pain. This may be the result of intrarenal fluid accumulation such as occurs with inflammation, infected or bleeding cysts, hemorrhage from blunt trauma, or neoplastic expansion. In addition, whenever the renal capsule is penetrated (e.g., during biopsy or trauma), a dull pain or intense pressure may be felt. The renal pelvis and the rest of the urinary tract are innervated by many pain receptors. Obstruction of the intrarenal collecting system causes pain if the obstruction leads to distention of the renal pelvis or capsule. Large calculi, however, can develop insidiously in the renal pelvis or calices and may be painless until they start to move into the ureteral junction. Ischemia caused by the occlusion of renal blood vessels (e.g., from an embolus, atherosclerotic disease, or neoplasm) results in a constant dull or sharp pain.

Pain associated with intrarenal disorders affecting the capsule is classically assessed by palpation or light percussion over the costovertebral angle posteriorly and is recorded as **CVA tenderness** or **flank pain.** Sympathetic nerves transmit information from renal and ureteral nociceptors to the spinal cord between the T10 and L1 levels. Because these sympathetic nerves enter the spinal cord at this level, the pain can be felt throughout the corresponding T10-L1 dermatomes. A **dermatome** is an area of skin innervated by a specific spinal cord segment (Figure 27-1). Visceral and cutaneous afferent fibers enter the spinal cord in close proximity and converge on some of the same neurons at the spinal, thalamic, and cortical levels of the central nervous system. When visceral pain fibers are stimulated, concurrent stimulation of cutaneous fibers occurs and the visceral pain is perceived as though it had originated in the skin. Nerve fibers from the renal plexus communicate with the spermatic plexus, and because of this association, scrotal pain in males and labial pain in females may accompany renal pain.

Abnormal Urinalysis Findings

Urinalysis is an essential laboratory test for all suspected problems of the genitourinary system[1] (see Chapter 26). After history taking and a physical examination, urinalysis generally serves as a starting point for the differential diagnosis. First, urine is examined grossly, encompassing both the solvent and the solutes. The color, odor, and turbidity of the urine offer the first clues. Dark, strong-smelling urine may be an

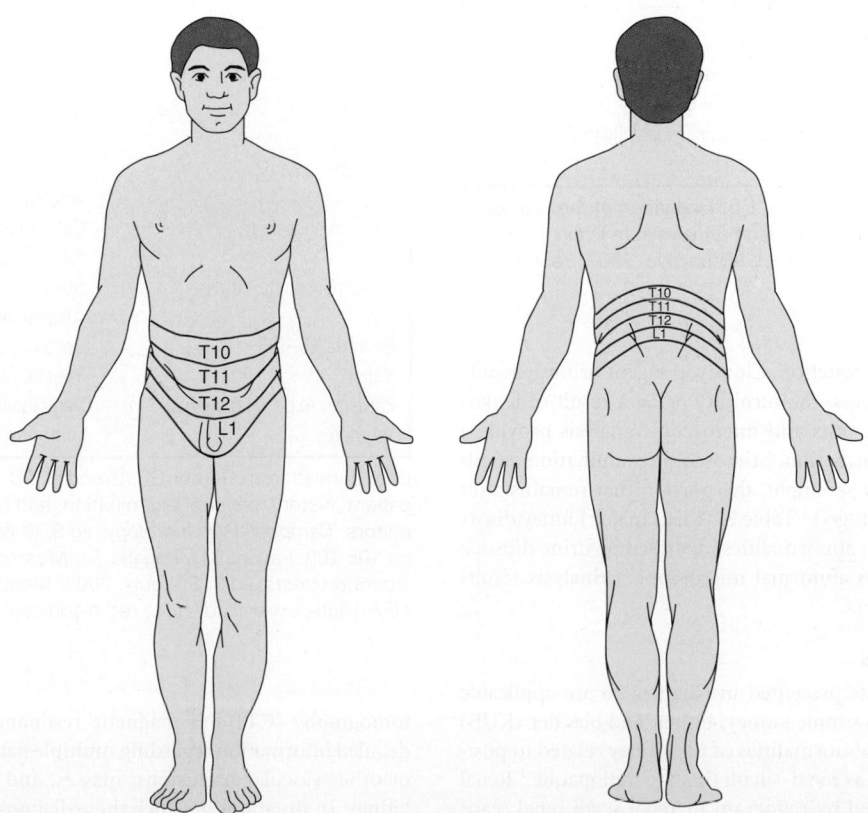

FIGURE 27-1 Dermatomes T10 (thoracic) to L1 (lumbar) correspond to areas that innervate the renal structures.

TABLE 27-1	URINE DIPSTICK FINDINGS ASSOCIATED WITH KIDNEY DISORDERS
URINE DIPSTICK FINDING	**ASSOCIATED KIDNEY DISORDERS**
Specific Gravity	
Decreased	Chronic kidney disease (decreased concentrating ability)
	Diabetes insipidus
Increased	Diabetes mellitus
	Syndrome of inappropriate secretion of antidiuretic hormone
pH	
Increased (6.5-8.0)	>7.5 Urinary tract infection with urea-splitting bacteria (e.g., *Proteus*)
	Renal tubular acidosis
	Calcium or struvite calculi
Decreased (4.5-5.5)	Uric acid or cystine calculi
Hematuria	Renal cell carcinoma
	Tubulointerstitial renal disease
	Urinary tract infection
	Trauma
	Glomerulonephritis
	Obstructive processes (e.g., calculi, neoplasms)
Proteinuria	Diabetic nephropathy
	Renal hypertension
	Glomerulopathies
	Nephrotic syndrome
	Renal arterial or venous obstruction
Glycosuria and Ketones	Diabetes mellitus
	Protein-energy malnutrition
White Blood Cells/ Leukocyte Esterase	Urinary tract infection
Nitrites	Urinary tract infection (especially with gram-negative bacteria)

Data derived from Gerber GS, Brendler CB: Evaluation of the urologic patient: history, physical examination, and urinalysis. In Wein JA et al, editors: *Campbell-Walsh urology*, ed 9, Philadelphia, 2007, Saunders, pp 97-105.

TABLE 27-2	MICROSCOPIC URINALYSIS FINDINGS AND ASSOCIATED KIDNEY DISORDERS
MICROSCOPIC URINALYSIS FINDING	**ASSOCIATED KIDNEY DISORDERS**
Cells	
RBCs (circular shaped)	Urinary tract infection
	Trauma
	Obstructive disorders (e.g., calculi, neoplasm)
RBCs (irregularly shaped)	Glomerulopathies
WBCs (>1-2/HPF)	Infection or inflammation (e.g., urinary tract infection, neoplasm, calculi)
Irregular transitional epithelial cells	Malignancy
Casts	
Hyaline	Usually no pathologic significance
	Chronic kidney disease
	Pyelonephritis
Fatty	Nephrotic syndrome
	Nephrosis
RBC	Glomerulonephritis
WBC	Acute glomerulonephritis
	Acute pyelonephritis
	Acute tubulointerstitial nephritis
Waxy	Chronic kidney disease
	Diabetic nephropathy
	Glomerulonephritis
Crystals	
Cystine	Cystinuria
	Acidic urine
Uric acid	Uric acid calculi
	Acidic urine
Calcium oxalate	Calcium calculi
	Acidic urine
Calcium phosphate	Calcium calculi
	Alkaline urine
Triple phosphate/struvite	Struvite calculi
	Alkaline urine
Bacteria ≥5/HPF	Bacterial urinary tract infection
Yeast	Yeast urinary tract infection
Parasites (e.g., *Trichomonas vaginalis*)	Vaginitis in women
	Urethritis in men

Data derived from Gerber GS, Brendler CB: Evaluation of the urologic patient: history, physical examination, and urinalysis. In Wein JA et al, editors: *Campbell-Walsh urology*, ed 9, Philadelphia, 2007, Saunders, pp 105-109; Pagana KD, Pagana TJ: *Mosby's manual of diagnostic and laboratory tests*, ed 3, St Louis, 2006, Mosby, pp 1007-1014. *HPF*, High-power field; *RBC*, red blood cell; *WBC*, white blood cell.

indicator of decreased renal function. Cloudy, pungent urine generally indicates an infectious process, the turbidity being a result of leukocytes in the urine. Dipstick tests and microscopic analysis provide a great deal of additional information. Microscopic examination entails the assessment of the urine sediment, the portion that remains after the urine specimen is centrifuged.[1] Table 27-1 lists major kidney disorders that are associated with abnormalities identified by urine dipstick testing. Table 27-2 provides abnormal microscopic urinalysis results indicative of kidney disorders.

Other Diagnostic Tests

Many of the diagnostic tests presented in Chapter 26 are applicable to intrarenal disorders. The simple kidney, ureter, and bladder (KUB) radiograph identifies gross abnormalities of the kidney related to position, size, and shape as well as renal calculi that are radiopaque.[1] Renal vasculature can be examined by renogram or renal scan; renal scans will also identify neoplasms in the kidney. Ultrasonography differentiates the solid mass of a neoplasm from fluid-filled cysts. Computerized tomography (CT) and magnetic resonance imaging (MRI) provide detailed information regarding multiple pathologies including thrombi or other vascular occlusions, masses, and obstructions involving the kidney. In situations in which these diagnostic tests are insufficient and actual tissue examination is necessary (e.g., neoplasm assessment), a renal biopsy may be required.[1]

CONGENITAL ABNORMALITIES

A wide variety of anomalies in the development of the kidneys have been documented in the literature. One or both kidneys may be involved. In some cases, findings are associated with other abnormalities, whereas in others the renal abnormalities are isolated. Congenital kidney abnormalities may be exceptionally rare or may occur with considerable frequency. They may be identified prenatally during ultrasound assessment of the developing fetus, noted at birth, or manifest only in later life. Discussion here will focus on the more common congenital anomalies because a complete discussion of all these pathologies is beyond the scope of this text.

Renal Agenesis and Hypoplasia

Renal agenesis means a failure of one or both kidneys to embryonically develop at all.[2,3] On the other hand, **renal hypoplasia** describes a condition in which some fetal development of the kidneys has occurred. They both can be found as a single entity or in combination with other congenital malformations.

Bilateral renal agenesis (BRA) results from failure of the metanephros (renal buds) to develop in the fetus.[2] It is incompatible with extrauterine life and results in stillbirth or death shortly thereafter.[2,4] It is usually found in Potter syndrome, where severely inadequate quantities of amniotic fluid result in compression of the fetus within the uterus.[2] This pathology is characterized by a collection of associated anomalies that includes wide-spaced eyes with epicanthal folds, low-set ears with insufficient cartilage, a beaked nose, and a receding chin.[4]

Unilateral renal agenesis (URA) is more common than bilateral renal agenesis.[3] URA is often associated with concurrent urologic or nonurologic congenital anomalies. Nonurologic anomalies are usually cardiac or gastrointestinal in nature. Sometimes renal agenesis has been found to be familial and inherited as a dominant trait; screening by ultrasound of parents and siblings has been recommended when infants with agenesis or dysgenesis are involved. Poorly controlled diabetes and exposure to certain drugs (e.g., those affecting angiotensin II) and chemicals have been implicated as teratogens. In URA, the remaining kidney usually enlarges as a compensatory mechanism. Lifelong monitoring of renal function is recommended.[3]

Congenital renal hypoplasia is estimated to cause 40% to 60% of the pediatric cases of ESRD. Gene mutation is likely responsible for the incomplete development of the kidney. Hypoplasia may be insufficient for extrauterine life if both kidneys are involved or may not impact renal functioning until later in life.[2,4] When renal hypoplasia has been identified, lifelong monitoring is recommended.[2]

Cystic Kidney Diseases

Cystic disease of the kidneys incorporates a wide range of hereditary, developmental, and acquired conditions.[5-10] Depending on the classification, these fluid-filled craters may be present at birth or only visible later in life. They may involve one or both kidneys and be accompanied by other anomalies, or they may be the only pathology present.[8] More commonly found in men, and increasing in prevalence with aging, renal cysts have been reportedly identified in more than half of patients over the age of 50.[6] Cysts may be found in other organs, or limited to the kidneys, depending on the disorder. Within the kidney, cysts may be diffuse or confined to one anatomic area.[8] Renal cysts of significant size produce flank pain and hemorrhage.[6]

The two most common forms of cystic kidney disease are the autosomal recessive and autosomal dominant polycystic diseases.[5,8,9] Autosomal recessive polycystic kidney disease (ARPKD) is usually diagnosed in infants and young children, whereas autosomal dominant polycystic kidney disease (ADPKD) is generally diagnosed in adulthood.[8,9] Although the pathogenesis is similar, the ARPKD and ADPKD forms of the disease are genetically different, and their clinical courses are usually distinct (Table 27-3).

Autosomal Recessive Polycystic Kidney Disease

ARPKD is often identified in the neonatal period, and when accompanied by pulmonary hypoplasia, it may result in death.[9] In ARPKD, the kidneys retain their shape but are uniformly enlarged, and collecting ducts are dilated from the medulla to the cortex. Abnormal portal ducts are found in neonates, and portal fibrosis is noted in older patients.[9] The most common clinical signs in the neonatal period are respiratory distress or palpable kidneys on physical examination. Systemic hypertension is frequently most severe in infancy.[9] Those who live to reach adulthood typically retain some renal function, but experience a progressive decline in liver function.[9] There has been no documented evidence of ARPKD being linked with renal neoplasia.[11] A recessive pattern of inheritance within the family and pathology on liver biopsy are the best diagnostic data because both the clinical presentation and the results of ultrasounds, CT, or MRI can be similar to those of the autosomal dominant form of polycystic kidney disease.[10]

FEATURE	AUTOSOMAL RECESSIVE	AUTOSOMAL DOMINANT
TABLE 27-3 COMPARISON OF AUTOSOMAL RECESSIVE AND AUTOSOMAL DOMINANT POLYCYSTIC KIDNEY DISEASE		
Gene defect	Chromosome 6p	Gene *PKD1* on chromosome 16, or gene *PKD2* on chromosome 4, or gene *PDK3* location unknown
Incidence	1:20,000	1-2:1000
Age at diagnosis	Usually neonate to childhood	Usually fourth to fifth decade
Imaging findings	Symmetrically enlarged kidneys	Enlarged kidneys, often asymmetric
Histologic findings	Cysts derived from epithelial cells of collecting ducts	Entire nephron involved
Liver involvement	Abnormal portal ducts progressing to fibrosis	Multiple cysts
Other systemic findings	Usually none	Cysts in other abdominal organs, aneurysms, abnormal cardiac valves, hernias, and diverticuli

Autosomal Dominant Polycystic Kidney Disease

ADPKD is the most common of all the hereditary cystic kidney diseases.[5,7,10] Typically, both kidneys are involved, but in 17% of the cases, kidney disease is unilateral and these are most likely to be the pediatric cases. The other kidney is often affected by the time the child reaches adulthood.[5] For 5% of the end-stage kidney disease patients receiving hemodialysis in the United States, the etiology of their disease is ADPKD.[10] The disease affects both genders and has no racial preference.[7,11] Although prenatal and neonatal cases have been reported and ADPKD can present at any age, it usually manifests in patients who are 40 to 59 years old.[10,11] In less than 1% of cases, ADPKD is identified in the neonate or in utero.[7] ADPKD is marked by a great deal of variability in the rate of decline in renal function.[9,11] The disease process appears to advance more rapidly in men than in women.[7] The incidence of renal cell carcinoma is no greater in ADPKD than in the general population, but it does occur at an earlier age.[7]

There are two genetically distinct but phenotypically similar forms of ADPKD: *PKD1* and *PKD2*. Distribution of these genotypes is such that 85% of the cases are associated with *PDK1* and just less than 15% with *PDK2*.[5,7,11] Mutations of these genes add further complexity to ADPKD.[7] Approximately 10% of the cases of ADPKD are not familial in origin and appear sporadically.[5] Because of significant variability in clinical presentation within families, environmental modifying factors have been suggested, though not yet documented.[7] It does seem that the specific gene is responsible for the initiation of cystic development, but not necessarily for cyst expansion.[7]

While the cysts multiply and expand, the overall size of the kidneys increases and there is a progressive decline in glomerular filtration rate (GFR) as the amount of normally functioning tissue is slowly reduced.[7] Figure 27-2 provides a comparison of normal and polycystic kidneys. Renal perfusion decreases, and significant remodeling occurs in the renal circulation.[7] Expansion of the cysts compacts and distorts the vascular system, and the resulting local ischemia activates the intrarenal renin-angiotensin system. The progressive reduction in renal function appears to be primarily associated with an increase in the size of the kidney and the overall volume of the cysts.[7]

In contrast to its recessive form, ADPKD is associated with pathologies in other body systems.[5,9,11] The most common extrarenal presentation is in the liver. Additional extrarenal sites include the spleen, pancreas, lung, seminal vesicles, circle of Willis, skin, and heart.[5,7,11]

Involvement of these other organs and tissues results in additional clinical manifestations, each requiring attention by health care providers.[7] In the early phases of the disease, the ability to concentrate urine is decreased.[7] Hypertension is often diagnosed late in the disease process and increases the likelihood of escalated loss of renal function, proteinuria, and hematuria.[7] In 60% of adult patients with ADPKD, pain is the most frequent complaint.[7] Pain may be due to bleeding within the kidney, movement of kidney stones, or the development of urinary tract infections. Kidney stones develop in 20% of the cases and are usually uric acid–based or calcium oxalate–based. Urinary tract infections are most often attributable to *Enterobacter* organisms. Infection of the cysts themselves may also develop; these infections are more difficult to treat, and patients with this condition may require months of antimicrobial therapy. When it occurs, hemorrhage of cysts is usually self-limited.[7]

Diagnosis is based on genetic history and imaging techniques, most often ultrasonography.[7,9,11] When there is no family history of ADPKD, a presumption of the disease is made if imaging either identifies cysts and bilaterally enlarged kidneys or shows cysts in the liver and both kidneys. Genetic testing is then performed to substantiate the diagnosis.[7,10]

Treatment of ADPKD is primarily supportive, emphasizing the control of blood pressure and the management of any associated pathologic conditions.[7] Once ESRD is reached, dialysis or kidney transplantation is required.[7]

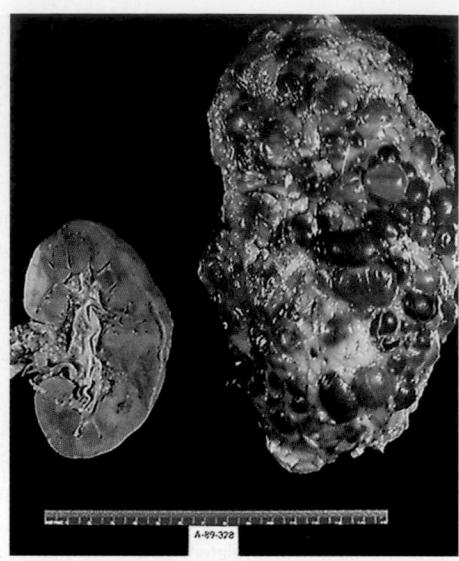

FIGURE 27-2 Comparison of normal and polycystic kidneys. (From Brundage DJ: *Renal disorders*, St Louis, 1992, Mosby.)

KEY POINTS

- Renal agenesis is relatively rare, and its presence is often associated with other congenital malformations. Bilateral renal agenesis is not compatible with life. Unilateral renal agenesis results in compensatory hypertrophy of the functional kidney. A single normal kidney is sufficient to maintain normal renal function.
- Polycystic kidney diseases are genetically transmitted kidney disorders. Autosomal recessive forms are evident at birth. In the autosomal dominant type, symptoms generally occur later in life. Expanding cysts disrupt urine formation and flow. The inevitability of renal failure necessitates dialysis or transplantation.

NEOPLASMS

Neoplasms found in the kidney may be benign or malignant primary tumors, or result from metastases from extrarenal sites. Because the kidney is encased in a tough, fibrous capsule, growing renal neoplasms will distort the architecture of the kidney and ultimately hinder kidney function. Malignant renal neoplasms also carry the threat of metastasis to distant sites.

Benign Renal Neoplasms

Several benign neoplasms may be found in the kidney, developing from the renal cortex, medulla, or capsule, but they are less common than malignant neoplasms.[6] Contrary to most benign neoplasms, those in the kidney are not truly encapsulated.[6] Table 27-4 summarizes the etiology and pathogenesis of some of these benign neoplasms.

Diagnosis and treatment. Renal neoplasms are typically detected incidentally during abdominal imaging for other reasons.[35] The neoplasm may attain sufficient size to be detected with abdominal palpation, produce flank pain, and cause hematuria. Generally, benign renal neoplasms are treated by removal of the kidney (**nephrectomy**) because they are space-occupying lesions and because of their propensity to undergo malignant changes.[6] More recently, laparoscopic and tissue-sparing approaches have been developed, allowing the retention of more functioning renal tissue.[14]

Renal Cell Carcinoma

The vast majority of renal cancer is due to renal cell carcinoma (RCC) (85% to 90%).[13,15,18] The remaining 10% to 15% of cases are primarily

TABLE 27-4	SUMMARY OF BENIGN RENAL NEOPLASMS
BENIGN NEOPLASM	**ETIOLOGY AND PATHOGENESIS**
Renal cortical adenomas	Small, solid growths that develop from cortical tissue; incidences of less than 1% up to 23%; typically <1 cm; patient is asymptomatic
Metanephric adenoma	Histologically related to Wilms tumor
Oncocytoma	Most difficult to differentiate from renal cell carcinoma; light brown to tan in color with well-defined borders
Angiomyolipoma	Composed of adipose, smooth muscle tissue, and blood vessels; believed to be hormone dependent because it is primarily found in postpubescent women
Nephroma	Cystic neoplasm not reliably differentiated from renal cell carcinoma in adults or nephroblastoma in children
Mixed epithelial stromal neoplasm	Most often found in perimenopausal women, most of whom are taking estrogen replacement therapy
Leiomyomas	Evolve from renal capsule, pelvis, or renal vein
Hemangiomas, fibromas, lipomas, lymphangiomas, and reninomas	Rare benign neoplasms

From Campbell SC, Novick AC, Bukowski RM: Neoplasms of the upper urinary tract. In Wein JA et al, editors: *Campbell-Walsh urology,* ed 9, Philadelphia, 2007, Saunders, pp 1575-1582.

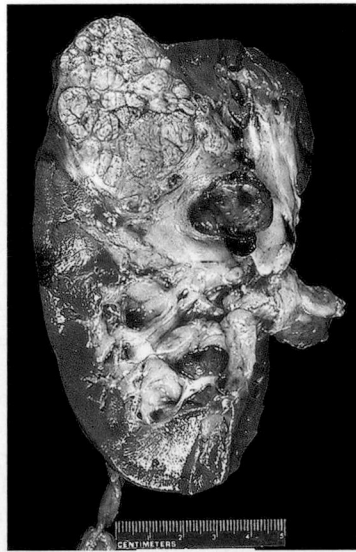

FIGURE 27-3 Cross-sectional view of renal cell carcinoma. (From Kumar V et al: *Robbins and Cotran pathologic basis of disease,* ed 8, Philadelphia, 2010, Saunders, p 965.)

transitional cell cancers of the pelvis. Figure 27-3 illustrates a cross-sectional view of RCC. In the United States in 2011, the number of new cases of renal cell and renal pelvis cancers combined was estimated to be 60,920, with 13,120 fatalities.[17] Approximately 57,760 new cases of RCC were diagnosed in 2009,[16] with about 14,000 deaths.[15] This represents only 2% of all adult malignancies.[15] Since the early 1970s, the incidence has progressively risen in the United States and most of Europe,[13,15] occurring two to three times

BOX 27-1	RISK FACTORS FOR RENAL CELL CARCINOMA

- Cigarette smoking
- Obesity
- Hypertension
- Diabetes mellitus
- Asbestos exposure
- Multiparous women
- Long-term renal dialysis
- Kidney transplantation

more frequently in men than in women.[6,13,15] Incident rates among African Americans are 20% higher[6] and continue to increase more rapidly than the incidence in Caucasians.[18] Rates among Hispanics are also rising.[18] Taken as a whole, these trends are gradually altering the overall distribution of the disease. Age at diagnosis averages the early sixties.[13,15]

Etiology and pathogenesis. Although only a small portion of the cases of RCC are attributed to genetic factors, the risk of its development is greater than twofold when there is a first-degree relative with the disease. These hereditary kidney cancers have been the source of most of the knowledge regarding RCC. Several specific genes have been identified in these cases and are associated with specific subtypes.[13,15,16,19]

The identification of risk factors has been derived from pooled data from a large number of studies worldwide[18] and these are listed in Box 27-1. The primary risk factors are obesity, cigarette smoking, and hypertension with risk reduction documented with weight loss, smoking cessation, and decreased blood pressure. Evidence linking trichloroethylene to renal cell cancer risk is accumulating.[18] Low fruit/vegetable intake has not been adequately substantiated.[18]

Renal cell carcinoma encompasses several subtypes, histologically differentiated from one another. This variability in histology complicates diagnosis. The World Health Organization (WHO) has established a system of terminology and differentiation of these subtypes.[15] The most common of these (approximately 85%) is **clear cell RCC.**[12,13] These tumors originate in the renal cortex from cells of the proximal tubule and are usually unilateral and random in occurrence with rare cases of familial patterns of inheritance.[12] Clear cell RCC is most frequently associated with metastatic disease.[15] Next in frequency is **papillary RCC,** representing 10% to 15% of all renal cell carcinomas.[12,16] Papillary RCC evolves from cells of the distal tubule. This type of RCC may also be sporadic or hereditary, and two subtypes of familial papillary RCC have been identified.[12,16] When compared to clear cell RCC, papillary RCC is less likely to metastasize and therefore has a better prognosis; however, if it does metastasize, the prognosis is poorer than that of clear cell RCC.[12] **Chromophobe RCC** represents 4% to 6% of all RCC cases.[12,16] This subtype originates from the renal parenchyma.[12] Because of slow growth and infrequent metastasis, 5-year survival rates exceed 90%.[12] Cell membranes are prominent. Finally, **medullary** and **collecting duct carcinomas** are the least common, representing less than 1% of all RCC cases.[12] Unfortunately, they occur in younger patients, develop rapidly, and carry only a 30% 5-year survival rate.[12] Medullary RCC has been found to be associated with the sickle cell trait.

Clinical manifestations. RCC is often asymptomatic until it is quite advanced. When it does present with signs and symptoms, the most common are CVA tenderness, hematuria, and a palpable abdominal mass. Dyspnea, cough, and bone pain develop secondary to metastasis.

Diagnosis and treatment. Renal ultrasound and CT of the abdomen may be of value. If cysts accompany RCC, renal ultrasound is 98% accurate in discerning them. Figure 27-4 illustrates the staging system used with RCC. When RCC is localized, it can be surgically removed in a nephrectomy, and this is the standard of treatment.[12,13] Unfortunately, metastasis occurs in more than one third of cases,[12,14] and metastatic RCC has been found to be unresponsive to cytotoxic

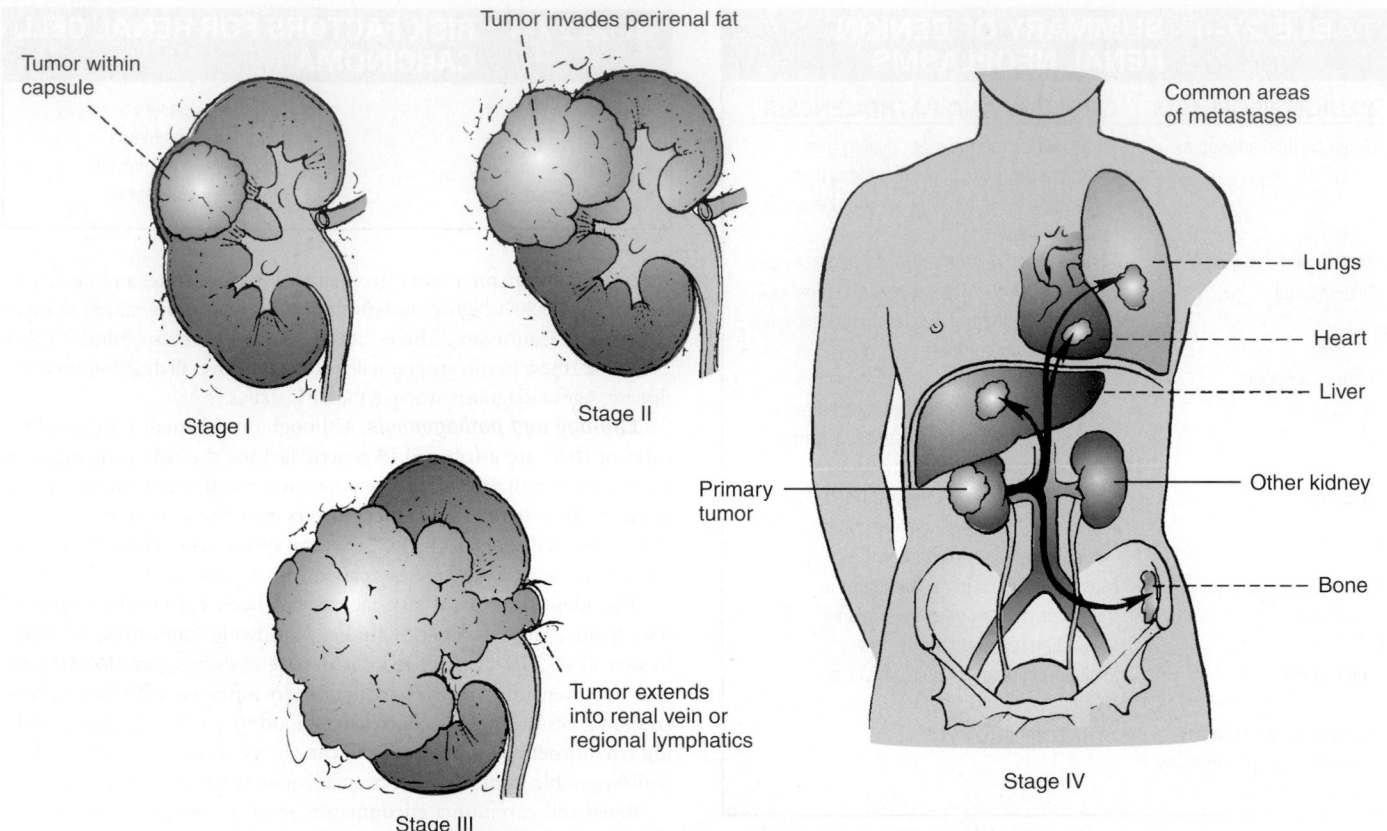

FIGURE 27-4 Staging system for renal cell carcinoma. (From Black JM, Matassarin-Jacobs E: *Medical-surgical nursing: clinical management for continuity of care,* ed 8, Philadelphia, 2009, Saunders, p 923.)

chemotherapy.[14,16] The standard nephrectomy is a major surgery, necessitating a large lateral incision. Other less radical approaches include nephron-sparing interventions and laparoscopic nephrectomy. In metastatic disease, spontaneous regression of metastases following nephrectomy occurs in less than 1% of cases. Conventional chemotherapeutic interventions have been found to elicit a poor response in advanced RCC. Interferon-α and interleukin-2 (IL-2) are cytokines used as tissue-specific therapies in these situations with clear cell RCC, with 6% to 27% response rates.[13,14] More targeted therapies, specifically angiogenic inhibitors and tyrosine kinase inhibitors, have been studied in clinical trials or are now available for selected patient situations.[13,14,20]

Nephroblastoma (Wilms Tumor)

Nephroblastoma is the fifth most frequently occurring pediatric malignancy and the most common childhood kidney cancer, affecting 8 out of 1 million children in the United States less than 15 years old.[23] Seventy-five percent of the cases occur in children less than 5 years old, with a peak incidence at 2 to 3 years of age.[23] Wilms tumor is very rarely found in children older than 15 years of age.[22] Incidence is equally distributed between genders,[21] it is primarily unilateral and sporadic, and only 1% to 2% of patients diagnosed with Wilms tumor have a relative who has been diagnosed with the disease.[22] In 5% to 10% of cases, the tumor presents bilaterally or multifocally.[21,22] Bilateral presentation is often associated with cysts in combination with the tumor.

Etiology and pathogenesis. Nephroblastomas develop from embryonic pluripotent kidney precursor cells.[21] Precursor lesions called *nephrogenic rests,* persistent clusters of embryonic cells, are notable histologic findings.[22] The first gene found to be associated with Wilms tumor was *WT1,* located on the short arm of chromosome 11.[21]

Nephroblastomas are typically large, well-encapsulated tumors that grow rapidly. They undergo hemorrhage and cystic changes; necrosis

that occurs because of hemorrhaging is responsible for the development of cysts. As the malignant cells proliferate, the normal architecture of the kidney is altered. The renal pelvis becomes compressed, and locally the tumor infiltrates into the renal veins and hilar nodes. Metastasis is typically via the bloodstream to the brain, liver, adrenal glands, and bone.

Clinical manifestations. A palpable abdominal mass is evident in about 80% of cases. Abdominal pain, hypertension, and hematuria are also common local manifestations. Nephroblastoma may produce a tumor thrombus in the inferior vena cava, which can lead to decreased venous return and lower extremity edema. Additional signs or symptoms may be noted reflective of the sites of metastasis.

Diagnosis and treatment. Most often the tumor is identified by the parents or during a routine physical examination. Renal ultrasound and/or CT scan will usually identify anatomic abnormalities associated with the tumor. Over the past 20 years, treatment protocols have improved to the point that this previously lethal disease now has a cure rate of more than 90%.[23] Key to treatment is the removal of the involved kidney (nephrectomy). Radiation and chemotherapy are routine following surgery. Radiation therapy may also be administered preoperatively to shrink tumors and reduce their vascularity.

KEY POINTS
- A number of benign and malignant primary neoplasms may develop in the kidney. Symptoms depend on the size of the neoplasm and the presence of metastasis. Neoplasms may be asymptomatic until quite large. At that time, a palpable abdominal mass, hematuria, and flank pain may be noted.

- Neoplasms are usually detected with renal ultrasound and/or CT scan. Nephrectomy remains the initial treatment of choice for both benign and malignant renal neoplasms. Nephron-sparing approaches are increasingly utilized.
- RCC is particularly resistant to radiation, immunotherapy, and chemotherapy. This resistance combined with the typical advanced stage at diagnosis makes the prognosis for late-stage disease and recurrent cancer quite poor. Recent advances based upon gene pathways hold future promise.
- Nephroblastoma, or Wilms tumor, is the most common kidney cancer in children. Nephrectomy, radiation therapy, and chemotherapy are used in the management of nephroblastomas. Cure rates are excellent.

INFECTION

Normally, a number of host defense mechanisms serve to protect the renal system from infection. Chemically, the acidic pH and the presence of urea in the urine produce a relatively hostile environment for bacterial growth. Bacteriostatic prostatic secretions in men also act as a protective mechanism against bacterial invasion. In women, glands in the distal urethra secrete mucus that captures bacteria, preventing progression to the bladder. Small numbers of bacteria that may enter the system are washed out by micturition. Normal unidirectional flow prevents **reflux** of urine from the bladder to the kidney via the ureter by contraction of the vesicoureteral junction that occurs with bladder filling. In children, urinary tract infections may be associated with vesicoureteral reflux or other anatomic malformations of the urinary tract[24] (see discussion of vesicoureteral reflux in Chapter 29). Epithelial cells of the urinary tract provide a physical barrier to infectious organisms, and indigenous proteins trap bacteria or block their adhesion to epithelial cells.[26] The inflammatory response to bacterial attachment encourages their destruction and removal. As is so often the case with the inflammatory response, it is the secondary injury associated with this response that is ultimately responsible for subsequent damage to urinary structures.[40]

Infection of the kidney is known as **pyelonephritis** or upper urinary tract infection and affects the renal parenchyma, pelvis, and calices. Although infectious organisms responsible for upper urinary tract infections may be delivered to the kidney via the bloodstream or lymphatic system, they most commonly reach the kidneys as an ascending infection from the lower urinary tract (urethra, bladder, and ureters)[26] (Figure 27-5). Infection of the lower urinary tract is discussed in Chapter 29.

The most common causative agents of renal system infection are serogroups of *Escherichia coli*, whereas *Enterobacter, Enterococcus, Proteus mirabilis,* and strains of *Klebsiella* are responsible for most of the other infections.[25,28,29] Most often, infections with these other organisms are linked to calculi or to anatomic abnormalities of the urinary tract. In certain populations, *Staphylococcus saprophyticus* and group B *Streptococcus* have been identified. Fungal infections, mycoplasmas, and other anaerobic bacteria are occasionally responsible. Infections attributable to *Neisseria gonorrhoeae* or *Chlamydia trachomatis* are associated with sexually transmitted diseases and are typically limited to the urethra.[25] Uropathogenic bacteria possess a substance that allows the bacteria to bind to epithelial cells of the urinary tract.[25-27] Some bacteria secrete proteins that aid in protection from phagocytosis by cells of the immune system.[25] At the same time, the bacteria responsible for urinary tract infections undergo continuous mutation in an effort to overcome both host defenses and antimicrobials used in their treatment.[28]

Risk factors for urinary tract infections are listed in Box 27-2. One of the most significant preventive interventions is the early removal of urinary catheters. Anatomically, women are at increased risk because of their shortened urethras, but the resulting infections are most often confined to the lower urinary tract.[25] In 2005, 1.8 million patients in emergency departments were diagnosed with urinary tract infections.[28]

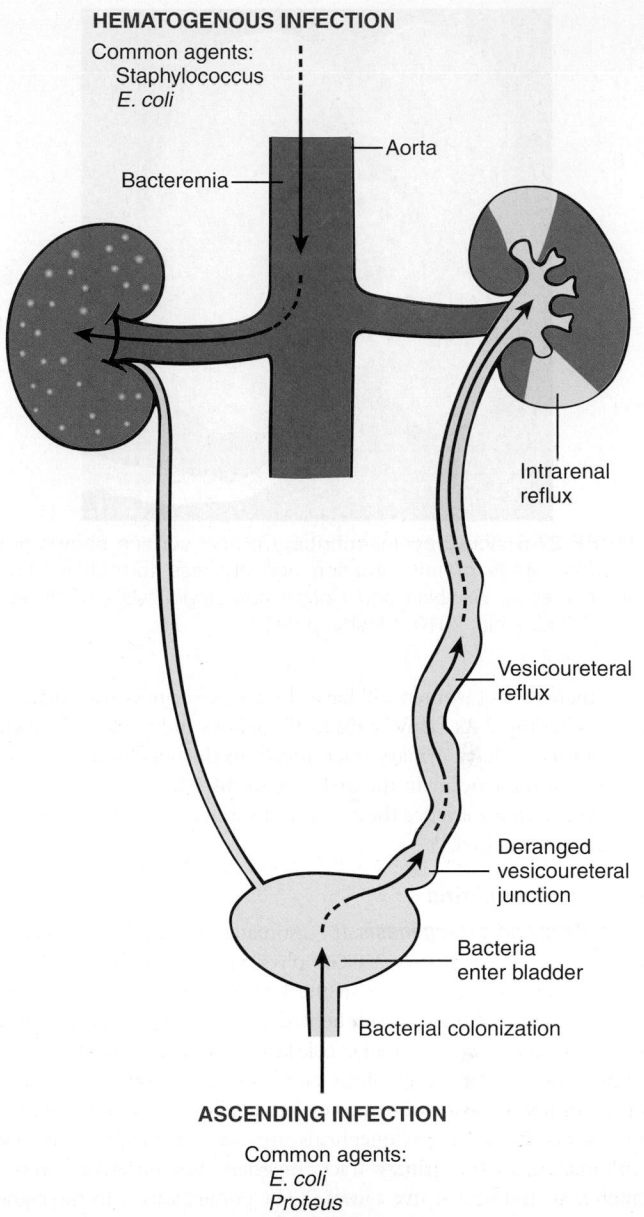

FIGURE 27-5 Pathways of renal infection. (From Kumar V et al: *Robbins and Cotran pathologic basis of disease,* ed 8, Philadelphia, 2010, Saunders, p 940.)

BOX 27-2 RISK FACTORS FOR URINARY TRACT INFECTIONS

- Increasing age
- Vesicoureteral reflux
- Congenital anatomic anomalies of the urinary tract
- Female gender
- Pregnancy
- Diaphragms with spermicidal agents for contraception
- Neurogenic bladder
- Instrumentation of the urinary tract (catheterization, cystoscopy)
- Urinary obstruction (calculi, benign prostatic hyperplasia)
- Glucocorticoids, radiation, or cytotoxic chemotherapy
- Immunodeficiency conditions such as AIDS
- Diabetes mellitus
- Obesity
- Sickle cell trait

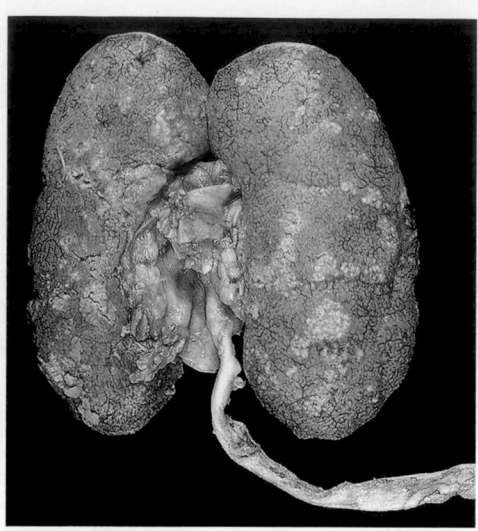

FIGURE 27-6 Acute pyelonephritis. Cortical surface shows grayish white areas of inflammation and abscess formation. (From Kumar V et al: *Robbins and Cotran pathologic basis of disease,* ed 8, Philadelphia, 2010, Mosby, p 941.)

More than 50% of women will have at least one urinary tract infection in their lifetime.[28] As many as 2% to 3% of boys and 8% to 11% of girls are reported to have urinary tract infections during childhood.[32] The majority of these occur in the first 12 months. Male children who are uncircumcised experience these infections more frequently than those who are circumcised.[24]

Acute Pyelonephritis

Etiology and pathogenesis. It is estimated that acute pyelonephritis accounts for approximately 250,000 physician office visits and 200,000 hospital admissions each year in the United States.[29] Recent research results suggest that there is an inherited susceptibility to acute pyelonephritis.[30] Pregnancy is the major risk factor for acute pyelonephritis in women because of the physiologic alterations that occur in the urinary tract.[25] In nonpregnant women, men, and children, the most common risk factors for acute pyelonephritis are diabetes mellitus, anatomic abnormalities of the urinary tract (especially vesicoureteral reflux in children[24]), and obstructive causes.[25] The populations with the highest incidence were young women, infants, and the elderly. *E. coli* is the causative organism in 80% of acute pyelonephritis cases involving women and 70% of those involving men.[31] Pyelonephritis is usually unilateral, involving the right kidney (>50%); 25% of the cases involve the left kidney, and pyelonephritis is bilateral 25% of the time.[24,25] Acute infection of the kidney usually originates as an ascending infection but may arrive at the kidney via the bloodstream. Once in the kidney, bacteria bind to epithelial cell receptors, initiating an inflammatory response. Inflammatory mediators and bacterial toxins are responsible for the parenchymal damage to the kidney.

Clinical manifestations. The onset of acute pyelonephritis is sudden; patients are acutely ill and present with fever, chills, and CVA tenderness, as well as symptoms of lower urinary tract infection (dysuria, urgency, and frequency).[25] Nausea, vomiting, and anorexia are frequent accompaniments, increasing the fever-induced dehydration.[25,28]

Complications of acute pyelonephritis include abscesses, septic shock, acute respiratory distress syndrome, recurrent/chronic pyelonephritis, and chronic kidney disease attributable to scarring produced by recurrent infections.[25,28] Renal scarring and the subsequent development of chronic kidney disease are more likely when there are preexisting anatomic or functional urinary tract abnormalities.[32] Chronic

kidney disease has been found to progress more rapidly following acute pyelonephritis. Preexisting chronic kidney disease can also increase the severity of an infection. Overall, however, the risk of decreased renal function subsequent to acute pyelonephritis is low, occurring in only 3% to 4% of cases. The term **urosepsis** describes organisms in the bloodstream originating from a urinary tract infection. Urinary tract infections are the cause of 20% to 30% of all septic patients.[33] Figure 27-6 illustrates acute pyelonephritis complicated by abscess formation.

Diagnosis and treatment. In addition to the clinical manifestations, diagnosis of acute pyelonephritis is confirmed by urinalysis results illustrating the presence of significant amounts of bacteria.[25] Elevated levels of white and red blood cells and leukocyte esterase are also noted. The urinalysis dipstick may be positive for nitrites, especially if gram-negative organisms are involved. White blood cell casts are common findings.[25] Barring complications, patients are treated with empirical antimicrobial therapy on an outpatient basis for 7 to 10 days.[25,28,29] If improvement is not noted within 48 to 72 hours or the patient's condition deteriorates, urine is cultured to allow targeted therapy and the patient may be further assessed for such problems as urinary obstruction or an extraurinary focus of infection. In cases of complicated acute pyelonephritis, such as septicemia, patients are hospitalized and treated with intravenous antimicrobials and fluids.[25,28,29]

Chronic Pyelonephritis

Chronic pyelonephritis is characterized by small atrophied kidneys with diffuse scarring and blunting of the calices secondary to persistent or recurrent infection of the kidney.

Etiology and pathogenesis. Reflux of infected urine into the renal pelvis is the typical cause of chronic pyelonephritis. The kidneys are usually smaller than normal with caliceal deformity, chronic inflammation, and parenchymal scarring.[34,35] Chronic pyelonephritis causes about 2% to 3% of the cases of end-stage renal disease.[35] Individuals at risk for developing chronic pyelonephritis have bacteriuria associated with obstructive disorders such as renal calculi, neurogenic bladder, vesicoureteral reflux, or underlying intrarenal disease. Chronic or recurrent pyelonephritis is one potential cause of chronic kidney disease (see Chapter 28).

Clinical manifestations. The symptoms of chronic pyelonephritis may be vague, inconsistent, or similar to those of acute pyelonephritis.[35] Patients may have flank or abdominal pain, fever, malaise or anorexia.[35] It is often diagnosed incidentally during the diagnostic evaluation.[35]

Diagnosis and treatment. Urinalysis results typically parallel the findings of acute pyelonephritis, but may not be as profound. Diagnostic testing includes renal ultrasound and other imaging tests that show one or both kidneys to be smaller than normal with distorted architecture and significant scarring. Renal tubules may be dilated or atrophied. Other diagnostic tests may be performed to determine underlying pathologies such as vesicoureteral reflux or obstruction caused by renal calculi. Treatment is based on the correction of these underlying causes, administration of antimicrobial therapy that may continue for several months, and support of compromised renal function, if it exists.

KEY POINTS

- Pyelonephritis is an infection of the renal pelvis and parenchyma that is usually due to an ascending urinary tract infection. Costovertebral angle tenderness is the classic symptom. It is frequently accompanied by fever, chills, nausea, vomiting, and anorexia. Urinalysis generally shows evidence of an infective process. The presence of WBC casts is specifically indicative of an upper urinary tract infection as opposed to a lower urinary tract infection. When managed promptly and effectively, acute pyelonephritis does not generally result in decreased renal function.

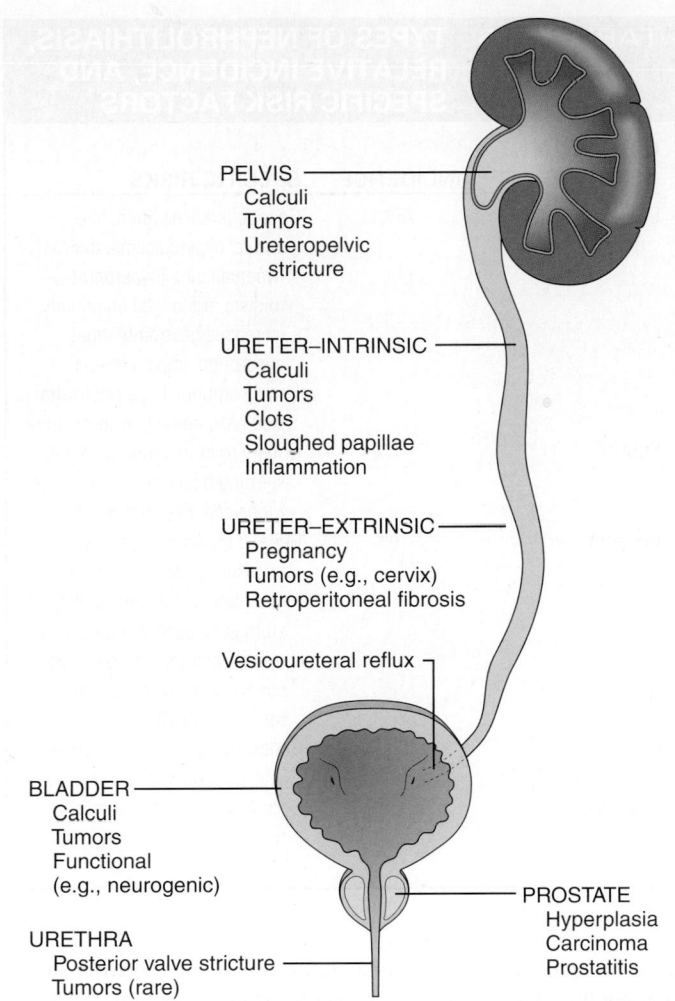

PELVIS
Calculi
Tumors
Ureteropelvic
 stricture

URETER–INTRINSIC
Calculi
Tumors
Clots
Sloughed papillae
Inflammation

URETER–EXTRINSIC
Pregnancy
Tumors (e.g., cervix)
Retroperitoneal fibrosis

Vesicoureteral reflux

BLADDER
Calculi
Tumors
Functional
 (e.g., neurogenic)

URETHRA
Posterior valve stricture
Tumors (rare)

PROSTATE
Hyperplasia
Carcinoma
Prostatitis

FIGURE 27-7 Obstructions of the urinary tract. (From Cotran RS et al: *Robbins pathologic basis of disease*, ed 6, Philadelphia, 1999, Saunders, p 988.)

- Chronic pyelonephritis can potentially result in chronic kidney disease. It is usually associated with vesicoureteral reflux or obstructive processes leading to persistent urine stasis. Ongoing inflammation causes fibrosis and scarring and loss of functional nephrons. The diagnosis is confirmed by renal imaging. Urinalysis results mirror those of acute pyelonephritis, but may not be as significant. Treatment includes correction of the underlying processes and often extended antimicrobial therapy.

OBSTRUCTION

Obstructive disorders of the urinary tract interfere with the flow of urine. Obstruction can occur at any point in the system from the renal pelvis to the urethral meatus (Figure 27-7). In general, it causes dilation of the tract proximal to the obstruction. Stasis of urine occurs and predisposes to urinary tract infection and structural damage. Prolonged obstruction results in postrenal acute kidney injury and can ultimately lead to acute tubular necrosis (intrarenal acute kidney injury) (Chapter 28).

Disorders resulting in urinary tract obstruction may be congenital or acquired. In children, urinary tract obstruction is usually due to anatomic abnormalities such as with ureteral valves, strictures of the urethral meatus, and stenosis at the ureterovesical or ureteropelvic junction. Obstruction in adults predominantly occurs as a result of acquired disorders and may be either intraluminal (e.g., renal calculi)

TABLE 27-5	CAUSES OF RENAL SYSTEM OBSTRUCTION	
TYPE OF OBSTRUCTION	**CAUSE**
Intraluminal	Calculi, clot
	Tumor: bladder, urethra, kidney
	Papillary necrosis
Extrinsic	Prostatic hypertrophy
	Retroperitoneal fibrosis
	Tumor: pelvic, retroperitoneal
Acquired	Neurogenic bladder
	Ureteral stricture
	Urethral stricture

or secondary to extrinsic compression (e.g., tumors). Acquired obstructions are due to anatomic anomalies of the urinary tract (Table 27-5). Complications of urinary obstruction include infection, sepsis, acute kidney injury, and, potentially, chronic kidney disease.

Changes that occur within the urinary tract as a result of obstruction are dependent on (1) location and degree of obstruction (i.e., partial or complete, unilateral or bilateral) and (2) the duration and timing (acute onset or chronic) of the obstruction. Initially, in complete or significant partial obstruction, hydrostatic pressure increases proximal to the obstruction as a consequence of continued glomerular filtration and simultaneous obstruction to the flow of urine. Other structures proximal to the obstruction then begin to dilate. The more distal to the kidney the obstruction is located, the less dilation is seen because the pressure is distributed over a greater surface area. Complete obstruction of a ureter results in its dilation (**hydroureter**). The renal pelvis and tubules enlarge with the increased pressure, and the renal papillae flatten. The enlarged kidney is called **hydronephrosis.** Glomerular filtration rate (GFR) and renal perfusion decline, and eventually portions of the kidney become ischemic. Over the course of several weeks, if the obstruction is not corrected, tubular atrophy and destruction of the medulla result in scar tissue and nonfunctioning or poorly functioning glomeruli. Hydronephrosis is found at postmortem examination in 2% to 4% of patients.[35] Postrenal acute kidney injury is discussed in detail in Chapter 28.

Partial obstruction is much more common. In this situation, the renal pelvis may become very dilated but the structural or functional disruption of the kidney may be minimal. If the obstruction is bilateral, however, clinical manifestations of fluid retention will be present. Patients often complain of symptoms such as weight gain, nausea, anorexia, malaise, headaches, increased abdominal girth, and ankle edema. Functionally, partial obstruction can produce a slight to moderate decrease in blood flow and GFR and an inability to concentrate urine or secrete potassium and hydrogen ions. Compensatory hypertrophy occurs in the unaffected kidney. Renal calculi are the most common cause of urinary tract obstruction.[31]

Renal Calculi (Nephrolithiasis)

Renal calculi, or lithiasis, are crystal aggregates composed of organic and inorganic materials located within the urinary tract. These calculi are thought to form within the kidney, in the tubules or the collecting system, and may then migrate to more distal structures. Occasionally, terminology is used to identify where these calculi are found (e.g., *ureterolithiasis,* located in the ureters), but more commonly, the terms *renal calculi* or **nephrolithiasis** are used to describe the formation and passage of calculi anywhere within the urinary tract.[38] The Greek term *lithiasis* means *stone,* so renal calculi are also referred to as *kidney stones.*

BOX 27-3 GENERAL CONTRIBUTING FACTORS TO NEPHROLITHIASIS

- Hyperparathyroidism
- Gout
- Certain medications
- Hypertension
- Urinary tract infections
- Chronic inflammatory bowel disease; irritable bowel disease; chronic diarrhea
- Excess dietary meat
- Excess dietary sodium
- Excess dietary oxalate
- Past medical history or family history of nephrolithiasis
- Obesity
- Insulin resistance/type 2 diabetes mellitus
- Dehydration
- Prolonged immobility
- Congenital kidney defects/anatomic alterations (e.g., abnormal kidney shape)
- Vesicoureteral reflux

TABLE 27-6 TYPES OF NEPHROLITHIASIS, RELATIVE INCIDENCE, AND SPECIFIC RISK FACTORS

CONSTITUENT OF STONE	INCIDENCE	SPECIFIC RISKS
Calcium oxalate (primarily)	75%	Genetic predisposition; idiopathic; hypercalcemia and/or hypercalciuria (hyperparathyroidism, prolonged immobility, increased gastrointestinal absorption, impaired renal reabsorption); hyperuricosuria (see risks below); hyperoxaluria
Struvite	7-10%	Urinary tract infection with urea-splitting bacteria (e.g., *Proteus, Klebsiella, Pseudomonas*)
Uric acid	7-10%	Genetic predisposition; hyperuricosuria associated with gout, acute leukemia, glycogen storage disease, malignancy; excessive intake of meat, fish, poultry; obesity; type 2 diabetes; urine pH <5.5
Cystine	1-3%	Genetic defect in renal cystine reabsorption
Ephedrine, guaifenesin, indinavir, xanthine	All <1%	Secondary to specific medications

Nephrolithiasis affects individuals throughout the world[36,37]and has been traced back as far as Egyptian mummies.[37] Worldwide prevalence is estimated to be between 2% and 20%, with the highest lifetime risk in the United Arab Emirates and Saudi Arabia.[41] It is estimated that 10% to 15% of Americans will experience a kidney stone during their lifetime.[39] Historically, kidney stones have been more common in men than women,[36] but rates in women are increasing.[41] Examining incidence according to race/ethnicity, the risk of stone disease is significantly lower among non-Hispanic African Americans and Mexican Americans than among non-Hispanic Caucasians for both genders.[38] Although little is currently known about genetic predisposition, it is clearly a factor given the ethnic distribution and the increased risk associated with family history,[41] and the fact that some stones are associated with congenital metabolic abnormalities. There seems to be an increased prevalence of calculi in areas of the United States characterized by mountains, desert, or tropical climates. Prevalence increases moving from the North to the South and from West to East; the Southeastern United States, therefore, has the highest rates in the country.[37,38,41] It has been postulated that this is due to increased fluid loss through perspiration resulting in decreased urine volume.[37,38] Occupations where there is increased exposure to high temperatures or sedentary levels of activity are also associated with an increased incidence of stone formation. Nephrolithiasis has been found to be uncommon before age 20.[37] Although the exact rates are unknown, the incidence of nephrolithiasis in childhood is believed to be approximately 10% of that in adults.[42] Approximately 40% of children with urolithiasis have a positive family history of kidney stones and most of the children have a metabolic background of stone disease.[42]

Etiology and pathogenesis. Crystallization and stone formation occurs with many solutes found in urine and may be promoted or inhibited by a number of factors.[38,41,43] Some of these factors are inherent to the urinary tract and the characteristics of urine, whereas others are unique to the individual and the type of renal calculi formed. Box 27-3 identifies general factors that contribute to the formation of renal calculi. The general process of stone formation, however, is a physiologic constant.

The pathogenesis of nephrolithiasis begins with urine becoming supersaturated with the specific solute.[36-38] Urine is a solution of solvent (water) and solutes (particles). Certain of these solutes have a tendency to form crystals if their concentration within the urine becomes great enough; this is the meaning of *supersaturation*.[36] Urinary supersaturation is an essential requirement for stone formation.[36-38] These crystals begin their development somewhere in the nephron's loop of Henle, distal tubule, or collecting duct.[41] Crystallization is enhanced when a person is dehydrated (decreased solvent).[36,38,41] Crystals are unable to aggregate into a calculus of sufficient size to obstruct the urinary tract if urine is moving freely through the system.[41] Adequate fluid intake is therefore an inhibitor to stone formation, and because urine flows by gravity, urinary stasis, as may occur with immobility and a sedentary lifestyle, facilitates calculus formation.[43]

In addition to a crystalline component, nephrolithiasis also consists of a noncrystalline, organic component termed the calculus *matrix*.[37] Matrix itself consists of protein, sugar, glucosamine, bound water, and organic ash.[37] The matrix represents approximately 2.5% of the overall weight of the calculus. For some stones, the matrix is the dominant component; this is primarily true for stones that form with chronic urinary tract infections, where 65% of the stone is matrix. The specific role matrix plays in genesis of calculi is unclear.[37]

The types of renal calculi are shown in Table 27-6, along with their relative incidence in adults, and primary risk factors. Calcium oxalate–based stones are by far the most common in both children and adults.[36-38] Calcium-based nephrolithiasis is primarily idiopathic in etiology (unknown cause), but a genetic component is implicated.[41] Primary risk factors for calcium-based calculi are hypercalciuria and/or hypercalcemia, hyperoxaluria, and hyperuricosuria.[35,36] Hypercalciuria and/or hypercalcemia is commonly due to increased gastrointestinal absorption, impaired renal tubular reabsorption, and primary hyperparathyroidism, and less often to prolonged immobility, metastatic bone cancer, multiple myeloma, prolonged metabolic acidosis, hypocitraturia, and excessive amounts of vitamin D.[35,36,43] Hyperoxaluria can increase the urinary saturation of calcium oxalate.[36] It may be due to a genetic defect that increases urinary oxalate excretion, a defect in liver metabolism, or increased gastrointestinal absorption of an oxalate-rich diet (rhubarb, spinach, chocolate, nuts, beer, coffee, tea, cocoa, or excessive vitamin C).[36,41] Hyperuricosuria facilitates precipitation of calcium oxalate stones or may produce uric acid stones.[35-37] There is a genetic predisposition for hyperuricosuria, which may be found in association with gouty arthritis or secondary purine excess attributable to overproduction in myeloproliferative disorders, excess ingestion of purine-rich foods, or errors of purine metabolism.[35,36] Foods high in purine include organ meats such as liver and kidney, sardines, anchovies, salmon, and foods high in yeast such as beer and bread. Uric acid and struvite calculi are the second most frequently occurring stones, following calcium oxalate stones. In addition to the risk factors previously identified for hyperuricosuria, an increased body mass index and glucose intolerance or type 2 diabetes are frequently associated with uric acid stones.[36] Calculi are uric acid–based in patients with diabetes 30% to 40% of the time compared with 10% or less in the nondiabetic population.[36] The basis of struvite stones is not metabolic, but rather the changes that occur within the urinary tract with some infectious processes, and often assisted by some underlying anatomic or functional abnormalities that facilitate urinary stasis.[36,38] Struvite stones are composed of magnesium, ammonium, and phosphate. Urinary tract infections with certain bacterial species capable of splitting urea into two ammonium ions and one bicarbonate ion neutralize the urine and support bacterial proliferation as well as stone formation. Struvite stones form around a bacterial nucleus, producing an antimicrobial barrier. They grow rapidly and assume a jagged formation known as *staghorn*.[36,38] Other types of nephrolithiasis are less common and are associated with familial defects in renal transport,[41] or are produced as adverse effects of certain drugs (e.g., indinavir, triamterene, and xanthine).[43]

Clinical manifestations. Signs and symptoms of renal calculi differ with their size and location and may mimic any number of other causes of abdominal pain.[39,43] Pain may be vague or, more commonly, acute renal colic or flank pain.[39,43] Stones within the kidney are responsible for flank pain that may be dull and localized. While the stone moves to the ureteropelvic junction and down into the ureter, spasmodic, intermittent sharp pain known as renal colic develops. The pain may radiate into the ipsilateral groin area, testicle, or labia. The pain induced by nephrolithiasis makes the patient acutely uncomfortable and is often accompanied by nausea and vomiting, diaphoresis, tachycardia, and tachypnea. When the stone reaches the bladder, there is often a noticeable reduction in the pain. If the stone results in a partial obstruction at the urethra, dysuria, urgency, and frequency are common findings. These findings may present earlier if there is a concomitant urinary tract infection.[43] Renal calculi may develop as a result of a urinary tract infection (struvite stones), or increase the risk of its development.[43] If the infection reaches the kidney itself (pyelonephritis), the patient will become acutely ill (see Acute Pyelonephritis section). Prolonged or repeated nephrolithiasis may result in scarring of the kidney and, if bilateral, chronic kidney disease.

Diagnosis and treatment. In addition to the clinical manifestations, a thorough family history should be obtained, risk factors for nephrolithiasis should be assessed, and any anatomic or functional urinary tract anomalies should be identified.[41] Urinalysis permits the identification of a concomitant infection, levels of specific stone-forming constituents (e.g., hypercalciuria), and urinary pH, which affects crystallization. Hematuria (gross or microscopic) may be present persistently or intermittently with or without other manifestations.[43] If a stone has been passed and is available, it is sent for analysis of its composition. Determination of a complete blood count; measurement of levels of serum electrolytes, serum creatinine, and BUN; and

---

BOX 27-4 GENERAL INTERVENTIONS FOR NEPHROLITHIASIS

- Narcotic analgesics for pain management
- Increased fluid intake (>2 L/day; oral and/or IV)
- Antimicrobials for urinary tract infection
- Shock-wave lithotripsy, ureteral stenting, ureteroscopy for removal of large stones unable to pass spontaneously
- Dietary modifications unique to stone composition
- Medications unique to stone composition (e.g., allopurinol for uric acid stones)

BOX 27-5 DIETARY MODIFICATIONS FOR NEPHROLITHIASIS

- Increase water intake (minimum of 2 L/day).
- Ensure adequate dietary calcium intake.
- Avoid calcium supplementation.
- Avoid foods with additional vitamin D (and vitamin C, if recommended).
- Avoid calcium-based antacids.
- Limit intake of coffee, tea, or colas to ≤2 per day.
- Reduce protein intake from meat, fish, and poultry.
- Limit dietary sodium and oxalate intake.
- Avoid high-purine foods for uric acid stones (and if recommended, for calcium).

---

assessment of parathormone level provide information related to risk factors and renal function.

The traditional gold standard for the assessment of renal calculi has been intravenous pyelogram (IVP), but it has been effectively replaced by computerized tomography (CT scans).[39,43] Basic abdominal x-rays identify only those stones that are radiopaque.[41,43] Ultrasonography is considered as effective as IVP, but provides limited data relative to renal function. It is second in choice for diagnosis to the CT scan.[41,43] CT scanning can identify renal calculi, other potential sources of flank pain, and anatomic anomalies.[41,43]

Treatment of nephrolithiasis may be medical or surgical and is determined by the size, position, and composition of the calculus; the presence or absence of urinary tract infection; and the involvement of one or both kidneys. Interventions are generally summarized in Box 27-4, and dietary changes are listed in Box 27-5. The goal is not only treatment of existing stones but also prevention of their recurrence.[35,43] Acute pain requires intervention with opiates. Morphine is especially useful because it reduces renal colic as well as affecting both transmission and perception of painful stimuli. With increased fluid intake, most stones pass out of the urinary tract spontaneously in both children and adults.[35,41] Stones less than 5 mm in diameter have a high chance of being passed, whereas those 5 to 7 mm in diameter have a 50% chance, and those >7 mm almost always require urologic intervention.[38] Other interventions that may be required include extracorporeal shock-wave lithotripsy, where the stone is broken into smaller pieces for passage, or percutaneous approaches to stone removal by endoscopy with basket retrieval or ultrasonic or laser lithotripsy.[41] Open surgical approaches are required when no other intervention is successful, but are usually avoidable and therefore uncommon. Unfortunately, depending upon the type of renal calculus, 30% to 50% of adults can expect a recurrence within 5 to 10 years.[35,43] Dietary modifications can decrease this risk.[41] Recommendations are designed for each individual patient, based upon the type of stone and specific risk factors.[41]

GLOMERULAR DISORDERS (GLOMERULOPATHIES)

Glomerular disorders result from alterations in the structure and function of the glomerular capillary circulation and are broadly delineated as **glomerulopathies.** The membranes of glomerular capillaries have three layers: endothelium, basement membrane, and a layer of specialized epithelial cells with footlike projections (podocytes) that encircle the basement membrane[40] (Figure 27-8). Together, this triple layer comprises the filtration barrier of the glomerulus. The glomerular filtrate passes through gaps (slit pores) between these podocytes, enters the space in Bowman capsule, and progresses into the proximal tubule. Glomerulopathies are responsible for 90% of the cases of end-stage renal disease.[44]

Pathologic changes to nephron glomeruli may occur insidiously, altering function over the course of months or years, or they may have an acute onset, with rapidly developing impairment. In some cases, there are no apparent signs or symptoms and glomerular dysfunction is identified serendipitously during routine physical examination or evaluation of some other health concern. The specific etiologies of glomerulopathies are often unknown. Hereditary and environmental factors are implicated; metabolic, infectious, hemodynamic, toxic, immune, genetic, and other mechanisms of injury are involved.[44] Immune or inflammatory processes are most often implicated.[44]

The challenge in any discussion of glomerulopathies lies in the often confusing range of clinical and pathologic approaches to their classification. One approach is to classify glomerular disorders according to primary and secondary etiologies.[35,45] *Primary glomerulopathies* are disease states in which the kidney is the only or the predominant organ involved, and *secondary glomerulopathies* result from drug exposure, infection, or glomerular injury in the setting of multisystem or vascular abnormalities. Goodpasture syndrome is an example of a secondary glomerulopathy, affecting the basement membranes of both the glomeruli of the kidney and the alveoli of the lung.[35] Systemic lupus erythematosus also causes a secondary glomerulopathy.[46] Diabetic nephropathy and renal damage attributable to undiagnosed or inadequately managed hypertension are also examples of secondary glomerulopathies.

The specific location and features of glomerular injury is another method of classification that has been used. Glomerular involvement may be characterized as *diffuse* (all glomeruli) or *focal* (some but not all glomeruli).[45-47] Within the affected glomeruli, lesions may be *global*, affecting all parts of the glomerulus, or present as patches *(segmental)* when only specific parts of the glomerulus are involved.[44,47,48] If thickening of glomerular capillary walls is present, the glomerulopathy is *membranous*. Membranous changes involve the basement membrane and are usually due to accumulated deposition of immunoglobulins (IgG) and complement components (C5).[35,45] *Sclerotic* changes refer to scarring attributable to persistent or recurrent injury and may occur within the capillaries, in the capillary space, or at the point of initiation of the proximal tubule. The site of deposition of noncellular materials as part of the glomerulopathic process may be described specifically as *mesangial, subendothelial,* or *subepithelial.*[45] Efforts to specify the glomerulopathy often result in combinations of terminology, such as *focal segmental*[47,48] or *membranoproliferative.*[35] Various glomerulopathies may be linked to more than one type of injury, however; so this lack of specificity makes absolute classification by this criterion less beneficial. Its primary value rests in providing a common vocabulary for the description of glomerulopathic lesions. Renal biopsy and histologic examination are required for this level of specificity. More recently, a method of classification according to the degree and type of dysfunction, injury, or loss of the glomerular podocytes has been proposed.[44]

Glomerulopathies may result in proteinuria, hematuria, abnormal urinary casts, decreased GFR, and hypertension; however, these manifestations may not all be present in a single pathology and/or they may present along a continuum of degree. Proteinuria is classically the clinical manifestation associated with glomerulopathy; other urinary or systemic conditions may present with hematuria, urinary casts, reduced GFR, or hypertension. Damage to the glomerulus will result in protein loss from the bloodstream into the urine.[1] Under normal circumstances, protein molecules are too large to pass through the slit pores of the glomerulus, so they are retained in the bloodstream. The very small Bence Jones protein associated with multiple myeloma is easily filtered and will appear in the urine in that condition. Transient proteinuria may be seen with diets high in protein, or as a result of excessive exercise or emotional stress. Normally, protein lost in the urine amounts to 50 to 80 mg in 24 hours (at rest).[1] Glomerulopathies may be classified according to the degree of proteinuria.[45] **Nephrotic syndrome** is specifically characterized by protein loss ≥3 to 3.5 g in 24 hours[1] and is most commonly associated with minimal change disease/lipoid nephrosis, focal segmental glomerulosclerosis, and membranous nephropathy, but can occur with any glomerulopathy if the injury is sufficient to allow significant protein loss.[51] **Nephritic syndrome** is also a reflection of glomerular inflammation. In this case, hematuria is seen on gross urinalysis, and red blood cell (RBC) casts are present in the sediment. Mild to moderate proteinuria, edema, hypertension, oliguria, and decreased GFR producing an elevation in serum creatinine level may also be noted.[1,35,51]

The most common types of glomerular disease are acute postinfectious glomerulonephritis, IgA nephropathy, rapidly progressive/crescentic glomerulonephritis, nephrotic syndrome (includes membranous glomerulonephritis, focal segmental glomerulosclerosis, minimal change disease/lipoid nephrosis), and chronic glomerulonephritis. By far the most common secondary glomerulopathies are diabetic nephropathy and glomerulopathy resulting from hypertension. These are addressed in Chapters 41 and 16, respectively.

Glomerulonephritis

Glomerulonephritis includes an assortment of immune-mediated conditions that produce inflammation of glomeruli and other areas of the kidney.[45] It may have a primary etiology, which is commonly believed to be autoimmune, or a secondary one, in which it is associated with a number of autoimmune, metabolic, malignant, or infectious systemic disorders.

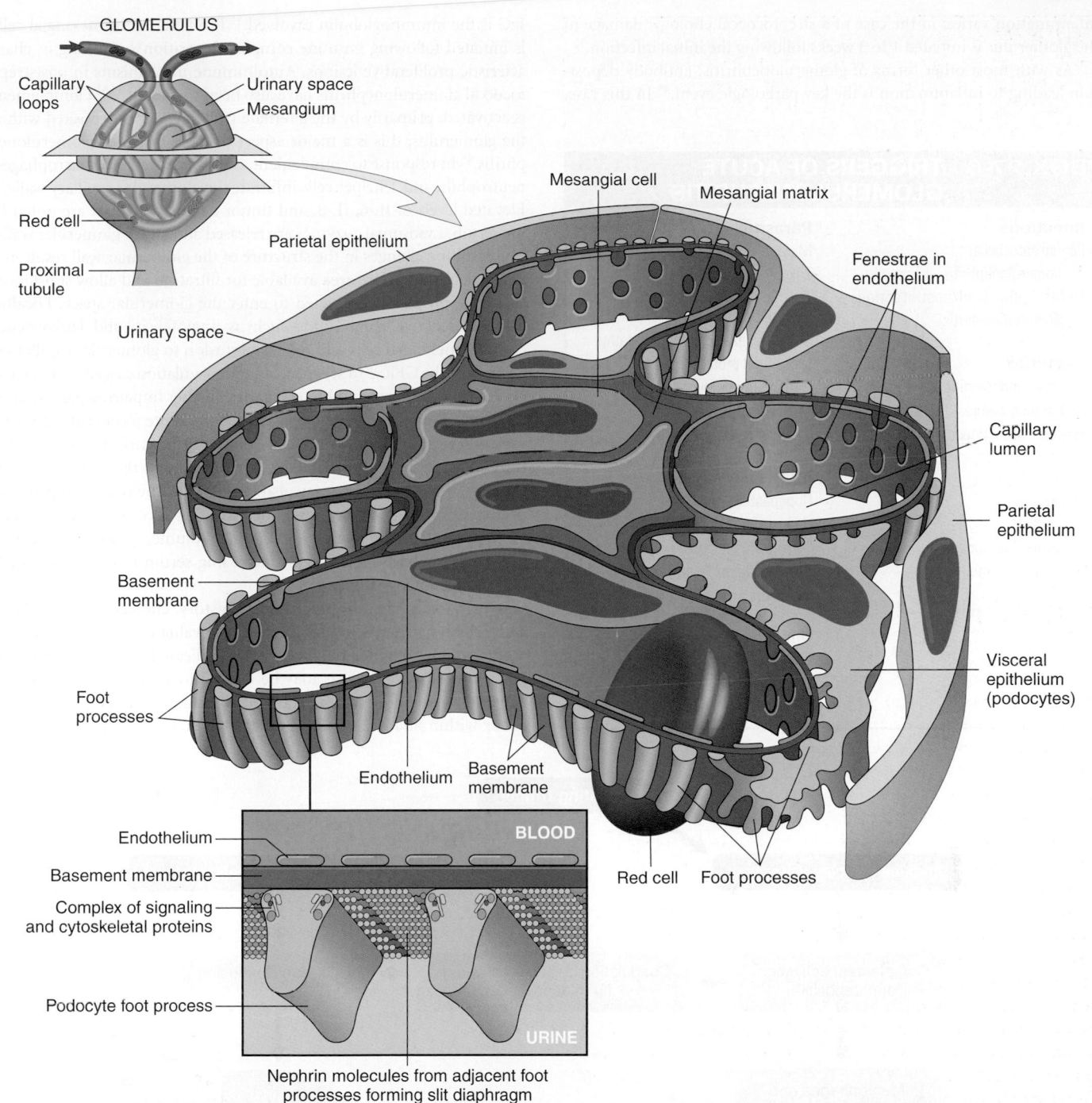

GLOMERULUS

Capillary loops
Urinary space
Mesangium
Red cell
Proximal tubule

Mesangial cell
Mesangial matrix
Parietal epithelium
Urinary space
Basement membrane
Foot processes
Endothelium
Basement membrane

Fenestrae in endothelium
Capillary lumen
Parietal epithelium
Visceral epithelium (podocytes)
Red cell   Foot processes

Endothelium
Basement membrane
Complex of signaling and cytoskeletal proteins
Podocyte foot process
BLOOD
URINE

Nephrin molecules from adjacent foot processes forming slit diaphragm

FIGURE 27-8 Schematic illustration of the lobe of a glomerulus. Note the foot processes of the podocytes, basement membrane, and endothelium of the glomerular capillary. (From Kumar V et al: *Robbins basic pathology,* ed 8, Philadelphia, 2007, Saunders, p 543.)

Although there is some variation, for the most part glomerulonephritis is more common among men than women.[45] More than 20 years ago, glomerulonephritis was believed to be the leading cause of the end-stage of chronic renal disease.[40] Although worldwide it remains the second most common cause,[45] in the United States the glomerulopathies associated with diabetes mellitus and hypertension hold that distinction.[40,45]

Acute Glomerulonephritis

The term *acute glomerulonephritis* encompasses a constellation of inflammatory glomerulopathies that are characterized by the abrupt onset of varying degrees of hematuria, proteinuria, oliguria and azotemia, edema,

and hypertension.[45] A wide variety of triggers may initiate the process (Box 27-6). The pathophysiologic process is summarized in Figure 27-9.

Postinfectious acute glomerulonephritis is historically most well-known to follow skin (impetigo) and throat infections with specific strains of group A β-hemolytic streptococci.[35,45,51] This etiology is common today only among children in impoverished areas of developed countries and developing countries,[45,51] where it is the basis of 4.6% to 51.6% of pediatric acute kidney injury admissions.[51] The reduction in incidence of this etiology elsewhere is most likely due to early diagnosis and treatment of streptococcal infections.[51] The infectious organism acts as the antigen, initiating an antibody-antigen reaction. The onset of glomerular inflammation varies; in the case of a streptococcal etiology, damage to the glomerulus is initiated 1 to 3 weeks following the initial infection.[35]

As with most other forms of glomerulonephritis, antibody deposition leading to inflammation is the key pathologic event.[45] In this case, IgG is the immunoglobulin involved.[51] Proliferation of mesangial cells is initiated following immune complex deposition[40] resulting in characteristic proliferative lesions. Autoimmune mechanisms in poststreptococcal glomerulonephritis have also been suggested.[35,51] Complement is activated, primarily by the alternate pathway.[51] It is deposited within the glomerulus; this is a major aspect of most forms of glomerulonephritis.[45] In response to complement, chemotaxic factors, macrophages, neutrophils, and T helper cells infiltrate the glomerular capillary walls.[51] Elevated levels of IL-6, IL-8, and tumor necrosis factor-α are noted in the serum. Lysosomal enzymes are released and attack glomerular walls. The resulting changes in the structure of the glomerular wall result in a decrease in the surface area available for filtration and allow substances that were previously restricted to enter the glomerular space. Locally-acting vasoactive compounds such as angiotensin and leukotrienes contract mesangial cells and reduce perfusion to glomerular capillaries, decreasing the GFR.[51] In severe cases, the coagulation cascade is activated and fibrin is deposited within capillaries, further impairing perfusion.[45]

Clinical manifestations of postinfectious acute glomerulonephritis vary in severity.[51] Smoky or coffee-colored urine attributable to hematuria and red cell casts (nephritic syndrome) are the most common findings. White cell casts may also be present. The degree of proteinuria is variable, and may reach nephrotic syndrome level. Reduced GFR presents as increased circulating volume, producing edema, hypertension, and oliguria with increasing serum levels of creatinine and nitrogenous wastes (BUN).[35,51]

Diagnosis is based on the patient's history, clinical manifestations, and urinalysis results. Renal function is evaluated by BUN and creatinine levels. A renal biopsy may be indicated. Care is supportive and symptomatic. Dialysis may be needed to support renal function. Especially in children, resolution of the inflammatory process may occur within about 2 weeks (poststreptococcal) with no sequelae or

BOX 27-6   TRIGGERS OF ACUTE GLOMERULONEPHRITIS

Infectious
Poststreptococcal glomerulonephritis
Nonstreptococcal/postinfectious glomerulonephritis

Bacterial
Infective endocarditis
Meningococcemia
Pneumococcal pneumonia
Sepsis

Viral
Hepatitis B
Hepatitis C (associated cryoglobinemia)
Mononucleosis
Mumps/measles
Varicella

Parasitic
Malaria
Toxoplasmosis

Primary Disease
Berger disease (IgA nephropathy)
Mesangial proliferative glomerulonephritis
Mesangiocapillary glomerulonephritis

Multisystem Disease
Goodpasture syndrome
Henoch-Schönlein purpura
Polyarteritis nodosa
Systemic lupus erythematosus
Vasculitis

Miscellaneous
Guillain-Barré syndrome
Serum sickness
Irradiation for Wilms tumor

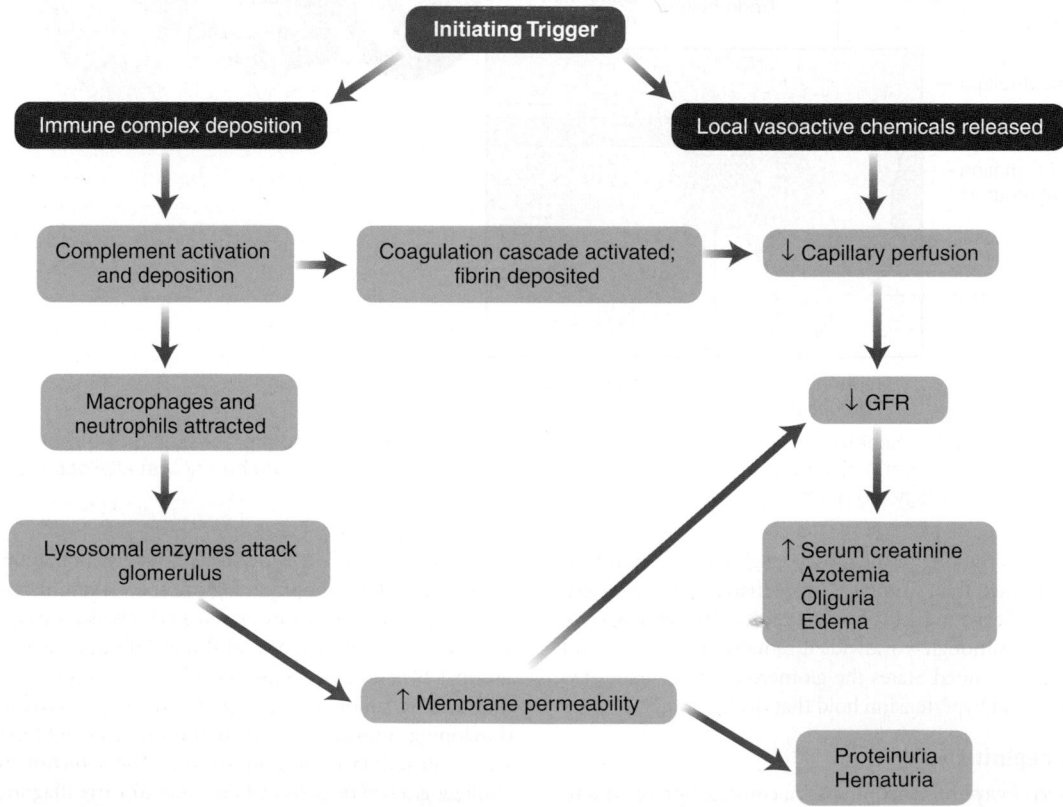

FIGURE 27-9 Summary of the pathophysiologic process of acute glomerulonephritis and associated clinical manifestations.

complications, or the deterioration of renal function may continue, resulting in chronic glomerulonephritis, nephrotic syndrome (glomerulosclerosis), and chronic kidney disease.[35,40]

IgA nephropathy (Berger disease) is the most commonly diagnosed type of primary glomerulonephritis worldwide.[35,50] It is more common in the adult population than among pediatric patients.[45] Upper respiratory tract or gastrointestinal viral infections appear to be the triggers, initiating the deposition of IgA in the glomerular mesangium.[35] Increased abnormal IgA_1 production and formation of IgA_1 complexes cause mesangial injury, leading to renal failure.[35,50] Hematuria is usually apparent within 1 to 2 days, but the proteinuria, edema, and hypertension common with other glomerulopathies are generally not evident. Prognosis is variable; as many as half the patients develop glomerulosclerosis and end-stage renal disease.[35,50]

Crescentic Glomerulonephritis/Rapidly Progressive Glomerulonephritis (RPGN)

The condition previously known as *rapidly progressive glomerulonephritis* is now more often called *crescentic glomerulonephritis* because of its characteristic lesions.[45] The lesions are proliferative in nature and composed of crescent-shaped depositions of accumulated epithelial cells, fibrin, and macrophages that are found in Bowman space.[45] Podocytes that are progressively losing their markers of differentiation are also a part of the process.[44] This form of glomerulonephritis may have an acute onset, with hematuria, proteinuria, and red cell casts followed by a swift decline in renal function within 6 months.[35] It occurs predominantly in patients 20 to 50 years old.[35] When not idiopathic, causes of crescentic glomerulonephritis fall into four general categories: (1) complication of an acute or subacute infection; (2) complication of a multisystem disease; (3) drug exposure; and (4) a primary disorder in the absence of other systemic disease. The most common infections associated with this disorder are poststreptococcal glomerulonephritis and infective endocarditis. Multisystem diseases associated with it are systemic lupus erythematosus, Henoch-Schönlein purpura, systemic necrotizing vasculitis, and Goodpasture syndrome. Examples of drugs identified as causative are penicillamine, hydralazine, allopurinol in the presence of vasculitis, and rifampin.[45]

Goodpasture syndrome is an autoimmune disorder that results from the combination of glomerulonephritis with alveolar hemorrhage and the presence of anti–glomerular basement membrane (anti-GBM) antibodies. It most often develops in genetically susceptible people who smoke cigarettes. Men are affected more than women.[35] Patients suffer with the clinical manifestations of glomerulonephritis and also shortness of breath and hemoptysis because of pulmonary involvement. Manifestations of pulmonary involvement may appear before those associated with glomerulonephritis. Prognosis is good when treatment is begun before onset of respiratory or renal failure.[35] Treatment is based on system support; plasmapheresis (therapeutic plasma exchange to decrease circulating antibodies), corticosteroids, and immunosuppression are the most common interventions.[35]

Chronic Glomerulonephritis

Glomerular diseases that assume a progressive course ultimately develop into chronic kidney disease.[45] These patients present with persistent proteinuria, with or without hematuria, and slowly declining renal function. In many cases, patients appear to have recovered from the initial insult. Proteinuria and hypertension are both capable of advancing renal damage. The pathophysiology is an extension of that seen in acute glomerulonephritis. Proliferative and membranous lesions are present but sclerotic injury dominates, resulting in ongoing fibrotic changes. Tubulointerstitial damage contributes to the reduction in renal function. Nephrons atrophy and ultimately the kidneys

become small, scarred, and nonfunctional. While the chronic kidney disease progresses, supportive interventions may retard the process (see Chapter 28), but the patient ultimately reaches end-stage renal disease and dialysis or transplantation is required.[45]

Nephrotic Syndrome

Nephrotic syndrome is a glomerulopathy in which there is a urinary elimination of >3 to 3.5 grams of protein per day due to glomerular damage.[52,53] Ultimately, most patients will develop the full constellation of nephrotic syndrome manifestations: hypoalbuminemia, hyperlipidemia, edema, and a propensity for thrombus formation. The most common primary causes are minimal change disease (lipoid nephrosis), idiopathic focal segmental glomerulosclerosis, and membranous nephropathy. Several systemic diseases, such as systemic lupus erythematosus and Henoch-Schönlein purpura, as well as infections, malignancies, and vasculitis have been found to be associated with nephrotic syndrome, but the most common cause in adults is diabetes mellitus.[52,53]

The pathophysiology of nephrotic syndrome is shown in Figure 27-10. The increased permeability of the glomerular membrane allows large quantities of protein to leave the bloodstream and exit the body in the urine. This produces hypoalbuminemia and proteinuria. The low serum albumin concentration serves to stimulate the liver to increase production of cholesterol and lipoproteins, producing hyperlipidemia.[52-54] The actual mechanism has not been fully elucidated but is clearly multifactorial and complex.[52-54] Levels of cholesterol and low-density lipoproteins (LDLs) are elevated; cholesterol levels are consistently greater than 300 mg/dl.[53] Lipid casts or fat droplets may appear in the urine.[1] Oval fat bodies, epithelial cells from the tubules, may also be sloughed.[1] There is an increased risk of thrombotic events in nephrotic syndrome.[52,53] This complication has many possible etiologies, but most likely the proteins required for hemostasis are lost in the urine, stimulating hepatic synthesis of clotting factors.[52,53] Edema is the most common clinical manifestation of nephrotic syndrome.[52,53] Two theories have been proposed to explain its development.[53] As the serum albumin is lost, the oncotic pressure within the blood vessels declines and the hydrostatic pressure is relatively increased, forcing fluid into the interstitial spaces. Reduction in circulating volume results in the activation of the renin-angiotensin-aldosterone system, causing sodium and then water retention and promoting more protein loss and edema. The second theory claims that the kidneys' intrinsic sodium-retaining mechanism is activated before the loss of protein, expanding circulating volume, and increasing capillary filtration and edema formation. A vicious cycle of protein loss, fluid retention, and edema is initiated.

Treatment of nephrotic syndrome, regardless of causation, includes gradual removal of fluid with diuretics to treat edema.[52,53] Elevated lipid levels are routinely treated with lipid-lowering therapy, if rapid recovery from nephrotic syndrome is not anticipated.[52,53] Hypertension is treated with angiotensin II receptor blockers and/or angiotensin-converting enzyme inhibition, as is recommended for chronic kidney disease. Treatment with immunosuppression or immunomodulation is standard for most primary etiologies, although response is variable.[52,53]

Membranous Nephropathy (MN)

MN accounts for about one third of the cases of adult-onset nephrotic syndrome.[49,55] Twenty percent of these cases have secondary causes such as infections, autoimmune diseases, and malignancies. For lack of any concrete evidence, the remaining 80% are said to be idiopathic.[49,55] Figure 27-11 illustrates the histologic findings with MN and the pathologic changes in the glomerulus. Immune deposits and as-yet unidentified antigens collect in the subepithelium of the distal portion of the basement membrane and produce a membranous thickening.[35,49,55] Spontaneous remission occurs in approximately 25% of cases, 25%

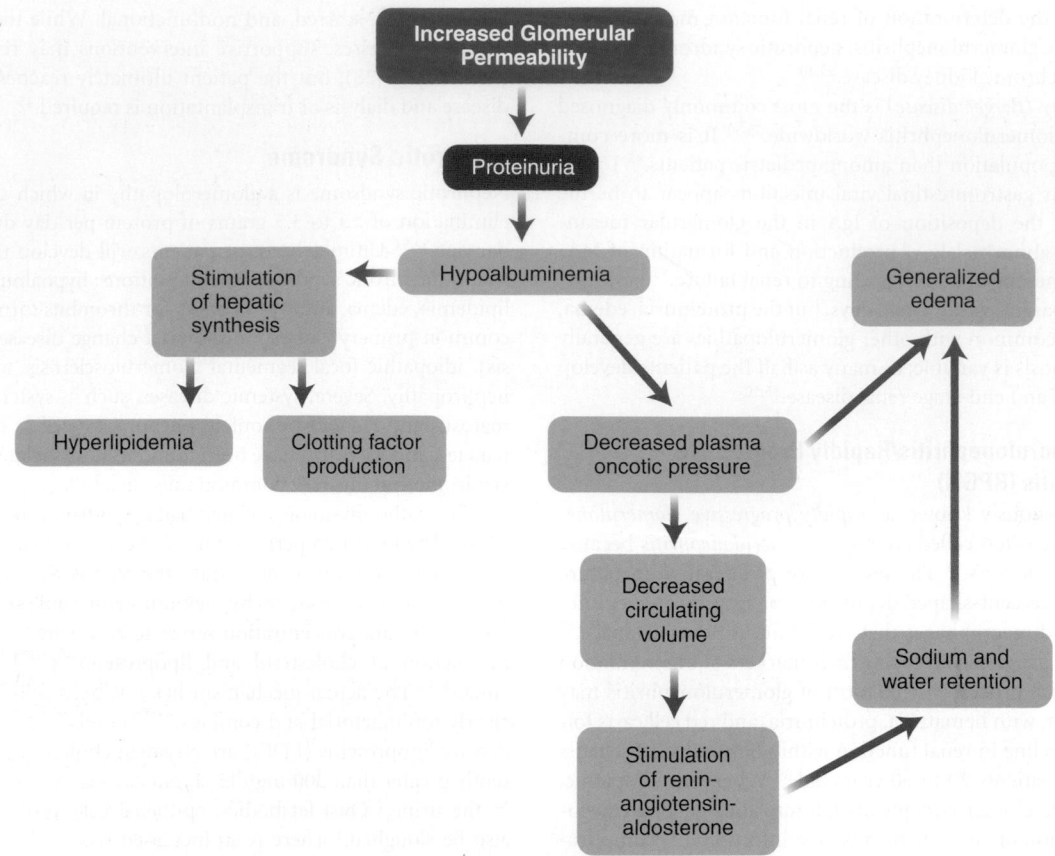

FIGURE 27-10 Pathophysiologic process of nephrotic syndrome.

develop persistent nonnephrotic-range proteinuria, 25% develop persistent nephrotic syndrome, and 25% of the individuals with MN progress to end-stage renal disease.[35]

Focal Segmental Glomerulosclerosis (FSGS)

FSGS is now the most common cause of idiopathic (or primary) nephrotic syndrome among adults in the United States.[35] It may develop secondarily to a number of immunologic, metabolic, interstitial, hemodynamic, or other conditions. Only a portion of the glomeruli are affected (segmental), and glomeruli within the kidney are not uniformly impacted (focal). This is a disease of glomeruli podocytes that over time progresses to scarred lesions. Epithelial injury and endothelial cellular injury initiate the protein loss across the glomerular membrane. In addition to proteinuria, patients can develop mild hematuria, hypertension, and azotemia.[35] Only 5% of patients will experience complete remission. Once proteinuria reaches nephrotic syndrome levels, 50% of those with FSGS will reach ESRD within 6 to 8 years.[48] Disproportionately, more blacks than other ethnic groups develop FSGS.[35]

Minimal Change Disease (MCD)

Previously called *lipoid nephrosis*, MCD is the primary cause of idiopathic nephrotic syndrome in children, accounting for 77% of nephrotic syndrome diagnoses by biopsy in children and adolescents.[56] It is usually initiated by an allergic or immune condition, including lymphomas. The result of the altered structure of the podocytes is a less effective glomerular filtration and the loss of copious amounts of albumin in the urine. Onset of edema, heavy levels of proteinuria, and hypoalbuminemia is sudden.[35] Although a longer course is usually needed in children, MCD responds well to treatment with corticosteroids.[35] Fewer patients progress to ESRD with MCD than the other common forms of nephrotic syndrome.

KEY POINTS

- Glomerulopathies alter glomerular capillary structure and function. Damage is mediated by immune processes. The glomerular damage may result in some combination of hematuria, proteinuria, abnormal casts, decreased GFR, edema, and hypertension.

- Glomerulonephritis is due to an immune response to a variety of potential triggers and may have a primary or secondary etiology. Attraction of immune cells to the area of inflammation results in lysosomal degradation of the basement membrane. The GFR may fall, in part because of contraction of mesangial cells resulting in decreased surface area for filtration.

- Glomerulonephritis may be classified as acute, crescentic, or chronic. Acute forms are usually triggered by infection. The cause of the crescentic form is often unknown, but it may be secondary to other disease processes such as Goodpasture syndrome. Chronic forms are those that progress to chronic kidney disease.

- Treatment of glomerulonephritis may include steroids, plasmapheresis, and supportive measures such as dietary and fluid management and management of systemic and renal hypertension. End-stage renal disease is a common outcome of chronic glomerulonephritis, necessitating dialysis or kidney transplantation.

- Nephrotic syndrome occurs because of increased glomerular permeability to proteins, which results in a urinary loss of 3 to 3.5 g of protein or more per day. Proteinuria leads to hypoalbuminemia and generalized edema as a result of decreased blood colloid osmotic pressure. Hyperlipidemia and hypercoagulability are thought to occur because of a generalized increase in liver activity stimulated by hypoalbuminemia.

- Treatment of nephrotic syndrome is conservative, consisting of management of symptoms and the underlying process that initiated the syndrome, when possible. Although many cases resolve spontaneously, others progress to end-stage renal disease.

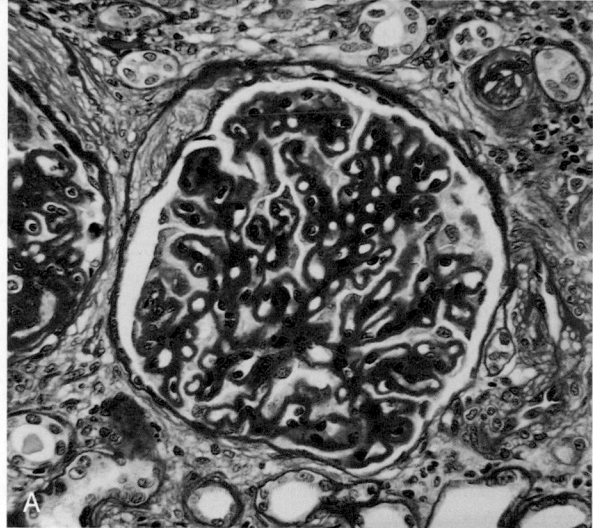
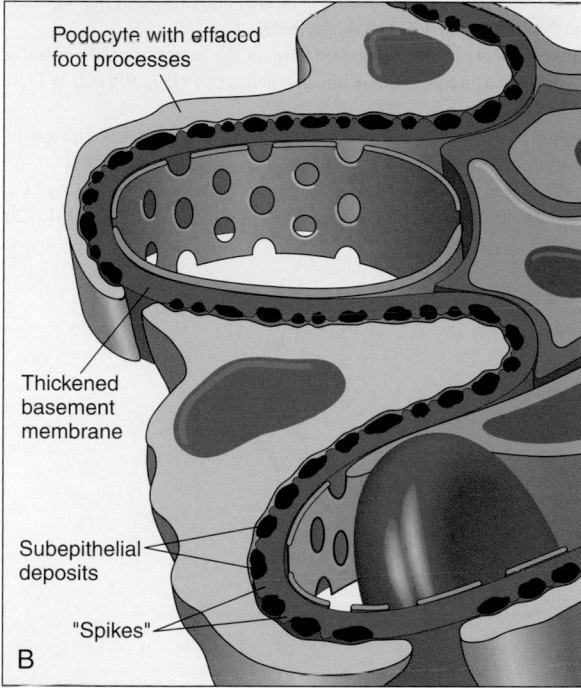

FIGURE 27-11 Membranous nephropathy. **A,** Diffuse thickening of the glomerular basement membrane. **B,** Schematic diagram illustrating subepithelial deposits, effacement of foot processes, and the presence of "spikes" of basement membrane material between the immune deposits. (From Kumar V et al: *Robbins basic pathology*, ed 8, Philadelphia, 2007, Saunders, p 552.)

SUMMARY

Many diseases can cause damage to the kidney. Any process that disrupts the normal architecture of the kidney will cause altered function, whether in the glomeruli, the vascular tree, or the collecting/draining system. Despite the kidney's resiliency and capacity to respond to treatment, ultimately any abnormality in the system has the potential to progress to chronic kidney disease.

REFERENCES

1. Pagana KD, Pagana TJ: *Mosby's manual of diagnostic and laboratory tests,* ed 4, St Louis, 2011, Mosby.
2. Dziarmaga A, Quinlan J, Goodyer P: Renal hypoplasia: lessons from Pax2, *Pediatr Nephrol* 21:26–31, 2006.
3. Woolf AS, Hillman KA: Unilateral renal agenesis and the congenital solitary functioning kidney: developmental, genetic and clinical perspectives, *BJU Int* 99:17–21, 2006.
4. Schwaderer AL, et al: Renal anomalies in family members of infants with bilateral renal agenesis/adysplasia, *Pediatr Nephrol* 22:52–56, 2007.
5. Balcells T, Ars Criach A: Molecular diagnosis of autosomal dominant polycystic kidney disease, *Nefrologia* 31:35–43, 2011.
6. Campbell SC, Novick AC, Bukowski RM: Neoplasms of the upper urinary tract. In Wein JA, et al, editors: *Campbell-Walsh urology,* ed 9, Philadelphia, 2007, Saunders, pp 1575–1582.
7. Torres WE, Harris PC, Pirson Y: Autosomal dominant polycystic kidney disease, *Lancet* 369:1287–1301, 2007.
8. Patel V, Chowdhury R, Igarashi P: Advances in the pathogenesis and treatment of polycystic kidney disease, *Curr Opin Nephrol Hypertens* 18:99–106, 2009.
9. Halvorson CR, Bremmer MS, Jacobs SC: Polycystic kidney disease: inheritance, pathophysiology, prognosis, and treatment, *Int J Nephrol Renovasc Dis* 3:69–83, 2010.
10. Pei Y, Watnick T: Diagnosis and screening of autosomal dominant polycystic kidney disease, *Adv Chronic Kidney Dis* 17:140–152, 2010.
11. Grantham JJ: Autosomal dominant polycystic kidney disease, *Ann Transplant* 14:86–90, 2009.
12. Nelson EC, Evans CP, Lara PN: Renal cell carcinoma: current status and emerging therapies, *Cancer Treatment Rev* 33:299–313, 2007.
13. Ljungberg B, et al: EAU guidelines on renal cell carcinoma: the 2010 update, *Eur Assoc Urol* 58:398–406, 2010.
14. Novick AC: Kidney cancer: past, present, and future, *Urol Oncol* 23:188–195, 2007.
15. Arai E, Kanai Y: Genetic and epigenetic alterations during renal carcinogenesis, *Int J Clin Exp Pathol* 4:58–73, 2011.
16. Tazi EM, et al: Advanced treatments in non-clear renal cell carcinoma, *Urol J* 8:1–11, Winter 2011.
17. National Cancer Institute: 2011. Cancer topics. Available at www.cancer.gov/cancertopics/types/kidney. Accessed 11/28/11.
18. Chow W, Dong LM, Devesa SS: *Epidemiology and risk factors for kidney cancer* 2010. doi: 10.1038/nerurol.2010.46. Accessed 11/28/11.
19. Linehan WM, et al: Identification of the genes for kidney cancer: opportunity for disease-specific targeted therapeutics, *Clin Cancer Res* 13(2 suppl):671s–679s, 2007.
20. Vira MA, et al: Genetic basis of kidney cancer: a model for developing molecular-targeted therapies, *BJU Int* 99:1223–1229, 2007.
21. Rivera MN, Haber DA: Wilms' tumour: connecting tumorigenesis and organ development in the kidney, *Nat Rev Cancer* 5(9):699–712, 2005.
22. Scott RH, et al: Syndromes and constitutional chromosomal abnormalities associated with Wilms tumour, *J Med Genet* 43:705–715, 2006.
23. Davidoff AM: Wilms tumor, *Curr Opin Pediatr* 21:357–364, 2009.
24. Chishti AS, et al: A guideline for the inpatient care of children with pyelonephritis, *Ann Saudi Med* 30:341–349, 2010.
25. Sheffield JS, Cunningham FG: Urinary tract infection in women, *Obstet Gynecol* 106(5 pt 1):1085–1092, 2005.
26. Chung A, et al: Bacterial cystitis in women, *Aust Fam Physician* 39:295–298, 2010.
27. Lane MC, Mobley HLT: Role of p-fimbrial-mediated adherence in pyelonephritis and persistence of uropathogenic *Escherichia coli* (UPEC) in the mammalian kidney, *Kidney Int* 72:19–25, 2007.
28. Lane DR, Takhar SS: Diagnosis and management of urinary tract infection and pyelonephritis, *Emerg Med Clin North Am* 29, August 2011. Retrieved from MD Consult 12/5/11.
29. Colgan R, et al: Diagnosis and treatment of acute pyelonephritis in women, *Am Fam Physician* 84, September 2011. Retrieved from MD Consult 12/5/11.

30. Lundstedt A, et al: Inherited susceptibility to acute pyelonephritis: a family study of urinary tract infection, *J Infect Dis* 195(8):1227–1234, 2007.

31. Czaja CA, et al: Population-based epidemiologic analysis of acute pyelonephritis, *Clin Infect Dis* 45(3):273–280, 2007.

32. Mathew JL: Antibiotic prophylaxis following urinary tract infection in children: a systematic review of randomized controlled trials, *Indian Pediatr* 47:599–605, 2010.

33. Wagenlehner FM, et al: Therapeutic challenges of urosepsis, *Eur J Clin Invest* 38:45–49, 2008.

34. Tolkoff-Rubin NE, Cotran RS, et al: Urinary tract infection, pyelonephritis, and reflex nephropathy. In Brenner BM, Levine SA, editors: *Bremmer and Rector's the kidney*, ed 8, Philadelphia, 2008, Saunders.

35. Porter RS, Kaplam JL: *The Merck manual*, ed 19, Whitehouse Station, NJ, 2011, Merck Sharp & Dohme.

36. Moe OW: Kidney stones: pathophysiology and medical management, *Lancet* 367:333–344, 2006.

37. Pearle MS, Lotan Y: Urinary lithiasis: etiology, epidemiology, and pathogenesis. In Wein JA, et al, editors: *Campbell-Walsh urology*, ed 9, Philadelphia, 2007, Saunders, pp 1363–1373.

38. Evan AP: Physiopathology and etiology of stone formation in the kidney and the urinary tract, *Pediatr Nephrol* 25:831–841, 2010.

39. Samplaski MK: Less invasive ways to remove stones from the kidneys and ureters, *Cleve Clin J Med* 76:592–598, 2009.

40. Guyton AC, Hall JE: *Textbook of medical physiology*, ed 12, Philadelphia, 2011, Saunders.

41. Johri N, et al: An update and practical guide to renal stone management, *Nephron Clin Pract* 116:159–171, 2010.

42. Hoppe B, Kemper MJ: Diagnostic examination of the child with urolithiasis and nephrocalcinosis, *Pediatr Nephrol* 25:403–413, 2010.

43. Hall PM: Nephrolithiasis: treatment, causes and prevention, *Cleve Clin J Med* 76:583–591, 2009.

44. Wiggins RC: The spectrum of podocytopathies: a unifying view of glomerular diseases, *Kidney Int* 71:1205–1214, 2007.

45. Chadban RC, Atkins RC: Glomerulonephritis, *Lancet* 365:1797–1806, 2005.

46. Davidson A, Aranow C: Pathogenesis and treatment of systemic lupus erythematosus nephritis, *Curr Opin Rheumatol* 18(5):468–475, 2006.

47. Reidy K, Kaskel FJ: Pathophysiology of focal segmental glomerulosclerosis, *Pediatr Nephrol* 22:350–354, 2007.

48. Glick AM: Focal segmental glomerulosclerosis: a case study with review of pathophysiology, *Nephrol Nurs J* 34(2):176–182, 2007.

49. Ronco P, Debiec H: New insights into the pathogenesis of membranous glomerulonephritis, *Curr Opin Nephrol Hypertens* 15:258–263, 2006.

50. Zhou Y, et al: Steroids in the treatment of IgA nephropathy to the improvement of renal survival: a systematic review and meta analysis, *PLoS*, published online 4/12/11, doi:10.1371/journal.pone.0018788.

51. Rodriguez-Iturbe B, Batsford S: Pathogenesis of poststreptococcal glomerulonephritis a century after Clemens von Pirquet, *Kidney Int* 71:1094–1104, 2007.

52. Seigneux S: Management of patients with nephrotic syndrome, *Swiss Med Wkly* 139:416–422, 2009.

53. Kodner C: Nephrotic syndrome in adults: diagnosis and management, *Am Fam Physician* 80:1129–1140, 2009.

54. Hinkes BG, et al: Nephrotic syndrome in the first year of life: two thirds of cases are caused by mutations in 4 genes *(NPHS1, NPHS2, WT1, and LAMB2)*, *Pediatrics* 119:907–919, 2007.

55. Waldman M, Austin HA: Controversies in the treatment of idiopathic membranous nephropathy, *Nat Rev Nephrol* 5:469–479, 2009.

56. Borges FF, et al: Is focal segmental glomerulosclerosis increasing in patients with nephrotic syndrome? *Pediatr Nephrol* 22:1309–1313, 2007.

Acute Kidney Injury and Chronic Kidney Disease

Robin Y. Beeman and Roberta J. Emerson

⊖volve WEBSITE

http://evolve.elsevier.com/Copstead/

- Review Questions and Answers
- Glossary (with audio pronunciations for selected terms)
- Animations

- Case Studies
- Key Points Review

KEY QUESTIONS

- How do the prerenal, intrinsic, and postrenal types of acute kidney injury differ in etiology, prognosis, clinical manifestations, and management?
- What are the characteristic clinical and laboratory findings in each of the three stages of acute tubular necrosis (acute intrarenal renal failure)?
- What is the relationship between the degree of nephron loss, reductions in glomerular filtration rate, and the stages of chronic kidney disease?

- What are the similarities and differences between acute kidney injury and end-stage chronic kidney disease?
- What are the characteristic findings of uremic syndrome?
- How can acute kidney injury be prevented, and how is it treated?
- How is the progression of chronic kidney disease retarded?
- How is end-stage renal disease treated?

CHAPTER OUTLINE

The kidneys have a number of regulatory roles within the body.[1] These key functions include the regulation of body fluid volume and osmolality, electrolyte balance, and acid-base balance. Additionally, the kidneys produce and secrete hormones, and excrete metabolic waste products and foreign materials.[1] When the kidneys are unable to carry out these functions on a temporary or permanent basis, the ramifications are significant to each body system.

ACUTE KIDNEY INJURY

Acute kidney injury (AKI), formerly known as acute renal failure (ARF), represents a broad spectrum of kidney diseases ranging from minor changes in renal function to complete renal failure requiring renal replacement therapy.[2-5] Acute kidney injury is the sudden reduction of kidney function causing disruptions in fluid, electrolyte, and acid-base balances; retention of nitrogenous waste products; increased serum creatinine level; and decreased glomerular filtration rate (GFR).[2-4] Classification criteria for AKI have been developed to identify kidney injury and improve patient outcomes. The 5-point system is known as the RIFLE classification system (R = Risk of injury, I = Injury, F = Failure, L = Loss of function, and E = End-stage kidney disease)[2,3] (Table 28-1). The first three stages indicate severity of kidney injury and the last two stages represent patient outcomes. Subsequent to the development of the RIFLE classification, The Acute Kidney Injury Network (AKIN) proposed modifications to the RIFLE criteria, namely, the addition of an absolute increase in serum creatinine concentration of ≥ 0.3 mg/dl and the specification that the reduction in kidney function occur within a 48-hour period.[2]

The incidence of AKI in hospitalized patients ranges from 2% to 7%, with higher rates in elderly patients.[2,3] Despite improvements in treatments, mortality rates range from 40% to 90%.[3] In critical care units, the incidence of AKI reportedly ranges from 1% to 25% with mortality rates between 15% and 60%.[6]

Etiology and Pathophysiology

The risk of developing acute kidney injury is increased by certain preexisting conditions. These comorbidities include preexisting kidney impairment, cardiovascular and peripheral vascular disease, hypertension, diabetes mellitus, heart failure, malignancies, and benign prostatic hypertrophy.[2] Not only are the elderly more likely to have one or more of these conditions, but also aging itself results in changes within the kidney that make it more susceptible to damage. Renal blood flow may drop by 50% between the ages of 20 and 80 and the GFR by about 8 ml/min/1.73 m² per decade after the age of 30.[2,8] These alterations in function increase the risk of AKI and can negatively impact overall prognosis. The aging kidney is less capable of concentrating and diluting urine, conserving sodium, producing prostaglandin, and maintaining renin and aldosterone levels.[2,8] See Chapter 26 for a discussion of the effects of aging on renal function.

Acute loss of renal function is attributed to conditions that affect renal perfusion (prerenal), factors that obstruct urine flow distal to the kidney (postrenal), or circumstances within the kidney blood vessels, tubules, glomeruli, or interstitium (intrinsic).[2,7] These anatomic delineations are broadly seen as the types or causes of AKI, but the specific etiology must also be identified. Determination of the specific etiology as well as the type of AKI is essential for effective management. Box 28-1 shows the types of AKI and some of their etiologies.

Prerenal Kidney Injury

When acute kidney injury develops because of diminished perfusion of the kidney, it is termed *prerenal* kidney injury because the etiology occurs before the kidney itself.[10] As seen in Box 28-1, this can be due to an

TABLE 28-1   RIFLE CLASSIFICATION FOR STAGING ACUTE KIDNEY INJURY

STAGE	GFR CRITERIA	URINE OUTPUT CRITERIA
Risk	Serum creatinine increased ×1.5 or GFR decreased by 25%	Urine output <0.5 ml/kg/hr for 6 hr
Injury	Serum creatinine increased ×2 or GFR decreased by 50%	Urine output <0.5 ml/kg/hr for 12 hr
Failure	Serum creatinine increased ×3 or GFR decreased by 75% or serum creatinine >4 mg/dl with acute rise ≥0.5 mg/dl	Urine output <0.3 ml/kg/hr for 24 hr (oliguria) or anuria for 12 hr
Loss	Persistent acute kidney failure; complete loss of kidney function >4 wk	
End-stage kidney disease	Complete loss of kidney function >3 mo	

From Lewis SL, Dirksen SR, Heitkemper MM, Bucher L, Camera I: *Medical-surgical nursing*, ed 8, St Louis, 2011, Mosby.

absolute or relative decrease in circulating volume, or abnormalities of renal hemodynamics. Actual or relative depletion of volume are the most common etiologies.[27] Fever, vomiting, diarrhea, burns, hemorrhage, and overuse of diuretic therapy produce fluid volume deficits that can lead to prerenal kidney injury. Decreased renal perfusion also results if large volumes of fluid collect in extravascular spaces as in edema (interstitial space) or ascites (peritoneal space). Any number of conditions reduces the ability of the heart to generate a cardiac output sufficient to meet the needs of body organ systems. Even though the kidney receives 20% to 25% of the cardiac output,[7] that volume may be inadequate when the cardiac output is markedly decreased by cardiogenic shock, heart failure, or lethal ventricular dysrhythmias.

Although most patients who develop prerenal kidney injury have an episode of decreased blood pressure that results in decreased perfusion to the kidney, in some cases perfusion drops without the blood pressure falling below normal.[9] These "normotensive" cases of prerenal kidney injury arise in susceptible individuals with very modest reductions in blood pressure who have preexisting impairments in renal autoregulation. Use of nonsteroidal antiinflammatory drugs (NSAIDs), angiotensin-converting enzyme inhibitors (ACEIs), and angiotensin II (AII) receptor blockers is known to interfere with renal vascular autoregulation and can precipitate prerenal kidney injury in certain populations of patients. This includes those who are older than 60 years of age with atherosclerotic cardiovascular disease or have preexisting renal insufficiency (elevated serum creatinine level), heart failure, advanced liver disease, or nephrotic syndrome.[2,9] These drugs cause either vasoconstriction of afferent arterioles (NSAIDs) or vasodilation of efferent arterioles (ACE inhibitors and AII blockers); either of these actions results in a decrease in glomerular perfusion pressure.[2,9] Thrombus, embolus, dissection, or stenosis of the renal arteries will also result in prerenal kidney injury,[2,9] and the risk increases significantly if ACE inhibitors or AII blockers are being used.[2,9]

Prerenal oliguria is the kidney's normal physiologic response to a decrease in perfusion,[7,9] and at least for a time the renal tissue is unharmed. Neurohumoral mechanisms of local autoregulation are activated as the kidneys attempt to autoregulate perfusion and maintain GFR, and systemic mechanisms such as the renin-angiotensin-aldosterone system (RAAS) act to increase the total

BOX 28-1   TYPES OF ACUTE KIDNEY INJURY

Prerenal
- Absolute decrease in circulating volume
  - Hemorrhage
  - Dehydration
  - Burns
- Relative decrease in circulating volume
  - Distributive shock (neurogenic, anaphylactic, septic)
  - Third-spacing and edema
  - Decreased cardiac output
    - Cardiogenic shock
    - Dysrhythmias
    - Cardiac tamponade
    - Heart failure
    - Myocardial infarction
- Primary renal hemodynamic abnormalities
  - Occlusion or stenosis of renal artery*
  - Drug-induced impairment of renal autoregulation in susceptible persons†

Postrenal
- Benign prostatic hyperplasia
- Kinked or obstructed catheters
- Intraabdominal tumors
- Strictures
- Calculi

Intrarenal/Intrinsic
- Tubular (acute tubular necrosis)
  - Ischemic
    - Prolonged prerenal failure
    - Transfusion reactions
    - Rhabdomyolysis
  - Nephrotoxic
    - Prolonged postrenal failure
    - Certain antimicrobials (antibiotics; antifungal and antiviral drugs)
    - Radiographic contrast media
    - Certain cytotoxic chemotherapy agents
    - Recreational drugs (amphetamines, heroin)
    - Environmental agents (heavy metals, carbon tetrachloride, insecticides)
    - Snake and insect venom
- Glomerular
  - Acute glomerulonephritis
- Interstitial
  - Acute allergic interstitial nephritis
  - Acute pyelonephritis
- Vascular
  - Vasculitis
  - Emboli
  - Nephrosclerosis (due to primary hypertension, hypertensive emergencies, and urgency)

*Use of ACE inhibitors or AII receptor blockers increases the risk.
†Preexisting chronic renal insufficiency, cirrhosis, heart failure, or elderly persons (>60 years) with atherosclerotic cardiovascular disease, hypotension, diuretic use, or nephritic syndrome.[11]

circulating volume.[2,7] The sensed decrease in renal blood flow results in a decrease in GFR and urine output. Because of the kidney's ability to tolerate significant reduction in perfusion (as long as it is not greater than 20% to 25% of normal), and as long as the hypoperfusion etiology is identified and corrected, prerenal oliguria will not affect the parenchyma of the kidney.[2,7] Efforts to restore adequate perfusion should be fully effective in restoring normal renal function within 1 to 2 days.[9] In the case of normotensive patients who have impaired perfusion, by far the smallest subset of prerenal kidney injury cases, interventions must be targeted to the specific etiology.[9] Regardless of the etiology, persistent prerenal kidney injury will result in hypoxic renal cells. If hypoxia continues and ischemia lasts more than a few hours, prerenal kidney injury will progress to acute tubular necrosis (intrinsic kidney injury).[7,8]

Postrenal Kidney Injury

Obstruction of the normal outflow of urine from the kidneys can result in postrenal kidney injury.[2,7,8] Box 28-1 lists the most common etiologies of this type of AKI. If only one kidney is affected, the activity of the remaining kidney will increase to maintain fluid and electrolyte balance.[2,7] Obstruction of the renal pelvis or ureters of both kidneys, of the bladder outlet, or of the urethra will result in discernible postrenal kidney disease. This type of AKI is the least common and the most amenable to intervention. Normalization of renal function depends on the length of time the obstruction persists.[7] Should obstruction persist, the increasing retrograde pressure of urine will result in acute tubular necrosis (intrinsic AKI), and if the obstruction continues over several days or weeks, irreversible damage to the kidney will result.[7,8]

Intrinsic/Intrarenal Kidney Injury

AKI intrinsic to the kidney itself is further classified by the specific anatomic area involved: vascular, interstitial, glomerular, or tubular[2]

(see Box 28-1). Some references incorporate the vascular and tubular classifications together because damage to one ultimately leads to damage of the other.[7] All of these etiologies are capable of producing the potentially reversible rapid decline in renal function that is AKI. When the small vessels within the kidney are inflamed, obstructed, or damaged by an acute hypertensive episode, the injury may be sufficient to impair nephron functioning. Acute glomerulonephritis is due to an abnormal immune reaction, whereby immune complexes are deposited in the basement membrane of the glomerulus, thereby damaging the glomeruli.[7] Normal renal function is disrupted to some degree during this acute inflammatory process, usually lasting about 2 weeks. Acute glomerulonephritis is discussed in detail in Chapter 27. Inflammation of interstitial tissues may be sufficient to result in intrinsic kidney injury. This is usually due to an infection of the kidney (pyelonephritis), an allergic reaction to medications, or an autoimmune disease.[2,5] Long-standing pyelonephritis causes damage to the renal medulla and progressive loss of functional renal tissue.[7]

By far the most common cause of intrinsic kidney injury is acute tubular necrosis (ATN), which itself has many potential etiologies.[2,7] Acute tubular necrosis is the result of tubular cell injury, primarily attributable to ischemia or exposure to nephrotoxic substances. Acute tubular necrosis accounts for nearly half of all cases of AKI in hospitalized patients. Sepsis is the most common cause of ischemic ATN and may develop in about 50% of critically ill patients. It causes vasodilation leading to hypoperfusion within the kidney.[10] In the elderly, about 30% of ischemic cases are due to sepsis and another third are due to surgical interventions.[2] Prolonged prerenal kidney injury, perioperative and postoperative hypotension, hemorrhage, gastrointestinal drainage, and preoperative cardiac complications also contribute to many case of ATN.[2]

The list of medications and chemicals toxic to the kidney is expansive,[2,7] each one inducing a specific toxic reaction in the tubular cells and causing the death of many of them.[7] Of all of these nephrotoxins, contrast medium is the most common offending agent.[2,7] Contrast-induced AKI (also known as contrast-induced nephropathy) is a major cause of AKI in hospitalized elderly patients, and can develop within 12 to 24 hours of contrast administration.[10] Risk factors for developing contrast-induced AKI are underlying kidney insufficiency, age greater than 70, volume depletion, repeated exposures to contrast media in a short time, and coexisting heart failure or diabetes mellitus.[10] Prevention is aimed at avoidance of unnecessary contrast administration to high-risk patients, avoidance of multiple procedures over a 24- to 48-hour period, and adequate administration of hypotonic and isotonic intravenous (IV) fluids before and after contrast administration.[2,10] ATN caused by contrast media results in prolonged hospitalization, increased health care costs, and an increased risk of death.[37] Other nephrotoxic agents include commonly used medications such as aminoglycosides, NSAIDs, amphotericin B, cisplatin, and tetracycline.[2,7,10]

In ATN, there are two pathophysiologic processes that result in the rapid decrease in glomerular filtration rate: a vascular process and a tubular process.[11] The two processes are interrelated, and the severity of one contributes to the severity of the other. Renal blood flow is decreased by 30% to 50% in ATN, and blood is shunted from the medulla to the cortex, further compromising the medullary cells.[11,12] Local vasoconstrictors such as prostaglandins and leukotrienes are released, and the effects of sympathetic nervous system (SNS) stimulation contribute further to the vasoconstriction.[12] Hypoxia or direct tubular damage, attributable to toxins, initiates an inflammatory response, activating the cascade of inflammatory mediators. When perfusion is restored, more inflammatory cells are enlisted and reperfusion injury perpetuates damage in some areas. Cells in part of the proximal tubule and outer cortex begin the repair process when perfusion is returned, but endothelial cells and those in the ascending limb continue to be injured, become necrosed, and commit apoptosis, resulting in a further decline in GFR.[11,12]

The pathogenesis of the tubular process is a reflection of the ischemia[11] and the inflammatory process (Figure 28-1). Damaged tubular epithelial cells, both viable and nonviable, are shed from the basement membrane and accumulate in the tubular filtrate, where they obstruct filtrate flow.[7,11] These cells combine with inflammatory cells and debris to form casts that contribute further to the urinary obstruction.[11] Obstructed urinary flow produces an increased pressure within the nephron that is communicated backwards to the glomerulus, further reducing the GFR. The increasing pressure generated by the tubular obstruction forces filtrate through the partially denuded tubular basement membrane into the interstitial space and even into the bloodstream, a process known as *tubular backleak*.[10] Half of the already limited quantity of glomerular filtrate may be lost to the interstitium by this process.

Recovery following ATN is highly dependent on the extent of injury and slower than in the other two types of AKI.[7,12] If sufficient destruction of the basement membrane occurs, there may be no recovery and the patient develops end-stage renal disease, the final stage of chronic kidney disease. But the tubules can repair themselves within 10 to 20 days when the basement membrane is intact and new epithelial cells are produced on that surface.[7] As with the other types of renal failure, the clinical presentation of ATN is primarily a reflection of the loss of the normal functions performed by the kidney.

Clinical Presentation of Acute Tubular Necrosis

Prerenal kidney injury can be reversed if treated before perfusion drops to below 20% of normal and ischemia occurs.[7] It is at this point that ATN develops. Prerenal or postrenal kidney injury will ultimately progress to intrinsic kidney injury if not corrected within a few hours.[7] The course of ATN is roughly divided into three phases, and the clinical presentation varies with the phase[16] (Figure 28-2). The laboratory findings that differentiate prerenal from intrinsic kidney injury are shown in Table 28-2. Table 28-3 provides the laboratory profile associated with renal failure; some of these findings are more likely to be noted in end-stage renal disease than in AKI. Though serum creatinine

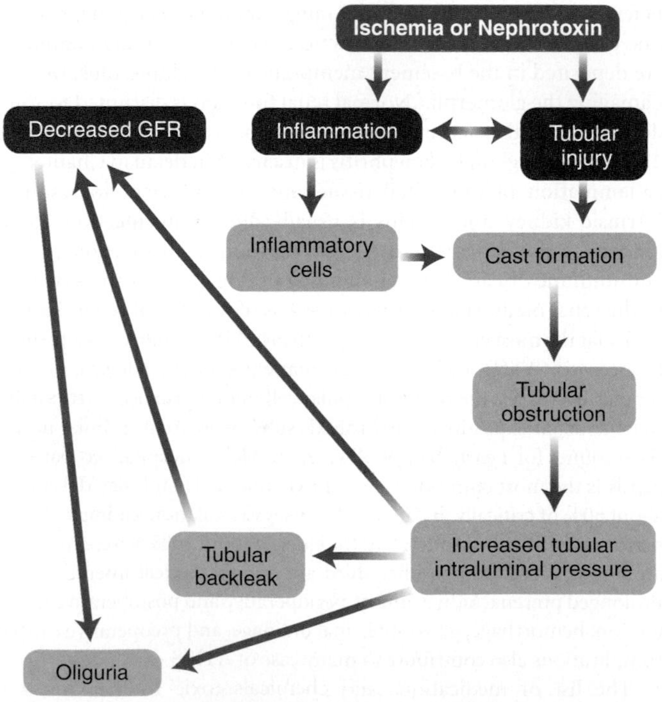

FIGURE 28-1 Pathogenesis of acute tubular necrosis.

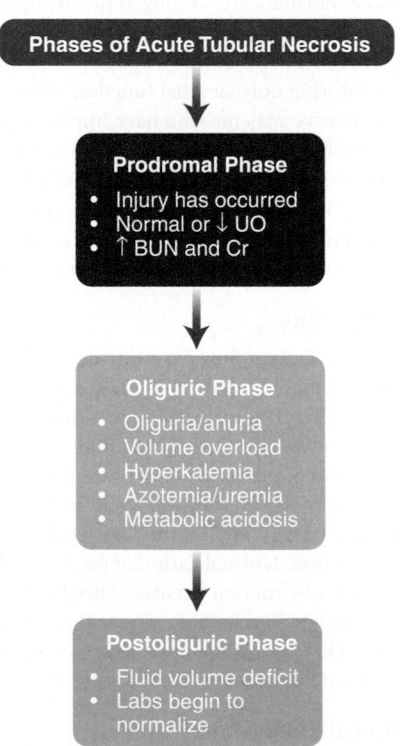

FIGURE 28-2 Phases of acute tubular necrosis and primary clinical issues. *BUN,* Blood urea nitrogen; *Cr,* creatinine; *UO,* urine output.

TABLE 28-2 LABORATORY VALUE DIFFERENCES IN PRERENAL AND INTRINSIC AKI

LABORATORY TEST	PRERENAL FINDINGS	INTRARENAL FINDINGS
FENa %	<1	>2
Proteinuria	Absent	Possible
Urine specific gravity	>1.020	1.010-1.020
Urine osmolality (mOsm/kg)	>500	300-500
BUN/creatinine ratio	>20:1	10-20:1
Urine sodium concentration (mmol/L)	<10	>20
Urinary sediment	Few hyaline casts	Tubular, RBC, and WBC casts

*Derived from Gammill HS, Jeyabalan A: Acute renal failure in pregnancy, *Crit Care Med* 33(10):S372-S384, 2005; Needham E: Management of acute renal failure, *Am Fam Physician* 72(9):1739-1746, 2005; Lameire N, Van Biesen W, Vanholder R: Acute renal failure, *Lancet* 365:417-430, 2005. *AKI*, Acute kidney injury; *FENa %*, fraction of excreted sodium, percent.

TABLE 28-3 LABORATORY PROFILE FOR RENAL DISEASE

TEST	NORMAL RANGE FOR ADULTS	VALUES IN RENAL DISEASE	COMMENTS
Test to Evaluate Removal of Nitrogenous Wastes			
Serum creatinine	*Male:* 0.6-1.2 mg/dl *Female:* 0.5-1.1 mg/dl *Older adults:* Decreased	**In Chronic Kidney Disease** May increase by 0.5-1.0 mg/dl every 1-2 yr May be as high as 15-30 mg/dl *before* symptoms of CKD are present **In Acute Kidney Injury** Gradual increase of 1-2 mg/dl every 24-48 hr May increase 1-6 mg/dl in 1 wk or less	Consistently elevated levels indicate decreased renal function. Serum creatinine levels are used to evaluate effectiveness of dialysis treatments.
Blood urea nitrogen	10-20 mg/dl *Older adults:* May be slightly increased	**In Chronic Kidney Disease** May reach 180-200 mg/dl *before* symptoms develop **In Acute Kidney Injury** Often increases by 1-20 mg/dl at same pace as serum creatinine level May reach 80-100 mg/dl within 1 wk	Increases depend on protein intake and other factors. Rate of increase is controlled by limiting protein intake. This intervention is believed to decrease the rate of onset of systemic symptoms, such as anorexia, nausea, and vomiting. Elevations have multiple causes, including diminished renal function, excessive protein intake, sepsis, GI bleeding, dehydration, and tissue catabolism.
Electrolyte Studies			
Serum sodium	136-145 mEq/L; 136-145 mmol/L (SI units)	Normal or decreased	Clients with renal disease retain sodium. With associated water retention, serum sodium levels seem normal. With excessive water retention, serum sodium levels seem decreased owing to hemodilution. Assess client for evidence of fluid volume excess: edema, weight increase, or elevation of diastolic blood pressure. Limit fluid intake as directed. Avoid excessive sodium intake. Monitor for signs of hypernatremia: dry skin, excessive thirst, dry mucous membranes, elevated body temperature, and flushed skin. Client may need diuretics or dialysis.
Serum potassium	3.5-5.0 mmol/L (SI units)	Increased	Advise client to avoid salt substitutes and to limit potassium-containing foods. Monitor for rapidly increasing serum potassium levels in AKI. ECG changes occur with serum potassium levels ≥6.5. Monitor for signs of hyperkalemia: dizziness, weakness, cardiac irregularities, muscle cramps, diarrhea, and nausea. May require administration of sodium polystyrene sulfonate (Kayexalate) or other treatment.

Continued

TABLE 28-3 LABORATORY PROFILE FOR RENAL DISEASE—cont'd

TEST	NORMAL RANGE FOR ADULTS	VALUES IN RENAL DISEASE	COMMENTS
Serum phosphorus (phosphate)	3.0-4.5 mg/dl, 0.97-1.45 mmol/L (SI units) *Older adults:* May be slightly decreased	Increased	Short-term increases have potential to cause rapid decrease in serum calcium level and cardiac rhythm disturbances. Long-term increases demineralize bones of calcium and enhance fracture potential. Phosphate-binding medications help control hyperphosphatemia and prevent calcium depletion from bones.
Serum calcium	Total calcium: 9.0-10.5 mg/dl; 2.25-2.75 mmol/L (SI units) Ionized calcium: 4.5-5.6 mg/dl; 1.05-1.3 mmol/L (SI units) *Older adults:* Slightly decreased	Decreased	Decreases in AKI may necessitate replacement. Decreases in CRF may only be slight and may or may not necessitate replacement. As serum phosphate level increases, serum calcium level decreases. Chronic calcium deficiency leads to renal osteodystrophy. Control of phosphate excess is usually essential before calcium replacement is initiated. Monitor for manifestations of hypocalcemia: abdominal cramps, hyperactive reflexes, tingling fingertips, and spasms in feet and wrists.
Serum magnesium	1.3-2.1 mEq/L; 0.65-1.05 mmol/L (SI units)	Increased	Advise patient to avoid compounds containing magnesium (e.g., laxatives).
Serum bicarbonate	23-30 mEq/L (venous); 23-30 mmol/L (SI units)	Decreased	Replace bicarbonate. Monitor respiratory rate and depth. Monitor for decreased orientation.
Arterial blood pH	7.35-7.45	Decreased (in metabolic acidosis) or normal	Respiratory system attempts to compensate by hyperventilation (increased rate and depth of respiration). Values are within normal range if blood buffers and lungs can compensate. Monitor breathing rate and depth. Monitor level of consciousness.
Arterial blood bicarbonate (HCO_3^-)	21-38 mEq/L	Decreased	Provide replacement oral, IV, or by hemodialysis or peritoneal dialysis.
Arterial blood ($Paco_2$)	35-45 mm Hg	Decreased	Monitor for respiratory fatigue (client breathes more rapidly and deeply to "blow off" carbon dioxide).
Other Blood Studies			
Hemoglobin	*Female:* 12-16 g/dl, 7.4-9.9 mmol/L (SI units) *Male:* 14-18 g/dl, 8.7-11.2 mmol/L (SI units) *Older adults:* Slightly decreased	Decreased	Decreased levels indicate anemia. Monitor for pallor, weakness, lethargy, dizziness, possible shortness of breath, and activity intolerance.
Hematocrit	*Female:* 37-47% *Male:* 42-52% *Older adults:* May be slightly decreased	Decreased to 20%	Same as for hemoglobin. With erythropoietin therapy, may be able to obtain levels as high as 36%.
Urinalysis*			
Specific gravity	Usually 1.010-1.025 Possible range: 1.005-1.030	Usually decreased and fixed	Reflects inability of tubules to produce concentrated or diluted urine in response to changes in plasma osmolarity. Monitor for fluid volume deficit or excess.
pH	Average: 5.5-6 Possible range: 4.6-8	May be fixed; pH does not change with dietary changes	Collect a freshly voided specimen for testing.
Glucose	None or <15 mg/dl Usually detectable in urine of nondiabetic clients when blood level is 160-180 mg/dl	Increased	Renal threshold is often increased; therefore blood glucose level may be >160-180 mg/dl before glucose is detectable in urine. Monitor *blood* glucose levels.

TABLE 28-3   LABORATORY PROFILE FOR RENAL DISEASE—cont'd

TEST	NORMAL RANGE FOR ADULTS	VALUES IN RENAL DISEASE	COMMENTS
Protein	0-8 mg/dl	Increased when there is glomerular damage or disease	Increases may be an incidental and benign finding. Transient increases occur with extreme exercise, fever, stress, or infection. Persistent proteinuria requires 24-hr collection for determination of total quantity excreted. Persistent proteinuria may indicate a serious renal problem. Instruct client about need for follow-up. Instruct client in correct procedure for collection of 24-hr specimen.
Occult blood	No RBCs or occasionally 2 or 3 RBCs per HPF No hemoglobin	More than 2 or 3 RBCs per HPF Detectable hemoglobin	Hemoglobin is detectable when hemolysis of RBCs has occurred. Intact RBCs are detectable only with microscopic examination. Collect a freshly voided specimen for testing.
WBCs	0-5 per HPF	Increased in urinary tract infection	Often indicates need for urine culture.
Bacteria	Fewer than 1000 colonies/ml	Increased in presence of infection, with or without an increase in WBCs	Obtain urine culture.
Casts	None or a few; composed of RBCs, WBCs, protein, or tubular cell casts such as hyaline	Casts present	Casts may be a benign occurrence or may signify that some renal injury or disease is present. Collect a freshly voided specimen for direct microscopic examination.
Creatinine clearance	*Male:* 107-109 ml/min *Female:* 87-107 ml/min *Older adults:* Progressively decreased with advancing age	Decreased	Change reflects decreases in GFR. Creatinine clearance is determined from a 24-hr urine collection and a serum creatinine value.

Adapted from Ignatavicius DD, Workman ML: *Medical-surgical nursing: critical thinking for collaborative care,* ed 5, Philadelphia, 2006, Saunders, pp 1733-1735.
AKI, Acute kidney injury; *CKD,* chronic kidney disease; *CRF,* chronic renal failure; *ECG,* electrocardiogram; *GFR,* glomerular filtration rate; *GI,* gastrointestinal; *HPF,* high-power field; *IV,* intravenous; *RBCs,* red blood cells; *SI,* Système International d'Unités; *WBCs,* white blood cells.
*Urine may become cloudy with heavy sediment. Urine output and appearance vary, depending on remaining renal function.

levels begin to increase within 12 hours to 2 days after injury,[3] new biomarkers are being investigated to detect AKI earlier than the rise in serum creatinine level, with the promise of leading to earlier detection and treatment. Examples of these new biomarkers currently being tested are interleukin-18, neutrophil gelatinase-associated lipocalin, and kidney injury molecule-1.[3,17] As with other aspects of the clinical presentation, laboratory findings are affected by the phase of ATN. Although the naming of the phases of AKI varies among resources, the clinical progression of ATN is consistent.

Prodromal Phase

Patients during this phase will typically have a normal or declining urine output. Serum blood urea nitrogen (BUN) and creatinine levels begin to rise.[10] The insult to the kidney has occurred and the duration of this phase will vary depending on the cause of the injury, the amount of the toxin ingested, or the duration and severity of the hypotension.[16]

Oliguric Phase

Most patients with ATN develop oliguria, though some will remain nonoliguric.[16] Those with severe injury often become anuric.[7,11,13] Renal function is monitored according to fluctuations in the serum creatinine level and the calculated GFR that is derived from it.[15] As urine output drops, metabolic waste products are retained and fluid and

electrolyte balance is disrupted.[7] These alterations are reflected in the physical assessment and laboratory data. Because it cannot be excreted, body water is retained. This hypervolemia results in the development of edema and hypertension.[7] Other signs and symptoms of fluid volume overload include distended neck veins (jugular venous distention [JVD]), weight gain, crackles, and possibly additional manifestations of heart failure.[16] Normally, as renal perfusion is reduced, the kidney responds by increasing the reabsorption of sodium and reducing its elimination. In ATN, this mechanism is impaired and sodium is lost in the reduced volume of urine that is produced.[16] Tubular casts are present in the urine, and white blood cells, red blood cells, and protein are also likely to appear.[8] Other electrolytes are typically retained in the blood (potassium, magnesium, and phosphorus) and their levels in the urine are decreased (see Table 28-3). Of all the potential electrolyte problems, hyperkalemia is of greatest concern because the normal range is narrow (3.5 to 5 mEq/L) and levels of less than double the normal values can be fatal.[7] Metabolic acidosis develops as a result of the kidney's decreased ability to excrete hydrogen ions (acid load).[7] The hydrogen ions shift into the cells in exchange for intracellular potassium. Thus hyperkalemia and metabolic acidosis often occur together. Changes in the levels of other electrolytes may not be seen unless the oliguric phase is prolonged. Anorexia, nausea, vomiting, weakness, seizures, acidosis, confusion, and coma are also possible.[16] Although these

TABLE 28-4 PATHOPHYSIOLOGY OF MANIFESTATIONS OF UREMIC SYNDROME

SYSTEM	MANIFESTATION	PATHOPHYSIOLOGIC BASIS
Central nervous system	Uremic encephalopathy	Brain cells shrink because of osmotic gradient
	• Disorientation	
	• Lethargy	
	• Coma	
Peripheral nervous system	Motor neuropathies	Toxin interference with nerve transmission
	• Weakness	
	Sensory neuropathies	
	• Numbness	
	• Tingling	
Cardiovascular system	Bleeding	Decreased platelet function and coagulation factor production
	Anemia	Decreased RBC life span; blood loss
	Decreased cardiac output	Negative inotropic effect
	Ischemic syndromes	Escalated coronary heart disease
	Pericarditis*	Uremic crystals deposited in pericardium
Immune system	Infections	Decreased immune cell production and immune response
Gastrointestinal system	Anorexia	Direct effect of toxins
	Nausea and vomiting	
Integumentary system	Impaired healing*	Decreased collagen production
	Pruritus; dermatitis*	Deposition of uremic crystals on skin
	Uremic frost*	
Acid-base balance	Metabolic acidosis	Accumulation of acidic metabolic wastes

*More likely to occur with chronic kidney injury.

manifestations are classically much more severe in end-stage renal disease, there is no identifiable point at which uremia presents, so some symptoms may be present in AKI. A GFR that is only slightly less than 50% of the normal for age may produce mild manifestations.[14]

As the GFR drops, organic metabolic waste products are retained. Urea represents the largest amount of these wastes. Other uremic solutes involved have been found to be responsible for many of the signs and symptoms that collectively are called uremic syndrome[14] (Table 28-4). This phase typically lasts 10 to 14 days, but can range from 1 day to 8 weeks. Development of uremia in AKI necessitates temporarily replacing renal function with dialysis. Nonoliguric patients have lower mortality and morbidity and less need for dialysis.[16]

Postoliguric Phase

Termination of the oliguric phase is marked by the beginning of renal recovery. The urine output gradually returns to normal.[16] Unfortunately, not all patients recover. In about 5% of cases, AKI is not reversible.[11] In the elderly, 31% of those with AKI may not regain renal function.[2] Tubular dysfunction may continue and is manifested by polyuria and sodium wasting, as well as depletion of electrolytes (especially potassium) previously retained.[16] Typically, urine output is more than 1 L per day, and may be as much as 4 to 5 L, causing a fluid volume deficit if fluids are not rapidly replaced. The elevated BUN level contributes to an osmotic diuresis, as the large molecules are filtered and draw more water into the tubules. Renal perfusion begins to increase, slowly advancing filtration ability and tubular function.

If full recovery of renal function does occur, it may take only 1 week but more often requires as much as 1 year. Full recovery is indicated when the serum creatinine level returns to within the normal range. This variation in recovery time is due to the diversity of ATN causes and degree of damage as well as the quality of interventions provided and patients' concomitant conditions. Even after recovery, progressive loss of renal function following AKI is a frequent finding, especially in pediatric cases. The loss of renal function following AKI in childhood has been found to result in progressive deterioration by adolescence or early adulthood.[11]

KEY POINTS

- AKI is an abrupt reduction in renal function producing an accumulation of waste materials in the blood. Oliguria is usually present. AKI is classified into three types according to the site of disruption: prerenal, postrenal, and intrinsic. Distinction between the types of AKI is necessary to determine appropriate therapy.

- Prerenal kidney injury is due to conditions that impair renal blood flow, such as hypovolemia, hypotension, cardiac failure, and renal artery obstruction. It is characterized by clinical manifestations of a low GFR, usually including oliguria, high urine specific gravity and osmolality, and low urinary sodium concentration. Signs and symptoms of fluid volume overload are present. Prolonged prerenal kidney injury results in intrinsic kidney injury.

- Postrenal kidney injury is due to obstruction within the urinary collecting system distal to the kidney. Obstruction results in elevated pressure in Bowman capsule, which impedes glomerular filtration. Clinical findings vary, based on the duration of the obstruction. Prolonged postrenal kidney injury results in intrinsic kidney injury.

- Intrinsic failure is due to a primary dysfunction of the nephrons. Although it may be due to glomerular, vascular, or interstitial etiologies, most often the problem is within the renal tubules, resulting in ATN. ATN may occur with nephrotoxic or ischemic insults. Clinical manifestations depend upon the phase of ATN.

- ATN has three characteristic phases. The first phase, prodromal, is characterized by normal or declining urine output and varies in duration depending on the causative factors. The oliguric phase may last up to 8 weeks with a usual urine output of 50 to 400 ml/day. Retention of nitrogenous wastes and certain electrolytes is likely. Fluid volume excess is expected. During the postoliguric phase, diuresis occurs, tubular function remains impaired, and azotemia continues. Fluid volume deficit is characteristic until the kidneys gradually recover. Recovery can last up to 12 months, and is characterized by gradual normalization of serum creatinine and BUN levels. Often a degree of renal insufficiency persists.

- AKI results in characteristic alterations in laboratory tests of the blood and urine. Renal function is monitored by serum creatinine level and calculated GFR. The retention of metabolic wastes (azotemia/uremia), which is monitored by the BUN level, produces widespread systemic effects (uremic syndrome).

BOX 28-2 RISK FACTORS FOR CHRONIC KIDNEY DISEASE

- Acute tubular necrosis (not progressing beyond the oliguric stage)
- Developmental/congenital conditions
  - Renal agenesis
  - Aplastic kidneys
  - Renal hypoplasia
  - Ectopic/displaced kidneys
  - Fused kidneys
- Cystic disorders
  - Polycystic kidney disease
  - Medullary cystic disease
- Neoplasms
  - Benign tumors of the kidney
  - Malignant tumors of the kidney (including Wilms tumor)
- Infections
  - Recurrent pyelonephritis
  - Renal tuberculosis
- Glomerulonephritis
- Systemic conditions
  - Diabetes mellitus*
  - Diabetes insipidus
  - Hypertension*
  - Hyperparathyroidism
  - Liver failure/cirrhosis
  - Gout
  - Amyloidosis
  - Scleroderma
  - Goodpasture syndrome
  - Systemic lupus erythematosus (produces glomerulonephritis)
- Other
  - Genetics
  - Increasing age
  - Race (blacks)
  - Overweight/obesity
  - Dyslipidemia
  - Family history of cardiovascular disease
  - Smoking

*Most common risk factors.

CHRONIC KIDNEY DISEASE

Chronic renal failure is the outcome of the progressive and irrevocable loss of nephrons.[7,16] The normal resiliency of the kidney means that more than 75% of the total number of nephrons must be lost before clinical manifestations appear.[7] What is termed *chronic renal failure* is the final outcome of chronic kidney disease (CKD). More commonly, this point is called *end-stage renal disease* (ESRD) in acknowledgment of the progressive process of deterioration of renal function. At some point in the CKD process, renal disease will proceed to ESRD progressively, irreversibly, and to the point where renal dialysis or transplantation is required for survival.[17-24]

Chronic kidney disease is a global health problem. Historically, the majority of the overall morbidity and mortality throughout the world was due to infectious disease. Today, chronic diseases are responsible for most of the world's illness and death.[23] More than 4 million people throughout the world have ESRD[23] and depend on dialysis. Many of them await renal transplantations that may not be available in time to save their lives. Every year, this number increases by nearly 250,000.[23] The highest incidence of untreated ESRD is found in North America, Japan, and Europe.[23] More than 20 million people ages 20 years and older in the United States have CKD, whereas another 547,982 people are being treated for ESRD.[18,19,21] Because of the rapidly escalating incidence of the two primary risk factors, diabetes and hypertension, the number of people afflicted with CKD is likely to increase in the years to come.[7,19]

Risk Factors

Chronic kidney disease is defined as either decreased kidney function or kidney damage of 3 months' or more duration based on blood tests, urinalysis, and imaging studies.[20,25] Alternatively, it may be defined as a glomerular filtration rate (GFR) <60 ml/min/1.73 m^2 for 3 months with or without indication of damage to the kidney.[25,26] CKD is a syndrome in that it can occur as a complication of many other conditions, such as diabetes and hypertension. This means that the etiologies and/or risk factors of these conditions are also risk factors for the development of CKD. Although some of the conditions and risk factors have been identified for many years, new research findings have added to the list and altered perceptions of their relative importance (Box 28-2).

In 2008 diabetes and hypertension accounted for more than 50% of the individuals in the United States with ESRD, followed by glomerulonephritis and cystic kidney disease.[19] Type 2 diabetes is projected to double in incidence worldwide within the next 25 years. Diabetic nephropathy is a major complication of that disease. Of those who develop diabetic nephropathy, about 30% ultimately progress to ESRD whereas the remainder most often die from cardiovascular disease before reaching that point.[20]

Hypertension is another major risk factor for CKD, and it also develops as a complication of it.[25] The majority of patients (70% to 80%) with CKD have hypertension, climbing to 90% in those treated with dialysis.[27,28] The aging of the population in the United States is predicted to escalate the incidence of systolic hypertension and resulting renal disease.[22,25] Some of the risk factors for CKD are not amenable to modification. These include a family history of CKD, a history of exposure to toxins (heavy metals, tobacco smoke, radiopaque dyes), age greater than 65 years, and ethnicity (non-Hispanic black, non-Hispanic white, and Mexican American).[26] It has been recommended that high-risk groups be screened for CKD (those with family histories, diabetes mellitus, hypertension, recurrent urinary tract infections, urinary obstructions, or other systemic conditions affecting the kidney) and that screening be extended to those without any other identified risks other than being older than age 65.[7,29] Research is under way to identify genes associated with CKD and diabetic nephropathy as well as biomarkers to assess for risk and likelihood of a positive response to treatment.[30]

Pathophysiology of Progression of Chronic Kidney Disease

Regardless of the origin of CKD, the decline in renal function is progressive and irreversible. The damaged nephrons are unable to function properly. The remaining nephrons initially compensate by enlarging and increasing their clearance capacity. Through this process, renal function remains relatively normal until 75% to 80% of the nephrons are damaged and nonfunctional. Over the course of several years, these compensatory changes may cause further injury to the remaining nephrons. Although the cause of this additional injury is unknown, some investigators believe that the increased workload of the remaining glomeruli and small arterioles may cause sclerosis of these vessels

TABLE 28-5 STAGES OF CHRONIC KIDNEY DISEASE ACCORDING TO NEPHRON LOSS AND CLINICAL PRESENTATION

STAGE	% NEPHRON LOSS	CLINICAL PRESENTATION
Decreased renal reserve	<75%	No signs or symptoms BUN and creatinine normal May not be diagnosed
Renal insufficiency	75-90%	Polyuria, nocturia Slight elevation in BUN and creatinine May be controlled by diet and medication
End-stage renal disease	>90%	Azotemia/uremia Fluid and electrolyte abnormalities Osteodystrophy Anemia Dialysis or transplantation essential

TABLE 28-6 STAGES OF CHRONIC KIDNEY DISEASE ACCORDING TO GLOMERULAR FILTRATION RATE*

STAGE	DESCRIPTION
Stage 1	Kidney damage with normal or increased GFR GFR >90 ml/min/1.73 m^2
Stage 2	Mildly decreased GFR GFR 60-89 ml/min/1.73 m^2
Stage 3	Moderately decreased GFR GFR 30-59 ml/min/1.73 m^2
Stage 4	Severely decreased GFR GFR 15-29 ml/min/1.73 m^2
Stage 5	End-stage kidney disease GFR <15 ml/min/1.73 m^2 (or dialysis)

*From National Kidney Foundation: *Kidney disease outcomes quality initiative,* 2002.
GFR, Glomerular filtration rate.

leading to further decline in kidney function and ultimately ESRD.[7] Progression of CKD is monitored by measuring changes in GFR, determining the presence and degree of proteinuria, examining urinary sediment for white or red blood cells, measuring serum creatinine levels, and performing imaging studies with renal ultrasonography to document kidney size.[25]

Stages of Chronic Kidney Disease

The progression of CKD is determined by monitoring GFRs. A five-stage system depicts severity of disease, with decreasing GFRs reflecting a higher stage of progression. The recommendation is that diagnosis of CKD not be based on a specific pathology (e.g., diabetes mellitus), but rather on the presence of damage to the kidney and the level of function according to the GFR measurement as shown in Table 28-5.[25] Screening for the complications of CKD is recommended to begin in stage 3.[31]

In stage 1 of the GFR staging system shown in Table 28-5, patients' blood pressures and laboratory values are usually normal and they are asymptomatic, though they have some form of kidney disease.[31] An initial reduction in GFR with or without documented kidney damage depicts stage 2. This would include, for example, a diabetic patient with proteinuria or an older person with the predictable age-related diminishment of renal function. Again, patients may be asymptomatic without laboratory value changes. The aims in stages 1 and 2 are to identify individuals at risk for progressive renal disease, and reduce those associated risks.

Beginning with stage 3, patients are classified as having chronic kidney disease, according to GFR, regardless of the existence of kidney damage. Although they may be otherwise asymptomatic in stage 3, hypertension is nearly always noted. At stage 4, diagnosis is made because manifestations are usually very apparent with the significant decline in renal function. Planning for ESRD should occur. By stage 5, manifestations of ESRD are present and renal function is so impaired that dialysis or transplantation is required.[31]

The staging system shown in Table 28-6 is useful because the terms *renal insufficiency* and *decreased renal reserve* are commonly used in clinical practice. Decreased renal reserve is not associated with signs or symptoms of renal failure, largely because the remaining nephrons

accommodate the additional workload. Electrolyte and fluid levels are maintained within normal limits.[7] Although not abnormally elevated, creatinine levels are usually at the high end of the normal range—a common finding in the elderly population. Interventions for those at risk for CKD (see Box 28-2) should be initiated to help slow disease progression. At this point, kidney function is already impaired and significant deterioration is possible if the kidney is stressed. There may be small amounts of protein in the urine. The stage of renal insufficiency is reached with further nephron damage. Although electrolyte levels remain within normal limits with the GFR decline, the metabolic wastes (creatinine and urea) are retained at levels proportional to nephron loss.[7] Impairment of the kidney's ability to concentrate the filtrate often results in increased urinary output (polyuria), often leading to nocturia. ESRD develops when more than 90% of the kidneys' nephrons have been destroyed. At this point, the patient typically demonstrates the sequelae and complications of renal failure, seen as laboratory alterations and signs and symptoms associated with the inability of the kidneys to fulfill their multiple roles within the body. Without interventions, when the remaining nephrons number less than 5% to 10% of normal, death is inevitable.[7]

Complications of Chronic Kidney Disease

The consequences of CKD are affected by the intake of food and water and the degree to which renal function is impaired.[7] Some of the complications of CKD begin to appear when the GFR falls below 60 ml/min/1.73 m^2 (stage 3 of the GFR-based classification).[25] Because of the widespread impact of the kidneys on nearly every part of the body, the effects of their failure are seen in every body organ system.[7] Complications impact the gastrointestinal, neurologic, musculoskeletal, dermatologic, cardiovascular, and endocrine systems. Immune function, acid-base regulation, and the coagulation cascade are affected as well. In many cases, complications are interrelated, one contributing to or exacerbating the development of others. Laboratory alterations become significant as CKD progresses; typical values are shown in Table 28-3. Major complications of CKD are discussed in the following sections.

Hypertension and Cardiovascular Disease

Cardiovascular disease and CKD have many risk factors in common: increasing age, black race, hypertension, diabetes mellitus, smoking, decreased GFR, proteinuria, obesity, and RAAS overactivity.[7,32,35] If hypertension was not a precursor to CKD, it inevitably develops with decreasing renal function,[27,28,32] appearing in stage 2 or 3.[31] The excess fluid volume and escalated atherosclerotic process along with heightened RAAS activity and evidence of increased SNS activity are all involved in the development of hypertension in CKD.[32,35] Most people with CKD do not die from kidney failure, but rather from the results of cardiovascular disease, which is both a risk factor for and a complication of CKD.[33,35] The incidence of cardiovascular morbidity and mortality is markedly increased in CKD.[34] In the elderly, death from cardiovascular disease is more common than progression to renal replacement therapy.[34] Although the risk of cardiovascular disease is greatest for those with end-stage disease, it has been found to be an issue at all stages of CKD.[34,35] A clear link exists between deterioration of kidney function and development of cardiovascular disease.[35] Multiple factors have been identified that are conducive to this, including, but not limited to, dyslipidemias, anemia, electrolyte-induced dysrhythmias, hypertension, endothelial dysfunction (including inflammation, alterations in nitric oxide activity, oxidative stress), proteinuria, premature atherosclerosis, activity limitations, and volume overload.[27,35]

Uremic Syndrome

As renal function declines, retention of metabolic wastes increases, creating a toxic environment within the body. Uremia produces signs and symptoms in many body systems (see Table 28-4). Compared to the presentation in AKI, uremic syndrome in CKD is far more severe and its effects are more widespread even though the serum levels often must be much higher for manifestations to be apparent.

Metabolic Acidosis

Normally, the human body produces 50 to 80 more millimoles of acids than bases during daily metabolism.[7] Metabolic acidosis occurs with the retention of acidic waste products of metabolism as part of uremia. It is also produced in association with hyperkalemia, when potassium ions in the blood are exchanged for intracellular hydrogen ions, lowering the pH of the blood (see Chapter 25). The kidneys lose their ability to secrete hydrogen ions or to produce bicarbonate, and with the limited capacity of the other buffers, pH can fall precipitously; coma develops and death will occur if the pH drops below 6.8.[7] Metabolic acidosis depresses cardiac as well as central nervous system function. The respiratory system attempts to compensate for metabolic acidosis by increasing the rate and depth of respirations.

Electrolyte Imbalances

The loss of renal mechanisms involved in electrolyte balance result in the retention of potassium, phosphorus, and magnesium in the blood. Each of these imbalances is associated with specific manifestations (see Chapter 24). Hyperkalemia is of special concern, as discussed with AKI, because it can be responsible for fatal cardiac dysrhythmias. The inability to eliminate phosphorus and the loss of the renal mechanisms involved in maintaining calcium balance result in mineral and bone disorders, which are discussed next.

Mineral and Bone Disorders

The inability of the kidney to excrete phosphorus in CKD results in elevated phosphorous levels in the blood. Because phosphorus and calcium maintain a reciprocal relationship in the body, as hyperphosphatemia develops in CKD, hypocalcemia likewise develops. The body's system of maintaining calcium balance is sophisticated, and involves the activation of parathyroid hormone (PTH) when the calcium level is low. When this occurs because of CKD, the result

is secondary hyperparathyroidism.[36] The normal response to PTH release is the increase in serum calcium levels by (1) increasing reabsorption by the kidney, (2) increasing absorption of dietary calcium, in the presence of vitamin D, which must be activated by the kidney, and (3) mobilizing calcium release from bone.[7,36] Vascular and soft-tissue calcifications as well as osteoporosis are the end results of the prolonged elevation of PTH level and altered bone and mineral metabolism.[36] The resulting bone pain, deformities, and fractures are significant long-term complications of CKD.[24,27,36] Additionally, abnormal PTH, calcium, and phosphorous levels are reported to have been identified as independent risk factors of cardiac-caused mortality during dialysis.[36]

Malnutrition

Protein-energy wasting (PEW) is the loss of muscle and visceral protein stores and is a common finding in advanced CKD.[36] Decreased nutrient intake is due to the anorexia of uremic syndrome, changes in taste sensation, and the depression of chronic illness, as well as the dietary limitations imposed by disease. Additionally, a negative-nitrogen balance exists because of escalated protein catabolism and decreased protein synthesis. Medications and concomitant diseases such as diabetes may cause nausea, vomiting, and slowed gastric emptying. The best serum marker of PEW is albumin level. Hypoalbuminemia in dialysis patients has a strong association with increased mortality and morbidity. However, caution must be used in interpreting these levels, because the serum level may be affected by the inflammatory response. Malnutrition has a negative impact on CKD prognosis.[36]

Anemia

The development of anemia is an anticipated problem as CKD progresses. The production of red blood cells by the bone marrow depends on numerous cofactors; perhaps the most significant of these is erythropoietin, which is produced by the kidneys.[7] Erythropoiesis, with all essential ingredients, requires about 5 days.[39] Lacking erythropoietin, fewer red blood cells are produced and anemia is a persistent problem. The problem is often further escalated by malnutrition, due to nutritional deficits of iron, folate, and vitamin B_{12}. Chronic inflammation and elevations of PTH level suppress bone marrow. At the same time, the uremia associated with CKD produces a toxic environment for red blood cells, reducing their normal life expectancy of 120 days. Blacks appear to have both a greater prevalence of anemia as well as more severe reductions in RBC counts and hemoglobin concentrations. By stage 5 and the initiation of dialysis, approximately 66% of patients have hemoglobin levels <11 g/dl.[39] The cardiovascular compensatory efforts for the chronic anemia of CKD can lead to myocardial dilatation, left ventricular hypertrophy, and remodeling.[27,39] The combination of worsening CKD, anemia, and heart failure is referred to as *cardiorenal anemia syndrome* and becomes a chain of escalating pathologies.[39]

Pain

The causes of pain in kidney disease are multifactorial. Surgery may be needed to create access for dialysis or to biopsy a kidney. Dialysis itself can be a painful experience with frequent needle sticks and accumulation of uremic toxins. The primary cause of kidney disease, such as cystic kidney or diabetes (due to neuropathies or ulcerations), may result in pain. Finally, comorbidities such as gout, bone disease, and peripheral vascular disease may also contribute to pain in the person with CKD.[24] The challenge lies in finding a balance between pain relief and the right analgesic and dose to avoid toxicity and drug-induced nephropathy.[24]

Depression

The prevalence of depression in patients with CKD is reported to be between 20% and 30%.[38] Reasons for depression stem from comorbid conditions as well as the process of kidney disease itself. Many patients with renal disease experience a high rate of cardiovascular events, which are also associated with higher rates of depression. In addition, the disruption of social interactions and relationships, possibly attributable to dialysis and fatigue, contributes to depressive symptoms. In patients with CKD, as in the general population, depression may lead to a decrease in quality of life, functional impairment, and sexual dysfunction.[38]

KEY POINTS

- CKD is characterized by a gradual, irreversible loss of functional nephrons. The two most common causes are diabetes mellitus and hypertension, followed by recurrent pyelonephritis, glomerulonephritis, and polycystic kidney disease.
- Progression of CKD is monitored by a staging system based on increasing severity of disease. There are five stages of CKD progression and with each higher stage, the GFR and kidney function decline. In stage 1, kidney function may be normal, though some disease exists. The patient is asymptomatic. The focus in stages 1 and 2 is minimizing risk factors. By stage 3 symptoms may be starting to appear and treatment may be needed. In stage 4, planning for dialysis or transplant should begin, and in stage 5 renal replacement therapy is needed or death will ensue. Complications of CKD include hypertension and increased cardiovascular risks, uremic syndrome, metabolic acidosis, electrolyte disturbances, bone and mineral disorders, malnutrition, anemia, pain, and depression.

CLINICAL MANAGEMENT

Clinical management of AKI and CKD requires a multidisciplinary approach. Collaboration among the nurse, physician, clinical pharmacist, and dietitian is essential to attain optimal patient outcomes. Prevention of the development of AKI is the goal. With CKD, prevention of the myriad of causes is certainly desirable; however, prevention also focuses on retarding the inevitable progression of the disease and reducing cardiovascular risk factors.

Acute Kidney Injury

AKI is often entirely preventable.[13] Prevention is highly dependent on recognizing patients who are at risk for the development of AKI and establishing prophylactic interventions to decrease this risk.

Etiologies and risk factors for prerenal kidney injury should be identified and, whenever possible, treated swiftly.[9] Early consultation with a nephrologist is recommended. Hypotension attributable to hypovolemia should be addressed; medications that might be contributing (antihypertensives, opioids) should be decreased or discontinued. Nutrition should be supported, and indwelling catheters and other invasive equipment should be removed as soon as possible to decrease the risk of infection. Development of infection should be monitored, and treated if it develops.[9] Maintaining adequate circulating volumes and supporting cardiac function, especially in those at risk for prerenal kidney injury, are the primary foci for prevention.

Should prerenal oliguria develop, efforts should be initiated to enhance renal perfusion before ATN can occur. Two interventions that were previously staples of treatment of prerenal oliguria have been deemed to be harmful, or at the very least ineffective.[40] Dopamine in the low-dosage range was previously believed to enhance

---

BOX 28-3 SELECTED CHEMICALS TOXIC TO THE KIDNEYS

Acetaminophen
Acyclovir (Zovirax)
Allopurinol
Aminoglycosides
Amphotericin B (Fungizone)
Angiotensin-converting enzyme inhibitors
Certain cytotoxic chemotherapeutic agents
Cocaine
Cyclosporine (Sandimmune)
Foscarnet (Foscavir)
Heavy metals
Hemoglobin; myoglobin
Heroin
Lithium
Nonsteroidal antiinflammatory drugs
Pentamidine (Pentam 300 and others)
Radiocontrast media*
Uric acid
Vasopressors (norepinephrine, high-dose dopamine)

Derived from McKenry L, Tessier E, Hogan M: *Mosby's pharmacology in nursing,* ed 22, St Louis, 2006, Mosby; Needham E: Management of acute renal failure, *Am Fam Physician* 72(9):1739-1746, 2005.
*Most common.

---

renal perfusion; evidence now indicates that use of this medication produces no difference from placebo therapy in the progression of AKI, the need for dialysis, or death. Again, compared to placebo therapy, loop diuretics made no difference in the recovery of renal function.[40] Aggressive management of conditions such as glomerulonephritis can prevent progression to intrinsic kidney injury.[13] Prevention of intrinsic kidney injury caused by chemicals begins with an awareness of the most likely harmful agents; these are listed in Box 28-3. Whenever possible their use should be limited, and if these agents must be prescribed, their serum levels may need to be monitored.[13] Single doses of aminoglycosides, rather than multiple doses, and liquid formulations of amphotericin B appear to be less nephrotoxic.[40] Of all the chemicals listed in Box 28-3, the most common culprit is radiocontrast media.

Prevention of contrast-induced AKI is aimed at initiating intravenous volume expansion with saline both before and after the contrast administration, administering the antioxidant N-acetylcysteine (Mucomyst) to patients at risk, measuring the serum creatinine concentration of patients with suspected renal dysfunction, and using either low-osmolar or iso-osmolar contrast media for all patients with renal insufficiency.[37] It is important to note that the evidence to support the effectiveness of Mucomyst in preventing contrast-induced AKI has demonstrated mixed results.[10,37] More research is needed. Postrenal etiologies should be avoided whenever possible, but if they occur they should be rapidly identified and corrected.[13] Postrenal kidney injury is the least common and most readily identifiable; promptly addressing it will prevent the progression to ATN.

Chronic Kidney Disease

Clinical management of CKD is complex and requires a multidisciplinary approach. Treatment is directed at slowing the progression to ESRD and managing the complications that are inevitable. This means that patient education regarding the trajectory of the illness, management of modifiable risk factors, and clinical management of

BOX 28-4 THERAPEUTIC GOALS IN CHRONIC KIDNEY DISEASE

- Maintain volume status.
- Prevent and treat acid-base and electrolyte disturbances.
- Prevent and treat uremia.
- Support nutritional needs.
- Prevent and treat infection.
- Prevent and treat anemia.
- Improve quality of life.
- Lower mortality and morbidity rates.
- Control pain.

TABLE 28-7 TARGET RANGES FOR CALCIUM AND PHOSPHORUS IN CKD

STAGE	CALCIUM	PHOSPHORUS
3	8.4-9.5 mg/dl	2.7-4.6 mg/dl
4	8.4-9.5 mg/dl	2.7-4.6 mg/dl
5	8.4-9.5 mg/dl	3.5-5.5 mg/dl

Data from Legg V: Complications of chronic kidney disease: a close look at renal osteodystrophy, nutritional disturbances, and inflammation, *Am J Nurs* 105(6):40-49, 2005.

the disease are essential. Because death is often due to cardiovascular pathologies, management of these risk factors assumes significant importance. At a community level, screening for hypertension, diabetes, and CKD is essential to stem the tide of these interrelated chronic diseases.[23] Underdiagnosis and undertreatment mediate the problem, and lack of awareness is the enemy of early diagnosis and treatment.

The speed with which CKD progresses varies significantly among individuals. Complications are typically evident by stage 3 or 4 and attention is directed to therapeutic interventions designed to minimize and treat these complications. Therapeutic and pharmacologic interventions are presented within the context of each complication listed in the following paragraphs. An in-depth presentation is beyond the scope of this text; discussion is simply an overview. Goals of therapeutic interventions for CKD are summarized in Box 28-4.

Hypertension and Cardiovascular Disease

Evaluation of risk factors for cardiovascular disease is an important part of intervention, because the risk of morbidity and mortality rises with the decline of GFR. Hypertension is associated with a more rapid progression of CKD; therefore control of blood pressure (BP) is critical. Lowering BP reduces the risk of proteinuria and prevents the development of cardiovascular and cerebrovascular events.[27] The BP goal with CKD patients is <130/80 mm Hg. An ACEI or an AII receptor blocker is considered the treatment of choice to delay progression, followed by a thiazide or loop diuretic.[27] ACEIs and AIIs have an additional benefit of reducing proteinuria by 40% to 45%.[27] However, it should be noted that effectively lowering BP does not necessarily improve survival.[28]

The benefits of using statins to treat dyslipidemia in patients with CKD have not been clearly established and remain controversial. Although a reduction in total and low-density lipoprotein (LDL) cholesterol levels occurs, and may be effective in decreasing cardiovascular events, there is no improvement in the GFR or the rate of CKD progression.[27,28] There is some evidence to indicate that there is a benefit from use of statins in stages 1 to 3, but not once patients start dialysis.[27] This is an area of ongoing research.

Metabolic Acidosis

Mild acidosis with a pH of 7.30 to 7.35 requires no therapy. Patients with chronic metabolic acidosis (<7.30) may be prescribed sodium bicarbonate.[16] In a single-center randomized trial, 134 adult patients with stage 4 CKD were treated with bicarbonate supplements. After 2 years of treatment, 6.5% of patients in the sodium bicarbonate group required dialysis compared to 33% in the control group.[27] Replication of this study is needed.

Fluid and Electrolyte Imbalances

Fluid restrictions are implemented when the sodium level drops below 135 mmol/L. Patients with edema, heart failure, or hypertension may need a 2 g/day sodium restriction.[16] Mild hyperkalemia (<6 mmol/L) can be treated by reducing potassium intake and correcting metabolic acidosis. Potassium levels >6 mmol/L require more urgent treatment, such as an IV infusion of calcium gluconate, 5% dextrose in water (D_5W), and insulin, or oral or rectal administration of sodium polystyrene sulfonate.[16]

Bone and Mineral Disorders

Hyperphosphatemia is addressed nutritionally, and later through drug management. Serum levels of parathyroid hormone (PTH), calcium, and phosphorus should be monitored in patients with a GFR less than 60 ml/min/1.73 m².[36] Calcium carbonate and calcium acetate effectively bind phosphorus, correct hypocalcemia, and are inexpensive,[27] though they are associated with hypercalcemia and vascular calcifications.[36] Lanthanum carbonate has potent phosphorous-binding ability and is generally well-tolerated.[36] Vitamin D therapies such as calcitriol, paricalcitol, and ergocalciferol are indicated for use in vitamin D deficiencies and to suppress PTH levels.[36] Calcimimetics, such as cinacalcet, have also been shown to decrease secretion of PTH. Target ranges for both calcium and phosphorous levels are shown in Table 28-7.

Malnutrition

Nutrition plays a large role in the treatment of CKD. Advanced CKD produces gastrointestinal manifestations, anorexia, nausea, and changes in the sense of taste, which further complicate the necessary modifications in diet.[16] Caloric requirements are increased. Sufficient carbohydrate and fat are needed to meet energy requirements.[16] Aspects of nutritional management of CKD include limiting intake of dietary phosphorus, protein, sodium, potassium, and water depending on lab values and other clinical manifestations. Avoiding malnutrition, preventing anemia, and countering disease- and drug-induced constipation are other aspects of nutritional management. Lists of foods high in sodium, potassium, and protein should be provided; patients can then be encouraged to identify their favorite foods and choose smaller portions or eat them less often. Additionally, diet-related risk factors for cardiovascular disease must be considered. This can all seem overwhelming to patients, so involvement of a dietitian and thorough education considering concomitant conditions, personal likes and dislikes, eating habits, and financial resources is essential.

Anemia

Erythropoiesis-stimulating agents, such as epoetin alfa and darbepoetin alfa, have dramatically improved the quality of life for patients with CKD, but have had little effect in reducing overall cardiovascular mortality or the rate of GFR loss.[27,28] Target hemoglobin (Hgb) levels have been the subject of much debate.[27,28] The National Kidney Foundation's *Kidney Disease Outcome Quality Initiative (KDOQI) Guidelines* recommend Hgb levels between 11 and 12 g/dl.[27,28] In addition to pharmacologic interventions, strategies for reducing fatigue, such as balancing rest and activity throughout the day, should be employed.

Pain

Pain in patients with CKD may be acute or chronic. Choice of medication and dosage needs to consider the patient's age, comorbidities, and degree of kidney failure; the pathway of elimination of the medication (i.e., through the liver, kidney, or dialysis); and the risk of drug-induced nephropathy.[24] Nonpharmacologic methods of pain relief should also be explored.

Depression

Studies have explored the use of pharmacologic and nonpharmacologic approaches to treat depressive symptoms in patients with CKD.[38] The safety of antidepressants in patients with decreased renal function is a significant concern. Psychotherapy, exercise therapy, cognitive behavioral therapy, and music therapy all have demonstrated varying degrees of success.[38]

Acute-on-Chronic Kidney Disease

Acute-on-chronic kidney disease describes a scenario in which acute kidney injury occurs in someone with preexisting chronic kidney disease. Incidence varies from 10% to greater than 30%, depending on the study population. Preexisting CKD is a strong risk factor for development of AKI.[50] The most common causes of AKI in someone with CKD include systemic infections, medications, dehydration, and urinary tract obstruction.[51] Management is directed towards identifying and treating the underlying cause of the acute deterioration, in order to prevent a possible irreversible drop in kidney function.[50,51]

Dialysis

The procedures, advantages, disadvantages, and expected outcomes of dialysis should begin to be discussed when the patient is in stage 4 of CKD.[31] When patients with CKD reach stage 5, dialysis is indicated.[45] The primary reason for the initiation of dialysis is the development of uremia.[14] Approximately two thirds of the total body urea content is removed by each dialysis treatment.[14] Dialysis may also be required if severe hyperkalemia is unresponsive to other interventions[13] or in cases of severe volume overload. If these conditions develop during the oliguric phase of ATN, dialysis may be required temporarily. Dialysis supports all the treatment goals in Box 28-4 and is the only therapeutic option for those with ESRD who are unable to obtain a transplant. Dialysis may be accomplished by hemodialysis, peritoneal dialysis, or continuous renal replacement therapy (CRRT).

Hemodialysis was first carried out on humans in 1924; before that time, patients with ESRD simply died. In 1972 the national ESRD program was signed into law, giving all Americans the right to treatment; ESRD is the sole recipient of this status.[45] In hemodialysis, an artificial kidney serves as the dialyzing semipermeable membrane. The patient's blood passes through a bundle of hollow capillary tubules and dialyzing fluid bathes these tubules.[7] Solutes that are present in high concentration in the uremic blood (i.e., phosphate, urea, creatinine, potassium) diffuse across the dialyzing tubule membrane into the dialyzing fluid and are discarded.[7]

Excess water in the uremic blood is eliminated through osmosis across the membrane. Preferred access for hemodialysis is established by creating an arteriovenous (AV) fistula, most commonly in the arm. AV grafts and specialized central venous catheters are other means of access. Most patients with ESRD go through hemodialysis treatments three times per week,[45] each treatment lasting about 4 hours. Although a life-saving intervention, dialysis treatments have complications, some of which are life-threatening, and long-term morbidity remains quite high.[45] Despite dialysis, cardiovascular disease remains the most common cause of death in ESRD patients.[41]

In peritoneal dialysis (PD), the peritoneum serves as the dialyzing membrane. A dialysis catheter is surgically placed in the abdomen for access. During the treatment, the peritoneal cavity is slowly filled with dialysate through the catheter. Extra fluid and waste products are drawn out of the uremic blood and into the dialysate.[42] There are two major types of PD: continuous ambulatory peritoneal dialysis (CAPD) and continuous cycling peritoneal dialysis (CCPD).

CAPD is carried out in the patient's home and without the use of machines. The patient instills about 2 quarts of dialysate into the peritoneum through the catheter. The dialysate remains there for 4 to 5 hours or longer, before it is drained and discarded. This is called an exchange.[42] While the dialysate resides in the peritoneal cavity, the patient has more freedom to continue his or her usual activities at work, at school, or at home.[42] Peritonitis is a potentially serious complication.

CCPD can also be performed at home, but uses a special machine called a cycler. This is similar to CAPD except that a number of cycles (exchanges) occur. Each cycle usually lasts 1½ hours and exchanges are done throughout the night while the patient sleeps.[42]

CRRT is limited to in-hospital acute kidney injury patients. Continuous hemofiltration and hemodialysis procedures filter and dialyze the blood without interruption. CRRT removes fluid and wastes from patients who are not hemodyamically stable enough (e.g., shock, multiple organ system failure) to tolerate the larger quantity of blood removed from the body during typical hemodialysis. This "gentler" continuous removal of wastes and blood helps avoid the hypotensive episodes caused by intermittent hemodialysis and its intermittent removal of large volumes of fluid.[16]

Kidney Transplant

Kidney transplantation is an alternative to dialysis for patients with ESRD. As with other conditions in which transplantation is indicated, the primary limiting factor is the availability of organs. Kidneys are obtained from deceased and living donors. For most of those who choose it, transplantation allows for increased independence, return to normal activities of daily living, and resumption of normal renal function. Thousands of patients receive kidney transplants each year in the United States, with a remarkable rise in transplant recipients over the last decade.[43,44] The 5-year patient survival rate (2003-2008) was estimated to be about 82% for a deceased donor and about 91% for a living donor transplant.[44] Given the number of transplant recipients and the improving patient survival rates, many patients need follow-up health care outside of transplant centers. This means that general health care providers will be caring for transplant recipients and the chronic medical conditions that accompany transplantation surgery. Common medical complications include cardiovascular disease, obesity, hypertension, dyslipidemia, diabetes, cerebrovascular disease, anemia, gout, depression, bone disease, malignancies, and infections.[43] Even with the best possible tissue matching, antirejection drug therapy is required and the adverse effects of these medications may have a significant impact on health and quality of life. Transplant recipients will be prescribed a combination of immunosuppressants, usually tacrolimus or cyclosporine, mycophenolate, and predisone.[43]

Chronic Kidney Disease in Older Adults

A decline in kidney function as one ages is well understood. What is less clear is whether the CKD that develops in older adults is a manifestation of the aging kidney or the associated cardiovascular disease and life exposure to vascular risk factors such as hypertension, diabetes, and smoking.[46,48] The majority of patients diagnosed with CKD are older adults,[30,48] and the rates of treated ESRD among the elderly (>80 years) have risen by more than 50% in the last decade.[49] Although progression of CKD to ESRD is costly and incurs significant health problems, it appears less frequently in older adults compared with cardiovascular mortality.[30] The majority will die as a result of cardiovascular disease.[30,48]

In the past 5 decades, increased numbers of older patients have initiated dialysis worldwide. Results from some studies indicate that elderly adults choosing peritoneal dialysis have higher mortality rates than those receiving hemodialysis.[49] With increased numbers of older adults on dialysis comes not only increased survival but also increased morbidity. Elderly patients who are on dialysis seem to have a higher burden of age-related problems, such as frailty, falls, and cognitive impairment. There is also emerging evidence that dialysis initiation may be associated with accelerated rates of functional and/or cognitive decline.[47,48] Primary care providers will be challenged with the complex care required of this population.

> ### KEY POINTS
>
> - Prevention of AKI includes early identification of those at risk, maintenance of fluid volume status and cardiac output, avoidance of exposure to nephrotoxic chemicals as well as subsequent treatment if necessary, and avoidance and aggressive treatment of infections. Prerenal and postrenal kidney injuries are treated by addressing their specific etiologies. Intrinsic kidney injury (ATN) is treated with many of the same interventions used to support renal function in CKD.
> - Slowing the progression of CKD is the focus of interventions until stages 4 to 5. Appropriate management of ATN, blood glucose control in patients with diabetes, use of ACE inhibitors or AII blockers to reduce proteinuria, and aggressive management of hypertension are the primary foci. Because cardiovascular disease both is a risk factor for CKD and accelerates progression, interventions are also included to retard it.
> - Nutritional needs for patients in renal failure include increased caloric intake as well as calcium and vitamin supplementation. Intake of fluids, phosphorus, potassium, sodium, and protein is usually restricted, depending on the underlying pathologic process and stage of the disease.
> - Drug therapy in CKD is used to control hypertension, anemia, and some of the electrolyte and acid-base imbalances.
> - Dialysis is used for some patients with ATN and for patients with CKD in stage 5 in order to remove metabolic wastes and correct fluid and electrolyte abnormalities.
> - Kidney transplantation is a potential option for patients with ESRD. Kidney transplantation has been associated with a high degree of success.
> - CKD is very prevalent in older adults. While many are initiating dialysis in ESRD, most will die of cardiovascular disease before reaching stage 5. The many comorbid conditions of this population require complex care.

■ SUMMARY

Renal failure can occur at any age. AKI has multiple causes that can be classified into one of three categories according to the physical location of the problem: prerenal, postrenal, or intrinsic. Each category has unique pathologic features and some variation in laboratory values. Intrinsic failure (ATN) is divided into three phases: prodromal, oliguric, and postoliguric. Interventions differ for each phase.

CKD is a progressive, irreversible process. It is characterized by stages of declining GFR producing increasing impairment in the ability of the kidney to maintain homeostasis. The clinical manifestations of CKD are determined by the degree of impairment of the kidneys' normal functions.

Key aspects of care include pharmacologic management of fluid overload, electrolyte abnormalities, and metabolic wastes; nutritional management; dialysis; and renal transplantation.

A clear understanding of the pathophysiology related to renal dysfunction is essential for any health care professional caring for patients in renal failure. Older adults with AKI, CKD, and ESRD add an additional layer of complexity to patient care. The impact that renal failure has on all other body systems presents many challenges.

REFERENCES

1. Koeppen BM, Stanton BA: *Renal physiology*, ed 4, Philadelphia, 2007, Mosby.
2. Abdel-Kader K, Palevsky PM: Acute kidney injury in the elderly, *Clin Geriatr Med* 25(3):1–20, 2009. doi: 10.1016/j.cger.2009.04.001.
3. Dirkes S: Acute kidney injury: not just acute renal failure anymore? *Crit Care Nurse* 31(1):37–49, 2011. doi: 10.4037/ccn2011946.
4. Bonventre JV, Lang L: Cellular pathophysiology of ischemic acute kidney injury, *J Clin Invest* 121(11):4210–4221, 2011.
5. Sabbahy ME, Vaidya VS: Ischemic kidney injury and mechanisms of tissue repair, *Wiley Interdisc Rev Syst Biol Med* 3(5):606–618, 2011. doi: 10.1002/wsbm.133.
6. Srisawat N, Hoste EEA, Kellum JA: Modern classification of acute kidney injury, *Blood Purif* 29:300–307, 2010. doi: 10.1159/000280099.
7. Hall JE: *Guyton and Hall textbook of medical physiology*, ed 12, Philadelphia, 2011, Saunders.
8. Weinstein JR, Anderson S: The aging kidney: physiological changes, *Adv Chronic Kid Dis* 17(4):302–307, 2010. doi: 10.1053/j.ackd.2010.05.002.
9. Abuelo JG: Normotensive ischemic acute renal failure, *New Engl J Med* 357:797–805, 2007.
10. Yaklin KM: Acute kidney injury: an overview of pathophysiology and treatments, *Nephrol Nurs J* 38(1):13–17, 30, 2011.
11. Lameire N, Van Biesen W, Vanholder R: Acute renal failure, *Lancet* 365:417–430, 2005.
12. Goldenberg I, Matetzky S: Nephropathy induced by contrast media: pathogenesis, risk factors and preventive strategies, *Can Med Assoc J* 172(11):1461–1471, 2005.
13. Needham E: Management of acute renal failure, *Am Fam Physician* 72(9):1739–1746, 2005.
14. Meyer TW, Hostetter TH: Uremia, *New Engl J Med* 357:1316–1325, 2007.
15. Pagana KD, Pagana TJ: *Mosby's manual of diagnostic and laboratory tests*, ed 4, St Louis, 2011, Mosby.
16. Porter RS, Kaplam JL: *The Merck manual*, ed 19, Whitehouse Station, NJ, 2011, Merck Sharp & Dohme.

17. Hawkins R: New biomarkers of acute kidney injury and the cardio-renal syndrome, *Korean J Lab Med* 31:72–80, 2011. doi: 10.3343/kjlm.2011.31.2.72.

18. Bastos MG, Kirsztajn GM: Chronic kidney disease: importance of early diagnosis, immediate referral and structured interdisciplinary approach to improve outcomes in patients not yet on dialysis, *Brazilian J Nephrol* 33, 2011. Available at http://dx.doi.org/10.1590/S0101-28002011000100013. Accessed 11/28/11.

19. U.S. Department of Health and Human Services: *National Kidney & Urologic Diseases Information Clearinghouse*. Available at http://kidney.niddk.nih.gov/KUDiseases/pubs/kustats/index.aspx. Accessed 1/15/12.

20. Weiner DE: Causes and consequences of chronic kidney disease: implications for managed health care, *J Manag Care Pharm* 13(suppl 3):S1–S9, 2007.

21. National Kidney Foundation Fact Sheet: *U.S. renal data system annual data report*, 2005. Available at www.kidney.org/news/newsroom/fs_new/esrdinus.cfm. Accessed 1/15/12.

22. Chobanian AV, et al: Seventh Report of the Joint National Committee on prevention, detection, evaluation, and treatment of high blood pressure: the JNC 7 complete report, *Hypertension* 42:1206–1252, 2003.

23. Atkins RC: The epidemiology of chronic kidney disease, *Kidney Int* 67(suppl 94):S14–S18, 2005.

24. Williams A, Manias E: A structured review of pain assessment and management of patients with chronic kidney disease, *J Clin Nurs*, 2007. doi: 10.1111/j.1365-2702.2007.01994.x.

25. National Kidney Foundation: *Kidney disease outcomes quality initiative*, 2002. Available at www.kidney.org/professionals/kdoqi/guidelines_ckd?p4_class_g1.htm. Accessed 1/28/12.

26. Centers for Disease Control and Prevention: *National chronic kidney disease fact sheet: general information and national estimates on chronic kidney disease in the United States*, Atlanta, GA, 2010, Author.

27. Brosnahan G, Fraer M: Management of chronic kidney disease: what is the evidence? *Southern Med Assoc* 103(3):222–230, 2010.

28. Stompór T, Olszewski A, Kierzkowska I: Can we prolong life of patients with advanced chronic kidney disease: what is the clinical evidence? *Polish Arch Int Med* 121(3):88–92, 2011.

29. Hallan SI, Stevens P: Screening for chronic kidney disease: which strategy? *J Nephrol* 23(2):147–155, 2010.

30. Anderson S, et al: Prediction, progression, and outcomes of chronic kidney disease in older adults, *J Am Soc Nephrol* 20:1199–1209, 2009. doi: 10.1681/ASN.2008080860.

31. The Renal Association. Available at www.renal.org/whatwedo/Information Resources/CKDeGUID. E/CKDstages.aspx. Accessed 1/28/12.

32. Eskridge M: Hypertension and chronic kidney disease: the role of lifestyle modification and medication management, *Nephrol Nurs J* 37(1):51–60, 2010.

33. Marin E, Sessa WC: Role of endothelial-derived nitric oxide in hypertension and renal disease, *Curr Opin Nephrol Hypertens* 16:105–110, 2007.

34. Clark LE, Kahn I: Outcomes in chronic kidney disease: what we know and what we need to know, *Nephron Clin Pract* 114:c95–c103, 2010.

35. Nanayakkara1 PWB, Gaillard CAJM: Vascular disease and chronic renal failure: new insights, *Neth J Med* 68(1):5–14, 2010.

36. Bonanni A, Mannucci I, et al: Protein energy wasting and mortality in chronic kidney disease, *Int J Environ Res Pub health* 8(5):1631–1654, 2011. doi: 10.3390/ijerph8051631.

37. Stanley G, McCullough P, et al: Contrast-induced acute kidney injury: specialty-specific protocols for interventional radiology, diagnostic computed tomography radiology, and interventional cardiology, *Mayo Clin Proc* 84(2):170–179, 2009.

38. Hedayati SS, Finkelstein FO: Epidemiology, diagnosis and management of depression in patients with CKD, *Am J Kidney Dis* 54(94):741–752, 2009.

39. Dowling TC: Prevalence, etiology, and consequences of anemia and clinical and economic benefits of anemia correction in patients with chronic kidney disease: an overview, *Am J Health Syst Pharm* 64(13 suppl 8):S3–S7, 2007.

40. Kellum J, LeBlanc M, Venkataraman V: Clinical evidence concise: acute renal failure, *Am Fam Physician* 76(3), 2007. Available at www.aafp.org/afp/20070801/bmj/html. Accessed 10/8/07.

41. Checherită IA, Turcu F, et al: Chronic complications in hemodialysis: correlations with primary renal disease, *Rom J Morphol Embryol* 51(1):21–26, 2010.

42. National Kidney Foundation: *Dialysis*. Available at www.kidney.org/atoz/content/dialysisinfo.cfm. Accessed 1/29/12.

43. Gupta G, Unruh ML, et al: Primary care of the renal transplant patient, *J Gen Intern Med* 25(7):731–740, 2010.

44. Organ Procurement and Transplantation Network (OPTN) and Scientific Registry of Transplant Recipients (SRTR): *OPTN/SRTR 2010 annual data report*, Rockville, MD, 2011, U.S. Department of Health and Human Services, Health Resources and Services Administration, Healthcare Systems Bureau, Division of Transplantation.

45. Rosner MH: Hemodialysis for the non-nephrologist, *South Med J* 98(8):785–791, 2005.

46. Abdelhafiz AH, Brown SHM, et al: Chronic kidney disease in older people: Physiology, pathology or both? *Nephron Clin Pract* 116:c19–c24, 2010. doi: 10.1159/000314545.

47. Jassal SV, Watson D: Dialysis in late life: benefit or burden? *Clin J Am Soc Nephrol* 4(12):2008–2012, 2009.

48. Ahmed AK, Brown SH, Abdelhafiz AH: Chronic kidney disease in older people: disease or dilemma? *Saudi J Kidney Dis Transpl* 21(5):835–841, 2010. Available at www.sjkdt.org/text.asp?2010/21/5/835/68876.

49. Tamura MK: Incidence, management, and outcomes of end-stage renal disease in the elderly, *Curr Opin Nephrol Hypertens* 18(3):252–257, 2009. doi: 10.1097/MNH.0b013e328326f3ac.

50. Madala ND: Acute renal failure in patients with chronic kidney disease, *CME* 25(8):395–398, 2007. Available at www.ajol.info/index.php/cme/article/viewFile/43804/27324. Accessed 3/24/12.

51. Willacy H: Acute on chronic renal failure, *Patient.co.uk*., 2010. Available at www.patient.co.uk/doctor/Acute-on-Chronic-Renal-Failure.htm. Accessed 3/24/12.

Disorders of the Lower Urinary Tract

Cheryl L. Brandt and Roberta J. Emerson

⊖volve WEBSITE

http://evolve.elsevier.com/Copstead/
- Review Questions and Answers
- Glossary (with audio pronunciations for selected terms)
- Animations
- Case Studies
- Key Points Review

KEY QUESTIONS

- How do the pathophysiologic characteristics and management of stress, urge, mixed, overflow, and functional incontinence differ?
- How are congenital abnormalities of the urinary collecting system detected and treated?
- What are the risk factors and clinical manifestations for bladder cancer?
- How do the manifestations of urethritis, cystitis, and interstitial cystitis/bladder pain syndrome differ?
- How do stones in the lower urinary tract present clinically?

CHAPTER OUTLINE

The lower urinary tract encompasses several structures that together are responsible for the transport and elimination of urine from the body. These structures include the ureters, bladder, urethra, and associated urinary sphincters. The male prostate gland is anatomically located in this area, but is functionally involved in male reproduction; the role and disorders of the prostate gland are presented in Chapters 30 and 31, respectively.

Ureters collect the urine formed in the kidneys from the renal pelvises and transport it to the bladder. The bladder is a hollow, muscular reservoir for urine that expands to store it and then contracts to expel urine through the urethra. Urine storage depends on intact spinal reflexes. The process of micturition (voiding) involves both reflex and voluntary mechanisms, mediated by the micturation center in the pons. Voiding is a result of coordinated function of bladder mechanoreceptors, neurologic impulse transmission, bladder muscle contraction, and urethral sphincter relaxation.[1]

In addition to voiding dysfunction, disorders of the lower urinary tract can generally be classified as congenital, neoplastic, infective, inflammatory, or obstructive. These disorders are often interrelated. For instance, stasis of urine, which occurs with a variety of disorders, often leads to urinary tract infection (UTI). Infection of the kidney, pyelonephritis (see Chapter 27), and acute postrenal kidney injury (see Chapter 28) can be caused by any number of pathologies affecting the lower urinary tract. Lower urinary tract disorders can result in significant health problems that have tremendous physical, psychosocial, and economic ramifications on patients and their families.[2-5]

LOWER URINARY TRACT

The role of the lower urinary tract is to transport urine formed by the kidneys and allow its appropriate removal from the body. The anatomy of the lower urinary tract is presented in Chapter 26. Urine movement from the kidneys to the bladder is due to the effect of gravity facilitated by peristaltic movement of the ureters. The bladder stores the urine until it is released through the urethra, ultimately by conscious decision. Anatomic integrity of the ureters and bladder, competent urethral sphincters, and an appropriately functioning nervous system are required for the lower urinary system to properly carry out its role.

Diagnostic Tests

Several of the procedures presented in Chapter 26 are used to diagnose urologic disorders discussed in this chapter. Other, more specialized diagnostic tests are often even more appropriate. A urinalysis (U/A) is the simplest and least costly test that can provide a wealth of information. For the lower urinary tract, it is primarily used in the diagnosis of infection.

Although the abdominal radiograph known as a KUB (kidneys, ureters, and bladder) provides information regarding anatomy and may detect neoplasms or urinary stones, it is not the most frequently used procedure for this purpose. Ultrasonography, which is painless, does not involve radiation, and provides excellent visualization of the urinary system, is the most common initial screening study for infants and children with urinary problems. Cystography may be required to yield more specific information about the bladder than can be obtained by ultrasound.[6] Voiding cystourethrography (VCUG) involves placing a catheter in the bladder and then filling it with sterile, iodinated, dilute contrast material. The catheter is then removed and the patient voids. Images of the bladder are taken before voiding to detect a ureterocele or tumor, and images taken during voiding can identify reflux or urethral abnormalities. Radionuclide voiding cystography also requires catheterization but involves the use of a small amount of radioactive material. A technetium-99m–labeled radiopharmaceutical is instilled in the bladder through the catheter, followed by sterile normal saline to fill the bladder. Once the catheter is removed, images are taken with the bladder full and during voiding, but this procedure does not allow visualization of the urethra.

The term *urodynamic testing* is used for procedures associated with diagnosing voiding dysfunction.[6] There are multiple urodynamic tests and procedures and the choice of tests is based on clinical presentation and begins with the least invasive of the desired tests. The most common tests are cystometry (measurement of intrabladder pressure during filling); urethral pressure profilometry (measurement of intraluminal pressure along the length of the urethra); uroflowmetry (noninvasive method of measuring characteristics of urine flow); and pressure-flow micturition studies (invasive method of measuring characteristics of urine flow). Electrophysiologic testing may also be done to determine pathologic processes underlying voiding dysfunction. Neurophysiologic tests provide information about the coordination between the bladder and the external sphincter. Neurophysiologic tests are much more involved and are completed only in very specialized laboratories.

Physiology of Micturition

Micturition is often taken for granted by health care providers and patients, but is a complicated process. Understanding of the process

begins with a review of the significant role the nervous system plays in controlling the functions of the lower urinary tract structures.

Nervous System Innervation of the Lower Urinary Tract

The central, autonomic, and peripheral nervous systems are all involved in urinary elimination. The pontine micturition center coordinates relaxation of the internal sphincter and contraction of the bladder to enable urination, whereas the cerebral cortex primarily inhibits the process through conscious control of the external sphincter.[1] Any disease process affecting these areas can interfere with urination. This includes such pathologies as Parkinson disease, multiple sclerosis, traumatic brain injury, spinal cord injury, or stroke.

The smooth muscle of the bladder is innervated by both the sympathetic and parasympathetic branches of the autonomic nervous system (Figure 29-1). This innervation controls the detrusor muscle in the bladder wall and the bladder neck, ultimately controlling filling and emptying of the bladder. In other words, the bladder itself does not respond to voluntary control, but rather to neurologic reflexes. The nerves responsible for these reflexes have both autonomic efferent motor and afferent sensory roles; efferent nerves control bladder smooth muscle, and afferent fibers transmit sensations of bladder stretch—distention and fullness—and pain. Injury or disease of the spinal cord in this region profoundly affects lower urinary tract function.

Sympathetic outflow of the autonomic nervous system to the bladder originates from the spinal cord region of L1-L2; the release of norepinephrine causes relaxation of the bladder and contraction of the bladder neck, allowing the storage of urine. Parasympathetic innervation of the urinary tract is supplied via the pelvic nerves, which exit the spinal cord at S2-S4. Their stimulation causes contraction of the detrusor muscle and relaxation of the internal sphincter (bladder neck). Parasympathetic signals from the posterior urethra in response to stretch of the bladder lining (urothelium) and bladder musculature are primarily responsible for initiating bladder emptying.

The somatic nerve fibers of the peripheral nervous system control the voluntary skeletal muscle of the external bladder sphincter via the pudendal nerve. The peripheral nervous system is primarily responsible for muscle function at the pelvic floor.

Mechanism of Micturition

The softness, pliability, mucosal secretions, and submucosal cushioning of the urethra are responsible for the maintenance of a water-tight seal or "compression" of the urethra. The *internal sphincter* is located at the proximal portion of the urethra, where the convergence of the detrusor muscle fibers provides pressure to keep it closed. When the internal sphincter has normal tone, the bladder is prevented from emptying until the pressure in the body of the bladder rises above a specific threshold. The sequence of urination begins with the bladder filling with urine until a first sensation of fullness is felt. This causes the internal bladder pressure to trigger stretch receptors in the bladder wall. Activation of these receptors results in afferent communication to the nervous system to cause contraction of the bladder detrusor muscle. The internal sphincter simultaneously relaxes, taking on a funnel shape.

The very noticeable urge to urinate causes an individual to consciously tighten the external sphincter. The *external sphincter* is located at the distal end of the urethra, surrounded by a ring of skeletal muscle from the pelvic floor. This musculature provides the necessary tension needed to maintain continence at normal resting bladder pressures. The external sphincter allows voluntary emptying of the bladder or the prevention of urination. Usually, enough pressure to hold the urine in the bladder can be voluntarily generated until about 350 to 400 ml of urine has collected in the bladder. At this point an urgent sensation to void

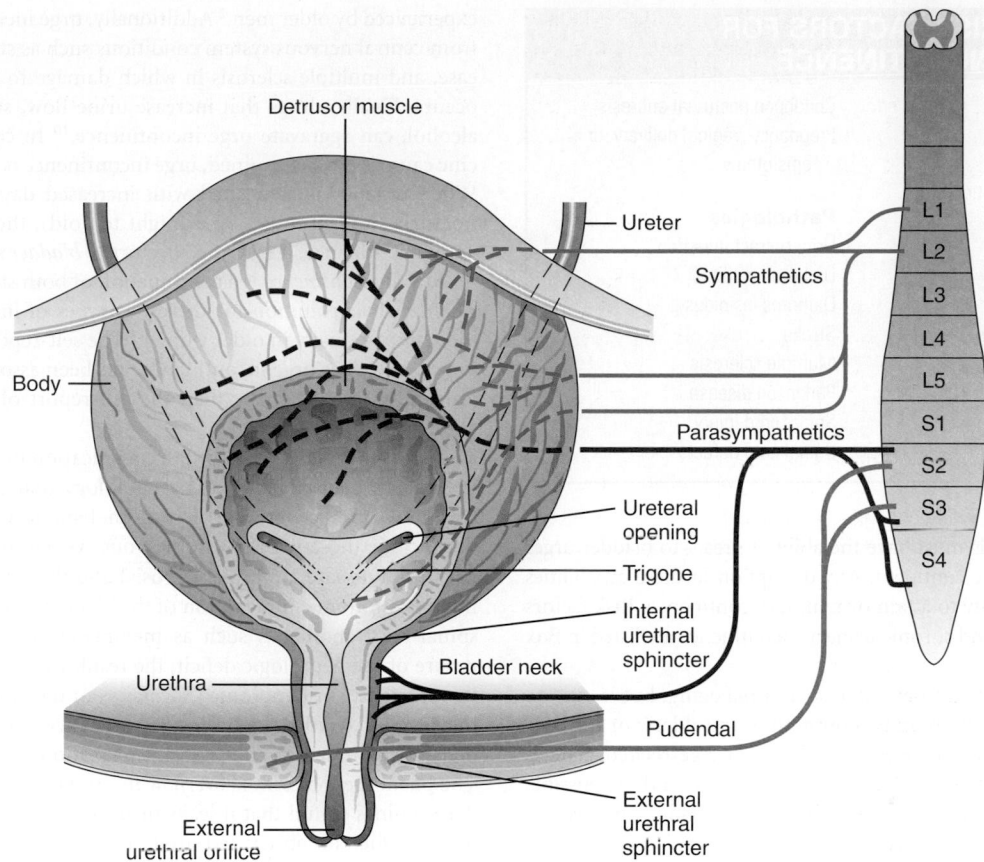

FIGURE 29-1 Bladder structure and innervation.

occurs and the resulting activation of the voiding centers in the brain (central nervous system) also helps inhibit the bladder from emptying. At the appropriate time, a coordinated nerve response allows the detrusor muscle to contract and both urethral sphincters to relax, and voiding occurs. If an individual is able to coordinate urination at a suitable location and desired time, we consider the individual to be **continent.**

Normal adult bladder capacity is 300 to 500 ml; the urge to void usually develops when 150 to 250 ml are present.[2] With an average fluid intake, this typically results in a voiding pattern of every 4 to 5 hours, with no need to awaken at night in order to void. With aging, bladder capacity declines to 200 to 350 ml; urination becomes more frequent (every 3 to 4 hours), and awakening at night to urinate is common. Under normal circumstances, the adult bladder contains less than 50 to 100 ml following voiding.[2] This volume of postvoiding urine is called **residual urine.** Certain pathologies are associated with incomplete bladder emptying, and increased residual urine volumes.

KEY POINTS

- The lower urinary tract transports urine from the kidneys and facilitates its removal from the body. A variety of laboratory tests are used in the diagnosis of lower urinary tract disorders.
- Bladder innervation is supplied by sympathetic nerves that exit the spinal cord at L1 and L2 and allow relaxation and filling. Stimulation of parasympathetic nerves from S1 to S4 results in bladder contraction and relaxation of the internal sphincter. The somatic pudendal nerve innervates the external bladder sphincter.
- Micturition requires central, autonomic, and peripheral nervous system functioning. It is a result of parasympathetic and voluntary motor control.

VOIDING DYSFUNCTION

Voiding dysfunction can be associated with pathologies affecting the central, autonomic, and peripheral nervous systems. However, voiding dysfunctions may also be associated with other factors affecting control of micturition, including medications and access to toileting facilities. Disorders of the lower urinary tract, such as infection, can cause secondary problems with voiding. Voiding dysfunction encompasses several types of incontinence, and enuresis.

Incontinence

The International Continence Society defines the symptom of urinary incontinence as the report of any involuntary urine loss.[7] Issues of urinary incontinence in adults are two times more common among women than men until age 80; after that point rates are equal.[2] The prevalence of urinary incontinence increases across women's lifetimes: 12% to 42% of middle-aged and younger women report urge incontinence, with these values increasing to 17% to 55% in older women.[7] However, incontinence is not normal under any circumstances and is not a normal part of aging. In 2000 the overall cost of incontinence in the United States was nearly $20 billion.[8] Itemization of these costs illustrates the complexity of the problem: 3% for diagnostic testing, 9% for routine care, 32% for treatments, and 56% for the indirect costs of nursing home admissions and loss of productivity.[8] The personal financial cost is high as well; median weekly out-of-pocket costs for women with severe incontinence have been estimated at more than $10 in 2005 terms.[9]

Pathogenesis. Continence requires both physiologic and cognitive capabilities. Physiologic requirements include an appropriately functional nervous system, and intact bladder and urethral function.

BOX 29-1 RISK FACTORS FOR INCONTINENCE

Risk Factors
Immobility
Impaired cognition
Medications (e.g., diuretics)
Morbid obesity
Smoking
Fecal impaction
Delirium
Environmental barriers to toileting
High-impact physical activities
Estrogen depletion
Low fluid intake
Pelvic muscle weakness

Childhood nocturnal enuresis
Pregnancy, vaginal delivery, or
   episiotomy

Pathologies
Urinary tract infection
Diabetes mellitus
Diabetes insipidus
Stroke
Multiple sclerosis
Parkinson disease
Spinal cord injury
Spinal cord defects

Cognitively, individuals must have the ability to react to bladder urges and be motivated to be continent. Any disruption in these capabilities can result in an inability to attain or maintain continence. Risk factors associated with acute and chronic urinary incontinence are listed in Box 29-1.

Urinary incontinence is not a part of normal aging, but it may be a result of disorders that are more common in the elderly or medications that induce urinary changes (e.g., diuretics). Age-related changes in the function or structure of the lower urinary tract and the possible limitations in the mobility and independence of the elderly predispose them to incontinence.[8]

Acute incontinence has a sudden onset and is due to potentially reversible, more easily treatable conditions. Examples of such conditions include urinary tract infections and constipation or fecal impactions.[2] Chronic urinary incontinence is usually classified by type, based on the specific characteristics of presentation. These types are urge, stress, mixed, overflow, and functional incontinence. The etiologies and treatments vary, so identification of the type of incontinence is clinically important.

Stress incontinence, the most prevalent type of chronic incontinence, occurs when urine is involuntarily lost with increases in intraabdominal pressure.[2,10] It is precipitated by effort or exertion, such as by lifting heavy objects, or by coughing or sneezing. Stress incontinence is thought to occur as a result of loss of pelvic muscle and/or fascial support of the bladder and urethra. Without this support, whenever there is an increase in intraabdominal pressure the normal angle between the bladder and posterior urethra is disrupted, forces that support urethral closure are reduced, and urine is lost.[2,10] Decreased estrogen availability with menopause also contributes by reducing urethral closing pressure.[11] Age-related loss of pelvic floor muscle fibers decreases muscular support. Other factors that favor the development of stress incontinence include obesity, childbirth-related trauma, urologic or retropubic surgery, pelvic radiotherapy, and the presence of conditions such as diabetes or degenerative neurologic diseases that impair nerves innervating the structures involved in micturition.[2,10]

Urge (urgency) incontinence involves the involuntary leakage of urine suddenly along with or immediately following the sensation of a need to urinate (urgency).[7,12] This condition is most often due to an overactive detrusor muscle that suddenly contracts without the patient's desire for it to do so.[2] Aging is known to increase the frequency of spontaneous involuntary detrusor contractions.[10] Contributing factors may include bladder infections that irritate the bladder lining and bladder outlet obstruction attributable to prostate enlargement. Urge incontinence is the most common type of incontinence

experienced by older men.[2] Additionally, urge incontinence may result from central nervous system conditions such as stroke, Parkinson disease, and multiple sclerosis in which damage to inhibitory pathways occurs. Finally, drugs that increase urine flow, such as diuretics and alcohol, can aggravate urge incontinence.[10] In cases in which a specific cause is not determined, urge incontinence is said to be *idiopathic*. When urgency is associated with increased daytime frequency and **nocturia** (a need to get up at night to void), though not necessarily with incontinence, it is termed *overactive bladder syndrome*.[12]

Mixed incontinence is a combination of both stress and urge incontinence.[7] It is common for these two types of incontinence to occur together, especially in older women. The self-report of mixed incontinence, as well as urge incontinence, has been associated with a greater impact on quality of life than the self-report of stress incontinence alone.[5]

Neurogenic bladder is a broad classification of voiding dysfunction in which the specific cause is a pathology that disrupts the nervous communication governing micturition. Patients with neurogenic bladder include those with central nervous system disorders (e.g., stroke, Parkinson disease, multiple sclerosis) and those with disorders affecting the autonomic innervation of the bladder (e.g., spinal cord injury, spinal cord anomalies such as meningocele). Depending upon the nature of the neurologic deficit, the result may be detrusor overactivity (spasticity) or hypotonia (flaccidity) of the bladder. Those affected may exhibit overflow incontinence, urge incontinence, uncoordinated detrusor contraction and urethral relaxation, or urinary retention.[10] The phenomenon termed *overflow incontinence* occurs when the bladder becomes so full that it leaks urine, or "overflows."[8] This can also happen when an obstructed urethra prevents the bladder from emptying normally, such as with an enlarged prostate, urethral stricture, cystocele, or prolapsed uterus.

Some experts describe *functional incontinence* as incontinence related to physical or environmental limitations resulting in an inability to access a toilet in time.[8] The urinary system may work well, but inaccessible toilets, mobility disorders, cognitive dysfunction, or mental disabilities prevent normal toilet usage. Health care workers can be critical in manipulating the environment to facilitate the patient's timely access to the toilet to maintain "dependent continence."[12]

Diagnosis. Patients should be assessed for reversible issues affecting the function of the lower urinary tract. These include potential drug-induced effects, UTIs or obstructions, fecal impaction, overuse of alcohol or caffeine, and excess intake of fluid. Impaired cognitive function may be due to chronic illness, depression, or delirium. All disorders associated with cognitive or neurologic function (e.g., stroke, Parkinson disease) should be identified. Circumstances or conditions affecting mobility should also be acknowledged.[13]

Patients may be asked to keep a bladder diary, recording the time, frequency, and volume of micturition as well as incidents of incontinence.[7] In addition to the physical examination, such diagnostic tests as residual urine measurement, filling cystometry studies, and pressure flow studies during voiding may be used to establish the diagnosis of incontinence.[6,7]

Treatment. Management of incontinence begins by addressing reversible contributing factors. Lifestyle changes such as losing weight, reducing caffeine intake, and avoiding constipation may be useful. Additional treatment may include behavioral, pharmacologic, and surgical interventions, depending on the cause of incontinence. Pelvic floor muscle training (PFMT), a behavioral intervention, is recommended for urge incontinence in both men and women. PFMT may be as simple as the performance of exercises to strengthen pelvic muscles, or more complex to include techniques with vaginal weights, pelvic floor electrical stimulation, and biofeedback. Bladder training incorporates education, scheduled voiding with systematic delay of voiding to conform with the schedule, and positive reinforcement.

Pharmacologic agents may be used to promote or inhibit physiologic activities associated with micturition, depending on the cause of incontinence. This may include anticholinergic agents (e.g., oxybutynin), vaginal or oral estrogen, and α-adrenergic blockers (e.g., prazosin, tamsulosin) or 5α-reductase inhibitors (e.g., finasteride) for men with bladder outlet obstruction.[14,15] The addition of drug therapy often increases the effectiveness of behavioral interventions. Injections with botulinum toxin are being used for detrusor overactivity. Surgical procedures for incontinence, used if nonsurgical interventions are ineffective, vary depending on the underlying anatomic or physiologic problems. Several surgical options are available to treat urge incontinence in women. The anterior colporrhaphy involves ther repair of a weakened anterior vaginal wall that has allowed the bladder to prolapse into the vagina. A colposuspension is performed by using sutures to tighten the muscles of the pelvic floor that support the uterus and bladder; the procedure may be performed via laparoscope. Sling procedures involve implanting strips of synthetic or natural material around the bladder neck and urethra to support urethral closure. Surgical options for men may include artificial urinary sphincter implantation for sphincter incompetence and placement of a perineal compression sling for post-prostatectomy incontinence.[16]

Incontinence that is not resolved by behavioral, pharmacologic, or surgical treatment occasionally may be managed by supportive approaches such as intermittent catheterization, indwelling catheterization, or use of incontinence undergarments.[2] Each of these devices creates the potential for further complications. UTIs are more likely with stasis of urine in the bladder and, in the case of catheterization, with continuous or intermittent introduction of a foreign object into the normally sterile bladder. Catheterization is never an appropriate solution solely for caregiver convenience. Stasis of urine also increases the risk for bladder and renal calculi. Management of incontinence with incontinence undergarments predisposes patients to skin breakdown.

Enuresis

Enuresis as defined by the International Children's Continence Society means intermittent incontinence while asleep.[17] Nocturnal enuresis is a common childhood condition, more common in boys than girls. One study, conducted using a strict definition of enuresis as incontinence twice a week for a minimum of 3 consecutive months, estimated a prevalence of 4.45% in children in the United States ages 8 to 11.[18] *Primary nocturnal enuresis* describes a child who has never achieved continence, whereas *secondary enuresis* refers to enuresis that develops after a period of at least 6 months of dryness.[17] In *monosymptomatic nocturnal enuresis,* the child has nocturnal incontinence but no other signs of lower urinary tract malfunction such as urgency, postvoid dribbling, and daytime incontinence. *Nonmonosymptomatic nocturnal enuresis* is diagnosed when the child has symptoms of urgency, frequency, or daytime incontinence in addition to nighttime enuresis.

Pathogenesis. Primary *monosymptomatic nocturnal enuresis* is thought to be present in less than half of the cases of nocturnal enuresis.[19] Three main mechanisms are considered to contribute to the condition. Some children exhibit nocturnal polyuria, linked in many cases to a deficiency in vasopressin (antidiuretic hormone [ADH]). Other children exhibit nocturnal overactivity of the detrusor muscle, which contributes to incontinence. Finally, immature or abnormal arousal mechanisms may explain why the child does not awaken.[19,20]

The fact that parents and siblings of children with nocturnal enuresis also report a history of the problem has led to the establishment of a genetic contribution.[21] Enuresis is associated with such conditions as constipation, attention-deficit hyperactivity disorder, and sleep-disordered breathing.[19,22,23]

Diagnosis. Clinical workup for enuresis includes a thorough history of elimination patterns via a bladder diary and a physical examination to identify gross anatomic abnormalities. Children with monosymptomatic nocturnal enuresis (MNE) should also be tested for diabetes mellitus.[19] Additional diagnostic tests, including flow cystometry and urinary tract imaging, are warranted for children who present with nonmonosymptomatic nocturnal enuresis (NMNE).[24]

Treatment. Treatment for MNE, not recommended before age 6, begins with education about appropriate daytime and bedtime voiding patterns.[24] If constipation is present it is managed with fiber intake, physical activity, and stool softeners. Enuresis alarms, designed with a moisture sensor in the bed linen or nightclothes, arouse and/or condition children to contract pelvic muscles; alarm therapy is effective for approximately two thirds of children. A second course of alarm therapy may be required if there is relapse.[19] "Overlearning" is recommended as a technique to strengthen the child's response to a full bladder; after dryness is established the child is instructed to drink liquids an hour before bedtime.

Pharmacotherapy may be added if nonpharmacologic treatments are ineffective. Desmopressin, a vasopressin analogue, effects a full response in 30% of children and a partial response in 40%.[19] Imipramine, a tricyclic antidepressant, is effective in about half of the children but its risk of cardiotoxicity mandates careful use in selected children. Anticholinergics such as oxybutynin and tolterodine are sometimes used, in combination with desmopressin or alone, and are effective in about 40% of cases. Urinary retention and constipation are side effects of anticholinergics that are worrisome in the setting of enuresis.[19] In children who remain enuretic after many months of standard treatment, additional diagnostic testing such as ultrasound is recommended. Efforts to manage enuresis without treating an underlying pathology are likely to be unsuccessful.

KEY POINTS

- Voiding dysfunction may be secondary to disorders of the lower urinary tract, attributable to pathologies affecting the central, autonomic, and peripheral nervous systems, or associated with a wide variety of factors affecting control of micturition, including medications and access to toileting facilities.
- Urge incontinence may be idiopathic or attributable to bladder infections that irritate the bladder lining, radiation therapy, tumors or stones in the urinary tract, or central nervous system damage to inhibitory pathways (as would occur with stroke, dementia, Parkinson disease, and multiple sclerosis).
- Weakening of pelvic muscles or intrinsic urethral sphincter deficiency results in stress incontinence.
- Mixed incontinence is a combination of both stress and urge incontinence.
- Obstruction of the urethra, or an underactive or inactive detrusor muscle causes overflow incontinence.
- Functional incontinence is related to physical or environmental limitations in reaching a toilet in time to void.
- *Neurogenic bladder* is a broad classification of voiding dysfunction in which the specific cause is a pathology that produces a disruption of neurologic communication governing micturition.
- Treatment options for voiding dysfunction include behavioral, pharmaceutical, and surgical interventions.
- Enuresis is inappropriate wetting of clothing or bedding, with the term usually reserved for incontinence in children, particularly at night.
- Treatment for enuresis is usually behavioral modification with or without pharmacologic intervention.

CONGENITAL DISORDERS

Vesicoureteral Reflux

Reflux of urine from the bladder to the ureter and renal pelvis, known as **vesicoureteral reflux (VUR)**, is usually due to incompetence of the valvular mechanism at the ureter-bladder junction.

The incidence of vesicoureteral reflux in asymptomatic children (without a UTI) is low, estimated at 1%.[25] However, the incidence in infants and children with UTIs is much greater, between 30% and 40%. More common in females, a genetic component is also present.[26] In siblings of children in whom reflux had been diagnosed, the incidence is 27% to 51%. There is a 66% rate of VUR in the children of parents who have been diagnosed with reflux. The specific mode of inheritance has not yet been identified; a major, dominantly inherited allele, multifactorial or polygenic traits, and an X-linked pattern have all been postulated.[27]

Pathogenesis. VUR is usually due to incompetence of the valvular mechanism at the ureter-bladder (ureterovesical) junction. Normally, the ureters enter the bladder at an oblique angle and then continue for 1 to 2 cm under the bladder mucosa before exiting inside the bladder cavity. As the bladder fills, pressure within it increases against the muscle wall and closes the ureteral passageway. In the case of VUR, closure of the ureteral passage is unsuccessful, and the urine flows backward into the ureters, sometimes reaching the kidney.

Vesicoureteral reflux is classified as being of either a primary or a secondary etiology. Congenital abnormalities at the ureterovesical junction are a chief cause of primary reflux.[28] One such abnormality is a shortened ureteral tunnel through the bladder wall, which decreases the efficiency of the valvular mechanism. Impaired bladder dynamics may be a contributing factor; the prevalence reports of bladder dysfunction in children with primary VUR have ranged from 18% to 75%.[28,29] Primary reflux is also associated with other abnormalities of the urinary system, among them ureteral duplication, ureterocele with duplication, ureteral ectopia, and paraurethral diverticula. Secondary reflux can occur from increased pressure within the bladder (neurogenic bladder, bladder outlet obstruction), inflammatory processes, or surgical procedures at or near the ureterovesical junction. Reflux may be bilateral or unilateral; the extent of reflux is graded from I to V (Figure 29-2).

Reflux of urine may cause increased renal pelvis pressure; additionally, migration of bacteria from the bladder to the kidneys may result in pyelonephritis or renal scarring that may cause hypertension or renal insufficiency.[26,30] In the 1970s, in 50% of the cases of hypertension in children, VUR was documented as the specific etiology. At that time, up to 40% of the children treated at renal failure clinics had VUR. More recent data indicate that VUR is noted as the etiology of hypertension or renal insufficiency in only about 6% of the children. These differences may be due to changes in disease-coding procedures, and/or better diagnosis and treatment.[30]

Diagnosis and clinical manifestations. Reflux may be discovered prenatally, during ultrasonography, when hydronephrosis is identified.[30] The other most common time of diagnosis is during the screening of children with a family history of VUR.[31] It may also be identified during evaluation for recurrent UTI, voiding dysfunction, renal insufficiency, or hypertension in children. Diagnostic tests such as voiding cystourethrography (VCUG), intravenous pyelography (IVP), and computed tomography (CT) are performed to evaluate the status of the kidney and bladder system. Nuclear medicine scans of kidney function such as the technetium-99m–labeled dimercaptosuccinic acid (DMSA) renal scanning may be warranted.[32]

Treatment. In nearly 80% of cases, reflux resolves spontaneously as the child grows.[33] The factors predictive of spontaneous resolution are younger age at diagnosis, classification as grade I or II reflux, higher bladder capacity at the onset of reflux manifestations, and a history of prenatal hydronephrosis. This information is helpful in determining when and how to treat patients, given questions about safety and efficacy of long-term prophylactic antimicrobial therapy and surgical interventions.[33]

For those with VUR most likely to resolve spontaneously, observation and medical management when necessary are recommended.[32] Continuous antibiotic prophylaxis is an appropriate option for children with a history of UTI. Observation with regular urinalysis and culture is an option for children without recurrent infection, with antibiotic therapy initiated for a diagnosed UTI.[32] Children who experience breakthrough UTI despite continuous antibiotic therapy are considered for surgical intervention; both endoscopic and open ureteral reimplantation procedures may be used.[32]

Obstruction of the Ureteropelvic Junction

Ureteropelvic junction obstruction (UPJO) is defined as a blockage (partial or complete) in urinary flow from the renal pelvis at the entry point of one or both ureters.[34] It is diagnosed more often in males, and more frequently presents unilaterally at the left ureter.[35] Bilateral UPJO has an incidence of 10% to 40% and is usually diagnosed in infants under the age of 6 months.[35] It may be either congenital or acquired; acquired UPJO may be due to such conditions as urinary tract stones, postoperative or inflammatory strictures, or neoplasms of the ureters.[34]An autosomal dominant model of inheritance has been proposed but not verified.[35] An increased incidence in premature infants and twins has been noted, as well as an increased incidence of other urologic abnormalities in conjunction with UPJO.[35]

Pathogenesis. The exact etiology of UPJO remains unknown, but in the majority of cases, stenosis (narrowing) of the junction by either intrinsic or extrinsic factors is the cause of the obstruction. Excessive collagen in the muscle cells of the junction is a usual intrinsic source of UPJO, whereas compression from renal veins or arteries, "crossing vessels," is a possible external cause. Because uncrossing the vessels never solves the obstruction, it is likely that an intrinsic factor changes the structure of the renal pelvis producing these variations in the vasculature. The result of intrinsic and extrinsic UPJO is inefficient ureter drainage leading to progressive dilation of the renal pelvis and hydronephrosis. Eventually, structural damage to the renal parenchyma and kidney dysfunction will occur.

Diagnosis and clinical manifestations. The majority of UPJO diagnoses are made prenatally during maternal ultrasonography.[34,35] Neonates with hydronephrosis attributable to UPJO frequently have elevated serum creatinine levels and reduced urinary output, but it is not common for renal failure to be present in neonates with either unilateral or bilateral UPJO.[35] Other early signs and symptoms include a palpable flank mass in a newborn infant; abdominal, flank, or back pain; a UTI with fever; or hematuria without significant trauma. UPJO may also be asymptomatic and discovered incidentally on renal ultrasonography. A VCUG may be performed to rule out other conditions such as vesicoureteral reflux.

Treatment. Surgical intervention for UPJO has decreased in recent decades, in favor of more conservative approaches.[34] In the case of prenatally diagnosed UPJO, observation is considered most appropriate.[34,36] Conservative, observational management consists of frequent renal ultrasound to assess for hydronephrosis.

The intent of surgery is to relieve symptoms and/or maintain renal function, but for some asymptomatic cases, monitoring the patient has been found to be most appropriate.[34] The percentage of surgical interventions in children younger than 6 months of age has decreased from

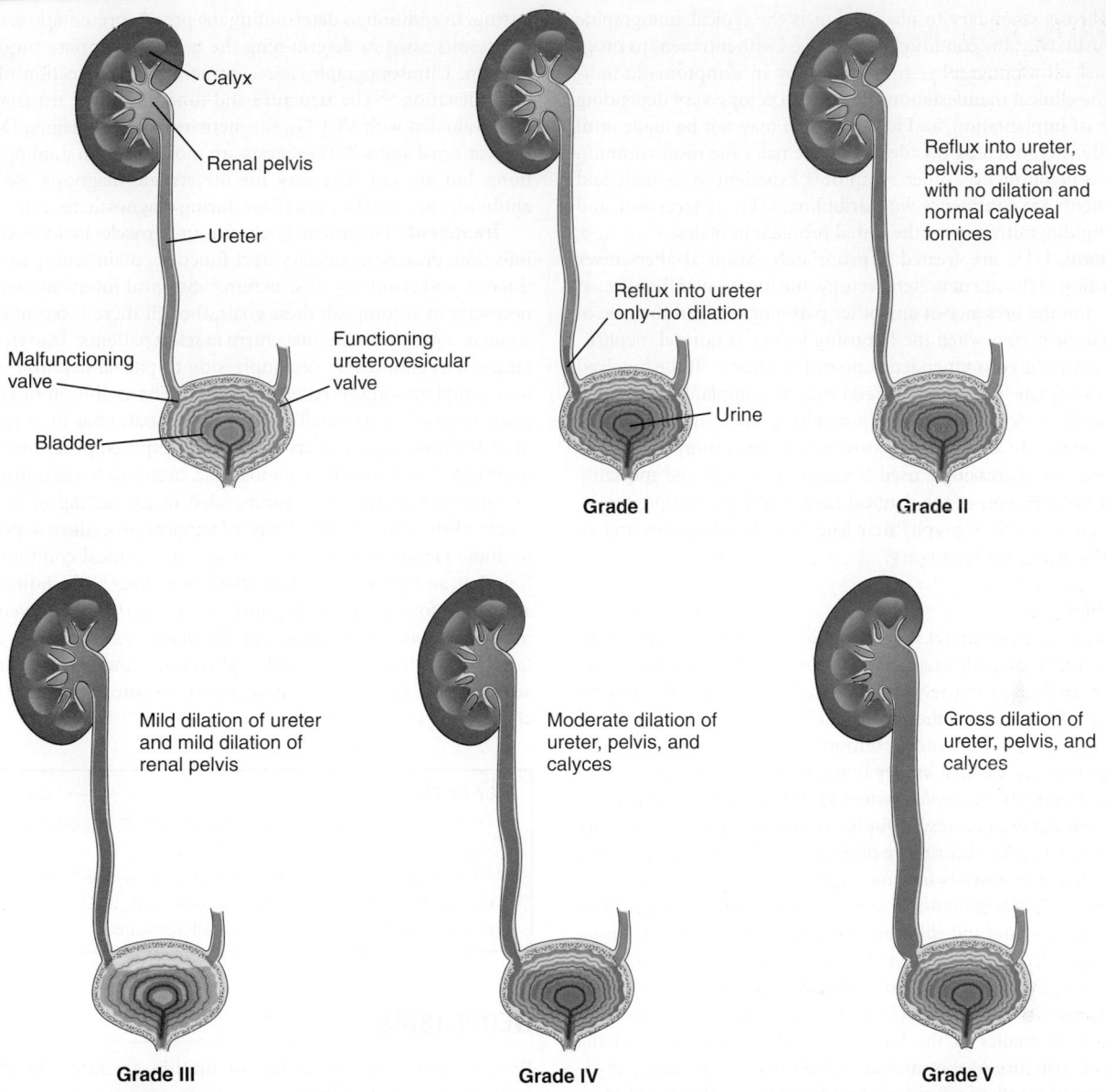

FIGURE 29-2 International classification of vesicoureteral reflux. (From James SR et al: *Nursing care of children: principles and practice,* ed 4, Philadelphia, 2013, Saunders, p 576.)

34.2% in an assessment from 1988 to 1991 to 25.2% in a similar review from 1997 to 2000.[36]

The timing of surgical intervention to correct UPJO is also controversial. Ultimately, it is a clinical decision based on the degree of obstruction, a careful analysis of kidney function, and the overall health of the infant or child. Early surgical repair is usually warranted if function of the affected kidney decreases, in cases of bilateral obstruction, and in cases of congenital single kidney with obstruction.

Pyeloplasty is the surgical reconstruction of the UPJ. It usually involves removal of the stenosed area of the junction and anastomosis of the ureter and renal pelvis. Endoscopic and laparoscopic techniques are being utilized widely in the United States.[36,37] An improvement in renal function is likely, although a small percentage of patients require a second surgical intervention because of the postoperative development of urine leakage or a return of the obstruction.[37] The use of a robotic endoscopic approach to surgery is increasingly popular in locations where it is available.[38]

Ureteral Ectopy

An **ectopic ureter** is a single ureter implanted in an abnormal location or a duplicate ureter. Alternative or duplicate sites of ureter implantation predispose the patient to infection and a potential reduction in renal function.

Pathogenesis. Ureters may implant anywhere along the route of migration of the mesonephric duct during fetal development. Ectopic ureters are significantly more common in females than in males.[39,40] In males, the ectopy is usually unilateral and is most frequently found implanted in the urethra; the bladder neck, seminal vesicle, and vas deferens are also common sites. In females, ectopic ureters may be implanted in the urethra, vagina, cervix, ovarian tubes, or uterus.[39,40]

Diagnosis and clinical manifestations. An ectopic ureter is often found in conjunction with other genitourinary pathologies, including renal dysgenesis or agenesis, ectopic kidneys, abnormal ovaries or fallopian tubes, or abnormalities in the seminal vesicles.[39,40] The diagnosis of ureteral ectopy is frequently made during maternal ultrasonography.

Hydronephrosis secondary to obstruction is the typical sonographic finding. Postnatally, the condition is diagnosed with intravenous urography, renal ultrasonography, and endoscopy in symptomatic individuals. The clinical manifestations of ureteral ectopy vary depending on the site of implantation, and identification may not be made until significantly later, often by decades.[39-42] In females the most common symptom is incontinence; other symptoms experienced by male and female patients are continence with dribbling, UTIs, obstruction, and pain.[39-41] Epididymitis may be the initial problem in males.

Treatment. UTIs are treated appropriately. Surgical alternatives vary according to the site of ureteral ectopy, the function of the affected kidney(s), and the presence of any other pathology.[39-42] In the case of a single ectopic ureter, when the opposing kidney is normal, nephroureterectomy is the recommended course of treatment. If the involved kidney has adequate function, the ureter may be reimplanted in a more physiologically acceptable site. Heminephrectomy and ureteropyelostomy are not uncommon. Laparoscopic nephrectomy and heminephrectomy are increasingly used because of the reduced mortality and better visualization of the surgical field with laparoscopic procedures.[39-42] Antenatal sonography may lead to earlier diagnosis and an increase in kidney-sparing surgery.

Ureterocele

A **ureterocele** is a congenital cystic dilation of the distal end of the ureter. These cystic dilations are called *intravesical* or *orthotopic* ureteroceles when they are entirely within the bladder itself and *extravesical* or *ectopic* when found in the neck of the bladder or in the urethra.[43] Ectopic ureteroceles are the more common form in the pediatric population. A ureterocele with a kidney that has just one ureter is called a *single system* ureterocele; *duplex system* ureteroceles are found with a kidney possessing two ureters.[43] Duplex system ureteroceles are more common. Ureteroceles occur more often in females than in males (6:1 ratio) and almost exclusively in Caucasians.

Etiology and pathogenesis. Ureteroceles are most often identified prenatally or in infants and children; however, they may not be found until adulthood.[44] It is most likely that the etiology of ureteroceles is complex rather than unified. Most certainly there are multiple points in embryogenesis when ureterocele formation could occur, often with concomitant anomalies of the kidney(s).[43] On histologic exam the microscopic structure of the muscle is abnormal, with smaller myocytes, decreased numbers of muscle bundles, and an absence of thick myofibrils.

Ureteroceles may be classified as simple structures when they are not associated with duplicate collecting systems, but the majority present as duplicate systems with ectopic implantation. They are infrequently bilateral. When identified in adults, they are typically intravesical, simple, and unilateral.[44] The small orifice of the ureter poses an obstruction in the collecting system and results in ureteral and renal calyx dilatation and often facilitates reflux and infection. If the ureterocele is large, obstruction of the bladder outlet may occur.[45]

Diagnosis and clinical manifestations. Ureteroceles are increasingly identified serendipitously during prenatal ultrasonography by the appearance of hydronephrosis and evidence of cystic dilation.[45] After birth, confirmation with further assessment is necessary. UTIs are the most common manifestation in infants. In addition to the manifestations of UTI, patients with ureteroceles may present with either urinary retention or urinary incontinence if the bladder outlet is obstructed, ureteral calculus, hematuria, urosepsis, or a general failure to thrive. Ureteroceles discovered in adults are often asymptomatic.

Anatomically, ureteroceles present with significant variability, requiring a thorough history, physical examination, and diagnostic testing. In addition to determining the precise presentation, diagnostic test results assist in determining the most appropriate surgical intervention. Ultrasonography is recommended for detection of the ureteral dilatation.[46] The structure and function of the urinary tract are also evaluated with VCUGs, magnetic resonance imaging (MRI), and nuclear renal scans.[46] These tests are most useful in guiding interventions, but are not necessary for ureterocele diagnosis. Prophylactic antibiotics are usually prescribed during diagnostic testing.

Treatment. Treatment goals for ureterocele include controlling infection, preserving urinary tract function, maintaining urinary continence, and removing obstruction.[47] Surgical interventions are often necessary to accomplish these goals, though there is recent discussion about using expectant management in select patients.[48] Surgical options range from endoscopic decompression to partial nephroureterotomy to a complete surgical reconstruction.[46] The evolution of endoscopic instruments that are small enough for neonates has increased the use of endoscopic surgery to accomplish the required procedures with less morbidity.[45,47] Immediate endoscopic ureterocele decompression by incision or puncture is recommended in the setting of infection or severe obstruction.[46] The choice of surgical procedure depends upon multiple factors including patient age and clinical condition, kidney function, and presence of obstruction or reflux.[46] Depending upon the anomalies found during diagnostic evaluation, the intervention may include transurethral incision of the defect, excision with reimplantation of the ureter, or partial nephrectomy and ureterectomy. In an acutely septic patient, a percutaneous nephrostomy to drain the upper collecting system may be needed.

> **KEY POINTS**
> - Congenital abnormalities of the bladder include misimplantation of ureters, strictures, an extra ureter, and ureterocele.
> - These disorders cause problems by obstructing normal urine flow and predisposing to retrograde urine flow, urinary stasis, and secondary infection; they are usually treated with surgical interventions.

NEOPLASMS

Primary cancers of the ureters or urethra are rare. Bladder cancer, however, is quite common.

Bladder Cancer

The American Cancer Society estimated there would be approximately 69,250 new bladder cancer patients diagnosed in the United States in 2011—52,020 men and 17,230 women.[49] Bladder cancer is the fourth most common cancer diagnosed in men in the United States (following prostate, lung, and colon cancers) and the ninth most common cancer in U.S. women. The male/female ratio of incidence is 3:1.[3] The mortality rate for 2011 was estimated to be about 10,670 men and 4320 women.[49] The rates of both incidence and mortality attributable to bladder cancer have been quite stable across the last 20 years. Like most cancers, the risk of developing bladder cancer increases with age; median age at diagnosis for men is 69 years and for women is 71 years. From 2004 to 2008, the incidence in white males was nearly twice that in black males, and slightly lower in Hispanic males than in blacks.[50] Blacks, however, have more advanced stages of bladder cancer than whites at the time of diagnosis. At diagnosis, about half of bladder cancer patients have superficial cancers, and about 35% have bladder muscle–invasive cancer. In the remainder of patients, the cancer has spread outside the bladder, rarely to distant sites.[49]

There are four general types of bladder cancer, differentiated by their histologic appearance.[49] Some of these bladder cancer histologies are also found in malignancies of the renal pelvis, ureters, and/or urethra. More than 95% of all cases of bladder cancer are *urothelial (transitional cell)* carcinomas originating in the transitional epithelium, or urothelium, which is the lining found throughout the urinary tract. There are two subtypes of urothelial carcinomas (UCs); the majority exhibit a papillary appearance with the remainder having a flat appearance. Flat lesions tend to be more muscle-invasive and thus have a poorer prognosis.[3] *Squamous cell* carcinoma of the bladder represents only approximately 1% to 2% of the overall cases. This type of bladder cancer is microscopically very similar to skin cancer, and is quite invasive. About 1% of bladder cancers are *adenocarcinomas*. These tumors, arising from glandular tissue, are also invasive in nature. *Small cell* bladder cancers account for less than 1% of all bladder cancers; these cancers arise from neuroendocrine cells.[49] These diverse types of malignancies may respond differently to the interventions for bladder cancer. A very rare muscle cancer called *rhabdomyosarcoma* is not usually included in discussions of bladder cancer. It may originate in the bladder but more frequently involves other organs and tissues.

Risk factors. Bladder cancer risk usually is divided into environmental and inherited classifications. Environmental risk factors for bladder cancer are shown in Box 29-2. Smoking is the greatest risk factor, increasing risk by about threefold; smoking cessation has been shown to decrease bladder cancer risk.[3] Carcinogenic chemicals in cigarette smoke are inhaled, enter the bloodstream, and then are filtered and concentrated in the urinary tract. About 66% of deaths from bladder tumors in men and 30% in women are attributable to smoking.[3] Occupational exposure to carcinogens and smoking may increase bladder cancer risk synergistically.[49] People with occupational exposure to aniline (an aromatic amine) textile dyes, hair dyes (especially for greater than 10 years), paint and leather, carpet, rubber, and cement are at increased risk for bladder cancer.[3] Chronic inflammation of the bladder by UTIs is associated with an increased risk of bladder cancer, especially the invasive squamous cell type. Other causes of inflammation, such as stones, have also been associated with the disease. Certain chemotherapy agents (e.g., cyclophosphamide, ifosfamide) used in the treatment of other malignancies as well as radiation therapy to the pelvis increase the risk of bladder cancer. Low fluid intake is a risk factor for bladder cancer.[3] A family history of bladder cancer increases a person's risk, likely through inherited gene syndromes and/or shared exposure to environmental carcinogens. One heritable risk factor is a mutation of the retinoblastoma gene responsible for an infantile cancer of the eye that is associated with increased bladder cancer risk.[49]

BOX 29-2 ENVIRONMENTAL RISK FACTORS FOR BLADDER CANCER

Tobacco smoking (aromatic amines)
Certain types of dyes, including hair, medical, and industrial dyes (aromatic amines)
Certain chemicals used in rubber tire production
Certain pesticides that contain aromatic amines
Certain chemotherapeutic agents (e.g., cyclophosphamide)
Diesel exhaust (polycyclic aromatic hydrocarbons)
Arsenic in drinking water
Low fluid intake
Pelvic radiation therapy

In children, the congenital anomaly of exstrophy of the bladder (bladder outside the abdominal cavity) may predispose to the development of bladder tumors, particularly adenocarcinomas.[3,49] Parasitic infections from schistosomiasis, prevalent in the Middle East and Africa (especially Egypt), have been associated with squamous cell carcinoma as a result of urine-borne carcinogens formed during the infectious process and irritation by the parasitic ova.[49]

Pathogenesis. Bladder cancer metastasis occurs directly through the bladder wall to adjacent organs (e.g., prostate, bowel, vagina, uterus) or via lymph nodes in the pelvis and abdomen. Once treated, tumors can recur at the original site, or an entirely new tumor may develop at another site. The sites of metastasis most commonly include the lymph nodes, liver, lungs, and bone.[3] Specific details of the pathogenesis of cancer are found in Chapter 7.

Clinical manifestations. Painless hematuria is usually the initial symptom of bladder cancer.[3] However, in the early stages of bladder cancer, both gross and microscopic hematuria are often intermittent, and hematuria is associated with numerous urinary tract pathologies. Other manifestations related to bladder cancer include urinary frequency and urgency; dysuria is an uncommon finding. But again, all these symptoms are also seen with other conditions involving the urinary tract.[3,49] Because these signs and symptoms are so general, early diagnosis of bladder cancer requires a thorough workup by the health care provider, especially in persons more than 40 years of age.[3]

Diagnosis. In most cases, diagnostic evaluation for bladder cancer is initiated because of the development of one or more of the previously listed clinical manifestations. A thorough history may reveal risk factors for bladder cancer, or physical examination and diagnostic testing may indicate another etiology.

The recommended diagnostic test for suspected bladder cancer is cystoscopy, with biopsy of any questionable tissue and washings of free cells for cytologic examination.[51] White light cystoscopy allows direct visualization of tumors. Newer fluorescent cystoscopy uses a photosensitive substance such as 5-aminolevulinic acid (5-ALA) to enhance the ability to detect small high-grade urothelial lesions.[52] Urine specimens will be tested for the presence of tumor markers. The sensitivity and specificity of available tumor markers varies widely; at this time, no tumor marker is reliable enough to replace cystoscopy.[3,51] Tumor markers may also be used to monitor response to treatment.[49] Recommended imaging tests include intravenous pyelogram (IVP), computerized tomography (CT) scan, and transabdominal ultrasound.[51] Other tests such as bone scans may be performed to determine the presence of metastasis. The stage of the malignancy is an important contributor to treatment decisions, and also aids in the determination of prognosis. The TNM (tumor, node, metastasis) staging system is commonly used for bladder cancer.[3]

The examination of biopsied tissue, cells obtained during cystoscopy, and cells that might be found in the urine is essential to the determination of the specific type and grade of the tumor. (See Chapter 7 for a thorough discussion of staging and grading.) The World Health Organization grading system for non–muscle-invasive UC addresses risk for invasion and recurrence.[51] Examination of the biopsy also allows determination of the depth to which the tumor has penetrated the bladder wall and facilitates staging. All of this information is used to guide the selection of the specific treatment approach.

Treatment. Treatment protocols are based on the tumor's features: the type of bladder cancer and its grade and stage. The primary options are surgery, radiation therapy, chemotherapy, and immunotherapy. Treatment selection is evidence-based, with available information continuously being updated.[51,53] Surgery as the single treatment, or with other adjuvants, is the intervention for the majority of bladder cancers. The specific approach to surgery varies with the stage of the tumor. For non–muscle-invasive carcinoma, endoscopic transurethral resection of bladder tumors (TURBT) with appropriate cystoscopic and cytologic follow-up is recommended.[51] Intravesical immunotherapy with Bacillus Calmette-Guérin (BCG) is also recommended, either as a single dose or as a course of doses over time, depending upon risk of recurrence and progression.[51] Adjuvant intravesical instillation of chemotherapeutic agents (e.g., mitomycin C, doxorubicin) has been shown to reduce recurrence.[51]

If the tumor is at high risk for progression, unresponsive to BCG, or muscle-invasive, more extensive surgical procedures are employed. Chemotherapy or radiation therapy may be performed preoperatively to reduce tumor size and improve survival.[51,53] Surgical removal of the bladder (cystectomy), either partial or total, may be performed; a total cystectomy requires urinary diversion to provide for storage and elimination of urine.[49] Urinary diversions typically involve the creation of a reservoir, using a portion of the intestine, into which the ureters are implanted. Urine is drained from the reservoir often through a stoma created through the abdominal wall; however, substitute bladder reservoir (neobladder) procedures involve connecting the urethra to the reservoir, allowing the patient to void normally. In cases where the tumor is large or there are multiple bladder tumors, a radical cystectomy is performed, in which the bladder and surrounding nodes are removed; in men the prostate gland is also removed, and in women the uterus, ovaries, fallopian tubes, and part of the vagina are also often removed.[51,53]

Therapies that preserve the bladder may be selected, even for muscle-invasive carcinomas, if the disease is bladder-localized. External beam radiation therapy may be an acceptable alternative for patients who are not sufficiently strong for radical surgical procedures. Systemic chemotherapy may be an option for people with metastatic bladder cancer.[53]

The prognosis for stage 0 (noninvasive papillary carcinoma or carcinoma in situ [CIS]) is excellent, with a relative 5-year survival rate of 98%.[49] As the tumor invades deeper into the bladder wall or metastasizes beyond the bladder, the survival rate begins to decline. The 5-year relative survival rate for muscle-invasive (stage II) bladder cancer is 63% and drops to 15% for metastatic (stage IV) cancer.[49] Risk of recurrence of bladder cancer is high, even for superficial malignancies; ongoing follow-up with periodic diagnostic tests is necessary.[3]

KEY POINTS

- Bladder cancer is the fourth most common cancer diagnosed in men in the United States and the ninth most common in women.
- Risk of developing bladder cancer increases with age; smoking and occupational exposure to carcinogenic chemicals are thought to be the main predisposing factors.
- There are four general types of bladder cancer, differentiated by their histologic appearance. About 95% of bladder tumors originate from the transitional epithelium (urothelium) lining the urinary tract.
- Bladder cancer is primarily manifested as hematuria. Frequency and urgency may also be present. Dysuria is not common.
- The most frequently used invasive test in the diagnosis of bladder cancer is cystoscopy, with biopsy of any questionable tissue and washings of free cells for cytologic examination.
- Treatment protocols are based on the tumor's features: the type of bladder cancer and its grade and stage. The primary options are surgery, radiation therapy, chemotherapy, and immunotherapy.

INFLAMMATION AND INFECTION

Most inflammations of the lower urinary tract are due to infection. The normal defense mechanisms of the urinary tract are presented in detail in Chapter 27 with the discussion of pyelonephritis (infection of the kidney). Urinary tract infections (UTIs) are typically ascending in nature; they begin in the lower urinary tract and may progress to the kidney (upper urinary tract). By the time infection reaches the kidneys, the bladder and urethra are already infected. Involvement of the ureters does not seem to present with clinical manifestations.

Urethritis

Urethritis is an inflammation of the urethra. Inflammation of the urethra may lead to pain, burning, and urinary incontinence, and if it is attributable to an infectious organism, it may progress to infective cystitis. Urethritis can be caused by infection, external irritants, or, in women, insufficient estrogen levels.

Infection of the urethra may be due to a wide variety of organisms, most often including *Neisseria gonorrhoeae* and *Chlamydia trachomatis*.[4] Urethritis is the most commonly occurring sexually transmitted infection (STI) in men.[54] Symptoms include dysuria, urgency, and frequency, often but not always accompanied by urethral discharge. Some people are asymptomatic; if the cause is an STI, they may not know they are infected until notified that their partner has an infection. The urethra is an estrogen-dependent structure, and postmenopausal women are at increased risk for irritation and inflammation of the urethra. Application of topical estrogen to the urethral opening helps maintain mucosal health.[11] If urethritis is due to a sexually transmitted organism, targeted pharmacologic therapy is indicated. Otherwise, urethritis attributable to infection is often asymptomatic until the organism progresses to the bladder, causing cystitis.

Cystitis

Cystitis, or inflammation of the bladder lining, may result from bacterial, fungal, or parasitic infections, chemical irritants, foreign bodies (e.g., stones), or trauma. By far the most common cause of cystitis—and the focus of this discussion—is bacterial infection.

Etiology and pathogenesis. Normally, bacteria are cleared from the bladder by the flushing and dilutional effects of voiding. The high urea concentration and osmolarity and the low pH in urine act as natural barriers, killing invading bacteria in a normal bladder environment.

UTIs are highly prevalent, accounting for 8 million office and emergency department visits, about 100,000 hospital admissions, and over $3 billion in treatment costs annually.[4,55] Incidence is higher in women but men tend to have more complicated infections. Risk factors are listed in detail in Box 29-3. In the pediatric population, uncircumcised male infants less than 6 months of age and females less than 12 months of age have the highest prevalence.[56] Recurrent UTIs are common in women.[57] A shorter urethra as well as a colonization route from both the rectum and the vagina to the urethra is thought to explain the increased rate of infections in women. They are common occurrences during pregnancy, and have been associated with an increased risk of premature delivery and low birth weight.[4] Use of spermicidal agents, with diaphragms or coated condoms, increases the risk of UTIs.[4] Prostatic secretions, which are antibacterial, inhibit cystitis in men younger than 50 years. *Escherichia coli* is responsible for 80% of cases of bacterial cystitis, with *Staphylococcus saprophyticus* as the next most common causative pathogen.[57] The microbial characteristics of *E. coli*

BOX 29-3 RISK FACTORS FOR CYSTITIS

Factors Increasing Urinary Stasis
Intrinsic obstruction (stone, tumor of urinary tract, urethral stricture, BPH)
Extrinsic obstruction (tumor, fibrosis compressing urinary tract)
Urinary retention (including neurogenic bladder and low bladder wall compliance)
Renal impairment

Foreign Bodies
Urinary tract calculi
Catheters (indwelling, external condom catheter, urethral stent, nephrostomy tube, intermittent catheterization)
Urinary tract instrumentation (cystoscopy, urodynamics)

Anatomic Factors
Congenital defects leading to obstruction or urinary stasis
Fistula (abnormal opening) exposing urinary stream to skin, vagina, or fecal stream
Shorter female urethra and colonization from normal vaginal flora
Obesity

Factors Compromising Immune Response
Aging
Human immunodeficiency virus infection
Diabetes mellitus

Functional Disorders
Constipation
Voiding dysfunction with detrusor sphincter dyssynergia

Other Factors
Pregnancy
Hypoestrogenic state
Multiple sex partners (women)
Use of spermicidal agents or contraceptive diaphragm (women)
Poor personal hygiene

From Lewis S et al: *Medical-surgical nursing: assessment and management of clinical problems*, ed 8, St Louis, 2011, Mosby.
BPH, Benign prostatic hyperplasia.

promote its adherence to bladder mucosa and ability to evade the host's immune response.[4] Fungal infections, mycoplasmas, and other anaerobic bacteria are occasionally responsible. Infections attributable to *Neisseria gonorrhoeae* or *Chlamydia trachomatis* are associated with sexually transmitted diseases but are typically limited to the urethra.[4] Additional risk factors include sexual activity, diabetes mellitus, poor personal hygiene, any type of bladder dysfunction causing urine stasis, urinary catheterization and indwelling catheters, antimicrobial therapy in the previous month, postmenopausal status, and a family history of UTIs.[4]

Clinical manifestations. The majority of patients with cystitis experience an acute onset of frequency, urgency, dysuria, and pain, often in the suprapubic area.[4,55] The urine may appear pink because of hematuria or cloudy as a result of the infectious organism. Common symptoms of cystitis in children include fever, irritability, poor feeding, vomiting, diarrhea, and ill appearance.[58,59] Children who are able to talk may also indicate dysuria, suprapubic pain, or incontinence, but even older children sometimes have difficulty localizing signs and symptoms.[58,59] Untreated cystitis may lead to renal damage secondary to ascension of the infection to the upper urinary tract. Therefore, prompt intervention is essential.

Diagnosis and treatment. Screening for suspected UTI is often performed using a clean-catch urine specimen and a simple nitrite and leukocyte esterase dipstick test.[6] Nitrites are present in UTI because many urinary pathogens produce enzymes that reduce nitrates to nitrites; the presence of leukocyte esterase is indicative of **pyuria** (white blood cells in the urine). The dipstick test is quite sensitive in detecting UTIs.[6] However, the sensitivity of dipstick urinalysis combined with visual appearance has been reported to be decreased in children; microscopic analysis is recommended.[58,59] A urine culture is not always necessary for the diagnosis of UTI. Uncomplicated infections, caused by common organisms, may be diagnosed on the basis of symptoms and a positive dipstick. Culture is recommended in situations in which the patient has manifestations suggesting pyelonephritis, fails to respond to empirical pharmacologic therapy, is pregnant, or has urinary calculi. A culture should be considered if the patient is immunosuppressed (because of the likelihood of atypical organisms) or has diabetes mellitus.[56] Under these circumstances, cultures precisely identify organisms and permit targeted pharmacologic therapy.

Men, children, and those women with recurrent infections, unresolved infections, atypical manifestations, or other problems previously identified have complicated UTIs and require physical examination and diagnostic testing.[4,55] *Recurrent UTIs* are repeated infections within a short period after verified resolution of the earlier infection. Recurrent UTIs are fairly common in women but rare in healthy adult men. Recurrent infections in men should trigger a urologic examination that may include endoscopy and a CT scan. *Unresolved infections* are those in which bacteriuria remains after the initial treatment.[4]

Treatment algorithms for acute cystitis and recurrent UTIs are shown in Figures 29-3 and 29-4, respectively. Acute, uncomplicated UTIs in women with no anatomic anomalies of the urinary tract, with no recent history of cystitis, and with no symptoms suggestive of either vaginitis or cervicitis may be treated empirically with a 3-day course of trimethoprim-sulfamethoxazole or a 5-day course of nitrofurantoin.[4,60]

Cystitis in healthy younger men is managed with a 7-day course of antibiotics.[55] In older men, a minimum of 14 and up to 28 days of antibiotic therapy is recommended. Unresolved infections are usually treated with targeted antimicrobials for 7 to 10 days. Urine culture and sensitivity are also necessary to ensure antibiotic effectiveness.[56] Some women with recurrent UTIs are treated with low-dose prophylactic antibiotics or given the option of a self-start antibiotic regimen in which the woman initiates antibiotic therapy with symptoms.[57] In elderly women, topical estrogen can be effective to prevent recurring infection because bacteria colonize in the urethra as a result of deestrogenization of the tissue attributable to menopause. In some women, recurrent infections are related to sexual intercourse, and a postcoital prophylactic antibiotic program is an effective treatment option.[57] Persistent bacterial infections are nearly always due to an anatomic abnormality or pathology in the urinary tract.[57] Such problems include calculi, prostatitis, foreign bodies, and duplicated or ectopic ureters.

In children, administration of broad-spectrum antibiotics for 7 to 14 days is the treatment of choice.[58] The specific choice of therapy, including the initiation of parenteral fluids, is contingent on many factors including age, illness severity, illness duration, and ability to drink adequate fluids. However, children younger than 5 years should keep taking prophylactic doses of antibiotics until radiographic evaluation is completed. UTIs in children are often indicative of an underlying pathologic process (e.g., vesicoureteral reflux, ureteropelvic junction obstruction [UPJO]) and warrant prompt urologic evaluation.[58]

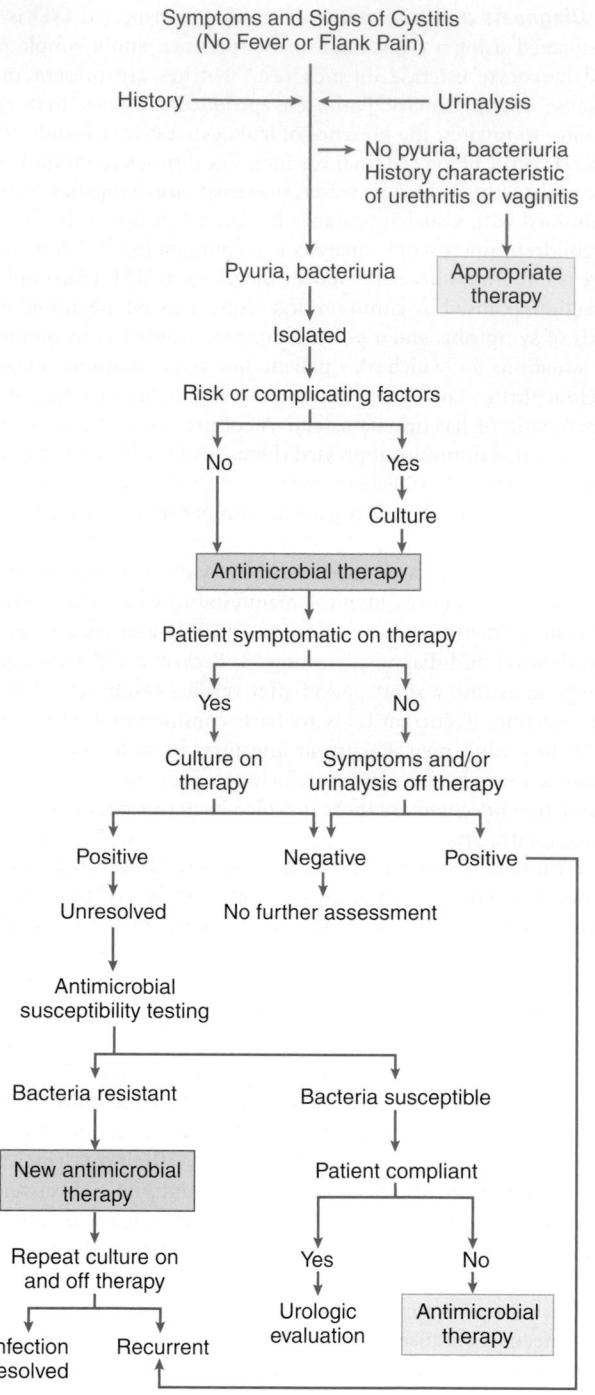

FIGURE 29-3 Management of acute cystitis. (From Wein AJ et al, editors: *Campbell-Walsh urology*, ed 10, St Louis, 2012, Saunders.)

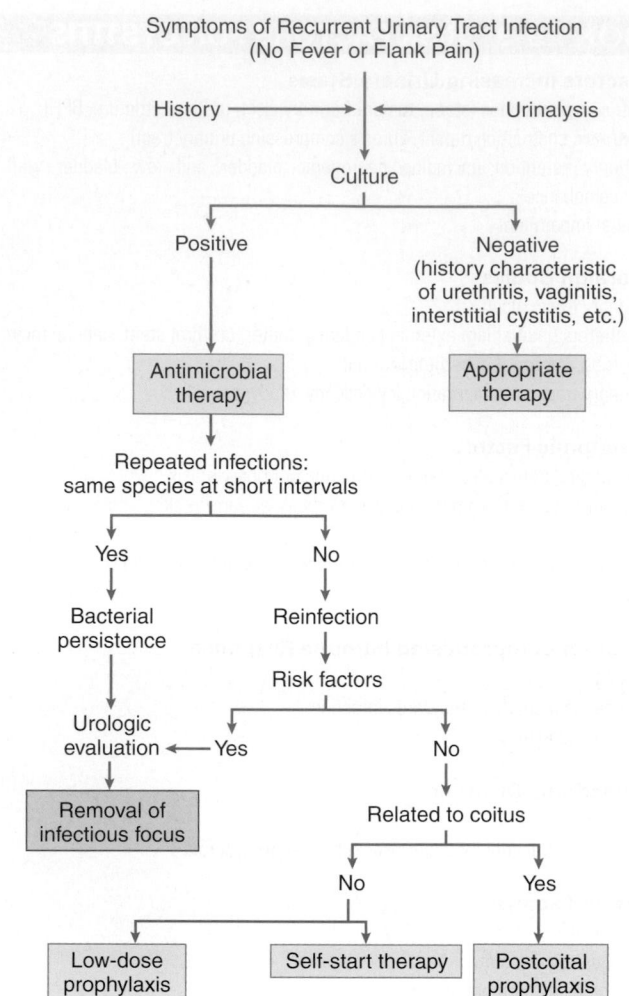

FIGURE 29-4 Management of recurrent UTI. (From Wein AJ et al, editors: *Campbell-Walsh urology*, ed 10, St Louis, 2012, Saunders.)

Pregnant women have the same prevalence of bacteriuria as nonpregnant women, but diagnosis and treatment are critical in pregnant women because of their greater propensity for pyelonephritis as a result of pregnancy-induced physiologic alterations.[4] Antibiotic therapy must be carefully chosen to avoid fetal harm.

Rates of bacteriuria significantly increase with age. Factors that predispose the elderly to cystitis include genitourinary abnormalities (e.g., calculi, benign prostatic hyperplasia, prostatitis), chronic illnesses (particularly diabetes mellitus and neurologic diseases), changes in urinary pH, decreased estrogen production in women, bowel incontinence, and greater prevalence of catheterization.[4,55] A 7- to 10-day course of

antibiotic treatment and close monitoring for adverse effects are recommended for symptomatic UTIs. Symptoms associated with bacteriuria in the elderly may include anxiety, confusion, lethargy, and anorexia as opposed to dysuria and fever. The diagnosis is often one of exclusion, and urinalysis and culture are included in the diagnostic evaluation. Antibiotics are not recommended for asymptomatic bacteriuria in the elderly.

Interstitial Cystitis/Bladder Pain Syndrome

Interstitial cystitis/bladder pain syndrome (IC/BPS) is a pain syndrome characterized by pelvic pain lasting longer than 6 months, perceived to be stemming from the bladder, and accompanied by other lower urinary tract symptoms such as frequency, urgency, dysuria, and dyspareunia.[61,62] The pain may worsen with a full bladder as well as with consumption of certain foods and drinks.[61] Pain is often relieved with voiding. The syndrome is more prevalent in women; an estimated 1.2 million U.S. women and 82,000 men suffer from IC/BPS.[62] This condition can have a serious impact on quality of life, interfering with work, daily activities, sleep, family life, and sexual activities.

The specific etiology is unknown and the pathophysiology is unclear, but a fundamental mechanism appears to be urothelial damage. Inflammation is activated and the damaged urothelium is less able to serve its protective functions, including production of mucus.[62] People with BPS are more likely to be diagnosed with other pain syndromes such as fibromyalgia and with autoimmune conditions such as inflammatory bowel disease.[61]

Diagnosis of BPS is challenging because of the nonspecific nature of the syndrome. The diagnostic workup should include a history, physical exam, urinalysis, and possibly a urine culture and cytology to rule out subclinical infection and bladder cancer.[63] Pain is usually present in several locations, but physical exam is often negative. The foods and drinks most often associated with pain are alcohol, citrus fruits, coffee, carbonated beverages, tea, chocolate, and tomatoes. Hydrodistention of the bladder and instillations of potassium chloride will often reproduce the pain. Cystoscopy and urodynamic studies are unnecessary unless there is diagnostic uncertainty; IC/BPS is diagnosed as a symptom-based syndrome after eliminating other pathologies.[63] Treatment begins with lifestyle modifications such as avoiding known bladder irritants. Pelvic floor muscle training and bladder retraining may be helpful in moderating urgency.[63] Pentosan polysulfate sodium is approved for treating IC; the drug presumably coats and protects the urothelium. Amitriptyline and hydroxyzine are other drugs that have been prescribed for symptom management.[62] For people with intractable pain, major surgery such as cystectomy with urinary diversion may be performed as a last resort.[63]

KEY POINTS

- Urethritis is inflammation of the urethra. It is most often due to infection, either from the bladder or associated with a sexually transmitted disease. Sexually transmitted diseases are confined to the urethra; infections of other etiologies may ascend to the bladder before symptoms present. Urethritis may also be due to external factors such as frequent catheterizations or poor personal hygiene. Treatment depends on the cause.

- Cystitis is an inflammation of the bladder lining that may be due to infection, chemical irritants, stones, or trauma. Most cases have an infectious etiology and result from infection originating in the urethra.

- Factors predisposing to cystitis include female gender, increased age, catheterization, diabetes mellitus, bladder dysfunction, poor personal hygiene, and any disorder causing urinary stasis. Manifestations include frequency, urgency, dysuria, possible suprapubic pain, and cloudy urine, although the infection may be asymptomatic. Most female patients are treated based only on this information. More complicated situations, and cystitis in men and children, may require urine culture and/or further assessment.

- Symptoms of cystitis in older adults may be atypical and include lethargy, anorexia, confusion, and anxiety. Symptomatic cystitis in the elderly should be managed with close drug monitoring to avoid toxicity. Asymptomatic bacteriuria in the elderly should not be treated.

- Interstitial cystitis/painful bladder syndrome is a chronic condition consisting of bladder pain and often urgency, frequency, and nocturia, when no other etiology can be identified. It is diagnosed based on this information. Treatment is based on the identification of contributory lifestyle factors, such as some foods and beverages. Avoidance of these factors is the primary intervention; medication may be added to manage IC/BPS.

OBSTRUCTION

Obstruction of the lower urinary tract develops when a stone obstructs urine transport. Stones in the lower urinary tract produce some manifestations that are similar to stones formed and lodged in the kidney.

Lower Urinary Tract Urolithiasis

Stones, or calculi, usually form in the kidneys *(nephrolithiasis)*. Nephrolithiasis is discussed in Chapter 27. The term **urolithiasis** is used for stones forming anywhere in the urinary tract, primarily in the kidney or ureters, as well as those that form or travel into the ureters, bladder, or urethra. The manifestations of stones in the ureters and bladder vary somewhat from those associated with kidney stones, but the risk factors, stone composition, diagnostic tests, and treatment aspects are essentially the same. Refer to Chapter 27 for a detailed discussion of these topics. If diagnosis and treatment are not completed in a timely manner, the patient is at risk for the development of postrenal acute kidney injury (Chapter 28).

Ureterolithiasis

Calculi in the ureters are usually those that were able to pass through the junction of the renal pelvis and ureters, as opposed to being formed there. In many cases, these stones are small, pass easily through the ureters, and cause no clinical manifestations. When a larger stone becomes wedged at the junction, manifestations are those characteristic of nephrolithiasis. Other stones enter the ureters and instigate an inflammatory process that increases prostaglandin synthesis. Prostaglandins increase renal blood flow, aggravating inflammation and edema.[64] Ureteral spasm contributes to pain that is termed ureteral colic. This is an acute, sharp, spasmodic pain, experienced in the flank area, possibly radiating into the umbilical region. Irritation of the ureters may result in hematuria. When the stone approaches the distal portion of the ureters, the pain may continue to be sharp in quality, but intermittent in nature. Or, instead of this presentation, the pain may increase, with radiation into the groin region, testicles, or labia. Manifestations associated with ureteral colic include tachycardia, tachypnea, diaphoresis, nausea, and vomiting.

Diagnostic approaches are the same as those used for nephrolithiasis, being sure to include the lower urinary tract region in scans. Ureteral calculi may be spontaneously expelled; the probability of and time to passage vary depending upon the size and location of the stone.[64] Stones ≤2 mm were reported as taking an average of 8.2 days to pass; stones 4 to 6 mm in size averaged 22.1 days.[64] Smaller stones warrant observation with pain management while waiting for spontaneous passage; however, failure of the stone to move or unrelenting pain is an indication for stone removal.[65] Medical expulsion therapy using α-adrenergic blockers such as tamsulosin may facilitate passage of stones <10 mm.[64,66] Larger stones (>10 mm) may necessitate stone removal; shock-wave lithotripsy and ureteroscopy are first-line treatments for both adults and children. Either laparoscopic or open surgical removal of stones is recommended in cases of first-line treatment failure.[65] Therapeutic and preventive interventions are otherwise the same as those presented in Chapter 27. These interventions will affect stones formed anywhere in the urinary tract.

Bladder (Vesical) Urolithiasis

Formation of stones in the bladder is rare in the developed world though more common in developing countries, including in children.[67] Ammonium acid urate is the main substance in bladder stones in the developing world.[67] Urinary stasis, infection, and foreign bodies in the bladder contribute to stone formation. Some patients are asymptomatic; those with symptoms may experience dysuria, suprapubic pain, and urinary hesitancy. A stone in the bladder may irritate the urothelium and result in hematuria; once the bladder neck or urethral orifice is reached, manifestations of obstruction may appear.

Diagnostic tests are similar to those for calculi in other segments of the urinary tract. Stone expulsion is often spontaneous; stones causing obstruction pose a risk for postrenal acute kidney injury and require prompt intervention. Stone removal procedures include transurethral lithotripsy for stones smaller than 1 cm, percutaneous cystolithotomy for stones up to 5 cm, and open cystolithotomy for stones ≥5 cm.[67]

KEY POINTS

- Urolithiasis is most often due to stones traveling to the ureters, bladder, or urethra from the kidney. They may also originate in the bladder or ureters. Manifestations are associated with tissue irritation and obstruction.
- Manifestations of ureterolithiasis include ureteral colic, hematuria, tachycardia, tachypnea, diaphoresis, nausea, and vomiting. Individuals with stones that approach the bladder may experience pain that is sharp in quality but intermittent in nature. Otherwise, the pain may increase and radiate into the groin region, testicles, or labia.

- Bladder urolithiasis is usually due to stones traveling from the ureters, but stones may form in the bladder, usually as a result of urinary stasis.
- Manifestations of bladder stones are often limited to dysuria and frequency; hematuria is possible. Obstructive signs and symptoms will present if stones obstruct the bladder neck or urethral orifice.
- Ureterolithiasis and bladder urolithiasis are similar to nephrolithiasis in terms of risk factors and stone characteristics. If infection is present, it is treated with appropriate antimicrobials, based on culture and sensitivity tests. Intervention for stones that do not pass spontaneously is endoscopic (transurethral) lithotripsy.

SUMMARY

Disorders involving the lower urinary tract are quite common. In adults, the most prevalent pathologic conditions are voiding dysfunction, malignancies, infections, and urinary stones. Incontinence as a result of bladder dysfunction affects millions of adults. The prevalence of incontinence increases with age and is more common in women than men. However, incontinence is not a result of the normal aging process, and patients should be urged to seek evaluation and treatment. Behavioral, pharmacologic, and surgical approaches may be used to manage voiding dysfunction. Interstitial cystitis/painful bladder syndrome is a chronic condition consisting of bladder pain and a variety of other manifestations typically associated with other bladder pathologies. However, these patients have no other identifiable pathology. Urgency, frequency, and nocturia are other common findings. In the United States, bladder cancer is the fourth most common type of cancer in men and the ninth most common type in women. The primary clinical manifestation of bladder cancer is hematuria. Treatment is based on stage, grade, and type of cancer. Interventions include surgery, radiation, and chemotherapy.

Both childhood UTIs and enuresis should trigger more detailed urologic evaluation to rule out congenital disorders such as UPJO, ectopic ureters, ureterocele, and vesicoureteral reflux. Vesicoureteral reflux is the most prevalent congenital lower urinary tract disorder. It predisposes children to UTIs, which can result in kidney scarring and permanent renal impairment. Most cases of vesicoureteral reflux resolve spontaneously as the child ages. Before resolution, close medical management is necessary to prevent upper UTI and kidney damage.

Stones in the lower urinary tract usually arrive there after being formed in the kidney. Risk factors and treatment are much the same as those for nephrolithiasis; however, manifestations of urolithiasis in the ureters or bladder differ.

REFERENCES

1. Benarroch EE: Neural control of the bladder: recent advances and neurologic implications, *Neurology* 75:1839–1846, 2010.
2. Casey G: Incontinence and retention—how the bladder misfunctions, *New Zealand Nurs J* 17:26–31, 2011.
3. Tanaka MF, Sonpavde G: Diagnosis and management of urothelial carcinoma of the bladder, *Postgrad Med* 123:43–55, 2011.
4. Dielubanza EJ, Schaeffer AJ: Urinary tract infections in women, *Med Clin North Am* 95:27–41, 2011.
5. Frick AC, et al: Mixed urinary incontinence: greater impact on quality of life, *J Urol* 182:596–600, 2009.
6. Pagana KD, Pagana TJ: *Mosby's manual of diagnostic and laboratory tests*, ed 4, St Louis, 2010, Mosby.
7. Abrams P, et al: The standardization of terminology of lower urinary tract function, *Neurourol Urodyn* 21:167–178, 2002.
8. Gibbs CF, Johnson TM, Ouslander JG: Office management of geriatric urinary incontinence, *Am J Med* 120:211–220, 2007.
9. Subak LL, et al: The "costs" of urinary incontinence for women, *Obstet Gynecol* 107:908–916, 2006.
10. Rahn DD, Roshanravan SM: Pathophysiology of urinary incontinence, voiding dysfunction, and overactive bladder, *Obstet Gynecol Clin North Am* 36:463–474, 2009.
11. Hillard T: The postmenopausal bladder, *Menopause Int* 16:74–80, 2010.
12. Abrams P, et al: Reviewing the ICS 2002 Terminology Report: the ongoing debate, *Neurourol Urodyn* 28:287, 2009.
13. Sand PK, Appell R: Disruptive effects of overactive bladder and urge urinary incontinence in younger women, *Am J Med* 119:16S–23S, 2006.
14. Mappilakkandy R, Mistri AK: Anticholinergics for urge incontinence, *Rev Clin Gerontol* 20:30–41, 2010.
15. Stothers L: Should hormone replacement therapy be used in postmenopausal women for voiding dysfunction? *Can Urol Assoc J* 3:150–152, 2009.
16. National Guideline Clearinghouse (NGC): *Guideline summary: guidelines on urinary incontinence, incontinence in men,* Rockville, MD, Agency for Healthcare Research and Quality (AHRQ). Available at www.guidelines.gov/content.aspx?id=14817&search=urinary+incontinence+in+men. Accessed 11/18/11.
17. Neveus T, et al: The standardization of terminology of lower urinary tract function in children and adolescents, *J Urol* 176:314–324, 2006.
18. Shreeram S, et al: Prevalence of enuresis and its association with attention-deficit/hyperactivity disorder among U.S. children: results from a nationally representative study, *J Am Acad Child Adolesc Psychiatry* 48:35–41, 2009.
19. Neveus T, et al: Evaluation of and treatment for monosymptomatic enuresis, *J Urol* 183:441–447, 2010.
20. Hoban TF: Sleep disorders in children, *Ann N Y Acad Sci* 1184:1–14, 2009.
21. von Gontard A, Heron J, Joinson C: Family history of nocturnal enuresis and urinary incontinence: results from a large epidemiological study, *J Urol* 185:2303–2306, 2011.
22. Bascom A, et al: High risk of sleep disordered breathing in the enuresis population, *J Urol* 186:1710–1714, 2011.
23. Burgu B, et al: Lower urinary tract conditions in children with attention deficit hyperactivity disorder, *J Urol* 185:663–668, 2011.
24. Ramakrishnan K: Evaluation and treatment of enuresis, *Am Fam Physician* 78:489–496, 2008.
25. Hannula A: Vesicoureteral reflux in children with suspected and proven urinary tract infection, *Pediatr Nephrol* 25:1463–1469, 2010.
26. Coulthard MG: Vesicoureteric reflux is not a benign condition, *Pediatr Nephrol* 24:227–232, 2009.
27. Pirker ME: Familiar vesicoureteral reflux: influence of sex on prevalence and expression, *J Urol* 176:1776–1780, 2006.
28. Demirbag S: Bladder dysfunction in infants with primary vesicoureteric reflux, *J Int Med Res* 37:1877–1881, 2009.

29. Peters C, Rushton HG: Vesicoureteral reflux associated renal damage: congenital reflux nephropathy and acquired renal scarring, *J Urol* 184:265–273, 2010.

30. Pohl HG, et al: Vesicoureteral reflux and ureteroceles, *J Urol* 177:1659–1666, 2007.

31. MacNeily AE, Afshar K: Screening asymptomatic siblings for vesicoureteral reflux: sound science or religious rhetoric? *Can J Urol* 13:3309–3316, 2006.

32. National Guideline Clearinghouse (NGC): *Guideline summary: management and screening of primary vesicoureteral reflux in children. AUA guideline, management of vesicoureteral reflux in the child over one year of age,* Rockville, MD, Agency for Healthcare Research and Quality (AHRQ). Available at www.guidelines.gov/content.aspx?id=23923&;search= vesicoureteral+reflux. Accessed 12/30/11.

33. Knudson MJ, et al: Predictive factors of early spontaneous resolution in children with primary vesicoureteral reflux, *J Urol* 178:1684–1688, 2007.

34. Lam JS, Breda A, Schulam PG: Ureteropelvic junction obstruction, *J Urol* 177:1652–1658, 2007.

35. Karnak I, et al: Prenatally detected ureteropelvic junction obstruction: clinical features and associated urologic abnormalities, *Pediatr Surg Int* 24:395–402, 2008.

36. Nelson CP, et al: Contemporary trends in surgical correction of pediatric ureteropelvic junction obstruction: data from the nationwide inpatient sample, *J Urol* 173:232–236, 2005.

37. Sheu JC, et al: Ureteropelvic junction obstruction in children: 10 years' experience in one institution, *Pediatr Surg Int* 22:519–523, 2006.

38. Casale P: Robotic pediatric urology, *Expert Rev Med Devices* 5:59–64, 2008.

39. Hernandez-Rey AE, Vitenson J, McGovern PG: Duplicated ectopic hydroureter presenting as a hydrosalpinx, with chronic pelvic pain and recurrent urinary infections, *Fertil Steril* 88:1677–1679, 2007.

40. Elzayat EA, Al-Mandil MS, Ethilali MM: Renal agenesis associated with ipsilateral ectopic ureters entering a large seminal vesicle cyst, *Can J Urol* 14:3463–3466, 2007.

41. Gordon M, Cervellione RM, Hennayake S: Constant urinary dribbling due to an ectopic ureter and delays in diagnosis, *Clin Pediatr* 46(6):544–546, 2007.

42. Funahashi Y, et al: Radical prostatectomy for prostate carcinoma with ectopic ureters: a case report, *Nippon Hinyokika Gakkai Zasshi* 98:580–582, 2007.

43. Jaiman S, Ulhoj BP: Bilateral intravesical ureterocele associated with unilateral partial duplication of the ureter and other anomalies, *APMIS* 118:809–814, 2010.

44. Spatafora S, Pierfrancesco B, Leoni S: Combined percutaneous-transurethral incision for treatment of ureterocele in adults, *Urology* 68(6):1333–1335, 2006.

45. Nonmura K, Kakizaki H: Recent trends of genitourinary endoscopy in children, *Int J Urol* 12:607–614, 2005.

46. National Guideline Clearinghouse (NGC): *Guideline summary: guidelines on paediatric urology, obstructive pathology of renal duplication: ureterocele and ectopic ureter,* Rockville, MD, Agency for Healthcare Research and Quality (AHRQ). Available at www.guidelines.gov/content.aspx?id=12604&search=ureterocele. Accessed 12/30/11.

47. Kajbafzadeh A, et al: Evolution of endoscopic management of ectopic ureterocele: a new approach, *J Urol* 177:1118–1123, 2007.

48. Pohl HG: Recent advances in the management of ureteroceles in infants and children: why less may be more, *Curr Opin Urol* 21:322–327, 2011.

49. American Cancer Society: *Bladder cancer.* Available at www.cancer.org/acs/groups/cid/documents/webcontent/003085-pdf. Accessed 12/31/11.

50. National Cancer Institute: *Surveillance Epidemiology and End Results (SEER) stat fact sheets: bladder.* Available at http://seer.cancer.gov/statfacts/html/urinb.html. Accessed 12/31/11.

51. Babjuk M, et al: EAU guidelines on non-muscle-invasive urothelial carcinoma of the bladder, the 2011 update, *Eur Urol* 59:997–1008, 2011.

52. Goh AC, Lerner SP: Application of new technology in bladder cancer diagnosis and treatment, *World J Urol* 27:301–307, 2009.

53. Stenzl A, et al: Treatment of muscle-invasive and metastatic bladder cancer: update of the EAU guidelines, *Eur Urol* 59:1009–1018, 2011.

54. Brill JR: Diagnosis and treatment of urethritis in men, *Am Fam Physician* 81:873–878, 2010.

55. Raynor MC, Carson CC III: Urinary infections in men, *Med Clin North Am* 95:43–54, 2011.

56. Car J: Urinary tract infections in women: diagnosis and management in primary care, *BMJ* 332:94–97, 2006.

57. Kodner CM, Thomas Gupton EK: Recurrent urinary tract infections in women: diagnosis and management, *Am Fam Physician* 82:638–643, 2010.

58. Shaikh N, et al: Prevalence of urinary tract infection in childhood: a meta-analysis, *Pediatr Infect Dis J* 27(4):302–308, 2008.

59. Mak RH, Kuo H: Pathogenesis of urinary tract infection: an update, *Curr Opin Pediatr* 18:148–152, 2006.

60. National Guideline Clearinghouse (NGC): *Guideline summary: international clinical practice guidelines for the treatment of acute uncomplicated cystitis and pyelonephritis in women: a 2010 update by the Infectious Diseases Society of America and the European Society for Microbiology and Infectious Diseases,* Rockville, MD, Agency for Healthcare Research and Quality (AHRQ). Available at www.guidelines.gov/content.aspx?id= 25652&search=uncomplicated+cystitis. Accessed 1/1/12.

61. Hanno P, et al: Bladder Pain Syndrome Committee of the International Consultation on Incontinence, *Neurourol Urodyn* 29:191–198, 2010.

62. French LM, Bhambore N: Interstitial cystitis/painful bladder syndrome, *Am Fam Physician* 83:1175–1181, 2011.

63. Hanno PM, et al: AUA guideline for the diagnosis and treatment of interstitial cystitis/bladder pain syndrome, *J Urol* 185:2162–2170, 2011.

64. Seitz C: Medical expulsive therapy of ureteral calculi and supportive therapy after extracorporeal shock wave lithotripsy, *Eur Urol Suppl* 9:807–813, 2010.

65. National Guideline Clearinghouse (NGC): *Guideline summary: 2007 guideline for the management of ureteral calculi,* Rockville, MD, Agency for Healthcare Research and Quality (AHRQ). Available at www.guidelines.gov/content.aspx?id=12209&search=ureteral+calculi. Accessed 1/1/12.

66. Arrabal-Martin M, et al: Treatment of ureteral lithiasis with tamsulosin: literature review and meta-analysis, *Urol Int* 84:254–259, 2010.

67. Al-Marhoon MS, et al: Comparison of endourological and open cystolithotomy in the management of bladder stones in children, *J Urol* 181:2684–2688, 2009.

Male Genital and Reproductive Function

Marvin Van Every

⊝volve WEBSITE

http://evolve.elsevier.com/Copstead/
- Review Questions and Answers
- Glossary (with audio pronunciations for selected terms)
- Animations

- Case Studies
- Key Points Review

KEY QUESTIONS

- What is the role of Sertoli cells in spermatogenesis?
- What is the function of Leydig cells?
- Which branch of the autonomic nervous system is responsible for penile erection? Ejaculation?
- Which genitourinary structures develop embryologically from the wolffian ductal system in males?

- How do the hypothalamic-pituitary gonadotropic hormones influence male reproductive function?
- How do the processes of capacitation and acrosome reaction affect the fertilization process?

CHAPTER OUTLINE

This chapter provides a foundation for comprehending male genital and reproductive disorders, which are presented in Chapter 31. The anatomy and embryology of the male genitourinary tract—those organs involved in the processes of sexual reproduction and elimination of nitrogenous wastes—will be presented first. Because these organs are derived from common embryologic structures, the anatomy and embryology of the male genitalia and urinary system will be emphasized, and the differences in embryologic development between males and females will be considered when pertinent. The remainder of this chapter will deal with the physiologic processes of male reproduction.

ANATOMY

Upper Genitourinary Tract

The upper genitourinary tract consists of the kidneys and ureters. The kidneys receive their blood from the renal arteries, which arise directly from the aorta. They are usually solitary but will at times be duplicated. The ureteral blood supply is derived from multiple sources. The renal pelvis and upper part of the ureter receive blood from branches of the renal artery. The arterial blood supply of the middle ureter segment comes from the internal spermatic artery (gonadal artery), and the lowermost ureter sections receive blood from the branches of the common iliac, internal iliac, and vesical arteries (Figure 30-1). The veins of the renal pelvis and ureter are usually paired with the arteries.

Lower Genitourinary Tract
Bladder

The bladder is a hollow muscular organ that serves as a reservoir for urine. The adult bladder normally has a capacity of 450 to 500 ml. When empty, the bladder lies behind the pubic symphysis and is mainly a pelvic organ. With overdistention or chronic urine retention, the abdomen may bulge, allowing easy palpation of the bladder in the suprapubic region.

The ureters enter the bladder posteroinferiorly. The ureteral orifices are situated on a crescent-shaped ridge and are approximately 2.5 cm apart. The triangular area demarcated by this interureteric ridge and bladder neck is called the *trigone* (Figure 30-2). As will be discussed later in the chapter, the **trigone** has a different embryologic origin from the rest of the bladder body, or fundus. The trigone is composed of mesoderm, and the fundus is composed of endoderm.

In males, the bladder lies anterior to the seminal vesicles, vasa deferentia, ureters, and rectum. The dome and part of the posterior bladder surfaces are covered by peritoneum and are thus in close proximity to the small bowel and the sigmoid colon. The neck of the bladder, which is the most inferior part, leads to the urethra. In males, the prostate lies between the bladder and the muscle layers of the pelvic floor that composes the urogenital diaphragm.

The arterial blood supply of the bladder comes from the superior, middle, and inferior vesical arteries, which originate from the anterior division of the hypogastric artery. Venous drainage occurs by a rich plexus of veins that surround the bladder and ultimately drain into the hypogastric veins.

The bladder and urethra receive their nerve supply from both the sympathetic and the parasympathetic divisions of the autonomic

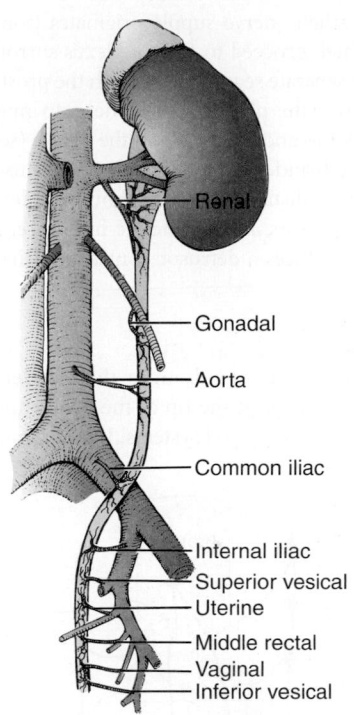

FIGURE 30-1 Sources of ureteral blood supply. (From Wein AJ et al, editors: *Campbell-Walsh urology,* ed 10, Philadelphia, 2012, Saunders.)

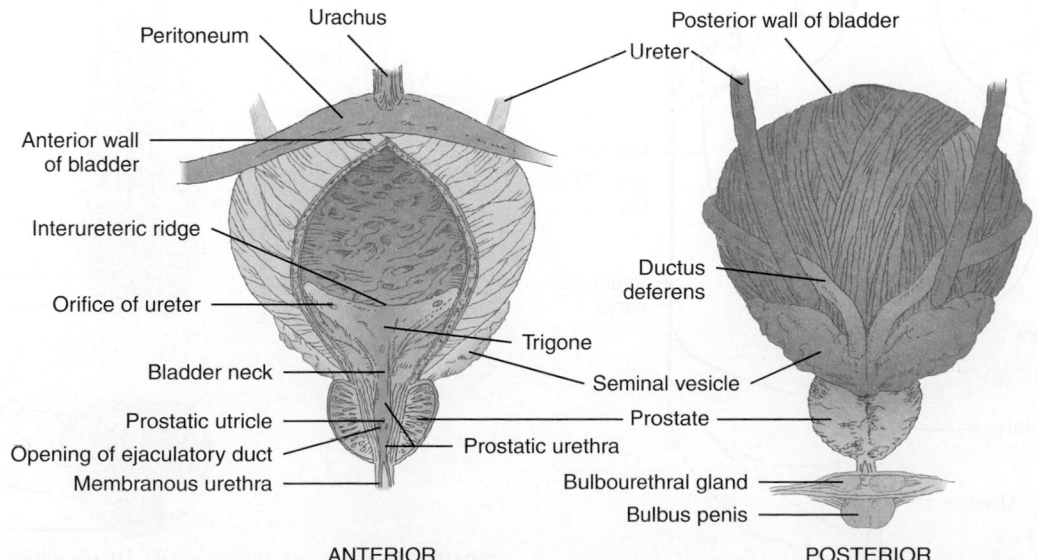

FIGURE 30-2 Anterior and posterior views of the prostate gland and related structures. The triangular area demarcated by the interureteric ridge and the bladder neck is the trigone. (From Black JM et al: *Medical-surgical nursing: clinical management for positive outcomes,* ed 6, Philadelphia, 2001, Saunders, p 940.)

nervous system. The sympathetic fibers, originating mainly from the lower thoracic and upper lumbar segments (T11-T12 and L1-L2), innervate the bladder and urethra as the hypogastric nerves. These sympathetic fibers are distributed more densely in the bladder base and proximal end of the urethra than in the bladder dome. The sympathetic nerves facilitate storage of urine. Studies have revealed differences in the bladder muscle receptors, with cholinergic receptors concentrated in the fundus and adrenergic receptors present in the trigone and proximal end of the urethra (Figure 30-3).

The parasympathetic nerve supply originates from the sacral segments (S2-S4), which proceed to form a plexus surrounding the bladder. In the male, a separate segment will reach the prostate and form the prostatic plexus. From this plexus, nerves emerge to innervate the erectile tissue of the male penis and the clitoris of the female (see Figure 30-3).

Branches of the bladder plexus penetrate the muscular coat of the bladder and become distributed throughout the detrusor. Parasympathetic muscle receptors are cholinergic in nature, and parasympathetic stimulation induces a detrusor contraction that causes bladder emptying.

Urethra

The male urethra, which extends from the bladder to the external opening (urethral meatus) at the tip of the penis, functions as a conduit for both urinary and genital systems. It is commonly divided into

three segments: the *prostatic*, the *membranous*, and the *penile* or *spongy urethra* (Figure 30-4).

Auxiliary Genital Glands

The auxiliary genital glands of the male consist of the *prostate*, the *seminal vesicles*, and the *bulbourethral glands*. These glands secrete products that contribute to the seminal fluid.

Prostate

The **prostate** lies below the bladder and has both a muscular and a glandular component. The normal prostate weighs about 20 g and measures about 3.5 cm transversely and about 2.5 cm in its vertical and anteroposterior dimensions. The prostate is conical and is anterior to the rectum. Its base is continuous with the bladder neck, and the inferior aspect of the prostate gland, or apex, lies adjacent to the urogenital diaphragm (Figure 30-5).

The prostate consists of a thin fibrous capsule with internally circular smooth muscle fibers and collagenous tissue that surround the urethra. Deep in this layer of connective and elastic tissue lies the prostatic stroma, which contains the prostatic epithelial glands. These glands drain into excretory ducts, which open chiefly on the floor of the urethra between the verumontanum and the vesical neck. The prostate is primarily a reproductive organ. In conjunction with the seminal vesicles, the prostate produces the fluid that supports the sperm. In

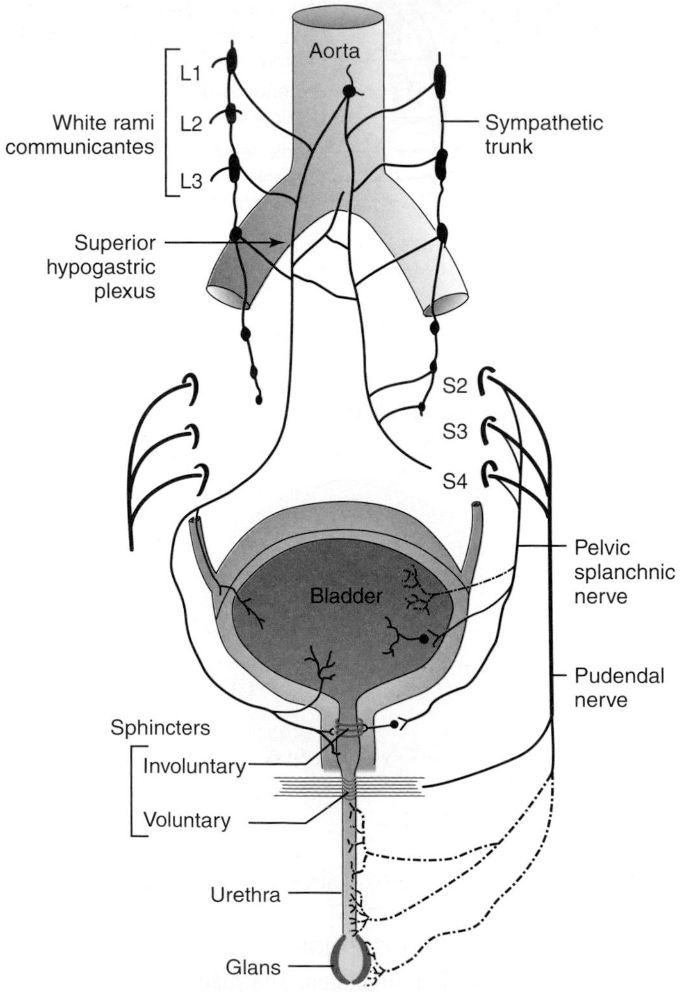

FIGURE 30-3 Diagram of nerve supply to bladder and urethra. (From Sauerland EK: *Grants dissector,* ed 10, Baltimore, 1991, Williams & Wilkins, p 66.)

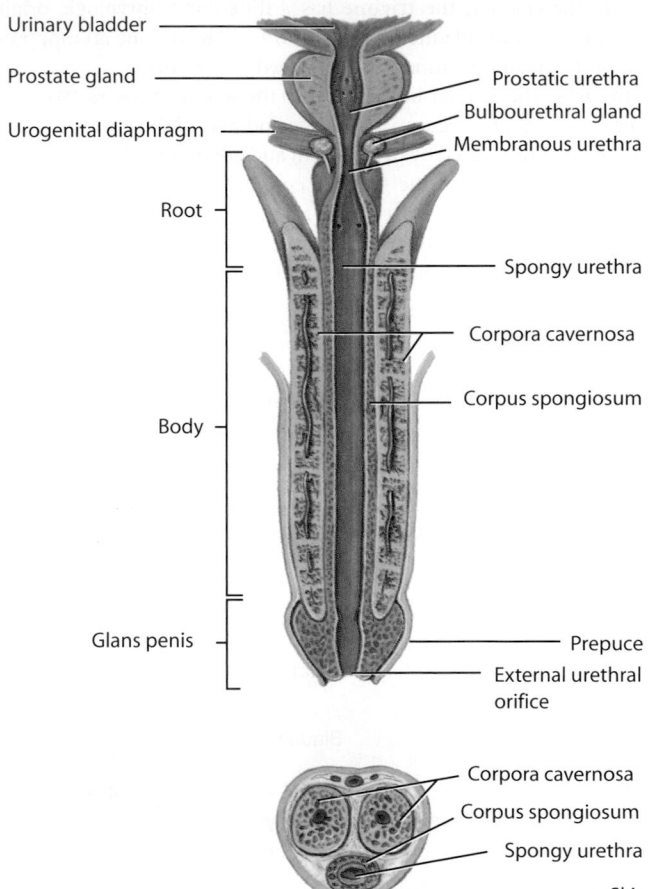

FIGURE 30-4 Cross-sectional view of the penis emphasizing the membranous urethra, the urogenital diaphragm, the bulbourethral or cowper gland, and the orifices of the bulbourethral glands. (From Applegate EJ: *The anatomy and physiology learning system: textbook,* ed 4, St Louis, 2011, Saunders.)

fact, the sperm constitute a small amount of the semen with the vast majority of the seminal fluid coming from the prostate and seminal vesicles. A further function of the prostate gland is to act as a valve for the bladder.

The main blood supply of the prostate is derived from the inferior vesical artery, a branch of the hypogastric artery. Besides the prostate, this artery also supplies the distal portion of the ureter, the seminal vesicles, and part of the bladder. A complex plexus situated between the prostate and overlying tissue freely communicates with the inferior hypogastric veins and provides venous drainage to the prostate.

Seminal Vesicles

The **seminal vesicles** are paired organs that lie next to the prostate under the base of the bladder (see Figure 30-5). Their coiled pouches secrete a fluid important to the survival of spermatozoa.

Bulbourethral Glands

The **bulbourethral** or **Cowper glands** are located on each side of the membranous urethra within the urogenital diaphragm. They add a mucoid secretion to the semen.

External Genitalia
Scrotum

The **scrotum** (see Figure 30-5) is a pouchlike sac that lies below the penis and pubic symphysis. A septum of connective tissue divides the sac into two compartments. Each compartment contains a male gonad, or testis, with its associated epididymis and the lower portion of

the vas deferens protected by the spermatic cord and its coverings. The scrotum not only supports the testes but also, by relaxation and contraction of its muscular layer, helps regulate temperature of the testes.

The scrotal sac consists of several tissue layers. The scrotal skin overlies the dartos muscle layer, whose smooth muscle fibers are embedded in loose connective tissue. The dartos muscle functions to contract the scrotal pouch when cold and expand it when warm. Under the dartos layer are several fascial layers (see Figure 30-5) that are continuous with the muscular layers of the abdominal wall and make up the covering of the spermatic cord. The external spermatic fascia is continuous with the external oblique aponeurosis of the abdominal wall. A few slips of skeletal muscle derived from the internal oblique muscle layer make up the cremasteric muscle, which adds to the upper part of the cord. The internal spermatic fascia is a continuation of the transverse fascia of the abdominal wall, with the transversus abdominis muscle not contributing to the cord layers. Finally, the peritoneum provides the tunica vaginalis layers, which are actually separated from the abdominal cavity by obliteration of the processus vaginalis.

The scrotum receives its blood supply from the external pudendal artery, a branch of the femoral artery. In addition, the scrotum receives blood from portions of the internal pudendal artery (a branch of the hypogastric artery) and the cremasteric and testicular arteries that transverse the spermatic cord.

Testes

The **testes** are the male reproductive organs responsible for sperm production. They average about 4 to 5 cm in length and 2 to 3 cm in

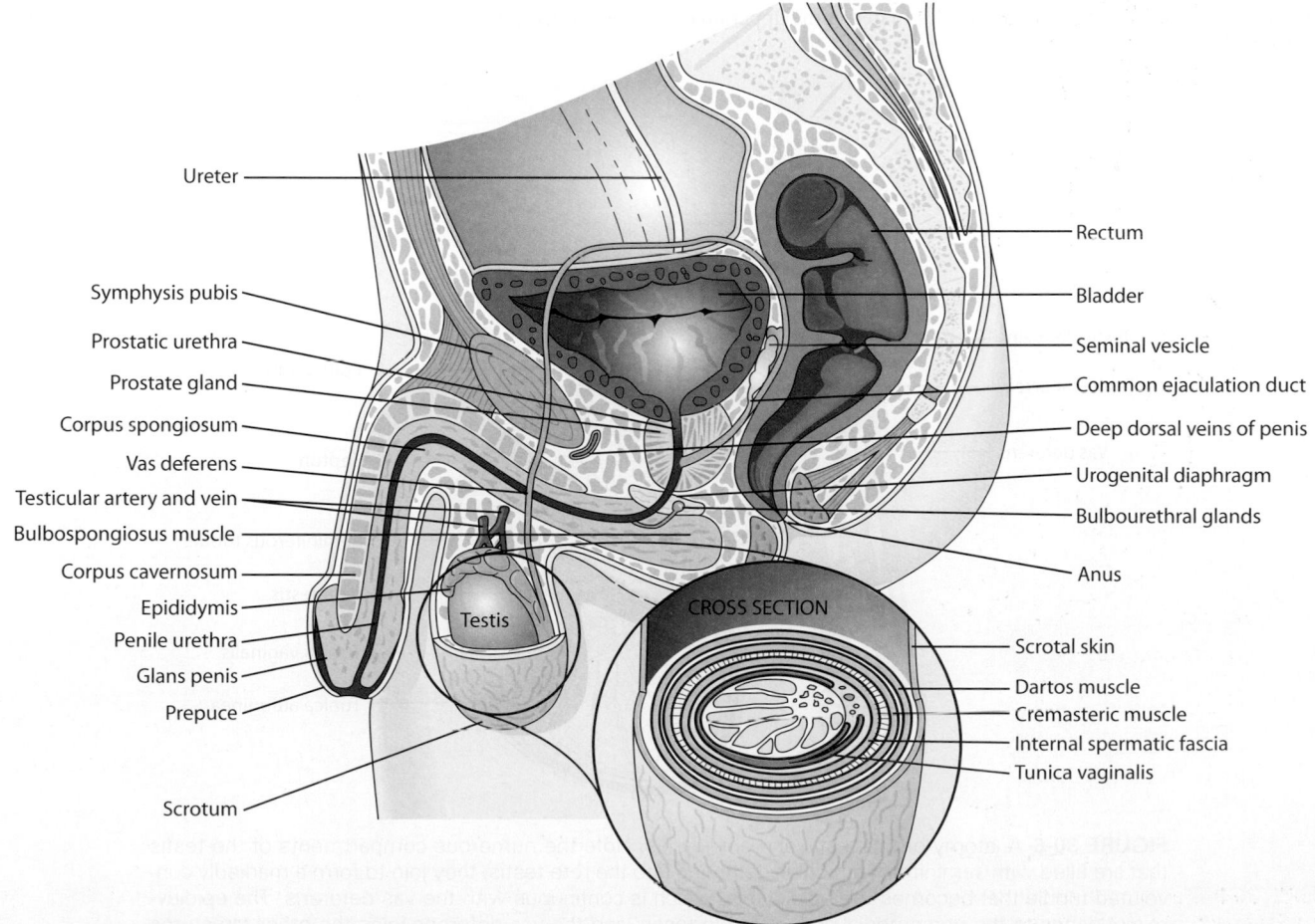

FIGURE 30-5 Male genitourinary anatomy, including a cross-section of the scrotum and its layers.

thickness. The testes lie within the scrotum and are suspended by the spermatic cord. The testes are covered by a thick fascial layer called the tunica albuginea. This layer invaginates posteriorly to form the mediastinum testis. This fibrous mediastinum sends fibrous septa into each testis that separate it into many different lobules. Each lobule contains one to four seminiferous tubules that if stretched to full length would measure approximately 60 cm. Spermatozoa production occurs within the epithelial lining of the seminiferous tubules (Figure 30-6).

The seminiferous tubules have a basement membrane consisting of elastic and connective tissue that supports the seminiferous cells. The seminiferous cells are either **Sertoli cells** (supporting cells) or spermatogenic cells. Found between the seminiferous tubules and embedded in connective tissue, the interstitial **Leydig cells** produce and secrete testosterone, a hormone involved in the development of male sexual characteristics (Figure 30-7). The seminiferous tubules converge on the mediastinum testis. The tubules, which are connected by the straight efferent ducts, drain into the head of the epididymis.

The testicular blood supply is derived from the internal spermatics, which arise directly from the aorta below the renal arteries. They course inferiorly through the spermatic cord and anastomose with the cremasteric arteries and the arteries of the vas; these vessels also contribute to the blood supply. The blood from the testis returns through a plexus of veins in the spermatic cord (the pampiniform plexus) that forms the spermatic veins. The left internal spermatic vein enters the left renal vein, which subsequently enters the vena cava. The right internal spermatic vein enters the vena cava directly.

Epididymis and Ductus Deferens

The **epididymis** is a tightly coiled tube that lies along the top of and behind each testis. It is divided into the head, situated at the upper pole of the testes; the body, lying posterior to the testes; and the tail, which is attached to the inferior pole of the testes (see Figure 30-6). The body and the tail of the epididymis form one continuous tube that serves as a conduit for maturing spermatozoa. In the epididymis, sperm develop the ability to swim.

As the convoluted tube of the tail leaves its testicular attachments, it increases in diameter to become a thick, muscular tube called the **ductus deferens,** also called the **vas deferens.** Leaving the spermatic cord, the vas deferens follows an extraperitoneal course and passes caudally and laterally along the pelvic wall. As it passes medial to the distal end of the ureter, it bends caudally to reach the midline and lies on the posterior wall of the bladder just medial to the seminal vesicles. It terminates in a dilated ampulla that courses underneath the base of the prostate. At this point the duct of the seminal vesicle joins with the duct of the ampulla, and the ejaculatory duct is formed. The ejaculatory ducts open in the prostatic urethra at the level of the verumontanum.

Penis

The **penis** is the male organ of copulation and urinary excretion. It is composed of three erectile bodies—two paired **corpora cavernosa,** which lie dorsally, and the *corpus spongiosum,* which contains the urethra (Figure 30-8). Grossly, the penis is divided into three segments. The root of the penis consists of the proximal ends of the corpora cavernosa, which attach to the pelvic bones, and the proximal end of the corpus spongiosum, which connects to the undersurface of the urogenital diaphragm. Together these attachments provide fixation and stability to the penis. The shaft or body of the penis consists of all three erectile bodies: the two cavernous bodies lying on the dorsum, and the corpus spongiosum, which occupies a depression on their ventral

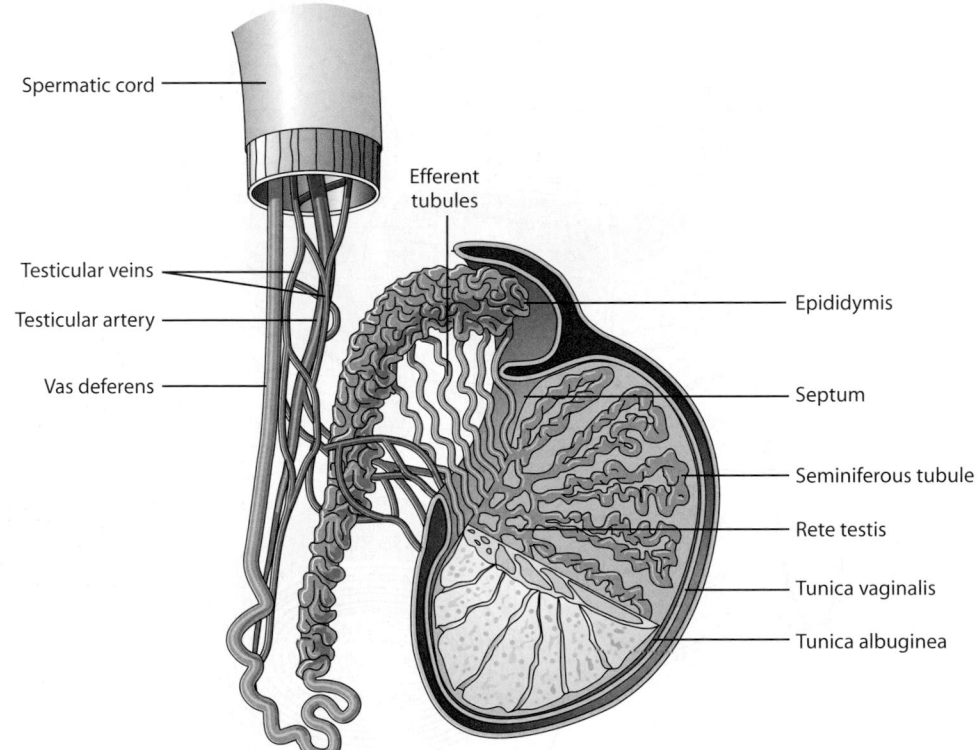

FIGURE 30-6 Anatomy of the testis and epididymis. Note the numerous compartments of the testis that are filled with seminiferous tubules gathering into the rete testis; they join to form a markedly convoluted tubule that becomes the epididymis, which is continuous with the vas deferens. The epididymis attaches to the dorsomedial aspect of the testis, and the vas deferens joins the other structures of the spermatic cord.

surface. Finally, the glans of the penis forms the distal segment of the corpus spongiosum (see Figure 30-4).

The three erectile bodies have the capability to become engorged with blood and enlarge considerably with erection. Microscopically, these bodies have an internal spongelike network that consists of endothelium-lined spaces surrounded by smooth muscle.

Each corpus is enclosed in a fascial sheath, the tunica albuginea, and all are subsequently surrounded by a thick fibrous envelope known as the **fascia of Buck.** The overlying skin of the penis is remarkable for its thinness and looseness of connection with the fascial sheath of the penis. The skin of the penis is folded upon itself to form the **prepuce,** or **foreskin.** It is this penile skin overlying the glans that is removed with circumcision.

The arterial blood supply is primarily derived from the paired internal pudendal arteries, which are branches of the hypogastric arteries. Each internal pudendal artery branches several times in the penis. The deep or cavernous artery supplies the entire corpus cavernosum. The urethral artery supplies the corpus spongiosum, and the bulbar artery supplies the bulb of the corpus spongiosum. The dorsal artery continues along the dorsum of the penis and lies below the fascia of Buck and between two dorsal veins. It provides additional supply to the glans (Figure 30-9).

Venous drainage of the penis is through several channels. The cavernous veins drain the corpora cavernosa, and the circumflex veins join the deep dorsal vein of the penis to also drain the corpora. The superficial dorsal vein drains the glans and part of the distal portion of the corpora. Finally, a bulbar branch drains the bulbous urethra and proximal portion of the corpus spongiosum (see Figure 30-9). Together these branches coalesce and pass through the urogenital diaphragm into the retropubic venous plexus of Santorini.

The nerve supply of the penis is formed from both parasympathetic and sympathetic components. The parasympathetic fibers arise from S2-S4, and the sympathetic component is derived from the hypogastric

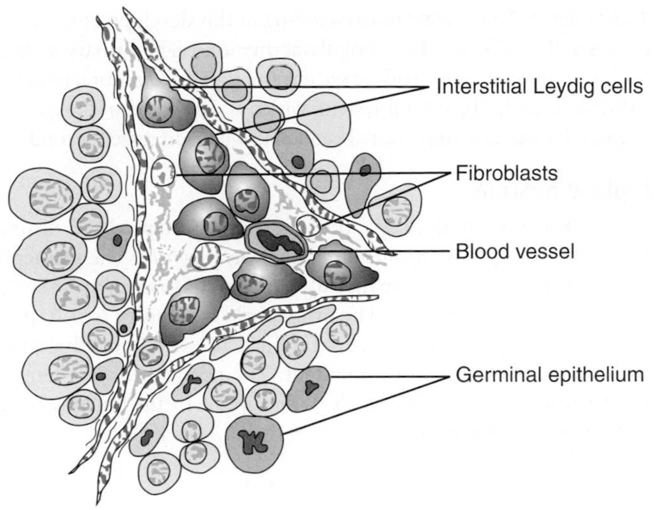

FIGURE 30-7 The interstitial Leydig cells that secrete testosterone are located in the interstices between the seminiferous tubules. (From Hall JE, editor: *Guyton and Hall textbook of medical physiology,* ed 12, Philadelphia, 2011, Saunders.)

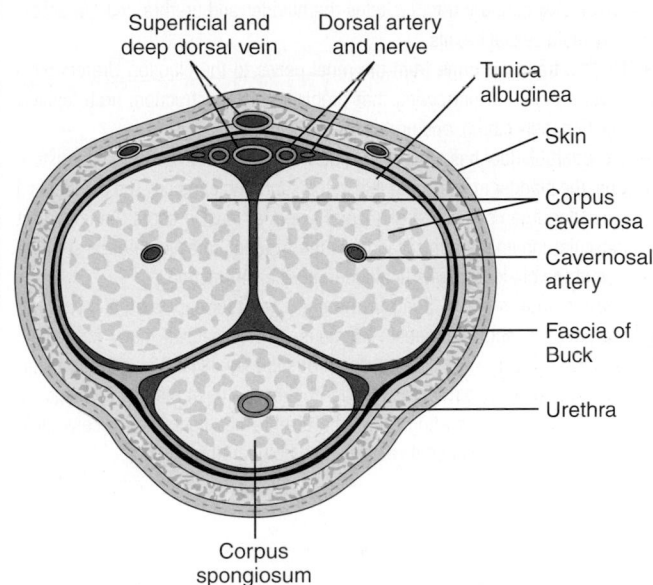

FIGURE 30-8 Transverse section through the penis. The paired upper structures are the corpora cavernosa. The single lower body surrounding the urethra is the corpus spongiosum.

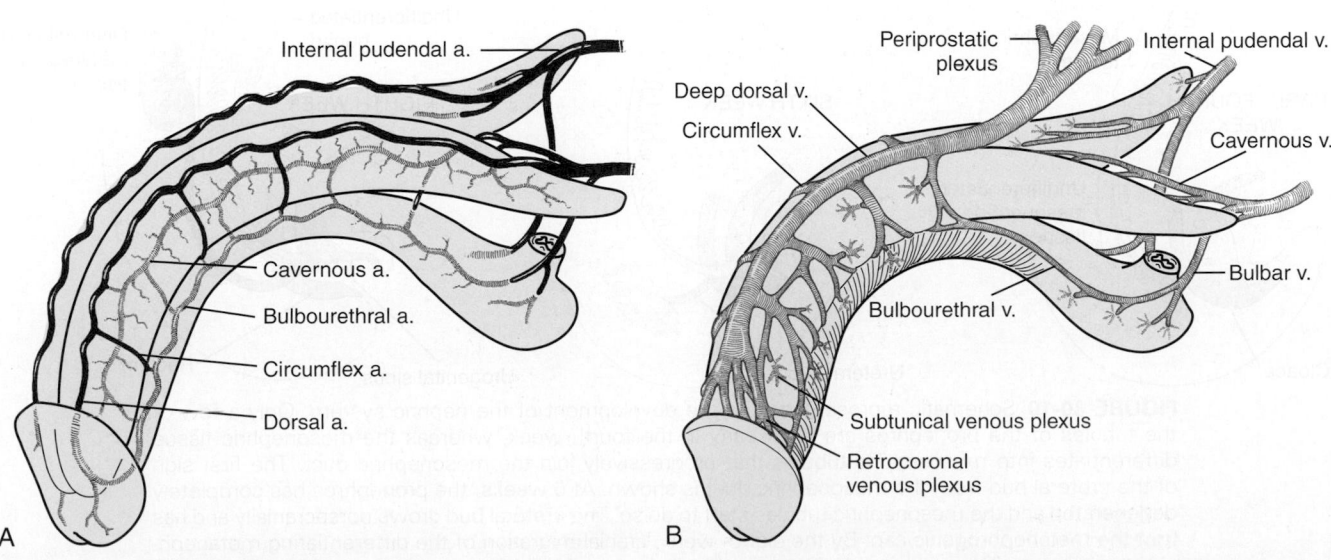

FIGURE 30-9 Penile arterial supply **(A)** and venous drainage **(B),** longitudinal views. *a.,* artery; *v.,* vein. (From Walsh PC et al, editors: *Campbell's urology,* ed 7, Philadelphia, 1998, Saunders, p 1160.)

plexus. Parasympathetic stimulation from the pudendal nerve results in relaxation of vascular resistance, which increases blood flow to the penis and creates an erection. The pudendal nerve also carries sensory fibers from the penis and enters the sacral spinal cord to contribute to penile erection.

Sympathetic nerve fibers may contribute to erectile capacity, but their role has not been proved conclusively. They do innervate the proximal involuntary sphincter of the bladder neck, where contraction prevents retrograde ejaculation of semen from the prostatic urethra into the bladder. They also innervate the muscles of the seminal vesicles and prostate, which when stimulated cause ejaculation of seminal fluid into the urethra.

KEY POINTS

- The upper genitourinary tract is composed of the kidneys and ureters. The lower genitourinary tract includes the bladder and urethra and the accessory male sexual organs.
- Ureters transport urine from the renal pelvis to the bladder. Ureters have several points of narrowing that predispose to obstruction: ureteropelvic junction, pelvic brim, and ureterovesical junction.
- The adult bladder has a normal capacity of 450 to 500 ml. With overdistention, the bladder may be palpable in the suprapubic region. The bladder is a muscular organ composed of several layers of muscle fibers. An important muscular landmark in the bladder is the trigone. Parasympathetic stimulation of the bladder results in bladder muscle contraction.
- The prostate is a key organ in the male genitourinary system with both reproductive and continence functions. It also causes many pathologic conditions as men age such as prostatitis, benign hyperplasia, and cancer.
- The urethra extends from the bladder to the meatus at the end of the penis. In addition to transporting urine, the urethra has ducts that receive fluid from the prostate, seminal vesicles, and bulbourethral glands.

- The scrotal sac supports the testes and regulates their temperature. Testes contain several cell types important in sperm production and the development of secondary sex characteristics. Spermatogenic cells produce sperm in the testes. Sertoli cells serve to support and nurture spermatogenesis. Leydig cells produce and secrete testosterone.
- Situated next to the testes, the epididymis serves as a collecting conduit for sperm. The epididymis is continuous with the ductus (vas) deferens. The vas travels along the pelvic wall and joins with the seminal vesicle duct at the prostate to form the ejaculatory duct. The ejaculatory ducts open into the urethra.
- Skin overlying the penis is very loose, which facilitates significant enlargement when the penis is engorged with blood during erection. Parasympathetic fibers forming the pudendal nerve are responsible for erection. Ejaculation is a function of the sympathetic nerve fibers.

EMBRYOLOGY

Developmental processes in the genital and urinary systems are intimately related. To facilitate understanding of this development, the two systems will be discussed in several subdivisions. The urinary system, which is composed of the nephric system and the vesicourethral unit, will be discussed first. The genital system, which is composed of the gonads, the genital ducts, and the external genitalia, will be discussed second.

Nephric System

The nephric system develops progressively through three distinct phases: the *pronephros*, *mesonephros*, and *metanephros*. The **pronephros** is the earliest state in humans but corresponds to the mature structure in primitive vertebrates. The pronephros consists of 6 to 10 pairs of tubules connected by a pronephric duct. It grows caudally to join the cloaca, a blind end of the hindgut. The pronephros is a temporary structure and, except for its duct, disappears by the fourth week of intrauterine life (Figure 30-10).

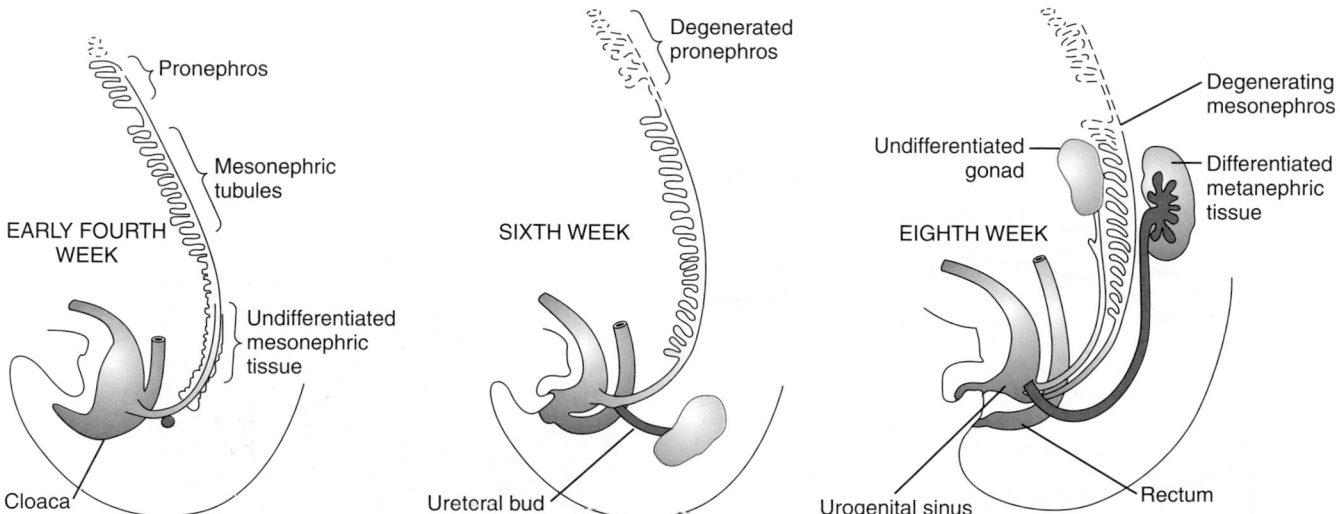

FIGURE 30-10 Schematic representation of the development of the nephric system. Only a few of the tubules of the pronephros are seen early in the fourth week, whereas the mesonephric tissue differentiates into mesonephric tubules that progressively join the mesonephric duct. The first sign of the ureteral bud from the mesonephric duct is shown. At 6 weeks, the pronephros has completely degenerated and the mesonephric tubules start to do so. The ureteral bud grows dorsocranially and has met the metanephrogenic cap. By the eighth week, cranial migration of the differentiating metanephros can be seen. The cranial end of the ureteric bud expands and starts to show multiple successive outgrowths. (From Tanagho EA, McAninch JW, editors: *Smith's general urology*, ed 13, East Norwalk, CT, 1992, Appleton & Lange, p 18.)

The **mesonephros** corresponds to the mature excretory organ of some amphibians. In humans it begins developing at about the fourth to fifth week of gestation.[1-4] The tubules of the mesonephros are more numerous and form a cuplike outgrowth into which capillaries push to form a primitive glomerulus. The tubules communicate with the mesonephric duct, which is derived from the preceding pronephric duct. The number of mesonephros tubules reaches a maximum by about 8 weeks' gestation and then degenerates.

The final stage of development, the **metanephros,** begins in the fourth week when the ureteral bud grows out of the mesonephric duct. The bud elongates in a dorsocranial direction, where it meets a mass of mesoderm, the nephrogenic blastema, and begins to differentiate into the ureter and renal collecting system.[1,4] The metanephros is derived from the nephrogenic blastema and eventually differentiates into the mature mammalian kidney.

Vesicourethral Unit

The blind end of the caudal hindgut forms the cloaca, which is separated from the outside by a thin membrane of tissue, the urogenital membrane. At about 4 weeks' gestation a septum grows downward and separates the cloaca into a posterior compartment, which will become the rectum, and an anterior compartment, which will form the urogenital sinus.

The urogenital sinus receives the mesonephric duct, which is progressively absorbed into this structure. The mesonephric duct distal to the ureteral bud is absorbed into the sinus, and its mesenchyme subsequently forms the bladder trigone. The ureter, which is derived from the ureteral bud, and the mesonephric duct, which differentiates into

the vas deferens, merge into the sinus as well. In a complex pattern of development, the opening of the ureteral bud, which will eventually become the ureteral orifice, migrates upward and laterally. The opening of the mesonephric duct, which will become the ejaculatory duct, migrates downward and medially (Figure 30-11).

The urogenital sinus can be divided into two main segments. The ventral and pelvic portion, which receives the ureter, forms the bladder, part of the urethra in males, and the whole urethra in females. A phallic or urethral portion will receive the mesonephric ducts and in males will form a second part of the urethra. In females, this portion receives the müllerian ducts, which fuse distally to form the uterus and upper part of the vagina. The lower portion of the female urogenital sinus forms the lower part of the vagina and vaginal vestibule (Figure 30-12).

Gonads

The undifferentiated and primitive **gonads** are derived from the urogenital ridge, a dorsal region of thickening from which the primitive kidney also forms. The gonads serve as precursors to the testes in males and the ovaries in females. During the seventh week, an individual gonad begins to assume the characteristics of either a testis or an ovary.

In the presence of testis-determining factor, which is located on the Y chromosome, a gonad develops into a testis. The gland increases in size, and the cells of the epithelium grow centrally into the organ's mesenchyme. These ingrowths become radially arranged, form cords, and begin to converge on the posterior aspect of the testis. The cords eventually differentiate into the seminiferous tubules, which produce spermatozoa. The testes descend behind the abdominal cavity in the

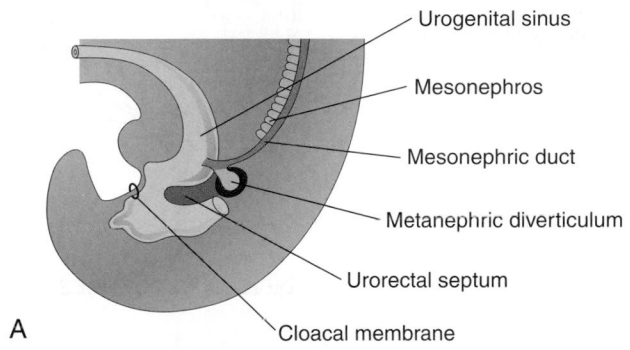

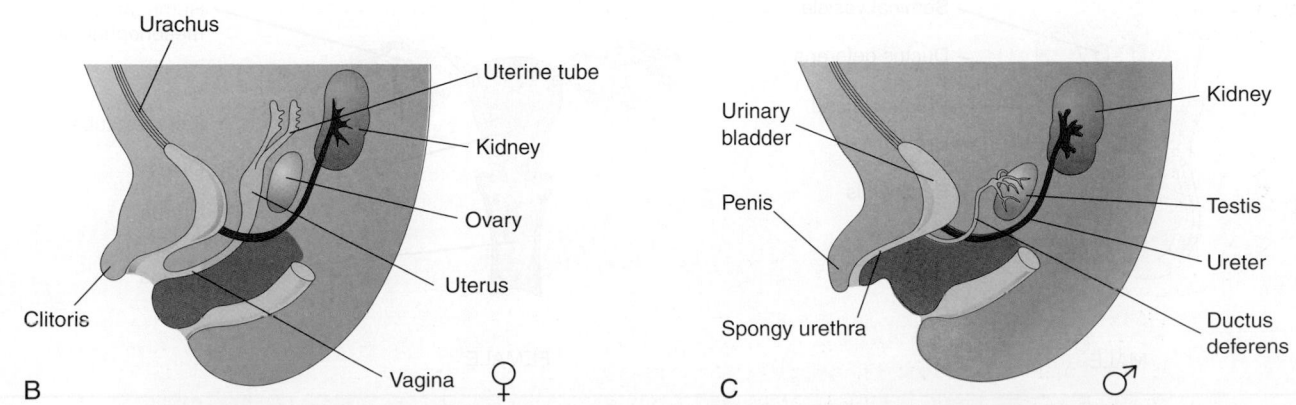

FIGURE 30-11 Diagrams showing division of the cloaca into the urogenital sinus and rectum; absorption of the mesonephric ducts; development of the urinary bladder, urethra, and urachus; and changes in location of the ureters. **A,** Lateral view of the caudal half of a 5-week embryo. The stages shown in **B** and **C** are reached by the 12th week. (From Moore KL et al, editors: *The developing human: clinically oriented embryology,* ed 9, Philadelphia, 2013, Saunders.)

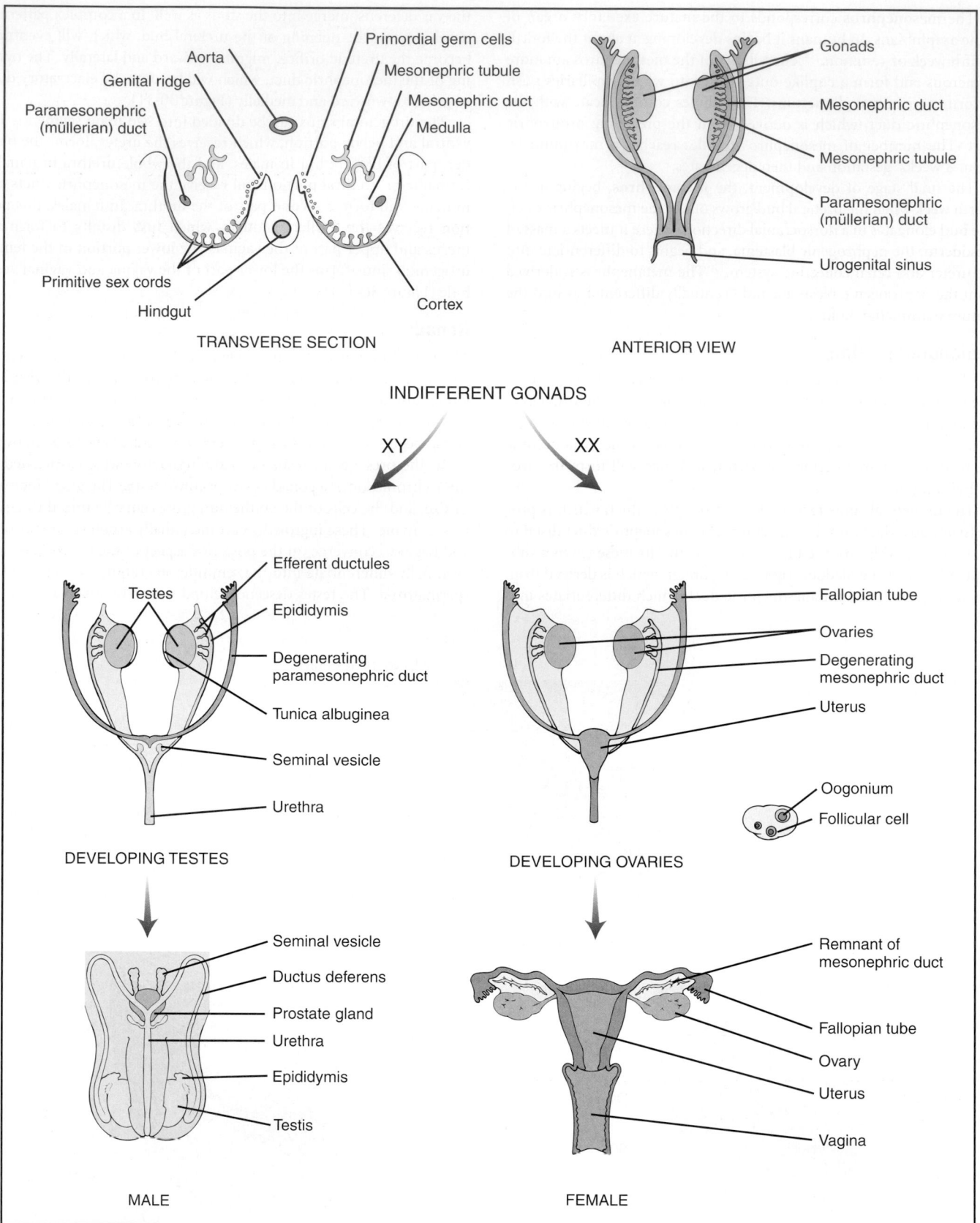

FIGURE 30-12 Transformation of the undifferentiated genital system into the definitive male and female systems. (From Nichols FH, Zwelling E: *Maternal-newborn nursing: theory and practice,* Philadelphia, 1997, Saunders, p 174.)

retroperitoneal space and into the scrotum, usually by the eighth month of gestation.

In the absence of testis-determining factor, a gonad differentiates into an ovary, and a cortex forms from the germinal epithelium and ultimately gives rise to ovarian follicles containing ova. It descends only partially through the abdominal cavity and eventually lies adjacent to the fallopian tubes.

Genital Duct System

As the embryo develops, two different but related kinds of ducts form beside the undifferentiated gonads. The mesonephric ducts, or **wolffian ducts,** as previously explained, develop as nephric ducts but will go on to form the male genital ducts. The **müllerian ducts** develop alongside the mesonephric ducts (paramesonephric) and are genital structures from the start.

Early in development, each of the two müllerian ducts arises lateral to the mesonephric ducts, either directly from the mesonephric ducts themselves or possibly from the adjacent epithelium of the primitive abdominal cavity. Both ducts grow caudally to enter the urogenital sinus.

If a gonad differentiates into a testis, the wolffian ducts subsequently develop into the male duct system consisting of the epididymis, vas deferens, seminal vesicles, and ejaculatory ducts. The müllerian ducts, except for a few rudimentary fragments, rapidly atrophy.

If, on the other hand, a gonad develops into an ovary, the müllerian ducts proceed to form the uterus, fallopian tubes, and upper part of the vagina. The mesonephric, or wolffian, ducts fail to develop further and remain rudimentary (see Figure 30-12).

External Genitalia

Development of the external genitalia begins at about 12 intrauterine weeks. Before this point, three small protuberances appear on the external aspect of the cloacal membrane. The genital tubercle is located anteriorly and the genital swellings are situated on either side of the membrane. In the seventh week, rupture of the urogenital membrane gives the urogenital sinus a separate opening on the undersurface of the genital tubercle.

In males, the genital or labioscrotal swellings migrate and fuse centrally to form the scrotum. The fused genital tubercles elongate. The elongated fused tubercles form a cylindric shape with a ventral groove communicating with the urogenital sinus. This groove subsequently becomes covered by folds of tissue and forms the penile urethra (Figure 30-13).

The female external genitalia closely resemble those of the male until about the eighth intrauterine week. At this time the genital tubercle lags behind in growth and becomes the clitoris. The urogenital sinus shortens and widens somewhat to form the vaginal vestibule, and the genital swellings form the labia majora. The urethral folds become the labia minora.

KEY POINTS
- The fetal gonads can become either a testis or an ovary. The presence of the testis-determining factor on the Y chromosome causes the testis to develop in the male fetus, whereas the absence of this factor allows the gonad to become an ovary in the female. Once the gonad has differentiated, it then is responsible for the cascade of events that lead to the formation of the female or male sexual organs and genitalia.
- During early embryonic development, the genital structures of males and females are similar. Two important ductal systems are the mesonephric (wolffian) ducts and the paramesonephric (müllerian) ducts. The mesonephric ducts develop to form the kidneys and the genital duct in males. In the

---

presence of a testis, the wolffian ducts develop into the epididymis, vas deferens, seminal vesicles, and ejaculatory ducts. In the presence of an ovary, the müllerian ducts develop into the uterus, fallopian tubes, and upper part of the vagina, and the wolffian ducts fail to develop.
- Development of the external genitalia begins at about 12 weeks' gestation. In males the labioscrotal tissue fuses and elongates to form the scrotum and penis. In females, this tissue remains separated and forms the labia minora.

MALE REPRODUCTIVE PHYSIOLOGY

Hypothalamic-Pituitary-Testicular Axis

To fully understand male reproductive function, one must consider the endocrine function of the hypothalamic-pituitary-testicular axis. The components of this system function to maintain a constant level of the circulating hormones responsible for normal male sexual development and behavior, as well as the maturation of sperm necessary for fertility (Figure 30-14).

The hypothalamus is the integrating center for this hormonal axis. This organ coordinates neural messages from the central nervous system and humoral (bloodborne) messages from the testis to control the secretion of a small peptide hormone: gonadotropin-releasing hormone (GnRH). The pituitary stalk provides the route for GnRH to travel to the pituitary gland, which lies caudal to the hypothalamus. A system of veins, the pituitary portal system, traverses the pituitary stalk and maintains responsibility for transporting GnRH to the anterior portion of the pituitary gland.

In response to the secretion of GnRH, the pituitary synthesizes and releases two hormones: luteinizing hormone (LH) and follicle-stimulating hormone (FSH). Although these hormones carry names related to their function in females, they are produced by both genders through a feedback mechanism with GnRH for reproductive purposes.[5]

By binding to receptors on the surface of the testicular Leydig cells, LH mediates testosterone synthesis. Binding of LH produces an increase in the conversion of adenosine triphosphate to cyclic 3,5-adenosine monophosphate. This activity stimulates the production of other intracellular enzymes with subsequent increased synthesis of testosterone. Testosterone is then released into the bloodstream and adjacent seminiferous tubules.

Besides testosterone, other steroid hormones are synthesized, among them dihydrotestosterone, 17-hydroxyprogesterone, and estradiol. Dihydrotestosterone functions to differentiate and mature the male external genitalia and prostate.[6] In early puberty the production of androgen begins to increase, with normal adult plasma levels of testosterone and dihydrotestosterone being 300 to 1200 ng/dl and 30 to 60 ng/dl, respectively.

The function of FSH in male reproduction remains somewhat unclear. However, it appears that the production of sperm in the seminiferous tubules (spermatogenesis) requires the presence of high levels of both androgen and FSH.[7]

A feedback inhibition mechanism controls the secretion of both LH and FSH. Production of LH occurs in response to serum levels of testosterone and estradiol. The mechanism of the regulation of FSH is more hypothetical, but the existence of a nonsteroid factor called inhibin produced by Sertoli cells in response to FSH has been proposed.[8] In addition to inhibin, sex steroids also modulate FSH secretion through feedback inhibition on the pituitary.[7]

Spermatogenesis

To understand spermatogenesis, one must briefly consider the histology of the testis and its seminiferous tubules. As previously stated,

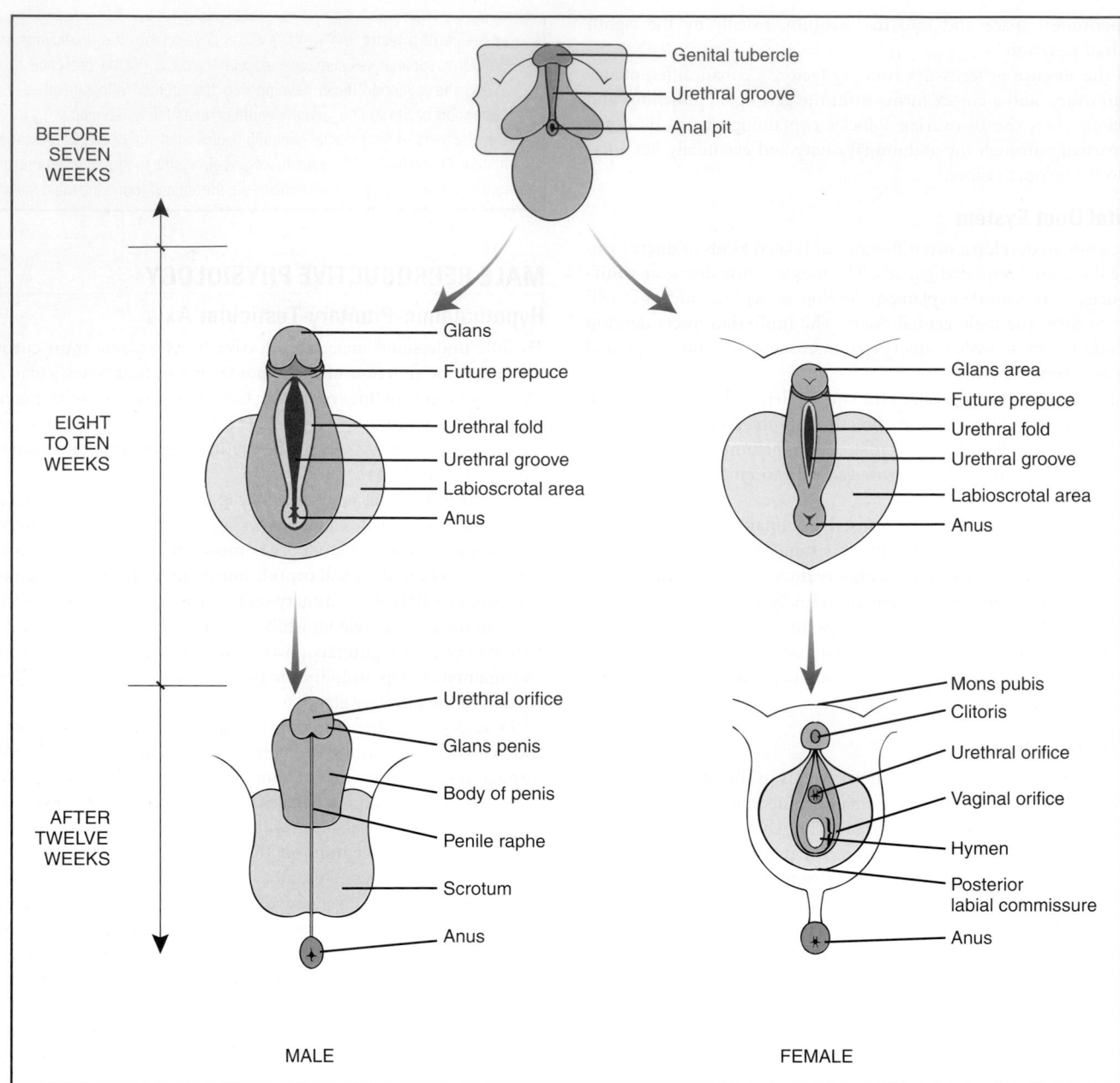

FIGURE 30-13 Development of the external genitalia from the indifferent stage (before 7 weeks) to fully differentiated stages (after 12 weeks of gestation). (From Nichols FH, Zwelling E: *Maternal-newborn nursing: theory and practice,* Philadelphia, 1997, Saunders, p 175.)

Leydig cells occur in clusters in the interstitial tissue between the seminiferous tubules. These Leydig cells are responsible for the testicular production of testosterone.

The seminiferous tubules contain both germinal elements and supporting cells, which include the sustaining cells of the basement membrane and the Sertoli cells. The Sertoli cells rest on the basement membrane of the tubule and form a unique impermeable junction with each adjacent Sertoli cell. It is through this junction that the young germinal cells, or primary spermatocytes, migrate and pass from the basal compartment to the basement membrane and then to the central or adluminal compartment of the seminiferous tubule. The junction is also responsible for maintenance of the blood-testes barrier. This barrier ensures that the more mature spermatocytes and spermatids located in the adluminal compartment are behind the barrier and theoretically maintained in a constant intratubular environment to support the development of maturing sperm cells.[8]

The process of sperm production is called **spermatogenesis** and involves several phases (Figure 30-15). The proliferative phase involves division of the young germinal cells near the basement membrane (spermatogonia) either to replace their numbers or to produce daughter cells that will form spermatocytes. Next, a meiotic phase occurs in which spermatocytes undergo a reduction division. This division reduces the number of chromosomes to the monoploid number of 23 from the diploid number of 46. Finally, haploid spermatids undergo change to form mature **spermatozoa.**

While sperm cells mature and move from the basement membrane to the adluminal compartment, the Sertoli cells have an important nutritional role in the spermatogenic process. As the spermatid matures,

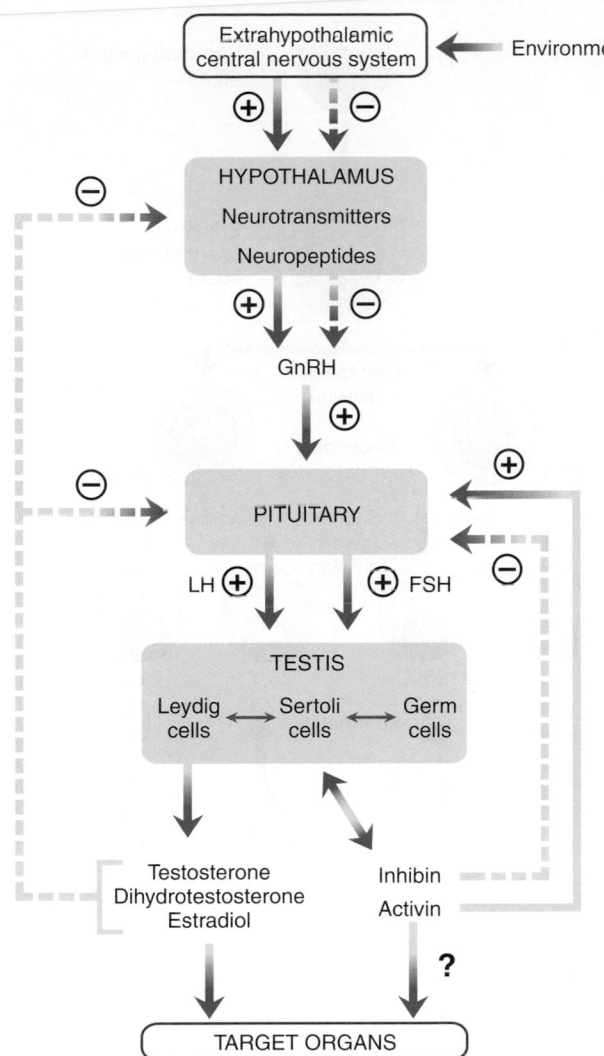

FIGURE 30-14 Diagram of the hypothalamic-pituitary-testicular axis. *FSH,* Follicle-stimulating hormone; *GnRH,* gonadotropin-releasing hormone; *LH,* luteinizing hormone. (Redrawn from Walsh PC et al, editors: *Campbell's urology,* ed 7, Philadelphia, 1998, Saunders, p 1240.)

it elongates and develops a tail, or **flagellum,** that attains a form similar to that of the mature spermatozoon. Mature spermatozoa are released into the tubular lumen and rapidly flow out to the rete testis and into the epididymis. Although each spermatogonium, one of the primitive male germ cells, requires about 70 days to develop into a mature sperm cell, or spermatozoon, within each tubule are spermatozoa in all stages of development. This characteristic allows new spermatozoa to be continuously produced across the male life span. The effects of aging on the male reproductive system are described in the Geriatric Considerations box.

Anatomy of Spermatozoa

The human spermatozoon is approximately 60 μm in length. The oval head contains a nucleus that is highly condensed and stabilized by cross-links between its molecules, which makes it very resistant to physical injury during its passage and storage in the epididymis. An outer membrane, the acrosome, contains the enzymes required for penetration of the female egg before fertilization.

The tail accounts for 90% of the length of the spermatozoon and is divided into a middle piece, principal piece, and end piece. The spermatozoon derives its motile ability from the motor apparatus of the

tail, which is called the **axoneme.** The axoneme, which runs the length of the tail, is composed of a central pair of tubules surrounded by a ring of nine pairs of tubules (the 9 + 2 pattern). This ring of tubules is surrounded by a supporting structure of nine noncontractile dense fibers. Within the middle piece, a circular sheath of mitochondria[9] (Figure 30-16) surrounds these outer dense fibers.

The mitochondria contain the enzymes required for the production of adenosine triphosphate, the energy source for the cell. Within the axoneme are enzymes and structural proteins. These enzymes convert chemical energy from adenosine triphosphate to the mechanical energy of sperm cell movement to aid in fertilization of the egg.

Transport of Spermatozoa

Once mature spermatozoa are released from the Sertoli cells into the seminiferous tubules, they must pass through approximately 6 m of duct in the male reproductive tract before leaving the urethral meatus and being deposited in the vagina during sexual intercourse. From the seminiferous tubules, the spermatozoa are deposited into the rete testis, a collecting chamber for all the seminiferous tubules. From the rete testis, the sperm travel through the efferent ductules, 12 to 20 channels that pass into a single compact duct, the epididymis. The epididymis is a tightly convoluted duct that is divided into three regions: the caput (globus major), the corpus (body), and the cauda epididymis (tail, or globus minor). Unfolded and stretched, the epididymis would measure 12 to 15 feet.

After leaving the epididymis, the sperm enter the ductus or vas deferens. Embryologically, this duct is derived from the mesonephric duct. It passes through the scrotum, traverses the inguinal canal into the pelvis, and then passes behind the bladder to enter the prostatic urethra at the ejaculatory ducts of the verumontanum. The terminal portion of the vas deferens is known as the **ampulla.** It is joined by the ducts of the seminal vesicle before entering the ejaculatory ducts.

As one passes in a proximal-to-distal direction from the efferent ducts to the vas deferens, the thickness of the muscle gradually increases. In the vas deferens, three interconnected smooth muscle layers form a thick muscular wall, with the ratio of wall thickness to lumen being the greatest in any human structure.[7] This thick muscular wall facilitates rapid sperm transport at the time of ejaculation.

Aside from serving as a conduit and storage depot for spermatozoa, the epididymis probably sustains maturational processes. Most studies have demonstrated that sperm taken directly from the testes

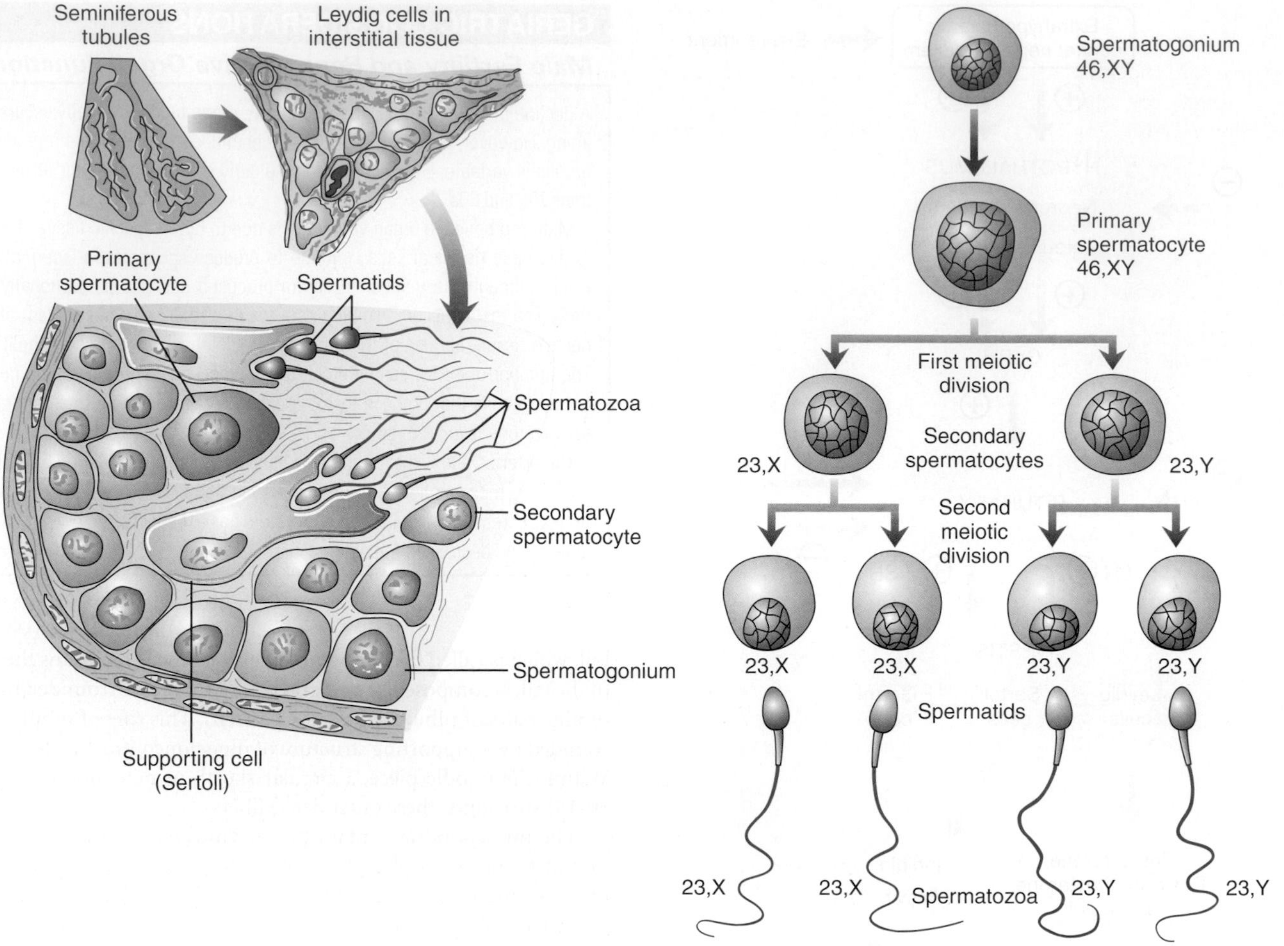

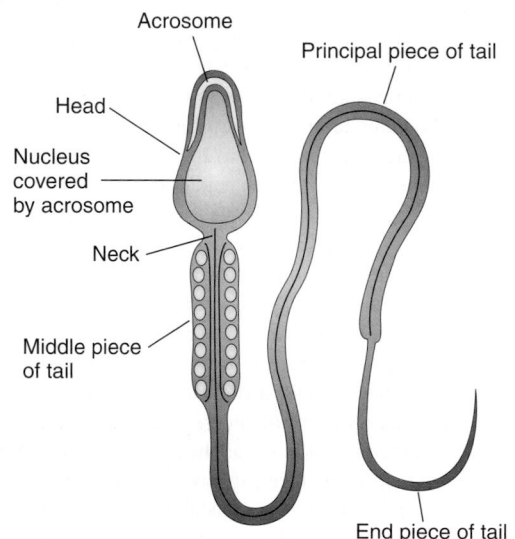

Seminiferous tubules

Leydig cells in interstitial tissue

Primary spermatocyte

Spermatids

Spermatozoa

Secondary spermatocyte

Spermatogonium

Supporting cell (Sertoli)

Spermatogonium
46,XY

Primary spermatocyte
46,XY

First meiotic division

Secondary spermatocytes

23,X

23,Y

Second meiotic division

23,X   23,X   23,Y   23,Y

Spermatids

23,X   23,X   Spermatozoa   23,Y   23,Y

FIGURE 30-15 Process of meiosis in spermatogenesis.

Acrosome

Principal piece of tail

Head

Nucleus covered by acrosome

Neck

Middle piece of tail

End piece of tail

FIGURE 30-16 Anatomy of a mature sperm cell. (From Moore KL et al, editors: *The developing human: clinically oriented embryology*, ed 9, Philadelphia, 2013, Saunders.)

are incapable of fertilizing eggs. It appears that the development of motility and increased fertility are acquired during transit through the epididymis.[7]

Because epididymal sperm are probably immotile, other mechanisms must be involved in their transport. Initially, spermatozoa are carried into the efferent ducts by fluid from the rete testis. Within the efferent ducts, motile cilia within the lumen function to reabsorb testicular fluid and help move spermatozoa into the epididymis. Within the epididymis, the spermatozoa are probably transported by rhythmic contraction of the smooth muscle cells.[7]

Ejaculation accelerates the passage of spermatozoa through the vas deferens and distal end of the epididymis. In young men, approximately 200 million sperm can be found in the reservoir of the epididymis. About 50% are found in the cauda region. With ejaculation, sperm from the distal part of the epididymis and vas deferens are deposited into the prostatic urethra, where they account for less than 10% of the normal ejaculate.[10]

Erection, Emission, and Ejaculation

To penetrate the vagina and deposit sperm, the penis must be erect. The physiology of **erection** is a complicated interaction of vascular, neurologic, and hormonal factors. Although erection has classically been thought of as a parasympathetic function, it is more complex. Erection may be mediated by either local stimulation, which causes a reflexogenic erection through the sacral spinal cord, or psychological stimulation, which causes a psychogenic erection through cerebral centers. The presence of erections in patients with spinal cord injuries attests to the presence of reflex erections. Such patients have an intact sacral spinal cord and its reflex arc of afferent and efferent nerves below the site of spinal cord injury.

The penis receives sensory innervation from the pudendal sensory nerves entering the sacral spinal cord. The pudendal nerve is a mixed nerve that provides motor innervation to the pelvic floor musculature and penile sensory fibers. The efferent nerve to the erectile tissue is provided by sacral parasympathetic fibers. Although erection is possible in patients with spinal cord injuries, in intact men it is a much more controlled process influenced to a great extent by the cerebral cortex. Impulses may traverse the spinal cord from the cerebral cortex in the lateral columns and exit the spinal cord through sacral parasympathetic and possibly the thoracolumbar sympathetic nerves as well.[7]

During erection, the vascular spaces that make up the spongy vacuous tissues of the corpora cavernosa and corpus spongiosum fill with blood. The relaxation of smooth muscle tone in these structures that allows filling and subsequent penile erection is modulated by an undetermined neurotransmitter, most likely nitric oxide (NO). Research indicates that erectile function cannot be fully explained by parasympathetic or sympathetic mechanisms; this observation has led to consideration that nonadrenergic and noncholinergic neuromodulators may be involved in such function.[11] For example, penile injection of certain prostaglandins has been shown to induce smooth muscle relaxation and has been used to induce erections in some men experiencing erectile dysfunction.[12]

Ejaculation may be divided into two phases: *emission* and *ejaculation*. During **emission,** secretions from the periurethral glands, seminal vesicles, and prostate are deposited with sperm from the vasa deferentia and the cauda epididymis into the prostatic urethra. Control of emission is mediated primarily through the sympathetic nerves, which stimulate contraction of smooth muscle in these genital structures.

With **ejaculation,** the bladder neck or internal sphincter closes. This closure is also mediated through the sympathetic nervous system. Next, the external sphincter relaxes and the perineal and bulbourethral muscles surrounding the bulb of the corpus spongiosum contract and expel the ejaculate from the posterior urethra and through the urethral meatus.

The physiologic function of the secretory products of the accessory sex glands is uncertain. These secretions make up most of the seminal plasma, with the sperm and testicular fluid probably composing less than 10% of the final ejaculated semen volume. Although some investigators have demonstrated that sperm removed directly from the epididymis are capable of fertilization, these secretions most likely optimize conditions for sperm motility, survival, and transport in both the female and the male reproductive tracts.

Capacitation

Capacitation of the spermatozoa refers to the multiple changes that activate the sperm and enhance their ability to participate in the final process of fertilization. Although sperm are anatomically complete and highly motile when ejaculated, the complex process of capacitation is necessary before the sperm are actually capable of fertilizing the egg. The capacitation process occurs over a period of 1 to 10 hours and occurs in sperm only after they have been introduced into the vagina of the female. Once the sperm are inside the female, the uterine and fallopian tube fluids wash away the various inhibitory factors that had suppressed sperm activity in the male genital ducts. During the time that the spermatozoa were in the fluid of the male genital ducts, they were continually exposed to many floating vesicles from the seminiferous tubules containing large amounts of cholesterol. This cholesterol,

continually donated to the cellular membrane covering the sperm acrosome, toughens the outside membrane and prevents release of its enzymes. After ejaculation, the sperm that are deposited in the vagina swim away from the cholesterol vesicles upward into the uterine fluid, and they gradually lose much of their excess cholesterol during the next few hours. As the cholesterol is lost, the membrane at the head of the sperm becomes much weaker.

The membrane of the sperm head also becomes much more permeable to calcium ions. Large amounts of calcium enter the sperm to increase the powerful whiplike motion of the flagellum beyond its previously weak, undulating motion. In addition, the calcium ions probably also alter the intracellular membrane covering the leading edge of the acrosome, thus making it possible for the acrosome to release its enzymes very rapidly and easily as the sperm penetrates the granulosa cell mass surrounding the ovum. These enzymes are released even more rapidly and easily as the sperm attempts to penetrate the zona pellucida of the ovum itself.[13]

KEY POINTS

- Normal male sexual development and spermatogenesis depend on the appropriate secretion of reproductive hormones. GnRH, secreted by the hypothalamus, induces the anterior pituitary gland to secrete LH and FSH. The bloodstream receives these hormones, which then travel to the testes where they bind to testicular cells.

- Leydig cells in the testes possess LH receptors and respond by increasing production of testosterone. Testosterone and related androgens are necessary for maturation of the male external genitalia. The function of FSH is less well understood, but appears to be necessary for spermatogenesis.

- Spermatogenesis occurs when germinal cells within the seminiferous tubules undergo meiosis to form haploid (23 chromosomes) spermatids. Spermatids then develop into mature spermatozoa with the assistance of Sertoli cells. Sperm require 70 days to mature, and they are continuously produced and released into the epididymis.

- Sperm are well formed to perform their function in that they have a highly stabilized nucleus that is resistant to physical trauma, a mobile tail (axoneme) for swimming, and specialized enzymes to enhance penetration of the egg.

- Sperm traveling from their site of origin in the testes must pass through approximately 6 m of tubules before arriving at the penile meatus. This tubular system includes the seminiferous tubules in the testes, epididymis, vas deferens, and urethra. About 200 million sperm may be stored in the epididymal reservoir. Increased motility and fertility appear to be acquired by sperm as they pass through the epididymis. Sperm account for less than 10% of the ejaculate volume.

- The physiologic process of erection is a complex interplay of vascular, neurologic, and hormonal factors. The sacral parasympathetic nerves provide important innervation to the penis. Acetylcholine from parasympathetic nerves causes relaxation of penile smooth muscle with subsequent engorgement. Injected prostaglandins may also induce penile erections.

- The sympathetic nervous system mediates the process of ejaculation. Sympathetic actions include contraction of the internal sphincter to prevent retrograde ejaculation and relaxation of the external sphincter to allow emission.

- Sperm deposited in the vagina undergo further changes in a process known as capacitation. This process improves the chances of sperm successfully producing fertilization of an egg. Enzymes are released (acrosome reaction) to facilitate penetration of the ovum, a process that further increases the chances of successful fertilization.

Acrosome Reaction

The head of a sperm is essentially a highly compact package of genetic chromatin material covered by a specialized **acrosome** and acrosomal (head) cap. Stored in the acrosome of the sperm are large quantities of hydrolytic (water-splitting) enzymes that are released during capacitation. The specialized acrosomal enzymes first break down cervical mucus to allow sperm to pass into the uterus and uterine tubes. If an ovum is present in the female reproductive tract when semen is introduced, continued release of acrosomal enzymes results in digestion of proteins in the structural elements of the outer covering of the egg. A high sperm count is essential for male fertility because the female ovum, once it is expelled from the ovarian follicle into the abdominal cavity and fallopian tube, contains multiple layers of granulosa cells. Before a sperm can fertilize the ovum, it must first pass through the granulosa cell layer, and then it must penetrate the thick covering of the ovum itself, the **zona pellucida.** It is believed that the acrosomal enzyme hyaluronidase plays an important role in opening pathways between the granulosa cells so that the sperm can reach the ovum.

On reaching the zona pellucida of the ovum, the anterior membrane of the sperm binds specifically with a receptor protein in the zona pellucida. Then the entire anterior membrane of the acrosome rapidly dissolves, and all the acrosomal enzymes are immediately released. Within minutes, these open a penetrating pathway for passage of the sperm head through the zona pellucida.

The head at first enters the perivitelline space lying beneath the zona pellucida but outside the membrane of the underlying oocyte. Within 30 minutes, the membranes of the sperm head and the oocyte fuse; the sperm genetic material enters the oocyte to cause fertilization, and the embryo begins to develop.

SUMMARY

The male genitourinary tract may be divided into upper and lower tracts, with the upper tract composed of the kidneys and ureters and the lower tract composed of the bladder and urethra. Auxiliary genital glands that lie adjacent to or surround the urethra include the prostate, seminal vesicles, and bulbourethral glands. The external genitalia of the male consist of the scrotum, testes, epididymis, and penis.

Embryologic development of the male and female genital and urinary systems is closely related. The nephric system develops progressively through three distinct phases: the pronephros, mesonephros, and metanephros. The gonads are derived from the urogenital ridge, from which the primitive kidney also forms. Finally, the genital duct systems develop from two different but related ducts adjacent to the undifferentiated gonads, the müllerian ducts and the mesonephric, or wolffian, ducts.

Male reproductive function depends on an intact hypothalamic-pituitary-testicular endocrine axis. Spermatogenesis takes place in the seminiferous tubules. Spermatozoa mature in their transit through the male reproductive tract. Through erection, emission, and ejaculation, sperm enter the vagina. Through capacitation and the acrosome reaction, spermatozoa acquire the ability to fertilize ova residing in the female reproductive tract.

REFERENCES

1. Bullock N, Sibley G, Whitaker R: *Essential urology*, ed 2, Edinburgh, 1994, Churchill Livingstone, pp 1–2.
2. Zderic SA, Levin RM, Wein AJ: Voiding function and dysfunction. In Gillenwater JY, et al, editors: *Adult and pediatric urology*, ed 3, vol 2, St Louis, 1996, Mosby, pp 1159–1219.
3. Redman JF: Anatomy of the genitourinary system. In Gillenwater JY, et al, editors: *Adult and pediatric urology*, ed 3, vol 1, St Louis, 1996, Mosby, pp 3–61.
4. Kissane JM: Development and structure of the urogenital system. In Murphy WM, editor: *Urological pathology*, ed 2, Philadelphia, 1997, Saunders, pp 1–3.
5. Hoffman GE, Berghorn KA: Gonadotropin-releasing hormone neurons: their structure and function, *Semin Reprod Endocrinol* 15(1):5–17, 1997.
6. Grayhack JT, Kozlowski JM: Benign prostatic hyperplasia. In Gillenwater JY, et al, editors: *Adult and pediatric urology*, ed 3, vol 2, St Louis, 1996, Mosby, pp 1501–1574.
7. Meacham RB, Lipschultz LI, Howards SS: Male infertility. In Gillenwater JY, et al, editors: *Adult and pediatric urology*, ed 3, vol 2, St Louis, 1996, Mosby, pp 1747–1802.
8. Pyror JP: Male infertility. In Sant GR, editor: *Pathophysiologic principles of urology*, Blackwell, 1994, Oxford, pp 155–179.
9. Gondos B, Wong TW: Non-neoplastic diseases of the testis and epididymis. In Murphy WM, editor: *Urological pathology*, ed 2, Philadelphia, 1997, Saunders, pp 277–341.
10. Pabst RZ: Investigations of the construction and function of the human ductus deferens, *Z Anat Entwicklungsgesch* 129(20):154–176, 1969.
11. Lerner SE, Melman A, Christ G: A review of an erectile dysfunction: new insights and more questions, *J Urol* 149(5):1246–1255, 1993.
12. O'Leary MP, Lue TF: Penile function. In Sant GR, editor: *Pathophysiologic principles of urology*, Blackwell, 1994, Oxford, pp 181–207.
13. Guyton AC, Hall JE: Reproductive and hormonal functions of the male (and the pineal gland). In Guyton AC, Hall JE, editors: *Textbook of medical physiology*, ed 9, Philadelphia, 1996, Saunders, pp 1003–1016.

Alterations in Male Genital and Reproductive Function

Marvin Van Every

⊜volve WEBSITE

http://evolve.elsevier.com/Copstead/
- Review Questions and Answers
- Glossary (with audio pronunciations for selected terms)
- Animations
- Case Studies
- Key Points Review

KEY QUESTIONS

- What are the common causes of and clinical findings in priapism?
- What are the common causes of primary and secondary impotence?
- What are the usual clinical manifestations and significance of testicular cancer, testicular torsion, cryptorchidism, and hydrocele or spermatocele?
- What clinical manifestations would lead to a suspicion of prostatitis, and how would confirmed prostatitis be treated?
- How can benign prostatic hyperplasia be distinguished from prostate cancer?
- What clinical manifestations are indicative of prostatic enlargement?

CHAPTER OUTLINE

The male genital system is susceptible to numerous congenital, acquired, and infectious conditions and, to a lesser extent, neoplasms. These disorders may interrupt the normal functions of urinary excretion and sexual function and fertility and directly affect the quality of life. This chapter will identify and explain the most common conditions that come to the attention of practitioners.

DISORDERS OF THE PENIS AND MALE URETHRA

CONGENITAL ANOMALIES

Micropenis

Micropenis is defined as a small, normally formed penis with a stretched length more than two standard deviations below the mean.[1] The normal range in newborns is 2.0 to 3.5 cm, so micropenis may be defined as a stretched length of less than 1.9 cm.[2]

Etiology and pathogenesis. Penile development and growth are both testosterone dependent. Therefore, micropenis may result from defects in testosterone production or a deficiency that results in poor growth of the organs that are targets of this hormone.

Diagnoses and treatment. Patients with micropenis must be evaluated for endocrine abnormalities. To check for these, one should measure serum levels of testosterone, luteinizing hormone, and follicle-stimulating hormone (FSH). Depending on the results of these measurements, the problem may be determined to involve the hypothalamic-pituitary axis (Prader-Willi and Kallmann syndromes) or to be some form of a testicular disorder (Klinefelter syndrome).[3]

Treatment depends on administering testosterone, either intramuscularly (IM) or topically, to stimulate penile growth. Such treatment requires caution because growth may be altered by premature closure of the epiphyseal growth plates in the long bones. In rare cases, when micropenis fails to respond to testosterone, a female sex assignment is indicated.[3]

Urethral Valves

The vast majority of **urethral valves** are posterior in location and occur in the distal prostatic urethra. They are the most common cause of urinary obstruction in male newborns and infants. These valves are mucosal folds that resemble thin membranes and cause obstruction when the child attempts to void (Figure 31-1).

Etiology. Many theories have been given to explain how valves develop. It has been suggested that several different processes may occur to form different posterior valves. Most commonly, posterior valves may result from abnormal insertion and persistence of the distal wolffian ducts. Less frequently, a persistent urogenital membrane may result in valves and obstruction.[4]

Clinical manifestations. Children with posterior valves may have variable degrees of obstruction. In the most severe cases, intrauterine renal failure may cause oligohydramnios (decreased amniotic fluid), pulmonary hypoplasia (incomplete lung development), and either stillbirth or extreme distress at the time of delivery. More frequently, inability to void is noted shortly after birth (normal voiding occurs within 48 hours after birth), or the infant has abdominal masses representing a thickened palpable bladder or hydronephrotic kidneys. Varying degrees of azotemia and renal failure occur with this scenario. Finally, urinary ascites (extravasated urine in the peritoneum) may result from a urinary leak that is usually difficult to localize. In an infant with abdominal distention, the diagnosis of urethral valves is confirmed by a plain abdominal radiograph showing the bowel "floating" in the center of the abdomen. Prenatal ultrasounds often suggest the diagnosis before birth so immediate evaluation and treatment can take place upon delivery.

Older infants with a urethral valve are less likely to have a palpable kidney or ascites. Rather, urinary tract infection, poor stream with straining to void, or occasionally hematuria may be present. Urethral valves in these older male infants may not produce much obstruction, thus making the diagnosis more difficult.[5]

Treatment. Management of posterior valves involves initial management of the metabolic abnormalities with appropriate fluid management and electrolyte replacement. In patients with a urinary tract infection, drainage of urine with a urethral or occasionally a suprapubic catheter is necessary. Finally, ablation of the valves with an endoscopic resectoscope should be performed. In infants, this step may be delayed and a cutaneous vesicostomy made to temporarily divert and drain the urine. This approach reduces the risk of traumatizing the infant's delicate urethra, which may create urethral stricture disease.

Rarely, urethral valves are located anteriorly in the penile urethra. Valves in this location are a very rare congenital anomaly and most likely represent urethral dilation or a diverticulum proximal to the valve.[6] Endoscopic resection will correct the problem.

Urethrorectal and Vesicourethral Fistulas

Etiology. **Urethrorectal** and **vesicourethral fistulas** are rare and almost always associated with an imperforate anus. Failure of the urorectal septum to develop completely leads to persistent communication between the rectum posteriorly and the urogenital tract anteriorly.

Clinical manifestations and treatment. Children with a urethrorectal or vesicourethral fistula may pass fecal material and gas through the urethra. If the anus has formed normally with an external opening, urine may drain through the rectum. The diagnosis is made with cystoscopy and contrast-enhanced radiography to delineate a blind rectal pouch or communication. Surgery is needed to resect the fistula and open the imperforate anus.

Hypospadias

In **hypospadias,** the urethral meatus is located on the ventral undersurface of the penis or on the perineum (Figure 31-2). The condition may occur with varying degrees of severity. In the least severe cases, the meatus is located distally on the penis, either at the corona or on the undersurface of the glans. With increasing severity of the condition, the meatus assumes a more proximal location and is more often associated with chordee, or curvature of the penile shaft (Figure 31-3).

Etiology and treatment. Hypospadias is the result of incomplete fusion of the urethral folds, so the meatus may be found anywhere

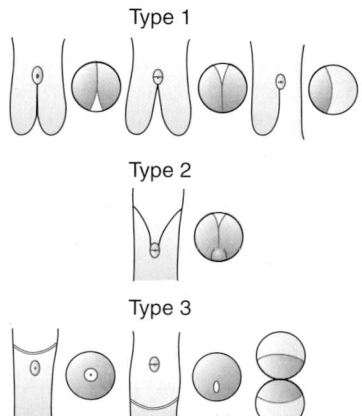

Type 1

Type 2

Type 3

FIGURE 31-1 Posterior urethral valves. (Redrawn from Young HH, Frontz WA, Baldwin JC: Congenital obstruction of the posterior urethra, *J Urol* 3:289, 1919.)

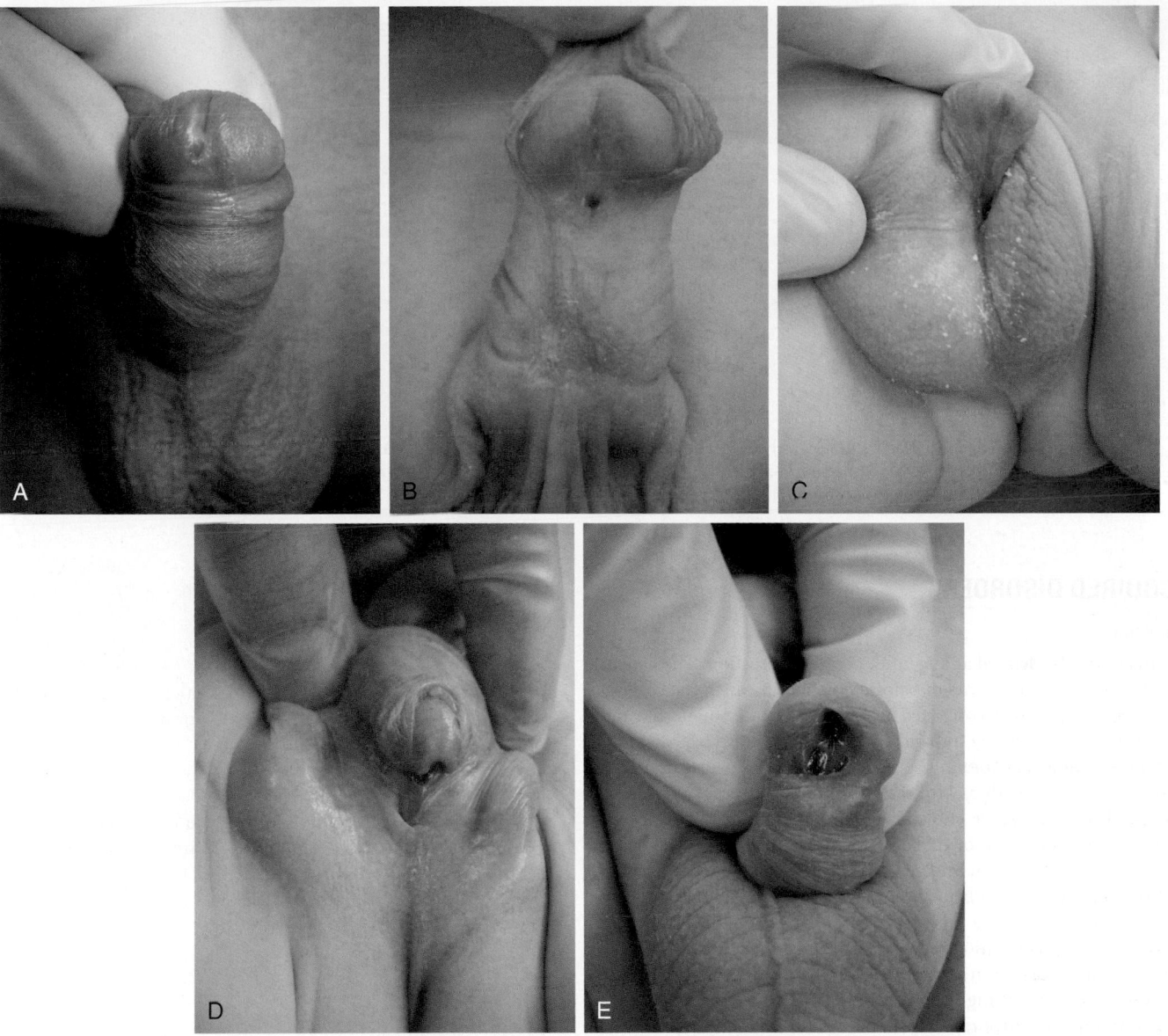

FIGURE 31-2 Varying forms of hypospadias. **A,** Glanular hypospadias. **B,** Subcoronal hypospadias. Note the dorsal hood of foreskin. **C,** Penoscrotal hypospadias with chordee. **D,** Perineal hypospadias with chordee and partial penoscrotal transposition. **E,** Megameatal variant of hypospadias diagnosed following circumcision; note absence of hooded foreskin. (From Kliegman RM et al: *Nelson textbook of pediatrics,* ed 19, Philadelphia, 2011, Saunders.)

along the phallus from the perineum to the glans. In the majority of cases hypospadias occurs distally, with about 85% of all cases involving the glans or corona.[7] Because incomplete fusion of urethral folds may indicate insufficient masculinization, it is recommended that the more severe penoscrotal and perineal openings be evaluated for conditions of intersex.[8]

Management of hypospadias involves surgical repair. Many procedures are available, with several repairs indicated for each type of hypospadias. The goal of surgery is a good overall cosmetic appearance that will allow the patient to stand and direct his urinary stream and will also allow normal sexual function.

Epispadias

In **epispadias,** the urethra opens on the dorsal aspect of the penis at a point proximal to the glans (see Figure 31-2). Although much less common than hypospadias, it can be considerably more disabling.

Etiology and treatment. The embryogenesis of epispadias is related to another congenital condition, exstrophy of the bladder. In this condition, the abdominal wall fails to form below the level of the umbilicus. At birth, the back wall of the bladder is exposed to the external environment.[9] The development of epispadias is simply a mild degree of exstrophy, with a deficiency of abdominal wall formation present inferiorly. Most commonly, the defect extends proximally to involve the urinary sphincter and results in urinary incontinence. Less commonly, the urethral meatus is located more distally along the dorsum of the penis and is accompanied by urinary continence because the sphincter is not affected (see Figure 31-3).

Management of exstrophy and proximal epispadias with incontinence is difficult and involves staged surgical procedures to reconstruct a continent bladder neck and a functional urethra. The less common distal epispadias is usually managed with tubular reconstruction procedures similar to those used for repair of hypospadias.

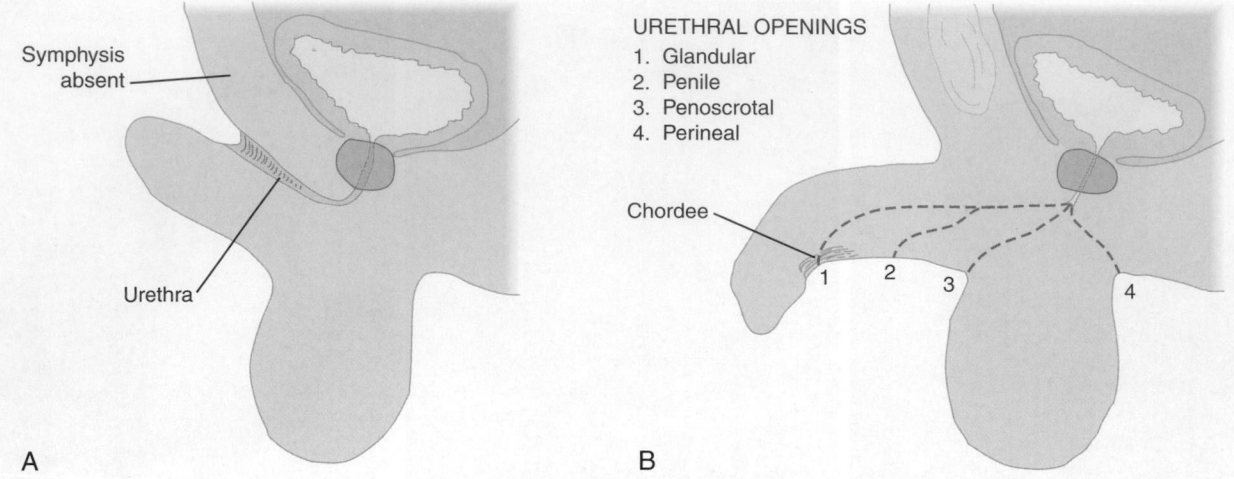

FIGURE 31-3 Epispadias **(A)** and hypospadias **(B)** showing possible locations of the urethral meatus. (From Black JM, Matassarin-Jacobs E: *Medical-surgical nursing: clinical management for continuity of care,* ed 6, Philadelphia, 2001, Saunders, p 971.)

ACQUIRED DISORDERS

Priapism

Priapism may be defined as a painful, persistent erection. The patient usually reports several hours of painful erection in which the corpora cavernosa are tense with congested blood. The corpus spongiosum and glans are characteristically soft and uninvolved.

Etiology and treatment. The causes of priapism are multiple. Most cases are idiopathic, with the next most common cause being sickle cell disease. Other etiologic factors include use of anticoagulant therapy, presence of diabetes mellitus or leukemia, and use of certain antidepressant medications.[10] Recently, intracavernosal injection of vasoactive substances for the management of impotence has been noted to cause priapism. On a rare occasion, oral erectile dysfunction medications can cause priapism. Although multiple causes exist, the common abnormality is probably an obstruction of venous drainage resulting in the buildup of viscous, poorly oxygenated blood in the corpora.[11] If the process is allowed to continue, fibrosis of the corpora cavernosa will eventually occur and may cause impotence.

Management of priapism may involve a combination of measures, depending on the cause and duration of the condition. Initial therapy for priapism secondary to sickle cell disease includes sedation and oxygen.[12] For the management of priapism secondary to other causes, initial measures may include aspiration of blood from the corpora, as well as injection of α-adrenergic agents.[13] If the priapism remains refractory to these initial measures, a surgical shunting procedure may be necessary in which a shunt is created between the erect corpora cavernosa and the detumesced corpus spongiosum.

Phimosis and Paraphimosis

Etiology, clinical manifestations, and treatment. **Phimosis** occurs when the uncircumcised foreskin cannot be retracted over the glans of the penis (Figure 31-4, *A*). Phimosis is usually the result of chronic inflammation and infection from poor hygiene. Calculi and squamous cell carcinoma may occur, although it is usually the presence of erythema, tenderness of the phimotic foreskin, or a discharge that prompts the patient to seek medical attention.[14] Management involves treating the infection with antifungal agents or antibiotics, followed by circumcision.

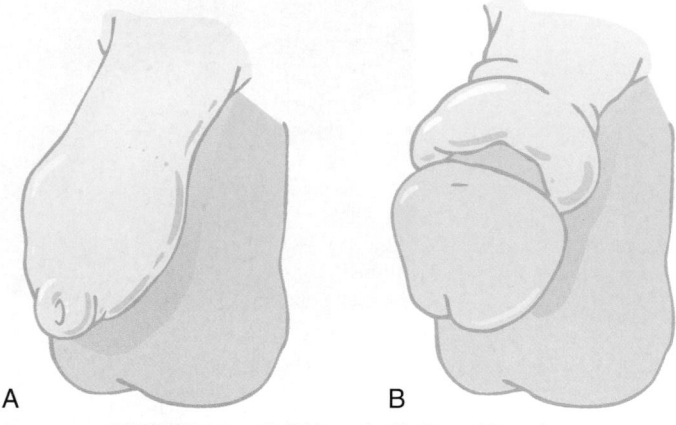

FIGURE 31-4 A, Phimosis. **B,** Paraphimosis.

Paraphimosis, on the other hand, occurs when a foreskin that has been retracted over the glans up onto the shaft of the penis cannot be replaced in its normal position (see Figure 31-4, *B*). In this condition, which is usually secondary to chronic inflammation under the foreskin, a constricting ring of skin forms around the base of the retracted glans. The constriction causes venous congestion of the glans, with further swelling and edema making the condition worse. Treatment entails reducing the paraphimotic foreskin back over the glans, which can usually be accomplished by compressing the glans to reduce the edema. Occasionally, a slit or formal circumcision is needed to manage the problem.

Peyronie Disease

Etiology and treatment. **Peyronie disease** refers to the formation of palpable, fibrous plaque on the surface of the corpora cavernosa. This plaque subsequently causes curvature of the penis with painful, incomplete erections. No satisfactory treatment for this disease is available, although some cases may remit with time. Conservative therapies that have had limited success include the use of vitamin E or aminobenzoate potassium (Potaba), colchicine, and pentoxifylline (Trental). In addition, several operative procedures have been developed. These procedures involve excising the plaque and repairing the corporal defect with a graft or plicating the corporal bodies.[15]

Urethral Strictures

Etiology. **Urethral strictures** are fibrotic narrowings of the urethra and are usually composed of scar tissue. Most acquired strictures are due to a prior infection such as gonorrhea or trauma. Traumatic causes can be both iatrogenic, such as large urethral catheters and instrumentation, and noniatrogenic, such as straddle injuries.

Clinical manifestations and treatment. A decreased urinary stream is the most common complaint. Other common complaints include urethral discharge, infection, and urine retention. Urethral strictures are usually diagnosed by cystoscopy or retrograde urethrography, which would demonstrate a narrowing of the urethra. Management of urethral strictures involves procedures to dilate, incise, or reconstruct the urethra, depending on the extent and duration of the stricture.

Erectile Dysfunction

Erectile dysfunction (ED) is the inability to achieve or maintain an erection sufficient for satisfactory sexual performance.[17] It is highly prevalent in aging men, affecting approximately 50% of men older than 60 years of age.[16] Its prevalence and incidence are highly connected with risk factors such as hypertension, elevated cholesterol level, presence of diabetes mellitus and/or metabolic syndrome, and lifestyle choices such as smoking, obesity, and lack of exercise.[18]

The physiologic process of penile erection is a complex interaction of the vascular, hormonal, and neurologic systems. **Impotence** may be primary or secondary. Primary impotence refers to the inability to attain an erection throughout life and is often related to deep-seated psychiatric problems of some duration. Occasionally, vascular trauma sustained during early childhood or adolescence may account for primary impotence.[18]

There are many causes of secondary ED ranging from psychogenic to traumatic. As our knowledge of the disease has advanced, we understand that most ED is due to physiologic changes in the vasculature of the corporal bodies of the penis. These changes may be due to surgery (e.g., radical prostatectomy or cystectomy), trauma (penile or neurologic), disease (diabetes mellitus, hypertension, pelvic irradiation, hyperlipidemia, hypogonadism), and aging.[19]

Etiology. Far more common than primary impotence is secondary impotence. An individual with secondary impotence is no longer able to achieve normal erections but did have normal erections in the past. The causes of secondary impotence are multiple and may be discovered by examining the patient's medical history. Common causes of secondary impotence are peripheral vascular disease, the use of certain medications, endocrine problems, trauma, iatrogenic causes, and psychological causes. To differentiate organic causes from psychogenic impotence, one relies on the history, physical, and basic laboratory testing such as measurement of serum glucose and testosterone levels. Penile tumescence testing can also be utilized to make this distinction.

Arterial insufficiency of the penis may occur from obstruction of the arterial supply. Several processes may account for this obstructive arteriosclerosis. Stenosis of the arteries secondary to atheromatous plaque may be the most common etiologic factor. Diabetes mellitus not only may result in occlusion of arterial vessels but also may cause a neuropathy of the pudendal nerve that might result in erectile dysfunction.[20] Most investigators have suggested that erectile dysfunction may result from excessive venous drainage from the penis. This occurs because the blood is not adequately trapped in the corpora.

The list of medications that may cause erectile dysfunction is long. Several antihypertensive agents, including propranolol, monoamine oxidase inhibitors, and thiazides, have been associated with varying degrees of impotence. Other medications linked to erectile dysfunction include phenothiazines, antihistamines, and some antidepressants.[21]

Endocrinopathy accounts for a small percentage of impotence cases.[22] Pituitary dysfunction resulting in decreased or no secretion of luteinizing hormone may result in decreased secretion of testosterone. Primary failure of the testes may also occur, resulting in decreased secretion of testosterone. Finally, excessive secretion of the hormone prolactin by the pituitary gland may result in low testosterone levels.

Trauma to the penis resulting in penile fractures and damage to penile erectile tissue may occasionally lead to partial or complete impotence. More common injuries include pelvic fractures with subsequent damage to the penile vascular and nervous supply. Iatrogenic trauma secondary to several commonly performed operations, including aortoiliac vascular surgery, and radical pelvic cancer operations may also result in impotence.

A newer concept in erectile dysfunction is the idea of vascular endothelial damage, which can be diffuse throughout the body. Some researchers believe impotence may be an indicator of coronary artery disease.

Finally, it must be remembered that successful sexual function depends not only on intact vascular, hormonal, and neurologic systems but also on intact psychological and social responses. Several psychological factors may be manifested as problems of low desire, erectile failure, or premature ejaculation. A discussion of the psychological contribution to impotence is beyond the scope of this book.

Treatment. Management of erectile dysfunction requires an initial evaluation to differentiate organic causes from psychogenic causes. Further evaluation to distinguish among the various organic causes may then be needed. Once a psychogenic cause has been ruled out, several therapeutic options exist. Surgical options include the insertion of an inflatable or semirigid prosthetic device into the corpora cavernosa. In the past few years, several investigators have discovered that intracavernous injection of various vasoactive substances can cause an erection. Several of these substances, including papaverine, phentolamine, and prostaglandin E_1, are commonly used and afford a nonsurgical treatment option.

Viagra, the first oral therapy for erectile dysfunction, is the citrate salt of sildenafil, a selective inhibitor of cyclic guanosine monophosphate (cGMP)–specific phosphodiesterase type 5 (PDE5). To understand its clinical pharmacology, a review of some of the physiologic mechanisms of erection follows. Briefly, erection of the penis involves release of nitric oxide in the corpus cavernosum during sexual stimulation. Nitric oxide then activates the enzyme guanylate cyclase, and the subsequently increased levels of cGMP produce smooth muscle relaxation in the corpus cavernosum and allow inflow of blood. Sildenafil has no direct relaxant effect on isolated human corpus cavernosum, but it enhances the effect of nitric oxide by inhibiting PDE5, which is responsible for degradation of cGMP in the corpus cavernosum. When sexual stimulation causes local release of nitric oxide, inhibition of PDE5 by sildenafil causes increased levels of cGMP in the corpus cavernosum, smooth muscle relaxation, and inflow of blood to the corpus cavernosum, which results in erection (Figure 31-5). Sildenafil citrate at the recommended doses appears to have no effect in the absence of sexual stimulation and affords another nonsurgical treatment option. Two newer agents for erectile dysfunction are Levitra and Cialis. In any particular patient, one of the three available oral medications may work better than the others. None of these agents should be used in conjunction with nitrate medications.

Another nonsurgical alternative entails the use of a vacuum device to sustain an erection. Finally, in very specific cases of erectile dysfunction, surgical procedures may be done to revascularize the arterial supply of the penis or ligate the penile venous drainage.

Premature Ejaculation

Premature ejaculation (PE) is the most common male sexual dysfunction and is present in up to 30% of all males. The World Health

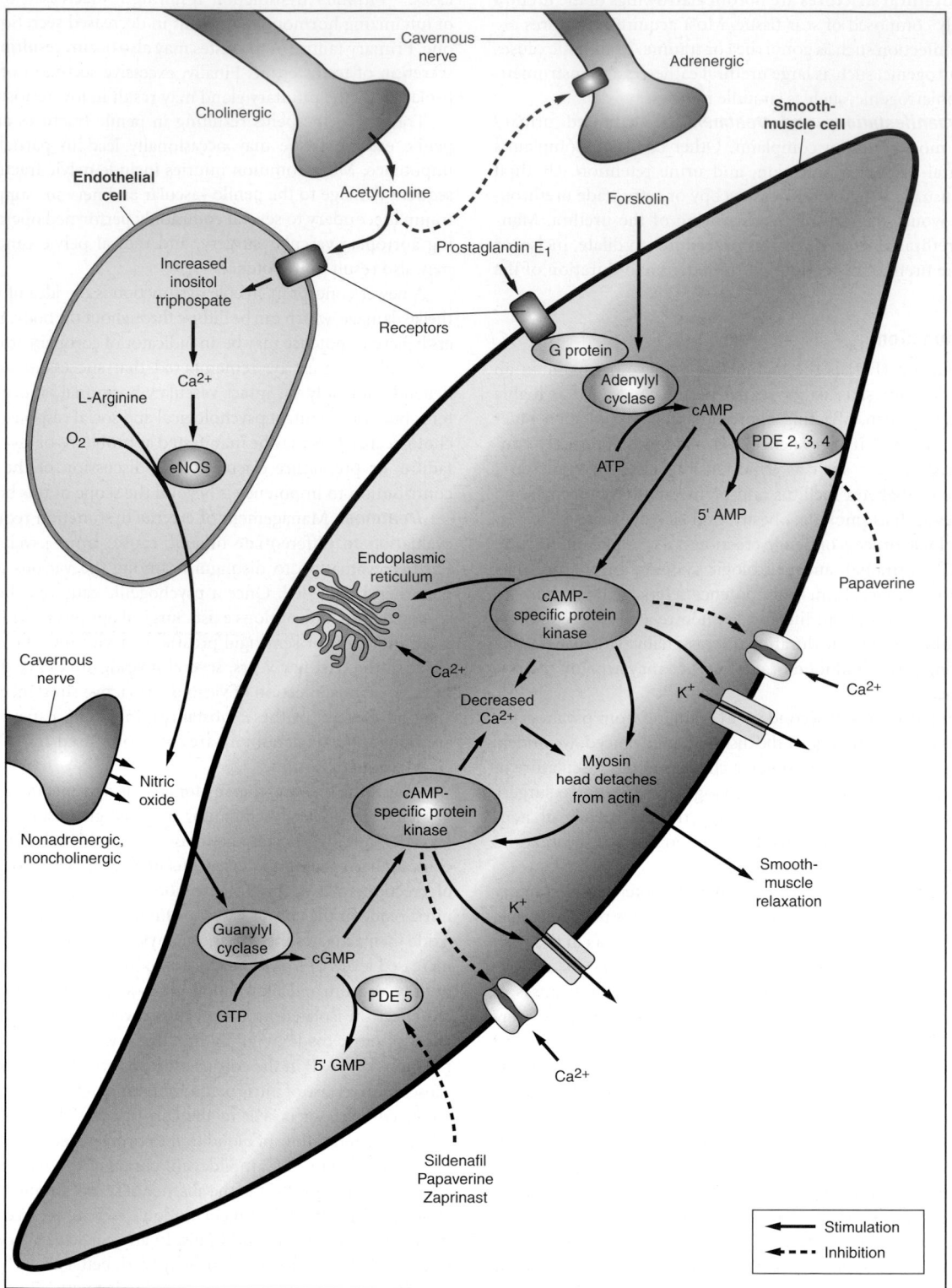

FIGURE 31-5 Mechanism of corpus cavernosum smooth muscle relaxation. Smooth muscle relaxation in the corpus cavernosum is the underlying mechanism of erection. The principal neurotransmitter is NO acting through cGMP and G-protein. Pharmacologic agents that produce erection act through this pathway by regulation of the intracellular balance of Ca^{2+} and K^+ concentrations. *ATP,* Adenosine triphosphate; *cAMP,* cyclic adenosine monophosphate; *cGMP,* cyclic guanosine monophosphate; *GTP,* guanosine triphosphate; *NO,* nitric oxide; *eNOS,* nitric oxide synthase; *PDE₅,* phosphodiesterase type 5. (Redrawn from Lue TF: Erectile dysfunction, *New Engl J Med* 342:1802-1813, 2000.)

TABLE 31-1   MEDICAL THERAPY OPTIONS FOR THE TREATMENT OF PREMATURE EJACULATION*

ORAL THERAPIES	TRADE NAMES[†]	RECOMMENDED DOSE[‡§]
Nonselective Serotonin Reuptake Inhibitors		
Clomipramine	Anafranil	25-50 mg/day *or* 25 mg 4-24 hr preintercourse
Selective Serotonin Reuptake Inhibitors		
Fluoxetine	Prozac, Sarafem	5-20 mg/day
Paroxetine	Paxil	10, 20, 40 mg/day *or* 20 mg 3-4 hr preintercourse
Sertraline	Zoloft	25-200 mg/day *or* 50 mg 4-8 hr preintercourse
Topical Therapies		
Lidocaine/prilo-caine cream	EMLA cream	Lidocaine 2.5%/prilocaine 2.5% 20-30 min preintercourse

*This list does not reflect order of choice or efficacy.
[†]Trade names listed may not be all-inclusive.
[‡]Peak plasma concentrations occur 2 to 8 hours (hr) postdose and half-lives range from 1 to 3 days.
[§]Titrate doses from low to high based on response.

Organization (WHO) defines PE as "persistent or recurrent ejaculation with minimal stimulation before, on, or shortly after penetration and before the person wishes it, over which the sufferer has little or no voluntary control, which causes the sufferer and/or partner bother or distress."[23]

Etiology and treatment. The etiology of PE is not well-defined but can be both biological and psychosocial. The diagnosis is achieved with a careful medical and sexual history and physical examination.

There are no FDA-approved medications for treatment but several are currently being used off label (Table 31-1). Further research will elucidate the causes and allow for better treatment in the future.

INFECTIOUS DISORDERS

Sexually transmitted infections (STIs) are common in the male genital system. A more in-depth discussion of STIs is provided in Chapter 34.

NEOPLASTIC DISORDERS

Neoplasms of the Penis

Etiology. Although cancer of the penis is rare in the United States and accounts for fewer than 0.2% of cancer deaths, its prevalence fluctuates widely among various locations. The causes are poorly understood, but phimosis of the foreskin accompanied by chronic inflammation has been thought to be the primary etiologic factor. The incidence of penile cancer among circumcised men is extremely low.[24]

The majority of penile cancer cases are squamous cell carcinoma (97%). They usually occur on the glans or the inner surface of the foreskin. Metastasis occurs by lymphatic dissemination, with initial involvement of the palpable inguinal lymph nodes. Death from penile carcinoma is a result of uncontrolled lymphatic spread and subsequent necrosis of the overlying skin, debilitation, and sepsis.

Penile carcinoma is staged as follows[25]:

Stage I: The lesion is limited to the glans or foreskin.
Stage II: The tumor involves the shaft of the penis.
Stage III: The inguinal nodes are involved but the lesion is operable.
Stage IV: The disease is disseminated.

The lesion of penile cancer is usually ulcerative and fungating in appearance and may be associated with pain, bleeding, and urethral discharge. Inguinal adenopathy is present in more than 50% of patients at the time of diagnosis, although frequently the adenopathy represents an inflammatory response secondary to the lesion rather than metastasis.

Treatment. Therapy for penile carcinoma depends on the stage of the lesion. Topical chemotherapy and radiation therapy may be considered for certain small superficial lesions. Larger distal penile lesions usually require partial penectomy, whereas proximal lesions may require total penectomy with creation of a perineal urethrostomy. Finally, removal of the involved inguinal lymph nodes by inguinal lymphadenectomy may be performed in cases of suspected stage III disease. Systemic chemotherapy is also used to treat metastatic disease.

The prognosis of penile carcinoma depends on the stage of disease. The 5-year survival rate for men with tumors localized to the penis is 65% to 90%. With inguinal node involvement, 5-year survival rates drop to about 30% to 50%, and if distant metastases are present, the 5-year survival rate is virtually zero.[25]

KEY POINTS

- Congenital disorders of the penis may result from hormonal deficiencies or abnormalities in embryonic development. Micropenis, for example, is usually a result of testosterone deficiency. Urethral valves, fistulas, and malpositioning of the urinary meatus (hypospadias, epispadias) are related to abnormal embryonic development.

- Priapism is a persistent, painful erection, most commonly of unknown cause. Priapism may occur in conditions that cause obstruction of venous drainage, including sickle cell anemia, anticoagulant therapy, diabetes mellitus, certain antidepressant medications, and PDE5 inhibitors such as Viagra.

- Phimosis and paraphimosis are disorders of the foreskin. Phimosis is associated with chronic inflammation and poor hygiene and results in a foreskin that cannot be retracted. Paraphimosis refers to a foreskin that remains retracted and cannot be returned to its normal position.

- Urethral strictures may be congenital or acquired. Most acquired strictures are secondary to gonorrheal infection or urethral trauma. Weak urinary stream, bladder infections, and retained urine are common manifestations.

- Impotence is the inability to achieve a sustained erection. Causes of impotence are categorized as primary and secondary. Primary impotence is rare and usually related to adolescent vascular trauma or psychiatric problems. Secondary impotence may be due to a variety of factors, including vascular disease, medications, endocrine disorders, trauma, and psychological distress.

- A number of infections are sexually transmitted and affect the penis and urethra, including gonococcal urethritis, nongonococcal urethritis, syphilis, herpes, and genital warts. Gonococcal and nongonococcal urethritis and syphilis are effectively managed with antibiotics. Herpes and genital warts are associated with viruses and tend to be chronic, with intermittent recurrence.

- Penile neoplasms are rare, particularly in circumcised males. Phimosis and chronic inflammation may be important etiologic factors. Like other neoplasms, penile cancer has a better prognosis if managed before dissemination.

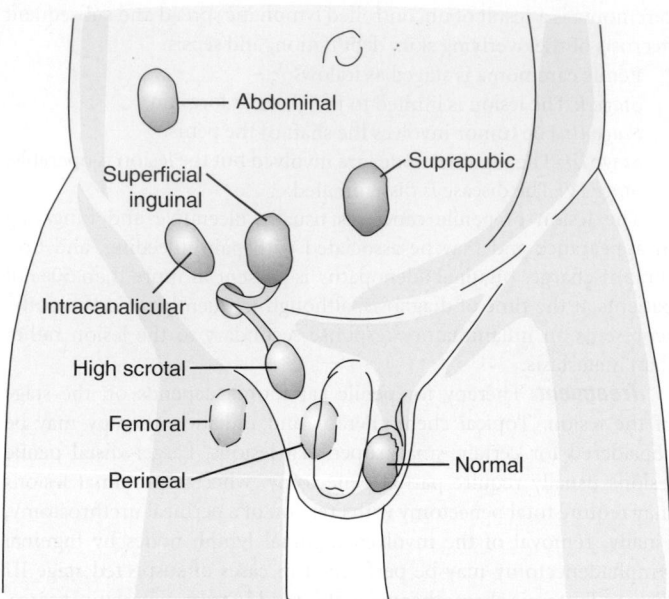

FIGURE 31-6 Sites of ectopic testes.

DISORDERS OF THE SCROTUM AND TESTES

CONGENITAL DISORDERS

Cryptorchidism

Cryptorchidism means "hidden testis" and refers to any testis that occupies an extrascrotal position. The cryptorchid testis may be incompletely descended and as such be located intraabdominally, within the inguinal canal, or just external to the canal but above the scrotum. Occasionally the testis may emerge from the external ring of the inguinal canal and be misdirected into an abnormal extrascrotal position. In this situation the testis may be called ectopic. An ectopic testis may be located in any of several locations but is most commonly found in a superficial inguinal pouch[26] (Figure 31-6).

The incidence of cryptorchidism is about 0.7% to 1.0% of male infants at 1 year of age. The cause of the condition is uncertain but may be related to an intrinsic testicular defect or a subtle hormonal deficiency.[26]

The incompletely descended, cryptorchid testis undergoes deleterious changes. The tubules become fibrotic, with a deficiency of spermatogenesis and subsequent infertility. More important is the increased incidence of testicular malignancy in cryptorchid testes.[27] Several studies have revealed an increased prevalence of testicular tumors in subjects with a history of cryptorchidism.

Treatment. Because of the increased risk of malignancy and infertility, treatment at an early age to bring the testis into a normal scrotal position is recommended. An operative procedure *(orchiopexy)* is usually required, although in certain situations descent may be stimulated by the administration of human chorionic gonadotropin, which is given in a series of intramuscular injections.[28]

ACQUIRED DISORDERS

Hypogonadism

Androgen deficiency in the aging male (ADAM)—or andropause—is increasingly recognized as a problem for American men. The U.S. Food and Drug Administration estimates that between 4 and 5 million men suffer from hypogonadism.[29] There are multiple causes (Box 31-1) but primary testicular failure is the most common etiology.

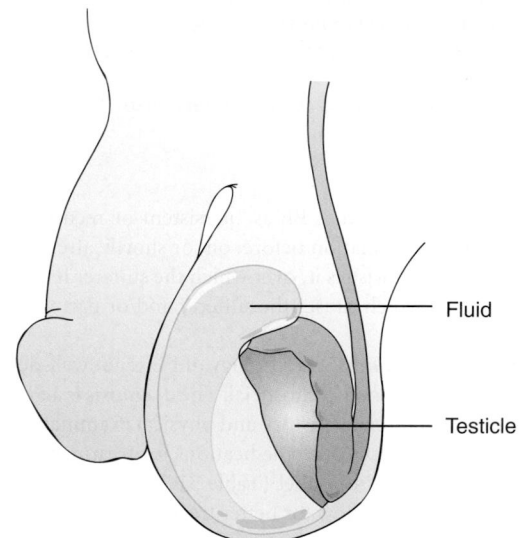

FIGURE 31-7 Hydrocele.

The effects of ADAM include erectile dysfunction (ED), loss of muscle tone, osteoporosis, and lipid metabolism changes. It is also associated with metabolic syndrome.

The diagnosis is made by determining the serum testosterone level. Other laboratory tests may include measurement of prolactin and luteinizing hormone (LH) levels.[29]

Treatment. Fortunately, it is quite easy to treat because there are multiple forms of testosterone that can be administered, including IM injections, patches, gels, and subcutaneous pellets. Patients receiving replacement therapy need to be monitored for prostate cancer and polycythemia.

Hydrocele

Etiology and clinical manifestations. A **hydrocele** consists of a fluid collection surrounding the testicle or spermatic cord and contained within the tunica or processus vaginalis (Figure 31-7). Scrotal

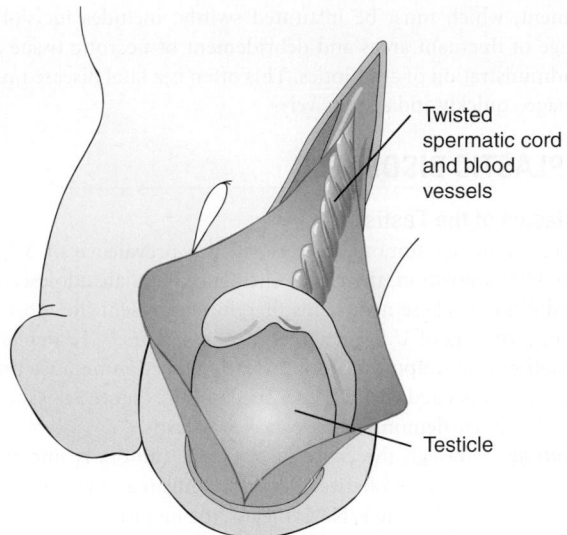

FIGURE 31-8 Testicular torsion.

Labels in figure: Twisted spermatic cord and blood vessels; Testicle

BOX 31-2 CORRECTABLE CAUSES OF MALE INFERTILITY

Endocrinologic causes	Obstruction
Testicular abnormalities	Vasal
Retractile testes	Epididymal
Cryptorchidism	Ejaculatory
Torsion	Disorders of ejaculation
	Sexual dysfunction
	Varicocele

From Galarneau GJ, Nagler HM: Cost-effective infertility therapies in the '90s: to treat or to cure? *Contemp Urol* 11:32-45, 1999.

swelling in infants or young boys may indicate a hydrocele. These congenital hydroceles exist because of communication between the abdominal cavity and scrotum through the processus vaginalis. The scrotum is characteristically small and soft in the morning but larger and tense at night as it fills with fluid from the abdominal cavity.

Hydroceles may also develop secondary to scrotal injury, radiation therapy, infection of the epididymis, or testicular neoplasms. More commonly, however, the cause is uncertain, with the hydrocele developing slowly over time and occurring in middle-aged or elderly men. These acquired hydroceles may vary in size and consistency from small and soft to large and tense. The fluid is usually clear and yellow.

Treatment. Because hydrocele is a benign condition, treatment is required only if the fluid collection becomes uncomfortable for the patient. Occasionally, a tense hydrocele might restrict circulation to the testicle. Management usually involves a surgical procedure to drain the fluid with either resection or plication of the hydrocele sac to prevent reaccumulation of the fluid. Aspiration of the hydrocele may be performed, although fluid often reaccumulates.

Spermatocele

Etiology and treatment. **Spermatoceles** are painless, cystic masses containing sperm. Although they are usually small, they may be quite large and difficult to distinguish from a hydrocele. The cause of spermatoceles is uncertain; they may arise from the tiny tubules that connect the epididymis to the testis (vasa efferentia) or from the epididymis itself. Like hydroceles, spermatoceles need not be treated unless they become large enough to trouble the patient, in which case an operative procedure to excise the spermatocele may be performed.

Testicular Torsion

Torsion of the testicle is described as a twisting of the spermatic cord with subsequent compromise of the testicular vascular supply and testicular ischemia, followed by infarction (Figure 31-8). Although torsion may occur in the neonatal period, the majority of cases occur in prepubertal boys.

Clinical manifestations. The diagnosis is suggested by the onset of severe pain in one testis, followed by swelling of the scrotum. Lower abdominal pain accompanied by nausea and vomiting may also occur. The condition may be differentiated from epididymitis (inflammation of the epididymis), which is also associated with scrotal swelling, by the presence of vascular echoes detected with a Doppler ultrasound.

A testis made ischemic by torsion will not demonstrate blood flow, whereas the inflammation of epididymitis and its hypervascularity show increased vascular flow. Testicular nuclear scanning is another way to diagnose testicular torsion.

Treatment. Management of torsion involves an operation to open the scrotum, untwist the testis, and "pex" (secure) it to the scrotal wall. Because the chance of torsion also involving the contralateral testis is increased, the contralateral testicle is "pexed" to the scrotal wall as well. If detorsion is accomplished within 12 hours of the event, the prognosis for testicular viability is usually good. If torsion has been present for more than 24 hours, viability of the testis is doubtful.

Male Infertility

Etiology and pathogenesis. Approximately 15% of couples are unable to conceive after 1 year of unprotected intercourse.[30] A male factor is solely responsible in about 20% and contributory in another 30% to 40% of infertility cases.[1] An abnormal semen analysis is present in almost all cases of male infertility, but other factors may also be involved. Some causes of male infertility are identifiable and can be corrected, such as ductal obstruction varicocele or hypogonadotropic hypogonadism (a hormone abnormality)[31] (Box 31-2). Other problems can be diagnosed but not corrected such as bilateral testicular atrophy. Many cases are simply idiopathic or unexplained.

Diagnosis and treatment. The purpose of evaluating the male partner in infertility couples is to determine the cause of the infertility if possible so appropriate treatment and counseling can be accomplished. In some couples, treatment can result in pregnancy through intercourse. In others more advanced treatments are necessary.

In some patients there is no effective treatment and they can be appropriately counseled. Other patients will have a risk of transmitting genetic abnormalities and will need to be made aware of that potential. In some patients a life- or health-threatening condition may underlie the infertility and need treatment.[30]

As with all medical evaluations there should be a complete and specific history and physical examination. Lab testing includes two semen analyses (Box 31-3), and usually an endocrine evaluation (testosterone and FSH). More evaluation could include postejaculatory urinalysis, transrectal ultrasound, scrotal ultrasound, specialized semen tests, and karyotyping.

There are multiple treatments for male factor infertility. In men with varicoceles surgical repair or embolization can often improve fertility. Ductal obstruction can sometimes be surgically treated. In other cases more advanced treatment is necessary such as microsurgical epididymal sperm aspiration (MESA) or percutaneous testicular sperm extraction (TESE). This allows for retrieval of sperm that can then be used for in vitro fertilization (IVF) or intracytoplasmic sperm injection (ICSI). Some patients will improve their semen analysis with endocrine therapy and in some couples intrauterine insemination (IUI) will be successful. For some couples the best option may be donor sperm or adoption.

INFECTIOUS DISORDERS

Epididymitis

Etiology. **Epididymitis,** or inflammation of the testis, has several causes. It may occur as a result of trauma or the reflux of sterile urine up the vas deferens. However, the majority of cases are probably secondary to a bacterial cause, with both sexually transmitted organisms (*Neisseria gonorrhoeae* and *Chlamydia trachomatis*) and non–sexually transmitted organisms (*Pseudomonas* and *Escherichia coli*) involved.

Clinical manifestations and treatment. With epididymitis the scrotum may be enlarged, reddened, and tender. The pain may radiate along the spermatic cord into the inguinal area. Fever may also occur, as may urethral discharge, cystitis, and cloudy urine. Laboratory testing usually reveals an elevated white blood cell (WBC) count, and urine culture may reveal the infecting organism.

Treatment for the condition involves bed rest, scrotal support, and administration of antibiotics. In advanced cases, incision and drainage with the intravenous administration of antibiotics may be needed to effectively manage a resulting scrotal abscess. On rare occasions, the testicle may need to be removed.

Fournier Gangrene

Etiology, clinical manifestations, and treatment. **Fournier gangrene** is a severe but rare condition involving gangrenous necrosis of the scrotum. Symptoms are pain and swelling of the scrotum, fever and chills, and sepsis.[32] The diagnosis can often be made by history and physical examination. Additional tests such as ultrasound, computed tomography (CT), or magnetic resonance imaging (MRI) can also be helpful in diagnosis. Usually, an underlying disease such as diabetes, alcoholism, or another general debility predisposes the patient to such an aggressive infection. Extravasation of infected urine from urethral trauma, a perforated urethral diverticulum, or a non–urinary tract source such as a perirectal abscess may act as the source of infection.

Treatment, which must be instituted swiftly, includes incision and drainage of fluctuant areas and debridement of necrotic tissue along with administration of antibiotics. This often is a fatal disease unless it is managed quickly and aggressively.

NEOPLASTIC DISORDERS

Neoplasms of the Testis

Although testicular tumors are rare, with a prevalence of 3.7 cases per 100,000 population, their peak incidence is in late adolescence to early adulthood. These neoplasms therefore represent the most common solid tumors of U.S. men ages 20 to 34 years.[33] Testicular self-examination is an important tool for early detection because prompt treatment is associated with a higher success rate. Figure 31-9 shows an ultrasound image demonstrating cancer in a testis.

Etiology. Although the cause of testicular tumors is uncertain, a strong association is seen between cryptorchidism and the subsequent development of malignancy. Nevertheless, the majority of patients with testicular tumors have no history of cryptorchidism, which suggests that several unrecognized factors may be contributing to the pathogenesis.

Histologically, testicular tumors may be considered in two groups. In the first group are nongerminal neoplasms, including tumors that originate from either the Leydig cells or other stromal tissue cells of the testis. In the second group are germinal neoplasms, which are derived from the germinal cells of the testis. This group accounts for the vast majority (95%) of testicular tumors. Germinal neoplasms may be further subdivided into two groups: seminomas and nonseminomas.

Treatment. Although germinal tumors may consist entirely of one histologic subtype, many contain elements of more than one subtype. Treatment and prognosis vary according to the subtype of germinal tumor. For example, seminoma in its early stages is exquisitely sensitive to and easily cured with radiation therapy. On the other hand, nonseminomatous germ cell tumors in the early stage are usually successfully managed with surgery. The prognosis is also variable. Pure choriocarcinomas are usually first seen at an advanced stage with distant metastases. Treatment is usually less effective for this aggressive lesion. However, the majority of germ cell tumors may be effectively managed even if lymph node metastases are present.

Except for choriocarcinomas, which disseminate by vascular means, testicular germ cell tumors usually metastasize through the lymphatic system. They usually disseminate in a stepwise manner, first involving the retroperitoneal lymph nodes lying adjacent to the great vessels.

BOX 31-3 SEMEN ANALYSIS: REFERENCE VALUES

On at Least Two Occasions

Ejaculate volume 1.5-5.0 ml

pH >7.2

Sperm concentration >20 million/ml

Total sperm number >40 million/ejaculate

Percent motility >50%

Forward progression >2 (scale 0-4)

Normal morphology:

   >50% normal*

   >30% normal[†]

   >14% normal[‡]

And

Sperm agglutination <2 (Scale 0-3)

Viscosity <3 (Scale 0-4)

From Jarow J, Sigman M, Kolettis PN, Lipshultz LR, McClure RD et al: *The optimal evaluation of the infertile male: AUA Best Practice Statement,* Linthicum, MD, 2010, American Urological Association Education and Research, pp 1-38.

*World Health Organization, 1987.[8]

[†]World Health Organization, 1992.[9]

[‡]Kruger (Tygerberg) Strict Criteria, World Health Organization, 1999.[1,5]

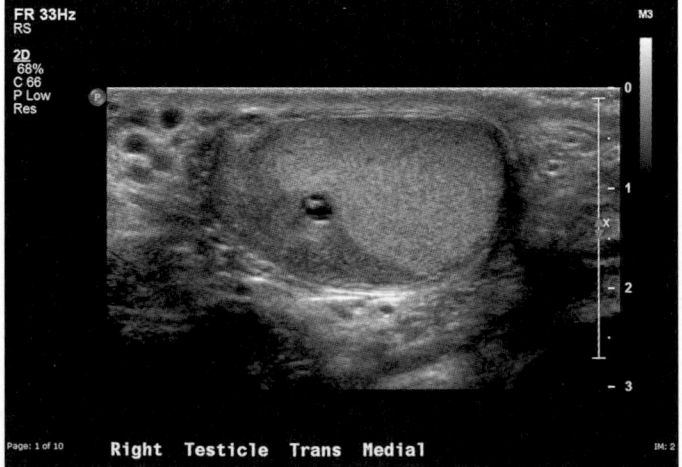

FIGURE 31-9 Testis ultrasound demonstrating cancer.

If unmanaged, the disease may progress to involve other lymph nodes and other organs such as the lungs.

Multiple staging systems have been devised to classify the extent of this disease. Most are a variation of the system proposed by Boden and Gibb in 1951.[33] One commonly used system is as follows:

Stage I: The tumor is confined to the testis.
Stage II: The tumor has spread to retroperitoneal lymph nodes.
Stage III: The tumor has spread to nodes above the diaphragm.
Stage IV: The tumor has spread to other organs.

Because the management of testicular tumors is complicated and somewhat controversial, a complete discussion is not possible here; however, several issues can be highlighted. After diagnosis of a testicular tumor, an operation to remove the testicle is performed. This procedure involves an inguinal incision with removal of the testis from the scrotum, followed by ligation and removal of the spermatic cord and testicle together. Histologic classification, additional staging studies, and other factors then determine further treatment. This treatment may involve close observation with frequent radiologic studies to determine new progression, surgery to remove the retroperitoneal lymph nodes (Figure 31-10), chemotherapy, or radiation therapy. Some situations may call for a combination of these measures.

KEY POINTS

- Cryptorchidism refers to a testis located in a position other than the scrotum. Often the testis has failed to descend completely and is located in the inguinal canal. Undescended testes are associated with infertility and an increased risk of testicular malignancy.
- A hydrocele is a collection of fluid in the testicle or spermatic cord. In the pediatric age group it is associated with a communication between the abdominal cavity and the scrotum (hernia). Hydroceles are benign and treated only if they become uncomfortable. A spermatocele is a cyst that contains sperm. Like hydroceles, they are benign and do not require treatment unless they cause discomfort.
- Testicular torsion refers to a twisting of the spermatic cord with subsequent testicular ischemia and infarction. Sudden onset of severe testicular pain is common. If the torsion is reduced within 12 hours, the testicle may be viable.

- Inflammation of the epididymis, called epididymitis, is most commonly associated with infectious agents. Manifestations include a swollen, tender, reddened scrotum with associated bladder infection and cloudy urine. Antibiotics are indicated. Aggressive infections of the scrotum may result in Fournier gangrene manifested by gangrenous necrosis of the scrotum.
- Although rare in the population, testicular cancer is the most common solid tumor in men ages 20 to 34 years. The great majority of testicular neoplasms originate in the germ cells. Most germ cell tumors can be effectively managed even after lymph node metastasis. Management includes surgical removal of the testis and spermatic cord, with irradiation and chemotherapy as indicated.

DISORDERS OF THE PROSTATE

Benign Prostatic Hyperplasia

Benign prostatic hyperplasia, also referred to as benign prostatic hypertrophy (BPH), is a very common disorder. An estimated 80% of men older than 60 years experience some degree of BPH. It is important to recognize that BPH and prostate cancer are not related entities, and no study has conclusively demonstrated that BPH predisposes to the development of prostate cancer.[34]

Etiology. Although the exact cause of BPH is unknown, the occurrence of the disease with aging suggests a relationship to changes in the aging male endocrine system. The process involves hyperplasia of the glands surrounding the prostatic urethra (Figure 31-11). As this tissue increases in size, it compresses the urethra and produces symptoms of bladder outlet obstruction.

Clinical manifestations. Symptoms of obstruction may be minimal at first but may eventually progress to complete obstruction and urinary retention. A decrease in the force of the urinary stream, hesitancy or difficulty in initiating a urinary stream, and interruption of the stream may occur. Because the bladder may fail to empty completely, infection associated with residual urine may occur. Figure 31-12 illustrates possible complications of benign prostatic enlargement.

The diagnosis of BPH usually involves recognition of the characteristic symptoms. Rectal examination disclosing an enlarged prostate, urethral catheterization or bladder scanning to document a large postvoid urinary residual, and radiographic evidence of hypertrophy and

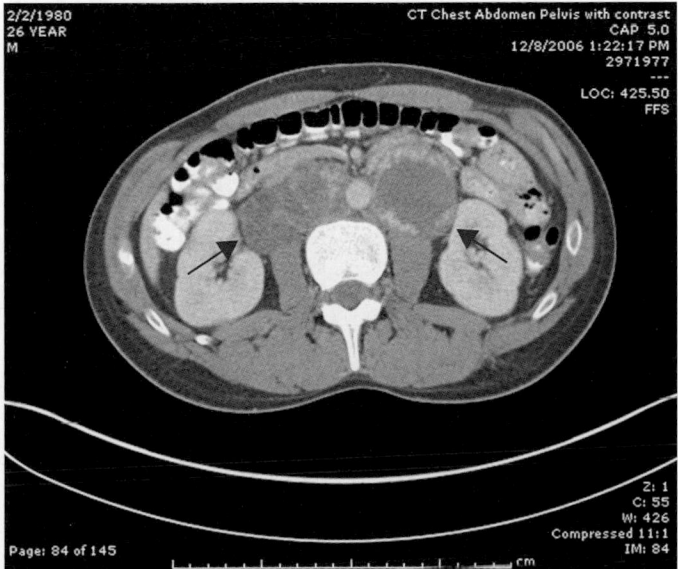

FIGURE 31-10 CT scan demonstrating large retroperitoneal lymph nodes.

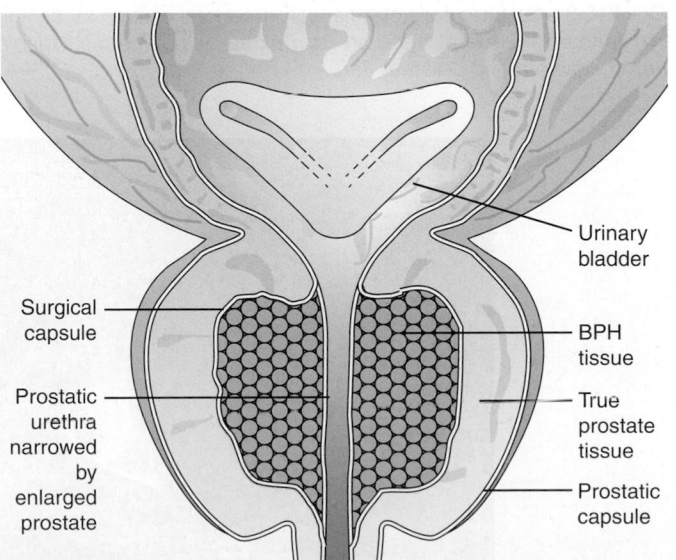

FIGURE 31-11 Gross appearance of hyperplastic prostatic tissue obstructing the prostatic urethra. *BPH,* Benign Prostatic Hypertrophy.

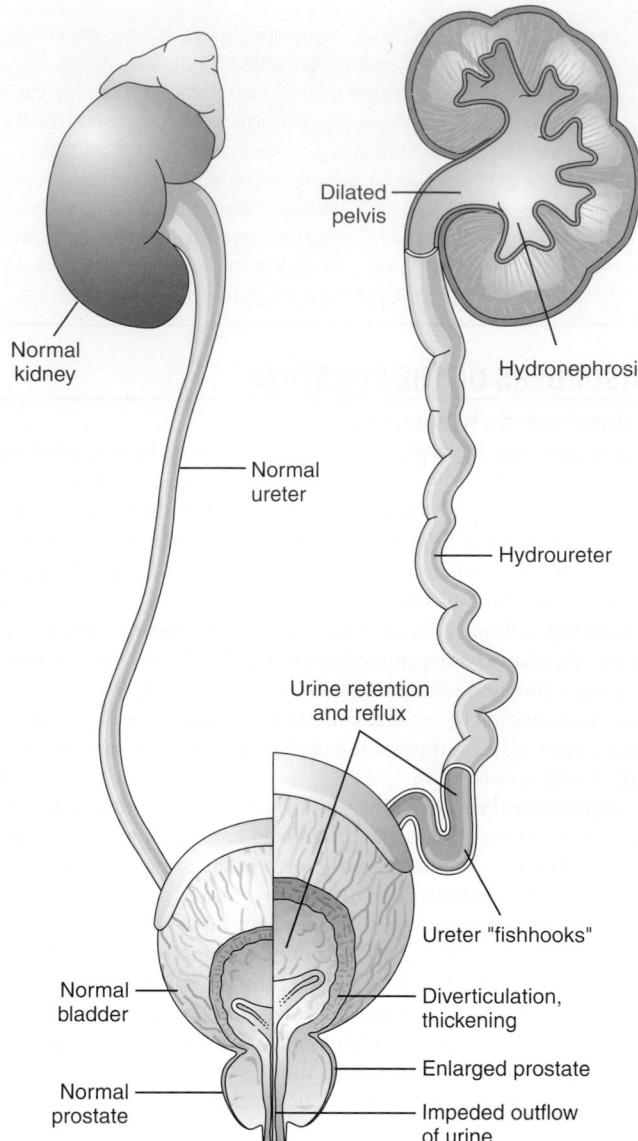

FIGURE 31-12 Sites for potential complications caused by benign prostatic enlargement *(right)* are compared with a normal kidney, ureter, bladder, and prostate *(left)*.

Normal kidney

Normal ureter

Dilated pelvis

Hydronephrosis

Hydroureter

Urine retention and reflux

Normal bladder

Normal prostate

Ureter "fishhooks"

Diverticulation, thickening

Enlarged prostate

Impeded outflow of urine

obstruction on CT scan (Figure 31-13) or abdominal ultrasound are some of the measures that may be used to confirm the diagnosis. Urodynamics are sophisticated measures of urinary function that can help confirm the diagnosis.

Treatment. The treatment of BPH has changed markedly over the last several years. The first line of treatment is with medication such as α-blockers or 5α-reductase inhibitors. The former treatment decreases the tension in the prostate by relaxing the muscle fibers in the gland. This reduces pressure in the bladder neck and urethra, allowing easier flow. The latter treatment actually decreases the size of the gland by blocking the conversion of testosterone to dihydrotestosterone. This can shrink the gland by up to one third and thereby reverse the years of growth that have caused impingement of the urethra.

The next forms of treatment are the minimally invasive treatments that are usually performed in the physician's office. These include microwave therapy, needle ablation, and some other forms of treatment to decrease the tissue squeezing the urethra closed. They are usually well tolerated but may not cause total relief of the obstruction, and the long-term results are variable.

The last form of treatment is surgery. The classic operation for BPH is called a transurethral resection of the prostate (TURP). This procedure uses a resectoscope that is passed through the penis and into the prostate. An electric wire is then used to resect chips of tissue from the interior of the gland to form an open channel for urination.

A newer alternative to the TURP is laser therapy. In this approach, a scope is passed via the urethra into the prostate, and the tissue is vaporized with a laser fiber to create an open channel.

In some patients with extremely large glands or other bladder pathology, an incision is made and an open simple prostatectomy can be performed to remove the adenoma (inner portion of the gland). This creates a large cavity and channel for the urine to pass through.

All of the treatments have various side effects and risks. Therefore, each patient should have his treatment tailored to his specific situation.

Prostatitis

Prostatitis, or inflammation of the prostate, has several causes and encompasses several syndromes. A common classification of prostatitis proposed by Drach and colleagues[34] in 1978 considers four types: acute bacterial prostatitis, chronic bacterial prostatitis, nonbacterial prostatitis, and prostatodynia.[35-38]

The causative organism in bacterial prostatitis is usually *E. coli*, with species of *Proteus, Klebsiella, Enterobacter, Pseudomonas, Serratia,*

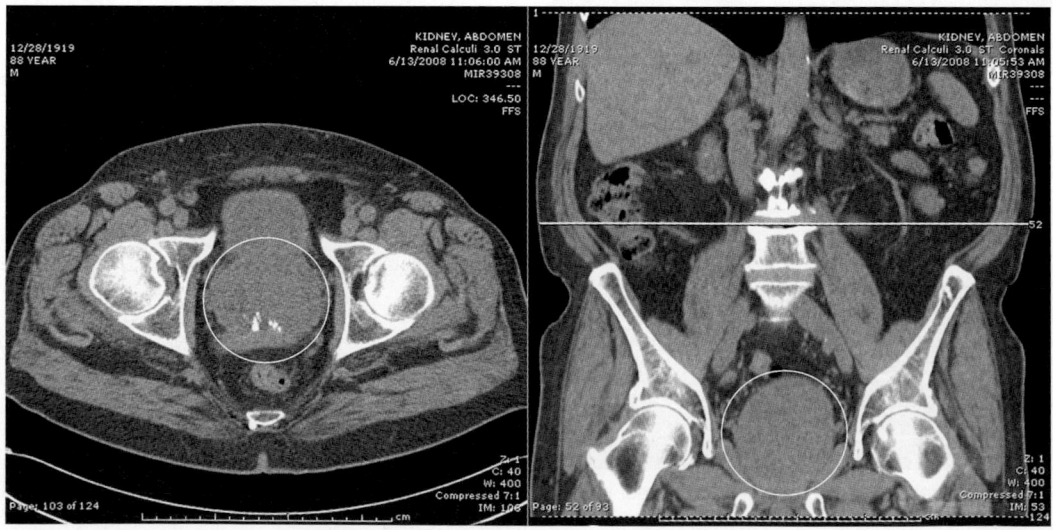

FIGURE 31-13 CT scan demonstrating BPH.

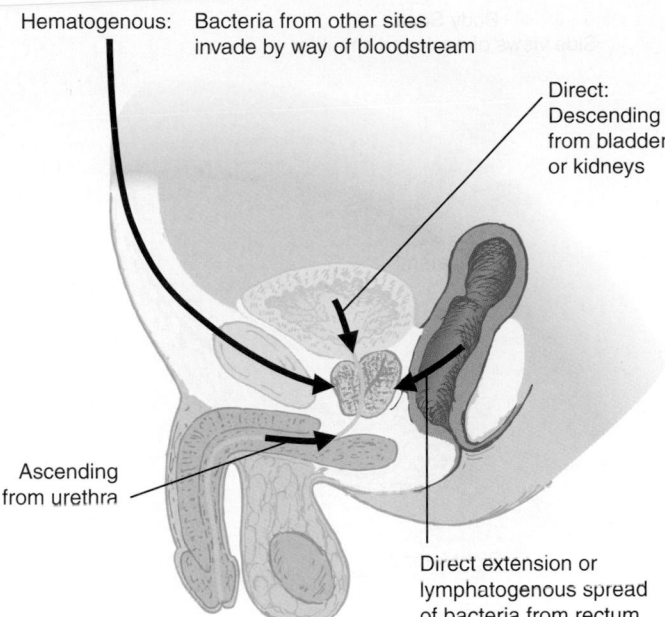

Hematogenous: Bacteria from other sites invade by way of bloodstream

Direct: Descending from bladder or kidneys

Ascending from urethra

Direct extension or lymphatogenous spread of bacteria from rectum

FIGURE 31-14 Postulated pathways of infection to the prostate gland. (From Black JM, Matassarin-Jacobs E: *Medical-surgical nursing: clinical management for continuity of care*, ed 6, Philadelphia, 2001, Saunders, p 963.)

Staphylococcus, and *Enterococcus* occurring less commonly.[35-36] Possible routes of infection include ascending infection up the urethra, reflux of infected urine into the prostatic ducts, hematogenous infection, and invasion of rectal bacteria by direct extension or lymphogenous spread (Figure 31-14). Many cases of prostatitis result from periurethral infection associated with an indwelling urethral catheter.[36-37]

Clinical manifestations, diagnosis, and treatment. Acute bacterial prostatitis is characterized by the onset of fever, chills, low back pain, and the voiding symptoms of frequency, urgency, and dysuria. Rectal examination usually reveals a tender, swollen prostate, and subsequent urinalysis may show the presence of WBCs and bacteria.

The diagnosis of bacterial prostatitis is usually suggested by the initial symptoms and signs. Microscopic inspection of the urine and expressed prostatic secretions may reveal WBCs and bacteria. A urine culture with sensitivity testing for the offending organism is recommended to direct therapy with an appropriate antibiotic. In the event of high fever and an elevated WBC count, intravenous antibiotics are recommended.

Chronic bacterial prostatitis may be associated with variable symptoms. Although some men with chronic bacterial prostatitis may report a history of acute bacterial prostatitis, many have no history of this problem. Most men complain of voiding symptoms with pain localized to various areas, including the perineum, back, suprapubic area, and, occasionally, the testis. High-grade fever and chills are uncommon with this entity, as opposed to acute bacterial prostatitis.

In chronic bacterial prostatitis, pathogenic organisms may persist in prostatic tissues unaltered by the administration of several antibiotics. Because most antibiotics accumulate poorly in prostatic secretions, discontinuation of antibiotic use often results in reinfection and recurrence of symptoms. It is this occurrence of relapsing infections, often caused by the same organism, which is typical of chronic bacterial prostatitis. Several antibiotic agents, such as trimethoprim-sulfamethoxazole (Septra, Bactrim), when used for a prolonged period (4 to 6 weeks) have a better cure rate because of their capability to penetrate prostatic tissue.

Prostatitis may also occur secondary to nonbacterial inflammation. In fact, nonbacterial prostatitis probably accounts for the majority of cases of prostatitis. The symptoms of this entity are variable but usually include irritative voiding; symptoms of urgency, frequency, and

nocturia; as well as occasional perineal and suprapubic pain. Although these symptoms are similar to those of bacterial prostatitis, patients have no history of positive urine cultures or urinary tract infections. Treatment may include a course of antibiotics, oral antiinflammatory agents (e.g., ibuprofen), α-blockers, prostatic massage, and, occasionally, sitz baths. Symptoms are often intermittent, and patients should be reassured that the disease is not contagious and does not predispose to the development of cancer or other serious disease.

The final classification of prostatitis, **prostatodynia,** is typified by symptoms of prostatitis but no history of urinary tract infection and no evidence of inflammation in prostatic secretions. The cause of this entity is uncertain and may involve spasm of the pelvic floor musculature. Treatment may involve the use of α-adrenergic receptor–blocking agents and occasionally diazepam (Valium).[37-38]

Prostate Cancer

Other than skin cancers, prostate cancer is now recognized as the most prevalent form of cancer in men. About 200,000 cases are diagnosed annually in the United States, with approximately 30,000 deaths annually attributed to the disease. Prostate cancer ranks as the second leading cause of cancer death among men. Cancer of the prostate rarely occurs in men younger than 50 years, and its incidence increases with age. The majority (95%) of prostate cancers are adenocarcinomas with abnormal proliferation of prostatic glandular structures.[38-39]

Etiology. The precise cause of prostate cancer is undetermined, although genetic, hormonal, dietary, and viral factors have all been suggested. Varying degrees of aggressiveness of prostate cancer have been recognized, with different tumors expressing different malignant potential and ultimately carrying a different prognosis. Attempts to classify prostate cancer into separate groups of cancer have been made, with different tumors expressing different malignant potential and ultimately carrying a different prognosis. Such attempts to classify prostate cancer into different groups consider the structure and internal architecture of tumor cells and their pattern of proliferation. For example, cells of the more aggressive or poorly differentiated prostate cancers have more indistinct cell borders, larger nuclei, and loss of acinar (gland) formation.

Prostate cancer is staged as follows:

Stage 1: The tumor is microscopic and intracapsular.

Stage 2: The tumor is palpable on rectal examination but confined to the prostate.

Stage 3: The tumor has extended beyond the capsule of the prostate.

Stage 4: The tumor has metastasized to distant organs.

Diagnosis. The diagnosis of prostate cancer may involve several clinical scenarios. The disease may be diagnosed after microscopic inspection of prostate tissue removed for the management of presumed BPH. Prostate cancer may also be detected on rectal examination in patients with or without voiding symptoms. Occasionally, patients have urinary retention or even azotemia and renal failure secondary to obstructive nephropathy. Much interest has focused on the search for effective measures to detect prostate cancer in its early and most easily manageable stages. Two new techniques, a blood test for serum prostate-specific antigen (PSA) and transrectal ultrasonography, have generated considerable excitement within the field of urology. Several initial investigations have shown efficacy in the early detection of prostate cancer.

The diagnosis of adenocarcinoma of prostate cancer is usually made by checking the PSA level. This simple blood test has been a major factor in the early detection of adenocarcinoma of the prostate. Although it is not very accurate, it is helpful in identifying men who are at risk of having cancer. Since the adoption of its widespread use, most patients have been diagnosed before becoming symptomatic. However, many patients will have symptoms of BPH because of a benign enlargement of the gland, which is common in the age group that also is at risk for prostate cancer. If a patient has symptoms from his cancer, it is

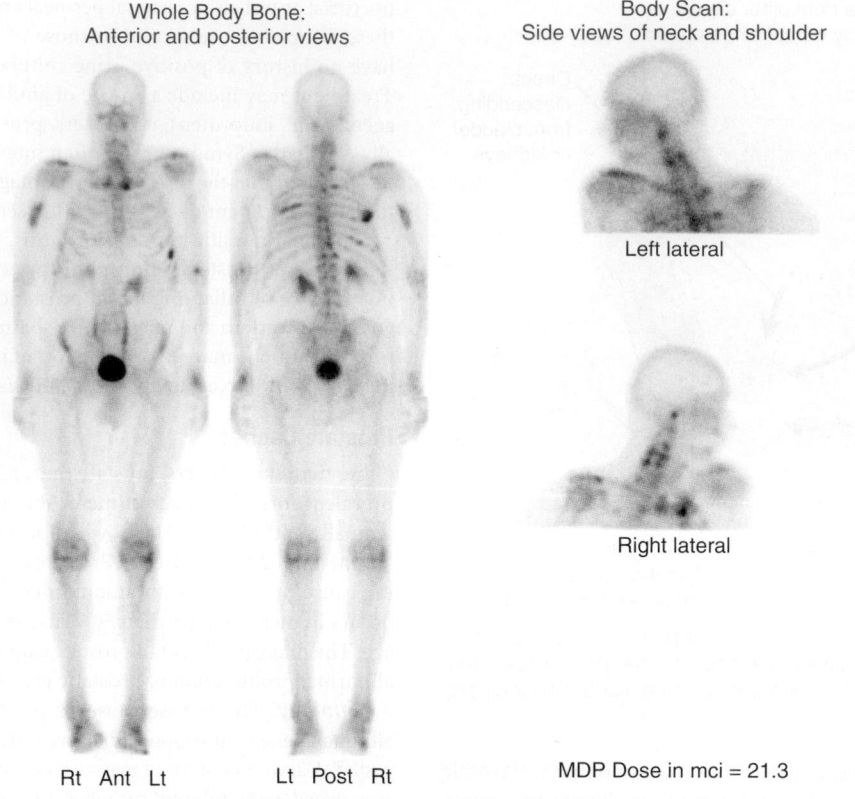

Whole Body Bone:
Anterior and posterior views

Body Scan:
Side views of neck and shoulder

Left lateral

Right lateral

Rt Ant Lt   Lt Post Rt

MDP Dose in mci = 21.3

FIGURE 31-15 Bone scan demonstrating skeletal metastases.

often too late for cure because the symptoms usually indicate extensive disease. These symptoms include hematuria, weight loss, malaise, anorexia, and back pain.

Most patients will be diagnosed on the basis of an abnormal PSA blood test result, which usually leads to a transrectal ultrasound (TRUS) and biopsy of the prostate.

Since most patients are now diagnosed at an early stage there is little need for further staging tests. However, if there is concern for more extensive cancer, then they can be evaluated with a bone scan (Figure 31-15) or CT scan of the abdomen and pelvis.

Treatment. Management of prostate cancer depends on several factors, including the stage of the tumor, as well as the age and health of the patient. Debate exists over treatment for men with localized disease, with options ranging from aggressive therapy to "watchful waiting." Watchful waiting may be an option for older men with asymptomatic stage A prostate cancer. Younger men may be candidates for the more aggressive approach, which includes surgery to remove the prostate and surrounding tissue (radical prostatectomy), radiation therapy, or cryotherapy (freezing the gland). It is important to note that approximately 70% to 90% of men who undergo radical prostatectomy will experience impotence. Urinary incontinence may also occur. Given the effects of surgical intervention, it is important that patients have access to preoperative and postoperative counseling about issues arising from their diagnosis and the effect of various treatments and potential complications.

In addition to radical prostatectomy or radiation therapy, in some cases lymph nodes in the pelvis are also removed (pelvic lymph node dissection). Advanced lesions may respond to hormonal manipulation. Orchiectomy, oral administration of estrogens, or intramuscular injection of luteinizing hormone–releasing hormone agonist and antagonist may reduce the patient's serum testosterone level. Many prostate cancers are androgen sensitive and may be temporarily controlled with androgen ablation. In more advanced cases that are no longer hormonally responsive, palliative measures such as spot radiation treatment of painful areas of bone metastasis and analgesics may be required.

In the last several years there have been advances in chemotherapy for the treatment of hormone-resistant prostate cancer. One of the latest treatments is Sipuleucel-T. This therapy is based on autologous cellular immunotherapy to induce the patient's immune system to attack the prostate cancer cells.[39] A great deal of research is being conducted to identify vaccines and other therapies to prevent and cure this highly prevalent cancer.

GERIATRIC CONSIDERATIONS

Prostate Cancer

Cancer of the prostate rarely occurs in men younger than 50 years, and its incidence increases with age. Symptoms vary depending on the stage of the disease. Men who are older and have stage A prostate cancer may be monitored closely without any treatment. Men with more advanced stage disease may be treated more aggressively.

KEY POINTS
- Symptoms of BPH include diminished force of the urinary stream, hesitancy, and poor bladder emptying. Transurethral resection of the obstructing prostatic tissue is the usual treatment.
- Inflammation of the prostate, or prostatitis, is characterized by low back pain, urinary frequency, urgency, and dysuria. Fever and chills may also be present with acute bacterial prostatitis. *E. coli* is the most commonly associated organism. Prostatitis may also occur in the absence of infection.
- Prostate cancer is usually detected as a lump or enlargement of the prostate gland. As with other cancers, early, accurate diagnosis is important for effective therapy. Surgical resection, radiation therapy, and hormone therapy (to reduce androgen levels) may be used. The choice of treatment depends on the grade and stage of the disease and the individual's age, general health, and life expectancy.

SUMMARY

Disorders of the penis and male urethra may be grouped into congenital and acquired anomalies, infections, and neoplasms. Common congenital anomalies include urethral valves and hypospadias. Common acquired disorders involve phimosis, urethral strictures, and impotence. Sexually transmitted diseases are some of the most common infections involving the penis and urethra; they include gonococcal urethritis, nongonococcal urethritis, syphilis, genital herpes, and genital warts. Neoplasms of the penis and urethra are relatively rare.

Congenital disorders of the scrotum and testes include cryptorchidism. This condition is one of the most common problems seen by pediatric urologists. Testicular torsion and Fournier gangrene are two of the more immediate urologic emergencies. Finally, neoplasms of the testes, although rare, may afflict younger men in the prime of life.

Disorders of the prostate account for a majority of the visits to a practicing urologist. Briefly, these disorders can be divided into problems of benign prostatic hyperplasia, prostatitis, and prostatic cancer. Prostate cancer is the most frequently diagnosed cancer in men, with more than 200,000 cases diagnosed and approximately 30,000 deaths yearly.

REFERENCES

1. Underwood LE, Van Wyk JJ: Normal and aberrant growth. In Wilson JD, Foster DW, editors: *Williams textbook of endocrinology*, ed 9, Philadelphia, 1998, Saunders, pp 1117–1124.
2. Feldman KW, Smith DW: Fetal phallic growth and penile standards for newborn male infants, *J Pediatr* 86(3):395–398, 1975.
3. Kogan SJ, Williams DI: The micropenis syndrome: clinical observations and expectations for growth, *J Urol* 118(2):311–313, 1977.
4. Greenfield SP: Posterior urethral valves: new concepts, *J Urol* 157(3):996–997, 1997.
5. King LR: Posterior urethra. In Kelalis PP, King LR, editors: *Clinical pediatric urology*, ed 3, Philadelphia, 1992, Saunders.
6. Van Savage JG, et al: An algorithm for the management of anterior urethral valves, *J Urol* 158(3 pt 2):1030–1032, 1997.
7. Zaontz MR, Packer MG: Abnormalities of the external genitalia, *Pediatr Clin North Am* 44(5):1267–1297, 1997.
8. Albers N, et al: Etiologic classification of severe hypospadias: implications for prognosis and management, *J Pediatr* 131(3):344–346, 1997.
9. Beaudoin S, Simon L, Bargy F: Anatomical basis of a common embryological origin for epispadias and bladder or cloacal exstrophies, *Surg Radiol Anat* 19(1):11–16, 1997.
10. Mulhall JP, Honig SC: Priapism: etiology and management, *Acad Emerg Med* 3(8):810–816, 1996.
11. Powars DR, Johnson CS: Priapism, *Hematol Oncol Clin North Am* 10(6):1363–1372, 1996.
12. Fitzpatrick TJ: Spongiograms and cavernosograms: a study of their value in priapism, *J Urol* 109(5):843–846, 1973.
13. deHoll JD, et al: Alternative approaches to the management of priapism, *Int J Impot Res* 10(1):11–14, 1998.
14. Golubovic Z, et al: The conservative treatment of phimosis in boys, *Br J Urol* 78(5):786–788, 1996.
15. Licht MR, Lewis RW: Modified Nesbit procedure for the treatment of Peyronie's disease: a comparative outcome analysis, *J Urol* 158(2):460–463, 1997.
16. Droupy S, Ponsot Y, Giuliano F: How, why and when should urologists evaluate male sexual function? *Nat Clin Pract Urol* 3(2):84, 2006.
17. Montague DK, et al: The management of erectile dysfunction: an AUA update, *J Urol* 174:230, 2005.
18. Bortolotti A, et al: The epidemiology of erectile dysfunction and its risk factors, *Int J Androl* 20(6):323–334, 1997.
19. Dean RC, Lue TF: Physiology of penile erection and pathophysiology of erectile dysfunction, *Urol Clin North Am* 32:379–395, 2005.
20. McMillan DE: Development of vascular complications in diabetes, *Vasc Med* 2(2):132–142, 1997.
21. Fabbri A, Aversa A, Isidori A: Erectile dysfunction: an overview, *Hum Reprod Update* 3(5):455–466, 1997.
22. Roy JB: Advances in the management of impotence, *J Okla State Med Assoc* 91(1):14–16, 1998.
23. Wayne J, Hellstrom G: Premature ejaculation: out of the Dark Ages and into the 21st century, *Urol Times* 33(Suppl 7):5, 2005.
24. Micali G, et al: Squamous cell carcinoma of the penis, *J Am Acad Dermatol* 35(3 pt 1):432–451, 1996.
25. Schellhammer PF, Grabstald H: Tumors of the penis. In Walsh PC, et al, editors: *Campbell's urology*, ed 7, Philadelphia, 1997, Saunders.
26. Kogan SJ: Cryptorchidism. In Kelalis PP, King LR, editors: *Clinical pediatric urology*, ed 3, Philadelphia, 1992, Saunders.
27. Cortes D: Cryptorchidism: aspects of pathogenesis, histology and treatment, *Scand J Urol Nephrol Suppl* 196:1–54, 1998.
28. Gill B, Kogan S: Cryptorchidism. Current concepts, *Pediatr Clin North Am* 44(5):1211–1227, 1997.
29. Carson CC: Evolving concepts in the management of androgen deficiency in the aging male, *Contemp Urol* 15(Suppl 4), 2003.
30. Jarow J, et al: *The optimal evaluation of the infertile male: AUA Best Practice Statement*, Linthicum, MD, 2010, American Urological Association Education and Research, pp 1–38.
31. Galarneau GJ, Nagler HM: Cost-effective infertility therapies in the '90s: to treat or to cure? *Contemp Urol* 11:32–45, 1999.
32. Morpurgo E, Galandiuk S: Fournier's gangrene, *Surg Clin North Am* 82(6):1213–1224, 2002.
33. Morse MJ, Whitmore WF: Neoplasms of the testis. In Walsh PC, et al, editors: *Campbell's urology*, ed 7, Philadelphia, 1997, Saunders.
34. Drach GW, et al: Classification of benign diseases associated with prostatic pain: prostatitis or prostatodynia, *J Urol* 120(2):266, 1978.
35. Nickel JC: Prostatitis: myths and realities, *Urology* 51(3):362–366, 1998.
36. Meares EM: Prostatitis and related disorders. In Walsh PC, et al, editors: *Campbell's urology*, ed 7, Philadelphia, 1997, Saunders.
37. Walsh PC: Benign prostatic hyperplasia. In Walsh PC, et al, editors: *Campbell's urology*, ed 7, Philadelphia, 1997, Saunders.
38. Catalona WJ: Carcinoma of the prostate. In Walsh PC, et al, editors: *Campbell's urology*, ed 7, Philadelphia, 1997, Saunders.
39. Hall SJ, et al: Integrated safety data from a randomized, double-blind, controlled trial of autologous cellular immunotherapy with Sipuleucel-T patients with prostate cancer, *J Urol* 186:877–881, 2011.

Female Genital and Reproductive Function

Rosemary A. Jadack

ⓔvolve WEBSITE

http://evolve.elsevier.com/Copstead/
- Review Questions and Answers
- Glossary (with audio pronunciations for selected terms)
- Animations
- Case Studies
- Key Points Review

KEY QUESTIONS

- What are the major structures of the internal and the external female reproductive tract?
- What are the major hormonal events of the female reproductive cycle?
- Which hormones are involved in breast development during pregnancy and lactation, and what are their specific functions?
- What are the physiologic changes associated with pregnancy?
- What gestational events occur in the fetus during each of the three trimesters of pregnancy?
- What hormonal changes lead to menopause?
- What physiologic changes and complications may result from menopausal hormone deficiencies?

CHAPTER OUTLINE

The female reproductive system is complex both in structure and in function. From birth to senescence, the organs of the female reproductive system function in concert with each other, with the brain, and with other endocrine organs. This integrated functioning constitutes some of the most intricate and elegant processes of the human body. This chapter presents an overview of these functions, beginning with the development of the female reproductive tract.

The major processes related to the reproductive tract throughout life, including the menstrual cycle, pregnancy, lactation, and menopause, are then described with an emphasis on recent research findings. Health care providers must also consider the developmental, cognitive, functional, social, and financial aspects of women's reproductive lives.[1-3] Because the functioning of the female reproductive system has an enormous impact on the life of the individual woman, increased importance has been placed on the active involvement of women in understanding their own health care needs. Health care professionals are encouraged to include women as collaborators in decisions about their reproductive health.[4,5]

REPRODUCTIVE STRUCTURES

Organization of the Female Reproductive Organs

The internal organs of the female reproductive system include the ovaries, **oviducts** (fallopian tubes), uterus, cervix, and vagina (Figure 32-1). These organs are situated in the pelvic cavity and are supported and anchored in place by a series of ligaments (Figure 32-2).

Ovaries

The two ovaries, which are the female gonads, are located close to the lateral walls of the pelvic cavity. When the ovary is in its normal position, its long axis is nearly vertical with respect to the horizontal axis of the body. The size of the ovary varies with age and with the stage of the menstrual cycle. It is somewhat larger before than after pregnancy and further reduces in size with the aging process.[6]

The ovary is covered with a single layer of epithelium. Underneath the epithelium is a layer of dense fibrous connective tissue called the tunica albuginea. The tunica albuginea constitutes the outer portion of the cortex of the ovary. The remainder of the cortex consists of connective tissue called the *stroma,* which contains ova in various stages of maturation. The innermost part of the ovary, the medulla, consists of loose connective tissue that is richly supplied with blood and lymph vessels and nerve fibers.[7]

Before birth, hundreds of thousands of **oogonia** (cells that develop into ova) are present in the ovaries. Thus the entire lifetime supply of ova is established during embryonic development; no new oogonia arise after birth. Each oogonium is surrounded by a cluster of granulosa cells. The oogonium and its granulosa cells constitute a follicle. During prenatal development, the oogonia increase in size and become primary oocytes. By the time of full gestational development, the primary oocytes are in the prophase of the first meiotic division. Ovarian follicular development is shown in Figure 32-3. During childhood and into adult life, the oocytes enter a nonactive phase. After puberty, a few of the oocytes develop in follicles each month in response to follicle-stimulating hormone (FSH) secreted by the anterior pituitary gland. The vast majority of follicles and their oocytes die by atresia. Generally, each month, only one mature follicle will develop to eject an oocyte through the wall of the ovary in the process of ovulation, which is described in more detail in the Menstrual Cycle section.

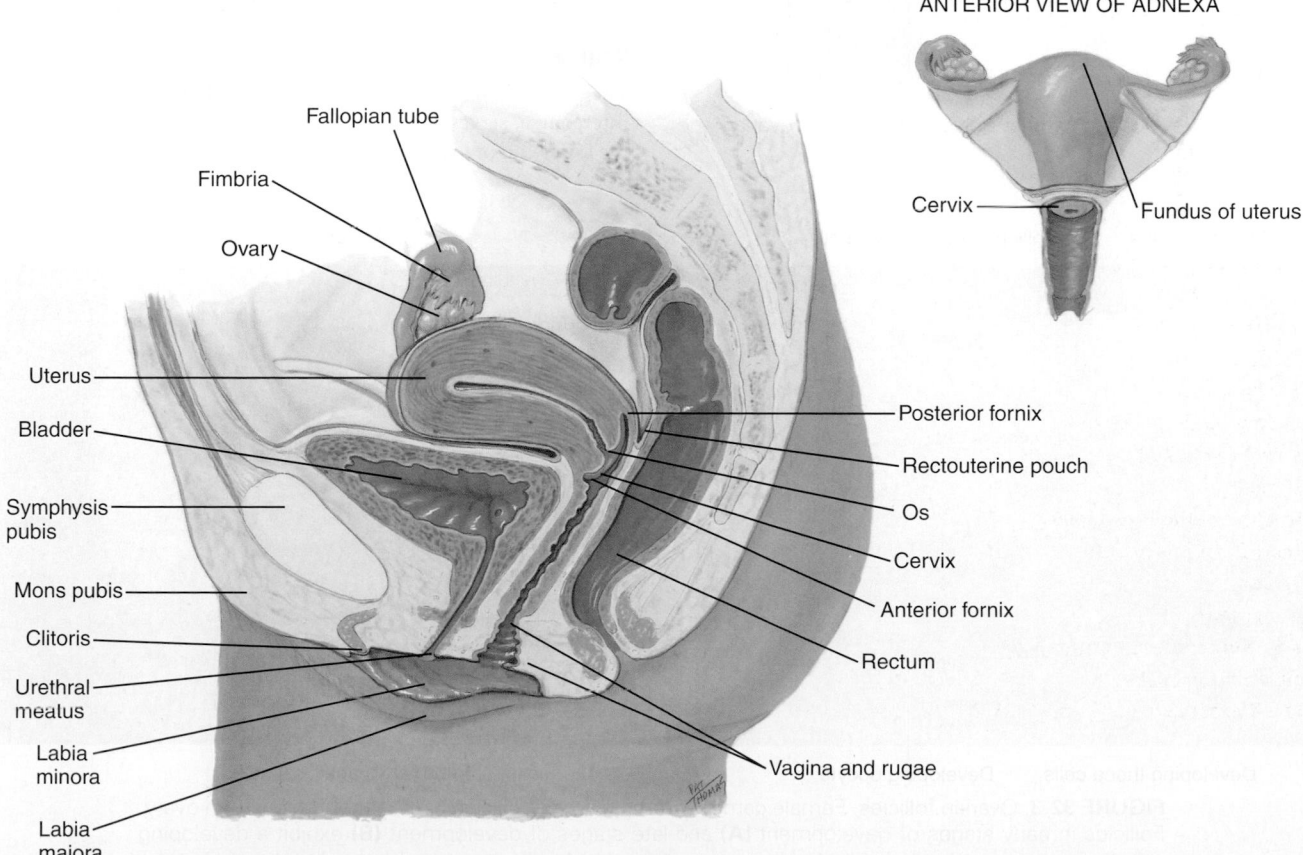

ANTERIOR VIEW OF ADNEXA

FIGURE 32-1 Cross-sectional view of the female genitourinary system. (From Jarvis C: *Physical examination and health assessment,* ed 6, St Louis, 2012, Elsevier, p 728.)

Oviducts

The two **oviducts,** also called the fallopian or uterine tubes, are each about 10 cm long and located in the upper margin of the broad ligament. Each oviduct runs laterally from the uterus to the uterine end of the ovary. The free end of the oviduct adjacent to the ovary is called the *infundibulum.* It is shaped like a funnel with long, fingerlike projections termed *fimbriae.* The ampulla, the longest part of the oviduct, has an inner lining consisting of ciliated mucous membrane arranged in longitudinal folds. Beneath this ciliated lining is a double layer of smooth muscle with a thick outer layer of peritoneal serosa. The oviduct has an active role in propelling the ovum toward the uterus; the current created by the beating cilia and the peristaltic contractions of

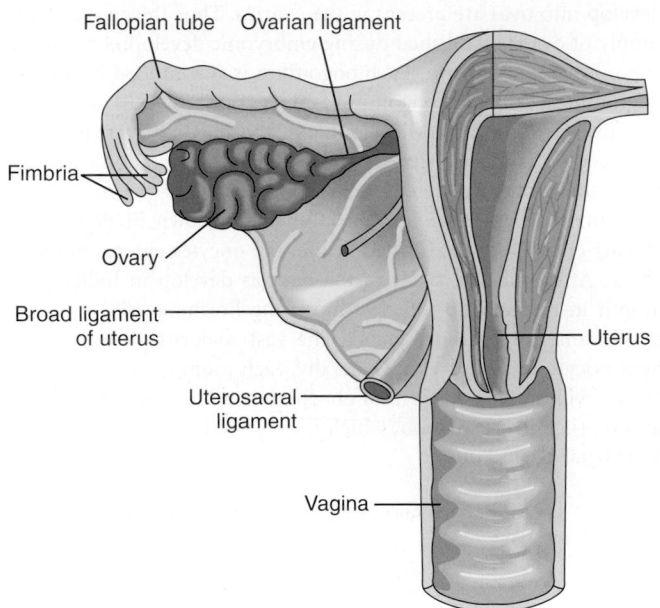

FIGURE 32-2 View of the female pelvis showing the ovarian and uterine ligaments.

the muscular wall are powerful forces that move ova along the oviduct. Once inside the oviduct, the ovum is moved through the ampulla to the isthmus (the short, narrow portion near the uterus) and finally through the intramural passageway to the uterus. Fertilization of the ovum occurs in the upper third of the oviduct, and the **zygote** (fertilized ovum) begins developing as it moves through the oviduct. If no fertilization occurs, the ovum undergoes degeneration in the oviduct.[7]

Uterus

The uterus varies in size, shape, location, and structure during various phases of a woman's life and reproductive status. In the nonpregnant state, the uterus is about 8 cm long, 4 cm wide in its upper part, and 2 cm thick. The rounded part of the uterus, which lies above and in front of the openings of the oviducts, is called the *fundus;* the main portion of the uterus is the *corpus,* or body. The lower, narrow portion of the uterus is the *cervix,* which extends downward to the opening within the vagina. The cervix contains a narrow canal that joins the uterine cavity at the internal os and opens into the vagina at the external os.

The wall of the body and fundus of the uterus consists of three layers: endometrium, myometrium, and serosa (Figure 32-4). The outermost layer of the uterus, the serosa, consists of a single layer of mesothelial cells supported by a thin layer of loose connective tissue. The middle layer, the myometrium, consists of three layers of smooth muscle with the muscle fibers arranged in a different direction in each layer. The innermost lining of the uterus, the **endometrium,** consists of two layers: a thin deep layer called the *basilar layer* and a thick superficial layer referred to as the *functional layer.* During a woman's reproductive years, the endometrium displays a constant cyclic activity of alternate proliferation and sloughing of the functional layer in response to **estrogen** and **progesterone** secretion.[8] These changes will be discussed in more detail in the Menstrual Cycle section.

Vagina

The vagina is the sexual organ that enfolds the penis during sexual intercourse, serves as an exit for discarded endometrium, and forms the lower end of the birth canal. It is located anterior to the rectum and

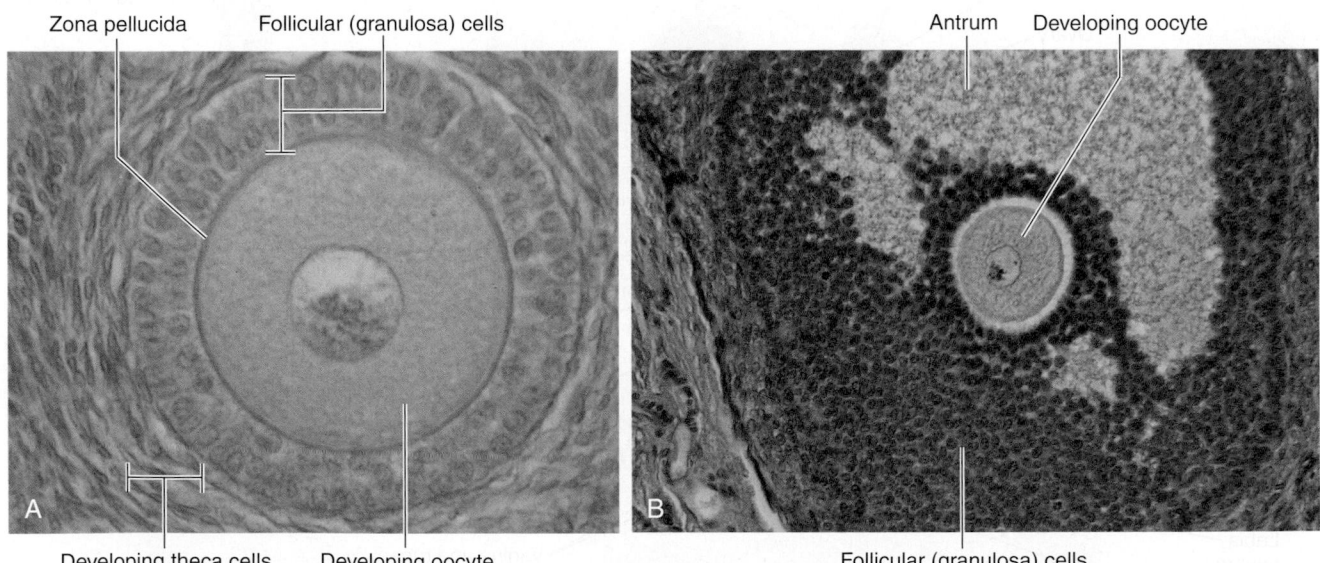

FIGURE 32-3 Ovarian follicles. Female gametes mature within follicles in the outer region of an ovary. Follicles in early stages of development **(A)** and late stages of development **(B)** exhibit a developing oocyte (immature ovum) surrounded by hormone-secreting follicular (granulosa) cells. Notice that the more mature ovarian follicle in **(B)** has a fluid-filled cavity called the antrum. (From Patton KT, Thibodeau GA: *Anatomy & physiology,* ed 8, St Louis, 2013, Elsevier, p 1067.)

posterior to the urethra and urinary bladder. The vagina surrounds the cervix at one end and opens to the vestibule at its other end. The vagina is a highly elastic muscle that is capable of considerable distention. Two longitudinal ridges run along the anterior and posterior walls, with numerous transverse folds called *rugae*. The vagina is lined by a mucous membrane of stratified squamous epithelium overlying a layer of connective tissue.[7] The vaginal wall is subject to thinning with aging; this and other age-related changes in the female sexual organs are described in the Menopause section.

External Genitalia

The external female genital structures include the mons pubis, labia majora, labia minora, clitoris, and vestibule of the vagina (Figure 32-5). The stages of development of the female external genitalia are depicted in Figure 32-6. The mons pubis is a rounded elevation in front of the pubis symphysis. It consists primarily of an accumulation of fat. After puberty, the skin over it is covered by coarse hair. The labia majora, which are

homologous (i.e., corresponding in structure) with the scrotum of the male, are folds of skin that run downward and backward from the mons pubis to the area behind the vaginal opening. After puberty, the labia majora become pigmented and covered with hair. The labia minora are two small folds of skin located between the labia majora on either side of the vaginal opening. The vestibule of the vagina is the cleft between the labia minora and contains the openings of the vagina, the urethra, and the ducts of the greater vestibular glands (also called *Bartholin glands*). These glands, along with the lesser vestibular or Skene glands, secrete mucus to provide lubrication during sexual intercourse.[7]

The clitoris is a body of erectile tissue that projects from the anterior end of the vulva at the anterior junction of the labia minora. It is about 2 cm long and 0.5 cm in diameter and is covered by a fold of tissue called the prepuce, which is formed by the merging of labial tissue. The glans of the clitoris is the rounded elevation on the free end of the body and is highly sensitive to stimulation. During sexual arousal, the erectile tissue of the clitoris becomes engorged with blood.[7,8]

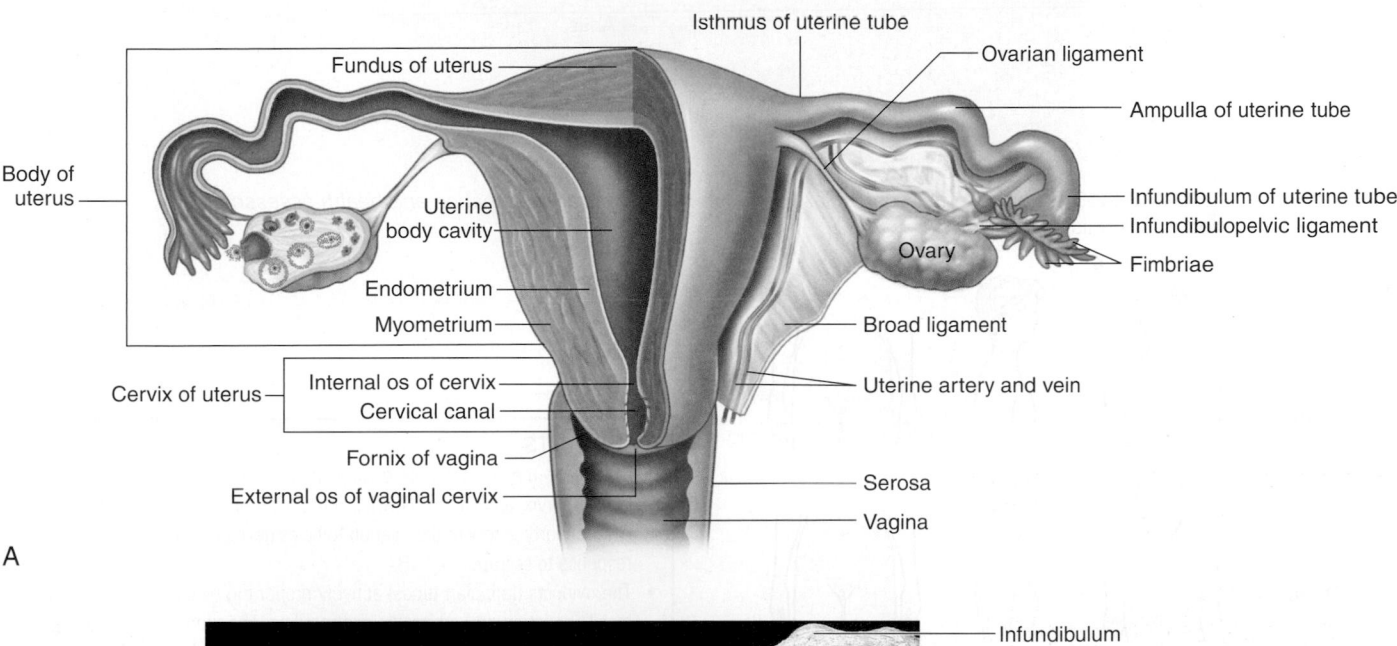

A

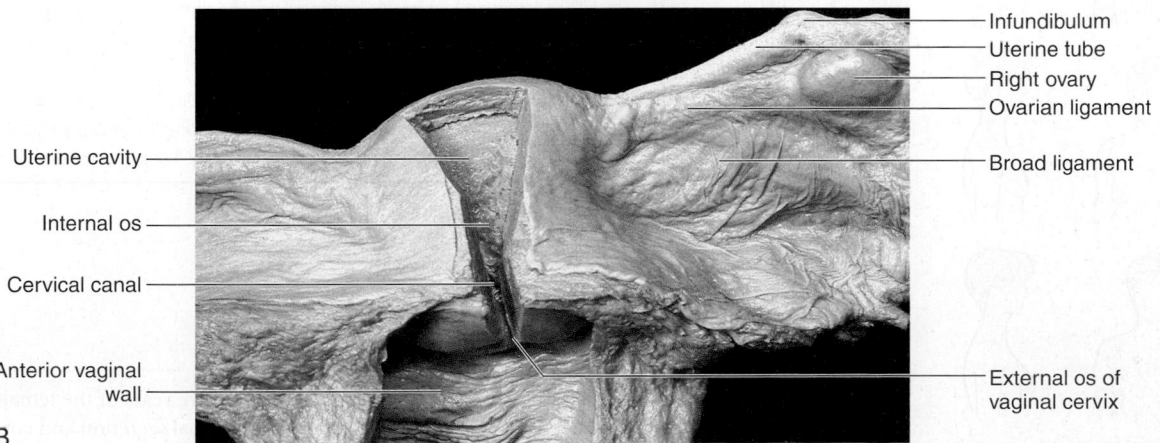

B

FIGURE 32-4 Internal female reproductive organs (posterior view). **A,** Diagram shows left side of uterus and upper portion of the vagina and the left uterine tube and ovary in a frontal section. The broad ligament has been removed from the posterior surface of the uterus and adjacent structures. **B,** Cadaver dissection showing uterine cavity and cervical canal, exposed by removal of parts of their posterior walls. Note that the uterine wall consists of an epithelial lining from which uterine glands extend through the full thickness of the mucosa. Beneath the endometrium, a portion of myometrium is shown. (**A,** From Patton KT, Thibodeau GA: *Anatomy & physiology*, ed 8, St Louis, 2013, Elsevier, p 1066. **B,** From Gosling J et al: *Human anatomy*, ed 4, Philadelphia, 2005, Mosby.)

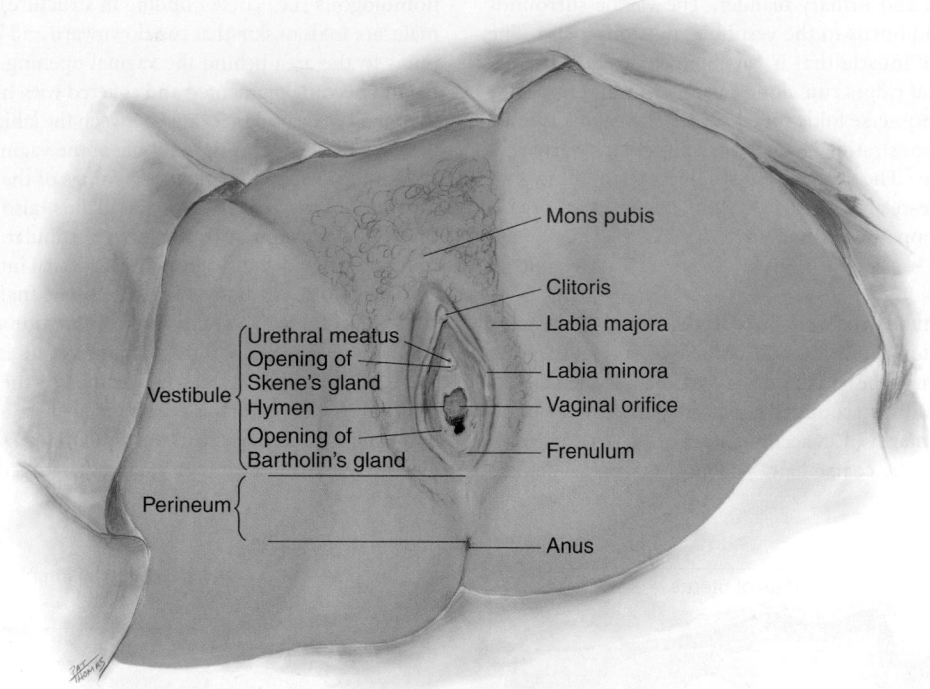

FIGURE 32-5 External female genitalia. (From Jarvis C: *Physical examination and health assessment*, ed 6, St Louis, 2012, Elsevier, p 726.)

Labels in figure:
- Mons pubis
- Clitoris
- Labia majora
- Labia minora
- Vaginal orifice
- Frenulum
- Anus
- Vestibule { Urethral meatus, Opening of Skene's gland, Hymen, Opening of Bartholin's gland
- Perineum

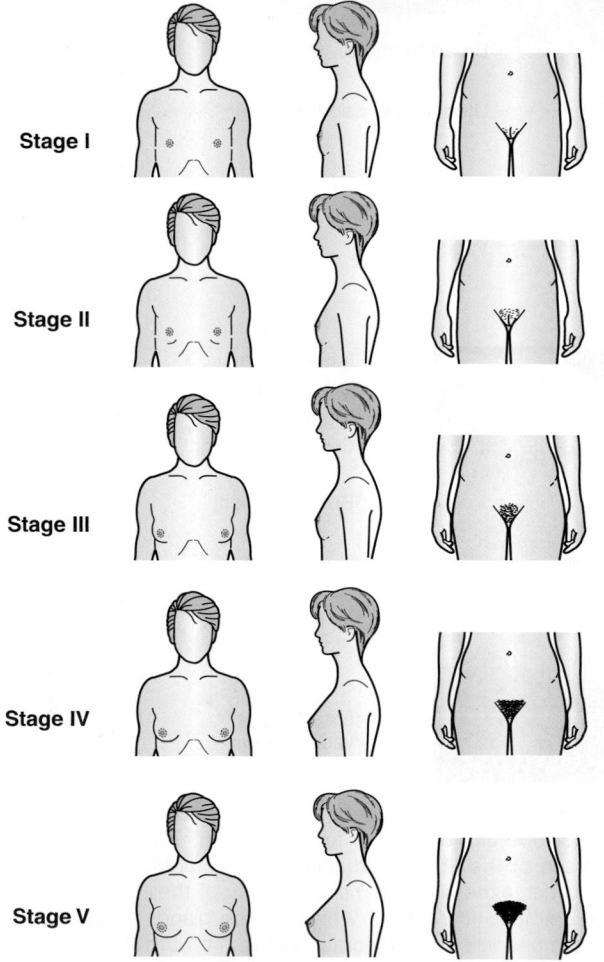

Stage I
Stage II
Stage III
Stage IV
Stage V

FIGURE 32-6 Five tanner stages of sexual maturity ratings (SMRs) in girls.

> **KEY POINTS**
> - Organs of the female reproductive tract include the ovaries, oviducts, uterus, cervix, and vagina. Ovaries contain a lifetime supply of ova at birth. After puberty, a few of the ovarian follicles develop about every 28 days in response to secretion of FSH.
> - The oviducts (fallopian tubes) actively propel the ovum toward the uterus by ciliary action and peristaltic contractions. The uterine lining undergoes a cyclic process of proliferation and then sloughing in response to estrogen and progesterone.
> - External genitalia in the female include the mons pubis, labia majora, labia minora, clitoris, and vestibule of the vagina. The urinary meatus, vaginal opening, and vestibular gland ducts are located in the vaginal vestibule.

MENSTRUAL CYCLE

From **menarche** onward, the normal reproductive years of the female are characterized by rhythmic changes in hormonal secretion and corresponding changes in the sexual organs, which are called the *target organs* of the female hormones. This rhythmic pattern is called the **menstrual cycle** (Figure 32-7). Two significant results of the menstrual cycle are stimulation of the production of an ovum and preparation of the uterine endometrium for the implantation of a fertilized ovum at the appropriate phase of the cycle.[8]

Although considerable variation can be found in human females, an average menstrual cycle is 28 days long, with cycles as short as 20 days or as long as 45 days occurring in normal women. The first day of menstruation is considered the first day of the menstrual cycle. Ovulation occurs approximately 14 days before the next cycle begins; thus in a 28-day cycle, ovulation occurs on about day 14 of the cycle.

The release of hormones and the accompanying response of the female sexual target organs are depicted in Figure 32-7. The principal female reproductive hormones are summarized in Table 32-1. As shown in Figure 32-7, the events of the menstrual cycle require precise synchronization between the activities of the pituitary gland, ovary, and uterus. Beginning at the first day of the menstrual cycle, or the first day of menstruation, these events can be summarized as follows. The thickened functional layer of the endometrium of the uterus is gradually sloughed off, and about 35 ml of blood is lost. During this phase of the menstrual cycle, follicle-stimulating hormone (FSH) is released by the pituitary gland and stimulates a group of follicles to develop in the ovary.

In the preovulatory phase, also called the proliferative phase, theca and granulosa cells in the developing follicles in the ovary secrete estrogen, which stimulates growth of the uterine endometrium once again. At about the midpoint of the cycle, an increase in estrogen secretion from the follicles occurs. This increase in estrogen level is thought to render the anterior pituitary more responsive to luteinizing hormone–releasing hormone secreted by the hypothalamus.[9] The anterior pituitary gland then produces a burst of luteinizing hormone (LH). The FSH level also increases about twofold at the same time, and these two hormones act synergistically to cause the extremely rapid swelling of the follicle that culminates in ovulation.[10] During the process of ovulation, the secondary oocyte is ejected through the wall of the ovary into the peritoneal cavity. The free end of the oviduct is strategically located so that the ovum enters its fimbriated end almost immediately.[7]

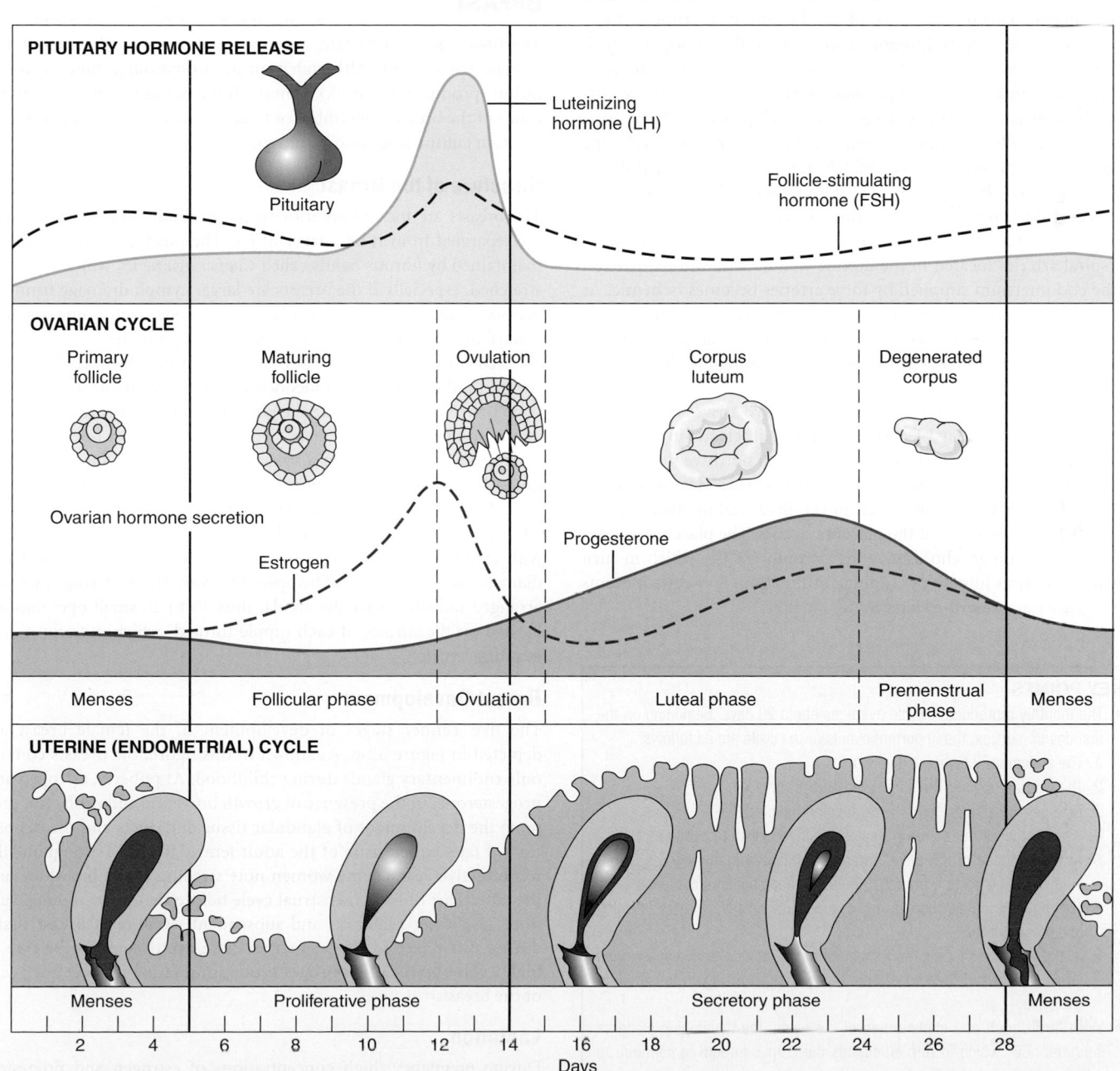

FIGURE 32-7 Menstrual cycle. The events that take place within the pituitary, ovary, and uterus are precisely synchronized. When fertilization does not occur, the cycle repeats itself about every 28 days.

TABLE 32-1 PRINCIPAL FEMALE REPRODUCTIVE HORMONES

HORMONE	TARGET ORGANS	SIGNIFICANT ACTIONS
Estrogen	Multiple sites throughout body, including reproductive structures, bone, fat, and muscle tissues	Development of reproductive organs during puberty Development of secondary sex characteristics, including breast maturation, widening of pelvis, and distribution of fat and muscle tissues in a distinctively female pattern Cyclic preparation of endometrium for implantation of an ovum
Progesterone	Primarily uterus and breasts	Cyclic preparation and maintenance of endometrium for implantation of an ovum Stimulation of development of breast lobes and alveoli
Follicle-stimulating hormone	Ovary	Stimulates ovarian follicle development; with luteinizing hormone, stimulates secretion of estrogen and ovulation
Luteinizing hormone	Ovary	Stimulates final development of ovarian follicle, process of ovulation, and development of corpus luteum

After ovulation, the postovulatory phase (also called the luteal phase) begins. During the luteal phase the site of the ruptured follicle becomes a **corpus luteum** (Latin for "yellow body"), which secretes estrogen and progesterone. These hormones stimulate continued thickening of the uterine endometrium. The cells of the corpus luteum become greatly enlarged and develop lipid, or fatty, areas that give the cells a distinctive yellow color. In a normal cycle, the corpus luteum grows to approximately 1.5 cm, with maximal development attained about 7 to 8 days after ovulation. If pregnancy does not occur, the corpus luteum begins to degenerate, and progesterone and estrogen levels in the blood fall markedly. Constriction of the spiral arteries located in the uterine wall occurs, and the portion of the endometrium supplied by these arteries becomes ischemic. As the cells in the endometrium die, tissue is sloughed off and menstruation begins again. It is presently thought that prostaglandins liberated in the endometrium may have a role in stimulating the sloughing of endometrial tissue.[7,11]

If fertilization of the ovum occurs, the embryo arrives in the uterus on about the fourth day of development. Small glands in the endometrium stimulated by progesterone produce a nutritive fluid for the developing embryo. On approximately the seventh day after fertilization, the embryo implants itself in the thick endometrium of the uterus, and development of the **placenta** occurs. The placenta secretes the hormone human chorionic gonadotropin (hCG), which in turn signals the corpus luteum to continue to function. Subsequent events in pregnancy are described later in this chapter.

KEY POINTS

- The monthly reproductive cycle averages about 28 days. Beginning on the first day of menses, the important events of the cycle are as follows:
  1. The endometrial layer is sloughed.
  2. The ovarian follicles are stimulated by pituitary FSH.
  3. Estrogen is secreted from the developing follicles.
  4. Proliferation of the endometrium occurs in response to estrogen.
  5. At the midpoint of the cycle, a burst of luteinizing hormone and a doubling of FSH secretion from the pituitary gland stimulate ovulation.
  6. The ruptured follicle changes into a corpus luteum and secretes estrogen and progesterone.
  7. In the absence of pregnancy, secretion of estrogen and progesterone drops rapidly and the endometrial lining sloughs off again to complete the cycle.
- With fertilization and implantation of the ovum, the developing placenta secretes hCG, which in turn stimulates the corpus luteum to continue to secrete estrogen and progesterone and thus prevent endometrial sloughing.

BREAST

The breast is an important accessory organ in sexual function and human reproduction. Although its primary physiologic function is **lactation** (production of milk) to nourish the human infant, the significance of the breast as a symbol of feminine sexuality in contemporary Western culture must also be recognized.

Structure of the Breast

The breasts are located anterior to the pectoralis major muscle and are separated from it by a layer of fat. The position of the breasts is maintained by fibrous bands called *Cooper ligaments,* which are easily stretched, especially if the breasts are large. Lymph drainage from the breasts is mainly toward the axillary lymph nodes, with some drainage toward the substernal and diaphragmatic lymph nodes.[12]

Each breast consists of 15 to 20 lobes of glandular epithelial tissue and a ductal system embedded in interstitial tissue and fat. The secretory cells that constitute the glandular epithelium are arranged in grapelike clusters called *alveoli* (Figure 32-8). Ducts or openings from each alveolus unite to form a single duct from each lobe. These main ducts then enlarge slightly into ampullae immediately before opening onto the surface of the nipple. The nipple, located at the center of the adult female breast, is composed of bundles of smooth muscle fibers with erectile properties. The areola that surrounds the nipple has a diameter of 1.5 to 2.5 cm. The openings from the lactiferous ducts are arranged radially under the areola; thus 15 to 20 small openings are located on the surface of each nipple through which milk flows in a lactating female.[7]

Breast Development

The five Tanner stages of development of the female breast are depicted in Figure 32-6. As shown in this figure, the breasts contain only rudimentary glands during childhood. At puberty, estrogen and progesterone, in the presence of growth hormone and prolactin, promote the development of glandular tissue and ducts and the deposition of fat characteristic of the adult female breast. Throughout the reproductive years, some women note swelling of the breast around the latter part of each menstrual cycle before the onset of menstruation. The water retention and subsequent swelling of breast tissue during this phase of the menstrual cycle are thought to be due to high levels of circulating progesterone stimulating the secretory cells of the breast.[12]

Lactation

During pregnancy, high concentrations of estrogen and progesterone produced by the corpus luteum and the placenta stimulate the

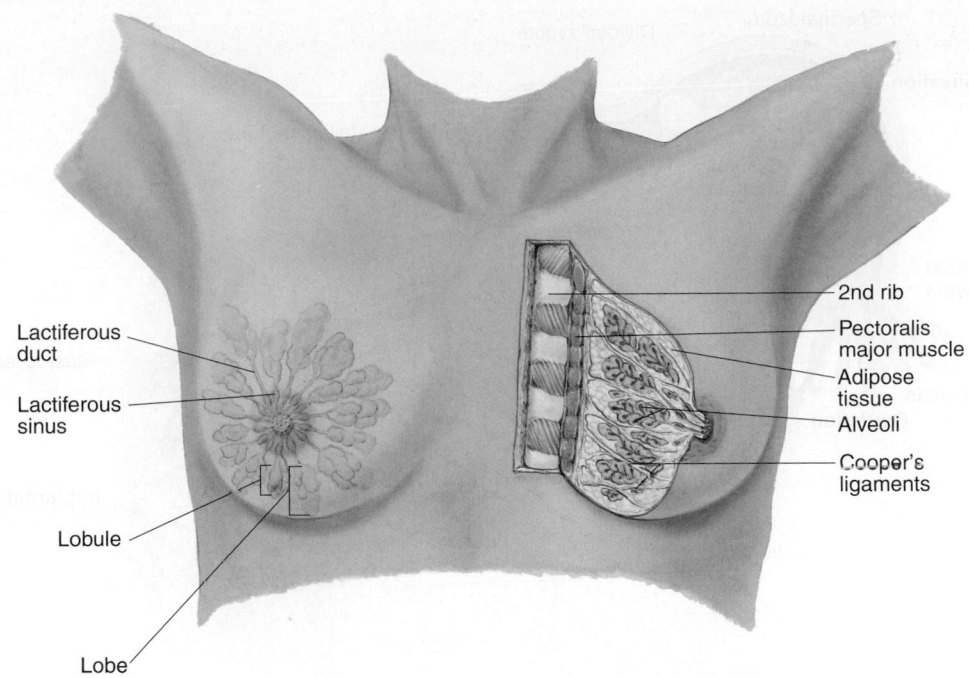

FIGURE 32-8 Mature female breast. (From Jarvis C: *Physical examination and health assessment,* ed 5, St Louis, 2008, Elsevier, p 409.)

development of glands and ducts in the breast. During the first trimester of pregnancy, the ducts proliferate; in the second trimester, the ducts group together to form large lobules with new alveoli formation. In the third trimester, the existing alveoli dilate in preparation for lactation. Toward the end of pregnancy and until 1 to 3 days after childbirth, the mammary glands form colostrum, which contains protein and lactose but little fat. After birth of the infant, the hormone **prolactin** secreted by the mother's anterior pituitary gland stimulates milk production, and milk is produced by the third day after delivery. The initiation and maintenance of lactation are a complex neuroendocrine process involving sensory nerves in the nipples and breast tissue, the spinal cord and hypothalamus, and the pituitary gland. The suckling movements of the infant on the breast stimulate the release of prolactin from the anterior pituitary gland and **oxytocin** from the posterior pituitary gland. These hormones in turn stimulate lactation and ejection of milk from the alveoli into the ducts, where it is accessible to the infant. Oxytocin then promotes the actual release of milk, called the "milk ejection reflex."[7,13]

KEY POINTS
- At puberty, breast development occurs in response to estrogen and progesterone in cooperation with growth hormone and prolactin. During pregnancy, high estrogen and progesterone levels stimulate further development of the mammary glands and ducts.
- Milk production and release are stimulated by the pituitary hormones prolactin and oxytocin in response to suckling.

PREGNANCY

During the 9 months of human gestation, the single-celled zygote gives rise to an infant with a complex set of physiologic systems.

The fertilized ovum contains the entire genetic complement—or encoded genetic instructions—to develop into a fully functioning term infant, given adequate nutrition and time. Three basic developmental processes—growth, **morphogenesis,** and cellular differentiation—are involved in this transformation.[14] Growth denotes the proliferation of new cells by mitosis, a necessary but not sufficient process for development. The arrangement of cells in a particular order is called *morphogenesis* and is essential to the elaboration of higher forms of life. In addition to growth and morphogenesis, cellular differentiation is needed for cells to specialize structurally and biochemically in a myriad of ways. This section describes the sequence of events in which growth, morphogenesis, and cellular differentiation function to transform a human zygote with encoded genetic information into a human infant. In addition, this section will describe the response of the mother's body to pregnancy. Information on genetic control of inheritance and genetic disorders is contained in Chapters 5 and 6, respectively, and the reader may wish to refer to these chapters for specific content in these areas.

Early Human Development

Fertilization of the ovum occurs in the oviduct. Within 24 hours after fertilization, the zygote begins a series of divisions by the process of mitosis; this process is referred to as *cleavage* (Figure 32-9). From a two-cell entity the zygote soon divides multiple times, and its cytoplasm begins to be partitioned into specific cells that will serve as the building blocks of the embryo. As more cleavage takes place, the embryo is transported through the oviduct to the uterus. This process takes about 4 days. The embryo receives nutrition during this time from secretions released by the epithelial cells lining the oviduct. After the embryo enters the uterus, the zona pellucida, the membrane surrounding the embryo, dissolves. About day 4, the embryo arrives in the uterus and floats freely while receiving nutrition from secretions from the endometrial glands stimulated by progesterone.

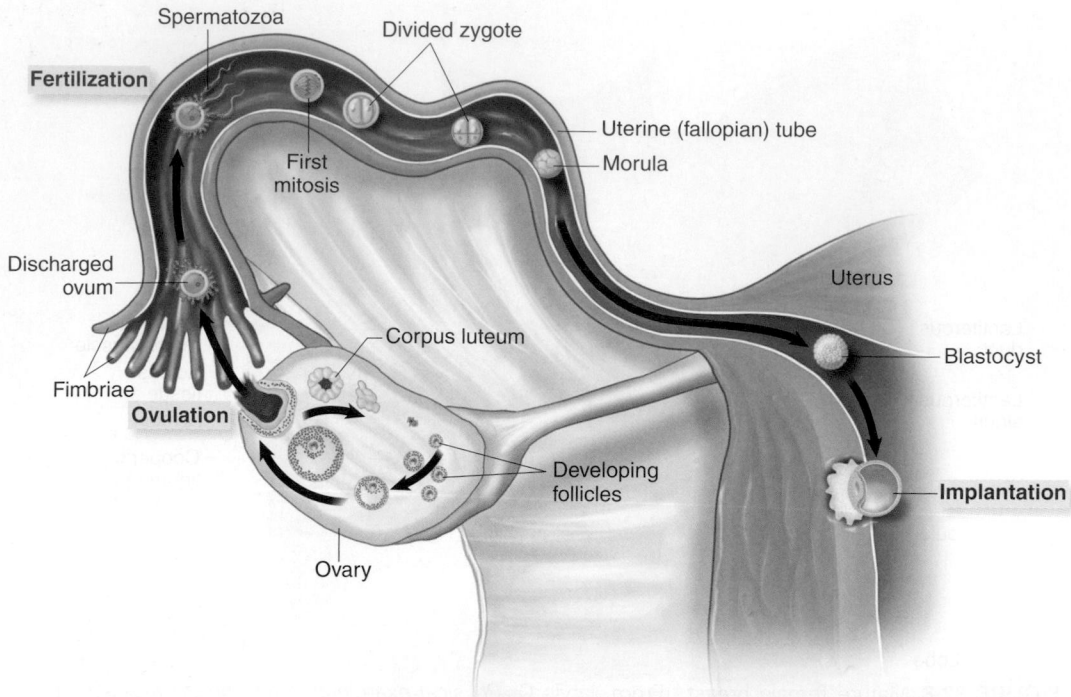

FIGURE 32-9 Early human development. Drawings illustrate cleavage of the zygote and formation of the blastocyst. At ovulation, an ovum is released from the ovary and begins its journey through the uterine tube. While in the tube, the ovum unites with a sperm to form the single-celled zygote. After a few days of rapid mitotic division, a ball of cells called a morula is formed. After the morula develops into a hollow ball called a blastocyst, implantation occurs. (From Patton KT, Thibodeau GA: *Anatomy & physiology*, ed 8, St Louis, 2013, Elsevier, p 1102.)

At this point the cells of the embryo have arranged themselves into a hollow spherical structure called the *blastocyst* (Figure 32-9). The outer cells of the blastocyst, called the *trophoblast,* will ultimately become the protective and nutritive membranes (chorion and placenta) that surround the developing embryo. The inner cell mass, a small cluster of cells that projects into the cavity of the blastocyst, will develop into the structures of the embryo itself. If at this point the inner cell mass divides into two separate groups of cells, identical twins with an identical genetic complement will result. Fraternal twins develop when two ova are fertilized by two sperm cells and do not have an identical genetic complement.[14]

Implantation

On approximately day 7 after fertilization, the embryo attaches to the uterine lining and then implants itself in the endometrium (Figure 32-10). Enzymes secreted by the trophoblast erode a small portion of the uterine lining, and by day 10 of development the embryo has completely penetrated the endometrium. The opening in the uterine lining is closed, initially by a blood clot and then by regeneration of uterine epithelium; all subsequent development of the embryo occurs in the wall of the uterus.[7]

Fetal Membranes and Placenta

Fetal membranes protect the developing embryo or fetus and provide needed substrates for growth and development, particularly oxygen and nutrition. In addition, they serve the purpose of elimination of waste products of metabolism. All terrestrial vertebrates have four fetal

membranes: amnion, yolk sac, chorion, and allantois.[14] In the developing human, the yolk sac is usually thought to be a vestigial structure, although it serves as an important temporary center for the formation of blood cells between the second and sixth weeks. The allantois is also considered vestigial, although its blood supply contributes to formation of the umbilical vessels.

The amnion begins to develop at a very early stage and eventually expands to surround the entire embryo. The space between the amnion and the embryo is called the **amniotic cavity.** It is filled with a clear amniotic fluid that keeps the embryo moist and provides a measure of protection against mechanical injury.

The **placenta** serves two basic functions. It is the organ of exchange between the developing fetus and the mother; it also provides nutrients to the fetus and removes wastes. It is also an endocrine organ and produces several hormones, most notably hCG. The placenta develops from both the chorion and the maternal uterine tissue. After implantation, the chorion develops rapidly and forms highly vascularized villi while the embryonic circulation develops. The umbilical cord develops and connects the embryo with the placenta. Two umbilical arteries arise in the umbilical cord and connect with a rapidly proliferating network of capillaries in the villi. The umbilical vein, also located in the umbilical cord, carries blood from the villi back to the fetus.

The placenta eventually consists of the portion of the chorion in which villi develop, along with the uterine tissue between the villi that contains maternal capillaries and small pools of maternal blood. The placenta brings maternal blood adjacent to fetal blood, although the two circulatory systems are completely separate from each other. Thus

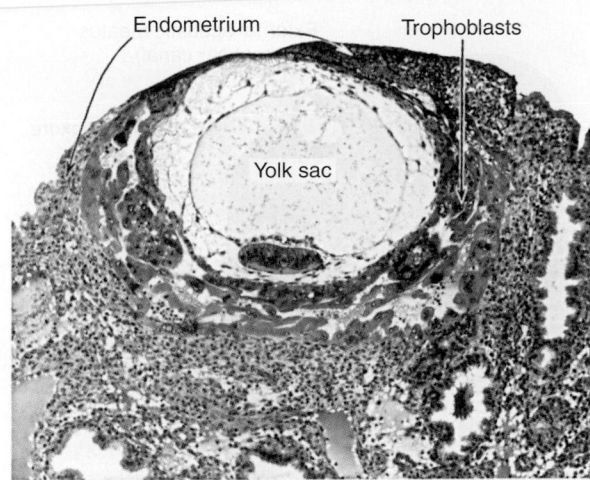

FIGURE 32-10 Implantation of the early human embryo showing trophoblastic digestion and invasion of the endometrium. (From Guyton AC, Hall JE: *Textbook of medical physiology*, ed 12, St Louis, 2010, Elsevier. Courtesy Arthur Hortig, MD.)

TABLE 32-2	SUMMARY OF DEVELOPMENTAL EVENTS IN HUMAN FETAL LIFE
TIME FROM FERTILIZATION	**KEY EVENTS**
36 hours	Embryo has achieved two-cell stage
4 days	Embryo reaches uterus
7 days	Implantation of embryo in uterine wall
2.5 weeks	Differentiation of heart tissue
	Blood cell formation in yolk sac and chorion
	Formation of notochord and neural plate
3.5 weeks	Formation of neural tube
	Heart tubes begin to beat
	Primordial eye and ear visible
	Respiratory system begins development
	Liver bud differentiates
	Blood vessels established
4 weeks	Formation of three primary brain vesicles
	Limb buds appear
2 months	Embryo capable of movement
	Cerebral cortex differentiating
	Gonad identifiable as testis or ovary
	Bones begin ossification and muscles are differentiating
	Major blood vessels in final positions
3 months	Fetus performs breathing and sucking movements
	Gender is clearly identifiable
5 months	Heartbeat is audible with a stethoscope
	Fetus moves freely through amniotic cavity
6-9 months	Rapid growth with final differentiation of tissues and organs
266 days	Birth

oxygen and nutrient substrates pass from the maternal blood through the placental tissue and diffuse into the blood of the fetus, where these substances can be used for growth and development of various body tissues. Waste products of fetal metabolism from fetal blood then pass through the placenta into the maternal blood supply and are eventually transported to the maternal kidneys for disposal.[14]

The placenta, like the corpus luteum, secretes both estrogen and progesterone during pregnancy. These hormones serve a variety of purposes in pregnancy. Estrogen promotes enlargement of the uterus and growth of the ductal structure of the breast, as well as alters the elasticity of various pelvic ligaments and the symphysis pubis to allow passage of the infant through the pelvic structures during delivery. In addition to its role in providing early nutrition for the embryo, progesterone has the special effect of decreasing contractility of the gravid uterus, thus preventing spontaneous abortion. In addition, progesterone may have a role in preparing the breasts for lactation, as described earlier in the Lactation section.

Of major importance in the role of the placenta as an endocrine gland is its production of hCG. From the time of implantation, the trophoblastic cells begin to secrete hCG, which sends a signal to the corpus luteum that a pregnancy has begun. The corpus luteum responds by increasing its size and its secretion of estrogen and progesterone, which then promote continued development of the endometrium and the placenta. In the absence of hCG, the corpus luteum would disintegrate, as it does in a nonfertilized menstrual cycle, and the endometrium would deteriorate and be sloughed off along with the embryo. Thus, hCG is an essential element in continuation of the pregnant state.[14]

Development of the Human Embryo and Fetus

From fertilization to the end of the eighth week, the developing organism is referred to as an *embryo*; from the ninth week until birth, the developing baby is referred to as a *fetus*. Development of the fetus proceeds in an orderly sequence of complex events. With recent developments in fetal physiology, it is possible to predict which structures will begin their development or function on a particular day of development after conception. Table 32-2 depicts some important developmental events from the time of fertilization to birth. Detailed information on the development of organ systems during fetal life is

contained in the chapters in this book that focus on these organ systems; for example, Chapter 35 contains a description of the development of the gastrointestinal tract.

First Month

Rapid growth, morphogenesis, and cell differentiation occur early in development of the human embryo. By 2.5 weeks of development, the notochord and neural plate are formed; these structures eventually give rise to the central nervous system. In addition, the tissue that will form the heart has differentiated. By the end of the first month, an S-shaped heart beats about 60 times per minute, and the three primary vesicles of the brain have formed.

Second Month

Until the sixth week of gestation, the gonads in both genders are *bipotential*, which means that the gonads present in the embryo may become either testes or ovaries. Beginning about the seventh week, the so-called indifferent gonad begins to develop into either a male or a female derivative.[15] Recent research has demonstrated that *SRY* (sex-determining region of the Y chromosome) is the gene that influences the indifferent gonad to organize into a testis.[15] In a genetically female embryo, the gonad organizes into an ovary under the influence of one or more ovary-determining genes, which have not yet been well characterized. The cortex of the gonad accumulates nests of cells that differentiate into ovarian follicles, each containing a primary oocyte.

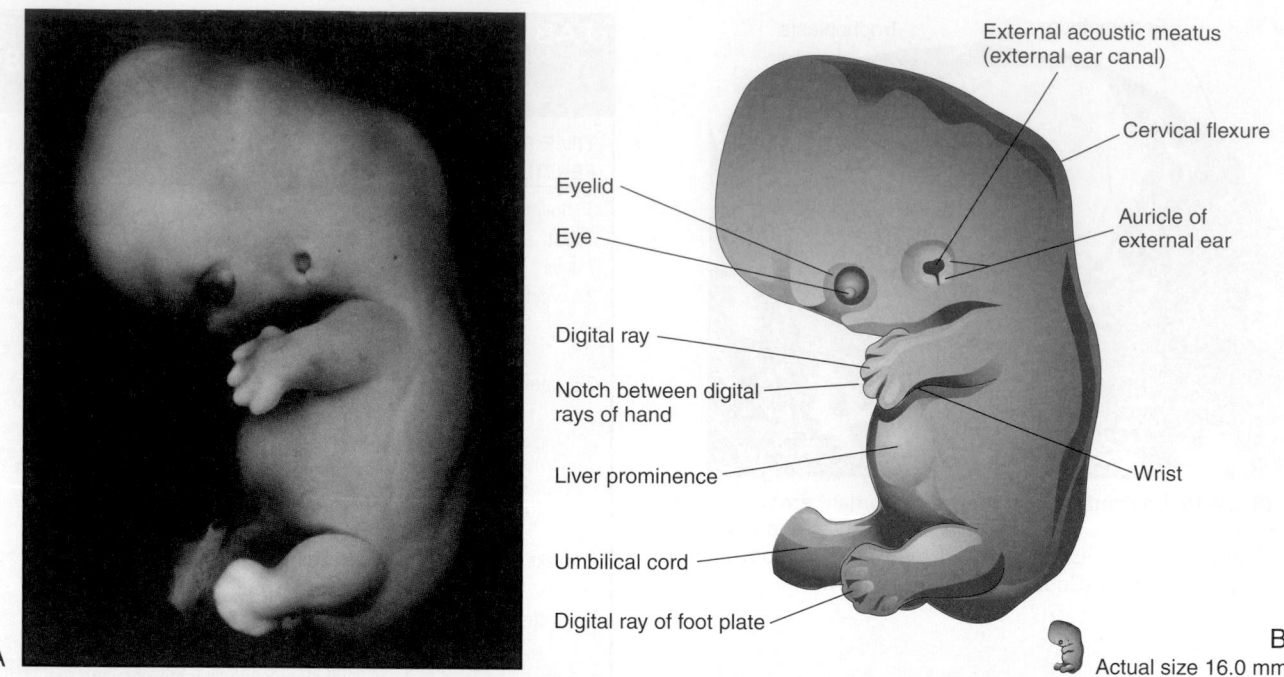

External acoustic meatus (external ear canal)

Cervical flexure

Eyelid

Eye

Auricle of external ear

Digital ray

Notch between digital rays of hand

Liver prominence

Wrist

Umbilical cord

Digital ray of foot plate

A

B

Actual size 16.0 mm

FIGURE 32-11 Human embryo in the seventh week of development. (**A,** From Moore KL et al: *Color atlas of clinical embryology*, ed 2, Philadelphia, 2000, Saunders. **B,** From Moore KL, Persaud TVN, Torchia MG: *The developing human: clinically oriented embryology*, ed 9, Philadelphia, 2013, Saunders, p 85.)

The wolffian ducts, the primordial structures that are precursors to the male internal reproductive organs, begin to disappear, and the müllerian ducts, the structures that will develop into the female internal reproductive organs, become dominant.[16]

The external genitalia of both the male and the female are identical until the eighth week of gestation. Like the gonads, the genitalia are bipotential until this time, with the capability of developing into organs of either gender. In a genetically male embryo, dihydrotestosterone, a metabolite of testosterone, binds to androgen receptors in the external genitalia and effects the differentiation of these structures into the male external genitalia. Without the influence of dihydrotestosterone, the bipotential external genitalia will spontaneously develop into female external genitalia.[15]

Figure 32-11 shows an embryo on day 49. All of the organs continue to develop during the second month, and the embryo becomes capable of movement. The major blood vessels assume their final positions, and the heart assumes its final shape. The brain begins to transmit impulses to regulate function of the organ systems, and a few reflexes are now present. At the end of the second month, the rudiments of all organs are present and the embryo is referred to as a *fetus*.[7]

Third Month

During the third month, the ears and eyes approach their final positions, and some of the bones become distinct. The fetus performs breathing movements consisting of moving amniotic fluid in and out of the lungs and can carry on sucking movements. By the end of the third month, the fetus is almost 56 mm in length and weighs about 14 g (Figure 32-12).

Second Trimester

A *trimester* refers to a period of 3 months during pregnancy. During the second trimester, or months 4 to 6 of development, the fetus achieves independent mobility and can move freely through the amniotic cavity. The heartbeat of the fetus is now audible through a stethoscope and averages 150 beats per minute. By the fifth month of development, the fetus measures 250 mm (10 inches) in length, which is half its total length at birth.[14] Figure 32-13 shows a fetus in the second trimester at 4 months of development.

Third Trimester

By far the greatest growth of the fetus occurs during the third trimester. The weight of the fetus almost doubles during the last 2 months.[12] In addition, final differentiation of tissues and organs takes place. Survival of infants born prematurely during this time has increased markedly in the past few years because of an enhanced ability to sustain vital functions such as respiration and regulation of body temperature in neonatal intensive care settings.

Parturition

Parturition refers to the process by which the infant is born. Toward the end of pregnancy, the uterus becomes progressively more excitable until it begins strong rhythmic contractions that ultimately expel the infant.[10] At the present time, the exact cause of the increased uterine activity remains unknown. However, two sets of effects have been suggested as contributing to the increased excitability of uterine musculature at this time: progressive hormonal changes and progressive mechanical changes.[12,17]

Hormonal Changes

During the latter part of pregnancy, large amounts of estrogen, which has a definite tendency to increase uterine contractility, are secreted. Concurrent with this enhanced estrogen release, the secretion of progesterone, which inhibits uterine contractility, remains constant or may decrease slightly. Thus it is hypothesized that the increased ratio of estrogen to progesterone secretion in the latter part of pregnancy may promote the increased contractility of the uterus.[12]

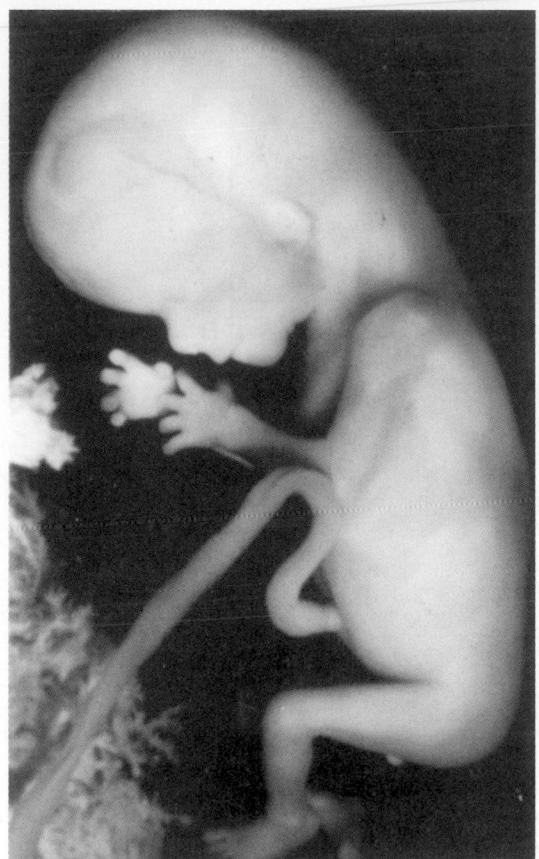

FIGURE 32-12 Photograph of the human fetus at 11 weeks of development. (From Moore KL, Persaud TVN, Torchia MG: *The developing human: clinically oriented embryology*, ed 9, Philadelphia, 2013, Saunders, p 97. Courtesy Professor Jean Hay [Retired], Department of Anatomy, University of Manitoba, Winnipeg, Canada.)

Oxytocin is a hormone secreted by the posterior pituitary gland that specifically causes uterine contraction and is thought to have a major role in promoting increased uterine contractility during parturition. The rate of oxytocin secretion is considerably increased at the time of labor (see the following discussion of Mechanical Changes), and the uterus displays increased responsiveness to a given dose of oxytocin at this time.[12,17]

Mechanical Changes

Stretching smooth muscle organs increases their contractility; in addition, intermittent stretching of smooth muscle can elicit contraction. Thus it is hypothesized that the stretch or irritation of the fetal head against the cervix begins a reflex action that causes the uterus to contract. As the cycle of stretching and contraction is repeated again and again, increased contractions result. In addition, stretching of the cervix causes the release of oxytocin from the posterior pituitary. Oxytocin then stimulates additional uterine contractions, thus initiating another positive feedback cycle of stretching and contraction.[17-19]

Response of the Mother's Body to Pregnancy

The presence of a developing fetus in the uterus creates an extra physiologic load for the pregnant woman, with resulting effects on her basal metabolism and specific organ systems. Normal physiologic responses

to pregnancy are described here; complications of pregnancy are discussed in Chapter 33.

Metabolism During Pregnancy

As a result of increased secretion of many hormones, including thyroxine, adrenocortical hormones, and the sex hormones, the basal metabolic rate increases by about 15% during the latter half of pregnancy.[12] This increase in metabolism results in alterations in many organ systems, including the circulatory, respiratory, and urinary systems.

Changes in the Female Reproductive Organs

The hormones secreted during pregnancy, either by the placenta or by the endocrine glands, directly promote alterations in body structures. In particular, the organs of the female reproductive tract increase markedly in size, with the uterus increasing from 30 to 1100 g and the breasts approximately doubling in size. Concurrently, the vagina enlarges with a widening of the vaginal introitus.

Changes in the Circulatory System

In the latter stages of pregnancy, about 625 ml of blood flows through the maternal circulation of the placenta each minute. This factor, along with a general increase in metabolism, causes an increase in maternal cardiac output to 30% to 40% above normal by week 27 of pregnancy. However, for reasons not understood at the present time, cardiac output decreases to a little above normal during the last 8 weeks of pregnancy, although the high uterine blood flow continues.[12] As shown in Figure 32-14, an increase in maternal blood volume occurs mainly during the latter half of pregnancy. This increase is mainly due to hormonal factors. Both aldosterone and estrogens, which are greatly increased in pregnancy, promote increased fluid retention by the kidneys. In addition, bone marrow increases its activity to produce an excess of red blood cells to accompany the excess vascular volume. At the time of parturition, the mother has an additional 1 to 2 extra liters of blood in her circulatory system.[12]

Changes in the Respiratory System

The increased basal metabolic rate and size of the pregnant woman result in an increase in oxygen utilization, with utilization of oxygen being 20% above normal at the time of birth. Concurrently, a commensurate amount of carbon dioxide is formed. In addition, the growing uterus is pressing upward against the abdominal organs, which in turn press against the diaphragm and cause a decrease in diaphragmatic excursion. The net result of these changes is an increase in minute ventilation of approximately 50% and a decrease in arterial P_{CO_2} to slightly below normal.[12]

Changes in the Urinary System

Because of an increased load of excretory products, the rate of urine formation in pregnancy is usually slightly increased. In addition, other alterations in urinary function occur. Renal tubule reabsorption of sodium, chloride, and water is increased as a result of increased production of steroidal hormones by the placenta and adrenal cortex. Concurrently, the glomerular filtration rate often increases by as much as 50%, a change that serves to increase the rate of water and electrolyte loss in the urine. These two events tend to balance each other out, with the result that only a moderate excess of water and salt accumulation occurs under normal circumstances.[10] However, in the condition of toxemia of pregnancy, excess water and salt accumulation may occur with life-threatening consequences.

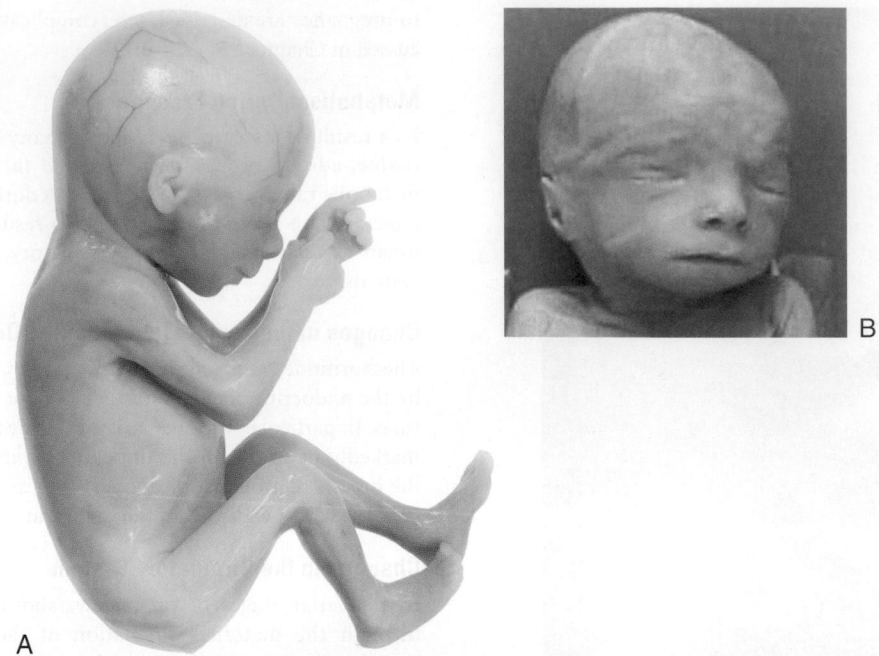

A

B

FIGURE 32-13 A, Side view of human fetus at 17 weeks. **B,** Frontal view of 17-week fetus. (**A,** From Moore KL et al: *Color atlas of clinical embryology*, ed 2, Philadelphia, 2000, Saunders. **B,** Courtesy Dr. Robert Jordan, St. Georges University Medical School, Grenada.)

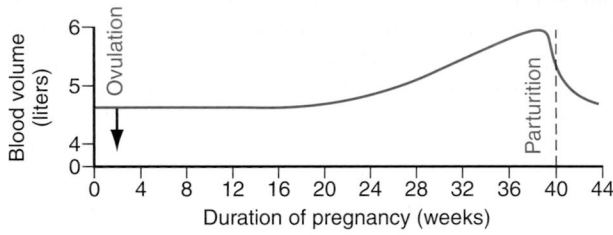

FIGURE 32-14 Effect of pregnancy on the mother's blood volume. (From Guyton AC, Hall JE: *Textbook of medical physiology*, ed 12, St Louis, 2011, Elsevier.)

Weight Gain and Nutrition During Pregnancy

The average weight gain during pregnancy is about 24 lb, with most of this gain occurring during the last two trimesters. Approximately 7 lb of this weight gain is the fetus; 4 lb of the increased weight is amniotic fluid, placenta, and fetal membranes; 2 lb represents an increase in uterine tissue; and another 2 lb of the weight gain is an increase in breast tissue. Thus an average 9-lb increase in weight occurs in the remainder of the woman's body. Approximately 6 lb of fluid may be excreted during the days following birth, after loss of the fluid-retaining hormones of the placenta.[12]

Appetite may be greatly increased during the latter part of pregnancy, in part because of fetal removal of food substrates from the mother's blood and partly because of hormonal factors. The developing fetus assumes priority in regard to many of the nutritional substrates of the mother's body fluids and will continue to grow even when maternal nutrition is inadequate. However, although fetal length may increase normally in the absence of adequate maternal nutrition, fetal weight will be considerably decreased, and abnormal

bone formation and decreased size of many bodily organs of the fetus may result.[12]

If the intake of nutritional elements during pregnancy is inadequate, a number of deficiencies can be present in the mother. In particular, deficiencies of calcium, phosphates, iron, and vitamins may be present. As an example, approximately 375 mg of iron is needed by the fetus to form its blood, and an additional 600 mg is needed by the mother to form her own extra blood supply. Because the normal store of nonhemoglobin iron in the mother at the beginning of pregnancy is often about 100 mg and seldom greater than 700 mg, anemia will develop in a pregnant woman without sufficient iron intake in her food.[12] Important also is adequate folic acid intake, which has been shown to help prevent neural tube defects.[20,21]

KEY POINTS

- At about the seventh day after fertilization, the embryo attaches to the uterine lining. The placenta is the fetal lifeline that provides nutrients and oxygen and eliminates wastes. The placenta also secretes hCG, which is important in maintaining pregnancy.
- Normal gestation is about 9 months. Each 3-month period is called a trimester. By the end of the first trimester, fetal structures and organ systems are present. During the second and third trimesters, the fetus grows in size and weight.
- Near the end of the third trimester, an increase in estrogen production and mechanical stretching of the uterus and cervix are thought to induce parturition. Cervical stretching stimulates the release of oxytocin from the pituitary gland. Oxytocin stimulates uterine contractions.
- Pregnancy is associated with many physiologic changes, including an increased basal metabolic rate (15%), increased cardiac output (30% to 40%) and blood volume (1 to 2 L), increased oxygen consumption (20%) and minute ventilation (50%), increased glomerular filtration rate and tubular reabsorption of sodium and water, and increased body weight (24 lb).

MENOPAUSE

Although **menopause** is defined specifically as the last menstrual period in a woman's reproductive life, the term is often used to denote the entire period of years before and after this event in which the function of the ovaries is in transition. The terms *climacteric* and *perimenopause* are used in the health care literature to describe this transitional period. At about 45 to 52 years of age the supply of ovarian follicles declines, with the majority becoming atretic or degenerated. With the depletion of ovarian follicles, secretion of estrogen and progesterone by the ovaries declines, and the menstrual cycle becomes irregular. When too little estrogen is secreted to cause endometrial growth, menstrual periods stop permanently.[12]

The decline in ovarian hormone production that occurs in the perimenopausal period causes important physiologic changes in a woman's body. The decline in plasma estrogen levels may result in a number of distressing symptoms, although some women experience no symptoms during this time. Hot flashes, described by women as an unpleasant sensation of sudden warmth sweeping upward over the abdomen, chest, neck, and face, are experienced by nearly 75% of postmenopausal women. Although the precise cause of hot flushes is unknown, it is thought that decreased estrogen levels have an effect on the temperature-regulating center in the hypothalamus. Hot flushes are often accompanied by other symptoms of autonomic nervous system instability such as tachycardia, palpitations, and feelings of faintness. Other distressing symptoms, including pain and stiffness in the joints, sleep pattern disturbances, and changes in gastrointestinal function, have been noted by women in the perimenopausal period. These symptoms are presently the focus of many nursing research projects examining the health of aging women. Although such psychological symptoms as increased nervousness have been reported in the medical literature as being related to hormonal imbalance in menopause, it has been established that psychological symptoms are not directly related to estrogen deficiency.[22] There is an increasing awareness of the importance of role of culture and other social factors in the understanding of how women view and experience menopause.[23]

With the decline in estrogen level associated with perimenopause, many structural changes occur in various organs. These changes are summarized in Geriatric Considerations: Changes in the Female Reproductive System. The epidermis of the skin becomes thinner and less elastic throughout the entire body. The breasts may decrease in size; the labia may also lose their underlying fat and become thinner.[24] The vaginal epithelium may become thin and atrophied, with the result that sexual intercourse may be painful. The decline in estrogen level also leads to osteoporosis and decreased bone density, particularly in white women, with resulting bone fractures. Exercise and supplemental calcium and vitamin D are recommended for postmenopausal women to prevent accelerated bone loss.[25] At present, most authorities recommend estrogen therapy during the perimenopausal period only to prevent and relieve symptoms such as hot flashes and vaginal atrophy.[26] This is due to strong evidence showing that supplemental estrogen and progestin therapy has been associated with an increased risk of breast cancer and cardiovascular disease.[27,28] Newer treatments that have been developed for

GERIATRIC CONSIDERATIONS

Changes in the Female Reproductive System

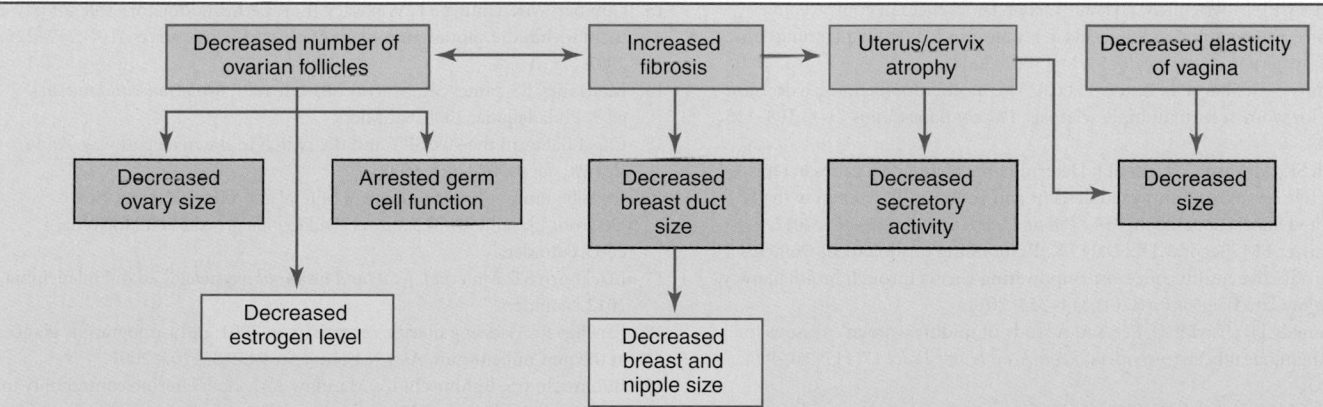

Female reproductive system function declines with organ-specific tissue changes. The number of active female germ cells declines over time with variable function before they are arrested in menopause. The ovaries become smaller and increasingly fibrotic and have fewer ovarian follicles.

The secretion of estrogen by the ovaries stops at menopause, resulting in a marked estrogen level decrease. The ovarian follicles become insensitive to gonadotropins (FSH and luteinizing hormone). However, the peripheral conversion of androgens to estrogen causes a small maintenance level of estrogen to persist at 10% to 30% of previous levels. The androgen-producing ovarian cells (hilar and thecal) continue to secrete testosterone in postmenopausal women.

The follicles, uterus, and cervix undergo atrophy with a decrease in size and secretory action. The vagina is reduced in size with a loss of elasticity and atrophy of the vaginal epithelium. The vascular supply to the vaginal walls decreases with reduced amounts of glycogen and mucopolysaccharide. The pH of Bartholin gland secretions is increased (i.e., more alkaline) because of the loss of estrogen.

The breasts decrease in size. Breast ducts become smaller and are replaced by fat tissue. Some fibrosis and calcification may occur within the ducts. The nipples are smaller with less nipple pigmentation. The aging female nipple may be normal or retracted.

osteoporosis include bisphosphonates, calcitonin nasal spray, and raloxifene.[29,30] Work continues on the development of selective estrogen receptor modulators that may retain some of the beneficial effects of estrogen while avoiding the negative effects.[31] Women in perimenopause may wish to discuss the risks and potential benefits of hormone replacement therapy and other menopausal therapies with their health care providers before making an informed decision about these medications.

> **KEY POINTS**
> - Menopause begins at 45 to 52 years of age and denotes the cessation of menstruation. A declining supply of ovarian follicles with decreased estrogen and progesterone production results in irregular menses and then complete cessation of menstruation.
> - Declines in estrogen production are associated with hot flushes, tachycardia, palpitations, faintness, joint pain, and sleep disturbances. Structural changes associated with menopause include osteoporosis, thinning of the skin, and atrophy of the vaginal structures and breast tissue.

SUMMARY

This chapter has described the major processes related to the human female reproductive tract, including the menstrual cycle, pregnancy, lactation, and menopause. In approaching this material, the reader must view the information presented within the current context of social change in which women are taking an active role in meeting their health care needs. In addition, recent research in the area of reproductive endocrinology has yielded a rapidly expanding understanding of the reproductive structures and their function.

The female reproductive structures are a complex set of organs with multiple, integrated functions. Careful review of the section on reproductive structures, including their embryologic development, will assist the reader in understanding the various alterations in these structures that occur throughout a woman's life. Although the hormonal and structural changes occurring in the female reproductive organs may at first seem overwhelmingly complex to the student, some

basic concepts will help in organizing this material. First, the menstrual cycle has two significant results: production of an ovum and preparation of the uterus for implantation of the fertilized ovum. Second, the fertilized ovum contains the entire encoded genetic instructions to produce a unique human individual. Third, pregnancy consists of three basic developmental processes—growth, morphogenesis, and cellular differentiation—to bring about this transformation, which will also result in multiple changes in the body of the mother. The breast, with its function of lactation, is also a component of the reproductive system and is subject to alterations throughout a woman's life span. Finally, menopause is not a discrete event but rather a process during which the supply of ovarian follicles declines. A review of these concepts will prepare the student for a better understanding of women's health concerns and provide a basis for approaching the next chapter, which considers alterations in reproductive functioning.

REFERENCES

1. Heavey EJ, Moysich KB, Hyland A, et al: Differences in contraceptive choice among female adolescents at a state-funded family planning clinic, *J Midwifery Womens Health* 53(1):45–52, 2008.
2. Prunty MC, Sharpe L, Butow P, et al: The motherhood choice: a decision aid for women with multiple sclerosis, *Patient Educ Couns* 71(1):108–115, 2008.
3. Hall SK, Moreau C, Trussell J: Determinants of and disparities in reproductive service use among adolescent and young adult women in the United States, 2002-2008, *Am J Public Health* 102(2):359–367, 2012.
4. Banister EM, Begoray DL, Daly LK: Responding to adolescent women's reproductive health concerns: empowering clients through health literacy, *Health Care Women Int* 32(4):344–354, 2011.
5. Kennedy HP, Taylor D, Lee KA: A study of midlife women's reasons for changing healthcare providers, *J Am Acad Nurse Pract* 17(11):480–486, 2005.
6. Sokalska A, Valentin L: Changes in ultrasound morphology of the uterus and ovaries during the menopausal transition and early postmenopause: a 4-year longitudinal study, *Ultrasound Obstet Gynecol* 31(2):210–217, 2008.
7. Solomon EP: *Introduction to human anatomy and physiology*, ed 3, Philadelphia, 2008, Saunders.
8. Hacker NF, Gambone JC, Hobel CJ: *Essentials of obstetrics and gynecology*, ed 5, Philadelphia, 2009, Saunders.
9. Apter D: Development of the hypothalamic-pituitary-ovarian axis, *Ann N Y Acad Sci* 17(816):9–21, 1997.
10. Barrett KE, Barman SM, Boitano S, Brooks H: *Ganong's review of medical physiology*, ed 23, New York, 2005, McGraw-Hill.
11. Genazzani AR, et al: Neuroendocrinology of the menstrual cycle, *Ann N Y Acad Sci* 17(816):143–150, 1997.
12. Hall JE: *Guyton and Hall textbook of medical physiology*, ed 12, Philadelphia, 2010, Saunders.
13. Cumbers MR, Chung ST, Wakerley JB: A neuromodulatory role for oxytocin within the supramammillary nucleus, *Neuropeptides* 41(4):217–226, 2007.
14. McKinney ES, James SR, Murray SS, Ashwill J: *Maternal-child nursing*, ed 3, Philadelphia, 2008, Saunders.
15. Capel B: Sex in the 90s: SRY and the switch to the male pathway, *Annu Rev Physiol* 69:497–523, 1998.
16. Josso N: Embryology and control of fetal sex differentiation. In DeGroot LJ, Jameson JL, editors: *Endocrinology*, ed 5, Philadelphia, 2005, Saunders.
17. Blackburn ST: *Maternal, fetal, and neonatal physiology*, ed 4, Philadelphia, 2012, Saunders.
18. Fanchin R: Assessing uterine receptivity in 2001: ultrasonographic glances at the new millennium, *Ann N Y Acad Sci* 943:185–202, 2001.
19. Buhimschi CS, Buhimschi IA, Manilow AM, et al: Uterine contractility in women whose fetus is delivered in the occipitoposterior position, *Am J Obstet Gynecol* 188(3):734–739, 2003.
20. Green NS: Folic acid supplementation and prevention of birth defects, *J Nutr* 132(8 suppl):23565–23605, 2002.
21. Hermoso M, Vollhardt C, Bergmann K, Koletzko B: Critical micronutrients in pregnancy, lactation, and infancy: considerations on vitamin D, folic acid, and iron, and priorities for future research, *Ann Nutr Metab* 59(1):5–9, 2011.
22. Nelson HD: Menopause, *Lancet* 371(9614):760–770, 2008.
23. Hall L, Callister LC, Berry JA, et al: Meanings of menopause: cultural influences on perception and management of menopause, *J Holist Nurs* 25(2):106–118, 2008.
24. Farage M, Maibach H: Lifetime changes in the vulva and vagina, *Arch Gynecol Obstet* 273(4):195–202, 2006.

25. North American Menopause Society: Management of osteoporosis in postmenopausal women: 2010 position statement of the North American Menopause Society, *Menopause* 17(1):25–54, 2010.

26. North American Menopause Society: Estrogen and progesterone use in postmenopausal women: 2010 position statement of the North American Menopause Society, *Menopause* 17(2):242–255, 2010.

27. Writing Group for the Women's Health Initiative Investigators: Risks and benefits of estrogen plus progestin in healthy postmenopausal women: principal results from the Women's Health Initiative randomized controlled trial, *JAMA* 288:321–333, 2002.

28. North American Menopause Society: Estrogen and progestogen use in peri- and post-menopausal women: March 2007 position statement of the North American Menopause Society, *Menopause* 14(2):168–182, 2007.

29. National Osteoporosis Foundation: *Clinician's guide to prevention and treatment of osteoporosis*, Washington, DC, 2010, Author.

30. Johnell O, et al: Additive effects of raloxifene and alendronate on bone density and biochemical markers of bone remodeling in postmenopausal women with osteoporosis, *J Clin Endocrinol Metab* 87:985–992, 2002.

31. Riggs BL, Hartmann LC: Selective estrogen-receptor modulators: mechanisms of action and application to clinical practice, *New Engl J Med* 348:618–629, 2003.

Alterations in Female Genital and Reproductive Function

Rosemary A. Jadack

evolve WEBSITE

http://evolve.elsevier.com/Copstead/
- Review Questions and Answers
- Glossary (with audio pronunciations for selected terms)
- Animations
- Case Studies
- Key Points Review

KEY QUESTIONS

- What are the differentiating factors of the common menstrual disorders?
- What are the common etiologic factors leading to uterine prolapse, uterine retrodisplacement, cystocele, and rectocele?
- How can the pain of endometriosis be differentiated from that of dysmenorrhea?
- What is the rationale for routine Papanicolaou testing for cervical cancer?
- What factors contribute to the high mortality rate of ovarian cancer?
- What clinical findings would indicate the development of pregnancy-induced hypertension, placenta previa, and abruptio placentae in a pregnant woman?
- How can benign and malignant breast lumps be clinically differentiated?

CHAPTER OUTLINE

The complex functioning of the female reproductive system described in Chapter 32 may be subject to alterations in structure and function throughout a woman's life that can have far-reaching effects on her health and well-being. This chapter is a survey of these alterations and describes the pathophysiologic basis of the most common disorders of the female reproductive system. In addition, current therapeutics for these alterations, including pharmacologic therapy, will be summarized. The information presented here is an introduction to these complex areas, and the reader may wish to consult in-depth gynecology and obstetrics texts for more detailed information.

Perhaps no other function of the human body is so closely linked to psychological, social, and spiritual concerns as reproductive function. Any alteration in reproductive status (or the perceived threat of such an alteration) may have profound effects on an individual. Clinicians caring for women experiencing alterations in functioning of the reproductive system should bear in mind the profundity of such alterations for the individual woman and must also maintain an awareness of the context in which women seek help for such problems. A clinical approach in which information is freely shared between caregiver and client and in which mutual decision making is an integral part of the therapeutic environment is a necessary component of care for women seeking help for reproductive concerns. Previous clinical approaches in which women's concerns were labeled as unimportant or merely psychogenic often resulted in anger, frustration with health

care providers, and withdrawal from the health care delivery system. Women consumers of health care are now seeking active involvement in their own care, and clinicians who care for women experiencing the alterations described in this chapter need to approach women's health concerns with sensitivity and openness.

MENSTRUAL DISORDERS

Alterations in the normal functioning of the menstrual cycle include amenorrhea (no menses), abnormal uterine bleeding patterns, and dysmenorrhea (painful menstruation). Although many pathologic conditions can cause these alterations, an obvious cause is often not found.

Amenorrhea

Etiology and pathogenesis. **Amenorrhea** is the absence or suppression of menstruation in a female age 16 years or older; it occurs if a woman misses three or more consecutive periods. Amenorrhea is categorized as either primary or secondary. Primary amenorrhea is the failure to begin menses by the age of 16 years. Secondary amenorrhea is the cessation of established, regular menstruation for 6 months or longer. Figure 33-1 shows causes of primary and secondary amenorrhea.

Amenorrhea is normal before menarche (the first menstrual period at the time of puberty), after menopause, and during pregnancy and

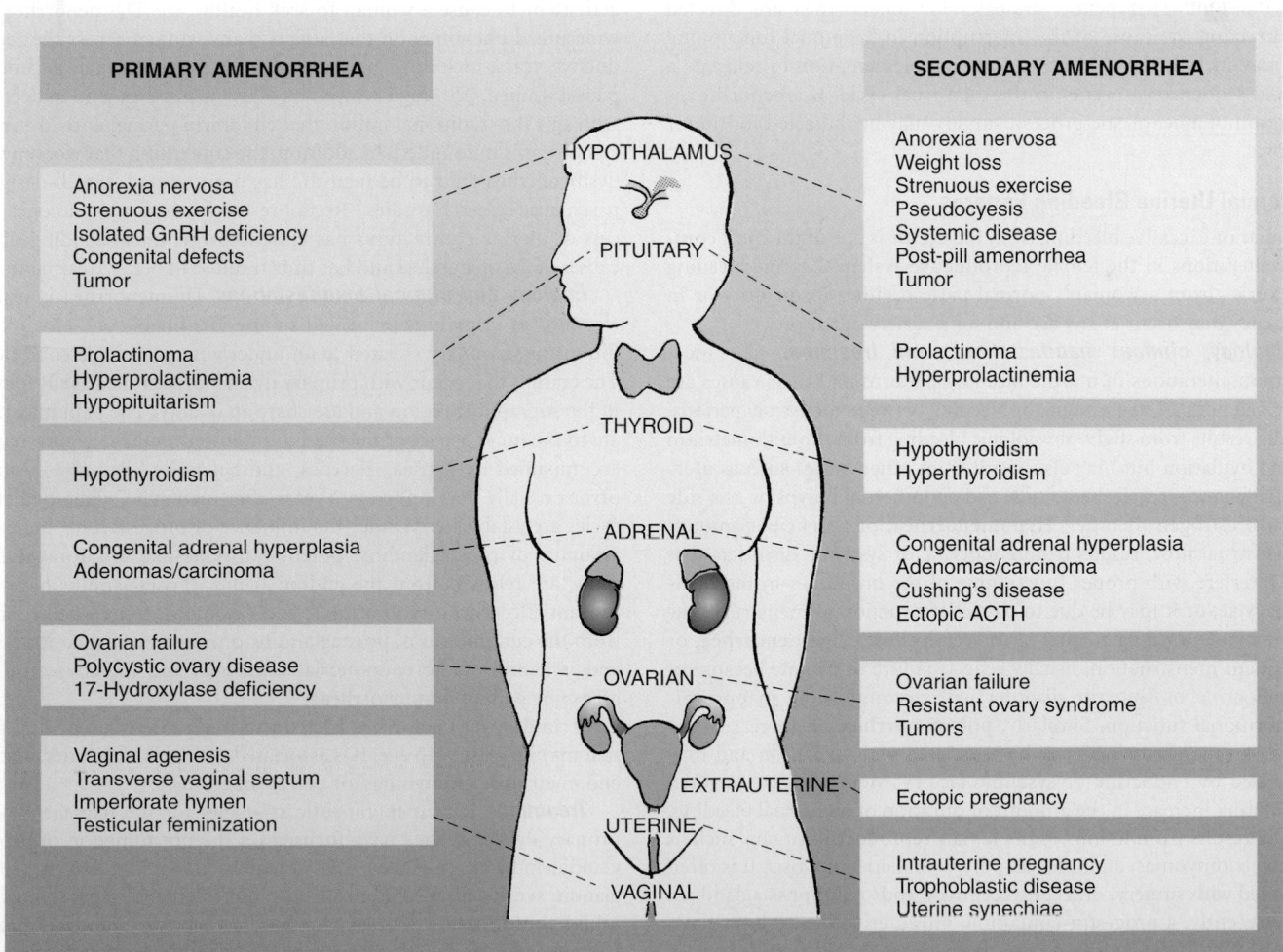

FIGURE 33-1 Causes of amenorrhea. *ACTH,* Adrenocorticotropic hormone; *GnRH,* gonadotropin-releasing hormone. (From Black JM, Hawks JH: *Medical-surgical nursing: clinical management for positive outcomes,* ed 8, Philadelphia, 2009, Saunders, p 915.)

lactation.[1] At other times, it is considered pathologic and may result from a wide range of pathophysiologic causes (see Figure 33-1). In the majority of cases, amenorrhea is due to an abnormal pattern of hormonal functioning that interrupts the normal sequence of events in which the endometrial tissue lining the uterus proliferates and then is sloughed. The endometrial tissue must be stimulated and regulated by the correct quantity and sequence of the female sex hormones estrogen and progesterone and the gonadotropic hormones follicle-stimulating hormone (FSH) and luteinizing hormone (LH). As described in Chapter 32, the menstrual cycle is dependent on the sequential changes in estrogen and progesterone levels. The initial rise in LH and FSH levels in the menstrual cycle occurs in response to a decline in estrogen and progesterone levels; estrogen levels then rise again in response to actions of the gonadotropic hormones, and the endometrium proliferates again in response to estrogen secretion. Thus events that prevent estrogen production, interfere with the normal fluctuations in estrogen levels, or block the action of estrogen on the endometrium will result in abnormal or absent menstrual flow.[2,3] Such events may include physical or emotional stress, which can interfere with normal production of the gonadotropic hormones and alter the pattern of estrogen functioning. In addition, ovarian, adrenal, or pituitary tumors may interfere with the normal production of female sex hormones or LH and FSH. Neoplasms of the ovaries or adrenal and pituitary glands may result in excess or deficient production of these hormones, with a consequent interruption in normal menstrual flow.

Treatment. Therapeutic strategies for amenorrhea are directed to correcting the cause of the interruption in hormonal functioning and may include the use of hormonal supplementation to reinstate a normal sequence of events in the menstrual cycle. If amenorrhea is the result of a neoplastic process, surgery may be indicated for tumor removal.

Abnormal Uterine Bleeding Patterns

Irregular or excessive bleeding from the uterus is one of the most common alterations in the female reproductive system. Uterine bleeding that varies from a woman's normal pattern either in quantity or in frequency may occur at any age and for a variety of reasons.

Etiology, clinical manifestations, and treatment. The most common alterations in uterine bleeding patterns and their causes are described here. **Metrorrhagia,** or bleeding between menstrual periods, usually results from slight physiologic bleeding from the endometrium during ovulation but may also result from other causes such as uterine malignancy, cervical erosions, and endometrial polyps or as a side effect of estrogen therapy.[1] **Hypomenorrhea,** or a deficient amount of menstrual flow, results from endocrine or systemic disorders that may interfere with proper functioning of the hormones in the menstrual cycle, or it may be due to partial obstruction of menstrual flow by the hymen or a narrowing of the cervical os. **Oligomenorrhea,** or infrequent menstruation, usually reflects failure to ovulate because of an endocrine or systemic disorder with accompanying inappropriate hormonal function. Similarly, **polymenorrhea,** an increased frequency of menstruation, may be associated with ovulation and may be caused by endocrine or systemic factors. **Menorrhagia,** an often debilitating increase in the amount or duration of menstrual bleeding, usually results from lesions of the female reproductive organs such as uterine leiomyomas, endometrial polyps, and adenomyosis. It is often managed with surgery, oral contraceptives, and/or antiprostaglandins. More recently, a progestin-containing intrauterine device has shown promise in reducing menorrhagia, dysmenorrhea, and anemia.[4,5]

The term **dysfunctional uterine bleeding** is used to describe abnormal endometrial bleeding not associated with tumor, inflammation, pregnancy, trauma, or hormonal effects. Dysfunctional uterine bleeding is most common around the time of menarche and menopause and not as common in women before menopause.[6] In adolescents, dysfunctional uterine bleeding is most often due to immaturity in functioning of the pituitary and ovary, which have not yet properly orchestrated their activities.[7] Thus an imbalance may be present in the ratio of estrogen to progesterone. Absent or diminished levels of progesterone will result in a thick and extremely vascular endometrium that lacks structural support. As a result of this fragile structure, spontaneous and superficial hemorrhage occurs randomly throughout the endometrium. In addition, the blood vessels in the endometrium fail to constrict to limit the extent and duration of bleeding.[7] Uterine bleeding that is abnormal in both quantity and frequency can therefore occur in a noncyclic pattern.

In perimenopausal women, dysfunctional uterine bleeding may be the result of progressive degeneration and failure of the ovary to produce estrogen. As the number of ovarian follicles diminishes, the production of estrogen by the ovary becomes unpredictable, and the secretion of LH and FSH may also assume an unpredictable pattern. As in adolescents with dysfunctional uterine bleeding, diminished or absent production of progesterone may result in unopposed stimulation of the endometrium by estrogen, with subsequent unpredictable bleeding from a fragile endometrium.[6,7]

Dysmenorrhea

Dysmenorrhea is menstruation that is painful enough to limit normal activity or to cause a woman to seek health care. Dysmenorrhea is a widespread phenomenon that affects many women across the reproductive years, including girls of high school age through perimenopausal women. Although symptoms of dysmenorrhea tend to decrease with age, the traditional notion that childbirth permanently decreases symptoms is unfounded. In addition, the contention that women with dysmenorrhea tend to be neurotic has been refuted in well-designed psychiatric research studies.[7] Recent research into the physiologic process of uterine contractions has enhanced our understanding of the causes of dysmenorrhea and has thus resulted in better treatment.

Etiology and clinical manifestations. Dysmenorrhea is usually classified as primary (not related to any identifiable pathologic condition) or secondary (related to an underlying pathologic condition). The cramps that occur with primary dysmenorrhea are usually located in the suprapubic region and are sharp in quality. The pain may radiate to the inner aspect of the thighs and lower sacral area and may be accompanied by nausea, diarrhea, and headache.[2] Primary dysmenorrhea usually develops 1 or 2 years after menarche, when ovulatory cycles are established. Under the influence of progesterone, increased amounts of prostaglandins, potent hormone-like unsaturated fatty acids, are released from the endometrium. Prostaglandins have significant effects on smooth muscle and vasomotor tone; when released from the endometrium, prostaglandins promote uterine contractions and ischemia of the endometrial capillaries and thereby cause the cramping pain of dysmenorrhea.[8,9]

Secondary dysmenorrhea is characterized more often by dull pain that may increase with age. It is associated with pelvic disorders such as endometriosis, leiomyomas, or pelvic adhesions.[8,9]

Treatment. Recent therapeutic strategies for the management of primary dysmenorrhea have focused on the phenomenon of prostaglandin-induced enhanced uterine contractility. The use of prostaglandin synthetase inhibitors such as ibuprofen and naproxen, which inhibit the formation of prostaglandins, has been very effective in many women experiencing dysmenorrhea.[10] Other approaches that use steroid hormones, such as progestins or combined high-progestin/low-estrogen oral contraceptives, have also been advocated. The rationale is that production of the high menstrual levels of prostaglandins needed to produce dysmenorrhea requires high levels of estrogen without progesterone in the proliferative phase of the menstrual cycle. Progestin administration therefore inhibits the production of prostaglandins and relieves the symptoms of dysmenorrhea.[7] However, the use of steroid hormones may involve significant risks, which the individual client must weigh against the benefits of such therapy.

Therapeutic strategies for secondary dysmenorrhea may involve diagnostic operative procedures such as laparoscopy, as well as medical and surgical therapy for the underlying condition.[9]

KEY POINTS

- Amenorrhea, the absence of menstruation, is most commonly due to hormonal disturbances. Stress and neoplasms (ovarian, adrenal, or pituitary tumors) may interfere with the normal patterns of hormone secretion. Treatment is aimed at the underlying cause of the hormonal imbalance.
- Irregular or excessive uterine bleeding is a common problem. Metrorrhagia is bleeding between periods, hypomenorrhea is reduced menstrual flow, oligomenorrhea is infrequent menstruation, polymenorrhea is an increased frequency of menstruation, and menorrhagia is prolonged and heavy bleeding during menstruation. These disorders may be associated with hormonal imbalances or primary lesions of the reproductive tract.
- Dysfunctional uterine bleeding is common at menarche and menopause and is due to irregular secretion of reproductive hormones. Other causes of abnormal bleeding, such as tumor, trauma, inflammation, and endocrine diseases, are ruled out before a diagnosis of dysfunctional uterine bleeding is made.
- Dysmenorrhea is painful menstruation, generally described as sharp supra pubic cramping severe enough to limit activity. Dysmenorrhea may be treated with prostaglandin inhibitors. Dysmenorrhea secondary to pelvic disorders (endometriosis, adhesions) generally has a dull quality and may increase with age.

ALTERATIONS IN UTERINE POSITION AND PELVIC SUPPORT

Alterations in uterine position and pelvic support may occur anytime during a woman's reproductive years. The major support for the uterus and upper part of the vagina is provided by the thickenings of the endopelvic fascia known as the *cardinal ligaments.* Although tearing of the cardinal ligaments during labor and delivery is rare, they can be stretched abnormally during a difficult or prolonged delivery

and subsequently fail to support the pelvic organs adequately.[7] In addition, congenital defects in the muscles of the pelvic floor may promote alterations in position of the uterus and other pelvic structures. The two most common alterations in uterine position are **uterine prolapse** and **retrodisplacement** of the uterus. Other commonly occurring alterations resulting from a weakening of the vaginal and pelvic floor musculature are **cystocele** and **rectocele.**

Uterine Prolapse

Etiology. The axis of the uterus normally forms an acute angle with the axis of the vagina. This anatomic feature itself tends to prevent a prolapse, or sinking, of the uterus from its normal position. Descent of the uterus occurs when supporting structures, such as the uterosacral ligaments and the cardinal ligaments, relax and allow the relationship of the uterus to the vaginal axis to be altered. This relaxation permits the cervix to sag downward into the vagina. If the support of the vaginal wall is also compromised, the pressure of the abdominal organs on the uterus will gradually force it downward through the vagina into the introitus.[11] Uterine prolapse may occur at any age. In female infants and in women who have never given birth, congenital defects in the basic integrity of the pelvic supporting structures are usually responsible. Trauma to the ligaments during childbirth is the cause of uterine prolapse in women who have given birth, particularly if multiple deliveries have occurred. Uterine prolapse is classified as first-degree, second-degree, or third-degree according to the level to which the uterus has descended (Figure 33-2). In first-degree prolapse, the uterus is approximately halfway between the vaginal introitus and the level of the ischial spines. In second-degree prolapse, the end of the cervix has begun to protrude through the introitus. In third-degree or complete prolapse, the body of the uterus is outside the vaginal introitus. Figure 33-3 shows a third-degree, or complete, uterine prolapse.

Clinical manifestations. The symptoms of uterine prolapse depend on the degree of severity of prolapse. The woman may become increasingly aware of a sensation of bearing down and discomfort in the vagina. If the prolapse has advanced to the second or third degree, she may note discomfort while walking or sitting and have difficulty urinating. In addition, as the end of the cervix begins to protrude outside the body, it may be subject to trauma from friction and ulceration. Bleeding and ulceration of the cervix may be present.

Treatment. Uterine prolapse is one of the most common reasons for hysterectomy, usually from the vaginal approach.[12] In patients who are at poor risk for surgery or who choose not to have a hysterectomy, a pessary, which is a small supportive device, is inserted to hold the uterus in place.[11]

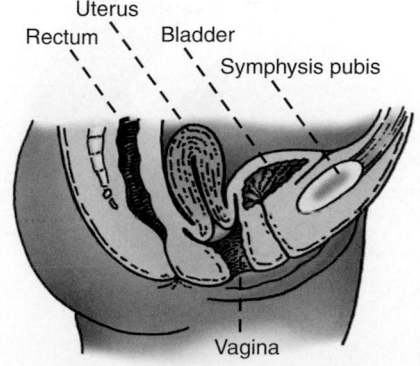
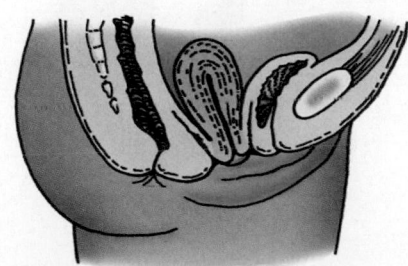
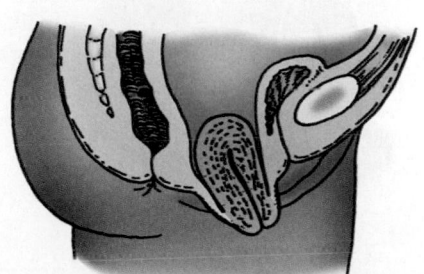

FIRST-DEGREE PROLAPSE   SECOND-DEGREE PROLAPSE   THIRD-DEGREE PROLAPSE

FIGURE 33-2 Degrees of uterine prolapse. (From Black JM, Hawks JH: *Medical-surgical nursing: clinical management for positive outcomes,* ed 8, Philadelphia, 2009, Saunders, p 931.)

Retrodisplacement of the Uterus

The term **retrodisplacement** refers to situations in which the body of the uterus is displaced from its usual location overlying the bladder to a position in the posterior of the pelvis.[13] As shown in Figure 33-4, the uterus may be in one of five positions: anteverted, midposition, anteflexed, retroflexed, or retroverted.

Etiology and clinical manifestations. Retrodisplacement can be detected in 20% to 30% of all women.[14] It may be a normal variation and therefore be present throughout a woman's entire life, or it may develop after childbirth when the supporting structures are injured.

In many women, no symptoms occur from uterine retrodisplacement. In some women, symptoms of pelvic pain or pressure, dysmenorrhea, and dyspareunia (painful intercourse) may be present. In addition, infertility has been associated with retrodisplacement.[7]

Treatment. If the woman has no symptoms, no treatment is indicated. The use of a pessary to support the uterus in a normal position may relieve the symptoms, but surgical correction is sometimes indicated when symptoms are severe.[7] If surgery is indicated, less invasive, laparoscopic surgical procedures are often preferred.[13,14]

Cystocele

Etiology. A *cystocele* is a protrusion of a portion of the urinary bladder into the anterior of the vagina at a weakened part of the vaginal musculature (Figure 33-5, *A*). The defect in the vaginal wall is usually caused by injury during childbirth or surgery but may also result from the aging process or develop as an inherent weakness. Other predisposing factors include obesity and a history of lifting heavy objects. The pressure created by this protrusion causes the anterior vaginal wall to bulge in a downward direction.

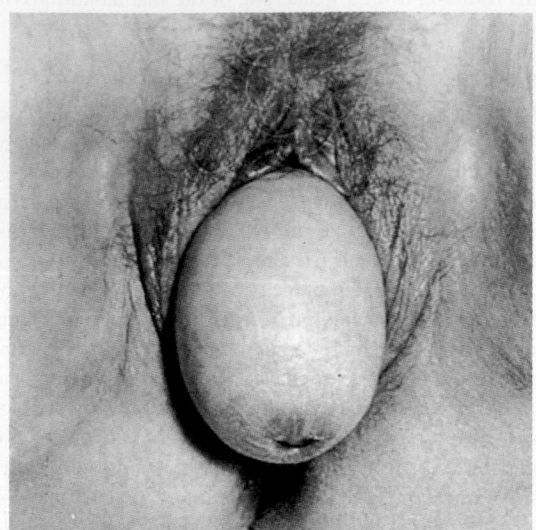

FIGURE 33-3 Complete uterine prolapse. (From Parsons L, Sommers SC: *Gynecology*, ed 2, Philadelphia, 1978, Saunders, p 1443.)

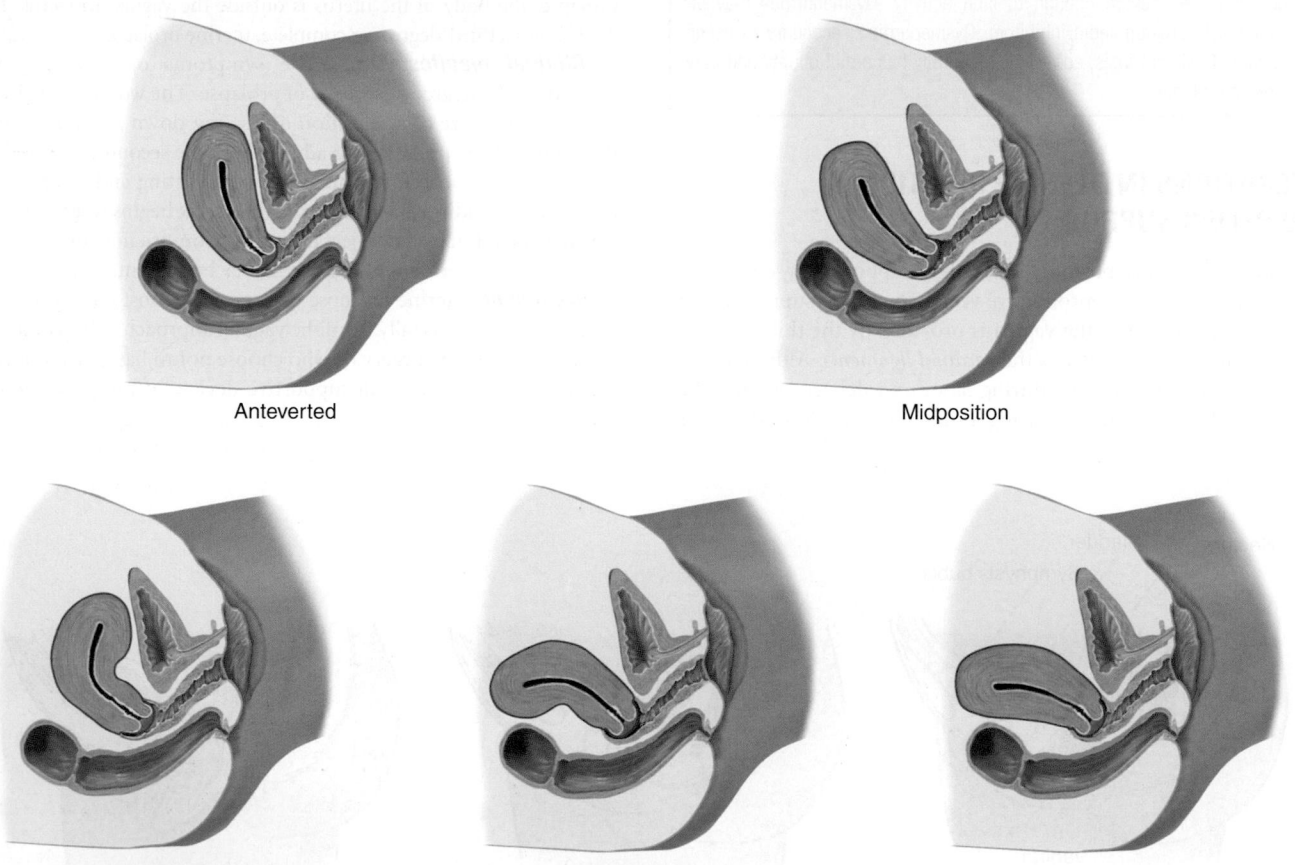

Anteverted

Midposition

Anteflexed

Retroflexed

Retroverted

FIGURE 33-4 Various positions of the uterus. Note that the classifications describe the position of the long axis of the uterus with respect to the long axis of the body. (From Jarvis C: *Physical examination and health assessment*, ed 6, St Louis, 2012, Elsevier, p 745.)

Clinical manifestations and treatment. A wide range of symptoms may be present, depending on the degree of severity of the cystocele. A mild degree of protrusion of the bladder may result in no symptoms. In moderate to severe cases, a sensation of pressure can be felt in the vagina, along with dysuria, incontinence, and back pain. Fullness at the vaginal opening may be observed, as may a soft, reducible mucosal mass bulging into the anterior of the vaginal introitus.

Surgical repair of the vagina is done to correct the cystocele and reestablish support of the anterior vaginal wall. The bladder is restored to a normal position by reinforcement of the weakened portion of the anterior vaginal wall. Prosthetic mesh may also be inserted to further support the bladder during the repair of the cystocele.

Rectocele

Etiology. A **rectocele** (also called *proctocele*) is a protrusion of the anterior rectal wall into the posterior of the vagina at a weakened part of the vaginal musculature (see Figure 33-5, *B*). As for a cystocele, the defect in the vaginal wall is usually caused by injury during childbirth or surgery but may also occur with aging or arise as an inherent weakness. Other predisposing factors for a rectocele include multiparity, obesity, and postmenopausal status. The rectocele forms a bulging mass beneath the posterior vaginal mucosa and pushes downward into the lower vaginal canal. Gradually, the rectum may be torn from its

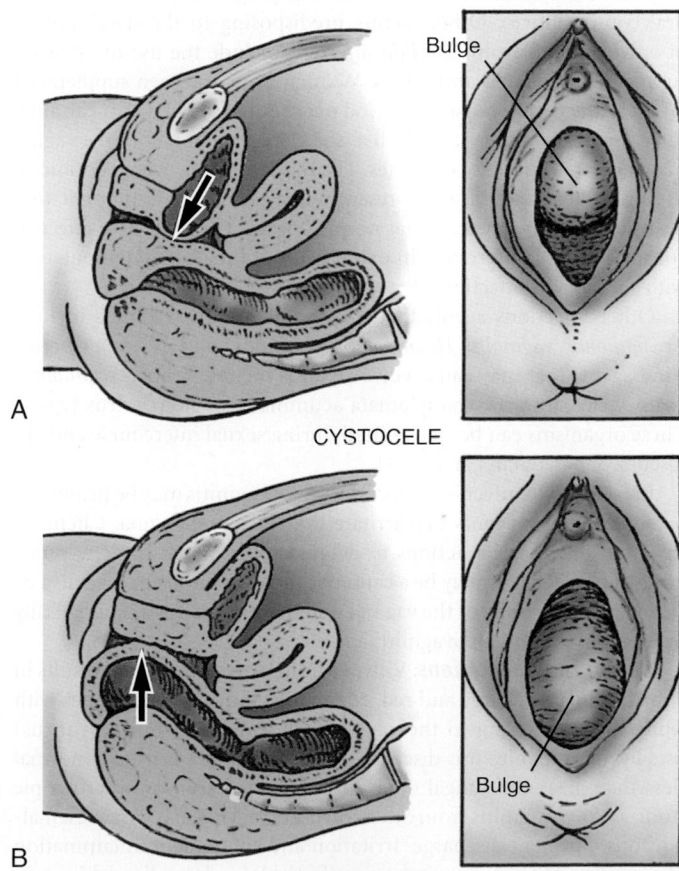

A
CYSTOCELE

B
RECTOCELE

FIGURE 33-5 A, Cystocele. Note the bulging of the anterior vaginal wall. The urinary bladder is displaced downward. The cystocele pushes the anterior wall downward into the vagina. **B,** Rectocele. Note the bulging of the posterior vaginal wall. (From Black JM, Hawks JH: *Medical-surgical nursing: clinical management for positive outcomes,* ed 8, Philadelphia, 2009, Saunders, p 930.)

fascial and muscular attachments to the pelvic wall. The levator ani muscles may also become stretched or torn.

Clinical manifestations and treatment. A wide range of symptoms may be present, depending on the degree of severity of the rectocele. The patient may report a history of difficulty in bowel evacuation and may have experienced chronic constipation with laxative and enema dependency. A feeling of pressure may also be reported, along with painful sexual intercourse. Physical examination reveals a mass bulging into the posterior of the vaginal introitus.[5]

Surgical repair of the vagina is done to correct the rectocele and reestablish support of the posterior vaginal wall. The rectum is restored to its normal location, and the levator ani muscles are realigned in proper position.

> ### KEY POINTS
> - Uterine prolapse occurs when supporting pelvic structures relax and the cervix sags downward into the vagina. Congenital defects, pregnancy, and childbirth are the usual contributing factors. Prolapse may be accompanied by a sensation of pelvic fullness and vaginal discomfort.
> - Retrodisplacement of the uterus is common (20% to 30% of women) and may be congenital or due to pregnancy and childbirth. The body of the uterus is flexed or rotated into the posterior of the pelvis, which sometimes leads to varied symptoms of pelvic pain or pressure, dysmenorrhea, and dyspareunia.
> - A cystocele may result from weakness in the vaginal musculature that allows the urinary bladder to protrude into the anterior of the vagina. Contributing factors include childbirth, surgery, aging, obesity, and heavy lifting. Vaginal pressure, dysuria, and back pain may be present.
> - A rectocele may result from weakness in the posterior vaginal musculature that allows the rectum to protrude into the vagina. Contributing factors are similar to those for cystocele. Symptoms include constipation, painful bowel evacuation, and painful intercourse.

INFLAMMATION AND INFECTION OF THE FEMALE REPRODUCTIVE TRACT

Inflammatory and infectious processes of the female reproductive tract may have effects that range from discomfort to life-threatening situations. Because the infectious agents responsible for inflammation and infection of the female genital tract may be sexually transmitted, some overlap in the discussion of these processes and sexually transmitted diseases is necessary. This chapter will describe the two principal inflammatory and infectious processes of the upper and lower female reproductive tract: pelvic inflammatory disease (PID) and vulvovaginitis. The reader may wish to refer to Chapter 34 for additional information on sexually transmitted infections.

Pelvic Inflammatory Disease

Pelvic inflammatory disease (PID) is any acute, subacute, recurrent, or chronic infection of the oviducts and ovaries with involvement of the adjacent reproductive organs (Figure 33-6). It includes inflammation of the cervix (cervicitis), uterus (endometritis), oviducts (salpingitis), and ovaries (oophoritis). When the connective tissue underlying these structures between the broad ligaments is also involved, the condition is called *parametritis*.[1]

Hospitalizations for PID have declined between 2001 and 2009.[15,16] The CDC reports approximately 113,000 initial physician visits for PID in 2010.[15,16] Significant reproductive health problems may occur as a result of PID. A substantial number of women with a history of PID eventually experience one or more long-term health problems.

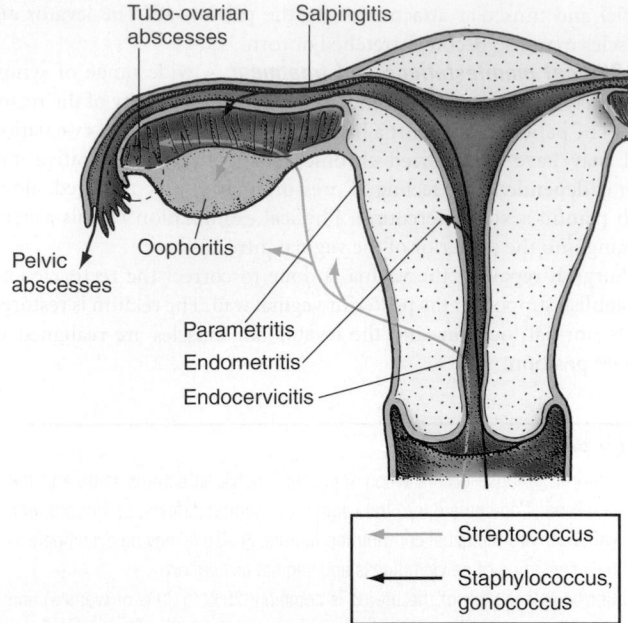

Tubo-ovarian
abscesses

Salpingitis

Pelvic
abscesses

Oophoritis

Parametritis

Endometritis

Endocervicitis

← Streptococcus

← Staphylococcus,
   gonococcus

FIGURE 33-6 Spread of pelvic inflammatory disease. (From Ignata-vicius DD, Workman ML: *Medical-surgical nursing*, ed 6, St Louis, 2010, Elsevier, p 1748.)

Infertility is present in 10% to 15% of women who have experienced PID, and the incidence of ectopic pregnancy is increased six to ten times.[17] Chronic pelvic pain, dyspareunia, pelvic adhesions, and chronic inflammation and abscesses of the oviducts and ovaries may all occur in women after PID.[7]

Etiology. Normally, cervical secretions provide protective and defensive functions for the reproductive organs. By providing a bacteriostatic barrier, cervical mucus prevents bacterial agents present in the cervix or vagina from ascending into the uterus. Therefore, conditions or surgical procedures that alter or destroy cervical mucus may impair this bacteriostatic mechanism. PID may follow the insertion of an intrauterine device, pelvic surgery, abortion procedures, and infection during or after pregnancy. Bacteria may also enter the uterine cavity through the bloodstream or from drainage from other foci of infection such as a pelvic abscess, ruptured appendix, or diverticulitis of the sigmoid colon.[1]

PID can result from infection with aerobic and anaerobic organisms. *Neisseria gonorrhoeae* and *Chlamydia trachomatis* are the most common causative agents because they readily penetrate the bacteriostatic barrier of cervical mucus. However, a variety of bacterial organisms may contribute to the development of PID, including staphylococci, streptococci, diphtheroids, and coliforms such as *Pseudomonas* and *Escherichia coli*. These bacteria are commonly found in cervical mucus, and PID can result from infection by one or several of these bacteria. In addition, PID may occur after multiplication of bacteria in the endometrium that are normally nonpathogenic. During parturition, the traumatized endometrium favors the multiplication of bacteria.[1]

Clinical manifestations. The associated signs and symptoms of PID vary with the affected part of the reproductive tract but generally include abdominal tenderness and tenderness or pain of the cervix or adnexa on palpation. In addition, the temperature may be elevated higher than 38° C and the white blood cell count elevated greater than 10,000/mm³. A pelvic abscess or inflammatory mass may be present on physical examination or ultrasound, and purulent vaginal discharge may be noted.[1,7]

Treatment. Early and aggressive use of antibiotic agents best suited for the causative organisms is essential in preventing the progression of PID. Various antibiotic regimens involving the use of multiple antimicrobial agents have been suggested by the Centers for Disease Control and Prevention for use in PID.[18] Inpatient hospitalization may be indicated for patients with rapidly progressing PID and for those requiring surgical drainage of pelvic abscesses. Rupture of a pelvic abscess is a potentially life-threatening condition, and a total abdominal hysterectomy (removal of the uterus) with bilateral salpingo-oophorectomy (removal of both oviducts and ovaries) may be indicated in this situation.

Vulvovaginitis

Vulvovaginitis is an inflammation of the vulva (vulvitis) and vagina (vaginitis). Because the vulva and vagina are anatomically close to each other, inflammation of one location usually precipitates inflammation of the other. Vulvovaginitis may occur at any time during a girl's or woman's life and affects most females at some point in life.[1]

Etiology. Infection by *Candida albicans* (formerly called *Monilia*) accounts for approximately half of all reported cases of vulvovaginitis. (Infection by *Candida* is referred to as *candidiasis*.[18]) *C. albicans* is a fungus that requires glucose for growth; thus its growth may be promoted during the secretory phase of the menstrual cycle when glycogen levels increase in the vaginal environment. In addition, other conditions in which the glycogen content of the vagina is enhanced may favor candidiasis, such as diabetes, pregnancy, and the use of oral contraceptives. Other factors predisposing to the development of vulvovaginitis from *Candida* infection include the use of estrogen supplementation and antibiotics. Women using estrogen supplementation in the perimenopausal period may be at greater risk for candidal infection of the vagina inasmuch as the glycogen content of the vagina may increase with these therapies. The mechanism by which antibiotic use promotes candidiasis is presently unclear, but it is thought that destruction of the bacteria that normally exert the protective effect of consuming *Candida* results in overgrowth of the *Candida* population with subsequent infection.[1,7]

Other infectious agents that may result in vulvovaginitis include *Trichomonas vaginalis, Haemophilus vaginalis,* and *N. gonorrhoeae.* Viral agents that may cause vulvovaginitis include human *papillomavirus* (venereal warts, condylomata acuminata) or herpesvirus type 2. These organisms can be transmitted during sexual intercourse and are discussed in detail in Chapter 34.

In addition to infectious processes, vulvovaginitis may be promoted by conditions or agents that irritate the vulva and vagina. Chemical irritation or allergic reactions to detergents, feminine hygiene products, and toilet paper may be a causative factor. Trauma to the vulva or vagina or the atrophy of the vaginal wall that occurs postmenopausally may predispose to vulvovaginitis as well.[1]

Clinical manifestations. Vulvovaginitis from candidiasis results in a thick, white discharge and red, edematous mucous membranes with white flecks adhering to the vaginal wall. Intense itching (pruritus) usually accompanies this discharge. The vaginal pH is usually normal (less than 4.5), and fungal organisms are often seen on microscopic studies. Vulvovaginitis from other infectious agents may involve a malodorous, purulent discharge. Irritation and subsequent inflammation of the vulva and vagina may be manifested by red, swollen labia, pain on urination and intercourse, and itching.

Treatment. Appropriate medical therapy for the causative organisms is usually instituted, including local antifungal preparations for vaginal candidiasis and local and systemic antibiotic therapy for vulvovaginitis caused by bacterial agents. Cool compresses and sitz baths provide relief of itching and burning of inflamed tissues. Avoidance of factors that promote irritation of the vulva, such as drying soaps, nonabsorptive underwear, and tight clothing, is also of therapeutic benefit.[1]

Bartholinitis

Bartholinitis is an inflammation of the Bartholin glands, which are located on either side of the vaginal orifice and lubricate the vaginal introitus with a clear, viscous secretion. The location of Bartholin glands renders them susceptible to access by bacteria such as *N. gonorrhoeae*, *C. trachomatis*, and other organisms.

Clinical manifestations and treatment. Once bacteria are established, an abscess (also referred to as a *Bartholin cyst*) may form and cause tenderness and swelling at the site. Pus may be observed exuding from the duct orifice leading to the affected gland, and symptoms of fever and malaise are present in some individuals. Laboratory culture with proper diagnosis of the causative organism is performed, and appropriate antibiotic therapy is usually instituted. Surgical incision and drainage of the abscess may be necessary for effective management.

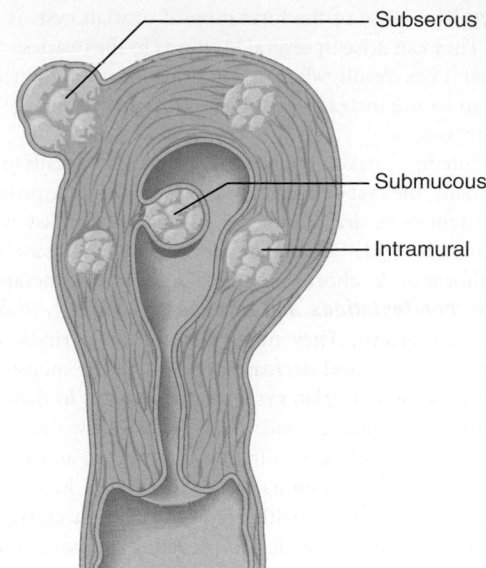

FIGURE 33-7   Uterine leiomyomas. (From Huether SE, McCance KL: *Understanding pathophysiology*, ed 5, St Louis, 2012, Mosby, p 812.)

> **KEY POINTS**
> - PID refers to any infection of the oviducts, ovaries, and adjacent reproductive organs. It includes cervicitis, endometritis, salpingitis, and oophoritis. Manifestations and complications of PID include infertility, ectopic pregnancy, pelvic pain, dyspareunia, and abscesses.
> - Intrauterine devices, abortion, and pelvic surgery predispose to PID. *N. gonorrhoeae* and *C. trachomatis* are the most common causative organisms, and treatment centers on aggressive antibiotic therapy.
> - Inflammation of the vulva and vagina, or vulvovaginitis, is a common problem in women. Most cases are associated with fungal infection by *C. albicans* and are manifested as a white vaginal discharge and an irritated, itchy mucosa. Predisposing factors include chemical irritation from feminine hygiene products, trauma, allergic reactions, and antibiotic therapy that inhibits the growth of normal flora.
> - Inflammation of the Bartholin glands, or bartholinitis, is typically a result of the entry and subsequent infection of the glands by *N. gonorrhoeae* or *C. trachomatis*. Tenderness, swelling, and pus may be present and signify the formation of an abscess within one of the Bartholin glands. Antibiotic therapy and surgical drainage are used to manage the abscess.

BENIGN GROWTHS AND ABERRANT TISSUE OF THE FEMALE REPRODUCTIVE TRACT

Benign growths and aberrant tissue in the female reproductive tract are not uncommon; for example, uterine leiomyomas develop in approximately 50% of all premenopausal women.[19] The presence of benign growths or aberrant tissue in the reproductive tract may cause no symptoms and remain entirely unnoticed, or symptoms ranging from debilitating to life threatening may be present. The diagnosis of these growths or tissue abnormalities may cause anxiety in women experiencing them; in spite of their benign classification, their presence can have devastating effects on the underlying reproductive structures.[19] This section focuses on three of the most common forms of benign growths and aberrant tissue in the female reproductive organs: uterine leiomyomas, ovarian cysts, and endometriosis.

Uterine Leiomyomas

Uterine **leiomyomas,** which are also called *myomas* or *fibroids,* are the most common form of uterine growths that appear in women. Their

actual incidence is difficult to establish because many myomas are either too small or inaccessibly placed to be palpated. Uterine leiomyomas occur in approximately 50% of all premenopausal women and affect black women three times more often than white women.[20,21] Age appears to be a factor in their development inasmuch as myomas are not found before the onset of puberty and rarely exhibit growth activity after menopause.

Etiology. Uterine leiomyomas make their appearance and exhibit growth activity during the reproductive years. Therefore, although the actual cause of myomas is presently unknown, it is thought that estrogen and human growth hormone may influence tumor formation by stimulating susceptible fibromuscular elements in the uterine wall. This theory is supported by the finding that tumor growth is enhanced with the administration of large doses of estrogen and during the later stages of pregnancy, when human growth hormone and estrogen levels are high. In addition, uterine leiomyomas usually shrink or disappear after menopause, when estrogen levels decrease.[1]

Clinical manifestations. Uterine leiomyomas can grow to a large size (Figure 33-7). Obviously, the presence of such a large mass within the uterus will cause symptoms of abdominal pain and pressure, but smaller myomas can result in such symptoms as well. Other symptoms associated with leiomyomas may include abnormal vaginal bleeding and discharge, depending on the location of the mass. If the myoma is sufficiently large to cause pressure on surrounding abdominal organs, backache, constipation, and urinary frequency or urgency may also be present. Finally, uterine leiomyomas can prevent pregnancy, and make carrying a pregnancy to term difficult.

Treatment. Treatment for uterine leiomyomas depends on such factors as the severity of symptoms, the size and location of the leiomyoma, and the patient's age. Small myomas that cause no health problems are generally monitored carefully for growth patterns. Large or multiple masses that promote severe uterine bleeding or interfere with functioning of the gastrointestinal or urinary tract are surgically removed, and hysterectomy may be indicated.[1]

Ovarian Cysts

Ovarian cysts are sacs on an ovary that contain fluid or semisolid material. Ovarian cysts can develop at any time between puberty and menopause, including during pregnancy.

Etiology. The cause of the formation of ovarian cysts is presently unknown. They can arise in several locations in the ovaries:

1. Follicular cysts result when a maturing ovarian follicle fails to release an ovum; instead, the follicle continues to enlarge and produce estrogen.
2. Corpus luteum cysts occur when the corpus luteum fails to degenerate normally; the cyst continues to grow and produce progesterone.
3. Theca-lutein cysts are commonly bilateral and filled with clear, straw-colored fluid. Often their development is associated with hydatidiform mole, choriocarcinoma, or hormone therapy.[6]

Clinical manifestations and treatment. Normally, ovarian cysts produce no symptoms. They may be noted on periodic examination and may increase and decrease in size with the menstrual cycle. Asymptomatic simple ovarian cysts less than 10 cm in diameter have a probability of malignancy and can be followed without intervention. However, when a larger ovarian cyst ruptures, an ovarian vessel may tear, with variable amounts of intraperitoneal hemorrhage and abdominal pain. In persons with recurrent ovarian cysts, oral contraceptives may be recommended to prevent ovulation. Oral contraceptives do not promote resolution of cysts that are already formed. Occasionally, immediate surgical intervention is indicated to control the hemorrhage and repair the site of rupture.[22,23]

Endometriosis

Endometriosis is the presence of endometrial tissue outside the lining of the uterine cavity. Because the only normal location for endometrial tissue is the endometrial lining of the uterus, the presence of this abnormal growth is associated with a variety of side effects ranging from mild symptoms to life-threatening consequences. These foci of abnormal endometrial tissue are called **endometriomas,** or endometrial implants, and usually occur within the pelvis. The most common sites of occurrence of endometriosis within the pelvis are the ovary, peritoneum of the cul-de-sac or pouch of Douglas, uterosacral ligaments, round ligament, oviduct, and the peritoneal surface of the uterus.[7] Less frequently, endometrial implants occur in other body sites such as the bladder or large intestine. Although endometriosis is a benign disease, it possesses certain characteristics of malignant disease, such as the ability to grow, infiltrate, and spread. Symptoms of endometriosis may have an abrupt onset or may develop over many years.

The actual incidence of endometriosis is unknown because it can exist without any significant symptoms. Conservative population estimates show that approximately 11% of women have undiagnosed endometriosis.[24] Active endometriosis usually occurs between 30 and 40 years of age, particularly in women who have never given birth. Endometriosis is rare in women younger than 20 years or after menopause. Although some authorities report a higher incidence of endometriosis in white women of higher socioeconomic levels,[4] these impressions may not be accurate given the tendency of this group to delay childbearing and to have enhanced access to health care. The infertility rate for women in whom endometriosis is diagnosed is about 30%.[25]

Etiology. At the present time, three major theories on the etiology of endometriosis have been proposed:

- *Transportation.* Endometrial tissue flows backward through the oviducts during a normal menstrual period. After this retrograde flow, endometrial fragments implant on the ovary, peritoneal surfaces, and other areas.
- *Metaplasia.* Inflammation or a hormonal change triggers metaplasia (conversion of one kind of tissue to a form that is not normal for that tissue). Thus, coelomic epithelium at certain sites converts to endometrial epithelium.
- *Induction.* In this theory, a combination of transportation and metaplasia takes place, and regurgitated endometrium

chemically induces mesenchyma to form endometrial epithelium. (At present, this theory is thought to be the most likely explanation for endometriosis.[1])

Once the endometrial implants arise in their abnormal locations, they continue to be under hormonal influence, just as the endometrial lining of the uterus responds to hormonal influence. Thus they periodically proliferate and bleed in response to hormonal stimulation. In some instances they may rupture, usually immediately before or after a menstrual period. Endometriomas are filled with brown blood debris; when they rupture, their contents spill onto the sensitive pelvic peritoneum. This irritative discharge establishes a local chemical peritonitis, followed by the formation of fibrous tissue in the injured location. Dense tissue adhesions in the pelvis may result as the pelvic peritoneum undergoes repeated irritation by the cyclic activities of the endometrial implants.

Clinical manifestations. The most prominent symptom of endometriosis is acquired dysmenorrhea, which produces pain in the lower part of the abdomen and in the vagina, posterior of the pelvis, and back. The pain usually begins 5 to 7 days before the peak of menses and lasts for 2 to 3 days. It differs from the pain of primary dysmenorrhea, which is more cramplike and concentrated in the abdominal midline. Pain may be extremely severe, although the degree of pain does not necessarily indicate the extent of disease. Dyspareunia and pain with defecation may also be present.[1,25] Significant changes in the pattern of menstrual flow may occur, with excessive bleeding that may progress to anemia and fatigue.

Treatment. Treatment varies according to the extent of disease, and the primary goals of therapy are to relieve pain symptoms and restore or maintain fertility.[26] Many women with endometrial implants never experience symptoms and require no treatment; others experience a rapidly progressive set of severe symptoms requiring immediate intervention. Both medical and surgical treatment modalities may be used. Therapies to reduce endometriosis-associated pain symptoms include use of nonsteroidal antiinflammatory drugs (NSAIDs) and hormonal agents, including progestins, androgenic agents, and gonadotropin-releasing hormone (GnRH).[26,27] Because endometriosis responds to cyclic hormonal functioning, it is thought that the use of hormones to interrupt this cyclic pattern may result in atrophy of the endometrial implants. Surgical intervention includes removal or destruction of the endometriosis. If damage to the pelvic organs is widespread and the disease is progressing rapidly, total abdominal hysterectomy with removal of the oviducts and ovaries is performed.[26,27]

KEY POINTS

- Benign fibroid tumors, or leiomyomas, are the most common uterine tumor, affecting about 20% of women older than 35 years. Depending on their size, uterine leiomyomas may be characterized by abnormal vaginal bleeding, pelvic pain, constipation, and urinary frequency.
- Ovarian cysts are usually asymptomatic and may change in size with the menstrual cycle. Rupture of an ovarian cyst may result in severe abdominal pain and hemorrhage, which occasionally necessitates immediate surgical intervention.
- Endometriosis occurs when endometrial tissue grows in areas other than the uterine lining. Endometriosis may involve the ovary, peritoneum, oviduct, outer layer of the uterus, bladder, and intestine. Although considered benign, endometriosis tends to infiltrate and spread to adjacent tissues. Endometriosis may be initiated by reflux of the uterine lining through the oviducts into the abdominal cavity during menses.
- Ectopic endometrial tissues periodically proliferate and bleed in response to fluctuations in the levels of reproductive hormones. Dysmenorrhea, with pelvic, back, and lower abdominal pain, usually begins 5 to 7 days before the peak of menses and lasts 2 to 3 days. The pain is more diffuse than that of primary dysmenorrhea. Treatment may include induction of a menopause-like state with hormone administration or the surgical excision of affected structures.

CANCER OF THE FEMALE GENITAL STRUCTURES

Malignant neoplasms occur in every part of the female reproductive system. This section describes the incidence and pathophysiologic aspects of the most common types of malignancies in female genital structures. For further information about the process of neoplasm development, the reader may wish to refer to Chapter 7 of this text.

Cancer of the Cervix

Etiology. Cancer of the uterine cervix is a neoplasm that can be detected in the early, curable stage by the Papanicolaou (Pap) test.[23] The main cause of cervical cancer is certain human papillomavirus (HPV) types. Other factors include having intercourse at a young age or with multiple sexual partners, becoming pregnant multiple times, or being infected by herpesvirus type 2 and other sexually transmitted infections.[1] The incidence of cervical cancer is decreasing in the United States; there are approximately 10,800 new cases of HPV-related cervical cancer diagnosed each year.[28] In 2007, 4021 women in the United States died from cervical cancer.[28] Widespread screening with a yearly Pap test in women at risk has continued to decrease the mortality of cervical cancer. The American Cancer Society now recommends that all women should begin cervical cancer screening about 3 years after they begin having vaginal intercourse, but no later than 21 years of age. After three consecutive negative Pap tests, women older than 30 years who are not at high risk can be tested every 2 to 3 years. Sexually active women younger than 21 years should also be tested within 3 years of first coitus. For women who have had a hysterectomy unrelated to cervical neoplasia, the Centers for Disease Control and Prevention no longer recommends Pap screening, unless surgery was done as treatment for cervical cancer or precancer.[29] Low-risk women who have been screened regularly may also stop screening at age 70.

Clinical manifestations. Preinvasive cervical cancer produces no symptoms, although the Pap test can detect changes in cells of the cervical epithelium, which may be present for 10 years before invasive cancer develops.[1] Early invasive cancer causes abnormal vaginal bleeding, persistent vaginal discharge, and pain and bleeding after intercourse.[1] When symptoms appear, the cancer has usually progressed beyond its early stages. Squamous cell carcinoma accounts for 95% of all invasive cervical cancers diagnosed, and adenocarcinomas account for most of the rest. Invasive carcinoma of the cervix spreads by direct extension to the vaginal wall, laterally into the parametrium toward the pelvic wall, and anteroposteriorly into the bladder and rectum. Metastasis to the pelvic lymph nodes is more common than spread to distant lymph nodes.[7]

Treatment. The treatment strategy depends on the clinical stage of the tumor at the time of diagnosis. Surgery— including cryotherapy, excision, and laser surgery for precancerous conditions and hysterectomy for invasive carcinoma—may be indicated. Chemotherapy and radiation therapy may be used in invasive disease. Radical surgery, including *pelvic exenteration,* or removal of all the pelvic organs, can now be performed with limited morbidity. Treatment works best at early stages of cancer. The 5-year survival rate for stage I cervical cancer is 93%. The 5-year survival rate for stage IV cancer is only 15%.

Prevention. In 2006 the Food and Drug Administration (FDA) licensed the first vaccine developed to prevent cervical cancer and other diseases in females caused by certain types of human papillomavirus (HPV). The quadrivalent vaccine Gardasil protects against four HPV types (6, 11, 16, 18) that are responsible for 70% of cervical cancers and 90% of genital warts. A bivalent vaccine, Cervarix, is also available, and protects against HPV types 16 and 18. The HPV vaccine is recommended for 11- to 12-year-old girls, but can be administered to girls as young as 9 years of age. The vaccine also is recommended for 13- to 26-year-old females who have not yet received or completed the vaccine series. Ideally, the vaccine should be administered before onset of sexual activity. However, females who are sexually active also may benefit from vaccination.[29,30] Experts have recently also suggested similar vaccination recommendations for males.[31]

Endometrial Cancer

Cancer of the endometrial lining of the uterus is less common than cervical cancer in young women, but both types of cancer occur with equal frequency in postmenopausal women.[7] Related factors include infertility, late menopause (older than 55 years), obesity, diabetes, and hypertension. Unopposed estrogen therapy also increases the frequency.

Clinical manifestations and treatment. The most common initial symptom is bleeding between menstrual periods or postmenopausal bleeding. The diagnosis of endometrial cancer is based on histologic tissue examination. Treatment strategies for endometrial cancer include radiation therapy and total hysterectomy with possible removal of the ovaries and oviducts. The 5-year survival rate for patients in whom early endometrial cancer is diagnosed early at a local stage is approximately 96%.[32] The 5-year survival rate drops to 17% if the cancer has metastasized before diagnosis.

Ovarian Cancer

Ovarian cancer has replaced cervical cancer as the leading cause of death from genital cancer. The peak incidence is between 60 and 80 years of age.[7] Because no symptoms are noted until late in the disease, the mortality rate is high, with only a 45% 5-year survival rate.[32]

Clinical manifestations and treatment. When symptoms occur, they are related to intraabdominal metastasis and include increasing abdominal girth, weight loss, abdominal pain, dysuria or urinary frequency, and constipation. Management of ovarian cancer includes removal of the uterus, ovaries, and oviducts. Radiation therapy and chemotherapy may be used in conjunction with surgery. Increasingly, prophylactic oophorectomy or salpingo-oophorectomy is being recommended in high-risk women.[33]

Vaginal Cancer

Cancer of the vagina generally occurs in women in their early- to mid-fifties, although it has an increased incidence in young women whose mothers took diethylstilbestrol during pregnancy.[1] Because the vagina is a thin-walled structure with rich lymphatic drainage, vaginal cancer may metastasize to the bladder, rectum, vulva, pubic bone, and other surrounding structures.

Clinical manifestations and treatment. The primary signs and symptoms of vaginal cancer are vaginal spotting and discharge, pain, groin masses, and changes in urinary pattern.[7] Early-stage therapy is designed to treat the malignant area while preserving normal parts of the vagina. Radiation therapy or surgery varies based on the size, depth, and location of the tumor.[1] Preservation of a functional vagina is generally possible only in the early stages, although grafting from other body sites may be performed to avoid vaginal stenosis, particularly in younger women.[7]

Cancer of the Vulva

Clinical manifestations and treatment. Cancer of the vulva accounts for approximately 5% of all gynecologic malignancies. It can occur at any age, including infancy, but has a peak incidence in the mid-sixties. Factors that seem to predispose to the disease include sexually transmitted infections, chronic pruritus of the vulva with swelling and dryness, obesity, hypertension, diabetes, and never having been pregnant.[1]

Leukoplakic changes (the presence of whitish plaquelike or ulcerated lesions) in the vulva may precede the development of carcinoma. Once the carcinoma develops, vulvar masses may be present, with groin masses and abnormal urination and defecation manifesting later in the disease.[1] Management of vulvar cancer includes partial excision of the vulva to remove precancerous leukoplakic lesions and total vulvar excision for advanced disease.[7] Local relapse is common whether conservative or radical procedures are undertaken.[34]

> **KEY POINTS**
> - Cervical cancer may be detected by evaluation of cervical cells (Pap test). Early-stage cervical cancer may be asymptomatic. When they appear, symptoms include abnormal vaginal bleeding and discharge. Cervical cancer may spread to the vaginal wall, pelvis, bladder, rectum, and pelvic lymph nodes. The quadrivalent vaccine Gardasil protects against four HPV types (6, 11, 16, 18), which are responsible for 70% of cervical cancers and 90% of genital warts.
> - Other cancers of the female reproductive tract include endometrial, ovarian, vaginal, and vulvar cancers. No routine screening tests are available for these cancers. Ovarian cancer has a high mortality rate because it is usually diagnosed after it has metastasized.

DISORDERS OF PREGNANCY

Pregnancy results in a number of physiologic alterations in the mother that are usually well tolerated, particularly if adequate prenatal care is available. However, pregnancy can result in a number of conditions that may be life threatening to the mother and the developing fetus. The most common pregnancy-related disorders are described here; in addition, for information concerning diabetes in pregnancy, the reader may wish to consult Chapter 41, which covers the topic of diabetes in depth.

Pregnancy-Induced Hypertension

Pregnancy-induced hypertension (PIH) is known by other names such as *toxemia* and *preeclampsia-eclampsia*. Hypertension complicates 0.5% to 10% of pregnancies in the United States and is one of the leading causes of pregnancy-related deaths.[35] PIH is characterized by a rapid rise in arterial blood pressure associated with the loss of large amounts of protein in the urine. Women at risk for the development of PIH include teenagers and women in their late thirties and early forties. In addition, the presence of multiple fetuses and the preexistence of hypertension, renal and cardiovascular disease, and diabetes may predispose to the development of PIH.[35]

Etiology, clinical manifestations, and treatment. The exact causes of PIH are presently unknown, although poor nutrition and genetic and immunologic factors have been suggested. PIH is characterized by salt and water retention by the kidneys, weight gain, and edema. In addition, arterial spasm occurs in many parts of the body, most significantly in the kidneys, brain, and liver. Both renal flow and the glomerular filtration rate are decreased, a condition exactly opposite the normal changes in pregnancy. The renal effects are caused by thickening of the glomerular tufts, which contain a fibrinoid deposit in the basement membranes.[1]

The severity of symptoms of PIH is closely related to the retention of salt and water and the degree of the increase in arterial pressure. The increasing arterial pressure seems to promote a vicious cycle in which arterial spasm and other pathologic effects give rise to further increases in arterial pressure. Milder forms of the disease are managed with bed rest. Fetal well-being is periodically assessed, and the infant is delivered if conditions deteriorate or maturity is achieved.

In its severe form, PIH is characterized by extreme vascular spasticity throughout the body, clonic convulsions followed by coma, renal failure, liver malfunction, and extreme hypertension. Usually, this severe form occurs shortly before parturition. The mortality rate in women with severe PIH who are left untreated is high. However, the immediate use of rapidly acting vasodilating drugs, seizure prophylaxis, and rapid delivery have reduced the mortality rate from PIH to less than 1%.[36]

Hyperemesis Gravidarum

Hyperemesis gravidarum is a Latin term for excessive vomiting in pregnant women. Although transient nausea and vomiting occur in about half of women in the first trimester of pregnancy, in a few women these symptoms continue throughout the entire course of pregnancy. Intractable vomiting, or hyperemesis gravidarum, occurs in about 1 in 1000 pregnancies, sometimes with life-threatening consequences.[1] Severe dehydration and electrolyte imbalance, hepatic and renal damage, encephalopathy, and ultimately death may ensue if the vomiting cannot be controlled.

Clinical manifestations and treatment. The causes of hyperemesis gravidarum are unknown, but it is thought that an abnormal response to the production of large amounts of human chorionic gonadotropin hormone by the placenta may be implicated. Intravenous therapy to correct metabolic and nutritional abnormalities, antiemetic agents, and supportive care in a hospital environment may be needed to resolve the symptoms.

Placenta Previa and Abruptio Placentae

Etiology and clinical manifestations. **Placenta previa** is a condition in which the placenta is implanted abnormally over the internal cervical os. **Abruptio placentae** is premature separation of the placenta before delivery of the fetus. Placenta previa occurs in approximately 1 in 200 deliveries and is more common in women with multiple pregnancies and previous cesarean section; its cause is unknown. Placenta previa may occur in varying degrees of severity ranging from partial to entire coverage of the internal cervical os. Abruptio placenta, or premature separation of the placenta, occurs after 20 weeks of gestation in about 1% of deliveries. The detachment may be partial or complete and may cause overt or concealed hemorrhage.[7] Abruptio placentae can be caused by trauma, a short umbilical cord, occlusion of the inferior vena cava, PIH, or abnormal uterine anatomy.

Treatment. Therapeutic strategies for placenta previa and abruptio placentae include cesarean section for fetal distress or hemorrhage control. Medications designed to control preterm labor may also be administered.

Spontaneous Abortion

Spontaneous abortion is expulsion of the products of conception from the uterus before the period of fetal viability. It is usually called a *miscarriage* by laypersons, and it is differentiated from elective abortion. Although the precise incidence is unknown, it is estimated that 50% of all pregnancies end in spontaneous abortion. Among those women who know they are pregnant, the rate of spontaneous abortion is 15% to 20%.

Etiology. Abnormal development accounts for a large percentage of aborted pregnancies. Nearly 61% of abortuses expelled in the first trimester demonstrate chromosomal abnormalities.[6] In addition, abnormal development may result from faulty implantation of the fertilized ovum or from an abnormality in the uterine environment. Maternal factors responsible for spontaneous abortion include both systemic and localized conditions. Infectious processes that may contribute to spontaneous abortion include cytomegalovirus, herpesvirus, and rubella infections. Abnormalities of the reproductive organs, immune disorders, endocrine malfunction, and physical and psychic trauma may all contribute to spontaneous abortion.[7]

Clinical manifestations and treatment. Associated signs and symptoms of spontaneous abortion include vaginal bleeding and abdominal cramps. The cramps may intensify as the cervix dilates for expulsion of the uterine contents. If the entire contents are expelled, the bleeding and cramps subside. However, if any contents remain, an incomplete abortion has occurred and intervention may be needed to control bleeding and to surgically remove the remaining uterine contents.

KEY POINTS

- PIH is characterized by a rapid rise in blood pressure and proteinuria. Renal blood flow and the glomerular filtration rate are reduced, and the kidneys retain salt and water. When severe, PIH may be associated with convulsions and coma. Antihypertensive therapy may be indicated.
- Excessive vomiting during pregnancy is termed *hyperemesis gravidarum.* Dehydration, electrolyte imbalance, hepatic and renal damage, and death may ensue.
- Placenta previa occurs when the placenta is implanted over the cervical os. Abruptio placentae is premature separation of the placenta. Both conditions may interrupt fetal oxygen supply and cause maternal hemorrhage. Cesarean section is indicated.
- It is estimated that 10% to 15% of known pregnancies end in spontaneous abortion. Fetal abnormalities, faulty implantation, infections, and trauma increase the risk of spontaneous abortion.

DISORDERS OF THE BREAST

The breast is considered an accessory organ of the female reproductive tract and is affected by many of the same factors that promote alterations in the other reproductive organs. Women's breast health has become a critical concern in the United States because the breast is the most common site of cancer in women between 25 and 75 years of age.[32] In addition, women are playing an increasingly important role in recognizing the symptoms of breast disease and are seeking earlier intervention with improved outcomes. It is essential that health care professionals continue to encourage this enhanced role and provide accurate information about breast health to their clients. This section includes information on specific breast disorders involving reactive-inflammatory breast disorders, benign breast disorders, and carcinoma of the breast. Before reading this information, the reader may wish to review the section on the structure and function of the breast in Chapter 32 of this text and the specific information on neoplasm development in Chapter 7.

REACTIVE-INFLAMMATORY BREAST DISORDERS

Breast disorders in which an inflammatory response occurs in reaction to irritation, injury, or infection include mammary duct ectasia, breast abscess, fat necrosis, and reactions to injections or implantation of foreign materials in the breast.

Mammary Duct Ectasia

Mammary duct ectasia is a chronic inflammatory process occurring in and around the terminal subareolar ducts of the breast (it is also referred to as *periductal mastitis*). It is more prevalent in older women, primarily postmenopausal women.[37] The Latin word **ectasia** means dilation, and in mammary duct ectasia the collecting ducts

beneath the nipple and areola become dilated, thinned, and filled with secretions.

Pathogenesis. Over time, the ducts become distended with cellular debris, and the debris begins to have an irritating effect on the duct walls. The inflammatory response is initiated, and a zone of granulation tissue is created around a small cavity filled with thick yellowish or brownish material. This area will be palpable as a mass in the central area of the breast, beneath or near the areola. By the time the duct ectasia has grown into a palpable mass, a reactive fibrosis will also have formed in the tissue around the mass. This fibrous thickening of the surrounding breast tissue causes dimpling and distortion of the breast and nipple inversion (Figure 33-8). However, a congenital inverted nipple is already present in some women with mammary duct ectasia, and it is thought that the presence of this nipple anomaly may in some way contribute to ductal wall irritation.[37]

Clinical manifestations and treatment. In addition to a palpable mass and dimpling or distortion of the breast or areola, women with mammary duct ectasia may have a persistent nipple discharge. These signs must be evaluated carefully because they may also be indicative of a malignant breast mass. A biopsy is usually performed to rule out the presence of a malignancy. After confirmation of the diagnosis of mammary ductal ectasia, surgical excision of the dilated subareolar ducts is performed.[37]

Breast Abscess

The majority of abscesses occurring in the breast are not associated with breast feeding and are referred to as *nonlactational* breast abscesses (for a complete description of abscesses or mastitis related to lactation, the reader may wish to refer to an obstetric or maternity nursing text). Nonlactational breast abscesses are most often a recurring problem and usually affect persons with conditions that predispose to infections, such as having diabetes mellitus, undergoing steroid therapy, or being afflicted with other skin lesions.

Etiology. Multiple factors may contribute to the formation of nonlactational breast abscesses. In some women, the presence of a congenital inverted nipple may predispose to abscess formation. Abscesses may also be part of the syndrome of mammary duct ectasia; in addition, women with the aforementioned preexisting conditions that predispose to infections may be at increased risk for the development of an infectious process in the breast tissue. Unlike breast abscesses

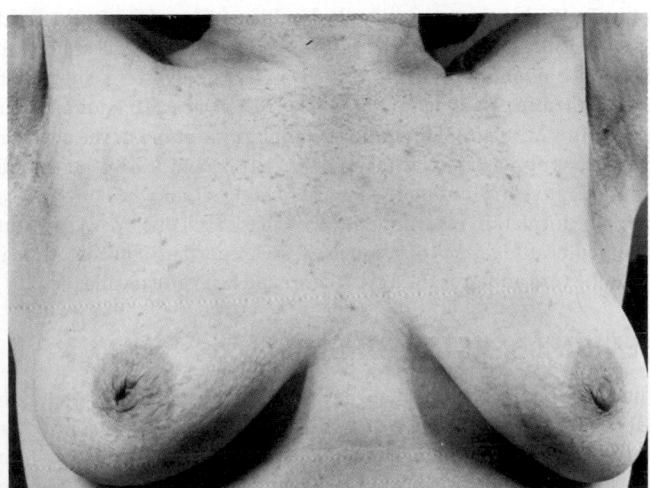

FIGURE 33-8 Nipple retraction in the right breast as a result of mammary duct ectasia. (From Haagensen CD: *Diseases of the breast,* ed 3, Philadelphia, 1986, Saunders, p 359.)

occurring during breast feeding, in which *Staphylococcus aureus* is the most common causative organism, nonlactational breast abscesses usually yield multiple organisms when cultured.

Clinical manifestations and treatment. Signs and symptoms of these abscesses include an area of tenderness, redness, and induration under the periareolar skin.[37] Unfortunately, nonlactational breast abscesses do not respond well to antibiotic therapy and often recur, and it is sometimes necessary to excise the major duct system beneath the areola to prevent further recurrence.[37]

Fat Necrosis

Necrosis refers to the death of a portion of tissue, and fat necrosis in the breast is the death of fat tissue after trauma or injury to the breast. The position of the breasts makes them vulnerable to trauma, particularly in larger women with pendulous breasts. This phenomenon is important for health care professionals to assess because fat necrosis may mimic or obscure carcinoma of the breast.

Clinical manifestations and diagnoses. Fat necrosis of the breast may have many of the same clinical signs as breast malignancy, including a painless mass in the breast that is firm, ill-defined, and poorly mobile. Skin thickening and retraction may also be present. In addition, a mammogram may not provide a clear diagnosis. Unfortunately, many women with pendulous breasts frequently sustain injuries to the breast and may be unable to recall any specific trauma; thus a diagnosis of fat necrosis may be difficult to make. If fat necrosis cannot be reliably distinguished from carcinoma based on clinical observation or mammography, excisional biopsy must be performed.[37]

Reactions to Foreign Material

Surgery to enlarge the female breast has become one of the most popular of all cosmetic surgical procedures in recent years.[37] Since the early twentieth century, a variety of materials have been used for breast augmentation. Silicone implants, which consist of silicone gel encased in polyurethane or other materials, have been the most widely used devices for breast enlargement and have been implanted in more than 1 million women.[37] At present, controversy surrounds the use of silicone breast implants because some side effects, including irritation at the implantation area and other symptoms suggestive of an immune system response, have been reported. Currently, the recommendations surrounding silicone breast implants are conflicting. The use of silicone implants for routine cosmetic breast augmentation is specifically controlled in the United States, favoring implants filled with a saline solution. Health care professionals should be aware of the reported side effects of silicone breast implants inasmuch as a substantial segment of the female population in the United States and Western Europe has undergone breast augmentation with these devices. In addition, persons with silicone implants who sustain blunt trauma to the chest are at risk for rupture of the implant, with subsequent leakage of the silicone gel into surrounding tissue. After chest trauma, the communication of information regarding the presence of silicone breast implants to other health care professionals is an important consideration in planning care and preventing further tissue exposure to silicone.

BENIGN BREAST DISORDERS

The term **benign breast disorders** encompasses a group of lesions affecting the breast. These disorders are usually divided into two categories: (1) fibrocystic breast disease and (2) specific benign neoplasms of the breast such as fibroadenomas, adenomas, and papillomas. It is important for health care professionals to understand the clinical significance of these benign disorders. Although these entities are "benign" in the sense of being differentiated from malignant breast neoplasms, clients experiencing them may be at risk for experiencing a psychological crisis and may need to be educated regarding their potential risk for breast malignancy.

Fibrocystic Breast Disease

Although the term **fibrocystic breast disease** is frequently used by health care professionals, it is important to understand that it is not a distinct disease entity.[37] Instead, it is a diagnosis classification that is applied to a condition in which the presence of palpable breast masses fluctuates with the menstrual cycle and may be associated with pain or tenderness. Laboratory examination of this breast tissue shows macroscopic and microscopic cysts, along with a variety of alterations in tissue structure such as fibrosis or overgrowth of stromal fibrous tissue. However, these alterations in breast tissue are present to some degree in all female breasts, which has led some authorities to question use of the term "disease" for such a widespread condition. Until a more precise system for classifying this type of benign breast disorder is widely adopted, fibrocystic breast disease will probably continue to be used to describe this phenomenon of tender breast masses that occur on a cyclic basis. A comparison of normal and fibrocystic breast tissue is shown in Figure 33-9.

Etiology and clinical manifestations. Hormonal imbalance in the reproductive years is thought to contribute to fibrocystic breast disease. Fibrocystic breast disease is more common in women ages 30 to 50 years. It is usually characterized by tenderness or pain in one or both breasts immediately before onset of the menstrual period. On palpation, the cysts tend to be firm, regular in shape, and mobile. They are located most often in the upper outer quadrant of the breasts, and their size may fluctuate throughout the menstrual cycle.[37]

Although it was previously thought that all women with fibrocystic breast disease were at increased risk for breast cancer, recent research has disproved this theory.[37] It is now known that only certain types of tissue changes may predispose a woman with fibrocystic breast disease to the development of breast malignancy. The vast majority of women with fibrocystic disease do not have these alterations in breast tissue and therefore are not at a substantially increased risk for breast cancer.[37]

Diagnoses and treatment. Diagnostic studies can include ultrasound and needle aspiration of a cyst for histologic analysis. Danazol, a weak androgen, has shown efficacy in the treatment of fibrocystic

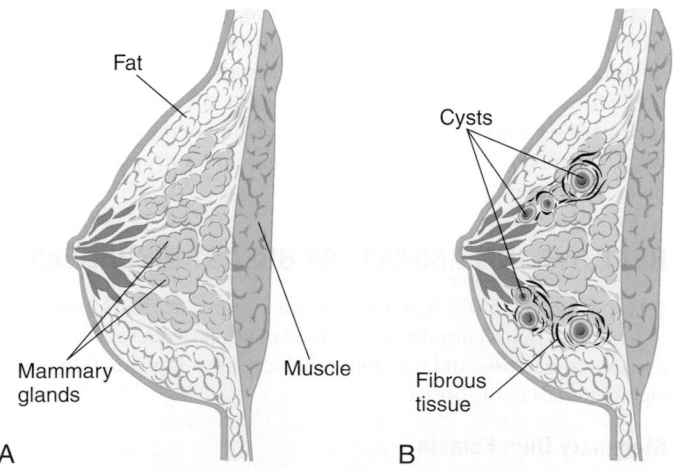

Fat

Cysts

Mammary glands

Muscle

Fibrous tissue

A   B

FIGURE 33-9 A, Normal breast. **B,** Fibrocystic breast tissue. Note image of cysts showing typical smooth margins, dark center, edge shadows, and a bright posterior wall. (From Lewis SL et al, editors: *Medical-surgical nursing: assessment and management of clinical problems*, ed 8, St Louis, 2011, Elsevier.)

breast disease. Oral contraceptives have also been recommended to control symptoms of fibrocystic breast disease. Other supportive measures include the application of local heat and use of a support bra. Nutritional therapies have shown success in some women, particularly avoidance of foods with methylxanthines, such as tea, coffee, cola, and chocolate. It is thought that methylxanthines tend to stimulate cyclic adenosine monophosphate and thus increase metabolic activity in the breast.[37] A low-fat, high-carbohydrate diet has been shown to decrease breast swelling and tenderness.

Specific Benign Neoplasms

Specific benign neoplasms of the breast, such as fibroadenomas, adenomas, and papillomas, may occur at any time during a woman's life from childhood through old age. These neoplasms behave in a clinically "benign" fashion; that is, they do not invade the surrounding tissue or metastasize to other sites. They generally appear as freely movable, encapsulated masses that are sharply delineated from the surrounding breast tissue.[37] However, it is important to have any breast mass evaluated because biopsy and histologic examination may be needed to differentiate these benign neoplasms from breast carcinoma.

MALIGNANT DISORDER OF THE BREAST

Cancer of the Breast

Carcinoma of the breast remains the most common form of cancer in women between the ages of 25 and 75 years.[26] In the United States it is the leading cause of death from all causes in women between the ages of 40 and 44 years. The incidence of breast carcinoma appears to be increasing in the United States, with an estimated 178,000 newly diagnosed cases per year.[32] Although the disease is more common in white women, its incidence in blacks and Asians is rising.[32] Breast cancer does occur in males but is 100 times less common.[32] Even though recent advances in early detection and treatment have afforded longer survival after diagnosis, invasive breast carcinoma remains an incurable disease that continues to take the lives of a large segment of the population.

Etiology. A substantial number of studies conducted in the past 30 years have begun to establish the risk factors and possible causes of breast cancer. Some factors that may place a woman at risk for breast cancer include hormonal influences, reproductive factors, dietary factors, family history, age, radiation exposure, and a history of cancer.[37] It should be noted that helping a client understand and interpret her personal breast cancer risk is a difficult task for a health care professional. The public media have given much attention to some of the risk factors for breast cancer but have not provided much context in which to interpret evaluations for individual risk factors.

Risk factors are characteristics related to the probability of a certain outcome—in this case, breast cancer. These risk factors may be either causally or correlatively associated with an outcome. For example, a factor may directly *cause* an outcome (as the smallpox virus causes smallpox) or may be *correlated* with an outcome (as not wearing a seat belt is correlated with an increased degree of injury in a motor vehicle accident). The distinction between causality and correlation is an important concept to impart to clients when discussing risk factors. A client may express concern, for example, that a certain risk factor will directly cause the development of breast cancer. The ability of a health care professional to describe and discuss risk factors in a knowledgeable way will greatly enhance the client's ability to make decisions regarding such issues as hormonal replacement therapy after menopause.

Hormonal factors. Several hormonal factors have been shown to be linked to the development of breast cancer.[37] Length of exposure to the hormones secreted by the ovary (estrogen and progesterone) has been shown to affect the risk for breast cancer in the following way. If a woman has had an early (younger than 12 years) onset of menses and a late (older than 55 years) menopause, her risk is increased. Stated another way, women with 40 or more years of menstrual activity have twice the breast cancer risk as women with fewer than 30 years of menstrual activity.[37] Postmenopausal hormone replacement therapy may increase the risk of breast cancer, and recent data show that the risk may be greater for women taking estrogen/progesterone combination therapies than for women taking estrogen-only therapies.[38,39] For some women, the known benefits of these medications may outweigh effects on cancer risk. Future research is needed to clarify the way in which hormonal exposure may foster breast cancer development and the many interactive factors associated with taking hormonal medications.

Reproductive factors. It has been observed in many research studies that giving birth at a young age (less than 18 years) is associated with a decreased risk of breast cancer and that giving birth for the first time at 35 years or older increases the risk.[37] In addition, parity (the number of viable children a woman has borne) has been associated with risk, with low parity increasing risk and high parity having a protective effect.[37] Breast feeding is also associated with a decrease in breast cancer.[40]

Dietary factors. It has been suggested that the amount of fat in the diet is a risk factor for breast cancer.[37] Researchers who favor this theory point to the relatively low rates of dietary fat ingestion in countries with low rates of breast cancer. Although the media have given a great deal of attention to this issue, scientific data have been inconclusive thus far.[37] Countries in which low-fat diets are widespread are typically nonindustrialized countries in which other factors, such as age at first delivery or parity, differ from those in industrialized countries. No single dietary pattern or food has been shown to "cause" cancer, just as no specific food has been shown to prevent or cure cancer.

Family history. The role of heredity in contributing to breast cancer has long been recognized. Specific gene mutations such as *BRCA1* and *BRCA2* have been identified in high-risk families. Research studies have indicated that women with a mother or sister with breast cancer have an increased risk of developing breast cancer, even if specific gene mutations are not identified. Women with family risk factors and gene mutations need careful care and accurate information in order to make informed choices. Women with *BRCA1* and *BRCA2* gene mutations are at risk for both breast cancer and ovarian cancer and may benefit from prophylactic salpingo-oophorectomy to reduce their risk.[41] Another controversial option for some high-risk women is bilateral mastectomy. Finally, chemoprevention with selective estrogen receptor modulators (SERMs) may be an option for some high-risk women.[42] SERMs may not be recommended in low-risk to average-risk women because they have their own adverse effects such as thromboembolic events and endometrial cancer.

Age. Breast cancer is extremely rare in young women. The incidence of breast cancer begins to increase by 25 to 30 years of age and continues to increase with advancing age.[37]

Other factors. Other factors, such as radiation exposure and a history of cancer, have been shown to be risk factors for the development of breast cancer.[37] Several potential factors have been suggested, such as exposure to low-frequency electric or magnetic fields and a virus transmitted through lactation. More research is required to establish the role of these potential factors.[42]

Clinical manifestations. Many breast cancers are discovered by the woman herself through self breast examination (SBE). She usually finds a single lump that is painless, hard, and poorly movable. Yearly clinical breast exams by trained clinicians are also recommended

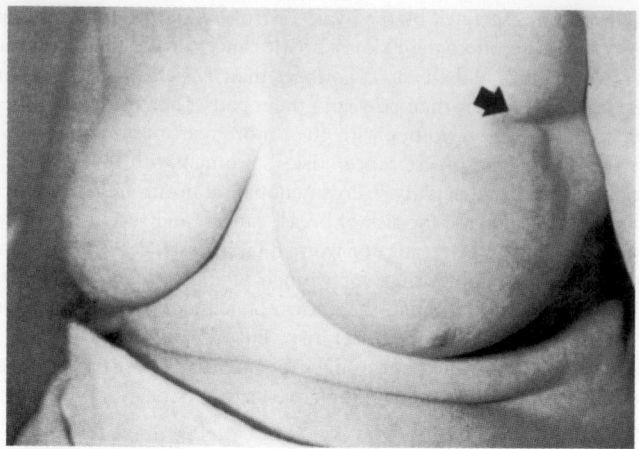

FIGURE 33-10 Skin dimpling caused by an underlying malignant tumor. (From Donegan WL, Spratt JS: *Cancer of the breast*, ed 5, Philadelphia, 2002, Saunders, p 321.)

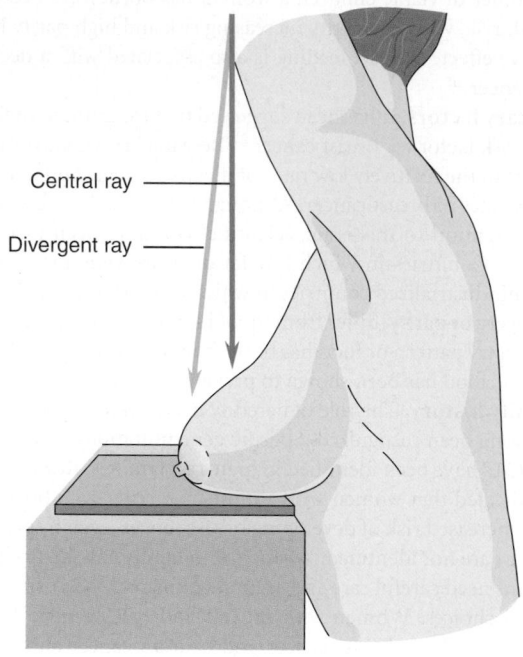

FIGURE 33-11 Placement of the breast for mammography, along with the direction of the x-rays.

Central ray

Divergent ray

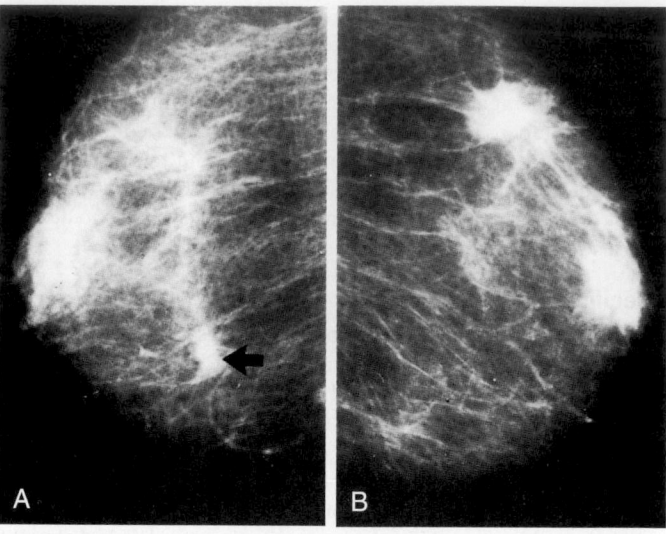

FIGURE 33-12 Mammogram showing bilateral invasive ductal carcinoma. **A,** Left breast. The larger mass was palpable. The smaller right mass was not palpable *(arrow).* **B,** Right breast. Multiple masses are shown. (From Powell DE, Stilling CB: *Diagnosis and detection of breast diseases*, St Louis, 1993, Mosby.)

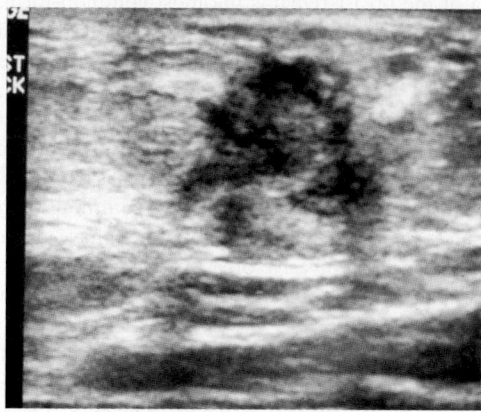

FIGURE 33-13 Ultrasound scan of a carcinoma. Note the ragged appearance of this invasive, malignant lesion. (From Donegan WL, Spratt JS: *Cancer of the breast*, ed 5, Philadelphia, 2002, Saunders, p 332.)

after the age of 40. Mammography is an important clinical tool, and according to current screening guidelines, most women should have yearly mammograms beginning at age 40. Other technologies, such as magnetic resonance imaging (MRI), are showing promise as screening tools. Improvements in technology, such as digital mammography and MRI, have greatly increased the ability to identify breast cancers.

Half of malignant tumors occur in the upper outer quadrant of the breast.[37] Other signs of advanced tumor development include dimpling of the skin (Figure 33-10), retraction of the nipple, changes in breast contour, and bloody discharge from the nipple. Breast cancer is diagnosed by a number of techniques that use films (mammography, xerography) (Figures 33-11 and 33-12), by computerized technologies (digital mammography), and by thermography, a technique in which "hot spots" indicate increased metabolic activity. A person of any age with a suspected breast mass should undergo mammography and biopsy.

Most breast carcinomas arise in the epithelium of the glandular ducts of the breast. The lesion(s) have infiltrating edges that begin to invade normal breast tissue (Figure 33-13). After this invasion, malignant cells begin to scatter or disseminate into the lymph system of the axilla (Figure 33-14). The breast is in close proximity to the large system of axillary lymph nodes, which makes easy dissemination of malignant cells possible. The major way by which breast carcinoma causes morbidity and death is through the dissemination of malignant cells to other body sites, most commonly lung, liver, and bone.[37] **Metastasis** (or spread of carcinoma) to these other body sites signifies a poorer prognosis. The prognosis is vastly better for persons with no evidence of spread of malignant cells to the regional lymph nodes. The 5-year survival rate is 98% when no lymph node involvement is found at surgery but averages 84% when lymph node involvement is present.[26] For women with distant spread (metastases), the rate drops to 23%.[32] The greater the number of positive lymph nodes (nodes with malignant cells) found at surgery, the less favorable the prognosis.

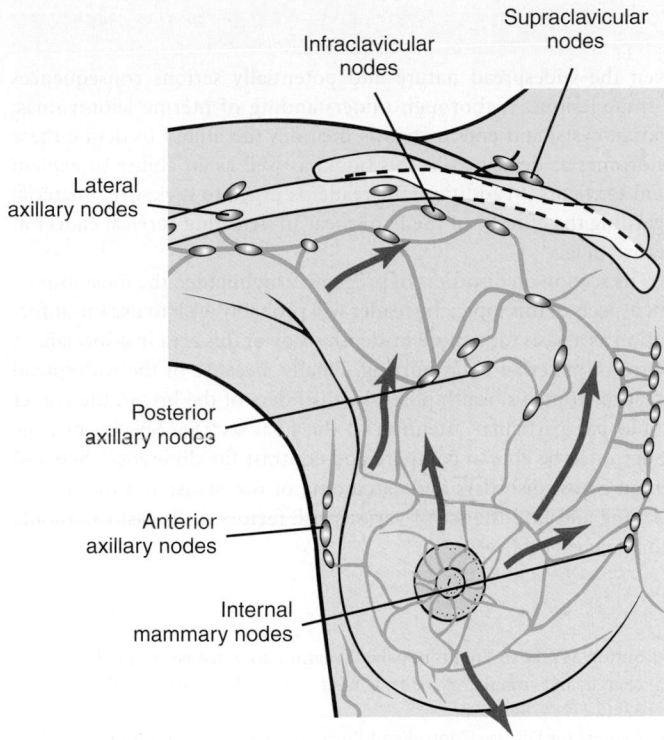

FIGURE 33-14 Lymphatic drainage of the breast. In general, lateral lesions in the breast metastasize to axillary and supraclavicular nodes, whereas medial tumors tend to metastasize to the internal mammary and mediastinal lymph nodes, as well as the supraclavicular nodes. (From Lewis SL et al, editors: *Medical-surgical nursing: assessment and management of clinical problems*, ed 7, St Louis, 2007, Elsevier, p 1327.)

Treatment. Treatment for breast cancer includes surgery, chemotherapy, radiation therapy, and supportive measures. Surgical therapy is a controversial area, and various options are available. Breast conserving therapy, which includes removal of only the lesion, is called a **lumpectomy.** Lumpectomy or lumpectomy in conjunction with either chemotherapy and/or radiation is becoming increasingly preferred. Removal of only the breast is a simple **mastectomy.** Other surgical interventions include a **modified radical mastectomy,** in which the breast is removed and a portion of the axillary lymphatic system is dissected, and a **radical mastectomy (rare),** in which the breast, lymphatic drainage, and underlying pectoral muscles are removed.[37]

Chemotherapy entailing a variety of hormonal and antineoplastic agents is also used. Malignant cells appear to have cytoplasmic hormone receptors that bind to hormone molecules and promote cellular division and growth. Selective estrogen receptor modulators (SERMs), estrogen antagonists, are the most common agents used. Popular examples of SERMs include tamoxifen and raloxifene. Antineoplastic agents are given to control the spread of malignant cells.[37]

Radiation therapy may be used as an adjunct to the aforementioned therapy and to control pain by shrinking large tumor masses. Other supportive measures in advanced disease include operations to reduce the bulk of tumors.[37]

Continuum of care. Breast cancer is characterized by a wide variation in clinical course. Many patients who undergo therapy for breast carcinoma are able to achieve a satisfying quality of life. Educational and support programs for breast cancer patients and their families, both preoperatively and postoperatively, have been an important means of providing emotional support. Programs for continuing care after mastectomy have helped patients and families face the adaptive challenges of living with breast cancer. Follow-up care includes early detection of recurrent disease, with an emphasis on breast self-examination, yearly mammography, and regular examination by health care professionals.

KEY POINTS

- Chronic inflammation of the subareolar ducts may result in mammary duct ectasia. Fibrous thickening results in a palpable central mass, breast distortion and dimpling, and nipple inversion. Persistent nipple discharge may occur. These signs are similar to those of malignancy and are carefully evaluated by biopsy. Surgical excision may be performed.

- Breast abscesses in nonlactating women are commonly associated with chronic infection, diabetes, and steroid therapy. These abscesses respond poorly to antibiotics and tend to recur.

- Fibrocystic breast disease is a condition in which palpable breast masses are present and fluctuate with the menstrual cycle. Breast cysts are firm, mobile, and tender, and are usually located in the upper outer quadrant. There is no evidence that women with fibrocystic breasts are at higher risk for breast cancer. A low-fat, high-carbohydrate diet; danazol; heat therapy; and avoidance of methylxanthines may be recommended.

- Breast cancer is the most common cancer in women between 25 and 75 years of age. Malignant tumors tend to be painless, hard, and fixed in place, in contrast to benign breast tumors, which are mobile and encapsulated. Risk factors for breast cancer include a high-fat diet, a first-degree relative with breast cancer, increasing age, radiation exposure, and a previous malignancy. In addition, reproductive factors such as the age at first pregnancy and the number of pregnancies may be associated with altered cancer risk.

- Breast cancer may spread to the regional lymphatics and disseminate to other sites. Localized breast cancer, without lymph node involvement, has a 98% 5-year survival rate. The survival rate falls to 84% when lymph nodes are cancerous and to 23% when there are distant metastases. Depending on the extent of tumor spread, surgery may be performed to remove the tumor only (lumpectomy), the affected breast only (simple mastectomy), the affected breast and involved lymph nodes (modified radical mastectomy), or the breast, lymphatics, and underlying muscle (radical mastectomy). In addition, radiation therapy and chemotherapy may be initiated.

SUMMARY

This chapter has described the most prevalent women's reproductive health problems at the present time. Any alteration in reproductive status may have profound implications for the individual; thus the reader should review this material carefully to acquire the ability to distinguish the differences and similarities in these alterations.

Commonly occurring alterations in reproductive health for women may have serious consequences and require immediate intervention. Menstrual disorders may have multiple manifestations, and such disorders as amenorrhea and abnormal uterine bleeding may occur at any time throughout a woman's life. Alterations in uterine position and pelvic support, including uterine prolapse, retrodisplacement of the uterus, cystocele, and rectocele, may result in severe symptoms and require surgical correction. Inflammation and infection of the female reproductive tract, including PID and vulvovaginitis, may have far-reaching effects for the individual experiencing them.

The reader should pay particular attention to the section on benign growths and aberrant tissue of the female reproductive tract given the widespread nature and potentially serious consequences of these lesions. A thorough understanding of uterine leiomyomas, ovarian cysts, and endometriosis includes the ability to define these syndromes as described in this book, as well as an ability to explain them to clients. In addition, the reader is urged to review the material regarding the efficacy of the Pap smear in detecting cervical cancer at an early stage.

The section on disorders of pregnancy highlighted the most important aspects of this topic; the reader will probably wish to use this information as a basis for a more in-depth study of this area in a specialized course in maternal-child nursing. Finally, because of the widespread threat to women's health posed by disorders of the breast, the reader should pay particular attention to the final section. Specifically, the reader must be able to compare and contrast the differences between benign breast disorders and carcinoma of the breast and discuss the meaning and importance of various risk factors for breast carcinoma in a knowledgeable way.

REFERENCES

1. Hacker NF, Gambone JC, Hobel CJ: *Essentials of obstetrics and gynecology*, ed 5, Philadelphia, 2009, Saunders.
2. Fritz M, Speroff L: *Clinical gynecologic endocrinology and infertility*, Philadelphia, 2011, Lippincott Williams & Williams.
3. Practice Committee of the American Society for Reproductive Medicine: Current evaluation of amenorrhea, *Fertil Steril* 87(5 suppl):S148–S155, 2006.
4. Hubasher D, Grimes DA: Noncontraceptive health benefits of intrauterine devices: a systematic review, *Obstet Gynecol Surv* 57:120–128, 2002.
5. Marret H, et al: CNGOF College National des Gynecologues et Obstetriciens Français: Clinical practice guidelines on menorrhagia: management of abnormal uterine bleeding before menopause, *Eur J Obstet Gynecol Reprod Biol* 152(2):133–137, 2010.
6. Albers JR, Hull SK, Wesley MA: Abnormal uterine bleeding, *Am Fam Physician* 69(8):1915–1926, 2004.
7. Curtis MG, Overholt S, Hopkins MP: *Glass's office gynecology*, ed 6, Baltimore, 2005, Lippincott Williams & Wilkins.
8. Lentz G: Primary and secondary dysmenorrheal, premenstrual syndrome, and premenstrual dysphoric disorder. In Katz V, et al, editors: *Comprehensive gynecology*, Maryland Heights, MO, 2007, Mosby Elsevier, pp 901–914.
9. Karnath B, Breitkopf D: Acute and chronic pelvic pain in women, *Hospital Physician* 43(7):41–48, 2007.
10. Lefebvre G, et al: Primary dysmenorrhea consensus guideline, *JOGC* 27(12):1117–1146, 2005.
11. Lentz G: Anatomic defects of the abdominal wall and pelvic floor: abdominal and inguinal hernias, cystocele, urethrocele, enterocele, rectocele, uterine and vaginal prolapse, and rectal incontinence: diagnosis and management. In Katz V, Lentz G, Lobo R, Gershenson D, editors: *Comprehensive Gynecology*, Maryland Heights, MO, 2007, Mosby Elsevier, pp 501–536.
12. Whiteman MK, et al: Inpatient hysterectomy surveillance in the United States, 2000-2004, *Am J Obstet Gynecol* 198(1):34, e1-7, 2008.
13. Lentz G, et al: Differential diagnosis of major gynecologic problems by age group: vaginal bleeding, pelvic pain, pelvic mass. In Katz V, et al, editors: *Comprehensive gynecology*, Maryland Heights, MO, 2007, Mosby Elsevier, pp 153–176.
14. Yen CF, et al: Combined laparoscopic uterosacral and round ligament procedures for treatment of symptomatic uterine retroversion and mild uterine decensus, *J Am Assoc Gynecol Laparosc* 9(3):359–366, 2002.

15. Sutton MY, et al: Trends in pelvic inflammatory disease hospital discharges and ambulatory visits, United States, 1985-2001, *Sex Transm Dis* 32(12):778–784, 2005.
16. Centers for Disease Control and Prevention: *Sexually transmitted disease surveillance 2010*, Atlanta, 2011, U.S. Department of Health and Human Services.
17. Centers for Disease Control and Prevention: *STD facts—pelvic inflammatory disease (PID)*. Accessed 12/2/11 at cdc.gov.
18. Centers for Disease Control and Prevention: Sexually transmitted diseases treatment guidelines, 2010, *MMWR Morb Mortal Wkly Rep* 59(no. RR-12): 1–110, 2010.
19. Day Baird D, et al: High cumulative incidence of uterine leiomyomas in black and white women: ultrasonic evidence, *Am J Obstet Gynecol* 188(1):100–107, 2003.
20. Wallach EE, Vlahos NF: Uterine myomas: an overview of development, clinical features, and management, *Obstet Gynecol* 104(2):393–406, 2004.
21. Wise LA, et al: Age-specific incidence rates for self-reported uterine leiomyomata in the Black Women's Health Study, *Obstet Gynecol* 105(3):563–568, 2005.
22. Knudsen UB, et al: Management of ovarian cysts, *Acta Obstet Gynecol Scand* 83(11):1012–1021, 2004.
23. Durnell Schuiling K, Likis FE: *Women's gynecologic health*, Burlington, MA, 2013, Jones & Bartlett.
24. Buck Louis GM, et al: ENDO Study Working Group: incidence of endometriosis by study population and diagnostic method: the ENDO study, *Fertil Steril* 96(2):360–365, 2011.
25. Farquhar C: Endometriosis, *BMJ* 334(7587):249–253, 2007.
26. Mao A, Anastasi J: Diagnosis and management of endometriosis: the role of the advanced practice nurse in primary care, *J Am Acad Nurse Pract* 22(2):109–116, 2010.
27. Leyland N, et al: Endometriosis: diagnosis and management, *J Obstet Gynaecol Can* 32(7 suppl):S1–S32, 2010.
28. U.S. Cancer Statistics Working Group: *United States cancer statistics: 1999-2007 incidence and mortality web-based report*, Atlanta, 2010, CDC and National Cancer Institute. Available at www.cdc.gov/uscs.
29. Smith RA, Cokkinides V, Brawley OW: Cancer screening in the United States, 2008: a review of current American Cancer Society guidelines and cancer screening issues, *CA Cancer J Clin* 58:161–179, 2008.
30. Markowitz LE, et al: Quadrivalent human papilloma virus vaccine: recommendations of the advisory committee on immunization practices, *MMWR Morb Mortal Wkly Rep* 56(RR02):1–24, 2007.
31. Centers for Disease Control and Prevention: Recommendations on the use of quadrivalent human papillomavirus vaccine in males—advisory committee on immunization practices (ACIP), *MMWR* 60(50):1705–1708, 2011.

32. American Cancer Society: *Cancer facts and figures*, Atlanta, 2011, Author.

33. Rebbeck TR, et al: Prophylactic oophorectomy in carriers of BRCA1 or BRCA2 mutations, *N Engl J Med* 346:1616–1622, 2002.

34. Rouzier R, et al: Local relapse in patients treated for squamous cell vulvar carcinoma: incidence and prognostic value, *Obstet Gynecol* 100:1159–1167, 2002.

35. Chang J, et al: Pregnancy-related mortality surveillance. United States, 1991-1999, *MMWR Morb Mortal Wkly Rep* 52(SS02):1–8, 2003.

36. American College of Obstetricians and Gynecologists: *Diagnosis and management of preeclampsia and eclampsia*, ACOG Practice Bulletin No. 33, Washington, DC, 2002, The College.

37. Harris JR, Lippman ME, Kent Osborne C, Morrow M: *Diseases of the breast*, ed 4, Philadelphia, 2009, Lippincott Williams & Wilkins.

38. Stefanick ML, Anderson GL, Margolis KL: Effects of conjugated equine estrogens on breast cancer and mammography screening in postmenopausal women with hysterectomy, *JAMA* 295:1647–1657, 2006.

39. Writing Group for the Women's Health Initiative Investigators: Risks and benefits of estrogen plus progestin in healthy postmenopausal women: principal results from the Women's Health Initiative randomized controlled trial, *JAMA* 288:321–333, 2002.

40. Collaborative Group on Hormonal Factors in Breast Cancer: Breast cancer and breastfeeding: collaborative reanalysis of individual data from 47 epidemiological studies in 30 countries, including 50,302 women with breast cancer and 96,973 women without the disease, *Lancet* 360:187–195, 2002.

41. Kauff ND, et al: Risk-reducing salpingo-oophorectomy in women with a BRCA1 or BRCA2 mutation, *N Engl J Med* 346:1609–1615, 2002.

42. U.S. Preventative Services Task Force: Chemoprevention of breast cancer: recommendations and rationale, *Ann Intern Med* 137:56–58, 2002.

Sexually Transmitted Infections

Rosemary A. Jadack

℮volve WEBSITE

http://evolve.elsevier.com/Copstead/

- Review Questions and Answers
- Glossary (with audio pronunciations for selected terms)
- Animations
- Case Studies
- Key Points Review

KEY QUESTIONS

- What are the characteristic clinical manifestations and lesions of gonorrhea and chlamydial infection?
- How do the pathologic changes and clinical manifestations of syphilis differ during the incubation, primary, secondary, and tertiary phases?
- How do the lesions of herpes simplex, syphilis, and lymphogranuloma venereum differ?
- Which sexually transmitted diseases remain localized, and which have systemic consequences?
- What are the causative organisms and characteristic lesions of the following localized sexually transmitted diseases: chancroid, granuloma inguinale, molluscum contagiosum, and condylomata acuminata (genital warts)?

CHAPTER OUTLINE

An epidemic of sexually transmitted infections (STIs) currently exists in the United States.[1,2] The Centers for Disease Control and Prevention (CDC) estimate that there are 19 million new infections every year.[3] More than 300,000 cases of gonococcal infections and 1.3 million chlamydial infections were reported in 2010.[3] However, the true incidence of these infections is likely to be significantly higher inasmuch as many sexually transmitted infections are unreported. The cost of STIs is extremely high. It is estimated that STIs cost the health care system $17 billion every year.[3] In addition, the personal costs to the individual experiencing an STI may include pain, disfigurement, psychosocial difficulties, and reproductive problems. Because of the epidemic status of these diseases and the enormous costs associated with them, it is imperative that health care providers become sufficiently knowledgeable to assess their patients' STI status and educate them about STIs in an accurate and compassionate manner.

The term **sexually transmitted infections** refers to a large group of disease syndromes that can be transmitted sexually, regardless of whether the disease has manifestations in genital structures.[1] In older texts, STIs are referred to as *sexually transmitted diseases* (STDs) and *venereal diseases*. Although STIs are more prevalent in the 15- to 25-year-old age group, they can occur at any age. These diseases are sometimes contracted by nonsexual transmission, as when a newborn infant contracts an STI from an infected mother during passage through the birth canal.[1]

BOX 34-1 SEXUALLY TRANSMITTED ORGANISMS

Bacterial Pathogens
Calymmatobacterium granulomatis
Chlamydia trachomatis
Gardnerella vaginalis
Haemophilus ducreyi
Mycoplasma hominis
Neisseria gonorrhoeae
Shigella
Group B streptococci
Ureaplasma urealyticum
Treponema pallidum

Fungal Pathogens
Candida albicans
Candida glabrata

Viral Pathogens
Human immunodeficiency virus
Cytomegalovirus
Herpes simplex virus
Hepatitis virus
Human papillomavirus
Molluscum contagiosum virus

Protozoan Pathogens
Entamoeba histolytica
Giardia lamblia
Trichomonas vaginalis

TABLE 34-1 SEXUALLY TRANSMITTED INFECTIONS CATEGORIZED ACCORDING TO DISEASE MANIFESTATIONS

DISEASE MANIFESTATIONS	DISEASE
Urethritis, cervicitis, and salpingitis	Gonorrhea
	Nongonococcal urethritis
	Pelvic inflammatory disease
Ulcerative lesions with systemic involvement	Syphilis
	Lymphogranuloma venereum
	Herpes simplex virus
Ulcerative lesions only	Chancroid
	Granuloma inguinale (donovanosis)
Nonulcerative lesions	Molluscum contagiosum
	Genital warts (condylomata acuminata)
Vulvovaginitis	Trichomoniasis
	Candidiasis
	Gardnerella vaginalis vaginitis
Systemic infections	Cytomegalovirus
	Hepatitis
	AIDS
Enteric infections	Giardiasis
	Campylobacter enteritis
	Shigellosis
	Amebic dysentery

A list of sexually transmitted organisms grouped according to type of pathogen is found in Box 34-1. A useful approach to learning the complex pathophysiologic processes of STIs is to group STIs according to the disease manifestations that the patient is most likely to exhibit when first seen by the health care provider. These categories of STIs and the disease manifestations associated with them are listed in Table 34-1. This chapter describes each of these categories and the pathophysiologic processes associated with each relevant STI.

Some diseases listed in Table 34-1 are discussed elsewhere in this text but have been included here for completeness. In particular, the reader may wish to refer to Chapter 33 for more detailed information on pelvic inflammatory disease and vulvovaginitis. Also, certain systemic infections are potentially transmitted by sexual contact. Cytomegalovirus infection, hepatitis A and hepatitis B, and human immunodeficiency virus (HIV) have the potential for sexual transmission. These diseases are covered in detail in Units III and IX, along with more in-depth information concerning infectious processes and immune responses. Before studying this chapter, the reader may wish to refer to Chapters 8 and 9 for a review of basic terminology such as *incubation period* and *period of communicability*. Health care providers caring for persons at risk for STIs should be aware of the potential for acquisition of systemic diseases by sexual contact and include assessment of these diseases as part of their overall clinical evaluation.

URETHRITIS, CERVICITIS, SALPINGITIS, AND PELVIC INFLAMMATORY DISEASE

Three types of STI are manifested by *urethritis* (inflammation of the urethra), *cervicitis* (inflammation of the uterine cervix), and/or *salpingitis* (inflammation of the oviduct or fallopian tube). **Gonorrhea** is an inflammation of epithelial tissue by the organism *Neisseria gonorrhoeae*. In men, nongonococcal urethritis refers to urethritis resulting from a pathogen other than the gonococcus, which is usually *Chlamydia trachomatis*. In women, mucopurulent cervicitis refers to an inflammation of the cervix, which is usually caused by either *Chlamydia trachomatis* or *Neisseria gonorrhoeae*. Pelvic inflammatory disease, which was described in Chapter 33, is usually the result of acute salpingitis caused by gonococcal or chlamydial infection that has extended into nearby pelvic tissue.[1,3,4]

Gonococcal Infection

Gonorrhea is associated with the gram-negative diplococcus *Neisseria gonorrhoeae*.

Etiology and clinical manifestations. In gonorrhea, disease transmission occurs through contact with exudates from the mucous membranes of infected persons, usually by direct contact. The gonococcus then attaches to and penetrates columnar epithelium and produces a patchy inflammatory response in the submucosa. Although usually asymptomatic in women, gonorrhea may produce purulent vaginal discharge, dysuria, and abnormal vaginal bleeding. The most commonly affected areas in women are the cervix, the urethra, the Skene and Bartholin glands, and the anus. Among females, adolescents (ages 15 to 19 years) and young adults (ages 20 to 24 years) now have the highest rates of gonorrhea.[3] In men, symptoms of urethritis, including dysuria and a purulent urethral discharge accompanied by redness and swelling at the site of infection, usually occur after a 3- to 6-day incubation period. Among males, young adults (ages 20 to 24 years) have the highest rates of gonorrhea.[3] In both genders, infection and inflammation of the pharynx, conjunctivae, and anus may be present. Direct extension of the infection with gonococci occurs by way of the lymphatic system. In the female, extension may spread unilaterally or bilaterally to the oviducts, with subsequent salpingitis. In the male, direct extension of the infection most frequently occurs to the epididymis.[1,3]

Once gonococcal infection has spread to other areas, localized infection occurs and may cause the formation of cysts and abscesses. Purulent exudate containing the organism causes damage to tissue, and fibrous tissue replaces inflamed tissue. This hardened, fibrous tissue may result in scarring and narrowing of the urethra, epididymis, or oviducts. In women, partial or complete closure of the oviducts results in sterility. Infection of the oviducts may also result in pelvic inflammatory disease if exudate is released into the peritoneal cavity.[1,5,6] As described in Chapter 33, pelvic inflammatory disease may be an acute or chronic condition causing widespread damage to the pelvic organs in the female.

Nongonococcal Infection

Etiology. Nongonococcal urethritis and cervicitis are often caused by strains of *C. trachomatis* that act on columnar epithelium in a manner similar to that noted for the gonococcus. The symptoms of infection with *Chlamydia* are generally less severe than those of gonorrhea. As with gonorrhea, the infection may spread by extension to the oviducts, and pelvic inflammatory disease may eventually result. Upper reproductive tract infection, whether symptomatic or subclinical, is an important cause of infertility and ectopic pregnancy.[7] Transmission of *Chlamydia* during birth may result in **ophthalmia neonatorum,** or infection of the eyes in the newborn.[1]

Treatment. The resistance of *N. gonorrhoeae* to antimicrobial agents continues to spread and intensify. Newer antimicrobial agents such as ceftriaxone, cefixime, spectinomycin, and cephalosporin are now being used to manage uncomplicated gonococcal infections. In 2007 the Centers for Disease Control and Prevention no longer recommended fluoroquinolones for treatment of gonococcal infections because of fluoroquinolone resistance to *N. gonorrheae*.[8,9] Increased resistance to cephalosporin is also currently being monitored.[10,11] Unless chlamydial infection is ruled out, dual therapy for gonococcal and chlamydial infection consisting of azithromycin or doxycycline added to one of the aforementioned agents is recommended.[8] Pelvic inflammatory disease is also generally managed with two agents to cover potential chlamydial and gonorrheal infection. A number of organizations now recommend *Chlamydia* (as well as gonorrhea) screening for sexually active adolescents and women through age 25 who have no symptoms in order to reduce the sequelae of infection.[12]

> **KEY POINTS**
> - Urethritis, cervicitis, salpingitis, and pelvic inflammatory disease are commonly due to gonorrheal or chlamydial infection. Transmission is usually by direct contact with infected mucous membranes. The symptoms of chlamydial infection are similar but usually less severe than those of gonorrhea.
> - Gonorrhea may produce purulent discharge, dysuria, and abnormal vaginal bleeding. Cysts and abscesses may form in localized areas of infection, followed by scarring and fibrosis. Inflammation of the pharynx, conjunctivae, and anus may be present. Antibiotic therapy is indicated.

DISEASES WITH SYSTEMIC INVOLVEMENT

Several STIs cause a distinctive ulcerative lesion and disseminate throughout the body to affect multiple organ systems. Most prominent of this type of STI are syphilis, herpesvirus infections, and lymphogranuloma venereum.

Syphilis

Syphilis is a systemic infection of the vascular system consisting of five distinct stages: incubation, primary and secondary stages, latency, and late syphilis.[3] Syphilis is communicable by persons with primary, secondary, or early latent syphilis.[1,3] The incidence of syphilis has varied in the United States since reporting began in 1941. The rate of primary and secondary syphilis decreased during the 1990s to its lowest levels since 1941. However, overall rates increased again between 2001 and 2009, before decreasing again in 2010.[4] Increased incidence rates were attributed primarily to men who have sex with men (MSM) and to men and women who engage in high-risk sexual behavior.[4] An

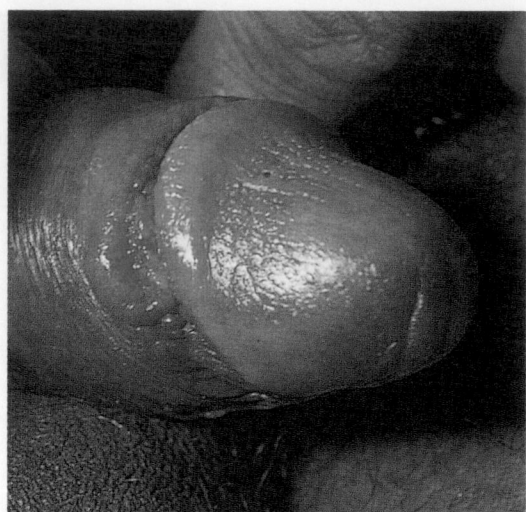

FIGURE 34-1 Typical syphilitic chancre, a painless, ulcerative lesion that arises at the original spirochete portal of entry. (From Morse SA et al: *Atlas of sexually transmitted diseases and AIDS*, ed 4, St Louis, 2010, Elsevier.)

estimated 1.1 cases of primary and secondary syphilis per 100,000 population occurred in 2010.[4]

Etiology. Syphilis is caused by *Treponema pallidum*, an anaerobic spirochete. Syphilis is acquired when *T. pallidum* penetrates intact mucous membranes or abraded skin during sexual contact. (The process of transmission of congenital syphilis is described later.) Some of the *T. pallidum* pathogens remain at the original invasion site, whereas others migrate to regional lymph nodes within hours. During this incubation phase, *T. pallidum* is disseminated throughout the body and can invade and multiply in any organ system.[1,3]

Pathogenesis. During all stages of syphilis, invasion of tissue by *T. pallidum* results in pathologic changes in the vascular system. The inflammatory response in endothelial tissue causes the infiltration of lymphocytes and plasma cells, with subsequent endothelial swelling. The terminal arterioles and small arteries may become obliterated and no longer functional. Finally, long-term inflammation of vascular tissue results in the formation of hardened, fibrous thickening in the blood vessels and eventually tissue necrosis.[1,3]

After the initial incubation period of 10 to 90 days, the primary phase begins with the formation of a **chancre,** a painless, ulcerative lesion that arises at the original spirochete portal of entry (Figure 34-1). The chancre may remain unnoticed in a female if it occurs on the cervix or in the vagina; in fact, most cases of syphilis in women are undiagnosed until recognized by positive testing of the blood in the latent phase. In males, the chancre may form on the genitalia; in both genders, chancres may erupt on the anus, fingers, lips, tongue, nipples, tonsils, or eyelids.[1,3]

Untreated chancres will resolve spontaneously within 3 to 6 weeks and are followed by the secondary stage of syphilis, which is characterized by a low-grade fever, malaise, sore throat, headache, lymphadenopathy, and mucosal or cutaneous rash (Figure 34-2). This secondary stage occurs as *T. pallidum* is spread throughout the bloodstream and lymphatic system. The secondary stage is also self-limiting and is followed by a latent phase in which no symptoms are present. During the latent stage, the affected person will test positive for syphilis on serologic assays and may still experience infectious mucocutaneous lesions during the early latent stage. Thus, the early latent stage is considered contagious. The latent stage is of variable length and may last more than 40 years.[2] In approximately two thirds of patients, the infection

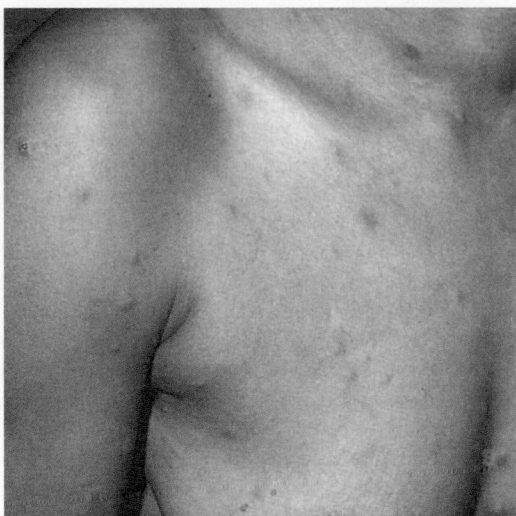

FIGURE 34-2 Typical generalized skin rash of secondary syphilis. (From Morse SA et al: *Atlas of sexually transmitted diseases and AIDS*, ed 4, St Louis, 2010, Elsevier.)

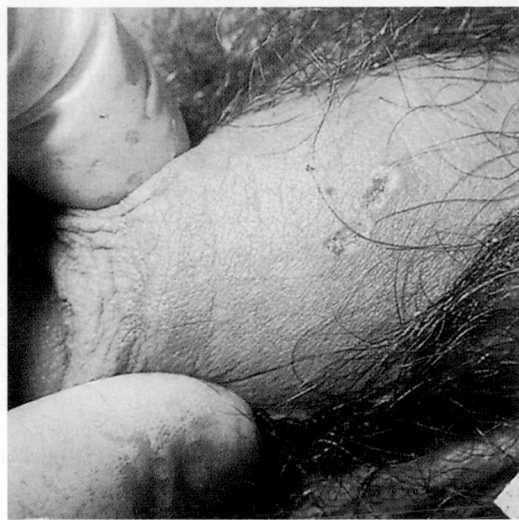

FIGURE 34-3 Lymphogranuloma venereum is characterized by a small, transient genital ulcer with swollen, extremely painful inguinal lymph nodes. (From Lewis SM et al: *Medical surgical nursing*, ed 6, St Louis, 2004, Mosby, p 1392.)

remains asymptomatic and never causes a recurrence of symptoms. If syphilis remains untreated, then late syphilis—the final, destructive phase of the disease—will eventually develop in approximately one third of affected people.[1,3] The manifestations of late syphilis depend on the area of arterial lesions and the extent of circulatory insufficiency.[3] Body systems particularly at risk are the cardiovascular and central nervous systems. Damage to the cardiovascular system may include aortic necrosis and subsequent aortic insufficiency; damage to the central nervous system may be progressively widespread, with degeneration of the cortical neurons and, eventually, paresis, blindness, and mental deterioration.[1,3]

Transmission of *T. pallidum* from the mother to the fetus may occur transplacentally at any point during pregnancy, but an inflammatory response to the pathogen does not develop in the fetus until around the fifteenth week of gestation. Therefore, treatment of infected women before the fifteenth week may prevent damage to the fetus. Infection with syphilis before birth may result in physical deformities and developmental disabilities in the infant. Infants born to untreated or inadequately treated mothers will have active infection and must be treated.[1] A presumptive diagnosis of syphilis is generally based on a positive result of a serologic screening test, such as the Venereal Disease Research Laboratories (VDRL) or rapid plasma reagin (RPR) test, followed by a positive result of a treponemal serologic test.[9] Dark-field examination of tissue and exudates or direct fluorescent antibody tests are also useful.

Treatment. Penicillin G is the first choice for the management of syphilis. If the affected person is allergic to penicillin, tetracycline or doxycycline is given. Treatment is administered to all individuals with positive evidence of syphilis on laboratory testing and to people who have had sexual contact with infected individuals.[1,4] Response to antibiotic treatment is monitored by repeating laboratory testing for evidence of syphilis at regular intervals up to 24 months after therapy.[8] Management during pregnancy is complex, but it focuses on maternal cure and prevention of congenital syphilis.[13]

Lymphogranuloma Venereum

Lymphogranuloma venereum (LGV) is a highly contagious systemic infection caused by a number of closely related strains of *Chlamydia*. The disease occurs more commonly in the tropics but has been

reported rarely in the United States.[14] LGV develops more often in males than in females and has a higher incidence among sexually active young adults.

Etiology and pathogenesis. Like syphilis, LGV has stages of development in which an initial lesion forms and systemic disease occurs after dissemination via the lymphatic system. After invasion of the mucosa by *Chlamydia* during sexual contact, a painless lesion appears on the genitalia after a 1- to 3-week incubation period. The lesion may range from a slight erosion to a small papule and often remains undetected (Figure 34-3). This lesion heals spontaneously in a few days. During this period, the pathogens are disseminated to regional lymph nodes, primarily the inguinal lymph nodes.

About 2 weeks after appearance of the primary lesion, the inguinal lymph nodes begin to swell, and the systemic symptoms of fever and malaise develop. The nodal swelling is a manifestation of inflammation of the lymphatic system in which lesions filled with polymorphonuclear leukocytes are forming in the lymph nodes. Spread of the inflammation throughout adjacent lymph nodes causes multiple nodes to become matted together and form a large abscess. These abscesses are said to be regional because they develop in one or more areas along the lymphatic system. If a person with LGV remains untreated, the abscesses rupture through the skin and other body cavities to create chronic fistulas. Thus, as the regional lymphadenitis progresses, complications such as perianal and rectovaginal fistulas develop, along with strictures of the rectum. Other complications include extreme swelling of the genitalia; this occurs because the normal lymph drainage of this area is impeded.[9] The diagnosis is usually made by serologic testing (antibody titers).

Treatment. Doxycycline is the recommended antibiotic with erythromycin being the alternative. Surgical treatment may include aspiration of lymph nodes as needed; rectal strictures and fistulas may require surgical correction.[9]

Herpesvirus Infections

Herpesviruses are an important group of viral agents that produce infection in humans. Two types of herpes simplex virus (HSV)—type 1 and type 2—may be sexually transmitted and are discussed in this section. HSV type 1 is most often associated with herpetic infections above the waist, typically in the oral cavity and on the lips, but also in the eyes or on the epidermis. HSV type 1 can be transmitted sexually and can cause genital herpetic infections. It is present in saliva, stool, and urine. The vesicles resulting from type 1 infection in the oral cavity are commonly referred to as *cold sores* or *chancres* and often affect children younger than 5 years.[1,3] HSV type 2 is implicated in most genital, anal, and perianal herpes and is sometimes referred to as *genital herpes* for this reason. Type 2 HSV can also result in oral lesions after sexual contact. Serologic studies indicate that one in five individuals in the United States have been infected with type 2 HSV.[4] Although type 2 is primarily transmitted through sexual contact, pregnant mothers can transmit the infection to newborns during vaginal delivery.[1,3]

Etiology. HSV types 1 and 2 have certain characteristics in common. Both produce an initial infection that is self-limiting. The lesions produced by this infection heal, but HSV continues to be present in the body. Recurrence of the lesions, usually in the area of the initial infection, may take place as the virus is reactivated. Recurrence of either type may be triggered by an infectious disease, emotional stress, or immunosuppression.[1,3] The exact mechanism for reactivation of the virus is presently unknown, but it is thought that ganglion neurons may contain latent forms of the virus and then receive a trigger to stimulate replication of the virus under certain conditions.[1,3]

Clinical manifestations. Genital infection with HSV type 2 is manifested by the appearance of fluid-filled vesicles after a 3- to 7-day incubation period. In the female, the cervix is usually the primary infection site, although the labia, perianal skin, vulva, or vagina may also be involved (Figure 34-4). In the male, the vesicles are located on the glans penis, foreskin, or penile shaft (Figure 34-5). Extragenital lesions may appear on the mouth or anus. In both males and females, the vesicles, which are usually painless at first, may rupture and develop into extensive shallow, painful ulcers. The virus may enter the lymphatic system and create localized lesions there; thus, the inguinal lymph nodes may be edematous and tender. Rarely, the virus spreads to visceral organs and can produce areas of necrosis in the liver, adrenal glands, lungs, and central nervous system.[3] In newborns and people with weak immune defenses (particularly people with acquired immunodeficiency syndrome [AIDS]), HSV type 2 may result in severe damage to these organ systems, with high related mortality.[1] Most human immunodeficiency virus (HIV)-infected individuals are HSV-2 seropositive, and perirectal involvement is common.[15,16]

HSV type 1 infections may appear as single or multiple fluid-filled, tender vesicles in the oral cavity or on the lips. Usually, the appearance of the lesions is preceded by 1 or 2 days of paresthesia before the chancre or "cold sore" erupts. These lesions will generally crust and heal within 3 to 10 days. HSV infections are usually diagnosed by cell culture.[2] Exudate from early lesions gives the most positive results.

Treatment. Normally, HSV type 1 lesions are self-limiting and respond to measures that promote good oral hygiene. HSV type 2 genital lesions are usually self-limiting but may be extremely painful. The use of antiviral agents such as acyclovir, famciclovir, and valacyclovir has been shown to accelerate healing time and reduce the duration and severity of symptoms in initial episodes of HSV type 2 infection.[8,16-18] Long-term or episodic suppression may also be used to reduce the number or severity of recurrent episodes.[8,18] Consistent use of condoms reduces transmission from men to women.[15,19] Prevention teaching should include the possibility of asymptomatic shedding of the virus.[16-19] If HSV type 2 lesions are active in a pregnant mother at term, a cesarean section may be recommended to reduce the risk of transmission to the newborn.[8]

KEY POINTS

- Syphilis is caused by an anaerobic spirochete that is transmitted sexually but disseminates throughout the body during incubation. Manifestations of early syphilis include chancre formation at the portal of entry, which spontaneously resolves in 3 to 6 weeks if untreated. General malaise, fever, sore throat, and rash may then occur, followed by an asymptomatic latent phase. The latent phase may last more than 40 years. Late syphilis is characterized by central nervous system degeneration, blindness, and paresis.

- LGV is a highly contagious systemic infection caused by strains of *Chlamydia*. An initial painless genital lesion appears after 1 to 3 weeks of incubation. The infection spreads to regional lymph nodes and is accompanied by fever and malaise. Infected lymph nodes become abscessed and may rupture through the skin and body cavities, causing fistula formation.

- HSV types 1 and 2 are implicated in cases of genital herpes. Herpes lesions are fluid-filled vesicles that appear 3 to 7 days after infection. The virus may enter the lymphatics and cause inguinal lymph node tenderness. Although the lesions may disappear, the virus remains in the body, thus predisposing to recurrence. Herpes may be transmitted from mother to newborn during the birth process.

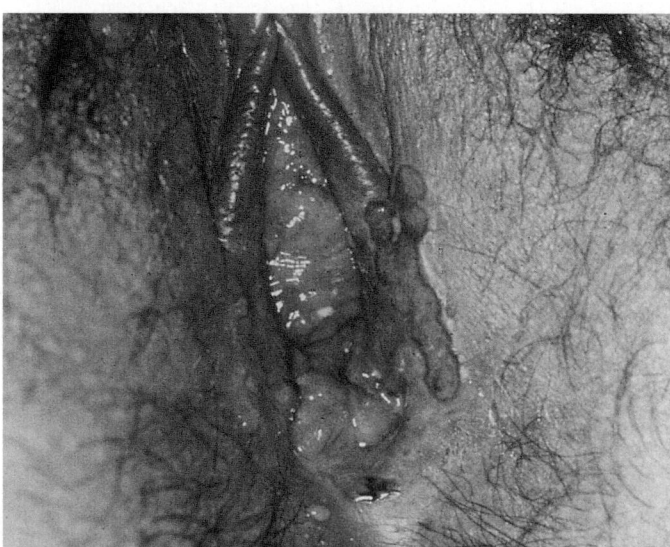

FIGURE 34-4 Primary genital herpes in the female showing herpetic vesicles and tender ulcerations. (From Morse SA et al: *Atlas of sexually transmitted diseases and AIDS*, ed 4, St Louis, 2010, Elsevier.)

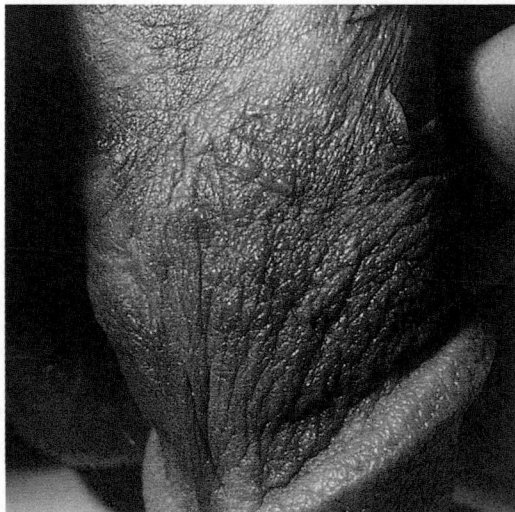

FIGURE 34-5 Recurrent genital herpes in the male showing erythema, groups of vesicles, erosions, and edema on the shaft of the penis. (From Morse SA et al: *Atlas of sexually transmitted diseases and AIDS*, ed 4, St Louis, 2010, Elsevier.)

DISEASES WITH LOCALIZED LESIONS

Ulcerative Lesions

Two types of STIs result in the formation of ulcerative lesions but do not progress to systemic involvement. **Chancroid** (also called soft chancre) and **granuloma inguinale** are both manifested by ulcerative lesions, although their pathophysiologic courses differ.

Chancroid

Etiology. Chancroid is an ulcerative, infectious disease of the genital tract caused by the sexually transmitted anaerobic bacillus *Haemophilus ducreyi*. Chancroid is relatively rare in the United States.[4] Chancroid is a cofactor for human immunodeficiency virus infection.

Pathogenesis and clinical manifestations. *Haemophilus ducreyi* initially invades the genital skin or mucous membranes at sites traumatized by sexual contact. The patient generally has one or more painful genital ulcers, unlike the chancre in syphilis, which is generally solitary and painless. Fresh lesions may occur from autoinoculation (self-infection). The ulcerated lesions may enlarge, continue to erode (Figure 34-6), and produce destruction of surrounding tissue. In addition, inguinal lymph nodes may become tender and painful as the infection is disseminated to this region. If the infection goes untreated, the enlarged lymph gland (called a *bubo*) may rupture, draining pus and leaving a large inguinal ulcer. The infection is communicable until the lesions heal, which may be a period of weeks.[1] Scarring may occur in advanced cases. Diagnosis is usually made by culture for *H. ducreyi*.

Treatment. Antiinfective agents recommended for management of chancroid include azithromycin, erythromycin, ceftriaxone, and ciprofloxacin.[8] Large ulcers may not heal for more than 2 weeks. As with all STIs, sexual partners should be treated simultaneously and reexposure avoided until therapy is completed.

Granuloma Inguinale

Etiology. *Calymmatobacterium granulomatis* is the causative agent of granuloma inguinale. This intracellular bacterium is also referred to as a *Donovan body* and the disease as *donovanosis*. Granuloma inguinale is rare in the United States.[4]

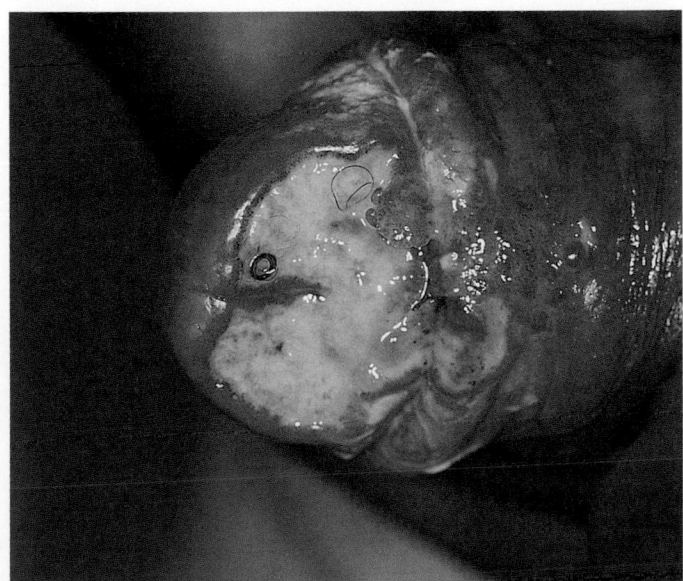

FIGURE 34-6 Eroded, purulent ulcer of chancroid. (From Morse SA et al: *Atlas of sexually transmitted diseases and AIDS*, ed 4, St Louis, 2010, Elsevier.)

Pathogenesis and clinical manifestations. Transmission of granuloma inguinale is not clearly understood. It is generally thought to be an STI, but the disease is also seen in adults who are not sexually active and in young children, possibly as a result of autoinoculation. The causative bacterium is found in the rectum of nondiseased persons, which suggests that the organism may be part of the normal gastrointestinal flora in some persons.[1]

The incubation period is variable and ranges from a few days to months. The initial sign of the disease may be a painless papule or nodule that subsequently ulcerates into an enlarging, granulomatous, red velvety ulcer. The raised mass of granulation tissue may look more like a tumor than an ulcer. The lesions are highly vascular and bleed easily with minor contact. Single or multiple lesions may coalesce, or lesions may spread to nearby tissue.[1,3] Secondary infection of the ulcers and expanding tissue necrosis in lesions may lead to erosion of the genitals.[3] Diagnosis is by identification of the dark-staining Donovan bodies on biopsy or tissue crush preparations.

Treatment. Doxycycline is given for at least 3 weeks or until all lesions are healed.[8] Alternative agents include trimethoprim-sulfamethoxazole, ciprofloxacin, erythromycin, and azithromycin.[8]

Nonulcerative Lesions

Molluscum contagiosum and infections caused by human papillomavirus (HPV) (also called genital warts) are two prevalent types of STIs that produce nonulcerative lesions. Both are caused by viral agents that invade superficial layers of the epidermis during sexual contact.

Molluscum Contagiosum

Etiology. **Molluscum contagiosum** is a viral skin disease caused by a member of the poxvirus family.[3] (The term *poxvirus* refers to a viral agent that causes an eruption, or "pox," on the skin.) The manifestations are much milder than those of smallpox or chickenpox. Two forms of the disease exist. One affects children and is transmitted by skin-to-skin contact and indirect contact; the other affects young adults and is transmitted during sexual contact.

Pathogenesis and clinical manifestations. After invasion of the epidermis by the virus, pink to white lesions with an exudative core appear on the genitalia. The lesions are multiple, are slow to develop, and remain stable for long periods. The disease is usually asymptomatic.

Treatment. The goal of treatment is primarily to prevent spread of the infection for cosmetic reasons. The lesions can be removed by minor surgery or frozen with liquid nitrogen. Sexual contacts of affected persons should be examined to prevent further spread.[3]

Human Papillomavirus Infections

Etiology. **Human papillomavirus (HPV) infections** cause epithelial lesions of the anogenital region.[1] Also called *genital warts* or *Condylomata acuminata*, HPV is predominantly transmitted sexually in young adults, with the highest prevalence in the 16- to 25-year-old age group.[4] The risk of contracting the disease by sexual contact with an infected person is high; lesions will develop in up to two thirds of the sexual contacts of affected persons. Nonsexual transmission has also been documented, and lesions have been found in infants.[1] The period of communicability is unknown but is thought to last as long as the lesions persist, and perhaps even after they are clinically removed.[1,3]

Pathogenesis and clinical manifestations. After invasion of the epidermis by HPV, an incubation period of 1 to 20 months (usually about 4 months) precedes the appearance of lesions. It is thought that the virus infects single epithelial cells and stimulates the cells to divide and proliferate into the wartlike lesions. The lesions can be single or multiple, and may have a soft pink to brown coloring. They can be small or large, and raised or flat (Figure 34-7). The lesions are generally

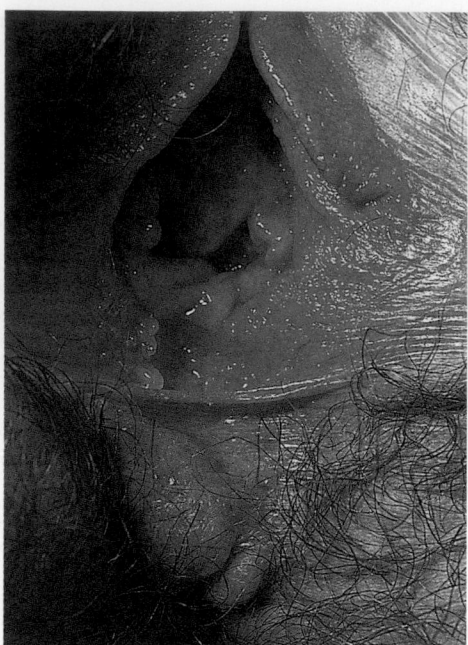

FIGURE 34-7 Human papillomavirus of the vulva. (From Morse SA et al: *Atlas of sexually transmitted diseases and AIDS*, ed 4, St Louis, 2010, Elsevier.)

asymptomatic but may be pruritic (itchy), painful, or friable (bleed easily). In females, HPV may be found in the vagina and cervix, as well as in the anogenital area.[1] In males, HPV lesions may occur in the anterior urethra and anogenital area.

Treatment. External genital warts may be treated with patient-applied podofilox or imiquimod topical preparations.[8] Providers can perform cryotherapy; administer podophyllin, trichloroacetic acid, or bichloroacetic acid; or carry out surgical excision of the warts.[8] Patient-applied preparations are also available, and include podofilox (0.5%) and imiquimod (5%) cream. Alternative regimens include intralesional interferon and laser surgery. Malignant transformation to invasive carcinoma has been observed with some types of genital warts. Persistent infections of HPV types 6, 11, 16, and 18 are thought to be responsible for 70% of cervical cancers and 90% of genital warts. Therefore, it is generally agreed that affected persons should be treated or monitored carefully.[8] Because HPV has been associated with cervical cancer, there has been an increasing use of human *papillomavirus* testing in evaluating abnormal Papanicolaou smears.[3]

In 2006 the Food and Drug Administration (FDA) licensed the first vaccine developed to prevent cervical cancer and other diseases in females caused by certain types of human papillomavirus (HPV) (see Chapter 33). The HPV quadrivalent vaccine is recommended for 11- to 12-year-old girls, but can be administered to girls as young as 9 years of age. The vaccine also is recommended for 13- to 26-year-old females who have not yet received or completed the vaccine series. Ideally, the vaccine should be administered before onset of sexual activity. However, females who are sexually active also may benefit from vaccination.[20,21] Recent 4-year follow-up research suggests that the vaccine is safe and tolerated well.[22] Researchers are also reporting promising results of studies examining the efficacy of the HPV quadrivalent vaccine in males.[23]

> **KEY POINTS**
> - Chancroid is caused by infection with an anaerobic bacillus. Initially the lesion is a small erythematous papule, and after 2 to 3 days the painful lesion ulcerates. Lesions resemble those of syphilis; however, the lesions of syphilis are painless.
> - Granuloma inguinale is caused by an intracellular bacterium. The initial papule is painless and subsequently ulcerates into a growing granulomatous ulcer resembling a tumor.
> - Molluscum contagiosum is associated with infection by a poxvirus. Genital lesions are pink to white with an exudative core. The disease is usually asymptomatic and self-limiting.
> - Condylomata acuminata, or genital warts, are associated with infection by human papillomavirus. Warts are pink to brown and painless and may occur in clusters. Persistent human papillomavirus infection is an important risk factor for cervical cancer.

ENTERIC INFECTIONS

Until recently, information regarding the transmission of enteric infections of the gastrointestinal tract through sexual contact was limited. Enteric pathogens may be transmitted sexually among any individuals who engage in direct or indirect fecal-oral contact. Enteric organisms that may be transmitted through sexual contact include *Giardia, Campylobacter, Shigella,* and the agents causing amebic dysentery.[8]

The pathophysiologic process of enteric infections of the gastrointestinal tract is described in Chapter 36, and the reader may wish to refer to this material. In general, persons who have acquired enteric infections by sexual contact will have variable manifestations. Some individuals may experience no symptoms, whereas others will have marked symptoms of enteritis or proctitis. All individuals who engage in oral-anal sexual practices should be monitored for the presence of enteric infections with laboratory studies and diagnostic examinations. Education for persons at risk for sexually transmitted enteric infections includes an emphasis on protective hygienic practices. Infected persons should avoid all sexual contact until all partners are examined and treated if necessary. After completion of appropriate therapy for enteric infections, affected individuals should be retested for assessment of therapeutic effectiveness.

▮ S U M M A R Y

Because of the epidemic nature of STIs, it is essential for readers preparing for careers in the health sciences to have a complete grasp of the material in this chapter. The STIs considered in the chapter are grouped according to the disease manifestations that the patient is most likely to exhibit. Gonorrhea, most chlamydial infections, and pelvic inflammatory disease are manifested by urethritis, cervicitis, or salpingitis. A second group of STIs cause ulcerative lesions with systemic involvement. Syphilis, herpes, and LGV all cause a distinctive ulcerative lesion and may disseminate throughout the body to affect multiple organ systems.

In reviewing the material on STIs related to ulcerative and nonulcerative lesions, the reader should compare and contrast the appearance of these lesions and consider the differing pathophysiologic characteristics of each type. Finally, the reader should consider how he or she would incorporate this material into an overall assessment process. Nurses and other health care providers caring for persons at risk for STIs should be aware of the potential for acquisition of these diseases as well. The overall goal in learning the material in this chapter is to be able to assess and educate clients with STIs in a comfortable and accurate manner.

REFERENCES

1. Holmes KK, et al, editors: *Sexually transmitted diseases*, ed 4, New York, 2007, McGraw-Hill.
2. Eng TR, Butler WT, editors: *The hidden epidemic: confronting sexually transmitted diseases*, Washington, DC, 1997, Institute of Medicine.
3. Zenilman JM, Shahmanesh M: *Sexually transmitted infections: diagnosis, management, and treatment*, Sudbury, MA, 2011, Jones and Bartlett Learning.
4. Centers for Disease Control and Prevention: *Sexually transmitted disease surveillance 2010*, Atlanta, 2011, U.S. Department of Health and Human Services.
5. Horner PJ, et al: Gonorrhoea: signs, symptoms, and serogroups, *Int J STD AIDS* 3(6):430–433, 1992.
6. Hacker NF, et al, editors: *Essentials of obstetrics and gynecology*, Philadelphia, 2009, Saunders.
7. Jossens MO, Schacter J, Sweet RL: Risk factors associated with pelvic inflammatory disease of differing microbial etiologies, *Obstet Gynecol* 83(6):989–997, 1994.
8. Centers for Disease Control and Prevention: Sexually transmitted diseases treatment guidelines, 2010, *MMWR Morb Mortal Wkly Rep* 59(no. RR-12):1–110, 2010.
9. Centers for Disease Control and Prevention: Update to CDC's sexually transmitted diseases treatment guidelines, 2006: fluoroquinolones no longer recommended for treatment of gonococcal infections, *MMWR Morb Mortal Wkly Rep* 56(14):332–336, 2007.
10. Kirkcaldy RD, Ballard RC, Dowell D: Gonococcal resistance: are cephalosporins next? *Curr Infect Dis Rep* 13:196–204, 2011.
11. Centers for Disease Control and Prevention: Cephalosporin susceptibility among *Neisseria gonorrhoeae* isolates—United States, 2000-2010, *MMWR Morb Mortal Wkly Rep* 60:873–877, 2011.
12. U.S. Preventive Services Task Force: Screening for chlamydial infection: recommendations and rationale, *Am J Prev Med* 20(3S):90–94, 2001.
13. Wendel GD, et al: Treatment of syphilis in pregnancy and prevention of congenital syphilis, *Clin Infect Dis* 35(suppl 2):S200–S209, 2002.
14. Centers for Disease Control and Prevention: Lymphogranuloma venereum among men who have sex with men: Netherlands, 2003-2004, *MMWR Morb Mortal Wkly Rep* 53(42):985–988, 2004.
15. Centers for Disease Control and Prevention: Guidelines for prevention and treatment of opportunistic infections in HIV-infected adults and adolescents, *MMWR Morb Mortal Wkly Rep* 58(no. RR-4), 2009.
16. Schacker T, et al: Frequency of symptomatic and asymptomatic herpes simplex type 2 reactivations among human immunodeficiency virus-infected men, *J Infect Dis* 178:1616–1622, 1998.
17. Mostad MB, et al: Cervical shedding of herpes simplex virus in human immunodeficiency virus–infected women: effects of hormonal contraception, pregnancy, and vitamin A deficiency, *J Infect Dis* 181:58–63, 2000.
18. Corey L: Challenges in genital herpes simplex virus management, *J Infect Dis* 186(suppl 1):S29–S33, 2002.
19. Wald A, et al: Effect of condoms on reducing the transmission of herpes simplex virus type-2 from men to women, *JAMA* 285:3100–3106, 2001.
20. Koutsky LA, et al: A controlled trial of a human papillomavirus type 16 vaccine, *N Engl J Med* 347:1645–1651, 2002.
21. Markowitz LE, et al: Quadrivalent human papilloma virus vaccine: recommendations of the advisory committee on immunization practices, *MMWR Morb Mortal Wkly Rep* 56(RR02):1–24, 2007.
22. Schwarz TF, et al: Four-year follow-up of the immunogenicity and safety of the HPV-16/18 AS04-adjuvanted vaccine when administered to adolescent girls aged 10-14 years, *J Adolesc Health* 50(2):187–194, 2012.
23. Giuliano AR, et al: Efficacy of quadrivalent HPV vaccine against HPV infection and disease in males, *N Engl J Med* 363(5):401–411, 2011.

Gastrointestinal Function

Jeffrey S. Sartin

evolve WEBSITE

http://evolve.elsevier.com/Copstead/
- Review Questions and Answers
- Glossary (with audio pronunciations for selected terms)
- Animations
- Case Studies
- Key Points Review

KEY QUESTIONS

- What are the major structures of the gastrointestinal tract and their corresponding functions?
- How does the autonomic nervous system influence gastrointestinal motility?
- How do segmental and propulsive movements influence the digestive and absorptive functions of the small intestine?
- What are the major secretions of each of the following secretory cells and glands: salivary, gastric, intestinal epithelium, pancreas, and gallbladder?
- How and where are complex carbohydrates, proteins, and lipids digested and absorbed?
- How and where are water and electrolytes absorbed?
- What alterations in gastrointestinal function occur in association with very young or very old age?

CHAPTER OUTLINE

CHAPTER OUTLINE—cont'd

The gastrointestinal (GI) system represents a remarkable interface between the human organism and the external environment for the purpose of providing nutrients for the body. The components of the GI tract can be thought of as a continuous tube about 7 m in length extending from the mouth to the anus. Beginning with the mouth and pharynx, the GI tract includes the esophagus, stomach, and small and large intestines (Figure 35-1). Other parts of the GI system located outside the GI tract include the salivary glands, the pancreas, and the biliary system (liver, gallbladder, and bile ducts).

The process of ingesting nutrients, propelling them through the GI tract, and transforming them into a form capable of absorption into the body's internal milieu is remarkably complex. The general functions of the GI tract can be divided into (1) movement of nutrients, including propulsive and mixing movements; (2) secretion of digestive

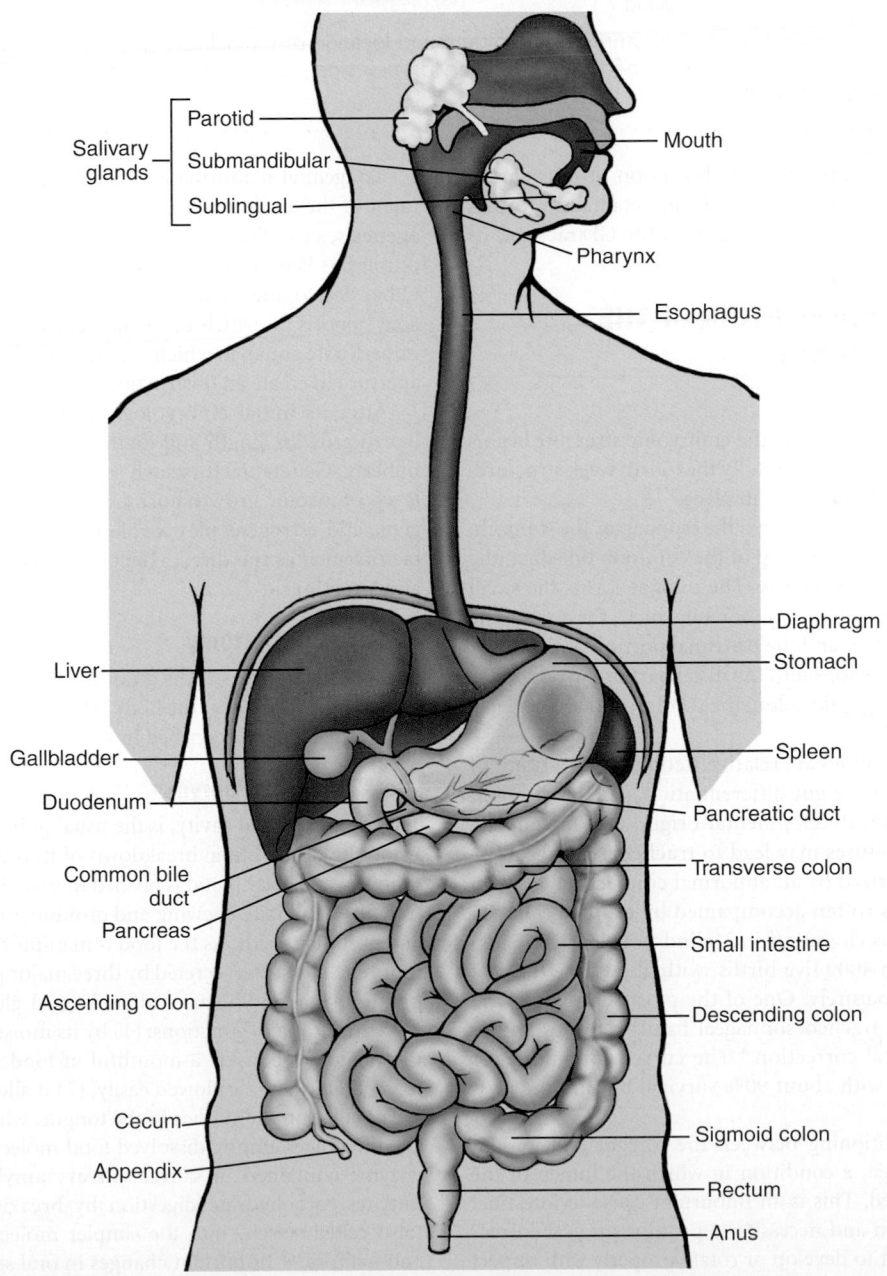

FIGURE 35-1 The gastrointestinal system. (From Monahan FD, Neighbors M: *Medical surgical nursing: foundations for clinical practice*, ed 2, Philadelphia, 1998, Saunders, p 950.)

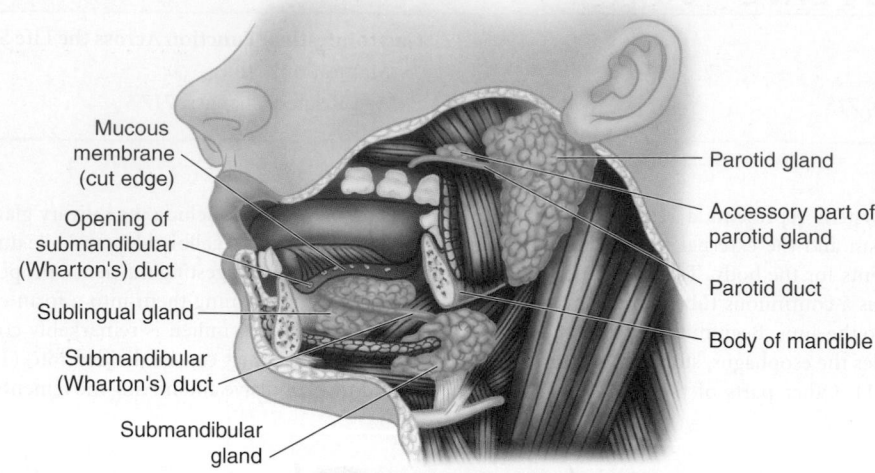

FIGURE 35-2 Oral cavity. Structures of the mouth and location of the salivary glands. (From O'Toole M, editor: *Miller-Keane encyclopedia and dictionary of medicine, nursing, and allied health*, ed 7, Philadelphia, 2003, Saunders.)

juices; (3) digestion of nutrients; and (4) absorption of nutrients.[1,2] This chapter describes each of these functions in detail and provides an overview of the structure and organization of the GI tract and its growth and alteration across the life span.

STRUCTURE AND ORGANIZATION OF THE GASTROINTESTINAL TRACT

Embryology

As early as the third week of gestation, the embryonic structure begins to fold inward to create the primitive gut. By the fourth week structures of the foregut, midgut, and hindgut are in place.[3]

The foregut develops into the pharynx, the esophagus, the stomach, the duodenum proximal to the opening of the common bile duct, the hepatobiliary system, and the pancreas. The midgut forms the small intestine (below the opening of the common bile duct), the cecum, the appendix, the ascending colon, and the proximal portion of the transverse colon. The hindgut develops into the distal part of the transverse colon, the descending and sigmoid colon, the rectum, and the superior portion of the anal canal.

Developmental abnormalities are relatively common as a result of incomplete partitioning during gut differentiation. The trachea and esophagus share a common developmental origin, and incomplete development of these structures may lead to **tracheoesophageal fistula,** an anomaly characterized by an abnormal connection between the trachea and esophagus (often accompanied by **esophageal atresia,** where the esophagus is closed off in a blind pouch). These disorders occur in about 1 in 4000 live births, with about one third of affected infants born prematurely. One of the most serious surgical emergencies in newborns, tracheoesophageal fistula requires immediate diagnosis and surgical correction.[4] The current prognosis for such infants is very good, with about 90% survival beyond the neonatal period.

Failure of normal partitioning between the foregut and midgut can lead to intestinal atresia, a condition in which the lumen of the small intestine is obliterated. This is an important cause of intestinal obstruction in the newborn and necessitates prompt surgical correction.[4] Failure of the midgut to develop or rotate properly with respect to the umbilical cord can result in omphalocele, a congenital herniation of viscera into the base of the umbilical cord.

Congenital malformations resulting from inappropriate development of the anorectal portion of the GI tract include **colonic** or **anal agenesis,** a condition in which the rectal pouch ends blindly. This condition has been rarely reported with congenital varicella syndrome.[4] Other developmental anomalies of this portion of the GI tract include anal stenosis, in which the anal aperture is small, and anal atresia (or imperforate anus), in which the anal membrane persists and covers the aperture to create an obstruction.

After its initial embryologic development, the GI tract continues to grow in length and diameter until somatic growth ends with puberty. General factors such as adequate nutrition and appropriate levels of insulin, growth hormone, thyroid hormone, cortisol, androgens, and estrogens play a role in GI development, as well as local factors such as the direct effect of ingested nutrients, GI hormones, and secretions.[5]

Functional Anatomy

Each part of the GI tract is uniquely adapted for a specific function in providing nutrients for the body. The role of each major component of the GI tract will be described in some detail.

Oral Cavity and Pharynx

The mouth, or oral cavity, is the usual point of entry for nutrients and is the site of the initial breakdown of nutrient substances into a form usable by the body. Food is pushed toward the side of the mouth by the tongue to facilitate chewing and grinding on the surfaces of the molar and premolar teeth. As the food is manipulated and broken down, it is moistened by saliva secreted by three major pairs of salivary glands: the parotid, submandibular, and sublingual glands (Figure 35-2). Saliva serves three major functions: (1) by its moistening action, saliva allows the tongue to convert a mouthful of food into a bolus, or semisolid mass, that can be swallowed easily; (2) it allows for taste perception by the papillae on the surface of the tongue, which are sensitive to chemical differences among dissolved food molecules; and (3) the digestive enzyme contained in saliva, **salivary amylase** (also called ptyalin), initiates carbohydrate digestion by breaking down polysaccharides (also called starch) into the simpler molecular structures of dextrin and maltose.[6,7] Important changes in oral structure and function that occur with aging are detailed in Geriatric Considerations: Changes in the Mouth.

GERIATRIC CONSIDERATIONS

Changes in the Mouth

Elderly people experience a decline in taste. This decline is due to both an increase in the sensation threshold for all four tastes and a decrease in the number of papillae. For example, children have more than 200 taste buds, whereas the elderly have fewer than 100. Of the four basic tastes, elderly people experience a particular decrease in salt and sugar tastes.

Older individuals also experience a decrease in the number of acinar cells in the salivary glands, leading to a reduction in salivary secretion. These changes can contribute to halitosis (bad breath).

Loss of teeth in the elderly is due to atrophy of gum and bone tissue as well as actual tooth deterioration. As tooth enamel is destroyed, dentin is exposed, allowing development of caries (cavities). Gingival epithelial loss may occur as a result of pathologic processes as well as normal aging.

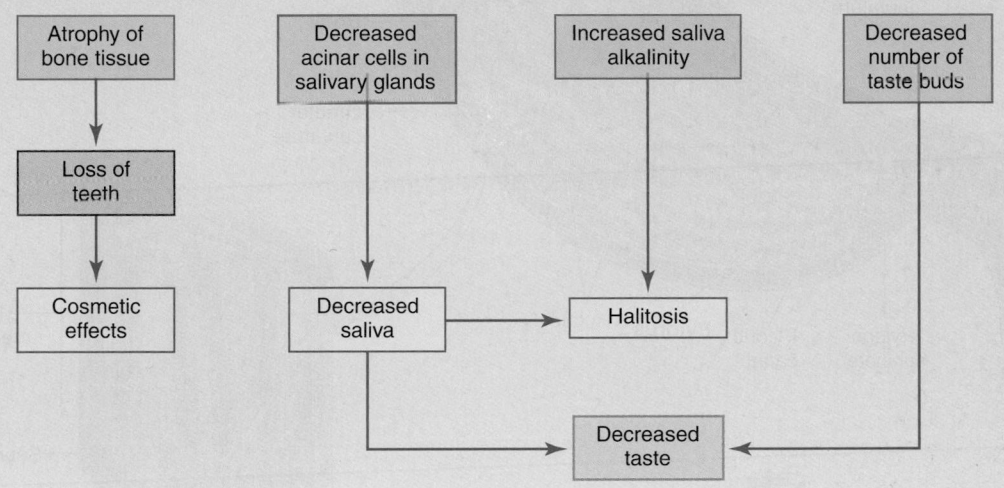

The pharynx, or throat, is about 12 cm long and serves as the entryway for both the respiratory and the GI systems. The oropharynx, the portion of the pharynx posterior to the mouth, is separated from the nasopharynx, the portion of the pharynx posterior to the nose, by the soft palate. The laryngopharynx is the portion of the pharynx that opens into the larynx and the esophagus. During swallowing, the soft palate is pulled upward to close off the nasopharynx. The bolus of food being swallowed is propelled by reflex movements of muscles in the pharynx through the laryngopharynx and into the esophagus. Simultaneously, the opening to the larynx is closed by the epiglottis. This coordinated set of actions prevents food substances and liquids from inadvertently entering the respiratory system, a potentially life-threatening occurrence referred to as aspiration.

Esophagus

The esophagus is a muscular tube approximately 25 cm in length that initiates the progress of food through the gut after ingestion. Passage of food through the esophagus is greatly facilitated by mucus secreted by cells in the epithelial lining. Extremely rough or fibrous foods may potentially penetrate the mucous lining of the esophagus and cause damage. The stratified squamous epithelium lining the esophagus is constantly renewed by cells moving to the surface from below, thus providing a means of epithelial renewal. The esophagus propels nutrients to the stomach by means of strong muscular contractions. (**Presbyesophagus,** or abnormal esophageal motility occurring with advanced age, is described in detail in the Age-Related Changes section.) When the body is in an upright position, gravity assists in the downward movement of food to the stomach. However, the muscular contractions of the esophagus are extremely strong and are sufficient to transport nutrients to the stomach even in the absence of gravity, as

persons living (and eating) in the weightless conditions of space have demonstrated.[1,3]

At the lower end of the esophagus, about 2 to 5 cm above its juncture with the stomach, the circular muscle of the esophagus functions as a sphincter; this region is referred to as the **lower esophageal sphincter (LES).** Although anatomically this sphincter is no different from the remainder of the esophagus, it remains tonically constricted, in contrast to the middle and upper portions of the esophagus, which are completely relaxed under normal conditions.[2] Thus the LES serves to prevent the highly acidic gastric contents from moving in a retrograde motion back into the esophagus. Under certain conditions the LES does not function properly, and reflux of gastric contents into the esophagus gastroesophageal reflux disease (GERD) may occur. The resulting subjective sensation of irritation and spasms of the distal portion of the esophagus is often referred to as heartburn or dyspepsia.

Stomach

The stomach (Figure 35-3) is essentially an elastic food reservoir. Under normal circumstances, its capacity is 1000 to 1500 ml, although a capacity of as much as 6000 ml is possible.[2] The portion of the stomach immediately below the LES is called the cardia. The fundus is the part of the stomach that continues lateral to and above the cardia; the body of the stomach extends from the cardia to the antrum, which stretches from the angulus to the pylorus. The antrum differs markedly from the rest of the stomach in function and is distinguished by the absence of rugae, the folds present in the mucous membrane of the other areas of the stomach. The **pylorus** is a muscular sphincter between the stomach and duodenum that serves to control gastric emptying and limits the reflux of bile from the small intestine.

The stomach is lined with simple columnar epithelium containing millions of gastric glands that extend down to the mucosa.

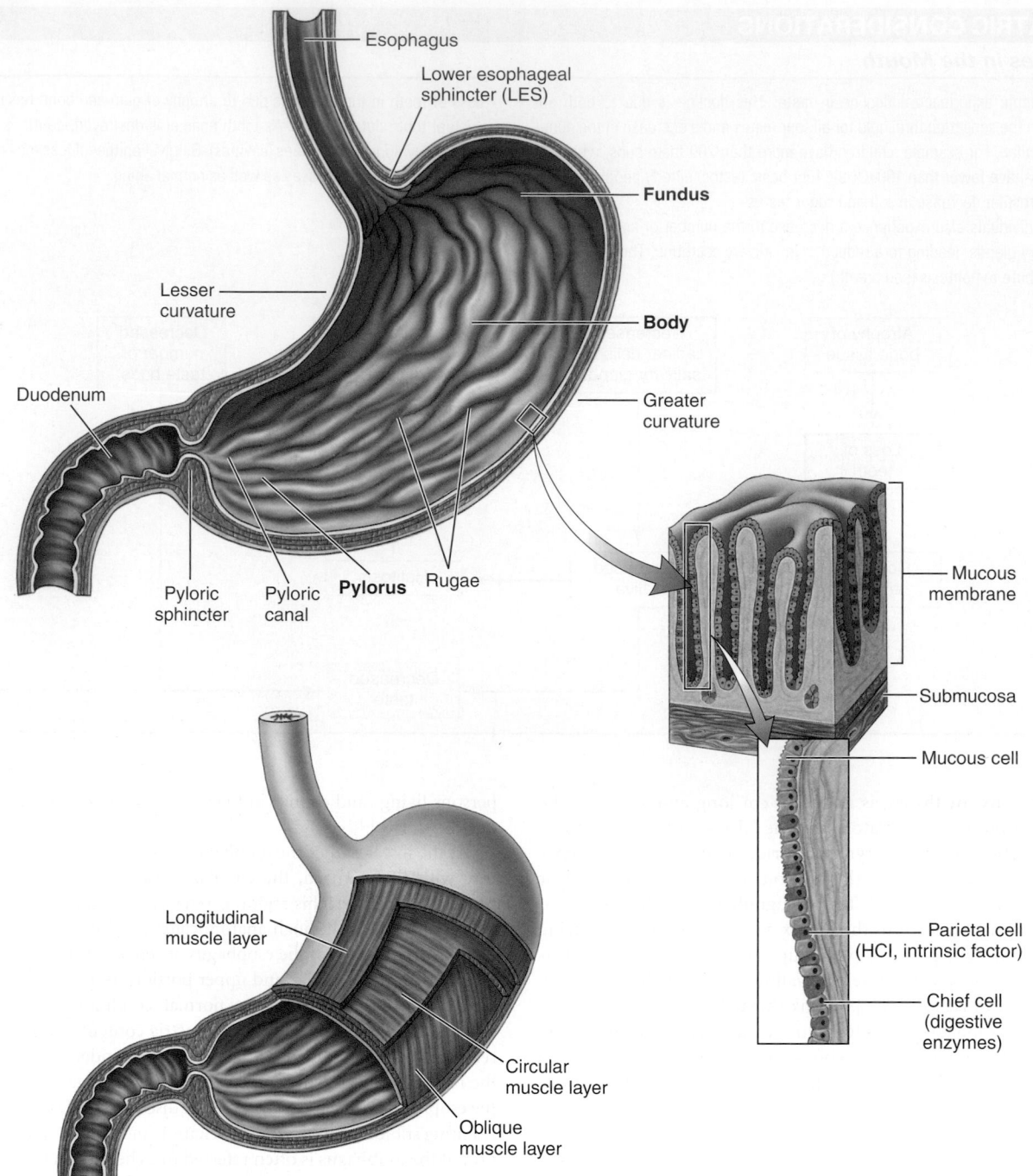

FIGURE 35-3 Physiologic anatomy of the stomach. *HCl,* Hydrochloric acid. (From Herlihy B: *The human body in health and illness,* ed 4, Philadelphia, 2011, Saunders.)

A typical gastric gland is shown in Figure 35-4. As shown in this illustration, gastric glands are lined by several types of specialized cells. Chief cells produce pepsinogen, the inactive form of the enzyme pepsin; parietal cells produce hydrochloric acid and also a substance called intrinsic factor that is needed for adequate intestinal absorption of vitamin B_{12}.[8] Mucous cells produce an alkaline mucus that serves to shield the stomach wall and neutralize the acidity in the immediate area of the lining. A layer of mucus more than 1 mm thick continuously bathes the free surfaces of the gastric epithelial lining. In addition to these cells, gastrin cells are located in the antral epithelium and have surface microvilli that monitor intragastric pH. The role of these cells and the substances they secrete in the digestion of nutrients are described in detail in the Secretory Function section.

Small Intestine

The small intestine of an adult is approximately 5 to 6 m long (the longest portion of the GI tract). The first 22 cm of the small intestine is called the duodenum; the jejunum constitutes the next 2 m, and the ileum forms the remainder. The entire inner wall of the small intestine is marked by circular folds of a mucous membrane called the plicae circulares, permanent ridges that do not lose their elasticity when the intestine is distended.

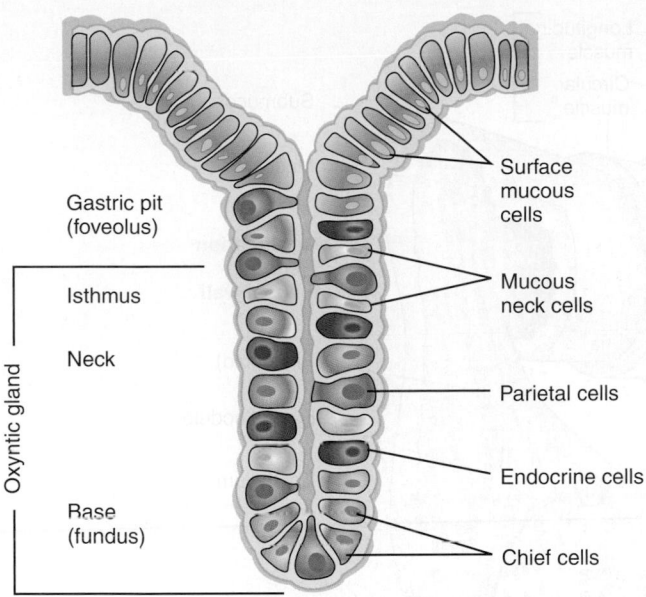

FIGURE 35-4 Gastric mucosa and gastric glands.

On microscopic examination, the lining of the small intestine contains millions of fingerlike projections called **intestinal villi** (Figure 35-5). Like the circular folds just described, these villi serve to increase the surface area of the intestine for digestion and absorption of nutrients. Each villus has its own microscopic projections called microvilli, which in turn are covered by a fuzzy coat (called the **brush border** because of its brushlike appearance when viewed with an electron microscope) containing many digestive enzymes. The combined effect of the circular folds, villi, and microvilli is to increase the surface area of the small intestine by about 600 times, thereby creating a remarkably efficient interface for nutrient digestion and absorption. Figure 35-6 shows a microscopic section of the small intestine.

Between the villi are situated the intestinal glands, or crypts of Lieberkühn. The intestinal glands secrete about 2 L of fluid daily into the lumen of the intestine, but most of the fluid is quickly reabsorbed by the villi. Goblet cells throughout the intestinal mucosa secrete large amounts of mucus. In addition, specialized mucous glands located in the first few centimeters of the duodenum, called Brunner glands, release a thick coating of mucus to protect the mucosa from the potentially damaging effects of acidic gastric juice that may enter through the pylorus.

Although the details of the process of digestion and absorption of nutrients in the intestinal mucosa will be covered in greater detail in subsequent sections, a unique and salient feature of the villus epithelial cells is described here. Villus epithelial cells have both digestive and absorptive functions, apparently dependent on their current stage of maturation. The rapidly dividing cells at the base of the intestinal glands are responsible for secretion, but as they migrate to the villus, they mature into absorptive cells and are eventually pushed out of the villus tip. Turnover of cells in the small intestine occurs in 48 to 72 hours, one of the fastest cell turnover rates in the body. Therefore, conditions such as malnutrition or substances that interfere with cell replication or protein synthesis, such as chemotherapeutic agents, may adversely affect intestinal function.

The **ileocecal valve,** a sphincter between the small and large intestines, is normally closed so that the contents of the large intestine cannot reflux back into the small intestine. As peristaltic contractions move intestinal contents toward the large intestine, the ileocecal valve opens.

Large Intestine

The large intestine (Figure 35-7) is a muscular tube 1.5 m long and 6.5 cm in diameter that forms a frame around the small intestine. The portion of the large intestine from the cecum to the rectum is known as the colon. The ascending colon extends from the cecum straight up to the lower border of the liver; the transverse colon then extends across the abdomen, anterior to the small intestine. The descending colon turns downward on the left side of the abdomen, finally becoming the S-shaped sigmoid colon, which empties into the rectum. The rectum has its outlet at the anus, the opening for elimination of feces (see Figure 35-7).

The vermiform appendix, attached to the cecum, is a worm-shaped blind tube containing specialized lymphatic structures. It contains T and B lymphocytes, secretes immunoglobulin A (IgA), and contributes to gut-associated lymphoid function.[9] Inflammation of the appendix, or appendicitis, is a life-threatening occurrence that can lead to peritonitis if not diagnosed and managed promptly.

The mucosa of the large intestine has no villi and does not produce digestive enzymes (Figure 35-8). The epithelial surface of the colon consists of absorptive cells that predominantly absorb water and electrolytes.[10] Mucus-producing goblet cells line the glandular crypts present in the surface epithelium. Endocrine cells are also present, perhaps helping coordinate colon neurologic activity, but at present the function of hormones in the large intestine is poorly understood. The turnover time of cells in the colonic mucosa is 3 to 8 days, comparatively longer than that of cells in the small intestine.

> **KEY POINTS**
> - Tracheoesophageal fistula, esophageal and duodenal atresia, and anal agenesis are congenital disorders that occur with abnormal development of the GI tract. These disorders are usually manifested as obstructions.
> - The major structures and corresponding functions of the GI tract can be summarized as follows:
>   - **Mouth and salivary glands:** Mastication, moistening, and the beginning of starch digestion (by the enzyme salivary amylase) of foodstuff.
>   - **Pharynx:** Transport of food to the esophagus and protection of the airway from aspiration of food particles.
>   - **Esophagus:** Movement of food to the stomach by peristaltic waves. The LES prevents reflux of stomach contents.
>   - **Stomach:** Reservoir for food, mixing, and initial digestion of proteins (by the enzyme pepsin); secretion of hydrochloric acid, intrinsic factor, and gastrin. The pyloric sphincter prevents reflux of intestinal contents.
>   - **Small intestine:** Digestion and absorption of nearly all nutrients in the duodenum and jejunum; absorption of bile salts in the terminal ileum. The brush border contains numerous digestive enzymes. The enzymes secretin and cholecystokinin are secreted by intestinal mucosa.
>   - **Pancreas and gallbladder:** The pancreas delivers digestive enzymes and bicarbonate to the duodenum. The gallbladder delivers bile salts to the duodenum.
>   - **Large intestine:** Reabsorption of water and storage of feces. Feces are delivered to the rectum for defecation.

GASTROINTESTINAL MOTILITY

The way in which nutrients and their eventual waste products are propelled through the GI tract is a complex and fascinating process, involving an exquisitely timed set of autoregulatory actions and responses. A summary of the characteristics of the intestinal wall, innervation of the gut, and hormonal control of GI motility will provide a basis for a description of how nutrients move through the GI tract.

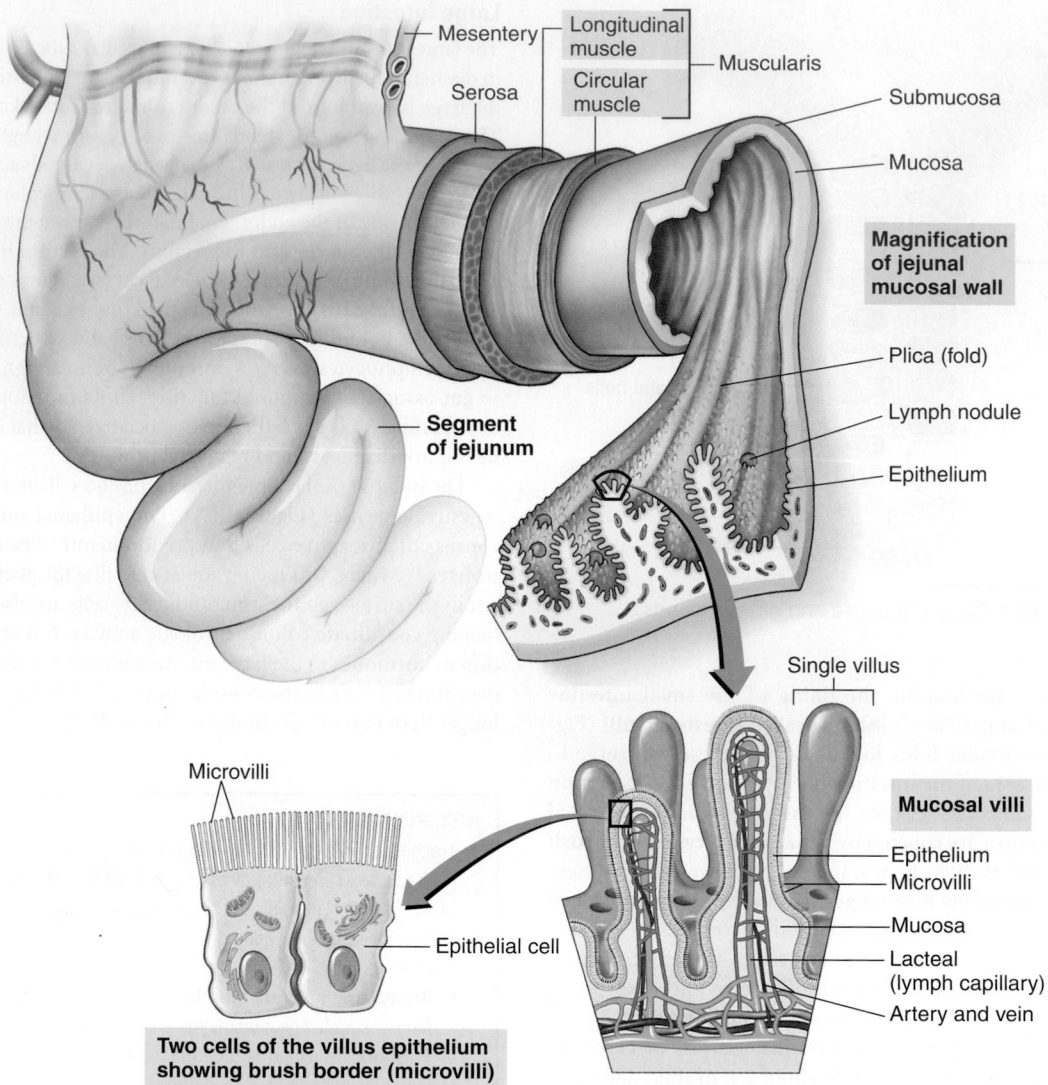

FIGURE 35-5 The intestinal wall showing the layers of muscle, mucosal villi, and the brush border microvilli. Villi contain blood capillaries and a lacteal (lymph capillary). Villi and microvilli significantly increase the surface area available for absorption. (From Patton KT, Thibodeau GA: *Anatomy and physiology,* ed 8, St Louis, 2013, Mosby, p 876.)

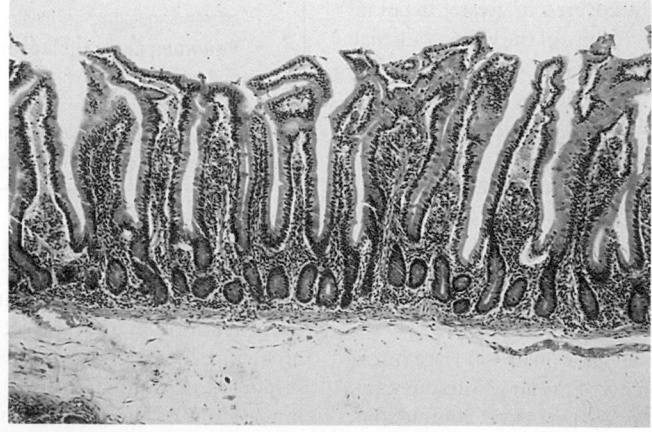

FIGURE 35-6 Microscopic section of the small intestine. (From Kumar V et al: *Robbins basic pathology,* ed 7, Philadelphia, 2003, Saunders, p 803.)

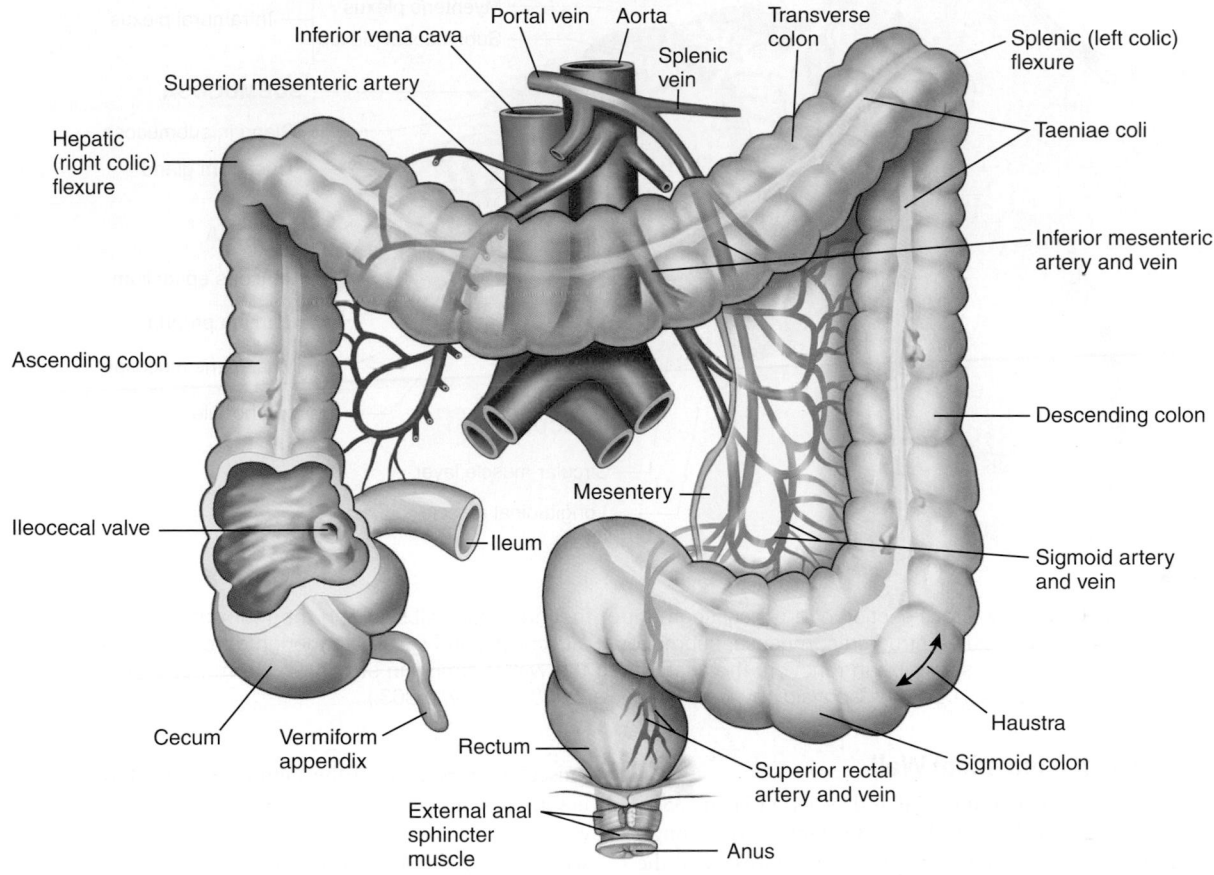

FIGURE 35-7 Divisions of the large intestine. (From Patton KT, Thibodeau GA: *Anatomy & physiology,* ed 8, St Louis, 2013, Mosby, p 878.)

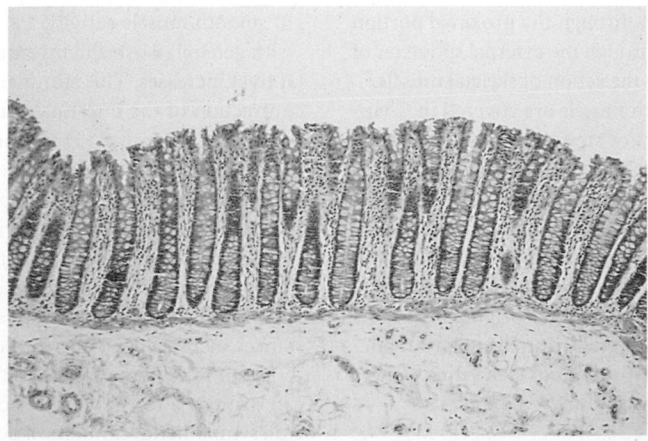

FIGURE 35-8 Normal colon histology showing a flat mucosal surface and abundant vertically oriented crypts. (From Kumar V et al: *Robbins basic pathology,* ed 7, Philadelphia, 2003, Saunders, p 803.)

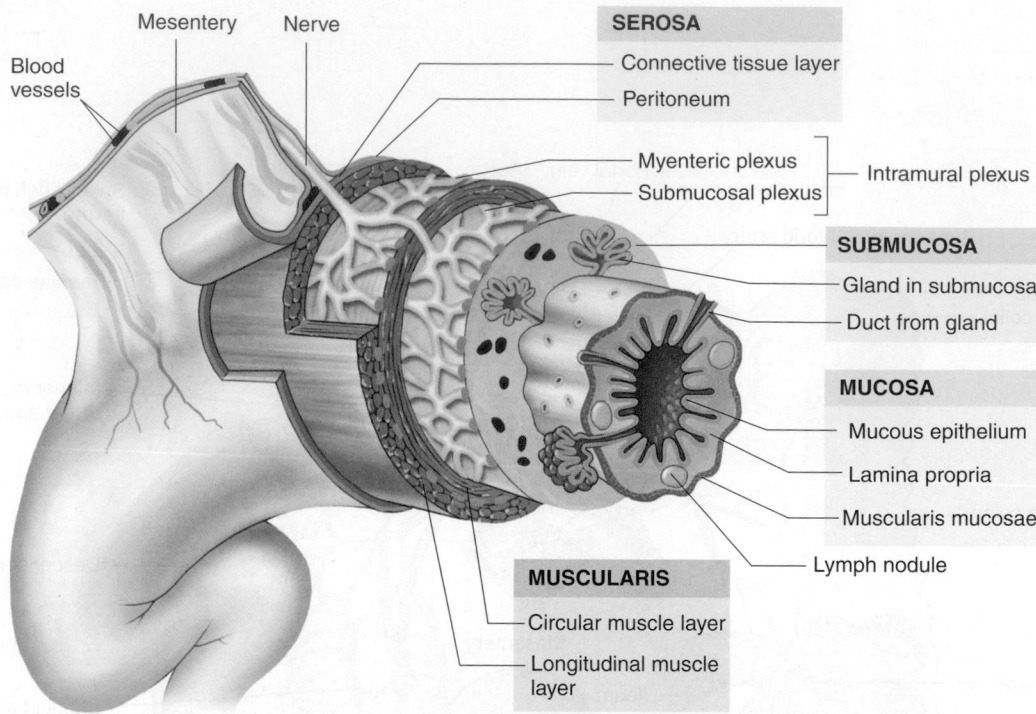

FIGURE 35-9 Cross-section of a typical segment of the intestinal wall showing the four principal layers and associated structures: mucosa, submucosa, muscularis, and serosa. Although different areas of the GI tract specialize in function, the anatomy of the wall is similar in structure. (From Patton KT, Thibodeau GA: *Anatomy & physiology*, ed 8, St Louis, 2013, Mosby, p 863.)

Characteristics of the Intestinal Wall

A typical cross-section of the intestinal wall is depicted in Figure 35-9. From the outer surface inward are five main layers: the serosa, a longitudinal muscle layer, a circular muscle layer, the submucosa, and the mucosa. A small layer, the muscularis mucosa, is located between the mucosa and submucosa. The muscular movements of the GI tract are performed mostly by the different layers of the smooth muscle, which extends from the distal end of the esophagus through most of the large intestine. However, skeletal muscle has a key role in motility at both ends of the GI tract; motility from the mouth through the proximal portion of the esophagus at the upper end and through the external sphincter of the anus at the lower end is mediated by the action of skeletal muscle.[2]

The general characteristics of smooth muscle are covered in Chapter 5. One of the specific characteristics of smooth muscle in the gut that enables its unique function is the close proximity of these fibers to each other. In most areas of the GI tract, smooth muscle fibers are extremely close; about 12% of their membrane surfaces are actually fused with the membranes of other adjacent muscle fibers to form a nexus, or junction. This allows intracellular current to travel very easily from one muscle fiber to another. Action potentials originating in one smooth muscle fiber in the GI tract are generally propagated from fiber to fiber; therefore, the GI tract acts as a **functional syncytium,** where separate cells have the ability to function in a unified manner.[1]

Neural Control

Movement of nutrients through the GI tract is controlled by the central nervous system through its autonomic division and is modulated by numerous hormonal interactions.[2,3,8] In addition, the GI system has an intrinsic nervous system of its own affecting most GI functions.[9-12] The intrinsic nervous system is composed of two layers: (1) the myenteric, or Auerbach, plexus, which lies between the longitudinal and circular muscular layers; and (2) the submucosal, or Meissner, plexus, which lies in the submucosa. The myenteric plexus is largely responsible for control of GI movements; the submucosal plexus serves to control secretion and is also involved in many sensory functions, with information being received from the gut epithelium and stretch receptors in the intestinal wall. The entire intrinsic nervous system, including both the myenteric plexus and the submucosal plexus, is responsible for many reflexes that occur locally in the GI tract, such as the localized secretion of digestive juices by the submucosal glands or an increase in gut smooth muscle activity.

In general, when the myenteric plexus is stimulated, activity in the GI tract increases. This stimulation has four principal effects: (1) tonic contraction of the intestinal wall increases; (2) rhythmic contractions increase in intensity; (3) rhythmic contractions increase in rate; and (4) the velocity of conduction of excitatory waves along the intestinal wall increases. As part of the parasympathetic nervous system, these excitatory fibers of the myenteric plexus are primarily cholinergic (i.e., secrete acetylcholine), in addition to one or more other excitatory transmitter substances. However, some myenteric plexus fibers have an inhibitory effect and may secrete purine-based transmitter substances such as adenosine triphosphate (ATP).

Input from the sympathetic and parasympathetic nervous systems can strongly affect the activity of the intrinsic nervous system. In general, sympathetic stimulation decreases the activity of the intrinsic nervous system whereas parasympathetic stimulation increases its activity.

Parasympathetic Innervation

The parasympathetic supply to the GI tract is divided into cranial and sacral divisions. Cranial parasympathetic stimulation is transmitted almost entirely by the vagus nerves, which provide extensive innervation to the esophagus, stomach, pancreas, and the first half of the large intestine (with little innervation of the small intestine). The sacral parasympathetic division originates in the second, third, and fourth sacral segments of the spinal cord and innervates the distal half of the large intestine. The sigmoid, rectal, and anal regions of the large intestine are especially well supplied with parasympathetic fibers; these fibers have a key role in the defecation reflex.

Sympathetic Innervation

The sympathetic fibers that innervate the GI tract have their origin in the spinal cord between T8 and L3. After exiting the cord, the preganglionic fibers enter the sympathetic chains and then pass through these chains to various ganglia adjacent to the GI tract, such as the celiac ganglion and the mesenteric ganglia. From these locations, postganglionic fibers radiate out to all parts of the gut. These sympathetic fibers supply essentially all parts of the GI tract (in contrast to the concentration of parasympathetic innervation at locations close to the entry and exit points of the gut).[2] The sympathetic nerve endings in the GI tract secrete norepinephrine, which promotes the inhibitory effect of the sympathetic nervous system on the GI tract in the following ways: Norepinephrine acts directly on smooth muscle in the GI tract to inhibit activity; in addition, norepinephrine has an inhibitory effect on the neurons of the intrinsic nervous system of the GI tract. Strong stimulation of the sympathetic nervous system can effectively stop motility in the gut and therefore block the movement of nutrients through the GI tract. Gastrointestinal sympathetic activity can also initiate vomiting through a complex sequence of events mediated by various neurotransmitters.[13-15]

Afferent Nerve Fibers

The GI tract is richly supplied with afferent nerve fibers arising from the gut that transmit important information about the status of the GI tract. Afferent fibers that have their cell bodies in the submucosal plexus and terminate in the myenteric plexus transmit signals in response to irritation of the gut mucosa, excessive distention, or the presence of specific chemical substances. These signals can result in excitation or, in some circumstances, inhibition of intestinal motility or secretion. Other afferent fibers with cell bodies in the dorsal root ganglia of the spinal cord or cranial nerve ganglia can transmit signals to higher levels of the central nervous system by traveling along sympathetic or parasympathetic pathways. For example, the vagus nerves contain many afferent fibers that transmit signals to the medulla; this information is then used to initiate and modulate vagal signals that control many important functions of the GI tract.

Electrical Activity of Gastrointestinal Smooth Muscle

Electrical activity is almost constantly present in the smooth muscle layers of the GI tract. Two basic types of electrical wave activity have been identified in the gut: slow waves and spikes (the latter named for the spiking appearance of these sudden increases in membrane potential).[1,2] These two types of electrical wave patterns are shown in Figure 35-10. **Slow-wave electrical activity** represents an ongoing basic oscillation in membrane potential that occurs in the smooth muscle of the GI tract, especially in the muscle in the longitudinal layer. Normally, between 3 and 12 slow waves occur per minute, ranging from 40 to 50 millivolts (mV) in amplitude. Slow waves can be any degree of intensity and are not the "all-or-nothing" type of action potential seen in other smooth muscle fibers in the body. In contrast to these nearly continuous slow waves, spikes occur under certain circumstances. When the muscle layer in the GI tract is stimulated by being stretched or by the effects of acetylcholine or parasympathetic excitation,

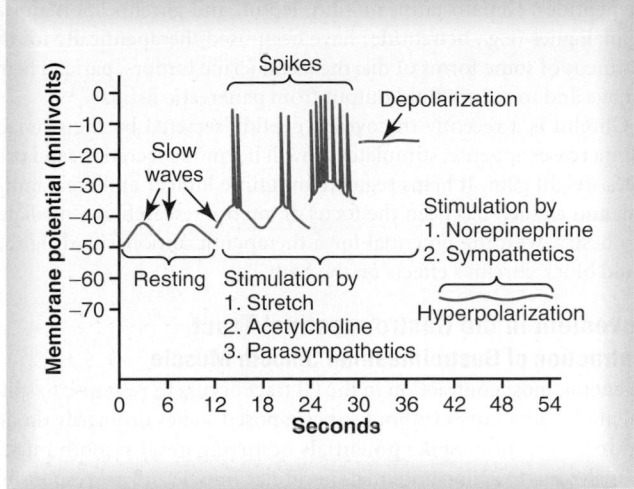

FIGURE 35-10 Membrane potentials in intestinal smooth muscle (From Hall JE: *Guyton and Hall textbook of medical physiology*, ed 12, Philadelphia, 2011, Saunders.)

the intracellular resting membrane potential of the muscle fibers becomes relatively more positive. The entire potential level of the slow waves is raised—an effect called depolarization.[1] As shown in Figure 35-10, when depolarization rises above a certain level (around −40 mV), sudden increases in the membrane potential, or spikes, start to appear on the peaks of the slow waves. If the resting potential rises further, spikes appear more frequently. With very strong stimulation, the spikes generally disappear because the membrane now remains entirely depolarized. Figure 35-10 also illustrates the response of smooth muscle fibers to stimulation by norepinephrine or sympathetic excitation. In this situation, the resting membrane potential is decreased, or hyperpolarized, and electrical activity is almost abolished.

Hormonal Control

The following section on secretory function of the GI tract describes in detail the role of hormones in controlling GI secretion. It is important to note that many of these same hormones are involved in controlling motility in different portions of the GI tract. Gastrin, which is secreted by specialized endocrine cells (G cells) of the stomach mucosa in response to food entry, increases stomach motility and is the primary mediator of gastric acid secretion. In addition, it promotes increased constriction of the LES, which serves to prevent reflux of stomach contents into the esophagus. Gastrin may also have a small effect in increasing motility of the small intestine and gallbladder.[2,3]

Cholecystokinin, which is secreted mainly by I cells of the jejunum in response to the entry of fatty substances, has an extremely strong effect on gallbladder contractility. This stimulation of gallbladder activity results in an outpouring of bile, which plays an important role in fat digestion and absorption. Cholecystokinin also stimulates pancreatic secretion, helps regulate gastric emptying and bowel motility, and induces satiety.[3]

Secretin, which is produced by the mucosa of the duodenum in response to the entry of acidic gastric juice from the stomach, stimulates pancreatic fluid and bicarbonate secretion, with the effect of neutralizing the acidity of intestinal contents. It also has a mild inhibitory effect on motility in most of the GI tract.[2,3]

Other important gastrointestinal polypeptide hormones include vasoactive intestinal polypeptide (VIP), glucagon, glucose-dependent insulinotropic polypeptide (GIP, also called gastric inhibitory polypeptide), somatostatin, motilin, leptin, and ghrelin.[3] Somatostatin analogues (e.g., octreotide) have been used therapeutically for the treatment of some forms of diarrhea, endocrine tumors, parietal hemorrhage and to reduce fluid output from pancreatic fistulas.[14]

Ghrelin is a recently discovered peptide secreted by the stomach that increases appetite, stimulates growth hormone secretion, and produces weight gain. It helps regulate mealtime hunger and meal initiation, and as such has been the focus of intense research as a mediator for obesity, with the potential for a therapeutic antiobesity drug that would block ghrelin's effects on the body.[16-21]

Movement in the Gastrointestinal Tract
Contraction of Gastrointestinal Smooth Muscle

In general, most contraction in the GI tract occurs in response to spike potentials; slow waves without superimposed spikes ordinarily do not lead to contraction. **Spike potentials** occurring in GI smooth muscle are analogous to action potentials in cardiac muscle and are responsible for the membrane changes that initiate contraction. As calcium enters the cell membrane and passes to the interior of the smooth muscle, it initiates a reaction between actin and myosin,[1] a process described in detail in Chapter 17.

The electrical activity occurring in the smooth muscle of the gut develops into tonic contractions and rhythmic contractions, both of which occur in most types of smooth muscle. Tonic contraction is continuous, instigated by pacemaker cells that reside at the interface between the longitudinal and circular muscle layers. The intensity of tonic contraction varies with the frequency of spike potentials and determines the amount of pressure in that segment. Thus, the degree of contraction exerted by the pyloric, ileocecal, and anal sphincters serves to regulate the movement of nutrients through the GI tract.

The degree of rhythmic contraction varies in different parts of the GI tract. These differing rhythmic frequencies are dependent on the rate of slow wave activity in a particular segment and may occur at rates of 3 to 12 times per minute. These slow wave–dependent contractions are responsible for the mixing and peristaltic propulsive movements present in the GI tract.

Two types of muscular activity are involved in the digestive and absorptive functions of the GI tract: mixing movements and propulsive movements. In different portions of the GI tract these movements may serve different functions to achieve proper digestion and absorption of nutrients. For example, mixing movements in the stomach and small intestine promote digestion by mixing the digestive juices with the food that enters from the esophagus. In the small intestine and proximal segment of the large intestine, mixing movements facilitate absorption by exposing newly arrived intestinal contents into contact with absorbing surfaces. In the case of propulsion, the rate at which nutrients are propelled through the GI tract depends on the function of the different organs of the tract. For example, the passageway for nutrients from the mouth through the pharynx and esophagus is simply a conduit; essentially no digestive or absorptive function occurs there and the transit of nutrients is quite rapid. In contrast, transit from the stomach and through the small and large intestines is quite slow. This slow rate of passage allows for completion of the digestive and absorptive processes that occur in these portions of the GI tract.

Although the characteristics of mixing and propulsive movements differ in various parts of the GI tract and will be described separately in the next section, a description of the general characteristics of these movements is presented here.

Propulsive Movements

The basic propulsive movement of the GI tract is called peristalsis (Figure 35-11). Nutrients are propelled by the slow advancement of

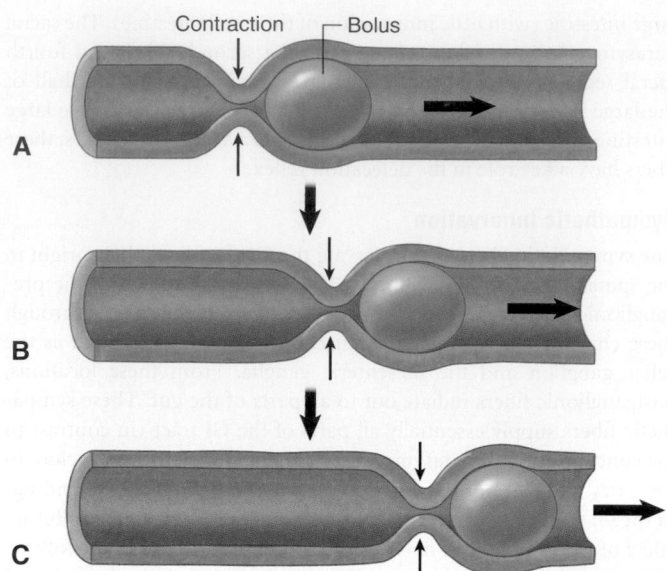

FIGURE 35-11 Peristalsis is a progressive type of movement, propelling material from point to point along the GI tract. **A,** A ring of contraction occurs where the GI wall is stretched, pushing the bolus forward. **B,** The moving bolus triggers a ring of contraction in the next region, which pushes the bolus even farther along. **C,** The ring of contraction moves like a wave along the GI tract, pushing the bolus forward. (From Patton KT, Thibodeau GA: *Anatomy & physiology*, ed 8, St Louis, 2013, Mosby, p 906.)

a circular constriction that squeezes the materials in front of the constricted area forward. Peristalsis is an inherent property of any smooth muscle tube that, like the intestine, is a functional syncytium. However, effective intestinal peristalsis requires the presence of an intact myenteric nerve plexus. The usual stimulus for peristalsis is distention of the intestinal walls. The entry and subsequent stretching of the intestinal wall by a bolus of food will have the effect of stimulating the gut wall 2 to 3 cm above this point, and a circular constriction will then occur and propel the food with a peristaltic movement. Although peristalsis can move in both directions in the gut, it normally moves toward the anus. It is thought that the myenteric plexus is organized in such a way that preferential transmission of signals downward occurs simultaneously with relaxation of the distal portion of the intestine below the distended stimulus point.

Mixing Movements

Segmental contractions serve to keep the intestinal contents thoroughly mixed on a constant basis. These movements may vary according to the specific function of each portion of the GI tract (see the Secretory Function section).

Movement of Nutrients

The path taken by foods ingested into the GI tract, as these nutrients travel down the tract and are digested and absorbed, will be traced beginning with the mouth. Although this process is described here as a linear sequence, it is important to note that several steps may occur simultaneously. The individual steps involved in nutrient ingestion constitute a synergistic process, and an inability to perform one phase of the process will ultimately have a profound effect on the entire GI tract. In addition, individuals manifest a great deal of variability in such aspects of digestive function as tolerance of certain nutrients and defecation patterns. Such variations may represent age-related differences or conditioned responses to environmental cues.

Chewing

The entry of solid food into the mouth results in the action of chewing, an important first step in the process of nutrient digestion. The process of moving the food around in the mouth and mixing it with saliva results in stimulation of the taste buds and olfactory epithelia; this sensory input greatly increases the subjective enjoyment of eating. As the food is mixed with saliva, it becomes softened and formed into a mass of appropriate size (bolus) that can be swallowed. The action of the molars and premolars in crushing more rigid forms of foods serves to prepare rough substances for transport down the esophagus. Although the act of chewing is under voluntary control, it is also partly reflexive in nature. The entry of food into the mouth has been shown to stimulate chewing in animals in the absence of full cerebral function. The movements of the skeletal muscles responsible for chewing are coordinated by impulses traveling through cranial nerves V, VII, IX, X, XI, and XII. Interruption of the proper transmission of impulses through these nerve tracts places an individual at risk for decreased voluntary control of the chewing function, with a resultant risk of aspiration (improper entry of oral or esophageal contents into the airways).

Swallowing

Swallowing is the transport of material from the mouth to the stomach. The process of swallowing has been divided into three stages that describe the regions through which the bolus of nutrients passes on its way to the stomach: (1) the oral stage, (2) the pharyngeal stage, and (3) the esophageal stage.[2,3,9]

During the oral stage, the bolus is passed from the mouth to the pharynx through the space called the fauces. The bolus, either solid or liquid, is rolled toward the back of the tongue, and the front of the tongue is then pushed up against the hard palate. Respiration is inhibited briefly in this phase, while the pharyngeal muscles constrict to force the bolus of food into the pharynx. In the pharyngeal stage the bolus is passed through the pharynx into the esophagus, a process taking about 0.2 seconds. Continued contraction of the pharyngeal muscles and the position of the tongue prevent reentry of the bolus into the oral cavity. The soft palate is pulled upward to block the nasopharynx; simultaneously, food is prevented from entering the larynx by elevation of the larynx and approximation of the vocal cords, both actions serving to close the glottis. As these openings are blocked, the pharyngeal constrictors contract and force the bolus of food into the esophagus. Respiration is now resumed, and pressure in the pharynx rises as a result of the muscular activities that have occurred.

The muscular characteristics of the esophagus are of particular importance in effecting the third, or esophageal, stage of swallowing. The upper one third of the esophagus consists of skeletal muscle, whereas the lower two thirds consists of predominantly smooth muscle. In the normal resting stage, the upper part of the esophagus is closed by the tonic contraction of a band of skeletal muscle that serves as the pharyngoesophageal sphincter. The pressure exerted by the pharyngoesophageal sphincter in this region is normally about 20 to 40 cm H_2O above atmospheric pressure; this zone of high pressure keeps air from entering the esophagus during inspiration. Almost immediately after initiation of a swallow, the sphincter relaxes and pressure in the region drops to atmospheric pressure, thus allowing the bolus to be forced into the esophagus by the pressure generated in the pharynx. Pressure in the pharyngoesophageal junction region then rises as a result of contraction of skeletal muscle in this area, thus preventing reflux of food from the esophagus back to the pharynx. Pressure in this region then gradually subsides to a resting level while muscular relaxation occurs.

If the bolus being swallowed is a liquid, it is propelled through the esophagus by the initial force of swallowing and travels by gravity to the stomach in about 1 second. If the bolus is a semisolid mass, it is propelled

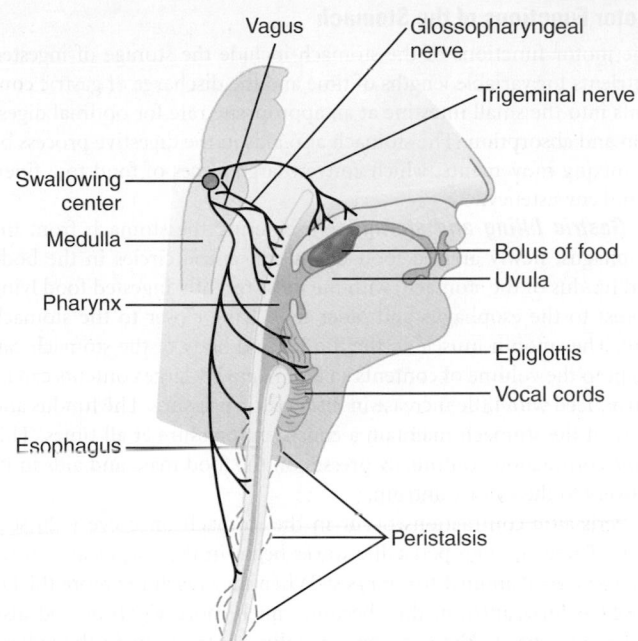

FIGURE 35-12 Neural pathways of the swallowing mechanism. (From Hall JE: *Guyton and Hall textbook of medical physiology,* ed 12, Philadelphia, 2011, Saunders.)

down the esophagus by means of a peristaltic wave. This esophageal peristalsis is caused by a contraction of circular muscle that forces the bolus ahead of it toward the stomach, with a transit time of about 4 to 6 seconds.

Although no well-differentiated muscular structure is located in the area where the esophagus joins the stomach, the region approximately 2 to 5 cm above the juncture with the stomach is referred to as the LES and is described in the Esophagus section. Almost immediately after initiation of a swallow, pressure at the LES drops and remains low during the time that a peristaltic wave is passing down through the lower end of the esophagus. Once the bolus has passed through the lower esophageal region and pressure in the lower portion of the esophagus has fallen to a resting level, the pressure in the LES rises and remains elevated for about 10 seconds before declining to a resting level once again.[2]

Neural control of swallowing. Figure 35-12 illustrates the neural pathways involved in the swallowing mechanism. Swallowing receptors in the posterior of the mouth and throat transmit impulses in response to a stimulus to the mucous membranes in the mouth, such as the presence of a moderate amount of fluid. These impulses travel mainly through the trigeminal nerve (cranial nerve V) into the reticular substance of the medulla oblongata, where the swallowing center is located. Once this center has been activated, the sequence of muscular reactions described earlier occurs automatically and usually cannot be voluntarily stopped. The swallowing center then sends impulses over a number of efferent nerves to the numerous skeletal and smooth muscles involved in the swallowing process to allow the complete act of swallowing to occur in the appropriate sequence. The glossopharyngeal (cranial nerve IX) and hypoglossal nerves (cranial nerve XII) are primarily concerned with the oral and pharyngeal stages, whereas the vagus nerve (cranial nerve X) is important in activating the esophageal stage.

The gag reflex is an important protective mechanism that aborts the normal swallowing response and helps eliminate potentially harmful ingestions. The afferent limb of the reflex is controlled by the glossopharyngeal nerve, and the efferent limb is regulated by the vagus nerve. Disorders of the gag reflex such as stroke or neuropathy can lead to life-threatening obstruction or aspiration.

Motor Functions of the Stomach

The motor functions of the stomach include the storage of ingested nutrients for variable lengths of time and the discharge of gastric contents into the small intestine at an appropriate rate for optimal digestion and absorption. The stomach also aids in the digestive process by its mixing movements, which convert large pieces of food to a finer, liquid consistency.

Gastric filling and storage. On entering the stomach from the esophagus, newly arrived food forms concentric circles in the body and fundus of the stomach, with the most recently ingested food lying closest to the esophagus and older food lying closer to the stomach wall. The smooth muscle in the fundus and body of the stomach can adapt to the volume of contents so that relatively large contents can be introduced with little increase in intragastric pressure. The fundus and body of the stomach maintain a consistent pressure at all times. This tonic contraction continually presses on the food mass and aids in its delivery to the pyloric antrum.

Peristaltic contractions occur in the stomach once every 20 seconds. These rippling peristaltic waves begin in the corpus and move at a velocity of about 1 to 2 cm/sec. When they reach the more thickly walled pyloric antrum, they become much more vigorous and also increase in speed. These strong peristaltic contractions in the pyloric antrum are largely responsible for mixing ingested nutrients with gastric secretions. As ingested food is churned and mixed to a greater degree of fluidity, the mixture takes on a milky white sludge appearance and is then called **chyme.**

Emptying. As pressure in the antrum rises momentarily because of peristaltic contraction, a pressure differential exists between pressure in the antral pylorus and pressure in the duodenal bulb. The higher pressure in the antrum is sufficient to overcome the resistance of the pyloric sphincter, and the contents of the stomach are then propelled into the duodenum. Concurrently, the degree of constriction of the pyloric sphincter may increase or decrease, depending on several factors discussed in the next section. Because this process is dependent on the muscular activity of the antrum as well as the muscular tone of the pylorus, gastric emptying is largely regulated by mechanisms that affect each of these regions.

Regulation of gastric emptying. Factors that may affect the rate at which the stomach empties include the degree of distention of the gastric wall and the release of the hormone **gastrin** in response to certain types of food in the stomach. Both of these factors increase the rate of gastric emptying by increasing the force of antral contractions, while simultaneously inhibiting pyloric constriction. Distention of the gastric wall results in stimulation of mechanoreceptors in the stomach with subsequent activation of reflexes over the vagus and the intrinsic nerve plexuses. These neural influences, along with contractile activity as a direct response to the stretch of gastric muscle, constitute a major stimulus for gastric emptying. Gastric emptying time can vary depending upon the food ingested (e.g., whether solid or liquid) and generally ranges from 1 to several hours.[3]

Gastrin is released from the antral mucosa in response to stretching of the gastric wall, as well as the presence of certain foods, particularly meat. The role of gastrin in promoting the secretion of highly acidic gastric juices will be discussed later. With respect to stomach emptying, gastrin has a key role in enhancing peristalsis while at the same time relaxing the pylorus.

In addition to these influences, many of the mechanisms that affect gastric emptying are initiated in the duodenum. Reflex nervous signals are transmitted from the duodenum back to the stomach in response to intraluminal stimuli; these signals likely help control both peristaltic activity and the degree of pyloric constriction. Stimulation of the duodenum in a variety of ways has the effect of slowing gastric emptying; both the chemical and the physical properties of chyme entering the duodenum may affect the rate of gastric emptying. A variety of both duodenal cells and duodenal receptors, including osmoreceptors, mechanoreceptors, and chemoreceptors, respond to intraluminal stimuli to produce hormonal and reflex inhibition of gastric motor activity and enhancement of pyloric tone. The presence in the duodenum of chyme containing the breakdown products of proteins, and to a lesser extent fats, may impede gastric emptying. Also, the presence of highly acidic or highly hypertonic or hypotonic chyme in the duodenum may inhibit the rate of gastric emptying. The degree of distention of the duodenum, as well as the presence of any degree of irritation of the duodenum, may also slow emptying of the stomach. These inhibitory mechanisms have a protective function and are effective in preventing the intestinal mucosa from overloading its digestive and absorptive abilities and potentially being damaged by chemical or mechanical sources.

Although regulation of gastric emptying is largely dependent on factors in the stomach and duodenum, gastric motility may be stimulated or inhibited reflexively from a variety of regions of the body. For example, stomach emptying is inhibited when the ileum is full and when the anus is mechanically distended. Stimulation of visceral and somatic pain receptors may result in inhibition of gastric motility. Various strong emotions such as anger, fear, and anxiety may produce changes in motility of the stomach, but whether these states tend to predispose an individual to inhibition or excitation of gastric motility is not always predictable.[3]

Vomiting. Vomiting is rapid emptying of the contents of the stomach through the esophagus and into the mouth. The major force for vomiting is supplied by the skeletal muscle of the diaphragm and abdomen, rather than by contraction of the muscles of the stomach wall. Vomiting is the result of an extremely complex set of neural events coordinated by the nucleus tractus solitarius (NTS), a center located in the medulla. Afferent impulses from receptors in various regions of the body, including the sensory nerve endings of the pharynx, abdominal viscera, and the labyrinths, arrive at this center to initiate the vomiting reflex. This reflex causes closure of the glottis and trachea, relaxation of the gastroesophageal sphincter, and contraction of the diaphragm and the abdominal muscles, which forcibly expels the contents of the stomach.

Motility of the Small Intestine

After intact food entering the mouth has been liquefied and partially digested in the stomach, it enters the small intestine, where the major part of digestion and absorption occurs. As in other parts of the GI tract, movements of the small intestine can be described as propulsive and mixing movements, which in the small intestine generally occur simultaneously.

Propulsion. Chyme is propelled through the small intestine by peristaltic waves that move at a rate of 0.5 to 2 cm/sec, with a faster rate at the proximal part of the intestine and a slower rate in the terminal portion. Approximately 3 to 5 hours is normally needed for the passage of chyme from the pyloric sphincter to the ileocecal valve, but this period may vary in some disease states. Peristaltic activity in the small intestine is greatly increased after the ingestion of a meal. The increase in contractile activity in the stomach caused by distention of the stomach wall is conducted principally through the myenteric plexus down along the wall of the small intestine. This so-called gastroenteric reflex serves to increase the activity of the small intestine, with an enhancement of both intestinal motility and intestinal secretion.

The usual stimulus for peristalsis in the small intestine is distention of the intestinal walls; stretch receptors in the gut wall are sensitive to circumferential stretch and initiate a local myenteric reflex in response to this stimulation. The resulting contraction of longitudinal muscle, followed by the contraction of circular muscle, spreads downward in a peristaltic motion.

The peristaltic waves in the small intestine not only propel chyme downward toward the ileocecal valve but also spread the chyme along

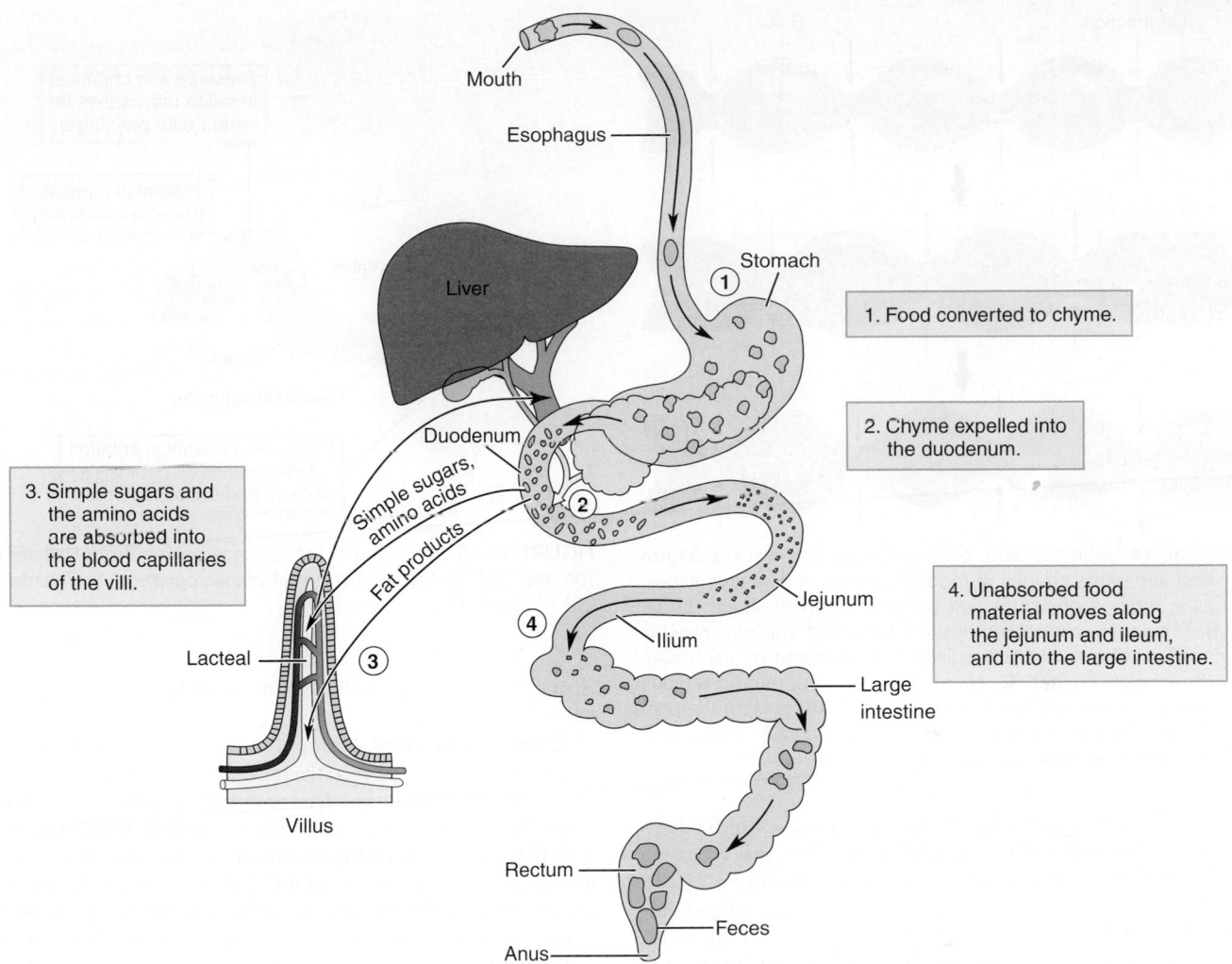

FIGURE 35-13 Chyme and the process of absorption of nutrients. (Modified from Herlihy B: *The human body in health and illness,* ed 4, Philadelphia, 2011, Saunders.)

the intestinal mucosa, thus facilitating the process of absorption of nutrients (Figure 35-13). As additional chyme enters the small intestine, this spreading process intensifies while peristalsis increases. When chyme reaches the ileocecal valve, it is sometimes stationary for several hours until the individual eats another meal and a new gastroenteric reflex intensifies the peristaltic process and propels the remaining chyme through the ileocecal valve.

Certain disease states, particularly those that involve intense irritation of the intestinal mucosa, may result in a peristaltic rush, a powerful peristaltic wave that travels long distances in the small intestine in a short period. The peristaltic rush clears the contents of the small intestine into the colon, thus relieving the small intestine of either irritating substances or excessive distention.[2,9]

Mixing. In addition to propulsive peristaltic movements, a set of movements characterized as **segmentation contractions** also occur in the small intestine. The primary effect of these contractions is progressive mixing of solid chyme particles with secretions of the small intestine. As their name implies, segmentation contractions involve contraction of the small intestine in regularly spaced segments that have the appearance of sausages (Figure 35-14). As one set of segmentation contractions is completed, a new set begins, with contractile points located at different locations along the small intestine. Segmentation contractions occur at a rate of 7 to 12 times per minute and effectively chop and mix the chyme, as

well as assist in propelling the chyme toward the ileocecal valve (see Figure 35-14).

Control of motility. The electrical and mechanical activities of the small intestine are closely associated. Slow waves, as described previously in this chapter, occur at the membranes of the longitudinal smooth muscle, with frequencies of 11 to 12 per minute in the duodenum decreasing to 7 to 9 per minute in the terminal ileum. Slow waves do not directly produce muscular contractions in the small intestine but provide the conditions under which contractions can occur. Although slow waves determine the velocity and direction of peristalsis, other factors determine whether action potentials and thus contraction will occur. Local mechanical and chemical stimulation by chyme is probably largely responsible for the initiation and continuance of contraction in the small intestine. Thus when the intestinal tract becomes overly distended or when the mucosa becomes irritated, myenteric reflexes enhance the electrical activity of the gut and spike potentials are superimposed on the slow waves. These spike potentials then spread through both longitudinal and circular muscle, and contraction results.

Intestinal motility may also be influenced by stimulation from sources extrinsic to the colon. Stimulation of the vagus nerve generally causes increased intestinal motility, with sympathetic stimulation resulting in inhibition. Intestinal motility can be altered reflexively by stimulation of many sensory areas. For example, trauma to organs outside the GI tract, such as irritation of the peritoneum or urinary tract, may cause

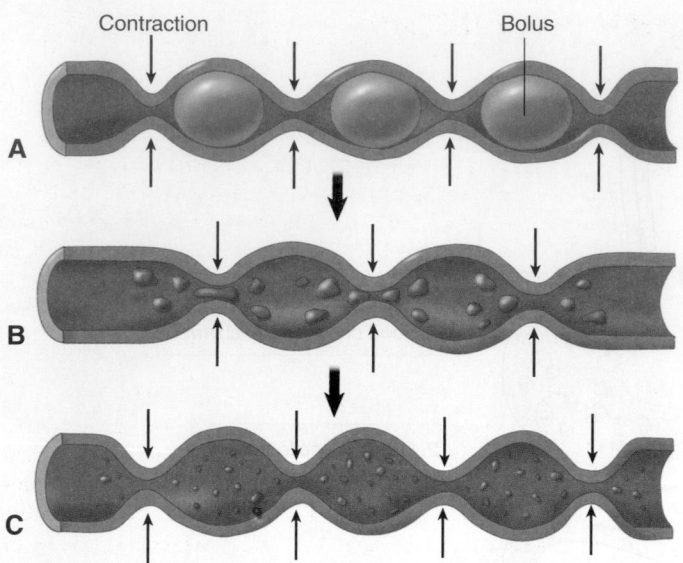

FIGURE 35-14 Segmentation. Segmentation is a back-and-forth action that separates chunks of food and mixes in digestive juices. **A,** Ringlike regions of contraction occur at intervals along the GI tract. **B,** Previously contracted regions relax and adjacent regions now contract, effectively "chopping" the contents of each segment into smaller chunks. **C,** Locations of the contracted regions continue to alternate back and forth, chopping and mixing the contents of the GI lumen. (From Patton KT, Thibodeau GA: *Anatomy & physiology*, ed 8, St Louis, 2013, Mosby, p 906.)

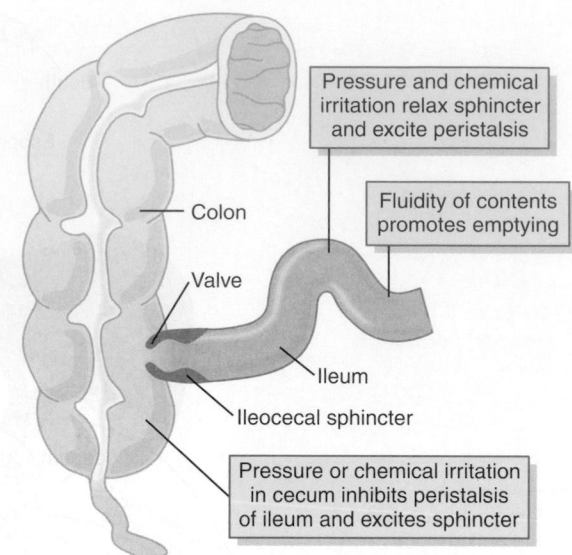

FIGURE 35-15 Emptying of the ileocecal valve. (From Hall JE: *Guyton and Hall textbook of medical physiology*, ed 12, Philadelphia, 2011, Saunders.)

intestinal inhibition. A condition called paralytic ileus, in which intestinal motility is inhibited as the result of reflex inhibition, may occur as a response to intraabdominal infection or surgery in this area.[3]

Much current research is focused on the involvement of gastrointestinal hormones in the regulation of GI tract motility.[2,3] Cholecystokinin, a hormone released from the mucosa of the jejunum in response to fatty substances in chyme, has been shown to block the increased gastric motility caused by gastrin. Another hormone, secretin, which is released mainly from the duodenal mucosa in response to gastric acid entering the duodenum, has the general effect of decreasing GI motility. The hormone gastric inhibitory polypeptide (GIP), which is released from the upper portion of the small intestine in response to fat in chyme, as well as to carbohydrates, is known to inhibit gastric motility under some conditions. These hormones will be described in more detail in the Secretory Function section.

Ileocecal Sphincter

Chyme from the small intestine is eventually propelled downward to the terminal ileum immediately proximal to the cecum, where the last 2 to 3 cm of the muscular coat is thicker than that in the rest of the ileum. This region, called the ileocecal sphincter, has a high resting pressure (about 20 cm H_2O above atmospheric pressure) and is normally closed. Distention of the distal ileum lowers the pressure in the ileocecal sphincter. Thus, when intestinal contents are present in the terminal ileum at sufficient quantity and are ready to be propelled into the cecum, the sphincter reflexively relaxes and the intestinal contents are pushed into the cecum by the propulsive movements of the distal small intestine. Conversely, distention of the cecum after it is filled with contents passing through the ileocecal valve results in increased pressure in the sphincter, which prevents reflux back into the ileum (Figure 35-15).

Motility of the Colon

The movements of the colon are effective in promoting the two major functions of the colon: (1) absorption of water and electrolytes from

chyme and (2) storage of the fecal mass until it can be expelled from the body by defecation.

Colonic movements. For most of the time, the large intestine in humans is inactive. However, the presence of material in the proximal end of the colon results in a type of mixing movement in the haustra (the outpouchings in the colon wall), termed **haustral churning,** that is similar to the segmenting movements in the small intestine. This movement is the major type of motility in the large intestine. Haustral churning exposes the contents of the large intestine to the mucosa, thus promoting the absorption of water. Normally, about 500 ml of chyme enters the proximal part of the colon each day. Out of this total volume, 400 ml—mostly water and electrolytes—is reabsorbed before defecation takes place, with an average volume of 100 ml of feces remaining for eventual disposal from the body.[1]

At infrequent intervals of about three to four times a day, a strong peristaltic movement termed a mass movement occurs and propels the fecal material long distances. These strong contractions may reach a peak of 100 cm H_2O pressure in the segment undergoing the contraction. Fecal material may be transported all the way from the ascending colon to the descending colon by a mass movement. Feces are then stored in the distal end of the colon until defecation occurs.

Defecation. Under normal conditions, it takes about 18 hours for intestinal contents to reach the distal end of the colon after leaving the small intestine. Fecal material is stored in the distal part of the colon for varying lengths of time; defecation may take place 24 hours or longer after the ingestion of food. Ordinarily the rectum is empty, but fecal material is occasionally shifted into it after one of the mass movements, and the resulting distention of the rectum initiates the urge to defecate. The act of defecation is a combination of voluntary and involuntary movements. Contraction of the distal end of the colon and relaxation of the internal anal sphincter, which are regions composed of smooth muscle, are involuntary movements. Relaxation of the external anal sphincter, which consists of striated muscle, is a voluntary movement. Other voluntary movements that may assist in the act of defecation are contraction of the abdominal muscles and forcible expiration with closure of the glottis (the Valsalva maneuver, often referred to as "bearing down").

Regulation of colonic motility. Movements in the proximal portion of the colon are largely initiated by distention in the colonic walls, which stimulates contractile activity by triggering short reflexes through the intrinsic nerve plexuses. Although the proximal part of the colon receives extrinsic innervation via the vagus nerve, it functions in a relatively autonomous manner in the absence of extrinsic motor innervation and is thus a somewhat self-regulating structure. Extrinsic nerves may occasionally modify proximal colonic activity, however; for example, entry of food into the stomach or duodenum may result in a mass contraction in the proximal end of the colon. Sometimes termed the gastrocolic or duodenocolic reflexes, these strong mass movements are most evident after the first intake of nutrients in the morning and are often followed by a strong need to defecate.

In contrast, the distal part of the colon is somewhat more dependent on its extrinsic nerve supply, so movements in this region, including the act of defecation, may be entirely abolished after injury to these nerves. However, weak movements return eventually, and defecation can still occur without voluntary control after the initial response to injury has passed.[3]

> **KEY POINTS**
> - Movements of the GI tract are due to contraction of two layers of smooth muscle (i.e., the longitudinal and circular layers). Smooth muscle exhibits two types of electrical potentials: basic oscillations (slow waves), which do not result in contraction, and action potentials (spikes), which trigger calcium entry and result in contraction. Contraction of smooth muscle results in two types of intestinal motility: propulsive (peristalsis) and mixing (segmental).
> - GI motility is regulated by the enteric nervous system, the autonomic nervous system, and hormonal mediators. The enteric nervous system has two branches—myenteric and submucosal—that coordinate reflexive contraction and relaxation along the entire GI tract.
> - Luminal distention is an important stimulus for reflexive motility. Sympathetic nervous system activity is generally inhibitory to GI motility (and secretion). Parasympathetic nervous system activity generally enhances motility. Regulatory hormones include gastrin (increases gastric motility), GIP (decreases gastric motility), cholecystokinin (stimulates gallbladder contraction), and secretin (decreases GI motility).
> - Swallowing is a complex function coordinated by a swallowing center in the medulla.
> - Swallowing is partially voluntary and partially involuntary. Cranial nerves IX, X, and XI mediate the various stages of swallowing.
> - Regulation of gastric emptying involves gastric and duodenal factors. Gastric distention and the release of gastrin from gastric mucosa promote gastric emptying. Duodenal distention, acidity, hypertonicity, and high protein and fat concentrations inhibit gastric emptying.
> - Chyme remains in the small intestine for 3 to 5 hours, where it is continually mixed by segmental contractions and slowly propelled toward the ileocecal valve by peristalsis. Distention of the terminal ileum results in relaxation of the ileocecal sphincter, which allows contents to enter the large intestine.
> - Segmental contractions (haustra) in the large intestine promote water absorption. About 18 hours is required for the contents to traverse the large intestine and reach the distal end of the colon. Three to four times a day a peristaltic mass movement sweeps fecal material along the colon. Mass movements may be initiated by entry of food into the stomach and duodenum (gastrocolic reflex).
> - An urge to defecate occurs when feces enters the rectum. Contraction of the distal end of the colon and relaxation of the internal anal sphincter occur involuntarily as feces enter the rectum. The external anal sphincter is under voluntary control and inhibits defecation until voluntarily relaxed.

SECRETORY FUNCTION

Secretion of Gastrointestinal Juices

The many glands associated with the GI tract generally produce enzymes that participate in the digestive process to break down the major nutrient components of carbohydrates, fats, and proteins. The somewhat archaic term juices is still used to describe the fluids secreted in the GI tract, which contain a complex mixture of salts and protein enzymes. Secretion of these digestive juices is stimulated by various factors, including mechanical and chemical stimulation by chyme, parasympathetic stimulation (in certain regions of the GI tract), and various hormones.

Gastrointestinal Hormones

Table 35-1 lists the major hormones of the GI tract and their sources, target organs, major actions, and factors that stimulate release. These hormones are released from the GI mucosa in response to distention or the presence of certain nutrient substances. They are then absorbed into the blood and carried to glands in target tissues (i.e., tissues on which they exert their effects), where they stimulate secretion. Chemically, GI hormones are polypeptides or polypeptide derivatives. Receptors for the peptide hormones are widely distributed throughout the body, including in the brain and central nervous system, and much current research is focused on the varied effects of these complex chemicals.[17,18]

In addition to their effects on motility, as mentioned previously, gastrin, secretin, cholecystokinin, and GIP have critical roles in mediating secretion of gastrointestinal juices. Gastrin is secreted by the stomach mucosa and stimulates the exocrine (secretory) cells of the gastric glands to produce their specific products, including hydrochloric acid (HCl). Research over the last two decades has shown that gastrin exerts its primary effect on enterochromaffin-like cells (ECL cells), provoking them to release histamine.[19-21] Histamine, an amine with multiple roles in human physiologic processes, including an ability to constrict bronchial smooth muscle, diffuses readily into nearby parietal cells to induce acid release (Figure 35-16). The development of specific medications that block the action of histamine (H_2 antagonists) led to the first effective treatment for peptic ulcers by reducing gastric acid secretion.

Secretin was one of the first of the body's many hormones to be discovered. The most potent stimulus for secretin release is hydrochloric acid, and the presence of acidic chyme in the duodenum promotes its release into the blood from the duodenal mucosa. It is carried to the pancreas, where it stimulates the secretion of a large volume of alkaline juice rich in sodium bicarbonate. In the duodenum, sodium bicarbonate then neutralizes the HCl of the chyme, thus protecting the duodenal mucosa from potential damage and creating a slightly alkaline medium that is optimal for chemical digestion by pancreatic intestinal enzymes. Although the liver produces bile continuously, secretin is effective in increasing the rate of bile secretion. Hormonal regulation is the most important mechanism governing the activity of the pancreas, and cholecystokinin has a key role in stimulating the release of large amounts of digestive enzymes from the pancreas. Cholecystokinin also stimulates the gallbladder to release the bile it stores. GIP acts to slow stomach emptying by decreasing gastric motor activity.[1]

Stimulation of the parasympathetic nerves to certain regions of the GI tract will also increase the rates of glandular secretion. Those glands in the upper portion of the GI tract that are innervated by the vagus and other cranial parasympathetic nerves (particularly the salivary, esophageal, and gastric glands; the pancreas; and some duodenal glands) are especially subject to parasympathetic stimulation. Glands in the distal portion of the large intestine are also affected by parasympathetic stimulation because this region is innervated by the pelvic

TABLE 35-1 MAJOR HORMONES OF THE GASTROINTESTINAL TRACT

HORMONE	SOURCE	TARGET ORGAN	MAJOR ACTIONS	STIMULATED BY
Gastrin	Stomach (mucosa)	Stomach (gastric glands)	Stimulates gastric glands to secrete specific substances	Distention of stomach by food; other specific substances (e.g., partially digested proteins, caffeine)
Secretin	Duodenum (mucosa)	Pancreas	Stimulates release of alkaline component of pancreatic juice	Acidic chyme acting on duodenal mucosa
		Liver	Increases bile secretion rate	
Cholecystokinin	Duodenum (mucosa)	Pancreas	Stimulates release of digestive enzymes	Presence of fatty acids and partially digested proteins in duodenum
		Gallbladder	Stimulates gallbladder contraction and emptying	
Glucose-dependent insulinotropic polypeptide (gastric inhibitory peptide)	Duodenum (mucosa)	Stomach	Reduces motor activity of stomach; slows rate of gastric emptying	Presence of fat or carbohydrate in duodenum

parasympathetic nerves. In the small intestine, the major stimulus for intestinal secretion is local and mechanical stimulation of the intestinal wall, which initiates the excitation of local myenteric reflexes and subsequent release of secretions.

KEY POINTS

- Major secreting glands and secretions in the GI tract can be summarized as follows:
  - **Salivary glands:** Secrete salivary amylase.
  - **Gastric glands:** Chief cells secrete pepsinogen; parietal cells secrete HCl and intrinsic factor. HCl activates the conversion of pepsinogen to pepsin, and intrinsic factor enhances vitamin B_{12} absorption. Parietal cell secretion is stimulated by acetylcholine, histamine, and gastrin. G cells secrete gastrin into the bloodstream. Gastrin increases gastric motility and stimulates chief and parietal cell secretion.
  - **Intestinal epithelium:** Secretes brush border enzymes (peptidases, lipases, sucrase, lactase), secretin (stimulates pancreatic secretion), and cholecystokinin (stimulates gallbladder contraction).
  - **Pancreas:** Secretes bicarbonate-rich fluid containing amylase, trypsin, chymotrypsin, and lipase into the duodenum when stimulated by secretin.
  - **Gallbladder:** Secretes concentrated bile salts into the duodenum when stimulated by cholecystokinin.

DIGESTION AND ABSORPTION

Substances contained in foods that are important to maintenance of the body include carbohydrates, fats (also called lipids), proteins, vitamins, inorganic salts, and water. Many of the nutrient constituents that compose intact food substances are structurally complex and cannot be easily absorbed from the GI tract in their original forms. During the process of digestion, digestive juices and the enzymes contained in these secretions convert these complex organic molecules to smaller molecules (Figure 35-17). These simpler compounds are then capable of absorption—transfer across the wall of the small intestine into the blood and lymph, and subsequent transfer to the cells. This complex task of digestion and absorption of nutrients is the primary task of the GI tract, and an inability to perform this function would be life threatening. This section describes the mechanisms of digestion of the three major groups of nutrients—carbohydrates, lipids, and proteins—and then considers the absorption of these substances.

Digestion of Carbohydrates

In terms of calories, carbohydrates account for approximately half of the American diet. The major digestible carbohydrate in food is the polysaccharide plant starch, a large molecule composed of straight and branched chains of glucose. A summary of carbohydrate digestion is presented in Table 35-2.

Digestion of starch begins in the mouth as salivary amylase breaks down polysaccharides to the much smaller disaccharide molecules maltose and dextrin. In the stomach, this action of salivary amylase continues until the enzyme is eventually inactivated by acidic gastric juice. In the duodenum, the pancreatic enzyme amylase completes the task of splitting any remaining undigested polysaccharides and dextrins to small maltose units. Then maltase, an enzyme located in the brush border of the epithelial cells lining the duodenum, hydrolyzes each maltose molecule to two molecules of glucose. Other carbohydrates that are present in the diet in smaller quantities are the disaccharides sucrose, which is table sugar (glucose-fructose), and lactose, which is milk sugar (glucose-galactose). These two carbohydrates remain chemically unaltered until they reach the duodenum, where the enzyme sucrase in the brush border converts sucrose to the monosaccharides glucose and fructose. The enzyme lactase hydrolyzes lactose into the monosaccharides glucose and galactose.[5]

Glucose, the major product of carbohydrate digestion, accounts for about 80% of the monosaccharides obtained from food, whereas fructose and galactose account for the other 20%. Humans do not secrete an enzyme capable of digesting cellulose—a plant polysaccharide found in the cell walls of plants and present in large amounts in fibrous vegetables. Although cellulose consists of glucose molecules, it contains molecular linkages different from those of starch. Consequently, much of this complex carbohydrate passes through the digestive tract without being digested and is excreted in the feces.

Digestion of Lipids

Lipids in the diet are mostly in the form of triglycerides but also include phospholipids, cholesterol, and the fat-soluble vitamins A, D, E, and K. Digestion of lipids occurs in the small intestine, where fats are emulsified by the action of bile; neither salivary nor gastric enzymes appear to have any effect on triglycerides. As the lipid particles enter the duodenum from the stomach, bile exerts a detergent action on them in which the surface tension of the particles is decreased. This decrease in surface tension promotes fragmentation of the particles into smaller particles as they are blended by the mixing movements of the small intestine. The emulsification process is an

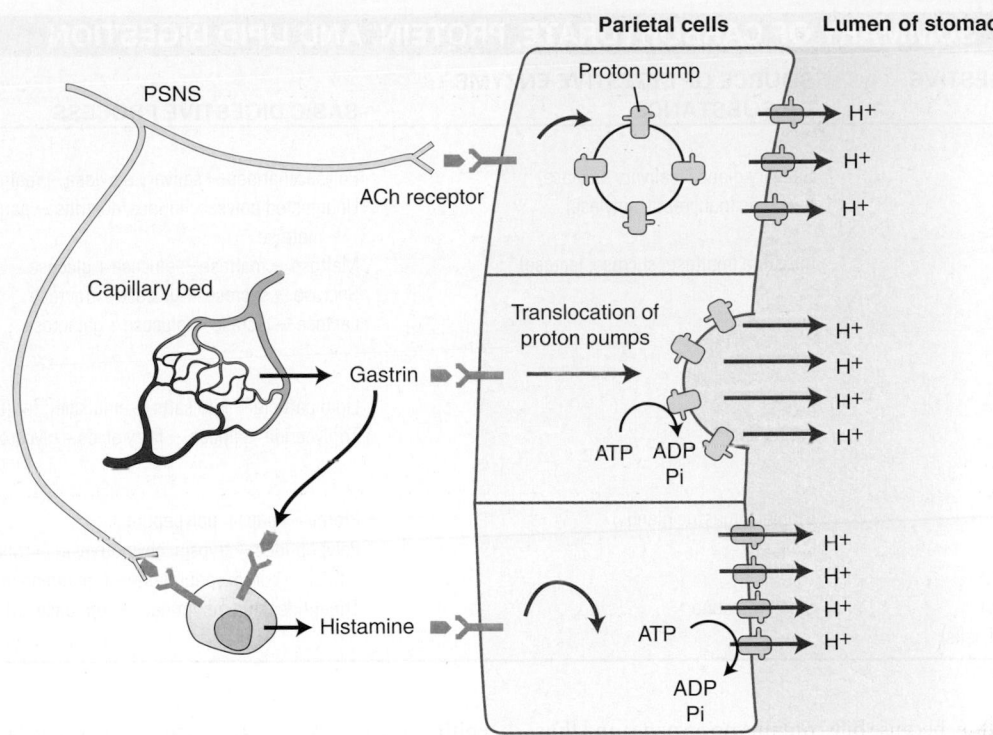

FIGURE 35-16 Schematic diagram of the complex regulation of acid (h+) secretion from parietal cells in the gastric pits. Gastrin stimulates enterochromaffin-like cells (ECL cells), which in turn release histamine onto H_2 receptors on the parietal cell. Gastrin also stimulates acid secretion directly as does acetylcholine. *ACh,* Acetylcholine; *ADP,* adenosine diphosphate; *ATP,* adenosine triphosphate; *Pi,* inorganic phosphate; *PSNS,* parasympathetic nervous system.

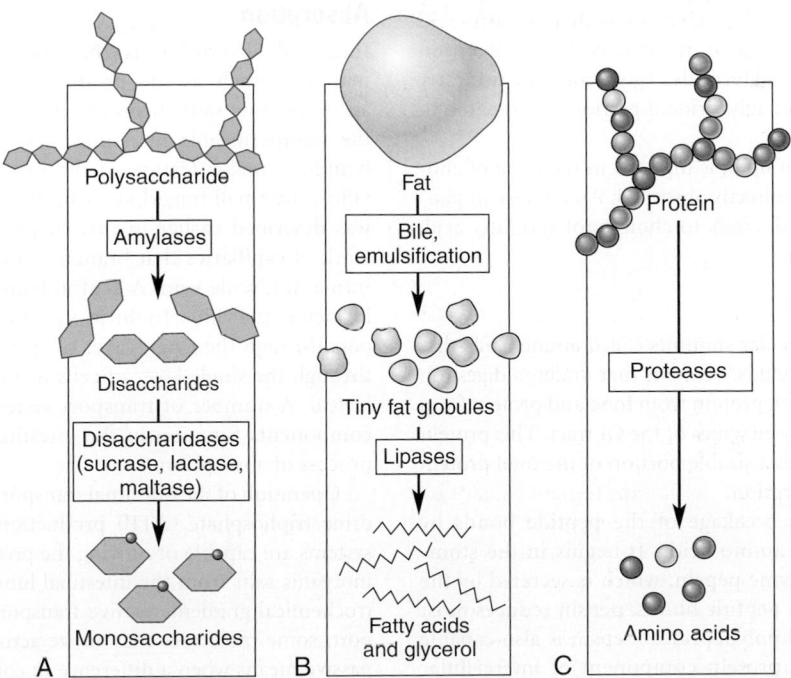

FIGURE 35-17 Chemical digestion. **A,** Amylases and disaccharidases break carbohydrates down into monosaccharides. **B,** Lipases break fats down to fatty acids and glycerol. The large fat globule must first be emulsified by bile. **C,** Proteases and peptidases break proteins down into amino acids. (From Herlihy B: *The human body in health and illness,* ed 4, Philadelphia, 2011, Saunders.)

TABLE 35-2 SUMMARY OF CARBOHYDRATE, PROTEIN, AND LIPID DIGESTION

LOCATION OF DIGESTIVE PROCESS	SOURCE OF DIGESTIVE ENZYME OR SUBSTANCE	BASIC DIGESTIVE PROCESS
Carbohydrates		
Mouth, stomach	Salivary glands (salivary amylase)	Polysaccharides → salivary amylase → maltose + dextrin
Small intestine lumen	Pancreas (pancreatic amylase)	Undigested polysaccharides/dextrins → pancreatic amylase → maltose
Brush borders	Intestine (maltase, sucrase, lactase)	Maltose → maltase → glucose + glucose
		Sucrose → sucrase → glucose + fructose
		Lactose → lactase → glucose + galactose
Lipids		
Small intestine	Liver	Lipid particle → bile salts → emulsified fat (triglycerides)
	Pancreas	Triglyceride → lipase → fatty acids + glycerol
Proteins		
Stomach	Stomach (gastric glands)	Protein → pepsin polypeptides
Small intestine lumen	Pancreas	Polypeptides → trypsin, chymotrypsin → tripeptides + dipeptides → carboxypeptidase → free amino acids
Brush borders (and within cytoplasm of epithelial cells)	Small intestine	Tripeptides and dipeptides → peptidase → free amino acids

entirely mechanical action, because bile contains no enzymes and thus performs no chemical digestion.

Eventually, the detergent action of bile salts reduces the particles of fat to tiny droplets so that their surface area is greatly increased. This enhancement of surface area allows for maximal exposure to pancreatic lipase, an enzyme that (along with intestinal lipase, to a lesser extent) hydrolyzes the triglycerides to free fatty acids and glycerol. Some monoglycerides (glycerol with one fatty acid still attached) may remain; in fact, some fat may escape digestion entirely or be reduced only to diglycerides (glycerol with two fatty acids attached). A summary of triglyceride digestion is presented in Table 35-2.

Cholesterol, a steroid type of lipid, is ingested in the form of cholesterol esters, which cannot be directly absorbed. An esterase in pancreatic juice degrades cholesterol esters to cholesterol and fatty acid, which then undergo absorption.

Digestion of Proteins

Proteins are composed of molecular subunits called amino acids that are linked together by peptide bonds. Proteins that undergo digestion in the small intestine include both protein from food and protein from desquamated cells and the many enzymes of the GI tract. This protein of endogenous origin constitutes a sizable portion of the total protein subjected to digestion and absorption.

Protein digestion involves breakage of the peptide bonds by hydrolysis and release of free amino acids. It begins in the stomach with the action of the enzyme pepsin, which is secreted by the gastric glands. By its action on peptide bonds, pepsin reduces most proteins to intermediate-sized polypeptides. Pepsin is also capable of breaking down collagen, a protein component of intercellular connective tissue, thus rendering cellular proteins more accessible to enzymatic action in the GI tract. In the duodenum, the trypsin and chymotrypsin contained in pancreatic juice reduce the polypeptides to small peptides (tripeptides and dipeptides). Carboxypeptidase, which has its source in the pancreas, and peptidases in the brush borders of the intestinal epithelial cells split some of these peptides into free amino acids. Free amino acids, in addition to dipeptides and tripeptides, are absorbed into the intestinal

epithelial cells. Within the cytoplasm of epithelial cells the small peptides are then hydrolyzed by various peptidases into free amino acids before their passage into the circulation. Numerous proteolytic enzymes are involved in protein digestion, and each enzyme acts on a slightly different type of peptide linkage. Protein digestion is summarized in Table 35-2.

Absorption

Intestinal absorption is the movement of water and dissolved materials, such as the products of nutrient digestion, vitamins, and inorganic salts, from the inside of the small intestine through the semipermeable intestinal membrane and into the blood and lymph. A major feature of the intestinal absorptive surface is the villus, the small fingerlike projection lined with epithelial cells that was described earlier in this chapter. Within each villus is a network of capillaries that branch from a miniscule artery and empty into a miniscule vein. A central lymph vessel called a lacteal is also located in the villus. In the process of absorption, nutrient molecules pass through the single layer of epithelial cells lining the villus and through the single layer of cells forming the wall of the capillary or lacteal. A number of transport systems specific to certain nutrient components function in the intestinal epithelium to promote this process of absorption.[4]

Operation of the intestinal transport systems is dependent on adenosine triphosphate (ATP) production by the epithelial cells. These systems are capable of moving the products of nutrient digestion and inorganic salts from the intestinal lumen into the blood against electrochemical gradients (active transport). In addition to active transport, some molecules may move across the intestinal epithelium by passive means when a difference in concentration on the two sides of the epithelium exists. The rate of molecular transfer based on diffusion gradients is dependent not only on the magnitude of the difference in concentration but also on the size of the molecules and the lipid solubility of the substances involved.

Almost all substances capable of intestinal absorption disappear from the lumen of the small intestine by the time that the intestinal contents reach the mid-jejunum. The ileum is not involved in absorption to any significant degree, because the proximal regions of the small intestine have usually completed the process of absorption before the intestinal contents reach the ileal region. Nevertheless, the distal end of the small intestine has the capability of absorption and may do so in situations in which absorption has not taken place in the proximal part of the small intestine. Thus about 50% of the small intestine can be surgically removed without compromising absorptive ability. However, it is important to note that vitamin B_{12} and bile salts are absorbed specifically in the terminal ileum, and surgical removal of this portion of the small intestine will result in impaired absorption of these substances.[6] Intrinsic factor produced by the parietal cells of the gastric antrum is also required for B_{12} absorption; intrinsic factor deficiency leads to a condition known as pernicious anemia.[3]

The intestinal contents arriving at the terminal ileum contain no digestible carbohydrate, very little fat, and only 15% to 17% nitrogen-containing substances. Most of the contents of the terminal ileum consist of bacteria, desquamated epithelial cells, digestive secretions, and the residue of foods that are undigested and therefore unabsorbed, such as the cellulose walls of fibrous plants and connective tissue from animal sources.

Carbohydrates

Carbohydrates are absorbed in the form of monosaccharides. Polysaccharides and disaccharides lack the capacity for absorption; apparently the intestinal epithelium is impermeable to carbohydrates of such high molecular weight, and no transport systems exist for these types of carbohydrate molecules. The monosaccharides glucose and galactose are absorbed by an active, energy-requiring process in which a carrier molecule located on the luminal border of epithelial cells transports them across the border. It is theorized that the same carrier molecule that ferries glucose and galactose also carries sodium and that the carrier affinity for monosaccharides is greatest when sodium is bound to the carrier. In contrast to the other monosaccharides, the monosaccharide fructose is absorbed passively by means of a diffusion gradient.[5]

Lipids

Absorption of lipids occurs by a highly complex, unique process. As fatty acids and monoglycerides are freed during digestion, they become dissolved in bile salt micelles, which are colloidal particles composed of many molecules. Within the micelles, the products of lipid digestion are now soluble and can be absorbed far more efficiently. The bile salt micelles transport the lipid products to the epithelial brush borders, where the monoglycerides or fatty acids, which are highly soluble in the lipid cell membrane, diffuse into the epithelial cells and leave the micelle behind. The micelle is now emptied of its cargo and can pick up more fatty acids and monoglycerides and transport them to the cell membrane.

Bile salts, which are required for micelle formation, are absorbed mostly in the terminal ileum and then recycled in the liver. In the absence of bile, the amount of lipid absorbed in this manner is reduced by more than 25%. In this situation, the absorption of fat-soluble vitamins (vitamins A, D, E, and K) is compromised. Several cholestatic conditions, such as primary biliary cirrhosis (PBC) and primary sclerosing cholangitis (PSC), may be associated with deficiencies of fat-soluble vitamins.[20]

Monoglycerides may be further degraded into glycerol and fatty acids by the enzyme lipase within the epithelial cell. Short-chain fatty acids (those with fewer than 12 carbon atoms) can be absorbed directly into the blood at this point. Long-chain fatty acids and glycerol, however, are reassembled into triglycerides by the endoplasmic reticulum. These newly synthesized triglycerides are aggregated into droplets that become progressively larger during passage through the cell. These lipid droplets are stabilized by enclosure with absorbed cholesterol and phospholipids and encased by a protein coat. The final product, called a chylomicron, passes out of the cell and into the lacteal of the villus. From the lacteal, chylomicrons pass through a series of lymph vessels that eventually drain into the general circulation.

Proteins

Amino acids are transported across the epithelial membrane by means of an active transport carrier system in much the same way as monosaccharides. It is currently thought that different carrier systems exist to carry the different chemical classes of amino acids (i.e., neutral, basic, dicarboxylic, and imino acids). As is the case for the transport of monosaccharides, brush border membrane carriers are involved in the transfer of amino acids across the intestinal epithelial cell; these carriers require energy and are coupled to the transport of sodium. After being transported to the epithelial cells of the villi, amino acids diffuse through the base of the cell and into the blood. Both amino acids and monosaccharides are transported directly to the liver by the hepatic portal vein.

Water and Electrolytes

Water and inorganic ions, which are in the GI tract as a result of ingestion and secretion, are absorbed mainly from the small intestine and, to a lesser extent, from the colon. The process of absorption of water and ions is the same in both the small and large intestines: sodium is actively transported to the blood, and water follows passively in response to the osmotic gradient created by the removal of sodium from the intraluminal fluid. About 8000 ml of water is absorbed every day by the small intestine and about 300 to 400 ml by the colon. Frequently, diarrhea is the result of failure of the small intestine to absorb water appropriately. If large quantities of water are allowed to enter the colon from the small intestine because of some malfunction of the small intestine's absorptive ability, the colonic absorptive mechanism may be overwhelmed, and diarrhea is the result (Figure 35-18).

KEY POINTS

- Digestion, the process of converting large molecules to simpler forms, is accomplished by mechanical and enzymatic processes. Digestion is a necessary prelude to absorption because only simple molecules can cross the intestinal epithelia.

- Digestion of complex carbohydrates is initiated in the mouth, where salivary amylase begins to cleave polysaccharides into disaccharides. Pancreatic amylase continues this process in the small intestine. Disaccharides (e.g., maltose, sucrose, lactose) are cleaved into monosaccharides (e.g., glucose, fructose, galactose) by brush border enzymes (e.g., maltase, sucrase, lactase) on the intestinal epithelia. Glucose and galactose are absorbed across the intestinal epithelia by a sodium-dependent cotransporter. Fructose is absorbed passively by facilitated diffusion. Monosaccharides then travel via the bloodstream to the liver.

- Lipid digestion begins in the small intestine, where bile salts from the gallbladder mix and emulsify the fatty substances. Emulsification mechanically separates the lipids into small drops that are more accessible to enzymatic digestion. Pancreatic lipase and brush border lipases digest the lipids into free fatty acids and glycerol, which remain associated with the bile salts and form micelles. Cholesterol is digested by pancreatic esterase. Fatty acids are transported to the intestinal epithelia by micelles. Free fatty acids diffuse out of the micelle and into the epithelial cell passively. Epithelial cells synthesize large protein-lipid complexes (chylomicrons) that enter the lymphatic system.

- Protein digestion begins in the stomach, where HCl from parietal cells activates the conversion of pepsinogen to pepsin. Pepsin cleaves proteins into smaller polypeptides. Pepsin is neutralized in the duodenum, and pancreatic trypsin, chymotrypsin, and carboxypeptidase take over protein digestion. Brush border peptidases split tripeptides and dipeptides into single amino acids. Amino acid transport into intestinal epithelial cells is mediated by a sodium-dependent cotransport system similar to monosaccharide transport. Small peptides may also undergo endocytosis and be cleaved into amino acids within the epithelial cells.
- Amino acids pass into the bloodstream and travel to the liver.
- Absorption of water occurs passively by osmosis. An osmotic gradient for water absorption is created as electrolytes are absorbed.

GASTROINTESTINAL FUNCTION ACROSS THE LIFE SPAN

Maturation

During the first months of life, the newborn's GI tract undergoes many maturational changes. In the first 3 to 4 months of life, sucking reflexes are present, and extrusion reflexes protect against the ingestion of solids

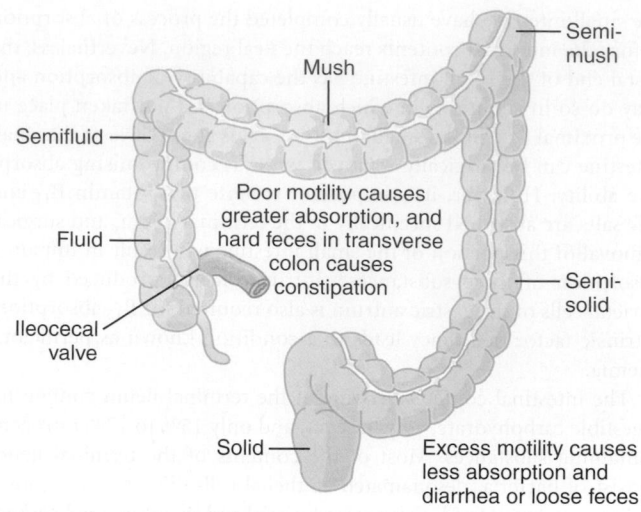

FIGURE 35-18 Absorptive function of the large intestine. (From Hall JE: *Guyton and Hall textbook of medical physiology,* ed 12, Philadelphia, 2011, Saunders.)

PEDIATRIC CONSIDERATIONS

Changes in the Gastrointestinal System in the Infant

The acid and enzymes present in the infant's gastrointestinal system are different than those in the adult's GI tract and affect the infant's ability to digest nutrients. The stomach depends on hydrochloric acid to begin digestion of human milk. Although hydrochloric acid is present, the acidity is low. This low acidity limits the gastrointestinal system's ability to destroy ingested bacteria, which causes the infant to be more susceptible to gastrointestinal infections. The acidity is also too low to digest protein in the stomach via the enzyme pepsin. As the child matures, the acidity of the gastric contents continues to increase until it reaches adult levels in the late school-age years.

Lipase and amylase in the stomach are limited for the first 4 months of the infant's life (Hockenberry & Wilson, 2011). The infant is unable to digest fats and complex carbohydrates until the levels of these enzymes are sufficient. Levels of the enzyme lactase, found in the small intestine, are extremely high in the newborn. This is essential for digestion of the human milk diet of the infant. The lactase levels decline during infancy and for most individuals lactase levels are absent by adulthood (MacGregor, 2008). Because of the enzyme composition in

the infant gastrointestinal system, human milk is the ideal food source for an infant.

Several factors of the gastrointestinal system predispose the infant to regurgitation. The lower esophageal sphincter is immature in the infant. This immaturity leads to inappropriate relaxation of the sphincter and the pressure of the sphincter is decreased. The infant also has a shorter esophagus, which results in less distance for gastric contents to travel and increases the likelihood of regurgitation. Muscle development is immature in the intestine. This immaturity leads to rapid peristaltic waves and simultaneous nonperistaltic waves. This inconsistency of the intestine to move food efficiently leads to delayed gastric emptying. As the gastric contents increase, the pressure of the stomach increases and exceeds the pressure of the lower esophageal sphincter. Once the pressure of the sphincter is exceeded, regurgitation occurs. The combination of all of these factors predisposes the infant to regurgitation. As the infant grows, the gastrointestinal system develops and is fairly complete by the beginning of toddlerhood (Hockenberry & Wilson, 2011).

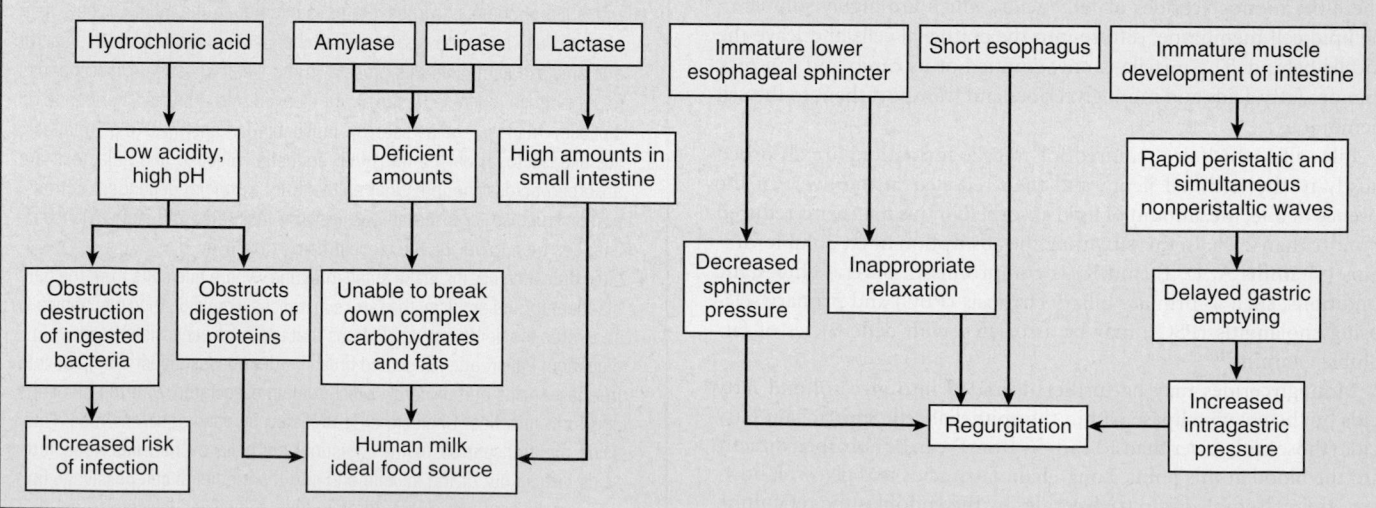

From MacGregor J: *Introduction to the anatomy and physiology of children: a guide for students of nursing, child care and health,* ed 2, New York, 2008, Routledge; Hockenberry MJ, Wilson D: *Wong's nursing care of infants and children,* ed 9, St Louis, 2011, Mosby.

that the immature GI tract is still unable to digest. The pressure in the LES remains low during this time, and "spitting up" of gastric contents is common because intragastric pressure often exceeds LES pressure. Gastric motility is not well coordinated for the first 3 to 4 months, so antral mixing is inadequate for the digestion of solid foods. At about 12 weeks of age, intestinal peristalsis similar to that in adults begins to develop, but it is one third slower. This slower transit in infants may serve to improve nutrient digestion and absorption by increasing the exposure of nutrients to the intestinal mucosa. The motor function of the large intestine appears to be fully developed at birth. During the first 2 years of life, the secretory and absorptive functions of the intestine mature and begin a pattern of functioning that continues into senescence.[5,10]

Age-Related Changes

Changes in GI function in older adults occur simultaneously with other age-related changes such as a decrease in lean body mass and impaired homeostasis of multiple body systems. Within the GI tract, a variety of changes occur that may place an aging individual at risk for health problems related to GI functioning and nutrition. Important elements of this process are summarized in Geriatric Considerations: Changes in the Gastrointestinal System.

Loss of dentition and reduced taste and smell acuity may promote a decreased interest in food intake as chewing becomes difficult and the sensory enjoyment associated with food becomes impaired. A condition called **presbyesophagus,** in which esophageal motility is slowed or disorganized, may develop in older adults. Presbyesophagus may be manifested as difficulty in swallowing and may cause discomfort as food passes through the esophagus. The incidence of hiatal hernia, where part of the stomach moves into the chest cavity through an enlarged diaphragmatic opening, is also increased in the aging population, affecting two-thirds of persons older than 70 years. The transit time for intestinal contents to pass through the GI tract is increased in older persons; this factor, coupled with a decreased perception of the sensory stimuli that produce the urge to defecate, may promote constipation in the aging population. Conversely, a confused or neurologically impaired older individual may experience fecal incontinence because the sensation and tone of the rectum diminish with aging.[5,21]

> **KEY POINTS**
> - Infants may experience GI dysfunction because of immaturity of the GI tract. Motility is not well coordinated until 3 to 4 months of age, making digestion of solids difficult in infancy. Pressure in the LES is low, which leads to "spitting up" and gastric distention. Maturation of the GI tract is complete by about 2 years of age.
> - Elderly individuals may experience GI dysfunction for a number of reasons. Poor dentition, loss of taste and smell acuity, and reduced esophageal motility may lead to poor intake of nutrients. Hiatal hernia and constipation are common in the elderly.

GERIATRIC CONSIDERATIONS

Changes in the Gastrointestinal System

As a person ages, gastrointestinal muscle strength and movement decrease, leading to reduced peristalsis and decreased gastrointestinal motility throughout the system.

In the esophagus, the elderly person experiences greater numbers of muscle movements that do not propel the contents onward. These nonperistaltic waves are common in the lower esophagus. The phenomenon of presbyesophagus—in which the esophageal sphincter fails to relax and the lower esophagus becomes dilated—may not necessarily be normal to the elderly.

In the stomach, decreased numbers of parietal and chief cells result in diminished acid (HCl) and pepsin secretion. This leads to increased pH and a more alkaline secretion. The amount of protective alkaline viscous mucus in the stomach is also decreased. The loss of smooth muscle in the stomach can delay emptying time, which increases and prolongs the exposure of gastric epithelial cells to the gastric contents.

The amount of small intestinal smooth muscle, Peyer patches, and lymphatic follicles is decreased. Normal intestinal absorption in the elderly is not well understood and may be influenced by a number of factors, including bowel motility, epithelial membranes, vascular perfusion, and gastrointestinal membrane transport. However, absorption of lipids, amino acids, glucose, calcium, and iron is known to be decreased. Normal changes in the large intestine have been difficult to determine. As a result of smooth muscle changes, anal sphincter tone decreases.

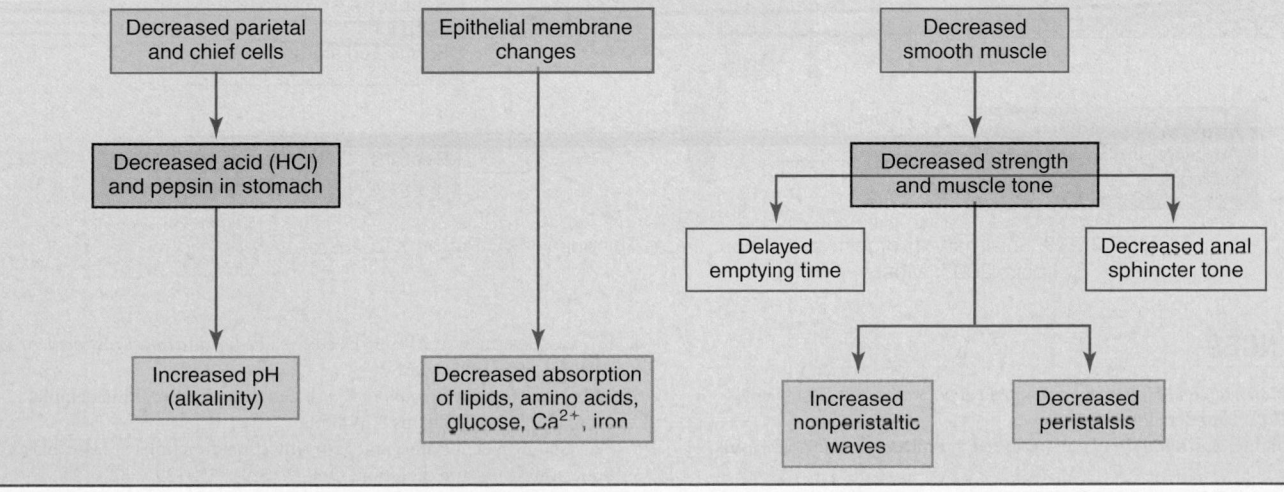

SUMMARY

This chapter describes the structure of the human GI system and the process by which it provides nutrients for the body. A thorough understanding of the structure and motility of the GI tract, secretion of digestive juices, and digestion and absorption of nutrients is needed as a basis for understanding other principles of health and disease.

GI motility is a complex process involving a set of carefully timed autoregulatory action responses (Figure 35-19). You may wish to trace the path and destiny of the apple you ate for lunch as an example of this process. As you track the movement of nutrients through the GI tract, consider the ways in which secretion of digestive juices occurs in response to the ingestion of your apple, which contains a great deal of carbohydrate (fructose), small amounts of protein, and minimal lipid. Consider also how digestion and absorption of these nutrients are occurring. What part of the apple will you use, for example, for energy to study this text? What part of the apple will your body "throw away," and how will this be accomplished? Finally, will your GI tract respond the same way to eating an apple when you are 85 years old? A careful review of the elegant and nearly automatic function of the human GI tract will prepare you to care for individuals experiencing interruptions in proper nutrient digestion and absorption.

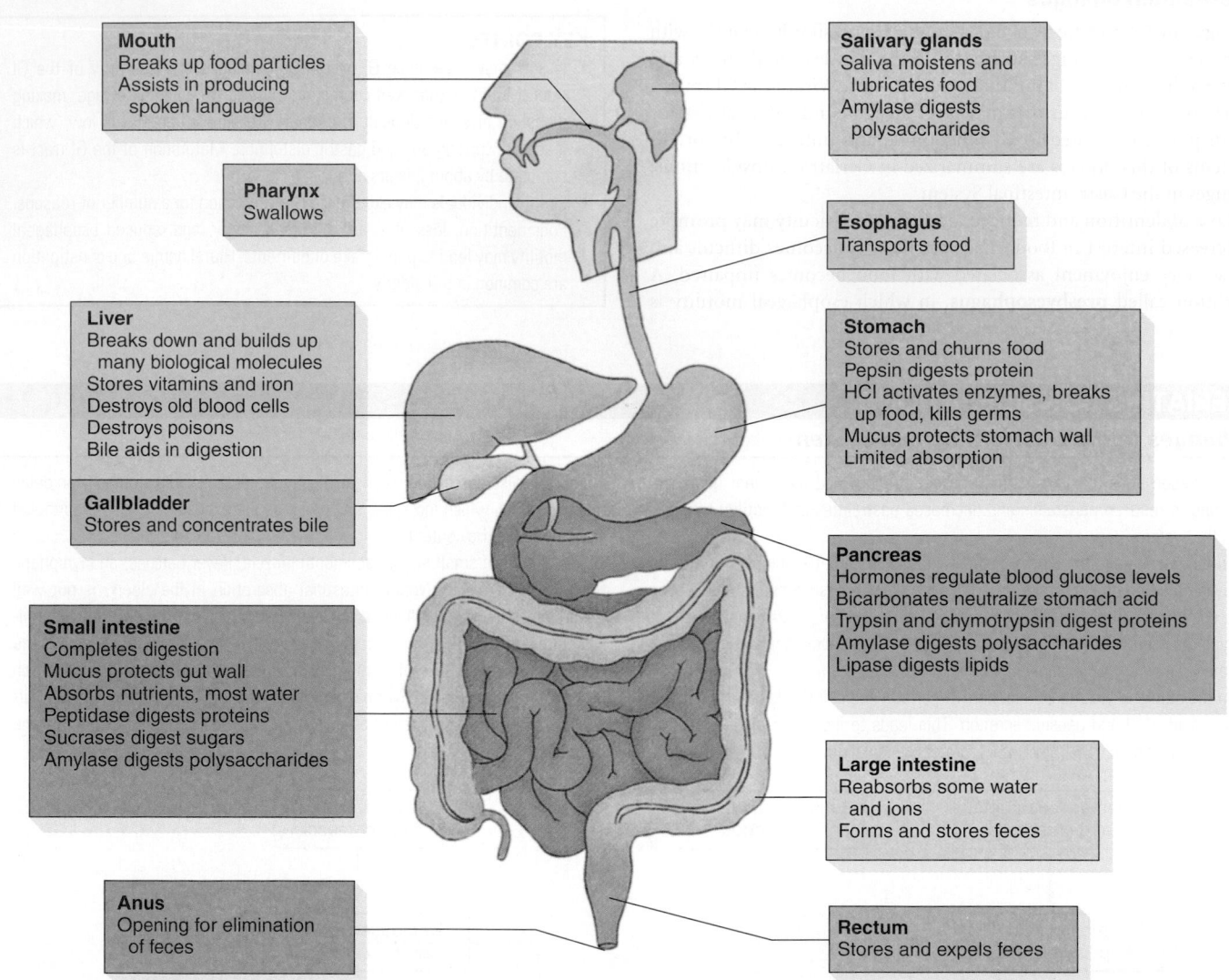

Mouth
Breaks up food particles
Assists in producing
spoken language

Pharynx
Swallows

Liver
Breaks down and builds up
many biological molecules
Stores vitamins and iron
Destroys old blood cells
Destroys poisons
Bile aids in digestion

Gallbladder
Stores and concentrates bile

Small intestine
Completes digestion
Mucus protects gut wall
Absorbs nutrients, most water
Peptidase digests proteins
Sucrases digest sugars
Amylase digests polysaccharides

Anus
Opening for elimination
of feces

Salivary glands
Saliva moistens and
lubricates food
Amylase digests
polysaccharides

Esophagus
Transports food

Stomach
Stores and churns food
Pepsin digests protein
HCl activates enzymes, breaks
up food, kills germs
Mucus protects stomach wall
Limited absorption

Pancreas
Hormones regulate blood glucose levels
Bicarbonates neutralize stomach acid
Trypsin and chymotrypsin digest proteins
Amylase digests polysaccharides
Lipase digests lipids

Large intestine
Reabsorbs some water
and ions
Forms and stores feces

Rectum
Stores and expels feces

FIGURE 35-19 Summary of digestive function. (From Thibodeau GA, Patton KT: *Anatomy & physiology,* ed 6, St Louis, 2007, Mosby, p 985.)

REFERENCES

1. Hall JE: *Guyton and Hall textbook of medical physiology,* ed 12, Philadelphia, 2011, Saunders Elsevier.
2. Johnson LR: *Gastrointestinal physiology,* ed 7, Philadelphia, 2006, Mosby Elsevier.
3. Feldman M, Friedman LS, Brandt LJ: *Sleisenger and Fordtran's gastrointestinal and liver disease,* ed 9, Philadelphia, 2010, Saunders Elsevier.
4. Roy CC, Siverman A, Alagille D, editors: *Pediatric clinical gastroenterology,* ed 4, St Louis, 1995, Mosby.
5. Shils ME: *Modern nutrition in health and disease,* ed 10, Philadelphia, 2006, Lippincott Williams & Wilkins.
6. Pedersen AM, et al: Saliva and gastrointestinal functions of taste, mastication, swallowing and digestion, *Oral Dis* 8(3):117–129, 2002.
7. Herrera JL, Lyons MF 2nd, Johnson LF: Saliva: its role in health and disease, *J Clin Gastroenterol* 10(5):569–578, 1988.

8. Yamada T, et al: *Textbook of gastroenterology*, ed 5, Oxford, 2011, Wiley-Blackwell.

9. Jaffe BM, Berger DH: The appendix. In Schwartz SI, Brunicardi CF, editors: *Schwartz principles of surgery*, ed 8, New York, 2005, McGraw-Hill.

10. Gebruers EM, Hall WJ: Role of the gastrointestinal tract in the regulation of hydration in man, *Dig Dis* 10(2):112–120, 1992.

11. Thomson AB, et al: Small bowel review: normal physiology part 2, *Dig Dis Sci* 46(12):2588–2607, 2001.

12. Burns AJ, Thapar N: Advances in ontogeny of the enteric nervous system, *Neurogastroenterol Motil* 18(10):876–887, 2006.

13. Hornby PJ: Central neurocircuitry associated with emesis, *Am J Med* 111(Suppl 8A):106S–112S, 2001.

14. de Herder WW, Lamberts SW: Somatostatin and somatostatin analogues: diagnostic and therapeutic uses, *Curr Opin Oncol* 14(1):53–57, 2002.

15. Nonogaki K: Ghrelin and feedback systems, *Vitam Horm* 77:149–170, 2007.

16. Wiedmer P, Nogueiras R, Broglio F, et al: Ghrelin, obesity and diabetes, *Nat Clin Pract Endocrinol Metab* 3(10):705–712, 2007.

17. Berna MJ, Jensen RT: Role of CCK/gastrin receptors in gastrointestinal/metabolic diseases and results of human studies using gastrin/CCK receptor agonists/antagonists in these diseases, *Curr Top Med Chem* 7(12):1211–1231, 2007.

18. Rehfeld JF, Friis-Hansen L, Goetze JP, et al: The biology of cholecystokinin and gastrin peptides, *Curr Top Med Chem* 7(12):1154–1165, 2007.

19. Barocelli E, Ballabeni V: Histamine in the control of gastric acid secretion: a topic review, *Pharmacol Res* 47(4):299–304, 2003.

20. Hofmann AF: Cholestatic liver disease: pathophysiology and therapeutic options, *Liver* 22(Suppl 2):14–19, 2002.

21. Orr WC, Chen CL: Aging and neural control of the GI tract, IV: clinical and physiological aspects of gastrointestinal motility and aging, *Am J Physiol Gastrointest Liver Physiol* 283(6):G1226–G1231, 2002.

Gastrointestinal Disorders

Jeffrey S. Sartin

evolve WEBSITE

http://evolve.elsevier.com/Copstead/

- Review Questions and Answers
- Glossary (with audio pronunciations for selected terms)
- Animations
- Case Studies
- Key Points Review

KEY QUESTIONS

- What are the common causes of the following general manifestations of gastrointestinal disorders: pain, nausea, vomiting, diarrhea, and constipation?
- What are the predisposing factors and characteristic manifestations common to inflammatory disorders of the gastrointestinal tract?
- What are the common causes of and clinical findings in functional and mechanical bowel obstructions?
- What are the common causes of and clinical findings in gastrointestinal malabsorption disorders?
- What warning signs may indicate cancer of the gastrointestinal tract?

CHAPTER OUTLINE

Alterations in function of the gastrointestinal (GI) tract may have far-reaching consequences in an individual's life. The ability to take in nutrients, convert them to usable forms for body functions, and dispose of their waste products goes beyond physiologic function and is intimately associated with social and psychological functioning. A person with an alteration in GI function may experience great emotional distress and be unable to participate fully in social activities, which in American society are often centered on food consumption. Certain symptoms that may accompany GI disorders, such as chronic diarrhea and abdominal pain, may severely limit an individual's ability to maintain employment. It has been estimated that 200,000 people miss work daily because of GI-related problems.[1] In addition, GI diseases account for more hospital admissions in the United States than any other category of disease. Because many chronic GI conditions begin in midlife and continue into old age, their prevalence will likely increase as the U.S. population continues to age.

This chapter describes the pathophysiologic processes of the most common disorders of the GI tract and summarizes current treatment for these conditions. Because knowledge about many GI disorders is expanding rapidly, some current research on selected GI conditions is described. Finally, because of the intimate relationship between GI function and the integrity and well-being of the person, a discussion of the psychological and emotional aspects of GI disorders across the life span is included.

MANIFESTATIONS OF GASTROINTESTINAL TRACT DISORDERS

As a basis for discussing individual types of GI disorders, a description of some common manifestations of these disorders and their pathophysiologic mechanisms is presented. Common manifestations include dysphagia, esophageal and abdominal pain, vomiting, intestinal gas, and alterations in bowel patterns.

Dysphagia

Dysphagia is a subjective difficulty in swallowing (Figure 36-1). It may include the inability to initiate swallowing or the sensation that the swallowed solids or liquids "stick" in the esophagus. In certain disorders, **odynophagia,** or pain with swallowing, may accompany dysphagia. The physiologic mechanism of normal swallowing is described in Chapter 35.

Categories

The pathophysiologic basis for dysphagia usually falls into three major categories: (1) problems in delivery of the bolus of food or fluid into the esophagus as a result of neuromuscular incoordination; (2) problems in transport of the bolus down the body of the esophagus as a result of altered esophageal peristaltic activity; and (3) problems in bolus entry into the stomach as a result of lower esophageal sphincter (LES) dysfunction or obstructing lesions.[2]

In the first category of dysphagia, individuals have a decreased ability to accomplish the initial steps of swallowing in an orderly sequence. The normal sequence of contraction of the pharynx, closure of the epiglottis, relaxation of the upper esophageal sphincter, and initiation of peristalsis by contraction of the striated muscle in the upper portion of the esophagus is altered, or certain steps in the sequence may be absent. Persons experiencing this type of dysphagia may cough and expel the ingested food or fluids through their mouth and nose or aspirate when they attempt to swallow. These symptoms are usually worse with liquids than with solids in this type of swallowing dysfunction.

The second type of dysphagia may be the result of any disorder, structural or neuromuscular, in which the peristaltic activity of the body of the esophagus is altered. The presence of (1) esophageal **diverticula,** or outpouchings of one or more layers of the esophageal wall; (2) **achalasia,** a disorder of esophageal smooth muscle function; or (3) structural disorders such as neoplasms or strictures may interfere with proper peristaltic activity in the esophagus.[2,3] This alteration in peristalsis may be simply weak peristaltic activity, aperistalsis (the absence of all peristaltic activity), or disorganized and therefore ineffective peristalsis. With this type of dysphagia the individual may have the sensation that food is "stuck" behind the sternum. Initially, dysphagia may be noted with solid foods; if the underlying pathologic process fosters a worsening of peristaltic ability, the passage of liquids may also become impaired.

The third category of dysphagia, which results from problems of bolus entry into the stomach, is secondary to any condition in which the LES functions improperly or is obstructed by a lesion. Tumors of the mediastinum, lower part of the esophagus, or gastroesophageal junction may invade the myenteric plexus or produce an obstruction at the LES, thus interrupting normal LES function by neural invasion or direct obstruction. In addition, motor disorders resulting from neuromuscular diseases or chronic lower esophageal inflammation from the reflux of acidic gastric contents may limit the ability of the LES to function properly. This type of dysphagia may be manifested as tightness or pain in the substernal area during the swallowing process.

Esophageal Pain

Two types of pain occur in the esophagus: (1) heartburn (also called **pyrosis**) and (2) pain located in the middle of the chest, which may mimic the pain of angina pectoris. Heartburn is caused by the reflux of gastric contents into the esophagus and is a substernal burning sensation that may radiate to the neck or throat. Two common mechanisms contribute to the development of heartburn. First, the highly acidic gastric contents may be a noxious stimulant to sensory afferent nerve endings in the esophageal mucosa. Second, spasm of the esophageal muscle instigated by acid stimulation may produce esophageal pain.

Chest pain other than heartburn may be the result of esophageal distention or powerful esophageal contractions. These stimuli may

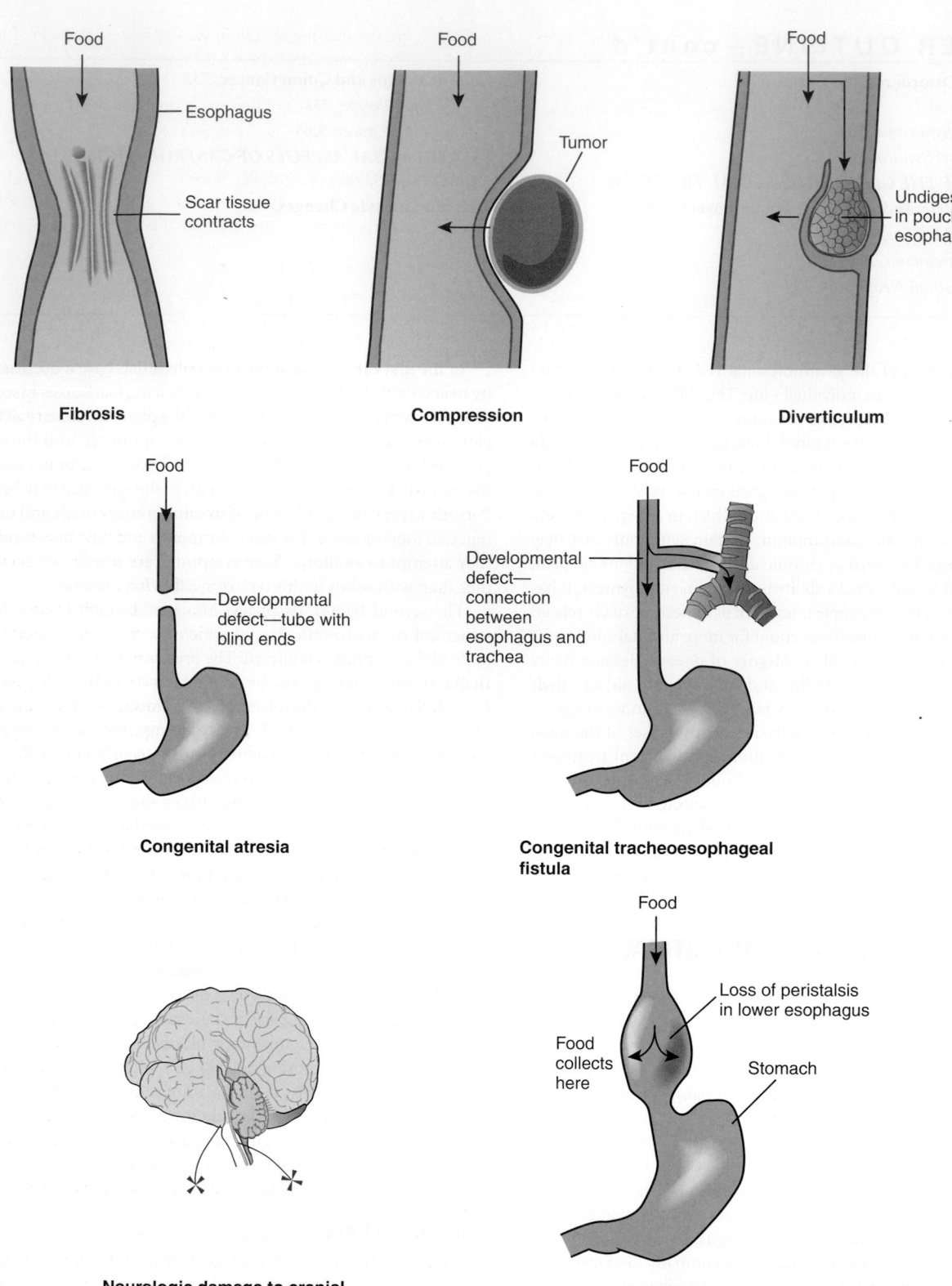

Fibrosis

Food → Esophagus

Scar tissue contracts

Compression

Food

Tumor

Diverticulum

Food

Undigested food in pouch obstructs esophagus

Congenital atresia

Food

Developmental defect—tube with blind ends

Congenital tracheoesophageal fistula

Food

Developmental defect— connection between esophagus and trachea

Neurologic damage to cranial nerves V, VII, IX, X, and XII

Achalasia

Food

Loss of peristalsis in lower esophagus

Food collects here

Stomach

FIGURE 36-1 Causes of dysphagia. (From Gould BE: *Pathophysiology for the health professions,* ed 4, Philadelphia, 2011, Saunders.)

arise from esophageal obstruction or a condition called diffuse esophageal spasm (DES), in which high-amplitude, simultaneous contractions in the smooth muscle portion of the esophagus alternate with normal peristalsis.[1] This type of esophageal pain is similar to that of

angina pectoris, particularly in its pattern of radiation into the neck, shoulder, arm, and jaw. Odynophagia may accompany diffuse esophageal spasm and can be indistinguishable from esophageal chest pain, except that it is triggered specifically by swallowing.

Infections of the esophagus attributable to herpes simplex virus, cytomegalovirus, or *Candida* species occur in immunocompromised patients. Patients with infectious esophagitis may experience a dull, aching chest pain. Swallowing generally worsens the sensation of heartburn or chest pain.

Abdominal Pain

Pain in the abdominal region may be the first sign of a disorder of the GI tract and is often an important impetus for seeking medical care. Although abdominal pain may result from GI tract disorders, it may also be the result of reproductive, genitourinary, musculoskeletal, or vascular disorders, as well as toxins or drug use. Abdominal pain is usually categorized into three types, which may manifest separately or in combination: (1) Visceral pain develops from stretching or distending an abdominal organ or from inflammation. The pain is diffuse and poorly localized and has a gnawing, burning, or cramping quality. (2) Somatic pain arises from injury to the abdominal wall, the parietal peritoneum, the root of the mesentery, or the diaphragm. In contrast to visceral pain, it is sharper, more intense, and generally well localized to the area of irritation. (3) Referred pain is felt at a location distant from the source of the pain but in the same dermatome or neurosegment. Referred pain is usually sharp and well localized and may be felt in the skin or deeper tissues.

Abdominal pain may be acute with instantaneous onset, such as pain caused by a perforated ulcer or a ruptured internal organ. A more gradual development of abdominal pain may accompany such chronic states as diverticulitis or ulcerative colitis (UC). Abdominal pain seldom occurs as a solitary manifestation of GI disorders; it is usually accompanied by other manifestations such as vomiting or alteration in bowel patterns to a variable degree.

Vomiting

Vomiting is the forceful expulsion of gastric contents through the mouth. Usually accompanied by a feeling of nausea, vomiting results from a coordinated sequence of abdominal muscle contractions and reverse esophageal peristalsis. Although vomiting is a common sign of GI disorders, it may also occur with metabolic, endocrine, vestibular (inner ear), and cardiac disorders, as well as with infection and fluid and electrolyte imbalances. It is also associated with such nonpathologic causes as pharmacologic agents, surgery, and the first trimester of pregnancy.

Vomiting associated with GI disorders may be the result of alterations in the integrity of the GI tract wall, such as gastroenteritis, or alterations in the motility of the GI tract, such as intestinal obstruction. The characteristics of the vomitus and the presence of blood or fecal matter may suggest the nature of the GI disorder and the level of the GI tract at which the disorder is located.

Intestinal Gas

Gas normally occurs in the GI tract and is the result of the swallowing of air, bacterial and digestive action on intestinal contents, diffusion from the blood, and the neutralization of acids by bicarbonate within the upper GI tract. The manifestations of excess intestinal gas may include excessive belching, distention of the abdomen, and excessive flatus. These manifestations may occur singly or in combination and may stem from a variety of causes. Belching is a normal phenomenon caused by the eructation of swallowed air but may also be the result of a motility disorder or gastric outlet obstruction. Abdominal distention may be due to failure to adequately digest a particular nutrient, such as the carbohydrate lactose. In the absence of adequate lactase (the digestive enzyme that breaks down lactose into glucose and galactose in the intestine), lactose undergoes bacterial fermentation, which results in gas production in the intestinal lumen. In some individuals, abdominal distention from excess gas may result from a defect in intestinal motility in which the intestinal contents are not propelled in a regular fashion, rather than from the production of too much gas. Excessive flatus may have causes similar to those of abdominal distention. Usually it is the result of increased amounts of gas produced by the action of bacteria on nutritional substrates that are particularly gas-producing, such as certain vegetables and legumes. Some individuals are particularly sensitive to the flatulent effects of beans, for instance.

Alterations in Bowel Patterns

Both constipation and diarrhea are difficult to define with precision, as a wide variation in bowel patterns can be found in different individuals. In addition, cultural and family socialization may play a role in the way in which an individual perceives bowel patterns. Alterations in bowel patterns may be the result of a change in GI tract motility or may be a component of a functional GI disorder such as irritable bowel syndrome (IBS).

Constipation

Constipation may be defined as small, infrequent, or difficult bowel movements.[2] Authorities have agreed on a norm of fewer than three stools per week as a guideline for defining constipation.[1] Dietary factors, particularly a diet low in fiber, have been shown to contribute to constipation. The presence of cellulose, the carbohydrate component of dietary fiber that is indigestible in the human intestine, may be effective in promoting regular peristaltic movement in the GI tract by forming bulk within the intestinal lumen to stimulate propulsion. In addition, because exercise stimulates intestinal peristalsis, a lack of exercise has been implicated in the development of constipation. In elderly persons the slowed rate of peristalsis that occurs with the aging process coupled with a decreased level of physical activity may promote chronic constipation. These factors may eventually contribute to the development of fecal impaction, a condition in which a firm, immovable mass of stool becomes stationary in the lower GI tract. Constipation may also be the result of pathologic conditions, including processes that alter the motility of the GI tract (such as intestinal obstruction) or processes that alter the integrity of the GI tract wall (such as diverticulitis).

Diarrhea

Diarrhea is defined as an increase in the frequency and fluidity of bowel movements and is often a primary sign of GI tract disorders. Although stool weight in excess of 200 g in 24 hours is an easily obtainable, objective definition of diarrhea,[3] most persons consider increased liquidity as the primary determinant. Diarrhea may be present as an acute or chronic manifestation. Acute diarrhea may be the result of an acute infection, emotional stress, or leakage of liquid stool around impacted feces. Chronic diarrhea is usually defined as symptoms lasting longer than 4 weeks and may be the result of a chronic GI tract infection (often associated with immune system compromise), alterations in the motility or integrity of the GI tract, malabsorption disorders, or certain endocrine disorders. Diarrhea that occurs on an episodic basis may be related to a food allergy or may be due to the ingestion of irritants to the GI tract, such as caffeine. Diarrhea in children frequently results from infection, although malabsorption disorders, anatomic defects, and allergy issues may also be causative factors.[4]

Pathophysiologic mechanisms. Four major pathophysiologic mechanisms have been identified in the development of diarrhea: (1) In osmotic diarrhea, increased amounts of poorly absorbable, osmotically active solutes such as a carbohydrate or magnesium sulfate cause sodium and water influx into the bowel lumen, resulting in diarrhea. (2) In secretory diarrhea, a pathophysiologic event such as the presence of a bacterial toxin causes enhanced secretion of chloride ion and water in the small intestine by simultaneously stimulating active secretion and inhibiting resorption. Diarrhea of 1 L or more per day may result from this inappropriate secretion of fluid across the intestinal mucosa.[2] Causes of secretory diarrhea include enterotoxins produced by such organisms as *Vibrio cholerae* and *Staphylococcus aureus*. (3) Exudative diarrhea is the result of exudation of mucus, blood, and protein from sites of active inflammation into the bowel lumen. This creates an increased osmotic load and a subsequent shift of water across the epithelium. In addition, if a large surface area of the bowel has an alteration in its integrity, intestinal absorption will be severely impaired, further compounding the diarrhea produced. Diarrhea associated with Crohn disease and UC may be the result of this exudative process.[2] (4) Diarrhea related to motility disturbances is a result of the decreased contact time of chyme with the absorptive surfaces of the intestinal lumen. If inadequate absorption takes place in the small intestine, large amounts of fluid will be delivered to the colon and may overwhelm the absorptive capability of the colon and cause diarrhea. In addition, if the fatty acids and bile salts present in chyme have not been adequately absorbed in the small intestine, they may induce a secretory diarrhea once they reach the colon, further compounding the process of diarrhea formation. Diarrhea associated with postgastrectomy dumping syndrome and IBS are examples of this type of diarrhea.

KEY POINTS

- Dysphagia is the perception of difficulty in swallowing. Dysphagia caused by neuromuscular disorders may be accompanied by coughing and aspiration, particularly with liquid ingestion. Altered esophageal peristalsis is associated with the sensation that food has become "stuck" behind the sternum. LES dysfunction may be manifested as substernal pain.

- Pain is a common symptom of GI disorders. A heartburn type of pain is associated with esophageal reflux. Chest pain similar to anginal pain may result from esophageal distention and obstruction. Abdominal pain may be visceral (diffuse, poorly localized), somatic (sharp, well localized), or referred (at a distance from the source but in the same dermatome).

- Nausea and vomiting are manifestations of many GI and other disorders. Alterations in bowel motility or integrity are causative factors. Excess gas may result from altered motility or lack of digestive enzymes. Gas is generated by swallowed air and bacterial action on nutritional substrates.

- Constipation is defined as small, infrequent (less than three per week), or difficult bowel movements. Lack of exercise, lack of dietary fiber, slowed peristalsis, and pathologic conditions that alter motility (e.g., obstruction) may produce constipation.

- Diarrhea is defined as an increased frequency and fluidity of bowel movements. Acute infection, stress, fecal impaction, malabsorption disorders, and ingestion of bowel irritants may produce diarrhea. Osmotic diarrhea is due to increased amounts of poorly absorbed solutes in the intestine. Secretory diarrhea is usually due to toxins that stimulate intestinal fluid secretion and impair absorption. Exudative diarrhea (mucus, blood, protein) results from inflammatory processes. A decreased transit time in the small intestine results in diarrhea because the absorptive capacity of the large intestine is exceeded.

DISORDERS OF THE MOUTH AND ESOPHAGUS

The mouth and the esophagus are the portals of entry for nutrients into the GI tract. An impairment in the proper functioning of these structures may have a profound effect on the ability of the individual to ingest adequate nutrients and begin the initial steps of the digestive process. Although disorders of the mouth and esophagus may not be acute, life-threatening emergencies, they may have severe long-term consequences for the well-being of the individual experiencing them.

ORAL INFECTIONS

Stomatitis

Etiology. Stomatitis is defined as an ulcerative inflammation of the oral mucosa that may extend to the buccal mucosa, lips, and palate. Among its many causes are pathogenic organisms, including bacteria and viruses; mechanical trauma; exposure to such irritants as alcohol, tobacco, and other chemical substances; certain medications, particularly chemotherapeutic agents; radiation therapy; and nutritional deficiencies, especially vitamin deficiencies. Stomatitis is a central manifestation of several autoimmune disorders, including Reiter syndrome and Behçet syndrome.[5] Stomatitis may also be idiopathic; that is, it has no identifiable cause.

One of the most commonly encountered types of stomatitis is acute herpetic stomatitis, also called herpetic gingivostomatitis, or more colloquially cold sores. It is caused by infection with herpes simplex virus (HSV), which has an affinity for the skin and nervous system. This type of stomatitis is commonly acquired by children between the ages of 1 and 3 years, although it may occur at any age. In primary infection, a brief period of prodromal tingling and itching may be present along with fever and pharyngitis. Vesicles may erupt on any part of the oral mucosa, particularly the tongue, gums, and cheeks. Vesicles form on an erythematous base, eventually rupture, and leave a painful ulcer. Once herpes simplex virus is acquired, it remains latent in the dorsal ganglia of the spinal cord and may be reactivated by physical or emotional stressors.

Treatment. The pharmacologic therapy used for stomatitis depends on its cause. The antiviral drugs acyclovir, famciclovir, and valacyclovir have been approved for treating acute herpetic stomatitis. Unfortunately, in a significant number of cases stomatitis is idiopathic or not amenable to specific therapy (e.g., stomatitis attributable to chemotherapy). In all types of stomatitis, measures designed to provide adequate oral hygiene and increase comfort in the oral cavity will be helpful in preventing decreased nutritional intake during the period of inflammation and assist in promoting the healing process. Topical mucosal barriers and corticosteroids may be of some benefit (e.g., triamcinolone [Kenalog] in Orabase)[5] whereas pentoxyphylline, colchicine, dapsone, and thalidomide have been used for recalcitrant cases of idiopathic stomatitis.[6]

ESOPHAGEAL DISORDERS

Gastroesophageal Reflux Disease

Gastroesophageal reflux disease (GERD) is the backflow of gastric contents into the esophagus through the LES. GERD may or may not produce symptoms.

Pathogenesis. The production of GERD is a multifactorial process. Any condition or agent that alters the closure strength and efficacy of the LES or increases intraabdominal pressure may predispose an individual to GERD. For example, the closure strength of the LES may be adversely affected by the intake of fatty foods, caffeine, and alcohol; cigarette smoking; sleep position; or obesity. In addition, pharmacologic agents such as progesterone-containing medications (e.g., birth control pills), narcotics, benzodiazepines, calcium channel blockers, and theophylline may decrease the pressure of the LES. Pregnancy increases the risk of reflux both by increasing intraabdominal pressure and by affecting hormonal mechanisms. Certain anatomic features, especially hiatal hernia, have been associated with GERD. The extent and severity of damage to the esophagus from GERD reflect the frequency and duration of exposure to refluxed material, as well as the volume and acidity of the gastric juices being refluxed.[2,3] The role of *Helicobacter pylori,* a cause of gastric and duodenal ulceration, in GERD is poorly understood and controversial.[7]

Clinical manifestations. The most common manifestations of GERD are heartburn, regurgitation, chest pain, and dysphagia. These symptoms are related to **reflux esophagitis,** which is esophageal inflammation caused by the highly acidic refluxed material. Complications of persistent GERD include esophageal strictures, Barrett esophagus (see Complications section), and pulmonary symptoms related to reflux esophagitis, such as cough, asthma, and laryngitis.

Treatment. Appropriate therapy is directed to increasing LES pressure, enhancing esophageal clearance, improving gastric emptying, and suppressing gastric acidity. Dietary and behavioral changes, such as avoiding tobacco and aggravating food and drink, are indicated for all patients, whereas over-the-counter antacids and histamine (H_2)-blocking medications may be effective for occasional GERD. Proton pump inhibitors (PPIs) are the mainstays of treatment for chronic GERD and have proven very successful in halting and even reversing the changes of chronic GERD.[8] If reflux esophagitis has progressed in severity, tissue damage, including ulceration, fibrotic scarring, and strictures, may be present in the distal third of the esophagus. Upper GI endoscopy is indicated for patients with ongoing symptoms, and some patients with stricture may require endoscopic dilatation. Surgical intervention, such as thoracoscopic Nissan fundoplication, may be helpful for intractable GERD.[9]

Complications. **Barrett esophagus** is a complication of chronic GERD and involves columnar tissue replacing the normal squamous epithelium of the distal esophagus. It carries a significant risk for esophageal cancer, and patients with Barrett esophagus should undergo regular endoscopic screening for cancer, along with pharmacologic control of their reflux.[10] For patients with documented dysplastic changes, endoscopic eradication therapy is a relatively low-morbidity option for treatment.[11]

Hiatal Hernia

A **hiatal hernia** is a defect in the diaphragm that allows a portion of the stomach to pass through the diaphragmatic opening into the thorax. Two types of hiatal hernia are commonly recognized: (1) a sliding hernia, in which both a portion of the stomach and the gastroesophageal junction slip up into the thorax so that the gastroesophageal junction is above the diaphragmatic opening; and (2) a paraesophageal hernia, in which a part of the greater curvature of the stomach rolls through

the diaphragmatic defect (Figure 36-2). "Mixed" hiatal hernias with features of both of these types may also occur. Sliding hernias are 3 to 10 times more common than paraesophageal and mixed hernias combined. The incidence of hiatal hernia increases with age and occurs more often in women than in men.

Etiology. Although the cause of the anatomic deformity leading to hiatal hernia is not well understood, certain conditions seem to predispose to loosening of the muscular band around the esophageal and diaphragmatic junction. Conditions in which intraabdominal pressure increases, such as ascites, pregnancy, obesity, and chronic straining or coughing, have been associated with the development of hiatal hernia.

Clinical manifestations and treatment. Individuals with hiatal hernia are predisposed to GERD and may experience symptoms such as heartburn, chest pain, and dysphagia. Ulcerations can develop along the mucosal surface of the stomach as it slides through the diaphragmatic opening, so-called Cameron ulcers. This is a fairly uncommon cause of chronic upper GI blood loss.[12] A potentially life-threatening situation can develop if a large portion of the stomach becomes caught above the diaphragm and is incarcerated, although this is extremely rare. Medical therapy for hiatal hernia is the same as that for GERD, detailed previously. Indications for surgery include acute incarceration or intractable reflux.

Mallory-Weiss Syndrome

Etiology. **Mallory-Weiss syndrome** is bleeding caused by a tear in the mucosa or submucosa of the cardia or lower portion of the esophagus. The tear is usually longitudinal and is primarily caused by forceful or prolonged vomiting in which the upper esophageal sphincter fails to relax during the vomiting process. Approximately 75% of individuals with Mallory-Weiss syndrome are men with a history of excessive ingestion of alcohol or salicylates.[2] Other factors and conditions that may contribute to the development of esophageal tearing in Mallory-Weiss syndrome are coughing, straining during bowel movements, trauma, hiatal hernia, esophagitis, and gastritis. Use of polyethylene glycol as a preparation for colonoscopy has also been associated with Mallory-Weiss tears.[13]

Clinical manifestations and treatment. Manifestations of Mallory-Weiss syndrome include vomiting of blood and passing of large amounts of blood rectally after an episode of forceful vomiting. Epigastric or back pain may also be present. Bleeding may range in severity from mild to massive. It is often profuse when the tear is near the cardia of the stomach and may proceed to fatal shock in this circumstance. Identification is made by endoscopic examination during an episode of acute upper GI bleeding. The majority of patients require at least one blood transfusion, but in most cases bleeding stops spontaneously.[14-19]

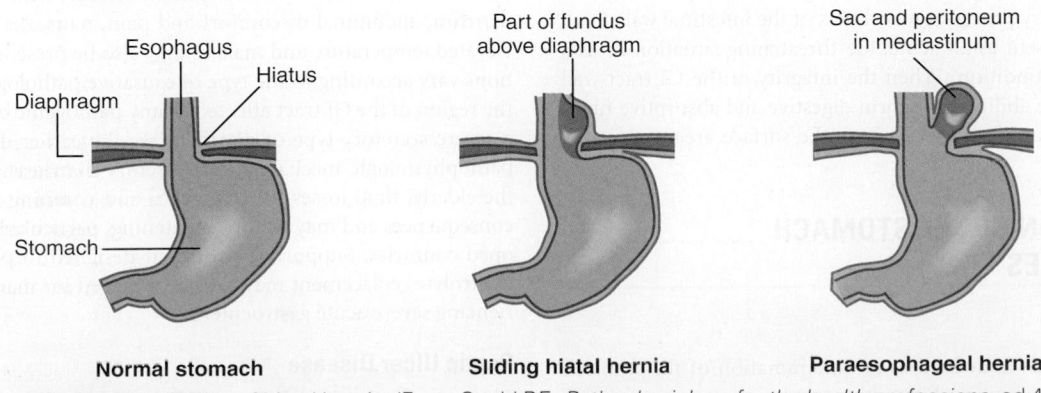

Normal stomach   **Sliding hiatal hernia**   **Paraesophageal hernia**

FIGURE 36-2 Types of hiatal hernia. (From Gould BE: *Pathophysiology for the health professions,* ed 4, Philadelphia, 2011, Saunders.)

Control of active bleeding may be achieved through endoscopic multipolar electric coagulation or similar techniques, epinephrine injection, or through interventional radiologic procedures (e.g., vasopressin infusion, Gelfoam embolization).[20] In selected cases, surgical intervention may be necessary.

Esophageal Varices

Esophageal varices represent a complication of portal hypertension, which in Western society is generally the result of cirrhosis attributable to alcoholism or viral hepatitis. In developing tropical countries, chronic infection with the *Schistosoma* species of liver flukes is a major cause of portal hypertension, along with cirrhosis attributable to chronic hepatitis B infection. Varices will affect more than half of cirrhotic patients, and approximately 30% of these patients experience an episode of variceal hemorrhage within 2 years of the diagnosis of varices.[21] The diagnosis and management of varices are discussed in detail in Chapter 38.

KEY POINTS

- Stomatitis is inflammation of the oral mucosa. It may result from pathogenic organisms, trauma, chemical irritants, chemotherapy, radiation therapy, or nutritional deficiencies.
- Common esophageal disorders are GERD with esophagitis, hiatal hernia, and bleeding. Reflux esophagitis is manifested as heartburn, chest pain, and dysphagia and may be precipitated by gastric overdistention or poor LES tone. Fatty foods, cigarettes, morphine, theophylline, and progesterone may inhibit LES tone.
- Hiatal hernias may be sliding or rolling (paraesophageal). Conditions that increase intraabdominal pressure predispose to the development of hiatal hernia. Esophageal reflux often accompanies hiatal hernia, and the manifestations are similar: heartburn, chest pain, dysphagia.
- Bleeding from the esophagus may pose a life-threatening situation. Mallory-Weiss syndrome is bleeding caused by tears in the lower end of the esophagus or upper part of the stomach. Alcohol and salicylate ingestion appear to be factors. Esophageal bleeding may also be precipitated by coughing, straining, or esophagitis. Rupture of esophageal varices is a dreaded complication of cirrhosis with portal hypertension and carries a high mortality.

ALTERATIONS IN THE INTEGRITY OF THE GASTROINTESTINAL TRACT WALL

Alterations in the integrity of the GI tract may occur at any location along the approximately 30 feet of its length, resulting from infection, an inflammatory process, or weakness of the intestinal wall. Such alterations may present as an acute, life-threatening situation or as a chronic, disabling condition. When the integrity of the GI tract wall is compromised, the ability to perform digestive and absorptive functions may also be compromised because the surface area or motility (or both) is altered.

INFLAMMATION OF THE STOMACH AND INTESTINES

Gastritis

Etiology. **Gastritis** is defined as an inflammation of the stomach lining. Acute inflammation of the stomach lining may occur after the ingestion of alcohol, aspirin, or irritating substances, as well as be caused by viral, bacterial, or autoimmune illnesses. (Some experts prefer use of the term gastropathy for toxic gastric inflammation, with gastritis defined as gastric inflammation attributable to infection or autoimmune disorders.[17]) In Western countries, overuse of nonsteroidal antiinflammatory drugs (NSAIDs) and overindulgence in alcohol and tobacco are preeminent causes of acute gastritis.

Pathogenesis. Chronic gastritis is currently the focus of extensive research. The factors promoting chronic gastritis have always been poorly understood. However, in 1983 identification of the bacterium *Helicobacter pylori* proved to be a landmark event.[18] Since that time, *H. pylori* has generated worldwide attention for its role in the promotion of chronic gastritis, peptic ulcer disease (PUD), and gastric carcinoma and lymphoma. Circumstantial evidence suggests that the mode of transmission of *H. pylori* is primarily person to person.[19] Some studies suggest a fecal-oral route, with the possibility of a reservoir in water sources.

It is now known that *H. pylori* causes chronic, superficial gastritis in virtually all infected persons.[2] Once established in the gastric mucosa, *H. pylori* establishes a destructive pattern of persistent inflammation. This persistent inflammation may resolve spontaneously, with clearance of the organism over time, leading to a decreased prevalence of *H. pylori* infection among older individuals. Consequences of *H. pylori* gastritis include PUD (discussed in a later section), atrophic gastritis, gastric adenocarcinoma, and mucosa-associated lymphoid tissue (MALT) lymphoma. The diagnosis and management of *H. pylori* infection will be discussed below.

Clinical manifestations. Although gastritis may be asymptomatic, manifestations of acute gastritis include anorexia, nausea, vomiting, and postprandial discomfort. Occasionally, **hematemesis** may occur in response to damage to the gastric epithelial mucosa. These manifestations usually disappear when the causative agent is removed, and the gastric epithelium undergoes a process of renewal after sloughing off the layer of damaged cells.

Gastroenteritis

Etiology. Gastroenteritis refers to inflammation of the stomach and small intestine, and may occur on an acute or chronic basis. Chronic gastroenteritis is usually the result of another GI disorder, such as Crohn disease, and is discussed in a later section. Acute gastroenteritis is the result of direct infection of the GI tract lining by a pathogenic organism such as the Norwalk virus, or it can occur from ingestion of preformed bacterial toxins (e.g., *Staphylococcus aureus, Bacillus cereus*) or bacteria that produce toxins (e.g., *Clostridium perfringens*). Acute gastroenteritis may also be caused by an imbalance in the normal bacterial flora of the GI tract precipitated by the introduction of an unusual bacterial strain, as may occur during travel.

Clinical manifestations and treatment. Acute gastroenteritis in adults is usually a self-limiting, nonfatal disease with manifestations of diarrhea, abdominal discomfort and pain, nausea, and vomiting. An elevated temperature and malaise may also be present. The manifestations vary according to the type of causative pathologic organism and the region of the GI tract affected. Many pathogenic organisms induce a severe secretory type of diarrhea (see the earlier discussion on the pathophysiologic mechanism of secretory diarrhea). In children and the elderly, fluid losses from diarrhea and vomiting can have serious consequences and may be life-threatening, particularly in underdeveloped countries. Supportive treatment designed to provide fluid and electrolyte replacement may thus be required for many patients experiencing severe acute gastroenteritis.

Peptic Ulcer Disease

The term **peptic ulcer disease (PUD)** refers to disorders of the upper GI tract caused by the action of hydrochloric acid and pepsin. These disorders may include injury to the mucosa of the esophagus, stomach, or duodenum and may range from a slight mucosal injury to severe ulceration (Figures 36-3 and 36-4). Peptic ulcer disease seems to be the result of an increase in factors that tend to injure the mucosa relative to factors that tend to protect it. The presence of an intact gastric mucosal barrier and the ability of the mucosa to renew its epithelium serve to protect it against injury. On the other hand, the presence of hydrochloric acid, which potentiates the actions of pepsin and other injurious substances such as aspirin and NSAIDs, will promote injury to the mucosa.

Previously, PUD was attributed to a stressful lifestyle and an irritating diet, and treatment revolved around removing spices from the diet and promoting a more relaxing lifestyle. In recent years, however, research has suggested that the organism *H. pylori* is a major precipitant of PUD, along with NSAIDs. A brief review of the current understanding of the pathogenesis of PUD is presented as a basis for further discussion of the manifestations and management of PUD.

Etiology and pathogenesis. Most peptic ulcers arise in the stomach and duodenum. Although the precise mechanisms of ulcer formation remain incompletely understood, the process involves the interplay of mucosal defense mechanisms, pepsin, and acid.[3] It is thought that a breakdown in the normally protective epithelial lining of the stomach occurs (Figure 36-5). In the formation of a gastric peptic ulcer, the barrier of the epithelial layer and the slightly alkaline layer of mucus may be interrupted by the chronic presence of such injurious substances as aspirin, NSAIDs, alcohol, and bile acids, which may be regurgitated from the duodenum. These substances apparently strip away the surface mucus and cause degeneration of the epithelial cell membranes, with diffusion of hydrochloric acid into the gastric epithelial wall.

Inappropriate excess secretion of acid is a major factor in the development of PUD in the duodenum (Figure 36-6). Studies have documented that the basal activity of the vagus nerve is increased in persons with PUD of the duodenum, particularly during a fasting state and at night. This stimulates the pyloric antrum cells to release gastrin, which travels via the bloodstream and acts on the gastric parietal cells to release hydrochloric acid (HCl). The result is an inappropriately high level of HCl in the duodenum. Interestingly, PUD patients also have lower bicarbonate levels in the duodenum as a consequence of the effect of *H. pylori* on the duodenal mucosa.[20]

H. pylori has a key role in promoting both gastric and duodenal ulcer formation (Figure 36-7). It has been reported that up to 75% of persons with duodenal ulcers and 60% of persons with gastric ulcers have *H. pylori* infection.[2] *H. pylori* thrives in acidic conditions; thus, infection with *H. pylori* renders a person with PUD subject to a slow rate of ulcer healing and a high rate of recurrence, and clearance of *H. pylori* promotes ulcer healing.[21] Although the precise mechanisms for the development of PUD remain complex and poorly understood, *H. pylori* virulence is associated with several factors, including the

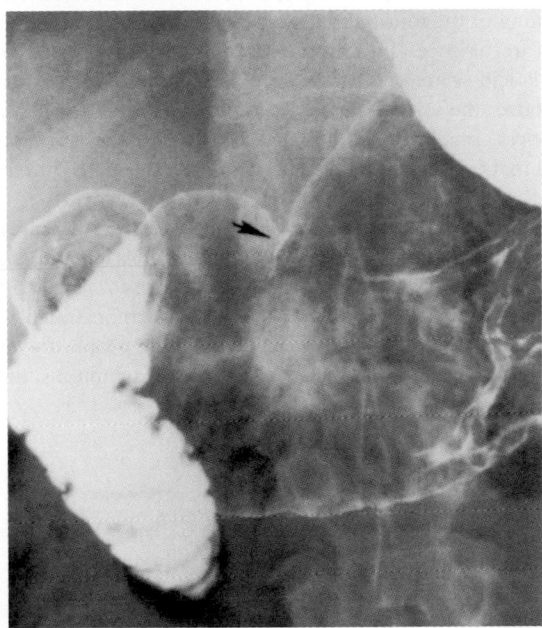

FIGURE 36-3 Radiograph of an ulcer in the lesser curvature of the stomach *(arrow).* (From Laufer I: *Double contrast gastrointestinal radiology with endoscopic correlation,* Philadelphia, 1979, Saunders.)

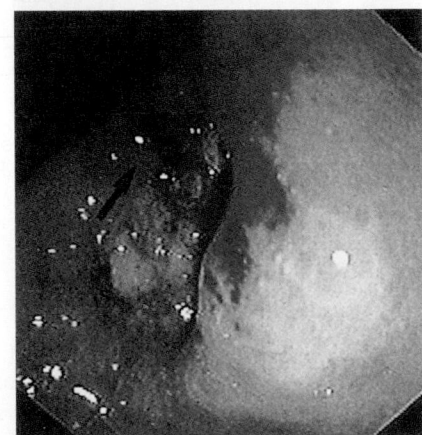

FIGURE 36-4 Photograph of an ulcer. (From Sleisenger MH, Fordtran JS, editors: *Gastrointestinal disease,* ed 5, Philadelphia, 1993, Saunders.)

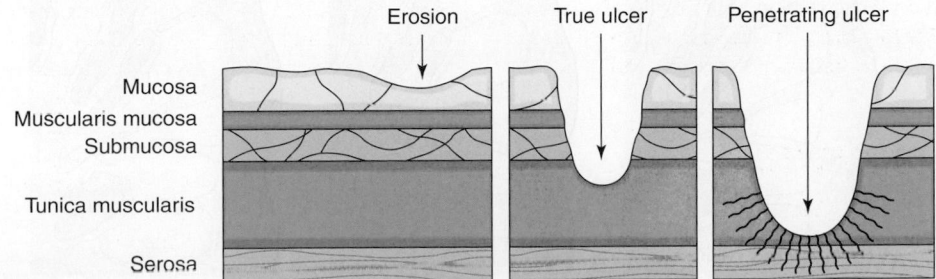

FIGURE 36-5 Lesions caused by peptic ulcer disease. (From Monahan FD, Sands JK, Neighbors M, Marek JF, Green-Nigro CJ: *Phipps medical-surgical nursing: health and illness perspectives,* ed 8, St Louis, 2007, Mosby.)

presence of unique, lengthy DNA sequences known as pathogenicity islands, particularly cytotoxin-associated gene A *(CagA)*.[22]

Other cofactors in the development of PUD have been investigated. Stress has long been considered a key factor in PUD. Glucocorticoids released in response to stress may have a role in the promotion of excess acid production or the destruction of gastric mucosal defenses. Smoking is an important risk factor, as identified by epidemiologic studies showing that PUD is twice as likely to develop in smokers as in nonsmokers.[23] In addition, smoking is related to poor ulcer healing and high rates of ulcer recurrence. Heredity is thought to have a role in the development of PUD. Certain patterns of gastrin release and pepsin secretion have been identified as genetic traits in families with an increased incidence of PUD.[9] Somewhat surprisingly, there is little evidence of a pathogenic role for alcohol, spicy foods, and caffeine.[2]

Clinical manifestations and diagnoses. Manifestations of PUD include epigastric burning pain that is usually relieved by the intake of food (especially dairy products) or antacids. The pain of gastric ulcers typically occurs on an empty stomach but may present soon after a meal. Duodenal ulcer pain classically occurs 2 to 3 hours after a meal and is relieved by further food ingestion. Other manifestations that may occur in individuals with PUD include nausea, abdominal upset, and chest discomfort. A significant proportion of ulcers are asymptomatic, and life-threatening complications, such as GI bleeding, may occur in patients with no warning. The symptoms of PUD are not specific enough to allow for a diagnosis, and malignant conditions can mimic benign PUD.

Diagnosis can be accomplished by upper GI barium contrast radiography or by endoscopy. The finding of a duodenal ulcer indicates a high probability of *H. pylori* and a low probability of malignancy, and the condition can be managed on this basis. All gastric ulcers should be visualized with endoscopy and biopsied to rule out malignancy and confirm the presence of *H. pylori*.[2] The necessity of testing for *Helicobacter* in patients with uncomplicated duodenal ulcers, given the very high pretest probability, is somewhat controversial. Most authorities do recommend testing for this organism in the case of gastric ulcers. Testing modalities include noninvasive tests such as the urease breath test, serologic analysis, and fecal antigen testing; invasive endoscopic tests include the tissue urease test, histologic analysis, and bacterial culture.[24]

Treatment. The major treatment objectives for PUD are to encourage healing of the injured mucosa by reducing gastric acidity and to prevent recurrence. Proton pump inhibitors are generally given to block acid secretion. Agents such as sucralfate form a protective coating over the injured mucosa and may be useful under some circumstances. Eradication of *H. pylori* infection with antibiotics has led to a marked reduction in the recurrence rate of PUD to less than 10%.[22,25,26]

In addition to these pharmacologic strategies, such measures as cessation of smoking, avoidance of aspirin and NSAIDs, and reduction of stress are all part of a comprehensive program to manage PUD. At the present time, no conclusive research has demonstrated that any specific diet has a therapeutic effect. Susceptible people are generally advised to avoid foods that seem to exacerbate symptoms, including caffeinated beverages and alcohol.

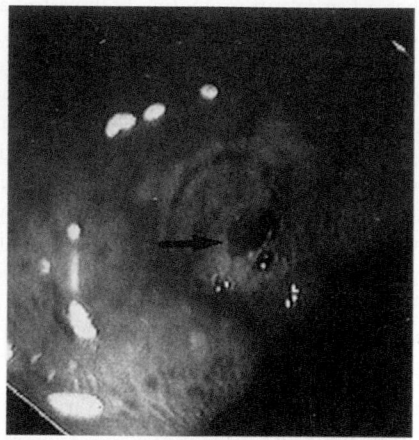

FIGURE 36-6 Duodenal bulbar ulcer. (From Sleisenger MH, Fordtran JS, editors: *Gastrointestinal disease,* ed 5, Philadelphia, 1993, Saunders.)

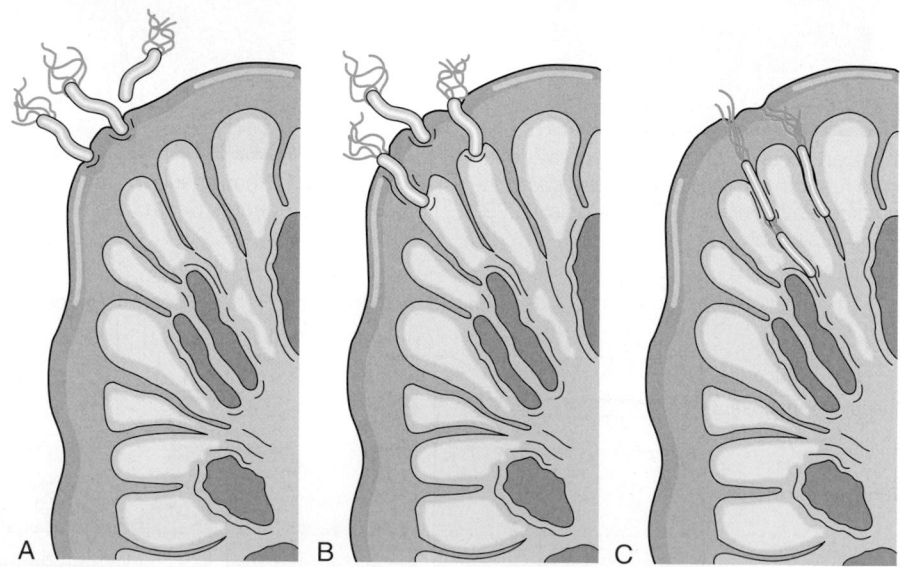

FIGURE 36-7 Penetration of the mucosal layer by *Helicobacter pylori.* **A,** After penetration, *H. pylori* forms clusters near membranes of surface epithelial cells. **B,** Some attach to the cell membrane. **C,** Others lodge between the epithelial cells.

INFLAMMATORY BOWEL DISEASE

The term **inflammatory bowel disease (IBD)** refers to the two separate disease entities of UC and Crohn disease. IBD is generally a life-altering chronic illness with serious consequences for people and their families who must cope with it. Both UC and Crohn disease have their onset most commonly in childhood and young adulthood, with obviously profound implications. This section describes the pathophysiologic aspects of UC and Crohn disease; a later section in this chapter discusses the psychosocial aspects of IBD.

Ulcerative Colitis

Ulcerative colitis (Figure 36-8) is an inflammatory disease of the mucosa of the rectum and colon. Approximately one fifth of patients have total colitis, one third have subtotal disease extending beyond the sigmoid, and one half have disease limited to the rectum and rectosigmoid.[2] The changes are usually most severe in the rectum and extend for a variable extent around the colon, although there are several exceptions to this general rule. IBD is typically characterized by exacerbations and remissions. Its causes are poorly understood, but recent research has focused on genetic, environmental, and immunologic factors.[27] The immunologic basis for the disease is supported by the fact that UC frequently accompanies other autoimmune conditions such as thyroid disease and pernicious anemia. The annual incidence in North America has been estimated between 2 and 14 per 100,000 persons.[28]

Etiology and clinical manifestations. Ulcerative colitis begins as an inflammation at the base of the crypts of Lieberkühn. Damage to the crypt epithelium results, with eventual invasion of leukocytes and the formation of abscesses in the crypts. When multiple abscesses form in close proximity and begin to coalesce, large areas of ulcerations develop in the epithelium. Concurrent with this destructive process are attempts at repair of damaged tissue, along with the development of fragile and highly vascularized granulation tissue. The manifestations of UC are the result of these processes and include abdominal pain, diarrhea, and rectal bleeding. Bleeding occurs as a result of mucosal destruction and ulceration, as well as damage to newly developed granulation tissue. Diarrhea is a result of the mucosal destruction in the colon, which leads to a decreased ability of the bowel to absorb water and sodium and thus to an increased volume of fluid in the intestinal contents.

The progression of UC may be highly variable. In some individuals it may have very mild manifestations; in others it may rapidly progress

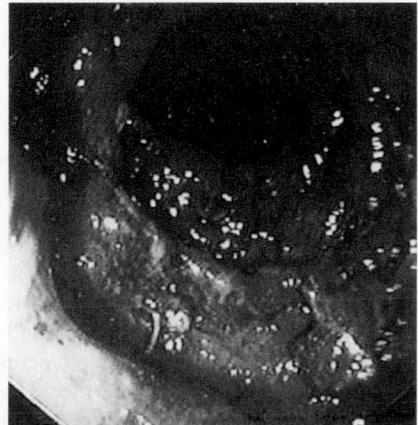

FIGURE 36-8 Ulcerative colitis. (From Sleisenger MH, Fordtran JS, editors: *Gastrointestinal disease*, ed 5, Philadelphia, 1993, Saunders.)

to a life-threatening disorder. Approximately 5% to 10% of persons with UC have only one attack, with no further recurrence. However, 65% to 75% of those with UC experience an intermittent series of exacerbations and remissions. Rarely, patients with UC will manifest toxic megacolon, a life-threatening condition in which the colon becomes massively enlarged. This condition generally requires urgent colectomy. A number of conditions in other organ systems complicate UC, the most devastating of which is the relentlessly progressive liver condition primary sclerosing cholangitis, which occurs in 3% of UC patients.[2]

An additional concern is increased risk for the development of colon cancer in persons who have had UC for more than 7 to 10 years. Authorities recommend monitoring these individuals carefully with regular endoscopy and biopsy. The presence of high-grade dysplasia should prompt consideration of prophylactic complete colectomy. Recent surgical advances, such as the ileoanal pouch, have allowed colectomy patients to avoid colostomy and have close to normal bowel function.

Treatment. Management of UC is complex and ever evolving. Corticosteroids have long been the mainstay of treatment of acute exacerbations, but side effects limit their long-term use. Patients with signs of systemic toxicity, especially those with impending or full-blown toxic megacolon, should receive broad-spectrum antibiotics. Important categories of disease-modifying agents include the salicylate analogues, and immunomodulating agents such as azathioprine and mercaptopurine. Intravenous followed by oral cyclosporine is a relatively new treatment for steroid-refractive UC that may help patients avoid colectomy.[29] Infliximab (Remicade) is another option for refractory UC whose exact role has yet to be determined.[30] It may help some patients with steroid-refractory UC who cannot take cyclosporine avoid colectomy.

Crohn Disease

Crohn disease, also called regional enteritis or granulomatous colitis, is an inflammation of the GI tract that extends through all layers of the intestinal wall (Figure 36-9). It most commonly affects the proximal portion of the colon and, less often, the terminal ileum. It may affect multiple portions of the colon, with intervening normal areas left between the affected regions. The manifestations of Crohn disease differ in some respects from those of UC, although some overlap may occur and distinction may be difficult. In Crohn disease, abdominal pain is often constant and in the right lower quadrant of the abdomen. A palpable abdominal mass may be present in the right lower quadrant, reflecting significant ileocecal involvement. The stool may be bloody, although not usually to the extent of that seen with UC. The cause of Crohn disease is unknown at the present time. There are fascinating parallels with UC as well as unexpected distinctions. For instance, smoking has been shown to protect against UC but to increase the risk of Crohn disease.[31] The annual incidence of Crohn disease in North America has been estimated from 3 to 15 per 100,000, and up to 5% of people with Crohn disease have 1 or more affected relatives.

Etiology and pathogenesis. Certain features of the pathogenesis of Crohn disease differ from those of UC. Crohn disease appears to be the result of a process in which the lymphoid and lymphatic structures of the GI tract become blocked. Subsequent engorgement and inflammation of surrounding tissue lead to the development of deep linear ulcers in the bowel wall. Eventually, all layers of the GI tract wall may become involved, and the portion of intestine that is affected may become thickened by fibrous scar tissue. Deep fissures may develop into fistulas, which may extend into adjacent tissue of other organs such as the bladder wall or even the skin. One of the cardinal features

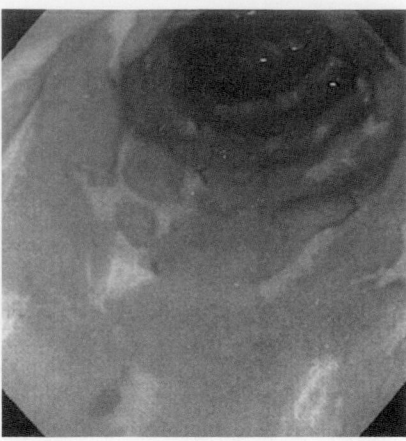

FIGURE 36-9 Crohn disease. (From Sleisenger MH, Fordtran JS, editors: *Gastrointestinal disease,* ed 5, Philadelphia, 1993, Saunders.)

of Crohn disease on histopathologic analysis is granulomas, which is generally diagnostic of this disorder.

Clinical manifestations. The manifestations of Crohn disease are the result of the pathologic changes just described, as the bowel becomes incapable of adequately absorbing the intestinal contents. Complications such as perianal fissures, fistulas, and abscesses are common in Crohn disease and may be the symptoms that lead individuals to seek health care. The onset and course of Crohn disease may vary a great deal; unlike UC, the symptoms present during a period of Crohn exacerbation may be subtle but persistent. At the present time, it is unclear whether a significantly increased incidence of intestinal cancer occurs in persons with Crohn disease. However, when Crohn disease involves the large bowel, the risk of colorectal cancer appears to be similar to that for UC of similar extent.[32] Toxic megacolon and primary sclerosing cholangitis also occur with Crohn disease but are much less frequent than in patients with UC. Many extraintestinal manifestations occur, including spondyloarthritis and uveitis.

The diagnosis of Crohn disease is typically made on the basis of the clinical history, radiographic changes, and typical biopsy findings of granulomatous intestinal inflammation. Several immunologic tests are also available, but these are expensive and generally reserved for cases where the diagnosis is uncertain.[2,3]

Treatment. Because the etiology of Crohn disease is unknown, therapeutic strategies are focused on alleviating and reducing inflammation. Therapeutic drug categories are similar to those for UC. Prednisone or sulfasalazine is generally used as initial therapy to achieve remission. The antibiotic metronidazole is particularly useful for colonic Crohn disease. Options for the treatment of refractory patients include azathioprine, 6-mercaptopurine, methotrexate, and biological therapies.

New types of treatments include the anti–tumor necrosis factor agents infliximab, adalimumab, and certolizumab, all of which have shown success in trials and are indicated for refractory Crohn disease.[33] Despite these advances, there is no cure for this challenging condition.

ENTEROCOLITIS

Antibiotic-Associated Colitis (Pseudomembranous Colitis)

Etiology. **Antibiotic-associated colitis (AAC),** also known as **pseudomembranous colitis,** is an acute inflammation and necrosis of the large intestine caused by *Clostridium difficile,* usually affecting the mucosa but sometimes extending to other layers.[34] Exposure

to antibiotics is the major factor predisposing to the development of this disorder, and patients with cancer or who have undergone abdominal surgery are at particular risk. The disease is mediated by bacterial toxins, leading to mucosal necrosis and the characteristic pseudomembrane composed of leukocytes, mucus, fibrin, and inflammatory cells.

Clinical manifestations and treatment. Resulting manifestations include diarrhea (often bloody), abdominal pain, fever, leukocytosis, and, rarely, colonic perforation. AAC is a major cause of fever and leukocytosis (elevated white blood cell count) among hospitalized patients receiving antibiotics. Treatment involves stopping the offending antibiotic, if possible, treating ischemia and other contributing conditions, and using antibiotics such as oral metronidazole or vancomycin. Recurrences are relatively common and may necessitate retreatment. In rare cases a fecal transplant (transfer of fecal material from another healthy person to the source patient via enema or gastric tube) or colectomy may be necessary to clear the infection.

Necrotizing Enterocolitis

Etiology. **Necrotizing enterocolitis (NEC)** is a disorder occurring most often in premature infants (less than 34 weeks' gestation) and infants with low birth weight (less than 5 lb or 2.25 kg). This disorder is characterized by diffuse or patchy intestinal necrosis accompanied by sepsis.

Clinical manifestations and treatment. Early manifestations include a distended abdomen and stomach. The major complication of NEC is intestinal perforation, which may necessitate surgery. Various theories regarding the etiologic progression of NEC include perinatal oxygen deficit with insufficient blood flow to the viscera, and the use of hypertonic feeding formulas in newborn infants. Greater than 90% of infants with NEC have a history of milk feeding as well. A special form of necrotizing enterocolitis, called typhlitis, may afflict adult cancer patients with neutropenia and carries a grave prognosis. Management of neonatal and adult forms of NEC includes careful supportive care, including fluid management and administration of broad-spectrum antibiotics. Early surgical consultation is essential for this syndrome, and surgery is necessary for patients with evidence of significant ischemia or perforation.

Appendicitis

Etiology. The most common cause of emergency surgery on the abdomen, **appendicitis** is an inflammation of the vermiform appendix. The classic hypothesis suggests that obstruction of the appendiceal lumen by a fecalith causes most cases of appendiceal inflammation. Less commonly, lymphoid hyperplasia or parasitic worms may lead to appendicitis. In an unknown number of cases appendiceal inflammation may be self-limited and may remit (e.g., with relief of the obstruction). If left unchecked, inflammation generally leads to necrosis of the appendix, with subsequent abscess formation and life-threatening peritonitis. Rarely appendicitis may occur in a subacute or stuttering fashion over several days or weeks.

Clinical manifestations and treatment. Appendicitis is two times more likely to occur in individuals younger than age 45 as compared to those 45 years and older, and it affects men somewhat more often than women. The peak incidence is between ages 10 and 19 years. The earliest manifestation of appendicitis is generalized periumbilical pain accompanied by nausea and, occasionally, diarrhea. The pain is often described as "migrating" or localizing to the lower right abdomen **(McBurney's point)** because of distention of the serosa from inflammatory edema, at which time fever usually manifests. Experienced surgeons generally operate in suspicious cases. Less typical cases should

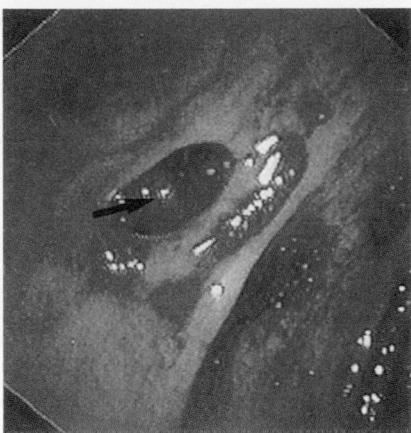

FIGURE 36-10 Colonic diverticula are evident as small outpouchings of colonic mucosa through the muscular tunicae *(arrow)*. (From Sleisenger MH, Fordtran JS, editors: *Gastrointestinal disease*, ed 5, Philadelphia, 1993, Saunders.)

be assessed with computed tomography (CT), or with ultrasound if the patient is a child or pregnant women or if CT is not readily available. Such an approach yields a relatively low false-positive surgical rate of around 5%.[2] Surgical removal of the appendix, either through an open procedure or laparoscopically, is the treatment of choice for appendicitis. Administration of antibiotics with replacement of fluid and electrolytes is usually necessary. Localized abscesses secondary to perforation may be managed with percutaneous tube drainage and antibiotics alone, if there are no signs of diffuse peritonitis.[35] Delayed appendectomy is usually carried out several weeks later, after the initial inflammation has subsided.

Diverticular Disease

Etiology. The term diverticular disease generally refers to **diverticulosis,** or the presence of diverticula in the colon. Diverticula are acquired herniations of the mucosa and submucosa through the muscular coat of the colon (Figure 36-10) that probably result from a combination of structural and functional factors. In particular, areas of weakness in the bowel wall, especially where blood vessels enter, are subject to damage from high intraluminal pressures. Colonic diverticulosis is very common in Western countries and is associated with a diet low in fiber; this lack of fiber presumably fails to provide enough bulk to dampen pressure variations in the intestine. The prevalence of diverticulosis increases with age; about 30% of the general population at 60 years of age and about 80% at 80 years will have diverticula in the colon.[1] Most persons experience no manifestations of diverticulosis, and by itself diverticulosis is not considered a pathologic condition. However, when diverticula become inflamed, the condition is referred to as diverticulitis (see Box 36-1 for the terminology of diverticulosis).

Clinical manifestations and treatment. Inflammation of diverticula can lead to serious consequences such as the development of abscesses in the bowel wall, peritonitis, and intestinal obstruction. Manifestations of diverticulitis include acute lower abdominal pain (usually left lower quadrant in location), fever, and leukocytosis. Constipation is common, but 25% of patients may have diarrhea. During an acute episode of diverticulitis, the administration of broad-spectrum antibiotics is indicated, and on occasion percutaneous or surgical drainage of an abscess may be necessary. Recurrence of diverticulitis is common. Long-term complications include colonic strictures and fistulas, which may necessitate surgery. Surgery is also recommended for patients with one or more recurrences of diverticulitis.

BOX 36-1 TERMINOLOGY OF DIVERTICULOSIS

Diverticulum: A single pouchlike herniation through the muscular layer of the colon
Diverticula: More than one diverticulum (Latin plural form)
Diverticulosis: The presence of one or more diverticula
Diverticulitis: Inflammation of one or more diverticula
Diverticular disease: Complications related to the presence of diverticula

---

KEY POINTS

- Alterations in intestinal wall integrity are generally a result of infection, inflammation, or weakness of the muscular layers. General symptoms include pain, bleeding, and diarrhea.
- Gastritis may be acute or chronic. Acute gastritis is generally precipitated by the ingestion of irritating substances, including alcohol and aspirin. Chronic gastritis may lead to atrophy of the gastric mucosa and the subsequent decreased production of HCl and intrinsic factor. Acute gastroenteritis is usually due to the ingestion of pathogenic organisms or preformed bacterial toxins and is characterized by self-limited vomiting, diarrhea, and abdominal pain.
- PUD may affect the esophagus, stomach, and duodenum. Gastric ulcers are thought to be due to breakdown of the protective mucous layer that normally prevents the diffusion of acids into gastric epithelia. Duodenal ulcers are caused by excessive acid secretion that is mediated by increased vagal activity. The organism *H. pylori* has been implicated in the pathogenesis of both gastric and duodenal ulcers. PUD is characterized by epigastric pain that is relieved by food or antacids. Perforation and bleeding are the major complications of PUD. Management of PUD is aimed at minimizing acid secretion and eradicating *H. pylori*.
- Ulcerative colitis and Crohn disease are chronic inflammatory disorders of the bowel. Ulcerative colitis (inflammation and ulceration of the colon and rectal mucosa) is manifested as bloody diarrhea and abdominal pain. There is an increased risk for colon cancer in persons who have had ulcerative colitis for more than 7 to 10 years. Crohn disease generally affects the proximal portion of the colon or the terminal ileum. Involvement of all layers of the intestinal wall predisposes to fistula formation and malabsorption. Crohn disease may result from blockage and subsequent inflammation of lymphatic vessels. Chronic abdominal pain and diarrhea are common. Management of ulcerative colitis and Crohn disease is aimed at reducing inflammation and subsequently trying to maintain remission.
- Acute inflammation of the intestinal wall may manifest as pseudomembranous enterocolitis or necrotizing enterocolitis. Abdominal pain, diarrhea, fever, and sepsis may result. The use of broad-spectrum antibiotics has been implicated in the etiologic development of pseudomembranous enterocolitis. Necrotizing enterocolitis, which occurs most often in infants, is thought to be due to bowel ischemia.
- Appendicitis is characterized by right lower quadrant pain, nausea and vomiting, and systemic signs of inflammation. Surgical removal of the appendix is necessary. Untreated appendicitis may result in rupture of the appendix and subsequent peritonitis; localized abscesses may be managed with tube drainage and antibiotics alone.
- Diverticula of the colon are very common in Western society because of a low intake of dietary fiber. Low-bulk stools result in the development of high intraluminal pressure, which predisposes to diverticula formation. Diverticulosis is generally asymptomatic. Inflammation of the diverticula, or diverticulitis, is manifested as fever and lower abdominal pain. Antibiotics and surgery may be required for management of complicated diverticulitis.

ALTERATIONS IN MOTILITY OF THE GASTROINTESTINAL TRACT

Disorders of the GI tract that alter its regular propulsive ability may have a negative effect on nutrient absorption. In the case of increased motility, the transit time of substances passing through the GI tract may be too fast to allow for adequate absorption. Conversely, a blockage or constriction of the GI tract may result in slowed or absent motility, which also prevents normal ingestion and processing of nutrient substances. As with alterations in the integrity of the GI tract wall, these alterations in GI motility may be acute or chronic, with many implications for the lifestyle of the patient.

MOTILITY DISORDERS

Irritable Bowel Syndrome

Irritable bowel syndrome is a complex entity that remains incompletely understood despite decades of intensive research. A clear definition of this syndrome has not yet been decided by all authorities; nevertheless, certain defining characteristics have been established. Typically, IBS is the presence of alternating diarrhea and constipation accompanied by abdominal cramping pain in the absence of any identifiable pathologic process in the GI tract.[2] (Other terms that have been used for this syndrome include spastic colitis and irritable colon syndrome.) Many authorities emphasize that the quantity of symptoms is not as important as their effect on the normal lifestyle of an individual. Persons with IBS may miss work, curtail their social life, and avoid sexual intercourse. This is an extremely common disorder, affecting up to 20% of the U.S. population.[2] It is important to differentiate IBS, in which no pathologic process of the GI tract has been identified, from inflammatory bowel disease, in which a specific pathologic process is identifiable.

Etiology and pathogenesis. The etiologic factors and pathogenesis of IBS are presently obscure. Most evidence seems to show that IBS is primarily a disorder of bowel motility. Studies have demonstrated that the myoelectric activity of the colon in persons with IBS is altered. In particular, the slow wave activity of the colon, which usually occurs at a rate of three to six times per minute, is markedly increased in IBS.[1,2] Moreover, the sensory response to distention and stimulation seems to be heightened. Whether these findings are the result of genetic factors or such environmental factors as episodic infection, psychological stressors, or dietary patterns remains unknown. The role of sensitivity to substances in ingested foods such as gluten and the contribution of bacterial overgrowth to symptoms are among current areas of exploration.

Clinical manifestations and treatment. The manifestations of IBS may vary greatly, with some persons experiencing only diarrhea or constipation and others experiencing an alternating pattern of both. In addition to cramping abdominal pain, manifestations such as nausea and mucus in the stool may also be present. The severity of manifestations ranges from barely noticeable to incapacitating. Current therapy focuses on the use of antidiarrheal agents and antispasmodic medications as appropriate. The 5-hydroxytryptamine (serotonin, 5-HT) 3 receptor antagonist alosetron has shown favorable results for the diarrhea-predominant form of IBS, whereas the 5-HT$_4$ receptor agonist tegaserod has been useful for patients with constipation as the main manifestation. However, both of these products have been associated with significant side effects, necessitating the Food and Drug Administration (FDA) to restrict their use. Lubiprostone is a locally acting chloride channel activator that enhances chloride-rich intestinal fluid secretion and is useful for patients with primarily constipative IBS.

Ingestion of a diet with increased amounts of fiber has proved useful in many cases and is thought to promote a more normal pattern of myoelectric activity by providing a regular propulsive stimulus in the gut. Perhaps more than with most GI disorders, patients with IBS may benefit from support groups, Internet-based resources, and alternative therapies.

Intestinal Obstruction

Intestinal obstruction is partial or complete blockage of the intestinal lumen of the small or large bowel. Mechanical obstructions are caused by blockage of the intestine by adhesions, hernia, tumor, inflammation, stricture (as in Crohn disease), impacted feces, volvulus, or intussusception. (Volvulus and intussusception are covered in more detail in the following sections.) Functional obstruction or ileus refers to the loss of propulsive ability by the bowel and may occur after abdominal surgery or in association with hypokalemia, peritonitis, severe trauma, spinal fractures, ureteral distention, and the administration of medications such as narcotics. Ogilvie syndrome is a rare severe motility problem characterized by recurrent bouts of ileus.

Etiology and pathogenesis. The most common location for gastrointestinal obstruction is the small bowel (90% of cases). The most frequent contributing factors are previous abdominal surgery with adhesions and congenital abnormalities of the bowel. Metastatic carcinoma, particularly cancer of the intestinal tract or female reproductive organs, is an important cause of obstruction and should be considered in patients with obstruction who have never had abdominal surgery. The severity and types of symptoms initially accompanying an intestinal obstruction vary with its cause and location.

With obstruction of the bowel lumen, fluid and gas begin to accumulate proximal to the obstructed location. The distention produced by trapped fluid and gas causes water and electrolytes to be secreted into the obstructed lumen of the small bowel. Distention also results in the impedance of venous return, and the bowel wall becomes edematous. The absorptive ability of the bowel wall is compromised, and fluid and gas continue to accumulate as additional water and electrolytes are secreted into the lumen. The pressure on the bowel wall exerted by the excess fluid and gas may result in leakage of fluid through the wall into the peritoneum, as well as necrosis of the bowel wall.

In addition to the process just described, other complications may be present with blockage of the intestinal lumen. Impairment of bowel circulation leads to ischemia, a process referred to as strangulation. Bacteria may translocate across the bowel wall into the bloodstream to produce fever and other signs of sepsis. As blood escapes from the engorged veins, significant loss of blood and plasma from the affected segment may result in the rapid development of shock. In addition, the strangulated segment may become gangrenous, with resulting peritonitis, or become perforated, with the leakage of highly toxic bacterial material into the peritoneal cavity.[2] If left untreated, a person with an intestinal obstruction of the small bowel has a high risk of death from shock and vascular collapse.

Clinical manifestations and treatment. The manifestations of an intestinal obstruction depend on its site and duration. Obstructions in the upper jejunal area usually result in vomiting, dehydration, and electrolyte depletion. In obstructions of the distal portion of the small bowel or ileum, constipation may be an early manifestation, with massive accumulation of fluid in the lumen occurring later. Dehydration may progress to hypovolemic shock if the obstruction is left untreated. In obstructions of the colon, massive gas distention may be present. The fluid and electrolyte losses associated with colonic obstruction may not be as severe as those seen in obstruction of the small bowel. Blockage of the colon by a tumor is the most common cause of colonic

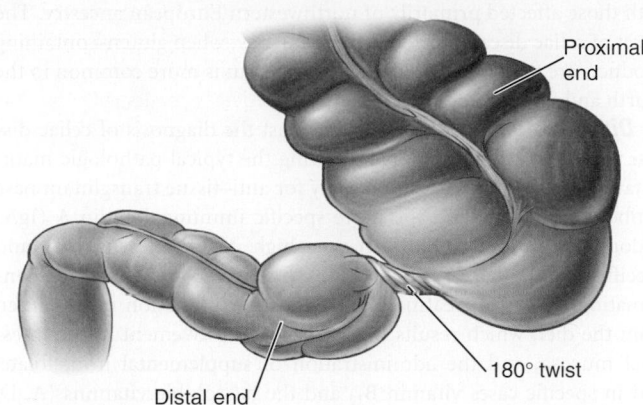

FIGURE 36-11 Volvulus. Intestine twists at least 180 degrees, causing obstruction and ischemia. (From Black JM, Hawks JH: *Medical-surgical nursing: clinical management for positive outcomes*, ed 8, Philadelphia, 2009, Saunders, p 714.)

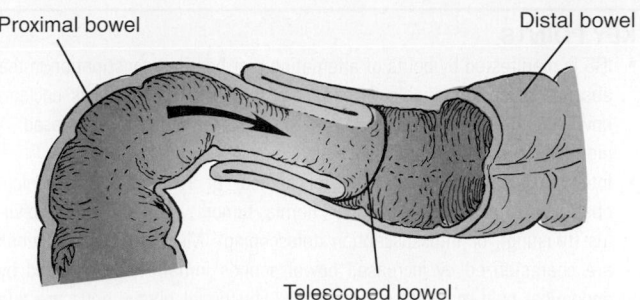

FIGURE 36-12 Intussusception. A portion of bowel telescopes into adjacent (usually distal) bowel. (From Black JM, Hawks JH: *Medical-surgical nursing: clinical management for positive outcomes*, ed 8, Philadelphia, 2009, Saunders, p 714.)

obstruction, and perforation of the bowel wall adjacent to the tumor may occur in association with an obstruction.

Therapeutic strategies for intestinal obstruction include surgical intervention to correct or remove the source of a mechanical obstruction. Supportive therapy, including decompression of the bowel with specialized tubes or endoscopy, and fluid and electrolyte replacement therapy, may be needed during an acute obstructive episode.

Volvulus

Volvulus is twisting of the bowel on itself, causing intestinal obstruction and blood vessel compression (Figure 36-11). The two most common sites for the development of volvulus are the cecum and the sigmoid colon.[2] A volvulus may be the result of an anomaly of rotation, an ingested foreign body, or an adhesion; however, the cause cannot always be determined. Volvulus tends to occur in elderly individuals with coexistent medical conditions. With the sudden tight twisting of the bowel on its mesentery, blood flow to the bowel is impeded. Gangrene, necrosis, and perforation may develop, resulting in a life-threatening situation. If both ends of a bowel segment are twisted, a closed-loop obstruction results, with the manifestations described earlier for intestinal obstruction. Treatment varies according to the severity and location of the volvulus and includes the therapeutic approaches described for intestinal obstruction.[2]

Intussusception

Intussusception is a telescoping or invagination of a portion of the bowel into an adjacent distal portion (Figure 36-12). It is most common in infants and occurs three times more often in males than in females.[2] In most cases involving infants, the actual cause is unknown, although intussusception has been linked to viral infections[36] and the use of some forms of rotavirus vaccine. In older children, it may be associated with alterations in intestinal motility or a condition called Meckel diverticulum, in which a congenital abnormality consisting of a blind tube is present in the distal end of the ileum. In adults, intussusception usually results from the presence of benign or malignant tumors.

As a bowel segment undergoes intussusception, peristalsis acts to pull more bowel along with it. The resulting area of tightened, invaginated bowel becomes edematous; venous engorgement with hemorrhage may occur. Intestinal obstruction of the bowel may develop, with eventual gangrene, shock, and perforation of the bowel if surgical treatment is delayed.

Megacolon

Megacolon can be congenital or acquired at any age. Perhaps the most common cause in Western countries is prolonged constipation/obstipation, usually chronic in nature. This is particularly common in younger children who are dealing with the psychological aspects of toilet training and bowel control. Although most of these children are psychologically normal, a small number of children with **encopresis** have experienced sexual abuse, and its presence should be considered.[37] Significant voiding issues also plague the other end of the age spectrum, and constipation/obstipation in the elderly may lead to megacolon, particularly when the sufferer has relied on regular enemas or laxatives for many years.

Hirschsprung disease (see following section) is characterized by the congenital absence of autonomic smooth muscle ganglia. The aganglionic bowel segment contracts but without the reciprocal relaxation needed to propel the intestinal contents forward. Stasis of stool and dilation of the proximal end of the colon result in megacolon, or massive dilation of the colon. Chagas disease caused by infection with *Trypanosoma cruzi* is a common cause of acquired colon neuronal dysfunction and megacolon in Central and South America, but is rarely seen in the United States, except among immigrants from endemic countries. As discussed earlier in the chapter, antibiotic-associated colitis (pseudomembranous colitis) may result in acute megacolon, which is a surgical emergency. Finally, the idiopathic syndrome of intestinal pseudoobstruction (**Ogilvie syndrome**) may rarely result in megacolon.

Hirschsprung Disease

Hirschsprung disease is a congenital disorder of the large intestine in which the autonomic nerve ganglia in the smooth muscle are absent or markedly reduced in number. In 90% of individuals with Hirschsprung disease, the aganglionic segment is in the rectosigmoid area, but occasionally the entire colon may be affected.[2] Hirschsprung disease occurs in approximately 1 in 5000 live births and is occasionally familial.[38] It is more common in males than in females, with a ratio of 3.8:1.[2] The disease often coexists with other anomalies, particularly Down syndrome. Although Hirschsprung disease is most commonly identified in infants and children, it may be present in adults as a long-standing undiagnosed condition.

In infants, Hirschsprung disease may have severe, life-threatening effects. Fecal stagnation may result in enterocolitis with bacterial overgrowth, profuse diarrhea, hypovolemic shock, and intestinal perforation. Interventions such as colonic lavage may be performed to empty the bowel until the infant is stable enough to withstand surgical intervention, which is the definitive treatment.

DISORDERS OF MALABSORPTION

Malabsorption refers to failure of the GI tract to absorb or normally digest one or more dietary constituents.[1] It is typically manifested as diarrhea, with the passage of inappropriately processed intestinal contents resulting in impaired fluid absorption. A variety of pathologic processes produce malabsorption syndromes, including intestinal enzyme abnormalities (e.g., lactase deficiency), infection (e.g., AIDS enteritis), and radiation enteritis, among others. The types of malabsorption syndromes discussed here result from a mucosal disorder of the small bowel or from the surgical removal of portions of the stomach or small bowel.

MUCOSAL DISORDERS

Myriad disorders affect the mucosa of the small intestine. Because the small intestine is the principal site of digestion and absorption of nutrients, a defect in this area has the potential for causing malabsorption of fat, protein, carbohydrate, vitamins, and minerals. Crohn disease, described earlier, may result in damage to the mucosa of the distal portion of the ileum, which is the site of vitamin B_{12} and bile acid absorption. Other important mucosal disorders of the small intestine are celiac disease and tropical sprue.

Celiac Disease

Etiology. **Celiac disease** (also called celiac sprue) is characterized by intolerance of gluten, a protein in wheat and wheat products. Current research suggests that celiac sprue is an immune disorder triggered by exposure to gliadin (a specific wheat gluten) in genetically predisposed persons.[2,39] Environmental, genetic, and immune factors play pivotal roles in determining the nature of symptoms. The main pathologic finding is villus atrophy, with a decrease in the activity and amount of surface epithelial enzymes. The resulting malabsorption of ingested nutrients may promote malnutrition and severe debilitation.

Celiac disease affects twice as many females as males and may have a familial inheritance pattern. More accurate serologic tests have shown the incidence in the general population to be much higher than previously believed; the current prevalence is about 1 in 300,

with those affected primarily of northwestern European ancestry. The onset of celiac disease may present in infancy, when gluten-containing products are first introduced into the diet, but is more common in the fourth and fifth decades.[2]

Diagnosis and treatment. In the past the diagnosis of celiac disease relied on intestinal biopsy showing the typical pathologic manifestations. New blood tests that assay for anti–tissue transglutaminase antibody (anti-ttG) and the more specific immunoglobulin A (IgA) endomysial antibody (EMA) have a high degree of sensitivity and specificity, although in general biopsy is still recommended for confirmation. Effective treatment includes the elimination of all gluten from the diet, which results in significant improvement in the intestinal mucosa, and the administration of supplemental iron, folate, and in specific cases vitamin B_{12} and the fat-soluble vitamins (A, D, E, K). Refractory cases may be treated with oral corticosteroids or other immunomodulating agents.[3] Ulcerative jejunitis and lymphoma should be suspected among refractory patients who do not respond to corticosteroids. Importantly, although the overall risk for malignancy is no higher than the general population, the incidence of certain types of intestinal malignancy, especially lymphoma, is modestly increased among sprue patients.[40]

Tropical Sprue

Etiology. **Tropical sprue** or **enteropathy** is a malabsorptive syndrome of unknown cause prevalent in equatorial countries. Current theory suggests that bacterial overgrowth of the large intestine produces products of fermentation that damage intestinal mucosa, although the exact etiology is obscure. In tropical sprue, the mucosa of the small intestine atrophies, with resulting malabsorption, malnutrition, and B_{12} and folic acid deficiency. Its incidence is high in persons living in or visiting tropical climates, and it appears to affect adults more often than children.[2] Although environmental factors seem preeminent, a genetic component may be present in some cases.

Clinical manifestations and treatment. The atrophy of the small intestinal mucosa may have severe effects. Massive malabsorption may result from failure of the mucosa to produce the enzymes needed for digestion. Manifestations include severe diarrhea with blood-tinged stools, abdominal distention, and steatorrhea (the presence of excess fat in the stool). In the Caribbean, tropical sprue is strongly linked to the presence of enterotoxin-producing coliforms and responds well to broad-spectrum antibiotics.[2] The response of patients from other areas (e.g., India) to treatment is less predictable than that of patients with Caribbean sprue. Treatment includes antidiarrheal medication and prolonged antimicrobial therapy as well as replacement of deficient vitamins, particularly folic acid.

MALABSORPTION DISORDERS AFTER SURGICAL INTERVENTION

Surgical procedures in which a portion of the stomach or small bowel is removed may result in loss of the ability to absorb nutrients properly, either through a loss of appropriate motility patterns or through a loss of the surface area of the small bowel needed for adequate absorption. Two types of disorders of malabsorption may occur after surgical intervention on the stomach or small bowel: dumping syndrome and short-bowel syndrome.

Dumping Syndrome

Etiology. **Dumping syndrome** is a term used to describe the literal dumping of stomach contents into the proximal portion of the small intestine because of impaired gastric emptying (Figure 36-13). This loss of normal, gradual pyloric emptying may occur after removal

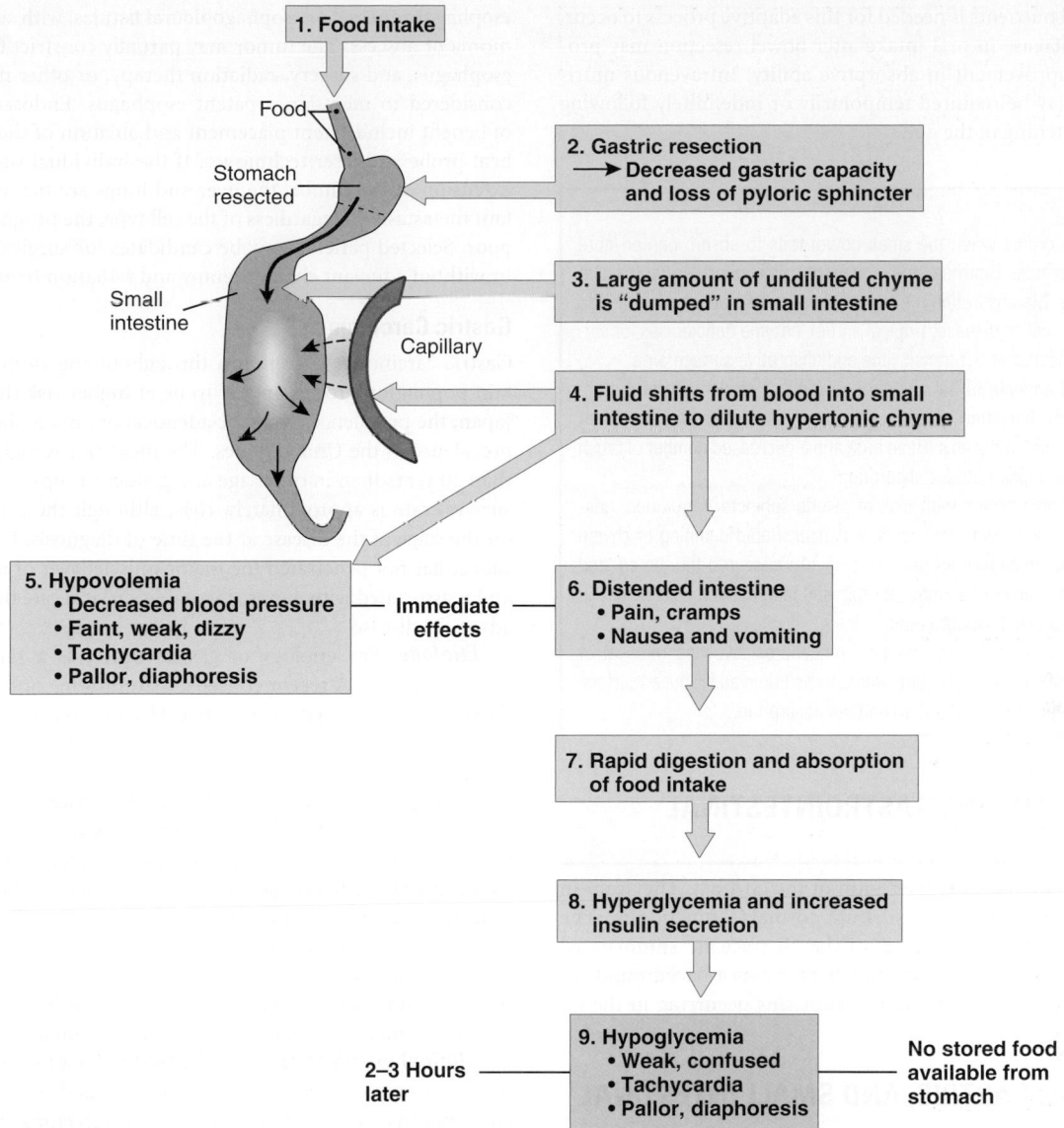

FIGURE 36-13 Dumping syndrome (postgastrectomy). (From Gould BE: *Pathophysiology for the health professions,* ed 4, Philadelphia, 2011, Saunders.)

of all or part of the stomach (gastrectomy), a procedure performed commonly for PUD in previous years, but more recently primarily for control of obesity. Interestingly, dumping seems to occur only with Roux-en-Y gastric bypass procedures.

Pathogenesis and clinical manifestations. With the normal reservoir function of the stomach now impaired, a large volume of hyperosmolar food is dumped rapidly into the small intestine, with consequences that may be severe. The hyperosmolar contents of the small intestine draw water into the lumen and stimulate bowel motility, with manifestations of diarrhea and abdominal pain. In addition, the rapid absorption of a large amount of glucose and a subsequent rise in blood glucose levels promote an excessive rise in plasma insulin level. The elevated insulin level then causes a rapid fall in blood glucose levels 1 to 3 hours after a meal. This sudden reversal is referred to as "rebound hypoglycemia."[2]

Treatment. Persons who have undergone a gastrectomy procedure will require specific instruction regarding eating small meals six to eight times a day rather than three large meals. Restriction of carbohydrate intake may be needed to limit glucose absorption. Medications to

reduce bowel motility have been helpful in promoting a more normal pattern of bowel function in this population.

Short-Bowel Syndrome

Etiology. **Short-bowel syndrome** refers to the severe diarrhea and significant malabsorption that develop after the surgical removal of large portions of the small intestine.

Pathogenesis and clinical manifestations. The severity of the manifestations depends on the amount and location of the bowel resected. In particular, removal of the distal two thirds of the ileum and the ileocecal valve may result in severe malabsorption. Because the ileocecal valve serves to regulate the transit time of intestinal contents, its removal may promote a transit time that is too rapid for adequate absorption of nutrients. In addition, loss of large portions of the small intestine will result in a diminished ability to absorb water, electrolytes, protein, fat, carbohydrates, vitamins, and trace elements.

Treatment. The small intestine displays an amazing ability to adapt after bowel resection. The remaining villi may enlarge and lengthen, thus increasing the absorptive surface area of the bowel. The presence of orally ingested nutrients is needed for this adaptive process to occur, and a gradual increase in oral intake after bowel resection may promote gradual improvement in absorptive ability. Intravenous nutritional support may be required temporarily or indefinitely following surgical foreshortening of the gut.

KEY POINTS

- Malabsorption occurs when the small bowel fails to absorb one or more dietary components. Diarrhea and abdominal discomfort are the usual manifestations. Malabsorption may occur because of mucosal dysfunction (Crohn disease, celiac disease, tropical sprue), enzyme deficiencies, or surgical alterations that affect transit time and absorptive surface area.
- Celiac disease appears to be caused by a familial intolerance of gluten-containing foods. Ingestion of gluten leads to inflammation and atrophy of the intestinal villi. A reduced surface area and a decreased number of brush border enzymes impair nutrient absorption.
- Dumping syndrome occurs with loss of pyloric sphincter regulation, generally after gastric surgery for ulcers or cancer. Rapid dumping of chyme into the duodenum causes an osmotic shift of water into the lumen, and diarrhea. Glucose absorption may be rapid and lead to overshoot of insulin secretion and rebound hypoglycemia.
- Short-bowel syndrome follows surgical procedures involving removal of large sections of the small intestine. Rapid transit time and reduced surface area for absorption lead to diarrhea and malabsorption.

NEOPLASMS OF THE GASTROINTESTINAL TRACT

Neoplasms may develop in every region of the GI tract. They vary in their severity and in their ability to disrupt normal GI functioning. The most common neoplastic processes of the GI tract are summarized here; the reader may wish to refer to Chapter 7 as a background for understanding these specific types of neoplasms occurring in the GI tract.

ESOPHAGEAL, GASTRIC, AND SMALL INTESTINAL CANCERS

Esophageal Cancer

Etiology. Esophageal cancer accounts for 1% to 2% of all cancers and affects men three times more often than women.[1] It usually develops in men older than 60 years, with a 5-year survival rate of about 15%.[41-45] Although the cause of esophageal cancer is presently unknown, several predisposing factors have been identified, including genetic predisposition, dietary habits (especially ingestion of foods high in nitrosamine content), environmental exposures, and chronic irritation of the esophagus from heavy smoking and alcohol use. Chronic severe reflux, especially that associated with **achalasia,** is a prominent risk factor for adenocarcinoma as well.

Most esophageal tumors worldwide are squamous cell carcinomas. The incidence of adenocarcinoma of the gastroesophageal junction has been increasing steadily in the United States and is now more common than squamous cell cancer. This shift seems to reflect an increased prevalence of **Barrett esophagus** (discussed earlier in the chapter). Interestingly, infection with *H. pylori* seems to protect against development of this form of esophageal cancer.[42]

Pathogenesis and treatment. Tumors of the esophagus are usually infiltrating, and the disease may spread extensively to surrounding organs by way of the esophageal lymphatics at an early stage. Invasion of surrounding structures may lead to the formation of esophagobronchial or esophagopleural fistulas, with subsequent pneumonia or abscess. The tumor may partially constrict the lumen of the esophagus, and surgery, radiation therapy, or other measures may be considered to maintain a patent esophagus. Endoscopic procedures of benefit include stent placement and ablation of the tumor through heat probe and laser techniques. If the individual survives the initial extension of the tumor, the liver and lungs are the usual sites of distant metastasis.[45] Regardless of the cell type, the prognosis is extremely poor. Selected patients may be candidates for surgical resection, with or without adjuvant chemotherapy and radiation treatment.

Gastric Carcinoma

Gastric carcinoma is common throughout the world; however, certain population groups appear to be at higher risk than others.[1,41] In Japan, the prevalence of gastric adenocarcinoma is about 10 times the prevalence in the United States. The incidence is higher in men older than 30 years than in other age and gender groups. The overall 5-year survival rate is approximately 10%, although the prognosis depends on the stage of the disease at the time of diagnosis. Early stage gastric cancer has not penetrated the major muscle layer of the stomach wall and is associated with a more favorable survival rate than seen in more advanced disease.

Etiology. The etiology of gastric cancer is a rapidly expanding area of research. A recent consensus Committee of the World Health Organization affirmed the role that *H. pylori* plays in development of gastric cancer, with a twofold increased risk for infected individuals compared to their uninfected peers.[2] In particular, the development of multifocal atrophic gastritis induced by persistent *H. pylori* infection is a critical step in the development of gastric cancer.[7] Epstein-Barr virus is another viral oncogene that has been identified as contributing to the global burden of gastric cancer.[43] Other risk factors are similar to those for esophageal cancer, with the exception that alcohol is not a significant contributor to gastric carcinoma.[2] Aspirin use seems to be protective against stomach cancer. Small numbers of gastric neoplasms may have different histologic characteristics, including lymphoma and carcinoid tumors, and have distinct clinical courses.

Clinical manifestations and treatment. Unfortunately, early gastric cancer typically has no manifestations and is rarely identified in countries that do not have a widespread screening program. Gastric carcinoma extends rapidly to the regional lymph nodes and surrounding organs by way of the lymphatic system and the bloodstream and by direct extension through the wall of the stomach. Advanced gastric cancer (Figure 36-14) has penetrated the muscle layer of the stomach and produces manifestations such as anorexia, weight loss, and GI bleeding.

Surgical resection of the tumor with appropriate surrounding margins remains the only effective treatment for this cancer, which, like esophageal cancer, has a dismal long-term survival.

Small Intestinal Neoplasms

Neoplasms of the small intestine may be benign or malignant. Fairly unusual, they account for fewer than 5% of GI tumors.[1] Tumors of the small intestine (usually adenocarcinomas) occur most often in persons older than 50 years. Carcinoid tumors, lymphoma, and sarcoma represent less common forms of intestinal tumors. Depending on the extent and type of tumor, partial or complete obstruction of the small bowel may occur.

Clinical manifestations and treatment. If the tumor is located near the ampulla of Vater, the common bile duct may become obstructed, with resulting biliary stasis and jaundice. Bleeding and ulceration of small intestinal tumors are common manifestations, as is obstruction and less commonly intussusception. Treatment may

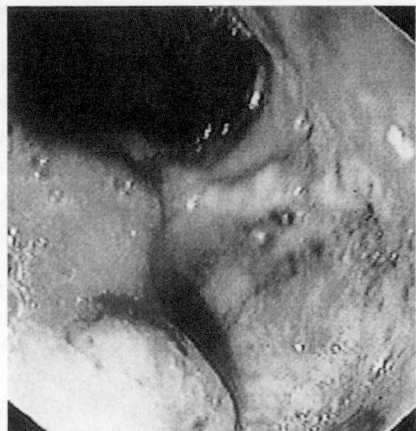

FIGURE 36-14 Ulcerating gastric cancer. (From Sleisenger MH, Fordtran JS, editors: *Gastrointestinal disease,* ed 5, Philadelphia, 1993, Saunders.)

include surgical intervention to remove the tumor and the affected portion of the small intestine, as well as chemotherapy for lymphomas and carcinoid tumors.

COLONIC POLYPS AND COLON CANCER

Cancer of the colon and rectum is identified in more than 140,000 men and women in the United States each year, with the incidence equally distributed between men and women.[3] It is second only to lung cancer as a cause of cancer deaths. It is well accepted that adenomatous colon polyps represent the major precursor lesion in the development of colon cancer.[2,41]

Colon Polyps

The term **polyp** refers to any protrusion into the lumen of the GI tract. Polyps may be benign or malignant, although most clinicians use the term polyp to refer to a benign or not-yet-malignant lesion. Polyps can have several forms; a sessile polyp is a raised protuberance with a broad base, whereas a pedunculated polyp is attached to the bowel wall by a stalk that is narrower than the body of the polyp. Benign adenomatous polyps of the colon predispose to malignant adenocarcinoma of the colon through dysplasia and neoplastic degeneration. In fact, some adenomatous polyps may already contain a focus of carcinoma (carcinoma in situ). Many people with polyps have no manifestations, although polyps may cause occult or gross bleeding and abdominal pain attributable to obstruction. Treatment will vary according to the size and type of polyp and its location in the colon. Biopsy and subsequent removal of polyps may be performed during sigmoidoscopy or colonoscopy. Figure 36-15 shows various colonic polyps. Several benign colon polyps, including the common hyperplastic variety, may be found on endoscopic biopsy and carry no cancer risk.

Colon Cancer

Etiology and risk factors. A number of risk factors have been identified for the development of colon cancer. The risk of colon cancer increases with advancing age. After age 40 the annual incidence of colon cancer accelerates, doubling every decade until age 80.[1] Dietary factors also seem to increase the risk; a high-fat, low-fiber diet has been proposed as an associated factor. Certain bowel conditions may predispose an individual to colon cancer, including ulcerative colitis and Crohn disease of the colon (see previous discussions). A hereditary predisposition may also be present; the probability of colorectal cancer

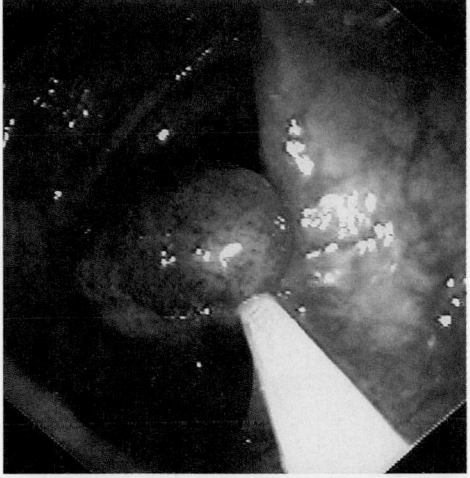
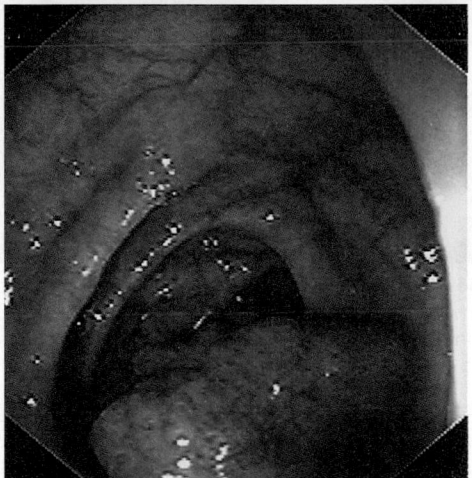
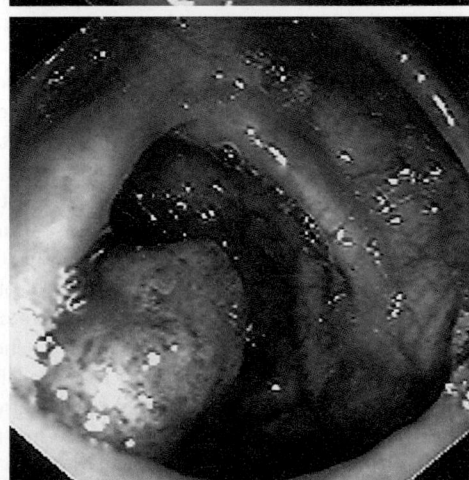

FIGURE 36-15 Photographs of colonic polyps. (Courtesy LE Copstead.)

in a person who has a first-degree relative with the disease is greater than 15%, compared with a 5% risk in the general population.[1]

An important hereditary condition is familial adenomatous polyposis (FAP), one form of which is Gardner syndrome. More common are the so-called hereditary nonpolyposis colorectal cancer syndromes. Clues to a familial syndrome include at least three close relatives with colorectal cancer, colorectal cancer involving at least two generations, and one or more cases of colorectal cancer occurring before age 50 years.[2] Colon cancer screening guidelines have recently

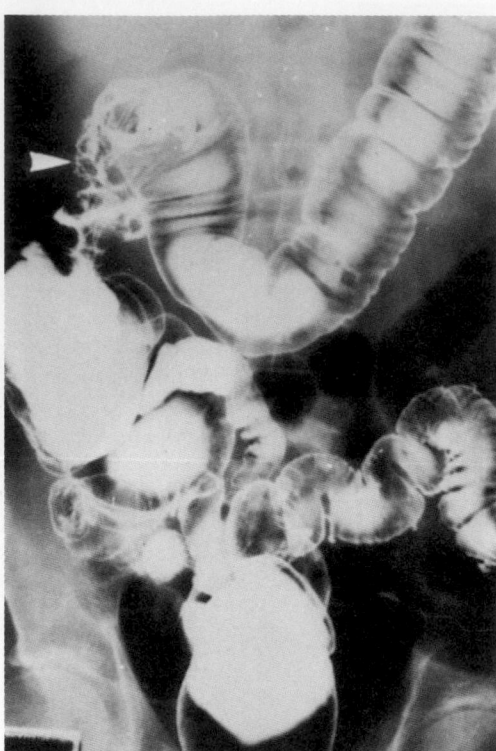

FIGURE 36-16 Barium enema demonstrating extensive mucosal destruction from a primary lymphoma of the right colon *(arrowhead)*. (From Sleisenger MH, Fordtran JS, editors: *Gastrointestinal disease,* ed 5, Philadelphia, 1993, Saunders, p 1484.)

TABLE 36-1	MODIFIED DUKES CLASSIFICATION FOR COLORECTAL CANCER	
DUKES CATEGORY	**DEFINITION**	**5-YR SURVIVAL (%) AFTER TREATMENT**
A	Cancer limited to mucosa or submucosa	90
B1	Cancer penetrates into but not through muscularis propria	80
B2	Cancer penetrates through muscularis	70
C1	Same as B1, plus lymph node metastases	50
C2	Same as B2, plus lymph node metastases	50
D	Distant metastases are present	<30

been updated; for the individual at average risk, colonoscopy every 10 years is recommended.[44] Persons with an increased risk for colon cancer based on family history should undergo more aggressive colon cancer screening.

Clinical manifestations. The manifestations of colon cancer depend on the anatomic location and function of the bowel segment containing the tumor. On the right side of the colon, the site of water and electrolyte absorption, tumor growth tends to extend along the bowel rather than surround the lumen (Figure 36-16). Although no signs of obstruction are present, black, tarry stools, which signify bleeding into the intestinal lumen, are a significant finding. On the left side of the colon, a tumor may cause manifestations of obstruction in the early stages of its growth. Feelings of intermittent abdominal cramping and fullness may be present, and "ribbon" or pencil-shaped stools may occur. Typically, the individual may note that the passage of stool or flatus relieves the abdominal pain. As tumor growth progresses, blood or mucus may be present in the stool. When the tumor is located in the rectum, early manifestations may include a change in bowel habits, often beginning with an urgent need to defecate upon awakening in the morning or alternating constipation and diarrhea. Later in the progression of tumor growth, a sensation of rectal fullness and a dull ache may be felt in the rectum or sacral region.

Treatment. The treatment and prognosis for colon cancer depend on several factors, including the extent of tumor invasion through the colon wall, cell type and degree of dysplasia, tumor genetics, and the presence or absence of local or distant tumor metastases.[2,41] The 5-year survival rate is directly related to the extent of tissue invasion. The traditional Dukes classification scheme (Table 36-1) has been modified and expanded over the last several decades; currently the tumor-node-metastasis (TNM) classification is accepted as the standard scheme. The most effective treatment is surgery to remove the malignant tumor

and adjacent tissue and lymph nodes that may contain cancer cells. The surgical formation of a **colostomy,** or an artificial opening of the colon on the abdominal wall, may be performed after removal of the affected bowel segment. Chemotherapy and radiation therapy are used as supportive measures in addition to surgical intervention. Chemotherapy in particular has advanced rapidly over the last 2 decades and has significantly improved the prognosis for moderately advanced (i.e., with nodal metastases) colon cancer.[41,45]

KEY POINTS

- Warning signs for cancer of the GI tract include black, tarry, bloody, or pencil-shaped stools and a change in bowel habits. Risk factors for GI cancer include a low-fiber, high-fat diet; polyps; and chronic irritation or inflammation.
- The prognosis for GI cancer is related to the extent of spread in the body. Surgical removal of tumors followed by chemotherapy, radiation therapy, or both is the usual treatment. Early detection is associated with a better prognosis.

PSYCHOSOCIAL ASPECTS OF GASTROINTESTINAL DISORDERS

STRESS OF LIFESTYLE CHANGES

GI disorders may have profound effects on the psychosocial functioning of the affected individual. Moreover, these disorders may place great stress on the family attempting to cope with the demands of that person's illness. Nutrition and bowel elimination are behaviors that are dependent on cultural norms; changes in these basic areas of human activity caused by a GI disorder may have a variety of meanings to different individuals. A teenager affected by a chronic GI disorder such as Crohn disease may be unable to participate in social activities that revolve around eating and thus may feel isolated from peers. IBS in a young adult who is beginning the most productive years of life may curtail the ability to function fully in the roles of spouse, parent, and wage earner. Finally, the onset of GI disorders, particularly a neoplastic process, in a middle-aged or older individual not only may limit that person's ability to perform activities of daily living but also may result in an increased awareness of aging and mortality.

In the past, much of the health care literature, including nursing texts, tended to stereotype individuals with chronic disorders of the GI tract as having behavioral disorders. Aberrant psychological characteristics, it was thought, were somehow associated with or even responsible for certain diseases of the GI tract, such as Crohn disease and UC. It is now recognized that the pathogenic process is almost never the result of primarily psychological causes, although some chronic diseases of the GI tract may be aggravated by emotional factors.[1,3] The stress of coping with a chronic, disabling illness may result in psychological trauma; in addition, any type of illness represents a threat to the integrity of the person. Individuals experiencing a chronic GI disorder may exhibit the psychological effects of such threats and will benefit from a sensitive approach to meeting their needs.

SUMMARY

This chapter has described the major alterations in the GI tract that may occur across the human life span. Because of the strong links between cultural and psychological functioning and activities associated with the GI tract, an in-depth understanding of these alterations is essential for health care professionals.

Disorders of the GI tract may have many manifestations, including dysphagia, pain, vomiting, gas, and alterations in bowel elimination patterns. Disorders may occur in any portion of the GI tract, from the mouth to the anus, and may be the result of alterations in the integrity of the GI tract wall (as in UC) or alterations in motility (as in IBS).

Disorders of malabsorption, such as celiac disease, may seriously limit the individual's ability to utilize dietary nutrients and are therefore potentially life threatening. Patients who have undergone surgery on the GI tract may also be at risk for malabsorption. Neoplasms of the GI tract are prevalent in the U.S. population, and the reader will want to review the associated risk factors for these neoplasms very carefully. Finally, readers who are preparing for a career in health care should carefully consider the information provided on the psychosocial aspects of GI disorders and identify ways to provide optimal care for patients with these disorders.

REFERENCES

1. Avunduk C: *Manual of gastroenterology*, ed 4, Philadelphia, 2008, Lippincott Williams & Wilkins.
2. Feldman M, Friedman LS, Brandt LJ: *Sleisenger and Fordtran's gastrointestinal and liver disease*, ed 9, Philadelphia, 2010, Saunders Elsevier.
3. Yamada T, et al: *Textbook of gastroenterology*, ed 5, Oxford, 2011, Wiley-Blackwell.
4. Kneepkens CM, Hoekstra JH: Chronic nonspecific diarrhea of childhood: pathophysiology and management, *Pediatr Clin North Am* 43(2):375–390, 1996.
5. Scully C, Gorsky M, Lozada-Nur F: The diagnosis and management of recurrent aphthous stomatitis: a consensus approach, *J Am Dent Assoc* 134(2):200–207, 2003.
6. Bruce A, Rogers RS: New and old therapeutics for oral ulcerations, *Arch Dermatol* 143(4):519–523, 2007.
7. Vakil N: Gastroesophageal reflux disease and *Helicobacter pylori* infection, *Rev Gastroenterol Disord* 3(1):1–7, 2003.
8. Coron E, Hatlebakk JG, Galmiche JP: Medical therapy of gastroesophageal reflux disease, *Curr Opin Gastroenterol* 23(4):434–439, 2007.
9. Liu JY, et al: Determining an appropriate threshold for referral to surgery for gastroesophageal reflux disease, *Surgery* 133(1):5–12, 2003.
10. Spechler SJ: Barrett's esophagus and esophageal adenocarcinoma: pathogenesis, diagnosis, and therapy, *Med Clin North Am* 86(6):1423–1445, vii, 2002.
11. Sampliner RE: Endoscopic ablative therapy for Barrett's esophagus: current status, *Gastrointest Endosc* 59(1):66, 2004.
12. Weston AP: Hiatal hernia with Cameron ulcers and erosions, *Gastrointest Endosc Clin North Am* 6(4):671–679, 1996.
13. Santoro MJ, Chen YK, Collen MJ: Polyethylene glycol electrolyte lavage solution-induced Mallory-Weiss tears, *Am J Gastroenterol* 88(8):1292, 1993.
14. Bharucha AE, Gostout CJ, Balm RK: Clinical and endoscopic risk factors in the Mallory-Weiss syndrome, *Am J Gastroenterol* 92(5):805–808, 1997.
15. Morales P, Baum AE: Therapeutic alternatives for the Mallory-Weiss tear, *Curr Treat Options Gastroenterol* 6(1):75–83, 2003.
16. Navarro VJ, Garcia-Tsao G: Variceal hemorrhage, *Crit Care Clin* 11(2):391–414, 1995.
17. Carpenter HA, Talley NJ: Gastroscopy is incomplete without biopsy: clinical relevance of distinguishing gastropathy from gastritis, *Gastroenterology* 108(3):917–924, 1995.
18. Marshall B: Unidentified curved bacilli on gastric epithelium in active chronic gastritis, *Lancet* 1:1273–1274, 1983. letter.
19. Malaty HM, et al: Transmission of *Helicobacter pylori* infection: studies in families of healthy individuals, *Scand J Gastroenterol* 26:927–932, 1991.
20. Hogan DL, Rapier RC, Dreilinger A, et al: Duodenal bicarbonate secretion: eradication of *Helicobacter pylori* and duodenal structure and function in humans, *Gastroenterology* 110(3):705, 1996.
21. Walsh JH, Peterson WL: The treatment of *Helicobacter pylori* infection in the management of peptic ulcer disease, *N Engl J Med* 333:984–991, 1995.
22. Atherton JC: CagA, the cag pathogenicity island and *Helicobacter pylori* virulence, *Gut* 44:307–308, 1999.
23. Kurata JH, Nogawa AN: Meta-analysis of risk factors for peptic ulcers: nonsteroidal anti-inflammatory drugs, *Helicobacter pylori*, and smoking, *J Clin Gastroenterol* 24:2–17, 1997.
24. Bickston SJ, Peura DA: Diagnostic tests for *Helicobacter pylori* infection. In Rose BD, editor: *UpToDate*. Available at www.utdol.com. Accessed 12/5/07.
25. Suerbaum S, Michetti P: Medical progress: *Helicobacter pylori* infection, *N Engl J Med* 347:1175–1186, 2002.
26. Shiotani A, Graham DY: Pathogenesis and therapy of gastric and duodenal ulcer disease, *Med Clin North Am* 86(6):1447–1466, 2002.
27. Podolsky DK: Medical progress: inflammatory bowel disease, *N Engl J Med* 347:417–429, 2002.
28. Loftus EV Jr: Clinical epidemiology of inflammatory bowel disease: incidence, prevalence, and environmental influences, *Gastroenterology* 126(6):1504, 2004.
29. Cohen RD, Stein R, Hanauer SB: Intravenous cyclosporin in ulcerative colitis: a five-year experience, *Am J Gastroenterol* 94(6):1587–1592, 1999.
30. Rutgeerts P, et al: Infliximab for induction and maintenance therapy for ulcerative colitis, *N Engl J Med* 353(23):2462–2476, 2005.
31. Cosnes J, et al: Smoking cessation and the course of Crohn's disease: an intervention study, *Gastroenterology* 120:1093–1099, 2001.
32. Lewis JD, Deren JJ, Lichtenstein GR: Cancer risk in patients with inflammatory bowel disease, *Gastroenterol Clin North Am* 28(2):459–477, 1999.
33. Peyrin-Biroulet L, Deltenre P, et al: Efficacy and safety of tumor necrosis factor antagonists in Crohn's disease: meta-analysis of placebo-controlled trials, *Clin Gastroenterol Hepatol* 6(6):644, 2008.
34. Hurley BW, Nguyen CC: The spectrum of pseudomembranous enterocolitis and antibiotic-associated diarrhea, *Arch Intern Med* 162(19):2177–2184, 2002.
35. Oliak D, et al: Initial nonoperative management for periappendiceal abscess, *Dis Colon Rectum* 44(7):936–941, 2001.

36. Buettcher M, Baer G, Bonhoeffer J, et al: Three-year surveillance of intussusception in children in Switzerland, *Pediatrics* 120(3):473–480, 2007.

37. Loening-Baucke Encopresis V: *Curr Opin Pediatr* 14(5):570–575, 2002.

38. Parisi MA, Kapur RP: Genetics of Hirschsprung disease, *Curr Opin Pediatr* 12(6):610–617, 2000.

39. Schuppan D: Current concepts of celiac disease pathogenesis, *Gastroenterology* 119(1):234–242, 2000.

40. Askling J, Linet M, Gridley G, et al: Cancer incidence in a population-based cohort of individuals hospitalized with celiac disease or dermatitis herpetiformis, *Gastroenterology* 123(5):1428–1435, 2002.

41. Kelsen DP, et al: *Principles and practice of gastrointestinal oncology*, Philadelphia, 2008, Lippincott Williams & Wilkins.

42. Chow WH, et al: An inverse relation between cagA+ strains of *Helicobacter pylori* infection and risk of esophageal and gastric cardia adenocarcinoma, *Cancer Res* 58:589–590, 1998.

43. Takada K: Epstein-Barr virus and gastric carcinoma, *Mol Path* 53(5):255–261, 2000.

44. Trowbridge B: Colorectal cancer screening, *Surg Clin North Am* 82(5):943–945, 2002.

45. National Comprehensive Cancer Network (NCCN): *Clinical practice guidelines in oncology.* Available at www.nccn.org/professionals/physician_gls/PDF/colon.pdf. Accessed 12/10/07.

Alterations in Function of the Gallbladder and Exocrine Pancreas

Jeffrey S. Sartin

⊝volve WEBSITE

http://evolve.elsevier.com/Copstead/
- Review Questions and Answers
- Glossary (with audio pronunciations for selected terms)
- Animations

- Case Studies
- Key Points Review

KEY QUESTIONS

- How is bile produced, stored, and secreted?
- How is pancreatic enzyme secretion regulated?
- What factors predispose to formation of cholesterol gallstones?
- What is the relationship between cholecystitis and cholelithiasis?
- What clinical and laboratory findings are indicative of acute pancreatitis?

- What serious complications may result from acute pancreatitis?
- How do the etiologic factors, clinical presentation, and management of chronic pancreatitis differ from those of acute pancreatitis?
- What are the signs, symptoms, and treatment for pancreatic cancer?

CHAPTER OUTLINE

Stones have been discovered in the gallbladders of Egyptian and Chinese mummies, suggesting that gallbladder disease has been present in humans for thousands of years. More than 700,000 operations to remove the gallbladder (cholecystectomy) are performed annually in the United States, and the incidence of new gallstones is 1 million to 2 million cases per year.[1,2] The incidence of acute pancreatitis varies according to geographic area but has been reported to range from 5 to 24 per 100,000 population in the United States and Europe.[1] Many health care professionals will encounter diseases of the pancreaticobiliary system frequently and need an in-depth understanding of the mechanisms that promote them. This chapter describes the

pathophysiology of diseases of the gallbladder, the biliary tree, and the exocrine pancreas, and summarizes current treatments. Cancers of the pancreas and biliary tree will be discussed briefly.

STRUCTURE AND FUNCTION OF THE PANCREATICOBILIARY SYSTEM

The pancreaticobiliary system is composed of the gallbladder and cystic duct; the intrahepatic, hepatic, and common bile ducts; and the endocrine and exocrine pancreas. The extrahepatic biliary tree and the gallbladder form a controlled system for delivering bile to the intestinal

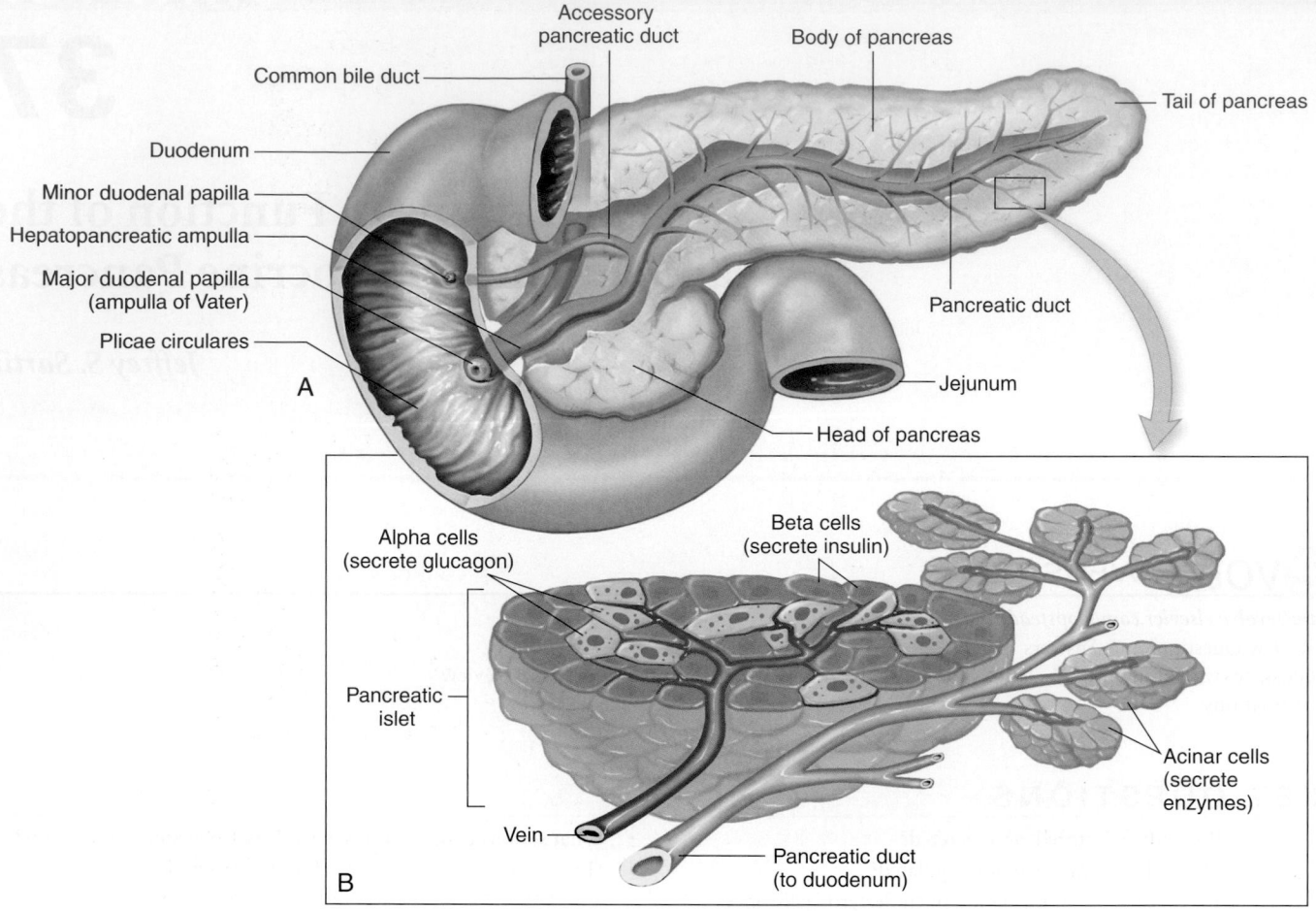

FIGURE 37-1 A, The pancreaticobiliary system showing the anatomic placement of the gallbladder and pancreas, the junction of the common bile duct and the pancreatic duct in the ampulla, and the ampulla of Vater. **B,** Exocrine acinar cells are arranged around pancreatic ducts and secrete enzymes and bicarbonate into the pancreatic juice that enters the duodenum, whereas endocrine cells of the pancreatic islets secrete hormones into the interstitial space where they diffuse into capillaries and enter the bloodstream. (From Patton KT, Thibodeau GA: *Anatomy & physiology,* ed 8, St Louis, 2013, Mosby, p 887.)

tract. (For additional background, refer to Chapter 35, which describes the physiology of digestion in the gastrointestinal lumen.)

The **gallbladder** is a distensible sack of about 30- to 50-ml capacity that connects via the cystic duct with the common hepatic duct to form the common bile duct. The common bile duct, which is about 3 inches long, extends behind the duodenum to terminate at the ampulla of Vater, a complex structure that also forms the terminating point of the main pancreatic duct. The pancreatic duct travels proximally in the pancreas and branches off dorsally to drain the tail of the pancreas. Thus, the ampulla of Vater forms the major aqueduct through which important digestive secretions enter the intestinal tract (Figure 37-1).

EMBRYOLOGY OF THE PANCREATICOBILIARY SYSTEM

In about the third or fourth week of gestation, the hepatic diverticulum forms from the primitive foregut.[3,4] It is composed of specialized progenitor liver cells that will eventually develop into the entire liver, biliary tree, and ventral pancreas. The dorsal pancreas forms from a separate outcropping of cells lying on the opposite side of the primitive foregut.

At 5 weeks of gestation, three buds can be seen in the hepatic diverticulum. The cranial bud contains specialized liver cells (hepatoblasts),

which will form the liver. The liver sinusoids develop and feed into the developing bile canaliculi, which drain into intralobular ductules and then into interlobular ducts. The caudal bud develops into the gallbladder, which joins the common hepatic duct via the developing cystic duct to form the common bile duct. The gallbladder and the hepatic ducts are initially hollow, but they solidify with development and become solid cords. With further differentiation, they become hollow once again to become the tubes and reservoir for bile flow. During the second trimester, the fetus produces bile, which gives color to the fetal meconium. Finally, the basal bud transforms into the ventral pancreas (Figure 37-2).[3,4]

PHYSIOLOGY OF BILE

Normal bile is composed primarily of water, electrolytes, and organic solutes. It has a low protein content, containing mainly bile acids, pigment, cholesterol, and phospholipids.[1] Bile acids consist mostly of primary bile salts (cholic and chenodeoxycholic acids) and secondary bile salts (deoxycholic, ursodeoxycholic, and lithocholic acids). Bile is formed in the liver and then modified and stored in the gallbladder and bile ducts before secretion into the intestinal tract. The major functions of bile are to aid in the digestion of lipids in the diet

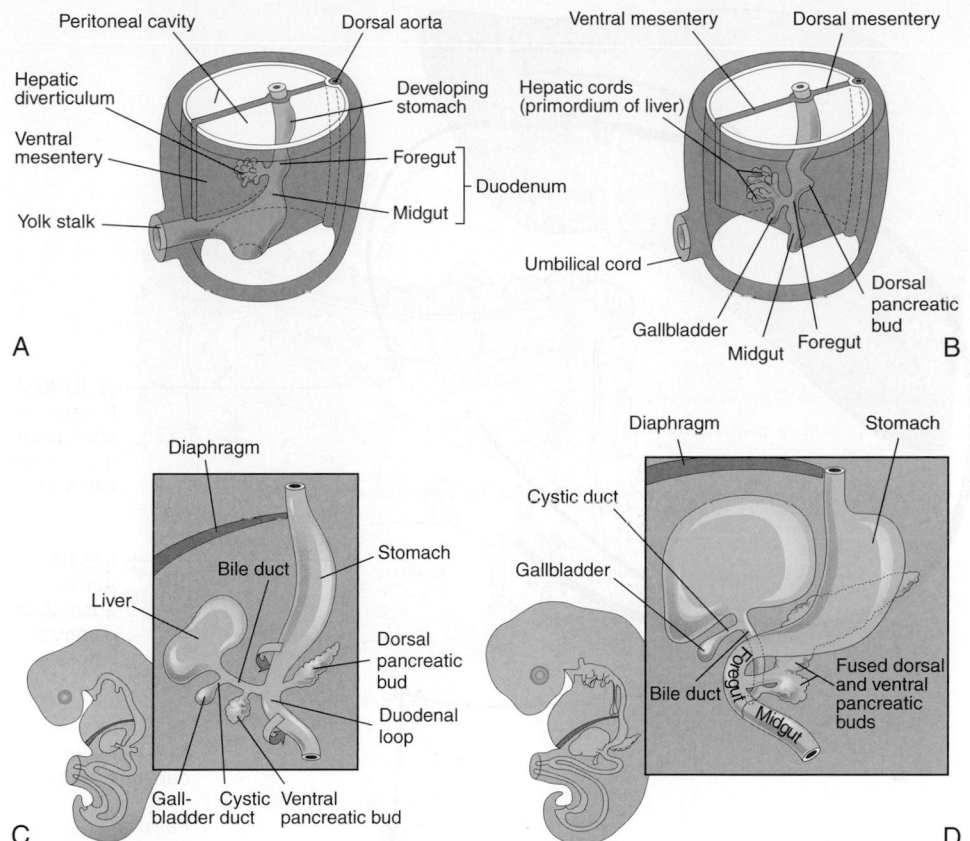

FIGURE 37-2 Stages in the embryonic development of the liver, pancreas, and duodenum at 4 weeks **(A),** 5 weeks **(B and C),** and 6 weeks **(D).** (From Moore KL, Persaud TVN, Torchia MG: *The developing human: clinically oriented embryology,* ed 9, Philadelphia, 2013, Saunders.)

and to transport waste products (particularly bilirubin), immunoglobulins (IgA), toxins, and cholesterol into the intestine for eventual disposal or reabsorption. After secretion into the bile canaliculi, bile flows through the canals of Hering, ductules, interlobular ducts, septal ducts, and right and left lobar ducts, and into the common bile duct (see Figure 37-1).[5]

The principal function of the gallbladder is the concentration and storage of bile. During the fasting state, the muscular sphincter at the ampulla of Vater is contracted, promoting flow of bile into the gallbladder. Only about half of the bile is stored during this time; the remainder flows into the duodenum. At the same time that bile is moving into the gallbladder, absorption is also occurring so that within 4 hours up to 90% of water in bile can be removed, leaving a very concentrated mixture of sodium, bile salts, and other electrolytes.[5]

With the first morning meal, a hormonally and neurally regulated contraction of the gallbladder occurs, releasing the concentrated bile into the duodenum. Bile acids eventually will be absorbed again in the terminal ileum and travel by the portal circulation to be secreted again into the bile. (Bile acids are reabsorbed on average two or three times daily.) A small amount of the bile acid pool (less than 5%) enters the colon, where primary bile salts undergo bacterial transformation into secondary bile salts (Figure 37-3).[6]

After secretion into the bile, bile salts have dual properties, being **hydrophilic** (soluble in water) at one end and **hydrophobic** (insoluble in water) at the other. Thus, these molecules tend to aggregate into clusters called micelles, which surround lipids such as cholesterol and allow them to solubilize (Figure 37-4). Micelles are not good stabilizers

of cholesterol alone, but another molecule, lecithin, also secreted in large amounts in the bile, is readily incorporated in the core of the micelle to greatly enhance the solubility of cholesterol. In this way, bile keeps cholesterol partly solubilized. Precipitation of cholesterol from bile occurs at high concentrations, predisposing to formation of gallstones.[6]

FUNCTIONAL ANATOMY OF THE PANCREAS

The pancreas is really two organs in one: it functions as both an endocrine and an exocrine organ. On the one hand, hormones such as insulin, glucagon, and somatostatin are produced and secreted into the vascular system (characteristic of an endocrine organ). On the other hand, every 24 hours the pancreas secretes more than 1 L of digestive juice into the digestive tract (characteristic of an exocrine organ).[5]

Embryologically, the pancreas is composed of two fused organs: a dorsal and a ventral pancreas (Figure 37-5). Microscopically, the pancreas is somewhat lobular and arranged into exocrine glands. The pancreatic juices are secreted into the glandular acini, which eventually drain into the main pancreatic duct and then enter the intestinal tract. The juices themselves are composed of both active digestive enzymes (e.g., amylase, lipase) and precursor or proenzymes (e.g., trypsinogen). Their release during a meal is controlled by hormones secreted from the small intestinal mucosa: **cholecystokinin (CCK)** and secretin. When this regulation is deranged, enzymes may be released within the gland and produce **acute pancreatitis.**

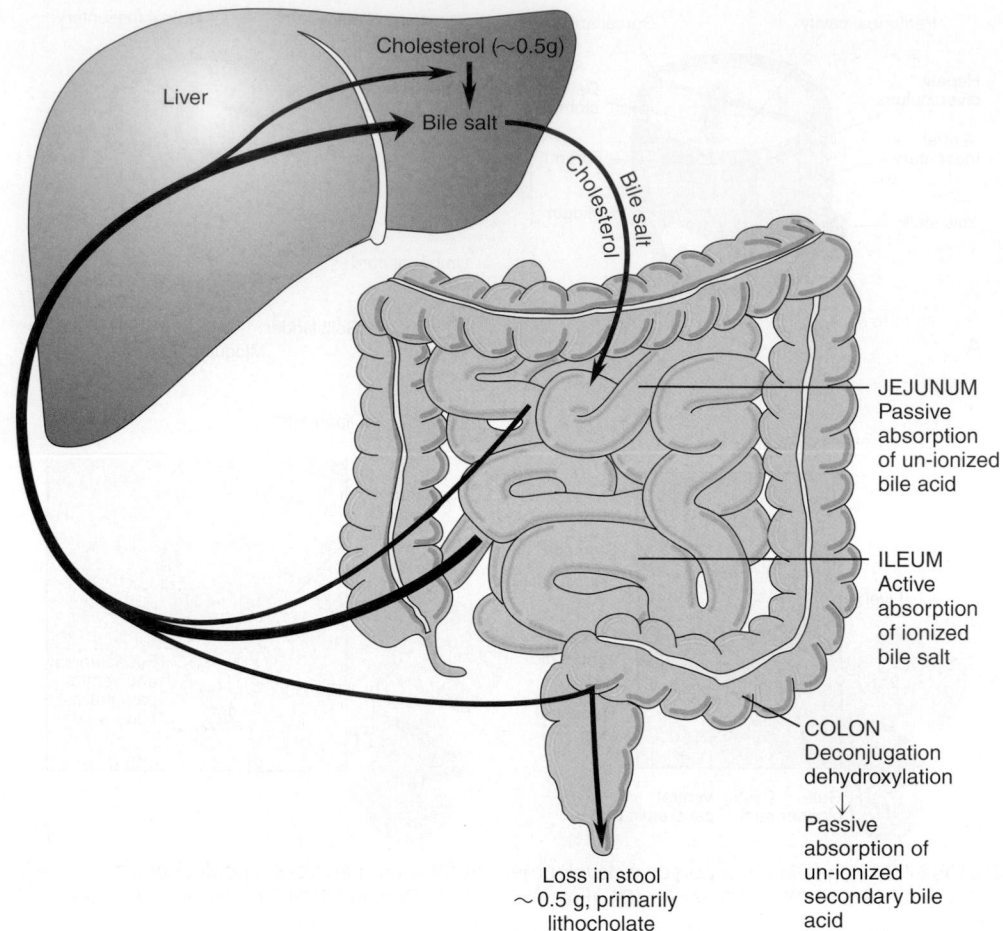

FIGURE 37-3 Enterohepatic bile salt recirculation is maintained by passive jejunal absorption of un-ionized bile salts, active ileal absorption of ionized bile salts, and colonic deconjugation and dehydroxylation of bile salts followed by passive absorption of lipid-soluble un-ionized secondary bile salt. The loss of unabsorbable bile salt is balanced by the de novo hepatic synthesis of bile salt from cholesterol. (From Cooper AD: Metabolic basis of cholesterol gallstone disease, *Gastroenterol Clin North Am* 20:34, 1991.)

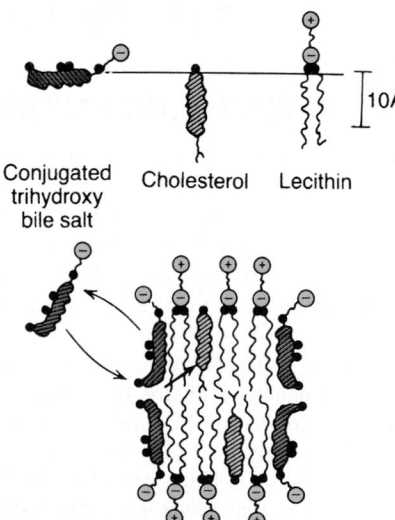

FIGURE 37-4 Bile acid–lecithin–cholesterol mixed micelle. Polar ends of bile acid and lecithin are oriented outward, whereas hydrophobic, nonpolar portions make up the interior. Cholesterol is solubilized within the hydrophobic, nonpolar center. (From Saunders KD et al: Pathogenesis of gallstones, *Surg Clin North Am* 70:1197-1216, 1990.)

KEY POINTS

- Bile is produced by hepatocytes in the liver and stored in the gallbladder. The main components of bile are bile acids, pigment, cholesterol, and phospholipids. Bile salts are important for digestion and absorption of fats from the small bowel. Bile is an important route for excretion of waste products, particularly bilirubin. The gallbladder receives bile from the liver, concentrates bile by absorbing water, and then contracts to expel stored bile into the common bile duct, which terminates in the duodenum.
- The pancreas is both an endocrine organ (secreting insulin, glucagon, and somatostatin into the bloodstream) and an exocrine gland (secreting digestive juice into the duodenum). Some pancreatic enzymes are secreted in active form (amylase, lipase), whereas others are proenzymes that are activated in the duodenum (trypsinogen). Release of pancreatic enzymes is stimulated by cholecystokinin and secretin.

DISORDERS OF THE GALLBLADDER

PATHOPHYSIOLOGY OF CHOLESTEROL GALLSTONE FORMATION

The majority of gallstones among patients in the United States are cholesterol stones.[1] In general, the formation of cholesterol stones

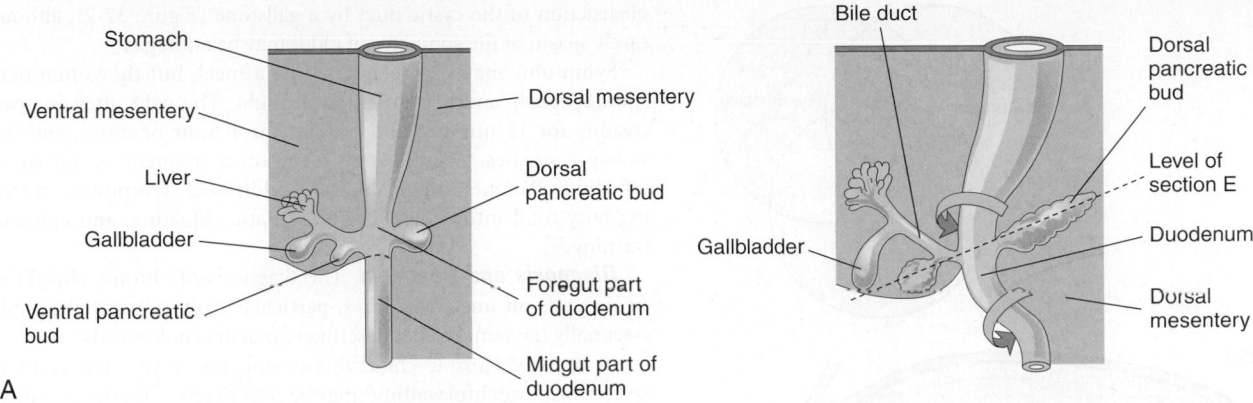

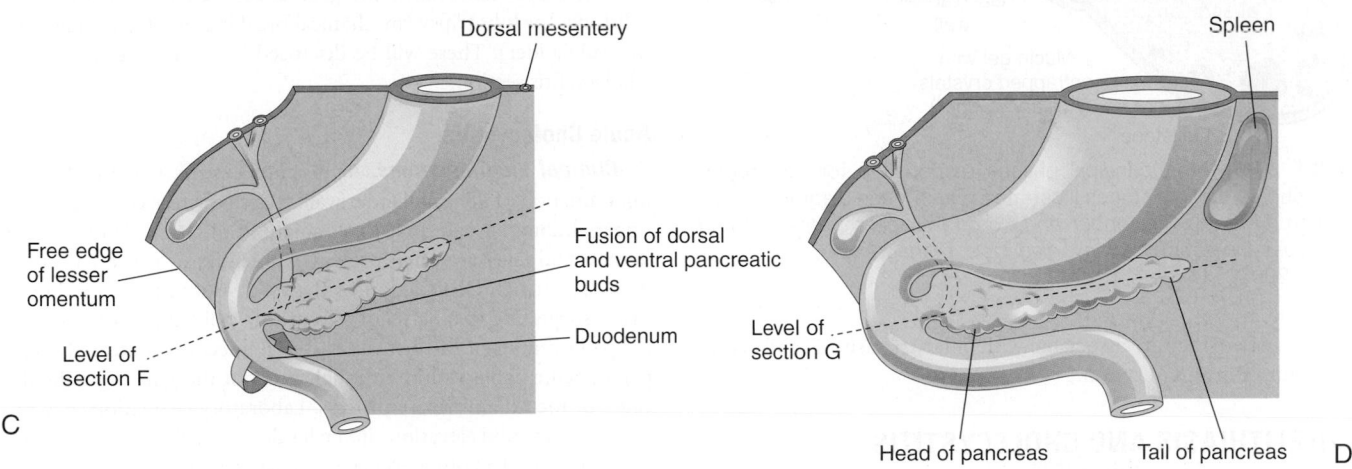

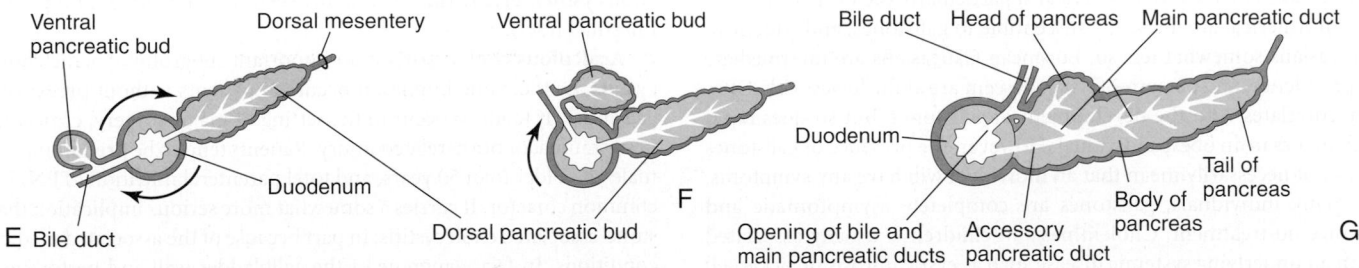

FIGURE 37-5 Stages in the embryonic development of the pancreas from the fifth to eighth week **(A-D),** and a diagram of the progressive development of the bile duct and main pancreatic duct **(E-G).** (From Moore KL, Persaud TVN, Torchia MG: *The developing human: clinically oriented embryology,* ed 9, Philadelphia, 2013, Saunders.)

in the gallbladder (**cholelithiasis**) can be broken down into three phases: (1) supersaturation of bile with cholesterol; (2) nucleation of crystals; and (3) hypomotility allowing stone growth (Figure 37-6).

As described previously, cholesterol eventually precipitates from supersaturated bile. If conditions are right for the formation of cholesterol gallstones, nucleation occurs in which the cholesterol crystals aggregate together. Continued growth of the crystals then depends upon the balance between cholesterol growth–promoting factors and factors that tend to cause stone dissolution. A significant factor that promotes the continued growth of stones is hypomotility or stasis of bile within the gallbladder. Patients with high spinal cord injuries,

patients receiving total parenteral nutrition, and persons who undergo prolonged fasting or rapid weight loss have impaired emptying and are at particular risk for development of cholesterol gallstones. Other risk factors for cholelithiasis include pregnancy, oral contraceptives, obesity, diabetes mellitus, and octreotide (somatostatin analogue) therapy.[1]

About 25% of gallstones in Western countries are due to pigment stones, which contain a mixture of pigment polymers and calcium salts. "Black" pigment stones are most common and may be idiopathic or associated with cirrhosis or hemolysis. "Brown" pigment stones differ in their composition and are much more common in developing

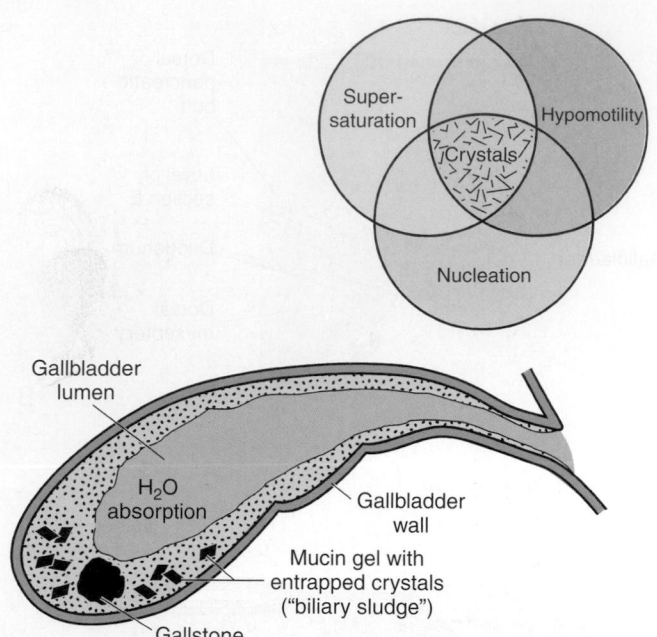

FIGURE 37-6 Three principal phases responsible for the formation of cholesterol gallstones illustrated with a Venn diagram. (From Feldman M et al: *Sleisenger and Fordtran's gastrointestinal and liver disease: pathophysiology, diagnosis, management,* ed 7, Philadelphia, 2002, Saunders, p 1069.)

countries, where they are associated with biliary parasitosis and bacterial colonization and infection.[1]

CHOLELITHIASIS AND CHOLECYSTITIS

Currently, about 20 million people in the United States have gallstones (cholelithiasis). The incidence of gallstones is related to age, gender, and a variety of medical factors. Gallstones are twice as common in women as in men. Native Americans, particularly the Pima Indians of North America, are markedly susceptible to gallstones, and American Caucasians somewhat less so. European Caucasians are intermediate in prevalence, and persons of Asian descent are at the lowest risk. Obesity correlates with the development of gallstones, but so does rapid weight loss in an obese individual. However, the presence of gallstones does not necessarily mean that an individual will have any symptoms. In many individuals, gallstones are completely asymptomatic and require no treatment. Cholelithiasis in children is usually associated with an underlying systemic disease such as cystic fibrosis or sickle cell disease. It is often symptomatic and requires treatment by gallbladder removal.

The term cholecystitis refers to inflammation of the gallbladder wall. The continued presence of gallstones in the gallbladder ultimately promotes inflammatory changes in the gallbladder wall, with fibrosis and thickening.[7] Cholecystitis is classified as acute or chronic, according to its clinical manifestations. The clinical manifestations of each are described, followed by diagnostic and treatment methods.

Chronic Cholelithiasis

Clinical manifestations. The chief complication of chronic cholelithiasis is intermittent biliary colic, a persistent epigastric or right upper abdominal pain. Often the pain radiates to the back and is accompanied by nausea, vomiting, sweating, and flatus. A typical episode lasts several hours. Biliary colic is typically caused by periodic obstruction of the cystic duct by a gallstone (Figure 37-7), although rarely spasm of the sphincter of Oddi may be etiologic.

Symptoms may be precipitated by a meal, but they often occur spontaneously and may manifest at night. The pain often increases steadily for 15 minutes and persists for 1 hour or more, and then slowly decreases. Attacks may recur on a frequent or infrequent schedule. Patients often describe additional symptoms, including fatty food intolerance, belching, flatus, bloating, and epigastric burning.[1,7]

Diagnosis and treatment. The diagnosis of chronic cholelithiasis depends on imaging studies, particularly ultrasonography, and is essentially the same as that described for acute cholecystitis.

In cases of chronic cholelithiasis with no or very few recurrent symptoms, "watchful waiting" may be considered.[1,7] However, patients with significant recurrences of biliary colic are candidates for one of the three current modes of treatment for cholecystitis: cholecystectomy (surgical removal of the gallbladder), chemical dissolution of gallstones, or lithotripsy (mechanical breaking up of gallstones within the gallbladder). These will be discussed in more detail in the Acute Cholecystitis section.

Acute Cholecystitis

Clinical manifestations. Acute **cholecystitis** is defined as acute inflammation of the gallbladder wall. It is characterized by severe right upper abdominal pain that may radiate to the back. Abdominal tenderness and fever are often present. Cholelithiasis is present in about 90% of patients. Obstruction of the cystic duct occurs in almost all cases, suggesting that stasis of bile in the gallbladder is important in the pathogenesis of the disease. Bacterial infection commonly accompanies acute cholecystitis, although it is not thought to be the direct cause of the inflammatory process. Laboratory evaluation may reveal leukocytosis, mild elevations in the levels of bilirubin and serum transaminases, and, less often, elevated amylase levels.[7]

If left untreated, the inflammatory process often escalates, and gangrene of the gallbladder wall with rupture may occur. This can lead to peritonitis and septic shock, a localized abscess (**empyema**), or a **cholecystoenteric fistula** (fistula between the gallbladder and gastrointestinal tract).

Acalculous cholecystitis is an important subgroup of acute cholecystitis. As the name implies, it occurs in patients without preexisting gallstones. It tends to occur in the setting of major surgery, critical illness, trauma, or burn-related injury. Patients tend to be predominantly male and older than 50 years, and total parenteral nutrition (TPN) is a common cofactor. It carries a somewhat more serious implication than stone-associated cholecystitis, in part because of the associated medical conditions. In fact, gangrene of the gallbladder wall and perforation, **emphysematous cholecystitis,** and **empyema** all develop more rapidly than in calculous cholecystitis.[1]

Diagnosis. Evaluation for possible cholecystitis includes an appropriate history and physical examination, laboratory studies, and imaging studies designed to evaluate the gallbladder and biliary tree. Ultrasound of the abdomen is the procedure of choice early in the diagnostic evaluation. Typically, the ultrasound scan reveals the presence of stones, occasionally in the cystic duct, as well as thickening of the gallbladder wall and distention of the lumen. It may also point to another diagnosis of right upper quadrant pain, such as a liver neoplasm or renal lesions. The sensitivity and specificity of ultrasound for stones larger than 2 mm in diameter approach 95%.[7] Sensitivity rates for acalculous cholecystitis are somewhat lower.

However, the presence of cholelithiasis and a thickened gallbladder wall may not be diagnostic, and other diagnostic tests are used on occasion. Hepatobiliary scintigraphy (or cholescintigraphy) by hydroxyiminodiacetic acid (HIDA) scanning provides a good functional assessment of gallbladder excretion, which is markedly impaired with cholecystitis. Computed tomography (CT), magnetic resonance cholangiography (MRCA), and endoscopic retrograde cholangiopancreatography (ERCP) are useful for selected cases. The latter carries a risk of perforation and pancreatitis, and so is reserved for cases requiring intervention (stent placement, biopsy, or special contrast studies).

Treatment. Treatment for cholecystitis depends on the severity of symptoms and the patient's clinical status. Acute cholecystitis may necessitate intervention, but surgeons generally prefer to allow a "hot" gallbladder to "cool down" before performing surgery, particularly if the patient is considered a high surgical risk.[7] The benefit of antibiotics for uncomplicated cholecystitis remains unclear, but broad-spectrum antibiotics are generally administered in the setting of acute cholecystitis. Percutaneous catheter drainage or endoscopic drainage with stent placement may be performed to relieve obstruction, particularly if infection is involved. If the patient's condition precludes surgery, these may be the main treatments, and drains can be left in place indefinitely. Advanced acute cholecystitis complicated by empyema, gangrene, or emphysematous change is considered a surgical emergency.

Laparoscopic cholecystectomy was first performed in 1987 and has benefited from rapid improvements in video **laparoscopy** and instrumentation. Laparoscopic cholecystectomy is now the treatment of choice for symptomatic gallstones. The procedure is usually performed with four small incisions through which instruments are inserted. The gallbladder is freed either by electrosurgical or laser excision and is then withdrawn through one of the small incisions. Advantages of the laparoscopic technique include minimal scarring, less postoperative pain than after laparotomy, shortened hospital stays, and a rapid return to daily activities.[7]

Open cholecystectomy was first performed in the nineteenth century and remains an extremely safe operation with low morbidity and mortality. However, the length of the incision and accompanying postoperative pain render many patients immobile after the procedure. Altered anatomy or scarring from previous surgery or the presence of common bile duct stones may necessitate a traditional cholecystectomy. A laparoscopic procedure may be converted to an open one intraoperatively if necessary (e.g., upon finding a malignant tumor in the vicinity of the gallbladder). Complications of cholecystectomy (either laparoscopic or open) can include infection, inadvertent transection of the common bile duct, and the rare but debilitating syndrome of recurrent sclerosing cholangitis.

Some patients, such as elderly or debilitated persons, may be poor surgical risks and cannot undergo the stress of surgery. Nonoperative methods to manage gallstones, such as **chemodissolution** with a variety of bile acids or organic solvents and **lithotripsy,** have been tried as alternatives to surgery. Chemodissolution is the use of chemical substances, such as bile acids or organic solvents, to dissolve gallstones. Such agents as ursodeoxycholic acid (UDCA) and chenodeoxycholic acid (CDCA) are administered orally.[7] However, this approach has several major drawbacks, including diarrhea in about 50% of patients and a low overall efficacy. CDCA is also quite expensive. Extracorporeal shock wave lithotripsy (ESWL), which involves the breaking up of gallstones using shock waves, is another nonsurgical approach. The objective is to fragment stones into pieces small enough to be passed through the cystic duct, or small enough to allow dissolving agents to function. ESWL is safe and relatively effective, under proper circumstances. The disadvantages include strict selection criteria (e.g., stones less than 2 cm in diameter), resulting in a low percentage of eligible patients. The

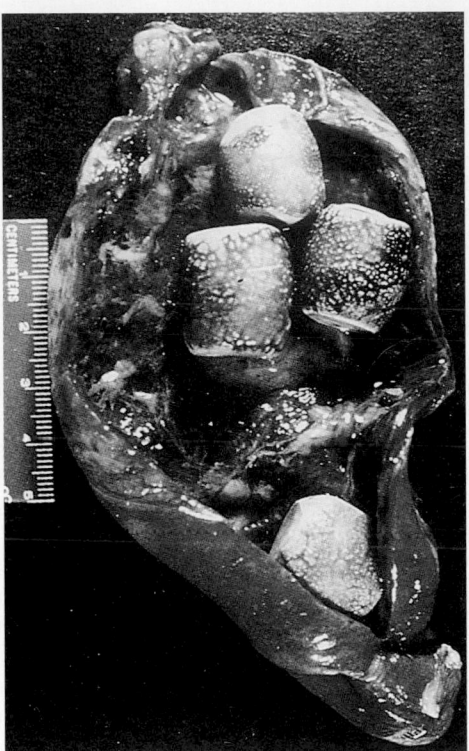

FIGURE 37-7 Chronic cholecystitis demonstrated by a thickened gallbladder wall and luminal cholesterol gallstones. (From Cotran RS et al: *Robbins pathologic basis of disease,* ed 6, Philadelphia, 1999, Saunders, p 897.)

gallbladder also is left in place, allowing for possible recurrence of gallstones and necessitating the concurrent use of dissolving agents such as UDCA or CDCA to prevent new stone formation.

For the most part, in the near future the management of gallstone disease is likely to remain surgical, with traditional or laparoscopic cholecystectomy being the major forms of intervention.

Chronic Cholecystitis

Clinical manifestations. Chronic cholecystitis is defined as chronic inflammation of the gallbladder wall attributable to persistent low-grade irritation from gallstones or to recurrent attacks of acute cholecystitis. Diabetes mellitus and obesity are important predisposing factors. Although many patients suffer from intermittent biliary colic or have symptomatic acute attacks, a surprising number of patients experience no symptoms.

Chronic cholecystitis may lead to many of the complications described earlier for acute cholecystitis, including biliary sepsis, as well as a specific type of scarring known as a calcified or porcelain gallbladder, which is associated with a higher risk of cancer.[1]

Biliary Malignancy

Cancers of the biliary system are relatively rare; in the United States it accounts for only 1 to 2 cases per 100,000 per year.[8-10] Unfortunately, they tend to be asymptomatic and progress insidiously until well advanced. Chronic cholecystitis predisposes sufferers to the very uncommon gallbladder cancer, but is only a minor risk factor for cancer of the biliary tract. **Primary sclerosing cholangitis** is a significant risk factor, and among immigrants from endemic countries infestation with liver flukes such as *Clonorchis* species can lead to biliary cancer. Typical symptoms at presentation include right upper quadrant pain and jaundice associated with biliary obstruction.

Surgery for cure is a treatment option in fewer than 10% of cases. Chemotherapy and radiation therapy are indicted for palliation, and certain patients may benefit from stenting and other procedures to alleviate biliary obstruction.

KEY POINTS

- Lecithin is an important component of bile that helps keep cholesterol from precipitating into crystals. Crystals of cholesterol may initiate gallstone formation. The relative concentrations of cholesterol, lecithin, and bile acids appear to determine the likelihood of cholesterol gallstone formation. Bile hypomotility or stasis contributes to growth of cholesterol stones.
- Gallstones occur more frequently in women than in men. Ethnicity, obesity, and rapid weight loss are predisposing factors. Gallstones may be asymptomatic or associated with symptomatic cholecystitis. Colicky pain attributable to intermittent obstruction of the cystic duct by a stone is the chief complaint. Symptoms of chronic cholecystitis include epigastric or right upper quadrant pain radiating to the back, nausea, vomiting, sweating, fat intolerance, bloating, and flatus.
- Acute cholecystitis is acute inflammation of the gallbladder associated with abdominal pain, leukocytosis, and fever. Cholelithiasis is present in about 90% of patients; obstruction of the cystic duct is present in nearly all patients.
- Treatment for cholecystitis includes surgical removal of the gallbladder (cholecystectomy), chemodissolution, ESWL (lithotripsy) for stones, antibiotics if indicated, and management of pain. Cholecystectomy is the mainstay of therapy.
- Biliary cancer is a rare malignancy with a poor prognosis. Surgery is the only curative therapy, but only available for a small minority of sufferers.

DISORDERS OF THE PANCREAS

PANCREATITIS

Acute Pancreatitis

Etiology and pathogenesis. Acute pancreatitis is an inflammatory process involving the pancreas that may range from mild and inconveniencing to severe and life threatening. After an attack, the exocrine and endocrine functions of the pancreas may remain impaired for a variable period. Pancreatitis affects between 1 and 5 per 10,000 individuals in the United States annually.[1,7] Predisposing factors for pancreatitis have been well-known for more than 100 years (Box 37-1); in the United States the most common causes are biliary tract disease, hypertriglyceridemia, and ethanol-associated pancreatitis. Although the exact mechanisms leading to pancreatitis are not fully understood, three possible pathways are known (Figure 37-8). The most prominent factor is obstruction of the pancreatic duct by a stone or other cause (usually unknown), with release of digestive enzymes within the parenchyma, followed by enzyme activation and then autodigestion of the pancreas.[10] Edema leading to vascular insufficiency and ischemic injury is a contributing factor. Other possible mechanisms include acinar cell injury from alcohol or drugs, trauma, or viral infection; and defective intracellular transport of proenzymes within acinar cells.

Up to 66% of first cases of pancreatitis are associated with alcoholism.[1] Although there is clearly an association of alcohol with pancreatitis, the causal mechanism has not been determined. Transient increases in pancreatic exocrine secretion, contraction of the sphincter of Oddi, and direct toxic effects on acinar cells have all been postulated from experimental studies.[7] Many authorities now believe that most cases of alcoholic pancreatitis are sudden exacerbations of chronic pancreatitis,

---

BOX 37-1   CONDITIONS PREDISPOSING TO ACUTE PANCREATITIS

Gallstones
Biliary sludge and microlithiasis
Other causes of mechanical ampullary obstruction
Alcohol
Hypertriglyceridemia
Hypercalcemia
Drugs
Infections and toxins
Trauma
Pancreas divisum
Vascular disease
Pregnancy
Post-ERCP
Postoperative pancreatitis
Hereditary pancreatitis
Structural abnormalities
- Duodenum/ampullary region
- Bile duct
- Sphincter of Oddi dysfunction
- Main pancreatic duct

From Feldman M et al: *Sleisenger and Fordtran's gastrointestinal and liver disease: pathophysiology, diagnosis, management,* ed 7, Philadelphia, 2002, Saunders, p 914.
ERCP, Endoscopic retrograde cholangiopancreatography.

---

presenting as apparent de novo acute pancreatitis.[10] According to this view, chronic alcohol ingestion causes secretion of protein-rich pancreatic fluid, leading to deposition of inspissated protein plugs and obstruction of small pancreatic ducts, followed by the train of events described previously. However, other pathologic studies show no evidence of chronic pancreatitis in up to 40% of acute alcoholic pancreatitis patients.

Clinical manifestations. The presentation of acute pancreatitis usually begins with steady, boring pain in the epigastrium or left upper quadrant, which gradually increases in intensity. It often radiates or penetrates through to the back and is accompanied by nausea and vomiting. Tenderness on palpation may be exquisite. Bowel sounds are reduced but not absent. Abdominal distention may be present. Fever is common but is usually low grade initially. In more severe pancreatitis, this clinical picture is accompanied by signs of circulatory instability, respiratory insufficiency, and shock.[11-12]

Diagnosis. The laboratory evaluation of acute pancreatitis begins with measurements of serum pancreatic enzymes. Serum lipase and amylase levels rise more or less in tandem during the first 12 hours and remain elevated for several days. Lipase is more specific and persists longer, and therefore has become the preferred test for most clinicians. Levels of serum aminotransferases (aspartate aminotransferase, alanine aminotransferase) may also be elevated. Marked elevation of the alkaline phosphatase and bilirubin levels suggests the possibility of biliary disease or obstruction, particularly by gallstones. Associated laboratory findings include leukocytosis, hyperlipidemia (which may be marked), and hypocalcemia.[1,7]

The diagnosis of acute pancreatitis is based on the signs and symptoms, laboratory data, and imaging studies of the pancreas and surrounding organs. Radiographs of the abdomen may reveal an ileus pattern or the "sentinel loop" (a distended loop of small bowel in the area of the pancreas). Ultrasound can provide a convenient bedside technique to visualize the pancreas, gallbladder, common bile duct,

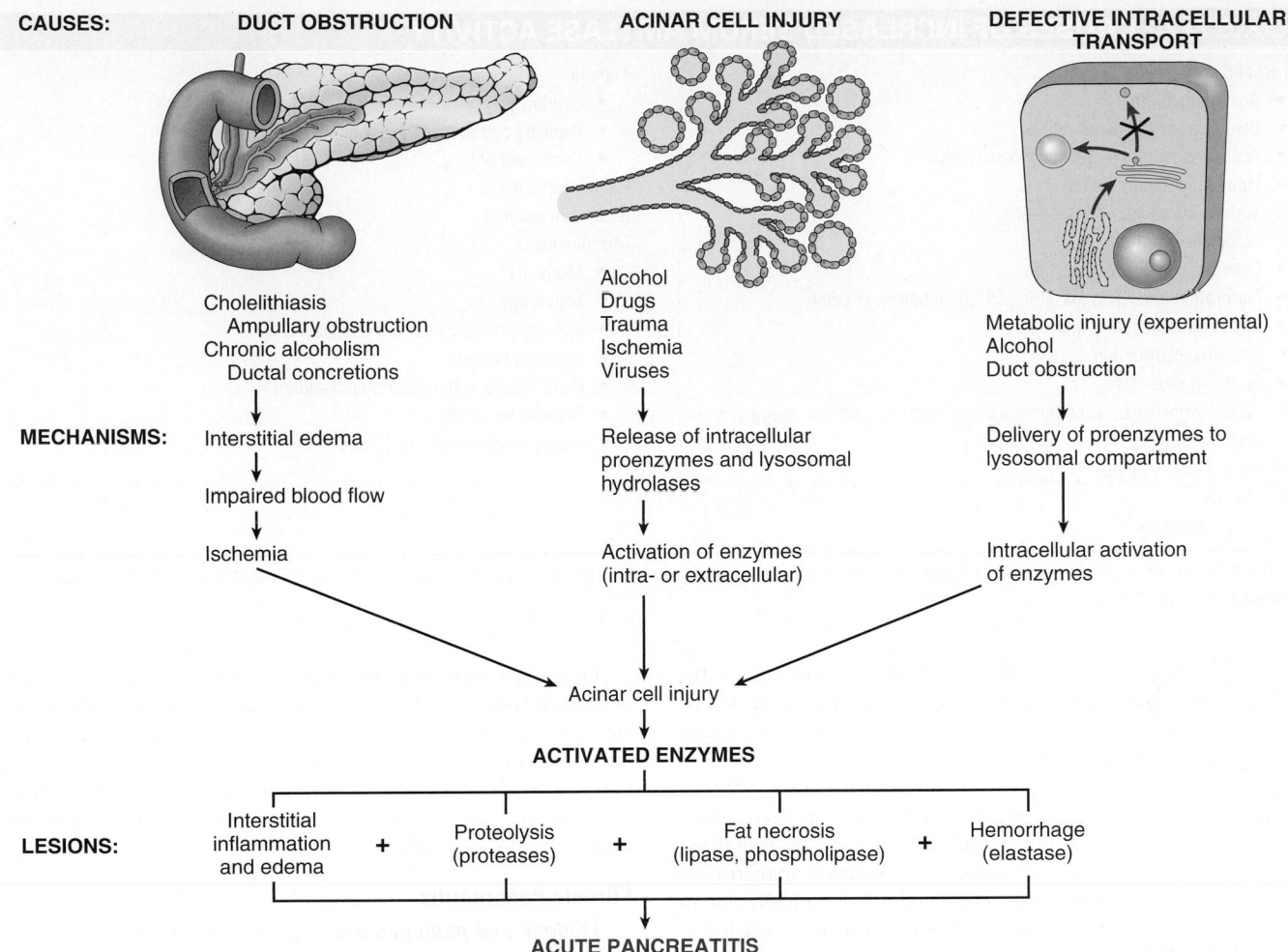

CAUSES: **DUCT OBSTRUCTION**   **ACINAR CELL INJURY**   **DEFECTIVE INTRACELLULAR TRANSPORT**

Cholelithiasis
  Ampullary obstruction
Chronic alcoholism
  Ductal concretions

Alcohol
Drugs
Trauma
Ischemia
Viruses

Metabolic injury (experimental)
Alcohol
Duct obstruction

MECHANISMS: Interstitial edema → Impaired blood flow → Ischemia

Release of intracellular proenzymes and lysosomal hydrolases → Activation of enzymes (intra- or extracellular)

Delivery of proenzymes to lysosomal compartment → Intracellular activation of enzymes

→ Acinar cell injury

ACTIVATED ENZYMES

LESIONS: Interstitial inflammation and edema   +   Proteolysis (proteases)   +   Fat necrosis (lipase, phospholipase)   +   Hemorrhage (elastase)

ACUTE PANCREATITIS

FIGURE 37-8 Three proposed pathways in the pathogenesis of acute pancreatitis. Obstruction of the duct, extrinsic injury, and intrinsic metabolic mechanisms lead to injury of pancreatic cells. Injured cells release activated pancreatic enzymes that cause autodigestion and inflammation of the pancreas. (From Kumar V et al: *Robbins and Cotran pathologic basis of disease,* ed 8, Philadelphia, 2010, Saunders.)

and other abdominal structures, but is limited by poor image resolution attributable to bowel gas. Computed tomography (CT) of the abdomen is the gold standard for evaluation of the pancreas and allows depiction of the pancreas in remarkable detail, including edema and abscess or cyst formation. The differential diagnosis of acute pancreatitis includes perforated peptic ulcer, acute cholecystitis, mesenteric vascular disease, and a variety of other illnesses (Box 37-2), most of which may be differentiated on the basis of biochemical and radiographic tests.

Grading systems allow prediction of the clinical course of acute pancreatitis. Ranson's criteria are a widely used benchmark for prognostic assessment, and are particularly useful with modifications based on CT scoring.[13-18] Early monitoring in the intensive care unit is indicated for patients with a high number of risk factors. One particularly important finding on contrast CT is the presence of significant pancreatic necrosis. Acute necrotizing pancreatitis carries a high risk for progression to infected pancreatic necrosis, a devastating complication with a high morbidity and mortality.

Treatment. Conservative management is indicated for mild to moderate cases of acute pancreatitis. In general, withholding oral feedings, providing nasogastric suction for significant adynamic ileus, and providing careful volume replacement with IV fluids are indicated.

Analgesics are administered parenterally. All narcotics should be used carefully because of the potential of sphincter of Oddi dysfunction, although recent studies show that no single agent is contraindicated.[14] This treatment is often sufficient when carried out for 3 to 7 days, after which the acute episode subsides and oral intake may gradually be resumed.

Severe pancreatitis, particularly in the setting of acute necrotizing pancreatitis, may result in multisystem organ dysfunction, requiring aggressive support in the intensive care unit setting. Nutritional deficits develop rapidly with extensive catabolism (tissue breakdown) and lack of caloric intake; total parenteral nutrition is usually indicated with pancreatitis of more than a few days' duration or if complications arise.[6] Additional supportive measures include calcium administration to reverse severe hypocalcemia, correction of magnesium deficiency, and control of hyperglycemia. Causes of death from severe pancreatitis include respiratory failure (usually associated with adult respiratory distress syndrome), acute renal failure, and acute intraabdominal sepsis. Mechanical ventilation and hemodialysis may be required in complicated cases.

Bacterial infection is a critical determinant of poor outcome in acute necrotizing pancreatitis. Although some authorities advocate broad-spectrum antibiotics (e.g., carbapenems) for all patients with

---

BOX 37-2   CAUSES OF INCREASED SERUM AMYLASE ACTIVITY

Pancreatic diseases
- Acute pancreatitis
- Complications of pancreatitis
- Acute exacerbation of chronic pancreatitis
- Pancreatic tumors, cysts

Other serious intraabdominal diseases
- Acute cholecystitis
- Common bile duct obstruction
- Perforation of esophagus, stomach, small bowel, or colon
- Intestinal ischemia or infarction
- Intestinal obstruction
- Acute appendicitis
- Acute gynecologic conditions such as ruptured ectopic pregnancy and acute salpingitis

Diseases of salivary glands
- Mumps
- Effects of alcohol

Tumors
- Ovarian cysts
- Papillary cystadenocarcinoma of ovary
- Carcinoma of lung

Renal insufficiency

Macroamylasemia

Miscellaneous
- Morphine
- Endoscopy
- Sphincter of Oddi stenosis or spasm
- Anorexia nervosa
- Head trauma with intracranial bleeding
- Diabetic ketoacidosis
- Human immunodeficiency virus

From Feldman M et al: *Sleisenger and Fordtran's gastrointestinal and liver disease: pathophysiology, diagnosis, management*, ed 7, Philadelphia, 2002, Saunders, p 914.

---

acute necrotizing pancreatitis, definitive studies are lacking.[1] In the patient with fever and signs of sepsis, empirical antibiotics should be administered, and any significant fluid collections found on CT scan should be aspirated for culture and sensitivity.

Abscess or hemorrhage may complicate pancreatitis with or without significant pancreatic necrosis and may necessitate surgical intervention. Open laparotomy with debridement of devitalized tissue (necrosectomy) and major pancreatic resection (pancreatectomy) are the main surgical options.[8] Drains are typically left in place postoperatively, and repeated debridement may be needed to remove infective debris and necrotic tissue. Pancreatic surgery is technically challenging and risky, and generally is only considered as a last resort.

Localized complications of acute pancreatitis may result in prolonged morbidity for the patient. The most common localized complication is pancreatic **pseudocyst.** This is a collection of fluid within or adjacent to the pancreas that often has a direct communication to the pancreatic duct. Unlike a true cyst, a *pseudocyst* contains no epithelial lining. It can develop rather acutely or more subacutely, as the patient recuperates from the acute illness. The presentation often includes fever, tachycardia, and an abdominal mass and tenderness. Complications of pseudocysts include infection (usually termed an infected pseudocyst, as opposed to the pancreatic abscess described earlier), spontaneous rupture, or hemorrhage. Management of pseudocyst includes endoscopic or surgical drainage of the cyst, either externally or internally, usually into the stomach or bowel.[1,8]

Pancreatic ascites may occur and may represent a persistent leak in the main pancreatic duct. It is usually painless and often massive. The fluid may find its way into unusual places, including the pleural space and mediastinum.[1] Pancreatic ascites may be detected by ultrasonography or CT, and diagnosis is confirmed by analysis of fluid obtained by aspiration, in particular the amylase level. Management is often conservative, with prolonged parenteral nutrition. Improvement may occur following the endoscopic placement of a stent (a thin-walled tube) into the main pancreatic duct.

Other complications of acute pancreatitis include common bile duct obstruction, portal or splenic vein thrombosis, peptic ulcer disease, and chronic fistula formation.

Endoscopic treatment may be carried out for gallstone pancreatitis in selected cases. Indications for urgent ERCP with ampullotomy (incision of the ampulla) include biliary sepsis, recalcitrant severe pancreatitis, and jaundice.[1] In milder cases, traditional conservative therapy followed by elective ERCP is acceptable. The risks of ERCP include exacerbation of pancreatitis, and therefore the need for this procedure must be carefully considered.

Chronic Pancreatitis

Etiology and pathogenesis. Chronic pancreatitis is defined histologically as the presence of chronic inflammatory lesions in the pancreas, and in practice is the persistence of symptoms secondary to pancreatic dysfunction over weeks and months. Destruction of exocrine parenchyma and fibrosis precede the destruction of endocrine parenchyma. After a variable time, most patients with chronic pancreatitis develop calcifications that become visible on radiologic films of the abdomen or CT. Chronic pancreatitis is most often associated with alcohol consumption, although a small percentage of cases are idiopathic, hereditary, or associated with hyperparathyroidism (hypercalcemia), trauma, or various other factors.[1,10]

The association of alcohol ingestion with chronic pancreatitis is profound. Autopsy studies have shown that the changes of chronic pancreatitis are present in 45% of alcoholics, even those without symptoms, and that this rate is 40 to 50 times higher than that in nondrinkers.[1,7] Exactly how alcohol causes chronic pancreatitis is not known (see the previous discussion of alcohol and acute pancreatitis). One recent theory suggests that the initial factors include an increase in the protein concentration in pancreatic juice coupled with reduction in a specific "pancreatic stone protein" that inhibits the formation of pancreatic protein plugs.[10] This biochemical situation allows the formation of protein plugs that can later calcify, in addition to causing obstruction to the flow of pancreatic juice. A key element seems to be necrosis, followed by fibrosis, perhaps analogous to cirrhosis of the liver. Ischemic and antioxidant damage may occur as well. Another facet of alcohol-associated chronic pancreatitis is its tendency to progress after alcohol consumption is stopped.

Clinical manifestations. The presentation of chronic pancreatitis may consist of bouts of acute pancreatitis with progressive signs of persistent pancreatic dysfunction after the acute attack subsides. Alternatively, an insidious onset of pain in the epigastrium that radiates to the back may be the first symptom. About 10% to 15% of patients will not present with pain but rather with the sequelae of chronic pancreatitis, including diabetes mellitus, malabsorption, and weight loss.[1,7] The mortality is 3% to 4% per year. Interestingly, the incidence of pancreatic carcinoma does not appear to be substantially increased in patients with chronic pancreatitis.

The pain of chronic pancreatitis is often the major form of debility. Nerve fibers from the pancreas pass to the celiac plexus and then to spinal sympathetic ganglia. The events that actually trigger the pain are not well understood. There may be a relation to ductal pressures or possibly to ischemia in the pancreas. The pain is often accompanied by nausea and is steady and boring in nature. The pain is usually located in the upper abdomen, particularly in the epigastrium, and radiates to the back in more than half of cases. In alcoholic pancreatitis, continued drinking affords temporary anesthesia but may foster recurrences of pain. Cessation of drinking may allow for a better long-term prognosis. After about 5 years of continual pain, many patients note a decrease in the symptoms (i.e., the pain "burns out").

Endocrine and exocrine pancreatic insufficiency lead to diabetes mellitus, malabsorption, and weight loss. Diabetes mellitus arises from progressive loss of endocrine cells in the pancreatic islets and usually requires exogenous insulin administration; diabetic ketoacidosis is an unusual finding. Weight loss may be aggravated by poor intake as a result of pancreatic pain. Malabsorption of fat does not occur until pancreatic enzyme output drops to 10% of normal. Along with the malabsorption of fat, the absorption of fat-soluble vitamins (A, D, E, and K) may be impaired, leading to such problems as coagulopathy and night vision impairment.[1]

Further complications of chronic pancreatitis are similar to those of acute pancreatitis and include pseudocyst, pancreatic ascites, and obstruction of the common bile duct. Obstruction of the bile duct may lead to elevated values on liver function tests and the need to intervene either surgically or endoscopically. Alkaline phosphatase and bilirubin levels may become markedly elevated if obstruction is severe. Unusual complications include thrombosis of the portal and splenic veins. This may lead to gastrointestinal hemorrhage from gastric varices.[12] Peptic ulcer disease is also increased in patients with chronic pancreatitis, although a definite causal relationship has not been established.

Diagnosis. The diagnosis of chronic pancreatitis is usually suggested by the clinical history, physical examination findings, and routine blood chemical analyses. Biochemical studies of pancreatic function may be helpful. Confirmation of the diagnosis is aided by plain radiographs showing calcifications in the area of the pancreas. Abdominal ultrasound, CT, or magnetic resonance cholangiopancreatography (MRCP) are usually performed with reasonable sensitivities and specificities. ERCP is reserved for suspicious cases that cannot be confirmed by other techniques, or for cases in which biopsy or cytologic examination is necessary to rule out malignancy.[1] It shows the pancreatic duct to range from almost normal in early cases, to markedly dilated or beaded—the "chain of lakes" appearance (Figure 37-9). A common finding is truncation of the secondary branches of the pancreatic duct.

Treatment. The treatment for chronic pancreatitis is directed toward controlling pain, addressing exocrine and endocrine insufficiency, and managing complications. By far the most challenging is the management of pain. Absolute abstention from alcohol is paramount to prevent worsening of symptoms. For almost 40 years, analgesics and surgical intervention have been the mainstay of pain control, and celiac plexus block is helpful for some patients. With the advent of ERCP,

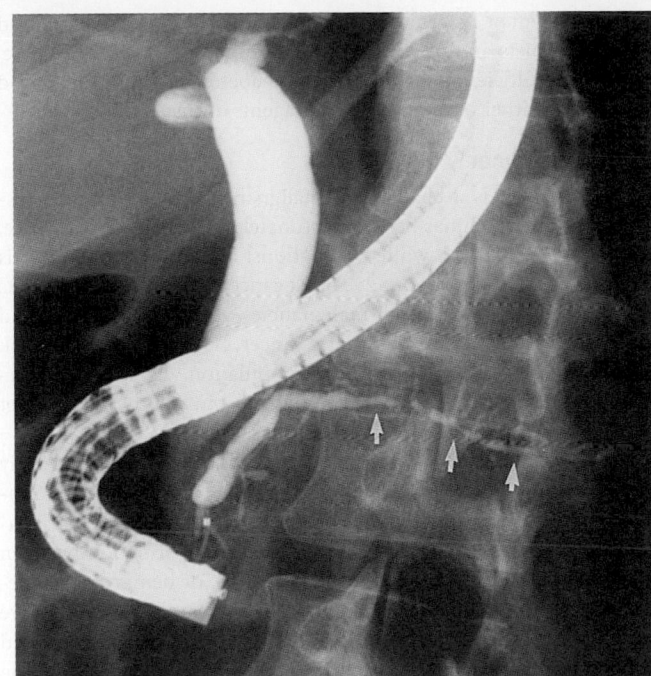

FIGURE 37-9 Endoscopic retrograde cholangiopancreatogram in a patient with chronic pancreatitis shows marked narrowing and irregularity of the main pancreatic duct body and tail *(arrows).* (From Feldman M et al: *Sleisenger and Fordtran's gastrointestinal and liver disease: pathophysiology, diagnosis, management,* ed 6, Philadelphia, 1998, Saunders, p 952.)

less drastic forms of intervention are now possible. Pancreatic sphincterotomy is indicated for the management of single or multiple stones. Endoscopic drains may be placed for pseudocysts of the pancreas if they are adjacent to the stomach or duodenum. Obstruction of the common bile duct can be managed with endoscopically placed biliary stents. Strictures of the main pancreatic duct can be managed with indwelling pancreatic stents.[1,7]

If endoscopic management fails or is not appropriate in a given patient, surgery may be indicated. Various procedures, such as the pylorus-preserving Whipple procedure (pancreaticoduodenectomy), may be used, generally with favorable results regarding relief of pain.[8] Complete and distal pancreatic resections are rarely used for this condition. As with management of acute pancreatitis, the judgment of the surgeon is paramount to prevent the catastrophic complications that can result from surgery on the pancreas.

Pancreatic enzyme replacement has become a standard therapy for chronic pancreatitis, both for its effects on steatorrhea and for the management of chronic pain.[1] Because proteases (e.g., trypsin, chymotrypsin, and elastase) exert a controlling influence on pancreatic secretion, feedback regulation should result in relief of pain following oral administration of pancreatic enzymes. Unfortunately, only 20% to 30% of patients with the typical alcohol-induced type of disease respond to such therapy. Responses seem to be higher in patients with small-duct disease. Acid suppression with an H_2-blocker or proton pump inhibitor is indicated to reduce inactivation of the enzymes from gastric acid. Medium-chain triglycerides (MCTs) can provide extra calories in patients with weight loss. Research on octreotide, a synthetic long-acting analogue of somatostatin that has been shown to inhibit CCK release and both basal and neural-stimulated pancreatic secretion, has generally been disappointing.[1,18]

Management of exocrine insufficiency can usually be accomplished with low-fat diets and pancreatic enzyme supplementation. Likewise, endocrine insufficiency in the form of diabetes mellitus is managed with diet and either oral hypoglycemic agents or insulin.[6]

Pancreatic Cancer

Pancreatic cancer is a challenging malignancy with a generally dismal prognosis, which has been unfortunately increasing in incidence, particularly among non-white populations. The current incidence is about 9 per 100,000, or about 2% of all cancers, but this cancer ranks fourth among deaths from all malignancies.[9] Cigarette smoking and obesity are risk factors for pancreatic cancer, both increasing the risk by about 50% compared to the general population.[1,10] The vast majority of pancreatic tumors are adenocarcinomas, but an important subset of neoplasms are neuroendocrine tumors.

Lesions of the head of the pancreas outnumber those in the body and tail 3 to 1. Symptoms of pancreatic head tumors include jaundice, malabsorption, and weight loss, whereas those of the tail generally include abdominal pain and nausea. The distinction between chronic pancreatitis, autoimmune pancreatitis, or benign cystic adenomas and pancreatic cancer may be difficult, and even a negative needle biopsy does not preclude cancer.[10] Most cancers are advanced at the time of presentation, with only 15% to 20% of cases being candidates for surgical resection.[8] Patients presenting with painless jaundice attributable to an obstructing pancreatic head lesion have the best prognosis. Even with surgery, most patients die of their disease. Chemotherapy plays a role in both attempts at surgical cure and palliation. The median survival among all patients is only 1 year, though there is some evidence that the cure rate may be improving somewhat because of new therapeutic modalities being employed at major medical centers.[9]

> ### KEY POINTS
> - Acute pancreatitis is commonly associated with biliary tract disease and excessive ethanol ingestion. Activation of pancreatic proenzymes to active forms within the pancreas leads to autodigestion and inflammation of the gland. The manifestations of acute pancreatitis may be mild or severe and include a steady, boring pain in the epigastrium or left upper quadrant, nausea, vomiting, a tender abdomen, reduced bowel sounds, and fever. In severe cases, circulatory shock may occur. Elevated serum amylase and lipase levels are indicative of pancreatitis.
> - Management of acute pancreatitis is aimed at reducing pancreatic secretion. Because chyme entering the duodenum is the primary stimulus for pancreatic secretion, food is withheld and nasogastric suctioning may be instituted. Complications of acute pancreatitis include hyperglycemia, nutritional deficit, and pancreatic hemorrhage, infection, abscess formation, or necrosis. Antibiotics, fluid management, total parenteral nutrition, and insulin may be indicated to manage complications.
> - Chronic pancreatitis is closely associated with alcohol use. Acute pancreatitis attributable to biliary obstruction rarely progresses to chronic pancreatitis. Chronic pancreatitis results in progressive destruction of endocrine and exocrine function. Manifestations of chronic pancreatitis are more insidious than those of acute pancreatitis. Epigastric pain, diabetes mellitus, malabsorption, and weight loss may be the presenting problems.
> - The complications of chronic pancreatitis are similar to those of acute pancreatitis. Therapy is directed to controlling pain, ameliorating endocrine and exocrine deficiency, and monitoring and managing complications. Surgery to correct obstruction of the pancreatic duct may be performed. Pancreatic enzyme therapy may be helpful in reducing pain by providing negative feedback, which reduces pancreatic secretion.
> - Pancreatic cancer is a highly fatal cancer that can be difficult to diagnose and treat. Median survival is 12 months.

SUMMARY

The pancreaticobiliary system is central to the digestion of food because it provides necessary digestive enzymes and lipid-emulsifying agents that allow the intestine to absorb nutrients. This chapter has considered alterations in the function of the gallbladder and exocrine pancreas. A major disease of the pancreaticobiliary system is the formation of cholesterol gallstones, which can lead to acute and chronic cholecystitis and acute and chronic pancreatitis. New forms of surgical and nonsurgical interventions for the management of gallstone disease have become available in the past few years, with conventional open surgery remaining a useful option. These interventions, as well as interventions for acute and chronic pancreatitis, are currently the focus of much clinical research.

REFERENCES

1. Yamada T, et al: *Textbook of gastroenterology*, ed 5, Oxford, 2011, Wiley-Blackwell.
2. Avunduk C: *Manual of gastroenterology*, ed 4, Philadelphia, 2008, Lippincott Williams & Wilkins.
3. Moore KL, Persaud TVN, Torchia MG: *The developing human: clinically oriented embryology*, Philadelphia, 2008, Saunders.
4. Moore KL, Persaud TVN, Shiota K: *Color atlas of clinical embryology*, ed 2, Philadelphia, 2000, Saunders.
5. Hall JE: *Guyton and Hall textbook of medical physiology*, ed 12, Philadelphia, 2011, Saunders Elsevier.
6. Shils ME: *Modern nutrition in health and disease*, ed 10, Philadelphia, 2006, Lippincott Williams & Wilkins.
7. Feldman M, Friedman LS, Brandt LJ: *Sleisenger and Fordtran's gastrointestinal and liver disease*, ed 9, Philadelphia, 2010, Saunders Elsevier.
8. Townsend CM, et al: *Sabiston textbook of surgery: the biological basis of modern surgical practice*, ed 18, Philadelphia, 2007, Saunders Elsevier.
9. Kelsen DP, et al: *Principles and practice of gastrointestinal oncology*, Philadelphia, 2008, Lippincott Williams & Wilkins.
10. Kumar V, et al: *Robbins pathologic basis of disease*, ed 8, Philadelphia, 2010, Saunders.
11. Laoser C, Faolsch UR: A concept of treatment in acute pancreatitis: results of controlled trials and future developments, *Hepatogastroenterology* 40:569–573, 1993.
12. Sole ML, Klein DG: *Introduction to critical care nursing*, Philadelphia, 2009, Saunders Elsevier.
13. Chatzicostas C, et al: Computed tomography severity index is superior to Ranson criteria and Apache II and III scoring systems in predicting acute pancreatitis outcome, *J Clin Gastroenterol* 36(3):253–260, 2003.
14. Thompson DR: Narcotic analgesic effects on the sphincter of Oddi: a review of the data and therapeutic implications in treating pancreatitis, *Am J Gastroenterol* 96(4):1266–1272, 2001.
15. Yamedera K, Moriyama T, Makino I: Identification of immunoreactive pancreatic stone protein in pancreatic stone, pancreatic tissue and pancreatic juice, *Pancreas* 5(3):255–260, 1990.
16. Haubrich WS, Schaffner F, Berk JE: *Bockus gastroenterology*, ed 5, Philadelphia, 1995, Saunders.
17. Treacy PJ, Worthley CS: Pancreatic stents in the management of chronic pancreatitis, *Aust N Z J Surg* 66:210–213, 1996.
18. Singh VV, Toskes PP: Medical therapy for chronic pancreatitis pain, *Curr Gastroenterol Rep* 5(2):110–116, 2003.

Liver Diseases

Jeffrey S. Sartin

⊖volve WEBSITE

http://evolve.elsevier.com/Copstead/

- Review Questions and Answers
- Glossary (with audio pronunciations for selected terms)
- Animations
- Case Studies
- Key Points Review

KEY QUESTIONS

- What role does the liver play in nutrient metabolism, bile synthesis, storage of vitamins and minerals, urea synthesis, clotting factor synthesis, and detoxification?
- Which manifestations of liver disease are due to hepatocellular failure, and which are due to portal hypertension?
- How do the different types of viral hepatitis vary with regard to mode of transmission and severity of symptoms?
- What clinical and laboratory findings would lead to a diagnosis of liver cirrhosis?
- What treatment modalities are available to patients with end-stage liver failure?

CHAPTER OUTLINE

The liver is a vital but vulnerable organ. Its role in digestion of fats, storage of carbohydrates, detoxification of blood, and production of proteins makes it indispensable; in contrast to the kidney and heart, there are no "artificial livers." Nevertheless, the liver is susceptible to a wide variety of metabolic, circulatory, toxic, microbial, and neoplastic insults. In some instances the disease is primary to the liver, as in viral hepatitis and hepatocellular carcinoma (HCC). More often the hepatic involvement is secondary, a consequence of some of the more common diseases of humans, such as cardiac decompensation, metastatic cancer, alcoholism, and infections. This chapter will focus on primary diseases of the liver.

STRUCTURE AND FUNCTION OF THE LIVER

The liver, the largest parenchymal organ of the body, averages 1500 grams (g). It is located in the right upper quadrant of the abdomen,

beneath the diaphragm, and is anatomically divided into right and left lobes and then further subdivided according to the pattern of its blood supply and biliary drainage. It is covered by a connective tissue capsule, the Glisson capsule, which in turn is covered by visceral peritoneum, reflections of which form the various suspensory hepatic ligaments. These structures demarcate the bare area of the liver directly in contact with the diaphragm (Figure 38-1).[1-3]

The liver has a dual blood supply. Arterial inflow from the aorta via the celiac trunk and hepatic artery provides 25% of the organ's blood supply, with the remainder from the portal vein, which drains the capillary bed of the alimentary canal and pancreas (Figure 38-2). This oxygen-depleted venous blood is rich in substances absorbed and secreted by the gut. These afferent blood vessels then branch throughout the liver in association with the bile ducts and form the portal triads (consisting of the portal veins, hepatic arteries, and bile ducts).

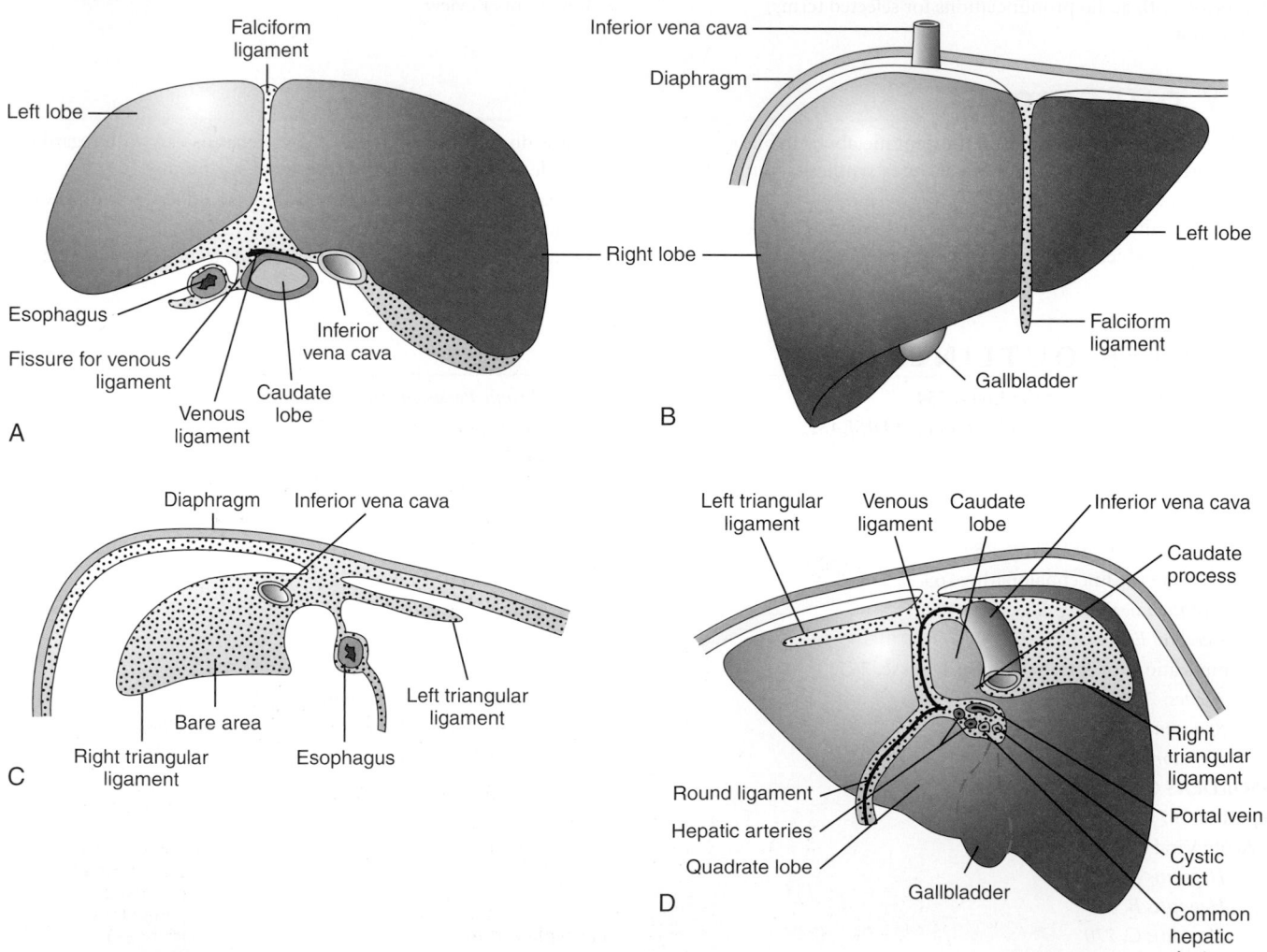

FIGURE 38-1 The liver and its peritoneal relations. Stippled areas represent surfaces not covered with peritoneum. **A,** Superior view. **B,** Anterior view. **C,** The diaphragm, viewed from the front, showing the position of the bare area of the liver. **D,** Visceral surface of the liver, viewed from behind. (Redrawn from Gardner E et al: *Anatomy: a regional study of human structure,* ed 3, Philadelphia, 1969, Saunders, p 414.)

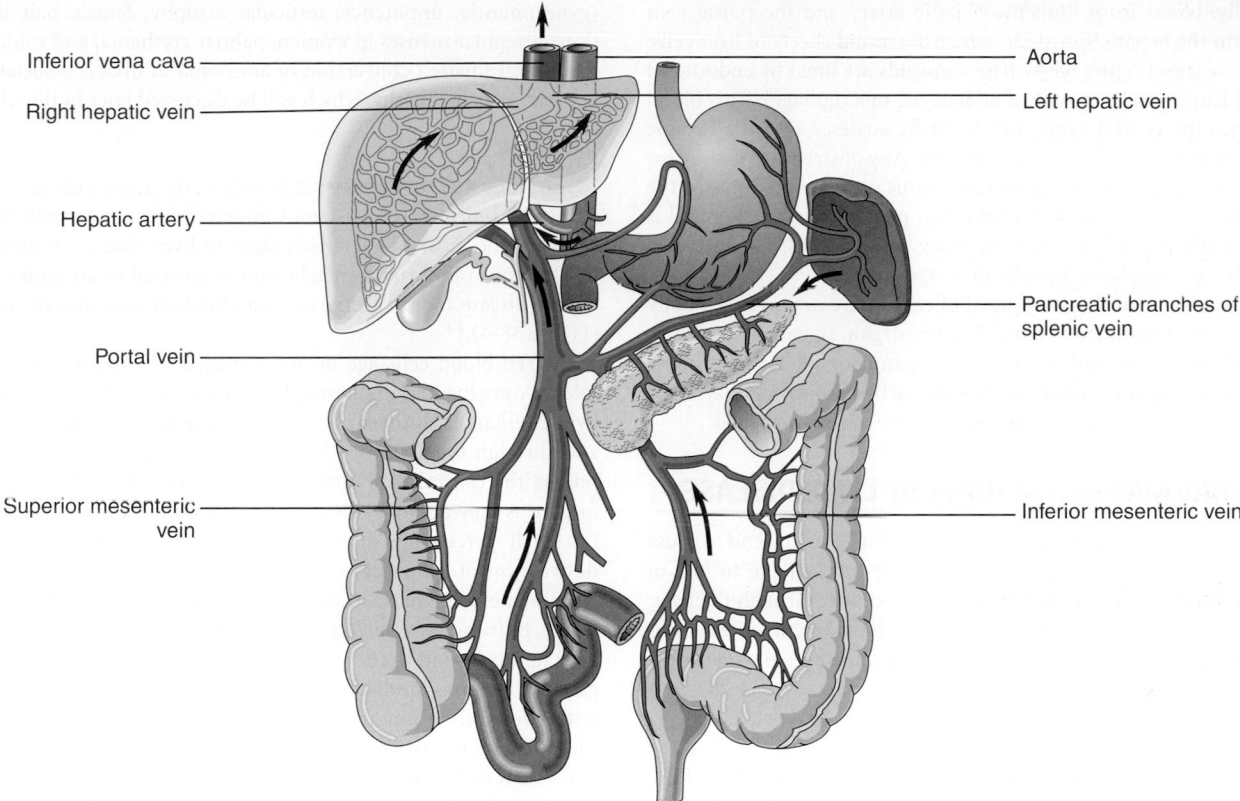

FIGURE 38-2 Schematic diagram of the portal circulation. Blood from the aorta supplies the alimentary canal. Venous blood from the intestine reaches the sinusoids of the liver by way of the portal vein. Venous blood from the liver reaches the inferior vena cava by way of the hepatic veins.

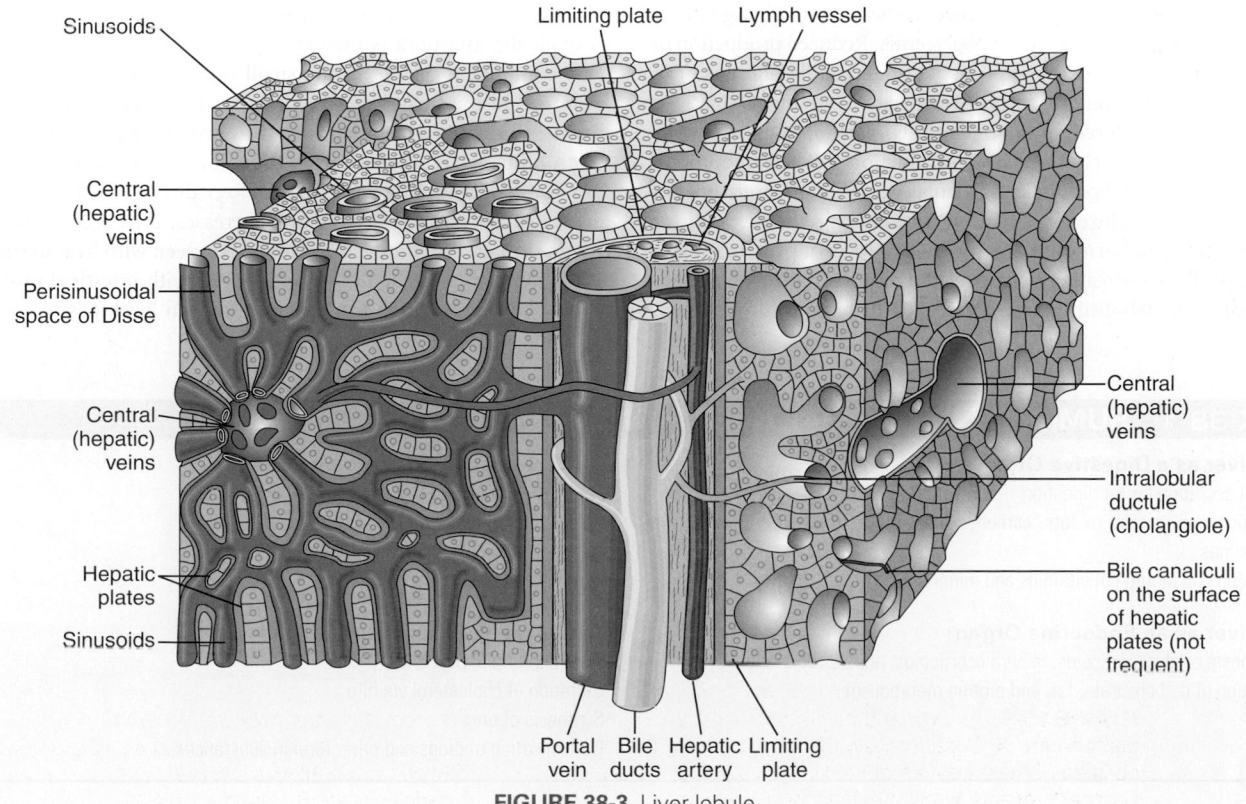

FIGURE 38-3 Liver lobule.

Eventually, blood from both the hepatic artery and the portal vein drains into the hepatic sinusoids, which surround sheets of liver cells, or hepatic plates (Figure 38-3). The sinusoids are lined by endothelial cells and Kupffer cells (a type of phagocytic macrophage). This blood drains into the central veins, which finally coalesce into the hepatic vein and empty into the inferior vena cava. Any obstruction to the flow of blood may result in a rise in portal venous pressure proximal to the level of blockage. This condition is called **portal hypertension** and is a central pathophysiologic event in many liver diseases. The liver also has a rich and complex lymphatic drainage system.

The liver is one of the most metabolically active organs in the body and functions simultaneously as a digestive organ, an endocrine organ, a hematologic organ, and an excretory organ (Box 38-1). All of these functions are elegantly interwoven with such redundancy that more than 80% of the liver may be destroyed before life is threatened.

GENERAL MANIFESTATIONS OF LIVER DISEASE

Whether primary or secondary, all hepatic derangements tend to cause similar signs and symptoms that are directly attributable to loss of hepatocellular function or disruption of blood flow through the liver. Because of the liver's considerable reserve, however, manifestations appear only when the injury is significant and diffuse or so strategically located that it obstructs biliary outflow.

Hepatocellular Failure

Hepatocellular failure results in a number of typical manifestations, including jaundice, muscle wasting, ascites, excessive bleeding, deficiencies of important blood proteins and vitamins, glucose imbalance, and impaired hormone production (Table 38-1). At its most basic the liver is a sophisticated biochemical factory, and these conditions all derive from problems with processing the essential molecules of the body. Inadequate protein metabolism leads to decreased production of clotting factors and hypoalbuminemia. Decreased serum albumin level in turn leads to generalized edema as a result of low serum oncotic pressure. Abnormal storage and release of glucose in the form of glycogen may result in bouts of either hyper- or hypoglycemia. Reduced production of bile salts by the liver impairs absorption of the fat-soluble vitamins A, D, E, and K from the gastrointestinal (GI) tract. Lack of vitamin D may lead to osteomalacia (impaired bone homeostasis); lack of vitamin K contributes to poor blood clotting factor production. Altered lipoprotein processing leads to dyslipidemias, particularly hypertriglyceridemia.

Hepatocellular failure is associated with impaired processing of endogenous steroid hormones and the by-products of protein metabolism, as well as decreased clearance of exogenous drugs and toxins. Impaired metabolism of estrogen leads to feminization in men

(gynecomastia, impotence, testicular atrophy, female hair distribution), irregular menses in women, palmar erythema, and spider telangiectasia. Impaired conversion of ammonia to urea is associated with hepatic encephalopathy, which will be discussed later in this chapter.

Jaundice

Etiology and pathogenesis. Jaundice, the green-yellow staining of tissues by bilirubin, results from impaired bilirubin metabolism and is one of the most characteristic signs of liver disease. A study of the mechanisms of bilirubin metabolism is essential to an understanding of liver disease and may serve as a paradigm for other hepatic processes (Figure 38-4).[4-6]

As red blood cells age or are damaged by disease, they lyse and release oxygen-carrying hemoglobin molecules. These are taken up by the reticuloendothelial system, which separates heme from globin, and through the action of heme oxygenase opens the heme ring to release the central iron atom. This process yields biliverdin, which in turn is converted by the enzyme bilirubin reductase to bilirubin. (A small percentage of bilirubin is derived from the premature destruction of immature cells in the bone marrow and spleen and from heme proteins such as myoglobin and the cytochromes in the liver.) Bilirubin is released into the plasma and transported to the liver tightly bound to the plasma protein albumin. The free unconjugated bilirubin is lipid soluble and can be displaced from albumin by fatty acids and certain organic anions (e.g., sulfonamides, salicylates). The neonate is particularly sensitive to free unconjugated bilirubin, which can diffuse into the brain and cause a type of encephalopathy known as **kernicterus** (see the Liver Diseases and Pediatric Considerations section).

Liver cells are able to extract unconjugated bilirubin from the plasma with special transport proteins. In the cytosol, bilirubin is quickly bound, or conjugated, to water-soluble derivatives of glucuronic acid by the action of the enzyme uridine diphosphate glucuronosyltransferase (UDPGT) located in the endoplasmic reticulum. This process yields water-soluble bilirubin monoglucuronide and diglucuronide, which is then actively excreted into microscopic bile ducts (canaliculi). Bilirubin is then transported through the biliary system as a component of bile to the small intestine. Because it cannot be absorbed in the small intestine, it passes to the colon where bacterial β-glucuronidase enzymes convert it to urobilinogen. A small fraction of urobilinogen is absorbed from the colon and re-excreted by the kidneys and the liver. In the presence of liver disease, the hepatic fraction decreases and the urinary fraction increases, thus accounting for the rise in urinary urobilinogen concentration seen with liver dysfunction. With complete obstruction to bile flow or with intestinal obstruction above the colonic level, urinary urobilinogen level falls to zero, since

---

BOX 38-1　SUMMARY OF NORMAL LIVER FUNCTION

The Liver as a Digestive Organ
Bile salt secretion for fat digestion
Processing and storage of fats, carbohydrates, and proteins absorbed by the intestines
Processing and storage of vitamins and minerals

The Liver as an Endocrine Organ
Metabolism of glucocorticoids, mineralocorticoids, and sex hormones
Regulation of carbohydrate, fat, and protein metabolism

The Liver as a Hematologic Organ
Temporary storage of blood
Removal of bilirubin from the bloodstream
Hematopoiesis in certain disease states
Synthesis of blood clotting factors

The Liver as an Excretory Organ
Excretion of bile pigment
Excretion of cholesterol via bile
Synthesis of urea
Detoxification of drugs and other foreign substances

no bilirubin reaches the colon. (The function of bile salts and the other components of bile flow are discussed in Chapter 37.)

Therefore, jaundice may result from dysfunction anywhere along this complex pathway. Classically, it is divided into prehepatic, hepatic, and posthepatic or cholestatic, but much overlap occurs.

Prehepatic. The most common causes of prehepatic jaundice are hemolysis and ineffective erythropoiesis. The resorption of large hematomas in patients with mild liver disease is a frequent and harmless cause of mild jaundice attributable to unconjugated hyperbilirubinemia.

Hepatic. Dysfunction of each of the hepatic steps in bilirubin metabolism may cause jaundice. In the neonate, immature UDPGT levels may result in physiologic jaundice of the newborn. Various genetic disorders of UDPGT synthesis are characterized by high levels of unconjugated bilirubin in the blood. Mutant UDPGT enzymes can produce the common and benign Gilbert syndrome, in which low levels of unconjugated bilirubin may be increased by fasting or illness (e.g., viral gastroenteritis). Other UDPGT mutations cause the Crigler-Najjar type I and II syndromes with severe neonatal unconjugated hyperbilirubinemia (see the Liver Diseases and Pediatric Considerations section). Most of the liver diseases to be discussed later, such as viral hepatitis, alcoholic liver disease, and autoimmune hepatitis, result in jaundice because dysfunction within the liver cells result in elevated levels of conjugated bilirubin.

Posthepatic. At the level of canalicular bilirubin transport, the rare inherited Dubin-Johnson and Rotor syndromes cause conjugated hyperbilirubinemia. Both conditions have an excellent prognosis. At the canalicular posthepatocytic level, many drugs such as the phenothiazines and the sex hormones may cause jaundice.[1] In susceptible women, the high sex hormone levels of normal pregnancy can cause benign cholestasis of pregnancy.[1] This condition is also associated with defective transport of bile salts and is characterized by jaundice and intense pruritus (i.e., itching).

Mechanical obstruction of the bile ducts from obstructing tumors, strictures, or gallstones is the most common cause of cholestatic jaundice. Some experts differentiate obstructive jaundice caused by a gross mechanical blockage to bile flow in the biliary tract from intrahepatic cholestatic jaundice, the latter implying a defect at the microscopic level.

Evaluation. Evaluation of a jaundiced patient may be used as a model for investigation of any patient with liver disease. After a complete history and physical examination are obtained and routine laboratory data reviewed, specific liver-related tests may be performed (Table 38-2). The underlying cause, such as alcoholic liver disease, a drug reaction, or metastatic or primary malignancy, is often suggested by the history and physical examination. Physical stigmata of chronic liver disease include telangiectasia, ascites, palmar erythema, gynecomastia, testicular atrophy, hair loss (in men), and central obesity with peripheral muscle wasting.

Diagnostic tests. Biochemical test abnormalities usually fall into one of several categories. A significant elevation in the levels of transaminases out of proportion to the other liver enzymes indicates a primarily hepatocellular disorder (i.e., hepatitis). Alcoholic and other toxic hepatitides virtually always show the aspartate aminotransferase

TABLE 38-1 PATHOPHYSIOLOGY UNDERLYING THE SYMPTOMS AND SIGNS OF LIVER DISEASE

SYMPTOMS/SIGNS	PATHOPHYSIOLOGIC MECHANISM
Weakness, fatigue, anorexia, weight loss, muscle wasting	Failure of multiple metabolic functions
Fever	Liver inflammation, decreased reticuloendothelial function with increased risk of infection
Bruising, increased bleeding	Thrombocytopenia secondary to splenic enlargement, decreased synthesis of clotting factors I, II, V, VII, VIII, IX, and X
Palmar erythema, cutaneous spider telangiectases, irregular menses, gynecomastia, impotence, female body hair distribution in men, testicular atrophy	Altered metabolism of sex hormones, chronic debilitation
Hepatic encephalopathy	Abnormal protein metabolism
Fetor hepaticus	Decreased detoxification
Pruritus	Decreased bile salt excretion
Cyanosis	Arteriovenous shunts in lungs, liver
Jaundice	Biliary obstruction, decreased bilirubin synthesis, decreased bilirubin excretion
Hyperdynamic circulation, wide pulse pressure, tachycardia	Generalized vasodilation (? Hormonally mediated)
Ascites, peripheral edema	Portal hypertension, sodium and water retention, low serum albumin secondary to decreased hepatic synthesis
Splenomegaly	Portal hypertension
Hepatomegaly	Cirrhosis (liver may be small), hepatitis, vascular congestion, bile duct obstruction, infection, benign infiltrative disease (e.g., fatty liver, amyloidosis, hemochromatosis), malignant infiltrative disease (e.g., metastatic cancer, lymphoma, large space-occupying lesions such as neoplasm, abscess)
Varices (esophageal, gastric, rectal, ectopic) or abnormal abdominal vascular pattern (caput medusae, umbilical bruit)	Portal hypertension with collateral blood flow around hepatic blockage
Osteomalacia, hypocalcemia, night blindness, coagulopathy	Fat-soluble vitamin malabsorption and loss of fat-soluble vitamin reserves A, D, and K; loss of vitamin K metabolism (a cofactor for I, II, VII, VIII, IX, and X)
Anemia	Multifactorial: blood loss, chronic disease, vitamin B_{12} deficiency, splenic sequestration
Leukopenia	Hypersplenism secondary to portal hypertension
Hypoglycemia	Altered glycogenolysis, gluconeogenesis
Hyperglycemia	Portosystemic shunting with delayed hepatic uptake of absorbed glucose
Hypercholesterolemia	Obstructive jaundice with decreased cholesterol excretion

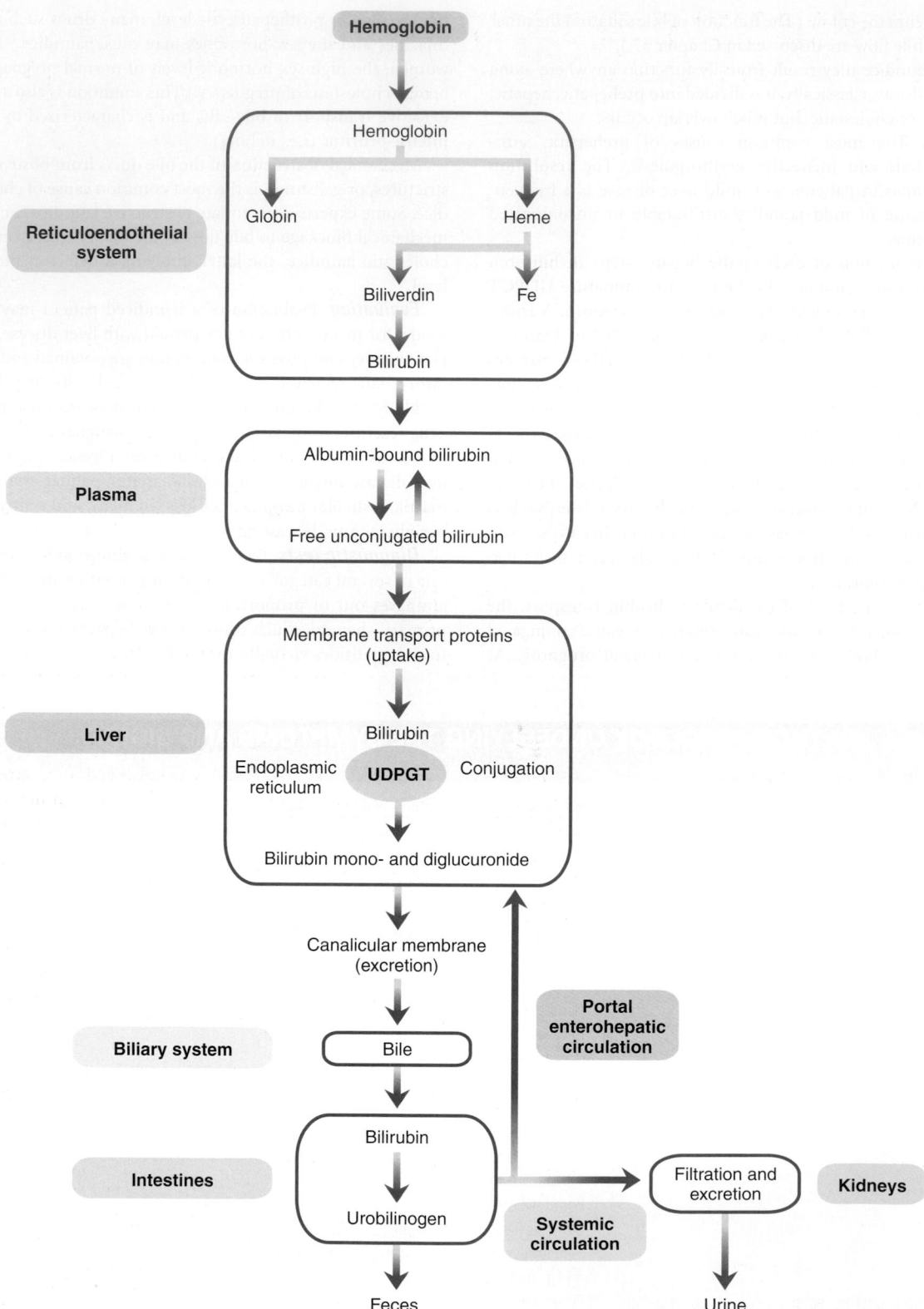

FIGURE 38-4 Summary of bilirubin metabolism (see text for explanation). *UDPGT,* Uridine diphosphate glucuronosyltransferase.

TABLE 38-2 COMMON LABORATORY TESTS IN LIVER DISEASE

TEST	NORMAL RANGE	SIGNIFICANCE
AST/SGOT	5-40 units/ml	Elevated levels indicate hepatocellular inflammation or necrosis
ALT/SGPT	5-35 units/ml	AST much greater than ALT in alcoholic liver disease
		AST less specific; may be of skeletal muscle, myocardial, kidney, or liver origin
		ALT more specific for liver disease
Alkaline phosphatase	35-150 units/ml	Elevated in cholestasis, infiltrative liver disease (e.g., cancer, granulomas)
		May be of bone origin
γ-Glutamyltranspeptidase	10-48 units/ml	Elevated in cholestasis and hepatocellular disease
		Used to confirm that elevated alkaline phosphatase is of hepatic origin
		Disproportionately elevated in alcoholic liver disease
		May be induced by many drugs (e.g., phenobarbital)
5'-Nucleotidase	2-11 units/ml	Elevated in cholestasis
		Very specific to liver
Total bilirubin	<1.0 mg/dl	Elevated levels diagnose jaundice
Indirect bilirubin	<0.8 mg/dl	Elevated in hemolysis, Gilbert disease
Prothrombin time	11.5-14 sec	Prolongation suggests decreased hepatic synthetic function
Serum albumin	3.5-5.5 gm/dl	Decreased level suggests decreased hepatic synthesis
Serum globulin	2.5-3.5 gm/dl	Elevated in autoimmune hepatitis
Urine bilirubin	0	Increased with elevation of serum conjugated (direct) bilirubin, zero in unconjugated (indirect) hyperbilirubinemia
Urinary urobilinogen	0-4 mg/24 hr; spot test ± on urine dipstick	Zero in complete biliary or proximal bowel obstruction Increase may suggest liver disease
		Nonspecifically insensitive
		Primary utility because its presence on urine dipsticks allows simple office/bedside testing or screening with one-time urinalysis

(AST) concentration markedly elevated in comparison with the alanine aminotransferase (ALT) concentration, whereas in viral hepatitis the reverse is usually true. Predominant elevations of alkaline phosphatase (ALP) level indicate intrahepatic cholestasis and are often due to an infiltrative process (e.g., metastatic carcinoma, sarcoidosis). Elevated levels of bilirubin can result from either direct (conjugated) or indirect (unconjugated) causes. Although an overwhelming liver process in an adult will produce elevations of both forms of bilirubin, as a practical matter unconjugated hyperbilirubinemia points to significant hemolysis. Predominant conjugated bilirubin level elevation points to extrahepatic cholestasis attributable to biliary obstruction. It is noteworthy that jaundice in patients with cirrhosis often shows elevations in all parameters, reflecting the widespread liver dysfunction and obstruction of the bile canals and small vessels caused by scarring.

Evaluation of hepatocellular and cholestatic disorders may include assessment for viral hepatitis (Table 38-3), performance of various biochemical assays (see the specific disorders discussed later), or conduction of a needle biopsy of the liver. Needle biopsies may be carried out "blind" or may be directed by ultrasound or computed tomography (CT), allowing examination of a specific target such as a mass lesion.

Radiologic imaging with ultrasonography is often helpful for significant liver disease. This is particularly true given the fact that structural liver abnormalities such as tumors may present with any of the aforementioned enzyme patterns or with a mixed picture. CT provides more information and has a special role in evaluating the content of iron in the liver in cases of suspected hemochromatosis. Specific visualization of the bile ducts may necessitate percutaneous transhepatic cholangiography or endoscopic retrograde cholangiopancreatography (ERCP; see Chapter 37), although magnetic resonance cholangiopancreatography (MRCP) has rapidly gained acceptance as a noninvasive way of evaluating the liver and biliary tree in great detail.

Portal Hypertension

Manifestations of liver disease not attributed to hepatocellular failure are mainly due to impaired blood flow through the liver as a result of increased resistance from fibrosis and degeneration of liver tissue. Sluggish blood flow through the liver results in increased pressure in the portal circulation (**portal hypertension**) (Figure 38-5). In this condition, venous drainage of much of the gastrointestinal tract is congested. Symptoms are surprisingly few early in the course, but as abnormal vascular patterns progress anorexia may result. The end results of elevated venous pressure are varices, particularly esophageal, but also gastric and hemorrhoidal. A pathognomic feature of advanced liver disease is superficial periumbilical varices, known as caput medusae, or the head of Medusa. Portal hypertension may present as an accumulation of peritoneal fluid, or **ascites.** A serious consequence of portal hypertension is uncontrolled bleeding from esophageal varices, which are prone to rupture.

Gastroesophageal Varices

Etiology. Esophageal varices result mainly from portal hypertension, which in Western society is generally the result of cirrhosis attributable to the chronic effects of alcoholism or viral hepatitis. In developing tropical countries, chronic infection with the *Schistosoma* species of liver fluke is a major cause of portal hypertension. Recently, it has been recognized that vasoactive hormones, as well as increased splanchnic blood flow and increased vascular resistance in the liver, have a prominent role in the formation of variceal esophageal veins.[1] Gastric varices may occur in conjunction with or independently from esophageal varices, the latter if splenic vein obstruction or thrombosis occurs.

Pathogenesis. Gastroesophageal varices are merely one of a number of collateral venous pathways that dilate in response to elevated portal pressure in an attempt to transport blood from the

TABLE 38-3 IMMUNOLOGIC MARKERS IN VIRAL HEPATITIS

MARKER	DESCRIPTION
Hepatitis A	
Anti-HAV IgM	Acute infection with HAV, but may persist for months
Anti-HAV IgG	Past infection with HAV
	Implies immunity to the virus
Hepatitis B	
Hepatitis B surface antigen (HBsAg)	Surface protein coat of HBV
	Implies active infection
	Detectable 2-6 wk after infection
	Remains present as long as infection is active
Hepatitis B surface antibody IgM (HBsAb IgM)	Antibody to surface protein of HBV
	Detectable shortly after or with clearance of HBsAg
	Implies resolution of infection and immunity to HBV
Hepatitis B core antibody IgM (HBcAb IgM)	Antibody to inner core protein of HBV
	Detectable 3-5 wk after infection
	Implies recent infection
Hepatitis B core antibody IgG (HBcAb IgG)	Same as for HBcAb IgM, but implies past infection
Hepatitis Be antigen (HBeAg)	Soluble fraction of HBV
	Detectable 2-6 wk after infection
	Implies ongoing infection with high infectivity
	May resolve independently of HBsAg
Hepatitis Be antibody (HBeAb)	Antibody to soluble fraction of HBV
	Detectable when HBeAg clears
	Implies decreased infectivity
HBV DNA polymerase activity	Same significance as HBV DNA
Hepatitis C	
Anti-HCV	Antibody to HCV antigens
	May not be detectable early in infection
	Does not indicate immunity to the virus
	Rapidly evolving area; many commercially available assays of different sensitivity and specificity
	Many false-positive and false-negative results
HCV RNA by PCR	Assay for level of viremia
	Correlates positively with activity of infection
	Clears with resolution of infection
	Technically difficult; available through reference laboratories
Hepatitis D (Delta)	
Hepatitis delta antigen (HDAg)	Assay for 35-nm RNA virus
	Detectable 2-10 wk after infection
	Implies early infection
Anti-HDV	Implies past or chronic infection
	Does not indicate immunity to the virus
Hepatitis E	
HEV RNA by PCR	Detects presence of virus
HEV antibody IgG and IgM	Not well standardized
Hepatitis G	
HGV by PCR	Measures level of viremia

PCR, Polymerase chain reaction.

splanchnic bed around the cirrhotic obstructed liver and back to the heart. Other common pathways include a variety of spontaneous deep and usually entirely asymptomatic portosystemic shunts, such as splenorenal shunts; dilated veins in the small intestine, colon, and rectum are also not uncommon.[1] Unfortunately, part of the very complex venous network that surrounds the proximal part of the stomach and esophagus lies just beneath the mucosa, rendering it especially liable to rupture when portal pressures reach a critical level. Rupture often results in massive, life-threatening upper GI bleeding (Figure 38-6).

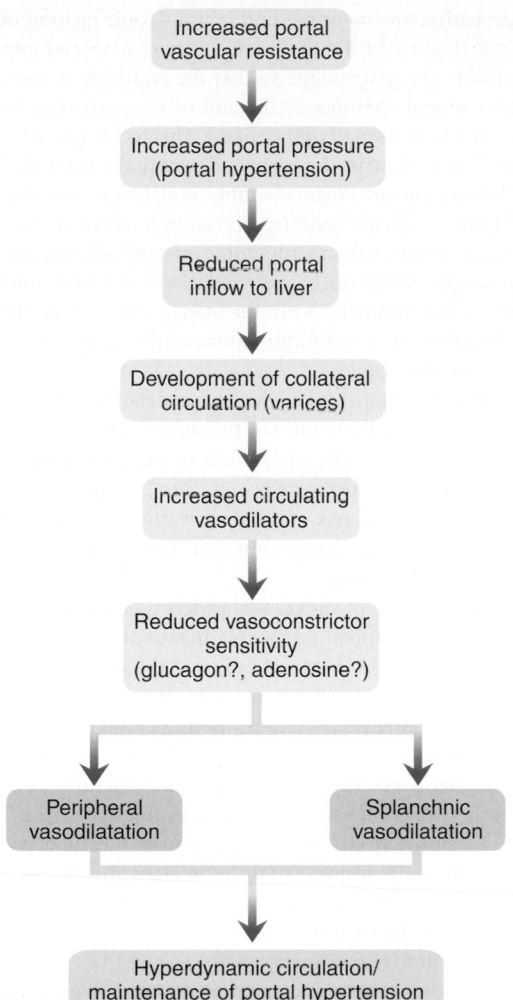

FIGURE 38-5 Pathophysiologic process of portal hypertension. (Redrawn from MacMathuna P: The pathogenesis of variceal rupture, *Gastrointest Endosc Clin North Am* 2[1]:1-8, 1992.)

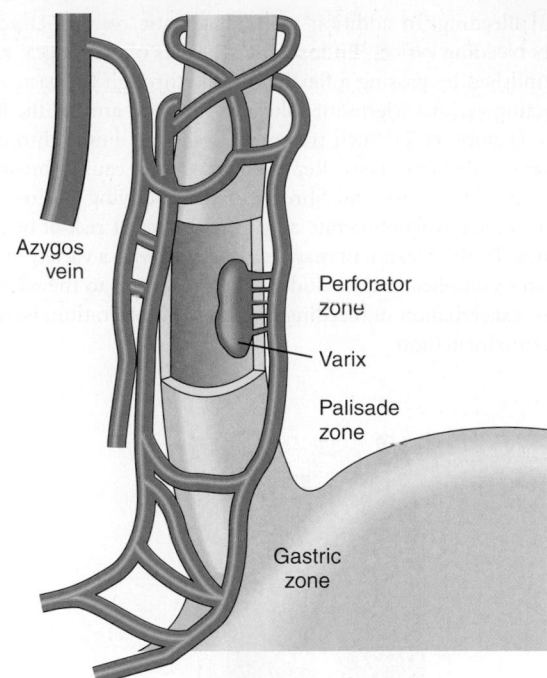

FIGURE 38-6 Gastroesophageal venous anatomy. (Redrawn from MacMathuna P: The pathogenesis of variceal rupture, *Gastrointest Endosc Clin North Am* 2[1]:1-8, 1992.)

Clinical features. Varices will affect more than half of cirrhotic patients, and approximately 30% of them experience an episode of variceal hemorrhage within 2 years of the diagnosis of varices.[1] Variceal size is the main determinant of risk for bleeding, which is one of the main causes of death (20% to 33%) in persons with long-standing cirrhosis. The mortality after an episode of significant variceal bleeding is as high as 50%. The diagnosis is made mainly endoscopically, but varices may be seen on CT scans of the abdomen, as well as on upper GI barium examinations.

The initial symptoms and signs of bleeding from gastroesophageal varices include hematemesis, melena, and even bright red rectal bleeding. These characteristics may be associated with profound anemia and symptoms and signs of shock. In most cases, concomitant evidence of chronic liver disease and portal hypertension is seen on physical and laboratory examination. There are two distinct phases of the variceal hemorrhage process: one, coincident with and shortly after the bleeding; and two, a period of 6 to 8 weeks following the initial bleed, when there is a high risk of rebleeding. The greatest risk of rebleeding occurs in the first 72 hours.

Treatment. Initial treatment is directed at performing fluid resuscitation, correcting the coagulopathy, and stopping further bleeding. Large-bore intravenous lines are placed, and fluid resuscitation is carried out with normal saline. Blood components and clotting factors are replaced as needed. Any coagulopathy may necessitate administration of parenteral vitamin K, fresh frozen plasma, and platelet infusions if profound thrombocytopenia is present. Recombinant factor VIIa is helpful in reversing the coagulopathy associated with advanced liver disease and may be considered for patients whose prothrombin time (PT) fails to normalize after the previously stated measures have been performed.[7-9]

Primary acute pharmacologic management rests on drugs that can effectively lower portal pressure by dilating alternative collateral pathways, reducing splanchnic blood flow, or both. Until recently, the agent of choice in the United States was vasopressin, an analogue of antidiuretic hormone, administered by continuous intravenous infusion along with nitroglycerin. Although effective in controlling variceal bleeding, vasopressin use may be associated with angina pectoris, severe abdominal cramping, and hyponatremia, side effects that limit its usefulness.[3]

In recent years, octreotide acetate, a synthetic analogue of the naturally occurring hormone somatostatin, has been effectively used as a replacement for vasopressin.[1] It is administered as an initial intravenous bolus followed by continuous infusion, which may be administered for as long as 3 to 5 days. In the doses used, the drug is remarkably free of side effects and more effective than vasopressin. However, it should be noted that no drug treatment has shown a mortality benefit for this condition.

Metoclopramide and β-blockers have been used as ancillary treatments in the past and may be considered for selected patients. Intravenous H_2-blockers or proton pump inhibitors are also often administered. The use of prophylactic antibiotics is recommended by the American Association for the Study of Liver Diseases; intravenous ceftriaxone or an oral quinolone for a 1-week course is the preferred regimen.[8]

Emergency esophagogastroduodenoscopy (EGD) is crucial in determining the site of bleeding, as well as excluding other causes of upper GI bleeding. In addition to its diagnostic role, EGD actively addresses bleeding varices. **Endoscopic sclerosis** of esophageal varices is accomplished by passing a flexible needle through the gastroscope and injecting various sclerosant solutions into and around the bleeding varix (Figure 38-7). Such treatment results in initial thrombosis of the vein with hemostasis. Repeated injections cause fibrosis and obliteration of the varix and fibrosis of the overlying mucosa. This process can effectively obliterate all of the varices at risk of bleeding. Unfortunately, this treatment may be associated with a variety of acute and chronic complications, including drug reactions to the sclerosing solutions, exacerbation of bleeding, perforation, ulceration, infection, and stricture formation.[5]

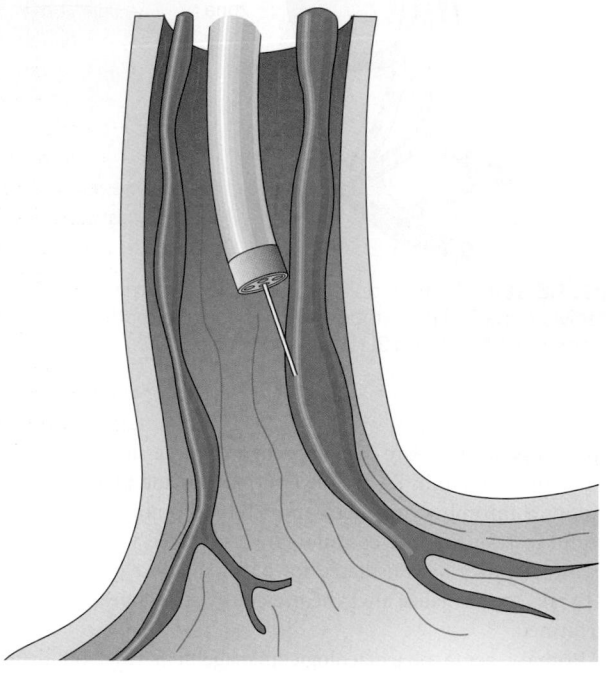

FIGURE 38-7 Endoscopic sclerosis of varices.

An alternative treatment method is endoscopic ligation of esophageal varices (Figure 38-8). In this technique, a special apparatus is preloaded onto the gastroscope so that the endoscopist can suction a varix into a special chamber at the end of the gastroscope and then ligate the varix with a small rubber band. This technique also results in immediate loss of flow in the varix and eventually leads to thrombosis and fibrosis. The area ligated simply sloughs off over the next few weeks without significant residual ulceration or scarring. This method requires fewer sessions than endoscopic sclerosis to completely obliterate the varices, seems to be associated with a lower complication rate, and may be more effective in the management of bleeding gastric varices.[1] However, it is technically more challenging and is generally reserved for elective use.

Endoscopic techniques have shown a mortality benefit relative to treatment with drugs alone but fail to control acute bleeding in 10% to 20% of patients. Unfortunately, both of these methods may result in an increase in venous pressure proximal to the area treated, perhaps resulting in an increased risk of bleeding from congestive gastroenteropathy (a diffuse venous congestion that may result in both chronic and acute severe blood loss).

Balloon tamponade of varices was widely used before the availability of endoscopic treatment.[1] This treatment consists of a gastric balloon that is passed orally or transnasally into the stomach, inflated, and held in gentle traction against the gastric varices in the fundus, thus tamponading bleeding vessels and restricting blood flow from the fundus up into the esophageal varices (Figure 38-9). Suction of oropharyngeal and gastric secretions is accomplished with integral or separate drainage tubes. Balloon tamponade carries frequent risks, including aspiration of stomach contents, migration of the tube with airway compression, pressure necrosis of the esophagus and stomach, rupture of the balloon, and rebleeding after the maximal inflation period of 24 hours. These limit the usefulness of balloon tamponade to a temporizing role until definitive treatment.

Chronic pharmacologic management of portal hypertension is frequently successful with nonselective β-blockers such as propranolol or nadolol. The drug is carefully titrated to reduce the initial resting heart rate by 25%. These drugs may be used prophylactically in patients with known portal hypertension and are often prescribed following

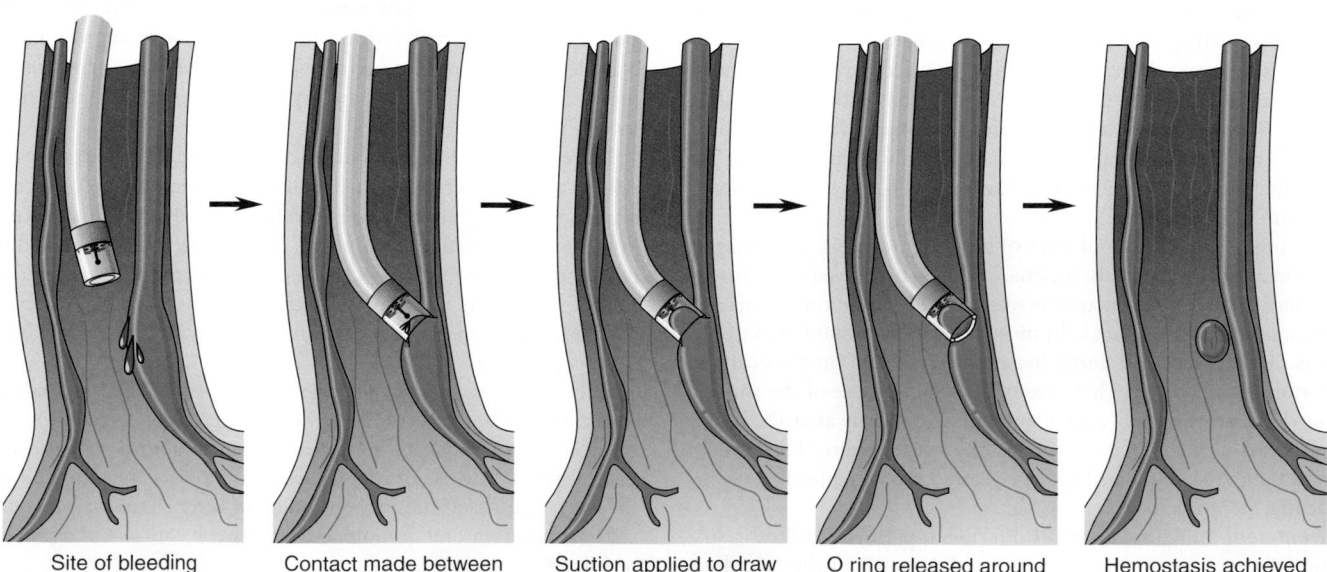

| Site of bleeding identified | Contact made between ligator and varix | Suction applied to draw varix into ligator lumen | O ring released around neck of varix | Hemostasis achieved |

FIGURE 38-8 Endoscopic band ligation of varices.

endoscopic therapy as part of a combined approach to variceal bleeding prevention. It should be noted that studies have not yet shown a consistent survival benefit for this intervention, however. In addition to β-blockers, oral long-acting nitrates such as isosorbide mononitrate act synergistically with β-blockers to reduce portal pressure and have been studied for prevention of variceal hemorrhage.[9,10] Side effects limit use of nitrates as primary prophylaxis, but these agents could be considered for secondary prophylaxis in patients who do not respond to β-blockers alone.

If the aforementioned measures are ineffective, a number of surgical and radiologic procedures are possible. Although rarely used in the United States, esophageal transection and reanastomosis with ligation of other collateral channels has been used in other countries.[1] Surgery to reduce portal pressure is very effective in decreasing the rate of rebleeding, but it may not alter overall survival. A variety of surgical techniques are used, all of which create an alternative connection between the splanchnic and systemic circulations. These techniques include portacaval, mesocaval, splenorenal, and distal splenorenal shunts (Figure 38-10). A discussion of the specific indications and technical aspects of these shunts is beyond the scope of this text, but each has certain specific indications, advantages, and disadvantages.[1]

In recent years a radiographic procedure called transjugular intrahepatic portosystemic shunting (TIPS) has been developed that combines angiographic and ultrasonographic techniques.[1] The hepatic vein is cannulated by the transjugular route. A needle is then passed into a main portal vein branch. Catheters are passed over this guidewire along with balloon dilation of the tract just created. This step is then followed by placement of an expandable metallic stent, thus creating a portosystemic shunt (portal vein to hepatic vein) within the liver itself. This procedure is technically very demanding and may be complicated by hemorrhage, infection, stent migration, stent stenosis, and occlusion, both acute and chronic. In addition, hepatic encephalopathy and congestive heart failure may result. The primary use of this modality is as a bridge to allow stabilization of patients who are candidates for liver transplantation.[17]

Treatment of esophageal varices is often unsatisfactory. Ideally, the underlying condition for varices (i.e., portal hypertension) should be reversed. The only consistently effective way to accomplish this goal is by liver transplantation (see the Transplantation section), which is limited in its application to a select group of patients.

Portal Systemic Encephalopathy
Hepatic Encephalopathy

Pathogenesis. Hepatic encephalopathy is a complex neuropsychiatric syndrome characterized by symptoms ranging from mild confusion and lethargy to stupor and coma. Some patients exhibit dementia, psychotic symptoms, spastic myelopathy, and cerebellar or extrapyramidal signs. The classic physical finding is asterixis, or "liver flap," a spastic jerking of the hands held in forced extension. Hepatic encephalopathy is associated with fulminant hepatic failure or severe chronic liver disease, conditions in which liver function is severely depressed and blood is shunted around the liver. The arterial ammonia level correlates positively with the level of encephalopathy in most patients, consistent with its central role in the pathogenesis of hepatic encephalopathy as one of the primary causes of neuronal dysfunction. The exact cause is unclear, and other contributing factors such as elevated mercaptan levels, enhanced activation of certain neurotransmitter receptors (including γ-aminobutyric acid and benzodiazepine receptors), and elevated levels of aromatic amino acids (false neurotransmitters) remain under investigation.[1,18]

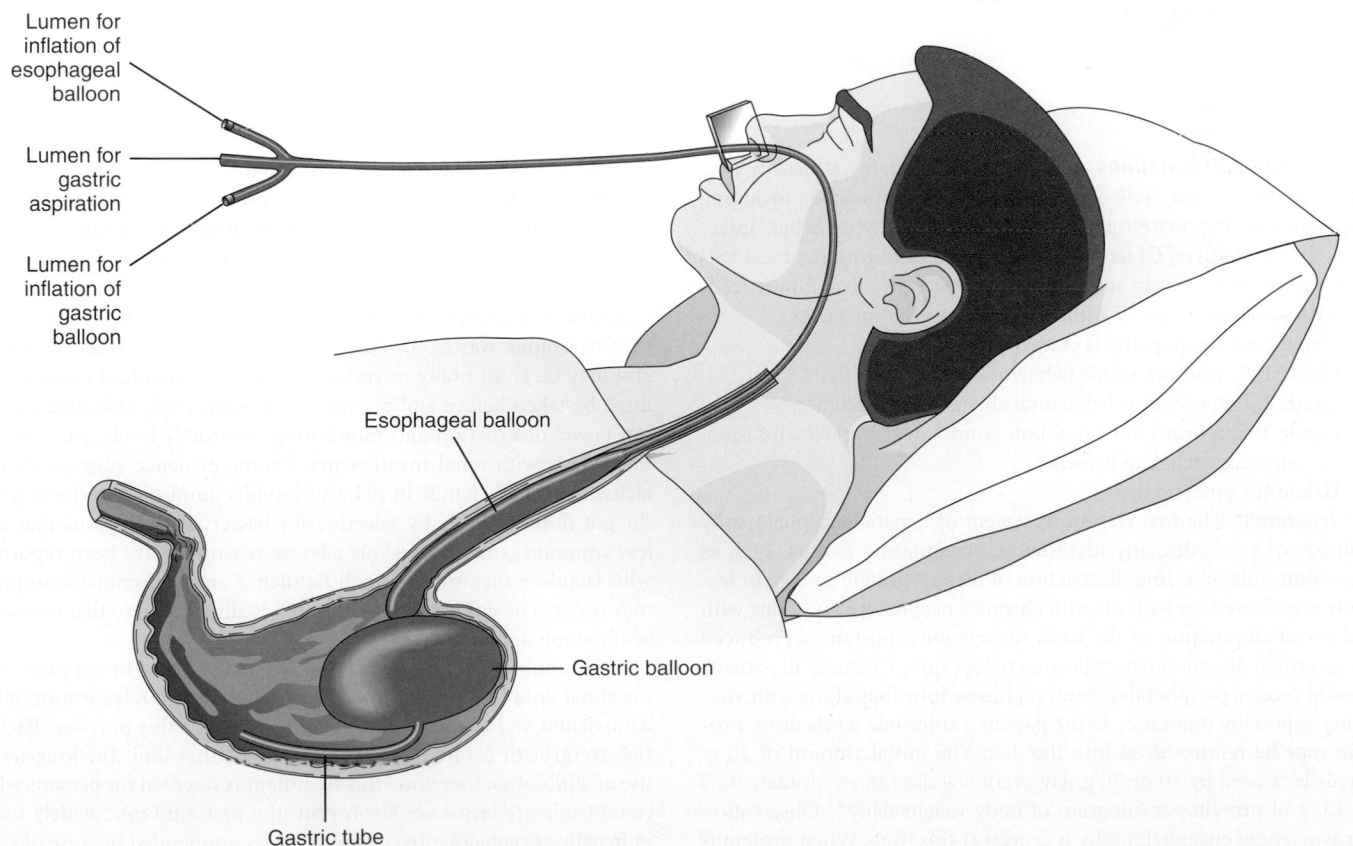

FIGURE 38-9 Sengstaken-Blakemore tube.

Lumen for inflation of esophageal balloon

Lumen for gastric aspiration

Lumen for inflation of gastric balloon

Esophageal balloon

Gastric balloon

Gastric tube

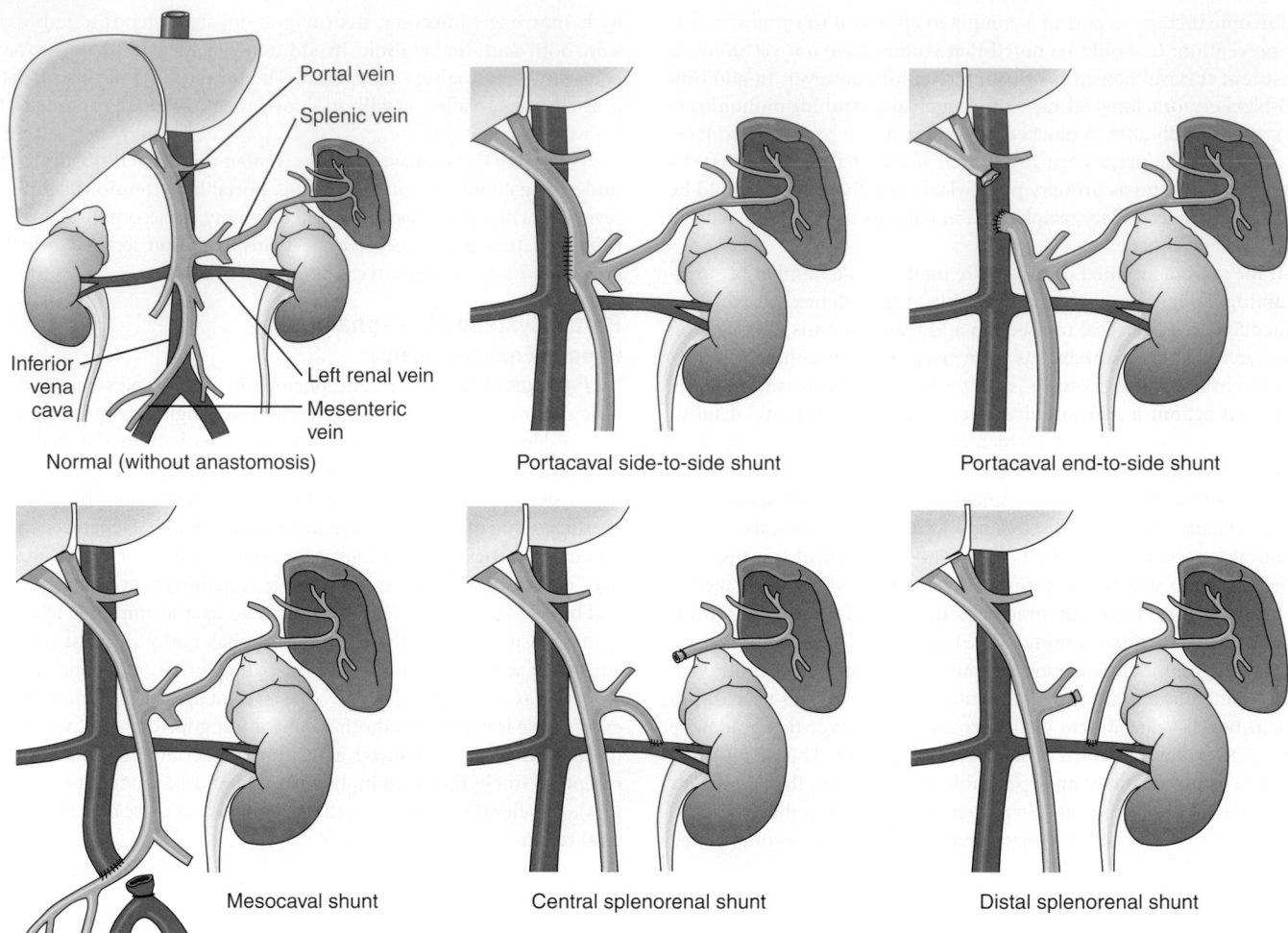

Normal (without anastomosis)

Portal vein
Splenic vein
Inferior vena cava
Left renal vein
Mesenteric vein

Portacaval side-to-side shunt

Portacaval end-to-side shunt

Mesocaval shunt

Central splenorenal shunt

Distal splenorenal shunt

FIGURE 38-10 Portosystemic shunt operations.

Clinical manifestations. Hepatic encephalopathy is usually precipitated by certain well-defined clinical developments, including hypokalemia, hyponatremia, alkalosis, hypoxia, hypercarbia, infection, use of sedatives, GI hemorrhage, protein meal gorging, renal failure, and constipation. In some patients, progressive liver failure leads to chronic encephalopathy without other exacerbating factors.

Hepatic encephalopathy is graded 1 to 4:

Grade 1: Confusion, subtle behavioral changes, no flap
Grade 2: Drowsy, clear behavioral changes, flap present
Grade 3: Stuporous but can follow commands, marked confusion, slurred speech, flap present
Grade 4: Coma, no flap

Treatment. The first step in treatment of hepatic encephalopathy consists of correcting any identifiable precipitating factors, such as gastrointestinal bleeding. Restriction of dietary protein to 60 g or less daily is indicated for patients with chronic encephalopathy, along with enhanced elimination of the toxic nitrogenous substances produced by intestinal digestion (see following paragraph). Critically ill patients should receive peripheral or central glucose infusions along with vitamins, especially thiamine. As the patient's ammonia levels drop, protein may be reintroduced into the diet. The initial amount of 20 g/day is increased by 10 or 20 g/day every few days to an ultimate 0.75 to 1.0 g of protein per kilogram of body weight daily.[13] Observation for worsening encephalopathy is crucial at this time. When protein is restricted, it is essential to provide at least 400 g of carbohydrate daily.

Vegetable protein may be better tolerated than animal protein. High dietary fiber intake may help by decreasing constipation. If dietary measures fail, oral defined-formula feedings containing essential amino acids and enriched with branched-chain amino acids may be indicated.

Osmotic diuretics or antibiotics are used to enhance elimination of nitrogenous wastes. Lactulose is the standard osmotic cathartic and may be given orally or rectally by enema. (Standard precautions must be taken before any cathartic is administered, including ruling out bowel obstruction and monitoring electrolyte levels, particularly in patients with renal insufficiency.) Some evidence suggests that a lactulose-related change in pH also inhibits ammonia production by the gut flora, possibly by selecting for bacterial populations that are less ammoniagenic. No serious adverse reactions have been reported with lactulose therapy, although flatulence and abdominal cramping may occur. The dosage should be individually titrated so that two soft, acidic stools are passed daily.

Oral antibiotics have been used for many years to suppress the intestinal flora that break down dietary protein and release ammonia. Amoxicillin and rifaximin are currently used for this purpose. Bacterial overgrowth is one of the complications that limit the long-term use of antibiotics; therefore, this treatment is reserved for persons who cannot tolerate lactulose. Neomycin, the first antibiotic widely used in hepatic encephalopathy, is no longer recommended because of side effects.[1]

Cerebral Edema

Pathogenesis. Swelling of the brain (cerebral edema) often develops in patients with grade 3 or 4 hepatic encephalopathy and results in an increase in intracranial pressure. Both vascular and toxic mechanisms have been implicated as etiologic factors. With increasing intracranial pressure, blood perfusion of the brain is decreased (cerebral perfusion pressure = carotid artery pressure − intracranial pressure) with resulting cerebral hypoxia. Cerebral edema is a major cause of death in patients with acute hepatic failure.[1]

Clinical manifestations. Clinically, cerebral edema is suggested by deepening coma, systolic hypertension, and extensor rigidity (decerebrate posture), followed by pupillary dilation and, if brainstem herniation occurs, respiratory arrest. Some highly specialized referral centers monitor patients with advanced hepatic encephalopathy by extradural pressure monitors to permit early detection. Unfortunately, complications of extradural monitors occur up to 20% of the time and include infection and intracranial bleeding.[1]

Treatment. Cerebral edema is managed primarily by the intravenous infusion of mannitol, which by increasing serum osmolarity draws water from the brain and thus reduces the swelling. Patients should be kept in the semi-Fowler position (head and trunk elevated 30 degrees). The barbiturate sodium pentothal is used as a second-line agent for patients with recalcitrant intracranial hypertension and those who cannot tolerate the fluid volume component of mannitol therapy (e.g., those in heart or kidney failure). Moderate hypothermia with the use of cooling blankets has looked promising in preliminary trials as well.[14] Aggressive treatment allows patient survival in 60% of cases, until liver failure resolves or liver transplantation can be accomplished.

Complications of Advanced Liver Disease
Ascites

Etiology, pathogenesis, and clinical manifestations. Ascites, or the pathologic accumulation of fluid in the peritoneal cavity, can occur in patients with advanced liver disease complicated by portal hypertension and hypoalbuminemia (Figure 38-11). Abdominal distention results from an inappropriate osmotic gradient across the pleura, with the intraabdominal accumulation of sodium, water, and protein.[1,15] Other causes of ascites are malignancy, infection, pancreatitis, hypothyroidism, vasculitis, nephrosis, cardiac failure, constrictive pericarditis, Budd-Chiari syndrome, and portal vein thrombosis. The specific chemical and cellular composition of the ascites varies with its cause.

Abdominal paracentesis should be performed in all patients with new ascites and in those with known ascites who have experienced significant worsening of their condition.[1] The fluid should be examined for total protein level, albumin level, and cell count. Optional tests include culture for bacteria, fungi, and mycobacteria; cytologic studies; and measurement of amylase, glucose, and lactate dehydrogenase levels. A small amount of ascites may not require specific therapy. However, with increasing volumes, abdominal discomfort, abdominal or umbilical herniation, respiratory embarrassment, or infection may occur.

Treatment. Dietary sodium should be restricted to 88 mEq (2000 mg) per day in patients with ascites. In motivated patients, this is perhaps the most helpful intervention that can be undertaken. Bed rest is useful, although strict bed rest can result in decubitus ulcers, deconditioning, and other problems. Diuretics are necessary for the majority of patients. The aldosterone antagonist spironolactone works in the distal nephron as a weak diuretic that also inhibits potassium secretion, thus sparing serum potassium. A delay of 2 to 3 days may occur before the full effect of the drug is seen, and the dosage should not be increased more frequently. Many authorities suggest adding a loop diuretic such as furosemide from the beginning and increasing

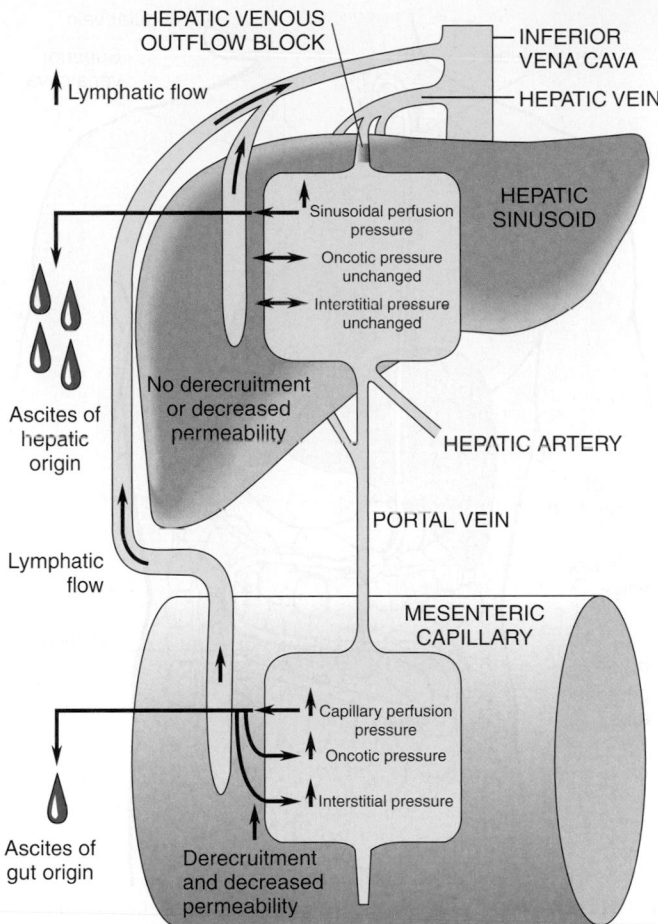

FIGURE 38-11 Pathophysiologic process of ascites. (Redrawn from Dudley FJ: Pathophysiology of ascites formation, *Gastroenterol Clin North Am* 21:215-235, 1992.)

the dose at a ratio of 4:10 with spironolactone.[1] It is helpful to monitor both urinary sodium and potassium levels periodically. When the urinary sodium level exceeds the urinary potassium level, spironolactone is exerting its maximal effect. Serum potassium levels must be carefully controlled.

The goal is the loss of approximately 0.5 kg of body weight daily, although in patients with peripheral edema, slightly more rapid weight loss is tolerable. More rapid losses may result in diuretic-induced renal impairment, intravascular volume depletion and severe electrolyte abnormalities, and hepatic encephalopathy. Diuresis should be continued until the ascites is barely detectable. Free water restriction is prescribed if hyponatremia is present or develops during treatment, although compliance with a strict regimen is unlikely.

In patients who do not respond to both diuretic therapy and sodium restriction, the use of 25% albumin infusions may help initiate diuresis. However, the effect of this treatment is often short lived and not without a risk of overexpansion of the intravascular volume, with congestive heart failure, pulmonary edema, and precipitation of variceal hemorrhage all possible. Alternatively, large volumes of ascitic fluid can be removed from the peritoneal space through paracentesis. This "large-volume therapeutic paracentesis" is a very rapid and effective treatment that can be safely instituted if the intravascular volume is maintained by appropriate measures.[1] Diuretic and dietary treatment should be continued, but in severe cases, large-volume paracentesis may be repeated as needed.

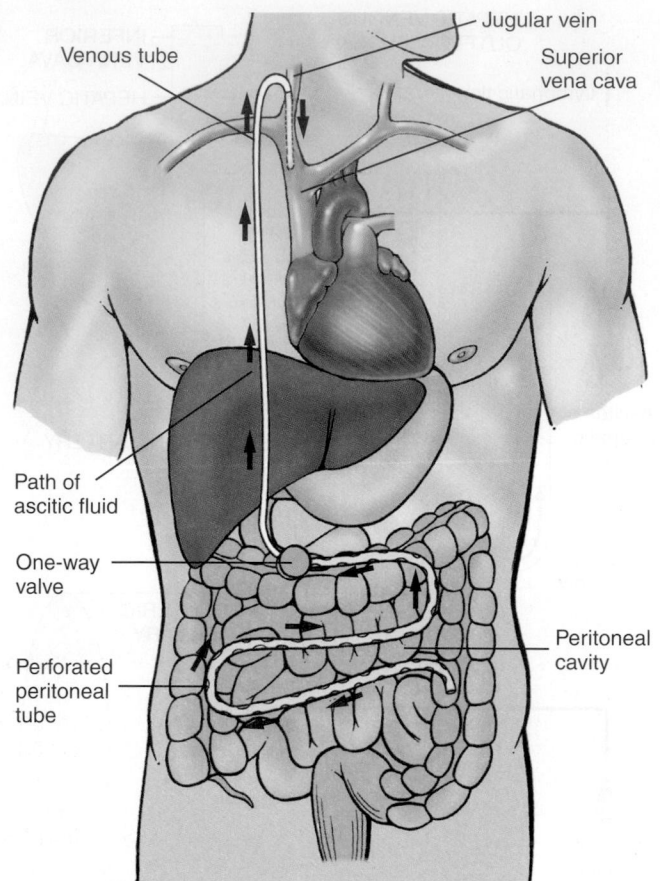

FIGURE 38-12 LeVeen shunt. Arrows show direction of flow of ascitic fluid out of the peritoneal cavity, through the shunt, into the superior vena cava. (From Monahan FD, Neighbors M: *Medical-surgical nursing: foundations for clinical practice*, ed 2, Philadelphia, 1998, Saunders, p 1146.)

Shunting procedures such as the LeVeen (Figure 38-12) and Denver shunts have been used. These one-way valves connect the peritoneal space with the venous system, usually at the jugular vein. These shunting procedures, although useful, carry significant risks and are best reserved for a small subset of ascites patients who have refractory ascites and are not candidates for liver transplantation.[1] The use of transjugular intrahepatic portosystemic stenting (TIPS) has largely replaced traditional surgical procedures for treatment of refractory ascites (see earlier discussion). Diuretic-resistant ascites is also an indication for liver transplantation in the patient who meets other criteria.

Spontaneous Bacterial Peritonitis

Pathogenesis and clinical manifestations. Patients with cirrhosis and ascites suffer from a variety of defects in host defense that predispose to infection in the peritoneal cavity. This observation is especially true in patients who have ascites with a low protein concentration. These defects include diminished opsonic activity of the ascitic fluid, diminished reticuloendothelial function, and transmigration of gut bacteria across the intestinal wall and into the ascites.[1] Chronic alcoholics demonstrate abnormal white blood cell function as well (Figure 38-13).

Typically, patients with spontaneous bacterial peritonitis (SBP) have a single infecting organism of gut origin in the fluid. This pattern is in marked distinction to patients with secondary infection of the ascites, as may occur after traumatic gut perforation, for instance, in which a polymicrobial infection is typical. The onset of spontaneous bacterial peritonitis may be subtle, with only mild abdominal discomfort or general clinical deterioration, including worsening hepatic encephalopathy, renal failure, or a nonspecific "septic" picture. Significant fever may be lacking. The most important diagnostic study is abdominal paracentesis. An ascitic polymorphonuclear leukocyte count greater than $250/cm^3$ suggests the diagnosis, although it should be noted that a low count does not rule out the diagnosis, and bacterial culture remains the gold standard.

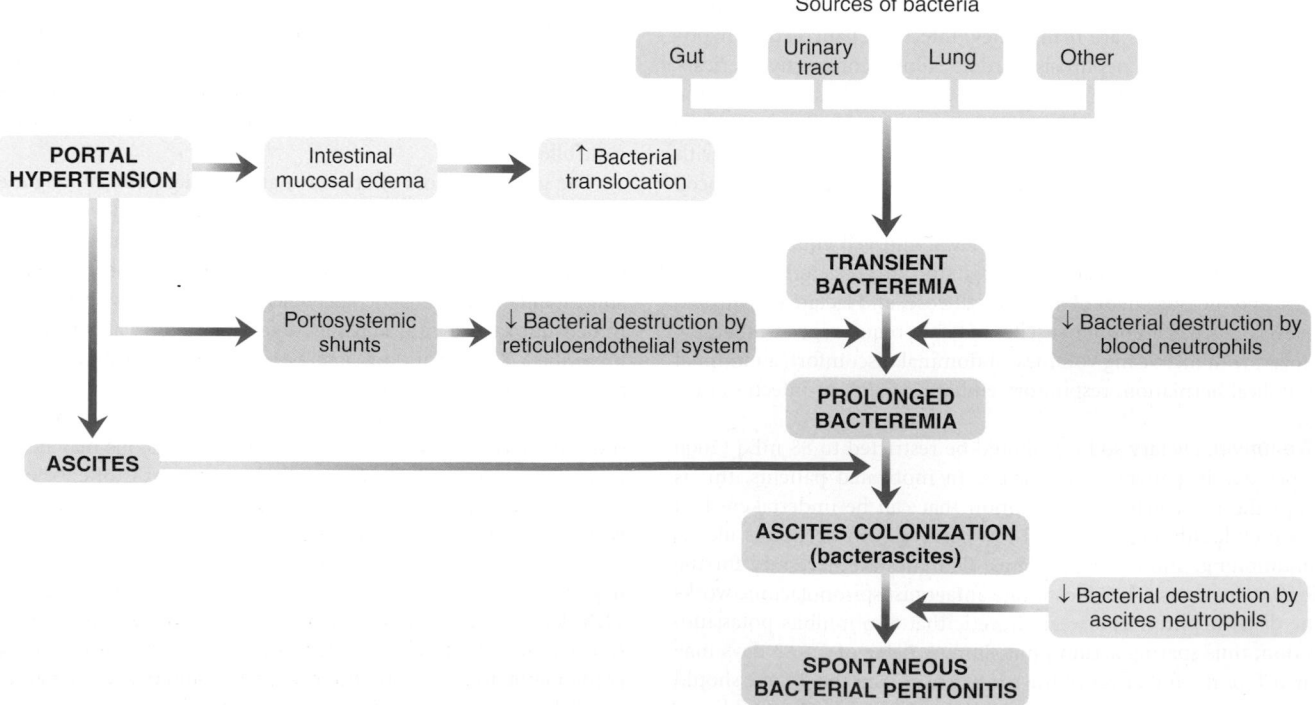

FIGURE 38-13 Pathophysiologic process of spontaneous bacterial peritonitis. (Redrawn from Garcia-Tsao G: Spontaneous bacterial peritonitis, *Gastroenterol Clin North Am* 21:257-275, 1992.)

Treatment. Antimicrobial therapy should be initiated promptly in suspected cases of spontaneous bacterial peritonitis pending culture results. Third-generation cephalosporins and quinolone antibiotics are effective empirical therapy. Use of long-term oral antibiotics for prophylaxis in at-risk patients with cirrhosis is controversial but may be considered for selected patients. Use of a narrow-spectrum agent such as trimethoprim-sulfamethoxazole therapy is preferable to agents of the quinolone class.[1] Overall, the occurrence of spontaneous bacterial peritonitis is a poor prognostic sign, because it is typically associated with end-stage liver disease.

Hepatorenal Syndrome

Etiology and pathogenesis. Patients with liver failure may experience acute kidney failure with rising serum creatinine levels and oliguria. The kidney itself is normal, but intrarenal blood flow is seriously disturbed. This disturbance in blood flow appears to be due to an imbalance between vasoconstricting and vasodilating mechanisms related to the liver disease.[1,16] The course is usually acute and progressive, but chronic cases are occasionally seen. Differentiation from reversible causes of renal failure is essential. Hepatorenal syndrome may be precipitated by overly vigorous diuretic therapy or paracentesis, severe diarrhea, nonsteroidal antiinflammatory drugs, variceal bleeding, and sepsis.

Prognosis and treatment. The prognosis depends on the severity of the liver disease and is generally poor.[17] Treatment is primarily preventive and supportive; hemodialysis should be considered only as a bridge to definitive therapy. Fortunately, liver transplantation generally results in return of normal renal function, providing no undue delay has occurred.

KEY POINTS

- The liver is a vital, multifunctional organ located in the right upper quadrant beneath the diaphragm. Blood is supplied to the liver by the hepatic artery and the portal vein. The portal vein drains the capillaries of the alimentary canal and pancreas. Arterial and portal blood flows into the hepatic sinusoids, which have direct contact with hepatic cells.

- The functions of the liver are multiple and include metabolism of fats, proteins, and glucose; synthesis and secretion of bile salts; storage of vitamins and minerals; metabolism and detoxification of endogenous and exogenous substances; and synthesis of urea.

- Manifestations of liver disease are attributable to hepatocellular failure and portal hypertension. Jaundice, decreased levels of clotting factors, hypoalbuminemia, decreased levels of vitamins D and K, and feminization are attributed to hepatocellular failure. Portal hypertension may result in GI congestion with the development of esophageal or gastric varices, hemorrhoids, splenomegaly, and ascites. Bleeding from varices is often massive and life threatening; various pharmacologic, endoscopic, and surgical treatments are now available.

- Symptoms of hepatic encephalopathy range from confusion and lethargy to coma. A spastic flapping tremor of the hands, called asterixis, is a classic finding. The severity of the encephalopathy correlates positively with serum ammonia levels. Encephalopathy may be precipitated by conditions that increase protein metabolism, such as GI hemorrhage and increased protein consumption, and by conditions that further impair hepatocyte function. Treatment may include restriction of protein intake, administration of antibiotics to reduce ammonia production by intestinal organisms, and utilization of lactulose to enhance ammonia excretion in the stool. Cerebral edema is a common cause of death in patients in deep hepatic coma.

- Ascites is a pathologic accumulation of fluid in the peritoneal cavity. It occurs commonly in liver disease because of the increased fluid transudation that occurs with portal hypertension and hypoalbuminemia. In severe ascites, treatment may be instituted to ameliorate pain and respiratory difficulty. Sodium restriction, diuretics, and intermittent paracentesis are commonly prescribed. Surgical shunting procedures that allow accumulated peritoneal fluid to flow back into the circulation through a one-way valve may be effective.

- Spontaneous bacterial peritonitis is infection of ascites by a single organism unrelated to bowel perforation or surgical procedures. Antibiotic therapy alone is usually curative.

- Hepatorenal syndrome is a type of functional renal failure caused by severe liver disease. The prognosis is poor and is contingent on the outcome of the liver disease.

DISORDERS OF THE LIVER

HEPATITIS

Acute Viral Hepatitis

Hepatitis is inflammation of the liver parenchyma. Acute hepatitis may be caused by many viruses, among them cytomegalovirus and Epstein-Barr virus. However, the term viral hepatitis is usually applied to illnesses caused by hepatitis A, hepatitis B, and hepatitis C viruses (Table 38-4). A fourth virus, known as the delta agent, is a defective RNA virus that requires the helper function of hepatitis B virus and so occurs only as a coinfection with that agent. Hepatitis E virus is a recently described agent common mainly in developing countries.

Despite variation in the symptoms, signs, and epidemiologic progression of these diseases, it is often clinically impossible to differentiate them in a given patient without appropriate serologic tests (Figure 38-14) (see Table 38-2).

Hepatitis A

Pathogenesis and clinical manifestations. Hepatitis A virus (HAV) is an RNA virus that is usually spread by the fecal-oral route. The infection has a 2- to 7-week incubation period (see Figure 38-14). The illness may be asymptomatic or mildly symptomatic without jaundice (anicteric); the latter occurs especially in children, with the patient exhibiting nonspecific GI symptoms. The majority of adults develop hepatitis with jaundice. The prodromal symptoms of icteric hepatitis consist of malaise, anorexia, nausea, low-grade fever, and right upper quadrant pain. This is followed by jaundice lasting 2 weeks on average. The clinical course is generally self-limited, although fulminant and fatal attacks occur rarely, particularly in patients with preexisting chronic active hepatitis B or C infection. Two uncommon prolonged syndromes are recognized: prolonged cholestasis and relapsing hepatitis.[1]

Diagnosis, treatment, and prevention. HAV infection is diagnosed through serologic testing. The presence of anti-HAV immunoglobulin G (IgG) indicates previous infection, and the presence of immunoglobulin M (IgM) indicates acute infection. The test is highly reliable within several weeks of exposure.

Treatment does not change the course of acute HAV infection. Supportive management includes rest and a nutritious diet. Alcohol, acetaminophen, and other potential hepatotoxins should be avoided. HAV is a common infection control concern, particularly in the community setting. The usual fecal-oral precautions, such as careful hand washing, segregation, and cleaning of laundry and personal items, should be undertaken by patients and contacts.

TABLE 38-4 COMPARISON OF HEPATITIS VIRUSES

VIRUS	HEPATITIS A	HEPATITIS B	HEPATITIS C	HEPATITIS D	HEPATITIS E
Type of virus	ssRNA	Partially dsDNA	ssRNA	Circular defective ssRNA	ssRNA
Viral family	Hepatovirus; related to picornavirus	Hepadnavirus	Flaviviridae	Subviral particle in Deltaviridae family	Calicivirus
Route of transmission	Fecal-oral (contaminated food or water)	Parenteral, sexual contact, perinatal	Parenteral; intranasal cocaine use is a risk factor	Parenteral	Fecal-oral
Mean incubation period	2-4 weeks	1-4 months	7-8 weeks	Same as HBV	4-5 weeks
Frequency of chronic liver disease	Never	10%	≈80%	5% (coinfection); ≤70% for superinfection	Never
Diagnosis	Detection of serum IgM antibodies	Detection of HBsAg or antibody to HBcAg	PCR for HCV RNA; third-generation ELISA for antibody detection	Detection of IgM and IgG antibodies; HDV RNA serum; HDAg in liver	PCR for HEV RNA; detection of serum IgM and IgG antibodies

From Washington K: Inflammatory and infectious diseases of the liver. In Kumar V et al, editors: *Robbins basic pathology*, ed 8, Philadelphia, 2007, Saunders, p 640.

dsDNA, Double-stranded DNA; *ELISA,* enzyme-linked immunosorbent assay; *HBcAg,* hepatitis B core antigen; *HBsAg,* hepatitis B surface antigen; *HBV,* hepatitis B virus; *HCV,* hepatitis C virus; *HDAg,* hepatitis D antigen; *HDV,* hepatitis D virus; *HEV,* hepatitis E virus; *PCR,* polymerase chain reaction; *ssRNA,* single-stranded RNA.

Active immunization is indicated for risk groups (e.g., foreign travelers, persons with chronic active hepatitis B or C, persons in institutions) using an inactivated whole-virus vaccine that is highly immunogenic and effective in preventing acute hepatitis A.[18] An intramuscular dose is followed by a booster 6 to 12 months later, providing lifelong immunity in at least 98% of recipients.[19] The vaccine is ideally administered at least 2 weeks preexposure (e.g., before travel to a developing country) but can also be administered in the setting of a community outbreak. It is effective even among persons with advanced chronic liver disease. Hepatitis A vaccination was added to the routine childhood vaccination schedule by the Advisory Committee on Immunization Practices (ACIP) of the Centers for Disease Control and Prevention (CDC) in 2006.

Patients exposed to HAV who are anti–HAV antibody negative should receive passive immunization with pooled human immunoglobulin, in addition to active vaccination. An intramuscular dose should be given within 2 weeks of exposure. Passive immunity lasts 4 to 6 months and does not diminish vaccine effectiveness. However, subclinical or symptomatic but attenuated infections may develop in some exposed patients.

Hepatitis B

Pathogenesis and clinical manifestations. Hepatitis B virus (HBV) is a partially double-stranded DNA virus that is highly prevalent worldwide. Probably 300 million persons, or 5% of the world population, have chronic HBV infection. Chronic infection in the United States affects approximately 1 to 1.25 million people, most of them immigrants from endemic countries. In contrast to HAV, HBV is spread by parenteral contact with infected blood or blood products, including contaminated needles, and by sexual contact. Perinatal infection is a major route in endemic (mainly developing) countries. Other risk factors for HBV infection include working in a health care setting (3% of cases in the United States), undergoing transfusions and dialysis (1% each), having acupuncture treatments, tattooing, travelling for extended time overseas, and residing in an institution.[1]

HBV has an incubation period of 2 to 6 months. The prodrome of HBV infection is often longer and more insidious than that of HAV infection and may involve a variety of immune complex–related phenomena, including urticarial (i.e., hives) and other rashes, arthralgia and arthritis, angioedema, serum sickness, and glomerulonephritis. Severity of illness ranges from no symptoms to moderate illness to fulminant hepatitis (1% of cases). The jaundice phase for most HBV infections is similar in degree and duration to that of HAV infections, although serious extrahepatic illness occurs more frequently.

Diagnosis. The serologic diagnosis is somewhat complicated (see Figure 38-14). A typical screening panel for HBV infection includes surface antigen (HBsAg), surface antibody (HBsAb), core antigen (HBcAg), and core antibody (HBcAb). In brief, with acute infection HBV core antigen (HBcAg) appears first, followed by seroconversion to core antibody (HBcAb). Presence of HBV surface antigen (HBsAg) shows up early and may persist, indicating active infection; development of surface antibody (HBsAb) points to resolution and immunity. (It should be noted that conversion from surface antigen to surface antibody positivity can take as long as 1 year after acute infection, so treatment should not be considered immediately after infection.) In chronic infection, hepatitis B e antigen (HBeAg) is associated with viral replication and infectivity, whereas hepatitis B e antibody (HBeAb) indicates minimal replication and infective potential.

Chronic infection is indicated by HBsAg positivity. There are two important features of chronic infection: ongoing liver inflammation and active viral replication. Liver damage may be deduced from persistently elevated levels of liver enzymes and confirmed by liver biopsy. Viral replication can be measured by molecular testing (HBV DNA by quantitative polymerase chain reaction) and is associated with a positive HBeAg. Persons who have a detectable virus and are HBeAg positive can readily transmit the virus to their contacts, and should be counseled regarding appropriate sexual and blood exposure precautions (including no blood donation). Patients with chronic HBV and cirrhosis are at risk for development of hepatocellular carcinoma (HCC), and periodic screening (e.g., at 6- to 12-month intervals) with ultrasound and α-fetoprotein determinations is recommended. Screening for other blood-borne pathogens such as human immunodeficiency virus (HIV) and hepatitis C virus (HCV) is recommended.

Treatment. Fulminant hepatitis is a life-threatening illness with high mortality. Care for patients with acute hepatitis is largely supportive, and those with fulminant hepatitis may require aggressive treatment for coagulopathy, encephalopathy, cerebral edema, and other manifestations. Liver transplantation is the only definitive treatment

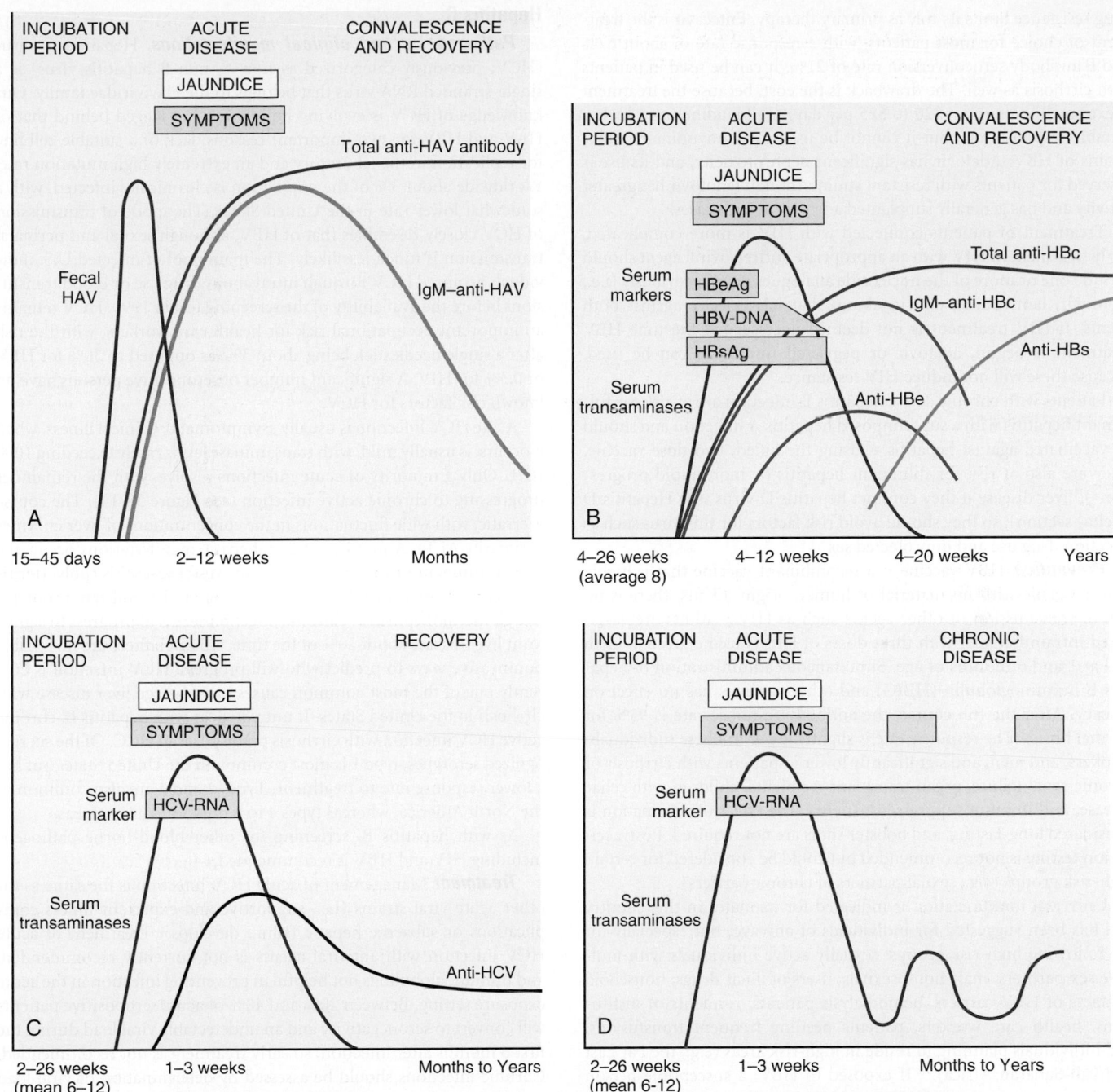

FIGURE 38-14 Comparison of clinical course and serologic tests in viral hepatitis. **A,** Hepatitis A only occurs in an acute form. **B,** The acute phase of hepatitis B—a small number of patients may not clear the virus during this stage and become chronic carriers. **C,** Acute hepatitis C is often not diagnosed because the symptoms tend to be mild. **D,** Most patients with hepatitis C infection are unable to clear the virus and develop chronic hepatitis C. (From Kumar V et al: *Robbins basic pathology*, ed 8, Philadelphia, 2007, Saunders, pp 641, 642, 644.)

for progressive liver failure in acute hepatitis. Most nonfulminant HBV infections resolve spontaneously, although about 5% of acute hepatitis cases progress to chronic infection. Management of acute HBV infection is similar to that of HAV infection in terms of supportive care.

Management of chronic HBV infection has advanced dramatically over the last decade.[20-22] Endpoints are defined as elimination of hepatitis B DNA from the blood and conversion from E antigen positivity to E antibody positivity. Currently available therapies are interferon-α, lamivudine, adefovir, entecavir, tenofovir, and telbivudine. Interferon-α

was the first effective treatment available and may be given daily or weekly (in the pegylated form) for 24 to 48 weeks with a response rate of about 33%. A significant proportion of patients experience a flare-up of acute hepatitis, and therefore this treatment cannot be used for patients with advanced liver disease (e.g., cirrhosis) or significant comorbidities. Lamivudine, emtricitabine, adefovir, entecavir, tenofovir, and telbivudine are oral nucleoside analogues that are generally given for several years. Lamivudine has the advantage of being significantly cheaper than the other options and is safe during pregnancy, but increasing drug resistance limits its role as primary therapy. Entecavir is the treatment of choice for most patients, with a response rate of about 67% and E antibody seroconversion rate of 21%. It can be used in patients with cirrhosis as well. The drawback is the cost, because the treatment is extremely expensive ($20 to $25 per day). Telbivudine has a higher durable response rate, but it cannot be used for lamivudine-resistant strains of HBV. Adefovir has significant nephrotoxicity, and its use is reserved for patients with resistant strains, though tenofovir has greater activity and has generally supplanted adefovir in such cases.

Treatment of patients coinfected with HIV is more complicated. Early treatment of HIV with an appropriate antiretroviral agent should include one or more of the nucleoside analogues noted previously (i.e., tenofovir, lamivudine, emtricitabine) that has activity against both agents. If HIV treatment is not deemed necessary at the time HBV treatment is begun, adefovir or pegylated interferon can be used, because these will not induce HIV resistance.

Patients with chronic active hepatitis B infection are at risk for fulminant hepatitis with a superimposed hepatitis A infection and should be vaccinated against hepatitis A using the killed, two-dose vaccine. They are also at risk for fulminant hepatitis or more rapid progression of liver disease if they contract hepatitis D virus (see Hepatitis D [Delta] section), so they should avoid risk factors for this virus such as injection drug use and unprotected sex.

Prevention. HBV vaccine is a recombinant vaccine that is highly immunogenic with no material of human origin. (Thus, there is no risk of transmission of other agents such as HIV.) Adults are vaccinated intramuscularly with three doses of HBV vaccine given at birth and at 1 and 6 months of age. Simultaneous administration of hepatitis B immunoglobulin (HBIG) and other vaccines has no effect on efficacy. After the full course, the antibody response rate is 95% for normal hosts.[1] The response rate is slightly lower in obese individuals, smokers, and men, and significantly lower in patients with cirrhosis or chronic renal failure, organ transplant recipients, children with celiac disease, and immunosuppressed patients. The effect of vaccination is considered long-lasting, and booster shots are not required. Postvaccination testing is not recommended but could be considered for certain high-risk groups (e.g., sexual partners of chronic carriers).

Universal immunization is indicated for neonates in this country and has been suggested for individuals of any age, but especially for the following high-risk groups: sexually active individuals with multiple sex partners, male homosexuals, users of illicit drugs, household contacts of HBV carriers, hemodialysis patients, residents of institutions, health care workers, patients needing frequent transfusions, and individuals planning to reside in high-risk areas (e.g., the Far East and sub-Saharan Africa).[18] If exposed to HBV, a susceptible person should receive one dose of HBIG and HBV vaccine as soon as possible after exposure and then complete the vaccination program. The issue of how to deal with persistent nonresponders, especially health care workers, is unsettled, but most authorities recommend a full three-injection course according to the usual schedule.[23-26]

The administration of immunoglobulin containing high levels of hepatitis B surface antibody (HBIG) affords effective postinoculation prophylaxis if given within 7 days of exposure. The indications for HBIG are as follows: (1) neonates born to HBsAg-positive mothers; (2) prophylaxis after needlestick or sexual exposure in nonimmune persons; and (3) after liver transplantation in patients who are HBsAg positive before transplantation.[1,37] The usual dose is 0.05 to 0.07 ml/kg given intramuscularly, with the same dose repeated 25 to 30 days later. (See Foster and colleagues for dosing recommendations for perinatal vaccination.[37]) The immune status of the recipient may be determined before treatment to avoid unnecessary administration. HBV vaccine should be given concomitantly with HBIG in most cases.

Hepatitis C

Pathogenesis and clinical manifestations. Hepatitis C virus (HCV; previously categorized as non-A, non-B hepatitis virus) is a single-stranded RNA virus that belongs to the Flaviviridae family. Our knowledge of HCV is evolving rapidly but has lagged behind that of HAV and HBV for two important reasons: lack of a suitable cell line for replication in the laboratory and an extremely high mutation rate. Worldwide about 3% of the population is chronically infected, with a somewhat lower rate in the United States. The mode of transmission of HCV closely resembles that of HBV, although sexual and perinatal transmission is much less likely. The main pool of infected U.S. individuals acquired HCV through intravenous drug use or blood transfusions before the availability of the screening test in 1990. HCV remains an important occupational risk for health care workers, with the risk after a single needlestick being about 3%, as opposed to 30% for HBV or 0.3% for HIV. A significant number of seropositive persons have no known risk factors for HCV.

Acute HCV infection is usually asymptomatic. Clinical illness, when it occurs, is usually mild, with transaminase levels rarely exceeding 1000 IU/L. Only a minority of acute infections resolve, with the remainder progressing to chronic active infection (see Figure 38-14). The course is erratic, with wide fluctuations in the concentrations of liver enzymes (primarily ALT). A number of extrahepatic manifestations occur, the most prominent of which are a medium-vessel vasculitis (polyarteritis nodosa), essential mixed cryoglobulinemia, and membranoproliferative glomerulonephritis.[1] Chronic infection seems to progress to significant liver disease about 20% of the time, although there are no reliable noninvasive ways to predict who will progress. HCV infection is currently one of the most common causes of end-stage liver disease with cirrhosis in the United States. If untreated, as with hepatitis B, chronic active HCV infection with cirrhosis predisposes to HCC. Of the six recognized serotypes, type 1 is most common in the United States but has a lower response rate to treatment. Types 2 and 3 are also common in the North America, whereas types 4 to 6 predominate overseas.

As with hepatitis B, screening for other blood-borne pathogens including HIV and HBV is recommended.

Treatment. Management of acute HCV infection is the same as for other acute viral strains (i.e., supportive and expectant unless complications or subacute hepatic failure develops). Treatment of acute HCV infection with antiviral agents is not currently recommended, and immunoglobulin is not helpful in preventing infection in the acute exposure setting. Between 20% and 40% of acute seropositive patients will convert to seronegativity and an undetectable viral load during the first 6 months after infection, so early treatment is not recommended. Chronic infections should be assessed by determination of viral load and viral genotype, and a liver biopsy to stage disease activity should be considered for those with a type 1 virus.[1]

The current standard of treatment for chronic HCV infection depends on virus type. Treatment of type 1 consists of pegylated interferon-α, given intramuscularly once weekly, and ribavirin orally twice daily. Treatment of acute HCV infection with antiviral agents is recommended two times daily.[1,24] Since the advent of effective protease inhibitor therapy the response rate for type 1 virus has improved from 45% to as much as 80%.[25,26] Important factors influencing a sustained virologic response include baseline viral load (i.e., a viral load greater than 800,000 copies per milliliter indicates a poorer response) and presence of the TT genotype of the *IL28B* gene. The latter is much more common among African Americans (and to a lesser extent Hispanics) than other ethnic groups and likely accounts for a significantly poorer response rate among these groups.[27]

For the less common types 2 and 3, the response rate is 85%. Side effects of interferon-based therapy are significant and include cytopenias, malaise, and flulike symptoms, as well as induction or aggravation of depression and anxiety. In fact, in many patients the latter side effects are severe and have resulted in suicides. About 5% to 10% of recipients drop out of treatment because of side effects. The expense is considerable—from $10,000 to $50,000 for a treatment course. Treatment for type 1 virus lasts 48 weeks, and for other types 24 weeks. New treatments for HCV infection are currently a burgeoning area of research.

Patients with chronic active hepatitis C infection should be vaccinated against hepatitis A and hepatitis B and counseled regarding blood-borne precautions. Because the issue of sexual transmission is unsettled, the Centers for Disease Control and Prevention does not currently recommend barrier methods for patients with long-term sexual partners because of the apparent low risk of infection.

Coinfection with HIV significantly complicates the treatment of both conditions. Optimal treatment of HIV is recommended, along with standard therapies for hepatitis C as discussed previously. Treatment responses are similar, though side effects and drug interactions are significant. Use of the newer anti-HCV protease inhibitors boceprevir and telaprevir has not been well studied in coinfected patients.

Hepatitis D (Delta)

Pathogenesis and clinical manifestations. Hepatitis D virus (HDV) is an incomplete viral organism that requires the presence of HBV for replication. It may occur coincident with or subsequent to initial infection with hepatitis B. The disease is primarily transmitted by parenteral routes and by intimate personal contact, like hepatitis B.[1] In the United States and northern Europe, HDV infection is most prevalent in persons exposed to blood and blood products (e.g., drug addicts and hemophiliacs). HDV infection tends to accelerate the progress of liver disease associated with HBV infection. In fact, fulminant hepatitis may result from HDV infection superimposed on chronic HBV infection. Because HDV is a deficient virus, its persistence is determined by the duration of the HBV infection. Diagnosis is by anti-HDV IgM and IgG enzyme-linked immunosorbent assays (ELISAs).

Treatment and control. HDV infection is controlled through the same measures used to prevent transmission of other hepatitis viruses: following safe sexual practices, screening blood products, avoiding intravenous drug use, and vaccinating susceptible persons with the HBV vaccine. There is no specific vaccine or treatment for HDV.

Hepatitis E

Pathogenesis and clinical manifestations. Hepatitis E virus (HEV) is one of the most common causes of acute hepatitis in developing countries. Cases in developed countries are usually related to recent travel. HEV is an RNA virus spread via the fecal-oral route, especially through contaminated water. Parenteral transmission may occur.

The incubation period is 2 to 9 weeks. The prodrome and icteric illnesses are similar to those of HAV infection but usually last only 2 weeks. It is assumed that many subclinical cases occur, but in the absence of widely available serologic testing, subclinical infection is difficult to determine. Fulminant hepatic failure may occur, especially in pregnant women (see the Liver Diseases and Pediatric Considerations section).

Treatment. Treatment is supportive. Because no vaccine is available, the only prophylaxis is avoiding undercooked foods, performing careful hand washing, and drinking safe water and beverages (i.e., canned, bottled, or purified through the usual means). The antiviral drug ribavirin has been studied as a potentially effective treatment but is not currently recommended.

Chronic Hepatitis

Chronic hepatitis encompasses a group of diseases characterized by inflammation of the liver that lasts 6 months or longer. The most prominent of these conditions is chronic active viral hepatitis, but chronic hepatitis may be due to toxic, autoimmune, or metabolic causes as well.

Chronic Persistent Hepatitis

Chronic persistent hepatitis, often called triaditis or transaminitis, is an archaic term for a chronic, low-grade liver inflammation of any cause. The inflammation is confined to the portal triads without destruction of normal liver structures, but serum transaminase levels are elevated. The condition may be asymptomatic or may be associated with mild, nonspecific symptoms. Progressive liver disease does not usually develop, and no drug treatment is indicated. The illness has an excellent prognosis. However, other more serious liver diseases may pass through a phase that is histologically indistinguishable from chronic persistent hepatitis and may progress (e.g., chronic viral hepatitis).

Current classification schemes emphasize (1) etiologic factor, (2) histologic grade, and (3) stage in terms of fibrosis. Therefore, chronic persistent hepatitis would generally correspond to a liver condition with mild disease activity and minimal or no fibrosis by biopsy.

Chronic Active Hepatitis

Pathogenesis and clinical manifestations. On the other hand, **chronic active hepatitis** is a progressive, destructive inflammatory disease that extends beyond the portal triad to the hepatic lobule (piecemeal necrosis). In current nomenclature, grade and stage span the spectrum from mild to severe. The natural history of chronic active hepatitis (CAH) is variable, since the disease could spontaneously arrest with any degree of fibrosis or could progress to cirrhosis and end-stage liver disease.

Symptoms typical of acute hepatitis are often seen, including fatigue, malaise, nausea, anorexia, ascites, hepatomegaly, abdominal pain, and jaundice.

Patients with chronic active hepatitis may be grouped into several categories based on etiology. First, as discussed earlier, a minority of newly infected HBV patients but a majority of those with HCV will progress to chronic active hepatitis. The second subgroup (mainly young women) manifests autoimmune hepatitis and exhibits a variety of immunologic markers, including antinuclear antibodies and anti–smooth muscle antibodies. In addition, these patients frequently suffer from a second autoimmune disease such as Hashimoto thyroiditis. In the third subgroup are patients with chronic hepatitis induced by alcohol or other toxins, including therapeutic agents such as minocycline or nitrofurantoin. In the fourth subgroup are patients with a metabolic liver disorder such as Wilson disease or hemochromatosis. A small number of patients have neither a suggestive history nor any detectable markers to suggest an etiology; advanced liver disease in this group is usually termed **cryptogenic cirrhosis.**

Diagnosis. The diagnosis of chronic hepatitis is made on the basis of the clinical setting and abnormal values for liver enzymes. Serologic studies are indicated to screen for viral hepatitis and autoimmune hepatitis. Serum iron and ferritin studies are performed to diagnose hemochromatosis, and a serum ceruloplasmin level is determined to screen for Wilson disease. A liver biopsy may be performed to confirm the diagnosis and to exclude other specific causes, if the etiology is not forthcoming. Biopsy also allows for grading and staging, as discussed earlier in the chapter.

Management of chronic active hepatitis. Treatment of CAH depends on the cause; management of HBV and HCV infection has already been discussed. Managing toxic hepatitis involves discontinuing the offending drug, including alcohol. Specific antidotes or treatments are available for some of these conditions.[1] Specific treatments for Wilson disease and hemochromatosis are discussed later in the chapter in the Metal Storage Diseases section.

Diagnosis. Autoimmune hepatitis is characterized by the presence of several autoantibodies as well as a polyclonal hypergammaglobulinemia. Antinuclear antibody (ANA) is generally positive at a high level. Anti–smooth muscle antibodies (ASMAs) are a less sensitive indicator than ANA level but highly specific for autoimmune hepatitis. The finding of highly positive autoimmune markers in the presence of significant hepatitis, in the absence of other tests indicative of viral or metabolic liver disease, is pathognomonic for this condition. There is some overlap between conditions, however, and in questionable cases a liver biopsy is indicated.

Management of autoimmune hepatitis. Corticosteroids and immunosuppressive drugs have been used since the early 1960s for the management of autoimmune chronic active hepatitis. Their use is based on the assumption that immunologic mechanisms either cause or maintain ongoing hepatic inflammation. Corticosteroids alone or in combination clearly lower mortality in chronic active hepatitis, most noticeably in symptomatic patients and those with very severe pathologic lesions demonstrated on liver biopsy. Current guidelines recommend prednisone with azathioprine until a remission is induced (usually within 18 to 24 months, as indicated by significant improvement in liver function test results).[28] Subsequently, steroids can be tapered over 6 weeks or more, with azathioprine tapered more slowly; 65% to 80% of patients will respond to this initial regimen. Cyclosporine is another treatment option for nonresponders. Treatment with corticosteroids is generally accompanied by well-known complications: arterial hypertension and fluid retention, hypokalemia, glucose intolerance, mental status changes, cataracts, thinning of skin and bones, suppression of the adrenal gland, avascular necrosis of the joints, rounding of the face (moon facies), loss of muscle mass, and central adiposity, as well as increased risk for certain infections. Suddenly stopping long-term treatment with corticosteroids may result in acute adrenal insufficiency with hypotension and shock.

KEY POINTS

- Acute viral hepatitis is generally classified as hepatitis A, B, C, D (delta), and E infection. Modes of transmission and severity of symptoms differ among types.
- HAV infection is also known as enteric hepatitis because it is generally transmitted by ingestion of contaminated substances. Symptoms are flulike and tend to be less severe than those of HBV infection. Early treatment with γ-globulin and vaccination after exposure may be effective in preventing disease.
- HBV infection is also known as serum hepatitis because its usual route of transmission is through infected blood. The incubation period is longer and the severity of symptoms (particularly jaundice) is greater than in HAV infection. Hepatitis B immunoglobulin (HBIG) is effective after inoculation if given within 7 days of exposure. HBV vaccine is recommended as part of the childhood vaccination regimen and for high-risk individuals, and after exposure. Treatment is with intramuscular interferon-α for 6 to 12 months, or with one of several nucleoside analogues for 1 to several years.
- HCV, also known as non-A, non-B hepatitis virus, resembles HBV in its routes of transmission. Chronic HCV infection develops in 85% of cases and is usually asymptomatic until advanced liver disease intervenes. Immunoglobulin does not protect against HCV infection. Treatment is with intramuscular pegylated interferon and oral ribavirin for 6 to 12 months, with the addition of one of two recently approved protease inhibitors for type 1 virus.

- HDV coinfects with HBV and requires the presence of HBV to be active. Infection appears to accelerate and worsen HBV infection symptoms. Prevention of HBV infection also prevents HDV infection.
- HEV is a common virus in the developing world that causes an illness similar to HAV infection but has a relatively high mortality in pregnant women.
- Chronic hepatitis is characterized by persistent inflammation of the liver lasting 6 months or more. Autoimmune disease, viral hepatitis (B and C), toxins, and metabolic diseases may result in chronic hepatitis. Chronic active hepatitis may progress to cirrhosis. Corticosteroids (prednisone) and immunosuppressants (azathioprine) are common therapeutics for autoimmune hepatitis.

CIRRHOSIS

Cirrhosis represents the irreversible end stage of many different hepatic injuries, including severe acute hepatitis, chronic hepatitis, the metal storage diseases, alcoholism, and toxic hepatitis. It is characterized by diffuse hepatic fibrosis surrounding nodules of liver tissue and results in permanent alteration in hepatic blood flow and liver function. The pathophysiology of cirrhosis and its complications have been reviewed earlier in this chapter. We will discuss briefly the sequelae of chronic biliary disease and alcoholic liver disease.

Biliary Cirrhosis

Etiology and pathogenesis. **Biliary cirrhosis** represents the end result of continuous, ongoing inflammation of the bile ducts, which may be due to macroscopic or microscopic biliary obstruction. Persistent biliary obstruction results in inflammation and scarring of the liver, with obliteration of the bile ductules. The consequence is diffuse and widespread fibrosis with regenerative nodule formation (islands of healthy liver tissue within a background of fibrosis), and the consequences of portal hypertension described earlier. The prototypical form of microscopic biliary disease is **primary biliary cirrhosis (PBC),** an autoimmune condition often associated with systemic lupus erythematosus and other autoimmune illnesses. It is usually associated with positive tests for ANA and antimitochondrial antibodies (AMAs).

Examples of large-duct obstruction include gallstone disease, chronic biliary fluke infestation, and primary sclerosing cholangitis (PSC). The biliary flukes endemic in Asia, *Opisthorchis* and *Clonorchis* species, are acquired by eating raw fish that carry larval cyst forms.[29] *Fasciola hepatica* is found in all sheep-producing and cattle-producing areas of the world and infects humans as accidental hosts; it is acquired by eating fecally contaminated watercress and other aquatic plants that harbor the immature cysts. Immigrants from infected areas may be at risk for these chronic infestations.

Diagnosis and treatment. The diagnosis of PBC depends upon appropriate serologic and liver biopsy results. Ursodeoxycholic acid (ursodiol, UDCA) is the only approved treatment for PBC and may delay development of end-stage liver disease. Methotrexate and colchicine are other therapies whose efficacy has yet to be elucidated in studies, but which may be added to UDCA in certain cases. Supportive care is similar to that for other conditions with impaired bile metabolism, including supplementation with fat-soluble vitamins. In spite of these measures, most patients will eventually require liver transplantation for prolonged survival.

The diagnosis of biliary flukes in immigrants and (less commonly) foreign travelers can usually be made by serial stool examinations for parasitic ova, and serologic testing is often helpful. Treatment with antiparasitic agents (praziquantel, mebendazole, or albendazole) will eliminate the live worms but will not necessarily prevent recurrent episodes of cholangitis and other consequences.

Primary Sclerosing Cholangitis

Etiology and pathogenesis. Primary sclerosing cholangitis (PSC) is an autoimmune condition generally seen in patients with ulcerative colitis; 80% of PSC patients have coexistent ulcerative colitis, whereas 3% to 5% of ulcerative colitis patients develop PSC.[1] It is characterized by recurrent episodes of cholangitis, with progressive biliary scarring and obstruction. Secondary forms of sclerosing cholangitis, such as that following bile duct injury during surgery, behave in a similar fashion.

Diagnosis and treatment. A majority of patients with PSC will have a positive perinuclear antinuclear cytoplasmic antibody (p-ANCA) test, though this is not necessarily pathognomonic. Diagnosis is primarily by means of endoscopic retrograde cholangiopancreatography (ERCP) or magnetic resonance cholangiopancreatography (MRCP) showing the typical beaded and atrophic appearance of the biliary tree; liver biopsy is often performed for staging reasons. Although a variety of treatments have been investigated, medical and endoscopic treatments (for relief of strictures) are merely palliative, and the only effective recourse is liver transplantation.[30] The end result of recurrent cholangitis of any cause is cirrhosis, and such patients are predisposed to cholangiocarcinoma.

Alcoholic Liver Disease

Alcoholic liver disease is manifested by fatty liver, hepatitis, and cirrhosis. One or more of these manifestations may be found in alcoholic patients.

Alcoholic Fatty Liver

Etiology. **Alcoholic fatty liver** (alcoholic steatohepatitis) is an accumulation of fat in the liver cells. It is caused by more fat being delivered to the hepatocyte than it can normally metabolize or by a defect in fat metabolism within the cell.

Diagnosis and treatment. Steatohepatitis is not exclusively alcohol-related. Indeed, diabetes mellitus, obesity, protein malnutrition, total parenteral nutrition, drugs, and many other factors may result in a similar pathologic process. It is usually mild and asymptomatic, and is often diagnosed incidentally on ultrasound or CT examination or by liver biopsy for another reason. Levels of liver enzymes are often mildly abnormal, generally serum transaminases. Hypertriglyceridemia is commonly found and at times may be dramatically elevated (e.g., greater than 1000 mg/dl). Occasionally, there is significant liver enlargement, abdominal discomfort, and even portal hypertension. Treatment involves stopping alcohol intake and providing appropriate nutrition. Nonalcoholic steatohepatitis (NASH) may be managed with reduction of weight, control of diabetes and hyperlipidemia, or other treatment directed at the underlying cause. Although the exact risk is unclear, it has been estimated that between 3% and 15% of persons with untreated NASH will eventually develop progressive liver fibrosis and cirrhosis.[1]

Alcoholic Hepatitis

Pathogenesis and clinical manifestations. **Alcoholic hepatitis** is an active inflammation of the centrilobular region of the liver. The liver cells show pathologic changes of hepatocyte necrosis with neutrophilic infiltration and intracellular inclusions known as Mallory bodies. This form of liver disease often occurs in chronic alcoholics who "go on a bender" and binge on quantities much greater than their usual intake. Clinically the illness ranges from mild to very severe, with the worst cases characterized by hepatomegaly, fever, signs of acute liver failure, and encephalopathy. Hepatitis may be complicated by acute alcohol withdrawal and delirium tremens. Mortality rates as high as 33% are seen with this condition.[1]

Diagnosis and treatment. The diagnosis is supported by the history, if the patient is reliable. The finding of a serum AST (SGOT) level markedly higher than a serum ALT (SGPT) level strongly suggests a toxic etiology, rather than acute viral hepatitis. Viral serologies, serum acetaminophen levels, and tests for certain metabolic disorders (e.g., determination of serum ceruloplasmin level for Wilson disease) may help sort diagnostic dilemmas.

Because one of the pathogenetic factors in alcoholic hepatitis is malnutrition and vitamin deficiencies, special attention should be given to nutrition. Thiamine 100 mg daily and a multivitamin should be administered routinely, and vitamin B_{12} and folate levels should be measured and replenished as necessary. Patients with an elevated prothrombin time or International Normalized Ratio (INR) should receive subcutaneous vitamin K. Corticosteroid therapy with prednisolone is recommended for seriously ill patients, especially those with declining liver function and coma.[28-32]

TOXIC LIVER DISORDERS

Metal Storage Diseases
Hereditary Hemochromatosis

Pathogenesis and diagnosis. **Hereditary hemochromatosis** (**HH**) is one of the most common autosomal recessive disorders in the world. In European populations, approximately 1 in 10 persons is a heterozygous carrier, and 0.5% are homozygous persons with disease.[45] Studies in the United States show a prevalence of HH homozygosity of 0.44% for Caucasians, 0.027% for Hispanics, and 0.014% for African Americans.[33] The prevalence among Asians is extremely low. However, despite the high prevalence of the gene, the number of persons with clinical hemochromatosis is considerably smaller—less than 1% of homozygotes. This is due to incomplete penetrance of the gene and environmental factors.

The disease is caused by the activity of a mutant gene called *HFE*, which allows excessive and uncontrolled iron absorption by the GI tract. The usual *HFE* mutation has been identified as C282Y, but other mutations can occur and act in a similar way. A small number of patients with HH are heterozygotes for *HFE;* disease in this population may result from as-yet-unidentified mutations or other factors. The result of these mutations is iron deposition in numerous organs; in advanced disease, the body may contain 20 g or more of iron, mainly in the liver, pancreas, and heart. Because of menstruation and perhaps endocrinologic factors, hemochromatosis is much less common in women than in men (ratio of 1:5 to 1:10 female to male ratio).[1]

The liver is usually the first organ to show evidence of involvement, with hepatomegaly and elevated levels of liver enzymes. Specific manifestations in organ systems other than the liver include diabetes mellitus, hyperpigmentation, polyarthritis, hypogonadism, and heart failure. (Archaically the condition was known as bronze diabetes, polyarthritis, hypogonadism, heart failure and bronze discoloration of the skin.) In advanced disease, fibrosis and macronodular cirrhosis of the liver develop insidiously and represent the major cause of death. Splenomegaly is common, although portal hypertension and its complications (see earlier discussion) occur less frequently than with other forms of liver disease. HCC develops in about 30% of persons with hemochromatosis, exclusively in the setting of cirrhosis.[1] Therefore, early diagnosis and treatment are critical.

Clinical manifestations and diagnosis. The diagnosis is suggested by clinical features and family history. Plasma iron and transferrin saturation is increased, and serum ferritin level is dramatically elevated, often to several thousand micrograms per liter (normal 10 to 200 mcg/L). The diagnosis of hereditary hemochromatosis is confirmed by genetic analysis for the *HFE* gene. In selected cases liver biopsy may be performed, demonstrating iron deposition in periportal hepatocytes.[1] The diagnosis of hereditary hemochromatosis should prompt investigation of other family members for carriage and expression of the *HFE* gene.

It should be noted that a second large category of iron overload syndromes exists—that of secondary hemochromatosis. This may occur with chronic hereditary dyserythropoietic states (e.g., sideroblastic anemia and thalassemia), in alcoholic patients with liver disease, and in patients with excessive iron ingestion over a period of many years. Hemochromatosis related to anemias is generally the result of repeated blood transfusions and iron intake. Of mainly historical interest is an interesting condition called Bantu siderosis, which occurred among South African tribesmen who imbibed beer fermented in iron pots. All of these secondary forms of hemosiderosis are not associated with the *HFE* gene.

Treatment. Recently, observational studies have shown that asymptomatic patients with a relatively low iron load have an essentially normal lifespan.[34] Therefore treatment is reserved for those patients with a ferritin level greater than 1000 mcg/L. The mainstay of treatment for hemochromatosis is repeated phlebotomy. The typical protocol is weekly phlebotomy of 500 ml (1 unit) of whole blood until the hematocrit drops below 37%, at which time maintenance phlebotomy of 1 unit is carried out every 2 to 3 months. Patients who do not tolerate phlebotomy may be treated with subcutaneous or intramuscular deferoxamine, a drug that chelates iron and facilitates its renal excretion. Deferoxamine is much less efficient than phlebotomy and requires adequate renal function. If identified early, hereditary and acquired hemochromatosis carries an excellent prognosis in terms of preventing heart failure and liver disease. Diabetes may still develop, however, and iron removal does not change hypogonadism or arthritis. Liver transplantation is available for patients with irreversible cirrhosis whose heart involvement does not preclude surgery.

Wilson Disease (Hepatolenticular Degeneration)

Etiology. **Wilson disease,** or hepatolenticular degeneration, is a rare autosomal recessive disorder in which excessive amounts of copper accumulate in the liver and other organs. As with hereditary hemochromatosis, it has now been linked to a specific abnormal protein mutation in the Wilson disease protein ATP7B gene, which results in retention of copper in the liver as well as impaired incorporation of copper into ceruloplasmin. Most patients are compound heterozygotes with more than one of several mutations involving the *ATP7B* gene. The condition may present at any time before age 30, generally with either significant hepatic dysfunction or neuropsychiatric illness. Patients with a neuropsychiatric presentation virtually always have occult compensated cirrhosis at the time of diagnosis.

Clinical manifestations. Hepatic disease is more common in children than adults and begins as hepatomegaly, fatty infiltration of the liver, and elevated levels of liver enzymes. Great variability in liver disease is seen, and Wilson disease may manifest as acute hepatitis progressing to fulminant hepatic failure, a condition very similar to autoimmune hepatitis with numerous extrahepatic symptoms, or insidious development of macronodular cirrhosis with portal hypertension. Neurologic involvement presents as a movement disorder or rigid dystonia, or occasionally as primarily psychiatric symptoms. Other manifestations include renal tubular acidosis with a Fanconi-like syndrome, cardiomyopathy, hypogonadism, metabolic bone disease (i.e., vitamin D–resistant rickets), and arthritis.

Diagnosis. Clinical signs and symptoms suggest the diagnosis, in particular the finding on slit-lamp examination of the brownish Kayser-Fleischer rings at the margin of the cornea. However, lack of Kayser-Fleischer rings does not exclude the diagnosis. Unlike hereditary hemochromatosis, genetic analysis is not the primary diagnostic pathway; it should be reserved for those with proven metabolic abnormalities because of variability in the genetic mutations that cause copper overload syndromes. The combination of low serum ceruloplasmin level and elevated 24-hour urinary copper excretion is highly suggestive of Wilson disease.[1] Results of 24-hour urinary copper excretion after penicillamine administration provide additional diagnostic proof in ambiguous cases. The liver biopsy technique for copper determination is technically demanding and is not routinely performed. As with hereditary hemochromatosis, genetic screening of close relatives should be carried out.

Treatment. Treatment involves dietary modification and copper removal therapy. Patients should try to eliminate copper-rich foods from their diet, including organ meats, shellfish, nuts, chocolate, and mushrooms.[1,13] (Vegetarians require specific dietary counseling.) Dietary measures include testing home water sources and filtering water with a high copper content. Oral chelation therapy is the mainstay of treatment for Wilson disease, and the currently preferred agent is trientene. Alternative agents include penicillamine and zinc. Patients receiving this treatment early in the course of the disease will show marked improvement and protection against liver and neurologic disease.[1] Even patients with advanced Wilson disease may expect some functional recovery. Treatment is lifelong, and noncompliance leads to definite progression.

Side effects are less common with trientene than with the older therapy, penicillamine. A mild anemia and gastritis may occur with this medication, also a transient worsening of neurologic symptoms. Finally, ammonium tetrathiomolybdate is occasionally used for severe neurologic Wilson disease because, unlike penicillamine, it is not associated with early transient neurologic deterioration.[35] As with hemochromatosis, liver transplantation has a limited but useful role.

Toxic Metabolic Agents
Acetaminophen Poisoning

Etiology. Many drugs and toxins cause liver damage. Unfortunately, treatment is often limited to withdrawal of the offending agent and administration of supportive care. Standard measures, including gastric lavage, induced emesis, and activated charcoal, are used in cases of acute ingestive poisoning. Specific antidotes are few, although heavy metal intoxication may be managed with chelating drugs. Acetaminophen overdose is an important exception that bears further discussion.

Pathogenesis and clinical manifestations. Acetaminophen (paracetamol in Britain and Europe) is a widely used, nonprescription analgesic and antipyretic that is frequently implicated in suicide attempts and accidental poisonings. In fact, a multicenter study recently showed that acetaminophen overdose was responsible for 39% of cases of acute hepatic failure in the United States.[36] Oral acetaminophen is rapidly absorbed and metabolized (Figure 38-15). A toxic metabolite, *N*-acetyl-*p*-benzoquinone imine, is formed and rapidly detoxified by reaction with glutathione. However, acute ingestion of at least 140 mg of acetaminophen per kilogram of body weight may expose the liver to high levels of the toxic metabolite with resultant hepatic necrosis. Importantly, repeated ingestion of smaller amounts may cause harm in children, the elderly, patients with pre-existing liver disease, persons abusing alcohol, and persons taking other possibly hepatotoxic drugs. Significant liver damage is rare if serum acetaminophen levels are less than 150 and 37 g/ml, respectively, 4 and 12 hours after ingestion. Given the many variables affecting acetaminophen toxicity, it is imperative for clinicians evaluating a suspected case to refer to a published nomogram and obtain periodic drug levels of acetaminophen.[37] (Screening for ingestion of other drugs, such as tricyclic antidepressants, should also be done.)

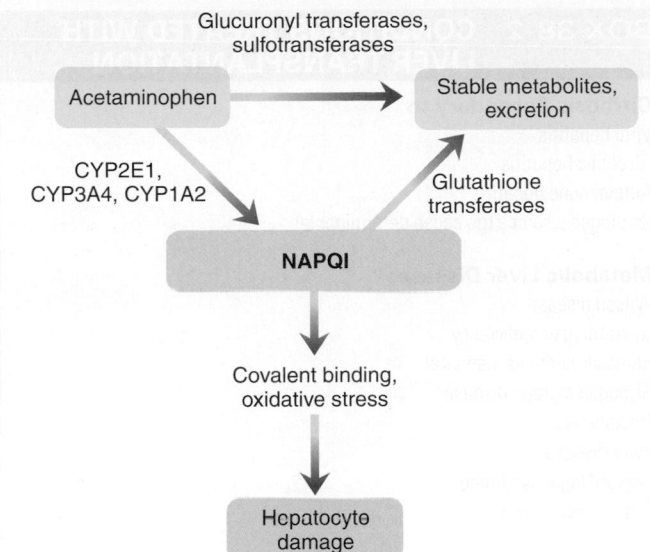

FIGURE 38-15 Mechanism of acetaminophen toxicity. The majority of an administered dose of acetaminophen is conjugated with sulfate or glucuronic acid to form stable metabolites that are promptly excreted in urine. Under most circumstances, only a minority of the total acetaminophen dose undergoes bioactivation to the reactive intermediate *N-acetyl-p-benzoquinone imine (NAPQI).* This species is capable of binding to intracellular proteins and mediating cell injury or death. The liver enzymes capable of bioactivating acetaminophen to NAPQI are CYP2E1, CYP3A4, and CYP1A2. Accumulation of NAPQI in the liver does not generally occur because the liver has sufficient ability to detoxify this metabolite through glutathione conjugation. (Redrawn from Fontana RJ, Watkins PB: Genetic predisposition to drug-induced liver disease, *Gastroenterol Clin North Am* 24:811-823, 1995.)

Within several hours of ingestion, the patient generally experiences nausea, vomiting, and diarrhea. After these symptoms, there is often a temporary "window" period, in which the patient feels well and may wish to withdraw from medical care. Within 24 to 48 hours, signs of hepatic injury occur, including abnormal liver enzyme levels. If untreated, progressive liver failure with jaundice, encephalopathy, hypoglycemia, coagulopathy, and even death may occur, generally within the first week. Patients surviving 1 week generally experience complete recovery of normal liver function without sequelae.

Treatment. Initial treatment, as for any poisoning, involves decontamination with induced emesis or lavage and activated charcoal (which will not interfere with use of acetylcysteine). The proper use of acetylcysteine for patients with clearly toxic levels can effectively prevent hepatic necrosis and its fatal consequences if started in a timely fashion. Acetylcysteine, a mucolytic solution often used in patients with bronchial diseases, stimulates liver production of reduced glutathione, which can then keep up with blood levels of toxic metababolites.[37] Acetylcysteine is nontoxic but may cause rash and frequently induces vomiting because of its foul odor and taste. It is often given by nasogastric tube in conjunction with antinausea medications. It can also be given intravenously, although this preparation is associated with a 10% incidence of anaphylactic-type reactions requiring immediate attention.

OTHER STRUCTURAL LIVER CONDITIONS

Liver Abscess

Pathogenesis, clinical manifestations, and diagnosis. Pyogenic liver abscess is a very common condition worldwide. In the United States it represents most commonly a complication of ascending cholangitis with or without gallstones, from anaphylactic-type reactions associated with intestinal infection (e.g., appendicitis, through the portal vein), or from hematogenous seeding caused by an endovascular infection.

Liver abscess should be considered in any patient with fever and right upper abdominal pain. Nausea and vomiting are common, and jaundice from biliary obstruction may rarely be present. Frequently, tender hepatosplenomegaly and sometimes a palpable mass are noted. Typical signs of pyogenic infection are usually present, including leukocytosis, an elevated erythrocyte sedimentation rate, and elevated levels of liver enzymes, usually in a "mixed" pattern. Because the primary diagnostic considerations include acute cholecystitis, cholangitis, or liver tumor, imaging of the liver with ultrasonography or CT is usually carried out. Ultrasound-guided or CT-guided thin-needle aspiration of abscesses is recommended to provide the necessary material for Gram stain and cultures; blood cultures should also be obtained.

Pyogenic liver abscess from abdominal sources generally contains enteric aerobic and anaerobic gram-negative bacteria. *Escherichia coli, Klebsiella* species, and *Bacteroides fragilis* are particularly important. Abscesses of hematogenous origin are more heterogeneous. *Streptococcus viridans* and related streptococcal species are commonly seen. *Staphylococcus aureus* is seen in the setting of endocarditis or widespread bacteremia.

Other uncommon causes of cystic liver abnormalities should be considered, in particular hydatid liver cysts secondary to *Echinococcus* species and amebic liver abscess. These conditions are virtually always seen among persons who have lived in developing countries for many years. Their appearance on ultrasound and CT is usually characteristic, and serologic values are available to assist with diagnosis. (Aspiration of probable echinococcal cysts is contraindicated because of the possibility of anaphylactic shock attributable to leakage of immunogenic cyst material.) Fungal and mycobacterial infections of the liver are usually granulomatous and diffuse, but in certain settings, such as in neutropenic patients, localized infection with an organism such as *Aspergillus* may be seen.

Treatment. Large (2.0 cm) solitary or multiple liver abscesses require drainage, formerly a surgical procedure. However, at present CT-guided and ultrasound-guided percutaneous drainage tubes are the standard of care and may be placed with minimal morbidity and discomfort. These should be kept in place until drainage has essentially resolved.

Antibiotic coverage should be directed at likely organisms. A third-generation cephalosporin such as ceftriaxone can be used alone or in combination with metronidazole, if anaerobic bacteria are likely. A β-lactam with β-lactamase inhibitor (e.g., ampicillin/sulbactam) is an excellent choice, but it must be given four times daily. Ertapenem is a once-daily carbapenem with broad aerobic and anaerobic coverage and is a good choice for outpatient administration. Since 3 to 4 weeks of antibiotic administration is generally required, the latter part of the treatment course could be given orally, using an oral quinolone such as levofloxacin with or without oral metronidazole. Therapy should be adjusted depending on culture results.

Trauma

Etiology and clinical manifestations. The liver is the most common solid organ to be injured by penetrating abdominal trauma (such as gunshot wounds, stab wounds, or rib fractures) and the second most commonly injured organ in blunt trauma. Damage or injury to the liver should be suspected when any upper abdominal or lower chest trauma is sustained. The liver is frequently injured by steering wheels in vehicular accidents. Common injuries to the liver include simple lacerations, multiple lacerations, avulsions, and crush injuries.

The gravity of liver wounds arises from the fact that the liver is a highly vascular organ receiving approximately 29% of the body's cardiac output. When hepatic trauma occurs, blood loss can be massive. The patient generally exhibits the typical signs of hemorrhagic shock: hypotension, tachycardia, tachypnea, pallor, diaphoresis, and confusion. Hemoglobin/hematocrit levels may be normal early following the trauma but eventually will reflect significant blood loss. Clinical manifestations include right upper quadrant pain with abdominal tenderness, distention, guarding, and rigidity. Abdominal pain exaggerated by deep breathing and referred to the shoulder may indicate diaphragmatic irritation.

Treatment. Treatment entails the administration of fresh whole blood or packed red blood cells and fresh frozen plasma, as well as massive fluid infusion to maintain adequate intravascular volume and hematocrit. Most patients require surgical management, although some may be treated angiographically or expectantly with medical support. Postoperatively, a patient with hepatic trauma is usually admitted to a critical care unit and monitored for persistent bleeding. The complete blood cell count and coagulation parameters must be closely monitored for trends in changes.

Malignancy

Etiology. Malignancy in the liver usually develops as a metastatic process. Because of the vascularity and lymphatic drainage of the liver, the organ is a common site for metastasis from primary cancers of the esophagus, stomach, colon, rectum, breast, and lung—among many other possibilities.

Primary hepatic malignancy (cancer originating within the liver) is rare in the United States, though increasing in frequency.[38] However, in other parts of the world such as Africa, it is one of the most common sites of malignancy because of a high prevalence of chronic hepatitis B virus infection. Primary liver tumors include HCCs (discussed in the next section), cholangiocarcinoma, and angiosarcoma. Hepatoblastoma is the most common malignant tumor in children. Lymphoma, especially T-cell lymphoma, may occasionally arise primarily in the liver. Benign liver tumors are much less common, with the exception of cavernous hemangioma.

Clinical manifestations and diagnosis. The most common form of primary hepatic malignancy is **hepatocellular carcinoma (HCC),** often referred to as hepatoma. HCC is a malignancy of middle-aged persons, more frequent in men than in women. The incidence is increasing in the United States, in part as a result of increasing HBV and HCV prevalence. (It is always preceded in these situations by cirrhosis.) Approximately 28,000 cases were diagnosed in the United States last year. Signs and symptoms of HCC include hepatomegaly, abdominal pain, weight loss, nausea, and, in advanced cases, jaundice and ascites. HCC has an extraordinary number of paraneoplastic syndromes, including hypercalcemia, erythrocytosis, hypoglycemia, thyrotoxicosis, and hypertrophic osteoarthropathy (finger clubbing).[1]

Space-occupying masses of the liver may first be suggested by abnormal measurements of liver-related enzymes, especially alkaline phosphatase. α-Fetoprotein level is often dramatically elevated in cases of HCC, although some false-positive results can occur. Definitive diagnosis requires imaging of the liver with ultrasonography, CT, or magnetic resonance imaging, although on occasion the tumor may be diffuse and difficult to image. These studies also allow guided needle biopsy of the liver lesion.

Treatment. The only treatment for HCC is hepatic resection. Unfortunately, because of advanced diffuse liver disease or multifocal tumors, such treatment is not usually possible. Partial resection is preferred, but complete hepatectomy followed by liver transplantation is a radical option for tumor localized to the liver. Other treatments

---

BOX 38-2   CONDITIONS TREATED WITH LIVER TRANSPLANTATION

Cirrhosis Secondary to
Viral hepatitis
Alcoholic hepatitis
Autoimmune hepatitis
Cryptogenic source (no cause determinable)

Metabolic Liver Diseases
Wilson disease
α₁-Antitrypsin deficiency
Hemochromatosis, neonatal
Glycogen storage disease
Tyrosinemia
Byler disease
Crigler-Najjar syndrome
Other miscellaneous

Cholestatic Liver Diseases
Primary biliary cirrhosis
Sclerosing cholangitis
Biliary atresia
Other miscellaneous

Acute Liver Failure
Drug reactions
Toxins (e.g., mushroom poisoning)
Viral hepatitis
Acute Budd-Chiari syndrome, other ischemic insult

---

include systemic chemotherapy and chemotherapy directed selectively to the liver via portal vein or hepatic artery cannulation.[1] Other novel palliative treatments include hepatic artery ligation, direct percutaneous injection of alcohol into hepatic tumors, cryotherapy, and other thermal techniques. A new drug, sorafenib, has been approved for treatment of HCC not amenable to curative surgery and has shown a modest survival benefit. Nevertheless, the 5-year survival for this cancer is only 14%.

TRANSPLANTATION

Patients with end-stage liver disease that has not responded to conventional medical or surgical intervention are potential candidates for **liver transplantation** (Boxes 38-2, 38-3, and 38-4). In adults, diseases currently managed by orthotopic (in-place) liver transplantation (OLT) include end-stage cirrhosis from chronic active hepatitis, alcoholic liver disease, primary biliary cirrhosis, and primary sclerosing cholangitis; and hepatic metabolic diseases such as hemochromatosis and Wilson disease.[1,39] Liver transplantation is rarely performed for patients with malignant neoplasms, although there is clearly a subset of patients with HCC who are candidates for this procedure.[40] The major indication for pediatric OLT is biliary atresia following a failed Kasai procedure (portoenterostomy) or delayed recognition of the diagnosis. Other major pediatric indications include α₁-antitrypsin deficiency and other metabolic disorders. Currently about 5000 liver transplantations are performed yearly, although the waiting list contains about three times that number.

Evaluation of the Transplantation Patient

Potential transplantation patients undergo extensive physiologic and psychological evaluation by physicians, nurses, psychologists, and

BOX 38-3 INDICATIONS FOR LIVER TRANSPLANTATION

Acute Liver Disease

Fulminant liver failure with progressive encephalopathy

Prothrombin time >10 sec above control

Bilirubin <15 mg/dl and rising

Chronic Liver Disease

Bilirubin >15 mg/dl

Intractable hepatic encephalopathy

Intractable ascites

Serum albumin <2.5 mg/dl

Prothrombin time ≥20 sec

Hepatorenal syndrome

BOX 38-4 CONTRAINDICATIONS TO LIVER TRANSPLANTATION

Absolute Contraindications

End-stage cardiopulmonary disease

Metastatic cancer

Active sepsis

Acquired immunodeficiency syndrome

Psychiatric illness preventing compliance with treatment

Relative Contraindications (Vary Greatly Among Transplant Centers)

Renal failure

Hepatitis B infection

Liver cancer

Portal vein thrombosis

Active alcoholism

social workers to identify potential contraindications to the procedure. Conditions that would normally preclude OLT include uncontrolled bacterial sepsis, failure of other major organ systems, extrahepatic malignancy, and more. Additional identified risk factors include portal vein thrombosis, previous portosystemic shunt operations, current alcohol or drug addiction, a poor psychosocial support system, and psychological instability. Many of these conditions are relative contraindications that diminish the chance of a successful outcome, but they do not always preclude transplantation. One group whose numbers are growing is patients with HIV and end-stage liver disease, and this group is increasingly being considered for OLT.[1]

Patients with viral hepatitis are particularly susceptible to recurrence in the transplanted organ and must be managed with care. Recent data show that patients transplanted for HBV who are treated indefinitely with high-dose HBIG have low recurrence rates, with acceptable survival and quality of life.[41] In contrast to HBV, it has not been possible to develop an effective regimen to prevent recurrent HCV infection. A promising approach is preemptive antiviral therapy started shortly after OLT but before histologic recurrence is established; in particular, the use of long-acting pegylated interferons is currently the focus of ongoing clinical trials.[42]

After the patient has been identified as a candidate and a donor organ has been procured, the actual surgical procedure can take 8 to 22 hours to complete. The procedure involves five anastomoses between recipient and donor organs, including the following vascular anastomosis sites: suprahepatic inferior vena cava, infrahepatic vena cava, portal vein, hepatic artery, and biliary tract. The biliary anastomosis site varies, depending on the patient's extrahepatic biliary tract.

Posttransplantation Management

A cornerstone of posttransplantation management is immunosuppression to prevent rejection of the transplant graft. The rejection response after liver transplantation most often occurs between postoperative days 4 and 10. Clinical manifestations of acute rejection include tachycardia, fever, right upper quadrant or flank pain, diminished bile flow through the T tube drain or a change in bile color, and increasing jaundice. Laboratory findings include elevated serum bilirubin, transaminase, and alkaline phosphatase levels and increased prothrombin time. Following the successful use of cyclosporine, a number of immunosuppressive drugs have appeared and provide several choices for improving outcome. Immunosuppressives may be broadly categorized into three groups: initial immunosuppression, maintenance immunosuppression, and management of acute cellular rejection.[1] Prednisone is the primary posttransplantation immunosuppressive and is steadily tapered in favor of maintenance drugs. The calcineurin inhibitors cyclosporine or tacrolimus are begun during anesthesia induction and represent the mainstays of maintenance therapy. In most centers, tacrolimus has supplanted cyclosporine as the preferred immunosuppressive. Adjunctive maintenance agents include either mycophenolate mofetil or the older drug azathioprine. Acute rejection is generally managed with high-dose corticosteroids. Patients who fail to respond to steroids can be treated with infusion of one of several agents, including muromonab (OKT3), mycophenolate mofetil (MMF), or an interleukin-2 receptor blocker (e.g., basiliximab).

Side effects limit the usefulness of all these drugs and are a main source of morbidity and mortality among transplant recipients. The main nonimmunologic side effects of cyclosporine and tacrolimus are hypertension and renal insufficiency. Blood levels must be carefully monitored. Side effects of mycophenolate mofetil and azathioprine include bone marrow suppression with cytopenias. Problems with the acute antirejection infusions include hypersensitivity and cytokine reactions, and a heightened risk of opportunistic infection, especially cytomegalovirus, immediately after use. Among the many side effects of prednisone are hypertension and hyperglycemia. The main consequence of all these treatments is immune suppression and increased risk for infection.

Early infections are generally due to issues involving surgical technique and pre-existing infection (e.g., cholangitis) and have declined significantly in recent years.[1] They usually represent nosocomially acquired pathogens. Infections in the middle period from 1 to 6 months often represent viral infection or reactivation. Trimethoprim-sulfamethoxazole (TMP-SMX) is usually prescribed for prophylaxis against bacterial infection and *Pneumocystis jiroveci* for the first year. Of particular concern and the focus of several prophylactic strategies is cytomegalovirus. Cytomegalovirus occurs at a high rate among seronegative recipients who receive a liver from a seropositive recipient, and reactivation rates are significant as well. In the middle and late periods fungal infection is important, especially *Aspergillus* species, and lymphoproliferative disorder attributable to Epstein-Barr virus is seen. OLT recipients should be instructed to avoid exposure to environmental or food-borne mold, which could increase their risk for fungal infection. Another important preventive strategy is appropriate vaccination, particularly annual influenza shots. (Live virus vaccinations, such as varicella and yellow fever, should be avoided.)

Critical issues in the posttransplantation period include the following: hypertension, renal dysfunction, hyperlipidemia and cardiovascular disease, obesity, osteoporosis, and increased risk for cancer. Psychological issues are especially prominent, and caregivers and family should be alert for signs of depression and anxiety. Many of the antirejection medications exacerbate these symptoms. With careful follow-up, OLT recipients can live productive lives for many years after transplantation. Chronic rejection, often in the setting of progressive ductopenia, and recurrence of primary pretransplantation liver disease tend to cause graft failure with time. Actuarial survival at 5 years is approximately 88% for persons with cholestatic liver disease, 78% for patients with noncholestatic liver disease who are HCV negative, and 70% for persons with HCV.[43]

AGE-RELATED LIVER DISORDERS

LIVER DISEASES AND PEDIATRIC CONSIDERATIONS

Liver disease in infants and children not only encompasses pediatric variations of adult liver diseases but also includes conditions unique to that age group. Many of these conditions present at birth or shortly thereafter, although several may appear in later life.

Abnormal Bilirubin Metabolism in the Neonatal Period

Physiologic jaundice of the newborn is a harmless condition lasting no longer than 2 weeks after delivery. (Bilirubin metabolism in the neonatal period has already been discussed; see earlier Jaundice section.) Immature bilirubin conjugation and transport mechanisms are the primary causes, along with increased gut absorption of bilirubin. Hyperbilirubinemia is not considered physiologic or normal if the bilirubin level is greater than 5 mg/dl on the first postpartum day, 10 mg/dl on the second day, or 13 mg/dl at any time.[44] It should be noted that breast-fed babies have a higher incidence of hyperbilirubinemia than do bottle-fed babies because the β-glucuronidase in breast milk results in increased unconjugated bilirubin in the gut, which can be absorbed. If significant hyperbilirubinemia occurs, breast feeding can be stopped.

Pathologic bilirubin levels should lead to an immediate evaluation to exclude congenital hemolytic disorders, Crigler-Najjar syndrome, hypothyroidism, congenital pyloric stenosis, sepsis, resorbing hematomas, and other conditions associated with an elevated serum bilirubin level.

Kernicterus refers to brain injury as a result of hyperbilirubinemia. It is a serious complication of the neonatal period, generally occurring in the setting of premature birth, neonatal jaundice, and especially hemolytic disease of the newborn.[45] In brief, the immature blood-brain barrier allows free unconjugated bilirubin to enter the brain, leading to encephalopathy. The term kernicterus refers to yellowish staining of permanently damaged brain tissue, primarily in the basal ganglia and thalamus. Despite decades of research, the exact pathophysiologic mechanisms by which elevated levels of bilirubin cause brain damage have not been elucidated, although evidence points toward premature programmed cell death (i.e., apoptosis). Unfortunately, most infants die of this condition, and survivors often suffer from cerebral palsy, movement disorders, and mental retardation. Drugs that displace bilirubin from albumin seriously worsen the condition.

If recognized early, treatment with exchange transfusions, phenobarbital (to increase the levels of UDPGT; see previous discussion), and phototherapy ("bili-lights") may prevent these catastrophic consequences.[46] Phototherapy with light in the 450-nm wavelength band is used to treat unconjugated hyperbilirubinemia in infants. Light at this wavelength converts unconjugated lipid-soluble bilirubin into water-soluble photoisomers that can be excreted by the kidneys, thus lowering the bilirubin level.

Infectious and Acquired Hepatitides in Children

Acute hepatitis A virus infection is often mild or asymptomatic in children. The prevalence of childhood infection correlates inversely with the quality of sanitation and hygiene. Treatment is supportive, and prevention guidelines parallel those for adults. Universal childhood vaccination is recommended in the United States and in many countries around the world.

Globally, **hepatitis B virus infection** is a common childhood disease, with vertical transmission from an HBsAg-positive mother to the infant being the most common mechanism of dissemination. Infected blood products and drugs are modes of infection in less developed areas. Features suggesting immune complex disease such as arthritis, fever, papular acrodermatitis (a rash not seen in adults), renal disease, and hematologic complications are more common in children. The incidence of chronic infection is also much higher after neonatal or childhood infection, which has grave long-term consequences because of the late sequelae of cirrhosis and HCC.

Passive immunization with HBIG should be given within 12 hours of birth to children of HBsAg-positive mothers. Active immunization with HBV vaccine should be administered as a series of intramuscular injections at birth and at 1 and 6 months of age. Identical prophylaxis should be given to children of high-risk mothers even if not screened for HBsAg and to children otherwise exposed to HBV. In 1991 the U.S. Public Health Service recommended universal childhood HBV vaccination.[22] Strategies include infant vaccination, possibly with a booster dose in young adulthood, or adolescent vaccination.

Unlike HBV, **hepatitis C** virus is less commonly spread vertically, and effective screening of blood products has greatly reduced the risk of childhood infection. **Hepatitis delta virus** may be transmitted by the intrafamily route as a coinfector with hepatitis B.

Acute **hepatitis E virus** is especially virulent in adolescents and young adults, with a high mortality in pregnant women. In endemic regions, it is the most common cause of childhood hepatitis and is indirectly a cause of infant mortality.

Many systemic viruses may cause biochemical or clinical hepatitis in the pediatric population, including Epstein-Barr virus, cytomegalovirus, herpesvirus, and adenovirus. Neonatal hepatitis is part of the so-called TORCH syndrome and may be caused by a variety of congenital infections, including cytomegalovirus, herpesvirus, varicella, *Toxoplasma,* and syphilis. Encephalitis and retinitis may accompany these conditions, with lifelong sequelae. An enlarged liver and elevated levels of transaminases in the newborn should necessitate a search for congenital infection.

Reye syndrome is primarily a disease of children, although adult cases are reported. The syndrome usually occurs shortly after a viral illness such as influenza or chickenpox, and begins with nausea and vomiting rapidly progressing to coma. The exact pathophysiologic mechanism is unknown, but significant mitochondrial dysfunction of hepatocytes occurs.[47-63] Reye syndrome is characterized by fatty infiltration of the liver with severe hepatic dysfunction, including encephalopathy, coagulopathy, and elevated levels of hepatocellular enzymes. Mortality may be as high as 40%. A strong association with aspirin use during the preceding viral illness has been noted, but other drugs may be causative as well.[47] (Because of the risk of Reye syndrome, aspirin is contraindicated for childhood viral illnesses.) Treatment of Reye syndrome is supportive, and if the child survives, recovery is complete. As with other toxic hepatitides, liver transplantation is reserved for irreversible disease.

Congenital Liver Disease

Many heritable diseases of the liver occur in childhood. These may be broadly characterized as enzyme deficiencies affecting multiple organ systems including the liver (e.g., α_1-antitrypsin deficiency), disorders of bilirubin metabolism (e.g., Crigler-Najjar syndrome), inborn errors affecting other metabolic pathways, intrahepatic ductopenic conditions, and extrahepatic ductopenia (biliary atresia).

Multisystem Enzyme Deficiencies

α-Antitrypsin deficiency is an autosomal recessive condition that commonly affects children and young adults, although it may not become obvious until later in life. α_1-Antitrypsin is an enzyme inhibitor found in many tissues that prevents normal enzymes, such as elastase and collagenase, from causing damage to those tissues. Production of this enzyme is genetically controlled by a gene that has many allelic variations (gene types). Although numerous abnormal alleles have been identified, the most common pathologic form, which causes both liver and lung disease, is the protease inhibitor Z variant PiZZ, which produces α_1-ATZ protein.[1] This defective α_1-antitrypsin protein accumulates in the liver and produces the diagnostic granules seen microscopically, although the exact mechanism of liver damage is unclear. A characteristic centrilobular emphysema, pancreatic insufficiency, and cirrhosis may occur. Treatment by liver transplantation is often precluded by these other problems. Gene therapy for α_1-antitrypsin deficiency is an area of active investigation.[1]

Cystic fibrosis (CF) is an autosomal recessive condition primarily known as a cause of lung disease in children. CF results from one of many mutations in a single large gene on chromosome 7 that encodes the cystic fibrosis transmembrane conductance regulator (CFTR) protein. Clinical disease requires disease-causing mutations in both copies of the *CFTR* gene.

In addition to pulmonary disease, this relatively common genetic condition (1 in 3000 Caucasian births; 1 in 15,000 African-American births) may also cause pancreatic insufficiency, intestinal obstruction, gallstone disease, neonatal giant cell hepatitis, bile duct obstruction, and biliary cirrhosis. Treatment is directed at complications.[1] Administration of ursodeoxycholic acid improves the biochemical indices of liver injury; however, conclusive evidence that the drug halts the progression to cirrhosis is lacking. Gene therapy for CF is in the experimental phase.

Wilson disease and **hemochromatosis** are single gene mutation illnesses with significant liver involvement and have been discussed earlier in the chapter.

Disorders of Bilirubin Metabolism

Inherited defects in bile acid metabolism can manifest as impaired synthesis or transport. The first group includes **cerebrotendinous xanthomatosis,** a steroid hydroxylase deficiency that leads to premature atherosclerosis and encephalopathy. However, manifestations do not generally include liver disease. Children treated with chenodeoxycholic acid have shown marked improvement. Peroxisomes are responsible for β-oxidation in the final steps of bile acid synthesis, and numerous hereditary peroxisomopathies have been described. The most well-known of these conditions is X-linked adrenal leukodystrophy, which is manifested by progressive neurologic dysfunction and adrenal insufficiency. Treatments for this and related conditions remain generally ineffective, but investigational therapies, including bone marrow transplantation and gene therapies, continue to be developed.[48] One interesting if controversial therapy for X-linked adrenal leukodystrophy is dietary therapy with the so-called "Lorenzo's oil"—a mixture of glycerol trioleate and glycerol trierucate.[49]

Disorders of bile acid transport include **Gilbert syndrome,** a very common (about 10% of the Caucasian population in the United States), entirely benign, autosomal dominant condition that results in mild unconjugated (indirect) hyperbilirubinemia. It is caused by

decreased bilirubin glucuronidation. Awareness of this disorder is important to avoid inappropriate evaluation of these patients.

Crigler-Najjar syndrome is a rare autosomal recessive disorder marked by significant unconjugated hyperbilirubinemia.[50] In type I Crigler-Najjar syndrome, the near–total absence of bilirubin conjugation results in high levels of unconjugated bilirubin crossing the immature blood-brain barrier. This condition presents shortly after birth, and neonates usually die of kernicterus or suffer irreversible neurologic damage. Liver transplantation following phototherapy and plasma exchange transfusion has been lifesaving in rare instances. In type II Crigler-Najjar syndrome, some conjugating capability exists, and it is enhanced by the administration of phenobarbital. These patients rarely experience bilirubin encephalopathy and can lead normal lives. Treatment consists of phototherapy, phenobarbital administration, and potentially liver transplantation. Gene therapy is an active area of research for Crigler-Najjar syndrome.

Progressive familial intrahepatic cholestasis (PFIC) is a rare autosomal recessive disorder involving severe jaundice, pruritus, and malabsorption attributable to a defect in bile salt excretion. PFIC type I, or **Byler syndrome,** is caused by a single-gene mutation and traces back to an Amish kindred descended from Jacob Byler. Other genetic defects cause different types of PFIC with similar manifestations. Medical therapy with ursodeoxycholic acid is helpful in some children, and biliary diversion procedures have given symptomatic relief to some patients by decreasing the bile acid pool.[1] In the past the disease was uniformly fatal, but liver transplantation has been shown to normalize bile acid synthesis and growth in selected patients.[51]

Other rare disorders of bile salt transport exist and are generally fatal in infancy. These chronic cholestatic diseases, such as North American Indian childhood cirrhosis and cholestasis-lymphedema syndrome (Aagenaes syndrome), are undergoing investigation at the molecular genetic level and are generally linked to single-gene mutations.

Inborn Errors of Metabolism

A very broad range of enzyme abnormalities resulting from single-gene mutations, generally autosomally recessive, may appear in children. These result in abnormal processing of lipids, glycogen, amino acids and proteins, lipopolysaccharides, and other substances. The pathologic process generally results from excessive accumulation of precursor substances in target organs, such as the brain and spinal cord. The liver is often the primary site of processing and may be the target of toxic accumulation as well. The latter may result in signs of liver disease, including hepatomegaly, elevation in levels of liver enzymes, and jaundice. Inborn errors that manifest in the neonatal period are usually fatal unless immediate treatment is undertaken. Inborn errors presenting in infancy and later years may be amenable to specific therapies. Liver or bone marrow transplantation may be effective for some of these conditions, and many of these conditions are foci of intense research regarding gene therapy.[52] The diagnosis of any inborn error of metabolism should prompt a thorough investigation of family history and the provision of appropriate genetic counseling and testing of family members.

As noted previously, given the heterogeneity and rarity of these conditions, they will not be discussed further in this chapter, and the interested reader is referred to a standard text on the subject.

Intrahepatic Cholestatic Conditions

Intrahepatic cholestasis may be defined as cholestatic liver disease in which the pathologic process is confined to the liver (i.e., the extrahepatic biliary system is normal).[53] One cause of this condition is neonatal hepatitis, which can be idiopathic, viral, or secondary to an inborn error of metabolism. (Viral hepatitis and inborn errors were discussed earlier in this chapter.) The second category of these illnesses includes conditions in which the number of bile ducts is decreased and inadequate to accommodate normal bile metabolism and transport.

Alagille syndrome, or arteriohepatic dysplasia, is the most common form of inherited intrahepatic cholestasis. This autosomal dominant condition has incomplete penetrance and expressivity, and is associated with typical bony and cardiovascular malformations, as well as a paucity of intrahepatic bile ducts. The disease generally progresses slowly; pruritus, hypercholesterolemia, xanthomas, and neurologic complications due to vitamin E deficiency may occur if untreated. Patients may be maintained on ursodeoxycholic acid until liver transplantation, which is the current treatment of choice.[54]

Several other conditions manifest a paucity of intrahepatic bile ducts. Some of these arise from defective bile transport mechanisms and are discussed in the Inborn Errors of Metabolism section.

Extrahepatic Cholestatic Conditions (Biliary Atresia)

Extrahepatic ductopenia is often referred to as **biliary atresia.** Biliary atresia or, as some authors prefer, progressive obliterative cholangiopathy can be either congenital or acquired. The latter occurs in the setting of certain autoimmune illnesses and is one of the principle forms of chronic rejection of a transplanted liver allograft. Biliary atresia is a rather common birth defect, occurring in 1:10,000 to 1:15,000 live births (and is therefore much more common than intrahepatic cholestatic conditions).[1] Distinguishing between this disorder and idiopathic neonatal hepatitis can be challenging, but the liver biopsy findings are usually characteristic. Infants and children with biliary atresia have progressive cholestasis with all the usual concomitant features: pruritus, malabsorption with growth retardation, fat-soluble vitamin deficiencies, hyperlipidemia, and eventually cirrhosis with portal hypertension. Some children have recurrent episodes of bacterial cholangitis as well. A cholangiogram should be obtained to assess the possibility of a correctable obstruction. The Kasai procedure is often performed to create a hepatoportoenteric connection, which may allow adequate bile drainage. This procedure is not usually curative but ideally does "buy time" for growth of the child until an appropriate time for liver transplantation.

KEY POINTS

- Cirrhosis is the irreversible end stage of many different hepatic injuries. The liver is fibrotic, scarred, and nodular. Symptoms of cirrhosis are due to hepatocellular failure and portal hypertension.
- Biliary cirrhosis is associated with chronic bile duct obstruction with resultant accumulation of bile in the liver. Gallstones and extrahepatic and intrahepatic bile duct inflammation are common causes.
- Alcoholic cirrhosis is associated with chronic alcohol ingestion, which may precipitate fatty liver, hepatitis, and, finally, cirrhosis.
- The liver is subject to damage because of its role in storing and detoxifying potentially injurious substances. Metal storage diseases are genetic disorders in which excessive minerals are absorbed and subsequently deposited in the liver. Hemochromatosis is characterized by excessive iron absorption and is manifested by elevated serum ferritin and iron levels. Phlebotomy is the usual treatment. Wilson disease is due to excessive accumulation of copper in the liver and other organs. Copper chelators are effective in preventing liver damage.
- Acetaminophen is converted to a toxic metabolite in the liver that is normally rapidly detoxified by liver enzymes. In acetaminophen overdose, the detoxification reaction may be overwhelmed and liver necrosis results. Treatment is with acetylcysteine.

- Liver abscesses are suspected in patients with fever, nausea, vomiting, and right upper quadrant pain. Ascending biliary infection, abdominal infections transported by the portal vein, and direct extension of infection from neighboring structures are usual sources of infection. Antibiotics and drainage are commonly prescribed.
- The liver commonly sustains injury during penetrating and blunt trauma to the abdomen. Because the liver is highly vascular, trauma may produce extreme blood loss and hemorrhagic shock. Liver trauma is manifested by abdominal tenderness, distention, guarding, and rigidity.
- In the United States, cancer of the liver is usually metastatic and rarely primary. Tumors of the esophagus, stomach, colon, rectum, breast, and lung commonly seed in the liver. HCC is more common in other parts of the world but its incidence is increasing in the United States, with HBV and HCV as important contributing factors.

LIVER DISEASES AND GERIATRIC CONSIDERATIONS

Liver size and blood flow decrease with aging, but this observation has little functional significance. Drugs whose metabolism is primarily related to hepatic blood flow and drugs processed by the mixed-function oxidase system (cytochromes) may have a prolonged serum half-life requiring careful monitoring and dose adjustment. Routine blood test results of liver-related enzymes are not changed by aging.

In the United States, HCC is usually the result of years of injury from alcohol or chronic viral hepatitis and is therefore more often seen in older people. The prognosis is unfortunately dismal (see discussion earlier in the chapter).

Ischemic hepatitis is usually associated with underlying cardiovascular disease and episodes of hypotension, as during surgery or sepsis, and is more common in older patients. Typically, the levels of serum transaminases rise rapidly and the prothrombin time is prolonged. Recovery may be rapid, but the prognosis depends on the severity of the underlying disorder. Ischemic hepatitis alone is rarely a cause of death in such patients. Right-sided heart failure may result in passive hepatic congestion with ascites and (rarely) liver failure. In developing countries, constrictive pericarditis and uncorrected valvular heart disease attributable to rheumatic fever are still significant causes of intractable ascites and should be considered in the differential diagnosis.

Metabolic liver diseases rarely present in the geriatric population. **Hemochromatosis** in women often occurs after menopause and may present as new-onset diabetes mellitus, heart failure, arthritis, cirrhosis, or HCC. Typically, **autoimmune liver diseases** are seen in young to middle-aged people. However, autoimmune chronic active hepatitis may be a cause of "cryptogenic" cirrhosis in older women. **Primary biliary cirrhosis** is uncommon in later life. **Primary sclerosing cholangitis (PSC)** may afflict older persons with long-standing ulcerative colitis, even those who had colectomies many years, even decades, earlier.

Because **alcohol abuse** generally starts early in life, older patients bear the cumulative injury of years of exposure and are likely to show signs of advanced liver disease. Treatment is the same as in younger patients, but attention must be given to the older patients' social circumstances and intercurrent medical problems. Symptoms and signs of alcohol intoxication and hepatic encephalopathy may be confused with senile dementia and made worse by concomitant drug use (e.g., minor tranquilizers, opiates).

The diagnosis of **acute viral hepatitis** may be more difficult in older people because of nonspecific symptoms in mild cases and decreased clinical suspicion. Acute HAV infection is less common as a result of the higher incidence of immunity, but it may be more severe with higher mortality rates in the elderly. The end results of HBV and HCV infection often become evident in elderly persons, and in the United States the increased prevalence of persons living with these viruses will mean more elderly patients with liver disease in coming decades.

Older patients with chronic HBV and HCV infection may be treated with the standard treatments, but comorbid medical problems, intolerance to the side effects of treatment, and advanced liver disease may preclude treatment in many persons. The indications for **liver transplantation** do not change with advancing years, and no arbitrary age limits have been set on transplantation. However, there may be subtle barriers in effect, and the allocation of organs remains a highly controversial issue. Each patient must be evaluated individually regarding the propriety of transplantation and the likelihood of success.

SUMMARY

Disorders of the liver are diverse and complex. Because the liver is vital to most life processes, even mild disorders can cause life-threatening alterations. Health care professionals need a good understanding of hepatobiliary anatomy and physiology to appreciate the effects of these disorders on patients.

Many liver disorders are the consequence of lifestyle choices such as alcoholism and drug abuse. Health care professionals are in a position to explain the risks of detrimental lifestyles and their relationship to liver diseases so as to prevent occurrence of these diseases.

Medical treatment entails the use of drugs from many different classes. Because the liver is central to the metabolism of many of these drugs, their use requires special attention. Before any drug is given to a patient with liver disease, it is essential to become completely familiar with it by consulting a good pharmacology text or drug information source.

REFERENCES

1. Feldman M, Friedman LS, Brandt LJ: *Sleisenger and Fordtran's gastrointestinal and liver disease*, ed 9, Philadelphia, 2010, Saunders Elsevier.
2. Moore KL, Persaud TVN, Torchia MG: *The developing human: clinically oriented embryology*, Philadelphia, 2008, Saunders.
3. Moore KL, Persaud TVN, Shiota K: *Color atlas of clinical embryology*, Philadelphia, 2000, Saunders.
4. Hall JE: *Guyton and Hall textbook of medical physiology*, ed 12, Philadelphia, 2011, Saunders Elsevier.
5. Johnson LR: *Gastrointestinal physiology*, ed 7, Philadelphia, 2006, Mosby.
6. Kamisako T, et al: Recent advances in bilirubin metabolism research: the molecular mechanism of hepatocyte bilirubin transport and its clinical relevance, *J Gastroenterol* 35(9):659–664, 2000.
7. Bosch J, et al: Recombinant factor VIIa for upper gastrointestinal bleeding in patients with cirrhosis: a randomized, double-blind trial, *Gastroenterology* 127(4):1123–1130, 2004.
8. Garcia-Tsao G, et al: Prevention and management of gastroesophageal varices and variceal hemorrhage in cirrhosis, *Hepatology* 46:922, 2007.
9. Gournay J, et al: Isosorbide mononitrate and propranolol compared with propranolol alone for the prevention of variceal rebleeding, *Hepatology* 31(6):1239–1245, 2000.
10. Bosch J, Garcia-Pagan JC: Prevention of variceal rebleeding, *Lancet* 361(9361):952–954, 2003.
11. Escorsell A, et al: TIPS versus drug therapy in preventing variceal rebleeding in advanced cirrhosis: a randomized controlled trial, *Hepatology* 35(2):385–392, 2002.
12. Butterworth RF: The astrocytic ("peripheral-type") benzodiazepine receptor: role in the pathogenesis of portal-systemic encephalopathy, *Neurochem Int* 36(4-5):411–416, 2000.
13. Shils ME: *Modern nutrition in health and disease*, ed 10, Philadelphia, 2006, Lippincott Williams & Wilkins.
14. Jalan R, et al: Moderate hypothermia prevents cerebral hyperemia and increase in intracranial pressure in patients undergoing liver transplantation for acute liver failure, *Transplantation* 75, 2034, 2003.
15. Schrier RW, Gurevich AK, Cadnapaphornchai MA: Pathogenesis and management of sodium and water retention in cardiac failure and cirrhosis, *Semin Nephrol* 21(2):157–172, 2001.
16. Watt K, Uhanova J, Minuk GY: Hepatorenal syndrome: diagnostic accuracy, clinical features, and outcome in a tertiary care center, *Am J Gastroenterol* 97(8):2046–2050, 2002.
17. Arroyo V, Guevara M, Gines P: Hepatorenal syndrome in cirrhosis: pathogenesis and treatment, *Gastroenterology* 122(6):1658–1676, 2002.
18. General recommendations on immunization: recommendations of the Advisory Committee on Immunization Practices (ACIP) and the American Academy of Family Physicians (AAFP), *MMWR Morb Mortal Wkly Rep* 51(RR02):1–36, 2002.
19. Braconier JH, Wennerholm S, Norrby SR: Comparative immunogenicity and tolerance of Vaqta and Havrix, *Vaccine* 17(17):2181–2184, 1999.
20. Marcellin P: Advances in therapy for chronic hepatitis B, *Semin Liver Dis* 22(Suppl 1):33–36, 2002.
21. Wai CT, Lok AS: Treatment of hepatitis B, *J Gastroenterol* 37(10):771–778, 2002.
22. A comprehensive immunization strategy to eliminate transmission of hepatitis B virus infection in the United States: recommendations of the Immunization Practices Advisory Committee (ACIP), *MMWR Morb Mortal Wkly Rep* 54(RR16):1–23, 2005.
23. Updated U.S. Public Health Service guidelines for the management of occupational exposures to HBV, HCV, and HIV and recommendations for postexposure prophylaxis, *MMWR Morb Mortal Wkly Rep* 50(RR11):1–42, 2001.
24. McHutchison JG, Fried MW: Current therapy for hepatitis C: pegylated interferon and ribavirin, *Clin Liver Dis* 7(1):149–161, 2003.
25. Zeuzem S, et al: Telaprevir for retreatment of HCV infection, *N Engl J Med* 364(25):2417–2418, 2011.
26. Poordad F, et al: Boceprevir for untreated chronic HCV genotype 1 infection, *N Engl J Med* 364(13):1195–1206, 2011.
27. Ge D, et al: Genetic variation in IL28B predicts hepatitis C treatment-induced viral clearance, *Nature* 461(7262):399–401, 2009.
28. Czaja AJ, Freese DK: Diagnosis and treatment of autoimmune hepatitis: American Association for the Study of Liver Disease recommendations, *Hepatology* 36(2):479–497, 2002.
29. Gorbach SL, Bartlett JG, Blacklow NR: *Infectious diseases*, ed 3, Philadelphia, 2004, Lippincott Williams & Wilkins.
30. Lee YM, Kaplan MM: Management of primary sclerosing cholangitis, *Am J Gastroenterol* 97(3):528–534, 2002.
31. Crosse KI, Anania FA: Alcoholic hepatitis, *Curr Treat Options Gastroenterol* 5(6):417–423, 2002.
32. O'Shea RS, McCullough AJ: Treatment of alcoholic hepatitis, *Clin Liver Dis* 9(1):103–134, 2005.
33. Adams PC, et al: Hemochromatosis and iron-overload screening in a racially diverse population, *N Engl J Med* 352(17):1769–1778, 2005.
34. Olynyk JK, et al: Evolution of untreated hereditary hemochromatosis in the Busselton population: a 17-year study, *Mayo Clin Proc* 79(3):309–313, 2004.

35. Brewer GJ, et al: Treatment of Wilson disease with ammonium tetra-thiomolybdate, III: initial therapy in a total of 55 neurologically affected patients and follow-up with zinc therapy, *Arch Neurol* 60(3):379–385, 2003.

36. Ostapowicz G, et al: Results of a prospective study of acute liver failure at 17 tertiary care centers in the United States, *Ann Intern Med* 137(12):947–954, 2002.

37. Foster C, et al: *The Washington manual of medical therapeutics*, ed 33, Philadelphia, 2010, Lippincott Williams & Wilkins.

38. American Cancer Society: *Cancer facts and figures 2012*. Available at www.cancer.org/Research/CancerFactsFigures/CancerFactsFigures/cancer-facts-figures-2012.

39. Keeffe EB: Liver transplantation: current status and novel approaches to liver replacement, *Gastroenterology* 120(3):749–762, 2001.

40. Yu AS, Keeffe EB: Management of hepatocellular carcinoma, *Rev Gastroenterol Disord* 3(1):8–24, 2003.

41. Shouval D, Samuel D: Hepatitis B immune globulin to prevent hepatitis B virus graft reinfection following liver transplantation: a concise review, *Hepatology* 32:1189–1195, 2000.

42. Samuel D, et al: Interferon-alpha 2b plus ribavirin in patients with chronic hepatitis C after liver transplantation: a randomized study, *Gastroenterology* 124(3):642–650, 2003.

43. Wiesner RH, et al: Recent advances in liver transplantation, *Mayo Clin Proc* 78(2):197–210, 2003.

44. Sherlock S, Dooley J: The liver in infancy and childhood. In *Diseases of the liver and biliary system*, ed 10, Blackwell, 1997, Oxford.

45. Hansen TW: Mechanisms of bilirubin toxicity: clinical implications, *Clin Perinatol* 29(4):765–778, 2002.

46. Bratlid D: Criteria for treatment of neonatal jaundice, *J Perinatol* 21(suppl 1):S88–S92, 2001. discussion, S104-S107.

47. Casteels-Van Daele M, et al: Reye syndrome revisited: a descriptive term covering a group of heterogeneous disorders, *Eur J Pediatr* 159(9):641–648, 2000.

48. McGuinness MC, Wei H, Smith KD: Therapeutic developments in peroxisome biogenesis disorders, *Expert Opin Investig Drugs* 9(9):1985–1992, 2000.

49. Suzuki Y, et al: The clinical course of childhood and adolescent adreno-leukodystrophy before and after Lorenzo's oil, *Brain Dev* 23(1):30–33, 2001.

50. Ishak KG: Inherited metabolic diseases of the liver, *Clin Liver Dis* 6(2):455–479, 2002.

51. Ismail H, et al: Treatment of progressive familial intrahepatic cholestasis: liver transplantation or partial external biliary diversion, *Pediatr Transplant* 3(3):219–224, 1999.

52. Yeager AM: Allogeneic hematopoietic cell transplantation for inborn metabolic diseases, *Ann Hematol* 81(Suppl 2):S16–S19, 2002.

53. Bezerra JA, Balistreri WF: Cholestatic syndromes of infancy and childhood, *Semin Gastrointest Dis* 12(2):54–65, 2001.

54. Balistreri WF: Intrahepatic cholestasis, *J Pediatr Gastroenterol Nutr* 35(Suppl 1):S17–S23, 2002.

Endocrine Physiology and Mechanisms of Hypothalamic-Pituitary Regulation

Jacquelyn L. Banasik

evolve WEBSITE

http://evolve.elsevier.com/Copstead/
- Review Questions and Answers
- Glossary (with audio pronunciations for selected terms)
- Animations
- Case Studies
- Key Points Review

KEY QUESTIONS

- How does the lipid or water solubility of hormones affect their transport in the circulation?
- What are the general mechanisms of action of lipid-soluble and water-soluble hormones on target cells?
- How do target cells regulate their responsiveness to endocrine hormones?
- How do feedback mechanisms control the secretion of hormones?
- What are the anterior and posterior pituitary hormones, their target tissues, and their negative feedback mechanisms?
- How are thyroid and steroid hormones synthesized?
- What are the normal actions on target cells of antidiuretic hormone, growth hormone, thyroid hormone, and steroid hormones?

CHAPTER OUTLINE

The endocrine system is composed of cells and organs that are specialized to synthesize and secrete hormones into the bloodstream to act at distant target cells. The nervous and endocrine systems are closely integrated, and many of their actions are coordinated at the level of the hypothalamus. Endocrine systems are particularly suited for regulating complex functions that involve numerous tissues and organs such as growth, metabolism, fluid balance, responses to stress, and reproduction.[1] It is now appreciated that all cells in an organism are involved in cell-to-cell communication, not just the specialized endocrine cells; therefore the term *classical* endocrine systems is sometimes used to designate specialized endocrine glands. This chapter describes general principles of endocrine communication systems and explores the details of hypothalamic-pituitary regulation of antidiuretic hormone, oxytocin, growth hormone, prolactin, gonadotropins, thyroid hormone, and corticosteroid hormones. Disorders of these systems are discussed in Chapters 40 and 41. Reproductive function and disorders can be found in Unit IX.

HORMONE STRUCTURE AND ACTION

An endocrine **hormone** may be defined as a blood-borne chemical messenger that has an effect on target cells anatomically distant from the secreting cell (Figure 39-1). Chemical messengers may also act in a **paracrine** or **autocrine** fashion; the hormone molecule is secreted by one cell and affects adjacent cells, or the original secreting cell. Paracrine and autocrine actions of hormones are not traditionally included in endocrine system physiology; however, the same signaling molecules can have autocrine, paracrine, and distant actions. As an example, estrogen acts locally within the ovary potentiating maturation of ova but is required systemically for outward female sexual differentiation.[2] Secretion of hormones into the bloodstream by neurons may be termed **neurocrine** signaling, a process common to the hypothalamic-pituitary communication system.

Chemical Structure of Hormone Classes

Hormones may be classified according to chemical structure as peptides, tyrosine-derived catecholamines and thyroid hormones, and steroids (Box 39-1). The great majority of endocrine hormones are peptides (small proteins) and are water-soluble and easily transported through the circulation to target cells.[3] The catecholamines (dopamine, epinephrine, and norepinephrine) are also water-soluble. Water-soluble hormones usually travel free in solution in the plasma, although some are partially protein-bound. Water-soluble hormones are unable to cross the plasma membrane to enter cells and therefore must exert their actions by binding to receptors located on the surface of target cell membranes.[1]

Thyroid hormones (T_3 and T_4) are derived from tyrosine amino acids to which iodine has been attached. The steroid hormones are derived from cholesterol. Thyroid and steroid hormones require transport proteins (globulin) to convey them through the circulation because they are poorly soluble in the blood. In some cases these transport proteins are specialized to carry a certain hormone (thyroxine-binding globulin, cortisol-binding globulin), but hormones can also be carried by nonspecific proteins, such as albumin.[1] Transport proteins are manufactured by the liver. At the target cell, the hormone detaches from the transport protein and moves through the cell membrane to activate intracellular receptors in the cytoplasm or nucleus.[1]

Mechanisms of Hormone Action
Hormones with Cell Membrane Receptors

Hormones exert their actions by binding to target cell receptor proteins. The target cell receptors for water-soluble hormones have a

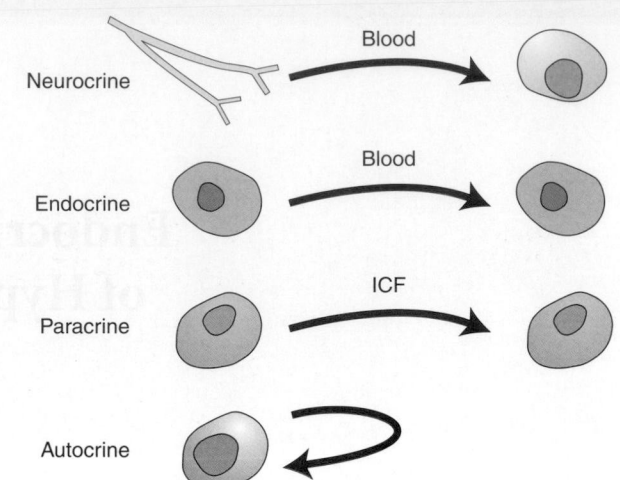

FIGURE 39-1 Terminology and comparison of cell-to-cell signaling pathways. *ICF,* Intracellular fluid.

BOX 39-1   CHEMICAL CLASSIFICATION OF HORMONES

Water-Soluble

Peptides
Adrenocorticotropic hormone (ACTH)
Angiotensin II
Atrial natriuretic hormone
Antidiuretic hormone (vasopressin) (ADH)
Calcitonin
Cholecystokinin
Follicle-stimulating hormone (FSH)
Growth hormone (GH)
Glucagon
Hypothalamic-releasing hormones
Insulin
Insulin-like growth factor-1 (IGF-1)
Luteinizing hormone (LH)
Oxytocin
Parathyroid hormone (PTH)
Prolactin
Secretin
Thyroid-stimulating hormone (TSH)

Tyrosine-Derived Amines
Dopamine
Epinephrine
Norepinephrine

Lipid-Soluble
Tyrosine-Derived Thyroid Hormones
Triiodothyronine (T_3)
Thyroxine (T_4)

Steroids
Aldosterone
Cortisol
Corticosterone
Estrogen
Progesterone
Testosterone
Vitamin D

---

hormone-binding site located on the external portion of a specific cell-surface receptor. Once hormone-receptor binding takes place, a change in the conformation of the receptor protein conveys a signal to the interior of the cell. Some receptors generate second messengers, such as cyclic adenosine monophosphate (cAMP), within the cell whereas others become activated enzymes. The intracellular activities occurring after hormone-receptor binding may include changes in cell membrane permeability; activation or inactivation of enzymes; cellular maintenance, growth, and differentiation; protein synthesis; and genetic expression via RNA and DNA synthesis in the cell nucleus.[4] A more detailed explanation of receptor mechanisms can be found in Chapter 3.

G-protein–linked receptors. Hormones can be described as "first messengers"; the hormone carries a message from the secreting cell to the target cell. A **second messenger** is generated within the cell

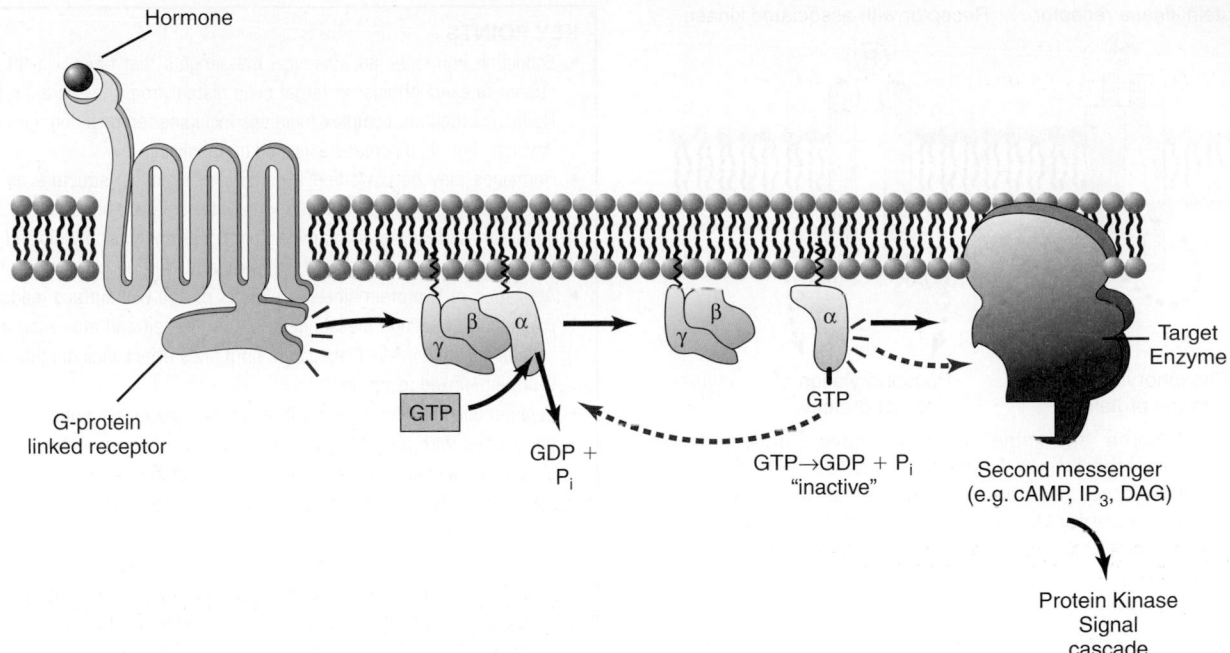

FIGURE 39-2 Mechanism of G-protein–linked receptor signaling in endocrine cells. Activation of the receptor by a hormone on the outside of the cell changes the conformation of the receptor and activates its target G-proteins. Common G-proteins in endocrine systems are G_s (which activates adenylyl cyclase to produce cAMP) and G_q (which activates phospholipase C to produce DAG and IP_3).

in response to the first message. The term *second messenger* is usually applied to the products generated by a class of receptors called G-protein–linked (or G-protein–coupled) receptors. These receptors undergo a conformational change upon binding to a hormone that allows them to interact with a class of proteins, called G-proteins, located on the inner side of the cell membrane (Figure 39-2). G-Proteins have three subunits and when activated by the receptor, one of these subunits (α) binds to a GTP molecule and then dissociates from the other subunits (β, γ).[3] The activated α subunit is able to move along the inner membrane and interact with target enzymes, inducing them to produce the second messenger. There are several different forms of G-proteins that have different target enzymes and produce different sets of second messengers (see Chapter 3). The most important of these for endocrine systems are the G_s and the G_q subtypes. Hormones that bind to receptors that are linked to G_s increase the production of cAMP within the cell. The usual downstream target of cAMP is an enzyme called protein kinase A. Kinases are enzymes that attach phosphates (phosphorylation) to target proteins to change their activity. Enzymes within the cell called phosphorylases work to remove the attached phosphates. Phosphorylation-dephosphorylation is a common strategy for controlling enzyme activity in cells. Activation of protein kinase A causes varied cellular effects depending on the cell type. Important examples of hormones that are linked to increased cAMP production through activation of the G_s pathway include adrenocorticotropic hormone (ACTH), thyroid-stimulating hormone (TSH), follicle-stimulating hormone (FSH), luteinizing hormone (LH), epinephrine (β receptors), parathyroid hormone, antidiuretic hormone (ADH), and glucagon.[1]

The G_q pathway is linked to production of two second messengers, diacylglycerol (DAG) and inositol trisphosphate (IP_3). Norepinephrine and epinephrine can activate the G_q pathway by binding to α_1 receptors on target cells. DAG and IP_3 work together to increase the activity of protein kinase C, which then phosphorylates downstream target proteins to change cell behavior.

Protein kinase receptors. A second class of surface receptors important in endocrine signaling is the protein kinase receptor family. These receptors either become activated kinases themselves or are associated with cytoplasmic kinases on their inner domain (Figure 39-3). Both types of receptors phosphorylate their target proteins upon binding of the hormone to an external binding site. An important example of a receptor kinase is the insulin receptor that phosphorylates tyrosine amino acids in its targets and activates several different intracellular signaling cascades (Chapter 41). Growth hormone and prolactin receptors are associated with Janus kinase (JAK) on the cytoplasmic side and become activated when the hormone binds to the outside of the receptor, causing a conformational change that pulls two JAK enzymes closer together.[1] The JAK enzymes become activated and phosphorylate their target proteins, initiating a signaling cascade.

Amplification of Hormone Activity

The process of intracellular activation by secondary signals occurs via a cascade effect. Progressively larger numbers of chemical reactions occur at each step, so that activation of one receptor at the cell surface can activate numerous G-proteins.[3] Each activated G-protein may interact with 100 or more target enzyme molecules, such as adenylyl cyclase. Each activated enzyme produces many molecules of a second messenger (cAMP), and each second messenger molecule activates many molecules of protein kinase, and so forth. This mechanism of signal *amplification* explains why minute amounts of circulating hormone cause significant and rapid cellular and systemic effects.

Hormones with Intracellular Receptors

Receptors for thyroid and steroid hormones are located in the cytoplasm or the nucleus of the target cell (Figure 39-4). For decades the transport of thyroid hormone across the cell membrane was thought to be a passive process of diffusion through the bilayer; however, recent discoveries indicate that special protein carriers in the

Protein kinase receptor   Receptor with associated kinase

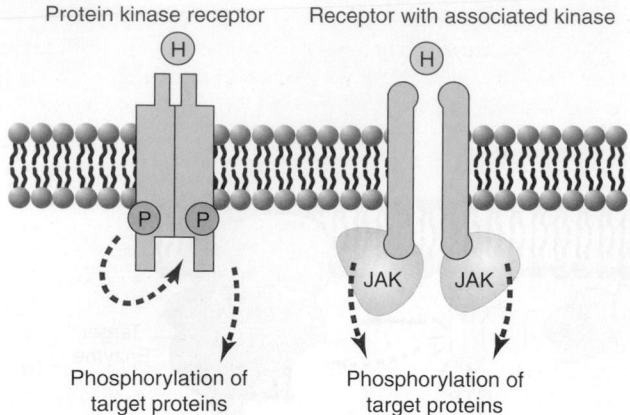

Phosphorylation of
target proteins

Phosphorylation of
target proteins

FIGURE 39-3 Some endocrine receptors have intrinsic kinase activity, whereas others have kinases associated with their inner domain. In either case, hormone binding to the outer part of the receptor triggers a conformational change in the receptor that initiates kinase activities. Kinases phosphorylate target proteins and alter their activity.

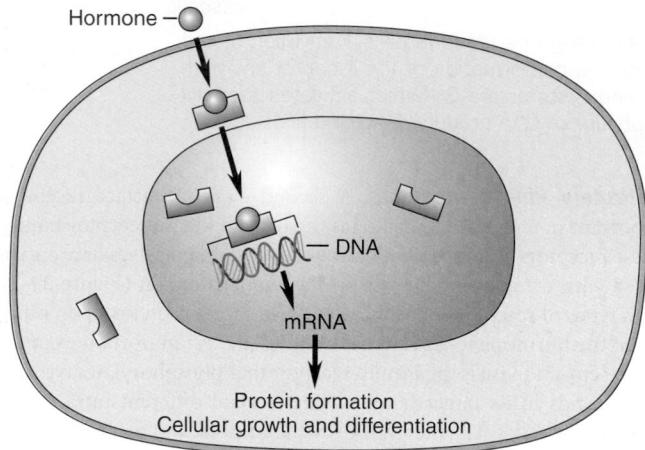

FIGURE 39-4 Thyroid and steroid hormones are transported through the plasma membrane and bind to intracellular receptors (located in the cytoplasm or nucleus). The hormone-receptor complexes are DNA-regulatory proteins that regulate messenger RNA transcription, processing, and translation into proteins.

membrane are necessary to transport thyroid hormone into the cell.[5] Steroid hormones are still believed to be able to pass directly across the plasma membrane to interact with intracellular receptors.[6] However, they may also bind cell-surface receptors as evidenced by the discovery that estrogen can bind to a G-protein–linked receptor on some cells. These G-protein receptors achieve a more rapid change in cell behavior than those associated with intracellular receptors. Binding of the hormones to intracellular receptors causes a change in affinity of the receptor for binding sites on DNA in the cell nucleus.[4] Gene expression is changed by binding of the hormone-receptor complex to specific DNA-binding sites. The events that result from the interaction between nuclear DNA and the receptor include messenger RNA transcription, processing, and translation into specific proteins (see Chapter 5 for a review of protein synthesis). In general, the onset of action of thyroid and steroid hormones is slow compared with that of the water-soluble hormones described previously, and there is no amplification cascade. Changes in DNA transcription and protein synthesis occur over hours to days.

HORMONE REGULATION

Hormone Synthesis, Secretion, and Metabolism

Hormone synthesis and secretion may take place in several different cell types, but one site is generally considered to be the primary endocrine tissue and is responsive to feedback about the need for the hormone or its effects. For example, endothelial cells throughout the vascular system produce small amounts of angiotensin II (AII); however, the primary endocrine control is through the renin-angiotensin-aldosterone cascade in which specialized cells in the kidney trigger AII production in response to changes in extracellular volume and pressure.

Most endocrine hormones are polypeptides manufactured on the rough endoplasmic reticulum and stored in vesicles within the cells. A review of protein synthesis can be found in Chapter 5. The initial forms of the polypeptide hormones are usually larger molecules called *prohormones* or *pre-prohormones*. These must be cleaved by specific enzymes to release the active form of the hormone.[1,3] Sometimes this cleavage occurs after the hormone is packaged into vesicles and the fragments are released into the bloodstream along with the hormone. In some cases, such as with insulin secretion, this is clinically useful as a marker of hormone synthesis. Insulin and its C-peptide fragment are produced in a 1:1 ratio and the concentration of C-peptide, which is more stable in the circulation, can be used as a measure of insulin production.

Because they are water-soluble, peptide hormones can be contained within the lipid bilayer of the vesicles and stored until a trigger results in exocytosis of the hormone into the extracellular space. Catecholamines are also water-soluble and stored in vesicles until they are released by exocytosis. However, they are formed by enzymes within the cytoplasm that begin with tyrosine and through a series of steps convert it first to dopamine; depending on the cell type, dopamine may be the final hormone or it can be converted to norepinephrine and then to epinephrine.

Steroid and thyroid hormones are not stored within vesicles because they are lipid-soluble and might leak from the vesicle. The strategy for synthesis and storage is much different for each of these hormones. When a steroid hormone is needed, increased production of the hormone closely precedes hormone release into the circulation.[2] Steroid hormones are formed on demand from cholesterol that is either stored in the cell or retrieved from the circulating lipoproteins. The stimuli that trigger steroid secretion induce the enzymes in the pathway to synthesize the necessary hormones from cholesterol. Once formed, steroid hormones can simply diffuse through the plasma membrane and into the circulation. The strategy for trapping thyroid hormones within the thyroid gland until they are needed is quite different. Hormone synthesis precedes secretion by weeks or months. Triiodothyronine (T_3) and thyroxine (T_4) are synthesized in the thyroid follicle, bound to a protein called *thyroglobulin*.[7] Thyroglobulin is a large water-soluble protein that is trapped within the thyroid follicle. Secretion occurs via cleavage of the thyroid hormone from thyroglobulin in response to systemic needs determined by the hypothalamus and the pituitary gland. Free T_3 and T_4 are released from the thyroid cells through membrane carrier proteins. Thyroid and steroid synthesis and release are detailed later in this chapter.

Factors Affecting Hormone Secretion

Secretion of endocrine hormones is dependent on the interplay of many factors. Most of the hormones controlled by the anterior pituitary gland are secreted in cyclical patterns. These cycles are regulated by the hypothalamus and may occur in response to feeding-fasting cycles, light-dark cycles, sleep-wake cycles, or in a 24-hour (circadian) period. Cycles also occur over longer periods (e.g., the 28-day menstrual cycle) or over years (e.g., the hormones that control reproductive differentiation and maturity).[1,2] Acute systemic needs or stressors can partially override cyclical patterns and modify hormone secretion. An example of this is activation of the stress response that alters the normal circadian pattern of cortisol secretion. Knowledge of the cyclical nature of hormone release is important when comparing measured serum concentrations to normal ranges and when attempting to provide hormone replacement therapy that mimics the normal physiologic pattern.

Feedback Control of Secretion

The most common mechanism regulating hormone production and secretion is *negative feedback* control in which some aspect of the secreted hormone is sensed and regulates further secretion.[4] An example of negative feedback is the interaction between the hypothalamic-pituitary system and the respective hormone-releasing glands controlled by this system. For example, thyrotropin-releasing hormone (TRH) is secreted by the hypothalamus when the central nervous system senses an inadequate supply of thyroid hormones in the circulation. TRH stimulates the synthesis and release of thyroid-stimulating hormone (TSH) from specific cells in the anterior pituitary gland; TSH then stimulates the synthesis and release of the thyroid hormones T_3 and T_4 from the thyroid follicle. The resulting increase in plasma thyroid hormone concentration exerts an inhibitory effect, or negative feedback, on the release of TSH by the anterior pituitary gland and TRH from the hypothalamus.[7,8] The negative feedback loop is a mechanism for maintaining hormone activity within a normal range or *set point* of normal activity. The set point is genetically determined and influenced by age, gender, circadian cycles, and current internal and environmental conditions. The regulatory influences are multiple and complex, but often there is a particular variable that is influenced by the hormone's activity and provides most of the feedback regulation. These feedback systems are detailed for the hormones of the pituitary system in later sections of this chapter. Knowledge of feedback controls is helpful when evaluating patients for endocrine diseases (see Chapter 40).

Hormone Metabolism and Excretion

The plasma concentration of a hormone depends not only on the rate of synthesis and release of the hormone but also on how rapidly the hormone is metabolized and excreted. Like other compounds, hormones are frequently degraded and excreted by the liver and kidneys. Water-soluble hormones may be excreted in the urinary filtrate. Lipid-soluble hormones, which are bound to plasma proteins and stored in adipose tissue, are less readily metabolized and remain in the circulation for a more prolonged period.[4] In addition to metabolism by the kidneys and liver, hormones are often degraded by the target cell after binding to receptors. *Half-life* is a term used to describe the duration of hormone activity in the circulation and may be expressed in minutes, hours, or days. The half-life is the time for a hormone to reach half of its original concentration in the blood and is influenced by the rate of uptake by cells, degradation, and excretion.

Pharmacologic Hormone Concentrations

It is important to differentiate between physiologic and pharmacologic hormone activity. Physiologic hormone concentrations are extremely low in most cases, and pharmacologic levels of hormones are usually several-fold greater than would normally be secreted by endocrine tissues. Pharmacologic levels occur as a consequence of either pathologic processes or the administration of large doses of hormones. The tissue response to pharmacologic hormone concentrations may be significantly different from that caused by physiologic levels of hormones.[4]

Regulation of Receptor Responses

Tissue response to circulating hormone is only partially determined by the amount of hormone present in the circulation. Although virtually all body tissues are exposed to circulating hormones, specific hormones elicit a response only from certain cells and tissues. The ability of a cell to respond to a particular hormone depends on the presence of specific receptors for that hormone on or in the cell. Target cells are able to regulate their responsiveness to hormones by altering the receptor number, affinity, and efficiency of coupling to intracellular responses.[3]

Receptor Specificity and Affinity

The concept of *receptor specificity* is important for understanding the targeted responses of the endocrine system. Specificity refers to the molecular "fit" of a hormone within a receptor-binding pocket. Specificity cannot easily be separated from the concept of *affinity*. Affinity describes the degree of "tightness" of the hormone-receptor bond, or the inclination of the hormone to remain bound to the receptor. Specificity and affinity determine whether a cell with a receptor will respond to a hormonal stimulus and the hormone concentration at which the receptor effectively can bind the hormone. The potency of the hormone, or the amount of hormone required to elicit a cellular response, is dependent in part on the affinity of the receptor for a particular hormone. The higher the affinity of the receptor for a hormone, the lesser the amount of hormone needed to produce a response.[3] Therefore, hormones that circulate in very minute amounts may have a large effect on cellular activity because of the tightness of the hormone-receptor bond.

"Cross-specificity" between hormones of similar structure may occur. For example, prolactin and growth hormone both can bind to the prolactin receptor, but with differing affinities. Under normal circumstances, the plasma concentration of growth hormone is not adequate to bind a significant number of prolactin receptors. However, in the condition called *acromegaly,* in which excessive concentrations of growth hormone lead to massive bone and tissue overgrowth, milk may be secreted from the mammary glands secondary to growth hormone stimulation of prolactin receptors.[9,10]

Receptor Down-Regulation and Up-Regulation

A factor determining the degree of response to a circulating hormone is the number of cell receptors available for hormone binding. When cells are exposed to high concentrations of hormone for a prolonged period, a common result is that the cell decreases the number of receptors. This phenomenon is known as *down-regulation*. An example of down-regulation occurs with insulin receptors in obese individuals. An increase in the plasma insulin level commonly occurs in obese individuals. This increased concentration of insulin does not result in an increase in cellular activities in most cells because the number of insulin receptors is down-regulated in response to the high plasma insulin concentration.[3] Down-regulation probably serves a protective function: the cells are protected against excessive activity despite pathologic processes that cause excessive hormone levels. *Up-regulation*, or an increase in the number of receptors in response to chronically low hormone concentrations, may also occur. Up-regulation would make the cell more sensitive to the hormone, and hormone-dependent cellular activity could occur at normal or nearly normal levels despite a lower than normal hormone concentration.[3]

Another mechanism for altering hormone responsiveness is through regulation of the coupling mechanism between receptor activation and its intracellular responses.[3] For example, the cytoplasmic domain of a receptor can be phosphorylated or otherwise altered so that it cannot effectively interact with its target G-protein. Additionally, enzymes such as phosphorylases, which remove phosphates from proteins, and phosphodiesterases, which degrade cyclic nucleotides, can be up-regulated or down-regulated to turn off the cellular responses more or less quickly. Many of these regulatory mechanisms are not fully understood.

Permissiveness

One effect that hormones may have on target cells is to increase the number of receptors for other hormones, thus enhancing the effect of the second hormone. This phenomenon is known as *permissiveness*. For example, one effect of thyroid hormone on adipose cells is to increase the number of receptors for epinephrine. When the adipose tissue is subsequently exposed to epinephrine, a greater release of fatty acids (used in providing energy for cellular processes) takes place than would occur in the absence of thyroid hormone.[4] Permissiveness also allows cellular events to occur in sequence. One effect of estrogen, secreted early in the menstrual cycle, is to increase the number of uterine receptors for progesterone. The uterus is therefore sensitive to progesterone when it is present during the last part of the menstrual cycle, and normal proliferative changes take place.[2,11]

Hormone Agonists and Antagonists

To produce a cellular effect, a hormone must bind to the receptor and initiate a series of events that lead to a change in cellular activity. A chemical may bind to a receptor without initiating the typical intracellular changes; this chemical is described as a hormone **antagonist** or **blocking agent. Agonists,** on the other hand, bind hormone receptors and cause the same intracellular events that would occur with hormone-receptor binding. A large number of pharmacologic agents have agonist or antagonist effects on receptors for hormones. For example, hormone antagonists that compete with epinephrine and norepinephrine for receptor sites are frequently used to block the cardiac stimulatory properties of these hormones and thus decrease cardiac workload. Conversely, agonist medications that mimic hormone activity are frequently given as hormone replacement therapy in deficiency syndromes.

HYPOTHALAMIC-PITUITARY ENDOCRINE SYSTEM

The pituitary gland is located beneath the hypothalamus in the sella turcica, a pocket of bone at the base of the skull (Figure 39-5).[12] In adults, the pituitary gland is composed of distinct anterior and posterior lobes. The pituitary gland is connected to the hypothalamus by the pituitary stalk, which contains a portal system that transports capillary blood from the hypothalamus to the capillaries of the anterior pituitary gland. Neurons whose cell bodies lie within the hypothalamus send their axons down the pituitary stalk and terminate in the posterior pituitary gland. Synthesis and secretion of the various pituitary hormones are controlled, directly or indirectly, by the hypothalamus. Release of posterior pituitary hormones occurs when action potentials generated in the hypothalamic neurons travel down the axons of the pituitary stalk and trigger exocytosis of hormone from the nerve terminals in the posterior pituitary gland. The hypothalamus regulates endocrine function of the anterior pituitary gland by secreting releasing hormones and inhibiting hormones from hypothalamic neurons that are subsequently carried to anterior pituitary endocrine cells by the pituitary portal system.

The pituitary gland is also called the *hypophysis*, and the anterior and posterior lobes are sometimes referred to as the *adenohypophysis* and the *neurohypophysis*, respectively. The posterior pituitary gland secretes two important peptide hormones: antidiuretic hormone (vasopressin) and oxytocin. The anterior lobe of the pituitary gland has five endocrine cell types that secrete six different peptide hormones: (1) somatotropes, which secrete growth hormone (GH); (2) gonadotropes, which secrete gonadotropins (luteinizing hormone [LH], follicle-stimulating hormone [FSH]); (3) thyrotropes, which secrete thyroid-stimulating hormone (TSH, thyrotropin); (4) corticotropes, which secrete adrenocorticotropic hormone (ACTH); and finally (5) lactotropes, which secrete prolactin (PRL).[9,10] The hormones produced by the anterior pituitary gland have direct actions on other endocrine tissues and the liver (Table 39-1).

Hormones of the Posterior Pituitary Gland

The posterior pituitary gland consists of nerve axons whose neuronal cell bodies originate in the supraoptic and paraventricular nuclei of the

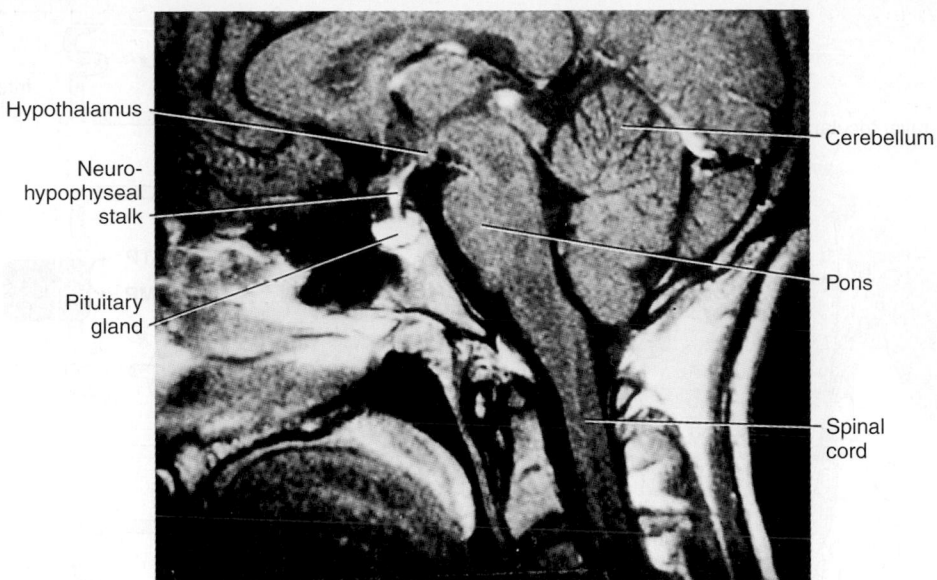

FIGURE 39-5 Cross section showing anatomic relationship of the hypothalamus and pituitary gland. (From Koeppen BM, Stanton BA, editors: *Berne & Levy physiology*, ed 6 [updated edition], Philadelphia, 2010, Mosby, p 707.)

TABLE 39-1 ENDOCRINE CELL TYPES OF ADENOHYPOPHYSIS

	CORTICOTROPE	THYROTROPE	GONADOTROPE	SOMATOTROPE	LACTOTROPE
Primary hypothalamic regulation	Corticotropin-releasing hormone (CRH) (41-aa peptide) (stimulatory)	Thyrotropin-releasing hormone (TRH) (3-aa peptide) (stimulatory)	Gonadotropin-releasing hormone (GnRH) (10-aa peptide) (stimulatory)	Growth hormone–releasing hormone (GHRH) (44-aa peptide) (stimulatory); somatostatin (14-aa peptide) (inhibitory)	Dopamine (catechol-amine) (inhibitory); prolactin-releasing factor (stimulatory)
Tropic hormone secreted	Adrenocorticotropic hormone (ACTH) (39-aa peptide)	Thyroid-stimulating hormone (TSH) (28-kDa glycoprotein hormone)	Follicle-stimulating hormone and luteinizing hormone (FSH and LH) (28- and 33-kDa glyco-protein hormone)	Growth hormone (GH) (ca. 22-kDa protein)	Prolactin (ca. 23-kDa protein)
Receptor	MC2R (G_s-linked GPCR)	TSH receptor (G_s-linked GPCR)	FSH and LH receptors (G_s-linked GPCRs)	GH receptor (JAK/STAT-linked cytokine receptor)	PRL receptor (JAK/STAT-linked cyto-kine receptor)
Target endocrine gland	Zona fasciculata and zona reticularis of adrenal cortex	Thyroid epithelium	Ovary (theca and granu-losa*) and testis (Leydig, Sertoli)	Liver (but also direct actions, especially in terms of metabolic effects)	No endocrine target organ; not part of an endocrine axis
Peripheral hormone involved in negative feedback	Cortisol	Triiodothyronine (T_3)	Estrogen,[†] proges-terone, testosterone, inhibin[‡]	IGF-1	None

From Koeppen BM, Stanton BA, editors: *Berne & Levy* physiology, ed 6 [updated edition], Philadelphia, 2010, Mosby, p 712.
aa, Amino acid(s); *IGF-1,* insulin-like growth factor-1; *GPCR,* G-protein–coupled receptor; kDa, kilodalton(s).
*Both follicular and luteinized thecal and granulosa cells.
[†]Estrogen can also have positive feedback in women.
[‡]Inhibin selectivity inhibits FSH release from the gonadotrope.

hypothalamus (Figure 39-6). Posterior pituitary hormones, oxytocin and antidiuretic hormone, are produced in the neurons of the hypothalamus and, packaged in vesicles, travel along the length of the nerve axons to the posterior pituitary gland. Release of antidiuretic hormone or oxytocin occurs as a result of depolarization of the appropriate hypothalamic neurons and conduction of action potentials to the nerve terminals in the posterior pituitary gland. Antidiuretic hormone is released in response to altered serum osmolality and hypotension and causes water retention by increasing water reabsorption by the renal collecting duct. Oxytocin is released during sexual activity, childbirth, and breast feeding and causes uterine and milk duct contractions.[10]

Antidiuretic Hormone

Antidiuretic hormone is a 9–amino acid peptide that differs by 2 amino acids from oxytocin, another 9–amino acid peptide. The circulating half-life of ADH is about 15 to 20 minutes, and it is destroyed by

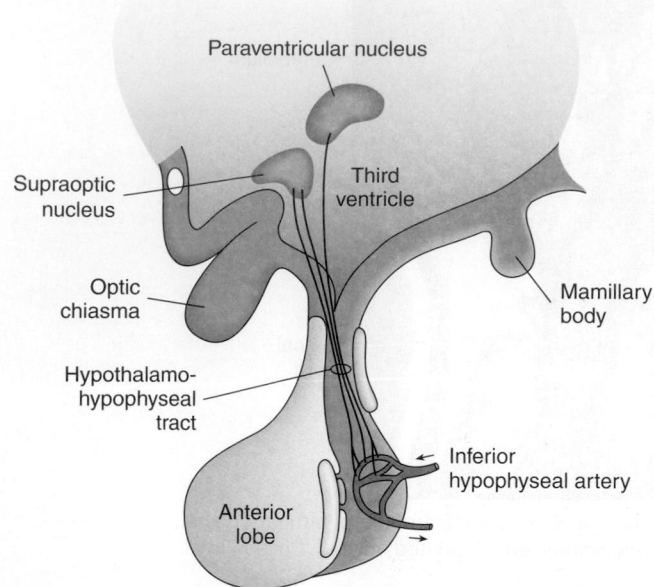

FIGURE 39-6 Axons from the paraventricular and supraoptic nuclei in the hypothalamus project down the pituitary stalk, and the axon terminals lie within the posterior pituitary gland. Oxytocin and antidiuretic hormone are produced in the hypothalamic neuron cell bodies and then transported to the axon terminals, where they are released into the bloodstream in response to action potentials. (From Porterfield SP, White BA: *Endocrine physiology*, ed 3, Philadelphia, 2007, Mosby, p 110.)

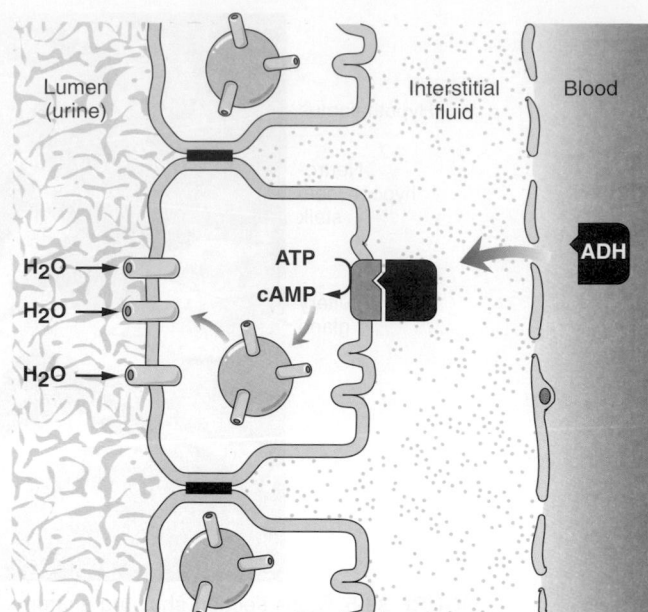

FIGURE 39-7 Antidiuretic hormone (ADH) acts on renal tubule G_s-protein–linked receptors to trigger movement of water channels (aquaporins) to the apical cell membrane. The aquaporins increase membrane permeability to water, allowing it to be absorbed through the process of osmosis. ADH thus decreases the osmolality of the extracellular fluids and creates a more concentrated urine. *ATP*, Adenosine triphosphate; *cAMP*, cyclic adenosine monophosphate.

proteolysis in the kidney and liver.[10] The most important regulator of ADH release is the osmolality of plasma, which is detected by specialized neurons called *osmoreceptors* that are found in the hypothalamus. The osmoreceptors have a set point that influences the stimulation and suppression of ADH. When body fluids become too concentrated, ADH is released, leading to increased reabsorption of water in the kidneys. ADH secretion is also stimulated by the baroreceptors in response to hypovolemia and low arterial blood pressure.

The primary targets for ADH are vasopressin 2 (V2) G-protein–linked receptors on the basolateral membrane of distal renal tubule cells. ADH causes pores, called *aquaporins,* to move from the cytoplasm to the cell membranes of apical tubular epithelial cells (Figure 39-7). These pores allow free diffusion of water from the tubular fluid into the cell. Water then flows out the basolateral membrane and into the interstitium. The enhanced reabsorption conserves water in the body, creates concentrated urine, and reduces serum osmolality (see Chapter 26).

Oxytocin

Oxytocin is structurally similar to ADH, and there is some overlap in biological activity. Oxytocin can inhibit diuresis. Oxytocin has a half-life of 3 to 5 minutes. Oxytocin is known for its actions on the breast and uterus. Sexual intercourse can stimulate oxytocin release in men and women. Its role in men is not well understood, but in women it is proposed to affect sperm motility through uterine contractions. Oxytocin also stimulates uterine contractions during labor. It is not thought to initiate labor, but once labor has begun, stretching of the cervix increases oxytocin release, which increases the intensity of uterine contractions.[10] This is an example of a positive feedback loop in which stretching of the cervix induces oxytocin release, resulting in

more forceful uterine contractions and further stretching of the cervix. Oxytocin has been characterized as the "tend and befriend" hormone because of its effects on social interaction and its participation in the stress response in men and women.

Oxytocin release is triggered by stimulation of the nipple and areola, which have sensory receptors that send neuronal signals to the hypothalamic nuclei. Oxytocin then binds to myoepithelial cells surrounding the milk ducts, causing them to contract and eject milk during breast feeding. This reflex can be triggered centrally without breast stimulation as a conditioned response to the sight or sound of an infant.

Hormones of the Hypothalamus and Anterior Pituitary Gland

The hypothalamic-pituitary endocrine system is a three-tiered axis that includes hypothalamic releasing and inhibiting hormones, anterior pituitary hormones, and target organ hormones (Figure 39-8). Releasing and inhibiting factors are secreted into a capillary bed that is contained within the hypothalamus by hypothalamic neurons having short axons. Hypothalamic hormones diffuse into the capillary network, travel down the portal vein, and then diffuse from the anterior pituitary capillary network into the tissue where they bind receptors on pituitary cells.[12] All of the hypothalamic releasing and inhibiting factors are peptides, with the exception of dopamine, and all are water-soluble. Therefore all releasing and inhibiting factors interact with cell-surface receptors on the target pituitary cells.

The three-tiered hypothalamic-pituitary-target system provides an opportunity for fine modulation of hormone action on target tissues. The hypothalamic and pituitary hormones exemplify the complexity of endocrine interactions. In addition to feedback from target organ hormones, the hypothalamus processes numerous neuronal signals into an integrated response by the anterior pituitary gland. The hypothalamic releasing and inhibiting hormones are typically secreted in

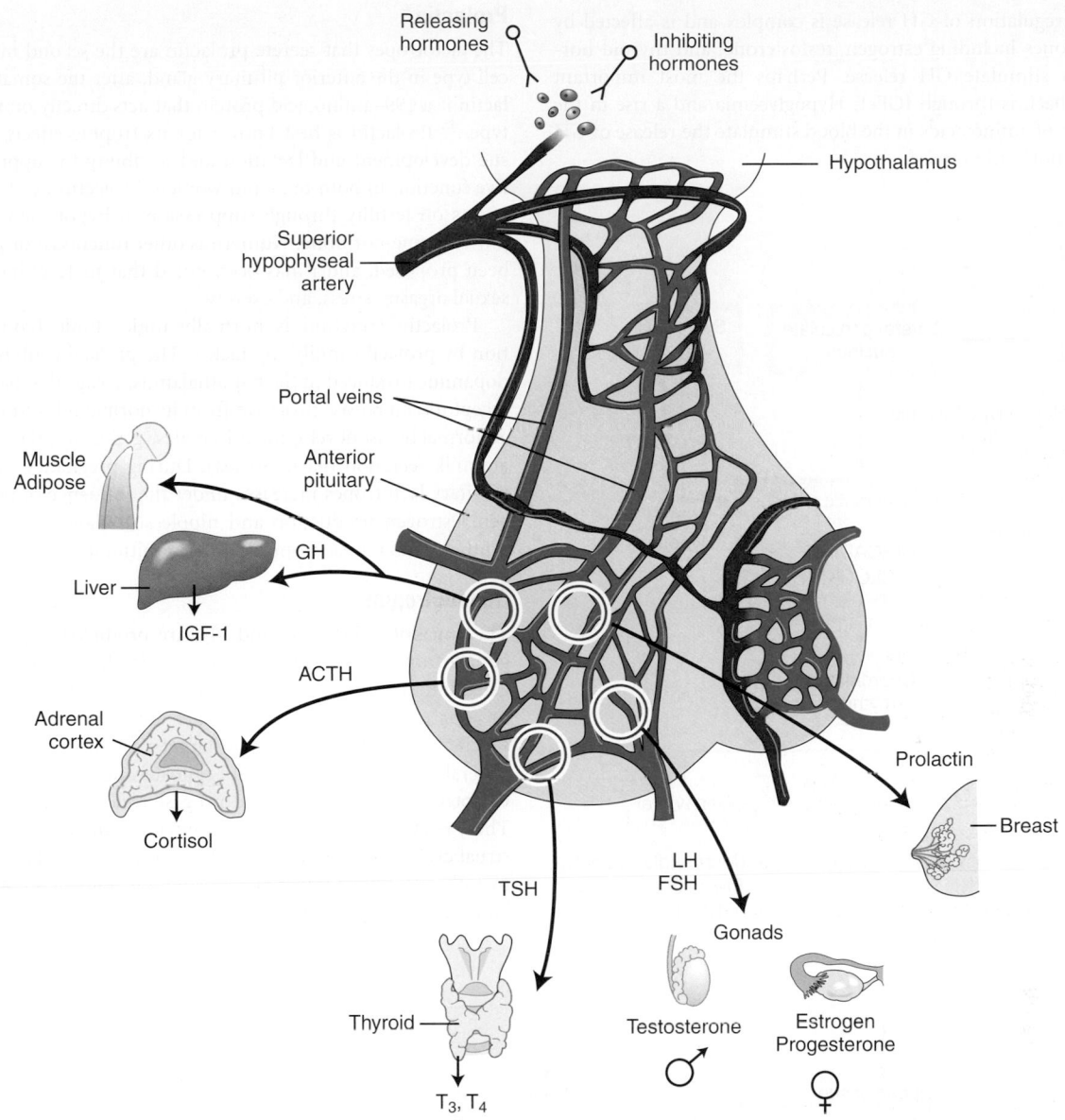

FIGURE 39-8 Relationship of the hypothalamic releasing and inhibiting hormones, anterior pituitary hormones, and target gland hormones. *ACTH,* Adrenocorticotropic hormone; *FSH,* follicle-stimulating hormone; *GH,* growth hormone; *IGF-1,* insulin-like growth factor-1; *LH,* luteinizing hormone; *TSH,* thyroid-stimulating hormone; *T₃,* triiodothyronine; *T₄,* thyroxine.

a pulsatile and circadian rhythm. Two structures thought to modulate this activity are the suprachiasmatic nucleus (SCN) and the pineal gland. Changes in light and dark patterns influence the SCN and pineal gland, resulting in a diurnal (daily) pattern of hormone secretion (Figure 39-9).[9] Each of the major anterior pituitary hormones is briefly described next.

Growth Hormone

Pituitary GH secretion is controlled by hypothalamic release of growth hormone–releasing hormone (GHRH) and growth hormone–inhibiting hormone (somatostatin). GHRH binds to receptors on pituitary somatotropes and stimulates release of GH, whereas somatostatin inhibits GH release. Under normal physiologic conditions, the anterior pituitary gland secretes small pulsatile amounts of GH each day. Sleep studies indicate a circadian pattern to GH secretion, with secretion being greatest during deep, slow-wave sleep (stage 3 or 4). GH secretion is greatest during adolescence and decreases in the elderly.[10]

GH is a 191–amino acid protein that is similar in structure to prolactin. A major target for GH is the liver, where it affects liver metabolism and also induces the production of another endocrine hormone called *insulin-like growth factor-1* (IGF-1). Previously, IGF-1 was called *somatomedin*. IGF-1 is an anabolic hormone that increases the growth of bone and cartilage tissues of the body. GH is not the only stimulus for the production of IGF-1, nor is the liver the only source. Insulin is an important costimulator of IGF-1 along with GH.[10] GH also has direct effects on some cells and binds to receptors on muscle and adipose tissue, increasing muscle mass and decreasing fat mass by inducing lipolysis. It affects metabolic processes by increasing the rate of protein synthesis, decreasing protein catabolism, slowing carbohydrate utilization, and increasing mobilization of fats and the use of fats for energy (Figure 39-10).[4] An insufficient level of GH is exhibited as short stature in children, whereas excesses may lead to increased height in children and excessive growth of nonadipose tissues in adults (see Chapter 40).

Feedback regulation of GH release is complex and is affected by several hormones including estrogen, testosterone, and thyroid hormone, which stimulate GH release. Perhaps the most important negative feedback is through IGF-1. Hypoglycemia and a rise in the concentration of amino acids in the blood stimulate the release of GH as does starvation and exercise.

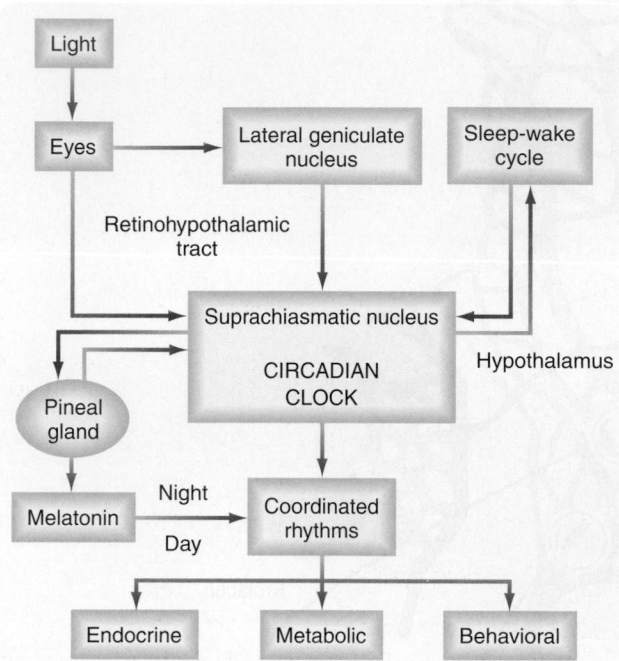

FIGURE 39-9 Origin of circadian rhythms in endocrine gland secretion. (From Koeppen BM, Stanton BA, editors: *Berne & Levy physiology*, ed 6 [updated edition], Philadelphia, 2010, Mosby, p 656.)

Prolactin

The lactotropes that secrete prolactin are the second most numerous cell type in the anterior pituitary gland, after the somatotropes. Prolactin is a 199–amino acid protein that acts directly on numerous cell types.[10] Prolactin is best known for its trophic effects on breast tissue development and lactation and its ability to suppress reproductive function in both men and women. Prolactin exerts its inhibitory effects on fertility through suppression of hypothalamic gonadotropin-releasing hormone. Numerous other functions for prolactin have been proposed, and it has been noted that its level increases during sexual orgasm, stress, and exercise.

Prolactin secretion is normally under tonic (constant) inhibition by prolactin-inhibiting factor. The prolactin-inhibiting factor is dopamine produced in the hypothalamus. Drugs that block dopamine receptors can release prolactin from its normal inhibition, resulting in abnormal breast development in males (gynecomastia) or inappropriate milk secretion (galactorrhea). During pregnancy, the number of pituitary lactotropes increases under the influence of placental estrogen. Estrogen production and nipple stimulation increase prolactin synthesis and release from the anterior pituitary gland.

Gonadotropins

The gonadotropins, FSH and LH, are produced together within the gonadotropes in the anterior pituitary gland; however, they are segregated into different packaging vesicles and are not necessarily released in equal amounts.[2,10] FSH and LH are proteins and bind to their specific respective receptors on target cells in the ovary or testes. In general, FSH and LH stimulate testosterone production in men (see Chapter 30) and estrogen and progesterone production in women.[11] These relationships are complex in women and change over the menstrual cycle (see Chapter 32). Release of FSH and LH is stimulated by hypothalamic gonadotropin-releasing hormone in a pulsatile fashion, and inhibited by negative feedback from sex steroids (except for the

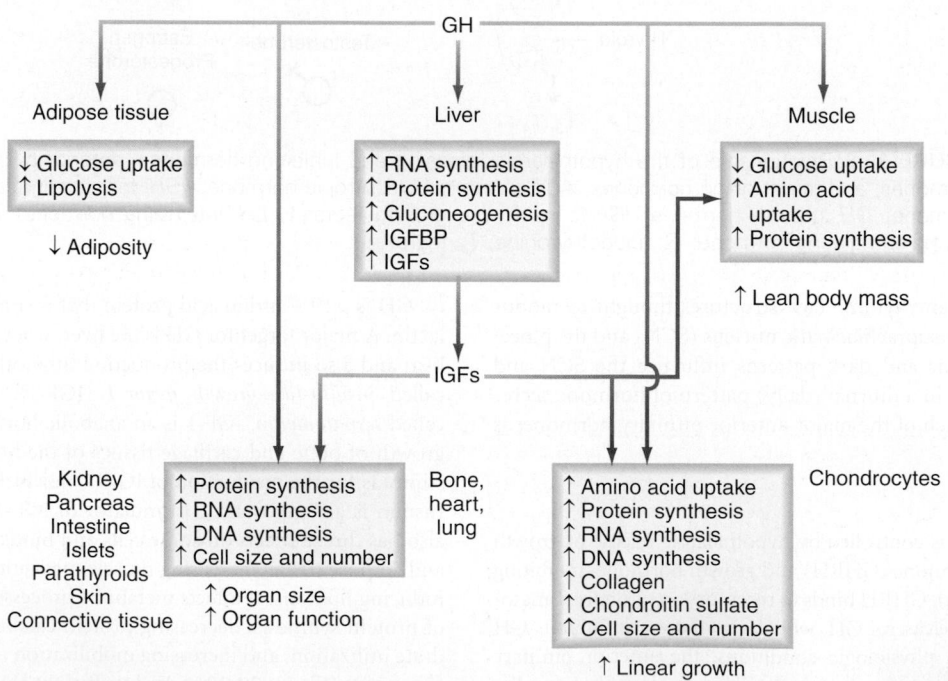

FIGURE 39-10 Biological actions of growth hormone (GH). *IGF*, Insulin-like growth factor; *IGFBP*, insulin-like growth factor binding protein. (From Koeppen BM, Stanton BA, editors: *Berne & Levy physiology*, ed 6 [updated edition], Philadelphia, 2010, Mosby, p 721.)

midcycle positive feedback LH surge induced by estrogen at the time of ovulation in women).

Thyroid-Stimulating Hormone

Thyrotropes release TSH in response to hypothalamic thyrotropin-releasing hormone (TRH). TSH is a glycoprotein that binds to TSH receptors on follicle cells of the thyroid gland. TRH is released according to a diurnal (daily circadian) rhythm with its lowest period in the evening. Stress, starvation, and infection reduce the secretion of TRH. Negative feedback regulation of TRH and TSH is achieved primarily by the concentration of circulating T_3. TSH regulates all aspects of thyroid function, including growth of the gland and synthesis and secretion of hormone.[8,10] The details of thyroid hormone synthesis and action on target tissues are described later in this chapter.

Adrenocorticotropic Hormone

ACTH is produced by corticotropes in the anterior pituitary gland in response to hypothalamic corticotropin-releasing hormone (CRH). ACTH is a 39–amino acid peptide that is derived from cleavage of a large pre-prohormone called pro-opiomelanocortin (POMC). Although POMC has the protein sequences for melanocyte-stimulating hormone and endorphin in its structure, human corticotropes express only the enzyme for cleaving ACTH as the sole hormone from this pre-prohormone.[6,10] ACTH circulates unbound in the circulation and has a half-life of about 10 minutes. It binds to G_s-coupled receptors on cells in the adrenal cortex and stimulates the production of cortisol and adrenal androgens. ACTH also has trophic effects on the adrenal cortex and supports the structure and synthetic enzymes of the gland. Withdrawal of ACTH results in adrenal cortical atrophy. ACTH in high concentration stimulates darkening of the skin by stimulating melanocyte receptors on skin cells. Normally keratinocytes in the skin produce melanocyte-stimulating hormone (MSH) in response to ultraviolet light, which can bind to MSH receptors on neighboring skin melanocytes in a paracrine fashion. ACTH can cross-react with melanocyte MSH receptors, and in high concentrations ACTH can produce abnormal skin pigmentation.

CRH and ACTH secretion demonstrate a significant diurnal pattern, with a peak upon wakening and a valley during the usual time of sleep (Figure 39-11). The diurnal pattern can be altered when there are chronic changes in sleep-wake patterns. Negative feedback regulation of ACTH is accomplished by the actions of cortisol, which suppress CRH and ACTH release. Regulation of the hypothalamic-pituitary-adrenal (HPA) axis is complex and is affected by acute and chronic stress (see Chapter 2). The adrenal cortex produces three types of steroid hormones: glucocorticoids, mineralocorticoids, and androgens. The details of adrenocortical steroid hormone synthesis and action on target tissues are described later in this chapter.

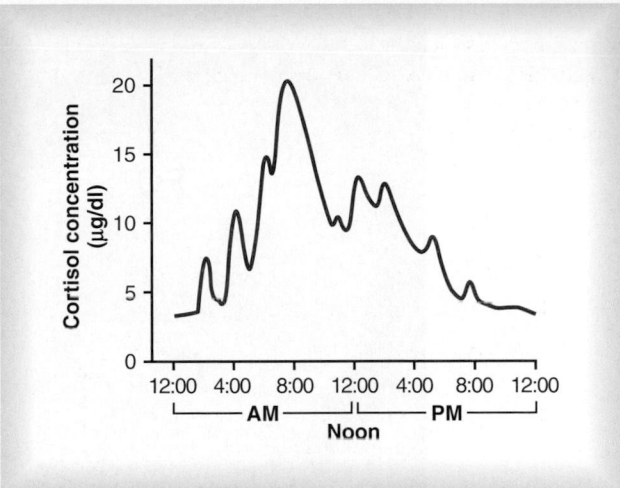

FIGURE 39-11 Typical pattern of cortisol secretion showing a diurnal (circadian) rhythm, with highest secretion occurring in the morning upon awakening and lowest levels in the late evening. The pattern can change when the usual wake and sleep times are altered, for example, in night-shift workers. (In Hall JE, editor: *Guyton and Hall textbook of medical physiology*, ed 12, Philadelphia, 2011, Saunders, p 933.)

THYROID HORMONES

Thyroid Hormone Synthesis and Secretion

The thyroid gland, a two-lobed gland, lies in the neck region on either side of and anterior to the trachea. It secretes the thyroid hormones thyroxine (T_4) and triiodothyronine (T_3).[7,12] The thyroid gland is composed of microscopic follicles made up of a single layer of epithelial cells forming a ball, with their apical surfaces toward a pocket in the middle filled with colloid and their basal surfaces facing the interstitial fluid and capillary system (Figure 39-12). Follicular cells perform all the functions required to make and secrete thyroid hormones.[7,8] They trap dietary iodine and transport it into the colloid, synthesize thyroglobulin protein, and transport it into the colloid along with the enzyme thyroid peroxidase. Thyroid peroxidase acts on thyroglobulin to produce thyroid hormones (Figure 39-13). First it oxidizes iodide and couples it to tyrosine amino acids in thyroglobulin. Some tyrosines receive two iodides (diiodotyrosine, DIT) and others have only one (monoiodotyrosine, MIT). Two iodotyrosines are then attached to each other by thyroid peroxidase to form T_4 (two DIT) or T_3 (one DIT and one MIT). Approximately 90% of the thyroid hormone is in the form of T_4, and 10% is in the form of T_3. The thyroid hormones remain attached to thyroglobulin, a storage protein, which accumulates in the thyroid follicles. By remaining attached to thyroglobulin, T_3 and T_4 are trapped within the water-soluble colloid. When stimulated by TSH, the follicular cells endocytose a portion of the colloid containing thyroglobulin with its attached thyroid hormones. The endocytic vesicle combines with a lysosome, and the thyroid hormones are cleaved from thyroglobulin. Released T_4 and T_3 are transported from the follicle and into the circulation through carriers on the basal membrane.

Thyroid Action on Target Cells

Thyroid hormones are carried in the circulation bound to thyroid-binding proteins. Ninety percent of the circulating thyroid hormone is T_4, and 10% is T_3 (Figure 39-14). A small percentage of thyroid hormone (less than 1%) is dissolved in the plasma as free hormone and is able to

---

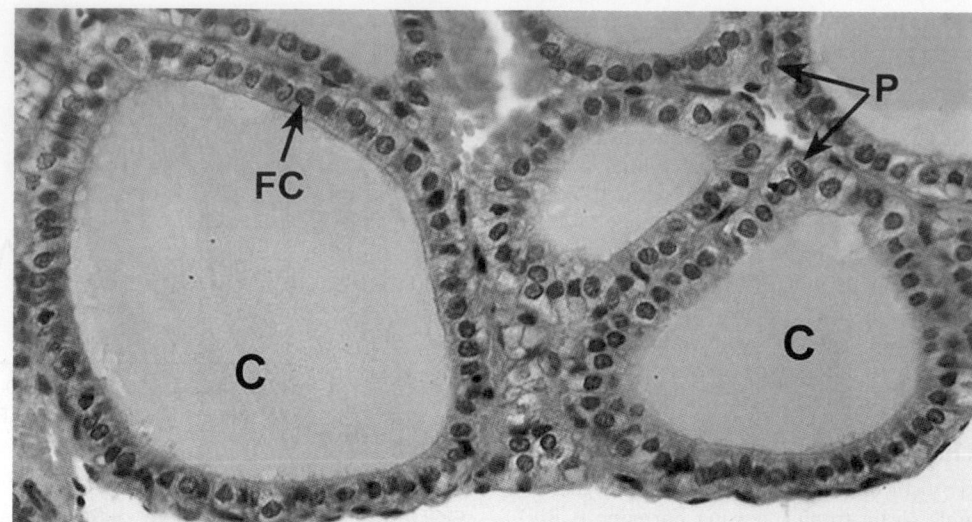

FIGURE 39-12 Histology of thyroid follicle demonstrating single layer of epithelial follicular cells *(FC)* surrounding a core of colloid *(C)*. The parafollicular cells *(P)* produce another hormone called *calcitonin*, which is involved in calcium regulation. (From Porterfield SP, White BA: *Endocrine physiology*, ed 3, Philadelphia, 2007, Mosby, p 142.)

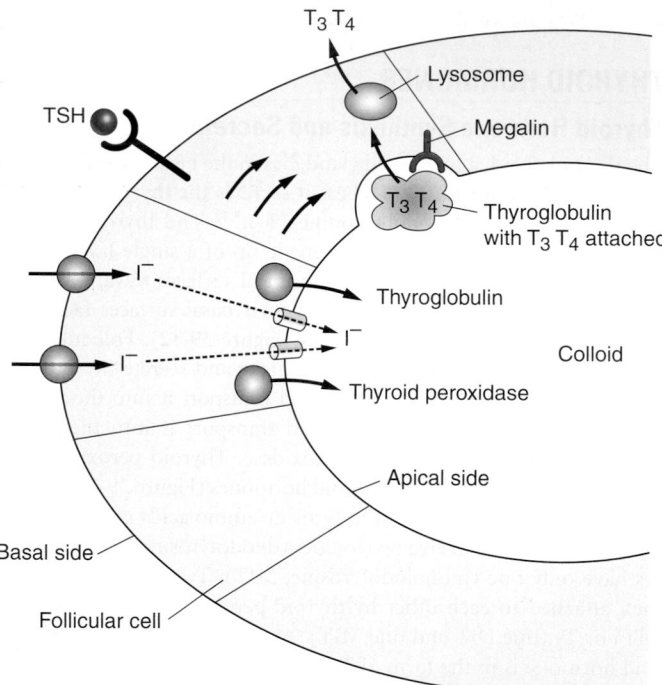

FIGURE 39-13 The follicular cells in the thyroid gland perform all of the functions required for thyroid hormone synthesis. Iodide is transported from the circulation into the inner core along with the protein thyroglobulin, which is synthesized within the cells. Follicles also produce a thyroid peroxidase enzyme and secrete it from the apical surface next to the colloid. Thyroid peroxidase activates and attaches iodides to tyrosine amino acids in the thyroglobulin. Two iodotyrosines are then coupled together, but remain attached to thyroglobulin. Stimulation by TSH initiates a cascade that induces the follicle cell to endocytose some of the colloid, followed by combining it with a lysosome that cleaves the T_3 and T_4 from the thyroglobulin. T_3 and T_4 can then leave the cell into the circulation.

cross into the target cells through specific membrane carrier proteins. Once in the cell, T_3 is able to bind to its receptor and exert its actions. T_4 is acted upon by cellular enzymes that cleave one of the iodine molecules to form either the active T_3 or a mirror image of T_3 called *reverse T_3*. This stereoisomer of T_3 has no known biological activity. The ratio of production of T_3 and reverse T_3 is normally about 1:1, but is influenced by altered metabolic states such as starvation.[8] Most of the actions of thyroid hormone on target cells are mediated through alterations in gene transcription. The nuclear thyroid receptor has much higher affinity for T_3 than T_4 and primarily binds T_3 to form a complex that binds to specific DNA sequences and alters gene activity. Many of these genes influence the metabolic rate of the cell. The general physiologic effects of thyroid hormones are shown in Table 39-2. Excesses and deficits of thyroid hormone are exhibited by alterations in growth, development, and metabolic rate (see Chapter 40).

KEY POINTS

- Follicular cells in the thyroid gland perform all the functions required to make and secrete thyroid hormones. They trap dietary iodine and transport it into the colloid, synthesize thyroglobulin protein, and transport it into the colloid along with the enzyme thyroid peroxidase.
- Thyroid peroxidase oxidizes iodide and couples it to tyrosine amino acids in thyroglobulin. Two iodotyrosines are then attached to each other to form T_4 (two DIT) or T_3 (one DIT and one MIT). Approximately 90% of the thyroid hormone is in the form of T_4, and 10% is in the form of T_3.
- When stimulated by TSH, the follicular cells endocytose a portion of the colloid. The endocytic vesicle combines with a lysosome, and the lipid-soluble T_4 and T_3 are released and leave the follicle where they are more than 99% bound to proteins in the circulation. Only free hormone is physiologically active.
- Actions of thyroid hormone on target cells are mediated through alterations in gene transcription. The nuclear thyroid receptor binds T_3 to form a complex that binds to specific DNA sequences and alters gene activity.
- Thyroid hormone increases metabolic rate and is essential for normal growth and development.

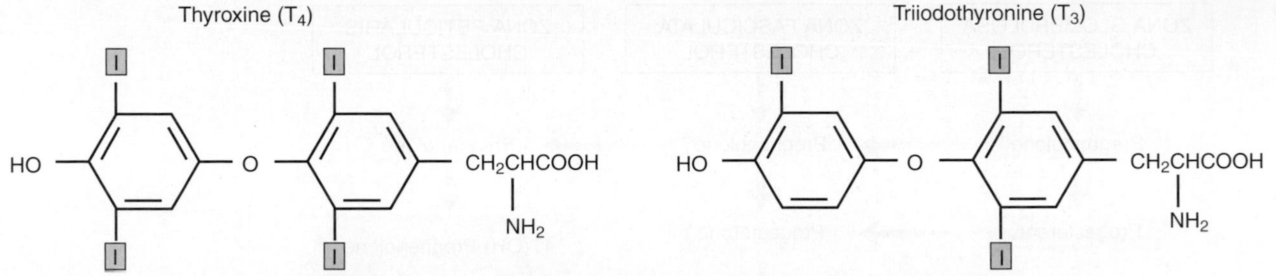

Thyroxine (T₄)

Triiodothyronine (T₃)

FIGURE 39-14 Structures of thyroxine (T₄) and triiodothyronine (T₃).

TABLE 39-2 PHYSIOLOGIC ACTIONS OF THYROID HORMONES

	HYPOTHYROID	EUTHYROID	HYPERTHYROID
Metabolic rate	Decreased BMR	—	Increased BMR
Proteins	↓ Synthesis, ↓ degradation, ↓ turnover (% BW as protein will ↓)	Protein anabolic	↑ Synthesis, ↑ degradation, ↑ turnover (catabolic if insufficient dietary protein)
Lipids	↓ Synthesis, ↓ degradation, ↓ turnover (% BW as lipid increases), ↓ serum cholesterol	↑ Beta oxidation, ↑ lipolysis, ↑ lipogenesis	↑ Synthesis, ↑ degradation, ↑ turnover (% of BW as lipid decreases), ↓ serum cholesterol
Glucose	Normal	Normal	Normal serum glucose; abnormal glucose tolerance test
Glycogen	↓ Synthesis, ↓ degradation, ↓ turnover, glycogen accumulates	—	↑ Synthesis, ↑ degradation, ↑ turnover; glycogen is depleted
Actions with SNS	—	—	Excess mimics effects of ↑ β-adrenergic stimulation; can ↑ number and affinity of β-receptors and ↑ adenylyl cyclase sensitivity
Direct cardiovascular actions	↓ Amplitude of ECG waves	↑ HR, ↑ CO, ↑ contractility, ↑ pulse pressure, ↑ actin and myosin	↑ Amplitude of ECG waves

From Porterfield SP, White BA: *Endocrine physiology,* ed 3, Philadelphia, 2007, Mosby, p 155.
BMR, Basal metabolic rate; *BW,* body weight; *CO,* cardiac output; *ECG,* electrocardiogram; *HR,* heart rate; *SNS,* sympathetic nervous system.

STEROID HORMONES

Steroid Hormone Synthesis and Secretion

The adrenal glands are located atop the kidneys and are composed of an inner medulla and an outer cortex. The adrenal medulla secretes epinephrine and norepinephrine in response to sympathetic nervous system stimulation and is discussed in Chapter 40. The hormones produced by the adrenal cortex are called **steroids** and include (1) glucocorticoids (cortisol), (2) mineralocorticoids (aldosterone), and (3) sex steroids (DHEAS, androgen).[13,14] The synthesis and secretion of these hormones, especially cortisol, are considered essential for life, regulating the body's response to normal and abnormal levels of physiologic and psychological stress. The activities of these three hormones can be remembered as regulating the "three S's": sugar, salt, and sex.

The adrenal cortex has distinct zones that differ in histologic appearance, hormonal regulation, and enzyme pathways available for steroid synthesis (Figure 39-15). The outer *zona glomerulosa* produces the mineralocorticoid (aldosterone) in response to stimulation by AII. The middle *zona fasciculata* produces the glucocorticoid (cortisol) in response to stimulation by ACTH from the pituitary gland.[14] The inner *zona reticularis* is adjacent to the adrenal medulla and produces the androgen (DHEAS). All of these hormones are synthesized from cholesterol, and some of the cholesterol-derived precursors feed enzymatic pathways in all three zones (Figure 39-16) This is an important concept because it explains why an enzyme deficiency in one pathway (e.g., cortisol synthesis) may lead to an overproduction in another pathway (e.g., DHEAS) as precursors are shunted. This is what happens in a disorder called *congenital adrenal hyperplasia* (see Chapter 40).

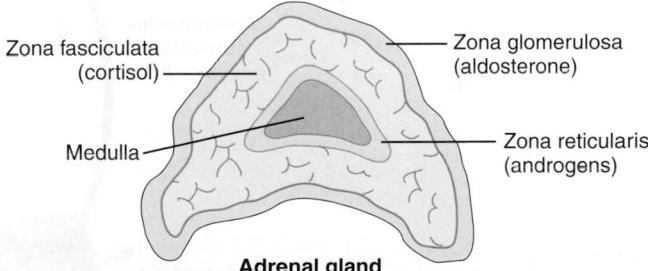

FIGURE 39-15 The adrenal gland is composed of the adrenal medulla at the innermost core, surrounded by the cortex. The adrenal cortex is composed of three anatomically and physiologically distinct layers: the zona glomerulosa, the zona fasciculata, and the zona reticularis. Each zone produces a different adrenocortical hormone.

As previously noted, steroid hormones are lipid-soluble and diffuse from the adrenocortical cells as they are synthesized, so they are made on demand and not stored in the cells. The stimulus for both cortisol and androgen synthesis and secretion is ACTH, whereas aldosterone synthesis and secretion is under control of AII (Figure 39-17). The activity of aldosterone synthase, the enzyme that performs the last step to produce aldosterone, is stimulated by AII binding to G_q receptors on adrenocortical cells in the zona glomerulosa.[6]

Steroid Action on Target Cells

Steroid hormones travel in the circulation bound to proteins, including corticosteroid-binding globulin (transcortin) and albumin. Cortisol

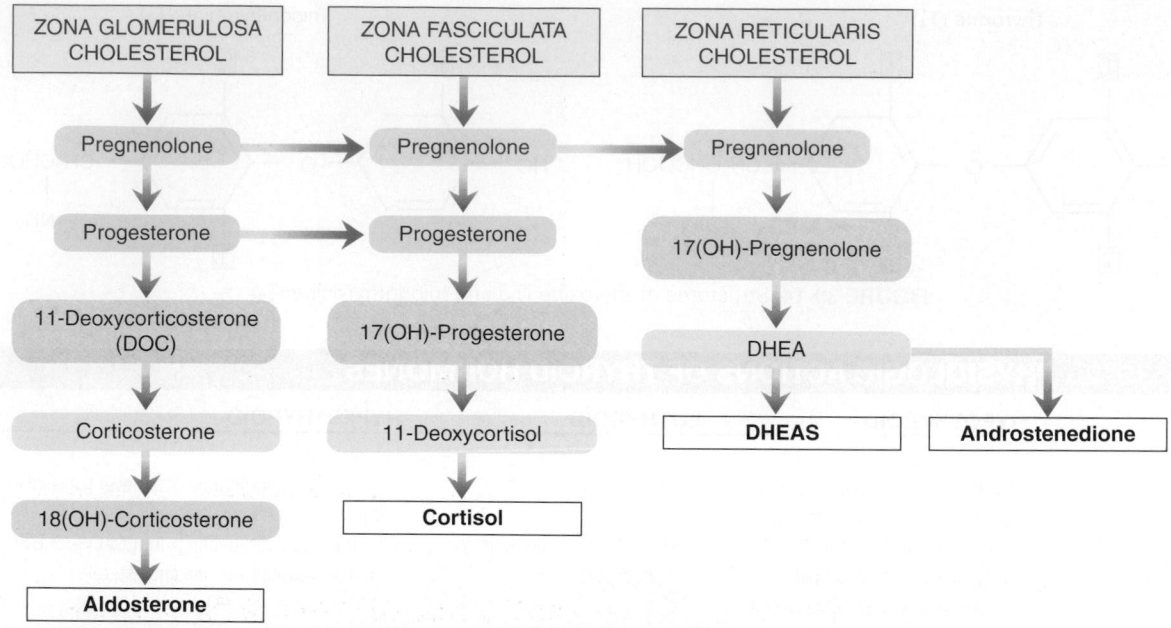

FIGURE 39-16 Adrenal cortex steroid hormone synthesis. Steroid hormones are synthesized from cholesterol and have some common precursors. *DHEAS,* Dehydroepiandrosterone.

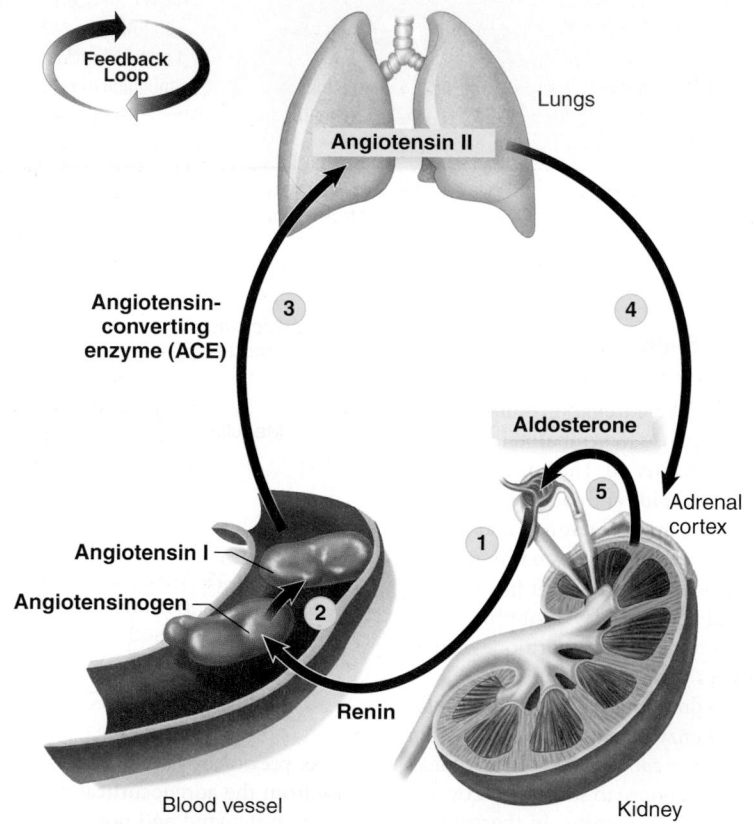

FIGURE 39-17 Renin-angiotensin mechanism for regulating aldosterone secretion. *(1)* When the incoming blood pressure in the kidneys drops below a certain level, the juxtaglomerular apparatus secretes **renin** into the blood. *(2)* Renin, an enzyme, causes angiotensinogen (a normal constituent of blood) to be converted to angiotensin I. *(3)* Angiotensin I circulates to the lungs, where converting enzymes in the capillaries split the molecule, forming angiotensin II. *(4)* Angiotensin II circulates to the adrenal cortex, where it stimulates the secretion of aldosterone. *(5)* Aldosterone causes increased reabsorption of sodium, which causes increased water retention. As water is retained, the volume of blood increases. The increased volume of blood creates higher blood pressure, which then causes the renin secretion to stop. (From Patton KT, Thibodeau GA: *Anatomy & physiology,* ed 7, St Louis, 2010, Mosby, p 561.)

BOX 39-2 BIOLOGIC ACTIONS OF CORTISOL

Hyperglycemic
Gluconeogenic
Lipolytic
Protein catabolic
Insulin antagonist in muscle and adipose tissue
Inhibits bone formation, stimulates bone resorption
Necessary for vascular response to catecholamines
Antiinflammatory
Suppresses immune system
Inhibits antidiuretic hormone secretion and action
Stimulates gastric acid secretion
Necessary for integrity and function of gastrointestinal tract
Stimulates red blood cell production
Alters mood and behavior
Permissive for calorigenic, lipolytic effects of catecholamines

Adapted from Porterfield SP, White BA: *Endocrine physiology,* ed 3, Philadelphia, 2007, Mosby, p 175.

- Steroids diffuse through their target cell membranes and bind with their respective cytoplasmic (or nuclear) receptors. The hormone-receptor complex rapidly translocates into the nucleus where it binds to specific DNA sequences to alter responsive genes. More rapid actions of steroid hormones have been noted and are mediated by cell membrane–associated receptors.
- Cortisol affects nearly every tissue in the body and exhibits a broad range of effects on metabolism including increasing plasma glucose level, regulating immune and inflammatory reactions, and inhibiting bone and collagen synthesis. Cortisol is an important hormone in the response to acute and chronic stress.
- Aldosterone secretion increases in response to low blood pressure and reduced perfusion of the kidney, which stimulate the renin-angiotensin-aldosterone cascade. Aldosterone increases sodium and water reabsorption in the distal tubule of the kidney and promotes the excretion of potassium in the urine.

and androgens bind tightly with their binding proteins, but aldosterone does not and has a shorter half-life in the circulation. Steroids have long been known to diffuse through their target cell membranes and bind with their respective cytoplasmic receptors, and then the hormone-receptor complex rapidly translocates into the nucleus. The complex binds to specific DNA sequences to alter responsive genes. In addition to this classic pathway, steroid hormones may also bind to receptors already located in the nucleus or to cell membrane–associated receptors. Membrane-associated receptors mediate more rapid changes in cell function than the classic DNA-binding pathway.

Glucocorticoids, principally cortisol, are named for their primary effect on glucose metabolism. Cortisol affects nearly every tissue in the body and exhibits a broad range of manifestations (Box 39-2). Glucocorticoids oppose the effects of insulin and raise the blood glucose level. This is accomplished by decreasing glucose uptake by many body cells, and increasing glucose synthesis in the liver from glycogen and amino acid and glycerol substrates in protein and fat stores. Glucocorticoids also contribute to protein catabolism by releasing muscle stores of proteins, providing amino acids for glucose production in the liver. Glucocorticoids promote lipolysis and increased blood cholesterol level. Glucocorticoids protect against the damaging physiologic effects of stress (see Chapter 2) and regulate the inflammatory and immune responses.[13,14]

Mineralocorticoids, principally aldosterone, function to maintain normal salt and water balance by promoting sodium retention and potassium excretion at the distal renal tubules. Aldosterone production is regulated primarily by the renin-angiotensin system associated with the juxtaglomerular cells of the kidney in response to a reduction in renal perfusion, and by a high serum potassium level (see Chapter 26).

KEY POINTS

- The hormones produced by the adrenal cortex are called steroids and include (1) glucocorticoids (cortisol), (2) mineralocorticoids (aldosterone), and (3) sex steroids (androgens).
- The adrenal cortex has distinct zones. The outer *zona glomerulosa* produces aldosterone, in response to stimulation by AII. The middle *zona fasciculata* produces cortisol in response to stimulation of ACTH from the pituitary gland. The inner *zona reticularis* is adjacent to the adrenal medulla and produces androgens.

CATEGORIES OF ENDOCRINE DISEASE

Endocrine pathologic processes can be divided into three general categories: disorders of hyposecretion, hypersecretion, and target cell hyporesponsiveness. These are discussed in relation to specific endocrine diseases in Chapter 40.

Hyposecretion

Primary hyposecretion occurs when an endocrine gland, such as the thyroid or adrenal cortex, releases an inadequate amount of hormone to meet physiologic needs. Secondary hyposecretion occurs when secretion of a tropic hormone, such as TSH or ACTH, is inadequate to cause the target gland to secrete adequate amounts of hormone. The diagnosis of hormone deficiency is complex because knowledge of tropic and releasing hormone levels, as well as the deficient hormone level, is necessary. For example, in a *primary* thyroid hormone deficiency (common), serum thyroid hormone level would be low but TSH levels would be high because the anterior pituitary gland would not be receiving negative feedback from thyroid hormone. However, in *secondary* thyroid hormone deficiency (rare), both thyroid hormone and TSH concentrations would be abnormally low.

Hypersecretion

Hypersecretion disorders can also be either primary or secondary.[14] When a diseased endocrine gland secretes an abnormally high amount of its hormone, the tropic pituitary hormone will be at an unusually low plasma level because of excessive negative feedback. Alternatively, if hypersecretion is secondary to elevated tropic hormone levels (rare), the plasma concentration of both hormones will be elevated. For example, in Cushing disease, the pituitary gland becomes hyperactive and oversecretes ACTH, which induces the adrenal cortex to produce too much cortisol (causing symptoms of cortisol excess). Excessive plasma hormone levels can also occur from hormone secretion by an ectopic source, as sometimes occurs with malignancies.

Hyporesponsiveness

Hyporesponsiveness (hormone resistance) of the target tissues will cause the same set of clinical symptoms as hyposecretion. The usual reason for hyporesponsiveness is lack of or a deficiency in cellular receptors, although postreceptor mechanisms such as second-messenger dysfunction can also cause decreased cellular response. If the target cell does not have appropriate receptors for a hormone, the clinical symptoms will be the same as if inadequate hormone levels were reaching the target cells. However, plasma concentrations of hormone would be expected to be normal or high because of the lack of negative feedback to hormone-secreting organs. Nephrogenic diabetes insipidus is an example of kidney tubule resistance to the effect of ADH because of defective receptors on the tubular cells.[15] Some forms of diabetes mellitus also are characterized by tissue resistance to the effects of insulin (see Chapter 41).

> **KEY POINTS**
> - Endocrine disorders occur because of hyposecretion, hypersecretion, or lack of responsiveness by target cells. Hyporesponsiveness is clinically similar to hyposecretion and usually results from a lack of functional receptors or a defect in postreceptor signaling.
> - Endocrine disorders may be due to abnormal tropic signals from the pituitary gland (secondary disorder) or to dysfunction of target glands (primary disorder).

SUMMARY

The endocrine system, together with the nervous system, is responsible for coordination of cellular activity between many body systems and organs. Hormone secretion occurs in response to a variety of stimuli, including psychological or physiologic stress, electrolyte and metabolite levels, and normal circadian cycles. Increases or decreases in the quantity of a particular circulating hormone tend to regulate levels of that hormone through negative feedback mechanisms. The cellular responses to hormones are complex and controlled by many other factors in addition to the circulating hormone levels.

REFERENCES

1. Porterfield SP, White BA: Introduction to the endocrine system. In Porterfield SP, White BA, editors: *Endocrine physiology*, ed 3, Philadelphia, 2007, Mosby, pp 1–24.
2. Koeppen BM, Stanton BA: The male and female reproductive systems. In Koeppen BM, Stanton BA, editors: *Berne & Levy physiology*, ed 6, Philadelphia, 2010, Mosby, pp 758–798.
3. Alberts B, et al: Mechanisms of cell communication. In Alberts B, et al, editors: *Molecular biology of the cell*, ed 5, New York, 2008, Garland Science, pp 879–964.
4. Hall JE: Introduction to endocrinology. In Hall JE, editor: *Guyton and Hall textbook of medical physiology*, ed 12, Philadelphia, 2011, Saunders, pp 881–906.
5. Van der Deure WM, Peeters RP, Visser TJ: Molecular aspects of thyroid hormone transporters, including MCT8, MCT10 and OATPs, and the effects of genetic variation in these transporters, *J Mol Endocrinol* 44:1–11, 2010.
6. Porterfield SP, White BA: The adrenal gland. In Porterfield SP, White BA, editors: *Endocrine physiology*, ed 3, Philadelphia, 2007, Mosby, pp 163–196.
7. Koeppen BM, Stanton BA: The thyroid gland. In Koeppen BM, Stanton BA, editors: *Berne & Levy physiology*, ed 6, Philadelphia, 2010, Mosby, pp 725–737.
8. Porterfield SP, White BA: The thyroid gland. In Porterfield SP, White BA, editors: *Endocrine physiology*, ed 3, Philadelphia, 2007, Mosby, pp 141–162.
9. Koeppen BM, Stanton BA: The hypothalamus and pituitary gland. In Koeppen BM, Stanton BA, editors: *Berne & Levy physiology*, ed 6, Philadelphia, 2010, Mosby, pp 706–724.
10. Porterfield SP, White BA: The hypothalamus-pituitary complex. In Porterfield SP, White BA, editors: *Endocrine physiology*, ed 3, Philadelphia, 2007, Mosby, pp 107–140.
11. Costanzo LS: Reproductive physiology. In Costanzo LS, editor: *Physiology*, ed 3, Philadelphia, 2006, Saunders, pp 441–462.
12. Patton KT, Thibodeau GA: Endocrine system. In Patton KT, Thibodeau GA, editors: *Anatomy and physiology*, ed 7, St Louis, 2010, Mosby, pp 533–580.
13. Hall JE: Adrenocortical hormones. In Hall JE, editor: *Guyton and Hall textbook of medical physiology*, ed 12, Philadelphia, 2011, Saunders, pp 921–938.
14. Koeppen BM, Stanton BA: The adrenal gland. In Koeppen BM, Stanton BA, editors: *Berne & Levy physiology*, ed 6, Philadelphia, 2010, Mosby, pp 738–757.
15. Ball SG: Vasopressin and disorders of water balance: the physiology and pathophysiology of vasopressin, *Ann Clin Biochem* 44(pt 5):417–431, 2007.

Disorders of Endocrine Function

Jacquelyn L. Banasik

evolve WEBSITE

KEY QUESTIONS

- How can primary and secondary endocrine disorders be differentiated?
- What etiologic factors would lead to clinical manifestations of hormone excess or deficiency?

- What are the etiologic factors, clinical findings, and management of excess and deficiency of the following endocrine hormones: growth hormone, thyroid hormone, adrenocortical hormones, adrenal medullary hormones, parathyroid hormone, and antidiuretic hormone?

CHAPTER OUTLINE

Together with the nervous system, the endocrine system (the glands and the hormones they secrete) regulates body processes involving growth, maturation, metabolic functions, fluid balance, responses to stress, and reproduction.[1,2] This regulation is carried out through the actions of the hormones produced and secreted by the endocrine cells. **Endocrine hormones** are chemical messengers that travel through the bloodstream to exert physiologic effects on specific target cells and tissues. In the healthy state, hormones are released by endocrine glands when their action is needed and inhibited when their effect is attained.

Endocrine disease is marked by either hyperfunction (excessively high blood concentrations of a hormone, or conditions that mimic high hormone levels) or hypofunction (depressed levels, or conditions that mimic low hormone levels). Some endocrine disorders have such striking characteristics that recognition is obvious. Other symptoms of endocrine disease may be nonspecific and more difficult to detect. Observing and interviewing skills are important because, with the exception of the thyroid and testicles, the endocrine glands cannot be directly examined. Laboratory diagnostic tests are especially important in assessing the endocrine system.

This chapter describes alterations in the anterior pituitary regulatory system, including growth hormone, thyroid hormone, and adrenal hormones, as well as parathyroid hormone disorders and posterior pituitary disorders of antidiuretic hormone (vasopressin) secretion. Disorders of prolactin and the gonadotropins (follicle-stimulating hormone and luteinizing hormone) are discussed in Unit IX. Disorders of insulin secretion are discussed in Chapter 41.

BASIC CONCEPTS OF ENDOCRINE DISORDERS

Etiology of Endocrine Disorders

Dysfunction, either hyposecretion or hypersecretion, may originate in the hypothalamus/pituitary, the hormone-producing gland, or the target tissue (Figure 40-1). The etiology of endocrine disorders may be congenital, infectious, autoimmune, neoplastic, idiopathic, or iatrogenic. The onset of the disorders can be slow and insidious or abrupt and life threatening. The age at onset may range from birth to old age.

Abnormal hormone production occasionally results from an inborn genetic defect. Such defects may cause excessive production of hormone precursors because of an enzymatic block in the synthetic pathway, and enzyme deficiencies that impair hormone synthesis. An important example is congenital adrenal hyperplasia in which infants develop enlarged adrenal glands, but have a deficiency of cortisol production. If genetic defects do not cause a complete block of synthesis, increased pituitary stimulus may compensate by causing glandular hyperplasia, resulting in near-normal hormone levels.

Autoimmune disorders commonly cause endocrine dysfunction, particularly in women. The pathogenesis of autoimmunity is incompletely understood, but involves both a genetic predisposition and an environmental trigger (see Chapter 10). Antibodies are produced against certain antigens on self tissue cells, resulting either in hyperfunction of the endocrine gland (e.g., hyperthyroidism of Graves disease) or in immune destruction of the gland, eventually leading to hypofunction (e.g., adrenal insufficiency of Addison disease).

Hormones may be produced by abnormal tissue sites. Such *ectopic* hormone production is usually associated with a malignant tumor. Although different tumors can produce hormones, some cell types are more commonly associated with specific tumors. For example, some lung tumors produce antidiuretic hormone (ADH), leading to water intoxication and hyponatremia. Endocrine disorders can also be classified as functional disorders caused by nonendocrine disease such as chronic renal failure, liver disease, or heart failure.

In some cases endocrine disease occurs when the target tissue fails to respond to a hormone. The presence of normal or elevated hormone levels without normal hormonal action indicates target tissue resistance. This problem is also demonstrated by diminished or absent response to the administration of exogenous hormones. The mechanisms of hormone resistance may be genetic or acquired and may include defects at receptor sites, antibody reaction to hormone receptors, and defective postreceptor hormone action.

Finally, some endocrine disorders may be induced by medical treatments, such as therapy for a nonendocrine disorder. These iatrogenic disorders can be caused by chemotherapy, radiation therapy, or surgical removal of glands. Commonly, a treatment for endocrine hyperfunction involves removal or destruction of glandular tissue with resultant chronic hypofunction. Long-term hormone replacement therapy may then be needed.

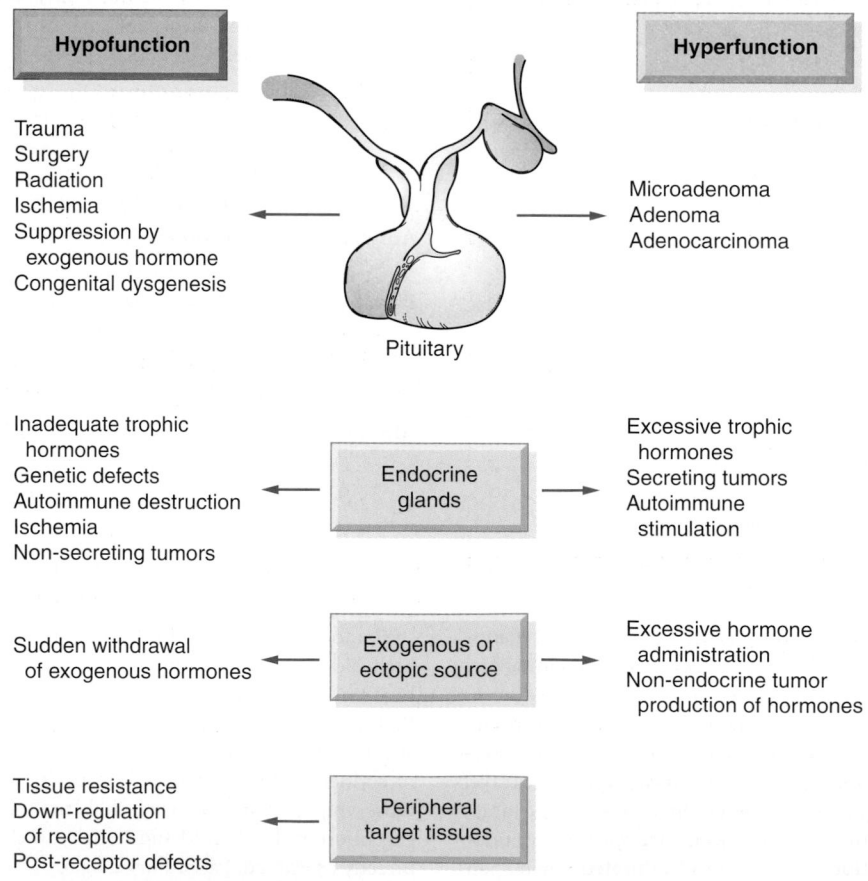

FIGURE 40-1 Common etiologies of endocrine disorders.

Classification of Endocrine Disorders

Endocrine disorders involving control by the anterior pituitary gland commonly are classified as *primary* (intrinsic malfunction of the hormone-producing target gland) or *secondary* (malfunction of the hypothalamus/pituitary cells that control the hormone-producing target gland). The clinical presentation of an endocrine disorder of primary or secondary etiology is similar; however, diagnosing the source of the problem may be important in determining the best treatment. Measurement of serum concentrations of pituitary and target gland hormones allows differentiation between primary and secondary endocrine etiologies.

Clinically useful laboratory measures are available for diagnosing and monitoring hormone disorders including those affecting thyroid and adrenal function. Laboratory diagnosis is based on an understanding of the feedback loop communication between the hypothalamic-pituitary system and the target gland. When the *primary* gland fails, inadequate hormone is produced and low levels of hormone are present in the circulation, but blood levels of the corresponding trophic pituitary hormone become very elevated (Figure 40-2). For example, in primary hypothyroidism, the thyroid fails to secrete thyroid hormones and serum levels of thyroxine (T_4) become lower. Thyroid-stimulating hormone (TSH) levels rise as the pituitary gland attempts to stimulate the malfunctioning thyroid. In contrast, in secondary hypothyroidism, the pituitary gland fails to release TSH, secondarily reducing thyroid gland production, so both thyroxine and TSH levels are abnormally low in the circulation. It is important to recall that the hormones released by the target gland are the ones that produce clinical signs and symptoms and that they are the starting point for interpretation of laboratory test results.

KEY POINTS

- Endocrine disorders occur because of hypersecretion, hyposecretion, or nonresponsiveness by target cells.
- *Hypersecretion* is usually due to secreting tumors, autoimmune disease, or excessive stimulation of the gland by trophic signals.
- *Hyposecretion* may be due to failure or congenital absence of glandular tissue, autoimmune destruction, surgical removal of the gland, or lack of normal trophic signals.
- *Hyporesponsiveness* is clinically similar to hyposecretion and is due to target tissue dysfunction. This phenomenon is called *tissue resistance*.
- Endocrine disorders involving the hypothalamic-pituitary system are often classified as primary or secondary.
- Primary endocrine disorders result from intrinsic defects within the hormone-secreting gland.
- Secondary disorders result from abnormal hypothalamic-pituitary secretion of trophic signals. Manifestations of an endocrine disorder are due to abnormal target gland function and are therefore similar whether the etiologic classification is primary or secondary.

GROWTH HORMONE DISORDERS

Growth hormone (GH) is produced in the anterior pituitary gland under the influence of hypothalamic releasing (growth hormone–releasing hormone) and inhibiting (somatostatin) factors. Its primary target organ is the liver, but GH also has direct effects on several tissue types. In general, GH increases lean body mass, reduces fat mass, and induces the liver to release glucose under conditions of hypoglycemia. Many of the effects of GH are mediated by a peptide called IGF-1 (insulin-like growth factor-1) that is released from the liver when stimulated by GH. Please refer to

Chapter 39 for details of GH synthesis, regulation, and activity. The major signs and symptoms of GH imbalance are summarized in Box 40-1.

Growth Hormone Deficiency

Etiology and pathogenesis. Deficiencies in GH secretion can be classified into several major categories: (1) decreased GH secretion, (2) defective GH action (structurally abnormal GH or defective GH receptor), and (3) defective IGF-1 (somatomedin) generation.

Growth hormone deficiency is most clinically relevant in children. A birth history of prolonged labor or breech delivery is common, but GH deficiency may also be present in children who are born with midline craniocerebral defects, most likely attributable to congenital malformations or as sequelae of a chromosomal anomaly. Deficiencies in

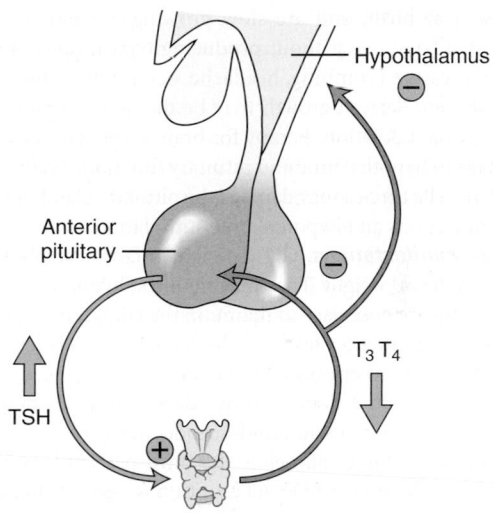

FIGURE 40-2 Diagnosing endocrine disorders as primary or secondary is based on the hypothalamic-pituitary and target tissue feedback loops. In this example, the low T_3 and T_4 levels are indicative of hypothyroidism. The elevated TSH level indicates that the pituitary gland is responding appropriately and is not the source of the hypothyroidism. A diagnosis of primary hypothyroidism would be made on the basis of these laboratory results.

BOX 40-1	SIGNS AND SYMPTOMS OF GROWTH HORMONE IMBALANCE	
GROWTH HORMONE EXCESS		**GROWTH HORMONE DEFICIENCY**
Children		
Increased linear growth and tall stature		Delayed growth
		Fine features
		Short stature, proportionate
Adults		
Soft-tissue hyperplasia		May be associated with hyposecretion
Increased bone density		of other pituitary hormones
Large hands, feet		
Coarse facial features		
Thick, leathery skin		
Weight gain		
Glucose intolerance		

GH and other pituitary hormones should be considered in any child with nystagmus, retinal abnormalities, and other midline or midfacial abnormalities, such as cleft lip or palate. The association between GH deficiency and other midline abnormalities appears to occur because the pituitary gland is developing during the same stage of fetal life as the other midline structures.

Children with GH deficiency have a variety of presentations, depending on the cause of the deficiency, the age at onset, and the severity of the disorder. The basis for this defect may be failure of the hypothalamus to stimulate pituitary GH secretion or failure of the pituitary to produce GH.

The most common tumors to influence hypothalamic-pituitary function are midline brain tumors. These include gliomas of the optic nerve and craniopharyngiomas. Craniopharyngiomas arise from cells at the junction of the anterior and posterior pituitary gland, are believed to be present at birth, and are slow growing. Craniopharyngiomas may grow to a large size without producing typical signs of increased intracranial pressure (vomiting, headache, oculomotor abnormalities). In older children, delayed growth may be the first symptom of a craniopharyngioma. Radiation therapy for brain tumors or leukemia may cause damage to hypothalamic and pituitary function. Traumatic insult to the skull or sella turcica may damage the pituitary gland, interrupting vascular connections and hypothalamic stimulation.

Clinical manifestations. GH-deficient infants usually have normal birth length and weight. They may manifest hypoglycemia because GH and cortisol are necessary to maintain the euglycemic state. Hypoglycemia may present after fasting, which could be as brief as 3 hours in an infant. Recurrent episodes of hypoglycemia may lead to seizures and permanent cerebral damage. Boys developing GH deficiency in utero may have micropenis and undescended testicles.

GH-deficient children fall below the third percentile of growth in comparison with their peers. Dental eruption is delayed, and the development and setting of the permanent teeth are irregular. The hair is thin, and the nail growth is poor. Older children have greater fat mass and decreased muscle mass, with delayed bone formation. Delayed puberty is common if other anterior pituitary hormones are also affected.

Children's growth should be evaluated annually. If growth velocity is abnormal, an endocrinologic evaluation and physiologic tests to stimulate GH release can be planned. Many pharmacologic agents are available that stimulate GH secretion in children, including insulin, arginine, levodopa, and clonidine. Children's neurosecretory GH patterns can be studied by obtaining timed serum GH samples during a normal nighttime sleep cycle.

Treatment. Hormonal replacement therapy for GH-deficient children has been available for several decades. The most obvious effect of GH replacement is stimulation of linear growth in children whose bones have not fused. With treatment, children experience an increase in growth velocity as well as depletion of the excess fat stores noted in GH-deficient children.

Acquired GH deficiency in adults has only recently been recognized and treatment approved by the Food and Drug Administration.[3] Adults may become GH deficient after resection of pituitary tumors or after traumatic head injuries. There is controversy regarding the manifestations of GH deficiency acquired in adulthood. There appears to be increased mortality attributable to cardiovascular causes when adults do not receive GH replacement following pituitary damage. GH-deficient adults may have diminished lean body mass, hypercholesterolemia, and decreased bone density.

Growth Hormone Excess

Etiology and pathogenesis. GH excess is nearly always due to uncontrolled production of the hormone by a benign somatotropic tumor in the pituitary gland adenoma. GH stimulates the liver to produce IGF-1, and these two hormones act in concert to cause up-regulated growth of soft and bony tissues. Because GH secretion varies significantly over the course of the day, the serum level of IGF-1, which is more stable, may be measured as an indicator of GH secretion. An elevated IGF-1 level is a useful indicator of GH hypersecretion. If the tumor presents in childhood before the skeletal epiphyses are closed, rapid growth results in *pituitary giantism*. These children experience markedly accelerated growth velocity and quickly exceed the 95th percentile on pediatric growth charts. When the disorder is allowed to progress untreated, some of these children may grow to 8 feet or more in height and usually suffer an early cardiovascular death related to cardiomegaly and heart failure.

In adults, GH excess is called *acromegaly* and may be clinically subtle. Acromegaly occurs with equal frequency in men and women during the fourth and fifth decades of life. After the skeletal epiphyses close, bony growth increases bone density and thickening of the short bones, such as the hands and feet.

Clinical manifestations of acromegaly. Patients usually notice increased ring and shoe size, which progressively advances over several years. Enlargement of the frontal sinus causes a prominent brow, and growth of the mandible results in progressive underbite *(prognathism)* (Figure 40-3). Soft tissues also slowly hypertrophy, causing coarsening of facial features and skin tags. Internal organs increase in size, resulting in goiter (thyroid enlargement) and cardiomegaly. Other manifestations include deepening of the voice secondary to vocal cord thickening and enlargement of the tongue, resulting in sleep apnea. Colonic polyps become more common, with the potential for malignant degeneration. It is estimated that the average patient with acromegaly has an active pituitary tumor for 7 or more years before seeking evaluation. Most often the changes are attributed by the patient and his or her family as "just growing older." Abnormalities in bone and soft-tissue growth are mostly irreversible. Patients may develop symptoms of increased intracranial pressure if the pituitary tumor enlarges significantly, including headache and visual disturbances. Some patients may develop glucose intolerance or hyperglycemia, and GH has been called a *diabetogenic* hormone for this reason.

Treatment. Effective therapy for acromegaly involves surgically removing the tumor while counteracting the effects of excess GH. Octreotide, a synthetic form of somatostatin, suppresses production of GH. Surgery is usually performed using a transsphenoidal approach, but often the tumor is too large to completely resect. Radiation may be used postoperatively in these cases.

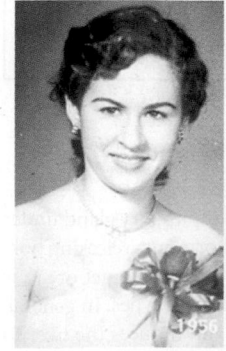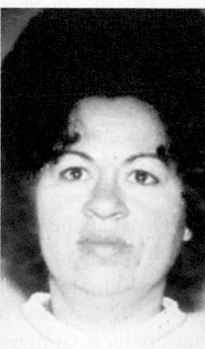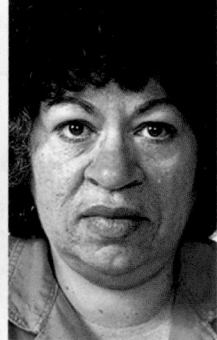

FIGURE 40-3 Progressive development of facial features of acromegaly. (From Lewis SM et al: *Medical-surgical nursing*, ed 8, St Louis, 2011, Mosby. Courtesy Linda Haas, Seattle, WA.)

THYROID HORMONE DISORDERS

Secretion of the thyroid hormones, triiodothyronine (T_3) and thyroxine (T_4), is under control of thyroid-stimulating hormone (TSH) secretion from the anterior pituitary gland. In turn, TSH secretion from the pituitary is under control of thyroid-releasing hormone (TRH) from the hypothalamus. Thyroid hormones are important for normal growth and development of tissues throughout the body and an important regulator of metabolism. The details of thyroid hormone synthesis, regulation, and activity are described in Chapter 39.

Hypothyroidism

Etiology and pathogenesis. Hypothyroidism may be congenital in origin or acquired later in life. The great majority of cases of hypothyroidism are primary, due to intrinsic dysfunction of the thyroid gland. Congenital hypothyroidism may result from a variety of causes. Thyroid dysgenesis (lack of thyroid gland development) accounts for most of the cases of congenital hypothyroidism. Abnormal TSH receptors and defective synthesis of thyroid hormone are other mechanisms causing congenital hypothyroidism.[4] Congenital hypothyroidism that results in significant defects in mental and physical development may be referred to as cretinism.

Lymphocytic thyroiditis (Hashimoto thyroiditis, or autoimmune thyroiditis) is the most common cause of acquired hypothyroidism. Lymphocytic thyroiditis is characterized by an enlarged thyroid gland (Figure 40-4) caused by lymphocytic infiltration. Thyroid hormone production decreases, stimulating the release of TSH from the pituitary gland and resulting in elevated serum TSH levels. Hypothyroidism and its clinical symptoms progress as the gland becomes fibrotic.

Other causes of acquired hypothyroidism include irradiation of the thyroid gland, surgical removal of thyroid tissue, and iodine deficiency. Iodine is essential for the formation of T_4 and T_3. Lack of iodine prevents production of both T_4 and T_3 but does not stop the formation of thyroglobulin. As a result, insufficient hormone is available to inhibit production of TSH by the anterior pituitary gland. The elevated TSH level then causes the thyroid cells to secrete excessive amounts of thyroglobulin (colloid) into the follicles, and the gland grows larger and larger, producing a **goiter** (see Figure 40-4). An enlarged thyroid (goiter) is not always associated with hypothyroidism and can be present in euthyroid and hyperthyroid states.

Some foods contain "goitrogenic" substances that interfere with thyroid hormone synthesis. Such goitrogenic substances occur in some varieties of turnips and cabbage, but the clinical significance of these goitrogens is considered to be minimal. The drug lithium inhibits thyroid hormone synthesis and secretion and causes hypothyroidism in up to 20% of patients.[5]

Secondary hypothyroidism is caused by defects in TSH production and is uncommon. Individuals who have been exposed to severe head trauma, cranial neoplasms, brain infections, cranial irradiation, and neurosurgery can be left with secondary hypothyroidism.

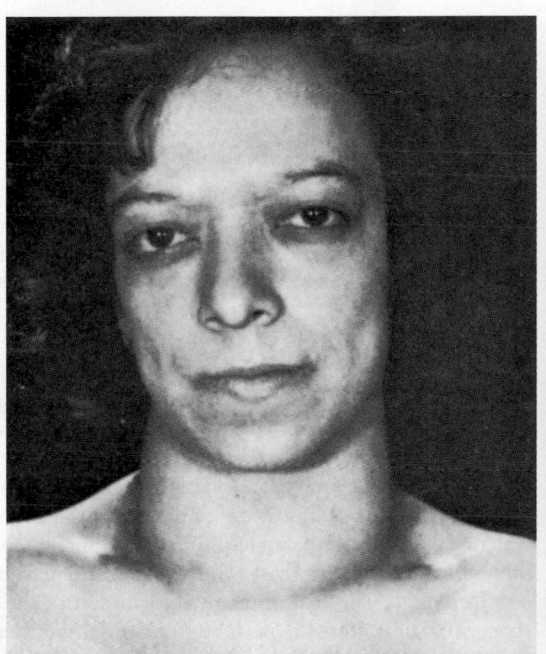
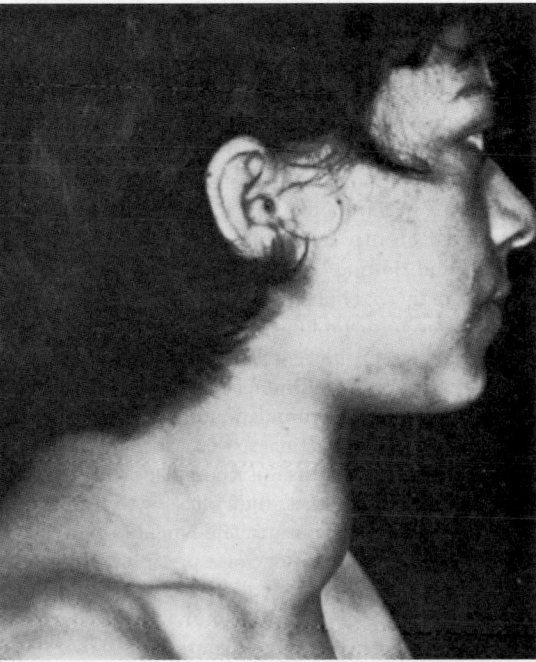

FIGURE 40-4 An enlarged thyroid gland (goiter) can be present in hypothyroid, hyperthyroid, and euthyroid states. Note enlargement at the base of the neck. (From Wilson JD, Foster DW, editors: *Williams textbook of endocrinology*, ed 8, Philadelphia, 1992, Saunders, p 425.)

BOX 40-2 TYPICAL SIGNS AND SYMPTOMS OF THYROID IMBALANCE

HYPERTHYROIDISM	HYPOTHYROIDISM
Sleeplessness, nervousness	Lethargy
Muscle weakness, fatigue	Weakness
Susceptibility to infection	Dry, pale, cool, coarse skin
Skin texture warm, silky, damp	Cold intolerance
Heat intolerance	Weight gain
Increased appetite with weight loss	Constipation
Increased gastric emptying, increased intestinal motility	Bradycardia, wide pulse pressure
Tachycardia, narrow pulse pressure, palpitations, angina	Dyspnea, chest pain
Dyspnea	Thyroid may be diffusely enlarged (goiter) or may not be palpable
Enlarged thyroid, may be diffuse or nodular	Hair coarse
Hair silky, nail loose or detached from nail bed	Sluggish return of reflexes; mental impairment: slowed cognitive ability, poor memory, forgetfulness, depressed affect; deafness (in one third of population)
Hyperreflexia, fine tremor	Facial edema (especially periorbital); thinned lateral aspect of eyebrows
Eye symptoms: burning, tearing, diplopia, lid lag, prominent eyes (exophthalmia with Graves disease), stare, eyelid tremors when closed	Heavy, prolonged menses; infertility; decreased libido
Absence of forehead wrinkling on upward gaze	
Decreased or absent menses	

Clinical manifestations. Routine screening of newborns has resulted in early treatment of most infants with congenital hypothyroidism. Few clinical manifestations are present at birth. In untreated infants, symptoms appear in the first months of life and include a dull appearance; a thick, protuberant tongue; and thick lips (leading to feeding difficulties). Other signs include prolonged neonatal jaundice, poor muscle tone, bradycardia, mottled extremities, umbilical hernia, and a hoarse cry. Thyroid hormone is essential for normal central nervous system development; significant and irreversible intellectual disability will occur unless thyroid hormone replacement therapy is started early in infancy. Older children who acquire hypothyroidism have essentially the same clinical manifestations as seen in adults. In addition, growth retardation, delayed bone development, and delayed or precocious puberty may occur.

In general, individuals with hypothyroidism have decreased basal metabolic rates as the basis for many of their signs and symptoms. Patients report subjective feelings of weakness, lethargy, cold intolerance, and decreased appetite. Bradycardia, narrowed pulse pressure, and mild to moderate weight gain may occur. Elevated levels of serum cholesterol and triglycerides are common as is an increased incidence of atherosclerosis. The thyroid gland may become enlarged (goitrous), the skin may be cool and dry, and constipation may be present. Depression and difficulties with concentration and memory occur. Women with acquired hypothyroidism may experience menstrual irregularities, with increased flow and clotting.[6] Box 40-2 summarizes the general signs and symptoms of thyroid imbalance.

Myxedema occurs in severe or prolonged thyroid deficiency. The term *myxedema* is in reference to the generalized, nonpitting edema that patients with long-term hypothyroidism tend to demonstrate. The edematous-looking skin is from the accumulation of glycosaminoglycans (mucopolysaccharides) in the interstitial spaces, which then retain fluid. Thyroid hormone normally prevents the accumulation of glycosaminoglycans within subcutaneous tissues. Individuals with hypothyroid-induced myxedema usually present in an altered mental state, with alterations in thermoregulation and a history of a precipitating event such as sepsis, trauma, or the use of certain medications.[6] Without medical intervention, patients may lapse into so-called myxedema coma, a medical emergency with significant mortality. Figure 40-5 shows the typical features of patients with myxedema.

The diagnosis of hypothyroidism can be confirmed by measuring serum TSH and thyroid hormone levels. Because the most common

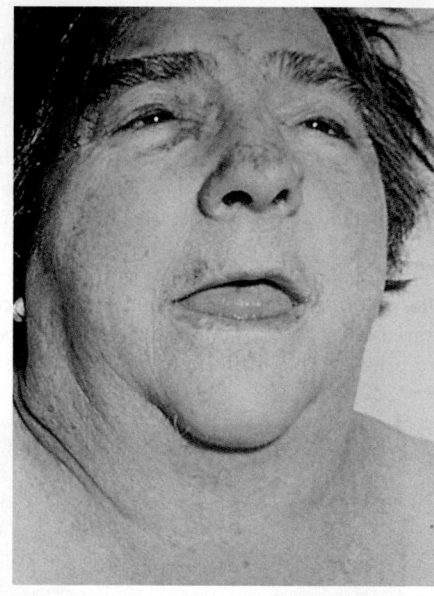

FIGURE 40-5 Typical facial puffiness and dull expression of patients with myxedema. (From Seidel HM et al: *Mosby's guide to physical examination,* ed 6, St Louis, 2006, Mosby. Courtesy Paul W. Ladenson, MD, The Johns Hopkins University and Hospital, Baltimore, MD.)

cause of hypothyroidism is thyroid failure (primary hypothyroidism), nearly all patients will have elevated TSH levels because of the lack of negative feedback exerted by T_3 and T_4.[6] The serum TSH level is a sensitive indicator of thyroid hypoactivity, and an increase in TSH level often is detectable long before many symptoms develop. A decline in T_4 and T_3 levels may not occur until later in the course of disease. In the rare case of hypothalamic-pituitary dysfunction, both serum TSH and serum T_4 concentrations will be inappropriately low (Table 40-1).

Treatment. The goal of treatment is to return the individual with congenital or acquired hypothyroidism and thyroiditis to a euthyroid state. When serum thyroid levels are replaced too quickly, patients may experience insomnia, anxiety, and mood lability. Once treatment has begun, those individuals with a goiter usually experience a regression in glandular enlargement.

TABLE 40-1 THYROID HORMONE LEVELS IN VARIOUS STATES

STATE	SERUM T_4 (µg/dl), RANGE	SERUM T_3 (ng/dl), RANGE	SERUM TSH (µU/ml), RANGE
Euthyroid	4.5-11.5	60-180	0.5-4.5
Infants (<2 wk)	8.0-15.0	—	0.5-4.5
Children (prepubertal)	6.5-11.5	80-220	0.5-4.5
Hyperthyroid	>11.5	—	<0.15
Hypothyroid	<1.0-5.0	—	>5.0

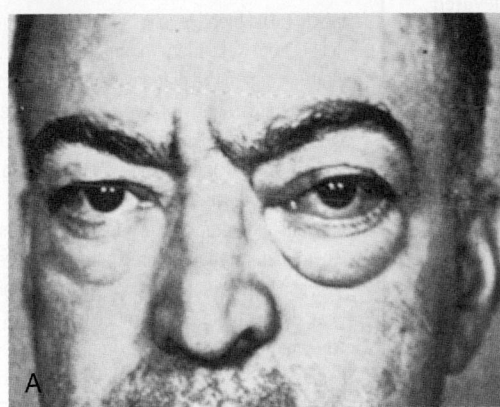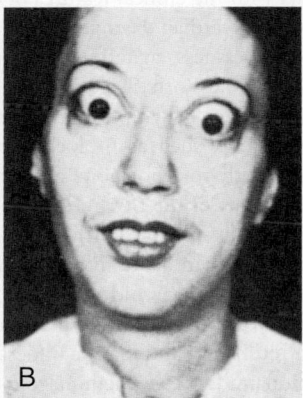

FIGURE 40-6 Patients with the usual ophthalmopathy found in Graves disease. **A,** Patient with periorbital swelling, exophthalmos, and chemosis (edema). **B,** Woman with widening of the palpebral fissures owing to lid retraction and proptosis. (From Larsen PR, Ingbar SH: The thyroid gland. In Wilson JD, Foster DW, editors: *Williams textbook of endocrinology,* ed 8, Philadelphia, 1992, Saunders, p 426.)

Oral levothyroxine is used to replace or supplement hormone production from an underactive thyroid. Patients notice an increase in exercise tolerance, decreased fatigue, and improved mentation with therapy. Resolution of symptoms occurs gradually over weeks. As therapy returns the patient to a "euthyroid" state, the serum TSH level should return to the normal range. Overtreatment with thyroid hormone can be detected by a serum TSH level that is below the normal range. Overtreatment should be avoided in part because it contributes to osteoporosis.

Hyperthyroidism

Etiology and pathogenesis. Mechanisms that produce hyperthyroidism include thyroid follicular cell hyperfunction with increased synthesis and secretion of T_4 and T_3 (e.g., Graves disease); thyroid follicular cell destruction with release of preformed T_4 and T_3 (e.g., Hashimoto thyroiditis); and ingestion of excessive thyroid hormone. The increased serum levels of thyroid hormones increase the metabolic rate (see Table 40-1).

Hyperfunction of thyroid follicular cells can be either autonomous (primary) or mediated through stimulation of TSH receptors by TSH (secondary). Primary hyperfunction can be caused by adenomas and, rarely, thyroid carcinoma. Inflammation of thyroid follicular cells, with release of preformed thyroid hormone, can be associated with viral or autoimmune processes. Examples are the toxic thyroiditis of Hashimoto disease and subacute thyroiditis. Hashimoto thyroiditis typically presents first with hyperthyroid symptoms because the injured thyroid gland releases stored hormone and then progresses to a hypothyroid state when the autoimmune process destroys the gland. Acute or chronic ingestion of thyroid hormone preparations can produce excess levels of thyroid hormones.

The most common etiology of hyperthyroidism is from autoantibodies that bind and stimulate TSH receptors on the thyroid gland.[6]

This stimulation leads to a diffuse toxic goiter and a type of primary hyperthyroidism called **Graves disease.** The etiology of Graves disease is autoimmune, and it has been associated with certain genetic markers (e.g., *HLA B8, HLA DR3*). There is an increased incidence during the second and third decades of life. In response to the high circulating T_3 and T_4 levels that are stimulated by autoantibodies, the pituitary gland stops producing TSH, and serum TSH falls to very low levels.

Clinical manifestations. Symptoms of hyperthyroidism are from an increase in metabolic rate and enhanced sympathetic nervous system activity. Symptoms may be mild to severe and include insomnia, restlessness, tremor, irritability, palpitations, increased heart rate, heat intolerance, diaphoresis, and an inability to concentrate that interferes with work performance (see Box 40-2). Increased basal metabolic rate may result in weight loss, even though appetite and dietary intake increase. In women, amenorrhea or scant menses is a frequent finding. The term thyrotoxicosis is used to describe a hyperthyroid condition that is associated with significant symptoms of the disorder.

Individuals with Graves disease usually present with thyromegaly (diffusely enlarged thyroid), thyrotoxicosis, and, often, **exophthalmos** (enlargement of retro-orbital muscles causing protrusion of the eyes) (Figure 40-6). Spasm and retraction of the eyelids leads to widening of the palpebral fissure, resulting in exposed sclera. Lid lag develops, and severe, progressive exophthalmos may occur. Eye complaints may include vision changes and photophobia. The exophthalmos of Graves disease is not from elevated levels of thyroid hormones but is thought to develop as a result of autoimmune injury to retro-ocular structures. Tissues behind the eye become infiltrated with immune cells, followed by release of inflammatory cytokines that stimulate local cells to secrete excessive glycosaminoglycans. The tissue behind the eye swells and pushes the eyeball forward. Reduction of circulating thyroid hormone levels often does not prevent progression of the exophthalmos.

Undetectable TSH levels are the best indicator of primary hyperthyroidism. Serum T_4 and T_3 levels are elevated. A 24-hour radioactive iodine uptake study can confirm the diagnosis of Graves disease, when the scan shows diffuse homogeneous uptake of tracer, and can exclude the presence of thyroid neoplasms.

Thyroid storm (accelerated hyperthyroidism) is a form of life-threatening thyrotoxicosis that occurs when excessive amounts of thyroid hormones are acutely released into the circulation. This may occur under conditions of psychological or physiologic stress or with physical manipulation of the gland during diagnostic or surgical procedures. Thyroid storm presents with the clinical features of elevated temperature, significant tachycardia, cardiac dysrhythmias, and congestive heart failure.[7] Extreme restlessness, agitation, and psychosis may occur. Prompt treatment of thyroid storm is required.

Treatment. Depending on the degree of symptoms, hyperthyroidism may be treated with medications, such as β-blockers to block acute symptoms or drugs to inhibit thyroid hormone production, or with radioactive iodine to destroy part of the thyroid gland. Surgical removal of the thyroid gland usually is reserved for hyperthyroidism associated with tumors and may result in acute hypocalcemia from inadvertent resection of one or more parathyroid glands. In the rare case of hyperthyroidism secondary to pituitary adenoma, surgical or laser destruction of the anterior pituitary gland may be undertaken.

Antithyroid drugs called thionamides (e.g., methimazole, propylthiouracil) block the activities of the enzyme thyroid peroxidase and inhibit thyroid hormone production by follicular cells. These drugs do not prevent release of hormone, and because the typical thyroid gland contains a 2- to 3-month supply of previously synthesized hormone, the onset of symptom reduction is slow. Thionamides produce a gradual reduction in the basal metabolic rate and reduction of symptoms. Relapse frequently occurs once medications are stopped.

Radioactive iodine treatment to ablate the gland, thereby curtailing its ability to produce excess thyroid hormones, is the treatment of choice for Graves disease. Hypothyroidism occurs following radioactive iodine therapy in 50% to 80% of patients, so patients should be prepared for the likelihood of lifelong thyroid hormone replacement therapy.

Because thyroid storm is a life-threatening form of thyrotoxicosis, urgent management is needed. Antithyroid drugs such as methimazole may be used, followed by iodine administration to further inhibit release of T_3 and T_4. High-dose iodine paradoxically inhibits thyroid hormone synthesis. β-Blockers used for their antiadrenergic effects on the heart also inhibit the peripheral conversion of T_4 to T_3. Antipyretic therapy (e.g., use of cooling blankets or ice packs, administration of acetaminophen) may be started to achieve peripheral cooling. Fluid replacement may be needed and the cardiovascular status should be monitored. Thyroid storm can be fatal if untreated. With treatment, the mortality is between 20% and 30%.[7]

KEY POINTS

- Thyroid hormone (T_3, T_4) is produced in follicular cells of the thyroid gland. The synthesis and secretion of thyroid hormone are stimulated by TSH from the pituitary gland. TSH release from the pituitary gland is stimulated by TRH from the hypothalamus. Thyroid hormone is an important stimulator of growth and cellular metabolism.
- Hypothyroidism may be primary (due to congenital agenesis, autoimmune destruction, irradiation, trauma, surgical removal of the gland, or iodine deficiency) or secondary to pituitary hyposecretion of TSH.
- TSH level is helpful in differentiating between primary (high TSH level) and secondary (low TSH level) causes of hypothyroidism. Low serum T_3 and T_4 levels confirm the diagnosis of hypothyroidism. Hypothyroidism is nearly always from a primary etiology.

- Manifestations of hypothyroidism are attributable to a generalized decrease in metabolism and include nonpitting edema (myxedema), slowed mentation, weight gain, dry skin, constipation, decreased heart rate, decreased pulse pressure, lethargy, and loss of the outer third of the eyebrow. Severe hypothyroidism may lead to myxedema coma, characterized by bradycardia, hypothermia, hypotension, and decreased level of consciousness. Untreated congenital hypothyroidism results in profound mental and physical retardation (cretinism). Treatment centers on hormone replacement therapy.
- Hyperthyroidism may be primary (Graves disease, autoimmune, tumor related, inflammatory) or secondary, attributable to pituitary hypersecretion of TSH. The blood level of TSH is helpful in differentiating primary (low TSH level) from secondary (high TSH level) hyperthyroidism. High levels of T_3 and T_4 confirm the diagnosis of hyperthyroidism.
- The manifestations of hyperthyroidism result from a generalized increase in metabolism. Hyperactivity, irritability, insomnia, weight loss, increased appetite, heat intolerance, diarrhea, and palpitations are common. Most individuals have a detectably enlarged thyroid gland. Exophthalmos is immune mediated and occurs with Graves disease.
- Thyroid storm may be precipitated by stress or manipulation of the gland. It is characterized by tachycardia, hypertension, high temperature, and cardiac dysrhythmias. Treatment includes β-blockers to control cardiovascular symptoms, antithyroid drugs to reduce thyroid production, radioactive iodine to ablate the gland, and surgical removal of tumors.

ADRENOCORTICAL HORMONE DISORDERS

The adrenal cortex synthesizes three different classes of steroid hormones including glucocorticoids, mineralocorticoids, and androgens. Cortisol is the primary glucocorticoid, and its concentration in the circulation provides negative feedback regulation of the hypothalamus and pituitary gland to suppress corticotropin-releasing hormone (CRH) and adrenocorticotropic hormone (ACTH) release. Aldosterone secretion is not regulated by the hypothalamic-pituitary system and is instead regulated by the presence of angiotensin II in the circulation. **Androgenic** hormone secretion by the adrenal cortex plays a relatively minor role in the development and maintenance of secondary sex characteristics, except in children with adrenogenital syndromes, which produce virilization in the female and precocious sexual development in the male. Physiologically, adrenal androgens are the main source of androgens in the female. As with mineralocorticoids, there is no known feedback mechanism to suppress ACTH production associated with adrenal sex hormone plasma levels. The details of adrenocortical hormone synthesis, regulation, and activity are discussed in Chapter 39.

Adrenocortical Insufficiency

Etiology and pathogenesis. Hyposecretion of adrenocortical hormones can result from disease of the adrenal cortex (primary adrenocortical insufficiency, **Addison disease**), from the inadequate secretion of ACTH from the anterior pituitary gland (secondary adrenal insufficiency), or from a lack of CRH secretion from the hypothalamus attributable to hypothalamic malfunction or injury (tertiary adrenal insufficiency). Although hyposecretion of all the adrenocortical hormones may occur, the most severe clinical manifestations of adrenocortical insufficiency occur because of inadequate levels of circulating cortisol.

The syndrome of **congenital adrenal hyperplasia,** a rare cause of adrenal insufficiency in pediatric populations, is due to specific enzymatic defects in the biosynthesis of cortisol by the adrenal glands. The lack of negative feedback results in overproduction of ACTH, leading to hyperplasia of the adrenal glands and excessive androgen secretion.[8]

Congenital adrenal hyperplasia is discussed at the end of the section on adrenal insufficiency.

Primary adrenal insufficiency (Addison disease) is caused by destruction of the adrenal cortex through idiopathic or autoimmune mechanisms, tuberculosis, trauma or hemorrhage of the adrenals (often associated with anticoagulant therapy), fungal disease (e.g., histoplasmosis), and neoplasia. Because of the high functional reserve, symptoms of adrenal insufficiency may not be recognized until 90% of the cortical tissue has been rendered nonfunctional.

Secondary adrenal insufficiency (hypothalamic-pituitary dysfunction) is usually iatrogenic in origin because of the large numbers of patients receiving corticosteroid therapy for chronic illnesses. Prolonged exposure to pharmacologic doses of exogenous corticosteroids suppresses CRH and ACTH stimulation of the adrenal gland through negative feedback. A lack of ACTH results in atrophy of the adrenal cortex. If corticosteroid administration is suddenly halted, or if the individual experiences a sudden stress-induced increase in need for cortisol, the adrenal gland will be unable to respond by increasing cortisol secretion. Acute and severe manifestations of adrenal insufficiency ensue. Secondary adrenal insufficiency occurs because of damage to the anterior pituitary gland or hypothalamus by tumors, infection, radiation, postpartum necrosis, trauma, or surgery.[8]

Addisonian crisis or acute adrenal insufficiency represents a true medical emergency caused by inadequate levels of glucocorticoids and mineralocorticoids in the circulation. This may result from a slowly developing and unrecognized ACTH or cortisol deficiency in which secretion is adequate for the normal demands of life but inadequate for increased stress or trauma. Diminished vascular tone, reduced cardiac output, and inadequate circulating blood volume all contribute to potentially lethal vascular collapse. Hypotension, tachycardia, and symptoms of shock may occur.

Clinical manifestations. The clinical manifestations of adrenal insufficiency (Box 40-3) occur because of inadequate levels of circulating cortisol and aldosterone (Figure 40-7). Clinical manifestations may appear gradually, especially if adrenal destruction is slow and incremental, such as in autoimmune adrenal insufficiency. Symptoms are more dramatic if adrenal destruction is sudden (hemorrhage) or if a stressor, such as trauma, causes sudden decompensation in a patient with chronic adrenal insufficiency.

Early signs of primary adrenal insufficiency include anorexia, weight loss, weakness, malaise, apathy, electrolyte imbalances, and hyperpigmentation of the skin caused by unsuppressed ACTH production (Figure 40-8). ACTH is able to stimulate receptors on melanocytes and promote pigment development in the skin.[2] Salt craving may be present as a result of sodium deficit. If the condition is unrecognized or left untreated, gastrointestinal symptoms can develop, including nausea, vomiting, diarrhea, and dehydration. The patient may be hypotensive or tachycardic. The sudden onset of symptoms suggests acute adrenal insufficiency, which is a medical emergency.

Diagnosis. The diagnosis of acute adrenal insufficiency is assisted by the patient's medical history (use of steroids and/or anticoagulant therapy, previous trauma), physical examination, and laboratory findings. Decreased plasma cortisol levels assist in the diagnosis; however, since acute decompensation progresses to death so rapidly, cortisol samples are obtained for lab analysis and therapy is initiated

BOX 40-3	SIGNS AND SYMPTOMS OF ADRENOCORTICAL HORMONE IMBALANCE	
CUSHING SYNDROME	**ADRENOCORTICAL INSUFFICIENCY**	
Truncal obesity	Weakness	
Moon face	Hypotension	
Dorsocervical fat pad	Hypoglycemia	
Hirsutism	Hyperpigmentation (Addison disease)	
Muscle wasting		
Striae	Hyperkalemia	
Petechiae	Weight loss	
Glucose intolerance		
Hypertension		
Hypokalemia		

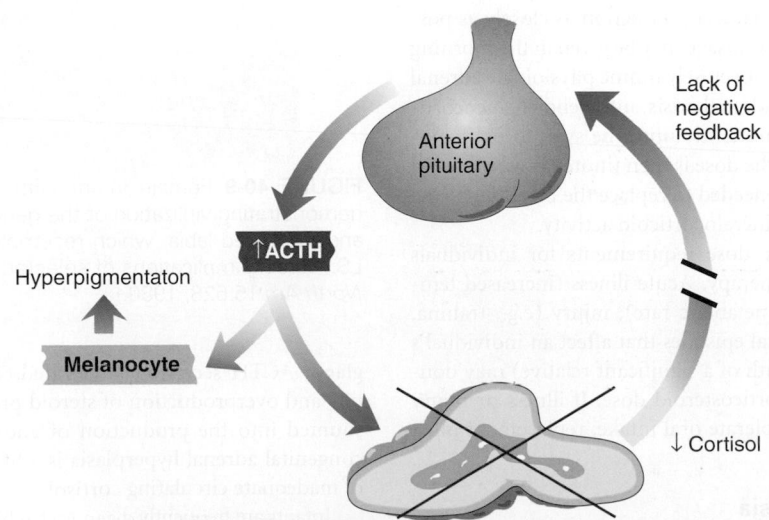

FIGURE 40-7 Primary adrenocortical insufficiency (decreased cortisol production) leads to hypersecretion of adrenocorticotropic hormone *(ACTH)* because of lack of negative feedback. ACTH binds to receptors on melanocytes and stimulates pigment development in the skin. Even though ACTH levels are high, the adrenal gland is unable to produce adequate levels of cortisol.

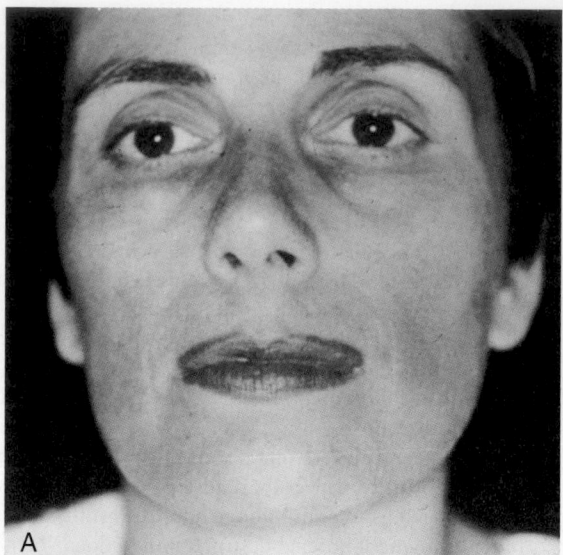
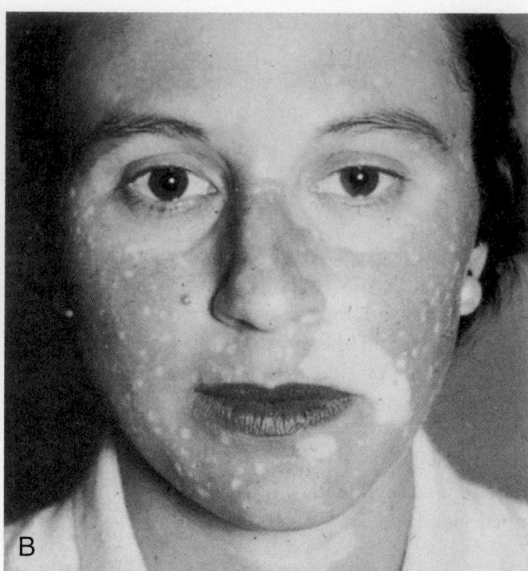

FIGURE 40-8 Altered pigmentation in adrenocortical insufficiency. **A,** Increased pigmentation across the bridge of the nose. **B,** Generalized hyperpigmentation with vitiligo. (From Bondy PK, Rosenberg LE: *Metabolic control and disease,* ed 8, Philadelphia, 1980, Saunders, p 1462.)

presumptively. Resolution of symptoms may be remarkably rapid with administration of intravenous glucocorticoids.

In cases of chronic adrenal insufficiency, an ACTH provocation test can be given. Cosyntropin, synthetic ACTH, is given, and serum samples of cortisol are measured 30 and 60 minutes after administration. Serum cortisol levels should increase following this stimulus if the adrenal cortex is functioning normally. A failure to produce cortisol indicates a primary adrenal insufficiency. Abdominal computerized tomography (CT) or magnetic resonance imaging (MRI) may be performed to determine the size of the adrenal glands. Small adrenal glands occur with autoimmune destruction, whereas tuberculous glands are large and calcified and hemorrhagic glands are large and smooth.

Treatment. The treatment for adrenal insufficiency entails replacing the absent or deficient hormones usually produced by the adrenal cortex in a manner that mimics natural production as closely as possible. About two thirds of the daily dosage may be given in the morning and one third in the evening to more closely mimic physiologic adrenal cortical function. In the case of adrenal crisis, intravenous glucocorticoids can be administered intermittently until the symptoms (hypotension, hypoglycemia) resolve; the dose is then titrated downward. In addition, volume replacement is needed to replace the increased urine output associated with lack of mineralocorticoid activity.

Stress situations increase the dose requirements for individuals receiving chronic replacement therapy. Acute illness (increased temperature causes an increase in metabolic rate), injury (e.g., trauma, surgery, burns), and psychological episodes that affect an individual's ability to function normally (death of a significant relative) may double or triple the needed daily corticosteroid dose. If illness or injury restricts the patient's ability to tolerate oral intake, replacement must be given parenterally.

Congenital Adrenal Hyperplasia

Congenital adrenal hyperplasia is also called *adrenogenital syndrome* and occurs when an enzyme needed for cortisol production is lacking because of a gene defect. The disorder usually follows an autosomal recessive inheritance pattern. Because circulating cortisol levels are inadequate to provide negative feedback to the anterior pituitary

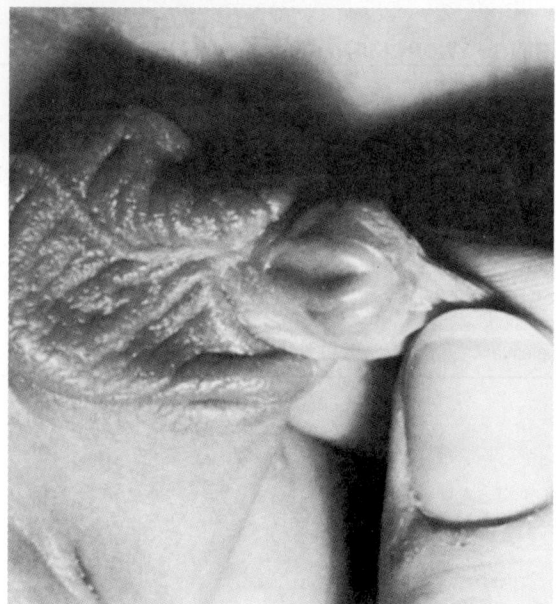

FIGURE 40-9 Female infant with congenital adrenal hyperplasia demonstrating virilization of the genitalia. Note the enlarged clitoris and the fused labia, which resemble a scrotal sac. (From Hurwitz LS: Nursing implications of selected endocrine disorders, *Nurs Clin North Am* 15:528, 1980.)

gland, ACTH secretion is elevated. This leads to adrenal hypertrophy and overproduction of steroid precursors in the gland, which are shunted into the production of androgens. In the newborn, classic congenital adrenal hyperplasia is a life-threatening condition because of inadequate circulating cortisol.

Infants are frequently diagnosed at birth because of the effects of excessive androgens on the genitals of the newborn. Virilization of the genitalia of a female fetus occurs. The female infant may be born with an enlarged clitoris and fused labia, resembling a scrotal sac (Figure 40-9). Male infants with congenital adrenal hyperplasia may have an enlarged penis and hyperpigmented scrotum, but the examiner may not recognize these subtle signs.

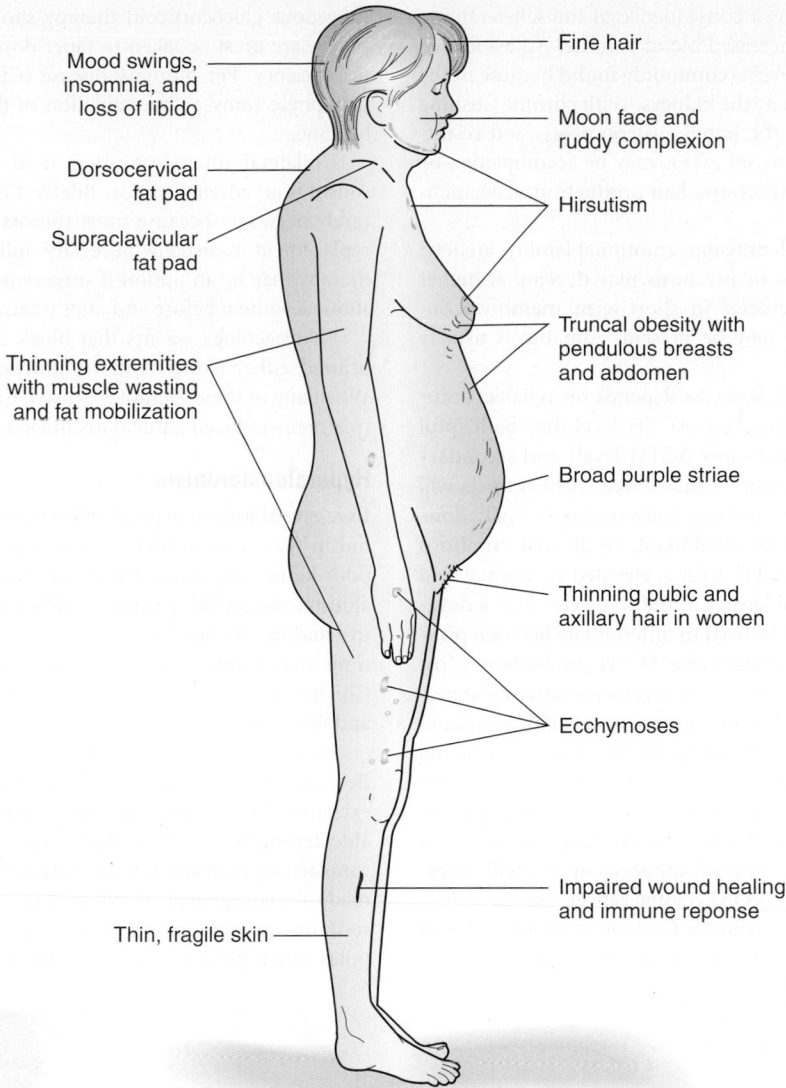

Fine hair

Mood swings, insomnia, and loss of libido

Moon face and ruddy complexion

Dorsocervical fat pad

Hirsutism

Supraclavicular fat pad

Truncal obesity with pendulous breasts and abdomen

Thinning extremities with muscle wasting and fat mobilization

Broad purple striae

Thinning pubic and axillary hair in women

Ecchymoses

Impaired wound healing and immune reponse

Thin, fragile skin

FIGURE 40-10 Common clinical manifestations of Cushing syndrome.

Depending on the enzymes affected, androgen overproduction may occur at any time from birth to early adult life. If it occurs in an adult female, she may develop such virile characteristics as a beard, a much deeper voice, baldness, masculine distribution of pubic hair, growth of the clitoris to resemble a penis, and deposition of proteins in the skin and muscles to yield typical masculine characteristics.

In adult men, the virilizing characteristics of adrenogenital syndrome are less obvious because masculine characteristics are normal and associated with testosterone secreted by the testes. Therefore, the diagnosis is more difficult. In the prepubertal male, adrenogenital syndrome usually causes precocious puberty.

In all cases, treatment with glucocorticoids is necessary to avoid the complications associated with adrenal insufficiency as previously described. In addition, exogenous glucocorticoid therapy suppresses pituitary secretion of ACTH, allowing the adrenal cortex to atrophy and the overproduction of adrenal androgens to cease.

Hypercortisolism

Etiology and pathogenesis. Hyperfunction of the adrenal cortex results in conditions characterized by hypercortisolism. Primary adrenocortical hyperfunction is caused by disease of the adrenal cortex (adrenal adenoma). Secondary disease is caused by hyperfunction

of the anterior pituitary ACTH-secreting cells, and tertiary disease is caused by hypothalamic dysfunction or injury. The term Cushing *syndrome* is used to describe the clinical features of hypercortisolism, regardless of cause. Cushing *disease* is the diagnosis reserved for pituitary-dependent conditions.

In pediatric and adult populations, hypercortisolism is frequently caused by the excessive production of pituitary ACTH by microadenomas or adenomas. Ectopic ACTH production by nonpituitary tumors can also stimulate the adrenal glands. In the United States, exogenous steroids used in the management of various diseases, such as allergic and autoimmune diseases, are the most common cause of Cushing syndrome.

Clinical manifestations. An individual with excess circulating glucocorticoids typically develops a round face with prominent, flushed cheeks, often referred to as "moon face" (see Box 40-3). There is a noticeable weight gain with increasing total body fat, especially in the abdomen. A dorsocervical fat pad, capillary friability, and thinning of the skin with the formation of purple striae and ecchymoses over the abdomen, arms, and thighs develop. Muscle mass decreases and muscle weakness develops. Cortisol increases tissue resistance to the effects of insulin and may contribute to glucose intolerance or hyperglycemia. Figure 40-10 shows the common clinical manifestations of Cushing syndrome.

Hypertension may develop as a consequence of the salt-retaining activity of cortisol and of the increased blood volume. An associated reduction of serum potassium level is commonly found because of the excessive excretion of potassium by the kidneys. With chronic Cushing syndrome, demineralization of the bones (osteoporosis) and resulting fractures may occur. The cortisol excess may be accompanied by increased androgen production (excessive hair production, acne, menstrual irregularities).

Emotional changes include depression, emotional lability, anxiety, and irritability. Rarely, euphoria or psychosis may develop at higher concentrations of cortisol. Decreases in short-term memory, concentration, and attention span may be present. Appetite is usually increased.

The diagnosis of adrenocortical excess depends on reliable, accurate laboratory measurements. A serum ACTH level may be helpful in differentiating between primary (low ACTH level) and secondary (high ACTH level) hypercortisolism. Urinary free cortisol levels will be elevated in all forms. A 24-hour urine collection is typically done to exclude inappropriate diagnoses attributable to diurnal variations in cortisol production. If the ACTH level is elevated or normal and the 24-hour urinary free cortisol level is found to be elevated, a dexamethasone suppression test may be used to differentiate between pituitary causes and ectopic causes of excessive ACTH production. Most pituitary adenomas (Cushing disease) demonstrate a relative resistance to feedback inhibition by cortisol. When a more potent glucocorticoid is given (dexamethasone), the pituitary gland responds by reducing ACTH production. Sometimes Cushing syndrome is a result of ectopic production of ACTH by cancer cells. In this case, the suppression test will fail to reduce ACTH production because the cancer cells do not respond to feedback control. A negative suppression test will necessitate a diagnostic evaluation to find the ectopic cancer source.

Treatment. The choice of treatment for Cushing syndrome is based on its etiology. Patients who have Cushing syndrome as a result of exogenous glucocorticoid therapy should have doses reduced if possible. Care must be taken to taper doses slowly to avoid acute adrenal insufficiency. For pituitary disease (Cushing disease), transsphenoidal hypophysectomy or laser ablation of the anterior pituitary gland may be done.

Unilateral adrenalectomy is used if the cause of the hypercortisolism is an adrenal tumor. Bilateral removal of the adrenal glands is rarely necessary because most tumors are unilateral. Lifelong steroid replacement is usually necessary following this surgery. Radiation therapy may be an option if surgery is contraindicated.[8] Figure 40-11 shows a woman before and after treatment for Cushing syndrome.

Pharmacologic agents that block cortisol production can also be utilized either alone or in conjunction with surgery and radiation. When any of these therapies is used, the patient should be assessed for treatment-induced adrenal insufficiency.

Hyperaldosteronism

Excessive aldosterone production may be from primary hyperaldosteronism (Conn syndrome) or secondary to conditions associated with poor kidney perfusion. Conn syndrome usually occurs as a result of aldosterone-secreting tumors. Aldosterone is not under pituitary control and in this case "secondary" refers to disease processes or conditions that stimulate the renin-angiotensin-aldosterone cascade (see Chapter 39). These include heart failure, reduced kidney perfusion, and liver cirrhosis.

Aldosterone facilitates salt and water retention by the kidney. Because aldosterone acts on the distal renal tubule to promote sodium exchange for the potassium lost in the urine, individuals with hyperaldosteronism may have decreased potassium levels. The drug spironolactone is an aldosterone antagonist and therefore is useful in the medical management of aldosterone excess. Spironolactone increases sodium excretion and potassium retention. Sodium restriction and potassium replacement may also be necessary.

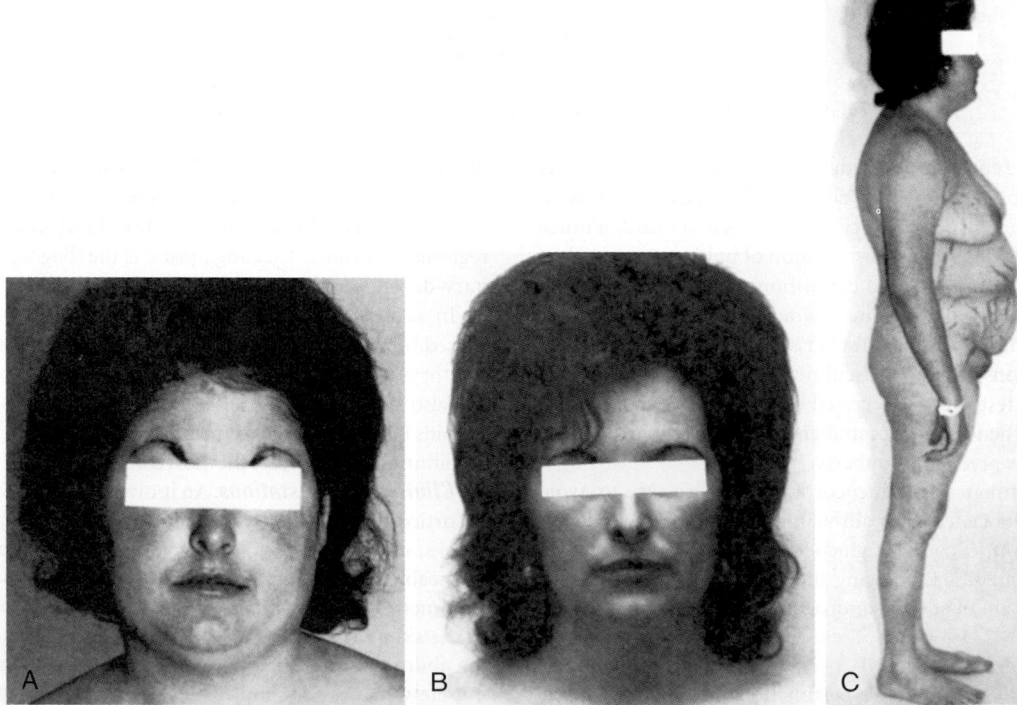

FIGURE 40-11 A woman with Cushing syndrome before **(A** and **C)** and after **(B)** removal of an adrenal adenoma. (From Wyngaarden JB et al: *Cecil textbook of medicine,* ed 19, Philadelphia, 1992, Saunders, p 1285.)

ADRENAL MEDULLA DISORDER

Pheochromocytoma

Etiology and pathogenesis. The adrenal medulla secretes two important catecholamine hormones in response to stimulation by the sympathetic nervous system. Epinephrine, or adrenaline, accounts for about 80% of the adrenal medulla's secretion; norepinephrine accounts for the other 20%. Norepinephrine is also the neurotransmitter produced by the postganglionic sympathetic fibers. Sympathetic effectors such as the heart, smooth muscle, and glands have adrenergic receptors for norepinephrine and epinephrine. Both epinephrine and norepinephrine can bind to adrenergic receptors to prolong and enhance the effects of sympathetic stimulation.

Pheochromocytoma is a tumor of chromaffin tissue that results in the excessive production and release of catecholamines. It is usually benign, but in about 10% of cases the tumor exhibits malignant behavior. It is usually found in the adrenal medulla, but it may also arise in

other sites where there is chromaffin tissue, such as the sympathetic ganglia. Like adrenal medullary cells, the tumor cells of a pheochromocytoma produce and secrete the catecholamines epinephrine and norepinephrine in response to sympathetic stimulation. Intermittent excessive release of these catecholamines results in periods of hypertension.[9] The hypertension in individuals with pheochromocytoma is influenced by the level of sympathetic nervous system stimulation, the circulating catecholamine levels, and the cardiovascular response to these changes.

Clinical manifestations. The most common problem experienced by individuals with pheochromocytomas is intermittent or persistent hypertension. Bouts of the classic triad of headache, tachycardia, and diaphoresis strongly suggest the diagnosis of pheochromocytoma. Sporadic hypertensive episodes may occur with stress, excitement, physical activity, ingestion of certain drugs, and the smoking of tobacco products. Other symptoms may include tremor, nervousness, emotional lability, pallor, fatigue, generalized gastrointestinal complaints, and orthostatic hypotension. Signs of a hypermetabolic state may be present, such as fever and weight loss. CT and MRI are commonly employed diagnostic tools to locate tumors on the adrenal glands.

Treatment. Uncontrolled hypertension can lead to end-organ damage and stroke, so prompt diagnosis and aggressive therapy are necessary. The usual treatment for this condition is surgical removal of the tumor. Before surgery, sympathetic blocking medications may be prescribed to manage blood pressure and relieve symptoms.

If surgery is contraindicated, treatment with drugs to block catecholamine production is possible. However, surgery is the only curative therapy. After a period of stabilization, the sympathetic nervous system is able to compensate for the loss of adrenal medullary function and hormone replacement is no longer necessary. Because there is an increased risk of recurrence of the tumor in later years, annual follow-up is recommended.

PARATHYROID GLAND DISORDERS

Regulation and Actions of Parathyroid Hormone

The parathyroid glands are small glands located at the upper and lower poles of the thyroid. There are usually four parathyroid glands, although there are reports of fewer or more than four being found during surgery. The parathyroid glands detect serum calcium concentration and help maintain constant levels through the regulation of calcium absorption and resorption from bone (Figure 40-12). The absorption of calcium from the intestine and renal tubules is dependent on vitamin D and is impaired in conditions such as renal failure, in which active vitamin D is deficient (see Chapter 28).

Serum calcium levels provide the feedback necessary to regulate parathyroid hormone (PTH) secretion. A decrease in serum calcium level causes a release of PTH. An elevated serum calcium level leads

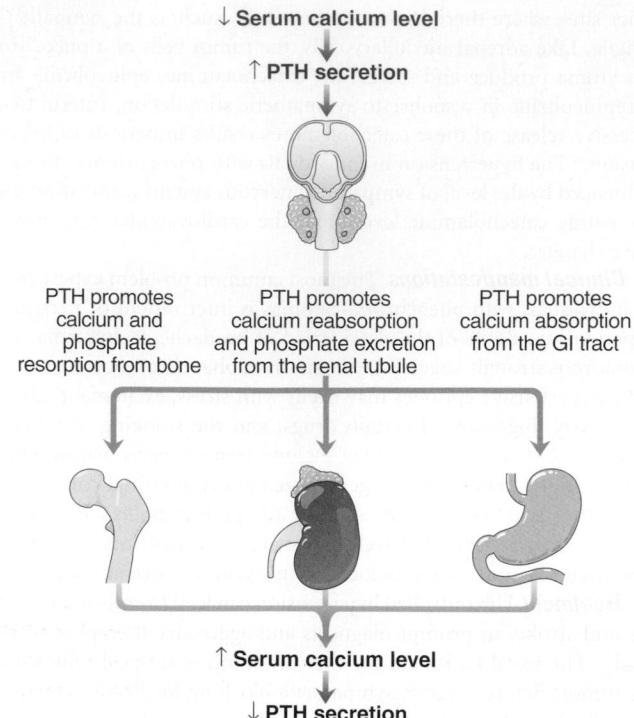

FIGURE 40-12 Parathyroid hormone *(PTH)* increases serum calcium level through its effects on bone, renal tubules, and intestine. *GI,* Gastrointestinal.

to suppression of PTH secretion. PTH is not under control of the hypothalamic-pituitary system. Parathyroid hormone acts on bones, intestine, and renal tubules to increase serum calcium levels. In the bone, PTH increases osteoclastic activity, resulting in the release of calcium (and phosphate) from bone into extracellular fluid. Renal calcium reabsorption increases under the effect of PTH, thus decreasing urinary calcium excretion.

Calcitonin, produced by thyroid parafollicular cells (C-cells), also influences the processing of calcium by bone cells. Calcitonin increases bone formation by osteoblasts and inhibits bone breakdown by osteoclasts. Although the role of calcitonin in calcium homeostasis is not entirely clear, calcitonin tends to decrease blood calcium levels and promote conservation of hard bone matrix.

The clinical manifestations of parathyroid hormone dysfunction are those of hypercalcemia and hypocalcemia and related changes in neuromuscular excitability. A discussion of serum calcium regulation and disorders can be found in Chapter 24.

Hyperparathyroidism

Etiology and pathogenesis. The causes of primary hyperparathyroidism remain unclear. Despite an elevated serum calcium level, PTH continues to be secreted. Some forms of hyperparathyroidism can have a genetic origin. Hyperparathyroidism from a single parathyroid adenoma occurs in 80% of surgically proven cases. Hyperplasia of the parathyroid is found in the remainder of the cases.

In hyperparathyroidism, bone resorption and formation rates are increased. Serum calcium levels do not rise uncontrollably; indeed, excessive parathyroid gland secretion rarely causes hypercalcemic crisis. Malignant tumors elsewhere in the body can also release PTH-like hormones and are a more frequent cause of extreme hypercalcemia and hypercalcemic crisis.

A hyperparathyroid state during pregnancy leads to perinatal and neonatal complications. The newborn's PTH production will be suppressed by maternal hypercalcemia, and neonatal hypocalcemia and tetany can develop. This presentation in a newborn may be the first indication of the need for investigative studies in the mother if the disorder was asymptomatic during pregnancy.[10] In chronic renal failure, hyperparathyroidism may result from reduced production of active vitamin D (which impairs calcium absorption) and from impaired glomerular filtration (which limits excretion of phosphate in the urine). Some drugs, such as lithium and thiazides, may increase serum calcium levels, leading to a misdiagnosis of hyperparathyroidism.

Clinical manifestations. The presentation of hyperparathyroidism is related to the level of hypercalcemia and the hyperparathyroid state. Hyperparathyroidism may present as asymptomatic hypercalcemia. Individuals are prone to kidney stones and to bone demineralization (osteoporosis). Severe hypercalcemia causes a wide variety of effects, including polyuria and dehydration. Anorexia, nausea, vomiting, and constipation may develop. Various cardiac problems can arise including bradycardia, heart block, and cardiac arrest.

Often, asymptomatic cases of hyperparathyroidism are found on screening serum chemistry laboratory reports that note mild elevations in serum calcium levels. In primary hyperparathyroidism (not secondary to renal disease), serum calcium levels are elevated and serum phosphorous levels are low to low-normal. Urinary excretion of calcium and phosphate is elevated, as are serum PTH levels.

Treatment. Surgical removal of the abnormal parathyroid gland(s) is the treatment of choice. Individuals with asymptomatic hyperparathyroidism may defer surgery. In such cases, medical management may work for a time. Medical management includes hydration (to prevent kidney stone formation) and ambulation to maintain bone density.

For hypercalcemic crisis, rapid volume expansion with normal saline reverses dehydration. Volume replacement also results in improved glomerular filtration rate and increased calcium excretion. Diuretics, other than thiazide diuretics, may be used to increase calcium excretion by the kidney.

Hypoparathyroidism

Etiology and pathogenesis. Hypoparathyroidism most frequently occurs as a consequence of parathyroid or thyroid surgery or radiation in the area. Transient or permanent hypoparathyroidism may develop following thyroidectomy because of damage to parathyroid gland blood supply, postsurgical swelling, or fibrosis.

Hypoparathyroidism can occur following the removal of one hyperfunctioning parathyroid gland. The hyperfunctioning gland had been suppressing the function of the other parathyroid glands, and when removed a temporary state of deficiency may follow until the remaining parathyroid glands resume function. Congenital lack of parathyroid tissue and idiopathic hypoparathyroidism are causes of hypoparathyroidism in infants and children. Autoimmune processes may also target and damage the parathyroid glands.

Clinical manifestations. Clinical manifestations of hypoparathyroidism occur as a result of low serum calcium levels. The manifestations of acute hypocalcemia include circumoral numbness, paresthesias of the distal extremities, muscle cramps, fatigue, neuromuscular irritability, anxiety, nonspecific electroencephalographic changes, and prolongation of Q-T intervals on the electrocardiogram. Severe manifestations of hypocalcemia include carpopedal spasm, laryngospasm, and seizures. Neuromuscular irritability can be elicited by a positive Chvostek sign (ipsilateral contraction of the facial muscles that occurs from tapping the facial nerve anterior to the ear) or Trousseau sign (carpal spasm produced by pressure ischemia of the nerves in the upper arm during inflation of a blood pressure cuff for 3 to 5 minutes above the systolic blood pressure).

The serum calcium level is low, and the phosphorous level is elevated. Antibodies to the parathyroid gland are present if an autoimmune mechanism is operant.

Treatment. Emergency treatment with intravenous (IV) calcium is needed if an individual presents in acute hypocalcemic crisis (tetany, laryngospasm, and convulsions). Calcitriol, an activated form of vitamin D, may be useful. Long-term treatment includes administration of an oral calcium supplement with vitamin D.

KEY POINTS

- PTH is an important regulator of serum calcium levels. Low serum levels of ionized calcium are a potent stimulus for PTH release. PTH increases calcium absorption from the gastrointestinal (GI) tract in concert with vitamin D, resorption of calcium and phosphate from bones, and reabsorption of calcium from the urine filtrate. PTH also increases the excretion of phosphate by the kidney. Disorders of PTH secretion are manifested as alterations in serum Ca^{2+} levels.
- Hyperparathyroidism may be idiopathic or may be due to a parathyroid adenoma. Its manifestations result from high serum calcium levels and bone demineralization. High serum calcium levels decrease neuromuscular excitability. Treatment entails removing the abnormal glands. Adequate hydration may help prevent the formation of kidney stones.
- Hypoparathyroidism may be idiopathic, autoimmune, or secondary to surgical removal of the parathyroid gland. The manifestations result from low serum calcium levels, which increase neuromuscular excitability. Paresthesias, cramps, spasms, tetany, and seizures may result. Elicitation of Chvostek and Trousseau signs indicates neuromuscular hyperexcitability. Treatment entails calcium (and vitamin D) supplementation rather than PTH replacement.

ANTIDIURETIC HORMONE DISORDERS

ADH (vasopressin) is secreted from the posterior pituitary gland in response to changes in blood osmolality. The details of ADH synthesis, regulation, and activity are described in Chapter 39. Concepts related to physiologic effects on renal water handling can be found in Chapter 26; Chapter 24 includes details of body fluid regulation and osmolality.

Diabetes Insipidus

Etiology and pathogenesis. **Diabetes insipidus (DI)** is a disorder of insufficient ADH activity characterized by excessive loss of water in the urine. ADH acts directly on the renal collecting ducts and distal tubules, increasing membrane permeability to and reabsorption of water. Damage to the ADH-producing cells in the hypothalamus can occur with closed head trauma, intracranial tumors, and neurosurgery. Some pharmacologic agents can lead to abnormalities in ADH secretion (Box 40-4). For example, the diuresis that follows alcohol ingestion occurs because of decreased ADH secretion.

Diabetes insipidus (DI) is a term meaning *a large diuresis of inappropriately dilute urine.* In adults with DI, 30% of cases are idiopathic, 20% are caused by the surgical treatment of brain tumors, 16% result from nonsurgical brain trauma, 25% are secondary to brain tumors, and 9% follow a hypophysectomy.[11] ADH deficiency may be accompanied by other hypothalamic-pituitary hormone deficiencies. Damage to the posterior pituitary gland may cause temporary or permanent deficiency of ADH. With insufficient amounts of ADH, urine cannot be concentrated and free water is lost, causing hyperosmolality and hypernatremia. This is called *central DI* because the ability to produce and release ADH from the pituitary gland is lost. *Nephrogenic DI* occurs when the kidney is unable to respond to ADH because of

---

BOX 40-4	**AGENTS THAT CAUSE ALTERATIONS IN ANTIDIURETIC HORMONE SECRETION**
AGENTS THAT ENHANCE RELEASE	**AGENTS THAT SUPPRESS RELEASE**
β-Adrenergic agents	α-Adrenergic agents
Barbiturates	Alcohol
Carbamazepine	Phenytoin
Clofibrate	
Cyclophosphamide	
Histamine	
CO_2	
Morphine and narcotic analogues	
Nicotine	
Prostaglandin E_2	
Vincristine	

---

chronic renal disease, receptor defects, serum electrolyte abnormalities, or drugs (e.g., lithium). The clinical presentation of both forms of DI is similar, and measurement of serum ADH level may be helpful in determining the etiology.

Clinical manifestations and diagnosis. The development of **polyuria** (excessive urination) and **polydipsia** (excessive drinking) is the hallmark of DI. The patient may void as much as 15 L of urine daily. The specific gravity of the urine will be greatly decreased. If the thirst center of the hypothalamus is functional, the patient will consume up to 15 L of water to maintain osmolar balance. Symptoms persist at night (**nocturia**), interrupting normal sleep patterns. If the thirst center has been damaged, DI becomes a life-threatening illness because increased water losses from the kidneys (resulting from the absence of ADH) are not counteracted by increased thirst and fluid intake.

DI results in hypernatremia (water deficit) from loss of water without concurrent loss of sodium. Hypernatremia is associated with serum sodium concentrations in excess of 145 mEq/L and indicates a body water deficit relative to sodium. Signs and symptoms include thirst, dry mucous membranes, poor skin turgor, decreased saliva and sweat production, disorientation, lethargy, and seizures. The early neurologic symptoms are thought to be due to shrinkage and dehydration of neuronal cells, which are more sensitive to osmolality changes than other cell types.

Most sudden, critical presentations are straightforward, with documented hypotonic polyuria, hypernatremia, and hypertonicity indicating a defect in secretion of ADH. Individuals presenting with the sudden onset of polyuria and polydipsia should undergo laboratory studies, including tests for glucose, urine and serum electrolytes, serum creatinine, and blood urea nitrogen (BUN) levels. The results of these tests should exclude diabetes mellitus and kidney disease as the basis for the presenting complaints. A comparison of serum and urine osmolality is needed, as is a urine specific gravity measurement. Dilute urine in the presence of water deficit and hypernatremia along with abnormally low serum ADH levels are diagnostic of central DI.

A water deprivation test may be used to confirm the diagnosis. Water intake is restricted, and the urine osmolality is measured hourly. When a plateau in urine osmolality is reached, vasopressin is administered. With central DI, urine concentration increases following vasopressin administration. Polyuria and polydipsia also resolve. In the case of nephrogenic DI, little or no response to vasopressin occurs.

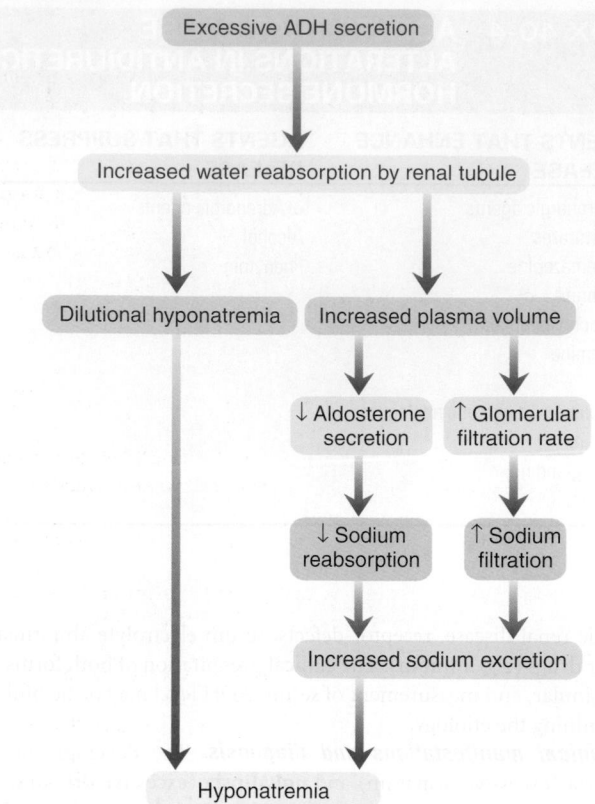

FIGURE 40-13 Syndrome of inappropriate antidiuretic hormone secretion leads to hyponatremia by two mechanisms: (1) dilution of plasma and (2) increased excretion of sodium by the kidneys. Sodium excretion is increased because of the expanded plasma volume, which enhances sodium filtration and reduces sodium reabsorption. *ADH*, Antidiuretic hormone.

Treatment. Daily replacement of ADH is needed for the management of DI. DDAVP (1-deamino-8-D-arginine vasopressin), a synthetic analogue of ADH, can be given to replace vasopressin deficiency. Free access to fluids is necessary, and home testing of urine specific gravity may be useful for some individuals to allow them to adjust their dose independently.

Syndrome of Inappropriate Antidiuretic Hormone Secretion

Etiology and pathogenesis. Inappropriate secretion of excessive amounts of ADH is referred to as *syndrome of inappropriate antidiuretic hormone* (SIADH). The excessive ADH is from ectopic production and has been noted in association with several types of tumors, the most common of which are primary lung malignancies. Nonmalignant lung disorders are also capable of ADH synthesis, or stimulation of central ADH production, especially pulmonary tuberculosis. Drug-induced ADH secretion occurs with the administration of a number of medications, including (but not limited to) chlorpropamide, carbamazepine, morphine, and barbiturates.

SIADH results in hyponatremia when free water is inappropriately conserved and "dilutes" the serum to a sodium concentration below the normal range (<135 mEq/L). In hyponatremia there is an excess of water relative to solute. Cells swell, and the effects of cellular swelling on neurons can be profound. Adrenal insufficiency and hypothyroidism may also cause increased ADH secretion, and hyponatremia. Both of these hormonal deficiencies must be excluded before SIADH is diagnosed.

Clinical manifestations. Clinical manifestations are due to the hypotonicity of body fluids. SIADH is characterized by hyponatremia. Urine osmolality is inappropriately high because of increased water reabsorption in the renal tubules and collecting ducts. Serum osmolality is low because of dilution by the reabsorbed water (Figure 40-13). The symptoms of SIADH include weakness, muscle cramps, nausea and vomiting, postural blood pressure changes, poor skin turgor, fatigue, anorexia, and lethargy. In very severe cases, confusion, hemiparesis (motor weakness on one side of the body), seizures, and coma may occur. Laboratory findings include low serum sodium, hematocrit, and blood urea nitrogen (BUN) levels as a result of dilution of the extracellular fluid.

Treatment. Free water restriction is implemented for individuals with SIADH. Water restriction should result in a slow, steady rise in serum sodium levels and osmolality. If severe symptoms develop, intravenous (IV) administration of saline, combined with diuretic therapy, may cause loss of free water. Hyponatremia should be corrected slowly to avoid rapid changes in brain cell volume. If hyponatremia is persistent, drugs such as lithium may be used to block the effects of ADH.

KEY POINTS

- ADH secretion is regulated primarily by osmoreceptors in the hypothalamus that respond to changes in extracellular osmolality. An increase in serum osmolality stimulates secretion of ADH. Renal distal and collecting tubules respond to ADH by becoming more permeable to water. In the presence of ADH, water is reabsorbed from the urine filtrate, resulting in a concentrated urine.
- Central DI is due to lack of production of ADH by the hypothalamus or release by the posterior pituitary gland. Central DI may be idiopathic or related to brain surgery, trauma, or tumor.
- Nephrogenic DI is caused by lack of renal collecting tubule responsiveness to ADH. Nephrogenic DI may be caused by receptor abnormalities, renal disease, medications, or electrolyte imbalance.
- Most commonly, DI causes polydipsia accompanied by thirst, polyuria, increased serum sodium level, and increased osmolality. Increased osmolality may cause cellular shrinkage with neurologic signs and symptoms. The diagnosis is confirmed when dilute urine is formed during water deprivation, which is promptly corrected with administration of vasopressin.
- DI is treated with ADH hormone replacement therapy and fluid therapy.
- SIADH is associated with pulmonary tumors, central nervous system disease, and certain drugs. Excess ADH stimulates the renal tubules to reabsorb water despite decreased blood osmolality.
- Clinical manifestations of hyponatremia are associated with cellular swelling and neurologic dysfunction (e.g., confusion, coma). Water restriction and diuretic administration may be used to manage hyponatremia. Detection and management of the underlying cause are paramount.

SUMMARY

Endocrine disorders present as hyperfunction or hypofunction of hormone actions. An understanding of the usual actions of hormones is useful in predicting the signs and symptoms that will be apparent with excesses and deficits (see Chapter 39). Several important hormone systems are controlled by the hypothalamic-pituitary system and disorders may occur from intrinsic defects in the target gland (primary) or abnormalities in pituitary secretion of trophic hormones (secondary). Diagnosis relies on laboratory evaluation of pituitary gland and target gland hormone levels because the signs and symptoms are similar regardless of primary or secondary etiology. The etiologies of endocrine disorders are similar regardless of the particular gland involved and include tumors and autoimmune disorders as well as destruction, suppression, removal, or inadequate development of the gland. Treatment strategies are few and for hyperfunction include surgical removal, ablation, or drugs to block hormone synthesis. Replacement therapy is available for most endocrine deficiency disorders and is tailored to mimic normal secretion as much as possible.

REFERENCES

1. Porterfield SP, White BA: The hypothalamus-pituitary complex. In Porterfield SP, White BA, editors: *Endocrine physiology*, ed 3, Philadelphia, 2007, Mosby, pp 107–140.
2. White B: The hypothalamus and pituitary gland. In Koeppen BM, Stanton BM, editors: *Berne and Levy physiology*, ed 6, Philadelphia, 2010, Mosby, pp 706–724.
3. Biller BM: Concepts in the diagnosis of adult growth hormone deficiency, *Horm Res* 68(Suppl 5):59–65, 2007.
4. Deladoëy J, et al: Is the incidence of congenital hypothyroidism really increasing? A 20-year retrospective population-based study in Québec, *J Clin Endocrinol Metab* 96(8):2422–2429, 2011.
5. Porterfield SP, White BA: The thyroid gland. In Porterfield SP, White BA, editors: *Endocrine physiology*, ed 3, Philadelphia, 2007, Mosby, pp 141–162.
6. Maitra A: The endocrine system. In Kumar V, et al, editors: *Robbins and Cotran pathologic basis of disease*, ed 8, Philadelphia, 2010, Saunders, pp 1097–1164.
7. Nayak B, Burman K: Thyrotoxicosis and thyroid storm, *Endocrinol Metab Clin North Am* 35(4):663–686, 2006.
8. Porterfield SP, White BA: The adrenal gland. In Porterfield SP, White BA, editors: *Endocrine physiology*, ed 3, Philadelphia, 2007, Mosby, pp 163–196.
9. Karagiannis A, et al: Pheochromocytoma: an update on genetics and management, *Endocr Relat Cancer* 14(4):935–956, 2007.
10. Jain A, et al: Hypocalcemia in the newborn, *Indian J Pediatr* 77(10):1123–1128, 2010.
11. Ball SG: Vasopressin and disorders of water balance: the physiology and pathophysiology of vasopressin, *Ann Clin Biochem* 44(pt 5):417–431, 2007.

Diabetes Mellitus

Benjamin J. Miller

evolve WEBSITE

http://evolve.elsevier.com/Copstead/
- Review Questions and Answers
- Glossary (with audio pronunciations for selected terms)
- Animations
- Case Studies
- Key Points Review

KEY QUESTIONS

- Which hormones are involved in the regulation of serum glucose level, and under what physiologic conditions would each be secreted?
- What are the differentiating characteristics of type 1 and type 2 diabetes?
- How do the pathophysiologic processes differ among the various types of diabetes?
- What clinical findings are associated with hyperglycemia, and how do they differ from those of hypoglycemia?
- How is diabetes mellitus diagnosed, monitored, and managed?
- What are the acute and chronic complications of diabetes mellitus?

CHAPTER OUTLINE

CHAPTER OUTLINE—cont'd

The public health impact of diabetes mellitus is enormous. In the United States, nearly 25.8 million persons (8.3% of the population) have diabetes mellitus, although it is estimated that only 72% are aware of their diagnosis. Should this trend continue unabated, worldwide the number of persons with diabetes will rise to 366 million by 2015.[1] The annual cost of diabetes to the U.S. medical care system was estimated to be $176 billion in 2007, with half of the total cost attributed to inpatient diabetes care.[2] Diabetes mellitus is the seventh leading cause of death and a major cause of disability in the United States. It increases the risk for heart disease, end-stage renal disease, blindness, amputation, and complications of pregnancy. The disease disproportionately affects non-Caucasian and elderly individuals.[3]

REGULATION OF GLUCOSE METABOLISM

Because diabetes mellitus affects the utilization of all energy nutrients, it is helpful to review energy nutrient metabolism to understand the disease process of diabetes mellitus. The energy requirements of humans are predominantly met by glucose and fats. Produced from endogenous glycogen stores in the muscles and liver or manufactured from such substrates as amino acids and lactate, glucose is supplied to the bloodstream from the gastrointestinal tract and liver. Glucose is typically present in greater quantities in extracellular fluid than within cells.[3]

Cells are variously permeable to glucose, and the diffusion of glucose into them is accomplished by glucose transporters (GLUT 1-4) specific to each tissue. GLUT 1-3 transporters are insulin independent; they remain in the plasma membrane whether or not insulin is present. GLUT 1 is the major glucose transporter at the blood-brain barrier and GLUT 3 is the dominant glucose transport molecule for neurons. GLUT 2 is the primary glucose transporter in the liver and is present in small quantities in the pancreatic β cells.[4] GLUT 1 and GLUT 3 are the predominant glucose transport molecules in the pancreatic β cells.[5]

GLUT 4, found in muscle and adipose cells, is insulin dependent. In the absence of insulin GLUT 4 is sequestered in vesicles located within the cell. When insulin binds to insulin receptors, an intracellular signaling cascade occurs that causes the vesicles with GLUT 4 in their membranes to move (translocate) to the plasma membrane, enabling glucose entry into the muscle cell or adipocyte. When insulin no longer binds to its receptor, GLUT 4 is removed from the plasma membrane.[4,6]

Hormonal Regulation

Protein and fat metabolism is regulated by the anabolic effects of insulin. Insulin is synthesized in the pancreas by the β cells of the islets of Langerhans. The islets are groups of cells dispersed throughout the pancreas. Within the islets can be found β cells that produce insulin in the form of proinsulin, α cells that produce glucagon, δ cells that produce somatostatin, and F cells that produce pancreatic polypeptide. The primary stimulus for release of insulin from the pancreatic β cells is glucose. Glucose enters the β cells by facilitated diffusion through GLUT 1 and GLUT 3 carriers in the plasma membrane (Figure 41-1). The concentration of glucose in the extracellular fluids determines how much enters the cell. Glucose within the β cell triggers a cascade

of events that results in exocytosis of vesicles containing insulin (see Figure 41-1). Proinsulin is produced and packaged into vesicles along with enzymes that cleave proinsulin into insulin and C-peptide (Figure 41-2). Insulin binds to its receptor on insulin-sensitive cells and triggers glucose uptake through GLUT 4 carriers (Figure 41-3). These carriers are sequestered within the cell when insulin levels are low and then sent to the plasma membrane to transport glucose when insulin levels are higher. Insulin mediates other effects besides glucose uptake. Insulin appears to increase the uptake and to decrease the release of

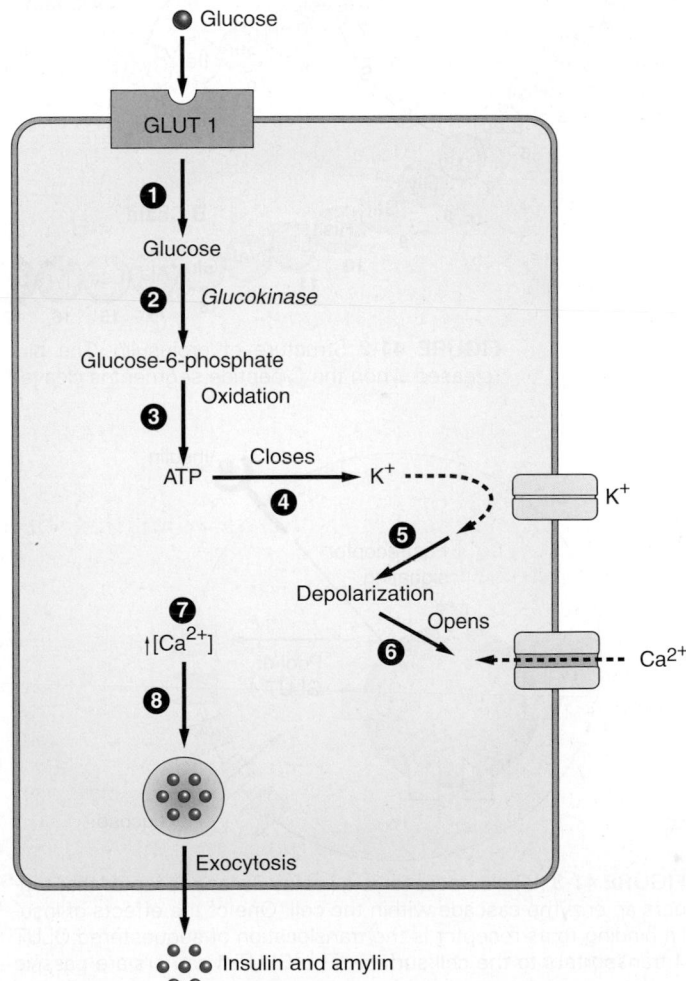

FIGURE 41-1 Processes of glucose-stimulated exocytosis of insulin from β cells of the pancreas. Glucose enters the β cells by facilitated diffusion through GLUT 1 in the plasma membrane. Glucose triggers production of ATP, which closes ATP-sensitive K+ channels and promotes depolarization of the cell. Depolarization triggers opening of voltage-sensitive Ca2+ channels, allowing calcium ions to enter the cell. Calcium ions interact with release-site proteins and trigger exocytosis of stored insulin and amylin.

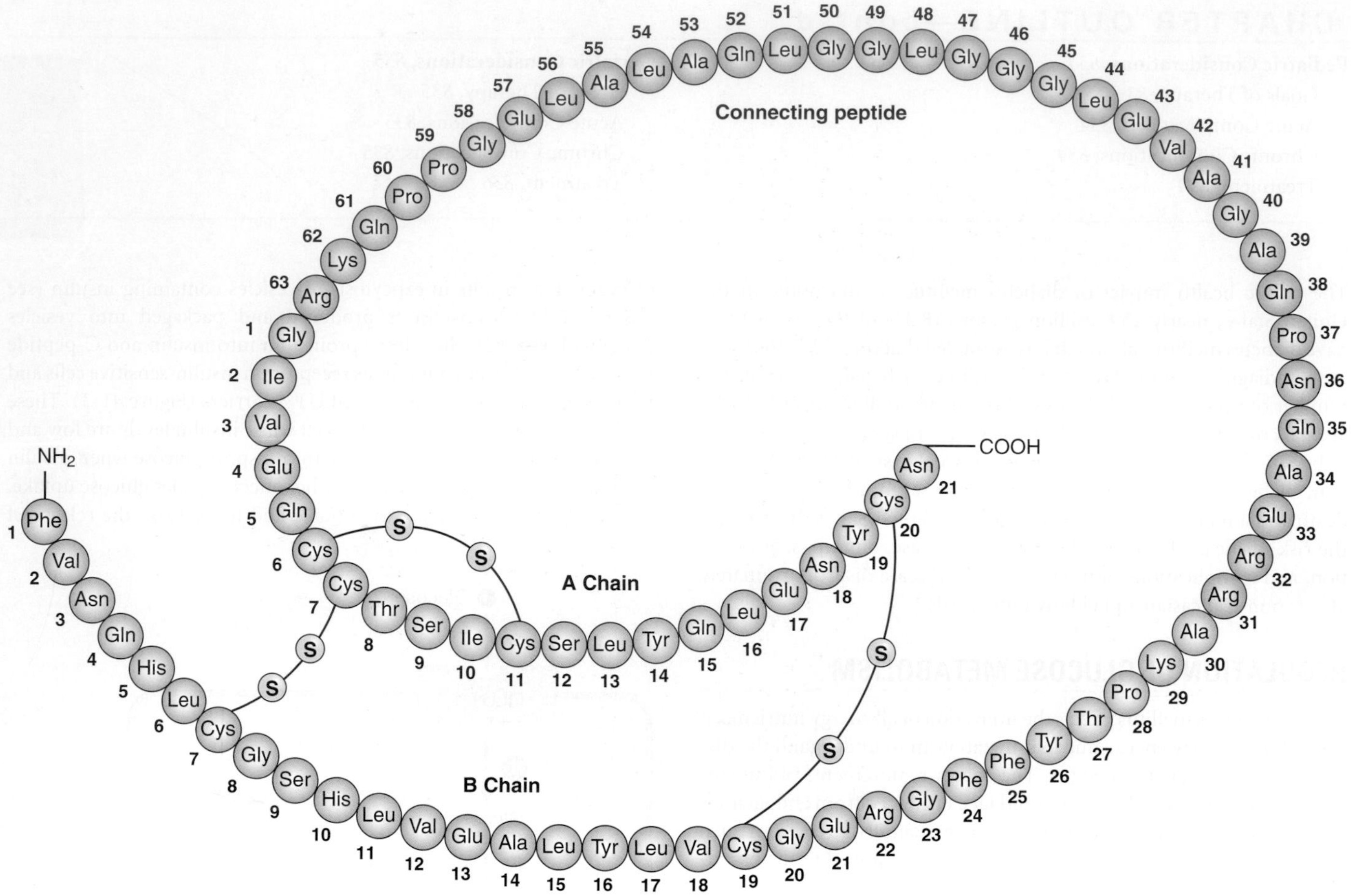

Connecting peptide

A Chain

B Chain

NH₂

COOH

FIGURE 41-2 Structure of proinsulin. The blue-colored amino acids represent the insulin that is released when the C-peptide segment is cleaved.

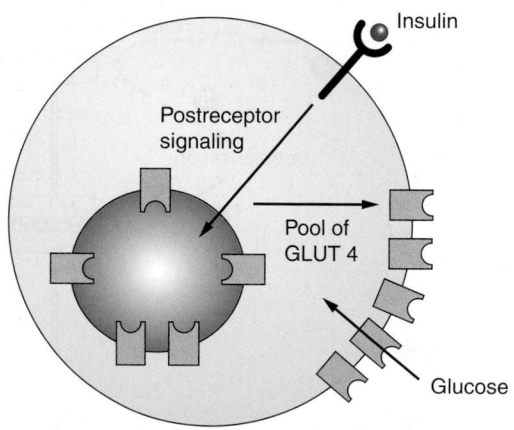

FIGURE 41-3 Insulin receptor is a protein kinase receptor that triggers an enzyme cascade within the cell. One of the effects of insulin binding to its receptor is the translocation of sequestered GLUT 4 transporters to the cell surface. The GLUT 4 carriers are passive and transport glucose down its concentration gradient.

amino acids by skeletal muscle, thus inducing protein synthesis and preventing muscle breakdown. The amount of stored fats in the form of triglyceride is potentiated by the action of insulin in preventing fat breakdown and inducing lipid formation. Insulin also appears to have a role in growth by stimulating the secretion of insulin-like growth factor 1 (IGF-1, somatomedin).[7]

Normal glucose metabolism is usually described in reference to the fed and fasting (or absorptive and postabsorptive, respectively) states. The fed state occurs after ingestion of a meal and is characterized by utilization and storage of ingested energy nutrients. The fasting state is characterized by utilization of stored nutrients for the energy needs of the body.[7]

In the fed state, glucose from ingested food provides the primary energy source (Figure 41-4). The postprandial rise in blood glucose level and the presence of certain gastrointestinal hormones stimulate the production of insulin. Initial stimulation produces a brief rise in insulin secretion, termed the *first phase*. The continued presence of increased concentration of glucose produces the second phase of insulin secretion, a state characterized by insulin synthesis. Amylin is a peptide hormone produced by pancreatic β cells and cosecreted with insulin. Amylin acts upon the area postrema (AP) in the brain to inhibit gastric emptying, induce satiety, and prevent postprandial spikes in blood glucose levels.[8-10] Suppression of glucagon release by amylin is from a paracrine effect within the pancreatic islets and does not require any participation by the area postrema.[11]

The ingestion of nutrients stimulates the release of incretin hormones, which include glucose-dependent insulinotropic polypeptide (GIP) and glucagon-like peptide 1 (GLP-1) from cells in the gut. Both hormones stimulate production of insulin in the presence of glucose, promote proliferation of β cells, and inhibit apoptosis. The presence of these hormones and their effect on blood glucose level is known as

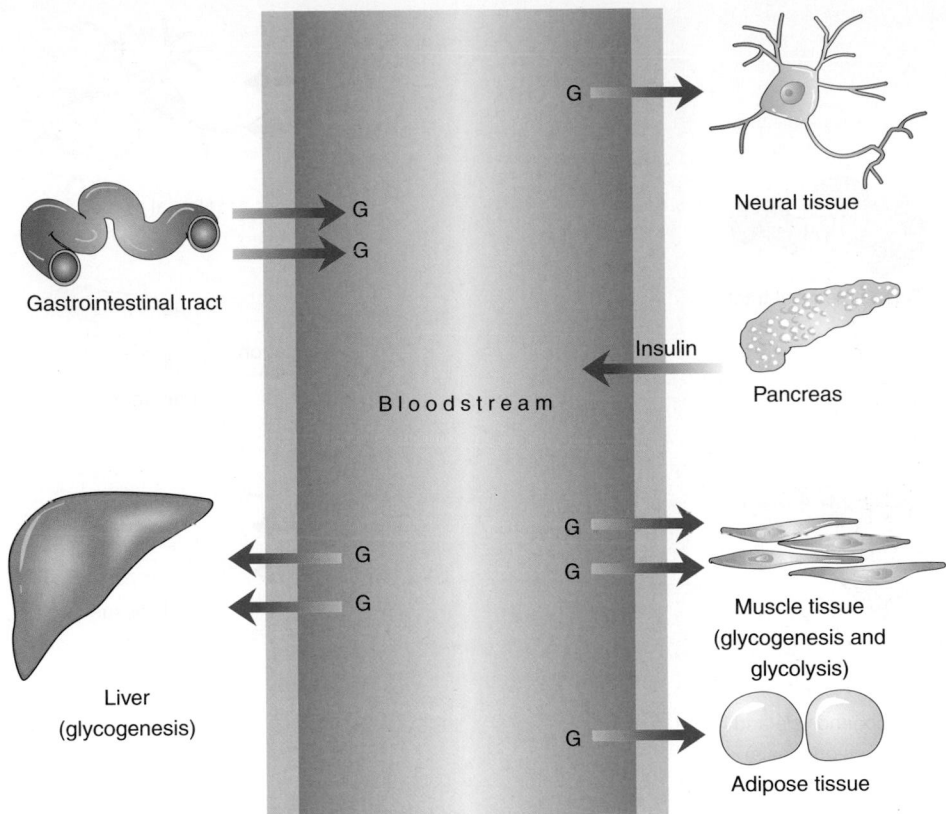

FIGURE 41-4 Energy metabolism in the fed state. *G*, Glucose.

the *incretin effect*. With parenteral nutrition, the incretin effect is not observed. In addition, GLP-1 delays gastric emptying, inhibits glucagon production, and increases satiety.[12]

The presence of insulin stimulates the diffusion of glucose into adipose and muscle tissue and inhibits the production of glucose by the liver. After diffusion into the cell, glucose may be oxidized for the energy needs of the cell, a process termed *glycolysis*. Most ingested glucose is utilized in *glycogenesis* (production of glycogen in the muscle and the liver) (see Metabolic Syndrome section in Chapter 42).

In the fasting state, glucose is produced by *glycogenolysis* (breakdown of stored glycogen) in the liver and muscles and by *gluconeogenesis* (production of glucose from amino acids and other substrates) in the liver (Figure 41-5). Insulin levels, no longer stimulated by an influx of ingested glucose, fall to a basal level. The catabolic effects of the absence of insulin are evident in the stimulation of glycogenolysis and are accompanied by a rise in glucagon levels. If insulin is the hormone that dominates the fed state, glucagon dominates the fasting state. Glucagon-stimulated glycogenolysis and gluconeogenesis are responsible for up to 75% of glucose production in the fasting state. The primary source of energy to muscle tissue in the fasting state is free fatty acids produced by lipolysis (breakdown of fat from adipose tissue). Lipolysis is stimulated by the decline in plasma insulin levels.[13]

Other hormones referred to as *counter-regulatory hormones* have a role in glucose metabolism in the fasting state. Corticosteroids stimulate gluconeogenesis and counteract the hypoglycemic action of insulin. Growth hormone increases peripheral insulin resistance and prevents insulin from suppressing hepatic glucose production. Catecholamines augment glucose production by prompting hepatic glycogenolysis and gluconeogenesis.[13]

Neural Regulation

There is a strong connection between the neural regulatory pathways and the enteric function of digestion, motility, secretion, absorption, and defense. Neural influences from the sympathetic and parasympathetic nervous system are directly involved with carbohydrate metabolism and glucose utilization.[14] There are glucose-sensitive receptors in the brain, mouth, and pancreatic β cells and also in the hepatic portal vein. Once food is placed in the mouth, there is stimulation of the parasympathetic nervous system with stimulation of the β cells for insulin release. This is referred to as first-phase insulin release.[14,15] Glucose-sensitive cells are located in many areas of the brain. These are activated by a decline in glucose levels (glucose-inhibited neurons [GI neurons]) or by a rise in glucose concentrations (glucose-excited neurons [GE neurons]). Under the control of the vagus pathway, the parasympathetic nervous system not only stimulates the release of insulin but also can influence the secretion activity and β-cell mass.[15]

Glucagon is predominantly regulated by the sympathetic nervous system in response to hypoglycemia. The hepatoportal vein contains glucose-sensitive nerve fibers; when stimulated they release norepinephrine and, along with epinephrine released from the adrenals, activate α cells to release glucagon.[15,16]

Exercise

Increasing activity requires increased fuel for muscle tissue. At the onset of exercise, insulin levels drop and glucagon and catecholamine levels initially rise and increase the production of free fatty acids, the primary energy source of resting muscle (Figure 41-6). Falling insulin levels and increased glucagon levels stimulate glycogenolysis. Under the influence of catecholamines, muscle tissue shifts

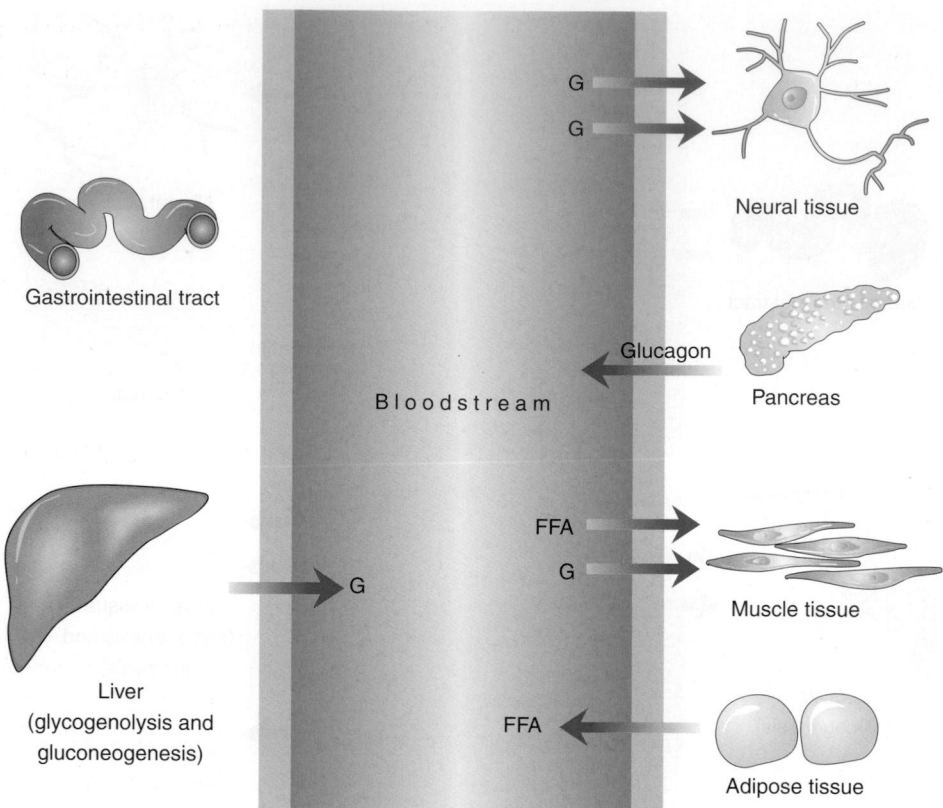

FIGURE 41-5 Energy metabolism in the fasting state. *FFA,* Free fatty acid(s); *G,* glucose.

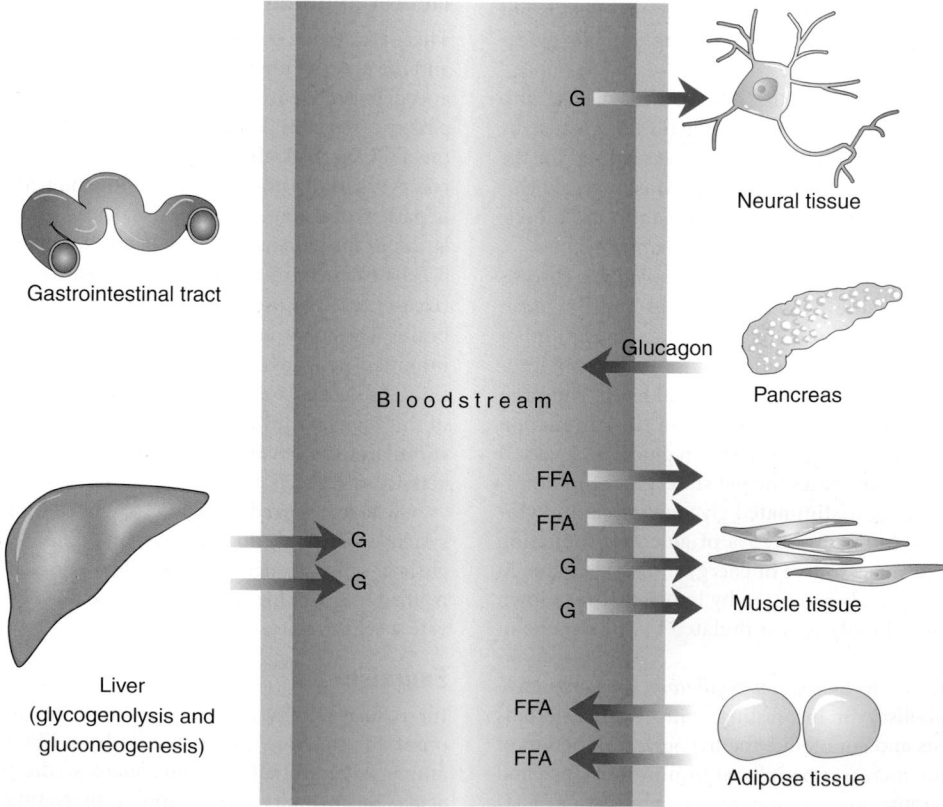

FIGURE 41-6 Energy metabolism during exercise. *FFA,* Free fatty acid(s); *G,* glucose.

from using primarily fatty acids for fuel to using stored glycogen. The relative absence of insulin and the increased production of glucagon also stimulate hepatic glycogenolysis. Glucose released by the liver increasingly meets the energy needs of muscle tissue while exercise continues. After 10 to 40 minutes of exercise, blood glucose use by muscle tissue increases 7 to 20 times. The interactions of hormones thus produce the mixture of glucose and free fatty acids used by muscle tissue during exercise.[13]

Muscle tissue is affected not only by the influence of hormones but also by exercise itself. The resulting increase in insulin sensitivity can last as long as 16 hours. Thus in normal metabolism, increased insulin sensitivity allows normal blood glucose values in the presence of lower levels of circulating insulin.

Stress

During stress such as injury, illness, and pain, stress hormones, including corticosteroids and catecholamines, interact to ensure continuous supplies of glucose. Corticosteroids increase the production of glucose in the liver and elevate the production of glucagon. Glucocorticoids also decrease the utilization of glucose by muscle tissue by diminishing the effect of insulin on glucose transporters and by generating a decline in the number of insulin receptors and their function.

Catecholamines increase plasma glucagon levels, increase glucose production by the liver, and decrease the use of glucose by muscle and fat tissue. The production of fatty acids that is triggered by the action of catecholamines further inhibits glucose uptake in the periphery. The series of events produced by traumatic stress is referred to as *stress hyperglycemia*.[13]

Psychological stress can produce metabolic changes comparable with those of physical stress. Deterioration in metabolic control has been noted in stressed diabetic subjects. However, the response is by no means universal. An increase in blood glucose levels has frequently been observed during acute stress reflecting responses to psychological stress (e.g., disordered eating).[17]

KEY POINTS

- Plasma membrane permeability to glucose is determined by the type and density of glucose transport proteins in the membrane. In some tissues, particularly muscle and fat, the density of facilitative glucose transporters is regulated by insulin. Insulin binding to receptors on the cell surface results in translocation of glucose transporters to the cell surface. Glucose enters the cell passively by facilitated diffusion. Neurons, endothelial cells and erythrocytes have glucose transporters that do not require insulin.
- The metabolic effects of insulin include enhancing protein synthesis and inhibiting gluconeogenesis, enhancing fat deposition and inhibiting lipolysis, and stimulating cellular growth by enhancing somatomedin secretion. Insulin is synthesized in pancreatic β cells as proinsulin. Proinsulin is stored in granules, where it is cleaved into insulin and C-peptide. A postprandial rise in the levels of glucose and other substrates stimulates the release of insulin into the bloodstream. During fasting, when blood glucose levels fall, the decrease in insulin production and the increase in glucagon secretion lead to lipolysis, glycogenolysis, and gluconeogenesis.
- Exercise has complex effects on glucose metabolism. The decrease in production of insulin and the increase in secretion of glucagon and catecholamines lead to elevated blood glucose levels. However, exercising muscle has increased insulin sensitivity, which facilitates glucose uptake.
- A number of hormones released during stress increase blood glucose levels and oppose the effects of insulin. Catecholamines, glucocorticoids, and glucagon may precipitate stress hyperglycemia.

GLUCOSE INTOLERANCE DISORDERS

Classification of Glucose Intolerance Disorders

Diabetes mellitus is not a single disease entity; as many as 30 different disorders may be called diabetes. Criteria for diagnosing the different conditions, all associated with glucose intolerance, were established by the Expert Committee on the Diagnosis and Classification of Diabetes Mellitus in 2011.[18]

Classifications include two pre-diabetes classes and four clinical classes (Box 41-1). Pre-diabetes classes are impaired glucose tolerance and impaired fasting glucose tolerance. The four clinical classes are type 1 diabetes mellitus, type 2 diabetes mellitus, other specific types of diabetes mellitus, and gestational diabetes mellitus.

Pre-Diabetes
Impaired Glucose Tolerance and Impaired Fasting Glucose Tolerance

Guidelines for diagnosing the categories of impaired glucose tolerance (IGT) and impaired fasting glucose tolerance (IFG) are listed in Box 41-2. Impaired glucose tolerance and IFG are intermediate stages between normal glucose metabolism and the onset of diabetes. The pathophysiology of pre-diabetes is complex with a distinct relationship of elevated glucose levels and the development of insulin resistance. Glucose release is stimulated by the mass of metabolically active tissues, including fat free mass and fat mass. The signals to stimulate gluconeogenesis are greater than the counter-regulatory effects, resulting in hepatic insulin resistance.[19]

When glucose levels remain high, the fat-free tissues such as muscle become supersaturated with glucose and start to down-regulate the glucose transporters, accelerating systemic insulin resistance.[19-21]

Diabetes Mellitus
Type 1 Diabetes Mellitus

Type 1 diabetes mellitus (type 1 DM) is, by definition, characterized by destruction of the β cells of the pancreas. Type 1 diabetes can occur at any age but peaks at the ages of 2, 4-6, and 10-14 years of age. Type 1 diabetes accounts for 10% of all diabetes and affects 1.4 million people in the United States and approximately 10 to 20 million people globally.[22-24] The incidence is 1 in every 300 to 600 children and adolescents. Caucasian populations are more susceptible to type 1 diabetes mellitus than are African-American, Hispanic, Asian, or Native American populations. Little difference is noted in the incidence of type 1 diabetes mellitus in children younger than age 15.[23,24] However, more men than women are affected in the population.[24]

Etiology. The two forms of type 1 diabetes are type 1A immune-mediated diabetes, which is the most common, and type 1B idiopathic, which is rare. Immune-mediated type 1A can be further delineated into three subcategories. Polygenic type 1 diabetes involves two or more genetic loci and accounts for 80% to 90% of type 1 cases. Monogenic causes of type 1 diabetes are rare and associated with IPEX syndrome (*immune dysfunction, polyendocrinopathy, enteropathy, X-linked*). The final subgroup of type 1 diabetes is latent autoimmune diabetes in adults (LADA).[25] LADA is linked to the development of T-cell reactivity to islet antigens and autoantibodies to glutamic acid decarboxylase 65 (GADA65). LADA accounts for 2% to 12% of all cases of diabetes and is typically diagnosed after the age of 35. Often initially misdiagnosed as type 2 diabetes, LADA involves destruction of the pancreatic β cells, resulting in insulinopenia.[25-27]

Type 1A diabetes is the result of an autoimmune attack on the β cells of the pancreas. A strong association with the presence of a gene

BOX 41-1   CLASSIFICATIONS OF GLUCOSE METABOLISM DISORDERS

Pre-Diabetes (Increased Risk for Diabetes Mellitus)
Impaired fasting glucose levels
Impaired glucose tolerance

Type 1 Diabetes Mellitus
Type 1A: Immune mediated
- Polygenic
- Monogenic
- Latent autoimmune diabetes in adults
Type 1B: Idiopathic

Type 2 Diabetes Mellitus
Other Specific Types of Diabetes
1. Genetic defects of β-cell function
   a. Chromosome 12, *HNF1A* (formerly *MODY3*)
   b. Chromosome 7, glucokinase (formerly *MODY2*)
   c. Chromosome 20, *HNF4A* (formerly *MODY1*)
   d. Chromosome 13, insulin promoter factor 1 (IPF-1, *MODY4*)
   e. Chromosome 17, *HNF-1β* (*MODY5*)
   f. Chromosome 2, *NeuroD1* (*MODY6*)
   g. Mitochondrial DNA
   h. Others
2. Genetic defects in insulin action
   a. Type A insulin resistance
   b. Leprechaunism
   c. Rabson-Mendenhall syndrome
   d. Lipoatrophic diabetes
   e. Others
3. Diseases of the exocrine pancreas
   Pancreatitis
   a. Trauma/pancreatectomy
   b. Neoplasia
   c. Cystic fibrosis
   d. Hemochromatosis
   e. Fibrocalculous pancreatopathy
   f. Others
4. Endocrinopathies
   a. Acromegaly
   b. Cushing syndrome

   c. Glucagonoma
   d. Pheochromocytoma
   e. Hyperthyroidism
   f. Somatostatinoma
   g. Aldosteronoma
   h. Others
5. Drug or chemical induced
   a. Pyriminil (Vacor)
   b. Pentamidine
   c. Nicotinic acid
   d. Glucocorticoids
   e. Thyroid hormone
   f. Diazoxide
   g. β-Adrenergic agonists
   h. Thiazides
   i. Phenytoin (Dilantin)
   j. Interferon-α
   k. Others
6. Infections
   a. Congenital rubella
   b. Cytomegalovirus
   c. Others
7. Uncommon forms of immune-mediated diabetes
   a. Stiff-man syndrome
   b. Anti–insulin receptor antibodies
   c. Others
8. Other genetic syndromes sometimes associated with diabetes
   a. Down syndrome
   b. Klinefelter syndrome
   c. Turner syndrome
   d. Friedreich ataxia
   e. Huntington chorea
   f. Laurence-Moon-Biedl syndrome
   g. Myotonic dystrophy
   h. Porphyria
   i. Prader-Willi syndrome
   j. Others

Gestational Diabetes Mellitus

Data from American Diabetes Association: Diagnosis and classification of diabetes mellitus, *Diabetes Care* 35(suppl 1):S64-S71, 2012, doi: org/10.2337/dc12-s064; Dib S, Gomes M: Etiopathogenesis of type 1 diabetes mellitus: prognostic factors for the evolution of residual beta cell function, *Diabet Metab Syndrome* 1(1):25, 2009.

or genes in the major histocompatibility complex on chromosome 6 has been observed. Genes in the major histocompatibility complex (MHC) are responsible for the creation of cell-surface proteins (human leukocyte antigens, or HLAs) influencing the lymphocytes to stimulate or suppress antibody production. Recent evidence demonstrates that two primary loci (DR and DQ) confer a genetic predisposition whereas other loci may have a protective effect on the development of type 1 diabetes mellitus.[25,28]

Viral infection or exposure to a toxic agent may be the responsible environmental influence for triggering the autoimmune process in susceptible individuals. The immune system activation is a complex process of antigen recognition (please see Chapter 9 for a detailed explanation).

The etiologic progression of type 1B diabetes mellitus is not known. Idiopathic diabetes is associated with β-cell destruction without autoimmune markers or HLA association.

Pathogenesis and clinical manifestations. Type 1A diabetes is the result of destruction of the pancreatic β cells. The process is mediated by macrophages and T lymphocytes with detectable autoantibodies to various β cells. The T lymphocytes infiltrate the islets and destroy the β cells through the secretion of cytokines (CD4 cells) and direct cytotoxic action (CD8 cells). The preclinical β-cell autoimmunity is variable and precedes the clinical diagnosis. Specific antibodies that develop against glutamic acid decarboxylase 65 (GADA65), insulinoma-antigen 2 (IA-2), or insulin frequently appear early in the onset of immune-mediated diabetes. Antibodies may be present for as long as 13 years before diagnosis and the order of antibody appearance is not significant; however, the presence of multiple antibodies is highly predictive of type 1A diabetes.[23] The presence of these antibodies results in the destruction of the pancreatic β cells. The presence of hyperglycemia indicates that autoimmune destruction of β cells has reached the point at which insulin secretion is inadequate.[29]

Type 1A and 1B diabetes mellitus is characterized by an absolute insulin deficiency, and thus glucose cannot enter muscle and adipose tissue (Figure 41-7). Production of glucose by the liver is no longer opposed by insulin. Overproduction of glucagon by pancreatic α cells stimulates glycogenolysis and gluconeogenesis. Plasma blood glucose levels rise. When the maximal tubular absorptive capacity of the kidney is exceeded, glucose is lost in the urine, and the resulting glycosuria and osmotic fluid loss eventually lead to profound hypovolemia. Tissues dependent on insulin for glucose transport do not have glucose available as a substrate. Neural tissue in the brain responds to this emergency by promoting eating behavior. The increased thirst (polydipsia), increased urination (polyuria), and increased hunger (polyphagia) resulting from the aforementioned processes are the classic symptoms of diabetes.[13]

Type 2 Diabetes Mellitus

Etiology. Individuals with type 2 diabetes mellitus are resistant to the action of insulin on peripheral tissues. Type 2 diabetes mellitus affects 90% to 95% of individuals with diabetes in the United States. Non-Caucasian and elderly populations are disproportionately affected. The prevalence of diabetes is 7.1% in the non-Hispanic white population, 12.6% in non-Hispanic blacks, and 11.8% in Hispanic/Latino-Americans. The age-adjusted prevalence of diabetes in Native American populations ranges from 5.5% among Alaska Native adults to 33.5% in American Indians in southern Arizona. Overall, close to 26.9% of American individuals older than 65 years have diabetes mellitus. In people under the age of 20, diabetes affects 25.6 million people in the United States or 11.3% of the population. The greatest at-risk population is adolescent Native Americans.[3]

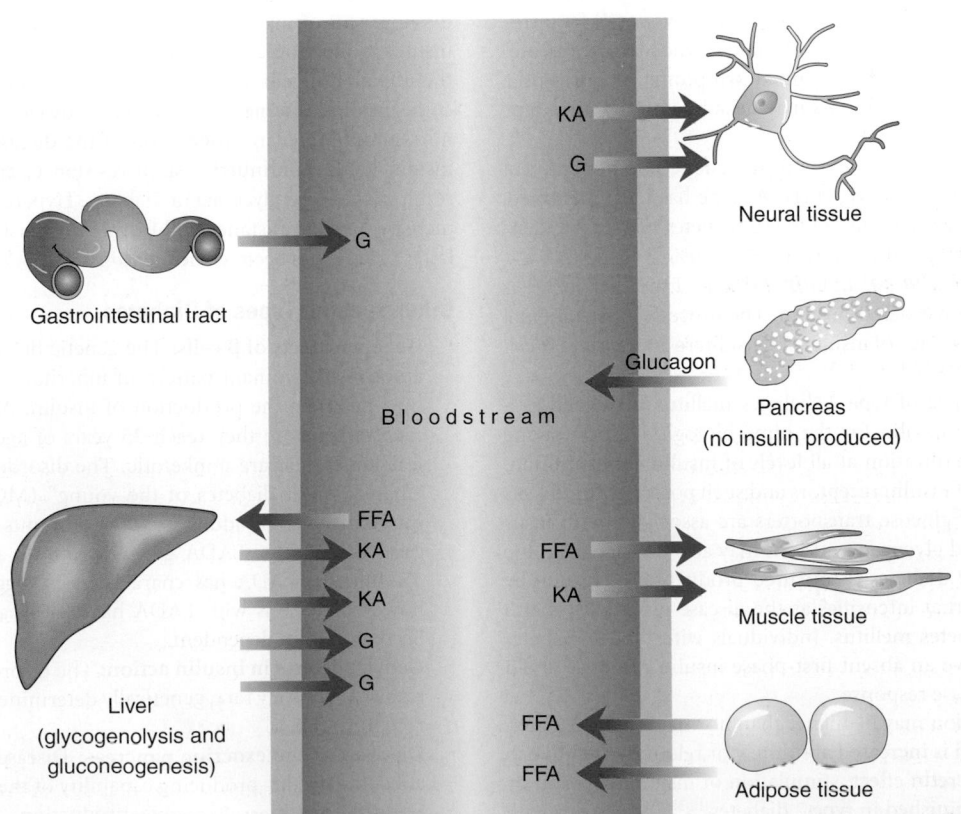

FIGURE 41-7 Pathophysiology of energy metabolism in type 1 diabetes mellitus. *FFA,* Free fatty acid(s); *G,* glucose; *KA,* ketoacid(s).

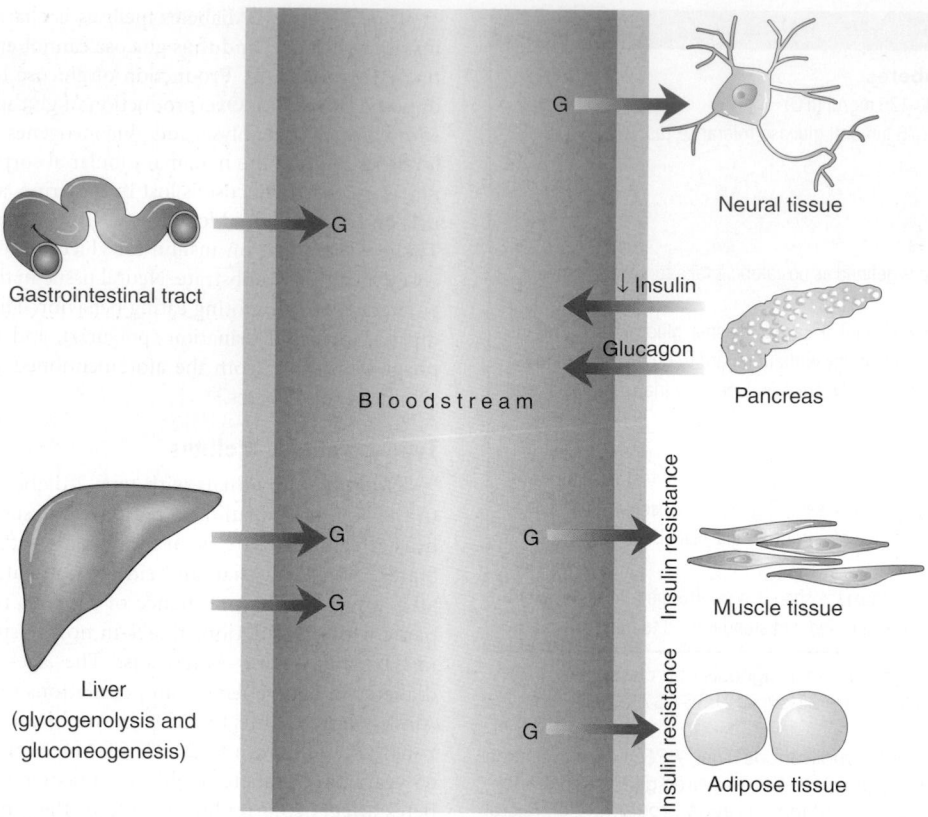

FIGURE 41-8 Pathophysiology of energy metabolism in type 2 diabetes mellitus. *G,* Glucose.

Risk factors include aging and a sedentary lifestyle, but the most powerful predictor is obesity. Excessive abdominal (visceral) fat introduces a greater threat of diabetes mellitus (and cardiovascular disease) than does lower body obesity. The initial symptoms of polydipsia, polyuria, polyphagia, and weight loss may be subtle or absent in type 2 diabetic patients.[3]

Epidemiologic studies indicate a strong genetic component, but no specific human leukocyte antigen (HLA) type has been identified. Studies indicate that the prevalence of type 2 diabetes mellitus in identical twins when one twin is affected is close to 100%.[30]

Pathogenesis and clinical manifestations. Type 2 diabetes is characterized by a relative lack of insulin. The processes instrumental in producing the relative lack of insulin are insulin resistance and β-cell dysfunction (Figure 41-8).[3,30]

The insulin resistance of type 2 diabetes mellitus is defined as a requirement for more insulin for the same biological action, along with lowered glucose utilization at all levels of insulin concentration. A decreased number of insulin receptors and such postreceptor defects as decreased action of glucose transporters are associated with insulin resistance. Impaired glycogen synthesis may also be a factor in the development of type 2 diabetes.[31] Impaired production of insulin by the pancreatic β cells that intensifies as the disease progresses is also present in type 2 diabetes mellitus. Individuals with type 2 diabetes mellitus ultimately have an absent first-phase insulin response and a diminished second-phase response.

Basal insulin secretion may be higher than normal in type 2 diabetes. Glucagon secretion is increased absolutely or relatively (relative to insulin levels). The incretin effect, stimulation of insulin secretion by GLP-1 and GIP, is diminished in type 2 diabetes.[12,30] Individuals with type 2 diabetes may be predominantly insulin resistant or predominantly insulin deficient.

Type 2 diabetes mellitus is a progressive disease characterized by the development of insulin resistance, at first compensated by increased insulin production and hyperinsulinemia. Decompensation occurs as the impaired β cells are unable to produce sufficient insulin to overcome insulin resistance. Insulin levels, however, remain elevated above normal until later in progression of the disease. Relatively decreased insulin levels, continued insulin resistance, and hyperglucagonemia result in the hyperglycemia of diabetes. Hyperglycemia itself may then increase insulin resistance and further diminish insulin secretion. The latter process has been termed *glucose toxicity.*[30]

Other Specific Types of Diabetes

- **Genetic defects of β cells:** The genetic defects of β cells follow an autosomal dominant pattern of inheritance and are characterized by a defect in the production of insulin. Affected individuals are identified before they reach 25 years of age, respond to oral sulfonylureas, and are nonketotic. The disorder is also referred to as "mature-onset diabetes of the young" (MODY). Latent autoimmune diabetes in adults (LADA) accounts for 2% to 12% of all cases of diabetes. LADA generally affects adults after the age of 35. Initially, LADA has characteristics suggestive of type 2 DM; however, persons with LADA have β-cell antibodies and quickly become insulin dependent.
- **Genetic defects in insulin action:** The disorders listed in Box 41-1 result in relatively rare, genetically determined defects of the insulin receptor.
- **Diseases of the exocrine pancreas:** Diseases of the pancreas can affect the insulin-producing capability of the organ (see Box 41-1).
- **Endocrinopathies:** Excessive production of insulin antagonists (e.g., cortisol, growth hormone, glucagon, and epinephrine) affects glucose metabolism (see Box 41-1).

- **Drug- or chemical-induced diabetes:** Many chemicals can affect the ability of the pancreas to produce insulin (see Box 41-1).
- **Infections:** Destruction of the β cells of the pancreas has been linked to various infectious agents (see Box 41-1).
- **Uncommon forms of immune-mediated diabetes:** Certain auto-immune disorders are linked to glucose intolerance (see Box 41-1).
- **Other genetic syndromes sometimes associated with diabetes:** Certain genetic syndromes are linked to glucose intolerance (see Box 41-1).

GESTATIONAL DIABETES MELLITUS. Gestational diabetes mellitus (GDM) is by definition a disorder of glucose intolerance of variable severity with onset or first recognition during pregnancy. Approximately 4% (may range from 1% to 14% depending on population) of pregnancies are affected by gestational diabetes. GDM represents 90% of all pregnancies complicated by diabetes.[18]

Etiology. In its pathophysiologic characteristics, gestational diabetes mellitus closely resembles type 2 diabetes mellitus. As in type 2 diabetes, tissue insulin resistance is present during normal pregnancy. Insulin resistance in normal pregnancy is most likely precipitated by the presence of placental hormones: human chorionic somatomammotropin, estrogen, and cortisol. The weight gain of pregnancy is also responsible for an increase in insulin resistance. During pregnancy, women require two to three times as much insulin as they do in the nonpregnant state. Women with gestational diabetes are unable to produce sufficient insulin to meet their needs during pregnancy.[18]

Risk factors for gestational diabetes mellitus include severe obesity, history of gestational diabetes, previous offspring weighing more than 9 lb at birth, presence of glycosuria, or a strong family history of type 2 diabetes. High-risk individuals should be screened as soon as possible after confirmation of pregnancy. Because insulin needs rise sharply in the twenty-fourth to twenty-eighth weeks of pregnancy, it is recommended that all pregnant women older than 25 years be screened for gestational diabetes during the twenty-fourth to twenty-eighth weeks with either 50 or 100 grams (g) of oral glucose. Younger pregnant women who are obese, have a first-degree relative with diabetes, are members of an ethnic/racial group with a high prevalence of diabetes (e.g., African American, Hispanic, Asian, Native American), have a history of abnormal glucose tolerance, or have a history of poor obstetric outcome should also be screened. If the venous plasma glucose concentration is 140 mg/dl or greater with 50 g of glucose, an oral glucose tolerance test is performed using 100-g load (Table 41-1).[32] Untreated gestational diabetes can result in metabolic abnormalities and stillbirth. However, the most common complications of gestational diabetes are macrosomia and neonatal hypoglycemia. Macrosomia (birth weight greater than 4000 g or >90% for gestational age) is a result of increased glucose, free fatty acids, and amino acids delivered to the fetus. Neonatal hypoglycemia is due to increased production of insulin by the fetal pancreas in response to the chronic stimulation of hyperglycemia while in utero.[33,34]

Treatment. Management of gestational diabetes mellitus includes education regarding appropriate dietary choices, implementation of an exercise regimen, and observation of blood glucose and urine ketone levels. If hyperglycemia persists, insulin therapy should be initiated. Only glyburide does not cross the placenta to cause fetal hypoglycemia; this sulfonylurea may be used in gestational diabetes mellitus.[32,33]

Glucose tolerance will return to normal after parturition in 97% of women with gestational diabetes mellitus. Women with gestational diabetes mellitus have a markedly increased risk for the development of type 2 diabetes mellitus or impairment in glucose tolerance later in life, especially within the first 5 years postpartum.[34] In subsequent

TABLE 41-1	DIAGNOSIS OF GDM WITH A 100- OR 75-g GLUCOSE LOAD*	
	100-g GLUCOSE LOAD	**75-g GLUCOSE LOAD**
Fasting	95 mg/dl	95 mg/dl
1 hour	180 mg/dl	180 mg/dl
2 hours	155 mg/dl	155 mg/dl
3 hours	140 mg/dl	**

Data from American Diabetes Association: Diagnosis and classification of diabetes mellitus, *Diabetes Care* 34(suppl 1):S62-S69, 2011.
*Two or more blood glucose level determinations must be equal to or greater than these values to establish the diagnosis. The test should be done in the morning after an overnight fast of between 8 and 14 hours and after at least 3 days of unrestricted diet (150 g of carbohydrate per day) and unlimited physical activity. The subject should remain seated and should not smoke throughout the test.

BOX 41-3 SCREENING FOR DIABETES

Testing should be considered in all adults older than age 30 who are overweight (BMI ≥25 kg/m^2) and have additional risk factors:
Physical inactivity
- First-degree relative with diabetes
- Members of a high-risk ethnic population (e.g., African American, Latino, Native American, Asian American, and Pacific Islander)
- Women who delivered a baby weighing >9 lb or were diagnosed with GDM
- Hypertension (≥140/90 mm Hg) or receiving therapy for hypertension
- HDL cholesterol level <35 mg/dl and/or triglyceride level >250 mg/dl
- Women with polycystic ovarian syndrome

IGT or IFG on previous testing
Other clinical conditions associated with insulin resistance (e.g., severe obesity and acanthosis nigricans)
History of CVD
In the absence of the above criteria, testing for pre-diabetes and diabetes should begin at age 45 years.
If results are normal, testing should be repeated at least at 3-year intervals, with consideration of more frequent testing depending on initial results and risk status.

Data from American Diabetes Association: Standards of medical care in diabetes, *Diabetes Care* 34(suppl 1):S11-S61, 2011.
CVD, Coronary vascular disease; *HDL,* high-density lipoprotein; *IFG,* impaired fasting glucose; *IGT,* impaired glucose tolerance.

pregnancies, recurrence varies between 30% and 84% in women with a history of gestational diabetes mellitus.[35]

Screening for Diabetes

Because of the high prevalence of undiagnosed type 2 diabetes mellitus, current recommendations are to screen all adults older than age 45 for diabetes at least every 3 years. There is some controversy regarding screening individuals with asymptomatic disease. Individuals with risk factors should be screened at more frequent intervals (Box 41-3).[32]

Screening for gestational diabetes is discussed in the Gestational Diabetes Mellitus section. It is not recommended that routine screening for type 1 diabetes mellitus be performed. No agreement has been reached on the blood level of immune markers that represents a risk for type 1 diabetes or on treatment after identification of the presence of such markers.[32]

KEY POINTS

- Diabetes mellitus is an endocrine disorder diagnosed by the presence of chronic hyperglycemia. Diabetes is diagnosed if any two of the following conditions occurs: a random sampling of blood glucose level higher than 200 mg/dl with classic signs and symptoms, a fasting blood glucose level of greater than 126 mg/dl on two occasions, a blood glucose concentration greater than 200 mg/dl 2 hours after a 75-g oral glucose load, or a hemoglobin A_{1c} (HbA_{1c}) level greater than 6.5%.
- The classification of diabetes mellitus includes two broad categories: (1) actual glucose intolerance and (2) risk of glucose intolerance. Disorders of actual glucose intolerance include type 1, type 2, other specific types, and gestational diabetes. Pre-diabetes categories include individuals with impaired glucose tolerance and those with impaired fasting glucose tolerance. Individuals at risk for glucose intolerance include those with a history of glucose intolerance and those with a positive family history, obesity, or other risk factors.
- Persons with type 1 diabetes have an absolute insulin deficiency caused by pancreatic β-cell failure. Immune-mediated type 1A diabetes is associated with a specific HLA genetic makeup and is autoimmune. Idiopathic type 1B diabetes is not an autoimmune process. Type 1 diabetes may affect people of any age. Classic manifestations include polyuria, polydipsia, polyphagia, and weight loss.
- Persons with type 2 diabetes have a relative insulin deficiency caused by decreased tissue sensitivity and decreased responsiveness to insulin. A decreased number of insulin receptors or abnormal translocation of glucose transporters is suspected. As the disease progresses, pancreatic insulin production may become impaired. Obesity, female gender, family history, older age, and lack of exercise are risk factors.
- Gestational diabetes is a disorder of glucose intolerance that is diagnosed during pregnancy. Placental hormones and weight gain are contributing factors. High infant birth weight and neonatal hypoglycemia are common complications. Gestational diabetes is a risk factor for the later development of type 2 diabetes.

CLINICAL MANIFESTATIONS AND COMPLICATIONS

Acute Hyperglycemia

Etiology. Acute hyperglycemia is most commonly caused by alterations in nutrition, inactivity, inadequate use of antidiabetic medications, or any combination of these factors. Persistent fasting hyperglycemia can occasionally be attributed to the dawn phenomenon, which is a rise in blood glucose concentration in the early morning hours attributed to increased growth hormone, cortisol, glucagon, and epinephrine release.[13,30]

Complications. A primary concern both of health care providers and of individuals with diabetes is avoiding the acute and chronic complications of diabetes. Acute complications of diabetes include the signs and symptoms of hyperglycemia—polydipsia, polyphagia, and polyuria—and concomitant metabolic and fluid problems. Prolonged insulinopenia can result in ketoacidosis and nonketotic hyperglycemic coma with the accompanying more severe electrolyte and fluid derangements.[32]

Acute complications of diabetes also include infections, most commonly of the skin, urinary tract, and vagina. Infections that particularly affect elderly diabetic patients include malignant otitis externa, necrotizing fasciitis, and persistent candidal infections. Tuberculosis infection and reactivation can be a particular problem in diabetic residents of extended care facilities.[32]

Nausea, fatigue, and a generally decreased sense of well-being frequently accompany hyperglycemia. Blurred vision is a common

PARAMETER	DIABETIC KETOACIDOSIS	NONKETOTIC HYPERGLYCEMIC HYPEROSMOLAR SYNDROME
Glucose	>300 mg/dl	>600 mg/dl
Urine ketones	Moderate to high	None
pH	6.8-7.3	Normal
Na^+, K^+	Low, normal, or high	Low, normal, or high
Hct, Hb, protein, WBC count, Cr, BUN, serum osmolality	High	High

TABLE 41-2 DIABETIC KETOACIDOSIS AND NONKETOTIC HYPERGLYCEMIC HYPEROSMOLAR SYNDROME

BUN, Blood urea nitrogen; *Cr,* creatinine; *Hb,* hemoglobin; *Hct,* hematocrit; *WBC,* white blood cell.

short-term problem of acute hyperglycemia. These symptoms can be quite distressing and uncomfortable. Acute complications are directly linked to hyperglycemia and recede as euglycemia is approached.[32]

Diabetic Ketoacidosis

Continued insulin deficiency and other hormonal influences (increased levels of catecholamines, cortisol, glucagon, and growth hormone, in part caused by hypovolemia, physical stress, or insulin deficiency itself) lead to lipolysis in body tissues. As the catabolic process continues, metabolism of fats stored in adipose tissue leads to the production of fatty acids. The resulting fatty acids undergo transformation to ketoacids in the liver. Hepatic gluconeogenesis in response to tissue glucose deprivation is also responsible for the increased production of ketoacids. Under normal circumstances, ketoacids can be used by neural and muscle tissue in energy metabolism. When the normal pathway is saturated, the pH falls (6.8 to 7.3) and ketone bodies are present in the urine, thus sharply increasing osmotic fluid loss. Metabolic acidosis ensues as the bicarbonate concentration decreases, and diabetic ketoacidosis results. In response to the metabolic acidosis, extracellular hydrogen ions are transported intracellularly. Physiologically, potassium is constantly leaking into the vascular space through diffusion and is transported intracellularly via the sodium-potassium pump. This active transport mechanism requires insulin, and in the presence of ketoacidosis, the absence of insulin results in hyperkalemia. Serum potassium levels rise (transient hyperkalemia) and excess potassium is excreted into the urine, eventually leading to a net potassium loss. Losses of sodium, magnesium, and phosphorus also occur as the amount of total body water decreases. Serum levels of the ions may be normal or elevated owing to hypovolemia. Hypovolemia and dehydration also account for increased values of the following: hematocrit, hemoglobin (Hb), protein, white blood cell count, creatinine, and serum osmolality (Table 41-2). Lactic acidosis, or an excessive amount of lactate, a product of glucose metabolism, can also be present because of hypovolemia and possibly reduced uptake of lactate by the liver as a result of acidosis. Hypovolemia and muscle catabolism are present in persons with ketoacidosis and often at diagnosis of type 1 diabetes. Hypovolemic shock can lead to death if the patient is not promptly treated.[13]

Respiratory compensation for the metabolic acidosis in the form of deep, labored respirations that are "fruity" in odor (Kussmaul respirations) results in lowered Pco_2 values (compensatory respiratory alkalosis). Ketoacidosis may be the initial symptom of a new diagnosis of type 1 diabetes. Other factors that may precipitate ketoacidosis are intercurrent illness and inadequate treatment. The need for hospitalization for diabetic ketoacidosis is greatest for individuals less than 45 years of age (39.7 per 1000 individuals with diabetes).[13]

Nonketotic Hyperglycemic Hyperosmolar Syndrome

The relative lack of insulin seen in individuals with type 2 diabetes mellitus leads to similar but not identical sequelae as the absolute lack of insulin of type 1 diabetes mellitus. The initial symptoms of polyuria, polydipsia, and polyphagia may be present, possibly in a more subtle form. Ketoacidosis is an uncommon occurrence in type 2 diabetes. The presence of endogenous insulin in type 2 diabetes suppresses the lipolysis that leads to the production of ketone bodies and subsequently ketoacidosis. More common in type 2 diabetes mellitus, especially in older individuals, is nonketotic hyperglycemic hyperosmolar syndrome (NHHS), characterized by severe hyperglycemia with no or slight ketosis and striking dehydration. Nonketotic hyperglycemic hyperosmolar syndrome is more likely to occur in institutionalized patients, especially patients unable to recognize or respond appropriately to thirst. Diabetic ketoacidosis and NHHS can be life-threatening events, especially in the elderly. Seventy percent of all cases of NHHS coma occur in individuals older than 64 years. The mortality rate is approximately 11%.[36]

Chronic Hyperglycemia

Chronic complications associated with diabetes are extensive and are generally placed into two categories: vascular and neuropathic. The vascular complications are further subdivided into macrovascular and microvascular components. Microvascular complications affect the capillaries, and macrovascular complications involve damage to large vessels.[32]

Vascular Complications
Macrovascular Complications

Macrovascular complications of diabetes mellitus are defined as damage to the large blood vessels providing circulation to the brain, heart, and extremities. Although atherosclerosis is an age-dependent process, the presence of diabetes results in accelerated atherosclerosis. These complications include cardiovascular disease and stroke (38.1% of all individuals with diabetes mellitus over the age of 35), as well as peripheral arterial disease. The presence of heart and blood vessel disease is increased twofold to fourfold in individuals with diabetes and is responsible for more than half of all deaths.[3] Ischemic cerebrovascular accidents (strokes) are more prevalent in individuals with diabetes and are associated with poorer outcomes. Cerebrovascular accidents are responsible for almost 1% of hospitalizations of individuals with diabetes mellitus.[3]

Several studies have investigated whether intensive glycemic control (HbA$_{1c}$ <6.5%) would result in a decrease in cerebrovascular events, cardiovascular events, and all-cause mortality. The ACCORD study was the only study to suggest an increase in overall mortality but a significant reduction in nonfatal coronary events.[37] Other studies have demonstrated improved overall mortality with aggressive glycemic control (mean HbA$_{1c}$ of 6.5%) and a 14% reduction in cardiovascular events for a 1% decrease in HbA$_{1c}$. Despite the reduced mortality, the risk of severe hypoglycemic events significantly increased.[38-41]

Diabetes is an independent risk factor for coronary artery disease. However, several important risk factors for coronary artery disease—dyslipidemia, hypertension, and impaired fibrinolysis—are present in uncontrolled diabetes and decrease with improved blood glucose level control. The latter risk factor may be linked to the presence of the compensatory hyperinsulinemia of type 2 diabetes mellitus.[30,32] Reduction of insulin resistance by such hygienic measures as caloric restriction

and exercise, and possibly by pharmacologic means, may be of principal importance in reducing the incidence of macrovascular complications. Conventional measures of risk reduction, including measures to control dyslipidemia and hypertension, continue to be considered essential. Improved glycemic control is thought to affect the microvasculature rather than the macrovascular complications.

Microvascular Complications

The microvascular complications of diabetes—retinopathy and nephropathy—are thought to result from abnormal thickening of the basement membrane in capillaries. Capillary basement membrane thickening has been shown to increase with the length of time after diagnosis and with persistent hyperglycemia.[32]

Hyperglycemia has been shown to disrupt platelet function and growth of the basement membrane. The presence of proteins altered by high glucose levels (advanced glycation end products) is also believed to play a part in the pathogenesis of microvascular complications. Thickening of capillary basement membranes has been shown to decrease with improved glycemic control.[42] Other risk factors for microvascular disease include hypertension and smoking.

Retinopathy is evident in less than 10% of those diagnosed with diabetes for less than 5 years. However, greater than 50% of patients diagnosed with diabetes for more than 20 years are found to be suffering with some degree of retinopathy. Because of the prevalence of long-standing undiagnosed diabetes mellitus, as many as 21% of individuals with newly diagnosed type 2 diabetes are affected by retinopathy.[30]

Retinopathy is the primary cause of new cases of blindness in adults in the United States. The incidence of diabetic retinopathy appears to correlate with the duration of diabetes. Retinopathy is a progressive disease involving three stages: background retinopathy, preproliferative retinopathy, and proliferative retinopathy. Background retinopathy is characterized by microaneurysms and small hemorrhages in the retinal capillaries. Background retinopathy usually does not affect visual acuity. Preproliferative and proliferative retinopathies involve further damage to retinal capillaries, with the latter condition characterized by capillary neovascularization. The small new capillaries are particularly prone to hemorrhage. Proliferative retinopathy is managed with laser photocoagulation.[13,30,43,44]

Nephropathy affects 20% to 40% of individuals with type 1 diabetes. Fewer individuals with type 2 progress to end-stage renal disease.[42] Diabetic nephropathy accounts for 40% of cases of end-stage renal disease. Ethnic origin is a risk factor in the development of diabetic nephropathy, with African-American, Hispanic, and Native American diabetic individuals experiencing an increased rate of end-stage renal disease as compared with Caucasians.[42,44] The characteristic lesion of diabetic nephropathy is glomerulosclerosis, or thickening and hardening of the basement membrane of capillaries in the glomeruli. Filtration, an essential component of kidney function, occurs in the glomerulus. The first stage of diabetic nephropathy is an increase in the glomerular flow rate, or the rate of blood flow through the glomerulus. This increased flow rate leads to hyperfiltration in the glomerulus, or a rise in the rate at which blood is filtered. The mechanisms leading to the increase in glomerular flow rate are unclear but are evidently related to poor glycemic control. As hyperfiltration progresses, the glomeruli become damaged. The resulting glomerulosclerosis leads to blockage and leaking of the capillaries. Protein is characteristically seen in the urine, at first in small amounts (microalbuminuria) and then grossly. As diabetic nephropathy advances, the glomerular filtration rate drops and chronic kidney disease ensues. Hypertension is an important contributing factor to diabetic nephropathy. Management of hypertension with medications that inhibit angiotensin-converting enzyme has been shown to reduce the rate of chronic kidney disease, end-stage renal disease, and mortality.[43]

Neuropathic Complications

Diabetic neuropathy produces symptoms in 60% to 70% of individuals with diabetes and is responsible for 6.8 per 1000 diabetic population hospitalizations. Neuropathic complications are divided into autonomic dysfunction and sensory dysfunction. Autonomic complications include gastrointestinal disturbances, bladder dysfunction, tachycardia, postural hypotension, and sexual dysfunction. Approximately 35% to 50% of men with diabetes experience erectile dysfunction. Sensory disturbances include carpal tunnel syndrome and paresthesias or lack of sensation in the feet and lower legs. Neuropathy is largely responsible for the increased risk of serious foot problems in individuals with diabetes. The rate of lower extremity amputation in individuals with diabetes is 15 to 40 times higher than in nondiabetic individuals. More than 60% of all nontraumatic amputations in the United States are performed on individuals with diabetes.[44-46]

Diabetes in humans and experimentally induced diabetes in animals are associated with decreased levels of myoinositol in peripheral nerves. Myoinositol is a cell membrane component normally found in abundance in nerve tissue. Several theoretical explanations have been proposed for the myoinositol link to neuropathy. Glucose appears to compete with myoinositol in transport into the cell. Degradation of glucose to sorbitol and fructose (the polyol pathway) occurs in the nerves in the presence of hyperglycemia and insulinopenia. Increased activity of the polyol pathway also appears to be linked to reduced amounts of myoinositol in the peripheral nerves. Focal ischemic lesions of the nerves may also have a role in diabetic neuropathy. Pathologic findings include degeneration or loss of nerve fibers resulting in decreased nerve function.[13]

Glycemic control has been shown to improve nerve function in animals and in humans and to decrease perceived pain. In addition to hyperglycemia, hypertriglyceridemia, obesity, smoking, and hypertension are modifiable vascular risk factors for the development of neuropathy.[44] Other risk factors associated with neuropathy include male gender, white race, older age, and possibly height >175.5 cm.[45] In addition, the elderly, non-Hispanic blacks, and Mexican Americans are disproportionately affected.[46] Strong evidence linking prolonged hyperglycemia to neuropathy and the microvascular complications of diabetes was provided by the Diabetes Control and Complications Trial, a 9-year multicenter prospective study designed to examine the effect of intensive insulin therapy on the development of retinopathy. Renal and neurologic indices were also examined. Subjects in this trial were individuals with type 1 diabetes and no or mild retinopathy at baseline.[47] The experimental group was intensively treated with three or more insulin injections daily or with insulin delivered by a pump. The incidence of initial retinopathy was reduced by 76%, and progression of existing retinopathy was reduced by 54% in the experimental group. Indices of beginning nephropathy such as microalbuminuria and albuminuria were reduced in the experimental group by 39% and 54%, respectively. Symptomatic neuropathy was reduced by 60% in the experimental group. Dilemmas presented by the Diabetes Control and Complications Trial include the presence of a significant increase in severe hypoglycemia in the experimental group and some question about the validity of extrapolating all results to individuals with type 2 diabetes. A large study on the effect of lowering blood glucose level in type 2 diabetes has also yielded data on decreased morbidity and mortality with improved glycemic control (United Kingdom Prospective Diabetes Study).[48]

Complications in Pregnancy

Pregnancy in women with type 1 diabetes has been complicated by an increased risk for perinatal infant mortality and congenital anomalies. Metabolic control during pregnancy reduces the risk of perinatal mortality to a rate approximating that of the general population. An increased rate of congenital malformations continues to attend pregnancies in women with type 1 diabetes. Because the affected organs develop early in the first trimester, excellent glycemic control before conception is recommended.[32] Untreated maternal hyperglycemia can result in increased rates of macrosomia, shoulder dystocia, and preeclampsia as well as death, fractures, and nerve palsies.[49,50]

KEY POINTS

- The acute complications of diabetes are hyperosmolar coma, ketoacidosis, and infection. Hyperglycemia may be associated with nausea, fatigue, and blurred vision.
- Ketoacidosis occurs primarily in type 1 diabetes mellitus as a result of increased lipolysis and conversion to ketone bodies. Excessive ketones result in metabolic acidosis, which is recognized by a fall in pH and bicarbonate levels. Ketoacidosis may occur in patients with type 2 diabetes mellitus under severe stress, such as concomitant sepsis, stroke, or myocardial infarction. Acidosis-induced hyperkalemia and compensatory hyperventilation (Kussmaul respirations) resulting in reduced levels of arterial carbon dioxide are associated findings.
- Nonketotic hyperosmolar syndrome is more common in type 2 diabetes because endogenous insulin suppresses ketone formation and thus prevents ketoacidosis. Hyperglycemia may go untreated for a time and result in persistent glycosuria with osmotic diuresis. Dehydration may be manifested as high osmolality and hemoconcentration of erythrocytes, proteins, and creatinine.
- The chronic complications of hyperglycemia are primarily caused by vascular and neuropathic dysfunction. Individuals with diabetes are prone to vascular complications, including coronary artery disease, stroke, and peripheral arterial disease. These complications are related to dyslipidemia, hypertension, and impaired fibrinolysis. Retinopathy and nephropathy are thought to be due to hyperglycemia-induced thickening of retinal and glomerular basement membranes. Neuropathy is manifested as pain and loss of sensation. Excessive glucose is thought to interfere with myoinositol in neurons.

TREATMENT AND EDUCATION

The usual treatment goals in diabetes are achieving metabolic control of blood glucose levels and preventing acute and chronic complications. The American Diabetes Association recommends as goals a preprandial blood glucose level between 70 and 130 mg/dl and a postprandial blood glucose level less than 180 mg/dl for adults with diabetes.[32] A glycemic control algorithm to guide treatment is presented in Figure 41-9. The goals of treatment are accomplished by diet, exercise, medication, and such hygiene practices as daily foot care and smoking cessation. Each treatment involves lifestyle changes that are difficult to accomplish initially and challenging to maintain. Treatment must be individualized to the type of diabetes and the unique traits of each patient.[51]

Nutrition

Nutrition has often been called the cornerstone of diabetes therapy. Ideas about the optimal dietary prescription have been far from constant throughout recorded history. From wheat, fruit, and beer in ancient Egypt through blood pudding and rancid meats in nineteenth

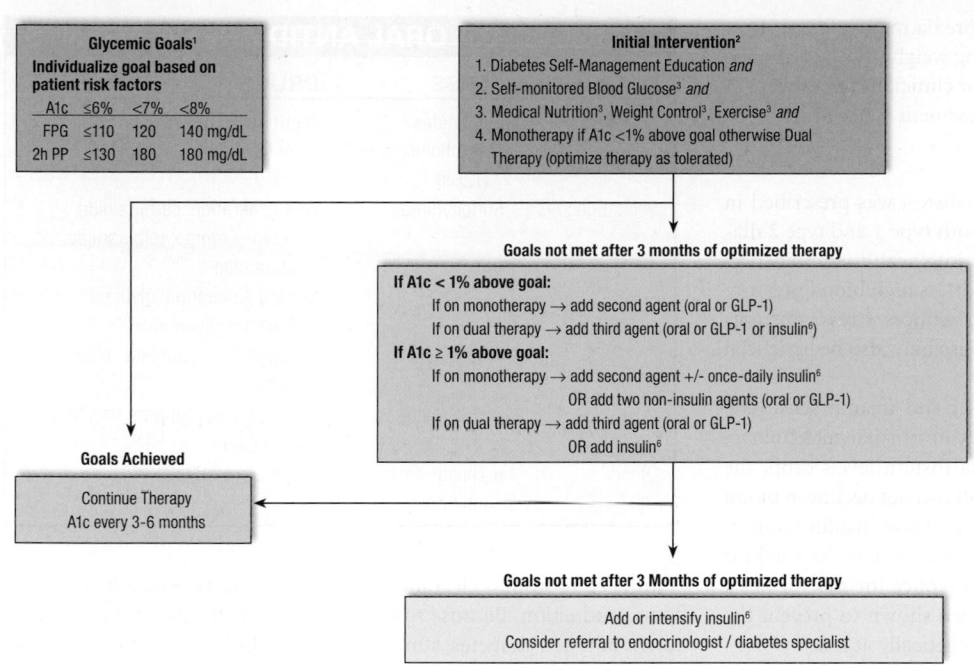

Footnotes

1. **Intensify management if:** Absent/stable cardiovascular disease, mild-moderate microvascular complications, intact hypoglycemia awareness, infrequent hypoglycemic episodes, recently diagnosed diabetes. **Less intensive management if:** Evidence of advanced or poorly controlled cardiovascular and/or microvascular complications, hypoglycemia unawareness, vulnerable patient (ie, impaired cognition, dementia, fall history). Refer to TDC "A1c Goal" treatment strategy for further explanation. A1c is referenced to a non-diabetic range of 4-6% using a DCCT-based assay. ADA Clinical Practice Recommendations. *Diabetes Care* 2010;33(suppl 1):S19-20.

2. If initial A1c on presentation is ≥10%, consider the use of insulin, with or without oral agents, as the initial intervention (see Insulin Algorithm). Other agents may be introduced as glycemic control improves. If ketoacidosis or recent rapid weight loss, consider Type 1 diagnosis.

3. These interventions should be maintained life-long; (refer to Medical Nutrition, Weight Loss, and Exercise Algorithms).

4. Refer to the Diabetes Medications Supplement: Working Together to Manage Diabetes found in the Texas Diabetes Council's Diabetes Toolkit.

5. If a SU is selected, low dose glipizide ER or glimepiride are recommended because they have a lower incidence of hypoglycemia than glyburide.

6. Refer to Insulin Algorithm for Type 2 Diabetes Mellitus in Children and Adults / Initial Insulin Therapy for Type 2 Diabetes Mellitus in Children and Adults: A Simplified Approach

FIGURE 41-9 Algorithm to achieve glycemic control for type 2 diabetes mellitus in adults. *ER,* Extended release. (Reprinted with permission from the Texas Diabetes Council, Texas Department of State Health Services. www.tdctoolkit.org.)

century France to more recent investigations of fiber and fat, nutritional controversies are far from over.

In a position statement, the American Diabetes Association has listed four recommendations for nutritional therapy in patients with diabetes (Box 41-4).[51] Accomplishing the goals can involve changes in composition of the diet, meal patterns and timing, and caloric consumption. All the energy nutrients—carbohydrates, fats, and protein—have an essential role in optimal nutrition. Obesity and eating disorders such as bulimia have an important impact on nutritional status.

Obesity and Eating Disorders

Obesity is the strongest risk factor for type 2 diabetes, in addition to being a risk factor for cardiovascular disease in women. Obesity is defined as a body mass index (BMI) of greater than 30 kg/m². BMI is calculated by dividing body weight in kilograms by the square of the height in meters. Increased risk for health problems occurs at a body mass index of equal to or greater than 25.2 kg/m². A body mass index of 18.5 to 24.9 kg/m² is considered normal. Weight management is a chronic and difficult problem for many individuals. No single strategy has been shown to be effective for all individuals. Current recommendations for management of obesity include the use of a nutritionally complete diet, a maintenance routine, and an exercise program.[51] Consult Chapter 42 for additional nutritional risk factors related to obesity.

BOX 41-4 AMERICAN DIABETES ASSOCIATION RECOMMENDATIONS FOR NUTRITIONAL THERAPY

Achieve and maintain

- Blood glucose levels in the normal range or as close to normal as is safely possible
- A lipid and lipoprotein profile that reduces the risk for vascular disease
- Blood pressure levels in the normal range or as close to normal as is safely possible

To prevent, or at least slow, the rate of development of the chronic complications of diabetes by modifying nutrient intake and lifestyle

To address individual nutrition needs, taking into account personal and cultural preferences and willingness to change

To maintain the pleasure of eating by only limiting food choices when indicated by scientific evidence

Data from American Diabetes Association: Nutrition recommendations and interventions for diabetes, *Diabetes Care* 31(suppl 1):S61-S78, 2008.

Eating disorders such as bulimia and anorexia may be more common in women with type 1 diabetes. Inducing weight loss by reducing insulin levels has also been noted. In order for clinicians to be aware of eating disorders in their patients, careful assessment is necessary.

Exercise

Exercise, one of the oldest treatments for diabetes, was prescribed in India in 500 BC. Exercise can have a role in both type 1 and type 2 diabetes to lower blood glucose levels and promote health maintenance. Exercise lowers such cardiovascular risk factors as high blood pressure and dyslipidemia, increases work capacity, reduces stress, prevents bone loss, and improves reaction time. Exercise may also be beneficial in weight reduction.[52-54]

The effects of exercise on fuel utilization and insulin sensitivity are comparable to exercise-induced changes in normal metabolism. As glucose production increases and plasma insulin levels drop, the reduction in tissue insulin resistance can result in a net decline in blood glucose levels. Exercise has the potential to decrease insulin requirements in type 1 diabetes, decrease and possibly eliminate the need for pharmacologic agents in type 2 diabetes, and reduce the risk for heart disease in all persons with diabetes. It has been shown to prevent the onset of type 2 diabetes in persons who are genetically at risk.[52-54]

Although the benefits of exercise are numerous, there are associated risks. Individuals with type 1 diabetes are at risk for hypoglycemia and ketoacidosis. Exercise in individuals with type 2 diabetes can be associated with hypoglycemia, cardiac dysfunction, orthopedic injury, and worsening of some complications.

When insulin or an oral hypoglycemic agent is used in the management of diabetes, the usual fuel metabolism of exercise is disturbed. Inappropriately high insulin levels result in decreased hepatic glucose production and increased tissue insulin sensitivity. The latter processes can lead to hypoglycemia. Replacement of expended glycogen and continued insulin sensitivity can result in hypoglycemia as long as 24 hours after activity.[52-54]

Hyperglycemia and ketosis may be a result of exercise under insulinopenic conditions. Safeguards must be built into exercise programs to prevent hypoglycemia, ketoacidosis, injury, cardiac compromise, and exacerbation of diabetic complications.

The exercise prescription is as essential in diabetes management as the medication or nutrition prescription. The Centers for Disease Control and Prevention recommend an exercise program of moderate intensity for at least 30 minutes, 5 or more days per week or vigorous intensity for 20 minutes, 3 or more days per week.[52-54]

Exercise should be avoided if ketosis is present, because it can indicate an acute shortage of insulin. Exercise under the latter conditions can lead to increased hyperglycemia. Exercise when blood glucose values are greater than 250 mg/dl is safe if ketosis is not present.[51]

Pharmacologic Agents
Oral Antidiabetic Agents

Along with diet and exercise as initial treatment of type 2 diabetes, numerous medications may be used. Current guidelines call for timely implementation and titration of oral agents as well as insulin to achieve euglycemia.[55] Sulfonylurea drugs have been used in the management of type 2 diabetes for more than 40 years. These drugs have been joined by other agents with different mechanisms of action. Table 41-3 includes a list of common antidiabetic agents.

Sulfonylureas exert their hypoglycemic effect by binding to the ATP-dependent potassium channels on the cell membrane of β cells. This inhibits efflux of potassium, resulting in a rise in intracellular calcium concentration and the secretion of proinsulin. Sulfonylureas are effective in augmenting the action of insulin in glucose disposal,

TABLE 41-3 ORAL ANTIDIABETIC AGENTS

CATEGORY	CLASS	DRUGS
Sensitizers	Biguanides	Metformin
	Thiazolidinediones (TZDs)	Pioglitazone, rosiglitazone
Secretagogues	Sulfonylureas	First generation: carbutamide, chlorpropamide, tolbutamide, tolazamide
		Second generation: glyburide, glipizide, glimepiride
	Meglitinides	Nateglinide, repaglinide, mitiglinide
	DDP-4 inhibitors	Linagliptin, saxagliptin, sitagliptin, vildagliptin
Other	α-Glucosidase inhibitors	Acarbose, miglitol

diminishing insulin clearance by the liver, and reducing hepatic glucose production. Because sulfonylureas are ineffective in the management of type 1 diabetes, stimulation of β cells is known to be a crucial factor in the action of these oral agents. Enhanced insulin secretion appears to be a short-term effect, possibly caused by a reduction in insulin requirements as a result of the other hypoglycemic activities of sulfonylurea agents.[55]

The so-called *first-generation agents* (those formulated earliest) are tolbutamide, chlorpropamide, and tolazamide. Second-generation agents include glyburide, glipizide, and glimepiride. Use of first-generation agents is not recommended unless patients have a well-established history of previous use with good results. Second-generation agents are more potent than first-generation agents, possibly because of increased capacity to bind to the plasma membrane of the β cell. In addition, they are more predictable, have fewer side effects, and represent more convenient dosing.

The side effects of sulfonylureas include hypoglycemia, nausea, dizziness, headache, allergic reactions, and flushing with alcohol use (disulfiram effect). Sulfonylureas that are metabolized to inactive compounds by the liver are considered safer for use in renal disease. Duration of action is another safety issue. After insulin, sulfonylureas are the major cause of severe hypoglycemia caused by a drug. The longer acting sulfonylureas chlorpropamide and glyburide are responsible for the majority of cases of severe hypoglycemia and fatal hypoglycemic coma.

Metformin, classified as a biguanide, suppresses hepatic gluconeogenesis and enhances glucose uptake by peripheral tissues without causing hypoglycemia. Metformin has been used alone and in combination with a sulfonylurea drug and sitagliptin. Metformin is associated with improvement in dyslipidemia and weight loss. Side effects include nausea and diarrhea. Serious side effects of metformin include acute renal injury and metabolic acidosis. In a large review of several thousand patient-years, the incidence of metformin-associated lactic acidosis is rare and most commonly associated with acute kidney injury. Caution should be employed when using metformin in patients with liver disease.[56] Administration of radiographic iodine dyes has potential risk for causing acute renal injury. Patients who are taking metformin have an increased risk of developing metabolic acidosis. Depending on the creatinine clearance value, some patients should hold their metformin for 24 hours before and 48 hours after receiving IV contrast medium.[57]

Acarbose and miglitol, α-glucosidase inhibitors, diminish postprandial hyperglycemia by delaying carbohydrate absorption. They can be used alone and in combination with sulfonylurea drugs, metformin, or insulin. Side effects include symptoms related to decreased gastrointestinal absorption (e.g., flatulence and diarrhea). They do not cause hypoglycemia but can complicate management of hypoglycemia if used in combination with a sulfonylurea. Sulfonylurea-induced hypoglycemia cannot be managed with sucrose when acarbose is being used because of drug-induced delayed sucrose absorption.[32,55]

Thiazolidinedione drugs increase tissue sensitivity to insulin and inhibit hepatic gluconeogenesis. Thiazolidinediones are thought to decrease insulin resistance, increase glucose uptake, and redistribute fat. In addition, they are believed to preserve β-cell function, decrease vascular inflammation, and minimally decrease hepatic glucose production. Currently pioglizatone is the only commercially available thiazolidinedione available; rosiglitazone is available only through selective distribution points because of the cardiovascular risks.

When prescribed along with an appropriate meal plan, oral antidiabetic agents can be very effective in the management of type 2 diabetes mellitus. Primary failure of the drug is considered to have occurred when initiation of oral agent therapy does not result in a significant decline in blood glucose levels. Primary failure can be due to misdiagnosis of type 1 diabetes mellitus or inadequate adherence to the diet and exercise regimen. Secondary failure, or hyperglycemia after an effective initial response to the drug, is often due to dietary nonadherence but may also be due to the progressive β-cell dysfunction of type 2 diabetes mellitus.[32,55]

Incretin Enhancers, Incretins, and Amylins

A newer group of oral agents for management of diabetes are the incretins, incretin enhancers, and amylins.

Dipeptidylpeptidase-4 (DPP-4) is a widely expressed enzyme that is responsible for rapidly degrading glucagon-like peptide 1 (GLP-1) and glucose-dependent insulinotropic polypeptide (GIP). Both of these substances are critical factors in the development and treatment of type 2 diabetes. DPP-4 inhibitors block the secretion of DPP-4, causing sustained action of incretin hormones that results in satiety,[58-60] lower serum glucose levels, and enhanced β-cell mass and function.[61] DPP-4 inhibitors prevent the release of glucagon from α cells through the release of incretin while increasing insulin secretion. Medications in this class include sitagliptin, saxagliptin, linagliptin, and vildagliptin.

The incretin class of medications focuses on glucagon-like peptide 1 (GLP-1). GLP-1 mimetics delay gastric emptying, inhibit release of glucagon, and increase satiety. GLP-1 mimetics are injectable medications with the common side effects of nausea and hypoglycemia. Exenatide can be used alone or in combination with sulfonylureas, metformin, or thiazolidinediones. Medications in this class include exenatide, liraglutide, and lixisenatide.[61]

Pramlintide is an amylin analogue and can be used in conjunction with insulin for the management of glycemia. It may not be mixed with insulin and should be injected separately. Insulin requirements are usually decreased by 50% with pramlintide; in addition, minimum carbohydrate and caloric intake is required for its use. It is contraindicated in patients with hypoglycemia unawareness or gastroparesis. Both incretin and amylin mimetics have been effective in weight loss and lowering HbA_{1c} values when used in conjunction with metformin or a sulfonylurea (both) or insulin (pramlintide only).[62]

Insulin

Insulin therapy is required in all persons with type 1 diabetes mellitus and in 35% of persons with type 2 diabetes mellitus.[13] Persons with type 1 diabetes mellitus require replacement of the deficient hormone in a manner that most closely resembles normal physiologic mechanisms. The role of insulin in type 2 diabetes mellitus is more complex.[30,32]

Because type 2 diabetes mellitus is a progressive disease, many (if not most) individuals will need insulin at some time, either because of increasing insulin resistance or because of β-cell dysfunction. Glucose toxicity, a phenomenon in which insulin resistance and decreased production of insulin are worsened by hyperglycemia, may respond to insulin therapy. Insulin may be necessary in type 2 diabetes intermittently during times of physiologic stress that increase insulin requirements (e.g., concomitant illness, surgery, inactivity, weight gain). However, with resolution of the stress, the individual may be able to discontinue insulin use.[30,32]

Types of insulin are classified by a variety of features, but from a practical standpoint are grouped according to the duration of action: rapid acting, short acting, intermediate acting, and long acting (Table 41-4). The most commonly used insulins in the rapid-acting category are aspart, glulisine, and lispro. Regular insulin is considered short acting. Intermediate-acting agents include isophane. Glargine and detemir are in the long-acting category.[32] There are novel forms of insulin and incretins being developed, including oral insulin tablets, oral insulin spray, and oral incretins.[55]

Patterns of insulin use vary with the type of diabetes and the degree of desired metabolic control. For patients with type 1 diabetes mellitus, a minimum of two or more daily injections of rapid-acting and long-acting insulins has been used to control postprandial and fasting hyperglycemia. A popular regimen includes use of long-acting glargine with preprandial injections of a rapid-acting insulin.[32]

In the management of type 2 diabetes, insulin is initiated early in the course of the disease to achieve and maintain glycemic control. It can be used concomitantly with other antidiabetic agents. The intensity of the regimen is based on the needs of the patient. Long-acting insulin or rapid-acting insulin can only be used to improve fasting or postprandial glycemia, respectively, depending upon the patient's needs. Normally, fasting glucose is targeted first; if HbA_{1c} goals are not met, prandial insulin is initiated. Mixed formulations are beneficial, and require only one to two injections per day, in type 2 diabetes as well.[13,32]

The action of insulin is affected by many elements, including climate, alteration in blood flow, tobacco use, and the injection site. Insulin is absorbed most rapidly from the abdomen, less rapidly from the arm, and most slowly from the legs and buttocks. Insulin is absorbed more rapidly from areas that are exercised or massaged after injection.[13,32]

Hypoglycemia complications. Hypoglycemia is the most common complication of hyperglycemic therapy and the most hazardous. Neural tissue depends on a constant supply of glucose for normal function. When insufficient food intake, unplanned activity, or an inappropriate insulin or sulfonylurea dose lowers the blood glucose concentration excessively, counter-regulatory mechanisms are activated to ensure a continued supply of glucose to the brain. The counter-regulatory mechanism that commences with the activation of the sympathetic nervous system is a response to hypoglycemia that results in the release of glucagon, corticosteroids, and growth hormones.[19]

Symptoms of hypoglycemia produced by counter-regulatory mechanisms include pallor, tremor, diaphoresis, palpitation, and anxiety. Neuroglycopenic symptoms noted in hypoglycemia are hunger, visual disturbance, weakness, paresthesias, confusion, agitation, coma, and death. In long-standing diabetes, neuropathy can alter the counter-regulatory mechanisms. Hypoglycemic unawareness, in which the diabetic patient does not experience counter-regulatory symptoms, can be the result.[32]

Other complications of insulin therapy. Another typical complication of insulin therapy is lipodystrophy. Lipoatrophy has been linked to the use of insulin from animal and human sources and is manifested as hollows in the surface of the skin caused by the destruction of subcutaneous adipose tissue. The exact mechanism is not clear

TABLE 41-4   INSULIN AND OTHER INJECTABLE ANTIHYPERGLYCEMIC MEDICATIONS

DRUG CLASS	ACTION	BRAND NAME	GENERIC NAME	APPEARANCE	RX OR OTC	DRUG TYPE
Insulin	Rapid	Humalog	Insulin lispro	Clear	Rx	Insulin analogue
		NovoLog	Insulin aspart	Clear	Rx	Insulin analogue
		Apidra	Insulin glulisine	Clear	Rx	Insulin analogue
	Short	Humulin R Novolin R	Regular insulin; injectable	Clear	OTC	Regular insulin; injected
	Intermediate	Humulin N Novolin N	Isophane insulin	Cloudy	OTC	Isophane insulin
	Long	Levemir	Insulin detemir	Clear	Rx	Long-acting insulin analogue
		Lantus	Insulin glargine	Clear	Rx	Long-acting insulin complex
	Combination products	Humulin 70/30 Novolin 70/30	70% isophane/ 30% regular	Cloudy	OTC	NPH and regular combination
		NovoLog 70/30	70% aspart protamine/ 30% aspart	Cloudy	Rx	NPH-like and rapid-acting combination
		Humalog mix 75/25	75% lispro protamine/25% lispro	Cloudy	Rx	NPH-like and rapid-acting combination
		Humalog mix 50/50	50% lispro protamine/ 50% lispro	Cloudy	Rx	NPH-like and rapid-acting
		Humulin 50/50	50% isophane/50% regular	Cloudy	OTC	NPH and regular combination
Non-Insulin Injectables						
Incretin mimetic	Adjunct therapy	Byetta	Exenatide	Clear	Rx	GLP-1 analogue
	Adjunct therapy	Victoza	Liraglutide	Clear	Rx	GLP-1 analogue
Amylin analogue		Symlin	Pramlintide		Rx	Amylin analogue

Data from Dipiro JT et al: *Pharmacotherapy: a pathophysiologic approach,* New York, 2008, McGraw-Hill, pp 1216-1217.
NPH, Neutral protamine hagedorn.

but is suggested to be derived from an immune-mediated response. Lipohypertrophy is characterized by an increase in subcutaneous tissue because of insulin-stimulated growth of adipose tissue at the injection sites. Avoiding repeated injections at the same site is recommended to prevent lipodystrophy.[63]

An acute complication of insulin use can be insulin edema, or a localized or generalized accumulation of fluid. Weight gain can accompany initiation of insulin therapy, especially when glycemic control is improved. A third complicating factor in insulin therapy is insulin resistance. Insulin resistance is exacerbated by obesity and can necessitate the use of large insulin doses. An appropriate diet and exercise program is as important to insulin-treated individuals as it is to other patients with diabetes.[32,51]

Stress Management

Living with diabetes can be stressful. The tasks of blood glucose monitoring, medication administration, meal planning, and implementing preventive care to avoid complications can be demanding. Fearing the onset of complications and their impact in addition to living with complications are parts of the psychological impact of diabetes. Depression is more likely to be diagnosed in individuals with diabetes and is correlated with deterioration of glycemic control.[64] Stress management can have an important role in diabetes care by improving quality of life and reducing the possible impact of stress on glycemic control.

Assessment of Efficacy

Several measures are used by clinicians to determine the adequacy of glycemic control. One indirect but very useful indication of blood glucose levels is the level of glycated hemoglobin. Hemoglobin becomes glycated when glucose is nonenzymatically attached to one of its terminal amino acids. Four glycated hemoglobin products are formed: HbA_{1a1}, HbA_{1a2}, HbA_{1b}, and HbA_{1c}. The latter is produced in the largest quantity and is used in most assays.[32]

Because erythrocytes are freely permeable to glucose, the quantities of glycated hemoglobin formed are proportional to the quantity of glucose in the blood plasma. Glycated hemoglobin values will reflect mean blood glucose levels for the life of the average erythrocyte (100 to 120 days).

ONSET (IN HOURS UNLESS NOTED)	PEAK (HOURS)	DURATION (HOURS)	COMPATIBLE MIXED WITH	STORAGE/ EXPIRATION	TYPICAL DOSING/ COMMENTS
15-30 min	1-2	3-4	NPH	Refrigerate/28 days at room temp	15 min before meal or immediately after meal
15-30 min	1-2	3-5	NPH	Refrigerate/28 days at room temp	5-10 min before meal
15-30 min	1-2	3-4	NPH	Refrigerate/28 days at room temp	15 min before or within 20 min after meal
0.5-1	2-3	3-6	NPH	Refrigerate/28 days at room temp	30 min before meal
2-4	4-6	8-12	Insulin analogues/ injectable regular insulin	Refrigerate/28 days at room temp	One, two, or three times daily
2	6-9	14-24	None	Refrigerate/42 days at room temp	Once or twice daily
4-5	Peakless	22-24	None	Refrigerate/28 days at room temp	Once daily, at same time each day
30 min	1.5-16	24	None	Refrigerate/28 days at room temp	30 min before meal
15 min	1-4	24	None	Refrigerate/28 days at room temp	15 min before meal
15 min	1-6.5	24	None	Refrigerate/28 days at room temp	15 min before meal
15- 30 min	1-13	14-24	None	Refrigerate/28 days at room temp	15 min before meal
30 min	2-5.5	24	None	Refrigerate/28 days at room temp	30 min before meal
	2	10	None	Refrigerate/30 days after opening	Within 60 min before morning and evening meals *When initiating, taking close to meals may minimize side effects
	8-12	13+	None	Refrigerate/30 days after opening	Initial dose is 0.6 mg SubQ daily × 1 week, then 1.2 mg SubQ daily
	20 min	3	None	Refrigerate/28 days at room temp or refrigerated	Immediately before each major meal (≥250 kcal or 30 g of carbohydrate)

Highly significant correlations have been found between HbA_{1c} levels and mean blood glucose level.[65,66] The presence of abnormal hemoglobins or hemolytic anemia can skew results. The normal value for HbA_{1c} varies with the laboratory technique but is usually less than 7%. Results of the A1C-Derived Average Glucose (ADAG) Trial published in 2008 correlated an HbA_{1c} number to average glucose levels rather than a percentage. This change has little impact on clinical management; however, it decreases patient confusion regarding glycemic control.[67,68]

HbA_{1c} values are used clinically to estimate long-term control and to establish and evaluate therapeutic goals. Values of less than 7% or as close to normal as possible without adverse effects are considered desirable. Depending upon individual circumstances and life expectancy, less stringent goals may be appropriate. HbA_{1c} values cannot be used for daily management of therapy.[32]

Assessment of glycemia on a daily basis was attempted in the past by the use of testing for glycosuria. However, the blood glucose level at which glucose is measurable in the urine, the glycemic threshold, varies from individual to individual, is usually unacceptably high, and cannot be used to establish the presence of hypoglycemia.

The First and Second Consensus Development Conference on Self-Monitoring of Blood Glucose, convened by the American Diabetes Association and other involved agencies, formulated several goals for the use of capillary blood glucose monitoring. The goals included use of capillary blood glucose monitoring to achieve and maintain a specific level of glycemic control, prevent and manage hypoglycemia, avoid severe hypoglycemia, adjust care in response to changes in lifestyle in individuals requiring pharmacologic therapy, and determine the need for initiating insulin therapy in women with gestational diabetes mellitus.[65,66]

Capillary blood glucose monitoring has been shown to be an accurate reflection of venous blood glucose level when performed by health professionals and by individuals with diabetes. Accuracy can be affected by such performance errors as underloading or overloading of the strip, incorrect placement of the sample, and improper handling of the sample. Training improves performance.[65,66,69]

Diabetic individuals using capillary blood glucose monitoring have frequently reported enthusiasm and increased insight into the relationship between blood glucose level and such factors as diet, exercise, and stress and also have expressed increased feelings of well-being. Capillary blood glucose monitoring has been associated with improved glycemic control. Monitoring of capillary blood glucose levels is simply a feedback mechanism that provides immediate information on the effects of a change in therapy.[65,66,69]

In the replacement of testing for glycosuria with capillary blood glucose monitoring, testing for ketonuria should not be neglected. The presence of ketones in the urine can be an indication of diabetic ketoacidosis and may be harmful to a developing fetus in diabetes complicated by pregnancy. All individuals with diabetes should be tested for ketonuria when blood glucose values are greater than 300 mg/dl, during concomitant illness, during pregnancy, and in the presence of symptoms of diabetic ketoacidosis (nausea, vomiting, abdominal pain).

KEY POINTS

- The mainstays of diabetic treatment are diet, exercise, and drug therapy. Education is an integral part of treatment, enabling individuals with diabetes to follow the diabetic regimen and avoid complications. The efficacy of therapy can be assessed by monitoring blood glucose and HbA$_{1c}$ levels. Blood glucose monitoring is useful for assessing short-term efficacy. HbA$_{1c}$ is a better measure of the long-term efficacy of therapy. A mean blood glucose level less than 170 mg/dl (HbA$_{1c}$ level of 7% or less) is desirable.

- Exercise has several benefits for an individual with diabetes. Insulin requirements may be reduced, weight loss facilitated, and the risk of cardiovascular complications decreased. Exercise may precipitate hypoglycemia, so insulin injections or dietary intake may have to be adjusted. Oral antidiabetic agents may be successfully used in type 2 diabetes. The sulfonylureas exert their effects primarily by stimulating the release of endogenous insulin. They also reduce insulin degradation and suppress the release of glucose from the liver. Metformin suppresses hepatic gluconeogenesis and enhances glucose uptake by peripheral tissue; thiazolidinediones enhance glucose uptake by peripheral tissue; and acarbose delays absorption of ingested carbohydrate. Newer agents such as incretin mimetics, incretin enhancers, and amylin analogues will also be impacted by exercise.

- Insulin replacement therapy is required in all patients with type 1 diabetes and in about one third of patients with type 2 diabetes mellitus. Insulin is classified according to its onset, peak, and duration of action. A combination of insulins may be given to produce optimal control. Long-acting insulin (glargine or detemir) and a rapid-acting insulin (aspart, lispro, glulisine) are commonly used to mimic basal and prandial insulin levels, respectively.

- Hypoglycemia is the most common complication of pharmacologic therapy. Symptoms are mediated primarily by activation of the sympathetic nervous system stress response. Secretion of catecholamines, glucagon, corticosteroids, and growth hormone rises in an attempt to increase blood glucose levels. Pallor, tremor, diaphoresis, weakness, and decreased consciousness are the usual manifestations of hypoglycemia.

PEDIATRIC CONSIDERATIONS

Diabetes has been diagnosed in approximately 176,500 children and adolescents younger than 20 years. One in every 400 to 600 children and adolescents has type 1 diabetes, and 18 new cases per population of 100,000 are diagnosed yearly. The overwhelming majority have type 1 diabetes, with an approximate 5% prevalence of genetic defects in β cells.[1,3,13]

Type 1 diabetes is characterized by destruction of the β cells of the pancreas with resulting insulinopenia. Type 1 diabetes in children is often manifested acutely as diabetic ketoacidosis when insulin secretion falls below insulin needs. A condition termed the "honeymoon period" can develop if the diagnosis occurs during a time of increased insulin needs, such as during a viral illness. When the illness is resolved, insulin needs can fall below residual insulin production and normoglycemia results without the use of exogenous insulin. The honeymoon period rarely lasts more than 1 year and is usually shorter.[13,18]

Goals of Therapy

Goals of therapy for children include achieving normal growth and development, avoiding acute and chronic complications of diabetes, addressing psychosocial issues, and educating children regarding self-care.[32]

Acute Complications

Whenever children with type 1 diabetes mellitus experience hyperglycemia, the resulting glycosuria can precipitate dehydration. The threat of dehydration is especially severe during episodes of diabetic ketoacidosis. Supplemental fluids and insulin may be necessary during these times.[32]

Diabetic ketoacidosis can occur when insulin administration is inadequate for needs. Diabetic ketoacidosis frequently accompanies the diagnosis of type 1 diabetes mellitus. Avoiding diabetic ketoacidosis involves knowledge of appropriate care during times of increased insulin need, such as during concomitant illness. To ensure early detection of incipient diabetic ketoacidosis, children and adolescents should be tested for ketonuria when the blood glucose concentration is greater than 240 mg/dl and during concomitant illness.[13,32]

Hypoglycemia can be difficult to detect in very young children. Caregivers should be alert for behavioral changes such as lethargy, pallor, and sleep disturbances.

Chronic Complications

Chronic complications of diabetes are rarely manifested during adolescence. Screening for neuropathy and nephropathy and determinations of serum lipid levels should occur on a regular basis. Adolescent girls must be counseled on the importance of excellent metabolic control before initiation of pregnancy.[32,49]

Treatment

Insulin requirements are approximately 1.0 unit/kg per day. An intensive regimen of at least three injections per day is recommended to prevent chronic complications. The administration of very small doses of insulin in infants and children may necessitate the use of a diluent.[13,32]

Insulin needs increase during times of physiologic stress, such as during concomitant illness or puberty. Children who are inadequately treated with insulin will not grow or mature normally.

Children are usually able to begin administering insulin and performing capillary blood glucose monitoring with supervision when they are of school age. The age may vary with different children. When administering insulin, the abdomen is the least preferred site because of insufficient abdominal subcutaneous fat.

Diabetic teaching of such self-management skills as insulin injection, capillary blood glucose monitoring, and recognition and treatment of hypoglycemia should include all caregivers. Baby-sitters and teachers will need information on prevention, recognition, and management of hypoglycemia. All educational materials used with children should be age appropriate.[32,69]

Children must be provided with a caloric intake adequate to meet needs for energy expenditure, growth, and maturation. Calorie intake is usually calculated as 1000 calories/day plus 100 added calories for each year until age 11 years. From ages 11 to 18 years, an additional 100 calories is added for girls and an additional 200 calories for boys. Growth should be plotted at each medical appointment to assess adequate nutrition and adequate insulinization. After the age of 2 years, recommended dietary guidelines for percentage of fat, carbohydrate, and protein intake are the same as those for adults.[32,51]

Exercise is encouraged, with careful attention to adequate nutritional intake. Insulin doses may need to be adjusted to plan for unusual levels of activity, such as during long-distance bike riding or hiking.[52-54]

Following a regimen designed to prevent acute and chronic complications of diabetes is difficult under the best of conditions. The goals of treatment are best accomplished when meals, medication, exercise, and blood glucose monitoring are consistent. Achieving consistency while also achieving developmental goals of separation and independence is very difficult. Peer pressure during adolescence can lead to poor adherence to therapeutic regimens. Concern regarding weight can lead to omission of insulin injections or the manifestation of eating disorders.

The child and family need support and counseling to develop effective strategies for achieving desired goals. Disturbed family functioning can have an impact on children and adolescents with diabetes and can lead to an increased frequency of hospitalization for diabetic ketoacidosis.

Genetic defects of the β cell are usually diagnosed in individuals younger than 25 years. These individuals are not likely to become ketotic. Management is identical to that of type 2 diabetes in young adults.

KEY POINTS

- Children and adolescents with diabetes overwhelmingly have type 1 diabetes mellitus (5% have genetic defects of the β cell). In type 1 diabetes, insulin is required at diagnosis or shortly thereafter.
- Goals of therapy for children include achieving normal growth and development, avoiding acute and chronic complications of diabetes, addressing psychosocial issues, and educating children regarding self-care.
- Acute complications of diabetes in children and adolescents include hyperglycemia leading to dehydration, possible diabetic ketoacidosis, and hypoglycemia. Hypoglycemia may manifest differently in children than in adults.
- Chronic complications in children and adolescents are rare. Screening for complications should nevertheless be initiated. Adolescent girls should be counseled on issues regarding diabetes and pregnancy.
- Insulin needs will vary according to growth stages, exercise, and concomitant illness. Regular capillary blood glucose monitoring is crucial for determining the efficacy of treatment. The age at which children can perform insulin measurement and administration as well as capillary blood glucose monitoring independently will vary. Nutritional needs are calculated at 1000 calories/day, with 100 added calories per year until age 11 and then an additional 100 calories for girls and an additional 200 calories for boys ages 11 to 18.
- Education in self-care activities should be appropriate for age and include other family members. Support both for the person with diabetes and for the family is important. Counseling may be helpful in some circumstances.

GERIATRIC CONSIDERATIONS

The prevalence of type 2 diabetes mellitus increases with age. Adults older than 60 years constitute nearly 50% of the diabetic population of the United States. The prevalence of diabetes in the elderly is almost 21% for individuals age 60 or older and more than doubles that of younger adults ages 40 to 59.[1]

The increase in risk for type 2 diabetes in older adults is multifactorial. Aging often involves increased adiposity and a decrease in lean body mass and activity levels. The latter factors contribute to insulin resistance. Insulin secretion also diminishes with age. The risk of diabetes in the elderly is likewise increased by surgery, illness, and the use of such medications as steroids and diuretics.[1]

Diabetes in the elderly can be difficult to diagnose because of fluctuating blood glucose values in response to food intake and activity and because of inconsistent or absent symptoms of hyperglycemia. Chronic complications of diabetes such as neuropathy and retinopathy are frequently present at diagnosis and indicate glucose intolerance of long duration.[32]

Goals of Therapy

Goals of treatment for the elderly include prevention of acute complications, prevention and management of chronic complications, attention to psychosocial issues, and education regarding self-care.[32,69]

Acute Complications

Uncontrolled hyperglycemia in the elderly may be asymptomatic or may produce such classic symptoms as polyuria and fatigue. Polydipsia is less common because of decreased thirst perception. Hyperglycemia can result in increased perception of pain and slowing of intellectual processes. The risk of infection is greater when blood glucose values are greater than 200 mg/dl. Such infectious disease processes as malignant otitis externa and reactivation of chronic tuberculosis are linked to hyperglycemia. Elderly individuals with diabetes are two times as likely to be hospitalized for kidney infections as elderly individuals without diabetes.[32,47]

Chronic hyperglycemia can cause mild to moderate dehydration in the elderly that can be exacerbated by age-related changes in kidney function and water conservation. The resulting postural hypotension and electrolyte imbalances can increase the risk of falls.

Elderly people with type 2 diabetes mellitus are not prone to ketosis, but they are at risk for nonketotic hyperglycemic hyperosmolar coma. Particular risk factors include impaired thirst recognition, polypharmacy, dementia, and concurrent illness. Profound dehydration can occur and lead to a significant mortality rate for this complication (10% to 50%).[34]

Older individuals with type 2 diabetes mellitus must be instructed in care during periods of concomitant illness and advised to perform capillary blood glucose monitoring on a regular basis to avoid undetected hyperglycemia.[69]

Hypoglycemia can occur when an elderly individual with diabetes is treated with a sulfonylurea or insulin. Hyperglycemia can occur atypically with symptoms of lethargy or focal neurologic dysfunction. Elderly individuals may have age-related decreases in counterregulatory function or an inability to report hypoglycemic symptoms. Glycemic targets for these individuals may be higher. The risk of injury during a hypoglycemic episode warrants careful observation of blood glucose values and regular evaluation of treatment of all elderly individuals with diabetes.[32]

Chronic Complications

The increased prevalence of heart and blood vessel disease, kidney disease, eye disease, and foot disease in patients with diabetes overlaps with the increased prevalence of these conditions in the general elderly population. Diabetes increases the incidence and severity of these diseases.

Aging-related changes can present a particular problem in the performance of diabetic foot care. Orthopedic deformity, loss of protective subcutaneous fat, and atherosclerotic changes are all common problems of the elderly. Inspection of the feet and nail care can be compromised by changes in visual acuity and joint function. Assistance with foot care is often necessary to minimize the risk of diabetic complications involving the feet.[32,40,42]

Treatment

Oral antidiabetic agents must be chosen carefully to avoid age-related adverse effects. Oral agents with a shorter duration of action are preferable. Elderly individuals with diabetes should be evaluated for changes in renal and hepatic function. Oral agents metabolized in an impaired system should be avoided. Metformin is not appropriate for individuals with decreased liver and renal function because of the increased risk of lactic acidosis.[32]

Insulin is safe to use with caution in the elderly. Thin elderly individuals can be highly sensitive to insulin and may require very small amounts to control hyperglycemia. Some elderly individuals are quite sensitive to regular insulin. Daily or twice-daily dosing of long-acting insulin may be preferable.

Age- or illness-related changes in vision, manual dexterity, and cognition can diminish the ability to measure and administer insulin. Magnification devices and the use of prefilled syringes can be of assistance.

Exercise is of benefit to individuals of all ages. Exercise plans must often be modified to account for orthopedic or other mobility problems. Armchair exercise can be an excellent way for elderly individuals to stay active.[52-54]

Appropriate food intake can help control hyperglycemia and reduce the risk of chronic complications in the elderly, as in all individuals with diabetes. The quality and quantity of nutrients must be assessed carefully in the elderly. Elderly individuals may be obese, malnourished, or both. Increasing the nutritional value of a meal plan that is low in calories because of choice or a desire to lose weight is an important and difficult goal. Dental and other oral disease or dysfunction can have an impact on nutritional intake.[51]

Education of the elderly in diabetic self-care practices can be challenged by age-related changes in vision, hearing, and cognition.

Simple, clearly written educational materials and less complex therapeutic regimens can be of assistance. Caretakers and family members should be included in education sessions if possible. Family or other assistance can ensure safe performance of diabetic self-care activities while maintaining as much independence as possible.[32]

KEY POINTS

- The increased prevalence of type 2 diabetes mellitus in the elderly is multifactorial and due to increased adiposity, decreased lean body mass, decreased activity levels, decreased insulin secretion, the hyperglycemic effect of certain medications, concurrent illness, and surgery. Varying blood glucose values can lead to difficulty in diagnosis.
- Goals of treatment for the elderly include prevention of acute complications, prevention and management of chronic complications, attention to psychosocial issues, and education regarding self-care.
- Acute complications of diabetes in the elderly include hyperglycemia, often asymptomatic, which can lead to dehydration; increased risk of infection; and nonketotic hyperglycemic hyperosmolar coma. Hypoglycemia can occur atypically and may lead to injury.
- Heart and blood vessel disease, foot problems, visual disabilities, and kidney disease have a significant presence in the aging population in general, as well as being chronic complications of diabetes. Avoiding foot problems can be particularly challenging given the frequent presence of orthopedic deformity and other common aging-related changes, as well as the decreased ability to perform appropriate foot care.
- Oral antidiabetic agents should be carefully chosen with consideration of renal and hepatic function. Short-acting agents are preferable. When insulin treatment is necessary, visual or orthopedic and other changes may hinder measurement of insulin. Adaptive devices can be helpful. Exercise should be encouraged and may have to be modified for people with limited mobility or other limiting factors. Meal planning for elderly individuals should emphasize appropriate amounts of foods with high nutritional value.
- Simple, clearly written educational material can be helpful for individuals with visual or cognitive impairments. Caretakers or family members should be included in education sessions if necessary.

SUMMARY

Diabetes mellitus, the most common endocrine disorder, affects millions of Americans.[1] Diabetes is characterized and diagnosed by chronic hyperglycemia, the result of a relative or absolute deficiency of insulin; however, the metabolism of all energy nutrients is altered. Of the four clinical classes of diabetes, the most common are type 2 and type 1 diabetes. Type 2 diabetes is characterized by insulin resistance and a reduction in insulin production leading to a relative insulin deficiency.[30] Type 1 diabetes is the result of destruction of the insulin-producing β cells of the pancreas because of an autoimmune or idiopathic process.[13]

Sequelae of insulin deficiency include the acute and chronic complications of diabetes. Acute complications include diabetic ketoacidosis in type 1 and nonketotic hyperglycemic hyperosmolar coma in type 2 diabetes. Chronic complications include cardiovascular disease, retinopathy, nephropathy, and neuropathy.

The goals of treatment are glycemic control and prevention of complications. Treatment is individualized and encompasses an

individualized diet, regular exercise, and appropriate use of medications such as oral antidiabetic agents, incretin and amylin mimetics, and insulin. The efficacy of treatment and the presence of complications of therapy are evaluated by capillary blood glucose monitoring. Patient education is an essential component in teaching skills associated with treatment.[32]

Special considerations attend the treatment and education of individuals with diabetes in the pediatric and geriatric age groups. Children and adolescents require careful monitoring to adjust insulin levels for variations in maturation, exercise, and concomitant illness. The elderly may have chronic complications of diabetes or other impairments of mobility, vision, or cognition that affect treatment.[32]

Educational materials must be appropriate for age in children and be accessible for elderly individuals with visual or cognitive impairments.[32,41]

REFERENCES

1. Wild S, Roglic G, Green A, et al: Global prevalence of diabetes: estimates for the year 2000 and projections for the year 2030, *Diabetes Care* 27:1047–1053, 2004.

2. American Diabetes Association: Economic costs of diabetes in the U.S. in 2007, *Diabetes Care* 31:1–20, 2008.

3. Centers for Disease Control and Prevention: *National diabetes fact sheet: national estimates and general information on diabetes and prediabetes in the United States, 2011,* Atlanta, 2011, U.S. Department of Health and Human Services, Centers for Disease Control and Prevention.

4. Augustin R: The protein family of glucose transport facilitators: it's not only about glucose after all, *IUBMB Life* 62(5):315–333, 2010. doi: 10.1002/iub.315.

5. McCulloch IJ, et al: GLUT2 (SLC2A2) is not the principal glucose transporter in human pancreatic beta cells: implications for understanding genetic association signals at this locus, *Mol Genet Metab* 104(4):648–653, 2011. doi: 10.1016/j.ymgme.2011.08.026(4).

6. Thorens B, Mueckler M: Glucose transporters in the 21st century, *Am J Physiol Endocrinol Metab* 298(2):E141–E145, 2010. doi: 10.1152/ajpendo.00712.2009.

7. Spiegel A, Carter-Su C, Taylor SI, et al: Mechanism of action of hormones that act at the cell surface. In Wilson RH, et al, editors: *Williams textbook of endocrinology,* ed 11, Philadelphia, 2008, Saunders.

8. Hartter E, Svoboda T, Ludvik B, et al: Basal and stimulated plasma levels of pancreatic amylin indicate its co-secretion with insulin in humans, *Diabetologia* 34:52–54, 1991.

9. Trevaskis JL, Parkes DG, Roth JD: Insights into amylin–leptin synergy, *Trends Endocrinol Metab* 21(8):473–479, 2010.

10. Plum L, Belgardt BF, Brüning JC: Central insulin action in energy and glucose homeostasis, *J Clin Invest* 116(7):1761–1766, 2006.

11. Guillo C, Roper MG: Simultaneous capillary electrophoresis competitive immunoassay for insulin, glucagon, and islet amyloid polypeptide secretion from mouse islets of Langerhans, *J Chromatogr A* 1218(26):4059–4064, 2011.

12. Drucker DJ: The biology of incretin hormones, *Cell Metab* 3:153–165, 2006.

13. Eisenbaeth GS, Polonsky KS, Buse JB: Diabetes mellitus. In Wilson RH, et al, editors: *Williams textbook of endocrinology,* ed 11, Philadelphia, 2008, Saunders.

14. Mourad FH, Saadé NE: Neural regulation of intestinal nutrient absorption, *Prog Neurobiol* 95(2):149–162, 2011.

15. Thorens B: Brain glucose sensing and neural regulation of insulin and glucagon secretion, *Diabetes Obesity Metab* 13:82–88, 2011.

16. D'Alessio D: The role of dysregulated glucagon secretion in type 2 diabetes, *Diabetes Obesity Metab* 13:126–132, 2011.

17. Kovalaske M, Gandhi GY: Glycemic control in the medical intensive care unit, *J Diabetes Sci Technol* 3(6):1330–1341, 2009.

18. American Diabetes Association: Diagnosis and classification of diabetes mellitus, *Diabetes Care* 35(suppl 1):S64–S71, 2012.

19. Ferrannini E, Gastaldelli A, Lozzo P: Pathophysiology of prediabetes, *Med Clin North Am* 95(2):327–339, 2011.

20. Nolan CJ, Damm P, Prentki M: Type 2 diabetes across generations: from pathophysiology to prevention and management, *Lancet* 378(9786):169–181, 2011.

21. Stumvoll M, Goldstein BJ, van Haeften TW: Type 2 diabetes: principles of pathogenesis and therapy, *Lancet* 365(9467):1333–1346, 2005.

22. International Diabetes Federation: *Diabetes atlas,* ed 5, Belgium, Brussels, 2011, Author.

23. Green A: Descriptive epidemiology of type 1 diabetes in youth: incidence, mortality, prevalence, and secular trends, *Endocr Res* 33(1-2):1–15, 2008.

24. Rewers M, Norris J, Kretowski A: *Epidemiology of type 1 diabetes. Type 1 diabetes: cellular, molecular & clinical immunology,* ed 3, London, 2010, Oxford University Press. Retrieved from www.ucdenver.edu/academics/colleges/medicalschool/centers/BarbaraDavis/OnlineBooks/Pages/Type1Diabetes.aspx.

25. Dib S, Gomes M: Etiopathogenesis of type 1 diabetes mellitus: prognostic factors for the evolution of residual beta cell function, *Diabetol Metab Syndrome* 1(1):25, 2009.

26. Nambam B, Aggarwal S, Jain A: Latent autoimmune diabetes in adults: a distinct but heterogeneous clinical entity, *World J Diabetes* 1(4):111–115, 2010.

27. Rolandsson O, Palmer JP: Latent autoimmune diabetes in adults (LADA) is dead: long live autoimmune diabetes, *Diabetologia* 53(7):1250–1253, 2010.

28. Esienbarth SC, Homann D: *Primer: immunology and autoimmunity type 1 diabetes: molecular, cellular, and clinical immunology,* ed 3, Denver, 2011, Barbara Favis Center for Diabetes.

29. Eisenbarth GS, Jeffrey J: The natural history of type 1A diabetes, *Arquivos Brasileiros Endocrinologia Metabologia* 52:146–155, 2008.

30. Buse JB, Polonsky KS, Purant CF: Type 2 diabetes mellitus. In Wilson RH, et al, editors: *Williams textbook of endocrinology,* ed 11, 2008, Saunders.

31. Nikoulina SE, Ciaraldi TP, Carter L, et al: Impaired muscle glycogen synthase in type 2 diabetes is associated with diminished phosphatidylinositol 3-kinase activation, *J Clin Endocrinol Metab* 86:4307–4314, 2001.

32. American Diabetes Association: Standards of medical care in diabetes—2011, *Diabetes Care* 34:S11–S61, 2011.

33. Coustand DR: Pharmacological management of gestational diabetes: an overview, *Diabetes Care* 30(S2):S206–S208, 2007.

34. Kim C, Newton KM, Knopp RH: Gestational diabetes and the incidence of type 2 diabetes—a systematic review, *Diabetes Care* 25:1862–1868, 2002.

35. Kim C, Berger DK, Chamany S: Recurrence of gestational diabetes mellitus: a system review, *Diabetes Care* 30:1314–1319, 2007.

36. Kitabchi AE, Umpierrez GE, Murphy MB, et al: Hyperglycemic crisis in adult patients with diabetes, *Diabetes Care* 29:2739–2748, 2006.

37. The ACCORD Study Group: Long-term effects of intensive glucose lowering on cardiovascular outcomes, *N Engl J Med* 364(9):818–828, 2011.

38. Kelly TN, Bazzano LA, Fonseca VA, Thethi TK, Reynolds K, et al: Systematic review: glucose control and cardiovascular disease in type 2 diabetes, *Ann Intern Med* 151(6):394–403, 2009.

39. MacIsaac RJ, Jerums G: Intensive glucose control and cardiovascular outcomes in type 2 diabetes, *Heart Lung Circ* 20(10):647–654, 2011.

40. Mannucci E, Monami M, Lamanna C, Gori F, Marchionni N: Prevention of cardiovascular disease through glycemic control in type 2 diabetes: a meta-analysis of randomized clinical trials, *Nutr Metab Cardiovasc Dis* 19(9):604–612, 2009.

41. Turnbull F, Abraira C, Anderson R, et al: Intensive glucose control and macrovascular outcomes in type 2 diabetes, *Diabetologia* 52(11):2288–2298, 2009.

42. American Diabetes Association: Nephropathy in diabetes, *Diabetes Care* 27:S79–S83, 2004.

43. Vijan S, Hayward RA: Treatment of hypertension in type 2 diabetes mellitus: blood pressure goals, choice of agents, and setting priorities in diabetic care, *Ann Intern Med* 138:593–602, 2003.

44. Tesfaye S, Chaturvedi N, Eaton SE, et al: Vascular risk factors and diabetic neuropathy, *N Engl J Med* 352:341–350, 2005.

45. Cheng YJ, Gregg EW, Kahn HS, et al: Peripheral insensate neuropathy—a tall problem for U.S. adults? *Am J Epidemiol* 164:873–880, 2006.

46. Gregg EW, Sorlie P, Paulose-Ram R, et al: Prevalence of lower-extremity disease in the U.S. adult population 40 years of age with and without diabetes, *Diabetes Care* 27:1591–1597, 2004.

47. American Diabetes Association: Implications of the diabetes control and complications trial, *Diabetes Care* 26:25–27, 2003.

48. American Diabetes Association: Implications of the United Kingdom prospective diabetes study, *Diabetes Care* 26:28–32, 2003.

49. Kwik M, Seeho SKM, Smith C, et al: Outcomes of pregnancies affected by impaired glucose tolerance, *Diabetes Res Clin Pract* 77:263–268, 2007.

50. Crowther CA, Hiller JE, Moss JR, et al: Effect of treatment of gestational diabetes mellitus on pregnancy outcomes, *N Engl J Med* 352:2477–2486, 2005.

51. American Diabetes Association: Nutrition recommendations and interventions for diabetes. A position statement of the American Diabetes Association, *Diabetes Care* 31:S61–S78, 2008.

52. Malin SK, Gerber R, Chipkin SR, Braun B: Independent and combined effects of exercise training and metformin on insulin sensitivity in individuals with prediabetes, *Diabetes Care* 35(1):131–136, 2012.

53. Linmans J, Spigt M, Deneer L, et al: Effect of lifestyle intervention for people with diabetes or prediabetes in real-world primary care: propensity score analysis, *BMC Fam Pract* 12(1):95, 2011.

54. Jenkins NT, Hagberg JM: Aerobic training effects on glucose tolerance in prediabetic and normoglycemic humans, *Sports Exercise* 43(12):2231–2240, 2011.

55. Nathan DM, Bus JB, Davidson MB, et al: Management of hyperglycemia in type 2 diabetes: a consensus algorithm for the initiation and adjustment of therapy. Update regarding thiazolidinediones: a consensus statement from the American Diabetes Association and the European Association for the Study of Diabetes, *Diabetes Care* 31:173–175, 2008.

56. Senior PA: Type 2 diabetes, metformin and lactic acidosis—defining the risk and promoting safe practice, *Diabet Med* 29(2):161–163, 2012.

57. Stacul F, van der Molen A, Reimer P, et al: Contrast induced nephropathy: updated ESUR Contrast Media Safety Committee guidelines, *Eur Radiol* 21(12):2527–2541, 2011.

58. Drucker DJ, Nauck MA: The incretin system: glucagon-like peptide-1 receptor agonists and dipeptidyl peptidase-4 inhibitors in type 2 diabetes, *Lancet* 368(9548):1696–1705, 2006.

59. Kyriakos K: Incretin effect: GLP-1, GIP, DPP4, *Diabetes Res Clin Pract* 93(suppl 1[0]):S32–S36, 2011.

60. Langley AK, Suffoletta TJ, Jennings HR: Dipeptidyl peptidase IV inhibitors and the incretin system in type 2 diabetes mellitus, *Pharmacotherapy* 27(8):1163–1180, 2007.

61. Neumiller JJ: Differential chemistry (structure), mechanism of action, and pharmacology of GLP-1 receptor agonists and DPP-4 inhibitors, *J Am Pharm Assoc* 49(5 suppl 1):S16–S29, 2009.

62. Jones MC: Therapies for diabetes: pramlintide and exenatide, *Am Fam Physician* 75:1831–1835, 2007.

63. Cabrera-Freitag P, Escalada J, Goikoetxea MJ, et al: A severe case of lipoatrophy due to human insulin and insulin analogs in a patient with diabetes: is an immunological mechanism involved? *J Investig Allergol Clin Immunol* 21(5):410–421, 2011.

64. Rustad JK, Musselman DL, Nemeroff CB: The relationship of depression and diabetes: pathophysiological and treatment implications, *Psychoneuroendocrinology* 36(9):1276–1286, 2011. doi: 10.1016/j.psyneuen.2011.03.005.

65. Jacobson AM: The psychological care of patients with insulin-dependent diabetes mellitus, *N Engl J Med* 334:1249–1253, 1996.

66. American Diabetes Association: Tests of glycemia in diabetes, *Diabetes Care* 26:106–108, 2003.

67. Goldstein DE, Little RR, Lorenz RA, et al: Tests of glycemia in diabetes, *Diabetes Care* 27:1761–1773, 2004.

68. Syed I: Glycated haemoglobin; past, present, and future: are we ready for the change? *J Pakisatin Med Assoc* 61(4):383–388, 2011.

68a. Lenters-Westra E, Slingerland R: Hemoglobin A1c determination in the A1C-derived average glucose (ADAG) study, *Clin Chem Lab Med* 46(11):1617–1623, 2008.

69. American Diabetes Association: National standards for diabetes self-management education, *Diabetes Care* 34:S89–S96, 2011.

Alterations in Metabolism and Nutrition

Daniel J. Guerra and Carrie W. Miller

evolve WEBSITE

http://evolve.elsevier.com/Copstead/
- Review Questions and Answers
- Glossary (with audio pronunciations for selected terms)
- Animations

- Case Studies
- Key Points Review

KEY QUESTIONS

- How do chronic and acute physiologic stress affect body metabolism?
- What are some useful biochemical diagnostic tests for malnutrition?

- How do insulin, glucagon, catecholamines, thyroid hormone, cortisol, and growth hormone affect the metabolism of fats, carbohydrates, and protein?
- What role does epigenetics play in metabolic disease?

CHAPTER OUTLINE

Throughout its life span, the human body is differentially adjusted and maintained by a complex and connected network of biochemical reactions embedded in pathways that are involved in both energy balance and the interconversion of metabolites to meet ever-changing physiologic needs. This process, known as **metabolism,** uses energy to sustain the body's vital functions.[1] Metabolism utilizes the favorable thermodynamics of biochemical reactions to carry out the physiologic processes of the body in a systematic and tissue-specific manner. These interrelated and dynamic reactions meet the unique requirements of each independent cellular activity.[2] To fuel this system, adequate supplies of digestible foodstuffs with the appropriate organic chemical structure must be acquired on a regular basis or malnutrition and eventual starvation will result. Adequate nutrition is needed for growth and metabolism, organ function, tissue repair, and response to infection. Excess nutrition without a compensatory energy expenditure leads to many diseases and may also make the body more susceptible to pathogens.

Many hospitalized patients enter the care center with a significant degree of physiologic stress and sometimes multiple organ dysfunctions, both of which can alter essential and general nutritional needs. Treatment modalities, altered intake, and restricted mobility may also require nutritional adjustment. In many cases, these problems can be averted, or at least addressed appropriately, if nutritional assessment and therapy are started early.[3,4] This chapter reviews normal nutrient metabolism and nutritional assessment and then progresses to a discussion of physiologic and metabolic dysfunctions.

It is clear that many diseases are fundamentally metabolic, even those typically associated with biological clock mechanisms[5] or ascribed to endocrine hormone dysfunction, such as insulin resistance in metabolic syndrome.[6] Although not discussed here, heritable diseases are almost exclusively inborn errors of metabolism (see Chapter 6).

METABOLIC PROCESSES

Metabolism is the dynamic phenomenon in biological systems involving the physical and chemical processes that produce and maintain (anabolic), and also transform (catabolic), molecules into energy and waste products. Metabolism may be functionally examined along interconnecting biochemical pathways, which fall into three discrete cellular programs:

1. **Intermediary metabolism,** which can be defined as the biochemical process involved with the interconversions of molecules through pathways that are controlled by multiple layers of regulation
2. **Primary metabolism,** which includes biochemical pathways and the cellular machinery of DNA replication, recombination, transcription, RNA processing, translation, and protein processing
3. **Secondary metabolism,** which refers to the synthesis, accumulation, and degradation of molecules that are not specifically essential for normal cellular processes

Nutrition and disease can impact all metabolic programs but the precise nature of this response must be carefully determined using the methods of biomedical screening and interpretation of results. Underlying these medical practices are the basic experimental sciences of biochemistry, genetics, cell physiology, pathology, and microbiology.

The key to metabolism is the control or regulation of the concentrations of metabolites in given cell types such that the system is poised to deal with nutritional and signaling phenomena. Cells must be receptive to membrane-associated signaling so that lipids (or glucose or amino acids) can be transferred or a suite of "messenger" molecules can be recruited and secreted by the activated cell. At the same time, the cell must be in an energetically favorable state; this requires both production and utilization of energy, usually in the form of

adenosine triphosphate (ATP), although many nucleotides take part in this energy transfer (e.g., cyclic AMP [cAMP], guanosine triphosphate [GTP], reduced nicotinamide adenine dinucleotide phosphate [NAD(P)H], flavin adenine dinucleotide [FAD]).

The reactions leading to the assimilation of organic molecules are organized into metabolic pathways. A pathway can be considered a sequential vectorial transfer of substrate to product where the individual catalytic events are carried out by specific enzymatic reactions. The following is a brief account of how metabolic pathways are organized.

- Enzymes in a pathway can be organized in clusters sometimes via simple compartmentalization and sometimes via more specific protein-protein interactions such as multisubunit and polyprotein complexes. Intermediates in a pathway are specifically transferred to the next enzyme active site, even though this process may be nothing more than simple diffusion. The rates of the reactions are such that flux through the pathway is guaranteed and intermediates do not simply diffuse away from the catalysis.
- Soluble and discrete enzymes carry out glycolysis within the cytosol. When this pathway design is utilized, it may be enhanced catalytically by compartmentalization, as the tricarboxylic acid (TCA) cycle is sequestered in the mitochondrial matrix. Another pathway that is utilized in eukaryotic cells is the same as that found in plant fatty acid synthesis (FAS). Here, the proteins are aggregated but not covalently attached. They can be separated as individual catalysts but are believed to exist as protein aggregates in the stroma of the chloroplast. FAS I, as found in mammals and yeast, is a multiprotein or polyprotein covalently linking all of the component proteins in a highly efficient multienzyme complex. Another form of order is that found in the oxidative phosphorylation reactions of the inner mitochondrial membrane leading from the utilization of NADH and the subsequent electrochemical proton pumping coupled to ATP synthesis. These are membrane-bound complexes.

Pathways are functionally separated and regulated:

- *Catabolism and degradative metabolism.* Dietary foods are combusted or oxidized to the final end products CO_2 and H_2O. The electrons from these reactions are largely driven to molecular oxygen, and the production of ATP is coupled to this reduction of oxygen (see Chapter 3). Some of the electrons driven off during the oxidation of carbon are used to make NADPH that in turn provides reducing power for biosynthesis. Glycolysis and the TCA cycle are the major metabolic routes, as well as fatty acid β oxidation, amino acid catabolism to ketogenic (TCA) or glucogenic products, purine degradation to uric acid, and pyrimidine degradation to β-alanine, NH_3, and CO_2. Along these degradation pathways, intermediates for biosynthesis are formed and used (e.g., oxidative pentose phosphate pathway, flavin nucleotides).
- *Biosynthesis or anabolism.* This metabolism involves several unique biosynthetic routes each coupled to the energy state of the cell and the specific cell type, age, and degree of stimulation/signaling. NADPH is the preferred bioreductant in biosynthesis. ATP is also usually required to overcome thermodynamic unfavorability of biosynthetic reactions. Thioester intermediates are also commonly used in biosynthesis. During biosynthesis, substrates are replenished from the catabolite pools, as are NADPH and ATP. Examples of biosynthetic pathways include gluconeogenesis, fatty acid synthesis, amino acid and nucleotide biosynthesis, and protein synthesis. DNA replication and transcription are anabolic pathways as is covalent modification of proteins.

Anabolism and Catabolism

Anabolism refers to the constructive phase of metabolism and involves the synthesis of organic molecules by cells. More complex or larger molecules are built from simple ones, and in the process energy is consumed. Anabolism occurs continuously along with catabolism, but is more prominent during times of rest, healing, pregnancy, lactation, and growth. Hormonal secretions such as insulin and sex hormones may also trigger anabolism. Obesity, with the accumulation of adipose tissue via net synthesis of lipids such as triacylglycerol, is a form of anabolism.[7] Conversely, **catabolism** is the degradative phase of metabolism. Complex molecules are broken down into simpler substances, often with the concurrent release or production of chemical energy. During times of disease, stress, fever, or starvation or during the release of certain hormones such as thyroid hormone and cortisol, catabolism dominates the body's metabolic processes. The resultant tissue wasting may lead to cellular injury or death if excessive catabolism is left unregulated.[8] Anabolism and catabolism occur simultaneously and together create the dynamic, homeostatic balance of chemical substance and energy known as metabolism. In humans, both processes are most efficient in the presence of molecular oxygen although it is not required in active muscle. In some disease states such as cancer, oxygen may be present but is not used in the metabolism found in the tumor (anaerobic glycolysis, *Warburg effect*),[9] although this has recently been challenged and may not be universal in breast cancer.[10]

The metabolic process requires nutrients in the form of carbohydrates, lipids, and proteins. Each of these three nutrients is altered or broken down into simpler substances. Lipids may be directly sequestered into adipose cells after limited lipolysis and synthesis into lipoproteins for transport. Enzymes and coenzymes mediate the metabolism of glucose, fatty acids, amino acids, and nucleic acids. In this fashion, the body's continual cellular energy requirements are met.[8] Energy produced by metabolic processes is used to create the energy currency of the body known as ATP (see Chapter 3).[8]

Cells use energy to perform essential physiologic and biochemical processes. **Energy** can be measured in kilocalories (kcal); 1 kcal represents the amount of energy required to raise the temperature of 1 kg of water from 15° to 16° C. For comparison, a medium-sized baked potato without butter is about 200 kcal whereas a glass of wine is about 100 kcal and a lean filet mignon (8 oz, 227 g) is about 400 kcal.

During catabolism of fuel molecules, approximately 40% of the available energy ultimately is converted to ATP or NADPH (nicotinamide adenine dinucleotide phosphate, reduced form), with the remaining 60% producing heat.[2] The energy released as heat is important for maintaining body temperature.

Metabolic Rate

Several factors determine the body's energy requirements or metabolic needs, including basal metabolic rate (BMR), growth, stress, activity level, and energy necessary for digestion.[8]

The **basal metabolic rate** refers to the rate of energy consumption by resting tissue. It is a measurement of the energy used in maintenance of the body at rest after a 12-hour fast.[8] It represents the energy used in maintaining basic body processes such as respiration, cellular metabolism, circulation, glandular activity, and the maintenance of body temperature.[8] The body's BMR is determined by calculating oxygen use during a specific period. The normal range for BMR is generally between 0.8 and 1.43 kcal/min.[8] Several factors that affect an individual's BMR are described in Table 42-1. Body stature and size affect BMR by the amount of heat lost from the body surface. BMR also is an important determinant of total daily energy expenditure (TEE).[5] Age is also an important determinant of BMR. A growing child's BMR is significantly higher than an adult's, primarily because of an increased rate of cellular activity, surface-to-volume ratio, and generation of new tissue.[8] Conversely, as one ages, the BMR gradually declines by about 2% per decade. Body composition, determined

TABLE 42-1	**EXAMPLES OF FACTORS AFFECTING BASAL METABOLIC RATE**
INCREASING METABOLISM	**DECREASING METABOLISM**
Childhood growth	Aging process
Exercise	End-stage illness
Sympathetic stimulation	Starvation
Shivering	Sleep
Fever	Tropical climates
Thyroid hormone	Calorie-restricted diets
Muscle tissue	Reduced muscle mass
Pregnancy	
Stress	
Male sex hormone	

by the amount of fat and lean tissue, also affects BMR. Muscle tissue requires more oxygen than adipose tissue, which explains why athletes have an approximately 5% higher BMR than nonathletes.[2] One contribution to this observation among athletes is the enhanced β oxidation of fatty acids in this group.[11] Women typically have a metabolic rate 5% to 10% less than that of men, probably because of differences in body mass. Women also tend to have more adipose tissue than men, and fat is less metabolically active than muscle.[7] Pregnancy increases the BMR by about 20% to 28%, or 300 kcal/day, as a consequence of increased uterine and mammary gland size, fetal development, and additional cardiopulmonary workload.[8] Other factors affecting BMR include nutritional status, muscle tone, sleep, fever, environmental temperature, and stress.[2] Metabolic thermoregulation in newborns is described in the Pediatrics Consideration box.

Almost any alteration in the body's normal homeostatic state will alter its energy requirements and BMR. Many diseases are known to dramatically increase the body's energy requirements, including chronic obstructive and restrictive pulmonary disease, hyperthermia, burns, cancer, diabetes, and Graves disease (hyperthyroidism).

KEY POINTS
- Anabolism refers to energy-requiring processes involving synthesis of biomolecules. Catabolism refers to energy-producing processes during which biomolecules are broken down into simpler forms. Metabolism refers to the dynamic state of simultaneously occurring anabolism and catabolism.
- The BMR is the rate of energy utilization when the body is at rest. Examples of factors affecting the BMR include body size and composition, age, nutritional status, muscle mass, fever, stress, and pregnancy.

NUTRIENT METABOLISM

Metabolism is dependent upon energy balance, which is defined as the relationship between nutritional intake and expenditure. In general, metabolism is controlled by both the nervous system and the endocrine system. There are several hormones secreted from these systems that are triggered by the nutritional and energy status of the body, which may become rapidly altered during times of acute stress or chronic disease. Four major hormones involved in nutrient metabolism are insulin, glucagon, catecholamines, and cortisol. The effects of these four hormones on carbohydrate, fat, and protein metabolism are summarized

PEDIATRIC CONSIDERATIONS

Thermoregulation in Newborns

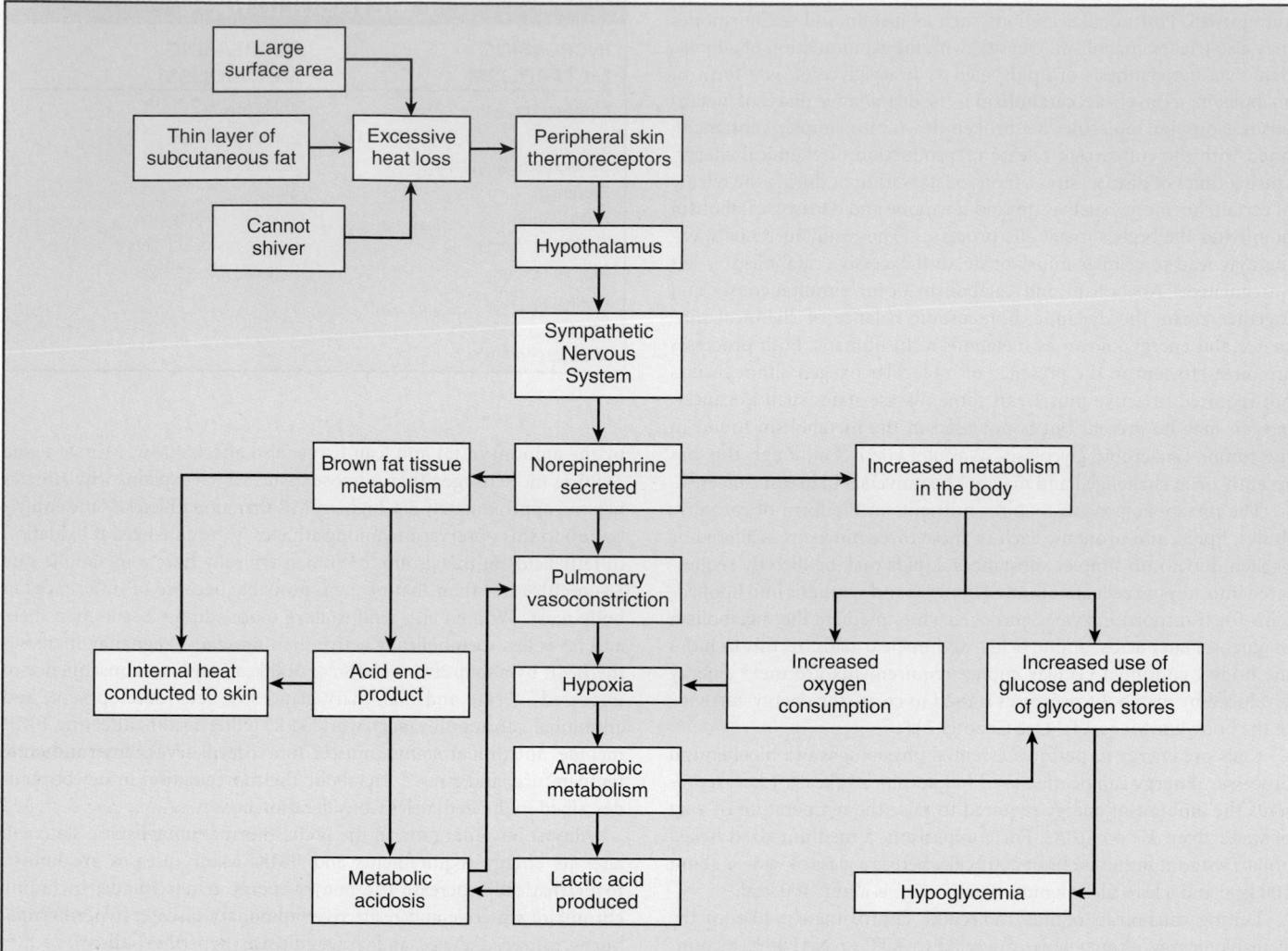

Newborns are more susceptible to excessive heat loss because of several factors. Newborns have a large surface area of skin relative to their weight; they are born with a thin layer of subcutaneous fat, and they cannot shiver. These factors can lead to excessive heat loss if the newborn is not kept warm by other means, such as appropriate clothing.

When heat is lost, the peripheral skin thermoreceptors sense the heat change and signal the hypothalamus. The hypothalamus is responsible for coordinating temperature control in the body. The sympathetic nervous system is signaled by the hypothalamus to secrete norepinephrine. Norepinephrine increases the body's metabolic rate. Metabolism first occurs in the brown fat tissue of the newborn. Brown fat, or adipose, tissue is extremely vascular, has increased glycogen stores, and has more mitochondria within the tissue. As blood passes through the brown fat tissue it absorbs heat from the metabolic process. The

heat is then conducted through the blood to the skin, warming the newborn. Brown fat tissue metabolism creates acidic end-products. Norepinephrine also increases general metabolism in the body, increasing consumption of oxygen, and glucose and glycogen stores. Norepinephrine secretion also results in pulmonary vasoconstriction that can contribute to hypoxia. The lack of oxygen forces the body to use anaerobic metabolism to create energy. Anaerobic metabolism depletes glycogen stores faster than aerobic metabolism, contributing to hypoglycemia. Anaerobic metabolism also produces lactic acid, which combined with the acidic end-products from brown fat metabolism leads to metabolic acidosis. Metabolic acidosis in turn contributes to pulmonary vasoconstriction, which further propagates the cycle. It is critical to keep the newborn warm to minimize cold stress because the newborn is ill equipped for a significant stress response.

in Tables 42-2 to 42-4. Both the nervous system and the endocrine system directly affect metabolism by the release of the catecholamines epinephrine and norepinephrine, which during times of stress inhibit insulin activity. The pancreatic hormones insulin and glucagon have a crucial role in the metabolic processes that govern the body's energy requirements. These hormones function in diametric opposition, with insulin lowering blood glucose levels and glucagon ultimately increasing blood glucose levels.[2] Each of these hormones is controlled by

another hierarchy of regulation. For example, growth hormone (GH) affects metabolism by decreasing cellular uptake and use of glucose. High levels of GH tend to decrease the affinity for insulin at the receptor site such that even increased secretion of insulin by the pancreas has diminutive effects on blood glucose levels. GH, in part, follows a circadian rhythm via stimulation by ghrelin, a gut peptide hormone.[12] Ghrelin concentration is highest after several hours of fasting. Thus, after an extended period of fasting (as during normal sleep) ghrelin is

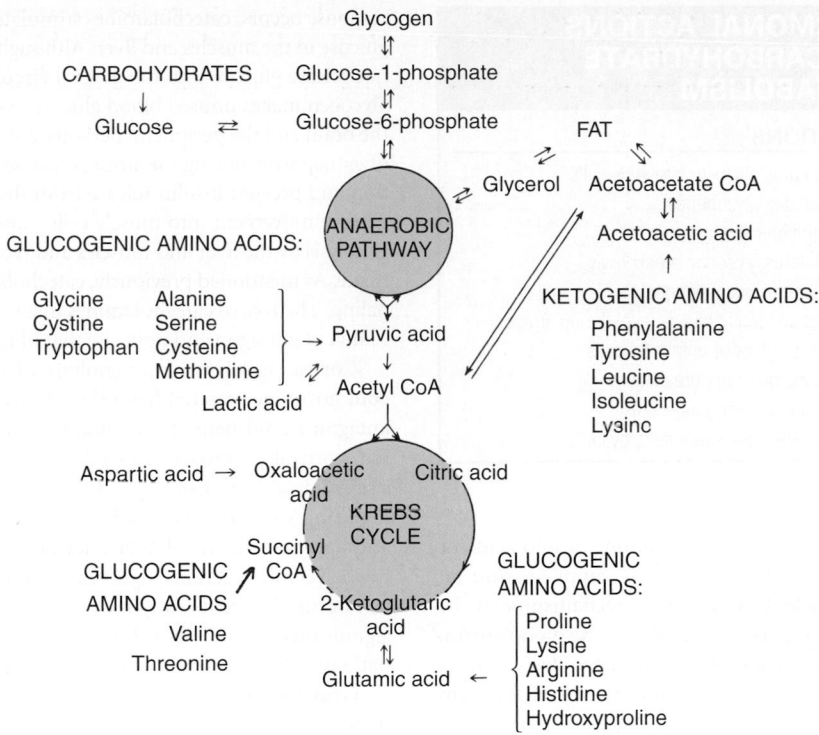

FIGURE 42-1 Metabolic integration of carbohydrate, fat, and protein metabolism. Anaerobic pathway: glycolysis moves with downward arrows; gluconeogenesis moves with upward arrows. *CoA*, Coenzyme A. (From Mahan LK, Arlin MT: *Krause's food, nutrition and diet therapy*, ed 8, Philadelphia, 1992, Saunders, p 345.)

released into the circulation, where it ultimately travels to the hypothalamus and triggers GH release. GH then travels to the periphery (e.g., muscle), where it stimulates lactic acid production for transport to the liver for gluconeogenesis. The release of ghrelin actually starts by catecholamine binding to adrenergic receptors in the gut.[13]

Glucocorticoid hormones, primarily cortisol, stimulate gluconeogenesis by the liver. Blood glucose levels 6 to 10 times normal may occur with significant cortisol secretion. Left uncorrected, diabetes mellitus type 2 may develop (see Chapter 41).[7] Metabolic syndrome, which is well correlated to obesity, may be a precondition for type 2 diabetes (see Metabolic Syndrome section).

Carbohydrates

Carbohydrates are the main energy source for the body. Approximately 45% to 65% of the recommended diet should consist of carbohydrates.[14] Dietary carbohydrates are starches or sugars. Carbohydrates are classified into the three categories of **monosaccharides** (simple sugars), **oligosaccharides** (2 to 10 joined monosaccharide units), and **polysaccharides** (10 to 10,000 monosaccharide units). They range from very simple sugars consisting of three to seven carbons to incredibly complex polymers made up of repeating units of thousands of monosaccharides.[8]

Dietary monosaccharides are the six-carbon sugars of glucose, mannose, fructose, and galactose. Glucose, the most physiologically important of the group, is the form of sugar normally found in the bloodstream. Glucose is derived from the catabolism of more complex carbohydrates during the process of digestion. Fructose and galactose are also eventually converted to glucose by the liver, although fructose can directly enter the metabolism via phosphorylation.[15] Once in the bloodstream, glucose is transported throughout the body where (depending on the location) it is either oxidized to provide cellular energy and reducing power, metabolized to fatty acids, utilized in

amino acid and nucleotide metabolism, or stored in the liver and muscles as glycogen. Blood sugar levels then reflect the difference between the amount of glucose released into the bloodstream by the liver and the amount of glucose taken up by the cells for energy.[7]

Intracellular Glucose Metabolism

Once in the cell, glucose undergoes various biochemical transformations including a form of anaerobic oxidation called glycolysis (see Chapter 3). Glycolysis is the metabolic sequence that converts glucose to pyruvate and, depending on several variables including oxygen availability and energy needs, eventually yields the end products of carbon dioxide and water.[8] Catabolism of glucose may occur anaerobically along the Embden-Meyerhof pathway (glycolysis), which is a 10-step process altering the chemical composition of glucose to pyruvic acid and results in a net gain of two ATP molecules for each molecule of glucose that enters the pathway. Pyruvic acid has two important roles in the catabolic process of carbohydrates. It provides the body with acetyl coenzyme A (acetyl CoA), which is required for conversion to fatty acids or to energy, and it is the initial step for the second stage of carbohydrate metabolism, the tricarboxylic acid (TCA) cycle (also called the *citric acid cycle* or the *Krebs cycle*) and oxidative phosphorylation. The TCA cycle occurs in the mitochondrial matrix. Oxidative phosphorylation (see Chapter 3) produces a total of about 30 molecules of ATP for each molecule of glucose. Although other pathways exist, the interrelated glycolytic, TCA cycle, and respiratory chain enzymes can produce nearly all of the energy required for cellular functioning.[8] Figure 42-1 illustrates the metabolism of carbohydrate, fat, and amino acids through the anaerobic glycolytic pathway and the TCA cycle. The TCA cycle and the respiratory chain require molecular oxygen (aerobic) to function.

Depending on needs, glucose is catabolized for the production of energy, synthesized into lipid, stored as polymers of glycogen, or resynthesized. **Gluconeogenesis** refers to the process by which glucose

TABLE 42-2 HORMONAL ACTIONS ON CARBOHYDRATE METABOLISM

HORMONE	ACTIONS
Insulin	Stimulates glucose uptake by cells
	Stimulates glycogenesis
	Inhibits gluconeogenesis
Glucagon	Stimulates glycogen breakdown
	Increases gluconeogenesis
Catecholamines	Maintain blood glucose level during stress
	Diminish glucose uptake by cells
	Increase glycogen breakdown
Cortisol	Stimulates gluconeogenesis
	Diminishes glucose uptake by cells

is formed from non-carbohydrate sources, including amino acids or lactic acid supplied by muscle tissue and glycerol supplied from fat breakdown.[14] The glucose made through this mechanism may be either stored in the liver as glycogen or released into the bloodstream. During periods of fasting, gluconeogenesis and glycogenolysis provide the necessary glucose to meet the metabolic requirements of the brain and other glucose-dependent tissues.[7]

Hormonal Control of Glucose Metabolism

Many hormones affect glucose levels by altering carbohydrate metabolism. The only hormone known to lower blood glucose levels is insulin. Hormones that tend to raise blood glucose levels include glucagon, growth hormone, glucocorticoid hormones, epinephrine and norepinephrine, and thyroid hormone. Table 42-2 describes the major hormonal effects on glucose metabolism.

Insulin, a peptide hormone formed from its precursor preproinsulin and synthesized by β cells in the pancreas, is secreted in response to increased blood glucose levels. Minutes after ingestion of a meal, insulin levels in the blood rise significantly, peak in 30 minutes, and plateau in about 3 hours. Between meals, when blood glucose levels tend to drop, insulin levels also remain low. At that time, glucose and amino acid stores are used for cellular energy requirements.[7]

Insulin directly affects glucose metabolism by promoting glucose uptake by the liver, which then favors the synthesis of glycogen. Glucose formation (**gluconeogenesis**) and the breakdown of glycogen to form glucose (**glycogenolysis**) are inhibited by insulin. The transport of glucose across cellular membranes into muscle and adipose tissue is facilitated by insulin and has a direct lowering effect on blood glucose levels.[16]

Glucagon is a peptide hormone secreted by α cells in the pancreas and also by some cells lining the gastrointestinal tract. Acting in a manner opposite that of insulin, glucagon increases blood glucose levels.[17] As blood glucose levels begin to drop, plasma glucagon levels begin to rise. Therefore, the two primary effects of glucagon are to promote the breakdown of liver glycogen with subsequent release of glucose into the bloodstream and to promote liver gluconeogenesis. These actions tend to bring serum glucose levels back to normal. Conversely, as glucose levels rise, glucagon secretion is diminished and serum glucose levels drop toward normal. The diametric actions of insulin and glucagon partially explain why increased glucagon secretion may also have a role in the elevated blood glucose levels seen in people with diabetes mellitus.[2]

Catecholamines (i.e., epinephrine and norepinephrine) are derived from the amino acid tyrosine and serve a role in carbohydrate metabolism to maintain blood glucose levels during times of stress. As the stress response occurs, catecholamines stimulate the conversion of glycogen to glucose in the muscles and liver. Although muscles, unlike the liver, cannot release glucose into the general circulation, mobilization of muscle glycogen makes unused blood glucose available for other tissues such as the brain and the peripheral nervous system. The second primary action of epinephrine during the stress response is to stimulate glucagon secretion and prevent insulin release from the pancreas, thereby preventing glucose movement into muscle cells. Epinephrine also promotes glycogenolysis by the liver and muscles and reduces glucose uptake by muscle tissue. As mentioned previously, catecholamines also control ghrelin signaling. The role of catecholamines in glucose metabolism is very similar to that of glucagon and opposite that of insulin.[2]

Cortisol is derived from cholesterol and is the primary **glucocorticoid** hormone secreted from the adrenal cortex. Cortisol is an insulin antagonist and helps to maintain serum glucose levels. During fasting, cortisol permissively enables other hormonal changes to occur, such as decreased insulin production and increased glucagon and epinephrine secretion. The end result is promotion of gluconeogenesis and lipolysis. If cortisol deficiency occurs simultaneously with fasting, hypoglycemic reactions significant enough to alter brain functioning can occur. A recent study indicated that cortisol deficiency may be a significant cause of morbidity and mortality in critically ill surgical patients, who frequently are poorly nourished.[18]

Growth hormone has a role in carbohydrate metabolism, although it may be indirect in comparison with its role in growth regulation and protein anabolism; however, it can have a significant impact on glucose regulation under certain circumstances. Growth hormone's effects parallel those of cortisol: growth hormone increases gluconeogenesis in the liver and inhibits glucose uptake by muscle cells.[2] Growth hormone disinhibits gene expression in the liver in favor of transcription of **phosphoenolpyruvate (PEP)** carboxykinase, a key enzyme in hepatic gluconeogenesis.[12] Elevated serum growth hormone levels tend to increase blood glucose levels. As a result, the insulin-secreting β cells in the pancreas are stimulated. If this process is not corrected, the β cells will eventually be exhausted. It is for this reason that diabetes mellitus eventually develops in individuals with excessive growth hormone, as in acromegaly.[7]

Thyroid hormone tends to raise blood glucose levels. In carbohydrate metabolism, the primary mode of action is to increase glucose absorption from the intestines and stimulate the release of epinephrine. Thyroid hormone also promotes the rate of insulin destruction. Ultimately, thyroid hormone causes an increase in cellular oxygen consumption and the basal metabolic rate of tissues. An alteration in thyroid hormone signaling because of activating mutations of its receptor causes a reduction in body weight and decreased amounts of adipose tissue.[19]

Lipids

Lipids or fats, the most concentrated form of energy, are derived de novo and from animal fats and vegetable oils. Fats supply 9 kcal of energy per gram, as compared with 4 kcal from glucose and 4 kcal from protein. Fats are 98% **triacylglycerol (TAG)**. Like carbohydrates, fats are made up of carbon, hydrogen, and oxygen. The bulk of each TAG molecule in humans consists of fatty acids containing 12 to 22 carbon atoms. Fatty acids are categorized as *saturated* or *unsaturated*. The degree of hydrogen **saturation** refers to the number of double bonds between the carbon atoms in the chain. If a fatty acid chain contains all the hydrogen atoms possible with no double bonds, it is called a **saturated fatty acid.** Those fatty acids with one double bond are termed **monounsaturated,** and those with several double bonds are called **polyunsaturated.**[8]

Fats in the form of TAG supply approximately two thirds of the cell's total energy requirements. Whereas the human body is able to economically store approximately 140,000 kcal of usable fats in adipose tissue, it can store only 24,000 kcal of protein and a mere 800 kcal of carbohydrate in an adult male.[17] Carbohydrates and amino acids not immediately used by the tissues are converted to fat and stored, along with ingested fat, as adipose tissue. Fat deposits are extremely important in the economical use of metabolites. If intake of calories exceeds expenditure, obesity develops over time. During times of fasting, the body quickly reverts to the breakdown and use of fats as its energy source.[18] All tissues in the body, with the exception of brain cells, can metabolize and use fatty acids as an energy source as effectively as glucose.[17]

Almost all fats are absorbed into the lymph system from the intestinal mucosa. They are then converted to a chylomicron consisting of 80% triglyceride, 9% cholesterol, 7% phospholipid, and 4% lipoprotein coat.[20] Chylomicrons empty into the venous blood at the thoracic duct and are carried to the liver for metabolism or assimilated into adipose tissue. Once in the liver, TAG is stored and eventually mobilized via lipoprotein secretion. TAG can also be hydrolyzed to glycerol and free fatty acid in a process known as **lipolysis.** When released into the circulation, the fatty acids, bound to albumin, are quickly assimilated into tissue. Oxidation in tissue begins when coenzyme A forms a thioester bond with the free carbonyl of the fatty acid. Progressing through a series of reactions known as β oxidation, the fatty acid chain is shortened by two carbon units until all is converted to acetyl CoA. During this process the reduced form of flavin adenine dinucleotide ($FADH_2$) and the reduced form of nicotinamide adenine dinucleotide (NADH) are formed, which can be used by the electron-transport chain to make ATP. Acetyl CoA can be used to make ketone bodies or it may enter the TCA cycle and oxidative phosphorylation, with each 2-carbon segment producing 2 molecules of carbon dioxide and 12 molecules of ATP. During prolonged fasting, the ketone bodies can traverse the blood-brain barrier and provide energy to the brain (see following paragraph). The average fatty acid contains approximately 18 carbon atoms, with 146 ATP molecules being produced during catabolism.[2] Unlike fatty acids, glycerol (the other component of triacylglycerol) can be further metabolized (primarily in the liver and in adipose and muscle tissue).[21,22] Free glycerol is generally carried to the liver, where it can be used to form glucose or recycled to generate new triglycerides.

As mentioned, within the liver, fatty acids are generally transformed to acetyl CoA, which is further processed into one of three compounds collectively known as **ketone bodies.** These are acetoacetate, β-hydroxybutyrate, and acetone. Once released into the bloodstream, ketone bodies have a critical role as an energy source for tissues able to oxidize them in the Krebs cycle. During the fasting state, tissues use ketone bodies as a primary energy source, with glucose reserved for brain metabolism. If the fasting state continues, many areas of the brain begin to use ketone bodies as an energy source. As the brain begins to use ketone bodies, less protein is broken down to provide glucose. For this reason, the body is able to withstand periods of fasting with minimal protein breakdown and associated lean body mass degeneration.[2] However, excessive acute ketogenesis is harmful and produces a condition known as ketoacidosis, which is prevalent in type 1 diabetes (Chapter 41).

The liver is the major organ responsible for lipid metabolism and regulation of serum lipid levels. The five primary functions of the hepatic system in regard to lipid metabolism are: (1) synthesis of triacylglycerol from carbohydrates and protein, (2) synthesis of phospholipids and cholesterol from dietary TAG, (3) desaturation and elongation of fatty acids, (4) utilization of TAG as an energy source, and (5) transport of lipids to the periphery, especially to adipose tissue.[8] Liver disease can significantly alter any of these processes and

TABLE 42-3	HORMONAL ACTIONS ON LIPID METABOLISM	
HORMONE	**ACTIONS**
Insulin	Increases fatty acid uptake by fat cells
	Promotes glucose uptake by fat cells
Glucagon	Promotes lipolysis in fat cells
Catecholamines	Increase fat mobilization
	Increase serum free fatty acid levels
Cortisol	Increases fat cell membrane permeability

cause serious metabolic dysfunction. A fatty liver is characterized by fat deposits in the liver cells caused either by ingestion of hepatotoxic substances such as alcohol or halocarbons or by consumption of diets significantly low in protein for a prolonged period (see Chapter 38). Infections managed with protein synthesis–inhibiting antibiotics, such as tetracycline, and malignancies may also lead to increased fat deposits within the liver by adversely affecting the hepatic cells or biliary tract. Increased mobilization of fatty acids from adipose tissue to the liver occurs in certain conditions, such as metabolic syndrome, diabetes mellitus, starvation, and obesity, where lipogenesis exceeds the ability of the liver to export the fat as lipoproteins.[23] Metabolic studies of critically ill patients indicate that fatty acid breakdown occurs at a much higher rate than required by patient caloric needs. This excess lipolysis may cause fatty liver.[24]

Hormonal Control of Lipid Metabolism

Carbohydrates can be metabolized along the anaerobic glycolytic pathway and this process can lead to mitochondrial production of citrate (via acetyl CoA and oxaloacetic acid [OAA]; both produced from pyruvate), which may reenter the cytosol for lipid synthesis. Therefore, hormones that affect carbohydrate metabolism also affect lipid metabolism. Table 42-3 describes the hormones considered to have the greatest effect on lipid metabolism. These hormones include insulin, thyroid hormone, glucocorticoids, mineralocorticoids, growth hormone, epinephrine, and norepinephrine. Insulin prevents fat utilization by indirectly causing fatty acids to be taken up by adipose tissue and by decreasing the activity of hormone-sensitive lipase, which promotes the movement of fat out of adipose tissue. Glucocorticoids increase fat cell membrane permeability, whereas mineralocorticoids and glucagon increase the activity of hormone-sensitive lipase. Epinephrine and norepinephrine increase fat mobilization by stimulating the activity of hormone-sensitive lipase, thus increasing the serum free fatty acid level. Growth hormone increases fatty acid mobilization and use by tissues as an energy source.[8]

Lipids also comprise the bulk of cellular membranes and they serve as paracrine and autocrine hormones. Because of their complex structure and elaborate function, including dietary and bioenergetic considerations, lipids are quite possibly the most significant class of organic compounds in metabolism.

Proteins

Proteins are composed of nitrogen, carbon, hydrogen, oxygen, and, occasionally, sulfur. When hydrolyzed, they yield amino acids. A total of 22 amino acids have been identified in protein, 8 of which are essential—meaning that they must be supplied through the diet.[20] These include phenylalanine, valine, threonine, tryptophan, isoleucine, methionine, leucine, and lysine. The distinction between essential and nonessential amino acids is somewhat unclear, because some amino acids can be produced from others via transamination. Several amino acids are considered to be conditionally essential and must be supplied by the diet under conditions of reduced ability to synthesize them in the body. For example, tyrosine can be synthesized from phenylalanine, but when a patient is receiving a phenylalanine-restricted diet, then tyrosine cannot be synthesized and must be provided in the diet. Muscle tissue, skin, and hair are composed primarily of protein. Proteins also serve as the major enzymatic catalysts. To function properly, most body processes require an adequate supply of proteins, many of which must be obtained through a balanced diet. Children, because of their rapid growth, require more protein per kilogram of body weight than adults. In addition, when compared with adults, children also need a larger percentage of their dietary intake of protein to contain essential amino acids.

Once ingested, proteins are broken down into amino acids or peptides and are absorbed through the intestinal lumen. They are then carried to the liver through the portal vein. The liver regulates protein metabolism through enzymatic breakdown of amino acids, formation of nonessential amino acids from simple precursors, and detoxification or elimination of ammonia, urea, uric acid, and other catabolic end products. Proteins are rapidly metabolized by the liver, which enables a quick response to changing metabolic demands. Amino acids supplied in excess of metabolic requirements are degraded to by-products such as urea, uric acid, or creatinine, and the remaining carbon skeletons are converted to carbohydrate and fat or oxidized for energy.[25] Of particular importance is the conversion of amino acids to ketoacids, which are carbohydrate-like in structure and created by removal of the amino group during deamination. These ketoacids may then enter the TCA cycle, where they provide energy for liver metabolism, or they may be converted to fatty acids by the liver.

Protein metabolism can be measured in terms of **nitrogen balance.** If nitrogen (protein) intake approximates output, an equal nitrogen balance exists. If dietary intake of proteins exceeds output, a **positive nitrogen balance** occurs. Protein anabolism exceeds catabolism during periods of rapid growth, pregnancy, and the formation of new tissue. Experimentally, positive nitrogen balance has been induced in malnourished patients through the administration of growth hormone.[26] A **negative nitrogen balance** occurs when protein breakdown exceeds daily protein intake and synthesis. If the daily caloric intake is insufficient, the body catabolizes dietary and tissue protein for energy, as is the case after severe burns and during fever, illness, or stress.[2]

Hormonal Control of Protein Metabolism

Anabolic and catabolic protein metabolism is controlled by various hormones. Table 42-4 lists the major hormonal effects on protein metabolism. Hormones that also promote protein synthesis include growth hormone, especially during growth spurts; testosterone in specific reproductive organs during puberty; and thyroid hormone indirectly, by increasing the metabolic rate. Insulin also promotes the active transport of amino acids across cell membranes and accelerates protein synthesis within the cell. Insulin, in concert with growth hormone, is required for normal growth and development of children

and adolescents. Glucagon, whose actions diametrically oppose those of insulin, promotes gluconeogenesis by stimulating the breakdown of protein into amino acids and increasing their transport into hepatic cells. Glucagon also enables the conversion of amino acids into glucose precursors.

KEY POINTS

- Metabolism of carbohydrate, lipid, and protein supplies energy to support the cell's energy-requiring processes and provides building blocks for the synthesis of cellular biomolecules. The primary hormonal regulators of nutrient metabolism are insulin, glucagon, catecholamines (i.e., epinephrine and norepinephrine), cortisol, thyroid hormone, and growth hormone.

- Insulin is secreted from pancreatic β cells in response to elevated serum glucose levels. Binding of insulin to receptors on target cells (muscle, adipose tissue) facilitates the transport of glucose into cells and reduces blood glucose levels. Insulin inhibits lipolysis and gluconeogenesis.

- Glucagon is secreted from pancreatic α cells in response to low blood glucose levels. Glucagon promotes glycogenolysis and gluconeogenesis (from lactate, amino acids, and glycerol) by the liver, thereby increasing blood glucose levels.

- Catecholamines increase glycogenolysis and gluconeogenesis by the liver, thereby increasing blood glucose levels. Catecholamines also stimulate lipolysis in adipose cells by enhancing the action of hormone-sensitive lipase. Glucagon secretion is enhanced and insulin secretion is inhibited by catecholamines.

- Cortisol enhances the actions of glucagon and catecholamines and promotes glycogenolysis, gluconeogenesis, and lipolysis, thus raising blood levels of glucose and fatty acids.

- Thyroid hormone tends to raise blood glucose levels. In carbohydrate metabolism, the primary mode of action is to increase glucose absorption from the intestines and stimulate the release of epinephrine. Thyroid hormone also enhances the rate of insulin destruction. Ultimately, thyroid hormone causes an increase in cellular oxygen consumption and the general metabolic rate of tissues.

- Growth hormone increases blood glucose levels by inhibiting uptake by muscle cells and by stimulating gluconeogenesis in the liver. Growth hormone enhances the cellular uptake of amino acids and stimulates protein synthesis. Catecholamine stimulation of ghrelin partially controls growth hormone secretion.

- The main sources of cellular energy are glucose and fatty acids. Glucose is the primary energy source for the brain, although the brain can use ketone bodies. Ketone bodies are produced from fatty acids by the liver, particularly under conditions of decreased carbohydrate intake or fasting.

OBESITY

Obesity is defined as excessive accumulation of adipose tissue and is considered to be one of the leading contributors to preventable death in the United States. The body mass index (BMI) is calculated as weight (kg) divided by height squared (m²). In the United States, estimates suggest 68% of adults have a BMI of 25 kg/m² or more. Overweight is defined as a BMI of 25 to 29.9 kg/m². Obesity is defined as a BMI greater than 30 kg/m² with morbid obesity 40 kg/m² or more. Obesity is a major health issue associated with higher rates of heart disease, kidney disease, hypertension, type 2 diabetes, polycystic ovary disease, and stroke. Obesity also creates challenges with activities of daily living from increased risk of osteoarthritis, chronic pain, gallbladder disease, sleep apnea, and psychosocial impairments.

Obesity involves complex interactions among a large number of factors, including lifestyle choices, environment, and genetics. Obesity

TABLE 42-4	**HORMONAL ACTIONS ON PROTEIN METABOLISM**
HORMONE	**ACTIONS**
Insulin	Actively transports amino acids into cells
	Accelerates cellular protein synthesis
Glucagon	Stimulates protein breakdown into amino acids
	Increases amino acid transport into hepatic cells
Cortisol	Increases protein catabolism

is associated with low-grade chronic inflammation from proinflammatory cytokines and acute-phase reactants affecting adipose tissue, skeletal muscle, and the vascular-renal systems.[27]

Family and twin studies have suggested that genetic heritability can be linked to 30% to 70% of body mass index variations.[28,29] However, most experts agree that genetics contributes only a modest factor to an individual's BMI.[28,29] There is increasing attention being paid to epigenetic control over obesity and related diseases (see Epigenetics in Metabolism and Nutrition).

Health care expenditures related to obesity were estimated to cost $147 billion in 2008.[27,30] The majority of individuals seek to lose weight through exercise, caloric reduction, or pharmacologic therapies; however, these approaches rarely achieve optimal long-term results.

Another option for weight loss is surgical intervention, known as bariatric surgery. The main focus of surgical interventions is either to reduce the stomach size, thus creating a small pouch for the stomach that severely restricts caloric intake, or to alter the absorptive capacity of the small intestine. In many cases, surgery provides patients with long-term results of weight loss and reduction or remission of chronic illness, including diabetes type 2, hypertension, and improvement with chronic pain issues.

Metabolic Syndrome

Metabolic syndrome, previously known as "syndrome X," occurs in 24% of the obese population.[28,31] Clinically, patients with metabolic syndrome have increased amounts of abdominal adiposity, increased levels of plasma free fatty acids, insulin resistance with or without type 2 diabetes, low serum high-density lipoprotein (HDL) concentrations, hypertriglyceridemia, and hypertension. The prevalence of metabolic syndrome has a linear relationship with age, approaching 45% for people in the seventh decade of life.[31]

Abdominal fat accumulation is the most recognized symptom of metabolic syndrome and when combined with hypertension, hyperlipidemia, and insulin resistance can create a "deadly cocktail" of health risk and increased mortality.[28] In most situations, metabolic syndrome is influenced by tissue resistance to hormones, particularly insulin, caused by excess energy intake that disrupts endocrine function.[28]

Numerous hormones are involved in the development of metabolic syndrome and type 2 diabetes including resistin, leptin, ghrelin, and apelin. Resistin is a hormone expressed in response to cellular inflammation and results in insulin resistance and activation of other proinflammatory cytokines linked with obesity. Leptin is produced in adipocytes and normally influences the hypothalamus to inhibit appetite. Resistance to the effects of leptin and hyperleptinemia are associated with the development of obesity.[27,32,33]

Ghrelin is a hormone produced by the epithelial cells of the stomach that appears to regulate appetite.[34] Apelin is expressed by a number of organs including the gastrointestinal tract. Researchers have identified apelin deficiency in type 2 diabetes and insulin resistance.[35] Excessive apelin level is associated with increased serum glucose level, leading to a proinflammatory state resulting from activation of cytokines.

Research suggests that fatty acids released during lipolysis of visceral fat are a key factor of insulin resistance because fatty acids enter the portal vein and are directly deposited in the liver.[31] Data from research suggest that visceral fat metabolism contributes approximately 20% of free fatty acids to the liver and 15% to skeletal muscle.[31] Excessive visceral fat contributes to hepatic insulin resistance.

Obesity and metabolic syndrome are chronic conditions with complex interactions between caloric intake, energy expenditure, genetics, and hormonal influences. Complications of obesity include type 2 diabetes, cardiovascular disease, and sleep apnea. Metabolic syndrome may precede the diagnosis of diabetes and cardiac disease and if treated early can slow the progression of these diseases.

> **KEY POINTS**
> - Obesity is a major contributor to several chronic disorders including type 2 diabetes, hypertension, and cardiovascular diseases.
> - Obesity rates are increasing with an estimated 68% of adults in the United States having BMIs greater than 25 kg/m^2.
> - Metabolic syndrome is characterized by excess abdominal adipose tissue, insulin resistance, hypertension, hyperglycemia, and dyslipidemia.

AGING AND METABOLIC FUNCTION

There is no question that the aging process has an effect on normal metabolism. It is sometimes difficult, however, to distinguish the effects of aging from the effects of chronic illness, dementia, drug therapy, or obesity. Essentially all metabolic processes begin a slow decline with increased aging until such morbidity ultimately leads to the end of life. The degree to which metabolism fails in the elderly and the precise targets for these dysfunctions are correlated to genetics, epigenetics (see Epigenetics in Metabolism and Nutrition), and the impact of chronic inflammation and disease.

There seems to be little difference in the ability of healthy people, young or old, to metabolize glucose and little difference in insulin secretion by the β cells in the pancreas. What does appear to occur with the aging process is a change in tissue sensitivity to insulin. Although many possible causes for this phenomenon have been proposed, such as reduced carbohydrate intake, decreased muscle mass, and lowered activity levels, the reason appears to lie in an alteration in the molecular composition of insulin. Compared to younger adults, the elderly population have higher levels of circulating serum proinsulin and there tends to be a decrease in insulin clearance, leading overall to insulinemia.[36] It is also believed that the aging process alters insulin receptor sites and thus renders insulin less effective (insulin resistance).[37]

The aging process may also affect lipid metabolism as proportionate body fat increases. Although caloric intake generally decreases, a concurrent loss of lean body mass and a decline in energy expenditure begin in middle age and continue through life. A decline in the resting metabolic rate also occurs with the aging process. This change is related to several factors, such as reduced lean body mass, reduced lipogenic enzyme response to glucose, and decreased catecholamine secretion after a meal. Although cross-sectional studies demonstrate that cholesterol and triglyceride serum levels tend to increase with age, evidence is increasing that this change may be due more to obesity than to the aging process itself. However, as a risk factor, hyperlipidemia poses less threat for coronary artery disease and atherosclerosis than aging alone.[38]

A decrease in the quantity of skeletal muscle also normally occurs with aging. Although this decrease in muscle is associated with factors such as physical inactivity and a decrease in the number of neurons to muscle cells, endocrine factors also influence the loss of muscle mass. The decreased growth hormone secretion noted in elderly individuals leads to decreased protein synthesis and a decline in insulin-like growth factor 1 (IGF-1), a condition called somatopause.[39]

KEY POINTS
- With aging there is a change in tissue sensitivity to insulin because of an alteration in the molecular composition of insulin. Compared to younger adults, elderly persons have higher levels of circulating serum proinsulin. The aging process may also alter insulin receptor sites and thereby render insulin less effective.
- The aging process may affect lipid metabolism as proportionate body fat increases. Although caloric intake generally decreases, a concurrent loss of lean body mass and a decline in energy expenditure begin with adulthood.
- A decline in the resting metabolic rate also occurs with aging. This change is related to several factors, such as reduced lean body mass, reduced lipogenic enzyme response to glucose, and decreased catecholamine secretion after a meal.

NUTRITIONAL ALTERATIONS OF PHYSIOLOGIC STRESS

Metabolic Response

The response of the body to starvation is different from the response to other forms of physiologic stress such as exhaustion from exercise.[40] In a study with healthy young males it was shown that exercise performed in the fasting state enhanced glucose tolerance by increasing the transport of GLUT 4 to the membrane. This was observed even when a diet rich in lipid was provided before fasting.[40] In contrast, a similar group of study participants who were fed and then immediately tested did not show enhanced glucose tolerance. This study suggests that intense physical exercise, which corresponds to a physiologic stress, has a greater impact on glucose and lipid metabolism when the body is fasting and that insulin resistance may be decreased via a regimen of exercise following fasting.[40] Starvation is a gradual process in

which the metabolic rate decreases as storage carbohydrate reserves are metabolized. As insulin levels decline during fasting, free fatty acids are released for energy use. Despite the available free fatty acids, protein is also used for energy by means of gluconeogenesis because certain tissues prefer glucose as an energy source and because oxygen is required for fatty acid β oxidation whereas anaerobic glycolysis can function in the absence of abundant oxygen. This preference creates a negative nitrogen balance. As starvation continues, overall energy needs are reduced and the tissues that usually require glucose for function adapt by using ketone bodies for energy. Then lipolysis provides the source of needed energy, and the use of protein as an energy source decreases. This change is an adaptive response through which the body strives to conserve lean body mass. Overall, the result is minimal depletion of the body's protein. Decreased serum glucose levels and urinary nitrogen excretion, along with elevation in the levels of ketone bodies and free fatty acids, characterize starvation. Fasting (voluntary starving) alone is not associated with a high mortality unless it is prolonged, as it is in anorexia nervosa. Figure 42-2 provides a summary of the physiologic effect of starvation.

With physiologic stress not associated with exercise or starvation, conservation of lean body mass does not occur. The metabolic rate increases rather than decreases, and a high sustained rate of catabolism (breakdown of protein to meet energy needs) results. Protein is used as an energy source via hepatic gluconeogenesis through release of muscle stores of protein-derived amino acids. This adaptation quickly results in a negative nitrogen balance. Cell mass is redistributed in response to the stressor, with an increase in the production of acute-phase proteins.[41] The degree of hypermetabolism, hypercatabolism, and negative nitrogen balance associated with physiologic stress depends on the type, duration, and severity of the stressor present. It has been shown that certain apolipoproteins of the HDL class are specifically targeted for hypermetabolism when levels of very low density

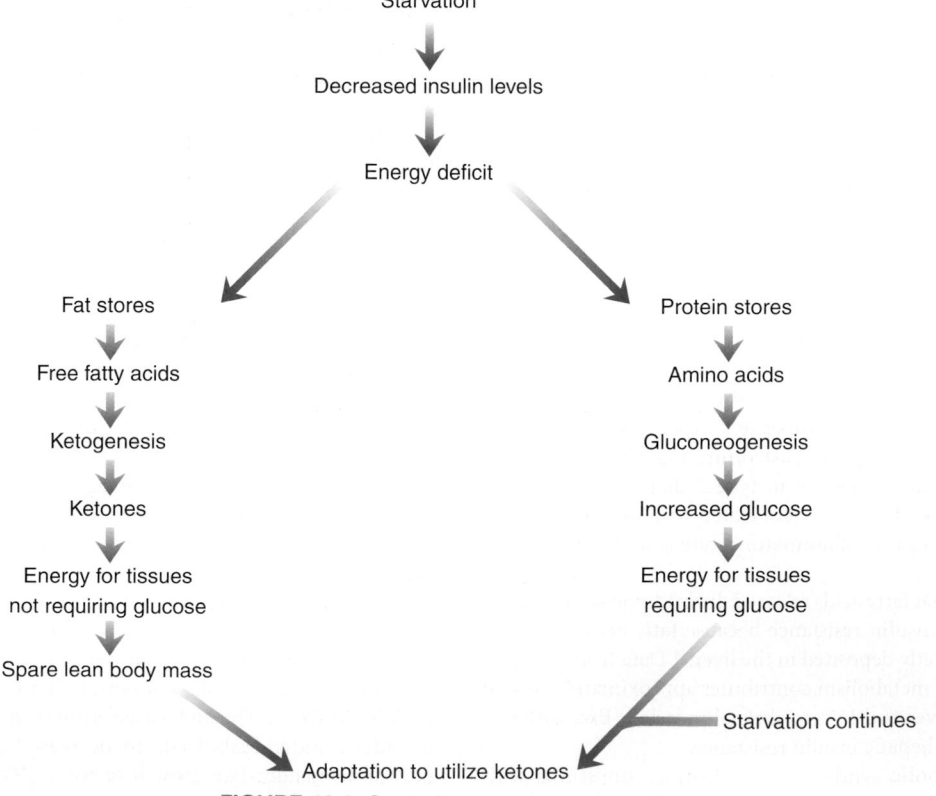

FIGURE 42-2 Catabolic response to starvation.

lipoprotein (VLDL) apolipoprotein increase and this change is linked to hypertriglyceridemia and insulin resistance in obese males.[42]

Phases of Catabolic Response

Typically, the catabolic response to stress occurs in two phases: the immediate phase, lasting 5 to 8 days, and the subsequent adaptive phase. The physiologic effects of each phase are summarized in Figures 42-3 and 42-4.

The immediate phase of **catabolism** is characterized by increased sympathetic nervous system stimulation with release of glucagon, glucocorticoids, and catecholamines. The resultant decreased production and circulation of insulin cause a pseudo-diabetic state. Hyperglycemia develops from decreased levels of circulating insulin and decreased utilization of glucose by muscle and other tissues (insulin resistance). An energy deficit is created, and alternative mechanisms of glucose production are then required. The oxidation of branched-chain amino acids occurs for two reasons: to meet energy requirements and to provide the liver with amino acids for the synthesis of acute-phase proteins (C-reactive protein, mannose-binding protein, complement factors, ferritin, ceruloplasmin, amyloid A, and haptoglobin). As the amino acids are mobilized to meet energy needs, alanine is formed and used as a carbon source in hepatic gluconeogenesis. Sodium and water are retained secondary to an increase in aldosterone level, which results in potassium loss. The mineralocorticoid aldosterone is released as a result of stimulation of the sympathetic nervous system. During this phase, adipose is not well used as an energy source because some level of insulin is present and has an antilipolytic action.

The nutritional result of the immediate phase of stress on the body is hyperglycemia, negative nitrogen balance, and retention of fluid and sodium. This protective mechanism uses skeletal muscle to meet energy requirements and protects the rest of the body's tissue from breaking down during periods of high-energy need. An overall loss of nitrogen and other electrolytes, including magnesium, phosphorus, and zinc, takes place.

The adaptive phase occurs if the sympathetic nervous system response can selectively persevere with the stressors present. Hypermetabolism, a condition caused by excessive trauma, helps keep the system active, thus providing essential energy needs and new protein synthesis during severe stress.[43] If the stressors overwhelm the body's response system, the effect on prognosis will be negative. In the adaptive phase, the body begins to use ketone bodies and reducing power from the oxidation of fatty acids, thus limiting protein catabolism. As the sympathetic nervous system response diminishes, insulin resistance decreases and glucose utilization improves. Return of aldosterone levels to normal results in diuresis. The overall result is an improvement in negative nitrogen balance as the serum glucose level improves. This phase is similar to the response of the body during starvation, when fat is used to meet energy requirements. Chronic conditions such as diabetes, liver disease, or renal disease restrict the body's ability to move into the adaptive phase during physiologic stress. Chronic system failure or inadequate treatment of any current disease complicates the course of recovery. Nutritional input is used more efficiently by the body's tissue during the adaptive phase than during the immediate phase. It is in this phase that nutrition can have a vital role in recovery. The combination of starvation and physiologic stress increases the risk for morbidity and mortality. When poor nutritional status coincides with physiologic stress, the body's response is weakened. The ability to mobilize the immune response also decreases with impaired cell-mediated immunity and humoral immunity as well as altered response of the tissue barriers to infection.

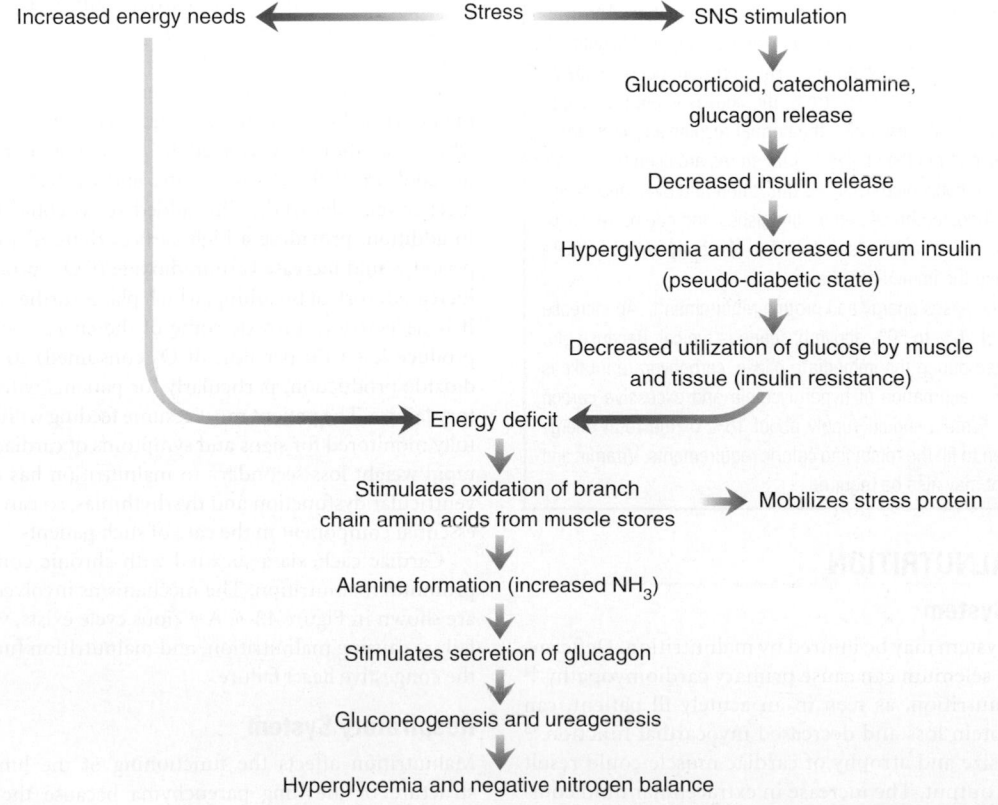

FIGURE 42-3 Immediate catabolic response to stress. *NH₃,* Ammonia; *SNS,* sympathetic nervous system.

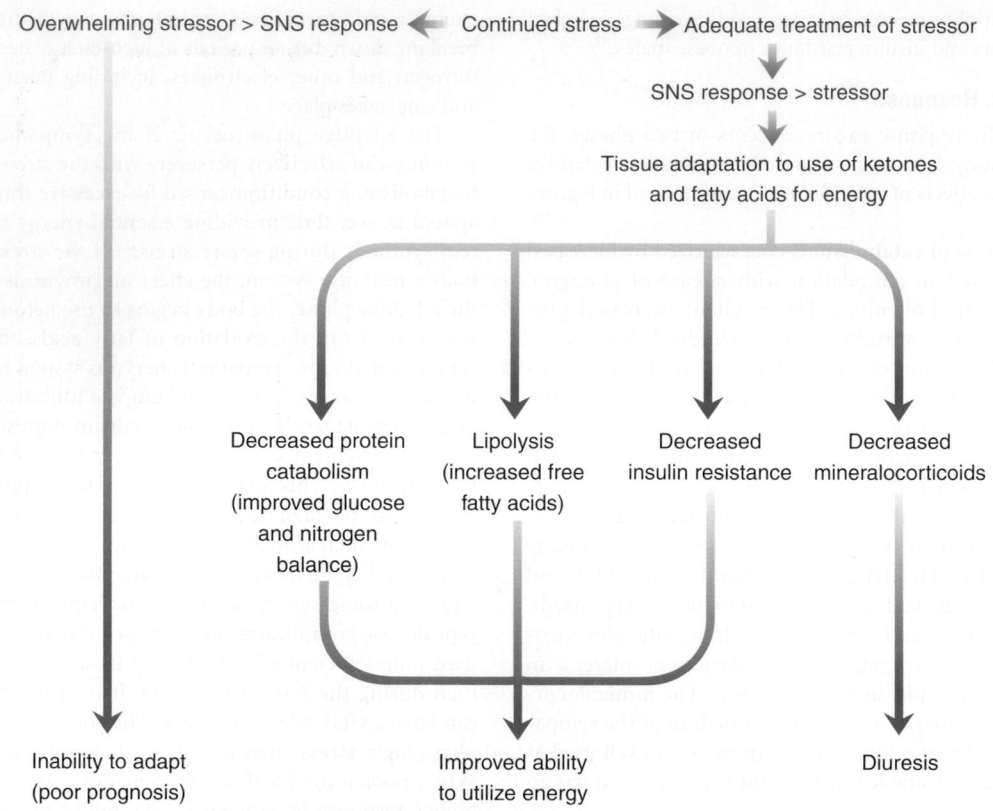

FIGURE 42-4 Adaptive phase of the catabolic response to stress. *SNS,* Sympathetic nervous system.

KEY POINTS

- Acute physiologic stress results in activation of the sympathetic nervous system. The immediate phase is characterized by a high metabolic rate, sustained catabolism, hyperglycemia, and salt and water retention. The sympathetic response promotes the use of protein stores for gluconeogenesis, which results in a negative nitrogen balance. Fat stores are poorly utilized.

- After 5 to 7 days of acute physiologic stress, the body may enter an adaptive phase that more closely resembles the normal response to starvation. Ketones and fatty acids from the lipolysis of fat stores are used for energy, and body proteins are conserved. Glucose utilization improves and hyperglycemia resolves. Aldosterone secretion diminishes and edema resolves. During the adaptive phase, nutrients supplied to the body are used more efficiently than during the immediate phase.

- Physiologic stress increases energy and protein requirements. An increase in needed calories of 20% to 50% above baseline is typical. Because glucose is poorly utilized during the immediate phase, carbohydrate intake is controlled to avoid exacerbation of hyperglycemia and excessive carbon dioxide production. Protein should supply about 16% of the total energy needs. Fats are given to fill the remaining caloric requirements. Vitamin and mineral replacement may also be required.

EFFECTS OF MALNUTRITION

Cardiovascular System

The cardiovascular system may be injured by malnutrition. Deficiencies in thiamine and selenium can cause primary cardiomyopathy.[44] Protein-energy malnutrition, as seen in an acutely ill patient, can result in visceral protein loss and decreased myocardial function.[45] A decrease in heart size and atrophy of cardiac muscle could result in decreased cardiac output. The increase in extracellular fluid commonly associated with physiologic stress could further compromise

cardiac output. In compensation, the cardiac muscle fibers lengthen in response to increased workload. This compensation, together with a decreased oxygen demand secondary to decreased intake, curtails the development of cardiac failure. However, if the cardiac muscle is diseased, malnutrition will contribute to uncompensated heart failure.

Even though the body compensates to prevent heart failure in a malnourished patient, heart failure is common even in a healthy heart when starvation is corrected by refeeding. Refeeding increases the metabolism of the stressed state, and cardiac output is increased to meet oxygen demands. This added stress could lead to heart failure. In addition, providing a high-carbohydrate diet during the refeeding period would increase carbon dioxide (CO_2) production and result in increased work of breathing, which places further demand on the heart. It is necessary to provide some of the energy needs with fats (which produce less CO_2 per unit of O_2 consumed) to decrease the carbon dioxide production, particularly for patients with concurrent respiratory failure. The patient must resume feeding with caution and be carefully monitored for signs and symptoms of cardiac failure. In addition, rapid weight loss secondary to malnutrition has been associated with ventricular dysfunction and dysrhythmias, so cardiac monitoring is an essential component in the care of such patients.

Cardiac cachexia associated with chronic congestive heart failure promotes malnutrition. The mechanisms involved in cardiac cachexia are shown in Figure 42-5. A vicious cycle exists, with congestive heart failure causing malnutrition, and malnutrition further contributing to the congestive heart failure.

Respiratory System

Malnutrition affects the functioning of the lungs. It decreases the structure of the lung parenchyma because the use of protein for energy reduces protein synthesis. This structural alteration can cause

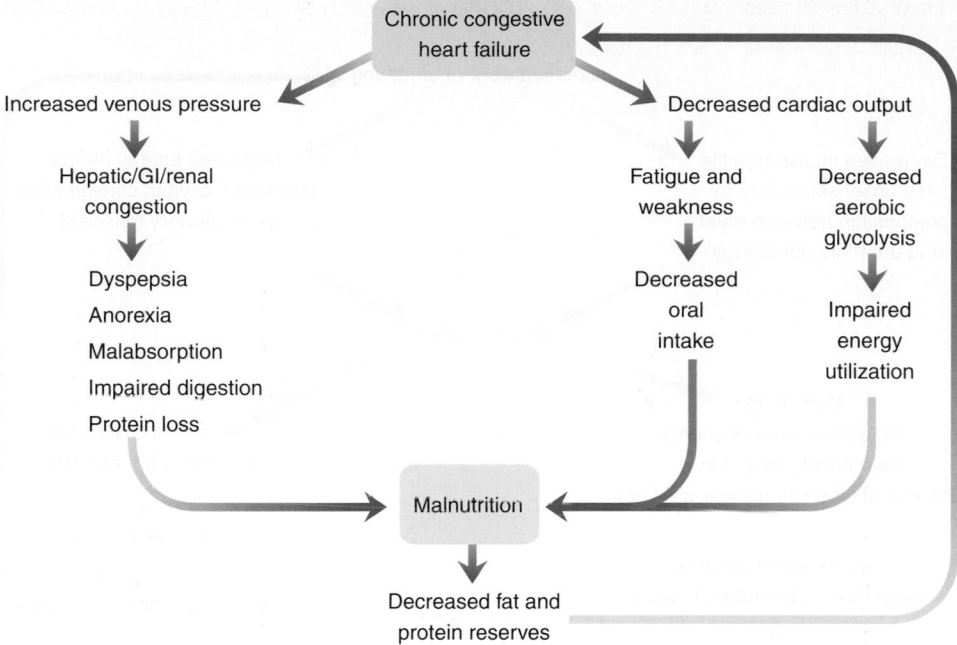

FIGURE 42-5 Cyclic effect of malnutrition on chronic congestive heart failure. *GI*, Gastrointestinal.

excessive lung compliance and result in increased work of breathing.[46] Respiratory muscle function is decreased as a result of visceral protein loss, and both endurance and contractility are affected.

Malnourished patients often suffer from decreased vital capacity and respiratory muscle strength. If vital capacity and muscle strength fall below 50% of predicted norms, respiratory failure is probable owing to retention of carbon dioxide. Malnutrition also decreases the immune response in the lung. Surfactant stability is decreased, contributing to decreased lung compliance and microatelectasis. The result of an alteration in immune function and structural changes is an increase in the likelihood of respiratory tract infections. Infections develop easily and are not controlled by the protein-deficient immune system. The consequences of energy deficit in chronic obstructive pulmonary disease (COPD) are summarized in Figure 42-6. When a patient has respiratory distress and must work harder to breathe, the caloric requirement for breathing alone can increase to 10 times normal levels. Inadequate intake and increased utilization further contribute to the effects of malnutrition on the respiratory system.

Immune System

Increased rates of infection in malnourished patients secondary to depression of the immune system and defense mechanisms are caused by nutrient deficiency. Changes in the immune system vary according to the type of nutrient lacking (Table 42-5). For example, lack of protein can impair the immune response from lack of amino acids necessary for immunoglobulin and interleukin synthesis.[47] As previously mentioned, cellular immunity (delayed cutaneous hypersensitivity), which is needed for reaction to an antigen in skin testing, is often depressed in undernourished patients. In addition, the total lymphocyte count decreases. Thus the normal reaction that occurs with antigen stimulation is absent or decreased in malnutrition secondary to both a decrease in synthesis of immune system cells and a decrease in antibody response to stimulation (humoral immunity).

Malnutrition also causes a decrease in the amount of lymphoid tissue mass, a decrease in the number of circulating T and B lymphocytes, a depression of phagocytic function, and a decrease in complement activity. The overall result is a decrease in resistance and an increased infection rate. In the critical care setting, the high number of invasive procedures and indwelling lines increases the potential for infection and complicates the patient's recovery.

KEY POINTS

- The cardiovascular, respiratory, and immune systems are particularly susceptible to the effects of malnutrition.
- Cardiac atrophy and reduced cardiac output may be associated with heart failure, particularly during refeeding, which increases the myocardial workload.
- Respiratory muscle atrophy and fatigue and deficient surfactant production impair effective respiration.
- Immune system depression is associated with an increased risk of infection.

EPIGENETICS IN METABOLISM AND NUTRITION

Genetic and epigenetic mechanisms shape metabolic activity and can respond negatively to produce the pathophysiologic state. Whereas the genome establishes the template for developmental and metabolic patterns, an adaptational phenomenon helps to produce the final phenotype. This latter epigenetic mechanism has become a key subject of developmental and cell biology, gene expression, and pathology. The biochemistry of epigenetics involves several covalent modifications of nuclear chromatin (DNA and histones) as well as posttranscriptional RNA-based gene silencing. These modifications can be reversibly administered by interactions with the genome caused by, and resulting in, poor nutrition and disease.

Covalent epigenetic modifications have a profound influence over gene expression and the mechanism for this effect requires environmental input and readily available substrates including target DNA and associated histones plus the methylating agent. During fetal development, it has been shown that obese pregnant mothers can transfer a pro-obese phenotype to their offspring.[48] It has been known for some time that maternal metabolism during gestation has an imprinting effect on fetal gene expression. Indeed, this epigenetic regulation controls the divergent expression of paternal over maternal genes, including

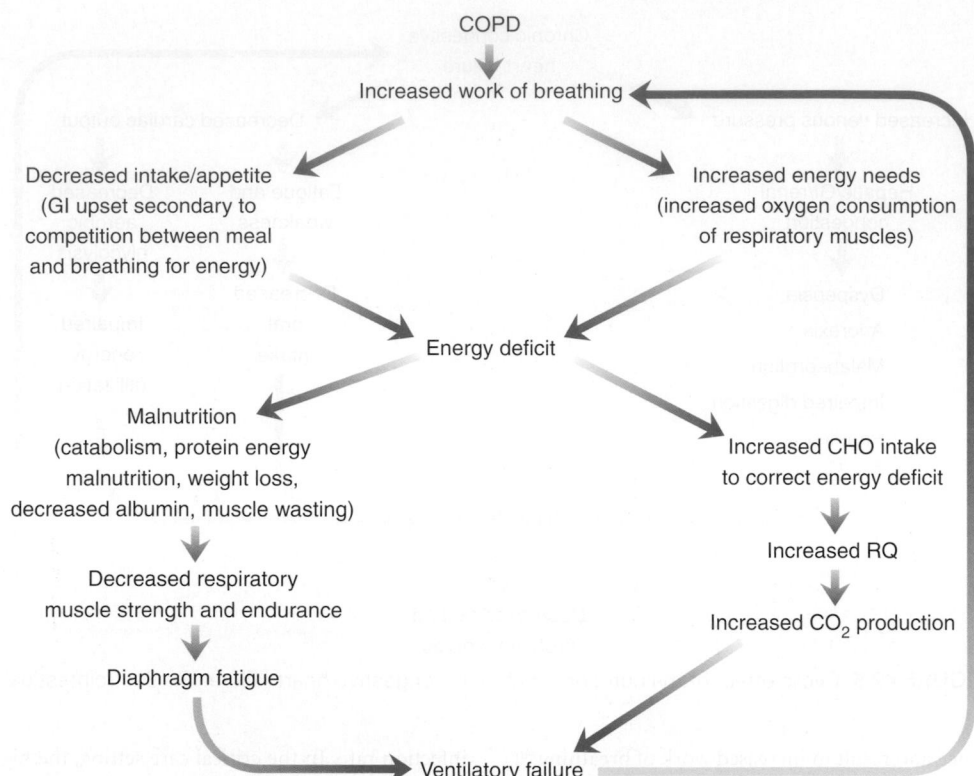

FIGURE 42-6 Increased work of breathing with chronic obstructive pulmonary disease. *CHO,* Carbohydrate; *COPD,* chronic obstructive pulmonary disease; *GI,* gastrointestinal; *RQ,* respiratory quotient.

TABLE 42-5	**EFFECTS OF DEFICIENCY OF SELECTED NUTRIENTS ON IMMUNITY**
DEFICIENT NUTRIENT	**IMMUNE SYSTEM CHANGE**
Vitamin C	Decreased mobility of neutrophils
Vitamin A	Lymphoid tissue atrophy
Vitamin B group	Lymphoid tissue atrophy
Amino acids	Decreased immunoglobulins, interferons, and acute-phase proteins
Fatty acids	Impaired lymphocyte function
Iron	Decreased bacterial activity of phagocytes
Zinc	Lymphoid tissue atrophy
Selenium	Decreased antibody production

one involved in glucose metabolism and growth—insulin-like growth factor 2 (IGF-2). This fetal imprinting is the result of maternal metabolism, which is indirectly linked to maternal diet. This epigenetic effect is presumably advantageous during a specific stage of gestation.[49] However, if these epigenetic modifications persist into later stages of gestation, they may increase the risk of being a component of "maintenance methylation" that persists after parturition and into infancy, childhood, and even adult development. This may predispose the individual to new environmental pressures leading to chronic disease such as obesity, metabolic syndrome, and cardiovascular and renal dysfunction.

Besides the gestational effects of maternal obesity on subsequent metabolic dysfunction in the offspring, nutritional deficiencies or excesses can also specifically alter the epigenome. Dietary sources of methylating agents, such as bioavailable folic acid, methionine, choline, betaine, and homocysteine, may have a permanent effect on the epigenetic methylation patterns of CpG islands and the coherence of histones in locus- and temporal-dependent genes. If these gene products are involved in normal development and have been arbitrarily altered, the fetus may not develop correctly or there may be infant diseases linked to these methylation patterns. As the individual matures to adulthood, the maternal exposure to methyl group–containing nutrients may have a lifelong effect on basic physiology, response to nutrition, and, sometimes, the manifestation of pathologic and disease states.[50] Clearly diet plays a major role in both general and specific epigenomic patterns and these can cause significant metabolic disease. Diet (both at the caloric level and at the essential nutrient level) controls metabolic flux in a dynamic way. Excess chronic caloric intake can induce several disease states including obesity and metabolic syndrome. Insufficient caloric intake can also cause disease as can inappropriate nutrition or excessive ingestion of vitamins and certain growth-promoting molecules. Besides a direct effect on metabolic rate and function, diet can also introduce these epigenetic changes to the endocrine hormone system.

Epigenetic changes can arise within a single generation and remain fixed there; alternatively, as in the case of maintenance methylation, the changes can also be preserved and inherited. Therefore, the distinction between the two forms of modification lies more in the degree of alteration in gene expression than in the mechanisms of acquisition or potential for inheritance. Indeed, environment plays a very significant role in epigenesis of the endocrine system and may be the more robust factor in variations around this physiologic axis.

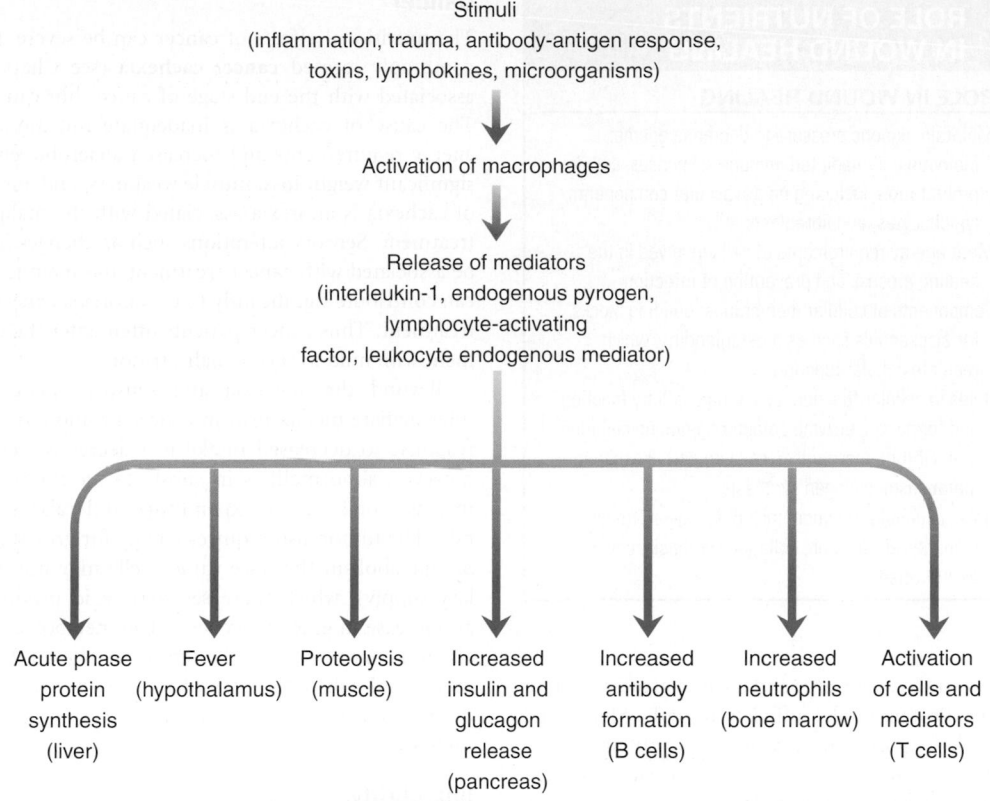

Stimuli
(inflammation, trauma, antibody-antigen response,
toxins, lymphokines, microorganisms)

↓

Activation of macrophages

↓

Release of mediators
(interleukin-1, endogenous pyrogen,
lymphocyte-activating
factor, leukocyte endogenous mediator)

| Acute phase protein synthesis (liver) | Fever (hypothalamus) | Proteolysis (muscle) | Increased insulin and glucagon release (pancreas) | Increased antibody formation (B cells) | Increased neutrophils (bone marrow) | Activation of cells and mediators (T cells) |

FIGURE 42-7 Mediator-stimulated response.

KEY POINTS
- Epigenetic modification of nuclear chromatin can occur throughout life and includes reversible methylation of promoter regions of DNA as well as various covalent modifications of histones and production of interfering RNA.
- Epigenetic modifications can have profound effects on gene expression that may cause nutritional and metabolic dysfunction or conversely may be caused by malnutrition, including that associated with obesity.
- Bioavailability of methyl group–containing nutrients such as folic acid and choline can directly affect DNA methylation patterning that may be acquired in utero and subsequently cause metabolic disease in the adult.

NUTRITIONAL REQUIREMENTS OF ALTERED HEALTH STATES

Infection, Sepsis, and Fever

A complex interaction exists between the development of infection, the immune system, and nutritional intake.[51] Malnutrition contributes to the infectious process by directly depressing the immune system. This depression impairs the patient's defense mechanism and opens a pathway for the development of unimpeded infection. Infection then potentiates malnutrition through inhibition of nutrient assimilation and stimulation of metabolic rate (fever).

Fever is a common symptom accompanying infection. Fever increases metabolic needs by 7% for each 1° F increase (13% for each 1° C increase). Energy requirements can increase by 40% when a high fever (above 104° F) is present. The metabolic response to fever is both anabolic and catabolic, which greatly increases nutrient requirements.

It is known that peptide mediators secreted by macrophages and other immune cells initiate the metabolic alterations associated with infection. The mediator-stimulated response is summarized in Figure 42-7. This process is complex, with the need for protein synthesis requiring the

availability of amino acids.[52] Although catabolism may be detrimental in some aspects, it is also a protective mechanism that provides needed substrates for activation of the immune response to infection. Nutritional support is often aimed at decreasing catabolism, but it is also important to provide substrates (amino acids) for the protective mechanisms that catabolism supports.

Infection is a stressor that increases energy expenditure as a result of fever, increased immune cell demand, and catabolism. The body's metabolic response to the infection is to increase the amount of available glucose. Often the demand is too great for the body to manage; for example, sepsis can increase energy expenditure 20% to 60% above basal energy requirements. Nutritional support is needed to supply additional energy and the necessary substrates so that body stores are not excessively depleted.

Surgery

Adequate nutrition before and after surgery promotes wound healing, prevents infection, and decreases complications and mortality. A patient should be in the best nutritional condition possible before surgery.[53] A common cause of protein-energy malnutrition in postoperative patients is starvation. The combination of poor presurgical nutrition and postoperative starvation may increase complications after surgery, such as separation of the layers of the surgical wound. Obesity, malnutrition, and dehydration are among the causes of this serious postoperative problem.

Nutritional needs in the postoperative period depend on the extent and type of surgery, as well as the presurgical nutritional status. The postoperative energy requirement can increase from 10% to 35% above BMR. Frequently, postoperative oral intake is delayed in critically ill patients well beyond the return of bowel function. This combination of increased need with decreased intake can have a major impact on wound healing. The functions of various nutrients in wound healing have long been established and are listed in Table 42-6. In addition,

TABLE 42-6   ROLE OF NUTRIENTS IN WOUND HEALING

NUTRIENT	ROLE IN WOUND HEALING
Proteins (amino acids and albumin)	Maintain osmotic pressure to decrease edema; maintain cell-mediated immune responses; cellular proliferation, including neurovascular components, lymphocytes, and fibroblasts
Carbohydrates (glucose)	Meet energy requirements of cells involved in the healing process and prevention of infection
Fats (essential fatty acids)	Components of cellular membranes; building blocks for eicosanoids such as prostaglandins, which regulate cellular function
Vitamins	Roles in cellular function, including capillary function and formation, enzyme cofactors, immune cell function, clotting mechanism, calcium and phosphorus metabolism, collagen synthesis
Minerals	Roles in cellular function, including oxygen transport, immune cell function, collagen synthesis, cellular proliferation

nitrogen loss through wounds can be large and create a greater need for increased protein intake. Protein intake sufficient to replace losses and promote anabolism will be required, together with nonprotein calories for energy requirements. As with every patient, individual assessment and determination of exact needs are required.

Trauma

The general catabolic response to stress is also seen in trauma patients.[54] Energy expenditure is increased by 15% to 30%. Increased carbohydrate intake will be needed, but patients must be observed for complications of high carbohydrate intake, such as glucose intolerance. Nitrogen loss secondary to catabolism and to cellular damage can be high. Circulating hormones in the immediate phase have an anti-insulin effect that decreases glucose utilization; therefore, gluconeogenesis is increased to meet energy needs. As with other stress states, the catabolism of protein provides a source of amino acids for acute-phase protein synthesis by the liver (see Chapter 9). Because trauma is a sudden stress, catabolism is much greater than anabolism because the body has not had enough time to replenish the proteins lost. This dominance of catabolism results in excessive negative nitrogen balance and significant loss of skeletal muscle, which is a problem in posttrauma rehabilitation.

Burns

A burn is an extreme physiologic stressor that results in significant hypermetabolism.[55] In addition, the destruction of skin increases energy expenditure through evaporative heat loss. The energy needs of a burn patient increase 50% to 100% from the basal metabolic requirement. Because of individual variations such as preburn nutritional status, the presence of other physiologic stresses, activity level, stage of burn, and patient age, indirect calorimetry is the best method for determination of individual nutrition needs.

As with other stressors, negative nitrogen balance is increased by catabolism and by the use of amino acids to form stress proteins. In addition, burn wounds directly contribute to protein loss because soluble proteins leak from the wound and proteolysis is activated. Fatty acids are also increased in response to the release of stress hormones and breakdown of lipoproteins. The effective utilization of this available energy source in the immediate postburn phase may be impaired.

Cancer

The nutritional effects of cancer can be severe and result in what is commonly termed **cancer cachexia** (see Chapter 7).[56] Cachexia is associated with the end stage of cancer but can also develop earlier. The cause of cachexia is inadequate nutritional intake relative to energy requirements and increased anaerobic glycolysis. It results in significant weight loss, muscle weakness, and anorexia. A major cause of cachexia is anorexia associated with the malignancy and with the treatment. Sensory alterations such as changes in smell or taste may be associated with cancer treatment and malnutrition. These changes can contribute significantly to the anorexia experienced during cancer treatment. Thus cancer patients often enter the critical care environment with mild to severe malnutrition.

Beyond the anorexia and sensory changes, abnormalities of intermediate metabolism in cancer promote tissue loss. The normal response to decreased intake is a decreased resting metabolic rate; however, abnormalities in substrate metabolism in cancer patients increase total energy expenditure and raise the resting metabolic rate. The tumor also requires energy for growth, often using anaerobic metabolism (because tumor cells may not have sufficient capillary supply), which increases lactic acid production and promotes an increase in gluconeogenesis. The metabolism of vitamins, minerals, and enzymes is also thought to be altered. Because both nutrient intake and substrate metabolism are altered, nutritional support is difficult to achieve and frequently ineffective in reversing the existing cachexia.

Immobility

The main nutritional effect of immobility is loss of calcium from nonstressed bone, a process that can elevate serum calcium and phosphorus levels. This demineralization is best managed with weight-bearing exercise as early as possible rather than calcium supplementation. Calcium supplementation during immobility may increase the risk of developing renal calculi. A physical therapist should be consulted early to assist in prevention of demineralization. Because negative calcium balance can increase in a catabolic state, serum calcium levels must be monitored and abnormalities treated.

A second effect of immobilization is nitrogen loss while tissue mass is decreased from disuse atrophy. This loss can total 2 to 3 g/kg per day and require up to 10 to 15 g of protein to replenish the daily loss, which further emphasizes the need for early physical therapy and aggressive range-of-motion exercises.

KEY POINTS

- Infection is associated with fever and an increased metabolic rate. For each 1° F increase in body temperature, metabolic needs increase 7%. The synthesis of acute-phase proteins and immune factors requires sufficient amino acid substrates.
- A major nutritional problem in postoperative patients is starvation. In addition, nitrogen loss through wounds may be significant.
- Major trauma is associated with a 15% to 30% increase in energy expenditure. Glucose utilization is maintained. Trauma victims are usually in good nutritional health before admission.
- Major burns are extreme physiologic stressors that result in an increase in energy expenditure of 50% to 100% above baseline. Protein loss from burned areas is high.
- Cancer cachexia is a result of several factors, including anorexia, poor intake, and preferential nutrient utilization by tumor cells.
- Immobility is associated with muscle atrophy and bone demineralization.

SUMMARY

Metabolism is a dynamic and continuous process affecting every organ and physiologic process in the human system. The building phase of anabolic metabolism occurs concurrently with the energy-consuming and destructive phase of catabolic metabolism. Phases of metabolism either release or require energy in the form of ATP. The rate at which metabolism occurs in the resting human system is referred to as the basal metabolic rate, and the process releases both heat and energy. The metabolic fate of carbohydrate, protein, and fat depends on cellular needs and systemic regulatory functions. The endocrine system greatly affects metabolism. Only one hormone, insulin, is known to lower serum glucose levels by decreasing liver glucose production and promoting the transfer of glucose into cells. Although each works in a unique manner, growth hormone, cortisol, epinephrine, thyroid hormone, and glucagon all act in concert to maintain or raise blood glucose levels.

Physiologic stress is accompanied by changes in metabolism that alter nutrient utilization and increase nutrient requirements. The degree to which these changes occur varies with the type and severity of the particular stress. If the patient is not provided with adequate nutrition when one or more stressors are present, the hypermetabolism, hypercatabolism, and negative nitrogen balance associated with the physiologic stress will have detrimental effects on recovery.

Health care professionals must be aware of the impact of stressors on the nutritional status of the body, as well as the impact of nutrition on the well-being of body systems. If this point is well understood, appropriate interventions can be taken to prevent some of the complications that can develop when nutritional support is inadequate. Most well-nourished patients can tolerate a short period of inadequate intake (about 5 days) without untoward effects. However, critically ill patients require early nutritional support because of the magnitude and intensity of the stressors. Identification of the various risk factors and the nutritional needs of patients is an essential part of nursing care for critically ill patients. Overfeeding of patients should also be avoided because specific complications can develop with inappropriate nutritional support. Nurses must also understand nutritional interventions so that decisions regarding nutritional support for the patient can be based on specific nutritional assessments and knowledge of individual needs.

REFERENCES

1. Ryan DH, et al: Nonsurgical weight loss for extreme obesity in primary care settings: results of the Louisiana obese subjects study, *Arch Intern Med* 170:146–154, 2010.
2. Widmaier EP, Raff H, Strang KT: *Vander, Sherman & Luciano's human physiology: the mechanisms of body function*, ed 9, New York, 2004, McGraw-Hill.
3. Kalupahana NS, Moustaid-Moussa N: Overview of symposium, "Systems Genetics in Nutrition and Obesity Research," *J Nutr* 141:512–514, 2011.
4. Sultan MI, Leon CDG, Biank VF: Role of nutrition in pediatric chronic liver disease, *Nutr Clin Pract* 26:401–408, 2011.
5. Bray MS, Young ME: Regulation of fatty acid metabolism by cell autonomous circadian clocks: time to fatten up on information? *J Biol Chem* 286:11883–11889, 2011.
6. Hu W, et al: Differential regulation of dihydroceramide desaturase by palmitate versus monounsaturated fatty acids: implications for insulin resistance, *J Biol Chem* 286:16596–16605, 2011.
7. Mahan LK, Escott-Stump S: *Krause's food and nutrition therapy*, ed 12, St Louis, 2008, Saunders.
8. Guyton AC, Hall JE: *Textbook of medical physiology*, ed 11, Philadelphia, 2006, Saunders.
9. Christofk HR, et al: The M2 splice isoform of pyruvate kinase is important for cancer metabolism and tumour growth, *Nature* 452:230–233, 2008.
10. Fogal V, et al: Mitochondrial p32 protein is a critical regulator of tumor metabolism via maintenance of oxidative phosphorylation, *Mol Cell Biol* 30:1303–1318, 2010.
11. Cooper JA, et al: Maximal sustained levels of energy expenditure in humans during exercise, *Med Sci Sports Exerc*, 2011 May 20. [Epub ahead of print].
12. Osterstock G, et al: Ghrelin stimulation of growth hormone-releasing hormone neurons is direct in the arcuate nucleus, *PLoS One* 5(2):e9159, 2010, doi.org/10.1371/journal.pone.0009159.
13. Zhao T-J, et al: Ghrelin secretion stimulated by β1-adrenergic receptors in cultured ghrelinoma cells and in fasted mice, *Proc Natl Acad Sci USA* 107:15868–15873, 2010.
14. U.S. Department of Health and Human Services: *The Report of the Dietary Guidelines Advisory Committee on Dietary Guidelines for Americans*, 2005. Available at www.health.gov/DietaryGuidelines/dga2005/default.htm.
15. Jijakli H, et al: Anomeric specificity of the stimulatory effect of D-glucose on D-fructose phosphorylation by human liver glucokinase, *J Biol Chem* 278(7):4531–4535, 2003.
16. Ignatavicius DD, Workman ML: *Medical-surgical nursing: critical thinking for collaborative care*, ed 5, Philadelphia, 2006, Elsevier Saunders.
17. Laddu D, et al: A review of evidence-based strategies to treat obesity in adults, *Nutr Clin Pract* 26(5):512–525, 2011.
18. Debono M, et al: Assessing adrenal status in patients before and immediately after coronary artery bypass graft surgery, *Eur J Endocrinol* 164:413–419, 2011.
19. Santiago LA, et al: The Δ337T mutation on the TRβ causes alterations in growth, adiposity, and hepatic glucose homeostasis in mice, *J Endocrinol* 211:39–46, 2011.
20. Kumpf V, Chessman K: Enteral nutrition. In DiPiro JT, Talbert RL, Yee GC, et al, editors: *Pharmacotherapy: a pathophysiologic approach*, ed 7, New York, 2008, McGraw-Hill, pp 2399–2415.
21. Wallis GA, et al: Substantial working muscle glycerol turnover during two-legged cycle ergometry, *Am J Physiol Endocrinol Metab* 293(4):E950–E957, 2007. [Epub 2007 Jul 10].
22. Mitrou P, Raptis SA, Dimitriadis G: Insulin action in hyperthyroidism: a focus on muscle and adipose tissue, *Endocr Rev* 31(5):663–679, 2010.
23. Griffin JE, Ojeda SR: *Textbook of endocrine physiology*, ed 3, Oxford, 1996, Oxford University Press.
24. Klein S, et al: Lipolytic response to metabolic stress in critically ill patients, *Crit Care Med* 19(6):776–779, 1991.
25. Goldman L, Ausiello D: *Cecil textbook of medicine*, ed 23, Philadelphia, 2008, Elsevier Saunders.
26. Ziegler TR, et al: Metabolic effects of recombinant human growth hormone in patients receiving parenteral nutrition, *Ann Surg* 208(1):6–16, 1988.
27. Thaler J, Schwartz M: Inflammation and obesity pathogenesis: the hypothalamus heats up, *Endocrinology* 151(9):1–7, 2010.
28. Gade W, et al: Beyond obesity: the diagnosis and pathophysiology of metabolic syndrome, *Clin Lab Sci* 23(1):51–61, 2010.
29. O'Rahilly S, Farooqi IS: Genetics of obesity, *Philos Trans R Soc B* 361:1095–1105, 2006.
30. Finkelstein EA, et al: Annual spending attributable to obesity: payer- and service-specific estimates, *Health Aff (Millwood)* 28:w822–w831, 2009.
31. Kirk E, Klein S: Pathogenesis and pathophysiology of the cardiometabolic syndrome, *J Clin Hypertens* 11(12):761–765, 2009.

32. Park H, et al: Inflammatory induction of human resistin causes insulin resistance in endotoxemic mice, *Diabetes* 60:775–783, 2011.

33. Aizawa-Abe M, et al: Pathophysiological role of leptin in obesity-related hypertension, *J Clin Invest* 150(9):1243–1252, 2000.

34. Pulkkinen L, et al: Ghrelin in diabetes and metabolic syndrome, *Int J Pept* 1–11, 2010.

35. Dray C, Knauf C, Daviaud D, Waget A, et al: Apelin stimulates glucose utilization in normal and obese insulin-resistant mice, *Cell Metab* 8:437–445, 2008.

36. Gama R, et al: Hyperproinsulinaemia in elderly subjects: evidence for age-related pancreatic β-cell dysfunction, *Ann Clin Biochem* 37(3):367–371, 2000.

37. Manzato E, et al: Metabolic syndrome and cardiovascular disease in the elderly: the Progetto Veneto Anziani (Pro.V.A.) Study, *Aging Clin Exp Res* 20(1):47–52, 2008.

38. Pohlel K, et al: Treating dyslipidemia in the elderly, *Curr Opin Lipidol* 17(1):54–57, 2006.

39. Giordano R, et al: Review: growth hormone treatment in human ageing: benefits and risks, *Hormones* 7(2):133–139, 2008.

40. Van Proeyen K, et al: Training in the fasted state improves glucose tolerance during fat-rich diet, *J Physiol* 588(21):4289–4302, 2010.

41. Bautmans I, et al: Circulating acute phase mediators and skeletal muscle performance in hospitalized geriatric patients, *J Gerontol A Biol Sci Med Sci* 60(3):361–367, 2005.

42. Chan DC, et al: Very low density lipoprotein metabolism and plasma adiponectin as predictors of high-density lipoprotein apolipoprotein A-I kinetics in obese and nonobese men, *J Clin Endocrinol Metab* 94(3):989–997, 2009.

43. Cartwright MM: The metabolic response to stress: a case of complex nutrition support management, *Crit Care Nurs Clin North Am* 16(4):467–487, 2004.

44. Van Heerebeek L, et al: Myocardial structure and function differ in systolic and diastolic heart failure, *Circulation* 113:1966–1973, 2006.

45. Pecoits-Filho R, Lindholm B, Stenvinkel P: The malnutrition, inflammation, and atherosclerosis (MIA) syndrome—the heart of the matter, *Nephrol Dial Transplant* 17(suppl 11):28–31, 2002.

46. Mattison S, Christensen M: The pathophysiology of emphysema: considerations for critical care nursing practice, *I Crit Care Nurse* 22(6):329–337, 2006.

47. Zimmer KP: Nutrition and celiac disease, *Curr Probl Pediatr Adolesc Health Care* 41(9):244–247, 2011.

48. Simmons D, Breier BH: Fetal overnutrition in Polynesian pregnancies and in gestational diabetes may lead to dysregulation of the adipoinsular axis in offspring, *Diabetes Care* 25(9):1539–1544, 2002.

49. Tabano S, et al: Epigenetic modulation of the IGF2/H19 imprinted domain in human embryonic and extra-embryonic compartments and its possible role in fetal growth restriction, *Epigenetics* 5(4):313–324, 2010.

50. Zeisel SH: Epigenetic mechanisms for nutrition determinants of later health outcomes, *Am J Clin Nutr* 89(suppl):S1488–S1493, 2009.

51. Sultan S, Forsmark CE: Therapeutics. Review: enteral nutrition reduces mortality, multiple organ failure, and systemic infection more than TPN in acute pancreatitis, *Ann Intern Med* 153(2):JC1–JC6, 2010.

52. Sanchez JA, Sanchez LL, Dudrick SJ: Nutritional considerations in adult cardiothoracic surgical patients, *Surg Clin North Am* 91(4):857–875, 2011.

53. Dudrick SJ, Sanchez JA: Nutrition and metabolism of the surgical patient, part II, *Surg Clin North Am* 91(4):xv–xvii, 2011.

54. Aronowski J, Zhao X: Molecular pathophysiology of cerebral hemorrhage: secondary brain injury, *Stroke* 42(6):1781–1786, 2011.

55. Wischmeyer PE, Heyland DK: The future of critical care nutrition therapy, *Crit Care Clin* 26(3):433–441, vii, 2010.

56. Holmes S: Nutrition in the care of patients with cancer cachexia, *Br J Commun Nurs* 16(7):314, 316, 318, 2011.

Structure and Function of the Nervous System

Jacquelyn L. Banasik

⊖volve WEBSITE

http://evolve.elsevier.com/Copstead/
- Review Questions and Answers
- Glossary (with audio pronunciations for selected terms)
- Animations
- Case Studies
- Key Points Review

KEY QUESTIONS

- How do the central nervous system (CNS), peripheral nervous system, and autonomic nervous system interrelate?
- How is the CNS protected and supported?
- What structures are located in each of the four principal areas of the brain: cerebrum, diencephalon, cerebellum, and brainstem?
- What neurologic functions have been mapped to particular locations in the brain?

- How do the properties of neuronal action potentials and neuronal communication through synapses relate to the functions of the nervous system?
- How is the somatotopic organization of sensory receptors and muscles maintained in the CNS?
- How is voluntary muscle activity initiated and executed?
- How do the properties of the mind, including thought, memory, learning, consciousness, and sleep, relate to the physiologic substance of the nervous system?

CHAPTER OUTLINE

The nervous system is a complex network of neurons and supportive cells that enables rapid communication between sensory receptors, central processing neurons, and functional responses. Much has been discovered about the mechanisms of sensory input and motor output, but the physiologic bases of thought, consciousness, emotion, and learning remain elusive. The idea that the mind is within the biological realm has been generally accepted, and the effects of mind-altering drugs on emotions, appetite, sleep, thought, and sensory perception have long been recognized. Research continues to reveal the great complexity of neurologic function. A bewildering array of neurotransmitter signaling molecules and an even greater number of neurotransmitter receptors have been identified. Recently, the long-held notion that neurons cannot regenerate in the mature brain has been disproved, and neuronal stem cells have been identified in certain areas. Each discovery brings us closer to understanding neural physiologic processes and gives hope for finding effective therapies for the devastating diseases that affect them. This chapter provides an overview of neural structure and function and is the basis for understanding the neurologic disorders in the chapters that follow.

STRUCTURAL ORGANIZATION

The nervous system is traditionally divided into three principal anatomic units: the central nervous system (CNS), the peripheral nervous system (PNS), and the autonomic nervous system (ANS). These systems are not anatomically or functionally distinct, and they work together as an integrated whole. Therefore, when function, rather than anatomy, is the topic of concern, the nervous system is more conveniently divided into the sensory, motor, and higher brain functions. This chapter begins with a review of the major anatomic features of the nervous system, then addresses neurologic function at the cellular and synaptic level, and concludes with a summary of sensory, motor, and cognitive functions.

CENTRAL NERVOUS SYSTEM

The CNS includes the brain and spinal cord. Its primary functions are receiving and processing sensory information and creating appropriate responses to be relayed to muscles and glands. It is the site of emotion, memory, cognition, and learning. The CNS is bathed in cerebrospinal fluid (CSF) and shielded from the periphery by the blood-brain barrier. The CNS interacts with the neurons of the PNS through synapses in the spinal cord and cranial nerve **ganglia.** The cranial and spinal nerves constitute the PNS.

Support and Protection of the Central Nervous System

Nervous tissue has the consistency of gelatin, so measures to support and protect its fragile structure are necessary. In addition, the CNS must be shielded from circulating substances that would interfere with neurotransmission. These protective functions are provided by the skull and vertebral column, meninges, CSF, and blood-brain barriers. The bony structures of the skull and vertebral column encase the brain and cord and protect them from external trauma, whereas the CSF and meninges provide buoyancy and shock-absorbing capacity.

The meninges are composed of three layers that serve to suspend and maintain the shape and position of the nervous tissue during head and body movements. The brain is suspended within layers of meninges that are fixed to the skull. In this manner, the brain turns with the movement of the skull. The CSF circulates within the subarachnoid space, giving buoyancy to the brain neud making an average 1500-gram brain mass resistant to distortion, which could occur from gravity

alone were it not for the buoyancy effect.[1] The three meningeal layers are the *dura mater, arachnoid,* and *pia mater* (Figure 43-1).

The dura mater, the outermost meningeal layer, is a thick, tough, collagenous membrane. It is composed of two layers, one contiguous with the periosteum of the skull and the other, which is adherent to the first, covering the surface of the brain. The tough dura protects the soft tissue of the brain. Support and stability are also provided by dural septa that invaginate into the cranial cavity. The falx cerebri is a thin wall of dura that folds down the cortical midline, separating the two hemispheres (see Figure 43-1). The tentorium cerebelli is a septum that separates the cerebellum and brainstem from the rest of the cerebrum. The dural septa fix the brain in place by their tentlike structure and limit its movement within the skull. Venous sinuses that collect venous blood from cerebral veins are located between the two layers of the dura at the base of the septum.

Beneath and continuous with the dura is the arachnoid layer. The spaces between the dura and the skull and between the dura mater and the arachnoid are potential spaces. Only in the presence of pathologic processes, notably epidural and subdural hemorrhages, do these spaces become evident (see Chapter 44). Unlike the dura mater, the arachnoid is a thin, delicate membrane. It is semitransparent and weblike in appearance, hence its name. Strands of collagenous connective tissue called *trabeculae* extend from the arachnoid layer down to the pia mater, forming a subarachnoid space. The CSF flows in this space.

The pia mater, the third meningeal layer, is also very thin. However, unlike the other meningeal layers, the pia is attached to the brain and closely follows its contours over every **sulcus** and into every **gyrus.** Consequently, the subarachnoid space between the arachnoid and the pia mater is not evenly distributed. The arachnoid meshes with the pia via the trabeculae in such a subtle manner that it is often difficult to differentiate one from the other. Consequently, the two layers together are often referred to as the *leptomeninges.*

The meninges that cover and provide protection to the spinal cord are similar to those of the brain, with a few variations (Figure 43-2). The spinal dura has no periosteal layer, so it is a single rather than a double layer. It is continuous with the foramen magnum at the base of the skull and is separated from the spinal vertebral periosteum by an epidural space. Thus, in the spinal cord, the epidural space is a true space, unlike its counterpart in the cranium, which is only a potential space. Within this space lie fatty connective tissue and a vertebral venous plexus.

The spinal arachnoid, much like that covering the cerebrum, is closely adherent to the spinal dura. Between the arachnoid layer and the pial lining is the CSF-filled subarachnoid space. The spinal meninges end at approximately the second sacral vertebra. However, the spinal cord ends between the first and second lumbar vertebrae (L1 to L2). This results in a large subarachnoid cistern, called the *lumbar cistern,* which is a favored place to obtain CSF samples (see Figure 43-2). The spinal pia is much tougher and thicker than the cerebral pia. Projecting along the length of each side is the dentate ligament, which anchors the spinal cord to the arachnoid and through it to the dura. Another pial projection connects the tail of the spinal cord (the cauda equina) at level L1 to L2 to the **caudal** end of the spinal dural sheath, where it is tethered to the end of the vertebral column. This projection is called the *filum terminale.*

The majority of CSF is produced by the choroid plexus, located in the lateral and third ventricles of the brain, at a rate of approximately 500 ml/day.[2] The composition of normal CSF is compared to plasma in Table 43-1. CSF is absorbed at about the same rate at which it is produced, so that only 150 to 175 ml is in circulation at any time. The large C-shaped lateral ventricles occupy the center of each hemisphere. They communicate with the third ventricle in the

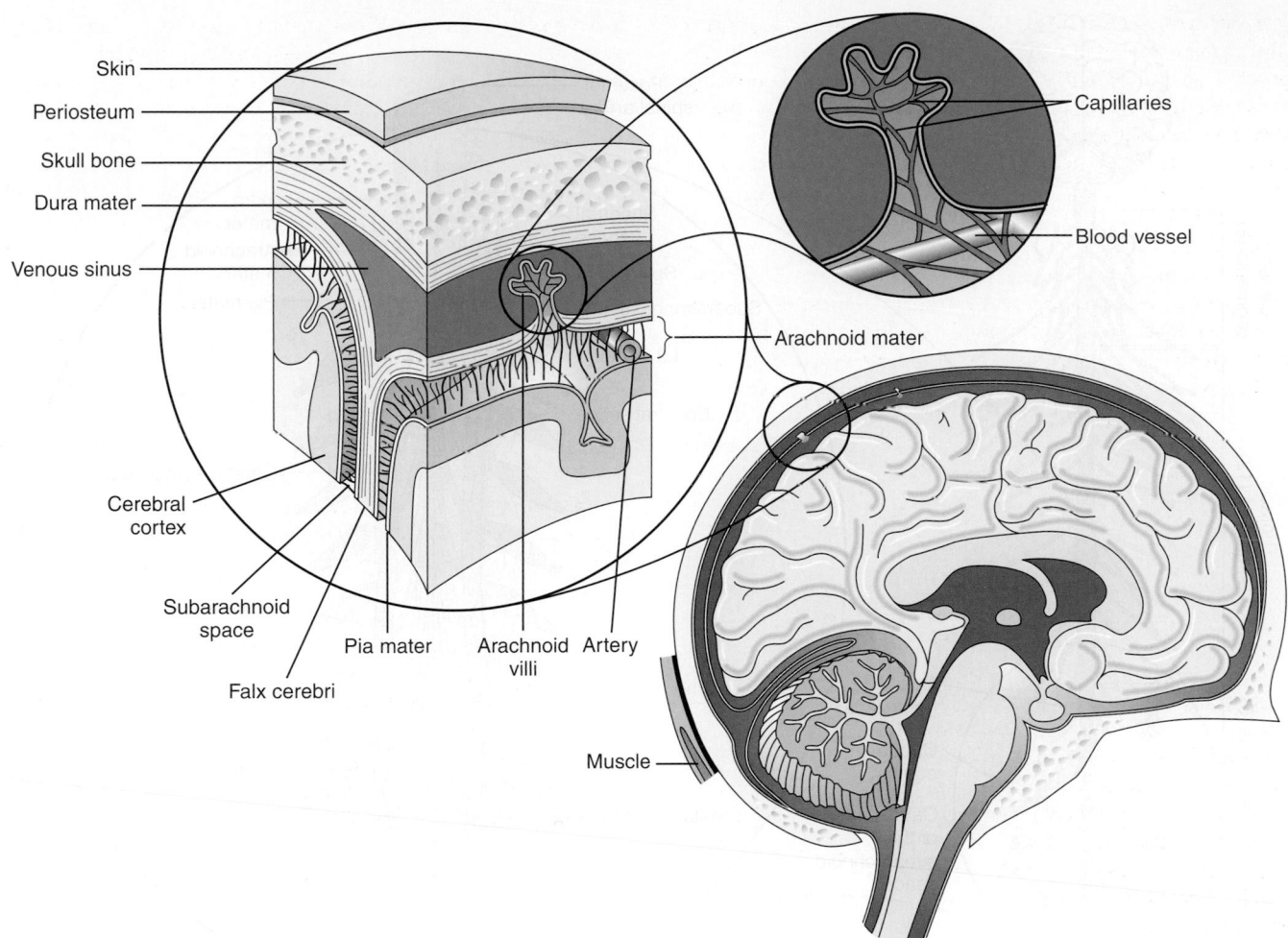

FIGURE 43-1 Principle membranes of the cranial meninges. Cerebrospinal fluid flows in the subarachnoid space and is reabsorbed by arachnoid villi within the dural sinuses.

diencephalon by way of the intraventricular foramen. The third ventricle is linked to the fourth ventricle by way of the cerebral aqueduct, which lies between the pons and the medulla (Figure 43-3). The CSF flows from the fourth ventricle through the median or lateral aperture and into the subarachnoid space. It flows around the spinal cord and up over the cerebral hemispheres to the arachnoid villi, where it is absorbed into the venous system.

CSF is absorbed by the arachnoid villi, which are small tufts of the arachnoid that invaginate into the dural sinus. These tufts bring CSF into close approximation with venous blood. CSF flows into the venous system through one-way valves because of pressure gradient differences. Although the CSF flows readily into the venous sinus, flow in the opposite direction cannot occur[2]; that is, the fluid in the venous sinus cannot flow into the subarachnoid space. This mechanism is part of a system of barriers between the extracellular space in the nervous system and the rest of the body.

The rate of production of CSF is independent of blood pressure or intraventricular pressure.[2] Thus, CSF will continue to be produced even when its path of circulation or absorption is blocked. If this occurs, the amount of CSF increases, as does the size of the ventricles. This pathologic process is called *hydrocephalus*. Although hydrocephalus is usually caused by blockage of CSF pathways, it can also be caused by overproduction and malabsorption of CSF (see Chapter 45).

Blood supply to the brain is provided by two pairs of arteries; the anterior circulation is supplied by the internal carotid arteries, and the posterior circulation is supplied by the vertebral arteries (Figure 43-4). The cerebral circulation is discussed in detail in Chapter 44 as it relates to stroke. The internal carotid arteries have three principal branches: the anterior and middle cerebral arteries and the posterior communicating arteries. The vertebral arteries enter the skull at the foramen magnum and join at the level of the pons to form the basilar arteries. The ring of vessels that unites the anterior and posterior circulation at the base of the brain is known as the *circle of Willis* (see Figure 43-4, *B*). The cerebral veins drain into large vascular channels called *sinuses* that are formed by folds in the dura. From the sinuses, venous blood returns to the heart by way of the jugular veins (see Figure 43-4, *C*).

The extracellular fluid that bathes the neurons is carefully shielded from elements in the CSF and blood by cellular barriers. Specialized tight junctions between the cells that line the CSF spaces and between the endothelial cells of brain capillaries prevent leakage of molecules through the spaces between the cells (Figure 43-5). Therefore, substances must move through the plasma membranes of these barrier cells to access the CNS. Lipid-soluble molecules move through more easily than water-soluble ones. Thus, the flow of ions, nutrients, drugs, proteins, and other charged or polar substances is highly restricted.[2] The blood-brain barrier (BBB) is a crucial structure for protecting the brain, but it may also restrict access of beneficial molecules, such as antibiotics and cancer drugs, making treatment more difficult.

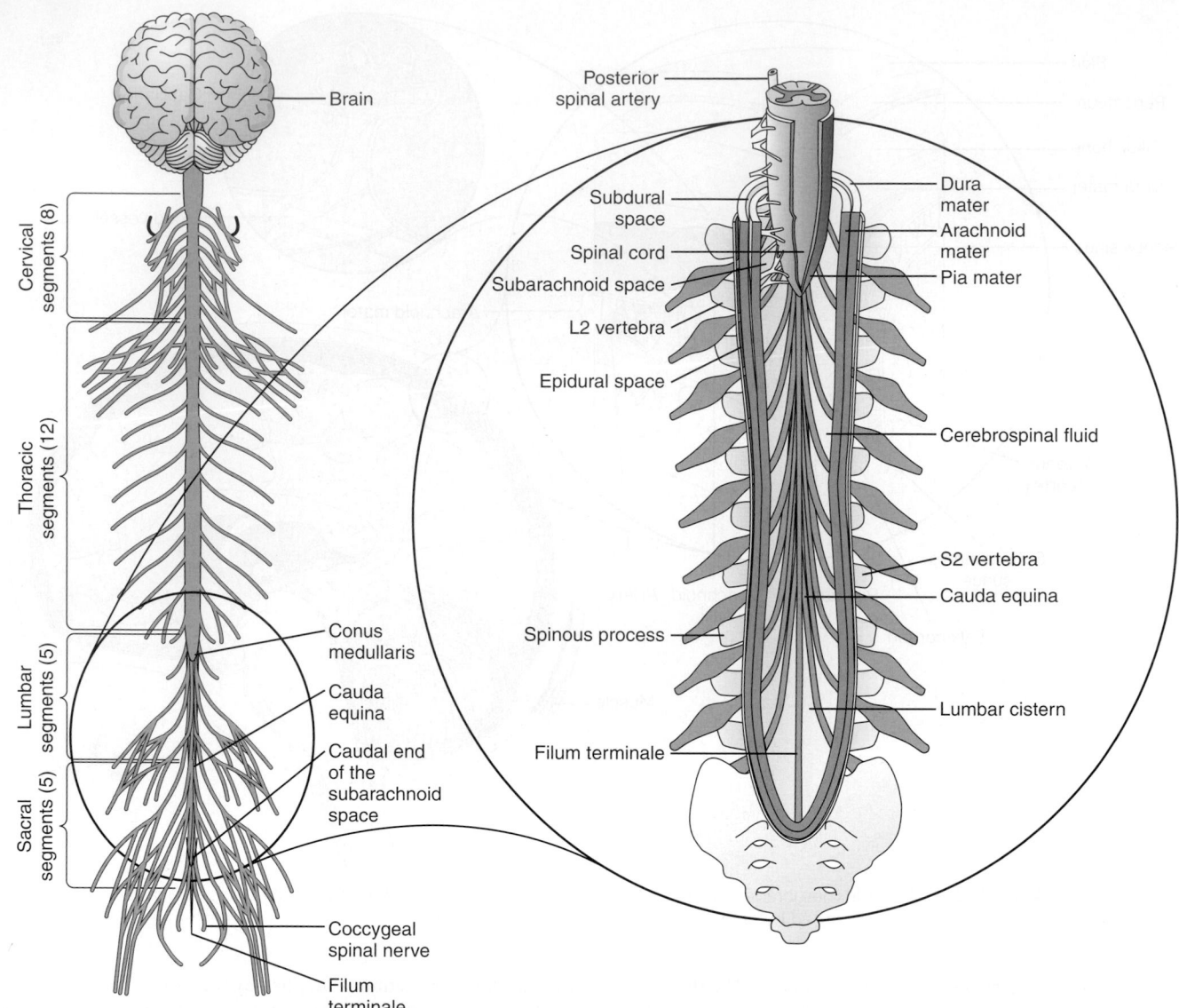

FIGURE 43-2 Spinal cord, spinal nerves, and meninges. Spinal meninges are similar to cranial membranes. Spinal meninges end at S2, creating a CSF-filled cistern below the spinal cord. The cauda equina (horse tail) is formed by the lumbar and sacral nerves, which protrude from the end of the spinal cord.

TABLE 43-1	COMPOSITION OF CEREBROSPINAL FLUID COMPARED TO PLASMA AND SELECTED CEREBROSPINAL FLUID ABNORMALITIES		
SUBSTANCE	**NORMAL CSF**	**ABNORMAL CSF**	**PLASMA**
Na^+ (mEq/L)	148	—	136-145
K^+ (mEq/L)	2.9	—	3.5-5.0
Cl^- (mEq/L)	120-130	—	100-106
Glucose (mg/dl)	50-75	↓ Infection	70-100
Protein (mg/dl)	15-45	↑ Inflammation	6800
pH	7.3	—	7.4
Red blood cells (high-power field)	None	↑ Trauma, subarachnoid hemorrhage	—
White blood cells (high-power field)	<5	↑ Infection (e.g., meningitis)	—
Pressure (mm H_2O)	70-180	↑ Mass lesions	—

CSF, Cerebrospinal fluid.

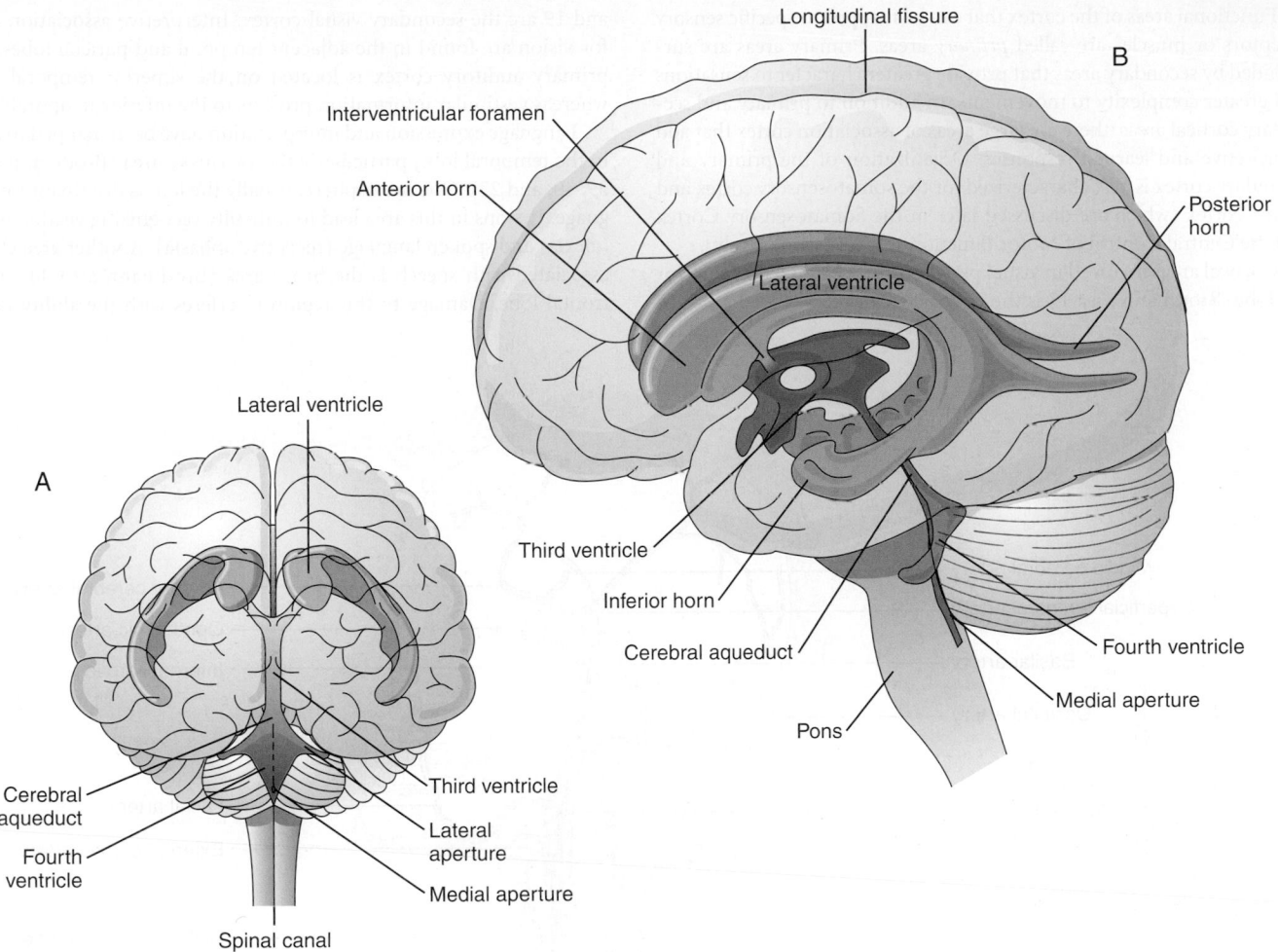

FIGURE 43-3 Ventricles within the brain from frontal (**A**) and lateral (**B**) views.

The integrity of the blood-brain barrier is maintained in part by CNS cells called *astrocytes*. These specialized **glial** cells have foot processes that contact the brain capillaries and are thought to help regulate transport across the capillary endothelium[3] (see Figure 43-5). The blood-brain barrier is less effective in infancy and can also be compromised by ischemia and chemical injury in adults.

A similar barrier exists between the circulating CSF and the interstitial fluid of the CNS—the CSF-brain barrier. The ependymal cells that line the ventricles are tightly joined and regulate the movement of water-soluble elements between the CSF and neurons. In addition, these cells serve the important function of removing unwanted substances from the CNS and secreting them into the CSF for eventual removal by the venous system.

Some areas of the brain need to sample the contents of the blood or CSF more directly to make regulatory adjustments in respiratory, autonomic, or endocrine functions, and these areas therefore have more permeable barriers (leaky BBB). These areas include the hypothalamus, pituitary, and other circumventricular organs (around the ventricles).

The Brain

Various schemes have been used to subdivide the structures of the brain using embryologic, evolutionary, and anatomic frameworks (Table 43-2). In this section, an anatomic framework is used that includes the cerebrum, diencephalon, cerebellum, and brainstem (Figure 43-6).

Cerebrum

The cerebrum is divided into left and right hemispheres by the longitudinal fissure and is the largest part of the brain. The cerebral cortex is the outermost layer of the cerebrum and is composed of gray matter arranged in six histologically distinct layers[4] (Figure 43-7). Each layer makes connections with other parts of the brain. The cortex is characterized by its convoluted exterior having ridges (gyri), grooves (sulci), and deeper depressions (fissures). The sulci and fissures are used as landmarks to divide the cerebral cortex into lobes. The central sulcus separates the frontal and parietal lobes, the lateral sulcus separates the temporal lobe from the parietal and frontal lobes, and the parieto-occipital line defines the occipital lobe (Figure 43-8).

Some anatomic locations are particularly associated with certain brain functions. These functions have been characterized through lesion studies in which an area of brain is damaged and then the functional losses studied, and by mapping procedures during which the cerebral cortex is stimulated and responses are recorded. The functional areas of specialization of brain loci are listed in Table 43-3. A partial map of Brodmann areas is shown in Figure 43-9. Although the concept of functional anatomic areas is clinically useful, one should realize that even though an area may be critical for a particular function, it is not wholly responsible for that function, and many brain areas may be involved. A certain degree of reassignment of brain function from one area to another can occur, allowing the brain to adapt to loss of normal neural function (neural plasticity).

Functional areas of the cortex that can be mapped to specific sensory receptors or muscles are called *primary* areas. Primary areas are surrounded by secondary areas that provide greater character to sensations and greater complexity to movements. In addition to primary and secondary cortical areas, there are large areas of association cortex that add interpretive and learned responses. Organization of the primary and secondary cortex is best characterized for the somatosensory cortex and motor cortex (which are discussed later in the Somatosensory Cortex and the Central Control of Motor Function sections, respectively).

Cortical areas involved in visual perception are located in the occipital lobe. Brodmann area 17 is the primary visual cortex, and areas 18 and 19 are the secondary visual cortex. Interpretive association areas for vision are found in the adjacent temporal and parietal lobes. The primary auditory cortex is located on the superior temporal lobe, whereas vestibular information projects to the inferior temporal lobe.

Language expression and interpretation have been mapped to areas in the temporal lobe, particularly the Wernicke area (Brodmann areas 39, 40, and 22). One hemisphere, usually the left, is dominant for language. Lesions in this area lead to difficulty recognizing written words (alexia) and spoken language (receptive aphasia). Another area closely associated with speech is the Broca area (Brodmann area 44) in the frontal lobe. Damage to this region interferes with the ability to use

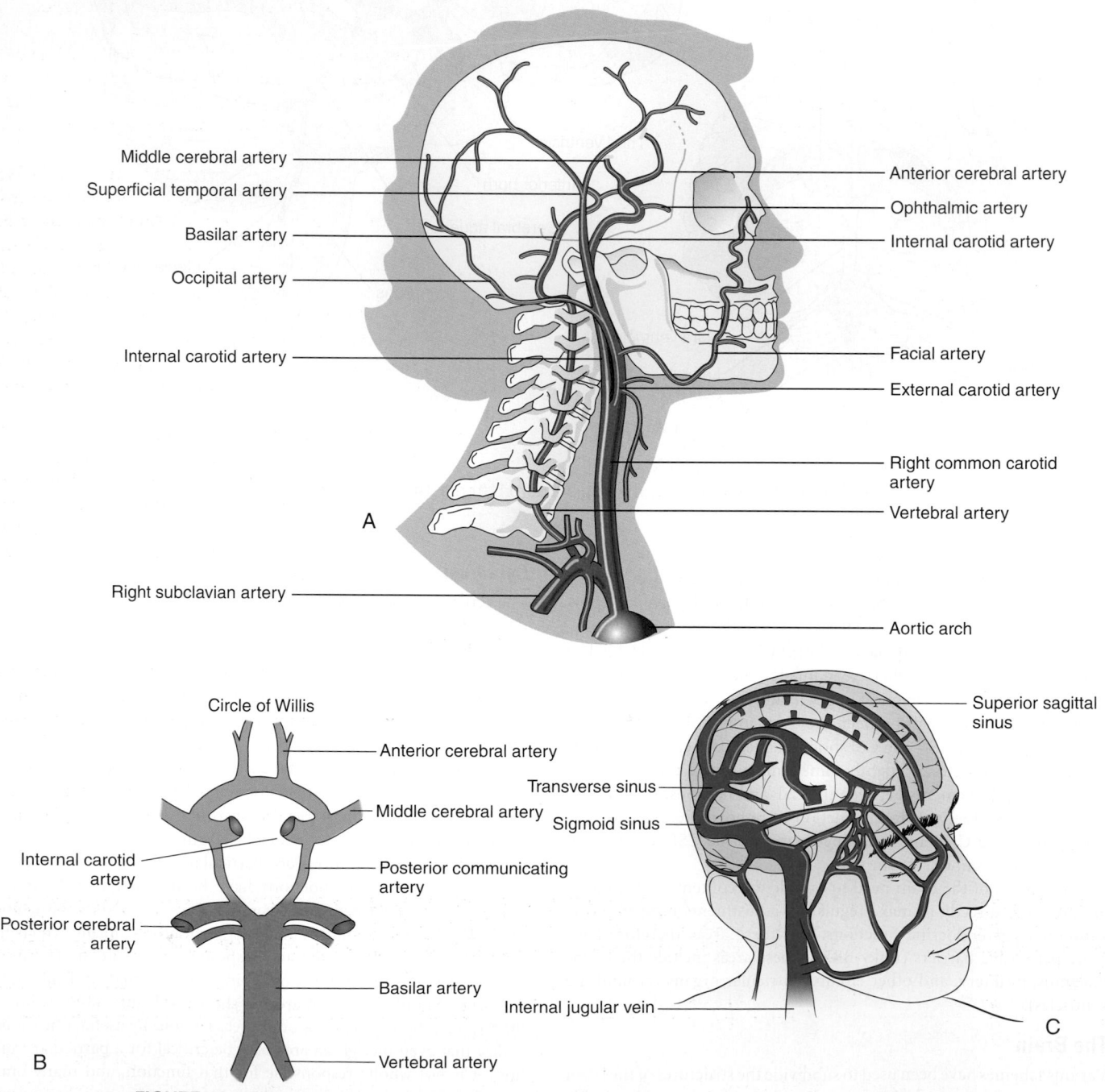

FIGURE 43-4 Blood supply to the brain. **A,** The internal carotid and vertebral arteries supply blood to the anterior and posterior aspects of the brain, respectively. **B,** At the base of the brain, the internal carotid and vertebral arteries join to form the circle of Willis. **C,** Major venous drainage from the brain.

language (expressive aphasia). In most cases, receptive and expressive aphasia occur together (see Chapter 44).

The frontal lobe is usually credited with control over emotional responses, ethical behavior, and morality. It is also the site of initiative and motivation. Patients with lesions of the frontal lobe may fail to conform to societal behavioral norms.

Another small cortical lobe, the central lobe or insula, lies deep in the lateral cerebral fissure under the junction of the frontal, parietal, and temporal lobes. Little is known about its specific functions, although it is thought to regulate visceral and intestinal functions.

The limbic lobe and **limbic system** are the parts of the cerebrum most closely associated with memory and emotion. The limbic lobe is a ring of cortex on the medial surface of each hemisphere containing the cingulate gyrus, isthmus, and parahippocampal gyrus (Figure 43-10). Olfaction (the perception of smell) occurs within the limbic cortex. The limbic system is a group of structures that encircle the brainstem. In addition to the limbic lobe, the limbic system includes the amygdala, fornix, hippocampus, and portions of the thalamus (see Figure 43-10). Lesions of the limbic system, particularly the hippocampus, cause impairment of short-term memory.

The **basal ganglia** are large masses of gray matter that lie deep within the cerebral hemispheres. They are intimately involved in the initiation, coordination, and execution of movement.[5,6] The basal ganglia include the caudate nucleus, putamen, globus pallidus, subthalamus, and substantia nigra (Figure 43-11). The caudate nucleus and putamen

together are called the *striatum*. The five basal ganglia structures occur in pairs, with each cerebral hemisphere containing a set.

The basal ganglia are connected by complex neural circuits that incorporate sensory information about the current muscle conditions, cortical input about desired motor activities, and cerebellar signals about timing and coordination. Much of what is known about the function of basal ganglia has been learned from studying Parkinson disease. Parkinson disease is characterized by difficulty initiating voluntary movements (akinesia), stiff muscles (rigidity), and a tremor of the hands when idle (rest tremor). Improvement in symptoms occurs when the patient is given a precursor of dopamine (DA, levodopa), which can cross the blood-brain barrier. Studies of these patients revealed degeneration of DA-secreting neurons that project from the substantia nigra to the striatum. As these neurons slowly degenerate over many years, the amount of DA secreted decreases, downstream γ-aminobutyric acid (GABA) pathways become dysregulated, and the relative activity of acetylcholine-secreting neurons in the basal ganglia is increased.[7] A number of drugs (those that block DA) are known to produce a similar clinical syndrome (see Chapter 45).

In addition to the gray matter of the cerebral cortex and the basal ganglia, the cerebrum contains thick layers of white matter that consist of myelinated axons. Some of these axons connect the two cerebral hemispheres (commissural fibers), some connect one area of cortex to another within the same hemisphere (association fibers), and others connect the cortex with lower brain centers, including the thalamus, basal ganglia, brainstem, and spinal cord (projection fibers). The corpus callosum and the anterior commissure connect the two hemispheres. The corpus callosum is a massive bundle of fibers crossing the brain just above the lateral ventricles and is the principal means of communication between the hemispheres.

In summary, the cerebrum is the largest brain structure, garnering about 70% of the neurons and supporting cells of the brain to accomplish its diverse and complex functions. Each of the 100 billion neurons in the brain may make hundreds of synaptic connections with other neurons, providing an incomprehensible number of potential interactions. Discovering the ways in which the substance of the cerebrum relates to the workings of the mind is one of the great remaining mysteries of science.

Diencephalon

The diencephalon lies deep in the brain, forming a connecting structure between the upper brainstem (midbrain) and the cerebral hemispheres. The principal structures of the diencephalon are the thalamus, hypothalamus, pineal gland, epithalamus, and ventral thalamus (Figure 43-12). The third ventricle also traverses the diencephalon.

The thalamus is the principal receiving site and relay center for impulses traveling to the cerebral cortex from the spinal cord,

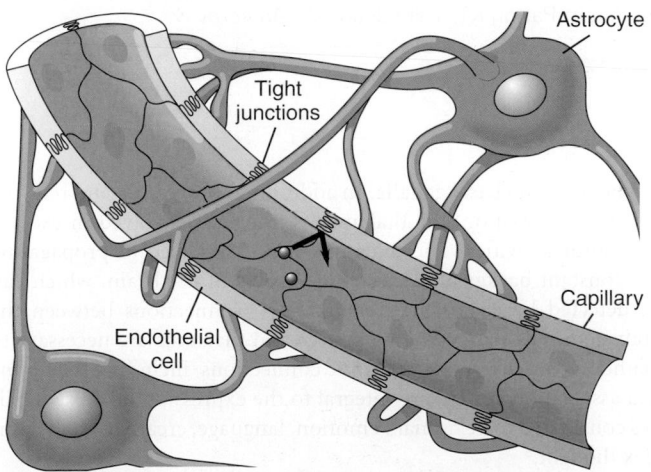

FIGURE 43-5 Tight junctions between brain capillary endothelial cells prevent polar and charged molecules from passing between cells. Astrocytes have foot processes on the capillary that help to maintain integrity of the blood-brain barrier.

TABLE 43-2	**SUBDIVISIONS OF THE BRAIN USING EMBRYOLOGIC, EVOLUTIONARY, AND ANATOMIC FRAMEWORKS**		
	FRAMEWORK		
STRUCTURE	**EMBRYOLOGIC**	**EVOLUTIONARY**	**ANATOMIC**
Cerebral hemisphere	Telencephalon	Forebrain (includes diencephalon)	Cerebrum
Thalamus	Diencephalon	—	Diencephalon hypothalamus
Midbrain	Mesencephalon	Midbrain	—
Cerebellum	Metencephalon (includes pons)	Cerebellum	Cerebellum
Medulla	Myelencephalon	Hindbrain	Brainstem (includes midbrain, pons)

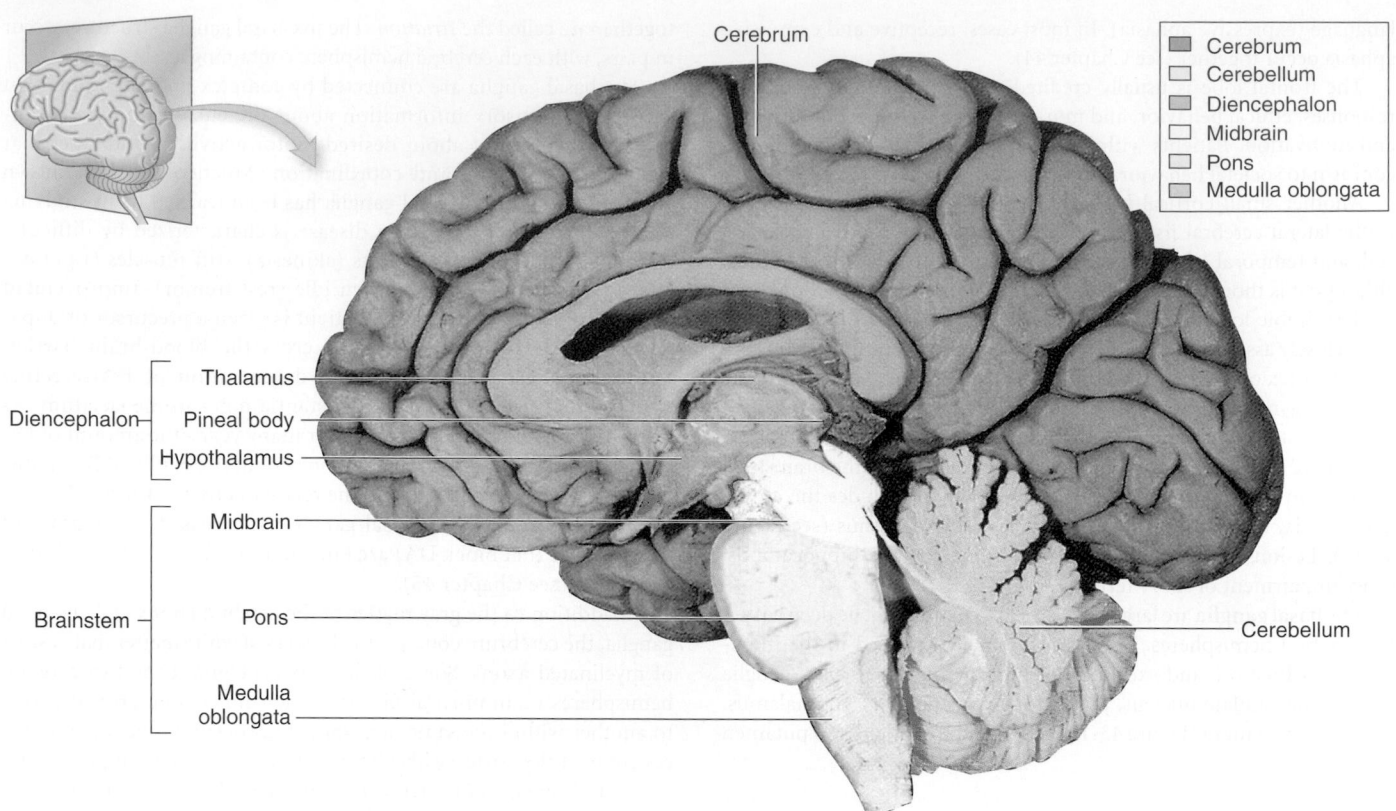

Cerebrum

- ■ Cerebrum
- □ Cerebellum
- ■ Diencephalon
- □ Midbrain
- □ Pons
- ■ Medulla oblongata

Diencephalon — Thalamus
— Pineal body
— Hypothalamus

Brainstem — Midbrain
— Pons
— Medulla oblongata

Cerebellum

FIGURE 43-6 Four principal anatomic areas of the brain. (From Patton KT, Thibodeau GA: *Anatomy & physiology*, ed 8, St Louis, 2013, Mosby, p 429.)

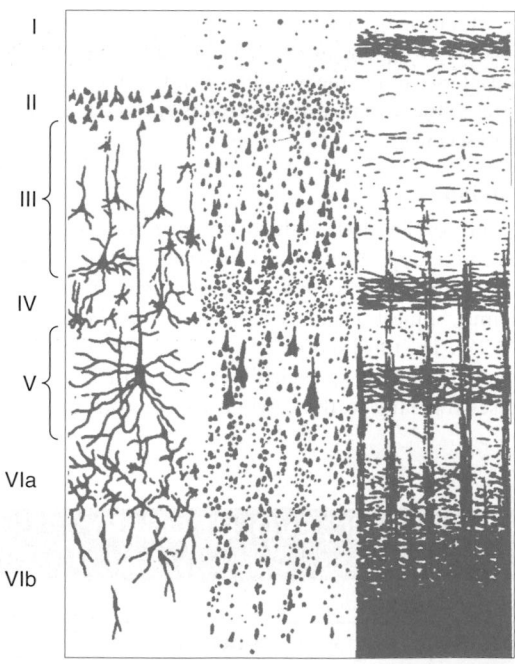

I
II
III
IV
V
VIa
VIb

FIGURE 43-7 The cortex of the brain is histologically divided into six layers that differ in their connections to other parts of the nervous system. (From Ransom SW, Clark SL [after Brodmann]: *Anatomy of the nervous system*, Philadelphia, 1959, Saunders.)

cerebellum, and basal ganglia. In addition to processing and relaying sensory information, the thalamus is integrally involved in executing motor activities. The thalamus also is involved in propagating the constant background electrical activity of the brain, which can be detected by electroencephalography. Connections between the brainstem reticular activating system and thalamus are necessary to maintain consciousness. Thalamic connections, including the limbic and association cortex, are integral to the expression of those qualities considered to be human: emotion, language, creativity, and complex thought.[8]

The hypothalamus is located just beneath the thalamus on the floor of the diencephalon. The inferior aspect of the hypothalamus extends downward to form the pituitary gland (hypophysis). The posterior pituitary gland is an extension of the neuronal tissue of the hypothalamus, whereas the anterior pituitary gland is derived from glandular tissue (Figure 43-13). Hormones secreted by the pituitary gland enter the systemic circulation and influence target cells at a distance. Neurons in the hypothalamus regulate the secretion of anterior pituitary hormones by releasing and inhibiting hormones (see Chapter 39 for a discussion of the endocrine system).

The hypothalamus is also an important regulatory center for the ANS and for basic functions, such as sleep, body temperature, appetite, and sex drive. Input from sensors of blood pressure, osmolarity, blood oxygen concentration, carbon dioxide level and pH, and temperature is received and integrated into appropriate regulatory responses. The hypothalamus is responsible for homeostasis of life-sustaining functions, including cardiovascular, respiratory, metabolic, fluid and electrolyte, and stress responses.

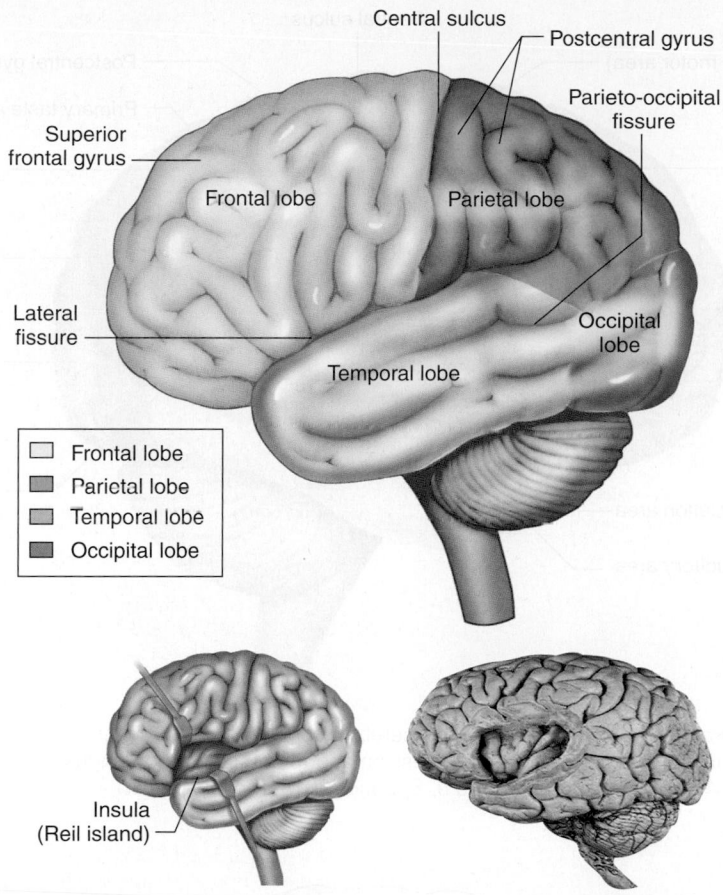

FIGURE 43-8 Four principal lobes of the cerebral cortex. (From Patton KT, Thibodeau GA: *Anatomy & physiology*, ed 8, St Louis, 2013, Mosby, p 437.)

TABLE 43-3 FUNCTIONAL AREAS OF BRAIN SPECIALIZATION

AREA	SPECIALIZED FUNCTION
Occipital lobe	Visual cortex and association areas
Parietal lobe	Somatosensory cortex and association areas
Temporal lobe	Hearing and equilibrium, emotion, and memory
Frontal lobe	Motor cortex and association areas; prefrontal cortex involved in complex thought, ethical behavior, and morality
Limbic structures	Emotions, short-term memory, olfaction
Basal ganglia	Initiation and planning of learned motor activities
Broca and Wernicke areas	Interpretation and expression of language

The epithalamus contains the pineal gland, thought to be important in regulating circadian rhythms in response to light-dark cycles. The ventral thalamus contains the basal ganglia structure called the *subthalamic nucleus*.

Cerebellum

The cerebellum is located in the posterior fossa behind the pons. It is separated from the cerebrum by the tentorium cerebelli. The main roles of the cerebellum are to coordinate and smooth movements and to maintain posture and balance. The cerebellum compares the desired motor program with the moment-to-moment execution of the movement and makes instantaneous adjustments to improve the match.[9] The cerebellum receives information from proprioceptors in muscles and joints and from the vestibular apparatus in the inner ear about the position of the head in space. Some of the fastest-conducting neurons in the nervous system are involved in relaying sensory information to the cerebellum.

The cerebellar cortex is folded much as the cerebral cortex is folded, in a way that significantly increases surface area. Its tightly folded shape gives it a banded appearance. The cortical ridges on the surface of the cerebellum are called *folia*. The white matter beneath is called the *medullary* center and is made up of fibers running to and from the cerebellar cortex.

The cerebellum is divided anatomically, first by the posterolateral fissure, which separates the flocculonodular lobe (the region immediately inferior to the middle cerebellar peduncles) from the main body (Figure 43-14). The midline body is called the *vermis*, and it is straddled on either side by the cerebellar hemispheres.

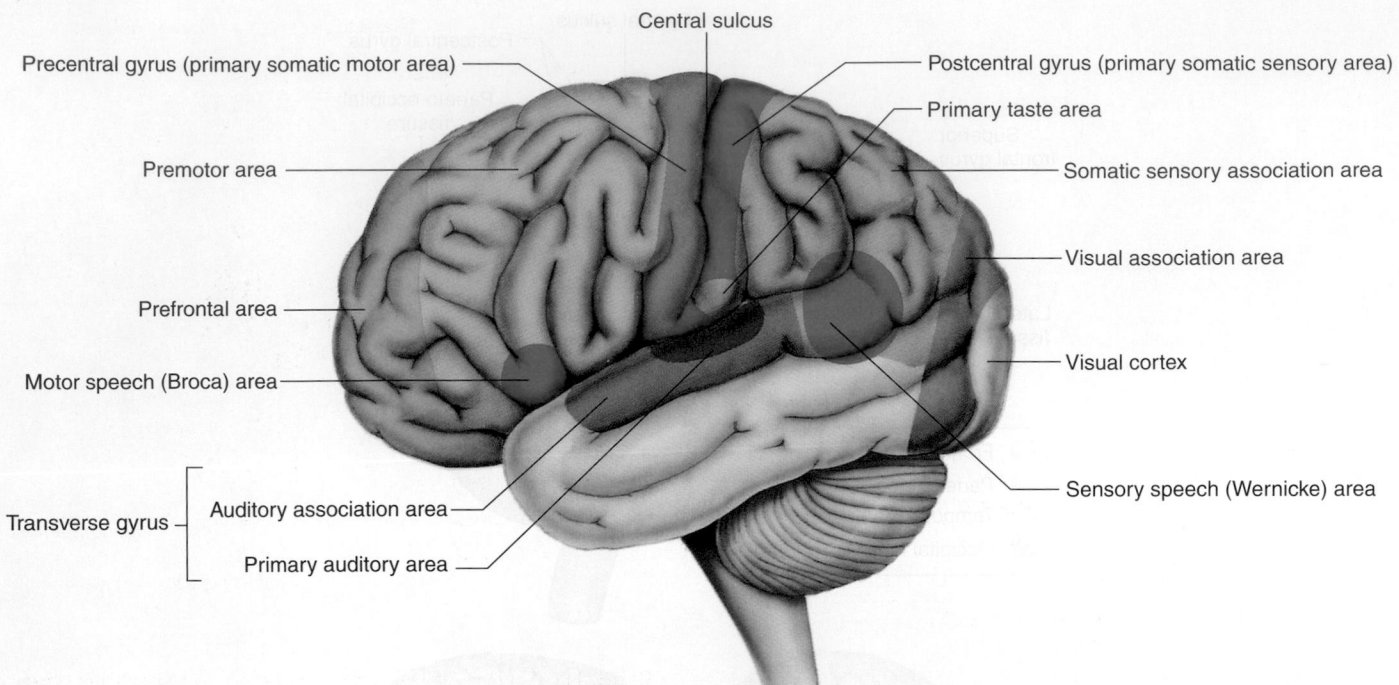

FIGURE 43-9 Partial Brodmann map of the cerebral cortex. Note the locations of Broca and Wernicke areas, which are important in the expression and understanding of language. (From Patton KT, Thibodeau GA: *Anatomy & physiology*, ed 8, St Louis, 2013, Mosby, p 441.)

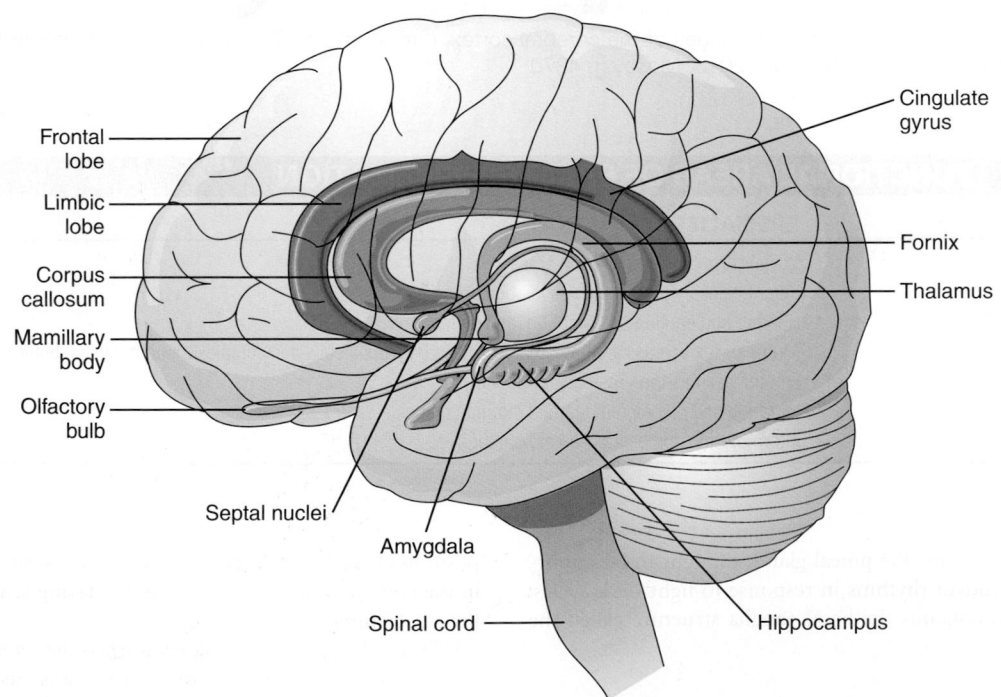

FIGURE 43-10 The limbic system is composed of a group of structures deep in the brain that are important in memory and emotion. These structures include the limbic lobe, amygdala, fornix, hippocampus, olfactory bulb, and portions of the thalamus.

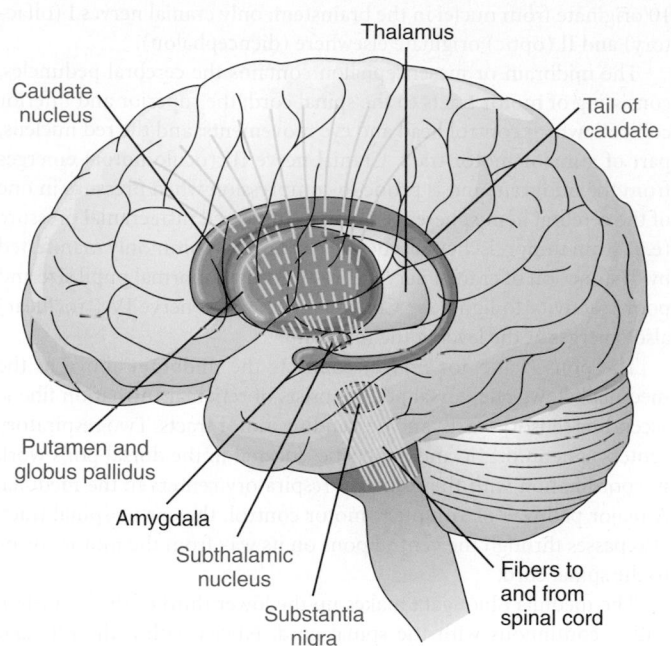

FIGURE 43-11 The basal ganglia include the caudate nucleus, putamen, globus pallidus, subthalamic nucleus, and substantia nigra (labeled in blue).

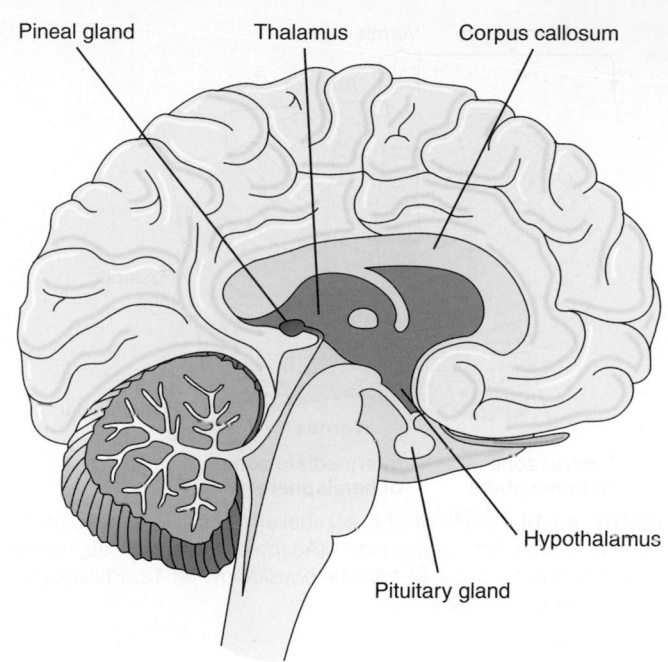

FIGURE 43-12 The diencephalon includes the thalamus, hypothalamus, pineal gland, and hypothalamic extension to the pituitary gland.

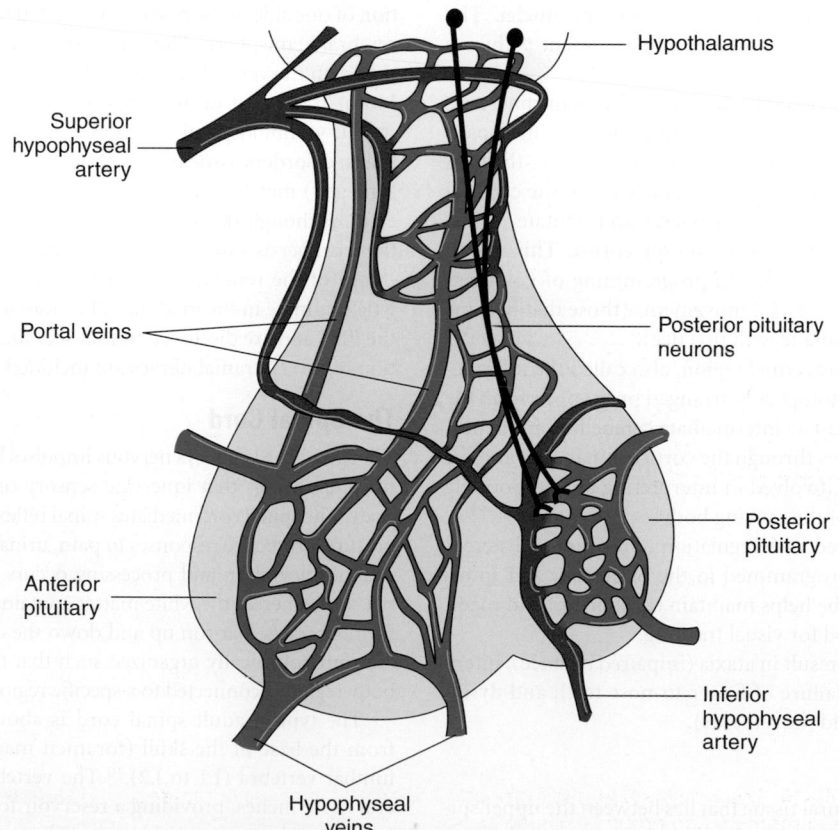

FIGURE 43-13 Anatomy of the hypothalamus and pituitary gland. Note that the posterior pituitary gland is connected to the hypothalamus by neuronal axons, whereas the anterior pituitary gland receives signals by way of a portal vein system. The portal veins drain blood from the capillaries of the hypothalamus and take it to the capillaries of the anterior pituitary gland.

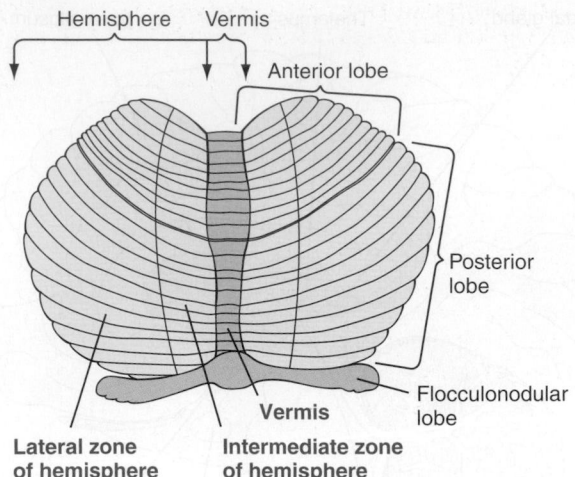

Hemisphere · Vermis · Anterior lobe · Posterior lobe · Flocculonodular lobe · Vermis · Lateral zone of hemisphere · Intermediate zone of hemisphere

FIGURE 43-14 Lobes of the cerebellum from a posteroinferior view. See text for explanation. (Adapted from Hall JE, editor: *Guyton & Hall textbook of medical physiology*, ed 12, Philadelphia, 2011, Saunders, p 682.)

The prominent tracts that attach the cerebellum to the brainstem are called the *inferior, middle,* and *superior* cerebellar peduncles. The inferior cerebellar peduncle is composed primarily of afferent fibers coming from the spinal cord and the brainstem. The middle peduncle contains afferent fibers from the contralateral pontine **nuclei.** The superior cerebellar peduncle is composed of major efferent pathways leaving the cerebellum.

Deep within the medullary center in each cerebellar hemisphere are the cerebellar nuclei. These include the dentate nuclei, the interposed nuclei, and the fastigial nuclei. The deep cerebellar nuclei are the final pathway of cerebellar output. Input from several areas of the cerebral cortex is received by the cerebellar hemispheres and dentate nuclei, and then sent back to the motor and premotor cortex. This circuit is believed to influence the planning and programming of voluntary movements, especially learned, skilled movements (those that become more rapid, precise, and automatic with practice).

The major input to the paravermal region, also called the intermediate cortex, consists of somatotopically arranged projections from the motor cortex and spinal cord. The intermediate cerebellum influences spinal cord and motor neurons through the corticospinal tract and the rubrospinal tract, where it is involved in interpreting and responding to the position and velocity of the moving body.

The vermis is most involved with regulation of posture and stereotyped movements that are programmed in the brainstem and spinal cord. The flocculonodular lobe helps maintain equilibrium and mediate the eye movements needed for visual tracking.

Lesions of the cerebellum result in ataxia (impaired balance), intention tremor, past pointing (failure of finger-to-nose test), and dysdiadochokinesia (failure of rapid movements).

Brainstem

The brainstem is a stalk of neural tissue that lies between the upper spinal cord and the diencephalon. It has three parts: from top to bottom these are the *midbrain, pons,* and *medulla oblongata.* The brainstem is critical for transmission of impulses between the brain and spinal cord. Vital centers for regulating respiratory and cardiovascular function are located in the medulla and pons. In addition, the reticular activating neurons that maintain consciousness and alertness traverse the brainstem to reach the thalamus. Of the 12 pairs of cranial nerves,

10 originate from nuclei in the brainstem; only cranial nerves I (olfactory) and II (optic) originate elsewhere (diencephalon).

The midbrain or mesencephalon contains the cerebral peduncles, consisting of motor tracts to the spinal cord; the superior and inferior colliculi, which control head and eye movements; and the red nucleus, part of a major motor tract. Cranial nerve III (oculomotor) emerges from the midbrain and is prone to compression when pressure in one of the cerebral hemispheres is elevated. Increased intracranial pressure (e.g., from tumor, ischemia, edema, bleeding) is commonly manifested by dysfunction of cranial nerve III resulting in abnormal pupil size and poor reactivity to light (see Chapter 44). Cranial nerve IV (trochlear) also emerges at the level of the midbrain.

The pons (Latin for *bridge*) connects the midbrain above to the medulla below. The dorsal pons consists of reticular formation fibers, ascending sensory tracts, and descending motor tracts. Two respiratory centers (pneumotaxic and apneustic) located in the dorsal pons work in coordination with the principal respiratory centers in the medulla. A major pathway of voluntary motor control, the corticospinal tract, also passes through the ventral pons on its way from the motor cortex to the spinal cord.

The medulla oblongata makes up the lower third of the brainstem and is continuous with the spinal cord. Nuclei within the reticular formation of the medulla form the vital centers that regulate cardiac, vascular, and respiratory function. The medulla also contains centers that coordinate swallowing, vomiting, coughing, and sneezing. The medulla is the site of decussation (crossing over) of the major sensory (dorsal column) and motor (corticospinal) tracts such that innervation of one side of the body is connected to the opposite (contralateral) cerebral hemisphere. The corticospinal tract neurons decussate within ridges on the ventral surface of the medulla called *medullary pyramids.* Motor tracts that do not cross over within the pyramids (e.g., tectospinal, vestibulospinal) are sometimes referred to as extrapyramidal tracts; disorders associated with function of these tracts (balance, posture, gait) may be called *extrapyramidal disorders* (e.g., Parkinson disease). Although the anatomic correlation is not quite accurate, use of the term persists in a clinical context.

All of the remaining cranial nerves (VI, VII, VIII, IX, X, XI, and XII) originate in the medulla. The cranial nerves themselves are part of the PNS and are discussed in that section. The name, origin, and function of the 12 cranial nerves are included in Table 43-4.

The Spinal Cord

The spinal cord conveys nervous impulses between the brain and 31 pairs of spinal nerves that innervate sensory organs and muscle cells of the body. The spinal cord mediates spinal reflexes involved in maintenance of posture, protective responses to pain, urination, and muscle tone. A great deal of integration and processing occurs in the gray matter of the spinal cord, whereas the white matter contains bundles of myelinated axons forming tracts that run up and down the cord. Tracts in the spinal cord are **somatotopically** organized such that the innervation of a particular body region is connected to a specific region in the cerebral cortex.

The typical adult spinal cord is about 18 inches long, extending from the base of the skull (foramen magnum) to the first or second lumbar vertebra (L1 to L2).[10] The vertebral column extends for several more inches, providing a reservoir for CSF and exit points for the lumbar and sacral spinal nerves. The vertebral column is formed by interlocking sections of bone separated and cushioned by intervertebral disks. At the lateral aspect of the intersection of two vertebrae is an opening (intervertebral foramen) that provides a passageway for spinal nerves to exit the cord. The spinal cord travels in a small lumen (1 cm) in the center of the vertebral column and is itself only slightly larger than the diameter of a pencil[10] (Figure 43-15).

TABLE 43-4 CRANIAL NERVES

CRANIAL NERVE	ORIGIN	FUNCTION
I (olfactory)	Nasal mucous membrane	Olfaction
II (optic)	Retina	Vision
III (oculomotor)	Midbrain	Movement of eyeball, eyelid, constriction of pupil
IV (trochlear)	Lower midbrain	Lateral eye movements
V (trigeminal)		
Ophthalmic	Forehead, eyes	Sensation from forehead, eye, scalp
Maxillary	Upper jaw, lip	Sensation from cheek, upper lip
Mandibular	Lower jaw area	Sensation from chin and lower jaw, motor chewing
VI (abducens)	Lower pons	Lateral eye movements
VII (facial)	Pons	Taste from anterior tongue, control of muscles of face
VIII (vestibulocochlear)	Cochlea	Hearing
	Inner ear	Equilibrium
IX (glossopharyngeal)	Medulla	Taste from posterior tongue, secretion of saliva, swallowing
X (vagus)	Medulla	Monitors oxygen, carbon dioxide, and pH levels in blood; senses blood pressure; inhibits cardiac action and has extensive gastrointestinal activities
XI (spinal accessory)	Medulla and cervical cord	Voice production, movement of head and shoulders
XII (hypoglossal)	Medulla	Movements of tongue during speech and swallowing

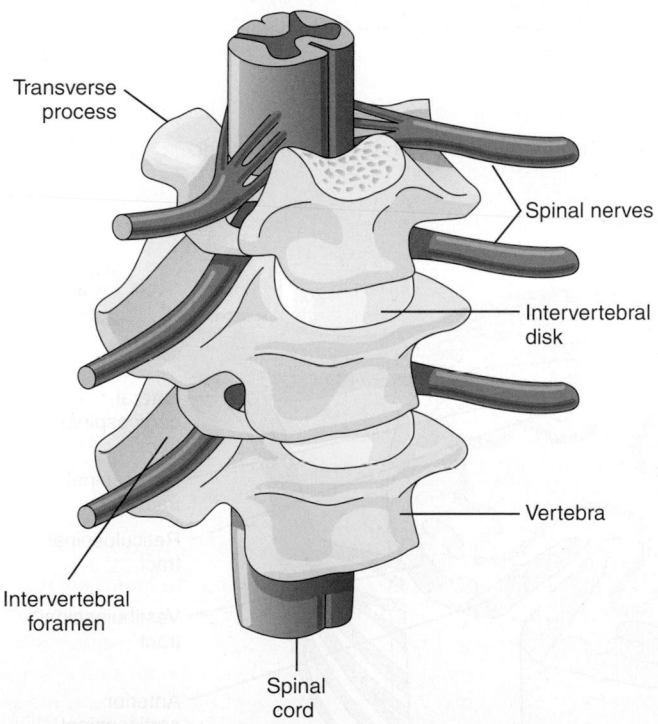

FIGURE 43-15 Spinal cord travels down the center of the vertebral column. A foramen at the intersection of two vertebrae forms an exit point for the spinal nerves.

On cross-section the spinal cord has a butterfly pattern of gray matter surrounded by white matter (Figure 43-16). Three bumps on the butterfly wings are called *horns:* the ventral horn (motor neurons), the dorsal horn (sensory neurons), and the lateral horn (sympathetic neurons). The horns consist of neuron cell bodies, synapses, and small unmyelinated interneurons. The white matter is divided into columns that contain tracts of nerve fibers traveling to and from the brain. These are the posterior (dorsal) columns, anterior columns, and lateral columns. Some of the neurons in the columns convey signals from one level of the cord to another and are important in reflex and postural

adjustments. The principal ascending sensory tracts include the dorsal column–lemniscal and the anterolateral (spinothalamic) tracts, which send **afferent** signals to the brain. The principal descending motor tracts include the corticospinal, rubrospinal, reticulospinal, and vestibulospinal tracts. These tracts are located in specific regions of the cord (Figure 43-17). Sensory and motor pathways are discussed in later sections of this chapter.

Spinal nerves divide into two sections as they make contact with the spinal cord: the ventral and dorsal roots (Figure 43-18). Ventral roots contain motor neurons that originate in the anterior horn and travel in the spinal nerve to skeletal muscles. Dorsal roots carry sensory information from somatic receptors to neurons in the posterior horn. The cell bodies of sensory afferents collect together in the dorsal root ganglion. Autonomic nerves also travel in the spinal cord and exit and enter the cord by way of the ventral and dorsal roots.

The points at which sensory neurons enter the cord and at which motor neurons exit represent the separation of the CNS and PNS.

PERIPHERAL NERVOUS SYSTEM

The PNS consists of the 31 pairs of spinal nerves and the 12 pairs of cranial nerves. These nerves are myelinated with Schwann cells, which differ somewhat from the oligodendrocytes that form the myelin sheaths of CNS neurons. By convention, groups of cell bodies are called *ganglia* in the PNS and *nuclei* in the CNS. A major exception to this naming rule is the basal ganglia of the CNS. The PNS is not protected by CSF, meninges, or bony coverings as is the CNS; however, a sheath of connective tissue covers the nerves and provides support.

The PNS serves both afferent sensory functions and efferent motor functions of the somatic and autonomic systems. Cranial nerves III, VII, IX, and X and spinal nerves S2 and S3 contain parasympathetic neurons, and spinal nerves T1 to L2 contain sympathetic neurons.[11]

Cranial Nerves

As previously noted, all of the cranial nerves originate in the brainstem except cranial nerves I and II, which originate in the diencephalon[12] (Figure 43-19). Cranial nerve I is strictly sensory, transmitting olfactory signals from the 10 million to 20 million olfactory neurons in the nasal cavities to the olfactory bulbs. The olfactory bulb neurons then

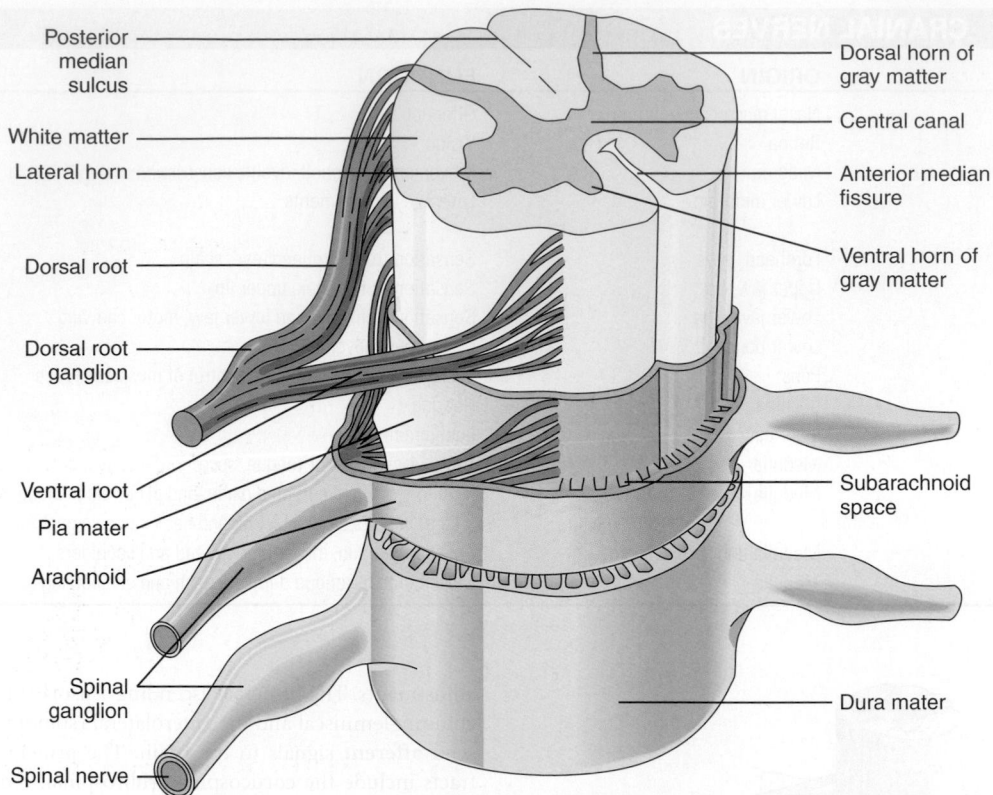

Posterior median sulcus

White matter

Lateral horn

Dorsal root

Dorsal root ganglion

Ventral root

Pia mater

Arachnoid

Spinal ganglion

Spinal nerve

Dorsal horn of gray matter

Central canal

Anterior median fissure

Ventral horn of gray matter

Subarachnoid space

Dura mater

FIGURE 43-16 Spinal cord in cross-section, showing the butterfly pattern of white and gray matter.

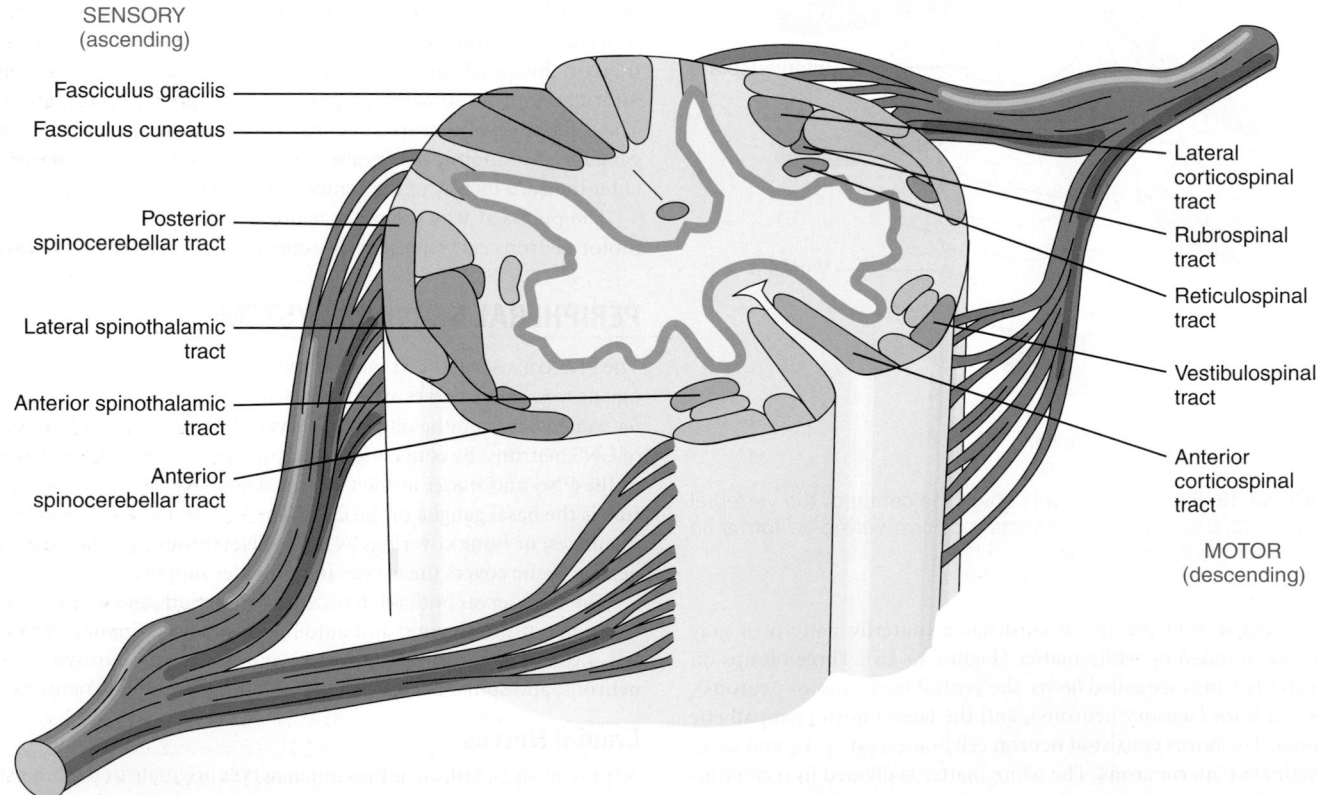

SENSORY (ascending)

Fasciculus gracilis

Fasciculus cuneatus

Posterior spinocerebellar tract

Lateral spinothalamic tract

Anterior spinothalamic tract

Anterior spinocerebellar tract

Lateral corticospinal tract

Rubrospinal tract

Reticulospinal tract

Vestibulospinal tract

Anterior corticospinal tract

MOTOR (descending)

FIGURE 43-17 Main ascending (left) and descending (right) tracts of the spinal cord.

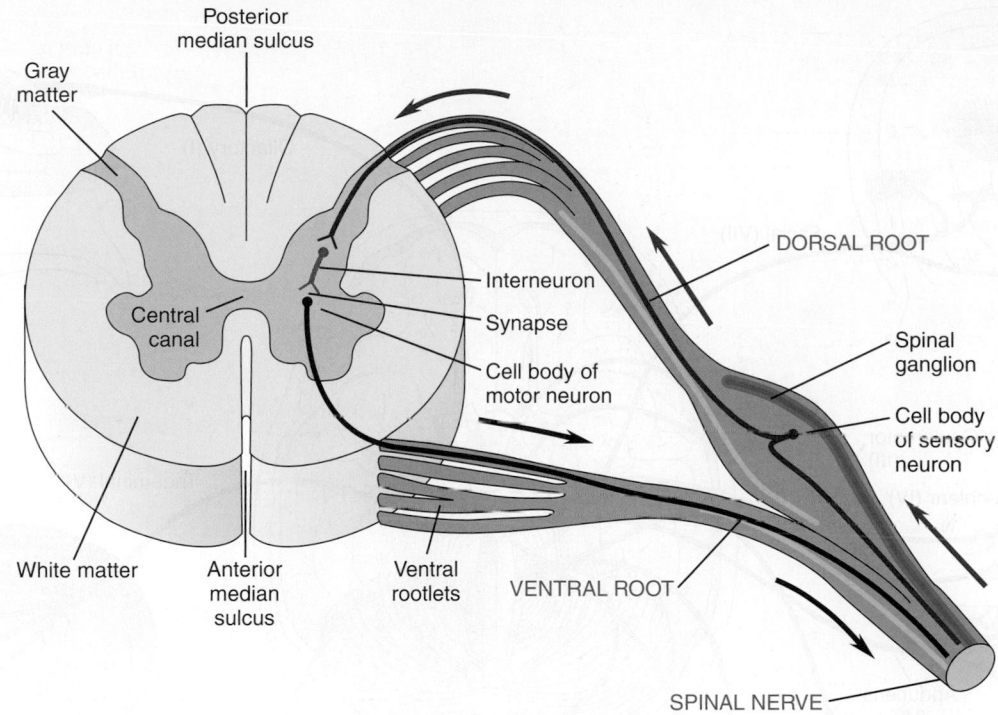

FIGURE 43-18 Spinal nerves split to form dorsal and ventral roots as they emerge from the spinal cord. Ventral roots carry motor efferent neurons, whereas dorsal roots carry sensory afferent neurons. See text for explanation.

project to the olfactory cortex. Cranial nerve II is also sensory, conveying visual information from the retina to the brain. The optic nerve is unusual in that it is an extension of the CNS, myelinated by oligodendrocytes rather than Schwann cells. The neurons from the medial retina decussate in the optic chiasm, whereas the lateral retina neurons do not. Thus, the right visual field projects to the left hemisphere and the left visual field projects to the right hemisphere. Damage to one hemisphere, as occurs in stroke, often interrupts visual signals from the corresponding sides of each retina—a condition known as homonymous hemianopsia (see Chapters 44 and 46).

Cranial nerves III, IV, and VI innervate motor structures in the eyes. Cranial nerve III mediates pupil constriction. The trigeminal nerve (cranial nerve V) is so named because it has three branches, which provide sensory innervation of the forehead and eyes (ophthalmic branch); upper lip, teeth, and palate (maxillary branch); and lower jaw (mandibular branch). The mandibular branch is both sensory and motor. Cranial nerve VII is also mixed sensory and motor, detecting taste in the anterior two thirds of the tongue and innervating muscles of facial expression. Cranial nerve VII also contains autonomic fibers that innervate salivary and lacrimal (tear) glands.

Cranial nerve VIII has two important sensory functions: transmitting auditory information from the cochlea and vestibular information from inner ear structures. The vestibular neurons of cranial nerve VIII interact with the neurons of cranial nerves III and VI to reflexively control eye movements during head rotation such that a visual image can remain fixed on the retina. This reflex, the oculovestibular reflex, is commonly assessed in the unconscious patient to evaluate brainstem function (see Chapter 44).

Cranial nerve IX innervates tongue and pharyngeal muscles, conveying taste from the posterior tongue and controlling pharyngeal

motion during swallowing. Cranial nerve IX also has autonomic functions and transmits sensory information from the carotid baroreceptors and carotid bodies to the brainstem. Cranial nerve X, the vagus nerve, contains parasympathetic afferent and efferent fibers that innervate many visceral structures, including the heart, lungs, and gastrointestinal (GI) tract from pharynx to anus. Sensory information from aortic baroreceptors and aortic bodies is conveyed to the brainstem by the vagus nerve.

Cranial nerve XI innervates muscles of the larynx, neck, and shoulders and mediates voice production and neck and head movements. Cranial nerve XII innervates tongue muscles and controls their action during speech and swallowing.

Spinal Nerves

The 31 pairs of spinal nerves are named after the vertebral segments from which they emerge. There are 8 cervical, 12 thoracic, 5 lumbar, 5 sacral, and 1 coccygeal pair of spinal nerves. The first cervical nerve exits above C1, whereas the others all exit below the vertebral segment; thus there is one more pair of cervical spinal nerves (8) than there are cervical vertebrae (7).

Except for spinal nerves T2 to T12, the spinal nerves travel a distance from the cord and then merge into a large group called a *plexus*.[12] In the plexus, nerve fibers are recombined into different groups and emerge as peripheral nerves (Figure 43-20). There are five plexuses: (1) the cervical plexus (C1 to C4), (2) the brachial plexus (C5 to C8, T1), (3) the lumbar plexus (L1 to L4), (4) the sacral plexus (L4 to L5, S1 to S3), and (5) the coccygeal plexus (S4 to S5, coccygeal) (Table 43-5). Because of this recombination of nerve fibers in the plexus, the spinal nerves and peripheral nerves have different somatic distributions. The segment of the body innervated by a spinal nerve is called a *dermatome*, whereas the peripheral nerve innervates a peripheral

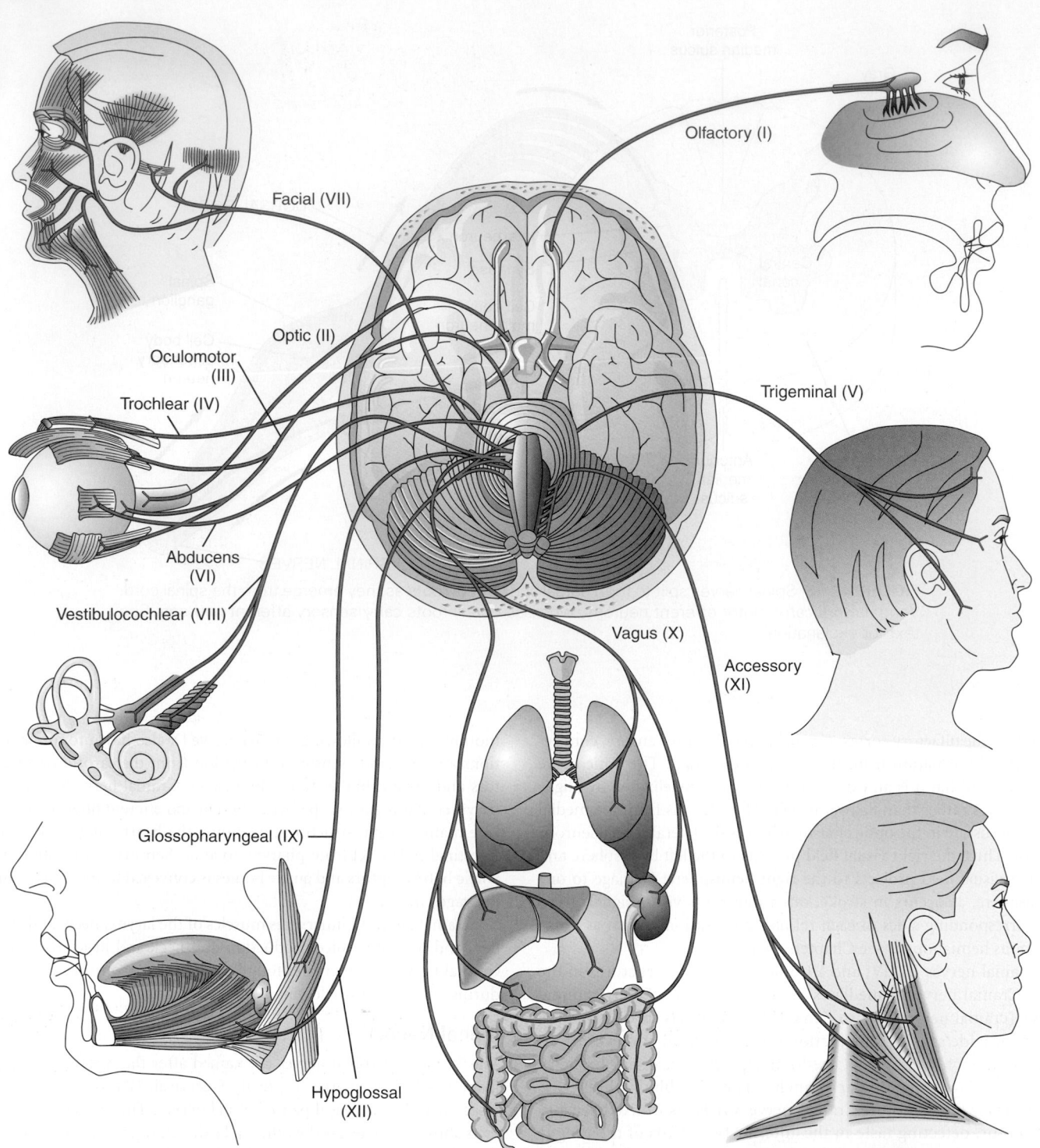

FIGURE 43-19 View of the inferior aspect of the brain showing the origin and distribution of the 12 cranial nerves. Only one of each pair is shown.

Olfactory (I)

Facial (VII)

Optic (II)

Oculomotor (III)

Trochlear (IV)

Trigeminal (V)

Abducens (VI)

Vestibulocochlear (VIII)

Vagus (X)

Accessory (XI)

Glossopharyngeal (IX)

Hypoglossal (XII)

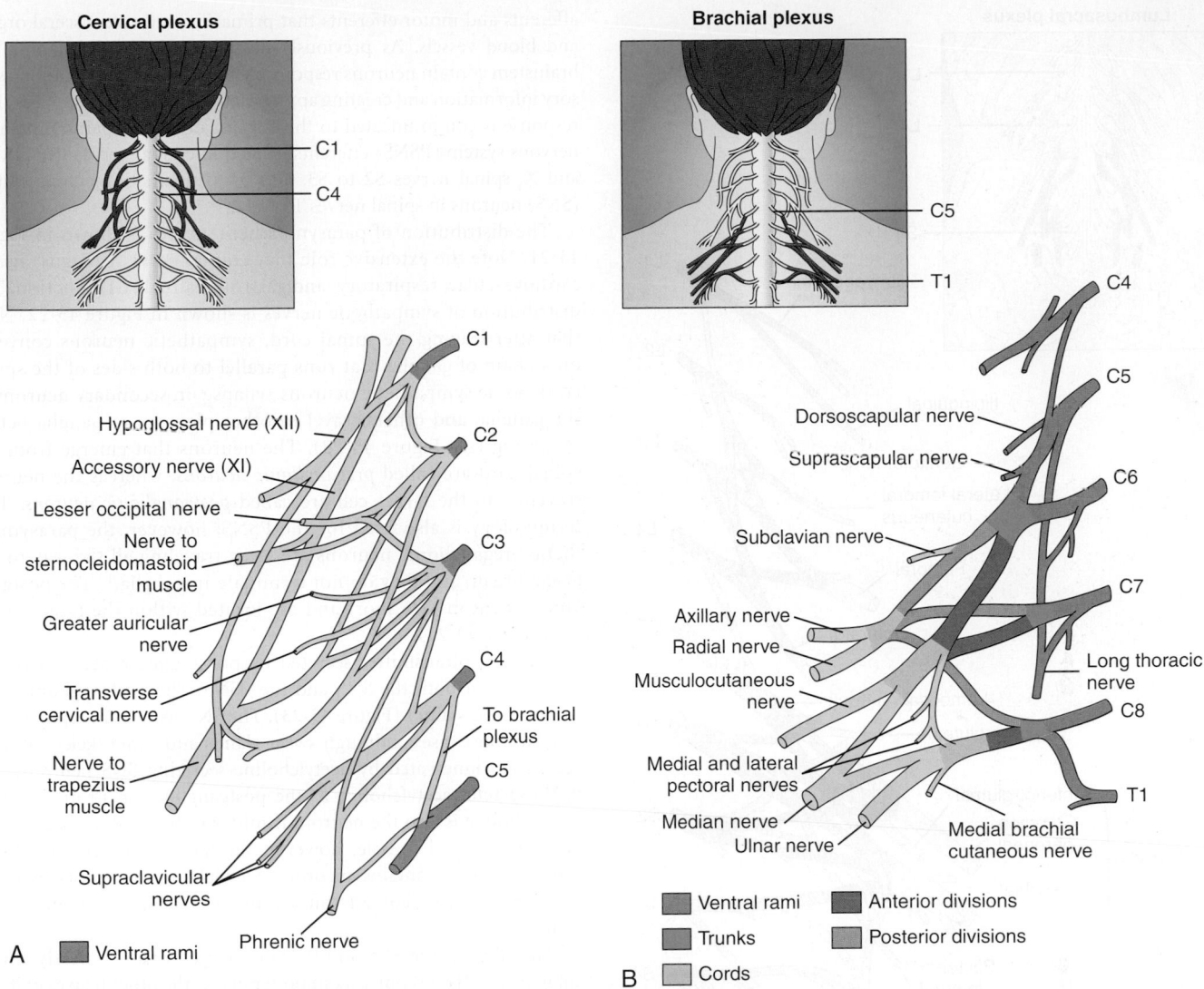

FIGURE 43-20 Examples of neuronal organization at the plexuses showing reassortment of spinal nerves into peripheral nerves. **A,** Cervical plexus. **B,** Brachial plexus. (From Patton KT, Thibodeau GA: *Anatomy & physiology*, ed 8, St Louis, 2013, Mosby, pp 468-470.)

(Continued)

TABLE 43-5 SPINAL NERVE PLEXUSES

PLEXUS	SPINAL NERVES	PERIPHERAL NERVES	DISTRIBUTION
Cervical	C1-C4	Phrenic	Diaphragm
		Cutaneous	Neck
		Ansa cervicalis	Hyoid bone
Brachial	C5-C8, T1	Axillary	Upper arm
		Ulnar	Forearm, wrist, fifth digit
		Median	Second through fourth digits
		Radial	Thumb
		Musculocutaneous	Upper arm
Lumbar	L1-L4	Femoral (saphenous)	Hip, knee (lower leg)
		Obturator	Inner thigh
Sacral	L4-L5, S1-S3	Superior gluteal	Gluteus medius, minimus
		Inferior gluteal	Gluteus maximus
		Sciatic (tibial, peroneal)	Thigh, leg, foot
		Pudendal	Perineum
Coccygeal	S4-S5, coccygeal	Coccygeal fibers	Skin on coccyx

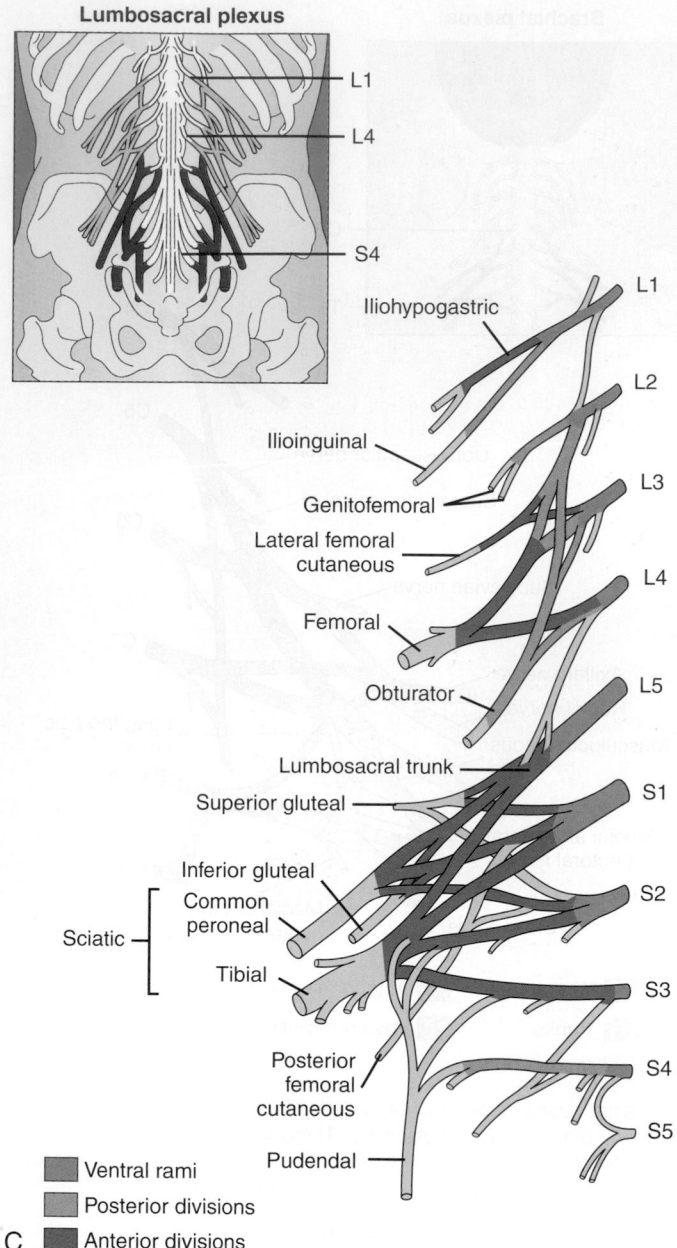

Lumbosacral plexus

L1
L4
S4

L1
Iliohypogastric
L2
Ilioinguinal
L3
Genitofemoral
Lateral femoral
cutaneous
L4
Femoral
Obturator
L5
Lumbosacral trunk
Superior gluteal
S1
Inferior gluteal
Common
peroneal
S2
Sciatic
Tibial
S3
Posterior
femoral
cutaneous
S4
S5
Pudendal

■ Ventral rami
■ Posterior divisions
C ■ Anterior divisions

FIGURE 43-20, cont'd C, Lumbosacral plexus (because of their overlap the lumbar and sacral plexuses are often considered together as in this example).

nerve field. Knowledge of dermatomes and peripheral nerve distribution can help the clinician differentiate between radiculopathy from spinal nerve compression (dermatomal sensory changes) and peripheral neuropathy. (Dermatomal and peripheral nerve maps are located in Chapter 47.)

The intercostal nerves (T2 to T12) do not form plexuses; they travel in a course parallel to the ribs to innervate intercostal muscles and skin on the trunk and abdomen.

AUTONOMIC NERVOUS SYSTEM

The ANS is composed of neurons in the CNS and PNS that mediate automatic or involuntary functions. The ANS has both sensory

afferents and motor efferents that primarily innervate visceral organs and blood vessels. As previously described, the hypothalamus and brainstem contain neurons responsible for integrating autonomic sensory information and creating appropriate homeostatic responses. This response is communicated to the effector organs by parasympathetic nervous system (PSNS) efferents located in cranial nerves III, VII, IX, and X, spinal nerves S2 to S3, and by sympathetic nervous system (SNS) neurons in spinal nerves T1 to L2.[11]

The distribution of parasympathetic nerves is shown in Figure 43-21. Note the extensive role that cranial nerve X (vagus) has in cardiovascular, respiratory, and gastrointestinal (GI) function. The distribution of sympathetic nerves is shown in Figure 43-22. Note that after leaving the spinal cord, sympathetic neurons converge on a chain of ganglia that runs parallel to both sides of the spinal cord. Some sympathetic neurons synapse on secondary neurons in the ganglia, and others travel to other plexuses or ganglia before synapsing (see Figure 43-22). The neurons that emerge from the spinal cord are called *preganglionic neurons,* whereas the neurons traveling to the target cell are called *postganglionic neurons.* This terminology is also used for the PSNS; however, the parasympathetic preganglionic neurons are long, traveling all the way to the target organ, and they do not terminate in ganglia.[11] The postganglionic neurons are short and are located within the target organ (see Figure 43-21).

The neurotransmitter secreted by preganglionic neurons is acetylcholine for both the SNS and the PSNS. The postganglionic neurotransmitters differ (Figure 43-23). The SNS secretes norepinephrine (NE) in most cases, although sweat glands and some skeletal muscle vessels are innervated by acetylcholine-secreting SNS neurons. The PSNS secretes acetylcholine as the postganglionic neurotransmitter. Acetylcholine is also the neurotransmitter of the motor neurons that innervate skeletal muscle; however, the target cell receptors differ. Skeletal muscle contains nicotinic acetylcholine receptors, whereas autonomic organs contain muscarinic acetylcholine receptors (see Figure 43-23).

The effect of the SNS and PSNS on target organs is nearly always antagonistic. If one contracts smooth muscle, the other relaxes it; if one stimulates glandular secretion, the other inhibits it; if one speeds up a process, the other slows it down. The effects of SNS and PSNS stimulation on major target organs are shown in Table 43-6.

A specialized extension of the SNS is found in the adrenal gland. The adrenal medulla receives preganglionic neurons from SNS neurons emerging from the spinal cord, which stimulate the gland to secrete epinephrine (and smaller amounts of NE) into the bloodstream. These hormones have effects similar to those of direct SNS stimulation.

The manner in which target cells respond to SNS stimulation depends on the types of receptors they possess. Several subtypes of receptors bind and respond to NE and epinephrine; these include α_1, α_2, β_1, β_2, β_3, and several DA receptors (see Table 43-6). (The details of autonomic regulation of cardiac, genitourinary, and GI function can be found in Chapters 17, 29, and 35, respectively.)

The coordination of SNS and PSNS activity within a target organ is accomplished by centers in the brainstem and hypothalamus with input from sensory neurons and cortical neurons. Most of these systems work on a negative feedback principle to achieve homeostasis. Negative feedback requires accurate sensory input about the conditions being regulated. Much of this feedback is provided by the vagus nerves that obtain extensive sensory information from receptors in the GI tract and aorta. This sensory input is processed in lower brain centers and does not reach the level of perception.

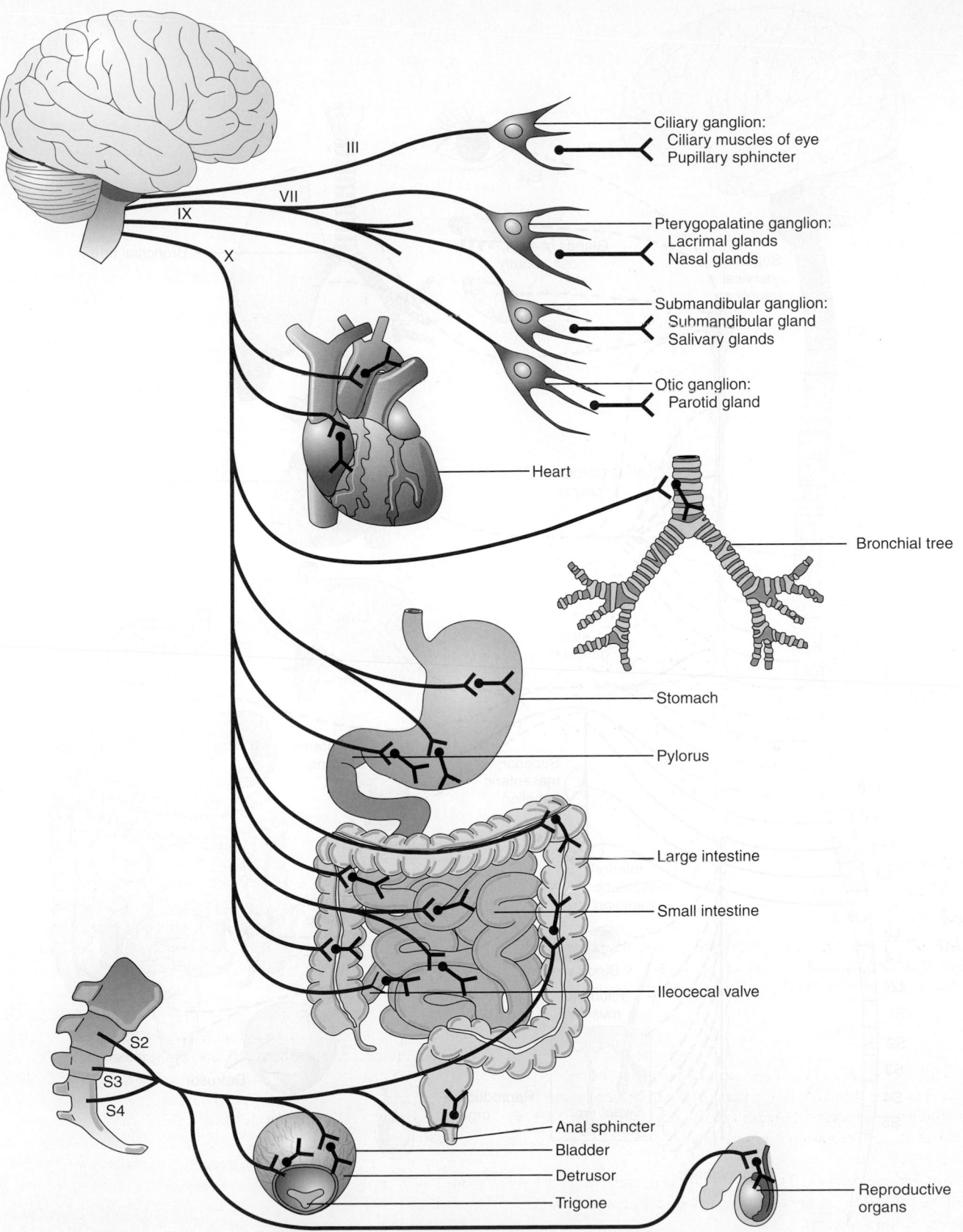

FIGURE 43-21 Distribution of parasympathetic nerves.

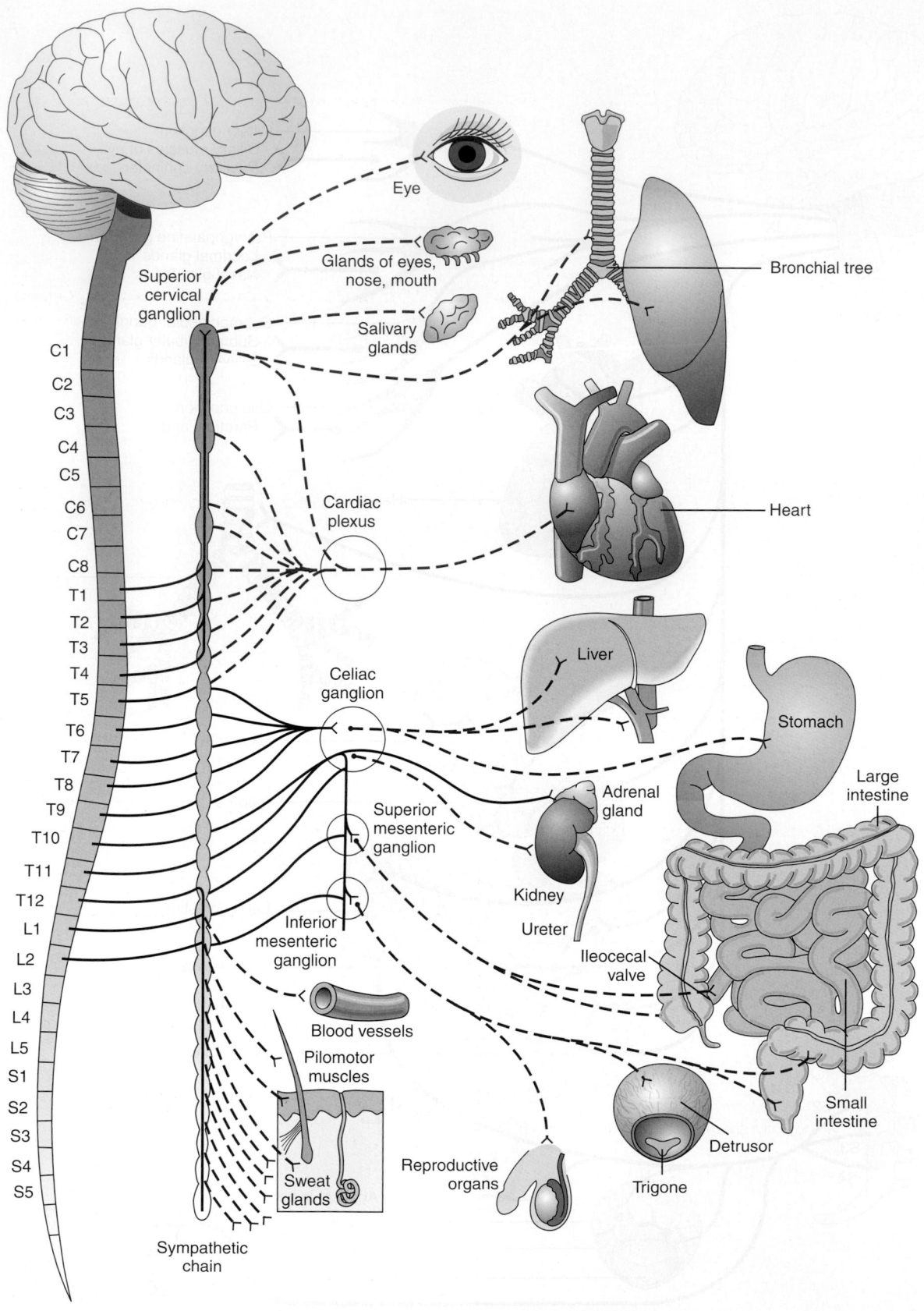

FIGURE 43-22 Distribution of sympathetic nerves.

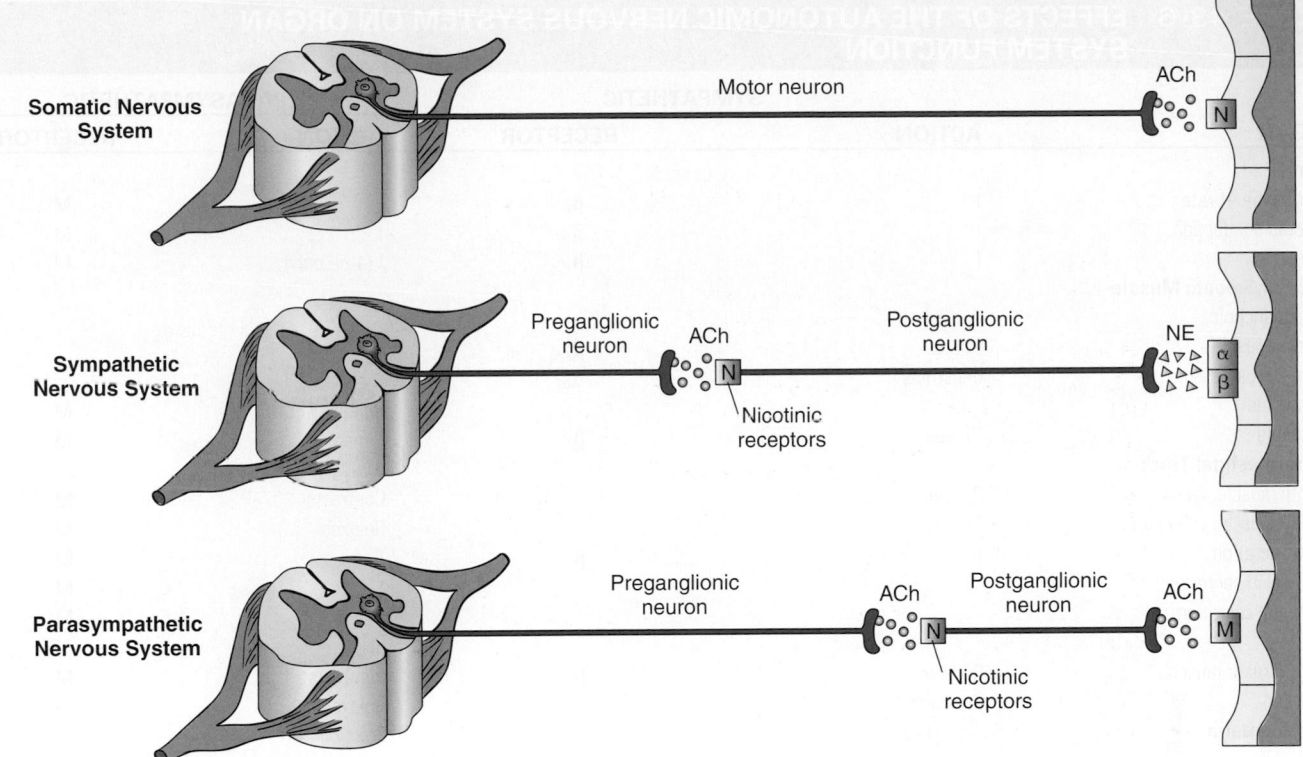

FIGURE 43-23 Comparison of preganglionic and postganglionic neurotransmitters in the sympathetic and parasympathetic systems. Acetylcholine *(ACh)* is the neurotransmitter of the motor neuron, but its receptor differs from that of the parasympathetic terminations. *N*, Nicotinic receptors; *NE*, norepinephrine; *M*, muscarinic receptors.

KEY POINTS

- The nervous system can be divided into three principal systems: (1) the central nervous system (CNS), consisting of the brain and spinal cord; (2) the peripheral nervous system (PNS), consisting of 31 pairs of spinal nerves and 12 pairs of cranial nerves; and (3) the autonomic nervous system (ANS), consisting of the sympathetic and parasympathetic branches.
- Meninges affix the brain to the skull so that the brain is suspended and supported. Meninges have three layers: (1) The dura mater is the tough outer layer attached to the periosteum of the skull. (2) The arachnoid is a delicate weblike membrane spanning the space between the dura mater and the pia mater. (3) The pia mater covers the contours of the brain surface. The spinal cord has a similar arrangement of meningeal coverings.
- Cerebrospinal fluid (CSF) is produced in the brain ventricles and circulates in the subarachnoid spaces, providing cushioning and nutritive functions.
- The brain is protected by specialized tight junctions between the cells of the capillary endothelium (blood-brain barrier) and between the ependymal cells that line the ventricles (CSF-brain barrier).
- The brain can be anatomically divided into four principal structures: (1) the cerebrum (cerebral cortex, basal ganglia, limbic cortex, and corpus callosum); (2) the diencephalon (thalamus and hypothalamus); (3) the cerebellum; and (4) the brainstem (midbrain, pons, and medulla).
- Certain cortical areas are closely associated with specific functions: the frontal lobe contains the motor cortex and is involved in complex thought, motivation, and morality; the temporal lobe contains the auditory and vestibular centers and parts of the language center; the occipital lobe contains the visual cortex; the parietal lobe contains the somatosensory cortex; the limbic area is involved in memory and emotion.
- Basal ganglia are located deep within the cerebral hemispheres and are important in the control of skeletal muscles. Parkinson disease is an important example of basal ganglia dysfunction characterized by akinesia, rigidity, and rest tremor.

- The thalamus is a centrally located structure that processes and relays most of the signals traveling to and from the cortex and lower centers. Connections between the thalamus and the brainstem and cortex are needed to maintain consciousness and allow higher brain functions.
- The hypothalamus and brainstem are important structures regulating the ANS. The sympathetic nerves originate in spinal cord segments T1 to L2. The parasympathetic nerves emerge from the sacral segments and also travel in cranial nerves III, VII, IX, and X.

NEURONAL STRUCTURE AND FUNCTION

The ways in which the nervous system achieves its rapid communication function can be understood by examining the structure and behavior of neurons and neuronal synapses.

NEURONS AND SUPPORTIVE CELLS

The nervous system is composed of two principal cell types: neurons, which generate and transmit nerve impulses; and glial cells, which provide supportive functions to neurons but do not transmit action potentials. There are approximately 10 glial cells per neuron and about 100 billion neurons in the CNS.[13]

Neurons

A neuron has three basic components: (1) the cell body containing cellular organelles, (2) the dendrites that receive signals and conduct them to the cell body, and (3) the axon that generates and conducts action potentials. Neurons can be categorized according to their structure or by the neurotransmitters they secrete. Neurons are present in three basic configurations based on the location of the cell body and the relative length and number of dendrites and axons[13] (Figure 43-24).

TABLE 43-6 **EFFECTS OF THE AUTONOMIC NERVOUS SYSTEM ON ORGAN SYSTEM FUNCTION**

| ORGAN | SYMPATHETIC | | PARASYMPATHETIC | |
	ACTION	RECEPTOR	ACTION	RECEPTOR
Heart				
SA node, heart rate	↑	β_1	↓	M
AV nodal conduction	↑	β_1	↓	M
Contractility	↑	β_1	↓ (atria only)	M
Vascular Smooth Muscle				
Skin; splanchnic	Constricts	α_1		
Skeletal muscle	Dilates	β_2		
Skeletal muscle	Constricts	α_1		
Endothelium			Releases EDRF	M
Bronchioles	Dilates	β_2	Constricts	M
Gastrointestinal Tract				
Smooth muscle, walls	Relaxes	α_2, β_2	Contracts	M
Smooth muscle, sphincters	Contracts	α_1	Relaxes	M
Saliva secretion	↑	β_1	↑	M
Gastric acid secretion			↑	M
Pancreatic secretion			↑	M
Bladder				
Wall, detrusor muscle	Relaxes	β_2	Contracts	M
Sphincter	Contracts	α_1	Relaxes	M
Male Genitalia	Ejaculation	α	Erection	M
Eye				
Radial muscle, iris	Dilates pupil (mydriasis)	α_1		
Circular sphincter muscle, iris			Constricts pupil (miosis)	M
Ciliary muscle	Dilates (far vision)	β	Contracts (near vision)	M
Skin				
Sweat glands, thermoregulatory	↑	M*		
Sweat glands, stress	↑	α		
Pilomotor muscle (goose bumps)	Contracts	α		
Lacrimal glands			Secretion	M
Liver	Gluconeogenesis; glycogenolysis	α, β_2		
Adipose tissue	Lipolysis	β_1		
Kidney	Renin secretion	β_1		

*Sympathetic cholinergic neurons.
AV, Atrioventricular; *EDRF*, endothelial-derived relaxing factor; *M*, muscarinic receptor; *SA*, sinoatrial.

Multipolar neurons have a large number of dendrites extending from the cell body and one axon. Most neurons are of this type. Bipolar neurons have only one dendrite and one axon extending from the cell body. These neurons are prevalent in the retina, cochlea, and olfactory structures but are rare elsewhere. Unipolar neurons have a single process protruding from the cell body, which splits to form a dendrite and axon. This arrangement makes the cell body appear to be off-center. Unipolar neurons are prevalent in the somatosensory nerves in which the cell bodies are grouped in the dorsal root ganglia. The dendrites extend to the sensory receptors and the axons enter the spinal cord.

Neurons also can be grouped as excitatory or inhibitory based on the nature of the neurotransmitter they secrete. Each neuron secretes one principal neurotransmitter, which is excitatory if it depolarizes the target neuron or inhibitory if it results in hyperpolarization.

Glia

Glial cells in the nervous system (neuroglia) serve a number of supportive functions, but they are not capable of generating action potentials. Four major types of neuroglia are recognized: oligodendrocytes, astrocytes, microglia, and ependymal cells (Figure 43-25). The Schwann cells of the PNS are similar to oligodendrocytes. Both of these cell types form the myelin sheath that wraps around nerve axons to insulate and speed the rate of action potential conduction (Figure 43-26). Myelin gives the white matter its color.

Astrocytes serve many functions in the CNS. Some astrocytes have foot processes that contact the brain capillaries and help maintain the integrity of the blood-brain barrier. Astrocytes regulate ionic balance of the interstitial fluid and may influence the transfer of nutrients from capillaries to neurons. Astrocytes also participate in nervous system signaling and have been shown to take up and release molecules, such as neurotransmitters and cotransmitters that modulate neurotransmission.[3]

Microglia are derived from the monocyte-macrophage cell type and provide phagocytic functions within the CNS.[14] Ependymal cells line the ventricles and central canal of the spinal cord, producing CSF and maintaining the CSF-brain barrier.

Terminally differentiated neurons are not capable of cell division and cannot replace themselves if they die. However, certain areas of the brain, particularly the hippocampus and ventricles, are populated by neural stem cells. These cells are capable of cell division to produce two daughter cells, one of which retains stem cell characteristics whereas the other may differentiate into a neuron or glial cell (Figure 43-27). Specific signals are thought to guide the new cell as it migrates to the brain tissue and begins differentiation. Approximately half of the newborn cells will not find a suitable place and undergo apoptosis

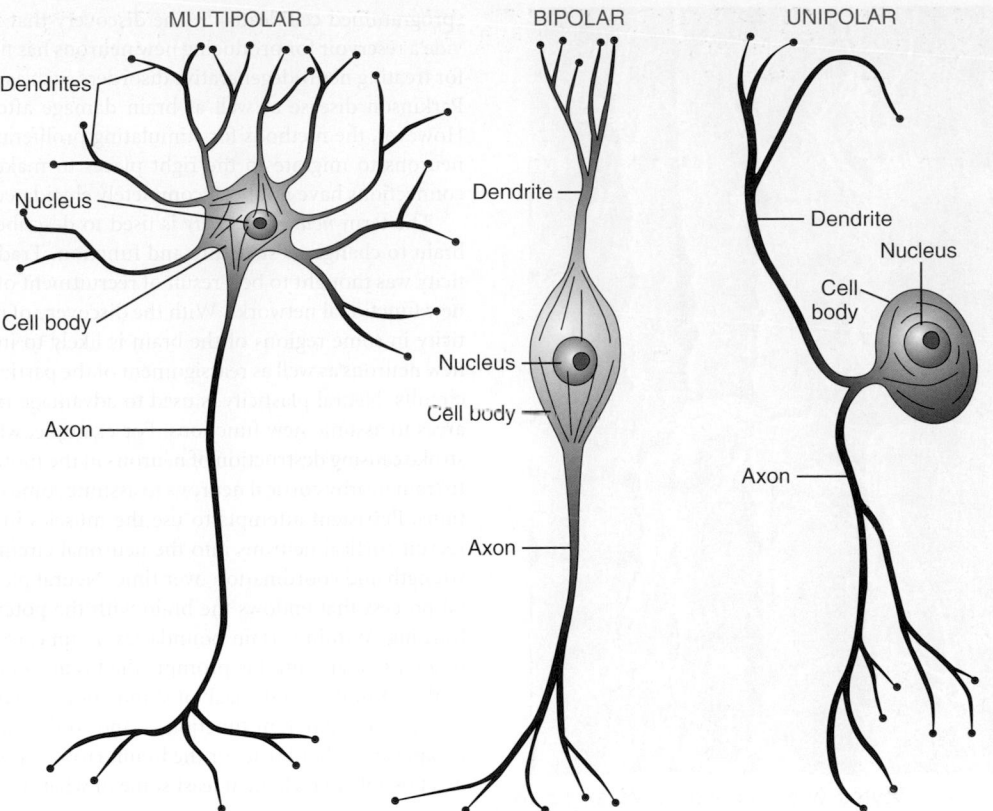

FIGURE 43-24 Three basic types of neurons: multipolar, bipolar, and unipolar.

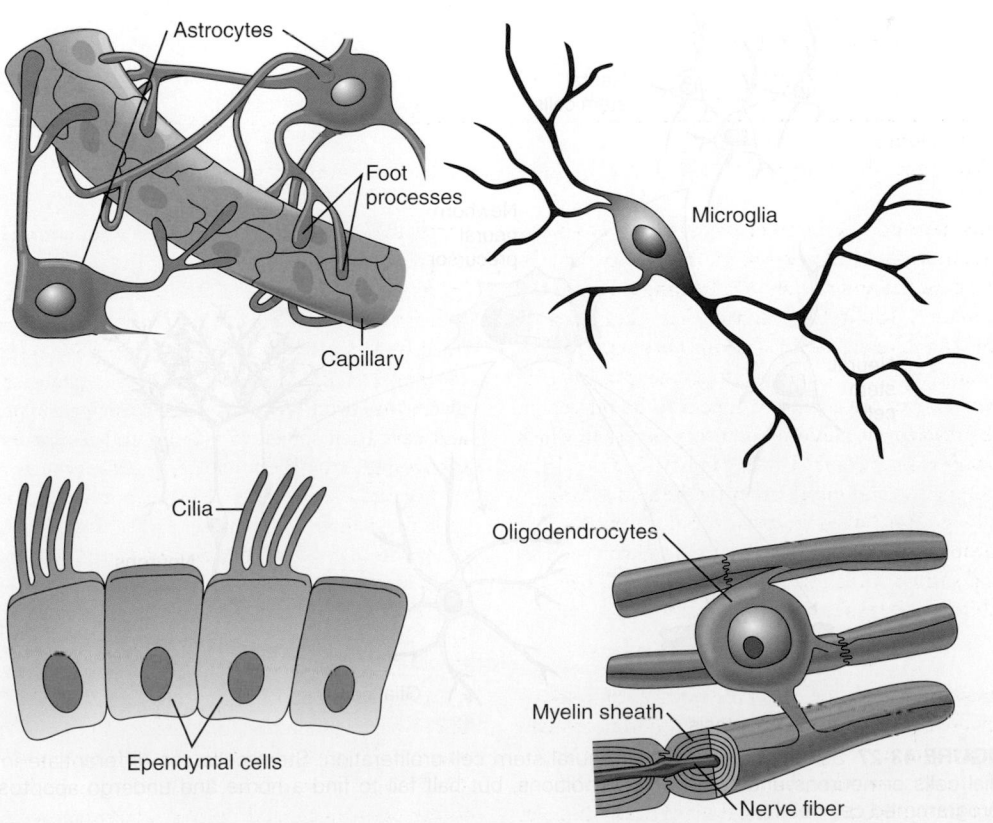

FIGURE 43-25 Four types of neuroglial cells: astrocytes, microglia, ependymal cells, and oligodendrocytes.

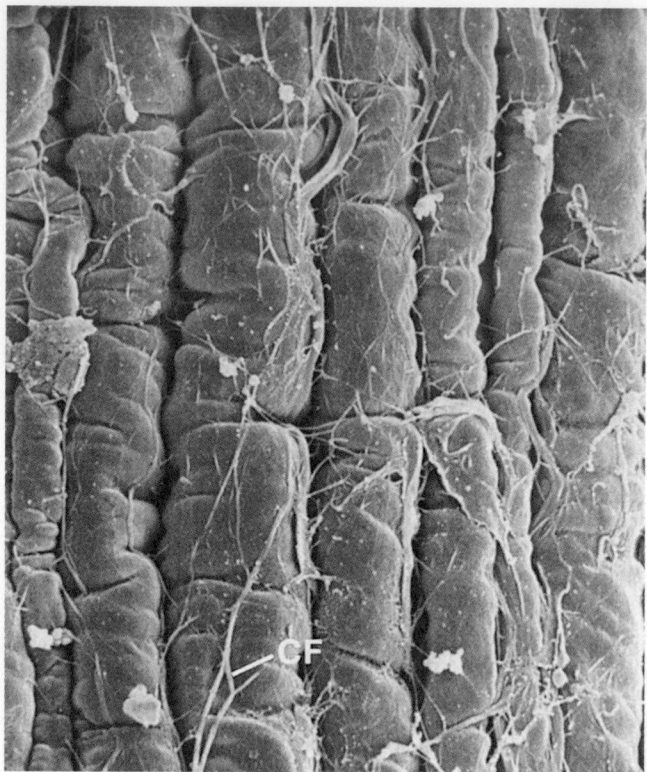

FIGURE 43-26 Oligodendrocytes wrap around nerve axons to form a myelin sheath. The nodes of Ranvier are the small spaces between the oligodendrocytes. *CF*, C-fiber (unmyelinated). (From Kessel RG, Kardon RH: *Tissues and organs: a text-atlas of scanning electron microscopy*, San Francisco, 1979, Freeman, p 80.)

(programmed cell death).[15] The discovery that neural stem cells provide a reservoir for producing new neurons has numerous implications for treating neurodegenerative disorders such as Alzheimer disease and Parkinson disease as well as brain damage after stroke and trauma. However, the methods for stimulating proliferation and coaching the neurons to migrate to the right places to make the correct synaptic connections have not been completely elucidated.

The term *neural plasticity* is used to describe the potential for the brain to change its structure and function. Traditionally, neural plasticity was thought to be a result of recruitment of formed neurons into new functional networks. With the discovery of neural stem cells, plasticity in some regions of the brain is likely to include the addition of new neurons as well as reassignment of the participants in the neuronal circuits. Neural plasticity is used to advantage to train different brain areas to assume new functions. For example, when a person suffers a stroke causing destruction of neurons in the motor cortex, it is possible to train nearby cortical neurons to assume some of the lost motor functions. Persistent attempts to use the muscles in an affected area may recruit cortical neurons into the neuronal circuit and improve motor strength and coordination over time. Neural plasticity is a fundamental process that endows the brain with the potential for memory and learning. Within certain boundaries, it appears that greater exposure to a particular stimulus prompts the brain to dedicate more neurons to that stimulus (and a lack of stimulation allows the brain to reassign neurons to a different function)—and so the old adage "use it or lose it" appears to hold true for the brain. However, with significant effort, it is possible to reclaim at least some of what was lost.

NEURONAL COMMUNICATION

Neurons communicate primarily through the release of neurotransmitters into the synapses adjacent to target neurons. Postsynaptic neurons

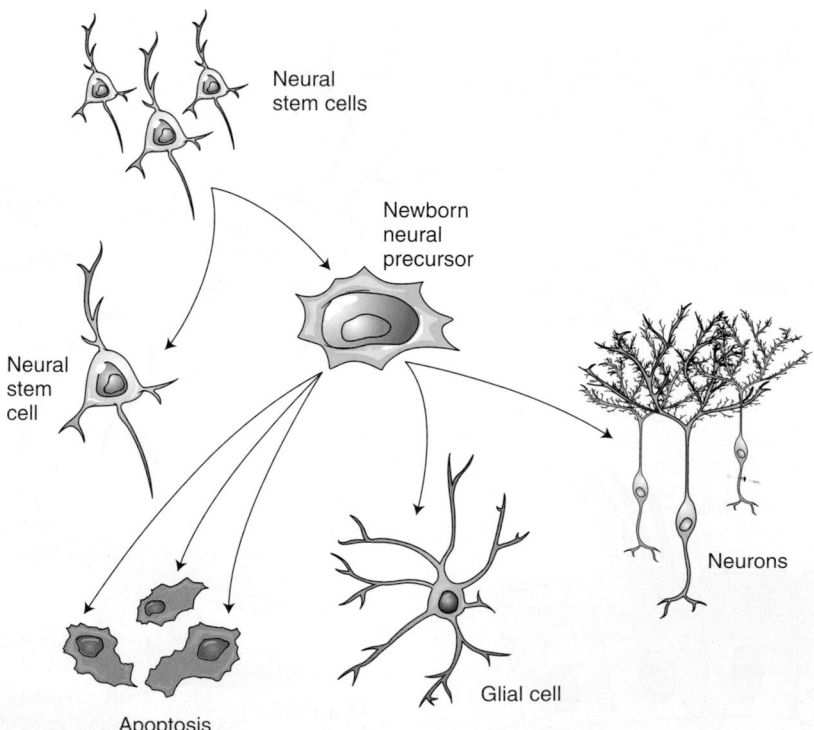

Neural stem cells

Newborn neural precursor

Neural stem cell

Neurons

Glial cell

Apoptosis

FIGURE 43-27 Schematic drawing of neural stem cell proliferation. Stem cells can differentiate into glial cells or neurons under the right conditions, but half fail to find a home and undergo apoptosis (programmed cell death).

have receptors for these neurotransmitters and respond by changing the flow of ions through channels in the cell membrane. Some neuronal communication occurs through gap junctions that connect the cytoplasm of one neuron to the next, forming electrical synapses (see Chapter 3).

Sufficient depolarization of the neuronal membrane results in the generation of action potentials, which transmit signals quickly from one end of the neuron to the other. Action potentials reaching the axon terminal open voltage-gated Ca^{2+} channels and stimulate the release of neurotransmitter into the synapse. Not all neurotransmitters are excitatory; some are inhibitory and suppress the formation of action potentials in the postsynaptic neuron. Most neurons have many contacts, some inhibitory and some excitatory, such that the response of the postsynaptic neuron is a summation of all the input.

Membrane Potentials

A detailed discussion of membrane potentials can be found in Chapter 3, and the major points are reviewed here. All cells of the body contain slightly more negatively charged molecules than positively charged ones. These negative ions are trapped intracellularly because they cannot pass through the plasma membrane. Positive ions are attracted to the cell membrane by the negatively charged intracellular ions. Because the cell membrane is permeable at rest to K^+ ions, but not to Ca^{2+} or Na^+ ions, potassium accumulates in the cell to neutralize the intracellular anions. The unequal distribution of K^+ across the cell membrane creates a concentration gradient, pulling K^+ back out of the cell. At equilibrium, the electrical gradient pulling K^+ into the cell and the chemical gradient pulling it out are balanced. This equilibrium point leaves a few extra negatively charged ions inside the cell with no positive ion to neutralize them. The negative ions line up on the inside of the cell membrane to interact with positive ions on the other side (Na^+, K^+, Ca^{2+}). This separation of charge across the membrane at rest creates a membrane potential that can be measured and is about -65 to -90 mV.[16] The membrane potential changes when the concentration of K^+ changes and when the permeability of the membrane to other ions changes.

Excitable cell types, like nerve and muscle, have ion channels in their cell membranes that open and close in response to fluctuations in membrane voltage. The most important voltage-gated ion channels in nerves are the fast Na^+ channels and the K^+ channels. Fast sodium channels allow Na^+ influx during the upstroke of the action potential, whereas potassium channels allow K^+ to leave the cell and help repolarize the membrane (see Chapter 3).

An action potential is initiated when neurotransmitters bind to receptors on the dendrite and cell body and allow cations, especially Na^+, to leak in. These channels are not voltage-gated channels; they are ligand-gated channels that open in response to a neurotransmitter binding to their receptor domain. If sufficient Na^+ leaks into the cell to raise the membrane potential to threshold, the fast voltage-gated Na^+ channels open and an action potential results. Opening of fast Na^+ channels in one section of the membrane allows Na^+ to flow in and bring the next section to threshold, thus opening the fast Na^+ channels in that section. This pattern repeats over and over again down the length of the axon. Threshold represents the amount of membrane depolarization required to cause fast Na^+ channels to flip into their open conformation (see Chapter 3). The axon hillock, the point at which the axon emerges from the cell body, is the usual site of action potential initiation because it has a high density of fast Na^+ channels and, therefore, a lower threshold.

Voltage-gated K^+ channels assist with repolarization because K^+ is allowed to flow out of the cell. During an action potential, the electrical gradient holding K^+ in the cell temporarily disappears as the membrane voltage moves toward zero. Potassium flows out of the cell passively down its concentration gradient. The Na^+-K^+ pumps work continuously to remove Na^+ from the cell interior and bring K^+ back in. The majority of a nerve cell's energy expenditure is used to power the Na^+-K^+ pumps.

The speed at which an action potential travels is determined by axonal diameter and myelination. Larger and myelinated neurons conduct impulses more quickly (Figure 43-28). In myelinated neurons, action potentials are generated only at the nodes of Ranvier, allowing the impulse to hop quickly from node to node down the axon. This is called *saltatory conduction.*

Synaptic Transmission

The great majority of synapses responsible for signal transmission in the CNS function by using neurotransmitters. A neurotransmitter is released from the synaptic terminal of one neuron, proceeds across the synaptic cleft, and acts on the receptor proteins in the membrane of the second neuron to excite, inhibit, or modify its activity. The response at the postsynaptic membrane depends on the type of ion channel that is opened or closed when the neurotransmitter binds to the receptor. Once neurotransmitters are released into the synaptic cleft, their potential to activate the postsynaptic receptors is limited by deactivation processes. Neurotransmitters are either actively transported back into the axon terminals for reuse or destroyed by enzyme activity.

An *excitatory postsynaptic potential* (EPSP) results when a neurotransmitter has a depolarizing effect on the postsynaptic membrane. The EPSP may be too small to bring the axon hillock to threshold, and EPSPs from several presynaptic neurons may be required to generate an action potential. Thus postsynaptic potentials are not all-or-none phenomena, as are action potentials. Neurotransmitters that produce EPSPs do so by opening channels in the membrane that allow Na^+ influx. In some cases, the receptor itself is a channel (*ionotropic receptor);* in others, the receptor is linked to the channel through a second messenger cascade (*metabotropic receptor)* (Figure 43-29). The ion channels regulated by metabotropic receptors may participate in action potential generation, but receptor activation also exerts more long-lasting effects on cell structure and behavior.

Some neurotransmitters inhibit depolarization and may produce hyperpolarization of the postsynaptic membrane by opening Cl^- or K^+ channels. Chloride ions leaking into the cell or potassium ions leaking out of the cell serve to short-circuit the effect of sodium ion influx, thus making it more difficult to reach threshold. This effect is called an *inhibitory postsynaptic potential* (IPSP). Neurotransmitters that result in IPSPs include γ-aminobutyric acid (GABA) and glycine.

Most synapses in the CNS have many presynaptic neurons, some producing EPSPs and some producing IPSPs. The membrane potential of the postsynaptic membrane is an algebraic sum of all the IPSPs and EPSPs occurring at any one moment in time. This is called *summation* and is the basis of neuronal processing and integration (Figure 43-30). The term *spatial summation* is applied when multiple presynaptic neurons release their neurotransmitters onto one postsynaptic neuron at the same time. The IPSPs and EPSPs sum algebraically to produce the overall postsynaptic potential. *Temporal summation* occurs when one presynaptic neuron fires in rapid succession so that it releases more neurotransmitter onto the postsynaptic cell before the postsynaptic neuron has completely recovered from a previous dose.

Neurotransmitters

Neurotransmitters are grouped according to their chemical structure into six principal categories[16] (Box 43-1). *Acetylcholine* (ACh) is the sole neurotransmitter in its class and is prevalent in numerous areas in the CNS. It is the neurotransmitter in autonomic ganglia, postganglionic parasympathetic synapses, and neuromuscular junctions. There are two major types of acetylcholine receptors: the nicotinic receptors (N) are of the ionotropic variety and the muscarinic receptors (M) are metabotropic (Table 43-7). When acetylcholine is released into the synapse, it is quickly degraded by acetylcholinesterase to limit the duration of action (Figure 43-31). Choline is actively taken back up into the presynaptic membrane for resynthesis. Acetylcholine receptors located on the presynaptic membrane provide a negative feedback loop, whereby the presynaptic neuron monitors the amount of acetylcholine in the synapse. Acetylcholinesterase inhibitor drugs are used for treating diseases such as Alzheimer disease and myasthenia gravis in which there is a deficiency of acetylcholine in the synapse and for reversing the effect of neuromuscular blocking drugs.

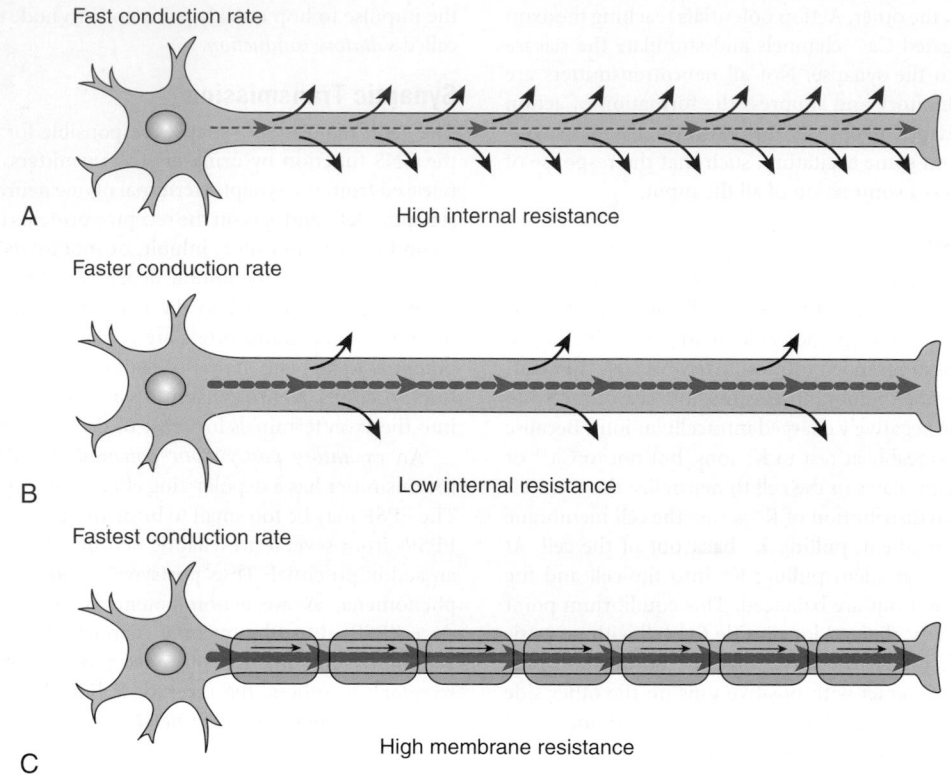

FIGURE 43-28 Rate of action potential conduction down an axon depends on the relative degree of internal resistance to current flow. When the diameter is small **(A),** there is higher internal resistance and slower conduction than in large-diameter neurons. A larger diameter **(B)** reduces internal resistance and accelerates the rate of conduction. Myelination **(C)** produces the fastest rate of conduction by increasing membrane resistance and decreasing internal resistance.

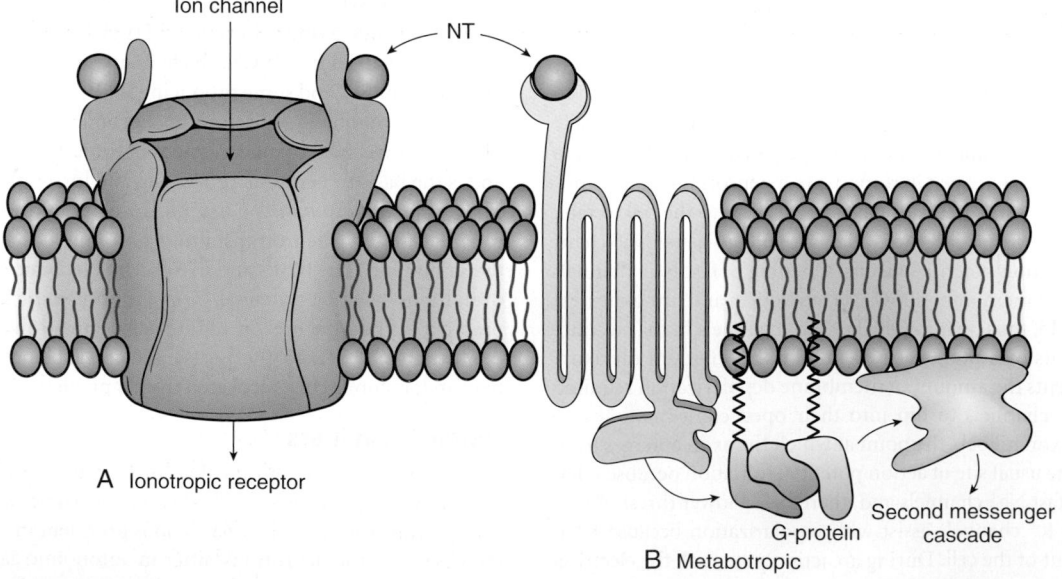

FIGURE 43-29 Neurotransmitter *(NT)* receptor classes. **A,** Ionotropic receptors are channel proteins that open when a neurotransmitter binds to them. **B,** Metabotropic receptors activate intracellular signaling cascades that generate second messengers in the cell when the neurotransmitter binds.

Spatial summation

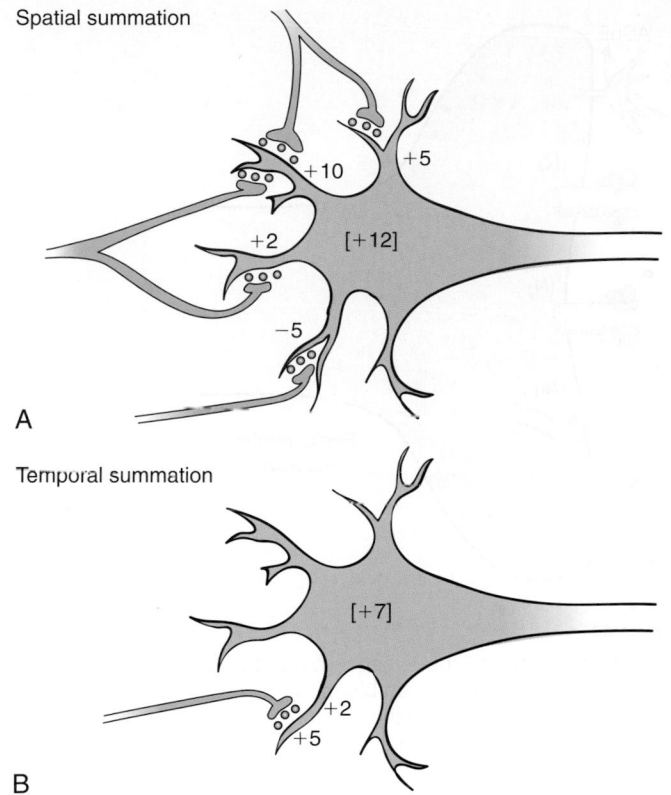

A

Temporal summation

B

FIGURE 43-30 Summation. **A,** Spatial summation occurs when two or more presynaptic neurons release neurotransmitter onto one postsynaptic cell at the same time. The various excitatory postsynaptic potentials and inhibitory postsynaptic potentials add algebraically to determine the overall postsynaptic potential (PSP) reaching the axon hillock. **B,** Temporal summation occurs when one presynaptic neuron fires in rapid succession such that a previous PSP has not fully dissipated before the next PSP is added to it.

BOX 43-1   SIX MAJOR CLASSES OF NEUROTRANSMITTERS

Acetylcholine

Amines
Dopamine
Norepinephrine
Epinephrine
Serotonin
Histamine

Amino Acids
Excitatory
Glutamate
Aspartate

Inhibitory
Glycine
γ-Aminobutyric acid (GABA)

Polypeptides
Substance P, other tachykinins
Vasopressin
Oxytocin
Corticotropin-releasing hormone
Thyrotropin-releasing hormone
Growth hormone–releasing hormone
Somatostatin
Gonadotropin-releasing hormone
Endothelins

Enkephalins
β-Endorphin, other derivatives of pro-opiomelanocortin
Cholecystokinin
Vasoactive intestinal polypeptide
Neurotensin
Gastrin-releasing peptide
Gastrin
Glucagon
Motilin
Secretin
Calcitonin gene–related peptide α
Neuropeptide Y
Activins
Inhibins
Angiotensin II
Galanin
Atrial natriuretic peptide
Brain natriuretic peptide

Purines
Adenosine
Adenosine triphosphate

Gases
Nitric oxide
Carbon monoxide

TABLE 43-7   MECHANISM OF ACTION OF SELECTED NONPEPTIDE NEUROTRANSMITTERS

TRANSMITTER	RECEPTOR	SECOND MESSENGER OR ION CHANNEL
Acetylcholine	Nicotinic	Cation channel
	M_1, M_3, M_5	↑ IP_3, DAG
	M_2, M_4	↓ cAMP
Dopamine	D_1, D_5	↑ cAMP
	D_2, D_3, D_4	↓ cAMP
Norepinephrine	α_{1A}, α_{1B}, α_{1D}	↑ IP_3, DAG
	α_{2A}, α_{2B}, α_{2C}	↓ cAMP
	β_1, β_2, β_3	↑ cAMP
5HT (serotonin)	$5HT_{1A}$, $5HT_{1B}$, $5HT_{1D}$, $5HT_5$	↓ cAMP
	$5HT_{2A}$, $5HT_{2C}$	↑ IP_3, DAG
	$5HT_3$	Na^+ channel
	$5HT_4$, $5HT_6$, $5HT_7$	↑ cAMP
Adenosine	A_1, A_3	↓ cAMP
	A_2	↑ cAMP
Glutamate	Metabotropic ($mGluR_1$ to $mGluR_8$)	Some ↑ cAMP, some ↓ cAMP, some ↑ IP_3, DAG
	AMPA, kainate	Na^+ channel
	NMDA	Ca^{2+} channel
GABA	$GABA_A$	Cl^- channel
	$GABA_B$	↓ cAMP

AMPA, α-Amino-3-hydroxy-5-methyl-4-isoxazolepropionate; *cAMP,* cyclic adenosine monophosphate; *DAG,* diacylglycerol; *GABA,* γ-aminobutyric acid; *5HT,* serotonin; *IP₃,* inositol trisphosphate; *NMDA,* N-methyl-D-aspartate.

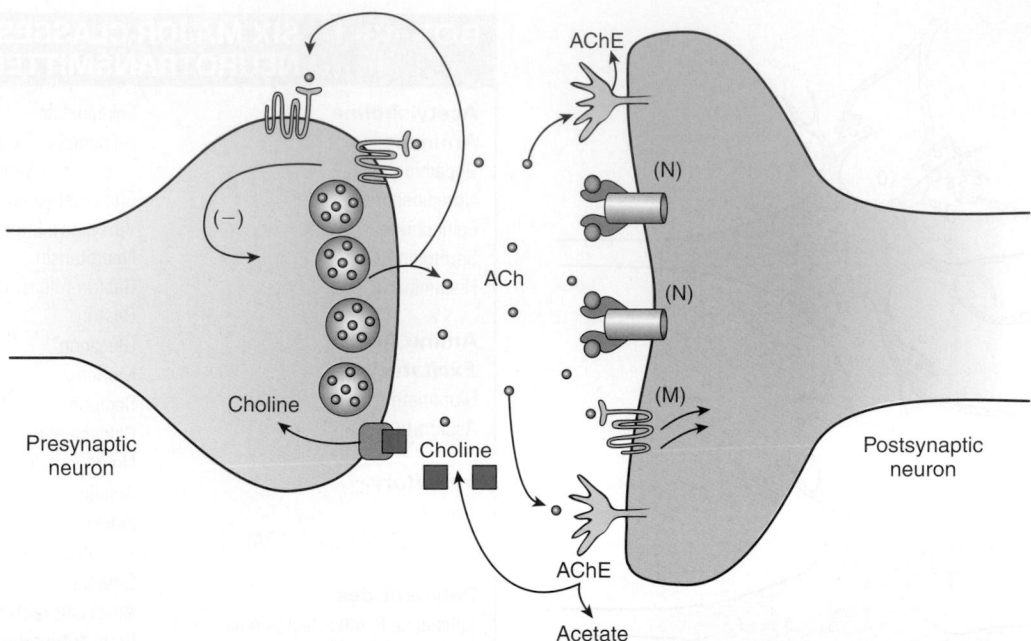

FIGURE 43-31 Acetylcholine synapse. Acetylcholine *(ACh)* released into the synapse binds to nicotinic *(N)* or muscarinic *(M)* receptors on the postsynaptic membrane. ACh also can bind to presynaptic receptors that are linked to a decrease in ACh release (negative feedback). Acetylcholinesterase *(AChE)* quickly degrades the ACh into acetate and choline. Choline is actively taken back into the presynaptic neuron for resynthesis.

The *amines* include dopamine (DA), norepinephrine (NE), epinephrine, serotonin (5-hydroxytryptamine, 5HT), and histamine. Amines are particularly involved in the limbic system, hypothalamus, and basal ganglia. NE is the neurotransmitter released at SNS postganglionic nerve endings. DA, NE, and serotonin are important in regulating thought processes and mood. Antipsychotic and mood-altering drugs change the activity of one or more of these amines in the brain (see Chapters 48 and 49). DA-secreting neurons project to the striatum (basal ganglia), pituitary gland, limbic system, and frontal cortex (Figure 43-32, *A*). DA can be degraded by enzymes in the extracellular fluid (catechol-*O*-methyltransferase, COMT) or by enzymes in the presynaptic nerve (monoamine oxidase, MAO). The primary means of clearing DA from the synapse is by active reuptake into the presynaptic membrane (see Figure 43-32, *B*). There are at least five DA receptor subtypes; all of these subtypes are metabotropic and linked to the production of second messengers (see Table 43-7). Abnormality of DA metabolism is apparent in various diseases, including Parkinson disease and schizophrenia.

Some neurons have an enzyme for the hydroxylation of DA to form NE. The NE-secreting neurons originate in the brainstem (locus caeruleus) and project widely throughout the brain including the cerebral cortex, cerebellum, limbic structures, brainstem, and spinal cord (see Figure 43-32, *C*). Most of the NE released into the synapse is cleared by active reuptake into the presynaptic neuron, where it can be repackaged for release or broken down by MAO. A number of receptor subtypes can bind NE in the synapse, and all are of the metabotropic variety and linked to second messenger cascades (see Table 43-7). The receptor subtype α_2 is commonly located on the presynaptic membrane where it provides a negative feedback loop for the presynaptic cell to monitor the amount of NE in the synapse (see Figure 43-32, *D*). Stimulation of the presynaptic α_2 receptor by NE or by α_2-agonist drugs reduces the amount of NE released into the synapse by the neuron.

Serotonin is another amine that affects numerous areas of the brain in a pattern similar to that of NE (see Figure 43-32, *E*). Numerous serotonin receptor subtypes have been identified, including one ionotropic

($5HT_3$) and several metabotropic subtypes (see Table 43-7). Like NE and DA, serotonin is cleared from the synapse by an active reuptake carrier on the presynaptic membrane (see Figure 43-32, *F*). It is also subject to degradation by MAO in the presynaptic cell. Like other neurotransmitters (NTs), serotonin can bind to presynaptic receptors that regulate its release. Numerous drugs have been developed to manage disorders associated with serotonin pathways, including depression, anxiety, and migraine headache. The class of medications known as selective serotonin reuptake inhibitors blocks the reuptake carrier for serotonin. The tricyclic antidepressants also block reuptake of serotonin, but they are less specific than the selective serotonin reuptake inhibitors and also affect reuptake of other amines.

The category of *amino acids* can be subdivided into excitatory and inhibitory mechanisms of action. Glutamate and aspartate are the principal excitatory amino acids. Glutamate neurons are widely distributed throughout the brain, and it is considered to be the primary excitatory neurotransmitter. Glutamate is involved in memory and has been implicated as a neurotoxin when released in excessive amounts (Chapter 44). Glutamate is removed from the synapse by active reuptake transporters on the presynaptic membrane. When energy stores are low because of interrupted blood supply or hypoxia, the transporters do not function effectively and glutamate remains in the synapse where it can behave as a neurotoxin. Most glutamate receptors are ionotropic; the metabotropic types are poorly understood. The α-amino-3-hydroxy-5-methyl-4-isoxazolepropionate (AMPA) receptors are classic ligand-gated sodium channels that depolarize the postsynaptic membrane. The *N*-methyl-D-aspartate (NMDA) receptors are interesting because they will not open unless the binding of glutamate is paired with a cotransmitter (such as glycine or D-serine) and concurrent depolarization of the membrane (Figure 43-33).[3] The NMDA receptor is a ligand-gated calcium ion channel, but it is blocked by a magnesium ion when the postsynaptic membrane is polarized. It only opens in response to glutamate binding if a depolarization is produced at the same time by another neurotransmitter-receptor

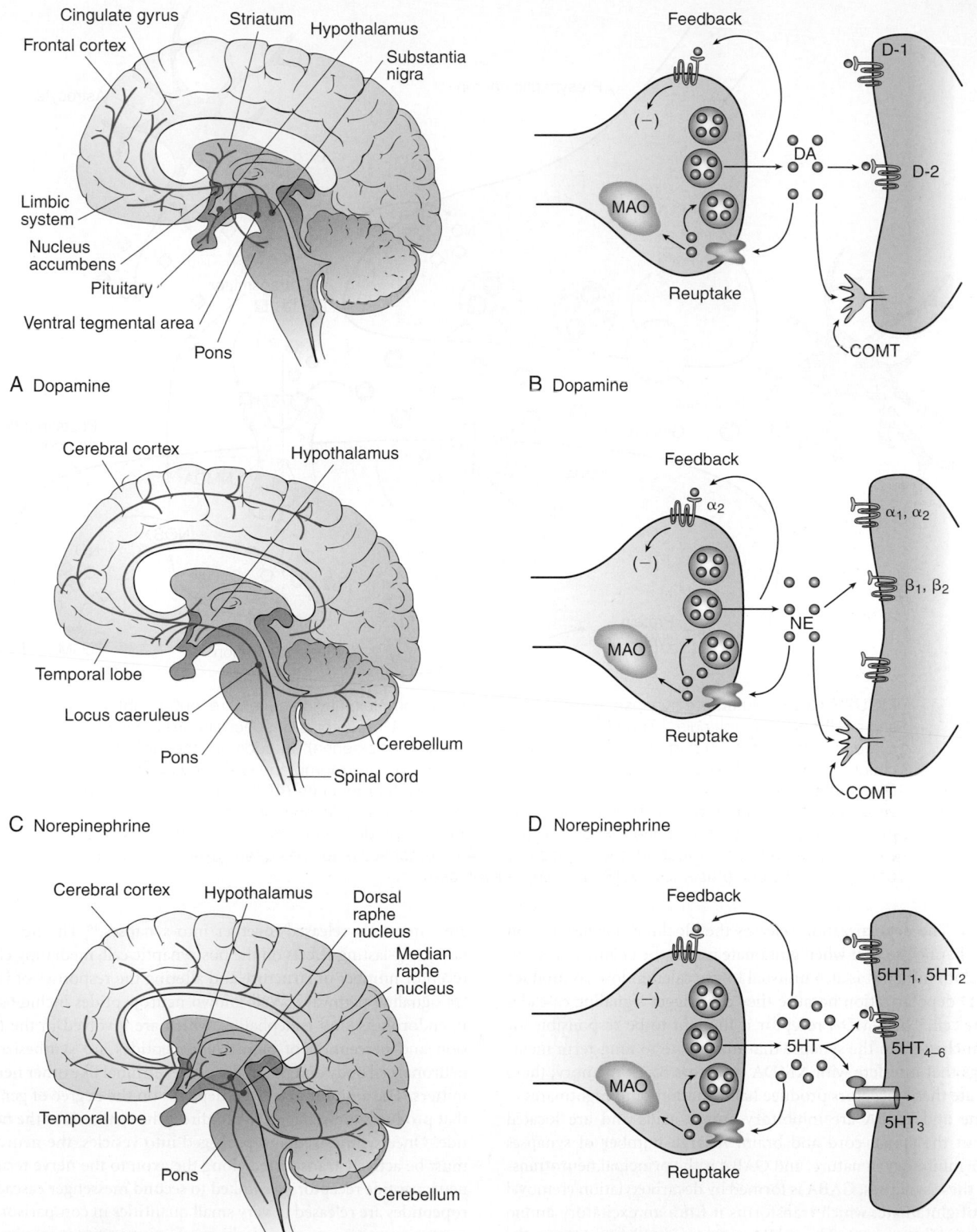

FIGURE 43-32 Amine synapses. **A,** Dopamine *(DA)* distribution in the brain. **B,** The DA synapse. **C,** Norepinephrine *(NE)* distribution in the brain. **D,** The NE synapse. **E,** Serotonin *(5HT)* distribution in the brain. **F,** The 5HT synapse. *COMT,* Catechol-O-methyltransferase; *MAO,* monoamine oxidase.

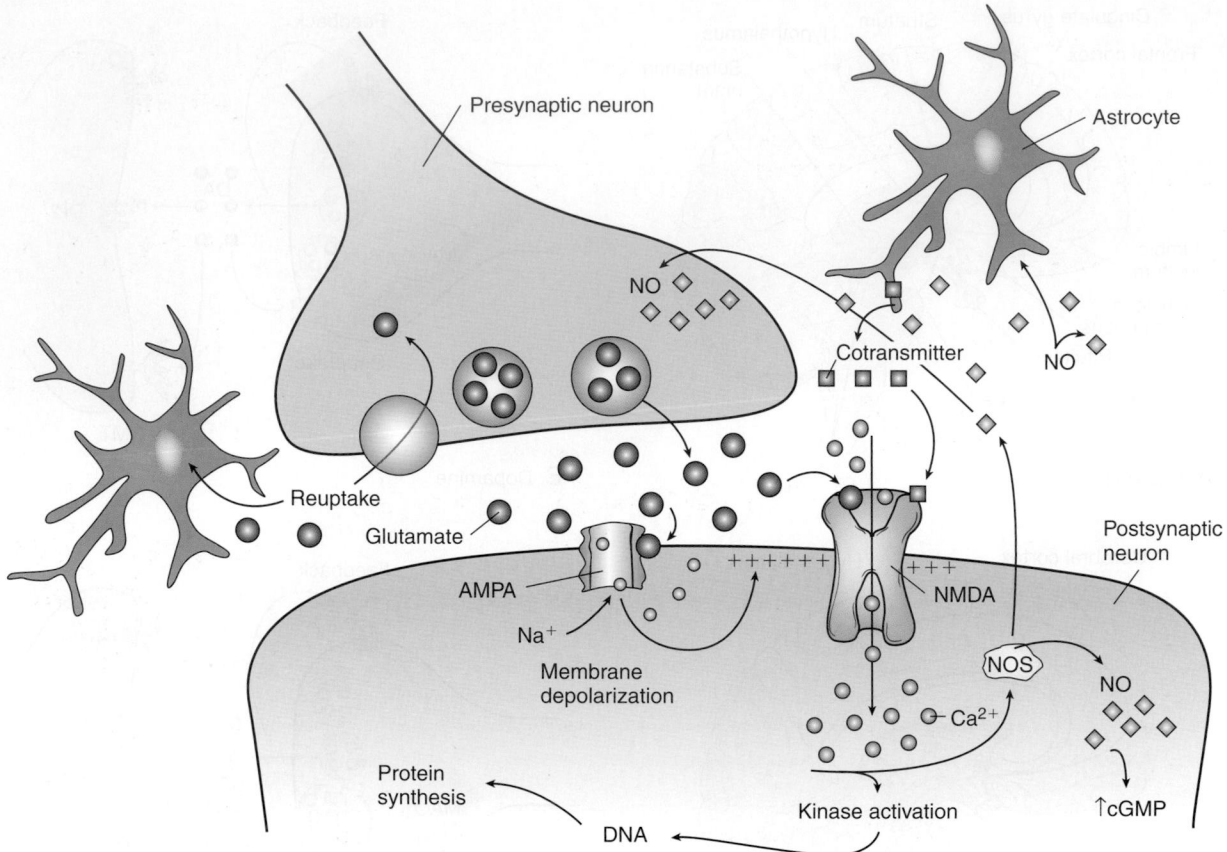

FIGURE 43-33 Glutamate synapse. Glutamate signaling is complex, having several receptor subtypes and costimulating molecules. The *N*-methyl-D-aspartate *(NMDA)* receptor is of special interest because it requires binding of glutamate and a cotransmitter (glycine or D-serine). In addition, the NMDA ion channel is blocked by Mg^{2+} and cannot open unless the postsynaptic membrane is already depolarized. Glutamate binding to its α-amino-3-hydroxy-5-methyl-4-isoxazolepropionate *(AMPA)* receptors can provide this depolarization by allowing sodium influx. When the NMDA channel opens, it allows calcium ions to flow in, triggering intracellular signaling cascades that produce nitric oxide *(NO)*. Nitric oxide is a gas that can diffuse throughout the synapse. NMDA receptor activation has been linked to long-term changes in synaptic efficiency. *NOS,* Nitric oxide synthase.

interaction. The depolarization releases the blocking magnesium ion from the channel, so that when glutamate binds, the channel opens to allow calcium influx. It is also unusual to use calcium ions to produce membrane depolarization because they can trigger signaling cascades within the cell. The NMDA receptor is thought to be responsible for long-term changes in the synapse that may relate to long-term memory. Drugs that interfere with NMDA receptors block memory; those that activate these receptors produce hallucinations and nightmares.

Glycine and GABA are inhibitory amino acids and are located throughout the spinal cord and brain. A large number of synapses (30%) are inhibitory in nature, and GABA is the principal neurotransmitter in these synapses. GABA is formed by decarboxylation (removal of CO_2) of glutamate, which transforms it from an excitatory amino acid to an inhibitory one. The GABA receptors are of two types: the $GABA_A$ is a classic ligand-gated chloride channel that produces an IPSP when activated. The $GABA_B$ receptor is a metabotropic receptor that also produces an IPSP and is linked to a reduction of cAMP concentration in the cell. Barbiturates and benzodiazepines are thought to exert their depressive effects by increasing GABA activity.

A long list of neurotransmitters is found in the *neuropeptide* category (see Table 43-7). Neuropeptides may function as the primary neurotransmitter in the synapse, but more often they are released together with another neurotransmitter. Amines and neuropeptides

are commonly released together into synapses.[16] The neuropeptides have long-lasting effects on the postsynaptic cell, mediating changes in receptor number or structure and altering the responses of intracellular signaling pathways. Well-known neuropeptides include substance P, endorphins, and enkephalins, which are involved in the transmission and perception of pain. Neuropeptides are synthesized in the neuronal cell body and not in the nerve terminal like other neurotransmitters. The amount produced depends on the degree of gene activity that produces messenger RNA to direct the synthesis of the neuropeptide. Once synthesized and packaged into vesicles, the neuropeptides must be actively transported along the axon to the nerve terminal. All neuropeptide receptors are linked to second messenger cascades. Neuropeptides are released in very small quantities in comparison to other neurotransmitters, and reuptake mechanisms are not required to turn off their activity. The neuropeptide with its bound receptor may be internalized into the postsynaptic cell, where the receptor is degraded or recycled to the synaptic membrane.

Purines, including adenosine triphosphate (ATP) and adenosine, function as neurotransmitters in various brain regions. Adenosine is thought to be continuously released by most neurons and modulates neurotransmission by blocking neurotransmitter release. Adenosine may be important in preventing seizure activity. The role of ATP as a neurotransmitter continues to be elucidated. There are at least three

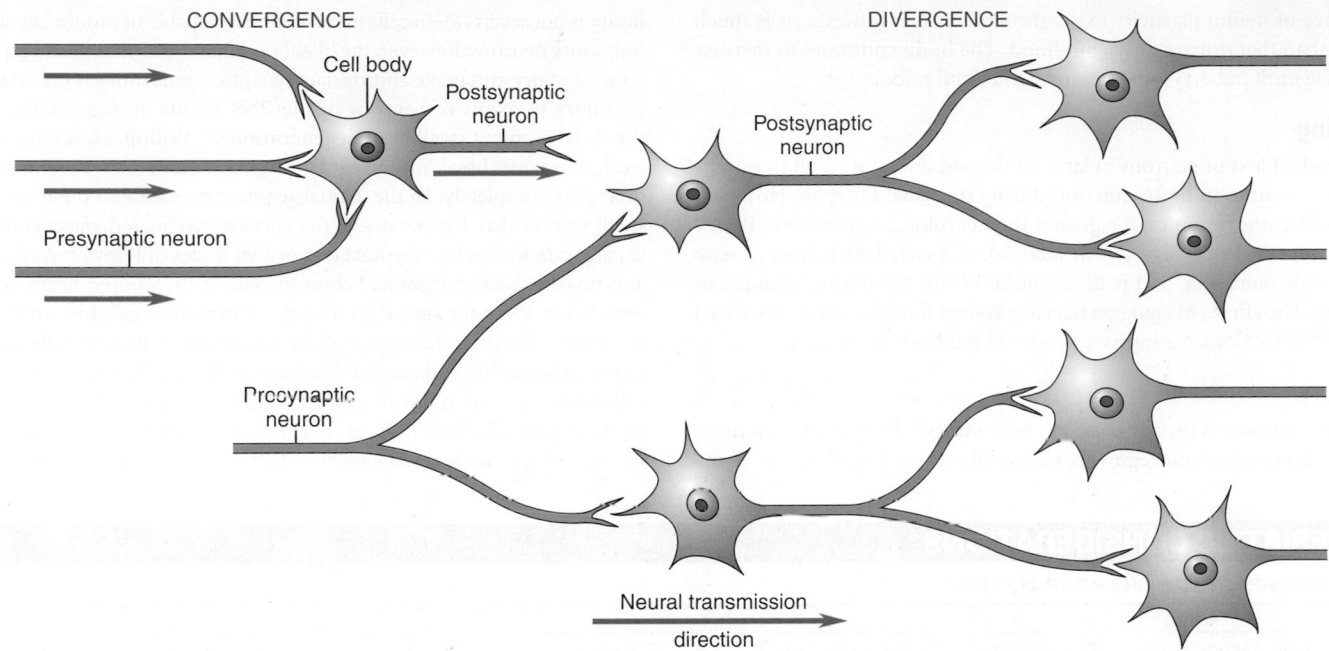

CONVERGENCE   DIVERGENCE

Cell body
Postsynaptic neuron
Postsynaptic neuron
Presynaptic neuron
Presynaptic neuron

Neural transmission direction

FIGURE 43-34 Convergence of several presynaptic neurons on one postsynaptic neuron is compared with divergence of one presynaptic neuron to several postsynaptic neurons.

ATP receptor subtypes, two that decrease cAMP production and one that increases cAMP production.

Nitric oxide (NO) is a gas that can diffuse through cell membranes and therefore does not require a synaptic receptor for its activity. NO has several different potential targets within cells. For example, NO can bind and stimulate guanylyl cyclase, an enzyme that produces cyclic guanosine monophosphate (cGMP), a second messenger in the cell, or it can alter the activity of ion pumps, metabolic enzymes, and DNA transcription factors.[16] Unlike other neurotransmitters that are produced and released by presynaptic neurons, NO can be synthesized in the postsynaptic neuron and diffuse locally to affect presynaptic neurons and nearby glial cells. The functions of NO are not completely known, but it is thought to be important in memory and pain perception. One trigger known to stimulate NO is activation of the previously described NMDA receptor. The calcium ions that flow in through the open NMDA receptor cause activation of an enzyme called nitric oxide synthase (NOS), which produces NO. NO may be the messenger that alerts the presynaptic membrane that the paired stimuli required to open the NMDA receptor were received.[17]

Neuronal Circuits

Patterns of neuronal synaptic connections are called *neuronal circuits*. Activity in particular groups of neurons in one or more circuits is the basis of nervous system function: thoughts, memories, sensations, movements, and learning.

Divergence is a term used to describe neuronal circuits in which one presynaptic neuron makes contact with more than one postsynaptic neuron (Figure 43-34). Divergence is a strategy used to send sensory input to a large number of receiving neurons. *Convergence* occurs when many presynaptic neurons synapse with one postsynaptic neuron (see Figure 43-34). This arrangement is typical in the motor pathways, in which sensory, reflex, and voluntary inputs must be integrated into a response by the motor neurons that innervate skeletal muscle. Convergence is a mechanism of processing and integration of input.

The efficiency of circuits can be altered by changes in synaptic function. Synaptic transmission can be facilitated or inhibited in various ways. Alteration in the ease of synaptic transmission is the basis of memory and is discussed in more detail in the Consciousness, Memory, and Sleep section at the end of this chapter.

NEURAL DEVELOPMENT, AGING, AND INJURY

Development

The nervous system starts to take shape during the third week of embryonic development. At this time, three primary tissues of the embryo are distinguishable: the ectoderm, endoderm, and mesoderm. A thickened plate of ectoderm, running longitudinally on the dorsal surface of the embryo (neural plate), gives rise to the CNS and PNS. By the end of the third week, the neural plate folds to form a neural tube. Openings at either end of the neural tube are called *neuropores*. The neural tube is the precursor of the future brain and spinal cord.

Fusion of cells and formation of the neural tube start in the cervical region of the future spinal cord and then progress rapidly in a **rostral** direction toward the future brain. Failure of the neural tube to close properly is a cause of congenital malformation of the nervous system. Anencephaly (absent brain) results from failure of the rostral portion to close, whereas failure of closure of the caudal portion results in myelomeningocele. In this defect, the spinal cord and meninges are displaced into a sac on the back (see Chapter 45). A reduction in neural tube defects has been achieved through prenatal maternal supplementation with folic acid.[18]

Neurons grow and divide at an incredible rate during embryologic development and make primitive synaptic connections according to a basic architecture that is genetically programmed. The number of neurons and synapses ultimately dedicated to particular functions is determined in large part by their use. For example, if no visual sensory input is relayed to the primary visual cortex (as occurs with congenital cataracts), the cortical neurons will be reassigned to other functions. Similarly, a person born without arms will lack representation of these structures in the primary somatosensory cortex. In contrast, greater stimulation appears to increase the number of neurons dedicated to a particular function. Critical periods in the early neonatal period have been identified when neuronal assignment to specific functions is determined.[19,20] In recent years it has been recognized that a significant degree of neural plasticity exists throughout life; however, it is much less than that during early childhood. The brain continues to increase in size until puberty and remains stable until middle age.

Aging

A gradual loss of neurons in later adulthood does not result in significant alteration in brain function during the usual life span. However, the older one becomes, the greater the neurologic impairment. Excessive neuronal degeneration in adulthood is called Alzheimer disease or senile dementia, and is distinguished from the normal changes of aging. The effects of aging on nervous system function are summarized in Geriatric Considerations: Changes in the Nervous System.

Injury

Injury to neurons usually results in neuronal cell death and loss of function; however, some regrowth is possible in peripheral nerves if the injury is not severe. Stem cells in the brain are capable of producing new, immature neurons; however, the likelihood that they will find and repair a site of injury and make appropriate synaptic connections is uncertain.

Injury to axons of neurons in the PNS results in degeneration of the distal segment (**wallerian degeneration**).[18] Within a few days to a week, the axons break into irregular fragments, and after 3 weeks they disappear completely. In the axonal segment proximal to the injury, a small section also degenerates. If the nerve is myelinated, degeneration usually extends back to the next one or two nodes of Ranvier. As axons and myelin sheaths degrade, Schwann cells of the injured nerve swell and divide. Over the next 2 to 3 weeks, continuous columns of short Schwann cells mark the course of the lost axons. If there is little separation between the ends of a divided nerve, the proliferating Schwann cells bridge the gap. If the divided ends are further apart, the proliferating Schwann cells form bulbous swellings at the end of the nerves and the surviving axons form fine fibrils, which extend into the surrounding

GERIATRIC CONSIDERATIONS

Changes in the Nervous System

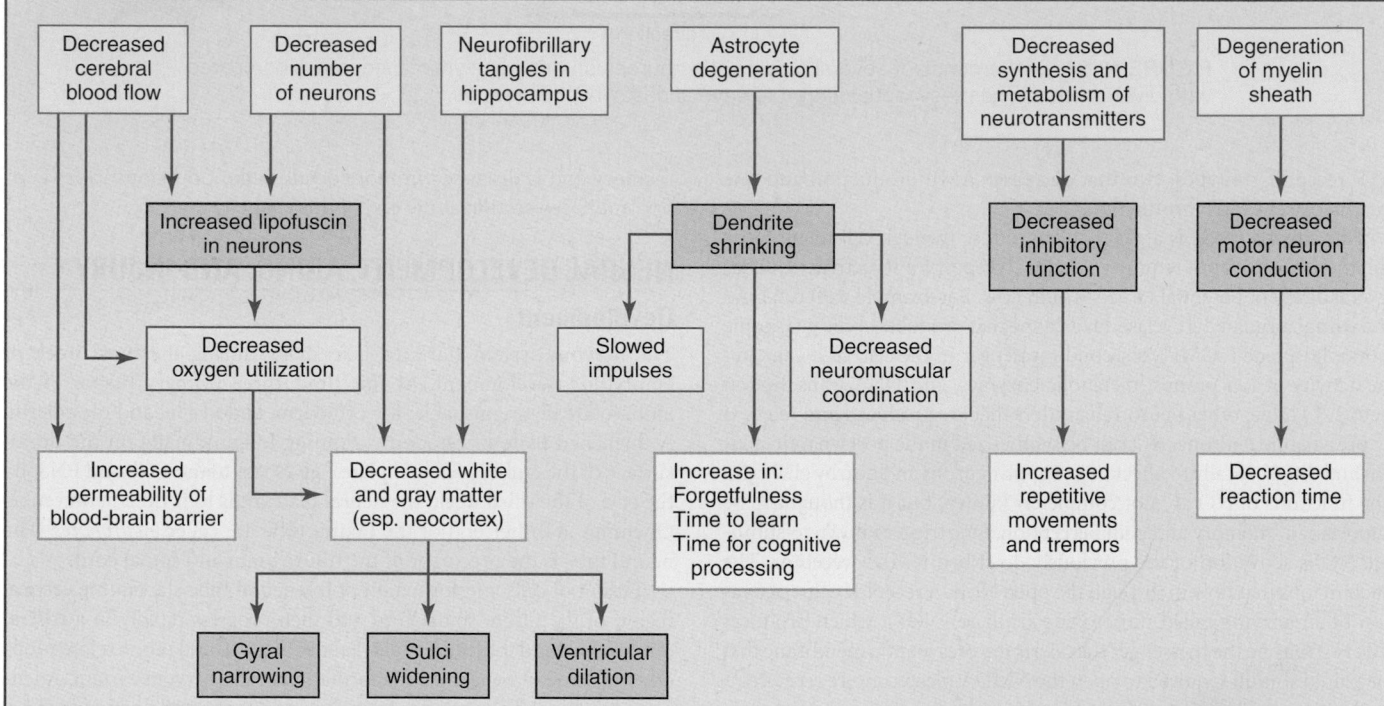

With aging, brain atrophy and a decrease in brain weight occur. This is evidenced by a decrease in the amount of white matter and gray matter up to 0.5% per year, with gyral narrowing, sulci widening, and ventricular dilation. There is a gradual atrophy and loss of neurons in the brain and spinal cord over time; but neuron loss is not uniform within the brain. Most of the neuron loss is in the neocortex (20%), Purkinje cells of the cerebellum, substantia nigra, and locus caeruleus. Some parts of the brain, such as the vestibular nucleus, have no neuron loss. Blood supply to the brain is decreased because of the decreased metabolic demands and brain atrophy. There is also increased permeability of the blood-brain barrier.

Intracellularly there is an increase in the amount of lipofuscin, which hampers cellular oxygen use, crowds intracellular organelles, and reduces the number of mitochondria. There are also neurofibrillary tangles in the hippocampus and neuritic plaques that are found only in the elderly.

Nerve fibers in the brain decrease in number and show signs of splitting or fragmentation. The cortex, subcortex, and cerebellar astrocytes degenerate. Nerve axons develop swellings near their ends called neuroaxonal dystrophy.

The relevance of these swellings is unknown. Dendrites shrink, decreasing the number of messages received from other cells and synaptic linkages. This causes slowing of impulses and decreases neuromuscular coordination. These changes result in decreased short-term memory, reduced speed of learning, prolonged new information processing, increased reaction time, diminished abstract reasoning, and impaired perception.

Changes in the secretion and metabolism of neurotransmitters also impact the aging brain. There is a decrease in norepinephrine and dopamine secretion with an increase in monoamine oxidase secretion. The reduction of dopamine levels leads to decreased inhibitory motor functions.

In the spinal cord, posterior root fibers and sympathetic nerve fibers of the autonomic nervous system decline in number. Peripherally, there is degeneration of the motor nerve fibers and myelin sheath. Motor neuron axons remain intact. Decreasing motor neuron conduction velocity and prolonged muscle action potentials lead to decreased reaction times. Reflexes may be decreased or absent. There is an increased risk of falls.

Schwann cells at random. Those fibrils that find a column of Schwann cells in the distal part of the nerve grow down the column. There is often good functional return to the nerve secondary to this process. If continuity is not restored, the distal end gradually becomes replaced by collagenous scar tissue.

Damaged axons in the CNS show a pattern of degeneration that is similar to that of peripheral neurons. Damaged axons become irregular and beaded, break up, and disappear, but the process is significantly slower. Methods using stains for β-amyloid precursor protein to identify axonal injury in the CNS have revealed that axonal injury is a common event even in mild concussion.[21] Axonal damage impairs axonal streaming and causes a buildup of β-amyloid precursor protein proximal to the injury. This buildup is taken as evidence of axonal injury. Contrary to previously held notions, a significant degree of axonal repair appears to occur in CNS neurons when the injury is not too severe.[21] If neurons that were the principal source of stimulation to some other group of neurons are damaged and die, that other group of neurons may also degenerate because of the loss of trophic (growth and survival) signals. Researchers continue to discover new nerve growth and survival factors. Eventually they may find ways to minimize neuronal degeneration after injury and encourage repair or replacement.

KEY POINTS

- The fundamental unit of the nervous system is the neuron. Neurons have three basic parts: the cell body, dendrites, and axons. The dendrites receive signals and transmit them to the cell body. The axon generates and conducts action potentials. Conduction of action potentials is faster in large and myelinated axons.
- Neuronal communication through chemical synapses can be summarized as follows: Stimulation from other neurons occurs primarily at the dendrite and cell body. Action potentials are initiated at the axon hillock and conducted down the axon to the axon terminal, where neurotransmitter is stored. Depolarization of the terminal opens voltage-gated calcium channels. Calcium influx mediates exocytosis of neurotransmitter into the interneuronal synapse. Neurotransmitter binds and activates specific receptors on the postsynaptic cell, changing its ion conductance. With sufficient depolarization of the postsynaptic cell, an action potential is generated.
- There are six categories of neurotransmitters based on their chemical structure: acetylcholine, amines, amino acids, neuropeptides, purines, and gases.
- Excitatory neurotransmitters create excitatory postsynaptic potentials (EPSPs) in the postsynaptic neuron attributable to opening of channels that allow Na^+ or Ca^{2+} influx. Inhibitory neurotransmitters create inhibitory postsynaptic potentials (IPSPs) in the postsynaptic neuron attributable to opening of channels that allow Cl^- influx or K^+ efflux. The summation of EPSPs and IPSPs at the axon hillock determines whether an action potential will be initiated.
- Neuroglial cells are supportive cells in the CNS. Oligodendroglial cells form insulating myelin sheaths, astroglial cells moderate extracellular fluid composition and synaptic conditions, microglial cells are derived from circulating monocytes and destroy foreign materials, and ependymal cells form CSF.
- Development of the nervous system follows a basic architecture that is genetically programmed. However, the brain is quite plastic, especially during infancy, and alters the assignment of neurons to certain functions based on the degree of stimulation.
- Neurons in the CNS that are severely injured generally do not regenerate. Peripheral neurons may regenerate if the Schwann cells provide a pathway for growth. Neural stem cells in the ventricles and hippocampus of the brain can proliferate to produce either glial or neuronal cells depending on specific cues, most of which have yet to be elucidated.

SENSORY FUNCTION

The discussion of sensory function in this chapter is restricted to the somatosensory system. The special senses of hearing, vision, taste, and olfaction are discussed in Chapter 46. Neural pathways related to pain transmission are discussed in detail in Chapter 47.

Transmission of sensory signals begins with activation of specialized dendritic processes, called *sensory receptors*, at the ends of sensory afferents that project to the spinal cord (or brainstem in the case of some cranial nerves). Secondary neurons in the cord are activated and carry the signals up the cord to the brain. The thalamus is the principal receiving site for somatosensory signals, which are then relayed to various brain areas, including the somatosensory cortex in the parietal lobe.

An important principle of sensory transmission is that somatotopic organization is maintained from receptor to somatosensory cortex. This property allows for precise localization of the origin of sensory signals. The somatosensory system conveys a number of different sensory modalities, including fine touch, vibration sense, pressure, temperature, itch, crude touch, and pain. In general, different modalities are sensed by different types of sensory receptors.

SENSORY RECEPTORS

Sensory receptors are specialized terminations of the dendrites of primary sensory neurons. The receptor may be a free nerve ending or may have various connective tissue elaborations that affect its responsiveness (Figure 43-35). All types of receptors respond to stimuli by altering their membrane permeability to ions, thus creating a change in the membrane voltage. These receptor potentials are similar to the EPSPs generated in postsynaptic neurons, except that the stimulus is not a neurotransmitter. Different receptor types respond to different kinds of stimuli: mechanical stretch, changes in temperature, or the binding of chemicals. When a stimulus depolarizes the receptor sufficiently, voltage-gated fast Na^+ channels in the membrane open and an action potential is generated. The rate of action potential generation by the receptor depends on the intensity of the stimulus (Figure 43-36).

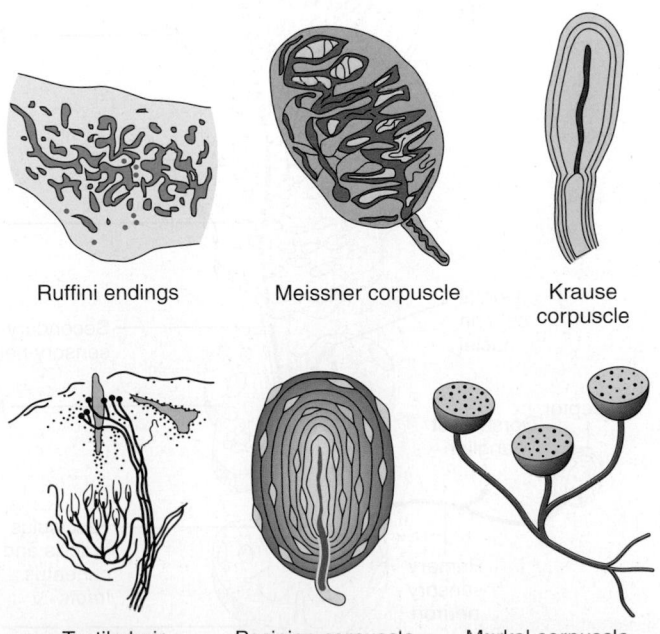

Ruffini endings   Meissner corpuscle   Krause corpuscle

Tactile hair   Pacinian corpuscle   Merkel corpuscle

FIGURE 43-35 Common types of somatosensory receptors. Sensory receptors are specialized to respond to particular types of stimuli.

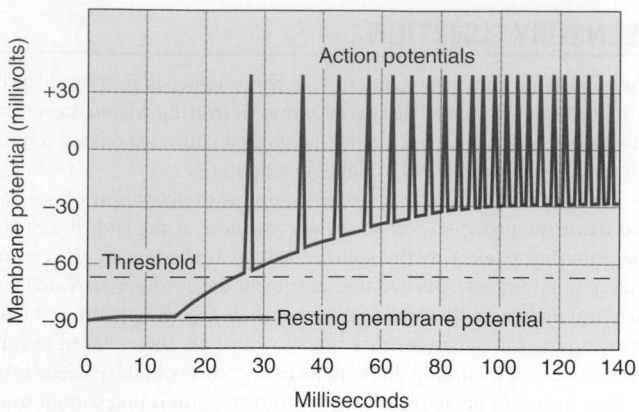

FIGURE 43-36 Relationship between stimulus intensity and action potential generation. As the stimulus increases, the receptor potential is greater, and action potentials are generated at a faster rate. (From Hall JE, editor: *Guyton & Hall textbook of medical physiology*, ed 12, Philadelphia, 2011, Saunders, p 561.)

Some receptors are rapidly adapting and generate action potentials only when a change in the stimulus intensity occurs. The pacinian corpuscle is a classic example of a rapidly adapting receptor that is well suited to transmitting the sense of vibration. Tonic receptors adapt slowly and are good for conveying information about stimulus intensity over time. Free nerve endings, such as pain receptors, are usually tonic receptors.

Impulses generated by receptors are transmitted to the dorsal root of the spinal nerve. Depending on the sensory modality, the nerve impulses may travel up the **ipsilateral** side of the cord or may cross the spinal cord to travel up the **contralateral** side. In general, the well-localized sensations of touch, pressure, and vibration travel up the ipsilateral side of the cord, whereas the sensations of pain, itch, and temperature usually cross over and travel to the brain on the contralateral side. Regardless of pathway taken, somatosensory signals eventually converge on the somatosensory cortex in the hemisphere opposite from the location of the primary receptor.

SENSORY PATHWAYS

Two major tracts, the dorsal column–medial lemniscal tracts and the anterolateral tracts, carry information from the spinal segments to the brain[22] (Figure 43-37). The dorsal column–medial lemniscal tract

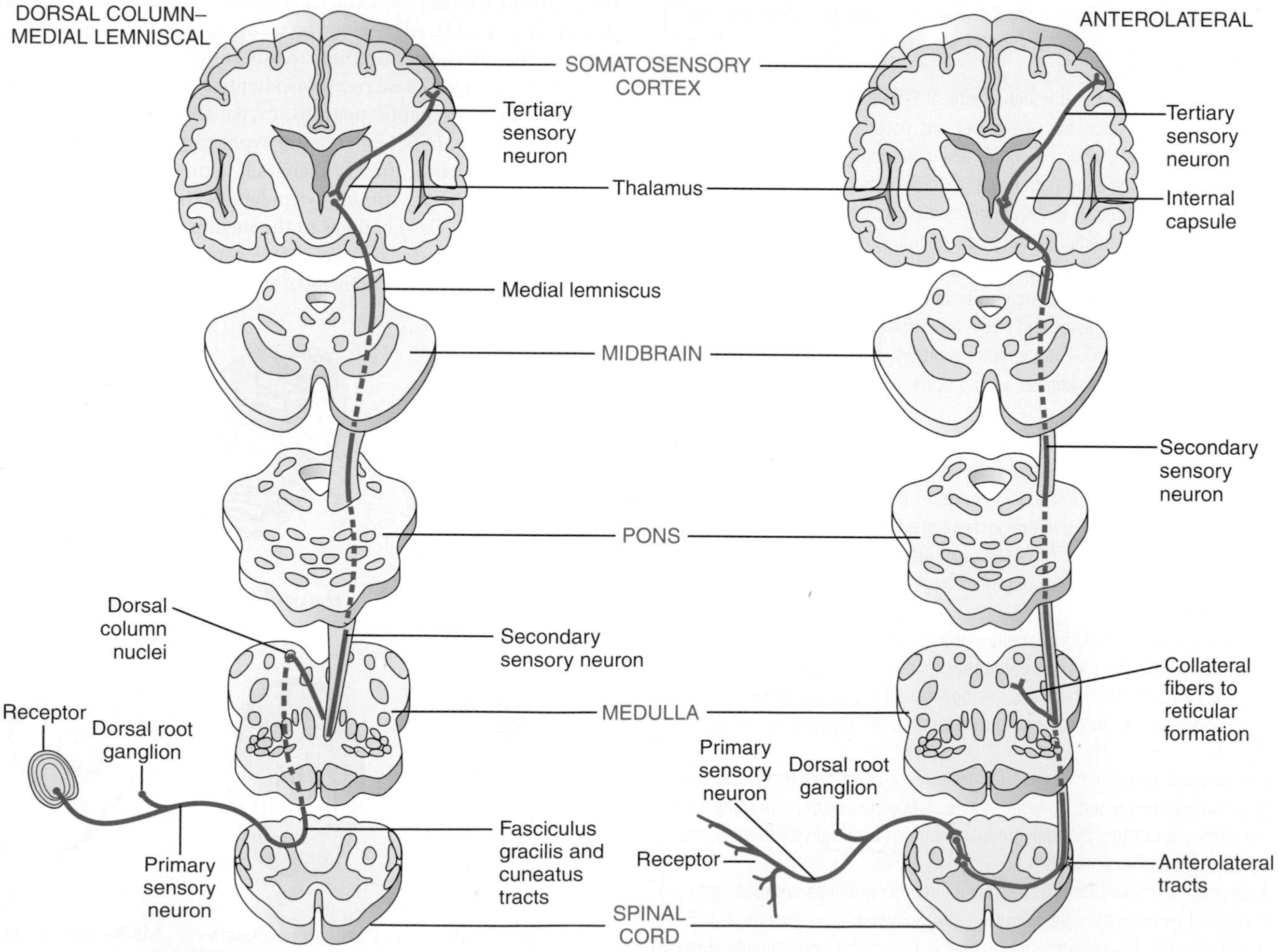

FIGURE 43-37 Comparison of the two major ascending somatosensory tracts. *Left*, Dorsal column–medial lemniscal tract. *Right*, Anterolateral tract. Note that the dorsal column tracts do not cross the midline until the level of the medulla, whereas the anterolateral tracts cross at the spinal cord level.

carries fine touch, vibration sense, and proprioception and remains ipsilateral until the level of the medulla. As the fibers progress upward, they gradually move toward the midline, so that those corresponding to the lower extremities occupy the medial white column and those representing the arm are more lateral. From the nuclei in the medulla, neurons of the dorsal column pathway cross to the opposite side and travel up the brainstem, where they form the medial lemniscus, and then on to the thalamus. In the thalamus, fibers synapse with tertiary neurons, which in turn pass upward in a great band of fibers known as the *internal capsule,* and then travel on to the primary sensory cortex.

The anterolateral tract (previously called the *spinothalamic tract*) carries impulses for sensations of pain, itch, and temperature from small myelinated (Aδ) and unmyelinated (C-fiber) neurons. These neurons ascend one or more spinal segments before entering the posterior horn and synapsing with their secondary neuron. A few secondary fibers ascend ipsilaterally in the Lissauer fasciculus all the way to the thalamus. However, the majority of fibers cross the midline and ascend as the anterolateral tract. Fibers from the lower extremities and trunk are pushed laterally as they ascend in the spinal cord by the addition of fibers from the upper extremities and upper body, which enter medially.

On their way to the thalamus, these fibers give off collaterals to the reticular formation of the brainstem and the periaqueductal gray matter in the midbrain, where it is believed that one of their functions is pain inhibition (see Chapter 47). Secondary fibers of the anterolateral tract terminate in several thalamic regions. Tertiary neurons project from the thalamus to the somatosensory cortex. Thus, although the sensations of fine touch and pain are separated in the cord, they reunite in the somatosensory cortex that lies in the cerebral hemisphere opposite the site of sensory receptor origin.

SOMATOSENSORY CORTEX

The primary somatosensory cortex is organized in columns of gray matter that correspond to specific body locations. All modalities of sensation are grouped together in adjacent sections. The somatotopic representation of the body along a strip of cortex creates a distorted picture of the human body, called a homunculus map[22] (Figure 43-38). Body areas with a greater density of receptors garner a larger part of the homunculus map. The homunculus map was created by stimulating discrete areas of the cortex in awake subjects and recording the sensations that they reported. It is now known that several different cortical areas contain somatotopically organized maps in addition to the well-known one in the primary somatosensory cortex. The *perception* of sensation from the body occurs at the level of the cortex.

KEY POINTS

- The body is somatotopically represented in the spinal cord and cerebral cortex. Stimulation of points in the primary somatosensory cortex results in discrete sensations in the contralateral side of the body.
- Projections to the somatosensory cortex begin in sensory receptors throughout the body. Receptors send axons to the spinal cord through the dorsal root. Stimulation of receptors by mechanical deformation, temperature, or chemicals alters membrane permeability, resulting in receptor potentials. The intensity of the stimulus is reflected in the rate of action potentials generated.
- Sensations of touch and proprioception (dorsal column–medial lemniscal tract) project up to the medulla on the ipsilateral side, then cross over and project to the thalamus.

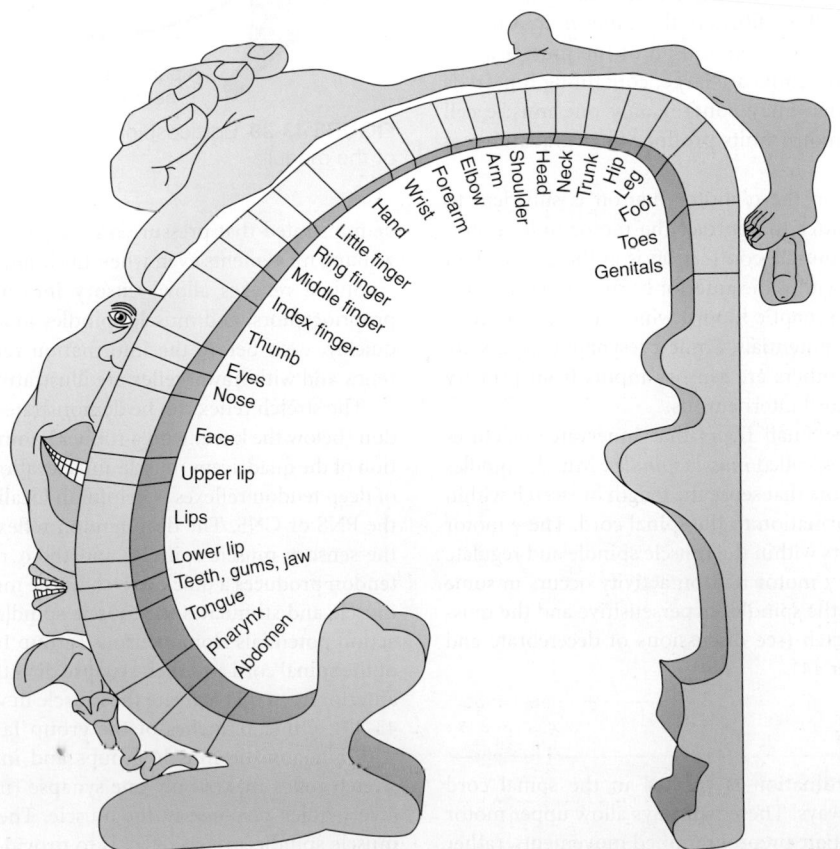

FIGURE 43-38 Topographic organization of the body on the somatosensory cortex, forming a homunculus map.

- Sensations of pain, temperature, and itch (anterolateral tract) usually cross the cord near the level of entry and travel to the brain on the contralateral side.
- Sensory information from both tracts is transmitted from the thalamus to the same areas of the somatosensory cortex by way of the internal capsule.

▌MOTOR FUNCTION

The execution of voluntary movement requires interaction among basal ganglia, the cerebellum, and several regions of the cortex. The final program of voluntary muscle activity is transmitted from the brain down the spinal cord by way of the lateral corticospinal tracts. As previously noted, the corticospinal tract decussates in the medullary pyramids and travels down the spinal cord to control muscles on the contralateral side of the body (Figure 43-39). The corticospinal tract primarily controls distal muscles of the arms, wrists, fingers, lower legs, feet, and toes. These are the muscles capable of fine-motor control. Another group of motor tracts innervate large proximal muscle groups and axial muscles that control posture and balance. These tracts include the vestibulospinal, reticulospinal, and tectospinal tracts. Motor tracts descending from the brain synapse on the cell bodies of motor neurons that lie in the anterior horn of the spinal cord and project to skeletal muscles.

MOTOR NEURONS

Motor neurons travel from the anterior horn of the spinal cord through the ventral root and within the spinal and peripheral nerves to finally innervate target muscles. The α motor neurons release acetylcholine into neuromuscular junctions, depolarizing skeletal muscle cells and contracting all the fibers in the *motor unit*. A motor unit consists of a single motor neuron and all of the muscle fibers under its control. Some motor units are large, containing hundreds of muscle cells, whereas others may contain only one muscle cell per motor neuron. Smaller motor units produce finer gradations of muscle control.

A single action potential in the α motor neuron is sufficient to release enough neurotransmitter to contract the motor unit. Therefore, the point of control of muscle contraction is at the cell body of the α motor neuron that lies within the anterior horn. A typical motor neuron receives hundreds of synaptic inputs, which summate to control the generation of action potentials. Some presynaptic inputs are from corticospinal neurons; others are sensory inputs from primary sensory afferents and spinal cord interneurons.

The γ motor neurons are small fibers that innervate structures within the body of the muscles, called *muscle spindles*. Muscle spindles are specialized sensory receptors that sense the length or stretch within the muscle and relay the information to the spinal cord. The γ motor neurons contract muscle fibers within the muscle spindle and regulate spindle sensitivity. Excessive γ motor neuron activity occurs in some types of brain coma, making the spindles hypersensitive and the muscles stiff and resistant to stretch (see discussions of decerebrate and decorticate rigidity in Chapter 44).

SPINAL REFLEXES

A great deal of motor coordination is exerted in the spinal cord through complex reflex pathways. These pathways allow upper motor neurons from the brain to initiate preprogrammed movements, rather than having to excite and inhibit each and every lower motor neuron individually. For example, experiments in lower animals have

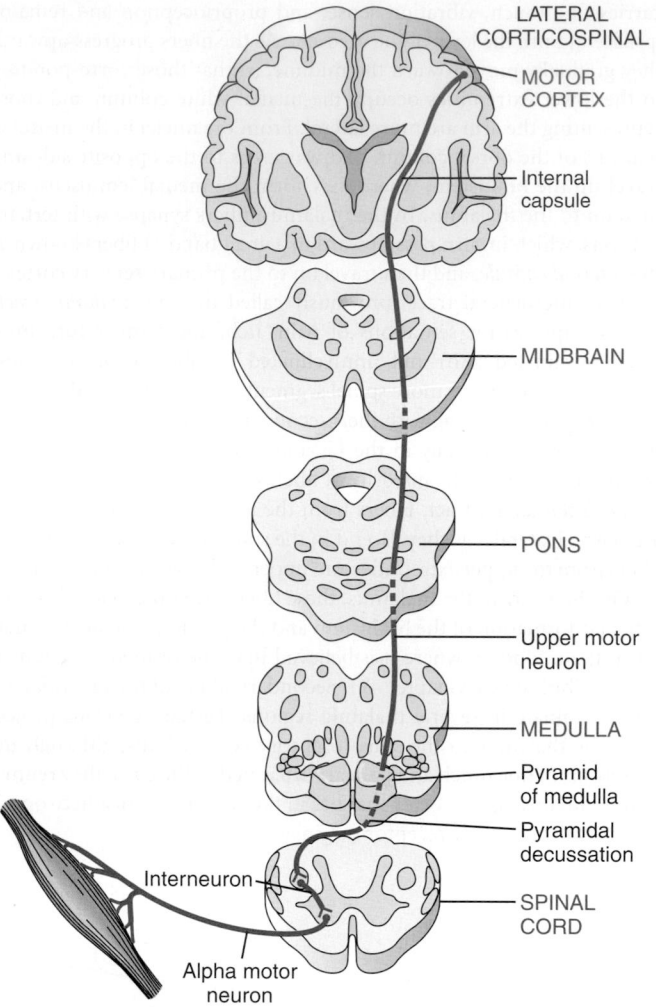

FIGURE 43-39 Corticospinal tract showing decussation at the level of the medulla.

demonstrated that pressure on the pads of the feet initiates complex walking movements even when the brain is no longer functional.

Spinal reflexes allow sensory information from pain receptors, proprioceptors, and muscle spindles to alter muscle contraction very quickly, even before the information reaches the brain. The stretch reflex and withdrawal reflex are illustrative examples.

The stretch reflex can be demonstrated by tapping the patellar tendon (below the knee) with a rubber hammer, which results in contraction of the quadriceps muscle and elevation of the lower leg. Evaluation of deep tendon reflexes is helpful in localizing a motor abnormality to the PNS or CNS. The deep tendon reflex tests the reflex arc between the sensory muscle spindles and the α motor neurons. Tapping the tendon produces a quick stretch in the muscle fibers of the quadriceps muscle and stimulates the muscle spindles. The muscle spindle sends action potentials along neurons (group Ia) that enter the dorsal horn of the spinal cord and then synapse directly on α motor neurons in the anterior horn that activate the muscle in which the spindles lie (Figure 43-40). Other branches of the group Ia neurons make connections with antagonistic muscle groups and inhibit their contraction. The stretch reflex makes only one synapse (monosynaptic) and produces a very quick response in the muscle. The physiologic function of the muscle spindle stretch reflex is to provide feedback to α and γ motor neurons to adjust the strength of muscle contraction to match the load on the muscle.

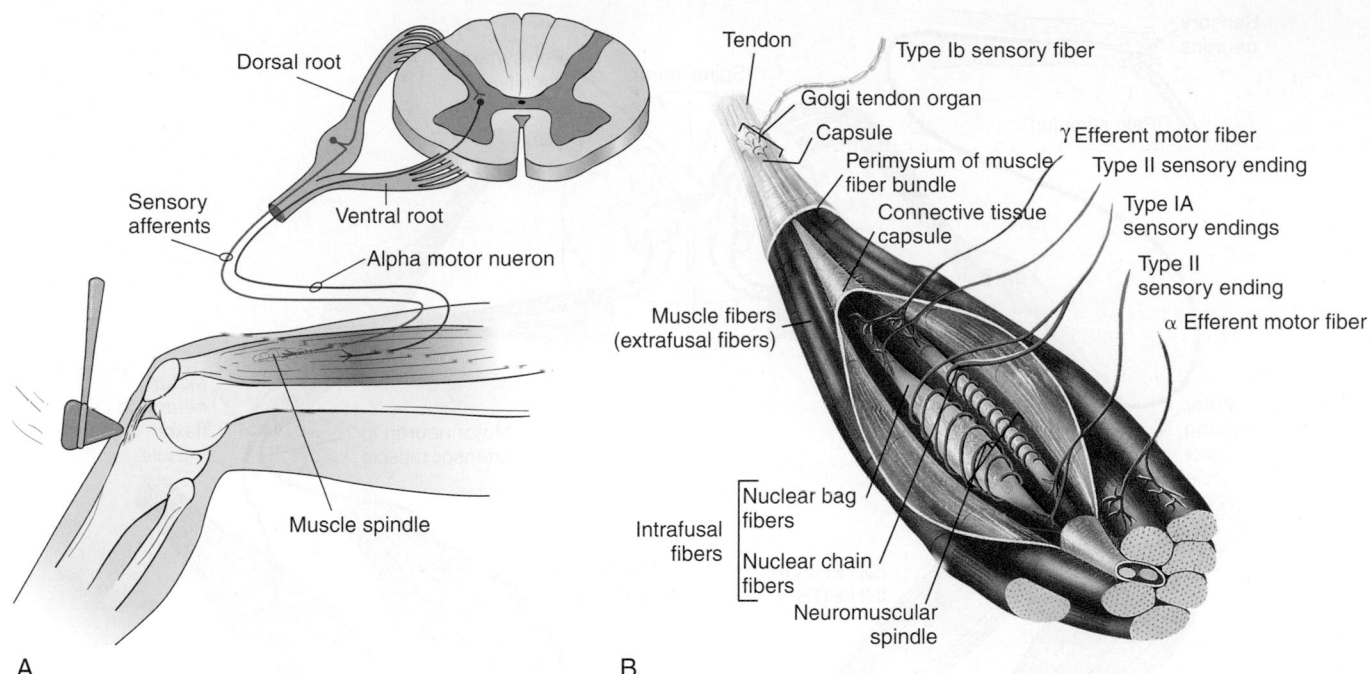

FIGURE 43-40 Diagram of the stretch reflex in which activation of the muscle spindle stimulates contraction of the stretched muscle. **A,** Stretch of the muscle sends action potentials to the cord, which make a monosynaptic connection to motor neurons from the same muscle fibers. **B,** Detailed view of the muscle spindle apparatus showing type 1 and type 2 sensory fibers that are large, myelinated, and rapidly conducting neurons that detect stretch. The γ motor neurons contract the spindle to keep it taut and sensitive to further stretch, while the α motor neurons contract the muscle fibers. Also shown in this figure is another stretch receptor located at the juncture between the muscle and the tendon called the *Golgi tendon organ*. Muscle shortening during contraction stimulates the Golgi tendon organ, causing it to send signals to the cord that inhibit muscle contraction. This is thought to protect the muscle from excessive contraction that could tear it from its tendon insertion points on the bone.

The withdrawal reflex is an important protective mechanism that allows reflexive withdrawal of a body part from a physical threat while simultaneously making postural adjustments to avoid loss of balance. The withdrawal reflex is polysynaptic, making connections with interneurons in the cord to affect muscles on both sides of the body. A simplified model of the withdrawal reflex is shown in Figure 43-41. Note that a painful stimulus to one extremity results in activation of flexor muscles and inhibition of extensor muscles on the ipsilateral side. This allows quick withdrawal of the extremity from the source of injury. Connections with muscle groups on the opposite side of the cord stimulate extensors and inhibit flexors to stabilize posture.

CENTRAL CONTROL OF MOTOR FUNCTION

Corticospinal tract neurons originate in the primary motor cortex, which is arranged in a similar manner to the somatosensory cortex. The motor homunculus map (Figure 43-42) shows that muscles of the face, lips, tongue, and hands occupy most of the cortical neurons. These areas have small motor units and produce fine-motor control. Corticospinal neurons from the primary motor cortex, in association with neuronal output from the premotor area and the supplemental motor cortex, activate α motor neurons to execute voluntary motor commands.

First, a motivation to move is needed to spur an individual to action. Little is known about motivation; however, signals from the limbic system are thought to be important. Circuits between the basal ganglia and association areas of the cerebral cortex plan the intended movement. Somewhat different circuits are involved in new situations, such as first learning to type, than are involved in the execution of learned, but subconscious, patterns of movement (e.g., typing 100 words per minute).[5] An important part of the planning process involves the somatosensory cortex, which provides information about the spatial coordinates of body parts in relation to the physical surroundings (e.g., placement of the fingers on the keyboard).

The cerebellum serves to adjust the timing and intensity of movements to improve the similarity between the intended and actual movements. Neurons in the cerebellum learn with practice. Visual, proprioceptive, and vestibular information is used by the cerebellum to make adjustments in the execution phase of the movement. In addition, the cerebellum functions with the cerebral cortex to make muscle adjustments in advance of the movement. For example, if a person is asked to lift what appears to be a pile of bricks, but the bricks are made of lightweight Styrofoam, the unsuspecting subject will throw the pile up into the air. Visual cues and past learned experiences are used to gauge the intensity of muscle contraction. The brain learns quickly, however, and if the subject is asked to repeat the maneuver, the intensity of muscle contraction will exactly match that needed to lift the load smoothly. Once a motor activity is well-learned and can be performed "automatically," the cerebellum participates less and the basal ganglia and cortical neurons are most active.[5]

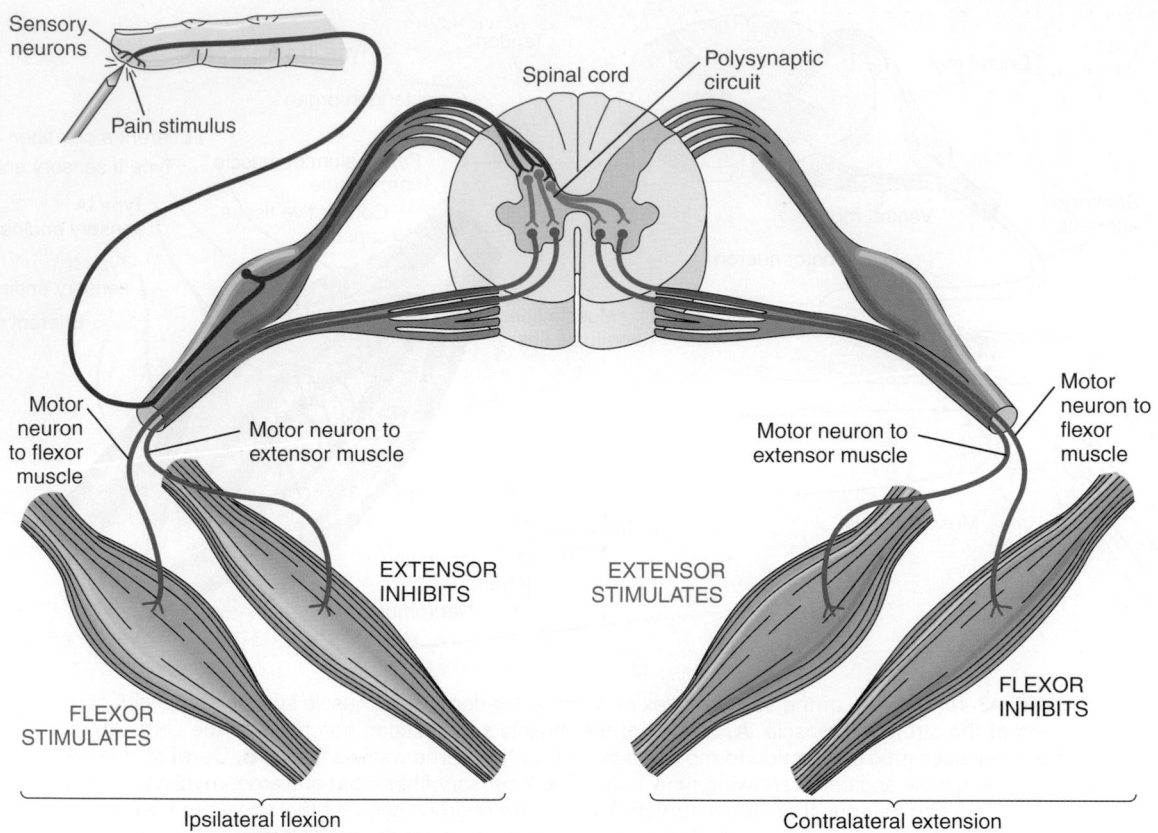

FIGURE 43-41 Neural connections mediating the flexor-withdrawal reflex.

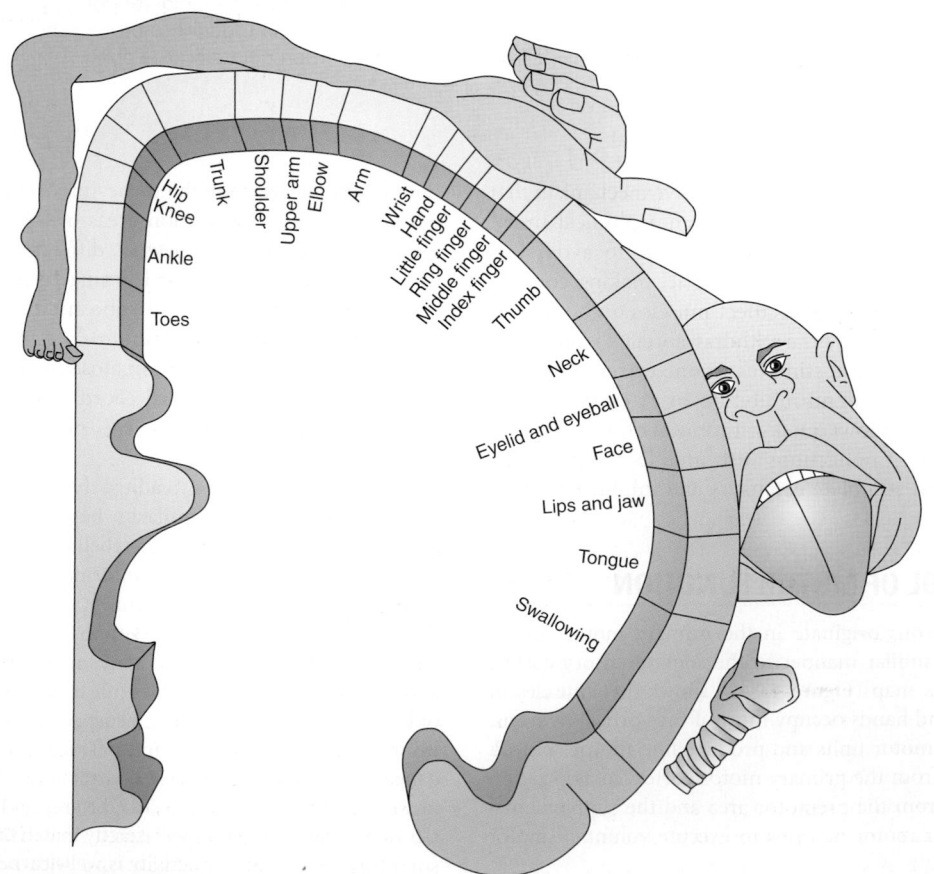

FIGURE 43-42 Cortical representation of the muscles of the body. Note the large area devoted to control of the hands and face.

KEY POINTS

- The body is somatotopically represented in the motor cortex. Stimulation of points in the primary motor cortex results in discrete movements in the contralateral side of the body.
- Projections from the motor cortex (corticospinal tract) travel by way of the internal capsule, cross over at the medulla, and travel down the contralateral spinal cord to synapse on α motor neurons in the anterior horn. The α motor neurons innervate skeletal muscle.
- Extrapyramidal tracts (tectospinal, vestibulospinal, reticulospinal) from subcortical nuclei innervate antigravity muscles and are primarily involved in balance, posture, and movement of large proximal muscle groups.
- A great deal of motor activity is preprogrammed into neuronal connections in the spinal cord. These connections produce reflexive alterations in muscle contraction in response to sensory information about the tension on the muscle or the need to move a body part away from a painful stimulus.
- The planning and execution of movements is accomplished through neuronal circuits between the basal ganglia and the premotor and association areas of the motor cortex. The cerebellum contributes primarily to the learning phase of a motor skill by making instantaneous adjustments in muscle force and timing to improve the match between the intended and the actual movement.

CONSCIOUSNESS, MEMORY, AND SLEEP

That the cerebral cortex is integral to the elaboration of complex thought, learning, memory, and so-called higher brain functions is well supported by lesion studies, yet little is known about the ways in which these higher functions are accomplished. Each thought involves neuronal circuits in portions of the cerebral cortex, thalamus, limbic system, and reticular formation of the brainstem. A thought or memory is not stored in any one place; rather, it is the outcome of a pattern or circuit of neuronal activation.[23] Neurons in the limbic system, especially the amygdala, are thought to determine the general emotional value of the thought as being pleasant, painful, or neutral, whereas neurons in the cerebral cortex add the specific details, including remembered sensations and visual and auditory images. Consciousness and memory are prerequisites to thinking.

CONSCIOUSNESS AND MEMORY

Consciousness can be defined as awareness of the surroundings and of one's own thoughts and sensations. The neural correlates of consciousness are not known; however, continuous activation of neuronal circuits between the thalamus and cortex and between the thalamus and brainstem are believed to be necessary.[24] Consciousness is assessed by the expression of motor behaviors, such as speech, response to questions, and body movements. However, behavioral responses are not necessarily an outcome of consciousness. A person completely paralyzed with neuromuscular blocking agents is still conscious even though all outward behaviors are suppressed. It is difficult to know the level of brain activity in an individual who cannot move. Brain waves are frequently measured in an attempt to assess brain activity, and a correlation with consciousness is assumed; α waves are thought to reflect search and retrieval functions and θ waves are associated with memory encoding tasks. Groups of neurons firing synchronously produce the regular oscillations of brain waves that seem to underlie consciousness. Much remains to be discovered before the phenomenon of consciousness and its counterpart, unconsciousness, are understood.

To think and learn, one must be able to remember past events and link them to current circumstances. Memory is a synaptic phenomenon in which neurons in the memory trace or circuit alter the efficiency of synaptic transmission. Greater stimulation of neurons in the memory circuit results in longer-lasting effects. Once the memory trace is established, it can be reactivated by the thinking mind to reproduce the memory. Reactivation by the mind is called *retrieval* and may be enhanced by rehearsal or by strategies to link the memory trace with associated circuits that are already established. Experiences that have important consequences, such as pain or pleasure, are usually enhanced and stored as memory traces, whereas experiences of little consequence may be suppressed. The value of a memory is determined primarily by the limbic system, which helps the brain learn to ignore information of little consequence (which can be construed as a form of negative memory, or remembering to ignore). This is an important function, because it prevents preoccupation and overload of brain circuits with useless stimuli.

Some memories last for a short time, and others persist for a lifetime. The mechanisms for different types of memory are mostly unknown; however, it is believed that short-term alteration of *presynaptic* neurons in the memory trace is responsible for short-term memory, whereas long-term memory requires more permanent changes in the *postsynaptic* neurons.[23] A certain time period is required for memories to be consolidated into long-term memory. An interruption of the consolidation phase, by head trauma, for example, results in loss of memory for events occurring just before the injury.

Some examples of presynaptic modulation are shown in Figure 43-43. The interaction between the presynaptic and postsynaptic neurons is modified by the activity of the modulating neuron. For example, the modulating neuron could send a signal from the limbic system to indicate that the incoming signal was important. The modulating neuron would then enhance neurotransmitter release from the presynaptic neuron to facilitate transmission to the postsynaptic cell. Presynaptic inhibition could suppress synaptic transmission by preventing or reducing the amount of neurotransmitter released from the presynaptic neuron.

Longer-term memory is thought to occur because of long-term changes in synaptic efficiency. In some cases memory may incorporate new neurons into the memory circuit. The hippocampus is an important limbic structure that must be intact for memory to be consolidated. It is also a site of neural stem cell proliferation, leading some to conclude that memory involves the growth of new neurons.[15] Changes in synaptic efficiency could include alterations in receptor number or structure and changes in the components of second messenger cascades. Protein synthesis in the involved neurons is necessary to consolidate long-term changes in synaptic efficiency.[23] Memories are thought to be stored in the brain in association with memories of similar qualities that share some of the same neuronal circuits. Information is added to the memory circuit that is already in place. This makes it easier to learn information that is connected to previously learned material. Learning something completely new, such as a foreign language, requires a great deal of rehearsal.

SLEEP

Sleep is a state of decreased arousal from which a person is easily awakened. Different levels of brain activity from wakefulness to deep sleep are characterized by different electroencephalographic waveforms. Brain waves become progressively slower and more synchronized with deeper levels of sleep. These waveforms are called α, β, θ, and δ waves (Figure 43-44). The α and β waves are found in awake individuals: α waves predominate during a relaxed state with the eyes closed; β waves occur during visual stimulation and with active problem solving. β waves are also apparent during a stage of sleep called *rapid eye movement* (REM) sleep. Both θ and δ waves occur during deep sleep.

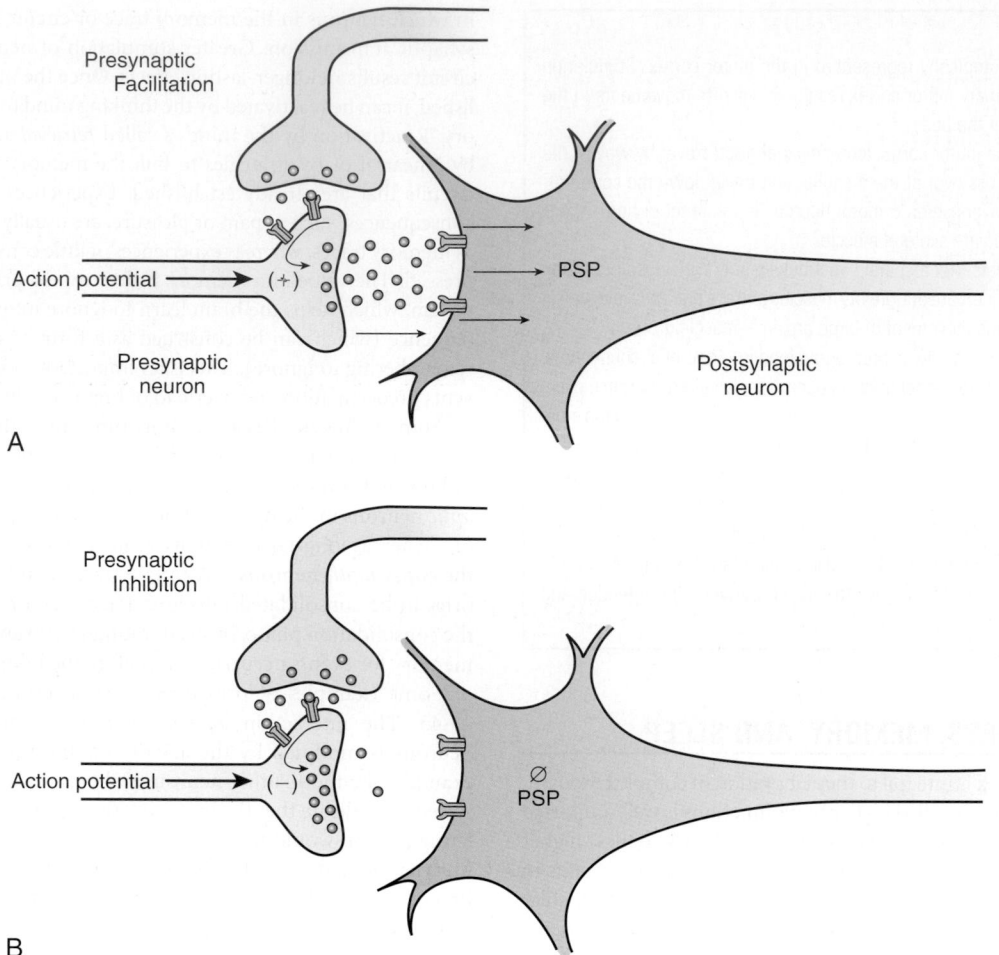

FIGURE 43-43 Example of a modulating neuron that terminates on the presynaptic cell and alters its response. **A,** Facilitation: The presynaptic neuron releases more neurotransmitter into the synapse when an action potential arrives. **B,** Inhibition: The presynaptic neuron releases less neurotransmitter into the synapse with each action potential. *PSP,* Postsynaptic potential.

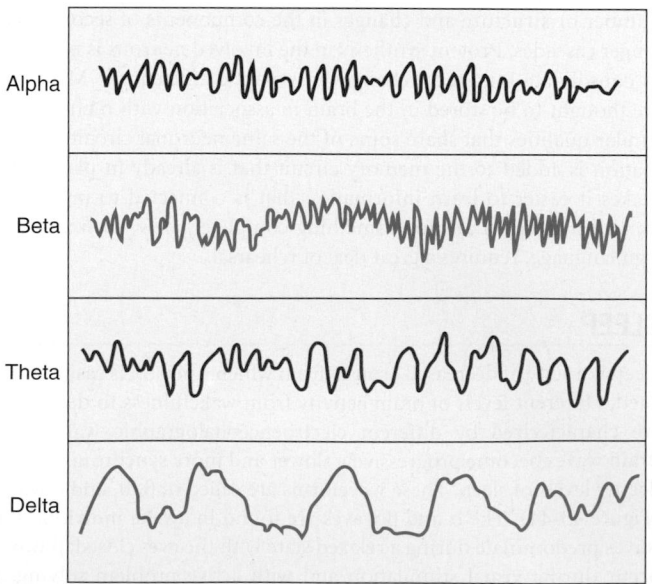

FIGURE 43-44 Brain waves are categorized according to frequency and synchrony as α, β, θ, and δ.

Most sleep is of the restful, slow-wave type of deep sleep. Interspersed at about 90-minute intervals are episodes of REM sleep, which last 5 to 30 minutes. REM sleep is characterized by irregular breathing and heartbeat, rapid eye movements, depressed muscle tone, and active dreaming.[25] The number and length of REM episodes usually increases over the course of the night. Individuals who have been awake for a prolonged period spend more time in deep sleep at the beginning of sleep and begin to have more REM sleep as the brain becomes more rested.[25] Dreams occur in both types of sleep but are more likely to be remembered when they occur during REM sleep.

The mechanisms of the sleep-wake cycle and the reason the brain needs to sleep are not well understood. Experiments in animals have demonstrated that sleep is an active process initiated by sleep-inducing substances within the brain. CSF removed from sleep-deprived animals promptly produces sleep when injected into another animal. Production of sleep-inducing substances within the brain occurs during wakefulness; they gradually accumulate, producing a desire to sleep. A period of sleep is thought to inhibit production of sleep-inducing chemicals, and they are cleared from the CNS.

The physiologic significance of sleep may be to rebalance synaptic transmission strength and to avoid the behavioral consequences of sleep deprivation.[25] Prolonged sleep deprivation produces hallucinations, disordered thought processes, and personality changes. It has been noted that the smaller the animal and the higher the metabolic rate, the greater the sleep requirement. Non-REM sleep is associated with lowering of metabolism and body temperature and may provide an opportunity to avoid or repair metabolism-induced brain damage. REM sleep is associated with an active brain; however, certain types of neurons—those that secrete amines—are turned off during REM sleep. The younger and more immature brain spends more time in REM sleep, and some have speculated that the brain is laying down circuits for genetically programmed or instinctive neural pathways.[25]

KEY POINTS

- Thoughts and memories are not stored in a particular location in the brain; rather, they are the outcome of activation of neurons in a neuronal circuit.
- Memories are stored by altering the synaptic efficiency of neurons in the memory trace. Short-term memory is thought to result from presynaptic mechanisms, whereas long-term memory is consolidated by more permanent changes in the postsynaptic neurons.
- Sleep is characterized as REM sleep (β waves) and deep sleep (θ and δ waves). Most sleep is of the deep-sleep variety, interspersed with periods of REM activity at about 90-minute intervals. Sleep is an active process produced by sleep-inducing chemicals in the brain. The reason that the brain requires sleep remains unknown.

SUMMARY

The nervous system is a complex network of neurons and supporting cells that provides the body with a rapid means of communication. The anatomy of the nervous system has been extensively studied, but the functional mechanisms of thought, memory, emotion, and sleep are poorly understood. The nervous system can be partially understood by examining the function of individual neurons and their synaptic connections. Neural communication occurs primarily through the secretion of neurotransmitters into synapses between neurons. Neurotransmitters bind to specific receptors to exert their effects on the membrane potential of the target cell.

Activation of groups of neurons in a particular circuit is the basis for neuronal processing of information, thoughts, and memories and for learning. Although certain brain locations have been associated with particular functions, most brain activities require participation by neurons in widespread locations. The ability of the nervous system to learn and adapt is remarkable in the early childhood period, and a significant degree of neural plasticity is maintained throughout life. However, damage to large numbers of neurons in a particular location usually results in significant disability because mature neurons cannot regenerate and neural stem cells may not survive or establish appropriate connections.

REFERENCES

1. Nolte J: *The human brain: an introduction to its functional anatomy*, ed 6, St Louis, 2008, Mosby.
2. Hall JE: Cerebral blood flow, cerebrospinal fluid, and brain metabolism. In Hall JE, editor: *Guyton & Hall textbook of medical physiology*, ed 12, Philadelphia, 2011, Saunders, pp 743–750.
3. Liebner S, Czupalla CJ, Wolburg H: Current concepts of blood-brain barrier development, *Int J Dev Biol* 55:467–476, 2011.
4. Hall JE: Somatic sensations: I. General organization, the tactile and position senses. In Hall JE, editor: *Guyton & Hall textbook of medical physiology*, ed 12, Philadelphia, 2011, Saunders, pp 571–582.
5. Rothwell JC: The motor functions of the basal ganglia, *J Integr Neurosci* 10(3):303–315, 2011.
6. Penhune VB, Steele CJ: Parallel contributions of cerebellar, striatal and M1 mechanisms to motor sequence learning, *Behav Brain Res* 226(2):579–591, 2012.
7. Chen JJ, Nelson MV, Swope DM: Parkinson's disease. In Dipiro J, et al, editors: *Pharmacotherapy: a pathophysiologic approach*, ed 8, New York, 2011, McGraw-Hill, pp 1033–1044.
8. Smith Y, et al: The thalamostriatal systems: anatomical and functional organization in normal and parkinsonian states, *Brain Res Bull* 78(2-3):60–68, 2009.
9. Oberdick J, Sillitoe RV: Cerebellar zones: history, development, and function, *Cerebellum* 10(3):301–306, 2011.
10. Patton KT, Thibodeau GA: Central nervous system. In Patton KT, Thibodeau GA, editors: *Anatomy & physiology*, ed 7, St Louis, 2010, Mosby, pp 412–454.
11. Hall JE: The autonomic nervous system and the adrenal medulla. In Hall JE, editor: *Guyton & Hall textbook of medical physiology*, ed 12, Philadelphia, 2011, Saunders, pp 729–742.
12. Patton KT, Thibodeau GA: Peripheral nervous system. In Patton KT, Thibodeau GA, editors: *Anatomy & physiology*, ed 7, St Louis, 2010, Mosby, pp 455–492.
13. Patton KT, Thibodeau GA: Nervous system cells. In Patton KT, Thibodeau GA, editors: *Anatomy & physiology*, ed 7, St Louis, 2010, Mosby, pp 372–411.
14. Saijo K, Glass CK: Microglial cell origin and phenotypes in health and disease, *Nat Rev Immunol* 11(11):775–787, 2011.
15. Zhao C, Deng W, Gage FH: Mechanisms and functional implications of adult neurogenesis, *Cell* 132(4):645–660, 2008.
16. Hall JE: Organization of the nervous system, basic functions of synapses and neurotransmitters. In Hall JE, editor: *Guyton & Hall textbook of medical physiology*, ed 12, Philadelphia, 2011, Saunders, pp 543–558.
17. Vincent SR: Nitric oxide neurons and neurotransmission, *Prog Neurobiol* 90(2):246–255, 2010.
18. Anthony DC, Frosch MP, De Girolami U: Peripheral nerve and skeletal muscle. In Kumar V, et al, editors: *Robbins and Cotran pathologic basis of disease*, ed 8, Philadelphia, 2010, Saunders, pp 1257–1277.
19. Hensch TK: Critical period plasticity in local cortical circuits, *Nat Rev Neurosci* 6(11):877–888, 2005.
20. LeBlanc JJ, Fagiolini M: Autism: a "critical period" disorder? *Neural Plast* 921680, 2011. (Epub).
21. Medana IM, Esiri MM: Axonal damage: a key predictor of outcome in human CNS diseases, *Brain* 126:515–530, 2003.
22. Rubinson K, Lang E: The somatosensory system. In Koeppen BM, Stanton BA, editors: *Berne & Levy physiology*, ed 6, Philadelphia, 2010, Mosby, pp 105–122.
23. Richter-Levin G, Akirav I: Emotional tagging of memory formation—in the search for neural mechanisms, *Brain Res Rev* 43:247–256, 2003.
24. Ward LM: The thalamic dynamic core theory of conscious experience, *Conscious Cogn* 20(2):464–486, 2011.
25. Hanlon EC, et al: Synaptic potentiation and sleep need: clues from molecular and electrophysiological studies, *Curr Top Med Chem* 11(19):2472–2482, 2011.

Acute Disorders of Brain Function

Joni D. Marsh and Jacquelyn L. Banasik

℮volve WEBSITE

KEY QUESTIONS

- What are the proposed mechanisms and potential consequences of secondary brain injury?
- Which brain components determine intracranial pressure, and under what conditions might each contribute to elevated intracranial pressure?
- How are level of consciousness and cranial nerve reflexes used to assess changes in neurologic status in the brain-injured patient?
- What are the common manifestations of types of traumatic brain injury (focal, polar, diffuse) and hemorrhage (epidural, subdural, subarachnoid)?
- How do the three most common causes of stroke (thrombi, emboli, and hemorrhage) differ with regard to risk factors, prevention strategies, and acute management?

- How do the clinical manifestations of ischemic stroke vary depending on the location of cerebral artery obstruction?
- What are the common long-term sequelae of stroke, and how are they managed?
- What are the causes and usual presentations of cerebral aneurysm and arteriovenous malformation?
- How do meningitis and encephalitis differ with regard to usual infective organisms, cerebrospinal fluid analysis findings, clinical manifestations, and treatment?

CHAPTER OUTLINE

CHAPTER OUTLINE—cont'd

Disorders of brain function can result from a wide variety of pathophysiologic processes. The focus of this chapter is on primary causes of acute brain injury including brain trauma, cerebrovascular disease, brain hemorrhage, and central nervous system (CNS) infections. These conditions are acute because they generally have a sudden onset and progress rapidly. Thus, early detection and prompt management are necessary to prevent death and minimize morbidity. However, the majority of patients who survive acute injury to brain structures will be left with some degree of permanent neurologic damage and chronic dysfunction. The designation of acute and chronic disorders is, therefore, somewhat arbitrary. The chronic aspects of neurologic diseases, including seizure disorders and dementias, are discussed in Chapter 45. Acute neurologic dysfunction often is a complication of diseases primarily affecting other systems. Hypoglycemia, renal failure, liver failure, human immunodeficiency virus infection, drug overdoses, fluid imbalances, and many other abnormalities may cause acute brain dysfunction. Accurate determination of the source of acute alterations in brain function is an important step in developing an appropriate treatment plan. However, there are many common elements in the pathogenesis of acute brain injuries, regardless of etiologic factors. These cellular aspects are presented as a foundation for understanding the specific disorders that follow.

MECHANISMS OF BRAIN INJURY

The mechanisms of brain injury are varied, complex, and incompletely understood. Mechanical trauma, ischemia, cellular energy failure, reperfusion injury, excitotoxins, edema, vascular failure, and injury-induced apoptosis (programmed cell death) are all factors thought to be operative in most kinds of acute brain injury. These mechanisms are often separated into two categories: *primary injury* and *secondary injury*.

The primary injury is that which occurs immediately at the onset of brain injury. This definition implies that there is little that can be done to reverse the process once it has occurred. For example, in the case of head trauma, some tissues will be irreversibly damaged at the time of impact owing to mechanical forces. This damage represents the primary injury. Similarly, with the sudden cessation of blood flow to an area of brain tissue, as occurs in stroke, an area of irreversible ischemia in cells may develop quickly, and this constitutes the primary injury. Brain tissue necrosis occurs rapidly as cells lose membrane integrity, rupture, and release their intracellular contents into the extracellular space. Cytotoxic edema quickly follows, which can cause deleterious effects to surrounding brain tissue.

Secondary injury refers to the development of further neurologic damage subsequent to the primary injury, and this may progress over days or weeks. Delayed cell death may involve necrosis from further acute injury or may be a delayed consequence of the primary injury. Cells that die slowly after injury are said to undergo apoptosis or programmed cell death. Apoptosis requires energy and protein synthesis, and the cells shrink and die in a tidy fashion without releasing their internal contents. Necrosis follows severe ischemic injury, whereas apoptosis is associated with moderate injury. A critical factor in determining the neuronal cell fate after injury is the degree of adenosine triphosphate (ATP) depletion. If ATP levels fall profoundly, increased membrane permeability and necrosis ensue. If the ATP level is partially maintained for a period of time after the injury, apoptosis is the likely consequence. Mild reductions in the amount of ATP are associated with reversible injury and cellular recovery.[1] ATP level reduction is a consequence of ischemia and hypoxia, which accompany many types of acute brain injury including trauma and stroke.

Mechanisms of secondary injury are the subject of much interest because of the potential to effectively intervene to limit brain damage. Unfortunately, effective means of preventing secondary damage have remained elusive, leading to high rates of mortality and morbidity. The effort to elucidate mechanisms of secondary injury and develop effective treatments would seem worthwhile because the degree of primary injury is thought to be small in most cases.[2] Thus, the high rates of mortality and morbidity may be attributed in large part to mechanisms of secondary injury.

Ischemia and Hypoxia

Ischemia occurs when the delivery of oxygenated blood is below the level needed to meet metabolic demands of the brain tissue. Ischemia is a contributing factor in most forms of acute brain injury, either as the primary insult (e.g., stroke) or as part of the secondary response to injury (e.g., vasospasm, vascular compression, or abnormal autoregulation). Hypoxia is a deficiency of oxygen at the cellular level, which may occur as a result of decreased blood flow (ischemia) or decreased blood oxygenation (hypoxemia). In practice, ischemia and hypoxia usually occur together and are considered together in this discussion. Ischemia results in immediate neurologic dysfunction because of the inability of neurons to generate the ATP needed for energy-requiring processes. In addition, ischemia sets the stage for secondary injury by oxygen free radicals, excitatory amino acids, and inflammatory cells.

Cellular Energy Failure

Neuronal tissue is highly sensitive to oxygen deprivation because it has great ATP requirements and limited capacity for anaerobic metabolism during ischemia. The normal brain receives about 15% of the total cardiac output and garners 20% of the body's oxygen consumption (750 ml/min), despite contributing only 2% of the body weight.[1] Neurons are dependent on glucose for production of ATP; however, they store little in the form of glycogen. Thus, when oxygen supply is decreased, not only is oxidative phosphorylation impaired, but also the low supply of stored glucose restricts anaerobic production of ATP. Brain cells tolerate loss of ATP for several minutes; about 5 to

10 minutes of complete occlusion is necessary for irreversible brain damage in humans. Complete occlusion of blood flow is rare but even a partial occlusion, if allowed to continue for a sufficient amount of time, may produce irreversible brain damage. Once blood flow to cerebral neurons diminishes, two mechanisms can independently lead to brain cell death: anaerobic metabolism and deterioration of ion gradients.

A general sequence of events following acute brain ischemia has been proposed (Figure 44-1).[3] The critical event is mitochondrial dysfunction owing to lack of cellular oxygen. Recall that oxygen is required to accept electrons from the mitochondrial electron transport chain. In the absence of oxygen, the transport proteins and cytochromes remain reduced and unable to accept any more electrons from the Krebs cycle (tricarboxylic acid cycle). Anaerobic glycolytic pathways are initiated in the affected region to compensate for the loss of oxygen and to provide a source of energy. Glycolysis may continue for a short time, producing pyruvate, which is converted to lactate. However, this conversion releases H^+ and contributes to cellular acidosis, a damaging by-product of glycolysis. Toxicity of hydrogen ions leads to loss of neuronal integrity.

Inadequate energy supply leads to deterioration of ion gradients. Most of the ATP used by neurons is for maintenance of ion gradients across the plasma membrane. The sodium-potassium (Na^+-K^+) pump consumes three fourths of the ATP in a typical neuron. Anoxic depolarization causes potassium to leave the cell and sodium, chloride, and calcium ions to enter. Energy also is required to maintain calcium balance and regulate neurotransmitter synthesis and reuptake. Not surprisingly, energy failure results in neuronal dysfunction, injury, and, if severe or prolonged, necrotic cell death. Ischemia also is the probable inciting factor for apoptosis (see Chapter 4).

The mitochondria are also important regulators of calcium ion concentration in the cell. The mitochondrial membrane contains calcium transporters that sequester calcium ions within the mitochondria when cytoplasmic calcium levels are elevated. Mitochondrial energy failure impairs the ability of mitochondria to perform this sequestering function. Thus, the mitochondria become severely overloaded with calcium, which activates enzymes (phospholipases) that damage mitochondrial membrane structures. Ischemic cells are prone to calcium overload because pumps that move calcium out of the cell are energy dependent. Calcium ions have a large electrochemical gradient for diffusion into the neuron and tend to accumulate intracellularly.

Unfortunately, the activity of many intracellular enzymes is regulated by intracellular calcium. Calcium overload is thought to be a critical factor leading to activation of enzyme cascades, which disrupt function and cause irreversible damage to cell membranes (lipid peroxidation). One might speculate that measures to inhibit calcium entry into damaged cells would be of therapeutic benefit. One way to reduce calcium influx is by administration of calcium channel–blocking agents. These drugs block voltage-gated calcium channels. Unfortunately, clinical trials with calcium channel–blocking agents have failed to show benefit.[2] Other avenues for inhibiting calcium overload are being investigated, including those that block the effect of glutamate receptors as described in the following section.

Excitatory Amino Acids

Calcium may gain entry into cells by portals other than voltage-gated channels. Glutamate is an excitatory amino acid neurotransmitter thought to be important in learning and memory. Overstimulation of neurons by glutamate is associated with cell injury, leading to its designation as an *excitotoxin*. Glutamate binds two kinds of receptors that

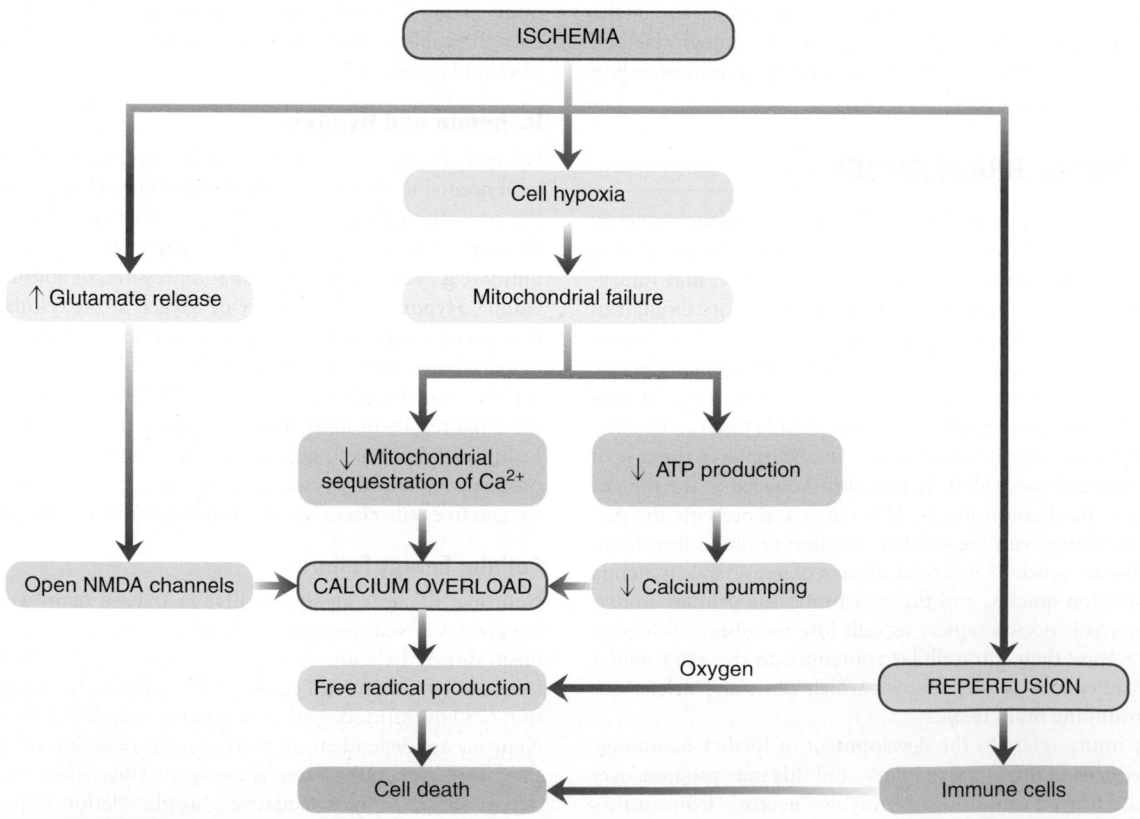

FIGURE 44-1 Sequence of neuronal cell injury following acute ischemia. Calcium overload is a key event in producing cellular damage.

are linked to the opening of ion channels in the plasma membrane of neurons. N-methyl-D-aspartate (NMDA) receptors have received the most attention, but α-amino-3-hydroxy-5-methyl-4-isoxazolepropionate (AMPA) channels are also thought to contribute to the neurotoxic effects of glutamate. Activation of AMPA receptors results in opening of Na^+ channels in the membrane, which leads to depolarization. Depolarization then affects the NMDA channels by removing a Mg^{2+} ion that usually blocks the NMDA channel (Figure 44-2). Subsequent binding of glutamate to the NMDA receptor opens it and allows Ca^{2+} to enter the cell accompanied by inflow of water, which results in cytotoxic edema, a rapid swelling of neurons. As previously described, calcium overload mediates a cascade of events leading to cell injury.

The amount of glutamate in the synapses is usually tightly regulated by release and reuptake controls. In the presence of neuronal injury, excessive glutamate may be released because of impaired membrane integrity. With concomitant ischemia, reuptake mechanisms fail to remove excess glutamate from the synapse because they are energy-dependent processes. Excess glutamate stimulates nearby neurons, which then take up large amounts of injurious calcium ions. Small neurons in the cerebral cortex and hippocampus are particularly prone to glutamate excitotoxicity, and selective damage in these areas may occur. In addition to the calcium overload mechanism of injury, NMDA receptor activation stimulates nitric oxide (NO) production in neurons. NO is a neurotransmitter, but in excess it may increase the production of reactive nitrogen species (RNS), which function as free radicals to damage cellular components. The potential neuroprotective effects of controlling glutamate release or activity have been investigated but have not clearly shown efficacy in improving outcomes.[2]

Reperfusion Injury

Reestablishing perfusion to an area of prior ischemia is a matter of great urgency if neuronal tissue is to be salvaged. The longer and more

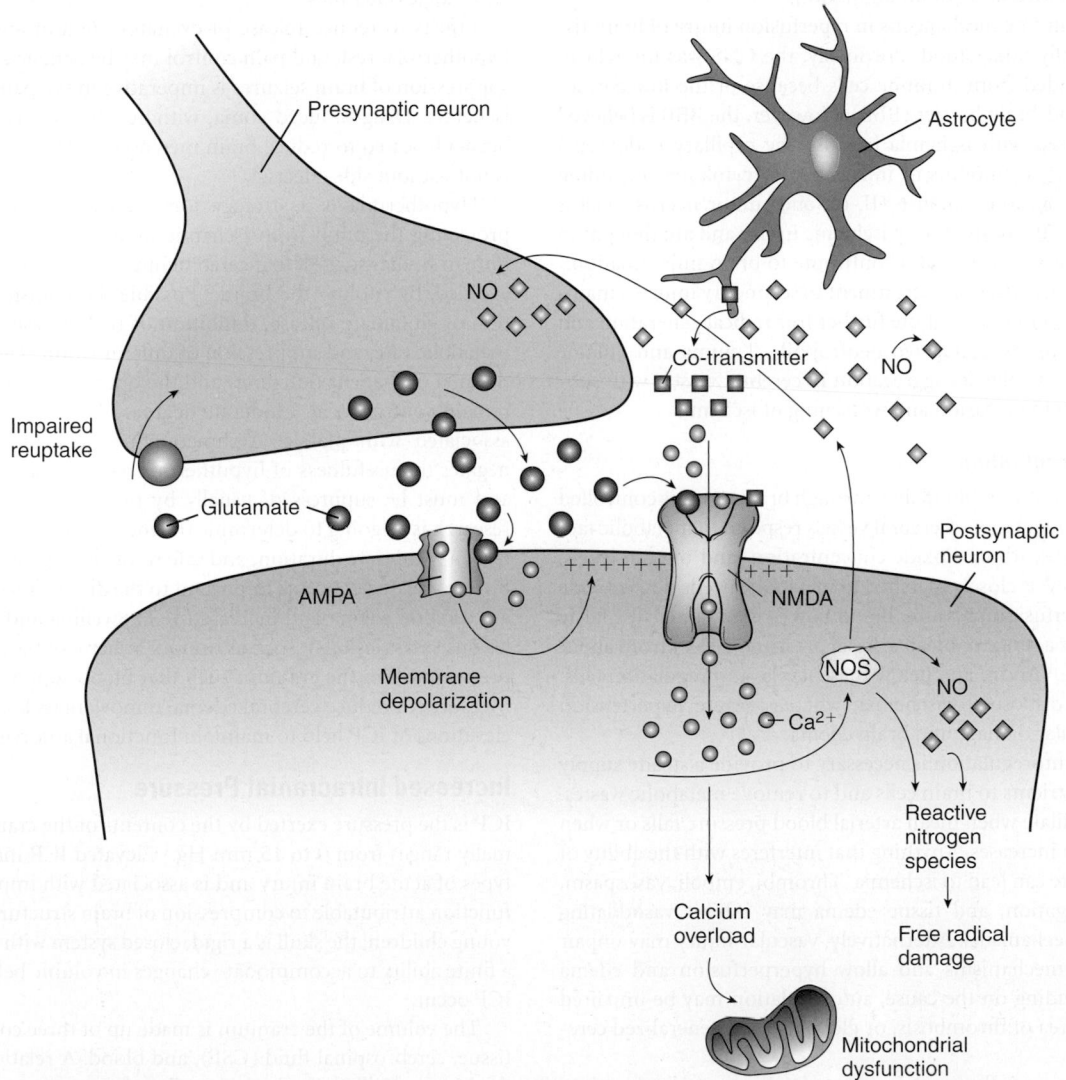

FIGURE 44-2 Mechanism of glutamate-mediated calcium influx. Impaired removal of glutamate from the synapse by energy-requiring reuptake mechanisms on the presynaptic membrane contributes to excessive glutamate in the synapse. Glutamate binds to the N-methyl-D-aspartate (NMDA) channel, causing it to open and allow calcium influx. A previous depolarization is necessary to remove the Mg^{2+} that normally blocks the channel. Excessive calcium entry impairs mitochondrial function and triggers nitric oxide production. Excessive nitric oxide can increase cell damage through free radical production. AMPA, α-Amino-3-hydroxy-5-methyl-4-isoxazolepropionate; NO, nitric oxide; NOS, nitric oxide synthase.

severe the period of ischemia, the greater the extent of necrosis. However, previously ischemic cells face new dangers with the return of blood flow. In particular, the return of oxygen brings the potential for oxygen free radical formation, and the flow of blood allows inflammatory cells to invade the area. The secondary injury that occurs after reestablishing blood flow has been termed *reperfusion injury* and has been studied extensively in cardiac tissues. The mechanisms in the brain appear to be similar. During the period of ischemia, brain cells accumulate substrates for oxidative phosphorylation, including the free radical–forming metabolites of adenosine monophosphate (AMP), xanthine, and hypoxanthine. When oxygen reenters the cell, erratic transfer of electrons to oxygen can produce a number of reactive oxygen products that behave as free radicals, damaging cell structures. These include hydroxyl radicals ($OH^{\cdot}$), superoxide (O_2^-), and peroxide (H_2O_2). Cell membranes may undergo lipid peroxidation in response to free radical damage, with subsequent formation of arachidonic acid. The arachidonic acid cascade yields more oxygen free radicals as well as mediators of inflammation.[2]

The role of immune mechanisms in reperfusion injury of brain tissue is only partially understood. Previously, the CNS was thought to be relatively shielded from immune cells because of the low permeability of the blood-brain barrier (BBB). However, the BBB is believed to be compromised with ischemia because the capillary endothelial cells are injured. The amounts of inflammatory cytokines, including interleukin-1 (IL-1), interleukin-6 (IL-6), and tumor necrosis factor (TNF), increase in the brain during ischemic injury and are thought to attract neutrophils to the area and contribute to brain inflammation.[4] The importance of neutrophil recruitment to secondary injury remains controversial, but it may contribute further free radical generation and vascular obstruction by aggregated neutrophils. Trauma and inflammation also promote platelet aggregation in cerebral vessels with subsequent reduction in perfusion and worsening of ischemia.

Abnormal Autoregulation

Under normal conditions, blood flow through brain tissue is controlled primarily by autoregulation. Cerebral vessels respond to metabolic factors including pH, carbon dioxide concentration, and oxygen levels. Cerebral blood flow is closely matched to metabolic needs despite wide fluctuations in perfusion pressure. Blood flow is maintained at a fairly constant rate over a range of mean arterial pressure (MAP) from about 50 to 150 mm Hg.[1] Above and below these levels, autoregulation fails. Hypotension predisposes to ischemia, whereas severe hypertension may lead to vascular damage and brain edema.

Appropriate autoregulation is necessary to provide a steady supply of oxygen and nutrients to brain cells and to remove metabolic wastes. Cerebral vessels dilate when mean arterial blood pressure falls or when brain metabolism increases. Anything that interferes with the ability of the vessels to dilate can lead to ischemia. Thrombi, emboli, vasospasm, neutrophil aggregation, and tissue edema may inhibit vasodilating autoregulatory mechanisms. Alternatively, vascular injury may impair vasoconstricting mechanisms and allow hyperperfusion and edema formation. Depending on the cause, autoregulation may be impaired locally, as in an area of thrombosis, or globally, as in generalized cerebral edema.

Autoregulation is influenced by the partial pressures of carbon dioxide ($Paco_2$) and oxygen (Pao_2) in the arterial blood. The response to a change in $Paco_2$ is very brisk: as $Paco_2$ levels fall, cerebral vessels constrict, and as $Paco_2$ levels rise, the cerebral vessels dilate. A rise in $Paco_2$ can increase cerebral blood flow significantly. The response to changes in Pao_2 is much less dramatic.

The autoregulatory response to $Paco_2$ remains robust, except in severely brain-injured patients, and can cause detrimental increases in

cerebral blood flow when respiratory compromise leads to hypercapnia. Excessive cerebral blood volume can exacerbate cerebral edema. Conversely, hyperventilation to produce low $Paco_2$ results in prompt vasoconstriction and, often, a reduction in intracranial pressure (ICP). Hyperventilation had been used for many years as standard therapy in the treatment of patients with increased ICP. However, prolonged hyperventilation does more harm than good because it critically reduces cerebral blood flow to responsive vessels and triggers tissue ischemia in these areas.

Loss of matching between oxygen supply and demand occurs when autoregulatory mechanisms fail. Cerebral oxygen demand is correlated with the degree of neuronal activity and may vary widely in different regions within the brain. Excessive levels of catecholamines or excitatory amino acids can significantly increase cerebral metabolism. In the context of impaired blood flow, these neurotransmitters may contribute to ischemia by increasing cerebral oxygen demand. Likewise, seizure activity increases neuronal metabolism and leads to worsening neurologic outcomes.[5]

Efforts to reduce release of excitatory neurotransmitters through hypothermia, rest, and pain control may be beneficial. Pharmacologic suppression of brain seizures is imperative in the patient with cerebral ischemia. Drug-induced coma, with agents such as barbiturates, has been advocated to reduce brain metabolism. However, this treatment is not without side effects.[2]

Hypothermia is a strategy for reducing brain metabolism and protecting the brain from ischemic injury. A number of animal and human studies suggest that cerebral injury can be delayed, and possibly avoided, by cooling the brain.[6] Possible mechanisms include inhibition of glutamate release, inhibition of IL-1 release, reduced cerebral metabolic rate, and suppression of inflammation. The effects of hypothermia on patient outcomes and the optimal degree of hypothermia remain controversial. Moderate degrees of cooling (28° to 32° C) are associated with platelet dysfunction and coagulopathy.[6] Shivering negates the usefulness of hypothermia by increasing oxygen demand, and must be suppressed, usually by pharmacologic means. Further research is ongoing to determine the therapeutic window for effectiveness, appropriate duration, and safe rewarming protocols.[6,7]

Two related concepts important to the discussion of autoregulation are cerebral edema and increased ICP. Swelling and space-occupying lesions (mass lesions), such as tumors or hematomas, may increase the pressure within the cranium such that blood supply is compromised. Measures to reduce cerebral edema, remove mass lesions, and prevent elevations of ICP help to maintain functional autoregulation.

Increased Intracranial Pressure

ICP is the pressure exerted by the contents of the cranium, and it normally ranges from 0 to 15 mm Hg.[1] Elevated ICP may occur in most types of acute brain injury and is associated with impaired neurologic function attributable to compression of brain structures. In all but very young children, the skull is a rigid, closed system with a set volume and a finite ability to accommodate changes in volume before elevations in ICP occur.

The volume of the cranium is made up of three components: brain tissue, cerebrospinal fluid (CSF), and blood. A relationship known as the Monro-Kellie hypothesis describes the compensatory responses to a change in volume in any of the three components.[8] A slight increase in one component can be offset by a reduction in the volume of the other two. An increase in brain volume, as might occur with cerebral edema, can be offset by a reduction in the CSF space and the space occupied by the cerebral vasculature. The ability to accommodate changes in volume without significant increases in pressure is called *compliance*. Intracranial compliance is limited because of the rigid skull; although

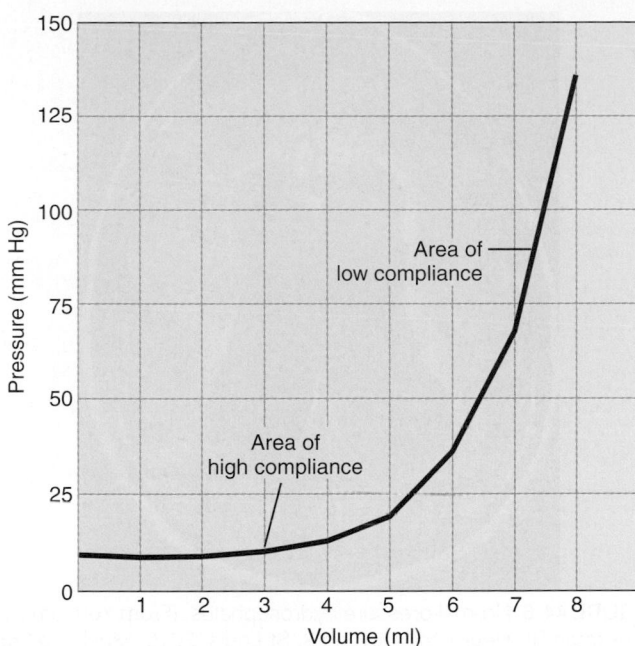

FIGURE 44-3 A volume-pressure curve showing intracranial compliance. Small increases in volume have little effect on pressure, but larger increases exceed the ability to compensate, and pressure rises dramatically.

small increases in intracranial volume may be absorbed, moderate changes result in significant increases in ICP (Figure 44-3).

Each of the cranial components has a varying capability to compensate for the others. Cerebral blood vessels can reduce their volume through vasoconstriction. The CSF compartment is capable of significant reduction in volume by shunting CSF to the spinal cord or into the venous system via the arachnoid villi. The brain parenchyma has little ability to reduce its volume to compensate for CSF or blood volume expansion. In young children, an increase in ICP may manifest as an increase in head circumference. This occurs because the cranial bones have not yet fused, and the skull can expand to accommodate the increased intracranial volume.

In the healthy brain, transient changes in ICP are common and well tolerated. Sneezing, coughing, straining, and head-dependent positions all cause elevated ICP, but they are without consequence because ICP quickly returns to normal. In the brain-injured person, however, transient elevations in ICP can be very dangerous and poorly tolerated.

Etiology. The most common causes of increased ICP include stroke, trauma, and tumors, but many other primary and secondary disorders can cause significant elevations in ICP (Box 44-1). These disorders have common features in that they all affect the volume of CSF, blood, or brain tissue. An increase in brain tissue volume commonly occurs from conditions that cause cerebral edema. Edema of brain tissues is due to accumulation of fluid in interstitial or intracellular spaces.

Interstitial edema is usually secondary to an increase in capillary pressure, damage to the capillary endothelium from a chemical injury, or a sudden increase in vascular pressure beyond autoregulatory limits. This type of edema has been termed *vasogenic*, and it results in extravasation of electrolytes, proteins, and fluid into the intercellular space. Vasogenic edema is a consequence of stroke, ischemia, and severe hypertension, and may occur surrounding brain tumors. The edema is often localized to a particular brain region where the BBB has been disrupted. Thus the swelling may be unilateral, occurring in one brain hemisphere or the other. Unilateral swelling often is poorly tolerated

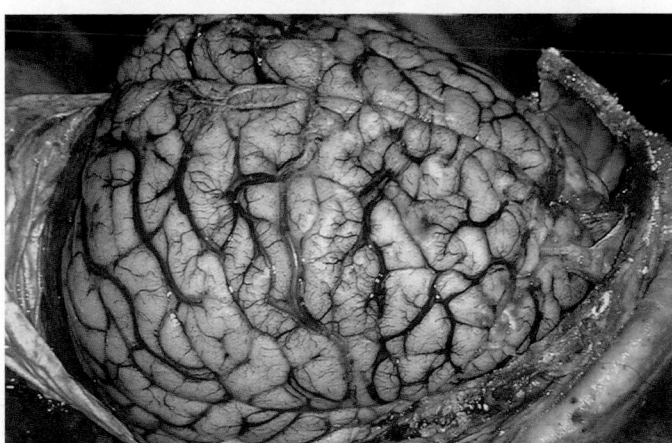

FIGURE 44-4 Generalized brain edema with increased intracranial pressure. The convolutions of the brain surface (gyri) are flattened, and the space between them is reduced. (From Kumar V, Cotran R, *Robbins S: Robbins basic pathology*, ed 9, Philadelphia, 2013, Saunders.)

because midbrain structures are compressed, and can lead to shifting of cerebral tissue or brain herniation.

Intracellular edema, called *cytotoxic edema*, occurs when ischemic tissue swells because of cellular energy failure. A lack of ATP allows Na^+ to accumulate in the cell, creating an osmotic force to draw in water. Cytotoxic edema predominates in cases of global ischemia. Global ischemia occurs when oxygenation of the whole brain is impaired, as would occur with cardiac arrest or severe hypoxemia. Generalized brain edema flattens the gyri and reduces the spaces between them (Figure 44-4).

In many cases of acute brain injury, vasogenic and cytotoxic edema occur together. Cerebral edema, when severe, can start a cyclic process that promotes further edema of increasing severity and contributes to increased ICP. As edema fluid collects, it compresses local vessels, preventing adequate blood and oxygen from reaching the cells. This results in ischemia, which in turn triggers vasodilation and increased capillary pressure, further fluid leakage into the injured tissue, and increased edema. Vasogenic edema tends to be a delayed process in terms of the secondary effects of brain injury, progressively worsening during the first several days after injury. Clearance of brain edema occurs primarily by absorption into the CSF system.[1]

In addition to edema, a number of space-occupying processes, such as tumors, hematomas, and abscesses, can increase intracranial volume

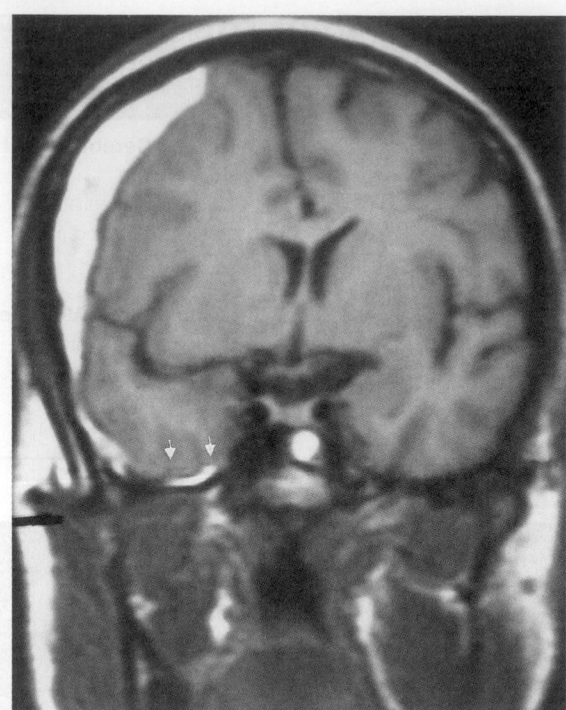

FIGURE 44-5 Right subacute subdural hematoma on weighted CT scan. Note the shift in midline structures. (From Yousem DM, Grossman RI: *Neuroradiology*, ed 3, St Louis, 2010, Mosby, p 174.)

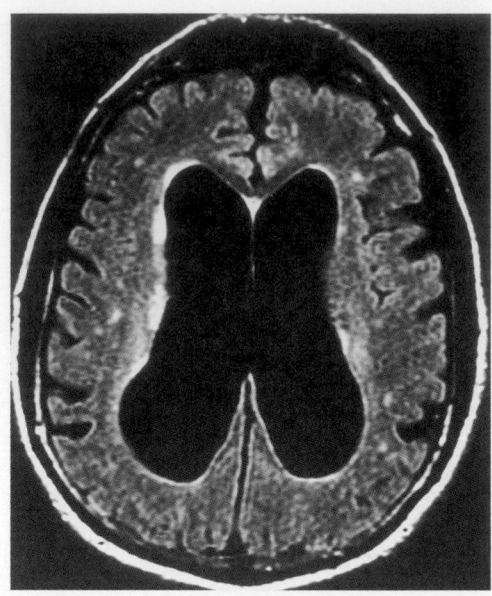

FIGURE 44-6 Normal-pressure hydrocephalus. (From Yousem DM, Grossman RI: *Neuroradiology*, ed 3, St Louis, 2010, Mosby, p 255.)

and contribute to elevated ICP. These mass lesions are often unilateral and may result in severe compression of vital brain structures. Attempts by the brain to accommodate the expanding mass result in typical findings on computed tomography (CT) scans (Figure 44-5). The ventricles are reduced in size, and midline structures are displaced.

Excessive accumulation of CSF (hydrocephalus) is another important cause of increased ICP. Elevated CSF volume causes the ventricles to enlarge and press on cerebral brain structures (Figure 44-6). Hydrocephalus may be a primary disorder or may develop as a result of obstruction proximal to the arachnoid granulations (obstructive; noncommunicating hydrocephalus) or at the level of the arachnoid granulations (communicating; nonobstructive hydrocephalus). Obstructive hydrocephalus commonly occurs when a lesion blocks the flow of CSF out of the ventricle, whereas nonobstructive hydrocephalus is common following subarachnoid hemorrhage because residual blood clogs the arachnoid villi and prevents the CSF from being reabsorbed.

Increased intravascular cerebral blood volume is unlikely to be a primary cause of high ICP, but it may contribute to pressure elevations initiated by ischemia or trauma. High $Paco_2$ or loss of autoregulatory controls can lead to vasodilation and increased cerebral blood volume.

Manifestations. Manifestations of elevated ICP include headache, vomiting, and altered level of consciousness (drowsiness). The patient may complain of blurry vision, and evaluation of the fundi may reveal edema of the optic disk (papilledema). As ICP rises to higher levels, the level of consciousness decreases, and pupil responsiveness to light becomes impaired. Eventually the patient will exhibit altered respiratory patterns and will become unresponsive to stimulation and unable to move, verbalize, or open the eyes. Prolonged elevations of ICP are thought to damage brain structures by compressing the blood supply and causing ischemia.

Patients exhibiting manifestations of elevated ICP, or those with significant risk for elevated ICP, may be monitored with a pressure device inserted into the brain parenchyma through an opening in the skull (burr hole). The pressure device is connected to an electrical transducer, and the ICP waveforms can be monitored continuously (Figure 44-7). In general, a high ICP is associated with poor outcome. Different ICP waveforms are thought to carry different prognoses. The normal ICP waveform is characterized by three pressure peaks called P1, P2, and P3. These waves are reflections of changes in ICP associated with each arterial pulsation. Normally P1 is higher than P2, and P2 is higher than P3 (see Figure 44-7). As ICP begins to increase, the pattern of waves remains normal, but the peak and mean pressures are higher. Further increases in ICP are characterized by a P2 wave that exceeds P1 and a dampening of the individual waveforms (plateau or rounded waves).[9]

Rounded or monotonous waves reflect severe pathologic increases in ICP attributable to changes in cerebral volume. Plateau waves can reach 50 to 100 mm Hg. After the plateau period the ICP slowly decreases, but it usually remains elevated above baseline. These waves reflect a potentially life-threatening situation, and if the pathologic process is not stopped, a cycle of increased ICP followed by vasodilation to maintain constant blood flow through swollen tissues continues, which in turn further increases ICP. An extreme increase in ICP can precipitate an intense reaction by the sympathetic nervous system as it attempts to maintain cerebral perfusion through the compressed blood vessels. This has been termed an *ischemic response* or *Cushing reflex*. The systolic blood pressure can jump to values exceeding 200 mm Hg, accompanied by bradycardia and a widening pulse pressure. The Cushing reflex generally is viewed as a "last ditch" effort by the brain to reestablish cerebral perfusion.[8]

Brain Compression and Herniation

A dreaded complication of elevated ICP is brain compression and herniation. Compression of midbrain and brainstem structures is associated with rapid neurologic demise unless corrected quickly. Important midline structures include the reticular activating system (RAS), which is necessary for maintaining consciousness, and vital regulatory centers for cardiovascular and respiratory control. Radiologic examination by computerized tomography (CT) scan or other means (e.g., magnetic resonance imaging [MRI]) is useful in evaluating the patient with increased ICP who exhibits a change in neurologic

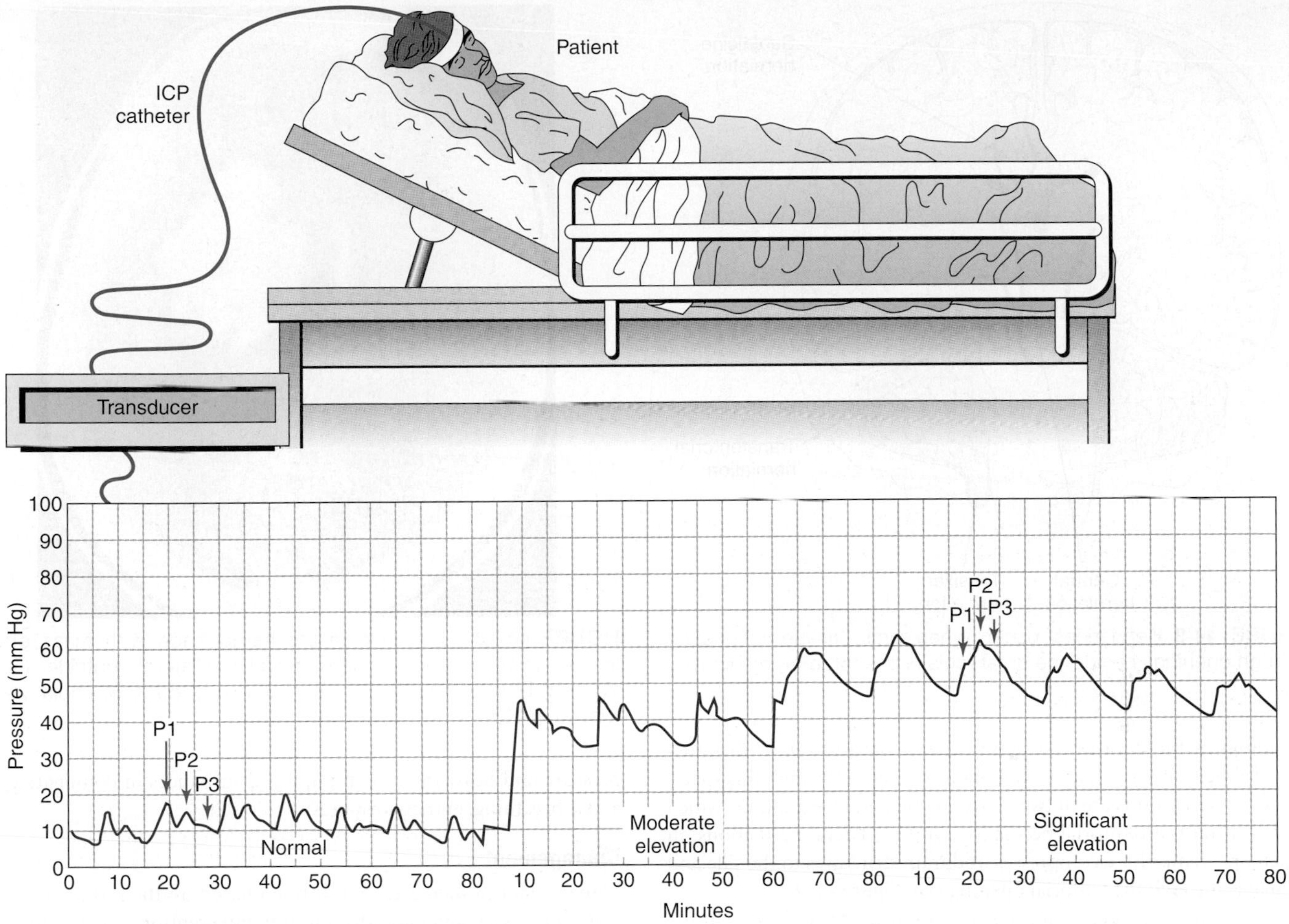

FIGURE 44-7 Intracranial pressure *(ICP)* monitoring can be used to continuously measure ICP. The ICP tracing shows normal, elevated, and plateau waves. At high ICP the P2 peak is higher than the P1 peak, and the peaks become less distinct and plateau.

status. CT scans may show midline shifts and herniations when ICP is sufficiently elevated.

Herniation refers to the protrusion of brain tissue through an opening in the supporting dura of the brain. Several types of brain herniation have been described according to their anatomic locations. The brain parenchyma is divided into compartments by the supporting structure of the dura. The dura folds into the space between the cerebral hemispheres to form the falx cerebri and folds in from the lateral aspects to form the tentorium, which separates the cerebellum from the cerebral hemispheres (Figure 44-8). The most common herniations occur through openings in these structures (Figure 44-9).

There is a small space between the tip of the falx cerebri and the corpus callosum through which the neurologic lobe of the cerebral cortex can herniate (Figure 44-10). This is called a *subfalcine hernia*. Subfalcine herniation occurs when a lesion in one hemisphere is large enough to cause a lateral shift across the midline of the intracranial cavity, forcing the neurologic gyrus under the falx cerebri. This results in distortion and compression of the internal cerebral vein. Subfalcine herniation can be asymptomatic and generally carries a better prognosis than other types of brain herniation. The greatest danger results from compression of blood vessels, particularly the ipsilateral anterior cerebral artery, which can cause further cerebral ischemia and edema and contribute to the ICP elevation.

The tentorium is a rigid dural fold that separates the cerebellum and cerebral hemispheres. Midbrain structures pass between the

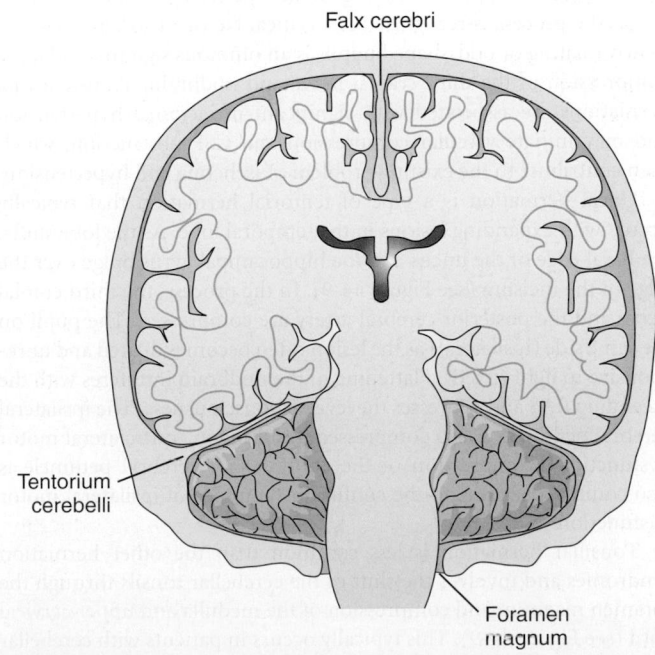

FIGURE 44-8 Schematic drawing of the normal brain compartments showing the dural folds that form the falx cerebri and the tentorium.

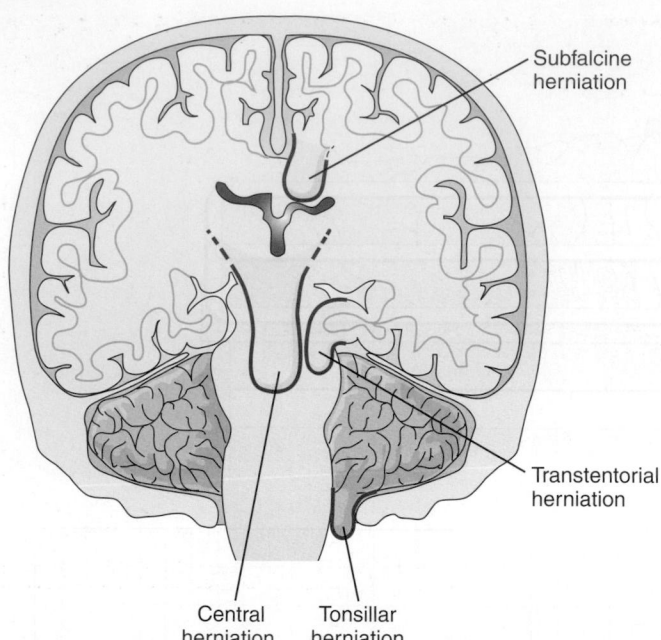

FIGURE 44-9 Herniations occur when brain tissue is pushed through openings beside the dural folds or the foramen magnum.

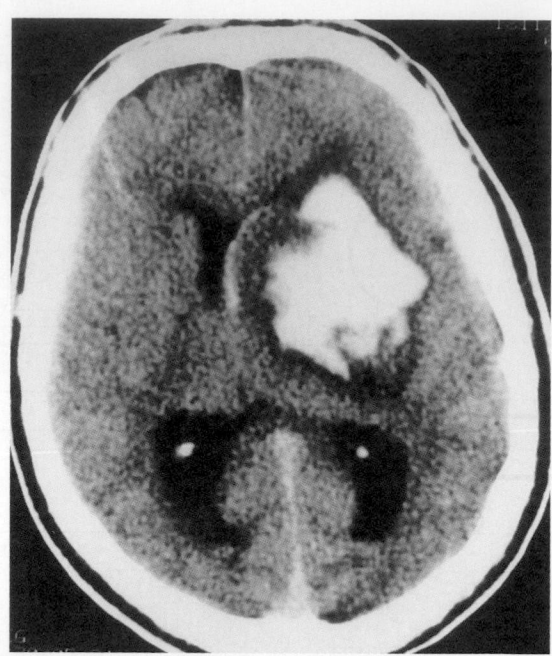

FIGURE 44-10 CT scan of acute hemorrhage with mass effect and subfalcine herniation and shift of the lateral ventricle. (From Yousem DM, Grossman RI: *Neuroradiology*, ed 3, St Louis, 2010, Mosby, p 185.)

infoldings of the dura in a structure called the *incisura*. With transtentorial herniations, a part of the brain protrudes through this space. Tentorial herniations are of two types: (1) bilateral herniations, which cause central transtentorial herniation, and (2) lateral herniations, in which one hemisphere compresses midbrain structures to the side and herniates through the tentorial opening (see Figure 44-9).

Central tentorial herniation results from expanding lesions in the frontal, parietal, and occipital lobes that force a downward displacement of the hemispheres and basal nuclei with compression of the diencephalon and adjoining midbrain. Transtentorial herniation can occur rapidly or slowly, depending on the type of lesion. The speed with which the process is recognized is a critical factor in patient survival. Slowly dilating or odd-shaped pupils is an ominous sign that indicates compression of the third cranial nerve and midbrain. Transtentorial herniations are associated with significant intracranial hypertension and may initiate vascular compression and CSF obstruction, which then contribute to the existing problem of ischemia and hypertension.

Uncal herniation is a type of tentorial herniation that typically occurs with expanding lesions in the temporal lobe. As the lobe shifts, the basal edge of the uncus and the hippocampal gyrus bulge over the edge of the incisura (see Figure 44-9). In the process, the third cranial nerve and the posterior cerebral artery are compressed. The pupil on the same side (ipsilateral) as the lesion often becomes dilated and unresponsive to light (fixed). Flattening of the midbrain interferes with the ascending RAS and depresses the level of consciousness. The ipsilateral cerebral peduncle is also compressed, resulting in contralateral motor dysfunction. Compression of the contralateral cerebral peduncle is also common, leading to the confusing symptom of ipsilateral motor dysfunction.

Tonsillar herniation is less common than the other herniation syndromes and involves the shift of the cerebellar tonsils through the foramen magnum and compression of the medulla and upper cervical cord (see Figure 44-9). This typically occurs in patients with cerebellar lesions. Because of the proximity of the cerebellum to the brainstem, tonsillar herniation evolves very rapidly and can result in death in a matter of minutes. Signs usually include precipitous changes in blood pressure and heart rate, small pupils, disturbances in conjugate gaze, ataxic breathing, and quadriparesis.

Management

Management of increased ICP is often based on the results of CT or MRI. Processes amenable to surgical intervention can be detected and treated. Removal of excess CSF, tumors, abscesses, and hematomas can dramatically improve ICP. Nonsurgical processes such as cerebral edema, intracerebral bleeding, and infections are managed medically. ICP measurements and determinations of cerebral perfusion pressure (CPP) are used to guide therapy. Controversy regarding the appropriate treatment of increased ICP continues, and the focus of management has shifted from ICP control to management of cerebral oxygenation. The roles of previously established therapies such as hyperventilation, brain dehydration with diuretics, head-up and neutral body positions, and corticosteroid administration have been called into question. Previously discarded therapies, such as hypothermia, hypertonic saline infusion, and drug-induced comas, have been reintroduced. Despite these controversies in medical management, the value of careful observation and assessment of neurologic function is unquestioned. Many times subtle changes in neurologic function are detectable early in the process of evolving brain injury. Several tools have been developed to help standardize neurologic examination and are discussed in the following section.

KEY POINTS
- Primary brain injury occurs as a direct result of the initial insult. Secondary injury refers to progressive damage resulting from the body's physiologic response to the initial insult.
- Ischemia is an important mechanism of brain injury that occurs when the blood supply is inadequate to meet metabolic needs. A lack of oxygen results in mitochondrial failure, ATP depletion, and accumulation of intracellular calcium ions.

- Excessive release of excitatory amino acids, like glutamate, is thought to contribute to calcium overload during acute brain injury. Calcium overload is a critical event leading to cell dysfunction, membrane damage, and cell necrosis.
- Reperfusion injury occurs when blood flow is reintroduced to previously ischemic but viable cells. Free radicals are generated, which damage cell structures. Inflammatory cells are recruited to the area and may increase edema, block vessels, and contribute to free radical production.
- Autoregulation of cerebral blood flow achieves appropriate flow to meet metabolic needs despite changes in blood pressure and metabolism. Auto-regulation is effective over a range of mean arterial blood pressure from 50 to 150 mm Hg. Hypoxia and high $Paco_2$ result in dilation of cerebral vessels. Hyperventilation with low $Paco_2$ results in cerebral vasoconstriction.
- Pressure in the cranium is a product of the volume of brain tissue, blood, and CSF. Increases in any one component are partially offset by reductions in the others to maintain ICP.
- Brain swelling is a common cause of increased ICP. Edema may result from changes in vascular competency that lead to transudation of fluid into inter-cellular spaces (vasogenic), or from cellular swelling (cytotoxic) owing to a deficiency in cellular ATP.
- Normal ICP ranges from 0 to 15 mm Hg. Transient increases are well toler-ated, but chronically increased ICP results in compression of vessels and brain tissue, leading to cellular ischemia and brain damage. High ICP may precipitate herniation of brain tissue through dural compartments.

TABLE 44-1 TERMS USED TO DESCRIBE ALTERED LEVEL OF CONSCIOUSNESS

TERM	DESCRIPTION
Confused	Unable to think clearly or engage in effective problem solving; orientation to time, place, person impaired; easily aroused by verbal stimuli
Delirious	Restless and disoriented, may have hallucinations; easily aroused, but may have difficulty with attention
Lethargic	Uninterested in surroundings or events; sluggish in thought and motor activities; does not engage spontaneously in activities
Obtunded	Falls asleep unless stimulated; arousable with voice or touch, but quickly returns to sleep
Stuporous	In a deep state of sleep; vigorous stimulation is required to arouse, and a wakeful state is not maintained
Comatose	Unable to be aroused, even with vigorous painful stimuli; mo-tor responses, such as withdrawal or posturing, may occur

BOX 44-2 GLASGOW COMA SCALE

Eye Opening
4. Spontaneously (eyes open, does not imply awareness)
3. To speech (any speech, not necessarily a command)
2. To pain
1. Never

Verbal Response
5. Oriented (to time, person, place)
4. Confused speech (disoriented)
3. Inappropriate (swearing, yelling)

2. Incomprehensible sounds (moaning, groaning)
1. None

Motor Response
6. Obeys commands
5. Localizes pain (deliberate or purposeful movement)
4. Withdrawal (moves away from stimulus)
3. Abnormal flexion (decortication)
2. Extension (decerebration)
1. None (flaccidity)

MANIFESTATIONS OF BRAIN INJURY

Depending on the severity and location of brain injury, a wide vari-ety of clinical manifestations may occur. Patients may present with symptoms ranging from minor headache and visual disturbances to complete loss of consciousness. Patients with significant acute injuries require frequent neurologic assessments to detect changes that may evolve rapidly. Level of consciousness (LOC), cranial nerve reflexes, and brain hemodynamics provide important clues to neu-rologic status.

Level of Consciousness

A change in level of consciousness is one of the most sensitive indi-cators of altered brain function. Efforts have been made to standard-ize the terms used to describe level of consciousness (Table 44-1). In practice, however, it is best to use a full description because of lack of consistency in interpretation of the terms. Consciousness is a state of alertness and attentiveness to one's environment and situation. A fully conscious individual is awake, alert, and oriented to time, person, place, and current circumstances. Consciousness is thought to be dependent on activity in the RAS neurons, which project to the thalamus, and in tracts between the thalamus and cortex.[1] Although consciousness may be suddenly and completely lost, the decline is usually progressive. Cortical neurons are most sensitive, and cognitive and memory functions are impaired early, leading to confusion.

Delirium, a primary disorder of attention, is characterized by an acute onset of severe confusion, motor signs, slurred speech, altered consciousness, and hallucinations. As RAS function is compromised, the patient becomes difficult to arouse and requires increasingly nox-ious stimuli to produce verbal or motor responses. Eventually com-plete loss of consciousness may occur, a condition called *coma*. The **Glasgow Coma Scale (GCS)** can be used to assess level of conscious-ness with greater reliability among different observers (Box 44-2). Sud-den or progressive changes in level of consciousness should prompt a thorough neurologic examination to determine the cause and best course of therapy.

Glasgow Coma Scale

The Glasgow Coma Scale (GCS) is a standardized tool developed for the purpose of assessing the level of consciousness in acutely brain–injured patients. It can also be used to evaluate patients with an altered level of consciousness as a result of other neurologic insults such as hemorrhage or craniotomy. Numeric scores are given to arousal-directed responses of eye opening, verbal utterances, and motor reac-tions. The best response is scored, bilateral responses are recorded for motor reactions, and consistent application of a painful stimulus is required for accuracy. When used correctly, the GCS has a high degree of interrater reliability.

The eye opening response is a simple measure of alertness. Nor-mally, the eyes open spontaneously in response to verbal stimuli. If the eyes do not open in response to verbal stimuli, noxious stimuli, such as compression of the nail beds, may be applied. It is important to be consistent and vigorous enough to achieve the best response from the patient. In patients with acute space-occupying lesions, eye open-ing is usually depressed in conjunction with impaired response to pain and motor function. Spontaneous eye opening in the acute phase is

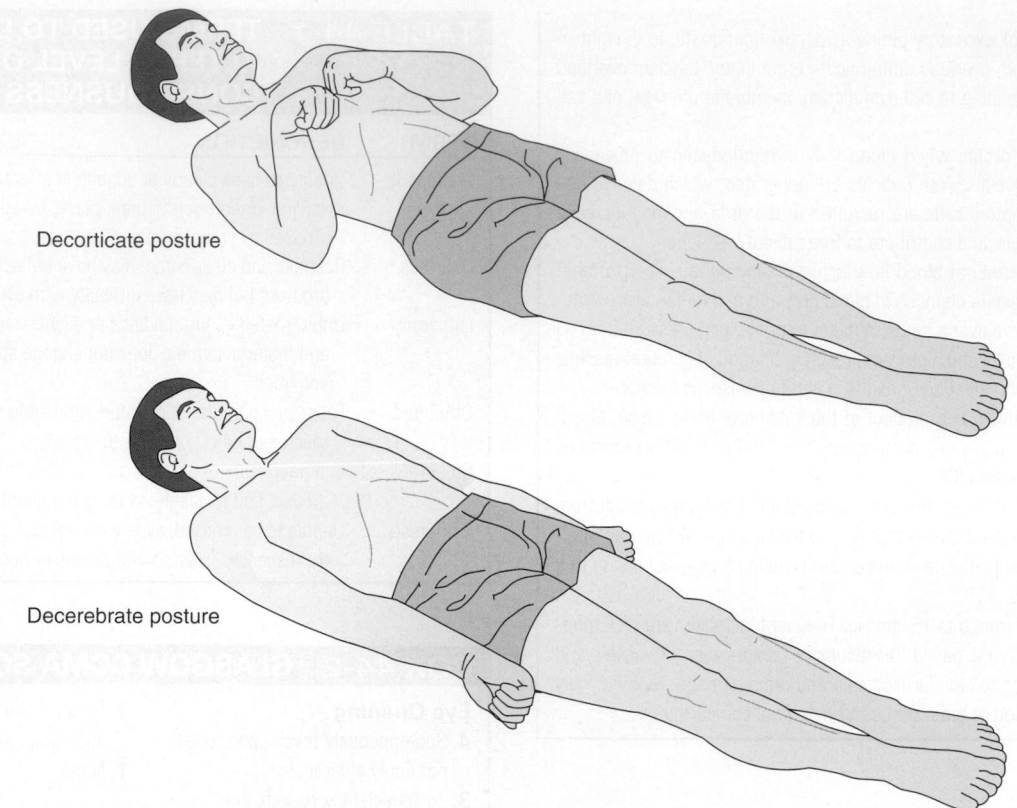

Decorticate posture

Decerebrate posture

FIGURE 44-11 Abnormal motor activity with coma. Decorticate posturing is indicated by flexed wrists and arms and extended legs and feet. Decerebrate posturing is indicated by arm and leg extension.

an encouraging sign, as it implies that the arousal mechanism in the brainstem is intact.

The verbal response on the GCS reflects orientation. A full score (i.e., 5) in this category indicates that the patient is alert and fully oriented: the patient knows his or her name, current location, and the time of day. In the next level (score 4), the patient is awake and can pay attention to a certain degree, but is confused about his or her identity and does not know the time or the location. If attention is poor and the verbal responses consist of yelling and swearing, it is scored as an inappropriate response (i.e., score 3). Incomprehensible verbalizations are unintelligible sounds or mumbling (i.e., score 2). Absence of verbalization is given a score of 1. As in the eye opening category, noxious stimuli are applied to achieve the best verbal response from the patient.

Motor response is a powerful predictor of outcome. Motor response is scored as the best level of response the patient is able to perform. Each extremity is evaluated to avoid misinterpretation secondary to muscle paralysis. At the highest level (score 6), the patient can obey a command to move. At the next level down (score 5), the patient does not obey commands, but when a painful stimulus is applied, the patient moves in a purposeful manner to avoid the stimulus; the patient is able to localize the source of pain. As status deteriorates, the patient withdraws only the extremity from the painful stimulus (score 4). This is not considered a purposeful response. Further deterioration results in abnormal posturing movements. *Decorticate* posturing (score 3) is characterized by an abnormal flexor response of the arms and wrists. The legs and feet extend and internally rotate (Figure 44-11). The level below decorticate posturing is called *decerebrate* or *abnormal extension* (score 2). The arms extend with external rotation of the wrists. The legs and feet

extend and rotate internally (see Figure 44-11). The lowest level of motor response is no response to painful stimuli (i.e., flaccidity in all four limbs, score 1). It is important to emphasize that all limbs must be tested separately, because motor responses may be preserved on one side only, and levels of involvement may vary from side to side. Higher initial scores tend to predict better recovery. On the GCS, the level of coma occurs on a continuum from mild (>12), to moderate (9 to 12), to severe (<8). The lowest total score of 3 indicates likely fatal damage, especially if both pupils fail to respond to light and oculovestibular responses are absent; however, the severity and prognosis are predicted more accurately by also considering diagnostic imaging and other factors.

Cranial Nerve Reflexes

The GCS score alone is not sufficient to accurately determine the status of the patient with an acute insult to the brain. Assessment of the integrity of brainstem function is also important and is indicated by various brainstem reflexes including the pupil light reflex, oculovestibular reflex, and corneal reflex.

Pupil Reflex

Pupillary assessment provides important information about the function of the brainstem and cranial nerves II and III. The normal pupillary response to light results from an intact afferent cranial nerve II (optic) detecting the light and stimulating the intact efferent cranial nerve III (oculomotor) to constrict the pupils. The response of the pupil to light, in terms of both its shape and the speed of reaction, is a function of cranial nerve III.

The pupillary response is recorded by noting pupil size in millimeters, shape, and reactivity to light. Careful monitoring of the pupillary response to light during the acute phase is critical, because a failing response may be the first indication of brain compression from increasing ICP. Mild dilation of a pupil with sluggish or absent light response is ominous. This phenomenon results from pressure on the oculomotor nerve (cranial nerve III) by lateral displacement of midbrain structures. An oval pupil may be an early indicator of dangerously poor compliance and transtentorial herniation. The oval pupil represents a transitional pupil that can return to normal responsiveness if ICP is controlled.

Other pupillary responses indicate damage to the optic nerve. The afferent pupillary defect is a paradoxical response that is detected with the swinging-light test. As the examiner swings a light from the normal eye to the abnormal eye, the abnormal pupil responds by dilating instead of constricting. This occurs because the light signals transmitted to the Edinger-Westphal nucleus in the midbrain through the injured optic nerve are insufficient to maintain constriction triggered by stimulation of the normal eye.

Bilaterally small pupils suggest a destructive lesion in the pons or the presence of certain drugs. Bilaterally fixed and dilated pupils suggest inadequate cerebral perfusion. This could be related to hypotension or increased ICP. If perfusion is not interrupted for too long, a normal pupillary response returns with adequate flow.

Eye movements are important indicators of brainstem function. Cranial nerves III, IV, and VI are responsible for normal eye movements. Abnormalities of eye movement are useful in localizing the site of brain dysfunction. Abnormal eye movements seen in the brain-injured patient can include nystagmus, dysconjugate eye movements, and ocular palsies. **Nystagmus** is a persistent rhythmic or jerky movement in one or both eyes. **Dysconjugate movements** occur when the eyes do not move together in the same direction. Ocular palsies occur when one or more cranial nerves are dysfunctional such that motor paralysis of the eye muscles impairs movements in one or more directions.

Oculovestibular Reflex

The oculovestibular reflex normally detects head movements (via receptors in the semicircular canals) and causes appropriate adjustments of eye position such that an object can remain fixed on the retina even though the head is moving. An impaired oculovestibular reflex implies brainstem dysfunction. Two tests can be performed to evaluate this reflex in the unconscious patient: the doll's eyes test and the cold calorics test.

The oculocephalic or doll's eyes test is performed only in patients in whom a lateral spine radiograph has been obtained to rule out spinal injury. The test is performed by holding open the patient's eyelids and rotating the head from one side to the other (Figure 44-12). If the brainstem is intact, the eyes will turn in a direction opposite to the direction of head rotation. If the eyes do not move in conjugate fashion or are asymmetric, the response is abnormal and brainstem function is impaired. If the eyes remain fixed at the midline and do not move, the response is said to be absent. An absent response indicates severe brainstem impairment.

The oculovestibular response, or cold calorics, is a similar test of brainstem function using cold water instillation into the ear. Cold against the tympanic membrane causes action potentials from the vestibular apparatus to change and simulates the neuronal response to head rotation. If the brainstem is intact, the normal response will be a tonic deviation of both eyes toward the side that is irrigated. Dysconjugate or asymmetric eye movement is abnormal. If there is no eye movement, the response is absent. Testing of the oculovestibular response is one of the essential examinations performed in patients thought to be brain dead. Patients with depression of brain

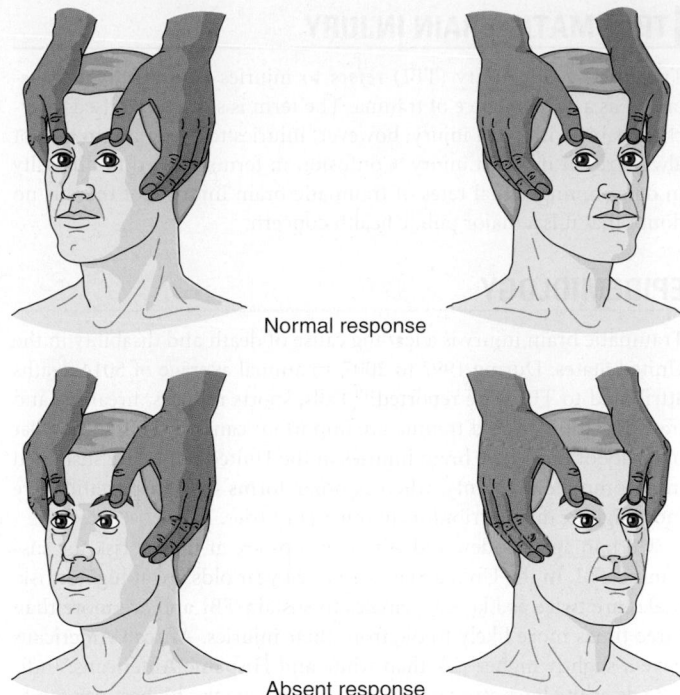

Normal response

Absent response

FIGURE 44-12 Doll's eyes response is indicated by an absent (abnormal) response to the oculocephalic head turning test and indicates brainstem damage. In the normal response, the eyes turn in a direction opposite to head rotation. In the absent response, the eyes stay midline and do not turn when the head is rotated.

function attributable to metabolic abnormalities usually retain an intact oculovestibular response. Certain drugs, such as barbiturates and high doses of phenytoin, can severely depress the oculovestibular response. In the absence of drug effect, an absent response to cold calorics is a poor prognostic sign indicating minimal chance of brain recovery.

Corneal Reflex

A simple test of cranial nerve function is the corneal reflex. A wisp of cotton is touched to the cornea of the eye to elicit a blink response. Absence of blink is another indicator of severely impaired brain function.

KEY POINTS

- A change in level of consciousness often is an early indicator of compromised neurologic status. Normal consciousness is apparent as alertness and orientation to time, person, place, and situation.
- The Glasgow Coma Scale is used to assess level of coma by scoring alertness (eye opening response), orientation (verbal response), and motor control (movements). The highest score is given to demonstrating spontaneous eye opening, showing full orientation, and obeying motor commands.
- Pupillary responses indicate the function of the brainstem and cranial nerves II and III. Changes in size, shape, and reactivity of the pupil may be an early indicator of impending brain herniation. Eye movements controlled by cranial nerves III, IV, and VI may be impaired with increased ICP. Nystagmus, dysconjugate gaze, and ocular palsies may be evident.
- An absent doll's eyes response when the subject's head is turned and an abnormal response to activation of the oculovestibular reflex upon installation of cold water in the ear are very poor prognostic signs.

TRAUMATIC BRAIN INJURY

Traumatic brain injury (TBI) refers to injuries of brain tissues sustained as a consequence of trauma. The term is sometimes used interchangeably with head injury; however, injuries to the cranium do not always result in brain injury. Confusion in terms has led to difficulty in determining actual rates of traumatic brain injury, but there is no doubt that it is a major public health concern.

EPIDEMIOLOGY

Traumatic brain injury is a leading cause of death and disability in the United States. During 1997 to 2007 an annual average of 5014 deaths attributed to TBI were reported.[10] Falls, sports injuries, firearms, and transportation-related trauma are important causes of TBI. The great majority of traumatic brain injuries in the United States are sustained in automobile accidents, whereas other forms of transportation are more significant contributors in other countries.

Certain age, gender, and ethnic groups are at higher risk for sustaining TBI. In the United States, 15 to 24 year olds are at highest risk. Males are twice as likely as females to sustain TBI and are more than three times more likely to die from their injuries. African Americans have a slightly higher risk than white and Hispanic Americans. Individuals at the lowest socioeconomic levels have the highest per capita rates of brain injury.[10]

It is difficult to quantify the social, medical, and economic impact of TBI. The cost of acute hospital care for a moderately to severely brain-injured patient is substantial, and the long-term care, rehabilitation, and loss of productivity for survivors add significantly to the cost. One in five patients who are hospitalized for TBI and survive will have a substantial long-term disability. Prevention of TBI is an important initiative for public health.

Early rescue from the trauma scene and immediate emergency management are important in the effort to reduce morbidity and mortality after TBI. Many TBI fatalities occur within minutes of the traumatic event. Victims who survive until hospitalization require expert monitoring and intervention.

TYPES OF TRAUMATIC BRAIN INJURY

TBI is often characterized according to severity, location of injury, and mechanism of injury. There are different prognoses and management strategies for the different types of TBI.

Severity of TBI usually is based on the patient's GCS score on admission to the hospital or the lowest score in the first 48 hours following admission. A GCS score of 8 or less is defined as a severe injury; moderate injury is defined by a GCS score of 9 to 12; mild injury is associated with a GCS score greater than 12. Injury severity can also be estimated by the degree of brain injury detected on CT examination.

In general, an increased severity score is thought to be associated with a poorer prognosis; however, the predictive value of these tools is not very high. Some authors have suggested that the duration of postinjury amnesia is a useful predictor of outcome, but this measure often cannot be made early in the course of treatment and may not be timely enough to be helpful.[11]

Injury severity and outcome are somewhat dependent on the physiologic state of the brain before the trauma. Physical factors such as bone thickness, dural stability, brain atrophy, drug effects, previous brain damage, preexisting dementia, and cerebral atherosclerosis have an impact on the outcome of TBI. There is so much individual variation in brain response to injury that making a prognosis statement is often guesswork. After 48 to 72 hours following the injury, a better estimate of outcome is possible because the degree of secondary injury will be manifested.

PRIMARY INJURY

Primary injury is the result of the initial trauma on neural tissue. Primary injuries are commonly described as *focal, polar,* or *diffuse.* Although such injuries rarely occur in pure form, they are discussed separately for the sake of simplicity.

Focal injuries (coup) are those that are localized to the site of impact to the skull. The extent of the damage is quite variable. They may be superficial or extend deep into the brain matter. Local injury to the brain can result in specific neurologic symptoms, depending on the site. An injury over the motor cortex may result in contralateral weakness of the face and arm, whereas an injury to the frontal lobe can lead to **apraxia,** impulsive behavior, and poor judgment. However, localized hemorrhages or significant edema may act as space-occupying lesions and result in increased ICP, brain shifting, and herniation. In such cases, symptoms may include a decreased level of consciousness, cranial nerve dysfunction, and contralateral muscle weakness.

Polar injuries (coup contrecoup) occur as a consequence of the brain shifting within the skull and meninges during the course of an acceleration-deceleration movement, resulting in local injury at two opposite poles of the brain. This is commonly the case in motor vehicle accidents in which the head, traveling at the same high speed as the motor vehicle, is abruptly stopped by an obstacle such as the windshield. As a result, the frontal and temporal poles are crushed against the anterior and middle cranial fossae, damaging the tips and inferior surface of the temporal and frontal lobes. Damage may cause bruising or bleeding and, in combination with edema, may result in significant intracerebral mass lesions. Most forces to the head have a lateral rotational component; thus, one side of the brain typically is more severely injured than the other. Patients with polar injuries may or may not need significant acute care, depending on the severity of the injury. Polar injuries can, however, be a significant factor in the extent of subsequent cognitive impairment, affecting rehabilitation and long-term recovery.

Diffuse injuries occur when movement of the brain within the cranial cavity causes widespread neuronal damage. The brain is often subject to shifting and rotational forces during injury. The combined force causes stretching and shearing of the axonal white matter, known as *diffuse axonal injury.* Patients with severe diffuse axonal injury frequently are comatose from the time of injury. Coma is a consequence of axonal damage in the cerebral cortex or reticular activating center in the brainstem and can be prolonged. Recovery may be limited to a severely disabled or vegetative state. In addition to falls and motor vehicle accidents, diffuse injury is an unfortunate consequence of vigorous shaking, particularly of babies and the elderly, who have greater mobility of the brain within the skull.

In addition to categorizing primary injuries according to location as focal, polar, or diffuse, they can be differentiated by the mechanism of injury: concussion, contusion, and intracranial hematoma. *Concussion,* otherwise known as mild traumatic brain injury (MTBI), is the most common injury encountered by military personnel and athletes. In this type of injury there is an alteration or loss of consciousness (<30 minutes) but no evidence of brain damage on CT. Symptoms associated with MTBI present immediately and may resolve quickly after the traumatic event. In some instances they may last much longer: headache, nausea, vomiting, dizziness, fatigue, blurred vision. Cognitive and emotional disturbances may also be present. Grades of concussion and management are currently under much debate by the Department of Defense and schools/colleges alike (Boxes 44-3 and 44-4).[12] The effects of MTBI may be cumulative with additional trauma.[13] Long-term behavioral and cognitive changes are seen in individuals with repeated "mild" injuries. Severe intracerebral bleeds have been reported in young athletes returning to practice/play before completely recovering from a MTBI.[13] Contusion is present when CT or MRI reveals an area of brain tissue damage (necrosis, laceration, bruising). An intracranial hematoma is a localized collection of blood within the cranium resulting from vascular damage.

Intracranial Hematomas

Three types of hematoma can occur after traumatic head injury: epidural (extradural), subdural, and subarachnoid (Figure 44-13). Hematomas may expand slowly or rapidly, progressively compressing brain structures and increasing ICP. The types of hematoma differ in their clinical presentation and significance. Recognition and prompt management of intracranial hematomas can significantly improve outcome in the patient with TBI.

Epidural Hematoma

Epidural hematomas are collections of blood in the epidural space, which lies between the inner surface of the skull and the dura mater (extradural). Vessels that travel within the dura are susceptible to injury in conjunction with skull fractures. Fracture of the temporal bone commonly disrupts the middle meningeal artery, resulting in an

acute epidural hemorrhage. Because the source of bleeding in most epidural hematomas is arterial, the hematoma can expand rapidly, causing acute deterioration of neurologic function. Often, the severity of the primary injury is minor, and the patient may suffer only a brief period of disturbed consciousness followed by a period of normal cognition (lucid interval). Then consciousness rapidly deteriorates as the epidural hematoma expands and compresses brain structures.

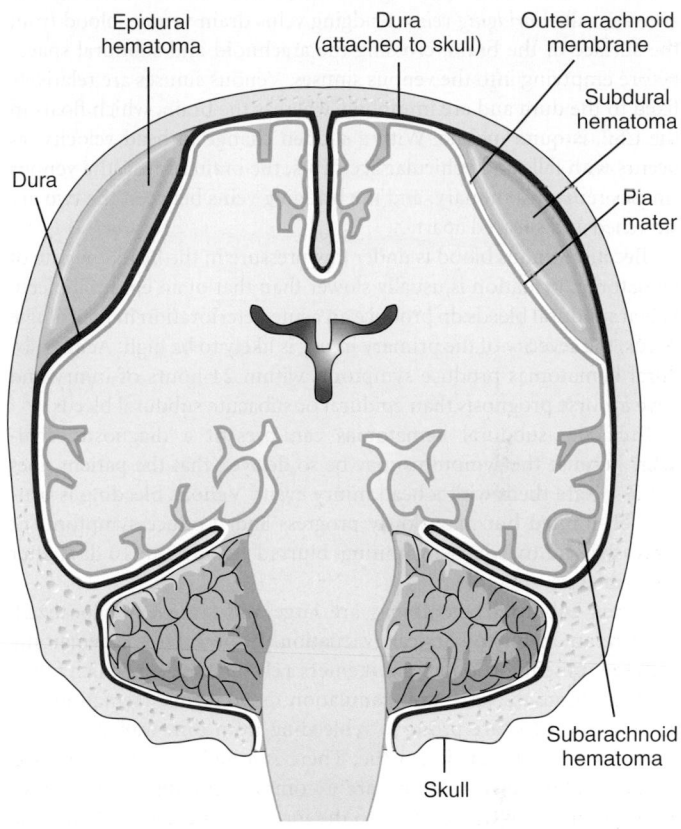

FIGURE 44-13 Locations of epidural, subdural, and subarachnoid hematomas.

BOX 44-3 GRADES OF CONCUSSION

Grade 1

Transient confusion (inattentiveness, inability to maintain a coherent stream of thought and carry out goal-directed movements)

No loss of consciousness

Concussion symptoms or mental status abnormalities on examination resolve in less than 15 minutes

Grade 2

Transient confusion

No loss of consciousness

Concussion symptoms or mental status abnormalities (including amnesia) on examination last more than 15 minutes

Grade 3

Any loss of consciousness

Brief (seconds)

Prolonged (minutes)

BOX 44-4 MANAGEMENT RECOMMENDATIONS FOR CONCUSSION

Grade 1

Remove from contest.

Examine immediately and at 5-minute intervals for the development of mental status abnormalities or postconcussive symptoms at rest and with exertion.

May return to contest if mental status abnormalities or postconcussive symptoms clear within 15 minutes. A second grade 1 concussion eliminates player for 1 week, with return contingent upon normal neurologic assessment at rest and with exertion.

Grade 2

Remove from contest and disallow return for at least 1 week.

Examine on-site frequently for signs of evolving intracranial pathologic process.

A trained person should reexamine the athlete the following day.

A physician should perform a neurologic examination to clear the athlete for return to play after 1 full asymptomatic week at rest and with exertion. If headache or other symptoms persist for 1 week or longer, CT or MRI scan is indicated. A second grade 2 concussion eliminates player for at least 2 weeks following complete resolution of symptoms at rest or with exertion. If imaging shows abnormality, player is removed from play for the season.

Grade 3

Transport the athlete from the field to the nearest emergency department by ambulance if still unconscious or if worrisome signs are detected (with cervical spine immobilization, if indicated).

Perform a thorough neurologic evaluation emergently, including appropriate neuroimaging procedures when indicated.

Admit to hospital if any signs of pathologic process are detected or if the mental status of the athlete remains abnormal. If findings are normal at time of initial medical evaluation, the athlete may be sent home, but daily exams as an outpatient are indicated. A brief (loss of consciousness for seconds) grade 3 concussion eliminates player for 1 week, and a prolonged (loss of consciousness for minutes) grade 3 concussion for 2 weeks, following complete resolution of symptoms. A second grade 3 concussion should eliminate player from sports for at least 1 month following resolution of symptoms. Any abnormality on CT or MRI should result in termination of the season for the athlete and return to play at any future time should be discouraged.

LOC, Loss of consciousness.

Rapid evaluation by CT is recommended to detect the hematoma, and surgical intervention to remove the hematoma is necessary in most cases. Patients with promptly managed epidural hematomas usually have an excellent prognosis because the associated primary injury is minimal.

Subdural Hematoma

Subdural hematomas form in the space between the dura and the outer arachnoid membrane (see Figure 44-5). The vessels traversing this area are called *bridging veins.* Bridging veins drain venous blood from the surface of the brain, crossing the arachnoid and subdural spaces before emptying into the venous sinuses. Venous sinuses are relatively fixed to the dura and are immobile, whereas the brain, which floats in the CSF, is quite mobile. With a sudden change in head velocity, as occurs with falls and vehicular accidents, the brain moves, the venous sinuses remain stationary, and the bridging veins between the two are stretched and sheared apart.

Because venous blood is under low pressure in the head, the rate of hematoma formation is usually slower than that of an epidural bleed. When subdural bleeds do produce an acute deterioration in neurologic status, the severity of the primary injury is likely to be high. Acute subdural hematomas produce symptoms within 24 hours of injury and have a worse prognosis than epidural or subacute subdural bleeds.

Subacute subdural hematomas can present a diagnostic challenge because the symptoms may be so delayed that the patient does not associate them with a head injury event. Venous bleeding is usually self-limited but may slowly progress and produce symptoms of increased ICP (headache, vomiting, blurred vision) 2 to 10 days after the primary event.

When subdural hematomas are large and sufficiently localized, they are amenable to surgical evacuation. If the subdural hematoma has been present for some time, it enters a chronic stage in which fibroblasts infiltrate the area and granulation tissue forms. Hematomas at this chronic stage are prone to rebleeding from thin-walled capillaries in the new granulation tissue. There is a high risk of rebleeding. Chronic subdural hematomas are a common finding at autopsy of elderly individuals. In addition to the increased incidence of falls, the elderly usually have some degree of cerebral atrophy, which makes the brain more mobile within the skull. In the elderly, the likelihood of damage to bridging veins is high even with minor trauma. Alcoholics and those taking anticoagulant medications are also at high risk.

The manifestations of chronic subdural hematoma may be subtle and remain undiagnosed. In the elderly, changes in mentation may be erroneously attributed to dementia. Chronic subdural hematomas are detectable by CT and MRI, and if they are symptomatic they may be managed by surgical removal of the clot and surrounding reactive tissue.

Subarachnoid Hemorrhage

The space between the outer arachnoid membrane and the pia mater is the subarachnoid space. The pia mater is tightly bound to the surface of the brain. The subarachnoid space is filled with CSF. Traumatic subarachnoid bleeding is due to rupture of the bridging veins that pass through the space, in a manner similar to subdural bleeding. Although trauma is an important cause of subarachnoid hemorrhage, it is more commonly associated with rupture of cerebral aneurysms or arteriovenous malformations (AVMs). In that case, bleeding is arterial in origin.

Blood in the CSF manifests with meningeal irritation and a bloody spinal tap. Blood in the subarachnoid space can spread throughout the CSF spaces and may not organize into a confined hematoma. Blood in the CSF produces severe headache in the conscious person and predisposes to secondary vasospasm neural ischemia. It also predisposes to clogging of ventricular drainage, which leads to hydrocephalus.

Further discussion of manifestations and management of subarachnoid hemorrhage is included in the Cerebral Aneurysm section.

SECONDARY INJURY

TBI often initiates mechanisms of secondary injury, resulting in ischemia, increased ICP, and altered vascular regulation. Most of the research on secondary mechanisms of injury has been conducted in the TBI model. Often the damage done by secondary mechanisms far exceeds that of the primary trauma.

In contrast to other types of brain injury, patients with TBI must be carefully evaluated for skull fractures, epidural and subdural hematomas, and injuries to other body systems. Concomitant trauma may complicate the brain injury. For example, uncontrolled hemorrhage can lead to hypovolemia and hypotension, which contribute to brain ischemia. Injuries to the chest can compromise ventilation and produce hypoxemia and hypercarbia, which contribute to cerebral vessel dilation and increased ICP. Attention to other life-threatening injuries may extend the time until radiologic examination of the head can be accomplished, thus delaying surgical management of lesions.

Once the TBI patient's condition is stabilized, many other sources of secondary injury still loom. Brain swelling from both cytotoxic and vasogenic edema may increase for 48 to 72 hours after injury. Ruptured vessels may rebleed or spasm, and CSF drainage can become clogged. Open skull fractures predispose to CNS infections, as do ICP monitors, burr holes, and surgical incisions. Seizures and fever may develop, significantly increasing the brain's metabolic rate and further contributing to brain ischemia. Inflammation and free radical damage continue to cause injury to cells even after ischemia has resolved. Monitoring and managing a patient's course through the myriad perils of secondary injury requires expert knowledge and skill.

TREATMENT

After cardiopulmonary stabilization, the first priority in the TBI patient is radiologic screening of the brain for surgically correctable lesions. Hematomas, depressed skull fractures, and bleeding vessels require prompt surgical intervention. Surgical decompression by performing a craniotomy or craniectomy and insertion of ICP monitors and/or CSF drainage devices may be done. Further therapy is individualized, seeking to maintain ICP, cerebral blood flow, and cerebral oxygen utilization within optimal ranges. Treatment recommendations are controversial, but in patients with acceptable cerebral blood flow, maintenance of normal body temperature or mild hypothermia, normal $Paco_2$, normal serum glucose levels, and normal intravascular volume is suggested.[2,3] In the acute period of injury, elevated ICP can be managed with administration of mannitol (osmotic diuretic), sedation, hypothermia, and mild hyperventilation. Repeat radiologic examination is indicated to determine if a new surgical lesion has developed. If a new lesion is not present and the patient continues to exhibit high ICP, more aggressive measures may be attempted, including diuretics, hypertonic saline, moderate hyperventilation, and barbiturate coma; however, the outcome is likely to be poor.

Patients with open head injuries may be treated with prophylactic antibiotics to prevent CNS infection. Sometimes fractures at the base of the skull are not visible on the routine CT scan but allow drainage of CSF into the nasal sinuses. Head-injured patients who have drainage of clear fluid from the ears or nose should be evaluated for basilar skull fracture. CSF drainage differs from normal nasal mucus because it has a high glucose content and tends to separate into layers (halo) on tissue paper. Other findings with basilar skull fracture are bilateral periorbital hematomas (black eyes, "raccoon sign") and bruising under the ear (Battle sign). The presence of basilar skull fracture increases the risk of CNS infection.

Although morbidity and mortality after acute TBI remain high, significant advances in prehospital, hospital, and rehabilitative care continue to occur. The care received during the first hour of injury can dramatically affect outcome. Efforts to improve prehospital management are likely to have the greatest impact on patient outcomes.

KEY POINTS

- Most head injuries are incurred in motor vehicle accidents, falls, and sports accidents. Young males ages 15 to 24 years are the most common victims. The seriousness of head injury can be classified according to Glasgow Coma Scale scores as mild (>12), moderate (9 to 12), or severe (<8).
- Injury that is directly due to the initial impact is called *primary injury.* Primary injuries are classified as focal, polar, or diffuse. Focal injuries are localized to the site of skull impact. Polar injuries are due to acceleration-deceleration movement of the brain within the skull, resulting in double injury. Diffuse injury is due to movement of the brain within the skull, resulting in widespread axonal injury.
- Disruption of the vasculature can result in intracranial hemorrhage. Epidural hematomas are associated with skull fracture and progress rapidly because they are arterial in origin. Subdural hematomas are associated with shearing of bridging veins and may develop slowly. Traumatic subarachnoid hemorrhage is also due to trauma to bridging veins.
- Secondary injury is a consequence of the body's response to the primary injury. Mechanisms are similar to those described for nontraumatic brain injury. In addition, concomitant injuries and cardiopulmonary impairment may contribute.
- The management of brain injury is directed primarily to detecting and managing surgical lesions and reducing brain damage from secondary injury. Normovolemia, normothermia (or mild hypothermia), normal glucose level, and normal Pao_2 and $Paco_2$ values are recommended for most patients. In those with high ICP, diuretics, hyperventilation, and drug-induced coma may be tried. Open head injuries constitute a risk for CNS infections, and prophylactic antibiotics may be used.

CEREBROVASCULAR DISEASE AND STROKE

Cerebrovascular diseases cause abnormalities of cerebral perfusion including transient ischemic attack (TIA), ischemic stroke, and hemorrhagic stroke. *Stroke* is a term applied to cerebrovascular events that result in a localized area of brain infarction and was previously termed *cerebrovascular accident* (CVA). The term *brain attack* has been popularized to educate the public about the importance of seeking care early, as is recommended for heart attack.

The symptoms of stroke usually are sudden in onset and may include the following: (1) numbness or weakness of the face, arm, or leg, especially affecting only one side of the body; (2) confusion, trouble in speaking or in understanding others; (3) visual disturbances in one or both eyes; (4) dizziness, loss of balance, and difficulty with walking; and (5) severe headache. Persons experiencing any of these symptoms, even temporarily, should seek medical care immediately.

EPIDEMIOLOGY

More than 700,000 new and recurrent strokes occur each year in the United States, making stroke the third leading cause of death.[14] The majority of these victims survive, with most requiring long-term care and rehabilitation. Currently, there are about 5 million stroke survivors living in the United States. Stroke is the leading cause of serious disability. Among long-term survivors (>6 months), 50% have **hemiparesis,** 30% cannot walk, 26% are unable to independently perform activities of daily living, 19% are aphasic, 35% are clinically depressed, and 26% are institutionalized in a nursing home. Each year approximately 55,000 more women than men have a stroke.[4] Stroke death rates are significantly higher for black males and females than for their white counterparts.

Risk factors for stroke are similar to those for other atherosclerotic vascular diseases and include hypertension, diabetes, hyperlipidemia, cigarette smoking, advancing age, and family history. A previous stroke significantly increases the risk for suffering a subsequent stroke. Cardiac disease complicated by atrial fibrillation is an important risk factor for embolic types of strokes. Strokes can be categorized according to cause as ischemic and hemorrhagic strokes. Ischemic strokes are by far the most common (87%) and include thrombotic and embolic types.[14]

ISCHEMIC STROKE

Ischemic strokes result from sudden occlusion of a cerebral artery secondary to thrombus formation or embolization. Thrombotic and embolic strokes are grouped together because the clinical presentation and treatment are similar. However, etiologic risk factors and preventive measures are different and are discussed separately.

Thrombotic strokes are associated with atherosclerosis and hypercoagulable states. Risk reduction strategies for thrombotic stroke are those aimed at reducing atherosclerosis and platelet aggregation. Significant atherosclerotic plaques in the carotid arteries are sometimes evident as carotid bruits. Assessment for the presence of carotid bruits in all individuals older than 50 years may help identify persons at risk so that prevention strategies can be initiated early.

Emboli usually are from a cardiac source, although disruptions in carotid artery plaques may lead to downstream embolization. Cardiac sources include thrombi formed in the cardiac chambers (mural thrombi) and thrombi or vegetations on valve leaflets. Because atrial fibrillation allows stagnation of blood in the left atrium, it is associated with a high risk of mural thrombi, which can dislodge and travel to the cerebral circulation. Patients with chronic atrial fibrillation commonly receive anticoagulant medications to prevent this occurrence.

Sudden blockage of a cerebral artery by a thrombus or embolus produces acute ischemia in the territory served by the artery. Insufficient blood flow to brain tissue results in oxygen deprivation and rapid cerebral deterioration. Neurologic deficits become evident after just 1 minute of insufficient oxygen. If the ischemia continues for several minutes, irreversible cellular damage can occur. With further progression, the local area becomes infarcted and necrotic. Surrounding the infarct is a much larger area of ischemic but viable cells, called the **penumbra.** The penumbra receives some partial or collateral flow and may recover if the ischemia is mild or perfusion is restored in a timely manner. Salvaging the penumbra is the aim of early thrombolytic therapy; however, treatment must be instituted within 3 hours of stroke onset to be maximally effective.

In some cases, the obstructing clot is efficiently lysed by the endogenous fibrinolytic system before permanent tissue damage occurs. If the associated neurologic deficits completely resolve, the episode is called a *transient ischemic attack* (TIA). The neurologic symptoms of a TIA typically last only minutes, but they may last as long as 24 hours. Symptoms resolve completely without evidence of neurologic dysfunction. TIAs are important warning signs of thrombotic disease and carry a significant risk for subsequent stroke. Approximately 15% of strokes are preceded by TIA.[14]

Patients who present with TIAs should undergo evaluation to determine the origin of their symptoms. Unless contraindicated, these patients are started on daily aspirin therapy to prevent thrombus formation. Carotid endarterectomy or angioplasty may prevent stroke in a subset of patients experiencing TIAs who have carotid artery plaques occluding more than 70% of the arterial lumen.[15]

Manifestations of ischemic stroke are related to the cerebral vasculature involved (Figure 44-14) and the area of brain tissue the vessel supplies. The middle cerebral artery is most commonly occluded, resulting in damage to the lateral hemisphere. Contralateral **hemiplegia,** hemisensory loss, and contralateral visual field blindness are usual. If the dominant hemisphere is affected, global aphasia will occur. Occlusions of smaller branches of the middle cerebral artery produce more limited neurologic findings. Occlusions of the other cerebral arteries have different neurologic manifestations depending on the brain area they normally perfuse (Table 44-2).

Occlusion of the small penetrating arterioles can produce small lesions called *lacunar infarcts.* The basal ganglia, pons, cerebellum, and internal capsule are common sites of lacunar infarcts. These lesions are sometimes not observable on CT scan. The prognosis for recovery from a lacunar infarct is usually good, and neurologic manifestations are more circumscribed, often affecting purely motor or sensory functions.

HEMORRHAGIC STROKE

Intracerebral hemorrhage is a hemorrhage within the brain parenchyma and usually occurs in the context of severe and often long-standing hypertension. It carries a 38% mortality, with death usually

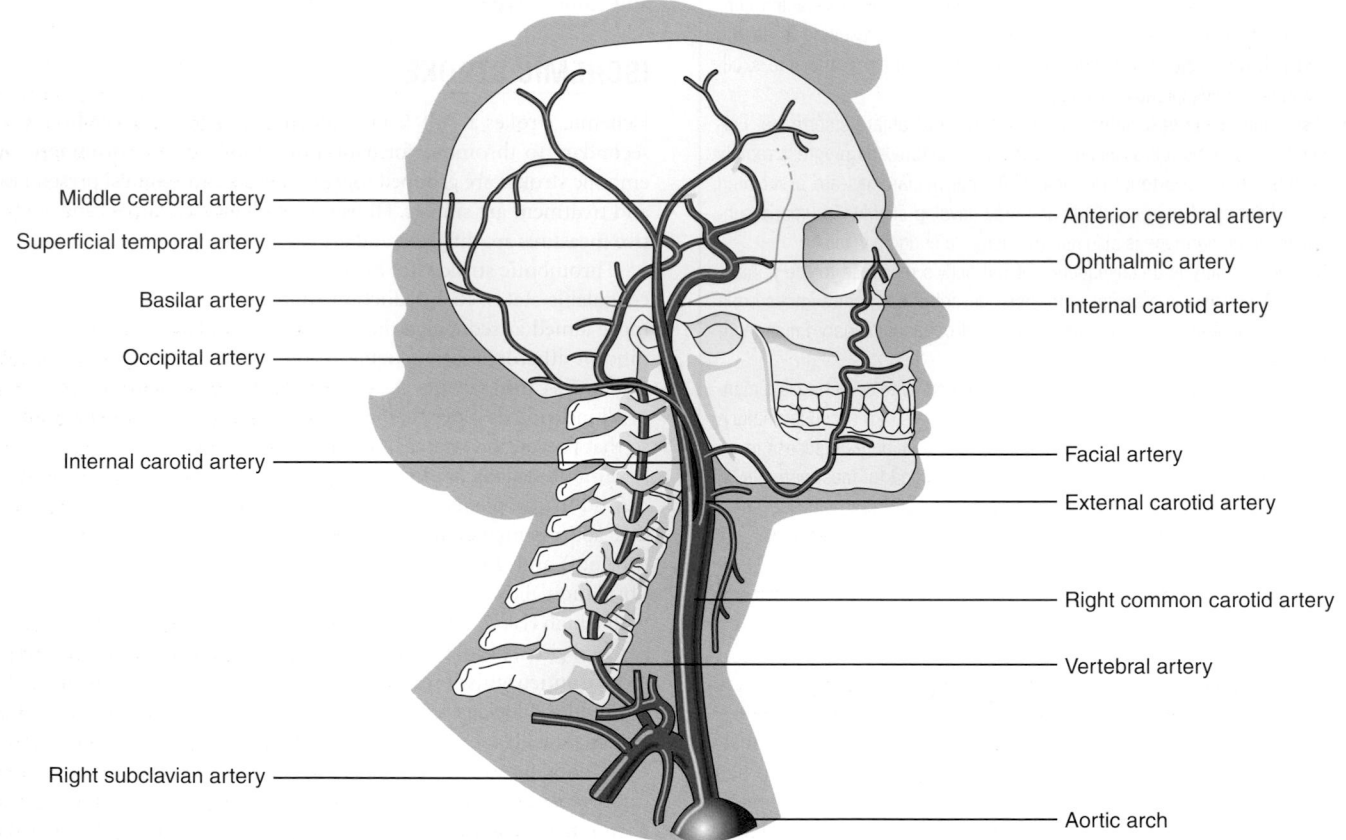

Middle cerebral artery
Superficial temporal artery
Basilar artery
Occipital artery
Internal carotid artery
Right subclavian artery

Anterior cerebral artery
Ophthalmic artery
Internal carotid artery
Facial artery
External carotid artery
Right common carotid artery
Vertebral artery
Aortic arch

FIGURE 44-14 Cerebral vasculature showing fields of perfusion.

TABLE 44-2	MANIFESTATIONS OF ISCHEMIC STROKE ACCORDING TO LOCATION OF ARTERIAL BLOCKAGE	
CEREBRAL ARTERY	**TERRITORY OF PERFUSION**	**CLINICAL MANIFESTATIONS**
Anterior cerebral	Medial aspect of frontal lobes	Contralateral hemiparesis; contralateral sensory loss; impaired cognition and decision making; aphasia (left-sided stroke); incontinence
Middle cerebral	Most of lateral cerebral hemisphere, internal capsule, and basal ganglia	Contralateral hemiplegia; contralateral sensory loss; aphasia (left-sided stroke); homonymous hemianopsia; altered consciousness; neglect syndrome
Posterior cerebral	Occipital lobe and medial aspect of temporal lobe	Visual defects including homonymous central blindness and color blindness; memory impairment
Basilar and vertebral	Thalamus, cerebellum, and brainstem	Sensory loss; mild hemiparesis; disturbances of gait, speech, swallowing, and vision

occurring within minutes to hours.[14,16] In contrast, subarachnoid hemorrhage occurs under the arachnoid membrane and above the pia mater. Two common structural abnormalities that can cause subarachnoid hemorrhage (cerebral aneurysms and arteriovenous malformations) are discussed in the Cerebral Aneurysm and Arteriovenous Malformation sections. Most intracerebral hemorrhagic strokes occur in the basal ganglia or thalamus (see Figure 44-10). If the hemorrhage is large, it may significantly increase ICP, which can lead to herniation and death. The prognosis for hemorrhagic stroke depends on the patient's age, the location and size of the hemorrhage, and the speed at which the hemorrhage produces brain distortion and shift. The degree of secondary injury and associated morbidity and mortality is significantly higher for hemorrhagic stroke than for ischemic stroke.

TREATMENT

Initially, after the patient's airway, respiratory status, and cardiovascular function are assured, an assessment of stroke severity and associated neurologic deficits is made. An initial CT scan is used to determine the type of stroke and treatment, because treatment pathways differ between ischemic and hemorrhagic stroke. Patients who have experienced a hemorrhagic stroke secondary to hypertensive disease often have extremely high blood pressure. Returning their blood pressure into normotensive ranges could result in ischemia. In these circumstances it is best to keep the patient mildly hypertensive with the goal of normalizing the blood pressure once the patient is medically stable.[16,17] Patients who have experienced a hemorrhagic stroke are at risk for increased intracranial pressure and are assessed and treated similar to patients with a traumatic brain injury. Thus, the remaining discussion will focus on treatment of ischemic stroke.

The goals of therapy for acute ischemic stroke are to minimize infarct size and preserve neurologic function. Aspirin may be administered following negative findings of hemorrhagic stroke on CT scan. The administration of 325 mg of aspirin immediately affects platelet aggregation and may help inhibit thrombus size. Thrombolytic therapy is most effective in limiting infarct size if it is initiated early.

It is critical to prevent further cerebral hypoxia or ischemia after ischemic stroke. Thus, volume depletion, hemoconcentration, hypotension, and arterial obstruction must be avoided. As with the hemorrhagic stroke patient, careful blood pressure management is critical. Overhydration can result in cerebral edema in the ischemic area of the brain and raise ICP. Patients should have their ability to swallow evaluated *before* they take any food or liquids orally. Injury to cranial nerves V, VII, IX, X, or XII can place a patient at risk for respiratory aspiration and further compromise the individual's health and potential for recovery.

Anticoagulation therapy may be used in ischemic stroke, especially if the event is progressive. A stroke is termed *progressive* if an initial focal deficit worsened or fluctuated before hospital admission or deteriorated on serial examinations after admission. Patients who receive thrombolytic therapy should not receive anticoagulation therapy because the risk of bleeding is high. Throughout the course of therapy, it is essential to monitor clotting parameters and recognize the potential for hemorrhage into the ischemic area. Even in the absence of thrombolytic or anticoagulant therapy, a significant number of ischemic strokes convert to hemorrhagic lesions. A sudden change in neurologic function should prompt reevaluation by CT. Trials of medications called free radical scavengers appear promising for reducing lesion size for certain CVA types.[18]

Management of the stroke patient also must include efforts to prevent stroke recurrence. Evaluation and management of risk factors is an essential part of prevention. The survivor of a stroke is at high risk for a subsequent stroke if precipitating factors are still present. Patients who have experienced thrombotic strokes are also at significant risk for other vascular events, such as myocardial infarctions. Secondary prevention varies according to the cause of the stroke. For hemorrhagic strokes, careful monitoring and control of blood pressure is essential. For ischemic strokes of embolic origin, identifying and removing the source of emboli is crucial. Usually the source is the heart, and therapy includes control of dysrhythmias, implementation of anticoagulation therapy, and administration of antiplatelet drugs such as aspirin. The most common cause of embolic stroke is atrial fibrillation. Conversion of this dysrhythmia to normal sinus rhythm can sometimes be accomplished with antidysrhythmic agents or electrical cardioversion. Measures to improve left ventricular function may help to reduce atrial pressure and correct atrial fibrillation. Patients with long-standing atrial fibrillation require anticoagulation therapy. When abnormal valves are suspected to be the source of emboli, evaluation for surgical replacement may be indicated.

Secondary prevention for thrombotic stroke includes lifestyle modifications to address modifiable risk factors, including smoking cessation and lowering of serum lipid levels. In addition, the long-term daily use of aspirin or other antiplatelet agents (e.g., clopidogrel bisulfate) has been recommended. Some patients may benefit from surgical removal of carotid artery plaque by endarterectomy or angioplasty. Placement of rigid tubes, called *stents,* in the area of plaque removal may be helpful in preventing reocclusion.

STROKE SEQUELAE

Recovery after stroke depends on the size and location of the cerebral infarct, comorbid conditions, and rehabilitative efforts. Stroke rehabilitation begins during the acute hospitalization phase and continues after the patient has returned to the community. Many patients have residual or permanent deficits in motor, sensory, language, and cognitive functions that necessitate intensive strategies to maximize the likelihood of return to a productive life.

Motor and Sensory Deficits

Motor impairment from a stroke is initially characterized by flaccidity, which is a decrease in or absence of muscle tone in the affected extremities. Most commonly, motor paralysis is contralateral to the side of the brain in which the stroke occurs. Thus a stroke on the right side of the brain results in left-sided body paralysis, whereas left brain strokes result in right-sided body paralysis. Footdrop, outward rotation of the leg, and dependent edema are common features in the lower extremity. In the upper extremity, the arm may separate from the shoulder if not supported. Muscles in the affected limbs tend to atrophy from lack of tone and use. Many of the complications can be limited with therapeutic interventions, including performing frequent range-of-motion exercises, elevating edematous limbs, wearing elastic stockings, and maintaining body alignment.

Starting at about 6 weeks after the stroke, recovery of motor function is evident by the onset of spasticity. Spasticity is the resistance of muscle groups to passive stretch with an increase in tone. Increased flexor tone is usually seen in the upper extremities and increased extensor tone in the lower extremities. Performing passive or active range-of-motion exercises and maintaining proper body position are critical to maintenance of function, because uncontrolled spasticity can result in contractures of the limbs, including adduction of the shoulder, pronation of the forearm, and flexion of the fingers. In the lower extremity, the patient may have problems with hip and knee extension. If spasticity in a paretic extremity is not evident within 3 months, motor function is not likely to return to the affected limb.

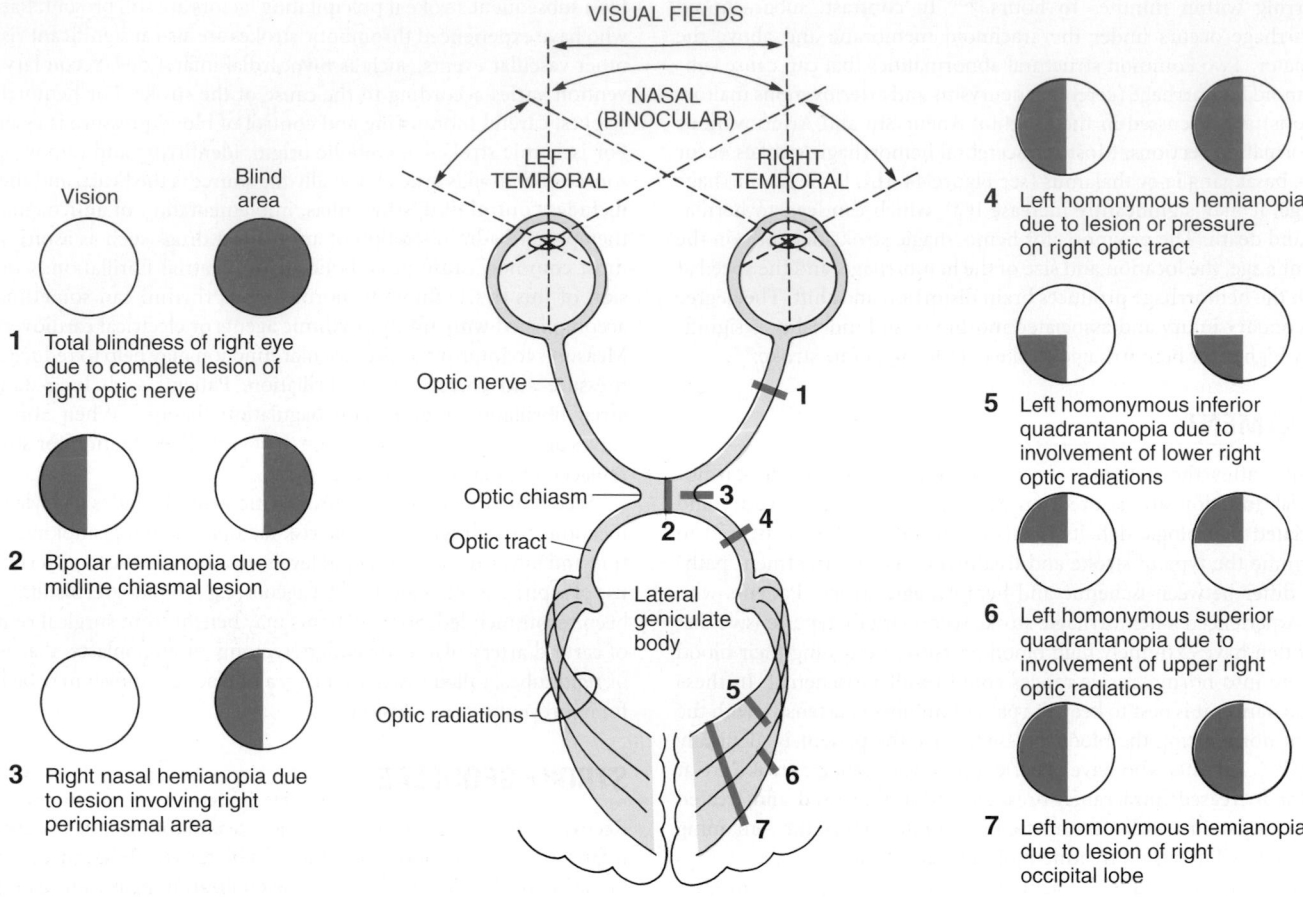

FIGURE 44-15 Homonymous hemianopsia (also called hemianopia). A right-sided brain stroke may cause lesions that disturb visual fibers and result in blindness in the left visual field. The optic pathway from the other side remains intact. (From Black JM, Hawks JH: *Medical-surgical nursing: clinical management for positive outcomes*, ed 8, Philadelphia, 2008, Saunders, p 1850.)

Sensory impairment occurs in the same locations as the motor paralysis. A lack of sensory information from the paralyzed side contributes to the phenomenon of *neglect* (also called *hemiattention*). The patient seems unaware that the affected body parts belong to him or her. Loss of the visual field on the paralyzed side also contributes to neglect. Contralateral field blindness is called *homonymous hemianopsia* (also called hemianopia) because the same side of the retina in each eye is blinded (Figure 44-15). Patients with neglect may crush, burn, or otherwise injure the neglected body parts without realizing it. Poor hygiene of affected extremities may be apparent. Neuropsychological studies have shown that objects in the field of neglect are usually ignored. For example, when asked to draw the numbers on the face of a clock, all 12 are drawn on one side. Self-portraits may be conspicuous for the distortion or omission of structures on the neglected side. Neglect is associated with a high risk for falls and other injuries.

Language Deficits

Aphasia is an integrative language disorder that occurs with brain damage to the dominant cerebral hemisphere (usually left) and involves all language modalities. Characteristics of aphasia include a reduced vocabulary, reduced verbal attention span, and reduced ability to use learned linguistic rules. Aphasia is associated with lesions in the primary language centers (Broca and/or Wernicke areas) as well as in adjacent cortical areas. Aphasia is categorized according to the location of the lesion and the linguistic deficit. The following is a brief description of those categories.

Broca aphasia, also known as verbal motor or expressive aphasia, results from a lesion in the third frontal convolution of the left hemisphere in most persons. Patients speak with poorly articulated and sparse vocabulary and in the simplest grammatical constructions.

Wernicke aphasia, also known as sensory, acoustic, or receptive aphasia, is characterized by impaired auditory comprehension and speech that is fluent but empty of content. This form of aphasia is caused by lesions in the posterior portion of the first temporal gyrus of the left hemisphere. Speech is frequently circumlocutory or tangential and contains paraphasic errors and jargon. Word finding and naming difficulties are a prominent feature of this disorder. Patients with Wernicke aphasia are unable to monitor their own language production and cannot comprehend or monitor the language production of others.

Anomic aphasia results from lesions in the parietotemporal area in proximity to the angular gyrus. This is a fluent aphasia with intact grammatical structure. Patients have greater word finding difficulties than those with Wernicke aphasia but do not make paraphasic errors and have intact comprehension. However, their speech is typically constructed of simple words.

Conduction or central aphasia is associated with increased paraphasic errors and a reduced ability to repeat words. It is associated with a lesion in the arcuate fasciculus in the left hemisphere. Patients are well aware that they are making language errors. However, the more they struggle to find the correct words, the more likely they are to repeat paraphasic errors.

Cognitive Deficits

Patients experience impairments of cognition attributable to diffuse cortical or subcortical injuries that affect the ability to be alert, to concentrate or attend to stimuli, to remember, and to reason. Cognitive impairment varies according to the area of brain affected and the severity of the injury. Injuries that disturb an individual's ability to maintain an alert status are the most severe. Increasing cognitive skill is necessary for the function of memory and the ability to learn and associate, to discriminate, to separate, and to categorize various stimuli. The highest levels of cognitive function include analysis, synthesis, and reasoning abilities.

Cognitive impairment is commonly evidenced as language deficit, impaired spatial relationship skills, short-term memory impairment, and poor judgment. Patients who do not retain the ability to learn are unlikely to benefit from rehabilitative services.

> **KEY POINTS**
> - Stroke is the sudden onset of neurologic dysfunction attributable to cerebrovascular disease. The most common cause of stroke is thrombosis, followed by embolization and intracranial hemorrhage.
> - Thrombi form at atherosclerotic plaques, causing sudden occlusion of an already narrowed vessel. If the clot is quickly lysed, the deficits may completely disappear, a phenomenon associated with a TIA. Emboli are usually a consequence of clots from within the heart chambers caused by disease or dysrhythmia. Hemorrhagic stroke is usually associated with uncontrolled hypertension.
> - Stroke symptoms depend on the area of brain affected, which in turn depends on the vessel occluded: internal carotid, anterior cerebral, middle cerebral, or posterior cerebral artery. Common manifestations include contralateral motor and sensory loss, aphasia, and contralateral visual field loss.
> - Treatment is aimed at limiting the size of the brain infarction, supporting bodily functions, and initiating aggressive rehabilitation strategies. Acute therapy with thrombolytic agents may limit infarct size in patients with ischemic stroke.
> - Stroke is associated with long-term deficits in motor, sensory, language, and cognitive abilities. Initially, affected muscles are flaccid, with spasticity occurring after about 6 weeks. Prevention of contractures is a major concern. Aphasia may be described as expressive or receptive. Most individuals with aphasia have impaired integrative ability involving all language modalities. Concentration, memory, and reasoning may be impaired.

CEREBRAL ANEURYSM AND ARTERIOVENOUS MALFORMATION

Structural abnormalities of the cerebral arteries predispose individuals to intracerebral bleeding and hemorrhagic stroke. Cerebral aneurysms and arteriovenous malformations (AVMs) are the two most common causes of subarachnoid hemorrhage. Early recognition and surgical management of these conditions are necessary to prevent significant mortality and morbidity associated with rupture.

Cerebral Aneurysm

Etiology. An aneurysm is a lesion of an artery that results in dilation and ballooning of a segment of the vessel. Aneurysm rupture occurs in about 30,000 Americans each year; 60% of these individuals will either die or suffer permanent disability.[19] The prevalence is higher in women than in men, and rupture most often occurs between the ages of 30 and 60 years. Intracerebral aneurysms are found in about 6% of the general population, and more than half remain unruptured

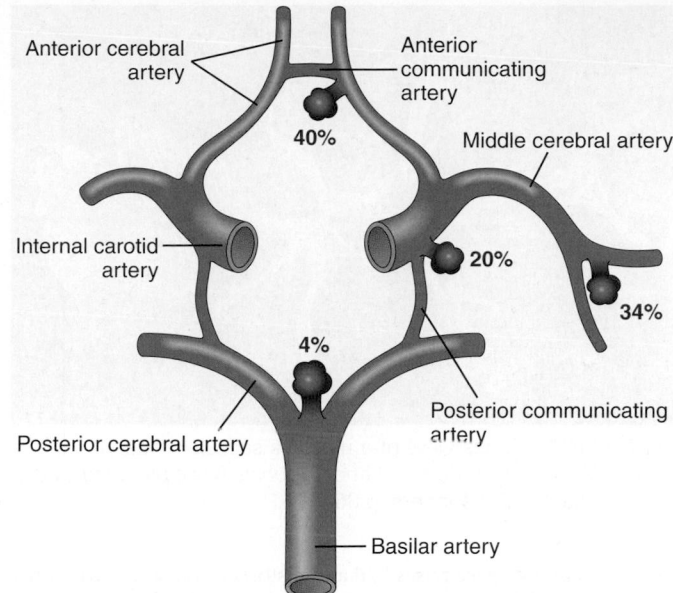

FIGURE 44-16 Saccular (berry) aneurysms are most commonly found in the circle of Willis, particularly at arterial bifurcations. (From Kumar V et al: *Robbins and Cotran pathologic basis of disease*, ed 8, Philadelphia, 2010, Saunders, p 1297.)

and undiagnosed.[19,20] Thus, other factors are likely to be important in precipitating aneurysm rupture. High blood pressure, acute alcohol intoxication, and recreational drug use (especially cocaine) have been implicated. The annual risk of rupture in persons with aneurysms is 1% to 2%. Larger aneurysms and those located in the posterior circulation are more prone to rupture.

Pathogenesis and manifestations. Although the exact pathogenesis is not understood, saccular aneurysms are believed to result from congenital defects of the medial layer of the artery. This structural weakness permits gradual ballooning at the site as a consequence of arterial pressure effects over years. A common location for saccular aneurysms is arterial bifurcations, where turbulent blood flow might have a greater impact on a weakened vessel wall. Ninety-five percent of cerebral aneurysms are located in the circle of Willis; 10% to 20% of affected individuals have more than one aneurysm.

Saccular aneurysms (berry aneurysms) are round and are the most common (Figure 44-16). The aneurysmal sac is composed of thickened intima and adventitia layers, with the medial layer having abruptly ended at the sac edge (Figure 44-17). Rupture of the aneurysm generally occurs from the dome of the sac or at the edge of the atheromatous plaque.

The development of aneurysms is a multifactorial interaction of acquired factors, such as atherosclerosis or hypertension, and congenital predisposition, and aneurysm development is associated with various vascular abnormalities. Multiple conditions have been associated with cerebral aneurysms including autosomal dominant inherited polycystic kidney disease, Marfan syndrome, Ehler-Danlos syndrome, lupus, and bacterial endocarditis, among others.[19]

Warning leaks may occur before an aneurysm ruptures and often produce severe headache, which is typically described by the patient as "the worst headache I have ever had." The frequency of true "warning leaks" is unknown, but rapid evaluation of patients presenting with new onset of severe generalized headache is warranted.[20] Patients may also complain of photophobia (visual sensitivity to light), nausea/vomiting, and stiff neck. A stiff and painful neck results from meningismus caused by the irritating properties of blood in the CSF. After rupture, the onset of symptoms is very rapid. Sudden injection of blood into

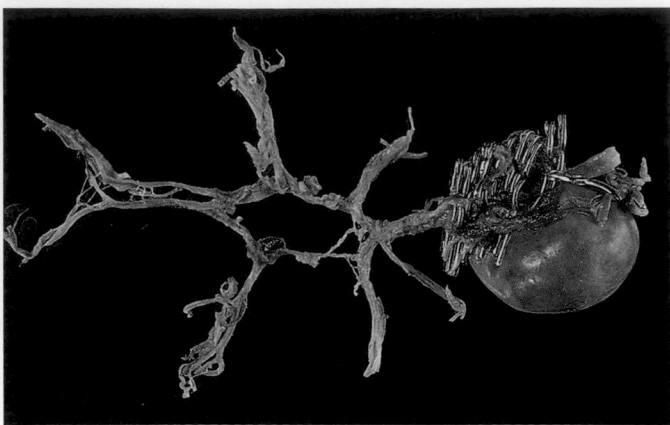

FIGURE 44-17 Gross view of a massive saccular aneurysm in the circle of Willis. (From Kumar V et al: *Robbins basic pathology*, ed 8, Philadelphia, 2007, Saunders, p 867.)

the subarachnoid space raises ICP and distorts intracranial structures. Secondary cerebral vasospasm, a pathologic narrowing of the major vessels around the area of rupture, typically occurs from day 4 to day 14. This process significantly reduces cerebral blood flow and results in increased cerebral ischemia and possibly infarction. Vasospasm is due to the presence of blood in the CSF. The next most serious consequence of the initial rupture is rebleeding. The risk for rebleeding is highest in the first 14 days. Patients are also at risk for developing hydrocephalus from clogging and obstruction of CSF flow through the ventricular system.

Diagnostic procedures for detecting a ruptured aneurysm include CT or MRI to confirm a subarachnoid hemorrhage. If the scan is negative but suspicion of subarachnoid hemorrhage is high, a lumbar puncture for CSF analysis can be done. Blood in the CSF is indicative of subarachnoid hemorrhage. A cerebral angiogram is obtained to demonstrate the location of aneurysms in preparation for surgical management.

Treatment. The primary treatments for aneurysms are surgical stabilization by clipping or placement of endovascular coils for embolization. Prognosis is favorable if the aneurysm is detected and managed before significant rupture occurs. In most cases, the aneurysm is not diagnosed until after subarachnoid or intracerebral hemorrhage has occurred, and mortality is higher. Early surgery in stable patients with subarachnoid hemorrhage is associated with a lower overall mortality. Aneurysm clipping is accomplished by placement of a permanent vascular clip at the neck of the aneurysm. Coil devices may be inserted under radiographic guidance to thrombose or sclerose the area.

In patients experiencing subarachnoid hemorrhage as a consequence of a ruptured aneurysm, the complications of cerebral vasospasm and hydrocephalus must be monitored and managed. Vasospasm can be managed by keeping blood volume and blood pressure at normal to high levels. Calcium channel blockers may be used to reduce vasospasm. In addition to hemodynamic monitoring, careful and frequent neurologic assessments are essential to monitor stability and indicate the first signs of deterioration so that rapid intervention can be undertaken.

Arteriovenous Malformation

Etiology. AVMs are the second most common cause of spontaneous subarachnoid hemorrhage, but can also cause intracerebral hemorrhage. The majority of AVMs are diagnosed in patients between 10 and 30 years, and are located in the cerebral hemispheres.[20,21] AVMs are vascular lesions thought to be congenital; however, they are rarely

diagnosed in the pediatric population. AVMs are more frequent in men and rarely follow a familial pattern.[21]

The risk of clinically recognizable hemorrhage from an AVM is 2% to 4% per year.[21] The risk of rebleeding within the first year after an initial hemorrhage is approximately 2% to 4%.[21]

Pathogenesis and manifestations. In the normal vascular system, the capillaries are situated between the arterioles and the venules. In an AVM, the capillary system fails to develop appropriately, and arterial blood is shunted directly into the venous system. Exposure of the high-capacitance venous system to the high pressure of the arteries causes the vessels to progressively enlarge, as do the arteries and veins that feed and drain the lesion. The blood vessels that comprise the AVM proliferate and enlarge over time. AVMs were once considered purely a congenital abnormality, however, numerous endothelial growth factors and vascular substances have been identified that continue to affect the structure and function of these abnormal vessels and contribute to the risk of rupture and hemorrhage.[22]

Because of their abnormal structure and the high vascular pressure, AVMs are vulnerable to hemorrhage. Hemorrhage is the initial manifestation in 50% of cases of AVM; 30% are manifested by seizures and the rest by varying degrees of vascular steal syndrome. The abnormal shunting of blood into the AVM, called *vascular steal syndrome*, causes progressive neurologic dysfunction as a result of ischemia in normal tissue.

Treatment. Once the AVM and vascular bed are evaluated, the AVM may be surgically removed. Alternatively, gamma knife or stereotactic radiosurgery can be used to deliver precisely aligned beams of gamma radiation to shrink the abnormal vascular tissue. For deep or very large AVMs, other approaches (e.g., irradiation and glue embolization) may be used.[20] Supportive therapy for AVMs that rupture and cause subarachnoid hemorrhage is similar to that described for ruptured cerebral aneurysms.

KEY POINTS

- Cerebral aneurysms and arteriovenous malformations are the two most common causes of subarachnoid hemorrhage. Aneurysm is most common and has a higher mortality rate.
- Blood in the subarachnoid space is associated with headache, stiff neck, and secondary cerebral vasospasm. Vasospasm, which leads to cerebral ischemia, is an important cause of morbidity and mortality.
- Aneurysms are congenital weaknesses in the arterial walls that lead to dilation and ballooning of the wall. Treatment includes surgical stabilization by clip ligation and aggressive management of secondary vasospasm.
- AVMs are congenital malformations in which arterial blood is shunted directly into the venous system, causing high venous pressure. The AVM enlarges and may compress adjacent structures or rupture. Surgical management, radiation, or glue embolization to occlude the AVM may be done to prevent bleeding.

CENTRAL NERVOUS SYSTEM INFECTIONS

Infections of the CNS include meningitis, encephalitis, and abscesses. Organisms gain access to the CNS by various portals of entry. These include via the bloodstream, by direct extension from a primary site (e.g., sinuses), by extension along peripheral and cranial nerves, and through maternal-fetal exchange. Factors contributing to infections include such conditions as immunocompromised status, debilitation, poor nutrition, radiation therapy, steroid therapy, and contact with vectors. Meningitis and cerebral abscess are most commonly associated with bacterial infections, whereas encephalitis is usually viral.

Meningitis

Meningitis is the most common sequela to microbial invasion of the CNS. Most frequently, meningitis is bacterial in origin, but it can also be viral or fungal. Persons with acquired immunodeficiency syndrome (AIDS) have an increased susceptibility to infection and have an increased prevalence of meningitis of viral, fungal, or parasitic origin.

Etiology. The bacterium most frequently involved in causing meningitis in adults is *Streptococcus pneumoniae. Haemophilus influenzae* type B (HIB) incidence has fallen dramatically since the introduction of the HIB vaccines.[23] The bacteria that cause meningitis usually reach the CNS by way of the bloodstream or by extension from cranial structures, such as the paranasal sinuses or ears. Some of the organisms responsible for causing meningitis may be normal inhabitants of the nasopharynx. Pathogens can also gain access to the CNS through breaks in the barrier system, as occur with penetrating head wounds or skull fractures or following neurosurgery in which the dura is penetrated. The overall mortality rate for meningitis is highest for individuals 65 years of age and older (23%) whereas that for infants is 7%. Survivors of meningococcal disease have an 11% to 19% chance of ongoing neurologic deficits.[24]

Pathogenesis and clinical manifestations. Bacterial meningitis is a **pyogenic** infection that invades the **leptomeninges** and the subarachnoid space. Because of its involvement in the subarachnoid space, the infection travels readily around the brain and spinal cord. The accumulation of inflammatory exudate frequently results in obstructive hydrocephalus and exudative invasion into the sheaths of the blood vessels and spinal and cranial nerves.

The combination of headache, fever, stiff neck (meningismus), and signs of cerebral dysfunction (confusion, delirium) is the classic presentation of meningitis. Deterioration in level of consciousness is progressive and often rapid. Patients who deteriorate rapidly often demonstrate dramatic tachypnea. About one third of patients experience seizures. Cranial nerve involvement is also common and is most often seen as ocular palsies, facial weakness and/or deafness, and vertigo.

The diagnosis of meningitis is usually made by lumbar puncture. Typical CSF findings are shown in Table 44-3. Gram stain of the CSF will reveal the causative organism in most patients. In addition to the causative organism, classic CSF findings include white blood cell counts between 1000 and 10,000/mm³ with a predominance of neutrophils. The CSF glucose level is reduced and often extremely low, and patients with bacterial or fungal meningitis have increased protein levels.

Treatment. Recovery from bacterial meningitis depends largely on how quickly effective treatment is started. Treatment includes general supportive care, intravenous antibacterial drug therapy targeting the specific pathogen, and management of any complications. Complications from meningitis can include visual impairment, optic neuritis, deafness, headache, seizures, personality changes, motor weakness, hydrocephalus, endocarditis, and pneumonia. Much of the damage to CNS structures is not a direct result of the pathogen; rather, it is the immune response that is injurious. Antibiotic therapy, with resultant bacterial cell wall lysis, can increase the immune-mediated injury. This has led some investigators to recommend the use of corticosteroids during the antibiotic treatment phase. However, treatment with dexamethasone remains controversial.[23,24]

Prevention strategies include public education promoting prompt and appropriate management of sinusitis, mastoiditis, ear infections, and pneumonia. Strict aseptic techniques for all procedures involving a break in the CNS barrier system may help prevent nosocomial CNS infections. Vaccination against *Neisseria meningitidis* provides short-term protection (a few years) and may be useful before situations in which exposure is more likely, such as during the college years.

TABLE 44-3	**TYPICAL CEREBROSPINAL FLUID FINDINGS IN BACTERIAL MENINGITIS**	
CSF VARIABLE	**TYPICAL FINDINGS**	**NORMAL**
White blood cell count	1000-5000 cells/mm³ (up to 10,000) (high)	<5 cells/mm³
Neutrophils	≥90% (high)	60-80%
Protein	80-500 mg/dl (high)	30 mg/dl
Glucose	≤40 mg/dl (low)	50-80 mg/dl
Gram stain	Positive (60-90% of cases)	Negative
Culture	Positive (70-85% of cases)	Negative
CSF opening pressure	>20 cm H₂O (high)	<15 cm H₂O

CSF, Cerebrospinal fluid.

Encephalitis

Etiology. Encephalitis, an inflammation of the brain, can be caused by a variety of agents including viruses, bacteria, fungi, and parasites. Viral causes account for the vast majority of encephalitis cases. According to the Centers for Disease Control and Prevention (CDC), approximately 20,000 cases of acute viral encephalitis are reported annually in the United States.[25] Death occurs in 5% to 20% of affected individuals and another 20% are left with residual neurologic deficits of varying severity. In herpes simplex encephalitis, approximately 50% of patients die or are left with impairment. Western/eastern equine and West Nile infections only cause death or neurologic deficit in 5% to 15% of patients.[25] Herpesviruses are by far the most common viral cause. It is almost always associated with herpes simplex virus type 1 (HSV-1), which is also the cause of herpetic lesions of the oral mucosa; however, it can also be caused by HSV-2. Western equine and West Nile viruses are arthropod-borne viruses transmitted to humans primarily through the bites of infected mosquitoes or insects.[25,26]

Pathogenesis and manifestations. HSV-1 encephalitis occurs sporadically in healthy and immunocompromised adults. The HSV-1 virus lies dormant in the trigeminal nerve and is reactivated, or infects the nose and travels along the olfactory tracts. HSV-2 can be transmitted to neonates during vaginal delivery. Once across the blood-brain barrier, the virus enters the neurons and disrupts cellular functioning, causing bleeding and inflammation. HSV forms intense hemorrhagic necrosis of the inferior and medial temporal lobes and mediorbital parts of the frontal lobe.[25]

Clinical manifestations of HSV encephalitis typically evolve over several days and commonly include fever, headache, seizure, confusion, stupor, and coma. Hallucinations, personality changes, and psychotic behavior also may occur. Lumbar puncture shows increased opening pressure with elevated numbers of white blood cells (WBCs). Rarely do red blood cells (RBCs) appear in the CSF despite the hemorrhagic nature of the lesions. CSF protein level may be elevated and glucose level will likely be normal. CT and MRI may show characteristic scattered hemorrhages with surrounding edema.

Western/eastern equine virus is transmitted by mosquitoes—birds serve as a host as well as humans. It is primarily a disease of summer months. It most often infects the very young and those older than 50. Once inside the CNS these viruses infect neurons and cause severe immunopathology and apoptosis. The mechanism used by these viruses to cross the blood-brain barrier and invade the CNS is unclear. However, case studies show that underlying hypertension and vascular disease may predispose individuals to neuroinvasive disease.[26]

Onset of symptoms is generally rapid and includes malaise, mild headache, and often nausea and vomiting. A moderately elevated temperature develops and the headache usually becomes more severe. In an uncomplicated infection, symptoms persist about 10 days and gradually resolve. In severe cases, lethargy progresses to stupor alternating with extreme restlessness. In fatal cases the progression of the disease is rapid, culminating in coma and death.

Treatment. In general, the management of encephalitis is supportive and symptomatic. As with all severe illnesses, respiratory and cardiovascular support is imperative. Patients with encephalitis must be carefully hydrated because they frequently show signs and symptoms of excessive antidiuretic hormone secretion and water retention. Those with moderate to severe disease require careful and ongoing neurologic assessment. Seizures are a common complication in encephalitis secondary to hypoxia, tissue destruction, toxic encephalopathy, inflammatory vasculitis, and hyponatremia. All patients with moderate to severe illness should be monitored for intracranial hypertension. Although there is no definitive drug treatment, steroids may be given to control edema, anticonvulsants to prevent seizures, analgesics to relieve headaches, and antipyretics to control hyperthermia. Patients in whom herpes simplex encephalitis has been diagnosed should be treated with antiviral medications such as acyclovir.

Brain Abscess

Etiology. A brain abscess is a localized collection of pus within the brain parenchyma. **Pyogenic** (pus-producing) pathogens reach the brain by a number of routes, including (1) penetrating wounds, (2) direct extension or retrograde thrombophlebitis of an infected neighboring structure (e.g., mastoiditis, sinusitis), or (3) bloodborne dissemination from a distant infected site (e.g., the lungs). Most brain abscesses are bacterial. The most common infective organisms are streptococci, staphylococci, and anaerobes.[27]

Pathogenesis and manifestations. Brain abscess presents as a space-occupying lesion in the brain. Most patients experience symptoms 1 to 4 weeks after the initial infection. The abscess has a focal infected core in which the central portion contains an abundance of neutrophils and tissue debris (pus). The peripheral portion of the abscess consists of inflammatory granulation tissue. Around the abscess is perifocal edema with proliferation of surviving astrocytes. In the chronic phase, the core of the abscess is liquefied and the peripheral portion forms a collagenous capsule that in turn is surrounded by fibrous gliosis. A CT scan typically shows an outer ring surrounding a low-density core (Figure 44-18).

Treatment. Management of a brain abscess depends on its location and accessibility, and usually involves drainage or excision. A critical feature in management is the administration of intravenous antibiotics, which is required for several weeks. Recently, the treatment of patients with brain abscess has become increasingly challenging because of the increase in unusual bacterial, fungal, and parasitic infections, particularly in immunosuppressed patients. Postinfection care must address residual neurologic deficits of cognitive, motor, or sensory function.

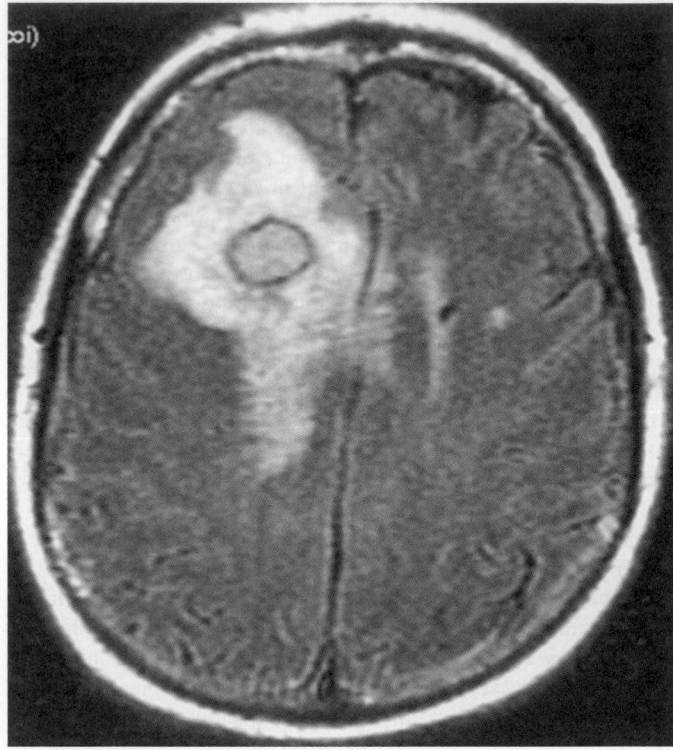

FIGURE 44-18 CT scan of a cerebral abscess showing typical ring with decreased core density and an edematous area surrounding the abscess. (From Yousem DM, Grossman RI: *Neuroradiology*, ed 3, St Louis, 2010, Mosby, p 199.)

> **KEY POINTS**
> - Meningitis is usually a consequence of bacterial infection in the CNS. Infection may be introduced through the bloodstream or by invasion from infected sinuses or ears. Fever, stiff neck, and headache are common. Seizures may occur. The diagnosis is based on an elevated CSF white blood cell count and the presence of bacteria in the CSF.
> - Obstructive hydrocephalus is a serious complication of meningitis that leads to increased ICP. Antibiotics are used for treatment.
> - Encephalitis is inflammation of the brain that is most commonly due to viral infection. Common causes of viral encephalitis in the United States include West Nile virus, Western equine encephalitis, and herpes simplex virus. Management is based on symptoms and may include steroids, anticonvulsants, analgesics, and antipyretics. Antiviral agents (e.g., acyclovir) are helpful in the treatment of herpes simplex encephalitis.
> - Brain abscesses are usually due to pus-forming bacteria. Abscesses may be asymptomatic at first, later showing manifestations of a progressive space-occupying lesion. Drainage or excision and antibiotics are indicated.

SUMMARY

Acute disorders of brain function are characterized by rapidly progressing neurologic deficits and life-threatening complications. The cellular pathophysiologic process is similar for most types of brain injury and includes mechanisms of ischemia, cellular calcium overload, and free radical and immune-mediated damage. The development of increased ICP with compression of vital brain structures is a potential complication of all types of brain injury.

Efforts to minimize brain damage focus on recognizing and managing secondary brain damage. Careful monitoring and management of body temperature, blood pressure, volume status, and respiratory function are essential. Efforts to reduce brain ischemia are important because it is thought to be a critical factor in acute brain injury.

The acute brain injury disorders presented in this chapter, including TBI, stroke, vascular rupture, and CNS infections, are all largely preventable. Efforts at prevention are paramount because often the outcome of acute brain injury is poor.

REFERENCES

1. Hall JE, editor: *Guyton and Hall textbook of medical physiology*, ed 12, Philadelphia, 2011, Saunders.
2. Xiong Y, Mahmood A, Chopp M: Emerging treatments for traumatic brain injury, *Expert Opin Emerg Drugs* 14(1):67–84, 2009.
3. Cecil S, Chen PM, Callaway SE, et al: Traumatic brain injury: advanced multimodal neuromonitoring from theory to clinical practice, *Crit Care Nurse* 31(2):25–36, 2011.
4. Rhind SG, Crnko NT, Baker AJ, et al: Prehospital resuscitation with hypertonic saline-dextran modulates inflammatory, coagulation and endothelial activation marker profiles in severe traumatic brain injured patients, *J Neuroinflammation* 7:5, 2010. Available at www.jneuroinflammation.com/content/7/1/1. Accessed 9/1/2011.
5. Silverstein FS: Do seizures contribute to neonatal hypoxic-ischemic brain injury? *J Pediatr* 155(3):305–306, 2009.
6. Sinclair HL, Andrews PJ: Bench-to-bedside review: hypothermia in traumatic brain injury, *Crit Care* 14:204, 2010. Available at http://ccforum.com/content. Accessed 9/1/2011.
7. Fox JL, Vu EN, Doyle-Waters M, et al: Prophylactic hypothermia for traumatic brain injury: a quantitative systematic review, *CJEM* 12(4):355–364, 2010.
8. Cushing H: *Studies in intracranial physiology and surgery,* London, 1926, Oxford University Press, pp 19–23.
9. Fan J, Kirkness C, Vicini P, et al: Intracranial pressure waveform morphology and intracranial adaptive capacity, *Am J Crit Care* 17(6):545–554, 2008.
10. Centers for Disease Control and Prevention: *Surveillance for traumatic brain injury—related deaths—United States, 1997-2007.* Available at www.cdc.gov/mmwr/preview/mmwrhtml/ss6005a1.htm.
11. Ropper AH, Samuels MA: Craniocerebral trauma. In Ropper AH, Samuels MA, editors: *Adams and Victor's principles of neurology*, ed 9, New York, 2009, McGraw-Hill. Available at www.accessmedicine.com.proxy.heal-wa.org/content.aspx?aID3638543. Accessed 12/8/2011.
12. Ropper AH: Concussion and other head injuries. In Longo DL, Fauci AS, Kasper DL, et al, editors: *Harrison's principles of internal medicine*, ed 18, New York, 2012, McGraw-Hill. Available at www.accessmedicine.com.proxy.heal-wa.org/content.aspx?aID9147447. Accessed 12/9/2011.
13. Cantu RC, Gean AD: Second-impact syndrome and a small subdural hematoma: an uncommon catastrophic result of repetitive head injury with a characteristic imaging appearance, *J Neurotrauma* 27(9):1557–1564, 2010.
14. American Heart Association: *Heart disease and stroke statistics—2011 update: a report from the American Heart Association, 2011.* Available at http://circ.ahajournals.org. Accessed 12/9/2011.
15. Rothwell PM: Endarterectomy for symptomatic and asymptomatic carotid stenosis, *Neurol Clin* 26(4):1079–1097, 2008.
16. Elliott J, Smith M: The acute management of intracerebral hemorrhage: a clinical review, *Anesth Analg* 110(5):1419–1427, 2010.
17. Gingrich C, Carroll WE: Neurology. In Rakel RE, Rakel DP, editors: *Textbook of family medicine*, ed 8, Philadelphia, 2011, Saunders. Available at www.accessmedicine.com.proxy.heal-wa.org/das/book/pdf/3. Accessed 1/8/2012.
18. Nakese T, Yoshioka S, Suziki A: Free radical scavenger, edaravone, reduces the lesion size of lacunar infarction in human brain ischemic stroke, *BMC Neurol* 11:39, 2011. Available at www.biomedcentral.com/1471-2377/11/39. Accessed 9/1/2011.
19. Liebeskind DS, Lutsep HL: *Cerebral aneurysms.* Available at http://emedicine.medscape.com/article/1161518-overview.
20. Ropper AH, Samuels MA: Cerebrovascular diseases. In Ropper AH, Samuels MA, editors: *Adams and Victor's principles of neurology*, ed 9, New York, 2009, McGraw-Hill. Available at www.accessmedicine.com.proxy.heal-wa.org/content.aspx?aID=3635560. Accessed 1/8/2012.
21. Smith WS, English JD, Johnston SC: Cerebrovascular diseases. In Longo DL, Fauci AS, Kasper DL, et al, editors: *Harrison's principles of internal medicine*, ed 18, New York, 2012, McGraw-Hill. Available at www.accessmedicine.com.proxy.heal-wa.org/content.aspx?aID=9145753. Accessed 1/8/2012.
22. Kim H, Su H, Weinsheimer S, et al: Brain arteriovenous malformation pathogenesis: a response-to-injury paradigm, *Acta Neurochir Suppl* 111:83–92, 2011.
23. Mertz L: Meningococcal disease: early recognition is vital to patient outcomes, *Nurse Pract* 36(7):13–20, 2011.
24. Yogev R, Pelton S: To treat or not to treat is the nagging question, *Pediatrics* 125(1):e188–e190, 2010.
25. Ropper AH, Samuels MA: Viral infections of the nervous system, chronic meningitis and prion diseases. In Ropper AH, Samuels MA, editors: *Adams and Victor's principles of neurology*, ed 9, New York, 2009, McGraw-Hill. Available at www.accessmedicine.com.proxy.heal-wa.org/content.aspx?aID=3635253. Accessed 1/13/2012.
26. Murray KO, Mertens E, Despres P: West Nile virus and its emergency in the United States of America, *Vet Res* 41:67, 2010. Available at www.vetres.org. Accessed 1/8/2012.
27. Aminoff JM, Kerchner GA: Nervous system disorders. In McPhee SJ, Papadakis MA, Rabow MW, editors: *Current medical diagnosis & treatment 2012*, New York, 2012, McGraw-Hill. Available at www.accessmedicine.com.proxy.heal-wa.org/content.aspx?aID=12507. Accessed 1/23/2012.

Chronic Disorders of Neurologic Function

Joni D. Marsh

evolve WEBSITE

KEY QUESTIONS

- How are the various types of seizures recognized, classified, and treated?
- How is Alzheimer dementia diagnosed and managed?
- What are the similarities between Alzheimer dementia and vascular dementia?
- What are the proposed neurotransmitter alterations in Parkinson disease, and how are drugs used to restore balance?
- What are the similarities and differences between multiple sclerosis and amyotrophic lateral sclerosis?

- How are congenital disorders, such as cerebral palsy, hydrocephalus, and spina bifida, manifested in the newborn?
- How does the level of spinal cord injury relate to expected functional losses and clinical manifestations?
- What are the roles of immune mechanisms in Guillain-Barré syndrome, amyotrophic lateral sclerosis, and multiple sclerosis?
- What are the causes of facial paralysis in Bell palsy, and how is this condition different from other chronic disorders of neurologic function?

CHAPTER OUTLINE

Patients experiencing neurologic dysfunction from chronic disease states present a challenge to health care professionals, who must strive to maximize the patient's function and quality of life. This chapter focuses on common chronic disabilities of neurologic function including those primarily affecting the brain such as seizures, dementia, Parkinson disease, cerebral palsy, and hydrocephalus. Disorders of the spinal cord or peripheral nervous system include multiple sclerosis (MS), spina bifida, and spinal cord injury. Guillain-Barré syndrome and Bell palsy are examples of disorders affecting the peripheral nervous system.

BRAIN AND CEREBELLAR DISORDERS

Seizure Disorder

Seizures are a transient neurologic event of paroxysmal abnormal or excessive cortical electrical discharges that are manifested by disturbances of skeletal motor function, sensation, autonomic visceral function, behavior, or consciousness. Symptoms are not constant, and the length of time between seizure episodes is extremely variable. A seizure may only occur once in a person's lifetime. Epilepsy or seizure disorder refers to recurrent seizures. Seizures are a component of many diseases. Epilepsy affects 2 million Americans. It is predicted that 44 per 100,000 new cases will be diagnosed each year.[1]

Etiology. Seizures have many causes, and under the right circumstances anyone can experience a seizure. A seizure disorder can be acquired as a consequence of cerebral injury or other pathologic process, including structural lesions such as tumors, blood clots, or infection. Other causes include metabolic and nutritional disorders such as electrolyte and water imbalance, hypoxia, acidosis, pyridoxine deficiency, acute withdrawal from alcohol, therapeutic medication overdose or medication adverse effect, and exposure to toxins such as heavy metals or street drugs. If seizures develop as a result of a structural change such as head injury or stroke, the onset is not predictable. In some cases, seizures may not develop for months or years after the structural change has occurred. In some cases, no explanation for the seizure disorder can be found. These individuals are classified as having **idiopathic** seizures.

A seizure event is often triggered by specific stimuli, usually unique for each individual. Physical inducements include specific sensory stimuli such as flashing lights, loud noises, and rhythmic music. Fever, physical exhaustion, sleep deprivation, fatigue, inadequate nutrition, hormonal changes of the menstrual cycle, hyperventilation, injury, and drugs can also prompt seizure activity. Psychosocial factors include family and environmental stress, shock, and emotional stress.

Pathogenesis. Seizures are due to an alteration in membrane potential that makes certain neurons abnormally hyperactive and hypersensitive to changes in their environment. These physiologically abnormal neurons form an **epileptogenic focus** (i.e., an area of the brain from which the seizure emanates). The epileptogenic focus functions autonomously, emitting excessively large numbers of paroxysmal electrical discharges. Results from animal studies suggest that neuroinflammation may be a cause or consequence of these electrical abnormalities.[2] Nerve cells in this area can recruit neurons in adjacent areas as well as synaptically related neurons in distant areas of the brain, greatly increasing the number of neurons involved in the seizure activity. Recruitment can also incorporate neurons in the opposite hemisphere. Clinical symptoms become evident when a sufficient number of neurons have been excited. Seizures are classified according to clinical symptoms and the electroencephalographic (EEG) features. Clinical manifestations depend on the area of the brain involved, the area of origin, and the areas to which the seizure spreads.

Clinical manifestations. Seizures may be classified as partial, in which only part of the brain surface is affected (also known as focal seizures), or generalized, in which the whole brain surface is affected during the seizure (Box 45-1).

Generalized seizures. Episodes in which the entire brain is involved from the onset of the seizure are referred to as **generalized seizures.** Involvement of the thalamus and reticular activating system results in loss of consciousness. Metabolic or toxin-induced seizures tend to be generalized. This category includes the following: absence (petite mal), atypical absence, myoclonic, atonic (drop attack), or tonic-clonic (grand mal) seizures.

Absence or petite mal seizures usually occur only in children and are sometimes identified in children manifesting poor academic performance. They are very brief (2 to 10 seconds), and episodes are characterized by staring spells that last only seconds. Onset and termination of attacks are abrupt. During the spell, the individual is unaware of the surrounding environment and is usually motionless; however,

it is not unusual for the person to continue walking or performing a routine motor task. If the seizure activity occurs during conversation, the individual may pause or miss a few words. Absence seizures almost always occur during childhood and resolve by age 20 years, although another seizure type may occur later in life.[3] Atypical absence seizures have accompanying myoclonic jerks and automatisms (such as lip smacking or repetitive semi–purposeful movements) with the staring spell. The electroencephalographic patterns are unique to each syndrome. Myoclonic seizures are extremely brief and are characterized by a single jerk or multiple jerks of one or more muscle groups. Atonic seizures or drop attacks are characterized by a sudden and complete loss of muscle tone. Falls and injuries are common with this type of seizure activity. Myoclonic episodes may also be associated with atonic seizures. Tonic-clonic seizures involve stiffening and repetitive jerking of muscle groups.

Tonic-clonic or grand mal seizures are characterized by a sudden loss of consciousness followed by muscle rigidity (tonic phase). The individual falls, and initial motor signs include opening of the mouth and eyes, extension of the legs, and adduction of the arms. There may be tongue biting or a high-pitched cry while the whole musculature is in spasm and air is forced out of the lungs through closed vocal cords. Respiration is arrested, and cyanosis may occur. Bowel and bladder incontinence frequently occurs. The tonic phase may last 10 to 15 seconds and is followed by clonic activity, in which there is often violent but rhythmic muscular contractions. During this phase the eyes roll, the face grimaces, and the pulse rate accelerates. Salivation increases and the patient may become diaphoretic. The clonic phase usually lasts 1 to 2 minutes with a gradual decline in the amplitude of the clonic jerks. The individual remains apneic until the end of the clonic phase that is marked by a deep inspiration.

During the terminal or postictal phase, the individual may regain consciousness or drift into a deep coma-like state. Disorientation and confusion are common. If allowed, the individual may sleep for several hours. Other findings include headache, drowsiness, nausea, muscle soreness, no memory of the seizure event, and retrograde amnesia. During the seizure, the person is at risk for injury from the initial fall as well as from the muscle contractions of the clonic phase.

A potentially life-threatening situation known as **status epilepticus** occurs in some seizure disorders. Status epilepticus is a continuing series of seizures without a period of recovery between seizure episodes. It can occur with all types of seizures but is of greatest concern in tonic-clonic seizures. Irreversible brain damage and possible death from hypoxia, cardiac dysrhythmias, or lactic acidosis can occur if the airway is not maintained and seizure activity is not halted. Whether nonconvulsive status epilepticus causes neuronal damage is still a

---

BOX 45-1 CLASSIFICATIONS OF SEIZURES

Generalized Seizures: Entire Brain Surface Is Affected During Seizure	Partial Seizures: Part of Brain Surface Is Affected During Seizure
Absence (petit mal)	Simple partial: There is no impairment of consciousness during the seizure.
Atypical absence	
Myoclonic	
Atonic (drop attack)	Complex partial: There is impairment of consciousness during the seizure.
Clonic	
Tonic	
Generalized tonic-clonic (grand mal)	With secondary generalization: Onset begins as simple partial, and then progresses to impairment of consciousness.

matter of debate. Studies of elderly patients with nonconvulsive status epilepticus show very high mortality rates and ongoing research is suggesting that EEG be part of the evaluation for patients with altered levels of consciousness that cannot be otherwise explained.[3,4]

Partial seizures. Partial seizures are those in which activity is restricted to one brain hemisphere. They are further divided into three categories: simple partial, complex partial, and partial seizures that are secondarily generalized.

In simple partial seizures, the individual does not have a change in level of consciousness. The symptoms may be motor, sensory, or autonomic, or any combination of the three. Motor symptoms may be limited to one part of the body. Sensory seizures may result in tingling or numbness that spreads or "marches" to different parts of the limb or body (depending on the location of the seizure activity in the brain) or may involve the special senses, producing auditory (buzzing sounds), olfactory, or visual manifestations (flashing lights). Autonomic symptoms may include pupillary (pupil dilation), skin (diaphoresis, flushing), or respiratory changes.

Complex partial seizures have many different combinations of cognitive, affective, and psychomotor symptoms. Either loss or alteration of consciousness may occur when the seizure begins. After the attack, the individual may feel drowsy or confused. At the onset of impairment of consciousness, the individual often displays automatisms. Aggressive behavior may be displayed as well, especially if bystanders attempt to restrain the individual. Complex partial seizures often last several minutes and may be followed by a postictal state.

Partial seizures that are secondarily generalized are the third subtype of partial seizures. This category comprises seizures that begin as simple partial seizures and then progress to involve both brain hemispheres. Once generalized, these seizures are clinically similar to primary generalized seizures.

Aura/prodrome. Some people may have a subjective sense of an impending seizure. This **prodromal period** may be characterized by any one of several phenomena such as a type of myoclonic jerking, headache, lethargy, mood alterations, palpitations, or epigastric sensations, which may precede the actual seizure by several hours. In about half of cases there is some type of movement or odd sensory experience (visual, auditory, olfactory, or gustatory) that occurs seconds before consciousness is lost and that is remembered by the individual after recovery from the seizure. This experience is known as an *aura*. Although the individual may interpret the aura as an indication that a seizure is about to occur, in fact it is the beginning of the seizure episode. Auras can be significant, because they may be a clue to the location of the epileptogenic focus.

Diagnosis and treatment. The diagnosis and management of seizure disorders are based on the patient's history, physical, and neurologic examination results as well as the results of electroencephalographic studies. Electroencephalograms (EEGs) may be normal between seizures, so activation techniques (sleep deprivation, hyperventilation) may be used to elicit the pathologic mechanism. Laboratory studies are frequently used to investigate possible metabolic abnormalities as well as therapeutic serum levels in those already using anticonvulsant drugs. Lumbar puncture may be utilized when there is a suspicion of a central nervous system (CNS) infection.[3] Initial studies ruling out structural causes may include computed tomography (CT) or magnetic resonance imaging (MRI).

Treatment of an individual experiencing a seizure is concentrated on maintaining an airway and protecting the individual from injury. Recording the course of the seizure episode is useful for identifying the location of the epileptogenic focus and for noting any change in the patient's seizure pattern. These data are useful in treatment planning. The information recorded should include the time of onset and duration of the seizure, precipitating factors, presence of a prodrome or aura, sequence of seizure activity, autonomic signs, level of consciousness, and postictal state.

Long-term treatment depends on the cause of the seizure disorder. In seizures resulting from a metabolic abnormality, infection, or tumor, the precipitating source is removed. If the seizures are due to irreversible or unidentifiable factors, anticonvulsant medications specific to the type of seizure are the best management. The decision to treat after one seizure is controversial when an identifiable cause has not been found.[5] The objective of therapy is to achieve seizure control with a minimum of side effects. Medication is continued until there have been no seizures for at least 2 years and is then gradually withdrawn.[3] If seizures continue despite treatment at a maximal dose of a single medication, a second agent is added and the dosage is increased depending on patient tolerance. The first drug is then gradually discontinued. Anticonvulsant medication is a form of control, not a cure.

Treatment also includes patient education in the avoidance of activating factors (e.g., stress, loud noise, alcohol). Patients should be advised to avoid situations that could be dangerous or life threatening if seizures should reoccur (e.g., driving or swimming). State laws defining when patients with seizure disorders are allowed to resume driving vary widely.[5] Compliance to the treatment plan is sometimes difficult because of side effects of pharmacologic interventions. However, most patients are able to achieve optimal seizure control and lead active and productive lives. For some patients with seizure disorder uncontrolled by medications, surgical excision of the seizure focus may be an option. Neurostimulation is an appropriate therapy for certain patients with refractory seizures.[6]

KEY POINTS

- Seizure disorder is characterized by recurrent episodes of abnormal electrical impulses in the brain. Some individuals appear to have a lower-than-normal threshold for seizure activity. Seizure activity may occur in anyone, given the right conditions. Head injury, meningitis, brain tumors, and metabolic disorders (electrolyte imbalance, fever, acidosis) may predispose an individual to having seizures.
- Initiation of seizure activity may occur in a particular brain area (the epileptogenic focus). Nearby and distant neurons may then be recruited into the seizure. When sufficient neurons are involved, the seizure becomes clinically evident as involuntary movement or unusual sensations.
- Seizures are classified as partial or generalized. Partial seizures involve a part of the brain; generalized seizures involve the entire brain at the onset. Partial seizures are further classified as simple, in which consciousness is retained, and complex, in which consciousness is impaired. Seizures may begin as partial and then generalize to affect the entire brain. Generalized seizures include absence, myoclonic, atonic, and tonic-clonic types. Consciousness is always impaired in generalized seizures.
- Status epilepticus is a serious condition in which seizures occur continuously, resulting in intense brain metabolism. Ischemic brain damage may result. Management of a seizure in progress is aimed at maintaining the individual's airway and protecting the person from trauma. Close attention is given to the quality and progression of seizure activity. Anticonvulsant medications are used to suppress seizure activity.

Dementia

Dementia is not a specific disease but rather a syndrome associated with many pathologic processes. It is characterized by progressive deterioration and continuing decline of memory and other cognitive changes. Personality and behavior changes accompany the cognitive deterioration. Judgment, abstract thinking, and complex task performance are all affected. The onset of dementia may be insidious, and the affected individual may initially appear uninterested or lacking initiative. Many demented patients have **agnosia** or lack of insight into their cognitive deficiencies.

Alzheimer disease accounts for 60% to 80% of all dementias, whereas vascular dementia is the second most common cause. An estimated 1 in 8 people older than 65 have Alzheimer disease. It affects nearly half of those 85 years of age and older.[7]

Etiology. Multiple causes/types of dementia exist, and a full discussion of each is beyond the scope of this chapter. Some examples of dementia-causing illness include alcoholism, intracranial tumor, normal-pressure hydrocephalus, Parkinson disease, Lewy body disease, Huntington disease, multiple sclerosis, Pick disease, Creutzfeldt-Jakob disease, and bovine spongiform encephalopathy (mad cow disease). Unfortunately, these also can occur in combination, causing severe disease. Because Alzheimer- and vascular-type dementias are the first and second most common causes of dementia, they will be discussed in detail. The subsequent discussion of treatment of individuals with dementia will be more general because the care issues are similar regardless of type of dementia.

It is important to consider all potential causes of cognitive change when dealing with patients with mental status change. Both delirium and depression in the elderly can cause signs and symptoms that resemble those of dementia. Delirium is a global mental dysfunction that includes disturbed consciousness, decreased awareness of the environment, inability to maintain attention, disrupted sleep-wake cycles, drowsiness, restlessness, emotional lability, incoherence, and hallucinations.[8] Symptoms of delirium tend to have an abrupt onset and may fluctuate often, becoming worse at night. Delirium can result from numerous causes such as medication/polypharmacy, metabolic abnormalities, nutritional deficiencies, and infection, among others. Delirium may occur more frequently in individuals with an underlying dementing illness.

Pathogenesis. The hallmark pathophysiologic changes associated with Alzheimer disease include intracellular neurofibrillary tangles and extracellular amyloid (senile) plaques (Figure 45-1). As a result of these changes, diffuse neuronal damage and brain atrophy occur. The brain of a patient with advanced Alzheimer disease often weighs up to 20% less than a normal brain.[9] The temporoparietal and anterior frontal regions of the brain are chiefly affected, exhibiting enlarged sulci and ventricles and atrophic gyri (Figure 45-2). Neurofibrillary tangles are composed of helical filaments formed from hyperphosphorylated

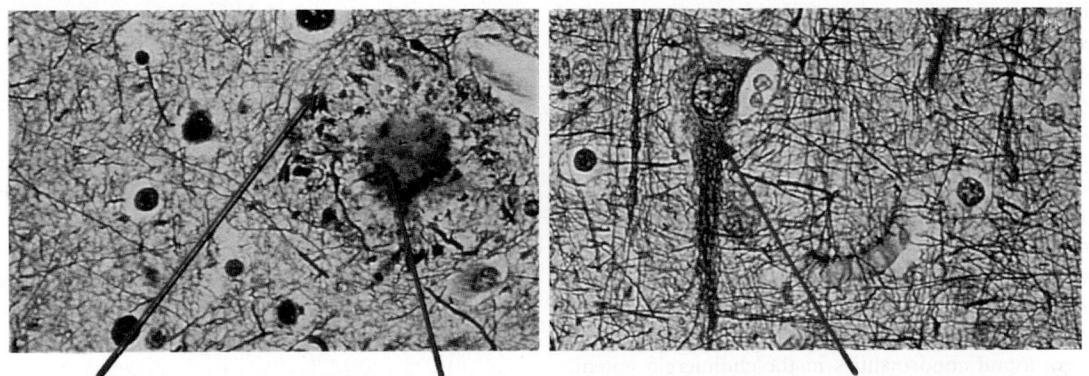

Plaque surrounding amyloid deposit | Neurons filled with neurofibrillary tangles

FIGURE 45-1 Amyloid plaques and neurofibrillary tangles. (Courtesy James King-Holmes and Science Photo Library.)

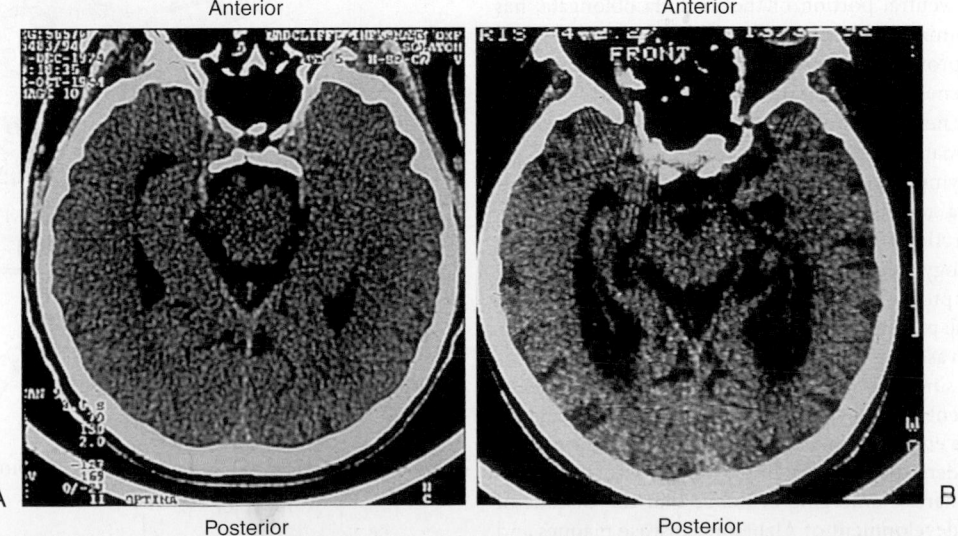

Anterior | Anterior

Posterior | Posterior

A | B

FIGURE 45-2 Axial (horizontal) CT scan section through the temporal lobes. **A,** Normal. **B,** Alzheimer disease. (Courtesy James King-Holmes and Science Photo Library.)

protein tau, also known as neural thread protein.[9] In the central nervous system, neural thread proteins bind and help stabilize microtubules (the cell's internal support structure or skeleton). Inflammatory changes, lipid abnormalities, and aging are among the processes thought to be responsible for activating the phosphorylating enzymes altering the structure of the tau proteins.[10] The presence of neurofibrillary tangles is well correlated with dementia; however, neurofibrillary tangles are not specific just to Alzheimer disease and are found in other neurodegenerative disease processes.[11] The second, but most specific, change in the brain of patients with Alzheimer disease is the deposition of extracellular amyloid plaques.

It is not known whether amyloid plaques cause Alzheimer disease or result from it. The number of senile plaques seems to correlate with the severity of disease. In plaques, β-amyloid is a protein fragment snipped from a larger protein—**amyloid precursor protein (APP)**—during metabolism. APP is a member of a large family of proteins that are associated with cell membranes. During metabolism, APP becomes embedded in the membrane of the nerve cell, partly inside and partly outside the cell. While APP is embedded in the cell membrane, proteases cleave APP apart. β-Amyloid is produced only when the cleavage happens at the wrong place in APP.

After β-amyloid is formed, it is not known how it moves through or around the nerve cells. In the final stages of its journey, it joins with other β-amyloid filaments and fragments of dead and dying neurons to form the dense, insoluble plaques that are a hallmark of Alzheimer disease in brain tissue. Inflammatory processes including acute-phase response, complement activation, and accumulation of activated microglia and astrocytes accompany the amyloid deposition and neurofibrillary tangle formation.[10,11] The accumulation of β-amyloid also causes oxidation of lipids, activation of apoptotic genes, disruption of cell membranes, and excitotoxicity from the neurotransmitter glutamate.[10]

Much interest exists in the neurotransmitter systems in relation to Alzheimer disease. Damage in Alzheimer disease involves changes in three mechanisms: nerve cell communication, metabolism, and repair. Several studies have found abnormalities in the cholinergic system, including reduced activity of choline acetyltransferase (the enzyme necessary for acetylcholine synthesis) and decreased acetylcholine synthesis (Figure 45-3). Some researchers believe that β-amyloid may be responsible for lower choline levels in nerve cells and decreased acetylcholine levels. The degeneration of cells in the nucleus basalis, a band of gray matter in the ventral portion of the medulla oblongata, has also been linked to diminished levels of acetylcholine in the cerebral cortex, a finding that provides further evidence for the significant role of the cholinergic system in Alzheimer disease.[9] Along with alterations in acetylcholine, other neurotransmitters are also affected. Imbalances in the activity of glutamate, dopamine, and serotonin contribute to the behavioral signs and symptoms of Alzheimer disease.[12]

Vascular dementia results from single cerebrovascular insults (such as cerebral infarction), from multiple lacunar infarcts, or from microvascular pathology. Microvascular insults may not show any localizing clinical symptoms and may be found incidentally on brain imaging. However, the presence of these also does not automatically mean a diagnosis of vascular dementia.[13] The symptoms of vascular dementia may be similar to those of Alzheimer dementia. Most research/reports present vascular dementia and Alzheimer dementia as entirely separate entities; however, there is increasing evidence that particularly in elderly patients the brain lesions associated with both often coexist. There is emerging evidence that the cascade of events leading to the development of Alzheimer disease plaques and tangles may be due to ischemic and inflammatory insults of cerebrovascular disease.[10,13]

The primary risk factors for the development of Alzheimer disease include age and family history. Epidemiologic studies show that individuals who have an affected first-degree relative with Alzheimer disease have a fourfold greater risk of developing the disease. The risk is greater if there are individuals in more than one generation with the disease.[7] Three main genes have been identified and are thought to be responsible for autosomal dominant familial Alzheimer disease. *Presenilin 1, presenilin 2,* and *APP* are believed to increase the amount of β-amyloid protein.[11] These genes are rare, accounting for only 3% of Alzheimer disease cases, usually the early-onset variant.[11] The major gene associated with late-onset Alzheimer disease is apolipoprotein e4 *(APOe4).* By age 85, those who are homozygous for the *APOe4* allele have a 50% to 90% chance of developing Alzheimer disease. Those who are heterozygous have a 45% chance of developing the disease. Carrying the *APOe4* gene has also been associated with increased risk of atherosclerosis and cerebrovascular disease, strengthening the link between Alzheimer disease and vascular dementia.[10,13] Lifestyle has also been linked to the risk of Alzheimer disease. Head trauma, diabetes, and depression have been linked to an increased incidence of the disease as well as marital status, urban living, and inactive mental and physical lifestyle.[13] Risk factors for vascular dementia include those for stroke, hypertension, and diabetes.[13,14] Clearly, both vascular dementia and Alzheimer disease include a complex interplay of genetic, environmental, and lifestyle factors.

Clinical manifestations. Regardless of when patients first present with dementia, it is likely that brain disease has been present for quite some time. Most patients experience a gradual onset with a chronic progressive decline in cognitive functioning. There is memory loss, especially in short-term memory, whereas long-term memory may be preserved. Thinking ability declines, and there is a decreasing ability to function at work and in social settings. Anxiety and agitation are common. As the disease progresses, individuals have increasing difficulty with judgment, problem solving, and communication. Assistance may be necessary for completing activities of daily living (ADLs). Difficulty with eating and swallowing, and weight loss are common. Loss

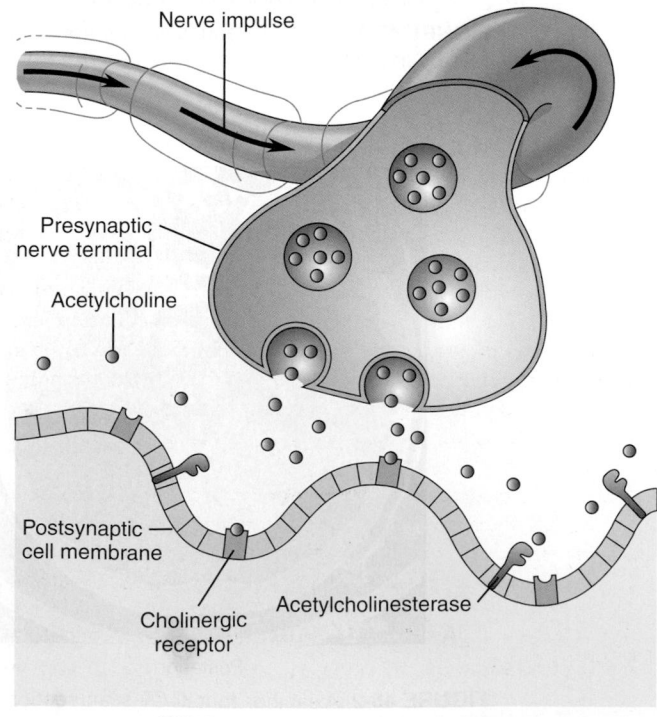

FIGURE 45-3 Cholinergic synapse.

of bladder and bowel control and eventual complete loss of the ability to ambulate occur in the late stages. Accidents and infection are common causes of death.[7]

Diagnosis and treatment. The initial evaluation of a patient thought to have dementia of any type begins with a complete history and physical examination. This should address the patient's overall general health and any coexisting medical conditions. All manageable causes for dementia or delirium should be ruled out. It is recommended that the evaluation should include a complete blood cell count, chemistry panel, thyroid function, vitamin B_{12} levels, and syphilis serology. Other testing such as Lyme serology, human immunodeficiency virus (HIV), urinalysis with culture/sensitivity, heavy-metal assays, sedimentation rate, and other vitamin levels may be warranted in certain patient situations. Other evaluations such as a chest x-ray and lumbar puncture may also be helpful. Neuroimaging may include computerized tomography (CT) and magnetic resonance imaging/magnetic resonance angiography (MRI/MRA), which may identify vascular disease, normal-pressure hydrocephalus, tumors, abscesses, or subdural hematoma. PET (positron emission tomography) scans are not routinely recommended at this point, but show promise in identifying Alzheimer disease when combined with a history of genetic risk. Mental status examinations, the clock drawing test, and tests of functional status are recommended.[9,11,14] A current list of the patient's medications, including over-the-counter medications, must also be reviewed. Medications with anticholinergic actions/side effects are a common cause of changes in cognitive functioning in the elderly.

Early diagnosis and intervention are key in the management of dementia. The financial and legal ramifications of dementia can be devastating to patients and their families and caregivers. If the diagnosis is made before the onset of severe cognitive disability, the patient can be involved in decisions regarding long-term care, power of attorney, and living will issues. Early diagnosis is also vital to initiating therapy as early as possible.

Currently, two classes of drugs are approved by the Food and Drug Administration for the treatment of Alzheimer disease. The first class is the acetylcholinesterase inhibitors: tacrine (Cognex), donepezil (Aricept), rivastigmine (Exelon), and galantamine (Reminyl). These agents are indicated for use in patients with mild to moderate Alzheimer disease. Although not a cure, the acetylcholinesterase inhibitors have been shown to stabilize cognitive function and slow progression of the illness.[14,15] Acetylcholinesterase inhibitors have also been shown to improve cognitive functioning in patients with vascular dementia.[15]

The second class of drugs used in the treatment of Alzheimer disease is known as the *N*-methyl-D-aspartate (NMDA) receptor antagonists. Currently only one drug in this class is available in the United States. Memantine (Namenda) is indicated for the treatment of moderate to severe Alzheimer-type dementia. This drug blocks stimulation by the neuroexcitatory transmitter glutamate. Again, this medication is not a cure, but slows progression of the disease.[16] Studies using combination therapy of acetylcholinesterase inhibitors and NMDA antagonists are showing modest improvement in cognitive functioning.[15,16] Studies using NMDA antagonists for vascular dementia have not shown conclusive benefit.[17]

Many other medications, although not approved for use in treating Alzheimer disease, are used to manage the symptoms, such as depression, sleep disturbance, agitation, and psychosis. These medications include antidepressants, anxiolytics, antipsychotics, and mood stabilizers.[16]

A variety of medications and nutritional supplements have been used in the prevention and management of Alzheimer disease, including gingko biloba; antioxidants such as vitamin E, α-lipoic acid, omega-3 fatty acids, and coenzyme Q_{10}; and nonsteroidal antiinflammatory drugs (NSAIDs). The blood pressure drugs angiotensin-converting enzyme (ACE) inhibitors and angiotensin receptor blockers (ARBs) are showing slowed progression of disease beyond just lowering blood pressure. However, all the research has been completed on hypertensive individuals.[18-20] Research findings regarding nutritional supplements are inconsistent and therefore ongoing.[18]

Other treatments for dementia include optimal management of other coexisting illnesses, interventions aimed at wellness, regulation of optimal nutritional intake, and protection from injury. In early stages of the disease, most patients are cared for at home, often by family members. It is important that the home environment be safe and that there be measures in place to control wandering. Consistent routines and familiar surroundings allow the patient to feel more comfortable and experience less confusion. As the disease progresses, the individual with dementia may have to be placed in an alternative living situation such as a nursing home or assisted-living program. Caring for the caregivers of patients with dementia is important.

> **KEY POINTS**
> - Dementia refers to progressive degeneration of cognitive function attributable to organic causes. In many instances the cause is unknown. There are limited definitive treatments for dementia, none of which is a cure. It is important to first rule out manageable causes of mental impairment.
> - The dementia of Alzheimer disease is characterized by degeneration of neurons in the temporal and frontal lobes, atrophy of the brain, and the formation of amyloid plaques and neurofibrillary tangles. The synthesis of brain acetylcholine is deficient. The cause of Alzheimer disease remains unknown, although genetic factors and environmental triggers are suspected.
> - The behavioral problems of individuals with Alzheimer disease progress from forgetfulness to total inability for self-care. Depression and psychosis may be significant.

Parkinson Disease

Parkinson disease is a disorder of mobility that affects 1 million Americans. It is estimated that 60,000 new cases are diagnosed each year. Although it usually develops after age 65, 4% of those diagnosed are younger than age 50.[21]

Etiology. Parkinson disease may be idiopathic or acquired. Idiopathic Parkinson disease is that in which no demonstrable cause is identified. Common causes of acquired **parkinsonism** include infection, intoxication, and trauma.[3] Typically, parkinsonism attributable to drug toxicity evolves rapidly, unlike the slow, insidious onset of the idiopathic form of the disease. Side effects of drugs of the phenothiazine class (e.g., chlorpromazine, prochlorperazine, and thioridazine) and butyrophenone class (e.g., haloperidol) may manifest in a parkinsonian syndrome at toxic levels. Discontinuing the medication generally results in improvement in the symptoms. However, the additional use of the anticholinergic antiparkinsonian drugs may aid in more rapid recovery. The rest of this discussion of Parkinson disease refers to the most common idiopathic type.

Pathogenesis. Parkinson disease results from degeneration of the pigmented dopaminergic neurons found in the substantia nigra (Figure 45-4) and, to a lesser extent, neurons elsewhere in the brain. Eosinophilic cytoplasmic inclusions known as Lewy bodies may be found in the surviving neurons. Incidentally, Lewy bodies are found along with amyloid plaques at autopsy in the brains of some patients with a severe form of dementia. This suggests a possible link with Alzheimer disease. The exact cause of this degeneration is unknown,

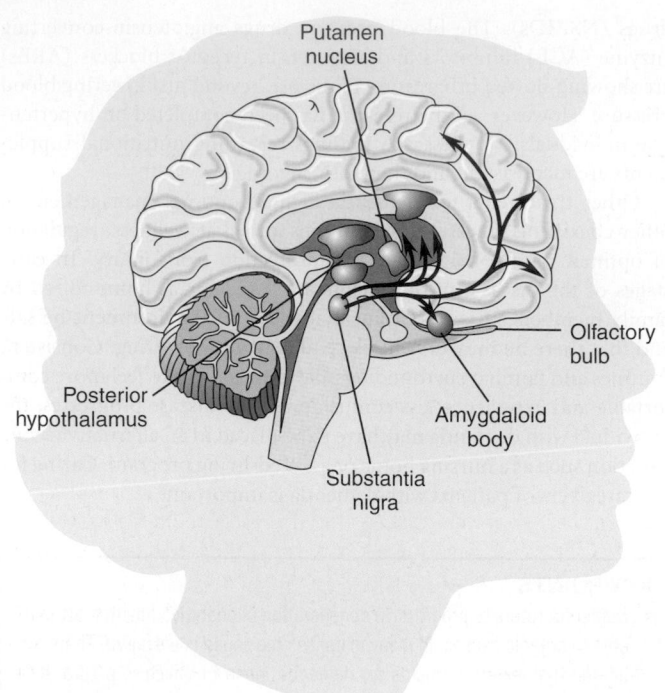

FIGURE 45-4 Dopaminergic neurons and their pathways in the human brain.

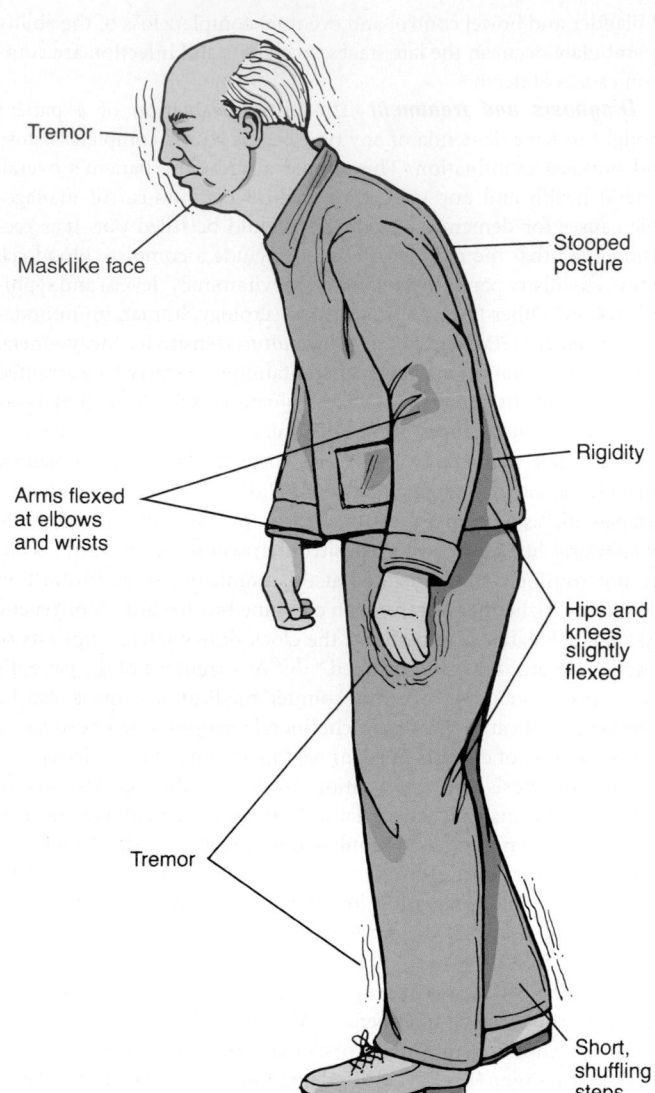

FIGURE 45-5 Clinical manifestations of Parkinson disease. (From Monahan FD, Neighbors M: *Phipps' medical-surgical nursing: health and illness perspectives*, ed 8, Philadelphia, 2007, Saunders, p 1446.)

but mitochondrial dysfunction from oxidative stress, genetics, and environmental toxins has been implicated.[22] Adaptive immunity may play a part in the progression of Parkinson disease by reacting to the abnormal proteins and causing neuroinflammation.[23]

At least 13 different gene groups have been identified as having a role in the development of Parkinson disease. In particular, identification of a mutation in the *α-synuclein* gene has become the focus of much interest. Although mutations of the gene are a rare cause of Parkinson disease, *α-synuclein* is abundant in neurons, specifically in presynaptic terminals, and is a major component of Lewy bodies.[22] Another gene identified in the development of Parkinson disease is *parkin*. Mitochondrial quality control is mediated by *parkin*. When functioning normally, it selectively recognizes and eliminates damaged mitochondria from the cell by autophagy. *Parkin* mutations are associated with monogenic forms of Parkinson disease.[24] Although genes have received much attention in Parkinson disease research, environmental factors have also been studied. High caffeine intake has been found to have an inverse relationship to the risk of developing the disorder.[22,25] Long-term exposure to the pesticide rotenone and the herbicide paraquat have been linked to increasing risk for Parkinson disease.[26] Whatever the cause of the degeneration of the dopaminergic cells, 75% to 80% of the neurons have died before any symptoms of the disease become apparent.

Clinical manifestations and treatment. Because of the insidious onset, earlier evidence of Parkinson disease may be discovered in a thorough health history. Frequently, the very early signs of the disorder (loss of flexibility, aching, and fatigue) are overlooked by the patient or are attributed to the aging process. Initially, symptoms are usually worse on one side of the body and then progress to involve both sides. Tremor is often the first symptom recognized that prompts patients to seek treatment. The tremor is generally at rest, unilaterally affecting distal extremities. Hand tremors may be described as pill-rolling movements. Attempts to passively move the extremities are met with cogwheel rigidity. As Parkinson disease progresses, the tremor will

often become bilateral/more generalized. Additional early signs of the disease include bradykinesia, rigidity, hypokinesia, loss of facial expression, and infrequent eye blinking (Figure 45-5). Again, these symptoms may be overlooked by patients but are usually apparent to observant family members.

As the disease progresses, additional functional changes are noted. The patient's handwriting may become small (micrographia) and cramped, with evidence of tremor. Speech may become low in volume, monotonous, and dysarthric. There may be a mumbling quality to the speech. The effects of bradykinesia are evident in the patient's swallowing function, ability to initiate activity, and level of mobility. Swallowing becomes delayed so much so that the individual may drool, and patients are at risk for aspiration. The effect of the disease on the ability to initiate activity is evident when the individual rises from a chair or begins to walk from a standing-still position. However, many people with Parkinson disease are able to act quickly in times of emergency, such as fire. This phenomenon is known as paradoxical kinesia.

Additional difficulties in mobility are evident from the lack of spontaneous position changes while the individual is sitting in one position, from the decreased or absent arm swing while the individual is walking, and from the shuffling gait. Impairment of postural reflexes presents particular safety problems for the individual with Parkinson disease in maintaining balance, as evidenced by propulsive or retropulsive gaits. Involvement of the autonomic nervous system may result in orthostatic hypotension, which adds yet another risk to the individual's health. Because of these various impairments, falls are a common problem. Depression is present in many patients with Parkinson disease. Daytime sleepiness is also common as well as sleep disturbances and restless leg syndrome.[27] Dementia is prevalent in patients with Parkinson disease.

There is no known cure for Parkinson disease. Treatments are aimed at slowing the progression of the disease and managing symptoms. The mainstay of Parkinson therapy has been aimed at increasing the level of dopamine in the CNS. Dopamine precursors such as levodopa are one approach to increasing dopamine levels. Dopamine itself cannot be used because it does not cross the blood-brain barrier efficiently. Outside the CNS, levodopa is metabolized to dopamine and then to adrenaline and noradrenaline, which can cause altered blood pressure. To minimize these side effects, levodopa is combined with carbidopa. This agent blocks the conversion of levodopa to dopamine in the periphery, allowing it to cross the blood-brain barrier.[27,28] Long-term use of levodopa has been associated with "on-off" phenomena (in which the action of the drug suddenly stops, leaving the patient with sudden onset of symptoms) or abnormal movements called *dyskinesias*. Other medications aimed at increasing the level of dopamine in the CNS include dopamine agonists (pramipexole, ropinirole); medications to slow the metabolism of dopamine (monoamine oxidase inhibitors such as selegiline, catechol-*O*-methyltransferase inhibitors); and medications shown to be helpful with akinesia and dyskinesia (such as amantadine).[27,28] Anticholinergic medications may help with tremor, rigidity, or drooling. The Alzheimer drug rivastigmine (Exelon) may be used to slow the progression of Parkinson-induced dementia.[28]

Surgical options for the management of Parkinson disease have received much recent attention. Tissue transplantation of embryonic stem cells in an attempt to increase the level of dopamine in the CNS is very controversial and has not been consistently shown to improve the symptoms of Parkinson disease.[29] Deep brain stimulation involves the surgical implantation of a high-frequency thalamic electrical stimulator that interrupts the tremor-causing nerve impulses, minimizing dystonia. This can decrease the need for Parkinson medication.[28,30]

Ablative surgical techniques of thalamotomy and pallidotomy create small lesions in the thalamus or pallidum; these can improve rigidity, tremor, and bradykinesia.[31] Symptoms are better controlled with medication following the surgery. These surgical techniques are considered for patients who have been unresponsive to the medical treatments or who are unable to tolerate the side effects. These surgical techniques have high morbidity associated with them and are rarely used. Genetic research on Parkinson disease continues.

KEY POINTS

- Parkinson disease may be idiopathic or a consequence of the use of certain drugs. Dopamine deficiency in the basal ganglia (substantia nigra, caudate, and putamen) is associated with symptoms of motor impairment. Difficulty initiating and controlling movements results in akinesia, tremor, and rigidity. Tremor occurs at rest, and hand tremors may be described as pill-rolling movements. Attempts to passively move the extremities are met with cogwheel rigidity. There is a general lack of movement, loss of facial expression, drooling, propulsive gait, and absent arm swing.

- Treatment is aimed at restoring brain dopamine levels or activity by administration of dopamine precursors, dopamine agonists, monoamine oxidase inhibitors, and anticholinergics. Antidepressant therapy may also help alleviate depression, and surgical procedures may be helpful for motor symptoms.

Cerebral Palsy

Etiology and pathogenesis. **Cerebral palsy** refers to a diverse group of crippling syndromes that appears during childhood and involves permanent, nonprogressive damage to the developing brain. Such damage occurs during fetal development; before, during, or shortly after birth; or during early infancy. Damage occurs in the upper motor neurons that control voluntary and involuntary muscle movement. The symptoms of this damage remain for life. The majority of these children will survive until at least early adulthood. Although cerebral palsy is not considered a progressive disorder, these adolescents and adults are challenged by a variety of health problems and functional decline including chronic pain, scoliosis, and respiratory dysfunction along with a host of other symptoms.[32]

Cerebral palsy is classified on the basis of neurologic signs and symptoms, with the major types involving spasticity, ataxia, or dyskinesia, or a combination of these symptoms. Cerebral palsy is one of the most common crippling disorders of childhood, with an incidence of between 2 and 2.5 per 1000 births.[33] Etiologic factors include prenatal infections or diseases of the mother; mechanical trauma to the head before, during, or after birth; or exposure to nerve-damaging poisons or a period of reduced oxygen supply to the brain. Neonatal hypoglycemia, **kernicterus,** prematurity, and low birth weight are also risk factors. Often the cause is multifactorial, and in many cases a single cause cannot be identified.[34]

Clinical manifestations. Spastic cerebral palsy manifests with hypertonia, prolonged primitive reflexes, exaggerated deep-tendon reflexes, clonus, rigidity of the extremities, scoliosis, and contractures. This type of cerebral palsy is the most common. Spastic paralysis often affects one entire side of the body (hemiplegia), both legs (paraplegia), both legs and one arm (triplegia), or all four extremities (quadriplegia). A "scissors" gait and toe walking are common. Dyskinetic/athetoid cerebral palsy manifests with extreme difficulty in purposeful movement and fine-motor coordination. Movements are slow, jerky, uncontrolled, and abrupt, resulting from injury to the **basal ganglia** or **extrapyramidal tracts.** The uncontrolled movements may increase during times of stress and disappear during sleep.[34,35] Ataxic cerebral palsy is associated with gait disturbances and instability. The infant with this type of cerebral palsy may have hypotonia at birth, but stiffness of the trunk muscles develops by late infancy. Persistence of truncal stiffness affects the child's gait and ability to maintain equilibrium. Pure ataxic cerebral palsy is rare. This palsy denotes maldevelopment of the cerebrum or its pathways, which if severe may be associated with significant cognitive impairment.[34,35] More typically, a child will have a mixed disorder with clinical manifestations of each of the types.

Children with cerebral palsy often have neurologic complications such as seizures, intellectual difficulties ranging from mild to severe, and visual problems.[33,34] Other associated clinical manifestations include hearing impairment, communication disorders, respiratory problems, bowel and bladder problems, and orthopedic disabilities.

Treatment. There is no cure for cerebral palsy, and the goal of management is to increase functionality. Treatment varies according to the nature and extent of brain damage. As a result of problems with muscle spasticity and contracture, muscle relaxation is a large part of therapy. Muscle relaxant medications are common. Several studies have also supported the use of botulinum toxin type A (Botox) to reduce pain and increase joint range of motion.[36] Anticonvulsant drugs are necessary when seizures are among the symptoms of the disorder.

Orthopedic surgery, casts, braces, and traction may be useful to correct some types of associated disability. A comprehensive rehabilitation program including early muscle training and special exercises may help the child with cerebral palsy lead a more productive life.

KEY POINTS

- Cerebral palsy refers to a diverse group of crippling syndromes that appear during childhood and involve permanent, nonprogressive damage to motor control areas of the brain.
- Cerebral palsy may be classified on the basis of neurologic signs and symptoms, with the major types involving spasticity, ataxia, or dyskinesia, or a mix of two or more of these three symptoms.
- Etiologic factors include prenatal infections or diseases of the mother; mechanical trauma to the head before, during, or after birth; or exposure to nerve-damaging poisons or a period of reduced oxygen supply to the brain.
- Treatment varies according to the nature and extent of brain damage. Muscle relaxants, anticonvulsant drugs, orthopedic surgery, casts, braces, and traction are among the therapies used.

Hydrocephalus

Etiology. **Hydrocephalus** is a condition caused by abnormal accumulation of cerebrospinal fluid (CSF) in the cerebral ventricular system. Figure 45-6 illustrates the normal flow of CSF. Hydrocephalus is generally associated with a congenital defect, usually a neural tube defect. Viral infections or other neurotoxic agents acquired during pregnancy have been implicated with the congenital forms. It also occurs occasionally in adults and elderly persons as a consequence of mass lesions, trauma, hemorrhage, or infections such as meningitis. There are three types of hydrocephalus: (1) normal-pressure hydrocephalus; (2) obstructive/noncommunicating hydrocephalus; and (3) nonobstructive/communicating hydrocephalus.

Normal-pressure hydrocephalus is a condition in which CSF volume increases without change in intracranial pressure because brain tissue has been lost. The cause of normal-pressure hydrocephalus remains unknown, but it is thought to be from an abnormality of the normal absorption of CSF. Ventricles become distended, compressing brain tissue and the cerebral vessels. There is no net change in intracranial pressure. Patients with this form of hydrocephalus demonstrate a triad of symptoms: gait instability, urinary incontinence, and dementia.[37] If the problem is identified quickly, symptoms may improve/resolve with appropriate treatment.

Obstructive/noncommunicating hydrocephalus is most common in children and attributable to an abnormality of the cerebral aqueduct or a lesion in the fourth ventricle. The cause is usually a congenital abnormality, such as stenosis of the foramina of the fourth ventricle or spina bifida cystica.[38]

Nonobstructive/communicating hydrocephalus (sometimes referred to as *acquired communicating hydrocephalus*) is identified by an abnormality in the capacity to absorb fluid from the subarachnoid space. There is no obstruction to the flow of fluid between the ventricles. Infections, trauma, and tumors have been identified as etiologic factors.[38] In premature infants this usually results from an intraventricular hemorrhage.

Pathogenesis and clinical manifestations. Usually the obstructive type of hydrocephalus is caused by a block in the aqueduct of Sylvius, resulting from premature closure before birth in affected babies or

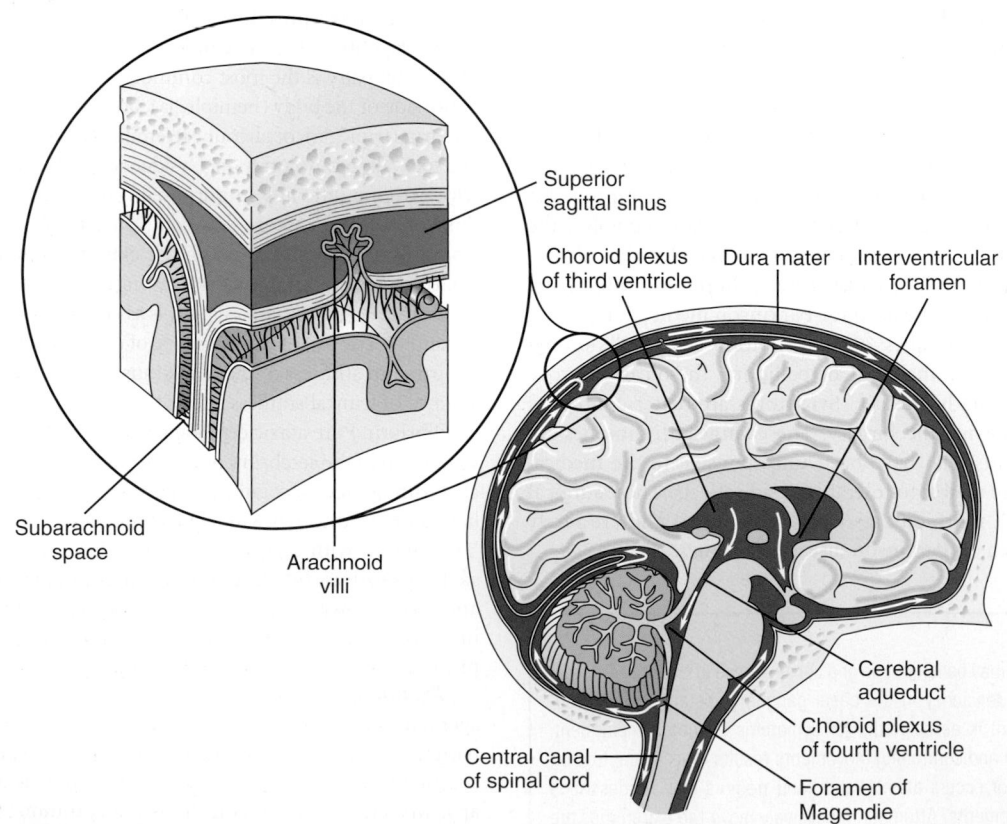

FIGURE 45-6 Ventricular system of the brain and distribution of cerebrospinal fluid (CSF). CSF is formed in the ventricles, passes to the subarachnoid space outside the brain and spinal cord, and moves through small valvelike structures into the large veins of the head.

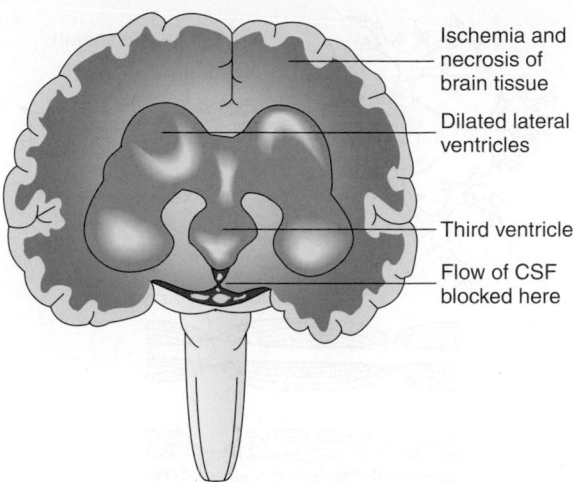

FIGURE 45-7 Hydrocephalus. *CSF*, Cerebrospinal fluid. (From Gould BE, Dyer R: *Pathophysiology for the health professions*, ed 4, Philadelphia, 2011, Saunders.)

from a brain tumor at any age (Figure 45-7). As fluid is formed by the choroid plexus in the two lateral and the third ventricles, the volumes of these three ventricles increase greatly. This flattens the brain into a thin shell against the skull. In neonates, the increased pressure also causes the entire head to swell because the skull bones have not fused.

The communicating type of hydrocephalus is usually caused by blockage of fluid flow in the **subarachnoid space** around the basal regions of the brain or blockage of the **arachnoid villi** themselves. Fluid therefore collects both inside the ventricles and on the outside of the brain. If it occurs in infants when the skull is still pliable and can be stretched, the head swells tremendously.

Treatment. Medical treatment has been used with only limited success in controlling the secretion of CSF and relieving hydrocephalus. The most effective treatment is surgical correction employing a shunting technique. The basic components of the shunt are a ventricular catheter, a valve, and a distal catheter. Multiple perforations along the ventricular catheter permit the drainage of fluid from the ventricle. The valve is constructed so that fluid will flow in one direction only, and some valves have a pumping chamber to facilitate drainage. The distal catheter may be positioned at any of a number of sites, the most common being the peritoneal cavity (ventriculoperitoneal shunt) (Figure 45-8). The shunt thus extends all the way from one of the ventricles to the peritoneal cavity where the fluid can then be absorbed and excreted. Another surgical approach is endoscopic third ventriculostomy. This involves making a hole in the third ventricle to allow free flow of CSF into the basal cisterns for reabsorption. This surgery is used for obstructive hydrocephalus.[38] It should be emphasized that the correlation between degree of hydrocephalus and impaired cognitive function often results from additional complications, such as severe congenital malformations, acute or chronic infections, or progressive brain tumors.

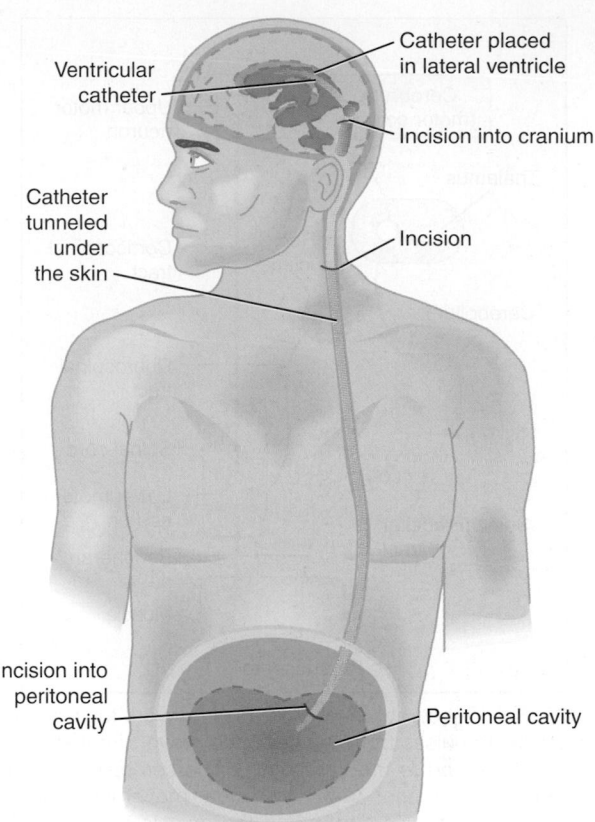

FIGURE 45-8 Ventriculoperitoneal shunt placed for chronic hydrocephalus. (From Black JM et al: *Medical-surgical nursing: clinical management for positive outcomes*, ed 8, Philadelphia, 2008, Saunders, p 1933.)

Cerebellar Disorders

The cerebellum performs three general functions in the control of skeletal muscles: (1) together with activity of the cerebral cortex, it coordinates the activities of muscle groups to produce skilled movement; (2) it functions below the level of consciousness to maintain posture and make movements smooth, steady, efficient, and coordinated; and (3) it controls skeletal muscles to maintain balance (see Chapter 43). Figure 45-9 illustrates the cerebrum and cerebellum working together to coordinate muscle movement. Impulses from the motor control areas of the cerebrum travel down the corticospinal tract and through peripheral nerves to skeletal muscle tissue. Simultaneously, the impulses go to the cerebellum. The cerebellum compares the motor commands of the cerebrum to information coming from receptors in the muscle. In effect, the cerebellum compares the intended movement to the actual movement. Impulses then travel from the cerebellum to both the cerebrum and the muscle tissue to adjust or coordinate the movements to produce the intended action.[39]

Etiology and clinical manifestations. Cerebellar disorders may have myriad causes. Abscess, hemorrhage, tumors, trauma, viral infection, and chronic alcoholism have been implicated. Identification and eradication of the causal agent determine treatment and prognosis. The clinical manifestations of cerebellar disorders primarily include **ataxia** (muscle incoordination), hypotonia, intention tremors, and disturbances of gait and balance.[39] Disturbances of gait and balance vary, depending on the muscle groups involved. The walk, for instance, is often characterized by staggering or lurching and by a clumsy manner of raising the foot too high and bringing it down with a clap. Loss of cerebellar function does not result in paralysis.[39]

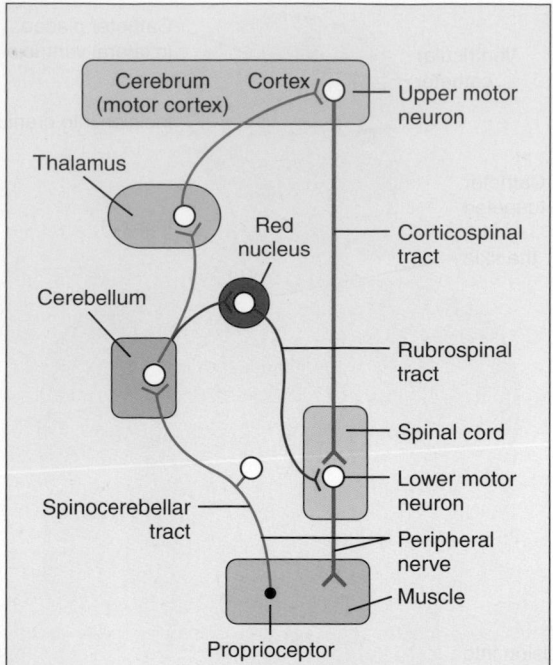

FIGURE 45-9 The cerebrum and cerebellum work together to control muscles. Impulses from the cerebrum travel simultaneously to skeletal muscle and to the cerebellum. The cerebellum compares the intended movement with the actual movement and sends impulses to both the cerebrum and the muscle tissue, coordinating and smoothing muscle activity. (Redrawn from Thibodeau GA, Patton KT: *Anatomy & physiology*, ed 5, St Louis, 2003, Mosby.)

KEY POINTS
- The cerebellum is responsible for coordinated control of muscle action, excitation and inhibition of postural reflexes, and maintenance of balance.
- Etiologic factors in cerebellar disorders may include the following: abscess, hemorrhage, tumors, trauma, viral infection, or chronic alcoholism.
- Clinical manifestations of cerebellar disorders primarily include ataxia, hypotonia, intention tremors, and disturbances of gait and balance.

SPINAL CORD AND PERIPHERAL NERVE DISORDERS

Multiple Sclerosis

Etiology. **Multiple sclerosis (MS)** is a chronic demyelinating disease of the CNS that causes significant disability in young adults. It is thought to be an autoimmune disorder that results in inflammation and scarring (sclerosis) of the myelin sheaths covering nerves. It is estimated that 400,000 Americans have MS. The age of onset ranges from 20 to 50 years, and MS is two to three times more common in women than in men. Epidemiologic studies show that MS occurs at a higher rate among individuals from Caucasian northern European descent and those who live in northern latitudes. Several studies indicate that those who were born and spent the early years of life (first 15 years) in northern areas carry an increased risk of MS even if they migrate south at some time later in their lives.[40]

MS is an unpredictable disease with a wide variety of clinical presentations. Symptoms can vary daily, and the disease may cause only mild disability with occasional exacerbations. In some individuals, however, MS may cause extreme progressive disability. Despite great

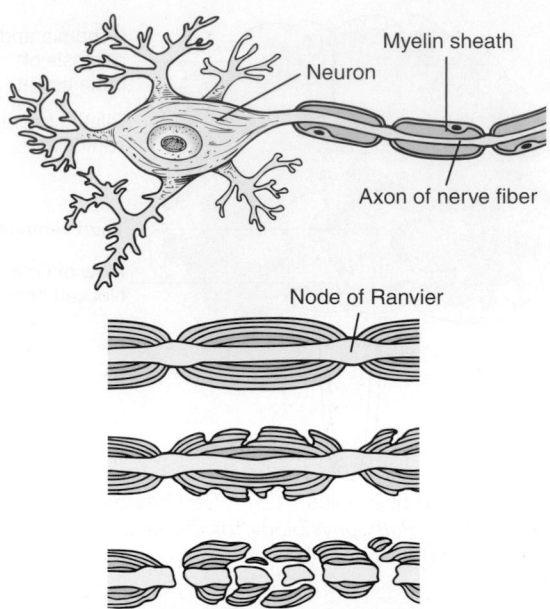

FIGURE 45-10 Changes in the nerve sheath, as seen in multiple sclerosis. Myelin is made by oligodendrocytes and coats nerves, facilitating nervous impulse. In patients with multiple sclerosis, the myelin degenerates in patches, causing nerve transmission to become erratic. (From Black JM et al: *Medical-surgical nursing: clinical management for positive outcomes*, ed 8, Philadelphia, 2008, Saunders, p 1909.)

advances in research, the exact cause of MS is unknown. Genetics may have a role. Non-twin first-degree relatives have a 1 in 40 risk of developing MS.[40]

Pathogenesis. In MS, the **demyelination** of nerves can occur anywhere in the CNS. There does not seem to be any predictable pattern in the timing or location of the lesions. However, structures most frequently affected are the optic nerves; the oculomotor nerves; and the corticospinal, cerebellar, and posterior column systems. Figure 45-10 illustrates demyelination. Myelin facilitates nerve conduction; the inflammation and scarring that occurs with MS slows or interrupts the conduction of nerve impulses. The triggering event for this process is not understood. It is theorized that an exposure to a viral infection or environmental toxin initiates the autoimmune attack in a genetically predisposed individual. Both humoral and cellular immune factors have been implicated in demyelination. Antibodies to specific myelin proteins have been found in both the serum and the CSF of MS patients. T-cell lymphocyte–mediated injury to the myelin has also been implicated in causing the autoimmune damage and sustaining inflammation.[41,42]

Clinical manifestations and treatment. Symptoms of MS vary widely and depend upon the location of damage to the myelin. They include impaired visual acuity or blurred vision, diplopia, weakness, numbness, tingling, extreme fatigue, imbalance, movement disorders, spasticity, coordination difficulties and gait disturbance, bladder and/or bowel difficulties, vertigo, pain, and paresthesia. Neurobehavioral symptoms may include depression, emotional lability, sexual dysfunction, as well as memory and cognitive impairment (Table 45-1). In later stages of the disease, spastic paralysis of the limbs may be present because of upper motor neuron damage. Symptoms may be exacerbated by heat, infection, trauma, and stress. Relapses are also common in the postpartum period following pregnancy.[43] There are four main categories to classify the clinical course of MS (Table 45-2).

There is no conclusive diagnostic test for MS. The diagnosis is based on clinical characteristics, imaging studies, and laboratory evidence. The current diagnostic criteria for MS require documentation of two or more episodes of symptoms and two or more signs that reflect pathology in anatomically different areas of the CNS.[42,43] Advances in neuroimaging techniques have become quite useful in the diagnosis of MS. MRI of the brain and spinal cord may show the presence of demyelination (plaques). CNS lesions that are disseminated in time and space with no better explanation is one diagnostic criterion for MS.[33] Evoked potential recording of nerve stimulation in the visual and other nerve pathways may be helpful. Laboratory tests may show mild lymphocytosis and elevated serum protein levels, especially following an acute relapse. Elevated levels of immunoglobulin G (IgG) in the CSF with the presence of discrete bands of IgG (oligoclonal bands) may also be present.[44]

There is no cure for MS. Treatment centers not only on managing the symptoms of the disease but also on minimizing the damage inflicted by the autoimmune attack on myelin. Corticosteroids such as prednisone are used to reduce edema and the inflammatory response in acute exacerbations. Recovery may be hastened by the use of these agents; however, the extent of recovery is unchanged.[42] Five drugs are currently approved by the FDA as disease-modifying agents for use in treating MS. Four are administered by injection: interferon beta-1a (Avonex and Rebif), interferon beta-1b (Betaseron), and glatiramer acetate (Copaxone). These medications reduce the number of attacks in relapsing-remitting MS. A fifth medication, mitoxantrone (Novantrone), is an antineoplastic medication that has been shown to be most helpful in decreasing symptoms of progressive-relapsing MS. Natalizumab (Tysabri) is a monoclonal antibody that has been shown to decrease the movement of myelin-damaging autoantibodies across the blood-brain barrier. Its use is limited under a special prescription program when benefits outweigh the risks of side effects.[43,44]

Management of symptoms frequently requires participation from multiple disciplines, including medicine, nursing, speech pathology, neuropsychiatry, social services, and vocational services. Treatment with an array of medications such as antispasmodics, anticholinergics,

TABLE 45-1 MULTIPLE SCLEROSIS SYMPTOMS

AREA OF DYSFUNCTION	SYMPTOMS
Cranial nerve dysfunction	Blurred central vision; faded colors; blind spots (optic neuritis)
	Diplopia
	Dysphagia
	Facial weakness, numbness, pain
Motor dysfunction	Weakness
	Paralysis
	Spasticity
	Abnormal gait
Sensory dysfunction	Paresthesias
	Lhermitte sign (electric shock–like sensation radiating down spine into extremities)
	Decreased proprioception
	Decreased temperature perception
Cerebellar dysfunction	Dysarthria
	Tremor
	Incoordination
	Ataxia
	Vertigo
Bowel and bladder dysfunction	Fecal urgency, constipation, incontinence
	Urinary frequency, urgency, hesitancy, nocturia, retention, incontinence
Cognitive dysfunction	Decreased short-term memory
	Difficulty learning new information
	Word-finding trouble
	Short attention span
	Decreased concentration
	Mood alterations (depression, euphoria)
Sexual dysfunction	Women: decreased libido, decreased orgasmic ability, decreased genital sensation
	Men: erectile, orgasmic, and ejaculatory dysfunction
Fatigue	Overwhelming weakness not overcome with increased physical effort

Adapted from Calabresi PA: Multiple sclerosis and demyelinating conditions of the central nervous system. In Goldman L, Schafter AI, editors: *Goldman's Cecil medicine*, ed 24, Philadelphia, 2012, Elsevier; Goodin DS, Hauser LS: Multiple sclerosis and other demyelinating diseases. In Longo DL, Fauci AS, Kasper DL et al, editors: *Harrison's principles of internal medicine*, ed 18, New York, 2012, McGraw-Hill. Available at www.accessmedicine.com.proxy.heal-wa.org/content.aspx?aID=9147780. Accessed 3/24/12.

TABLE 45-2 CLINICAL COURSE OF MULTIPLE SCLEROSIS

COURSE	CHARACTERISTICS
Relapsing-Remitting Most common form; approximately 85% of MS patients have this form	Clearly defined exacerbations (relapses) with acute decline in neurologic function; followed by periods of partial/complete recovery and remissions; remissions may last months to years
Primary-Progressive Relatively rare; approximately 10% of MS patients have this form	Slow but almost continuous decline in neurologic function; plateaus or temporary minor improvements may occur; relapses/remissions not present; severe disability develops early
Secondary-Progressive Before use of disease-modifying drugs; approximately 50% of relapsing-remitting patients develop this form	Begins as relapsing-remitting; followed by steady decline in neurologic function with or without occasional relapses, remissions, or plateaus
Progressive-Relapsing Relatively rare; approximately 5% of patients have this form	Progressive from outset, but with clear exacerbations with or without recovery

Adapted from Goodin DS, Hauser LS: Multiple sclerosis and other demyelinating diseases. In Longo DL, Fauci AS, Kasper DL et al, editors: *Harrison's principles of internal medicine*, ed 18, New York, 2012, McGraw-Hill. Available at www.accessmedicine.com.proxy.heal-wa.org/content.aspx?aID=9147780. Accessed 3/24/12. From Kerchner GA: Chapter 24: Nervous system disorders. In McPhee SJ, Papadakis MA, Rabow MW, editors: *Current medical diagnosis and treatment 2012*, New York, 2012, McGraw-Hill. Available at www.accessmedicine.com.proxy.heal-wa.org/content.aspx?aID=12507. Accessed 3/24/12.

antidepressants, and antimicrobials helps to manage symptoms. Treatment also includes avoidance of complications such as urinary tract infections, constipation/impactions, respiratory tract infections, and pressure sores.

Research in MS continues to examine the immune system role. Viruses such as the Epstein-Barr virus have been implicated.[45] Low levels of vitamin D have also been implicated as an associated risk factor, because this is a common finding in people living in higher latitudes.[46]

KEY POINTS

- MS is a demyelinating disease of the CNS that primarily affects young adults. The risk of contracting MS is greater for persons living in higher latitudes. The cause of MS is unknown, but immunologic abnormalities and environmental factors are suspected.
- Demyelination can occur throughout the CNS but most frequently affects the optic and oculomotor nerves and spinal nerve tracts.
- In most cases symptoms are slowly progressive, and the disease is marked by exacerbations and remissions.
- Symptoms include double vision, weakness, poor coordination, and sensory deficits. Bowel and bladder control may be lost. Memory impairment is common.
- Management is symptomatic. Short-term steroid therapy may be helpful during acute exacerbations, and immune-modifying drugs may slow the progression of symptoms.

Spina Bifida

Etiology and pathogenesis. **Spina bifida** is a developmental anomaly characterized by defective closure of the bony encasement of the spinal cord (neural tube) through which the spinal cord and meninges may or may not protrude. If the anomaly is not visible, the condition is called *spina bifida occulta*. If there is an external protrusion of the saclike structure, the condition is called *spina bifida cystica* and is further classified according to the extent of neural involvement (e.g., meningocele, meningomyelocele, or myelomeningocele) (Figure 45-11).

Both environmental factors and genetics appear to be a factor in the etiologic development of neural tube defects.[47] These include alcohol, vitamin deficiency (folate), congenital rubella, anti-acne (Accutane) and anticonvulsant drugs, and chromosomal abnormalities. Increased maternal age, obesity, and diabetes are also risk factors.[47,48] Substituting another anticonvulsant drug may be recommended for pregnant women or for those considering pregnancy. Supplementation of folic acid before conception and during pregnancy also appears to decrease the prevalence of neural tube defects.[47,48]

Clinical manifestations. In spina bifida occulta, the posterior vertebral laminae have failed to fuse. The defect is extremely common and occurs to some degree in 10% to 20% of the population.[49] The vast majority of these vertebral defects are located in the lumbosacral regions, most commonly in the fifth lumbar vertebra and the first sacral vertebra, and may be detected prenatally through ultrasound and α-fetoprotein testing.

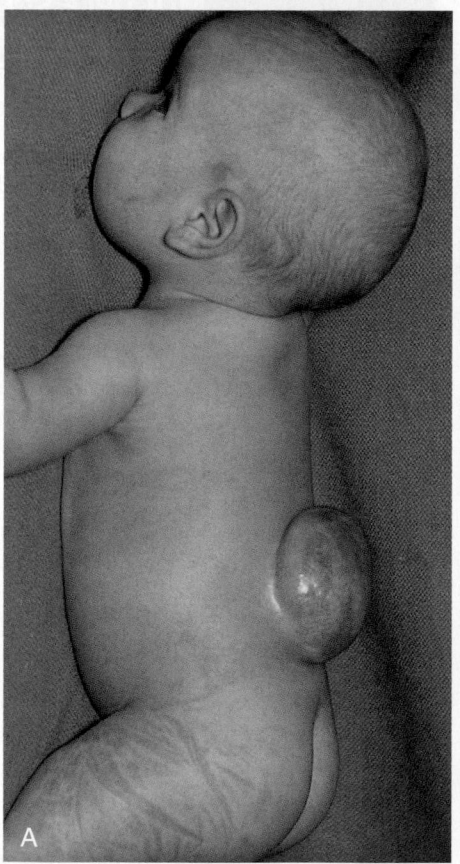
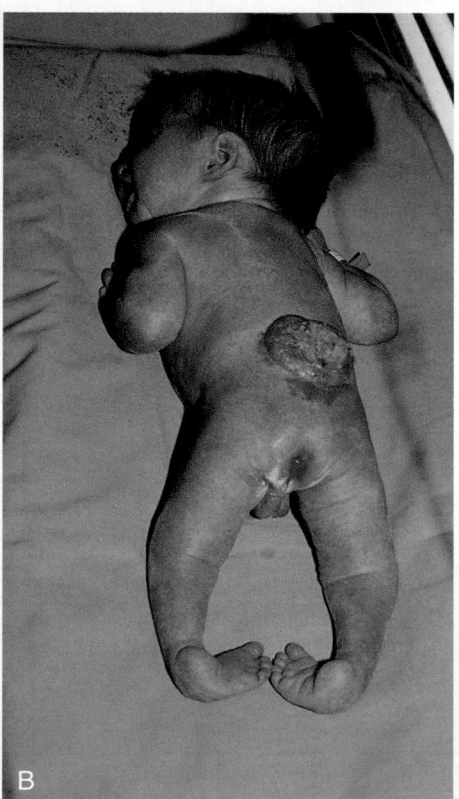

FIGURE 45-11 Photographs of infants with spina bifida cystica. **A,** Spina bifida with meningomyelocele in the lumbar region. **B,** Spina bifida with myeloschisis in the lumbar region. Note that the nerve involvement has affected the lower limbs. (In Moore KL, Persaud TVN: *The developing human: clinically oriented embryology*, ed 8, Philadelphia, 2008, Saunders. Courtesy Dr. Dwight Parkinson, Department of Surgery and Department of Human Anatomy and Cell Science, University of Manitoba, Winnipeg, Manitoba, Canada.)

Spina bifida occulta may be manifested by changes in the skin and body hair: either very coarse or silky hair along the spine; a midline dimple with or without a sinus tract; a cutaneous port-wine angioma; and/or a subcutaneous mass typically representing a lipoma or dermoid cyst.[49] Spina bifida occulta usually causes no serious neurologic problems. Common lumbosacral defects can cause gait disturbances, positional deformities of the feet, or bladder/bowel dysfunction. These symptoms become evident in childhood during periods of rapid growth.

In the **meningocele** form of spina bifida cystica, a saclike cyst filled with CSF protrudes through the spinal defect but does not involve the spinal cord. Meningoceles occur with equal frequency in the cervical, thoracic, and lumbar areas. A **myelomeningocele** or **meningomyelocele** deformity contains meninges, CSF, and a portion of the spinal cord that protrude from the vertebral defect in a cystlike sac. These defects most often occur in the lumbar or lumbosacral region of the spine, since these are the last areas of the neural tube to close during fetal development. These defects may be detected in prenatal ultrasound and with α-fetoprotein testing.[50] The bony prominences of the unfused neural arches are palpable at the lateral borders of the defect. The sac includes a transparent membranous covering that may have neural tissue attached to its inner surface. This membrane may be intact at birth or leak CSF, thereby increasing the risk of infection and neural damage. These infants are delivered via cesarean section to decrease the trauma to the exposed neural tissue, and surgical closure is attempted soon after delivery.[51] Affected infants often suffer from permanent neurologic damage resulting in motor weakness or paralysis and sensory deficit below the level of the spinal defect; bowel and bladder dysfunction; scoliosis; hydrocephalus; and seizures. Often the problems worsen as the child grows and the cord ascends within the vertebral canal, pulling primary scar tissue and thereby tethering the cord.[49] Attempts at closing the defect surgically in utero before delivery are currently being studied, and early results appear promising.[51]

Treatment. Treatment for this common disorder is based on the severity of the defect and neurologic dysfunction. Supplementation with folic acid during the period before conception has been shown to significantly decrease the risk of having a child with a neural tube defect. It is recommended that all women of childbearing age take 0.4 mg of folic acid daily for prevention. In fact, in the United States common foods are being supplemented with folic acid to decrease the incidence of this deformity.

KEY POINTS

- Spina bifida is a developmental anomaly characterized by defective closure of the bony encasement of the spinal cord (neural tube) through which the spinal cord and meninges may or may not protrude.
- If the anomaly is not visible, the condition is called *spina bifida occulta.* If there is an external protrusion of the saclike structure, the condition is called *spina bifida cystica,* and is further classified according to extent of neural involvement (e.g., meningocele, myelomeningocele).
- The natural history of myelomeningocele supports an early and aggressive operative approach before significant clinical deterioration begins. A cesarean section before rupture of amniotic membranes and onset of labor may decrease the degree of paralysis.
- Folic acid supplementation taken before conception and during pregnancy appears to decrease the prevalence of neural tube defects.

Amyotrophic Lateral Sclerosis

Etiology and pathogenesis. Amyotrophic lateral sclerosis (ALS) is a progressive degenerative disease affecting both the upper and the lower motor neurons characterized by muscle wasting and atrophy of the hands, arms, and legs. There are pathologic changes in the spinal cord that include degeneration of the lateral columns where the corticospinal tracts are located. ALS is also known as Lou Gehrig disease after the famed "Iron Man" of the New York Yankees who died from the disease. ALS affects an estimated 30,000 Americans at any given time. It most commonly strikes between the ages of 40 and 60 with a higher incidence in men than women. The majority of ALS cases occur at random; however, 5% to 10% of cases are familial.[52] There is also a higher incidence of the disease in military veterans, especially those of the Persian Gulf.[53] Although ALS is classified as a single disease entity, emerging evidence suggests that it is a clinical syndrome with several possible causes. It appears that sporadic cases of ALS are multifactorial and related to several environmental factors and a genetic predisposition. Smoking is the only probable risk factor identified at this point. Several unproven risk factors have been considered. These include lead or agricultural chemical exposure, viral infection, lymphoproliferative disease, and physical prowess.[54]

Genetic research has determined at least four different genetic mutations that are involved in ALS. One in particular involves a gene responsible for coding the free radical–scavenging enzyme superoxide dismutase 1 (*SOD1*). *SOD1* is the basis for much ALS research, and there seem to be multiple intracellular enzymatic pathways affected and causing premature programmed cell death, or **apoptosis** (see Chapter 4), of the neurons. Like Alzheimer and Parkinson diseases, ALS has been linked with oxidative stress and cellular damage. Neurons are highly susceptible to damage from oxygen free radicals and the activation of immune cells that propagate further cellular injury. High levels of the neurotransmitter glutamate have also been found in the CSF of ALS patients and are thought to be associated with the neuronal degeneration.[55,56] Other factors that may be involved in the pathogenesis include protein aggregation, mitochondrial dysfunction in motor neurons, and defective axonal transport.[55]

Clinical manifestations and treatment. Most patients with ALS demonstrate muscle weakness and atrophy. The earliest symptoms may be muscle twitching, cramping, and stiffness. Often the hands or upper extremities are affected first. The weakness is progressive and eventually affects the muscles that control speech, swallowing, and breathing. Finding hyperreflexia in a weak atrophied extremity is highly suggestive of ALS. Most individuals die from respiratory failure within 3 to 5 years from the onset of symptoms.[54] Despite the marked physical disability, most patients maintain their sensory and cognitive functions.

ALS is a diagnosis of exclusion, based on the patient's clinical signs and symptoms. Electromyography (EMG), nerve conduction studies, MRI, and serum laboratory testing may be used to rule out other causes of weakness, such as MS, brain and spinal tumors, human immunodeficiency virus, and Lyme disease.

The only FDA-approved treatment for ALS is riluzole (Rilutek), a glutamate inhibitor. This medication is not a cure, but its use can prolong life for several months and may delay the need for mechanical ventilation.[54] Patients with ALS benefit from a multidisciplinary approach to care to prevent complications from immobility as well as to address both physical and psychological needs.

KEY POINTS

- ALS is a progressive disease affecting both the upper and the lower motor neurons. The cause of ALS remains unknown. Weakness and wasting of the upper extremities usually occur, followed by impaired speech, swallowing, and respiration.
- ALS usually strikes between the ages of 40 and 60, and it is more common in men than in women. The mean survival time is about 3 years from the time of diagnosis.

- Clinical manifestations include weakness, atrophy, cramps, stiffness, and irregular twitching of muscle fibers.
- Diagnosis is based on clinical signs and symptoms, EMG results, nerve conduction studies, MRI studies, and serum laboratory testing.
- Riluzole (Rilutek) is a glutamate inhibitor, which may be helpful in management of ALS.

Spinal Cord Injury

Spinal cord injuries are among the most devastating and costly problems faced by patients and their families. Marked changes in lifestyle are required for survivors. Medical advances in the emergent management of spinal cord injuries and their associated complications have been responsible for increasing survival rates. Continuing research is focused on minimizing the incidence of injury and the mortality/morbidity of spinal cord injury.

Etiology. Spinal cord injury is primarily a problem of the young. Males are three to four times more likely to have suffered a spinal cord injury, and these injuries are most common on the weekends and during the summer months. Motor vehicle crashes contribute the highest number of spinal cord injuries, followed by violence (primarily gunshot wounds), falls, and recreational accidents.[57] Alcohol use and risk-taking behavior are often involved. Other causes of spinal cord injuries include birth injuries, herniated intravertebral disk, or bone spurs related to degenerative changes of aging and osteoporosis. Injuries to the spinal cord are classified by level, degree (complete or incomplete), and mechanism of injury (Box 45-2).

Pathogenesis. Spinal cord injury results from compression (tumor, hematoma, or bony encroachment) and from blunt trauma causing contusion or penetration/transection of neural tissue. The major mechanisms of injury are hyperflexion, hyperextension, and compression (Figure 45-12). Flexion injury with tearing of the posterior ligaments and dislocation is the most unstable injury and is often associated with severe neurologic deficits. Hyperextension injury is the most common. Aside from the primary injury to the spinal cord, damage also results from secondary injury. Secondary events result in edema, ischemia, excitotoxicity, and inflammation, causing increased cell death, disruption of the blood-brain barrier, cavitation, and demyelination, which are detrimental to functional recovery. Not all of these processes are well-understood, but substantial damage occurs because of these events. Neutrophils are the first immune cells to appear at the primary injury site.[58] Oxidative and proteolytic enzymes produced by the neutrophils sterilize the damaged area and prepare it for "repair." However, these neutrophils can cause further damage. Macrophages also infiltrate the area and contribute to further damage by releasing proinflammatory cytokines, reactive oxygen species, nitric oxide, and proteases. T lymphocytes, which are responsible for cell-mediated immunity, have also been identified in the site of injury. Whether T lymphocytes cause secondary injury or help with healing is still a matter of debate.[58]

The systemic hemodynamic changes that occur after spinal cord injury are a major factor in the resulting damage to the spinal cord. Because of the injury to the spinal cord, autoregulation is lost, resulting in a profound drop in systemic blood pressure. This adds to the ischemia of the tissue. In addition, spinal cord injuries are often accompanied by trauma to other organ tissue causing hypoxia, hypotension, hyperthermia/hypothermia, and hypoglycemia/hyperglycemia.

Clinical manifestations. Immediately following injury to the spinal cord, there is complete loss of function below the level of injury. This may occur even in incomplete injuries to the spinal cord, causing the injury to appear more severe than it actually is. This phenomenon,

BOX 45-2 AMERICAN SPINAL INJURY ASSOCIATION IMPAIRMENT SCALE

A = Complete: No motor or sensory function is preserved in the sacral segments S4 to S5.

B = Incomplete: Sensory function (but not motor function) is preserved below the neurologic level and includes the sacral segments S4 to S5.

C = Incomplete: Motor function is preserved below the neurologic level, and more than half of key muscles below the neurologic level have a muscle grade less than 3.

D = Incomplete: Motor function is preserved below the neurologic level, and at least half of key muscles below the neurologic level have a muscle grade of 3 or more.

E = Normal: Motor and sensory function are normal.

Standards for Neurological Classification of SCI Worksheet (Dermatome Chart), 2011. From American Spinal Injury Association. Available at http://www.asia-spinalinjury.org/publications.

known as **spinal shock,** can last from a few hours to a few weeks. Symptoms below the level of injury include flaccid paralysis of all skeletal muscles; loss of all spinal reflexes; loss of pain, proprioception, and other sensations; bowel and bladder dysfunction with paralytic ileus; and loss of thermoregulation. A return of spinal reflexes indicates the end of spinal shock. As reflex function returns, spastic paraplegia or quadriplegia develops with hyperreflexia and extensor plantar responses, but a flaccid atrophic (lower motor neuron) paralysis may be found depending on the segments of the cord affected. The bladder and bowel may regain some reflex function.

In patients with cervical or upper thoracic cord injury, **neurogenic shock** is a life-threatening complication. Neurogenic shock is a form of distributive shock caused by the loss of brainstem and higher center control of the sympathetic nervous system. The loss of sympathetic outflow results in hypotension caused by peripheral vasodilation. Bradycardia occurs (secondary to the overriding parasympathetic influence), and there is a loss of the cardiac accelerator reflex. The loss of impulses from the temperature regulatory center in the brain prevents the ability to sweat below the level of injury.

A chronic, ongoing complication of spinal cord injuries occurring at or above the T6 vertebra is **autonomic dysreflexia.** This is a potentially life-threatening complication that may occur any time after spinal shock has resolved. It is characterized by a sudden episode of hypertension, headache, bradycardia, upper-body flushing and lower body vasoconstriction, piloerection (goose bumps), and sweating. The usual stimulus initiating autonomic dysreflexia is activation of visceral or cutaneous pain receptors below the level of injury. A full bladder or constipation is a common cause.

Stimulation of afferent pain receptors causes activation of sympathetic efferents in the cord and reflex vasoconstriction. Sustained activation of sympathetic neurons below the level of cord injury increases blood pressure significantly. The hypertension initiates the baroreceptor response. Baroreceptors mediate inhibition of heart rate and vasodilation of vessels above the level of injury. This is responsible for the upper body flushing. Descending signals from the brain cannot pass the cord injury, so inhibition of sympathetic neurons below the level of injury does not occur. Blood pressure may be dangerously high, and may require aggressive treatment.

Treatment. Management of spinal cord injuries includes appropriate stabilization of spinal vertebra components to prevent further trauma to the spinal cord. This may be accomplished surgically with internal fixation; or with external fixation and bracing.[59] During

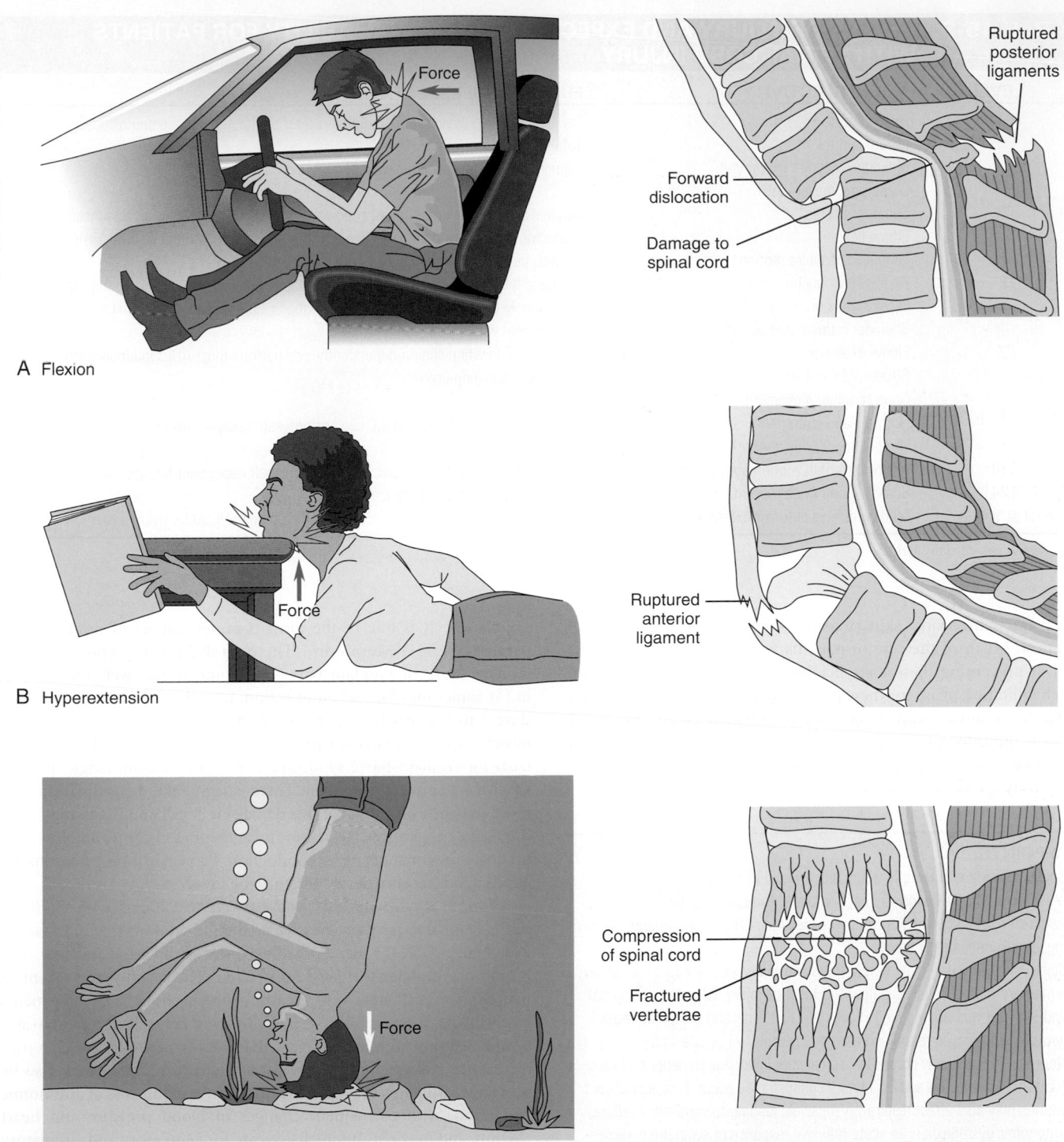

FIGURE 45-12 Mechanisms of spinal cord injury. Many situations may produce these consequences. This figure shows examples only. **A,** Flexion injury of the cervical spine ruptures the posterior ligaments. **B,** Hyperextension injury of the cervical spine ruptures the anterior ligaments. **C,** Compression fractures crush the vertebrae and force bony fragments into the spinal canal.

neurogenic shock, patients require intensive care to maintain oxygenation and blood pressure. The use of high-dose methylprednisolone initiated within the first 8 hours after injury and continued for 24 hours may preserve some function by decreasing the secondary injury to the spinal cord.[60] The benefit of this medication is modest at best, but it offers some hope of improving function. Ongoing assessment is critical. Methodical neurologic evaluations are important in determining improvement or deterioration in function. Treatment for autonomic dysreflexia includes removing or alleviating the painful stimulus, and in certain situations the use of adrenergic receptor–blocking medications to manage the hypertensive crisis.

Individuals suffering from spinal cord injuries have chronic and ongoing problems with spasticity and contracture related to upper motor neuron damage. They are also at high risk for respiratory and

TABLE 45-3 LEVELS OF INJURY AND EXPECTED FUNCTIONAL ABILITY FOR PATIENTS WITH SPINAL CORD INJURY

LEVEL	NORMAL ACTIVITY	FUNCTIONAL EXPECTATION
C4	Head control Mouth control Shoulder/scapular movement Diaphragm movement	Can use adaptive devices (i.e., mouth stick) for phone, reading, computer Total dependence for transfers/ADLs Pulmonary hygiene concerns; skin care issues
C5	Shoulder flexion Elbow flexion Increased scapular motion	Can use adaptive devices for self-feeding; can move wheelchair short distances (electric wheelchair preferred); can perform ADLs and bed mobility with assistance; needs pulmonary hygiene assistance
C6	Good elbow flexion Wrist extension Shoulder rotation and abduction	Independent with grooming/feeding with adaptive devices; weak hand grasp; can roll over in bed; can drive with car adaptations; can transfer with assistance; can self-propel wheelchair
C7	Elbow extension Strong wrist extension Good shoulder movement	Can transfer to wheelchair independently; can perform most ADLs independently; excellent bed mobility
T1	Normal hand strength Normal upper body strength	Bed and wheelchair independent; can perform self-catheterization
T10	Normal strength/motion above umbilicus	May stand for exercise with braces; still wheelchair dependent for ambulation
L2-L5	Some leg and thigh movement	Can ambulate indoors with braces/canes
Sacral segments	Mild weakness in lower extremities	Can ambulate with braces/canes; still significant bowel/bladder dysfunction

ADLs, Activities of daily living.

urinary tract infections, skin pressure sores, septicemia, and fecal impaction. Much of the care of patients with spinal cord injuries is aimed at preventing these complications and maximizing function. The rehabilitation phase for these patients is lengthy with emphasis on independence and self-care. Ongoing care of patients with spinal cord injuries is multidisciplinary and should also address the psychosocial impact of this life-changing event. Levels of injury and expected functional ability are summarized in Table 45-3.

> **KEY POINTS**
> - Spinal cord injury is usually traumatic, a result of motor vehicle accidents, falls, penetrating wounds, or sports injuries. The cord may be compressed, transected, or contused. Further injury may result from hemorrhage, swelling, and ischemia after injury.
> - Spinal shock occurs immediately following injury and is characterized by temporary loss of reflexes below the level of injury. Muscles are flaccid, and skeletal and autonomic reflexes are lost. The end of spinal shock is noted when reflexes return and flaccidity is replaced by spasticity.
> - Neurogenic shock may occur after spinal cord injury due to peripheral vasodilation. Hypotension and circulatory collapse may occur. High spinal cord injuries may also affect respiratory muscles, leading to ventilatory failure.
> - Autonomic dysreflexia is an acute reflexive response to sympathetic activation below the level of injury. Visceral stimulation (full bladder or bowel) and activation of pain receptors below the injury are common initiating stimuli. Manifestations include hypertension, bradycardia, flushing above the level of injury, and clammy skin below the level of injury. Prompt removal of the offending stimulus is indicated.

Guillain-Barré Syndrome

Etiology and pathogenesis. Guillain-Barré syndrome, also known as *acute idiopathic polyneuropathy* or *polyradiculoneuropathy,* is an inflammatory demyelinating disease of the *peripheral* nervous system or a lower motor neuron disorder. Between 1 and 4 cases per 100,000 individuals occur annually, with an increasing incidence in the aging

population. It is one of the most common causes of nontraumatic paralysis in the Western world. There is a slight male preponderance.[61]

The cause of Guillain-Barré syndrome is not well understood, but it sometimes follows an infection, inoculation, or surgical procedure 1 to 8 weeks before the onset of signs and symptoms. *Campylobacter jejuni* enteritis has been associated with the syndrome.[61] The basis for Guillain-Barré syndrome is probably immunologic, but the exact mechanism is unknown. There is segmental demyelination, and most evidence suggests that this damage is T-cell and B-cell mediated. Aggregates of lymphocytes are found at the sites of demyelination. This process slows or stops nerve conduction. Primarily motor neurons are affected, but sensory nerves may also be involved.[61]

Clinical manifestations and treatment. Patients with Guillain-Barré syndrome have progressive ascending weakness or paralysis. It usually begins in the legs, spreading often to the arms and face. The respiratory muscles may also be affected. The severity and extent of neurologic deficit may vary greatly between patients. Most patients reach the peak of disability in 10 to 14 days. Sensory nerves may also be affected, but to a lesser extent than motor neurons. Patients may experience paresthesia or dysesthesia; neuropathic pain may also be present. During this time, patients may demonstrate loss of autonomic regulation, with consequent changes in blood pressure and heart rhythm, and may require intensive care for ventilatory and circulatory support.

Diagnosis of Guillain-Barré syndrome is made through patient history, physical examination, and nerve conduction studies. The CSF characteristically contains high protein concentrations. Other laboratory studies and imaging are used to rule out other causes for neurologic dysfunction.

The majority of patients experience spontaneous recovery; however, 10% to 15% of patients may be left with a mild disability.[61] Gradually, neurologic function returns, often in a descending pattern with upper extremities recovering earlier than lower extremities. Treatment within 14 days of onset of symptoms with plasmapheresis, especially in those with severe or rapidly progressing symptoms, has been shown to have some value. Intravenous immunoglobulin is also helpful.

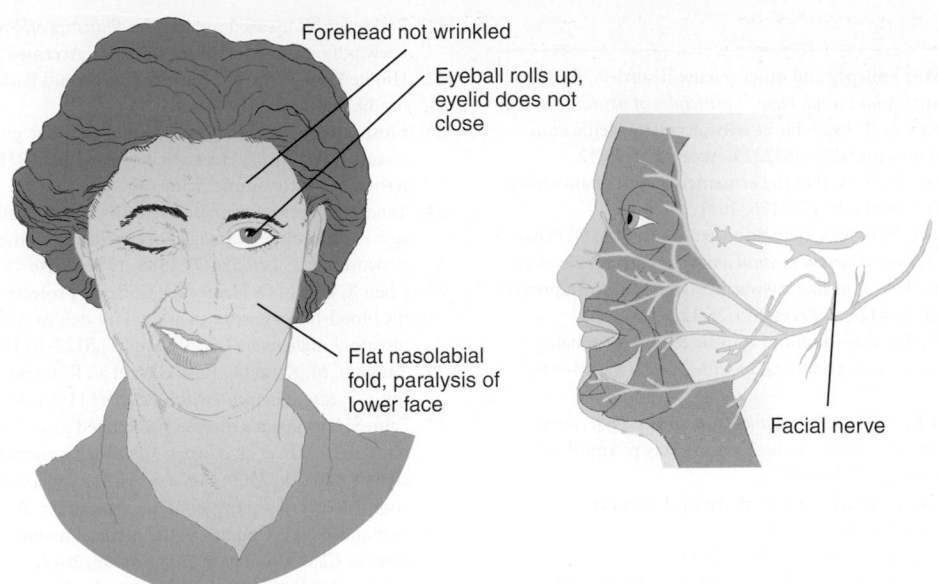

Forehead not wrinkled

Eyeball rolls up, eyelid does not close

Flat nasolabial fold, paralysis of lower face

Facial nerve

FIGURE 45-13 Bell palsy. Locations of the branches of the facial nerve (cranial nerve VII) correspond to the areas of peripheral facial paralysis. (From Black JM et al: *Medical-surgical nursing: clinical management for positive outcomes*, ed 8, Philadelphia, 2008, Saunders, p 1886.)

However, nearly 5% to 10% of patients may experience one or more exacerbations of symptoms.[62] Nursing care of these patients is aimed at preventing complications of immobility.

> **KEY POINTS**
> - Guillain-Barré syndrome is characterized by muscle weakness that begins in the lower extremities and spreads to the proximal spinal neurons.
> - The cause is unknown; however, a postinfectious immunologic mechanism is suspected.
> - Treatment is supportive, and spontaneous recovery usually occurs.

Bell Palsy

Etiology and pathogenesis. Bell palsy is an acute idiopathic paresis or paralysis of the facial nerve involving an inflammatory reaction at or near the stylomastoid foramen or in the bony facial canal with probable occurrence of compression, ischemia, and demyelination. The incidence peaks in the 40- to 49- year-old age group.[63] There is mounting evidence that Bell palsy is caused by a viral infection. Antibodies to the herpes simplex and herpes zoster viruses have been found in patients with Bell palsy.

Clinical manifestations and treatment. Symptoms of Bell palsy develop rapidly over 24 to 48 hours. Physical examination shows unilateral facial weakness with facial droop and diminished eye blink, **hyperacusis,** and decreased lacrimation (Figure 45-13). Patients may complain of a heavy sensation in their face as well as a decreased sense of taste, but sensation of the face is generally intact. Posterior auricular pain may be present. In the diagnosis of Bell palsy, other causes of facial paralysis, such as bacterial infection (otitis media), tumor, trauma, and cerebrovascular accident (stroke), must be ruled out. MRI, CT, and EMG can be helpful in certain situations. Laboratory testing is of limited value.

Management of Bell palsy is controversial. Most patients recover facial nerve function spontaneously within approximately 3 weeks. However, approximately 15% of patients are left with some level of residual disability.[63] Patients with the poorest prognosis for complete recovery are individuals older than 60 years, those with diabetes, and those who have had symptoms lasting longer than 3 months.[3] Prevention of corneal damage resulting from the inability of the eye to close is vital. Lubricating drops, ointments, and nighttime eye patching may be necessary. The use of corticosteroids has been shown to improve the likelihood of complete recovery. Because of the association of viruses with Bell palsy, the use of antiviral medications such as acyclovir or valacyclovir is recommended. Studies regarding the use of these medications have shown inconsistent results, but two recent studies show benefit when these drugs are combined with corticosteroids.[3] Surgical decompression of the nerve has not been shown to confer great benefit.[3]

> **KEY POINTS**
> - Bell palsy, or neuropathy of the facial nerve, results in paralysis of the muscles on one side of the face. Often a self-limiting condition with unknown cause, Bell palsy may last only a few days or weeks.
> - Treatment is supportive, and spontaneous recovery usually occurs.

SUMMARY

A traumatic event, such as a spinal cord injury, or a chronic neurologic disease, such as dementia, can transform an individual from a relatively healthy state to one of almost complete dependence. At best, some of the neurologic states described in this chapter may resolve spontaneously or require only minor lifestyle adjustment, but more commonly, chronic neurologic conditions require lifetime rehabilitation.

The process of life care planning includes taking stock of current health status, future health care concerns, appropriate resources, and associated costs to address lifelong disability and illness management.

In general, the goal of rehabilitation is to increase self-care and promote a meaningful lifestyle that incorporates the neurologic disability. The primary goal of such tertiary prevention is to help the affected individual maintain the highest possible level of wellness.

REFERENCES

1. Ropper AH, Samuels MA: Epilepsy and other seizure disorders. In Ropper AH, Samuels MA, editors: *Adams and Victor's principles of neurology*, ed 9, New York, 2009, McGraw-Hill. Available at www.accessmedicine.com. proxy.heal-wa.org/content.aspx?aID=3632229. Accessed 1/26/12.

2. Rajasekaran K, Goodkin HP: A swell in the armamentarium of antiepileptic drug targets, *Epilepsy Curr* 11(6):172–176, 2011.

3. Aminoff MJ, Kerchner GA: Nervous system disorders. In McPhee SJ, Papadakis MA, Rabow MW, editors: *Current medical diagnosis & treatment 2012*, New York, 2012, McGraw-Hill. Available at www.accessmedicine.com.proxy.h eal-wa.org/content. aspx?aID=12507. Accessed 1/26/12.

4. Seo KE, Choi Y, Kim W: The assessment of routine electroencephalography in patients with altered mental status, *Yonsei Med J* 52(6):933–938, 2011.

5. Alexopoulos AV, Wijdicks E, Sisson SD: *Epilepsy in adults. First consult.* Available at www.mdconsult.com.proxy.heal-wa.org/das/pdxmd/body/315751773-2/0?type=med. Accessed 2/2/12.

6. Schoenberg MR, Frontera AT, Pedro AB, et al: An update on epilepsy, *Expert Rev Neurother* 11(5):639–645, 2011.

7. Alzheimer's Association: *2011 Facts Fig* 7(2):12, 2011.

8. Johnston C, Harper G, Landefeld C: Geriatric disorders. In McPhee SJ, Papadakis MA, Rabow MW, editors: *Current medical diagnosis & treatment 2012*, New York, 2012, McGraw-Hill. Available at www.accessmedicine.com.proxy. heal-wa.org/content. aspx?aID=348. Accessed 2/4/12.

9. Ropper AH, Samuels MA: Degenerative diseases in the nervous system. In Ropper AH, Samuels MA, editors: *Adams and Victor's principles of neurology*, ed 9, New York, 2009, McGraw-Hill. Available at www.access medicine.com.proxy.heal-wa.org/content.aspx?aID3639002. Accessed 2/2/12.

10. Axelsen PH, Komatsu H, Murray IV: Oxidative stress and cell membranes in the pathogenesis of Alzheimer's disease, *Physiology* 26:54–69, 2011.

11. Carlsson CM, Gleason CE, Puglielli L, et al: Dementia including Alzheimer disease. In Halter JB, Ouslander JG, Tinetti ME, et al, editors: *Hazzard's geriatric medicine and gerontology*, ed 6, New York, 2009, McGraw-Hill. Available at www.access.medicine.com.proxy.heal-wa.org/content.aspx?aID=5122625. Accessed 2/13/12.

12. Chen KH, Reese EA, Kim HW, et al: Disturbed neurotransmitter transporter expression in Alzheimer disease brain, *J Alzheimers Dis* 26(4):755–766, 2011.

13. Grammas P: Neurovascular dysfunction, inflammation and endothelial activation: implications for the pathogenesis of Alzheimer's disease, *J Neuroinflammation* 8(6), 2011. Available at wwwjneuroinflammation. com/content/8/1/26.

14. Salamanca S: Treatment guidelines for Alzheimer-type dementia, *Clin Advisor* 14(6):47–55, 2011.

15. Standaert DG, Roberson ED: Treatment of central nervous system degenerative disorders. In Brunton LL, Chaber BA, Knollmann BC, editors: *Goodman and Gilman's the pharmacologic basis of therapeutics*, ed 12, New York, 2011, McGraw-Hill. Available at, www.accessmedicine.com.proxy. heal-wa.org/content.aspx?aID=16665863. Accessed 2/13/12.

16. Davis NJ, Hendrix CC, Superville JG: Supportive approaches for Alzheimer disease, *Nurse Practit* 36(8):22–29, 2011.

17. Thomas SJ, Grossberg GT: Memantine: a review of studies into its safety and efficacy in treating Alzheimer's disease and other dementias, *Clin Interv Aging* (4):367–377, 2009. Available at http://dx.doi.org/10.2147/CIA.S6666:www.dovepress.com/clincial-interventions-in-aging-journal.

18. Wollen KA: Alzheimer's disease: the pros and cons of pharmaceutical, nutritional, botanical, and stimulatory therapies, with a discussion of treatment strategies from the perspective of patients and practitioners, *Altern Med Rev* 15(3):223–224, 2010.

19. Sink KM, Leng X, Williamson J, et al: Angiotensin converting enzyme inhibitors and cognitive decline in older adults with hypertension: results from the cardiovascular health study, *Arch Intern Med* 169(13):1195–1202, 2009.

20. Li N, Lee A, Whitmer RA, et al: Use of angiotensin receptor blockers and the risk of dementia in a predominantly male population: prospective cohort analysis, *BMJ* 340:b5465, 2010.

21. Parkinson's Disease Foundation: *Statistics on Parkinsons.* Available at www.pdf.org/en/parkinson_statistics. Accessed 3/13/12.

22. Hindle JV: Ageing, neurodegeneration and Parkinson's disease, *Age Ageing* 39:156–161, 2010.

23. Mosley RL, et al: Inflammation and adaptive immunity in Parkinson's disease, *Cold Spring Harb Perspect Med* 2:a009381, 2012. Available at www.perspectivesinmedicine.org.

24. Tanaka A: Parkin-mediated selective mitochondrial autophagy, mitophagy: Parkin purges damaged organelles from the vital mitochondrial network, *FEBS Lett* 584(7):1386–1392, 2010.

25. Chen X, Ghribi O, Geiger JD: Caffeine protects against disruptions of the blood-brain barrier in animal models of Alzheimer's and Parkinson's disease, *J Alzheimers Dis* 20(suppl 1):S127–S141, 2010.

26. Tanner CM, Kamel F, Ross GW, et al: Rotenone, paraquat and Parkinson's disease, *Environ Health Perspect* 119(6):866–872, 2011.

27. Fahn S: Parkinson's disease and related disorders. In Halter JB, Ouslander JG, Tinetti ME, et al, editors: *Hazzard's geriatric medicine and gerontology*, ed 6, New York, 2009, McGraw-Hill. Available at www.accessmedicine. com.proxy.heal-wa.org/content. aspx?aID=. Accessed 3/17/12.

28. Fernandez HH: Updates in the medical management of Parkinson's disease, *Cleve Clin J Med* 79(1):28–35, 2012.

29. Pawitan JA: Prospect of cell therapy for Parkinson's disease, *Anat Cell Biol* 44:256–264, 2011.

30. Lyons MK: Deep brain stimulation: current and future clinical applications, *Mayo Clin Proc* 86(7):662–672, 2011.

31. Bronstein JM, Tagliati M, Alterman RL, et al: Deep brain stimulation for Parkinson's disease, *Arch Neurol* 68(2):165–171, 2011.

32. Hirsch AT, Gallegos JC, Gertz KJ, et al: Symptom burden in individuals with cerebral palsy, *J Rehabil Res Dev* 47(9):863–876, 2010.

33. Reddihough D: Cerebral palsy in childhood, *Aust Fam Physician* 40(4):192–196, 2011.

34. Merck Manual: *Cerebral palsy (CP) syndromes.* Available at www.merckman uals.com/professional/print/pediatrics/neurologic_disorders_in_children.

35. Sawyer JR: Cerebral palsy. In Canale ST, Beaty JH, editors: *Campbell's operative orthopedics*, ed 11, Philadelphia, 2008, Elsevier.

36. Friedman B, Goldman RD: Use of botulinum toxin A in management of children with cerebral palsy, *Can Fam Physician* 57:1006–1008, 2011.

37. Ropper AH, Samuels MA: Disturbances in cerebral spinal fluid and its circulation including hydrocephalus, pseudotumor cerebri and low pressure syndromes. In Ropper AH, Samuels MA, editors: *Adams and Victor's principles of neurology*, ed 9, New York, 2009, McGraw-Hill. Available at www.accessmedicine.com.proxy.heal-wa.org/content. aspx?aID=3635067. Accessed 3/16/12.

38. Kinsman SL, Johnston MV: Congenital abnormalities of the CNS. In Kliegman RM, Stanton BF, St. Geme JW, et al, editors: *Nelson's textbook of pediatrics*, ed 19, Philadelphia, 2011, Saunders.

39. Ropper AH, Samuels MA: Incoordination and other disorders of cerebellar function. In Ropper AH, Samuels MA, editors: *Adam's and Victors principles of neurology*, ed 9, New York, 2009, McGraw-Hill. Available at www.accessmedicine.com.proxy.heal-wa.org/content/aspx?aID=3630577. Accessed 3/24/12.

40. National Multiple Sclerosis Society: *Epidemiology of MS.* Available at www.nationalmssociety.org/about-multiple-sclerosis/what-we-know-about-ms/who-gets-ms/epidemiology-of-ms/index.aspx.

41. Brucklacher-Waldert V, Sturner K, Kolster M: Phenotypical and functional characterization of T helper 17 cells in multiple sclerosis, *Brain* 132:3329–3341, 2009.

42. Barten LJ, et al: New approaches in the management of multiple sclerosis, *Drug Design Dev Ther* 4, 2010. Available at www.dovepress.com/drug-design-development-and-therapy-journal.

43. Calabresi PA: Multiple sclerosis and demyelinating conditions of the central nervous system. In Goldman L, Schafer AI, editors: *Goldman's Cecil medicine*, ed 24, Philadelphia, 2012, Elsevier.

44. Goodin DS, Hauser SL: Multiple sclerosis and other demyelinating diseases. In Longo DL, Fauci AS, Kasper DL, et al, editors: *Harrison's principles of internal medicine*, ed 18, New York, 2012, McGraw-Hill. Available at www.accessmedine.com.proxy.heal-wa.org/content.aspx?aID=9147780. Accessed 3/24/12.

45. Conradi S, et al: Environmental factors in early childhood are associated with multiple sclerosis, *BMC Neurol* 11:123, 2011.

46. Disanto G, et al: Vitamin D: a link between Epstein-Barr virus and multiple sclerosis development? *Expert Rev Neurother* 11(9):1221–1224, 2011.

47. Ross EM: Gene-environment interactions, folate metabolism and the embryonic nervous system, *Wiley Interdiscip Rev Syst Biol Med* 2(4):471–480, 2010.

48. Au KS, Ashley-Koch A, Northrup H: Epidemiologic and genetic aspects of spina bifida and other neural tube defects, *Dev Disabil Res Rev* 16(1):6–15, 2010.

49. National Institute of Neurological Disorders and Stroke: *Spinal bifida fact sheet.* Available at www.ninds.nih.gov/disorders/spina_bifida/detail_spina_bifida.htm.

50. Fletcher JM, Brei TJ: Introduction: spina bifida—a multidisciplinary perspective, *Dev Disabil Res Rev* 16(1):1–5, 2010.

51. Adzick NS, Thom EA, Spong CY, et al: A randomized trial of prenatal versus postnatal repair of myelomeningocele, *N Engl J Med* 364(11):993 1004, 2011.

52. National Institute of Neurological Disorders and Stroke: *ALS (amyotrophic lateral sclerosis) fact sheet.* Available at www.ninds.nih.gov/disorders/amyotrophiclateralsclerosis/detail-ALS.htm.

53. ALS Association: Who gets ALS? Available at www.alsa.org/about-als/who-gets-als.html.

54. Davis M: Management of amyotrophic lateral sclerosis (ALS) by the family nurse practitioner: a timeline for anticipated referrals, *J Am Acad Nurse Pract* 23:464–471, 2011.

55. Wijesekera LC, Leigh PN: Amyotrophic lateral sclerosis, *Orphanet J Rare Dis* 4(3), 2009. Available at www.ojrd.com/content/4/1/3.

56. McCombe PA, Henderson RD: The role of immune and inflammatory mechanisms in ALS, *Curr Mol Med* 11:246–254, 2011.

57. Foundation for Spinal Cord Injury Prevention, Care and Cure: *Spinal cord injury facts,* Available at www.fscip.org/facts.htm.

58. Oyinbo CA: Secondary injury mechanisms in traumatic spinal cord injury: a nugget of this multiply cascade, *Acta Neurobiol Exp* 71:281–299, 2011.

59. Fehlings MG, Cadotte DW, Fehlings LN: A series of systematic reviews on the treatment of acute spinal cord injury: a foundation for best medical practice, *J Neurotrauma* 28:1329–1333, 2011.

60. Bracken MB: Steroids for acute spinal cord injury (review). In *The Cochrane collaboration*, 2012, John Wiley & Sons. Available at www.thecochranelibrary.com.

61. Amato AA, Hauser SL: Guillian-Barre syndrome and other immune-mediated neuropathies. In Longo DL, Fauci AS, Kasper DL, et al, editors: *Harrison's principles of internal medicine*, ed 18, New York, 2012, McGraw-Hill, Available at www.accessmedicine.com.proxy.heal-wa.org.content.aspx?aID=9148788. Accessed 3/24/12.

62. Ropper AH, Samuels MA: Diseases of the peripheral nerves. In Ropper AH, Samuels MA, editors: *Adam's and Victor's principles of neurology*, ed 9, New York, 2009, McGraw-Hill. Available at www.accessmedicine.com.proxy.heal-wa.org.content.aspx?aID=3641268. Accessed 3/24/12.

63. Ropper AH, Samuels MA: Diseases of the cranial nerves. In Ropper AH, Samuels MA, editors: *Adam's and Victor's principles of neurology*, ed 9, New York, 2009, McGraw-Hill. Available at www.accessmedicine.com.proxy.heal-wa.org.content.aspx?aID=3642006/. Accessed 3/24/12.

Alterations in Special Sensory Function

Joni D. Marsh

evolve WEBSITE

http://evolve.elsevier.com/Copstead/
- Review Questions and Answers
- Glossary (with audio pronunciations for selected terms)
- Animations
- Case Studies
- Key Points Review

KEY QUESTIONS

- What are the general manifestations of hearing impairment?
- How do conductive and sensorineural mechanisms of hearing loss differ in etiology and treatment?
- What are the predisposing factors, clinical manifestations, and management of otitis media?
- What are the general manifestations of visual impairment?
- What are the causes, clinical manifestations, and management of common visual disorders, including errors of refraction, strabismus, cataract, and retinopathies?
- How do open-angle and acute angle-closure glaucoma differ?
- How do the two forms of macular degeneration differ?

CHAPTER OUTLINE

The human body has countless sense organs that fall into two main categories: general sense organs and special sense organs. By far the most numerous are the general sense organs or receptors. The receptors function to produce the general or somatic senses. Examples of these senses are touch, temperature, and pain, and the receptors that initiate various reflexes necessary for maintaining homeostasis (see Chapter 43). The largest general sense organ in the body is the skin.

Special sense organs, by comparison, function to produce the unique sensations of hearing, balance, vision, smell, and taste. These senses allow humans to interact with their environment in a meaningful way.

Alterations in sensory function may be acute/short-term, chronic/long-term, or progressive in nature. They may result from such factors as genetics, disease, infection, trauma, and normal aging. Alterations in special sensory function require prompt assessment, evaluation, and treatment from appropriate health professionals. Equally important is an assessment of how the sensory impairment affects the individual's activities of daily living. This chapter discusses special sensory function with regard to physiologic processes, sensory impairment, and the diagnosis and management of these impairments.

HEARING AND BALANCE

STRUCTURE AND FUNCTION OF THE EAR

External Ear

Hearing results from normal functioning of several complex structures both external and internal to the body. Sound consists of waves of vibrations in the air, produced in the environment. These vibrations travel much like ripples in a pool of water. Externally, these vibrations are caught and funneled into the ear canal by the auricles (Figure 46-1). Even though the auricles are in a fixed position and lie close to the head, their shape serves to concentrate sound waves, especially high-frequency waves. The auricles also have an important role in sound localization.

The ear canal has a somewhat S shape from its opening to its termination at the tympanic membrane. This configuration affords both protection from airborne foreign objects and access to sound. The outer portion of the ear canal contains hair to filter out unwanted substances. Along the ear canal are also glands that secrete cerumen. This brown, waxlike substance coats the hairs in the canal to help prevent the entrance of foreign bodies into the ear canal. After entering the ear canal, sound waves strike the tympanic membrane (eardrum) and cause it to vibrate. The tympanic membrane is a thin, elastic membrane that is very sensitive to changes in pressure.

Middle Ear

The middle ear is a bony, air-containing space that functions primarily as a structure by which sound energy is transmitted from the air to the fluids of the inner ear. The tympanic membrane is connected to the first of the **ossicles,** the malleus (hammer), followed by the incus (anvil) and stapes (stirrup). The ossicles further amplify the sound waves and then transfer airborne sound waves to the fluid-filled inner ear at the oval window.

The eustachian tube is also part of the middle ear, and although it does not contribute directly to the transmission of sound through the ear, absence of proper function can greatly affect hearing. This tube has a mucosal lining and extends from the middle ear cavity to the nasopharynx. It makes equalization of pressure against the inner and outer surfaces of the tympanic membrane possible, thus improving mobility of the membrane for sound transduction. A patent eustachian tube prevents membrane rupture and discomfort that marked pressure differences can produce.

Inner Ear

The inner ear is composed of the oval window, the cochlea, and the semicircular canals. Within the cochlea are three parallel tubes: the scala vestibuli, the scala media, and the scala tympani. Movement of the perilymph, a fluid much like cerebrospinal fluid, in the scala vestibuli and the scala tympani is eventually dissipated by movement of the round window (Figure 46-2). The scala tympani and the scala vestibuli are continuous with one another at the apex of the cochlea through an opening called the *helicotrema.*

Transmission of the sound stimulus from the scala vestibuli to the vestibular membrane results in displacement of the endolymph, the fluid contained in the membranous labyrinth of the scala media and the basilar membrane. The organ of Corti, which contains the receptors for hearing, lies on the basilar membrane. Perilymph and endolymph transmit the mechanical vibrations from the footplate of the stapes to the organ of Corti. Endolymph also transports nutrients to the organ of Corti. No direct communication between endolymph and perilymph is normally present.

The organ of Corti consists of a series of sensory hair cells and supporting cells. These cells are innervated by the sensory fibers from the

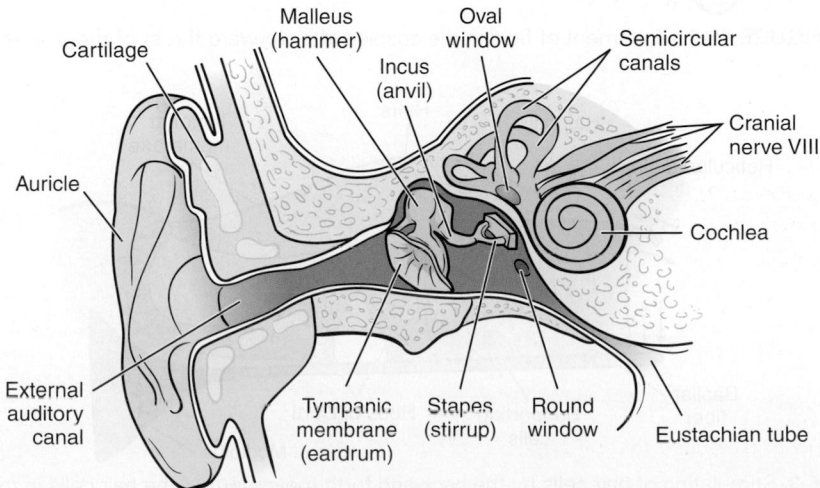

FIGURE 46-1 Anatomic structures of the ear.

vestibulocochlear nerve (cranial nerve VIII). Overhanging the organ of Corti is a flexible flap of tissue called the *tectorial membrane* (Figure 46-3). Hairs of the sensory cells of the organs of Corti are in contact with the tectorial membrane. The wave of perilymph induces movement of the basilar membrane, which causes a pull or shearing force on the hair cells in contact with the tectorial membrane. This action transforms the mechanical energy of sound into electrical impulses stimulating the vestibulocochlear nerve. Impulses are relayed through nuclei in the medulla, pons, midbrain, and thalamus before reaching the auditory area of the temporal lobe.

Balance

The ear has dual sensory functions. In addition to its role in hearing, it also functions as the sense organ of **equilibrium.** The stimulation or "trigger" responsible for balance involves activation of receptor hair cells contained in the semicircular canals. Movement of the head causes movement of the endolymph contained in the semicircular canals. The receptor hair cells in turn create a nerve impulse in the vestibular portion of the vestibulocochlear nerve (cranial nerve VIII), where the stimulus is transmitted to the brain. Signals from the inner ear are involved not only in keeping individuals upright but also in controlling the eye muscles so that the eyes can remain fixed on the same point despite changes in the position of the head.

Vertigo. Vertigo is a common symptom of vestibular disorders rather than a well-defined disease. It is either a sensation of motion without any actual motion or an exaggerated sense of motion; it is not simply a sensation of "spinning." Accompanying symptoms may include nausea, vomiting, pallor, and sweating. **Nystagmus** often is also noted. It is not associated with a loss of consciousness or a feeling of impending loss of consciousness more common to syncope. Vertigo can have a peripheral vestibular cause or central causes. In the case of

Meniere disease (discussed later in this chapter), a disorder in which vertigo is common, the cause is unknown.

Disorders of the brainstem or cerebellum that may also cause vertigo include tissue ischemia secondary to atherosclerosis, tumors, or conditions such as psychiatric disorders, migraine headaches, or multiple sclerosis. However, in these cases, additional neurologic signs and symptoms are typically present. Drugs may also cause vertigo (alcohol, anticonvulsants, sedatives). Management of vertigo is usually aimed at the cause if known. Medications such as antihistamines and anticholinergics can be helpful.[1]

GENERAL MANIFESTATIONS OF HEARING IMPAIRMENT

Hearing impairment is a very common disorder and a leading chronic health problem in the United States. Approximately 17% (36 million) of American adults report some degree of hearing loss. Out of 1000 U.S. children, 2 to 3 are born deaf or hard of hearing.[2]

Hearing may be impaired in many ways, and impairments can occur across the age spectrum. Disorders may affect the outer ear, such as impacted cerumen and foreign bodies in the ear canal. The middle ear may be affected by fluid **effusion,** infection (otitis media), tumors, or diseases such as otosclerosis. Hearing loss may also be caused by repeated exposure to loud sounds or **ototoxic** medications such as aminoglycoside antibiotics, chemotherapeutic agents, and high-dose loop diuretics. Some of these medications can cause hearing loss even when administered at therapeutic doses.[3] Other causes of hearing loss, especially in children, include infection (measles, meningitis), environmental teratogens (radiation), intrauterine infections (cytomegalovirus, herpes simplex virus, human immunodeficiency virus, and *Toxoplasma*), maternal metabolic disorders (diabetes,

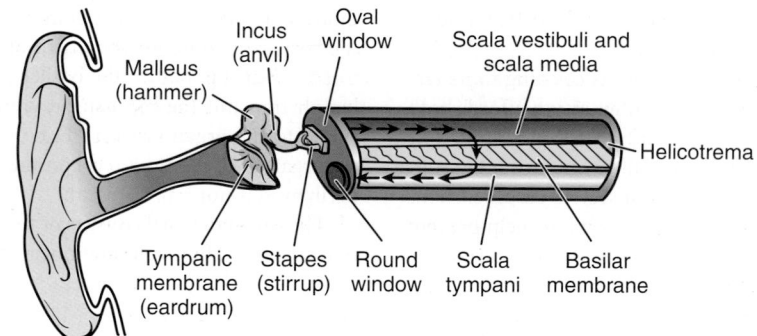

FIGURE 46-2 Movement of fluid in the cochlea after forward thrust of the stapes.

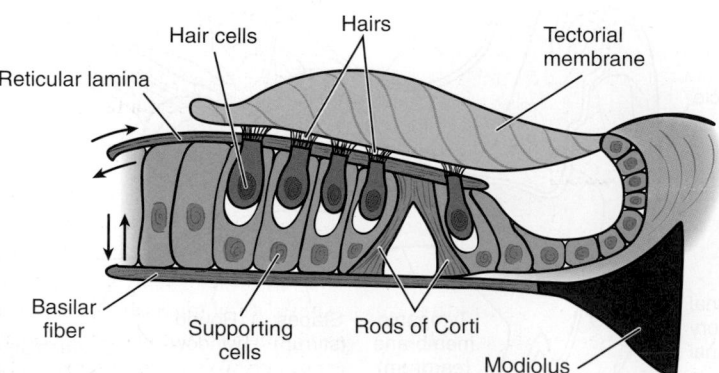

FIGURE 46-3 Stimulation of hair cells by the back-and-forth movement of the hair cells in the tectorial membrane.

hypothyroidism), and exposure to industrial chemicals (solvents or pesticides). In adults poor nutrition and smoking also contribute to hearing loss.[4,5] By whatever mechanism hearing impairment occurs, the signs and symptoms are similar.

Symptoms of hearing impairment may be manifested in behavior such as inattentiveness, speaking out of turn in conversations, withdrawal from social situations, increased volume of voice when speaking, increased volume of radio or television, confusion, loss of reaction to loud sounds, and emotional outbursts. Children with hearing impairment may demonstrate inattentiveness and difficulty with articulation and the development of speech. Alterations in hearing function can generally be classified into two categories, conductive and sensorineural, depending on the cause of the impairment. Some hearing impairments have a component of both. The following alterations in hearing function are categorized according to the primary cause of dysfunction.

HEARING IMPAIRMENT DISORDERS

Conductive Hearing Impairment

Conductive hearing loss occurs when sound cannot reach the cochlea. Individuals with conductive hearing impairment have a decreased sensitivity to sound. This type of hearing impairment is caused by dysfunction in the external or middle ear. Four mechanisms, each resulting in impairment of the passage of sound vibrations to the inner ear, lead to conductive hearing impairment: (1) obstruction (cerumen impaction), (2) mass loading (middle ear effusion), (3) stiffness effect (otosclerosis), and (4) discontinuity (ossicular disruption). Conductive hearing loss is generally correctable with medical or surgical therapy—or in some cases both.[3]

Loss Caused by Cerumen Impaction and Foreign Body Occlusion

Etiology. Cerumen impaction is a common and frequently overlooked cause of conductive hearing loss, especially in the elderly. In most cases, cerumen impaction is self-induced through attempts at cleaning the ear with objects such as cotton swabs. Foreign bodies in the ear canal occur most frequently in children. Objects such as small stones, pieces of wood, peas, beans, and paper are fairly common.

Clinical manifestations and treatment. Sometimes no symptoms are present and the foreign body is discovered on routine examination. If the foreign body is an insect, beating of its wings and movement may cause distress. When symptomatic, however, foreign bodies can cause pain or drainage of pus from the ear. The external ear canal is very sensitive to touch and bleeds easily, which increases the risk for subepithelial hematomas from minor trauma. Therefore, removal of solid foreign bodies carries a risk of additional trauma to the ear canal, as well as tympanic membrane rupture, if the individual is not completely cooperative or removal is difficult. Light anesthesia may be necessary. Firm materials may be removed from the canal with loop or hook instruments, taking care not to push the object further into the canal. Irrigation should not be performed on organic foreign bodies (beans, peas) because water may cause them to swell. Living insects may be immobilized with lidocaine before removal.[3] Excess cerumen may be removed with gentle irrigation.

Otosclerosis

Etiology. Otosclerosis is a progressive conductive, sensorineural, or mixed hearing impairment caused most often by stapedial fixation. Resorption of bone is followed by the formation of new sponge-like bony lesions usually occurring on and around the ossicles of the middle ear. Lesions involving the footplate of the stapes cause decreased transmission of sound waves to the oval window. However, when otosclerotic lesions impinge on the cochlea, permanent sensorineural hearing loss can occur. The basic initiating factors are unknown, but up to 50% of individuals with clinical otosclerosis have a history of the disease in the family.[6] Several types of inheritance patterns have been suggested. The disease is most common in Caucasian middle-aged women. Pregnancy may accelerate the otosclerotic process.[6] Viral infections and autoimmune processes are also thought to be possible causes. The age of onset is variable due to the insidious progression of the disorder, but the most common ages are between 15 and 45. There may be periods of symptom worsening, followed by times of little apparent change.

Diagnosis and treatment. The diagnosis of otosclerosis is made through careful history taking and radiologic studies, along with audiometric studies. Generally, hearing loss begins in one ear, but 80% to 90% of affected individuals will develop bilateral impairment.[6] Although hearing loss may be severe, speech discrimination is preserved except in the instance of cochlear involvement. The individual may report being able to hear better in a noisy environment than in a quiet one. **Tinnitus** is often present. Hearing tests reveal a conductive loss of varying severity.

Management of otosclerosis at this point is generally surgical, in an effort to prevent the conductive hearing loss. The limitation on treatment options for otosclerosis is related largely to the lack of exact knowledge regarding the cause and pathogenesis of the disease. The universally accepted operation for otosclerosis is stapedectomy, or removal of the focus of the disease by removing the stapes and inserting a prosthesis. In the case of otosclerosis involving the cochlea, treatment with oral sodium fluoride and bisphosphonates is associated with some decrease in development of the sensorineural hearing loss.[7] Amplification with hearing aids is another approach.

Sensorineural Hearing Impairment

In sensorineural hearing impairment, the hearing mechanism is disturbed in the inner ear in the cochlea or the vestibulocochlear nerve to the brain. Long-term exposure to loud sounds, ototoxic medication, trauma, metabolic causes, aging, and certain disease states cause sensorineural hearing impairment. Sensorineural hearing loss is usually irreversible. Progress, however, is being made in using novel approaches to protect the hair and supporting cells of the inner ear.[8]

Loss Caused by Ototoxic Medications

Drug toxicity is an increasingly important cause of sensorineural hearing loss. The drugs most well-known for this effect are the aminoglycoside antibiotics, salicylates, quinine and related antimalarials, and cytotoxic antineoplastic drugs. Most ototoxic drugs affect the hair cells of the cochlea. Unfortunately, these ototoxic effects may not become apparent during drug administration but may occur days to weeks after the therapy has been terminated. Ototoxicity may also be unilateral. Aspirin can produce a temporary hearing loss and tinnitus in individuals receiving high doses. In most cases, however, both of these symptoms disappear after aspirin use is terminated.

Loss Caused by Trauma

Etiology. Acquired sensorineural hearing loss caused by chronic, repeated exposure to loud sounds is common in the U.S. population. Four million people work each day in an environment with damaging levels of noise, and in 2008 approximately 2 million employees were exposed to workplace noise levels that put them at risk for hearing loss.[9] Noise-induced hearing loss can be associated with the use of firearms, personal stereo systems, and power tools and with occupations such as firefighting, construction, agriculture, mining, manufacturing, transportation, and the military.

The loudness of sound/noise is measured in the logarithmic units of decibels (dB). A normal whisper is measured at approximately 30 dB, a conversation at 3 feet at 50 to 60 dB. In contrast, ambulance sirens have been measured at 120 dB, lawnmowers and motorcycles at 90 dB.[10] Sounds exceeding 85 dB are considered potentially injurious, and chronic noise exposure is the most damaging. If exposure is severe enough, most structures of the inner ear can be damaged, including the organ of Corti. Sensory hair cells and supporting cells are lost because of overexposure. Noise-induced hearing loss typically is bilateral and affects higher (speech) frequencies first.[3]

Noise exposure has two phases: the first is a temporary *threshold* shift. When the ear is exposed to a loud sound, it will show a loss of sensitivity (a rise in the threshold for sound). If the hearing returns to normal after the sound has been removed, the shift was temporary and no permanent damage has occurred. If hearing does not return to normal, damage has occurred and the hearing impairment is permanent. Such a permanent threshold shift is the second phase of the damage. The ears of some individuals are more easily affected by noise, and considerable damage may occur before individuals are aware of the hearing loss.

Clinical manifestations. Individuals with hearing loss caused by noise trauma report that they are unable to discriminate words, particularly in noisy environments. Complaints about tinnitus are expressed more often than complaints about hearing loss. A diagnosis of noise-induced hearing loss is made through careful history and audiometric testing. Because noise-induced hearing loss is irreversible, no medical therapy can help once the problem has been established. Prevention is presently the only treatment for this type of hearing impairment.

Sensorineural hearing impairment can also occur with head trauma and subsequent damage to the structures of the inner ear. If blood is coming from the ear or the temporal bone is fractured, damage should be suspected. As a rule, hearing loss from trauma or head injury is permanent if the cochlea is damaged. A rare condition of sudden sensorineural hearing loss usually occurs in adults with middle ear problems. A viral or ischemic pathology is postulated. Prompt evaluation and treatment are necessary for these individuals. The prognosis is mixed but hearing may be recovered with intratympanic infusion of steroids.[3]

Presbycusis

Presbycusis is a sensorineural hearing loss and the most common form of hearing loss in older adults. Approximately 25% of people ages 65 to 75 and 50% of those older than 75 suffer from age-related hearing loss.[3] Typically, the hearing impairment is of gradual onset, is bilateral, and results in difficulty hearing high-pitched tones and conversational speech. Presbycusis can progress to involve the middle and lower tones. Frequently, individuals complain that people are mumbling to them but deny any other type of hearing loss.

Etiology. Four categories of presbycusis have been theorized: (1) sensory, characterized by atrophy and degeneration of the sensory and supporting cells; (2) neural, typified by loss of neurons in the cochlea and central nervous system; (3) metabolic, characterized by atrophy of the wall of the cochlea affecting central auditory processing; and (4) mechanical, in which the middle ear undergoes changes in properties with a resulting conductive hearing loss.[3,8,11,12] Some of these age-related changes are shown in the Geriatric Considerations: Changes in Hearing box. An endless list of genetic, environmental, and disease states can also cause hearing loss in an older adult, many of which may occur concurrently. Thus uncertainty remains regarding the exact cause of presbycusis.

Diagnosis. Assessment of an individual with suspected presbycusis should begin with exclusion of all other causes of hearing impairment. Diseases such as diabetes, stroke, and heart disease may produce effects similar to those seen with hearing loss and must be ruled out. The diagnosis is made by obtaining a thorough history and performing audiometric studies. Individuals with presbycusis respond well to hearing aids that amplify sound. Many simple lifestyle adjustments that will be mentioned at the end of this section can dramatically improve the quality of life for an individual experiencing presbycusis. It is important in these patients to avoid excessive noise exposure and ototoxic drugs, which may cause further deterioration of hearing loss.[8]

Meniere Disease

Etiology and pathogenesis. Meniere disease is an excessive accumulation of endolymph in the membranous labyrinth. The volume of endolymph increases with distention of the scala media until the

GERIATRIC CONSIDERATIONS

Changes in Hearing

Presbycusis, or age-related hearing problems, occurs after age 50 and is thought to be caused by structural changes in the organs of hearing. **Ankylosis** of the ossicles can lead to a functional decrease in transmission of sound to the inner ear.

In the inner ear or cochlea, degeneration of hair cells, changes in the basilar membrane, or atrophic changes can lead to decreased hearing of higher tones. With these changes is also noted a decline in pitch discrimination. As hearing is progressively lost, even lower pitch tones will be more difficult to hear.

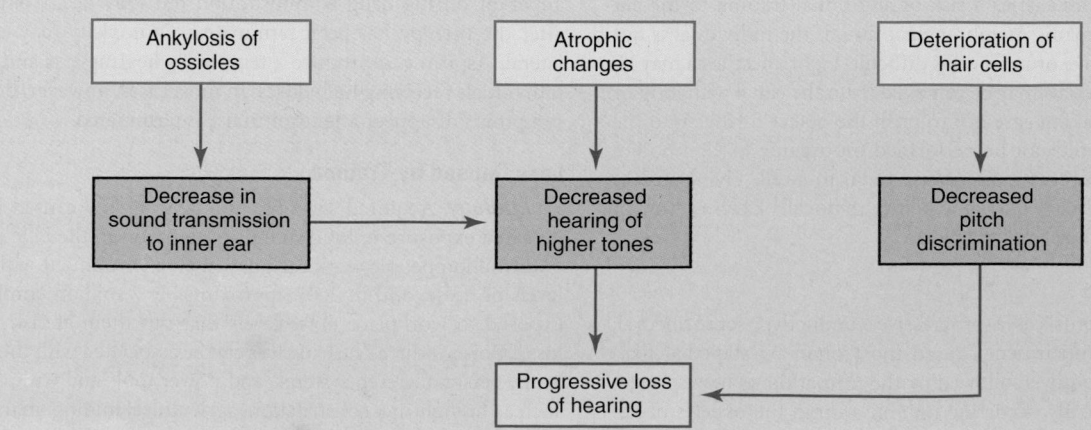

membrane ruptures. Consequently, the neural end organs of the cochlea degenerate. Many conditions including allergies, viral and bacterial infections (such as syphilis), head trauma, metabolic derangements, and chronic stress have been suggested as causative agents, but the precise cause cannot be established in most cases.[3,13] Men and women are equally affected by this disorder, and the onset of symptoms is typically in the fourth decade of life.[13]

Clinical manifestations. Clinical manifestations of Meniere disease include tinnitus, fluctuating sensorineural hearing loss, vertigo, and sensations of ear fullness. In the early stages, hearing loss fluctuates, with return to normal after the rupture heals. Remissions and exacerbations are typical. The hearing loss is usually in the low tones. As the disease progresses, hearing loss becomes permanent. Symptoms initially usually are unilateral; the mean time for the manifestation of bilateral symptoms is approximately 7 years.[13]

Episodes of vertigo may be immediately preceded by the sensation of pressure in the ear, increased hearing loss, increased tinnitus, or an alteration in the quality of these symptoms. The onset of vertigo is usually sudden, reaches maximal intensity within a few minutes, usually lasts for an hour or more, and either subsides completely or continues as a sensation of unsteadiness for several hours or days. The tinnitus is typically a low buzzing or blowing sound and is frequently louder before the attack of vertigo. The attacks are not precipitated by positional changes and may be several weeks or months apart. In the initial stages of the disease they may be years apart. If not treated, the episodes may become more frequent and severe. Nystagmus, which occurs only during acute attacks, may be directed to the side opposite the involved ear.

Diagnosis and treatment. Physical examination, including neurologic and otolaryngologic examination, is generally normal in those with Meniere disease. Radiologic studies are often used to rule out other causes of the symptoms of Meniere disease such as acoustic neuroma. Electrophysiologic studies, such as auditory brainstem response testing and electrocochleography, and audiometric tests as well as glycerol dehydration testing can lead to a diagnosis of Meniere disease.[13] Caloric testing (irrigating the ears with warm and cool water) commonly reveals loss or impairment of thermally induced nystagmus on the involved side.[13]

Treatment for Meniere disease consists of providing symptomatic relief during acute episodes with antiemetics and anticholinergics such as meclizine. Between acute attacks, eating a low-sodium diet and using diuretics may help reduce the volume of endolymph. Cessation of smoking, management of stress, and elimination of caffeine from the diet are also suggested.

Several surgical interventions are used to manage Meniere disease. Shunts can be placed to drain excess endolymph, and ablation of portions of the eighth cranial nerve and destruction of the labyrinth

are options. In refractory cases, patients may undergo intratympanic corticosteroid or gentamycin injections. These interventions have different indications, risks, and benefits associated with them. Almost all patients who choose surgical intervention have failed to respond to medical treatment.[3]

OTITIS MEDIA

Otitis media is an inflammation of the middle ear. It is almost always due to poor functioning of the eustachian tube and is often diagnosed by the presence of **effusion.** It is the most common reason for a child to require medical attention. In 2006 approximately 9 million children from newborns to 17 years of age were reported to have ear infections or otitis media.[14]

Otitis media is more common in the winter months when viral and bacterial infections are most prevalent. Upper respiratory tract infections can cause eustachian tubes to become blocked and predispose individuals to middle ear inflammation. Children are especially susceptible because of shorter, more flexible and horizontally positioned eustachian tubes. The dysfunction of the eustachian tube prevents middle ear secretions from draining and creates negative pressure in the middle ear space. Negative pressure leads to the introduction of infected nasopharyngeal secretions into the middle ear. Risk factors for otitis media include use of pacifiers, second-hand cigarette smoke exposure, gastroesophageal reflux, poor socioeconomic conditions, daycare attendance, and propped bottles. Males, Native Americans, Eskimo children, children with craniofacial abnormalities such as cleft palate, and individuals with Down syndrome have a higher incidence of otitis media.[15]

Much confusion surrounds the use of terminology in categorizing otitis media. This confusion relates to the presence of effusion and the length of illness (Table 46-1).

Acute Otitis Media

Acute otitis media is characterized by the sudden onset of ear pain in association with symptoms of upper respiratory tract infection. Most children have spontaneous resolution within 7 to 14 days.[15] Although older children and adults complain of pain, younger children may demonstrate irritability, difficulty eating and sleeping, or tugging at the affected ear, as well as fever. Physical examination reveals a reddened tympanic membrane that has poor mobility. Bulging or rupture of the tympanic membrane may also be present.

In 2004 the American Academy of Pediatrics and the American Academy of Family Physicians published guidelines for the management of acute otitis media. Antibiotic therapy was recommended for all children younger than 6 months of age, for children ages 6 to 24 months with a confirmed diagnosis, and for all children older

TABLE 46-1	COMPARISON OF OTITIS MEDIA TYPES		
TYPE	**ONSET/DURATION**	**SYMPTOMS**	**TREATMENT OPTIONS**
Acute otitis media	Sudden onset, associated with upper respiratory tract infections	Reddened tympanic membrane with poor mobility, may be bulging or ruptured, ear pain	Antibiotics, analgesics, antipyretics, or "watch and wait"
Recurrent acute otitis media	3 or more episodes in 6 months	Same as above	Daily doses of prophylactic antibiotics in some cases, ventilation tube placement
Chronic otitis media	Duration of more than 12 wk, may develop as consequence of acute otitis media	Thick immobile tympanic membrane, purulent drainage from ear, may have conductive hearing loss, pain is rare	Removal of debris from middle ear, ventilation tube placement
Otitis media with effusion	May precede or follow any type of otitis media	Ear popping, feeling of pressure in middle ear, hearing loss, retraction of tympanic membrane, fluid line or bubbles	Treat acute otitis media or "watch and wait"

than 2 years with severe infection. In children older than 2 years with milder symptoms, a "wait and see" approach may be used. Adequate pain relief and fever control are important as well as repeated evaluation. Providing the parent with a "rescue or safety net" prescription for antibiotics is one approach.[16] In children 6 to 23 months of age, amoxicillin-clavulanate is an appropriate choice.[17] Surgical placement of ventilation tubes in the tympanic membrane is also done in cases of recurrent otitis media. Complications of unresolved otitis media include hearing loss, mastoiditis, meningitis, osteomyelitis of the skull bones, and facial paralysis.

Chronic Otitis Media

Chronic otitis media is inflammation in the middle ear lasting longer than 12 weeks. Irreversible damage has occurred to structures in the middle ear. This damage manifests in many forms, including atrophy or perforation of the tympanic membrane or adhesions in the middle ear causing tympanic membrane retraction. Calcification of the ossicles may occur, as well as the formation of cholesteatomas (benign, slowly growing collections of skin tissue) within the middle ear space. The hallmark clinical sign of chronic otitis media is purulent drainage from the ear. Pain is an uncommon finding, and conductive hearing loss may occur. Chronic otitis media generally develops as a consequence of acute otitis media, but it may follow other diseases or trauma. Management of chronic otitis media generally includes surgical removal of debris in the middle ear, placement of ventilation tubes in the tympanic membrane, and adenoidectomy to assist with eustachian tube function.

INTERVENTIONS FOR INDIVIDUALS WITH HEARING IMPAIRMENT

In general, interventions for individuals with hearing loss are aimed at maximizing their residual hearing ability and allowing for compensation with other senses. To improve communication, adequate visual contact should be made. Lighting and positioning should be such that the individual can see the speaker's lips. Reductions should be made in background noise. Speech should be at a normal rate and rhythm and at normal volume. Shouting can distort sounds and actually make them more difficult to hear. The speaker should use shorter sentences and gestures such as pointing when appropriate.

Devices that amplify sound or transform sounds into tactile or visual signals may be helpful. Amplifiers for the telephone, television, or radio; closed-captioned television; and teletypewriters are examples of these devices. Others include doorbells and telephones that glow as well as ring, and flashing smoke detectors and alarm clocks.

Implanted hearing devices such as cochlear implants may be helpful for patients over the age of 2 years with profound hearing loss. Surgically implanted cochlear electrodes work together with an external processor that converts sound waves to electrical signals that can be recognized by the brain. These devices can improve communication and provide psychosocial benefits.

> **KEY POINTS**
> - Perception of sound requires that sound waves be transmitted through the outer ear canal, across the tympanic membrane, and through the ossicles to the oval window. Movement of the oval window initiates movement of perilymph, which causes movement of endolymph through the vestibular membrane. This fluid's motion stimulates the neurosensory organs of hearing—the hair cells. Bending of the hair cells induces action potentials in the cochlear nerve, which projects to the brainstem. Neural projections to the auditory area in the temporal lobe result in sound perception.

> - Balance is controlled by hair cells contained in the semicircular canals. Stimulation of these cells by head movement causes nerve impulses to be transmitted to the brain to keep individuals upright and control eye movement.
> - Vertigo, the sensation of motion or aggravation of motion, is a cardinal symptom of disorders of the vestibular system. Vertigo is often associated with nystagmus and nausea.
> - Hearing loss may result from interruptions in any part of the sound transmission pathway. Disorders of the outer and middle ear are generally termed *conductive* because sound waves are not reliably conducted to sensory organs of hearing. Accumulation of wax in the outer ear, ossification of bones, and middle ear infections and edema may result in conductive hearing loss. Conductive hearing loss is amenable to treatment.
> - Sensorineural hearing loss is due to dysfunction of the hair cells or neural pathways to the brain. Chronic exposure to loud noise, ototoxic drugs, head trauma, and aging changes may lead to sensorineural hearing loss. Sensorineural hearing loss is not as amenable to treatment as conductive loss.
> - Otosclerosis is a disorder characterized by resorption of healthy bone and deposition of weak, spongelike bone in the ossicles of the middle ear, most frequently the stapes. These bony lesions lead to progressive conductive hearing loss.
> - Presbycusis is a gradual sensorineural hearing loss common in older adults. Its cause is unclear and difficult to distinguish from other types of hearing loss, especially noise trauma.
> - Meniere disease is a chronic inner ear disease of unknown cause characterized by vertigo and progressive unilateral sensorineural hearing loss.
> - Otitis media, or inflammation of the middle ear, is most frequently seen in children and commonly results from eustachian tube dysfunction after upper respiratory tract infections. Otitis media can be both acute and chronic.

VISION

Healthy vision requires three basic processes to function appropriately: formation of an image on the retina, stimulation of rods and cones, and conduction of nerve impulses to the brain. Malfunction of any of these processes can disrupt normal vision.

STRUCTURE OF THE EYE

The eye is a spherical structure contained in the bony cavity of the eye socket, composed of three basic layers: the sclera, the choroid, and the retina (Figure 46-4). The sclera is white and opaque, and is made up of dense connective tissue. It aids in protecting the inner structures of the eye, and helps maintain the shape of the eye. The sclera merges with the coverings of the optic nerve on the posterior of the eye. The clear front portion of the sclera is the cornea. The cornea is also composed of dense connective tissue and has a greater curvature than the sclera that causes it to protrude from the sclera. No blood vessels are located in the cornea. Deep within the anterior portion of the sclera, at its conjunction with the cornea, lies a ring-shaped venous sinus: the canal of Schlemm. Affixed to the sclera are the **extraocular** muscles that control eye movement.

The choroid layer of the eye is highly vascularized and darkly pigmented. Attached to this layer is the iris. The iris is a muscular diaphragm whose pigments are responsible for eye color. The iris controls the size of the pupil, the opening through which light stimuli enter the posterior portion of the eye. Behind the pupil is a clear lens. The lens is a transparent, avascular elastic membrane. This elasticity assists in focusing light stimuli on the retina.

The eye is composed of anterior and posterior chambers separated by the lens and iris. The anterior chamber is filled with aqueous humor, the transparent protein-free liquid that is formed in the ciliary body and

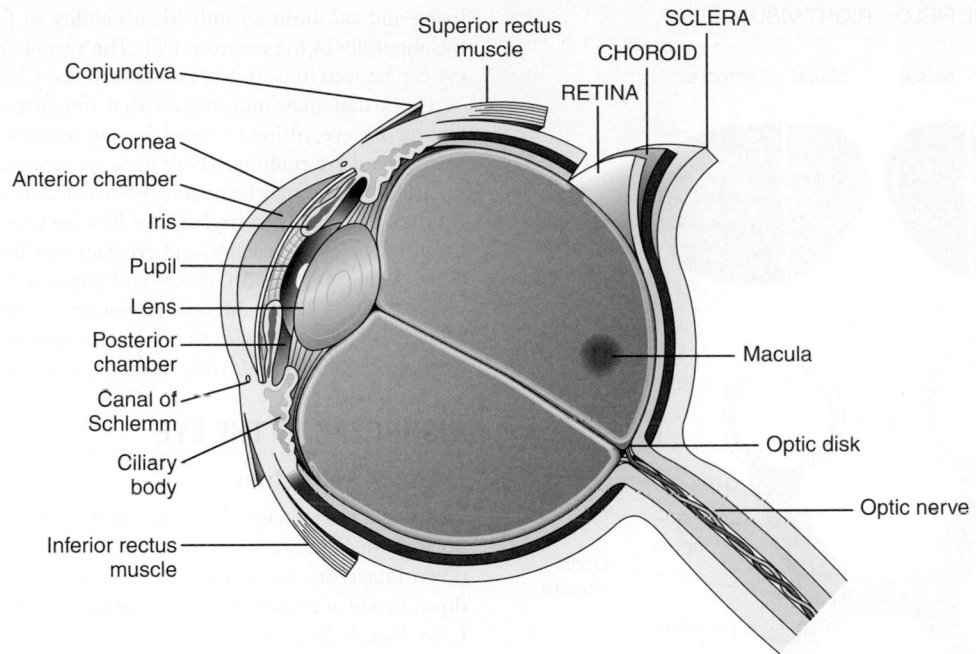

FIGURE 46-4 Anatomic structures of the eye.

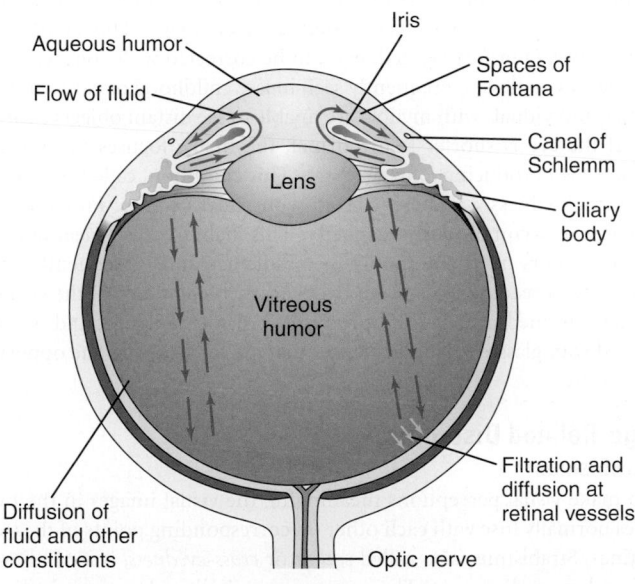

FIGURE 46-5 Circulation of the aqueous and vitreous humor of the eye.

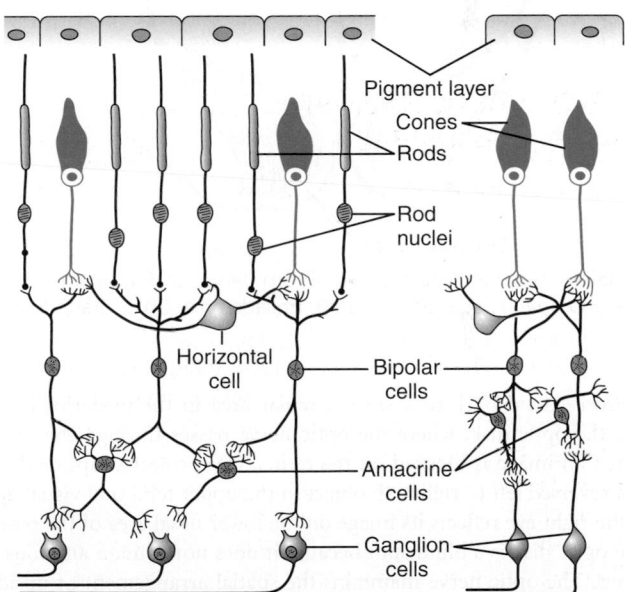

FIGURE 46-6 Three-neuron organization of the retina. (Redrawn from Hall JE: *Guyton and Hall textbook of medical physiology*, ed 12, Philadelphia, 2011, Saunders, p 617.)

drained through the canal of Schlemm (Figure 46-5). Aqueous humor provides oxygen and nutrients to the lens and cornea and is continually being formed and reabsorbed. The balance between formation and reabsorption of aqueous humor regulates the total volume and pressure of the **intraocular fluid.** The posterior chamber is the portion of the eye behind the lens that contains a thicker fluid, vitreous humor.

VISUAL PATHWAYS

The innermost layer of the eye is the retinal layer. It is here that light waves are transformed into nerve impulses. Three layers of neurons comprise the major portion of the retina (Figure 46-6). The outermost layer is composed of **photoreceptor** neurons, the rods and cones.

Cones are responsible for daylight vision, color vision, and visual acuity. The greatest concentration of cones occurs in the macula. This area is devoid of retinal vessels and is responsible for the most detailed vision. Rods are important for nighttime and peripheral vision and outnumber cones by nearly 20 to 1. The pigmented layer of the retina or the retinal pigment epithelium is one cell thick. It functions to protect and nourish the retina. The retinal pigment epithelium also removes metabolic cellular debris from the photoreceptor cells, prevents new blood vessel growth into the retina, and absorbs light to diminish scattering and thereby enhance vision.

Action potentials from the rods and cones are communicated throughout the other layers of the retina. All axons of the ganglion

LEFT VISUAL FIELD   RIGHT VISUAL FIELD

Temporal   Nasal   Nasal   Temporal

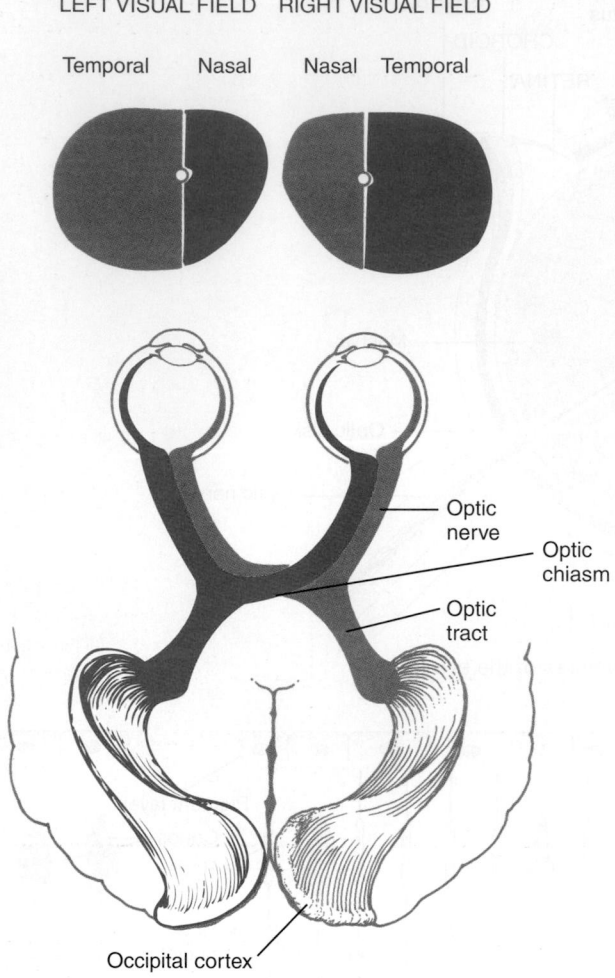

Optic nerve

Optic chiasm

Optic tract

Occipital cortex

FIGURE 46-7 Visual pathways. (From Jarvis C: *Physical examination and health assessment*, ed 6, Philadelphia, 2012, Saunders.)

neuron extend back to a small circular area in the posterior of the eye, the optic disk, where the optic nerve passes through the sclera. When an image is focused on the retina, it is projected upside down and reversed left to right. An object in the upper temporal visual field of the right eye reflects its image on the lower nasal area of the retina. The optic disk is a blind spot because it does not contain any rods or cones. The optic nerve maintains the spatial arrangement of upside-down and reversed images, and at the optic chiasm just anterior to the pituitary gland half of the nerve fibers cross over to the other side of the brain (Figure 46-7). The left optic tract contains fibers from the left half of each retina, and the right optic tract contains fibers from the right half of each retina. The nerve impulse travels through the optic nerves to connections in the thalamus and finally connects with the neurons of the occipital cortex.

GENERAL MANIFESTATIONS OF VISUAL IMPAIRMENT

Visual impairment may occur or become evident at any time during the life span. If these impairments occur during infancy or early childhood and are not immediately detected and managed, vision may not develop normally (see Pediatric Considerations: Development of Newborn Vision). In older children, academic performance may suffer. In adults and elderly individuals, poor eyesight affects activities of daily living and can limit an individual's ability to function normally and meaningfully in the environment. The various effects of aging on the eye can be seen in Geriatric Considerations: Changes in the Eyes.

Clues that may indicate a visual impairment include squinting, closing one eye, tilting the head, having redness of the eye or excessive tearing, and eye rubbing. These signs are especially helpful in identifying children who may be unable to verbalize visual difficulties. In older children and adults, complaints of blurred vision, halos, "floaters" in the visual fields, headaches, and eye pain may indicate a visual impairment. A thorough health history and physical examination along with *visual acuity testing* and *ophthalmoscopic examination* will provide health care providers with the necessary information to appropriately treat or refer individuals with visual impairment.

DISORDERS OF THE EYE
Errors of Refraction

Focusing a clear image on the retina is essential for good vision. In a normal eye, light rays enter the eye and are focused into a clear, upside-down image on the retina. The brain can easily "right" the upside-down image in conscious perception but cannot correct an image that is not sharply focused (Figure 46-8).

Myopia, Hyperopia, Presbyopia, and Astigmatism

If the eye is elongated, the image focuses in front of the retina rather than on it. The retina receives only a fuzzy image. This condition, called *myopia* or nearsightedness, can be corrected with concave contact lenses or glasses. Frequently seen in late childhood or early adolescence, individuals with myopia are unable to see distant objects clearly.

If the eye is shorter than normal, the image focuses behind the retina, also producing a fuzzy image. This condition, called *hyperopia* or farsightedness, can be corrected with convex lenses. *Presbyopia* is the loss of **accommodative capacity.** This inability to see near objects clearly occurs most commonly in middle age and is frequently corrected with reading glasses. An irregularity in curvature of the cornea or lens, termed *astigmatism,* produces a distorted image, and is corrected with glasses or contact lenses that are formed with the opposite curvature.

Age-Related Disorders
Strabismus

To make visual perceptions meaningful, the visual images in the two eyes normally fuse with each other on corresponding points of the two retinas. Strabismus, also called *squint* or *cross-eyedness,* is a condition of ocular misalignment. The eyes appear misaligned on examination. Symptoms include squinting and frowning when reading, closing one eye to see, having trouble picking up objects, being dizzy, and having headaches. Strabismus is often caused by an abnormal "set" of the fusion mechanism of the visual system and is most commonly found in children. Strabismus affects 2% to 4% of the population.[18] Studies have shown that advanced maternal age, cigarette smoking during pregnancy, and low birth weight contribute to the incidence of strabismus. There also may be a genetic link predisposing children to certain types of strabismus.[18]

In the early efforts of the child to fixate the two eyes on the same object, one of the eyes fixates satisfactorily but the other fails to fixate, or both eyes fixate satisfactorily but never simultaneously. Soon the patterns of conjugate movements of the eyes become abnormally set so that the eyes never fuse.

Treatment of strabismus includes occlusion therapy, or patching of the good eye to force use of the weak eye, use of corrective lenses, surgery on the eye muscles, use of prisms, and exercises for the eye. If

PEDIATRIC CONSIDERATIONS
Development of Newborn Vision

At birth, the newborn's visual acuity is 20/400. By 6 months of age, the infant's visual acuity is 20/30 because of increased synaptic density of the visual cortex and maturation of the retina, retinal photoreceptors, and optic nerves. The newborn has several reflexive eye movements such as the blink reflex, corneal reflex, and pupillary reactions to light. The newborn is unable to coordinate the head and eyes at birth, so the doll's eyes reflex is present. As the infant begins to explore the environment visually, the voluntary eye movements increase. The reflexive and voluntary movements begin to coordinate to create normal eye alignment. Eyes must be close to alignment for vision. If a strabismus (eyes not properly aligned) occurs, it can lead to blindness. The shapes of the eyeball, cornea, and lens change as the infant grows. The eyeball is less spherical than the adult eye and is too short for the lens. As the eyeball lengthens, convergence created by the cornea and the lens decreases, which helps create binocularity. Binocularity is perceived vision from both eyes simultaneously; it begins to develop at age 6 weeks and is established at 4 months. Stereopsis or depth perception develops by 7 months of age.

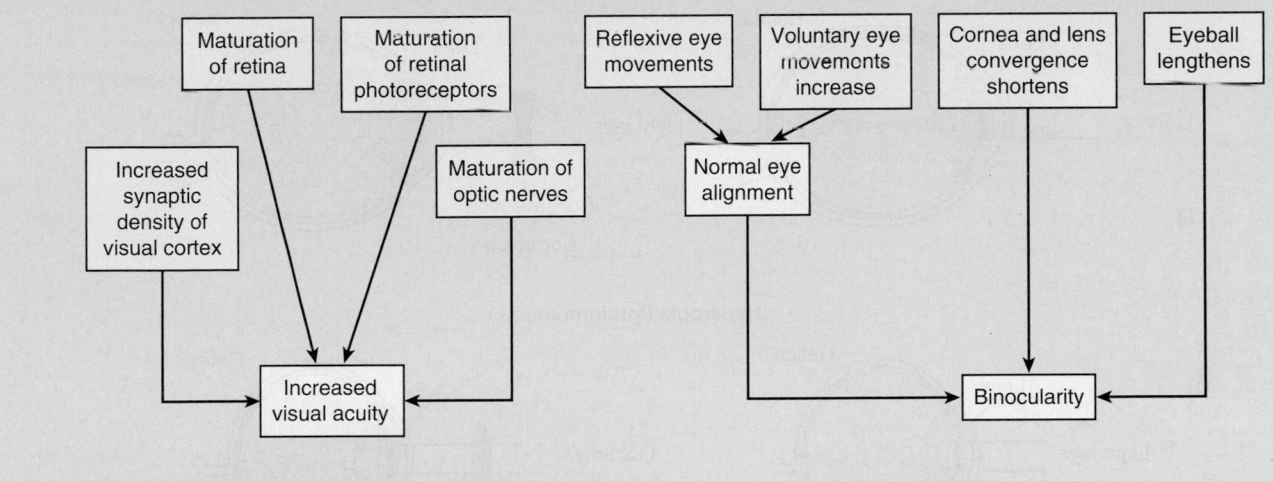

GERIATRIC CONSIDERATIONS
Changes in the Eyes

Aging affects all parts of the eye. Minor changes include decreased skin elasticity, alterations in lacrimal gland function, and shrinking of the vitreous body. The changes in the lens and retina of the eye are more significant. These changes cause decreased color vision and discrimination, reduced contrast sensitivity, and diminished accommodation. As a result, the elderly need brighter light to see and do not differentiate color well. The elderly also have less dynamic visual acuity.

The retina is affected by a loss of the luteal pigment in the macular areas, as well as reduced light-sensing thresholds of the rods and cones. These changes lead directly to a slowing of dark adaptation and a decrease in the ability to discern brightness and colors, particularly shorter light wavelengths such as blues and greens.

A primary change in the aging eye is the development of presbyopia. Presbyopia is caused by a decrease in the elasticity of the lens and a decrease in the effectiveness of the ciliary muscle, which lead to an inability to focus on near objects.

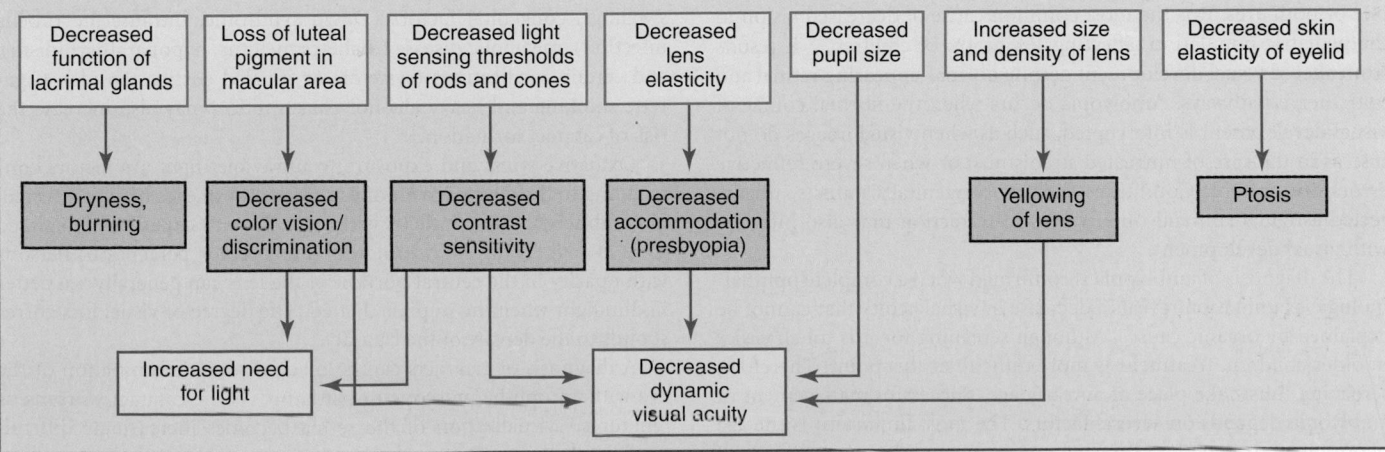

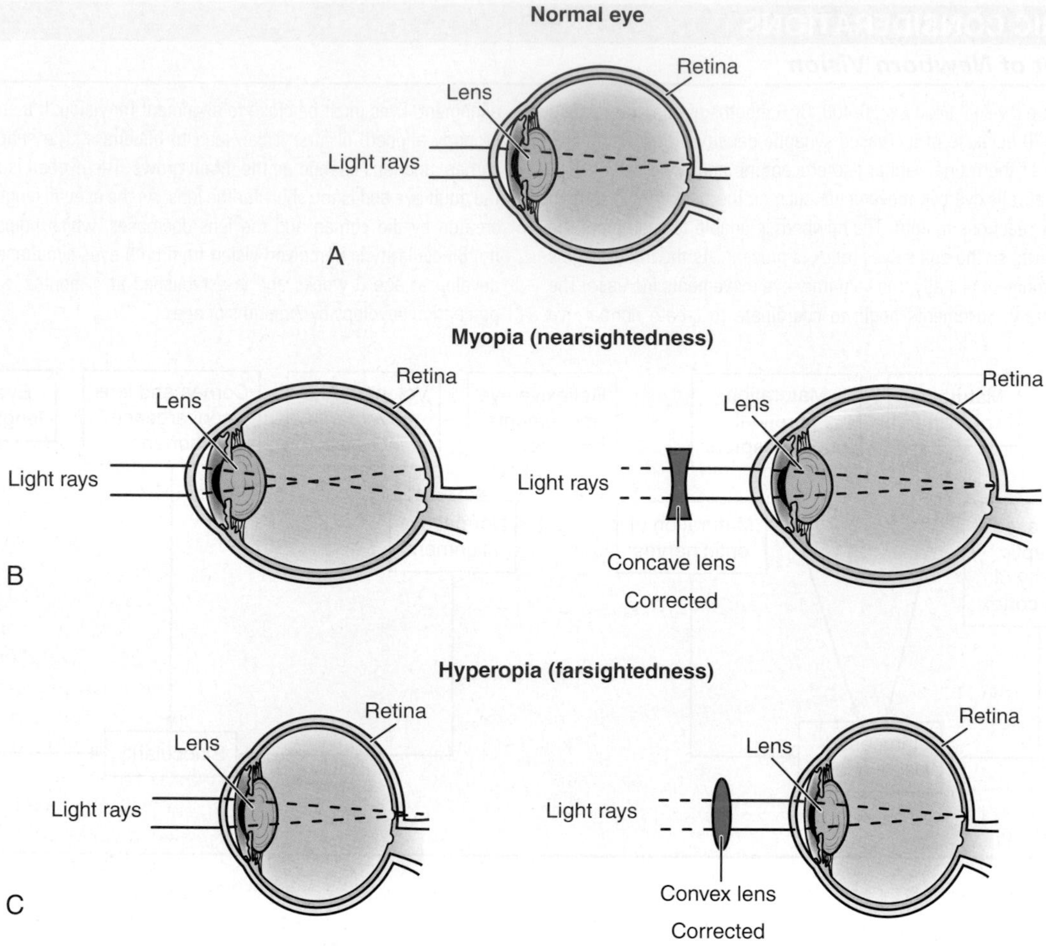

Normal eye

Myopia (nearsightedness)

Concave lens
Corrected

Hyperopia (farsightedness)

Convex lens
Corrected

FIGURE 46-8 A, Light rays are focused to produce a clear visual image (emmetropia). **B,** In myopia, light rays are focused in front of the retina. A concave lens moves the focus back onto the retina and results in a clear image. **C,** In hyperopia, light rays are focused behind the retina. A convex lens moves the focus forward so that the light rays fall directly on the retina.

management of strabismus is begun before 24 months of age, amblyopia may be prevented.

Amblyopia

Amblyopia is poor vision, even with the proper optical correction, in one or both eyes. It is the most common cause of decreased vision in the pediatric population, affecting 1% to 4% of children.[19] It results from altered visual development despite normal-appearing retinal and optic nerve pathways. Amblyopia occurs when the normal course of visual development is interrupted, such as when visual images do not fuse as in the case of untreated strabismus, or when severe refractive errors are present. Conditions such as congenital cataracts, uncorrected astigmatism, and other errors of refraction may also interfere with visual development.

The diagnosis of amblyopia is confirmed when a complete ophthalmologic examination reveals a decrease in visual acuity that cannot be explained by organic causes. Although screening for it is much easier in older children, treatment is more difficult at this point. Therefore, screening must take place at an early age. Successful management of amblyopia depends on several factors. The most important is the age of onset and the length of time between onset and the commencement of treatment. Management of amblyopia includes the use of atropine to blur vision or patching of the "stronger" eye. This forces the brain and weaker eye to work together to stimulate vision.[20]

Cataracts

Cataracts are a clouding or opacity of the lens that leads to gradual, painless blurring of vision and eventual loss of sight. Most people older than 60 years of age have some degree of cataracts.[20] Cataracts result from the process of aging (senile), trauma (causing lens rupture and swelling), congenital factors (Down syndrome, intrauterine rubella infection), metabolic disease (diabetes mellitus, hypoparathyroidism), and certain medications (systemic or inhaled corticosteroids). Cigarette smoking and heavy alcohol consumption may also increase the risk of cataract formation.[21]

Oxidative stress and exposure to ultraviolet light are factors contributing to the development of cataracts.[21] Both eyes may be affected, but at different rates. Patients with cataracts may experience increased glare at night, blurred vision, and altered color perception. Persons with opacity in the central portion of the lens can generally see better in dim light when the pupil is dilated. The degree of visual loss corresponds to the density of the cataract.

A diagnosis of cataracts can be made through examination of the eye with an ophthalmoscope or slit lamp. As the cataract worsens or "matures," visualization of the retina becomes increasingly difficult until finally the pupil appears white and the retina cannot be visualized at all. Treatment for cataracts involves surgical removal and replacement of the lens. This procedure is completed on an outpatient basis, with individuals returning home immediately after surgery.

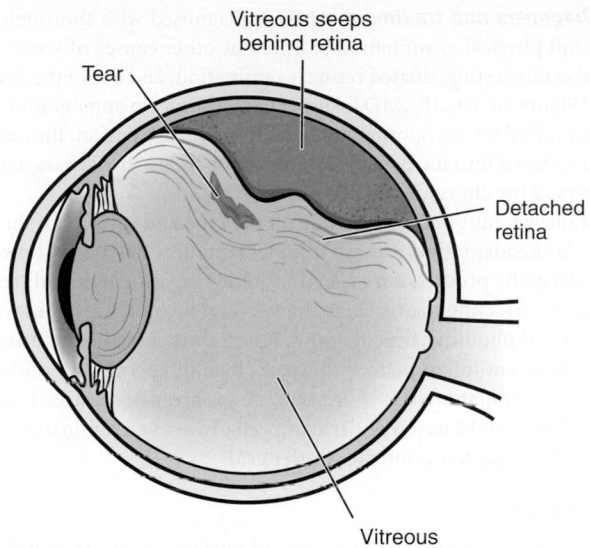

Vitreous seeps behind retina

Tear

Detached retina

Vitreous

FIGURE 46-9 Retinal detachment.

Retinopathy

Retinopathy is any disorder of the retina. Damage to the retina impairs vision because even a well-focused image cannot be perceived if some or all of the light receptors do not function properly. Retinopathies can result from a variety of causes, the most common being trauma and vascular disease, especially in individuals with diabetes mellitus and hypertension.

Retinal Detachment

Detachment of the retina is usually spontaneous but may be secondary to trauma such as sudden blows to the head. Spontaneous detachment occurs most frequently in individuals older than 50 years.[22] Eye tumors, myopia, and cataract extraction are other common predisposing factors. Retinal detachments are classified into three categories. Exudative (or serous) detachments result from accumulation of serous or hemorrhagic fluid in the subretinal space, generally due to hydrostatic factors (e.g., severe, sudden hypertension), inflammation (sarcoidosis), or neoplastic effusions. The second type, tractional retinal detachment, occurs when mechanical forces on the retina caused by fibrosis and scarring pull it away from the underlying epithelium (injury or surgery to the eye). The third type of retinal detachment is spontaneous or rhegmatogenous. As individuals age, the vitreous humor shrinks and traction develops, causing separation.[22]

Tearing of the retina allows vitreous fluid to flow behind the retina and cause traction and progressive detachment (Figure 46-9). The area of detachment increases rapidly, and visual loss is progressive. Common manifestations of retinal detachment include the sudden appearance of floating spots that may decrease over a period of weeks and odd flashes of light that appear when the eye moves. Other symptoms include blurring of vision in a single eye that appears as though "a curtain is being pulled down over the eye." If untreated, the retina may detach entirely and result in total blindness in the affected eye. However, if diagnosed and treated early, permanent vision loss can be prevented. Retinal detachments may also cause vitreous hemorrhage.[23]

Retinal detachments are diagnosed through ophthalmoscopic examination. The retina appears to hang in the vitreous humor like a gray cloud. One or more retinal tears, generally crescent-shaped, are usually present. Management of retinal detachment is aimed at closing tears in the retina and positioning the fragments of the retina so that reattachment can occur.

Diabetic Retinopathy

Etiology and pathogenesis. Diabetic retinopathy is one of the most common complications of diabetes, afflicting about 20% of adults with the disease.[24] Symptoms increase in prevalence and severity with increasing duration of illness and poorer control of blood glucose levels.[22] Diabetic retinopathy is a disease of the vasculature of the retina. In diabetes, the retinal capillary becomes diseased; it loses the ability to transport red blood cells and thus oxygen and nourishment to the retina, with consequent tissue hypoxia and ischemia. Diabetic retinopathy can be divided into two categories: nonproliferative and proliferative.

In nonproliferative diabetic retinopathy, retinal veins become dilated and microaneurysms develop. This effect is a result of damaged vascular epithelium. Small retinal hemorrhages and cotton-wool spots (infarctions in the nerve fibers) occur. Early in the process, visual changes may be minimal or resolve after a few days. As the disease progresses, retinal edema occurs. If the edema involves the macular area, visual acuity is noticeably affected. This form is more common in persons with type 2 diabetes.[25]

Proliferative diabetic retinopathy is characterized by the development of new but abnormal blood vessels (neovascularization) caused by the loss of retinal blood flow and ischemia. These new vessels affect vision in two ways: first, because they are abnormal, they are prone to leakage of blood into the vitreous cavity and may thus result in vitreous hemorrhage. Second, the vessels firmly attach themselves to the retina and grow out into the vitreous humor. The subsequent traction on the retina increases the risk for retinal detachment. This form is more common in persons with type 1 diabetes.[25]

Clinical manifestations. Diabetic retinopathy is associated with complaints of blurred, darkened, and distorted vision. Visual changes may fluctuate in severity. Some individuals complain of being unable to read or have vague changes in vision.

Diagnosis and treatment. The diagnosis of diabetic retinopathy is made through careful history taking, visual acuity testing, and performing ophthalmologic examination and retinal angiography. The most important factor in the management of diabetic retinopathy is prevention. Intensive blood glucose level control and blood pressure management have been shown to slow the progression or reduce the risk of developing diabetic retinopathy.[25] Laser treatments are also used to prevent further vision loss. Because the retina is nervous system tissue, it does not regenerate efficiently. Therefore, treatment may prevent any further injury to eye tissue, but it cannot restore vision.

Management of proliferative diabetic retinopathy must be instituted as soon as possible to prevent blindness. Surgical intervention and laser procedures are used in conjunction with the measures used for nonproliferative retinopathy. Because of the risk of diabetic retinopathy, it is recommended that individuals with diabetes mellitus have annual ophthalmologic examinations.

Age-Related Macular Degeneration

Etiology and pathogenesis. Age-related macular degeneration (AMD) is the leading cause of blindness among people ages 55 years and older.[26] The exact causes of macular degeneration are unknown, but the outcome is bilateral progressive macular deterioration with central vision loss. Risk factors for developing AMD include age, female gender, history of cigarette smoking, family history of AMD, increased serum cholesterol level, cardiovascular disease, hypertension, obesity, and previous cataract surgery. Oxidative stress and inflammatory chemicals appear to be key factors in development of the disorder.[22,26,27] There is also a strong relationship between AMD and nutrition.[28] Dietary supplements have been shown to delay progression from intermediate to advanced forms of the disease; however, some studies suggest they do not prevent the disease. AMD includes a wide spectrum of findings that can be divided into two subgroups. Manifestations, diagnosis, and management of each subgroup differ.

"Dry" or non-neovascular geographic atrophic AMD is the most common form, causing visual loss attributable to degeneration of the outer retina, the pigmented layer, and the choroidal layer. There are subretinal accumulations of cellular debris known as *drusen,* along with metabolic dysfunction of the retina. Hard drusen may be seen during ophthalmologic examination and appear as discrete yellow deposits on the retina. Atrophic AMD often affects just one eye initially but later develops in the unaffected eye. It causes a gradual decline in vision.

In "wet" neovascular or exudative AMD, visual loss is usually more rapid in onset and causes more severe visual disruption. Impairment of barrier function allows for subretinal fluid collections, which may cause retinal detachments and/or neovascularizations. These fluid buildups may be visualized on retinal examination.

Clinical manifestations. AMD is generally painless. In the atrophic form, the initial symptom is slightly blurred vision and decreased ability to see fine detail. Often patients need more light for completing fine tasks such as reading and needlework. As the disorder progresses, the area of central vision loss becomes larger and darker.

Exudative AMD may also be manifested by a progressive blurring of vision. A hallmark of this form of AMD is the wavy appearance of straight lines. This occurs because of distortion of the retina from fluid accumulations behind it. Vision may be lost rapidly or occur suddenly in previously undiagnosed patients attributable to retinal detachment or hemorrhage.

Diagnosis and treatment. AMD is diagnosed with thorough history and physical examination to rule out other causes of visual loss, visual acuity testing, dilated retinal examination, and use of the Amsler grid (Figure 46-10). If AMD is suspected, fluorescein angiography may be completed by the ophthalmologist. In this examination, fluorescein dye is injected into the patient. Photos of the retina show characteristic changes of the choroidal vascular layer.

Management of AMD depends on the type and severity of the disease. Antioxidant/zinc vitamin supplementation has been shown to slow/delay the progression of AMD.[22] Other treatment modalities are aimed at correcting the vascular changes and include laser photocoagulation and photodynamic therapy. Research is currently focusing on a variety of antiinflammatory therapies including corticosteroids and immune-modulating drugs.[27] As with all progressive diseases, patients with AMD should have regular comprehensive eye examinations and daily self-evaluation using the Amsler grid.

Glaucoma

Glaucoma is characterized by increased intraocular pressure and progressive loss of vision. As fluid pressure inside the eye and against the retina increases, blood flow through the retina slows. Reduced blood flow causes degeneration of the retina and thus loss of vision. Glaucoma can be categorized into two main types: chronic open-angle and acute closed-angle (narrow-angle) (Figure 46-11).

Glaucoma is more common in the elderly, African Americans, those with a family history, those with myopia, and individuals with

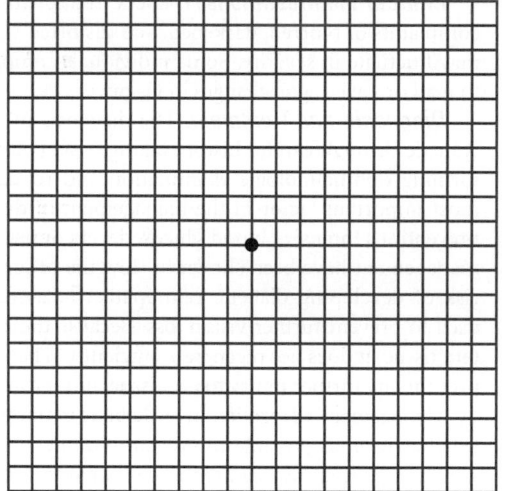 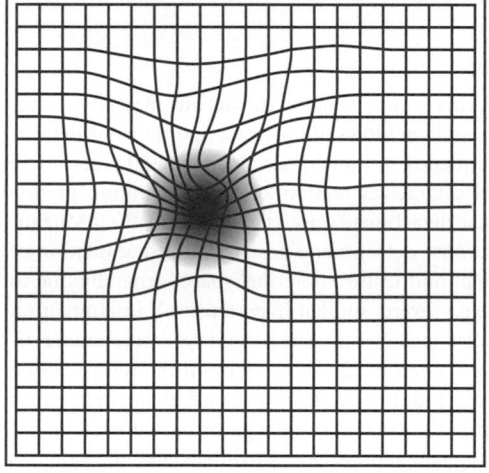

FIGURE 46-10 *Left,* What an Amsler grid looks like to an individual with normal vision. *Right,* What an Amsler grid might look like to an individual with macular degeneration. (From Macular Degeneration Network. Available at www.macular-degeneration.org/.)

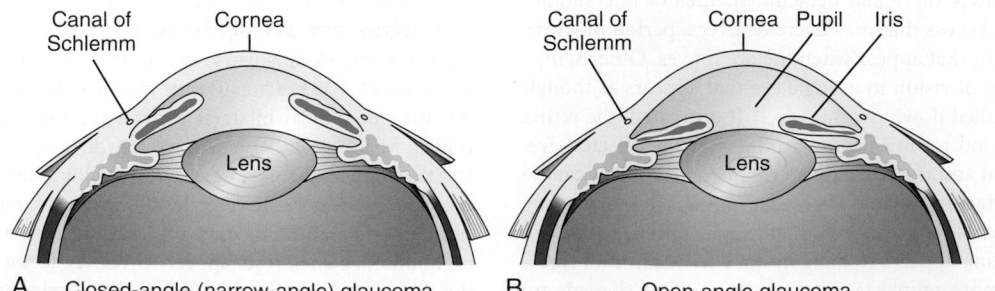

FIGURE 46-11 Closed-angle (narrow-angle) glaucoma compared with open-angle glaucoma. **A,** In closed-angle glaucoma, the outflow of aqueous humor is obstructed by the iris root of the dilated pupil. **B,** In open-angle glaucoma, the obstruction to outflow of aqueous humor is in the drainage canals.

diabetes. It may also occur as a result of trauma, inflammation, or exposure to corticosteroids.[22]

Chronic Open-Angle Glaucoma

Etiology and pathogenesis. The cause of open-angle glaucoma is not clear. The drainage channels for aqueous humor appear normal. The disease is often bilateral and has a genetic component. Open-angle glaucoma accounts for the majority of all cases of glaucoma.

Open-angle glaucoma has an insidious onset with no symptoms in the early stages. However, the intraocular pressure is consistently elevated, and, over a period of months or years, symptoms including gradual loss of vision in the periphery resulting in tunnel vision appear. Affected individuals may have complaints of vague but persistent dull eye pain or an inability to distinguish colors. Halos may appear around lights if the intraocular pressure is markedly elevated.

Diagnosis and treatment. The diagnosis of open-angle glaucoma is made through intraocular pressure measurement, ophthalmoscopic examination of the optic disk, and central visual field testing. Because of the insidious nature of the disorder, it is recommended that all individuals older than 40 years have an intraocular pressure measurement and ophthalmoscopic examination every 3 to 5 years. If a family history of glaucoma is present, more frequent examination is recommended.

Management of open-angle glaucoma is aimed at increasing drainage of aqueous humor and decreasing intraocular pressure. Prostaglandin analogue eye drops (latanoprost 0.005%, bimatoprost 0.03%) are first-line agents. β-Adrenergic–blocking eye drops, such as timolol, are used to help decrease intraocular pressure by decreasing aqueous humor production. Miotics such as pilocarpine are also useful in that they constrict the pupil and thereby stimulate the ciliary muscles to pull on the trabecular meshwork surrounding the canal of Schlemm to increase the flow of aqueous humor. If the intraocular pressure elevation persists or the optic nerve damage progresses despite treatment, laser surgery aimed at the trabecular meshwork may be done to lower intraocular pressure.[22]

Acute Angle-Closure Glaucoma

Etiology and pathogenesis. Primary acute angle-closure glaucoma is caused by abnormality of the angle between the pupil and lateral cornea. This angle is narrow and blocks outflow of aqueous humor when the pupil is dilated. Angle-closure glaucoma is much less common than open-angle glaucoma but is more prevalent in the elderly, hyperopes, and Asian populations.[22] This form of glaucoma has a rapid onset and is treated as an emergency. Angle-closure glaucoma is associated with pupillary dilation and thus might occur when an individual is sitting in a darkened room or during times of stress. Forward displacement of the iris toward the cornea with dilation narrows or closes the chamber angle, obstructing the outflow of aqueous humor (see Figure 46-11).

Manifestations of angle-closure glaucoma include severe eye pain, nausea and vomiting, blurred vision with halos around lights, redness of the eye, a steamy cornea, and a dilated pupil that is nonreactive to light. This form of glaucoma is an emergency situation because permanent blindness can occur within 2 to 5 days after onset of symptoms.[22]

Diagnosis and treatment. Diagnosis of angle-closure glaucoma involves the same tests as used for diagnosis of open-angle glaucoma. Treatment again in this case is aimed at decreasing intraocular pressure. Acutely, carbonic anhydrase inhibitors such as acetazolamide and miotics may be used to decrease aqueous humor production and blockage. Laser iridectomy usually results in a permanent cure. Novel therapies are currently being explored aimed at reducing cell death/apoptosis and improving retinal cell survival.[29]

Visual Field Deficits
Visual Field Loss

Etiology and pathogenesis. Visual field loss can be caused by changes in the eye itself, as is the case in cataracts, or result from tumors, vascular lesions, and demyelinating lesions near or in the neural pathways of the retina, optic nerve, or the visual cortex of the brain.

Damage to the visual pathway does not always result in a total loss of vision. Depending on where the damage occurs, only part of the visual field may be affected (Figure 46-12). Monocular field loss indicates disease of the retina or optic nerve. For example, a certain form of neuritis often associated with multiple sclerosis can cause loss of only the center of the visual field, called a *scotoma*.

Damage or lesions may also cause bilateral visual field losses or loss of half of the visual field, called **hemianopsia**. Lesions of the optic chiasm, usually caused by pituitary tumors, characteristically produce a bitemporal hemianopsia. Lesions occurring behind the optic chiasm cause a homonymous hemianopsia, which is a visual field loss involving the same side in both eyes. The more posterior the lesion in the visual pathway, the more congruous (similar size, shape, location) are the defects in the two eyes. Cerebrovascular accidents (strokes) and tumors are responsible for most of these lesions.

Diagnosis and treatment. Visual field deficits are easily and rapidly assessed through confrontation (i.e., comparison of the patient's vision to the examiner's vision). Visual field deficits should be suspected if patients demonstrate one-sided neglect of their environment or eye deviation toward the side of the lesion. Treatment for visual field loss includes managing the underlying cause (tumor removal), adapting the patient's environment, and teaching compensatory techniques.

INTERVENTIONS FOR INDIVIDUALS WITH VISION IMPAIRMENT

Once the visual impairment of an individual has been thoroughly investigated, specific interventions may be prescribed. Interventions may be classified into three general categories: assistive devices, environmental adaptations, and behavioral techniques. Proper care and cleaning of contact lenses and eyeglasses directly influences the effectiveness of the prosthesis. Tinted lenses are generally available and may be effective in reducing glare for some individuals. Pocket magnifiers are frequently useful for persons with an acuity impairment. Large print is now available on many household items (e.g., watches, playing cards, telephones, books), and various textures are used in further modifications for the visually impaired.

An unchanging, structured environment where items are kept in fixed locations familiar to the visually impaired person promotes safety and independence. Attempts to structure temporary environments, such as by introducing personal items into a hospital room, might yield positive results if consistently considered by the staff. Attention to adequate lighting, glare reduction, and appropriate use of contrasting colors enhances safety and independent function of those with visual impairment.

Behavioral techniques for the health care professional and visually impaired individuals can promote client comfort, safety, and independence. Such techniques for the professional include announcing oneself at all interactions and explaining sensory occurrences. Encouraging independence and social interaction often benefits individuals inasmuch as they may experience anger, frustration, or changes in self-concept as a result of their visual deficit.

Visually impaired individuals may be taught to wait several minutes for changes in dark-light adaptation and avoid abrupt changes in lighting. Individuals should be discouraged from looking directly into bright lights to reduce glare. Assessment of the visually impaired patient's ability to summon help in the health care and home settings is advised.

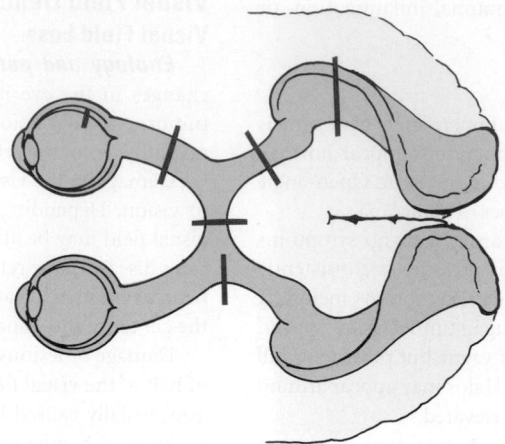

1. Retinal damage
   - Macula—central blind area (e.g., diabetes):

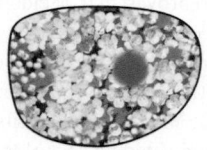 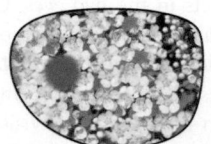

   - Localized damage—blind spot (scotoma) corresponding to particular area:

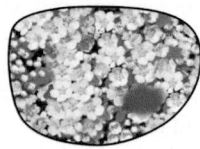 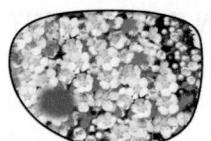

   - Increasing intraocular pressure—decrease in peripheral vision (e.g., glaucoma). Starts with paracentral scotoma in early stage:

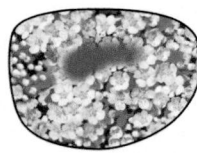 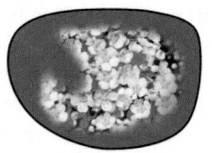

   - Retinal detachment. Person has shadow or diminished vision in one quadrant or one half of visual field:

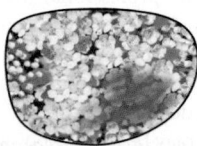 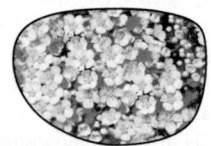

2. Lesion in globe or optic nerve. Injury here yields one blind eye, or unilateral blindness:

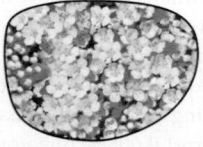 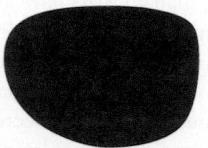

3. Lesion at optic chiasm (e.g., pituitary tumor)—injury to crossing fibers only yields a loss of the nasal part of each retina and a loss of both temporal visual fields. Bitemporal (heteronymous) hemianopsia:

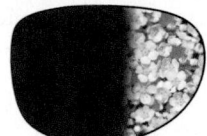 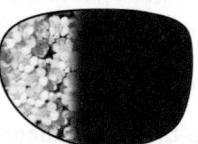

4. Lesion of outer uncrossed fibers at optic chiasm (e.g., aneurysm of left internal carotid artery exerts pressure on uncrossed fibers). Injury yields left nasal hemianopsia:

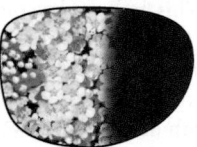 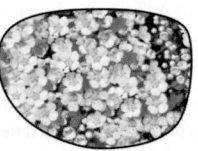

5. Lesion of right optic tract or right optic radiation. Visual field loss in right nasal and left temporal fields. Loss of same half of visual field in both eyes is homonymous hemianopsia:

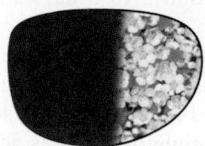 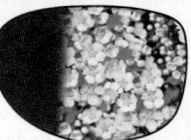

FIGURE 46-12 Visual field losses. (From Jarvis C: *Physical examination and health assessment*, ed 6, Philadelphia, 2012, Saunders.)

SMELL AND TASTE

The senses of smell and taste allow separation of noxious or even lethal agents from those that are desirable. The sense of smell has a protective function in signaling danger: animals use smell to recognize the proximity of other animals, and humans use smell to sense harmful substances, such as smoke or spoiled food items, in the environment. The sense of taste allows a person to select food in accordance with desire and perhaps also in accordance with tissue needs. Both senses are strongly tied to primitive emotional and behavioral functions of the nervous system. These chemical senses are interrelated and will be discussed together.

Nerve fibers of the **olfactory** system have their cell bodies in the mucous membrane of the upper and posterior parts of the nasal cavity. The sense of smell begins with chemical stimulation of these cells. Axons of these receptor cells pass through the cribriform plate and travel to the olfactory area of the cortex through the first cranial nerve. These nerves lie under the frontal lobes of the brain. It has been long thought that olfactory impulses reach the cerebral cortex without relay through the thalamus, making olfaction unique among the sensory systems. However, newer pathways have been identified that pass through the thalamus and are thought to aid in the conscious analysis of odor.[30]

Like stimuli for smell, stimuli for taste are chemical. Food particles dissolved in fluid stimulate sensory receptors (taste buds) located on the surface of the tongue and in lesser density on the palate, pharynx, and larynx.[30] Stimulation from the sensory receptors is conducted through the cranial nerves of taste (VII, IX, X) to connections in the brainstem and thalamus with eventual termination in the **gustatory** cortex in the parietal lobe. The gustatory sensory receptors have a heightened sensitivity for one of the primary taste sensations (sweet, salty, sour, or bitter); however, they can respond to a variety of stimuli. The number of sensory receptors for taste diminishes with age, often affecting nutritional status.

Disorders of Smell and Taste

Etiology and pathogenesis. Olfactory disorders range from loss or reduction in the sense of smell to distortions and olfactory hallucinations. Commonly the sense of smell is diminished in those who smoke and in individuals with conditions involving congestion and swelling of the nasal mucosa, such as allergies and sinusitis. Head trauma often results in the loss of smell because of actual shearing of the neuronal fibers as they traverse the cribriform plate. Tumors and large cerebral aneurysms of the anterior cerebral and anterior communicating arteries are lesions capable of diminishing olfactory sense. Epilepsy and psychiatric disorders may be associated with olfactory hallucinations.

A decreased gustatory sense can also result from heavy smoking, as well as extreme dryness of the tongue and mucous membranes. A variety of medications are known to alter the sense of taste, including certain antidepressant, antithyroid, antirheumatic, and anticancer medications. In addition, influenza-like illnesses and lesions on the thalamus and parietal lobe may impair taste sensation.

Clinical manifestations. Individuals with smell dysfunction frequently complain of a diminished ability to taste. They may experience a decreased appetite and use excessive amounts of salt, sugar, or other seasonings on their foods. These individuals may stop reacting to strong smells and not notice their own body odor. Smell dysfunction increases the risk of accidents in that these individuals may not detect signs of imminent danger such as gas or smoke. In addition, spoiled food may be ingested, and excessive use of salt is associated with health risks.

Diagnosis and treatment. Assessment of the sense of smell is done by asking the individual to smell different known odors while keeping the eyes closed. Irritating substances such as ammonia should be avoided because they stimulate the trigeminal nerve. Assessment of gustatory sense should include the primary taste sensations in appropriate areas of the tongue, with the surface of the tongue wiped clean between substances. Questions regarding weight loss and appetite add valuable information to the assessment data.

Interventions for those with smell and taste dysfunction focus on augmenting the stimulus, teaching the individual to rely on other senses, and changing the environment. Because their senses of smell and taste are unreliable in identifying spoiled foods, people with these dysfunctions are encouraged to adhere to a strict schedule for discarding leftovers and be aware of expiration dates on food products. Because significant nutritional problems may occur, it is important to educate and monitor the individual's diet. The creative use of seasonings and spices along with variations in the texture and presentation of food may enhance appetite. Individuals with taste impairments are encouraged to avoid blended foods and to practice frequent oral hygiene. Smoke detectors should be installed in all rooms where smell-impaired individuals sleep, and fire safety should be emphasized.

SUMMARY

Humans interact with their environment by means of the special senses of hearing, vision, smell, and taste. Through a variety of stimuli, including chemicals, light, and sound, individuals are able to enjoy everything from a symphony performance to a hot fudge sundae. The special senses also protect individuals from harm by allowing the perception of smoke or alarms. Only when these special senses are impaired does their importance become apparent.

Loss of these senses may result from congenital conditions, trauma, tumors, illness, or unknown causes. Loss may also be a consequence of aging. The mechanism of impairment may be a disruption of the mechanical aspect of the special sense, as in the obstruction of sound waves from cerumen impaction in the ears, or may be a neurologic event, as in the occurrence of homonymous hemianopsia after a stroke.

Regardless of the cause of loss of the sense of hearing, vision, smell, or taste, prompt intervention and treatment can make tremendous differences in outcome. The loss may be totally corrected, or its progression may be slowed. Treatment may be aimed at the underlying cause of the sensory impairment or at altering the individual's behavior or environment to maximize the remaining function. In working with individuals who have alterations in special sensory function, health care professionals have the opportunity to make a great difference in that person's quality of life.

REFERENCES

1. Post RE, Dickerson LM: Dizziness: a diagnostic approach, *Am Fam Physician* 82(4):361–368, 2010.
2. National Institute on Deafness and Other Communication Disorders: *Quick statistics*. Available at www.nidcd.nih.gov/health/statistics/Pages/quick.aspx.
3. Lustig LR, Schindler JS: Ear, nose & throat disorders. In McPhee SJ, Papadakis MA, Rabow MW, editors: *Current medical diagnosis & treatment 2012*, New York, 2011, McGraw-Hill. Available at www.accessmedicine/com/content.aspx?aID=2356. Accessed 11/11/11.
4. Centers for Disease Control and Prevention: *Hearing loss data and statistics*. Available at www.cdc.gov/ncbddd/hearingloss/data/html.
5. Mohammadi S, Mazhari MM, Mehrparvar AH, et al: Effect of simultaneous exposure to occupational noise and cigarette smoke on binaural hearing impairment, *Noise Health* 12(48):187–190, 2010.
6. Markou K, Goudakos J: An overview of the etiology of otosclerosis, *Eur Arch Otorhinolaryngol* 266:25–35, 2009.
7. Cureoglu S, Baylan MY, Paparella MM: Cochlear otosclerosis, *Curr Opin Otolaryngol Head Neck Surg* 18(5):357–362, 2010.
8. Shibata SB, Raphael Y: Future approaches for inner ear protection and repair, *J Commun Disord* 43(4):295–310, 2010.
9. Centers for Disease Control and Prevention: *Noise and hearing loss prevention*. Available at www.cdc.gov/niosh/topics/noise/stats.html.
10. The Mayo Clinic: *Hearing loss: risk factors*. Available at www.mayoclinic.com/health/hearing-loss/DS00172/DSECTION=risk-factors.
11. Bared A, Ouyang X, Angeli S, et al: Antioxidant enzymes, presbycusis and ethnic variability, *Otolaryngol Head Neck Surg* 143(2):263–268, 2010.
12. Gopinath B, Flood VM, Rochtchina E, et al: Consumption of omega-3 fatty acids and fish and risk of age-related hearing loss, *Am J Clin Nutr* 92:416–421, 2010.
13. Vassiliou A, Vlastarakos PV, Maragoudakis P, et al: Meniere's disease: still a mystery disease with difficult differential diagnosis, *Ann Indian Acad Neurol* 14(1):12–18, 2011.
14. Agency for Healthcare Research and Quality: *Medical Expenditure Panel Survey, Statistical brief #228*. Available at www.meps.ahrq.gov/mepsweb/data_files/publications/st228/stat228.shtml.
15. Ramakrishnan K, Sparks RA, Berryhill WE: Diagnosis and treatment of otitis media, *Am Fam Physician* 76(11):1650–1658, 2007.
16. Siegel RM: Acute otitis media guidelines, antibiotic use and shared medical decision-making, *Pediatrics* 125:384–385, 2010.
17. Hoberman A, Paradise JL, Rockette HE, et al: Treatment of acute otitis media in children under 2 years of age, *N Engl J Med* 364(2):105–115, 2011.
18. Engle EC: Genetic basis of congenital strabismus, *Arch Ophthalmol* 125(2):189–195, 2007.
19. Kanonidou E, Proudlock FA, Gottlob I: Reading strategies in mild to moderate strabismic amblyopia: an eye movement investigation, *Invest Ophthalmol Vis Sci* 51(7):3502–3508, 2010.
20. American Academy of Ophthalmology: *Amblyopia: lazy eye treatment*. Available at www.geteyesmart.org/eyesmart/diseases/amblyopia-treatment.cfm.
21. Beebe DC, Holekamp NM, Shui YB: Oxidative damage and the prevention of age-related cataracts, *Ophthalmic Res* 44:155–165, 2010.
22. Riordan-Eva P: Disorders of the eyes & lids. In McPhee SJ, Papadakis MA, Rabow MW, editors: *Current medical diagnosis and treatment 2012*, New York, 2011, McGraw-Hill. Available at www.accessmedicine.com/content.aspx?aID=2002. Accessed 11/11/11.
23. PubMed Health, a service of the National Library of Medicine, National Institutes of Health: *Retinal detachment*. Available at www.ncbi.nlm.nih.gov/pubmedhealth/PMH0002022/?report=printable.
24. Barber AJ, Gardner TW, Abcouwer SF: The significance of vascular and neural apoptosis to the pathology of diabetic retinopathy, *Invest Ophthalmol Visu Sci* 52(2):1156–1163, 2011.
25. Simo R, Hernandez C: Advances in the medical treatment of diabetic retinopathy, *Diabetes Care* 32(8):1556–1562, 2009.
26. Chakravarthy U, Wong TY, Fletcher A: Clinical risk factors for age-related macular degeneration: a systematic review and meta-analysis, *BMC Ophthalmol* 10: 31, 2010.
27. Wang Y, Wang VM, Chan CC: The role of anti-inflammatory agents in age related macular degeneration (AMD) treatment, *Eye (London)* 25(2):127–139, 2011.
28. Mares JA, Voland R, Sondel SA, et al: Healthy lifestyles related to subsequent prevalence of age-related macular degeneration, *Arch Ophthalmol* 129(4):470–480, 2011.
29. Fan BJ, Wiggs JL: Glaucoma: genes, phenotypes and new directions for therapy, *J Clin Invest* 120(9):3064–3072, 2010.
30. Hall JE: *Guyton and Hall textbook of medical physiology*, ed 12, Philadelphia, 2011, Saunders.

Pain

Joni D. Marsh

evolve WEBSITE

http://evolve.elsevier.com/Copstead/

- Review Questions and Answers
- Glossary (with audio pronunciations for selected terms)
- Animations

- Case Studies
- Key Points Review

KEY QUESTIONS

- How do the processes of transduction, transmission, perception, and modulation relate to the phenomenon of nociception?
- How is neurotransmission of pain signals modulated at the receptor, spinal cord, and brain?

- How do acute pain and chronic pain differ with regard to cause and clinical manifestations?
- Why are some painful sensations perceived at a distance from the site of injury (referred)?
- Why is it important to adequately manage pain?

CHAPTER OUTLINE

Pain is a complex physiologic and perceptual phenomenon. Because pain is very much a subjective experience, defining and assessing it are difficult. Merskey defined pain as "an unpleasant sensory and emotional experience associated with actual or potential tissue damage or described in terms of such damage."[1] McCaffery offered a clinically useful definition: "Pain is whatever the experiencing person says it is,

existing whenever the experiencing person says it does."[2] Accurate assessment and optimal management of pain are extremely important not only because relief of pain and suffering is ethically desirable but also because unrelieved pain is physiologically harmful. Studies have documented the benefits of adequate pain control on the rate of recovery, health care costs, and postoperative morbidity. In fact, The

Joint Commission (TJC) has developed standards of care regarding the assessment and management of pain that must be followed by all accredited agencies. Pain has been referred to as the fifth vital sign.

PHYSIOLOGY OF PAIN

The physiologic mechanisms involved in the pain phenomenon are termed **nociception**. Nociception can be divided into four stages: transduction, transmission, perception, and modulation. Transduction is the process of converting painful stimuli to neuronal action potentials at the sensory receptor. Transmission refers to the movement of action potentials along neurons that make their way from the peripheral receptor to the spinal cord and then centrally to the brain. Perception occurs when the brain receives pain signals and interprets them as painful. The complex mechanism whereby synaptic transmission of pain signals is altered is called modulation. It is clinically useful to conceptualize pain physiology according to these four processes because each stage provides an opportunity for intervention in the pain experience (Figure 47-1).

Transduction

Most pain begins in the periphery when free nerve endings called **nociceptors** are stimulated. Nociceptors transduce noxious stimuli into neuronal action potentials that progress centrally to the spinal cord and then the brain. Nociceptors are found in skin; muscle; connective tissue; the circulatory system; and the abdominal, pelvic, and thoracic viscera. Stimulation can be the result of direct damage to nerve endings, or it can result from release of chemicals at the site of injury.

Numerous substances participate in the initiation of nociceptive impulses. Some of these substances are released as a direct result of

tissue injury, whereas others may be produced as part of the inflammatory response to the injury. Important chemical mediators of pain include K^+, H^+, lactate, histamine, serotonin, bradykinins, and prostaglandins.[3] These chemicals alter the membrane potential of the pain receptor, and if depolarization is sufficient, action potentials are generated. When these impulses are conducted centrally, the second step (transmission) is initiated.

Prostaglandin involvement in the process of nociceptor stimulation is of particular interest because prostaglandin inhibitors such as aspirin and other nonsteroidal antiinflammatory drugs (NSAIDs) are commonly used to manage pain. Prostaglandins are formed when cells are damaged and an enzyme, phospholipase A, breaks down phospholipids in the cell membrane and converts them to arachidonic acid[4] (Figure 47-2). Arachidonic acid undergoes further breakdown by the enzyme cyclooxygenase to form prostaglandins. Sensitization by prostaglandins lowers the threshold of nociceptive fibers so that stimuli that would not cause pain under normal circumstances are now pain producing. NSAIDs prevent prostaglandin production by inhibiting the action of cyclooxygenase.

Transmission

Stimulated nociceptors transmit impulses to the central nervous system (CNS) by means of specialized sensory fibers. The primary sensory fibers involved in the transmission of nociceptive impulses are the Aδ and C fibers.[3] The characteristics and functions of these fibers are summarized in Table 47-1. In general, the larger, myelinated Aδ fibers transmit the nociceptive impulses very quickly as an initial response to tissue injury. The nature of the pain carried by the fast-traveling Aδ fibers is characterized as sharp, stinging, and highly

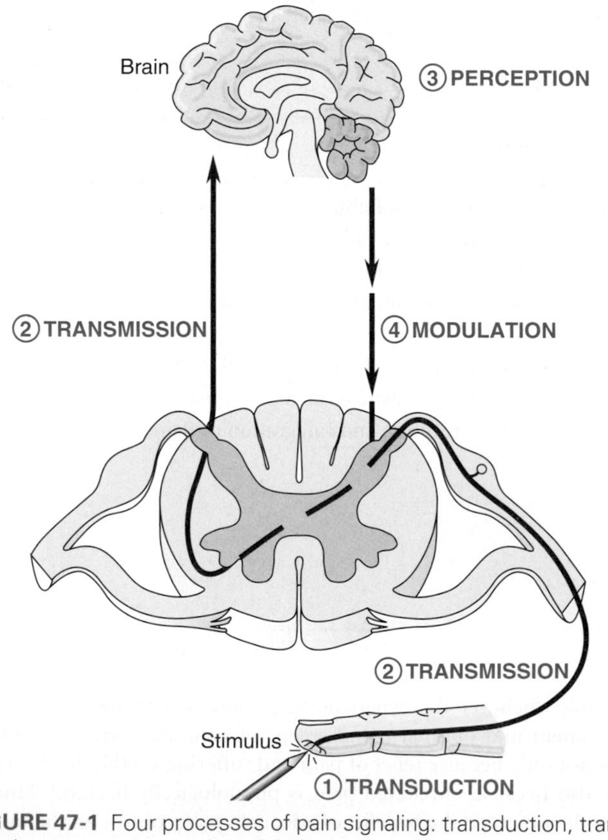

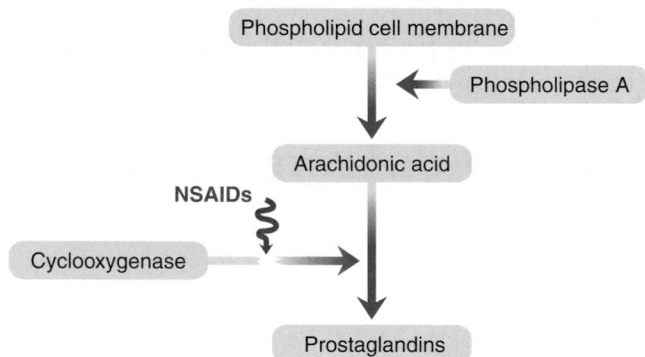

FIGURE 47-2 Tissue injury results in the release of prostaglandins from the breakdown of phospholipids in cell membranes. Nonsteroidal antiinflammatory drugs *(NSAIDs)* inhibit the cyclooxygenase enzyme and block the production of prostaglandins.

FIGURE 47-1 Four processes of pain signaling: transduction, transmission, perception, and modulation.

TABLE 47-1	AFFERENT SENSORY PAIN FIBERS	
FEATURE	**Aδ FIBERS**	**C FIBERS**
Structure	Myelinated	Unmyelinated
Amount	10%	90%
Source	Thermal, mechanical stimuli	Polymodal stimuli (mechanical, thermal, chemical)
Speed	Fast traveling, 5-10 m/sec	Slower traveling, 0.6-2 m/sec
Sensory quality of pain mediated	Sharp, stinging, cutting, pinching	Dull, burning, aching

localized. In contrast, unmyelinated C fibers transmit pain more slowly. Pain transmitted by C fibers is poorly localized and has a dull or aching quality that lingers long after the initial sharp pain abates. The majority of pain sensations travel via C fibers and project to areas of the brain that evoke emotional responses such as displeasure and anxiety.

Most sensory afferent pain fibers enter the spinal cord by way of the posterior nerve roots (Figure 47-3). The cell bodies of pain neurons are located in the dorsal root ganglion. As the afferent neurons enter the dorsal horn, collateral branches spread up and down the spinal cord for two to three segments by way of the tract of Lissauer. These spinal connections are important for reflex postural adjustments when a painful body part is suddenly withdrawn from the painful stimulus.

Sensory afferent neurons synapse with interneurons, anterior motor neurons, and sympathetic preganglionic neurons in specific regions of the spinal cord (see Figure 47-3). Aδ fibers and C fibers carry excitatory impulses from cutaneous pain receptors in small, localized areas of the skin to interneurons in lamina I. Many of the neurons originating in lamina I cross the spinal cord to activate neurons in the anterolateral tract.

Laminae II and III represent a key anatomic region of the cord involved in pain transmission known as the **substantia gelatinosa**. The substantia gelatinosa is characterized by multiple synaptic connections among primary sensory afferent neurons, interneurons, and anterolateral ascending fibers. There is much opportunity at this point for pain signal transmission to be modulated by other sensory input or from CNS activity. Pain signals can be either enhanced or blocked at these synapses.

Another key synaptic area involved in nociception is lamina V. Numerous Aδ and C fibers deliver somatic input from mechanical, thermal, and chemical receptors in the periphery to lamina V. Sensory afferent neurons from visceral receptors also terminate in lamina V. The convergence of both somatic and visceral fibers in lamina V may help explain the phenomenon of referred pain, in which pain from a visceral organ is perceived at the body surface.[3,5] The remaining, deeper laminae VI to VIII receive sensory input from muscles, joints, and visceral afferent fibers.

A number of neurotransmitters and neuropeptides are involved in synaptic transmission in the spinal cord. Substance P is a well-known example. Others include excitatory amino acids (glutamate), γ-aminobutyric acid (GABA), cholecystokinin, and calcitonin gene–related peptide. These neurotransmitters bind to the next neurons in the pathway and thereby initiate action potentials. The pain signal is propelled along its pathway toward the brain. Interruption of these synaptic processes can inhibit pain transmission. The synapses in the spinal cord are extremely important points of pain modulation by both endogenous and exogenous means.

The excitatory neurotransmitter glutamate is involved in carrying the nociceptive message from primary afferent fibers to secondary neurons. Glutamate binding to its N-methyl-D-aspartate (NMDA) receptors on the postsynaptic neuron is thought to induce a kind of synaptic memory in the pain pathway. Excessive or repeated stimulation of C fibers sensitizes the spinal cord neurons so that even mild stimulation may be perceived as painful.[5,6] This phenomenon has been termed "wind-up" and may be an important mechanism in the development of chronic pain syndromes. Drugs that inhibit glutamate production may impede the wind-up response, thereby controlling pain before synaptic memory of the pain develops in the pain pathways.

Pain signals transmitted by the spinal interneurons are then conducted to the brain by ascending spinal pathways (Figure 47-4). The major pathway for pain signal transmission up the spinal cord is the anterolateral tract, so named because it travels in the anterolateral portion of the white matter of the spinal column. This tract is also called the *spinothalamic tract* in some texts and has two divisions: the neospinothalamic tract and the paleospinothalamic tract. Both divisions cross at the spinal segment and carry pain signals up the contralateral (opposite) side of the cord. Thus nociceptor input from the right side of the body travels in the anterolateral tracts on the left side of the cord, whereas pain signals from the left side of the body travel on the right side of the cord.

The neospinothalamic division has fewer synapses in the cord and projects first to the thalamus and then to the primary somatosensory cortex. Aδ fiber signals are transmitted in this tract and reach the brain quickly to provide specific information about pain location with little emotional connotation. C fiber impulses travel mainly in the paleospinothalamic division, which makes a greater number of synapses and reaches the brain more slowly. The paleospinothalamic tract projects to widespread brain areas and stirs aversive emotional responses. The

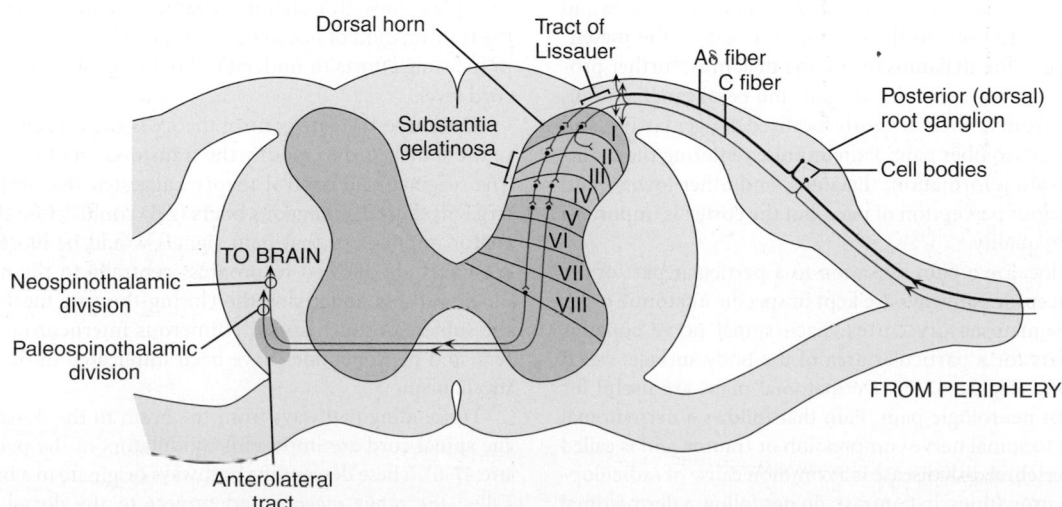

FIGURE 47-3 Spinal cord segment showing primary afferent pain fibers, Aδ and C fibers, entering the dorsal horn, synapsing on interneurons, crossing to the opposite side, and traveling to the brain in the anterolateral tract.

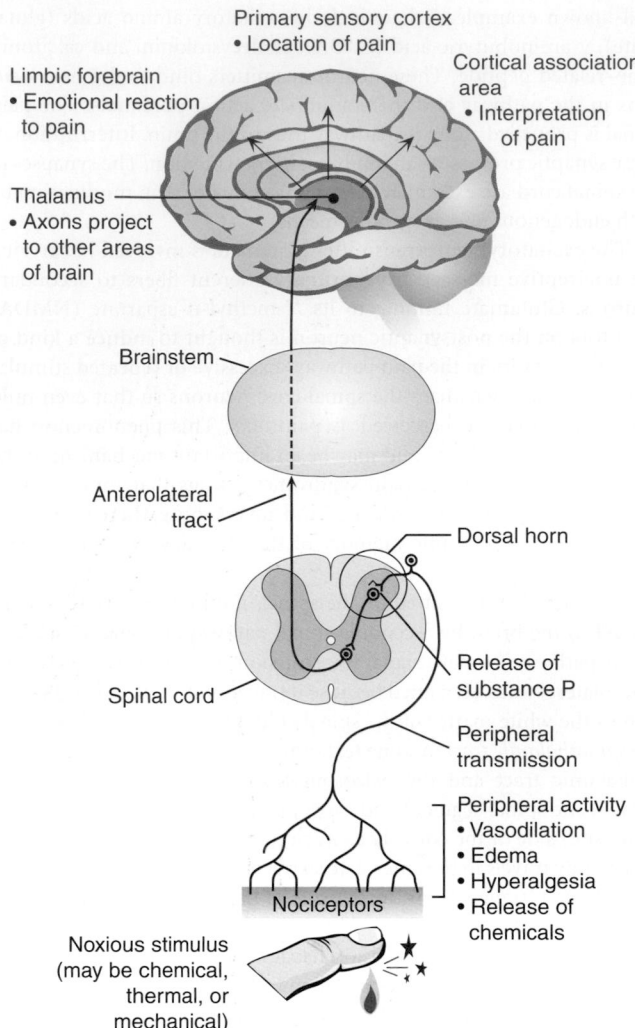

Primary sensory cortex
• Location of pain

Limbic forebrain
• Emotional reaction to pain

Cortical association area
• Interpretation of pain

Thalamus
• Axons project to other areas of brain

Brainstem

Anterolateral tract

Dorsal horn

Spinal cord

Release of substance P

Peripheral transmission

Peripheral activity
• Vasodilation
• Edema
• Hyperalgesia
• Release of chemicals

Nociceptors

Noxious stimulus (may be chemical, thermal, or mechanical)

FIGURE 47-4 Anterolateral nociceptive pathways travel up the spinal cord and project to the thalamus, somatosensory cortex, cortical association areas, and limbic structures.

paleospinothalamic tract travels with the neospinothalamic tract in the anterolateral portion of the spinal cord to the level of the medulla and then sends diffuse projections to the reticular formation, the mesencephalon, and, finally, the thalamus. From the thalamus, further projections to the cerebral cortex, limbic system, and basal ganglia occur. The pain sensation from C fibers is poorly localized, longer lasting, and more distressing than Aδ fiber pain. Pain impulses entering the brainstem reticular activating formation, thalamus, and other lower brain centers cause conscious perception of pain, but the cortex is important in interpreting pain quality.[3]

The brain can localize a pain sensation to a particular part of the body because nociceptor pathways are kept in specific anatomic order in the cord and somatosensory cortex. Each spinal nerve contains the nociceptor fibers for a particular area of the body surface, called a *sensory dermatome* (Figure 47-5). Dermatomal maps are useful for locating a source of neurologic pain. Pain that follows a dermatomal distribution is due to spinal nerve compression or trauma and is called a *radiculopathy*. Vertebral disk disease is a common cause of radiculopathy. Peripheral neuropathies, in contrast, do not follow a dermatomal pattern. Examples of peripheral neuropathies are carpal tunnel syndrome (median nerve) and diabetic neuropathy, which often affects both legs in a stocking-like pattern.

Perception

Perception is the result of neural processing of pain sensations in the brain. Perception includes an awareness and interpretation of the meaning of the sensation. Pain perception is influenced by attention, distraction, anxiety, fear, fatigue, and previous experience and expectations. Pain perception is not localized to a specific brain area.[3] Complete removal of the somatic sensory areas of the cerebral cortex does not destroy an animal's ability to perceive pain.[3] Numerous neuronal networks are necessary to localize, process, and interpret painful sensations. The primary somatosensory cortex, association cortex, frontal lobe, and limbic structures all participate in this processing.

Pain perception can be described in terms of pain threshold and pain tolerance. Pain threshold is the level of painful stimulation required to be perceived and is remarkably similar from one individual to another. Pain tolerance is the degree of pain that one is willing to bear before seeking relief. Pain tolerance varies widely among individuals and within the same individual under differing conditions. Age, culture, family upbringing, gender, and previous pain experience influence tolerance to pain. Environmental factors, including noise, bright light, and interrupted sleep, may affect pain tolerance.

Pain expression is the way in which the pain experience is communicated to others. Pacing, writhing, jaw clenching, facial grimacing, muscle guarding, crying, moaning, groaning, and verbal descriptions may be used to express pain. Thus the highly variable nature of pain expression among individuals makes accurate pain assessment difficult.

Modulation

Modulation of pain signals occurs at multiple sites along the pain pathway. A fair amount is known about pain modulation at the spinal cord, where neurons from nociceptors, somatosensory receptors, and descending neurons from the CNS all converge and interact. Modulation also occurs at the peripheral nociceptor ending and within the brain; however, these mechanisms are less well understood.

Attempts to decrease the perception of painful stimuli may be initiated spontaneously by the person experiencing pain. Rubbing, pressing, or shaking the painful area may reduce the intensity of pain. In 1965, Melzack and Wall proposed the gate control theory to explain how stimulation of large "touch" neurons could inhibit the transmission of nociceptor impulses.[7] This theory was very useful in focusing efforts to understand pain signal processing at the spinal cord level.

Central to the gate control theory is the capacity for interneurons in the spinal cord to modify the transmission of nociceptor impulses. The original gate control theory suggested that impulses carried by large myelinated cutaneous fibers (Aβ) could "close the gate" on nociceptor impulses so that pain signals would be blocked in the spinal cord and not allowed to progress centrally to the brain. The physiologic process underlying the closing-the-gate mechanisms has been the subject of much study. Numerous interneurons, neurotransmitters, and neuropeptides have been implicated in this complex gating mechanism.

Descending pathways from the brain to the dorsal horn region of the spinal cord are important modulators of the pain response (Figure 47-6). These descending pathways originate in a brainstem nucleus called the *raphe magnus* and project to the dorsal horn regions of laminae I, II, and IV.[3] Neurotransmitters released by these neurons can inhibit synaptic transmission of pain signals. One way to inhibit synaptic transmission is through presynaptic inhibition of substance

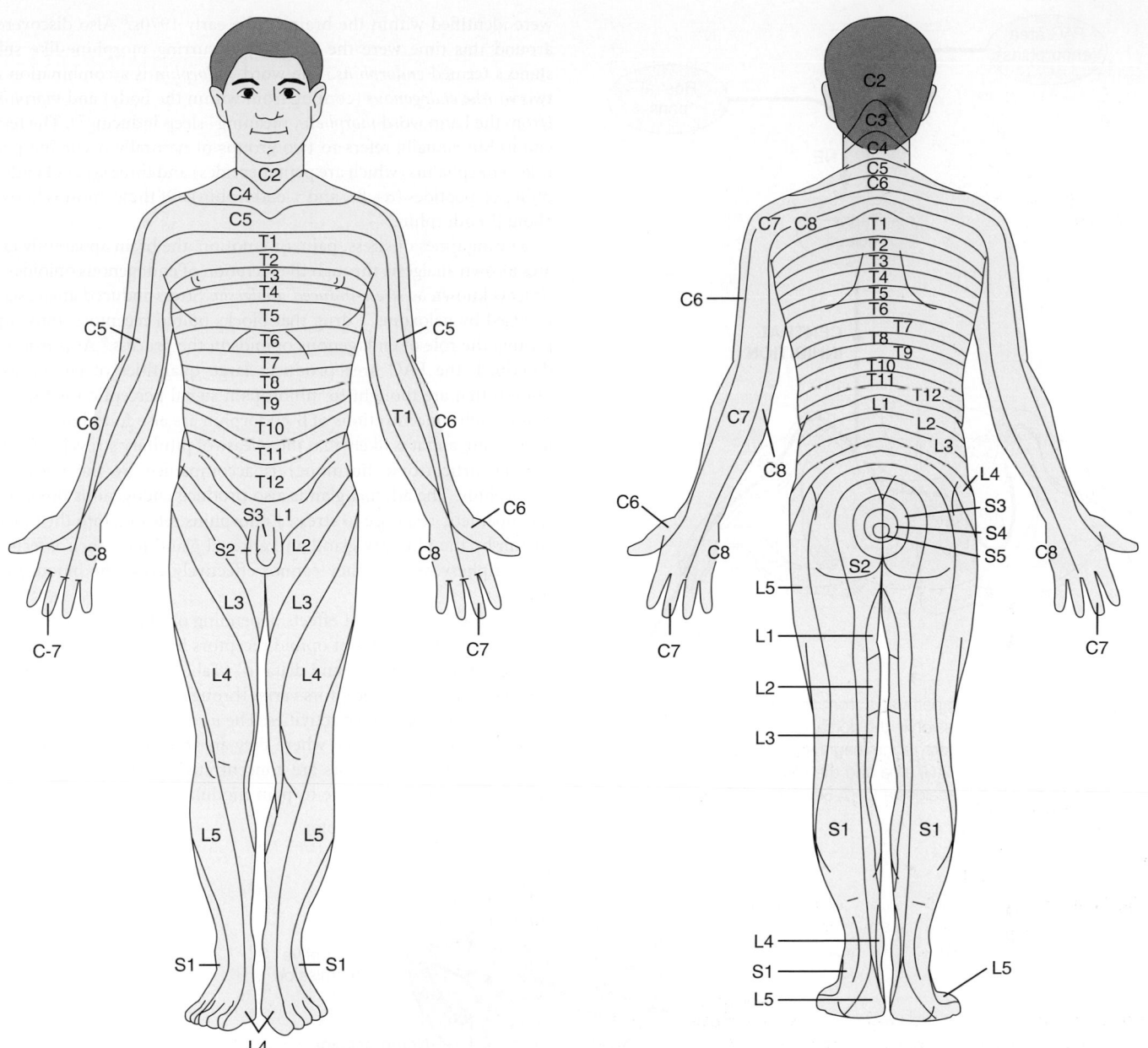

FIGURE 47-5 Sensory dermatomes. Pain located in the pattern of a dermatome occurs with spinal nerve injury and is referred to as *radiculopathy*.

P release from nociceptor neurons (Figure 47-7). **Opioids** such as **endorphins** are thought to be the mediators of presynaptic inhibition. A similar inhibitory effect can be achieved by administering opioid drugs, such as morphine, that bind to opioid receptors and mimic the effect of endorphins.

The raphe magnus receives input from two other brain areas important in the pain response: the periaqueductal gray (PAG) area in the midbrain and the rostral pons in the brainstem. The PAG area has a high concentration of endogenous opioids (endorphins and enkephalins) that are known to produce analgesic effects similar to narcotic drugs. Stimulation of the PAG area causes release of these endogenous opioids and also sends nerve impulses to the raphe magnus. Serotonin (5-hydroxytryptamine, 5HT) is the neurotransmitter that conveys analgesic signals from the PAG area to the raphe magnus. This finding helps explain the pain-relieving action of

drugs that enhance serotonin activity in the brain, such as tricyclic antidepressants.

The neurons projecting to the raphe magnus from the rostral pons secrete norepinephrine as the neurotransmitter. Stimulation of these neurons also produces an analgesic effect. Clonidine, a drug that mimics the effect of norepinephrine in the brain, has been shown to have pain-relieving properties.

The descending pathways from the brain provide an important means for gating the flow of pain impulses from the periphery to the brain. The PAG area is apprised of the flow of pain signals because it receives input by way of the thalamus and limbic structures.

Pain modulation occurs not only at the cord level but also in the brain itself. Opioids produced in the brain are thought to be important modulators of pain perception. Specific opioid receptors

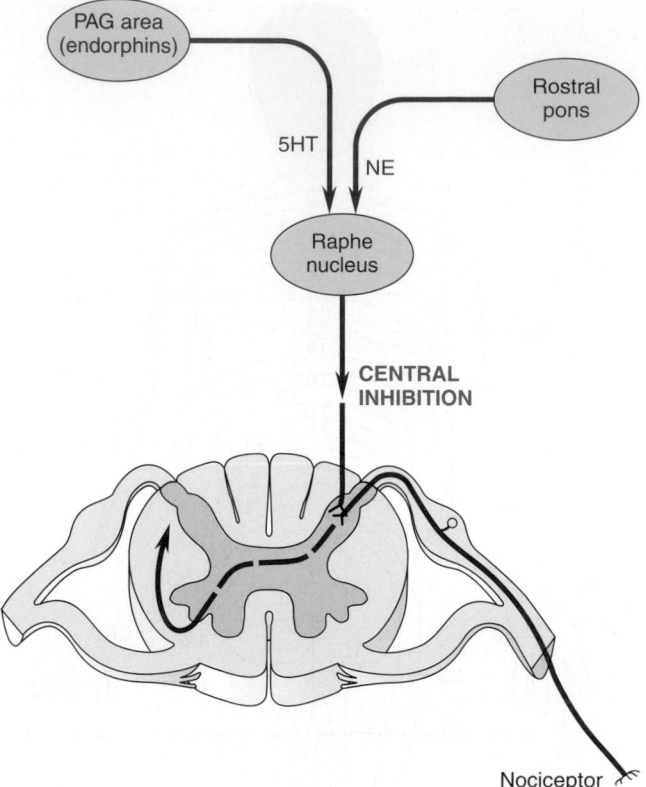

FIGURE 47-6 Descending pathways from the brain are thought to regulate pain impulse transmission in the dorsal horn. These regulatory neurons originate in the brainstem raphe magnus, which receives input from the periaqueductal gray *(PAG)* area and the rostral pons. Stimulation of these brain areas induces analgesia. *5HT,* Serotonin; *NE,* norepinephrine.

were identified within the brain in the early 1970s.[8] Also discovered around this time were the naturally occurring morphine-like substances termed *endorphins*. The word *endorphin* is a combination of two words: *endogenous* (coming from within the body) and *morphine* (from the Latin word *morpheus*, meaning "sleep inducing"). The term endorphin actually refers to two groups of naturally occurring peptides: enkephalins (which are pentapeptides) and three types of endorphin polypeptides (α-, β-, and γ-endorphin). Of these, most is known about β-endorphin.

During times of stress, pain, or emotion, the brain apparently creates its own analgesia through the secretion of endogenous opioids—a process known as *stress-induced analgesia.* Stress-induced analgesia is reversed by naloxone, a drug that blocks opioid receptors, thus supporting the role of endogenous opioids in the process.[9] As previously described, the PAG area produces large quantities of endogenous opioids that are thought to inhibit pain signal perception within the brain. High concentrations of β-endorphin are also found in the pituitary gland, and it is likely that the release of pituitary stress hormones (adrenocorticotropic hormone) is accompanied by the release of endorphins. The adrenal glands also produce endogenous opioids as a sympathetic response to stress. Endorphins released into the bloodstream by the pituitary gland and adrenal gland have their effects in the periphery because they cannot effectively cross the blood-brain barrier.

Opioids have different effects depending on the types of receptors they activate. Four types of opioid receptors have been identified: mu (μ), kappa (κ), sigma (σ), and delta (δ) (Table 47-2). The distribution of the specific opioid receptors varies throughout the body. The μ and κ receptors have analgesic activities. The μ receptors are found in high concentration in the brain, where they are thought to modulate pain perception. The κ receptors are concentrated primarily in the spinal cord, where they contribute to pain modulation by CNS descending

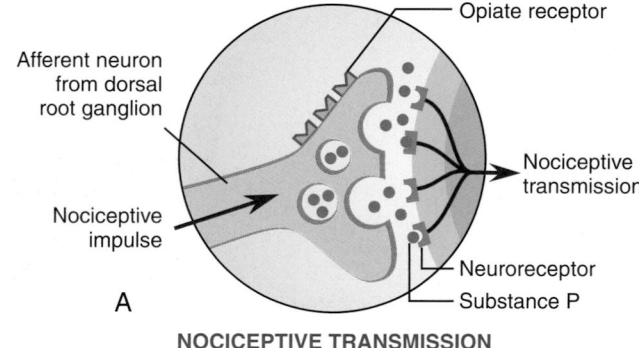

A

NOCICEPTIVE TRANSMISSION

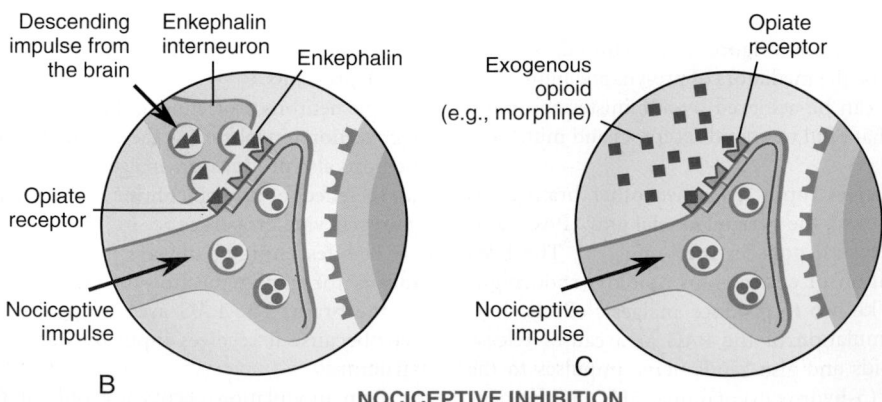

B   C

NOCICEPTIVE INHIBITION

FIGURE 47-7 Pain transmission and inhibition at the molecular level. **A,** Nociceptive transmission to higher levels of the central nervous system. **B,** Nociception inhibited through binding of endogenous opioids (e.g., enkephalin). The release of substance P is prevented. **C,** Nociception inhibited through binding of exogenous opioid (e.g., morphine). Release of substance P is prevented.

pathways. Each opioid receptor subtype is associated with a number of undesirable side effects. Depending on the affinity for certain receptors, different drugs may have differing analgesic potency and side effect profiles (Table 47-3).

TABLE 47-2 OPIOID RECEPTOR ACTIVITY

OPIOID RECEPTOR	ACTIVITY
Mu (μ)	Analgesia
	Sedation
	Respiratory depression
	Pupil constriction
	Nausea and vomiting
	Constipation
	Urine retention
	Pruritus
Kappa (κ)	Analgesia
	Sedation
	Respiratory depression
	Pupil constriction
	Diuresis
Sigma (σ)	No analgesia
	Vasomotor stimulation
	Tachypnea
	Pupil dilation
	Psychotomimetic effects (hallucinations, paranoia, delirium)
Delta (δ)	No analgesia
	Respiratory depression
	Nausea and vomiting
	Pruritus

KEY POINTS

- Nociception can be conceptualized as four interdependent processes: stimulus transduction, signal transmission, pain perception, and pain modulation.
- Nociceptor activity is transmitted to the spinal cord by two types of neurons: larger, myelinated Aδ fibers, which transmit sharp, localized sensations; and small, unmyelinated C fibers, which transmit dull, aching, poorly localized sensations.
- Pain signals are transmitted by afferent fibers that enter the spinal cord through the dorsal horn, synapse on interneurons, and then cross the cord and project centrally in the anterolateral tract.
- The anterolateral tract has two divisions: the neospinothalamic tract, which carries Aδ fiber input and projects to the thalamus and then the sensory cortex; and the paleospinothalamic tract, which carries C fiber input and projects diffusely to the reticular formation, mesencephalon, and thalamus.
- Perception of painful stimuli involves several brain structures, including the primary somatosensory cortex, association areas, and limbic structures. Pain perception is influenced by culture, environment, and physical status and varies widely among individuals.
- Afferent pain signals can be modulated at several levels. Descending pathways project from the PAG area and rostral pons by way of the raphe magnus to inhibit pain neurons in the dorsal aspect of the spinal cord. Pain is also modulated within the brain/spinal cord by endogenous opioids (enkephalins, endorphins).

TYPES OF PAIN

Pain can be categorized into two major subtypes: physiologic pain and pathologic pain. Physiologic pain occurs when tissue injury has occurred, and aides in prevention of further injury or in some cases survival. This is the pain felt when a person, for example, has touched a hot stove. This injury will likely heal, and the memory of the experience will hopefully prevent future similar injuries. Pain of acute appendicitis

TABLE 47-3 RECEPTOR AFFINITY OF COMMONLY USED OPIOIDS

DRUG	RECEPTOR AFFINITY	AGONIST		ANTAGONIST	
		PURE	PARTIAL	PURE	PARTIAL
Morphine, meperidine, hydromorphone, methadone, fentanyl	Mu (μ)	X			
	Kappa (κ) *(morphine only)*	X			
	Delta (δ)	X			
Buprenorphine	Mu (μ)		X		
	Kappa (κ)			X	
Butorphanol	Mu (μ)		X		
	Kappa (κ)	X			
Nalbuphine	Mu (μ)				X
	Kappa (κ)	X			
Pentazocine	Mu (μ)				X
	Kappa (κ)	X			
Naloxone	Mu (μ)			X	
	Kappa (κ)			X	
	Delta (δ)				X
Naltrexone	Mu (μ)			X	
	Kappa (κ)			X	

also may be considered physiologic pain because it alerts a person to a serious problem. In contrast, pathologic pain occurs after tissue injury, but long-term changes occur both within the peripheral and within the central nervous systems. These changes occur along somatosensory pathways from the periphery to the cortex. The pain sensation can be significantly enhanced (**hyperalgesia**), or non-noxious stimuli may cause pain (**allodynia**). These changes in pain perception and modulation serve no beneficial purpose to learning or survival. These underlying changes are theorized to be the cause of neuropathic pain, fibromyalgia, and other chronic pain syndromes.[6,10]

Pain most commonly is classified according to duration (acute, chronic), source (cancer, neuropathic, ischemic), or location and referral pattern. Pain is a symptom of an underlying problem rather than a primary disorder; attempts to alleviate pain should be accompanied by efforts to locate and manage the underlying etiology. The character, location, and duration of pain can provide helpful clues to aid the diagnostic process.

ACUTE PAIN

Pain is categorized as being acute or chronic, depending on the duration of symptoms. Acute pain results from tissue injury and resolves when the injury heals, usually in less than 3 months. Acute pain is typically accompanied by clinical signs and symptoms of pain that result from stimulation of the sympathetic nervous system. These signs and symptoms include an elevated heart rate, respiratory rate, and blood pressure, as well as pallor, sweating, and nausea (Table 47-4). Persons experiencing acute pain may express pain behavior such as pacing, grimacing, crying, or moaning. Short-term therapy with nonopioid and opioid agents is often helpful. The risk of becoming dependent on pain medications is minimal in persons experiencing acute pain. Adequate management of pain during an acute episode may help prevent the development of some types of chronic pain syndromes.

Headache

Etiology and pathogenesis. Headache is one of the most common causes of acute pain, accounting for approximately 13 million visits each year in the Unites States to physician's offices, urgent care clinics, and emergency departments.[11] Headaches are classified according to etiologic categories (e.g., tension, migraine, sinus). However, it is very common for headache type to be misdiagnosed, migraines frequently being labeled as tension or sinus headache. In the United States greater than 10% of the population, including children, suffer from migraines.[12] Previous theories of migraine included simply a vascular causation. It was believed that the spasm of cerebral vessels and the ensuing vasodilation caused the throbbing pain typical of migraine. Current theories involve stimulation of the trigeminal nerve in combination with changes in neurotransmitter levels in the CNS and alterations in blood vessel tone.

Migraines probably result from dysfunction of the brainstem areas involved with modulation of craniovascular afferent fibers. There is a release of inflammatory chemicals including local release of calcitonin gene–related peptide, which causes vasodilation. The inflammatory cascade that results in migraine can be initiated by many "migraine triggers." There is a genetic predisposition for sensitivity to these headache triggers. The brainstem becomes activated, causing stimulation of the trigeminal nucleus caudalis. This activation causes pain signals to be sent to the thalamus and cerebral cortex where pain is perceived and is responsible for many signs/symptoms of migraine. Any of the branches of the trigeminal nerve can refer pain signals along this pathway. If left untreated, continuous activation of the trigeminal nucleus caudalis may result in central sensitization and more refractory pain.

TABLE 47-4	PHYSIOLOGIC RESPONSES TO ACUTE PAIN
CRITERIA	**RESPONSE**
Signs and symptoms	↑ Heart rate
	↑ Blood pressure
	↑ Respiratory rate
	Dilated pupils
	Pallor and perspiration
	Nausea and vomiting
	Urine retention
Physiologic response	Blood shifts from superficial vessels to striated muscle, heart, lungs, and brain
	Bronchioles dilate to ↑ oxygenation
	↑ Gastric secretions
	↓ Gastrointestinal motility
	↑ Circulating blood glucose
	Hypomotility of bladder and ureters

Adapted from Merck Manual: *Pain*. Available at www.merckmanuals.com/professional/neurologic_disorders/pain/overview_of_pain.html; Mohn-Brown E, Burke KM, Eby L, editors: *Medical-surgical nursing care*, ed 3, Upper Saddle River, NJ, 2011, Pearson Education.

Clinical manifestations. Typical signs of a migraine headache include severe unilateral pounding or throbbing pain that may be accompanied by nausea, vomiting, photophobia, phonophobia, and lacrimation. The pain is increased by routine physical activity. Some migraines may be preceded by an aura such as flashing lights or other visual disturbances, and unilateral paresthesias. Other symptoms may include sinus/nasal congestion, neck muscle stiffness and pain, vertigo, and changes in bowel pattern.

Diagnosis and treatment. Headaches are diagnosed through careful history and physical examination. Brain tumors, infection, hydrocephalus, and increased intracranial pressure must be ruled out. Physical assessment should include the ears, nose and throat, sinuses, temporomandibular joint, neck musculature, cranial nerves, and retinal examination. General cognitive, neurologic, and motor function should also be examined. Headaches caused by trauma, following a worsening pattern, accompanied by other neurologic symptoms, or developing suddenly and described as the "worst headache ever" require neuroimaging. The International Headache Society has established criteria for a migraine diagnosis, and this has been adopted by many health care providers (Box 47-1).

Headaches are managed with a wide variety of therapies and medications, each aimed at a different piece of the pathophysiologic puzzle. Depending on the type and frequency of the headache, prophylactic medications may also be used. One mainstay of nonpharmacologic migraine therapy is the avoidance of headache triggers. Patients are encouraged to eliminate vasoactive substances from their diets including caffeine, cheese, chocolate, foods containing nitrates and nitrites, and monosodium glutamate. Adherence to regular sleep-wake schedules is helpful as is the use of stress management techniques in preventing the occurrence of migraines. Other nonpharmacologic therapies for headache include resting in a quiet, darkened room or applying cold packs to the head and back of the neck. There are numerous medications used to control migraines and other types of headaches. A key to successful treatment is the prompt use of these agents at the onset of pain. Prophylactic therapy employing administration of antiepileptics (topiramate), antidepressants (selective serotonin reuptake inhibitors, tricyclic antidepressants), β-blockers (propranolol), α-blockers

BOX 47-1 INTERNATIONAL HEADACHE SOCIETY DIAGNOSTIC CRITERIA FOR MIGRAINE

MIGRAINE WITHOUT AURA	MIGRAINE WITH AURA
Recurrent headache attacks lasting 4-72 hours and having at least two of the following: • Unilateral location • Pulsating quality • Moderate or severe intensity • Aggravation by routine physical activity At least one of the following characteristics is present: • Nausea and/or vomiting • Photophobia and phonophobia Can evolve to a very frequent (chronic) migraine condition with or without acute or analgesic medication overuse.	Recurrent disorder manifesting in attacks of reversible focal neurologic symptoms that usually develop gradually over 5-20 minutes and last for less than 60 minutes. Typical aura consists of visual and/or sensory and/or speech symptoms. Headache with the same features as migraine without aura usually follows the aura symptoms. Less commonly, headache lacks migrainous features or is completely absent.

Data from Headache Classification Subcommittee of the International Headache Society: The International Classification of Headache Disorders, ed 2, *Cephalgia* 24(supp 1):23-135, 2004.

(clonidine), or calcium channel blockers (verapamil); injections of botulinum toxin type A (Botox) into the scalp; or manipulation of hormone levels in younger female patients may be necessary. Refer to Table 47-5 for a comparison of pharmacologic therapies for the acute management of migraine headache.

CHRONIC PAIN

Pain is considered chronic when it lasts more than several months beyond the expected healing time (usually more than 6 months). When chronic pain is not due to a malignancy, its cause is often difficult to ascertain. In chronic pain, pain is no longer protective and appears to be self-perpetuating. Two concepts have emerged as probable mechanisms for this phenomenon. Peripheral sensitization represents a reduction in threshold and an amplification in the responsiveness of nociceptors that occur when the peripheral terminals of the primary sensory neurons are exposed to inflammatory mediators and damaged tissue. Increased peripheral transduction sensitivity develops.[10] Central sensitization results in changes in the properties of neurons in the CNS. It is an abnormal state of responsiveness or increased gain of the nociceptive inputs. When neurons in the dorsal horn of the spinal cord are affected by central sensitization, they develop increased spontaneous activity and a reduction in the threshold for activation by peripheral stimuli, show increased responsiveness to stimulation, and have an enlargement of receptor field.[6,10]

TABLE 47-5 ACUTE MIGRAINE THERAPIES

DRUG	ROUTE OF ADMINISTRATION	COMMENTS
Serotonin Receptor Agonists (Triptans)		
Sumatriptan (Imitrex) Zolmitriptan (Zomig) Rizatriptan (Maxalt) Naratriptan (Amerge) Eletriptan (Relpax)	PO, nasal spray, SubQ injection, dissolvable tablet	Increases serotonin; cannot be given with monoamine oxidase inhibitors; contraindicated in renal/hepatic failure; risk of serotonin syndrome if given with selective serotonin reuptake inhibitors
Ergot Alkaloids		
Ergotamine with caffeine (Wigraine, Ercaf, Cafergot)	IV, IM, SubQ, PO, rectal suppository, inhaler	Rarely used because of development of newer agents with less side effects; increases serotonin; causes intracerebral vasoconstriction; best if given early after onset; contraindicated in patients with cardiovascular disease and pregnancy; may cause nausea/vomiting
Dihydroergotamine mesylate (DHE, Migranal)		Rarely used now
Nonsteroidal Antiinflammatories and Nonopiates		
Acetaminophen (Tylenol) Ketorolac (Toradol) Naproxen sodium (Naprosyn, Aleve) Ibuprofen (Motrin, Advil) Aspirin	PO, IV, IM	May cause gastrointestinal upset/bleeding; frequent use may cause "rebound" headache
Barbiturate-Hypnotic Combinations		
Butalbital with aspirin and caffeine (Fioricet, Fioricet with codeine)	PO	High abuse/addictive potential; may cause sedation; rebound headache with frequent use; withdrawal potential
Opiates/Combinations		
Acetaminophen with codeine, oxycodone, or hydrocodone (Tylenol no. 3/4, Percocet, Lorcet) Butorphanol (Stadol)	PO Nasal spray	High abuse/addictive potential; may cause sedation; considered "rescue medications"

Adapted from Goadsby PJ, Raskin NH: Headache. In Ropper AH, Samuels MA, editors: *Adam's and Victor's principles of neurology*, ed 9, New York, 2009, McGraw-Hill. Available at www.accessmedicine.com.proxy.heal-wa.org/content.aspx?aID=9094791.
IM, Intramuscular; *IV*, intravenous; *PO*, oral; *SubQ*, subcutaneous.

Chronic pain is generally not associated with signs and symptoms of sympathetic activity. As the body becomes accustomed to pain, the sympathetic nervous system desensitizes itself to the noxious input; therefore, symptoms are more often psychological. Lack of sleep because of pain causes fatigue and irritability. Loss of a job or loss of body image because of pain causes personal and family difficulties. Treatment failures may create a sense of hopelessness or distrust of caregivers.

Depression is a common finding in individuals experiencing chronic pain. In many cases the cause of the chronic pain cannot be determined, and therefore treatment is difficult. The use of narcotic pain relievers is discouraged because of the necessity of long-term therapy and therefore a risk of dependency. Satisfactory treatment may require numerous coordinated approaches, and the patient may benefit from the services of a pain clinic that specializes in multimodal therapies.

Fibromyalgia Syndrome

Etiology and pathogenesis. Fibromyalgia syndrome (FMS) is a chronic pain syndrome affecting an estimated 2% of the population. Women are affected more frequently than men.[13] FMS is a collection of symptoms without a clear physiologic cause. It is neither degenerative nor progressive. Patients have a history of chronic widespread pain affecting all four extremities. FMS was once a controversial diagnosis classified as a psychosomatic illness. It can now be objectively identified using criteria established by the American College of Rheumatology.

The cause of FMS is unknown. However, etiologic studies have identified several risk factors for the development of the syndrome. Individuals with a medical history of excessive stress, trauma (both physical and emotional), sexual abuse, viral infections (parvovirus, hepatitis C, Epstein-Barr), and endocrine disorders (hypothyroidism) are more commonly affected. Disordered pain mechanisms in the CNS

are a suspected factor in FMS. Patients with FMS have a lower threshold for pain than those without the disorder. Pain maintenance and modulation mechanisms in the brain and spinal cord are also suspect. Central sensitization is thought to be a key factor.

Clinical manifestations. Patients complain of pain that waxes and wanes, and does not follow a dermatomal pattern. The pain tends to be exacerbated by physical exertion. Hyperalgesia and allodynia are common. Musculoskeletal examinations are generally normal. Other symptoms commonly seen associated with FMS include sleep disturbance/insomnia with nonrestorative sleep and irritable bowel syndrome. Fatigue is a hallmark of the syndrome. Depression and anxiety are also common along with cognitive difficulties such as problems with attention and short-term memory.

Diagnosis and treatment. FMS is a diagnosis of exclusion. Thyroid disorders, myopathies, rheumatoid arthritis, and chronic viral infections (e.g., human immunodeficiency virus) must be excluded. In FMS there is a lack of objective or laboratory findings. However, the American College of Rheumatology has established criteria to assist in the diagnosis of FMS. An individual must complain of widespread pain in all four extremities and the axial skeleton that has been present for at least 3 months without other reasonable explanation. The presence of pain in 11 of 18 "trigger" or "tender" points when pressure is applied to these areas (Figure 47-8) is also diagnostic.

Management of FMS begins with patient education. Although sometimes disabling, FMS is not a fatal illness and does not affect life span. Treatment includes a variety of medications including antidepressants, such as the selective serotonin reuptake inhibitors and the tricyclic antidepressants. Restoration of sleep patterns seems to be a key factor of successful treatment. NSAIDs and muscle-relaxing agents are also helpful. Opioid medications and corticosteroids are generally avoided because these are not effective long-term therapies.[14] There are three FDA-approved therapies for the pain of FMS. Pregabalin (Lyrica)

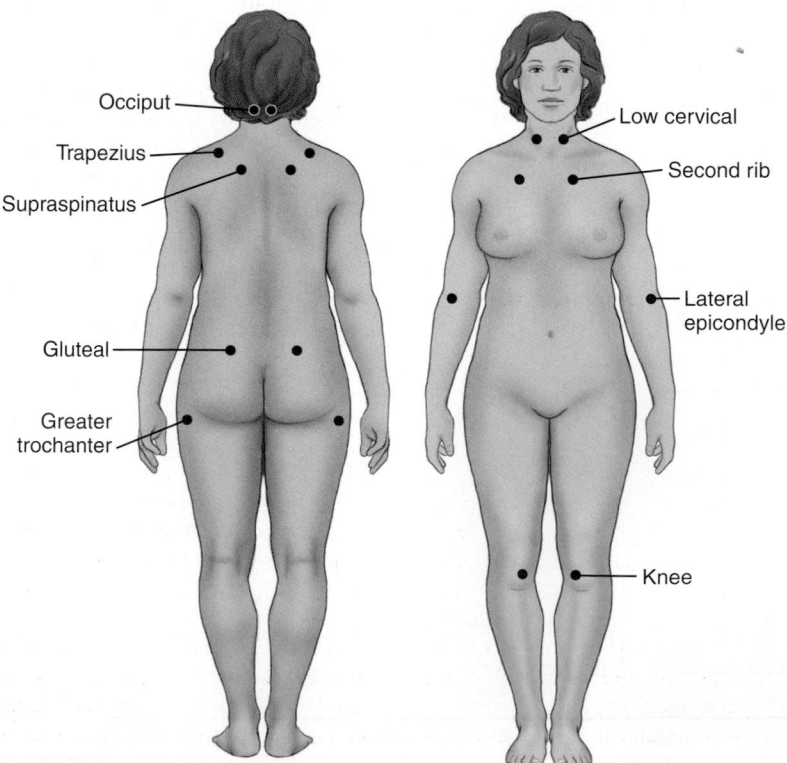

FIGURE 47-8 Posterior and anterior trigger points in fibromyalgia.

is an analogue of the neurotransmitter GABA (γ-aminobutyric acid). Milnacipran (Savella) and duloxetine (Cymbalta) are in the class of medications of serotonin-norepinephrine reuptake inhibitors.[15] Nonpharmacologic therapies include regular physical exercise, good nutrition, and psychological counseling.

CANCER-RELATED PAIN

Cancer pain is a subcategory of chronic pain, although it may be associated with acute pain episodes. Malignant pain differs from nonmalignant chronic pain in that it often has an identifiable cause. Pain associated with cancer may result from infiltration of organs or compression of structures by an expanding tumor, or it may occur as a result of treatments that damage tissue such as radiation therapy or chemotherapy. In patients with cancer pain, clinical signs and symptoms are often a mixture of sympathetic nervous system activation and behavioral changes. Unremitting cancer pain requires a multifaceted approach and use of potent medications. Often the quality of life is a larger consideration than the length of life, and adequate pain control is a major factor affecting the quality of life.

NEUROPATHIC PAIN

Neuropathic pain is a complex, often disabling chronic pain that results from tissue injury in which the nerves themselves become damaged or dysfunctional. This may occur in the peripheral or central nerves. The pain results from the actual damage or dysfunction of the nerves rather than stimulation of the pain receptors.[10] Nerve injury from surgery, tumor growth, metastasis, radiation therapy, chemotherapy, elevated blood glucose level, viral infection, or trauma often causes neuropathic pain. It is characterized by constant aching sensations that may be interrupted by bursts of burning or shocklike pain in the affected area. Allodynia is common. Neuropathic pain may not occur immediately after an injury. Days, weeks, or even months after the tissue-damaging source of pain has resolved, the onset of neuropathic pain can initiate a new and complex pain state. Pain often seems to be out of proportion to the area of tissue damage.

Neuropathic pain is thought to result from altered central processing of nociceptive input. Nerve injury may initiate excitotoxic and apoptotic cell death of neurons within the spinal cord dorsal horn. GABAergic interneurons are significantly depleted. GABA is an inhibitory neurotransmitter in the spinal cord, and a reduction in GABA-secreting neurons may be the cause of the hyperalgesia and allodynia. In some cases, excessive responsiveness to ongoing stimulation of afferent pain fibers appears to be important; however, central perception of pain may occur in the absence of any nociceptor input.[10] Examples of neuropathic pain include postherpetic neuralgia, diabetic neuropathy, trigeminal neuralgia, epidural spinal cord compression, cauda equina compression, plexus injuries, and phantom limb pain. Sympathetically maintained pain is a unique type of neuropathic pain that may occur in the absence of nerve injury. Sympathetically maintained pain is attributed to hyperactivity of the sympathetic nervous system. Release of norepinephrine from sympathetic nerve endings sensitizes nociceptors such that they respond to a lower level of nociceptor stimuli.[10] Not all patients affected by this type of pain exhibit the same symptoms; however, the most prevalent clinical manifestations are allodynia, hyperalgesia, atrophy of the affected extremity, coldness in the affected area, and dystrophic changes, most often manifested as hair loss and a shiny appearance of the skin. Neuropathic pain is difficult to manage. It is frequently unresponsive to opioid or other pharmacologic therapy.

Trigeminal Neuralgia

Etiology and pathogenesis. Trigeminal neuralgia is a form of neuropathic pain that can be quite disabling for patients. It appears as sudden, momentary, and excruciating pain along the second and third divisions of the trigeminal nerve. Trigeminal neuralgia is more common in women than in men, and occurs more frequently in middle-aged or older individuals.[16] If trigeminal neuralgia occurs at an earlier age, multiple sclerosis should be ruled out.[16] Other causes of trigeminal neuralgia include lesions or tumors of the brainstem. Chronic compression of the trigeminal nerve by a vessel is suspected in most cases. This causes demyelination of the trigeminal nerve and interruption and alteration in nerve signaling.

Clinical manifestations. The pain of trigeminal neuralgia is often described as sharp or shooting; some have compared it to the pain of an electrical shock. Patients may be pain free between episodes or complain of a dull ache in the affected area. Sometimes patients may only have a few episodes of pain followed by a long remission period. However, others may unfortunately experience an increase in frequency and duration of the pain. Anxiety is common, since patients worry about when their next attack may occur.

Diagnosis and treatment. Diagnosis of neuralgia is most frequently based on the clinical history. The results of neurologic evaluation are normal if there is no underlying lesion. Management of trigeminal neuralgia includes use of antiseizure medications such as carbamazepine (Tegretol), phenytoin (Dilantin), or gabapentin (Neurontin). Surgical nerve decompression has been used successfully for trigeminal neuralgia in patients who do not respond to or cannot tolerate the medications. Gamma-knife radiosurgery is the newest treatment for this condition.[16]

Diabetic Neuropathy

Etiology and pathogenesis. One of the most common complications of diabetes, diabetic neuropathy affects approximately 60% to 70% of all persons with diabetes.[17] Diabetic neuropathy is caused by damage to the peripheral nerves. The exact pathogenetic mechanism is unknown, but this damage is thought to be mediated by occult inflammation and demyelination of the larger peripheral nerves, leaving an excess of smaller myelinated fibers. This causes a loss of inhibitory input from the spinal cord with unopposed nociceptive afferent bombardment. Ischemic damage to nerves is also a contributing factor. Some also hypothesize that hyperglycemia and related biochemical changes in the nerve microenvironment cause nerve malfunction and injury. It is unclear why patients develop such varying levels of nerve dysfunction and pain. Strict blood glucose level control does not always prevent or improve the condition. More attention is now being focused on the role of peripheral and central sensitization.[18]

Clinical manifestations. Although pain is the most common feature, patients also complain of numbness and tingling, mild weakness, and loss of vibratory sense and proprioception. Fine touch and vibratory sensation are decreased. Patients complain of burning pain in the distal bilateral lower extremities, often with a symmetric distribution. Pain is frequently worse at night.

Diagnosis and treatment. Diabetic neuropathy is confirmed through careful physical examination. Diabetic patients are encouraged to maintain strict control of their blood glucose levels to prevent neuropathy. Management of this disorder includes the use of a wide variety of topical and systemic pain medications. Systemic therapeutic agents include tricyclic antidepressants, serotonin-norepinephrine reuptake inhibitors, and anticonvulsants.[18] Although opioids can help with pain relief of diabetic neuropathy, their use has been limited because of tolerance and dependence issues. Side effects of all of these medications can limit their usefulness, especially in elderly patients or those with other comorbid conditions. Many patients use a combination of topical and systemic therapies. An important nonpharmacologic treatment for diabetic neuropathy is the prevention of further complications. Diabetic patients are strongly encouraged to perform daily foot examinations, taking precautions against the development of foot sores and ingrown toenails. The combination of numbness and impaired circulation make diabetic patients at high risk for undetected injuries that do not heal and become easily infected. Amputation is a common outcome.[17]

Postherpetic Neuralgia

Etiology and pathogenesis. A common but disabling complication of the varicella virus is herpes zoster. Years after an individual has recovered from the chickenpox virus, herpes zoster (shingles) may occur. This is a reactivation of the latent virus that has lain dormant along the nerve roots.

Postherpetic neuropathy is persistent pain that lasts for more than 8 weeks after the onset of skin lesions. Approximately 10% to 15% of patients with herpes zoster develop postherpetic neuralgia.[19] Risk factors for the development of this neuralgia are advanced age and history of immune compromise.

Clinical manifestations. Herpes zoster is characterized by a burning pain that follows along a dermatomal pathway and is accompanied by a blistering rash. It occurs in individuals who have a history of varicella infection (chickenpox). Frequently the pain is present before the eruption of the blisters.

Diagnosis and treatment. The diagnosis is most often made clinically; however, cultures can be used to determine the presence of the virus. The early use (within 72 hours of eruption of rash) of antiviral medications such as acyclovir (Zovirax) can decrease the risk of developing postherpetic neuralgia.[19]

Management of the neuralgia includes both topical and systemic therapies. Transdermal lidocaine and capsaicin cream may be helpful in mild cases. Anticonvulsants and tricyclic antidepressants are also useful. NSAIDs and opioids may be mildly helpful as well.[19] There is also a vaccine that adults may receive that will prevent or lessen the severity of a varicella-zoster outbreak, and decrease the risk of postherpetic neuralgia.

ISCHEMIC PAIN

Pain resulting from a sudden or profound loss of blood flow to the tissues in a particular part of the body may result in ischemic pain. Decreased perfusion leads to tissue hypoxia and injury, with release of inflammatory and pain-producing chemicals. Ischemic pain is described as aching, burning, or prickling (paresthesia). The symptoms of ischemic pain depend on the origin of the ischemia. For example, pain of cardiac origin is visceral and radiates to the arm or jaw. This pain is perceived as being deep, aching, diffuse, and pressing. Ischemia resulting from acute deep venous occlusion is also aching and has a deep quality and gradual onset. Acute arterial occlusion may be felt as either burning or aching but has a sudden onset.

Chronic ischemic pain can occur in atherosclerotic syndromes. Arteriosclerosis obliterans occurs gradually as plaque develops in the intima of the arteries, most often arteries of the lower extremities. In the early stages, the pain, called *intermittent claudication,* is associated with physical activity, is alleviated with rest, and has a cramping quality. In severe cases, ischemic neuropathy may ensue and cause a more consistent burning, shooting pain in the leg or foot.

Management of ischemic pain is directed at improving blood flow and reducing tissue hypoxia. Acute ischemia is usually associated with a thrombus or embolus and can be managed with drugs to dissolve the clot or surgery to remove it. Chronic ischemia is most often associated with atherosclerosis and may be improved through lifestyle changes, including smoking cessation, weight loss, reduction of lipid levels, and

regular exercise. Surgical bypass procedures or placement of intravascular stents are other therapeutic modalities.

REFERRED PAIN

Referred pain is perceived in an area other than the site of the injury. It is often felt at some distance from the point of nociceptor activation. A familiar example is the pain of myocardial infarction that is felt in the jaw or left arm. Other examples of referred pain include shoulder pain after pelvic procedures, diaphragmatic irritation from peritonitis, and cutaneous abdominal pain experienced with visceral irritation or tension. Common patterns of referral are shown in Figure 47-9. Pain is generally referred to other structures in the same sensory dermatome. Convergence of nociceptors from internal organs with somatic afferents from the body surface occurs in the dorsal horn of the spinal cord.[3] The brain cannot differentiate the two sources of pain signals and tends to attribute the visceral pain to a body surface location. Patterns of referred pain are fairly uniform and can be used to help locate a source of visceral pathologic process.[3]

KEY POINTS

- Acute pain results from tissue injury and generally resolves when the injury resolves. The clinical manifestations result from activation of the sympathetic nervous system (elevated heart rate, blood pressure, and respiratory rate; dilated pupils; perspiration; and pallor).
- Headaches are a common but disabling cause of acute pain. Migraine headaches are caused by an interaction between neurotransmitters and cerebrovascular mechanisms and may be triggered by factors such as stress, foods, and sleep deprivation. There are a variety of treatments for headaches, but all must be initiated early in the course of the headache.
- Chronic pain lasts several months beyond the expected healing time and is often not associated with sympathetic manifestations of pain owing to physiologic adaptation. Instead, changes in personality or lifestyle may occur. Individuals may experience acute and chronic pain simultaneously, as commonly occurs in advanced cancer.
- Fibromyalgia syndrome (FMS) is a poorly understood cause of chronic pain. It is more common in women and has many associated signs and symptoms. FMS is best treated with multiple approaches, both pharmacologic and nonpharmacologic.
- Neuropathic pain results from injury to peripheral or central nerves as a consequence of surgery, tumor, trauma, or drugs and has a constant, achy, or shocklike quality. The sympathetic nervous system may maintain neuropathic pain by releasing norepinephrine onto nociceptors.
- Ischemic pain occurs when inadequate blood flow to tissues results in cellular injury and release of chemicals that stimulate and/or damage nociceptors.
- Referred pain is a painful sensation perceived at some distance from an injury but generally within the same dermatome. Referred pain is thought to occur because of the convergence of visceral nociceptor activity with primary somatic afferents in the posterior horn of the cord.

PHYSIOLOGIC RESPONSES TO PAIN

The autonomic nervous system, which is responsible for much of the physiologic response to pain, includes both the sympathetic and parasympathetic divisions. Activation of the sympathetic nervous system results in a predictable cluster of physical signs and symptoms, including an elevated heart rate, blood pressure, and respiratory rate, as well as dilated pupils, perspiration, and pallor[20] (see Table 47-4). Sympathetic stimulation results in constriction of superficial vessels to divert blood to striated muscle, heart, and lungs; bronchodilation; increased

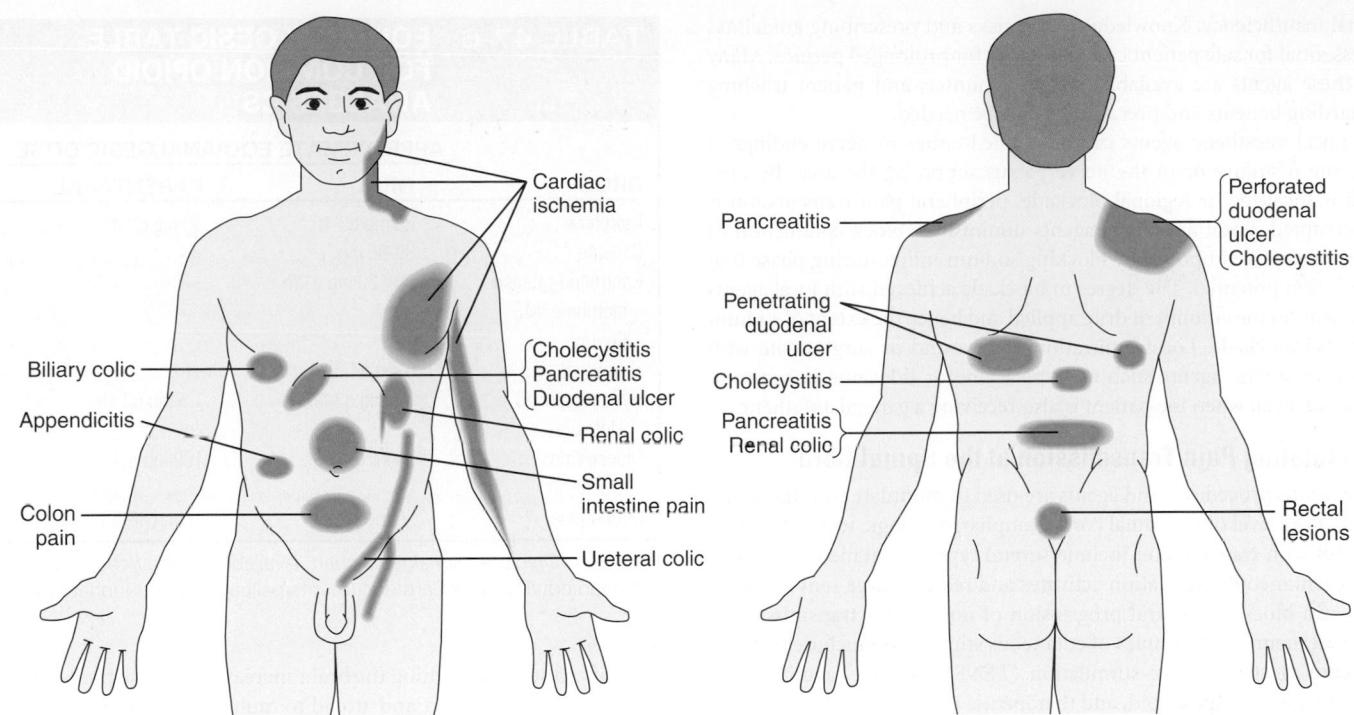

FIGURE 47-9 Areas of referred pain.

cardiac contractility; and increased levels of circulating blood glucose. In addition, although gastrointestinal motility and secretion decrease, sphincter tone increases. Nausea, vomiting, and even paralytic ileus may develop. Hypomotility of the bladder and ureters can also result from sympathetic activation and lead to urine retention. Pain stimulates the release of numerous stress hormones, including antidiuretic hormone, aldosterone, and cortisol. These hormones help the kidneys conserve fluid and stimulate the release of glucose from the liver.

The sympathetic responses to pain may be physiologically helpful in the short term but become deleterious if excessive or prolonged. The body cannot sustain this level of activation for long periods. Eventually, physiologic adaptation occurs and the observed sympathetic response to pain abates. Thus the heart rate, blood pressure, and respiratory rate return toward normal or baseline. Signs and symptoms of sympathetic nervous system activation may be an important clue in pain assessment when present, but their absence does not guarantee the absence of pain sensations.

PAIN IN THE YOUNG AND THE ELDERLY

Many myths and misconceptions surround the issue of pain, especially in the very young and the elderly. As a result, often the young and the old receive inadequate treatment of their pain. It was previously thought that neonates were unable to perceive pain. Because their central nervous systems had not yet fully developed and they were unable to recall painful events, neonates often did not receive pain medication or anesthesia for surgery. It has since been found that infants do indeed have pain perception and that inadequate pain control may lead to persistent behavioral changes and physical changes in the CNS.[21]

In the elderly, it has also been theorized that pain perception is decreased. Research in this area has been inconclusive.[22] Social expectations interfere with the adequacy of pain control in the elderly, because pain is often an expected part of aging. Cognitive factors also hinder pain treatment, especially in patients with dementia who are unable to communicate their need for pain medication. However, it has been found that pain has a significant effect on an elderly individual's quality of life. No matter what the age of the patient, adequate pain control is important to his or her care.

TREATMENT MODALITIES

PHARMACOLOGIC AND NONPHARMACOLOGIC PAIN MANAGEMENT

Many pain management strategies are available. By understanding the basic mechanisms of pain transmission, one can readily identify potential sites where various types of treatment modalities could interrupt pain transmission and perception. Pain management interventions can be directed at three points: (1) interrupting peripheral transmission of nociception; (2) modulating pain transmission at the spinal cord level; and (3) altering the perception and integration of nociceptive impulses in the brain.

Interrupting Peripheral Transmission of Pain

Modalities that interrupt the peripheral transmission of nociceptive impulses are often the first step in controlling pain. The basic action of splinting an injured limb or area of the body alters the peripheral transmission of pain by minimizing or reducing tissue injury. Applying heat or cold to an injured area also helps reduce peripheral nociception by altering blood flow to the area or by reducing swelling.

Pharmacologic treatments such as NSAIDs or local anesthetic agents also exert their analgesic effects by interrupting peripheral transmission at an early stage. NSAIDs and local anesthetic agents are used as a primary intervention for pain management. Inhibition of prostaglandin production by NSAIDs reduces the number of pain chemicals available to stimulate nociceptors in the peripheral tissues. NSAIDs include indomethacin, ibuprofen, naproxen, sulindac, piroxicam, ketorolac, and many others. Blocking the production and action of prostaglandins is not without side effects. For example, prostaglandins are responsible for maintenance of the gastric mucosa, and blocking their actions can result in gastrointestinal bleeding. Prostaglandin inhibition can also lead to decreased platelet aggregation and renal insufficiency. Knowledge of the risks and prescribing guidelines is essential for safe patient care, especially for prolonged periods. Many of these agents are available over-the-counter, and patient teaching regarding benefits and precautions may be needed.

Local anesthetic agents can be applied either to nerve endings at the site of injury or to the nerve plexus supplying the area. By providing localized or regional blockade, peripheral pain transmission is interrupted. Local anesthetic agents diminish or block conduction of the nociceptive impulses by blocking sodium influx during phase 0 of the action potential. The degree of blockade achieved with local agents depends on the amount of drug applied and hence the extent of sodium channel blockade. Local infiltration of a wound or surgical site with local anesthetic agents such as bupivacaine or lidocaine is common practice, even when the patient is also receiving a general anesthetic.

Modulating Pain Transmission at the Spinal Cord

Numerous procedures and agents are used to modulate pain transmission at the level of the spinal cord. Nonpharmacologic techniques that inhibit pain transmission include several types of cutaneous stimulation. Cutaneous stimulation activates and recruits large sensory fibers that can block the central progression of nociceptive transmission at the interneurons. Examples of cutaneous stimulation include transcutaneous electrical nerve stimulation (TENS), massage, acupuncture, application of heat or cold, and therapeutic touch.

Pharmacologic measures that act at the level of the spinal cord include epidural and intrathecal analgesia. Spinal analgesia can be achieved with opioids, local anesthetics, and α-adrenergic blocking agents. Intraspinal opioids work by binding with opioid receptors in the posterior horn of the spinal cord, thereby decreasing the release of neurotransmitters such as substance P. Intraspinal local anesthetic agents block nerve conduction at the posterior nerve root. Epidural administration of an α-adrenergic blocking agent such as clonidine is thought to achieve analgesic effects by blocking sympathetically mediated pain transmission.

Dorsal column stimulators, sometimes used in chronic pain management, also work at the level of the spinal cord to "close the pain gate" by modulating descending input from the brain to the spinal cord.

Altering the Perception and Integration of Pain

The traditional modality for managing moderate to severe pain is the administration of systemic opioids. This pharmacologic intervention has stood the test of time. Opioids work at specific receptor sites that are located throughout the body but are highly concentrated in the brain. Opioid analgesic agents such as morphine and other derivatives alter the perception of pain by the brain. Opioid analgesics have similar mechanisms of action but vary widely in potency. This difference in potency has led to the development of equianalgesic tables to help clinicians prescribe these drugs appropriately (Table 47-6).

Opioid administration is associated with numerous side effects that may limit effectiveness (nausea, vomiting, respiratory depression, constipation). Long-term use of opioids leads to physical dependence and tolerance. Although the incidence of opioid addiction in persons experiencing acute pain is very low, fears about addiction contribute to inadequate pain therapy. Physical dependence is characterized by withdrawal symptoms if treatment is stopped abruptly. Tolerance to opioids is characterized by the need for increasing dosages to achieve the same analgesic effect. Dependence and tolerance are expected responses to long-term opioid therapy. Drug addiction is a behavioral pattern characterized by craving and preoccupation with obtaining the drug.

Nonpharmacologic techniques of pain management include such activities and procedures as distraction, guided imagery, relaxation, biofeedback, and hypnosis. With distraction, the number of

TABLE 47-6	EQUIANALGESIC TABLE FOR COMMON OPIOID ANALGESICS	
	APPROXIMATE EQUIANALGESIC DOSE	
DRUG	ORAL	PARENTERAL
Morphine	30 mg q3-4h	10 mg q3-4h
Codeine	30-60 mg	—
Controlled-release morphine (MS Contin)	90-120 mg q12h	—
Hydrocodone	5 mg q4-6h	—
Hydromorphone (Dilaudid)	7.5 mg q3-4h	1.5 mg q3-4h
Meperidine (Demerol)	300 mg q2-3h	100 mg q3h
Methadone	20 mg q6-8h	10 mg q6-8h

Data from *Opioid equianalgesic chart.* Available at http://champ.bsd.uchicago.edu/PalliativeCare/documents/pallpaincard2009update.pdf.

generalized stimuli reaching the brain increases. Because the brain has a limited capacity to sort and attend to multiple and varied stimuli, it is less able to integrate the pain experience when other competition is present. Imagery may alter the perception of painful stimuli in the higher centers of the brain and produce relaxation as well as analgesia. Biofeedback is a conditioned response that can be learned as a pain-control strategy. Biofeedback is thought to control pain by increasing blood flow (usually as a consequence of relaxation) to targeted body areas. The increased blood flow decreases the concentration of pain-inducing chemicals in the area. Biofeedback may also increase the amount of endorphins produced and released.

A combination of nonpharmacologic and pharmacologic strategies may help reduce the need for high doses of medications. The choice of drug therapy should correspond to the severity of the pain. It has been recommended that mild pain be managed with nonopioid analgesics such as NSAIDs or acetaminophen, whereas moderate pain may require low-potency opioids such as codeine. Severe pain requires larger and more potent doses of opioids like morphine and fentanyl. The value of combination therapy in blocking pain transmission at multiple sites has been recognized. In the arena of chronic pain management, further research is delving into the central and peripheral sensitization theories. Questions remain as to why these develop and which patient populations are at highest risk for developing these complications. Great opportunity lies in the development of novel therapies for the control of chronic pain.

KEY POINTS
- Treatment is aimed at moderating pain transmission at specific points along the pain pathways. Potential sites of pain moderation are at the peripheral nociceptor, spinal cord, and brain.
- Nociceptor activation can be altered by prostaglandin inhibitors (NSAIDs), heat and cold, and local anesthetics that block sodium influx through fast channels.
- Spinal cord transmission can be altered by cutaneous stimulation (gate control theory), intraspinal analgesics (opioids, local anesthetics, α-adrenergic blockers), and dorsal column stimulators.
- The perception of pain can be altered within the brain by systemic opioids and by nonpharmacologic means such as hypnosis, distraction, and biofeedback.

SUMMARY

The human experience of pain, although unpleasant, is a normal and expected phenomenon in response to injury. Pain sensations alert the individual to a physiologic problem and help ensure that timely treatment is sought. However, prolonged severe pain serves no good purpose and can be physiologically and psychologically harmful.

Appropriate efforts to alleviate pain may enhance recovery from illness and prevent the development of some types of chronic pain syndromes. As understanding of pain physiologic mechanisms grows, treatment strategies can more effectively combine the best of pharmacologic and nonpharmacologic therapies.

REFERENCES

1. Pain terms: A list with definitions and notes on usage. Recommended by the IASP Subcommittee on Taxonomy, *Pain* 6(3):249, 1979.
2. McCaffery M: *Nursing practice theories related to cognition, bodily pain and man-environment interactions,* Los Angeles, 1968, University of California, (master's thesis).
3. Hall JE, editor: *Guyton and Hall textbook of medical physiology,* ed 12, Philadelphia, 2011, Saunders.
4. Boron WF, Boulpaep EL, editors: *Medical physiology: a cellular and molecular approach,* ed 2, Philadelphia, 2009, Saunders.
5. Ropper AH, Samuels MA: Pain. In Ropper AH, Samuels MA, editors: *Adam's and Victor's principles of neurology,* ed 9, New York, 2009, McGraw-Hill. Available at www.accessmedicine.com.proxy.heal-wa.org/content.aspx?aID=3632863. Accessed 3/24/12.
6. Woolf CJ: Central sensitization: implications for the diagnosis and treatment of pain, *Pain* 152(Suppl 3):S2–S12, 2011.
7. Melzack R, Wall PD: Pain mechanisms: a new theory, *Science* 150(699):971–979, 1965.
8. Melzack R, Wall PD, editors: *The challenge of pain,* ed 2, Harmondworth, U.K, 1988, Penguin.
9. Schoell ED, Bingel U, Eippert F, et al: The effect of opioid receptor blockage on the neural processing of thermal stimuli, *PLoS ONE* 5(8):e12344, 2010. Available at www.plosone.org.
10. Latremoliere A, Woolf CJ: Central sensitization: a generator of pain hypersensitivity by central neuroplasticity, *J Pain* 10(9):895–926, 2009.
11. Gonzales R, Nadler PL: Common symptoms. In McPhee SJ, Papadakis MA, Rabow MW, editors: *Current medical diagnosis and treatment 2012,* New York, 2012, McGraw-Hill. Available at www.accessmedicine.com. proxy.heal-wa.org/content.aspx?aID=79. Accessed 3/24/12.
12. Migraine Research Foundation: *About migraine.* Available at www. migraineresearchfoundation.org/print-friendly/about-migraine. html.
13. Williams DA, Schilling S: Advances in the assessment of fibromyalgia, *Rheum Dis Clin North Am* 35(2):339–357, 2009.
14. Hellmann DB, Imboden JB Jr: Musculoskeletal and immunologic disorders. In McPhee SJ, Papadakis MA, Rabow MW, editors: *Current medical diagnosis and treatment 2012,* New York, 2012, McGraw-Hill. Available at www.accessmedicine.com.proxy.heal-wa.org/content.aspx?aID=10083. Accessed 3/24/12.
15. Fibromyalgia. In DynaMed [database online] EBSCO publishing. Available at http://search.ebscohost.com.heal-wa.org.aspx?direct=true&site= DynaMed&ID=113862. Updated 3/8/12. Accessed 3/23/12.
16. Beal MF, Hauser SL: Trigeminal neuralgia, Bell's palsy, and other cranial nerve disorders. In Longo DL, Fauci AS, Kasper DL, et al, editors: *Harrison's principles of internal medicine,* ed 18, New York, 2012, McGraw-Hill. Available at www.accessmedicine.com.proxy.heal-wa.org.content.aspx?aID=9147168. Accessed 3/24/12.
17. American Diabetic Association: *Diabetes statistics.* Available at www.diabetes.org/diabetes-basics/diabetes-statistics/.
18. King SA: Diabetic peripheral neuropathic pain: effective management, *Consultant* 51(4):197–200, 2011.
19. Johnson RW, McElhaney J: Postherpetic neuralgia in the elderly, *Int J Clin Pract* 63(9):1386–1391, 2009.
20. Mohn-Brown E, Burke KM, Eby L, editors: *Medical-surgical nursing care,* ed 3, Upper Saddle River, NJ, 2011, Pearson Education.
21. Lago P, Garetti E, Merazzi D, et al: Guidelines for procedural pain in the newborn, *Acta Paediatr* 98:932–939, 2009.
22. Ferrell BA, Charette SL: Pain management. In Halter JB, Ouslander JG, Tinetti ME, editors: *Hazzard's geriatric medicine and gerontology,* ed 6, New York, 2009, McGraw-Hill. Available at www.accessmedicine.com. proxy.heal-wa.org/content. aspx?aID=5113633. Accessed 3/24/12.

Neurobiology of Psychotic Illnesses

Ann Futterman Collier

evolve WEBSITE

http://evolve.elsevier.com/Copstead/
- Review Questions and Answers
- Glossary (with audio pronunciations for selected terms)
- Animations
- Case Studies
- Key Points Review

KEY QUESTIONS

- What are the "positive" and "negative" symptoms of schizophrenia?
- What genetic, gestational, and neurologic risk factors are related to schizophrenia?
- How are the dopamine D_1 and D_2 receptors related to positive and negative symptoms of schizophrenia?
- How is schizophrenia managed?
- What are the hallmark symptoms of major depression?
- What is the neurobiology of major depression?
- What are the subtypes of bipolar disorder?
- How are major depression and bipolar disorder managed?

CHAPTER OUTLINE

Abnormal behavior is typically considered the opposite of mental well-being. Current internationally recognized clinical diagnostic schemes rely on categorical systems to define mental disorders and provide standardized criteria for each diagnosis. The two most widely established systems are: (1) *ICD-10,* Chapter V: Mental and Behavioural Disorders, which is part of the *International Classification of Diseases* published by the World Health Organization,[1] and (2) the *Diagnostic and Statistical Manual of Mental Disorders (DSM),*[2] published by the American Psychiatric Association. Although historically there have been significant differences between these systems, in recent years there has been convergence so that both sets of codes are broadly comparable. There are more than 300 different psychiatric disorders listed in the fourth text revision of *DSM (DSM-IV-TR),* with more added each revision. The fifth edition of *DSM (DSM-5)* will be published in May 2013.[3] Although there will be changes in nomenclature and disorder criteria in the newest version, *DSM-5* will continue its clinical utility, be guided more heavily by research evidence, and attempt to maintain continuity with previous editions.

The *National Survey on Drug Use and Health (NSDUH)* defines serious mental illness (SMI) as a mental, behavioral, or emotional disorder (excluding developmental and substance use disorders) that is diagnosable currently or within the past year, is of sufficient duration to meet diagnostic criteria specified within *DSM-IV-TR,* and results in serious functional impairment that substantially interferes with or limits one or more major life activities.[4] Using the SMI nomenclature, we now know that currently in the United States approximately 5% of all adults meet criteria for SMI. It is also known that 26.2% of the U.S. adult population will have experienced an SMI in the previous year, and 22.3% of these cases will be classified as "severe." In addition, 46.3% of adolescents between 13 and 18 years of age will be diagnosed with an SMI. Research also shows that SMIs occur more frequently in women than in men, are more prevalent in individuals between the ages of 18 to 49, and are least likely to be seen in American individuals of Asian descent. Table 48-1 provides a review of the most common SMIs by lifetime prevalence; 12-month health care service utilization is also provided for each disorder. Some SMIs have very high lifetime

TABLE 48-1 LIFETIME PREVALENCE OF SERIOUS MENTAL ILLNESS (IN U.S.)

NAME OF DISORDER	OVERALL CLASSIFICATION	LIFETIME PREVALENCE (%)	AVERAGE AGE OF ONSET (yr)	TREATMENT AND SERVICES USE (ANY TYPE) (%)
Social phobia	Anxiety disorders	29.9%	13	45.6%
Major depression	Mood disorder	16.5%	32	56.8%
Attention deficit disorder with hyperactivity (ADHD)	Attention deficit disorder (13-18 yr old)	9.8%	Not reported	Not reported
Posttraumatic stress disorder (PTSD)	Anxiety disorders	6.8%	23	57.4%
Generalized anxiety disorder	Anxiety disorders	5.7%	31	52.3%
Avoidant personality disorder	Personality disorders	5.2%	Not reported	Not reported
Panic disorder	Anxiety disorders	4.7%	24	65.4%
Bipolar disorder	Mood disorders	3.9%	25	55.5%
Obsessive-compulsive disorder	Anxiety disorders	1.6%	19	Not reported
Borderline personality disorder	Personality disorders	1.6%	Not reported	42.4%
Schizophrenia	Schizophrenia	1.1%	Not reported	64.3%
Antisocial personality disorder	Personality disorders	1.0%	Not reported	46.1%
Autism spectrum disorders	Autism spectrum disorders	0.9%	8	Not reported

From National Institutes of Mental Health (NIMH). Available at www.nimh.nih.gov/statistics/index.shtml. Accessed 4/25/12.

prevalence but only moderate treatment service use (e.g., social phobia). Alternately, other SMIs have low lifetime prevalence but very high treatment service utilization (e.g., schizophrenia). Based on a combination of the lifetime prevalence rates and health care service utilization, the *most frequently occurring SMI disorders* and those with the *highest health care utilization* will be reviewed in Chapters 48 and 49.

THOUGHT DISORDER, DELIRIUM, AND DEMENTIA

Psychosis is a term used to describe a serious and debilitating mental state. The most restricted definition refers to delusions and prominent hallucinations, which occur in the absence of insight into their pathologic basis.[2] The broadest definition of psychosis includes other positive symptoms that are characteristics of schizophrenia, such as disorganized speech and grossly disorganized or catatonic behavior. Hallmark symptoms of psychosis are delusions, hallucinations, cognitive disorganization, and altered reality. These symptoms characterize a small number of specific mental disorders; however, a wide range of different physical and mental conditions can produce psychotic symptoms. The neurobiological basis of psychosis can be summarized as acute or chronic alterations in neuron anatomy and physiology and cellular biochemical processes. Although psychosis occurs most often with schizophrenia and mood disorders, it may also manifest with substance disorders, delirium, dementia, amnestic disorders, and acute stress disorder. Groundbreaking research in brain imaging techniques and psychopharmacology now allows highly precise definitions of the various biochemical pathways associated with psychosis. This chapter addresses three disorders that are associated with psychosis: schizophrenia, major depressive disorder (MDD), and bipolar disorder (BD).

Schizophrenia

Schizophrenia refers to a chronic, remitting, and relapsing psychotic disorder that is associated with significant impairment in social and vocational functioning.[5,6] Literally, the term is defined as "split mind," and once was believed to be a disorder that caused the personality to split into multiple subtypes. Schizophrenia is now correctly understood as a split or separation among normally well-synchronized brain functions. This loss of synchronized brain functioning leads to thoughts, behaviors, and feelings that are disordered, disorganized,

and disconnected from reality—a condition generally referred to as psychosis.[7]

The global incidence rate of schizophrenia has consistently been estimated to be about 1% of the world population,[7] and is fairly equally distributed across genders. Unfortunately, schizophrenia appears to be associated with an average lifespan reduction of 15 to 25 years.[5,6,8] Women show symptom onset and are diagnosed typically between the ages of 25 and 35 years, men between the ages of 15 and 25 years. Women with schizophrenia appear to have better outcomes than men.[9] Possibly, the later age of onset, the protective nature of female hormones such as estrogens, or a better drug response accounts for this difference.[9] People with schizophrenia may be at increased risk for type 2 diabetes and cardiovascular disorders,[10-13] perhaps attributable to the side effects of antipsychotic medications, poorer overall physical health, less healthy lifestyles, and substandard health care. However, newer antipsychotic medications alone do not appear to account for the increased incidence of diabetes and cardiovascular disease.[10-12]

Etiology and neurobiology

Dopamine effects. Several decades ago it was hypothesized that abnormalities in dopaminergic pathways in specific regions of the brain were the cause of schizophrenia. This conclusion was reached after noting that dopamine antagonists (competitive) reduce symptoms of schizophrenia whereas dopamine agonists (complementary) produce schizophrenic symptoms. Dopamine-specific neurons in the brain primarily are located in the ventral tegmentum of the mesencephalon, medial and superior to the substantia nigra. These regions, as a whole, are referred to as the mesolimbic dopaminergic system. The long nerve fibers leaving this system mainly project into the medial and anterior portions of the limbic system. The limbic system contains three powerful centers of behavior control: the nucleus accumbens, the amygdala, and the anterior caudate nucleus.

Generally speaking, we now know that decreased neurotransmission and connectivity is the neurobiological basis of schizophrenia. Frankle and colleagues[14] reported that the core biochemical process of schizophrenia involved an excess of subcortical dopaminergic transmission at dopamine D_2 receptors and a deficit of glutamate transmission at N-methyl-D-aspartate (NMDA) receptors. The dopamine pathogenesis of schizophrenia can be thought of as disordered synaptic organization. In the brain, normal synaptic organization implies

Controls

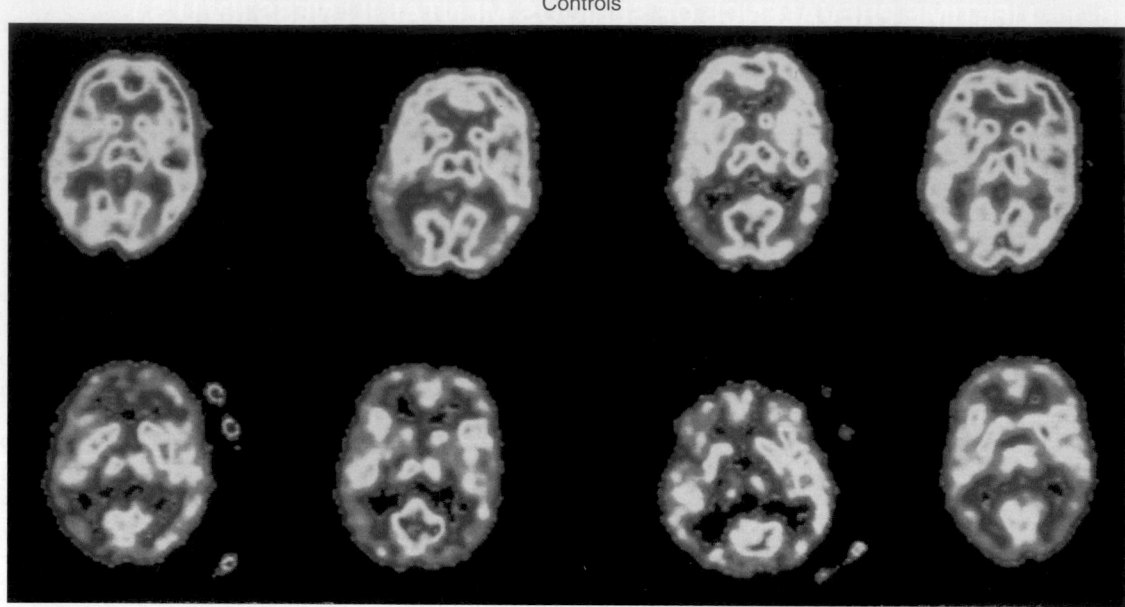

Schizophrenics

FIGURE 48-1 Individual variation in positron emission tomography (PET) scans. Four normal individuals *(top row)* and four schizophrenics *(bottom row)* show range of hypofrontality and diminished basal ganglia metabolism. (From Buchsbaum MS, Haier RJ: Functional and anatomical brain imaging: impact on schizophrenia research, *Schizophr Bull* 13[1]:115-132, 1987. Reproduced by permission of Monte S. Buchsbaum, MD.)

the provision for normal communication among brain cells. Specific schizophrenia symptoms have been associated with neurotransmission dysregulation that diminishes or elevates dopamine activity. Hyperdopaminergic states have primarily been associated with positive symptoms of schizophrenia, such as hallucinations, delusions, and psychosis. Hypodopaminergic states have primarily been associated with negative symptoms of schizophrenia, such as cognitive difficulties, lack of energy and motivation, and depression.[15] Dopamine D_2 receptors have been associated with positive symptoms and psychosis, whereas dopamine D_1 receptors have been associated with negative symptoms.

That said, dopamine receptor activity and synaptic transmission are subject to a variety of mediators such as brain-derived neurotrophic factor (BDNF), a neurotrophin that increases synaptic activity and neurotransmitter output.[16] Dopamine synaptic activity also has been closely linked with stress-related cortisol activity and drugs of abuse (cocaine, amphetamines, morphine, nicotine, and ethanol).[17] Although dopamine dysregulation clearly is the driving force behind the neurochemical processes of psychosis, other experts suggest considering the role of biopsychosocial contextual factors in shaping and aggravating the expression of biochemical dysregulation.[18]

Positron emission tomography (PET) brain images have enabled researchers to further examine the overall role of dopamine activity in psychosis and schizophrenia. PET studies have demonstrated low glucose metabolism rates in the frontal cortex and dopamine regions[19] of the brains of persons with schizophrenia (Figure 48-1). Of the many different types of dopamine brain cell receptors identified, dopamine D_2 receptors once again were found to be strongly associated with symptoms of schizophrenia. Similar research has shown that dopamine D_2 receptors are particularly responsive to antipsychotic drugs.

Thus, the dopamine hypothesis, which postulates that schizophrenia symptoms result from presynaptic dysregulation of dopamine transmission, continues to be the focus of neurobiological studies. The specific neuropathologic mechanism of schizophrenia appears to be caused by a functional excess of postsynaptic dopamine receptor activity and dopamine receptor hypersensitivity, either alone or in combination.

Genetic effects. In the absence of any other condition, a family history of schizophrenia by itself does not lead to schizophrenia: Schizophrenia can and does develop in persons with no family history of the disease. Initial interest in identifying possible genetic contributions to schizophrenia was based on early research on monozygotic (identical) and dizygotic twins, by studying twins born to parents with schizophrenia but reared apart from their parents. Results suggested that nearly 50% of these offspring developed schizophrenia.[20] Children of two parents with schizophrenia have a 40% to 68% risk of developing the illness, whereas children with one parent with schizophrenia have a 9% to 16% risk.[9] The risk of a non–twin sibling of a brother or sister with schizophrenia developing the disease is slightly less at 8% to 14%. The obvious limitation of these findings is that they do not explain why an at-risk offspring does not develop schizophrenia.

Several additional conditions are thought to be involved in the transformation from genetic risk to actual illness. Factors such as prenatal infections, malnutrition, birth complications, and brain injury have been associated with the development of schizophrenia in persons who have increased genetic risk.[21] Moreover, different gene locations are also relevant to the illness onset. Experts question whether inherited genetic risk for schizophrenia could explain observed differences in incidence and prevalence rates based on gender and race. Lastly, genetic models of schizophrenia typically do not address risk in terms of the subtype of schizophrenia, such as paranoid schizophrenia as opposed to schizophrenia without paranoia. Given the high standards of proof required for gene typing, a purely genetic explanation of an illness as complex as schizophrenia seems unlikely. Increased genetic risk of schizophrenia appears to be a critical part of a puzzle composed of many pieces. Thus, for individuals who are genetically predisposed, some aspects of schizophrenia will probably be determined

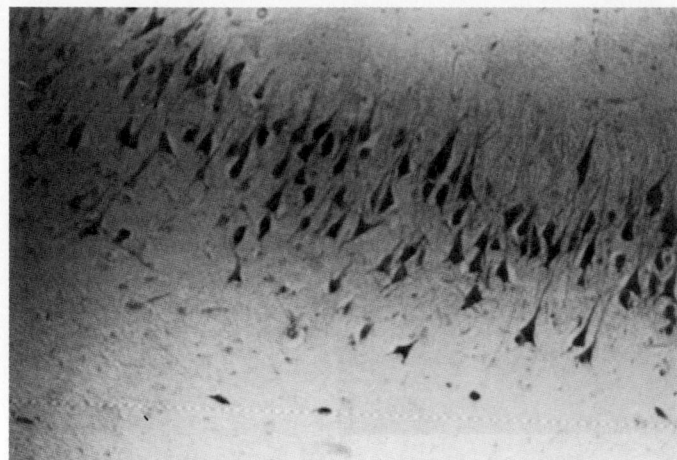

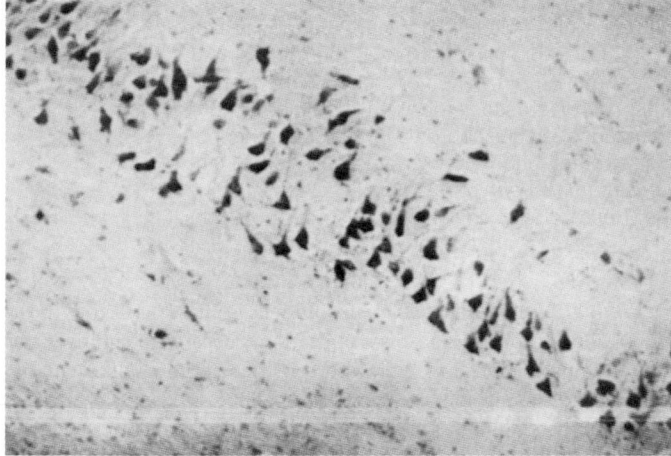

FIGURE 48-2 Photographic comparison of hippocampal tissue at CA 2/3 interface in a control *(top)* and in a person with chronic schizophrenia *(bottom).* (Original magnification of the Nissl-stained tissue, ×100. From Kovelman JA, Scheibel AB: A neurohistological correlate of schizophrenia, *Biol Psychiatry* 19:1601-1621, 1984.)

by biopsychosocial characteristics.[22] Researchers continue to study the actual versus potential genetic risks of schizophrenia.

Gestational effects. Early findings noted that in persons with schizophrenia, pyramidal cells in the hippocampus were not lined up like a "picket fence," as they were in control subjects (Figure 48-2). Instead, the cells appeared to be rotated at 70-degree to 90-degree angles.[23] Pyramidal cells migrate during the second trimester of gestation and later become fastened by neuronal cell adhesion molecules (N-CAMs). Researchers focused on the possibility of pyramidal cell misalignment and lost N-CAM adhesive effects as links between gestation and schizophrenia. Researchers noted that in pregnant women living in Scandinavia and England who were exposed to the 1957 flu epidemic during their second trimester, 300% more of their children were diagnosed with schizophrenia than those of women who experienced flu during the first or third trimester.

These findings were considered significant for two reasons: (1) neuronal migration peaks during the second trimester, and (2) the influenza virus is one of very few viruses that produce capsular neuraminidase, an enzyme that can change the adhesive properties of N-CAMs.[24] Hippocampal, parahippocampal gyrus, and amygdala neurons process information and emotional expression. Other researchers have suggested that delivery complications could be an additional factor, playing a mediating role between prenatal influenza exposure and later development of schizophrenia.[25]

More recent studies of gestational abnormalities focus on specific brain regions and stages of prenatal neurodevelopment.[26] This research is exemplified in a well-controlled Canadian study that examined the association of hippocampal formation abnormalities and first adult episode of schizophrenia. The main functions of the hippocampus are learning and new-memory formation. Both abilities may be lost when hippocampal functioning is impaired. Macroscopic cell abnormalities, such as fewer synapse connections and diminished synapse activity, result in reduced hippocampal volume. Reduced hippocampal volume has been associated with severe stress, mood disorders, and schizophrenia.[27] The Canadian researchers hypothesized that schizophrenia was associated with incomplete formation of the hippocampus during the second trimester of development. They used magnetic resonance images to compare the brains of newly diagnosed patients with healthy matched controls. Although the number of participants in the study was too small to allow for generalizations to be drawn, the magnetic resonance images of the newly diagnosed patients clearly showed enlarged hippocampal fissures or disrupted hippocampal formation. Interestingly, obstetric complications during pregnancy were not significant factors.

Neurologic effects. Observed neuroanatomic differences in persons with schizophrenia led researchers to study anatomic and functional abnormalities in the limbic region and frontal lobe parts of the brain. Structural abnormalities in these brain regions would suggest that abnormal functioning might contribute to the disrupted cognitive processes or symptoms of schizophrenia. Beginning in 1976, computed tomography (CT) studies revealed enlarged brain ventricles in persons with schizophrenia. A groundbreaking 1980 study showed that the neurochemical basis of schizophrenia might involve two processes: dopamine neurotransmission dysregulation and abnormal cerebral structure.[28]

Magnetic resonance imaging (MRI) studies of persons with chronic schizophrenia indicated larger-than-normal lateral and third ventricles and reduced temporal lobe gray matter[29] (Figure 48-3). MRI findings also showed reduced frontal lobe blood flow and relative decreases in frontal lobe metabolic activity. Prefrontal cortex structure and functioning deficits were consistently observed when the subject was simultaneously placed under stress. The stress used in the study was primarily psychological, such as contingency planning exercises or divergent thinking during performance of a cognitive task that utilized specific regions of the prefrontal cortex.[30]

Subsequent studies of brain structure in persons with severe schizophrenia replicated the earlier findings of abnormal limbic-cortical structures and smaller, misarranged hippocampal pyramidal cells. This includes replication of MRI findings of reduced bilateral temporal lobe volume, decreased hippocampal volume, and reduced volume in the parahippocampal gyrus region of the brain. Studies of brain regions other than the limbic system revealed frontal lobe structural alterations in the dorsolateral area of the prefrontal cortex and in the cingulate and motor cortices. The finding of decreased frontal lobe glucose metabolism associated with schizophrenia also has been replicated (Figure 48-4).[31]

Postmortem brain tissue studies indicated fewer nicotinic receptors present in the hippocampus of schizophrenics. Tobacco dependence is a common secondary disorder with schizophrenia. The finding of fewer nicotinic receptors was of particular interest to researchers in that previous studies had shown that smoking could temporarily normalize auditory sensory gating that typically becomes impaired with schizophrenia.[32] Since then, researchers found that a neurophysiologic deficit at chromosome 15, at the *OC7* nicotinic receptor gene, may partially explain the inheritance of this neurophysiologic symptom.[33] Although the development of schizophrenia is associated with any number of specific abnormalities, early neurodevelopmental alterations that result in dysfunction of the limbic and prefrontal regions of the brain appear to be critical.

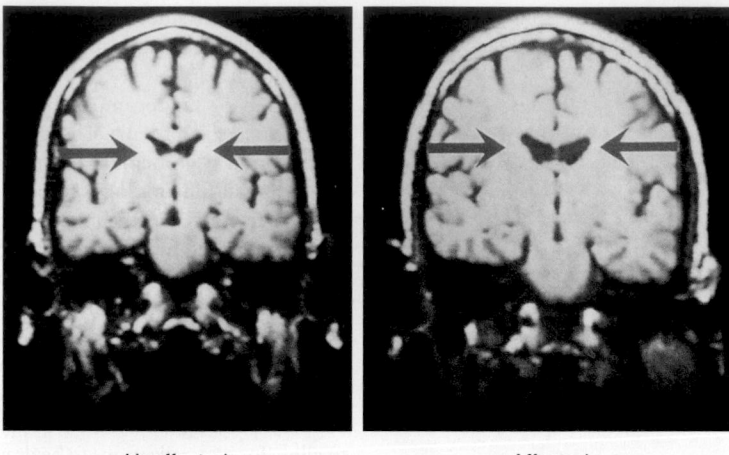

Unaffected

Affected

FIGURE 48-3 Loss of brain volume associated with schizophrenia is clearly shown by magnetic resonance images comparing the size of ventricles (butterfly-shaped, fluid-filled spaces in the midbrain) of 44-year-old male identical twins, one of whom has schizophrenia *(right)*. The ventricles of the person with schizophrenia are larger, suggesting structural brain changes associated with the illness. Note that such magnetic resonance images cannot be used to diagnose schizophrenia in the general population because of normal genetic variation in ventricle size; many unaffected people have large ventricles. (From Fortinash KM, Worret PA, editors: *Psychiatric mental health nursing*, ed 5, St Louis, 2011, Mosby, p 264. Courtesy Daniel R. Weinberger, MD, Chief Researcher, Clinical Brain Disorders Branch, National Institute of Mental Health, Bethesda, MD.)

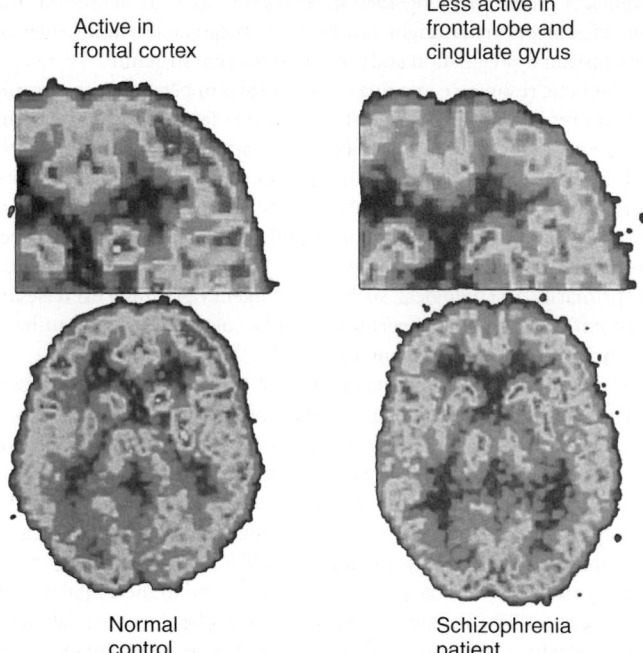

Active in
frontal cortex

Less active in
frontal lobe and
cingulate gyrus

Normal
control

Schizophrenia
patient

FIGURE 48-4 Positron emission tomography (PET) scan with ^{18}F-deoxyglucose shows metabolic activity in a horizontal section of the brain in a control subject *(left)* and in an unmedicated client with schizophrenia *(right)*. Red and yellow indicate lower activity in the white matter areas of the brain. The frontal lobe is magnified to show reduced frontal activity in the prefrontal cortex of the client with schizophrenia. (From Fortinash KM, Worret PA, editors: *Psychiatric mental health nursing*, ed 5, St Louis, 2012, Elsevier, p 279. Courtesy Monte S. Buchsbaum, MD, Mt. Sinai School of Medicine, New York.)

Clinical manifestations. Schizophrenia is characterized by positive (reality distortion and disorganization), negative, cognitive, and mood symptoms.[7] The types and severity of symptoms differ among patients and change over the course of the illness. Positive symptoms typically reflect an excess or distortion of normal functions. In contrast, negative symptoms reflect a decrease or loss of normal functions. *Positive symptoms* include the psychotic dimension, or distortions in thought content (delusions) and perception (hallucinations), as well as the disorganization dimension, or disorganization in speech and behavior. The resulting positive symptoms also include the inability to self-monitor behavior, which results in grossly disorganized or catatonic behavior. *Delusions,* or systematic, fixed, false beliefs, usually involve themes of persecution, reference, somatization, religiosity, or grandiosity. *Hallucinations* are sensory perceptions with no apparent stimulus. They occur in any sensory system (such as auditory, visual, olfactory, gustatory, or tactile) but usually auditory hallucinations are the norm. Auditory hallucinations are commonly experienced as voices, distinct from the person's own thoughts, and out of the range of normal experience. *Disorganized thinking* is usually evaluated by an individual's speech, and is frequently characterized by frequent derailment or loose associations, invented words, tangential ideas, and, when most severe, incomprehensible speech. *Grossly disorganized behavior* can range from childlike silliness to unpredictable agitation, and impairs the individual's ability to complete tasks of daily living. When individuals display catatonic motor behaviors, they show a decrease in reactivity to environmental events, to such an extreme that they can maintain a rigid posture and resist efforts to be moved. The positive symptoms[13] of schizophrenia are thought to result from excessive dopamine D_2 receptor activity in the brain. *Negative symptoms* are considered to be restricted affect, or avolition and asociality. Negative symptoms represent deficits in functioning and can be more difficult to recognize than positive symptoms. Negative symptoms[13] of schizophrenia are considered to be associated with dopamine D_1 receptor activity in the brain. Poor *cognitive functioning* in schizophrenia includes difficulties with memory, attention (e.g., poor concentration, distractibility, selective attention), and decision making.

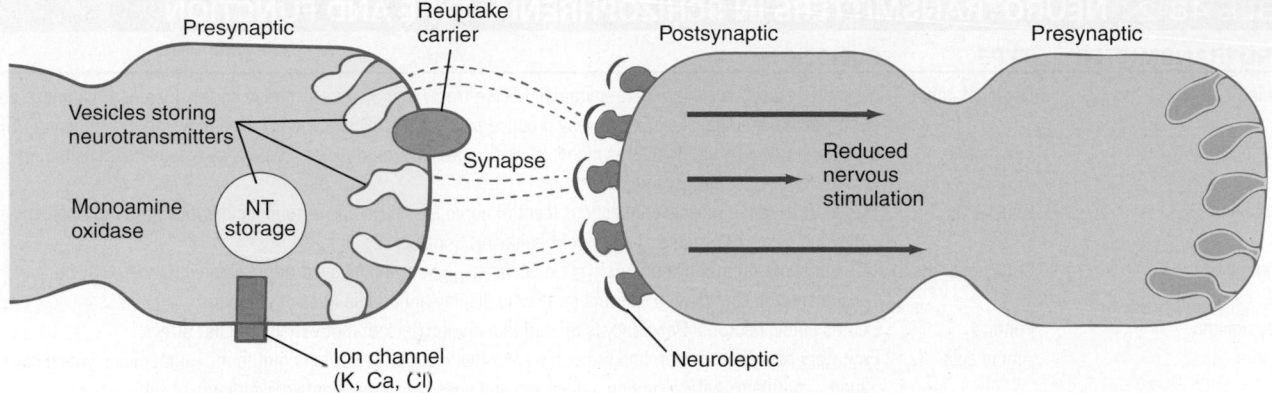

FIGURE 48-5 Neuroleptic (antipsychotic) action. Neurotransmitter *(NT)* action at the synapse is modified by neuroleptics, which block postsynaptic receptor sites to reduce nervous stimulation (reducing symptoms of schizophrenia). (From Fortinash KM, Worret PA, editors: *Psychiatric mental health nursing,* ed 5, St Louis, 2012, Elsevier, p 265.)

According to the workgroup responsible for developing *DSM-5,*[3] the active phase of schizophrenia is characterized by two or more of the following symptoms that must be present for a significant portion of time during a 1-month period (or less if successfully treated): (1) delusions; (2) hallucinations; (3) disorganized speech; (4) grossly abnormal psychomotor behavior; and (5) negative symptoms. At least one of these symptoms should include delusions, hallucinations, or disorganized speech. In addition, for a significant portion of the time since the onset of the disturbance, schizophrenia is also characterized by social/occupational dysfunction in one or more major areas: work, interpersonal relations, or self-care. All of these are markedly below the level achieved before the onset of the illness (or when the onset is in childhood or adolescence, failure to achieve expected level of interpersonal, academic, or occupational achievement). Regarding duration, typically continuous signs of the disturbance exist for at least 6 months, with at least 1 month of symptoms (or less if successfully treated) that meet criteria for the active phase (delusions, hallucinations, disorganized speech), and may include periods of prodromal or residual symptoms. During these prodromal or residual periods, the signs of the disturbance may be manifested by only negative symptoms or by two or more of the active-phase symptoms in an attenuated form (e.g., odd beliefs, unusual perceptual experiences). Finally, for an individual to receive the diagnosis of schizophrenia, the diagnoses of schizoaffective disorder and mood disorder with psychotic features must be ruled out. In addition, symptoms cannot be due to the direct physiologic effects of a substance (e.g., a drug of abuse, a medication) or a general medical condition.[7]

Schizophrenia has been divided into five subtypes in *DSM-IV-TR:*[2] paranoid; disorganized; catatonic; undifferentiated; and residual. In each subtype there is predominant symptomatology at the time of evaluation; these can change over time, such as at a subsequent diagnosis. In addition, an individual may have symptoms characteristic of more than one subtype. *DSM-V* may introduce a different classification of subtypes. The paranoid and disorganized types are the least severe (in that order). The undifferentiated type is essentially a catch-all category for individuals who do not meet criteria for any of the other subtypes. The residual type indicates that the disturbance has continued, but the active-phase symptoms are no longer met.

Pharmacologic treatment. When untreated, schizophrenia is associated with increased mortality, impaired vocational and social functioning, and reduced quality of life.[5] Unfortunately, the extent to which treatment does actually improve life span and psychosocial functioning is not specifically clear. Because antipsychotic medications do decrease the likelihood of relapse, they are encouraged.

When effective, antipsychotic medication can be expected to diminish or remit hallucinations or reduce their impact on functioning.[34] The ability to reason should improve; ambivalence, delusions, and suspiciousness should be greatly reduced; agitation and confusion should be relieved; and social behavior should improve. Antipsychotic medications are designed to have specific effects on targeted neurotransmitters. Newer antipsychotic medications, typically called second-generation agents (SGAs) (atypical), are intended to generally manage psychosis as well as both positive and negative schizophrenia symptoms.[5] Older antipsychotic medications, traditionally called first-generation agents (FGAs) (conventional), were less effective in managing negative schizophrenia symptoms. They mainly acted as dopamine antagonists, blocking the dopamine receptors (D_2). This action diminishes the amount of dopamine received by the receptor sites (Figure 48-5).

All FGAs and SGAs appear to be equally effective in reducing the positive symptoms and disorganization associated with schizophrenia, hence blocking the dopamine D_2 receptor.[5,34] Neither antipsychotic agent appears to improve the cognitive symptoms in patients with schizophrenia; in fact, findings suggest that they worsen cognitive impairment.[5] Although the maximum drug response may not be reached for many months, patient response over the first 2 to 4 weeks of antipsychotic medication use will typically predict long-term response. Antipsychotic response will vary as a result of the stage of illness, with first-episode patients responding faster and at a higher rate than those at later stages.[5] In addition, both FGAs and SGAs play a substantial role in decreasing the likelihood of relapse.

FGAs and SGAs differ most notably in their side effect profiles and their potential for interacting with other medications. FGAs (e.g., chlorpromazine) had relatively nonspecific neurotransmitter effects and numerous side effects, the most difficult being extrapyramidal symptoms (EPS). Haloperidol was the first FGA that had significantly less anticholinergic and hypotensive side effects. By 1990, SGAs became widely available; the SGAs have generally shown a lower risk of EPS but a higher risk of other metabolic adverse effects. The first SGA, clozapine, was quickly followed by a generation of new atypical antipsychotics (risperidone, olanzapine, quetiapine, ziprasidone), each promising still fewer side effects, better relief of both positive and negative schizophrenic symptoms, and minimal risk of EPS, specifically

TABLE 48-2 NEUROTRANSMITTERS IN SCHIZOPHRENIA: TYPE AND FUNCTION

NEUROTRANSMITTER	TYPE	FUNCTION
Dopamine	Catecholamine	Regulates motor behavior in extrapyramidal nerve tracts and also transmits in cortex. Increases vigilance and may increase aggression. Excess may produce psychosis; deficiency may cause movement disorders (EPS).
Serotonin	Indolamine	Brainstem transmitter; modulates mood; lowers aggressive tendencies. Deficiency may be responsible for some forms of schizophrenia.
Acetylcholine	Cholinergic	Transmits at nerve-muscle connections (central nervous system and autonomic nervous system). Deficiency may increase confusion and acting-out behavior. Controls EPS.
Norepinephrine	Catecholamine	Transmits in sympathetic nervous system. Induces "fight or flight" syndrome (hypervigilance). May be insufficient in clients with schizophrenia who display anhedonia (loss of pleasure).
Cholecystokinin	Peptide	Excites limbic neurons. Deficiency is related to avolition (lack of motivation) and flat affect.
Glutamate	Amino acid	Excitatory neurotransmitter. Impairment in N-methyl-D-aspartate affects glutamate metabolism, which can lead to problems with cognition, delusions, and possibly some negative symptoms of schizophrenia.
γ-Aminobutyric acid (GABA)	Amino acid	Inhibitory neurotransmitter; predominantly a brain transmitter. Promotes balance between dopamine and glutamate and thus inhibits impulsive behaviors.

From Fortinash KM, Worret PA: *Psychiatric mental health nursing,* ed 5, St Louis, 2012, Elsevier, p 265.
EPS, Extrapyramidal symptoms.

those associated with tardive dyskinesia. Some worrisome side effects are clinically significant weight gain, glucose dysregulation, and dyslipidemia.[35,36] Experts have speculated that hyperglycemia may have to do with dopamine receptor involvement in the regulation of insulin secretion. Numerous explanations for weight gain as a major side effect of antipsychotic medication continue to be developed and tested. The glutamate neurobiological model[37] of psychosis and schizophrenia, an alternative to the dopamine model, may be the basis for the next new generation of antipsychotic medications.

The glutamate deficit[37] model attempts to focus attention on the cause of excessive dopamine receptor activity rather than the excessive activity itself. γ-Aminobutyric acid (GABA) is the most important inhibitory brain neurotransmitter. GABA synthesis depends on and is controlled by the enzyme glutamic acid decarboxylase (GAD). GAD activity is modulated by the glutamate receptor NMDA. GAD dysregulation is thought to lead to insufficient GABA activity and, consequently, excessive dopamine activity. Reduced GAD activity has been observed in the dorsolateral prefrontal cortex and hippocampus of patients with schizophrenia. The interesting observation for pharmacologic researchers is that a broad range of different drugs has been shown to be capable of affecting GAD activity. Although the glutamate deficit model is not new, the model still may lead to a class of antipsychotic medications unlike any previous generation.

Dopamine D_2 continues to remain the lead neurotransmitter target of the atypical antipsychotics.[34] Researchers found that the most common side effects of antipsychotic medication could be reduced if the drug's impact on dopamine D_2 receptors was not excessive. Lower receptor occupancy, less receptor affinity, and faster release[38] of the receptor were methods shown to be associated with fewer side effects. More recently, the aim for effective antipsychotic medication is to stabilize rather than reduce dopamine activity. The newest SGAs, such as aripiprazole, paliperidone, iloperidone, asenapine, and lurasidone, show greater affinity for serotonin receptors (negative symptoms) and moderate affinity for dopamine and norepinephrine receptors (positive symptoms).[5,38] Effective antipsychotic medications have significant dopamine effects; however, schizophrenia symptoms are highly complex and likely to involve other neurotransmitters, particularly serotonin and norepinephrine (Table 48-2).

Nonpharmacologic treatment. Psychosocial treatments that offer integrated care are essential for all patients with schizophrenia. At a minimum this should include case management in order to maintain the system of care, permit the most efficacious treatment in the least restrictive setting, and optimize quality of life and social function. However, cognitive-behavioral therapy (CBT), cognitive remediation and rehabilitation, social skills–based therapies, vocational rehabilitation, and family therapy have all proven to be effective supplemental care for schizophrenia.[7]

KEY POINTS

- *DSM* and *ICD* are the two main systems for the classification of mental illness; *DSM-IV-TR* will be revised as *DSM-5*, which will be published in 2013. There are more than 300 different types of mental illness classifications today.
- Schizophrenia is characterized by altered perceptions of reality and disordered thinking. Genetic predisposition and environmental factors are thought to interact to produce biological changes in the brain, particularly in the hippocampus, temporal lobes, and dopaminergic pathways that project to the limbic system. Exposure to influenza virus during the fifth to sixth months of gestation appears to predispose to schizophrenia.
- The average age at onset for schizophrenia is 15 to 25 years for men and 25 to 35 years for women. There is a higher incidence in industrialized societies.
- The positive symptoms of schizophrenia are thought to be due to excessive dopamine D_2 receptor activation in the brain. Disorganized thinking (inability to connect thoughts logically), disorganized speech (rambling, tangentiality), delusions (fixed system of false beliefs), and hallucinations (sensory perceptions when no apparent stimulus exists) are typical positive symptoms. Delusions are often persecutory, grandiose, or controlling. Hallucinations are most often auditory but may also be visual, olfactory, gustatory, or tactile. Positive symptoms respond to drugs that decrease dopamine activity in the brain (e.g., olanzapine, quetiapine).
- Negative symptoms are thought to be mediated by dopamine D_1 receptors in the brain. Drugs that block D_1 receptors (e.g., clozapine) may alleviate some of the negative symptoms, which include social withdrawal, flat affect, poverty of speech, ritualistic posturing, and autism.

Major Depressive Disorder

Major depressive disorder (MDD), once referred to as endogenous depression (or depression that arises from innate characteristics of the person), is now understood to be a complex illness involving inherited genetic susceptibility and symptoms associated with specific alterations in brain structures and functioning. According to *DSM-IV-TR*[2] the diagnosis of MDD requires the presence of multiple symptoms that

TABLE 48-3	RISK FACTORS FOR MAJOR DEPRESSION AND BIPOLAR DISORDERS	
RISK FACTOR	**MAJOR DEPRESSION**	**BIPOLAR DISORDER**
Lifetime prevalence (%)	Overall: 5.2-17.1	Bipolar I: 0.9-1.6
	Females: 7.4-21.3	Bipolar II: 0.3-3
	Males: 2.8-12.7	Spectrum: 3-6
Female/male ratio (U.S.)	1.7-2.6	No significant differences
Age at onset (yr) (U.S.)	23.8-25.6	18-27
Social class	No clear relationship	Slight increase in upper classes
Marital status	Divorced and separated have 2× increase compared to married or never married	More frequent in people with multiple divorces and unmarried
Race and ethnicity	No relationship	No relationship
Family history	Ranges from 14.7 to 24.2 per 100 in probands; depends on severity and age of onset of depression	Bipolar I 7× more frequent in relatives of proband
		Twin studies suggest 50% to 60% increase
	For monozygotic twins, ranges from 31% to 71%; for dizygotic twins, ranges from 20% to 25%; higher for females	

From Hirschfeld RMA, Weissman MM: Risk factors for major depression and bipolar disorder. In Davis KL, Charney D, Coyle JT, Nemeroff C, editors: *Neuropsychopharmacology: the fifth generation of progress,* Brentwood, TN, 2002, American College of Neuropsychopharmacology, pp 1017-1025.

are intense enough to cause distress and to persistently impair psychosocial functioning. Depression with one or two symptoms that last 2 years or more is commonly referred to as *dysthymia*. More than 40% of adults with MDD remain untreated, probably because of underdetection.[39] Some people experience a seasonal pattern to depression (i.e., seasonal affective disorder *[SAD]*), where depression is more likely to occur in the fall or winter months. This occurs in one third of the cases, enough that SAD is a new entry for *DSM-IV-TR.*[2] MDD frequently occurs as a comorbid disorder to serious physical illness as well as other mental disorders. MDD can develop as a serious secondary illness or illness complication. For example, as early as 1937, researchers were able to show that cardiac patients with severe depression had higher cardiac death rates than their counterparts. Recent studies confirm that depression continues to be a significant risk factor for 1-year mortality rates in myocardial infarction patients.[40] Similarly, systematic reviews and longitudinal studies validate that patients with comorbid renal disease, cardiovascular disease, and cancer demonstrate significant improvement in overall morbidity and mortality when depressive symptoms are effectively treated.[41]

Significant rates of MDD are observed across all ages, races, education, and income groups.[42] Globally, females are diagnosed with MDD two times more often than males.[43] Depressed individuals with a family history of MDD have a onefold to twofold increased risk for developing dysthymia and anxiety disorders.[44] The complexity of managing severe depression in adolescents[45] and older adults[46,47] has made these population groups particularly concerning. As a result of the potentially serious disability, morbidity, and mortality risks directly associated with MDD, the World Health Organization (WHO) has ranked major depression among the top five global health problems.[48]

Etiology and neurobiology. Improved neurobiological research techniques have allowed for advances in the understanding of the neurobiological mechanisms of MDD. Nevertheless, the specific *cause* of MDD remains unknown. Table 48-3 summarizes mood disorder risk factors.

Cognitive processing models of depression describe dysfunctional thoughts and beliefs that occur during depression. These dysfunctional thoughts are believed to result from underlying schemas, or ways in which attention, memory, and information are organized with a negative bias. The depressed person focuses on negative information, emotions, and memories and selectively attends to negative material with automatic negative thoughts. This reinforces the continuation of the dysfunctional depressive schemas, creating a self-referent bias towards negative thoughts and expectations. When the

depressed person ruminates, everything is interpreted through a negative filter.[49-51] Research suggests that depressive states are indeed associated with slower cognitive processing, impaired attention, and bias towards negative stimuli; these appear to abate as depression goes into remission.[52,53]

Neurobiological changes associated with MDD are thought to involve neurotransmission dysregulation,[46] altered hippocampal and prefrontal cortex cell structure and functioning,[54] and impaired hypothalamic-pituitary-adrenal (HPA) system activation[55] (Table 48-4). Based on observations of low central nervous system levels of serotonin (Figure 48-6) in persons with severe symptoms of depression, the basic neurobiology of depression has been hypothesized to be reduced brain serotonin neurotransmission activity either through excessive presynaptic uptake or through stress-related down-regulation of postsynaptic receptors. Chronic or persistent vulnerability to depression is thought to be related to decreased hippocampal volume or capacity[56] and suppressed hippocampal neurogenesis.[57]

Some of the biological factors associated with depression are illustrated in Figure 48-7. HPA axis dysfunction has been associated with depression. Although no single gene has been identified as a cause of MDD,[49] both family studies[58] and twin studies[59] suggest an increased risk of heritability. Genetic susceptibility to depression may also mediate the link between stress and depression.[60,61]

Other theorists propose that increased stress hormone levels can lead to significant decreases in the expression of brain-derived neurotrophic factor (BDNF). Reduced BDNF activity has been shown to lead to hippocampal cell atrophy and, consequently, reduced neurotransmission activity in this area of the brain.[62] According to the researchers, effective antidepressant medications seemed to improve BDNF activity and thereby promote the growth and survival of serotonin neurons in this vital brain region. Significant reduction in BDNF activity, as a result of severe stress, has also been demonstrated in research animals. The HPA model of depression supports the development of novel treatments that can target cortisol activity (e.g., mifepristone) rather than serotonin activity (e.g., selective serotonin reuptake inhibitors [SSRIs]).[63]

Circadian rhythms (synchronizing cycles) are closely associated with symptoms of major depression.[49] The pineal gland in the brain produces the hormone melatonin. Brain melatonin levels can fluctuate significantly, with annual and daily increases and decreases in light and dark periods. Melatonin helps regulate circadian rhythms; in turn, these cycles govern body temperature changes and the urge to sleep. Depressed persons have been shown to suffer from low melatonin

TABLE 48-4	PREFRONTAL CORTEX AND SEROTONIN INTERCONNECTIONS: IMPLICATIONS IN DEPRESSION
INTERCONNECTED BRAIN STRUCTURES	**HYPOTHESIZED ROLE OF THESE INTERCONNECTIONS IN DEPRESSION**
Prefrontal cortex	Covering the frontal lobes, it is unique within the central nervous system for its strong interconnections with all other areas of the brain; it receives information that has already been processed by other sensory areas and then merges this information with other emotional, historical, or relevant information, thus attending to both feelings and intellect.
Limbic system structures • Hippocampus • Amygdala • Cingulate gyrus	Prefrontal cortex modulates limbic system activities (emotional and instinctive) by way of these three structures: • Major importance in cognitive function, including memory • Major importance in modulating feelings such as aggression, anger, love, and shyness • Involved in motivation and interest
Brainstem	Responsible for regulating the general state of arousal and tone of brain function; also the location of structures that manufacture various neurotransmitters, such as serotonin (5-HT), norepinephrine (NE), and dopamine (DA).
Raphe nuclei	Located in the brainstem, they manufacture 5-HT; they also modulate excessive stimuli, and the organization and coordination of appropriate responses to these stimuli.
Hypothalamus	This interconnection allows for direct prefrontal input into neuroendocrine function via the hypothalamic-pituitary axes.
Suprachiasmatic nucleus	Located in the hypothalamus, it regulates circadian (24-hr) rhythms and circannual rhythms; thus it is also implicated in seasonal affective disorder.

From Stuart GW, editor: *Principles and practice of psychiatric nursing*, ed 9, St Louis, 2009, Elsevier, p 292.

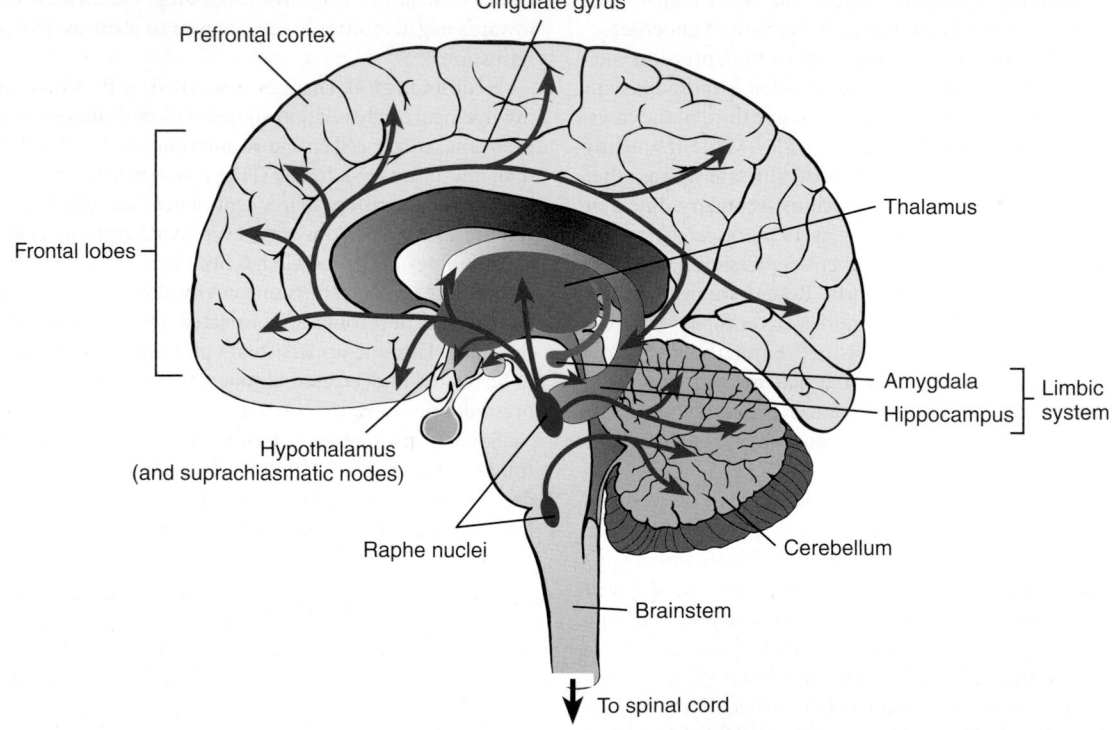

FIGURE 48-6 The serotonin neurotransmitter system implicated in depression. (From Stuart GW, editor: *Principles and practice of psychiatric nursing*, ed 9, St Louis, 2009, Elsevier, p 290.)

levels when their symptoms include disturbed sleep. In theory, natural light acts as a zeitgeber, or a biological clock synchronizer that is based on the 24-hour day-night cycle. It has been hypothesized that persons with seasonal affective disorder who are exposed to additional natural light will experience improvement in their sleep-wake cycle and, consequently, improved mental health.[49]

Clinical manifestations. To be diagnosed with MDD, an individual must experience five (or more) of the following criteria during the same 2-week period; this must also represent a change from previous functioning.[2] In addition, at least one of the symptoms must be either depressed mood or loss of interest or pleasure. *Depressed mood,*

occurring most of the day, nearly every day, is indicated by either subjective report (e.g., feels sad or empty) or observation made by others (e.g., appears tearful). In children and adolescents, depressed mood can be irritable mood. Depressed mood associated with MDD is qualitatively different from normal sadness or grief associated with loss; it is typically experienced as painful, numbing, and bottomless. Markedly *diminished interest or pleasure* in all, or almost all, activities most of the day, nearly every day (as indicated by either subjective account or observation made by others), is another hallmark symptom of MDD. Even if the depressed person does engage in activities that were previously enjoyable, interest and pleasure are not experienced. There is also significant *appetite disturbance* that results in weight loss (when not trying to diet) or weight gain (e.g., a change of more than 5% of body weight in a month). Depression is also associated with *insomnia or hypersomnia* nearly every day. Sleep symptoms include difficulty falling asleep and/or staying asleep, early-morning awakening, frequent awakenings, and waking feeling extremely tired. *Psychomotor agitation or retardation* can occur nearly every day (observable by others, not merely subjective feelings of restlessness or being slowed down). This can make normal daily activities difficult to perform. There is frequently *fatigue or loss of energy* nearly every day. Depressed people may associate their severe or sudden fatigue with serious physical illness such as cancer or cardiovascular disease. The fatigue can also make ordinary daily activities, once performed automatically, nearly impossible. Individuals experience *feelings of worthlessness or excessive or inappropriate guilt* (which may be delusional) nearly every day (not merely self-reproach or guilt about being sick). Negative self-appraisals range from pointless guilt to self-hate. In some cases, the guilt reaches delusional proportions or is markedly disproportionate to actual misdeeds or perceived failings. Negative thinking, expressed as negative views of self, life, and the future, is a common symptom of depression. There is often a *diminished ability to think or concentrate, or indecisiveness,* nearly every day (either by subjective account or as observed by others).

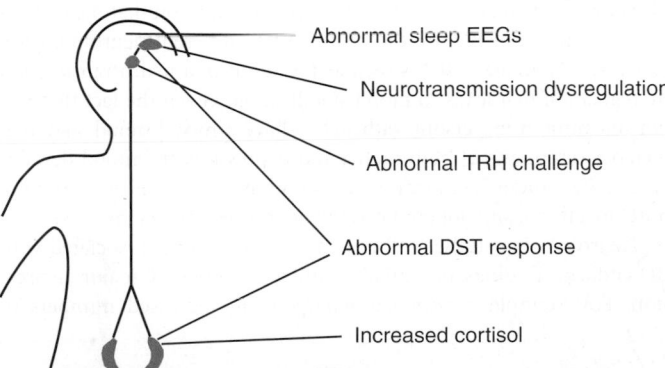

FIGURE 48-7 Biological factors related to depression. *EEGs,* Electroencephalograms; *DST,* dexamethasone suppression test; *TRH,* thyroid-releasing hormone. (From Stuart GW, editor: *Principles and practice of psychiatric nursing,* ed 9, St Louis, 2009, Elsevier, p 293.)

Finally, individuals with MDD have *recurrent thoughts of death (not just fear of dying),* display recurrent suicidal ideation without a specific plan, adopt a specific plan for committing suicide, or actually complete a suicide attempt.[49] Individuals may think about suicide passively, attempt suicide, or develop a specific plan for suicide. The clinician should ask directly about suicidal ideation to determine the presence of these thoughts, the intention to act on these ideas, and the extent of plans or preparation for suicide. If a method to complete suicide is identified, the lethality, the patient's expectation about the lethality, and the accessibility to the means of committing the plan (e.g., availability of firearms or medications) should be assessed. The client should also be interviewed to determine psychiatric risk factors, including agitation, pervasive insomnia, and impulsiveness; comorbidities, including substance abuse, psychosis (especially with command hallucinations), or personality disorder; family history of suicide; previous history of suicide attempts; and history of recent exposure to suicide.

Psychosis associated with MDD is thought to result from extreme symptoms, prolonged symptom duration, or comorbid illness complications. Hallucinations (especially auditory), delusions (especially nihilistic or somatic), and disorganization may become prominent in psychotic depression and require treatment with antipsychotic medications. Usually the psychosis is ego-syntonic, meaning that the hallucinations or delusions are consistent with their negative view of themselves, the world, and the future. Severely depressed older adults are at increased risk of depression-associated psychosis.

Pharmacologic treatment. Most antidepressants currently available act by improving brain norepinephrine and serotonin activity (Figure 48-8). Earlier generations of antidepressants had less specific effects on these neurotransmitters and significantly more side effects. Monoamine oxidase inhibitors (MAOIs) blocked the destruction of norepinephrine and serotonin once they were released into the synaptic cleft. Tricyclic antidepressants (TCAs) blocked the reuptake of norepinephrine and serotonin, thereby allowing more neurotransmitter activity. Selective serotonin reuptake inhibitors (SSRIs) include medications such as fluoxetine, paroxetine, and sertraline. Response rates vary across studies but range from 60% to 75%. No single SSRI is more effective than another. Although the side effect profile of SSRIs represents real improvement over earlier antidepressants, SSRIs are not side effect free.[64] Serotonin syndrome,[65] a serious side effect that results from excessive serotonin activity, includes altered mental status, restless agitation, myoclonus, hyperreflexia, sweating (diaphoresis), shivering, tremor, gastrointestinal upset, ataxia,

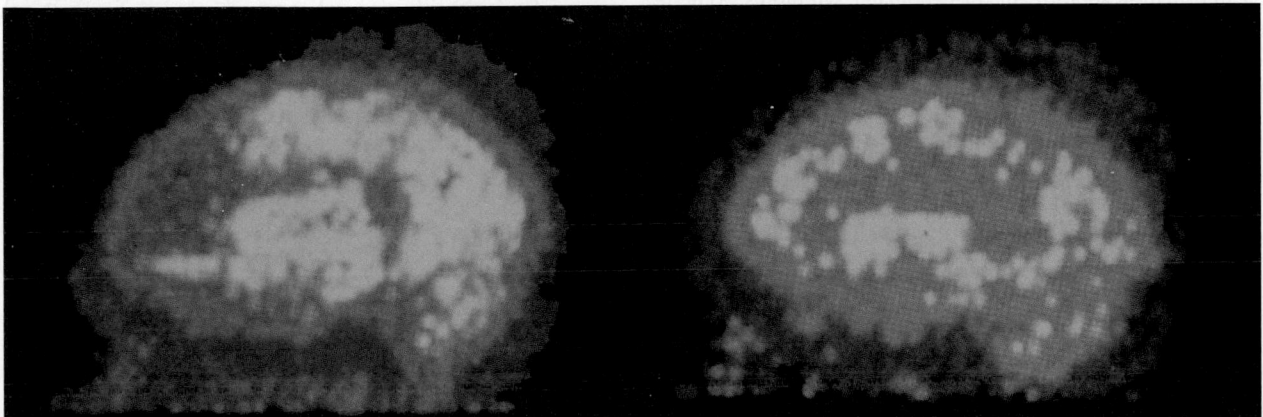

FIGURE 48-8 Positron emission tomography (PET) scan of glucose use in depressed subject *(figure on left)* showing frontal hypometabolism *(left side of figure).* This improves after treatment with antidepressant medication *(figure on right);* note increased glucose metabolism in frontal lobe *(left side of figure).* (From Stuart GW, editor: *Principles and practice of psychiatric nursing,* ed 9, St Louis, 2009, Elsevier, p 291.)

and headache. Sexual dysfunction, evidenced by loss of interest, impaired arousal, and anorgasmia, is also thought to result from SSRI-induced excessive serotonin activity. Less severe but equally troublesome side effects include gastrointestinal upset, headache, allergy, dry mouth, constipation, urination difficulties, diaphoresis, and significant weight gain. In general, it takes 3 to 6 weeks for depressed patients to notice improvements in symptoms after beginning any type of pharmacotherapy.

SSRI cellular and neurochemical mechanisms continue to be the subject of a great deal of basic and clinical research. It would appear that the SSRIs share the basic action of boosting neurotransmission activity of mood-related monoamines. More recent research findings suggest that SSRIs may also alter the genetics-based expression of BDNF and cell neurogenesis in the hippocampus.[47]

Nonpharmacologic treatment. *Electroconvulsive therapy (ECT)* has been shown to be useful for patients who have inadequate response to two to three other antidepressant treatment modalities or require intensive therapy because of psychotic features or active suicidality; ECT is also efficacious in pregnant women who cannot receive pharmacotherapy.[49] *Phototherapy,* which consists of 30 minutes per day of direct facial exposure to a 10,000-lux intensity full-spectrum white-light box, can augment antidepressant therapy or be used alone, especially when a seasonal pattern has been identified.[49] There are several *psychotherapeutic interventions* that have been shown to be effective with depression, namely, cognitive-behavioral therapy and interpersonal therapy. With mild to moderate uncomplicated MDD, these psychotherapies can be used as the first-line treatment option. When used in conjunction with pharmacologic agents, a more rapid therapeutic response can be found, especially when a client has severe, recurrent MDD.[66,67] In addition, behavioral therapies combined with maintenance pharmacotherapy appear more successful at preventing relapse than use of pharmacotherapy alone.[49]

Bipolar Disorder

Bipolar disorder (BD) is a highly complex mood disorder characterized by recurring symptoms of depression and elation that can become severe enough to produce psychosis. The most recognizable course of illness with BD is the sudden onset of severe mania lasting from weeks to months. Although mania is the hallmark of BD, the depressive phase actually represents the greatest burden on patients,[68] and it is more common for BD patients to present with depressive symptoms. BD patients experience three times more days with depression than do persons with any other mood disorders, and frequently have a continuous presence of subthreshold depressive symptomatology.[69] Because they are less likely to volunteer information about manic or hypomanic symptoms, accurate diagnosis of BD when the initial symptom profile is depression can be quite difficult or delayed. When the initial symptoms of mania are severe enough to produce psychosis, BD can be mistaken for schizophrenia.

Within the last decade, there has been a marked increase in the rate at which children are being assigned the diagnosis of BD.[70,71] BD in children is characterized by irritability, cyclical mood changes, and associated attentional deficit disorder with hyperactivity. The clinical course is often more chronic and undulating, with fewer discrete mood episodes. Some researchers have suggested that severe, nonepisodic temporal dysregulation is characteristic of pediatric BD.[72]

The two basic forms of bipolar disorder are bipolar I and bipolar II. A diagnosis of bipolar I disorder requires any past or present history of a full manic episode. There is usually a history of depressive episode(s) meeting criteria for MDD, but depression is not a requirement for the diagnosis of bipolar I disorder. Bipolar II disorder requires any past or present history of hypomania (never full mania), and a history of depression consistent with MDD. Thus what differentiates bipolar I from bipolar II disorder is the intensity of manic symptoms: bipolar I has a history of at least one full manic episode; bipolar II has a history of hypomanic

episodes (never a full manic episode). Three additional types of BD have been proposed (types II½, III, and IV), which further differentiate types I and II and better represent the clinical complexity of bipolar symptoms.[73] This suggests the concept of a bipolar spectrum and allows for earlier and more accurate diagnosis and treatment of persons who clearly suffer from mood dysregulation but who do not meet the narrow symptom criteria for bipolar I or bipolar II disorder. There are no known gender differences in the incidence of BD. The risk in the general population is 1%.

Etiology and neurobiology. Decades of clinical and genetic research findings indicate that the increased risk of developing BD is both inherited and acquired, with genetic risk reported to range from 60% to 85%.[2,74] Figure 48-9 illustrates a unified model of mood disorders. Efforts to identify the neurobiological factors that characterize BD have yielded mixed results. First, the similarities between psychosis associated with mania, psychosis associated with depression, and psychosis associated with schizophrenia are a major hurdle. Second, the depressive symptoms associated with BD differ very little from the depressive symptoms that characterize MDD (although response to treatment differs). Third, when bipolar symptom onset is gradual, changes in behavior can be mistaken for personality disorder or substance use disorder.

The neurotransmission model of BD follows the basic catecholamine hypothesis for major depression and schizophrenia. Neurotransmission activity deficits are thought to promote depression symptoms associated with BD, whereas excessive activity is believed to promote symptoms of mania and psychosis. There is a general assumption that the depression and mania of BD are the result of two different neurobiological processes. Alternately, BD is seen as the result of a neurotransmission dysregulation that leads to mood stabilization. Given the fact that it is not uncommon in persons with BD to have a mixed mood state that includes symptoms of both mania and depression, the mood destabilization hypothesis is of great interest. Both models focus on serotonin, norepinephrine, and dopamine as the neurotransmitters involved.[75]

Neuroimaging studies of brain structural changes associated with BD indicate findings potentially similar to those of major depression. For example, ventricular enlargement, increased numbers of

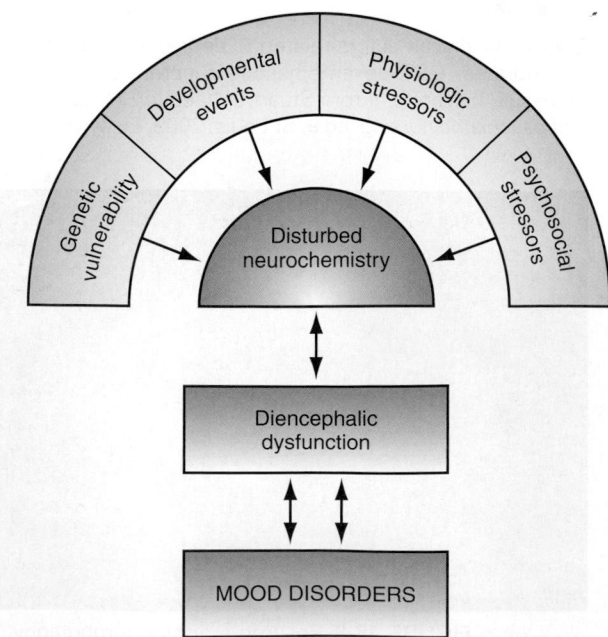

FIGURE 48-9 Unified model of mood disorders. (Redrawn from Stuart GW, Sundeen SJ: Disturbances of mood. In Stuart GW, Sundeen SJ, editors: *Principles and practice of psychiatric nursing,* ed 4, St Louis, 1991, Elsevier, p 429.)

T2 signal hyperintensities, and tissue loss in the basal ganglia, lateral and mesial temporal structures, and cortical regions have been observed. At the same time, other researchers have reported no significant tissue changes associated with BD. Experts suggest that tissue changes probably are linked with greater mania symptom severity and duration. For example, symptom onset in older age has been related to greater tissue changes.[49] Neurobiological studies of the evidence of tissue changes associated with BD thus far have not linked specific changes with depression, elation, or mania. Nevertheless, impaired functioning has consistently been associated with tissue changes. Findings such as these lend important support to the hypothesis of impaired emotion processing and impaired regulation of emotional behavior as the probable neurobiological mechanisms of BD.[75]

Clinical manifestations. *Mania* is characterized by an abnormally and persistently elevated, expansive, or irritable mood that lasts for 1 week or more (or any duration if hospitalization is required). During the period of mood disturbance, the person also typically experiences three to four of the following symptoms: *inflated self-esteem or grandiosity* (e.g., self-appraised importance, claims of limitless expertise, and insulting derogatory statements). This perceived self-importance can reach delusional proportions resulting in the person's attempting to act on his or her perceived importance, genius, and infallibility. Serious negative consequences of grandiose actions as well as financial and criminal schemes are not uncommon. Other manifestations that may become evident during the manic phase of BP include *decreased need for sleep; increased talkativeness or pressure* to keep talking; *flight of ideas or subjective experience that thoughts are racing; distractibility; increased goal-directed activity* (such as social, work or school, sexual) or *psychomotor agitation;* and *excessive involvement in pleasurable activities that have a high potential for painful, long-term consequences* (e.g., unrestrained buying spree, sexual indiscretions). The mood disturbance must be severe enough to cause marked impairment in functioning and/or maintaining relationships with others, or necessitate hospitalization to prevent harm to self or others; in addition, psychotic features in the mood disturbance may also be evident.

The *difference between mania and hypomania* can be characterized by a difference in severity and duration. For example, although the symptoms are the same, hypomanic symptoms persist for 4 days or more (instead of 7). Typically, hypomania does not include psychosis or impaired functioning. Instead, the individual experiencing hypomania has a sudden onset of increased energy, expanded self-esteem, and decreased anxiety; these symptoms typically are reported to have improved the affected individual's productivity and are experienced as an acceptable natural high. Unlike mania, it is possible for an episode of hypomania to run its course without being recognized as hypomania.

Hallucinations and delusions can occur with the psychosis that typically develops with severe, prolonged mania. Unlike the hallucinations and delusions associated with schizophrenia, the alterations in perceptions and thinking that occur with mania generally are mood congruent. In other words, grandiose mood is likely to be mirrored by grandiose delusions and hallucinations.

Pharmacologic treatment. BD is a complex condition. Although the "depression" in BD appears similar to unipolar depression, it is different with regards to pathology, outcome, and management. Caution needs to be taken to avoid manic switches or rapid-cycling induction with antidepressants.[76] Appropriate pharmacologic treatment for BD requires accurate diagnosis. Before BD diagnosis and treatment are considered, the possibility of a primary medical condition or drug reaction as the cause of depression, elation, mania, or psychosis must be considered. Because of the many overlapping symptoms, it is not uncommon for persons with BD to be misdiagnosed as depressed or schizophrenic for many years before a diagnosis of BD is made.[77]

Even though most BD patients present with symptoms of depression and do not volunteer information about mania, treatment guidelines typically focus on the management of hypomania and mania, rather than depression.[68] Most treatment guidelines since 2005 emphasize using antidepressant medications only in combination with antimanic agents. In general, medications presently indicated for use as mood stabilizers include lithium, anticonvulsants, and atypical antipsychotics. For patients not yet in treatment for BD, with severe mania or mixed episodes, lithium (most typically) or valproates are commonly used in combination with an antipsychotic to stabilize mood. Many individuals with severe BD symptoms require additional antidepressant and antipsychotic medications to achieve optimal symptom management. Antipsychotic medications have been found to be effective in remitting symptoms of psychosis as well as in preventing their recurrence. Managing the depression symptoms of BD can prove more complicated. In some cases antidepressant medications can trigger mood switching or destabilize mood; as such, antidepressant monotherapy is not recommended.

Growing numbers of anticonvulsants now are being considered for use as mood stabilizers. These include various reformulations of carbamazepine, divalproex, and lamotrigine. Several treatment guidelines suggest that lamotrigine can also be used as the first-line choice.[68] Many of the pharmacodynamic and pharmacokinetic properties of the commonly used mood-stabilizing medications have been well-defined.[78] A variety of potential mechanisms of action have been proposed for lithium. The neurotransmission effects of lithium have been attributed to calcium-dependent cell wall depolarization. Through this process, dopamine and norepinephrine are released, and major secondary messenger neurotransmitter signals are released. Lithium is absorbed in the gastrointestinal tract but is not metabolized; more than 90% is excreted by the renal system. Any interference with the excretion of lithium (e.g., fluid volume depletion, angiotensin-converting enzyme inhibitors, diuretics, ibuprofen) can lead to rapidly increasing plasma lithium levels and toxicity. Continuous patient education and routine plasma lithium level measurements help to reduce the risk of toxicity. Early symptoms of lithium toxicity include confusion, nausea, and fatigue. Prelithium assessment of liver, renal, and thyroid functioning is required. In some cases, lithium leads to hypothyroidism that requires treatment. Lastly, lithium treatment for BD requires multiple daily doses, generally twice a day or more often. Multiple daily doses can exacerbate patient ambivalence about taking lithium. Euphoria, mania, and long symptom-free periods typically are misperceived as signs that lithium no longer is needed. There is some evidence that the degree of response to lithium treatment is familial.[79]

Divalproex often is the next best choice when lithium cannot be taken. This anticonvulsant has been found to have neuroprotective effects similar to those of lithium.[78] Unlike lithium, divalproex is highly bioavailable, is metabolized by the liver, produces an active metabolite, has a long half-life, and can be used to manage acute mania. Persons with impaired liver functioning or liver disease cannot take divalproex, and the routine evaluation of plasma levels is required to reduce the risk of toxicity.

Several atypical antipsychotic medications show promise as potentially effective mood-stabilizing medications. Of these, olanzapine, risperidone, quetiapine, and ziprasidone have received considerable attention. These medications exhibit a range of dopaminergic, serotonergic, and norepinephrinergic effects that improve many bipolar symptoms, particularly when the symptoms include full mania rather than hypomania. Once-daily dosing is an important advantage. The two atypical antipsychotics that have emerged as the best treatment options for bipolar depression are either quetiapine monotherapy or quetiapine with olanzapine-fluoxetine combination (OFC);[68] if psychotic features are present, then an antipsychotic such as olanzapine, quetiapine, or risperidone is suggested. It is critical to discontinue medications that no longer seem effective, although most treatment guidelines provide little information about a specific time frame before interrupting or switching medications.

Nonpharmacologic treatment. Although pharmacotherapy is the first-line treatment choice, supplemental psychotherapy can be extremely helpful in the treatment of BP.[52] Psychoeducational approaches have been shown to reduce relapse rate by educating the patient about the illness and medication, gaining insight into early signs of relapse, and promoting regular sleep-wake cycles. Cognitive-behavioral therapy that focuses on treatment adherence and addressing barriers to treatment has been associated with fewer bipolar episodes, reduced hospitalizations, and reduced episode duration.[80] Family-focused treatment has also proven to be effective.[81] It is usually easier to engage patients during their depressive cycles than manic, because the mania itself is associated with lack of insight and motivation.

WOMEN AND MENTAL ILLNESS

Globally, women are more than twice as likely as men to suffer from depression (including unipolar depression, dysthymia, and bipolar disorder) and anxiety disorders (including panic disorder, posttraumatic stress disorder, generalized anxiety disorder, social anxiety, and phobias) (Table 48-5). These gender differences begin in adolescence and continue throughout midlife, occurring throughout childbearing years. There is very likely both a biological basis for this gender difference and an inherent vulnerability associated with the conditions of women's lives, including marital status, work and roles in society, and exposure to sexual abuse, assault, and physical violence.[43] Biologically, women and men have different physiologic responses to stress, and the hypothalamic-pituitary-adrenal axis (HPA) and sympathoadrenomedullary systems are known to play important roles in both depression and anxiety disorders. In addition, serotonin 1A (or 5-hydroxytryptamine, $5-HT_{1A}$) receptors have been implicated in both depression and anxiety, and there are known gender differences in $5-HT_{1A}$ receptor and 5-HT binding potentials.[43] Reproductive hormones also play an important role, because they impact HPA responsiveness, glucocorticoid feedback sensitivity, and brain GABA activity, and possibly destabilize homeostatic systems in vulnerable women, exacerbating anxiety and depression.[43] Thus, as hormonal levels change throughout the menstrual cycle (e.g., after parturition and during menopause), the balance and homeostasis of serotonin-specific neurotransmitter function are disrupted, and hence affect mood.

TABLE 48-5	GLOBAL HEALTH CONSIDERATIONS: PREVALENCE OF DEPRESSION AND ANXIETY IN WOMEN	
COUNTRY/ REGION	**PREVALENCE OF DEPRESSION AND ANXIETY**	**POSSIBLE CULTURAL FACTORS THAT CONTRIBUTE TO DEPRESSION AND ANXIETY**
Sub-Saharan Africa	18.2% Uganda 30.8% Zimbabwe	Female genital mutilation; abuse of women; PMDD (premenstrual dysphoric disorder) Multiple roles women fulfill in society: wives, mothers, caretakers, employees Continuing impact of HIV/AIDS
East Asia/China	24.2% older Chinese female	Female infanticide High suicide rate in Chinese Stressors of multiple roles (wives, mothers, caretakers, employees) Major social and economic changes
North America	8-11% perinatal depression 6-13% postpartum depression 36% all anxiety disorders (U.S.) 20% major depression	High incidence of rape Stressors of multiple roles (wives, mothers, caretakers, employees) Strong inverse relationship between social position and mental health outcomes Large socioeconomic inequalities linked to health inequalities
Western and Central Europe	18.2% Europe 44% Russia 40% Poland 34% Czech	High incidence of rape Stressors of multiple roles (wives, mothers, caretakers, employees) Strong inverse relationship between social position and mental health outcomes Large socioeconomic inequalities linked to health inequalities
South and South-East Asia	16.2% antenatal depression India 26.3% depression in Asia	Dowry death; domestic violence; other violence against women Burnings: in 1990, 87,000 women in India died in fires Stressors of multiple roles (wives, mothers, caretakers, employees) Major social and economic changes
Central and South America	Unclear; probably similar	Domestic violence, other violence against women Stressors of multiple roles (wives, mothers, caretakers, employees) Major social and economic changes
Middle East and North Africa	13-18% in Middle East and North Africa	Traditional arranged marriage; preference for males Stressors of multiple roles (wives, mothers, caretakers, employees)
Oceania	36% primary care have symptoms of psychological disorders; 20.5% of those have depression and anxiety symptoms	Australia: strong inverse relationship exists between social position and mental health outcomes Social disadvantage and discord, exposure to adverse life events

Data from WHO: *An evidence based review: a report to the World Health Organization (WHO),* Geneva, Nov 29, 2000. Available at http://whqlibdoc. who.int/hq/2000/who_msd_mdp_00.1.pdf. Accessed 4/25/12. *Action steps for improving women's mental health,* U.S. Department of Health and Human Services, Office on Women's Health, National Institutes of Health, National Institute of Mental Health, Rockville, MD, 2009. Available at http://store.samhsa.gov/shin/content/OWH09-PROFESSIONAL/OWH09-PROFESSIONAL.pdf. Accessed 4/25/12. Chandra PS, Herrman H, Fisher J et al: *Contemporary topics in women's mental health: global perspectives in a changing society,* West Sussex, UK, 2009, Wiley-Blackwell. Gomel MK: *A focus on women. Report for the Division of Mental Health and Prevention of Substance Abuse,* World Health Organization, Geneva, 1997. Available at http://whqlibdoc.who.int/hq/1997/WHO_MSA_NAM_97.4.pdf. Accessed 4/25/12.

CULTURAL CONSIDERATIONS

There are known differences in how cultures and regions around the world view mental health, and as such, how they express concerns about the body, self, and emotions. There are also aberrant behavioral patterns, indigenous to specific cultures that do not easily fit into *DSM-IV-TR* or *ICD-10* diagnostic categories. These aberrant behaviors, considered to be an "illness" by the indigenous population, are referred to as culture-bound syndromes in *DSM-IV-TR*. To be labeled as having a culture-bound syndrome in *DSM-IV-TR*, the disorder must be a discrete, well-defined syndrome; recognized as a specific illness in the given culture; expected, recognized, and sanctioned as a response to certain precipitants in the culture; and have a higher incidence or prevalence in societies where the disorder is culturally recognized, compared to other societies.

In addition to culture-bound syndromes, it is important for the clinician to consider the cultural identity of the individual and how that identity will influence cultural explanations of mental illness and their personal psychosocial environment. Cultural elements will also come into play in the relationship between the patient and the clinician, and in the patient's participation in diagnosis and care (e.g., adherence to psychotropic medication regimen). The clinician must consider all of these factors when formulating a treatment plan to be a culturally competent mental health provider.

GERIATRIC CONSIDERATIONS

Schizophrenia and delusional disorder may continue into old age or may appear later in life. Late-onset schizophrenia, which emerges after age 45 years, occurs more often in women than in men. Psychiatric admissions of older individuals are characterized by significantly more major depression and less dysthymia than that seen in younger adults. The incidence of BD in the geriatric age group should approach that of lifetime risk. It is extremely rare for BD to emerge after age 60 years, and all BD patients who survive to old age continue to be vulnerable to that illness.

Mood disorders in the elderly are likely to be associated with concomitant illnesses or their treatments.

Management of late-appearing psychoses is complicated by a number of factors. Older patients are more sensitive to medication than younger patients, and their response varies more than that of younger patients; they may suffer cognitive impairment; they may have visual or auditory impairment; they may be taking drugs for other chronic disorders; and they may forget to take their medications or take incorrect doses. In addition, older patients may suffer side effects such as tardive dyskinesia, a disorder related to antipsychotic drug dosage and duration and characterized by involuntary chewing motions and darting of the tongue. It is a generally accepted practice that antidepressants should be prescribed at lower dosages and titrated upward more slowly in the elderly (often referred to as "start low and go slow"). Some investigators have argued that this strategy delays response, and they suggest that as an alternative different TCAs should be used (such as nortriptyline). There has been little research on the effectiveness of SSRIs in the elderly; electroconvulsive therapy (ECT) has been shown to be effective and safe.[49]

KEY POINTS

- Mood disorders are due to disordered affect. Included in this category of psychoses are BD (periods of mania and depression) and MDD. The average age at onset is 30 years for BD and 40 years for MDD. Depression affects women twice as often as men.
- A biochemical basis for BD is supported by observations that levels of brain monoamines (norepinephrine, serotonin) are below normal or the ratio of norepinephrine to serotonin is altered. Depression is thought to occur when serotonin and norepinephrine activity in the brain is low. Mania may be due to a relative excess of norepinephrine in the context of low serotonin or acetylcholine activity. Plasma membrane transport of small molecules such as lithium also is different. BD has a familial pattern of expression, suggesting a genetic cause.
- Psychosocial factors that may affect the development and expression of mood disorders include loss (real, anticipated, or perceived) and low self-esteem. Sleep disorders accompany both extremes of mood. Depression is associated with altered rapid eye movement (REM) sleep and decreased slow-wave sleep. Mania is associated with short periods of sleep and reduced fatigue.
- Depression is manifested by low energy, inability to experience joy, difficulty initiating tasks, reduced decision-making ability, difficulty sleeping, poor appetite, weight loss, and decreased libido. Thoughts may focus on guilt, futility, emptiness, hopelessness, helplessness, and suicide.
- The management of MDD is aimed at increasing norepinephrine and serotonin activity in the brain. MAOIs reduce the rate of neurotransmitter destruction; TCAs inhibit reuptake; newer agents (fluoxetine) selectively prevent serotonin reuptake.
- Mania is manifested by high energy; inflated self-esteem; hyperactivity; inability to focus or concentrate; low sensitivity to fatigue, injury, or pain; rapid or incoherent speech; hallucinations; delusions; increased appetite and libido; decreased sleep; poor judgment; and poor impulse control. Mania is managed with lithium, a compound that inhibits the action of norepinephrine and serotonin in the brain.
- In general, BD is managed with mood stabilizers, including lithium, anticonvulsants, and atypical antipsychotics. Anticonvulsants as mood stabilizers are aimed at increasing norepinephrine and serotonin activity in the brain. MAOIs reduce the rate of neurotransmitter destruction; TCAs inhibit reuptake; newer agents (fluoxetine) selectively prevent serotonin reuptake. Depression, a common symptom in BD, is managed by using antidepressant medications only in combination with antimanic agents.

◼ SUMMARY

The clinical symptoms, causes, and neurobiological mechanisms of schizophrenia, MDD, and BD have been presented. Significant risk of psychosis is a common characteristic shared among these seemingly unrelated disorders. Brief overviews of the neurobiological basis of medications used to manage the symptoms of these disorders reflect the tremendous neurobiological advances that have been accomplished. Nevertheless, these three illnesses are potentially disabling conditions that all too often rob the affected person of academic goals, meaningful work, close relationships, self-actualization, and, in some circumstances, survival.

REFERENCES

1. International Statistical Classification of Diseases and Related Health Problems: *10th revision (ICD-10) Version for 2010: Mental and behavioural disorders.* Available at http://apps.who.int/classifications/icd10/browse/2010/en#/v. Accessed 4/27/12.

2. American Psychiatric Association: *Diagnostic and statistical manual of mental disorders (DSM-IV-TR)*, ed 4, text revision, Washington, DC, 2000, The Association.

3. American Psychiatric Association: *DSM-5 development.* Available at www.dsm5.org/proposedrevision/pages/default.aspx. Accessed 4/23/12.

4. National Institutes of Mental Health: *Serious mental illness in USA adults.* Available at www.nimh.nih.gov/statistics/index.shtml. Accessed 4/25/12.

5. Tandon R: Antipsychotics in the treatment of schizophrenia: an overview, *J Clin Psychiatry* (Suppl)72:4–8, 2011.

6. Tandon R, Nasrallah HA, Keshavan MS: Schizophrenia, "just the facts" 4. Clinical features and conceptualization, *Schizophrenia Res* 110(1-3):1–23, 2009.

7. Minzenberg MJ, Yoon JH, Carter CS: Schizophrenia. In Hales RE, Yudofsky SC, Gabbard GO, editors: *Textbook of psychiatry*, ed 5, Arlington, VA, 2008, American Psychiatric Publishing, pp 407–456.

8. Saha S, Chant D, McGrath J: A systematic review of mortality in schizophrenia—is the differential mortality gap worsening over time? *Arch Gen Psychiatry* 64(10):1123–1131, 2007.

9. Thara R, Padmavati R: Psychotic disorders and bipolar affective disorders. In Chandra PS, Herrman H, Fisher J, et al, editors: *Contemporary topics in women's mental health: global perspectives in a changing society*, West Sussex, UK, 2009, Wiley-Blackwell, pp 9–36.

10. Dixon L, Weiden P, Delahanty J, et al: Prevalence and correlates of diabetes in national schizophrenia samples, *Schizophr Bull* 26(4):903–912, 2000.

11. Schoepf D, Potluri R, Uppal H, et al: Type-2 diabetes mellitus in schizophrenia: increased prevalence and major risk factor of excess mortality in a naturalistic 7-year follow-up, *Eur Psychiatry* 27(1):33–42, 2012.

12. Bresee LC, Majumdar SR, Patten SB, et al: Prevalence of cardiovascular risk factors and disease in people with schizophrenia: a population-based study, *Schizophr Res* 117(1):75–82, 2010.

13. Fadem B: *High-yield behavioral science*, ed 2, Philadelphia, 2001, Lippincott Williams & Wilkins.

14. Frankle WG, Lerma J, Laruelle M: The synaptic hypothesis of schizophrenia, *Neuron* 39(2):205–216, 2003.

15. Keltner NL: Neuroreceptor function and psychopharmacologic response, *Issues Ment Health Nurs* 21(1):31–50, 2000.

16. Goggi J, Pullar IA, Carney SL, et al: Signaling pathways involved in the short-term potentiation of dopamine release by BDNF, *Brain Res* 968(1):156–161, 2003.

17. Saal D, Dong Y, Bonci A, et al: Drugs of abuse and stress trigger a common synaptic adaptation in dopamine neurons, *Neuron* 37(4):577–582, 2003.

18. Kapur S: Psychosis as a state of aberrant salience: a framework linking biology, phenomenology, and pharmacology in schizophrenia, *Am J Psychiatry* 160(1):13–23, 2003.

19. Portin P, Alanen YO: A critical review of genetic studies of schizophrenia: II. Molecular genetic studies, *Acta Psychiatr Scand* 95(2):73–80, 1997.

20. Rinomhota AS, Marshall P: *Biological aspects of mental health nursing*, Edinburgh, 2000, Churchill Livingstone.

21. Javitt DC, Coyle JT: Decoding schizophrenia, *Sci Am* 290(1):48–55, 2004.

22. Harrop C, Thrower P: *Why does schizophrenia develop at late adolescence? A cognitive-developmental approach to psychosis*, West Sussex, England, 2003, Wiley.

23. Weinberger DR: Implications of normal brain development for the pathogenesis of schizophrenia, *Arch Gen Psychiatry* 44(7):660–669, 1987.

24. Susser E, Lin SP, Brown AS, et al: No relation between risk of schizophrenia and prenatal exposure to influenza in Holland, *Am J Psychiatry* 151(6):922–924, 1994.

25. Venables PH, et al: Prenatal influenza exposure and delivery complications: implications for the development of schizophrenia, *Fam Community Health* 30(2):151–159, 2007.

26. Nasralla HA, Smeltzer DJ: *Contemporary diagnosis and management of the patient with schizophrenia*, Newtown, PA, 2002, Handbooks in Health Care.

27. Smith GN, Lang DJ, Kopala LC, et al: Developmental abnormalities of the hippocampus in first-episode schizophrenia, *Biol Psychiatry* 53(7):555–561, 2003.

28. Jampala VC, Taylor MA, Abrams R: The diagnostic implications of formal thought disorder in mania and schizophrenia: a reassessment, *Am J Psychiatry* 146(4):459–463, 1989.

29. Milev P, Ho BC, Amdt S, et al: Initial magnetic resonance imaging volumetric brain measurements and outcome in schizophrenia: a prospective longitudinal study with 5-year follow-up, *Biol Psychiatry* 54(6):608–615, 2003.

30. Jessen F, Scheef L, Germeshausen L, et al: Reduced hippocampal activation during encoding and recognition of words in schizophrenia patients, *Am J Psychiatry* 160(7):1305–1312, 2003.

31. Holden C: Neuroscience: deconstructing schizophrenia, *Science* 299(5605):333–335, 2003.

32. Schmitz Y, et al: Presynaptic regulation of dopaminergic neurotransmission, *J Neurochem* 87(2):273–289, 2003.

33. Evans JD, Heaton RK, Paulsen JS, et al: The relationship of neuropsychological abilities to specific domains of functional capacity in older schizophrenia patients, *Biol Psychiatry* 53(5):422–430, 2003.

34. Kapur S, Seeman P: Does fast dissociation from the dopamine D(2) receptor explain the action of atypical antipsychotics? A new hypothesis, *Am J Psychiatry* 158(3):360–369, 2001.

35. Nasrallah HA: Atypical antipsychotic-induced metabolic side effects: insights from receptor-binding profiles, *Mol Psychiatry* 13(1):27–35, 2007.

36. Aquila R: Management of weight gain in patients with schizophrenia, *J Clin Psychiatry* 63(Suppl 4):33–36, 2002.

37. Kalkman HO, Loetscher E: GAD(67): the link between the GABA-deficit hypothesis and the dopaminergic and glutamatergic theories of psychosis, *J Neural Transmission* 110(7):803–812, 2003.

38. Keltner NL, Folks DG: *Psychotropic drugs*, ed 4, St Louis, 2005, Elsevier.

39. Kessler RC, Berglund P, Demler O, et al: The epidemiology of major depressive disorder—results from the National Comorbidity Survey Replication (NCS-R), *JAMA* 289(23):3095–3105, 2003.

40. Frasure-Smith N, Lespérance F, Gravel G, et al: Social support, depression, and mortality during the first year after myocardial infarction, *Circulation* 101(16):1919–1924, 2000.

41. Halaris A: A primary care focus on the diagnosis and treatment of major depressive disorder in adults, *J Psychiatr Pract* 17(5):340–350, 2011.

42. Zubenko GS, Hughes HB 3rd, Stiffler JS, et al: D2S2944 identifies a likely susceptibility locus for recurrent, early-onset, major depression in women, *Mol Psychiatry* 7(5):460–467, 2002.

43. Kadri N, Alami K: Depression and anxiety among women. In Chandra P, Herrman H, Fisher J, Kastrup M, Niaz U, et al, editors: *Contemporary topics in women's mental health: global perspectives in a changing society*, Hoboken, NJ, 2009, Wiley-Blackwell, pp 37–64.

44. Verhagen M, van der Meij A, Franke B, et al: Familiality of major depressive disorder and gender differences in comorbidity, *Acta Psychiatr Scand* 118(2):130–138, 2008.

45. Brent DA, Birmaher B: Clinical practice: adolescent depression, *N Engl J Med* 347(9):667–671, 2002.

46. Insel TR, Charney DS: Research on major depression: strategies and priorities, *JAMA* 289(23):3167–3168, 2003.

47. National Association for the Mentally Ill: *Major depression fact sheet*, Arlington, VA. Available at www.nami.org/Template.cfm?Section=Depression&Template=/ContentManagement/ContentDisplay.cfm&ContentID=88956. Accessed 4/26/12.

48. Racagni G, Brunell N: Physiology to functionality: the brain and neurotransmitter activity, *Int Clin Psychopharmacol* 14(Suppl 1):S3–S7, 1999.

49. Joska JA, Stein DJ: Mood disorders. In Hales RE, Yudofsky SC, Gabbard GO, editors: *Textbook of psychiatry*, ed 5, Arlington, VA, 2008, American Psychiatric Publishing, pp 457–503.

50. Beck AT, Rush AJ, Shaw BF, et al: *Cognitive therapy of depression*, New York, 1979, Guilford.

51. Halberstadt L, Haeffel GJ, Abramson LY, et al: Schematic processing: a comparison of clinically depressed, dysphoric, and nondepressed college students, *Cognitive Ther Res* 32(6), 2008.

52. Phillips WJ, Hine DW, Thorsteinsson EB: Effortful information processing in patients with major depression—a 10-year follow-up study, *Clin Psychol Rev* 30(6), 2010.

53. Guro Å, Hammar Å: Is impairment in cognitive inhibition in the acute phase of major depression irreversible? Results from a 10-year follow-up study, *Psychol Psychother Theory Res Pract* 84(2):141–150, 2011.

54. Stockmeir CA, Shi X, Konick L, et al: Neurokinin-1 receptors are decreased in major depressive disorder, *Neuroreport* 13(9):1223–1227, 2002.

55. Young E, Korszun A: Psychoneuroendocrinology of depression: hypothalamic-pituitary-gonadal axis, *Psychiatr Clin North Am* 21(2):309–323, 1998.

56. Jacobs BL, van Praag H, Gage FH: Depression and the birth and death of brain cells, *Am Sci Online* 88(4):340–347, 2000.

57. Caspi A, Sugden K, Moffitt TE, et al: Influence of life stress on depression: moderation by a polymorphism in the 5-HTT gene, *Science* 301(5631):386–389, 2003.

58. Sullivan P, Kendler K: Genetic case-control studies in neuropsychiatry, *Arch Gen Psychiatry* 58:1015–1024, 2001.

59. McGuffin P, Rijsdijk S, Andrew M, et al: The heritability of bipolar affective disorder and the genetic relationship to unipolar depression, *Arch Gen Psychiatry* 60:497–502, 2003.

60. Posener JA, DeBattista C, Williams GH, et al: 24-hour monitoring of cortisol and corticotropin secretion in psychotic and nonpsychotic major depression, *Arch Gen Psychiatry* 57(8):755–760, 2000.

61. Shimizu E, Hashimoto K, Okamura N, et al: Alterations of serum levels of brain derived neurotrophic factor (BDNF) in depressed patients with or without antidepressants, *Biol Psychiatry* 54(1):70–75, 2002.

62. Manji HK, et al: Enhancing neuronal plasticity and cellular resilience to develop novel improved therapeutics for difficult-to-treat depression, *Biol Psychiatry* 53(8):707–742, 2003.

63. Phillips ML, Drevets WC, Rauch SL, et al: Neurobiology of emotion perception II: implications for major psychiatric disorders, *Soc Biol Psychiatry* 54(5):515–528, 2003.

64. Pearson G: Psychopharmacology. In Mohr WK, editor: *Psychiatric-mental health nursing*, ed 6, Philadelphia, 2006, Lippincott Williams & Wilkins.

65. Sheline YI: Neuroimaging studies of mood disorder effects on the brain, *Biol Psychiatry* 54(3):338–352, 2003.

66. Gelenberg A, Freeman M, Markowitz J, et al: *Practice guideline for the treatment of patients with major depression*, ed 3, Toronto, Ontario, Canada, 2010, Contact Resource Center.

67. Driessen E, Hollon SD: Cognitive behavioral therapy for mood disorders: efficacy, moderators and mediators, *Psychiatr Clin North Am* 33(3):537–555, 2010.

68. Nivoli AMA, Colom F, Murru A, et al: New treatment guidelines for acute bipolar depression: a systematic review, *J Affect Disord* 129(1-3):14–26, 2011.

69. Judd LL, Schettler PJ, Akiskal HS, et al: Residual symptom recovery from major affective episodes in bipolar disorders and rapid episode relapse/recurrence, *Arch Gen Psychiatry* 65(4):386–394, 2008.

70. Moreno C, Laje G, Blanco C, et al: National trends in the outpatient diagnosis and treatment of bipolar disorder in youth, *Arch Gen Psychiatry* 64(9):1032–1039, 2007.

71. Blader JC, Carlson GA: Increased rates of bipolar disorder diagnoses among U.S. child, adolescent, and adult inpatients, 1996-2004, *Biol Psychiatry* 62(2):107–114, 2007.

72. Biederman J, Faraone SV, Wozniak J: Further evidence of unique developmental phenotypic correlates of pediatric bipolar disorder: findings from a large sample of clinically referred preadolescent children assessed over the last 7 years, *J Affect Disord* 82:S45–S58, 2004.

73. Akiskal HS: The bipolar spectrum in psychiatric and general medical practice, *Prim Psychiatry* 11(9):30–35, 2004.

74. Hajek T, Gunde E, Slaney C: Striatal volumes in affected and unaffected relatives of bipolar patients—high-risk study, *J Psychiatric Res* 43(7):724–729, 2009.

75. Stahl SM: *Essential psychopharmacology: neuroscientific basis and practical applications*, ed 2, Cambridge, UK, 2000, Cambridge University Press.

76. Fountoulakis KN: The contemporary face of bipolar illness: complex diagnostic and therapeutic challenges, *CNS Spectrums* 13(9):763–774, 2008.

77. Tugrul K: The nurse's role in the assessment and treatment of bipolar disorder, *J Am Psychiatr Nurs Assoc* 9(6):180–186, 2003.

78. Keck PE, McElroy SL: Clinical pharmacodynamics and pharmacokinetics of antimanic and mood-stabilizing medications, *J Clin Psychiatry* 63(Suppl 4):3–11, 2002.

79. Cruceanu C, Alda M, Rouleau G, et al: Response to treatment in bipolar disorder, *Curr Opin Psychiatry* 24(1):24–28, 2011.

80. Lam DH, Watkins ER, Hayward P, et al: A randomized controlled study of cognitive therapy for relapse prevention for bipolar affective disorder: outcome of the first year, *Arch Gen Psychiatry* 60:145–152, 2003.

81. Milkowitz DJ, Hooley JM: Developing family psychoeducational treatments for patients with bipolar and other severe psychiatric disorders: a pathway from basic research to clinical trials, *Marital Fam Ther* 24:419–435, 1998.

Neurobiology of Nonpsychotic Illnesses

Ann Futterman Collier

℮volve WEBSITE

http://evolve.elsevier.com/Copstead/

- Review Questions and Answers
- Glossary (with audio pronunciations for selected terms)
- Animations

- Case Studies
- Key Points Review

KEY QUESTIONS

- What neurobiological alterations have been associated with panic disorder, generalized anxiety disorder, obsessive-compulsive disorder, and post-traumatic stress disorder?

- What neurobiological alterations have been associated with attention-deficit/hyperactivity disorder and autism spectrum disorder?

CHAPTER OUTLINE

Neurobiological mechanisms of mental disorders that do not cause psychosis may prove to be more similar than different from those of mental disorders associated with psychosis. These conditions already show similarity in that they are categorized by altered neuronal structures and functioning, genetic risk factors, and neurotransmission dysregulation. A major difference between psychotic and nonpsychotic illnesses is that individual variations in nonpsychotic conditions can be extensive. Greater individual variations increase the difficulty of defining the hallmark symptomatology and neurobiological basis of the condition. In addition, much has been learned about the neurobiological impact of stress response systems in psychotic illnesses, whereas the impact of stress response systems in nonpsychotic illnesses is less well understood. In the past, simple contrasts, such as comparing schizophrenia with eating disorders, invited the false assumption that one disorder may be more or less serious than another. For the affected person, such comparisons are unhelpful. Mental disorders, by definition, cause profound suffering and impairment.

ANXIETY DISORDERS

This section presents four anxiety disorders: panic disorder (PD), generalized anxiety disorder (GAD), posttraumatic stress disorder (PTSD), and obsessive-compulsive disorder (OCD).[1] Although anxiety disorders have many similar physical symptoms, they differ greatly in terms of symptom onset triggers, symptom duration, and symptom management. Because anxiety disorders are primarily characterized by physical symptoms, physical illnesses (e.g., hyperthyroidism) and medication reactions (e.g., antidepressants, steroids, anticholinergic medications) must be ruled out before a diagnosis of anxiety disorder can be made. Together with depression, anxiety disorders are the most common of all psychiatric illnesses, and aside from social phobia and OCD, occur two times more often in women than in men.

Panic Disorder (PD)

Panic disorder (PD) is characterized by acute episodes of anxiety symptoms that are unexpected, sudden, and recurrent and generate intense feelings of fear. Sudden symptom onset can cause affected persons to seek emergency health care for what they believe is a cardiac arrest, respiratory arrest, or "nervous breakdown." Panic attacks can be situation-bound, and hence occur in other anxiety disorders such as a specific phobias, social phobia, and PTSD.[2]

Depending on the subtype, panic disorder is diagnosed two to three times more often in women than in men.[1] Rates of 1% to 2% are most commonly reported. Initial onset usually occurs in late adolescence or young adulthood, with a mean age of onset of 26.6 years. Initial symptom onset in older age adults is less typical.

Etiology and neurobiology. The risk of anxiety disorder symptom onset has been associated with moderate genetic, psychological, and biological system alterations.[3] Family, twin, and adoptive family studies have consistently shown a strong genetic liability for these disorders. However, experts now speculate that the etiology question is no longer nature versus nurture. Current models seek to explain the *interactions* of nature and nurture that can create susceptibility to anxiety. Brain regions that underpin the experiences of fear, anxiety, and stress are thought of as circuits that can be shaped and altered by a wide range of forces. Neurobiological conditioning is one force shown to impact such circuits and thus is of particular importance to understanding the development of anxiety disorders.

Brain serotonin activity has been revealed to interact with both genes and environment, and these interactions contribute to what has come to be referred to as *synaptic plasticity*.[3] In this way, genes are linked with brain cell neurochemistry and psychological characteristics such as temperament. More specifically, evidence of genetic variability in negative emotions, such as anxiety, has been found in studies of serotonin transporter cells. In this research, gene variability is in gene allele length. For example, family studies have shown that siblings with serotonin transporter cells with the short-form gene allele had higher neuroticism scores than their siblings with the long-form gene allele. Research aimed at gene typing mental disorders clearly is in its infancy and findings such as these are inconclusive, but they demonstrate the possibility of genetics-based neurobiological models of anxiety.

Susceptible persons who breathe air with high levels of carbon dioxide will experience an acute onset of panic anxiety symptoms.[4] A small study of persons with panic anxiety disorder, using an infusion of doxapram (respiratory stimulant) to cause profound hyperventilation, examined the effectiveness of cognitive interventions to reduce respiratory anxiety symptoms.[5] Cognitive interventions were designed to minimize misinterpretation of drug-induced hyperventilation as a sign of danger and thereby reduce the odds of the respiratory stimulant triggering panic anxiety. Breath-by-breath analyses of the patients and healthy controls were performed. The researchers[5] hypothesized that if the respiration anxiety symptoms were the result of dysregulation within the brain respiratory control center, cognitive interventions would not be particularly effective. They found that less fearful thinking did reduce panic, but some respiratory anxiety symptoms persisted despite less fearful thinking. In other words, respiratory anxiety symptoms appeared to result both from anticipatory anxiety and from dysregulation within the brain respiratory center.

Surges of physiologic activation and physiologic instability are thought to be the hallmark neurobiological processes underlying panic anxiety disorder.[6] Multiple organ systems, including the cardiovascular and respiratory systems, are thought to be involved. Observations such as these help to explain why, for example, caffeine triggers panic anxiety symptoms in susceptible individuals. Physiologic instability may prove to be the key to identifying a genetics-based marker for susceptibility to panic. However, the biopsychological marker for the disorder is likely to be the overinterpretation of physical anxiety

symptoms (e.g., sudden increase in heart rate) as life threatening. This thinking, referred to as *learned panic,* is thought to result from inordinately high levels of life stress in early childhood.

Overwhelming life stress can increase the level of circulating glucocorticoids (stress hormones) and stimulate the release of glutamate (which inhibits neurogenesis).[7] Early-childhood life stress, specifically abuse and neglect, has been studied as a possible predictor of various adult-onset anxiety disorders. These models are based on altered serotonin, norepinephrine, and dopamine neurotransmission; glutamate release; and physiologic instability. Repeated and prolonged childhood exposure to overwhelming stress is thought to create adult susceptibility to anxiety disorders. The leading theory is that early life stress leads to an *overspecialized* or excessive stress response.

Early life stress is thought to produce adult susceptibility to anxiety by altering critical neuron structures and functioning during this critical stage of human growth and development. Brain regions most vulnerable to alteration as a result of early life stress include the hippocampus (glucocorticoid receptors), amygdala (γ-aminobutyric acid [GABA] and benzodiazepine receptors), corpus callosum (glial cells critical to myelination), cerebellar vermis (glucocorticoid receptors), and the prefrontal cortex (glucocorticoid receptors, dopamine projections, and inhibition of hypothalamic-pituitary-adrenal [HPA] axis activation).[7,8] When the developing brain of a young child is exposed to overwhelming life stress, the stress response system appears to adapt by overbuilding or building additional brain stress response pathways. Later, under less stressful adult circumstances, this overbuilt stress response system becomes maladaptive. Like a very large overpowered car on a small, winding road, the overbuilt stress response system could become the source of physiologic instability that has come to be associated with panic anxiety.[9]

Clinical manifestations. With panic disorder, no single experience consistently triggers symptom onset, although the first attack(s) frequently occur(s) during a life-threatening illness or accident, loss of a close interpersonal relationship, or separation from family. After that, they can occur during any routine activity, from reading to driving. When patients experience their first few panic attacks they frequently think they are either having a heart attack or losing their mind and it is common to seek emergency medical treatment.[2] *Physical* symptoms are most prominent and emphasized, and include respiratory distress, heart palpitations, tachycardia, pounding heart, chest pain, smothering or choking sensation, dizziness, lightheadedness, faintness, sweating, trembling, shaking, hot flushes, chills, numbness, tingling, nausea, abdominal distress, and urinary frequency.[2] *Psychological* and *cognitive* symptoms include expressed fears of dying, fear of cardiac arrest, fear of losing control, fear of nervous breakdown, derealization, depersonalization, and perceptual distortions. *Behavioral* symptoms include hyperkinesis, pressured speech, and exaggerated startle response. The attacks usually last between 5 and 20 minutes, although they can last as long as an hour. They can happen in a wavelike manner, so that they occur successively, or as described earlier, as part of another clinical disorder. Some people experience such severe anticipatory anxiety that it is hard to separate when the attack starts and ends, so that the panic attack is experienced as continuous.

Panic disorder is characterized by two important psychological symptoms: anticipatory anxiety and avoidance anxiety. *Anticipatory anxiety* refers to fearful expectation of panic anxiety onset. People with the disorder tend to develop a morbid dread of events or experiences that they come to believe *might* trigger panic anxiety. *Avoidance anxiety* refers to personal strategies used to increase feelings of control and thereby decrease the risk of panic anxiety. Persons with panic disorder strive to avoid situations and circumstances they associate with their symptoms. This helps to explain why panic disorder and agoraphobia (the phobic avoidance of public spaces beyond personal control, e.g., airports and shopping malls) often coexist.

Treatment. Panic anxiety disorder can be effectively managed with cognitive-behavioral therapy aimed at reducing fearful thinking and desensitization of cognitive and physical stress responses. When panic symptoms are disabling, medication for symptom management is recommended.[2] Long-acting benzodiazepines, such as clonazepam, are the sedatives of choice when short-term calming and symptom relief are mandatory. Tolerance to benzodiazepines develops with continuous use regardless of dosage. Misuse of benzodiazepines represents a serious health hazard. Although these drugs are useful in blocking the panic attack, they do not always decrease the anticipatory anxiety and avoidance, especially when drug regimens are initially undertaken. Many atypical psychiatric medications that can target serotonin, dopamine, or norepinephrine receptors have been clinically tested and shown to be effective treatment for anxiety symptoms. Examples of such medications found to be helpful include paroxetine, sertraline, citalopram, and fluoxetine. Unless contraindicated, β-blocker medications that dampen physical anxiety symptoms may also be helpful.

Generalized Anxiety Disorder (GAD)

GAD is characterized by chronic and persistent worry, as well as physical anxiety symptoms. The anxiety is excessive, pervasive, difficult to control, and associated with marked distress or impairment.[1] Typically, the patient experiences multiple anxiety symptoms including restlessness, fatigue, impaired concentration, irritability, muscle tension, muscle pain, and disturbed sleep.[10] Lacking clear symptom onset patterns, GAD is easily overlooked or misdiagnosed. GAD is a chronic condition, and earlier onset is associated with more overall impairment. There is high comorbidity with substance use and other anxiety disorders, depression, and personality disorders. Higher rates of GAD occur in women than men. The prevalence of GAD does not decline with age, and appears to account for most of the anxiety disorders in the elderly.[11]

Etiology and neurobiology. GAD[10] differs from other anxiety disorders in that the cognitive, psychological, and behavioral symptoms are relatively constant. Psychoanalysts developed most of the original etiologic theories concerning persistent worry. What now is referred to as persistent worry was then described as anxious expectation. Even at that early stage of discovery, it was apparent that generalized anxiety rarely occurred without comorbid conditions such as depression. This *psychodynamic* view of generalized anxiety prevailed until the late 1980s and early 1990s. More recently, *cognitive theorists* view GAD as having its origins in early attachment to the primary caretaker. Conceptually, worry is seen as an avoidance strategy for negative affect; as a distraction from realistic and proximal threats that need immediate solutions; and as a coping method to "prevent" the feared outcome, such as occurs with magical thinking. Unlike panic disorder, where the worry is more typically about physical catastrophes, in GAD, worries are more about interpersonal confrontation, competence, and acceptance. Technologically advanced research methods have now made it possible to precisely define GAD symptoms in terms of their actual qualities, intensity, and duration, but physical GAD symptoms continue to be viewed as *somatic* expressions of psychological problems.[10]

Unlike other anxiety disorders, GAD onset typically is gradual with symptom duration measured in years. As has been observed with other anxiety disorders, vulnerability to GAD likely is inherited. Twin and family study findings indicate a 30% increase in risk of GAD among the relatives of persons with the disorder.[2] Efforts to describe the neurobiological basis of GAD will no doubt be greatly advanced by theoretical models of inherited vulnerability as well as improved understanding of GAD symptoms. The most important unanswered question likely will have to do with the fact that the alterations in brain structure and functioning shown to be associated with GAD also are consistent with alterations observed with other disorders.

Preliminary positron emission tomography (PET) studies measuring brain glucose metabolism rates in GAD have shown higher than normal rates in patients at rest.[12] With GAD, apparently some brain regions undergo both increases and decreases in glucose metabolism rates. This mixed response is most apparent in the frontal and cingulate areas of the cortex, the brain region associated with worry and hypervigilance. Findings such as these lend support to the basic GAD explanatory hypothesis of anxiety symptoms as manifestations of hyperactive brain circuits. Just the opposite condition (hypoactive brain circuits) is thought to be the fundamental basis of depressive disorders.[12]

Neurotransmitter findings with GAD, as with other disorders that produce mood, thinking, and behavior symptoms, point to alterations in GABA receptors, benzodiazepine receptors, norepinephrine systems, serotonin systems, HPA axis activation, and plasma cortisol levels. Thus far, no specific alterations that can consistently explain GAD symptoms have been identified.[12] Nevertheless, one interesting observation shows considerable promise. At rest, no obvious alterations in neurotransmission are noted in GAD patients. Only when subjected to laboratory activities designed to induce stress responses is significant neurotransmitter overactivity observed. Evidence of norepinephrine receptor down-regulation lends additional support to this stress response model. Attempting to modulate overactive responses, receptor down-regulation is thought to occur automatically when subjected to prolonged, recurrent, excessive, or hyperactive neurotransmitter activity.

Whereas norepinephrine activity is thought to be associated with physical symptoms of GAD, anticipatory and avoidance symptoms are thought to be associated with activity along a key serotonin pathway linking the amygdala and frontal cortex. As might be expected, insufficient serotonin activity in specific brain regions is thought to be associated with GAD. Given the obvious symptom overlap between stress and anxiety, hyperactivity within the HPA axis and high plasma cortisol levels continue to be leading models in GAD research. Much of the difficulty in defining the neurobiological basis of GAD has to do with significant individual variations in GAD symptomatology. Uncontrollable worry (frontal cortex) is the only symptom likely to show meaningful consistency over time and from individual to individual. A second major research difficulty has to do with the frequency with which GAD symptoms co-occur with depression symptoms—so much so that some experts now view mixed depression-anxiety as a specific disorder.[2]

Clinical manifestations. The symptoms of GAD typically fall into two categories: apprehensive expectation and worry, and physical symptoms. The *worry* is often about minor issues, where the person anticipates the worst possible outcome, and finds it difficult to control. No areas of life are excluded, and worry is not limited to any single area of concern (e.g., children). *Physical* symptoms vary greatly, but people often feel "keyed up," which results in muscle tension, lightheadedness, sweating, palpitations, dizziness, and stomach distress. Concentration is typically severely impaired, and irritability is common. Diffuse anticipatory anxiety, avoidance anxiety, and dysphoria are common. Behavioral symptoms include severe sleep disturbance and fatigue. Although much of the behavior associated with GAD is likely to be the result of maladaptive methods of coping with physical and psychological GAD symptoms, impaired social and academic/employment functioning are common.

Pharmacologic treatment. Effective psychological and drug treatments for GAD can be relatively complex. When alcohol is comorbid, it may limit the effectiveness of treatment and/or delay the onset of benefits. Delayed onset of benefits from treatment is likely to be seen when GAD symptoms are long-standing and highly disabling. Lastly, neurobiological research findings indicate that effective drug treatment is likely to require one or more medications that are reliable modulators of multiple neurotransmission systems across multiple brain regions. Medications shown to relieve and in some cases remit GAD symptoms include long-acting benzodiazepines (e.g., clonazepam), partial serotonin (i.e., 5-hydroxytryptamine, 5-HT$_{1A}$) agonists (e.g., buspirone), tricyclic antidepressants (e.g., imipramine), selective serotonin reuptake inhibitors (e.g., sertraline), serotonin-norepinephrine reuptake inhibitors (e.g., venlafaxine), and long-acting β-blockers (e.g., propranolol).[13]

Nonpharmacologic treatment. Cognitive-behavioral therapy combined with relaxation training appears to be more effective than nondirective and supportive therapy for the treatment of GAD. In addition, cognitive-behavioral therapy is also superior to behavioral therapy alone.[2]

Obsessive-Compulsive Disorder (OCD)

Although listed here as an anxiety disorder, OCD will very likely be classified under a new category of disorders called *Obsessive Compulsive and Related Disorders* in the upcoming *DSM-5*.[14] The inclusion under *Anxiety Disorders* has occurred because anxiety is frequently associated with the symptoms and because yielding to compulsions temporarily decreases anxiety. However, recent research suggests that OCD more aptly belongs with a separate grouping of compulsive spectrum disorders.[2] Typically the disorder is characterized by persistent, involuntary thoughts that then provoke anxiety and involuntary anxiety management rituals. Unlike the acute onset and short duration of panic anxiety symptoms or the chronic symptoms of GAD, the obsessions and compulsions that characterize OCD are localized but nevertheless impact all areas of functioning.

More than 50% of patients diagnosed with OCD have a chronic and progressive course, 25% to 33% have a fluctuating course, and less than 15% have a phasic course with periods of complete remission.

Occasionally, there can be sudden onset of symptoms, especially when there is a neurologic basis for the illness. Predictors for poor prognosis include an early age of onset, longer duration of the illness, presence of obsessions and compulsions, poorer baseline social functioning, and presence of magical thinking.[2]

People with OCD typically strive to avoid disclosing their symptoms to relatives, friends, and health professionals. As such, accurate incidence and prevalence statistics are nearly impossible to determine. The lifetime OCD prevalence rate for the general population is 2.2%, whereas the risk in first-degree relatives is 9.2%.[2] Some experts consider this general-population estimate to be an underestimate. OCD is a severe disorder that typically begins in adolescence or early adulthood; the median age of symptom onset is about 23 years. However, 31% of the initial episodes have reportedly occurred between 10 and 15 years of age.[2] Although there is no gender difference in the prevalence rates of OCD, there is some indication that OCD might have its onset or worsen during pregnancy.[15] In addition, of children diagnosed with OCD, 70% are males.

Etiology and neurobiology. Neurobiological research findings indicate that there is a strong genetic or inherited risk of OCD.[2] Twin and family studies show a greater degree of concordance for OCD among monozygotic twins compared to dizygotic twins. Once an adult family member has been diagnosed with the disorder, child relatives are more likely to be diagnosed. Depression, anorexia, and Tourette syndrome are common OCD comorbid disorders. Close links between OCD and the hereditary neurologic disorder Tourette syndrome have been reported, but it is not clear whether this link represents an increased risk of OCD or whether Tourette syndrome and OCD are related in some other way.

OCD studies using PET brain scans have shown significant increases in glucose metabolism rates in the frontal lobes, caudate nucleus, and cingulate gyrus regions of the brain (Figure 49-1). These brain regions are directly associated with response to strong emotions. However, several OCD models of altered brain functioning have been hypothesized. One model proposes that a causal pathway for OCD exists between the frontal cortex region and basal ganglia region of the

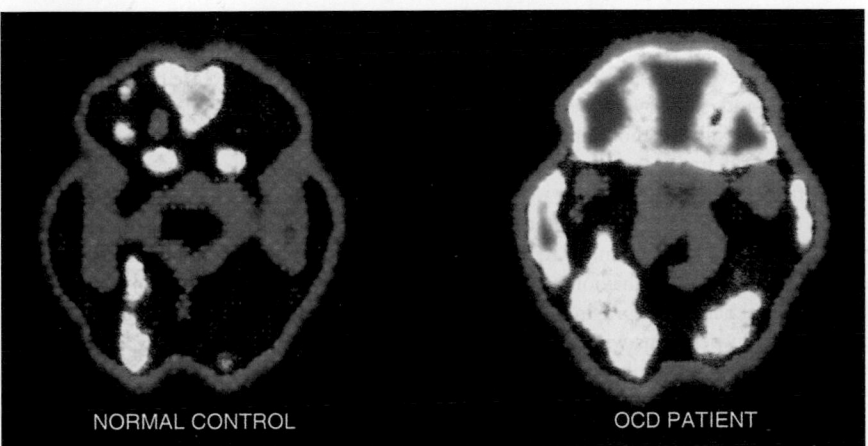

NORMAL CONTROL   OCD PATIENT

FIGURE 49-1 Hyperactivity of the orbitofrontal cortex has been a consistent finding in more than a decade of brain imaging research on patients with obsessive-compulsive disorder *(OCD)*. These positron emission tomographic images are from the initial report of this finding by a UCLA group. This excessive metabolic activity could generate spurious "error detection" signals that result in patients with obsessive-compulsive disorder experiencing repetitive adventitious feelings that "something is wrong." (Originally adapted from Baxter LR Jr, et al: Local cerebral glucose metabolic rates in obsessive-compulsive disorder: a comparison with rates in unipolar depression and in normal controls, *Arch Gen Psychiatry* 4[3]:211-218, 1987. As published in Schwartz JM: Obsessive-compulsive disorder, *Sci Med* 4:16, 1997.)

brain. This model draws on the observation that similar illnesses with well-defined etiologic factors have been shown to involve both cognitive and motor brain regions. Predictably, serotonin activity dysregulation and dysfunction also represent possible OCD models.

As shown in Figure 49-1, PET scans of the brain of a person with OCD reveal significant increases in glucose metabolism activity in the prefrontal cortex brain region. Magnetic resonance imaging (MRI) findings have suggested widely distributed cellular abnormalities such as significantly lower amounts of total white matter (connection fibers) and greater cortex cell volume. More recent models of OCD focus on the possibility of deficient serotonin inhibitory action in the basal ganglia region of the brain, which then permits excessive release of dopamine, a stimulating neurotransmitter.

PET, functional MRI (fMRI), and single-photon emission computed tomography (SPECT) studies of persons with OCD have confirmed the correlation between OCD symptoms and abnormal brain circuit activity in the orbitofrontal cortex, caudate nucleus, anterior cingulate cortex, and thalamus.[15-19] An fMRI study of medicated OCD patients and comparison subjects explored the possibility of meaningful links between anterior cingulate cortex activity and the severity of OCD symptoms by observing this activity under laboratory stress designed to trigger symptom onset. Hyperactivity was observed in one brain region (anterior cingulate cortex) and was significantly related to error making and expressed doubt, suggesting a neurobiological model for the disabling self-corrective urges associated with OCD.[19]

There are few prevailing psychological theories about the origin of OCD. Research on the cognitive thought processes suggests that cognitions do contribute to the maintenance of the disorder, even if they are not the genesis.[20] The following are some examples of faulty cognitions observed in patients with OCD: responsibility and overestimation of threat; perfectionism and intolerance of uncertainty; and importance and control of thoughts.[21] There is some evidence that people with OCD have deficits in selective attention,[22] memory bias towards disturbing themes,[23] and decreased confidence in memory.[24]

Clinical manifestations. The hallmarks of OCD are obsessions or compulsions. Symptom clusters are as follows: concern about dirt and contamination, counting, and a third group that is purely obsessional (with no compulsions). In the obsessional-only group, "slowness" is the main symptom, where patients often conduct daily activities at an extremely slow pace. Overall 90% of the patients have features of both obsessions and compulsions. However, 28% are most bothered by obsessions, 20% by compulsions and 50% by both.[2] *Obsessions* are strong, persistent, intrusive, uncontrollable thoughts. Obsessive thoughts manifest as ideas, images, and urges that dominate normal thinking and functioning. Affected persons recognize that their obsessions are products of their own mind and may judge them as senseless. Nevertheless, they are unable to stop, govern, or resist their obsessions. *Compulsions* are repetitive, ritualistic behaviors (e.g., hand washing, ordering, checking) or mental acts (e.g., praying, counting, repeating words silently) that the person performs with urgency and rigidity. They are typically content-related to the obsession. A recent meta-analysis with more than 2000 patients found four consistent "syndromes": symmetry/ordering; contamination/cleaning; hoarding; and obsessions/checking.[16] Other types of subtypes include sexual, religious, aggressive, or somatic obsessions. "Washers" comprise from 25% to 50% of the OCD samples and are concerned with dirt, contaminants, and germs. These people frequently spend hours each day washing hands or showering. "Checkers" compulsively check to see if they have done something, such as run over someone with a car or left the door unlocked. "Hoarding," the inability to dispossess of meaningless, worthless objects, is one example of the more complex compulsions.[17] Some investigators suggest that hoarding behaviors occur in

about 25% to 30% of individuals with OCD.[18] Mental compulsions should not be overlooked, because they are quite common and are often undetected since most clinicians only ask about behavioral rituals. Approximately 80% of OCD patients have both behavioral and mental compulsions; these are the third most common type of compulsions. Uncertainty is also hallmark of the compulsions: uncertainty results from a discrepancy between sensory information and internal beliefs.

Treatment. Either exposure therapy and response prevention (ETRP)[25] or CBT, when combined with effective medication treatment, can effectively diminish OCD obsessions and compulsions.[2] Nevertheless, the disorder itself makes entering treatment extremely difficult if not impossible. To be successful, CBT must target the person's obsessions and compulsions. This would require full disclosure, and as stated earlier, disclosure is very difficult. Higher doses of antianxiety and antidepressant medications (fluvoxamine, paroxetine, sertraline, venlafaxine, fluoxetine) have generally proven to be effective in reducing OCD symptoms.[2] Atypical antipsychotics, such as risperidone, in combination with antidepressants and β-blockers may be considered when OCD symptoms are disabling. Effective OCD symptom relief has been reported with the tricyclic antidepressant clomipramine, and some experts recommend the seizure medication gabapentin.[26]

Posttraumatic Stress Disorder (PTSD)

First introduced in *DSM-III*, PTSD validated that the constellation of symptoms experienced by war veterans did, in fact, cause real impairment. Although anxiety is the most prominent symptom of PTSD, depression and dissociation are common as well. PTSD is currently classified under *Anxiety Disorders* in *DSM-IV-TR*; however, many investigators believe that it should be included in a new section in *DSM-5*, titled *Trauma and Stressor-Related Disorders*.[14] Acute stress disorder is very similar to PTSD, because both are precipitated by a traumatic event. The main difference is in the time frame since the event: acute stress disorder occurs up to 1 month after the event; PTSD occurs beyond 1 month.

PTSD is typically a chronic condition. One longitudinal study with young adults reported that more than half of the sample showed no signs of remission after a 3- to 4-year period.[27] Other studies have indicated that as long as 5 years after trauma, 82% of the sample was not in remission.[28] Women appear to take four times longer to recover from PTSD than men, and are two times more likely to meet the criteria for PTSD than men.[29] Although this may be attributed to the higher rates of trauma and sexual violence that women have experienced as children, it is probably also because women respond to trauma differently than men. For example, women may be more likely to blame themselves for the event than men. There appears to be a strong relationship between PTSD and suicidal thoughts and behaviors[30] and PTSD is associated with poorer treatment outcome posttreatment.[31]

Etiology and neurobiology. Acute stress disorder is highly predictive of PTSD. Additional psychological risk factors include the following: past history of trauma (and PTSD), especially childhood trauma; depression; anxiety disorders; comorbid personality disorders; familial history of anxiety disorders, PTSD, and disrupted parental attachments; and severity of exposure to trauma.[2] High intelligence appears to be protective of PTSD. *DSM-5* is considering a special section for preschool children because their manifestation of the disorder is very different than that observed in adults.

One theory that has found support both in animal models and with patients is that during or after trauma, the stress response becomes dysregulated and chronic autonomic hyperactivity occurs. The result is hyperarousal and intrusive recollections, or the so-called "positive" symptoms of PTSD.[32-35] Evidence suggests that there is limbic hyperactivity in the amygdala and cingulate, cortical hyporesponsivity in both prefrontal and Broca areas, HPA axis dysregulation, noradrenergic activation, and heightened physiologic response to traumatic stimuli. Endogenous opioid systems also appear to be overreactive in PTSD; that is, individuals who have sustained prolonged or repeated trauma have endogenous opiates readily released with any reminder of the trauma, which leads to analgesia and psychic numbing.[36,37] Less is known about the role of the serotonergic system in PTSD, but the theory is that irritability and outbursts are related to serotonergic deficit. Some investigators have suggested that there are separate subgroups of PTSD subjects, where some show serotonin deficits and others exhibit noradrenergic sensitization.[38]

Multiple studies on brain neuroanatomy and neurocircuitry suggest that PTSD patients show decreased right and left hippocampus volumes compared to traumatized and nontraumatized control subjects.[39] It remains unclear whether hippocampi size plays a role in contributing to preexisting vulnerability to PTSD, acts as a developmental determinant, or is the outcome of traumatic stress. Limited research is available to compare brain neuroanatomy before and after PTSD treatment; some results do show that treatment using selective serotonin reuptake inhibitors (SSRIs) promotes hippocampal neurogenesis and increased volume.[40,41]

Cognitive and behavioral models of PTSD suggest that classical conditioning may play a role. Behaviorally, patients with PTSD could have higher sympathetic system arousal at the time of conditioning, which then allows them to be "more" conditionable then trauma-exposed individuals without PTSD.[42] Some studies suggest a higher incidence of PTSD after severe traumatic brain injury with loss of consciousness and few traumatic memories; this suggests that trauma itself could mediate PTSD at an implicit level.[43] There are also impairments in explicit memory associated with PTSD that could be attributable to hippocampal toxicity.[44]

Research on gender differences in the expression of PTSD suggests that women's response to stress is probably different than men's stress response, which sets the stage for women's higher incidence of PTSD. For example, women have lower cortisol levels, reduced HPA responses, and decreased serotonin transporter gene promoter polymorphism than men.[45] They also appear to have higher levels of nonsulfated dehydroepiandrosterone (DHEA) than men, who have higher levels of sulfated DHEA. The increased exposure of women to adverse events is also associated with depression and anxiety, and probably mediated by corticotropin-releasing factor (CRF).[46]

Clinical manifestations. There are five main characteristics of PTSD.[14] First, the person must have been *exposed to a traumatic event* (actual or threatened) by personally experiencing the event(s), witnessing the event(s), learning about the event(s), or experiencing repeated or extreme exposure to the event's details. Second, the person *experiences intrusive symptoms* associated with the traumatic event(s) including spontaneous or cued recurrent, involuntary, and intrusive distressing memories of the traumatic event(s); recurrent distressing dreams related to the event(s); dissociative reactions such as flashbacks that feel as if the traumatic event(s) was (were) recurring; intense or prolonged psychological distress at exposure to internal or external cues that symbolize or resemble an aspect of the traumatic event(s); and marked physiologic reactions to reminders of the traumatic event(s).

Third, the person persistently *avoids all stimuli* associated with the traumatic event(s) including internal reminders (thoughts, feelings, or physical sensations) and external reminders (people, places, conversations, activities, objects, situations) that arouse recollections of the traumatic event(s). Fourth, there are *negative cognitive and mood changes* associated with the traumatic event(s), including the inability to recall the event(s) (typically dissociative amnesia; not due to head

injury, alcohol, or drugs); persistent and exaggerated negative expectations about one's self, others, or the world; persistent distorted blame of self or others about the cause or consequences of the traumatic event(s); pervasive negative emotional state (e.g., fear, horror, anger, guilt, or shame); markedly diminished interest or participation in significant activities; feelings of detachment or estrangement from others; and persistent inability to experience positive emotions (e.g., unable to have loving feelings, psychic numbing). Finally, there is a *change in arousal and reactivity* associated with the traumatic event(s), including irritability, aggression, recklessness, self-destructiveness, hypervigilance, exaggerated startle response, problems with concentration, and sleep disturbance. None of these symptoms can be the direct physiologic effects of a substance (e.g., medication or alcohol) or a general medical condition (e.g., traumatic brain injury, coma)

Although both men and women report hyperarousal, reexperiencing, avoidance, and numbing, it is more common for women to feel anxious, to have more trouble feeling emotions, and to avoid things that remind them of the trauma. Women are also more likely than men to experience depression and general anxiety, whereas men with PTSD are more likely than women to have problems with alcohol or drugs. In contrast, men with PTSD are more likely to express anger and have anger management issues than women.[29]

Pharmacologic treatment. SSRIs are the first-line treatment for PTSD and are associated with marked improvement.[47] To date, most studies on SSRIs have been with fluoxetine,[48,49] sertraline,[50] and fluvoxamine.[51,52] Newer studies have reported success with venlafaxine extended release[53] and mirtazapine.[54] Tricyclic antidepressants (TCAs) have not been reported to be very effective, but adrenergic blockers show some improvement with both PTSD and acute stress disorder symptoms.[55]

Nonpharmacologic treatments. CBT approaches have been found to be helpful in the treatment of PTSD. Most treatment protocols include gradual or graded exposure to the trauma with imagination, real-life, and/or virtual reality therapy. Treatment also typically includes cognitive restructuring or reformulations[56] and relaxation techniques. One relatively new treatment is called eye movement desensitization and reprocessing (EMDR); results may be comparable to those achieved from use of exposure and stress inoculation.

KEY POINTS

- Anxiety disorders are characterized by irrational and debilitating fears. The four major categories of anxiety disorders are panic disorder, GAD, OCD, and PTSD. These disorders show some evidence of heritability, and biochemical correlates are suspected. Defects in serotonin pathways have been proposed as etiologic factors. Panic disorder, GAD, and PTSD are more likely to occur in females than males.

- Panic disorder is characterized by acute episodes of severe anxiety accompanied by dyspnea, chest pain, and a sense of impending doom. Palpitations, hyperventilation, dizziness, paresthesias, and diaphoresis may occur during an attack, which may last 5 to 30 minutes. Anticipatory anxiety and phobic avoidance may develop in individuals with panic disorder.

- GAD is characterized by a continuous but moderate degree of anxiety without discrete periods of acute attacks. Agoraphobia rarely develops, but chronic headaches, muscle tension, abdominal discomfort, and sleep disturbances are common.

- OCD is characterized by obsessive thoughts and compulsive behavior. Obsessive thoughts manifest as ideas, images, and urges that dominate normal thinking and functioning. Compulsions are repetitive, ritualistic behaviors (e.g., hand washing, ordering, checking) or mental acts (e.g., praying, counting, repeating words silently) that the person performs with urgency and rigidity. They are typically content-related to the obsession. There are four consistent syndromes: symmetry/ordering; contamination/cleaning; hoarding; and obsessions/checking, but they can also include sexual, religious, aggressive, or somatic content. Uncertainty is also a hallmark of the compulsions: uncertainty results from a discrepancy between sensory information and internal beliefs. OCD will not be categorized as an anxiety disorder in *DSM-5*.

- PTSD has previously been characterized as an anxiety disorder but in *DSM-5* it will likely be included in a section titled *Trauma and Stressor-Related Disorders*. It is usually precipitated by a traumatic event, after which the person typically experiences intrusive symptoms, avoids all stimuli associated with the event(s), has negative cognitive and mood changes, and experiences a change in arousal and reactivity. PTSD is frequently chronic, and women take longer to recover than men.

- Benzodiazepines and antidepressants may be used to manage all anxiety disorders; cognitive-behavioral therapy has proven to be quite successful.

NEURODEVELOPMENTAL DISORDERS

Under the proposed *DSM-5*, *Neurodevelopmental Disorders* will contain diagnoses that were previously listed in *DSM-IV* under the chapters of *Disorders Usually First Diagnosed in Infancy, Childhood, or Adolescence*.[14] Neurodevelopmental disorders are disabilities experienced by children that are primarily associated with the functioning of the neurologic system and brain. Examples include intellectual disability (previously known as mental retardation), attention-deficit/hyperactivity disorder (ADHD), autism spectrum disorder, and learning disabilities.[57] Children with these disorders typically experience problems in language and speech, motor skills, behavior, memory, learning, or other neurologic functions. Although the symptoms and behaviors can change as a person ages, many children with neurodevelopmental disorders will have permanent disabilities. As many as 12% of children in the United States ages 3 to 17 years are affected by at least one neurodevelopmental disorder, such as ADHD, learning disorders, or intellectual disability.[57] Some investigators believe that the prevalence of certain neurodevelopmental disorders, specifically autism and ADHD, has increased during the past 40 years. For example, the percentage of children reported to have ever been diagnosed with autism rose from 0.1% in 1997 to 0.7% in 2008. Because of a lack of long-term data and changes in awareness and diagnostic criteria, it is difficult to determine whether this is true.[57] Most neurodevelopmental disorders result from a combination of genetic, biological, psychosocial, and environmental risk factors, as well as behavioral risk factors such as alcohol, tobacco, or illicit drug use. There are also known environmental contaminants that can damage a child's developing brain and nervous system, such as lead, methyl mercury, and polychlorinated biphenyls.

Attention-Deficit/Hyperactivity Disorder (ADHD)

ADHD is the most common childhood psychiatric disorder. It typically begins in childhood and continues throughout adolescence and adulthood. ADHD is characterized by difficulty staying focused and paying attention, difficulty controlling behavior, and hyperactivity (overactivity). There are three subtypes: predominantly hyperactive-impulsive; predominantly inattentive; and combined hyperactive-impulsive and inattentive. Children with ADHD typically have poorer academic performance and higher rates of learning disabilities.[57] It is also common for these children to need special classroom placement, tutoring, or even to repeat a grade. When diagnosing ADHD, it is important to use several sources such as parent, child, and teacher ratings.

DSM-IV-TR estimates that ADHD occurs between 3% and 7% of school-age children, although the range varies widely across studies (e.g., 1.9% to 14.4%).[58] It accounts for as many as 3% to 50% of all mental health service referrals for children,[59] and occurs four times more often in males. In females, the inattentive type occurs more frequently than the hyperactive type. Interestingly, the gender ratio disappears in adults, but this could be due to methodological differences in studies.[57] Risk factors include family history of ADHD, psychosocial adversity, and comorbidity with oppositional defiant disorder (ODD) (50%) and conduct disorder (CD) (30%), mood disorder (15% to 20%), and anxiety disorders (20% to 25%) as well as tic disorders.[59] In fact, as many as two thirds of all individuals diagnosed with ADHD are diagnosed with other psychiatric disorders. When diagnosed with both ADHD and either ODD or CD, the child will typically have greater disability and longer persistence of symptoms. As the child grows into adolescence, ADHD is highly associated with substance use disorders. It can be difficult to differentiate ADHD symptoms from BD symptoms in children, because many of the symptoms overlap (e.g., distractibility, impulsivity, hyperactivity, mood swings, and irritability). Usually children with BD have elevated mood, decreased need for sleep, and grandiosity. As many as 75% of the children diagnosed with ADHD continue to have problems into adulthood, with the hyperactivity and impulsivity remitting and the inattention remaining.[60,61]

Etiology and neurobiology. There are a number of biological and environmental factors that have been implicated in ADHD, and a biopsychosocial model is best incorporated. Genetic models indicate that 25% to 50% of cases occur in families. First-degree relatives have a 15% to 25% chance of the disorder, and 50% if both parents have the disorder.[61] Research suggests that there are abnormalities in genes coding for proteins in central nervous system dopamine function,[62] and specific genes include the dopamine receptor gene, the dopamine transporter gene, and the dopamine-β-hydroxylase gene.[63] The specific pathophysiology of ADHD remains unclear, but research has shown that the neural circuits of the prefrontal cortex and striatum as well as the brainstem catecholamine systems that innervate these circuits show abnormalities. Exposure to toxins during pregnancy does appear to contribute to the development of ADHD, including maternal smoking[64] and lead and alcohol exposure. In addition, low birth weight, antepartum hemorrhage, prolonged labor, and low Apgar scores are associated with ADHD.[57] The role of diet (e.g., preservatives, artificial dyes, food allergies) on hyperactivity remains controversial.[57] Many scientists believe that this disorder is caused by a combination of factors, such as genetic susceptibility with exposure to environmental contaminants, rather than by any one factor.

Clinical manifestations. To be diagnosed with ADHD, a child must have symptoms for 6 or more months (symptoms within the cluster) and to a degree that is greater than that found in other children of the same age.[1] For either type of ADHD, symptoms are present by age 12 and are apparent in two or more settings (e.g., at home, school, or work; with friends or relatives; or in other activities). The symptoms must also interfere with or reduce the quality of social, academic, or occupational functioning.

Children who have symptoms of *inattention* are described in the following ways: (a) fails to give close attention to details; (b) has difficulty sustaining attention in tasks or play activities; (c) often does not seem to listen when spoken to directly; (d) frequently does not follow through on instructions; (e) often has difficulty organizing tasks and activities; (f) characteristically avoids, seems to dislike, and is reluctant to engage in tasks that require sustained mental effort; (g) frequently loses objects necessary for tasks or activities; (h) is often easily distracted by extraneous stimuli; (i) is often forgetful in daily activities, chores, and errands.[1]

Children who have symptoms of *hyperactivity and inattention* are described in the following ways: (a) often fidgets or taps hands or feet or squirms; (b) often restless during activities when others are seated; (c) often runs about or climbs on furniture and moves excessively in inappropriate situations; (d) is often excessively loud or noisy during play, leisure, or social activities; (e) often "on the go," acting as if "driven by a motor"; (f) often talks excessively; (g) often blurts out an answer before a question has been completed; (h) has difficulty waiting his or her turn or waiting in line; (i) often interrupts or intrudes on others; (j) tends to act without thinking; (k) often impatient; (l) uncomfortable doing things slowly and systematically; (m) finds it difficult to resist temptations or opportunities.[1]

Treatment. Most ADHD treatments focus on reducing the symptoms in order to improve functioning. Medication treatments especially do not cure the disorder but treat the symptoms, only while the medication is taken. Treatment typically includes medication, psychotherapy, education or training, or a combination of these treatment modalities.[57,59] *Medication treatments* most commonly comprise psychostimulants, which paradoxically have a calming effect, and are known to reduce inattention, impulsivity, and hyperactivity, and occasionally CD and anxiety disorders.[57] Stimulant medications are available in multiple forms (e.g., pill, capsule, liquid, skin patch) and in short-acting, long-acting, or extended-release varieties. The most commonly used psychostimulant is methylphenidate, which is available in both short-acting and long-acting agents (e.g., Concerta, Metadate CD, and Ritalin LA). Side effects are minor and typically disappear over time; these include delayed sleep, decreased appetite, and sometimes anxiety and irritability. Some children also report mild stomachaches or headaches. For children who do not respond well to psychostimulants, atomoxetine (Strattera) can be used, as well as TCAs, α-agonists, and some anxiolytic medications.[57]

Nonpharmacologic treatment. Psychosocial interventions are effective in teaching the child behavioral and social skills.[57,59] These can range from practical assistance (such as helping the child organize tasks or complete schoolwork) to assistance in crisis situations (such as helping the child cope with emotionally difficult events). Behavioral therapies can also teach children to monitor their own behavior, by controlling anger or by thinking before acting. Psychotherapy also can teach basic social skills, such as how to wait their turn, share toys, ask for help, or respond to teasing.

Autism Spectrum Disorder (ASD)

Autism was first introduced in the *DSM-III* in the early 1980s, and reclarified in the *DSM-IV* in the mid-1990s. In past versions of *DSM*, autism, Asperger disorder, and child disintegrative disorder were each separate disorders. Because of a wide research-base that is both reliable and valid, *DSM-5* will group these and similar disorders together under the category of *Autism Spectrum Disorder* (ASD).[14] ASD will be defined by a common set of behaviors: social/communication deficits and fixated interests and repetitive behaviors. For example, ASD patients may be interested in social interactions, but they lack the skills for reciprocal interaction. Normal attachment appears to be impaired and often there is a lack of social referencing, where others are seen and treated as objects. Individuals with autism frequently show difficulty with change and often perform ritualized, compulsive behaviors or thoughts that are reflected in repetitive questions and physical mannerisms. Clients with ASD also typically have unusual responses to sensory stimuli as well as poor

motor imitation, gait, and tone. In the past, language delays were a defining feature of the disorder. The *DSM-5* will consider language delays only as factors that influence the clinical symptoms; instead, they will be placed into the categories of social/communication or restricted, repetitive patterns of behavior. In addition, autistic symptoms must be present in early childhood (although they may not fully manifest until social demands exceed limited capacities), and symptoms must limit and impair everyday functioning. Autism has been associated with intellectual disability because between 66% and 75% of all individuals with autism have intellectual impairment. However, mental retardation and autistic disorder are considered distinct entities.

Based on past diagnostic criteria, investigators believe that the prevalence for autism is between 0.15 and 34.00 per 10,000[65] whereas that for Asperger syndrome is between 0.6 and 10.0 per 10,000 persons.[57] There appears to be a male predominance of 4:1, although females appear to be affected more severely and have greater cognitive impairment.[57] Prevalence rates for both disorders have increased since the mid-1990s. It is unclear whether this is due to an actual increase in incidence or because of an increase in both public awareness and more specific diagnostic criteria.

Etiology and neurobiology. To date, there is no known identifiable cause for autism. Popular media sources frequently suggest that measles-mumps-rubella vaccine or thimerosal exposure plays a role in the etiology; however, this has not been supported by research.[66,67] There are some medical illnesses that are associated with autism and these include tuberous sclerosis, fragile X syndrome, maternal rubella, congenital hypothyroidism, phenylketonuria, Down syndrome, neurofibromatosis, and Angelman syndrome.[57] There is also limited evidence for a genetic basis of autism, including higher concordance in monozygotic twins and low concordance in dizygotic twins, as well as greater than expected incidences of anxiety disorders, major depressive disorder (MDD), and motor tics in first-degree family members. In addition, parents of autistic children show higher rates of associated behaviors, such as rigidity, aloofness, anxiety, and restricted friendships.[68] It is fair to say that this is a very new area for research and future editions may shed more light on its neurobiology.

Clinical manifestations. First, in *DSM-5*, ASD will be defined by *persistent deficits in social communication and social interactions across contexts.*[14] This will include social-emotional reciprocity; deficits in nonverbal communicative behaviors used for social interaction; and deficits in developing and maintaining relationships, appropriate to developmental level (beyond those with caregivers). Second, ASD will be defined by *restricted, repetitive patterns of behavior, interests, or activities* including stereotyped or repetitive speech, motor movements, or use of objects; excessive adherence to routines, ritualized patterns of verbal or nonverbal behavior, or excessive resistance to change; highly restricted, fixated interests that are abnormal in intensity or focus; and hyperreactivity or hyporeactivity to sensory input or unusual interest in sensory aspects of the environment. Both the social communication and the restricted, repetitive patterns of behavior will be assigned a severity level, ranging from "1" (requiring support), to "2" (requiring substantial support), to "3" (requiring very substantial support). Thus, in the past, "milder" autism was often identified as Asperger disorder; under the new rubric, it would be assigned as level 1 ASD.

Treatment. To date, there are no established pharmacologic treatments for ASD. Research in the developmentally disordered population suggests that SSRIs may be effective in treating associated symptoms of ASD such as compulsive and repetitive behavior, behavioral rigidity, and aggression[69,70]; or that α-agonists may be effective in targeting impulsivity, hyperactivity, and poor concentration. Because there is anecdotal clinical evidence to suggest that individuals with ASD respond to very low doses (i.e., trivial) of psychoactive medications, clinicians recommend "starting low and going slow."[57]

There is a strong body of literature that supports the use of evidence-based behavioral interventions for children with ASD. These types of treatment are known to focus on social skills acquisition and environmental modifications, such as the use of schedules, visual cueing, and structured settings. One long-established method is the applied behavioral analysis approach, developed by Dr. Ivar Lovas, that starts with ASD children as young as 2 to 3 years of age and provides intensive, daily sessions. The goal of treatment is to focus on expansion of communication, emergence of new play skills, development of interactive relationships and more appropriate reaction to sensory input, and development of other pivotal skills such as imitation and requesting. Long-term results have proven successful in both raising IQ and adaptive behavior[71-73] with a sizable minority of children achieving normal educational and intellectual functioning by 7 years of age, especially with early intervention.

> **KEY POINTS**
> - There are a number of biological and environmental factors that have been implicated in both ASD and ADHD, and a biopsychosocial model is best incorporated. Early research on genetic models has suggested a limited basis of contribution to these disorders.
> - ADHD subtypes include symptoms of inattention or hyperactivity and impulsivity. The disorder typically continues into adulthood, with symptoms of inattention most common. Psychostimulant medications can effectively reduce the symptoms and improve daily functioning in most children and adults, but there is no "cure" for the disorder. Psychosocial interventions offer both practical assistance (such as help organizing tasks or completing schoolwork) and assistance in crisis situations (such as dealing with emotionally difficult events); in addition, these interventions teach behavioral self-control.
> - ASD captures the features of autism and Asperger syndrome. Children are given a severity rating from 1 (requiring support) to 3 (requiring substantial support) for symptoms that fall into the categories of (a) deficits in social communication and social interaction and (b) restricted, repetitive patterns of behavior, interests, or activities. There are no established pharmacologic treatments for ASD; however, behavior intervention, especially if provided early, assists children in developing behavioral, communication, and social skills.

SUMMARY

Hypotheses regarding the cause and pathogenesis, clinical manifestations, and implications for management of representative subsets have been presented. It is important to recognize that these disorders represent a mixture of biological, psychological, social, and environmental factors. Researchers have yet to unravel all of the mysteries surrounding the neurobiological mechanisms of nonpsychotic illnesses.

REFERENCES

1. American Psychiatric Association: *Diagnostic and statistical manual of mental disorders*, ed 4, text revision, Washington, DC, 2000, The Association.
2. Hollander E, Simeon D: Anxiety disorders. In Hales RE, Yudofsky SC, Gabbard GO, editors: *The American Psychiatric Publishing textbook of psychiatry*, Washington, DC, 2008, American Psychiatric Publishing, pp 505–608.
3. Lesch KP: Molecular foundation of anxiety disorders, *J Neural Transm* 108(6):717–746, 2001.
4. Gorman JM, Kent J, Martinez J, et al: Physiological changes during carbon dioxide inhalation in patients with panic disorder, major depression, and premenstrual dysphoric disorder: evidence for a central fear mechanism, *Arch Gen Psychiatry* 58(2):125–131, 2001.
5. Abelson JL, Weg JG, Nesse RM, et al: Persistent respiratory irregularity in patients with panic disorder, *Biol Psychiatry* 49(7):588–595, 2001.
6. Wilhelm FH, Trabert W, Roth WT: Physiologic instability in panic disorder and generalized anxiety disorder, *Biol Psychiatry* 49(7):596–605, 2002.
7. Mathew SJ, Coplan JD, Gorman JM: Neurobiological mechanisms of social anxiety disorder, *Am J Psychiatry* 158(10):1558–1567, 2001.
8. Heim C, Newport DJ, Bonsall R, et al: Altered pituitary-adrenal axis responses to provocative challenge tests in adult survivors of childhood abuse, *Am J Psychiatry* 158(4):575–581, 2001.
9. Teicher MH, Andersen SL, Polcari A, et al: The neurobiological consequences of early stress and childhood maltreatment, *Neurosci Biobehav Rev* 27(1-2):33–44, 2003.
10. Rickels K, Rynn MA: What is generalized anxiety disorder? *J Clin Psychiatry* 62(Suppl 11):4–12, 2001.
11. Sheikh JI: Anxiety in older adults. Assessment and management of three common presentations, *Geriatrics* 58(5):44–45, 2003.
12. Nutt DJ: Neurobiological mechanisms in generalized anxiety disorder, *J Clin Psychiatry* 62(Suppl 11):22–27, 2001.
13. Davidson JR: Pharmacotherapy of generalized anxiety disorder, *J Clin Psychiatry* 62(Suppl 11):46–50, 2001.
14. American Psychiatric Association: *DSM-5 development*. Available at www.dsm5.org/proposedrevision/Pages/Default.aspx. Accessed 4/23/12.
15. Kadri N, Alami K: Depression and anxiety among women. In Chandra P, Herrman H, Fisher J, et al, editors: *Contemporary topics in women's mental health: global perspectives in a changing society*, Hoboken, NJ, 2009, Wiley-Blackwell, pp 37–64.
16. Mataix-Cols D, do Rosario-Campos MC, Leckman JF: A multidimensional model of obsessive-compulsive disorder, *Am J Psychiatry* 162(2):228–238, 2005.
17. Winsber ME, Cassic KS, Koran LM: Hoarding in obsessive-compulsive disorder: a report of 20 cases, *J Clin Psychiatry* 60(9):591–597, 1999.
18. Brown WA: Hoarding, *Psychiatr Times* 24(13):50–52, 2007.
19. Ursu S, Stenger VA, Shear MK, et al: Overactive action monitoring in obsessive-compulsive disorder: evidence from functional magnetic resonance imaging, *Am Psychol Soc* 14(4):347–353, 2003.
20. Salkovskis PM, Wroe AL, Gledhill A, et al: Responsibility attitudes and interpretations are characteristic of obsessive compulsive disorder, *Behav Res Ther* 38(4):347–372, 2000.
21. Taylor S, McKay D, Abramowitz JS: Hierarchical structure of dysfunctional beliefs in obsessive-compulsive disorder, *Cogn Behav Ther* 34(4):216–228, 2005.
22. Clayton IC, Richards JC, Edwards CJ: Selective attention in obsessive-compulsive disorder, *J Abnorm Psychol* 108(1):171–175, 1999.
23. Radomsky AS, Rachman S: Memory bias in obsessive-compulsive disorder (OCD), *Behav Res Ther* 37(7):605–618, 1999.
24. MacDonald PA, Antony MM, MacLeod CM: Memory and confidence in memory judgments among individuals with obsessive compulsive disorder and non-clinical controls, *Behav Res Ther* 35(6):497–505, 1997.
25. Fisher PL, Wells A: How effective are cognitive and behavioral treatments for obsessive-compulsive disorder? A clinical significance analysis, *Behav Res Ther* 43(12):1543–1558, 2005.
26. Endler NS, Kocovski NL: Personality disorders at the crossroads, *J Pers Disord* 16(6):487–502, 2002.
27. Perkonigg A, Pfister H, Stein MB, et al: Longitudinal course of posttraumatic stress disorder and posttraumatic stress disorder symptoms in a community sample of adolescents and young adults, *J Am Acad Child Adolesc Psychiatr* 27:567–572, 2005.

28. Zlotnick C, Warshaw M, Shea MA, et al: Chronicity in posttraumatic stress disorder (PTSD) and predictors of course of comorbid PTSD in patients with anxiety disorders, *J Trauma Stress* 12(1):89–100, 1999.

29. Department of Veteran Affairs [online]: *Women, trauma, and PTSD.* Available at www.ptsd.va.gov/public/pages/women-trauma-and-ptsd.asp. Accessed 2/10/12.

30. Panagioti M, Gooding P, Tarrier N: Posttraumatic stress disorder and suicidal behavior: a narrative review, *Clin Psychol Rev* 29:471–482, 2009.

31. Tarrier N: The cognitive and behavioral treatment of PTSD: what is known and what is known to be unknown: how not to fall into the practice gap, *Clin Psychol Sci Pract* 17(2):134–143, 2010.

32. Anisman H, Pizzino A, Sklar LS: Coping with stress, norepinephrine depletion and escape performance, *Brain Res* 191(2):583–588, 1980.

33. Geracioti TD, Baker DG, Ekhator NN, et al: CSF norepinephrine concentrations in posttraumatic stress disorder, *Am J Psychiatry* 158(8):1227–1230, 2001.

34. Young EA, Breslau N: Cortisol and catecholamines in posttraumatic stress disorder—an epidemiologic community study, *Arch Gen Psychiatry* 61(4):394–401, 2004.

35. Young EA, Breslau N: Saliva cortisol in posttraumatic stress disorder: a community epidemiologic study, *Biol Psychiatry* 56(3):205–209, 2004.

36. van der Kolk BA: The psychobiology and psychopharmacology of PTSD, *Hum Psychopharmacol-Clin Exper* 16:S49–S64, 2001.

37. Pitman RK, Vanderkolk BA, Orr SP, et al: Naloxone-reversible analgesic response to combat-related stimuli in posttraumatic-stress-disorder—a pilot-study, *Arch Gen Psychiatry* 47(6):541–544, 1990.

38. Southwick SM, Krystal JH, Bremner JD, et al: Noradrenergic and serotonergic function in posttraumatic stress disorder, *Arch Gen Psychiatry* 54(8):749–758, 1997.

39. Lindauer RJL, Vlieger EJ, Jalink M, et al: Smaller hippocampal volume in Dutch police officers with posttraumatic stress disorder, *Biol Psychiatry* 56(5):356–363, 2004.

40. Bremner JD, Vermetten E: Neuroanatomical changes associated with pharmacotherapy in posttraumatic stress disorder, *Biobehav Stress Resp Protective Damaging Effects* 1032:154–157, 2004.

41. Vermetten E, Vythilingam M, Southwick SM, et al: Long-term treatment with paroxetine increases verbal declarative memory and hippocampal volume in posttraumatic stress disorder, *Biol Psychiatry* 54(7):693–702, 2003.

42. Orr SP, Metzger LJ, Lasko NB, et al: De novo conditioning in trauma-exposed individuals with and without posttraumatic stress disorder, *J Abnorm Psychol* 109(2):290–298, 2000.

43. Bryant RA, Marosszeky JE, Crooks H, et al: Posttraumatic stress disorder after severe traumatic brain injury, *Am J Psychiatry* 157(4):629–631, 2000.

44. Bremner JD, Randall P, Scott TM, et al: MRI-based measurement of hippocampal volume in patients with combat-related posttraumatic-stress-disorder, *Am J Psychiatry* 152(7):973–981, 1995.

45. Olff M, Langeland W, Draijer N, et al: Gender differences in posttraumatic stress disorder, *Psychol Bull* 133(2):183–204, 2007.

46. Heim C, Newport DJ, Heit S, et al: Pituitary-adrenal and autonomic responses to stress in women after sexual and physical abuse in childhood, *JAMA* 284(5):592–597, 2000.

47. Stein DJ, Isper JC, Seedat S: Pharmacotherapy for post traumatic stress disorder, *Cochrane Database Syst Rev* (1):CD002795, 2006.

48. Shay J: Fluoxetine reduces explosiveness and elevates mood of Vietnam combat vets with PTSD, *J Trauma Stress* 5(1):97–101, 1992.

49. Davidson JR, Conner KM, Hertzberg MA, et al: Maintenance therapy with fluoxetine in posttraumatic stress disorder: a placebo controlled discontinuation study, *J Clin Psychopharmacol* 25:166–169, 2005.

50. Davidson JR, Rothbaum BO, Tucker P, et al: Venlafaxine extended release in posttraumatic stress disorder: a sertraline- and placebo-controlled study, *J Clin Psychopharmacol* 26(5):473, 2006.

51. De Boer M, Op den Velde W, Falger PJ, et al: Fluvoxamine treatment for chronic PTSD: a pilot study, *Psychother Psychosom* 57:158–163, 1992.

52. Neylan TC, Metzler TJ, Schoenfeld FB, et al: Fluvoxamine and sleep disturbances in posttraumatic stress disorder, *J Trauma Stress* 14(3):461–467, 2001.

53. Davidson JR, Baldwin D, Stein DJ, et al: Treatment of posttraumatic stress disorder with venlafaxine extended release: a 6-month randomized controlled trial, *Arch Gen Psychiatry* 63:1158–1165, 2006.

54. Chung MY, Min KH, Jun YJ, et al: Efficacy and tolerability of mirtazapine and sertraline in Korean veterans with posttraumatic stress disorder: a randomized open label trial, *Hum Psychopharmacol-Clin Exper* 19(7):489–494, 2004.

55. Pitman RK, Sanders KM, Zusman RM, et al: Pilot study of secondary prevention of posttraumatic stress disorder with propranolol, *Biol Psychiatry* 51(2):189–192, 2002.

56. Resick PA, Nishith P, Weaver TL, et al: A comparison of cognitive-processing therapy with prolonged exposure and a waiting condition for the treatment of chronic posttraumatic stress disorder in female rape victims, *J Consult Clin Psychol* 70(4):867–879, 2002.

57. Ursano AM, Kartheiser PH, Barnhill LJ: Disorders usually first diagnosed in infancy, childhood, and adolescence. In Hales RE, Yudofsky SC, Gabbard GO, editors: *The American Psychiatric Publishing textbook of psychiatry*, Washington, DC, 2008, American Psychiatric Publishing, pp 861–920.

58. Scahill L, Schwab-Stone M: Epidemiology of ADHD in school-age children, *Child Adolesc Psychiatr Clin N Am* 9(3):541, 2000.

59. Arnold LE, Abikoff HB, Cantwell DP, et al: National Institute of Mental Health Collaborative Multimodal Treatment Study of children with ADHD (the MTA)—design challenges and choices, *Arch Gen Psychiatry* 54(9):865–870, 1997.

60. Biederman J, Wilens TE, Spencer T, et al: Diagnosis and treatment of adults with attention-deficit/hyperactivity disorder [Editorial Material], *CNS Spectrums* 12(4):A1–A14, 2007.

61. Wilens TE, Biederman J, Spencer TJ: Attention deficit/hyperactivity disorder across the lifespan, *Annu Rev Med* 53:113–131, 2002.

62. Gainetdinov RR, Mohn AR, Bohn LM, et al: Glutamatergic modulation of hyperactivity in mice lacking the dopamine transporter, *Proc Natl Acad Sci USA* 98(20):11047–11054, 2001.

63. Wilens TE, Dodson W: A clinical perspective of attention-deficit/hyperactivity disorder into adulthood, *J Clin Psychiatry* 65(10):1301–1313, 2004.

64. Rizwan S, Manning JT, Brabin BJ: Maternal smoking during pregnancy and possible effects of in utero testosterone: evidence from the 2D:4D finger length ratio, *Early Hum Dev* 83(2):87–90, 2007.

65. Tsai L, editor: *Autistic disorder*, ed 3, Washington, DC, 2003, American Psychiatric Publishing.

66. D'Souza Y, Fombonne E, Ward BJ: No evidence of persisting measles virus in peripheral blood mononuclear cells from children with autism spectrum disorder, *Pediatrics* 118(6):2608, 2006.

67. Shevell M, Fombonne E: Autism and MMR vaccination or thimerosal exposure: an urban legend? *Can J Neurol Sci* 33(4):339–340, 2006.

68. Piven J, Palmer P, Landa R, et al: Personality and language characteristics in parents from multiple-incidence autism families, *Am J Med Genet* 74(4):398–411, 1997.

69. McCracken JT, McGough J, Shah B, et al: Risperidone in children with autism and serious behavioral problems, *JAMA* 347(5):314–321, 2002.

70. McDougle CJ, Hollway J, Scahill L, et al: Risperidone for the core symptom domains of autism: results from the study by the autism network of the research units on pediatric psychopharmacology, *Am J Psychiatry* 162(6):1142–1148, 2005.

71. Eldevik S, Jahr F, Eikeseth S, et al: Cognitive and adaptive behavior outcomes of behavioral intervention for young children with intellectual disability, *Behav Modif* 34(1):16–34, 2010.

72. Eldevik S, Hastings RP, Hughes JC, et al: Meta-analysis of early intensive behavioral intervention for children with autism, *J Clin Child Adolesc Psychol* 38(3):439–450, 2009.

73. Eldevik S, Jahr E, Hastings R, et al: Behavioural intervention for children with autism in local mainstream pre-school settings, *J Appl Res Intellect Disabil* 23(5):440, 2010.

Structure and Function
of the Musculoskeletal System

Carol L. Danning

evolve WEBSITE

http://evolve.elsevier.com/Copstead/
- Review Questions and Answers
- Glossary (with audio pronunciations for selected terms)
- Animations
- Case Studies
- Key Points Review

KEY QUESTIONS

- What are the functions of osteoblasts and osteoclasts in bone remodeling?
- What is the relationship between joint structure and joint mobility?
- Why is articular cartilage particularly susceptible to degenerative changes?
- What factors determine tendon strength and compliance?
- How does the striated structure of skeletal muscle relate to its contractile function?
- How does an action potential in the α-motor neuron lead to a contraction in the muscle cells of the motor unit?

CHAPTER OUTLINE

Movement is one of the most characteristic and visible aspects of human life. Ease of movement adds to self-worth and well-being because the ability to move is closely connected to independence. A working knowledge of the system responsible for body movement is imperative to the health care provider. This chapter examines the basic characteristics of the firm support of bone and joint structures that make motion possible and the properties of skeletal muscles that are responsible for actually moving the body's framework.

STRUCTURE AND FUNCTION OF BONE

The primary purposes of the skeletal system are to protect internal organs, provide bony attachments for muscles and ligaments, present rigid levers to allow functional movement of the body and its separate parts, and store mineral and marrow elements for forming new blood cells. Bone is highly vascular and is metabolically active from birth to death.

Composition

Bone is comprised of three main components: an organic matrix, an inorganic mineral content, and water. Accounting for approximately 25% of bone weight is an organic matrix (called **osteoid**) that is composed mostly of collagen fibers (about 94% of matrix). These collagen fibers, extending along lines of tension, give bone its tensile strength and some flexibility. Also part of the organic matrix is a homogeneous ground substance composed of protein polysaccharides, particularly **proteoglycan,** which binds between collagen fibers. These proteins may serve to transfer mechanical information within the matrix to bone cells.[1]

The cellular component of the organic matrix includes predominantly osteoblasts, osteocytes, and osteoclasts. **Osteoblasts,** formed from osteoprogenitor cells that line bone surfaces, produce the organic matrix (osteoid), which is subsequently mineralized to form new bone. Osteoblasts communicate with each other in a network of cell extensions to exchange minerals, nutrients, and stimulatory signals. When an osteoblast becomes engulfed in its own calcified matrix, it becomes a mature **osteocyte** within the bone but is still connected with other cells via its extended cell processes. **Osteoclasts** migrate to the bone surfaces in response to certain stimuli and are responsible for bone resorption and mobilization of minerals.

The second and largest component of bone is the inorganic material (mineral salts such as calcium and phosphate), which accounts for approximately 70% of bone weight. This mineral content, bound and embedded within the matrix mostly in crystals of calcium hydroxyapatite, gives bone its hard, rigid structural strength while also serving as the body's main reservoir for calcium and phosphorus.[1]

Approximately 5% of bone weight is from water located within the organic matrix surrounding collagen fibers and ground substance and within the canals that carry nutrition to bone tissues.

Microscopically, the basic unit of bone is the **osteon** or the **haversian system** (Figure 50-1). The haversian canal lies at the center of each osteon and contains blood vessels and nerve fibers. A concentric series of lamellae of mineralized matrix surrounds the central canal. Bordering the lamellae are small cavities (lacunae) that contain a bone cell, the **osteocyte.** Many small channels, the canaliculi, connect adjacent lamellae with each other and eventually with the main haversian canal. This canal system allows nutrients from blood vessels in the haversian canal to reach osteocytes. Collagen fibers connect one lamella to another within the osteon and increase the mechanical strength of bone.[2]

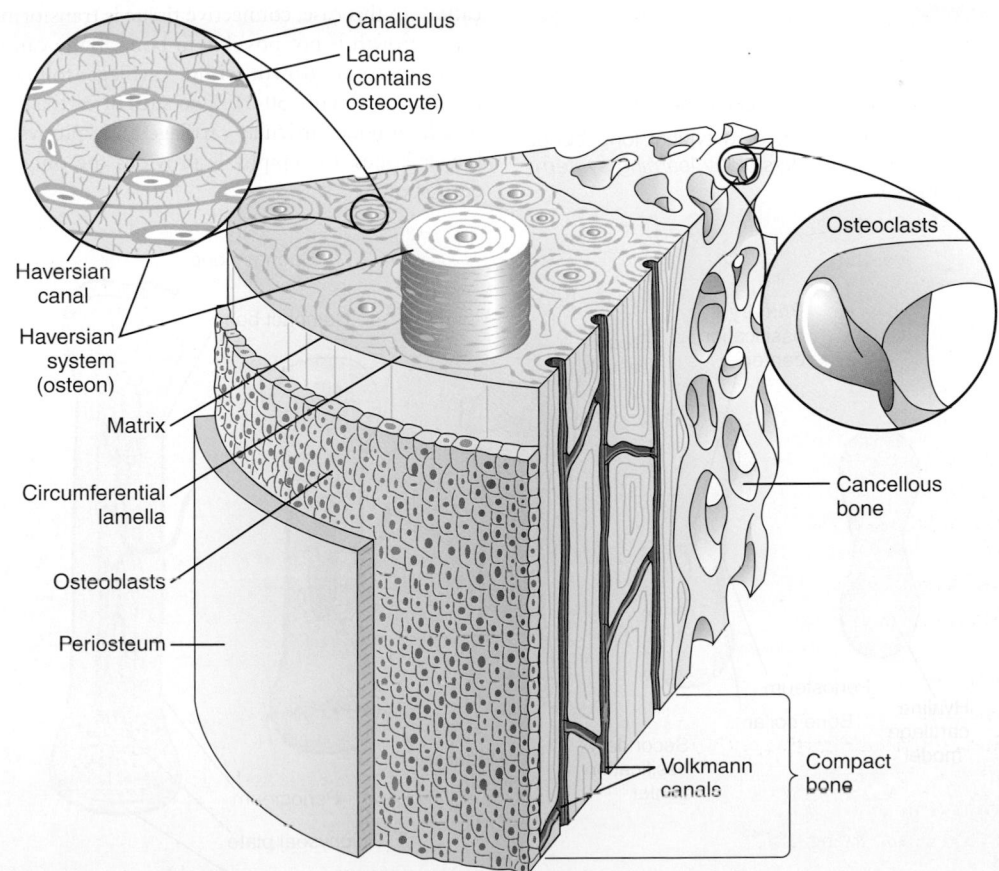

FIGURE 50-1 Microscopic anatomy of bone. The section has been enlarged to show the periosteum, osteoblasts, the haversian system, lacunae, and osteoclasts.

At the tissue level, bones are classified as two types: **cancellous** or **trabecular** bone and **compact** or **cortical** bone (Figure 50-2). **Cancellous bone** is formed in thin plates called trabeculae found within the center of long bones, vertebral bodies, and flat bones such as the pelvis. Trabeculae are laid down in response to stress and are shaped

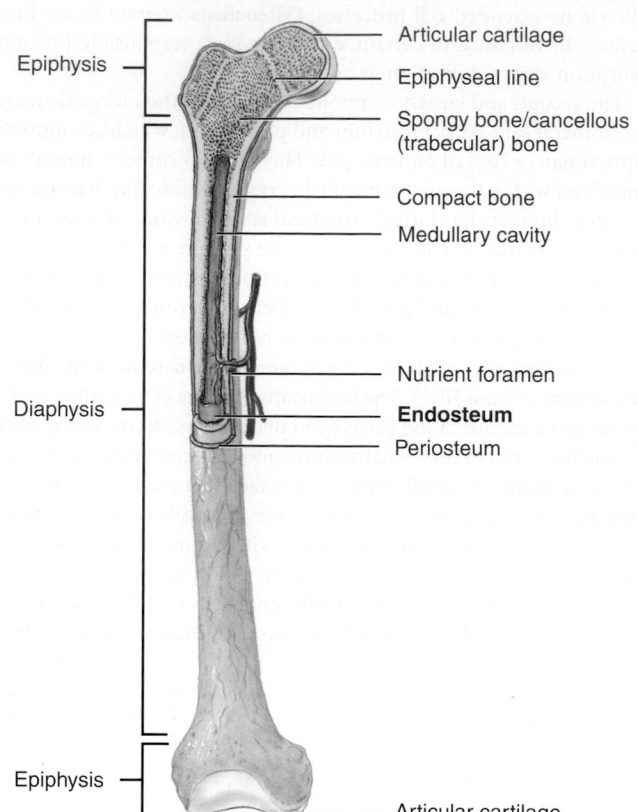

Epiphysis
— Articular cartilage
— Epiphyseal line
— Spongy bone/cancellous (trabecular) bone
— Compact bone
— Medullary cavity

Diaphysis
— Nutrient foramen
— **Endosteum**
— Periosteum

Epiphysis
— Articular cartilage

FIGURE 50-2 Structure and composition of a typical long bone. (From Applegate E: *The anatomy and physiology learning system,* ed 4, St Louis, 2011, Saunders.)

to accommodate loads placed on the bone. Cancellous bone is covered by compact bone. **Compact bone** is quite resistant to compression and is dense in structure. Compact bone is laid down in concentric layers. A tough fibrous membrane called the *periosteum* covers all bones. The periosteum is highly vascularized and provides nutrition for bone via Volkmann canals (see Figure 50-1). An inner layer of the periosteum contains **osteoblasts,** which are responsible for bone growth and repair. The periosteum covers the entire bone except for the ends, which are covered by hyaline cartilage.

In longer bones, a central cavity (**medullary cavity**) is present (see Figure 50-2). A thin membrane called the **endosteum** covers this cavity. The central cavity is filled with fatty marrow. Osteogenic cells are located in the endosteum.

Blood vessels are distributed through the haversian canals. Living cells in bone communicate with each other and the haversian system via threadlike processes.

Functional Properties
Growth and Ossification

The process of longitudinal bone growth involves endochondral ossification. In this type of growth, cartilage is replaced by bone; this process of growth is evident in embryonic development, fracture healing, and some bone tumor growth. In children, fracture through the shaft of a long bone stimulates bone growth, possibly because of increased nutrition to growth cartilage from the hyperemia associated with fracture healing. Particular attention to bone alignment or overlapping of fracture ends must be paid when managing a fracture in a child younger than 10 years of age because bone overgrowth or skeletal arrest can lead to limb length discrepancies.[3]

Circumferential bone growth occurs via intramembranous ossification. In this case, connective tissue is transformed into bone. Interstitial growth is not possible in bone. Bone can grow in length only by a process of growth within cartilage, followed by endochondral ossification (Figure 50-3). Two sites of cartilage growth are available in a long bone: articular cartilage and epiphyseal plate cartilage. In longer bones, the epiphysis provides the only growth plate for the entire bone.

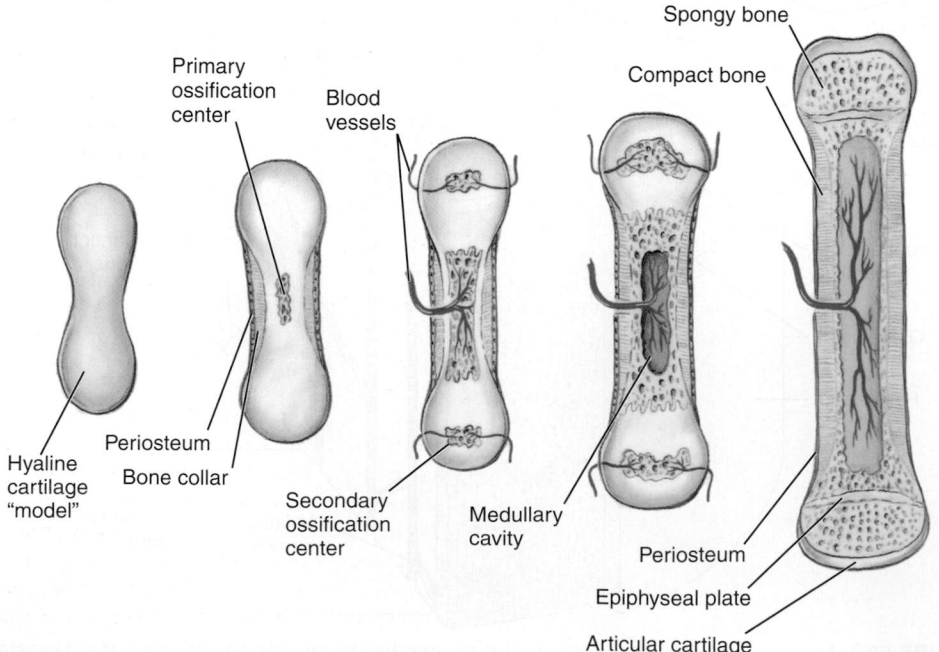

Primary ossification center
Blood vessels
Spongy bone
Compact bone

Hyaline cartilage "model"
Periosteum
Bone collar
Secondary ossification center
Medullary cavity
Periosteum
Epiphyseal plate
Articular cartilage

FIGURE 50-3 Events in endochondral ossification. (From Applegate E: *The anatomy and physiology learning system,* ed 4, St Louis, 2011, Saunders.)

Continuous Growth

The **epiphyseal plate** (see Figure 50-3) allows for lengthening of the metaphysis and diaphysis of a long bone and is the site of continuous growth. Growth and thickening of cartilage cells of the plate move the epiphysis away from the metaphysis. Calcification and replacement of cartilage occur on the metaphyseal surface (endochondral ossification). Injuries to this growth plate in children may lead to limb length discrepancies. In addition, inflammatory arthritis in children (particularly of the knee) can lead to increased blood flow to the epiphyseal plate, which also may accelerate growth or lead to premature plate closure. This also can lead to leg length abnormalities.

The function of the epiphyseal plate in the growth process may be illustrated by examining the specific zones of the plate (Figure 50-4) and determining how they contribute to the growth process. The **zone of resting cartilage** maintains adherence of the plate to the epiphysis. Immature chondrocytes and vessels penetrate this first zone from the epiphysis and nourish the plate. The **zone of young proliferating cartilage** demonstrates the most active cartilage cell growth. The **zone of maturing cartilage** contains the enlarged and mature cartilage cells as they migrate toward the metaphysis. The final zone is the **zone of calcifying cartilage,** which is a very thin line of chondrocytes and the weakest segment of the epiphyseal plate. These chondrocytes are no longer living because of calcification of the matrix.

Bone is also deposited quite actively on the metaphyseal side of the plate. With the addition of new bone, the metaphysis becomes longer.

Osteoblasts in the inner layer of the periosteum are responsible for growth in the width of bones. This process is called **intermembranous ossification.** Resorption of bone, through a process of osteoclastic resorption, causes the medullary cavity to enlarge, causing additional widening of bone.

Hormones influence bone growth. Inadequate secretion of thyroxine by the thyroid gland or insufficient growth hormone secretion from the pituitary gland results in dwarfism. Oversecretion of growth hormone results in giantism. Sex hormones, such as estradiol, are produced in higher amounts during and after puberty and can cause more rapid maturation and fusion of the epiphyseal plates. These hormones may limit the growth spurts of puberty, and early sexual maturity, especially in girls, can lead to shorter stature.

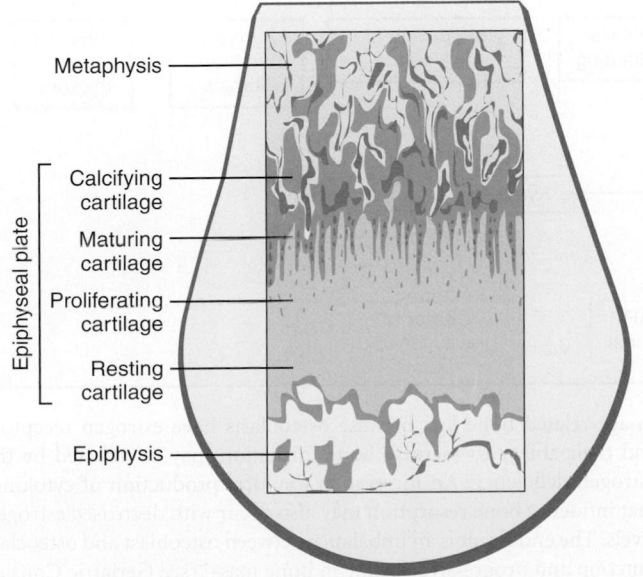

FIGURE 50-4 Zones of the epiphyseal plate.

Labels: Metaphysis; Calcifying cartilage; Maturing cartilage; Proliferating cartilage; Resting cartilage; Epiphysis; Epiphyseal plate

Bone Remodeling

Even in adulthood, bone is in a continuous state of turnover, a process that begins very early in skeletal development. This occurs in cycles of bone resorption and new bone formation called remodeling, with each complete cycle termed a **bone remodeling unit.** In a normal state, bone formation and resorption are closely coupled and balanced, serving to maintain the skeleton's peak strength by removal and repair of damaged areas, which contributes to osteocyte viability and impacts the body's calcium homeostasis.[2]

A bone remodeling unit occurs in a sequence of phases: stimulation and recruitment of osteoclasts to the area, resorption of bone, reversal and stimulation of osteoblasts, secretion of new matrix, mineralization of new bone, and completion of a resting phase.[4] The stimulation of a remodeling cycle is thought to occur with osteoblastic production of factors that stimulate the recruitment and activity of osteoclasts (such as osteoclast differentiating factor, also called receptor activator of nuclear factor κB ligand, or RANKL). One such signal of the need for bone remodeling could come from mature osteocytes within the bone sensing bone deformation or damage.[2] Osteoclasts gather at the site on the bone surface and form large multinucleated cells that begin the process of removal of bone matrix and minerals. This resorptive phase creates a pit in the bone, which is next filled with osteoblasts that begin to fill the space with bone matrix (osteoid). When the bone pit is filled, the new bone matrix is mineralized to complete the cycle (Figure 50-5).

Calcium Homeostasis

Almost all of the body's calcium supply is held within bone, but the small amount of calcium circulating in blood is essential for a wide variety of cellular functions and therefore its concentration is tightly controlled. Much of this regulation of calcium balance in bone and blood depends on hormonal effects. Parathyroid hormone maintains serum calcium levels by increasing bone resorption as well as calcium reabsorption from renal tubules. Vitamin D metabolites can increase bone mineralization by increasing calcium absorption from the intestinal tract; however, in the setting of calcium deficiency, vitamin D can stimulate bone resorption to help maintain mineral supply in the blood. Calcitonin can act as an inhibitor of bone resorption but likely only plays a minor role in adults. (See Chapter 51 for further discussion.[4])

Response to Injury, Stress, and Aging

The ability of bone to remodel after injury is important. Although remodeling of bone continues throughout life, death of the osteon or removal of calcium from bone requires that new bone be deposited to retain strength and function. Physical stresses lead to the realignment of bone trabecular systems and the deposition of additional bone at the site of increased stress. The response of bone to stress is summarized by **Wolff's law,** which states that bone is laid down where it is needed and resorbed where it is not needed.[5] If bone is immobilized or not subjected to mechanical stress, as occurs with prolonged bed rest, the activity of bone-resorbing cells increases.[6] Without external forces (or loads), osteoclast activity is greater than osteoblast activity and bone mass decreases. It is probable that during bed rest, age-related bone loss might be temporarily accelerated and may result in a greater decline in bone mass over time. Patients becoming mobile after prolonged bed rest are at risk for fractures because of a combined loss of muscle and bone strength. With loss of muscle, gait becomes unsteady and patients are more prone to falls.

Internal fixation of a fracture may also cause decreased bone strength. With metal implants, mechanical stress is dispersed from bone and carried by the implant. Bone under the plate is resorbed, and "stress relief" osteoporosis may occur. Care must be taken once implants are removed, and the bone must be protected until strength returns. Some implants are designed to compress fracture fragments to aid healing.

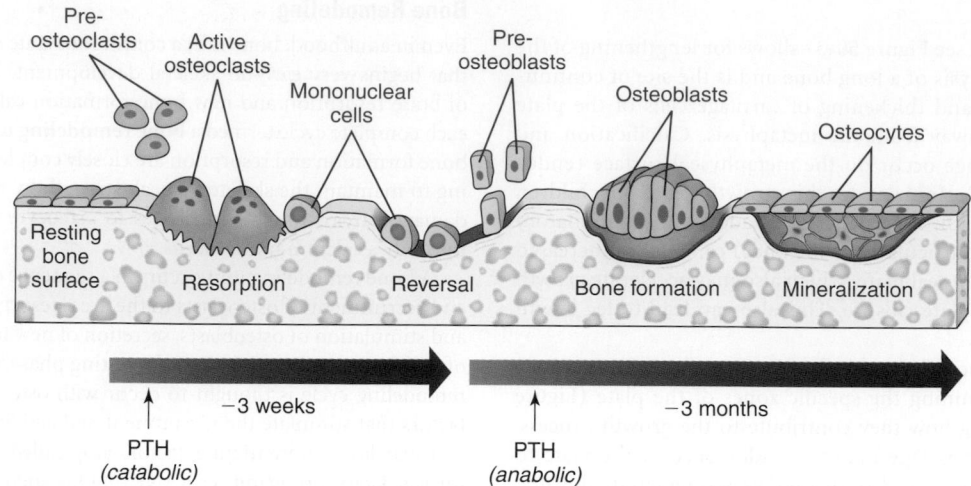

FIGURE 50-5 Bone remodeling cycle. First, osteoclasts begin bone resorption, creating the pit. Then osteoblasts enter the pit and produce bone matrix, which then calcifies. *PTH,* Parathyroid hormone. (From Garg AK: *Implant dentistry: a practical approach,* St Louis, 2010, Mosby.)

GERIATRIC CONSIDERATIONS

Changes in the Skeletal System

With aging, bone absorption exceeds bone formation. There is a net loss of bone mass and bone protein matrix. The interior of the long and the flat bones is absorbed faster than that of other bones. Trabecular bone destruction is greater than cortical bone loss. Compared to aging men, aging women have a greater amount of bone loss. The bone marrow space is decreased, with fat replacing marrow cells.

Although interior bone is lost, the circumference of the bones increases because osteoblasts on the exterior bone beneath the periosteum continue bone formation. The long bones, metacarpals, and ribs become bigger in circumference, whereas the pelvis becomes wider and the skull thicker.

The intervertebral disks become dehydrated, with narrowing of the disk space leading to a decrease in height of 3 to 5 cm. An increase in the thoracic curve occurs, resulting in kyphosis and anterior scapular displacement. This change leads to an increase in the anteroposterior diameter of the chest. A decrease in the lordotic curve results in lumbar flattening and a decrease in lumbar flexibility. Greater flexion of the knees and hips is noted. The relationship between the pelvis and the femoral head and neck also changes.

Fissuring, erosion, and thinning of cartilage occur. With the loss of cartilage, the greater pressure that subchondral bone must withstand results in increased density and the formation of joint margin osteophytes. The synovial membrane undergoes fibrosis and the synovial fluid thickens.

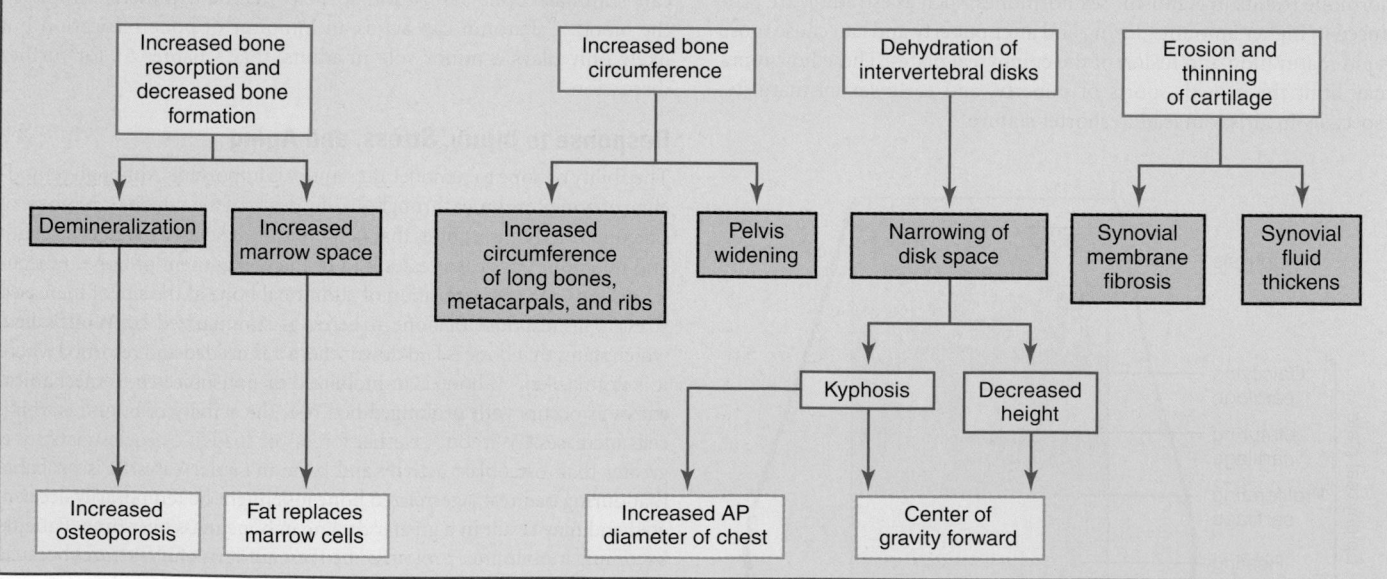

Bone mass decreases with age. Studies have shown that elderly individuals express higher levels of certain markers associated with bone resorption, whereas bone formation markers are much more variable. One common cause of increased bone resorption is calcium and vitamin D deficiency, which causes more rapid mobilization of calcium from bone. A secondary hyperparathyroidism can also result. Decreased levels of estrogen in elderly women and men can contribute to age-related bone loss because osteoblasts have estrogen receptors and their ability to increase bone formation may be affected by the estrogen deficiency. An increase in the local production of cytokines that influence bone resorption may also occur with decreased estrogen levels. The end result is an imbalance between osteoblast and osteoclast function and progressive decline in bone mass[4] (see Geriatric Considerations: Changes in the Skeletal System).

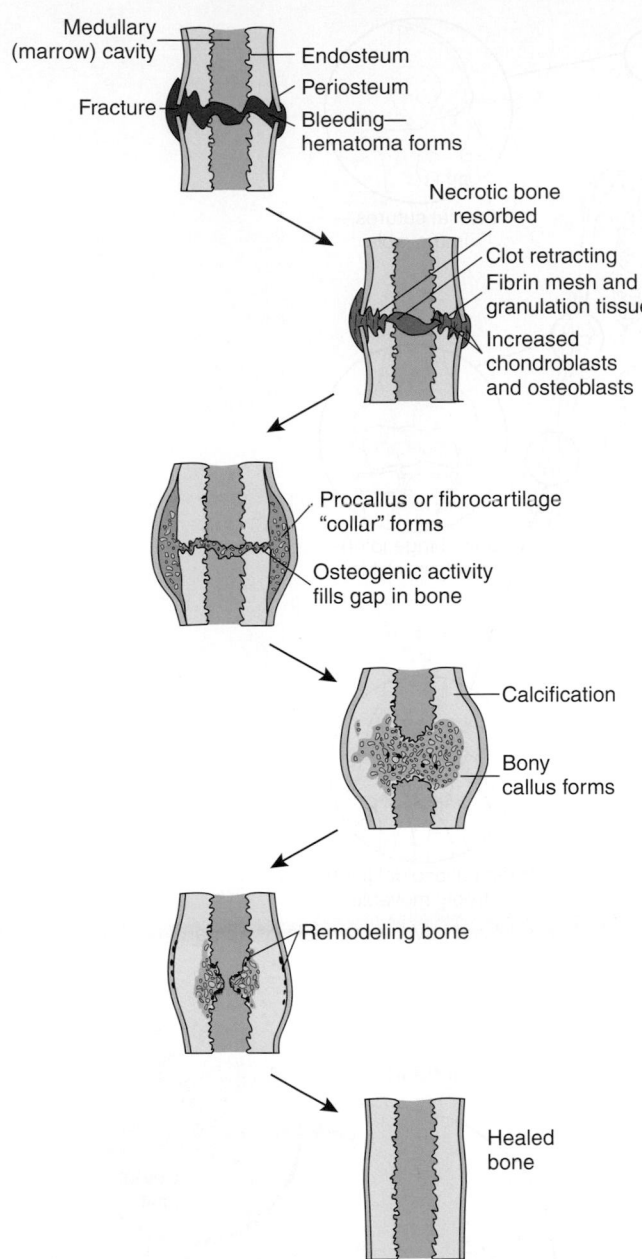

Medullary
(marrow) cavity
Endosteum
Periosteum
Fracture
Bleeding—
hematoma forms

Necrotic bone
resorbed

Clot retracting
Fibrin mesh and
granulation tissue
Increased
chondroblasts
and osteoblasts

Procallus or fibrocartilage
"collar" forms

Osteogenic activity
fills gap in bone

Calcification

Bony
callus forms

Remodeling bone

Healed
bone

FIGURE 50-6 Healing of a fracture. (From Gould BE, Dyer R: *Pathophysiology for the health professions,* ed 4, St Louis, 2011, Saunders.)

Bone mass can also decrease with certain disease processes. For example, osteoporosis is a metabolic bone disease characterized by a severe general reduction in skeletal bone mass and thus a susceptibility to fractures. In short, bone resorption is more rapid than bone formation.

Fracture Healing

Bone may heal in one of two ways after a fracture. A periosteal or external callus forms in fractures managed by closed methods. The blood supply to surrounding soft tissue and motion at the fracture site contribute to healing. Medullary callous formation takes place with rigid immobilization at the fracture site. The process of bone turnover contributes to healing.

The five stages of fracture healing are: (1) hematoma formation, 1 to 3 days; (2) fibrocartilage formation, 3 days to 2 weeks; (3) callous formation, 2 to 6 weeks; (4) ossification, 3 weeks to 6 months; and

(5) consolidation/remodeling, 6 weeks to 1 year (Figure 50-6). These five stages can be grouped into three phases: (1) inflammatory phase, (2) reparative phase (stages 2 to 4), and (3) remodeling phase.

Stage 1 begins when a hematoma forms at the fracture site. The size of the hematoma depends on the amount of damage at the fracture site. The hematoma offers some stability to fractured ends. Aseptic inflammation occurs at the fracture site.

Healing continues during *stage 2* with the formation of granular tissue containing blood vessels, fibroblasts, and osteoblasts. The hematoma provides the foundation for reparative tissue and bone healing. Vascular and mechanical factors such as motion and distraction of fragments influence stage 2.

Callous formation occurs during *stage 3* after the granulation tissue matures. If this stage is delayed or interrupted, the final stages cannot occur.

Stage 4, or ossification, occurs as the space in the bone is bridged and the fractured ends are united. The callus is slowly replaced by trabecular bone along the lines of stress, and unnecessary callus is reabsorbed.

During *stage 5,* consolidation and remodeling occur as the medullary canal is reestablished. Bone is resorbed and deposited along stress lines as bone reshapes to meet its mechanical requirements.

Fractures are usually considered healed when clinical healing is achieved. Clinical healing occurs when the fracture is stable and strong enough to resume its function, the fracture site is free of pain, no gross movement is seen across the fracture site, and radiographs show bone crossing the fracture site.

KEY POINTS

- Bone is capable of altering its shape and density in response to mechanical demands.
- The osteon is the basic unit of bone.
- Bone tissue may be dense and compact (cortical) or lighter and trabecular (cancellous).
- In long bones, the epiphyseal plate is the site of linear growth. Fracture through this plate may lead to limb length discrepancy after fracture healing in children. Increases in bone width are mediated by osteocytes in the periosteum.
- Bone cells responsible for deposition are called *osteoblasts;* osteoclasts mediate bone resorption. The balanced coupling of bone resorption and new bone formation is called remodeling.
- Absence of bone stress because of immobility or altered weight bearing leads to demineralization.

STRUCTURE AND FUNCTION OF JOINTS

Coordinated movement is only possible because of joint, bone, and muscle structure. Joints permit complex, highly coordinated, and purposeful movements. A **joint,** also called an **articulation,** is a point of contact between bones. Functional articulations between bones in extremities such as the shoulder, elbow, hip, and knee contribute to controlled and graceful movement.

The type and configuration of a joint depend on the functional demands placed on that joint. As is the case with all aspects of the musculoskeletal system, structure determines function (Figure 50-7). When considering the human joint, or articulation, it is also important to remember that once the articulation has developed, the configuration of the joint surface will determine the movement of the joint. Any aberrant joint movement has the potential to disrupt function and cause a breakdown in joint integrity.

Articulations can provide more than a single function, such as flexion and extension. Flexion, extension, adduction, abduction, rotation, opposition, and circumduction may all be functional movements of a joint. The more complex the movements, the more complex is the joint structure.

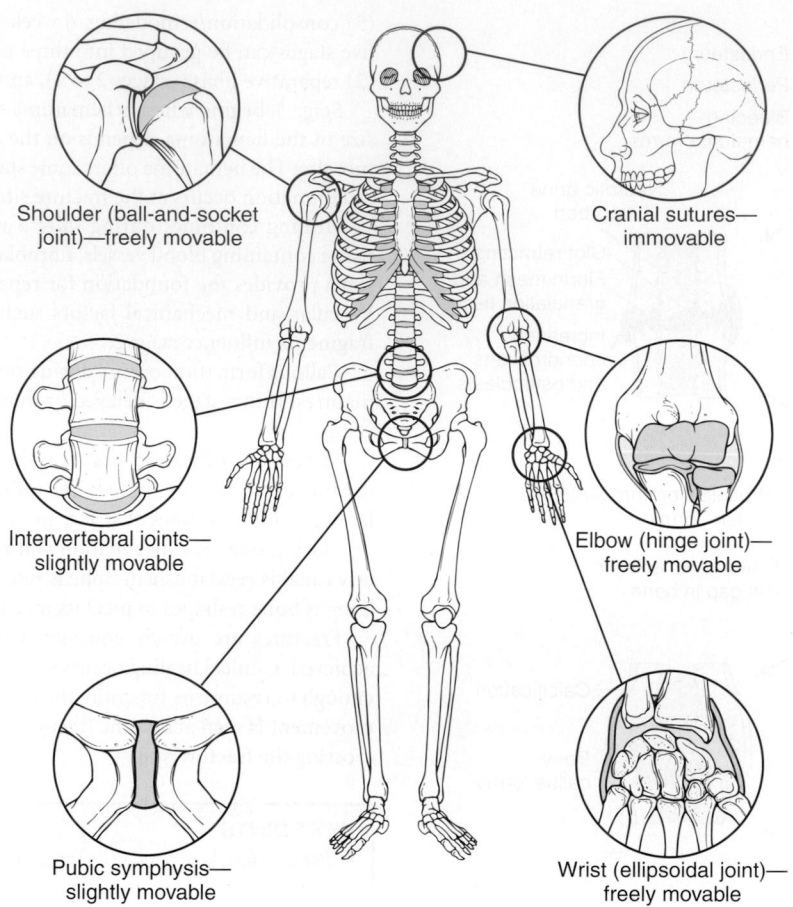

FIGURE 50-7 Examples of types of joints. (From Frazier MS, Drzymkowski JW: Essentials of human diseases and conditions, ed 5, Philadelphia, 2013, Saunders, p 302.)

Broadly speaking, articulations, or arthroses, in the human body may be divided into two categories based on the composition of the joint and the method in which the joints unite the body components. The two categories are **synarthroses,** or fibrous and cartilaginous (nonsynovial) joints, and **diarthroses,** or synovial joints.

Synarthroses

Synarthroses have two subdivisions based on the type of connective tissue used to form the joint. Fibrous and cartilaginous tissues give these joints their names.

Fibrous Structure

In a fibrous joint, bones are united by fibrous tissue. Three types of fibrous joints are found in the human body: suture joints, gomphosis joints, and syndesmosis joints. A suture joint unites bones with a thin but dense layer of fibrous tissue. Interlocking bony ends overlap and increase stability. Suture joints are found only in the skull (Figure 50-8). Fusion of the joint occurs later in life. This bony union is called a *synostosis*.[1]

The joint that is found between a tooth and the mandible or maxilla is the only gomphosis joint in the human body. The best description of a gomphosis joint is that of a peg implanted into a hole. Fibrous tissue stabilizes the two bony structures and permits little movement.

A syndesmosis joint is a joint in which the two bony components are joined by a ligament or interosseous membrane. These joints normally allow slight movement and are quite functional. The interosseous membrane joining the fibula and the tibia is an example of a syndesmosis joint (Figure 50-9).

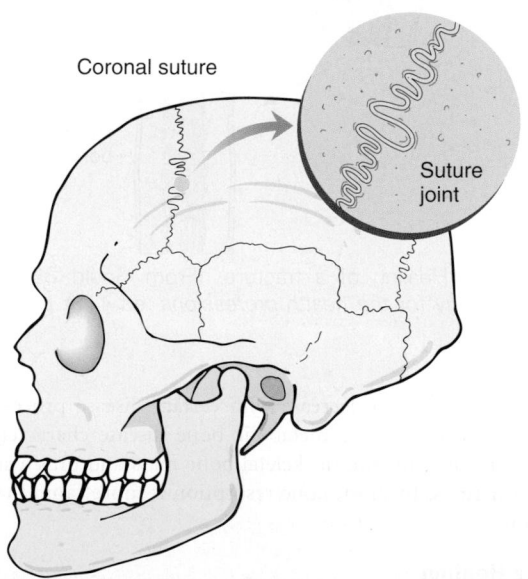

FIGURE 50-8 A suture joint is found only in the skull.

Cartilaginous Structure

Bony segments connected by fibrocartilage or hyaline growth cartilage are classified as **cartilaginous joints.** Symphysis joints and synchondrosis joints are the two types of cartilaginous joints in the body.

A **symphysis joint** connects bony segments by a fibrocartilaginous plate or disk. The symphysis pubis joint (Figure 50-10) joins the two

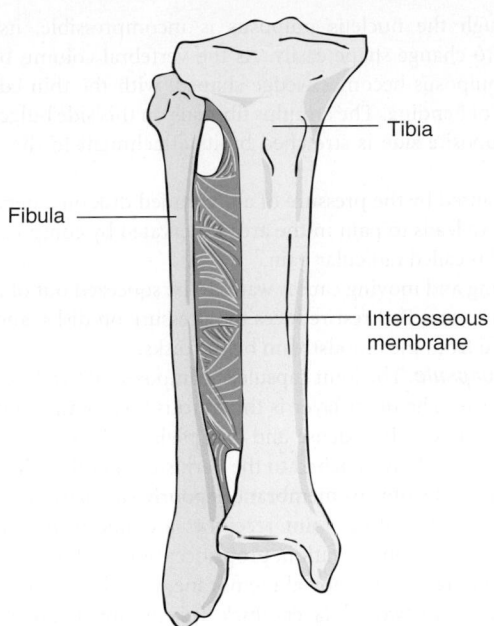

FIGURE 50-9 The interosseous membrane joining the fibula and the tibia is an example of a syndesmosis joint.

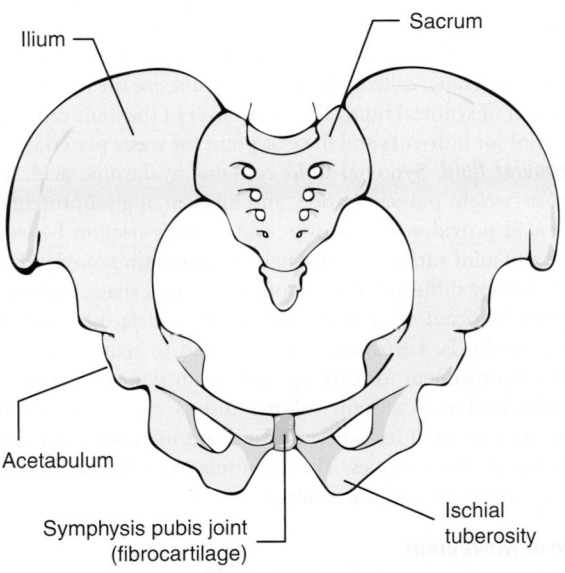

FIGURE 50-10 Symphysis pubis joint.

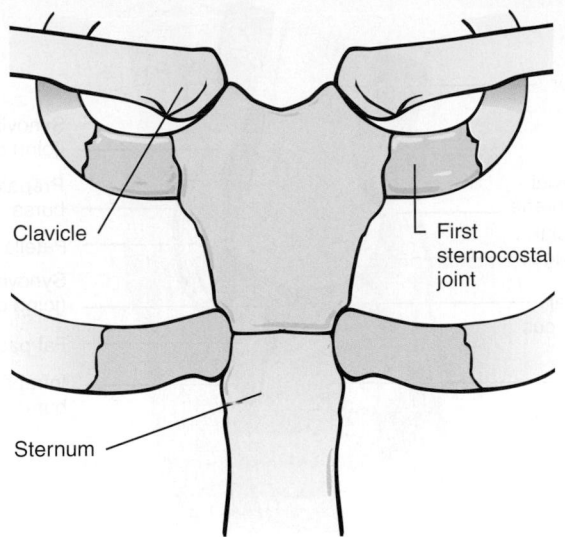

FIGURE 50-11 First sternocostal joint.

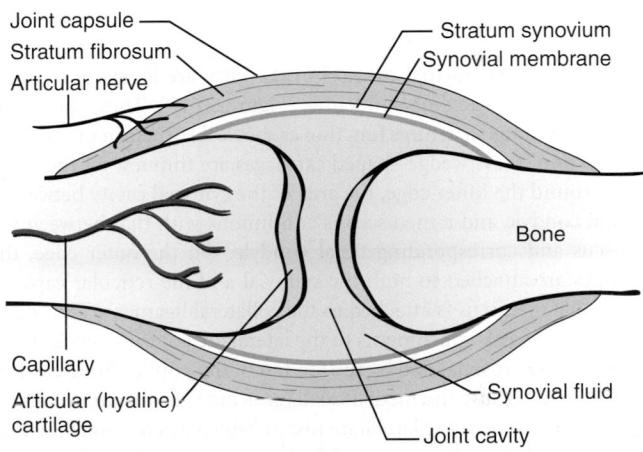

FIGURE 50-12 Typical synovial joint.

pubic bones of the pelvis. This joint is a weight-bearing structure and is important in transmitting stress and providing stability. Little or no motion is permitted or desired.

In a **synchondrosis joint,** cartilage connects bony components. This joint allows bone growth while providing stability. This type of joint can be found at growth sites of the body. The first sternocostal joint is an example of a synchondrosis joint (Figure 50-11). When bone growth is complete, these joints ossify and become unions (synostoses).

Diarthroses

Joints designed to allow mobility are classified as **diarthroses,** or **synovial joints.** These joints are covered with a **joint capsule,** or **synovial sheath.** Movement in these joints is provided by contraction of the muscle-tendon unit, and control depends on the joint

capsule and ligaments. Stability of the synovial joint is enhanced by additional soft-tissue structures—the menisci, disks, and labra. Synovial fluid is produced by fibroblast-like cells lining the joint capsule and is secreted into mobile joints to provide the lubrication necessary to reduce friction between articulating surfaces. In diarthrodial, or synovial, joints, the bony ends are free to move because no cartilaginous tissue connects the adjacent bony surfaces. The synovial joint connects adjacent bony surfaces through a joint capsule that surrounds the joint.

Synovial Structure

Features common to all synovial joints include: (1) a fibrous joint capsule, (2) a joint cavity enclosed by a joint capsule, (3) a synovial membrane that lines the inner surface of the capsule, (4) lubricating synovial fluid that coats joint surfaces, and (5) hyaline cartilage, which covers the joint surface (Figure 50-12).

Many synovial joints also have accessory structures within the joint capsule. Ligaments, fat pads, disks, and menisci are a few of the structures situated in the capsule that are important to proper function of the joint. Ligaments and tendons keep joint surfaces together and aid in joint motion. Menisci, disks, and synovial fluid limit excessive compression of articulating surfaces.

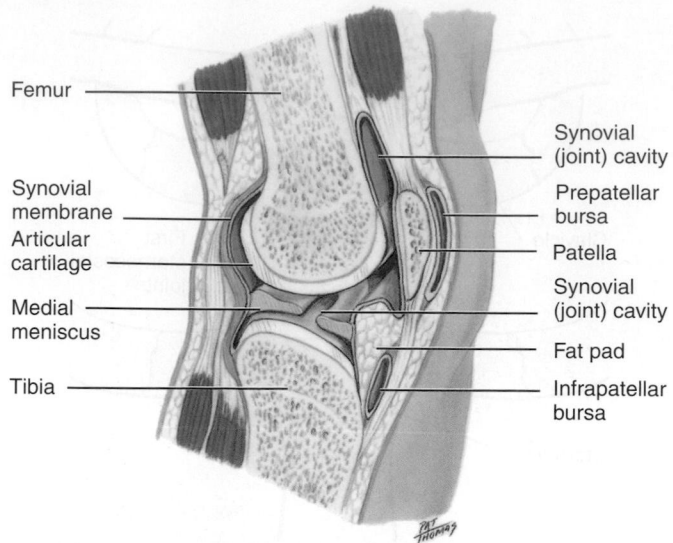

FIGURE 50-13 Schematic drawing of a typical diarthrodial (synovial) joint. (From Applegate E: *The anatomy and physiology learning system,* ed 4, St Louis, 2011, Saunders.)

The lateral and medial menisci of the knee are located on top of the tibia between the tibia and femur (Figure 50-13). These semilunar fibrocartilaginous structures function as shock absorbers in the knee. In cross-section, these wedge-shaped cartilages are thinnest on the inner edge. Around the inner edge, the area of the synovial cavity between a femoral condyle and a meniscus is continuous with that between the meniscus and corresponding tibial condyle. On the outer edge, the cartilages are attached to both the synovial and the reticular capsule. The medial meniscus is attached to the collateral ligament. The lateral meniscus has weak attachments to the lateral area of the capsule, from which it is in part separated by the tendon of the popliteal muscle. It is possible that because the medial cartilage is more firmly attached, it is torn more often than the lateral meniscus, which has no attachment to the fibular collateral ligament and is thus more mobile. Both menisci are anchored to the tibia via strong fibrous bands.

Menisci facilitate rotation at the knee by allowing better contact of the tibial surfaces with the femoral condyles. They function to evenly distribute load-bearing on the tibial plateau. Menisci are often torn by rotation of the femur when the knee is flexed.[1] The torn portion of the meniscus locks the joint, with accompanying pain and edema in the knee. If torn, the menisci can be removed; however, weight-bearing areas on the femur and tibia may then decrease by almost 50%.

Intervertebral disks are padlike structures between vertebrae that help bind vertebrae together and act as shock absorbers between adjacent vertebrae. These disks allow slight movement between any two adjacent vertebral bodies. Disks contribute to the natural curves of the spine in the cervical and lower lumbar areas.

Each intervertebral disk consists of an outer annulus fibrosus, or outer fibrous layer, and a nucleus pulposus, or soft center.[7] The annulus fibrosus consists of many layers of fibrous tissue and fibrocartilage that are strongly attached to the ends of the bodies adjoining the disks.

The nucleus pulposus is semigelatinous, containing a high percentage of water, and is located closer to the posterior edge of the disk. Because of its high water content, the intervertebral disk is prone to dehydration. Even when the vertebral column is not supporting the weight of the body, as in the supine position, intervertebral disks are maintained under pressure by ligaments connecting the arches.[7]

Although the nucleus pulposus is incompressible, its softness allows it to change shape easily. As the vertebral column bends, the nucleus pulposus becomes wedge-shaped, with the thin edge in the direction of bending. The annulus fibrosus on this side bulges out and on the opposite side is stretched by its attachment to the adjoining vertebrae.[7]

Pain caused by the pressure of a protruded disk on a nerve root or spinal nerve leads to pain in the area innervated by compressed nerve fibers and is called radicular pain.[7]

Standing and moving causes water to be squeezed out of disks into the bloodstream. Bed rest reduces the pressure on disks, and water is reabsorbed from the bloodstream by the disks.

Joint capsule. The joint capsule is composed of two layers of connective tissue. The outer layer is the fibrous membrane composed of collagenous tissue. It is dense and encapsulates the entire joint. This dense tissue is solidly attached to the periosteum of the adjacent bony components. The fibrous membrane is poorly vascularized and innervated by joint receptors. Joint receptors are able to detect motion, compression, tension, vibration, proprioception, and pain.[1]

The inner layer, or synovial membrane, is highly vascularized and often only one or two cell layers thick. It is minimally innervated and less pain-sensitive than other joint components. Because the outer joint capsule and the ligaments have more abundant nerve endings, pain can be caused by swelling and stretching of the capsule (as in arthritis or infection) or by injury to the ligaments (as in a strain).[1] Articular cartilage has no nerve fibers. A general rule notes that a joint is innervated by the major nerves that cross it. Specialized cells in the synovial membrane, called *synoviocytes,* synthesize the hyaluronic acid component of synovial fluid. The inner layer of the joint capsule is the entry point for nutrients and the exit point for waste material.

Synovial fluid. **Synovial fluid** contains hyaluronic acid, a high-molecular-weight polysaccharide, and lubricin, a glycoprotein. Hyaluronic acid provides for viscosity and reduces friction between the capsule and joint surfaces. It also helps to maintain synovial fluid volume by slowing diffusion of water out of the joint space. Lubricin is an important lubricant of cartilage and articular surfaces. Synovial fluid resists shear loads, keeps surfaces lubricated to reduce friction, and provides nourishment for cartilage. Although synovial fluid is generally maintained at a constant volume, disease states, such as inflammatory arthritis or infection, can stimulate increased synovial fluid production by synoviocytes. The accumulation of fluid outweighs its clearance, and joint swelling results.[1]

Range of Movement

Synovial joints can be divided into three main categories according to visible movement allowed at the joint: uniaxial, biaxial, and triaxial.

A **uniaxial joint** allows motion around a single axis of movement. Two types of uniaxial diarthrodial joint are **hinge joints** and **pivot joints.** A hinge, or **ginglymus,** joint permits flexion and extension; an example is the interphalangeal joint of the finger, the elbow, or the knee (Figure 50-14, *A*). A pivot, or trochoid, joint allows rotation as its single axis movement. The superior radioulnar joint of the elbow and the union between the first and second vertebrae are examples of a pivot joint (Figure 50-14, *B*).

A **biaxial joint** has two axes of movement and permits movement in two planes. Two kinds of biaxial joints are **condyloid joints** and **saddle joints.** The metacarpophalangeal joint of the hand is an example of a condyloid joint; it permits flexion and extension at one axis and adduction and abduction around another axis (Figure 50-15, parts *A* and B, respectively). A saddle, or sellar, joint is a joint in which the surfaces are convex in one plane and concave in the other. The surfaces of a saddle joint fit together as a saddle fits a horse. The carpometacarpal

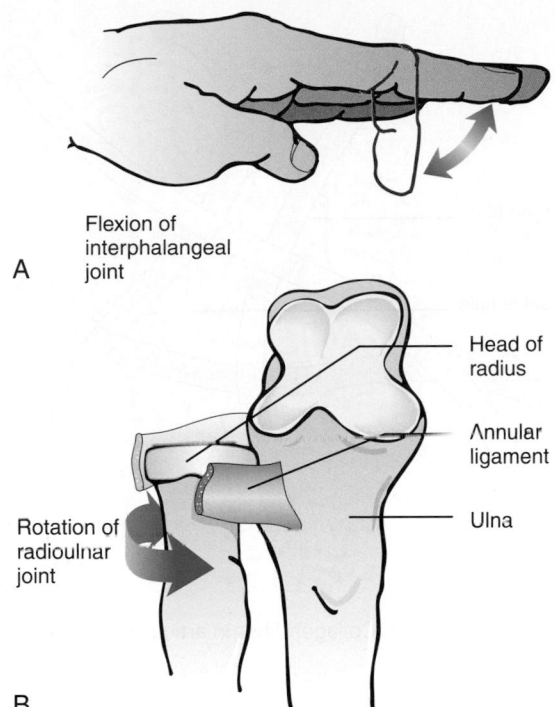

FIGURE 50-14 A hinge joint permits flexion and extension and is represented by the interphalangeal joint of the finger **(A)**. A pivot joint allows rotation and is represented by the superior radioulnar joint of the elbow **(B)**. Both the hinge joint and the pivot joint are considered uniaxial joints because they allow motion around a single axis.

joint of the thumb is a saddle joint; it permits both flexion-extension and adduction-abduction movements (Figure 50-15, *C*).

Triaxial joints permit movement around three axes so that motion can occur in three planes. A triaxial joint permits gliding movement between two bones and is exemplified by the carpal joints of the hand. The **carpal** joints may glide or rotate relative to the adjacent surfaces. A **ball-and-socket joint** is formed by a ball-like surface fitting into a concave socket. Ball-and-socket joints permit flexion-extension, adduction-abduction, and rotational movements. The hip and shoulder are examples of a ball-and-socket joint (Figure 50-16).

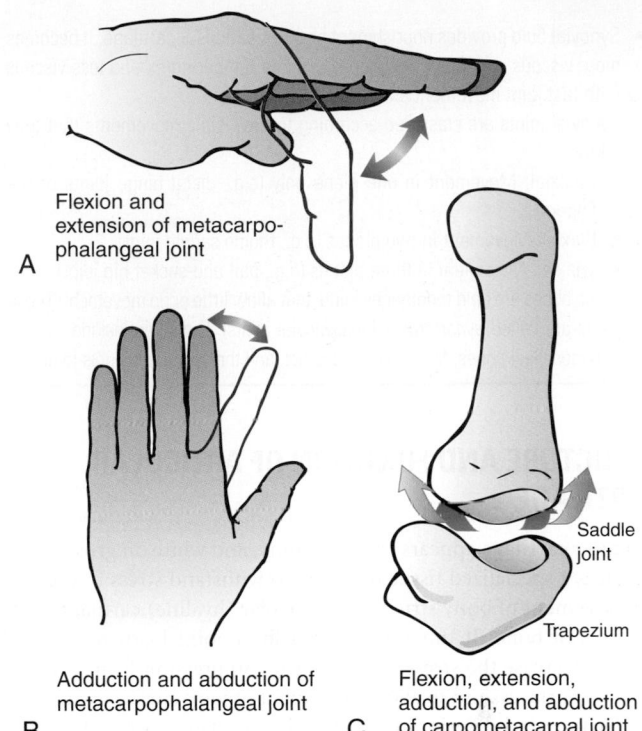

FIGURE 50-15 A condyloid joint permits flexion and extension at one axis and adduction and abduction around another axis; it is represented by the metacarpophalangeal joint of the hand **(A and B)**. Because of its convex and concave surfaces, a saddle joint allows for flexion and extension, as well as adduction and abduction; it is represented by the carpometacarpal joint of the thumb **(C)**. Both the condyloid joint and the saddle joint are considered biaxial joints because they have two axes of movement and permit movement in two planes.

KEY POINTS

- Joint configuration dictates possible motions of a joint. Types of joint movement include flexion, extension, adduction, abduction, and rotation. Joints that allow these types of movement are called *diarthroses* (synovial joints). The ends of bone in a synovial joint are held together by a joint capsule composed of two layers of connective tissue.
- The lateral and medial menisci in the knee serve as shock absorbers between the femur and tibia. The medial meniscus has strong attachments to the collateral ligaments, whereas the lateral meniscus has weak attachments to the lateral area of the joint capsule. Thus because of its strong attachment, the medial meniscus is more likely to be torn than the lateral meniscus.
- Intervertebral disks are padlike structures that act as cushions between vertebrae. A strong annulus fibrosus surrounds a gelatinous, high-water-content nucleus pulposus that can herniate and press on spinal nerves.
- The joint capsule is composed of two layers of connective tissue: an outer fibrous membrane and an inner synovial membrane.

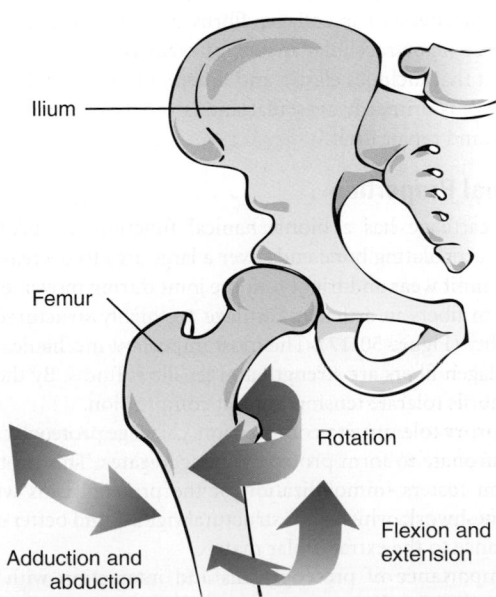

FIGURE 50-16 A ball-and-socket joint permits flexion and extension, adduction and abduction, and rotation; it is represented by the hip joint. A ball-and-socket joint is considered a triaxial joint because it permits movement around three axes; motion can occur in three planes.

- Synovial fluid provides nourishment and lubrication for cartilage. It becomes more viscous with slow movement and low temperatures and less viscous with fast joint movement and high temperatures.
- Synovial joints are classified according to the visible movements that they allow:
  - Uniaxial: Movement in one plane only (e.g., distal hinge joints of the fingers)
  - Biaxial: Movement in two planes (e.g., thumb saddle joint)
  - Triaxial: Movement in three planes (e.g., ball-and-socket hip joint)
- Some bones are held together by joints that allow little or no movement. These joints are called *synarthroses* (nonsynovial joints). Examples include sutures between skull bones, tooth-jawbone joints, and the symphysis pubis joint.

STRUCTURE AND FUNCTION OF ARTICULAR CARTILAGE

Articular cartilage appears smooth, shiny, and white on gross inspection. It is a specialized tissue designed to withstand stress imposed by the movement of bony structures. Articular (hyaline) cartilage covers the ends of bone. It functions to distribute joint loads over a wide area, to decrease the stress of prolonged compression from contracting joint surfaces, and to allow movement of joint surfaces with minimal friction and deterioration. Articular cartilage is devoid of blood vessels, lymph channels, and nerves. If a mechanical defect is present, however, this avascular structure can cause major disruption of joint movement.

Composition

Cartilage is hydrophilic in nature, with 65% to 80% of it being primarily water with some inorganic salts, proteins, glycoproteins, and lipids. Its extracellular matrix, which consists mostly of collagen fibers, accounts for almost all of the remaining weight. The cellular component of cartilage (chondrocytes) represents less than 2% of its weight.[2] Although sparsely distributed, chondrocytes manufacture the organic component of the matrix. This organic matrix, or ground substance, is composed of a network of collagen fibrils encased in a solution of **proteoglycans.** The extracellular matrix of cartilage consists of a fibrous component that includes elastin and different types of collagen. Articular cartilage is primarily avascular and is very limited in its ability to regenerate and repair itself.

Functional Properties

Articular cartilage has a biomechanical function. It spreads loads applied to articulating bone ends over a large area to decrease contact stress and limit wear and friction in the joint during movement.

Collagen fibers in articular cartilage are highly structured to provide stability (Figure 50-17). The most important mechanical properties of collagen fibers are strength and tensile stiffness. By themselves, collagen fibrils tolerate tension but not compression.

To improve tolerance to compression, cartilage proteoglycan works with hyaluronate to form proteoglycan aggregates. This proteoglycan aggregation fosters immobilization of the proteoglycans within the collagen meshwork, which adds structural rigidity and better compression tolerance to the extracellular matrix.

The importance of proteoglycans and interaction with collagen does not end with an increase in tolerance to compression. Proteoglycans also associate with collagen as a bonding agent to stabilize cross-links between collagen fibers. By maintaining ordered structure and the mechanical properties of collagen fibers, proteoglycans assist in increasing strength.

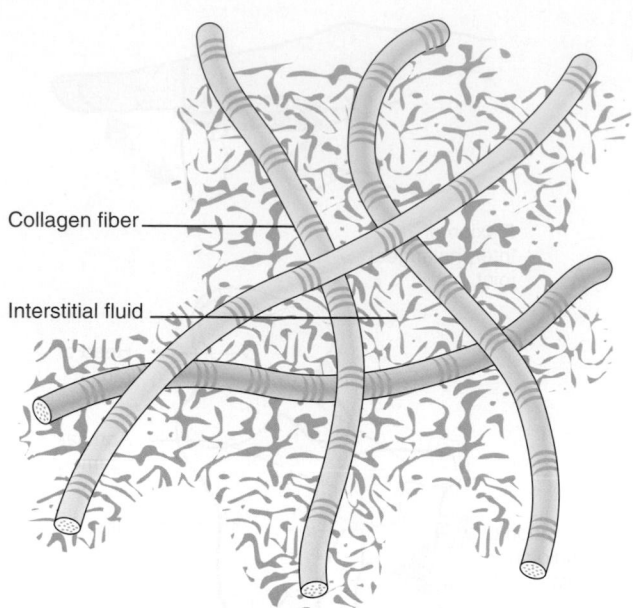

FIGURE 50-17 Collagen fiber in articular cartilage.

Articular cartilage requires a sophisticated lubrication process to ensure a decrease in friction between joint surfaces. Without correct lubrication by synovial fluid, articular cartilage will begin to break down as a result of mechanical action of the joint.

Joints are lubricated by two methods. One method is by the mechanics of joint physiology. A lubricating coating is formed between the joint surfaces when a weight-bearing force or load is applied to the cartilage and fluid is abstracted from the matrix. The movement of fluid under pressure acts as a self-lubricating mechanism. When the load is removed, liquid from the matrix is reabsorbed by the cartilage.[2] The second method is assisted by glycoproteins covering cartilage and providing a lubricated surface. Lubrication of cartilage from a combination of these two methods decreases friction in the joint. Weight bearing and joint motion are essential for healthy cartilage. Cartilage will atrophy if joints are not used because cells cannot be nourished by the synovial fluid.[2]

Response to Injury, Stress, and Aging

Articular cartilage can experience wear. Wear is the removal of material from solid surfaces by biomechanical action. Articular cartilage may begin to wear through two primary mechanisms: interfacial wear and fatigue wear. Interfacial wear results from the interaction of weight-bearing surfaces by either adhesive or abrasive action. Interfacial wear occurs when joint surfaces come into direct contact as a result of a lack of lubricating film. The nonlubricated surfaces are quite abrasive to each other, and joint surfaces may deteriorate. Fatigue wear results from repeated deformation secondary to weight bearing. Fatigue wear occurs as a result of the accumulation of microscopic injuries from repeated stress.

Because of the changes in the nature of glycoproteins with aging, cartilage becomes less able to retain water. This "drying out" effect can change the biomechanics of cartilage and lead to increased stress fractures or cracks in the collagen network. Over time and with joint wear, microcracks can accumulate and fragments of cartilage can detach into the joint space, creating "loose bodies." The resulting cartilage surface is rough and irregular and subject to further mechanical wear and degeneration. This process can form the basis of osteoarthritis or degenerative joint disease.[4] The effects of aging on the skeletal system are described in Geriatric Considerations: Changes in the Skeletal System.

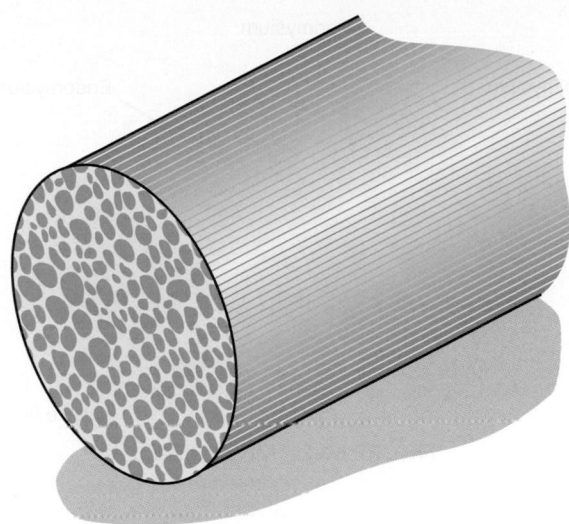

FIGURE 50-18 Parallel bundles of collagen fiber in tendons.

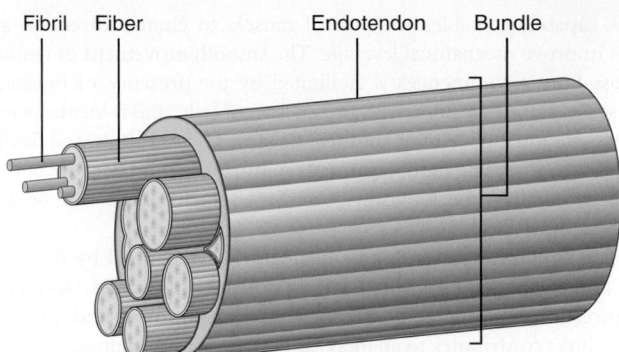

FIGURE 50-19 Schematic representation of a tendon.

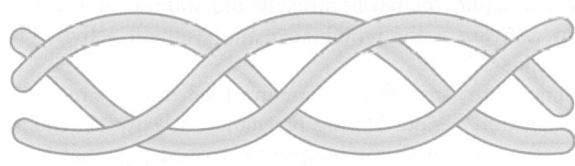

FIGURE 50-20 Triple-helix formation of collagen molecules.

> **KEY POINTS**
> - The ends of bones are covered with articular cartilage, which helps distribute mechanical loads placed on the joint and minimize friction and wear.
> - An important component of articular cartilage is collagen, which provides strength and tensile stiffness. A second component, proteoglycan, increases compression tolerance.
> - Articular cartilage is avascular and relies on synovial fluid for nutrition and waste removal.
> - Synovial fluid lubricates articular surfaces to reduce friction and minimize wear.
> - Articular cartilage has limited capacity for repair and regeneration.
> - Interfacial joint wear occurs because of insufficient lubrication.
> - Fatigue joint wear occurs because of repetitive stress injuries.
> - Sudden imposition of excessive stress may also cause trauma to the joint matrix.

STRUCTURE AND FUNCTION OF TENDONS AND LIGAMENTS

Approximately 200 bones in the human skeleton are connected by joints that provide movement and dynamic stability. Ligaments, tendons, and joint capsules provide joint stability but not movement because they are not contractile structures. Without joint stability, no movement of the limbs would be possible.

Ligaments and joint capsules connect bone to bone, provide mechanical stability to joints, and guide joint motion. Tendons, through attachment to a contractile structure (muscle) and a rigid object (bone), assist in the generation of movement. Injuries to ligaments and tendons are common, so an understanding of their function and properties is important.

Composition

Tendons and ligaments are dense connective tissue in which collagen fibers are positioned in generally parallel alignment (Figure 50-18). The arrangement of fibers provides greater tensile strength to these tissues. It has been noted that although most collagenous fibers of a tendon are aligned in the same direction, they are not solely parallel. They intertwine to form small bundles, which again intertwine to form the larger parallel bundles that give tendons their unique appearance.

As tendons near the bony attachments, larger tendon bundles also intertwine with each other. As a result, pull of any part of the muscle, instead of being limited to a tendon bundle, is spread widely through the tendon. Collagen fibers of the tendon nearest the bone blend into fibrocartilage and then become mineralized, merging into bone and forming a firm attachment.

Ligaments are similar in appearance to tendons, but they unite bone to bone rather than muscle to bone. Most ligaments are composed of dense collagenous tissue, whereas a few consist of almost pure elastic tissue.

Figure 50-19 shows a schematic representation of a tendon. Tendon and ligament tissue is composed of few cells (fibroblasts) and large amounts of extracellular matrix. Approximately 20% of the total tissue is fibroblastic and 80% of the structure consists of extracellular matrix. Of the matrix, 70% is water and 30% is solid material. The solids consist of collagen (75%), ground substance, and small amounts of elastin. Compared to ligaments, tendons contain more collagen.

Collagen molecules are in a triple-helix formation (Figure 50-20), with hydrogen-bonded water bridges or cross-links providing molecular stability. Cross-links give strength to tissue and increase tolerance to mechanical stress.

The protein **elastin** is found in tendons and ligaments. Elastin provides for some elasticity or extensibility. With the exception of the ligamentum flavum, the majority of tendons and ligaments contain very little elastin, and minimal stretch is allowed. Unlike these stiffer tendons and ligaments, the ligamentum flavum connects laminae of adjacent vertebrae and provides stretch and stability to the spine. The ratio of elastin to collagen fibers in the ligamentum flavum is 2:1.

Ground substance in ligaments and tendons consists of a large amount of proteoglycans, as well as glycoproteins and plasma proteins. The proteoglycan aggregate binds extracellular water in the matrix and acts to stabilize collagen fibers and strengthen ligaments and tendons.

Functional Properties

Tendons and ligaments are quite interesting relative to function. Tendons are extremely strong but can angulate around bony prominences.

This capability enables the pull of muscle to change direction and thus improve mechanical leverage. The smooth movement of tendons across bony prominences is facilitated by the presence of bursae. A bursa is a closed sac lined with mesenchymal cells, and is located where one tissue must glide over another.[2] Ligaments are supple and flexible but at the same time rigid. Ligaments stabilize the joint because of their rigidity but allow mechanically correct movement of the joint because of their suppleness.

The strength of a tendon or ligament is determined by the number and quality of cross-links within collagen molecules. As a child matures into a young adult, the increase in the number and quality of cross-links contributes to an increase in tendon and ligament strength.

Response to Injury, Stress, and Aging

With disuse of muscle, ligaments and tendons lose elasticity and resiliency. With aging, the tensile strength and stiffness of ligaments and tendons decrease as the proliferative and synthetic activity of fibroblasts declines.[8-9]

Tolerance to stress is also compromised during pregnancy and the postpartum period. During pregnancy, a laxity of tendons and ligaments is noted with a subsequent increased potential for injury. Estrogens relax various pelvic ligaments during pregnancy, and the sacroiliac joint and symphysis pubis become elastic. These alterations allow easier passage of the baby through the birth canal.

Similar to bone, ligaments and tendons respond to mechanical demands placed on them. Increased stress causes these structures to become stronger and tolerate higher mechanical loads. With a decrease in stress, ligaments and tendons become less taut, weaker, and potentially more susceptible to injury. Immobilization may also decrease the tensile strength of ligaments.

KEY POINTS
- Ligaments and joint capsules connect bones to bones and provide stability to joints.
- Tendons attach bones to muscles to allow movement.
- Tendons and ligaments are composed of dense connective tissue formed by fibroblasts.
- Collagen and elastin are the primary protein components in tendons and ligaments. Most tendons and ligaments have little elastin, which makes them strong but not very compliant. An exception is ligaments that connect adjacent vertebrae, which have more elastin than collagen.
- Tendons are composed of many very fine fibers, each of which originates on endomysium.
- Ligament and tendon strength is determined by the quantity and quality of collagen cross-links.
- Maximal strength is achieved in young adulthood; pregnancy and aging reduce collagen strength.
- Ligaments and tendons respond to increased functional demand by increasing strength. Disuse results in weakened structures.

STRUCTURE AND FUNCTION OF SKELETAL MUSCLE

Approximately 40% of the total body weight is composed of skeletal muscle.[1] Nearly another 10% is smooth and cardiac muscle. Although many of the same principles of contraction apply to these various muscle types, skeletal muscle will be the focus here. Skeletal muscle not only enables bones to move at the joint but also provides strength, stability, and protection of the skeleton by distributing loads and absorbing shock.

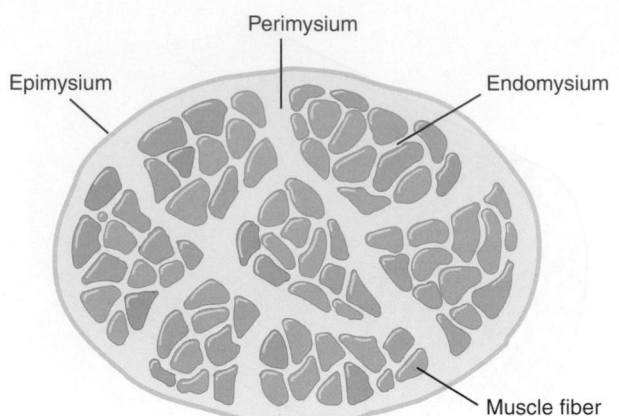

FIGURE 50-21 Muscle fiber.

Composition

The structural unit of skeletal muscle is the muscle fiber (Figure 50-21). A skeletal muscle is composed of thousands of muscle fibers. Each fiber is a single muscle cell, or myofibril, enclosed in a membrane called the **sarcolemma.** Muscle fibers are grouped together in bundles called **fasciculi.** Individual muscles are composed of many fasciculi. The sarcolemma of an individual muscle fiber is surrounded by connective tissue called the **endomysium.** Connective tissue surrounding the fasciculi is called the **perimysium.** Connective tissue surrounding the entire muscle is called the **epimysium.** The epimysium tracks continuously with the endomysium and the perimysium (Figure 50-22, A). Tendons are attached to bones by Sharpey fibers, which are continuous with the perimysium.

The arrangement of fasciculi varies among muscles and can present a specific visual effect of the muscle (Figure 50-22, B). Fasciculi that lie parallel to each other are often found in muscles that function to generate larger range-of-motion joints. Muscles designated as strap or spiral have fibers situated in parallel arrangements. Fibers situated in an oblique pattern relative to the long axis of the muscle are called **unipennate, bipennate,** or **multipennate** muscles. Pennate (Latin for "feather") muscles usually contain a large number of muscle fibers and can transmit a large amount of force to the muscle tendon. Examples of pennate muscles include the gastrocnemius (a bipennate muscle), the deltoid (a multipennate muscle), and the flexor pollicis longus found in the forearm and serving the thumb (a unipennate muscle).

The cytoplasm of the muscle fiber is called the **sarcoplasm.** Structures composing the sarcoplasm include ribosomes, glycogen, and mitochondria, which are required for cell metabolism. Muscle contraction is accomplished by protein filaments of the contractile apparatus.

Contractile Apparatus

Microscopic inspection of a skeletal muscle cell reveals a typical pattern of banding called **striation.** This striated appearance is due to an organized structure of proteins (myofibrils) of the contractile apparatus (Figure 50-22, C). The contractile proteins actin and myosin are called filaments because they are long and narrow. **Myosin** filaments are larger and are referred to as thick filaments. Thin filaments are actually composed of three different types of proteins bundled together. **Actin** is the primary constituent of thin filament, with smaller amounts of the proteins tropomyosin and troponin bound to it.

Thick and thin filaments are specifically arranged in contractile units called **sarcomeres** (Figure 50-23). Sarcomeres are defined by dark bands called **Z lines** that lie perpendicular to actin and myosin

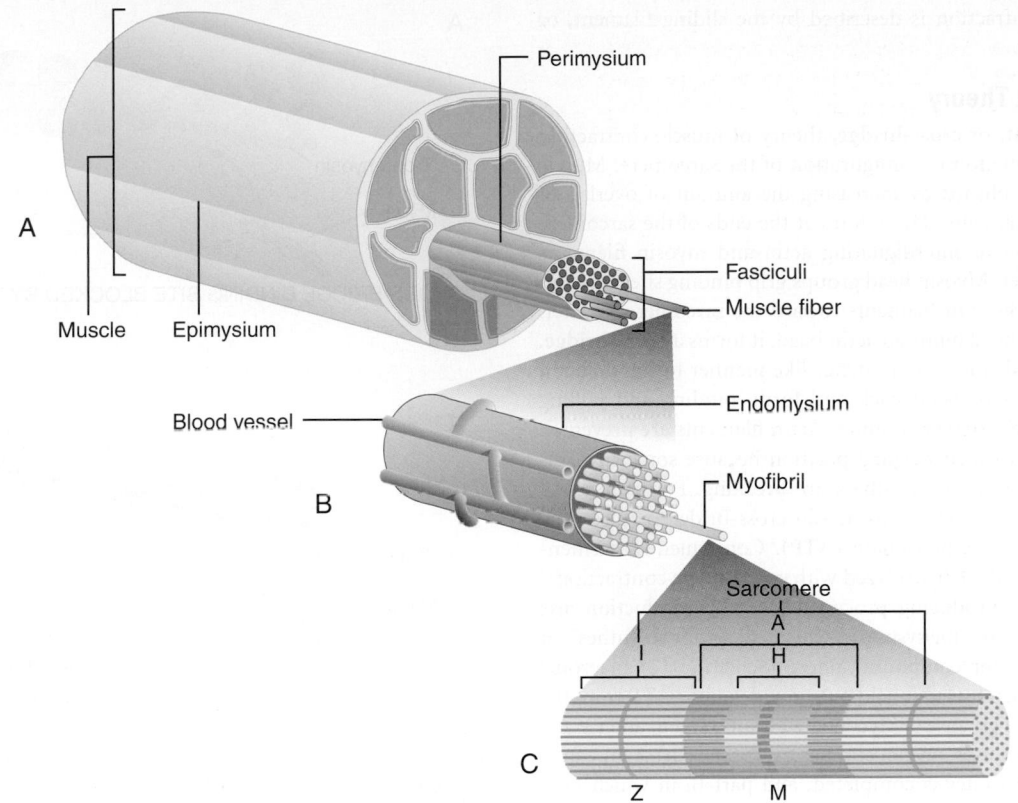

FIGURE 50-22 Structure of muscle fiber. **A,** The epimysium extends continuously with the endomysium and the perimysium. **B,** The arrangement of fasciculi varies among muscles. **C,** The banding pattern apparent on microscopic inspection of a muscle cell results from the organized structure of the proteins (myofibrils) of the contractile apparatus.

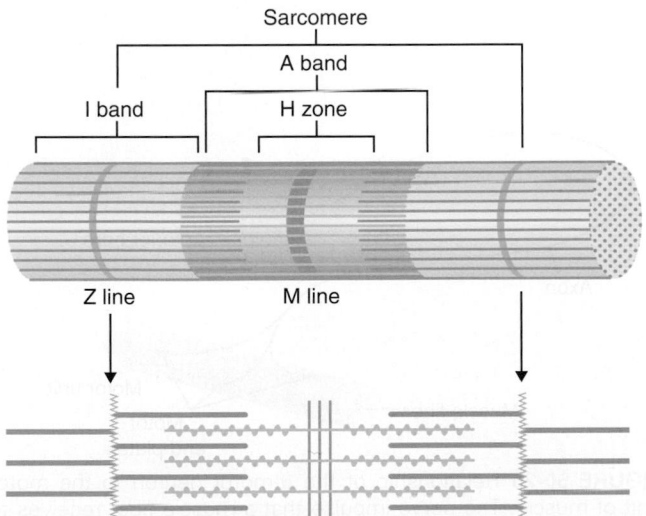

FIGURE 50-23 Thick and thin filaments are organized into contractile units called sarcomeres.

filaments. A sarcomere extends from one Z line to the next. Thin actin filaments are attached to Z lines and extend from them. The **I bands** (isotropic) are light in color and correspond to the position of thin actin filaments extending in both directions from the Z line. Thick myosin filaments lie parallel to and between the thin filaments. Each myosin filament is actually surrounded by six thin filaments. The dark **A band** corresponds to an area where actin and myosin filaments overlap. An **M line** marks the center of the A band and the midpoint of

myosin filaments. One other zone, the **H zone,** corresponds to a region occupied solely by myosin filaments with no actin filament overlap. An efficient, synchronized contraction is enhanced by this precise arrangement of contractile elements. (See Chapter 17 for a detailed description of contractile filament structure.[8])

> **KEY POINTS**
> - Muscles are composed of bundles of muscle fibers called fasciculi.
> - A single muscle fiber is one elongated muscle cell packed with contractile proteins and cytoplasmic organelles.
> - Connective tissue encases each fasciculus (endomysium) and the muscle as a whole (perimysium).
> - Tendons that attach muscle to bone are continuous with the perimysium.
> - The arrangement of fibers within a muscle may be parallel or oblique.
> - A parallel arrangement occurs in muscles having greater range of motion.
> - Oblique patterns occur in muscles with large force potential.
> - Skeletal muscle is striated because of an orderly arrangement of contractile proteins in muscle cells.
> - Myosin is the primary component of the thick filament. Thin filaments are composed mainly of actin, with smaller amounts of the regulatory proteins troponin and tropomyosin.

MECHANICS OF MUSCLE CONTRACTION

To accomplish the powerful shortening, or contraction, of a muscle fiber, several processes are necessary. Contraction allows muscle tissue to pull on bones and thus body movement is possible. The molecular basis of muscle contraction is described by the sliding filament, or cross-bridge, theory.

Sliding Filament Theory

The **sliding filament,** or **cross-bridge,** theory of muscle contraction is suggested by the anatomic configuration of the sarcomere. Muscle shortening is accomplished by increasing the amount of overlap of actin and myosin filaments. The Z lines at the ends of the sarcomere move closer together as interdigitating actin and myosin filaments slide past one another. Myosin head groups grip binding sites on actin filaments and pull the thin filaments toward the sarcomere's center. Each time a myosin head binds an actin bead, it forms a **cross-bridge.** Flexible myosin heads move in a ratchet-like manner to tug on actin filaments. Myosin heads bend back and forth, binding and pulling on actin filaments in a steplike fashion. Actin filaments are prevented from slipping back to their original position because some myosin-actin bonds are forming while others are breaking. Formation and subsequent breaking of each actin-myosin cross-bridge requires one molecule of adenosine triphosphate (ATP). Consequently, tremendous quantities of ATP are hydrolyzed with each muscle contraction.

The three energy-producing processes for ATP production are: (1) the ATP-phosphocreatine system in which energy for resynthesis of ATP is derived from one compound, phosphocreatine; (2) anaerobic glycolysis, which generates lactic acid but provides some ATP from the partial degradation of glucose or glycogen without oxygen; and (3) the aerobic system, which uses oxygen and has two parts: part A, in which oxidation of carbohydrates is completed, and part B, in which fatty acids and some amino acids are oxidized.

ATP is the immediate source of energy for muscle contraction. Glucose, obtained from glycogen in the muscles and liver, is the primary source of energy for muscle contraction. When enough oxygen is present, glucose is oxidized to carbon dioxide and water. The energy released is partly used to form more ATP. Some energy is wasted in heat. When enough oxygen cannot be supplied via the respiratory and vascular systems, as during intense exercise, glucose is converted to lactic acid. The smaller amount of energy liberated by this anaerobic reaction contributes to the formation of additional ATP. Lactic acid is basically a poison to muscle and oxygen is needed to remove it, so the muscle is said to have accumulated an oxygen debt. Resting muscle receiving enough oxygen uses the oxygen to re-form glucose and glycogen from lactic acid and oxidize the lactic acid to carbon dioxide and water.[1]

Role of Calcium

Muscle contraction depends on an adequate amount of calcium ion in the cytoplasm. In the absence of free intracellular calcium, no muscle contraction will take place even though myosin head groups have high affinity for actin binding sites. This phenomenon can be explained in the following way. Myosin heads are prevented from binding to actin by **tropomyosin proteins,** which lie on top of actin binding sites. The position of tropomyosin protein is controlled by **troponin.** When calcium is absent, troponin induces tropomyosin to cover the actin binding sites. When calcium is present, troponin allows tropomyosin to move and uncover the binding sites (Figure 50-24). Cross-bridge formation immediately ensues because myosin heads have a high affinity for these sites in the relaxed state.

Electromechanical Coupling

The nerve impulse that a muscle fiber receives to begin contraction is transmitted through the α-motor neuron (Figure 50-25). The neuron's cell body is located in the anterior horn of the spinal cord. The axon extends from the cell body to the muscle and divides into many small

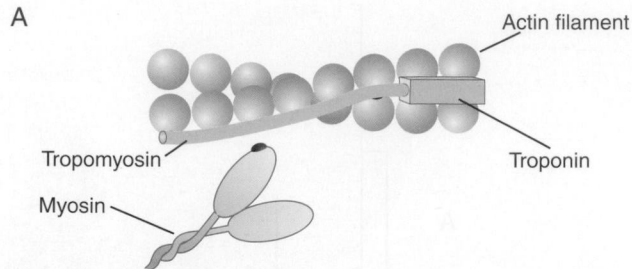

CROSS-BRIDGE BINDING SITE BLOCKED BY TROPOMYOSIN

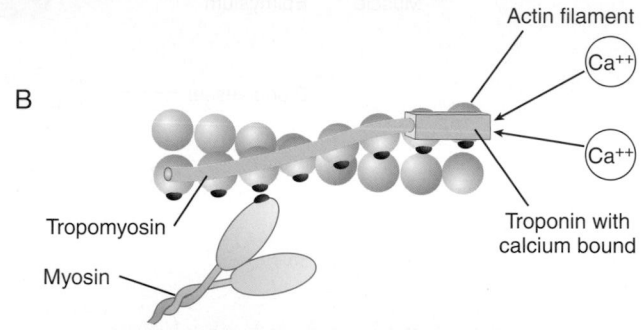

CROSS-BRIDGE BINDING SITE AVAILABLE

FIGURE 50-24 The proteins troponin and tropomyosin regulate the ability of actin and myosin to form cross-bridges. **A,** In the absence of calcium, tropomyosin covers the binding sites on actin and inhibits cross-bridge formation. **B,** In the presence of calcium, troponin induces the tropomyosin to uncover the actin binding sites and allows cross-bridge formation.

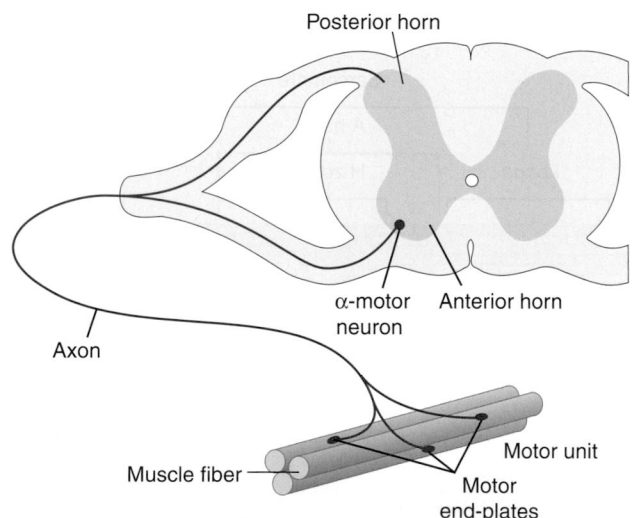

FIGURE 50-25 Relationship of the α-motor neuron to the motor unit of muscle. The nerve impulse that a muscle fiber receives to begin contraction is transmitted through the α-motor neuron. All muscle fibers innervated by a single motor neuron are part of one motor unit.

branches. Each branch ends in a structure called a **motor end-plate.** The end-plate is positioned near the sarcolemma of a single muscle fiber. All muscle fibers innervated by a single motor neuron are part of one motor unit (see Figure 50-25).

After the nerve impulse is transmitted from the cell body, it passes along the axon to the motor end-plate. Acetylcholine is released into the neuromuscular synapse and diffuses across to bind with receptors on the skeletal muscle cell. More than enough acetylcholine is released with a single action potential to ensure depolarization of the muscle cell. Acetylcholine binding opens channels in the membrane that allow sodium ions (Na^+) to flow into the cell. Depolarization of the motor end-plate area to threshold then opens voltage-gated channels and produces an action potential. An enzyme (acetylcholinesterase) in the synapse quickly degrades acetylcholine to stop receptor activation. The sarcolemma is depolarized, and an action potential spreads along the surface of the sarcolemma and into the interior of the fiber through the transverse tubules (T tubules). The **sarcoplasmic reticulum,** a calcium-storing structure, fills the space between myofibrils and forms sacs. The sacs, the terminal cisternae, are positioned close to the T tubules. When the action potential passes down the T tubules, free calcium from the terminal cisternae is released into the myofibrils. Release of the calcium ions stimulates the actin-myosin cross-bridge, thereby causing muscle tension. After depolarization, or when the sarcolemma becomes electrically stable, calcium ions rebind in the sarcoplasmic reticulum and the muscle fiber relaxes.

The motor unit is the functional unit of skeletal muscle and consists of the α-motor neuron and all of the muscle fibers that it innervates. When stimulated, all of the muscle fibers innervated by a motor unit will respond as one. This response is called the **all-or-none response,** which means that the motor unit will contract to its maximum or it will not contract at all. The size of the contraction of the muscle depends on the number of motor units recruited. The greater the demand placed on the muscle or the more stimuli provided, the greater the number of motor units firing. Fibers of each motor unit are not in contact with each other but are dispersed throughout muscle and intermixed with other fibers. If a single motor unit is stimulated, a large section of muscle visibly contracts. If additional motor units of the nerve are stimulated, the muscle can contract with greater force. **Recruitment** is the term used for calling in more motor units in response to an increase in stimulation of the motor nerves.

Types of Muscle Contraction

Electromyography is used to evaluate muscle contraction. With electromyography, aspects of the contractile process such as time relationships between the beginning of electrical activity and the actual contraction of the muscle may be studied. The mechanical response of a muscle to electrical stimulation causes movement in the joint, control of joint motion, or joint stabilization.

Twitch Contraction

The fundamental unit of recordable muscle activity on electromyography is the muscle twitch. A **twitch** is the mechanical response to a single stimulus of a motor unit. After stimulation, a latency period follows before tension in muscle fibers begins to increase. This **latency period** is the time required for elastic structures to tighten to prepare for the development of tension. The time from initial tension development to peak tension is called the **contraction time.** The period between peak tension and zero tension is the **relaxation time.**

An action potential in a muscle lasts only a fraction of a second. It is possible for a series of action potentials to be initiated before completion of the first twitch. The mechanical response to repetitive stimuli is known as **summation.** The period before a second stimulus can induce a twitch during the latency period of the first muscle twitch so no additional response of the muscle occurs is termed the **refractory period.**

The frequency of motor unit stimulation is quite variable. The greater the frequency of stimulation, the greater the tension produced in the muscle. A muscle may achieve higher levels of work when it shortens immediately after being stretched. The elastic components of muscle do not entirely account for this phenomenon. Some energy must be stored in the contractile component of muscle. If the stimulus is so great that the ability of the muscle to increase tension is exceeded, the muscle is said to be "in tetanus." In this situation, the speed of stimulation is faster than the contraction-relaxation time of the muscle. Little relaxation occurs before the next contraction.

The variable grade of contraction demonstrated by muscles is important. Repetitive twitching of all recruited motor units develops as a summation of contractions of the muscle, which is responsible for the smooth movements of skeletal muscle.

Based on the mechanical activity that they exhibit, muscles can be divided into two groups: **slow twitch** (type I, red) and **fast twitch** (type II, white). Slow-twitch fibers contract and relax more slowly. They support high levels of oxidative metabolism instead of using glycolytic processes to produce energy. Continual energy is provided by large amounts of myoglobin, which potentiates the action of stored oxygen. Slow-twitch fibers are modified for either prolonged or continuous muscle activity such as in the case of endurance marathon running and maintaining posture. These muscles have a high content of myoglobin.

Fast-twitch muscle fibers depend on energy released from the glycolytic process. Type II fibers are used for fast muscle contractions such as in sprinting, eye blinking, or jumping. Because of the lack of myoglobin in their fibers, they are white. Fast-twitch fibers fatigue more easily than slow-twitch fibers.[8]

Concentric, Eccentric, and Isometric Contractions

Contraction of a muscle exerts a force that causes a torque, or turning, effect on the joint involved. When muscle force generates sufficient tension to overcome the resistance of a limb, the muscle will shorten and joint movement occurs. This shortening contraction is called a **concentric contraction.** Lifting a cup of water to one's mouth is an example of concentric contraction of the biceps muscle. If the load is greater than the amount of tension that the muscle is able to generate, the muscle will lengthen even though it is contracting. A lengthening contraction is termed an **eccentric contraction.** Walking down stairs is an example of an eccentric contraction of the quadriceps muscles. A third type of contraction is an **isometric contraction.** No movement occurs, and the muscle maintains its specific length. Holding a weight in the hand with the elbow flexed is an example of an isometric contraction.

Combined actions of concentric, eccentric, and isometric contractions provide the body the ability to control movement and function in the environment. Walking, eating, and lifting require the interaction of various types of contractions to provide for smooth and coordinated activity. In a rehabilitative situation, it is interesting to note that isometric contractions generate greater tension than concentric contractions. Eccentric contractions may generate more tension than isometric contractions. When using strengthening programs in rehabilitation settings, a working knowledge of strengthening and tolerance of traumatized tissue is imperative to ensure safe reconditioning.

Mechanical Principles

The amount of tension that a muscle can generate is dictated by a number of mechanical concepts or principles of relationship. These principles include the length-tension relationship, the load-velocity relationship, the force-time relationship, and the effects of muscle temperature change and muscle fatigue. Muscle tension, fatigue, and prestretching are other important factors in muscle force production. A brief review follows.

Length-Tension Relationship

Maximal tension is produced when muscle is at its usual resting length because this position allows actin and myosin filaments to overlap and provide the maximal number of cross-bridges between filaments. At a short resting length, little tension or muscle shortening is possible inasmuch as myosin filaments abut the Z line. If muscle fiber is held at lengths beyond the resting length, tension decreases because actin and myosin do not overlap and therefore no active tension is present.

Load-Velocity Relationship

The velocity of shortening of a muscle contracting concentrically is inversely related to the weight of the applied load. The lower the weight, the higher the velocity of contraction. The greater the weight, the slower the contraction of the muscle. An isometric contraction occurs when the load equals the amount of force that the muscle exerts. If the load exceeds the force generated by the muscle, an eccentric contraction occurs. Greater load leads to faster eccentric lengthening.

Force-Time Relationship

The longer the time of contraction, the greater the force that the muscle can generate until the muscle reaches its point of maximal tension. An increase in the duration of force allows higher levels of tension to be produced by the contractile structures.

Effects of Temperature Change

Conduction velocity across the sarcolemma increases with a rise in muscle temperature. Temperature elevation increases the enzymatic activity of muscle metabolism and the elasticity of collagen in elastic components. For example, the warm-up exercises performed by athletes increases muscle temperature as a result of the increased blood flow and heat generated by metabolism. Both of these changes increase the amount of force that a muscle can produce.

Effects of Fatigue

The availability of ATP determines muscles' ability to contract and relax. Prolonged activity of muscles can be sustained only when the muscle has an adequate supply of nutrients and oxygen to synthesize ATP. If the activity is of sufficient intensity to deplete ATP faster than it can be replaced, muscle tension will gradually weaken and at some point drop to zero. When muscle returns to its original state, creatine phosphate, a major storage form of energy in muscle, must be resynthesized and glycogen stores replaced. This revitalization process requires energy, so the muscle will continue to consume oxygen at high rates even after termination of activity. Heavy, rapid breathing continues after a period of strenuous exercise to provide adequate oxygen for ATP synthesis. This oxygen is also essential for removing lactic acid from muscle. Resting muscle uses oxygen to re-form glucose and glycogen from lactic acid and to oxidize the lactic acid to carbon dioxide and water.

Response to Movement and Exercise

Early mobilization may prevent muscle atrophy after surgery or injury. With early motion, muscle fibers position themselves in a more parallel alignment as opposed to the fibers in an immobilized individual. With movement, capillarization occurs more rapidly and tensile strength improves more quickly. With immobilization, the cross-sectional area of muscles decreases and oxidative enzyme activity is reduced. Early mobility prevents atrophy. Afferent impulses from the muscle spindles are increased, thus improving the stimulation of some muscle fibers.

Physical training and conditioning increase the cross-sectional area of muscle fibers. An increase in area coincides with an increase in muscle bulk and strength. In addition, stretching exercises are effective in preventing injury and improving performance, as well as increasing muscle flexibility, maintaining and improving joint motion, and enhancing the elasticity and length of the musculoskeletal unit.

KEY POINTS
- The fundamental unit of muscle contraction is the sarcomere.
- A sarcomere extends from one Z line to the next and consists of interdigitating thick and thin filaments.
- Muscle contraction occurs when myosin head regions bind to sites on the actin filament to form cross-bridges.
  - After binding, myosin tugs on the actin filament, which causes thick and thin filaments to overlap more.
  - Myosin then releases and proceeds to bind at another point farther along the actin filament. Each cross-bridge cycle requires one molecule of ATP.
- For contraction to occur, the cytoplasm must have sufficient calcium ions.
  - In the absence of calcium, tropomyosin covers binding sites on the actin filament and prevents cross-bridge formation.
  - Another regulatory protein, troponin, controls the position of tropomyosin.
  - When calcium is bound to troponin, tropomyosin is moved to expose binding sites on actin, and cross-bridge formation ensues.
- Calcium ions are stored in the sarcoplasmic reticulum and released into the cytoplasm when the muscle cell depolarizes during an action potential.
- A group of skeletal muscle cells innervated by a single motor neuron is called a *motor unit*. All of the cells in the unit contract simultaneously when the motor neuron depolarizes.
  - An action potential in the α-motor neuron releases acetylcholine at the motor end-plate. Acetylcholine binds to receptors on the muscle cell membrane and triggers an action potential in the cell. To generate more force in the muscle, a greater number of motor units can be activated, a process termed *recruitment*.
- Activation of a motor unit by a single action potential results in a brief twitch contraction.
- A train of action potentials in the motor neuron results in a sustained contraction, in which calcium is released into the cytoplasm faster than it is removed.
- Sustained contraction in response to repetitive stimulation is termed *summation*.
- Muscle contraction does not always result in muscle shortening.
  - Isometric contraction refers to contraction with no change in muscle length.
  - Eccentric contraction occurs when the muscle lengthens while contracting (because of a high load).
  - Muscle shortening with contraction is termed *concentric*.
  - Isometric contraction generates greater tension than concentric contraction; eccentric contraction may generate the highest amount of tension.
- The behavior of contracting muscle is governed by several mechanical principles:
  - Length-tension relationship: Up to a point, a greater resting length of the muscle generates a greater force of contraction. Optimal actin-myosin overlap occurs at about the usual resting muscle length.
  - Load-velocity relationship: The velocity of muscle shortening is inversely related to the weight of the applied load.
  - Force-time relationship: A longer contraction is associated with a greater force of contraction.
- Creatine phosphate is a storage form of energy that is quickly converted to ATP when cellular ATP levels fall.
- Fatigue results when energy and nutrient supply are insufficient.
- A higher rate of muscle oxygen consumption occurs during and for a period after muscle activity.
- Lack of muscle use (disuse) leads to a reduction in muscle mass and slowing of oxidative enzyme activity.
- Early activity after injury is associated with quicker recovery of tensile strength, less atrophy, and better circulation.

GERIATRIC CONSIDERATIONS
Changes in the Muscular System

With aging, the size and number of muscle cells decrease. The remaining muscle cells undergo atrophy, resulting in decreased muscle fiber diameter and reduced amount of elastic tissue. These changes result in reduced muscle mass. Within muscle cells, amounts of extracellular sodium, chloride, water, and lipofuscin pigment increase, with diminished intracellular potassium concentration. The loss of muscle protein may not be obvious because of increased collagen and fat replacement.

Because fewer capillaries are available to supply the muscles, removal of metabolites is decreased. Hormonal stimulation of muscle by testosterone, somatotropin, and thyrotropin is decreased, in addition to reduced muscle uptake of glucose during exercise.

Muscle response to nervous system stimulation is decreased with reduced amounts of muscle norepinephrine. Muscles are also less responsive to neurotransmitters, including acetylcholine at the myoneural junction, and cholinesterase activity is decreased as well.

The muscle, neural, and hormonal changes of aging that affect the muscular system lead to a functional decrease in muscle strength of 30% to 50%, reduced muscle endurance, diminished muscle tone, and increased fatigability. Muscular decline rises with increasing age and usually occurs earlier in men; however, the extent of muscular system decline varies. An elderly individual with good nutritional balance and protein intake combined with adequate active exercise maintains muscle function and strength.[9]

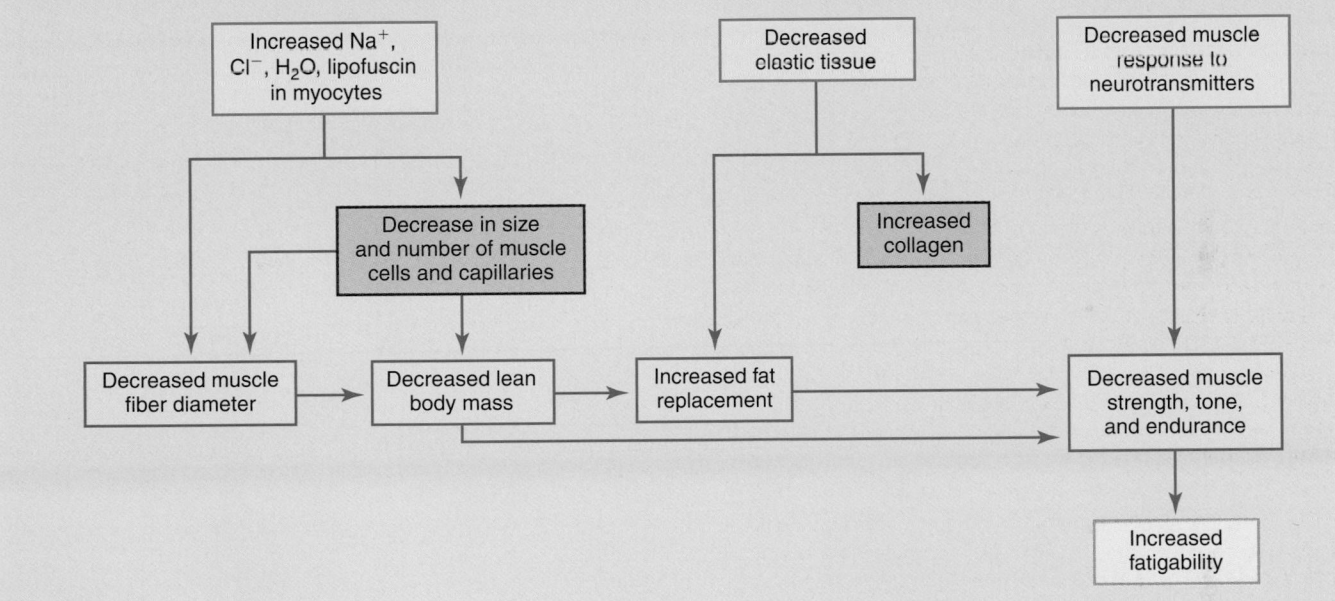

SUMMARY

The musculoskeletal system provides movement for the body. Alterations in function of the musculoskeletal system that decrease the efficiency of movement can often magnify the stress placed on uninvolved structures and increase the potential for degeneration, joint laxity, and pain.

A sound knowledge base of the anatomy, physiology, and mechanics of movement makes the diagnosis of aberrant movement and function easier and thus aids in planning the necessary care and education of patients. Too often, in attempts to provide relief for patients with musculoskeletal dysfunction, the tissue involved or the mechanism of activity causing the injury is not properly identified. Short-lived relief of pain may be provided through the use of analgesics. However, return to activity exacerbates pain and the restriction of movement present before medical care.

Familiarity with the musculoskeletal system also allows health care providers to identify basic tissues involved in injury or disease. Such awareness empowers the clinician to provide relief of pain as well as to address quality-of-life issues. Determination of the type of activity that creates the problem and identification of segments of the musculoskeletal system affected provide the basis to achieve positive long-lasting improvement. Weakness, instability, or decreased motion of structures involved in the dysfunction must be identified. Analysis of physical limitations can lead to patient education and referral to sources that can reduce the impact of physical limitations. In addition, use of recommended exercises, modification of living and working environments, and education of family members will help affected individuals achieve optimal motor function and prevent further injury. The effects of aging on the muscular system are described in Geriatric Considerations: Changes in the Muscular System.

REFERENCES

1. Firestein GS, Budd RC, Harris ED, et al, editors: *Kelley's textbook of rheumatology*, ed 8, Philadelphia, 2008, WB Saunders.
2. Seeman E, Delmas PD: Bone quality—the material and structural basis of bone strength and fragility, *N Eng J Med* 354(21):2250–2261, 2006.
3. Green NE, Swiontkowski MF, editors: *Skeletal trauma in children*, ed 4, Philadelphia, 2008, Elsevier.
4. Klippel JH, Stone JH, Crofford LJ, White PH, editors: *Primer on the rheumatic diseases*, ed 13, New York, 2008, Springer.
5. Wolff J: *Des gesetz der transformation der knochen*, Berlin, 1892, Hirschwold.
6. Giangregorio L, Blimkie CJ: Skeletal adaptations to alterations in weight-bearing activity: a comparison of models of disuse osteoporosis, *Sports Med* 32(7):459–476, 2002.
7. Hochberg MC, Silman AJ, Smolen JS, et al, editors: *Rheumatology*, ed 4, Philadelphia, 2008, Elsevier.
8. Barrett KE, Barman SM, Boitano S, Brooks HL, editors: *Ganong's review of medical physiology*, ed 23, New York, 2010, McGraw-Hill.
9. Beers MH, Berkow R, editors: *The Merck manual of geriatrics*, Rahway, NJ, 2000, Merck.

Alterations in Musculoskeletal Function: Trauma, Infection, and Disease

Carol L. Danning

⊖volve WEBSITE

http://evolve.elsevier.com/Copstead/

- Review Questions and Answers
- Glossary (with audio pronunciations for selected terms)
- Animations
- Case Studies
- Key Points Review

KEY QUESTIONS

- How are the mechanisms of injury different between noncontractile and contractile soft-tissue injuries?
- What are the key factors in the mechanisms of wound healing?
- What is the process and duration of normal bone healing after a fracture?
- What are the different complications that can occur following a fracture?
- What are the manifestations, dangers, and management of compartment syndrome?
- What are the clinical findings and management of bone infections?
- How are osteoporosis and osteomalacia or rickets similar, and how do they differ?
- What terminology is used to describe primary bone tumors?
- What are the cause and pathogenesis of muscular dystrophy and myasthenia gravis?
- Describe the clinical features and treatment options in fibromyalgia syndrome.

CHAPTER OUTLINE

A smoothly functioning musculoskeletal system facilitates a complete range of human actions, including walking, talking, running, breathing, and a myriad of voluntary physical activities. Any abnormality in the musculoskeletal system decreases the efficiency of movement and increases mechanical stress. Ballistic requirements of many sports and occupations, such as skiing and driving an automobile, have increased the potential for trauma. Diseases also disrupt the integrity of the musculoskeletal system. Infectious processes, genetic abnormalities, immune-mediated inflammatory disorders, and nutritional deficiencies may all affect movement.

Clinicians who work with patients experiencing dysfunctions of the musculoskeletal system must have a solid background in evaluation and management of such disorders. Without this preparation, interventions will not be sufficient to promote maximal functional return. This chapter discusses disorders particular to the musculoskeletal system as they affect the soft tissues, skeletal frame, and muscles.

SOFT-TISSUE INJURIES

In addition to injuries of the bony skeleton, soft tissue may also be traumatized. At times it is difficult to differentiate among the types of soft tissue. In an attempt to differentiate the exact site of a lesion, Cyriax[1] described two types of soft tissue: contractile and inert. **Contractile** tissue is composed of structures involved in the contraction of muscle and includes not only the muscle belly but also the tendon and bony insertion, called an enthesis. Although not involved in a pure contraction, as is the muscle belly, the tendon and its insertion into bone are mechanically linked to tension generated by the muscle. **Inert,** or **noncontractile,** tissue possesses no ability to contract or relax. Inert soft tissues include joint capsules, ligaments, bursae, fasciae, dura mater, and nerve roots. Passive stretching provokes pain from inert tissue. Evaluation of inert tissue lesions requires identification of all structures involved: the capsule of a joint, a section of a ligament or a nerve, or the mechanical displacement of the meniscus.

INERT SOFT-TISSUE INJURIES

Ligament Injuries

A **ligament** is a dense connective tissue with parallel-fibered collagenous tissues designed to connect bone to bone. Ligaments contribute to mechanical stability of the joint, guide motion, and prevent excessive motion. Injuries to ligaments occur when loading exceeds the physiologic range of motion. Microfailure precedes total failure of the ligament. With total failure of a ligament, damage to surrounding soft tissue occurs. Ligament injuries are classified by the extent of tear and may be described as mild, moderate, or severe.

    Grade 1 (mild) = stretching injury without instability
    Grade 2 (moderate) = severe injury with instability but some ligament fibers still intact
    Grade 3 (severe) = complete disruption of ligament[2]

Clinical manifestations. A common site of ligament injury, particularly among athletes, is the anterior cruciate ligament of the knee (Figure 51-1). Symptoms may include a sudden "tearing" sensation or "popping" in the knee followed by pain with weight bearing and often acute swelling of the knee. Another common site for ligament injury is the anterior ankle (talofibular ligament).

Treatment. Treatment is geared primarily toward relief of symptoms, and recovery is usually complete. A moderate ligament injury is a definite tear in some component of the ligament with loss of strength. The fibers are not widely separated. Treatment is primarily protection of the ligament. With a severe ligament injury, the ligament is completely torn and no longer functions. Potentially the fragments are widely separated. Treatment may require surgical restoration of ligament continuity, when possible.

Joint Capsule Injuries

Another inert structure that is intimately involved in stabilization of a synovial joint is the **joint capsule** (Figure 51-2). The joint capsule is composed of an inner layer and an outer layer. The inner layer is highly vascularized but has minimal innervation. It synthesizes the hyaluronic acid component of synovial fluid, produces matrix collagen, and is essential for joint nutrition.[3] The outer layer of the capsule is attached to the periosteum of the bones through Sharpey fibers. The capsule is reinforced by ligaments and musculotendinous structures. The outer layer of the capsule is poorly vascularized but richly innervated by joint receptors. Joint receptors are able to detect the rate and direction of motion, proprioception, compression and tension, vibration, and pain.[3]

After injury to the joint capsule, the ensuing increase in vascularity and development of fibrous tissue lead to a thickening of the capsule. Any effusion into the joint cavity may lead to stretching of the capsule and its associated ligaments. The joint capsule, like ligaments, provides joint stability. The capsule, however, has an interesting mechanical adaptation: capsular redundancy. An example of the importance of the redundancy has been identified by Hettinga[4]: "The inferior medial portion of the shoulder joint capsule is a loose, redundant sac that becomes tense only when the shoulder is fully abducted or flexed.

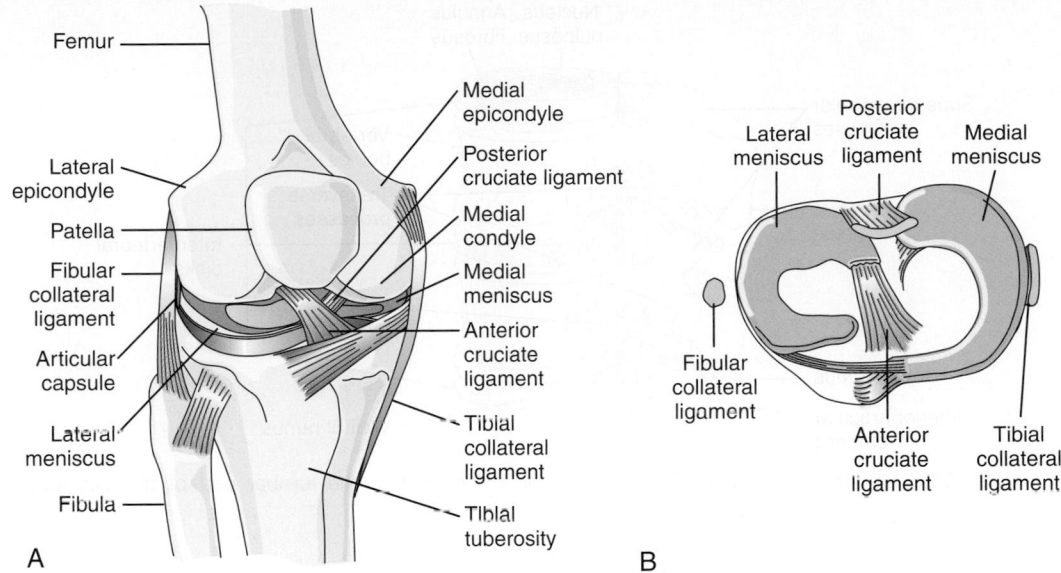

FIGURE 51-1 The principal structures of the interior of the knee joint. **A,** From the front. **B,** From above with the femur removed.

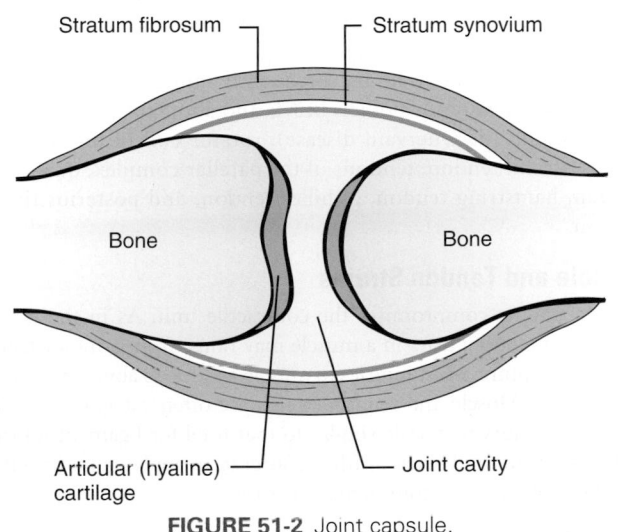

FIGURE 51-2 Joint capsule.

The posterior capsule of the knee is loose in flexion but so tight in extension that it becomes an important stabilizer."

Capsular redundancy provides for a stable joint at the end ranges of movement. Any injury or edema in the joint that causes scarring in the lax section of the capsule prevents full range of motion. Prolonged immobilization of a joint causes loss of mobility and extensibility of the capsule, with subsequent loss of motion. Immobilization of a joint causes an alteration in the flow of synovial fluid and contracture of the joint capsule and periarticular muscle. The altered flow of synovial fluid prevents fluid diffusion into and out of cartilage and causes compression and distention of cartilage. Nutrition of the joint components stagnates, leading to degenerative changes in the joint that become permanent. Contracture of the joint capsule and periarticular muscle results when fatty tissue proliferates in the joint space. This increase in the amount of connective tissue leads to adhesions that limit joint motion. The increase in connective tissue is due to failure to keep the latticework of tissue stretched open, which usually occurs by normal flexion and extension of muscle. The muscles bridging the immobilized joint also shorten.

Adhesive Capsulitis

An example of such a restriction is loss of function in the shoulder after even a minor injury, leading to a "frozen shoulder," also called adhesive capsulitis. With an injury to any component of the shoulder complex, inflammation occurs in the joint along with swelling and distention of the joint capsule. With prolonged immobilization, thickening of the capsule may ensue possibly attributable to proliferation of fibroblasts and capsular contraction. Capsular tightness leads to a loss of movement and an increase in pain, especially at night. Excessive joint motion may cause a tearing of the capsule, similar to a ligamentous tear, and render the joint unstable. Conservative treatment of the frozen shoulder is usually recommended with intraarticular corticosteroid injections, gentle stretching and physical therapy, and anti-inflammatory medication. Prevention of adhesive capsulitis involves avoiding prolonged or excessive immobilization of the shoulder after minor injuries and performing early, gentle stretching.[3]

Internal Joint Derangement

Internal joint derangement may be caused by injury to inert soft-tissue structures. Meniscal tears at the knee, labrum tears at the glenohumeral joint, and disk tears in the temporomandibular joint all cause restrictions of the joint and may lead to soft-tissue dysfunction in the form of weakness, loss of motion, or pain. Tears of the medial and lateral menisci in the knee are common causes of knee pain, with the medial meniscus being torn more often. A meniscal tear is usually the result of a twisting motion.

The anterior and posterior cruciate ligaments prevent anterior and posterior displacement of the tibia relative to the femur, respectively (see Figure 51-1). These ligaments can be torn in varying degrees of severity. Injury to either ligament leads to some degree of instability in the knee joint.

Injuries to Fasciae and Bursae

Fasciae and **bursae** may also be causes of pain and restriction of movement of the musculoskeletal system.

Fasciae

When connective tissues of the body are arranged in sheaths that envelop muscles, they are designated **fasciae**. Individual muscles are

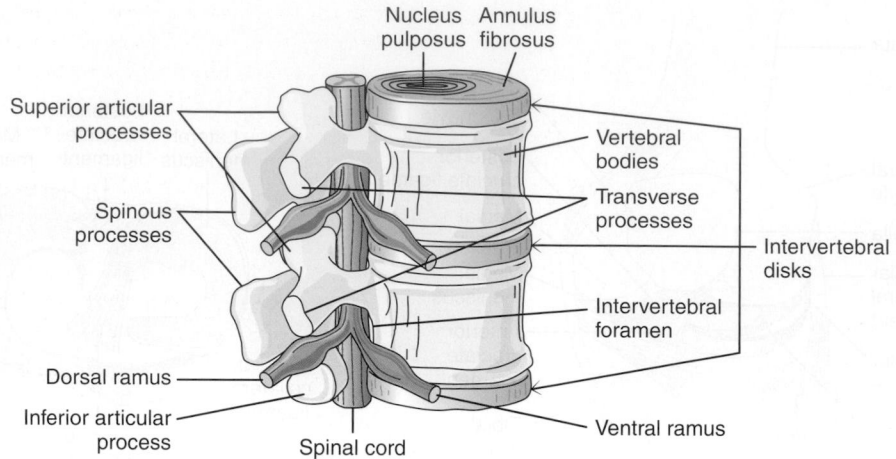

FIGURE 51-3 Lateral view (somewhat superior) of a segment of the lumbar part of the vertebral column.

surrounded by a thin fascia called the **perimysium.** Trauma to fascia, as with any soft tissue, may cause edema and scarring. Restrictions in fascia movement cause a restriction in joint function.

Bursae

In many locations between muscles or between muscle or tendon and bone, connective tissue forms a pocket lined with synovium that contains fluid. These pockets are identified as **bursae.** Bursae are located in areas of high friction and are designed to dissipate some of the stress. With faulty mechanics of the joint, repetitive movement, or direct trauma, the bursal sac may become inflamed (bursitis) and extremely painful. Bursitis, because of its strategic position at stress points of muscle function, causes major disruption of movement. An inflamed bursa may restrict any movement of the joint and lead to restriction in capsular function or muscle dysfunction as a result of edema. Some of the more common sites of bursitis include the trochanteric bursa (lateral hip), subacromial bursa (shoulder), pes anserine bursa (medial knee), and olecranon bursa (elbow).

Injuries to Nerves, Nerve Roots, or Dura Mater

Trauma to any soft tissue may lead to adhesive constriction of the nerve, nerve root, or dura mater. Irritation or entrapment of a nerve causes pain that radiates along the structures innervated by that nerve. Pain, altered sensation (numbness and tingling), motor weakness, and diminished reflexes may result from trauma to these essential soft-tissue components of the musculoskeletal system.[5]

An example is trauma to vertebrae in the lumbosacral area with nerve root impingement. Components of the intervertebral disk can herniate and cause pressure on nerve roots (Figure 51-3). The intervertebral disk is a shock absorber located between vertebrae. The center is a gelatinous-like material, the nucleus pulposus, which has a high water content. The nucleus pulposus is surrounded by the fibrous annulus fibrosus. Trauma to the back can cause unequal pressure on the disk leading to herniation. Common sites of disk problems are at L3 to L4, which affects the L4 nerve root; L4 to L5, which affects the L5 nerve root; and L5 to S1, which affects the S1 nerve root.

CONTRACTILE SOFT-TISSUE INJURIES

Injury to Tendons

Injury to tendons occurs along a continuum from a minor strain, in which a few fibers of the tendon are torn, to a complete tear or

rupture. The sheath in which a tendon slides may also be traumatized. Inflammation of the tendon within the sheath is called **tendinitis.** This inflammation may be due to infection, direct injury, or injury from repetitive motion. Tendons are injured when the stress placed on them is greater than the fibers can tolerate. Muscle tendons that are subjected to high tensile stress or compression are more prone to injury. Frequently injured tendons include the following: extensor pollicis brevis and abductor pollicis longus of the thumb (de Quervain disease), rotator cuff of the shoulder, biceps brachii tendon, tendons of the patellar complex, quadriceps tendon, hamstring tendon, Achilles tendon, and posterior tibialis tendon.

Muscle and Tendon Strains

Muscle trauma compromises the contractile unit. As in the case of injury to a tendon, tears in a muscle may range from a minor tear to complete rupture. Most injuries to muscle are due to abnormal muscle contraction. Muscle and tendon strains are often categorized by the severity of injury in a scale similar to that used for ligament injuries: mild, moderate, and severe, with the latter term applying in the setting of total rupture of the contractile structure.

Blunt Trauma

A soft-tissue contusion or crush injury also compromises the contractile structure. Any blunt trauma that causes bleeding into the muscle belly may lead to an inability to contract the muscle. Hemorrhage in a muscle belly has the potential to coagulate and calcify. This abnormal calcification in a muscle results in a painful condition called **myositis ossificans.** Calcification prevents a normal and strong contraction of the muscle involved.

Compartment Syndrome

Compartment syndrome is due to trauma to soft tissue caused by the unyielding structure of inert tissue. Causes of compartment syndrome may be divided into three categories: decreased compartment size, increased compartment content, or externally applied pressure. With an injury, edema causes an increase in pressure within the compartment. Because volume is expanding in a confined area, pressure reduces capillary flow. Muscle and nerves become ischemic, with a resultant excruciating pain and tissue damage. For a more detailed discussion of compartment syndrome, see the Complications of Fractures section later in this chapter.

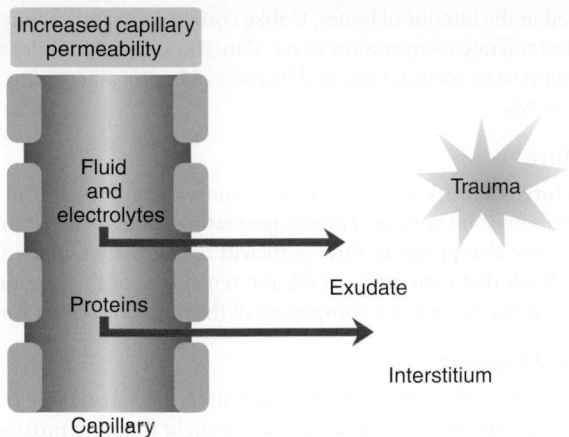

FIGURE 51-4 Edema formation. With trauma, increased capillary permeability and dilation cause leaking into tissue space. Initially clear, the exudate in the tissue space becomes more viscous with an increase in the amount of plasma protein.

Soft-Tissue Healing After Trauma

Trauma to soft tissue results in disruption of the circulatory and lymphatic systems. Hemorrhage, fluid loss, and cell death result. Blood vessels at the site of trauma constrict, which limits blood loss from the affected area. Norepinephrine mediates this initial constriction response, which may last a few minutes. Serotonin (from mast cells of connective tissue) and platelets prolong vasoconstriction. These processes may also contribute to vasodilation in inflamed tissue.

Platelets adhere to collagen fibers and release serotonin and adenosine diphosphate, which causes platelets to adhere to the traumatized endothelial wall and form a platelet plug that temporarily decreases bleeding. Trauma to the endothelial surface triggers release of an enzyme that initiates clotting by converting prothrombin to thrombin, which converts fibrinogen to fibrin. The endothelial surfaces of small vessels are also compressed, thereby ensuring that vessels remain closed after vasoconstriction has ceased. In the early stages of inflammation, the endothelial margins of the venules may be covered with neutrophilic leukocytes, a process called neutrophilic margination. At this point the release of histamine from mast cells, basophils, and platelets causes vasodilation and increased permeability of venules. With the increase in permeability, serous fluid containing cells and plasma proteins accumulates as edema in tissue spaces (Figure 51-4). This edema fluid contains fibrinogen, which forms fibrin through an interaction with thrombin. Fibrin seals damaged lymphatics and confines the inflammatory reaction to an area immediately surrounding the injury.

Wound Repair

The inflammatory response prepares injured tissue to progress to the healing process of repair and reorganization. Figures 51-5 and 51-6 provide a summary of the phases of wound repair. The acute response lasts about 2 weeks, and the subacute phase lasts another 2 weeks. When the wound is clear of foreign substances, an infiltrate of macrophages and fibroblasts is noted. A matrix of collagen, hyaluronic acid, and fibronectin develops. Lymphatics form in the matrix, prevent additional edema, and assist in preventing infection. This granulation tissue develops in the wound space. Macrophages have an important role in wound repair.

Next in the process of wound repair is reepithelialization of the wound surface. Epidermal cells migrate over established epidermal cells until the defect is closed. The formation of basement membrane follows. This membrane is first laid down at the wound periphery and then progresses to the center of the wound. A strong bond forms between epidermal cells and the newly formed basement membrane to complete reepithelialization (granulation tissue formation).

Wound tensile strength is a result of the deposition of collagen. Collagen production begins approximately 5 days after myofibroblast migration into the wound space. Hyaluronic acid, found in the extracellular matrix, assists glycosaminoglycans to stimulate fibroplasia. Myofibroblasts secrete an extracellular matrix, which induces cell migration and proliferation, and synthesize proteoglycans, which stimulate collagen formation and increase tissue resilience and tensile strength. By the end of the first month, tensile strength begins to increase, but several months are required to achieve the maximal level. Collagen reaches its maximal strength approximately 3 months after injury. Maximal tensile strength is only 70% to 80% of preinjury levels.

Revascularization (angiogenesis or growth of new blood vessels) must take place to ensure survival of the new tissue. Vascularization occurs through the development of new circulatory networks in the wound and reattachment of existing vessels. The formation of extracellular matrix, the development of endothelial cells, and the presence of lactic acid and heparin are a few of the factors that stimulate revascularization.

Wound closure or contraction is the final phase of healing in soft-tissue injuries. Contraction begins soon after injury and is completed in approximately 2 weeks. Myofibrils assist in wound closure. Interaction between extracellular matrix and granulation tissue results in a contractile unit called a *fibronexus*. Cytoplasmic actin binds to the fibronexus and draws tissue together to ensure a stable wound. As tension increases across the wound, collagen fibers are reoriented and collagen phagocytosis increases. Complete organization and concentration of collagen may require more than 40 weeks. In the case of rupture of soft-tissue structures, surgical intervention may be necessary to ensure that the traumatized tissue is in close enough proximity to allow healing.

KEY POINTS

- Soft-tissue injury refers to injuries of noncontractile elements (joint capsule, ligament, bursa, fascia, dura mater, and nerve root) and contractile elements (muscle and tendons).
- Ligament, tendon, and other soft-tissue injuries are classified on the basis of the severity of fiber disruption.
- Passive stretching causes pain in noncontractile tissue injury, whereas active contraction is painful in contractile injury.
- Noncontractile tissue injuries generally cause altered range of motion around a joint as a result of pain, edema, adhesion, or fibrosis.
- Contractile tissue injuries are characterized by decreased muscle strength.
- Compartment syndrome is a dangerous complication of soft-tissue injury that results from swelling of injured tissue within a restrictive fascia. Unless pressure is quickly reduced, compressed tissue may become ischemic and necrotic.
- Soft-tissue injury results in local inflammation and initiates the process of wound healing. Strength of the injured tissue is improved by the deposition of collagen. Normalization of collagen may require more than 40 weeks.

BONE INJURIES AND INFECTIONS

BONE AND JOINT TRAUMA

The skeletal system is subject to alterations in function from mechanical stress and infection. The purposes of the skeletal system are to protect internal organs, contribute to mineral homeostasis, produce blood cells, and provide muscle attachment sites and thus facilitate body movement. Bone is one of the body's hardest structures, as well as one of its most dynamic and metabolically active tissues. Bone is vascular with a capacity for repair. It adapts to mechanical demands placed on it and alters its configuration in response to those mechanical stresses.

Types of Bone

Two basic forms of bone are present in the human body: cortical bone and cancellous bone. **Cortical bone** forms the cortex, or outer shell, of the bone. Cortical bone is designed to tolerate compression and shearing forces, but tension forces may exceed the tolerance of cortical bone. Most fractures are due to tension failures in which bone is pulled apart. With bending, twisting, or straight tension, stress may exceed the bone's tolerance, and a fracture occurs on the convex side of the bend. **Cancellous bone,** which has a spongy or lattice-like appearance,

is found in the interior of bones. Unlike cortical bone, cancellous bone does not tolerate compression stress. Cancellous bone provides structural support to cortical bone and increases a bone's potential to withstand stress.

Fracture

A **fracture** is a break in continuity of a bone, an epiphyseal plate, or a cartilaginous joint surface. Trauma generating enough energy to fracture a bone also produces force sufficient to traumatize adjacent soft tissue. With that concept in mind, the remainder of this section will address injury to the bony component of the musculoskeletal system.

Types of Fracture

Fracture type reflects the type of tension stress placed on bone (Figure 51-7). A **transverse** fracture occurs in a straight line at approximately

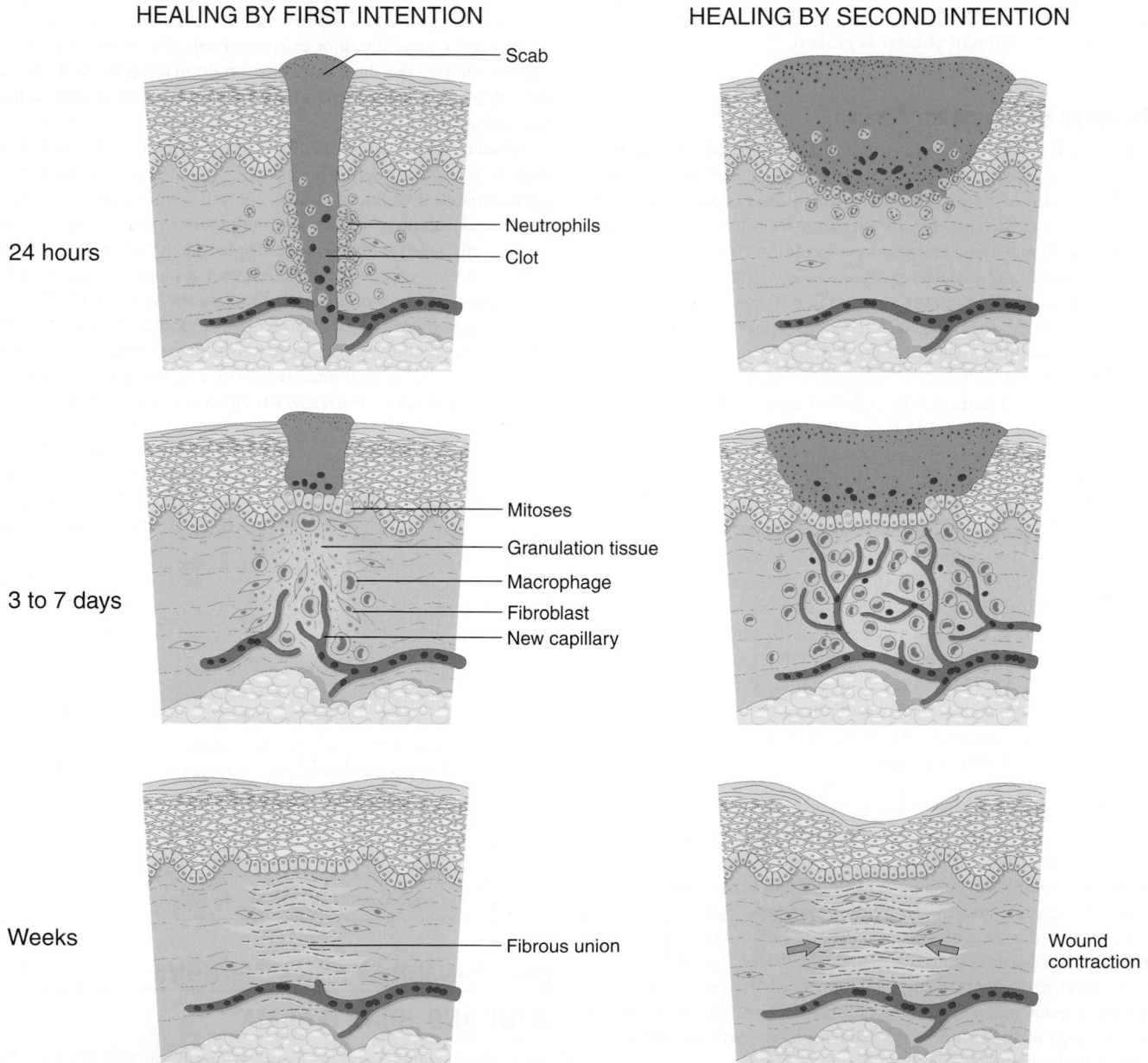

HEALING BY FIRST INTENTION

HEALING BY SECOND INTENTION

24 hours

3 to 7 days

Weeks

Scab

Neutrophils
Clot

Mitoses
Granulation tissue
Macrophage
Fibroblast
New capillary

Fibrous union

Wound contraction

FIGURE 51-5 Steps in wound healing by first intention and second intention. In the latter, the resultant scar is much smaller than the original wound because of wound contraction. (From Kumar V et al: *Robbins basic pathology*, ed 9, Philadelphia, 2013, Saunders.)

a 90-degree angle to the longitudinal axis of the bone. **Spiral** fractures are the result of rotational forces and cause bone to separate in the form of an S around the bone. **Longitudinal** fractures split bone along its length. **Oblique** fractures result from a rotational force, but unlike spiral fractures, the break is along an oblique course (45-degree angle) and does not rotate around the entire bone. **Comminuted** fractures consist of more than one fracture line and more than two bone fragments. These fragments may be shattered or crushed. Comminuted fractures often present considerable treatment problems because of associated soft-tissue damage and multiple bone fragments. An **impacted** fracture is caused by excessive force that telescopes or drives one fragment into another. A **greenstick** fracture is an incomplete break in the bone with the intact side of the cortex flexed. It is usually seen in children. A **stress** fracture is a failure of one cortical surface of the bone, often caused by repetitive activity such as running. Without proper treatment, a stress fracture can become a complete fracture with two distinct fragments. An **avulsion** fracture is the separation of a small fragment of bone at the site of attachment of a ligament or tendon.

Of special concern are fractures at or near a joint line in children. This location of a fracture may suggest an epiphyseal growth plate fracture (Figure 51-8). With epiphyseal injuries, the potential for

disruption of growth of the long bones is present. Proper reduction and fixation are necessary to avoid growth disturbance in fractures through the growth plate. Crush injury to the epiphyseal plate commonly leads to premature growth cessation. Cancellous bone does not tolerate compression stress; it buckles and then cracks. Therefore, **crush** or **compression** fractures (Figure 51-9) are consistent with cancellous bone trauma. In children, a compression injury to cancellous bone of the metaphysis of a long bone is identified as a **buckle** fracture, where bone buckles and eventually cracks. In adults, compression fractures are often found in a vertebral body of the spine, especially in older individuals with osteoporosis.

Extent of Fracture

Fractures can be classified according to extent and depth. A **displaced** fracture is one in which the ends of fracture fragments are separated. In a **nondisplaced** fracture, the fracture fragments remain in alignment and position. With a **depressed** fracture, the fragment is displaced below the level of the surface of the bone, usually in the skull. A **complete** fracture is one in which the fracture line disrupts bone continuity through the whole thickness of the bone, including the cortex (Figure 51-10). In an **incomplete** fracture, the cortex of the bone buckles or cracks; however, bone continuity is not disrupted. Incomplete fractures tend to occur in the more flexible, growing bones of children. Fractures can also be classified as **open** (compound) or **closed** (simple) (Figure 51-11). An open fracture occurs when bone is broken and an external wound leads to the fracture site. These fractures present an increased risk of infection and are therefore difficult to manage. A closed fracture is a fracture in which the fragments do not extend through mucous membrane or skin and skin is not broken.

In cases of open fractures, a wound classification system may be used that ranges from type I to type IIIC in increasing degree of severity. Type I is a wound smaller than 1 cm, moderately clean with minimal contamination. The fracture is a simple transverse or an oblique fracture with a bone spike piercing the skin. Soft-tissue damage is minimal. Type II wounds are larger than 1 cm with moderate contamination. The fracture might be a moderate comminution or crush injury with moderate soft-tissue damage. Type III wounds have a high degree of contamination. The fracture is severely comminuted and unstable. It is accompanied by much soft-tissue damage involving muscle, skin, and neurovascular structures. Traumatic amputations would be classified here. With type IIIA wounds, soft-tissue coverage of the fracture is sufficient. Segmental or severely comminuted fractures occur with these wounds. Type IIIB wounds with open fractures include extensive injury or loss of soft tissue, as well as periosteal stripping and bone exposure. Fractures are severely comminuted. Massive contamination

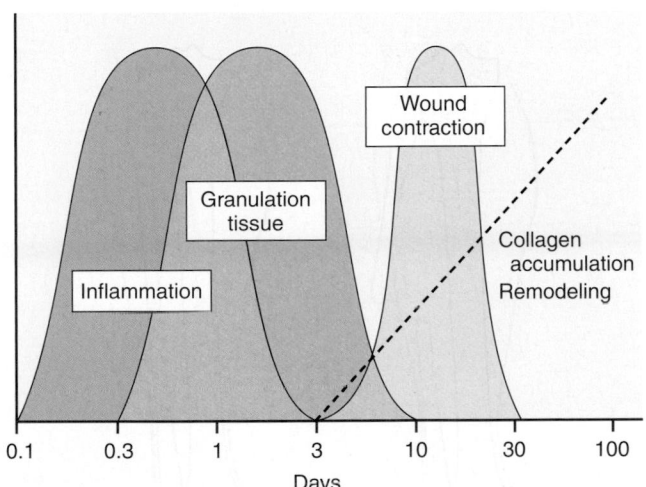

FIGURE 51-6 Orderly phases of wound healing. (Modified from Clark RA: Basics of cutaneous wound repair. In Goldsmith LA, editor: *Physiology, biochemistry and molecular biology of the skin,* ed 2, vol 1, New York, 1991, Oxford University Press, p 577. In Kumar V et al: *Robbins basic pathology,* ed 8, Philadelphia, 2007, Saunders, p 74.)

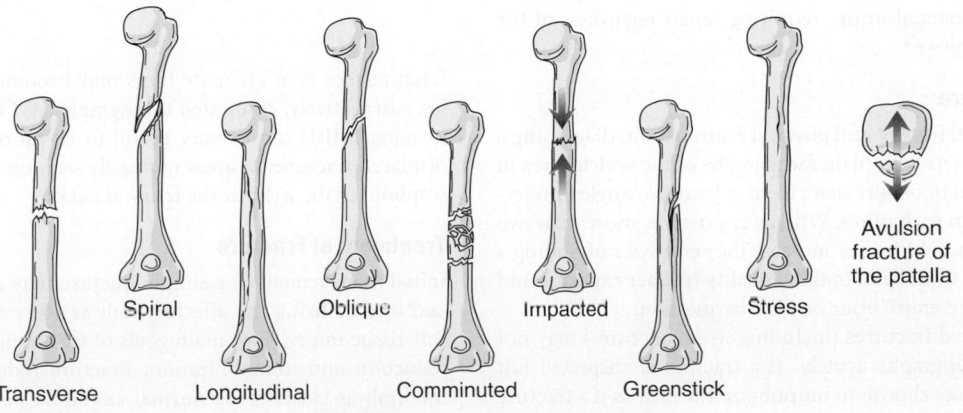

FIGURE 51-7 Types of fractures.

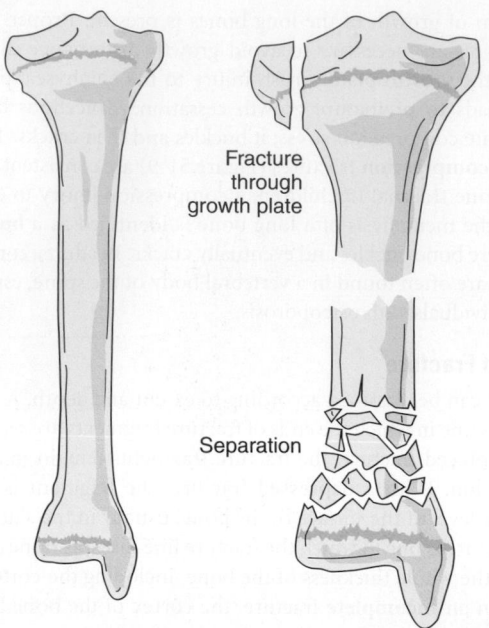

FIGURE 51-8 Epiphyseal injury. **A,** An uninjured long bone, showing the normal locations of growth plates in dark yellow. **B,** Two types of epiphyseal fractures.

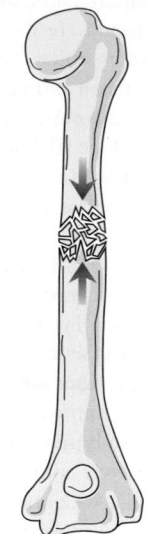

FIGURE 51-9 Compression fracture.

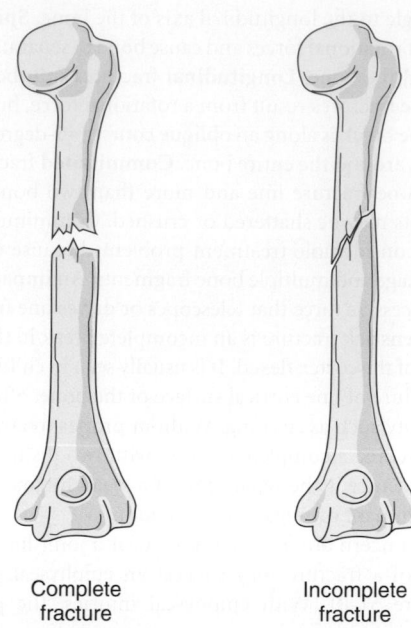

FIGURE 51-10 Comparison of complete and incomplete fractures.

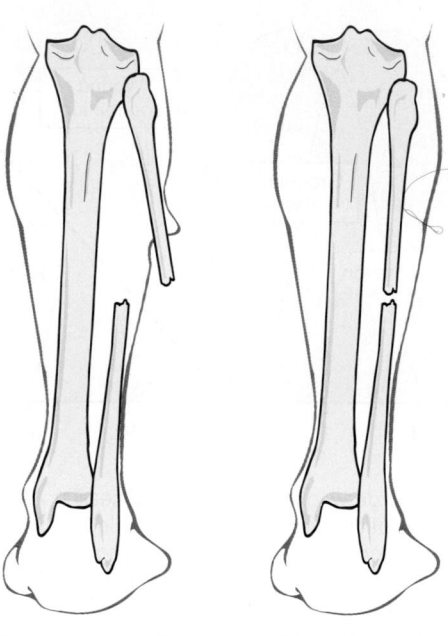

FIGURE 51-11 Comparison of open and closed fractures.

is found with such wounds. Type IIIC wounds include any open fracture associated with arterial injury requiring repair regardless of the extent of soft-tissue injury.[2]

Diagnosis of Fracture

In addition to a careful history and physical examination, diagnosing a fracture most often starts with plain radiographs of the skeletal area in question. It is essential to obtain views from at least two angles, preferably at 90 degrees from each other. Whenever possible, more than two views should be taken, which may increase the sensitivity of finding a fracture. Radiographs must be of optimal quality (proper exposure and angles) and include the entire bone or joint in question.

Occult nondisplaced fractures (including stress fractures) may not be seen on plain radiographs acutely. If a fracture is suspected but not easily seen, one may choose to immobilize the area as if a fracture was confirmed and then repeat the plain films in 1 to 2 weeks. Fine

fractures not seen on acute films may become evident on later studies. Alternatively, computed tomography (CT) or magnetic resonance imaging (MRI) can be very useful to reveal occult fractures or nondisplaced fractures in areas not easily seen on plain films (such as the scaphoid of the wrist or the femoral neck).[6]

Treatment of Fracture

Initial management of a simple fracture may include icing, elevating, and immobilizing the affected limb as soon as possible to minimize soft-tissue injury. Two main goals of treatment often include fracture reduction and immobilization. Fracture reduction means restoring the limb as close to the normal anatomic position as possible. This may need to be considered emergently if there are any concerns for

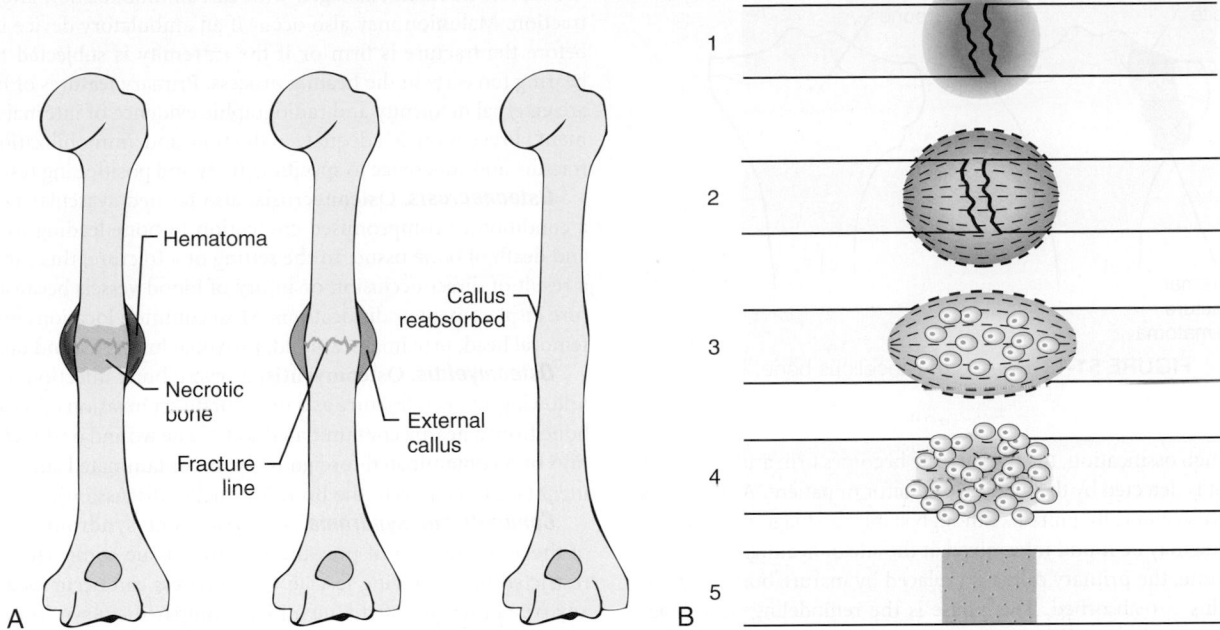

FIGURE 51-12 A, Stages of healing of cortical bone. **B,** Bone healing (schematic representation). *1,* Bleeding at broken ends of the bone with subsequent hematoma formation. *2,* Organization of hematoma into fibrous network. *3,* Invasion of osteoblasts, lengthening of collagen strands, and deposition of calcium. *4,* Callous formation: new bone is built as osteoclasts destroy dead bone. *5,* Remodeling is accomplished as excess callus is reabsorbed and trabecular bone is deposited. (**B,** From Lewis SM, et al: *Medical-surgical nursing,* ed 8, St Louis, 2011, Mosby.)

neurovascular compromise or potential for ischemia to the distal limb. The purpose of immobilization is to maintain the proper alignment of the reduced fracture until adequate bone healing occurs.[7]

Fracture immobilization may be accomplished through different means depending on the nature and severity of the fracture. For simple nondisplaced fractures, a hard cast may be the most useful. For injuries that involve considerable soft-tissue damage, splinting may be preferable over a cast because of the risk of compartment syndrome (see Complications of Fractures). Functional bracing can sometimes be used to allow joint movement while still securing the bone (such as in some types of humeral fractures).

In some circumstances, surgical intervention to reduce and immobilize the injured bone may be preferred or even required such as in cases of open fractures when debridement of the wound is needed or when multiple injuries are present. Intraarticular fractures often require surgical fixation to preserve joint motion and fractures with severely displaced bone may require surgical reduction and fixation. In other instances, when a rapid return to mobility is desired, surgical fixation may have an advantage over nonsurgical treatment.[7] Internal fixation may include plates and screws attached to bone or intramedullary nails placed within long bones. External fixation utilizes fixation devices applied temporarily until an injury or the patient is stabilized and a more permanent treatment initiated. This may be needed in the setting of multiple fractures, compromised blood supply, contaminated open fractures, or extensive surrounding tissue damage.

Further treatment options may also include bone grafting to bridge wider gaps in a displaced fracture or electrical bone stimulation, which utilizes negative current applied through the use of a bone stimulator to induce bone formation.

Other treatment considerations must include indications for antibiotic prophylaxis in the setting of open fractures, tetanus prophylaxis,

pain medication, and eventual rehabilitation of the soft-tissue structures surrounding the fracture.

Healing Process

When a fracture occurs, the continuity of both cortical and cancellous bone is usually compromised. The five stages of fracture healing are described in Chapter 50.

Healing in a cortical bone. At the time of fracture in a cortical bone, blood vessels in the haversian systems are torn. After a period of bleeding, clotting occurs at the fracture site and for a short distance on both sides of the fracture. Because of lack of circulation, a small section of bone distal to the fracture site undergoes necrosis (Figure 51-12). The avascular bone eventually is replaced by living bone through resorption and bone deposition. The majority of bleeding occurs from arteries in the periosteal sleeve.

The hematoma that forms becomes the medium for early stages of healing. Osteogenic cells, which develop from the periosteum, form the external and internal callus. If the periosteum is severely torn, healing cells must proliferate from the mesenchymal cells of surrounding soft tissue. During the early stages of repair, the amount of osteogenic tissue is extensive. Within the first few weeks, the thick mass of osteogenic tissue has formed a fracture callus.

During the initial stages of **callus formation,** no bone cells are present within the matrix. The callus is quite soft but becomes progressively firmer. With consolidation of the fracture callus, new bone formation begins. Initially, new bone forms at the edges of the periosteum, where the blood supply is more substantial. Where blood supply is sufficient, osteogenic cells differentiate into osteoblasts and primary woven bone. Near the fracture site, where the blood supply is less adequate, osteogenic cells initially differentiate into chondroblasts (cartilage).

As both the external callus (which unites cortical bone) and the internal callus (which unites cancellous bone) harden from the cartilage

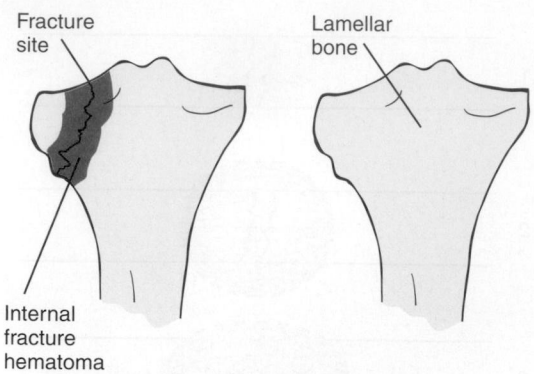

Fracture site

Lamellar bone

Internal fracture hematoma

FIGURE 51-13 Healing of cancellous bone.

stage through ossification, the fracture site becomes firm and stable. No movement is detected by the medical evaluator or patient. At this point the fracture is clinically united. Although stable, cartilage and primary woven bone may be found intermixed at the site of healing.

With time, the primary callus is replaced by mature bone, and any excess callus is reabsorbed. This phase is the remodeling (last) stage of bone healing. When all immature bone cells have been replaced by mature lamellar bone, the fracture is said to be consolidated (radiographic union).

Healing in a cancellous bone. Cancellous fracture healing occurs mainly through development of an internal callus. The rich blood supply present in cancellous bone prevents necrosis of bone at the fracture site. If the fracture is nondisplaced, the healing process is much more rapid than that of cortical bone. Osteogenic cells in the trabeculae form the primary woven bone in the internal fracture hematoma (Figure 51-13). The internal callus fills the open space of cancellous bone and crosses the fracture site. Woven bone develops and is eventually replaced by lamellar bone. As noted earlier, cancellous bone is susceptible to compression forces, and the majority of injuries incurred are compression-type fractures. With a compression fracture, fragments of bone are impacted together, which provides a more suitable environment for healing of cancellous bone. Rapid union occurs because fracture fragments move in unison.

Complications of Fractures

Delayed healing. Fracture healing may not always progress smoothly without complications. Delayed union, malunion, and nonunion of the fracture are all complications that might occur. Delayed union is usually identified anywhere from 3 to 6 months after the fracture, when bone pain and tenderness are continuously increasing beyond the expected healing period for the wound type. Healing is slowed. The cause of delayed union might be either distraction of fracture fragments or the consequence of systemic causes such as infection. Bone healing can be delayed by additional factors such as smoking, malnutrition, use of corticosteroids, and poor vascular circulation to the area. Elderly patients or those with disease comorbidities, such as diabetes, coronary artery disease, peripheral vascular disease, or osteoporosis, are at particular risk.[7]

Nonunion occurs when a fracture has not healed after 6 months. Failure to heal is due to poor blood supply and repetitive stress on the fracture site, and can be the result of interposition of muscle, tendon, or soft tissue between fracture pieces; prolonged or excessive traction; poor immobilization that allows motion at the fracture site; poor internal fixation; or wound infection after internal fixation.

Malunion results when unequal stresses of muscle pull and gravity lead to improper alignment of fracture fragments. It often happens in

the case of fractures managed with cast immobilization after skeletal traction. Malunion may also occur if an ambulatory device is applied before the fracture is firm or if the extremity is subjected to weight bearing too early in the healing process. Primary features of malunion are external deformity and radiographic evidence of internal derangement. Prevention is adequate reduction and immobilization of the fracture and adherence to specific activity and positioning restrictions.[7]

Osteonecrosis. **Osteonecrosis,** also termed avascular necrosis, is a condition of compromised circulation to bone leading to ischemia and death of bone tissue. In the setting of a fracture, this can occur as a result of direct occlusion or injury of blood vessels because of fracture displacement or dislocations. Most common locations include the femoral head, proximal scaphoid, proximal humerus, and talar neck.[7]

Osteomyelitis. **Osteomyelitis,** a severe bone infection, can occur following an open fracture as a result of direct invasion of bacteria into bone from a nearby contaminated soft-tissue wound or direct penetration by a contaminated foreign body or contaminated surgical equipment (see Infections of the Bone for further discussion).

Compartment syndrome. **Compartment syndrome** is a result of the accumulation of pressure in a soft-tissue compartment that is restricted by unyielding fasciae. This process can occur as a result of any type of severe soft-tissue injury. Compartment syndrome may be classified as acute, chronic, or crush. In the case of severe soft-tissue damage surrounding a fracture, the acute classification is of concern because it is the most severe form and often requires surgery urgently.

A compartment is a portion of the body where muscles, nerves, and blood vessels are enclosed within tissue such as fasciae. Compartment syndrome can be triggered by injury to the tissues surrounding bone with soft-tissue inflammation, swelling, and, in some cases, hemorrhage into the area. This increase in edema causes an increase in pressure attributable to the restriction of the surrounding compartment fasciae. Decreased blood flow from arterial damage can also occur, which leads to hypoxia of the cells of capillary walls. Capillary integrity is diminished and colloid proteins and fluid escape into the extravascular tissues, causing further swelling and escalation of the intracompartmental pressures. If the tissue pressure exceeds the intravascular pressure, blood vessels will collapse, impeding blood flow and leading to further hypoxia and worsening edema. Intracompartmental pressures of 30 to 40 mm Hg can compromise microcirculation in muscle. The excessive compartment pressures lead to hypoxia, damage, and eventual necrosis of the soft tissue, especially muscles and nerves. Emergent decompression is needed to preserve limb viability. Compartment syndrome can also occur as a result of extrinsic compression, such as that of a cast on an injured, swollen limb.[2] Symptoms of compartment syndrome are pain out of proportion to the injury, paralysis, paresthesia, pallor, and pulselessness. Compartment syndrome is noted most often with injuries to the leg (anterior, deep posterior, superficial posterior, and lateral), forearm, upper arm (deltoid, biceps), hand (interosseus), and thigh (quadriceps).

Fat emboli syndrome. Fat emboli syndrome occurs when, following a fracture, fat particles are released from bone marrow (especially from the pelvis or long bones) into the bloodstream and lodge in the vasculature of the lungs. Often occurring within 24 to 72 hours of the trauma, fat emboli syndrome may be subclinical or may lead to respiratory failure and death. The patient may be noted to have shortness of breath, rapid breathing, hypoxemia, and a fine petechial rash (especially on the torso and neck area) as well as altered mental status or focal neurologic deficits. A plain chest x-ray may be normal and often a CT scan or ventilation-perfusion scan of the chest is more useful in diagnosis. Treatment is predominantly with ventilatory support. Early mobilization of fracture patients is advisable when possible to reduce the risk of this complication.[2]

Deep venous thrombosis and pulmonary embolism. Deep venous thrombosis and pulmonary embolism should be considered in a patient who develops chest pain, dyspnea, and hypoxemia more than 5 days after a fracture. This occurs when a thrombus forms in a distal extremity and clot fragments break loose to enter the circulation, thereby lodging in the lung circulation. Those with highest risk include patients with multiple traumatic injuries, patients with pelvic or long bone fractures who require more than 5 days immobilization in bed, obese patients, patients with a prior history of deep venous thrombosis, or patients with other risk factors for coagulation disorders. Diagnostic testing is similar to that of fat emboli syndrome and treatment includes ventilatory support as well as anticoagulation therapy. Prevention of thrombosis often includes administration of anticoagulation prophylaxis, implementation of intermittent pneumatic compression devices, and early mobilization of the patient whenever possible.[2]

Neurovascular injury. **Neurovascular injury** after a fracture may be due to either the fracture or the treatment for the fracture. Neurovascular damage occurring at the time of fracture may be the result of any of the following: the force causing the fracture, fracture fragments, hemorrhage, joint dislocation, or the body position assumed after trauma. Neurovascular damage related to treatment may be due to moving or splinting the fracture, manipulation at the time of reduction of the fracture, application of stabilizing devices such as a cast or splint, or the presence of hemorrhage or edema.

Dislocations and Subluxations

Two additional mechanical alterations in the musculoskeletal system are dislocations and subluxations. A **dislocation** is displacement of a bone from its normal position to the extent that articulating surfaces completely lose contact.[7] A **subluxation** is displacement of a bone from its normal joint position to the extent that articulating surfaces partially lose contact.[7] A dislocation or subluxation can occur when forces cause one aspect of the joint complex to move beyond its normal anatomic limit. A considerable amount of tissue damage occurs in dislocation and subluxation, including possible ligament tear or rupture. With any dislocation, especially first-time dislocation, evaluation for a fracture is necessary. Although almost any joint may dislocate, some joints are more prone to dislocation than others. Joints most commonly dislocated are small joints of the fingers, the patella, and the shoulder. Symptoms of dislocation are pain, alteration in the normal contour of the joint, change in extremity length, and loss of normal mobility. Treatment must include consideration of local soft-tissue trauma and healing.

KEY POINTS
- Bones are subject to different types of fracture, depending on the type of tension stress imposed.
- Fractures can be classified according to the orientation of the break as transverse, longitudinal, oblique, or spiral.
- A comminuted fracture consists of more than one fracture line and more than two bone fragments.
- A greenstick fracture is an incomplete break.
- Fractures are classified as open or compound when the skin is penetrated and as closed or simple when the skin is not broken.
- Healing of fractured cancellous bone occurs more quickly than healing of cortical bone.
- Treatment goals of fractures are to minimize soft-tissue injury, maintain proper alignment until adequate bone healing can occur, and prevent complications as much as possible.

- Trauma causes hematoma formation, followed by callous formation; the callus is initially soft and cartilaginous; then it progressively ossifies to become firm and stable.
- Radiographically apparent union occurs when the callus has been completely replaced by mature bone.
- Delayed union, nonunion, and malunion are potential complications of a fracture that does not heal in a normal time period and with proper alignment.
- Compartment syndrome after a fracture can result when a buildup of pressure occurs in a soft-tissue compartment because of edema and inflammation within restrictive fascia layers. It is usually a surgical emergency.
- Symptoms of compartment syndrome include severe pain, pallor, paresthesias/paralysis, or pulselessness.
- Fat emboli syndrome and deep venous thrombosis with pulmonary emboli are two possible complications of a fracture that can lead to dyspnea, chest pain, hypoxemia, and respiratory failure.
- Complete separation of joint articulating surfaces is termed *dislocation*. Subluxation refers to partial separation. Soft-tissue damage is the primary problem.

INFECTIONS OF THE BONE

Osteomyelitis

Osteomyelitis is a severe pyogenic infection of bone and local tissue that requires immediate treatment. Organisms may reach bone by one of three routes: (1) via the bloodstream (hematogenous osteomyelitis), (2) from adjacent soft tissue (contiguous focus), and (3) by direct introduction of the organism into the bone.

Etiology and pathogenesis. *Hematogenous osteomyelitis,* in which the infectious agent may be introduced by blood from infection elsewhere in the body, is the most common type of osteomyelitis. It occurs most often in children younger than 16 years (mean age of 6 years old) and elderly adults, intravenous (IV) drug users, and patients with indwelling central lines.[8-9] It involves bone rich in red marrow. In children as well as infants, these are long bones and the infection usually begins acutely in the metaphyseal region of the bone. Bloodborne bacteria reach the marrow space via the nutrient artery, or after blunt trauma a hematoma develops; thus a pathway for the organism to reach the bone is present (Figure 51-14).

Clinical manifestations. In children, acute hematogenous osteomyelitis manifests as a high fever and pain at the site of bone involvement. The infection may remain localized if it becomes enclosed by fibrotic tissue reaction, a condition referred to as a *Brodie abscess.* Muscle spasms, redness, and swelling are common, and the child may refuse to move the limb. In adults, hematogenous osteomyelitis is more difficult to detect. Symptoms are vague and may include fever, malaise, anorexia, night sweats, and weight loss. Pain at rest is common. The diagnosis may be supported by radiographic signs of bone destruction. The most common causative organism is *Staphylococcus aureus* followed by *Streptococcus pneumoniae,* with gram-negative bacillary infections increasing in frequency. In children between 2 months and 3 years of age, *Haemophilus influenzae* can also be a cause though this is quite rare since the development of a vaccination.[9]

Osteomyelitis secondary to an introduced or contiguous focus of infection can occur after burns, sinus disease, trauma, malignant tumor necrosis, periodontal infection, or an infected pressure ulcer. Again, *S. aureus* is the most common pathogen; however, some infections are polymicrobial and include gram-negative and anaerobic agents.

Direct invasion of the organism into bone can occur as a result of open fractures; penetrating wounds; surgical contamination; or

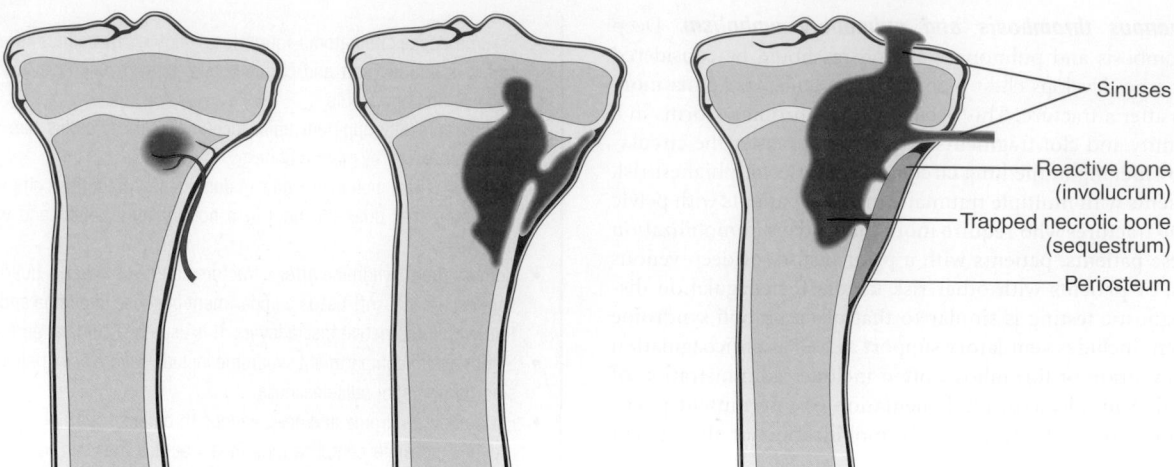

FIGURE 51-14 Osteomyelitis. The bacteria reach the metaphysis through the nutrient artery. Bacterial growth results in bone destruction and formation of an abscess. From the abscess cavity, the pus spreads between the trabeculae into the medulla, through the cartilage into the joint, and through the haversian canals of the compact bones to the outside. These sinuses traversing the bone persist for a long time and heal slowly. The pus destroys the bone and sequesters parts of it in the abscess cavity. Reactive new bone is formed around the focus of inflammation. (From Damjanov I: *Pathology for the health professions,* ed 4, Philadelphia, 2012, Saunders.)

insertion of surgical instrumentation such as prostheses, metal plates, or screws. Infections caused by surgical instrumentation can act as a focus for bacterial reproduction.

During the acute stage of osteomyelitis, bacteria remain in bone and proliferate where the circulation is not optimal. Before puberty the bacteria grow in the metaphyseal sinusoidal vein, which leads to infection of the metaphysis near the growth plate. The loose attachment of overlying periosteum permits exudate to accumulate in the subperiosteal area. Uncontrolled infection can disrupt the cortex and lead to joint infection or septic arthritis, which can cause osteoarthritis to develop later in life. In infants, medullary infection can reach the epiphysis and joint surfaces via capillaries crossing the growth plate, and stunted growth and angular deformities can result. The growth plate in children is avascular, so infection is limited. The inflammatory reaction leads to pus formation, edema, and vascular congestion. Pus collects and is confined within bone, thus increasing pressure and adding to vascular occlusion, ischemia, and, finally, necrosis of bone. Volkmann and haversian canals allow a route for release of pus and thus spread of bacteria. Blood and therefore antibiotics cannot reach bone tissue when vascular system pressure equals arteriolar pressure. As a result, the course and virulence of the osteomyelitis are affected. Even after meticulous treatment, the organism can reappear years later in a context of trauma or immunosuppression.

Healing complications. If osteomyelitis is not managed or if the treatment is not sufficient, the resulting necrotic bone can separate from healthy bone into dead segments called *sequestra.* A sequestrum is then a medium for the continued bacterial proliferation described as chronic osteomyelitis. Sequestra can enlarge and extrude through bone into soft tissue, where it is possible that they might revascularize and resolve as a result of the body's defense mechanisms.

Osteoblasts may try to heal infected bone by isolating the dead tissue and forming an involucrum (a layer of new bone around old bone). Involucrum formation prevents successful effects of antibiotics and phagocytosis and leads to chronic infection.

Any type of osteomyelitis may become chronic, especially if the treatment was inadequate during the acute phase. It may be manifested months or years after assumed cure, especially after acute hematogenous disease. Drainage via a sinus tract to the skin can occur.

Treatment. Treatment usually includes 4 to 6 weeks of parenteral antibiotic therapy for acute osteomyelitis, although in children a typical course may be about 3 weeks in some cases. A shorter period of parenteral therapy followed by oral antibiotics can be effective if the infection is under control, the patient is afebrile, and a therapeutic blood level of the antibiotic can be maintained. Antibiotic choice is based on culture and sensitivity results.

If acute osteomyelitis is complicated by an abscess or extensive necrosis, the involved area is debrided and antibiotic therapy is instituted. If a prosthesis is involved, it is usually removed. After debridement, dead space is usually filled with packing, bone grafts, muscle pedicles, or skin grafts. In osteomyelitis associated with peripheral vascular disease, amputation is performed if antibiotic therapy is unsuccessful.[2]

Tuberculosis

Etiology and pathogenesis. Bone and joint tuberculosis (TB) is an extrapulmonary form of TB that occurs after lymphohematogenous or sometimes contiguous spread from a primary lung lesion. It is estimated to occur in about 5% of patients with pulmonary TB worldwide.[8] As the incidence of TB increases in the United States, one can expect to see more cases of skeletal TB. Persons with skeletal TB may have a history of pulmonary TB, drug abuse, crowded and poor living conditions, diseases that depress the immune system, and immigration to the United States after 1991. Musculoskeletal TB is not communicable to others unless an open wound exists. *Mycobacterium tuberculosis,* the organism responsible for the destruction of bone and joint, is transmitted via the airborne route. Initially, infectious droplets are inhaled and infect lungs; then *M. tuberculosis* spreads hematogenously from lungs or lymphatic drainage to bone. The bacterium may lie dormant for a long time before it is detected.

Clinical manifestations. One of the more common sites of *M. tuberculosis*–infected bone (33% of skeletal TB cases) is in the vertebral column, particularly the lower thoracic and lumbar spine (called Pott's disease). Infection often begins at the anterior portion of the vertebral body and then spreads further into the bone, causing bony destruction, anterior wedging, and collapse. On x-ray, the appearance is of a lytic lesion in the bone without local sclerotic (new bone formation) reaction. In about 50% of cases, the infection spreads to adjacent disks and paraspinal fluid may accumulate as a "cold abscess" that can be seen on CT or MRI of the spine.[9] Symptoms may include local pain, low-grade fever, and possible neurologic symptoms (weakness of lower extremities) attributable to local inflammation of nerve tissue and its surroundings as well as impingement.

Other common sites of skeletal TB or tuberculous arthritis include weight-bearing joints such as the hips, knees, and ankles, although any joint or bone could be involved.[5]

Risk factors. Persons most at risk for TB are those at extremes of age or individuals who are immunosuppressed or undernourished. Children are at higher risk for skeletal TB because of extreme vascularity. In acquired immunodeficiency syndrome (AIDS), knowledge of the patient's human immunodeficiency virus status is critical to optimize the therapeutic plan for the patient.[5]

Treatment. Treatment for skeletal TB requires long-term combination antibiotic therapy. Agents such as isoniazid, rifampin, pyrazinamide, ethambutol, and others are used in combinations for at least 6 to 9 months with longer courses needed for certain drug combinations. Therapeutic response can be complicated by development of drug resistance. Surgical intervention may be indicated in cases of spinal TB when severe deformities or neurologic deficits are seen.[9]

KEY POINTS
- Bone infections may be from blood-borne organisms or direct traumatic infection.
- Osteomyelitis—organisms reach the bone by one of three routes: bloodstream (hematogenous osteomyelitis), adjacent soft tissue (contiguous focus), and direct introduction of the organism into the bone.
- *Staphylococcus aureus* and *Streptococcus pneumoniae* are the two most common organisms to cause bone infections in adults.
- Skeletal tuberculosis occurs when the TB infection spreads hematogenously or via the lung lymphatic drainage to bone and is most common in the vertebral bones, hips, and knees.
- Antibiotic therapy can help to reduce the progression of bone infection and is the first-line treatment; however, abscess formation and chronic infection may occur, requiring surgical intervention.

ALTERATIONS IN BONE STRUCTURE AND MASS

BONE STRUCTURE DISORDERS

Scoliosis

Etiology and pathogenesis. **Scoliosis** is a lateral curvature of the spine resulting in an S- or a C-shaped spinal column with vertebral rotation. Scoliosis can be a consequence of numerous congenital, connective tissue, and neuromuscular disorders. The majority of scoliosis cases are classified as idiopathic with an annual incidence in the general population of about 1%. The frequency is greater in children of women with scoliosis. The idiopathic form is more common in women.[2]

Clinical manifestations. Scoliosis may be described as either structural or nonstructural. Nonstructural scoliosis resolves when the patient bends to the affected side. No vertebral rotation or bony deformity of the vertebrae is present, and the condition is not progressive. When the patient bends laterally, the spine usually appears symmetric. The scoliotic curve will disappear on forward flexion. Nonstructural scoliosis may be related to postural problems, hysteria, nerve root irritation, inflammation, or compensation caused by leg length discrepancy or contracture (in the cervical spine).

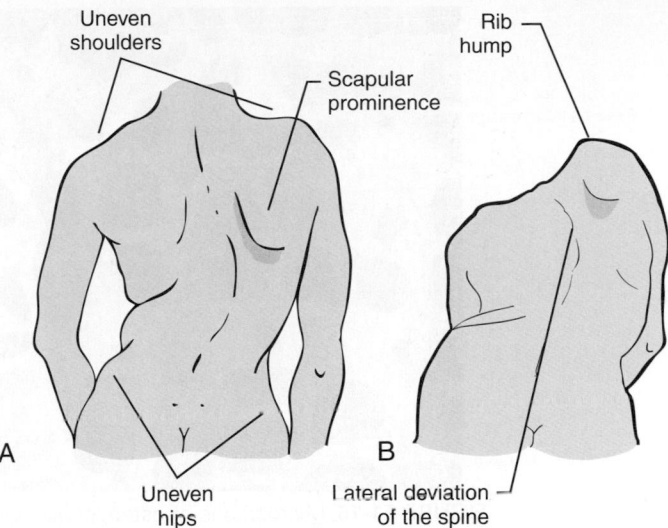

FIGURE 51-15 Structural scoliosis. **A,** The patient is standing erect, demonstrating the asymmetry of shoulder height as well as hip and scapular differences. **B,** The patient is bending forward at the waist, further emphasizing the spinal deviation and asymmetry of the shoulders and upper rib cage.

Structural scoliosis, often called congenital scoliosis, is a lateral curve of the spine that fails to correct itself on forced bending against the curvature and has vertebral rotation. This type of scoliosis is more serious and involves deformity of the vertebrae and asymmetric changes in hip, shoulder, and rib cage positions. The patient lacks normal flexibility, and side bending becomes asymmetric. This type of scoliosis is progressive, and the curve does not disappear on forward flexion. Severe structural scoliosis may require intensive therapy or surgical intervention to halt progression and correct deformities.[2]

Scoliosis is detected by typical asymmetric changes (Figure 51-15), including: (1) uneven shoulders or hips, (2) shoulder or scapular prominence, (3) rib or chest hump when bending over, and (4) a C- or S-shaped spine. A scoliometer can be used to assess the angle of trunk rotation when the patient is bent in a forward flexion position. Scoliosis is usually diagnosed after puberty because of a tendency for the curve to be accentuated during periods of rapid skeletal growth. The diagnosis is confirmed by radiographic examination of the spine. The degree of curvature is determined from radiographs and is classified as right or left, depending on the direction of convexity. Mild degrees of curvature may be managed conservatively with exercise and frequent reevaluation to assess progression to more significant deformity. Surgery is indicated for curvatures of 40 to 50 degrees or greater, or in cases of significant progression of scoliosis in spite of bracing and other conservative therapies.[2]

In addition to body image disturbances, scoliosis predisposes a patient to a number of physiologic problems. Respiratory difficulties from restricted expansion of the lungs may occur. Severe forms may be associated with significant pain. Gastrointestinal dysfunction can result from compression of abdominal organs. If uncorrected, scoliosis may progressively worsen with age owing to increased upper body weight and gravitational forces exacerbating the vertebral deformity. Over time, significant degenerative changes to the intervertebral disks can occur.

Treatment. Treatment for structural scoliosis is aimed at correcting spinal malalignment. Nonsurgical measures include primarily braces and exercises. Bracing applies constant pressure to the spinal convexity to straighten the curve. Braces must be worn for prolonged periods each day to be effective. Compliance is a major difficulty because the

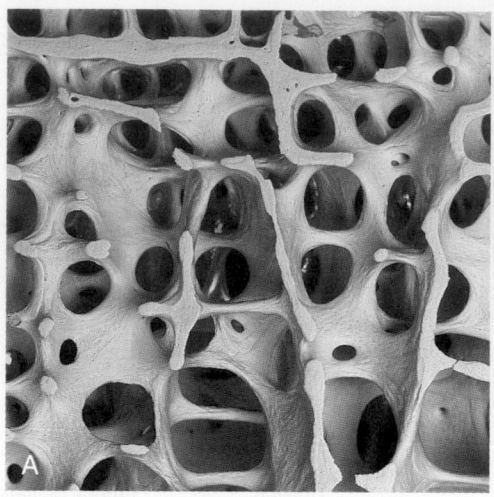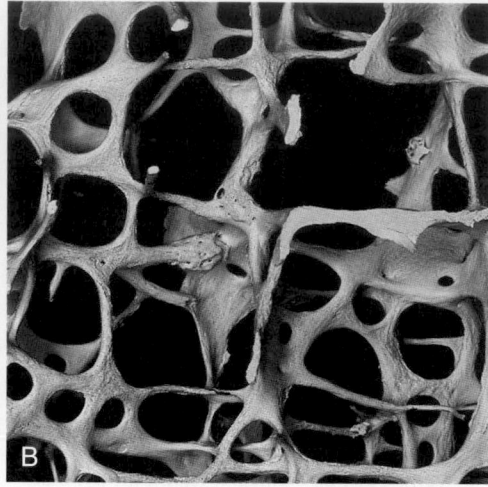

FIGURE 51-16 Micrographs of osteoporosis. On the left is normal bone. On the right is osteoporotic bone with decreased density and loss of trabeculae. (From Fillet HM: *Brocklehurst's textbook of geriatric medicine and gerontology,* ed 7, Philadelphia, 2010, Saunders. Courtesy of Professor A. Boyde, Department of Anatomy and Developmental Biology, University College, London.)

braces are stiff and uncomfortable. Spinal muscle strengthening should accompany brace therapy because trunk musculature loses tone after prolonged bracing.[2] Surgical intervention includes spinal realignment, fusion, and bracing with internal appliances, and most surgical procedures require prolonged body immobilization postoperatively.

Conditioning exercises to strengthen muscles and correct posture are used to treat nonstructural, or postural, scoliosis.

KEY POINTS
- Scoliosis is a lateral deformity of the spinal column that is detected from asymmetry of the shoulders, hips, and chest wall.
- Scoliosis may be described as structural or nonstructural.
- Severe scoliosis can compromise lung expansion and lead to a restrictive respiratory disorder.

METABOLIC BONE DISEASES

Osteoporosis

Etiology and pathogenesis. **Osteoporosis,** the most common metabolic bone disease, affects an estimated more than 10 million people in the United States and leads to more than 1.5 million osteoporotic fractures each year.[8] It occurs when the rate of bone resorption is greater than that of bone formation, osteoblastic and osteoclastic balance is disrupted, and the levels of mineral and protein matrix components are decreased (see discussion on Bone Remodeling in Chapter 50). The number of trabeculae is decreased and the width and mass of bone mass are reduced, which leads to fragile bone and thus fractures (Figure 51-16). Cancellous bone is lost faster than cortical bone, with fractures happening earlier in cancellous bone (vertebrae) than in cortical bone (femoral neck).

A current definition of osteoporosis is based on gradations of bone mineral density (BMD), which is most commonly measured by dual-energy x-ray absorptiometry (DXA). This yields a T score, which is the number of standard deviations the patient's BMD measurement is greater than or less than the young normal mean BMD value. A Z score is the number of standard deviations greater than or less than the mean BMD value of age-matched controls. The World Health Organization

(WHO) defines osteoporosis as bone mineral density (BMD) greater than or equal to 2.5 standard deviations below the mean peak BMD of young normal women (a T score less than −2.5).[8] Osteopenia, which also carries an increased risk of fracture, is defined as a T score between −1.0 and −2.5. Because hip fractures are not uncommon in women with BMD in the osteopenic range, other risk factors for fractures and progression to osteoporosis must be considered. The World Health Organization has developed a computer-based Fracture Risk Assessment tool (FRAX) that calculates a 10-year probability of hip fracture based on multiple variables, including age, body mass index, tobacco use, alcohol use, corticosteroid use, history of rheumatoid arthritis, and personal and parental history of fractures.

The specific cause of osteoporosis is not known. However, the rate of bone loss is influenced greatly by age, genetics, estrogen level, and risk factors. A family history of osteoporosis is a major risk factor. The normal bone loss that occurs with aging is accelerated during menopause, with the most rapid phase of loss occurring in the first 5 years because of the sudden decrease in estrogen concentration. The exact mechanisms of estrogen action are unclear, but estrogen derivatives may influence osteoblast activity and the production of local cytokines and growth factors that modulate the balance of bone resorption and formation. Estrogen deficiency increases the risk of osteoporosis by stimulating bone resorption over formation. Other risk factors include small frame, Caucasian or Asian race, early surgically induced menopause, high doses of thyroid hormone supplementation, use of corticosteroid drugs (such as prednisone), a diet low in sources of calcium and vitamin D, physical inactivity, and smoking or increased alcohol intake. Patients with chronic renal disease often have abnormal parathyroid function, as well as altered calcium and vitamin D metabolism, which can lead to a decline in bone mass. Furthermore, chronic inflammatory diseases, such as rheumatoid arthritis or systemic lupus erythematosus, can be associated with increased risk of osteoporosis, even independent of corticosteroid use (Box 51-1).[8]

Clinical manifestations. Evaluation of the patient must include an assessment of risk factors because osteoporosis is most often asymptomatic until a fracture occurs. On physical examination of someone with longstanding disease, the patient may have a Colles fracture, femoral or hip fractures, or vertebral compression fractures. Obvious kyphosis of the thoracic spine (dowager's hump) may be present. The patient often

BOX 51-1 RISK FACTORS FOR OSTEOPOROSIS

Common Risk Factors
Female gender
Ethnicity (Caucasian or Asian)
Family history
Increased age
Low calcium intake (<400 mg/day)
Low body weight
Smoking
Alcoholism
Prolonged immobilization

Comorbid Diseases Increasing Risk
Rheumatoid arthritis
Cushing syndrome
Hyperthyroidism and thyroid replacement therapy
Hyperparathyroidism
Anorexia nervosa or exercise-induced amenorrhea
Chronic obstructive pulmonary disease
Ankylosing spondylitis
Celiac disease
Hypogonadism
Type 1 diabetes

Genetic Disorders Increasing Risk
Osteogenesis imperfecta
Menkes syndrome
Ehlers-Danlos syndrome
Marfan syndrome
Homocystinuria

Medications Increasing Risk
Corticosteroids
Thyroid hormone supplements
Heparin
Antiepileptic agents
Gonadotropin-releasing hormone agents
Aromatase inhibitors
Cytotoxic/immunosuppressive drugs

Data from Klippel JH, Stone JH, Crofford LJ, White PH, editors: *Primer on the rheumatic diseases,* ed 13, New York, 2008, Springer.

has shortened stature, muscle wasting or spasms of back muscles, and difficulty bending over. The patient may complain of impaired breathing (because of deformities of the spine and rib cage) and poor dentition. Screening bone density measurement is also generally accomplished using DXA, assessing BMD of the hip (trochanter, femoral neck, and total hip), spine (L1 to L4 vertebral bodies), and sometimes the distal radius. Laboratory tests may show normal levels of urinary and serum calcium, phosphorus, and alkaline phosphatase but elevated serum osteocalcin levels. Radiographic and computed tomographic findings may show diffuse radiolucency of bones, sparse transverse trabeculae, normal vertical trabeculae, indistinct articular cortices, wedge-shaped thoracic vertebrae, biconcave lumbar vertebral bodies, and possibly old or new compression fractures.

Treatment. Treatment varies depending on the cause. Moderate, regular exercise such as walking or riding a stationary bicycle is valuable in prevention as well as treatment of osteoporosis. Physical therapy exercises for individuals who are immobilized or paralyzed are helpful as well.

Calcium and vitamin D. Both calcium and vitamin D are necessary for maintenance of bone mass. Calcium is needed as a constituent of bone and vitamin D is essential for increasing intestinal absorption of calcium and for calcium uptake into bone. In vitamin D deficiency states, calcium absorption can decrease from a normal rate of 30% to 40% to just 10% to 15%.[10] Vitamin D must be metabolized to its active form, 1,25-dihydroxyvitamin D_3, which is also regulated by the kidneys. Although sun exposure can increase vitamin D production in skin, this source is often inadequate, even in warm climates. Recommendations for calcium supplementation vary but most experts recommend 1000 to 1200 mg daily—preferring calcium citrate, which does not depend on an acidic environment in the gut for absorption. Vitamin D deficiency can be detected by measurement of blood levels, with a goal of at least 20 mg/ml. Many believe a level of 30 mg/ml not only increases BMD but may also decrease risk of falls by a stimulatory effect on muscle function.[10] The recommended doses of daily vitamin D_3 are 400 to 1000 IU; also, in a deficient state 2000 to 4000 IU daily appears to be safe.

Antiresorptive agents. The most often used antiresorptive agents are the bisphosphonates (alendronate, risedronate, ibandronate, and zoledronate), which increase BMD and decrease fracture risk by inhibiting bone resorption by osteoclasts while osteoblast-related bone formation continues. These agents bind to hydroxyapatite in the bone, thus blocking the enzymes needed for osteoclast cell structure stability during resorption.[11] Questions about long-term use (>5 years) of bisphosphonates have arisen with the concern that the longevity of bisphosphonate binding into the bone may decrease bone's ability to repair microtrauma and be associated with atypical fractures. One such complication is osteonecrosis of the jaw, which, though very rare, has been reported particularly in patients receiving intravenous bisphosphonates for the treatment of bone cancer. Another rare complication under study is the atypical femoral fracture, which occurs below the level of the trochanter and also may be at slightly increased risk in patients taking bisphosphonates for prolonged periods. Ultimately, the risk of a fracture attributable to untreated osteoporosis is 7- to 10-fold higher than the risk of these rare complications. It is recommended that after 5 years of bisphosphonate therapy, a drug "holiday" of 2 years or more be considered with subsequent BMD testing being used to determine need for further treatment.[11]

Other agents for the treatment of osteoporosis include teriparatide, a recombinant human parathyroid hormone, which is the only true anabolic agent. Parathyroid hormone, when given at intermittent doses, increases BMD by stimulating bone turnover with the rate of bone formation exceeding that of resorption. It is approved for daily subcutaneous administration, but its use is limited to 2 years because rat studies have shown an increase in risk for osteosarcomas.[11] Denosumab is a monoclonal antibody that inhibits the receptor activator of nuclear factor κB ligand (RANKL). By binding and inhibiting RANKL, osteoclast activity is suppressed and bone resorption is decreased. This agent is given subcutaneously every 6 months.

Other causes of osteoporosis. Disuse osteoporosis may occur with prolonged bed rest, which leads to an increase in osteoclast activity and resorption of bone greater than osteoblast accumulation. Stress placed on bone as a result of weight bearing is necessary for osteoblast function. The stress of exercise stimulates new bone growth as a result of changes in electrical charges on the bone surface.

The loss of bone density following a period of reduced weight bearing may be restored upon return to normal activity, although recovery may not be complete. Osteoporosis may also occur when collagen formation is impaired in such conditions as scurvy, protein deficiency, or Cushing syndrome.

Rickets and Osteomalacia

Clinical manifestations. **Rickets** and **osteomalacia** are characterized by deficits in mineralization of newly formed bone matrix either in the growing skeleton (rickets) or in the mature skeleton (osteomalacia) with resulting soft osteopenic bone. Deficiency of vitamin D prevents maintenance of normal levels of calcium and phosphorus. Children may have either vitamin D–resistant rickets or congenital hypophosphatasia. In rickets, cartilage in the growing epiphyses fails to calcify. Cartilage is not replaced by bone and continues to enlarge, leading to widening of epiphyseal plates and irregularity of the junction with the metaphyses. Bone is poorly calcified and less rigid. Kyphosis, genu valgum ("knock knee"), and genu varum ("bowleg") are common deformities as well as growth retardation. Delayed eruption of the teeth, enlargement of costochondral junctions, and decreased muscle tone can all be seen.[12]

Osteomalacia is the adult counterpart of rickets with defects occurring after closure of epiphyseal plates. Osteomalacia is always due to an inadequate concentration of vitamin D, calcium, and/or phosphorus in the body as a result of any of the following factors: decreased intestinal absorption of vitamin D and calcium attributable to poor intake or malabsorption; poor vitamin D metabolism attributable to decreased sun exposure; renal disease (especially chronic renal failure or nephrotic syndrome); or a combination of these conditions.[12] In the case of vitamin D deficiency, calcification fails to occur and the bone is soft. Patients may complain of bone pain and muscle weakness, and plain x-rays may show bowing of bones and "pseudofractures." All bones are affected, but weight-bearing structures may collapse and cause compression-type fractures.

Treatment. Treatment involves correction of the underlying deficiency with adequate intake of vitamin D supplementation (especially vitamin D_3). Adequate intake of calcium and phosphate is also indicated by dietary adjustments or supplements.

Paget Disease

Paget disease of bone (osteitis deformans) is a slowly progressive metabolic bone disease characterized by an initial phase of excessive bone resorption, mediated by osteoclasts, followed by excessive bone formation (Figure 51-17). The end product is a disorganized mosaic of bone matrix composed of woven and lamellar bone at affected sites of the skeleton. This new bone is less compact, more vascular, and more fragile, which accounts for the deformities and fractures of Paget disease.

Etiology and pathogenesis. The specific cause of Paget disease is unknown, but the disease has a familial tendency, suggesting a genetic component. It is prevalent in parts of northern Europe and the United States but rare in Africa or Asia.[12] It has also been theorized that a viral infection may affect osteoclastic function, leading to aberrant bone remodeling. Changes in certain cytokines produced in the local bone marrow environment may also influence the bone formation/resorption balance. In the United States, about 1% of individuals older than 40 years have Paget disease, with males being affected slightly more than females.[8]

Clinical manifestations. In the early stages the disease may not cause any symptoms; however, when pain develops, it can be severe and persistent bone pain. Fatigue and joint stiffness are also noted. In the initial stages of Paget disease, affected bones soften and tend to bend. As the disease progresses, irregular subperiosteal bone formation occurs and causes bone to become thick and hard. Thickening of cranial bones may cause compression of cranial nerves and result in vertigo, blindness, deafness (with or without tinnitus), headaches, and facial paralysis. Any bone can be affected, but the most common sites include the sacrum and spine (50%), femur (46%), skull (28%), and pelvis (22%).[12] Other complications may include hypertension, arthritis, calcific periarthritis, and pain.

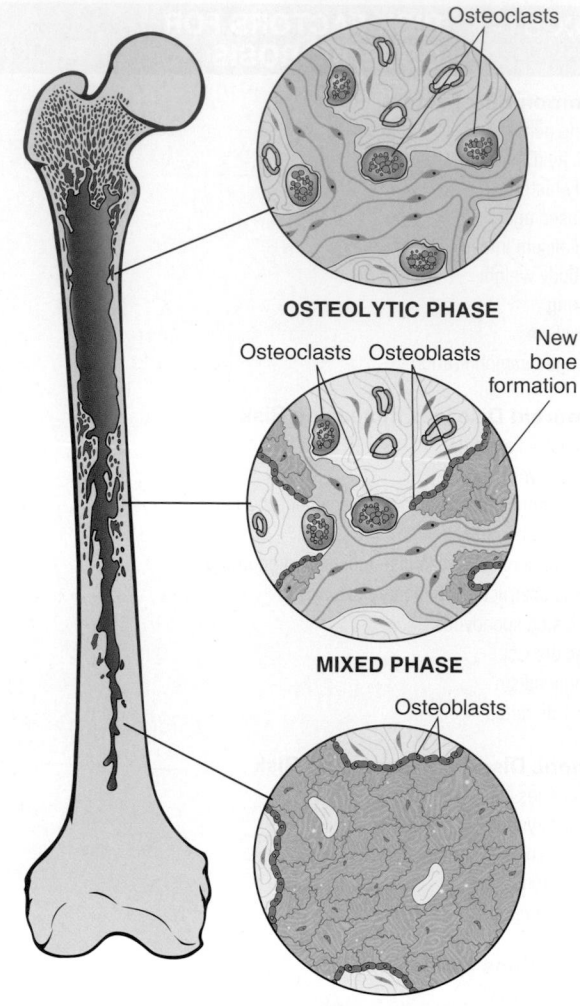

FIGURE 51-17 Diagrammatic representation of Paget disease of bone demonstrating the three phases in the evolution of the disease. (From Kumar V et al: *Robbins basic pathology,* ed 7, Philadelphia, 2003, Saunders, p 764.)

Treatment. During active stages of the disease, treatment focuses on preventing deformity and fracture, often with the use of calcitonin or bisphosphonates (such as alendronate, risedronate, or pamidronate, among others). These medications have been shown to decrease bone resorption, stabilize the fragile bone lesions, and reduce pain and the risk of fractures.[12]

KEY POINTS

- Bone density is a product of the rate of bone resorption and bone deposition.
- Osteoporosis occurs when the rate of bone resorption is greater than that of bone formation. A reduction in bone mass predisposes to fractures.
- Osteoporosis in women is defined by the WHO as a bone mineral density ≥2.5 standard deviations below the mean peak bone mineral density of young normal women.
- Hormone deficiencies (estrogen, androgen), poor calcium intake, and inadequate muscle use are common factors in the rate of bone loss.
- Treatment of osteoporosis should include adequate calcium and vitamin D supplementation along with a choice of antiresorptive agents (e.g., bisphosphonates), anabolic agents (e.g., teriparatide), or other inhibitors of bone resorption (e.g., denosumab) among others.

- Vitamin D deficiency is associated with rickets and osteomalacia, disorders characterized by soft, weak bones.
- Paget disease may be genetic. It has also been theorized that a viral infection may affect osteoclastic function, leading to aberrant bone remodeling. Painful deformities or bone fractures may result.

BONE TUMORS

Neoplasms occurring in the musculoskeletal system can be benign or malignant with a relative incidence ratio of benign to malignant lesions of 200 to 1.[2] Benign tumors often are undiagnosed because they cause no pain. These lesions typically do not grow aggressively or metastasize; also, they do not tend to recur. Malignant neoplasms that originate in bone are referred to as *sarcomas*. These lesions can be very destructive, tend to regrow, and may metastasize.[2] More common than sarcomas are metastatic lesions, which have spread to bone from a primary tumor elsewhere. Primary carcinomas that most commonly metastasize to bone are breast, prostate, lung, and kidney carcinomas. Other malignancies that can metastasize to bone include cancer of the thyroid, bladder, uterus, colon/rectum, and vagina. Common sites of bone metastases are the vertebral bodies, pelvis, proximal ends of the femur and humerus, and ribs. Metastases occur via direct spread within a body cavity or by hematogenous or lymphatic spread.

Thus although the majority of bone tumors are metastatic, a number of primary tumors of bone can be identified. Some bone tumors are benign (Figure 51-18).

Benign Tumors
Osteochondroma
Etiology, pathogenesis, and clinical manifestations. Osteochondroma is a common cartilage-forming benign tumor that is most often asymptomatic and may not be discovered until adulthood. Osteochondromas can be hereditary and are often found unintentionally.

The lesion arises from a growth plate defect that can become pedunculated or sessile. Bony projections on the external surface of the bone are capped with cartilage. Pressure on surrounding soft tissue may cause pain. These tumors are usually located on the metaphyses of long bones such as the proximal end of the tibia and the distal part of the femur, the shoulder, and the pelvis (see Figure 51-18).[2]

Chondroma
Chondroma or enchondroma is a cartilage-forming tumor in bone that can be located in the medullary cavity or in the subperiosteal layers of bone.[2] It is believed to arise from remnants of epiphyseal cartilage. Chondromas develop most often in the small bones of the hands and feet but can be found in other areas. Tumor growth may erode the cortex of bone and expand the contour. Chondromas may be found incidentally, sometimes not until adulthood.

Osteoid Osteoma
Osteoid osteoma is one of the more common types of benign bone-forming tumor and accounts for approximately 10% to 13% of symptomatic benign lesions.[2] The patient often complains of persistent, dull pain, which is often worse at night and alleviated by aspirin or other nonsteroidal antiinflammatory drugs. This small lesion is often found in the cortex of the tibia and femur, but any bone may be involved. Radiographs show the lesion enclosed in a sclerotic shell. This tumor usually occurs in persons in their twenties.[2]

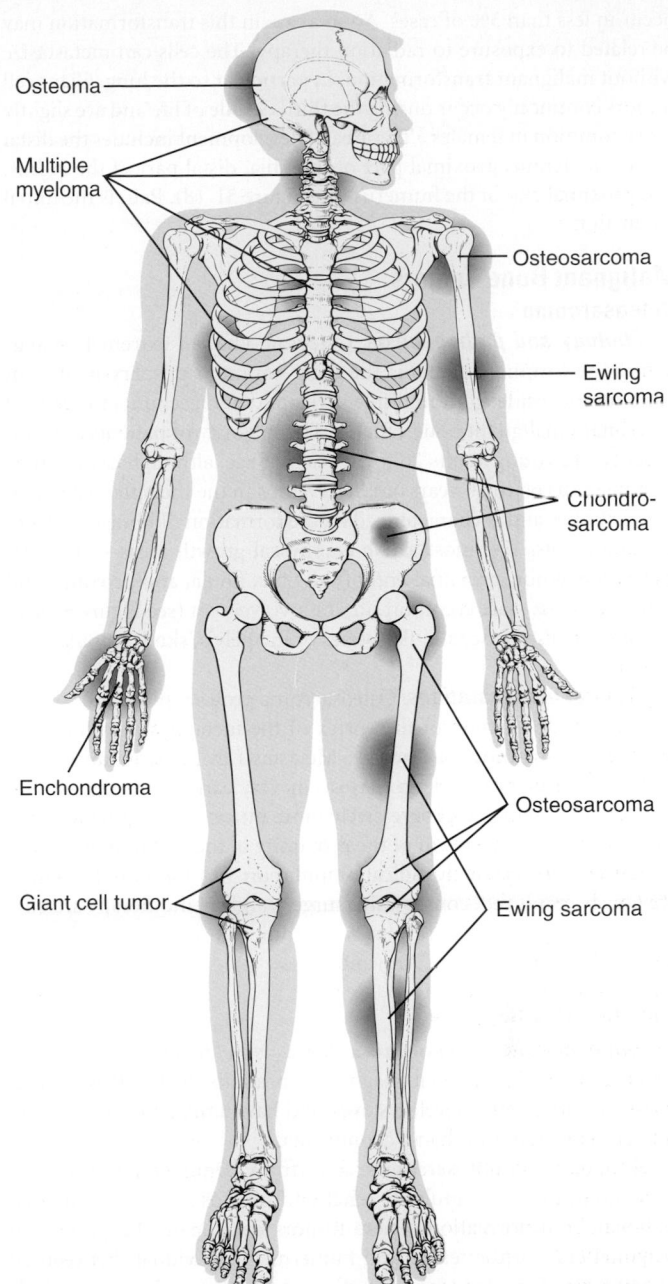

FIGURE 51-18 Schematic presentation of the most common sites of origin of bone tumors. Most often, osteosarcomas originate in the metaphyses of long bones, chondrosarcomas arise in the axial skeleton, Ewing sarcomas develop in the diaphyses of long bones, and giant cell tumors originate in the epiphyses of long bones. Osteomas occur most often in the skull and enchondromas in the small bones of the hand. Multiple myelomas involve the calvaria, vertebrae, and ribs, but also other bones that contain hematopoietic bone marrow. (From Damjanov I: *Pathology for the health professions,* ed 4, Philadelphia, 2012, Saunders.)

Giant Cell Tumor
Many different tumors can contain giant cells but are not true giant cell tumors. A **giant cell tumor,** or osteoclastoma, is benign but aggressive with richly vascularized tissue consisting of plump spindle-shaped cells and numerous giant cells. These lesions account for about 5% to 10% of all primary bone tumors.[2] In some cases, giant cell tumors undergo transformation to sarcomas, a complication that is thought to

occur in less than 5% of cases. An increase in this transformation may be related to exposure to radiation therapy. The cells can metastasize without malignant transformation, in particular to the lung. Giant cell tumors commonly occur during the third decade of life and are slightly more common in females.[2] The area of development includes the distal end of the femur, proximal part of the tibia, distal part of the radius, and proximal end of the humerus (see Figure 51-18). Pain is the initial complaint.

Malignant Bone Tumors
Osteosarcoma

Etiology and pathogenesis. Osteosarcoma, an extremely malignant bone-forming tumor, is the most common primary malignant bone tumor (aside from multiple myeloma) and accounts for 20% of all primary malignant bone cancers. The majority of patients are adolescents and young adults 20 to 30 years of age, although cases can be seen in adults 60 to 70 years old. It develops in the metaphyseal region of long bones and is characterized by the formation of bone or osteoid by tumor cells. The most active epiphyseal growth areas—the distal end of the femur, proximal end of the tibia, fibula, and proximal end of the humerus—are common sites of involvement (see Figure 51-18). Lesions can also be seen in flat bones of the pelvis, skull, scapula, ribs, or spine.[6]

Clinical manifestations. Osteosarcoma grows rapidly and is quite destructive; destruction of the cortex of the metaphyseal region predisposes it to pathologic fracture. Metastasis to lungs is noted early in disease development. Pain may occur very early in the disease and become consistent and progressively more intense. Joint function may be compromised as a result of the proximity of the metaphysis.

Treatment. Although radical amputation was the only treatment previously employed, conservative surgery and chemotherapy are currently providing positive results, with studies showing 5-year disease-free survival rates between 70% and 85%.[2]

Chondrosarcoma

Pathogenesis. A **chondrosarcoma** is a malignant cartilage-forming tumor most often diagnosed in adults 30 to 60 years old. These tumors usually develop slowly and have a higher cellularity and greater pleomorphism than a chondroma.

Secondary chondrosarcomas arise from benign lesions such as osteochondroma or multiple enchondromatosis, which undergo malignant transformation. These tumors develop in the pelvis and proximal ends of the femur and humerus in individuals between 20 and 40 years of age. Evidence of malignant transformation may include pain, an irregular border, or an increase in the proximal end of long bones after patient growth is complete.[2]

Clinical manifestations. Because of the slow growth of the tumor, pain is not usually a prominent clinical symptom. Even with a slow rate of development, the tumor will eventually metastasize, typically to the lung. Chondrosarcomas tend to develop in the pelvic and shoulder girdles as well as the ribs and the proximal ends of long bones such as the femur (see Figure 51-18).[2]

Ewing Sarcoma

Pathogenesis. Ewing sarcoma is the third most common primary sarcoma of bone and is characterized as a rapidly growing malignant round cell tumor. This tumor most often develops in the bones of children and young adults between the ages of 5 and 25 years. Ewing tumor is composed of densely packed small cells with round nuclei. It arises in the medullary canal of bone and perforates the cortex of the shaft, producing a painful soft-tissue mass (with a central lytic area) overlying the involved bone. The tumor favors pelvic bones followed by long tubular bones, such as the femur, tibia, humerus, or scapula (see Figure 51-18).[2]

Clinical manifestations and treatment. Ewing sarcoma metastasizes quite early in its development to the lungs and other bones, with 15% to 25% of cases being metastatic at diagnosis.[2] Because of the rapid rate of growth, pain is a dominant symptom that increases in severity. Ewing sarcoma is often confused with osteomyelitis because patients often appear systemically ill and may develop fever, anemia, leukocytosis, and an increased sedimentation rate.[2] Treatment with local resection and chemotherapy of an isolated lesion can have a 5-year survival approaching 70%. In patients with metastatic disease at diagnosis, 5-year survival drops to 30% even with surgery and radiotherapy or chemotherapy.[2]

Multiple Myeloma

Etiology and pathogenesis. Multiple myeloma is a slowly growing bone marrow malignancy with neoplastic proliferation of a single clone of plasma cells. The annual incidence is approximately 4 per 100,000 and represents about 1% of all malignant cancers.[13] It is usually a disease of elderly adults.

Clinical manifestations and treatment. Although multiple myeloma is not a sarcoma, its symptoms and radiographic findings are similar. On radiographs, evidence of bone destruction by a lytic, or bone-destroying, process and bone marrow involvement can be seen. Homogeneous immunoglobulin is also present in urine or serum. Because multiple myeloma is a slow-growing lesion, it takes a long time to become symptomatic. Bone pain is the most common symptom, particularly of the chest and back, and is related to excessive accumulation of abnormal plasma cells in the bone marrow (Chapter 11). Although it can affect any bone, multiple myeloma most commonly occurs in the thoracic and lumbar vertebrae. Patients experience hypercalcemia and pathologic fractures where bone has been destroyed. This disease can also cause kidney dysfunction, lung or pleural involvement, and neurologic symptoms attributable to nerve compression. Treatment often requires aggressive combination chemotherapy, although at times local radiation may be useful for refractory bone pain.

> **KEY POINTS**
> - Primary tumors of the bone are not common. Osteochondroma, chondroma, osteoid osteoma, and giant cell tumors are benign, primary bone tumors.
> - Malignant bone tumors include osteosarcoma, chondrosarcoma, and Ewing sarcoma.
> - Multiple myeloma is a slow-growing bone marrow malignancy in which plasma cells proliferate. This disease affects the kidneys and the immune and circulatory systems.

▌DISEASES OF SKELETAL MUSCLE

Skeletal muscle, the most abundant tissue in the human body, accounts for approximately 40% of total body weight.[3] Skeletal muscle performs dynamic work (locomotion) and static work (posture). As with other tissue of the musculoskeletal system, muscle atrophies in response to disuse and immobilization, and hypertrophies when subjected to increased stress.

MUSCULAR DYSTROPHY

Muscular dystrophy comprises a group of genetically determined myopathies characterized by progressive muscle weakness and degeneration as muscle tissue is replaced by fat and fibrous connective tissue.

The dystrophies are classified by their pattern of inheritance, age of onset, and distribution of muscular weakness.

Duchenne Muscular Dystrophy

Etiology and pathogenesis. **Duchenne muscular dystrophy,** the most common and most severe form of muscular dystrophy, is inherited as an X-linked trait and therefore afflicts only males. The incidence is 1 in 3500 male births. Because of a genetic mutation, muscle cells are deficient in the protein dystrophin, a deficiency that weakens the cell membrane and allows extracellular fluid to leak into the cell. Proteases and inflammatory processes are activated, leading to muscle fiber necrosis and muscle degeneration.[14]

The disease begins at birth and is usually apparent by the age of 3 years, with initial involvement of the pelvic girdle and progression to the shoulder girdle.

Clinical manifestations. The calf muscles of an individual with Duchenne muscular dystrophy are noticeably enlarged because of the infiltration of fat cells and degeneration of muscle fibers. Distal muscle involvement leads to frequent falling by the age of 5 or 6 years, and by age 12 to 14 years most children are confined to a wheelchair. Some muscles, such as those in the hands, face, jaw, pharynx, larynx, and eyes, are spared to the end. Survival to age 20 is rare. Cardiac failure or pulmonary infection is the usual cause of death.[14]

Treatment. Treatment of muscular dystrophy is focused on appropriate education for the patient and family, preservation of physical function as long as possible, and prevention of contractures. In some cases, corticosteroid therapy may be useful to delay loss of muscle strength and prolong independent ambulation, but eventual steroid-induced osteoporosis is a risk. Immunosuppressive therapies have also been tried but with limited success.

Becker Muscular Dystrophy

Etiology, pathogenesis, and clinical manifestations. Becker muscular dystrophy is a milder form of inherited muscle degeneration, somewhat less common than the Duchenne type. The genetic mutation leads to production of a reduced amount of an abnormal dystrophin protein and a slower muscular degeneration. Calf hypertrophy is still prominent and often painful with progressive loss of strength and ability to ambulate. The mean age of symptom onset is somewhat later (older than 5 years and even into adulthood) with patients requiring a wheelchair by the age of 30 years.[14]

Facioscapulohumeral Muscular Dystrophy

Etiology and pathogenesis. Facioscapulohumeral muscular dystrophy is an inherited autosomal dominant trait that affects the muscles of the shoulder girdle and the face. It is rare with an annual incidence of 1 in 20,000. The onset of disease can occur at any age, but it usually begins in the second decade. Facial muscles are involved early, with later involvement of scapular and upper arm musculature. It progresses slowly with periods of arrest and can ultimately involve more distal muscles of the upper and lower extremities. Both males and females are affected, and most live to a normal age.[14]

OTHER DISORDERS OF MUSCLE

Myasthenia Gravis

Myasthenia gravis is a chronic autoimmune disease affecting the neuromuscular function of voluntary muscles and characterized by profound muscle weakness and fatigability. Its peak onset in females occurs at 20 to 30 years of age although onset later in life is becoming more widely recognized. Women are affected more often than men with a prevalence of 15 per 100,000. Characteristically, weakness begins with ocular and cranial muscles, and then limb muscles can also be involved. During times of emotional stress, respiratory muscles may be included.[14]

In myasthenia gravis, acetylcholine receptor antibodies are produced that destroy or block acetylcholine receptors of the muscle end-plate of the neuromuscular junction. These antibodies impair the transmission of acetylcholine across the junction. The result is the muscle weakness and fatigability so prevalent in this disease.

Treatment. Anticholinesterase inhibitors (e.g., pyridostigmine bromide, neostigmine) may be used to inhibit breakdown of acetylcholine in the neuromuscular synapse. Increased synaptic acetylcholine enhances the activation of postsynaptic receptors and improves skeletal muscle contraction force. Because myasthenia gravis is an autoimmune disorder, corticosteroids, intravenous immunoglobulin, plasmapheresis, and immunosuppressive agents may be used to regulate the immune system. In severe cases, respiratory muscle fatigue may necessitate mechanical ventilation. Thymectomy is often recommended when patients fail to respond well to medications, particularly in patients less than 45 years old.[14]

Myasthenia crisis can be due to insufficient medication, emotional stress, trauma, infection, or surgery. A sudden increase in blood pressure and pulse rate is noted. Other symptoms include cyanosis from hypoxia, absent cough and gag reflexes, restlessness, increased secretions and lacrimation, diaphoresis, decreased urine output, bowel and bladder incontinence, dysarthria, and respiratory distress.

Cholinergic crisis is usually due to excessive medication. Patients experiencing such a crisis will have fasciculations, especially around the mouth; difficulty chewing, swallowing, and speaking; advancing muscle weakness approximately 1 hour after anticholinesterase medication; nausea and vomiting; cramps and diarrhea; increased secretions (salivary, perspiration, lacrimal, bronchial); headache; confusion; irritability and anxiety; syncope; and respiratory distress leading to respiratory arrest.

CHRONIC MUSCLE PAIN

Fibromyalgia Syndrome

Etiology and pathogenesis. The cause of **fibromyalgia syndrome** (**FMS**) is unknown. No laboratory abnormalities have been found, muscle biopsy findings are nonspecific, and patients are usually normal on psychological testing. The condition is not an inflammatory process but rather a "pain syndrome," with recent studies suggesting that changes in the central nervous system may lead to amplification of pain fiber impulses, a theory called *central sensitization.* This generalized increase in pain sensitivity may involve both ascending and descending neural pathways and a variety of neurotransmitters and neuropeptides.[15]

FMS is characterized by chronic pain in muscles and surrounding structures often of months' or years' duration. Additional symptoms include fatigue, sleep dysfunction, headache, numbness and tingling (i.e., paresthesia), joint pain, memory and concentration difficulties, irritable bowel syndrome, depression, edema of the hands, and sensitivity to cold. Patients either may have no other musculoskeletal disease or may have rheumatoid arthritis, osteoarthritis, Lyme disease, or sleep apnea. FMS is characterized by a strong female preponderance, with an estimated prevalence in the United States of more than 45% of the general population.[15]

Clinical manifestations. Patients with FMS complain of widespread musculoskeletal pain, stiffness, and fatigability. Joint pain and swelling may be perceived by the patient, but the swelling, if present, is usually soft-tissue "puffiness" and not a true inflammatory process. Complaints of muscle pain and weakness are expressed without objective demonstration. In addition to pain and fatigue, sleep disturbances are a common complaint. The examination of a patient with FMS is characterized by an excessive number of reported symptoms with minimal objective findings other than muscular tenderness. Proposed criteria for the diagnosis of FMS established by the American College of Rheumatology include widespread pain in combination with tenderness of at least 11 of 18 (9 bilateral sites) specific tender-point sites, especially of the cervical, paraspinal, trapezius, and parascapular muscles, as well as gluteal and trochanteric areas among others. However, these criteria were not meant to be used for diagnosis and FMS is diagnosed on a clinical basis. Although the specific tender points are the most common and are included in the criteria for fibromyalgia, in actuality, nearly any muscle in the human body could be tender to palpation.[8]

Treatment. FMS is a chronic pain condition that is not life threatening nor does it lead to destruction of musculoskeletal tissues. Because the cause of FMS is unknown, treatment focuses on maintaining functionality and reducing symptoms. Patient education is important and may be associated with improved outcomes and better prognosis. An exercise regimen is essential and should include regular stretching; improvement in physical conditioning via low-impact aerobic exercise (biking, swimming, walking); and measures of pacing, muscle protection, and relaxation. Because pain and fatigue may be aggravated by stress and other psychological factors, counseling may be helpful.[16]

Blinded, randomized, placebo-controlled studies of amitriptyline, cyclobenzaprine, zolpidem, and alprazolam administered at bedtime have indicated that all are effective FMS therapy. Treatment begins at the lowest possible doses and increases as tolerated, with the goal being to improve quality of sleep without drug side effects, such as daytime somnolence or excessive dry mouth. Other medications under investigation in FMS are meant to lower pain sensitivity. The selective serotonin reuptake inhibitors that have been studied in FMS include fluoxetine, sertraline, and citalopram. Although their efficacy as monotherapy is modest at best, they may prove beneficial in combination with other agents. Most recently, pregabalin (an anticonvulsant agent) has been shown to be effective in reducing pain and is the first FDA-approved drug for the treatment of FMS. Additional medications that may have a role include venlafaxine and duloxetine (both serotonin-norepinephrine reuptake inhibitors), and tramadol (an opioid-like analgesic) among many other agents being investigated.[8,16]

KEY POINTS

- Muscular dystrophy comprises a group of genetic disorders characterized by degeneration of skeletal muscle.
- Duchenne muscular dystrophy is inherited as an X-linked disorder and affects only males.
- Becker muscular dystrophy is a milder form of inherited muscle degeneration, somewhat less common than the Duchenne type. The genetic mutation leads to production of a reduced amount of an abnormal dystrophin protein and a slower muscular degeneration. Calf hypertrophy is still prominent and often painful with progressive loss of strength and ability to ambulate
- Facioscapulohumeral muscular dystrophy is an autosomal dominant disorder in which degenerating muscle fibers are replaced by connective tissue such that muscles may increase in bulk even though muscle strength is lost.
- Myasthenia gravis is an autoimmune disorder characterized by progressive weakness as the muscles are used. Antibodies against acetylcholine receptors in the motor end-plate interrupt neuromuscular transmission.
- FMS is a poorly characterized chronic disorder associated with generalized pain, stiffness, sleep dysfunction, and fatigability.

SUMMARY

A solid working knowledge of the anatomy, physiology, and biomechanics of movement is extremely important when dealing with any type of alteration in the musculoskeletal system. With a grasp of the mechanics involved in function, the clinician is able to approach each aberration with an awareness of the time requirements for healing, stress tolerances, and expected management outcomes.

The injuries and diseases discussed in this chapter are a small representation of the many dysfunctions that may afflict the musculoskeletal system. An ability to determine the specific type of tissue involved (contractile or inert) allows the clinician to be cognizant of activities that would aggravate trauma, types of injury that require supportive devices, and injuries that respond to medical intervention.

An awareness of the tissue response to healing enhances the clinician's evaluative skills and provides a signal regarding when intervention has achieved the expected results within an appropriate time frame. It is the responsibility of the practitioner to become knowledgeable about the variety of dysfunctions that occur. This knowledge base must continue to expand as technological advancements provide increasingly complex levels of information and new diagnostic tools become available.

REFERENCES

1. Cyriax J: *Textbook of orthopedic medicine: diagnosis of soft tissue lesions*, ed 8, London, 1982, Bailliere Tindall.
2. Skinner HB, editor: *Current diagnosis and treatment in orthopedics*, ed 4, New York, 2006, McGraw-Hill.
3. Firestein GS, Budd RC, Harris ED, et al, editors: *Kelley's textbook of rheumatology*, ed 8, Philadelphia, 2008, Saunders.
4. Hettinga DL: Inflammatory response of synovial joint structures. In Gould J, editor: *Orthopedic and sports physical therapy*, ed 2, St Louis, 1990, Mosby, p 100.
5. Hochberg MC, Silman AJ, Smolen JS, et al, editors: *Rheumatology*, ed 4, Philadelphia, 2008, Elsevier.
6. Ahn JM, El-Khoung GY: Occult fractures of extremities, *Radiol Clin North Am* 43(3):561–579, 2007.
7. Frassica FJ, Sponseller PD, Wilckens JH, editors: *5-Minute orthopaedic consult*, ed 2, Philadelphia, 2007, Lippincott Williams & Wilkins.
8. Klippel JH, Stone JH, Crofford LJ, White PH, editors: *Primer on the rheumatic diseases*, ed 13, New York, 2008, Springer.
9. Mandell GL, Bennett JE, Dolin R, editors: *Mandell, Douglas & Bennett's principles and practice of infectious disease*, ed 7, Philadelphia, 2009, Churchill Livingstone.
10. Silver DS: Calcium and vitamin D controversies, *Rheum Dis Clin North Am* 37(3):351–363, 2011.
11. Zhang J, Saag KG, Curtis JR: Long-term safety concerns of antiresorptive therapy, *Rheum Dis Clin North Am* 37(3):387–400, 2011.
12. Gardner DG, Shoback D, editors: *Greenspan's basic and clinical endocrinology*, ed 9, New York, 2011, McGraw-Hill.
13. Siegel R, Ward E, Brawley O, Jemal A: Cancer statistics, 2011: the impact of eliminating socioeconomic and racial disparities on premature cancer deaths, *CA Cancer J Clin* 61(4):212, 2011.
14. Goldman L, Schafer AI, editors: *Goldman's Cecil medicine*, ed 24, Philadelphia, 2011, Elsevier.
15. Staud R: Abnormal pain modulation in patients with spatially distributed chronic pain: fibromyalgia, *Rheum Dis Clin North Am* 35(2):263–274, 2009.
16. Mease PJ, Choy EH: Pharmacotherapy of fibromyalgia, *Rheum Dis Clin North Am* 35(2):359–372, 2009.

Alterations in Musculoskeletal Function: Rheumatic Disorders

Carol L. Danning

e_volve WEBSITE

http://evolve.elsevier.com/Copstead/
- Review Questions and Answers
- Glossary (with audio pronunciations for selected terms)
- Animations
- Case Studies
- Key Points Review

KEY QUESTIONS

- How are osteoarthritis and rheumatoid arthritis differentiated on the basis of cause, clinical findings, and treatment?
- What are the similarities and differences among rheumatoid arthritis, systemic lupus erythematosus, and scleroderma?
- What are the infective organisms associated with joint inflammation and Lyme disease?
- What is the pathogenesis of gouty arthritis?
- How do the three subtypes of juvenile rheumatoid arthritis differ?

CHAPTER OUTLINE

Arthritis is the most common disabling musculoskeletal condition in the United States. The National Arthritis Foundation estimates that approximately 46 million people have arthritis with the numbers increasing yearly as the population ages. More than 150 defined rheumatologic diseases have been identified. This chapter discusses the more common rheumatologic diseases.[1]

LOCAL DISORDERS OF JOINT FUNCTION

Osteoarthritis

Osteoarthritis (degenerative joint disease) is the most common arthritis worldwide. It is a progressive, noninflammatory disease of diarthrodial joints, especially those that bear weight. It is characterized by a progressive loss of articular cartilage and by formation of thick subchondral bone and new bone at the joint margins. Osteoarthritis (OA) becomes more prevalent with increasing age. Individuals older than 70 years have the highest incidence. In postmenopausal women, the knees and hands are most frequently affected by OA.[1] It is difficult to estimate the exact prevalence of OA because of difficulties associated with diagnosis, lack of longitudinal data, and problems in defining disease onset.

Etiology and pathogenesis. The etiologic progression of OA varies widely. Development of OA may be related to factors that increase the likelihood of abnormal "wear and tear" on joints such as obesity, joint trauma, and congenital disorders (e.g., hip dysplasia, joint laxity, leg length discrepancy). Other predisposing conditions include lifestyle factors and occupation (stress to joints), genetic predisposition, and hormonal status (postmenopausal).[1]

Biomechanical, biochemical, inflammatory, and immunologic factors may all be involved in the development of OA (Figure 52-1). An initial injury causes release of proteolytic and collagenolytic enzymes from chondrocytes. A breakdown of the matrix of proteoglycan and collagen occurs. The decreased hydration of cartilage that occurs with aging can increase the likelihood of wear and damage. Collagen fatigue and microfracture occur with the stress of weight bearing. The ability of the structure to absorb shock is decreased as a result of subcortical bone and cartilage microfractures. Breakdown of joint integrity overloads the capacity for repair, with resultant degenerative changes.

Structural deterioration of the cartilage involves fissuring, pitting, and erosion. Erosion can become so extensive that the articular surface denudes the full thickness of the cartilage. Osteophyte spur formation, subchondral bone sclerosis, and cyst formation are also examples of structural changes present in OA. Cartilage fragments may break off into joints and form "loose bodies" (Figure 52-2). Joint effusions are common in advanced cases. Synovium becomes inflamed and secretes an increased amount of synovial fluid, which causes the joint to distend.

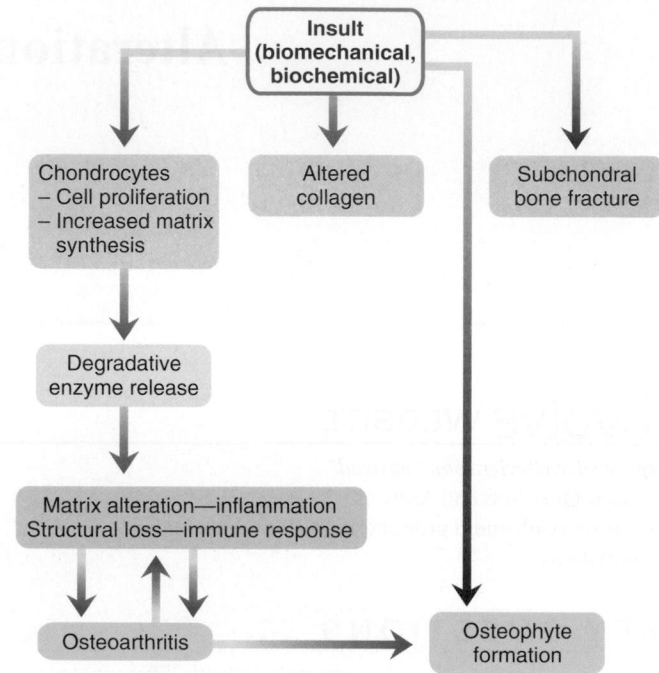

FIGURE 52-1 Pathogenesis of osteoarthritis.

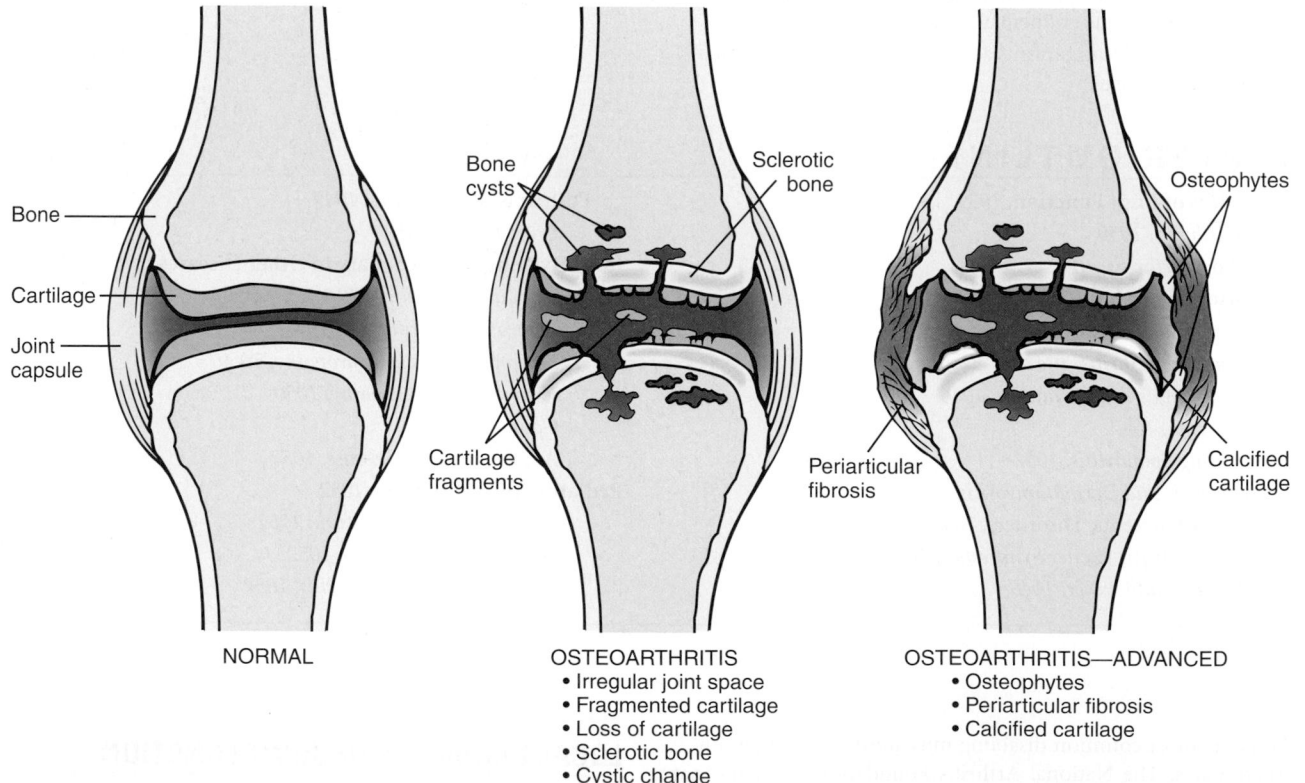

NORMAL

OSTEOARTHRITIS
- Irregular joint space
- Fragmented cartilage
- Loss of cartilage
- Sclerotic bone
- Cystic change

OSTEOARTHRITIS—ADVANCED
- Osteophytes
- Periarticular fibrosis
- Calcified cartilage

FIGURE 52-2 Schematic presentation of the pathologic changes in osteoarthritis. Fragmentation and loss of cartilage denude the subchondral bone, which undergoes sclerosis and cystic change. Osteophytes form on the lateral side and protrude into the adjacent soft tissues, causing irritation, inflammation, and fibrosis. (From Damjanov I: *Pathology for the health professions,* ed 4, Philadelphia, 2012, Saunders.)

Clinical manifestations. Bony enlargement of joints, crepitus with movement, morning stiffness lasting less than 30 minutes (that improves with joint mobility), and pain with function are typical clinical manifestations of OA. These signs and symptoms are usually local. Although any joint may be affected, weight-bearing joints such as the hips and knees, cervical and lumbosacral joints, and interphalangeal joints are most frequently involved. Degenerative arthritis or OA may occur in an isolated joint, or multiple joints can be involved, especially in the hand. Mechanical dysfunction, anatomic anomalies, or trauma may cause breakdown of the joint surface. It is imperative to establish a differential diagnosis and to eliminate a systemic or medical problem. Although OA is localized, rheumatoid arthritis (RA) is a systemic autoimmune disorder that causes a highly inflammatory, symmetric, peripheral arthritis.

Radiologic abnormalities are normally consistent with clinical symptoms. Classic findings include bony proliferation at the joint margins (i.e., osteophytes or bone spurs), asymmetric narrowing of the joint space, and sclerosis of the subchondral bone. Later, malalignment of the joints and cyst formation in subchondral bone can also be seen. When significant synovial fluid accumulates in the joint, it is usually translucent noninflammatory fluid containing less than 2000 white blood cells per cubic millimeter.[1]

The most common deformity of the hands occurs in the distal interphalangeal (DIP) joints (Figure 52-3). Enlargement is caused by bone spurs (*Heberden nodes*) that form on the dorsolateral and medial aspects of the joint. Similar enlargements in the proximal interphalangeal (PIP) joints are called *Bouchard nodes.* The knees and hips are also common locations for OA. Local pain over joint margins, tenderness, crepitus, and muscle atrophy are common findings. Loss of cartilage in medial or lateral compartments of the knee may lead to such structural changes as genu valgus or varus (Figure 52-4).

Pain is relieved by rest during initial stages, though stiffness can be a complaint after prolonged sitting. Because cartilage does not contain nociceptors (pain receptors), pain originates from intraarticular and periarticular structures. Although an acute inflammatory response is often the result of a specific traumatic incident and may cause synovitis in the joint capsule, acute inflammation is not commonly associated with OA. As breakdown in structure progresses, even light activity elicits discomfort, and pain at night is common.

Treatment. Initial treatment is designed to decrease stress on the joint and protect it from additional trauma. Acetaminophen is often the initial analgesic agent recommended for management of mild OA symptoms. Nonsteroidal antiinflammatory drug (NSAID) therapy decreases swelling and pain. Most NSAIDs are nonselective, but antiinflammatory agents that target the cyclooxygenase-2 (COX-2) enzyme have clinical benefit equal to traditional NSAIDs and may have potentially fewer gastrointestinal side effects. The only COX-2 inhibitor presently available in the United States is celecoxib (Celebrex). All NSAIDs (selective or nonselective) have the potential for renal toxicity and possibly even cardiovascular side effects. Visco-supplementation, the intraarticular injection of hyaluronan or its derivatives, may increase joint lubrication, reduce inflammation, and alleviate pain.

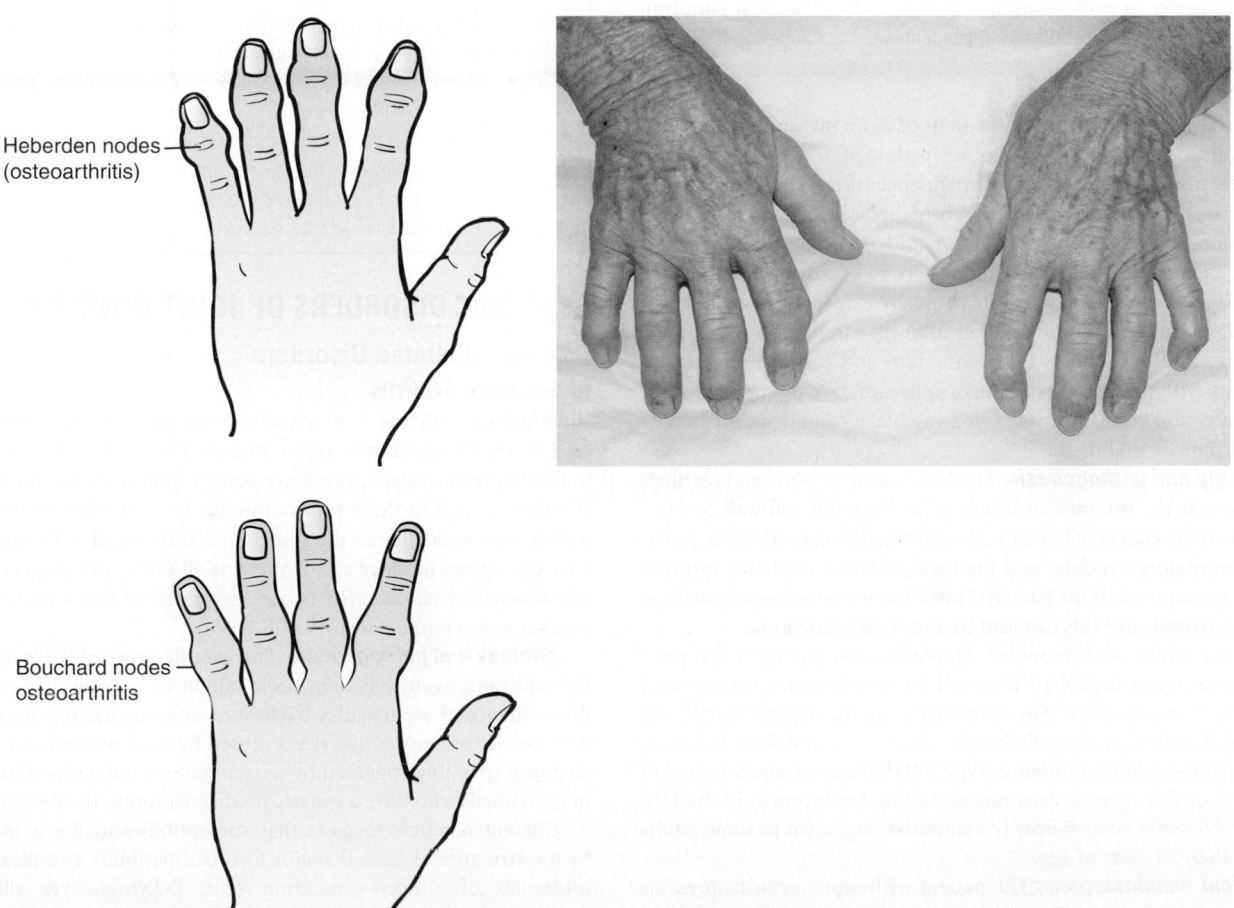

FIGURE 52-3 Comparison of Heberden nodes with Bouchard nodes (seen in patients with osteoarthritis).

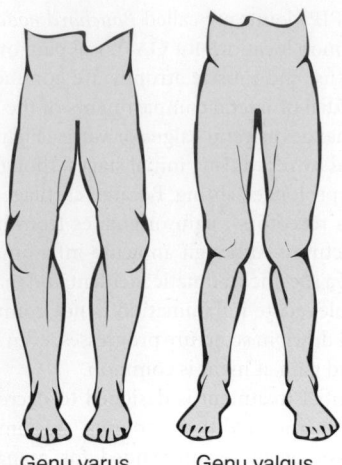

Genu varus   Genu valgus

FIGURE 52-4 Genu varus and genu valgus.

These agents are currently only available for use in knee OA. Intraarticular corticosteroid injections can provide temporary pain relief, but too frequent usage (i.e., more than three injections per year in the same joint) may accelerate cartilage deterioration.

Physical therapy to improve range of motion, muscle strength, and joint conditioning as well as weight reduction can improve symptoms and prevent loss of function. Assistive devices, such as a cane or walker, afford mechanical relief of weight-bearing stress as can supportive shoe wear. Surgical intervention may be necessary if the joint surface loses enough integrity to prevent joint function. OA is the most common cause for total hip and total knee replacement.

Infectious Arthritis

Infectious or septic arthritis may be defined as an invasion of the synovial membrane by bacteria or another pathogen, leading to a closed-space infection. A reported annual incidence of infection in a joint is 2 to 10 cases per 100,000, with much higher rates noted in patients with comorbid diseases such as rheumatoid arthritis, diabetes, osteoarthritis, chronic kidney disease, and others.[2] The pathogen can invade the joint space via a hematogenous route, by extension of an adjacent infection, or from direct inoculation following trauma or an invasive procedure. Infection causes both synovium and cartilage to deteriorate. Joints with underlying disease or inflammation are more susceptible to infection because of increased vascularity and defective barrier effects of the synovial tissue.

Etiology and pathogenesis. The basic cause of bone and cartilage destruction is the interaction of antigenic bacterial cell wall components, the toxic effects of bacteria, the destruction caused by the purulent inflammatory exudate, and the local immune-mediated synovial or cartilage response. If the bacterial infection is not managed, cartilage can be destroyed, and this can lead to ankylosis of the joint.

In most adults and neonates, *Staphylococcus aureus* is the most common causative organism followed by *Streptococcus pyogenes* and *Streptococcus pneumoniae.* Also in neonates, gram-negative bacilli can be cultured, including *Kingella kingae,* which is an oral flora. In young children, *Haemophilius influenzae* type B (HIB) was a frequent cause of infection but this agent is now rare since the development of the HIB vaccine.[2] *Neisseria gonorrhoeae* is a causative organism in some adults younger than 30 years of age.

Clinical manifestations. The patient with septic arthritis presents with joint pain, fever, chills, and leukocytosis. Fever may range from mild to high fever with shaking chills. A warm, red, and very swollen joint with limited range of motion attributable to pain is symptomatic

of any type of infectious arthritis. Usually only a single joint is involved, but polyarticular joint infections can occur in 10% to 20% of cases, most often in debilitated or immunosuppressed individuals. Synovial fluid analysis reveals a very high white cell count (often >50,000 cells/mm³), and diagnosis is established by recovery of bacteria from synovial fluid. Blood cultures are also used to provide a medical diagnosis.[2]

Treatment. Treatment of a septic joint should include appropriate antibiotic therapy (often initially intravenous and then oral) with the average duration required being 4 to 6 weeks. This therapy is most effective when the bacteria can be isolated and identified from the synovial fluid and antibiotic sensitivities can be used to determine the most effective antibiotic to be used. In addition, the infected joint usually requires repetitive drainage to facilitate bacterial clearance, decrease pain, and prevent loss of function. This can be accomplished by repeated joint aspiration, arthroscopy with tidal lavage, or open surgical drainage.

Joint prosthesis infection. Any bacteria can lead to infection in a prosthetic joint via the hematogenous route. *S. aureus* is still common, but *Staphylococcus epidermidis* can also result in prosthetic joint infection and is rarely seen in a native septic joint. Generally, a prosthetic joint infection requires removal of the prosthesis followed by a rigorous course of intravenous antibiotic therapy, often for 6 weeks or longer. Antibiotic beads may also be placed in the wound. The prosthesis is replaced when cultures from the wound show no growth.[2]

KEY POINTS

- Osteoarthritis is a local degenerative joint disorder associated with aging and wear and tear from repetitive stress.
- OA is characterized by loss of articular cartilage, deterioration of underlying bone, and the formation of bone spurs. The process is noninflammatory. Weight-bearing joints are often affected.
- Signs and symptoms of OA are localized (not systemic) and include joint pain and crepitus with movement.
- Joint infection may be due to a variety of infectious agents, but bacteria are the most problematic. The route of infection is usually by way of the bloodstream. Signs and symptoms are due to localized infection and the systemic manifestations of inflammation.

SYSTEMIC DISORDERS OF JOINT FUNCTION

Immune-Mediated Disorders
Rheumatoid Arthritis

Rheumatoid arthritis is a systemic autoimmune inflammatory disease. In the United States, approximately 1% to 2% of the population is affected with a lower prevalence being reported in Asian countries.[1] Women are two to three times more likely to develop RA than men, with a peak incidence in the fourth and fifth decades. Gender difference disappears in older age. RA affects all races, and its prevalence is not affected by climate. RA occurs two to three times more often in women with a familial history of RA.[1]

Etiology and pathogenesis. The specific cause of RA is unknown. An infectious agent has long been sought as a cause, but reproducible evidence of a particular bacterium or virus has not been found. A more likely theory is that RA is caused by an abnormal autoimmune response (possibly triggered by a bacterial or viral antigen) occurring in individuals who have a genetic predisposition to the disease.

Current research suggests that susceptibility to RA is influenced by the structure of class II major histocompatibility complex (MHC) molecules of antigen-presenting cells. β-Lymphocyte alloantigen human leukocyte antigen DR4 (HLA-DR4) has been noted in 70% of adult Caucasian patients with RA (compared with 30% in control patients), although it is likely that several genes are involved.[3] These genes possibly control humoral and cell-mediated immune mechanisms believed to contribute to the pathogenesis of RA. A particular amino acid sequence of the third hypervariable region of DR β chains (called the "shared epitope") is seen more commonly in RA patients. The cause and type of stimulus of immunologic abnormalities are not known, but they might be due to an infectious agent, environmental influences, or other lifestyle factors (such as tobacco use). An increase in physical and/or psychological stress has also been associated with precipitating acute exacerbation of the disease.

Initially, pathologic changes in RA occur when the immune response localizes in synovial tissue. Here lymphocytes (T and B cells) and macrophages are activated by an unknown antigen trigger. Activated B cells help to perpetuate the escalating inflammatory response by stimulating more lymphocytes and other immune cells. B cells also produce RF antibodies against immunoglobulin G (IgG) as well as anti–cyclic citrullinated peptide (anti-CCP) antibodies. Although immunoglobulins are natural human antibodies, the body produces an antibody (RF) against its own antibody (IgG). Anti-CCP antibodies target peptides modified by converting the amino acid arginine to citrulline.[1] Activated lymphocytes, macrophages, and antigen-antibody complexes activate the complement system, stimulate recruitment of other immune cells into the synovium, and produce an extensive array of inflammatory cytokines, metalloproteinases, and other mediators. These products of macrophages and lymphocytes are believed to be critical in RA pathogenesis because they stimulate and perpetuate the inflammation in the joint. Key proinflammatory cytokines demonstrated in the synovium include tumor necrosis factor-α (TNF-α); interleukin-1β (IL-1β); and interleukins 6, 8, 15, 17, 18, and 23, although many more are thought to be involved. Newer biological therapies are designed to target these cytokines as well as activated inflammatory cells and cell costimulatory markers.

The escalating inflammatory response in the rheumatoid joint leads to accumulation of dense aggregates of immune cells and infiltration of the synovium. The cells produce more cytokines and growth factors, which also stimulate edema, neovascularization, and proliferation of the synovium (which expands in a tumorlike manner). This hypertrophied synovium invades such surrounding tissue as cartilage, ligaments, joint capsules, and tendons. Granulation tissue forms, covering articular cartilage and leading to pannus formation. Pannus is vascularized tissue composed of lymphocytes, macrophages, histiocytes, fibroblasts, and mast cells. Pannus can erode and destroy articular cartilage, resulting in bone erosion, bone cysts, and fissures (Figure 52-5). The expansion and destruction of joint structures can lead to inflammation, shortening, and even rupture of tendons as well as ligament laxity, joint subluxations, contractures, and deformities.[1]

Clinical manifestations. RA has a wide range of clinical features, but the classic presentation is that of a bilateral symmetric polyarthritis involving smaller joints. Malaise, fatigue, and diffuse musculoskeletal pain are common manifestations during acute exacerbations of the disease. It is interesting to note that symmetric patterns involving the joints of the hands, wrists, elbows, and shoulders are evident. DIP joints are usually spared. This symmetry and the noninvolvement of the DIP joint assist in making the diagnosis of RA.

The hands, wrists, knees, and feet are most commonly involved. In the spine, the upper cervical area is most often affected. However, any diarthrodial joint is potentially at risk. The development of pannus followed by inflammatory destruction of the soft tissue leads to laxity of the ligaments and tendons and results in biomechanical dysfunction. This mechanical stress causes the typical deformities of RA.

Swelling in the hands is a typical sign of metacarpophalangeal (MCP) and proximal interphalangeal (PIP) joint involvement. Pain is elicited on palpation of the joints. Gradually, progressive synovial damage leads to characteristic ulnar deviation in the MCP joint

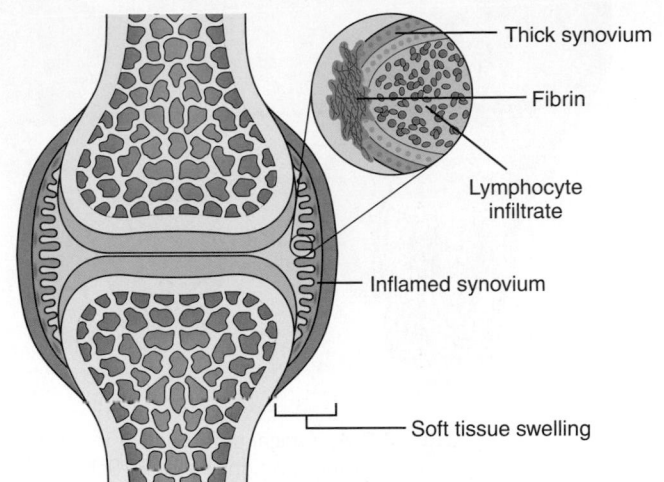

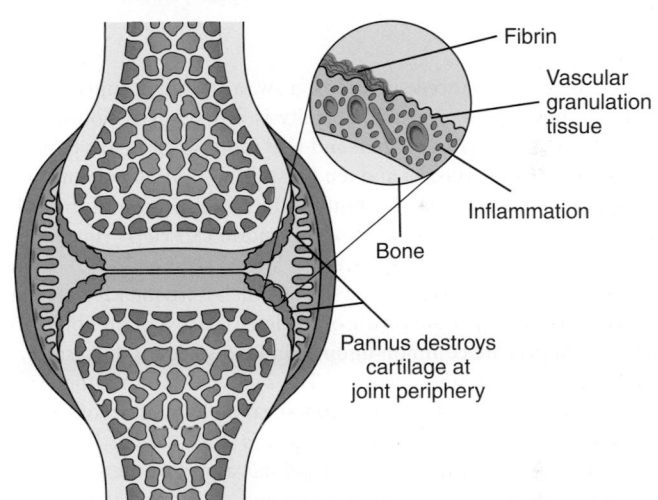

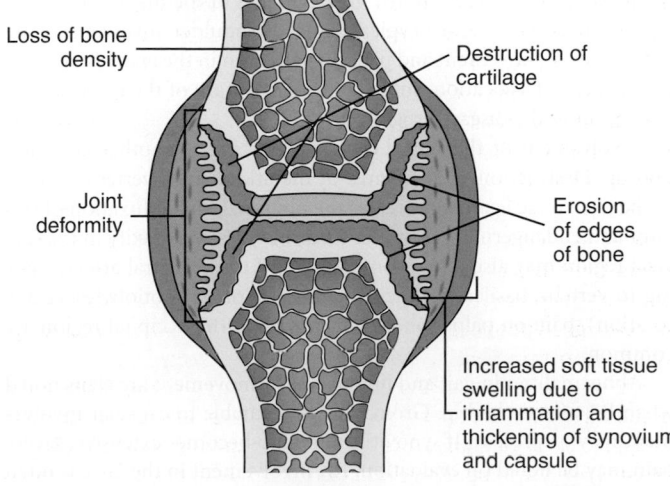

FIGURE 52-5 Schematic presentation of the pathologic changes in rheumatoid arthritis. The inflammation (synovitis) leads to pannus formation, obliteration of the articular space, and, finally, ankylosis. The periarticular bone shows disuse atrophy in the form of osteoporosis. (From Black JM et al: *Medical-surgical nursing: clinical management for positive outcomes*, ed 6, Philadelphia, 2001, Saunders.)

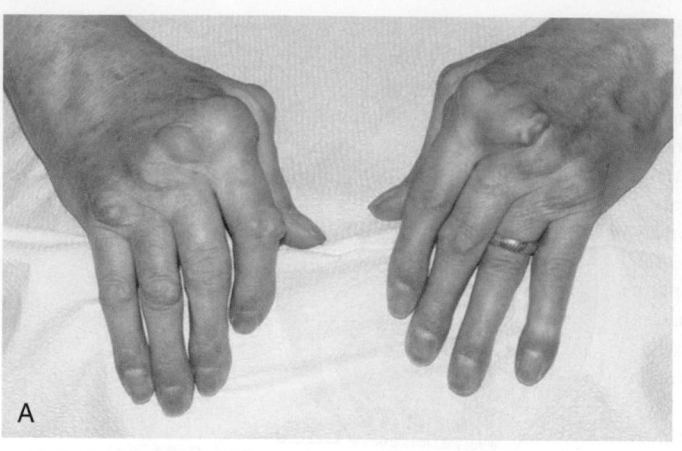

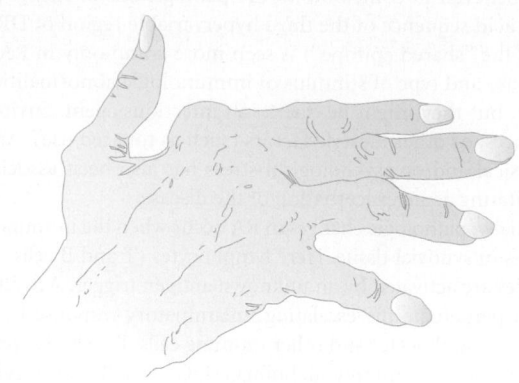

A   B

FIGURE 52-6 A, Typical deformity of the hand seen in patients with rheumatoid arthritis. Note ulnar deviation involving the right hand. **B,** Schematic of ulnar deviation. (From Black JM, Hawks JH: *Medical-surgical nursing: clinical management for positive outcomes*, ed 8, Philadelphia, 2009, Saunders, p 2058. Courtesy Dr. Douglas White.)

(Figure 52-6). In advanced situations, a swan-neck deformity develops in the fingers. Swan-neck deformity is a hyperextension of the PIP joint with flexion of the MCP and DIP joints attributable to contractures of intrinsic muscles and tendons.[4] A boutonnière deformity, consisting of flexion of the PIP joints and hyperextension of the DIP joints, is also a common dysfunctional position caused by rupture or excess laxity of extensor tendons over the fingers (Figure 52-7). Loss of strength and the ability to achieve a strong pinch is frequently noted in the hand affected by RA. A rupture of tendons and loss of the ability to extend the fingers are common findings in later stages of the disease.

The wrist is commonly involved. The synovium around the wrist becomes boggy and affects the tendon sheaths. Limitation of movement, especially dorsiflexion of the wrist, is often noted. Proliferation of the synovium on the volar or palmar aspect of the wrist may cause compression of the median nerve and development of carpal tunnel syndrome. Flexion contractures and swelling of the elbow are other common manifestations; in later stages of the disease, shoulder involvement may occur. Typical signs of shoulder involvement are limitations of movement and pain on palpation in the area of the coracoid process. Dislocation, subluxation, or rupture of the joint capsule may occur as the disease progresses.

Involvement of the upper cervical vertebrae is another common finding. Destruction of structures of the atlantoaxial vertebrae (such as the transverse ligament) creates the potential for subluxation of this joint and endangerment of spinal cord compression. Laxity in the cervical region may also allow compression of the vertebral artery, leading to vertebrobasilar insufficiency. Limitation of motion (especially rotation), pain on palpation, and headache in the occipital region are common.

Abnormalities in gait and limitations of movement are signs noted when RA affects the hip. Groin pain attributable to capsular involvement may be present. If synovitis of the hip becomes extensive, severe pain may be noted on evaluation. RA involvement in the knee is often extensive. Effusion, quadriceps atrophy, contractures, and synovitis of the semimembranous bursa (Baker cyst) may be observed. Destruction of the articular surface, bone, and soft tissue may result from joint instability. One common clinical sign of involvement of the foot is retrocalcaneal bursitis. Other features of foot involvement include swelling of joints, a cocking-up of the toes attributable to subluxation of the metatarsal heads (claw toes), and lateral deviation of the first through fourth toes.

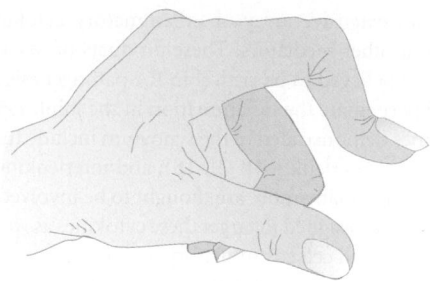

Boutonnière deformity

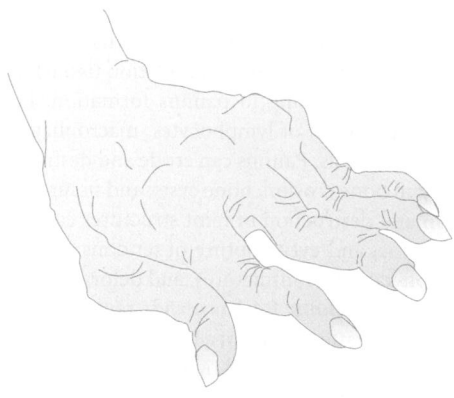

Swan-neck deformity

FIGURE 52-7 Boutonnière and swan-neck deformities. (From Black JM, Hawks JH: *Medical-surgical nursing: clinical management for positive outcomes*, ed 8, Philadelphia, 2009, Saunders, p 2058.)

These clinical manifestations may develop rapidly or progress over many years. Usually symptoms develop over weeks and months. Initially, the patient may feel fatigued or chronically tired and may complain of systemic aching in the musculoskeletal system. Specific joint pain, tenderness, swelling, redness, and nodules are quite common.

Prolonged inactivity, such as sitting, initiates complaints of stiffness and swelling. As the disease progresses, walking, climbing stairs, opening jars or doors, and precise movement of the digits become quite

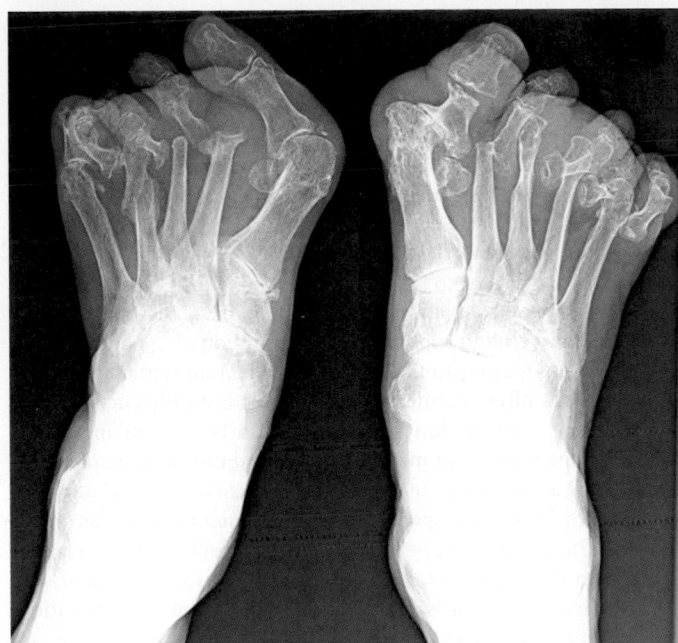

FIGURE 52-8 Rheumatoid arthritis. Radiographs of deformities of the feet, including bone erosions, osteopenia, lateral deviation, and subluxations, especially at the metatarsophalangeal joints. (Courtesy Dr. Douglas White.)

TABLE 52-1	2010 ACR/EULAR CLASSIFICATION CRITERIA FOR RHEUMATOID ARTHRITIS
CRITERION	**POINTS***
Joint Distribution (0-5 points)	
1 large joint	0
2-10 large joints	1
1-3 small joints	2
4-10 small joints	3
>10 joints (at least 1 small joint)	5
Serology (0-3 points)	
Negative RF *and* negative ACPA	0
Low-positive RF *or* low-positive ACPA	2
High-positive RF *or* high-positive ACPA	3
Symptom Duration (0-1 point)	
<6 weeks	0
≥6 weeks	1
Acute-Phase Reactants (0-1 point)	
Normal CRP *and* normal ESR	0
Elevated CRP *or* elevated ESR	1

Data from Aletaha D, Neogi T, Silman AJ, et al: 2010 Rheumatoid arthritis classification criteria, *Arthritis Rheum* 62(9):2574, 2010.
*A score ≥6 points indicates definite rheumatoid arthritis.
ACPA, Anti–citrullinated protein/peptide antibody; *ACR,* American College of Rheumatology; *CRP,* C-reactive protein; *ESR,* erythrocyte sedimentation rate; *EULAR,* European League Against Rheumatism; *RF,* rheumatoid factor.

difficult. Weight loss, depression, and a low-grade fever often are noted in these patients.

Unlike OA, RA is a systemic autoimmune disease. It is imperative that a definitive differential diagnosis be developed. RA may be confused with a number of disease entities such as Lyme disease, systemic lupus erythematosus (SLE), gout, and other inflammatory conditions. RA may also cause subcutaneous nodules and be associated with cardiac, pulmonary, and ophthalmologic manifestations.

Cardiac manifestations may include pericarditis, myocarditis, mitral valve disease, and conduction system disease or complete heart block. Pulmonary manifestations may occur as pleuritis, pulmonary fibrosis, pleural effusions, or pulmonary nodules. Ophthalmic manifestations might include episcleritis, scleritis, or secondary Sjögren syndrome (dry eyes and mouth).

A positive RF is found in the sera of approximately 75% to 85% of patients with RA. The titer of the RF does not fluctuate with disease activity and is not essential for the diagnosis of RA. Antibodies against cyclic citrullinated peptide (anti-CCP antibody) can be found with a sensitivity of 70% to 80% and a high specificity of 90% to 95% for RA. The presence of both RF and anti-CCP antibodies in a patient may signify a risk of more aggressive disease. Inflammatory markers (sedimentation rate, C-reactive protein) are often elevated. Other laboratory features may include hypergammaglobulinemia, thrombocytosis, and hypochromic microcytic anemia.[1]

Radiography may demonstrate structural damage caused by RA. Typical findings include erosions on the bony margins of joints, joint space narrowing, periarticular osteopenia, and eventual malalignment and subluxation of the bones (Figure 52-8).

Diagnosis. In 2010 the American College of Rheumatology (ACR) in collaboration with the European League Against Rheumatism (EULAR) published new guidelines for the classification and diagnosis of rheumatoid arthritis (Table 52-1). The criteria require the patient have at least one documented swollen joint, the absence of an alternative diagnosis that better explains the joint swelling, and a total

score on the criteria scale of 6 or more (out of 10). The diagnosis takes into account the number and size of the swollen joints, the presence or absence of the RF antibody or CCP antibody, and the level of the patient's markers of inflammation (sedimentation rate and C-reactive protein). The goal of these new criteria is to aid in the diagnosis of RA at an earlier stage of disease.[5]

Treatment. Goals of therapy should include alleviation of pain and swelling, prevention of structural damage, and preservation of function. Initial therapy with antiinflammatory medications may include NSAIDs, COX-2 inhibitors, or corticosteroids (oral, parenteral, or intraarticular injections). Corticosteroids are potent antiinflammatory agents, effective at quickly controlling the pain, stiffness, and swelling of RA activity; however, every effort is made to avoid long-term steroid use because of adverse consequences such as steroid-induced osteoporosis, diabetes mellitus, cataracts, and more.

Disease-modifying antirheumatic drugs (DMARDs) are used to achieve long-term control of RA activity and are recommended very early in the course of disease to minimize later damage. The most common first-line agent used is methotrexate (oral or subcutaneously once weekly), which is a folate analogue. Within cells, methotrexate (MTX) may exhibit its antiinflammatory and immunoregulatory effects by inhibiting several different enzymatic pathways, leading to decreased RNA and DNA synthesis (via decreased pyrimidine synthesis) and accumulation of intracellular and extracellular adenosine (which is a potent antiinflammatory agent). Leflunomide is another immune modulator that may work via decreased pyrimidine synthesis, although the mechanism of action of this agent is not well understood.[3]

Sulfasalazine and antimalarial drugs (especially hydroxychloroquine) have inhibitory effects on inflammatory cell function and may be useful in milder cases of RA or in combinations with methotrexate. Older immunosuppressive agents, such as azathioprine, gold (oral or intramuscular), or cyclosporine, are still available for management of RA but are much less commonly used.

In the last 10 years or more, the research into the use of biological agents in rheumatic disease, especially RA, has yielded a number of new and effective agents for controlling RA inflammation as well as preventing erosive and destructive mechanisms. Tumor necrosis factor-α is a central and potent stimulator of inflammation in the rheumatoid joint, and there are currently five TNF-α inhibitors available in the United States. Etanercept is a soluble TNF-α receptor fusion protein, whereas adalimumab, golimumab, and certolizumab are monoclonal antibodies or modified fragments of antibodies that can bind and inhibit TNF-α. These agents are all self-administered injections given once weekly to once monthly depending on the agent. Infliximab is a chimeric monoclonal antibody against human TNF-α and is given as an intravenous (IV) infusion every 6 to 8 weeks.

Another biological agent available for treatment of aggressive RA is abatacept, which is a fusion protein that binds to CD80/CD86 on the surface of antigen-presenting cells. This binding prevents CD80/86 from binding with CD28 on T cells, a process that is necessary for T-cell activation and increased activity in the inflammatory response. Abatacept is administered once every 4 weeks via IV infusion. Rituximab, a monoclonal antibody against the B-cell marker CD20, has been approved since 1997 for the treatment of non-Hodgkins lymphoma.[1] In RA, B cells are known to be active in several facets of the chronic inflammation and therefore the B-cell depletion caused by rituximab therapy can have very positive and sustained immunosuppressive effects. This agent is given as a series of two IV infusions administered 14 days apart every 6 months. The newest agent approved for RA is tocilizumab, a once monthly IV infusion, which binds the proinflammatory cytokine interleukin-6.

Systemic Lupus Erythematosus

Systemic lupus erythematosus (SLE) is a chronic, multisystem, inflammatory, autoimmune disease. It is characterized by periods of exacerbations and remission, with multiple organ systems being affected at different times.

Etiology and pathogenesis. Genetic involvement has been demonstrated in familial occurrences of SLE.[6] Although SLE occurs in all races, it occurs more often in the United States among African Americans than Caucasians and yet is uncommon in Africa.[6] Environmental factors such as sunlight, thermal burns, and other types of physical stress may initiate the development of SLE. SLE is more common in women, with peak incidence between 15 and 40 years of age, suggesting that hormonal factors may influence onset.

SLE is the result of an abnormal immune reaction of the body against its own tissues, cells, and serum proteins—the body has a decreased tolerance to itself. One of the main mechanisms is B-lymphocyte overactivity leading to excessive autoantibody production. SLE patients can express a myriad of antibodies directed against many self molecules and antigens located in cell nuclei and cytoplasm. Among these antibodies, those directed against nuclear antigens (antinuclear antibodies, or ANAs) are found in more than 98% of SLE patients.[6] Antigen-antibody complexes form within the basement membranes of glomeruli in the kidneys, heart, skin, brain, and joints. Immune complexes then activate complement and trigger the inflammatory responses, which are responsible for tissue destruction.

Clinical manifestations. SLE typically affects multiple organ systems such as the kidneys, heart, skin, nervous system, joints, lungs,

and gastrointestinal tract. Not all systems are affected simultaneously. The characteristic clinical course is one of exacerbation and remission. A remission may last for many years.

Arthralgias and synovitis are common features of SLE with most patients noting joint pain at some time during the course of the disease. In lupus arthritis, swelling, tenderness, pain on movement, and morning stiffness are noted. Involvement of the capsule, ligaments, and tendons can be extensive, causing reducible deformities in hands and feet (called Jaccoud arthropathy). Deformities range from contractures of the fingers, to hyperextension of the interphalangeal joint of the thumb, to subluxation of the MCP joint of the thumb. With steroid therapy, tendon rupture is not uncommon.

Skin lesions may be quite extensive in SLE. Acute cutaneous lupus erythematosus often manifests with a classic butterfly (malar) rash, though some form of skin involvement can be present in 80% of patients.[1] The skin lesion may be exacerbated during systemic flare-up. Swelling and redness are noted, and sunlight or artificial ultraviolet light may initiate a response. Skin involvement may occur on the shoulders, upper arms, upper back, chest, and neck. Scales or plaques develop on the scalp, ears, face, and neck. A latticelike venular skin change (livedo reticularis) is a very common skin manifestation. Alopecia may also occur.

A number of systemic manifestations may also be present. Cardiac complications include pericarditis, valvular heart disease, and rarely myocarditis with congestive heart failure. Premature atherosclerotic heart disease is recognized as an important cause of morbidity and mortality. Lung and pleural involvement includes pleuritis or pleural effusion. More aggressive lung involvement may include acute interstitial pneumonitis, pulmonary embolus, or pulmonary hypertension. Renal involvement is common (½ to ⅔ of lupus patients) and can vary in severity.[1] Glomerulonephritis (inflammation in the glomeruli of the kidneys) can be associated with proteinuria, hematuria, and progressive renal failure. Central nervous system involvement has also been recognized (ptosis, diplopia, ataxia, seizures, psychosis).[6] Lymphadenopathy or Raynaud phenomenon (small vessel vasospasm in response to cold) may also be noted at some time in the course of the illness.

When SLE involves autoantibodies against blood elements, laboratory testing can reveal hemolytic anemia, leukopenia, lymphopenia, or thrombocytopenia. Renal disease often causes proteinuria, hematuria, or cellular casts on microscopic urinalysis. Although many autoantibodies cannot be measured by conventional laboratory methods, testing for the ANA class of antibodies is most important in screening for SLE, although a positive ANA test result can be seen in about 2% of healthy young women and in an even higher number of elderly individuals.[1] Also found in the sera of some SLE patients are autoantibodies against double-stranded DNA and other extractable nuclear antigens such as SSA (Ro), SSB (La), Smith (Sm), and RNP. Complement levels (C3 and C4) can be low in the setting of active SLE because the complement proteins are "consumed" in the antigen-antibody–mediated immune activation.

Treatment. The choice of therapeutic agents often depends on disease manifestations. Application of topical corticosteroids, avoidance of the sun, and use of sunblock can help control skin disease. NSAIDs and/or antimalarial medications are useful for the management of arthritis and serositis. For more aggressive disease, including renal, hematologic, or neural involvement, oral or parenteral corticosteroids may be needed for initial control followed by immunosuppressive medications, such as azathioprine, methotrexate, mycophenolate mofetil, cyclophosphamide, and others. New biological therapies targeting activated B lymphocytes, cell costimulatory molecules, and cytokines are under investigation. The most recent agent to be FDA approved for the treatment of SLE is belimumab, which is a humanized monoclonal antibody that inhibits BLys (B-lymphocyte stimulator). Inhibition of BLys leads to a decreased number of activated B cells and lowered levels of autoantibody production (such as antibodies against double-stranded DNA).[7]

Scleroderma

Scleroderma is a multisystem inflammatory connective tissue disease characterized by skin thickening and a deposition of large quantities of collagenous tissue, which results in severe fibrosis.[3] Skin, blood vessels, synovium, skeletal muscle, and microvasculature of internal organs are all affected. Scleroderma may occur in a localized form that only involves areas of skin without any internal organ involvement, or it can be a systemic disease. Two major types of systemic scleroderma are limited systemic sclerosis (LSS) and diffuse systemic sclerosis (DSS). It affects women three to four times more frequently than men. Onset is most common between 30 and 50 years of age.

Etiology and pathogenesis. The cause of scleroderma is unknown. Early in the disease, inflammation and immune cell infiltration can be found in skin, lungs, and other tissues. Widespread vasculopathy is seen with proliferation of smooth muscle cells within vessels causing vascular wall thickening and eventual lumen obliteration, especially of small arteries, arterioles, and capillaries. Tissue ischemia results followed by diffuse tissue fibrosis. Increased amounts of collagen and other connective tissue components are produced by fibroblasts that are stimulated by local cytokines and mediators.[1]

Clinical manifestations. Clinical manifestations often begin with Raynaud phenomenon (blanching of the digits in response to cold) and puffiness of the fingers, which can precede the development of other clinical features by many months. Polyarthritis involving small joints of the hands is common early in the disease but can resolve later. Evaluation of the skin discloses initial bilateral swelling of the fingers, hands, and, periodically, feet. After a few weeks or months, edema is replaced by thick, tight skin that usually begins distally and progresses proximally, a feature called *sclerodactyly*. This tightening can eventually lead to severe contractures of the digits, skin ulceration at the tips, and severe loss of function. Skinfolds are lost, and a shiny appearance is noted. Hyperpigmentation or hypopigmentation may occur. In limited systemic sclerosis, the sclerodactyly involves just the distal extremities (below elbows and knees) with or without changes to the face, and other internal organ features can still occur. Diffuse systemic sclerosis involves the skin of proximal and distal extremities and can spread rapidly to the face and trunk. These patients are far more likely to have internal organ involvement early in the disease course. Tenosynovial involvement may be seen with tendon friction rubs, carpal tunnel syndrome, and very severe flexion contractures.

Patients with scleroderma may experience disuse atrophy of muscle because muscular motion is limited by involvement of skin and joints. A low-grade inflammatory myositis can be seen but this is uncommon. Gastrointestinal involvement is present in a majority of patients. Musculature of the esophagus is involved, with dysmotility leading to difficulties in swallowing. Involvement of the esophageal sphincter musculature may result in reflux of gastric contents and development of peptic esophagitis. Malabsorption problems may also result from gastroparesis, intestinal dysmotility, and bacterial overgrowth. Constipation related to hypomotility of the large colon can be severe.

Pulmonary involvement, particularly pulmonary fibrosis, is the leading cause of death in systemic sclerosis. Pulmonary arterial hypertension can also develop as a result of vasculopathy of the pulmonary vasculature or from cardiac dysfunction. Manifestations of myocardial involvement include congestive heart failure, pericarditis, and atrial or ventricular dysrhythmias. Renal involvement used to be the predominant cause of death before the availability of angiotensin-converting

enzyme inhibitors. In scleroderma *renal crisis,* sudden malignant arterial hypertension may rapidly progress to oliguric renal failure without immediate treatment.

A form of limited systemic sclerosis, abbreviated CREST, refers to *c*alcinosis (deposits of calcium in tissues); *R*aynaud phenomenon; *e*sophageal dysmotility; *s*clerodactyly; and *t*elangiectasias (capillary dilation that causes formation of vascular lesions on the face, lips, and fingers). Some patients with CREST syndrome develop pulmonary hypertension and intestinal malabsorption, often resulting in death.

Treatment. Treatment for scleroderma is largely organ-specific because systemic disease–modifying agents have had disappointing results. Raynaud phenomenon is managed with avoidance of cold exposure and use of vasodilator medications such as calcium channel blockers or, in severe cases, intravenous iloprost. Symptoms from gastrointestinal disease may be controlled with antacids, H_2 antagonists, proton pump inhibitors, and promotility agents. Previously associated with very high mortality, acute renal crisis (renal failure with malignant hypertension) can now be successfully managed with angiotensin-converting enzyme inhibitors. Pulmonary arterial hypertension is often managed with intravenous epoprostenol or trepostinil, which are two prostacyclin analogues. In some cases, an endothelin receptor antagonist (such as bosentan) can be tried.[1]

Ankylosing Spondylitis

Ankylosing spondylitis (AS) literally means fusion (ankylosis) of inflamed vertebra (spondylitis). It is arthritis of the sacroiliac joints that involves the axial skeleton and, in some cases, peripheral joints. The disease often begins in the spine of young males in their late teens or early twenties. The male to female incidence ratio is 2:1, with symptoms being somewhat more variable in women.[1]

Etiology and pathogenesis. A strong genetic component likely plays a role in the development of AS, because 90% to 95% of patients are positive for the HLA-B27 marker and the frequency of this arthritis in different ethnic groups roughly parallels the frequency of HLA-B27 presence.[4] The role of the HLA molecule in the pathogenesis of this arthritis is not clear, although antigen presenting cells (expressing these HLA markers) may interact with certain bacterial or environmental factors and cross-react with self antigens found in joint tissues. Activation of immune-mediated inflammation occurs within the sacroiliac joints of the pelvis and the ligaments supporting the vertebral column. This leads to persistent back pain, stiffness, and gradual loss of mobility.

Clinical manifestations. Clinical features include the insidious onset of low back pain that improves with exercise but is not relieved by rest and the presence of severe morning stiffness for more than 3 months. Back pain in the night is common. Initial evaluation of the spine suggests an increase in muscle tone, and a loss of normal lumbar lordosis that progresses to a marked limitation of mobility noted in both anterior and lateral planes. With this limitation of movement and a position of spinal flexion, the hips and knees must compensate, creating lower extremity joint degeneration and deformities. Because of restricted postural position and decreased chest expansion, tidal volume may be diminished. A typical postural position for advanced ankylosing spondylitis is shown in Figure 52-9.

Asymmetric peripheral arthritis with swelling of knees, ankles, or toes can also occur along with enthesitis (inflammation at the sites of ligament attachment to bone), with the plantar fascia and Achilles tendon being the most common sites. Persistent diffuse swelling of individual toes (called dactylitis or "sausage toes") can last weeks to months. Other organ systems that may be affected include the eyes (anterior uveitis, iritis), heart (aortitis, aortic valve insufficiency), and nervous system (nerve root or spinal cord impingement related to spinal deformities or fractures).

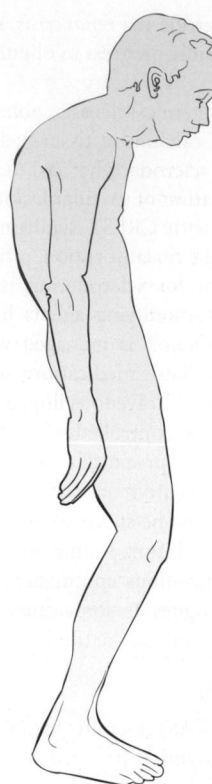

FIGURE 52-9 Typical posture of a patient with ankylosing spondylitis.

Treatment. The primary objectives of treatment are to relieve pain, decrease inflammation, and strengthen and maintain posture and function. Regular stretching and range-of- motion exercises are often recommended. Medication options include NSAIDs to reduce pain and swelling, or in severe cases, short-term corticosteroids. Disease-modifying agents, such as sulfasalazine or methotrexate, can be used. Agents that inhibit TNF-α (etanercept, adalimumab, golimumab, or infliximab) have been shown to slow disease progression.

Polymyositis and Dermatomyositis

Polymyositis and **dermatomyositis** are idiopathic inflammatory myopathies. With these diseases there is focal or extensive degeneration of muscle fibers attributable to inflammatory infiltrates of lymphocytes and macrophages.[3] Necrosis of muscle fibers occurs. Possible triggers of this immune-mediated inflammation include viruses, bacteria, parasitic organisms, neoplasms, drugs, vaccinations, and stress. A viral cause has been proposed because various researchers have noted virus-like inclusion bodies in muscle tissue of dermatomyositis patients.[3]

Proximal limb and neck weakness and associated muscle stiffness are clinical signs of these illnesses. Muscle pain is often mild. Most patients initially complain of hip and leg weakness and difficulty with climbing stairs and rising from a chair. Later in the progression of the disease, weakness in the arms prevents functional overhead activity. Anterior neck weakness makes lifting the head from the pillow very difficult. When classic skin changes occur with polymyositis, the disease is classified as dermatomyositis. Inflamed, injured skeletal muscle leaks several enzymes (creatine kinase, aldolase, aspartate aminotransferase) into the bloodstream and are found at high levels on laboratory testing.

Clinical manifestations. During the physical examination, manual muscle testing reveals weakness in the proximal limb muscles. Contractures are not usually present, but they may develop later. Facial and ocular muscle weakness seldom occurs, distinguishing myositis from myasthenia gravis. Diagnosis of myositis can be detected by electromyography and confirmed on skeletal muscle biopsy.

In dermatomyositis, cutaneous manifestations may develop with muscle involvement. Common findings are flat-topped papules overlying the dorsal surface of the small joints of the hands (Gottron papules). A more common finding is development of an erythematous smooth or scaly patch over other joints such as the elbow, knees, or medial malleoli areas (Gottron sign). Other skin changes may include the heliotrope rash (violaceous edema of the eyelids) or a dry erythematous rash over the anterior chest wall (V-sign) or the upper back and shoulders (shawl sign).

Cardiac involvement may occur but is often mild and asymptomatic. Dysrhythmias can occur, but development of congestive heart failure or pericarditis is less common. Weakness of the respiratory muscles can cause dyspnea as can interstitial lung disease, which can be severe in rare cases.

Treatment. Initial therapy with corticosteroids is usually used to decrease muscle inflammation and preserve function. Immunosuppressive agents, such as methotrexate, azathioprine, or mycophenolate mofetil, may be helpful in severe cases. Physical therapy is also important and should include passive range-of-motion activities, followed by assisted and then active strengthening exercises.

Postinfectious Systemic Disorders
Reactive Arthritis (Reiter Syndrome)

Historically, **Reiter syndrome** consisted of the triad of arthritis, urethritis, and conjunctivitis. Currently terminology renames this reactive arthritis (ReA), and it is defined as a seronegative arthritis preceded by urethritis, cervicitis, or dysentery. Additional problems may include inflammatory skin lesions, oral ulcers, and keratoderma. The onset is most common between 20 and 40 years of age. Onset following a gastrointestinal tract infection is equally common in males and females, but young men are more frequently affected following a sexually transmitted infection.[6] ReA is linked to the prevalence of HLA-B27. It develops in individuals who are genetically susceptible following an infection by bacteria such as *Chlamydia trachomatis* in the genitourinary tract, or *Salmonella*, *Shigella*, *Yersinia*, or *Campylobacter* in the gastrointestinal tract. It is thought that persistence of bacterial antigens and cross-reactivity of immune cells with these antigens trigger the inflammation seen in joints and tendons of persons affected by this syndrome.

Clinical manifestations. Clinically, oligoarthritis typically appears 2 to 6 weeks after the onset of the infectious episode. This acute arthritis onset predominantly affects knees and ankles. Three additional features of musculoskeletal manifestations are typical: diffuse swelling of toes (dactylitis); swelling at the Achilles tendon insertion or plantar fascia (enthesitis); and low back pain, especially associated with inflammation of the sacroiliac joints.

The most common eye involvement in ReA is noninfectious conjunctivitis in up to one third of patients.[6] Acute anterior uveitis (unilateral or bilateral) occurs in approximately 20% of cases and could lead to impairment of vision.[1]

Cutaneous lesions related to ReA include development of small, shallow, painless ulcers on the glans penis and urethral meatus (circinate balanitis). A hyperkeratotic skin lesion (keratoderma blennorrhagicum) may form on the soles of the feet and palms of the hands. Hyperkeratosis (thickening beneath the nails) can occur.

ReA patients may have elevated inflammatory markers (sedimentation rate, C-reactive protein) as well as a mild normocytic anemia, transient leukocytosis, and thrombocytosis. RF test results are usually negative.

Treatment. Antiinflammatory medications, particularly NSAIDs, are usually effective at controlling pain and swelling, although intraarticular corticosteroid injections may also help. Second-line immune-regulating agents, such as sulfasalazine or methotrexate and others, can be used in refractory cases.

Acute Rheumatic Fever

Acute rheumatic fever (ARF) is an inflammatory disease that follows a β-hemolytic group A streptococcal pharyngeal infection. The incubation period, or latent period from infection to onset of the disease, ranges from 2 to 6 weeks. The prevalence of ARF has been estimated at more than 15 million cases worldwide and may be increasing.[1] This might be due to the reappearance of heavily encapsulated, highly virulent rheumatogenic streptococcal strains and/or to the decrease in awareness of the disease and less stringent adherence to disease control measures, especially prevention.

Etiology and pathogenesis. One theory of disease occurrence is the cross-reactivity of a patient's immune cells within the lymphoid tissue of the pharynx. Lymphocyte activity and antibody production are stimulated by streptococcal antigens, and then these cells cross-react with proteins in the target organs such as joints, heart, skin, and nervous system, leading to inflammatory reactions in these areas.[1]

Clinical manifestations. The clinical aspects of ARF depend on the age of the affected individual. Peak incidence is between ages 5 and 15 years. Children and teenagers present with polyarthritis and carditis. Polyarthritis is usually the only manifestation in the adult. Fever is present in most patients.

Polyarthritis is the most common presenting symptom noted in patients with ARF. Pain may be quite severe over the initial few days to 1 or 2 weeks and then gradually subside. Synovial effusions and erythema may be noted. The knees, ankles, elbows, and shoulders are affected most often. Hips, wrists, and small joints of the hands and feet may also be compromised. Onset may be monoarticular with spread to numerous other joints. Joint symptoms usually respond rapidly to treatment with antiinflammatory medications, especially salicylates.

Children and teenagers with ARF are more likely than adults to develop carditis, with the youngest children (younger than 3 years) being the most likely affected. The signs of carditis include murmurs, cardiomegaly, congestive heart failure, and pericarditis. Mitral valve regurgitation is the most common murmur, followed by aortic regurgitation. Evidence of rheumatic heart disease may not be apparent for many years after the acute incident.

A rash is noted in less than 2% of individuals affected by ARF.[1] The rash, called *erythema marginatum*, begins as a pale erythematous, blanching macular rash over the trunk and proximal regions of the extremities. Painless nodules may cover the extensor surfaces.

Throat cultures may be negative by the time the symptoms of ARF are recognized, but certain antibody tests (antistreptolysin O, anti-DNase B) can be useful to aid in diagnosis.

Treatment. The most common therapy is NSAIDs, especially aspirin, and response can be rapid. Corticosteroids may be required in cases of severe cardiac involvement. Antibiotic therapy, including long-term prophylaxis in some cases, is generally recommended.

Postparasitic Disorders

Lyme Disease

Lyme disease is a complex illness caused by the *Borrelia burgdorferi* tick-borne spirochete. It is commonly carried by the deer tick, although other species serve as vectors as well. The process by which the presence of the spirochete leads to the later chronic clinical symptoms of Lyme disease is unclear. Theories suggest that persistent antigenic fragments of the dead or inactivated organism trigger the inflammatory responses, or the initial infection stimulates an autoimmune inflammatory response.

Clinical manifestations and treatment. The tick bite produces a red macule or papule that may expand to form an annular lesion. The lesion may expand and become quite red. The lesion is warm to the touch but not painful and is often accompanied by a flulike illness, headache, neck stiffness, fever, chills, myalgia, arthralgia, malaise, and fatigue. Systemic involvement may consist of lymphadenopathy, splenomegaly, hepatitis, nonproductive cough, testicular swelling, and conjunctivitis.

Musculoskeletal symptoms occur early in the illness and follow a pattern of migratory pain in joints, tendons, bursae, muscles, or bones. More than half of patients develop frank arthritis with involvement of the large joints. The knee is a particularly common site of Lyme arthritis and can be associated with large effusions. A persistent arthritis develops in about 10% of patients.

Neurologic abnormalities suggest meningeal irritation. Neurologic abnormalities may include meningitis, cranial neuritis, motor and sensory radiculoneuritis, and chorea.

Cardiac involvement may be noted, including atrioventricular blocks, left ventricular dysfunction, or cardiomegaly. Although cardiac involvement lasts only a few weeks, it can be fatal.

Treatment is with oral or parenteral antibiotics.

KEY POINTS

- A number of immune-mediated systemic connective tissue diseases result in joint dysfunction, including RA, SLE, and scleroderma. Most are classified as autoimmune disorders of unclear cause. The signs and symptoms of systemic joint disorders are generalized but involve multiple joints and usually other connective tissue structures.
- Differentiation among types of systemic joint disorders is based on patterns of joint dysfunction, immunologic factors (e.g., rheumatoid factor), and related lesions (e.g., the butterfly rash of SLE).
- Joint destruction in some systemic joint disorders is inflammatory in nature and involves the synovial membrane, cartilage, joint capsule, and surrounding ligaments and tendons.
- Rheumatic fever and Lyme disease are inflammatory joint disorders associated with a known organism.
- Rheumatic fever–related arthritis is a sequela of group A streptococcal infection. Lyme disease is associated with a spirochete carried by ticks.

JOINT DYSFUNCTION SECONDARY TO OTHER DISEASES

Psoriatic Arthritis

Psoriatic arthritis (PA) is an inflammatory arthritis associated with psoriasis occurring in 0.04% to 0.1% of individuals in the United States. Peak age of onset is 30 to 55 years of age, and the arthritis can occur in patients who have had psoriasis for many years.[6]

Etiology and pathogenesis. Studies have shown a strong familial tendency for psoriatic arthritis, suggesting that genetic factors may cause an increased predisposition to the disease. Environmental factors, such as infection or physical trauma, may trigger the onset of the arthritis. Immunologic features also have a dominant role, with activated T lymphocytes and macrophages infiltrating skin and joint tissue and producing multiple inflammatory cytokines (TNF-α, IL-1, and IL-15, among others). These immune reactions cause proliferation of synoviocytes within joints, angiogenesis (new blood vessel formation), and expansion of inflammatory tissue. In the skin, keratinocytes are stimulated and will proliferate extensively.

Clinical manifestations. The pattern of joint involvement seen clinically varies. The majority of patients have peripheral joint involvement in the form of asymmetric oligoarthritis. Fewer patients have a polyarthritis that is difficult to distinguish from RA. In some PA patients, the DIP joints of the hands can be affected, which is different from RA. Sacroiliac and spinal involvement can also occur.

Commonly, PA is characterized by a combination of soft-tissue and peripheral joint disease. Inflammation occurs in the joints as well as the periosteum, along the tendons, and at tendon insertions in bone (enthesitis). Fusiform swelling of the digits (dactylitis) is common.

Evidence of skin or nail changes, typical of psoriasis, is noted in psoriatic arthritis. These skin changes typical for psoriasis include erythematous papular lesions with characteristic scales. Nail involvement includes pitting and onycholysis (raised transverse thickening and longitudinal ridging). Subungual hyperkeratosis and oil droplet discoloration suggest psoriasis.

Inflammatory markers may be elevated, and rheumatoid factor (RF) and anti–cyclic citrullinated peptide antibody (anti-CCP) are usually negative. Radiographs may show minimal changes; however, some cases involve aggressive disease with bone erosion, fluffy new bone formation (periostitis), and marked loss of joint spaces.

Treatment. Psoriasis may respond to topical corticosteroids, emollients, and keratolytic agents. Light therapy, utilizing ultraviolet A radiation, can also be effective. Management of the arthritis centers on NSAIDs or corticosteroids to control pain and swelling, but in many cases, more aggressive immunosuppressive therapy is needed, including methotrexate, cyclosporine, or TNF-α antagonists (etanercept, adalimumab, infliximab).

Enteropathic Arthritis

Enteropathic arthritis refers to articular manifestations of two inflammatory bowel diseases (IBDs): **ulcerative colitis** and **Crohn disease.** A peripheral or axial arthritis can occur in 10% to 22% of patients with IBD, and in some cases the arthritis can precede the onset of gastrointestinal symptoms.[1]

As in the case of the other spondyloarthropathies, the cause of enteropathic arthritis is unclear, but it is postulated to be associated with immune cross-reactivity with bacterial antigens. In the setting of IBD, inflammation of the gut lining may permit entrance of bacteria from the bowel lumen into the lymphoid tissue and bloodstream, stimulating an autoimmune response that can target joints.

Clinical manifestations. Articular manifestations include peripheral arthritis, spondylitis, and involvement of muscle and bone. Peripheral arthritis is most commonly asymmetric and pauciarticular, usually in the knees and ankles. Synovial inflammation may be mild to severe, and in mild cases may be transient but prone to relapse. In severe cases, a chronic and potentially erosive arthritis can develop. In spondylitis, there is inflammation in the spinal ligaments and sacroiliac joints, similar to features seen in patients with ankylosing spondylitis. Like other spondyloarthropathies, enthesitis can also be noted.

Various cutaneous and ocular manifestations can occur in IBD. Skin lesions, such as erythema nodosum (painful inflamed nodules under the skin) or leg ulcers (pyoderma gangrenosum) may also be associated with the disease. Ocular manifestations, particularly acute anterior uveitis, occur in 3% to 11% of patients.[6] Amyloidosis with involvement of major organs can be observed in Crohn disease.

Anemia is common in IBD as well as leukocytosis. In the setting of arthritis, elevated inflammatory markers are often seen and HLA-B27, when positive, may identify patients at higher risk of developing spondylitis.

Treatment. Treatment focuses on management of the gastrointestinal disease with immunosuppressive agents. Control of the arthritis can be pursued with use of NSAIDs (when tolerated by the gut), COX-2 inhibitors, or corticosteroids. In severe cases, second-line medications may be required for treatment of the arthritis as well as

the bowel disease, particularly the use of TNF-α antagonists as in the setting of Crohn disease.

Neuropathic Osteoarthropathy

Commonly called *Charcot joint,* **neuropathic osteoarthropathy** is a neurologic disease that leads to bone and joint abnormalities. The mechanism is not clear, but because of a loss in normal proprioception and pain responses, damage occurs to the joint. The mechanics of disease development are probably a combination of neurovascular and neurotraumatic processes. Peripheral nerve injuries, diabetes mellitus, pernicious anemia, alcoholism, and multiple sclerosis can lead to Charcot joint.[1] Motor neuron involvement can affect both upper and lower motor neurons. Diabetes, tabes dorsalis, and syringomyelia are the three most prevalent disease processes that lead to neuropathic osteoarthropathy.

Clinical manifestations and treatment. Clinically, the patient presents with a swollen, deformed, and unstable joint. Radiographs reveal advanced joint destruction and pathologic fractures. Management requires protection of the involved joint through immobilization and less weight bearing. Surgical intervention has shown poor results attributable to nonunion, dislocation, or infection.

Hemophilic Arthropathy

Bleeding into joints, as noted in hemophilia, causes extension of the joint capsule and a limitation of movement. Hemorrhage stimulates a synovial proliferative response, chronic inflammation with a release of degradative proteinase, and changes in cartilage composition with less resistance to stress.[6] Chronic synovitis alters the synovial lining and eventually leads to joint destruction.

Clinical manifestations. Three stages of hemophilic arthropathy are described. The acute stage manifests with bleeding in the joint and occurs as the child begins to walk. Bleeding into the confined area of the capsule causes the joint to be positioned in flexion and increases stress to articular structures. Atrophy of muscles around the joint predisposes it to further hemarthrosis. The second stage is due to repetitive hemorrhages into the joint, resulting in chronic synovitis. The joint is edematous and warm but painless. The third stage is characterized by destruction of joint integrity.[3]

Larger joints are affected more frequently than smaller joints. Seldom are structures of the wrist involved. Elbows, hips, and knees are subject to major destruction. Muscle hemorrhage (iliopsoas, forearms, gastrocnemius), muscle cysts, and pseudotumors (attributable to osseous hemorrhage) may develop.[3] Medical treatment to enhance clotting is imperative. Education and prevention of joint deformity are essential in the management of hemophilia.

Gout

Gout is a heterogeneous disorder in which disturbance of uric acid metabolism leads to deposition of monosodium urate salts in articular, periarticular, and subcutaneous tissue (Figure 52-10). It is also characterized by hyperuricemia and urate crystal–induced arthritis. Gout arises in humans because of a lack of the enzyme uricase and subsequent inability to oxidize uric acid to a soluble compound. Uric acid is a normal waste product of purine metabolism and therefore must be filtered primarily by the kidneys. When production of uric acid exceeds removal, hyperuricemia results and the possibility of deposition of crystalline sodium urate increases. The acute attack is often triggered by a traumatic event, a surgical procedure, an acute illness, or use of alcohol or medications.

Clinical manifestations. The incidence of gout has been reported to be approximately 5.9%.[6] Risk of developing gout increases with age and with an increase in serum urate concentrations. Clinically, acute

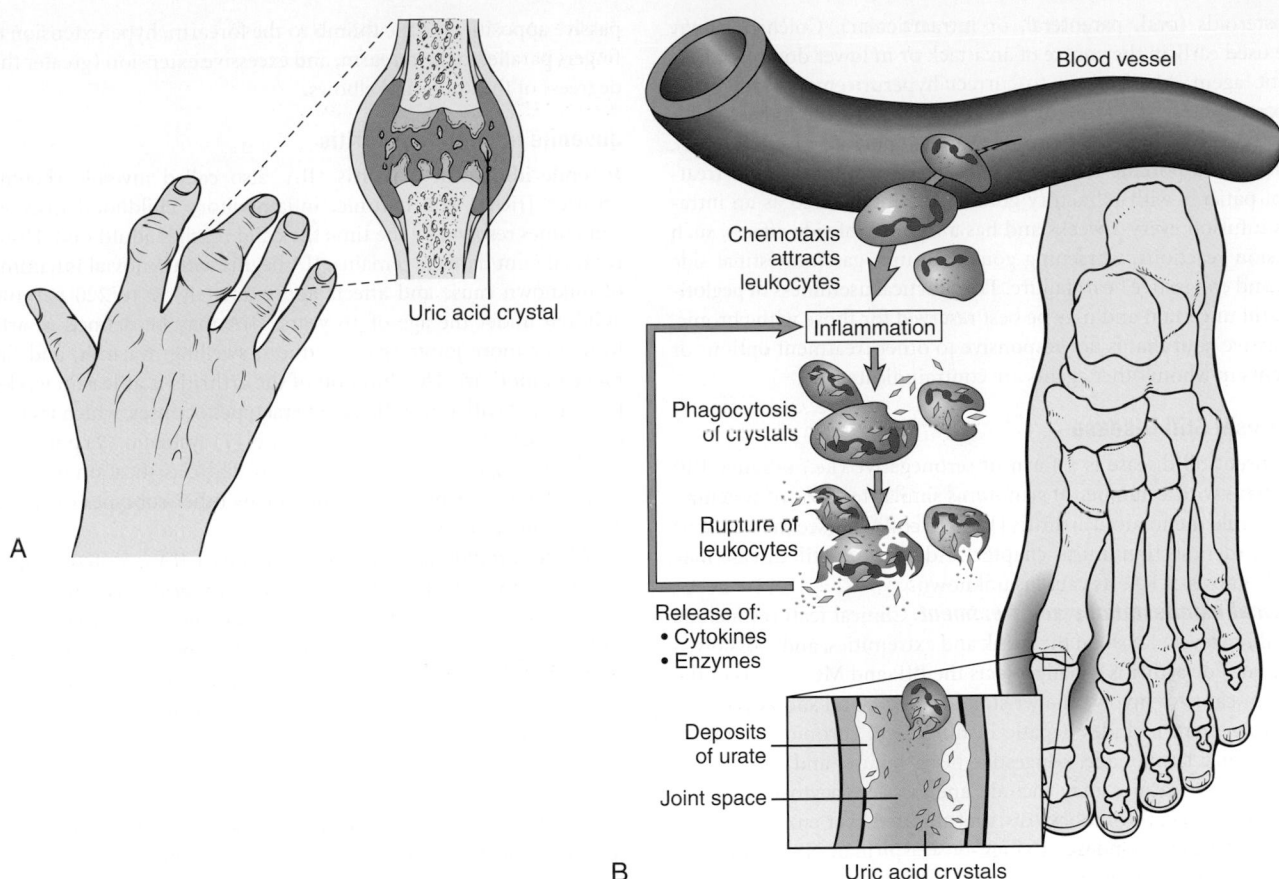

FIGURE 52-10 A, Gout. **B,** Gouty arthritis. Deposits of uric acid crystals in the connective tissue have a chemotactic effect and cause exudation of leukocytes into the joint. The inflammation most often affects the metatarsophalangeal joint. (**A,** From Frazier MS, Drzymkowski JW: *Essentials of human diseases and conditions,* ed 5, Philadelphia, 2013, Saunders. **B,** From Damjanov I: *Pathology for the health professions,* ed 4, Philadelphia, 2012, Saunders.)

gouty arthritis is the form most frequently observed. Gouty arthritis is common in middle-aged men and postmenopausal women. A familial tendency is often noted.

Manifestations of gout include recurrent episodes of articular and periarticular inflammation (acute gouty arthritis), accumulation of tophi (crystalline deposits) in bony and connective tissue, impairment of the renal system, and the presence of uric acid calculi. There are four phases in gout: asymptomatic hyperuricemia, acute gouty arthritis, intercritical gout, and chronic tophaceous gout.

ASYMPTOMATIC HYPERURICEMIA. Hyperuricemia has been estimated at highly variable rates in Americans, from 2% to 40% who are asymptomatic.[6] In this phase, there are no clinical signs; however, the serum urate level is elevated. In the male, hyperuricemia can begin at puberty. In women, hyperuricemia usually does not appear before menopause. No treatment is required at this stage.

ACUTE GOUTY ARTHRITIS. Gouty arthritis is the most common early clinical sign. Weight-bearing joints are usually affected and are warm, red, and tender to palpation. The metatarsophalangeal (MTP) joint of the great toe is most often involved. Ankle, tarsal, and knee joints are often affected, although attacks can occur in hands, wrists, and elbows. The first attack of acute gouty arthritis is often sudden onset with an intense pain that can awaken the patient from a sound sleep. Diffuse periarticular erythema often accompanies the attack. Diagnosis relies on classic clinical presentation, hyperuricemia, and the demonstration of urate crystals in synovial fluid of the involved joint.

Initial attacks subside within 1 or 2 days or may last 1 to 2 weeks, after which the patient is symptom free until the next episode. Later attacks tend to become more frequent, and mild arthralgia may occur between episodes.

INTERCRITICAL GOUT. Intercritical gout, the name for the disease in the intervals between acute attacks, presents no symptoms. Even during asymptomatic periods, urate crystals can be aspirated from involved joints.

CHRONIC TOPHACEOUS GOUT. This is an advanced stage of gout. Tophi begin to appear approximately 10 years after initial onset of gout. Tophi occur commonly in the synovium, subchondral bone, olecranon bursa, and infrapatellar and Achilles tendons. Tophi have been noted in walls of the aorta, valves of the heart, ear cartilage (pinna), corneas, sclerae, and kidneys.[1]

As a result of deposition of crystals and chronic inflammation, deforming arthritis can develop. Development of tophi in tendon sheaths of the hand and wrist can cause a trigger finger or carpal tunnel syndrome.

Patients with gout may have involvement of the kidneys and develop renal malfunction. These individuals have a higher incidence of arterial hypertension, diabetes mellitus, and cardiac and cerebral atherosclerosis. Hypertriglyceridemia occurs more frequently in the patient diagnosed with gout.

Treatment. Management of an acute gouty attack usually requires aggressive antiinflammatory medication such as NSAIDs or corticosteroids (oral, parenteral, or intraarticular). Colchicine may also be used early in the course of an attack or in lower doses as a prophylactic agent. Medications to correct hyperuricemia and prevent gout exacerbation may target uric acid excretion by the kidneys (uricosuric agents) or uric acid production (allopurinol or febuxostat). Pegloticase is a porcine uricase enzyme recently approved for treatment of patients with refractory gout. It is administered as an intravenous infusion every 2 weeks and has a number of side effects, such as infusion reactions, worsening gout flare-ups, gastrointestinal side effects, and congestive heart failure. The practical usefulness of pegloticase is still uncertain and may be best reserved for those with chronic, severe active gout that is not responsive to other treatment options or in patients in whom other agents are contraindicated.[8]

Adult-Onset Still Disease

Adult-onset Still disease is a form of seronegative (i.e., negative RF) polyarthritis with a number of symptoms similar to those of systemic-onset juvenile rheumatoid arthritis (JRA) in children (see the Pediatric Joint Disorders section in this chapter). Adult-onset Still disease may follow diagnosis of RA. Its cause is unknown.

Clinical manifestations and treatment. Clinical features include high-spiking fever, a rash on the trunk and extremities, and, possibly, a sore throat. Polyarthritis usually affects the PIP and MCP joints of the hands, but can also involve the wrist, knees, hips, and shoulders. Visceral involvement includes hepatic insufficiency, chronic respiratory failure, cardiac tamponade, congestive heart failure, and splenomegaly. Laboratory features may include anemia, leukocytosis, elevated sedimentation rate, thrombocytosis, and elevated liver enzymes.

Some patients respond well to high-dose aspirin or NSAIDs during the acute illness, although in severe cases corticosteroids are used.

KEY POINTS

- Psoriatic arthritis differs from rheumatoid arthritis in that PsA is more often asymmetric, is associated with psoriasis in the skin, and is not associated with autoantibody (RF or CCP) production. It can, however, lead to joint erosions and damage.
- Neurovascular, hematologic, and metabolic disorders may lead to associated disorders of joint function. Diabetes, for example, results in neurovascular changes that desensitize the joint and predispose it to traumatic joint dysfunction. Hemophilia predisposes to intraarticular bleeding.
- Altered uric acid metabolism leads to deposition of uric acid crystals in joints, causing inflammation and gouty arthritis.

PEDIATRIC JOINT DISORDERS

Pediatric rheumatic diseases include more than 100 illnesses associated with arthritis and musculoskeletal syndromes. Soft-tissue pain and restrictions constitute a major proportion of the complaints presented to pediatric rheumatologists.

Nonarticular Rheumatism

"Growing pain" or **nonarticular rheumatism** is a common soft-tissue syndrome in children. Nocturnal pain, usually occurring in the calves, shins, and thighs, is the most common symptom. Although this problem seems to be benign, medical consultation and education concerning the problem are essential.

Hypermobility of Joints

Hypermobility of joints is a common cause of complaints of pain in the joints. Mobility may be excessive in any joint, but it is most apparent in passive apposition of the thumb to the forearm, hyperextension of the fingers parallel to the forearm, and excessive extension (greater than 10 degrees) of the knees and elbows.

Juvenile Idiopathic Arthritis

Juvenile idiopathic arthritis (JIA; also called juvenile rheumatoid arthritis [JRA]) is a chronic, inflammatory childhood disease that sometimes resolves by the time the child reaches adulthood. However, residual joint damage remains. JIA begins with synovial inflammation of unknown cause and affects approximately 57 to 220 per 100,000 children under the age of 16 years.[1] JIA may be defined as arthritis in one or more joints (pain, redness, swelling, warmth, and limited range of motion). The duration of the arthritis is at least 6 weeks. JIA may present with one of three general types of onset, which is classified during the first 6 months of the disease: (1) systemic, (2) polyarticular, and (3) pauciarticular (oligoarticular).[1] The classification of JIA, however, is being expanded to include many other subtypes of childhood inflammatory arthritis.

Clinical manifestations. Systemic-onset JIA is noted in approximately 2% to 17% of children with JRA with peak onset at 1 to 6 years of age.[1] Clinical manifestations include spiking fevers (103° to 104° F), daily or twice daily and usually in the afternoon with return to baseline without antipyretics; transient, pale pink rash; lymphadenopathy; hepatosplenomegaly; and pericardial or pleural effusions. Fatigue, muscle atrophy, and weight loss can be severe. Anemia, leukocytosis, and thrombocytosis are common. RF is usually negative. Musculoskeletal findings in the early stages of the disease include recurrent arthralgia, myalgia, and transient arthritis, which are concurrent with fever spikes. Polyarthritis can develop weeks to months after the onset of the disease. Severe chronic arthritis may continue after the systemic symptoms subside.

A **polyarticular onset** of JIA (i.e., involving five or more joints) is seen in approximately 10% to 28% of patients (somewhat less when including only those who are RF positive), with peak onset at age 8 to 16 years. The female to male ratio is 3:1.[1] RF positivity is also more common in girls with later onset of disease that can resemble adult RA. These patients are at a higher risk of developing progressive bone erosions, nodules, and poor functional outcome. Malaise, growth retardation or weight loss, low-grade fever, and anemia are other clinical manifestations.

By definition, a child with **pauciarticular (oligoarticular) onset** of JIA has arthritis in four or fewer joints. One subset of this form of JIA includes patients who are very young at disease onset (1 to 5 years of age), can have a positive ANA test result, and are most often girls (female to male ratio is 4:1). Patients with a positive ANA test result are at highest risk for developing inflammatory ocular disease, a complication that may start with minimal or no symptoms yet can lead to severe irreversible vision impairment. A second group of patients with pauciarticular JIA have later disease onset. These children are more commonly boys, may be HLA-B27 positive (50%), and often develop large joint disease (hips, knees, shoulders, or spine). These patients may also develop eye inflammation, but this is less likely than in the early-onset group.

Treatment. All forms of JIA can cause general growth retardation, although it is more of a risk in children with systemic or polyarticular onset of disease. Inflammation close to the epiphyseal plates can result in altered growth of long bones. It is therefore imperative to achieve early diagnosis and implement appropriate treatment to minimize deformity and disability. Education and counseling are also important. Relief of symptoms and maintenance of joint position and muscle function are immediate goals of treatment.

Pharmacologic intervention is an important component of the treatment regimen. Drug therapy is instituted to decrease pain and arrest progression of the disease. The following categories of drugs are used: (1) antiinflammatory analgesics (aspirin or NSAIDs), (2) corticosteroids, (3) disease-modifying drugs (methotrexate, sulfasalazine, leflunomide), and (4) biological disease-modifying agents (such as the TNF-α inhibitors etanercept, adalimumab, and infliximab). An additional biological agent that can be used in severe JIA is tocilizumab, which inhibits activity of interleukin-6. Biological agents targeting other inflammatory cytokines, such as interleukin-1 (anakinra), have also shown some efficacy in JIA as well. Physical and occupational therapy assessment and treatment plans are important, and daily activity should be an integral part of the child's lifestyle. Joint support and physical activity help prevent joint contracture.

> **KEY POINTS**
> - JIA has three subtypes: systemic onset (which has more systemic manifestations, including rash, high fever, lymphadenopathy, splenomegaly, fatigue, and polyarthritis); polyarticular arthritis (in which symptoms are primarily localized to five or more joints); and pauciarticular arthritis (which involves four or fewer joints).

SUMMARY

This chapter has provided an overview of major rheumatic disorders. Broadly speaking, interventions must assist in controlling disease activity, managing pain, minimizing deformity, and maintaining or restoring function. Depending on the stage of the disease, correct intervention must be implemented using knowledge of joint physiology biomechanics and pathologic changes resulting from the disease.

The challenge to the health professional is to ensure that an inflammatory response is not exacerbated while the body structures are being stimulated to increase strength, enhance nutrition, and improve tolerance to stress. Long periods of immobilization, bed rest, and sedentary behavior are counterproductive in the patient with arthritis. Lack of activity poses particular problems in people with arthritis. Deleterious effects on muscle strength, reflexes, connective tissue extensibility, and cardiovascular fitness are identifiable in the immobilized arthritic patient. It is imperative that the health professional look beyond disease-specific interventions and prescribe a well-developed exercise program for patients with arthritis. Achievement or retention of as much function as possible is the ultimate goal for an individual with arthritis. Every level of intervention must be directed to achievement of specific performance goals cooperatively developed by clinician and patient.

REFERENCES

1. Klippel JH, Stone JH, Crofford LJ, White PH, editors: *Primer on the rheumatic diseases*, ed 13, New York, 2008, Springer.
2. Mandell GL, Bennett JE, Dolin R, editors: *Mandell, Douglas, and Bennett's principles and practice of infectious disease*, ed 7, Philadelphia, 2009, Churchill Livingstone.
3. Firestein GS, Budd RC, Harris ED, et al, editors: *Kelley's textbook of rheumatology*, ed 8, Philadelphia, 2008, Saunders.
4. Hunder GG, editor: *Atlas of rheumatology*, ed 2, Philadelphia, 2001, Current Medicine.
5. Aletaha D, Neogi T, Silman AJ, et al: 2010 Rheumatoid arthritis classification criteria, *Arthritis Rheum* 62(9):2569–2594, 2010.
6. Hochberg MC, Silman AJ, Smolen JS, et al, editors: *Rheumatology*, ed 4, Philadelphia, 2008, Elsevier.
7. Furie R, Petri M, Zamani O, et al: A phase III, randomized, placebo controlled study of belimumab, a monoclonal antibody that inhibits B lymphocyte stimulator, in patients with systemic lupus erythematosus, *Arthritis Rheum* 63(12):3918–3930, 2011.
8. Sundy JS, Baraf HSB, Yood RA, et al: Efficacy and tolerability of pegloticase for the treatment of chronic gout in patients refractory to conventional treatment, *JAMA* 306(7):711–720, 2011.

53

Alterations in the Integumentary System

Lee-Ellen C. Copstead, Ruth E. Diestelmeier, and Michael R. Diestelmeier

evolve WEBSITE

http://evolve.elsevier.com/Copstead/

- Review Questions and Answers
- Glossary (with audio pronunciations for selected terms)
- Animations
- Case Studies
- Key Points Review

KEY QUESTIONS

- How does the aging process affect the integumentary system?
- Why is it important to differentiate primary from secondary skin lesions?
- What lesion characteristics are assessed to aid in determination of the lesion's cause?
- How do systemic disorders affect nail and hair growth?
- Which skin disorders are more likely to occur more commonly in certain age groups, including infants, children, adolescents, and the elderly?
- How does ultraviolet radiation affect the skin?
- How do superficial and deep pressure ulcers differ in clinical and etiologic features?
- How can malignant melanoma be differentiated from other skin lesions?

CHAPTER OUTLINE

This chapter focuses on altered structure and function of the integumentary system. The etiologic factors, pathogenesis, and clinical manifestations of selected skin disorders as well as general considerations regarding treatment modalities and their therapeutic application are described.

AGE-RELATED CHANGES

The skin undergoes dramatic changes from birth through the mature years. Healthy infants and young children have relatively smooth and unwrinkled skin characterized by elasticity and flexibility. Because skin tissues are in an active phase of new growth, healing of skin injuries is often rapid and efficient. Young children and elderly individuals have fewer sweat glands than adults do, so their bodies rely more on increased blood flow to maintain a normal body temperature.

As adulthood begins at puberty, hormones stimulate the development and activation of sebaceous glands and sweat glands. After the sebaceous glands become active, especially during the initial years, they may overproduce sebum and thus give the skin an unusually oily appearance. Sebaceous ducts may become clogged or infected and form acne pimples or other blemishes on the skin. Activation of apocrine sweat glands during puberty causes increased sweat production, an ability needed to maintain an adult body properly, and also

the possibility of increased "body odor." Body odor is caused by wastes produced by bacteria that feed on the organic compounds found in apocrine sweat and on the surface of the skin.

Past early adulthood and into middle age, the sebaceous and sweat glands become less active. Although this can provide relief to those who suffer from acne or other problems associated with overactivity of these glands, it can affect the normal function of the body. For example, the reduction in sebum production can cause the skin and hair to become less resilient.

Changes in the appearance and function of the skin, perhaps more than in any other organ, reflect the continual aging process (see Geriatric Considerations: Changes in the Integumentary System). One need only look at a person to determine an approximate age. Evidence of advancing age includes wrinkling and sagging skin, gray hair, and baldness. Aging changes are also linked to environmental influences, genetic makeup, and other bodily changes (Figure 53-1).

Exposure to sunlight is one of the greatest factors in age-related skin changes. The result of such exposure can be seen in people who work outdoors in sunlight. Results are also evident when skin exposed to sunlight is compared with unexposed skin. Skin that is usually covered shows little change with age. Blue-eyed, fair-skinned individuals are more susceptible to solar skin damage than are people with darker, more heavily pigmented skin.

GERIATRIC CONSIDERATIONS

Changes in the Integumentary System

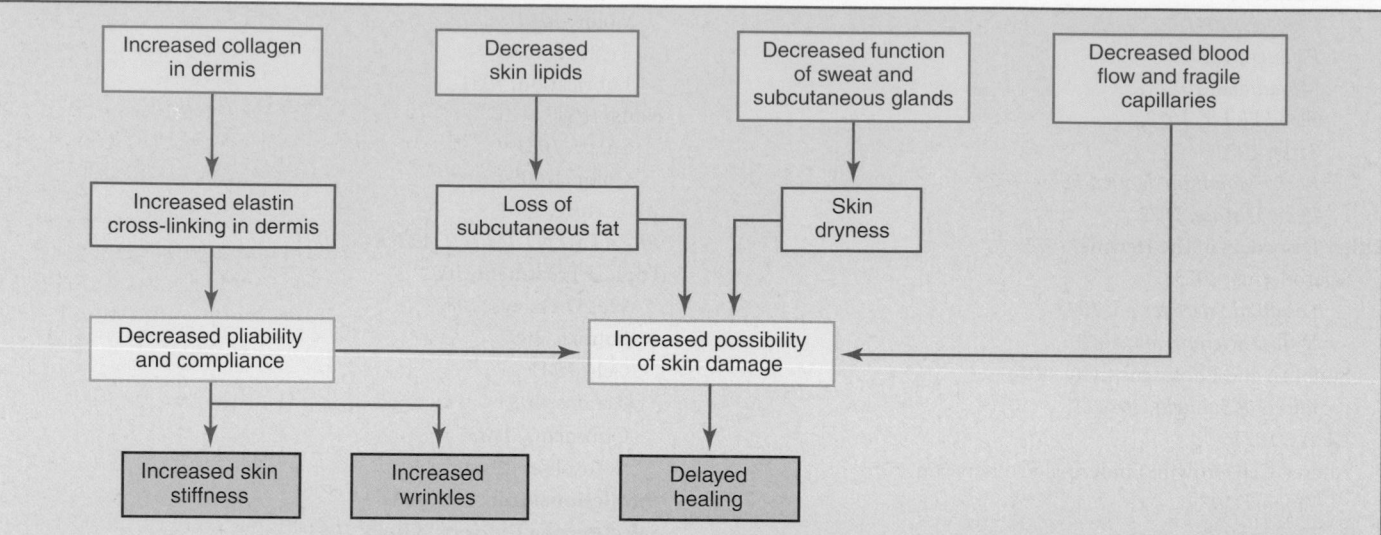

With aging, the skin's protective functions decline. Although the thickness of the stratum corneum remains the same, the properties of the water and chemical barriers in this layer of the integument are less effective. In the epidermis, mitosis decreases and cellular variation increases. The thickness of the epidermis is unchanged. The number of melanocytes decreases in Caucasians, with declining function. The melanocytes are less efficient and lack uniformity in pigment production with sun exposure.

There is a decrease in both the thickness and the amount of subcutaneous fat in the dermis, and there is an increase in the amounts of collagen and elastin with cross-linking and calcification of elastin fibers. These changes cause a loss of skin pliability, compliance, and resiliency. There is an accompanying escalation in skin stiffness and an increase in wrinkling of the skin. Sebaceous and sweat gland function declines, resulting in drier, less oily skin. The number of sensory nerves and blood vessels in the skin declines, resulting in decreased sensation and loss of effective vasoactivity by dermal arterioles.

Nail and hair growth declines. The nails may become yellowed and thickened. Graying of the hair is due to the loss of melanocytes at the hair follicle base. The degree and pattern of hair loss are affected by genetic and endocrine factors. Body hair patterns change, with thinning of leg, axillary, and pubic hair.

The cumulative effect of these skin changes is loss of the regulatory, secretory, and excretory properties of the skin. The skin becomes injured more easily, and, once injured, heals more slowly.

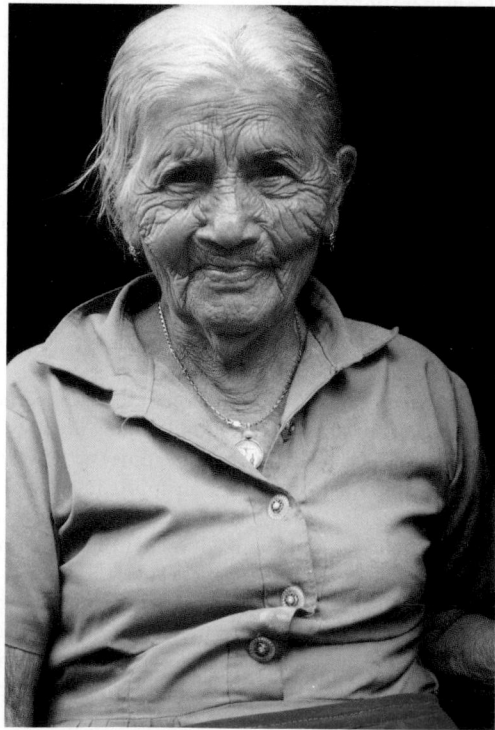

FIGURE 53-1 Physiologic signs of aging human skin. (Photo by Lee-Ellen C. Copstead.)

Epidermis

The epidermis shows a generalized thinning with advancing age, although there may be some thickening in sun-exposed areas. Although there is an increased variation in epidermal thickness, the average number of cell layers remains unchanged. The prickle cells of the inner layer of the epidermis show greater variation in nuclear and cytoplasmic size with a less orderly arrangement of cells. Cells reproduce more slowly and are larger and more irregular; however, exposed epidermal cells may divide more frequently than unexposed cells.

Dermis and Subcutaneous Tissue

The dermis contains blood vessels, nerves, hair follicles, and sebaceous glands, but the major portion is composed of collagen and elastin. The elasticity of the skin is largely due to dermal elastin. Decreased skin strength and elasticity with aging are attributed to a decreased amount of elastin and a proportionate increase in the collagen-to-elastin ratio. Collagen fibers change with age, becoming cross-linked and rearranged into thicker bundles. This condition is called **elastosis** and is closely associated with exposure to sunlight (**solar elastosis**). It produces a weather-beaten or tanned appearance.

Aging also produces a decrease in the vascularity of the dermal skin, as evidenced by decreasing numbers of epithelial cells and blood vessels. There is greater vascular fragility, leading to the frequent appearance of hemorrhages (senile purpura); cherry angiomas; venous stasis; and venous lakes on the ears, face, lips, and neck. The decreased vascularity and circulation in the dermis and the underlying subcutaneous tissue also have an effect on drug absorption. Drugs administered subcutaneously are absorbed more slowly, thus prolonging their half-life. The amount of subcutaneous fat tissue also decreases, especially in the extremities, so that arms and legs appear to be thinner.

Appendages

Hair

The most obvious change in aging hair is its color. Half of the population over age 50 years has at least 50% gray body hair, regardless of gender or hair color. Gray hair is determined by an autosomal dominant gene and results from a decreased rate of melanin production by the hair follicle. Hair color generally darkens with age, but this process is reversed with the onset of graying. Graying usually begins at the temples of the head and extends to the vertex of the scalp. It may not occur in the axilla, especially in women, and occurs to a lesser extent in the presternum or the pubis.

Changes in hair growth and distribution are also associated with aging. The amount and distribution of hair are determined by racial, genetic, and sex-linked factors; however, almost all older people have a diminution of body hair except on the face. Adults develop a full terminal hair pattern by age 40 years, and this is followed by a progressive loss of hair in reverse order of development. Postmenopausal Caucasian women lose trunk hair first, then pubic and axillary hair. Unopposed adrenal androgens produce coarse facial hair in 50% of Caucasian women older than 60 years, especially on the chin and around the lips.

Men also show a general thinning of hair distribution, with the hairs of the eyebrows, ears, and nose becoming longer and coarser. Baldness is often a concern, particularly in aging men, although women also tend to show some thinning of scalp hair. Frontal recession of the hairline occurs in 80% of older women and 100% of older men. Baldness in men is inherited from the mother and occurs only in the presence of testosterone. Onset is variable and is manifested by an M-shaped pattern of hair loss on either side of the midline or by a thinning patch over the vertex.

In general, the hair of both men and women changes from darker, thicker, and more numerous to lighter, thinner, and less numerous with aging. Hair changes begin in midlife and become highly noticeable in later life, especially after age 60 years. Women seem to manifest more hair loss on the trunk and extremities, whereas men have greater hair loss on the head.

Nails

With aging, nails become dull, brittle, hard, and thick. Most nail changes are due to a diminished vascular supply to the nail bed. There is approximately a 30% to 50% decrease in the growth rate of fingernails, from 0.1 mm/day in 30 year olds to 0.07 mm/day in 90 year olds. Aging nails show an increase in longitudinal striations, which can cause splitting of the nail surface.

Toenails are particularly prone to hyperkeratosis and resultant thickening. Pressure and trauma from poorly fitting footwear may be a significant factor, but onychomycosis, which affects approximately 20% of individuals over age 60, is the primary factor.[1]

Glands

Sebaceous glands show little atrophy or histologic change with age; however, their function tends to diminish, as evidenced by a decrease in sebum secretion. In men the decrease is minimal, but in women there is a gradual diminution in sebum secretion after menopause, with no significant changes after the seventh decade. There are fewer sebaceous glands in older individuals, which appear related to the loss of hair follicles. The decrease in sebum secretion and in the number of sebaceous glands results in the drier, coarser skin associated with aging.

Sweat glands generally decrease in size, number, and function with age. In the eccrine glands, the secretory epithelial cells become uneven

BOX 53-1 MORPHOLOGIC FEATURES OF AGING HUMAN SKIN

EPIDERMIS	DERMIS	APPENDAGES
Flat dermoepidermal junction	Atrophy	Graying of hair
Variable thickness	Fewer fibroblasts	Loss of hair
Variable cell size and shape	Fewer blood vessels	Conversion of terminal to vellus hair
Occasional nuclear atypia	Shortened capillary loops	Abnormal nail plates
Loss of melanocytes	Abnormal nerve endings	Fewer glands

From Gilchrest BA: Skin. In Rowe JW, Besdine RW, editors: *Health and disease in old age,* Boston, 1982, Little, Brown, p 383.

in size, ranging from normal to small, and there is a progressive accumulation of lipofuscin in the cytoplasm. In the very old, the secretory coils of many eccrine glands are replaced by fibrous tissue, which drastically diminishes their capacity to produce sweat. The thermal threshold for sweating is raised, so that the amount of sweat output at a body temperature of 38° C (100.4° F) decreases. This may be due to the fact that there are fewer blood vessels and nerve cells around the glands that enable the body to respond to temperature changes. Apocrine glands do not decrease in number or size, but they do decrease in function. An accumulation of lipofuscin has also been noted in apocrine glands. The diminished functioning of sweat glands in the elderly greatly impairs the ability to maintain body temperature homeostasis.

Box 53-1 summarizes the morphologic features of aging human skin, and Figure 53-2 summarizes the histologic changes associated with aging in normal human skin.

KEY POINTS

- The glandular function of skin varies considerably with age. Young children and elderly adults have fewer functional sweat glands and therefore less efficient evaporative heat loss capabilities. Sebaceous glands are particularly active during puberty, causing a predisposition to acne; they become less active with age, causing a predisposition to dry skin.
- The epidermis and dermis undergo degenerative changes with aging. The epidermis thins, and the dermis becomes less elastic and less vascular. The amount of subcutaneous fat decreases. Exposure to sunlight is an important factor in the development of aged skin.
- Graying of hair results from decreased melanin production by the hair follicle. After age 40 years, progressive hair loss occurs. Male pattern baldness is an inherited trait that is mediated by testosterone.

EVALUATION OF THE INTEGUMENTARY SYSTEM

A careful examination of the skin yields valuable information that may aid in identifying a systemic disease or a specific problem of the skin or appendages. Diagnostic evaluations include a careful history, and Table 53-1 provides a general guide. A proper skin examination also describes the objective signs of dermatologic disease, including all types of lesions and their distribution.

Primary and Secondary Lesions

Physical descriptions should include the lesions and their classification, generally **primary** (original appearance) or **secondary** (appearance modified by normal progress over time or by such external agents as scratching). Figure 53-3 shows clinical examples of primary and secondary lesions.

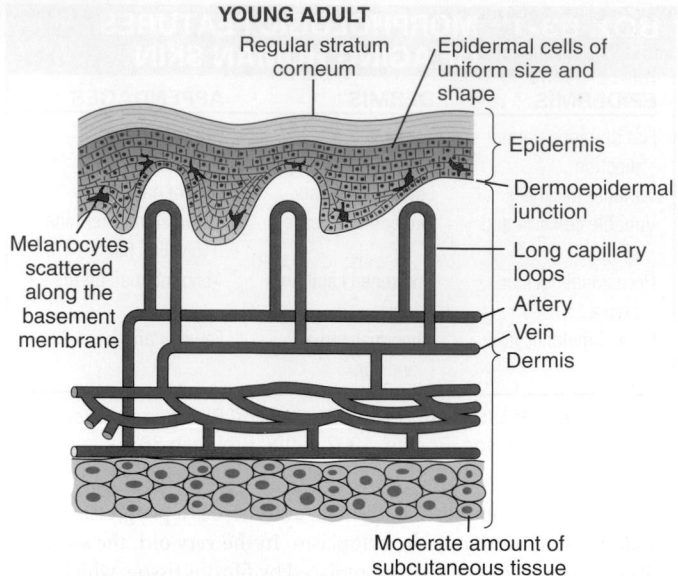

YOUNG ADULT

Regular stratum corneum — Epidermal cells of uniform size and shape

Melanocytes scattered along the basement membrane

Epidermis

Dermoepidermal junction

Long capillary loops

Artery

Vein

Dermis

Moderate amount of subcutaneous tissue

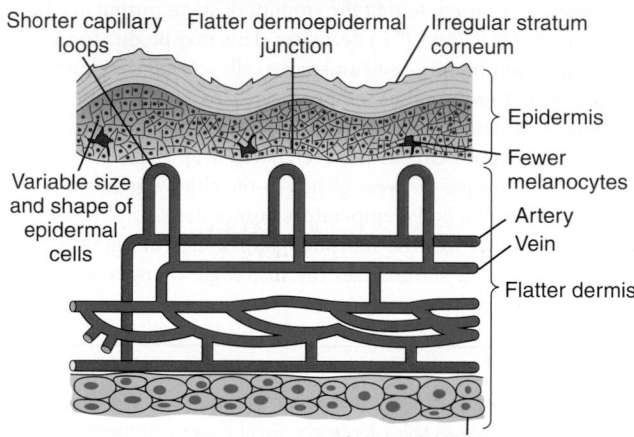

ELDERLY PERSON

Shorter capillary loops — Flatter dermoepidermal junction — Irregular stratum corneum

Variable size and shape of epidermal cells

Epidermis

Fewer melanocytes

Artery

Vein

Flatter dermis

Less subcutaneous tissue

FIGURE 53-2 Histologic changes associated with aging in normal human skin. Note the flattening of the dermoepidermal junction and the shortening of capillary loops in older skin. Variability in size and shape of epidermal cells, irregularity of stratum corneum, and loss of melanocytes are also apparent. Age-associated loss of dermal thickness and subcutaneous fat is also illustrated.

Lesion Descriptors

After a skin lesion has been classified as primary or secondary, other features should be noted, particularly size, symmetry of color and shape, and distribution if more than one lesion is present. Skin lesions may assume a wide range of colors—red–salmon pink, brown-black, blue-purple, bone white–slate gray, and yellow, to name a few. Each color suggests certain diagnoses. Skin lesions may be solitary, few, or profuse. When more than one lesion is present, the distribution pattern may be important in suggesting the diagnosis. Look for the following common patterns: symmetric (affecting mirror-image portions of the body), sun-exposed (affecting skin sites that routinely receive solar irradiation), intertriginous (affecting warm, moist, apposed skin sites), acral (affecting the distal extremities, ears, and nose), genital, and flexor or extensor predominance. Additional descriptors are often used to further characterize and describe a skin lesion or the relationship between various skin lesions such as confluent or clustered. Table 53-2 lists common morphologic and configurational terms.

TABLE 53-1	SUMMARY OF KEY ASSESSMENT ITEMS
ASSESSMENT ITEM	**PURPOSE AND RELEVANT QUESTIONS TO ASK**
Family history	Some skin diseases are familial or hereditary. When hereditary skin disease is ascertained, one may have the opportunity to both correct misconceptions and allay fears about the presence, absence, or prognosis of disease. What are the current familial dermatologic diseases?
Personal history	What was the age at onset of the problem? How has the patient adjusted to the problem? By social withdrawal? Cosmetic cover-up? Withdrawal from school athletic activities that require showers (e.g., football, tennis)? Does the problem threaten the patient's self-image of masculinity or femininity? What is the patient's ethnic origin? (Some skin diseases are more common in certain ethic groups.)
Geographic origin and present abode	Length of time spent living in each area? Some skin diseases are indigenous, which may be important because of increased exposure. Occasionally, a contact of only 5 min is all that is necessary for acquisition of a disease.
Season	Seasonal occurrence of a problem? Pollen? Sunlight?
Occupation	Type of work? Skin contact material (e.g., chemicals, dust, gas), excessive heat and abnormal lighting, unhygienic surroundings, possible infective insects, other family members' occupational exposures?
Leisure activities	Does the problem occur only on weekends? After yard activities? Painting? Woodworking? Camping? Fishing? Hiking? In association with children's play?
Accompanying diseases	Collagen disease? Drug therapy for collagen disease? Other diseases and their drug therapy?
Previous treatment	Self-treatment? Other drugs prescribed?
Special history	Onset of skin lesions (abnormality)? Remissions, exacerbations, or recurrences? Site of onset? Character of lesions? Original character and subsequent changes? Course or extension? Symptoms? Itching? Ability to perform duties? Topical therapy? Self-treatment? Psychological factor? What does the patient associate with exacerbations of the problem (e.g., stress of a family argument, tax time, report time)?

Data from Rosen T et al, editors: *Nurse's atlas of dermatology*, Boston, 1983, Little, Brown.

KEY POINTS
- Skin lesions may be categorized as primary or secondary.
- Primary lesions retain their original appearance, unmodified by time and external processes such as scratching.
- Secondary lesions are those whose appearance has been modified over time; they may look quite dissimilar to the original lesion. The differentiation of primary from secondary lesions aids in establishing a correct diagnosis.
- A description of lesion color, shape, number, and distribution is helpful in determining the cause of a lesion.

NONPALPABLE   **PRIMARY LESIONS** (Original Appearance)

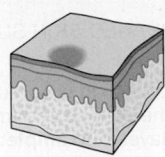

Macule: A spot, circumscribed, up to 1 cm; not palpable; not elevated above or depressed below surrounding skin surface; hypopigmented, hyperpigmented, or erythematous. **Example:** Freckles. Referred to as **patch** if greater than 1 cm. **Examples:** Café au lait spots, mongolian spots.

PALPABLE, SOLID

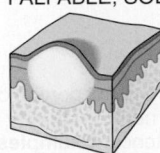

Papule: A bump, palpable and circumscribed, elevated and less than 5 mm in diameter; may be pigmented, erythematous, or flesh-toned. **Example:** Elevated nevus (mole).

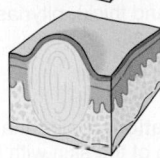

Nodule: A lesion similar to a papule, with a diameter of 5 mm to 2 cm; may have a significant palpable dermal component. **Examples:** Fibroma, xanthoma, intradermal nevi.

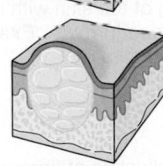

Tumor: Any mass lesion; generally larger than a nodule; may be either malignant or benign. **Example:** Lipoma.

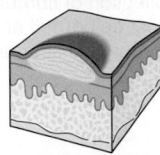

Plaque: Usually well-circumscribed lesion with large surface area and slight elevation. **Examples:** Psoriasis, lichen planus.

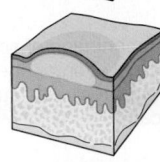

Wheal: An elevation in the skin, with a smooth surface, sloping borders, and (usually) light pink color; caused by acute areas of edema in the skin; may appear, disappear, or change form abruptly within minutes or hours; size ranges from 3 mm to 20 cm. **Example:** Mosquito bite.

PALPABLE, FLUID-FILLED

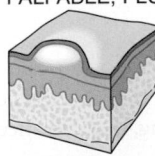

Vesicle: A small blister (up to 5 mm in diameter); fluid collection may be subcorneal, intraepidermal, or subepidermal. **Example:** Herpes simplex (early stages).

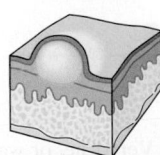

Bulla: A blister larger than 5 mm; fluid may be located at various levels. **Examples:** Pemphigus, pemphigoid.

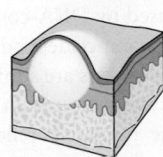

Pustule: An elevated, well-circumscribed lesion containing purulent exudate. **Example:** Acne vulgaris.

Continued

FIGURE 53-3 Characteristics of common skin lesions.

SELECTED SKIN DISORDERS

Diseases of the skin are divisible into two broad etiologic categories: inflammatory/infectious and proliferative/neoplastic. Inflammatory disorders of the skin often occur in individuals who have hypersensitivity reactions to substances in the environment. Infectious agents ranging from viruses to insects may infect the skin. Proliferative conditions include psoriasis, seborrheic keratosis, cysts, warts, and papillomas.

Other benign tumors arise from other cells in the skin: nevi, lipomas, dermatofibromas, neuromas, and hemangiomas. Kaposi sarcoma is a malignant, opportunistic neoplasm that occurs in persons with preexisting immunodeficiency.

Skin cancer is the most common malignancy in the United States; however, with the exceptions of malignant melanoma and a few squamous carcinomas, skin cancers are not life threatening. Ultraviolet light damages sun-exposed skin and is a major factor in development

SECONDARY LESIONS (Modification of Original Appearance)

DAMAGED OR DIMINISHED SKIN SURFACE

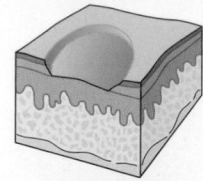

Erosion: Loss of epidermis that does not extend into dermis. **Example:** Ruptured chickenpox vesicle.

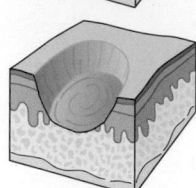

Ulcer: Loss of skin through the epidermis; healing results in scar formation. **Example:** Stasis ulcer.

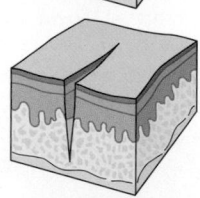

Fissure: A split in all epidermal layers of skin. **Example:** Athlete's foot.

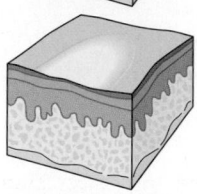

Atrophy: Diminution of epidermal surface; skin looks thinner and more translucent than normal; atrophy of the dermal layers may result in wasting or depression of the skin surface. **Example:** Arterial insufficiency.

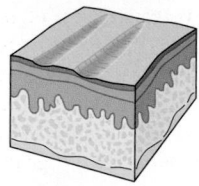

Excoriation: Loss of outer skin layers from scratching or rubbing. **Example:** Scratched insect bite.

AUGMENTED OR INCREASED SKIN SURFACE

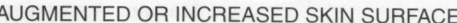

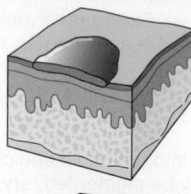

Crust: A collection of serous exudate and debris on the surface of damaged or absent outer skin layers. **Example:** Impetigo.

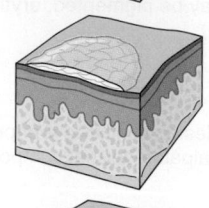

Scale: A compact portion of desquamating stratum corneum; may vary in size, thickness, and consistency. **Examples:** Psoriasis scale (compact and thick), pityriasis rosea scale (thin and small).

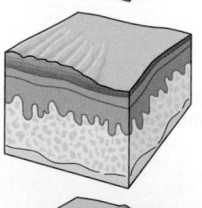

Lichenification: Epidermal thickening and roughening of the skin with increased visibility of skin surface furrows. **Example:** Chronic atopic dermatitis.

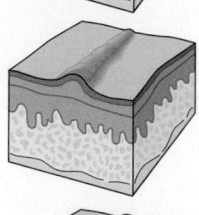

Scar: A collection of fibrous tissue that forms to replace lost epidermal and dermal tissue. **Examples:** Surgical scar, acne scar.

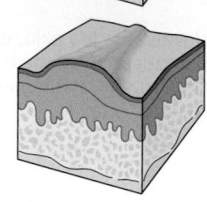

Keloid: Augmentation of scar tissue, creating a significant elevation on the skin surface after healing. **Examples:** Postsurgical scar, postacne scar.

FIGURE 53-3, cont'd Characteristics of common skin lesions.

TABLE 53-2	**LESION DESCRIPTORS**
TERM	**DEFINITION**
Confluent	Blending together
Diffuse	Generalized or widespread
Discrete	Remaining separate but close together
Eczematous	Vesicles with an oozing crust
Herpetiform	Closely grouped vesicles (herpeslike)
Linear	Set in a straight line
Localized	Found only in one area
Pedunculated	On a stalk
Reticulated	Netlike array
Round lesions	Annular (ring shaped, active edge, clear center)
	Arcuate (arc shaped, incomplete circle)
	Circinate (circular)
	Guttate (small droplet–like)
	Iris (concentric circles such as a bull's eye)
	Nummular (coin shaped)
	Ovoid (oval shaped)
Serpiginous	Wandering, snakelike
Telangiectatic	Characterized by dilated surface vessels
Verrucous	Rough, wartlike surface
Zosteriform	Similar to shingles, following along a nerve root dermatome

Data from Sauer GC: *Manual of skin diseases*, ed 6, Philadelphia, 1991, Lippincott.

of skin cancer. Although many of the disorders described in the following section are not life threatening, they can affect the quality of life.

INFECTIOUS PROCESSES

Viral Infections

Verrucae

Etiology and pathogenesis. **Verrucae,** or warts (Figure 53-4), are common benign papillomas caused by DNA-containing papillomaviruses. Although warts vary in appearance depending on their location, the histologic characteristics of all lesions are similar. A wart is actually an exaggeration of normal skin composition, with the stratum corneum being irregularly thickened. The human papillomaviruses, the subgroup of papovaviruses that causes human warts, are not found in other animals and invade only the skin and mucous membranes of humans.

Warts may resolve spontaneously if immunity to the virus develops, but the immune response can be delayed for years and is not reliably activated in every case. In 95% of cases, untreated warts will resolve within 5 years,[2] but they may multiply into hundreds of lesions and can involve any body site. Current surgical treatment may be directed at removal of the wart by laser. Liquid nitrogen or acid chemicals, cryotherapy, and salicylic acid paint or plasters have also been effective medical treatments. Topical blistering agents, immunomodulators, and intralesional injections of various agents may also be effective treatment modalities.

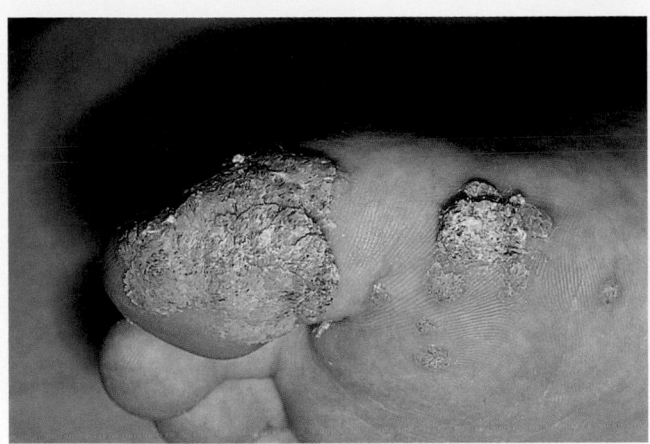

FIGURE 53-4 Plantar warts. (From Callen JP et al: *Color atlas of dermatology*, ed 2, Philadelphia, 2000, Saunders, p 92.)

Herpes Simplex Virus

Etiology and pathogenesis. **Herpes simplex virus** (HSV) infections of the skin and mucous membranes are common (Figure 53-5). Two types of herpesviruses infect humans: type 1 and type 2. Most HSV-1 infections occur above the waist.[3] HSV-1 may result when external infection is spread to the other parts of the body through the occupational hazards that exist in professions such as dentistry and medicine and some athletics. HSV-2 is responsible for most infections in the genital region.[3]

Herpesvirus lesions usually begin with a burning or tingling sensation. Vesicles and erythema follow and progress to pustules, ulcers, and crusts before healing. The lesion is most common on the lips, face, and mouth. Pain is common, and healing takes place in 10 to 14 days.[4] After the initial infection, the herpesvirus persists in latent form in the trigeminal nerve and other ganglia. Recurrent lesions are common and may be precipitated by stress, sunlight exposure, menses, or injury.[5,6] The vast majority of patients have at least 1 episode of herpesvirus reactivation, and some individuals may have 10 or more outbreaks per year. Recently, concern has arisen over the identification of infectious viral shedding in the absence of symptomatic lesions.[5]

Treatment. No cure for herpes simplex is known, and most treatment measures are palliative. Lidocaine (Xylocaine) or diphenhydramine (Benadryl) application and aspirin administration help relieve pain. Cold compresses help in the acute stages. Acyclovir, famciclovir, or valacyclovir is recommended to shorten the duration of active disease outbreaks; in certain situations, these drugs may be used for daily prophylaxis.

Herpes-Zoster Virus

Etiology and pathogenesis. **Herpes zoster** (**shingles**) is an acute localized inflammatory disease of a dermatomal segment of the skin (Figure 53-6). It is caused by the same herpesvirus that causes chickenpox (varicella-zoster virus). It is believed to be the result of reactivation of a latent varicella-zoster virus that has been present in the sensory dorsal ganglia since childhood infection. During an attack of shingles, the reactivated virus travels from the ganglia to the skin of the corresponding dermatome.

Clinical manifestations. The clinical manifestations of shingles include the eruption of vesicles with erythematous bases that are restricted to skin areas supplied by sensory neurons of a single or associated group of dorsal root ganglia. Eruptions generally follow a unilateral dermatomal distribution and most often occur on the thorax,

trunk, and face. In immunosuppressed persons, the lesions may extend beyond the dermatome. New crops of vesicles erupt for 3 to 5 days along the nerve pathway.[3] Lesions are deeper and more confluent than those of chickenpox. The vesicles dry, form crusts, and eventually fall off. Lesions usually clear in 2 to 3 weeks.[3] Severe pain and paresthesias are common. In the elderly, herpes-zoster virus is a particularly serious condition that may be long lasting. Pain reports from elderly individuals indicate an increased severity and lengthy episodes of up to 1 year.[3] Systemic treatment with acyclovir, famciclovir, or valacyclovir should be initiated as soon as possible, preferably within the first 48 to 72 hours.

Postherpetic neuralgia is the most important complication occurring in people older than 50 years.[3] Eye involvement can result in permanent blindness.

Treatment. Management of shingles includes oral antiviral drugs; acyclovir (Zovirax) is one example. Topical agents such as Burow compresses or aqueous alcohol shake lotions may also be used. Pain medication may be indicated in severe cases. Systemic corticosteroids have also been effective in healthy persons older than 50 years with severe pain, but their use remains controversial. High doses of interferon, an antiviral glycoprotein, have been used in persons with cancer when the herpetic lesions are limited to the dermatome.[7]

Additionally, vaccination is becoming an important tool in preventing herpes zoster (e.g., Zostavax).

Fungal Infections
Superficial Fungal Infections

Three genera of **fungi** (**dermatophytes**) commonly infect human skin: *Microsporum*, *Trichophyton*, and *Epidermophyton*. These organisms can cause an infection termed **tinea** in any cutaneous area, including the hair and nails. Infections in different locations are named after the location: tinea capitis (scalp) (Figure 53-7, *A*), tinea barbae (beard), tinea faciei (face) (Figure 53-7, *B*), tinea corporis (trunk) (Figure 53-7, *C*), tinea manus (hand), tinea cruris (groin), and tinea pedis (foot).

Clinical manifestations. The clinical signs of superficial fungal infection vary depending on the physical location and the host's response to the invading organism. Often fungal infections are manifested as erythematous macules or plaques with peripheral scaling and some central clearing. Vesicular lesions often accompany the dry scaling on the feet. Because of the variability of signs and symptoms, superficial dermatophytosis must be considered when evaluating even a weeping, crusted area more suggestive of eczema or impetigo. Dermatophyte infection of the nails, or onychomycosis, is usually seen as a white or yellow opaque discoloration that often progresses to a thickened, crumbled, or deformed nail (Figure 53-8).

Treatment. Topical management of localized superficial dermatophyte infections is very effective. Among the topical antifungal preparations available in cream and solution form are miconazole nitrate, clotrimazole, econazole nitrate, ciclopirox olamine, and terbinafine. A 4-week course of twice-daily applications will usually clear the symptoms. For more extensive infections involving the hair, nails, or resistant organisms, systemic therapy (e.g., griseofulvin or intraconazole and terbinafine) is required. Treatment duration ranges from 3 or 4 weeks (tinea corporis) to 12 months (onychomycosis).

Yeast Infections

The yeast *Candida albicans* is another common source of superficial infection (Figure 53-9). It is manifested in newborns as the white lesions of **thrush,** in infants and bedridden patients as **intertrigo,** and in immunoimpaired individuals as the systemic disorder **mucocutaneous candidiasis.** Mucocutaneous candidiasis may actually be the

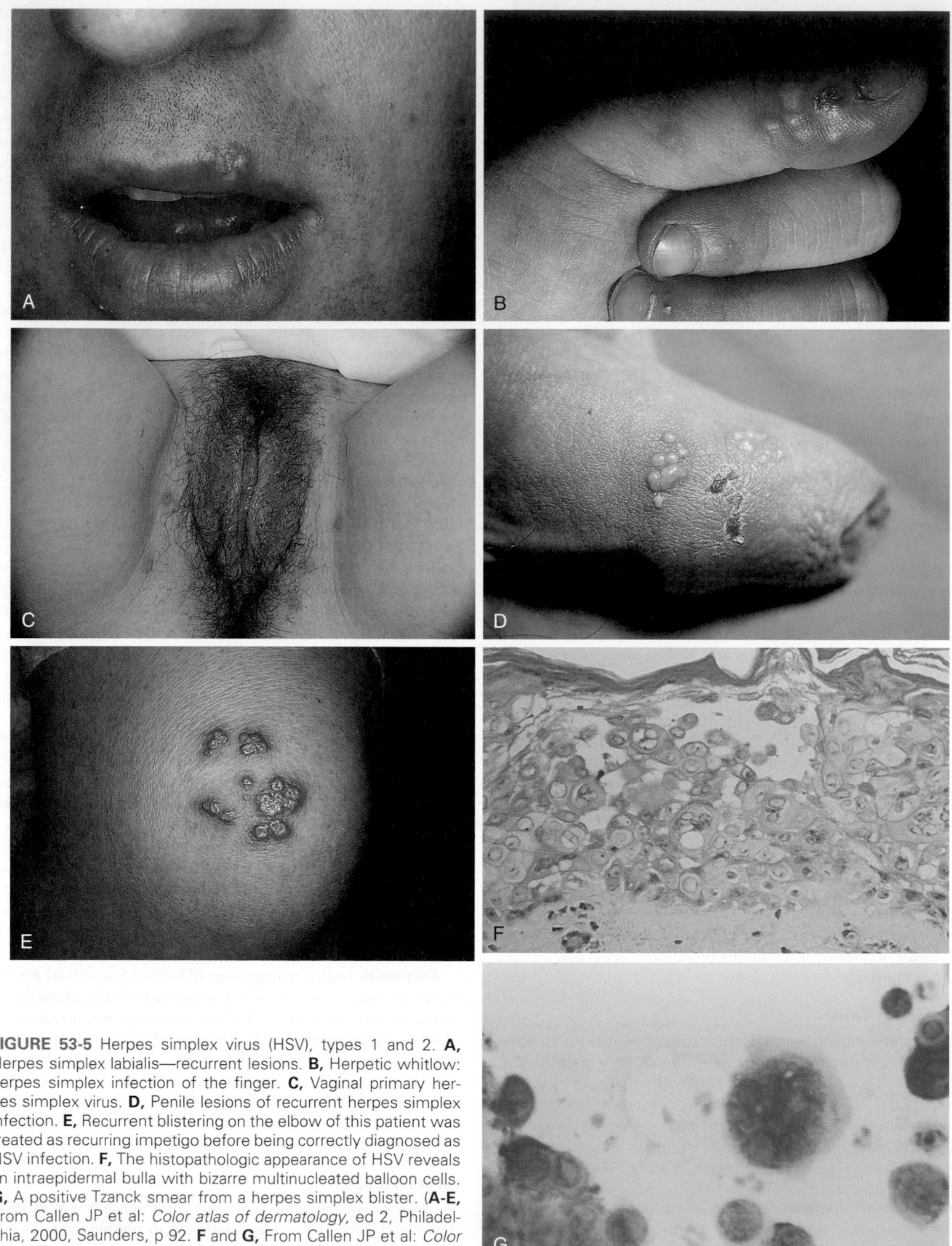

FIGURE 53-5 Herpes simplex virus (HSV), types 1 and 2. **A,** Herpes simplex labialis—recurrent lesions. **B,** Herpetic whitlow: herpes simplex infection of the finger. **C,** Vaginal primary herpes simplex virus. **D,** Penile lesions of recurrent herpes simplex infection. **E,** Recurrent blistering on the elbow of this patient was treated as recurring impetigo before being correctly diagnosed as HSV infection. **F,** The histopathologic appearance of HSV reveals an intraepidermal bulla with bizarre multinucleated balloon cells. **G,** A positive Tzanck smear from a herpes simplex blister. (**A-E,** From Callen JP et al: *Color atlas of dermatology,* ed 2, Philadelphia, 2000, Saunders, p 92. **F** and **G,** From Callen JP et al: *Color atlas of dermatology,* Philadelphia, 1993, Saunders, p 168.)

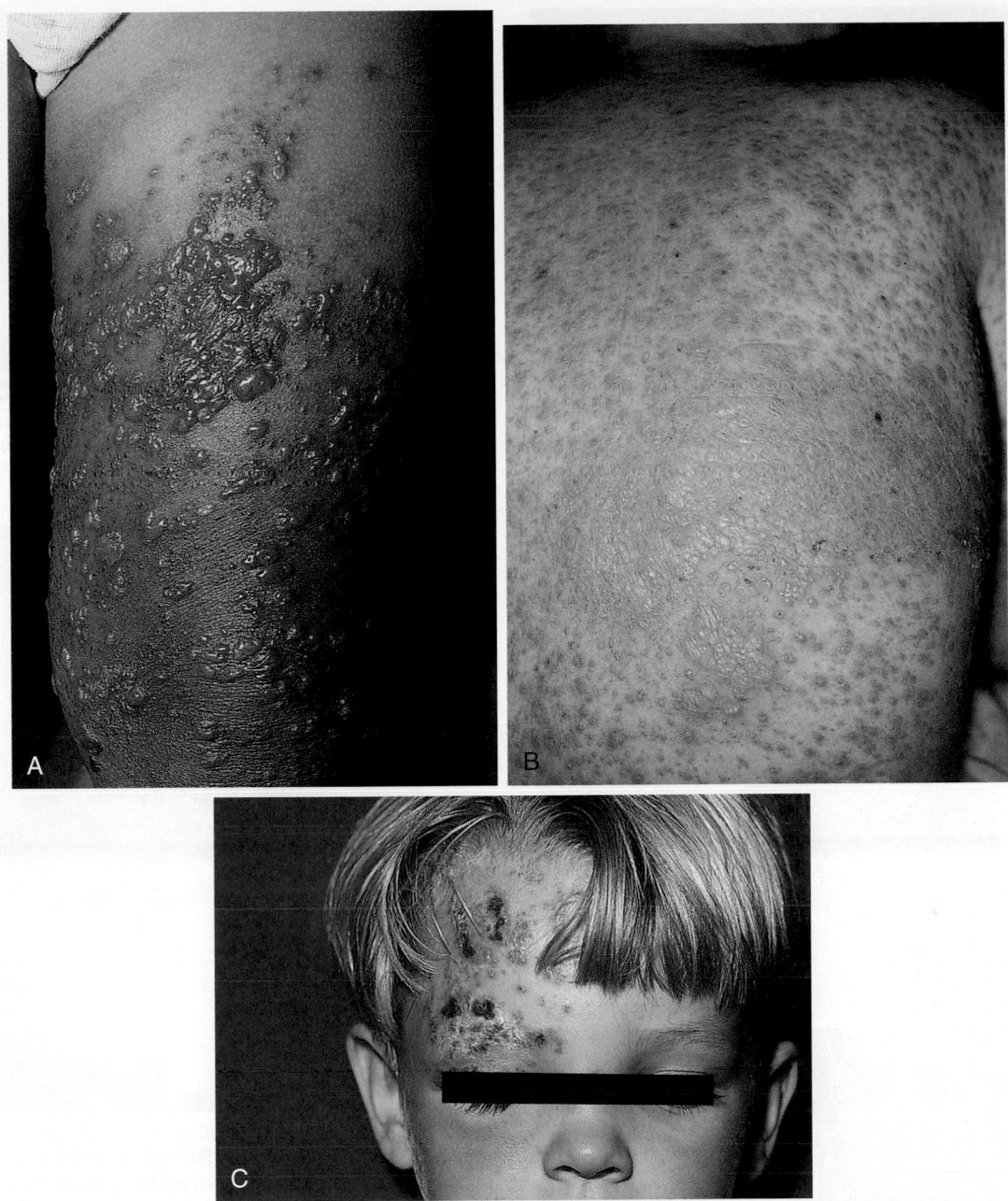

FIGURE 53-6 Herpes zoster. **A,** Recurrent infection with the varicella-zoster virus. The eruption is usually dermatomal but can become generalized. **B,** Disseminated herpes zoster. **C,** Herpes-zoster ophthalmicus. (From Callen JP et al: *Color atlas of dermatology,* ed 2, Philadelphia, 2000, Saunders, p 92.)

presenting sign in an individual with a previously undiagnosed immunodeficiency disorder.

Localized yeast infections such as oral candidiasis (thrush) may be managed with nystatin mouth rinse or clotrimazole troches (throat lozenges). The topical antifungal medications mentioned earlier may also be used in the management of localized yeast infections. Widespread or systemic infections respond well to oral ketoconazole or fluconazole (Diflucan).

Bacterial Infections
Impetigo

Etiology and clinical manifestations. **Impetigo** is an acute, contagious skin disease characterized by the formation of vesicles, pustules, and yellowish crusts (Figure 53-10). The most common cause of infection of the skin, impetigo is caused by staphylococci or streptococci. Approximately 5% of the population each year sustains staphylococcus infections of a severity sufficient to require medical attention.[8] Approximately 20% of adults are chronic carriers of the bacterium *Staphylococcus aureus,* and another 60% are intermittent carriers.[8] The bacterium is carried in the nasal area and may pass onto the skin and produce disease. Staphylococcal infections are a special problem for hospitalized patients, who may become infected from the infected hospital staff.

Treatment. Treatment for impetigo includes topical application of 2% mupirocin ointment (Bactroban) or 1% retapamulin (Altabax) ointment. If a large area of skin is involved or if the person is febrile, impetigo may be managed systemically with oral dicloxacillin, cephalexin, or erythromycin.

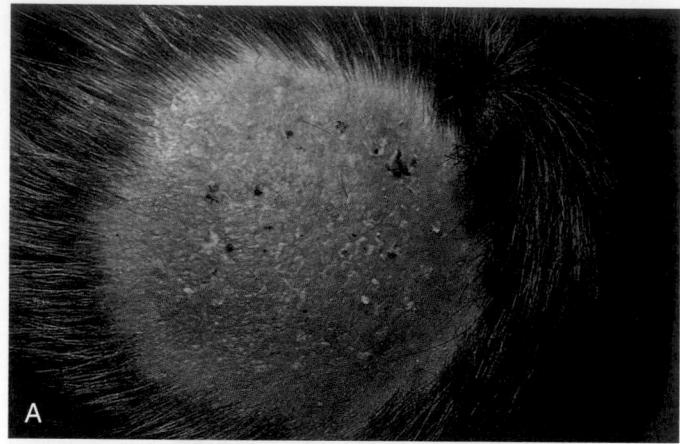

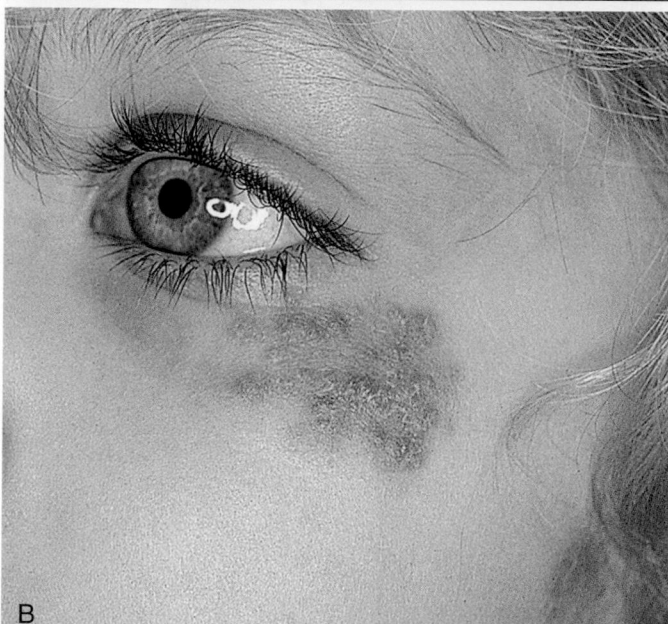

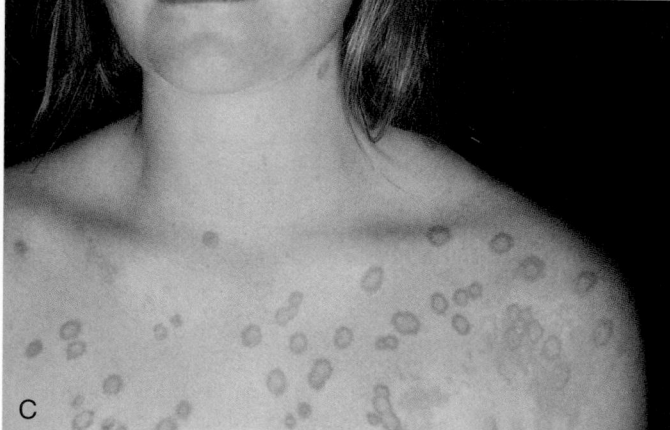

FIGURE 53-7 Tinea infections. **A,** Tinea capitis, localized patch. **B,** Tinea faciei. **C,** Tinea corporis. Annular scaly plaques in superficial basal cell epithelioma. (From Callen JP et al: *Color atlas of dermatology*, Philadelphia, 1993, Saunders, pp 89, 106.)

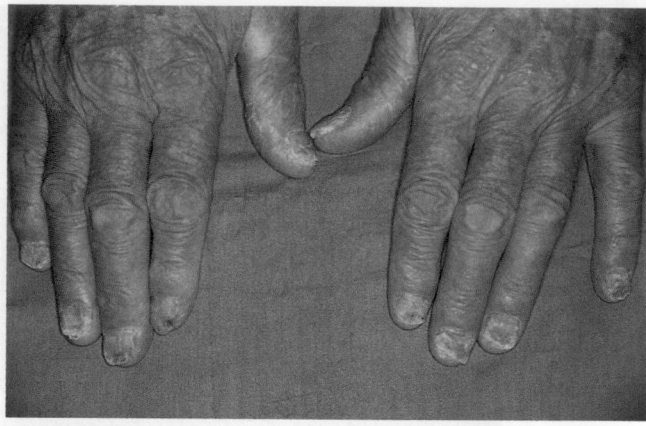

FIGURE 53-8 Dermatophyte infection of the nails resulting in onycholysis. (From Callen JP et al: *Color atlas of dermatology*, Philadelphia, 1993, Saunders, p 347.)

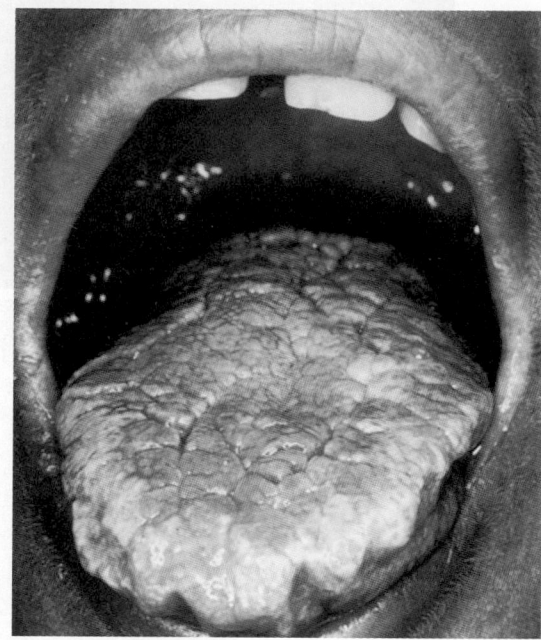

FIGURE 53-9 *Candida albicans* infection of the tongue in chronic mucocutaneous candidiasis. (From Berger TG et al: *Andrews' diseases of the skin: clinical dermatology*, ed 9, Philadelphia, 2000, Saunders, p 385.)

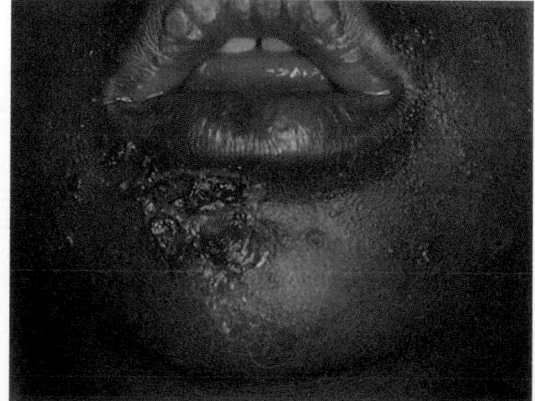

FIGURE 53-10 Impetigo. (From Swartz MH: *Textbook of physical diagnosis*, ed 6, Philadelphia, 2010, Saunders, p 785.)

TABLE 53-3　COMPARISON OF CHRONIC DISCOID WITH SYSTEMIC LUPUS ERYTHEMATOSUS

PARAMETER	CHRONIC DISCOID LE	SYSTEMIC LE
Primary lesions	Red, scaly, thickened, well-circumscribed patches with enlarged follicles and elevated border	Red, mildly scaly, diffuse, puffy lesions; purpura also seen
Secondary lesions	Atrophy, scarring, and pigmentary changes	No scarring; mild hyperpigmentation
Distribution	Face, mainly in the "butterfly" area, but also on the scalp, ears, arms, and chest. May not be symmetric.	Face in "butterfly" area, arms, fingers, and legs; usually symmetric
Course	Very chronic with gradual progression; slow healing under therapy; no effect on life	Acute onset with fever, rash, malaise, and joint pains; most cases respond rather rapidly to steroid and supportive therapy, but prognosis for life is poor
Season	Aggravated by intense sun exposure or radiation therapy	Same
Gender incidence	Almost twice as common in females	Same
Systemic pathology	None obvious	Nephritis, arthritis, epilepsy, pancarditis, hepatitis, etc.
Laboratory findings	Biopsy characteristic in classic case LE cell test negative, as are other laboratory tests	Biopsy less useful

From Sauer GC: *Manual of skin diseases,* ed 6, Philadelphia, 1991, Lippincott, p 253.
LE, Lupus erythematosus.

Syphilis

Etiology and clinical manifestations. A variety of sexually transmitted diseases caused by bacteria can infect the genitalia. The most serious is **syphilis,** which is caused by *Treponema pallidum.* If the person remains untreated, three stages can occur. In primary syphilis, a chancre (ulcer) generally occurs as a single lesion on the genitalia; the spirochetal microorganism that causes syphilis can be seen in a scraping of the chancre. Secondary syphilis is characterized by a disseminated rash that cannot be clearly distinguished from other rashes. Both the primary and the secondary stages of syphilis are contagious.

Treatment. Studies to detect serum antibodies against syphilis (such as the Venereal Disease Research Laboratories [VDRL]) and examination of the pustules for the spirochete are required to achieve a diagnosis. Penicillin is very effective in eradicating syphilis in the primary and secondary stages, but unfortunately damage caused by tertiary syphilis to the cardiovascular and central nervous systems is permanent.

Leprosy

Leprosy is a chronic infectious disease of the skin caused by the intracellular bacillus *Mycobacterium leprae.* Approximately 11 million people worldwide have leprosy.[8] The diagnosis is made with a skin biopsy. Leprosy has a low rate of infectivity and is usually responsive to sulfone drugs such as dapsone. For chronic deformities, corrective orthopedic surgery may be required.

INFLAMMATORY CONDITIONS

Lupus Erythematosus

Lupus erythematosus (LE) is an inflammatory disease that has cutaneous manifestations. Systemic LE and chronic discoid LE are clinically dissimilar but basically related diseases. The two diseases differ with regard to characteristic skin lesions, subjective complaints, other organ involvement, LE cell test findings, response to treatment, and eventual prognosis. Discoid lupus presents with scaly red plaques with scarring that involve sun-exposed skin. Classically, systemic lupus presents with a butterfly-shaped erythema involving the cheeks and nose; discoid lesions may be seen as well. A comparison of the two conditions is found in Table 53-3. Figure 53-11 illustrates characteristic skin lesions of both conditions.

Seborrheic Dermatitis

Clinical manifestations and treatment. Seborrheic dermatitis (Figure 53-12) is a papulosquamous skin disease manifested by various degrees of scaling and erythema in areas of high oil gland concentration such as the scalp, eyebrows, glabellae, eyelids, nasolabial folds, pinna and posterior sulcus of the ears, sternum, axillae, umbilicus, and anogenital area. Common manifestations of this disease are cradle cap in newborns and dandruff in adolescents and adults.

Although seborrheic dermatitis is not curable, it may be controlled with topical medication. The regular use of tar, zinc, selenium sulfide, or salicylic acid shampoos often clears the symptoms and signs of seborrheic dermatitis in the scalp; mild topical corticosteroids (e.g., 1% hydrocortisone) clear lesions on the face and ears.

Psoriasis

Etiology and clinical manifestations. **Psoriasis** is a common chronic skin disease characterized by papules and plaques with an overlying silvery scale. The specific cause of psoriasis is unknown, but it appears to be a multifactorial inherited condition in which minor aberrations of the immune system promote inflammation and hyperproliferation within the skin. The disease may affect, with varying degrees of severity, people of all ages. Lesions can appear on any area of the body; however, they seem to have a predilection for the knees, elbows, lower part of the back, scalp, and nails (Figure 53-13). Disease progression is unpredictable, and the patient may periodically experience spontaneous exacerbations or remission.

Treatment. No cure for psoriasis is known. Treatments, both topical and systemic, are directed at clearing and controlling the lesions. Therapies include topical corticosteroids (most commonly used), a vitamin D derivative (calcipotriene ointment [Dovonex]), ultraviolet light exposure, topical tar preparations, and combinations of ultraviolet light with topical tar or systemic psoralen. Systemic therapies with methotrexate and hydroxyurea are also effective in clearing psoriasis but carry considerable risk of toxicity. Newer, highly effective biological agents are now available for use by injection but are very expensive and also carry risks of significant side effects.

Lichen Planus

Etiology and pathogenesis. **Lichen planus** is a relatively common, chronic, pruritic disease involving inflammation and papular eruption of the skin and mucous membranes. Idiopathic lichen planus is of unknown cause but can be stimulated by a variety of drugs and chemicals in susceptible persons. The characteristic lesion is a shiny, white-topped, purplish, polygonal papule. Lesions appear on the wrists, ankles, and trunk (Figure 53-14). Mucous membrane

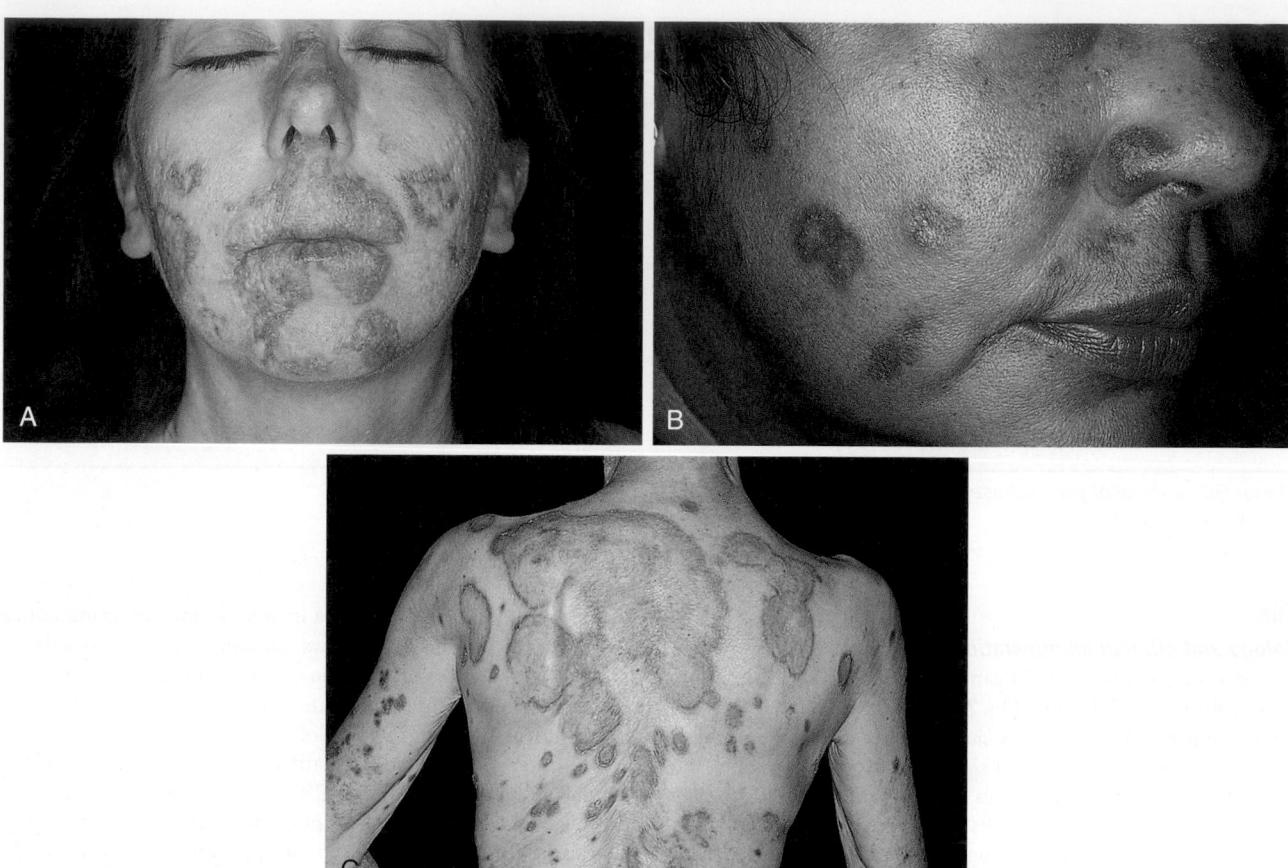

FIGURE 53-11 **A** and **B,** Discoid lupus erythematosus. Round or oval cutaneous lesions occurring in patients with lupus erythematosus. **C,** Subacute cutaneous lupus erythematosus. (From Callen JP et al: *Color atlas of dermatology*, ed 2, Philadelphia, 2000, Saunders, pp 15, 16.)

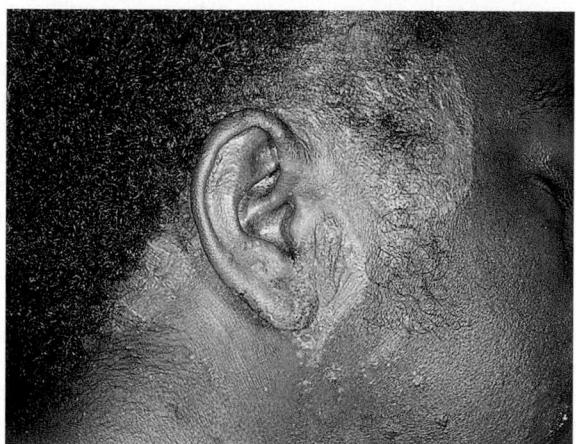

FIGURE 53-12 Annular seborrheic dermatitis of the ear. (From Callen JP et al: *Color atlas of dermatology*, ed 2, Philadelphia, 2000, Saunders, p 246.)

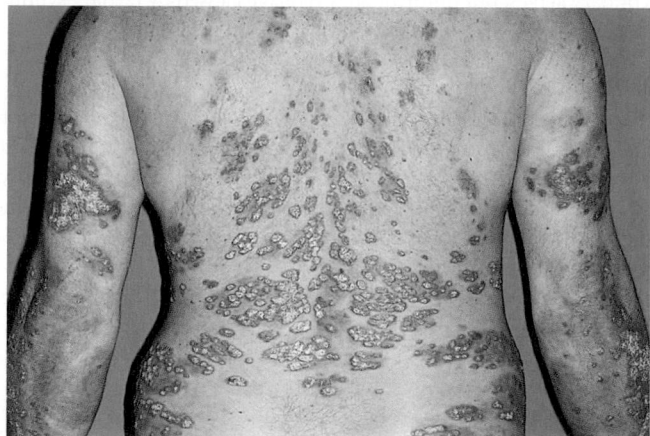

FIGURE 53-13 Psoriasis vulgaris. (From Callen JP et al: *Color atlas of dermatology*, ed 2, Philadelphia, 2000, Saunders, p 280.)

lesions are white and lacy and may become bullous. Pruritus is severe, and new lesions develop as a result of scratching (Koebner phenomenon). Nails are affected in approximately 10% of people with lichen planus.[9]

Treatment. In the majority of people, lichen planus is a self-limiting disease. Treatment measures include discontinuation of all medications, followed by the administration of topical corticosteroids and occlusive dressings. Systemic corticosteroids may be indicated in severe cases, and antipruritic agents are helpful in reducing the pruritus.

Pityriasis Rosea

Etiology, pathogenesis, and treatment. Pityriasis rosea is a rash of unknown origin that primarily affects young adults. The incidence is highest in the spring and fall seasons. It has been speculated to be viral in origin, but to date no virus has been isolated. The characteristic lesion is a macule or papule with surrounding erythema. The lesion spreads with central clearing, much like tinea corporis. This initial lesion is a solitary lesion, called the herald patch, and is usually located on the trunk or neck. As the lesion enlarges and begins to fade away

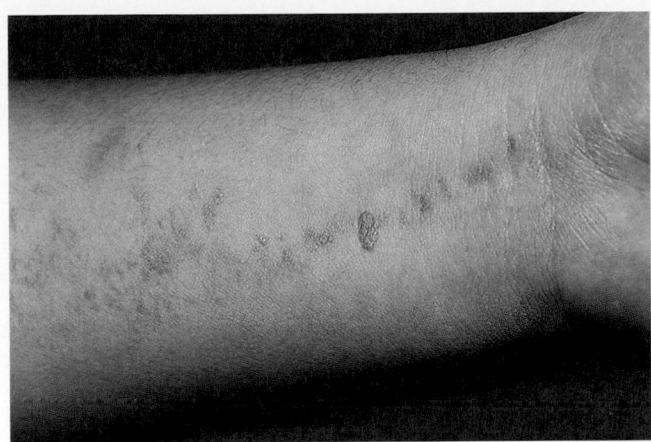

FIGURE 53-14 Linear lichen planus as a result of Koebner phenomenon. (From Callen JP et al: *Color atlas of dermatology*, ed 2, Philadelphia, 2000, Saunders, p 249.)

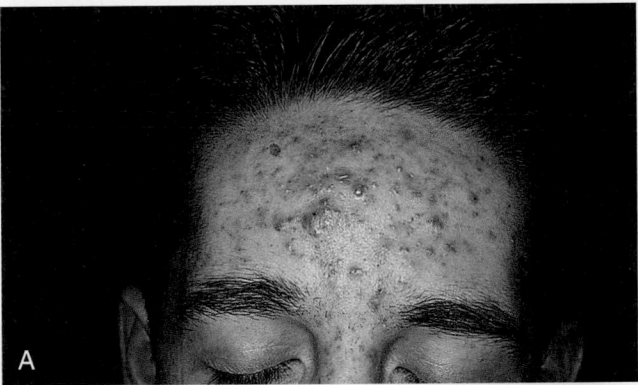

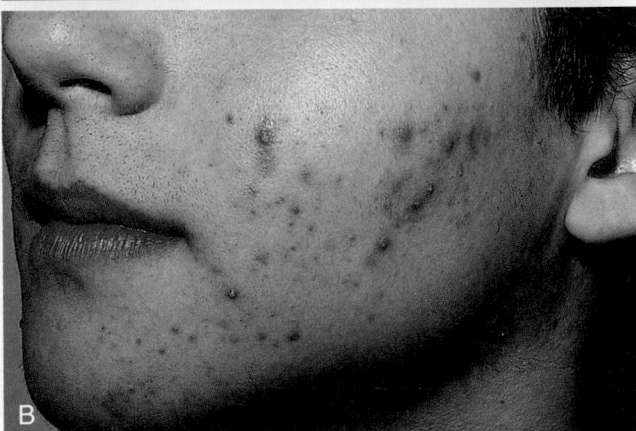

FIGURE 53-15 A and **B,** Acne vulgaris with papules and pustules. (From Callen JP et al: *Color atlas of dermatology*, ed 2, Philadelphia, 2000, Saunders, p 151.)

(2 to 10 days), successive crops of lesions appear on the trunk and neck.[10] The extremities, face, and scalp may be involved, and mild to severe pruritus may occur. The disease is self-limiting and usually disappears within 2 to 10 weeks.[10] Treatment is palliative and includes topical steroids, antihistamines, and colloid baths. Systemic corticosteroids may be indicated in severe cases. Systemic antibiotics, especially erythromycin, may also shorten the course.

Acne Vulgaris

Etiology and pathogenesis. Acne, an extremely common disease of the pilosebaceous unit, affects up to 90% of all individuals and produces unsightly lesions and sometimes permanent scarring and disfigurement[11] (Figure 53-15). Etiologically, acne involves multiple factors such as sex hormones, heredity, bacterial flora of the skin, stress, mechanical occlusion, and cosmetics' use. Acne arises when sludging of sebaceous oils and deposition of loose epithelial cells cause an obstruction of the follicular canal. Continued oil production and bacterial growth in this obstructed follicle may cause rupture of the wall or sebaceous gland and result in an inflamed lesion.

Treatment. No cure for acne is known. Treatment modalities are directed to clearing the lesions and maintaining a clear complexion. Topical therapy is effective for most patients. Such medications are designed to cause increased peeling of the stratum corneum and loosening of the follicular plugs.

Many products are available to achieve this goal. Soaps, lotions, and gels containing sulfur, resorcinol, salicylic acid, or benzoyl peroxide all enhance drying and peeling. Astringents, which are liquids primarily composed of alcohol with acetone, are used as solvents to remove the surface lipid and loose skin cells, as well as to enhance drying. Topical retinoids, of which there are several, are a mainstay of treatment. Retinoic acid, a derivative of vitamin A, is one example of this class of drugs.[4] Retinoic acid is an exfoliative agent and is very useful in dealing with open comedones and papules. Topical antibiotics are also available, the most effective being liquid preparations of erythromycin and clindamycin (Cleocin T) with an alcohol base.

For cases characterized by inflammatory lesions, pustules, or nodules, systemic therapy can be useful. Antibiotics, especially tetracycline and erythromycin, have long been used in such treatments. Concerns that continued use of systemic tetracycline group antibiotics may result in colonization with tetracycline-resistant *Staphylococcus aureus* have not been supported. This is significant because tetracycline group antibiotics are currently one of the primary options for outpatient treatment of methicillin-resistant *S. aureus* (MRSA).[12] In cases that are resistant, minocycline, sulfamethoxazole-trimethoprim, and sulfones are occasionally used. Isotretinoin, a vitamin A derivative, is effective in the management of nodular and cystic acne.[12] Birth control pills, especially the estrogen-dominant type, can be of value in managing severe recalcitrant acne in females. However, androgen-dominant contraceptives can aggravate or precipitate acne.

As with any medication regimen, both systemic and topical acne treatments can produce unwanted side effects in sensitive patients. Systemic tetracycline may cause gastrointestinal upset, nausea, diarrhea, and vaginal *Monilia* overgrowth. Tetracycline should not be used in children because their unerupted teeth may be severely and permanently discolored. Topical antibiotics can cause irritant or allergic contact dermatitis.

Other useful acne treatments include corticosteroid injection into cysts and nodules and surgery, which involves extraction of the comedones and drainage of fluctuant cystic lesions.[6]

Pemphigus

A group of related disorders (**pemphigus group** of vulgaris, vegetans, foliaceus, and erythematosus) is characterized by bullous eruptions (blisters). These disorders are thought to be caused by autoimmune reactions. Patients show antibodies against keratinocytes and basement membranes. The autoantibodies perhaps cause the keratinocytes to separate from one another to form blisters. Of the group of related diseases, **pemphigus vulgaris** has the worst prognosis (Figure 53-16). Bullae can erupt on the skin and mucous membranes (e.g., esophagus), and toxemia and infection can cause death if proper treatment (cortisone) is not administered.

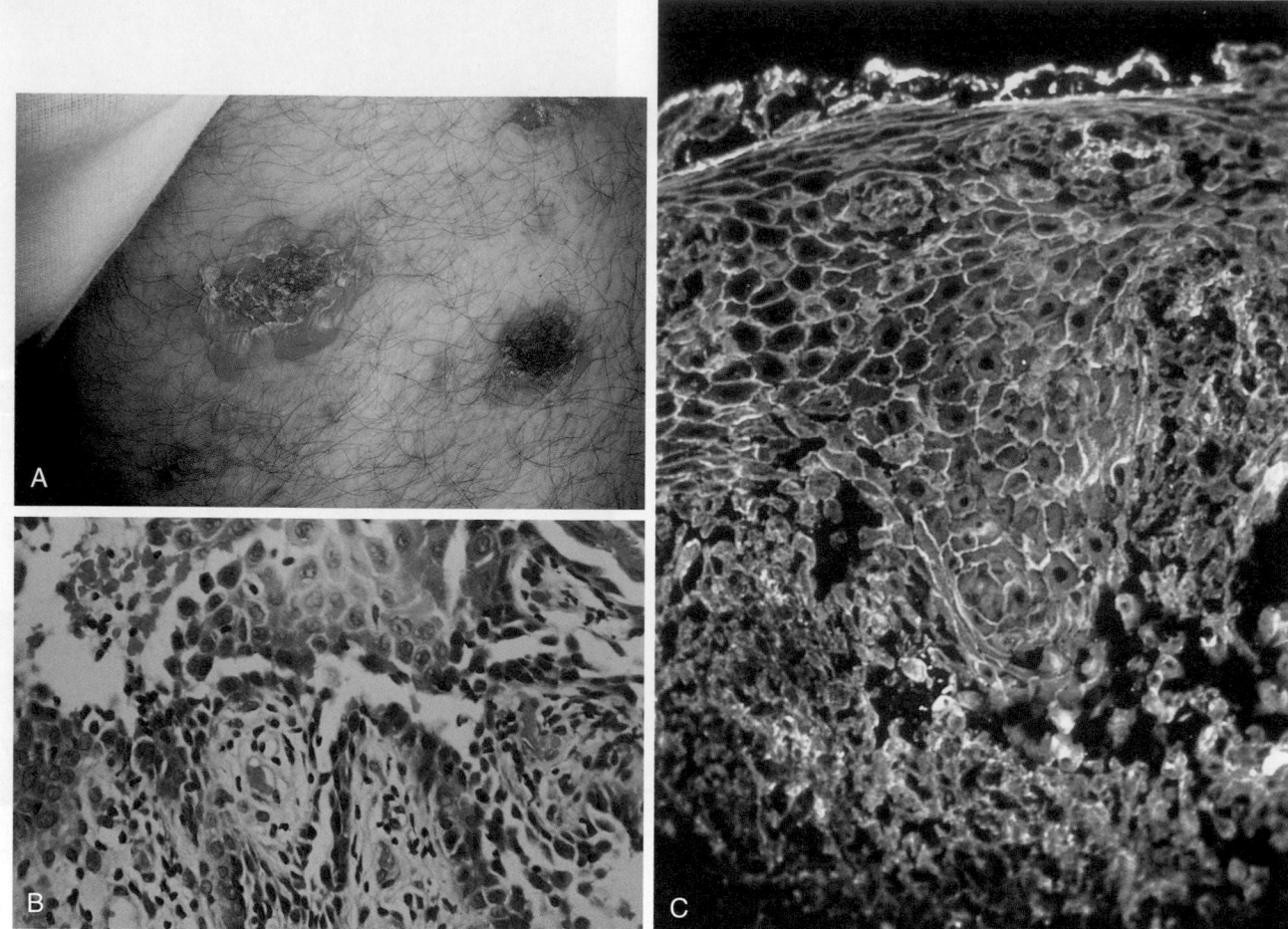

FIGURE 53-16 Pemphigus vulgaris. **A,** Bullae are transient in this disorder; erosion is more characteristic. **B,** The blister is suprabasilar within the epidermis. Individual cells are unattached within the bulla (acantholytic cells). **C,** Deposition of IgG in the intercellular areas of the epidermis is characteristic of pemphigus. (From Callen JP et al: *Color atlas of dermatology,* Philadelphia, 1993, Saunders, p 163.)

ALLERGIC SKIN RESPONSES

Atopic Dermatitis

Etiology and clinical manifestations. Atopic dermatitis is a complex genetic disease that results from gene-gene and gene-environment interactions. Genetic defects in the epidermal barrier protein filaggrin have been cited as a major cause of atopic dermatitis. It is suggested that the trait is inherited via a maternal gene located on chromosome 11. The stratum corneum layers of those individuals with loss-of-function mutations in the filaggrin gene have lower levels of natural moisturizing factor and also are deficient in extracellular lipids including ceramides. Repair of barrier function has become one of the important developments in treatment of atopic dermatitis; these treatments include emollients that contain ceramides.[13] **Atopy,** or **allergy,** is indicated by a personal and sometimes family history of asthma, allergic rhinitis, or the most commonly seen manifestation, eczematous dermatitis (Figures 53-17 and 53-18). The highest incidence of atopic dermatitis occurs in children, with most cases developing in those younger than 5 years.[13] The characteristic features depend on the age at onset, but pruritus is always present. In infants, the disease characteristically appears on the face, scalp, or extensor surfaces of the extremities; the predominant lesion is an oozing, crusting, coalescent papule. The disease in children is most often manifested as erythema, papules, and lichenification of the flexor surfaces of the extremities, especially the antecubital

and popliteal areas, the wrists, and the nape of the neck. Older children and young adults have thickening of the skin, or lichenification, along with fine, dry scaling and some papules. These changes are again seen on the flexor surfaces of the extremities and the scalp, face, and upper chest. Retrospective studies show that in nearly half of all patients with childhood atopic dermatitis, the disease improves or clears with age.[14]

Treatment. Treatment of atopic dermatitis is usually conducted on an outpatient basis. The most important considerations are moisturization of the skin and prevention of continued drying and water loss. The drying and scaling that are characteristic features of atopic dermatitis impair the skin's ability not only to retain moisture but also to repel such external invaders as chemical irritants and surface bacteria. Milder cases of atopic eczema can be managed conservatively by decreasing the frequency of bathing, using tepid water in baths, eliminating alkaline soaps, and using moisturizing creams (especially after baths and washing). In more severe cases that involve an inflammatory response to skin breakdown, topical steroids are an important part of therapy. Short courses of systemic antibiotics such as erythromycin have also been helpful in controlling the severity of atopic eczema by reducing the concentration of cutaneous bacterial flora. Even after all these measures have been executed, some patients with severe atopic dermatitis are hospitalized for application of continuous wet dressings and topical steroids.

An important feature of all atopic dermatitis cases that must be addressed is pruritus. The topical treatments mentioned previously

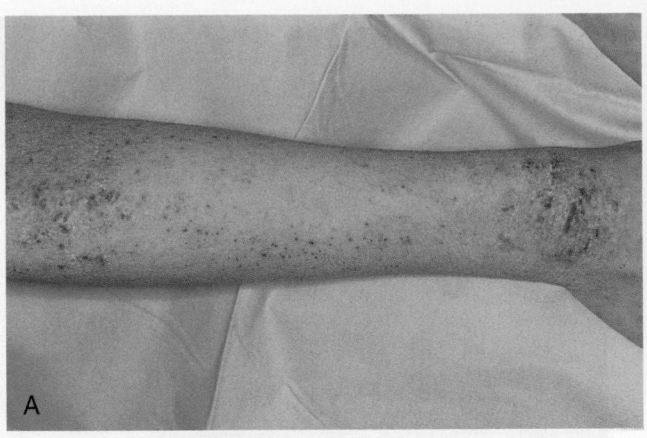
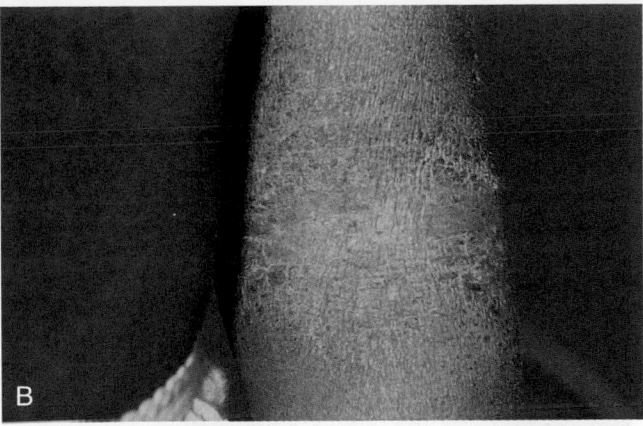

FIGURE 53-17 Atopic dermatitis. An extremely pruritic condition. **A,** Multiple excoriations, vesiculation, and marked lichenification are seen in this patient. **B,** Minute excoriations with marked lichenification in the antecubital fossa. (From Callen JP et al: *Color atlas of dermatology*, Philadelphia, 1993, Saunders, p 192.)

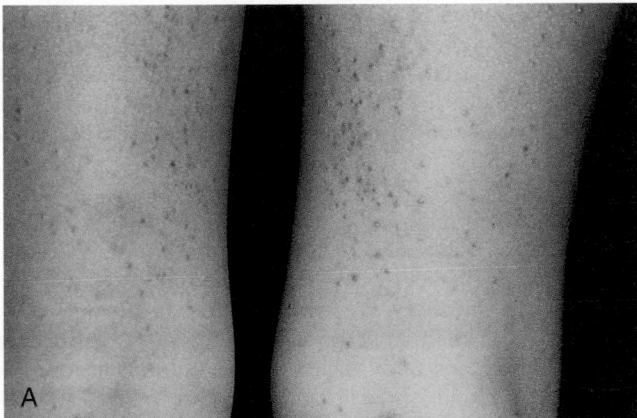
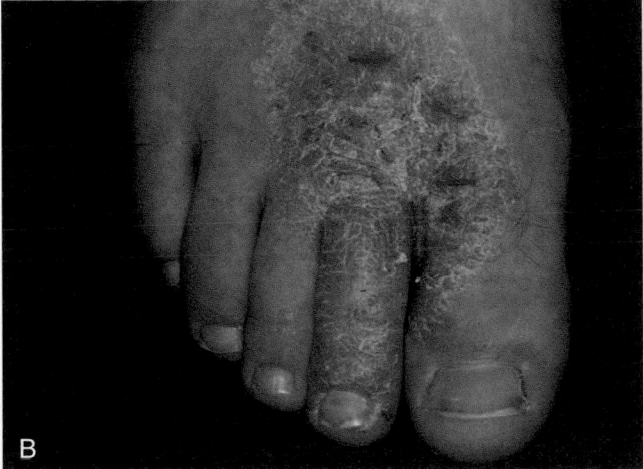

FIGURE 53-18 A, Papular eczema. **B,** Chronic eczema of the feet. (From Callen JP et al: *Color atlas of dermatology*, Philadelphia, 1993, Saunders, p 192.)

are helpful in reducing pruritus. If additional measures are needed, systemic antihistamines (e.g., hydroxyzine and diphenhydramine) are effective.

Contact Dermatitis

Etiologies and clinical manifestations. Contact dermatitis is a cutaneous reaction to topical irritation or allergy. Irritant contact dermatitis develops in any person exposed to a sufficiently high concentration of the irritating agent. Some of the more active irritants are acids, alkalis, and hydrocarbons.

Allergic contact dermatitis indicates delayed acquired hypersensitivity to a specific allergen. Dermatologic problems may appear after years of asymptomatic exposure to the precipitating agent. Chromates, nickel, ethylenediamine, paraphenylenediamine, neomycin, formaldehyde, and lanolin components may cause allergic contact dermatitis.

Aside from reactions to various industrial chemicals, the most common type of allergic contact dermatitis reaction is to plants. **Rhus dermatitis** encompasses allergy to poison ivy, poison oak, and poison sumac. Clinically, rhus dermatitis begins within 48 hours of contact. The first symptom is pruritus, followed by erythema and vesicle formation, sometimes in linear fashion (Figure 53-19). As long as the allergen remains on the surface of the skin, it can be spread to nonexposed areas. Therefore, thorough washing can help prevent spread by hand contact. Exposure to blister fluid does not spread poison ivy lesions.

Treatment. Contact dermatitis from exposure to poison ivy can range from mild to severe. For the mildest cases, application of topical steroids or cooling shake lotions of camphor and menthol may effectively decrease discomfort. Severe cases may require hospitalization for cooling baths and wet dressings, which dry the lesions and decrease the tense, pruritic blisters. Discomfort and generalized edema often respond to systemic steroids administered over a 10- to 14-day period.

Drug Eruptions

Etiology and clinical manifestations. Adverse or undesirable reactions to medically administered drugs are common, yet cutaneous reactions are uncommon (0.1%) within the overall prescription-taking population.[15] Cutaneous reactions to medication usually begin within a week of drug exposure, although reactions to penicillins may occur later. Women experience more cutaneous drug eruptions than men. The drugs that most frequently result in adverse cutaneous eruptions are ampicillin, penicillin, cephalosporins, and barbiturates. Blood transfusions also occasionally produce cutaneous reactions identical to those of a drug eruption.

The most common type of adverse cutaneous drug eruption is an erythematous maculopapular exanthem (rash). These often pruritic lesions are usually widely dispersed, and clearing is gradual and continues for several weeks after the drug has been discontinued. Other common drug reactions include urticaria (i.e., hives), erythema multiforme (including Stevens-Johnson syndrome), exfoliative dermatitis, photosensitivity, vasculitis, and fixed-drug eruption.

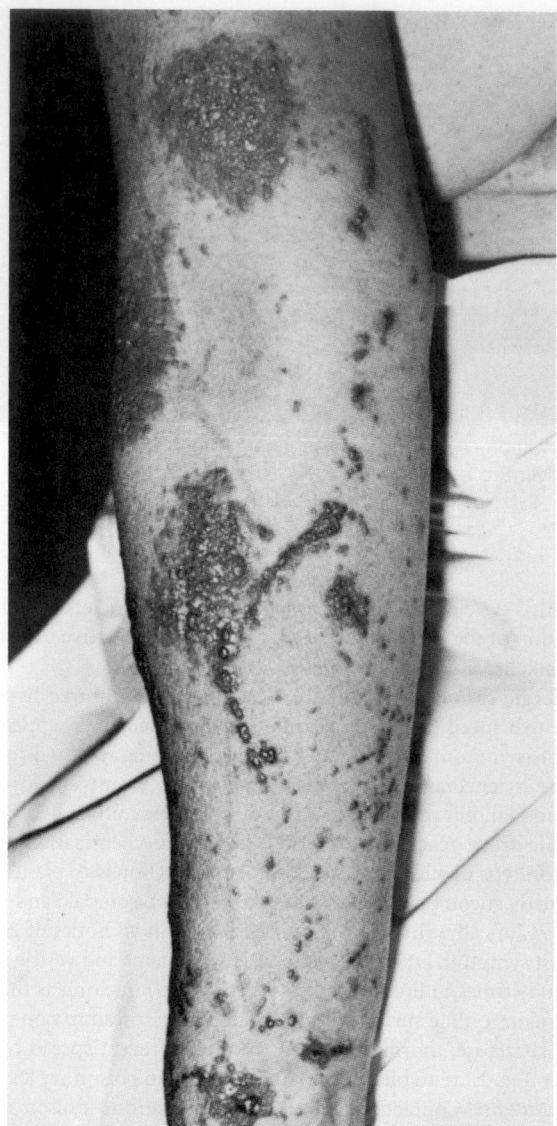

FIGURE 53-19 Rhus dermatitis with the characteristic linear groups of vesicles. (From Berger TG et al: *Andrews' diseases of the skin: clinical dermatology,* ed 9, Philadelphia, 2000, Saunders, p 101.)

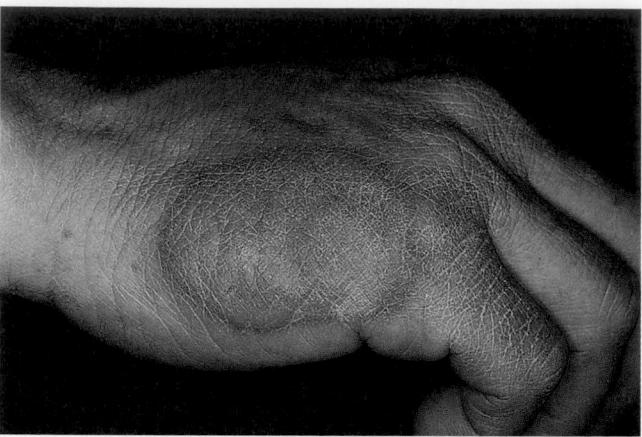

FIGURE 53-20 Fixed-drug eruption. An early lesion may be manifested as an urticarial plaque. This lesion frequently resolves with macular hyperpigmentation. (From Callen JP et al: *Color atlas of dermatology,* ed 2, Philadelphia, 2000, Saunders, p 217.)

Exanthem-type eruptions can be caused by such medications as barbiturates, griseofulvin, penicillin, thiazides, and sulfonamides. Urticarial eruptions may result from the use of barbiturates, penicillin, chloramphenicol, phenolphthalein, salicylates, sulfonamides, or tetracycline. Erythema multiforme is seen with erythromycin, penicillin, phenolphthalein, salicylate, diphenylhydantoin, and thiazides. Exfoliative dermatitis can be caused by barbiturates, gold, penicillin, phenothiazides, and sulfonamides, and photosensitivity is seen with chlordiazepoxide, fluoroquinolones, griseofulvin, phenothiazines, sulfonamides, tetracycline, and thiazides. Cutaneous vasculitis may be triggered by iodines, erythromycin, penicillin, quinidine, sulfonamides, and thiazides. A fixed-drug eruption (Figure 53-20) is a round to oval, violaceous macule or slightly palpable plaque that is often recurrent, especially in previously affected sites, on reexposure to the irritating medication. This effect can be caused by barbiturates, gold, phenolphthalein, sulfonamides, and tetracycline. These drug lists are not inclusive, and several substances are known to cause multiple adverse cutaneous reactions.[16]

Treatment. Management of drug eruptions includes discontinuation of the offending drug and administration of oral antihistamines and antipruritic lotions of hydrocortisone, menthol, camphor, or other proven substances for relief of pruritus. For more severe eruptions, a 2- to 3-week course of systemic corticosteroids should be considered. In addition, the patient should be counseled regarding use of the offending medication and an appropriate notation placed in the patient's medical record.

Vasculitis

Etiology. When antigen and antibody react in blood vessels in the skin, severe **necrotizing inflammation (vasculitis)** can appear. This condition can be caused by drug allergies; disorders such as systemic lupus erythematosus (SLE), rheumatoid arthritis, and glomerulonephritis; and certain infectious diseases such as hepatitis B. **Polyarteritis nodosa** is a form of systemic vasculitis that can cause inflamed arteries in visceral organs, brain, and skin.

Treatment. Immunofluorescent studies reveal antigens and serum immunoglobulins trapped in the wall of the blood vessel that is inflamed by neutrophils. Acute vasculitis can cause damage not only to skin but also to the brain and visceral organs. When the vasculitis is severe, systemic corticosteroids may be administered in high doses.

PARASITIC INFESTATIONS

Scabies

Sarcoptes scabiei is a mite, and infestation with this mite in humans is called **scabies.** Scabies begins with eggs laid in the stratum corneum. These eggs hatch into larvae within 3 to 4 days and grow to adulthood within 2 months. Scabies is usually contracted after close personal contact with an infested individual.

Clinically, scabies lesions are small (1 to 4 mm), erythematous papules, some with an overlying dry scale or crust (Figure 53-21). In some cases, linear burrows are seen. Scabies mites have a predilection for the finger webs, wrists, umbilicus, and groin area. The history related by most patients is an intensely pruritic eruption that spreads over a period of weeks from a single area of the body to other areas.

Scabies treatment consists of topical permethrin cream (Elimite), γ-benzene hexachloride (Lindane), or crotamiton (Eurax). For infants, 5% to 6% precipitated sulfur in petrolatum applied twice daily for 1 week is usually adequate.

Fleas

Three types of flea commonly bite and cause cutaneous reactions in humans: the human flea *(Pulex irritans),* the cat flea *(Ctenocephalides*

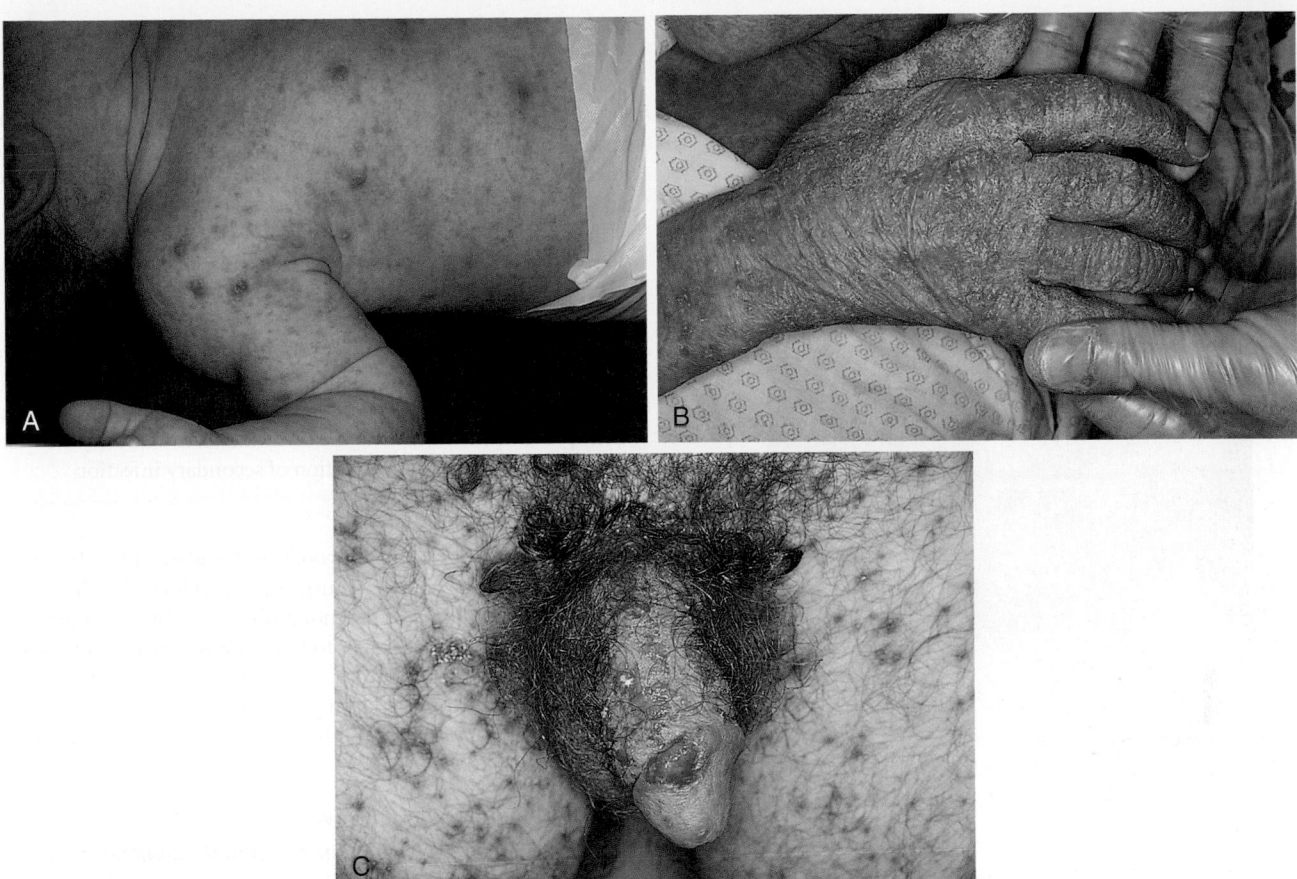

FIGURE 53-21 A, Scabies. **B,** An extremely pruritic infestation. **C,** Crusted (Norwegian) scabies. (**A,** From Callen JP et al: *Color atlas of dermatology,* ed 2, Philadelphia, 2000, Saunders, pp 170, 283.)

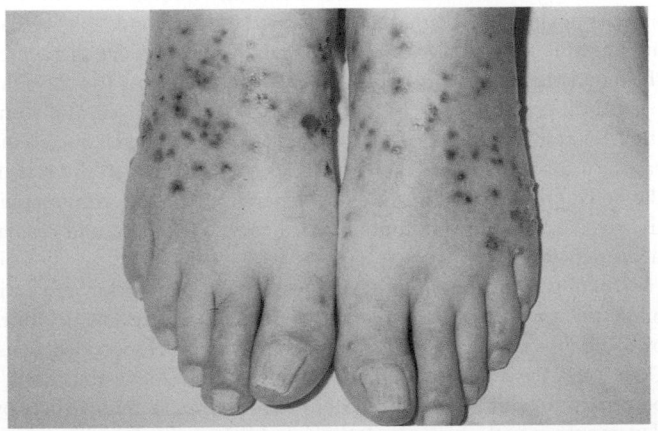

FIGURE 53-22 Insect bites (fleas) led this patient to scratch. (From Swartz MH: *Textbook of physical diagnosis,* ed 6, Philadelphia, 2010, Saunders, p 178.)

felis), and the dog flea *(Ctenocephalides canis).* Flea bites may appear as small erythematous macules, erythematous papules, wheals, or a vesicle (Figure 53-22).

Diethyltoluamide or pyrethrin insect repellents are effective in preventing flea infestation. Indoor carpeting, an ideal environment for fleas, should be treated with an appropriate insecticide.

The milder papular form of flea bites can be managed with soothing shake lotions of menthol and camphor or with topical steroids.

More severe reactions (e.g., vesicles or bullae) may require a course of systemic steroids.

Lice

Phthirus pubis (crab lice), *Pediculus humanus* var. *capitis* (head lice), and *Pediculus humanus* var. *corporis* (body lice) are the types of lice most often found on humans. They are surface dwelling, unlike the burrowing scabies mite, and they usually can be seen without magnification. Control and eradication are possible with one of the following: permethrin cream rinse or pyrethrin and piperonyl butoxide liquid, gel, or shampoo.

Chiggers

Chiggers are mites that reside in grass and bushes. They are common in the southern United States but can be found as far north as Canada. Puncture of the skin by the mite to obtain nourishment produces pruritic papules commonly seen wherever it encounters resistance, such as at the top of socks, at the belt line, or around the neckband area (Figure 53-23). Secondary lesions are excoriations from scratching that have become infected by bacteria. Treatment is palliative, and the use of insect repellent is encouraged for prevention.

Bedbugs

The common bedbug, *Cimex lectularius,* is a reddish-brown insect 3 to 6 mm long that turns purple after feeding. Like most parasites, bedbugs feed on human blood. Importantly, they can also alternate between human and animal hosts, and they live up to and sometimes beyond 1 year.[8] When not feeding, bedbugs stay hidden in the cracks and crevices

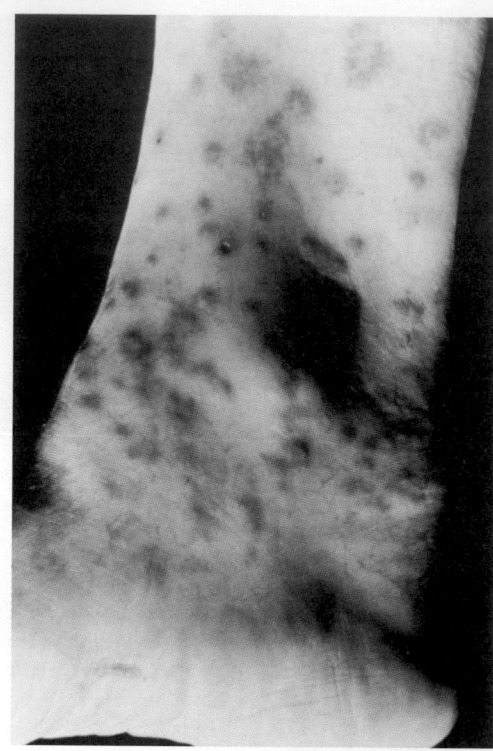

FIGURE 53-23 Chigger bites. (From Berger HL et al: *Andrews' diseases of the skin: clinical dermatology,* ed 9, Philadelphia, 2000, Saunders, p 569.)

of furniture, mattresses, wallpaper, picture frames, baseboards, flooring, door locks, or any darkened area. Unless their source is eliminated, recurrence is inevitable. Professional extermination is advised because of their many hiding places. Bedbugs have been known to feed on animal populations when forced from their living quarters. On rehabitation in the same quarters, the bedbug can easily return to human hosts.

They are nocturnal feeders, and, when crushed, they emit a foul odor. The bedbug bite is painless and produces a pruritic oval or oblong wheal with a small hemorrhagic punctum at the center. Bullous lesions are not uncommon. Usually, lesions are multiple and arranged in rows or clusters on the face, neck, hands, and arms. No area is exempt. The wheal is probably a type 1 sensitivity reaction to the anticoagulant saliva of the bedbug. Secondary excoriation and bacterial infections may occur.

The diagnosis depends on the time of the day when the lesions appear. Because of the painless bite, it is not uncommon for the victim to awake with one or several pruritic papules. Topical antipruritics are used as treatment.

Mosquitoes

Most people have experienced mosquitoes and are familiar with their bites. The typical lesion is a raised wheal on an erythematous base, accompanied by pruritus within 45 minutes of the bite. A second type of reaction is the delayed response: 8 to 12 hours after the bite, the lesion becomes raised, erythematous, and indurated, with extensive pruritus or pain. This reaction peaks 24 to 72 hours after the bite.[9] The saliva of the mosquito is believed to be the source of the skin reaction. Although severe skin reactions are possible, they are rare. Insect repellents are recommended for prevention; local antipruritics are used for treatment.

Blood Flukes

Bathers in the freshwater lakes of Wisconsin, Michigan, and Minnesota are prone to periodic attacks of inflammatory, papular, urticarial,

and vesicular eruptions on the uncovered areas of the body, mainly the legs. This pruritic eruption, commonly called "swimmer's itch," usually subsides within a week and is caused by invasion of the skin by cercariae (larvae) of the schistosomes (worms) of ducks and mammals. The life cycle of these various species of schistosomes includes the snail as an intermediate host. On invasion of the abnormal definitive host, the human skin, the cercariae die, and the resulting skin eruption is the skin's reaction in ridding itself of the foreign bodies. Repeated attacks are met with stronger resistance, and the dermatitis becomes increasingly severe. Secondary infection, edema, and lymphangitis can occur.

Swimmer's itch is best prevented by destruction of the snails through careful addition of a combination of copper sulfate and hydrated lime to the lake water. Rapid drying of the swimmer with a towel apparently prevents penetration of the cercariae. Active therapy is directed to relief of the itching and prevention of secondary infection.

Ticks

Ticks are insects that live in woods and underbrush. They attach to human and animal hosts and burrow in the epidermis, where they feed on blood. The tick bite itself is not problematic, but the infectious bacteria or viruses that ticks carry to human hosts create problems. Many tick-borne illnesses are known, including Central European encephalitis, Q fever, babesiasis, relapsing fever, Rocky Mountain spotted fever (RMSF), and Lyme disease. Both RMSF and Lyme disease are relatively common in the United States.

Rocky Mountain Spotted Fever

Etiology, pathogenesis, and clinical manifestations. Rocky Mountain spotted fever (RMSF) is caused by a tick that carries *Rickettsia rickettsii*. In the past RMSF was localized to the Rocky Mountain area, but by 1982 most states had reported a case of RMSF.[8]

The initial tick bite appears as a papule or macule, with or without a central punctate area. The tick burrows into the host and enlarges as it feeds. The tick must be attached to the human host for 4 to 6 hours before the rickettsiae are activated by the blood.[8] Rickettsiae are found in the tick feces and body parts. The rickettsiae then enter the bloodstream and multiply in body tissues. Within 4 to 8 days the patient experiences fever, headache, muscle aches, nausea, and vomiting.[8] A rash then appears on the wrist or ankle. The characteristic rash is a macular or maculopapular one that spreads to the rest of the body. Other symptoms include generalized edema, conjunctivitis, petechial lesions, photophobia, lethargy, confusion, and cranial nerve deficits.

Treatment. Treatment for RMSF requires hospitalization and antibiotic therapy. The most important measure is to prevent tick bites by using insect repellents while engaged in activities in wooded areas. Once a tick has attached itself, it is important to remove all the tick's body parts to limit the possibility of infection. One can remove ticks by dousing them with mineral oil or alcohol before slowly pulling them out with tweezers. The practice of applying a hot match to the end of the tick is not an effective method for removal because the tick may regurgitate into the open wound.[8]

Lyme Disease

Etiology. Lyme disease is caused by the bite of a tick that carries the spirochete *Borrelia burgdorferi*. White-tailed deer and white-footed mice are the main reservoirs of this disease-causing spirochete. Lyme disease causes multiple symptoms affecting the skin, nervous system, heart, and musculoskeletal system.

Pathogenesis, clinical manifestations, and treatment. The disease has three clinical stages. Stage I usually occurs in the summer and early fall with single or multiple erythematous papules that may itch, sting, or burn. The thighs, groin, and axillae are particularly common sites of involvement. This disease is often accompanied by flulike symptoms (fatigue, headache, chills, fever, sore throat, stiff neck, nausea, myalgias, and arthralgias). If the patient remains untreated, stage II Lyme disease appears weeks to months later. This stage is characterized by meningitis, cranial nerve palsies, and peripheral neuropathy; occasionally, cardiac involvement is noted. In stage III, oligoarticular arthritis occurs. In early Lyme disease, treatment includes administration of antibiotic therapy such as doxycycline, amoxicillin, or erythromycin for 10 to 21 days. Neurologic disease, arthritis, or cardiac

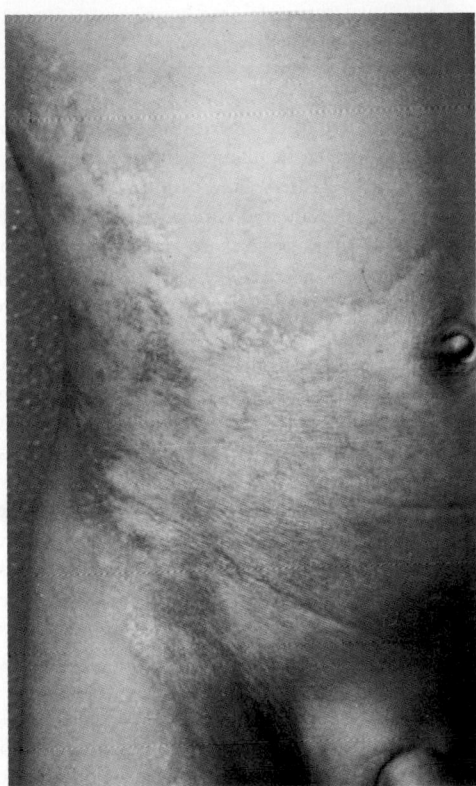

FIGURE 53-24 Extensive morphea (localized scleroderma). (From Berger TG et al: *Andrews' diseases of the skin: clinical dermatology,* ed 9, Philadelphia, 2000, Saunders, p 195.)

disease is managed with doxycycline or amoxicillin for 1 month or with intravenous penicillin for 10 to 14 days.

OTHER DISORDERS OF THE DERMIS

Scleroderma

Scleroderma is characterized by massive collagen deposition with fibrosis accompanied by inflammatory reactions and vascular changes in the capillary network. The process by which these changes occur is not known but may represent an autoimmune mechanism or primary vasculopathy.

The two forms of scleroderma, localized and diffuse, are clinically dissimilar except for some common skin histopathologic features. Localized scleroderma (morphea) is a benign disease; diffuse scleroderma (progressive systemic sclerosis) is serious, progressive, and fatal.

Localized Scleroderma

Localized scleroderma has an unknown etiology, no systemic involvement, and no known treatment. Disability is confined to the area involved. Lesions tend to involute (shrivel) slowly and spontaneously. Relapses are rare. Primary skin lesions are single or multiple, violet colored, firm, inelastic macules and plaques that enlarge slowly. The progressing border retains a violet hue while the center becomes whitish and slightly depressed beneath the skin surface. Bizarre lesions occur, such as long linear bands on extremities, "saber cut" lesions in the scalp, or lesions involving one side of the face or the body. Secondary lesions include mild or severe scarring after healing, permanent hair loss from the scalp lesions, and, rarely, ulceration. The trunk, extremities, and head are most frequently involved (Figure 53-24).

Diffuse Scleroderma

Diffuse scleroderma is a rare systemic collagen disease of unknown cause characterized by a long course of progressive disability resulting from lack of mobility of the areas and the organs affected. The skin becomes hardened like hide, the esophagus and the gastrointestinal tract semirigid, the lungs and heart fibrosed, the bones resorbed, and the overlying tissue calcified. Figure 53-25 illustrates the "hidelike" skin on the face of a woman with diffuse scleroderma.

Another rare collagen disorder, **dermatomyositis** is characterized by the acute or insidious onset of muscle pain, weakness, fever, arthralgia, and, in some cases, a puffy erythematous eruption that is usually confined to the face and the eyelids. Progression of the disease results in muscle atrophy and contractures, skin telangiectasias (vascular lesions formed by blood vessel dilation) and atrophy, and generalized organ involvement. Death occurs in 50% of cases.[12,17]

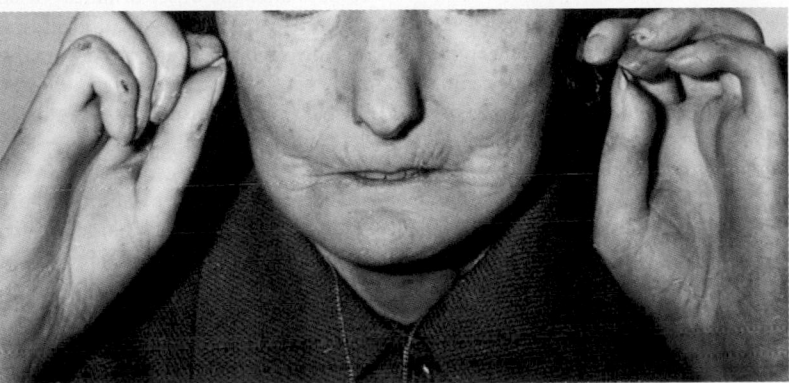

FIGURE 53-25 Hidelike skin on the face of a woman with diffuse scleroderma (progressive systemic sclerosis). (From Berger TG et al: *Andrews' diseases of the skin: clinical dermatology,* ed 9, Philadelphia, 2000, Saunders, p 197.)

TABLE 53-4 CLINICAL DESCRIPTION OF PRESSURE SORES

GRADE/STAGE	DESCRIPTION
1	Acute inflammatory response primarily in epidermis with minimal soft-tissue swelling and warmth; erythema of intact skin; is erythematous and, unless abraded, erythema will blanch; blancheable erythema (reactive hyperemia) can be expected to be present for 30-45 min following exposure to pressure; is usually very discretely bordered; reversible with intervention
2	Pressure sore representing an inflammatory and fibroblastic response extending through epidermis into dermis; is partial thickness or superficial skin loss involving epidermis and/or dermis; may present as blistering with erythema and/or induration; ulcer may also present as abrasion or shallow crater; wound base is moist and pink; wound is painful but free of necrotic tissue
3	Pressure sore clearly penetrating subcutaneous layers; often there is exposed muscle, fat, and tendons; full-thickness tissue loss extends through dermis to involve subcutaneous tissue; damage or necrosis of dermis may extend down to, but not through, underlying fascia; ulcer presents clinically as deep crater with or without undermining of adjacent tissue; stage may also include sinus tract formation, exudates, and/or infection; wound base is usually painful
4	Pressure sore extending beyond deep fascia, almost always to bone; deep-tissue destruction occurs, extending through subcutaneous tissue and fascia; is full-thickness skin loss with extensive tissue necrosis and damage to muscle, bone, and supporting structures (tendons and joint capsules); undermining sinus infection may be present; wound base is usually not painful

Sunburn and Photosensitivity

Effects of Sunlight

Sunlight is an extremely harmful environmental agent because it produces the short ultraviolet wavelength that is responsible for sunburn, thickening of the stratum corneum, suntan, and increased melanin production. Sunlight produces direct local effects on the skin in the form of elastotic syndromes, keratoacanthomas, premalignant diseases, basal cell epitheliomas, and squamous cell epitheliomas. Both indirect and direct effects can produce malignant melanomas.[18]

Sunburn is initially manifested as erythema, pain, heat, and occasionally blistering, edema, and tenderness. In severe sunburn, these symptoms may also be accompanied by the constitutional symptoms of chills, fever, nausea, and generalized discomfort.

The most effective treatment is to avoid or limit exposure to sunlight. Wearing protective clothing is effective; sunscreens are also quite useful in preventing sunburn and the chronic solar changes of the skin. *Para*-aminobenzoic acid is the most widely used sunscreen. People sensitive to *para*-aminobenzoic acid may use cinnamates and benzophenones as substitutes. Opaque screens such as zinc oxide and titanium dioxide also work well. However, these white preparations are not cosmetically elegant. Recently, titanium dioxide has been incorporated into foundation makeup for women.

Sunburn can be managed symptomatically with cold water baths or compresses; topical steroids are often effective in relieving the discomfort of localized severe burns. For widespread sunburn, a 10- to 14-day course of systemic steroids may suppress the symptoms.

Ulcers

An unfortunate problem for a bedridden person may be the development of **pressure sores,** or **decubitus ulcers.** Because thinning epithelial cells and blood vessels have a slower rate of repair in older adults, the incidence of decubitus ulcers is higher and the ulcer more severe in elderly individuals, and healing of damaged skin is slower.

Pressure sores are localized areas of cellular necrosis resulting from prolonged pressure between any bony prominence and an external object such as a bed or wheelchair. The tissues are deprived of blood supply and eventually die. Areas frequently affected in older persons include the heels, greater trochanter, sacrum, dorsal (especially in thin kyphotic persons) and scapular regions of the spine, and elbows. Long-term pressure increases vulnerability to decubitus ulcer development. High pressure maintained for a short time is less dangerous than low pressure continued for a long time. Predisposing factors include poor nutrition, aging, immobility, superficial sensory loss, and disturbed autonomic function (loss of bowel and bladder control).[19] Older people with dementia are particularly prone to the development of pressure sores because of arteriosclerotic changes in the vessels, loss of subcutaneous tissue and tissue elasticity, and clouding of the sensorium.[19]

Pressure sores can be evaluated clinically using the staging system described in Table 53-4. Pressure sores are superficial (benign) or deep (malignant). Superficial sores are reddened areas involving only the outer skin layers. They are less dangerous than deep sores and are caused by friction, shearing stresses, trauma, infection, and saturation with urine or other wet agents. The lesions are frequently painful but are easily treated and prevented. Treatment consists of keeping the area clean, dry, and free from infection or further pressure; covering the lesion with a nonstick dressing also promotes healing. Measures such as performing frequent body position changes (every 2 hours), transferring the person out of bed and into a chair, ensuring the vulnerable areas are clean and dry, and keeping the weight of the bed coverings off the feet are most effective in the prevention of superficial pressure sores.

Deep sores develop quickly as a result of thrombosis of the vessels in deep tissue overlying bony prominences. Muscle and fat layers are more vulnerable than the dermis, and involvement of these layers causes deep, large ulcers. The sore begins as a reddening of the skin with unobservable necrosis in the deep underlying tissue. In 1 to 2 days, the lesion bursts through the skin like an abscess to reveal a deep cavity full of black or infected slough, which may penetrate the bone.[19] Skin loss from such a large area results in extensive scarring. The development of deep pressure sores with an illness can delay recovery and may even be fatal.

Prevention is more difficult with deep pressure sores, especially in the elderly. The risk of these lesions developing is greatest during the 10 days after the onset of illness or admission to the hospital, which coincides with the period of greatest immobility.[19] A sore that develops early and penetrates deeply is most dangerous to an older person. Early signs of deterioration include apathy, loss of appetite, and incontinence. Some measures that can help prevent deep pressure sores are described in Box 53-2.

Treatment consists primarily of reinforcing preventive measures, including maintenance of fluid and protein stores that are lost through serous and purulent discharge, repair of tissues by administration of vitamin supplements, avoidance of general infections such as pneumonia or cystitis, and remediation of anemia. The lesions should be cleaned and dressed, with care taken to manage local infection. To promote granulation and healing, the wound should be irrigated with warm saline daily. Irrigation washes out the debris, reduces the growth of anaerobes, promotes separation of the slough, and decreases the pocketing of infection in deeper tissues. Infection must be eradicated and the slough must separate before healing can take place.

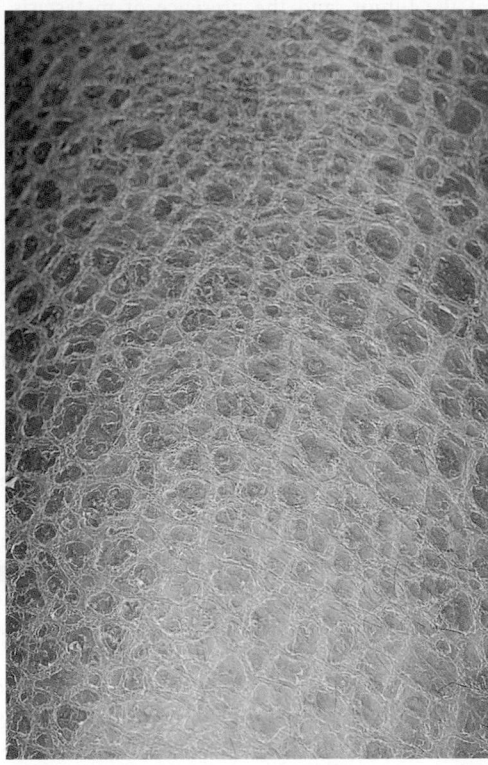

FIGURE 53-26 Ichthyosis. (From Callen JP et al: *Color atlas of dermatology*, ed 2, Philadelphia, 2000, Saunders, p 14. Courtesy Donald Hazelrigg, MD, Evansville, IN.)

Altered Cell Growth: Epidermal Proliferation

Keratinocytes produce keratin. Rare, inherited defects in keratinocytes can occur, and the inherited disease **congenital ichthyosis** is characterized by an excessive growth of keratinocytes and keratin, which gives the skin a fish-scale appearance (Figure 53-26).

Corns and **calluses** result from **hyperkeratosis.** Stimulation of the epidermis by intermittent pressure elicits hyperkeratosis (corn and callous formation). By contrast, *atrophy* of the epidermis can arise from a decreased blood supply.

Benign or malignant **neoplasms** commonly arise from keratinocytes. **Warts** (verrucae), for instance, are caused by a virus that provokes a benign proliferation of keratinocytes. **Squamous cell carcinomas** (arising from keratinocytes) often occur in areas of skin excessively exposed to sunlight.

Tumors

Each cell type of the skin can give rise to either benign or malignant tumors. Benign tumors, including squamous papillomas, arise from keratinocytes, common moles **(nevi)** from melanocytes, lipomas from

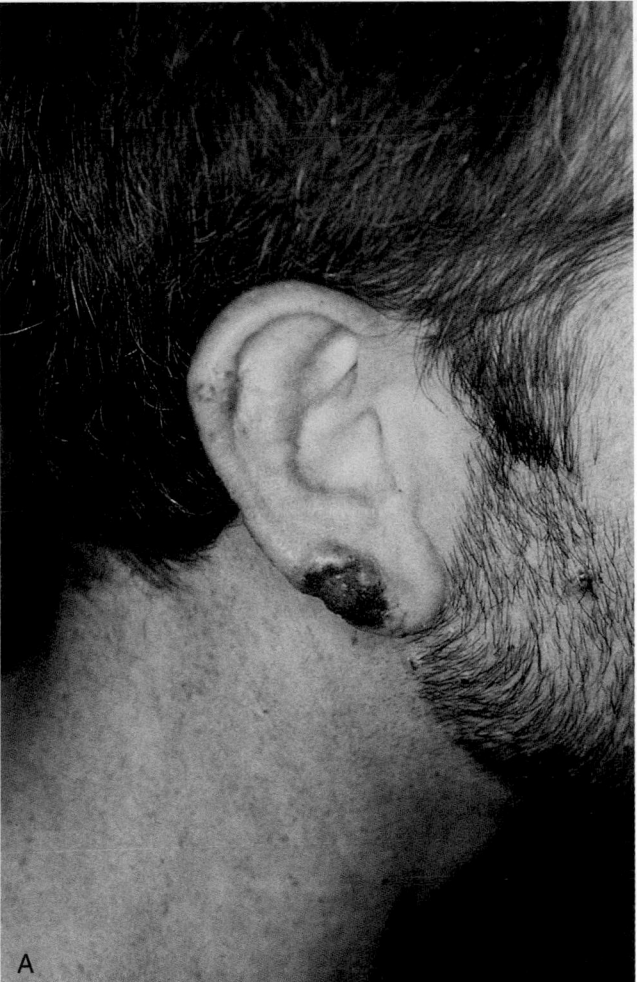

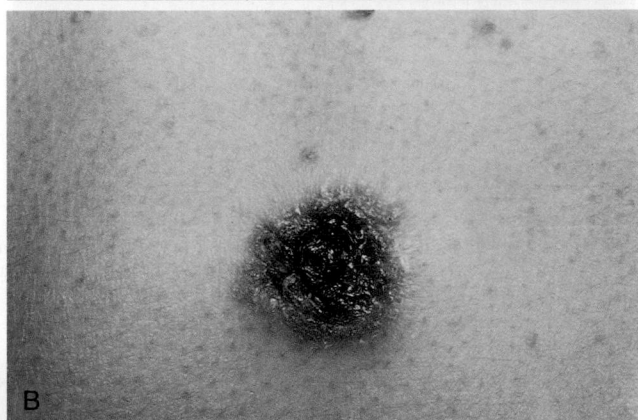

FIGURE 53-27 A and **B,** Cryptococcosis associated with HIV infection. (From Callen JP et al: *Color atlas of dermatology*, Philadelphia, 1993, Saunders, p 229.)

adipose cells, vascular tumors (hemangiomas) from blood vessels, dermatofibromas from fibroblasts, and neuromas from nerves.

Kaposi sarcoma arises from reticulocytes and is multifocal, metastasizing, and malignant. Kaposi sarcoma is classified as an opportunistic neoplasm because it occurs in persons with preexisting immunodeficiency, for example, in individuals with primary immunodeficiency, persons who undergo therapeutic immunosuppression, and persons with human immunodeficiency virus (HIV) infection. Figures 53-27 and 53-28 show some of the cutaneous diseases associated with HIV infection.

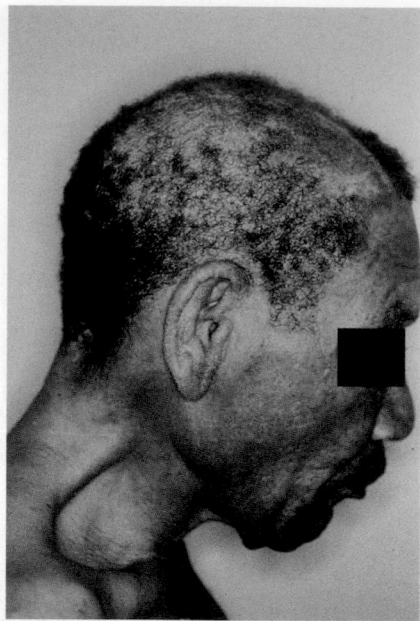

FIGURE 53-28 Seborrheic dermatitis associated with HIV infection. (From Callen JP et al: *Color atlas of dermatology*, Philadelphia, 1993, Saunders, p 372.)

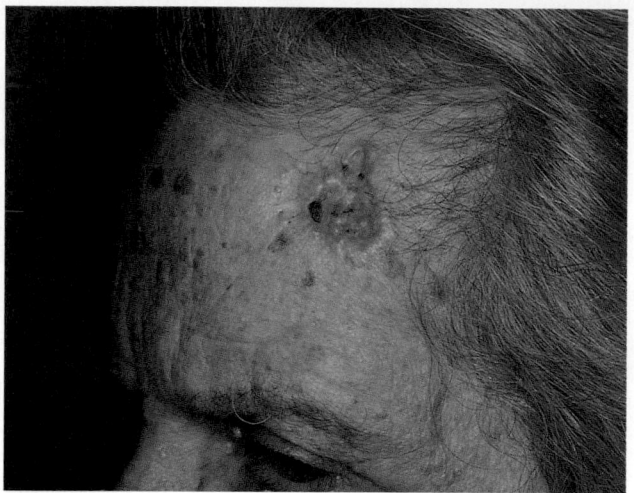

FIGURE 53-29 Basal cell carcinoma. Notice the rolled, well-defined margin. (From Swartz MH: *Textbook of physical diagnosis*, ed 6, Philadelphia, 2010, Saunders, p 159.)

Cancer

Cancer of the skin is common. Most skin cancers are slowly progressive, but certain types can be rapidly lethal. Excessive exposure to sunlight by a person with fair skin often leads to skin cancer. In addition to sunlight, exposure to irritating chemicals, recurrent trauma, and irradiation are associated with a high risk of skin cancer.

Basal cell carcinomas are the most common skin tumors and the most benign[20] (Figure 53-29). Squamous cell carcinomas are the second most common skin malignancy[20] (Figure 53-30). They can occasionally metastasize. By contrast, melanoma is rare but can be highly malignant (Figure 53-31). Melanoma is notoriously unpredictable; however, the prognosis is based on size, depth of invasion of the tumor, and the presence of metastasis.[21] Lumps that increase rapidly in size, change color, ulcerate, or bleed should undergo biopsy and be examined microscopically to rule out malignancy. Complete surgical excision is the treatment of choice for skin cancers.

Pigmentation Alterations
Vitiligo

Vitiligo (leukoderma) is a condition in which pigment disappears from a patch of skin. The onset is sudden and may be associated with pernicious anemia, hyperthyroidism, and diabetes mellitus.

Vitiligo is a concern to darkly pigmented individuals of all races. It also affects light-skinned individuals, but not as often. The lesion is a depigmented patch with definite borders on the face, axillae, neck, or extremities (Figure 53-32). The borders are smooth. Size varies from small to large macules involving large areas of the skin surface. The large macular type is much more common. Depigmented areas, which burn in sunlight, appear bone colored or grayish blue.

Vitiligo appears at any age, in men and women alike, and usually occurs before the age of 21.[22] Its incidence has been increasing in India, Pakistan, and Far Eastern countries.[22] Although the cause is unknown, inheritance and autoimmune factors have been implicated. Affected areas spread over time.

Treatment may consist of various topical immunomodulating agents as well as the use of various types of ultraviolet light. Cosmetics such as Dermablend may be used to camouflage the areas of depigmentation.

Albinism

Etiology and pathogenesis. Melanocytes produce melanin. A partial or total absence of melanin arises as an inborn error in metabolism in individuals with **albinism.** Albinism, also termed

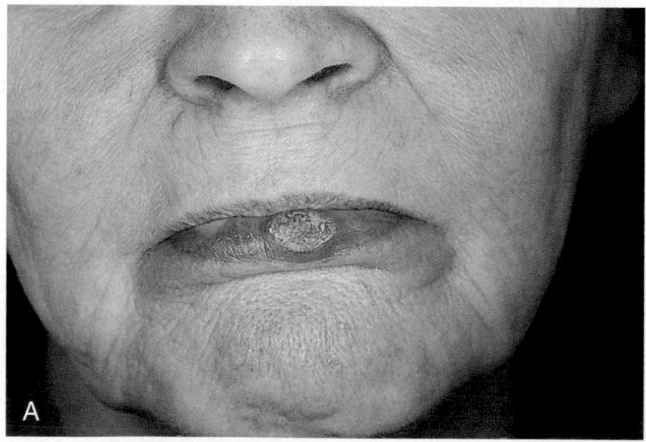
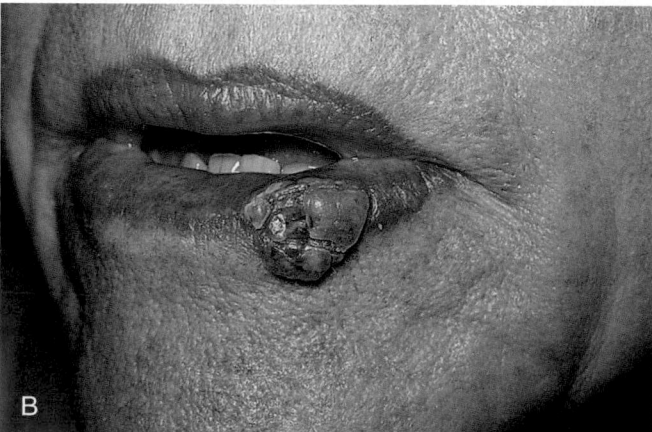

FIGURE 53-30 **A** and **B,** Squamous cell carcinomas. (From Callen JP et al: *Color atlas of dermatology*, ed 2, Philadelphia, 2000, Saunders, p 367.)

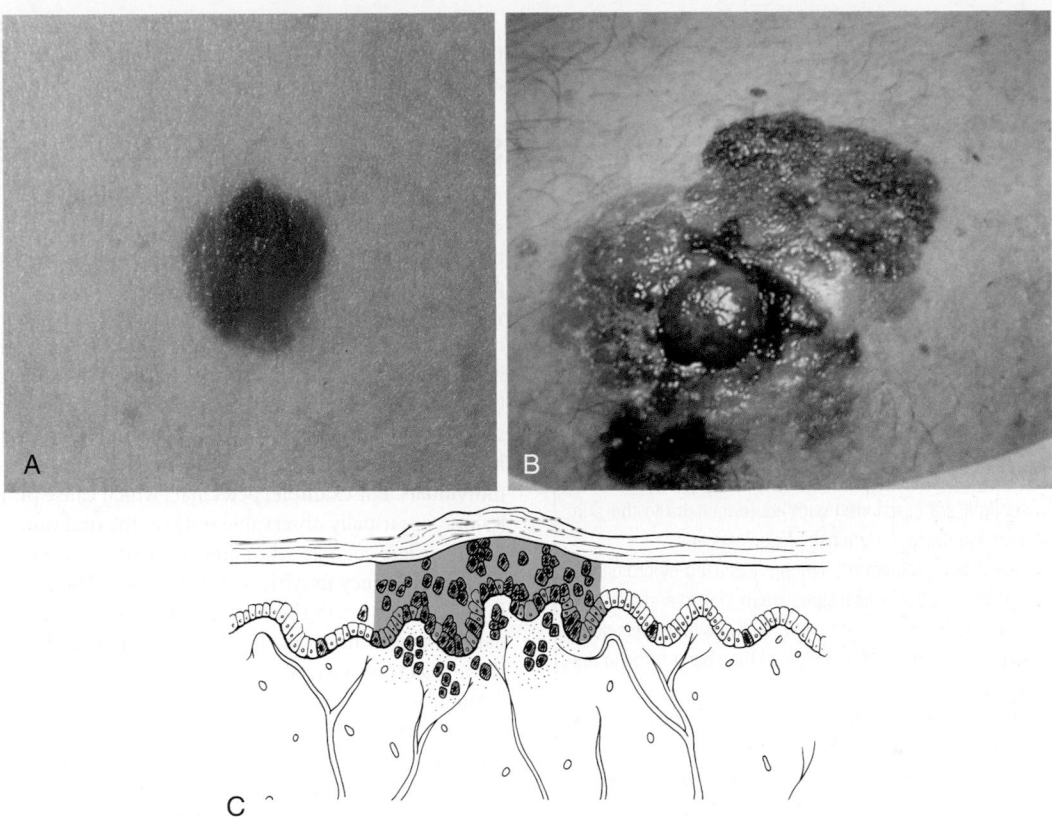

FIGURE 53-31 A and **B,** Superficial spreading malignant melanoma. **C,** Cross-section through a melanoma. Note the nests of melanoma cells in the dermis. (From Swartz MH: *Textbook of physical diagnosis,* ed 6, Philadelphia, 2010, Saunders, pp 160-161.)

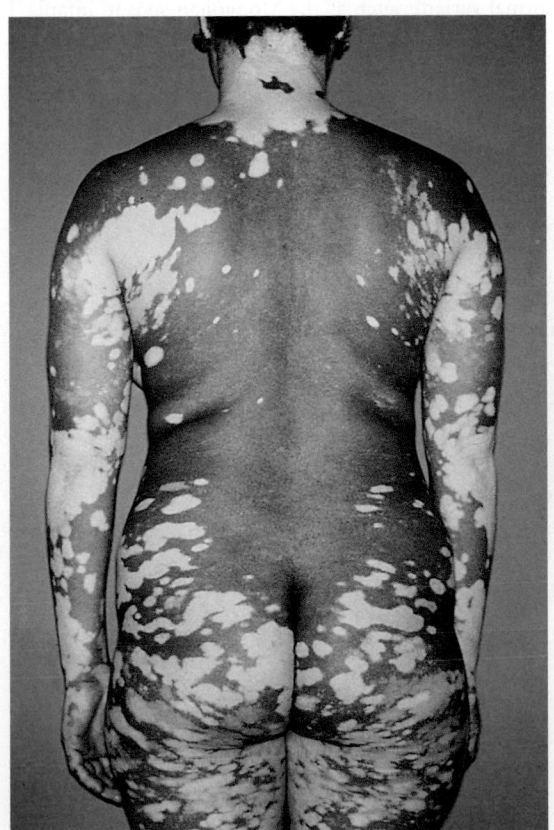

FIGURE 53-32 Vitiligo. (From Callen JP et al: *Color atlas of dermatology,* ed 2, Philadelphia, 2000, Saunders, p 282.)

oculocutaneous albinism, is characterized by a generalized lack of pigmentation of the skin and the hair. In addition, the eyes may show nystagmus and a lack of pigmentation of the fundi and translucent irises. The condition is recessively inherited. Biochemically, albinism occurs because of impaired or absent melanin synthesis. The long-term consequences of albinism may include solar keratoses and basal and squamous cell cancers.

KEY POINTS

- Skin infections may be caused by viral, fungal, or bacterial organisms.
- Viruses are associated with warts (human papillomavirus), cold sores (herpes simplex), and shingles (herpes zoster). Warts are painless. They may be surgically removed but often resolve spontaneously. Herpes simplex lesions are painful, may be managed symptomatically, and often recur in times of stress. Herpes zoster inhabits sensory dorsal ganglia neurons and causes pain along a dermatome.
- Superficial fungal infections (tinea, ringworm) are often characterized by central clearing and peripheral scaling. They may be effectively managed with topical antifungals. Yeast infections tend to occur in moist areas such as mucous membranes and are managed with systemic or topical drugs.
- Impetigo is caused by staphylococcal or streptococcal infection and is characterized by yellowish pustules and crusts. It responds to antibiotic therapy.
- The cause of noninfectious inflammatory diseases is usually unknown. Lupus erythematosus, seborrheic dermatitis, psoriasis, lichen planus, pityriasis rosea, and acne are in this category. Treatment is aimed at reducing inflammation rather than cure. Antibiotics may be used to prevent or manage lesion superinfections.

- Skin allergies are associated with substances that cause erythema and pruritus. Atopic dermatitis (eczema), commonly seen in young children, may be aggravated by substances to which the individual is allergic. Contact dermatitis can occur in anyone exposed to a sufficiently high concentration of an irritating substance. Drug reactions are allergic responses manifested as widely dispersed, often pruritic rashes. Antigen-antibody reactions within cutaneous blood vessels can result in severe necrotizing vasculitis.
- The skin is subject to invasion by a number of different bugs, ticks, and parasites. Lesions tend to be singular or grouped and in areas exposed to the particular pest. Scabies commonly occurs on the hands and wrists and may appear as linear burrows. Bites from fleas, mites, bedbugs, and mosquitoes often induce pruritic macules or papules. Tick bites are usually painless but may be problematic because ticks may carry diseases such as RMSF and Lyme disease.
- Scleroderma is a collagen disease of unknown cause. It may be localized to the skin or produce systemic involvement. The skin is discolored, thick, and hardened.
- Ultraviolet rays in sunlight are associated with acute damage to the skin (sunburn) and also increase the long-term risk of skin cancer.
- Pressure ulcer is a significant problem of immobility caused by prolonged pressure on bony prominences. Superficial sores are reddened areas involving the outer skin layers. Deep sores are due to thrombosis of vessels deep in tissue. Deep sores may be unnoticed initially and then burst through the skin like an abscess.
- Abnormalities of skin cell growth may result in such benign processes as corns and calluses or the more serious consequence of cancer. Basal cell and squamous cell carcinomas are slowly progressive and generally amenable to surgical excision. Malignant melanoma is more prone to metastasis and carries a poorer prognosis.
- Abnormal pigmentation may occur in response to skin injury, infection, or inflammation or may be genetically determined. Albinism is due to lack of melanin production. Vitiligo is a depigmented patch of skin that is most noticeable in dark-skinned individuals. The cause of vitiligo is unknown.

Education regarding the use of sunscreens and clothing for protection against ultraviolet light–induced damage is indicated. Sunglasses and magnifiers are beneficial for the ocular symptoms.

SPECIAL CHARACTERISTICS OF DARK SKIN

A number of disorders of the skin exclusively affect people with dark skin. Pigmentary disturbances from many causes, both hypopigmentation and hyperpigmentation, are common. Postinflammatory hyperpigmentation, for example, may occur in African-American individuals when melanocytes are stimulated by inflammation. Hyperpigmentation in any person with dark skin can occur after traumatic injury, skin infection, or inflammatory skin disease. Patchy areas of depigmentation (vitiligo), described earlier, are more noticeable in persons with dark skin because of the color contrast. Some lesions, such as those causing erythema, may show no visible color change in darkly pigmented individuals. For example, petechiae, which cause pinpoint purplish red lesions, are usually observable only on the oral mucosa or conjunctiva.

Disorders such as seborrheic dermatitis and keloids are seen with greater frequency in African Americans.[23] The custom of tightly plaiting the hair or using hot oil and tension on the scalp leads to gradual damage to hair follicles, hair thinning, and, eventually, hair loss. Known as **traumatic alopecia,** this condition is also seen with greater frequency in African Americans (Figure 53-33).

Conversely, many skin disorders that affect light-skinned people, such as squamous cell or basal cell carcinoma, senile keratoses, and psoriasis, only rarely affect darker-skinned persons.

Psoriasis is rare among the African-American population. If present, it may be difficult to detect. The typical bright red color is not present. The plaques assume a blue or violet hue because of stimulation of melanocytes. The characteristic silvery scale is often absent.

Literature related specifically to abnormalities of dark skin is also rare. Normal variants such as the Mongolian spot in infants, Futcher

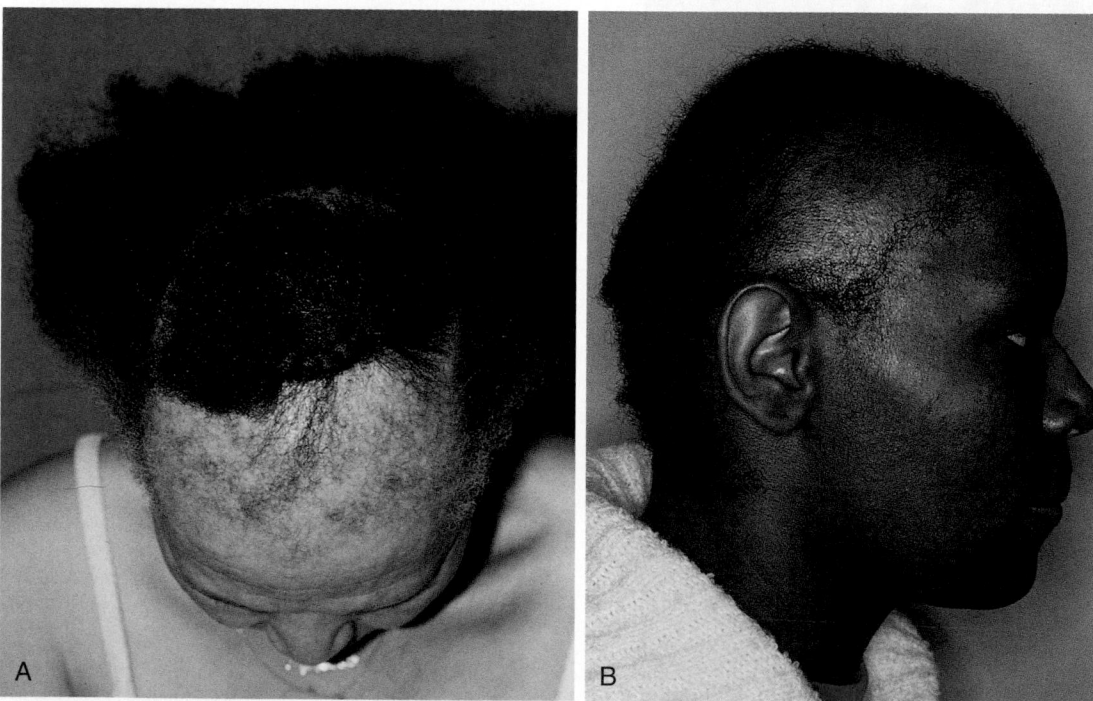

A

B

FIGURE 53-33 A, Traction alopecia from tight braiding and use of a hot comb. **B,** Hot comb damage resulting in scarring alopecia. (From Callen JP et al: *Color atlas of dermatology,* Philadelphia, 1993, Saunders, pp 363, 366.)

or Voigt lines, and linear nail pigmentation are frequently mistaken for disorders. Box 53-3 presents tips for assessing dark skin.

INTEGUMENTARY MANIFESTATIONS OF SYSTEMIC DISEASE

The skin reflects the status of many organ systems. For example, the endocrine, cardiovascular, renal, respiratory, and hepatic systems all have possible dermal manifestations. Metabolic disorders and internal malignancies also cause cutaneous alterations. Certainly, skin manifestations of internal malignancy can be obvious. The late-appearing features of **cachexia** (wasting), pallor, and cutaneous metastases are obvious signs of malignancy. Abnormalities in endocrine function also produce a myriad of cutaneous changes. In general, systemic disease states are expressed through altered color, sensation, texture, and temperature of the skin; altered growth, texture, color, and lubrication of the hair; and changes in nail shape, color, and texture.

SKIN

Color

Color changes in the skin can signal the presence of systemic disease. The entire color spectrum (red, orange, yellow, green, blue, indigo, and violet) is represented through possible coloration changes in the skin.

Redness (**erythema**) may be generalized, as with carbon monoxide poisoning, or localized, as with rashes or on the palms. Although erythema is often visible in lighter-skinned individuals, it may be less apparent in those whose skin is dark; however, the affected part may become an even deeper shade of brown. Redness may accompany inflammation.

When inflammation is suspected in a dark-skinned person, other parameters can be assessed by palpation, among them increased skin temperature, tight skin suggestive of edema, induration of deep tissue or blood vessels, and tenderness. Because the dorsal skin surface of the fingers is more sensitive to subtle skin temperature differences than the palmar surface, the examiner should use the dorsal portion of the fingers to move from one skin area to another for comparison. The patient's family and friends are also helpful in validating color change, particularly when it has occurred gradually.

Orange discoloration can occur from the deposition of carotene. Protein-calorie malnutrition can cause hypopigmentation in African-American children, with the hair and skin appearing orange.

Yellow discoloration can occur locally when lipids are deposited in skin secondary to a metabolic defect in blood lipids. More commonly, a generalized yellow (jaundiced) appearance arises because of liver disease. Bilirubin accumulates in blood and saturates the tissues. **Jaundice** is observed in the usual sites (e.g., mucous membranes, nail beds). Because many factors can alter these findings, one single positive finding should not be held as conclusive. Other parameters, such as environmental temperature, drug use, smoking, amount of hemoglobin, and the color of urine or stool, can support a description of cyanosis or jaundice. In both dark-skinned and light-skinned individuals, yellow sclerae may indicate jaundice, but other factors can cause yellow scleral pigmentation; fatty deposits that contain carotene are a common finding in dark-skinned individuals. To determine whether the yellow sclerae signify jaundice, observe the hard palate in bright daylight. Jaundice can be detected in this location quite early (i.e., when serum bilirubin level is 2 to 4 mg/100 ml) if the palate does not have heavy melanin pigmentation.[24] If the hard palate does not show jaundice when the sclerae are yellow, the pigmentation may be due to some other factor, such as carotene accumulation. All these factors support the importance of repeated observation and accurate description of what is seen. As often as possible, the same individual should perform the entire examination and confirm specific findings in one area with additional data from other areas.

When jaundice is severe, **biliverdin** also accumulates. A person with obstructed bile ducts can become green-yellow because of biliverdin.

Blueness of the skin (**cyanosis**) often occurs on the tips of the fingers, toes, nose, and lips in individuals with cardiac or respiratory problems that prevent oxygenation of blood. Localized blueness with pain of the fingers on exposure to cold is termed *Raynaud disease.* It frequently arises from the presence of cryoglobulins, which solidify in the cold, and is also associated with disorders of the immune system, such as lymphoma and acquired immunodeficiency syndrome.[25]

Indigo discoloration occurs locally, as in gangrene of the toes from severe generalized arteriosclerosis. The skin can darken from increased melanin synthesis, as in chronic adrenal insufficiency. Also, silver poisoning can make the skin dusky. Violet-colored palms (palmar erythema) can be seen in some individuals with liver disease and occasionally in pregnant women as a response to hyperestrogenism.

Shades of violet occur on the legs as a result of vascular insufficiency or when cardiopulmonary function is compromised.

The primary sites for assessing skin **pallor** are the nail beds, lips, and conjunctivae. When observing the lower eyelid (inferior palpebral conjunctiva) for pallor, the examiner should lower the lid sufficiently to see the conjunctiva near not only the outer canthus but also the inner canthus because the former is often darker. Greater perception is necessary when assessing a darkly pigmented individual for pallor because the changes are subtle. Red tones may be absent; a brown-skinned person may appear more yellowish brown, and a black-skinned person may appear ash gray. This variability supports the need for accurate baseline data for comparison.

Sensation

Sensory innervation is generally responsible for the itching (**pruritus**) and **pain** that accompany most skin diseases. *Itching* is often the initial symptom in such conditions as atopic eczema, allergic contact dermatitis, scabies, dermatophytosis, psoriasis, and varicella. It can also be associated with systemic disorders, including carcinoma, diabetes, thyroid disease, uremia, and obstructive biliary disease. Other dermatologic conditions, such as herpes simplex, aphthous stomatitis, herpes zoster, furuncles, and cellulitis, produce considerable *pain.*

Texture

Normal aging produces an alteration in the texture of skin. Loose and wrinkled skin that lacks tone may also indicate **dehydration** (an abnormal finding). Dehydration may also be apparent through inspection of the oral cavity. On inspection, a dry, leathery appearance of the tongue is *not* a reliable indicator of dehydration inasmuch as mouth breathing frequently makes the tongue look dry even when the individual is well hydrated. A more reliable method of assessing hydration of the oral cavity is to palpate the mucous membranes along the area of the gum and cheek where the membranes approximate. If the membranes are dry and the finger does not slide easily, dehydration is evident.

To evaluate **fluid excess,** palpate the skin over the hands, feet, ankles, and sacrum. If the skin is firm and indents easily (pitting edema) on moderate pressure from the fingertips, fluid excess is present.

Feeling the deeper portions of the skin may reveal areas of **induration** (hardness) such as those resulting from multiple intramuscular or subcutaneous injections of medication. **Lipodystrophies** consist of smooth, large depressions in the skin that indicate atrophy of the subcutaneous fat layer, which has a spongy consistency. Both induration and lipodystrophy are often seen at sites of repeated insulin injections.

Temperature

If the skin feels warm and dry in a person who is febrile (feverish), the blood temperature is probably rising, an indication that the thermoregulatory mechanism of sweating may not be functioning. Likewise, if the skin is warm and wet, the temperature can be expected to fall owing to the cooling mechanism of sweating.

Sweating can also occur when the blood glucose concentration falls rapidly with a resultant rise in the blood epinephrine level. Hypoglycemic sweating can usually be distinguished from other causes of sweating because of the additional symptoms of weakness, tachycardia, hunger, headache, and "inward nervousness" manifested as mental irritability and confusion.

Because skin temperature depends on the amount of blood circulating through the dermis, decreased localized blood flow (resulting in coolness), often to the feet, may indicate a peripheral vascular dysfunction. Generalized skin coolness may indicate decreased metabolism such as that occurring after administration of a general anesthetic. If the temperature is very low, signs of shock may be evident.

On the other hand, an increase in skin temperature may indicate a **hypermetabolic state,** such as that occurring in hyperthyroidism and after sun exposure or sunburn.

HAIR

Disturbances in body function are often reflected in changes in growth pattern, amount, texture, color, and lubrication of the hair.

Growth

The high speed of growth of the scalp hair makes it more susceptible to damage from systemic disease, toxic drugs, radiation, and stress. The rate of growth varies with general health and age, and hair growth is dependent on circulating hormonal factors (primarily testicular or adrenal androgens). Thus hormonal imbalances or shifts (e.g., those accompanying childbirth) may also result in disturbances in the hair growth cycle. Nutritional factors, although often promoted in the nonmedical literature, have little effect on hair growth except in cases of severe malnutrition.

Amount

Alterations in the amount of body hair can be extremely anxiety provoking for both males and females. In females with hypertrichosis, or **hirsutism,** hair growth is intensified on the upper lip, chin, cheeks, and chest; around the nipples; and from the pubic crest to the umbilicus (along the linea alba); the downy hair on the arms, legs, and back becomes coarse. The pubic hair often assumes the upright triangular distribution typical of the male as opposed to the female's usual inverted triangle. An endocrine malfunction such as excess androgen production may sometimes be associated with hirsutism, but ethnic background (Mediterranean groups predominantly) may also be responsible for the excessive hair growth. This propensity is especially true of the hair on the arms, legs, back, and face. Other ethnic group members such as full-blooded African-American females and male Native Americans rarely have facial hair. Distribution of the hair in family members and ethnic background are thus important considerations in ascertaining hair growth.

Hypertrichosis lanuginosa is typically a congenital, autosomal dominant disorder in which excessive hair is distributed over the entire body throughout life. The condition is usually associated with other congenital anomalies such as spina bifida.[26] In some cases, such as with certain internal carcinomas, hypertrichosis lanuginosa is an acquired disorder; the degree of hairiness is variable and usually involves the face.

Color

Perhaps the most common color change in the hair is the generalized graying that accompanies the aging process.

Texture

Normal aging also produces a decrease in hair thickness. Disturbances of the thickness of scalp hair are common. Baldness (**alopecia**) or

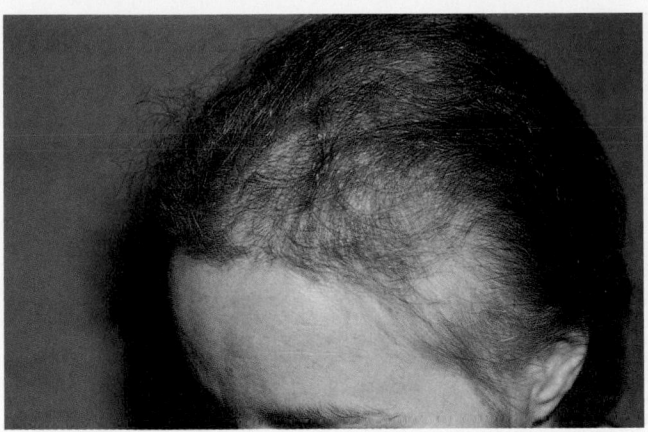

FIGURE 53-34 Male pattern baldness (androgenetic alopecia) in a woman. (From Callen JP et al: *Color atlas of dermatology*, Philadelphia, 1993, Saunders, p 365.)

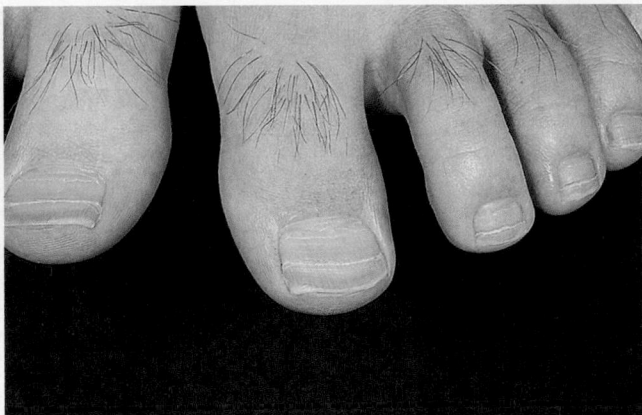

FIGURE 53-35 Beau lines. This patient had major surgery 5 months previously. (From Callen JP et al: *Color atlas of dermatology*, ed 2, Philadelphia, 2000, Saunders, p 334.)

thinning of the hair that is generalized or creates a receding hairline is often genetically determined (Figure 53-34). Some rare genetic defects in the hair shaft itself may produce breaking of the hairs and be erroneously diagnosed as alopecia. Generalized and localized baldness may result from treatment modalities such as radiation therapy or chemotherapy. In addition, various types of scalp diseases (e.g., fungal, lupus) and telogen effluvium (transient hair loss occurring 2 to 3 months after general anesthesia, febrile illness, or giving birth) can cause hair loss. Other traumatic types of hair loss may result from pulling of the hair because of a nervous habit, wearing hair styles such as tight braids or ponytails, or donning constrictive apparel such as a hat.

Lubrication

Hyperfunction of the sebaceous glands is associated with androgen stimulation such as occurs with the excessive scalp oiliness and facial acne in adolescence. Dry, brittle hair is commonly the result of excessive washing or the application of chemical agents (coloring, bleach, or detergent shampoos) to the hair.

In addition to direct observation of the scalp and face, correlation of the findings with data from the patient history helps determine dysfunctional states of health.

NAILS

Because nails are derived from a highly active tissue, they may be affected by any serious systemic illness. Moreover, any local skin disease that affects the epidermis may also affect the nail matrix (epidermal cells that give rise to the nail plate) and lead to an abnormal (**dystrophic**) nail. By measuring the distance between abnormalities (pits, grooves, and lines) and the proximal nail border, one may estimate the time of initial illness.

Shape

Transverse furrows (**Beau lines**) in the nail indicate that nail growth has been disturbed (Figure 53-35). These furrows can result from infection, systemic disease, or injury. Nails with a concave curve are known as spoon nails, or **koilonychia.** This may signal a form of iron-deficiency anemia and is also associated with other disorders such as coronary disease, syphilis, or the use of strong soaps. Destruction of the nails (**onycholysis**) may accompany a great variety of unrelated conditions ranging from the application of false nails to hyperthyroidism, fungal nail infection, or psoriasis (Figure 53-36). Certain medications may also cause onycholysis (Figure 53-36, D). **Splinter hemorrhages** may

be linked to bacterial endocarditis and trichinosis. These red or brown splinters or streaks run parallel to the finger in the nail bed (Figure 53-37). **Clubbing** of the fingers is characterized by a flattening of the angle of the base of the nail. It may occur in association with cardiovascular disease, subacute bacterial endocarditis, and pulmonary disease.

Color

Nail color indicates the amount of blood oxygenation. Bluish or purplish discoloration of the nail beds occurs with **cyanosis,** whereas **pallor** often indicates anemia. To compare color of the nail beds, apply slight pressure on the free edge of the second or third fingernail. The blanching that results is then compared with the normal color of the nail. The rate of color return also indicates the quality of peripheral vasomotor function.

Texture

Thickening of the nail may result from nutritional disturbances, repeated trauma, inflammation, and local infection. Along with thickening, toenails may become discolored and grooved, and debris may accumulate under the nail. This condition may be exacerbated as the distal portion of the nail works free from the underlying nail bed and more debris is accumulated; fungal infections may also follow. Treatment usually consists of periodic debridement of the nail plate; however, a return to normal nail structure rarely occurs after thickening.

> **KEY POINTS**
> - Many systemic diseases are associated with alterations in skin, hair, and nails. Skin reflects systemic inflammation and fever as erythema. A rising fever is manifested as warm, dry skin, whereas warm, moist skin indicates a fever beginning to decline. Poor oxygenation and circulation may be manifested by cyanosis, pallor, or coolness. Jaundice indicates altered bilirubin metabolism, usually caused by liver or biliary disease. Fluid balance may be manifested in the skin as decreased turgor or edema. Sympathetic activation may be indicated by cool, pale, diaphoretic skin.
> - Hair growth, strength, texture, and color are affected by systemic diseases such as endocrine abnormalities, extreme malnutrition, and drugs. Excessive androgen may result in hirsutism. Alopecia may result from chemotherapeutic drugs or radiation therapy.
> - Abnormalities of nail growth (pits, grooves, lines) occur as a result of nearly any serious systemic illness. Certain nail defects are characteristic of particular diseases: spoon nails may indicate iron-deficiency anemia; clubbing is associated with cardiopulmonary disease. Nail color is commonly assessed to determine the adequacy of oxygenation and perfusion.

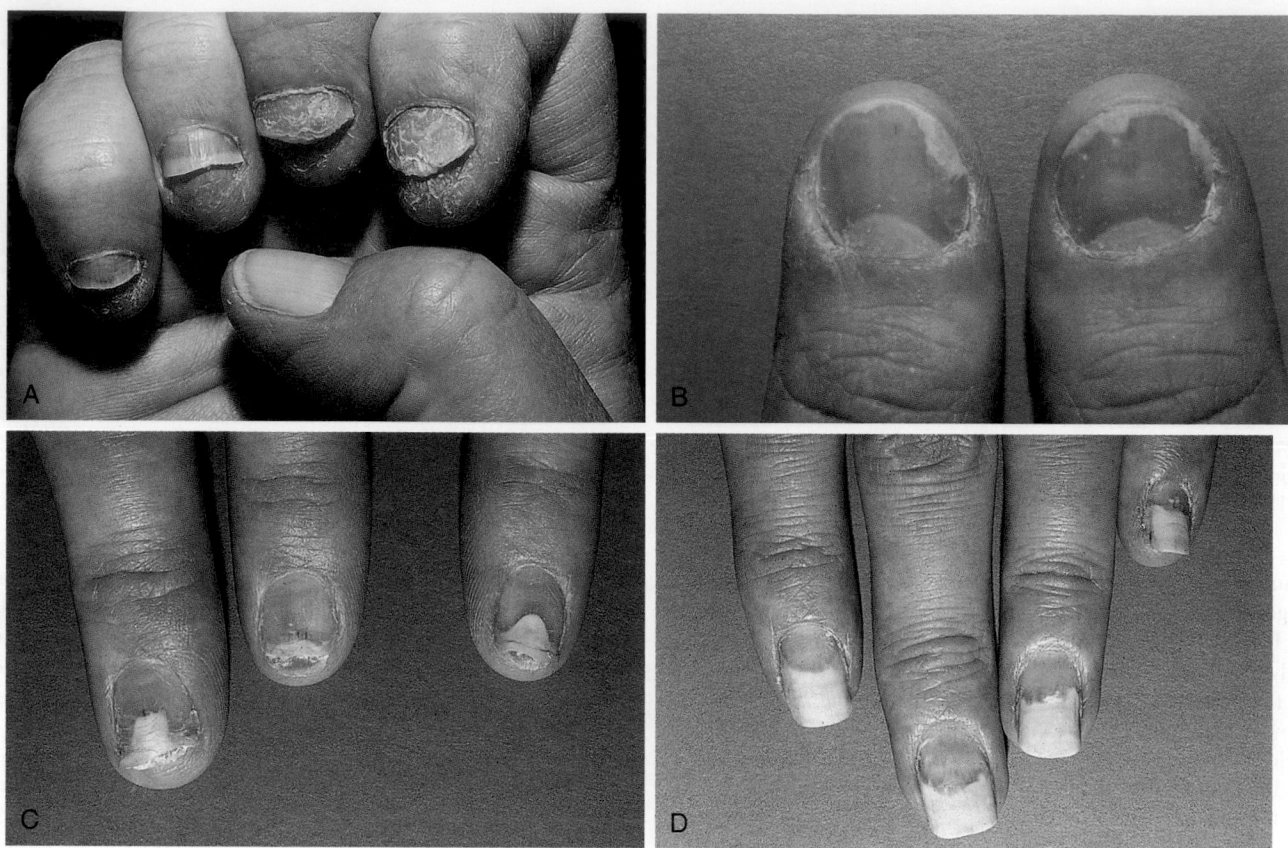

FIGURE 53-36 A, *Candida albicans* infection resulting in onycholysis. **B,** Psoriasis resulting in onycholysis. **C,** Onycholysis secondary to false "sculptured" nails. **D,** Drug-induced onycholysis. (From Callen JP et al: *Color atlas of dermatology,* ed 2, Philadelphia, 2000, Saunders, p 333, 334, 347, 367.)

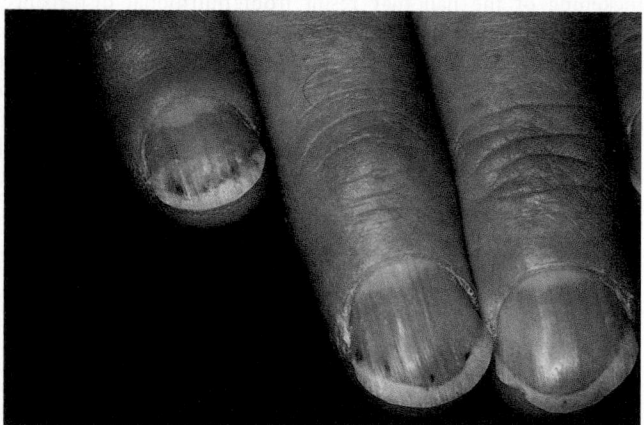

FIGURE 53-37 Splinter hemorrhages in a patient with leukocytoclastic vasculitis. (From Callen JP et al: *Color atlas of dermatology,* ed 2, Philadelphia, 2000, Saunders, p 337.)

▌TREATMENT IMPLICATIONS

A distinct advantage in treating the skin is the ease of direct observation of the pathologic process and the effects of treatment. Culture, macroscopic examination of skin scrapings, and biopsy also facilitate diagnosis. A correct diagnosis can help prevent complications from improper therapy but does not lessen the importance of choosing an appropriate delivery system.

TOPICAL TREATMENT

Wet Dressings

Wet dressings, the application of a liquid in compress form, are a very important part of the dermatologic therapy delivery system. The applied liquid can be plain water or water with additives (e.g., sodium, magnesium, or aluminum salts).

Wet dressings are a versatile, even paradoxical therapeutic approach in that they can dry or hydrate as necessary. Intermittently applied, they serve as an effective astringent for the weeping, oozing lesions that accompany stasis and decubitus ulcers and impetigo. Vesicular lesions, including those seen in dyshidrotic eczema, herpes zoster, and pemphigus, also respond nicely to treatment with intermittent wet dressings. By drying disease-related lesions, intermittent dressings help speed recovery.

Continuous wet dressings, on the other hand, are effective in rapidly hydrating the skin. This technique, used most often in severe cases of atopic eczema, normally requires hospitalization. Wet dressings of gauze soaked in tap water are applied directly to the skin and covered with an insulating agent such as towels, large thick gauze pads, or even long underwear to prevent evaporation. It is very important that the dressings remain moist. Therefore, they must be resoaked and changed every 3 hours around the clock throughout the course of treatment. Once the desired state of hydration has been achieved, the dressings can be discontinued and emollient creams used to prevent redrying of the treated area.

Lotions

Shake lotions are mixtures of small suspended particles in a liquid vehicle such as water or alcohol. These are especially useful for application directly to moist or exudative processes such as rhus dermatitis. As the liquid phase dissipates, the evaporative effect cools and dries the skin.[27]

Emollient lotions are a mixture of oil in water and have a slightly greasy consistency. These preparations are useful when skin moisturization is needed such as in xerotic conditions. Lotions are often used as a vehicle for other medications such as topical steroids that must be applied over large areas of skin.[27]

Gels

Most gels are clear, colorless, volatile substances. They generally penetrate better than creams. Gels are very convenient to use on wet lesions because of their astringent tendencies. Because they do not leave the white or oily residue of creams and ointments, they are appropriate for use on scalp lesions.

Creams

Creams are the most widely used dermatologic delivery system. Many different bases are used in creams, but the "vanishing" type is most common and allows application with no surface residue. Creams penetrate well and have some moisturizing capability. They are used most frequently in the management of dry to slightly moist dermatoses.

Ointments

The medication in most ointments is carried in a petrolatum-type base, which facilitates penetration into the upper skin layers. Ointments are frequently used on skin lesions that have overlying dry scaling and crusting, but they are also very effective on severe dermatoses requiring an increased medication dosage. Ointments are semiocclusive and often not appropriate for use on lesions that are oozing and discharging a transudate or exudate.

Aerosols and Foams

Aerosols, fine particle sprays of medication usually delivered by gas under pressure, are a cosmetically elegant way of treating dermatoses, especially on hairy areas of the body. Many topical medications are now available as foams that can be used in a similar fashion.

INTRALESIONAL INJECTION

Intralesional injection, or the deposition of medication directly into the lesion, can be done with a conventional needle and syringe or with an instrument (Dermojet) that injects fine particles of medication through the skin with air pressure. This delivery form is especially useful in delivering higher concentrations of corticosteroids to lesions (usually with deep dermal components) that do not respond to topical medication.

SELECTION OF A DELIVERY SYSTEM

Delivery system selection depends on the disease being treated, the type of lesions clinically present, and the practitioner's preferred medication routine. For instance, weeping exudative lesions require drying (wet dressings) and perhaps corticosteroids. Initial delivery as a gel would increase the drying tendency; as the lesion dries, a cream may be used to prevent overdrying and fissure formation.

In a disease state such as chronic atopic eczema with lichenoid or thickened skin, the prescriber may choose an ointment to enhance penetration of the medication into the lesion. The ointment's occlusive nature reduces moisture loss from the skin.

Seborrhea and psoriasis in the scalp may be treated with aerosols, which are quick and easy to use and are associated with a high degree of patient compliance. Patients often find them cosmetically superior to the identical medication in cream form. Keloids, which require highly concentrated medication to be delivered to a small area, are ideal candidates for intralesional injection of corticosteroids.

CORTICOSTEROIDS

Corticosteroids are a very important tool in the practice of dermatology. Dermatologists administer steroids systemically and topically. Steroids may be characterized as short acting (cortisone or hydrocortisone), intermediate acting (prednisone, prednisolone, methylprednisolone, or triamcinolone), or long acting (dexamethasone or betamethasone).

Systemic Steroids

Administration of systemic steroids in dermatologic disease is usually oral. Intermediate-acting steroids (prednisone, prednisolone, methylprednisolone) are used most often. The greatest benefit of oral administration is the ability to adjust dosage schedules quickly if required. Once-daily doses, divided daily dosage, or alternate-day regimens are all effective.

Intramuscular administration of corticosteroids is also common. Preparations such as triamcinolone acetonide are used most often. These drugs, which may reduce inflammation for more than 4 weeks, ensure that an unreliable patient will receive appropriate doses of medication.

Systemic corticosteroids are generally used for relatively short periods. Therefore, the complications commonly associated with corticosteroid use are not usually seen in dermatologic treatment. However, the long-term use of corticosteroids in diseases such as pemphigus and SLE often results in cushingoid features such as a round, puffy face and a "buffalo hump." Additional adverse effects include fatigue, weakness, and acne.

Topical Steroids

Corticosteroids can also be applied topically to suppress inflammation. Although this approach does not cure the disease, the reduction in erythema, edema, and pruritus promotes healing. Topical steroids are available in a variety of forms. Based on their capacity to cause cutaneous vasoconstriction, topical steroids are divided into seven groups, with group 1 being the most potent (augmented betamethasone dipropionate [Diprolene AF] and clobetasol dipropionate [Temovate]) and group 7 being the least potent (1% hydrocortisone).

KEY POINTS
- Selection of topical treatment depends largely on whether the goal is to moisturize or dry the affected area. Continuous wet dressings, lotions, creams, and ointments tend to be moisturizing. Intermittent wet dressings and gels tend to be astringents for weeping, oozing lesions.
- Corticosteroids are commonly administered to reduce inflammation. They may be given topically, intralesionally, or systemically.

DEVELOPMENTAL CONSIDERATIONS

The skin and the skin problems of special groups warrant consideration. Certain skin problems are seen only in infants and children (e.g., cradle cap and diaper rash) (Figure 53-38). Other dermatoses are seen in both children and adults, but in children these dermatoses may appear different from the adult counterpart. Still other dermatoses affect primarily older individuals.

INFANCY

Infancy connotes soft, flawless skin. In general, this is a true image. Several congenital skin lesions, such as Mongolian spots, hemangiomas, and nevi (moles), are nevertheless associated with the early neonatal period.

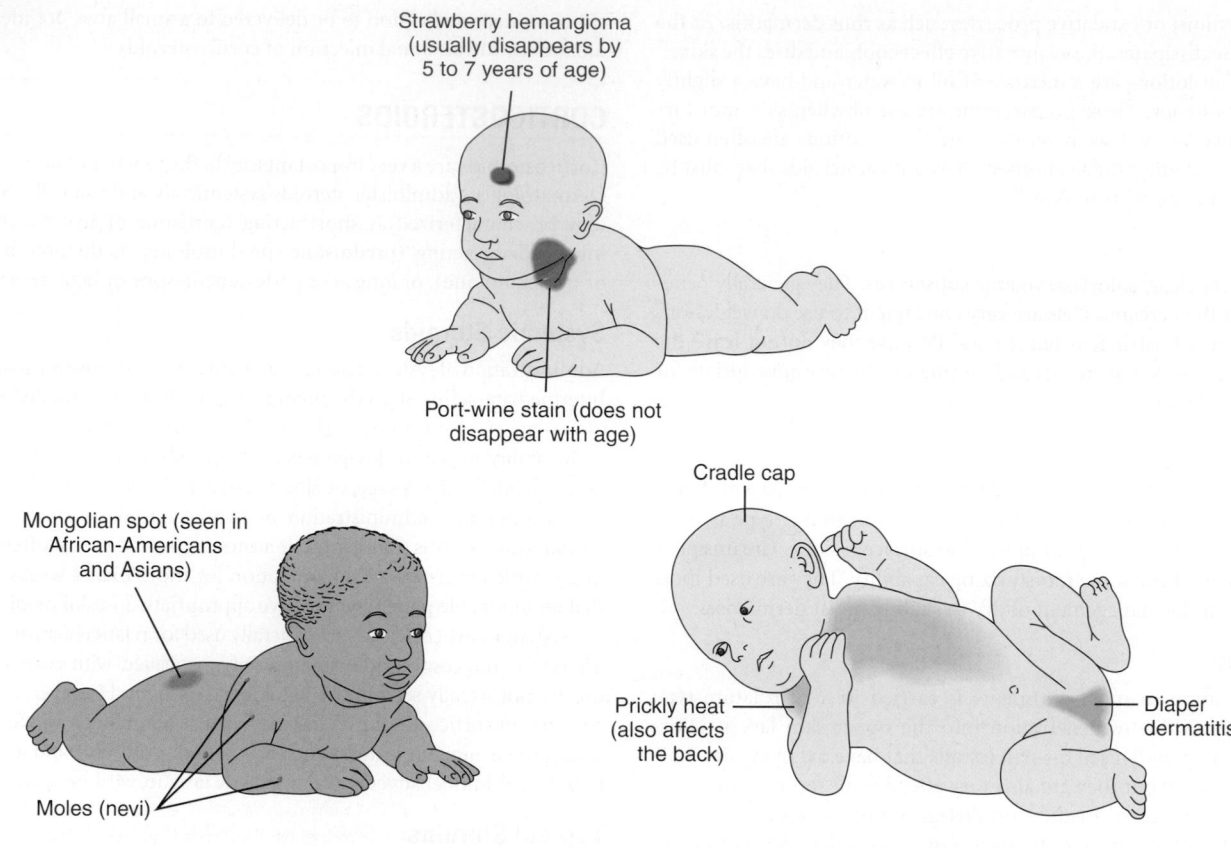

FIGURE 53-38 Sites of common dermatoses in infants and small children.

Mongolian spots are caused by selective pigmentation. They usually occur on the buttocks or sacral area and are commonly seen in Asian Americans or African Americans.

Hemangiomas are vascular disorders of the skin. Two types of hemangiomas are commonly seen in infants and small children: bright red, raised *strawberry hemangiomas* and flat, reddish purple *port-wine stain hemangiomas*. Strawberry hemangiomas begin as small red lesions shortly after birth. They may remain as small superficial lesions or extend to involve subcutaneous tissue. Strawberry hemangiomas usually disappear before the child reaches 5 to 7 years of age without leaving an appreciable scar.[28] Port-wine stain hemangiomas are rare, usually occur on the face and neck, and can be quite disfiguring. They do not disappear with age and no satisfactory medical treatment is available, although laser surgery may be effective in some cases. Coverage using cosmetic makeup such as Dermablend may sufficiently conceal their disfiguring effects.

Nevi may vary in shape or size, and they may be present at birth or develop later in life.

Infant skin is also exquisitely sensitive to irritation, injury, and extremes of temperature. Prolonged exposure to a warm humid environment can lead to **prickly heat,** and too frequent bathing can cause excessive dryness. Soiled diapers, left unchanged, can lead to **contact dermatitis** and bacterial infections. **Cradle cap** is a harmless and usually self-limited scaly condition of the scalp. Figure 53-38 illustrates common skin problems of infants and small children.

The primary factor in preventing infant skin disorders is careful and meticulous skin care. Baby lotions are helpful in maintaining skin moisture, whereas baby powder acts as a drying agent. Both are helpful aids when used selectively and according to the nature of the skin problem (excessive moisture or dryness).

Baby powders containing talc can cause serious respiratory problems if inhaled; therefore, containers should be kept out of the reach of small children. Corn starch is preferable to talc, and baby powders containing corn starch are readily available. Unnecessary bathing should be avoided, and clothing should be comfortable and appropriate for environmental conditions.

Diaper rash results from the ammonia and alkaline by-products of urine breakdown. Disposable diapers or diapers washed in gentle detergent and thoroughly rinsed to remove all traces of ammonia and alkali help prevent diaper rash. Treatment includes frequent diaper changes with careful cleansing of any irritated areas, especially in hot weather. Exposing irritated areas to air is also helpful. The use of plastic pants should be discouraged.

Prickly heat is caused by midepidermal obstruction and rupture of the sweat glands from prolonged exposure to a warm and humid environment. Treatment includes removing excessive clothing, cooling with warm water baths, drying with powders, and avoiding hot, humid environments.

Cradle cap is usually managed with mild shampooing and gentle combing to remove the scales.

CHILDHOOD SKIN DISORDERS

As infants grow and develop into active young children, they become susceptible to the many skin disorders affecting people of all age groups who encounter environmental agents. Children, because of their physiologic development and playful nature, may also be more prone to accidents that result in major skin trauma such as lacerations or burns. (See Chapter 54 for further discussion of burn injury.) Careful activity supervision helps prevent such accidental trauma.

PEDIATRIC CONSIDERATIONS
Integument in the Newborn

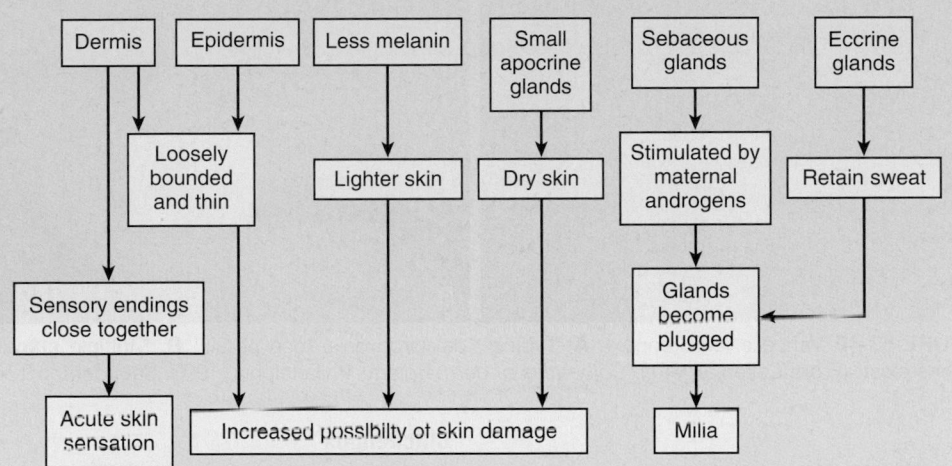

The integument in the newborn has sensory endings in the dermis that are closer together than seen in mature skin, creating more sensitive skin sensation. As the child develops the skin receptors begin to become more dispersed, decreasing skin sensitivity. There are several factors that lead to increased possibility of skin damage. The dermis and epidermis are present and functional at birth but the layers are thinner. The layers are loosely connected because rete pegs, which anchor the epidermis and dermis together, are not developed at birth. Therefore the dermis and epidermis are susceptible to skin damage with minimal friction. As a toddler, the dermis and epidermis become more closely linked. Another factor is that the newborn has less melanin at birth. The newborn will have lighter skin than he or she will have as a child. This lack of melanin makes the infant more susceptible to

harmful rays from the sun, increasing skin damage. The newborn also has small, nonfunctional apocrine glands. These glands, located on hair follicles, do not develop until puberty. The lack of functional glands can lead to dry skin.

Several other glands in the newborn help create milia—small, white acne found on newborns. The sebaceous glands can be found on the scalp, face, and genitalia of the newborn. The sebaceous glands are activated by maternal androgens in the fetus, producing vernix at birth, and becoming plugged and producing milia after birth. The eccrine glands respond to heat and emotional stimuli to create sweat that can obstruct the sebaceous glands and create milia. The eccrine glands will be activated at a higher temperature than in adults and are most active in the palms of newborns.

Besides interacting with the environment, children are frequently in close contact with other children. As a result, communicable diseases such as head lice, tinea capitis, and impetigo are more frequently seen in children (Figure 53-39). Epidemiologically, the incidence of rubella, roseola, rubeola (measles), chickenpox, and scarlet fever is also highest in this age group.

Rubella

Etiology, pathogenesis, and clinical manifestations. Rubella (3-day measles, German measles) is a childhood disease caused by the rubella virus. It is characterized by a diffuse punctate, macular rash that begins on the trunk and spreads to the arms and legs. Mild febrile states occur; generally the child's temperature is less than 100° F.[28] Postauricular, suboccipital, and cervical lymph node adenopathy is common. Coldlike symptoms usually accompany the disease in the form of cough, congestion, and coryza (profuse nasal mucous membrane discharge). Treatment is based on symptoms.

Rubella generally has no long-lasting sequelae; however, transmission of the disease to pregnant women early in the gestation period may result in severe teratogenic effects in the unborn fetus. Among the teratogenic effects are cataracts, microcephaly, mental retardation, deafness, patent ductus arteriosus, glaucoma, purpura, and bone defects.[25]

Prevention. Most states require immunization to prevent the transmission of rubella to pregnant women. Immunization is with a live virus vaccine called measles-mumps-rubella (MMR). One injection during infancy is followed by one booster dose when the child enters kindergarten or first grade or when the child enters middle school or junior high school. Administration of these two injections is considered adequate to prevent rubella. Cases of rubella in immunized children are rare.

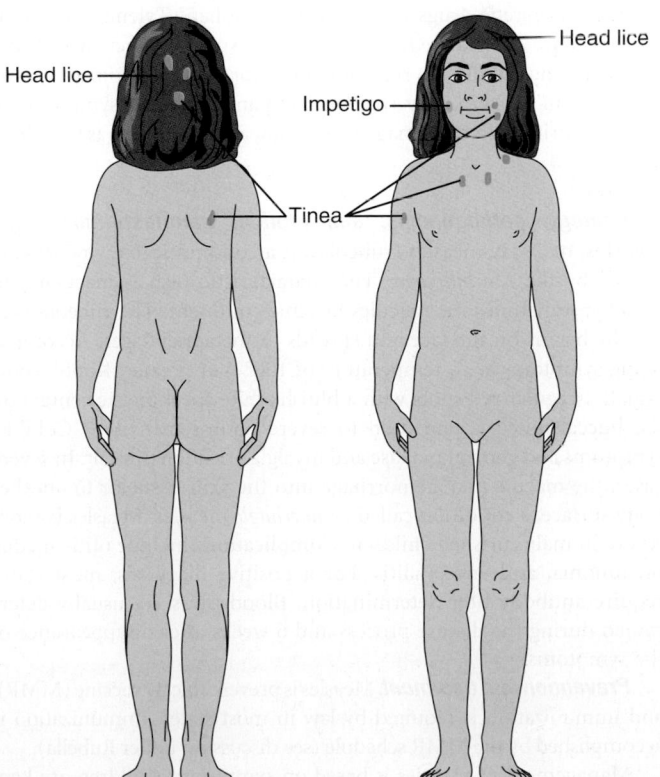

FIGURE 53-39 Sites of selected common communicable dermatoses affecting children.

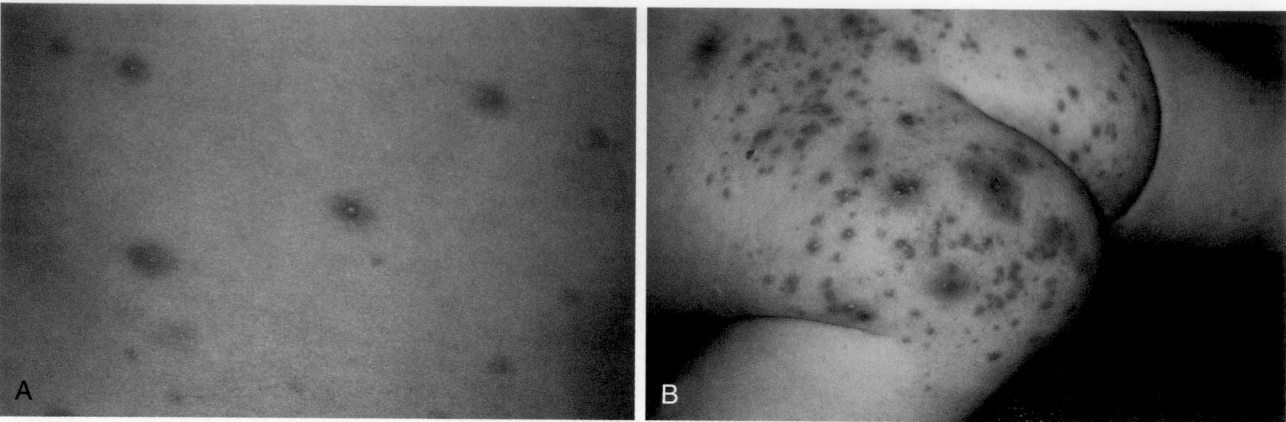

FIGURE 53-40 Varicella (chickenpox). **A,** Typical "dewdrop on a rose petal." **B,** Multiple stages of lesions exist. (From Callen JP et al: *Color atlas of dermatology*, Philadelphia, 1993, Saunders, p 170.)

Roseola Infantum

Pathogenesis and clinical manifestations. Roseola infantum is a contagious viral disease that generally affects children younger than 4 years and usually children about 1 year of age.[28] It produces a characteristic maculopapular rash covering the trunk and spreading to the appendages. A rapid rise in temperature to 105° F and the appearance of coldlike symptoms accompany the disease.[28] Unlike rubella, no cervical or postauricular lymph node adenopathy occurs. The symptoms usually subside within 3 to 5 days.[28] Roseola infantum is frequently mistaken for rubella, which can usually be ruled out by the age of the child, as well as by the absence of lymph node adenopathy. Generally, rubella does not develop in children younger than 6 to 9 months because of the presence of maternal antibodies.[28] Blood antibody titers may be assayed to determine the actual diagnosis. In most cases, no long-term effects from this disease are noted.

Treatment. Management of roseola infantum is palliative. As with rubella, antipyretic drugs such as acetaminophen (Tylenol) and cooling baths are used to reduce the fever. Ensuring sufficient rest and administering fluids are recommended for recuperation and body rehydration. Pruritus may rarely accompany the other symptoms. If severe, pruritus can be managed with topical lotions such as Caladryl.

Measles

Etiology, pathogenesis, and clinical manifestations. Hard **measles**, or 7-day measles (rubeola), is a communicable viral disease caused by the *Morbillivirus*. The characteristic rash is macular and blotchy; sometimes the macules become confluent. The rubeola rash usually begins on the face and spreads to the appendages. Accompanying symptoms are a temperature of 100° F or greater, Koplik spots (small, irregular red spots with a bluish white speck in the center) on the buccal mucosa, and mild to severe photosensitivity.[29] Coldlike symptoms and general malaise and myalgia are often present. In severe cases, the macule may hemorrhage into the skin tissue or to another body surface, a condition called *hemorrhagic* measles. Measles is more severe in malnourished children. Complications include otitis media, pneumonia, and encephalitis. For a positive diagnosis, most states require antibody titer determination. Blood titers are usually determined during the disease process and 6 weeks after disappearance of the symptoms.

Prevention and treatment. Measles is preventable by vaccine (MMR), and immunization is required by law in most states. Immunization is accomplished by the MMR schedule (see discussion under Rubella).

Management of measles is based on symptoms. Children are kept in darkened rooms. Antipyretic medications are given to reduce the fever, and rest and fluids are recommended.

Chickenpox

Etiology, pathogenesis, and clinical manifestations. Chickenpox (varicella) is a common communicable childhood disease. It is caused by the varicella-zoster virus, which is also the causative agent in shingles. The characteristic skin lesion occurs in three stages: macule, vesicle, and granular scab (Figure 53-40). The macular stage is characterized by the rapid development (within hours) of macules over the trunk of the body that spread to the limbs, buccal mucosa, scalp, axillae, upper respiratory tract, and conjunctivae. During the second stage, the macules vesiculate (blister) and may become depressed or umbilicated (raised blisters with depressed centers). The vesicles burst, and a scab forms during the third stage. Crops of lesions occur successively, so all three forms of the lesion are usually visible by the third day of illness. Mild to extreme pruritus accompanies these lesions and can be a complicating factor by leading to scratching and the subsequent development of secondary bacterial infection. Other symptoms that accompany chickenpox are coldlike symptoms, including cough, coryza, and sometimes photosensitivity. Mild febrile states usually occur. Complications such as pneumonia, sepsis, and encephalitis may occur but are rare among healthy children. Disease severity is age dependent, and the risk of visceral involvement is considerably higher in adults.

Prevention and treatment. Treatment is based on symptoms. Antipyretic drugs such as acetaminophen are given for fever reduction; they may also relieve local discomfort. Pruritus is relieved with lukewarm baths. Oral administration of diphenhydramine (Benadryl) or other antihistamines may be prescribed to alleviate itching. Application of topical antipruritics such as Caladryl lotion is also helpful. However, in young children, care must be taken to avoid topical preparations of Caladryl containing diphenhydramine to circumvent possible overdose of this agent through systemic absorption. (This consideration is especially important if the young child is also taking oral Benadryl.) Home remedies such as baking soda baths also relieve pruritus, and rest and fluids are important in recuperation and rehydration. Some authorities recommend acyclovir, an antiviral agent, for the management of chickenpox.[30,31]

Varicella-zoster immune globulin provides passive immunity against chickenpox and is recommended after exposure, especially for high-risk groups. A vaccine against chickenpox that will provide active immunity is also available. Vaccination is currently recommended for all children and sometimes required for school entrance.

Scarlet Fever

Etiology, clinical manifestations, and treatment. **Scarlet fever** is a systemic reaction to the toxins produced by group A β-hemolytic streptococci. It occurs when the individual is sensitized to the toxin-producing variety of streptococci. Scarlet fever frequently occurs in

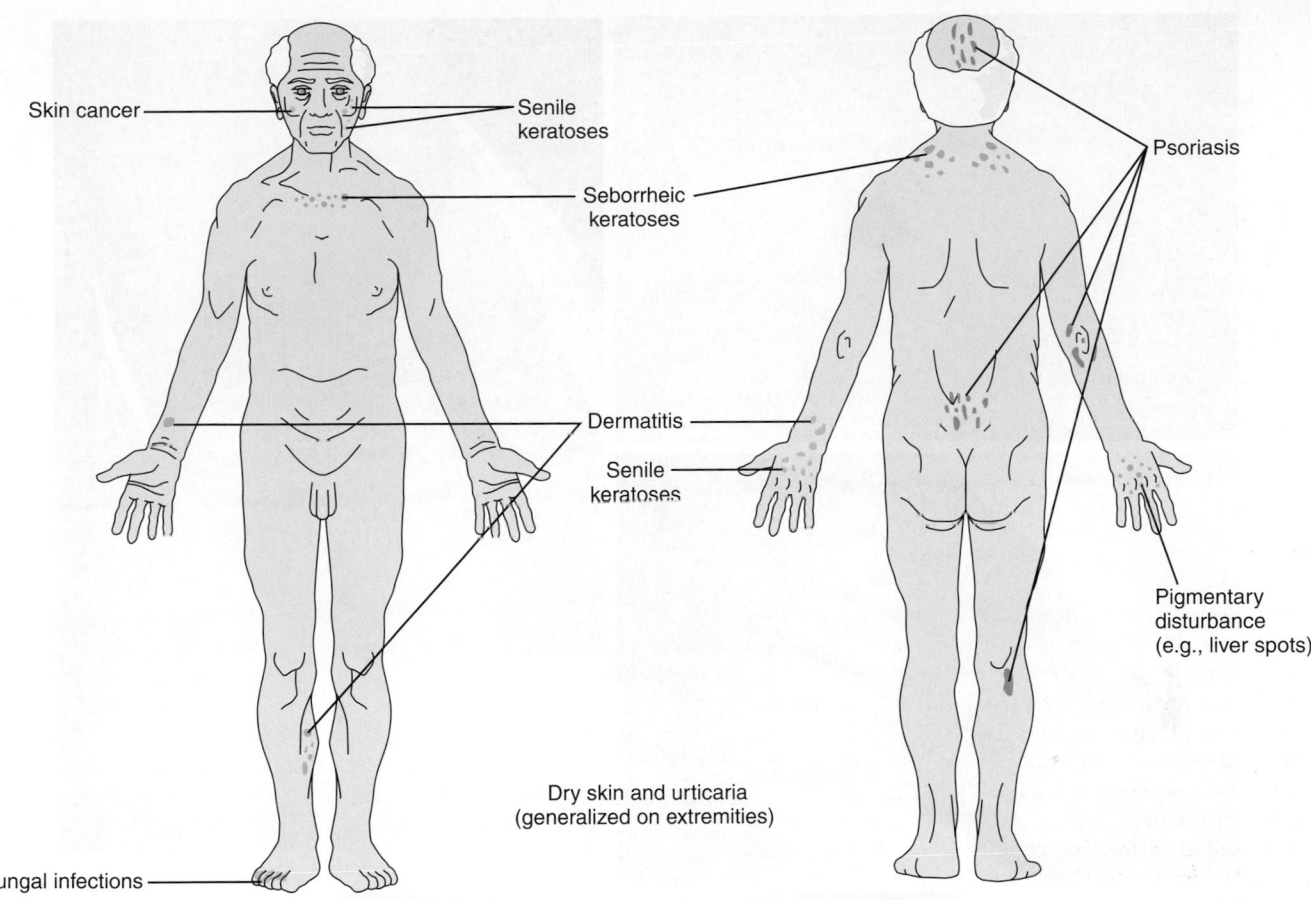

FIGURE 53-41 Sites of common dermatoses of the elderly.

association with streptococcal sore throat (strep throat), but it may also be associated with a wound, skin infection, or puerperal infection. Scarlet fever is characterized by a pink punctate skin rash on the neck, chest, axillae, groin, and thighs. When palpated, the rash feels like fine sandpaper. Flushing of the face with circumoral pallor is evident. Other symptoms include high fever, nausea and vomiting, strawberry- or raspberry-colored tongue, and skin desquamation. Complications of scarlet fever include otitis media, peritonsillar abscess, rheumatic fever, acute glomerulonephritis, and cholera. Penicillin is the treatment of choice.

ADOLESCENCE AND YOUNG ADULTHOOD

The most common skin disorder of adolescence and young adulthood is **acne vulgaris.** The increased production of sex hormones and oils contributes to the development of acne. Childhood diseases are less common in adolescence; however, chronic skin diseases may be exacerbated.

GERIATRIC CONSIDERATIONS

Skin disorders are so common in elderly individuals that it is difficult to distinguish normal from abnormal. More than 90% of elderly individuals have some kind of skin disorder[32,33] (Figure 53-41). The most common skin disorders in the elderly are keratoses and skin cancers, followed by fungal infections, dermatitis, pigmentary disturbances, psoriasis, and urticaria (hives). Other skin disorders frequently seen in the elderly are comedones (blackheads), asteatoses (scaling), cherry angiomas (small, red, benign tumors), nevi (moles), skin tags (pedunculated fleshy growths), and lentigines ("liver spots"). In addition, the incidence of senile purpura and senile warts (papillomas) significantly increases, especially among the very old. Senile purpura is related to loss of the

subcutaneous tissue that supports the skin capillaries. Minor trauma can cause small bruises or ecchymotic lesions, which largely occur on the extensor surface of the forearms. Approximately 40% of older men and 77% of older women show evidence of senile purpura.[34] Senile papillomas are small yellow, brown, or black warts located on the trunk, limbs, and face; 63% of all older individuals have some senile papillomas.[35]

Figure 53-42 illustrates several of the common skin lesions associated with aging. Most of these lesions are considered normal concomitants of aging and cause little discomfort. The greatest concern regarding body image is the appearance of the skin, which tends to look mottled and spotty. Disorders of the skin that tend to cause the most physical discomfort are pruritus, keratoses, epitheliomas, malignant melanomas, herpes zoster, psoriasis, and pressure sores.

KEY POINTS

- Certain skin disorders are more common in particular age groups.
- Infants are prone to irritating lesions, including prickly heat, contact dermatitis, and cradle cap. Altered areas of pigmentation are first noticed in infancy, including Mongolian spots, hemangiomas, and nevi.
- Children are prone to skin injuries and communicable diseases. A number of viral infections, including rubella, roseola, measles, and chickenpox, are associated with characteristic skin rashes. Fever and malaise are usually present. Treatment is symptomatic. Vaccinations are available to prevent rubella, measles, and chickenpox. Scarlet fever is due to a bacterial infection and is managed with antibiotics. Children are often exposed to superficial infections and infestations, including head lice, ringworm, scabies, and impetigo.
- Acne is the most common skin disorder of adolescents.
- Elderly skin is prone to a number of problems, including psoriasis, angiomas, and skin tags. Cancerous and precancerous lesions are common and require careful screening examination.

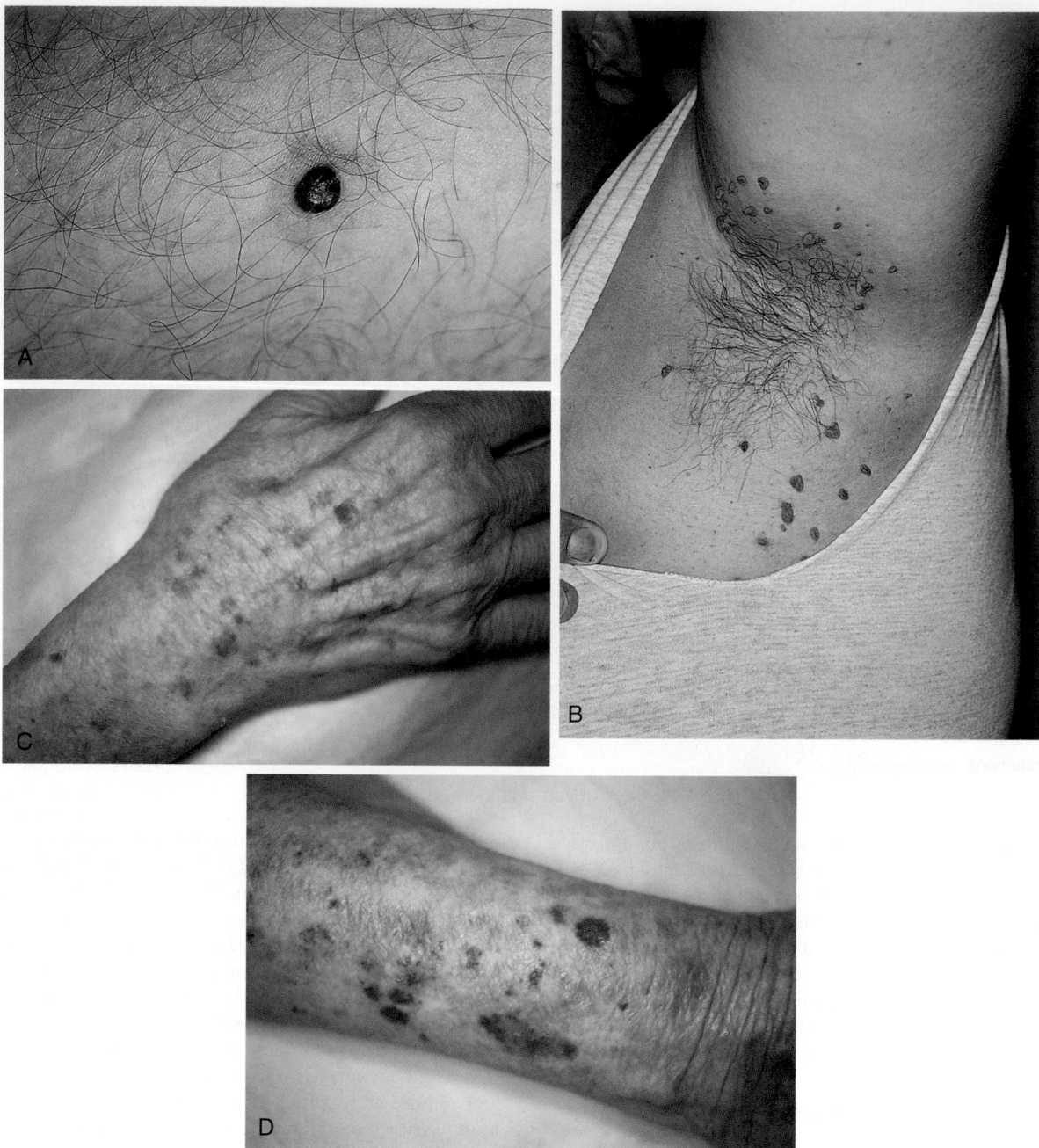

FIGURE 53-42 Common skin lesions associated with aging. **A,** Cherry angioma. **B,** Acrochordons (skin tags). **C,** Senile lentigines (liver spots) in an 87-year-old woman. Note the well-demarcated brownish black macules. **D,** Senile purpura. (**A** and **B,** From Callen JP et al: *Color atlas of dermatology*, ed 2, Philadelphia, 2000, Saunders, pp 83, 304. **C** and **D,** From Swartz MH: *Textbook of physical diagnosis*, ed 6, Philadelphia, 2010, Saunders, pp 807, 808.)

SUMMARY

In systemic diseases, the color, texture, and composition of the skin mirror and participate in widespread pathophysiologic events. For example, internal disease states such as acquired immunodeficiency syndrome; collagen diseases such as scleroderma and dermatomyositis; diabetes; gout; malignancies; neurologic diseases; liver disease; muscle weakness; and vascular, inflammatory, and metabolic disorders all exhibit cutaneous manifestations. Because the skin mirrors the interior condition of the body, it is important in the diagnosis of disease. Cutaneous manifestations may be caused by bodily changes such as

pregnancy or obesity. They may also be caused by external factors such as climate, industrial contamination, indoor heating systems, clothing, plant life, and toxic or allergic reactions to drugs and cosmetics.

A distinct advantage in treating individuals with skin disease is the ability to observe the pathology and the effects of treatment. In addition to a careful history, a culture, skin scraping, or biopsy provides good diagnostic information. A correct diagnosis can help prevent complications from improper therapy, but it does not lessen the importance of choosing an appropriate delivery system.

REFERENCES

1. Gupta AK, Jain HC, Lynde CW, et al: Prevalence and epidemiology of onychomycosis in patients visiting physicians' offices: a multicenter Canadian survey of 15,000 patients, *J Am Acad Dermatol* 43(2 pt 1):244–248, 2000.

2. Spanos NP, Williams V, Gwynn MI: Effects of hypnotic, placebo, and salicylic acid treatments on wart regression, *Psychosom Med* 52(1):109–114, 1990.

3. Gulick R: Herpes virus infections. In Arndt KA, et al, editors: *Cutaneous medicine and surgery: an integrated program in dermatology*, vol 1, Philadelphia, 1996, Saunders, pp 1074–1092.

4. Dicken CH: Retinoids: a review, *J Am Acad Dermatol* 11(4):541–552, 1984.

5. Yeung-Yue KA, Brentjens MH, Lee PC, et al: Herpes simplex viruses 1 and 2, *Dermatol Clin* 20(2):249–266, 2002.

6. Epstein JH: Phototherapy and photochemotherapy, *N Engl J Med* 322(16):1149–1151, 1990.

7. Groopman JE: Neoplasms in the acquired immune deficiency syndrome: the multidisciplinary approach to treatment, *Semin Oncol* 14(2 Suppl 3):S1–S6, 1987.

8. Benenson AS, editor: *Control of communicable diseases manual*, ed 16, Washington, DC, 1995, American Public Health Association.

9. Ackerman AB, Cockerell CJ: Papules, *Cutis* 37(4):242–245, 1986.

10. Gonzalez E: Pityriasis rosea. In Arndt KA, et al, editors: *Cutaneous medicine and surgery: an integrated program in dermatology*, vol 1, Philadelphia, 1996, Saunders, pp 218–220.

11. Strauss JS: Biology of the sebaceous gland and the pathophysiology of acne vulgaris. In Soter NA, Baden HP, editors: *Pathophysiology of dermatologic diseases*, New York, 1991, McGraw-Hill, pp 195–210.

12. Fanelli M, et al: Antibiotics, acne, and *Staphylococcus aureus* colonization, *Arch Dermatol* 147(8):917–921, 2011.

13. Kristal L, Clark RAF: Atopic dermatitis. In Arndt KA, et al, editors: *Cutaneous medicine and surgery: an integrated program in dermatology*, vol 1, Philadelphia, 1996, Saunders, pp 195–202.

14. Roth HL, Kierland RR: The natural history of atopic dermatitis. A 20-year follow-up study, *Arch Dermatol* 89:209–214, 1964.

15. Shear B, Stern RS: Cutaneous reactions to drugs and biologic response modifiers. In Arndt KA, et al, editors: *Cutaneous medicine and surgery: an integrated program in dermatology*, vol 1, Philadelphia, 1996, Saunders, pp 412–425.

16. Sober AJ, Fitzpatrick TB: Adverse drug reactions. In Sober AJ, Fitzpatrick TB, editors: *Yearbook of dermatology*, St Louis, 1990, Mosby, pp 109–120.

17. Rockerbie NR, Woo TY, Callen JP, et al: Cutaneous changes of dermatomyositis precede muscle weakness, *J Am Acad Dermatol* 20(4):629–632, 1989.

18. Gilchrest BA, Yaar M: Ageing and photoageing of the skin: observations at the cellular and molecular level, *Br J Dermatol* 127(Suppl 41):25–30, 1992.

19. Pieper B: Mechanical forces, pressure, shear, and friction. In Bryant RA, Nix DP, editors: *Acute and chronic wounds*, ed 3, St Louis, 2007, Mosby, pp 205–234.

20. Friedman RJ, et al: Skin cancer: basal cell and squamous cell carcinoma. In Holleb AI, Fink DJ, Murphy GP, editors: *Clinical oncology*, ed 7, New York, 1991, American Cancer Society, pp 290–303.

21. Sherman CD, et al: Malignant melanomas. In Rubin P, editor: *Clinical oncology: a multidisciplinary approach for physicians and students*, ed 7, Philadelphia, 1993, Saunders, pp 667–675.

22. Boissy RE, Nordlund JJ: Vitiligo. In Arndt KA, et al, editors: *Cutaneous medicine and surgery: an integrated program in dermatology*, vol 1, Philadelphia, 1996, Saunders, pp 1210–1218.

23. Berardesca E, Maibach HI: Sensitive and ethnic skin: a need for special skin-care agents? *Dermatol Clin* 9(1).89–92, 1991.

24. Martin S: Variants of normal skin in blacks. In Rosen T, Martin S, editors: *Atlas of black dermatology*, Boston, 1981, Little, Brown, pp 1–16.

25. Ackerman AB, Cockerell CJ: Cutaneous lesions: correlations from microscopic to gross morphologic features, *Cutis* 37(2):137–138, 1986.

26. Berger TG, Odom RB, James WD: Diseases of the skin appendages. In Berger TG, Odom RB, James WD, editors: *Andrew's diseases of the skin: clinical dermatology*, ed 9, Philadelphia, 2000, Saunders, pp 943–990.

27. Leyden JJ, Rawlings AV: *Skin moisturization*, New York, 2002, Marcel Dekker.

28. Cohen S: Programmed instruction: skin rashes in infants and children, *Am J Nurs* 78(Suppl 6):S1–S32, 1978.

29. Johnson ML: Skin diseases. In Wyngaarden JB, Smith LH Jr, Bennett CJ, editors: *Cecil textbook of medicine*, ed 19, vol 2, Philadelphia, 1992, Saunders, pp 2280–2330.

30. Dunkle LM, Arvin AM, Whitley RJ, et al: A controlled trial of acyclovir for chickenpox in normal children, *N Engl J Med* 325(22):1539–1544, 1991.

31. Arvin AM: Varicella-zoster virus, *Clin Microbiol Rev* 9(3):361–381, 1996.

32. Gilchrest BA: Dermatologic disorders in the elderly. In Rossman I, editor: *Clinical geriatrics*, ed 3, Philadelphia, 1986, Lippincott, pp 375–387.

33. Goldman R: Decline in organ function with aging. In Rossman I, editor: *Clinical geriatrics*, ed 2, Philadelphia, 1979, Lippincott, pp 23–52.

34. Smith L: Histopathologic characteristics and ultrastructure of aging skin, *Cutis* 43(5):414–424, 1989.

35. Cerimele D, Celleno L, Serri F: Physiological changes in ageing skin, *Br J Dermatol* 122(Suppl 35):S13–S20, 1990.

CHAPTER
54

Burn Injuries

Nirav Patel

evolve WEBSITE

http://evolve.elsevier.com/Copstead/

- Review Questions and Answers
- Glossary (with audio pronunciations for selected terms)
- Animations

- Case Studies
- Key Points Review

KEY QUESTIONS

- What are the most common causes of burn injuries?
- How are burn degree and severity determined?
- What are the principles that guide the management of burn injuries?

- What are the potential complications associated with burn injuries?
- What are the outcomes following burn injuries?

CHAPTER OUTLINE

Burns are injuries to tissues caused by contact with dry heat (flame or hot surfaces), moist heat (steam or hot liquids), electricity (current or lightning), chemicals (corrosive substances), friction, or radiant and electromagnetic energy. Approximately 450,000 individuals seek medical attention for burn injuries annually in the United States, with 10% necessitating acute hospitalization.[1] In recent decades, associated mortality rates have decreased significantly, with most patients achieving excellent functional and cosmetic outcomes. Improved outcomes have been attributed to the delineation of pathophysiologic mechanism of burns, advances in management, and the development of a comprehensive, treatment-oriented approach to care.[2-4] The American Burn Association in conjunction with the American College of Surgeons Committee on Trauma has been instrumental in promoting the development of burn centers.[5] Advanced burn life support prehospital and provider courses have also been developed to provide evidence-based guidelines for the assessment and treatment of burn victims.[6] To facilitate appropriate treatment decisions and recognize potential complications, an understanding of the pathophysiologic processes associated with the burn injury is vital.

THERMAL INJURY

Etiology, Incidence, and Mortality

Thermal injuries are burns caused by contact with or exposure to extremes of temperature. Over the past 6 decades the incidence of burn injuries in the United States has steadily decreased, with approximately 450,000 currently occurring annually,[1] resulting in approximately 40,000 hospitalizations and 3120 deaths.[7-10] The fire loss record in the United States is the worst in the industrialized world, with the fire-related mortality double that of most countries on a per capita basis. From 2005 to 2009, residential fires resulted in nearly $7 billion per year in property damage.[11]

A half century ago, burns over 50% of the total body surface area (TBSA) resulted in a greater than 50% mortality in pediatric patients.[12] Currently, most children survive burns of this size, and more than half survive burns of more than 90% of their TBSA.[13] Early mortality generally occurred as a result of inadequate initial resuscitation. As vigorous resuscitation protocols were developed, a significant reduction in mortality occurred. Additionally, many advances have also contributed to decreasing thermal burn–related mortality, including: a better understanding of the pathophysiologic mechanisms of burns, implementation of a multidisciplinary team–oriented approach, improvement of resuscitation strategies and infection control measures, use of early surgical excision and skin-grafting techniques, application of advances in skin substitute development, and employment of improved rehabilitation strategies.[14-18]

Unfortunately, the reduction in mortality was replaced by an increased number of survivors with wound sepsis. The development of improved topical and systemic antimicrobial agents, recognition of the importance of maintaining proper nutrition, and adoption of early wound excision and grafting techniques have resulted in a significant reduction in mortality. As a result of these advances, acute mortality in patients with thermal injuries remains relatively low. The primary cause of death in this population now occurs in the subacute setting as a result of pulmonary sepsis, often developing secondary to inhalation injury. More than 80% of patients sustaining burns have involvement of less than 20% of their TBSA and are treated on an outpatient basis. Despite burn degree, the associated physical and emotional sequelae are often extensive and prolonged. As a result, this unique population requires vigilant follow-up care.

Risk Factors

The U.S. Centers for Disease Control and Prevention (CDC) has identified the following groups as being at high risk for fire-related injuries and deaths: children younger than 4 years; adults 65 years and older; Native Americans and African Americans; economically challenged individuals; people living in rural areas; and those residing in manufactured homes or substandard housing. Children younger than 15 years old account for one third of all admissions to burn units and one third of all deaths from burns and burn-related injuries.[8] Scald injuries, primarily secondary to accidental spills, or in up to 20% from an element of abuse or neglect, account for up to 65% of all burn injuries.[4,12,19] See Figure 54-1 illustrating an abuse burn.

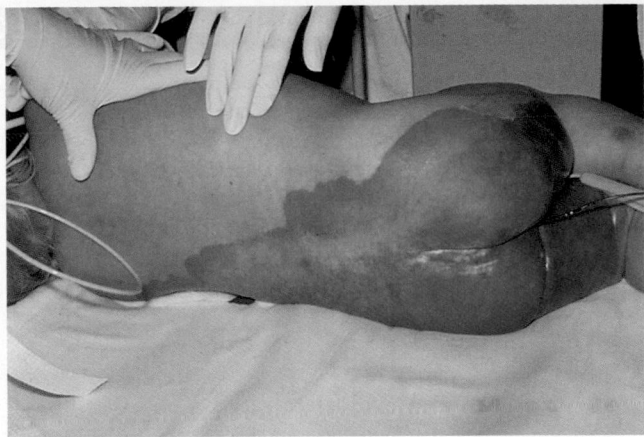

FIGURE 54-1 All burns in children must be carefully evaluated with a consideration for nonaccidental or intentional injury. This 2-year-old boy was immersed by his father in a bathtub of hot water and sustained burns over 55% of his total body surface area. One feature that characterizes abuse burns is a clear demarcation between burned and unburned skin and the absence of drip, spill, or splatter marks. (Courtesy Michael Peck, MD, University of North Carolina Burn Center, Chapel Hill.)

The population older than 65 years of age accounts for approximately 29% of all burn/fire-related deaths in the United States.[20] Burns in the elderly carry a high mortality rate as a result of preinjury disability, age-related immunosuppression, and impaired healing responses (Table 54-1).[8] Environmental and lifestyle factors influence the frequency and magnitude of thermal burn injuries. Alcohol and drug abuse contributes to approximately 40% of all residential fire-related deaths. Neurologic and psychiatric disorders have also been found to increase the risk of accidental burn injury, with one study finding 3% of patients admitted to the burn unit had thermal injuries associated with neurologic disorders.

Integument Effects

The skin is the largest organ of the body and constitutes approximately 20% of the total body weight. It consists of two layers, the epidermis and dermis, which rest on the hypodermis (or subcutaneous layer). The epidermis contains two main cell types, melanocytes and keratinocytes, as well as multiple appendages such as hair, nails, and glands (sweat and sebaceous). The appendages, although originating from the epidermal layer, are anatomically located in both the epidermis and the dermis. Keratinocytes synthesize keratin, and melanocytes scattered throughout the basal layer (stratum germinativum) produce melanin, a pigment that shields deeper structures of the skin from sunlight. Apocrine glands, the large sweat glands, are rudimentary structures with no known useful purpose. They respond to autonomic nerve stimulation rather than thermal stimulation to produce an odorless, viscous, milklike droplet from the hair shaft. Apocrine glands are more numerous in women and are located in the axilla, areola of nipples, groin, perineum, and perianal and periumbilical regions. Eccrine glands are small sweat glands distributed over the body that act as true secretory glands and produce the sweat responsible for heat regulation. At environmental temperatures greater than 31° or 32° C (90° F), sweating occurs over the entire body; at lower temperatures, microscopically visible droplets are secreted periodically as part of the total insensible water loss from the body. Sweat normally provides skin with an acid mantle (average pH, 5.7 to 6.4) that retards growth of the many bacteria that reside in the keratin layer, glands, and hair follicles.

TABLE 54-1 PHYSIOLOGIC CHANGES ASSOCIATED WITH AGE

BODY SYSTEM	PEDIATRIC	ELDERLY
Cardiovascular	**Symptoms of shock:** Increased heart rate Decreased blood pressure Decreased urine output Cardiac output dependent on heart rate Decreased myocardial compliance Stroke volume plateaus at lower filling pressures	Increased chronic disease processes Decreased vascular elasticity results in increased systolic blood pressure Decreased cardiac output Decreased β-adrenergic responsiveness Decreased cardiac stress response Decreased intrinsic heart rate Decreased blood flow Decreased vascular permeability Increased myocardial irritability Decreased myocardial perfusion Increased dysrhythmias Conduction system changes
	Peripheral cyanosis: Neonates: a normal finding Children: decreased cardiac output	
Pulmonary	Small trachea is easily obstructed Neck hyperextension leads to epiglottal or tracheal obstruction At <8 yr, cricoid cartilage is narrowest airway point At <8 yr, no cuff is needed on endotracheal tube Hypoxemia leads to decreased heart rate in neonates Hypoxemia leads to decreased heart rate in children Diaphragmatic breathing Lower airways are easily obstructed Decreased O_2 reserve	Increased need for ventilatory support Increased incidence of inhalation injury Increased pneumonia Decreased lung elasticity Decreased chest wall muscle Decreased oxygen saturation Decreased tidal volume Decreased vital capacity Decreased pulmonary capillary circulation
Thermoregulation and metabolism	Increased resting metabolic rate Increased resting O_2 consumption Increased BSA in relation to body weight Increased hypothermia Increased heat loss from evaporation and convection At <6 mo, inability to shiver to increase body heat Stress leads to hypoglycemia Glycosuria is a sign of infection At <2 yr, buffering capacity is decreased Increased metabolic demands of growth	Increased burn wound infection Increased sepsis Poor or delayed wound healing Increased preexisting malnutrition Decreased febrile response Increased hypothermia
Gastrointestinal and renal	Decreased endogenous calorie stores Increased diarrhea with fluid and calorie deficits At <2 yr, gastric emptying is delayed At <2 yr, increased gastric distention At <30% TBSA burn, can take sufficient caloric supplementation At >30% TBSA burn, requires caloric supplementation At <12 mo, poor renal filtration and absorption	Increased volume sensitivity Decreased nutritional status Increased likelihood of hypotensive or hypertensive renal damage Increased incidence of type 2 diabetes mellitus Decreased creatinine clearance
Neurocognitive	Increased incidence of cerebral edema with fluid resuscitation Increased irritability Increased regressive behavior Increased risk-taking behavior Immature judgment	Decreased brain mass Decreased cerebral nerve cells Decreased brain cortex layer Decreased cerebellar cortical cells Decreased nerve conduction velocity Decreased memory Decreased electroencephalographic activity Slower reaction time Decreased taste Decreased smell Decreased vision Decreased hearing Increased pain threshold Decreased judgment and cognitive abilities
Immune	Immature immune system Decreased immunocompetence	Decreased number of leukocytes Decreased immunocompetence Decreased T-cell response

From Carrougher GJ, editor: *Burn care and therapy*, St Louis, 1998, Mosby, p 100.
BSA, Body surface area; *mo*, month(s); *TBSA*, total body surface area; *yr*, year(s).

Sebaceous glands secrete sebum, a complex mixture of lipids that is emptied into the hair shaft. The rate of production of sebum and its location depend on androgens, which initiate and continue production. During the hypermetabolic state that follows major thermal injury, production of sebum is decreased, leading to the dry skin conditions commonly found after recovery.

Thermal injury to the integument occurs in two phases: (1) immediate, which is a result of direct cellular injury and (2) delayed, which occurs as a result of progressive dermal ischemia.

The duration of exposure and the temperature, or the amount of energy, to which the skin is exposed primarily determines the degree of tissue/cellular injury, which is characterized by three zones (from inner to outer): (1) zone of necrosis; (2) zone of stasis, which is a region with decreased blood flow that either can be returned to its normal state with appropriate resuscitation or can be converted to a necrotic state in the case of dehydration, infection, or decreased perfusion; and (3) zone of hyperemia, which is minimally injured tissue that usually recovers normal function within 1 week.[21]

In response to thermal injury, keratinocytes develop from cells in the basal layer of the epidermis and progress upward from the stratum germinativum to the stratum corneum over a 14-day period. During this time the wound develops a light pink or reddish coloration, with normal skin color restored in a delayed fashion by the melanocytes. Regeneration of hair and nails is dependent on viability of the hair follicle and nail matrix. With intact follicles, hair generally regrows at approximately 1 cm per month. New nail formation is often irregular and of abnormal thickness as regrowth occurs.

Depth Classification

Depth of burn injury is divided into four classifications: first-degree burns, also known as superficial burns, second-degree burns, also known as superficial and deep partial-thickness, third-degree burns (full-thickness), and fourth-degree burns (full-thickness with bone or muscle involvement), based on criteria established by the American Burn Association (Table 54-2).[22]

First-degree burns (also known as superficial burns) involve only superficial tissue destruction in the outermost layers of the epidermis, with no associated compromise of the function of the skin (see Table 54-2). These burns are often associated with local discomfort, erythema, and mild systemic responses such as headache, chills, nausea, and vomiting. Erythema, a thermovascular response that occurs in first-degree burns in the absence of direct trauma to the dermis, is probably related to the release of tissue contents into the superficial circulation. First-degree burns are generally self-limiting, require no fluid resuscitation, and are therefore not included in estimates of the percentage of TBSA burned. However, in infants and elderly adults, first-degree burns may lead to systemic dehydration, necessitating intravenous resuscitation. Therapy generally includes simple analgesia. These injuries typically heal in 3 to 6 days without scarring or pigmentation changes.

Second-degree (superficial partial-thickness) burns involve the epidermis to the level of the dermis and appear red to pale ivory. Moist, thin-walled blisters often form within minutes of the injury (Figure 54-2). Pain is a major clinical feature of this depth of injury because tactile and pain sensors remain intact (see Table 54-2). Injuries typically heal in 7 to 21 days in the absence of wound infection. The amount of scarring that follows is a genetically determined trait, with some groups of people tending to scar excessively (African Americans and Caucasians with red hair) or minimally (Native American and Asian groups). Hair follicles remain intact and will regrow hair in the area of injury. Hair usually reappears 7 to 10 days after injury.

Second-degree (deep partial-thickness) burns may involve the entire dermis and leave only the epidermal skin appendages located in the hair follicles. The area of injury has a mottled appearance, with large areas of waxy-white tissue surrounded by light pink or red tissue. The surface is generally dry, and blisters tend to resemble flat, dry tissue paper rather than the fluid-filled raised areas seen with superficial partial-thickness injury. Tactile and pain sensors are either absent or greatly diminished in the area of deepest tissue destruction, but this area is usually surrounded by margins of lesser depth of injury in which pain and tactile sensors remain intact. Deep partial-thickness

TABLE 54-2 BURN WOUND CLASSIFICATION

DEGREE OF BURN	CAUSE OF INJURY	DEPTH OF INJURY	WOUND CHARACTERISTICS	TREATMENT COURSE
First-degree burn	Prolonged ultraviolet light exposure, brief exposure to hot liquids	Limited damage to epithelium, skin intact	Erythematous, hypersensitive, no blister formation	Complete healing within 3-5 days without scarring
Superficial partial-thickness burn: second degree	Brief exposure to flash, flame, or hot liquids	Epidermis destroyed, minimal damage to superficial layers of dermis, epidermal appendages remain intact	Moist and weepy, pink or red, blisters, blanching, hypersensitive	Complete healing within 21 days with minimal or no scarring
Deep partial-thickness burn: second degree	Intense radiant energy, scalding liquids or hot semiliquids (e.g., tar) or solids, flame	Epidermis destroyed, underlying dermis damaged, some epidermal appendages remain intact	Pale, decreased moistness, blanching absent or prolonged; intact sensation to deep pressure but not to pinprick	Prolonged healing (often longer than 21 days), may require skin grafting to achieve complete healing with better functional outcome
Full-thickness burn: third degree	Prolonged contact with flame, scalding liquids, steam; hot objects; chemicals; electrical current	Epidermis, dermis, and epidermal appendages destroyed; injury through dermis	Dry, leatherlike; pale, mottled brown, or red; thrombosed vessels visible; insensate	Requires skin grafting
Full-thickness burn: fourth degree	Electrical current, prolonged contact with flame (e.g., unconscious victim)	Epidermis, dermis, and epidermal appendages destroyed; injury involves connective tissue, muscle, and possibly bone	Dry; charred, mottled brown, white, or red; no sensation; limited or no movement of involved extremities or digits	Requires skin grafting, amputation of involved extremities or digits likely

From Carrougher GJ, editor: *Burn care therapy*, St Louis, 1998, Mosby, p 138.

injury is visually and clinically indistinguishable from full-thickness injury at the time of injury. These wounds heal spontaneously in previously healthy individuals in about 4 weeks in the absence of secondary infection. As the length of healing time increases, so does the degree of scarring and depigmentation. As a result, these burns are often excised early and subsequently treated with a skin graft in an effort to diminish scarring and achieve early wound closure.

Third-degree (full-thickness) burns may also involve the entire epidermis, the dermis, and the underlying subcutaneous tissue. Immediately following injury, these areas appear white, cherry red, or black. Deep blisters may be present under a dry layer of dehydrated skin. Superficial blood vessels coagulated by the heat of injury may be visible through the skin as thrombosed veins. One of the physiologic characteristics of the skin that is lost (Box 54-1) is the elasticity of the dermis,

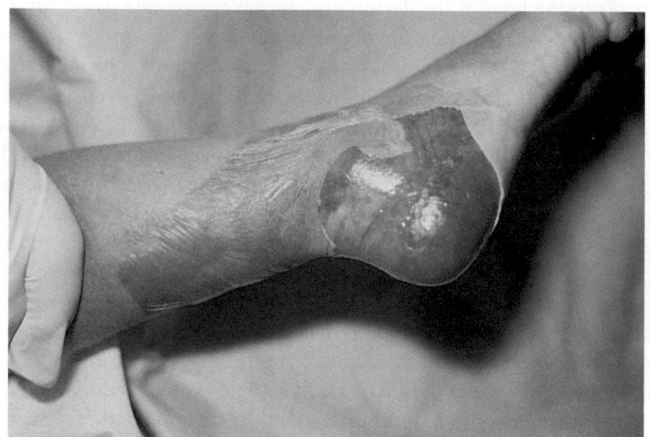

FIGURE 54-2 This young child sustained a hot water scald burn on the heel of the right foot that resulted in a superficial second-degree burn. A superficial second-degree (partial-thickness) burn will reepithelialize within 3 weeks. These burns are characterized by loss of epidermis (blistering) and by a shiny, sensate, vascularized dermis. (Courtesy Michael Peck, MD, University of North Carolina Burn Center, Chapel Hill.)

resulting in a wound with a dry, hard, leathery texture. The massive edema that accompanies major burn injury combined with the loss of elasticity may result in a tourniquet-like effect when the injury occurs circumferentially around a limb or torso. This often necessitates escharotomies or, rarely, fasciotomies to restore distal circulation.

These burns are painless to touch, because all superficial nerve endings in the skin have been destroyed. However, as with partial-thickness injuries, rarely are burn injuries totally uniform, and an area of lesser injury in which pain and tactile sensors are intact is usually located on the periphery. Areas of full-thickness injury require skin grafting with the patient's own skin because all dermal elements have been destroyed, leaving no residual tissue for regeneration. However, small injuries often heal by secondary intention as a result of ingrowth of dermal elements from the margins of the wound.

Fourth-degree (full-thickness) injuries that extend beyond the dermis to involve muscle, bone, or both are often classified as fourth-degree. These injuries often occur in victims of high-voltage electrical injury or in persons who have had prolonged exposure to intense heat, such as unconscious fire victims.

Extent of Injury

Extent of injury refers to the percentage of TBSA burned. Estimates can be calculated with the rule of nines (Figure 54-3) or the Lund and Browder chart (Figure 54-4). The rule of nines is commonly used in prehospital settings and emergency departments, and provides a rough estimate of TBSA involved. The Lund and Browder chart, or a variation of it, is generally used in burn centers and is more precise, particularly in assessing TBSA in children under the age of 10 years (see Figure 54-4).

Severity Classification

The severity of a burn injury is determined by the extent to which the physiologic functions of the skin are disrupted beyond the body's normal ability to respond with compensatory mechanisms. The American Burn Association[22] classifies burn injury as minor, moderate, and major (Table 54-3). The severity of the burn injury and the eventual morbidity and mortality associated with it are related to a combination of factors: the patient's medical history, the extent and depth of

---

BOX 54-1   NORMAL PHYSIOLOGIC FUNCTIONS OF THE SKIN ALTERED OR LOST AFTER THERMAL INJURY

Protection
Barrier between the internal organs and the external environment
Continuous with the mucous membrane at the external openings of organs of the digestive, respiratory, and urogenital systems
Acidic skin (pH 4.2 to 5.6) and perspiration protect against bacterial invasion
Thickened skin of palms and soles provides padding

Percutaneous Absorption
Epidermis is relatively impermeable to most chemical substances; some may be absorbed through the epidermis or the orifices of hair follicles

Sensory Processing
Receptor skin nerve endings allow constant monitoring of the environment by sensing warm and cold temperature, pain, touch, and pressure

Production
Endogenous production of vitamin D_3, which is necessary for synthesis of vitamin D

Barrier
Skin prevents water and electrolyte loss, maintains moist subcutaneous tissues, and prevents water absorption during immersion

Thermoregulation
Body continuously produces heat as a by-product of cellular metabolism; heat is dissipated through skin
Internal body temperature is regulated by radiation, conduction, or convection
Rate of heat loss depends primarily on the surface temperature of skin, which is a function of skin blood flow

Immunologic
Major location of immune complexes is at the dermal-epidermal junction and the dermal vessels of skin
Monocyte/macrophage system is mobilized by local tissue mediators

Circulatory
Skin temperature depends on the rate of blood flow through the skin
Circulatory system distributes pharmacologic agents to local tissues

Aesthetic
Provides the individual identity of a person

the burn, the body area involved, the presence of concomitant trauma sustained at the time of the burn, and the patient's age.

Acute Management

The first priority in burn management is the elimination of the source; however, extreme caution must be exercised to ensure that the rescuer does not become a victim. The fire should preferably be extinguished with water, because it not only eliminates the source of the heat but also enables cooling of the underlying skin. In the absence of water, flames may be smothered with a blanket, coat, or any other nonflammable covering that will aid in deprivation of the oxygen required for combustion. Once the flames are eliminated, the cover should

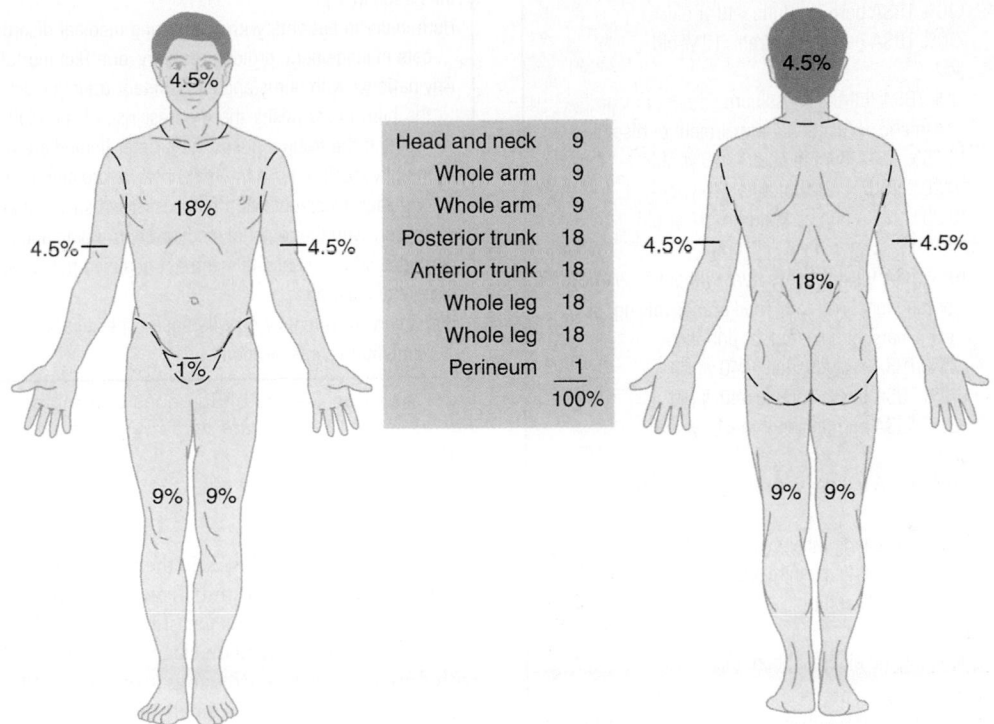

Head and neck	9
Whole arm	9
Whole arm	9
Posterior trunk	18
Anterior trunk	18
Whole leg	18
Whole leg	18
Perineum	1
	100%

FIGURE 54-3 The rule of nines is a commonly used assessment tool that permits a timely and useful estimate of the percentage of total body surface area burned.

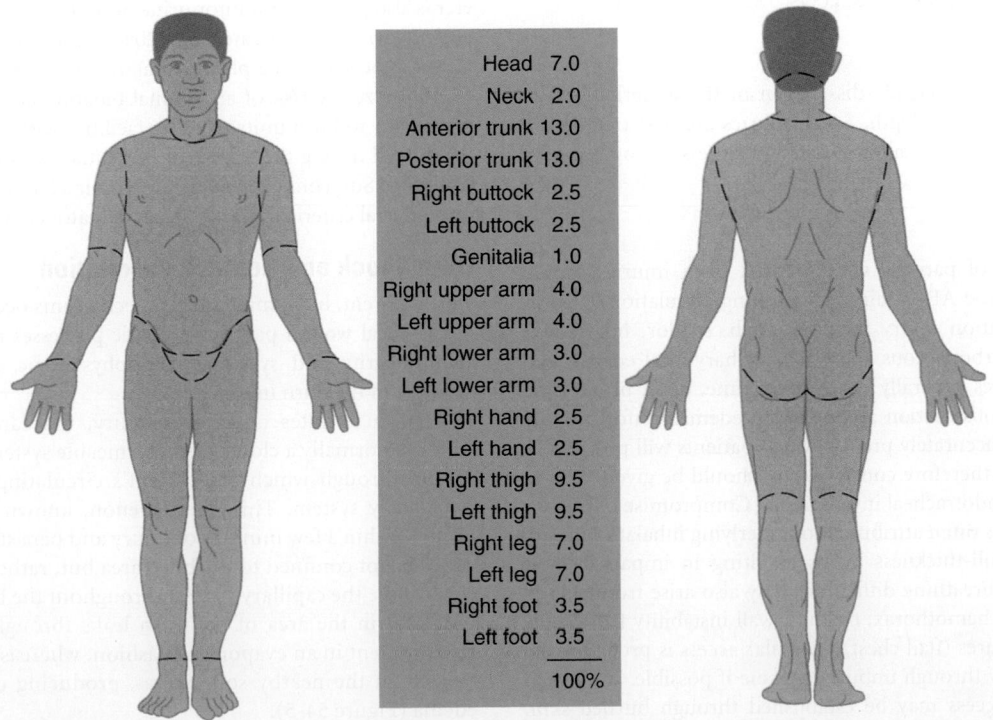

Head	7.0
Neck	2.0
Anterior trunk	13.0
Posterior trunk	13.0
Right buttock	2.5
Left buttock	2.5
Genitalia	1.0
Right upper arm	4.0
Left upper arm	4.0
Right lower arm	3.0
Left lower arm	3.0
Right hand	2.5
Left hand	2.5
Right thigh	9.5
Left thigh	9.5
Right leg	7.0
Left leg	7.0
Right foot	3.5
Left foot	3.5
	100%

FIGURE 54-4 The Lund and Browder chart. The areas of the body are presented in sections, which permits a more accurate estimation of burn size.

TABLE 54-3	AMERICAN BURN ASSOCIATION BURN SEVERITY CLASSIFICATION SCHEDULE
CLASSIFICATION	**ASSESSMENT CRITERIA**
Minor burn injury	<15% TBSA burn in adults <40 yr old
	<10% TBSA burn in adults >40 yr old
	<10% TBSA burn in children <10 yr old
	and
	<2% TBSA full-thickness burn without risk of cosmetic or functional impairment or disability
Moderate burn injury	12-25% TBSA burn in adults <40 yr old
	10-20% TBSA burn in adults >40 yr old
	10-20% TBSA burn in children <10 yr old
	and
	10% TBSA full-thickness burn without cosmetic or functional risk to burned area involving face, eyes, ears, hands, feet, or perineum
Major burn injury	>25% TBSA burn in adults <40 yr old
	>20% TBSA burn in adults >40 yr old
	>20% TBSA burn in children <10 yr old
	or
	>10% TBSA full-thickness burn (any age)
	or
	Injuries involving face, eyes, ears, hands, feet, or perineum likely to result in functional or cosmetic disability
	or
	High-voltage electrical burn injury
	or
	All burn injuries with concomitant inhalation injury or major trauma

Modified from American Burn Association guidelines. In Carrougher GJ, editor: *Burn care and therapy,* St Louis, 1998, Mosby, p 94.
TBSA, Total body surface area.

BOX 54-2	**BURN UNIT REFERRAL CRITERIA**

Partial-thickness burns greater than 10% TBSA
Burns that involve the face, hands, feet, genitalia, perineum, or major joints
Third-degree burns in any age group
Electrical burns, including lightning injury
Chemical burns
Inhalation injury
Burn injury in patients with preexisting medical disorders that could complicate management, prolong recovery, or affect mortality
Any patients with burns and concomitant trauma (such as fractures) in which the burn injury poses the greatest risk of morbidity or mortality; in such cases, if the trauma poses the greater immediate risk, the patient may be initially stabilized in a trauma center before being transferred to a burn unit; physician judgment will be necessary in such situations and should be in concert with the regional medical control plan and triage protocols
Burned children in hospitals without qualified personnel or equipment for the care of children
Burn injury in patients who will require special social, emotional, or long-term rehabilitative intervention

From American College of Surgeons Committee on Trauma: *Resources for optimal care of the injured patient,* Chicago, 1999, The College, p 55.
TBSA, Total body surface area.

be promptly removed to enable dissipation of the underlying heat, thereby minimizing injury depth. Scald injuries are best treated initially with cool water, which allows cooling of the scalding liquid as well as the underlying skin.

Assessment

Initial management of patients with thermal burn injuries should focus on stabilizing the ABCs (airway-breathing-circulation).[4] Common signs of inhalation injury include cough, stridor, hoarseness, singed nasal hair, carbonaceous sputum, oropharyngeal edema, and blisters. These injuries generally evolve over time, often progressing to complete airway obstruction secondary to edema. Unfortunately, no clinical variables accurately predict which patients will progress to airway compromise; therefore consideration should be given early to bronchoscopy and endotracheal intubation.[23] Compromise of breathing in burn patients is often attributed to underlying inhalation injury or circumferential full-thickness burns resulting in impaired chest excursion; however, breathing difficulties may also arise from associated pneumothorax, hemothorax, or chest wall instability from multiple segmental fractures (flail chest). Vascular access is preferentially obtained peripherally through unburned tissue if possible. If no such sites are available, access may be established through burned skin. The patient is then evaluated by a complete head-to-toe examination for any other associated traumatic injuries, which are identified and

managed as required. TBSA is then determined using a standardized chart such as the Lund and Browder chart (see Figure 54-4). Fluid resuscitation requirements are subsequently determined and initiated while the patient is placed on clean sheets and the burned areas covered with dry clean sheets or dressings. Coverage with cool wet sheets should be avoided, because these quickly become cold wet sheets, and with the loss of the burned skin's ability to regulate body temperature, hypothermia can quickly ensue. Application of topical agents in the acute setting outside of a burn center is not recommended. A Foley catheter is also placed to monitor urine output during resuscitation, and in patients with burns greater than 20% of the TBSA, if possible, a nasogastric tube should be placed to allow for gastric decompression and to minimize the risk of abdominal bloating and aspiration. Transfer of patients to burn units or other facilities with appropriate resources is initiated during the course of the initial assessment. The American College of Surgeons Committee on Trauma has developed a set of burn unit referral criteria to assist initial evaluators in triage (Box 54-2).

Burn Shock and Acute Resuscitation

Two different, but simultaneous mechanisms occur in cases of major burns: local wound pathophysiologic processes related to the loss of skin integrity and systemic pathophysiologic processes related to sequelae of the burn injury.

Within minutes of a burn injury, the cardiovascular system, which is normally a closed, semipermeable system, becomes an open system through which the patient's circulating volume leaves the circulatory system. This phenomenon, known as "capillary leak," occurs within a few minutes of injury and persists for 24 hours. Burn shock is not confined to the burn area but, rather, is a systemic process. While the capillary system throughout the body becomes leaky, fluid lost in the area of the burn leaks through the burn into the environment in an evaporative fashion, whereas fluid loss internally collects in the nearby soft tissues, producing extensive interstitial edema (Figure 54-5).

Restoration of the patient's circulating volume is an essential part of acute burn management. The rate and volume of fluids lost are related

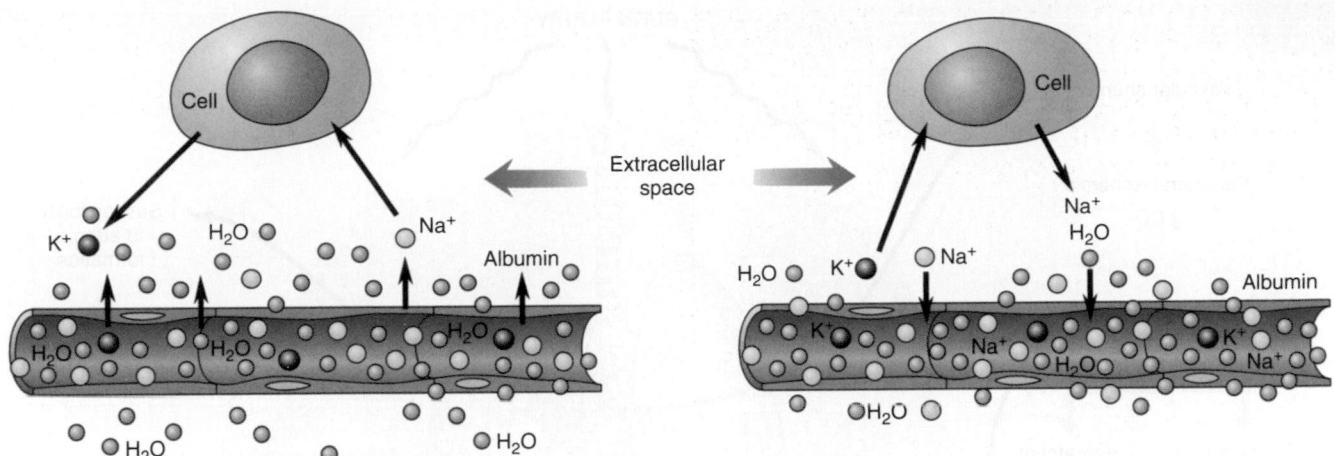

FIGURE 54-5 Direction of fluid and electrolyte shifts associated with burn shock. During burn shock, K^+ is exiting the cell, and Na^+ and H_2O are moving into the cell. After burn shock, K^+ enters the cell while and Na^+ and H_2O exit it.

BOX 54-3 PARKLAND FORMULA FOR FLUID RESUSCITATION IN BURN SHOCK

During the first 24 hours after a burn, administer intravenous LRS at the following rate:

4 ml LRS / % TBSA burn / kg body weight

where

- Time is calculated from the time of burn injury.
- TBSA is total body surface area.
- Half of the total fluid is administered in the first 8 hr after burn.
- One fourth of the total is administered in the second 8 hr.
- One fourth of the total is administered in the third 8 hr or in quantities to maintain adult urine output at 30 ml/hr or child urine output at 1 ml/kg/hr.

Example of formula calculation in a 70-kg patient with a 50% TBSA burn:

4 ml × 70 kg × 50 % TBSA burn = 14, 000 ml (14 L) LRS in 24 hr

- Administer 7000 ml in the first 8 hr at 875 ml/hr.
- Administer 3500 ml in the second 8 hr at 437 ml/hr.
- Administer 3500 ml in the third 8 hr at 437 ml/hr.

Data from Baxter CR: Guidelines for fluid resuscitation, *J Burn Care Rehabil* 2:279-286, 1981.
LRS, Lactated Ringer solution; *TBSA*, total body surface area.

BOX 54-4 PLASMA REQUIREMENTS AND EVAPORATIVE WATER LOSS AFTER BURN INJURY

Colloid Replacement
Twenty percent of blood volume given as fresh-frozen plasma or plasma expander
Adult males: 20% = 5 ml/kg body weight
Adult females and children: 20% = 8 ml/kg

Maintenance Fluids Until Wound Closure Is Achieved
Basal fluid requirements:
1500 ml of fluid/m² TBSA = 24-hr requirement
Evaporative water loss from burn wound until healed:
Adults: (25 + % TBSA burn) × m² BSA = ml/hr requirement
Children: (35 + % TBSA burn) × m² BSA = ml/hr requirement
Maintenance fluids equal basal fluid requirements plus evaporative water loss and may be administered intravenously, orally, or by nasogastric or jejunal tube, according to patient need.

BSA, Body surface area; *TBSA*, total body surface area burned.

---

directly to the severity of burn. Therefore, the extent and depth of the burn injury must be ascertained during the initial clinical assessment.

The most widely used formula to guide fluid resuscitation within the first 24 hours of burn injury is the Parkland formula (Box 54-3). The formula utilizes lactated Ringer solution as the resuscitation fluid, because it most closely approximates the fluid it is replacing and thereby minimizes the profound electrolyte imbalances often seen with large-volume resuscitation (Box 54-4). The standardized formulas provide an excellent guideline for initiating fluid resuscitation but do not ensure adequacy of resuscitation. In Cartotto's series, 30 patients with mean TBSA burns of 27% received 6.7 ± 2.8 ml/kg/% TBSA burn in the first 24 hours to ensure adequate resuscitation.[24] Adequacy of resuscitation is determined by the global response of the patient to the fluid administration and not by one single variable.[25] Markers commonly used to reflect adequacy of resuscitation include normalization

of mental status, blood pressure, pulse rate, capillary refill time, arterial pH, and base deficit and maintenance of urine output at 0.5 to1 ml/kg per hour for adults and 1 to 1.5 ml/kg per hour for children. In addition to the fluid volumes calculated by the standardized formulas, the patient should also receive appropriate maintenance fluid over the first 24-hour period.

Approximately 24 hours following the acute burn injury, the capillary leak syndrome begins to resolve as cardiovascular integrity is restored. At this time, a colloid solution such as albumin may be administered according to an appropriate formula, which differs by gender and age (see Box 54-4), in an effort to replace the protein lost during the acute burn shock phase. Resuscitation in the acute setting with colloid has been shown to decrease net volume of fluid administered and complications associated with large-volume resuscitation such as abdominal compartment syndrome.[26]

One of the major functions of intact skin is to serve as a barrier to water evaporation. With major burn injury, this ability of the skin to regulate evaporative loss is disrupted. In a classic study conducted in

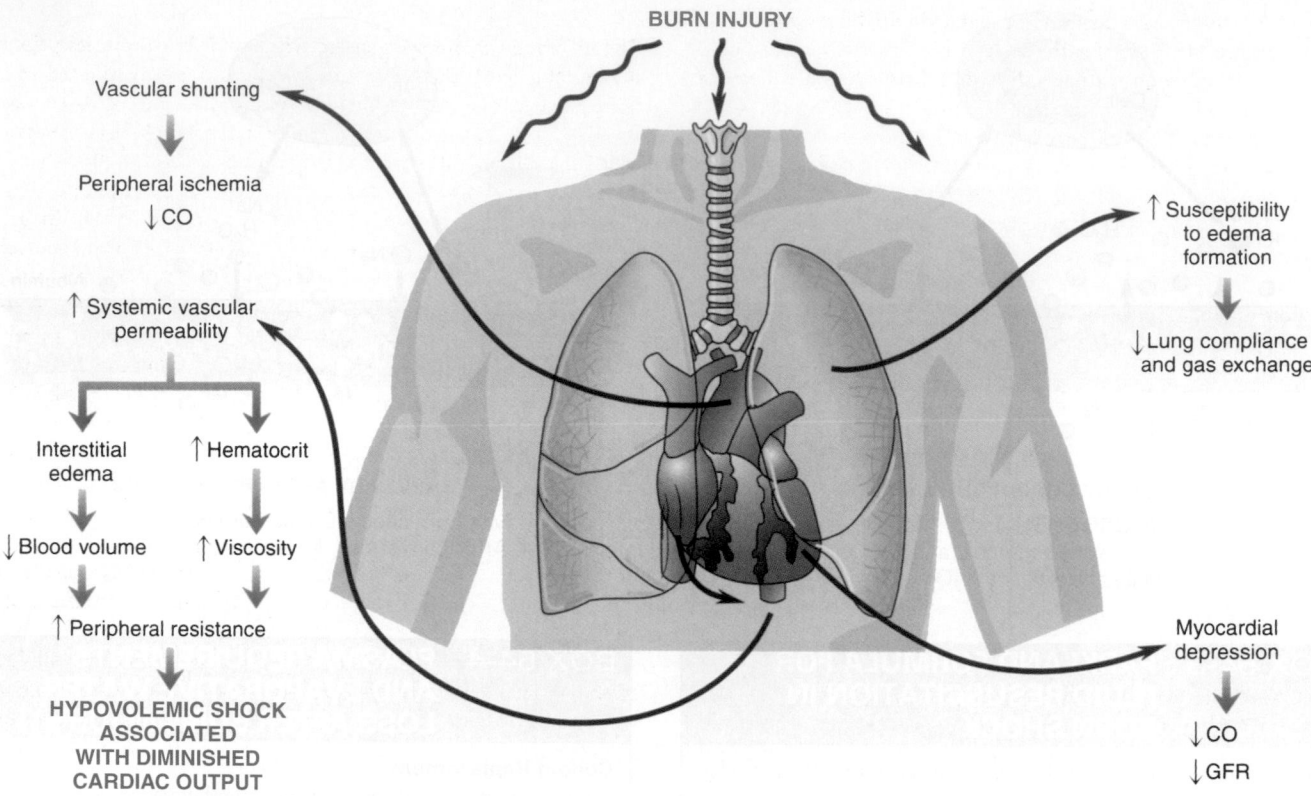

FIGURE 54-6 Cardiovascular and pulmonary effects of major burn injury within the first 24 hours after burn injury, during burn shock. *CO,* Cardiac output; *GFR,* glomerular filtration rate.

1962, Moncrief and Mason[27] attempted to determine the magnitude of such a loss and found that daily evaporative loss was in the range of 20 times normal during the early phase of burn injury, with gradual decreases as wound closure was achieved. Further studies revealed that the insensible water loss through burned skin is not caused by evaporation of water from sweat glands but rather by water vapor formed within the body and lost through the skin.[28,29] As the patient progresses to the subacute phase of resuscitation, it is imperative that attention be paid to these unaccountable losses.

Patients at the extremes of age groups require special considerations with respect to resuscitation. Table 54-1 summarizes the physiologic changes associated with age that increase the vulnerability of children and elderly persons.[30-32]

Organ Dysfunction
Cardiovascular Dysfunction

Burn shock is often accompanied by a precipitous drop in cardiac output that does not parallel the gradual reduction in blood volume and is refractory to restoration of the circulating volume. This finding of low cardiac output in the presence of vigorous intravenous fluid resuscitation and massive catecholamine release has led to the suggestion of a specific myocardial depressant factor.[33-38] The pathophysiologic mechanism behind this myocardial dysfunction is poorly understood. There appears to be no simple, specific myocardial depressant factor but rather a cascade of events involving metabolic and immunologic factors (Figure 54-6).[19]

Respiratory Dysfunction

Respiratory dysfunction following burn injury generally is the result of obstruction, interstitial alterations, and metabolic changes. Obstruction may occur as a result of edema of the upper airway secondary to

direct injury, or more often is attributable to the generalized edema that occurs following fluid resuscitation in the face of an ongoing capillary leak syndrome that accompanies burn injuries. On occasion, burns of the oral cavity and upper airway occur as superheated air is inhaled or scalding water enters the mouth. The pulmonary system is extremely efficient at dissipating heat and prevents the inhalation of superheated air beyond the bronchi, but steam may permeate further into the lung parenchyma (see Figure 54-6).[21,23]

Airway obstruction secondary to edema generally has its onset within the first few hours following burn injury but tends to manifest clinically 2 to 4 hours later as resuscitation is undertaken. Endotracheal intubation is recommended prophylactically when impending airway obstruction is identified. The endotracheal tube is preferably secured with cotton twill tape that enables readjustment to allow for the increase in head and face circumference related to increasing facial and soft-tissue edema.[39]

Smoke or fume inhalation often leads to acute hypoxia that is refractory to oxygen administration. Inhalation injury directly results in the chemical denaturing of pulmonary tissue, and the subsequent edema results in increased distances over which oxygen must diffuse to the capillaries. This may progress to acute respiratory distress syndrome (ARDS), which usually occurs within the first week. Whether the actual inhalation injury causes susceptibility towards ARDS is still a subject of debate. However, it is clear that many factors play a role in this condition because of the intense inflammatory response to the burn in addition to contributions from sepsis, shock, pneumonia, multiple organ failure, and increasing duration of mechanical support. Current ventilatory strategies emphasize use of low tidal volumes and increased frequency of breaths, which have resulted in decreased mortality.[36,40]

Smoke inhalation is also responsible for the majority of cases of inadvertent carbon monoxide poisoning. Carbon monoxide is in direct competition with oxygen for hemoglobin binding sites and has much greater affinity for the oxygen binding sites on hemoglobin. Once carbon monoxide has bound to hemoglobin, it becomes carboxyhemoglobin, which has decreased ability to off-load oxygen to peripheral tissues. It is also responsible for inactivation of cytochrome oxidase, an enzyme that aids in oxygen utilization. The vast range of clinical symptoms can include vague constitutional symptoms such as headache, nausea, and fatigue, or may be much more severe and lead to lactic acidosis, seizures, and coma. The degree of carboxyhemoglobinemia is largely dependent on the amounts of carbon monoxide and oxygen in the native environment, the duration of exposure, and the minute ventilation of the patient.

Carbon monoxide poisoning is diagnosed with a compatible history and physical in conjunction with the presence of elevated carboxyhemoglobin levels. Carboxyhemoglobin can be directly measured on arterial blood gas samples, although these levels may not correlate with the development of neurologic sequelae. In addition, pulse oximetry plays no role in monitoring patients with carbon monoxide poisoning because it cannot differentiate between oxyhemoglobin and carboxyhemoglobin.

Treatment involves removal of carbon monoxide from hemoglobin via its direct competition with oxygen. The normal half-life of carbon monoxide in a patient breathing room air is 300 minutes. If high-flow oxygen is delivered via face mask, the half-life can be decreased to 90 minutes. Therefore treatment involves removal of the patient from the source of inhalation and immediate institution of high-flow 100% oxygen via a nonrebreather face mask. In cases of severe poisoning manifested by a carboxyhemoglobin level greater than 25%, loss of consciousness, severe metabolic acidosis, or evidence of ischemic change in any organ system, the treatment should involve institution of hyperbaric oxygen therapy. This will reduce the half-life of carbon monoxide even further to approximately 30 minutes, and it also increases the amount of oxygen dissolved in the blood (unbound to hemoglobin) from 0.3 to 6 ml/dl. In addition to assisting with elimination of carbon monoxide, the addition of hyperbaric oxygen improves delivery of oxygen to peripheral tissues, even in the presence of elevated carboxyhemoglobin levels.[41,42]

Renal Dysfunction

Acute renal failure (ARF) after burn injury can be classified as early or late. Early renal failure occurs during the first 5 days postburn, secondary to low intravascular volumes and rhabdomyolysis-associated myoglobinemia. The etiology of renal failure in rhabdomyolysis is twofold: first, the shift of fluid into damaged muscle from the intravascular space (i.e., third spacing) causes reduced blood volume and less flow to the kidneys, with direct nephrotoxic effects of myoglobin by-products and possible renal failure. Second, the by-products of myoglobin can be toxic to the kidneys and cause damage by precipitation into the renal tubules. Development of early renal failure can be minimized by adequate fluid resuscitation and decompressive fasciotomy for compartment syndrome that may contribute to further muscle damage. Late ARF, defined as occurring after 5 days postburn, is less of a result of the initial burn and is generally attributable to infectious or direct nephrotoxic factors such as medications. Most patients will require renal supportive therapy. Continuous venovenous hemofiltration (CVVH) has been used with success in treating ARF in burns and is associated with less vascular complications than arteriovenous hemodialysis.[43] The prognosis is generally poor for the burn patient who develops ARF. Mortality rates from 50% to 100% have been described.[44] Survival is dismal for patients with early-onset ARF associated with rhabdomyolysis. However, even in the face of severe ARF, renal function will generally recover over time in those patients who survive.[45]

Metabolic Changes

The metabolic changes associated with major burn injuries primarily involve the sympathetic nervous system and are manifested as sustained tachycardia (120 to 140 beats/min range) and increased oxygen consumption (approximately 150% of normal). The hypermetabolic state generally persists until the burn wound is reduced to less than 20% of TBSA and poses a major challenge in the treatment of these patients. Modalities to attenuate the hypermetabolic response have included use of propranolol, administration of counterregulatory hormones such as insulin and insulin-like growth factor, and stimulation of anabolism using growth hormones and steroids (natural or synthetic). A study from Shriner's Burns Institute in Galveston, Texas, randomized 56 children with major burns to receive supplemental growth hormone, propranolol, or both. Propranolol markedly reduced resting heart rate and energy expenditure measured by indirect calorimetry and improved net muscle protein synthesis. Interestingly, the addition of growth hormone did not enhance these effects.[31] Muscle protein wasting appears to be caused primarily by accelerated protein breakdown. Although protein synthesis is also increased, it fails to keep pace with proteolysis and amino acid mobilization. Thomas and colleagues evaluated the effect of continuous infusions of insulin (to maintain blood glucose levels between 100 and 140 mg/dl) on preservation of muscle mass in a randomized controlled clinical trial in 18 children with major burns. Evaluation of each patient when the burn wounds were 95% healed showed that insulin-treated patients had improved lean body mass, diminished muscle wasting, and reduced length of hospital stay in comparison with controls.[41]

Gianotti and colleagues studied temporal fluctuations in insulin-like growth factor type I and its binding protein in a group of burn patients, and demonstrated that they both decline for the first 14 days after the burn, paralleling decreases in prealbumin and transferrin levels.[46] However, plasma levels of growth hormone remained unchanged. In a small study of burned children, administration of insulin-like growth factor type I and insulin growth factor binding protein appeared to exert widespread effects in ameliorating acute inflammation by reducing the synthesis of type 1 and type 2 acute-phase proteins and interleukin 6 (IL-6) while increasing the synthesis of constituted protein such as prealbumin and transferrin. Anabolic steroids, including testosterone and its analogues, such as oxandrolone, are widely used to ameliorate muscle wasting in patients with cancer and acquired immunodeficiency syndrome; however, they have had limited benefits in burn patients.

Cellular Changes

Major burn injury affects the entire body, but survival ultimately depends on its effects at the cellular level. The cellular response to burn injury occurs as a metabolic and an immunologic pathophysiologic process. The basic pathologic condition, named the "sick cell syndrome" by Welt[47] in 1967, is a cell membrane transport defect related to an alteration in the steady-state composition, characterized by high intracellular concentrations of sodium. Entry of sodium into the intracellular space occurs simultaneously with entry of water, which leads to cellular edema and possibly rupture of the cell wall. Trunkey and coworkers[48] demonstrated a marked decrease in the level of primate muscle extracellular water and an increase in the levels of intracellular sodium and water during burn shock. An associated decrease in resting membrane potential occurs as the transmembrane potential is disrupted and results in a decrease in amplitude of the action potential and prolongation of the repolarization and depolarization times.[49,50] As sodium and water enter the cell, the sodium-potassium pump is disrupted and potassium moves out, thus further exacerbating the electrolyte imbalance intracellularly.[51] Calcium channel transport is disrupted, along with a loss of intracellular magnesium and phosphate[43] and an increase in serum lactate dehydrogenase levels.[44] The cascade of events that occurs at the level of the cell membrane suggests impairments of basic cellular function as the underlying cause of the diminished membrane potentials. Although the pathophysiologic mechanism has not been completely described, data suggest a decrease in the efficiency of the sodium-potassium pump, a change that can be reversed over time with adequate fluid resuscitation.

Evidence suggests that the burn wound itself at least partially mediates the physiologic response to burn injury at both local and systemic levels. Burn tissue inflammation can lead to vasodilation, increased capillary permeability and edema, which are normal conditions that promote wound healing. Massive injury results in increased metabolic demands and consumption of inflammatory mediators by the wound, when the priority for survival should be transport of these mediators to healthy tissue.

The extensive evaporative water loss that accompanies burn injury is a heat-consuming process, with the energy need met in part by increased visceral heat production. This hypermetabolic state persists during rest, sleep, and external cooling. The increased oxygen consumption cannot be accounted for on the basis of elevated body temperature alone; thus, an increased basal metabolic rate, not a thermoregulatory drive, is responsible for the increased heat production.

Immune Response

Local and systemic physiologic changes are primarily mediated by the release of cytokines from burn wounds.[52] Cytokines act directly on the burn wound and also activate other agents, including those that release oxidants, arachidonic acid metabolites, and proteases, thereby contributing to further local and systemic inflammation and, potentially, multisystem organ dysfunction. Recent studies have shown a relationship between decreased cellular cytotoxicity in burned patients and increased production of the cytokines IL-4 and IL-10. Administration of immunopotentiators such as IL-12 has also demonstrated increased survival and resistance to bacterial infection.[53]

A host of chemicals found in altered concentrations in burn plasma may also play a role in burn shock. These substances include vasoactive amines (histamine, serotonin), products of complement activation (C3a, C5a), prostaglandins, kinins, endotoxins, and metabolic hormones (catecholamines, glucocorticoids). A decrease in the complement components C3a and C5a in the circulation after burn injury suggests nonspecific activation of the complement system. Activation of the complement system in injured tissue results in an inflammatory response caused by the release of histamine and serotonin by C3a and C5a. Because both histamine and serotonin alter capillary permeability, some investigators propose this mechanism as a cause for burn shock because these vasoactive amines initiate the inflammatory response along with kinin polypeptides and other chemical mediators. As a result of these vascular changes, fluid and fibrinogen leave the dilated, permeable vessels.

Elements of Burn Injury Survival

The emergent phase of burn care refers to the time between the end of burn shock and the closure of the burn wound to less than 20% of the TBSA. Three elements are essential for survival after a major burn injury: meticulous wound management, adequate nutritional support to establish positive nitrogen balance, and timely surgical excision and grafting of full-thickness wounds.

Management of Wounds

Optimal wound management strategies center around measures to limit bacterial proliferation on the wound and adjacent tissue following loss of the first line of defense—the skin. Burn wounds are sterile

initially as a result of thermal decontamination; however, bacterial flora soon re-establish colonies on the burned skin, or eschar. This medium is favorable for pathogenic growth because of the necrotic tissue and warm environment that exist within the burn wound dressing. Benign microorganisms normally found on skin, in the gastrointestinal tract, and in the pulmonary system become lethal as they colonize the burn wound, often resulting in burn progression, invasive sepsis, and death.

The most common source of burn wound bacteria is the patient's own hair follicles, sweat glands, pulmonary tract, and gastrointestinal system, although poor hand-washing technique by staff members can contribute to infection through cross-contamination from other patients.

The goals of wound care are to cleanse and debride the wound of necrotic tissue and debris that promote bacterial growth, minimize further destruction of viable tissue, prevent cross-contamination, preserve body heat and energy, and promote patient comfort. The excision of blisters is controversial and varies among institutions. Some argue that the blister provides a moist and protective environment for healing, whereas others state that large tense blisters apply pressure on the underlying wound bed (which impedes healing) and the contained fluid may serve as a nidus for infection. The decision to debride a blister should take into consideration the size and type of the blister. Blisters less than 6 mm in diameter are unlikely to rupture or place pressure on underlying tissue and should not be debrided. Thick-walled blisters attributable to thick skin, particularly on the hands and feet, should be left intact because they are not likely to become infected and debridement often leads to limited mobility of the affected extremity. Large tense blisters or those with thin walls that are likely to rupture and become infected can impede wound healing, and debridement of these lesions should be considered.[54] This debridement may also allow for further evaluation of the depth of injury in the underlying wound bed. Additional wound care requires daily observation and management, which includes bathing the patient at least once each day with mild soap and water. Burn wounds are washed to remove accumulated bacteria and previously applied ointments and to debride necrotic tissue. Cleansing of wounds is the most stressful and painful experience that burn patients endure. Pain medication diminishes the pain only marginally because the most effective analgesics work best on visceral or deep pain rather than pain at superficial skin nerve endings. Benzodiazepines are often added to decrease anxiety and provide a degree of amnesia.

After the wound is clean, topical antibacterial agents are applied and covered with a light dressing (Table 54-4). Systemic antibiotics are not helpful in controlling burn wound flora because the burn eschar has no blood supply, limiting local antibiotic bioavailability. Topical burn agents penetrate the eschar, thereby inhibiting bacterial invasion of the wound. Systemic antibiotics are administered when the patient demonstrates signs of systemic infection and are used prophylactically at times of surgical procedures. Appropriate antibiotic selection is based on laboratory cultures of the patient's wound tissue to identify and deliver antibiotics to which the bacteria are sensitive.

Healing of burn wounds begins when white blood cells have surrounded the burn wound and phagocytosis begins. Necrotic tissue begins to slough. Fibroblasts begin to build matrices of the collagen precursors that eventually form granulation tissue. Kept free from infection, a partial-thickness burn will heal from the edges and from below in a process that occurs over a 14- to 21-day period. Full-thickness burns require autografting to achieve wound closure because no dermal elements are available to form new skin.

Burn Surgery

The third element essential to survival after major burn injury is surgical excision of dead skin, or burn eschar, followed by skin grafting with the patient's own skin (autograft). Areas of full-thickness burn are

TABLE 54-4 TOPICAL ANTIBIOTIC THERAPY FOR THERMAL INJURY WOUNDS

DRUG	INDICATIONS FOR USE	ADVANTAGES	DISADVANTAGES	METHOD OF USE
Bacitracin	Bland ointment with minimal antibiotic properties used to promote comfort in patients with minor injury (<25% TBSA)	Prevents drying of wounds; keeps eschar soft and pliable; economical; works well on facial burns to promote healing and patient comfort without facial dressings; painless upon application	No major antibiotic properties; oil based, so it is difficult to remove	1. Apply to cleansed wound twice daily; cover with Adaptic and Kerlix 2. Apply to facial burns twice daily 3. Apply to recently grafted or healed areas twice daily; wrap with Adaptic and Kerlix
Silver sulfadiazine (Silvadene)	Partial- and/or full-thickness thermal injury (>25% TBSA); small wounds that require topical antibiotic therapy such as frostbite	Wide-spectrum bacteriostatic action and painless on application; organisms resistant to silver nitrate are usually sensitive to silver sulfadiazine; eschar remains soft and pliable; water miscible base promotes ease of removal	Not effective against fungal organisms; can cause leukopenia and is expensive; sulfa component can produce allergic reactions in sensitive patients; resistance can emerge with prolonged use	Apply to cleansed wound 1-3 times daily; may leave wound open or cover with light dressing
Silver nitrate	Partial- and/or full-thickness burns (>25% TBSA), fungal infections, patients with sulfa allergy	Wide-spectrum bacteriostatic action; effective against fungal infections; comfortable and economical; no sensitivity reported; painless on application; no resistant organisms	Can cause severe electrolyte imbalances (hyponatremia and hypochloremia), which are corrected with oral and intravenous NaCl; poor penetration into wound; requires bulky dressing, thereby severely limiting motion; messy and time consuming to use	0.5% solution in distilled water applied to wet dressing every 2 hr; dressing changes twice daily
Mafenide acetate (Sulfamylon)	Electrical injury, ear burns, wounds colonized with organisms resistant to other topical agents because it penetrates eschar more deeply	Wide-spectrum bacteriostatic action; active penetration allows delayed therapy to be effective; requires no dressing, thereby promoting motion; resistant organisms do not develop with prolonged use; drug of choice for all burns	Causes severe metabolic alterations within 72 hr when used on >20% TBSA wounds; carbonic anhydrase inhibition with excretion and chloride retention; compensation is by hyperventilation with subsequent CO_2 decreased or depletion	Apply to cleansed wound 1-2 times daily; leave open because wrapping produces maceration

From Kravitz M: Thermal injuries. In Cardona VD et al, editors: *Trauma nursing: from resuscitation through rehabilitation*, Philadelphia, 1988, Saunders, p 723.
TBSA, Total body surface area.

excised. In some cases, it is difficult to assess the depth of the burn. In these cases, it may be appropriate to wait 7 to 10 days to allow the area to declare its depth. This is especially true in young children with scald burns. In burns involving the face, scalp, and ears, it may be appropriate to wait as long as 3 weeks for the area to declare itself. These sites are particularly dense areas of dermal appendages and may heal without grafting if given time. Current surgical management of burn wounds has evolved from daily bathing and mechanical debridement of necrotic tissue for months, to early surgical excision and grafting, with significant associated decreases in attendant morbidity and mortality.

Excision and Grafting

Significant blood loss associated with burn excision traditionally resulted in local wound management until eschar separation, at which time grafting was undertaken. This often resulted in prolonged hospital stays of approximately 3 to 5 weeks, increased bacterial colonization of wounds, and subsequent higher incidences of sepsis and multiple organ failure. Current practice now favors early excision and grafting of wounds 2 to 7 days after injury. Although blood loss remains a concern with early excision, improvements in excision and hemostasis techniques have enabled a significant decrease in the degree of magnitude.

In tangential excision, eschar is removed in thin layers with an instrument called a *dermatome* until viable tissue is visible. Full-thickness excision using a surgical scalpel removes eschar to the level of fascia. Full-thickness excision often leaves an uneven contour post-excision, which is difficult to graft, with resultant poor cosmetic effects. After bleeding has been controlled in the area of excision, application of an autograft, skin substitute, or dressing follows. In some cases, the area may need to be covered with wet dressings soaked in antibiotic solutions for 24 hours with delayed autografting. Some studies have shown a benefit for use of a vacuum-assisted closure device to promote blood circulation in the wound bed, allowing for earlier placement of an epidermal graft.[55]

Ong and colleagues[56] conducted a meta-analysis of data from six randomized controlled trials published from 1966 through 2004 that compared early excision of burns with wound dressing and grafting after eschar separation. No difference in overall mortality was observed, except for a lower mortality in the subgroup without inhalation injury that underwent early excision. Early excision patients overall had higher blood transfusion requirements and shorter lengths of stay. No evidence of reduced sepsis or a better cosmetic or functional outcome was noted with early excision.

Skin Substitutes

In patients with burns that do not permit initial autografting, temporary coverage may be achieved by use of any of the following skin substitutes: biological (homograft—skin harvested from cadavers, xenograft—skin harvested from pigs); synthetic; and amnion (amniotic lining of human placenta harvested from afterbirth following delivery). Application often enhances patient comfort while partially restoring the water vapor barrier, thereby minimizing evaporative losses. Grafts often consist of a bilayer membrane that provides a dermal matrix of bovine collagen and an epidermal or silicone layer to prevent desiccation (drying), or the dermal and epidermal components may be replaced separately.[57] Bioactive dermal components added to the graft help to stimulate healing and include elastin, fibronectin, growth factors, glycosaminoglycans, and hyaluronic acid. The composition of a permanent skin substitute often includes the patient's own cells in either the dermal or the epidermal layer. The dermal matrix allows ingrowth of capillaries and fibroblasts. This matrix is slowly degraded as a neodermis develops. The silicone layer acting as the epidermal barrier is then removed and autograft is applied over the neodermis.[58]

The unburned area of the patient from which skin is harvested in a paper-thin sheet is referred to as the *donor site*. Donor sites heal in about 5 to 7 days in the presence of adequate nutritional support and the absence of infection and can be reharvested at that time. Donor sites can be repeatedly harvested depending on graft thickness, enabling increased wound coverage, which thereby permits survival in some patients with TBSA injury as large as 90%. To expand the surface area that a sheet of autograft will cover, harvested skin is cut in a manner that resembles a net or mesh by using an instrument called a *skin mesher*. The skin may then be expanded, depending on the size of the mesh, to cover two, three, four, or more times its original size. This combination of repeated harvesting and meshing allows autografting of massive burn injuries over a period of a few weeks. After grafting, the areas must be protected from infection, pressure, shearing, and trauma that produce bruising or bleeding under the graft. Major causes of graft loss include infection, blisters, or hematoma underneath the graft that interferes with revascularization. Negative-pressure dressings or vacuum-assisted closure (VAC) devices placed over a graft improve the contact surface of the graft as well as prevent underlying accumulation of serum or blood. When compared to standard bulky dressings, use of these devices has demonstrated a decrease in loss of graft, a decreased need for secondary grafting procedures on the same wound, and a resulting decrease in hospital stay for these procedures.[59]

The greatest risk of infection is after postoperative day 3, when the bacteria begin to recolonize the area. Grafts are usually stable by postoperative day 4, at which time physical and occupational therapy may begin.[10,60]

Surgical wound management of elderly burn patients is determined by the philosophy of the burn center. Elderly patients do not generally tolerate any surgical procedure as well as younger patients; this knowledge has been applied to the management of burn wounds in some patients, and conservative, nonsurgical wound management for weeks after injury has produced acceptable survival rates in elderly patients.[61] Others report that early excision of eschar and early wound closure are associated with increased survival and decreased length of stay for older patients with burns.[62] Children younger than 2 years have a high mortality with major burn injury, but older children recover at a high rate with proper medical management.[16,18,31] Table 54-5 summarizes physiologic changes related to the aging process that can affect surgical outcome.

Nutritional Support

One of the most significant advances in recent burn management is recognition of the critical importance of early nutrition to the wound-healing process. The magnitude of nutritional support required by burn patients depends on two factors: the patient's preburn nutritional status and the extent of the TBSA burn. Patients with minor burns require no nutritional support beyond a regular diet, whereas those with moderate and large burns require additional carbohydrate and protein supplementation. Patients with poor preburn nutritional status are classified as having a critical injury regardless of the burn size because of the associated immune deficiencies and limited metabolic reserves. The most easily recognized and documented finding in the absence of adequate nutritional support after burn injury is massive loss of body weight. Maintenance of body protein is critical for healing, minimizing complications, and survival. A 10% loss of total body mass leads to immune dysfunction; 20%, to decreased wound healing; 30%, to severe infections; and 40%, to death.[63]

Patients with greater than a 40% TBSA burn demonstrate the maximal stress response within predictable ranges of body mass. In these hypermetabolic patients, providing early protein and caloric support of at least the predicted energy requirement is necessary for optimal outcome and may be essential for survival. Providing early nutrition in enteral form may also help by blunting the hypermetabolic response to thermal injury.[64] Weight loss after thermal injury is not an obligatory component of the response to trauma but rather a reflection of the difference between the total energy requirements and the ability to supply them in the form of adequate caloric intake.[13] Kao and colleagues demonstrated that enteral feeding should begin within 18 hours of admission with a Dobhoff feeding tube.[65] These feedings should be continuous and should not be stopped when the patient goes to the operating room. With vigorous nutritional support, erosion of total body mass and subsequent starvation leading to immunologic alteration are not inevitable in a massively burned patient.[51,66,67]

General formulas are used to estimate the caloric requirements of burn patients, all of which are based on either preburn body weight and % of TBSA burn or square meters of body surface area and % of TBSA burn. The two most widely used formulas are the Curreri formula for adults and the Polk formula for children. Curreri and colleagues[68] demonstrated that caloric requirements in adult burn patients could be expressed by the following formula:

$$(25) \times (\text{body weight in kg}) + (40) \times (\% \text{ TBSA burn}) =$$
$$\text{Ideal 24-hour caloric needs}$$

The requirements in children[69] are predicted as follows:

$$(60) \times (\text{body weight in kg}) + (36) \times (\% \text{ TBSA burn}) =$$
$$\text{Ideal 24-hour caloric needs}$$

If the ideal daily caloric intake can be maintained, then the amount of postburn weight loss could be minimized. It is important to emphasize that these formulas represent more than just total caloric intake; they are used to predict positive nitrogen balance for each patient. Thus, if the patient is losing tremendous amounts of nitrogen or is not absorbing glucose, the net caloric utilization will be much less than the intake, even though the adult patient may be receiving as much as 5000 kcal/day. Monitoring of daily nitrogen balance by indirect calorimetry is essential throughout the course of burn treatment to ensure a positive nitrogen balance (nonprotein kilocalorie to nitrogen ratio of 100:1 and at least 2 grams of protein per kilogram per day). The serum prealbumin concentration is a useful indicator of nutritional progress.

The routes for initiating caloric support after major burn injury are either enteral or parenteral. Any patient with a functioning gastrointestinal tract should receive enteral nutrition orally, by tube feeding, or by a combination of both. Early enteral nutrition has been shown

TABLE 54-5 PHYSIOLOGIC CHANGES RELATED TO THE AGING PROCESS THAT CAN AFFECT SURGERY

PHYSIOLOGIC CHANGES	EFFECTS	POTENTIAL POSTOPERATIVE COMPLICATION
Cardiovascular		
↓ Elasticity of blood vessels	↓ Circulation to vital organs	Shock (hypotension), thrombosis with pulmonary emboli, delayed wound healing, postoperative confusion, hypervolemia, decreased response to stress
↓ Cardiac output	Slower blood flow	
↓ Peripheral circulation		
Respiratory		
↓ Elasticity of lungs and chest wall	↓ Vital capacity	Atelectasis, pneumonia, postoperative confusion
↑ Residual lung volume	↓ Alveolar volume	
↓ Forced expiratory volume	↓ Gas exchange	
↓ Ciliary action	↓ Cough reflex	
Fewer alveolar capillaries		
Urinary		
↓ Glomerular filtration rate	↓ Kidney function	Prolonged response to anesthesia and drugs, overhydration with intravenous fluids, hyperkalemia, urinary tract infection, urinary retention
↓ Bladder muscle tone	Stasis of urine in bladder	
Weakened perineal muscles	Loss of urinary control	
Musculoskeletal		
↓ Muscle strength	↓ Activity	Atelectasis, pneumonia, thrombophlebitis, constipation or fecal impaction
Limitation of motion		
Gastrointestinal		
↓ Intestinal motility	Retention of feces	Constipation or fecal impaction
Metabolic		
↓ γ-Globulin level	↓ Inflammatory response	Delayed wound healing, wound dehiscence or evisceration
↓ Plasma proteins		
Immune		
Fewer killer T cells	↓ Ability to protect against invasion by pathogenic microorganisms	Wound infection, wound dehiscence, pneumonia, urinary tract infection
↓ Response to foreign antigens		

From Keeling AW, Muro GA, Long BC: Preoperative nursing. In Phipps WJ et al, editors: *Medical-surgical nursing: concepts and clinical practice,* ed 5, St Louis, 1995, Mosby.

to effectively deliver caloric requirements (resting energy expenditure [REE]) by postburn day 3; diminish the hypermetabolic response; decrease circulating levels of catecholamines, cortisol, and glucagon; and preserve gut mucosal integrity, motility, and intestinal blood flow, which serves to decrease bacterial translocation and lower the incidence of intestinal ischemia.[70] Postburn ileus primarily affects the stomach and colon.[71] Patients with severe burn injuries may be fed through enteral tubes to the small bowel (duodenum or jejunum) as early as 6 hours' postburn, independent of total gastroduodenal function.[72] In a large meta-analysis conducted in critically ill patients that included a small number of burned patients, a grade B evidence-based recommendation was made for the use of parenteral nutrition for patients in whom enteral nutrition cannot be started within the first 24 hours of hospital admission. A subgroup analysis attributed a mortality risk reduction to parenteral nutrition versus delayed (>24 hours) enteral nutrition, despite an association with increased infectious complications with parenteral nutrition.[73,74]

Hart and colleagues demonstrated that the catabolic response may persist for up to 12 months in adults and 24 months in children.[75] Given this information, the nutritional status and dietary habits of burn patients should be continually evaluated for many months after their discharge from the burn unit.

Rehabilitation Phase

The rehabilitation phase begins when the burn size is reduced to less than 20% of the TBSA and the patient is capable of assuming some self-care. This phase may occur as early as 2 weeks or as long as 2 to 3 months after the burn and, in the case of a major debilitating or disfiguring injury, may last many years. Goals for this period are to assist the patient in resuming a functional role in society and to accomplish functional and cosmetic reconstruction.[10,15,17]

Wound Healing

During the rehabilitation phase, the pathophysiologic mechanism of hypermetabolism and the impaired immune function have begun to normalize, although some changes will persist beyond discharge from the hospital. The major pathophysiologic process of this phase is related to the dysfunctional results of wounds healing in a manner that causes flexor contractures, excessive scarring, and keloid formation. The burn wounds have healed either by primary intention or by autografting. Layers of epithelialization begin rebuilding the tissue structure destroyed by the burn injury. Collagen fibers present in the new scar tissue help healing and add strength to weakened areas. After healing, the new skin appears flat and pink, even in dark-skinned people.

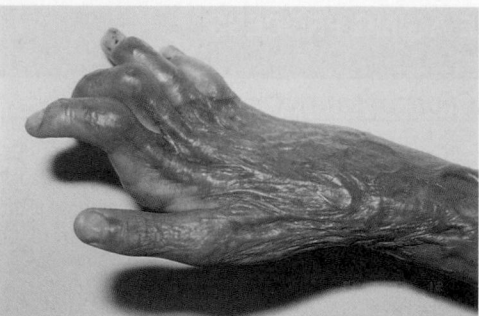

FIGURE 54-7 Physical and occupational therapy is necessary from the time of injury. This 8-year-old girl was burned 4 years previously in a house fire. Inadequate follow-up care because of parental neglect led to severe scar contractures and hand disability. (Courtesy Michael Peck, MD, University of North Carolina Burn Center, Chapel Hill.)

In approximately 4 to 6 weeks the area becomes raised and hyperemic. If adequate range-of-motion exercises are not instituted early in the hospital course, the new tissue will shorten and a contracture will result (Figure 54-7).[10,15] Mature healing is reached in 6 to 12 months, when suppleness has returned and the pink or red color has faded to a slightly lighter hue than the surrounding unburned tissue. It takes longer for darker skin to regain its color because many of the melanocytes were destroyed, and often the skin never returns to its original color. The mesh pattern in meshed autograft fades with time, but in larger expansions such as 4:1 or greater the pattern may persist.

Scarring has two components: discoloration and contour. The discoloration of scars fades with time and can be covered with makeup on visible body surface areas. However, scar tissue tends to develop altered contours; that is, the skin is no longer flat but becomes raised above the contour of the surrounding area (also known as hypertrophic scarring). Areas of the face tend to scar in an even plane—a process that distorts the natural contours around the nose, chin, and mouth and thus greatly alters a patient's appearance. Scarring on the cheeks can contract and pull the lower eyelid down sufficiently to prevent closure and protection of the eye normally afforded by the eyelid—a condition called ectropion. Burns on the eyelid can also result in ectropion and must be corrected by reconstructive surgery. Pressure can help keep a scar flat if the pressure is slightly greater than capillary pressure and is continuous during the healing process. This knowledge led to the development of burn garments, which are custom-made for each patient to contour with pressure over the area of burn for about 12 to 18 months after burn injury. Except for bath times, the garments must be worn continuously; patient compliance often becomes an issue (Figure 54-8).

Excessive and sometimes debilitating discomfort from pruritus occurs in the healing burn wound and persists for many months. The exact pathophysiologic process is not known but is related to the absence of sebaceous glands in the area and to the hyperactivity of sweat glands. Topical lotions and orally administered antihistamines provide partial relief of symptoms, but tolerance to the drugs develops and patients often require a series of different medications over time. The newly formed skin is extremely sensitive to trauma, and blisters form after very slight pressure or friction. The newly healed areas may be hypersensitive or hyposensitive to cold, heat, or touch. Ward and colleague[76] studied loss of cutaneous sensibility after grafting in 60 patients and found that 97% demonstrated markedly diminished or absent responses to sharp/dull, hot/cold, and light touch stimuli over the grafted areas. Grafted areas are more likely to be hyposensitive until peripheral nerve regeneration occurs, although donor sites harvested several times will show all the same healing pathologic process as healed burn wounds.

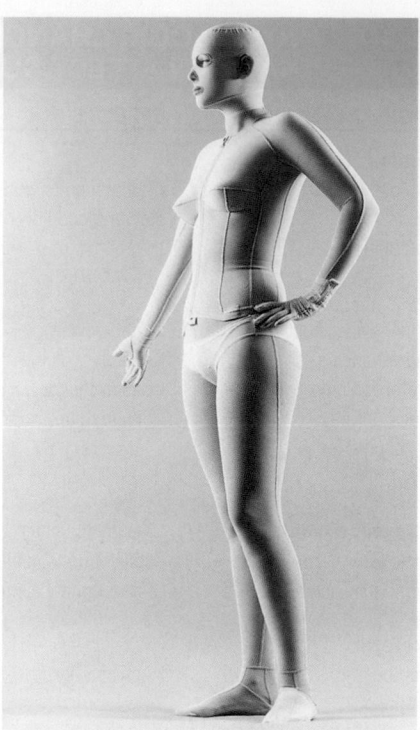

FIGURE 54-8 The custom-fitted anti-scar support garment modeled here effectively provides pressure therapy over wounds, which helps to minimize the development of hypertrophic scarring. (From Black JM, Hawks JH, editors: *Medical-surgical nursing: clinical management for positive outcomes,* ed 7, Philadelphia, 2005, Saunders. Courtesy Medical Z, San Antonio, TX.)

Scarring is a genetically inherited trait. Some people will have minimal scarring, whereas others, especially African Americans and Caucasians with red hair, tend to have significant scarring and keloid formation in which the scar tissue actually outgrows the boundary of the original wound. Healed burn wounds must be protected from direct sunlight for 1 year to prevent hyperpigmentation.

The most common complications during the rehabilitation phase are related to the formation of skin and joint contractures. Because of pain associated with movement, the patient will want to assume the position of comfort, which is with all extremities flexed, but this position predisposes to contracture formation. To minimize contracture formation, positioning in extension, splinting in the position of function, and performing active range-of-motion exercises are initiated on admission and continue throughout the course of treatment. The areas most subject to contracture formation include the anterior and lateral neck areas, axillae, antecubital fossae, fingers, groin areas, popliteal fossae, and ankles. Not only do contractures develop in the skin, but also the underlying tissues such as ligaments and tendons have a tendency to shorten during the healing process. Therapy is aimed at extension of body parts to ensure that the flexors are longer than the extensors.[10]

> **KEY POINTS**
> - The emergent phase is the time between the end of burn shock and closure of the wound to less than 20% of the TBSA. Wound management, nutritional support, and surgical grafting of full-thickness wounds are the priorities of treatment during the emergent phase.
> - Wound management is necessary to prevent bacterial colonization of the wound and subsequent septicemia. Early surgical wound management is

essential. Topical antibiotics are used because systemic antibiotics cannot reach the wound because of a lack of blood supply.

- Nutritional requirements after burn injury are high. A high-calorie, high-protein diet is needed. Persons with major burns usually cannot ingest sufficient nutrients and require parenteral and enteral supplementation. A positive nitrogen balance is essential for healing.

- Early surgical excision and skin grafting are the treatments of choice for deep burns. Excision procedures result in significant blood loss requiring blood transfusions. Skin grafts are taken from a healthy portion of the patient's skin. Temporary grafts (e.g., cadaver skin, synthetics, porcine skin) may be used to cover the wound until an autograft can be obtained.

- The rehabilitation phase begins when the burn is reduced to less than 20% of the TBSA. Problems during this phase include skin contracture and excessive scarring. Healing is complete at 6 to 12 months. Positioning in extension and performing range-of-motion exercises are important to prevent contracture.

ELECTRICAL INJURY

Incidence and Mortality

Electrical injury accounts for fewer than 2% of admissions to burn facilities; however, their incidence has been increasing in the United States.[77] Based on data from the National Institute for Occupational Safety and Health (NIOSH) National Traumatic Occupational Fatalities (NTOF) surveillance system, electrocutions were the fifth-leading cause of death from 1980 through 1992.[78]

Electrical injuries are classified as high-voltage (1000 volts or greater) or low-voltage. Household currents of 120 and 220 volts typically cause low-voltage electrical injury. High-voltage injuries are frequently due to high-tension sources, which commonly carry from 7200 to 19,000 volts (Figure 54-9) but may involve 100,000 to 1 million volts.[79]

According to the National Weather Service Storm Data, between the 1981-2010 the United States has averaged 55 *reported* lightning fatalities per year. Of all lightning strikes, only 10% are fatal, leaving 90% with various degrees of disability.[80] Lightning injuries kill between 150 and 300 people per year in the United States.[81] Lightning carries a direct current of 100 million or more volts and up to 200,000 amperes, and it can injure either by a direct strike or by a side flash as a result of the flow of current between the victim's body and a nearby object struck by lightning.[81]

Arnoldo and colleagues reviewed electrical injuries at a single institution over a 20-year period and reported that the highest mortality resulted from lightning strikes (17.6%) followed by high-voltage (5.3%) and low-voltage (2.8%) injuries, with the lowest electrical injury mortality resulting from electric arc injuries without passage of current through the patient (1.1%). Complication rates, mean length of hospital stay (18.9 ± 1.4 days), and number of operative procedures (3.0 ± 0.2) were increased in the high-voltage group. Work-related activity was responsible for the majority of these high-voltage injuries, with the most common occupations being linemen and electricians.[82]

Pathophysiology

The pathophysiologic mechanism of electrical injury is related to the subsequent tissue damage as electrical energy is converted to heat. Workplace electrocutions account for 5% of all worker deaths.[83] In children, electrical burns account for 2% to 3% of all burns, and 60% to 70% of these result from biting extension cords.[84,85]

Arcing electricity produces surface heat, which may ignite clothing and destroy superficial tissue, but internal damage is absent; this injury is actually a flame or thermal injury and not electrical. These injuries are properly classified as heat injuries, for which the treatment plan is identical to that for other heat injuries.[77] True electrical injury occurs as electrical current enters the body, traverses a portion of the body, and exits at another body site. Electrical injuries are usually deeper than full-thickness skin injury and are often classified as fourth-degree injury.

Voltage, type of current (direct or alternating), and length of contact all influence the extent of damage. Alternating current (AC) produces prolonged tetanic muscle contraction. At low voltages it can cause ventricular fibrillation, tetanic contraction of the respiratory muscles, superficial burns, and rhabdomyolysis. At lower voltage, AC is associated with low mortality. High-voltage AC or direct current (DC) causes ventricular fibrillation, a single sustained contraction, rhabdomyolysis, and higher overall mortality.[86]

Each true electrical injury produces an entrance wound and at least one exit wound, with the most extensive damage commonly occurring at the exit point. Electrical current follows the path of least resistance: in humans, this path is through blood vessels, nerves, tendons, and bone. Skin has high resistance; thus the current enters through the skin but goes deeper to travel the path of least resistance until it exits the body. The current rarely produces direct visceral damage, but severe injuries to the extremities are common. The amputation rate after severe electrical injury exceeds 90%. The pathophysiologic process, in addition to direct tissue destruction, involves heat coagulation of blood vessels, which leaves distal areas without blood supply. Electrical injuries produce both systemic and local alterations. The systemic changes produce three common complications during the acute period: dysrhythmias or cardiac arrest, metabolic acidosis, and myoglobinuria. Electrical injury may also cause direct myocardial necrosis. Dysrhythmias are exacerbated by any given voltage of AC. Higher voltage may also cause asystole. Locally, electrical injury produces direct cellular denaturation; areas of healthy tissue are devascularized as a result of heat coagulation of arteries and veins. These events are followed 48 to 72 hours after injury by gross tissue necrosis and subsequent gangrene resulting from lack of blood flow. Amputation is required early in electrical injury to prevent the development of deep soft-tissue infections and sepsis, leading to death.

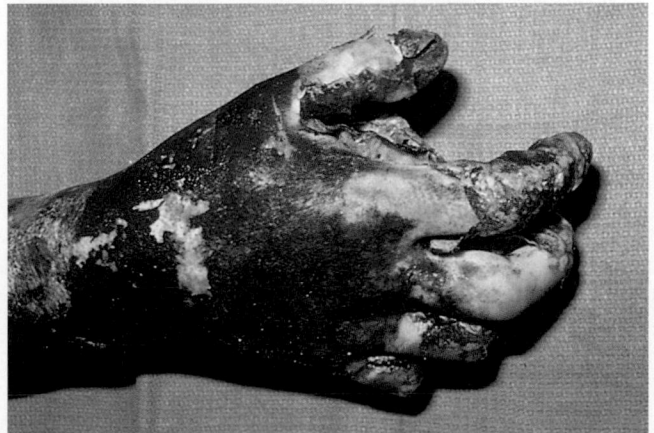

FIGURE 54-9 High-voltage electrical injuries produce devastating consequences, such as the damage to the right hand of this electrician who inadvertently contacted a 17,000 V line. The underlying muscle damage is often greater than that found in a thermal skin burn. Myoglobinuria, if inadequately managed, can lead to acute tubular necrosis. Early fasciotomies are mandatory, and amputation may be necessary to control rhabdomyolysis. (Courtesy Michael Peck, MD, University of North Carolina Burn Center, Chapel Hill.)

Management and Complications

Once the patient is admitted, airway management is the primary focus; patients with major electrical injury often require endotracheal intubation to ensure a patent airway. A condition similar to burn shock develops within a few minutes of major electrical injury and requires similar fluid resuscitation measures; however, there is no standardized formula to predict fluid requirements because often the only apparent damage is the entrance and exit wounds and no assessment of internal damage is possible. An adult patient is given a 1-L bolus of Ringer lactate solution intravenously within the first 15 minutes after intravenous line placement; children are given a smaller, size-appropriate amount. Thereafter, fluid is infused at a rate to produce a urine volume of 100 ml/hr in adults and 1 to 2 ml/kg/hr in children. Adult patients frequently require 1 to 2 L of fluid per hour to support the cardiovascular system.

Cardiovascular complications associated with lightning injury range from benign electrocardiogram (ECG) changes to sudden cardiac death. Atrial or ventricular fibrillation and T-wave inversions and prolonged QT intervals are the more common dysrhythmias and ECG findings. Traditionally, cardiac monitoring has been performed on these patients for the first 24 hours after injury. Bailey and colleagues determined that this is unnecessary, however, if the initial ECG is normal, there is no loss of consciousness at the scene, and the patient is an adult; 24-hour monitoring is indicated in adult patients with an abnormal initial ECG, a history of cardiac disease, positive loss of consciousness at the scene, and/or exposure to a voltage greater than 240 volts.[86] Measurement of the levels of cardiac enzymes initially reveals elevated values, also suggesting acute myocardial damage, but in such patients these findings are not indicative of a cardiac pathologic process.

Electrical injury also produces a profound, potentially lethal metabolic acidosis. These patients often have initial serum pH values of 6.8 to 7.2 on admission. Treatment consists of intravenous administration of sodium bicarbonate in amounts to correct the values toward normal. Metabolic acidosis is a recurring problem requiring ongoing treatment until it has been resolved for 24 to 48 hours after injury. The pathophysiologic mechanism is related both to the release of intracellular contents into the general circulation from areas of tissue damage and to the development of lactic acidosis that accompanies hypotensive shock states.

Myoglobinuria follows electrical injury as myoglobin, a component of muscle tissue, is released from muscles damaged by electrical current and enters the systemic circulation.[87] Myoglobin is a large protein that precipitates in the renal tubules and leads to cast formation. Subsequently, the tubules become obstructed and renal tubular acidosis develops. This accumulation is prevented by maintaining urine output at 100 to 200 ml/hr in adults and 2 ml/kg/hr in children until the urine clears. Mannitol, an osmotic diuretic, is administered along with large volumes of intravenous fluids to prevent the development of acute tubular necrosis, a totally preventable sequela of electrical injury with proper management. Sodium bicarbonate is often administered to alkalinize the urine, thereby increasing the solubility of myoglobin.

Local effects of electrical injury are related to alterations in tissue perfusion. Surgical decompression of areas of electrical burn by fasciotomy is performed for the purpose of releasing any increased compartment pressures that may be compromising blood flow. Amputation may be required during the initial surgery for devascularized areas. Because of the continued presence of necrotic tissue, areas of surgical decompression or initial amputation are not closed surgically.[88]

Central nervous system alterations can be noted in patients with major electrical injury. Memory deficits can occur for several weeks. This condition improves gradually and usually resolves within 4 to 6 weeks after injury. Other central nervous system deficits after electrical injury include ataxia and gait alterations accompanied by sensory deficits. These alterations may or may not improve over time. Electrically injured patients experience all the challenges of rehabilitation plus possible adjustments to amputation and gait instability related to central nervous system impairment. Skin grafting in areas adjacent to amputation presents challenging prosthetic problems that may delay independent ambulation and restoration of self-care abilities.[89] In general, patients with major electrical injury experience longer rehabilitation periods than do thermally injured patients.

A unique complication of electrical injury is the formation of corneal cataracts,[90] which can be detected as early as 1 month post injury. Ophthalmic examinations should be performed monthly for the first year and every 3 months for 1 year thereafter to enable early identification. Patients will usually complain of blurring vision, but young children may not report this visual change because they do not recognize the concept. Treatment consists of corneal transplantation.[90]

KEY POINTS

- Broadly speaking, persons wounded by major electrical burns have longer periods of rehabilitation than thermally injured patients. Systemic involvement is complex. Each true electrical injury produces an entrance wound and at least one exit wound, with the most extensive damage commonly occurring at the exit point.
- Management for electrical injury includes core practices of maintenance of airway, breathing, and circulation. Once the patient is admitted to the hospital for a serious electrical burn, airway management is the primary focus.
- A condition similar to burn shock develops within a few minutes of major electrical injury and requires similar fluid resuscitation measures; however, there is no standardized formula to predict fluid requirements because often the only apparent damage is the entrance and exit wounds and no assessment of internal damage is possible.
- Cardiovascular complications associated with electrical (lightning) injury range from benign electrocardiogram (ECG) changes to sudden cardiac death. Twenty-four-hour monitoring is indicated in adult patients with an abnormal initial ECG, a history of cardiac disease, positive loss of consciousness at the scene, and/or exposure to a voltage greater than 240 volts.
- Electrical injury also produces a profound, potentially lethal metabolic acidosis. These patients often have initial serum pH values of 6.8 to 7.2 on admission.
- Treatment for metabolic acidosis consists of IV administration of sodium bicarbonate. Metabolic acidosis is a recurring problem requiring ongoing treatment until resolved for 24-48 hours after injury. The pathophysiologic mechanisms are related both to the release of intracellular contents into the general circulation from areas of tissue damage and to the development of lactic acidosis that accompanies hypotensive shock states.
- Myoglobinuria follows electrical injury as myoglobin, a component of muscle tissue, is released from muscles damaged by electrical current and enters the systemic circulation. Myoglobin is a large protein that precipitates in the renal tubules and leads to cast formation. Subsequently, the tubules become obstructed and renal tubular acidosis develops.
- Accumulation of myoglobin is prevented by maintaining urine output at 100-200 ml/hr in adults and 2 ml/kg/hr in children until the urine clears. Mannitol, an osmotic diuretic, is administered along with large volumes of IV fluids to prevent the development of acute tubular necrosis. With proper treatment, acute tubular necrosis is totally preventable. Sodium bicarbonate is often administered to alkalinize the urine, thereby increasing the solubility of myoglobin.

- Local effects of electrical injury are related to alterations in tissue perfusion. Because of the continued presence of necrotic tissue, areas of surgical decompression or initial amputation are not closed surgically.
- Electrically injured patients experience all the challenges of rehabilitation plus possible adjustments to amputation and gait instability related to central nervous system impairment.
- A unique complication of electrical injury is the formation of corneal cataracts, which can be detected as early as 1 month post injury. Treatment consists of corneal transplantation.

CHEMICAL INJURY

Management and Complications

Chemicals are a mainstay in our everyday lives and encompass a diverse spectrum, ranging from occupational to household exposures. Chemical burns accounted for 3% of admissions to burn centers in the United States between 2000 and 2009.[91] Management protocols for these injuries share some basic core principles, yet have unique aspects depending upon chemical composition, making accurate knowledge of involved chemical(s) imperative.

Acids predominantly produce a coagulation necrosis by denaturing proteins and forming a coagulum (eschar) that limits the penetration of the acid. In contrast, alkalis produce a liquefaction necrosis that, in addition to involving denaturing proteins, also results in fat saponification, which does not limit tissue penetration and results in more severe injuries. The severity of a chemical burn is related to a number of factors including the agent's pH, concentration, volume, and physical form as well as the length of contact time. To minimize local and systemic toxic effects, it is critical that treatment be initiated immediately.

Initial management strategies include removing any contaminated clothing, brushing off dry agents, and irrigating with copious amounts of water. Care providers must ensure that they have taken the appropriate protection measures to avoid self exposure as established by the Occupational Safety and Health Administration (OSHA). Water irrigation is contraindicated for certain chemicals and metals such as lime, phenol, muriatic acid, concentrated sulfuric acid (52% to 100%), elemental potassium, and sodium,[92] because it may result in an exothermic reaction or release of hazardous by-products. Antidotes have a minor role in the management of most chemical burns except for those secondary to hydrofluoric acid.

The true extent of chemical burns is often difficult to appreciate in the acute setting given the nature of these injuries to continue to evolve over time following exposure. As a result, a lack of appreciation for unrecognized deep tissue involvement may result in inadequate initial management. Systemic toxicity associated with these injuries occurs primarily as a result of absorption through the skin and inhalation.

Comprehensive management guidelines for clinicians for specific chemical exposures are readily accessible online at www.osha.gov/dts/bestpractices/htm/hospital or by calling regional poison control centers. The World Health Organization provides a listing of international poison centers online at www.who.int/gho/phe/chemical safety/poisons centers/en/index.html.

Common Agents and Treatment
Hydrofluoric Acid

Hydrofluoric acid is a highly corrosive inorganic acid used in glass etching, electronic industries, and cleaning solutions. Symptomatic manifestation following exposure is dependent upon solution concentration, with concentrations greater than 15% manifesting more acutely. Because of the ability of hydrofluoric acid to penetrate tissue, poisoning can occur readily through exposure of skin or eyes, or when inhaled or swallowed. Symptoms of exposure to hydrofluoric acid may not be immediately evident. Hydrofluoric acid interferes with nerve function, meaning that burns may not initially be painful. Accidental exposures can go unnoticed, delaying treatment and increasing the extent and seriousness of the injury.

Hydrofluoric acid penetrates quickly into the dermis and deeper structures, where the fluoride ion forms complexes with calcium and magnesium. This complex formation in conjunction with the direct cardiotoxic effects of fluoride ions may contribute to the development of cardiac dysrhythmias, which are the primary cause of death in these patients.

Management of burn injuries consists of copious water irrigation and calcium administration. Calcium ions form complexes with free fluoride ions, thereby minimizing toxicity while also helping to correct any associated hypocalcemia. Calcium gluconate (2.5%) gel is massaged into affected areas for 30 to 60 minutes.[93,94] If discomfort persists, 5% calcium gluconate (0.5 ml/cm^2 wound area) may be injected intradermally directly into and around the affected areas. Injection directly into digits is not recommended. Burns refractory to these initial measures may necessitate intraarterial administration of calcium gluconate. This should only be undertaken in conjunction with the appropriate toxicology expert.[95] In cases where systemic toxicity is suspected (prolongation of QT interval, dysrhythmias) intravenous calcium and magnesium replacement should be considered.

Anhydrous Ammonia

Anhydrous ammonia is a colorless, pungent gas usually stored as a pressurized liquid at $-33°$ C ($-28°$ F) and used extensively as a fertilizer and in the manufacture of synthetic fibers and methamphetamine. Exposure generally results in a combination of alkali burns and cold injury.[96] It is extremely water soluble and immediate treatment consists of copious water irrigation after all clothing has been removed. Repeat irrigation should be performed every 4 to 6 hours for the first 24 hours. Inhalation injury is concentration-dependent and may range from minor airway irritation to laryngospasm, glottic edema, and pulmonary edema. Early intubation in patients with suspected or clinical evidence of significant inhalation exposure is critical. There is unfortunately no specific therapy for these inhalation injuries except supportive care.

Cement Burns

Wet cement is highly alkalotic, with the pH increasing as the cement sets. Burn symptoms are generally delayed, with partial- or full-thickness burns not becoming evident for up to 48 hours.[97] Immediate treatment with copious water irrigation is highly effective in preventing injury progression. Management of burns is similar to that used for secondary thermal injuries. Prevention education that promotes appropriate use of protective gear can be highly successful in minimizing these injuries.

Chemicals Associated With Automobile Airbag Burns

Airbag perforations during deployment have been reported to cause both thermal and alkaline burns (sodium azide or sodium hydroxide).[98] Lack of recognition of associated airbag rupture often results in failure to treat the potential alkali component of the burn and therefore concomitant injury progression. Management is simply irrigation with copious amounts of water.

Tar and Asphalt

In construction, both tar and asphalt are heated to high temperatures (approximately 140° C for paving; approximately 245° C for roofing); however, they cool rapidly. Initial treatment of injuries sustained by these substances consists of accelerating cooling by application of cold water. Subsequent removal of the substances, which may require multiple applications, can be facilitated by the application of several organic solvents (polymyxin-neomycin-bacitracin, petrolatum, sunflower oil, olive oil, butter, and baby oil).[99] Associated burns are treated in a fashion similar to that used in thermal burn treatment.

KEY POINTS

- Burn injuries can be caused by thermal, electrical, or chemical agents. Depending on the cause, burn injuries influence a variety of complex systemic, circulatory, and metabolic changes.
- Management protocols for chemical burns share some basic core principles with electrical and thermal wounds, yet chemical injuries have unique treatment aspects depending on the composition of the etiologic agent, making accurate knowledge of involved chemical(s) imperative.
- To assist the clinician in the treatment of burns, comprehensive current management guidelines for specific exposures are also accessible online.
- The true extent of chemical burns is often difficult to appreciate, given that the nature of these injuries continues to evolve over the time following exposure.
- Systemic toxicity associated with chemical injuries occurs primarily as a result of absorption through the skin and by inhalation.

▌SUMMARY

In recent decades, burn mortality rates have decreased significantly, with most patients achieving excellent functional and cosmetic outcomes. Improved outcomes have clearly been related to an improved understanding of the pathophysiologic mechanism of burns, advances in burn care management, and the development of a comprehensive, patient-centered, treatment-oriented approach.

Priorities for assessment and treatment of burn victims are no different than those of other trauma patients. However, accurate wound management depends upon precise identification of the cause of the burn injury.

As a result, patient care is extremely complex. In order to make appropriate treatment decisions and recognize potential complications, a clear understanding of the etiologic agent of the burn injury, the associated pathophysiologic processes, and the importance of supportive care, treatment, and rehabilitation for the involved person are essential.

REFERENCES

1. American Burn Association: *Burn incidence and treatment in the United States: 2011 fact sheet.* Available at www.ameriburn.org/resources_factsheet.php. Accessed 3/24/12.
2. Arturson G: Pathophysiology of the burn wound and pharmacological treatment, *Burns* 22(4):255–274, 1996.
3. Nguyen TT, et al: Current treatment of severely burned patients, *Ann Surg* 223(1):14–25, 1996.
4. Sheridan RL: Burns, *Crit Care Med* 30(Suppl 11):S500–S514, 2002.
5. American College of Surgeons Committee on Trauma: *Resources for optimal care of the injured patient*, Chicago, 2006, The College, p 79.
6. National Center for Injury Prevention and Control: *Fire deaths and injuries*. Available at www.cdc.gov/HomeandRecreationalSafety/Fire-Prevention/fires-factsheet.html. Accessed 3/24/12.
7. Karter MJ: *Fire loss in the United States during 2010*, Quincy, MA, 2011, National Fire Protection Association, Fire Analysis and Research Division. Available at www.nfpa.org/assets/files/PDF/OS.fireloss.pdf. Accessed 3/24/12.
8. Istre GR, et al: Residential fire related deaths and injuries among children: fireplay, smoke alarms, and prevention, *Inj Prev* 8(2):128–132, 2002.
9. Safe Kids USA: *Burn and scalds safety*, Washington, DC, 2007. Available at www.usa.safekids.org/assets/docs/ourwork/research/burn-scalds.pdf. Accessed 3/24/12.
10. Richard R: OT/PT forum, *J Burn Care Rehabil* 23(3):220, 2002.
11. Ahrens M: *Home structure fires*. Quincy, MA, 2011, National Fire Protection Association. Available at www.nfpa.org/assets/files/PDF/OS.Homes.pdf. Accessed 3/24/12.
12. Muller MJ, Pegg SP, Rule MR: Determinants of death following burn injury, *Br J Surg* 88(4):583–587, 2001.
13. Gore DC, et al: Hyperglycemia exacerbates muscle protein catabolism in burn-injured patients, *Crit Care Med* 30(11):2438–2442, 2002.
14. Ho WS, Ying SY, Burd A: Outcome analysis of 286 severely burned patients: retrospective study, *Hong Kong Med J* 8(4):235–239, 2002.
15. Young A: Rehabilitation of burn injuries (review), *Phys Med Rehabil Clin North Am* 13(1):85–108, 2002.
16. Stoddard FJ, et al: Treatment of pain in acutely burned children, *J Burn Care Rehabil* 23(2):135–156, 2002.
17. Partridge J: Psychosocial rehabilitation after burn injuries, *Nurs Times* 97(48):47, 2001.
18. Sheridan RL, et al: Long-term outcome of children surviving massive burns, *JAMA* 283(1):69–73, 2000.
19. Gibran NS, Heimbach DM: Current status of burn wound pathophysiology, *Clin Plast Surg* 27(1):11–22, 2000.
20. Flynn JD: *Characteristics of home fire victims.* Quincy, MA, 2010, National Fire Protection Association. Available at www.nfpa.org/assets/files/PDF/OS.SocFactors.pdf. Accessed 3/24/12.
21. Arturson G: Forty years in burns research—the postburn inflammatory response, *Burns* 26(7):599–604, 2000.
22. Kagan RJ, et al: *American Burn Association White Paper: surgical management of the burn wound and use of skin substitutes.* Available at www.ameriburn.org. Accessed 6/25/12.
23. Holm C, et al: The relationship between oxygen delivery and oxygen consumption during fluid resuscitation of burn-related shock, *J Burn Care Rehabil* 21(2):147–154, 2000.
24. Cartotto RC, et al: How well does the Parkland formula estimate actual fluid resuscitation volumes? *J Burn Care Rehabil* 23(4):258–265, 2002.
25. Tompkins RG: ABA 2002 presidential address: The American Burn Association in the new millennium, *J Burn Care Rehabil* 22:369–374, 2001.
26. O'Mara MS, Slater H, Goldfarb IW, Caushaj PF: A prospective, randomized evaluation of intra-abdominal pressures with crystalloid and colloid resuscitation in burn patients, *J Trauma* 58(5):1011–1018, 2005.
27. Moncrief JA, Mason AD Jr: Water vapor loss in the burned patient, *Surg Forum* 13:38–41, 1962.
28. Moncrief JA: Burns. In Schwartz SI, et al, editors: *Principles of surgery*, ed 2, New York, 1974, McGraw-Hill, pp 253–274.
29. Roe CF, Kinney JM: Water and heat exchange in third-degree burns, *Surgery* 56:212–220, 1964.
30. White DJ, et al: Cardiomyocyte intracellular calcium and cardiac dysfunction after burn trauma, *Crit Care Med* 30(1):14–22, 2002.
31. Sheridan RL, Schnitzer JJ: Management of the high-risk pediatric burn patient, *J Pediatr Surg* 36(8):1308–1312, 2001.

32. Wibbenmeyer LA, et al: Predicting survival in an elderly burn patient population, *Burns* 27(6):583–590, 2001.

33. Baxter CR, Cook WA, Shires GT: Serum myocardial depressant factor of burn shock, *Surg Forum* 17:1–2, 1966.

34. Lefer AM, Martin J: Origin of myocardial depressant factor in shock, *Am J Physiol* 218(5):1423–1427, 1970.

35. Ribeiro CA, et al: Association between early detection of soluble TNF-receptors and mortality in burn patients, *Intensive Care Med* 28(4):472–478, 2002.

36. No authors listed: Ventilation with lower tidal volumes as compared with traditional tidal volumes for acute lung injury and the acute respiratory distress syndrome. The Acute Respiratory Distress Syndrome Network, *N Engl J Med* 342(18):1301–1308, 2000.

37. Sukuki M, et al: Correlation between QT dispersion and burn severity, *Burns* 28(5):481–485, 2002.

38. Steinvall I, et al: Acute respiratory distress syndrome is as important as inhalation injury for the development of respiratory dysfunction in major burns, *Burns* 34(4):441–451, 2008. Epub ahead of print.

39. Turnage RH, et al: Mechanisms of pulmonary microvascular dysfunction during severe burn injury (review), *World J Surg* 26(7):848–853, 2002.

40. Liffner G, et al: Inhalation injury assessed by score does not contribute to the development of acute respiratory distress syndrome in burn victims, *Burns* 31(3):263–268, 2005.

41. Thomas JA, et al: IRAK contributes to burn-triggered myocardial contractile dysfunction, *Am J Physiol Heart Circ Physiol* 283(2):H829–H836, 2002.

42. Clardy PF, Manaker S: Carbon monoxide poisoning, Up To Date Online 20.2, October 19, 2011.

43. Sun IF, et al: Continuous arteriovenous hemodialysis and continuous venovenous hemofiltration in burn patients with acute renal failure, *Kaohsiung J Med Sci* 23(7):344–351, 2007.

44. Deets DK, Glaviano VV: Plasma and cardiac lactic dehydrogenase activity in burn shock, *Proc Soc Exp Biol Med* 142(2):412–416, 1973.

45. Mustonen KM, Vuola J: Acute renal failure in intensive care burn patients (ARF in burn patients), *J Burn Care Res* 29(1):227–237, 2008.

46. Gianotti L, et al: Activity of GH/IGF-1 axis in burn patients: comparison with normal subjects and patients with GH deficiency, *J Endocrinol Invest* 25(2):116–124, 2002.

47. Welt LG: Membrane transport defect: the sick cell, *Trans Assoc Am Physicians* 80:217–226, 1967.

48. Trunkey DD, et al: The effect of hemorrhagic shock on intracellular muscle action potentials in the primates, *Surgery* 74(2):241–250, 1973.

49. Cunningham JN Jr, Shires GT, Wagner Y: Changes in intracellular sodium and potassium content of red blood cells in trauma and shock, *Am J Surg* 122(5):650–654, 1971.

50. Rosenthal SM, Tabor H: Electrolyte changes and chemotherapy in experimental burn and traumatic shock and hemorrhage, *Arch Surg* 51:244–252, 1945.

51. Turinsky J, Gonnerman WA, Loose LD: Impaired mineral metabolism in post-burn muscle, *J Trauma* 21(6):417–423, 1981.

52. Ogura H, et al: Long-term enhanced expression of heat shock proteins and decelerated apoptosis in polymorphonuclear leukocytes from major burn patients, *J Burn Care Rehabil* 23(2):103–109, 2002.

53. Rose JK, Herndon DN: Advances in the treatment of burn patients, *Burns* 23(Suppl 1):S19–S26, 1997.

54. Sargent RL: Management of blisters in the partial-thickness burn: an integrative research review, *J Burn Care Res* 27(1):66–81, 2006.

55. Adamkova M, et al: First experience with the use of vacuum assisted closure in the treatment of skin defects at the burn center, *Acta Chir Plast* 47(1):24–27, 2005.

56. Ong Y, et al: Meta-analysis of early excision of burns, *Burns* 32(2):145–150, 2006.

57. Demling R, et al: *Use of skin substitutes.* Available at burnsurgery.org. Accessed 3/26/08.

58. Boyce ST, et al: The 1999 Clinical Research Award: cultured skin substitutes combined with Integra Artificial Skin to replace native skin autograft and allograft for the closure of excised full-thickness burns, *J Burn Care Rehabil* 20(6):453–461, 1999.

59. Llanos S, et al: Effectiveness of negative pressure closure in the integration of split thickness skin grafts, *Ann Surg* 244(5):700–705, 2006.

60. Latenser BA, Kowal-Vern A: Pediatric burn rehabilitation (review), *Pediatr Rehabil* 5(1):3–10, 2002.

61. Housinger T, et al: Conservative approach to the elderly patient with burns, *Am J Surg* 148(6):817–820, 1984.

62. Slater AL, Slater H, Goldfarb IW: Effect of aggressive surgical treatment in older patients with burns, *J Burn Care Rehabil* 10(6):527–530, 1989.

63. Rodriguez NA, et al: Nutrition in burns: Galveston contributions, *JPEN J Parenter Enteral Nutr* 35(6):704–714, 2011.

64. Wasiak J, et al: Early versus delayed enteral nutrition support for burn injuries, *Cochrane Database Syst Rev* (3):CD005489, 2006.

65. Kao CC, Garner WL: Acute burns, *Plast Reconstr Surg* 105(7):2482–2492, 2000.

66. Deveci M, et al: Comparison of lymphocyte populations in cutaneous and electrical burn patients: a clinical study, *Burns* 26(3):229–232, 2000.

67. Pratt VC, et al: Alterations in lymphocyte function and relation to phospholipid composition after burn injury in humans, *Crit Care Med* 30(8):1753–1761, 2002.

68. Curreri PW, et al: Dietary requirements of patient with major burns, *J Am Diet Assoc* 65(4):415–417, 1974.

69. Haynes BW Jr: The management of burns in children, *J Trauma* 5:267–277, 1965.

70. Chen Z, et al: A comparison study between early enteral nutrition and parenteral nutrition in severe burn patients, *Burns* 33(6):708–712, 2007.

71. Tinckler LF: Surgery and intestinal motility, *Br J Surg* 52:140–150, 1965.

72. Raff T, Hartmann B, Germann G: Early intragastric feeding of seriously burned and long-term ventilated patients: a review of 55 patients, *Burns* 23:19–25, 1997.

73. Simpson F, Doig GS: Parenteral vs. enteral nutrition in the critically ill patient: a meta-analysis of trials using the intention to treat principle, *Intensive Care Med* 31:12–23, 2005.

74. Singer P, et al: ESPEN guidelines on parenteral nutrition: intensive care, *Clin Nutr* 28:387–400, 2009.

75. Hart DW, et al: Persistence of muscle catabolism after severe burn, *Surgery* 128(2):312–319, 2000.

76. Ward RS, et al: Sensory loss over grafted areas in patients with burns, *J Burn Care Rehabil* 10(6):536–538, 1989.

77. Artz CP: Electrical injury. In Artz CP, Moncrief JA, Pruitt BA Jr, editors: *Burns: a team approach*, Philadelphia, 1979, Saunders, pp 351–362.

78. U.S. Department of Health and Human Services: *Worker deaths by electrocution*. Available at www.cdc.gov/niosh/docs/98-131/pdf. Accessed 3/24/12.

79. Luce EA, Gottlieb SE: "True" high-tension electrical injuries, *Ann Plast Surg* 12(4):321–326, 1984.

80. National Weather Service: *Lightning safety*. Available at www.lightning-safety.noaa.gov/medical/htm. Accessed 3/24/12.

81. Jain S, Bandi V: Electrical and lightning injuries, *Crit Care Clin* 15(2):319–331, 1999.

82. Arnoldo BD, et al: Electrical injuries: a 20-year review, *J Burn Care Rehabil* 25(6):479–484, 2004.

83. American Burn Association: *American Burn Association Committee on Specific Optimal Criteria for Hospital Resources for Care of Patients with Burn Injury*, San Antonio, 1976, The Association.

84. Leake JE, Curtin JW: Electrical burns of the mouth in children, *Clin Plast Surg* 11(4):669–683, 1984.

85. Port RM, Cooley RO: Treatment of electrical burns of the oral and perioral tissues in children, *J Am Dent Assoc* 112(3):352–354, 1986.

86. Bailey B, Gaudreault P, Thivierge RL: Experience with guidelines for cardiac monitoring after electrical injury in children, *Am J Emerg Med* 18(6):671–675, 2000.

87. David WS: Myoglobinuria, *Neurol Clin* 18(1):215–243, 2000.

88. Holliman CJ, Saffle JR, Kravitz M, et al: Early surgical decompression in the management of electrical injuries, *Am J Surg* 144(6):733–739, 1982.

89. Ward RS, et al: Prosthetic use in patients with burns and associated limb amputations, *J Burn Care Rehabil* 11(4):361–364, 1990.

90. Saffle JR, Crandall A, Warden GD: Cataracts: a long-term complication of electrical injury, *J Trauma* 25(1):17–21, 1985.

91. American Burn Association: *National Burn Repository 2010*. Available at www/ameriburn.org/2010NBRAnnualReport.pdf.

92. Berkowitz Z, et al: Hazardous substances emergency events in the agriculture industry and related services in four mid-western states, *J Occup Environ Med* 44(8):714–723, 2002.

93. Roblin I, et al: Topical treatment of experimental hydrofluoric acid skin burns by 2.5% calcium gluconate, *J Burn Care Res* 27:889, 2006.

94. Höjer J, et al: Topical treatments for hydrofluoric acid burns: a blind controlled experimental study, *J Toxicol Clin Toxicol* 40:861, 2002.

95. Wedler V, et al: Extensive hydrofluoric acid injuries: a serious problem, *J Trauma* 58:852, 2005.

96. Amshel CE, et al: Anhydrous ammonia burns case report and review of the literature, *Burns* 26:493, 2000.

97. Spoo J, Elsner P: Cement burns: a review 1960-2000, *Contact Dermatitis* 45:68, 2001.

98. Suhr M, Kreusch T: Burn injuries resulting from (accidental) airbag inflation, *J Craniomaxillofac Surg* 32:35, 2004.

99. Bozkurt A, O'Dey D, Pallua N: Treatment of hot bitumen-contact-burn injuries, *Burns* 34:1053, 2008.

Clinical and Laboratory Values

TABLE A-1 BLOOD, PLASMA, AND SERUM VALUES

TEST	NORMAL VALUES	SIGNIFICANCE OF CHANGE
Acid phosphatase	*Women:* 0.01-0.56 sigma U/ml *Men:* 0.13-0.63 sigma U/ml	↑ in kidney disease ↑ in prostate cancer ↑ after trauma and in fever
Alanine aminotransferase (ALT, SGPT)	7-56 U/L	↑ in liver damage
Albumin	3.5-5.0 g/dl	↓ in liver disease ↓ in malnutrition
Alkaline phosphatase	*Adult:* 38-110 IU/L *Child:* up to 104 IU/L	↑ in bone disorders ↑ in liver disease ↑ during pregnancy ↑ in hypothyroidism
Amylase	20-110 U/L	↑ in pancreatitis
α_1-Antitrypsin	110-270 mg/dl	↓ in genetic emphysema
Aspartate aminotransferase (AST, SGOT)	0-35 U/L	↑ in liver damage
Bicarbonate (arterial)	22-26 mEq/L	↑ in metabolic alkalosis ↓ in respiratory alkalosis ↓ in metabolic acidosis ↑ in respiratory acidosis
Blood urea nitrogen (BUN)	5-25 mg/dl	↑ with increased protein intake ↑ in kidney failure
Blood volume	*Women:* 65 ml/kg body weight *Men:* 69 ml/kg body weight	↓ during hemorrhage

Calcium
  Total
  Ionized
	
	8.4-10.5 mg/dl (2.1-2.6 mmol/L)
	4.6-5.3 mg/dl
		
		↑ in hypervitaminosis D
		↑ in hyperparathyroidism
		↑ in bone cancer and other bone diseases
		↓ in hypoparathyroidism
		↓ in avitaminosis D (rickets and osteomalacia)

Carbon dioxide content (venous bicarbonate)	24-32 mEq/L	↑ in severe vomiting ↑ in hypoventilation disorders ↑ in obstruction of intestines ↓ in metabolic acidosis ↓ in severe diarrhea ↓ in kidney disease

TABLE A-1   BLOOD, PLASMA, AND SERUM VALUES—cont'd

TEST	NORMAL VALUES	SIGNIFICANCE OF CHANGE
Chloride	98-110 mEq/L	↑ in hyperventilation ↑ in kidney disease ↑ in Cushing syndrome ↓ in severe diarrhea ↓ in severe burns ↓ in Addison disease
Cholesterol Total	<200 mg/dl	↑ in chronic hepatitis ↑ in hyperthyroidism ↑ in atherosclerosis ↓ in acute hepatitis ↓ in hypothyroidism
High-density lipoprotein (HDL) Low-density lipoprotein (LDL)	>40 mg/dl <130 mg/dl	↑ with regular exercise ↑ with high-fat diet ↑ in diabetes mellitus ↓ in chronic obstructive pulmonary disease
Triglycerides	<165 mg/dl	↑ in cardiovascular disease ↑ in diabetes mellitus ↓ in hyperthyroidism ↓ with exercise
Clotting time (bleeding time)	5-10 min	↓ in hemophilia ↓ in platelet deficiency or defects
Copper	100-200 µg/dl	↑ in some liver disorders
Cortisol (at 8 AM)	5-20 µg/dl	↑ in Cushing disease ↓ in Addison disease
Creatine phosphokinase (CPK)	32-260 U/L	↑ in Duchenne muscular dystrophy ↑ during myocardial infarction ↑ in muscle trauma
Creatinine	0.6-1.5 mg/dl	↑ in some kidney disorders
Ferritin	*Women:* 4-161 ng/ml *Men:* 16-300 ng/ml	↑ in hemochromatosis ↑ in iron deficiency
α-Fetoprotein	0-15 ng/ml	↓ in neural tube defects
Fibrinogen	175-433 mg/dl	↑ may increase risk of thrombus ↓ in disseminated intravascular coagulation
Folic acid (RBC)	165-760 ng/dl	↓ in macrocytic anemia
Glucose	60-100 mg/dl (fasting)	↑ in diabetes mellitus ↑ in liver disease ↑ during pregnancy ↑ in hyperthyroidism ↓ in hypothyroidism ↓ in Addison disease ↓ in hyperinsulinism
Glycosylated hemoglobin (HbA$_{1c}$)	3.9-6.9%	↑ in hyperglycemia
Hematocrit (packed cell volume)	*Women:* 38-47% *Men:* 40-54%	↑ in polycythemia ↑ in severe dehydration ↓ in anemia ↓ in leukemia ↓ in hyperthyroidism ↓ in cirrhosis of liver

TABLE A-1   BLOOD, PLASMA, AND SERUM VALUES—cont'd

TEST	NORMAL VALUES	SIGNIFICANCE OF CHANGE
Hemoglobin	*Women:* 12-16 g/dl *Men:* 13-18 g/dl *Newborn:* 14-20 g/dl	↑ in polycythemia ↑ in chronic obstructive pulmonary disease ↑ in congestive heart failure ↓ in anemia ↓ in hyperthyroidism ↓ in cirrhosis of liver
Iron	50-150 µg/dl (can be higher in men)	↑ in liver disease ↓ in iron-deficiency anemia
Total iron-binding capacity (TIBC)	250-460 µg/dl	↑ in iron deficiency
Lactate dehydrogenase (LDH)	88-230 U/L	↑ during myocardial infarction ↑ in anemia (several forms) ↑ in liver disease ↑ in acute leukemia and other cancers
Lipase	0-160 U/L	↑ in pancreatitis
Magnesium	1.8-3.0 mg/dl	↑ in excessive intake ↓ in alcoholism, renal disease
Mean corpuscular hemoglobin concentration	31-36%	↓ in iron-deficiency anemia
Mean corpuscular volume (RBC)	82-98 fl	↑ or ↓ in various forms of anemia
Osmolality	285-295 mOsm/L	↑ or ↓ in fluid and electrolyte imbalances
Paco$_2$	35-43 mm Hg	↑ in severe vomiting ↑ in hypoventilation disorders ↑ in obstruction of intestines ↓ in metabolic acidosis ↓ in severe diarrhea ↓ in kidney disease
Pao$_2$	75-100 mm Hg (breathing standard air)	↓ in cyanotic heart defects ↓ in chronic obstructive pulmonary disease
Partial thromboplastin time (activated PTT)	25-35 sec	↓ in intrinsic pathway defects
pH	7.35-7.45	↑ during hyperventilation ↑ in Cushing syndrome ↓ during hypoventilation ↓ in acidosis ↓ in Addison disease
Phosphorus	2.5-4.5 mg/dl	↑ in hypervitaminosis D ↑ in kidney disease ↑ in hypoparathyroidism ↑ in acromegaly ↓ hyperparathyroidism ↓ in hypovitaminosis D (rickets and osteomalacia)
Plasma volume	*Women:* 40 ml/kg body weight *Men:* 39 ml/kg body weight	↑ or ↓ in fluid and electrolyte imbalances ↓ during hemorrhage
Platelet count	150,000-400,000/µl	↑ in heart disease ↑ in some forms of cancer ↑ in cirrhosis of liver ↑ after trauma ↓ in anemia (some forms) ↓ during chemotherapy ↓ in some allergies

Continued

TABLE A-1   BLOOD, PLASMA, AND SERUM VALUES—cont'd

TEST	NORMAL VALUES	SIGNIFICANCE OF CHANGE
Potassium	3.5-5.1 mEq/L	↑ in hypoaldosteronism ↑ in acute kidney failure ↓ in vomiting or diarrhea ↓ in starvation
Prostate-specific antigen	0-4 ng/ml	↑ in prostate cancer
Protein		
Total	6-8.4 g/dl	↑ (total) in severe dehydration
Albumin	3.5-5 g/dl	↓ (total) during hemorrhage
Globulin	2.3-3.5 g/dl	↓ (total) in starvation
Prothrombin time (PT)	11-15 sec	↑ in extrinsic pathway defects
Red blood cell count	*Women:* 4.2-5.4 million/μl *Men:* 4.5-6.2 million/μl	↑ in polycythemia ↑ in dehydration ↓ in anemia (several forms) ↓ in systemic lupus erythematosus
Reticulocyte count	33,000-135,000/μl (0.5-1.5% of RBC count)	↑ in hemolytic anemia ↑ in leukemia and metastatic carcinoma ↓ in pernicious anemia ↓ in iron-deficiency anemia ↓ during radiation therapy
Sodium	135-145 mEq/L	↑ in dehydration ↑ in trauma or disease of the central nervous system ↑ or ↓ in kidney disorders ↓ in excessive sweating, vomiting, diarrhea ↓ in burns (sodium shift into cells)
Specific gravity	1.058	↑ or ↓ in fluid imbalances
Thyroid-stimulating hormone (TSH)	0.4-6 μU/ml	↑ in hypothyroidism (primary) ↓ in hyperthyroidism (primary)
Thyroxin (T_4)—total	5-11 μg/dl	↑ in hyperthyroidism ↓ in hypothyroidism
Transferrin	190-375 mg/dl	↓ in certain anemias
Troponin I	<0.05 ng/ml	↑ in myocardial infarction
Uric acid	*Women:* 1.5-6.0 mg/dl *Men:* 3-9 mg/dl	↑ in gout ↑ in toxemia of pregnancy ↑ during trauma
Viscosity	1.4-1.8 times the viscosity of water	↑ in polycythemia ↑ in dehydration
Vitamin B_{12}	140-820 pg/ml	↓ in pernicious anemia
White blood cell count		
Total	4500-11,000/μl	↑ in acute infections ↑ in trauma ↑ in some cancers ↓ in anemia (some forms) ↓ during chemotherapy
Basophils	0.5-1% of total	↓ in severe allergies
Eosinophils	2-4% of total	↑ in allergies
Lymphocytes	20-25% of total	↑ during antibody reactions
Monocytes	3-8% of total	↑ in chronic infections
Neutrophils	60-70% of total	↑ in acute infection

From Thibodeau GA, Patton KT: *Anatomy & physiology,* ed 5, St Louis, 2003, Mosby, pp 1023-1026.
*Values vary with the analysis method used.

TABLE A-2 CHARACTERISTICS OF URINE

TEST	NORMAL VALUES*	SIGNIFICANCE OF CHANGE
Routine Urinalysis		
Acetone and acetoacetate	0	↑ during fasting ↑ in diabetic acidosis
Albumin	0-trace	↑ in hypertension ↑ in kidney disease ↑ after strenuous exercise (temporary)
Ammonia	20-70 mEq/L	↑ in liver disease ↑ in diabetes mellitus
Bile and bilirubin	—	↑ during obstruction of the bile ducts
Calcium	<150 mg/day	↑ in hyperparathyroidism ↓ in hypoparathyroidism
Color	Transparent yellow, straw-colored, or amber	Abnormal color or cloudiness may indicate blood in urine, bile, bacteria, drugs, food pigments, or high solute concentration
Odor	Characteristic slight odor	Acetone odor in diabetes mellitus (diabetic ketosis)
Osmolality	500-800 mOsm/L	↑ in dehydration ↑ in heart failure ↓ in diabetes insipidus ↓ in aldosteronism
pH	4.6-8.0	↑ in alkalosis ↑ during urinary infections ↓ in acidosis ↓ in dehydration ↓ in emphysema
Potassium	25-100 mEq/L	↑ in dehydration ↑ in chronic kidney failure ↓ in diarrhea or vomiting ↓ in adrenal insufficiency
Sodium	75-200 mg/day	↑ in starvation ↑ in dehydration ↓ in acute kidney failure ↓ in Cushing syndrome
Creatinine	1-2 g/day	↑ in infections ↓ in some kidney diseases ↓ in anemia (some forms)
Creatinine clearance	100-140 ml/min	↑ in kidney disease
Glucose	0	↑ in diabetes mellitus ↑ in hyperthyroidism ↑ in hypersecretion of adrenal cortex
Urea	25-35 g/day	↑ in some liver diseases ↑ in hemolytic anemia ↓ during obstruction of bile ducts ↓ in severe diarrhea
Urea clearance	>40 ml blood cleared per min	↑ in some kidney diseases
Uric acid	0.6-1.0 g/day	↑ in gout ↓ in some kidney diseases

Continued

TABLE A-2 CHARACTERISTICS OF URINE—cont'd

TEST	NORMAL VALUES*	SIGNIFICANCE OF CHANGE
Microscopic Examination		
Bacteria	<10,000/ml	↑ during urinary infections
Blood cells (RBC)	0-trace	↑ in pyelonephritis
		↑ from damage by calculi
		↑ in infection
		↑ in cancer
Blood cells (WBC)	0-trace	↑ in infection
Blood cell casts (RBC)	0	↑ in pyelonephritis
Blood cell casts (WBC)	0	↑ in infection
Crystals	0-trace	↑ in urinary retention
		Very large crystalline masses are calculi
Epithelial casts	0-trace	↑ in some kidney disorders
		↑ in heavy metal toxicity
Granular casts	0-trace	↑ in some kidney disorders
Hyaline casts	0-trace	↑ in some kidney disorders
		↑ in fever

From Thibodeau GA, Patton KT: *Anatomy & physiology,* ed 5, St Louis, 2003, Mosby, pp 1027-1028.
*Values vary with the analysis method used.

A

A band A dark band corresponding to an area where actin and myosin filaments overlap in skeletal or cardiac muscle.

Abruptio placentae Premature separation of the placenta before delivery; the separation may be partial or complete and may result in overt or concealed hemorrhage.

Absolute anemia Anemia involving a decrease in the number of red blood cells (as opposed to a decrease in the percent of red blood cells).

Acalculous cholecystitis An important subgroup of acute cholecystitis. It tends to occur in the setting of major surgery, critical illness, trauma, or burn-related injury and does not occur in association with gallstones.

Accelerated (malignant) high blood pressure Rapidly progressing, potentially fatal form of hypertension in which the diastolic blood pressure exceeds 120 mm Hg.

Acclimatization A normal adaptive response to environmental changes, such as changes in altitude. For example, the red blood cell count increases when a person moves to a high altitude.

Accommodative capacity Ability of the eye to adjust to see objects at changing distances. This is a function of the ciliary muscle's ability to flatten or thicken the lens, thereby focusing the image on the retina.

Achalasia A disorder of esophageal smooth muscle function resulting in difficulty in swallowing both liquids and solids.

Acid A substance that releases hydrogen ions in solution and from which hydrogen may be displaced by a metal to form a salt. An increase in acid concentration produces a decrease in pH.

Acidemia The state in which the blood is overly acidic; usually defined as a pH <7.35.

Acidosis Presence of a condition that tends to make body fluids overly acidic.

Acne vulgaris A common disease of the skin in which sebaceous glands are numerous (face, upper back, and chest). Characteristic lesions include open (blackhead) and closed (whitehead) comedones, inflammatory papules, pustules, nodules, and cysts.

Acquired immunodeficiency syndrome (AIDS) A syndrome caused by the human immunodeficiency virus (HIV) in which the CD4 lymphocyte count is <200 cells/μL or an AIDS-indicator condition is present.

Acquired or secondary immunodeficiency An immunodeficiency that develops after birth and is the result of an illness rather than a genetic defect. Examples include impaired immune function secondary to poor nutrition or medication. This type of immunodeficiency may be reversible.

Acromegaly A chronic metabolic condition characterized by excessive growth of bone, soft tissues, and organs in adults due to abnormally high levels of growth hormone.

Acrosome Covering on the head of the sperm that contains large quantities of hydrolytic (water-splitting) enzymes that are released during capacitation.

Actin A cytoskeletal protein that comprises the thin filament of the muscle sarcomere in skeletal and cardiac muscle. It is also present in nonmuscle cells and is an important component of cell movement.

Actinic keratosis A horny premalignancy of skin epithelium caused by excessive exposure to sunlight.

Action potential An electrical impulse consisting of a self-propagating series of depolarizations and repolarizations, transmitted across the plasma membranes of excitable cells that have voltage-gated ion channels, such as nerve and muscle.

Active immunity A form of long-term, acquired immunity that protects the body against a new infection as the result of antibodies that develop naturally after an initial infection or artificially after a vaccination.

Active transport pumps The membrane proteins that move polar substances across lipid membranes against a concentration gradient.

Acute Relatively severe but running a short course.

Acute coronary syndrome (ACS) Sudden onset of cardiac ischemia from occlusion of coronary vessels resulting in unstable angina or myocardial infarction.

Acute HAV infection A viral hepatitis infection caused by the hepatitis A virus (HAV) characterized by jaundice and fatigue.

Acute renal failure An abrupt reduction of renal function that is potentially reversible.

Acute rheumatic fever An inflammatory disease following a group A β-hemolytic streptococcal pharyngeal infection.

Acute tubular necrosis Sudden onset of renal dysfunction from death of nephron tubule cells (tubular epithelium), usually resulting from nephrotoxicity, ischemia after major surgery, trauma, severe hypovolemia, sepsis, or burns.

Acute viral hepatitis Inflammatory liver disease usually caused by hepatitis A virus, hepatitis B virus, and hepatitis C virus.

Adaptation An alteration in structure or function in response to a changed environment, which enhances or promotes survival.

Adapting Making an adjustment to a change in internal or external conditions or circumstances.

Addison disease Primary adrenocortical insufficiency thought to be autoimmune in etiology.

Adenosine triphosphate (ATP) A nucleoside with three phosphate groups and an adenine base; it functions as the principal source of energy in cells.

Adherence The quality of clinging or being closely attached. The degree to which a patient complies with therapeutic interventions such as taking medications.

Adhesive capsulitis A shoulder condition characterized by stiffness, pain, and limited range of motion.

Adrenocortical insufficiency Abnormally diminished secretion of corticosteroids by the adrenal cortex, as in Addison disease.

Adrenocorticotropic hormone (ACTH) A hormone that stimulates growth of the adrenal cortex and the synthesis and secretion of corticosteroids.

Affect The outward expression of emotion associated with a mental state or in response to a stimulus.

Affective disorders Mood disorders consisting of a variety of conditions characterized by a disturbance in mood.

Afferent neuron A neuron that transmits impulses from the periphery (sensory receptors) to the central nervous system.

Affinity The "tightness" of a ligand-receptor bond; the tendency of ligand and receptor to remain bound at low ligand concentration.

Afterload The impedance or resistance that must be overcome in order to eject blood from a cardiac chamber. Systemic vascular resistance is the primary determinant of left ventricular afterload.

Age-related macular degeneration A progressive deterioration of the retina associated with abnormal retinal pigment epithelium that can progress to blindness.

Aggregates A total considered with reference to its constituent parts.

Agnosia Total or partial loss of the ability to recognize familiar objects or persons through sensory stimuli.

Agonist A substance with affinity for binding to receptors and mimicking the effect of the normal receptor-ligand interaction.

Agoraphobia Irrational fear of open spaces. In panic disorder, agoraphobia is a fear of any place or situation in which assistance would be unavailable in case of an unexpected panic attack. Agoraphobia is also known as *phobic avoidance*.

Airway resistance Relationship between pressure and flow of gas, as determined by the radius of the airway.

Alagille syndrome Also called *arteriohepatic dysplasia;* this autosomal dominant condition is associated with typical bony and vascular malformations and paucity of intrahepatic bile ducts.

Alarm The initial response to stress. The major features of the alarm reaction are attributable to activation of the sympathetic nervous system.

Albinism Partial or total absence of pigment in skin, hair, and eyes.

Alcohol abuse Overingestion of alcohol to the point of a person's being dependent on the substance.

Colored terms have audio pronunciation available on the Evolve site for this book. Visit http://evolve.elsevier.com/Copstead/.

Alcoholic fatty liver An accumulation of fat in the liver cells resulting from chronic alcohol consumption; also called *steatosis*.

Alcoholic hepatitis An active inflammation, especially of the centrilobular region of the liver, resulting from acute or chronic alcohol consumption.

Alcoholic liver disease Manifested by fatty liver, hepatitis, and cirrhosis. One or more of these manifestations may be found in alcoholic patients.

Aldosterone A mineralocorticoid synthesized by the adrenal cortex in response to angiotensin II that conserves sodium, producing increased water retention and consequently increased blood volume.

Alkalemia The state in which the blood is overly alkaline; usually defined as a pH >7.45.

Alkalosis Presence of a condition in which body fluids are overly alkaline.

Allele One of two or more alternative forms of a gene located at the same site on homologous chromosomes.

Allergic contact dermatitis Indicates delayed acquired hypersensitivity to a specific allergen on the skin. Chromates, nickel, ethylenediamine, *para*-phenylenediamine, neomycin, formaldehyde, and lanolin components may cause allergic contact dermatitis.

Allergic purpura A chronic disorder of the skin associated with urticaria, erythema, asthma, and rheumatic joint swellings. Platelet counts, bleeding times, and blood clotting are normal.

Allergy Type I hypersensitivity of the immune system to environmental agents. Antigens that trigger an allergic response are often called *allergens*.

Allodynia Perception of pain in response to normally nonpainful sensory stimuli.

Allogeneic Referring to transplanted tissue that was obtained from a closely matched donor, usually a sibling, parent, or child.

All-or-none response In a skeletal muscle, all of the muscle fibers innervated by a motor unit will respond as a single entity to its maximum or they will not contract at all. In a nerve, depolarization will result in either a full amplitude action potential or none at all.

Alopecia Loss of hair, usually referring to the scalp.

Allostasis The process of achieving stability, or homeostasis, through physiologic or behavioral change.

Allostatic load A term coined as a more precise alternative to the term *stress*; used to refer to environmental challenges that cause an organism to begin efforts to maintain stability.

α₁-Antitrypsin A plasma protein produced primarily in the liver; it is an acute-phase reactant that inhibits the activity of elastase, cathepsin G, trypsin, and other proteolytic enzymes.

Alveolar period The last stage in fetal lung development when alveolar ducts form from terminal sacs and alveoli mature by increasing both in size and in number.

Amblyopia Reduced vision in an eye not correctable by a fraction adjustment.

Amenorrhea Absence or suppression of menstrual bleeding, usually attributable to an altered pattern of hormonal functioning that interrupts the normal sequence of endometrial proliferation and sloughing.

Amniocentesis A procedure in which fluid is obtained from the amniotic cavity by an ultrasound-guided needle. The fluid contains fetal cells that can be used to screen for chromosomal and other defects.

Amniotic cavity The space between the amniotic sac and the developing embryo. It is filled with a clear amniotic fluid that keeps the embryo moist and provides a measure of protection against mechanical injury.

Amphipathic Having different characteristics. For example, membrane lipids are partly hydrophobic and partly hydrophilic, and hence are amphipathic.

Ampulla A flasklike cavity or dilatation of a tubular structure.

Amyloid plaque A microscopic lesion in the cerebral cortex composed of fragmented axon terminals and dendrites surrounding a core of β-amyloid, as found in Alzheimer disease.

Amyloid precursor protein A member of a large family of proteins that is associated with cell membranes and a precursor to β-amyloid, a component of brain plaques in Alzheimer disease.

Amyotrophic lateral sclerosis A progressive degenerative disease affecting both the upper and lower motor neurons characterized by muscle wasting and atrophy of the hands, arms, and legs; also called *Lou Gehrig disease*.

Anabolism The energy-requiring phase of metabolism through which molecules, cells, and tissues are created.

Anagen The growing phase of the hair cycle.

Anaphylactic shock A severe and sometimes fatal systemic allergic reaction to an allergen.

Anaplasia A lack of differentiated features in a tumor cell as evidenced by variations in cell size and shape and presence of abnormal nuclei.

Androgenic Producing masculine characteristics such as the androgenic hormone testosterone.

Anemia A decrease in the quantity of hemoglobin, hematocrit, and/or red blood cells.

Anergy Diminished immune responsiveness to antigens.

Aneuploidy An abnormal number of chromosomes—either too few (hypoploidy) or too many (hyperploidy, polyploidy).

Aneurysm Local dilation of an arterial wall or muscular chamber (e.g., cardiac ventricle).

Angina pectoris A paroxysmal chest pain most often due to cardiac ischemia associated with atherosclerotic coronary artery disease.

Angiogenesis The physiologic process involving the growth of new blood vessels from pre-existing vessels.

Angiomyolipoma The most common benign tumor of the kidney; composed of blood vessels, smooth muscle cells, and fat cells.

Angiotensinogen A serum glycoprotein produced in the liver that is the precursor of angiotensin I.

Anhedonia Loss of interest in and withdrawal from all regular and pleasurable activities, often associated with depression.

Ankylosis The fusion of a joint, often in an abnormal position, usually resulting from destruction of articular cartilage and subchondral bone, as occurs in rheumatoid arthritis.

Ankylosing spondylitis An arthritis of the axial skeleton including the sacroiliac joints, spine, hips, and shoulders. Marked limitation of motion develops, and a flexed spinal posture with flexed hips and knees may predominate.

Anorexia Loss of appetite.

Anorexia nervosa A refusal to eat or an aberration in eating patterns to the point of danger. The clinical syndrome may be due to an intense fear of becoming obese or to emotional states such as anxiety, irritation, or anger. Affected individuals become obsessed with the desire to become thin, and food intake is restricted even as weight falls well below minimal normal value for age and height. Periods of fasting may alternate with periods of bingeing.

Anosognosia Lack of insight or denial of a neurologic defect, or illness in general (especially paralysis), on one side of the body.

Antagonist or blocking agent A substance that has affinity to bind to a cellular receptor and blocks the activity of the normal receptor-ligand interaction.

Anthropometric Pertaining to measurements of the body or body parts such as height and weight for the purposes of understanding human physical variation.

Antibody Protein produced by B cells that destroys or inactivates a specific antigen.

Anticipatory anxiety Anxious anticipation of an anxiety-provoking event.

Anticodon Sequence of three nucleotides in a transfer RNA molecule that is complementary to the messenger RNA codon.

Antidiuretic hormone (ADH) A posterior pituitary hormone that induces renal collecting duct cells to become permeable to water, thus decreasing the production of urine and reducing the osmolality of the blood.

Antigen Macromolecule that provokes an immune system response.

Antimicrobial A chemical or agent that inhibits microbial activity.

Antisocial personality disorder A mental disorder characterized by failure to acquire the conditioned responses that are necessary for the learning of avoidance behaviors, conventional morality, and socialized positive responses to others. Also known as *antisocial reaction*.

Anuria Severe decrease or lack of urine output of less than 100 ml per day.

Anxiety disorders General group that comprises three major diagnoses: panic disorder, generalized anxiety disorder, and obsessive-compulsive disorder. Anxiety disorders are characterized by irrational fears and have great potential to cause disability in affected persons.

Aortic valve The cardiac valve that lies between the left ventricle and the aorta. It is open during ventricular systole and closed during ventricular diastole. Aortic valve closure contributes to heart sound S_2.

Aphasia A global disorder of language involving impaired speech (expressive aphasia) and impaired ability to understand the spoken word (receptive aphasia).

Aplastic anemia A deficiency of the formed elements of blood (specifically erythrocytes, leukocytes, and platelets) because of failure of the bone marrow to produce them.

Apocrine sweat gland A sweat gland that becomes functional only after puberty and discharges its products onto the skin through the hair follicle (hair pore).

Apoprotein A polypeptide chain not yet bound to its specific prosthetic group.

Apoptosis Programmed cell death; characterized by DNA degradation and cell dissolution, but without necrosis.

Appendicitis Inflammation of the vermiform appendix due to an obstruction. This inflammation may lead to necrosis of the appendix, with subsequent abscess formation and peritonitis.

Apraxia An inability to execute previously learned skills, usually following a stroke.

Arachnoidal villi Fingerlike projections in the delicate membrane between the dura mater and the pia mater of the brain.

Archaea A group of single-celled microorganisms, distinct from bacteria.

ARDS Acute respiratory distress syndrome; severe pulmonary dysfunction characterized by diffuse inflammatory injury to alveolar-capillary membranes.

Arnold-Chiari II malformation A congenital anomaly associated with meningomyelocele and hydrocephalus in which the cerebellum and medulla oblongata protrude into the cervical spinal canal through the foramen magnum.

Arterial pulse pressure The difference between systolic and diastolic blood pressures.

Arteriosclerosis Generalized term for pathologic conditions resulting in decreased distensibility of arteries; also known as *hardening of the arteries.*

Arteriovenous fistula Abnormal communication between an artery and a vein.

Arteriovenous malformation (AVM) A congenital disorder of the connections between veins and arteries in the vascular system.

Arteritis Inflammation of an artery. May be associated with an autoimmune reaction.

Arthralgia Joint pain.

Arthritis Any inflammatory condition of the joints; characterized by pain, swelling, heat, redness, and limitation of movement.

Articular (hyaline) cartilage Connective tissue that forms a smooth, resilient, low-friction surface for articulation of two bones. It is without nerves, is avascular in adults, and derives nourishment from synovial fluid. It tolerates extreme compression stress.

Articulation A point of contact between bones. Also called *joint.*

Ascites Abnormal accumulation of fluid in the peritoneal cavity. Causes include liver disease, heart failure, constrictive pericarditis, infection, malnutrition, pancreatitis, lymphatic obstruction or leakage, renal disease, hypothyroidism, collagen vascular diseases, and malignancy.

Aspiration Inadvertent entry of food substances, liquids, or gastric contents into the respiratory system. This potentially life-threatening occurrence is normally prevented by the coordinated set of actions performed by the muscles in the pharynx during swallowing.

Asthenia The lack or loss of strength or energy; weakness.

Asthma A respiratory condition characterized by increased responsiveness of the trachea and bronchi to various stimuli and manifested by widespread narrowing of the airways and inflammation.

Astigmatism An abnormal condition of the eye in which the light rays cannot be focused clearly in a point on the retina because the spherical curve of the cornea or lens is not equal in all meridians. Vision is typically blurred.

Ataxia Failure of muscular coordination, resulting in incoordination and disturbances in posture and gait.

Atelectasis Full or partial collapse of the lung alveoli.

Atherosclerosis A type of arteriosclerosis characterized by proliferation of smooth muscle cells and lipid collection within the walls of arteries, resulting in narrowed lumina and impaired ability to dilate.

Atopic Pertaining to a hereditary tendency to experience immediate allergic reactions because of the presence of an antibody.

Atopic dermatitis An intensely pruritic, often excoriated inflammation of skin in allergy-prone individuals.

Atopy A genetic predisposition to allergies.

Atresia Congenital failure to develop (absence) or abnormal closure of a normally open passage.

Atrial fibrillation A completely disorganized and irregular atrial rhythm accompanied by an irregular ventricular rhythm of variable rate.

Atrophy A reduction in size and function of a cell or tissue; wasting.

Attention-deficit/hyperactivity disorder (ADHD) A mental disorder involving impaired or diminished attention, and impulsivity, and hyperactivity.

Aura A peculiar sensation preceding the appearance of more definite symptoms, as in migraines and seizures.

Auscultatory gap The time during cuff deflation after systolic blood pressure when the Korotkoff sounds disappear.

Autism A mental disorder primarily characterized by abnormal development of social interaction and communicative skills. Affected individuals may manifest an inability to perceive or understand others' feelings or to express their own feelings, and may adhere to rigid, nonfunctional behaviors or rituals.

Autocrine Relating to hormone-like chemicals in which the target cell is the same cell that secretes the chemical.

Autocrine signaling The secretion of factors that feed back onto the cell that secreted them. Usually used in reference to growth factors.

Autografting Surgical procedure to move skin from one area of the body to an area of injury.

The purpose is to provide permanent skin coverage to the injured area.

Autoimmune liver disease Hepatic injury from self-reactive antibodies produced by errant B lymphocytes.

Autoimmunity An inappropriate and excessive response of the immune system to self antigens causing disease. Disorders that result from an autoimmune response are called *autoimmune diseases.*

Autologous Pertaining to a tissue or structure occurring naturally and derived from the same individual such as blood donated by a patient before surgery to be returned to the patient.

Automaticity A property of specialized excitable tissue that allows self-activation through spontaneous development of an action potential, as in the pacemaker cells of the heart.

Autonomic dysreflexia Hyperreflexia; an uninhibited and exaggerated reflex of the autonomic nervous system in response to stimulation in patients with spinal cord injuries.

Autoregulation The intrinsic tendency of an organ or tissue to maintain adequate blood flow despite changes in metabolism or blood pressure.

Autosomal dominant polycystic kidney disease Hereditary disorder associated with defects on chromosome 16 (95% of cases) or chromosome 4 (5% of cases), resulting in dilation of all collecting ducts and impaired renal function.

Autosomal recessive polycystic kidney disease Congenital disorder linked to a defect on chromosome 6 that results in dilations of the renal collecting ducts and hepatic fibrosis.

Autosome Any ordinary paired chromosome, as distinguished from a sex chromosome.

Avoidance Refers to conscious or subconscious defensive reactions used to increase feelings of control and decrease the risk of anxiety.

Avulsion fracture A separation of a small fragment of bone at the site of attachment of a ligament or tendon.

Axoneme 1. Central core of a cilium or flagellum, consisting of two central fibrils surrounded by nine peripheral fibrils. 2. Motor apparatus of the sperm's tail.

Azotemia Increased levels of nitrogenous waste products, especially urea nitrogen, in the blood indicative of impaired renal clearance.

B

B cell A type of lymphocyte that either produces antibodies to attack pathogens or directs other cells to attack pathogens. B cells that are actively producing antibodies are called *plasma cells.*

Bacillus A genus of aerobic or facultatively anaerobic, gram-positive, spore-bearing, rod-shaped bacteria that may or may not be motile.

Bacteria A domain of life existing as small unicellular microorganisms.

Bacterial enzyme An enzyme that aids in the microorganism's ability to spread or invade tissues; examples include fibrinolysin, coagulase, and hyaluronidase.

Ball-and-socket joint Formed by a ball-like surface fitting into a concave socket. Ball-and-socket joints permit flexion-extension,

adduction-abduction, and rotational movements, such as those of the hip and shoulder.

Baroreceptors One of the pressure-sensitive nerve endings in the walls of the atria of the heart, the aortic arch, and the carotid sinuses.

Barrett esophagus A complication of chronic gastroesophageal reflux disease that represents replacement of the normal squamous epithelium of the distal esophagus by columnar tissue. Considered to be a preneoplastic condition.

Bartholinitis An inflammatory condition of one or both Bartholin glands; caused by bacterial infection.

Basal energy expenditure A term used to describe the calculated basal metabolic rate—the metabolic rate at rest.

Basal ganglia Groups of cell bodies (nuclei) located deep within the cerebral hemispheres that help plan and execute motor activities, including the caudate, putamen, globus pallidus, substantia nigra, and subthalamus.

Basal metabolic rate The amount of energy required for an individual to maintain vital processes such as respiration, digestion, and circulation at rest.

Base 1. The nonacid part of a salt. 2. A substance that accepts hydrogen ions in solution to form salts and increases pH.

Basophil/basophilic granulocyte A leukocyte that is functionally and chemically related to the mast cell; it has a kidney-shaped nucleus and large, deep basophilic granules, which contain vasoactive amine and heparin and are important in IgE binding.

Beau line Transverse furrow in the nail that indicates a disturbance in nail growth.

Becker dystrophy A milder form of inherited muscle degeneration than the Duchenne type and somewhat less common, with an annual incidence of 5 per 100,000. The genetic mutation leads to production of a reduced amount of an abnormal dystrophin protein and slower muscular degeneration.

Bell palsy An acute idiopathic unilateral paresis or paralysis of the facial nerve (cranial nerve VII) involving an inflammatory reaction at or near the stylomastoid foramen or in the bony facial canal.

Bence Jones proteins Proteins found in the urine of patients with plasma cell (multiple) myeloma. They are derived from overproduction of light chain fragments of antibodies by malignant plasma cells. Bence Jones proteins are nephrotoxic and may contribute to development of kidney disease.

Benign breast disorders A group of lesions affecting the breast, which are usually divided into two categories: fibrocystic breast disease and benign neoplasms of the breast.

Benign prostatic hyperplasia or hypertrophy (BPH) A noncancerous enlargement of the prostate gland.

Benign tumor A type of tumor that is strictly local, is usually well differentiated, and does not metastasize.

β-Amyloid Protein fragment snipped from a larger molecule—called *amyloid precursor protein*—during metabolism. Abnormal β-amyloid is a component of neuritic plaques found in Alzheimer disease.

Biaxial joint A joint that has two axes of movement and permits movement in two planes.

Bile A substance produced by hepatocytes in the liver and stored in the gallbladder. It is composed primarily of water, electrolytes, bile salts, cholesterol, and phospholipids. The major functions of bile are to aid in the digestion of dietary lipids through emulsification and to transport waste products, particularly bilirubin, into the intestine for disposal or reabsorption.

Biliary atresia Also called *extrahepatic ductopenia* or *progressive obliterative cholangiopathy*; biliary atresia can be either congenital or acquired. The latter occurs in the setting of certain autoimmune illnesses and is one of the principal forms of chronic rejection of a transplanted liver allograft. Biliary atresia is a rather common birth defect, occurring in 1 of 10,000 to 15,000 live births.

Biliary cirrhosis A disease initiated by damage to the bile ducts, which may be due to macroscopic or microscopic biliary obstruction. Persistent biliary obstruction results in inflammation and scarring of the liver, with obliteration of the bile ductules.

Biliary colic Persistent epigastric pain related to intermittent obstruction of the cystic duct, usually by a gallstone. A typical episode lasts several hours.

Bilirubin A substance formed from the degradation of erythrocytic hemoglobin by reticuloendothelial cells.

Biliverdin A greenish bile pigment formed in the breakdown of hemoglobin and converted to bilirubin.

Bipennate Pertaining to a muscle with a central tendon toward which the fibers converge on either side like the barbs of a feather.

Bipolar disorder A mood disorder characterized by alternating periods of mania and depression.

Bladder calculus A solid mass (stone) formed from debris within the bladder.

Blast An immature precursor form of a lymphoid or myeloid white blood cell. Blasts are not normally found in the peripheral blood because they are retained in the marrow until mature. The presence of blasts in the peripheral blood indicates leukemia.

Blood pressure The pressure exerted by the circulating volume of blood on the walls of the arteries.

Blood urea nitrogen (BUN) Urea is an end product of amino acid metabolism, measured in the blood as BUN and excreted primarily by the kidney.

Blunted affect A severe reduction in the intensity of externalized feelings.

Body fluid The water contained in the body plus the substances dissolved in it.

Body mass index (BMI) A weight reference standard. The formula for BMI is weight (kg) divided by height squared (m²).

Body water All of the water contained in the body.

Bolus 1. A round mass of food that has been softened and formed into an appropriate size for swallowing by the action of chewing. 2. A concentrated mass of pharmaceutical preparation.

Bone and joint tuberculosis An extrapulmonary form of tuberculosis that occurs after lymphohematogenous spread from a primary lung lesion.

Bone marrow suppression Suppression of bone marrow activity, resulting in reduction in the number of platelets, red blood cells, and white blood cells, such as in aplastic anemia. Also called *myelosuppression*.

Borderline personality disorder Personality disorder that represents a pervasive and persistent disturbance in ways of handling events and situations. Personalities influenced by this disorder are unstable, unpredictable, impulsive, and often moody and self-deprecating. Some overlap with depression is suggested.

Brainstem Portion of the brain consisting of the midbrain, pons, and medulla oblongata and mesencephalon.

Branched-chain amino acids A group of amino acids that includes valine, leucine, and isoleucine; they are mainly metabolized in the muscle for energy.

Bronchiectasis A disorder characterized by destruction of the elastic and muscular structures; results in dilation of the bronchi.

Bronchiolitis Inflammation of small bronchi.

Bronchitis Widespread inflammation of bronchi and bronchioles attributable to infectious agents or allergic reactions.

Bronchospasm Narrowing of the bronchi and bronchioles because of abnormal contraction of the smooth muscles of the bronchial walls.

Bruit Sound generated by turbulent blood flow auscultated over a blood vessel.

Brush border Covering of the microvilli projecting from some types of epithelial cells, such as proximal renal tubule cells and the intestinal villi. This fuzzy coating contains many enzymes and transporters.

Buck fascia or fascia of Buck Thick fibrous envelope surrounding the tunica albuginea, which encloses each of the erectile bodies of the penis.

Buckle fracture A fracture in children whereby the bone buckles and eventually cracks as a result of a compression injury to cancellous bone of the metaphysis of a long bone.

Buffer A chemical that releases hydrogen ions when a fluid is too alkaline and takes up hydrogen ions when a fluid is too acidic.

Bulbourethral glands Also called *Cowper glands*, these two glands produce viscous fluid that is secreted into the urethra near the base of the penis.

Bulbous urethra The proximal portion of the penile urethra. The bulbous urethra is surrounded by the bulb of the urethra and the bulbospongiosus muscle.

Bulimia nervosa Recurrent episodes of binge eating followed by self-induced vomiting or diarrhea, excessive exercise, strict dieting, or fasting; person has an exaggerated concern about body shape and weight.

Bulla Large, thin-walled cyst. Commonly used in reference to lung or skin.

Bursa Pocket of connective tissue lined with liquid-containing synovium; located between muscles or between muscle or tendon and bone.

Byler syndrome A rare autosomal recessive disorder involving severe jaundice, pruritus, and malabsorption caused by an error in bile salt metabolism. Also called *progressive intrahepatic cholestasis* and *progressive familial intrahepatic cholestasis*.

C

Cachexia A combination of symptoms, including anorexia, weight loss, muscle wasting, and weakness, that is associated with the severe malnutrition of chronic diseases such as cancer.

Calcitonin A hormone produced by thyroid parafollicular cells, it influences the processing of calcium by bone cells.

Calculus A mass of solid mineral or metabolic substance. A stone.

Callus (bone) The bony deposit formed between and around the broken ends of a fractured bone during healing. Also called *keratoma*.

Calluses (skin) Common, usually painless thickenings of the stratum corneum at locations of external pressure or friction.

Cancellous bone Bone with a spongy or lattice-like appearance; found in the interior of bones. Cancellous bone does not tolerate compression stress.

Cancer cachexia The severe nutritional effects of cancer. See *cachexia*.

Capacitation The multiple changes that activate sperm and enhance their ability to participate in the final process of fertilization.

Capillary hydrostatic pressure The outward push of the vascular fluid against the capillary walls that is caused by blood pressure.

Capillary osmotic pressure The inward pull of particles in the vascular fluid from dissolved proteins in the blood; also called *oncotic pressure*.

Carbohydrates The main energy source for the body; consists of simple or complex sugars. They must be supplied in a fairly constant manner to meet the energy requirements for normal body functioning. Provides 4 kcal/gm of energy when metabolized.

Carbonic anhydrase The enzyme that catalyzes the reversible conversion of carbon dioxide and water to carbonic acid.

Carcinogen A substance that initiates or promotes the development of cancers. Most carcinogens cause cancer by damaging DNA to produce mutations.

Carcinoma in situ A premalignant neoplasm that has not invaded the basement membrane but shows cytologic characteristics of cancer.

Cardiac asthma Results from bronchospasm precipitated by congestive heart failure.

Cardiac catheterization A diagnostic procedure in which a catheter is introduced through an incision into a large vein or artery (cardiac angiography) and threaded through the circulatory system to the heart.

Cardiac cycle A cardiac cycle includes one diastolic and one systolic phase.

Cardiac index A measure of the heart's pumping ability taking into account body surface area. The cardiac index is calculated by dividing cardiac output by body surface area. A cardiac index less than 2.0 L/min/m^2 is considered to be insufficient for adequate peripheral perfusion.

Cardiac output A measure of the amount of blood pumped by the heart in 1 minute; usually expressed in liters per minute.

Cardiac tamponade Abnormal external pressure on the heart that results in poor cardiac filling and decreased cardiac output.

Cardiogenic shock A condition of low cardiac output and inadequate perfusion of tissues associated with acute myocardial infarction and congestive heart failure.

Cardiomyopathy Diseases that primarily affect myocardial cells, often of unknown cause. Three common types of cardiomyopathy are dilated, hypertrophic, and restrictive.

Carina A ridgelike structure at the base of the trachea that projects from the area that separates the left and right bronchi.

Carpal joint A synovial joint between the carpal bones.

Carrier A person who harbors a recessive gene for a particular trait. A recessive heterozygote.

Carrier proteins Proteins located in lipid bilayers that transport ions and small molecules through the membrane by first binding on one side and then moving to the other side by changing conformation.

Cartilaginous joint A joint that connects bony segments by fibrocartilage or hyaline growth cartilage.

Casts White or red blood cells that collect in a nephron tubule and conform to the shape of the tubule; their presence indicates infection or inflammation of the kidney.

Catabolism The process of converting large molecules of carbohydrate, protein, and fat to smaller molecules to be utilized for energy.

Cataracts An abnormal progressive condition of the lens of the eye that is characterized by loss of transparency.

Catecholamine A hormone (e.g., epinephrine and norepinephrine) that stimulates glycogenolysis and gluconeogenesis. An amine neurotransmitter (e.g., norepinephrine, dopamine).

Catecholamine hypothesis A hypothesis that abnormally low catecholaminergic neurotransmission leads to depression and abnormally high catecholaminergic neurotransmission leads to mania.

Caudal Signifying a position toward the distal end of the body, or an inferior position.

Caudate nuclei Portion of each cerebral hemisphere that, together with the lentiform nuclei, forms the corpus striatum of the basal ganglia.

Celiac disease Also called *celiac sprue*, this disease is characterized by intolerance of gluten, a protein in wheat and wheat products; ingestion of gluten causes abdominal distention and malabsorption.

Cell cycle The phases through which a cell progresses during cellular reproduction, including gap 1, synthesis, gap 2, and mitosis.

Central venous pressure The blood pressure in the large veins of the body measured in the right atrium of the heart.

Centromere Constricted region that holds two sister chromatids together. The centromere is the site of attachment to the microtubules, which pull the chromatids apart during mitosis.

Centrosome A centrally located organelle that organizes microtubules in the cell. It acts as the spindle pole during mitosis.

Cerebellum Portion of the brain attached to the brainstem; it has an essential role in maintaining muscle tone and posture and coordinating normal movements.

Cerebral dysrhythmia An abnormality in an otherwise normal rhythmic pattern, as seen on electroencephalography.

Cerebral edema An accumulation of fluid in the brain tissues. Causes include infection, tumor, trauma, or exposure to certain toxins. Because the skull cannot expand to accommodate the fluid pressure, brain tissues are compressed.

Cerebral palsy Refers to a diverse group of crippling syndromes that appears during childhood and involves permanent, nonprogressive encephalopathic damage to the developing brain.

Cerebrospinal fluid Fluid found in the cavities and canals of the brain and spinal cord.

Cerebrotendinous xanthomatosis A steroid hydroxylase deficiency that leads to premature atherosclerosis and encephalopathy. Also known as *van Bogaert disease*.

Cerebrovascular accident (CVA) An abnormal condition of the brain characterized by occlusion by an embolus, thrombus, hemorrhage, or vasospasm, resulting in ischemia of the brain tissues. Also called *stroke*, or *brain attack*.

Cerebrum Portion of the brain that controls consciousness, memory, sensations, emotions, and voluntary movements. The largest part of the brain, it consists of two hemispheres.

Ceruminous gland A special variety or modification of an apocrine sweat gland. The mixed secretions of sebaceous and ceruminous glands form a brown waxy substance called *cerumen*, which protects the ear canal from dehydration.

Chagas disease Caused by *Trypanosoma cruzi* and transmitted to humans by bloodsucking insects. It is a common cause of acquired myocarditis and megacolon in Central and South America but is rarely seen in the United States.

Chancre Painless, ulcerative lesion arising at the original port of entry of the spirochete that causes syphilis.

Chancroid An ulcerative, infectious disease of the genital tract caused by the sexually transmitted bacillus *Haemophilus ducreyi*. Unlike the chancre in syphilis, the lesion in chancroid is painful, tender, and often multiple.

Channel proteins Proteins located in lipid bilayers; they form porelike structures that allow ions to pass through by diffusion when appropriately stimulated.

Chemodissolution Use of chemical substances, such as bile acids or organic solvents, to dissolve gallstones. Used as a nonoperative method to treat gallstones.

Chemokines Any of a group of low-molecular-weight cytokines. They function as regulators of the immune system that help immune cells localize to areas of injury.

Chemotaxis The movement of cells according to chemical gradients (chemotaxins) that attract them.

Chemotherapy The treatment of cancer, infections, and other diseases with chemical agents. Chemotherapeutic agents are often cytotoxic.

Chest physiotherapy Use of percussion and postural drainage to mobilize secretions from specific segments of the lungs.

Chickenpox Also called *varicella*. Chickenpox is a common communicable childhood disease. It is caused by the varicella-zoster virus, which is also the causative agent in shingles. The characteristic skin lesion occurs in three stages: macule, vesicle, and granular scab.

Chlamydia Genus of a microorganism that lives as an intracellular bacterium. *Chlamydia trachomatis* inhabits the epithelium of the urethra and cervix and is responsible for the highly contagious systemic infection *lymphogranuloma venereum*.

Chloride shift An exchange of chloride ions for bicarbonate ions (HCO_3^-) in red blood cells in peripheral tissues as a response to changes in the Pco_2 of blood.

Cholecalciferol Precursor substance of active vitamin D.

Cholecystectomy Surgical removal of the gallbladder.

Cholecystitis Inflammation of the gallbladder wall; may be acute or chronic and usually is associated with cholelithiasis.

Cholecystokinin Hormone secreted from the small intestinal mucosa; two of its chief functions are stimulation of the release of pancreatic enzymes during a meal and contraction of the gallbladder.

Cholelithiasis Formation of stones in the gallbladder.

Cholesterol A lipid-soluble compound that facilitates the absorption and transport of fatty acids in bile and provides the building blocks for steroid hormone production.

Cholinergic-noradrenergic imbalance hypothesis A hypothesis that suggests that a relative increase in the ratio of acetylcholine activity to norepinephrine activity produces depression and that mania is the result of a relative increase in the ratio of norepinephrine activity to acetylcholine activity.

Chondroblasts Any one of the cells that develop from the mesenchyme and form cartilage. They play an important role in endochondral ossification and especially in longitudinal bone growth.

Chondroma Also called *enchondroma*; a cartilage-forming tumor located within bone that accounts for about 15% of benign bone tumors.

Chondrosarcoma A malignant cartilage-forming tumor; chondrosarcomas tend to develop in the pelvic and shoulder girdles and the proximal ends of long bones.

Chordae tendineae Bands of fibrous connective tissue that anchor the atrioventricular valves to the papillary muscles of the ventricular chambers.

Chorionic villus sampling A procedure in which tissue is obtained from the placenta by ultrasound-guided biopsy. Chorionic villus sampling can be performed earlier in pregnancy (10 to 12 weeks) than amniocentesis (16 weeks).

Chromatid One copy of a chromosome formed by DNA replication that may be joined to the other copy (sister chromatid) at the centromere.

Chromosome A linear thread of nuclear DNA that becomes visible under the microscope during cell mitosis.

Chronic Refers to a condition that lasts for a long time, generally from 6 months to years.

Chronic active hepatitis A progressive, destructive inflammatory disease that extends beyond the portal triad to the hepatic lobule (piecemeal necrosis).

Chronic bronchitis A condition characterized by excessive secretion of bronchial mucus and manifested by productive cough for 3 or more months in at least 2 consecutive years in the absence of any other disease process that may cause this symptom.

Chronic hepatitis Ongoing inflammation of the liver, usually of more than 6 months' duration, following viral hepatitis or attributable to autoimmune disease.

Chronic persistent hepatitis Also called *triaditis* or *transaminitis*. A benign disease in which the inflammation is confined to the portal triads without destruction of normal liver functions despite elevated serum transaminase levels.

Chronic renal failure Gradual loss of renal function that is progressive and irreversible.

Chronic venous insufficiency Varicosity of the deep veins that prevents effective return of blood from the periphery. Usually manifests as edema.

Chylothorax An accumulation of chylous fluid attributable to leakage of chyle (lymph fluid) from the thoracic duct or to rheumatoid pleural effusion or tuberculous pleuritis. Also called *chylous pleural effusion*.

Chyme Viscous, semifluid contents of the stomach following the mixture of ingested nutrients with gastric secretions. Chyme then passes through the pylorus into the duodenum, where further digestion occurs.

Cilia Motile hairlike processes on the surface of some cells.

Circadian rhythm The regular recurrence of certain biological phenomena in approximately 24-hour cycles, regardless of constant darkness or other conditions of illumination.

Circumferential burn A burn injury that wraps completely around an extremity or the trunk. Loss of elasticity of skin results in a tourniquet effect, compromising circulation to distal tissues or respiratory expansion of the chest. Escharotomy or fasciotomy is necessary.

Cirrhosis A diffuse, irreversible scarring of the liver resulting in abnormal nodules of liver cells surrounded by fibrosis.

Citric acid cycle A sequence of enzymatic reactions in the mitochondrial matrix that produces carbon dioxide and high-energy electrons from acetyl coenzyme A.

Clang association Association of words similar in sound but not in meaning, or words having no logical connection; may include rhyming and punning.

Clinical dehydration The combination of extracellular fluid volume deficit and hypernatremia.

Clinical manifestations The functional consequences of the structural and associated alterations in cells or tissues that are either characteristic of the disease or diagnostic of the process.

Clonic Characterized by alternating periods of involuntary muscular contraction and relaxation in rapid succession.

Closed fracture A type of fracture that occurs when fragments of a fracture do not extend through mucous membranes or skin and skin is not broken.

Closing volume Lung volume at which airways in the lower lung zones collapse and ventilation ceases.

Clotting factors Proteins that circulate in inactive forms and can be triggered to initiate a clotting cascade to produce insoluble fibrin clots.

Clubbing A process characterized by flattening of the angle of the base of the nail. It may occur in association with cardiovascular disease, subacute bacterial endocarditis, and pulmonary disease.

CO$_2$ Carbon dioxide; this gas is produced by cells during metabolism, is carried in the blood as carbonic acid, and is excreted by the lungs.

Coagulation The process of blood clot formation.

Coagulopathy An abnormality in blood clot formation.

Cocci Round nonmotile bacteria.

Codon Sequence of three nucleotides in DNA or messenger RNA that represents the instruction for a particular amino acid in a polypeptide chain.

Collagen Most abundant protein in the body. The major protein of the white fibers of connective tissue. Has tensile strength similar to that of steel and is responsible for functional integrity of connective tissue.

Colloid osmotic pressure Pressure produced by passage of fluid from an area of less concentration to an area of higher concentration of colloids (large charged molecules such as proteins).

Colonic or anal agenesis Imperforate anus.

Colonization Harmless inhabitation of the skin or mucous membranes by microorganisms.

Colostomy Establishment of an artificial opening of the colon on the abdominal wall; usually performed following removal of a diseased or injured bowel segment.

Comminuted fracture A fracture consisting of more than one fracture line and more than two bone fragments.

Compact bone Hard, dense bone that is usually found at the periphery of skeletal structures.

Compartment syndrome A syndrome resulting from trauma to soft tissue caused by swelling within the unyielding structure of a nonelastic tissue or device (e.g., a cast).

Compensation The counterbalancing of any defect of structure or function. For example, a process that tends to restore pH to normal by making other blood chemistry values abnormal.

Complement A protein that participates in a cascade of reactions resulting in inflammation and cell lysis. Complement activation can occur by the classical or the alternative pathways.

Complete fracture A fracture whose line disrupts bone continuity through the whole thickness of the bone, including the cortex.

Compliance A measure of the ease of elastic distensibility of a hollow organ.

Complication A new or separate process that may arise secondarily because of some change produced by the original entity. For example, bacterial pneumonia may be a complication of viral infection of the respiratory tract.

Compression fracture Consistent with cancellous bone trauma. Also called a *crush fracture.*

Compulsion Repetitive ritualistic behavior that has a driven quality.

Concentric contraction The shortening contraction of a muscle when the muscle force generates sufficient tension to overcome the resistance of the limb. One example is lifting a cup of water to one's mouth.

Condyloid joint A joint that permits flexion and extension at one axis and adduction and abduction around another axis, such as the metacarpophalangeal joint of the hand.

Condyloma acuminatum; condylomata acuminata Genital wart(s) caused by papillomavirus forms.

Conformational change A movement or alteration in the three-dimensional formation of a protein without any change in amino acid structure.

Congenital adrenal hyperplasia Overproduction of adrenal androgens attributable to a lack of an enzyme needed for cortisol production. Symptoms include virilization of the female infant's genitalia.

Congenital ichthyosis An inherited disease characterized by an excessive growth of keratinocytes and keratin, which gives the skin a fish-scale appearance.

Congenital immunodeficiency Rare condition that results from improper development of immune system components before birth.

Congenital malformation A general term meaning a defect in form or function that is present at birth.

Congestive heart failure Dysfunctional cardiac pumping that results in congestion of blood behind the dysfunctional cardiac pump. Right-sided heart failure is associated with systemic venous congestion. Left-sided heart failure is associated with pulmonary congestion.

Consanguinity Mating of blood-related individuals.

Consolidation The process of tissues becoming firm and solid, such as when the lung alveoli become firm while air spaces are filled with exudate in pneumonia.

Constipation A condition of having small, infrequent, and difficult bowel movements. Authorities have established a norm of fewer than three stools per week as a guideline for defining constipation.

Contact dermatitis A cutaneous reaction to topical irritation or allergy. Irritant contact dermatitis can develop in any person exposed to a sufficiently high concentration of the irritating agent. Some of the more active irritants are acids, alkalis, and hydrocarbons.

Contact hypersensitivity Allergy to a substance that produced a reaction in a previous contact. Usually occurs on the skin and may take several hours to develop (type IV hypersensitivity).

Continent The ability to control bladder or bowel function.

Contractile tissue Tissues involved in the contraction of muscle, including not only the muscle belly but also the tendon and bony insertion.

Contractility The force and velocity of cardiac muscle shortening in response to stimuli that increase cytoplasmic free calcium ion levels.

Contraction time The time from initial tension development to peak tension.

Contralateral Referring to the opposite side of the body.

Convalescence The stage of recovery after a disease, injury, or surgical operation.

Coombs antiglobulin test The direct test is an assay for antibody that is attached to red blood cells; the indirect test is an assay for antibody circulating in serum.

Coping A measure of the individual's resourcefulness and ability to deal with stress and stressors.

Corns Horny masses of condensed epithelial cells overlying bony prominences. Corns result from chronic friction and pressure.

Coronary angiography Radiographic visualization of the internal anatomy of the heart and blood vessels with the use of intravascular introduction of radiopaque contrast medium.

Cor pulmonale Right ventricular hypertrophy secondary to pulmonary diseases that increase right ventricular afterload.

Corpora cavernosa Two paired erectile bodies that lie dorsally in the penis.

Corpus luteum Anatomic structure on the surface of the ovary that grows in the ruptured ovarian follicle following ovulation and acts as a temporary endocrine organ that secretes progesterone.

Corpus spongiosum Erectile body in the penis containing the urethra.

Correction A process whereby normal values are restored when the underlying cause is addressed. An example would be restoring pH to normal by addressing the underlying cause of an acid-base imbalance.

Cortical bone The dense cortex or outer shell of bone; designed to tolerate compression and shearing forces.

Corticosteroid A hormone produced by the adrenal gland that stimulates gluconeogenesis and contributes to insulin resistance (e.g., cortisol); or a drug that has similar effects.

Cortisol A glucocorticoid (steroid hormone) released by the adrenal gland that causes an increase in blood glucose level by promoting liver gluconeogenesis.

Coryza A head cold with profuse nasal drainage.

Costovertebral angle Area lateral to the sacrospinalis muscle and beneath the twelfth rib used as an external landmark for the kidneys.

Cowper glands Also called *bulbourethral glands,* these two glands produce viscous fluid that is secreted into the urethra near the base of the penis.

Crackles Rales (pronounced "rahls"); discontinuous fine crackling sounds, usually heard on inspiration, that are indicative of air moving through fluid.

Cradle cap A seborrheic condition in infants characterized by scaling of the scalp. Occurs as a result of infrequent or inadequate washing of the scalp.

Cranial nerve reflexes The 12 pairs of nerves emerging from the cranial cavity that carry impulses for such functions as the senses.

Creatine kinase An enzyme that catalyzes the transfer of a phosphate group between adenosine triphosphate and creatine. The isoenzyme found in cardiac muscle is called *CK-MB* (the MB fraction of creatine kinase).

Creatinine End product of muscle metabolism that is filtered freely through the glomeruli and excreted by the kidney only. Creatinine clearance is used as a measure of glomerular filtration rate.

Cretinism Extreme hypothyroidism during infancy and childhood that causes mental and physical abnormalities.

Cricothyroidotomy Incision through the site below the thyroid cartilage for emergency opening of the tracheal passageway.

Crigler-Najjar syndrome A rare autosomal recessive disorder marked by severe unconjugated hyperbilirubinemia seen shortly after birth.

Crohn disease An inflammation of the gastrointestinal tract that extends through all layers of the intestinal wall, most commonly affecting the terminal ileum. It may affect multiple portions of the intestine, leaving intervening normal areas in between the affected regions. The manifestations of Crohn disease differ in some respects from those of *ulcerative colitis,* although some overlap may occur. In Crohn disease, abdominal pain is the predominant symptom.

Cross-bridge The interaction between thick and thin filaments of the contractile apparatus when myosin heads bind to actin.

Cross-bridge theory This theory of muscle contraction is suggested by the anatomic configuration of the sarcomere. Muscle shortening is accomplished by increasing the amount of overlap of actin and myosin filaments. Also called the *sliding filament theory.*

Croup An acute infection of the upper and lower respiratory tracts that occurs primarily in infants and young children; it is characterized by hoarseness and a distinctive harsh cough.

Crush fracture A fracture that is consistent with cancellous bone trauma. Also called *compression fracture*.

Cryptogenic cirrhosis Advanced liver disease in a small number of patients with neither a suggestive history nor any detectable markers that would place them in any of the four main groups of cirrhosis.

Cryptorchidism Undescended testes.

Culture An integrated pattern of customs, attitudes, values, and shared beliefs that bind people together to form a society.

Cushing disease Hyperfunctioning of the adrenal cortex with increased glucocorticoid (cortisol) secretion because of excessive secretion of adrenocorticotropic hormone (ACTH) from the anterior pituitary.

Cushing syndrome The clinical features of hypercortisolism, regardless of cause.

Cutaneous membrane Thin, flat organ, also known as *skin*. It is composed of two main layers: an outer, thinner layer, termed the *epidermis*; and an inner, thicker layer, termed the *dermis*.

CVA tenderness The costovertebral angle is one of two angles that outlines a space over the kidneys. Pain in this area is a common finding in pyelonephritis and other infections of the kidneys.

Cyanosis A blue coloration of the skin as a result of poor saturation of hemoglobin with oxygen. Cyanosis is usually not evident until saturation falls below 75%.

Cystectomy Surgical removal of all or part of the urinary bladder.

Cystic fibrosis An autosomal recessive condition with abnormal chloride channel function, producing lung and pancreatic disease in children.

Cystic kidney disease Acquired cystic kidney disease and polycystic kidney disease, where cysts form in the kidneys.

Cystitis Inflammation of the urothelium (lining of the bladder) resulting from infection, irritation, presence of foreign body, or trauma.

Cystocele Protrusion of a portion of the urinary bladder into the anterior vagina at a weakened part of the vaginal musculature. Predisposing factors include obesity, aging, inherent weakness, history of heavy-object lifting, or injury during childbirth or surgery.

Cytokine A peptide factor released by cells to influence the behavior of target cells. Cytokines have signaling, inflammatory, growth, and inhibitory functions.

Cytopathic Pertaining to significant cellular injury or death.

Cytoskeleton System of protein filaments in the cytoplasm of a cell that give the cell its shape and the capacity for purposeful movement.

D

Decubitus ulcer Localized area of cellular necrosis resulting from prolonged pressure between a bony prominence and an external object such as a bed or wheelchair. The tissues are deprived of blood supply and eventually die. Also called *pressure sore*.

Deep partial-thickness burn Second-degree burn characterized by destruction of entire dermis, leaving only epidermal skin appendages. All physiologic functions of skin are absent.

Deep vein thrombosis (DVT) A disorder involving a thrombus in one of the deep veins of the body, most commonly in the lower extremities.

Degranulate The release of granules by mast cells and basophils; the granules contain proinflammatory chemicals.

Degranulation Exocytosis of stored molecules contained in cytoplasmic vesicles.

Dehydration Excessive loss of water from body tissues, accompanied by an increase in serum osmolality and an increase in serum sodium level (hypernatremia).

Dehydroepiandrosterone (DHEA) An androgenic steroid hormone secreted largely by the adrenal cortex and found in human urine.

Deletion The loss of a piece of a chromosome.

Delirium An acute organic mental disorder characterized by confusion, disorientation, restlessness, and incoherence.

Delusion A fixed, false belief that is held despite considerable contradictory evidence.

Delusional disorder A behavioral constellation dominated by a system of fixed, false beliefs that are tenacious and typically refractory to contrary evidence.

Dementia Syndrome characterized by a general loss of intellectual abilities caused by either reversible or progressive disorders, most typically Alzheimer disease or multiinfarct dementia.

Demyelination Destruction, removal, or loss of the myelin sheath of a nerve or nerve fibers.

Dendritic cells A cell that captures antigens and migrates to the lymph nodes and spleen, where it presents the processed antigen to T cells.

Deoxyribonucleic acid (DNA) The biomolecule that carries genetic information in the cell. DNA is composed of covalently linked nucleotides that form long polymers.

Depressed fracture A fracture in which the fragment is displaced below the level of the surface of the bone, usually in the skull.

Depressed mood A hallmark symptom of major depression. This change in mood is relatively constant and is recognized both by the depressed person and by others.

Depression An abnormal mood disturbance characterized by exaggerated feelings of sadness and melancholy. Also known as *clinical depression*.

Dermatitis Inflammation of the skin.

Dermatome An area of skin that is innervated by a specific spinal cord segment.

Dermatomyositis A rare collagen disorder characterized by the acute or insidious onset of muscle pain, weakness, fever, arthralgia, and, in some cases, a puffy erythematous eruption that is usually confined to the face and the eyelids.

Dermatophyte A fungus that causes infection of the skin. The most common dermatophytes are *Microsporum, Trichophyton*, and *Epidermophyton*.

Dermatosis Any disorder of the skin, especially those not associated with inflammation.

Dermis Inner, thicker layer of the cutaneous membrane.

Dermoepidermal junction The specialized area where the cells of the epidermis meet the connective tissue cells of the dermis.

Desensitization The process of manipulating or "training" the hypothalamus to react less forcefully to a perceived threat or stressor. This technique works by changing the predominant brain waves of the individual from beta waves to alpha waves that are slower and more normal.

Desquamation The shedding of epithelial elements from the skin surface.

Detrusor muscle Smooth muscle of the bladder body.

Diabetes insipidus An endocrine deficiency of antidiuretic hormone manifesting as excretion of large quantities of very dilute urine and excessive thirst.

Diabetes mellitus An endocrine disorder characterized by impaired glucose entry into insulin-sensitive cells because of an absolute or relative deficiency of insulin.

Diabetic retinopathy A disorder of retinal blood vessels characterized by capillary microaneurysms. It occurs most frequently in patients with long-standing poorly controlled diabetes mellitus.

Dialysate fluid Prepared solution with varying concentrations of glucose and electrolytes used to aid dialysis.

Dialysis An artificial process that replaces the renal functions of diffusion and filtration necessary to maintain homeostasis.

Diaper rash A skin irritation resulting from feces or the ammonia and alkali by-products of urine breakdown.

Diarrhea An increase in the frequency and fluidity of bowel movements. It is usually a primary sign of gastrointestinal tract disorders.

Diarthrosis Also called *synovial joint*; a freely movable joint in which a contiguous bony surface is covered by articular cartilage and connected by a fibrous connective tissue capsule lined with a synovial membrane.

Diastole A phase of the cardiac cycle in which the ventricles are relaxing and filling with blood.

Diastolic blood pressure The lowest measured pressure in the arteries just prior to the next ventricular ejection.

Dicrotic notch A small, downward deflection observed on the downstroke of an arterial pressure waveform, representing closure of the aortic or pulmonic valves at the onset of ventricular diastole.

Diencephalon "Between" brain; part of the brain between the cerebral hemispheres and the midbrain.

Diffusion Passive movement of a gas or other substance from an area of high concentration to low concentration, or the process by which solutes move across a semipermeable membrane from an area of greater concentration to one of lesser concentration.

Diffusion coefficient A constant that depends on the properties of the tissue and the solute; the rate of movement of a solute is proportional to the diffusion coefficient.

Diploid Containing two sets of homologous chromosomes and, therefore, two copies of each gene—one from each parent.

Disconjugate An abnormal positioning of the eyes such that they deviate from one another in the direction of gaze.

Disease Sum of the deviations from normal structure or function of any part, organ, or system (or combination thereof) of the body manifested by a characteristic set of symptoms and/or signs and whose cause, pathogenesis, and prognosis may be known or unknown.

Dislocation Displacement of a bone from its normal position in a joint to the degree that the articulating surfaces lose contact.

Displaced fracture A fracture in which the ends of fragments are separated.

Disseminated intravascular coagulation (DIC) A grave coagulopathy resulting from the inappropriate stimulation of clotting and fibrinolytic processes within the vascular system; it is often precipitated by immune mechanisms.

Distributive shock State of insufficient perfusion of body tissues because of abnormal distribution of blood (for example, with anaphylaxis, sepsis, and spinal cord injury).

Disuse atrophy The tendency of cells and tissues to reduce size and function in response to lack of trophic stimuli.

Disuse osteoporosis Reduction in quantity of bone or atrophy of skeletal tissue in response to lack of weight-bearing activity. May occur with prolonged bed rest.

Diuresis Excretion of large amounts of urine as a result of the actions of a diuretic.

Diurnal variation The regular (24-hour) recurrence of certain biological phenomena under conditions of illumination; recurring during the daytime, or period of light.

Divergence A separation or movement of objects away from each other.

Diverticulitis Inflammation of one or more diverticula, or outpouchings, in the intestinal wall.

Diverticulosis The presence of diverticula, or outpouchings, in the wall of the colon.

Diverticulum Outpouching of one or more layers of the wall of a structure in the gastrointestinal tract, especially in the colon or esophagus.

DNA polymerase An enzyme complex that binds to DNA, using it as a template for synthesis of a complementary DNA strand.

Dominant Referring to the gene allele that is overtly expressed in the cell's phenotype. Opposite of recessive.

Dopamine hypothesis A hypothesis that postulates that schizophrenia is the result of neuronal overactivity dependent on dopamine.

Down-regulation A decrease in the number of cell receptors for a specific hormone resulting from the cell's prolonged exposure to high concentrations of the hormone. Down-regulation results in a decrease in the target cell response to a hormone.

Drug-induced asthma Asthma related to an ingested drug. An attack may occur within minutes of ingestion or may be delayed up to 12 hours. Nonsteroidal antiinflammatory drugs including indomethacin (Indocin) and ibuprofen (Motrin, Advil) are common causes.

Duchenne muscular dystrophy The most common and most severe form of muscular dystrophy; it is inherited as an X-linked trait and therefore afflicts only males.

Ductus deferens Thick, muscular tube that is continuous with the epididymis. The ductus deferens travels along the pelvic wall and joins with the seminal vesicle duct at the prostate to form the ejaculatory duct. Also called *vas deferens*.

Dumping syndrome The rapid emptying or "dumping" of stomach contents into the proximal small intestine attributable to loss of pyloric regulation of gastric emptying. This loss of function may occur following a gastrectomy.

Dysconjugate See *disconjugate*.

Dysfunctional uterine bleeding Abnormal endometrial bleeding not associated with tumor, inflammation, pregnancy, or trauma. It is most common around the time of menarche and menopause.

Dyslipidemia Abnormality in the concentrations of lipids and lipoproteins in the blood, especially an elevated low-density lipoprotein (LDL) level and a reduced high-density lipoprotein (HDL) level.

Dysmenorrhea Pain associated with menstruation; usually classified as primary (unrelated to an identifiable disease) or secondary (related to the presence of an underlying disease).

Dyspareunia Pain during sexual intercourse because of vaginal muscle spasms.

Dysphagia Difficulty in swallowing as perceived by the individual. It may include the inability to initiate swallowing and/or the sensation of ingested substances sticking to the esophagus.

Dysphoria The constant experience of unpleasant emotions.

Dysplasia An alteration in cellular growth in which cell morphologic characteristics are variable and disorderly. Dysplastic cells may become cancerous and therefore are often termed *preneoplastic*.

Dyspnea Breathlessness or difficulty breathing.

Dysrhythmia An abnormality of heart rhythm, including altered rates or sites of impulse initiation and abnormal conduction pathways.

Dysthymia A state of chronic depression.

Dystrophic Abnormal tissue growth that impairs function. May result from disordered growth (trophic) signals.

E

Eating disorder A group of behaviors often fueled by unresolved emotional conflicts symptomized by altered food consumption. Disorders include anorexia nervosa, bulimia, and binge eating.

Eccentric contraction A lengthening contraction that occurs when the load is greater than the amount of tension that the muscle is able to generate, such as walking down stairs (eccentric contraction of the quadriceps muscles).

Ecchymosis Bluish discoloration of the skin (bruise) caused by escape of blood into the tissues.

Eccrine sweat gland A sweat gland that opens directly onto the skin surface.

Echocardiogram A graphic representation of heart structures and movement produced by ultrasonography.

Ectasia Dilation of a tubular structure, as in mammary duct ectasia (in which the collecting ducts beneath the nipple and areola become dilated, thinned, and filled with secretions).

Ectopic In an abnormal location.

Ectopic ureter A single ureter that implants during fetal growth in any position other than normal, or an additional ureter.

Ectopy (cardiac) A cardiac impulse initiated at a site other than the sinoatrial node.

Edema An excess of fluid in the interstitial compartment.

Efferent neuron A neuron that carries information away from the central nervous system to the muscle cells, glands, or postganglionic neurons.

Effusion Presence of fluid in a contained space, causing pressure on structures within the space.

Ejaculation Expulsion of the ejaculate from the posterior urethra through the urethral meatus.

Ejection fraction Stroke volume divided by end-diastolic volume; indicates pumping efficiency of the ventricle.

Elastin A protein found in tendons and ligaments that provides some elasticity or extensibility.

Elastosis Skin wrinkling due to changes in collagen, with fibers becoming cross-linked and rearranged in thicker bundles.

Electrocardiogram A graphic record produced by an electrocardiograph, which records electrical conduction through the heart.

Electrochemical gradient A difference in concentration of charged particles across a membrane. Driving force that moves charged particles across a membrane as a result of the combined influences of concentration gradient and electrical charge gradient.

Electroconvulsive therapy (ECT) The induction of a brief convulsion by passing an electric current through the brain for the treatment of affective disorders.

Electroencephalogram Graphic tracing of the brain's action potentials; used to evaluate nervous tissue function.

Electrolyte Substance that releases charged particles (ions) when dissolved.

Electromyography A technique for evaluating muscle contraction. Using electromyography, aspects of the contractile process such as time relationships between the beginning of electrical activity and the actual contraction of the muscle can be studied.

Electron transport chain A series of proteins on the inner mitochondrial membrane that move an electron from a higher to a lower energy level and create a proton gradient.

ELISA Abbreviation for Enzyme-Linked Immunosorbent Assay, a test used in screening for HIV antibodies and measuring the quantity of numerous substances in blood and urine.

Embolectomy A surgical incision into an artery for the removal of an embolus.

Embolus A collection of material (thrombus, air, fat, tumor cells, bacteria, amniotic fluid) propelled by blood flow to another site, where it lodges and causes obstruction of flow.

Embryoscopy A procedure in which a scope is passed through the mother's abdominal wall and into the uterus to visualize and sample embryonic tissues.

Emission One of the two phases of ejaculation. During emission, secretions from the periurethral glands, seminal vesicles, and prostate are deposited with sperm into the prostatic urethra.

Emphysema A chronic obstructive respiratory condition characterized by abnormal, permanent enlargement of air spaces distal to the terminal bronchiole with destruction of their walls and without obvious fibrosis.

Empyema Accumulation of pus in a body cavity, especially the pleural space.

Encapsulation Physiologic process of enclosure in a sheath composed of a substance not normal to the part. Prevents opsonization (recognition and binding) by antibodies and thus prevents the microorganism from being phagocytized.

Encephalitis An inflammatory condition of the brain.

Encopresis Fecal holding with constipation and fecal soiling.

Endemic disease A physical or mental disorder caused by health conditions constantly present within a community.

Endocardium A layer of endothelial cells that lines the chambers of the heart. The layer of heart muscle immediately under the endocardium is called the subendocardium.

Endocrine organ Any organ that manufactures and secretes hormones into the bloodstream.

Endocrine system The cells and organs that produce and secrete hormones into the bloodstream.

Endocytosis Cellular ingestion of extracellular molecules.

Endogenous depression Mental depression arising from characteristics within the person as opposed to depression resulting from external events.

Endometrioma A mass of endometrial tissue that grows outside the lining of the uterine cavity in the condition known as endometriosis.

Endometriosis Growth of endometrial tissue outside the lining of the uterine cavity; an abnormal condition with potentially destructive effects on the pelvic organs.

Endometrium The innermost lining of the uterus, consisting of two layers: a thin deep layer, called the basilar layer; and a thick superficial layer, referred to as the functional layer. During a woman's reproductive years, the endometrium displays a constant cyclic activity of alternate proliferation and sloughing of the functional layer in response to hormonal secretion.

Endomysium The connective tissue that surrounds the sarcolemma of an individual muscle fiber.

End-organ damage Target organs refer to major organs fed by the circulatory system, such as the heart, kidneys, brain, and eyes. Damage may be from uncontrolled hyperglycemia, hypertension, hypotension, or hypovolemia.

Endorphin One of a group of potent endogenous opioid peptides derived from cells in the hypothalamus; also found in the periaqueductal gray matter of the brain. β-Endorphin has been found to have analgesic properties.

Endoscopic retrograde cholangiopancreatography (ERCP) A procedure whereby an optical scope is passed through the mouth, esophagus, stomach, and duodenum, and then guided in a retrograde fashion into the pancreaticobiliary system. Using this technique, physicians can complete a number of therapeutic procedures without performing a laparotomy.

Endoscopic sclerosis A procedure for the treatment of esophageal varices that is accomplished by passing a flexible needle through the gastroscope and injecting various sclerosant solutions into and around the bleeding varix.

Endospore A dormant, tough, and temporarily nonreproductive structure produced by a bacterium. It is not a true spore.

Endosteum The thin membrane that covers the medullary cavity in longer bones.

Endotoxin A heat-stable lipopolysaccharide derived from the cell wall of gram-negative bacteria that induces the release of pyrogens and inflammatory mediators from immune cells.

Energy The capacity to operate or work, measured in kilocalories (kcal); 1 kcal represents the amount of energy required to raise the temperature of 1 kg of water 1° C.

Enkephalins One of two types of pain-suppressing pentapeptides; they are produced in the body and located in the pituitary gland, brain, and gastrointestinal (GI) tract.

Enteropathic arthritis Refers to joint manifestations of inflammatory bowel diseases such as ulcerative colitis and Crohn disease.

Enuresis Involuntary voiding; the term is generally used when referring to inappropriate bed-wetting in children.

Eosinophil A leukocyte that is the same size as a neutrophil but contains a two-lobed nucleus and large, coarse, eosinophilic granules that fill the cell; eosinophils participate in allergic and inflammatory responses.

Epicardium A layer of epithelial cells that covers the outer surface of the heart and forms the inner (visceral) layer of the pericardial sac.

Epidemic An outbreak of a disease that occurs suddenly and affects numbers of people clearly in excess of normal expectancy.

Epidemiology The study of patterns of disease among human populations for the purpose of establishing programs to prevent and control their spread.

Epidermal proliferating unit Group of active basal cells, together with vertical columns of migrating keratinocytes, that are undergoing mitosis.

Epidermis Outer, thinner layer of the cutaneous membrane.

Epididymis Tightly coiled tube in which sperm mature and develop the ability to swim; lies along the top of and behind the testes.

Epididymitis Inflammation of the epididymis.

Epigenetics The transfer of heritable traits from parent cells to offspring that are not coded in the DNA.

Epiglottitis An inflammation of the epiglottis, characterized by fever and stridor. Can be a life-threatening condition.

Epileptogenic focus Cellular focus in the brain with the capacity to induce epilepsy.

Epimysium The connective tissue surrounding a muscle.

Epinephrine A neurotransmitter that produces some of the same effects as norepinephrine but has a greater influence on cardiac action. Epinephrine enhances myocardial contractility, increases heart rate, and increases venous return to the heart, thus increasing cardiac output and blood pressure.

Epiphyseal plate A segment of a long bone between the metaphysis and epiphysis developed from a center of ossification and distinct from the shaft. An area of growth in a bone.

Epispadias A congenital anomaly in which the urethra opens on the dorsal aspect of the penis at a point proximal to the glans.

Epistaxis Hemorrhage from the nose; nosebleed.

Epitope A site on the surface of an antigen that is specifically recognized by an immune cell, thus stimulating an immune response.

Equilibrium Sense of balance.

Erectile dysfunction Inability of the adult male to achieve or sustain a penile erection.

Erection A complicated interaction of vascular, neurologic, and hormonal factors that enables the penis to achieve penetration and deposit sperm.

Erythema Diffuse redness of skin.

Erythroblastosis Presence of erythroblasts in the blood due to premature release from the bone marrow.

Erythrocyte Mature biconcave red blood cell that has no internal organelles.

Erythromelalgia Painful erythema (redness of the skin) of the palms and soles due to congestion of the capillaries.

Erythron The blood as a single body system.

Erythropoiesis The process of red blood cell production.

Erythropoietin Hormone produced primarily by the kidneys that stimulates bone marrow to produce erythrocytes.

Eschar Burn tissue.

Escharotomy A surgical incision through eschar of a circumferential extremity burn for the purpose of restoring distal blood flow, or through eschar of the chest to restore respiratory expansion.

Esophageal atresia Congenital anomaly in which the esophagus is closed off in a blind pouch. It occurs in about 1 of every 4000 live births and requires immediate surgical correction.

Esophageal varix Abnormally dilated blood vessel lying immediately below the mucous membrane of the esophagus that connects the hypertensive portal system with the systemic circulation. Esophageal varices may rupture, causing massive hemorrhage.

Esophagitis Inflammation or infection of the esophagus.

Essential amino acids Amino acids that must be supplied in the diet because the body cannot manufacture them.

Estrogen One of a group of ovarian hormones that promote the development of female secondary sex characteristics. During the menstrual cycle, estrogen renders the female reproductive tract suitable for fertilization of the ovum, implantation of the zygote, and provision of nutrition for the early embryo.

Etiology Study of the assignment of causes or reasons for phenomena.

Euchromatin Chromatin that is less densely packed and potentially open to transcription, as opposed to heterochromatin that is condensed and not open to transcription. "Normal" chromatin.

Eukaryote A cell that has a true nucleus bounded by a nuclear membrane.

Euphoria Also called *expanded mood,* is a hallmark symptom of both mania and hypomania. Extreme cheerfulness, enthusiasm, and optimism are present, but the joyful, buoyant mood is disproportionate to events and surroundings.

Ewing sarcoma A malignant round cell tumor (marrow tumor) that is relatively uncommon but rapidly growing.

Exacerbation A relatively sudden increase in the severity of a disease or any of its signs and symptoms.

Exercise-induced asthma Asthma that manifests 5 to 10 minutes after the exercise period begins. The increased rate and depth of respiration during exercise, especially in cold air, leads to cooling and dehydration of the lower airways.

Exhaustion A stage in the stress response that occurs when the stressor is too great or prolonged, resulting in depletion of energy reserves.

Exocytosis The process of cellular secretion through the plasma membrane accomplished by opening vesicles into the extracellular space.

Exon The portion of an RNA transcript that remains after unwanted sections (introns) have been removed from the primary transcript. A linear section of DNA that serves as a template for synthesis of a particular RNA sequence.

Exophthalmos Protrusion of the eyeball.

Exotoxin Toxins, such as enzymes or pore-forming proteins, produced by bacteria that cause physiologic dysfunction in the host.

Extracellular fluid Body fluid that is not inside the cells; includes vascular, interstitial, and transcellular fluids.

Extraocular Outside the globe of the eyeball.

Extrapyramidal system Part of the brain that includes the corpus striatum, subthalamic nucleus, substantia nigra, red nucleus, and the interconnections with the reticular formation, cerebellum, and cerebrum.

Extrapyramidal tract Outside the pyramidal tract of the brain. Comprised of the nuclei and fibers involved in motor activities, extrapyramidal tracts control and coordinate postural, static, support, and locomotor mechanisms. Do not crossover in the medullary pyramid.

Extrinsic Originating from sources outside of the individual.

Extrinsic asthma Also called *allergic asthma,* it commonly affects children and young adults. Attacks are related to specific antigens and are mediated by immunoglobulin E.

Extrinsic pathway of clotting The mechanism that produces fibrin following tissue injury, beginning with formation of an activated complex between tissue factor and activated factor VII and leading to activation of factor X, which induces the reactions of the common pathway of coagulation.

Exudate Fluid of high protein content that moves into tissues or cavities as part of a reaction to inflammation or injury.

F

Fascia A sheath of connective tissue that envelops muscles or other parts of the body.

Fascia of Buck Layer of deep fascia covering the penis.

Fasciculus Bundle of muscle fibers that compose individual muscles.

Facioscapulohumeral muscular dystrophy A rare inherited autosomal dominant trait that affects the muscles of the shoulder girdle and the face and upper arms.

Fast twitch (type II, white) A muscle fiber that can develop high tension rapidly. It is usually innervated by a single α-motor neuron and has low fatigue resistance, low capillary density, low levels of aerobic enzymes, and low oxygen availability.

Fat The most concentrated dietary source of energy; derived from either animals or vegetables. Provides 9 kcal/gm of energy when metabolized.

Fat emboli syndrome A circulatory condition characterized by a plug of fat blocking an artery; it enters the circulatory system after the fracture of a long bone.

Fatigue A lack of physical or emotional energy or power.

Fatty acid An organic acid with a long, straight hydrocarbon chain that is a fundamental component of lipids. Some fatty acids are manufactured by the body; others are essential and must be supplied in the diet.

Fetotoxic Referring to a substance that is damaging to a developing fetus.

Fibrillation Cardiac dysrhythmia characterized by rapid, random myocardial contractions and uncoordinated pumping action.

Fibrinolysis Dissolution or breakup of a fibrin clot.

Fibroblast Connective tissue cells that produce collagen fibers, which compose the bulk of the dermis.

Fibrocystic breast disease A condition in which the presence of palpable breast masses (cysts) corresponds to fluctuations in the menstrual cycle; the masses may be associated with pain and tenderness.

Fibromyalgia syndrome A painful, noninflammatory musculoskeletal disorder associated with fatigue and multiple somatic complaints.

Fibrosis Condition of decreased elasticity because of excessive deposition of fibrin and collagen in the tissue (e.g., restrictive process characterized by thickening of the alveolar interstitium).

Fight-or-flight response The reaction of the body to stressors that is mediated by the sympathetic nervous system and produces elevated heart rate and release of glucocorticoids from the adrenal cortex.

Filaments or protein filaments Fine thread-like fibers found in most tissues and cells of the body.

Filtration Movement of fluid across capillary walls as a net result of opposing forces of hydrostatic and colloid osmotic pressures.

First-degree burn Superficial tissue destruction in the outermost layers of the epidermis. All physiologic functions of the skin remain intact.

Fistula An abnormal tubelike passage between two organs or between an internal organ and the body surface.

Flagellum Motile (whiplike) appendage that allows a cell to move or swim.

Flail chest A thorax in which there are two fractures on at least two adjacent ribs that cause instability in part of the chest wall and paradoxical breathing.

Flank pain Discomfort to the posterior portion of the body between the ribs and the ileum. Often associated with the ureters.

Flat affect Lack of appropriate emotional expression.

Focal segmental glomerulosclerosis A condition where only some of the glomeruli are involved, resulting in scarring of the glomerulus. It is a cause of nephrotic syndrome and renal failure.

Fomite An inanimate object that transmits a pathogen to a new host.

Foreskin Also called *prepuce;* penile skin that overlies the glans and is removed in circumcision.

Fossa navicularis Area of widening near the end of the penile urethra.

Fournier gangrene A rare condition involving a gangrenous necrosis of the scrotum, penis, or perineum.

Fourth-degree burn A full-thickness burn that penetrates the dermis to reach muscle or bone.

Fracture A break or disruption in the continuity of a bone, an epiphyseal plate, or cartilage.

Frank-Starling law of the heart Describes the relationship between diastolic stretch and subsequent increased strength of contraction. Also called the *length-tension relationship.*

Free-living bacteria Bacteria that can live outside the host cell.

Free radical An extremely reactive compound that avidly makes molecular bonds with other compounds.

Full-thickness burn Also called a *third degree burn,* this type of burn is marked by destruction of epidermis, dermis, and underlying tissue. All physiologic functions of the skin are absent. This burn will not heal and requires autografting.

Full-thickness excision Removal by surgical knife of complete eschar to fascia. Full-thickness excision often leaves an uneven contour, which presents difficulty with grafting, resulting in poor cosmesis.

Functional disorder of the endocrine system An endocrine disorder caused by a non-endocrine disease (e.g., chronic renal failure, liver disease, or heart failure).

Functional incontinence Loss of urine or feces as a result of factors external to the urinary or digestive tract, such as physical or cognitive impairment.

Functional syncytium A multinucleate mass of protoplasm that results from the merging of cells. It is characteristic of the gastrointestinal tract and heart, meaning that its separate cells have the ability to function in concert with one another in a unified manner.

Fungal infection Any inflammatory condition caused by a fungus.

Fungus A nonphotosynthetic, eukaryotic protist that is disseminated throughout the environment.

G

Gallbladder A distensible sac of about 30- to 50-ml capacity that connects the common hepatic duct to the common bile duct via the cystic duct.

Ganglion A group of neuronal cell bodies located outside of the central nervous system.

Gangrene Cellular death involving a large area of tissue; may be characterized as wet, dry, or gaseous.

Gap junction A cell-to-cell communication pore that allows small biomolecules to flow from the cytoplasm of one cell to the cytoplasm of an adjacent cell.

Gas exchange Diffusion of oxygen and carbon dioxide across the alveolar-capillary membranes of the lungs.

Gastrectomy Surgical removal of all or, more commonly, part of the stomach. This procedure may be used to remove a chronic peptic ulcer, to stop hemorrhage in a perforating ulcer, or to remove a malignancy.

Gastrin A stomach hormone that is released in response to certain types of food. Gastrin increases acid secretion by stomach parietal cells.

Gastritis Inflammation of the stomach lining. It may occur following the ingestion of irritating substances or in the presence of viral, bacterial, or chemical toxins.

Gastroenteritis Inflammation of the stomach and intestines; may occur on an acute or chronic basis and is commonly caused by viruses.

Gastroesophageal reflux disease (GERD) Backflow of gastric contents into the esophagus through the lower esophageal sphincter. GERD may or may not produce symptoms. The most common manifestations of GERD are heartburn, regurgitation, chest pain, and dysphagia.

Gastroesophageal varices A complex of longitudinal tortuous veins at the lower end of the esophagus, enlarged and swollen as the result of portal hypertension.

Gene A unit of heredity consisting of a segment of DNA nucleotides that encodes a messenger RNA capable of being translated into a protein.

General adaptation syndrome (GAS) The total organism's nonspecific response to stress. Term was coined by Hans Selye.

Generalized anxiety disorder (GAD) Characterized by the continual presence of a moderate degree of anxiety without discrete periods of acute attacks. GAD symptoms include chronic anxiety and tension accompanied by headaches, abdominal problems, or sleep disturbances. Agoraphobia is rarely seen in GAD.

Generalized seizure A seizure that involves the whole brain surface and impairs consciousness.

Genital herpes A chronic viral infection usually transmitted by sexual contact.

Genital warts A condyloma of the genitals; caused by sexual transmission of human papillomavirus.

Genome The entire complement of genes located on chromosomes in the nucleus of a cell.

Genotype The genetic constitution of an individual; often described by listing the allele types at a certain gene locus.

Gerontology The study of all aspects of the aging process.

Gestational diabetes mellitus A condition of glucose intolerance first diagnosed in the mother during pregnancy. Usually disappears after delivery of the infant.

Ghon tubercle A nodule or swelling containing *Mycobacterium tuberculosis.*

Giant cell tumor Also called *osteoclastoma;* a benign but aggressive tumor with richly vascularized tissue consisting of plump spindle-shaped cells and numerous giant cells.

Gilbert syndrome A common, benign autosomal dominant condition that results in mild unconjugated (indirect) hyperbilirubinemia.

Ginglymus A type of joint that permits flexion and extension; examples include the interphalangeal joint of the finger, the elbow joint, or the knee joint. Also called a *hinge joint.*

Glasgow Coma Scale Scale developed by G. Teasdale and B. Jennett for the purpose of objectively assessing coma and impaired consciousness.

Glaucoma An abnormal condition of elevated pressure within the eye.

Glial Supporting or nonneuronal cells within the central nervous system.

Glomerulopathies Diseases of the renal glomeruli.

Glomerular filtration rate The rate of fluid filtration through the glomeruli into Bowman capsule per minute; normally 125 ml/min.

Glomerulonephritis Inflammation of the glomerular capillary walls that causes impaired filtration and renal function.

Glucagon Hormone produced by the α cells of the pancreas that stimulates glycogenolysis and gluconeogenesis in the liver.

Glucocorticoid resistance model This model proposes a specific link between stress, immunity, and disease. Rather than viewing disease as a result of increased vulnerability due to stress, this model proposes that overwhelming stress reduces the sensitivity of the immune system to cortisol.

Glucocorticoids A class of steroid hormones secreted by the adrenal cortex; they are necessary for use of carbohydrates, fats, and proteins and for the body's normal response to stress.

Gluconeogenesis The production of glucose from amino acids and other substrates in the liver.

Glucose-6-phosphate dehydrogenase deficiency (G6PD) An inherited disorder characterized by red cells partially or completely deficient in G6PD, an enzyme critical in anaerobic glycolysis.

Glycogen A carbohydrate consisting of branched chains of glucose produced by muscles and the liver as a storage form of glucose.

Glycogenesis Production of glycogen from glucose in hepatic and muscle tissue.

Glycogenolysis Production of glucose from the breakdown of glycogen in hepatic and muscle tissue.

Glycolysis The anaerobic process of breaking down carbohydrates into simpler molecules, with the net production of two adenosine triphosphate and two pyruvate molecules per glucose molecule.

Glycosaminoglycan A protein polysaccharide contained in ground substances surrounded by collagen fibers in bone.

Glycosylated hemoglobin An index of glycemic control; the quantity of glucose attached to hemoglobin molecules (%), reflecting mean blood glucose values for a period of 120 days, usually reported as HbA_{1c}.

Goiter Enlargement of the thyroid gland.

Golgi apparatus A membrane-bound organelle in which the proteins and lipids that are synthesized in the endoplasmic reticulum are modified and sorted in preparation for transport to the lysosomes or plasma membrane.

Gomphosis joint An articulation created by the insertion of a conical process into a socket, such as the insertion of a root of a tooth into an alveolus of the mandible or the maxilla. Gomphosis is not a connection between true bones but is considered a type of fibrous joint.

Gonad An organ that produces sex cells. Derived from the urogenital ridge, the undifferentiated and primitive gonads become the testes in males and the ovaries in females.

Gonadotropins Hormones that stimulate the function of the testes and the ovaries (FSH and LH).

Gonorrhea Common sexually transmitted infection involving the inflammation of epithelial tissue by the organism *Neisseria gonorrhoeae.* Characteristic symptoms include urethritis, dysuria, purulent urethral discharge, and redness and swelling at the site of the infection.

Goodpasture syndrome A chronic relapsing autoimmune disease usually associated with glomerulonephritis.

Gout A condition caused by lack of the enzyme uricase and by inability to oxidize uric acid into a soluble compound; characterized by recurrent attacks of articular and periarticular inflammation, accumulation of tophi (crystalline deposits) in bony and connective tissue, renal impairment, and formation of uric acid calculi.

Grading Assignment of degree of differentiation of tumor cells by histologic examination. The degree of anaplasia usually correlates with the degree of malignancy, with higher grades conferring greater malignant potential.

Gram stain A process by which it is determined whether bacteria can retain a basic dye after iodine fixation. This ability is the basis for classifying bacteria into gram-negative and gram-positive organisms.

Granulocyte A leukocyte with polymorphic nuclei and cytoplasmic granules. Neutrophils, basophils, and eosinophils are types of granulocytes.

Granulocytopenia An abnormal decrease in the total number of granulocytes in the blood.

Granuloma Tissue that forms into a nodular mass as a result of inflammation, infection, or injury.

Granuloma inguinale An ulcerative disease of the genital tract caused by the bacterium *Calymmatobacterium granulomatis*. The communicability of the disease is relatively low, and it is generally believed that repeated exposure is necessary for infection.

Granulomatous Relating to granulomas; chronic inflammatory lesions characterized by an accumulation of macrophages; epithelioid macrophages, with or without lymphocytes; and giant cells into a discrete granule.

Graves disease Hyperthyroid state characterized by exophthalmos and goiter from autoimmune stimulation of the thyroid.

Greenstick fracture An incomplete break in the bone with the intact side of the cortex flexed; this is usually seen in children.

Ground substance A material composed of a hydrated network of proteins, mainly glycoproteins and proteoglycans, that serves as the "cement" between layers of collagen fibers. Also known as *matrix*.

Growing pain A common soft-tissue syndrome in children. The most common symptom is nocturnal pain that usually occurs in the calves, shins, and thighs. Also called *nonarticular rheumatism*.

Growth hormone A hormone secreted by the anterior pituitary gland with wide-ranging action, including effects on energy metabolism and increasing lean body mass.

Guillain-Barré syndrome Also called *acute idiopathic polyneuropathy* or *polyradiculoneuropathy;* Guillain-Barré syndrome is an inflammatory demyelinating disease of the peripheral nervous system.

Gustatory Pertaining to the sense of taste.

Gyrus A raised ridge or convolution on the surface of a structure (e.g., cerebral cortex).

H

H⁺ Hydrogen ion; released by acids; determines pH; also called a *proton*.

HCO₃⁻ Bicarbonate ion; a base that binds and buffers H⁺.

H₂CO₃ Carbonic acid; this acid is removed from the body in the form of carbon dioxide and water during exhalation.

H zone Corresponds to a region occupied solely by myosin filaments with no actin filament overlap in cardiac and skeletal muscle.

Hair Keratinized, threadlike outgrowth of the skin that covers most of the body.

Hair follicle Slender, cylindrical tube of epidermal cells in which hair grows.

Hallucination A perception for which there are no objective sensory data.

Haploid Containing only one set of chromosomes (as distinct from diploid), as in a sperm cell or egg cell.

Hapten Incomplete, lipid-soluble particle that is incapable of being an antigen by itself, but that becomes an antigen inside the body when it binds with a host protein called a carrier. When a hapten penetrates the epidermis and binds to a carrier, it can cause contact hypersensitivity.

Haustral churning The mixing movement of the haustra (the outpouchings in the colon wall) when material is in the proximal end of the colon.

Haversian system The basic unit of bone; also called *osteon*.

HBV infection Hepatitis B virus infection. Vertical transmission from an HBsAg-positive mother to the infant is a common mechanism of spread.

HCV infection Hepatitis C virus infection. A type of viral hepatitis that is usually chronic and transmitted most commonly by blood transfusion or percutaneous inoculation.

HDV infection Hepatitis D virus infection. A form of hepatitis that occurs only in patients co-infected with hepatitis B. HDV relies on HBV replication and cannot replicate independently. The disease usually progresses to a chronic state.

Heimlich maneuver An emergency procedure for dislodging an obstruction from the trachea. It consists of grasping the choking person from behind, placing the hands around the victim's waist just below the sternum (in a fist with the thumb toward the body), and pulling inward and upward with force to dislodge the obstruction. Now called *abdominal thrusts*.

Helicobacter pylori An infectious gastrointestinal tract bacterium first identified in 1982. Since then, *H. pylori* has generated worldwide attention for its role in the promotion of chronic gastritis, peptic ulcer disease, and gastric carcinoma. The mode of transmission of *H. pylori* is still unclear, although person-to-person, fecal-oral spread is suspected because of the tendency of *H. pylori* infections to cluster in families.

Hemangiomas Benign tumors consisting of a mass of blood vessels.

Hemarthrosis Blood in a joint cavity.

Hematemesis Blood in vomitus.

Hematochezia Feces containing bright red blood.

Hematoma A mass caused by extravasation of blood into a tissue or cavity (bruise).

Hematopoiesis Production of cells in the bone marrow, including red blood cells, white blood cells, and platelets.

Hematuria Blood in the urine.

Hemianopsia Partial loss of the same field of vision in both eyes.

Hemiparesis Motor weakness affecting one side of the body, usually occurring with lateral cerebral injuries.

Hemiplegia Paralysis of one side of the body.

Hemochromatosis A disorder (usually genetic) of iron metabolism characterized by excess absorption of iron, elevation of ferritin levels, and deposition of iron in organs such as the liver.

Hemodynamics Physical laws governing blood flow.

Hemoglobin Oxygen-carrying protein in the red blood cells.

Hemolysis Separation of hemoglobin from red blood cells and its appearance in the fluid in which the corpuscles are suspended; red blood cell lysis.

Hemophilia A group of hereditary disorders characterized by a deficiency of one of the factors necessary for coagulation of the blood, usually factor VIII or IX.

Hemoptysis Expectoration of blood, the origin of which is the lungs or bronchial tubes.

Hemostasis Arrest of bleeding; prevention of blood loss.

Hemothorax Accumulation of blood and fluid in the pleural space.

Hepatic encephalopathy A neuropsychiatric manifestation of extensive liver damage. Also known as *hepatic coma*.

Hepatitis An inflammatory condition of the liver. Potential causes include viral, bacterial, fungal, and protozoal infections; drugs and toxins; autoimmune disorders; and metabolic disorders.

Hepatocellular carcinoma A common form of primary hepatic malignancy. Signs and symptoms include hepatomegaly, abdominal pain, weight loss, nausea, and, in advanced cases, jaundice and ascites. Also called *hepatoma*.

Hepatocellular failure Acute or chronic loss of essential liver function resulting in portal systemic encephalopathy and a variety of other problems, including coagulopathy, renal failure, bleeding, infection, hypoglycemia, respiratory failure, and death.

Hepatorenal syndrome A type of kidney failure characterized by gradual loss of function without signs of tissue damage.

Hepatoma A primary liver cancer arising from cells normally found in the liver, not to be confused with cancer metastatic to the liver from a distant site.

Hereditary hemochromatosis An autosomal recessive disorder caused by the activity of a mutant gene called *HFE*, which allows excessive and uncontrolled iron absorption by the GI tract.

Herpes simplex virus A virus causing infection of the skin and nervous system; often associated with painful fluid-filled vesicles.

Herpesviruses Important group of viral agents producing infections in humans. Two types of herpes simplex viruses, referred to as types 1 and 2, may be sexually transmitted.

Herpes zoster (shingles) An acute localized inflammatory disease of a dermatomal segment of the skin caused by the same herpesvirus that causes chickenpox.

Heterochromatin A type of chromatin (DNA) that is tightly compacted and genetically inactive.

Heterozygous Having two different alleles for a specific gene product.

HEV infection Hepatitis E virus infection. A self-limited type of hepatitis acquired by ingestion of fecally contaminated water or food.

Hiatal hernia A defect in the diaphragm that allows a portion of the stomach to protrude through the diaphragmatic opening into the thorax.

High blood pressure A persistent elevation of blood pressure >140 mm Hg systolic/90 mm Hg diastolic. High blood pressure is an elevated blood pressure reading. If it is consistently >120/80 mm Hg but <140/90 mm Hg, then it is called *pre-hypertension*.

Hilum Concave portion of the kidney that faces the vertebral column through which nerves, blood vessels, and ureters enter and exit the kidney.

Hinge joint A joint that permits flexion and extension, such as the interphalangeal joint of the finger, the elbow joint, or the knee joint. Also called a *ginglymus joint*.

Hirschsprung disease A congenital disorder of the large intestine in which the autonomic nervous system ganglia in the smooth muscle are absent or markedly reduced in number, which causes poor or absent peristalsis.

Hirsutism Excessive growth of hair or the presence of hair in unusual places.

Histamine A compound found in cells, especially mast cells; it is produced by the breakdown of histidine. It is released in allergic inflammatory reactions.

Histiocyte A type of cell normally present in small numbers around blood vessels, but in pathologic conditions it can migrate in the dermis as a tissue monocyte. It can also form abundant reticulum fibers. When it phagocytizes bacteria and particulate matter, it is referred to as a *macrophage*.

Histone A protein around which linear DNA is wrapped.

Histrionic Theatrical, dramatic.

Hodgkin disease A progressive malignancy of the lymph node characterized by the presence of Reed-Sternberg cells and slow, predictable dissemination through the lymphatic vessels.

Homeostasis A dynamic steady state, representing the net effect of all the turnover reactions.

Homologous Corresponding in structure. For example, the labia majora are *homologous* with the scrotum of the male.

Homologous chromosomes A pair of chromosomes in a diploid cell that contain similar gene loci, each being derived from a different parent.

Homozygous Having two identical alleles for a specific gene product.

Hormone A blood-borne chemical messenger that affects target cells anatomically distant from the secreting cells.

Hormone agonist A chemical that binds to a hormone receptor and initiates intracellular activities identical to those caused by hormones. Some medications exert their therapeutic effects through this process.

Hormone antagonist A chemical that competes with hormones for cell receptors. Antagonists bind to cell receptors and prevent the occurrence of intracellular activities associated with hormone-receptor binding. Some medications produce their therapeutic effects through this process.

Hormone receptor A protein on or within a target cell that binds to circulating hormones and allows the cellular response to a specific hormone. Hormone-receptor binding is the first step in the cellular response to a particular hormone.

Host-parasite relationship The interaction between the host and the microorganisms that reside on or in it.

Human immunodeficiency virus (HIV) A general term for several types of retroviruses that affect the immune system, causing a defect in cell-mediated immunity and failure of the immune system to function properly.

Human leukocyte antigen (HLA) complex The major histocompatibility complex (MHC) in human leukocytes.

Human papillomavirus (HPV) infection A virus that is the cause of common warts of the hands and feet, as well as lesions of the oral, anal, and genital cavities. More than 50 types of HPV have been identified.

Humoral immunity A form of immunity mediated by circulating antibodies that coat the antigens and target them for destruction.

Hyaline membranes Membranes in alveolar tissue that look like glass. The alveoli are filled with proteinaceous fluid and epithelial cells.

Hydrocele Accumulation of fluid in the tunica vaginalis testis; one of the most common causes of scrotal swelling.

Hydrocephalus Increase in the amount of cerebrospinal fluid attributable to blocked circulation or absorption and the consequent enlargement of the ventricles.

Hydronephrosis Distention of the pelvis and calyces of the kidney by urine that cannot flow past an obstruction in the ureter.

Hydrophilic Soluble in water but not in lipid.

Hydrophobic Insoluble in water but soluble in lipid.

Hydropic swelling An increase in intracellular fluid volume and changes in intracellular organelles in association with cell injury. Also termed *oncosis*.

Hydrostatic pressure Pressure exerted by a liquid.

Hydroureter Distention of a ureter with urine, usually resulting from an obstruction process.

Hyperacusis Exceptionally acute hearing, the hearing threshold being unusually low. It may or may not be accompanied by pain.

Hyperaldosteronism A condition characterized by hypersecretion of aldosterone, occurring as a disease of the adrenal cortex or as a response to adrenal disease.

Hyperalgesia An increased sensitivity to painful stimuli characterized by a lower than normal pain threshold.

Hypercalcemia Serum calcium concentration greater than normal.

Hypercapnia An abnormally high amount of carbon dioxide in the blood.

Hypercortisolism Elevated serum level of cortisol.

Hyperemesis gravidarum A Latin term meaning "excess vomiting in pregnant women." Unlike the transient nausea and vomiting that occurs in about half of women in the first trimester of pregnancy, hyperemesis gravidarum continues throughout the entire pregnancy.

Hyperemia Localized redness produced by increased blood flow.

Hyperkalemia Serum potassium concentration higher than normal levels.

Hyperkeratosis Horny overgrowth of epidermis, such as callous formation.

Hypermagnesemia Serum magnesium concentration greater than normal levels.

Hypermetabolic state A condition of abnormally high basal metabolic rate. May be indicated by an increase in skin temperature, such as that occurring in hyperthyroidism and after sun exposure or sunburn.

Hypernatremia Serum sodium concentration greater than normal levels; results from a gain of salt relative to water or a loss of water relative to salt; water deficit.

Hyperopia Farsightedness or the inability of the eye to focus on nearby objects.

Hyperparathyroidism An abnormal endocrine condition characterized by hyperactivity of the parathyroid glands.

Hyperphosphatemia Serum phosphate concentration greater than normal levels.

Hyperplasia Abnormal multiplication or increase in the number of normal cells in normal arrangement in a tissue.

Hypersensitivity An abnormal excessive response to a sensitizing antigen.

Hypertension (see *High blood pressure*) A persistent elevation of blood pressure >140 mm Hg systolic/90 mm Hg diastolic.

Hypertensive crisis A sudden, severe increase in blood pressure that could be life threatening.

Hyperthyroidism Overactivity of the thyroid gland.

Hypertonic fluid Fluid that has a higher particle concentration (osmolality) than normal body fluid; causes a net flow of water across cell membranes out of cells.

Hypertrichosis lanuginosa Excessive hair growth over the entire body.

Hypertrophy An increase in cell or tissue size and function.

Hypocalcemia Serum calcium concentration below normal values.

Hypochromia An abnormal decrease in the hemoglobin content of the erythrocytes.

Hypodermis Loose subcutaneous layer rich in fat and areolar tissue lying beneath the dermis. Also known as *superficial fascia*.

Hypogonadism A deficiency in the size or function of the ovary or testis.

Hypoglycemic sweating Sweating caused by low blood glucose concentration. Usually distinguishable from other causes of sweating attributable to the additional symptoms of weakness, tachycardia, hunger, headache, and "inward nervousness" manifested as mental irritability and confusion.

Hypokalemia Serum potassium concentration less than normal levels.

Hypomagnesemia Serum magnesium concentration less than normal levels.

Hypomania Also called *partial mania*, can include any symptoms of mania but without the loss of reality testing, without psychosis (e.g., hallucinations, delusions), and without impaired functioning.

Hypomenorrhea A deficient amount of menstrual flow, usually the result of an endocrine or systemic disorder that interferes with hormonal function. It may also result from partial obstruction of the menstrual flow by the hymen or a narrowing of the cervical os.

Hyponatremia Serum sodium concentration less than normal levels; results from gain of water relative to salt or loss of salt relative to water; water intoxication.

Hypophosphatemia Serum phosphate concentration less than normal levels.

Hypophysis The pituitary gland, which consists of anterior and posterior lobes.

Hyposensitization Reduction in sensitivity to an allergen, accomplished by administering low doses of the allergen, which binds with immunoglobulin G.

Hypospadias A congenital anomaly in which the urethral meatus is located on the undersurface of the penis or on the perineum.

Hypothalamic-pituitary-adrenal (HPA) axis Refers to a hierarchy of control mechanisms whereby the hypothalamus regulates the anterior pituitary and the pituitary regulates the secretion of hormones from the adrenal cortex.

Hypothalamus A group of nuclei at the base of the brain concerned with regulation of body processes: temperature, thirst, hunger, satiety, and adaptive sexual behaviors.

Hypothyroidism Underactivity of the thyroid gland.

Hypotonic fluid Fluid that has a lower particle concentration (osmolality) than normal body fluid; causes a net flow of water across cell membranes into cells.

Hypoventilation Decreased exchange of air in the alveoli in relation to oxygen consumption; influenced by a decreased rate and depth of respiration, and evidenced by elevated $Paco_2$ values.

Hypovolemic shock A state of physical collapse and prostration usually caused by massive blood loss.

Hypoxemia An abnormally low amount of oxygen in the blood.

Hypoxia A reduction in oxygen at the tissue level that may lead to failure of aerobic production of adenosine triphosphate.

I

I bands "I" indicates "isotropic"; these bands are light in color and correspond to the position of thin actin filaments extending in both directions from the Z line in striated muscle.

Iatrogenic Resulting from the activity of a health care provider.

Icterus Also called *jaundice*. A yellow discoloration of the skin, mucous membranes, and sclerae of the eyes that is caused by greater than normal amounts of bilirubin in the blood.

Idiopathic Without known cause.

Idiopathic hypertension High blood pressure of unknown cause; also called *primary hypertension.*

Ileocecal valve Sphincter between the small and large intestines that is normally closed, so that the contents of the large intestine cannot move in a retrograde fashion back into the small intestine. It opens in response to peristaltic contractions in the small intestine, bringing intestinal contents toward it.

Illusion The misperception of a real sensory stimulus.

Immobilization A mechanical action of limiting or preventing movement of the body or a body part. Prolonged immobilization may cause a shortening of connective tissue, a breakdown of cartilage, a weakening of ligaments, and a decrease in the muscles' ability to contract, as well as increased bone resorption.

Immunity A state of active resistance to a particular pathogen, which requires functional T- and B-cell memory cells.

Immunization Exposure of a susceptible host to an altered pathogen that does not cause disease but instigates the host to create antibodies to that pathogen.

Immunodeficiency Failure of immune system mechanisms to defend against pathogens. There are two broad categories of immunodeficiencies, based on the mechanism of lymphocyte dysfunction: primary and acquired.

Immunogen Foreign substance, cell, toxin, or protein that causes the components of the immune system to react and respond, inducing the formation of antibodies. Also known as an *antigen.*

Immunogenicity The ability to stimulate an immune response.

Immunoglobulin Any of five structurally distinct classes of proteins that function as antibodies in the serum and secretions of the body.

Immunosuppression The inability to produce an immune response to an antigen, resulting in reduced resistance to infection.

Immunotherapy The use of immune products such as monoclonal antibodies to treat specific diseases.

Impacted fracture A fracture caused by excessive force that telescopes or drives one fragment into another.

Impaired fasting glucose A disorder of glucose tolerance, not diagnostic of diabetes, that is characterized by a fasting blood glucose value between 100 and 125 mg/dl.

Impaired glucose tolerance A disorder of glucose tolerance, not diagnostic of diabetes, that is characterized by a 2-hour postprandial blood glucose value of between 140 and 200 mg/dl.

Impetigo An acute, contagious skin disease characterized by the formation of vesicles, pustules, and yellowish crusts.

Impotence Failure to achieve and maintain an erection of the penis.

Impulsivity Spontaneous acting out of impulses accompanied by failure to plan ahead, predict consequences, or consider other possibilities.

Incomplete fracture A fracture in which the cortex of the bone buckles or cracks without disrupting bone continuity.

Incontinence The inability to control urination or defecation.

Induction The process of stimulating and determining morphogenetic differentiation in a developing embryo. Also the initial phase of cancer chemotherapy.

Induration Hardness, such as that resulting from multiple intramuscular or subcutaneous injections of medication.

Inert tissue Soft tissue that possesses no ability to contract or relax; this includes the joint capsule, ligament, bursa, fascia, dura mater, and nerve root.

Infectious disease A pathologic process caused by a microorganism that is transmissible from one host to another.

Infiltrate Fluid or material that has moved into tissues.

Inflammation The body's protective response at the site of injury or tissue destruction. It is important to recognize that although infectious agents can produce inflammation, infection is not synonymous with inflammation.

Inflammatory bowel disease A general term for inflammatory diseases of the bowel, such as ulcerative colitis and Crohn disease.

Inhalation injury Cellular injury to lung tissue as a result of inhalation of a toxic substance such as smoke. Smoke inhalation significantly increases the morbidity and mortality from burn injury.

Innate immune response Part of the host defense system that is composed of mechanical and biochemical barriers, phagocytes, and chemical mediators.

Inotropy The force or rate of cardiac contraction; similar to contractility.

Insulin Hormone produced by the β cells of the pancreas; has wide-ranging effects on energy metabolism and protein synthesis.

Insulin resistance The condition of requiring an increased amount of insulin for the same level of tissue glucose utilization.

Integrins A large family of transmembrane proteins that mediate adhesion of cells to the extracellular matrix.

Integument Covering; refers to the skin.

Integumentary system The skin and its appendages, including the hair and nails.

Intercurrent Occurring during the course of an already existing disease.

Interferons Natural glycoproteins formed by cells exposed to a virus.

Interleukins One of a large group of proteins produced mainly by T cells. Most direct other cells to divide and differentiate.

Intermembranous ossification The process in which osteoblasts in the inner layer of the periosteum are responsible for the increase in width of bones.

Interstitial cystitis Inflammation of the bladder that is believed to be associated with an autoimmune or allergic response.

Interstitial fluid Fluid that lies between the cells; a component of extracellular fluid.

Interstitial space The space between cells.

Intertrigo An erythematous irritation of opposing skin surfaces caused by friction.

Intestinal obstruction Failure of the contents of the intestines to progress through the lumen of the bowel because of mechanical blockage.

Intestinal villi Fingerlike projections, numbering in the millions, that line the small intestine and serve to increase the surface area of the intestine for digestion and absorption of nutrients.

Intraaortic Within the aorta. For example, in intraaortic balloon counterpulsation, a catheter with a balloon at the distal segment is inserted through the femoral artery and positioned in the aorta just distal to the left subclavian artery.

Intracellular fluid Fluid that is inside the cells.

Intracellular obligate parasites Bacteria that must live inside a living cell.

Intraocular Inside the globe of the eyeball.

Intrarenal Occurring within the kidney.

Intravenous pyelography A diagnostic procedure in which an iodine-based contrast material is injected into the vascular system to allow visualization of the kidneys and urinary tract.

Intrinsic Originating from within the individual.

Intrinsic asthma Asthma caused by pathophysiologic disturbances that do not involve IgE-mediated mechanisms. This type of asthma frequently develops in middle age. Psychological stress factors, pulmonary irritants, and exercise may precipitate an asthma attack.

Intrinsic (enteric) nervous system Neural structures belonging entirely to the gastrointestinal (GI) system that control most GI functions and are responsible for many reflexes occurring locally in the GI tract. Intrinsic nervous system is composed of two layers: the myenteric plexus and the submucosal plexus.

Intrinsic pathway of coagulation A sequence of reactions leading to fibrin formation, beginning with the contact activation of factor XII, followed by the sequential activation of factors XI and IX and resulting in the activation of factor X, which in activated form initiates the common pathway of coagulation.

Intron The portion of a primary RNA transcript that is removed prior to translation of the RNA message.

Intussusception A telescoping of a portion of the bowel into an adjacent distal portion. It is most common in infants and occurs three times more often in males than in females.

Invasion The process by which malignant cells move through the basement membrane and gain access to blood vessels and lymphatic channels.

Inversion An abnormal condition in which a section of chromosome is reversed and reinserted into DNA.

Involucrum A sheath or coating of new bone growth outside of existing bone seen in pyogenic osteomyelitis. It results from the stripping of the periosteum by the accumulation of pus within the bone, and new bone growing from the periosteum. It can be seen with x-rays, but is extremely rare in developed countries because osteomyelitis is rarely left untreated.

Ipsilateral Referring to the same side of the body.

Iron deficiency anemia A microcytic hypochromic anemia caused by inadequate supplies of iron needed to synthesize hemoglobin.

Irritable bowel syndrome The presence of alternating diarrhea and constipation accompanied by abdominal cramping in the absence of any identifiable pathologic process in the gastrointestinal tract.

Ischemia Inadequate blood flow through the arterial system, producing tissue hypoxia.

Ischemic hepatitis A lack of blood or oxygen supply to the liver that causes injury to liver cells.

Isoforms Isomeric forms of the same protein, with slightly different amino acid sequences but with the same function.

Isoimmunity The condition occurring when an individual's immune system reacts against antigens on tissues from other members of the same species, such as a blood transfusion reaction in which a person with type A blood reacts against a transfusion with type B blood.

Isolated systolic hypertension An elevation in systolic blood pressure greater than 140 mm Hg without an increase in diastolic blood pressure. Most commonly occurs in the elderly.

Isolated urinary tract infection A first infection or an infection that occurs more than 6 months after a previous infection.

Isometric contraction A contraction in which no movement takes place and the muscle maintains its specific length. For example, holding a weight in the hand with elbow flexed produces an isometric contraction.

Isotonic fluid Fluid that has the same particle concentration (osmolality) as normal body fluid.

Isovolumic contraction The early phase of systole, in which the myocardial muscle fibers have begun to shorten and all valves in the heart are closed.

J

Jaundice Yellowness of skin associated with elevated serum bilirubin levels.

Joint A point of contact between bones. Also called *articulation*.

Joint capsule A dense layer of connective tissue surrounding a synovial joint. The capsule is solidly attached to the periosteum of the adjacent bony components. The joint capsule provides strength to the joint and, through its neural receptors, detects motion, compression, tension, vibration, and pain.

Juxtaglomerular apparatus The collection of macula densa cells in the distal convoluted tubule and the afferent and efferent arterioles and also the juxtaglomerular cells located around the arterioles; they work together to control glomerular filtration rate.

Juxtamedullary nephron A nephron with long loops of Henle that extend deep into the medulla and create a concentrated interstitium via the countercurrent mechanism.

K

Keratin Tough, water-repellent protein produced by keratinocytes and found in hair, nails, and horny tissue.

Keratinocyte One of several types of epithelial cells. Keratinocytes are able to synthesize DNA and produce keratin.

Keratosis Any skin lesion in which there is overgrowth and thickening of the cornified epithelium.

Kernicterus An abnormal toxic accumulation of bilirubin in central nervous system tissues caused by hyperbilirubinemia.

Ketoacidosis Acidosis accompanied by an accumulation of ketones; it is usually associated with poorly controlled type 1 diabetes mellitus.

Ketone bodies The result of fatty acids in the liver that are transformed to acetyl coenzyme A, which is then processed into one of three compounds known as ketone bodies.

Kilocalorie The unit of measure for the energy value of foods.

Kinin A vasoactive peptide produced during inflammation and injury.

Koilonychia Dystrophy of the fingernails, in which the nails are concave; also known as *spoon nail*.

Korotkoff sounds Sounds heard during auscultation of arterial blood pressure. As the pressure in the blood pressure cuff is released, blood begins to flow turbulently through the artery, producing Korotkoff sounds.

Kyphoscoliosis An abnormal condition characterized by an anteroposterior and a lateral curvature of the spine.

L

Lactation Formation and secretion of milk from the breasts for the nourishment of the infant.

Lactic acidosis An increase in the anaerobic production of lactate, which, when released into the bloodstream, creates a condition of metabolic acidosis.

Laminar flow Flow of air or fluid in which there is no turbulence and the direction of flow is linear and parabolic.

Langerhans cell One of several types of epithelial cells. Langerhans cells are thought to have a role in immunologic reactions that affect the skin and may serve as a defense mechanism for the body.

Laparoscopic cholecystectomy Surgical removal of the gallbladder using an optical scope and instruments inserted through four small abdominal incisions.

Laparoscopy Examination of the abdominal cavity via a small incision to permit the insertion of a variety of optical scopes for diagnosis or therapy.

Latency period A period of time when there is no apparent change in status even though a process has begun to occur.

Leiomyoma Benign neoplasm of the smooth muscle of the uterus that is characteristically firm, well circumscribed, and round. Uterine leiomyomas usually appear and exhibit growth activity during the reproductive years.

Leprosy A chronic infectious disease of the skin caused by the intracellular bacillus *Mycobacterium leprae*.

Leptomeninges The combined structures of the pia mater and arachnoid mater.

Lesion A general term for a demonstrable structural change produced in the course of a disease. Lesions may be evident at a gross or microscopic level.

Leukemia A malignant disease of bone marrow stem cells, with accumulation of immature blasts in the marrow and peripheral blood.

Leukocyte A cell that mediates immune function. Leukocytes protect the body by phagocytosis of microorganisms and production of antibodies and memory cells. Also called *white blood cell*.

Leukoderma Patch of depigmentation, also called *vitiligo*.

Leukopenia A deficiency of white blood cells in the peripheral circulation, which is usually indicative of bone marrow failure.

Leukotrienes A class of biologically active compounds produced by leukocytes that trigger allergic and inflammatory reactions similar to those of histamine.

Leydig cell An interstitial cell in the testes that produces and secretes testosterone.

Libido Sexual drive; feeling of sexual desire.

Lichen planus A relatively common, chronic, pruritic disease involving inflammation and papular eruption of the skin and mucous membranes.

Ligament A dense connective tissue with parallel-fibered collagenous tissues designed to connect bone to bone.

Ligands A general term for a molecule, such as a hormone, neurotransmitter, or drug, that attaches to a receptor protein; usually involved in cell-to-cell communication.

Limbic system A group of structures surrounding the corpus callosum that produce various emotional feelings.

Lipid bilayer A double layer of lipid molecules that forms cellular membranes, including the plasma membrane, organelle membranes, and vesicles.

Lipodystrophy A group of conditions caused by defective metabolism of fat, resulting in atrophy of subcutaneous fat.

Lipolysis Production of free fatty acids resulting from the breakdown of fat in adipose tissue.

Lipoproteins A group of biomolecules composed of differing amounts of cholesterol, triglyceride, and protein, such as high-density lipoprotein (HDL) and low-density lipoprotein (LDL).

Lithotripsy Mechanical or chemical fragmentation of a calculus (stone).

Liver transplantation Surgical transfer of an appropriately matched donor liver into a host who has inadequate liver function to sustain life.

Longitudinal fracture Fracture in which a bone is split along its length.

Loose association Flow of thought in which ideas shift from one subject to another in a completely unrelated or noncohesive way. When severe, speech may be unintelligible.

Lower esophageal sphincter The circular band of muscular tissue at the lower end of the esophagus. It serves to prevent the highly acidic gastric contents from moving in a retrograde motion back into the esophagus.

Lumpectomy Surgical removal of only the malignant tumor or "lump" from an affected breast.

Lung compliance A measure of the ease of expansion of the lungs and thorax, determined by pulmonary elasticity (volume divided by pressure).

Lunula "Little moon"; the crescent-shaped white area nearest the root of the nail body.

Lupus erythematosus A chronic inflammatory disease affecting many systems of the body. It is an example of a collagen disease.

Lusitropy Rate of relaxation of cardiac muscle and chambers.

Lyme disease An infectious, immune-mediated multisystem disease caused by a tick-borne spirochete. It is characterized by an erythema migrans rash in which the area of redness begins at the site of the tick bite.

Lymphadenopathy A pathologic lymph node enlargement, which is usually painless and may be associated with malignancy, especially lymphoma. Lymphadenopathy must be distinguished from normal reactive lymph node enlargement in response to infection. Reactive nodes are usually tender and are situated "downstream" from a site of infection.

Lymphedema Swelling produced by an obstruction of lymphatic flow.

Lymphoblast A large, immature cell that develops into a lymphocyte. When found in the circulation lymphoblasts are indicative of leukemia.

Lymphocyte A white blood cell derived from the lymphoid stem cell that is not affected by diseases of the myeloid stem cell. Lymphocytes are of three basic types: T, B, and natural killer cells.

Lymphogranuloma venereum Highly contagious systemic infection caused by a number of strains of *Chlamydia*. It has progressive stages of development in which an initial lesion forms, and systemic disease occurs following dissemination via the lymphatic system.

Lymphoid group Dermal cells consisting of lymphocytes commonly found in inflammatory lesions of the skin.

Lymphopoiesis Formation of lymphocytes in the bone marrow.

Lysis Destruction or breakage of a cell membrane or molecule.

Lysosome An organelle containing hydrolytic enzymes that function to digest intracellular materials.

Lysozyme An enzyme secreted by macrophages and neutrophils to control foreign particle activity.

M

M line Marks the center of the A band and the midpoint of myosin filaments in striated muscle.

Macrocyte An abnormally large erythrocyte.

Macromolecule A molecule of colloidal size, such as a protein.

Macrophage A mature monocyte that migrates from the blood vessels to sites in the tissues. Macrophages are powerful phagocytes and secrete a number of cytokines that stimulate inflammation.

Major depressive disorder A mood disorder characterized by persistent dysphoria, anxiety, irritability, and fear.

Major histocompatibility complex (MHC) The regions on chromosome 6 that contain the genes for MHC proteins. Class I proteins are present on virtually all nucleated cells. Class II proteins are found mainly on antigen presenting cells: B cells, macrophages, and dendritic cells.

Malabsorption Failure of the gastrointestinal tract to absorb or normally digest one or more dietary constituents.

Maladaptation Ineffective, inadequate, or inappropriate change in response to new or altered circumstances.

Malignant tumor A type of tumor that has a tendency to invade local tissues and spread to distant sites (metastasis). Malignant tumors are generally poorly differentiated and are associated with a poor prognosis if not promptly managed.

Mallory-Weiss syndrome Mild to massive bleeding due to a tear in the mucosa or submucosa of the cardia or lower esophagus. The tear is usually longitudinal and is caused by forceful or prolonged vomiting during which the upper esophageal sphincter fails to relax.

Malnutrition A disorder of nutrition that may result from an unbalanced, insufficient, or excessive diet or from impaired absorption.

Malunion An imperfect union of previously fragmented bone or other tissue.

Mania Also called *full mania*, it is characterized by an overwhelming increase in energy and drive manifested as nonstop activity, grandiose thinking, impulsivity, euphoria, impaired judgment, acting-out behaviors, and hypersexuality.

Mass lesion Any lesion in the cranium that behaves like a space-occupying mass. Mass lesions tend to progress and cause signs and symptoms of increased intracranial pressure.

Mast cell Also called *histiocytic cell*. Mast cells have intracytoplasmic basophilic metachromatic granules containing heparin and histamine. The normal skin contains relatively few mast cells, but their number is increased in many different skin conditions, particularly the itching dermatoses.

Mastectomy Surgical removal of a breast. See *modified radical mastectomy* and *radical mastectomy*.

McBurney point Located in the lower right quadrant of the abdomen; situated in the normal area of the appendix midway between the umbilicus and the anterior iliac crest.

Mean arterial pressure The average pressure in the arterial system through the cardiac cycle. It is calculated by adding the systolic pressure to two times the diastolic reading and dividing the sum by 3.

Measles Known as *hard measles, 7-day measles,* or *rubeola.* This is a communicable viral disease caused by paramyxovirus of the genus *Morbillivirus* with a characteristic macular and blotchy rash; sometimes the macules become confluent.

Mediastinum The area of the chest between the sternum and vertebral column and between the lungs. Mediastinal structures include the trachea, esophagus, aorta, heart, and lymph nodes.

Medullary cavity Central cavity in longer bones.

Megacolon Abnormal massive dilation of the colon that may be congenital, toxic, or acquired.

Megakaryocyte A large bone marrow cell that sheds platelets into the circulation from its cytoplasm.

Megaloblastic dysplasia Abnormal development of large red blood cells and nonlymphocytic bone marrow cells.

Megaloblasts Large abnormal hematopoietic bone marrow cells.

Meiosis A type of cell division that results in daughter cells with one half the normal number of chromosomes. Meiosis occurs in gonadal germ cells.

Melanin Dark pigment found in melanocytes that gives color to hair and skin.

Melanocyte One of several types of epithelial cells. Melanocytes contribute color to the skin and serve to filter ultraviolet light.

Melena Tarry, black feces due to the action of gastrointestinal secretions on blood in the intestine.

Membranous urethra The urethral segment that passes through the muscular layers of the urogenital diaphragm.

Memory cells T and B lymphocytes that mediate immunologic memory through development of clones of long lived cells.

Menarche The first menstrual period at the time of puberty, usually occurring around age 12 years in North America.

Meniere disease A chronic disease of the inner ear characterized by recurrent episodes of vertigo.

Meninges Membranes surrounding the brain and spinal cord, which include the dura mater, arachnoid, and pia mater.

Meningitis Any infection or inflammation of the membranes covering the brain and spinal cord.

Meningocele Hernial protrusion of meninges through a neural tube defect in the skull or vertebral column.

Meniscus Curved, fibrous cartilage located in the knee and other joints. Menisci facilitate rotation at the knee by allowing better contact of the tibial surfaces with the femoral condyles.

Menopause A process by which the supply of ovarian follicles and estrogen hormones declines, usually beginning between the ages of 45 and 55 years.

Menorrhagia An increase in the amount or duration of menstrual bleeding, usually resulting from a lesion of the female reproductive organs.

Menstrual cycle The rhythmic pattern of changes in hormonal secretions and in sexual organs occurring approximately every 28 days during a female's reproductive years. The cycle culminates in the production of an ovum and the preparation of the uterus for implantation of a fertilized ovum.

Merkel cells One of several types of epithelial cells. Merkel cells consist of free nerve endings attached to modified epidermal cells. It is generally agreed that Merkel cells function as touch receptors.

Mesoblastic nephroma Benign congenital renal tumor.

Mesonephros One of three distinct stages in the development of the renal system. Mesonephros, which is the middle stage, corresponds to the mature excretory organ of some amphibians. In humans, it begins developing at about the fourth to fifth week of gestation.

Metabolic acidosis Any of the types of acidosis resulting from accumulation in the blood of noncarbonic, nonvolatile acids; characterized by a low HCO_3^- concentration.

Metabolic alkalosis A disturbance in which the acid-base balance shifts to alkaline because of uncompensated loss of acids, ingestion or retention of excess base, or depletion of potassium.

Metabolic syndrome A disorder of metabolism including at least three of the following: abdominal obesity, hypertriglyceridemia, low level of high-density lipoproteins, hypertension, and high fasting plasma glucose level. It is associated with an increased risk for development of diabetes mellitus and cardiovascular disease.

Metabolism Synthesis and breakdown of molecules in a living organism. Metabolism involves both the use and the release of energy.

Metanephros The final stage of development of the renal system. The metanephros begins in the fourth week of gestation when the ureteral bud grows out of the mesonephric duct.

Metaplasia Transformation of one kind of tissue to another fully differentiated tissue.

Metastasis Dissemination of cancer cells from the location of origin to other distant areas in the body.

Methemoglobin A transformation product of oxyhemoglobin that is formed when the iron of the hemoglobin molecule is oxidized to the ferric state (Fe^{3+}).

Metrorrhagia Bleeding between menstrual periods, usually the result of slight physiologic bleeding from the endometrium during ovulation. It may also result from other causes such as uterine malignancy, cervical erosions, endometrial polyps, or estrogen therapy.

Microbial adherence The ability of the microorganism to latch onto and gain entrance into the host.

Microcytic Referring to an abnormally small erythrocyte.

Micropenis A small, normally formed penis with an engorged length more than 2 standard deviations below the mean, or an engorged length less than 2.5 cm.

Micturition Urination.

Mineralocorticoids A class of steroid hormones secreted by the adrenal cortex that regulate the mineral salts (electrolytes) and water balance in the body.

Minimal change disease A kidney disorder characterized by subtle changes in glomerular structure.

Mitochondrion A membrane-bounded organelle that carries out oxidative phosphorylation to synthesize most of the adenosine triphosphate in a eukaryotic cell.

Mitosis A type of cell division that results in daughter cells with chromosomes that are identical to the parent cell. Mitosis occurs in somatic cells.

Mitral valve The cardiac valve that lies between the left atrium and left ventricle. The valve is normally closed during ventricular systole and open during ventricular diastole. Mitral valve closure contributes to heart sound S_1. Also called the *bicuspid atrioventricular valve.*

Mixed acid-base imbalance A combined disturbance of acid-base balance in which a primary respiratory disorder and a primary metabolic disorder coexist.

Mixed incontinence Loss of bladder control with symptoms of both stress and urge incontinence.

Mobility The ability to achieve purposeful movement.

Modified radical mastectomy Surgical removal of the breast accompanied by dissection of a portion of the axillary lymphatic system.

Molluscum contagiosum A viral skin disease with two forms. One form affects children and is spread through indirect contact; the other is sexually transmitted and occurs in young adults. It is characterized by pink and white lesions on the genitalia with an exudative core.

Mongolian spots Caused by selective pigmentation. They usually occur on the buttocks or sacral area and are commonly seen in Asian Americans and African Americans.

Monoclonal antibodies Identical antibodies produced in the body or in a laboratory from a single clone of B lymphocytes.

Monocyte An immature circulating macrophage.

Monosaccharide A simple sugar (e.g., glucose, fructose).

Monosomy Having only one member of a homologous chromosome pair, as in monosomy X, also called *Turner syndrome.*

Monounsaturated fatty acid A fatty acid with one double bond.

Mood Sustained expression of an emotion that affects one's outlook.

Mood disorder A disturbance of mood that may be caused by either organic damage to the brain or chemical alterations in neurotransmission. Mood disorders may also have no known biological basis.

Mood swings Oscillation between periods of euphoria (elevated mood) and depression or anxiety.

Morphogen A substance that triggers growth, proliferation, and differentiation of cells in a concentration-dependent manner.

Morphogenesis Arrangement of cells in a particular order during the development of complex organisms.

Morphologic changes Structural and associated functional alterations in cells or tissues that are either characteristic of the disease or diagnostic of the etiologic process.

Motor end-plate The points of contact between an α-motor neuron and the skeletal muscle cells it innervates.

Mucocutaneous candidiasis Candidal infection of the mucous membrane and the skin.

Mucosal edema Swelling of the membranes of the respiratory, gastrointestinal, or urogenital systems; usually a consequence of inflammation.

Müllerian ducts Genital structures, also called *paramesonephric ducts* because they develop alongside the mesonephric ducts. A pair of embryonic ducts that become the fallopian tubes, uterus, and vagina in females.

Multifactorial Pertaining to or characteristic of any condition or disease resulting from the interaction of many factors.

Multipennate muscle A muscle with several central tendons toward which the muscle fibers converge like the barbs of feathers.

Multiple myeloma (plasma cell myeloma) A malignant disorder of antibody-secreting plasma cells that produce large quantities of monoclonal antibodies and have a predilection to settle in the skeleton, where osteoclastic bone lesions are produced.

Multiple sclerosis A chronic demyelinating disease of the central nervous system that causes significant disability in young adults. It is thought to be an autoimmune disorder that results in inflammation and scarring (sclerosis) of the myelin sheaths covering nerves.

Muscular dystrophy Term referring to a group of genetically determined myopathies characterized by progressive degeneration of muscle fibers.

Mutagen A physical or chemical agent capable of causing alterations in an organism's DNA by inducing mutations.

Mutation A heritable change in the nucleotide sequence of a chromosome; it is passed on to daughter cells when the cell divides.

Myasthenia gravis A chronic autoimmune disease affecting the neuromuscular function of voluntary muscles and characterized by profound muscle weakness and fatigability.

Mycosis Infection caused by a fungus.

Myeloid group Cells of the dermis consisting of polymorphonuclear leukocytes and eosinophilic leukocytes. These cells occur commonly with allergic dermatoses.

Myelomeningocele or meningomyelocele Hernial protrusion of meninges, spinal fluid, and a portion of the spinal cord with its nerves through a defect in the skull and vertebral column.

Myocardial infarction Localized area of cardiac necrosis most often associated with coronary heart disease and sudden acute occlusion of a coronary artery by a thrombus.

Myocardium The middle layer of the heart, composed of cardiac muscle tissue.

Myopia A condition of nearsightedness caused by elongation of the eyeball or by an error in refraction so that parallel rays are focused in front of the retina.

Myosin A cytoskeletal protein that comprises the thick filament of the muscle sarcomere in skeletal and cardiac muscle. It is also present as a contractile filament in other types of cells. Myosin binds with actin during muscular contraction.

Myositis ossificans An abnormal calcification within a muscle.

Myxedema Nonpitting edema caused by advanced hypothyroidism in adulthood.

N

Narcissism Self-absorption; excessive self-love.

Natural killer cells A lymphocyte that is capable of binding to and killing virus-infected cells and some tumor cells by releasing cytotoxins.

Necrosis Death and degradation of body cells or tissues in response to irreversible injurious events.

Necrotizing enterocolitis A disorder occurring most often in premature infants (less than 34 weeks' gestation) and infants with low birth weight (less than 5 lb or 2.25 kg). This disorder is characterized by diffuse or patchy intestinal necrosis accompanied by sepsis.

Necrotizing inflammation Also called *vasculitis*. This response can occur when antigen and antibody react in blood vessels in the skin. Necrotizing inflammation can be caused by drug allergies; disorders such as systemic lupus erythematosus, rheumatoid arthritis, and glomerulonephritis; and certain infectious diseases such as hepatitis B.

Negative feedback A term used to explain homeostatic mechanisms. Negative feedback causes the controller to respond in a manner that opposes or negates deviation from normal level (set point). Most body systems operate on the principle of negative feedback.

Negative nitrogen balance The condition of protein catabolism (breakdown) exceeding daily protein intake and synthesis.

Negative symptoms (schizophrenia) Symptoms of schizophrenia that are thought to be mediated by dopamine D_1 receptors in the brain. Drugs that block D_1 receptors may alleviate some of the negative symptoms, which include social withdrawal, flat affect, poverty of speech, ritualistic posturing, and autism.

Neoantigen formation A new specific antigen that develops in a tumor cell.

Neologism New word, often created by combining syllables of other words; or a word given special or private significance.

Neoplasia New growth. The term implies an abnormality of cellular growth and may be used interchangeably with the term tumor.

Neoplasm A new and abnormal proliferation of cells. If malignant, the growth infiltrates

tissue, metastasizes, and often recurs, even after attempts at surgical removal.

Nephralgia Renal pain.

Nephrectomy The surgical removal of a kidney.

Nephritic syndrome A group of signs and symptoms of a urinary tract disorder, including hematuria, hypertension, and renal failure.

Nephroblastoma (Wilms tumor) The most common childhood malignant kidney tumor, resulting from a defect on chromosome 13.

Nephrogenic rests Remnants of embryonic tissue found in or around the kidney, retained after the period of embryonic development. Nephrogenic rests are sometimes precursors (forerunners) of Wilms tumor.

Nephrolithiasis The presence of a stone or calculus anywhere in the urinary tract.

Nephroma Tumor of the kidney or area of the kidney.

Nephron Functional unit of the kidney composed of epithelial cells forming the glomerulus, proximal convoluted tubule, loop of Henle, distal convoluted tubule, and collecting duct.

Nephropathy A pathologic process in the kidney, including inflammatory, degenerative, and sclerotic conditions. Many disorders can lead to nephropathy, as in diabetic nephropathy, toxic nephropathy, ischemic nephropathy, and obstructive nephropathy.

Nephrotic syndrome A common set of symptoms caused by damage to the glomeruli, in which proteins cross the glomerulus and are lost in the urine at a rate of >3.5 g/day.

Nephrotoxic Poisonous to the kidney.

Neural thread protein Microscopic protein thread that binds and helps stabilize microtubules (the cell's internal support structure or skeleton). In Alzheimer disease, the threads become chemically altered and twist into paired helical filaments, known as neurofibrillary tangles. See *tau protein*.

Neurocrine Secretion of hormone signaling molecules into the bloodstream from neurons.

Neurofibrillary tangle Abnormal bundle of twisted threads inside a nerve cell that is the collapsed remains of the neuron's microtubules, which normally provide structural support.

Neurogenic bladder Bladder dysfunction caused by a lesion at any level in the nervous system.

Neurogenic shock Often called "fainting," neurogenic shock may be caused by severe pain, fear, an unpleasant sight, or other strong stimuli that overwhelm the usual regulatory capacity of the nervous system.

Neuroglia, glia A group of cell types, including astrocytes, microglia, ependymal cells, and oligodendrocytes, that support nerve cells and do not themselves conduct action potentials.

Neurohormones A hormone secreted by a specialized neuron into the bloodstream, the cerebrospinal fluid, or the intercellular spaces of the nervous system.

Neuropathic osteoarthropathy A neurologic disease that leads to bone abnormalities and joint involvement. The mechanics of disease development are probably a combination of neurovascular and neurotraumatic processes.

Neurovascular injury An injury that affects the nerves that control the caliber of blood vessels.

Neutropenia A type of leukopenia in which the absolute neutrophil count is below 500 cells/µl. Neutropenia is associated with a high risk of bacterial sepsis.

Neutrophilia A high blood neutrophil count.

Neutrophil/neutrophilic granulocyte A cell that contains small lysosomal granules and a segmented nucleus with two to five lobes. These cells compose 60% to 70% of leukocytes.

Nevus Congenital discoloration of a circumscribed area of the skin; commonly called mole or birthmark.

Nociception Activation of nociceptors by potentially tissue-damaging stimuli, resulting in the perception of pain by the central nervous system. Nociception includes the processes of receptor transduction, signal transmission, perception, and signal modulation.

Nociceptor Pain receptor.

Nocturia Excessive urination at night.

Nonarticular rheumatism A common soft-tissue syndrome in children. The most common symptom is nocturnal pain that usually occurs in the calves, shins, and thighs. Also called *growing pain*.

Noncontractile tissue Soft tissue that possesses no ability to contract or relax; this includes the joint capsule, ligament, bursa, fascia, dura mater, and nerve root. Also called *inert tissue*.

Nondisjunction The failure of homologous chromosomes to separate normally during meiosis or mitosis, resulting in unequal distribution of chromosomes to daughter cells.

Nondisplaced fracture A fracture in which the fragments remain in alignment and position.

Non-Hodgkin lymphoma A varied group of malignant disorders of lymph node cells involving B cells, T cells, and natural killer cells. In comparison with Hodgkin disease, these lymphomas tend to spread unpredictably and metastasize early, and thus carry an overall worse prognosis.

Non–Q-wave infarct A subendocardial infarct affecting only the inner third to half of the ventricular wall and generally associated with less severe symptoms.

Nonspecific immune response Referring to a series of mechanical, biochemical, and phagocytic barriers to infection; also called the *innate immune system*.

Non-STEMI A myocardial infarction that does not have ST-segment elevation.

Nonunion Pertaining to a fractured bone that fails to heal properly.

Norepinephrine A major monoamine neurotransmitter of the sympathetic nervous system that is involved in the etiologic development of mood disorders.

Normochromic Pertaining to a blood cell having normal color resulting from the presence of an adequate amount of hemoglobin, measured by the mean corpuscular hemoglobin concentration (MCHC).

Normocytic Description of a typical adult red blood cell of average size, measured by the mean corpuscular volume (MCV).

Nuclei A cluster of neuronal cell bodies located in the central nervous system.

Nucleocapsid The core of the human immunodeficiency virus (HIV), which contains two strands or chains of RNA, protein, and enzymes.

Nucleotide A biomolecule composed of a purine or pyrimidine base linked to a ribose or deoxyribose sugar, with one or more phosphate groups attached to the sugar. DNA and RNA are polymers of nucleotides.

Nucleus A cellular organelle that contains chromosomal DNA.

Nutritional screening A method for quickly determining the nutritional status of an individual from a selected group of anthropometric and biochemical tests.

Nutritional status The state of an individual's nutrition, resulting from the consumption and utilization of nutrients to meet metabolic needs.

Nystagmus Involuntary, rapid, rhythmic movements of the eyeball; these occur commonly in a horizontal direction, but can also occur in a vertical or a rotational direction.

O

Oblique fracture Fracture resulting from a rotational force; however, unlike a spiral fracture, the break is along an oblique course (45-degree angle) and does not rotate around the entire bone.

Obsession A powerful, persistent, intrusive thought, impulse, or image that dominates the mental life of the individual to the extent of seriously interfering with normal living.

Obsessive-compulsive disorder (OCD) An anxiety disorder characterized by recurrent and persistent thoughts, ideas, and feelings or repetitive acts.

Obstruction Refers to an anomaly that compromises or prevents flow because of abnormal narrowings. Stenosis or atresia (failure to develop) of valves and coarctation of the aorta are examples of the most common cardiac obstructive defects.

Obstructive sleep apnea A form of sleep apnea involving a physical obstruction in the upper airways.

Occupational asthma Resembles allergic asthma and may be accompanied by positive skin test reactions to protein allergens in the work environment.

Odynophagia A severe sensation of burning, squeezing pain with swallowing; may accompany dysphagia, or difficulty with swallowing.

Ogilvie syndrome The idiopathic syndrome of intestinal pseudoobstruction; may result in megacolon.

Olfactory Pertaining to the sense of smell.

Oligomenorrhea Infrequent menstruation, usually the result of failure to ovulate as a result of inappropriate hormonal function.

Oligosaccharide A compound consisting of 2 to 10 joined monosaccharide units.

Oliguria Urine output of less than 500 ml/day.

Omphalocele Congenital anomaly in which a herniation of viscera at the base of the umbilical cord is present; requires surgical correction.

Oncocytoma Benign renal tumor consisting of large eosinophilic cells that have granular cytoplasm and round, uniform nuclei.

Oncogene A gene associated with the initiation of cancerous behavior in a cell.

Onycholysis Separation of the nail from its nail bed.

Oogonia The cells present in the female ovaries during prenatal development that ultimately develop into ova. The entire lifetime supply of ova is established prenatally; no new oogonia arise after birth.

Open fracture Fracture occurring when bone is broken and an external wound leads to the fracture site.

Ophthalmia neonatorum Purulent gonococcal conjunctivitis and keratitis in the newborn resulting from exposure of the infant's eyes to infected maternal secretions during the passage through the vagina at birth.

Ophthalmoscopic examination Examination of the structures of the eye, both extraocular and intraocular, using an ophthalmoscope.

Opioid Any of a group of drugs with an affinity for opioid receptors in the central nervous system. Morphine is the standard opioid with which others are compared for characteristics and potency.

Opportunistic infection An infection caused by organisms that are usually nonpathogenic but that become pathogenic because of decreased function of the immune system.

Opsonization The process of proteins, usually antibodies or complement fragments, binding to an antigen in order to make the antigen easier for phagocytic cells to locate. Phagocytic cells have receptors for opsonins.

Organelles The membrane-bound structures in the cell cytoplasm, including nucleus, mitochondria, endoplasmic reticulum, and Golgi apparatus.

Orthopnea Difficulty with breathing that is instigated or exacerbated by lying supine.

Orthostatic (postural) hypotension A form of low blood pressure that occurs after positional change from supine to standing. Diagnosed by an increase in heart rate of more than 15% and a decrease in either systolic blood pressure by more than 15 mm Hg, or diastolic blood pressure, by more than 10 mm Hg.

Osmolality A measure of degree of concentration; number of particles per kilogram of solvent.

Osmosis Movement of water across a semipermeable membrane to equalize the particle concentration of the fluid on both sides of the membrane.

Ossicle One of several small bones in the middle ear responsible for transmitting sound waves to the inner ear.

Osteoarthritis A common degenerative joint disease characterized by progressive loss of articular cartilage and by formation of new bone from subchondral bone at joint margins.

Osteoblast A bone-forming cell that is derived from the embryonic mesenchyme and, during the early development of the skeleton, differentiates from a fibroblast to function in the formation of bone tissue.

Osteochondroma A benign bone tumor consisting of bone and cartilage.

Osteoclast A cell responsible for bone resorption.

Osteocyte A mature bone cell.

Osteonecrosis The destruction and death of bone tissue, such as from ischemia, infection, malignant neoplastic disease, or trauma.

Osteoid osteoma A painful but benign bone-forming tumor that is often found in the cortex of the tibia and femur.

Osteomalacia An abnormal condition of lamellar bone, characterized by a loss of calcification of the matrix and consequent softening of the bone. The condition is the result of an inadequate amount of phosphorus and calcium available in the blood for mineralization of the bones.

Osteomyelitis A severe pyogenic infection of bone and local tissue that requires immediate management.

Osteon The basic unit of bone; also called the *haversian system*.

Osteoporosis A common metabolic bone disease in which reduction in bone mass results from bone resorption proceeding at a rate faster than that of new bone formation.

Osteoprogenitor A type of bone stem cell that lines bone surfaces.

Osteosarcoma A malignant bone-forming tumor and the most common primary malignant bone tumor that develops in the metaphyseal region of long bones.

Otosclerosis A hereditary condition of unknown cause in which irregular ossification occurs in the ossicles of the middle ear, causing hearing loss.

Ototoxic Damaging to the structures of the inner ear.

Ovarian cyst A sac on an ovary that contains fluid or semisolid material. It may develop at any time between puberty and menopause; the cause is presently unknown.

Overflow incontinence Loss of bladder control associated with urinary retention and bladder distention due to obstruction, detrusor underactivity or inactivity, or sphincteric malfunction.

Oviduct Another term for *fallopian tube*. Each oviduct runs laterally from the uterus to the uterine end of the ovary. The free end of the oviduct adjacent to the ovary is called the *infundibulum*.

Oxidative phosphorylation An ATP-generating process in which oxygen serves as the final electron acceptor. The process occurs in mitochondria and is the major source of ATP generation in aerobic organisms.

Oxygen consumption The amount of oxygen used by the tissues in 1 minute, usually expressed as $\dot{V}o_2$.

Oxygen delivery The amount of oxygen delivered to the tissues each minute. Oxygen delivery ($\dot{D}o_2$) is calculated by multiplying cardiac output and arterial oxygen content.

Oxytocin Hormone secreted by the posterior pituitary. It causes uterine contraction and is thought to have a major role in promoting increased uterine contractility during parturition. After birth, it is secreted in response to suckling by the infant and stimulates the release of milk, called the milk ejection reflex.

P

Paco₂ Partial pressure of carbon dioxide in arterial blood; an indicator of the effectiveness of respiratory excretion of carbonic acid.

Paget disease Also called *osteitis deformans*; a slowly progressive metabolic bone disease characterized by an initial phase of excessive bone resorption followed by a reactive phase of abnormal excessive bone formation.

Pain An unpleasant sensation caused by noxious stimulation of the sensory nerve endings, or perceived as such.

Pallor Paleness of skin, nail beds, lips, and conjunctivae. A possible symptom of anemia.

Pancreas Gland located in the abdomen; has both endocrine and exocrine functions. The endocrine pancreas produces insulin, glucagon, and somatostatin.

Pancreatitis Inflammation of the pancreas; may be acute or chronic.

Pancytopenia Decreased production of red blood cells, white blood cells, and platelets.

Pandemic An epidemic that affects large geographic regions, possibly spreading worldwide.

Panhypopituitarism A condition of deficiency in all pituitary hormones.

Panic disorder Psychiatric disorder characterized by recurrent, unexpected episodes of acute anxiety, fear, and panic; often accompanied by the subject's belief that he or she is having a heart attack, is unable to breathe, is losing control, or is dying.

Panmyelosis A pathologic condition characterized by excessive proliferation of bone marrow cells of all types.

Papillary layer One of two layers of the dermis. The papillary layer consists of bumps (papillae) that project into the epidermis.

Papillary muscles Muscles within the ventricles that connect the chordae tendineae to the ventricular wall. Papillary muscles contract during ventricular systole to place tension on the valves and prevent backflow through them.

Paracrine Referring to hormone-like chemicals, the target cell of which is located next to the cell secreting the chemical.

Parametritis An infection of the connective tissue between the broad ligaments underlying the female reproductive organs.

Paraneoplastic syndrome A cluster of systemic conditions associated with cancer, such as hypercalcemia, hyponatremia, or Cushing syndrome.

Paraphimosis Painful constriction of the glans penis by the foreskin, which has been retracted behind the corona.

Parasite One of a variety of protozoa (single-celled animals), nemathelminths (roundworms), platyhelminths (flatworms), and arthropods (invertebrate animals with jointed appendages). Parasites depend on another organism for survival.

Parkinsonism Parkinson disease symptoms; a neurologic disorder characterized by tremor, muscle rigidity, hypokinesia, a slow shuffling gait, and difficulty in chewing, swallowing, and speaking caused by various lesions in the extrapyramidal motor system.

Paroxysm A sudden outburst or change from the norm, as in a sudden burst of electrical activity seen on electroencephalography, as occurs with seizure activity.

Paroxysmal nocturnal dyspnea A sudden severe feeling of suffocation; usually occurs at night and awakens the person from sleep.

Partial seizure A seizure in which part of the brain surface is involved in the seizure.

Parturition The process by which an infant is born.

Passive immunity A form of acquired immunity resulting from antibodies that are transmitted naturally through the placenta to a fetus or through the colostrum to an infant, or artificially by injection.

Pathogen An agent that causes disease.

Pathogenesis Development or evolution of disease. A description of the pathogenesis includes the processes that occur in the body from the initial stimulus to the ultimate expression of manifestations of the disease.

Pathologic Pertaining to a condition that is caused by or involves a disease process.

Pathology Study of the causes, characteristics, and effects of disease.

Pathophysiology The study of the biological and physical manifestations of disease including etiology, pathogenesis, clinical manifestations, and treatment implications.

Pauciarticular onset Affecting four or fewer joints; used in association with juvenile rheumatoid arthritis.

Pedigree Genetic lineage or family history of traits; used to trace the pattern of inheritance.

Pelvic inflammatory disease Any acute or subacute recurrent or chronic infection of the oviducts and ovaries with involvement of the adjacent reproductive organs.

Pemphigus A group of disorders including vulgaris, vegetans, foliaccus, and erythematosus. The pemphigus group disorders are characterized by bullous eruptions (blisters) thought to be caused by autoimmune reactions.

Pemphigus vulgaris Included in the pemphigus group of disorders, pemphigus vulgaris has the worst prognosis. Bullae can erupt on the skin and mucous membranes (e.g., esophagus), and toxemia and infection can cause death if proper treatment (cortisone) is not administered.

Penile urethra The longest segment of the male urethra, extending about 15 cm in length from the membranous urethra to the external meatus.

Penis Male organ of copulation and urinary excretion.

Penumbra The margin or fringe surrounding a central part. In the case of stroke, a penumbra of viable tissue surrounds the necrotic core that can survive if optimal conditions exist and if it is not subject to further insults.

Peptic ulcer disease Disorder of the upper gastrointestinal tract caused by the action of acid and pepsin. This disorder may include injury to the mucosa of the esophagus, stomach, or duodenum, and may range from a slight mucosal injury to severe ulceration.

Percutaneous Referring to a procedural approach that traverses the skin and is less traumatic than open surgical methods.

Perfusion The delivery of blood flow to a specific organ or an area of the body.

Pericardial effusion The escape of blood or other fluid into the pericardial sac.

Pericarditis Inflammation of the pericardium associated with trauma, malignant neoplastic disease, or infection.

Pericardium A protective covering of the heart that is made of two layers separated by a fluid-filled space. The inner (visceral) layer is attached to the heart itself, whereas the outer (parietal) layer forms a sac around the heart.

Perimysium The connective tissue surrounding the fasciculi.

Peripheral vascular disease (peripheral arterial disease) Decreased localized blood flow, often to the feet, resulting in decreased arterial pressure and chronic ischemia.

Peristalsis The basic propulsive movement of the gastrointestinal (GI) tract. During normal functioning, this coordinated, rhythmic, serial contraction of smooth muscle propels the contents of the GI tract in a downward direction.

Peritoneal dialysis A procedure performed to correct an imbalance of fluid or electrolytes in the blood or to remove toxins by intermittent infusion and removal of dialysis fluid through a catheter in the peritoneal cavity.

Permissive hypothesis A hypothesis positing that poor dampening by serotonin of other neurotransmitter systems (e.g., norepinephrine and dopamine) allows wide variations in mood.

Permissiveness The process in which one hormone increases the number of cellular receptors for a second hormone, thus increasing the cellular response to the second hormone.

Peroxisome (microbody) Small membrane-bound organelle that uses molecular oxygen to degrade organic molecules.

Perseveration Persisting response to a previous stimulus after a new stimulus has been presented.

Personality disorder A disorder that represents immature, inflexible, and persistently maladaptive ways of dealing with the intrapersonal and interpersonal aspects of life.

Pessary A device inserted in the vagina to treat uterine prolapse.

Petechiae Nonblanching, pinpoint red or purple spots caused by capillary hemorrhages.

Peyronie disease Formation of palpable, fibrous plaques on the surface of the corpora cavernosa of the penis.

pH The negative logarithm of the hydrogen ion concentration; a measure of the acidity or alkalinity of a solution.

Phagocytosis Ingestion of pathogens by leukocytes using the process of receptor-mediated endocytosis.

Phagosome A cellular lysosome containing substances obtained by phagocytosis.

Phenotype The physical, biochemical, and biological composition of an individual; expressed as recognizable traits.

Pheochromocytoma Tumor of the adrenal gland that secretes catecholamines, resulting in elevated blood pressure. An example of a condition that causes secondary high blood pressure.

Phimosis A condition in which the penile foreskin fits so tightly over the glans that it cannot be retracted.

Phlebitis Inflammation of a vein.

Photoreceptor A receptor found in the eye that responds to light.

Photosensitivity An abnormal response to exposure to light. Certain medications are photosensitive and can cause a skin reaction if the person is exposed to excessive sunlight.

Physiologic jaundice of the newborn A harmless, short-term condition caused by immature bilirubin conjugation and transport mechanisms; characterized by yellowish staining of the skin and sclera.

Physiology The study of the specific characteristics and functions of a living organism and its parts.

Pigmentary disturbance Interruption of any organic coloring material produced in the body, such as melanin.

Pinocytosis A process of ingesting fluids and small particles that is common to most cell types. Also called *"cellular drinking."*

Pituitary gland A gland located at the base of the hypothalamus. It consists of anterior and posterior lobes. Also called *hypophysis*.

Pityriasis rosea A rash of unknown origin that primarily affects young adults. The characteristic lesion of a macule or papule with surrounding erythema is thought to be viral in origin, but no virus has been isolated to date.

Pivot joint A synovial joint that allows rotation as its single axis movement. Examples include the superior radioulnar joint of the elbow and the union between the first and second vertebrae. Also called *trochoid joint*.

Placenta A highly vascularized organ through which the fetus receives nutrients and by which wastes are removed. It also is an endocrine organ, producing several hormones, most notably human chorionic gonadotropin.

Placenta previa Condition of pregnancy in which the placenta is implanted abnormally over the internal cervical os. It occurs in varying degrees of severity and may result in sudden massive hemorrhage following dilatation of the internal os.

Plaque A flat patch on the skin or a patch of atherosclerosis.

Plasma A complex, aqueous liquid in blood and lymph containing a number of organic and inorganic substances from which blood cells have been removed.

Plasma cell 1. An antibody-secreting B lymphocyte. 2. A dermal cell rarely seen in normal skin secretions, occurring in small numbers in most chronic inflammatory diseases of the skin and in larger numbers in granulomas.

Plasmalemma Plasma membrane.

Plasma membrane The lipid bilayer that surrounds a living cell.

Plasmapheresis Removal of plasma from withdrawn blood, with retransfusion of the formed elements into the donor.

Platelet A circulating cytoplasmic fragment of megakaryocytes that is essential in the formation of blood clots and in the control of bleeding.

Pleural effusion A collection of fluid in the pleural cavity resulting from a disease process.

Pleurodesis Instillation of a chemically irritating drug (e.g., tetracycline, sterile talc, bleomycin, doxycycline) into the pleural space to stimulate inflammation and adhesion.

Pneumonia An acute inflammation of lung tissue caused by an infectious agent or by aspiration of chemically irritating fluid.

Pneumothorax Accumulation of air in the pleural space.

Poliomyelitis An infectious disease caused by one of three polioviruses.

Polyarteritis nodosa A form of systemic vasculitis that can cause inflamed arteries in visceral organs, brain, and skin.

Polyarticular onset (oligoarticular) Affecting five or more joints; used in association with juvenile rheumatoid arthritis.

Polycystic kidney disease A progressive genetic disease characterized by multiple dilations of the collecting ducts of the kidneys, which appear as if they are fluid-filled cysts, as a result of renal pathologic processes.

Polycythemia An excess of circulating red blood cells.

Polydipsia Excessive thirst.

Polygenic Referring to a trait determined by multiple genes at different loci, all having additive effects.

Polymenorrhea An increased frequency of menstruation, which may be associated with ovulation due to endocrine or systemic factors.

Polymorphism Inherited structural differences in proteins as a result of many alleles for a particular gene locus.

Polymorphonuclear neutrophil (PMN) A cell that contains small lysosomal granules and a segmented nucleus with two to five lobes. PMNs compose 60% to 70% of leukocytes.

Polymyositis Inflammation of many muscles, usually accompanied by deformity, edema, insomnia, pain, sweating, and tension.

Polyp A general descriptive term used for any mass of protruding tissue. Polyps may be either benign or malignant, although the term usually refers to the benign form.

Polyploidy Having more than two sets of homologous chromosomes.

Polysaccharide A saccharide containing 10 to 10,000 monosaccharide units.

Polysomy Having greater than the usual number of autosomal chromosomes.

Polyunsaturated fatty acid A fatty acid with several double bonds.

Polyuria Excretion of large amounts of urine.

Portal hypertension Abnormally high blood pressure in the blood vessels draining the intraabdominal alimentary tract, pancreas, gallbladder, and spleen. It may be due to increased resistance to blood flow, as in cirrhosis, or, rarely, to abnormally increased blood flow, as in arteriovenous communications.

Portal systemic encephalopathy A neuropsychiatric syndrome caused by liver dysfunction and resulting in mental status changes ranging from mild cerebral dysfunction to deep coma (hepatic coma) and death.

Positive end-expiratory pressure A method in which a ventilator is used to maintain positive airway pressure at the end of expiration, resulting in increased functional residual capacity and decreased shunt.

Positive feedback A term used to explain homeostatic mechanisms. Positive feedback increases deviation from the set point. Although most systems of the body operate on the principle of negative feedback, sneezing and childbirth are two examples of positive feedback.

Positive nitrogen balance The condition of dietary intake of proteins exceeding output.

Positive symptoms (schizophrenia) Symptoms of schizophrenia that are thought to be due to excessive dopamine D_2 receptor activation in the brain. Disorganized thinking (inability to connect thoughts logically), disorganized speech (rambling, tangentiality), delusions (fixed system of false beliefs), and hallucinations (sensory perception when no apparent stimulus exists) are typical positive symptoms.

Positron emission tomography (PET) A technique of brain imaging. PET studies measure changes in brain utilization of glucose.

Postictal phase The phase following a seizure during which the person is sleepy and confused.

Postobstructive diuresis Increased urinary output after resolution of partial or total obstruction of the urinary tract.

Postrenal A term referring to structures distal to the kidney, including the ureters and urethra, that may become obstructed and lead to kidney failure.

Posttraumatic stress disorder (PTSD) Psychiatric disorder characterized by an acute emotional response to a previous traumatic event.

Potter syndrome Congenital condition often associated with renal agenesis, but always manifesting with the following anomalies: widespaced eyes with epicanthal folds, low-set ears, broad and flat nose, hypoplastic lungs, and limb deformities.

Poverty of speech Speech that gives little information owing to vagueness, empty repetitions, or obscure phrases.

Predictive value A measure used by clinicians to interpret diagnostic test results, as in positive predictive value and negative predictive value

Preeclampsia-eclampsia Elevated blood pressure during pregnancy associated with edema and proteinuria. Blood pressure returns to normal after delivery. Eclampsia is present when preeclampsia progresses to seizures. Also known as *pregnancy-induced hypertension*.

Pregnancy-induced hypertension The rapid rise of arterial blood pressure associated with a loss of large amounts of protein in the urine occurring during pregnancy. Women at risk for pregnancy-induced hypertension include teenagers and women in their late 30s and early 40s (also known as *toxemia of pregnancy* and *preeclampsia-eclampsia*).

Preload The volume of blood in the cardiac chamber just prior to systole (end-diastolic volume).

Prepuce Also called *foreskin*; penile skin that overlies the glans and is removed with circumcision.

Prerenal Pertaining to the area proximal to the kidney, generally referring to blood flow to the kidney, which if disrupted can result in prerenal renal failure.

Presbycusis Hearing loss associated with aging.

Presbyesophagus Presence of slow or disorganized esophageal motility in the older adult.

Presbyopia A refractive condition in which the accommodative ability of the elderly eye cannot meet the accommodative demand for near vision.

Pressure sores Localized areas of cellular necrosis resulting from prolonged pressure between any bony prominence and an external object such as a bed or a wheelchair. The tissues are deprived of blood supply and eventually die. Also called *decubitus ulcers*.

Priapism Painful, persistent erection.

Prickly heat A rash caused by midepidermal obstruction and rupture of the sweat glands from prolonged exposure to a warm and humid environment.

Primary biliary cirrhosis A slowly progressive disease that destroys small to medium-sized bile ducts and results in cirrhosis and liver failure.

Primary dysthymia A long-term state of chronic depression not associated with any other disorder. It is neither a prelude to major depression nor a state existing between episodes of a cyclic form of mood disorder.

Primary endocrine disorder Direct malfunction of a hormone-producing gland not induced by the pituitary.

Primary glomerulopathy Disease states resulting from alterations in the structure and function of the glomerular capillary circulation, in which the kidney is the only or primary organ involved.

Primary (essential, idiopathic) hypertension High blood pressure of unidentified cause. Accounts for 90% of cases of high blood pressure.

Primary lesion Injury that originates in the skin and has not been altered by scratching or by treatment.

Primary prevention The first level of health promotion, designed to prevent disease.

Primary sclerosing cholangitis A progressive chronic fibrosing inflammation of the bile ducts of unknown cause, occurring most commonly in young men and frequently associated with chronic ulcerative colitis.

Prodromal period The period preceding the onset of a disorder. Symptoms indicate an impending seizure, migraine, or other problem.

Progesterone A hormone produced by the adrenal cortex and the corpus luteum during the luteal phase of the menstrual cycle; it promotes uterine changes essential for the implantation and growth of the fertilized ovum.

Prognosis A forecast about the probable outcome of a disease; the prospect of recovery from a disease indicated by the nature, signs, and/or symptoms of the case.

Progression (cancer) A phase of carcinogenesis when clones of cells that have undergone mutations begin to develop new properties that allow them to become increasingly malignant.

Progressive familial intrahepatic cholestasis A rare autosomal recessive disorder comprising severe jaundice, pruritus, and malabsorption attributable to a defect in bile salt excretion.

Proinsulin Precursor to insulin produced by the β cells of the pancreas.

Prokaryote A cell that does not have a membrane-bound nucleus or other membrane-bound organelles (e.g., bacteria).

Prolactin Hormone secreted by the anterior pituitary. Following birth of an infant, prolactin stimulates milk production.

Proliferation The reproduction or multiplication of similar forms. The term is usually applied to an increased number of cells as a result of mitosis.

Pronephros One of three distinct phases in the development of the renal system. The pronephros is the earliest state in humans, corresponding to the mature structure in primitive vertebrates.

Prostate Gland located below the bladder; its secretions help activate sperm and maintain their motility.

Prostatic urethra The widest and most distensible part of the male urethra.

Prostatitis Inflammation of the prostate.

Prostatodynia Pain in the prostate.

Protein A molecule composed of nitrogen, carbon, hydrogen, oxygen, and occasionally sulfur; when hydrolyzed, proteins yield amino acids.

Proteoglycan Any of a group of polysaccharide-protein conjugates occurring primarily in the matrix of connective tissue and cartilage; composed mainly of polysaccharide chains, particularly glycosaminoglycans, as well as minor protein components.

Proto-oncogene A normal cellular gene that is growth promoting and usually inhibited in nonproliferating cells. When erroneously activated, it becomes an oncogene and promotes cancer.

Provirus The viral DNA that is spliced into the host cell's DNA.

Pruritus Itching of the skin.

Pseudocyst A collection of fluid within or adjacent to the pancreas that often has a direct communication to the pancreatic duct. It is the most common localized complication of acute pancreatitis.

Pseudoglandular period The first stage in fetal lung development when the bronchial divisions are differentiated and the major elements of lung tissue are present except for those involved in gas exchange: the respiratory bronchioles and alveoli.

Pseudomembranous enterocolitis An acute inflammation and necrosis of the small and large intestines caused by *Clostridium difficile*, usually affecting the mucosa but sometimes extending to other layers.

Psoriasis A common chronic skin disease characterized by papules and plaques with an overlying silvery scale. Lesions can appear on any area of the body but especially the knees, elbows, lower part of the back, scalp, and nails.

Psoriatic arthritis An inflammatory arthritis associated with psoriasis occurring in approximately 0.1% of the population in the United States. Peak age of onset is 30 to 55 years of age, and the arthritis can occur in patients who have had psoriasis for many years.

Psychogenic Produced or caused by emotional or psychological factors rather than organic factors.

Psychosis The most serious and debilitating of mental disorders. The hallmarks of psychosis are delusions and hallucinations, thought disorders, and inappropriate emotional responses or social behavior.

Psychosomatic medicine The discipline involving the physiologic impact of psychic stress on the emergence of disease.

Pulmonary embolism (PE) The blockage of a pulmonary artery by fat, air, tumor tissue, or thrombus.

Pulmonary function testing (PFT) A procedure for determining the volumes and capacities of the lungs.

Pulmonary hypertension Abnormally high blood pressure within the pulmonary circulation.

Pulmonary tuberculosis Infection of the lungs by *Mycobacterium tuberculosis*.

Pulmonic valve The cardiac valve that lies between the right ventricle and the pulmonary artery. It is open during ventricular systole and closed during ventricular diastole. Pulmonic valve closure contributes to heart sound S_2.

Pulse pressure The difference between the systolic and diastolic blood pressures.

Purpura Hemorrhagic lesions 2 to 4 mm in diameter; petechiae that occur in groups or patches, caused by a vascular or bleeding disorder.

Putamen nuclei The larger, darker, and more lateral part of the lentiform nucleus.

Pyelonephritis An infection of the kidney medulla or cortex.

Pylorus Muscular sphincter between the stomach and the duodenum that controls gastric emptying and limits the reflux of bile from the small intestine.

Pyogenic Creating the formation of pus; typically at the site of an inflammation caused by bacterial infection.

Pyrogenic Producing or produced by fever.

Pyrosis A substernal burning sensation that may radiate to the neck or throat. It is caused by the reflux of gastric contents into the esophagus (also called *heartburn*).

Pyuria The presence of an excessive number of white blood cells in the urine. It is generally a sign of urinary tract infection.

R

Radiation Emissions of radioactive energy, rays, or waves. Can cause radiation sickness, but often used in the treatment of cancer.

Radical mastectomy Surgical removal of the entire breast, lymphatic drainage structures, and underlying pectoral muscles.

Radiculopathy A disease involving compression and dysfunction of a spinal nerve root.

Radiolysis Lysis or splitting of water molecules into H^+ and OH^- ions by the action of radioactive particles.

Rapidly progressing glomerulonephritis A syndrome that combines abrupt hematuria and proteinuria followed by a swift decline in renal function.

Rarefaction Decrease in density and weight of bone, but not in volume.

Raynaud phenomenon Blanching or cyanosis of fingers or hands on exposure to cold or emotional stress. The phenomenon is attributed to vasospasm and structural disease of blood vessels. Puffiness and swelling of the hands and fingers are noted clinically.

Reality testing The act of evaluating and considering the differences between internal experiences and external events.

Receptor activation Binding of a ligand to a cellular receptor, resulting in a change in intracellular cell signaling or function.

Receptor specificity The principle of allowing intracellular processes to be activated only by certain hormones. If a cell does not have the specific receptors for a hormone, it will not respond to the hormone.

Recessive Referring to a gene allele that fails to be expressed in the phenotype when a dominant allele is present. The trait carried in a recessive allele is apparent only when two identical copies are present.

Recruitment The process of calling in additional motor units in response to an increase in stimulation of motor nerves.

Rectocele Protrusion of the anterior rectal wall into the posterior vagina at a weakened part of the vaginal musculature. It usually results from an injury during either childbirth or surgery, and it may also be the result of the aging process or an inherent weakness in the vaginal wall.

Recurrent urinary tract infection Repeated infections within a short period of time following verified resolution of an earlier infection.

Red blood cell (erythrocyte) Cell responsible for transporting oxygen to the tissues, removing carbon dioxide from the tissues, and buffering blood pH.

Reed-Sternberg cell A malignant cell type found in affected lymph nodes of patients with Hodgkin disease. The presence of Reed-Sternberg cells differentiates Hodgkin disease from all other forms of malignant lymphoma.

Reentry The proposed mechanism for many dysrhythmias, including premature complexes and fibrillation. Reentry occurs when an impulse is able to activate the cardiac muscle more than once because of abnormalities in conduction through a portion of the heart.

Referred pain Pain felt at a site different from that of an injured or diseased organ or body part.

Reflex incontinence Urine loss that occurs without sensory warning or awareness.

Reflux (urinary) Retrograde flow of urine from the bladder to the kidney.

Refractory period The time during which a nerve or muscle membrane is unable to respond to a stimulus by generating an action potential.

Regurgitation (valvular) Retrograde blood flow through a cardiac valve when the valve is supposed to be closed.

Reiter syndrome Seronegative arthritis that appears 2 to 6 weeks after onset of an infection; characterized clinically by diffuse swelling of fingers and toes, swelling in the Achilles tendon or plantar fascia, and low back pain.

Relative anemia Anemia characterized by normal total red blood cell mass with disturbances causing excessive plasma fluid volume resulting in low hematocrit value.

Relative polycythemia Polycythemia characterized by normal total red blood cell mass with reduced plasma volume resulting in elevated hematocrit value.

Relaxation time The period between peak tension and zero tension.

Releasing hormone A hormone secreted by the hypothalamus that stimulates the anterior pituitary gland to secrete other hormones.

Reliability The extent to which a test measurement produces the same results with different investigators or with repeated measures over time.

Remission Disappearance of clinical manifestations of disease. In leukemia, complete remission is determined by the absence of leukemic blasts in the bone marrow aspirate and peripheral blood. Malignant stem cells still may be present, and remission does not imply cure.

Renal adenoma A tumor smaller than 3 cm with a cellular makeup similar to that of renal cell carcinoma.

Renal agenesis Failure of one or both kidneys to develop.

Renal angiomyolipoma (hamartoma) Benign renal tumor composed of abdominal blood vessels, clusters of fat cells, and sheets of smooth muscle.

Renal calculus Concretion of crystals of material (e.g., uric acid, calcium phosphate, struvite) that initially form in the calices or pelvis of the kidney. Calculi may migrate down the urinary tract and cause pain, obstruction, and infection.

Renal cell carcinoma Most common malignant tumor of the kidney.

Renal hypoplasia An abnormally small kidney that is morphologically normal but has either a reduced number of nephrons or smaller nephrons.

Renal or ureteral colic Intermittent flank or abdominal pain caused by spasms in the kidneys and/or ureters.

Renin An enzyme stored and released by the juxtaglomerular cells; converts angiotensinogen to angiotensin I.

Renin-angiotensin-aldosterone system (RAAS) The regulation of sodium balance, fluid volume, and blood pressure by the cascade of reactions beginning with release of renin, an enzyme that cleaves angiotensinogen to angiotensin I, followed by conversion of angiotensin I to angiotensin II by angiotensin-converting enzyme (ACE). Angiotensin II stimulates the release of aldosterone from the adrenal cortex.

Reperfusion injury Damage to tissues when blood flow is restored after a period of ischemia.

Resident flora Microorganisms that usually reside in a certain environment on the host without causing disease.

Residual urine Urine that remains in the bladder after urination.

Resistance In the stress response, resistance occurs when sympathetic activity declines while secretion of adrenocortical hormones is high.

Respiratory acidosis A pulmonary hypoventilation condition that tends to cause an excess of carbonic acid and results in acid-base imbalance.

Respiratory alkalosis A pulmonary hyperventilation condition that tends to cause a deficit of carbonic acid and results in acid-base imbalance.

Respiratory quotient The ratio of the volume of carbon dioxide produced to the volume of oxygen used in tissue metabolism.

Respiratory syncytial virus A member of a subgroup of myxoviruses that in tissue culture cause formation of giant cells or syncytia.

Resting membrane potential The transmembrane voltage that exists in nonexcitable cells and in neurons and muscle cells when not producing an action potential.

Reticular formation Fibers in the brainstem that arouse the cerebrum.

Reticular layer One of two layers of the dermis; consists of a more dense reticulum (network) of fibers than the papillary layer above it. The reticular layer is made of collagen and elastin and contains skeletal (voluntary) and smooth (involuntary) muscle fibers.

Reticulocytosis Increase in the number of circulating reticulocytes (immature red blood cells).

Reticulohistiocytic group Cells of the dermis consisting of fibroblasts, histiocytes, and mast cells. Immature cells of the reticulohistiocytic group are called reticulum cells.

Retinal detachment A separation of the retina in the back of the eye.

Retinopathy A group of noninflammatory eye disorders. Major contributing conditions include diabetes, hypertension, and atherosclerotic vascular disease.

Retrodisplacement Posterior displacement, such as an alteration in the position of the uterus in which the body of the uterus is displaced from its normal location overlying the bladder to a position in the posterior pelvis.

Retroperitoneal Referring to the anatomic space in the abdomen behind the peritoneal cavity, where the kidneys reside.

Retrovirus An RNA virus capable of transcribing its own RNA into DNA, which can be integrated into the host genome through the actions of a viral polymerase, also called *reverse transcriptase*.

Reverse transcriptase An enzyme that allows certain viruses to convert RNA to DNA and incorporate their genome into the DNA of the host cell.

Reye syndrome Primarily a children's disease, it is characterized by fatty infiltration of the liver with severe hepatic dysfunction.

Rheumatoid arthritis A systemic, inflammatory, autoimmune connective tissue disease. Enzymes are released into the joint fluid, causing inflammation, proliferation of synovium, and tissue damage. The hands, wrists, knees, and feet are most commonly involved. Joint involvement is symmetric. Other systems affected include integumentary, ocular, otolaryngologic, pulmonary, cardiac, gastrointestinal, renal, neurologic, and hematologic.

Rhinorrhea Drainage of a watery fluid from the nasal mucosa.

Rhonchus Coarse, bubbling sound usually heard on expiration, but which also can be heard on inspiration; it is caused by secretions in the airways.

Rhus dermatitis An inflammatory reaction to poison ivy, poison oak, and poison sumac. Clinically, rhus dermatitis begins within 48 hours of contact. The first symptom is pruritus, followed by erythema and vesicle formation, sometimes in linear fashion.

Rhythmicity The ability to beat regularly without external stimuli. Also called *automaticity*.

Ribonucleic acid (RNA) A nucleic acid, found in both the nucleus and the cytoplasm of cells, that has several roles in the translation of the genetic code and the assembly of proteins.

Ribosome A cellular structure containing ribosomal RNA and proteins that bind to mRNA and perform the task of translating the RNA message into a protein.

Rickets A condition caused by the deficiency of vitamin D; seen primarily in infancy and childhood and characterized by abnormal bone formation.

Rigor mortis The stiffening of muscles throughout the body after death resulting from the formation of persistent actin-myosin cross-bridges.

Risk factor Characteristic related to the probability of a certain outcome; a risk factor may be shown to cause an outcome or may be correlated with an outcome.

RNA polymerase An enzyme complex that binds to a gene segment of DNA, using it as a template for the synthesis of an RNA strand.

Rocky Mountain spotted fever An infection caused by a tick that carries *Rickettsia rickettsii*. The characteristic rash is a macular or maculopapular one that spreads to the rest of the body. Other symptoms include generalized edema, conjunctivitis, petechial lesions, photophobia, lethargy, confusion, and cranial nerve deficits.

Roseola infantum A contagious viral disease that generally affects children younger than 4 years and usually those about 1 year of age. It produces a characteristic maculopapular rash covering the trunk and spreading to the appendages.

Rostral A positional term referring to the head end.

Rough endoplasmic reticulum A portion of the endoplasmic reticulum that is studded by ribosomes. Ribosomes attached to the endoplasmic reticulum synthesize proteins that are destined for the plasma membrane or lysosomes.

Rubella Also known as *3-day measles* or *German measles*. Rubella is a childhood disease caused by the rubella virus. It is characterized by a diffuse punctate, macular rash that begins on the trunk and spreads to the arms and legs.

Rugae Folds in the lining of the body of the bladder (and stomach) that allow it to distend to accommodate volume at a low pressure.

S

Saddle joint A joint in which the surfaces are convex in one plane and concave in the other, permitting both flexion-extension and adduction-abduction movements; the surfaces of a saddle joint fit together as a saddle fits a horse. The carpometacarpal joint of the thumb is a saddle joint. Also called a *sellar joint*.

Saline deficit Extracellular fluid volume deficit.

Saline excess Extracellular fluid volume excess.

Saline imbalances Imbalances of extracellular fluid volume.

Salivary amylase Digestive enzyme (also called *ptyalin*) contained in saliva; initiates carbohydrate digestion in the mouth.

Sarcoidosis A chronic disorder of unknown origin characterized by the formation of tubercles of non-necrotizing epithelioid tissue.

Sarcolemma The plasma membrane that encloses a muscle cell.

Sarcomere The unit of muscle contraction in striated muscle. A sarcomere extends from one Z disk to another and consists of overlapping actin and myosin filaments.

Sarcoplasm The cytoplasm of the muscle fiber.

Sarcoplasmic reticulum A calcium-storing structure in muscle cells analogous to the endoplasmic reticulum; it fills the space between myofibrils and forms sacs.

Saturated fatty acid Having the maximal number of hydrogen atoms present so that only single bonds exist in the carbon chain, as in saturated fatty acids.

Saturation The condition of being saturated. The degree of hydrogen saturation refers to the number of double bonds between the carbon atoms in the hydrocarbon chain. Hemoglobin saturation occurs when all four ions in the hemoglobin molecule are bound to oxygen.

Scabies Infestation with the mite *Sarcoptes scabiei* in humans. Scabies begins with eggs laid in the stratum corneum. These eggs hatch into larvae within 3 to 4 days and reach adulthood within 2 months.

Scarlet fever A systemic reaction to the toxins produced by group A β-hemolytic streptococci. It occurs when the person is sensitized to the toxin-producing variation of streptococci. Scarlet fever frequently occurs in association with streptococcal sore throat (strep throat), but it may also be associated with a wound, skin infection, or puerperal infection.

Schizoaffective disorder A psychiatric disorder in which either a major depressive or manic episode develops concurrently with symptoms of schizophrenia.

Schizoid Indifferent to social interaction and possessing a limited range of emotional experience and expression.

Schizophrenia A syndrome or combination of mental disorders characterized by paranoia, delusions, and hallucinations associated with impaired interpretation of reality.

Scleroderma A disorder characterized by massive collagen deposition with fibrosis accompanied by inflammatory reactions and vascular changes in the capillary network.

Scoliosis A lateral deviation of the spine resulting in an S- or C-shaped spinal column. The disorder, most common in adolescent girls, can be a consequence of congenital, connective tissue, or neuromuscular disorders.

Scrotum Pouchlike sac containing the testes, epididymis, and spermatic cord.

Seasonal affective disorder A condition in which lethargy results from seasonal changes of decreased periods of daylight and longer nights.

Sebaceous gland Oil- or sebum-producing gland that anoints hair and skin.

Seborrheic dermatitis A common chronic inflammatory skin disease characterized by greasy scales and yellowish crusts.

Seborrheic keratosis Benign skin tumor common in the elderly; composed of immature epithelial cells.

Second messenger An intracellular signal that is produced in response to an extracellular signal binding to receptors on the cell membrane.

Secondary dysthymia A long-term state of chronic depression that is associated with some other non–mood disorder, which may be a classic mental disorder (e.g., anorexia nervosa) or a physical illness.

Secondary endocrine disorder A malfunction of the hypothalamus/pituitary cells that control the hormone-producing gland.

Secondary glomerulopathy Alterations in the structure and function of the glomerular capillary circulation resulting from drug exposure, infections, or glomerular injury in the setting of multisystem or vascular abnormalities.

Secondary hypertension High blood pressure in which the cause can be identified.

Secondary lesion Injury modified by normal progress over time or by such external actions as scratching.

Secondary prevention The second level of health promotion, based on early detection and screening.

Second-degree burn A burn that affects the epidermis and the dermis; classified as superficial or deep according to the depth of injury.

Secretin A digestive hormone that is produced by the S cells lining the duodenum and jejunum when protein of partially digested food enters the intestine from the stomach; it stimulates the pancreas.

Segmentation contractions A set of movements that occur in the small intestine. The primary effect of these contractions is progressive mixing of solid chyme particles with secretions of the small intestine.

Seizure A transient neurologic event of paroxysmal abnormal or excessive cortical electrical discharges that is manifested by disturbances of skeletal motor function, sensation, autonomic visceral function, behavior, or consciousness.

Self-identity disturbance In schizophrenic patients, self-identity disturbances can be profound, both in terms of the ability to differentiate one's physical self from the physical environment and in terms of the psychological discernment of self as distinct from others.

Semen Male reproductive fluid that contains spermatozoa; released with ejaculation.

Seminal vesicles Two glands that contribute rich nutrients to the seminal fluid.

Senile purpura A skin condition affecting older people and characterized by fragile blood vessels that rupture with minimal trauma.

Sensitivity Susceptibility to a substance, such as a medication or antigen.

Septic shock A form of distributive shock that occurs in septicemia when endotoxins or exotoxins are released from certain bacteria in the bloodstream causing inappropriate vasodilation.

Sequela, sequelae A condition or conditions caused by and following a disease.

Sequestra Fragment of dead bone that is partially or entirely detached from the surrounding or adjacent healthy bone.

Serotonin A major monoamine neurotransmitter that is an etiologic factor in mood disorders. See *norepinephrine*.

Sertoli cell An elongated cell that supports and provides nutrition to attached spermatids until they mature into spermatozoa.

Severe acute respiratory syndrome (SARS) An infectious respiratory illness first reported in Asia.

Sex chromosome A chromosome that confers gender to the individual. In humans, females are designated as 46XX, whereas males are 46XY. The Y chromosome confers male gender.

Sexually transmitted infection One of many infections that can be transmitted by sexual contact, regardless of whether the disease has manifestations in the genital organs (previously referred to as venereal disease or sexually transmitted disease).

Sharpey fibers Fibers that attach tendons to bones; they are continuous with the perimysium.

Shock A condition of severe hemodynamic and metabolic disturbance resulting in an imbalance between oxygen supply and oxygen demand at the cellular level. The common types of shock are cardiogenic, hypovolemic, obstructive, and distributive.

Short-bowel syndrome Severe diarrhea and significant malabsorption that develop following the surgical removal of large portions of the small intestine. The severity of the manifestations depends on the amount and location of the bowel resected.

Shunt (right-to-left) An abnormal route of blood flow through the heart or lungs that allows movement of blood into the arterial system without passing through areas of the lung.

Sickle cell A red blood cell containing abnormal hemoglobin that causes the cell to assume a sickle shape under decreased oxygen tension.

Sign Objectively identifiable manifestation of the disease. Fever, reddening of the skin, and a palpable mass are signs of disease.

Skeletal muscle Striated muscle that is attached to bone. Constituting 40% of total body weight, skeletal muscle enables bones to move at the joint and provides strength and protection to the skeleton by distributing and absorbing shock.

Skeletal system Rigid system of bony structures designed to protect internal organs and provide bony attachments for muscles and ligaments; presents rigid levers to allow for functional movement of the body and its separate parts.

Skin A relatively flat membrane composed of an outer, thinner layer (epidermis) and an inner, thicker layer (dermis).

Skin cancer A cutaneous neoplasm caused by ionizing radiation, certain genetic defects, or chemical carcinogens, including arsenics, petroleum, tar products, and fumes from some molten metals, or by overexposure to the sun or other sources of ultraviolet light.

Sleep study Recording of electroencephalograph (EEG) motor activity and respirations during sleep to determine duration and type of sleep and number of awakenings.

Sliding filament theory This theory of muscle contraction is suggested by the anatomic configuration of the sarcomere. Muscle shortening is accomplished by increasing the amount of overlap between actin and myosin filaments. Also called *cross-bridge theory*.

Slow twitch (type I, red) A muscle fiber that develops tension more slowly than a fast-twitch fiber. This fiber is usually fatigue resistant and relies on oxidative phosphorylation for energy.

Slow-wave electrical activity One of the basic types of electrical activity in the gut. Slow waves represent an ongoing basic oscillation in membrane potential occurring in the smooth muscle of the gastrointestinal tract between 3 and 12 times per minute.

Smooth endoplasmic reticulum A portion of the endoplasmic reticulum that has no ribosomes. Smooth endoplasmic reticulum is a site of lipid synthesis.

Soft-tissue injury Any trauma to soft tissue with disruption of circulatory and lymphatic systems.

Solar elastosis Wrinkled, weather-beaten appearance of skin caused by overexposure to sunlight.

Somatosensory receptors Specialized nerve endings located in the dermis of all skin areas. Receptors permit the skin to serve as a sensory organ, transmitting sensations of pain, pressure, touch, and temperature.

Somatotropic Referring to the sequential arrangement of neurons related to sensory or motor function in specific anatomic regions.

Specific immune response Creation of specific antibodies by the host against a specific pathogen that leads to the destruction of the pathogen.

Specificity The quality of being distinctive and the probability that the test will be negative among patients who do not have the disease.

Spermatid An immature sperm cell.

Spermatocele A painless, cystic mass containing sperm.

Spermatogenesis Production of sperm cells.

Spermatozoon A mature sperm cell.

Spherocyte An abnormal spherical (round) erythrocyte that is less biconcave than a normal erythrocyte.

Spherocytosis The presence of spherocytes in the blood.

Spike potential Sudden increase in membrane potential in the smooth muscle of the gastrointestinal tract that appears on the peaks of slow waves in response to certain conditions, including stimulation by stretching or the effects of acetylcholine or parasympathetic excitation.

Spina bifida A developmental anomaly characterized by defective closure of the bony encasement of the spinal cord (neural tube) through which the spinal cord and meninges may or may not protrude.

Spinal shock A temporary physiologic suspension of spinal cord function and reflexes below the level of cord injury.

Spiral (bacteria) Referring to any bacterium of the genus *Spirochaeta* that is motile and spiral-shaped with flexible filaments. See *spirochete.*

Spiral fracture A fracture resulting from rotational forces and causing bone to separate in the form of an S around the bone.

Spirochete Spiral-shaped bacterium.

Splinter hemorrhage A linear hemorrhage, appearing as a red or brown streak, running parallel to the finger in the nail bed; may be linked to bacterial endocarditis and trichinosis.

Spontaneous abortion Expulsion of the products of conception from the uterus before the period of fetal viability. It is usually called "miscarriage" by laypersons, and is differentiated from an elective abortion.

Squamous cell carcinoma A type of cancer that often occurs in areas of skin excessively exposed to sunlight and arising from keratinocytes.

Staging The process of determining the extent and location of cancer in an individual.

Standard deviations A mathematical statement of the dispersion of a set of values or scores from the mean.

Stasis A "staying" of a substance in an anatomic location. A reduction in the normal rate of flow. A *stasis* of bile in the gallbladder promotes an increase in gallstone formation.

Status asthmaticus Severe, prolonged asthma attack that does not respond to routine therapy.

Status epilepticus Rapid succession of seizures without intervals of consciousness. Brain damage may result.

Steatorrhea Passage of high fat content in the feces; seen in malabsorption diseases where there is lack of pancreatic enzymes, such as cystic fibrosis.

STEMI ST-segment elevated myocardial infarction.

Stenosis (valvular) Obstruction to blood flow through cardiac valves that open incompletely.

Steroid A hormone produced from cholesterol and secreted by the adrenal cortex and other cells. Includes glucocorticoids, mineralocorticoids, and androgens.

Still disease Systemic-onset juvenile rheumatoid arthritis.

Stomatitis An inflammation of the oral mucosa that may extend to the buccal mucosa, lips, and palate.

Strabismus An abnormal ocular condition in which the visual axes of the eyes are not directed at the same point.

Stratum Layer.

Stratum corneum Outermost layer of the epidermis; composed of flat, compact cells that have lost their nuclei.

Stratum germinativum Also known as the *basal cell layer,* the final (fifth) layer of the epidermis is a line of cuboidal cells that marks the lowest boundary of the epidermis and divides it from the dermis.

Stratum granulosum Third layer of the epidermis, comprising flatter cells that contain protein granules, called *keratohyalin granules.*

Stratum lucidum Second layer of the epidermis, appearing as a translucent line of flat cells. This layer of the skin is present only on the palms and the soles.

Stratum spinosum Fourth layer of the epidermis, composed of upwardly migrating and maturing keratinocytes. This layer forms the bulk of the epidermis over most of the body.

Strawberry hemangioma A soft vascular nevus, usually present on the face or neck, occurring at birth or shortly afterward.

Strawberry tongue Bright red papillated tongue, characteristic of scarlet fever.

Stress The sum of biological reactions produced when an organism's homeostasis is disrupted.

Stress fracture A fracture of one cortical surface of the bone; often caused by repetitive activity such as running.

Stress incontinence Loss of bladder control caused by increased intra-abdominal pressure combined with pelvic muscle laxity.

Stressor An agent or condition capable of producing stress. The term denotes both physical (gravity, mechanical force, pathogen, injury) and psychological (fear, anxiety, crisis, joy) forces that an individual may experience.

Striation (muscle) The typical pattern of banding apparent upon microscopic inspection of a skeletal or cardiac muscle cell.

Stricture A narrowing or constriction of the lumen of a tube, duct, or hollow organ, such as the intestine, ureter, or urethra.

Stroke volume The volume of blood ejected from the ventricle in one contraction (end-diastolic volume minus end-systolic volume).

Structural scoliosis The most severe form of scoliosis; can be progressive in which the mechanics of the curve are such that rotation of the vertebrae occurs in combination with lateral curvature. This usually produces a protuberance of one side of the rib cage, seen best when a person bends forward.

Subarachnoid space The space between the arachnoid and the pia mater.

Subendocardium The part of the myocardium lying in proximity to the endocardial surface.

Subluxation Displacement of a bone from its normal position (articulating surface) in a joint; less severe than dislocation.

Substantia gelatinosa Another term for areas in laminae II and III that are important in the transmission of pain signals in the spinal cord.

Substantia nigra The layer of gray matter separating the tegmentum of the midbrain from the crus cerebri; part of the basal ganglia.

Sudden cardiac death (sudden cardiac arrest) Death due to cardiac causes (or successful resuscitation) within 1 hour of symptom onset.

Sulcus A deep furrow or groove on the surface of a structure (e.g., cerebral cortex).

Summation The additive response to repetitive stimuli.

Superficial fascia Loose subcutaneous layer rich in fat and areolar tissue, which lies beneath the dermis. Also known as *hypodermis.*

Superficial partial-thickness burn Marked by destruction of the epidermis and dermis, a superficial partial-thickness burn is also a second-degree burn. The water vapor barrier is absent, but tactile and pain sensors are intact.

Suppurative disease A disease that produces purulent material (pus).

Surface film Thin film of emulsified material spread over the surface of skin.

Surfactant A surface tension–reducing agent produced by type II pneumocytes in the lung.

Suture joints A joint that unites bone with a thin but dense layer of fibrous tissue. Found only in the skull.

Sweat gland Most numerous of the skin glands. Sweat glands are of two types: apocrine and eccrine.

Symphysis joint A joint that connects bony segments by a fibrocartilaginous plate or disk.

Symptom Subjective feeling that an affected individual can report to an observer. Nausea, malaise, and pain are *symptoms* of disease.

Symptomatically Defined by symptoms.

Synarthrosis A fibrous or cartilaginous (nonsynovial) joint.

Synchondrosis A joint connecting cartilage to a bony component; allows bone growth while providing stability.

Syncytium A complex of fused cells that act in concert.

Syndesmosis A fibrous joint in which opposing surfaces that are relatively far apart are connected by ligaments.

Syndrome A collection of signs and symptoms that occur together.

Syndrome of inappropriate antidiuretic hormone (SIADH) secretion Excessive antidiuretic hormone secretion either from the posterior pituitary gland or from other tissues. SIADH results in retention of water, hemodilution, and hyponatremia.

Synostosis The bony union that results from the fusion of a suture joint.

Synovial fluid A clear, pale yellow, viscous fluid similar to blood plasma but containing hyaluronic acid and a glycoprotein called lubricin. Synovial fluid reduces friction between the capsule and joint surfaces, lubricates the surface of the cartilage, resists shear forces, and provides nourishment for cartilage. The viscosity of the fluid is inversely related to joint velocity or rate of shear. High temperature decreases viscosity and low temperature increases viscosity.

Synovial joint Freely movable joint in which contiguous bony surfaces are covered by articular cartilage and connected by a fibrous connective tissue capsule lined with a synovial membrane.

Synovial sheath Also called *joint capsule*. A dense layer of connective tissue surrounding synovial joints. The capsule is solidly attached to the periosteum of the adjacent bony components. The synovial sheath provides strength to the joint and, through its neural receptors, detects motion, compression, tension, vibration, and pain.

Synovitis An inflammatory condition of the synovial membrane of a joint as the result of an aseptic wound or traumatic injury.

Syphilis Sexually transmitted disease caused by the spirochete *Treponema pallidum* and characterized by distinct stages of effects over a period of years.

Systemic lupus erythematosus A chronic inflammatory autoimmune disease resulting from a type III hypersensitivity reaction. It is a multisystem relapsing disease that can affect skin, mucosa, lung, heart, kidneys, central and peripheral nervous systems, and blood components. Arthralgias and synovitis are common features. Skin lesions are often present as a butterfly rash. Renal failure is the leading cause of death with this disease.

Systemic vascular resistance The impedance to blood flow exerted by the arterioles; determined primarily by vascular diameter.

Systole A phase of the cardiac cycle in which the ventricles are contracting to develop force and eject blood.

Systolic blood pressure The maximal pressure in the aorta and major arteries during ventricular ejection of blood.

T

T cell Lymphocyte that provides cellular immunity, has regulatory functions, and attacks antigen in association with other cells. T cells have T-cell receptors (TCRs) and mature in the thymus.

Tangential excision Also called *full-thickness excision*. Done to remove eschar in thin layers until viable tissue is visible.

Target cell or target organ The cell or organ that is stimulated by the effects of a hormone.

Tau protein Neuronal protein that organizes microtubules. Also known as *neural thread protein,* tau protein becomes chemically altered in Alzheimer disease and twists into abnormal bundles, known as *neurofibrillary tangles*. See *neural thread protein.*

Telangiectasia A lesion created by dilated blood vessels.

Telogen The resting phase of hair growth.

Telomerase An enzyme that permits addition of nucleotides to the tips of the chromosomes to prevent progressive shortening of the telomeres during cell division. Telomerase is produced by cancer cells, enabling them to become immortal.

Telomere The end cap of the chromosome; this section shortens with each cell division.

Tendinitis Inflammation of the tendon within the sheath.

Tension pneumothorax Presence of air in the pleural space that develops a positive pressure and compresses mediastinal structures.

Teratogen An agent or factor that causes damage or physical defects in a developing embryo.

Terminal hair Long, coarse, thick, visible strands of tightly fused keratinized epidermal cells.

Terminal sac period The third stage in fetal lung development when terminal sacs become thinner, preparing the lung tissue for gas exchange. Proliferation of pulmonary capillaries is also prominent during this period.

Tertiary prevention The third phase of health promotion, based on supporting independent function and preventing further disease-related deterioration.

Testis The male gonad or reproductive gland that produces spermatozoa and houses the Leydig cells.

Testosterone Male sex hormone produced by interstitial cells in the testes.

Thalamus Portion of diencephalon; mass of gray matter involved in relay of sensory information, emotion, arousal, and complex reflexes.

Thalassemia An inherited form of anemia characterized by microcytic red blood cells that lack either α- or β-hemoglobin chains.

Thoracentesis Surgical perforation of the chest wall and pleural space with a needle to aspirate fluid for diagnostic or therapeutic purposes or to remove a specimen for biopsy.

Thoracotomy Surgical opening of the chest wall.

Threshold The lowest level at which a stimulus can produce a response.

Thrill Vibration palpated over a blood vessel or heart chamber reflecting turbulent blood flow.

Thromboangiitis obliterans (Buerger disease) An occlusive vascular condition, usually associated with smoking and affecting a leg or a foot, in which the small- and medium-sized arteries become inflamed and thrombotic.

Thrombocyte Circulating cytoplasmic fragment of a megakaryocyte that is essential in the formation of blood clots and in the control of bleeding. Also called *platelet.*

Thrombocytopenia A deficiency of platelets (thrombocytes) in the peripheral blood. Any reduction in platelet count below normal is called *thrombocytopenia,* but significant risk of bleeding does not occur until the count drops below about 20,000/μl.

Thrombocytosis An abnormal increase in the number of platelets in the blood.

Thromboembolus An embolus that originated as a thrombus, most commonly in the venous system of the lower extremities.

Thrombophlebitis Inflammation of a vein accompanied by the formation of a clot.

Thrombus Stationary blood clot formed within a vessel.

Thrush Candidiasis of the tissues of the mouth. The condition is characterized by the appearance of creamy white patches of exudates on an inflamed tongue or buccal mucosa.

Thyroid-stimulating hormone (TSH) A peptide secreted by the anterior lobe of the pituitary gland that controls the release of thyroid hormone and is necessary for the growth and function of the thyroid gland.

Thyroid storm Extreme thyrotoxicosis. Massively elevated levels of thyroid hormones cause an increased basal metabolic rate, tachycardia, hypertension, and fever, eventually leading to cardiovascular collapse.

Thyroxine (T_4) A hormone containing four iodine molecules secreted by the thyroid gland.

Tight junction Cell-to-cell junction that seals adjacent epithelial cells together and prevents the passage of most substances through the epithelial sheet.

Tinea The infection caused by fungal infections of the skin in any cutaneous area, including the hair and nails.

Tinnitus Ringing, buzzing, or roaring in the ears; commonly associated with exposure to loud noise or disorders such as Meniere disease.

Tonic Referring to continuous stimulation or muscular contraction.

TORCH complex An acronym used to describe the usual offending infectious agents that commonly cause congenital anomalies: *t*oxoplasmosis, *o*thers, *r*ubella, *c*ytomegalovirus, *h*erpesvirus.

Torsion Act of twisting or condition of being twisted. Applies to the state of the testes when abnormally rotated.

Trabecular bone Cancellous bone cells arranged in response to mechanical stress placed on the bone. Configuration of bone cells increases strength of bone.

Tracheoesophageal fistula Congenital anomaly in which an abnormal opening between the trachea and esophagus exists. It requires immediate diagnosis and surgical correction.

Transcellular fluid Body fluid contained in special compartments, such as the synovial or cerebrospinal compartments; a component of extracellular fluid.

Transcription The process by which a segment of DNA is used as a template to produce a complementary sequence of messenger RNA.

Transient flora Microorganisms that temporarily reside in a certain environment on the host.

Transient ischemic attack A temporary episode of cerebrovascular insufficiency that is usually associated with partial occlusion of a cerebral artery.

Transitional flow Airflow occurring in the larger airways, especially at bifurcations. Also known as *mixed pattern of airflow.*

Translation Formation of a polypeptide chain in a sequence dictated by messenger RNA.

Translocation Shifting of a segment of one chromosome into another chromosome.

Transmission of infection The process by which a pathogenic organism is transferred from one host to another.

Transmural Denoting the entire thickness of a wall (e.g., the myocardial wall). A transmural myocardial infarction extends throughout the entire cardiac muscle layer.

Transportation The movement or transference of biochemical substances from one site to another.

Transudate Fluid of low protein content that passes through membranes because of a difference in hydrostatic pressure.

Transverse fracture Fracture that occurs in a straight line at approximately a 90-degree angle to the longitudinal axis of the bone.

Traumatic alopecia Hair loss as a result of tight plaiting of hair or use of hot oil and tension on the scalp. Gradual damage to hair follicles occurs, leading to hair thinning and loss.

Traumatic brain injury Nondegenerative, non-congenital insult to the brain from an external mechanical force.

Triad asthma A subcategory of drug-induced asthma representing a combination of intrinsic asthma, aspirin sensitivity, and nasal polyposis.

Triaxial joint A joint that permits movement around three axes so that motion can occur in three planes. Permits gliding movement between two bones as exemplified by the carpal joints of the hand.

Tricuspid valve The cardiac valve that lies between the right atrium and right ventricle. The valve is normally closed during ventricular systole and open during ventricular diastole. Tricuspid valve closure contributes to heart sound S_1.

Trigeminal neuralgia A neurologic condition of the trigeminal cranial nerve, characterized by paroxysms of pain.

Triglyceride A simple fat compound consisting of three molecules of fatty acid and glycerol.

Trigone Triangular area, usually referring to the bladder muscle.

Triiodothyronine (T_3) A hormone containing three iodine molecules secreted by the thyroid gland and produced in tissues by the enzymatic deiodination of T_4.

Trisomy Having three homologous chromosomes instead of the usual pair, as in trisomy 21, also called *Down syndrome*.

Tropic/trophic hormone A hormone that stimulates the growth and maintenance of a tissue or gland.

Tropical sprue Inflammation of the mucosa of the small intestine secondary to infection.

Tropomyosin A structural protein involved in regulation of actin-myosin cross-bridge formation. Associated with the thin filament of the sarcomere in skeletal and cardiac muscle, where it blocks cross-bridge formation when intracellular calcium levels are low.

Troponin A regulatory protein involved in regulation of actin-myosin cross-bridge formation.

Associated with tropomyosin and actin in the thin filament of the sarcomere. Troponin binds calcium ion in the cell and regulates the position of tropomyosin, allowing muscle contraction when intracellular calcium levels rise.

Tuberculosis A chronic infection caused by the acid-fast bacillus *Mycobacterium tuberculosis*.

Tumor marker Biochemical substance, such as a specific enzyme, receptor, or surface protein, that helps identify the tumor cell.

Tumor suppressor gene A gene that regulates a group of growth-promoting genes and suppresses tumor formation. Mutation and underexpression of tumor suppressor genes are associated with the development of cancer.

Tunica albuginea Fascial layer covering the testes and erectile bodies of the penis.

Turbulent flow The friction and increased resistance caused by air movement from the nasal cavity through the large bronchi.

Turnover and regeneration time Time required for a population of cells to mature and reproduce. As the surface cells of the stratum corneum are lost, replacement of keratinocytes by mitosis must occur.

Twitch The mechanical response to a single stimulus of a motor unit.

Type 1 diabetes mellitus Insulin-dependent diabetes mellitus; characterized by an absolute deficiency of insulin.

Type 2 diabetes mellitus Non–insulin-dependent diabetes mellitus; characterized by tissue insulin resistance and impaired insulin production by the pancreas.

U

Ulcerative colitis An inflammatory disease of the mucosa of the rectum and colon. Most commonly it affects the most distal portions of the colon, but eventually it may affect the entire colon. It is typically characterized by exacerbations and remissions. The clinical manifestations of ulcerative colitis are abdominal pain, diarrhea, and rectal bleeding.

Ultrafiltration Filtration through a filter capable of removing colloidal particles from a dispersion medium, as in the filtration of plasma at the capillary membrane.

Ultrasound An imaging modality that uses sound waves to assess the size, structure, and function of internal organs, tissue, or the fetus.

Uniaxial joint A joint that allows motion around a single axis.

Unipennate A muscle with a lateral tendon to which the fibers are attached obliquely, like one half of a feather.

Unipolar depression Depression without periods of mania.

Unresolved urinary tract infection (UTI) A urinary tract infection in which bacteriuria remains after initial antibiotic treatment.

Unsaturated (fatty acid) Referring to an organic compound in which one or more pairs of carbon atoms are united by double or triple bonds, as in unsaturated fatty acids.

Up-regulation An increase in the number of cell receptors for a specific hormone resulting from chronically low concentrations of the

hormone. Up-regulation helps maintain the target cell response to a hormone, even when circulating hormone levels are low.

Urea Substance produced in the liver from the breakdown of protein and excreted in the urine.

Uremia A clinical syndrome related to the severe loss of renal function and resulting in the accumulation of metabolic waste products in the blood.

Ureter One of a pair of fibromuscular, mucosa-lined narrow tubes that connect the kidneys to the bladder.

Ureterocele Congenital cystic dilatation of the distal ureter.

Ureterolithiasis The presence of calculi (stones) in the urinary system, particularly the ureters.

Ureteropelvic junction obstruction Disruption of urinary flow from the kidney(s) into one or both ureters.

Urethral stricture A fibrotic narrowing of the urethra, usually composed of scar tissue.

Urethral valve The most common cause of urinary obstruction in male newborns and infants. Posterior in location, occurring in the distal prostatic urethra, urethral valves are mucosal folds that resemble thin membranes and cause obstruction when the child attempts to void.

Urethritis Inflammation of the urethra.

Urethrorectal fistula A rare congenital anomaly almost always associated with an imperforate anus. The fistula results from failure of the urorectal septum to develop completely, leading to a persistent communication between the rectum posteriorly and the urogenital tract anteriorly.

Urge incontinence A strong and immediate urge to void instigated by involuntary detrusor overactivity.

Urinary bladder Muscular sac located in the anterior inferior pelvic cavity that holds urine until it is excreted through the urethra.

Urodynamic testing The study of the mechanics of urinary bladder filling, emptying, and voiding.

Urolithiasis The presence of calculi in the urinary system.

Urothelial tumor A malignant tumor of the lining of the renal pelvis, calyces, ureter, and bladder.

Urothelium Epithelial lining of the urinary tract from the renal pelvis to the bladder.

Urticaria A pruritic (itchy) skin eruption characterized by transient wheals of varying shapes and sizes with well-defined erythematous margins and pale centers.

Uterine prolapse A sinking of the uterus from its normal position. It usually occurs when supporting structures, such as the uterosacral ligaments and cardinal ligaments, relax, altering the relationship of the uterus to the vaginal axis.

V

Validity The extent to which a test measures what it is intended to measure.

Valvular incompetence An acquired or congenital disorder of a cardiac valve resulting in regurgitation of blood through the valve because it doesn't close properly, also called *valvular insufficiency*.

Varicose veins Incompetency of the superficial veins of the extremities, producing engorgement.

Vas deferens Thick, muscular tube that is continuous with the epididymis. It travels along the pelvic wall and joins with the seminal vesicle duct at the prostate to form the ejaculatory duct. Also called *ductus deferens*.

Vascular fluid Fluid that is in blood vessels; a component of extracellular fluid.

Vasculitis Inflammation of the lining (intima) of a blood vessel.

Vasoconstriction A decrease in the diameter of a blood vessel, usually referring to an arteriole, caused by relaxation of vascular smooth muscle.

Vasodilation An increase in the diameter of a blood vessel, usually referring to an arteriole, caused by a relaxation of the smooth muscles in the vessel wall.

Vasospasm Sudden inappropriate constriction of a blood vessel, producing obstruction of flow.

Vellus Tiny hair strands that are almost unnoticeable. Vellus covers the whole body of a child, except the palms and soles. In contrast, terminal hair strands cover the arms and legs of adults.

Ventilation The process of moving air into the lungs and distributing air within the lungs to gas exchange units (alveoli) for maintenance of oxygenation and removal of CO_2.

Ventricle A fluid-filled compartment as in the brain or heart.

Ventricular ejection The forceful expulsion of blood from the ventricles into the aorta and the pulmonary arteries.

Ventriculoperitoneal shunt A shunt that extends all the way from the ventricular system of the brain to the peritoneal cavity of the body.

Verrucae Circumscribed elevations of the epidermis, commonly called *warts*.

Vertigo A sensation of loss of equilibrium, more than just dizziness.

Verumontanum A small elevation that is marked by a midline opening from the prostatic utricle, a remnant of the müllerian duct system.

Vesicle A portion of lipid bilayer membrane that forms a sphere and surrounds substances to be transported to a destination within the cell or plasma membrane.

Vesicoureteral reflux Retrograde movement of urine from the bladder to the kidney as a result of a disruption in the normal valvular mechanism at the ureter-bladder junction.

Vibrissae Large hairs of the nasal cavity.

Virion A virus particle.

Virulence The capacity of a microorganism to successfully evade host defenses and cause disease.

Virulent Referring to a microorganism's ability to evade host defenses and cause disease.

Viruses Tiny genetic parasites that are dependent on the host cell for replication. They take over the host cell "machinery" for energy and replication.

Visual acuity The ability of the eyes to focus clearly on an image at a known distance; it is assessed with a Snellen chart and often expressed as the ability of a person to accurately discern characters of various sizes at a distance of 20 feet.

Vitamin An organic substance that is essential in the diet and is required for the body's utilization of energy-containing nutrients.

Vitiligo Patch of depigmentation; also called *leukoderma*.

Voiding dysfunction A failure in the normal process of bladder emptying that results in urinary retention and/or incontinence.

Volvulus A twisting of the bowel on itself, which results in blood vessel compression.

Vulvovaginitis An inflammation of the vulva and vagina.

W

Wallerian degeneration Complete disintegration of the distal portion of an axon that has been severed from the cell body. The axon, myelin sheath, and terminal arborization all disintegrate.

Wart Also called *verruca*; caused by a virus that provokes a benign proliferation of keratinocytes.

Water imbalance Imbalance of body fluid concentration; osmolality imbalance; hypernatremia and hyponatremia.

Western blot A laboratory test to detect the presence of antibodies to specific antigens. It is regarded as more precise than the ELISA and is sometimes used to check the validity of ELISA tests.

White blood cell A cell that mediates immune function. White blood cells include granulocytes, monocytes, and lymphocytes. Also called *leukocyte*.

White-coat phenomenon Elevated blood pressure readings when measured in a clinic setting by a nurse or physician.

Wilson disease A rare autosomal recessive disorder in which excessive amounts of copper accumulate in the liver or other organs; also called *hepatolenticular degeneration*.

Wolffian ducts Mesonephric ducts that develop as nephric ducts but mature to form male genital ducts.

Wolff law States that bone is established where needed and resorbed where not needed.

X

Xerostomia Dryness of the mouth caused by cessation of normal salivary secretion.

Z

Z line A dark band that defines a sarcomere; Z lines are perpendicular to actin and myosin filaments. A sarcomere extends from one Z line to the next.

Zeitgeber A cue given by the environment, such as a change in light or temperature, to reset the internal body clock.

Zona pellucida The thick covering of the ovum.

Zone of calcifying cartilage A very thin line of chondrocytes and the weakest segment of the epiphyseal plate.

Zone of maturing cartilage Contains the enlarged and mature cartilage cells as they migrate toward the metaphysis.

Zone of resting cartilage Maintains adherence of the plate to the epiphysis.

Zone of young proliferating cartilage Demonstrates the most active cartilage cell growth.

Zygote The developing ovum, from the time it is fertilized until it is implanted in the uterus.

INDEX

Page numbers followed by *f* indicate figures; *t*, tables; *b*, boxes. **Bold entries** designate diseases or syndromes.

Asthma *(Continued)*
  exercise-induced, 476
  food additive-induced, 476
  non-allergic (intrinsic), 476
  occupational, 476
  pathogenesis of, 476–478, 477f–478f
  severity of
    classifying, 479, 479f–480f
    treatment based on, 481f, 493b–494b
  treatment of, 480–482
    severity-based, 481f, 493b–494b
Asthmatic bronchitis, 482–483
Astigmatism, 950, 952f
Astrocytes, 861, 863f, 878, 879f
Asystole, electrical, 423, 424f
Ataxia, in cerebral palsy, 929
Atazanavir (Reyataz), 253t
Atelectasis, 459
Atelectatic pulmonary disorders, 503–507
Atherosclerosis, 321–326
  clinical manifestations and diagnosis of, 326
  coronary
    coronary heart disease from, 379
    mechanisms of, 379–381, 380f, 383f
  etiology and pathogenesis of, 322–326, 322f, 324f
  hypertension and, 341
  pathogenesis of, 380–381, 383f
  risk factors for, 323–326, 325b
    modifiable, 324–326
    nonmodifiable, 326
  treatment of, 326
Atherosclerosis obliterans, 322–323
Athlete's foot, 152
Atmospheric pressure changes, cell injury from, 69
Atonic seizures, 923
Atopic dermatitis, 1068–1069, 1069f
Atopic hypersensitivity, 199–201. *See also* Type I hypersensitivity.
Atopy, 1068
ATP. *See* Adenosine triphosphate (ATP).
Atrial dysrhythmias, 424–425, 424f–425f
Atrial events, in cardiac cycle, 353f, 355
Atrial fibrillation, 424–425, 425f
Atrial flutter, 424–425, 424f
Atrial natriuretic peptides (ANPs)
  renal tubular fluid reabsorption and, 566, 566t
  secretion of, by cardiac myocytes, 372
Atrial septal defect, 396–398, 403f
Atrial tachycardia, paroxysmal focal, 424, 424f
Atrioventricular (AV) node, 366, 367f
Atrioventricular conduction disturbances, 426–427, 426f–427f
Atrioventricular valves, 350, 351f
Atrium(ia), 350–351
Atrophy, 60–61, 60f, 1059f–1060f
Attention-deficit/hyperactivity disorder (ADHD), 996–997
Atypical absence seizures, 923
Aura, in seizure disorders, 924
Auscultatory gap, in blood pressure measurement, 334–335, 335f
Autism spectrum disorder (ASD), 997–998
Autoantibody induction, in drug-induced immune hemolysis, 281
Autocrine signaling, 47, 48f, 120, 784, 784f
Autoimmune hepatitis, 771–772
  cirrhosis in older women, 780

Autoimmune polyendocrinopathy-candidiasis-ectodermal dystrophy, 211
Autoimmune thyroiditis, 803
Autoimmunity (autoimmune disorders), 196–198
  description of, 196
  endocrine dysfunction in, 800
  environmental triggers for, 197–198
  genetic factors in, 197, 197t
  pharmacotherapies for, 198
Autologous stem cell transplantation, 219, 219f
Autolysis, postmortem, 72
Automaticity, abnormal, in dysrhythmias, 420
Automobile airbag burns, chemicals associated with, 1107
Autonomic dysreflexia, in spinal cord injury, 936
Autonomic nervous system (ANS), 874–877, 875f–877f
  effects on organ system function, 878t
  parasympathetic division of. *See* Parasympathetic nervous system (PNS).
  in regulation of rhythmicity of heart, 367–368
  sympathetic division of. *See* Sympathetic nervous system (SNS).
Autoregulation
  abnormal, in acute brain injury, 902
  of blood flow, 319
    tissue pressure hypothesis of, 319
    vascular endothelium in, 319
  of coronary circulation, 356, 372
  myogenic, GFR and, 560
Autosomal chromosome disorders, 97
Autosomal dominant disorders, 100, 102t
Autosomal dominant polycystic kidney disease, 577t, 578, 578f
Autosomal recessive disorders, 101–102, 104t
Autosomal recessive polycystic kidney disease, 577, 577t
Autosomes, 101
Avascular necrosis, in fracture healing, 1028
Avoidance anxiety, in panic disorder, 991–992
Avulsion bone fracture, 1024–1025, 1025f
Axoneme, 635
Axons, 89, 89f

B-cell lymphoma, 229–231, 230t
B lymphocytes (B cells), 159, 168, 168f
  activated, class switching in, 183–184, 187f
  antigen recognition by, 182–183, 183f–185f
  immunodeficiency disorders involving, 209–212
  signaling pathways in, 184f
  theories of autoimmunity involving, 197
B-type natriuretic peptide, secretion of, by cardiac myocytes, 372
Bacilli, 147–149, 149f
Bacteremia, 442
  definition of, 442t
Bacteria
  antiphagocytic factors in, 146
  cell injury from, 67
  endospores produced by, 146
  enzymes produced by, 146
  gram staining of, 149–150
  morphology of, 147–149, 148f–149f
  other microorganisms compared with, 152t
  pathogenic, 147–150, 147b–148b, 148f–149f
    classified by body part targeted, 150f
  toxins produced by, 146

Bacterial emboli, 321
Bacterial infections
  autoimmunity triggered by, 197
  cutaneous, 1063–1065, 1064f
Bacterial meningitis, 919, 919t
Bacterial peritonitis, spontaneous, 766–767, 766f
Bacterial pneumonia, 512–513, 513t, 514f
Bacterial prostatitis, 648, 650–651
Balance, 944
Ball-and-socket joint, 1009, 1009f
Balloon tamponade, of gastroesophageal varices, 762, 763f
Band cells, in infection, 162, 163f
Barbiturate-hypnotic combinations, for migraine, 967t
Baroreceptors
  altered sensitivity to, in orthostatic hypotension, 345–346
  in blood pressure regulation, 336
  in control of respiration, 462f
  in response to heart failure, 410, 411f
  in response to shock, 435, 436f
Barrett esophagus, 725
Bartholin cyst, 677
Bartholin glands, 657
Bartholinitis, 677
Basal cell carcinoma, 1076
  in HIV infection, 1063
Basal ganglia, 863, 867f
  injury to, in cerebral palsy, 929
  in obsessive-compulsive disorder, 993–994
Basal metabolic rate (BMR), 841
  factors affecting, 841t
  in physiologic stress, 848–849
  in starvation, 848
Base pairs, in DNA, 75–76, 76f
Basophils, 163
  characteristics of, 258t–259t
  functions of, 162t
  in type I hypersensitivity, 199
Beau lines, in nail in systemic diseases, 1081, 1081f
Becker muscular dystrophy, 1037
Bedbug infestation, 1071–1072
Bell palsy, 939–940, 939f
Bence Jones protein, in plasma cell myeloma, 224–225
Benign prostatic hyperplasia (BPH), 649–653, 649f–650f
Benign tumors
  characteristics of, 114, 114t
  nomenclature for, 115t
Benzodiazepines, long-acting, for panic disorder, 992
Berger disease, 589
Bernard-Soulier syndrome, 303–304
Berry aneurysm, 327
β_2-Microglobulin test, in monitoring HIV disease status, 245
Biaxial joint, range of movement of, 1008–1009, 1009f
Bicarbonate, reabsorption of, in acid-base balance regulation, 563, 565f
Bicarbonate buffer system, 540
Bifascicular block, 429
Biguanides, for diabetes, 830
Bilateral renal agenesis, 577
Bile, physiology of, 742–743
Bile salts, 742–743, 744f
Biliary atresia, 780
Biliary cirrhosis, 772

P

PREFIXES AND SUFFIXES COMMONLY USED IN MEDICAL TERMINOLOGY

PREFIX	MEANING	SUFFIX	MEANING
a-	Without, not	-al, -ac	Pertaining to
a[d]-	Toward	-algia	Pain
all[o]-	[an]other, different		
an-	Without, not	-aps, -apt	Fit; fasten
ante-	Before	-arche	Beginning; origin
anti-	Against; resisting	-ase	Signifies an enzyme
auto-	Self	-blast	Sprout; make
bi-	Two; double	-centesis	A piercing
circum-	Around	-cide	To kill
co-, con-	With; together	-clast	Break; destroy
contra-	Against	-crine	Release; secrete
de-	Down from, undoing	-ectomy	A cutting out
dia-	Across; through	-emesis	Vomiting
dipl-	Twofold, double	-emia	Refers to blood condition
dys-	Bad; disordered; difficult	-flux	Flow
ectop-	Displaced	-gen	Creates; forms
ef-	Away from	-genesis	Creation, production
em-, en-	In, into	-gram	Something written
endo-	Within	-graph(y)	To write, draw
epi-	Upon	-hydrate	Containing H2O (water)
eu-	Good	-ia, -sia	Condition; process
ex-, exo-	Out of, out from	-iasis	Abnormal condition
extra-	Outside of	-ic, -ac	Pertaining to
hapl-	Single	-in	Signifies a protein
hem-, hemat-	Blood	-ism	Signifies "condition of"
hemi-	Half	-itis	Signifies "inflammation of"
hom(e)o-	Same; equal	-lemma	Rind; peel
hyper-	Over; above	-lepsy	Seizure
hypo-	Under; below	-lith	Stone; rock
infra-	Below, beneath	-logy	Study of
inter-	Between	-lunar	Moon; moonlike
intra-	Within	-malacia	Softening
iso-	Same, equal	-megaly	Enlargement
macro-	Large	-metric, -metry	Measurement, length
mega-	Large; million(th)	-oid	Like; in the shape of
mes-	Middle	-oma	Tumor
meta-	Beyond, after	-opia	Vision, vision condition
micro-	Small; millionth	-oscopy	Viewing
milli-	Thousandth	-ose	Signifies a carbohydrate (especially sugar)
mono-	One (single)	-osis	Condition, process
neo-	New	-ostomy	Formation of an opening
non-	Not	-otomy	Cut
oligo-	Few, scanty	-penia	Lack
ortho-	Straight; correct, normal	-philic	Loving
para-	By the side of; near	-phobic	Fearing
per-	Through	-phragm	Partition
peri-	Around; surrounding	-plasia	Growth, formation
poly-	Many	-plasm	Substance, matter
post-	After	-plasty	Shape; make
pre-	Before	-plegia	Paralysis
pro-	First; promoting	-pnea	Breath, breathing
quadr-	Four	-(r)rhage, -(r)rhagia	Breaking out, discharge
re-	Back again	-(r)rhaphy	Sew, suture
retro-	Behind	-(r)rhea	Flow
semi-	Half	-some	Body
sub-	Under	-tensin, -tension	Pressure
super-, supra-	Over, above, excessive	-tonic	Pressure, tension
trans-	Across; through	-tripsy	Crushing
tri-	Three; triple	-ule	Small, little
		-uria	Refers to urine condition

m Patton KT, Thibodeau GA: Anatomy & physiology, ed 8, St Louis, 2013, Mosby.